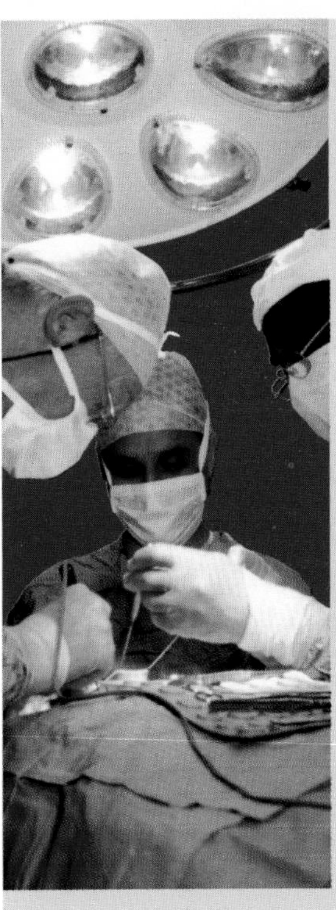

Bailey & Love's

Short Practice of Surgery

23rd edition

Edited by

R.C.G. Russell, MS, FRCS

Consulting Surgeon, The Middlesex Hospital, London, UK

N.S. Williams, MS, FRCS

Professor of Surgery and Director of The Academic Department of Surgery, St Bartholomew's and the Royal London School of Medicine and Dentistry, Royal London Hospital, London, UK

C.J.K. Bulstrode, MA, FRCS

Professor in Orthopaedic Surgery, John Radcliffe Hospital, Oxford, UK

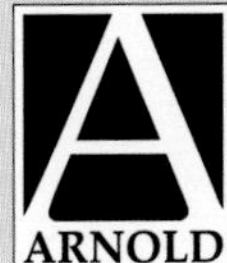

A member of the Hodder Headline Group
LONDON
Co-published in the USA by Oxford University Press Inc., New York

First published in Great Britain in 1932
Twenty-third edition published in 2000 by
Arnold, a member of the Hodder Headline Group,
338 Euston Road, London NW1 3BH

http://www.arnoldpublishers.com

Co-published in the USA by
Oxford University Press Inc.,
198 Madison Avenue, New York, NY 10016
Oxford is a registered trademark of Oxford University Press

British Library Cataloguing in Publication Data
A catalogue record for this book is available from the British Library

Library of Congress Cataloging-in-Publication Data
A catalog record for this book is available from the Library of Congress

ISBN 0 340 75924 0 (hb)
ISBN 0 340 75949 6 (pb – restricted territorial availability)

1 2 3 4 5 6 7 8 9 10

Publisher: Nick Dunton
Project Editor: Catherine Barnes
Production Editor: James Rabson
Production Controller: Iain McWilliams
Cover Design: Terry Griffiths

Typeset in 9.5/11.5 pt Sabon and produced by Gray Publishing, Tunbridge Wells, Kent
Colour separation by Tenon & Polert Colour Scanning Ltd
Printed and bound by Ajanta Offset Ltd, India

Contents

Contributors

Timothy G. Allen-Mersh MD, FRCS
Professor of Gastrointestinal Surgery, Imperial College School of Medicine, Chelsea & Westminister Hospital, London, UK

Jonathan R. Anderson FRCS
Senior Registrar, Cardiothoracic Unit, St George's Hospital, London, UK

John Bancewicz BSc, ChM, FRCS, FRCS(Glas)
Reader in Surgery, University of Manchester School of Medicine; Consultant Surgeon, Hope Hospital, Salford, UK

Grant J. E. M. Bates BSc, FRCS
Clinical Lecturer, University of Oxford School of Medicine; Consultant Otolaryngologist, John Radcliffe Hospital, Oxford, UK

Michael Baum ChM, MD, FRCS
Professor of Surgery, University College London Medical School, London, UK

David H. Bennett BSc, FRCS
Senior Registrar, Department of Surgery, Derriford Hospital, Plymouth, UK

Andrew W. Bradbury BSc, MD, FRCS(Ed)
Senior Lecturer and Consultant Vascular Surgeon, Vascular Surgery Unit, The Royal Infirmary of Edinburgh, Edinburgh, UK

J. Andrew Bradley PhD, FRCS(Glas)
Professor of Surgery, University of Cambridge School of Medicine, Addenbrooke's Hospital, Cambridge, UK

Keith Budd FRCA
Consultant in Pain Management, Bradford Royal Infirmary; Clinical Lecturer (Anaesthesia), University of Leeds School of Medicine, UK

Christopher J. K. Bulstrode MA, FRCS
Professor in Orthopaedic Surgery, John Radcliffe Hospital, Oxford; Associate Director of Postgraduate Medical & Dental Education, University of Oxford, UK

Andrew J. Carr ChM FRCS
Consultant Orthopaedic Surgeon, Nuffield Orthopaedic Centre, Oxford, UK

Jon C. Clasper FRCS(Ed)(Orth)
Consultant Orthopaedic Surgeon, Military Wing, Frimley Park Hospital, Frimley, Camberley, UK

David J. Coleman MS, FRCS(Plast)
Consultant Plastic Surgeon, The Radcliffe Infirmary, Oxford, UK

Philip D. Coleridge-Smith DM, FRCS
Reader in Surgery, University College London Medical School; Consultant Surgeon, The Middlesex Hospital, London, UK

Ara Darzi MD, FRCS, FRCSI
Professor of Surgery, Imperial College of Science and Technology and Medicine, London; Consultant Surgeon, St Mary's Hospital NHS Trust, London; Tutor in Laparoscopic Surgery, Minimal Access Therapy Training Unit, The Royal College of Surgeons of England, London, UK

Brian R. Davidson MD, FRCS(Glas)
Professor of Surgery, Royal Free Hospital School of Medicine, London, UK

Birgit Davies BA(Hons)
Research Co-ordinator, Gloucestershire Royal Hospital, Gloucester, UK

Len Doyal BA, MSc
Professor of Medical Ethics, St Bartholomew's and The Royal London School of Medicine and Dentistry, Queen Mary and Westfield College, University of London, UK

Jonathan J. Earnshaw DM, FRCS
Consultant Surgeon, Gloucestershire Royal Hospital, Gloucester, UK

Christopher Fowler BSc, MS, FRCP, FRCS(Urol), FEBU
Head of Academic Urological Unit and Director of Surgical Education, St Bartholomew's and The Royal London School of Medicine at Queen Mary and Westfield College, London; Consultant Urological Surgeon, The Royal London Hospital, London, UK

Simon P. Frostick MA, DM, FRCS
Professor of Orthopaedic and Accident Surgery, Department of Musculoskeletal Science, University of Liverpool Medical School, Liverpool, UK

Anthony W. Goode MD, FRCS
Professor of Endocrine and Metabolic Surgery, St Bartholomew's and The Royal London School of Medicine and Dentistry at Queen Mary and Westfield College, London, UK

Timothy E. J. Hems MA, DM, FRCS, FRCSEd(Orth)
Consultant Hand and Orthopaedic Surgeon, The Victoria Infirmary, Glasgow, UK

Robert A. Hill BSc, FRCS
Consultant Orthopaedic Surgeon, Great Ormond Street Hospital for Sick Children, London, UK

David J. Howard BSc, FRCS, FRCS(Ed)
Consultant Head and Neck Surgeon, Royal National Throat, Nose and Ear Hospital, London, UK

M. Dalvi Humzah BSc, AKC, FRCS(Plast), MBA
Consultant Plastic & Reconstructive Surgeon, Radcliffe Infirmary, Oxford, UK

David H. A. Jones FRCS, FRCS(Ed)(Orth)
Consultant Orthopaedic Surgeon, Great Ormond Street Hospital for Sick Children, London, UK

Richard P. Juniper FDSRCS
Regional Director of Postgraduate Dental Education, Oxford Postgraduate Medical & Dental Education, Oxford, UK

Catherine F. Kellett MRCS
Clinical Lecturer in Orthopaedics and Trauma, Nuffield Orthopaedic Centre, Oxford, UK

Richard C. S. Kerr MS, FRCS
Consultant Neurosurgeon, Radcliffe Infirmary, Oxford, UK

Andrew Kingsnorth BSc, MS, FRCS
Professor of Surgery, Plymouth Postgraduate Medical School, Derriford Hospital, Plymouth, UK

Zygmunt H. Krukowski PhD, FRCS(Ed)
Consultant Surgeon/Professor of Clinical Surgery, Aberdeen Royal Infirmary, Forersterhill, Aberdeen, UK

John D. Langdon MDS, FDSRCS, FRCS
Professor of Oral & Maxillofacial Surgery, Guy's, King's College & St Thomas' School of Medicine & Dentistry, London, UK

Richard M. Langford FRCA
Senior Lecturer, St Bartholomew's and The Royal London School of Medicine at Queen Mary and Westfield College, London; Consultant Anaesthetist, St Bartholomew's Hospital, London, UK

David J. Leaper MD, ChM, FRCS
Professorial Unit of Surgery, North Tees General Hospital, Stockton on Tees, Cleveland, UK

Valerie J. Lund MS, FRCS, FRCS(Ed)
Professor in Rhinology, Royal National Throat, Nose and Ear Hospital, London, UK

Nicholas F. Maartens FRCS
Senior Registrar, Department of Neurological Surgery, John Radcliffe Infirmary, Oxford, UK

Alison M. McLean MRCP, FRCR
Consultant Radiologist, St Bartholomew's Hospital, Royal Hospitals Trust, London, UK

Martin J. Martin MSc, MRCPath
Consultant Microbiologist, Royal Bournemouth Hospital, Bournemouth, UK

Bruce R. Mathalone FRCS, FRCS(Ed), FRCOphth
Consultant Ophthalmologist, Westminster & Chelsea Hospital, London, UK

Jean M. Millar FRCA
Consultant Anaesthetist, Nuffield Department of Anaesthetics, Oxford; Honorary Senior Clinical Lecturer, University of Oxford School of Medicine, UK

Neil J. McC. Mortensen MD, FRCS
Consultant Surgeon, John Radcliffe Hospital, Oxford; Reader in Colorectal Surgery, University of Oxford School of Medicine, UK

John A. Murie MA BSc MD FRCS
Consultant Surgeon, Vascular Surgery Unit, The Royal Infirmary of Edinburgh, Edinburgh, UK

Monty C. Mythen FRCA
Consultant Anaesthetist, University College Hospitals, London, UK

David E. Neal BSc, MS, FRCS, FRCS(Ed)
Head of Department of Surgery, School of Surgical Studies, The Medical School, University of Newcastle, Newcastle upon Tyne, UK

John P. Neoptolemos MA, MD, FRCS
Professor of Surgery, Royal Liverpool University Hospital, Liverpool, UK

P. Ronan O'Connell MD, FRCSI
Consultant Surgeon, Mater Misericordiae Hospital, Dublin, Ireland

Anthony L. G. Peel MA, MCh, FRCS, FRCS(Ed)
Consultant Surgeon, North Tees General Hospital, Stockton-on-Tees, UK

John N. Primrose MD, FRCS
Professor of Surgery, University of Southampton School of Medicine; Consultant Surgeon, Southampton General Hospital, Southampton, UK

R. David Rosin MS, FRCS, FRCS(Ed)
Consultant Surgeon, St Mary's Hospital, London, UK

Robert W. Ruckley FRCS
Consultant ENT Surgeon, Memorial Hospital, Darlington, UK

R. C. G. Russell MS, FRCS
Consultant Surgeon, The Middlesex Hospital, London, UK

James M. Ryan MCh, FRCS
Leonard Cheshire Professor of Conflict Recovery at University College London, UK

Christobel M. Saunders FRCS
Senior Lecturer, University College, London; Honorary Consultant Surgeon, University College Hospitals, London, UK

John H. Scurr BSc, FRCS
Senior Lecturer and Honorary Consultant Surgeon, The Middlesex and University College Hospitals, London, UK

William P. Smith FDS, FRCS(Ed) FDSRCS
Consultant Oral & Maxillofacial Surgeon, Kettering General Hospital, Kettering, UK

Jeremy Thompson MChir, FRCS
Consultant Gastrointestinal Surgeon, Chelsea & Westminister Hospital, London, UK

Tom Treasure MD, MS, FRCS
Professor of Cardiothoracic Surgery, St George's Hospital, London, UK

David J. Warwick MD, FRCS, FRCS(Orth)
Consultant Hand Surgeon, Southampton University Hospital, Southampton, UK

Jonathan M. Webb FRCS
Consultant Orthopaedic Surgeon, Southmead General Hospital, Bristol, UK

Norman S. Williams MS, FRCS
Professor of Surgery, Academic Department of Surgery, The Royal London Hospital, London, UK

James Wilson-MacDonald MCh, FRCS
Consultant Surgeon, Nuffield Orthopaedic Centre, Oxford, UK

Marc Christopher Winslet MS, FRCS, FRCS(Ed)
Professor of Surgery & Head of Department, University Department of Surgery, Royal Free Hospital School of Medicine, London, UK

Ian G. Winson FRCS(Ed)
Consultant Orthopaedic Surgeon, Southmead General Hospital, Bristol, UK

Preface

The 22nd edition of this famous book maintained its position as a bestselling international textbook of surgery. The success of *Bailey & Love's Short Practice of Surgery* reflected the wide appeal of its presentation of the fundamentals of surgical practice in a direct, concise way by surgeons who are recognised experts in their chosen fields. The 23rd edition maintains and develops the principles that underpinned the success of earlier editions.

In the 23rd edition emphasis continues to be placed on the importance of clinical observations at the bedside and the need to obtain accurate physical signs to make a sound diagnosis. Although the latest techniques for investigation are described, and their important contributions recognised, the book is based on the belief that sound surgical practice primarily depends on the skills and knowledge of the surgeon and secondarily on the strength of supporting departments and laboratories.

Despite the emphasis placed on the importance of clinical skills, each chapter has been carefully revised to ensure that the essential contribution made by specialist departments to modern surgical practice is fully documented. The huge strides that have been achieved by radiological techniques for diagnosis and treatment are described, including a new chapter on imaging, as are the advances in oncological, microbiological and biochemical methods, which ensure that the book caters for the requirements of up-to-the-minute surgical practice. Two completely new chapters stress the importance of the microbiological method in surgical practice, describing sterile precautions and theatre safety, which are now essential for good surgical practice. Further chapters on the principles of laparoscopic surgery and surgical ethics stress the importance of the fact that not only is the technique of surgery changing, but that the environment in which the surgeon practices is changing such that surgical ethics are now of major importance. These innovations, with the information provided in all chapters, keep the book abreast of the requirements of students, surgeons in training and practising general surgeons outside specialised departments.

To improve readability, the new format adopted for the 22nd edition has been enhanced to increase the use of colour and to improve the appearance such that the book now has a new look, but is still familiar. The wider use of colour has enabled more of the line drawings to be developed and ensures that the text remains lavishly illustrated by many clinical photographs in full colour. Despite these additions, the price of the book has been kept within the limits of a student's budget.

The 22nd edition was the last edited by Charles Mann, who has done much to develop this book and maintain its pre-eminence in surgical training. To replace Charles Mann, Professor Bulstrode, with his specialist knowledge of trauma and orthopaedics, has been enlisted, to emphasise that this specialty is now such an important part of general surgery that it deserves its own editor. He has completely revised the relevant sections and introduced innovative features developed from his wide experience in surgical education. This edition marks many changes and the editors have been aided by a wide list of distinguished specialists who have supervised the revision of its contents. Together with the continuing help of many overseas correspondents, the 23rd edition of *Bailey & Love's Short Practice of Surgery* caters in its very individual style for the needs of students and practising surgeons alike, and continues to provide the basis for sound surgical practice.

R.C.G. Russell
N.S. Williams
C.J. Bulstrode

Sayings of the Great

Both Hamilton Bailey and McNeill Love, when medical students, served as clerks to Sir Robert Hutchison, 1871–1960, who was Consulting Physician to the London Hospital and President of the Royal College of Physicians. They never tired of quoting his 'Medical Litany', which is appropriate for all clinicians, and, perhaps especially, to those who are surgically minded.

'From inability to leave well alone;
From too much zeal for what is new and
contempt for what is old;
From putting knowledge before wisdom,
science before art, cleverness before
common sense;
From treating patients as cases; and
From making the cure of a disease more
grievous than its endurance,
Good Lord, deliver.'

To which may be added.

'The patient is the centre of the medical universe around which all our works revolve and towards which all our efforts trend.' J.B. MURPHY, 1857–1916, Professor of Surgery Northwestern University, Chicago, Illinois, USA.

'To study the phenomenon of disease without books is to sail an uncharted sea, while to study books without patients is not to go to sea at all.' SIR WILLIAM OSLER, 1849–1919, Professor of Medicine, Oxford.

'A knowledge of healthy and diseased actions is not less necessary to be understood than the principles of other sciences. By an acquaintance with principles we learn the cause of disease. Without this knowledge a man cannot be a surgeon. ... The last part of surgery, namely operations, is a reflection on the healing art; it is a tacit acknowledgement of the insufficiency of surgery. It is like an armed savage who attempts to get that by force which a civilised man would by stratagem.' JOHN HUNTER, 1728–93, Surgeon, St George's Hospital, London.

'In investigating Nature you will do well to bear ever in mind that in every question there is the truth, whatever our notions may be. This seems perhaps a very simple consideration; yet it is strange how often it seems to be disregarded. If we had nothing but pecuniary rewards and worldly honours to look to, our profession would not be one to be desired. But in its practice you will find it to be attended with peculiar privileges; second to none in intense interest and pure pleasures. It is our proud office to tend the fleshy tabernacle of the immortal spirit, and our path, if rightly followed, will be guided by unfettered truth and love unfeigned. In the pursuit of this noble and holy calling wish you all God-speed.' 'Promotor's address, Graduation in Medicine, University of Edinburgh, August, 1876' by LORD LISTER, the Founder of Modern Surgery.

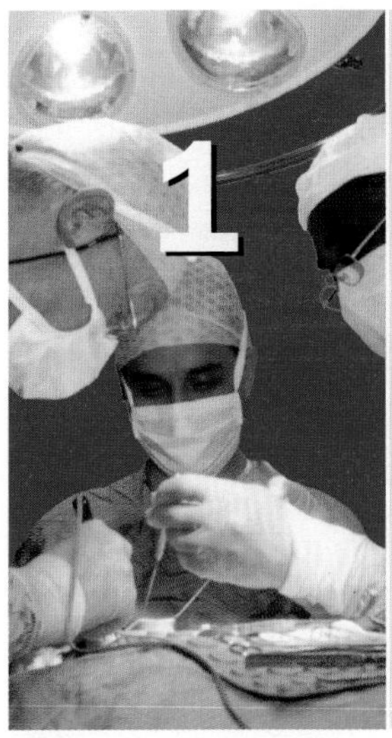

1 Introduction to surgery. Basic surgical principles

Introduction

Opening a surgical text has a forbidding feel, page after page of closely set print interspersed with pictures which sometimes help to explain the text but more often confuse on account of their lack of clarity. Didactic teaching required dull tomes to buttress the ethos of complexity so often promulgated by the professional. Bailey and Love set out to alter this trend by presenting a text that was colourful, readable and contained the precise information required by the student of surgery. Since the first publication of this book in 1932, surgery has become simpler to study. Greater knowledge simplifies and more exact diagnosis leaves less to supposition and opinion. It is now easy to verify an opinion, and even the most arrogant are worn down by the certainty of the newer imaging techniques in providing an exact diagnosis. The spleen palpated only by the consultant can soon be verified by computerised tomography (CT) (Fig. 1.1).

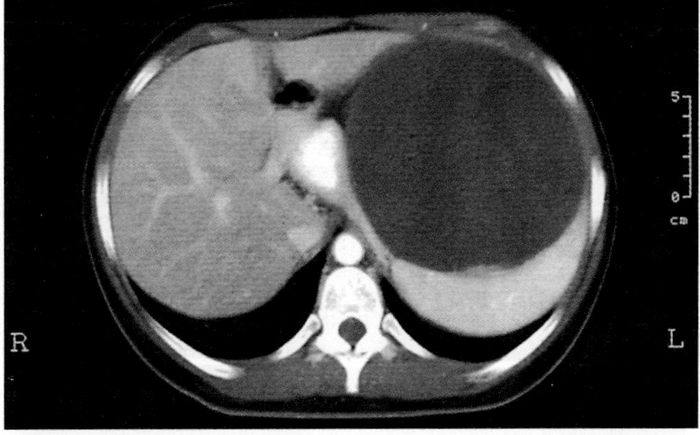

Fig. 1.1 Computerised tomogram of the upper abdomen showing a large cyst arising from the pancreas and pushing the spleen posteriorly in a 20-year-old girl. The signs were identical to those of an enlarged spleen but no splenic notch was palpable.

Surgical diagnosis is based on a sound knowledge of anatomy, physiology and pathology, a specific history and examination with confirmation by imaging and operative surgery. It is unnecessary to learn what can be deduced, and thus studying surgery concerns defining the basic facts on which the consequences of a disease process can be built (Fig. 1.2).

It is often surprising that a book entitled *Short Practice of Surgery* does not contain more about operative surgery. The actual operation in surgery is but one part of the process of surgical care; diagnosis, preoperative care and postoperative management being of equal importance in differing circumstances. No matter how good the operation, if it is performed for the wrong diagnosis, the benefit to the patient will be limited or void. In other situations, such as the patient who presents as a surgical emergency in association with severe illness, a common occurrence in this era of the elderly patient, skilled preoperative resuscitation and management, often in conjunction with the relevant physician, can turn a high-risk procedure into a routine operation. Similarly, the very ill patient can be salvaged by expert postoperative management. Nevertheless, the trend to denigrate the skills of operative surgery has been exposed as false by audit, which time and time again shows that a surgeon who does a procedure frequently outperforms in every parameter the surgeon who does an operation intermittently. The skills of operative

Hamilton Bailey, 1894–1961. Surgeon, Royal Northern Hospital, London, England.

Bailey & Love's Short Practice of Surgery, 23rd edition. Edited by R.C.G. Russell, N.S. Williams and C.J.K. Bulstrode. Published in 2000 by Arnold Publishers.

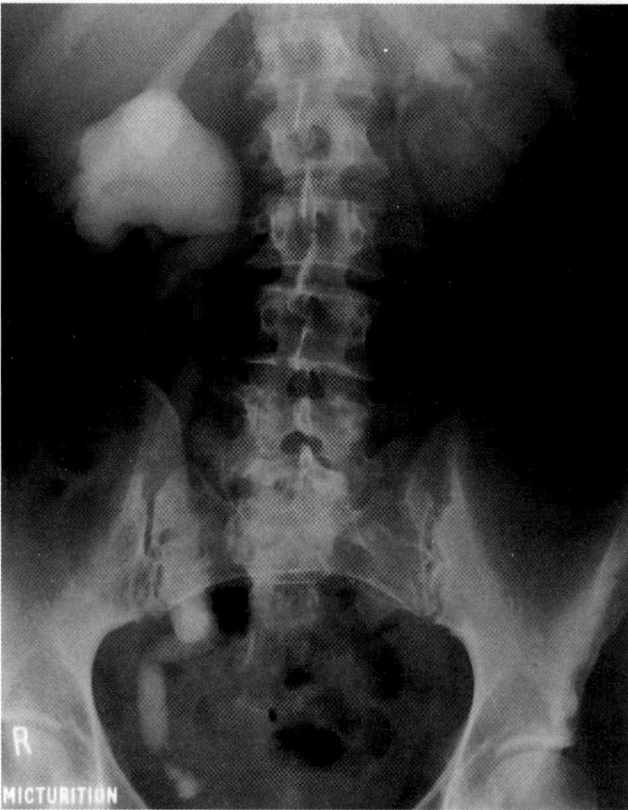

Fig. 1.2 Intravenous urogram showing the effect of obstruction by a stone at the lower end of the right ureter. The obstruction has caused dilatation of the renal pelvis with destruction of the parenchyma. Provided the left kidney is normal, there will be no change in renal function.

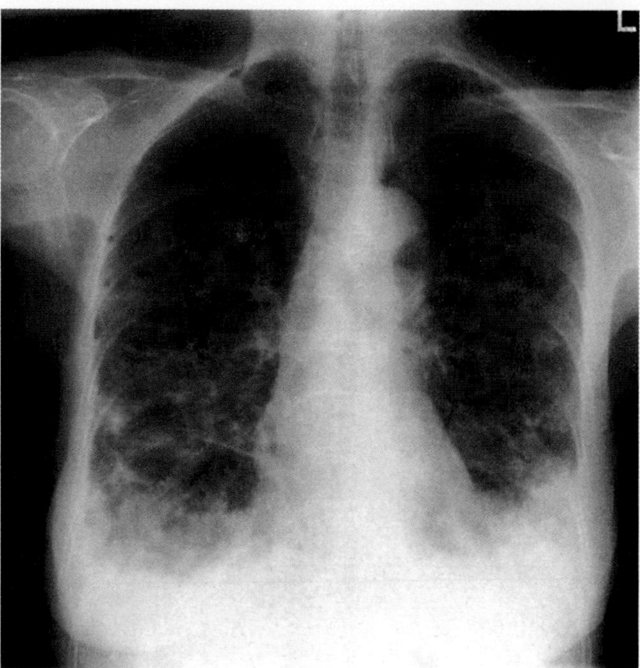

Fig. 1.3 Chest radiograph in a woman who was about to have an operation for cancer. The extensive chest disease due to malignant spread to the lungs rules out curative surgery.

surgery are primarily taught in the operating theatre and by supervised practice aided by specific illustrative texts on operative surgery. The objective of this book is to ensure that the surgeon understands the basis of the craft.

Surgical process

This starts with the patient from whom a careful history is taken. A focused physical examination is performed, and the complete medical status of the patient assessed. The likely diagnosis is considered on the basis of this clinical assessment, and confirmed by the appropriate test. Once confirmed, the specific treatment, be that medical or surgical, is advised. Should the likely diagnosis be wrong, attention is turned to the patient for further details of their ailment, and a more careful differential diagnosis considered as a basis for investigation. Continued observation over a limited period of time remains a powerful tool for achieving a diagnosis.

Despite current concepts, many patients with complaints requiring surgical treatment present with a simple history such as a lump or a pain for which a specific algorithmic approach will provide an answer. Experience will provide an answer for many patients who present with a physical sign, and no amount of history taking or examination will add to that visual assessment. A sebaceous cyst with its punctum standing proud is a simple surgical condition requiring a surgical exicision. The patient is operated upon, and the episode complete. Even the woman who presents with an ulcerating lump on her breast can be managed similarly in a diagnostic sense, but the knowledge attained in surgical study warns against a similar simplistic approach, and attention is turned to confirmation of the diagnosis noninvasively, so enabling full assessment of the whole patient on the basis of a confirmed pathology, often in co-operation with colleagues from other disciplines (Fig. 1.3).

Too little attention has been paid by the surgeon to the ancillary process of investigation, more so in some disciplines than others. Just as the stethoscope is helpful in diagnosis, so also ultrasonography, endoscopy and other forms of imaging will lead to a rapid confirmation of the clinical findings: an ultrasound scan is done to confirm gallstones (Fig. 1.4), a sigmoidoscopy to show a rectal carcinoma, a plain radiograph to confirm a fracture (Fig. 1.5), magnetic resonance imaging (MRI) to show a prolapsed disc (Fig. 1.6) and an angiogram to define the cause of anginal pain. Each has a specific place in the surgical process, and each makes the operative approach more specific, but none is the sole reason for operation as the clinical approach dictates that an operation is only performed for a condition causing symptoms in a patient fit to withstand the procedure.

Thus, surgery is about risk assessment. The diagnosis is made, the fitness of the patient assessed, the procedure determined and the outcome known. Will that outcome benefit the patient? A tumour in the head of the pancreas, if

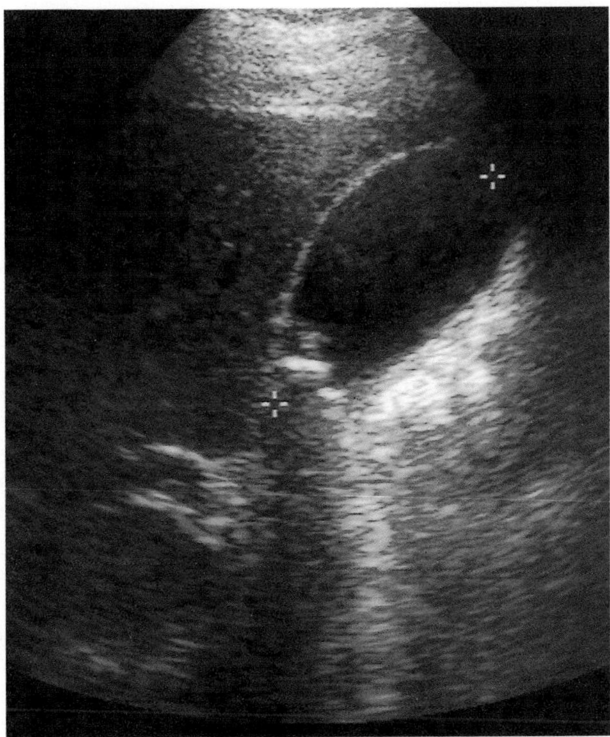

Fig. 1.4 Ultrasound image of the gallbladder showing an acoustic shadow caused by the gallstone.

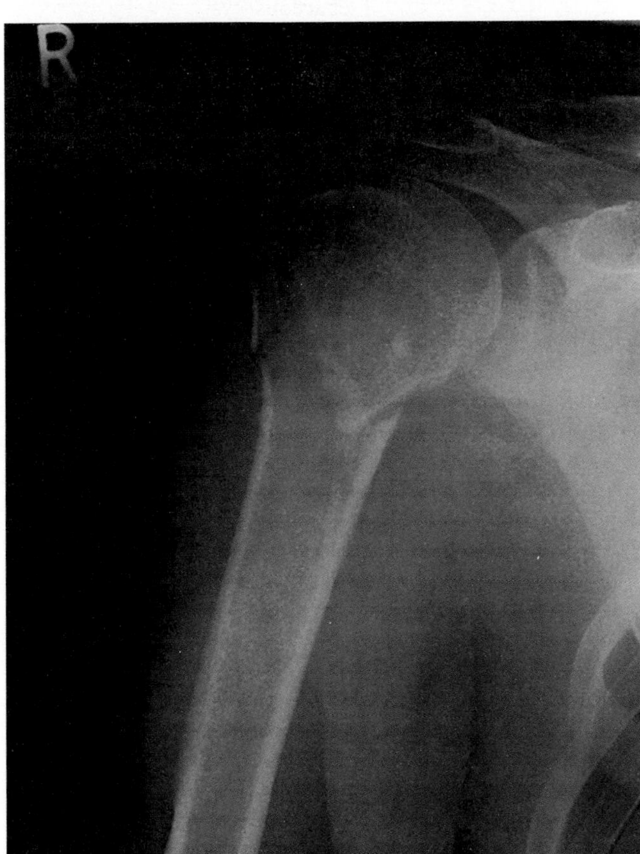

Fig. 1.5 Fracture of the neck of the right humerus.

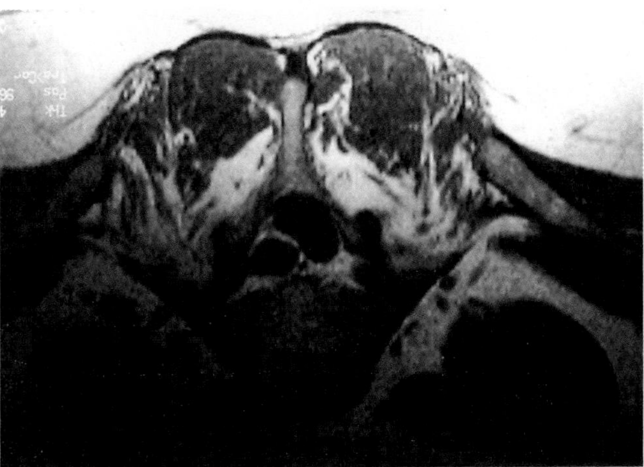

Fig. 1.6 Magnetic resonance image showing a prolapsed intervertebral disc filling part of the spinal canal and compressing the nerve root.

left untreated, will kill the patient in 6 months, so treatment appears mandatory, yet the operation has a mortality of 10 per cent, the median survival is only extended by 12 months and the comorbid factors are high, such that many patients will derive little benefit from the extensive surgery (Fig. 1.7). However, a patient with a strangulated femoral hernia, which in the elderly patient carries a mortality risk of 10 per cent, particularly if bowel is resected, faces the same comorbidity risk as the patient who has pancreatic cancer, but is cured by the procedure, and hence there is no doubt that the operation is worthwhile and the procedure is undertaken.

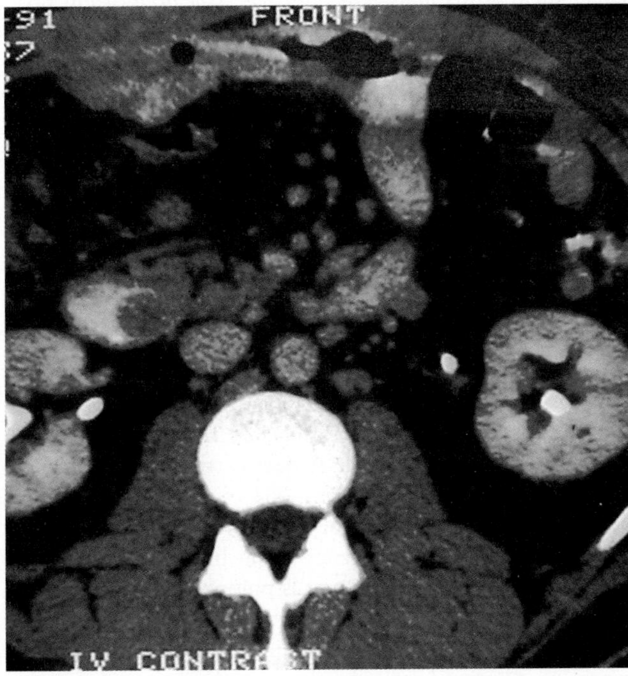

Fig. 1.7 Computerised tomogram showing a small ampullary tumour protruding into the duodenum. This 72-year-old man had successful surgery but died at home on day 35 of a coronary thrombosis.

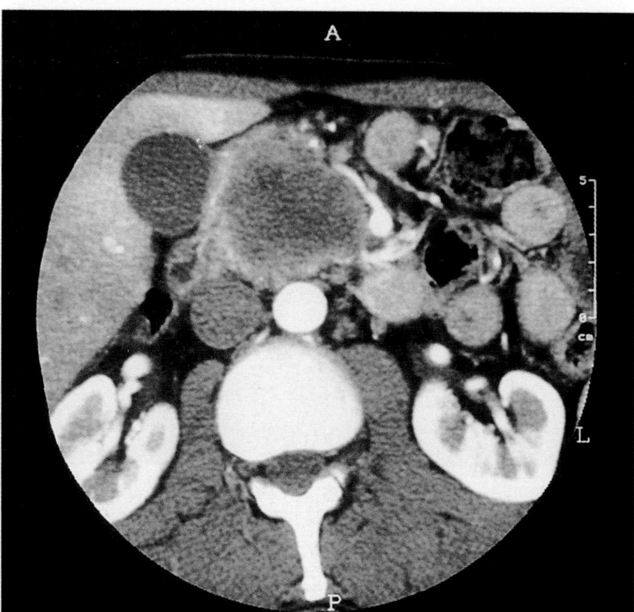

Fig. 1.8 Computerised tomogram of the upper abdomen in a 50-year-old man showing an inoperable cancer of the pancreas. A laparotomy to confirm the already proven histological diagnosis would merely add to the misery of this patient's remaining 3 months.

At present, such decisions are matters of judgement, but with increasing knowledge of risk assessment, the correct procedure or management can be more easily calculated and fewer errors of judgement made. By and large, it is errors of judgement that cause surgical misadventure. By avoiding these errors through better and more exact diagnosis, preoperative care and postoperative management, the surgical management of patients will improve. The premortem procedure to prove that everything was done for the patient that could be done is no longer acceptable, and a more humane approach to terminal illness is required (Fig. 1.8).

Surgical history

The history of the complaint is the key step in surgical diagnosis. It will vary according to the complaint, and be specific for particular complaints or systems. Such specific histories will be acquired as the particular surgical speciality is studied. There is no such thing as a standard surgical history as there is in medicine; it is for this reason that the student often adapts the medical history to the surgical clerking and misses many of the important points that are required in surgical decision making; thus, as the subject is studied, the form of history is acquired.

There are two types of history in surgical practice. The first is the out-patient or emergency room history in which the specific complaint of the patient is pinpointed; the second is the clerking of a patient admitted for elective surgery. The object of the first history is to obtain a diagnosis on which the treatment is ordered, whereas the second is to assess that the treatment planned is correctly indicated and to ensure that the patient is suitable for that operation.

Invariably the surgical patient presents in the out-patient department or the emergency room with a special problem such as pain or a lump. As opposed to most medical histories, the patient's story is limited and frequently the surgeon will focus the detail of the history, by a few specific questions. It is important to know when the symptom started, how it has progressed, whether there are associated features and whether the symptom is improving or getting worse. Time can be important, as are relationships to other symptoms. The effect of any treatment on the symptom is of value. Once the symptom complex has been resolved and clarified, the general health of the patient is defined to determine whether the complaint is local or part of a general disease. Questions are asked related to previous illness or concurrent illness, drug therapy, allergies and complications related to anaesthesia, to compose a picture of the patient's general status and determine suitability for treatment. The surgical history is a dynamic event, in that the pattern of questioning will change according to the answers of the patient, to compose the picture of that patient's illness.

The clerking history centres on direct questioning of the patient about specific points related to the complaint. For instance, it is important to record the symptoms of prostatism in the patient having prostatic surgery, so that these can easily be compared with the postoperative state to assess the effect of the surgical procedure. Further, in the patient who is referred by a physician for surgery, specific questions related to the indications for surgery are asked, and the surgeon decides whether or not the patient will benefit from the operation; this is particularly important in noncancerous conditions where continued medical management is an option.

Clinical examination

As with the history, so with the examination, there are two aspects of the examination: that concentrating on the specific complaint, the lump or the pain, and that reviewing the whole patient. Examination of the whole patient, particularly before an operation, should be as thorough as that performed in a routine medical examination. In examining a specific surgical feature, it is important to follow an accurate clinical description.

Diagnosis of a lump

First, determine in what anatomical plane the lump is situated: the skin, subcutaneous tissue, muscle, tendon, nerve or bone, or is it attached to some particular organ? Second, determine the physical characteristics of the lump: is it tender or nontender? If not acutely tender, determine: its size – measure in centimetres; shape – round or flattened, regular or irregular; and consistency – very soft (like a jelly), soft (as relaxed muscle), firm (like a contracted muscle), hard (as a contracted biceps) or stony hard.

Having completed the examination, it is a useful discipline to consider whether the lump is congenital, traumatic, inflammatory (acute or chronic), neoplastic (benign or malignant) and, if malignant, a primary or secondary neoplasm. If it is none of these, a degenerative, metabolic or hormonal disorder may provide the key.

Important specific signs

- *Thrill*: three fingers are placed on a swelling, the middle one being pressed firmly and the lateral ones lightly. The middle finger is percussed firmly, and after each stroke, the percussing finger is allowed to rest momentarily. The thrill felt by the adjacent fingers confirms the presence of fluid under pressure.
- *Sign of compression*: when the swelling is compressed it diminishes in size considerably or disappears. When the pressure is released it refills slowly. Characteristically the sign is related to vascular swellings.
- *Sign of indentation*: certain cysts containing putty-like material can be moulded – thus the swelling is indented by the finger. Faeces can be indented.
- *Sign of an aneurysm*: difficulty can be encountered in deciding whether the pulsation of a swelling is transmitted or whether the swelling itself is pulsating. If the swelling is expansile and pushes the fingers apart, then it is an aneurysmal swelling, while if the swelling is deflected by the pulsation it is transmitted.

Ulcers

An ulcer is a loss of epithelial lining; when examining an ulcer, attention should be paid to the following points.

- *Shape*: is it round, oval, irregular or serpiginous?
- *Edge*: this may slope downwards towards the crater, be undermined, punched out or everted.
- *Floor*: the most typical is a slough in the base of an ulcer.
- *Base*: whether indurated or attached to deeper structures.
- *Surrounding tissues*: examine for signs of inflammation, pigmentation or the presence of varicosities.

After an ulcer has been examined it is essential to consider the lymphatic drainage, and in particular the regional nodes.

Ulcers are of five main varieties:

- the septic ulcer with sloping edges;
- the tuberculous ulcer with undermined edges;
- the carcinomatous ulcer with everted hard edges;
- the rodent ulcer with barely visible pearly edges;
- the syphilitic punctated ulcer.

Terminology

In describing an examination, terms should be used specifically and correctly.

A *fistula* implies a tunnel connecting two epithelial surfaces.

A *sinus* is a blind track opening on to the skin or a mucous surface.

Fluid may discharge from a sinus or fistula; the discharge should be examined and noted: is it blood, blood-stained, clear, bile-like, serous, faecal or purulent? The type of fluid may give a clue to the possible diagnosis.

Lymphangitis is inflammation within a lymphatic vessel and appears as a red line often leading to an inflamed regional lymph node.

Phlebitis is a thrombosed and inflamed vein – it is more usual in superficial veins often associated with varicose veins, which are tender and hard.

Cellulitis is inflammation of tissues, usually superficial or subcutaneous tissue. The part affected is swollen, tense and tender. Later it becomes red, shiny and boggy. It may progress to an abscess, which is the presence of pus in the tissue concerned.

Inflammation, which is the earlier stage of cellulitis, is the presence of redness, swelling, heat and tenderness, often associated with the loss of function.

Crepitus is a term used in a variety of conditions but in each having a fundamental diagnostic importance. Bone crepitus is noted as coarse grating on movement of a bone – it is very painful to the patient, and an unmistakable diagnosis of a fracture of a bone. Joint crepitus is elucidated by placing one hand on a joint and passively moving the joint with the other hand: fine, evenly spaced crepitations are present in many subacute and chronic joint conditions. Coarse, irregular crepitations signify osteoarthritis.

The crepitus of tenosynovitis is found over an inflamed tendon sheath when effusion has occurred into the sheath.

The crepitus of subcutaneous emphysema is due to gas in the tissues: a peculiar crackling sensation is imparted to the examining fingers. It may be due to trauma when gas is released into the tissues after a rib fracture or damage to the oesophagus, or due to gas-forming organisms as in gas gangrene.

Translucency: there are occasions when swellings containing clear fluid lie adjacent to the skin. When a torch is shone through the swelling it lightens the area, confirming the diagnosis.

Ballotement is when a swelling can be tapped away from the examining finger, often due to fluid adjacent to the swelling. The term also describes the ability to palpate bimanually a renal swelling and to tap the kidney forward from the loin to the examining fingers of the other hand on the abdomen. A swelling may be balloted from the pelvis, by a finger in the vagina, to the examining abdominal hand.

Fluctuation is a specific term to elucidate the presence of fluid. Two watching fingers are placed on either side of a swelling and a central displacing finger presses momentarily. An impulse is felt by the watching finger confirming the presence of fluid, provided the sign is elicited in more than one plane.

Imaging

The reason for great emphasis on physical signs in the past was the absence of confirmatory imaging techniques. Because of the facility with which these facilities confirm or refute a physical sign, care in their interpretation is rarely taken. Yet, it is physical signs which may lead to a diagnosis, and the constant observation of the patient can delineate changes that are helpful to management.

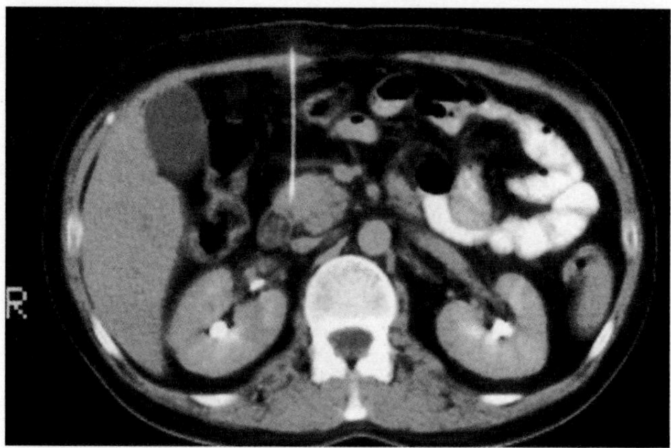

Fig. 1.9 Computerised tomography guided biopsy of a mass in the head of the pancreas.

Most physical signs can be confirmed by ultrasonography, plain radiography, CT or MRI. It is important to be aware of the appropriate test. If a swelling has been defined an ultrasound scan will usually confirm or refute the claim. It will define whether the swelling is solid or cystic, and whether it is aneurysmal, particularly with the aid of Doppler imaging. Biopsy using ultrasonography or CT guidance will give histological confirmation of the nature of the swelling (Fig. 1.9). Plain radiographs will define bony changes and fractures (Fig. 1.10), and gas shadows, such as in abdominal distension. MRI will define abnormalities in joints (Fig. 1.11) and within the skull, whereas CT, particularly with contrast enhancement, will outline solid organs (Fig. 1.12).

Imaging, to reach its full diagnostic potential, must be used correctly, and thus requires study within each surgical discipline.

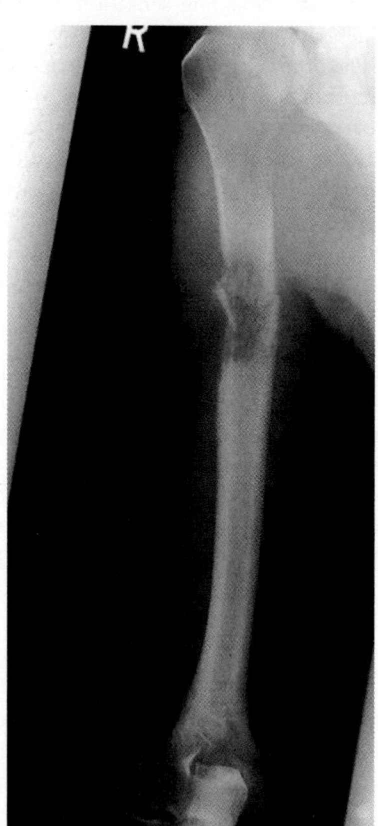

Fig. 1.10 A pathological fracture in the right humerus. A further metastasis is present above the fracture while periosteal thickening is present immediately below.

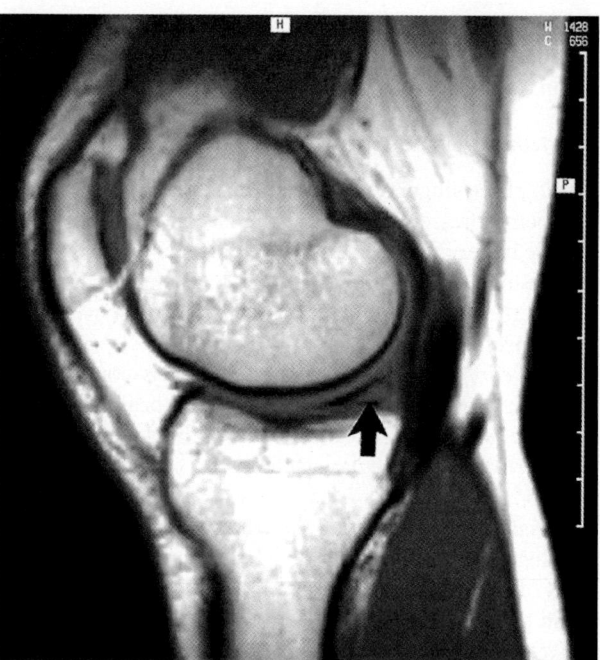

Fig. 1.11 Magnetic resonance image showing a torn meniscus (arrow).

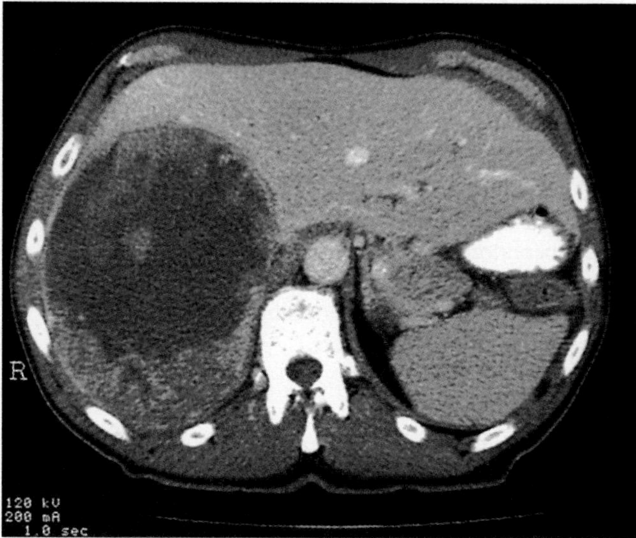

Fig. 1.12 The large mass on the right side of the abdomen is delineated by a contrast-enhanced computerised tomogram. The tumour is well defined and shows no sign of invasion. It was removed at operation.

Christian Johann Doppler, 1803–53. Austrian physicist.

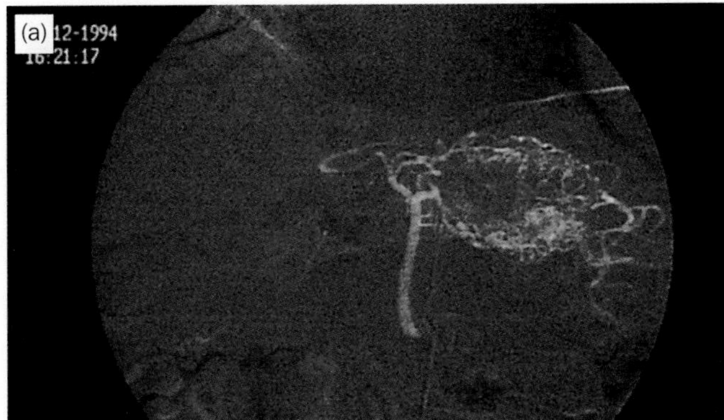

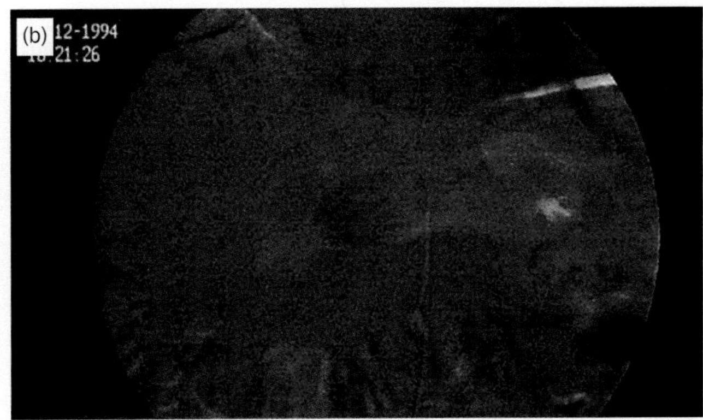

Fig. 1.13 (a) A selective angiogram of the left gastric artery defined bleeding varices in the fundus of the stomach. (b) A later film shows a blob of contrast (bleeding) in the stomach. Embolisation of the left gastric artery cured this man and prevented the need for surgical intervention.

Diagnostic process

The initial surgical process is complete when a diagnosis has been obtained by history, examination and imaging, supported by pathology. Experience enables correct weighting to be placed on each aspect of this process to define the correct treatment. All pieces of the jigsaw must fit together, and when they do not, great care must be exercised. Surgical conditions tend to follow a logic based on anatomy, physiology and pathology (Fig. 1.13); if that logic is transgressed, mistakes are made, and the patient may be wrongly treated.

Before submitting a patient to surgery, the diagnosis should be exact, the patient's condition carefully assessed and physiological variables corrected as far as possible. Any additional risks should be taken into account and allowance made for them in the surgical process.

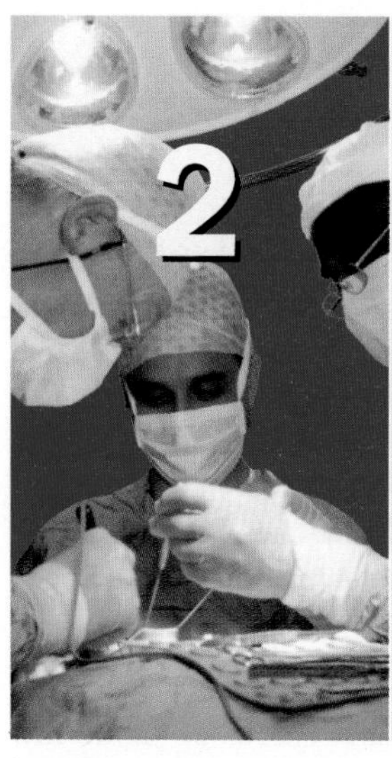

2 Diagnostic and interventional radiology

Introduction

Accurate diagnosis is the key to good surgical practice. Over the last two decades the introduction and increased availability of new imaging modalities have made the diagnostic process easier. Imaging helps to resolve the uncertainties of diagnosis based on physical signs and clinical judgement. To achieve the optimum diagnostic potential it is necessary to understand the complexities of modern imaging and to recognise the most appropriate test to fit the clinical context. Communication between the clinician and radiologist is vital for each to understand the clinical problem, and the strengths and weaknesses of the imaging test selected. An ability to interpret images gives a new depth of understanding of the disease process and of the nature and timing of surgical intervention.

There is no standard approach to imaging although some basic principles apply. It is generally good practice to perform the simplest and least expensive test first if this will provide the answer. For example, the plain abdominal film remains the diagnostic cornerstone in assessing the acute abdomen; in a patient with a clear history of biliary colic, a simple ultrasound examination may be sufficient to determine management. However, in a patient with a more complex clinical presentation, it may be more cost-effective to perform a more expensive test [e.g. computerised tomography (CT) scan] early in the diagnostic work-up as this may lead to a more confident diagnosis and management, and potentially shorten the hospital stay. Cost-effectiveness requires that more complex tests are not merely layered on top of existing more standard procedures. Through consultation, the best test must be determined. The selection of the best investigation for a particular clinical context has been made more complex by the rapid changes in existing technology. The development of spiral (helical) CT, for example, has created new diagnostic possibilities based on the patterns of arterial and venous blood flow providing information not previously available on older equipment. Decision making therefore must be tailored to both the available technology and local expertise. It is also essential to view the imaging results in conjunction with the clinical condition of the patient and to treat the patient rather than the X-rays. In a patient with inflammatory bowel disease, for example, the extent and severity of the abnormality demonstrated on a small bowel barium examination may have little correlation with the patient's clinical presentation (Fig. 2.1). In contrast, a patient with fulminant colitis may be clinically toxic but with only minimal signs on the plain film before the reflex dilatation signalling toxic megacolon develops.

There is a general increase in public awareness of the adverse effect of radiation in the induction of cancer and genetic defects. Most of the received ionising radiation comes from the sun and earth's core. However, medical radiation accounts for approximately 12 per cent of the total received by humans.

Bailey & Love's Short Practice of Surgery, 23rd edition. Edited by R.C.G. Russell, N.S. Williams and C.J.K. Bulstrode. Published in 2000 by Arnold Publishers.

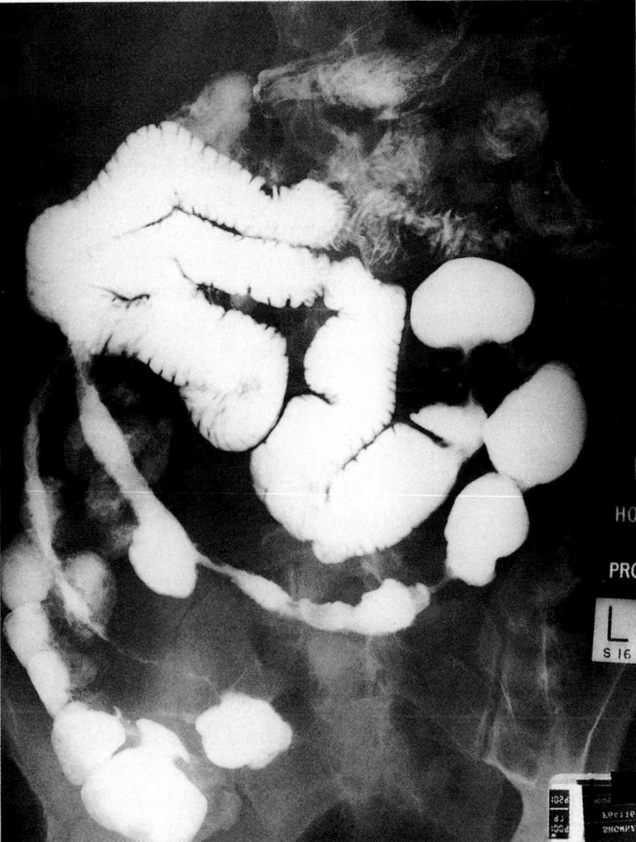

Fig. 2.1 Barium follow-through examination in a patient with Crohn's disease. Despite the presence of multiple strictures the patient was entirely asymptomatic.

Intravenous contrast
- Asthma, allergy, previous contrast reactions
  - May have increased incidence of adverse reaction. Usually require steroid premedication
- Renal failure, myeloma and diabetes (especially if treated with Metformin)
  - May have temporary adverse effect on renal function

MRI
- Absolute contraindications
  - Metallic foreign bodies
  - Pacemakers
  - Cochlear implants
  - Cranial aneurysm clips
- Relative contraindications
  - First trimester pregnancy
  - Claustrophobia

Barium enema
- Prosthetic valves
  - Risk of subacute bacterial endocarditis (SBE); require antibiotic prophylaxis
- Age/incontinence
  - Stressful examination for patient – consider CT – conventional or spiral pneumocolon

Fig. 2.3 Potential hazards in imaging.

As more nonradiation-dependent imaging techniques become more widely available [e.g. ultrasound, magnetic resonance imaging (MRI)], radiation hazard is an increasingly important factor influencing the selection of investigation, particularly in children and young people. The effective dose imparted by a CT scan, for example, is equivalent to 400 chest X-rays (CXRs). However, this theoretical risk must be balanced against the likely diagnostic yield of the examination in terms of benefit to the patient. The aim must be to reduce unnecessary investigations, which not only add needlessly to patient irradiation but also waste limited resources and increase waiting times. The Royal College of Radiologists has published a very useful booklet, *Making the Best Use of a Department of Clinical Radiology* (see Further reading section). This gives guidelines for investigations most likely to contribute to the clinical diagnosis and management in particular clinical situations. It highlights the chief causes of wasteful use of radiology (Fig. 2.2). Other factors must also be taken into consideration when deciding on the appropriate investigation, including the age and condition of the patient and their ability to undergo the chosen investigation (Fig. 2.3).

• *Results unlikely to affect patient management* – Positive finding unlikely – Anticipated finding probably irrelevant for management	Do I need it?
• *Investigating too often* – Before disease could be expected to have progressed or resolved	Do I need it now?
• *Repeating investigations done previously* – Other hospital? – GP?	Has it been done already?
• *Failing to provide adequate information* – Wrong test performed or essential view omitted	Have I explained the problem?
• *Requesting wrong investigation* – Discuss with radiologist	Is this the best test?

From: *Making the best use of a department of clinical radiology*, Royal College of Radiologists, 1998.

Fig. 2.2 Wasteful use of radiology.

Diagnostic imaging

Imaging techniques

Conventional radiology

Conventional radiographs depend on the differential absorption by soft tissue, bone, gas and fat of X-rays passing through the body. The unabsorbed rays blacken a photographic film, contained within light-sensitive screens, which is then processed to produce the hard copy. Modern radiology involves the use of many technical modifications to reduce the dose of X-rays to the patient. Plain X-rays remain the primary diagnostic tool in the chest and abdomen, and in trauma and orthopaedics. With careful interpretation, accurate diagnosis can be achieved and it is vital that the plain film is not jettisoned in favour of more complex and expensive imaging techniques.

When X-rays strike a fluorescent screen, light is emitted which, by means of an imaging intensifier, can be projected on a television screen. This is the basis of **fluoroscopy** (screening) which allows continuous monitoring of a moving process. It also provides guidance for many interventional and angiographic procedures and for barium investigations of the gastrointestinal tract. Barium studies remain a standard technique for evaluating disorders of swallowing and oesophageal function and for the small bowel. The role of the barium meal and enema is challenged by the expansion of endoscopy. However, there is little evidence to indicate that in the diagnosis of significant disease, e.g. ulcer/cancer, endoscopy is superior (Fig. 2.4). Choice of examination depends on local expertise and availability. Endoscopy is preferable where there is gastrointestinal bleeding (upper or lower) or inflammatory bowel disease.

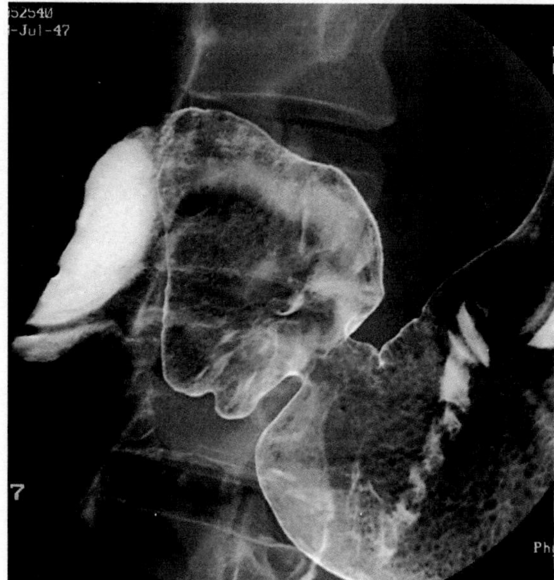

Fig. 2.4 Double contrast barium study of the duodenum demonstrating a central ulcer crater.

Intravenous contrast contains iodine which absorbs X-rays by virtue of its high atomic number. It provides arterial or venous opacification depending on the route and timing of injection. Contrast injected intravenously is excreted rapidly by the kidneys which forms the basis of the **intravenous urogram** (IVU) where the nephrographic (renal parenchymal) and pelvicalyceal (collecting system) phases, ureters and bladder are successively demonstrated and recorded over approximately 30 minutes following contrast injection. The IVU remains the best method for investigating renal stones and haematuria. No other technique can equally visualise the pelvicalyceal systems and ureters (Fig. 2.5).

Ultrasound

Ultrasound is inexpensive, quick, reliable and noninvasive and is an excellent initial investigation for a wide range of clinical problems. It is technically demanding and requires an experienced operator to maximise the potential of the examination. Despite the advances in technology, there are still problems with gas (which reflects sound completely) and obese patients, who are often unsuitable for ultrasound. As ultrasound is so accessible there is a tendency to overload departments with requests which may be on the margins of appropriateness. As with all investigations, clinicians should consider whether the request for ultrasound is justified as to its likely yield and its subsequent effect on patient management.

Ultrasound depends on the generation of high-frequency sound waves, usually of between 3 and 7 MHz, by a transducer placed on the skin. Sound is reflected by tissue interfaces in the body and the echoes generated are picked up by the same transducer and converted into an image which is then displayed in real time on a monitor. The scope of ultrasound has increased vastly over the last decade with higher frequency probes of diminishing size producing high-resolution images. The current range of ultrasound includes probes measuring only millimetres and operating at 20 MHz, which can be

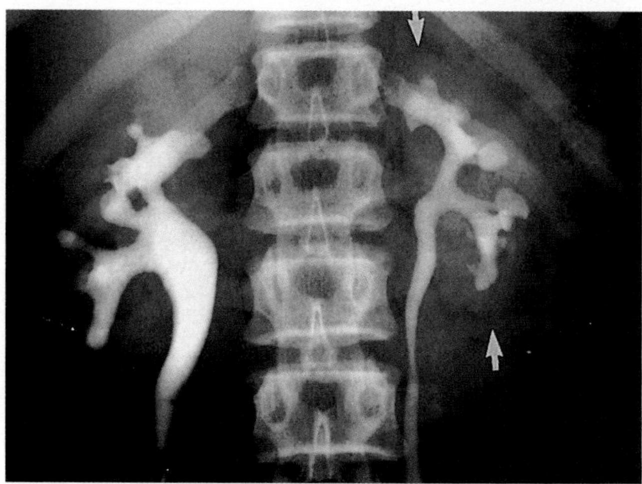

Fig. 2.5 IVU demonstrating a small left kidney with bilateral calyceal blunting and deformity in a patient with bilateral reflux nephropathy.

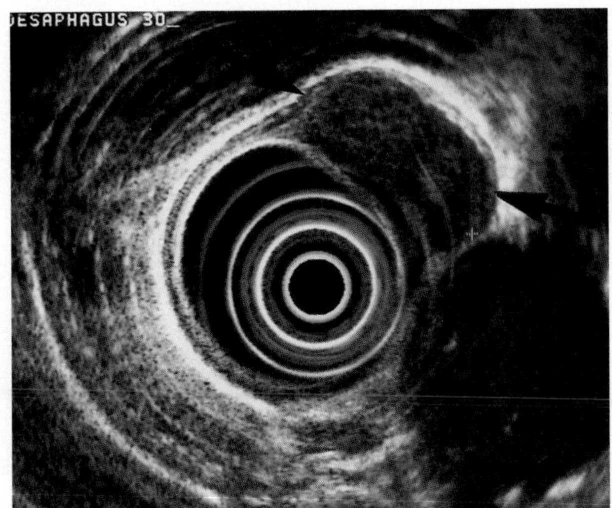

Fig. 2.6 Endoscopic ultrasound of the oesophagus showing a well-defined mass arising within the muscle wall (*arrows*) suggesting a leiomyoma.

introduced via a catheter into a blood vessel to image the vessel wall; probes combined with fibre-optic endoscopes to visualise the gut wall at echo endoscopy (EUS) (7.5–20 MHz) (Fig. 2.6); endoluminal probes for transvaginal and transrectal scanning (7.5 MHz); dedicated very-high-frequency probes of up to 15 MHz for scanning the breast, other superficial structures and musculoskeletal work; and an increasing array of specialised probes for abdominal scanning. Ultrasound is the first-line investigation in hepatobiliary disease, suspected pancreatic, aortic and many other intra-abdominal disorders (Fig. 2.7).

There is an increasing recognition of the value of intraoperative ultrasound scanning, acknowledging the fact that visualisation at surgery is frequently incomplete, the surgeon seeing only the exposed surfaces. These limitations are accentuated by the restrictions imposed by minimally invasive and laparoscopic surgery.

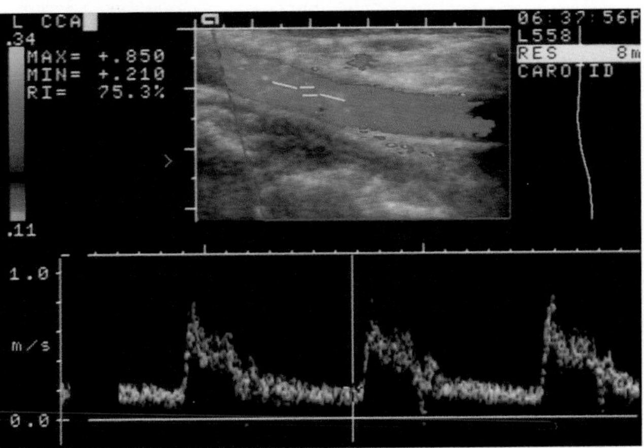

Fig. 2.8 Normal carotid artery. Colour Doppler showing the gate where the flow velocity waveform has been taken. Bottom: flow velocity waveform. The peaks represent systolic blood flow.

Doppler ultrasound measures the shift in frequency between transmitted and received sound and can therefore measure blood flow. The spectral Doppler wave form and ultrasound image are combined in duplex scanning. Colour Doppler imaging displays flowing blood as red or blue, depending on its direction, towards or away from the transducer (Fig. 2.8). Power Doppler is not dependent on frequency or direction of flow but is exquisitely sensitive to low flow and has the potential to demonstrate tissue perfusion (Fig. 2.9). Contrast agents have been developed based on micro-bubbles to enhance the Doppler effect. These techniques have revolutionised the diagnosis of both arterial and venous vascular disease.

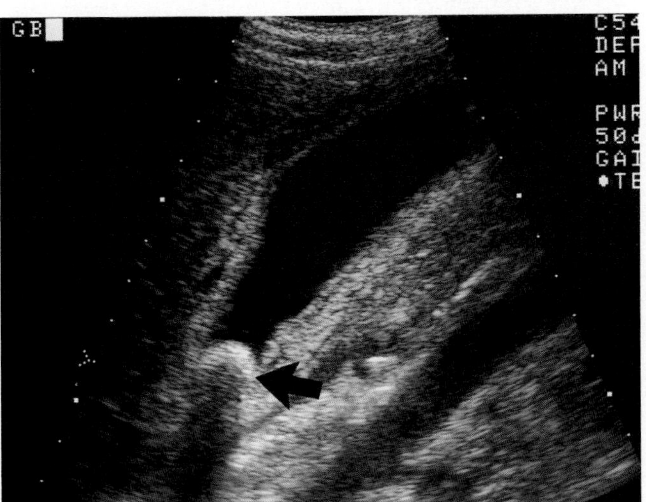

Fig. 2.7 Acute cholecystitis: ultrasound in a patient with acute right upper-quadrant pain and tenderness. The gall bladder is distended with a thickened wall and an impacted stone is seen in the gall bladder neck (*arrows*).

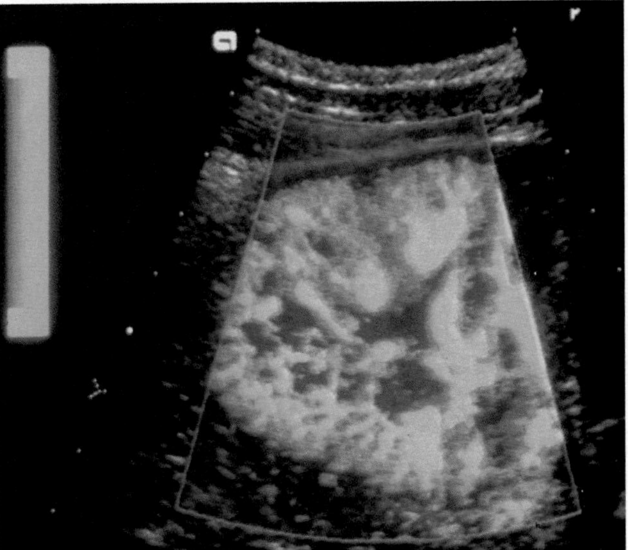

Fig. 2.9 Power Doppler perfusion scan of kidneys.

Christian Johann Doppler, 1803–1853. Austrian physicist.

Computerised tomography

To create a CT scan, a thinly collimated beam of X-rays passes through an axial 'slice' of tissue and strikes an array of very sensitive detectors which can distinguish very subtle differences in tissue density. By analysis of the collected data, the digital information is translated to a grey-scale image where the attenuation value of tissues is related to water, which is given a CT number of zero Hounsfield units (HU). Tissue densities range from +1000 (bone) down to −1000 (air). An observer working at a viewing console can, by varying the range and centering of densities represented (window width/level), display an image appropriate to the tissue being examined (Fig. 2.10).

In conventional CT, a series of individual scans is acquired during suspended respiration. Helical or spiral CT involves continuous rotation of the X-ray tube with the beam tracing a spiral path around the patient such that a volume of tissue is scanned. In this way, during a single breath-hold of up to 30 seconds, 30 cm or more of tissue can be covered in one acquisition. Further developments have allowed thinner collimation and stretching of the spiral to cover greater distances. The volumetric data can then be processed to produce conventional transaxial images or multiplanar (sagittal and coronal) and three-dimensional images (Fig. 2.11). The development of spiral scanning has greatly enhanced the diagnostic potential of CT (Fig. 2.12). It is now possible to exploit the enhancement characteristics of tissues in both the arterial and venous phases of imaging and this modification has opened up the fields of CT angiography, three-dimensional imaging and 'virtual endoscopy' of the bronchial tree and colon (Fig. 2.13).

CT scanning is usually performed after simpler investigations such as plain films or ultrasound. In many centres, however, CT is often used as a first-line examination in the evaluation of abdominal trauma and severe pancreatitis. It

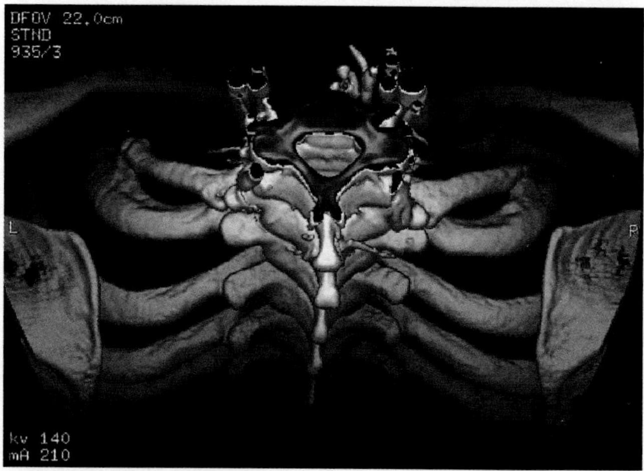

Fig. 2.11 Three-dimensional CT reconstruction of bilateral cervical ribs (*arrows*).

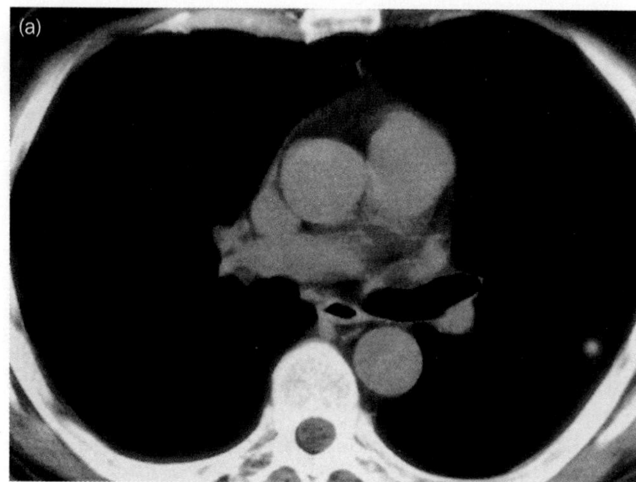

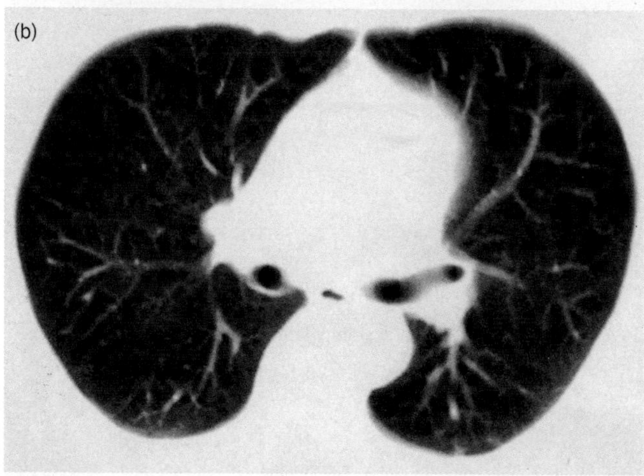

Fig. 2.10 The effect of varying window width and level. (a) At soft tissue settings (width 400 HU, level 40 HU) the normal mediastinal structures are shown; (b) at lung settings (width 1000 HU, level 700 HU), soft tissue and bone detail is lost but the lung parenchyma is seen.

- Reduced scan time: advantages in critically ill and children
- Imaging at peak levels of contrast: arterial and venous phase
- Overcomes the problem of 'mis-registration' – lesion 'missed' because of different depth of respiration
- Ability to review and reconstruct data retrospectively – improved lesion detection
- Multiplanar and three-dimensional analysis
  - CT angiography
  - Complex joints
  - Facial bones
  - 'Virtual endoscopy'
  - Spiral pneumocolon

Fig. 2.12 Advantages of helical (spiral) versus conventional CT.

Sir Godfrey Newbold Hounsfield, b. 1919. British engineer.

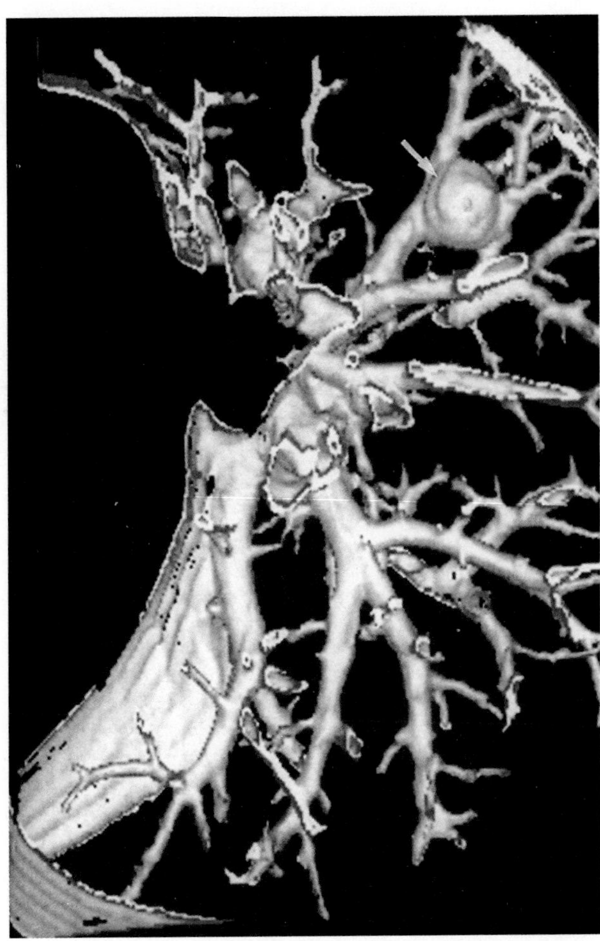

Fig. 2.13 Three-dimensional reconstruction of the pulmonary vasculature. The relationship of a small nodule to the adjacent vessels is clearly seen (*arrow*).

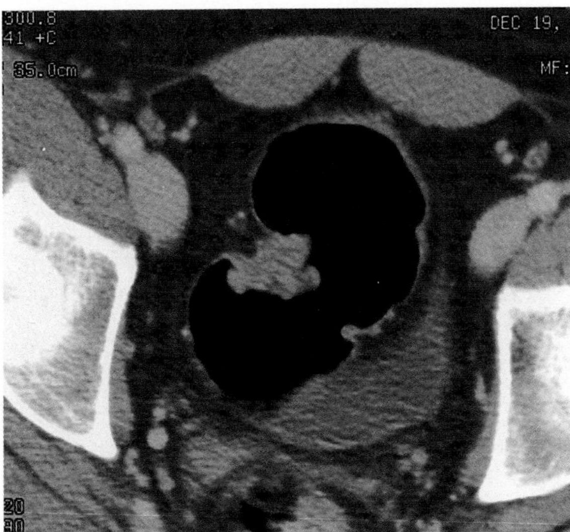

Fig. 2.14 CT spiral pneumocolon. A polypoid tumour of the sigmoid colon is clearly seen arising from the wall of the gas-distended bowel (*arrow*). The transmural extent of disease can be evaluated.

has a major role in cancer staging and an increasing role in 'problem solving' in the chest and abdomen. Some centres advocate early CT in assessment of the acute abdomen (*vide infra*). The development of the technique of CT spiral pneumocolon is challenging the barium enema and colonoscopy in the investigation of large bowel disorders (Fig. 2.14).

Magnetic resonance imaging

The basic principle of magnetic resonance imaging (MRI) centres on the concept that the nuclei of hydrogen, most prevalent in water molecules, behave like small spinning bar magnets and align with a strong external magnetic field. When knocked out of alignment by a radio frequency pulse, a proportion of these protons rotates in phase with each other and gradually returns to their original position, releasing small amounts of energy which can be detected by sensitive coils placed around the patient. The strength of the signal depends not only on the proton density but on the relaxation times, T1 and T2. T1 reflects the time taken to return to the axis of the original field and T2 on the time the protons take to de-phase. T1 images usually demonstrate exquisite anatomical detail because of the high soft tissue discrimination. Most pathological processes increase T2 relaxation times, producing a higher signal than the surrounding normal tissue on T2-weighted scans.

The complexity of the imaging process is compounded by the variety of pulse sequences available. In general, image acquisition time is longer than CT. Respiratory and cardiac motion degrade the image but this can be largely overcome with cardiac and respiratory gating. Technological developments are fast and scanning times are shortening. Intravenous gadolinium acts as a contrast agent by reducing T1 relaxation and enhancing lesions which then appear as areas of high signal intensity (Fig. 2.15). Specific sequences have been developed to demonstrate flowing blood and produce images resembling conventional angiography. This technique of **magnetic resonance angiography** (MRA) can be achieved without the risks of intravascular injection of contrast and may ultimately replace conventional studies (Fig. 2.16). Heavily T2-weighted sequences which demonstrate fluid-filled structures as areas of very high signal intensity have been developed to show the biliary and pancreatic ducts in **magnetic resonance cholangiopancreatography** (MRCP). It seems likely that this technique will take over from diagnostic endoscopic retrograde cholangiopancreatography (ERCP) (Fig. 2.17).

The major strength of MRI is in intracranial, spinal and musculoskeletal imaging, where it is superior to any other imaging technique because of its high contrast resolution and multiplanar imaging capability. Cardiac MRI is firmly established and the value of breast MRI, particularly in multifocal and recurrent cancer, is increasingly recognised. It is currently the best investigation for staging cervical cancer and for anorectal sepsis (Fig. 2.18).

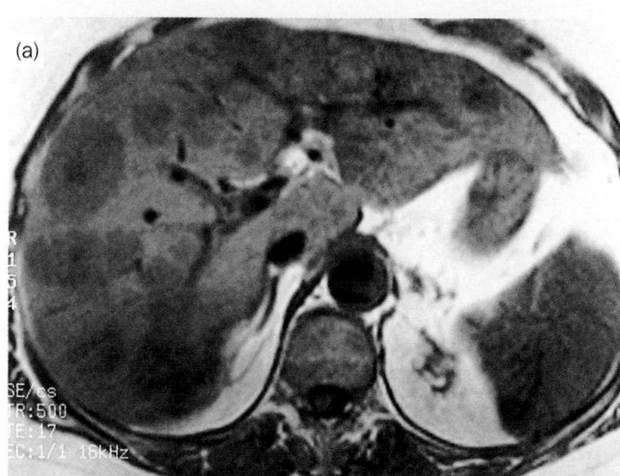

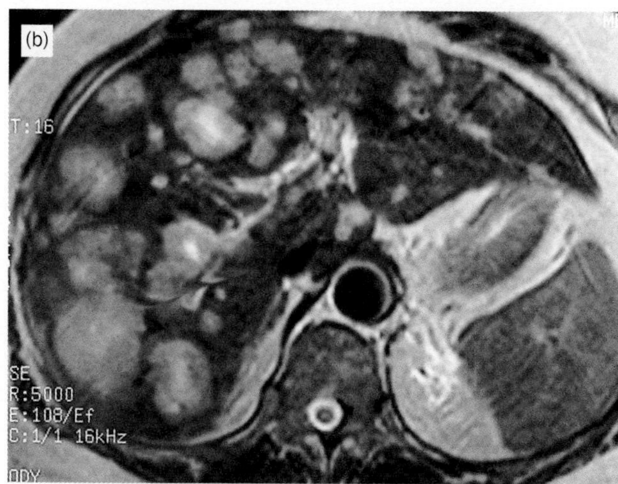

Fig. 2.15 MRI scan of the liver demonstrating multiple liver metastases as low signal on (a) T1- and high signal on (b) T2-weighted images.

Open access magnets have been developed which allow interventional procedures to be performed with MRI guidance and there is no doubt that this will revolutionise the operating room of the future (Fig. 2.19). There is a vast potential for MRI in the assessment of disease in the abdomen and pelvis and undoubtedly the role of MRI will continue to expand. However, because of the expense of the equipment and its installation, the provision of scanners cannot keep up with the demands for scanning time and most hospitals have to impose strict guidelines for access.

Radionuclide imaging

Radionuclides can be tagged to substances which concentrate selectively in certain tissues of the body. These radiopharmaceuticals are injected intravenously and, in general,

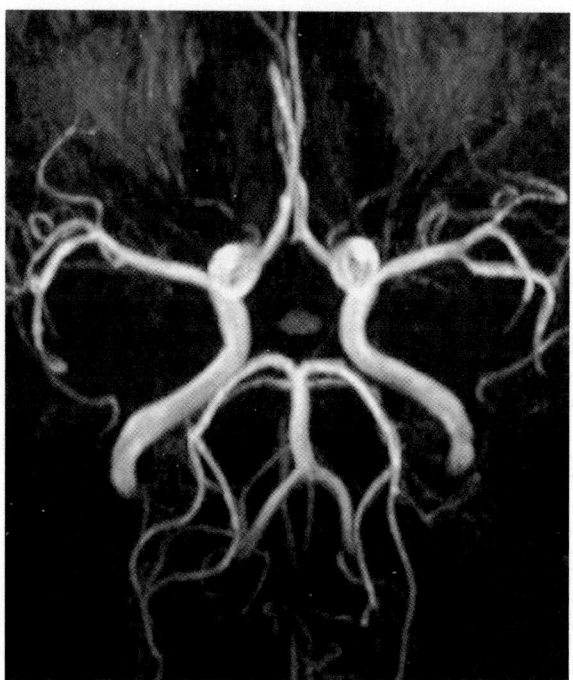

Fig. 2.16 MR angiogram of the cerebral arteries. This flow sequence produces images of the arteries forming the circle of Willis based on the signal obtained from flowing blood without the need for vascular contrast agents.

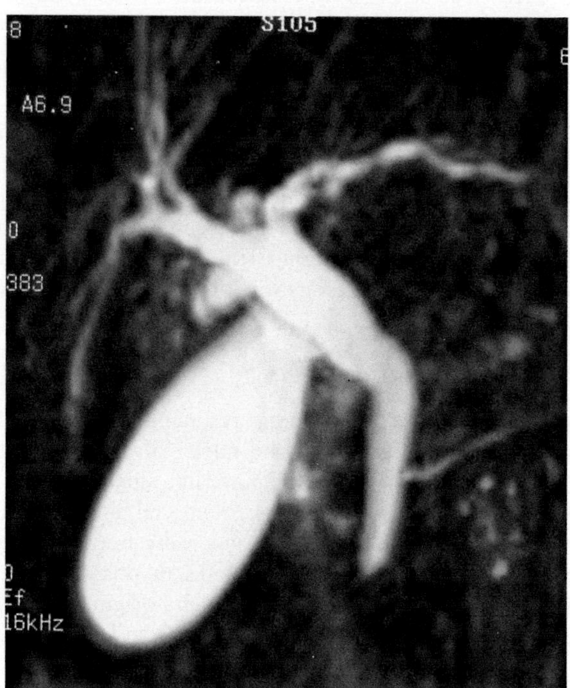

Fig. 2.17 MRCP. Heavily T2-weighted sequences detect the static fluid in the bile and pancreatic ducts and produce an image of the duct system, without the need for duct cannulation.

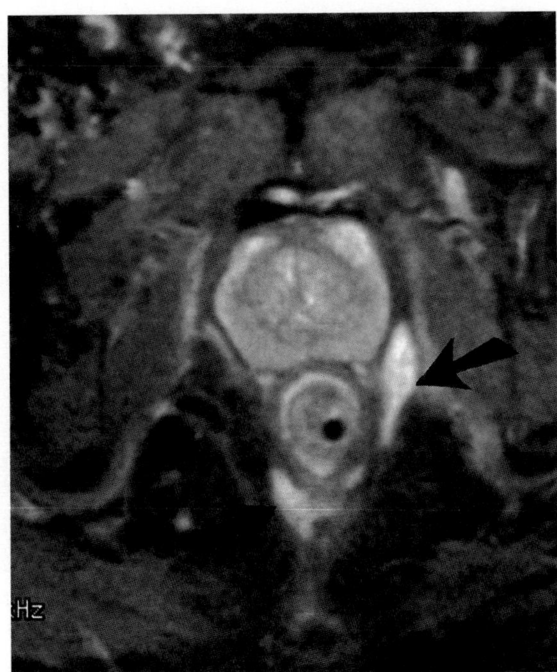

Fig. 2.18 Axial T2-weighted MRI showing extensive perianal fistula with intersphincteric tracking (*arrows*) in a patient with Crohn's disease.

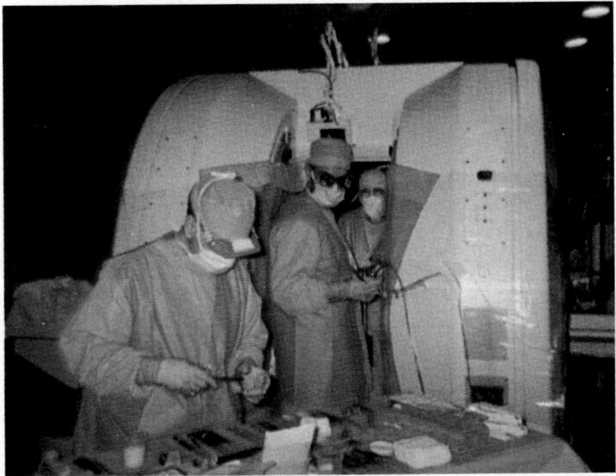

Fig. 2.19 A surgical procedure performed in the open configuration magnet (reproduced with permission of the Radiological Society of North America from *Radiology*, 1997, **204**, 605).

emit gamma radiation detected by a gamma camera. The emitted radiation strikes a sodium iodide crystal which generates a small flash of light which is then enhanced by photo-multiplier tubes to produce the image. Many studies employ technetium-99m (^{99m}Tc) which has a short half-life and imparts a radiation dose to the patient which is lower than many other imaging investigations.

In general, spatial resolution is poor as the technique demonstrates physiological and functional changes rather than anatomy (Fig. 2.20). A standard gamma camera provides only a two-dimensional display of activity. **Single photon emission computed tomography** (SPECT) creates a three-dimensional image by means of an array of photo-multiplier tubes that surround the patient in the same way as with CT and MRI. This technique uses conventional radionuclides. **Positron emission tomography** (PET) scanning is more sensitive, depending on the coincidence detection of annihilation protons resulting from radionuclides that decay by positron emission. However, these studies require specially designed, dedicated and currently expensive cameras and an in-hospital cyclotron to generate the radionuclide. These scans are therefore not widely available.

Cross-sectional imaging techniques have replaced many radionuclide studies (liver colloid scans, brain scans). Bone scanning remains a sensitive tool for detection of bone

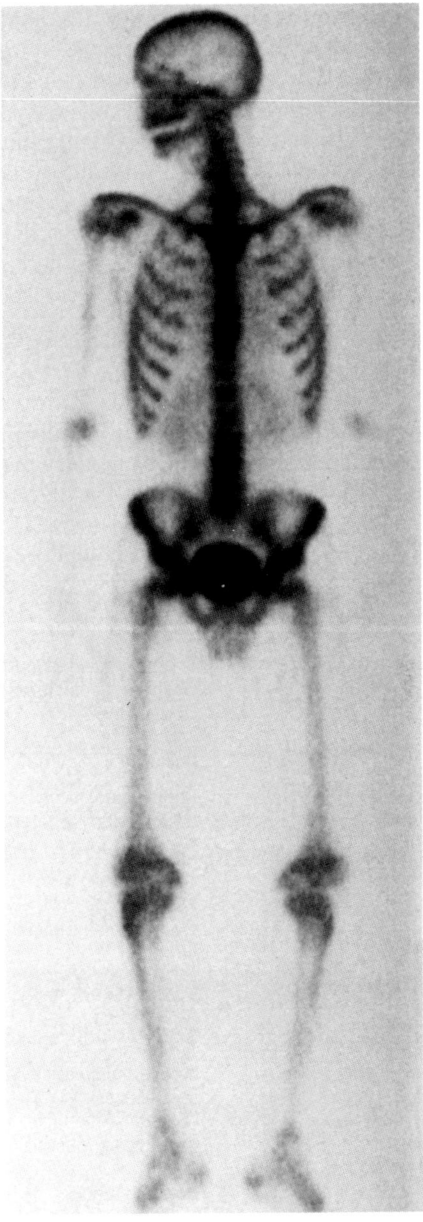

Fig. 2.20 Radionuclide bone scan. Following an intravenous injection of ^{99m}Tc-labelled organic phosphate, the agent is taken up into the skeleton in proportion to the rate of bone turnover and blood flow and an image of the skeleton is produced.

metastases and occult fractures. Ventilation–perfusion scans are widely used to detect pulmonary embolic disease, although contrast-enhanced spiral CT of the pulmonary vessels is challenging this role. New exciting techniques of radiopharmaceutical labelling of monoclonal antibodies are opening up possibilities of targeted cancer therapy and early detection of micrometastases.

Imaging in the acute abdomen

The term 'acute abdomen' encompasses many diverse entities. Imaging tests are selected based on the likely diagnosis (Fig. 2.21). The erect CXR and supine abdomen remain the investigation of choice where perforation or intestinal obstruction is suspected (Figs 2.22 and 2.23). In many patients this will provide sufficient information to determine further management. When the diagnosis is less clear, new imaging techniques are challenging the traditional approach. Both ultrasound and CT may contribute valuable information in inflammatory disease within the abdomen – notably in diverticulitis, appendicitis and in inflammatory bowel disease. In some centres – particularly in the USA – the use of spiral CT as a first-line investigation is being promoted as a cost-effective alternative to increase the specificity of primary diagnosis (Fig. 2.24).

Imaging in oncology

Modern surgical treatment of tumour requires an understanding of tumour staging systems, as in many instances this will define appropriate management. The development of stage-dependent treatment protocols involving neoadjuvant chemotherapy and preoperative radiotherapy relies on the ability to define tumour stage accurately by imaging before surgical and pathological staging. Once a diagnosis of tumour has been established, often by percutaneous or endoscopic

Imaging	*Indications/signs*
CXR (erect)	Gas under diaphragm
Abdominal X-ray (AXR) (supine)	Dilated bowel/gas pattern Gas inside/outside bowel Obstruction? Closed loop? Bowel wall oedema?
IVU	Renal colic Ureteric obstruction by stone?
Ultrasound (US)	Ascites Cholecystitis Abscess Obstruction? – dilated fluid-filled bowel
Focused high-resolution US	Diverticulitis Appendicitis Bowel wall thickening/abscess
CT	Severe pancreatitis Diverticulitis Abscess Small bowel obstruction (high grade) Bowel infarction
Focused CT	Appendicitis Ureteric colic (if contrast allergy)

Fig. 2.21 Imaging in the acute abdomen.

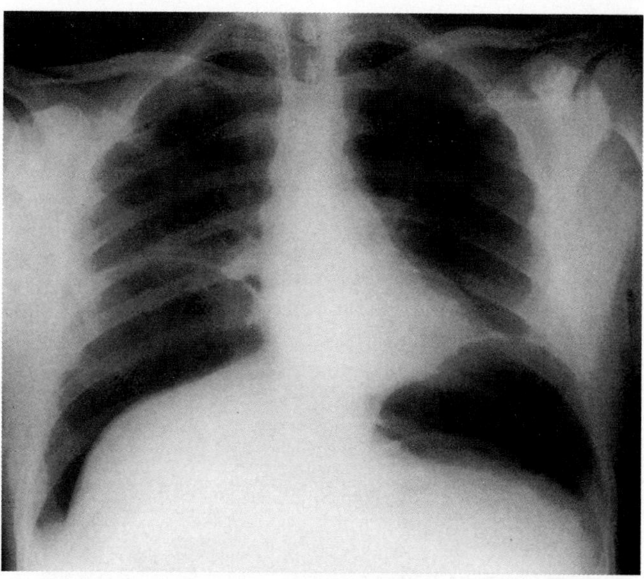

Fig. 2.22 Erect CXR showing marked bilateral elevation of the hemidiaphragms with a large volume of subdiaphragmatic free gas.

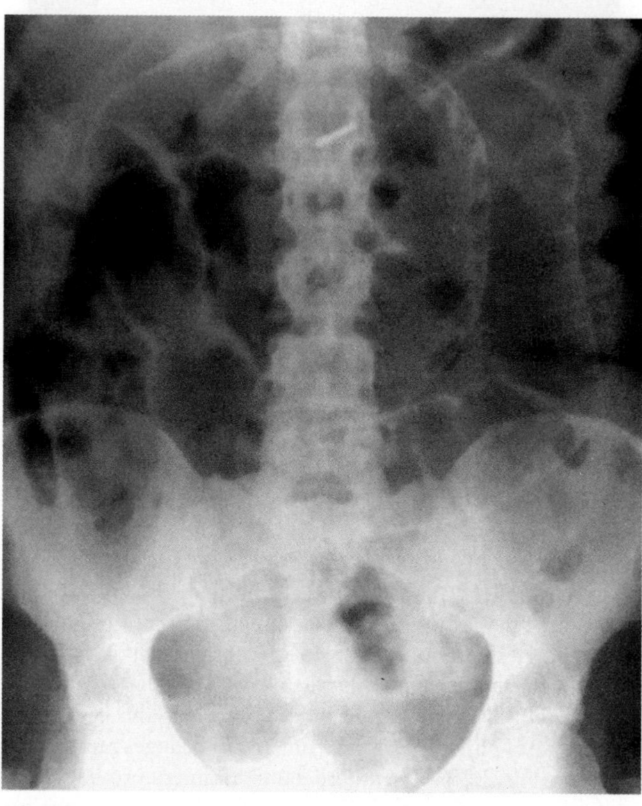

Fig. 2.23 Pneumoperitoneum. The presence of free intraperitoneal air outlines the bowel so that both sides of the bowel wall can be seen (Rigler's sign).

biopsy, new imaging techniques have considerably improved the ability to define the extent of tumour, although the pathological specimen remains the gold standard. Many staging systems are based on the TNM classification (tumour/node/metastasis).

Tumour

In most published studies, cross-sectional imaging techniques (CT, ultrasound, MRI) are more accurate in staging advanced (T3, T4) than early (T1, T2) diseases and the staging of early disease remains a challenge. In gut tumours, endoscopic ultrasound is more accurate than CT or MRI in staging early disease (T1 and T2) by virtue of its ability to demonstrate the layered structure of the bowel wall and the depth of tumour penetration (Fig. 2.25). Developments in MRI may also improve staging accuracy of early disease.

Nodes

Accurate assessment of nodal involvement remains a challenge for imaging. Most imaging techniques rely purely on size criteria to demonstrate lymph node involvement with no possibility of identifying micrometastases in normal sized nodes. A size criterion of 8–10 mm is taken but it is not usually possible to distinguish benign reactive nodes from infiltrated nodes. This is a particular problem with intrathoracic neoplasms where enlarged benign reactive mediastinal nodes

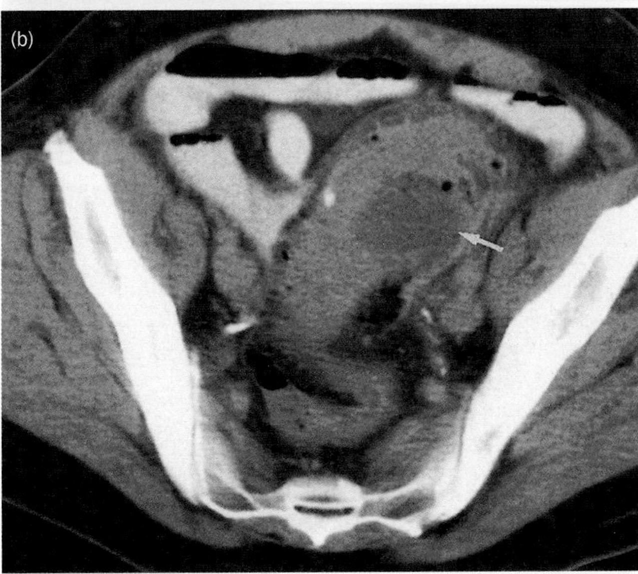

Fig. 2.24 (a) High-grade small bowel obstruction due to adhesions – CT scan showing multiple dilated fluid-filled loops of small bowel with collapsed distal ileal loops beyond the point of obstruction (*arrow*); (b) CT scan showing a segment of thickened sigmoid colon with a paracolic abscess (*arrow*) in a patient with diverticulitis.

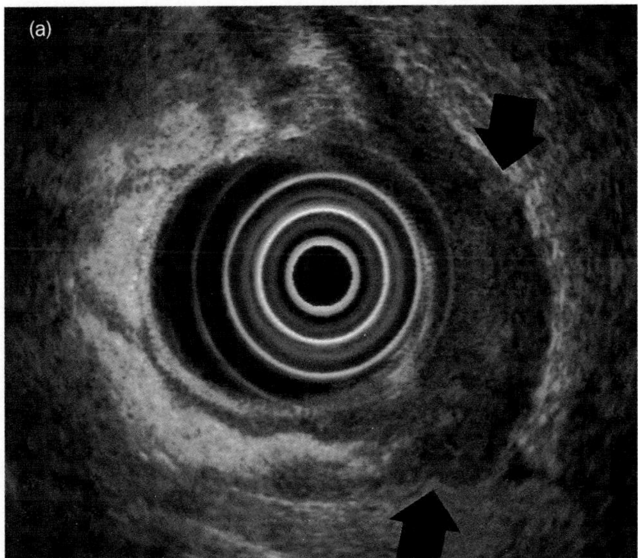

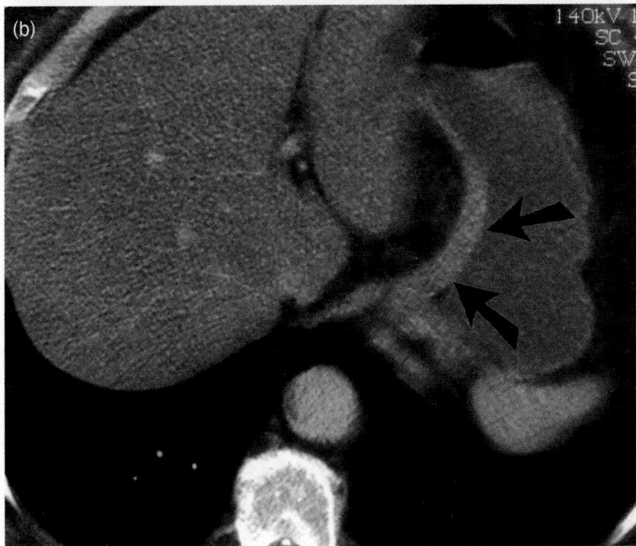

Fig. 2.25 (a) EUS in gastric cancer: the hypoechoic tumour (*arrows*) is destroying the layered structure of the bowel wall and extending out beyond the serosa; (b) CT scan demonstrates thickening and enhancement of the gastric wall in the same area. The stomach is distended with water to provide low-density contrast.

are common. The echo characteristics of nodes at endoscopic ultrasound have been used in many centres to increase the accuracy of nodal staging and nodal sampling, via either mediastinoscopy or transmural biopsy under EUS control. New radioisotope techniques are being developed using radiolabelled monoclonal antibodies against tumour antigens which may increase detection of nodal involvement by demonstrating micrometastases in nonenlarged nodes.

Metastases

The demonstration of metastatic disease will usually significantly affect surgical management. Modern cross-sectional imaging has greatly improved the detection of metastases but occult lesions will be missed in between 10 and 30 per cent of patients. CT is the most sensitive technique for detection of lung deposits, although the decision to perform CT will depend on the site of the primary tumour, its likelihood of intrapulmonary spread and the effect on staging and subsequent therapy of the demonstration of intrapulmonary deposits.

Ultrasound and CT are most frequently used to detect liver metastases. Contrast-enhanced CT can detect most lesions of greater than 1 cm, although accuracy rates of CT vary with the technique used and range from 70 to 90 per cent. Recent studies suggest that MRI may be more accurate than CT in demonstrating metastatic disease. While enhanced CT is used in most centres for screening for liver deposits, **CT AP (CT with arterial portography)**, which requires contrast injection via the superior mesenteric artery, is used in many centres as the most accurate technique for staging liver metastases if surgical resection is being considered. Preoperative identification of the segment of the liver involved can be determined by translation of the segmental surgical anatomy as defined by Couinaud to the cross-sectional CT images (Fig. 2.26).

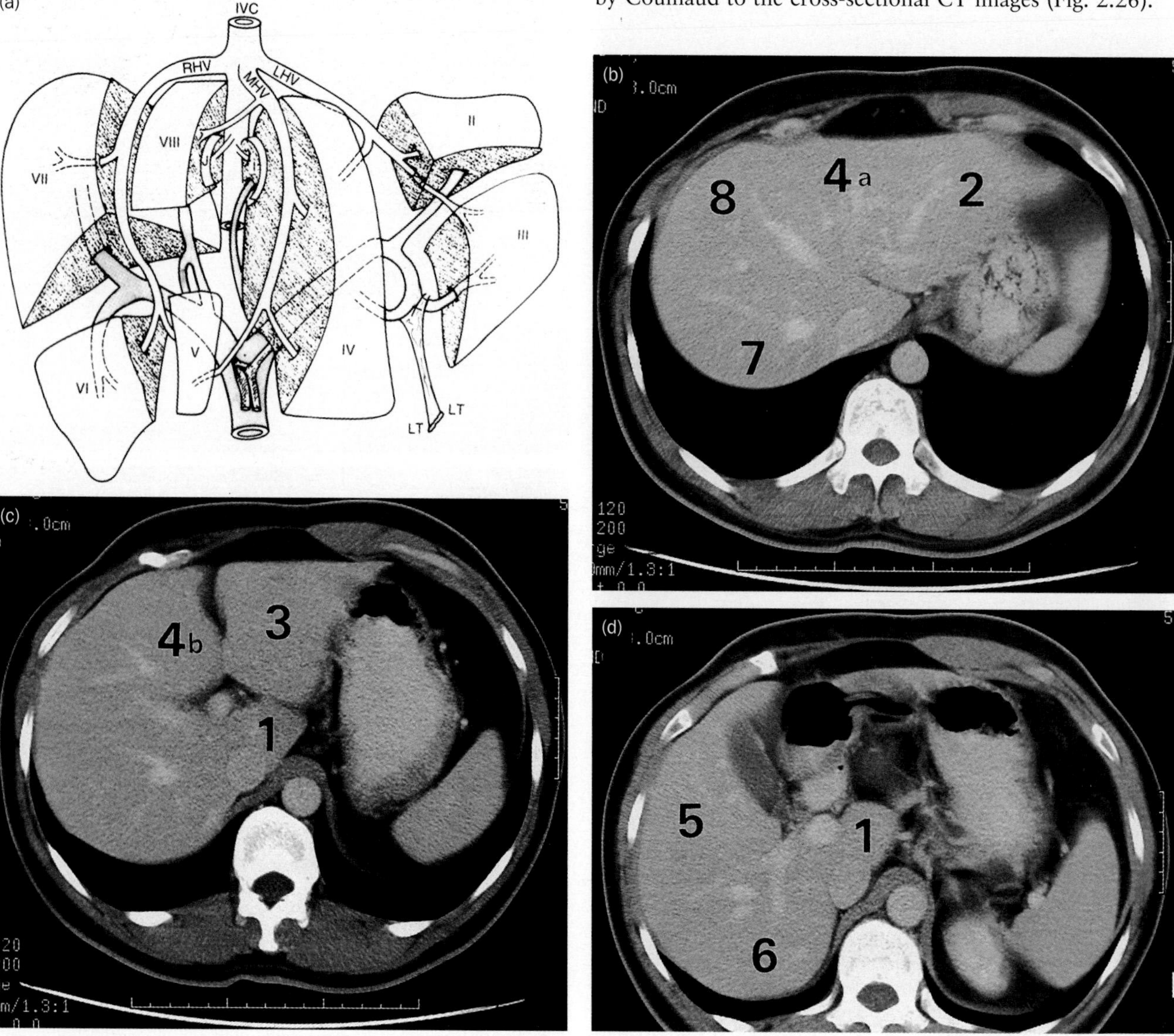

Fig. 2.26 (a) Surgical lobes of the liver (after Couinaud); (b) segmental anatomy on CT scan at level of hepatic veins; segmental anatomy at (c) and below (d) the level of the portal veins.

Intraoperative ultrasound is an alternative method of staging that provides superb high-resolution imaging of sub-centimetre liver nodules that may not be palpable at surgery.

Imaging in trauma

The response of the skeleton to trauma changes both with the nature and force of the injury and with the maturity and strength of the skeleton. In children the 'physis' or growth plate provides the weakest link and therefore epiphyseal injuries or apophyseal displacements are common. The skeleton is less brittle, resulting in buckling of the cortex or incomplete 'green-stick' fractures. In the mature adult skeleton the soft tissues – ligaments and muscular insertions – are the weakest link, and sprains and strains occur more commonly than fractures. The elderly osteopenic skeleton is brittle and susceptible to fracture often with minimal force.

Fracture radiographs should be performed in two planes and where possible should include the adjacent joint. Most fractures are easily diagnosed but some may be subtle and occult. Where a fracture is strongly suspected but not demonstrated, a repeat X-ray 5–10 days after the injury may identify the fracture line when bone absorption has begun. Stress fractures, either 'fatigue fractures' (normal bone) or 'insufficiency fractures' (abnormal bone), can be difficult to diagnose. Radionuclide bone scanning and more recently MRI are useful additional investigations if stress fractures are strongly suspected. The ability of CT to scan in the axial plane, together with excellent resolution of bony detail and the ability for multiplanar reconstruction, makes CT valuable in assessment of fractures of the spine, foot and pelvis (Fig. 2.27).

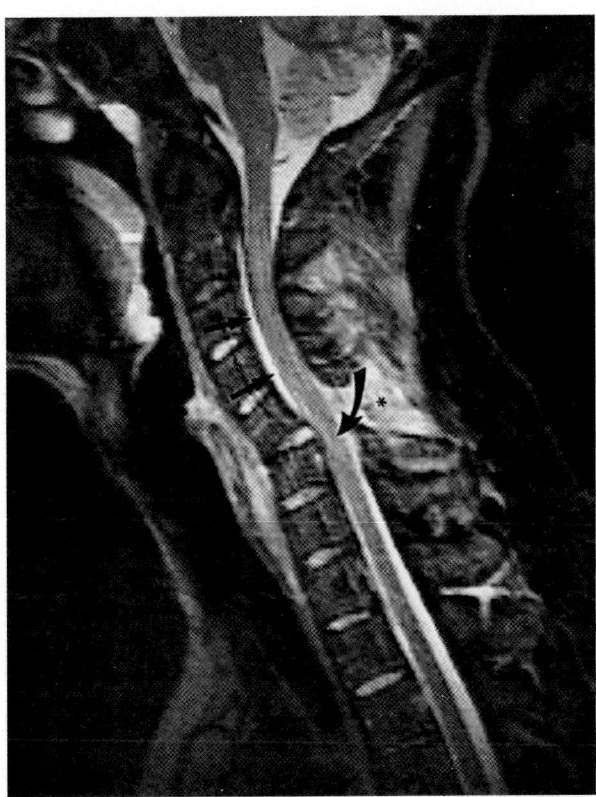

Fig. 2.28 T2-weighted sagittal MRI of an acute hyperflexion injury. Disruption of the C5/6 posterior annulus and posterior ligamentous complex (*) is present along with some cord contusion (*curved arrows*) seen as ill-defined high signal in the cord. There is an anterior extradural haematoma (*arrows*).

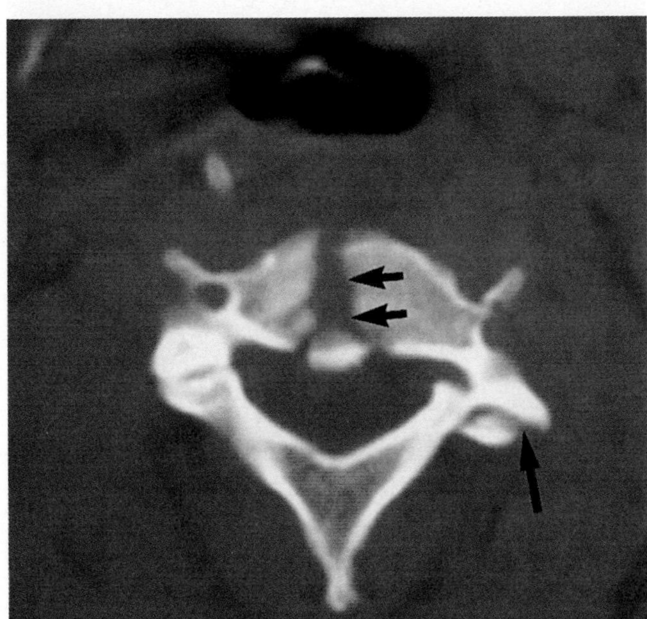

Fig. 2.27 CT scan of cervical axial burst fracture at C3 with vertebral body cleavage (*small arrows*) and left-sided facet joint dislocation (*arrow*).

Severe trauma

In patients who survive the immediate injury, imaging is considered after clinical evaluation and acute resuscitation. Acute spinal trauma is initially assessed by plain films. In approximately 10 per cent of patients there are multiple levels of injury. If spinal instability or spinal canal disruption is suspected, thin-section CT scanning with reconstruction of the images is required. Suspected cord damage may require an urgent MRI scan (Fig. 2.28). Evaluation of severe head, chest and abdominal trauma usually necessitates CT scanning after initial plain films (Fig. 2.29).

Interventional radiology

Over the last 20–30 years, interventional radiology has made an essential contribution to patient management. The speciality has developed from angiographic techniques, with guidewires and catheters as key ingredients. The parallel developments in cross-sectional imaging have provided enhanced guidance for interventional procedures and radiology has evolved from providing purely diagnostic information to

Clinical problem	*Investigation*
Head injury:	
Low risk of intracranial injury	Skull X-ray (SXR)/CT – NOT indicated
– Orientated/no LOC	
Medium risk	SXR – may proceed to CT
– LOC/amnesia	
– Swelling or laceration scalp	
– Inadequate history	
High risk	CT scan urgent
– Penetrating injury/ depressed fracture	
– Depressed or deteriorating consciousness	
– Focal signs/symptoms	
– Cerebrospinal fluid leak	
Chest trauma:	
Minor	CXR – not routinely required
Moderate	CXR
– Pneumothorax?	
– Lung contusion	
– Haemothorax	
– Mediastinal injury?	
– Aortic injury?	
Major	CXR
– Mediastinal haematoma?	CT scan ↓ Angiography
Renal/pelvic trauma:	
Haematuria	Urethrogram – exclude urethral injury
– Pelvic fracture	If normal – ?cystogram ?Bladder leak May need CT scan – ?CT cystography
Renal trauma:	
Mild to moderate	US (local injury) IVU – ?contralateral kidney normal ?Extent of injury
Severe	CT + contrast (obviates IVU)
Abdominal trauma:	
Severe (unstable)	Urgent surgery US (or peritoneal lavage) ?Haemoperitoneum ↓ Helical CT → Surgery
Stable	US (or peritoneal lavage) ↓ ?Haemoperitoneum ↓ Helical CT (if available) ?Organ injury ?Active bleeding ↓ Surgery, angiography (?embolisation), observe

Derived from: *Making the best use of a department of clinical radiology*, Royal College of Radiologists, 1998, 4th edn.

Fig. 2.29 Imaging in trauma (LOC, loss of consciousness).

therapy, offering effective alternatives in the treatment of abdominal and thoracic disorders. In some instances, interventional radiology techniques have replaced the conventional surgical approach, removing the need for a general anaesthetic with consequent decreased morbidity and length of hospital stay, with similar patient outcome. The increasing complexity and sophistication of both surgery and available interventional techniques requires close liaison in decision making between the surgeon and radiologist to choose the optimum method of treatment.

Percutaneous biopsy

Percutaneous biopsy is possible for most radiologically detected abnormalities. Small lesions immediately adjacent to major vessels or a biopsy path that traverses the colon may be regarded as relative contraindications but the decision often depends on local expertise. In general, the shortest route from skin to lesion is chosen if no vital structure intervenes. Fluoroscopy usually provides suitable guidance for biopsy of large parenchymal or perihilar masses in the chest. CT guidance may be necessary for small lesions. Ultrasound or CT guidance is most commonly employed in the abdomen. Ultrasound is quick and flexible and allows the needle path to be followed in real time without additional radiation burden to the patient. Small lesions and lesions which cannot be adequately imaged with ultrasound, particularly within the retroperitoneum, are more appropriately biopsied under CT control (Fig. 2.30).

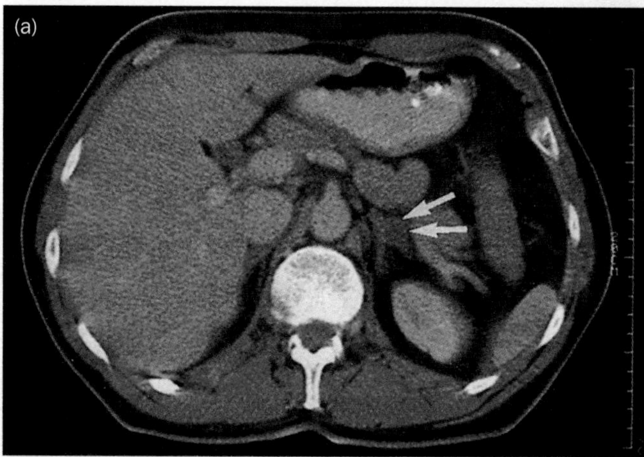

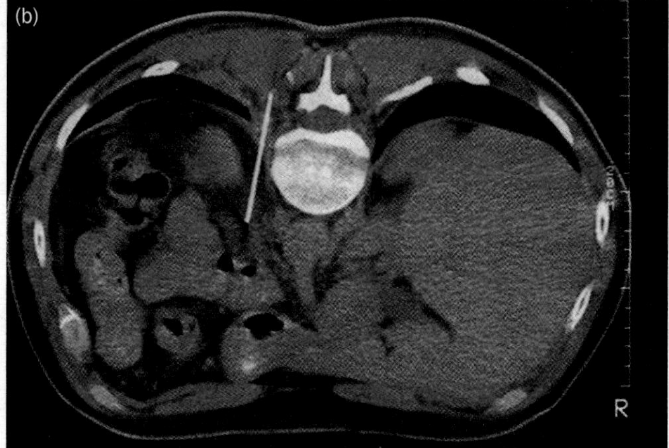

Fig. 2.30 CT guided biopsy. (a) CT scan demonstrates 2-cm mass on the lateral limb of the left adrenal (*arrows*); (b) prone CT scan with needle tip in the adrenal lesion. CT guidance enables lung puncture to be avoided.

A platelet count of less than 80 000 or an international normalised ratio (INR) of greater than 1.3 should be corrected where possible, by the administration of fresh frozen plasma and/or vitamin K, where appropriate, prior to biopsy. Gross ascites should be drained prior to liver biopsy unless biopsy via a transjugular approach is available. The choice of needles is wide. In general, an 18G automatic spring-loaded cutting needle provides an excellent core biopsy. Larger 14G needles may be useful where architectural assessment is required in patchy disease, e.g. cirrhosis. Cytological analysis via 22G needle is often adequate for the diagnosis of malignancy. Accuracy rates exceed 80 per cent. Negative biopsies may be due to faulty needle placement. Complications are unusual, occurring in less than 2 per cent of patients and include haemorrhage, pancreatitis, pneumothorax and occasional seeding of the needle track by tumour.

Drainage of abscesses and fluid collections

Almost any fluid collection in the chest, abdomen or pelvis may be considered for percutaneous catheter drainage, which has largely replaced surgery as the treatment of choice. Initially percutaneous drainage was confined to large superficial postoperative collections, but use has broadened to include complex multilocular collections, multiple abscesses and collections in difficult locations (e.g. presacral space, psoas muscle).

CT or ultrasound is used to define a safe access route avoiding the penetration of major vessels or bowel. Ultrasound is adequate for superficial collections and may be preferable where an angled approach is required, e.g. subphrenic collections (Fig. 2.31). Superficial collections, where there is little risk of misdirection, may be safely drained via a simple one-step trochar catheter system. More complex or deep collections often require the more precise guidance of CT, using the needle guidewire and catheter exchange system originally devised by Seldinger for arterial puncture (Fig. 2.32). Diagnostic fine needle aspiration should be performed before drainage to determine the nature and viscosity of the collection. Nonviscous fluid – ascites, cysts, seromas, bilomas, urinomas – can be satisfactorily drained via an 8–10 French catheter. Thick, inspissated, infected material often requires a larger bore catheter (10–14 French) with multiple side holes and, ideally, a double lumen for cavity irrigation. At catheter insertion, the cavity should be evacuated as completely as possible. Saline irrigation may help to decrease the viscosity of the contents and encourage drainage. Patients should be given broad-spectrum antibiotic cover before and after the procedure. Following catheter placement, regular saline irrigation (10–20 ml tds) is important to maintain catheter patency. The catheter should be left *in situ* for several days until drainage ceases. Continued drainage of 50 ml or more suggests possible fistulous communication which may be confirmed by a contrast study via the catheter. Prolonged catheter drainage over several weeks may be necessary in such cases to allow fistulae to close. Successful catheter drainage of simple postoperative collections or localised abscesses can be achieved in over 90 per cent of cases. The cure rate for more complex collections such as pancreatic abscesses, abscesses caused by leak from enteric, biliary or urinary anastomosis and thoracic empyaema is lower, between 70 and 85 per cent. The multilocular nature of many of these collections makes complete evacuation difficult. However, in many patients percutaneous drainage achieves palliation and allows the patient to undergo delayed, elective, single-stage surgery in a more stable condition with a relatively clean operative bed.

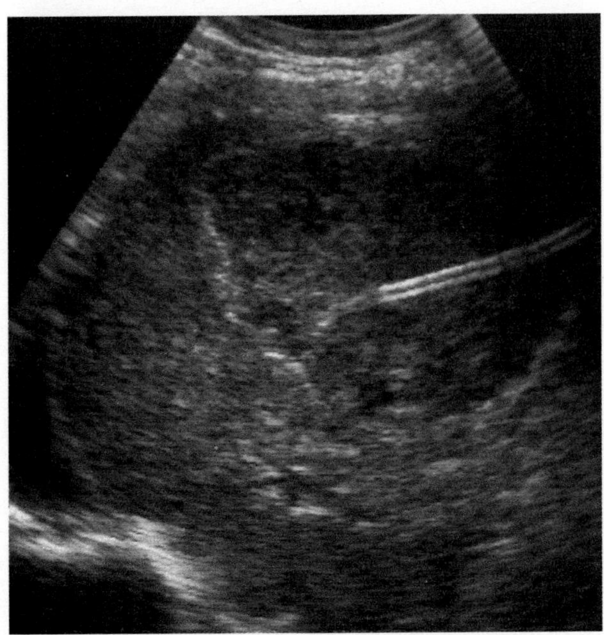

Fig. 2.31 US showing large amoebic abscess within the liver with a catheter inserted under US guidance for abscess drainage.

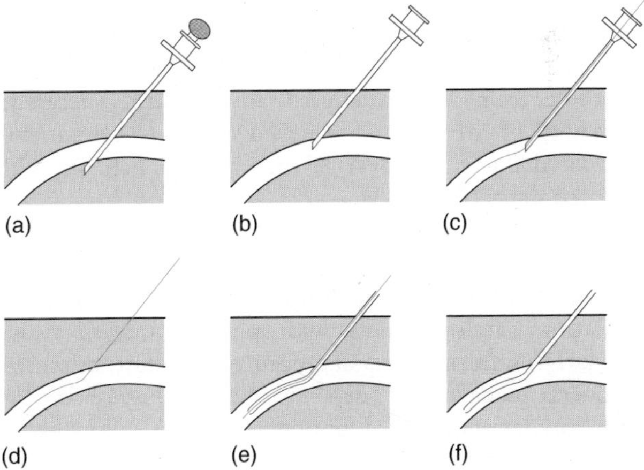

Fig. 2.32 Seldinger technique. (a) Both walls of vessel punctured; (b) stillette removed – needle withdrawn so that bevel is within lumen of vessel and blood flows from the hub; (c) guidewire inserted through needle; (d) needle withdrawn leaving guidewire *in situ*; (e) catheter threaded over wire; (f) guidewire withdrawn (reproduced from *A Guide to Radiological Procedures* (eds S. Chapman and R. Nakielny), 1986, by permission of W.B. Saunders Company Ltd, London).

S.I. Seldinger, b. 1921. Swedish radiologist and physician.

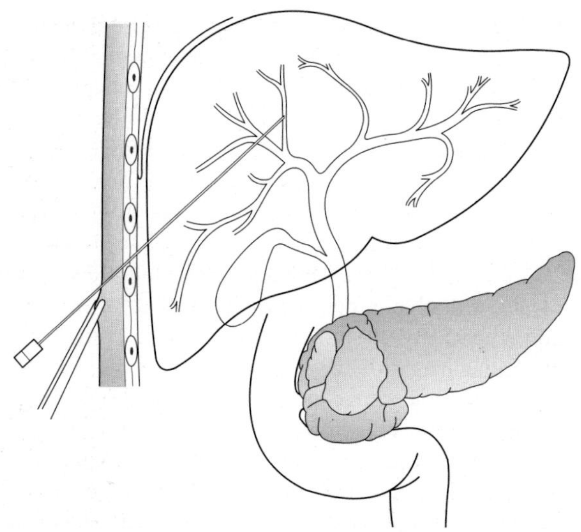

Fig. 2.33 Percutaneous transhepatic cholangiogram. A 22 gauge needle is advanced through the skin into the liver. Contrast is injected on withdrawal until a bile duct is opacified (reproduced with permission of W.B. Saunders Company Ltd, London).

Percutaneous biliary procedures

Drainage of an obstructed biliary system is usually achieved by **ERCP**. Endoscopic cannulation of the ampulla allows the passage of guidewires and catheters, and the majority of strictures can be bypassed and stented by this approach. In gallstone obstruction of the common bile duct, endoscopic stone removal can be achieved following sphincterotomy by basket retrieval, mechanical lithotripsy or balloon sweepage of the duct. A proportion of patients with obstructive jaundice is not suitable for this endoscopic approach, because of previous gastric surgery, difficulties with cannulation of the ampulla or a tight stricture which cannot be negotiated from below. In these patients, a percutaneous transhepatic approach is required. **Percutaneous transhepatic cholangiography** involves puncture of an intrahepatic bile duct with a fine needle from a right intercostal approach. Successful visualisation of the ducts is achieved in almost all patients with dilated ducts and over 85 per cent of patients with nondilated ducts (Fig. 2.33).

Dilated systems require drainage to reduce the risk of sepsis and relieve jaundice. A peripheral duct with a direct line of approach to the common hepatic duct is chosen for cannulation. Teflon-coated hydrophilic guidewires are particularly useful in traversing even the tightest strictures. Subsequent management depends on the nature of the obstruction demonstrated. Options include the following:

- balloon dilatation;
- simple external drainage;
- external/internal drainage;
- endoprosthesis – plastic or expanding metal.

Balloon dilatation

Over 90 per cent of benign biliary structures are post-operative, the remainder resulting from sclerosing cholangitis or pancreatitis. If there is biliary sepsis, balloon dilatation should not be attempted until this has been treated with antibiotics and a period of external biliary drainage. A 7–9 French balloon-tipped catheter is placed in the strictured segment with fluoroscopic guidance and the balloon inflated until the 'waist' of the balloon within the strictured segment is obliterated. Results suggest that 75–80 per cent of strictures will remain patent for at least 3 years.

External/internal drainage

The majority of biliary strictures is malignant and is due to carcinoma of the pancreas, primary bile duct tumours, nodal enlargement at the porta hepatis or encroachment on the major bile ducts by hepatic metastases. Treatment is aimed at palliation. If there is hilar obstruction, it is usually sufficient to drain only one side of the system as drainage of 30 per cent or more of the liver parenchyma will relieve the obstructing symptoms. If a stricture cannot be bypassed, a catheter may be left *in situ* with external biliary drainage. This will decompress the system, control the risk of sepsis and will result in resolution of oedema such that a second delayed attempt to traverse the stricture is often successful. A percutaneous catheter is manipulated through the obstruction, into the normal distal common duct or duodenum. Side holes in the catheter that are located above and below the obstruction permit the re-establishment of enterohepatic circulation of bile such that the catheter may be clamped (Fig. 2.34).

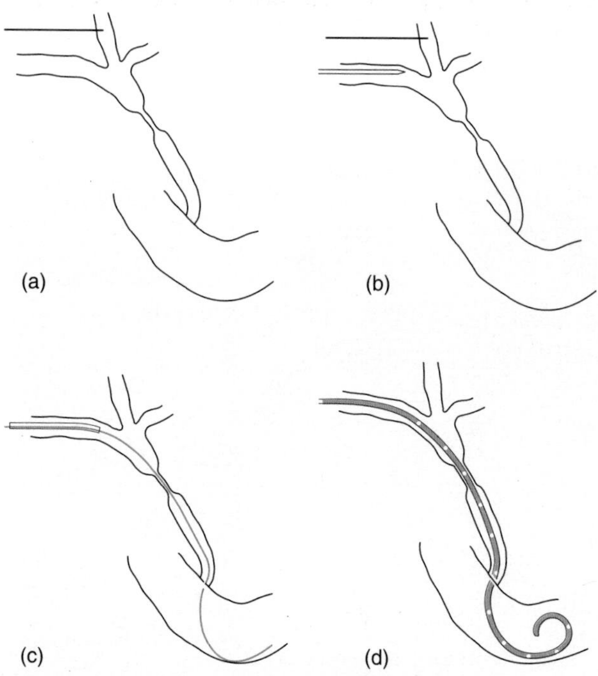

Fig. 2.34 Internal biliary drainage. (a) Initial diagnostic fine needle cholangiogram showing stricture; (b) selective 18G cannula sheath puncture of horizontal segment of right hepatic duct; (c) guidewire advanced through sheath across stricture and into duodenum; (d) multi-side hole 8.3F pigtail catheter inserted over guide into duodenum for internal drainage.

Endoprosthesis

An endoprosthesis may be placed into the bile duct to remove the inconvenience of a catheter protruding from the skin and reduce the risks of infection. Percutaneous placement of plastic endoprostheses requires a transhepatic track of 12 French or greater, which carries an increased morbidity (Fig. 2.35).

The recent introduction of self-expanding metallic prostheses means that a smaller percutaneous track is sufficient and the stent can often be inserted immediately without a period of external drainage. Often a percutaneous approach with guidewire manipulation through a stricture is combined with an endoscopic approach. The guidewire is 'grabbed' in the duodenum and a stent placed endoscopically. Stent occlusion, by either bile encrustation or tumour ingrowth or overgrowth, remains a problem, although the expanding metal stents have a longer life span than plastic endoprostheses (Fig. 2.36).

Major complications in these patients who generally have severe underlying disease have been observed in 2–5 per cent of patients (death, sepsis, haemorrhage).

Minor complications (pain, fever, catheter blockage or leakage) occur in 20–40 per cent of patients.

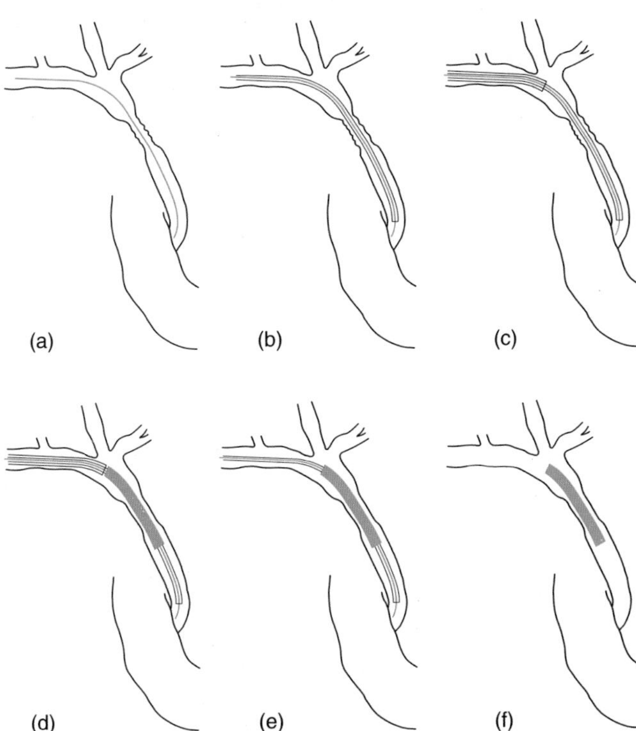

Fig. 2.35 Transhepatic placement of endoprosthesis. (a) Guidewire through stricture; (b) 8F internal drainage catheter placed; (c) 12F dilator passed over catheter and pushed through stricture for dilatation; (d) preshaped endoprosthesis (solid dark) pushed co-axially over 8F catheter by a 12F dilator catheter; (e) 12F dilator catheter withdrawn leaving endoprosthesis in place over protecting 8F drainage catheter (3–4 days of drainage allowed before removal); (f) endoprosthesis in place.

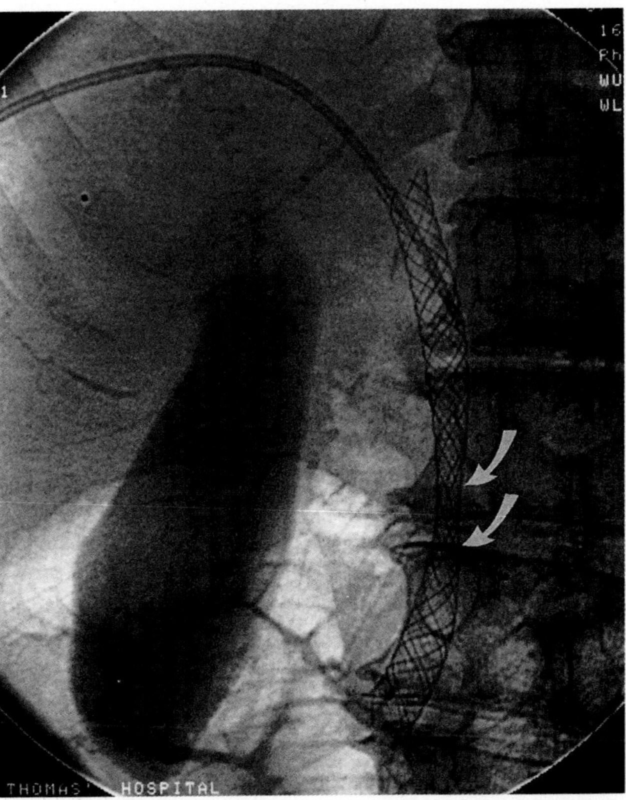

Fig. 2.36 Expanding metal stent *in situ* to relieve biliary obstruction due to a pancreatic head carcinoma.

Gall bladder drainage

Percutaneous gall bladder puncture and drainage may be beneficial in acute calculous or acalculous cholecystitis, or gall bladder empyema in patients who are high risk for surgery or whose medical condition is unstable. The procedure is usually performed under ultrasound guidance. A transhepatic route is advocated to reduce the risk of biliary peritonitis, although a transperitoneal approach is acceptable as the complication rate does not appear to be significantly increased. In severely ill patients the procedure can be performed at the bedside. Ideally, a self-retaining catheter with a locking loop should be left within the gall bladder. In septic patients, recovery is usually rapid and can be followed 2–3 weeks later by elective cholecystectomy. Complications are uncommon although vagal effects (bradycardia and hypotension) do occur and may be treated with atropine and intravenous fluid. Percutaneous gall bladder puncture and aspiration has been advocated in intensive therapy unit (ITU) patients who are pyrexial, without a demonstrable cause, in whom the gall bladder is distended and contains sludge, raising the possibility of acalculous cholecystitis. Approximately 50 per cent of such patients may improve following gall bladder drainage.

Percutaneous renal intervention

Percutaneous drainage of obstructed kidneys, **percutaneous nephrostomy**, is performed in patients who are septic or in renal failure due to ureteric obstruction by neoplasm, calculi or stricture. Other percutaneous techniques have evolved from this, including antegrade ureteric stent placement, balloon dilatation of ureteric strictures and the creation of a track for percutaneous stone removal (nephrolithotomy) in patients not suitable for lithotripsy.

In a patient presenting with renal failure, it is vital not to miss the presence of bilateral obstruction or an obstructed solitary kidney, and an ultrasound examination is mandatory. The decision to drain the kidney is usually straightforward, particularly in the presence of sepsis. In bilateral obstruction, the better functioning kidney (larger, thicker parenchyma) should be drained first to enable the uraemia and hyperkalaemia to be corrected. If known malignant pelvic disease is resulting in bilateral obstruction, then discussion and consideration of the likely prognosis of the underlying disease process is advisable before proceeding. The indications for percutaneous nephrostomy are shown in Fig. 2.37.

Nephrostomy tube placement may be performed under fluoroscopic or ultrasound guidance. The aim is usually to puncture a lower pole calyx rather than a direct central puncture which is more likely to cause vascular damage. A middle calyx approach may be preferred if antegrade stent placement is contemplated. Using a flexible sheathed needle and guidewire with dilatation of the track, final placement of a small pigtail catheter is achieved with minimal trauma to the kidney and discomfort to the patient (Fig. 2.38). The use of self-locking catheters reduces the risk of subsequent catheter dislodgement. Haemorrhage is usually venous and mild, lasting for up to 24 hours. Significant haemorrhage occurs in 1–2 per cent of patients and may occasionally require arteriography to identify a bleeding point or false aneurysm, which may then be treated with selective embolisation. Septic complications occur in 1–2 per cent. They can be minimised by appropriate prophylactic and antibiotic cover and minimising catheter/guidewire manipulation.

Ureteric J-J pigtail stent insertion is usually approached retrogradely by cystoscopy. It is of value where long-term drainage is required. Indications include calculous obstruction, often in relation to extracorporeal shock wave lithotripsy (ESWL) which produces many small fragments which may block the ureter; benign or malignant ureteric strictures and to allow ureteric perforations to heal. If a retrograde approach fails then an antegrade approach is possible. Most strictures can be traversed with modern flexible hydrophilic guidewires.

Urgent (within 12–24 hours)
- Obstructed infected kidney
- Obstructed solitary kidney with deteriorating renal function

Priority
- Obstruction with severe pain
- Obstruction with renal failure

Elective
- Pressure–flow studies – obstruction?
- Percutaneous access for stone removal or ureteric procedures, e.g. stent insertion

Fig. 2.37 Indications for percutaneous nephrostomy.

Gastrointestinal intervention

Enteric strictures

Dilatation of benign or malignant oesophageal strictures can be performed with either endoscopic or fluoroscopic guidance. The choice depends on local expertise but screening during dilatation is advisable to reduce the risk of oesophageal perforation. Balloon dilatation is achieved by the introduction of a balloon over a guidewire under fluoroscopic guidance. Balloon dilatation has the advantage of providing a controlled radial dilating force without the

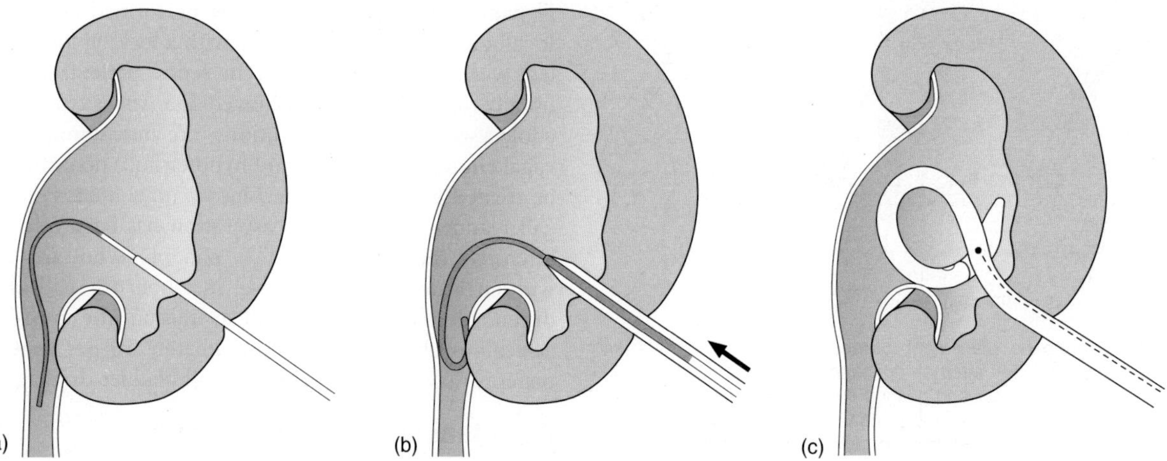

Fig. 2.38 Percutaneous nephrostomy technique. (a) A guidewire is threaded through a needle towards the ureter; (b) the track is dilated; (c) a pigtail catheter with a locking loop is left *in situ* in the renal pelvis.

longitudinal shearing forces associated with conventional oesophageal bougie dilatation, which is thought to predispose to oesophageal rupture. Obliteration of the waist of the balloon with inflation can be observed in real time and provides an indication of the likely success of the procedure.

In patients with malignant oesophageal disease, considered incurable by surgical intervention, oesophageal stent placement provides good palliation. The use of rigid plastic stents (Celestin or Atkinson tubes) has been gradually superseded by self-expanding metal stents (Fig. 2.39). Some of these are covered with plastic, minimising tumour ingrowth and sealing any associated perforation or fistula. Placement rapidly relieves symptoms, allowing the patient to return home to a relatively normal diet. These techniques are being expanded to strictures elsewhere in the gastrointestinal tract. Duodenal and colonic strictures have been satisfactorily stented although experience is currently limited and the long-term prospects for such procedures are currently unknown.

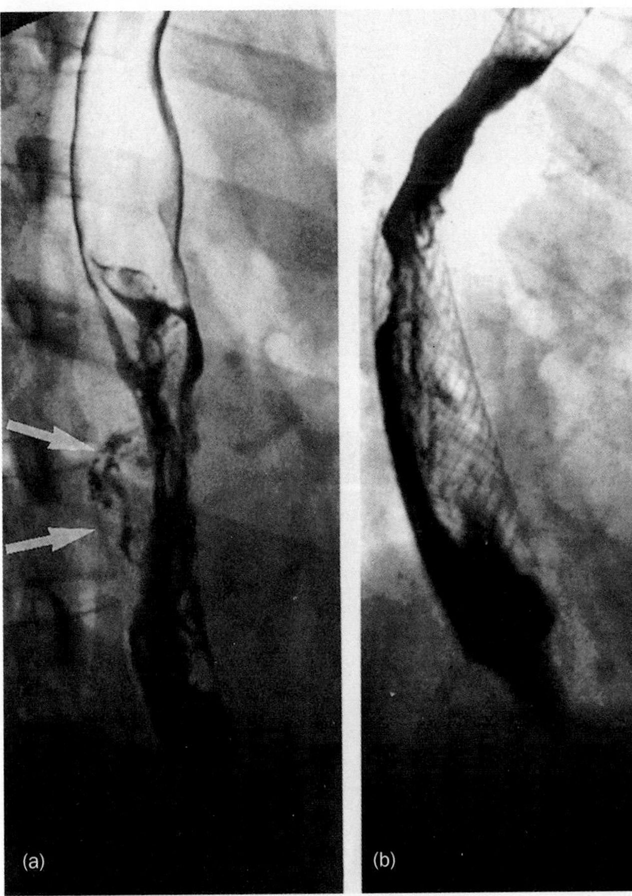

Fig. 2.39 Expanding metal stent in malignant oesophageal obstruction. (a) Contrast swallow demonstrating a malignant stricture in the lower oesophagus with evidence of fistulation (*arrows*); (b) a contrast swallow after placement of a self-expanding plastic-covered metal stent. There is a rapid free flow through the stent with no evidence of leakage.

Roger Celestin. Former surgeon, Frenchay Hospital, Bristol, England.
Michael Atkinson, Professor of Gastroenterology, University of Nottingham, England.

Percutaneous gastrostomy

Percutaneous gastrostomy placement provides a more comfortable alternative to long-term nasogastric feeding in patients who are unable to maintain nutrition with oral intake. This is usually as a result of upper aerodigestive tract malignancy or an inability to swallow as a result of a previous cerebrovascular accident. Percutaneous placement of gastrostomy feeding tubes can be achieved using either endoscopy or fluoroscopy. The choice again largely depends on local expertise and both methods are technically satisfactory. Fluoroscopic placement is essential in patients in whom nasopharyngeal or oesophageal narrowing is such that even the smallest endoscope cannot bypass the obstruction. The fluoroscopic technique requires insufflation of the stomach with air or CO_2 via a fine nasogastric tube. This renders it fluoroscopically visible and distends the stomach against the anterior abdominal wall. A puncture site is selected over the lower body of the stomach. Following guidewire placement, the track is dilated co-axially and a 12-French loop catheter finally positioned with a retention loop in the stomach. Minor complications include wound infection and tube dislodgement. Peritonitis does occasionally occur which may be minimised by gastropexy, i.e. fixation of the stomach to the anterior abdominal wall by removable sutures (Fig. 2.40).

Interventional vascular techniques

A wide range of interventional vascular techniques has developed from basic angiographic principles and has had a profound impact on many aspects of medicine and surgery.

Vascular therapy

By selective arterial cannulation it is possible to deliver a high local dose of a chemotherapeutic agent to the feeding vessels of a tumour. This technique has been used with success for liver tumours, particular hepatocellular carcinoma, metastatic colorectal cancer and ocular melanoma.

There has been a resurgence of interest in the potential of low-dose intra-arterial infusion of thrombolytic agents in peripheral arterial thromboembolic occlusion. The choice of therapy between surgical embolectomy and thrombolysis is controversial.

In patients with recurrent or threatened pulmonary embolisation from lower extremity or pelvic thrombus, **inferior vena caval filters** may be inserted percutaneously, from either a femoral or jugular approach to prevent the passage of a major embolus. A femoral approach is appropriate if the thrombus does not extend proximally into the inferior vena cava and if the contra-lateral femoral and pelvic veins are patent. Otherwise, a jugular approach is indicated, assuming the superior vena cava is patent.

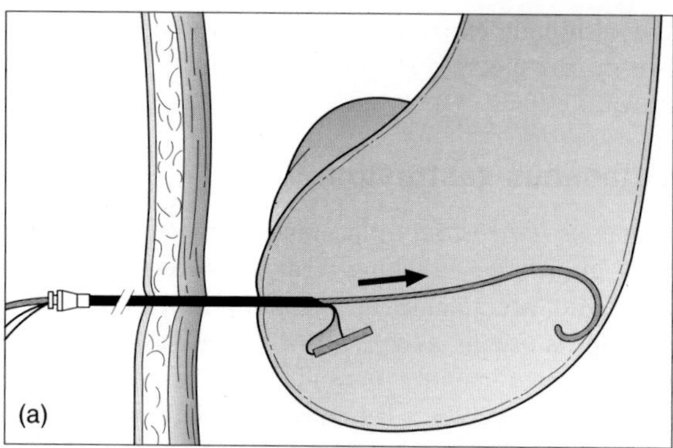

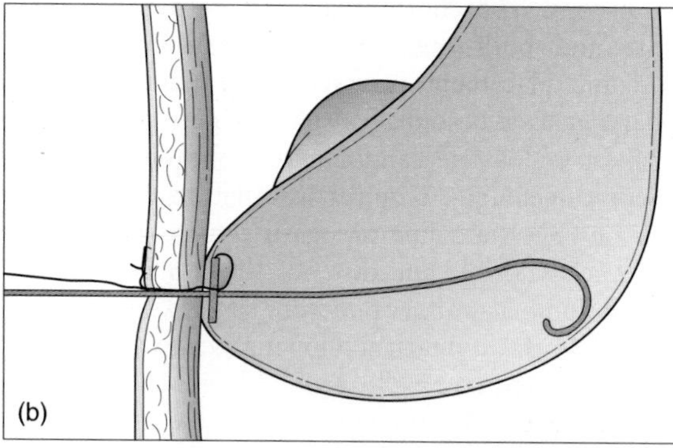

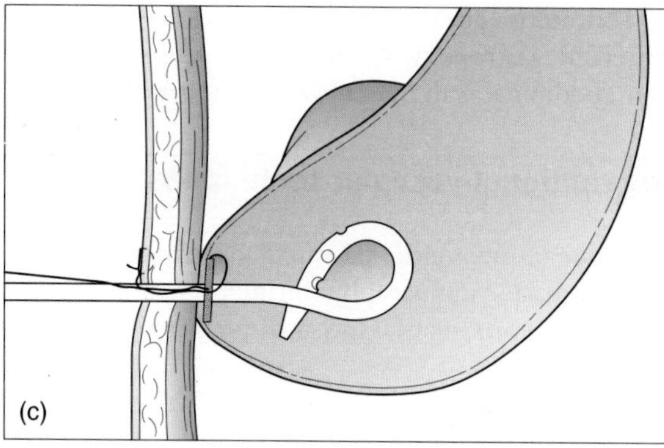

Fig. 2.40 Technique of percutaneous gastrostomy.

Management of vascular obstruction

Percutaneous transluminal angioplasty

This technique of balloon dilatation of a vascular stenosis, with the aim of increasing blood flow and improving perfusion, has had a profound impact on the treatment of vascular disease. Initially described by Dotter and Judkins in 1964, the technique has undergone many modifications and now provides a lower risk alternative treatment to surgical bypass graft. Indications include:

- peripheral vascular disease with relatively short occlusions (10–15 cm in length);
- ischaemic heart disease with coronary artery stenosis;
- hypertension or chronic renal failure with renal transplant artery stenosis;
- mesenteric/coeliac artery stenosis.

The technical success rate for femoral and popliteal angioplasty is between 85 and 95 per cent for stenoses with a 20–70 per cent patency rate at 5 years (Fig. 2.41). Complications include local haemorrhage and haematoma, false aneurysm formation at the puncture site, subintimal dissection and arterial perforation. The incidence of peripheral

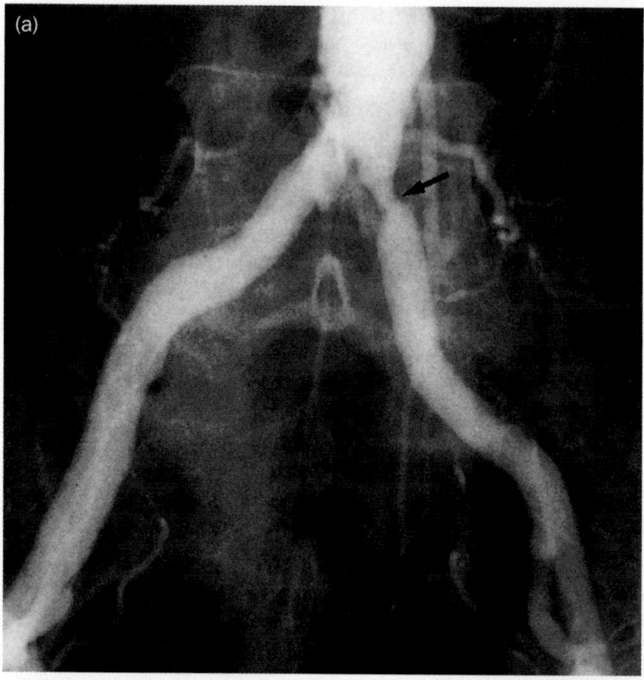

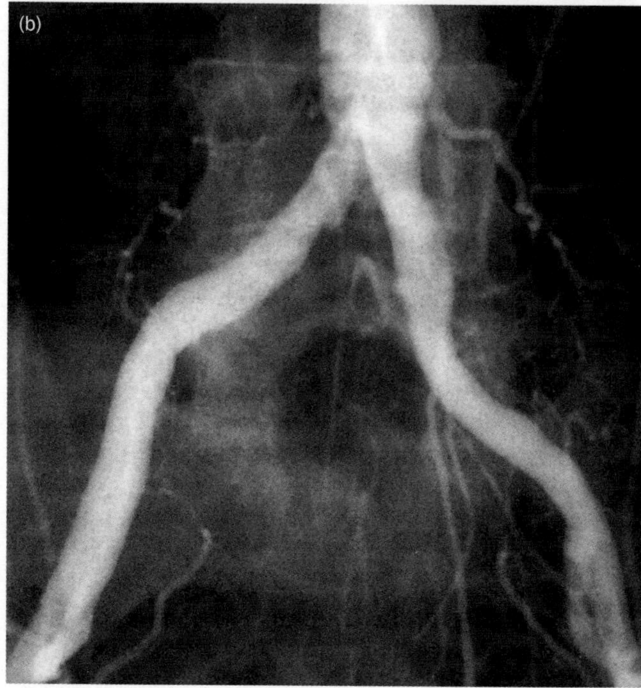

Fig. 2.41 Iliac arteriogram showing (a) a 50 per cent stenosis of the left common iliac artery (*arrow*) before angioplasty; (b) the result 2 years after angioplasty.

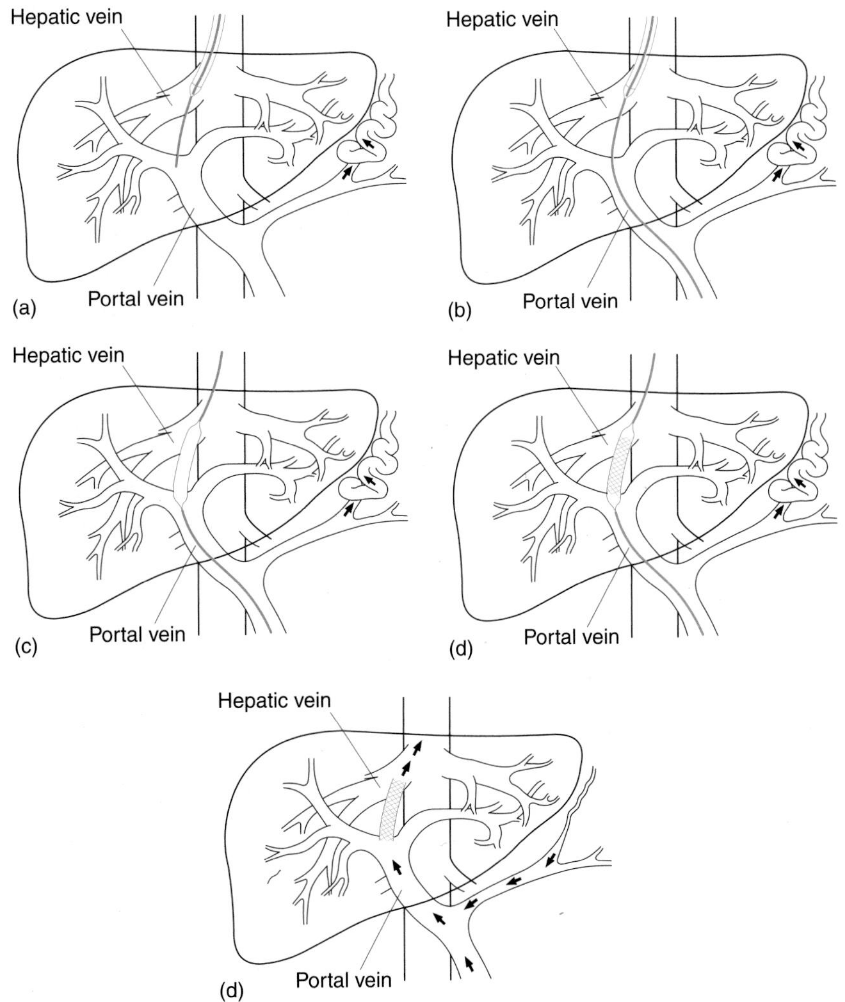

Fig. 2.42 Transjugular intrahepatic porto-systemic shunt procedure (TIPSS). (a) Needle advanced from hepatic to portal vein via transjugular approach; (b) guidewire passed through needle into superior mesenteric vein (note hepatofugal flow in enlarged coronary vein); (c) angioplasty balloon advanced over wire and expanded to create a parenchymal track; (d) metallic stent placed to bridge the track between hepatic and portal veins; (e) intrahepatic shunt created via stent. Hepato-petal flow created with decreased size of the coronary vein (reproduced with permission of W.B. Saunders Company Ltd, London).

embolisation of atheromatous deposits is low, reported as between 3 and 5 per cent of cases and rarely resulting in clinically apparent ischaemia.

Vascular stenting

In 1988, Palmaz reported the use of intravascular stents in atherosclerotic arterial stenosis. The therapeutic potential of expanding metal stents in vascular disease is great and stents are being successfully used in renal ostial stenosis, abdominal aortic aneurysm repair, coronary artery disease and other major peripheral vessels. A major problem of intravascular stents is their thrombogenic potential as fibrin and platelets are deposited within the mesh of the stent. This can be inhibited by anticoagulation and over a period of weeks endothelialisation of the stent occurs. It is likely that with further technical developments, stents will be developed that will be antithrombotic, encourage endothelialisation and inhibit neo-intimal hyperplasia.

Transjugular intrahepatic porto-systemic shunt (TIPSS)

A particular use of expanding metal stents has been in the development of TIPSS, which involves the percutaneous creation of a communication between the portal and hepatic venous systems for the relief of portal hypertension (Fig. 2.42). This procedure was first performed by Richter in 1988 and is now firmly established as an alternative to surgery in patients with recurrent variceal bleeding who are resistant to sclerotherapy or endoscopic banding. The technical success rate is over 90 per cent. The major complication is hepatic encephalopathy which can develop following the procedure. Shunt occlusion may develop, usually as a result of intimal hyperplasia. This may require re-intervention with balloon dilatation or a second stent insertion.

Burton Richter, b. 1931. US physicist.

Therapeutic embolisation

Deliberate vascular embolisation with the aim of occluding a vessel can be achieved using a variety of different materials including gelatin, sponge fragments, polyvinyl alcohol foam particles (PVA) and spiral metal coils. Arterial embolisation may be used in the treatment of:

- acute haemorrhage;
- tumour therapy;
- arterio-venous malformations;
- hypersplenism;
- priaprism.

Venous embolisation is used for treatment of:

- gastro-oesophageal varices;
- testicular varicocele.

The technique can be performed under local anaesthetic and requires a highly skilled radiologist to position selectively the catheter. The technique is not without risk as accidental embolisation of adjacent normal structures may occur. Tissue necrosis following the procedure may cause pain and fever due to tissue infarction and occasionally results in abscess formation.

Further reading

Armstrong, P. and Wastie, M. (eds) (1997) *Diagnostic and Interventional Radiology in Surgical Practice*, Chapman & Hall, London.

Mueller, P. and Van Sommenberg, E. (1990) Interventional radiology in the chest and abdomen. *New England Journal of Medicine*, **322**, 1364–74.

Royal College of Radiologists (1998) *Making the Best Use of a Department of Clinical Radiology: Guidelines for Doctors*, 4th edn, Royal College of Radiologists, London.

Shuman, W.P. (1997) CT of blunt abdominal trauma in adults. *Radiology*, **205**, 297–306.

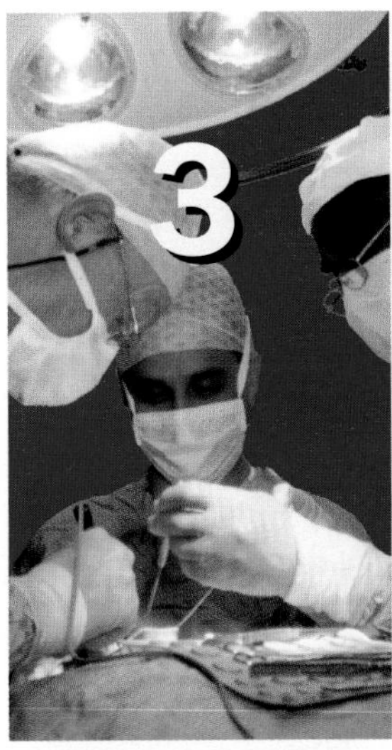

3 Wounds, tissue repair and scars

A wise physician skilled our wounds to heal is more than armies for the common weal[1]. (Homer)

Skin is the best dressing. (Lister)

Wounds

Wounds and their management are fundamental to the practice of surgery. Any elective surgical intervention will result in a wound in order to gain access to and deal with the underlying pathology. In the surgery of trauma the wound is the primary pathology. In both situations the surgeon's task is to minimise the adverse effects of the wound, remove or repair damaged structures and harness the processes of wound healing to restore function.

Wound healing

In human regeneration is limited to epithelium and the liver; most tissues heal by repair resulting in scarring. Wound healing is the summation of a number of processes which follow injury including coagulation, inflammation, matrix synthesis and deposition, angiogenesis, fibroplasia, epithelialisation, contraction, remodelling and scar maturation (Fig. 3.1). Where wound edges are apposed healing proceeds rapidly to closure; this is known as healing by first intention or primary healing (Figs 3.2 and 3.3). Where the wound edges are apart, such as when there has been tissue loss, the same biological processes occur, but rapid closure is not possible. Angiogenesis and fibroblast proliferation result in the formation of granulation tissue. This contracts to reduce wound area and allows epithelialisation across its surface to achieve wound

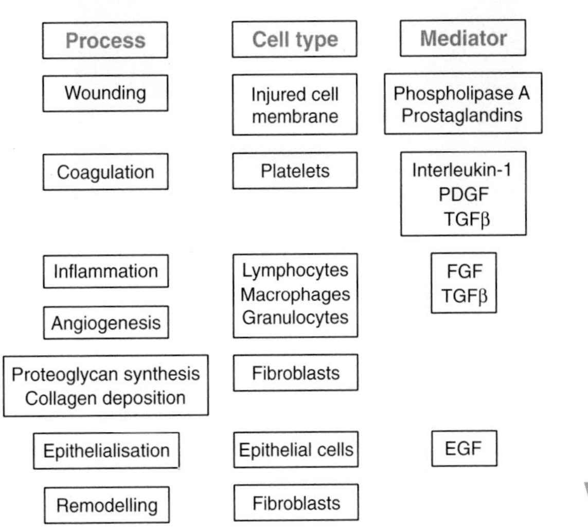

Fig. 3.1 Chart illustrating the biological processes involved in wound repair (PDGF, platelet-derived growth factor; TGFβ, transforming growth factor β; FGF, fibroblast growth factor; EGF, epidermal growth factor).

Homer, date of birth uncertain between 1050 and 850 BC, somewhere in Greece. Still regarded as the great epic poet and author of the 'Iliad' and the 'Odyssey'.

Joseph Lister (Lord Lister), 1827–1912. Professor of Surgery, Glasgow, Scotland (1860–69), Edinburgh, Scotland (1869–77) and King's College Hospital, London, England (1877–92).

[1]*Weal = the general good, the welfare of a country.*

Bailey & Love's Short Practice of Surgery, 23rd edition. Edited by R.C.G. Russell, N.S. Williams and C.J.K. Bulstrode. Published in 2000 by Arnold Publishers.

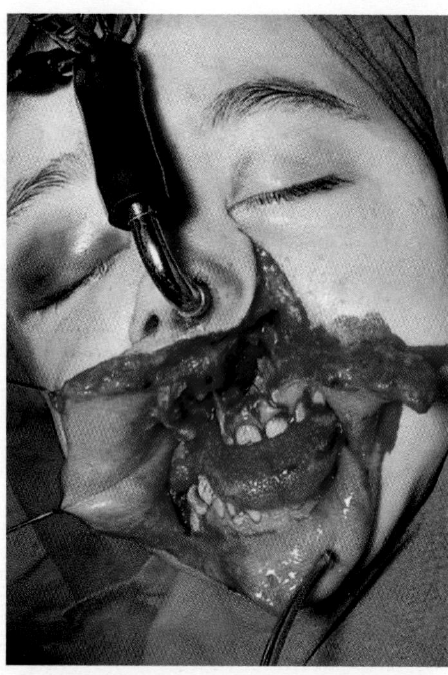

Fig. 3.2 Split-open face from a road traffic accident (*courtesy of the late Rainsford Mowlem, FRCS*).

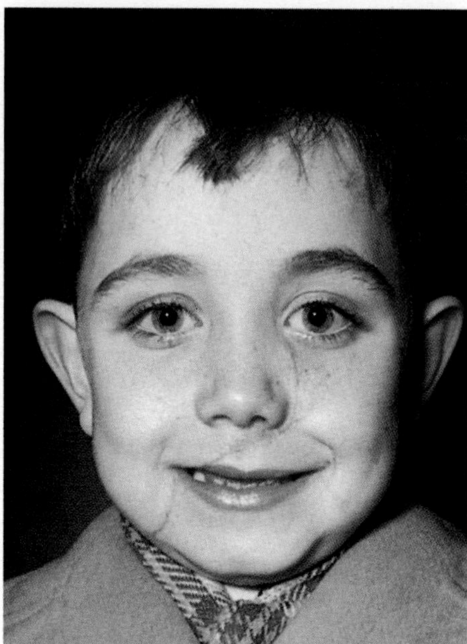

Fig. 3.3 Healing by first intention after primary suture of split-open face (*courtesy of the late Rainsford Mowlem, FRCS*).

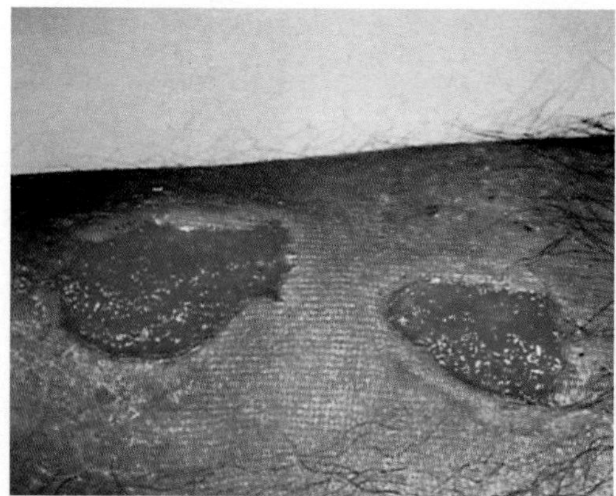

Fig. 3.4 Ulcers of the leg healing by second intention. Note the red granulation tissue.

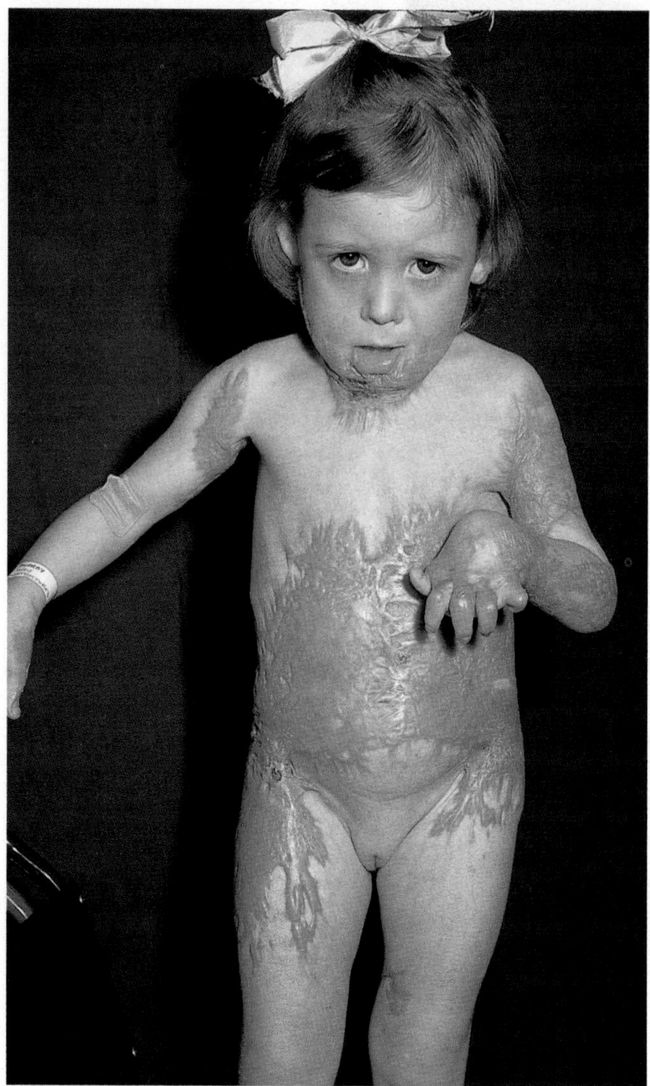

Fig. 3.5 Extensive hypertrophic scars following a burn injury. Note the contractures of the neck and dorsum of the hand.

closure. This is known as healing by second intention (Fig. 3.4). This process is slower, the contraction involved may cause contracture and functional restriction (Fig. 3.5), and the resultant healed surface is a thin layer of epithelium on scar tissue that may not prove durable in the long term. In general, healing by second intention will give a worse aesthetic outcome. It is because of the poor functional and aesthetic results of healing by second intention that surgical endeavour is usually directed towards achieving primary wound healing.

Classification of wounds

A wound can be caused by almost any injurious agent and can involve almost any tissue or structure. The most useful classification of wounds from a practical point of view is that of Rank and Wakefield into tidy and untidy wounds.

Tidy wounds

Tidy wounds are inflicted by sharp instruments and contain no devitalised tissue (Fig. 3.6); such wounds can be closed primarily with the expectation of quiet primary healing. Examples are surgical incisions, cuts from glass and knife wounds. Skin wounds will usually be single and clean cut. Tendons, arteries and nerves will commonly be injured in tidy wounds, but repair of these structures is usually possible (Fig. 3.7). Fractures are uncommon in tidy wounds.

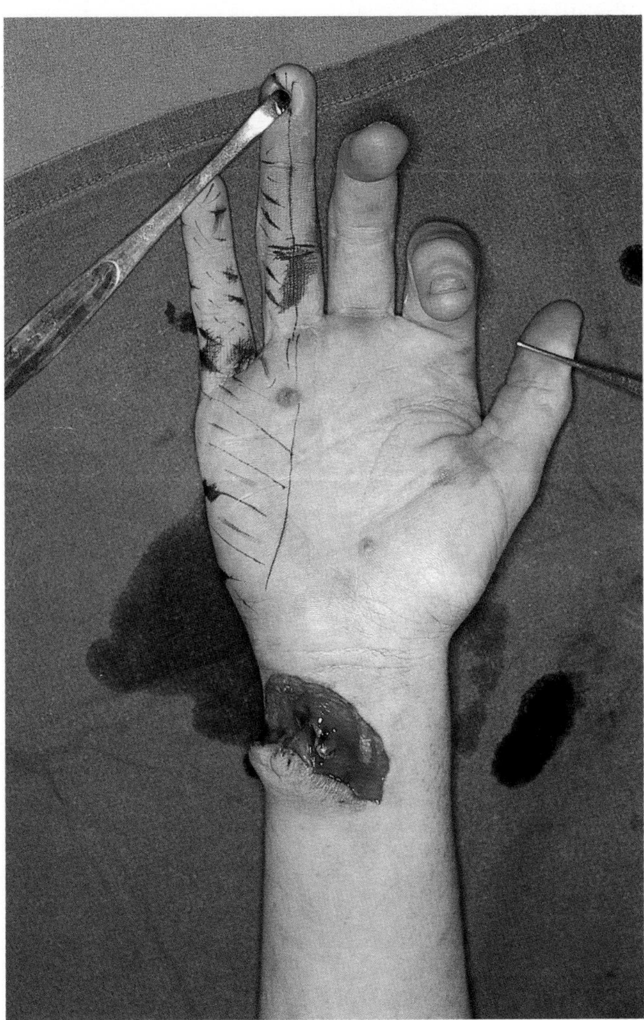

Fig. 3.6 A wrist laceration in a 14-year-old boy caused by falling through a glass door. Examination has revealed sensory loss and motor signs of an ulnar nerve injury. This is a *tidy* wound, it contains no devitalised tissue and after exploration it can safely be closed.

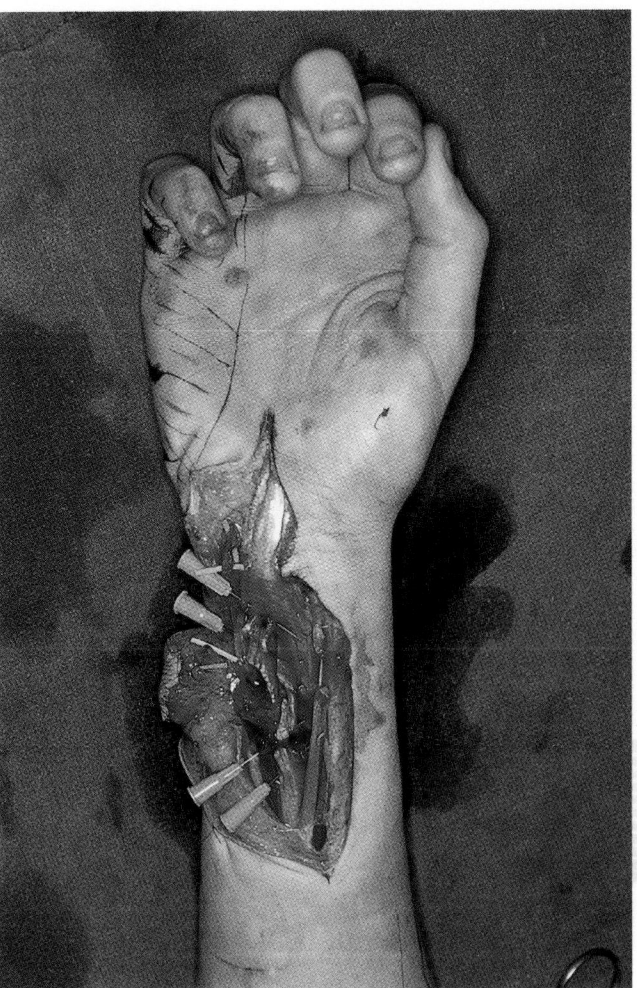

Fig. 3.7 After exploration the ulnar nerve, ulnar artery and several tendons were found to be divided. These structures will all be repaired primarily with the anticipation of quiet primary wound healing and a satisfactory functional result.

Untidy wounds

Untidy wounds result from crushing, tearing, avulsion, vascular injury or burns, and contain devitalised tissue (Fig. 3.8). Skin wounds will often be multiple and irregular. Tendons, arteries and nerves may be exposed, and might be injured in continuity, but will usually not be divided. Fractures are common and may be multifragmentary. Such wounds must not be closed primarily; if they are closed wound healing is unlikely to occur without complications. At best there may be wound dehiscence, infection and delayed healing, at worst gas gangrene and death may result. The correct management of untidy wounds is wound excision, by this is meant excision of all devitalised tissue to create a tidy wound. Once the untidy wound has been converted to a tidy wound by the process of wound excision it can be safely closed (Fig. 3.9) (or allowed to heal by second intention).

Sir Benjamin Keith Rank. Plastic surgeon, Royal Melbourne Hospital, Melbourne, Australia.

Allan Ross Wakefield. Plastic surgeon, Royal Children's Hospital, Melbourne, Australia.

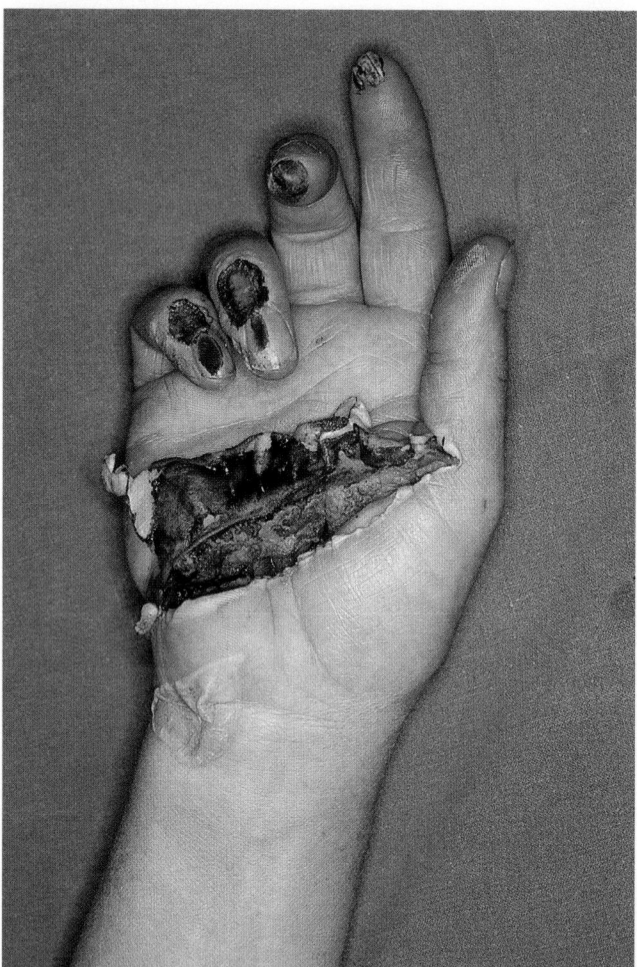

Fig. 3.8 This woman's hand was trapped in a moulding machine resulting in a combination of crush and burn mechanisms. This untidy wound must be excised.

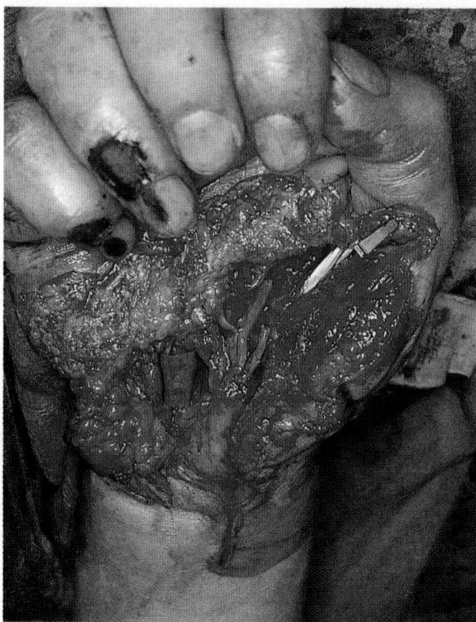

Fig. 3.9 A radical wound excision has been performed for the palmar wound. Most of the median nerve remains in-continuity. It is now safe to repair damaged structures and close this wound.

Wound excision

The most important step in the management of any untidy wound is wound excision. This process is sometimes called 'wound toilet' or 'debridement'. The former implies washing and the latter laying open or fasciotomy, all of which may be important in wound management but do not describe excision of devitalised tissue which is the most important process. For this reason the term 'wound excision' is preferred. In order to excise a wound adequate anaesthesia – local, regional or general – must be provided. Where possible a bloodless field also aids identification of structures. For superficial wounds the use of local anaesthetic with 1 in 200 000 adrenaline gives good haemostasis of skin edges. In the limbs a pneumatic tourniquet is used. It is helpful to use a skin-marking pen to plan the skin excision and any wound extensions. Excision should proceed in a systematic fashion dealing with each tissue layer in turn, usually starting superficial and moving deep. Longitudinal structures such as blood vessels, nerves and tendons are identified and exposed, but left in-continuity. With experience the surgeon learns to recognise dead tissues. Devitalised dermis is pink rather than white; devitalised fat is pink rather than yellow; devitalised muscle is a dark colour, has lost its usual sheen and turgor, and does not twitch when picked up with forceps. Bone fragments with no soft-tissue attachment or nonvital soft-tissue attachments are also discarded. This approach to radical wound excision is sometimes called a 'pseudotumour' approach, because the entire wound is excised with an appropriate margin back to healthy tissue (Figs 3.8 and 3.9). At the end of wound excision the wound should resemble an anatomical dissection. Normal bleeding should be observed from each layer. Occasionally in very extensive wounds this radical approach must be modified. Where radical wound excision would threaten the viability or function of the limb it is reasonable to excise what is definitely nonviable, carry out fasciotomy as appropriate and dress the wound, with a view to returning 48 hours later for a second look, and thereafter further serial wound excisions until a tidy wound is achieved.

Wound closure

Wound closure can be achieved by number of differing techniques. Most tidy wounds that do not involve loss of tissue can be closed directly. Where there is tissue loss a technique to import appropriate tissue is needed. Reconstructive plastic surgical techniques can range from simple skin grafts to complex composite free tissue transfers (Table 3.1). This list used to be described as a 'reconstructive ladder'; unfortunately this implies that the correct approach is to use the simplest technique and only when it fails move to a more complex technique. This approach is not appropriate in modern surgical practice. The available techniques should be regarded as a 'toolbox' from which to select the technique that provides most rapid healing, earliest return to function and superior aesthetic outcome.

Table 3.1 Toolbox of wound closure techniques

- Direct closure
- Partial-thickness skin graft
- Full-thickness skin graft
- Composite graft
- Skin flap
- Fasciocutaneous flap
- Musculocutaneous flap
- Free tissue transfer

Types of wound

Bruise, contusion and haematoma

A closed blunt injury may result in a bruise or contusion. There is bleeding into the tissues and visible discoloration. Where the amount of bleeding is sufficient to create a localised collection in the tissues, this is described as a haematoma. Initially this will be fluid, but it will clot within minutes or hours. Later, after a few days, the haematoma will again liquefy. There is a danger of secondary infection. Bruises require no specific management, and no treatment is of proven value. The patient should be advised that the time required for bruising to clear is extremely variable and in some individuals, in some sites, discoloration may persist for months. A haematoma should be evacuated by open surgery if large or causing pressure effects (such as intracranially), or aspirated by a large-bore needle if smaller or in a cosmetically sensitive site. It may be necessary to await liquefaction (which may take several days) and to perform repeated aspirations, with appropriate antiseptic precautions. A haematoma will generally reabsorb without scarring, but on occasions there may be persistent tethering of the skin. Blunt injuries may cause a variety of fat injuries. A blunt injury to the breast may result in an area of fat necrosis that can masquerade as a breast lump. Blunt injuries to the face may result in lumpy subcutaneous collections due to haematoma in subcutaneous fat that may persist for several months. A fat 'fracture' in the buttocks may result from a fall or sharp blow. This can result in separation of subcutaneous fat with an indentation that may not become apparent immediately due to haematoma.

Puncture wounds and bites

A puncture wound is an open injury in which foreign material and organisms are likely to be carried deeply into the underlying tissues. Common causes are standing on a nail or other sharp object. There may be little to see on the surface. Radiological examination may detect metal fragments or glass. Treatment is essentially by wound irrigation, antibiotic treatment and tetanus prophylaxis. Large foreign bodies should be removed, but small particles may be surprisingly difficult to find without a destructive dissection and are better left undisturbed. When a foreign body is visualised on a radiograph a surface marker should be taped to the skin to aid localisation. A metal detector may be helpful during exploration. The danger of puncture injuries is that they may give rise to an abscess deep within the tissues and on such occasions drainage may be required. It is likely that it will take 24–48 hours for an abscess to declare itself and arrangement should be made for review. Needle-stick injuries are a particular cause for concern. Although these are a particular hazard for hospital staff, discarded needles from drug abuse are becoming increasingly a cause of accidental injury in the community. Medical, nursing and ancillary staff should have hepatitis B immunisation. The chance of HIV infection from a needle-stick injury seems to be low but all such injuries should be recorded and, if dealing with a high-risk patient, HIV tests should be performed at 3 and 6 months after the episode. Bites are a particular type of puncture wound associated with a high incidence of infection, presumably from mouth organisms. Animal bites may result in small, sharp, incised wounds or in severe tissue crushing as in horse bites. Dog bites may also be associated with a degree of tissue avulsion (Fig. 3.10), and often there are puncture wounds from upper and lower teeth and contusion of the intervening tissue. Human bites may be associated with avulsion of pieces of the nose or ear. An accidental type of 'bite' injury may result from an attacker striking the victim's incisor teeth with the knuckles. This is a frequent injury that presents with a puncture wound over the metacarpophalangeal (MP) joints. It is important to recognise the nature of the injury as the history is often less than truthful. Radiological examination may demonstrate parts of a tooth within the MP joints. As all of the layers over the joints glide over one another on making a fist, the through-and-through nature of the puncture wound is often not appreciated with the hand extended. If there has been sufficient force to penetrate the skin, it must be assumed that the MP joint has been penetrated. Such wounds are best treated by open surgical exploration excision of skin margins, irrigation of the joint and antibiotic therapy.

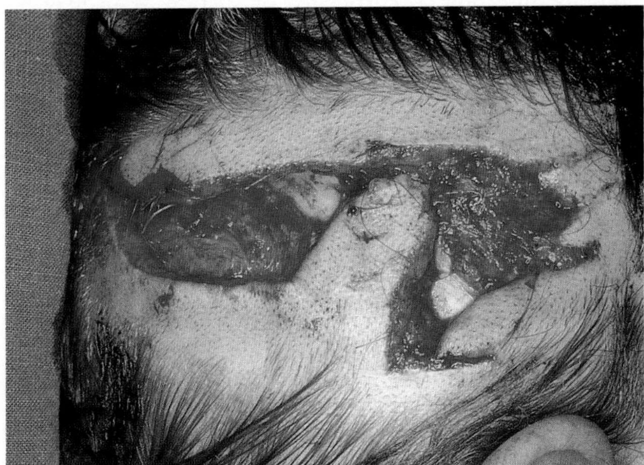

Fig. 3.10 A severe dog bite injury to the scalp.

Abrasions and friction burns

An abrasion is a shearing injury of skin in which the surface is rubbed off. Most are superficial and will heal by epithelialisation, but some may result in full-thickness skin loss. Abrasions may be dirt ingrained and if this dirt is not removed at the time of primary treatment permanent tattooing of the skin will result. Treatment is by cleaning with a scrubbing brush, gently brushing along the grain of the scratch lines. A friction burn is similar, but there will be an element of thermal damage as well as abrasion. Treatment is as for other types of burn.

Laceration

A laceration or cut is the result of contact with a sharp object (the surgical equivalent is an incised wound). Once the cutting implement has gone deep to the dermis, there is less resistance in the subcutaneous tissues and the cut may therefore penetrate to a considerable depth. It is important to ascertain from the history the amount of force involved. The clinical examination must therefore assess the integrity of all structures in the area: arteries, nerves, muscles, tendons and ligaments (Fig. 3.6). The ideal form of management of an incised wound is surgical inspection, cleaning and closure. The wound must be thoroughly inspected to ensure that there is no damage to deep structures or, where encountered, these must be repaired (Fig. 3.7). As a general rule, the damage to nerves and tendons is generally greater than suspected preoperatively. Once all of the damaged layers have been identified, each structure must be repaired individually by the appropriate technique. Haemostasis must be ensured throughout the exploration. There are precise suture placement techniques for nerves, tendons and blood vessels. Muscles can be apposed in layers by mattress sutures and fascia, and subcutaneous fat should be opposed by interrupted absorbable sutures to allow a firm platform for skin closure in such a way that the skin margins do not invert. It is an important principle to prevent collections of blood or other fluids in a wound as they separate tissues and act as a nidus for infection. A corrugated or suction drain may be required. In a simple incised laceration, a method of wound closure should be selected which is appropriate for the needs of function and appearance. On the face, fine (5/0 or 6/0) nylon sutures should be placed near to the wound margins, to be removed on the fifth day. Alternatively, subcuticular (intradermal) sutures avoid suture marks and can be left in place longer (2 weeks or more). An alternative to suturing is the application of adhesive tape strips. It is necessary to apply these with the same care as sutures ensuring that all bleeding has stopped and that the skin is dry. For limb and trunk wounds, a heavier suture is required but it is rarely necessary to use more than 4/0 or 3/0 sutures for skin closure. Monofilament sutures, such as nylon, are said to leave less obvious suture marks than braided material such as silk, but other factors contribute to stitch marks, such as inflammation (from infection or reaction to organic material such as silk), wound tension and late removal. All patients sustaining open wounds should have prophylaxis against tetanus, and antibiotics should be administered where there is significant contamination, commencing generally with a broad-spectrum antibiotic active against Gram-positive organisms.

Traction and avulsion

Avulsion injuries are open injuries where there has been a severe degree of tissue damage. Such injuries occur when hands or limbs are trapped in moving machinery, such as in rollers, producing a degloving injury. Degloving is caused by shearing forces that separate tissue planes, rupturing their vascular interconnections and causing tissue ischaemia. This most frequently occurs between the subcutaneous fat and deep fascia. Degloving injuries can be open or closed. Degloving can be localised or circumferential. It can occur only in the single, subcutaneous plane, but where present in multiple planes, such as between muscles and fascia and between muscles and bone, is an indication of a severe high-energy injury with a limited potential for primary healing. Similar injuries occur as a result of runover road traffic accident injuries where friction from rubber tyres will avulse skin and subcutaneous tissue from the underlying deep fascia (Fig. 3.11). The history should raise the examiner's suspicion and it is often possible to pinch the skin and lift it upwards revealing its detachment from the normal anchorage. The danger of degloving or avulsion injuries is that there is devascularisation of tissue and skin necrosis may become slowly apparent in the following few days. Even tissue that initially demonstrates venous bleeding may subsequently undergo necrosis if the circulation is insufficient. Treatment of such injuries is to identify the area of devitalised skin and to remove the skin, defat it and reapply it as a full-thickness skin graft. Avulsion injuries of hands or feet may require immediate flap cover using a one-stage microvascular tissue transfer of skin and/or muscle.

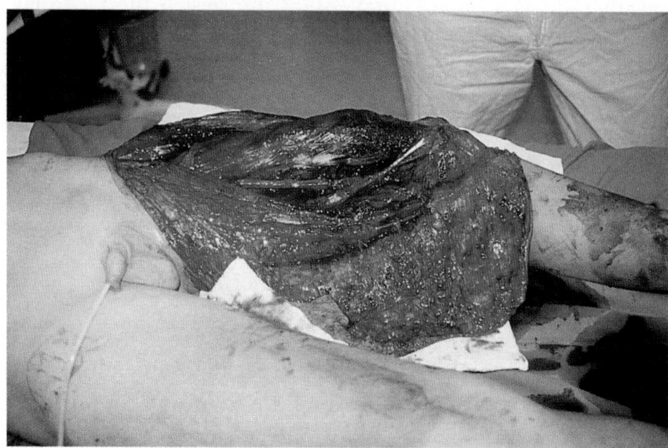

Fig. 3.11 A severe rollover injury to the left thigh. There is extensive multiplane degloving (*courtesy of Henk Giele, FRACS*).

Hans Christian Joachim Gram, 1853–1938. Professor of Medicine, Copenhagen, Denmark.

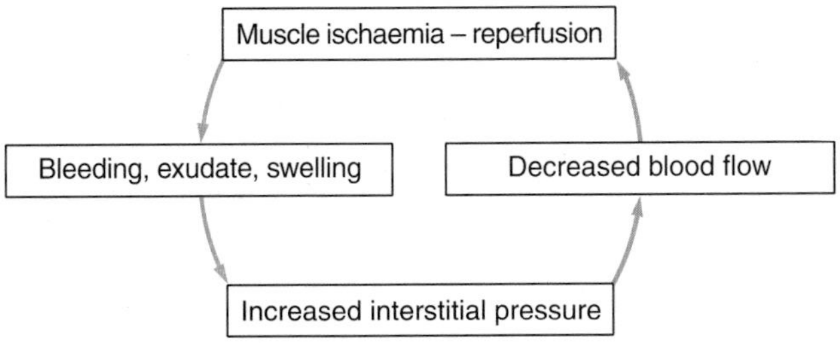

Muscle ischaemia – reperfusion

Bleeding, exudate, swelling

Decreased blood flow

Increased interstitial pressure

Fig. 3.12 Diagram illustrating the cycle of events in the developing compartment syndrome.

Crush

Crush injuries are a further variant of blunt injury and are often accompanied by degloving and compartment syndrome. Injury to tissues within a closed fascial compartment leads to bleeding, exudate and swelling of these tissues, and increased interstitial pressure. As the interstitial pressure rises above capillary perfusion pressure the blood supply to the viable tissues is reduced, resulting in further ischaemic tissue injury and swelling (Fig. 3.12). This cycle causes a worsening compartment syndrome with muscle ischaemia and nerve ischaemia progressing to muscle necrosis, skin necrosis and limb loss. Muscle necrosis may result in renal failure. This process can be arrested by early recognition and decompression of the affected compartment(s) by fasciotomy. The most reliable clinical sign of compartment syndrome is pain worsened by passive stretching of affected muscles. Where any doubt exists compartment pressure measurements can be carried out. Loss of peripheral pulses is not a sign of compartment syndrome, but indicates major vessel damage. Where compartment syndrome is suspected or confirmed fasciotomy is advised. Longitudinal incisions are made in the deep fascia and it may also be necessary to make extensive longitudinal releases in the skin. It is important to release the fascia over each individual compartment in a limb.

Injury to internal organs

Wounds such as stab wounds may be associated with damage to internal organs. Treatment of penetrating abdominal or thoracic wounds has been discussed elsewhere. The possibility of blunt or sharp abdominal trauma must not be overlooked when treating extensive injuries elsewhere, particularly in an unconscious patient.

War wounds and gunshot injuries

Gunshot injuries are associated with different severity of tissue damage depending upon whether the injury is of low or high velocity. Low-velocity injuries, such as from a hand gun, result in an entry and exit wound, the latter being the larger, and damage along the tract of the missile. Such injuries are often associated with severe tissue contamination from clothing, dirt or other foreign materials. High-velocity injuries (from modern assault rifles) cause explosive pressure and decompression effect, such that there is widespread tissue damage, with injury to major limb vessels and nerves situated some distance from the tract of the missile. Where a high-velocity missile strikes bone, the high-energy exchange results in fragmentation of the bone. Gunshot wounds and war wounds require careful surgical excision and such wounds should be left open. Following high-velocity injuries, fasciotomy of all of the fascial compartments of the limb should be undertaken. The damage from a shotgun wound depends on the scatter of the shot and therefore on the range. A large track of damage may result in severe bleeding or a pneumothorax, which requires immediate appropriate emergency management.

Injuries to bone and joints

Fractures may be *closed* where the skin is intact or *open* where there is a wound. Open fractures may have a skin wound due to penetration from the outside or, more frequently, due to bursting of the skin from within by bone fragments. The bone displacement is worst at the very moment of injury and bone fragments partially reduce spontaneously thereafter. It is important to appreciate that a puncture wound of the skin overlying a fracture is almost certainly evidence that the skin was penetrated by bone. The usual principles of wound management apply in that an adequate excision of the wound is necessary followed by antibiotic treatment and appropriate treatment of the fracture. Severe open lower limb injuries often have extensive damage to the skin and muscle in addition to fractures. It is best to treat the fracture and soft-tissue injuries simultaneously. Extensive removal of damaged soft tissue may be required and skin cover achieved by a one-stage microvascular tissue transfer.

Injury to nerves

Glass does not bruise nerves. Where there is an open wound, nerve division must always be suspected. Clinical examination should be undertaken to assess the motor and sensory function of every nerve in the region of the open wound, and it must be assumed that an underlying nerve has been divided until its function can be demonstrated to be intact. A sharp, wounding implement can travel a considerable distance in the soft tissues, and with limb injuries it is necessary to assess all the major nerve trunks at that level in the limb. Where there is doubt the nerve should be explored and visualised. Divided nerves should be repaired. Magnification and fine suture materials have improved results.

Injuries to arteries and veins

Where a wound is associated with much bleeding there is the possibility that a significantly large vessel has been divided. As a first-aid measure, bleeding will almost always be controlled by direct pressure, and elevation of the part where practicable. Limb tourniquets should not be applied as a first-aid measure. In the emergency department it is never desirable to plunge vascular damps or artery forceps into a wound without a proper view of the bleeding point, as grasping nerves can inflict great harm. Where a major limb vessel has been damaged it may be necessary to apply direct manual pressure while the patient is taken into an operating room. Under anaesthesia, the appropriate way to deal with bleeding in the limb is to explore the wound under pneumatic tourniquet control.

Chronic wounds

Several conditions are classified as varieties of chronic wounds, although they may not clearly follow mechanical trauma.

Ulcers

An ulcer is any breach in an epithelial surface. Chronic ulcers are wounds that fail to heal. In generally, they have a fibrotic margin and a bed of granulation tissue which may include areas of slough (necrotic tissue). Ulcers are particularly common in the lower third of the lower limb and foot. They have a number of different aetiologies, often being associated with arterial or venous insufficiency or a lack of normal skin innervation. The wound healing process is delayed by a variety of mechanisms including infection, mechanical irritation, ischaemia or other metabolic factors. Ulcers are common in diabetes and rheumatoid arthritis. Treatment consists of specific management of the underlying cause. The ulcer is managed either by dressings to allow healing by second intention or by surgical excision of granulation tissue and split-skin grafting. Recurrence is inevitable if the underlying cause is not corrected.

Pressure sores

These are chronic wounds following tissue necrosis from pressure. They occur over bony prominences. Their pathogenesis is identical to compartment syndrome in that they arise where there is unrelieved pressure in the soft tissues overlying bone such that the external pressure exceeds capillary perfusion pressure and ischaemic necrosis occurs. They occur in paraplegic individuals who lack the usual sensory input that tissue ischaemia is beginning and may lack the ability to move themselves and relieve this pressure. They also occur in situations where perfusion pressure is low, such as hypotension and peripheral vascular disease. Sacral and trochanteric sores occur in bed-bound patients, both paraplegic and nonparaplegic. Ischial pressure sores occur in chair-bound paraplegics. Patients with peripheral vascular disease are prone to heel pressure sores. On occasions almost any bony prominence may be involved. Prevention is better than cure. This depends on an awareness of pressure sore risk in all patients and the implementation of appropriate measures that may include turning or lifting the patient, pressure-relieving mattresses and beds, special seating and cushions, and educating the patient and their carers in taking responsibility for pressure relief. When a sore occurs it is essential to identify and correct the underlying cause. If this can be done most sores will heal by second intention. Incontinence should be managed appropriately and nutritional support provided if needed. Surgical treatment can accelerate healing. The sore is excised and closed using a flap. Pressure sore closure is indicated for nonparaplegics where the sore is delaying or complicating their recovery from an illness, and in paraplegics who have identified and corrected the precipitating cause and who are motivated to maintain adequate pressure relief. Surgery is usually inappropriate in those in the later stages of progressive neurological illnesses.

Scars

The most superficial wounds such as superficial burns and abrasions will heal by epithelialisation alone without scar formation. In these circumstances adnexal structures are preserved and the epithelium regenerates from these structures. This may leave alterations in keratinisation, texture or pigmentation of the healed area, but not scarring as such. A scar is the inevitable consequence of wound repair. The final phase of wound repair is the process of remodelling and scar maturation (Fig. 3.1). The fibroblasts, capillaries, glycosaminoglycans, and immature collagen of granulation tissue and the newly healed wound are replaced by relatively acellular, avascular scar tissue composed of mature collagen with scattered fibroblasts. This biological process is manifested by a change in appearance of the scar from a red, raised, firm, contracting, perhaps itchy nodule to a pale, flat, softer, static, symptomless plaque of mature scar. The rate at which any given scar passes through this process can vary widely depending on the age of the individual, the site of the wound, the time the wound took to heal, the direction of the scar and the tension across it (Fig. 3.13). In general, scars in younger patients with wounds on the trunk that heal slowly, perhaps with infection or dehiscence, and scars that have a lot of tension across them will take much longer to mature than scars in older people, in thin-skinned areas, that heal rapidly by first intention and that have minimal tension across them (Table 3.2). It is important to be aware of this variation in the natural history of scar maturation in order to counsel patients regarding the likely progress and outcome of

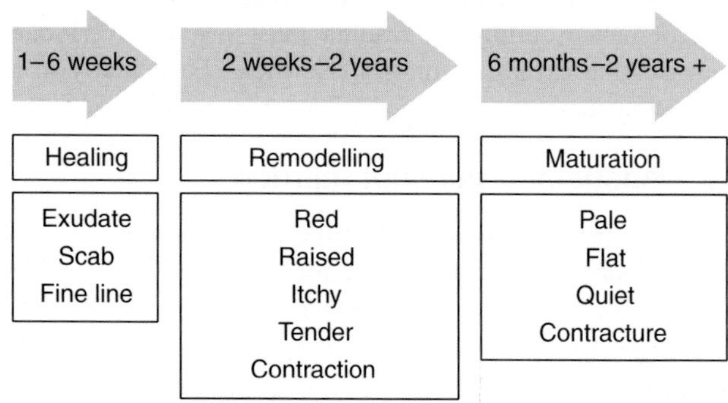

Fig. 3.13 Diagram showing the phases of wound healing remodelling and scar maturation. The times shown are approximate as they vary depending on a number of patient- and wound-related factors.

Table 3.2 How do you get an ideal scar?

- Achieve quiet primary healing
- Clean incised edges, no tissue loss
- Avoid dehiscence or infection
- Minimise tension
- Align scar with wrinkle, junction or relaxed skin tension line
- Site – eyelids, genitalia, palms, vermillion
- Old person
- Fine lax skin

their scar, advise those having elective surgery what the consequences in terms of scarring will be, and to recognise the various types of adverse scarring which can occur. One of the most frequent types of adverse scar, a hypertrophic scar, is one that remains red, raised, itchy and tender for longer than might generally be expected.

Adverse scars

There are many types of adverse scar (Table 3.3), many of which can be avoided or prevented by correct incision planning and adequate wound management. Some types, however, cannot be prevented and are unpredictable in their occurrence. The appearance of some scars can be improved by surgical or other means, but scars can never be removed totally. The types of adverse scar will be discussed and suggestions for avoidance or management made.

Wrong direction

Incisions that pass along ideal lines are more likely to leave acceptable scars. There are many types of 'lines of election' for incisions, most of which pass along skin wrinkles or along relaxed skin tension lines (that is a line along which maximal skin tension passes when the part is in a relaxed position). These lines have minimal tension across the wound edges. A scar which crosses these lines will have a greater tendency to stretch or become hypertrophic, and even if not hypertrophic will usually appear more conspicuous than one which follows a relaxed skin tension line. Other ideal positions for scars are at junctions between anatomical areas such as the nose and the cheek, the cheek and the ear or the junction between a hairy and hairless area.

Table 3.3 Types of adverse scar

- Wrong direction
- Poor alignment of features
- Stretched scar
- Contracted scar
- Pigment alteration
- Contour deformity
- Tattooing
- Stitch marks
- Hypertrophic scar
- Keloid scar

Poor alignment of features

Where a scar crosses the junction between distinct anatomical features, such as the vermillion of the lip, it is essential that these features are accurately realigned. Such malalignments result in conspicuous adverse scars.

Stretched scar

Scars from excisional wounds on the trunk and limbs often stretch. It has been shown that the width of a scar depends on the tension across the wound at the time of wound closure. In general, steps to avoid excessive tension across the wound will be rewarded with narrower scars. Where tension cannot be avoided there is evidence that prolonged wound support with buried nonabsorbable or long-term absorbable sutures can minimise scar stretching.

Contracted scar

The process of wound contraction continues in the remodelling phase of scar maturation such that a scar will always be shorter than the incision from which it results. Where a linear scar crosses a flexor surface this shortening may result in a scar contracture which may prevent full extension of that part. This will occur on the flexor surface of a finger if a straight-line incision is used. Curved or zigzag incisions will avoid this problem. Where scarring is extensive such as burn scars then scar contractures may be inevitable. Linear scar contractures can be corrected by realignment of the scar; there are various techniques to do this including Z-plasty and multiple Y–V-plasty. More extensive contractures will require release and introduction of additional skin by means of grafts or flaps.

Pigment alteration

The new epidermis of a scar will often not have the same degree of pigmentation as surrounding unscarred areas. Most scars are hypopigmented, but hyperpigmentation can also occur. The only ways to deal with this problem are cosmetic camouflage or tattooing.

Contour deformity

Where wound edges are not anatomically aligned in the vertical plane or where a bevelled cut is not repaired accurately there is a risk of contour irregularity in the healed scar. This can usually be avoided by accurate wound repair, if necessary excising bevelled edges to restore even vertical edges for repair. A variation of this problem occurs when a curved laceration heals, in that the scar shortens and that portion of skin within the concavity of the curved scar tends to become raised. This problem is known as trapdooring or mushrooming. It will often improve with time, but scar revision is sometimes indicated to correct it.

Tattooing

In traumatic wounds it is possible for particles of grit, dirt or soot to become implanted in the wound as it heals. This results in tattooed scars where the particles of foreign material show through as blue or black discoloration of the scar. Adequate primary wound management can avoid this. Abrasions with ingrained dirt should be scrubbed with a stiff brush; more deeply tattooed wounds should be excised. Late correction of tattooed scars can be very difficult.

Stitch marks

If skin sutures are left in place for more than 7 days then scars from the stitch marks will usually result. This problem can be avoided by using subcuticular sutures wherever possible, removing skin sutures before 7 days and, where prolonged wound support is needed, supplementing skin sutures with subcuticular sutures allowing early removal of the skin sutures. Adverse scars due to prominent stitch marks can rarely be improved by scar revision.

Hypertrophic scars

In some circumstances scars remain in the remodelling phase for longer than is usual. These hypertrophic scars are more cellular and more vascular than mature scars, there is increased collagen production and collagen breakdown, but the balance is such that excess collagen is produced. Clinically these scars are red, raised, itchy and tender (Fig. 3.14). Such scars will eventually mature to become pale and flat, and it is this spontaneous resolution which distinguishes hypertrophic scars from keloid scars. Hypertrophic scars typically occur in wounds where healing was delayed, perhaps where complications such as infection or dehiscence occurred. They are more common in children and where skin tension is high such as the tip of the shoulder or any scar that runs across relaxed skin tension lines.

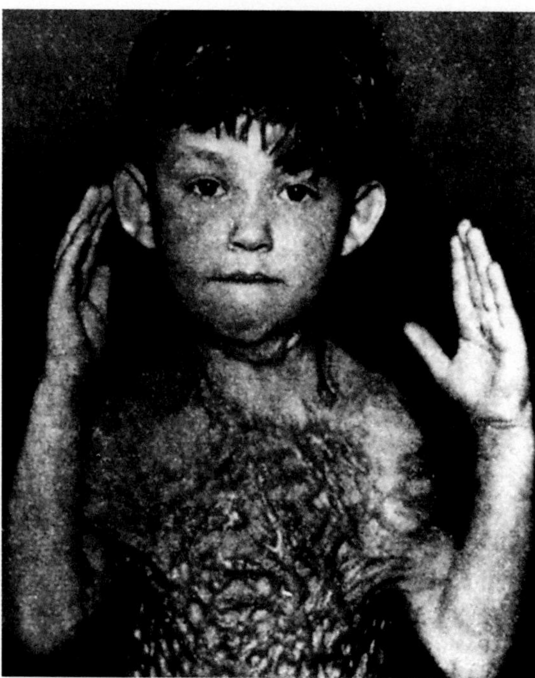

Fig. 3.14 Hypertrophic scars and contractures following burns (*courtesy of the late Patrick Clarkson, FRCS*).

The risk of developing a hypertrophic scar can be minimised by ensuring quiet primary healing. Where hypertrophy does occur patience is usually rewarded by improvement with time. Massage of the scar with moisturising cream or the application of pressure to the remodelling scar can accelerate the natural process of maturation. Patients with hypertrophic burn scars are supplied with custom-made Lycra pressure garments that promote acceleration of scar maturation. Revision of hypertrophic scars is appropriate where they cross skin tension lines or where a specific wound healing complication occurred. In the absence of these factors scar revision should be avoided as it will usually be met with recurrence.

Keloid scars

In some situations there is an extreme overgrowth of scar tissue that grows beyond the limits of the original wound and shows no tendency to resolve. Keloid scars are biologically identical to hypertrophic scars that in turn are an extension of normal scar behaviour. Whilst it is usually possible to make the distinction between these scar types, they are best regarded as a spectrum of scar behaviour (Table 3.4). Keloid scars are more frequent in Afro-Caribbean and oriental racial groups (Fig. 3.15). They often occur in wounds that healed perfectly

Table 3.4 Comparison of hypertrophic and keloid scars

Features	*Hypertrophic scar*	*Keloid scar*
Genetic	Not familial	May be familial
Race	Not race related	Black > white
Sex	Female = male	Female > male
Age	Children	10–30 years
Borders	Remains within wound	Outgrows wound area
Natural history	Subsides with time	Rarely subsides
Site	Flexor surfaces	Sternum, shoulder, face
Aetiology	Related to tension	Unknown

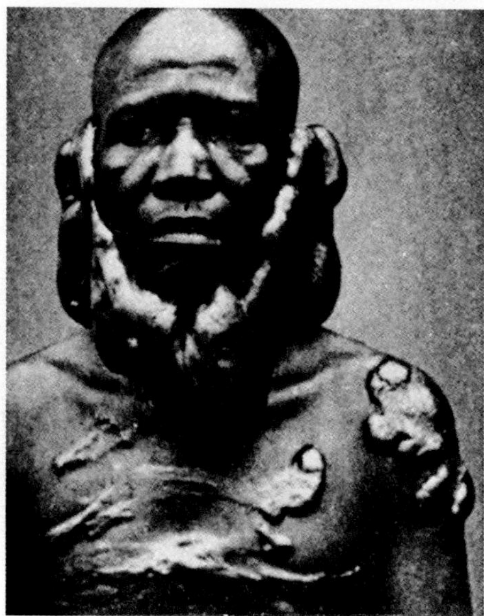

Fig. 3.15 Extensive keloid in a West African (*courtesy of C. Bowesman, FRCS, Kumasi, Ghana*).

without complications. They are more common in certain sites such as the central chest, the back and shoulders and the earlobes. Many keloid scars are untreatable and surgical treatment as a single modality will usually be met with recurrence. Some keloid scars will improve with the application of pressure. Intralesional injections of steroids such as triamcinolone can be helpful. The best cure rates are achieved with a combination of surgery and postoperative interstitial radiotherapy.

Further reading

BOA/BAPS (1997) *The Management of Open Tibial Fractures*, British Orthopaedic Association, London.

Granick, M.S., Long, C.D. and Ramasastry, S.S. (1998) Wound healing: state of the art. *Clinics in Plastic Surgery*, **25**, 321–483.

Lister, G. (1993) *The Hand: Diagnosis and Indications*, Churchill-Livingstone, Edinburgh.

Robson, M.C., Burns, B.F. and Phillips, L.G. (1994) Wound repair: principles and applications. In *Plastic Surgery: A Core Curriculum* (eds R.L. Ruberg and D.J. Smith), Mosby, St Louis, MO.

Watson, S. and Coleman, D.J. (1999) Soft tissue injury. In *Trauma Care Beyond the Resuscitation Room* (eds P.A. Driscoll and D.V. Skinner), BMJ Books, London.

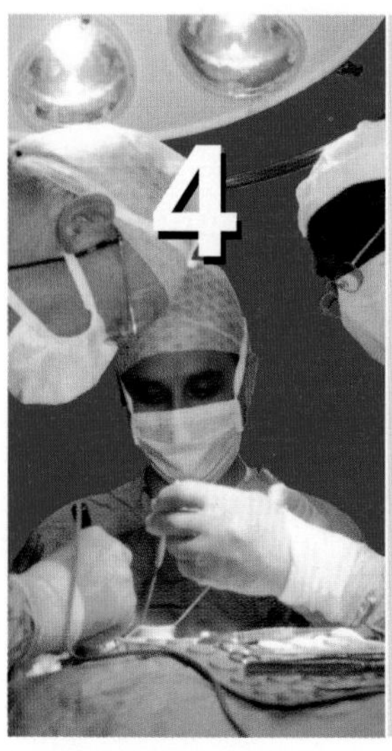

4 Critical care; fluid, electrolyte and acid–base balance; blood transfusion

Fluids

Fluid intake

Fluid intake is derived from two sources: (1) exogenous; and (2) endogenous.

Exogenous water is either drunk or ingested in solid food. The quantities vary within wide limits, but average 2–3 litres per 24 hours, of which nearly half is contained in solid food.

Taking into consideration their body weight, the water requirements of infants and children are relatively greater than those of adults because of: (1) the larger surface area per unit of body weight; (2) the greater metabolic activity due to growth; and (3) the comparatively poor concentrating ability of the immature kidney.

Endogenous water is released during the oxidation of ingested food; the amount is normally less than 500 ml/24 hours. However, during starvation, this amount is supplemented by water released from the breakdown of body tissues.

Table 4.1 Average daily water balance of a healthy adult in a temperate climate (70 kg)

Intake	*Output*
Water from beverage = 1200 ml	Urine = 1500 ml
Water from 'solid food' = 1000 ml	Insensible loss from skin and lungs = 900 ml
Water from oxidation = 300 ml	Faeces = 100 ml

Bailey & Love's Short Practice of Surgery, 23rd edition. Edited by R.C.G. Russell, N.S. Williams and C.J.K. Bulstrode. Published in 2000 by Arnold Publishers.

Fluid output

Water is lost from the body by four routes.

- *By the lungs*. About 400 ml of water is lost in expired air each 24 hours. In a dry atmosphere, and when the respiratory rate is increased, the loss is correspondingly greater (this also applies to the patient who has their trachea intubated).
- *By the skin*. When the body becomes overheated, there is visible perspiration, but throughout life invisible perspiration is always occurring. The cutaneous fluid loss varies within wide limits in accordance with the atmospheric temperature and humidity, muscular activity and body temperature. In a temperate climate the average loss is between 600 and 1000 ml/24 hours.
- *Faeces*. Between 60 and 150 ml of water are lost by this route daily. In diarrhoea this amount is greatly multiplied.
- *Urine*. The output of urine is under the control of multiple influences, such as blood volume, hormonal and nervous influences, among which the antidiuretic hormone plays a major role controlling tonicity of the body fluids, a function that it performs by stimulating the reabsorption of water from the renal tubules, thus varying the amount excreted after the requirements of the first three routes have been met. The normal urinary output is approximately 1500 ml/24 hours, and provided that the kidneys are healthy, the specific gravity of the urine bears a direct relationship to the volume. A minimum urinary output of approximately 400 ml/24 hours is required to excrete the end-products of protein metabolism.

Water depletion

Pure water depletion is usually due to diminished intake. This may be due to lack of availability, difficulty or inability to swallow because of painful conditions of the mouth and pharynx, or obstruction in the oesophagus. Exhaustion and paresis of the pharyngeal muscles will produce a similar picture. Pure water depletion may also follow the increased loss from the lungs after tracheostomy. This loss may be as much as 500 ml in excess of the normal insensible loss. After tracheostomy, humidification of the inspired air is an important preventive measure.

Clinical features

The main symptoms are weakness and intense thirst. The urinary output is diminished and its specific gravity increased. The increased serum osmotic pressure causes water to leave the cells (intracellular dehydration), and thus delays the onset of overt compensated hypovolaemia (see below).

Water intoxication

This can occur when excessive amounts of water, low sodium or hypotonic solutions are taken or given by any route. The commonest cause on surgical wards is the overprescribing of intravenous 5 per cent glucose solutions to postoperative patients. Colorectal washouts with plain water, instead of saline, have caused water intoxication during total bowel wash-through prior to colonic surgery. A major component of the TURP (transurethral resection of the prostate) syndrome is the water intoxication caused by excessive uptake of water (and glycine) from irrigation fluid.

Similarly, water intoxication can occur if the body retains water in excess to plasma solutes. This can be seen in the syndrome of inappropriate antidiuretic hormone (SIADH) secretion which is most commonly associated with lung conditions such as lobar pneumonia, empyema and oat-cell carcinoma of bronchus, as well as head injury.

Clinical features

These include drowsiness, weakness, sometimes convulsions and coma. Nausea and vomiting of clear fluid are common, and, with the notable exception of the SIADH, usually the patient passes a considerable amount of dilute urine. Laboratory investigations may show a falling haematocrit, serum sodium and other electrolyte concentrations.

Treatment

The intake of water having been stopped, the best course is water restriction. If the patient fails to improve, transfer to an intensive care or high dependency unit will be necessary for more invasive monitoring and controlled manipulation of fluids and electrolytes. The administration of diuretics or hypertonic saline should not be undertaken lightly as rapid changes in serum sodium concentration may result in neuronal demyelination and a fatal outcome.

Electrolyte balance

When inorganic salts are in solution, as in the extracellular or intracellular fluids of the body, they dissociate into ions. Ions are of two kinds: (1) *cations,* which are electropositive; and (2) *anions,* which are electronegative: collectively these are the electrolytes. The most accurate way of describing the chemical concentrations, reactivity and osmotic power of these ions is in SI units as millimoles per litre (mmol/litre). The cations include sodium, potassium, calcium and magnesium; the anions include chloride, phosphate, bicarbonate and sulphate. The distribution of the salts within the fluid compartments of the body controls the passage of water through the cell walls and maintains acid–base equilibrium.

Sodium balance

Sodium is the principal cation content of the extracellular fluid. The total body sodium amounts to approximately 5000 mmol, of which 44 per cent is in the extracellular fluid, 9 per cent in the intracellular fluid and the remaining 47 per cent in bone. The sodium housed in bone merits special notice: a little more than half of it is osmotically inactive and requires acid for its solution; the remainder is water soluble and exchangeable. Thus, there is a large storehouse of sodium ready to compensate abnormal loss from the body. The daily intake of sodium is inconstant. On average it is 1 mmol/kg sodium chloride or 500 ml of isotonic 0.9 per cent saline solution. An equivalent amount is excreted daily, mainly in the urine and some in the faeces. The loss in perspiration normally is negligible; however, in people not acclimatised to tropical heat, prolonged profuse sweating results in a considerable loss of sodium – as much as 85 mmol/hour. If water alone is given to counter-balance the fluid loss, serious sodium depletion can occur from excessive sweating. (See also mucoviscidosis, in Chapter 54 of this book on 'The gallbladder and bile ducts'.)

Control by adrenal corticoids

The output of sodium, governed by the variation in the avidity with which the renal tubules reabsorb sodium from the glomerular filtrate and the amount of sodium excreted by the sweat glands, is under the control of the adrenal corticoids, the most powerful conservator of sodium being aldosterone. When the adrenal glands have been destroyed by disease or extirpated, there is an unbridled loss of sodium in the urine.

The sodium excretion shut down of trauma

Following trauma/surgery there is a variable period of reduced excretion of sodium. For this reason it may be inadvisable to administer large quantities of isotonic (0.9 per cent) saline solution after an operation. The period of sodium excretion shut down can last for up to 48 hours and is due to increased adrenocortical activity.

Sodium depletion (syn. hyponatraemia)

The most frequent cause of sodium depletion seen in surgical practice is obstruction of the small intestine, with its rapid loss of gastric, biliary, pancreatic and intestinal secretions by antiperistalsis and ejection, whether by vomiting or aspiration. Duodenal, total biliary, pancreatic and high intestinal external fistulae also are all notorious for bringing about early and profound hyponatraemia. Severe diarrhoea due to dysentery, cholera, ulcerative colitis or pseudomembranous colitis will cause hyponatraemia with acidosis. The finding of hyponatraemia with elevated potassium would suggest adrenocortical insufficiency. Hyponatraemia is also seen in SIADH.

There is one other less obvious, and surreptitious, means whereby the patient is robbed of sodium and that is by gastric aspiration combined with allowing the patient to drink as he or she pleases and promptly aspirating the fluid swallowed. The act of drinking excites the flow of gastric juice, and this is also aspirated. During this form of therapy, should the patient be receiving intravenous dextrose solution to maintain fluid balance, he or she will soon become a victim of hyponatraemia.

Clinical features. Clinical features of hyponatraemia with salt and water depletion are due to extracellular dehydration. In established cases the eyes are sunken and the face is drawn. In infants the anterior fontanelle is depressed. The tongue is coated and dry; in advanced cases it is brown in colour. Unlike the dehydration produced by loss of water only, in water and salt depletion thirst is not particularly in evidence. The skin is dry and often wrinkled, making the patient look older than his or her years. The subcutaneous tissue feels lax. Peripheral veins are contracted and contain dark blood. The arterial blood pressure is likely to be below normal. The urine is scanty, dark in colour, of a high specific gravity and, except in cases of salt-losing nephritis, contains little or no chloride.

Presuming that the haemoglobin level before the dehydration commenced was normal, the haematocrit reading (PCV) provides an index of the degree of haemoconcentration. However, haemoconcentrations can be masked by pre-existing anaemia. Laboratory investigations would show normal or slightly reduced serum sodium with low urinary output and low urinary sodium.

Postoperative hyponatraemia

Hyponatraemia with a normal or increased extracellular fluid volume arises as a result of too prolonged administration of a sodium-free solution (cf. Water intoxication, above).

Sodium excess (syn. hypernatraemia)

This is likely to arise if a patient is given an excessive amount of 0.9 per cent saline solution intravenously during the early postoperative period when, as has been described, some degree of sodium retention is to be expected. The result is an overloading of the circulation with salt and its accompanying water.

Clinical features. Slight puffiness of the face is the only early sign. The patient makes no complaint. Pitting oedema should be sought, especially in the sacral region, but for pitting oedema to be present at least 4.5 litres of excess fluid must have accumulated in the tissue spaces. The patient's weight increases *pari passu* with the water-logging. Signs of overhydration in infancy (infants are very susceptible) are increased tension in the anterior fontanelle, increased weight, an increase in the number of urinations and oedema.

Potassium balance

Potassium is almost entirely intracellular. No less than 98 per cent is intracellular, and only 2 per cent is present in the extracellular fluid. Three-quarters of the total body potassium (approximately 3500 mmol) is found in skeletal muscles. When the body needs endogenous protein as a source of energy, potassium, as well as nitrogen, is mobilised. The mobilised potassium passes to the extracellular fluid, but the surplus over and above the normal content is so rapidly excreted by healthy kidneys that the concentration of potassium in the serum remains unaltered. Each day a normal adult ingests approximately 1.0 mmol/kg of potassium in food; fruit, milk and honey are rich in this cation. Except for a very small quantity in formed faeces, and a still smaller quantity in sweat, an amount corresponding to the intake is excreted in the urine.

Potassium depletion

The augmented potassium excretion of trauma. Following trauma, including operation trauma, there is a spell, varying directly with the degree of tissue damage, of increased excretion of potassium by the kidneys. This loss is greatest during the first 24 hours and lasts, for example in the case of partial gastrectomy, for about 3 or 4 days. So great are the body's reserves of potassium that, unless the patient was severely depleted at the time of the operation, hypokalaemia may not reveal itself for 48 hours. However, potassium is such a key intracellular cation that carefully monitored replacement should start early in the postoperative period in all patients, with the exception of those that have evidence of renal dysfunction.

Hypokalaemia. Hypokalaemia can occur suddenly or gradually.

Sudden hypokalaemia is unlikely to be encountered in surgical practice. It occurs most frequently in diabetic coma treated by insulin and prolonged infusion of saline solution.

Gradual hypokalaemia is the type encountered in surgical practice. It is most commonly seen in patients who present for surgery with chronic hypokalaemia as a result of potassium-losing medications such as diuretics. The diarrhoea from ulcerative colitis, villous tumours of the rectum (see Chapter 59 of this book on 'The vermiform appendix') and the loss from external fistulae of the alimentary tract are also common causes (e.g. duodenal fistula, ileostomy); the potassium content of the discharge from some of these fistulae is twice that of the plasma potassium concentration. Another frequent cause of hypokalaemia is prolonged gastroduodenal aspiration with fluid replacement by intravenous isotonic saline solution. It is also prone to occur in the postoperative period following extensive resections for carcinoma of the alimentary tract, because often the operation has to be undertaken after months of weight loss and potassium depletion.

Clinical features

Most patients are asymptomatic, but at risk of the sequelae of hypokalaemia such as cardiac arrythmias. Such consequences are more likely during surgery and anaesthesia, especially in the presence of pre-existing myocardial disease. Symptoms of severe hypokalaemia include listlessness and slurred speach, muscular hypotonia, depressed reflexes and abdominal distension as a result of a paralytic ileus. Weakness of the respiratory muscles may result in rapid, shallow, gasping respirations; these are conducive to postoperative pulmonary complications. The diagnosis is supported by electrocardiography (ECG), which may show a prolonged QT interval, depression of the ST segment and flattening or inversion of the T-wave.

Treatment

Oral potassium. Potassium can be given in the form of milk, meat extracts, fruit juices and honey. However, in hospital practice, effervescent tablets of potassium chloride 2 g can be given by mouth 6-hourly.

Intravenous potassium. Rapid intravenous supplementation (especially when renal function is impaired) carries the risk of dysrhythmias and cardiac arrest if the serum concentration rises to a dangerous level. Administration should be properly controlled; the level of potassium should be checked daily; the urine output must be adequate. *When there is no associated alkalosis*, the potassium deficit can be restored by adding 40 mmol potassium chloride to each litre of 5 per cent glucose, glucose–saline or 0.9 per cent saline solution, which is given 6–8-hourly. Severe hypokalaemia should be treated in a high dependency or intensive care environment.

For *hypokalaemic alkalosis* see later.

Estimation of electrolyte balance

Sodium

Sodium, with its equivalent anions, accounts for about 90 per cent of the osmotic pressure of the plasma. Changes in the sodium content coincide with changes in the osmolality of all the body fluids. The serum sodium value is normally between 137 and 147 mmol/litre. Whenever possible, the *serum chloride* and *bicarbonate* should be estimated simultaneously because variations in the one may be accompanied by opposite changes in the other. The normal level of chloride is 95–105 mmol/litre, and of bicarbonate 25–30 mmol/litre; the sum of the two remains roughly constant at 120–135 mmol/litre.

Potassium

Potassium deficiency is present if the serum potassium value is less than 3.5 mmol/litre. The normal range is 3.5–5.0 mmol/litre. It must be remembered that intracellular potassium deficiency may be present although the plasma concentration is normal, and that deficiency is to be expected if oral feeding has been withheld for more than 4 days. Estimation of potassium in the urine or aspirated gastrointestinal contents serves as a guide to the rate of depletion and the replacement necessary.

Calcium

Calcium is an extracellular cation with a plasma concentration of 2.2–2.5 mmol/litre. It exists in three forms: bound to protein, free nonionised and free ionised – the last form being the component necessary for blood coagulation and affecting neuromuscular excitability. The ionised proportion falls with increasing pH; thus in respiratory alkalosis due to hyperventilation there may be tetany – with an apparently normal total serum calcium level. In the urine, the ionisation and the solubility of calcium are similarly depressed if the pH is elevated, thus promoting stone formation. The serum level of calcium is likely to be modified by any factor promoting or inhibiting its absorption from the bowel, its storage in bone or its elimination by the kidneys: such factors include vitamin D and phytic acid, parathormone and calcitonin (see Chapter 44), and the state of renal and small-bowel function.

The management of abnormal calcium blood levels depends, where possible, on removal of the cause, for example removal of a parathyroid tumour (see Chapter 44), or in the coagulation disorder due to massive transfusion of blood containing acid citrate dextrose (ACD, see below), 10 ml of 10 per cent calcium gluconate may be injected slowly intravenously. If oral administration is possible, calcium aspirin is useful (see Chapter 44). On a long-term basis, the diet should be adjusted to provide a high calcium and a low phosphate intake.

Magnesium

Magnesium is an intracellular cation which shares some of the properties of potassium and some of calcium. The normal magnesium concentration is 0.7–0.9 mmol/litre. The average daily intake is approximately 10 mmol. Magnesium deficiency may occur when there is prolonged loss of gastrointestinal secretions due to fistulae or ulcerative colitis, very prolonged administration of intravenous fluids without magnesium supplements, following massive small bowel resections, and in some cases of cirrhosis of the liver or disease of the parathyroids. The clinical picture of magnesium deficiency is marked by central nervous system irritability, ECG changes, lowered blood pressure and lowered protein synthesis. Postoperative cardiac arrythmias (e.g. *de novo* atrial fibrillation) are commonly associated with both hypokalaemia and hypomagnesaemia.

Treatment. For the treatment of mild hypomagnesaemia 20 mmol as magnesium sulphate can be added to 5 per cent-dextrose or normal saline over a 24-hour period. Magnesium supplements are essential in hyperalimentation.

Acid–base balance

In health, blood hydrogen ion concentration lies within the range pH 7.36–7.44. The terms acidosis and alkalosis in clinical practice indicate a change or a tendency to a change in the pH of the blood in a particular direction. In acidosis, there is an accumulation of acid or a loss of a base causing a fall or a tendency to a fall in the pH. The converse occurs in alkalosis. The pH of the blood is regulated and controlled by various buffering systems essentially consisting of weak acids and bases, of which the most important is the bicarbonate:carbonic acid ratio HCO_3:H_2CO_3. It is also regulated by the removal of carbon dioxide by the lungs and by the excretion of both acids and bases by the kidneys.

The ratio of bicarbonate to carbonic acid is normally 20:1. Alteration in this ratio alters the pH regardless of the absolute values of the bicarbonate and carbonic acid. A decrease in the ratio leads to increased acidity and vice versa.

The bicarbonate level can be altered by metabolic factors, while the carbonic acid level is subject to alteration by respiratory factors. Alteration of one is followed automatically by a compensatory alteration in the other, so that the ratio (HCO_3:H_2CO_3) and therefore the pH of the blood remains constant.

Measurement of acid–base disturbances

These measurements are normally made on arterial or arterialised capillary blood. PCO_2 is a measurement of the tension or partial pressure of carbon dioxide in the blood. The normal arterial PCO_2 is 4.1–5.6 kPa (31–42 mmHg). PO_2 is a measurement of the tension or partial pressure of oxygen in the blood. The normal arterial PO_2 is 10.5–14.5 kPa (80–110 mmHg).

Standard bicarbonate is the concentration of the serum bicarbonate after *fully oxygenated* blood has been equilibrated with carbon dioxide at 40 mmHg (5.3 kPa) at 38°C. This eliminates respiratory causes and respiratory compensation for altered bicarbonate levels. Normal levels are 22–25 mmol/litre.

Base excess or deficit expresses, in mmol, the total buffer anions present in the blood in excess of deficit of normal. (Normal base excess or deficit + 2.5.) Base excess or deficit multiplied by 0.3 times the body weight in kg gives the total extracellular excess or deficit of base in mmol. Metabolic causes of acid–base disturbances are indicated by changes in the standard bicarbonate level and base excess or deficit. Respiratory causes of acid–base disturbances are indicated by changes in the PCO_2 and PO_2.

Alkalosis

Metabolic alkalosis

Metabolic alkalosis, a condition of base excess or a deficit of any acid other than H_2CO_3, can be caused by:

- excessive ingestion of absorbable alkali. This is not uncommon in patients who take proprietary indigestion remedies without medical supervision;
- loss of acid from the stomach by repeated vomiting or aspiration;
- cortisone excess, usually the result of over-administration of adrenal corticoids, but occasionally due to Cushing's syndrome (see Chapter 44).

Compensation is effected by: (a) retention of carbon dioxide by the lungs; and (b) excretion of bicarbonate base by the kidneys (alkaline urine).

Clinical features. Alkalosis due to loss of acid from the stomach is the most common and most important. In its most typical form, it is seen in patients with pyloric stenosis in whom the loss of acid by repeated vomiting is often accentuated by the taking of medicines containing sodium bicarbonate. The most striking feature of severe alkalosis is Cheyne–Stokes respiration with periods of apnoea lasting from 5 to 30 seconds. Tetany sometimes occurs. Latent tetany is more common, and can be unveiled by Trousseau's sign (see Chapter 44). Regarding other signs, the dual phenomenon of severe alkalosis and hypokalaemia is so interwoven that their clinical separation is well-nigh impossible. Subclinical degrees of alkalosis are recognisable only by a raised standard bicarbonate concentration and a positive base excess. Severe alkalosis may result in renal epithelial damage and consequent renal insufficiency.

Treatment. Metabolic alkalosis without hypokalaemia seldom requires direct treatment. The cause of the alkalosis should be removed where possible and a high urinary output encouraged.

Hypokalaemic alkalosis

Hypokalaemic alkalosis is seen in patients who have lost potassium and acid owing to repeated vomiting from pyloric stenosis. The low serum potassium causes potassium to leave the cell and be replaced by Na^+ and H^+ ions. The shift of H^+ ion into the cell causes intracellular acidosis and increases the cellular acidosis of the kidney cells.

Treatment. When hypokalaemia is sufficient to cause a metabolic alkalosis, the losses can be massive (> 1000 mmol). Replacement is a serious undertaking (see above). It can be

Harvey Cushing, 1869–1939. Professor of Surgery, Harvard University, Boston, Massachusetts. Described his syndrome in 1932.
John Cheyne, 1777–1836. Physician, Meath Hospital, Dublin, Ireland. First Professor of Medicine, Royal College of Surgeons in Ireland.
William Stokes, 1804–67. Physician, Meath Hospital, Dublin, Ireland.
Armand Trousseau, 1801–67. Physician, Hôtel Dieu, Paris, France.

achieved gradually and relatively safely by supplementing intravenous fluids with 40 mmol/litre of KCl if the urine output is adequate. More rapid replacement (up to 60 mmol/hour) will require intensive monitoring and supervision with continuous ECG monitoring in a high dependency or intensive care environment.

Respiratory alkalosis

Respiratory alkalosis, a condition where the arterial PCO_2 is below the normal range of 31–42 mmHg (4.1–5.6 kPa), is caused most commonly in surgical practice by excessive pulmonary ventilation carried out upon an anaesthetised patient. Other causes are hyperventilation occasioned by high altitudes, hyperpyrexia, a lesion of the hypothalamus and hysteria. Compensation, which depends on increased renal excretion of bicarbonate, usually is inadequate. During anaesthesia alkalosis is accompanied by pallor and a fall in blood pressure. In severe cases respiratory arrest follows.

Treatment. Respiratory suppression due to alkalosis is rectified by insufflation of carbon dioxide.

Acidosis

Metabolic acidosis

Metabolic acidosis, a condition where there is a deficit of base or an excess of any acid other than H_2CO_3, occurs as a result of:

- *increase in fixed acids* due to the formation of ketone bodies as in diabetes or starvation, the retention of metabolites in renal insufficiency, and the rapid increase of lactic and pyruvic acids by anaerobic tissue metabolism, following cardiac arrest, or the release of the clamped aorta in the surgery of abdominal aneurysm. Acute acidosis with pH levels of 7.1 is frequently encountered in such cases;
- *loss of bases* such as occurs in sustained diarrhoea, ulcerative colitis, gastrocolic fistula, a high intestinal fistula or prolonged *intestinal* aspiration.

Clinical features. In severe acidosis, the leading sign is rapid, deep, noisy breathing. The hyperpnoea is due to overstimulation of the respiratory centre by the reduction in pH of the blood, and the physiological purpose of overbreathing is to eliminate as much as possible of the acid substance H_2CO_3. Except in renal acidosis, the urine is strongly acidic. The standard bicarbonate level is lowered and there is a base deficit.

Treatment. The commonest cause of an acute peroperative metabolic acidosis is tissue hypoxia and the correct treatment is restoration of adequate tissue perfusion. Treament with bicarbonate solutions will correct the measured metabolic acidosis but not treat the problem. Indeed, as bicarbonate is rapidly converted into carbon dioxide intracellular acidosis may, in fact, get worse. The administration of bicarbonate solutions should be reserved solely for situations where bases have been lost or where the degree of acidosis is so severe that myocardial function is compromised (this is rare).

The acute acidosis seen in prolonged cardiac arrest may require the infusion of 50 mmol of 8.4 per cent sodium bicarbonate solution.

Acidosis due to transplantation of the ureters into the colon

Acidosis due to transplantation of the ureters into the colon is discussed in Chapter 63 of this book.

Respiratory acidosis

Respiratory acidosis, a condition where the PCO_2 is above the normal range, is caused by impaired alveolar ventilation.

In practice this problem most commonly occurs when there is inadequate ventilation of the anaesthetised patient, or when the effects of muscle relaxants have not worn off or been fully reversed at the end of the anaesthetic. There is also a risk of respiratory acidosis when the patient undergoing surgery already has pre-existing pulmonary disease (e.g. chronic bronchitis or emphysema), and this is accentuated by thoracic and upper abdominal incisions.

The anion gap

This is a calculated estimation of the undetermined or unmeasured anions in the blood. It is sometimes used to establish the cause of a metabolic acidosis. Anion gap = (Na + K) – (HCO_3 + Cl). The normal anion gap is 10–16 mmol/litre. An increased anion gap is seen in metabolic acidosis due to ketoacidosis, lactic acidosis, poisoning (salicylates) and renal failure. A normal anion gap is seen in metabolic acidosis due to renal tubular acidosis and loss of alkali due to diarrhoea, intestinal obstruction or intestinal fistula, and in the hyperchloraemia of ureterocolic anastomosis.

Haemorrhage

Recognition of types of haemorrhage

Arterial haemorrhage

Arterial haemorrhage is recognised as bright red blood, spurting as a jet which rises and falls in time with the pulse. In protracted bleeding, and when quantities of intravenous fluids other than blood are given, it can become watery in appearance.

Venous haemorrhage

Venous haemorrhage is a darker red, a steady and copious flow. The colour darkens still further from excessive oxygen desaturation when blood loss is severe, or in respiratory depression or obstruction. Blood loss is particularly rapid when large veins are opened, e.g. common femoral or jugular.

Venous bleeding can be under increased pressure as in asphyxia, or from ruptured varicose veins. Portal vein pressures (see Chapter 47) are high enough to cause rapid blood loss, especially in portal hypertension with oesophageal varices. Pulmonary artery haemorrhage is dark red (venous blood) at around 30 mmHg (4 kPa), whereas bleeding from the pulmonary veins is bright red (oxygenated).

Capillary haemorrhage

Capillary haemorrhage is a bright red, often rapid, ooze. If continuing for many hours, blood loss can become serious, as in haemophilia.

Primary haemorrhage

Primary haemorrhage occurs at the time of injury or operation.

Reactionary haemorrhage

Reactionary haemorrhage may follow primary haemorrhage within 24 hours (usually 4–6 hours) and is mainly due to rolling ('slipping') of a ligature, dislodgement of a clot or cessation of reflex vasospasm. The precipitating circumstances are: (1) the rise in blood pressure and the refilling of the venous system on recovery from shock; and (2) restlessness, coughing and vomiting which raise the venous pressure (e.g. reactionary venous haemorrhage within a few hours of thyroidectomy).

Venous haemorrhage, whether primary or reactionary, can tax the skill of even an experienced surgeon, for it may be exceedingly difficult to bring under control. Penetrating wounds involving main veins in the thigh or groin are potentially fatal, as exsanguination may follow the removal of a first-aid dressing which has apparently controlled the bleeding (butcher's thigh). Such a wound should never be treated in a perfunctory manner; it requires careful examination and closure in an operating theatre.

Secondary haemorrhage

Secondary haemorrhage occurs after 7–14 days, and is due to infection and sloughing of part of the wall of an artery. Predisposing factors are pressure of a drainage tube, a fragment of bone, a ligature in an infected area or cancer. It is also a complication of arterial surgery and amputations. It is heralded by 'warning' haemorrhages, which are bright red stains on the dressing, followed by a sudden severe haemorrhage which may be fatal. A warning haematemesis may occur in the case of a peptic ulcer, and is a danger signal which it is imprudent to ignore. In advanced cancer, the erosion of a main vessel (e.g. carotid or uterine) by a locally ulcerating growth becomes the way of a swift and merciful termination to the patient's suffering. Secondary haemorrhage is prone to occur with anorectal wounds, for example after haemorrhoidectomy.

External haemorrhage

External haemorrhage is visible, *revealed haemorrhage.*

Internal haemorrhage

Internal haemorrhage is invisible, *concealed haemorrhage.* Internal bleeding may be *concealed* as in ruptured spleen or liver, fractured femur, ruptured ectopic gestation or in cerebral haemorrhage. Concealed haemorrhage may become *revealed* as in haematemesis or melaena from a bleeding peptic ulcer, as in haematuria from a ruptured kidney, or via the vagina in accidental uterine haemorrhage of pregnancy.

Measurement of acute blood loss

Assessment and management of blood loss must be related to the pre-existing circulating blood volume, which can be derived from the patient's weight:

- infant = 80–85 ml/kg;
- adult = 65–75 ml/kg.

Measuring blood loss

- *Blood clot* the size of a clenched fist is roughly equal to 500 ml.
- *Swelling in closed fractures.* Moderate swelling in closed fracture of the tibia equals 500–1500 ml blood loss. Moderate swelling in a fractured shaft of femur equals 500–2000 ml blood loss.
- *Swab weighing.* In the operating theatre, blood loss can be measured by weighing the swabs after use and subtracting the dry weight. The resulting total obtained (1 g = 1 ml) is added to the volume of blood collected in the suction or drainage bottles. In extensive wounds and operations, the blood loss is grossly underestimated, due to evaporation of water from the swabs before weighing each batch. Prompt transfer of discarded swabs into polythene bags reduces this source of error. Blood, plasma and water are also lost from the vascular system because of evaporation from open wounds, into the tissues, sweating and expired water via the lungs. Indeed, for operations such as radical mastectomy or partial gastrectomy it may be necessary to multiply the swab weighing total by a factor of 1.5. For prolonged surgery via larger wounds, as in abdominothoracic or abdominoperineal operations, the total measured may need to be multiplied by 2.

Haemoglobin level

This is estimated in g/100 ml (g/dl), normal values being 12–16 g/100 ml (12–16 g/dl). There is no immediate change in haemorrhage, but after some hours the level falls by influx of interstitial fluid into the vascular compartment in order to restore the blood volume.

Measurement of central venous pressure

For measurement of central venous pressure (CVP) see later.

The treatment of haemorrhage

Minimise further blood loss by pressure and packing, position and rest, operative procedures (ligation, repair and excision) and then fluid resuscitation as described below.

Restore blood volume by blood transfusion, albumin 4.6 per cent, SAG-mannitol (SAG-M) blood, saline, gelatin, dextran and plasma infusions.

Pressure and packing

The *first-aid* treatment of haemorrhage from a wound is a pressure dressing made from anything handy which is soft and clean. The dressing or pack should be bound on tightly.

Other examples of *pressure* used to control haemorrhage include digital pressure, for example the use of forefinger and thumb or a clothes-peg for epistaxis. The use of a double balloon in the oesophagus and the stomach to control the bleeding from oesophageal varices is another example of pressure being applied.

Packing by means of rolls of wide gauze is an important standby in operative surgery. If several rolls are used, the ends must be tied together to ensure complete removal later.

N.B. If on removal of pressure or packing, bleeding appears to have ceased completely, one should not assume that all is well, especially when dealing with deep wounds involving large veins. Continued close observation is required and rapid operative action may be called for.

Position and rest

Elevation of limbs (e.g. in ruptured varicose veins) employs gravity to reduce bleeding. Elevation also causes helpful vasoconstriction (Lister). *A bed elevator* is often used to raise the foot of the bed, and thus increasing venous return to the heart also augmenting cardiac output. Gravity is also used in certain operations, as in thyroidectomy when the patient is tilted feet downwards (reverse-Trendelenburg position) or as in stripping of varicose veins when a head-down tilt is used (Trendelenburg).

Examples of operative techniques in haemorrhage

Artery forceps (haemostats) and clips are mechanical means of controlling bleeding by pressure. The clamped vessel can be ligated or it can be coagulated with diathermy. When an incision is made through the scalp for craniotomy, the profuse bleeding is not easily arrested by direct pressure, so the cranial aponeurosis is picked up by a series of forceps which are everted together, thus exerting pressure. Silver clips (Cushing) may be applied to cerebral vessels.

Suturing may be employed. The vessel can be underrun or transfixed by needle and suture, and then ligated, while if the continuity of a main vessel is to be restored 4/0 silk or polypropylene is used on a 20-mm atraumatic needle.

Pressure by packing, using rolls of wide gauze, has been previously mentioned, but temporary light pressure with a 'peanut' of gauze held by forceps aids the sealing of an arterial suture line after reconstruction following trauma, embolectomy or in artery grafting. About 5 minutes is required for the platelets to seal the join.

Patches of vein or Dacron mesh may be used to repair a vascular defect. A patch of muscle, lightly hammered, provides thrombokinase to stop a troublesome ooze.

Other topical applications for oozing include gauze or sponge, which is absorbed by the body. 'Oxycel' or gelatin sponge provides a network upon which fibrin and platelets can be deposited. This is the modern counterpart of the use of cobwebs by our forefathers, or sphagnum moss by our neolithic ancestors. Gauze soaked in adrenalin (1:1000) can be applied. Bone wax (Horsley) is used for oozing bone.

The whole or part of a bleeding viscus may have to be excised (e.g. splenectomy or partial hepatectomy). A ruptured kidney is treated conservatively if possible (see Chapter 63).

Natural blood volume and red cell recovery

The recovery of blood volume begins immediately by the withdrawal of fluid from the tissues into the circulation. There is haemodilution. Plasma proteins are replaced by the liver. Red cell recovery takes some 5–6 weeks. The iron content will be less than normal if stores are depleted or absorption is impaired, for example after gastrectomy.

Transfusion of blood and blood products

The indications for transfusion in surgical practice are as follows.

- Following traumatic incidents where there has been severe blood loss, or haemorrhage from pathological lesions, for example from the gastrointestinal tract.
- During major operative procedures where a certain amount of blood loss is inevitable, for example abdominoperineal or cardiovascular surgery.
- Following severe burns where, despite initial fluid and protein replacement, there may be associated haemolysis.
- Postoperatively in a patient who has become severely anaemic.
- Preoperatively, usually in the form of packed cells given slowly (see Blood fractions and Complications, later) in cases of chronic anaemia where surgery is indicated urgently, i.e. where there is inadequate time for effective iron or other replacement therapy, or where the anaemia is unresponsive to therapy, for example aplastic anaemia.
- To arrest haemorrhage or as a prophylactic measure prior to surgery, in a patient with a haemorrhagic state such as thrombocytopenia, haemophilia or liver disease (see Blood fractions, later).

Lord Joseph Lister, 1827–1912. Professor of Surgery, Glasgow, Edinburgh and King's College Hospital, London, England.

Friedrich Trendelenburg, 1844–1924. Professor of Surgery, Rostock (1875–82), Bonn (1882–95) and Leipzig (1895–1911).

Sir Victor Horsley, 1857–1916. Neurosurgeon, National Hospital, London, England. Performed the first operation for surgical management of epilepsy, aged 29, in 1886.

Preparation of blood products for transfusion

It is important that blood donors should be fit and with no evidence of infection, in particular hepatitis and human immunodeficiency virus (HIV) infection acquired immunodeficiency syndrome (AIDS), which are transmitted in donor blood.

Blood is collected into a sterile commercially prepared plastic bag with needle and plastic tube attached in a complete, closed sterile unit.

With the donor lying on a couch, a sphygmomanometer cuff is applied to the upper arm and inflated to a pressure of 70 mmHg (9.3 kPa) or 80 mmHg (10.6 kPa). After introducing 0.5 ml of local anaesthetic, a 15G needle is introduced into the median cubital vein and 410 ml of blood allowed to run into the bag containing 75 ml of anticoagulant solution (CPD – citrate potassium dextrose).

During collection, the blood is constantly mixed with the anticoagulant to prevent clotting, and at the end of the procedure the tube is clamped and the needle removed. Specimens for use in blood grouping and cross-matching procedures may be obtained by clamping off small sections of the plastic tubing containing the donor blood.

Blood storage

All blood for transfusion must be stored in special blood bank refrigerators controlled at 4°C ± 2°C. Blood allowed to stand at higher temperatures for more than 2 hours is in danger of transmitting infection.

CPD blood has a shelf-life of 3 weeks (CPDA 1–5 weeks). The red blood cells, or erythrocytes, suffer a temporary reduction (24–72 hours) in their ability to release oxygen to the tissues of the recipient, so if a patient requires an urgent and massive transfusion it is wise to give 1 or 2 units of blood which are less than 7 days old.

White blood cells

White blood cells are rapidly destroyed in stored blood.

Platelets

At 4°C the survival of platelets is considerably reduced, and few are functionally useful after 24 hours. Platelets which are separated (see Blood fractions below) show good survival even after 72 hours.

Clotting factors

Like platelets, clotting factors VIII and V are labile and their levels fall quickly.

Blood fractions

Whole blood may be divided into various fractions. This is not only more economical of blood donors, but certain fractions are more appropriate than whole blood transfusion for certain clinical conditions. Fractionation procedures are relatively safe and simple, using sealed sterile plastic bag units.

Packed red cells

Packed red cells are especially advisable in patients with chronic anaemia, in the elderly, in small children and in patients in whom introduction of large volumes of fluid may cause cardiac failure. Packed red cells are suitable for most forms of transfusion therapy, including major surgery, especially in association with clear fluids. Good packing can be obtained by letting the blood sediment and removing the plasma, or by centrifugation of whole blood at 2000–2300*g* for 15–20 minutes.

Platelet-rich plasma

Platelet-rich plasma is suitable for transfusions to patients with thrombocytopenia who are either bleeding or require surgery. It is prepared by centrifugation of freshly donated blood at 150–200 *g* for 15–20 minutes.

Platelet concentrate

Platelet concentrate for transfusion to patients with thrombocytopenia is prepared by centrifugation of platelet-rich plasma at 1200–1500 *g* for 15–20 minutes.

Plasma

This is removed after centrifugation of whole blood at 2000–2300 *g* for 15–20 minutes and it may be further processed or fractionated in various ways.

Human albumin 4.5 per cent. Repeated fractionation of plasma by organic liquids followed by heat treatment results in this plasma fraction, which is rich in protein but free from the danger of transmission of serum hepatitis. This may be stored for several months in liquid form at 4°C and is suitable for replacement of protein, for example following severe burns.

Fresh frozen plasma. Plasma removed from fresh blood obtained within 4 hours is rapidly frozen by immersing in a solid carbon dioxide and ethyl alcohol mixture. This is stored at –40°C and is a good source of all the coagulation factors. It is the treatment of choice when considering surgery in patients with abnormal coagulation due to severe liver failure. It may also be given in any of the congenital clotting factor deficiency diseases in their milder forms, especially *Christmas disease* (Factor IX deficiency) or haemophilia (Factor VIII deficiency).

Cryoprecipitate. When fresh frozen plasma is allowed to thaw at 4°C a white glutinous precipitate remains and, if the supernatant plasma is removed, this cryoprecipitate is a very rich source of Factor VIII. It is stored at –40°C and is immediately available for treatment of patients with haemophilia (Factor VIII deficiency). The advantage of cryoprecipitate treatment in haemophilia is the simplicity of administering large quantities of Factor VIII in relatively small volumes by intravenous injection. It is also a rich source of fibrinogen, of value in hypofibrinogenaemic states.

Factor VIII concentrate and Factor IX concentrate. Factor VIII concentrate and Factor IX concentrate are stored in freeze-dried form.

Fibrinogen. Fibrinogen is prepared by organic liquid fractionation of plasma and stored in the dried form. When reconstituted with distilled water, it is used in patients with severe depletion of fibrinogen (e.g. disseminated intravascular coagulation or congenital afibrinogenaemia). It does, however, carry a high risk of hepatitis.

SAG-mannitol blood. Because of the need for blood products, there will be an increasing use of SAG-M blood. A proportion of blood donations will have all the plasma removed, which will be replaced with 100 ml of a crystalloid solution containing: sodium chloride (877 mg), adenine (16.9 mg), glucose anhydrous (181 mg) and mannitol (525 mg).

This allows good viability of the cells, but there is practically no protein (albumin) present. For top-up transfusions for anaemia, this will not constitute a problem.

For healthy adults, the plasma albumin level will not be compromised by a replacement transfusion of up to 4 units of SAG-M blood, after which whole blood should be used. If this is not available, more SAG-M blood may be given, supplemented by 1 unit (400 ml) of 4.5 per cent human albumin solution BP for every 2 units of SAG-M blood. After 8 units of SAG-M red cells have been transfused, the need for fresh frozen plasma and platelets should be considered, after first checking the coagulation status and platelet count.

Blood grouping and cross-matching

Human red cells have on the cell surface many different antigens. For practical purposes, there are two groups of antigens which are of major importance in surgical practice: antigens of the ABO blood groups and antigens of the rhesus (Rh) blood groups.

Antigens of the ABO blood groups

These are strongly antigenic and are associated with naturally occurring antibodies in the serum. Individuals show four different ABO cell groups, as shown in Table 4.2.

Antigens of the rhesus blood groups

The antigen of major importance in this group is Rh(D), which is strongly antigenic and is present in approximately 85 per cent of the population in the UK. Antibodies to the D antigen are not naturally present in the serum of the remaining 15 per cent of individuals, but their formation may be stimulated by the transfusion of Rh-positive red cells. Such acquired antibodies are capable, during pregnancy, of crossing the placenta and, if present in a Rh-negative mother, may cause severe haemolytic anaemia and even death (hydrops fetalis) in a Rh-positive fetus *in utero*. The other minor blood group antigens may be associated with naturally occurring antibodies, or may stimulate the formation of antibodies on relatively rare occasions.

Table 4.2 The four different ABO red cell groups

Red cell group	*Serum contains*
A	Anti-B antibody
B	Anti-A antibody
AB	No ABO antibody
O	Anti-A and anti-B antibody

Incompatibility

If antibodies present in the recipient's serum are incompatible with the donor's cells, a transfusion reaction will result. This is the result of agglutination and haemolysis of the donated cells leading in severe cases to acute renal tubular necrosis and renal failure. For this reason, therefore, it is essential that all transfusion should be preceded by:

- *ABO and rhesus grouping* of the recipient's and donor's cells so that only ABO and Rh(D) compatible blood is given;
- direct matching of the recipient's serum with the donor's cells to confirm ABO compatibility and to test for rhesus and any other blood group antibody present in the serum of the recipient.

Blood grouping and cross-matching require full laboratory procedures and take 1 hour. In emergencies it may be necessary to reduce this time, but the risk of doing this must be weighed against the danger to the patient by the delay in transfusion entailed by the full procedures. In such emergencies, it may be advisable to restore the patient's blood volume by saline, gelatin (e.g. Haemaccel), dextran or human albumin 4.5 per cent until blood has been made available. Alternatively, donor blood, group O-negative, which is compatible with the majority of individuals, should be given and this should always be available in acute emergency situations.

Giving blood

Blood transfusion is commenced by:

- selection and preparation of the site;
- careful checking of the donor blood: this should bear a compatibility label stating the patient's name, hospital reference number, ward and blood group;
- insertion of the needle or cannula – the latter may be valuable if intravenous therapy is required for any length of time;
- giving detailed written instructions as to the rate of flow, for example 40 drops/min allows one 540 ml unit of blood to be transfused in 4 hours.

In acute emergencies, it may be necessary to increase the rate of flow and it is possible to give 1–2 units in 30 minutes using a pressure cuff around a plastic bag of blood.

Warming blood. During cardiopulmonary operations, the blood must be warmed before reaching the patient by passing it through a carefully temperature-regulated blood warming unit, thus reducing the risk of cardiac arrest from large volumes of cold blood direct from the refrigerator.

Filtering blood. A filter (Pall) with an absolute filtration rating of 40 μm will filter off platelet aggregates and leucocyte membranes in stored blood.

Autotransfusion

This is an old, well-tried method of immediately restoring a patient's blood volume, by transfusion with his or her own blood. In an emergency, for example, in a case of ruptured ectopic gestation, the blood is collected from the peritoneal cavity and put into a sterile container suitable for connecting to transfusion tubing. The classical method of filtration of this blood to prevent the transfusion of any small clots is to place a piece of sterile gauze within the container. Nowadays, special autotransfusion apparatus is being marketed. For major elective procedures, the patient may 'donate' his or her own blood, withdrawal and storage taking place up to 3 weeks before it is required. Natural blood volume and most of the red cell recovery will have taken place in that time.

Complications of blood transfusion

Congestive cardiac failure

This is especially liable to occur in the elderly or where there is cardiovascular insufficiency, and may result from too rapid infusion of large volumes of blood. It is advisable in the individual with chronic anaemia to give packed red cells and, at the same time, give diuretic drugs. The transfusion should be given slowly, i.e. 1 unit over 4–6 hours and, if necessary, on two separate occasions.

'Transfusion reactions'

These may be the result of the following problems:

- *Incompatibility.* This should be avoided if the correct procedures of grouping and cross-matching have been adopted but, in fact, it is nearly always due to human error in the collection, labelling or checking of the specimens and donor bags. The patient develops a rigor, temperature and pain in the loins, and may become extremely alarmed. The transfusion should be stopped immediately, and a fresh specimen of venous blood and urine from the patient sent together with the residue of *all* the used units of donor blood to the laboratory for checking.

  A close watch should be kept on the patient's pulse, blood pressure and urinary output. Frusemide 80–120 mg i.v. should be given to provoke a diuresis, and repeated if the urine output falls below 30 ml/hour. Dialysis may be necessary.
- *Simple pyrexial reactions* in which the patient develops pyrexia, rigor and some increase in pulse rate. These are the result of 'pyrogens' in the donor apparatus and are largely avoided by the use of plastic disposable giving sets.
- *Allergic reactions* in which the patient develops mild tachycardia and an urticarial rash; rarely an acute anaphylactic reaction may occur. This is the result of allergic reaction to plasma products in the donor blood. The reaction is treated by stopping the transfusion and giving an antihistamine drug (chlorpheniramine 10 mg or diphenhydrazine 25 mg).
- *Sensitisation to leucocytes and platelets.* This is not uncommon in those patients who have received many transfusions in the past, for example for thalassaemia, refractory anaemia or aplastic anaemia. The individual develops antibodies to donated white cells or platelets, which cause reactions with each transfusion. They may be minimised by giving packed red cells from which plasma and 'buffy coat layers' have been removed or by 'washing' of donor cells. Aspirin, antihistamines or steroids may also be given to the recipient if necessary.
- *Immunological sensitisation.* Only the ABO, Kell and Rh(D) groups are considered for blood transfusion. Immune antibodies may be stimulated by transfusion, and may give rise to difficulties with compatibility tests or to haemolytic transfusion reactions.

Infections

There are four main reasons for blood transfusion causing infection in the recipient.

- *Serum hepatitis virus* may be transmitted from the donor and is usually a severe hepatitis arising approximately 3 months after the transfusion. It should be avoided by adequate verbal screening of the blood donor and by testing for the presence of the hepatitis-associated antigen in the blood prior to transfusion.
- *HIV infection* can be transmitted by blood and blood products. All donors must be screened (see AIDS in Chapter 7). Haemophiliacs are at special risk because of their more frequent requirements for blood products.
- *Bacterial infection* may result faulty storage. This arises most commonly from the donor blood being left in a warm room for some hours before the transfusion is commenced. This allows proliferation of any bacteria, and transfusion of such infected blood may result in severe septicaemia in the recipient and rapid death.
- *Malaria* can be transmitted by blood transfusion in areas where the disease is endemic. Whenever possible, donors should be screened and the disease eradicated (by treatment of the donors who are positive) before blood is obtained or given. If the need for transfused blood is so urgent that precautions are impossible before transfusion, then the patient should be given prophylactic antimalarial drugs.

Thrombophlebitis

For more on thrombophlebitis see Chapter 16 of this book.

Air embolism

For more on air embolism see Chapter 15 of this book.

Coagulation failure

Coagulation failure is due to:

- *dilution of clotting factors/platelets* due to large volumes of stored blood being used to replace losses as stored blood is low in platelets, Factor VIII and Factor V;
- *disseminated intravascular coagulation* (DIC) following an incompatible blood transfusion, particularly ABO incompatibility. The further haemorrhage may be treated by replacement of the deficient factors (usually fibrinogen, Factors VIII, V and II, and platelets), with fresh frozen plasma, cryoprecipitate and platelet concentrates. Paradoxically, heparin may be used sometimes for the treatment of DIC.

Haemophilia and the congenital haemorrhagic diseases

Haemophilia

Haemophilia (haemophilia A) is a haemorrhagic diathesis caused by the congenital deficiency in the blood of Factor VIII [antihaemophilic globulin (AHG)]. It is a sex-linked characteristic, transmitted by the asymptomatic female carriers, and manifest only in males.

The levels of Factor VIII in the blood of severe haemophiliacs may be less than 1 per cent of the average normal level. In the case of spontaneous haemorrhage (e.g. into joints) treatment should aim at raising the level to at least 20 per cent. Should surgery be anticipated in the haemophiliac, the level should be raised to 50–100 per cent.

Factor VIII concentrates are superseding cryoprecipitates. The amount of either preparation depends on the problem and the level required for haemostasis, i.e. more for surgery than for a haemarthrosis. Frequent monitoring of the Factor VIII level will be necessary in cases involving surgery.

Additional forms of therapy may include fresh blood, if necessary for blood loss, fresh frozen plasma or, more rarely, dried concentrates of animal AHG (see also AIDS).

Christmas disease

Christmas disease (haemophilia B) is a congenital disease resulting from the deficiency of Factor IX (Christmas factor). Clinically, the manifestations of the disease are similar to haemophilia. Factor IX is replaced by the transfusion of fresh frozen plasma, or by reconstituted dried concentrates of human Factor IX.

Haemophilic joints

In both haemophilia and Christmas disease, haemorrhage into joints is very common, and persistent and recurrent haemarthrosis may result in permanent damage to the articular surfaces and disorganisation of the joint. The most important feature of treatment is that it should be prompt. Replacement of the clotting factor should be instituted immediately and before severe tension is allowed to build up in the joint.

Von Willebrand's disease

Von Willebrand's disease, with episodic bleeding manifestations, is a type of haemorrhagic disease, with low plasma levels of both Factor VIII complement and Factor VIII related antigen, and platelet abnormalities.

Sickle-cell disorders

Sickle-cell disorders can be a serious problem in surgery, especially with children. All patients of the negroid ethnic type should be screened for the presence of sickle haemoglobin. In *sickle-cell trait* (HbA + S) care to avoid hypoxia during anaesthesia is important. In *sickle-cell anaemia*, a preoperative partial exchange transfusion of packed cells to reduce the haemoglobin S level to less than 30 per cent may be required, depending on the procedure and the length of the operation. Oxygen is given for the prevention of hypoxia; hypothermia and dehydration must be strenuously avoided. Spinal anaesthesia and tourniquets are contraindicated. Pigments gallstone formation is common.

Blood substitutes – albumin, dextran, gelatin

One of the most urgent requirements in a patient suffering from acute blood loss is the re-establishment of a normal blood volume. This may be achieved satisfactorily with a number of plasma substitutes.

Human albumin 4.5 per cent has superseded the use of dried plasma and can be used whilst cross-matching is being performed. Two to three units (1.2 litres) are given intravenously over 30 minutes. It is valuable in patients with burns where there has been severe loss of protein. There is no risk of transmitting hepatitis.

Dextrans are polysaccharide polymers of varying molecular weight producing an osmotic pressure similar to that of plasma. They have the disadvantage of inducing rouleaux of the red cells and this interferes with blood-grouping and cross-matching procedures, hence the need for a blood sample beforehand. Dextrans interfere with platelet function and may be associated with abnormal bleeding, and for this reason it is recommended that the total volume of dextran should not exceed 1000 ml.

Low-molecular-weight dextran (40 000) (dextran 40, Rheomacrodex) has an immediate effect in a restoring plasma volume, but it is transitory because the small molecules are readily excreted by the kidney. It may be useful in preventing sludging of red cells in small blood vessels, for example of the kidney, and thus preventing the renal shutdown associated with severe hypotension. It is less likely to induce rouleaux formation than the high-molecular-weight compounds.

The *high-molecular-weight dextrans* (110 000 and 70 000) (dextran 110 and dextran 70) are less effective in the early phase of hypovolaemia but are longer acting as they are retained for some time within the circulation.

Gelatin in a degraded form (molecular weight around 30 000) is used increasingly as a plasma expander. Up to 1000 ml of a 3.4–4 per cent solution (containing anions and cations) is given intravenously (e.g. Haemaccel, Gelafusine).

Blood transfusion

After initial use of plasma expanders, major acute blood loss requires rapid blood transfusion. While it is vital to restore blood volume and oxygen-carrying capacity, rapid transfusion may produce problems over and above those which can occur with any administration of blood products (such as group incompatability and risk of infection).

Urgent provision by the transfusion laboratory and quick checking of multiple units of blood in an emergency inevitably enhances the chances of omission or error. However urgent the situation, unless one has resorted to giving uncross-matched or universal donor blood, safety standards must be maintained, if necessary by one member of staff dedicated to the checking and recording of blood units.

Other unwanted side effects result from the differences between fresh and stored blood. Some occur as a result of changes with time, and some relate to additives or extraction of plasma components. Blood is stored at 4°C and rapid transfusion has caused arrhythmias and worsened intraoperative hypothermia. Newer warming devices are able to raise the temperature satisfactorily even at very fast transfusion rates, but may require considerable pressure to force the blood through tortuous or narrow tubes. Cellular metabolism, membrane ion pump failure and haemolysis during storage lead to hyperkalaemia and acidaemia with rapid transfusion, compounding the effects of reperfusing ischaemic areas and again may impair cardiac performance.

Anticoagulant (usually citrate to chelate calcium) and early loss of clotting factors and active platelets result in dilutional coagulopathy during massive transfusion. Ideally clotting should be monitored (such as by thromboelastography in theatre, or in the laboratory), and specific defects identified and treated. However, the situation is often too fraught and rapidly changing, and it may be necessary to administer fresh frozen plasma and/or platelets on an empirical basis (per 6–10 units of blood transfused). Calcium is usually maintained by mobilisation from bone, except in severe circulatory failure; however, it too should be measured or empirical administration considered if clotting appears clinically inadequate.

Parenteral fluid therapy

The solutions mainly in use are given below and summarised in Table 4.3.

- *Plasma, albumin 4.5 per cent*;
- *dextrose 5 per cent* is an isotonic solution that supplies calories without electrolytes. It is useful in the postoperative period when sodium excretion is reduced. It is also valuable when the salt requirements of a patient needing much fluid have been satisfied on a particular day. Prolonged administration of 5 per cent dextrose solution alone is liable to result in hyponatraemia, and may cause thrombosis of the vein used;
- *isotonic (0.9 per cent) saline solution* is required to replace the normal sodium requirement (500 ml isotonic saline/day) and additional volume is required when a large amount of sodium has been lost by vomiting, or by gastric, duodenal or intestinal aspiration, or through an alimentary fistula. Possibly, on occasions, excessive sweating may justify its use;
- *dextrose 4.3 per cent with saline 0.18 per cent* (one-fifth isotonic saline) – this solution is isotonic. Usually it is referred to as dextrose–saline. *It must not be confused with 5 per cent dextrose in saline, which is hypertonic*;
- *Ringer's lactate solution* contains sodium, potassium and chloride in almost the same concentrations as they are in the plasma. It also contains some calcium and some lactate. This solution can be used in hypovolaemic shock while awaiting blood. It is also suitable for replacing lost intestinal secretions.

Table 4.3 Composition of commonly used intravenous fluids (mmol/litre)

	NA	*K*	*Cl*	*HCO_3*	*Lactate*
Plasma	137–147	4–5.5	95–105	22–25	–
Isotonic saline	153	–	153	–	–
1/5 Isotonic saline 4.3 per cent dextrose	30.6	–	30.6	–	–
Ringer's lactate	130	4	110	–	28

Shock

Shock is a life-threatening situation. In most cases, it is due to poor tissue perfusion with impaired cellular metabolism, manifested in turn by serious pathophysiological abnormalities.

Types of shock

While there is some practical wisdom in the saying 'shock means haemorrhage, and haemorrhage means shock', there are other causes of shock with different features.

Vasovagal shock

Vasovagal shock is brought about by pooling of blood in larger vascular reservoirs (limb muscles), and by dilatation of the splanchnic arteriolar bed, causing reduced venous return to the heart, low cardiac output and reflex bradycardia. Consequently, the reduced cerebral perfusion causes cerebral

Sydney Ringer, 1835–1910. English physician at University College Hospital, London (1863), England. Known for his work on the influence of organic salts on circulation and heartbeat.

hypoxia and unconsciousness, but prostration and reflex vasoconstriction so increases the venous return and cardiac output as to restore cerebral perfusion and consciousness. It must be remembered that if the patient is maintained in an upright or a sitting position (e.g. in a dental chair) permanent cerebral damage will occur.

Psychogenic shock

Psychogenic shock immediately follows a sudden fright (e.g. bad news) or accompanies severe pain (e.g. a blow to the testes). The expression 'I nearly died of fright' reflects the danger of the uncorrected faint.

Neurogenic shock

Neurogenic shock is caused by traumatic or pharmacological blockade of the sympathetic nervous system, producing dilatation of resistance arterioles and capacitance veins (see below) leading to relative hypovolaemia and hypotension. There is a low blood pressure, a normal or decreased cardiac output, a normal pulse rate and a warm dry skin. Trauma to the spinal cord and spinal anaesthesia lead to a systolic pressure of around 70 mmHg, which may be corrected by putting the patient in the Trendelenburg position, the rapid administration of fluids and/or a vasopressor drug.

Hypovolaemic shock

Hypovolaemic shock is due to loss of intravascular volume by haemorrhage, dehydration, vomiting and diarrhoea (e.g. cholera, acute enterocolitis). Until 10–15 per cent blood volume is lost, the blood pressure is maintained by tachycardia and vasoconstriction. Fluid moves into the intravascular space from the interstitial space – a 'transcapillary refill' which may exceed 1 litre in 1 hour in injured but otherwise fit patients. In addition, the venous capacitance vessels constrict, pushing blood into the arterial system and therefore compensating for the volume deficit.

Traumatic shock

Traumatic shock is due primarily to hypovolaemia from bleeding externally (open wounds), from bleeding internally (torn vessels in the mediastinal or peritoneal cavities, ruptured organs such as liver and spleen or fractured bones) or by fluid loss into contused tissue or into distended bowel. Traumatic contusion to the heart itself may cause pump failure and shock, while damage to the nervous system or to the respiratory system results in hypoxia.

Burns shock

Burns shock occurs as a result of rapid plasma loss from the damaged tissues, causing hypovolaemia. When 25 per cent or more of the body surface area is burnt, a generalised capillary leakage may result in gross hypovolaemia in the first 24 hours. Endotoxaemia due to infection makes matters worse and large volumes of colloidal and crystalloid fluids are required for resuscitation.

Cardiogenic shock

Cardiogenic shock occurs when more than 50 per cent of the wall of the left ventricle is damaged by infarction. Fluid overload, particularly when using colloids, can lead to overdistension of the left ventricle, with pump failure. The resultant high filling pressures exerted by the right ventricle make fluid leak out of the pulmonary capillaries, thereby causing pulmonary oedema and hypoxia. If an arrhythmia occurs this will reduce the pumping efficiency of the heart, while hypovolaemia from excess sweating, vomiting and diarrhoea will further diminish cardiac output.

Acute massive pulmonary embolism from a thrombus originating in a deep vein or an air embolus (more than 50 ml), if obstructing more than 50 per cent of the pulmonary vasculature, will cause acute right ventricular failure. This greatly reduces venous return to the left ventricle, and cardiac output falls catastrophically causing sudden death or severe shock.

Septic (endotoxic) shock

Hyperdynamic (warm) septic shock. This occurs in serious Gram-negative infections (see Chapter 5), for example from strangulated intestine, peritonitis, leaking oesophageal or intestinal anastomoses, or suppurative biliary conditions. At first, the patient has abnormal or increased cardiac output with tachycardia and a warm, dry skin, but the blood is shunted past the tissue cells, which become damaged by anaerobic metabolism (lactic acidosis). The capillary membranes start to leak and endotoxin is absorbed into the bloodstream, leading to a generalised systemic inflammatory state. The immediate and ready treatment of the cause, including the drainage of pus, is vital to the recovery of the patient at this stage (in strangulated hernia 'the danger is in the delay, not in the operation').

Hypovolaemic hypodynamic (cold) septic shock. This follows if severe sepsis or endotoxaemia is allowed to persist. Generalised capillary leakage and other fluid losses lead to severe hypovolaemia with reduced cardiac output, tachycardia and vasoconstriction. The systemic infection induces cardiac depression, pulmonary hypertension, pulmonary oedema and hypoxia which, in turn, reduce cardiac output still further. The patient becomes cold, clammy, drowsy and tachypnoeic, but still can be converted to hyperdynamic (warm) shock by the administration of several litres of plasma or other colloidal solution. The similar use of crystalloid solutions may give rise to systemic and pulmonary oedema because of the larger volumes necessary.

Anaphylactic shock

Penicillin administration is amongst the common causes of anaphylaxis. Other causes include anaesthetics, dextrans, serum injections, stings and the consumption of shellfish. The antigen combines with immunoglobin E (IgE) on the mast cells and basophils, releasing large amounts of histamine and SRS-A (slow-release substance-anaphylaxis). These compounds cause bronchospasm, laryngeal oedema and respiratory distress with hypoxia, massive vasodilatation, hypotension and shock. The mortality is around 10 per cent.

Notes on terms used

Resistance arterioles are the small-calibre vessels, 0.02–0.05 mm in diameter, containing abundant smooth muscle in their walls, the tone of which is controlled by local humoral factors and the sympathetic nerve fibres. The calibre of these small vessels gives rise to the peripheral vascular resistance, controlling blood pressure and blood flow through the capillary beds. The larger arteries merely serve to supply the arterioles with blood.

Capacitance veins comprise the entire venous network from the postcapillary venules to the large-calibre veins in limbs, abdomen and thorax and which normally contain 70 per cent of the circulating blood volume. Although thin walled with relatively little smooth muscle, sympathetic nerve stimulation contracts them, reducing their diameter and emptying the blood into the arterial side of the circulation.

A colloidal solution is one in which the majority of solute particles has a molecular weight greater than 30 000. The term includes all plasma solutions, including human plasma protein fraction (HPPF), dextrans, gelatin (e.g. Haemaccel) and hydroxyethyl starch. Blood is not usually included in this term.

Minute volume ventilation is the volume of air (or oxygen) which enters the patient's lungs in 1 (each) minute, and is the product of respiratory rate and tidal volume.

Hyperventilation occurs when the patient is 'overbreathing' due to pain, anxiety or shock, such that the arterial carbon dioxide tension ($PaCO_2$) is lowered from the normal 40 mmHg (5.5 kPa).

Aspects of the pathophysiology of haemorrhage and shock

Low cardiac output is an early feature in shock, except for warm septic shock and neurogenic shock. Vasoconstriction occurs in an attempt to maintain perfusion pressures to the vital organs, such as the brain, liver and kidneys, as well as the heart muscle itself. Venoconstriction pushes more blood into the dynamic circulation whilst tachycardia helps to maintain a falling cardiac output. The minute ventilation rises 1.5–2 times and the respiratory rate 2–3 times maintaining oxygenation (except in cardiogenic shock with pulmonary oedema). The renal blood flow is reduced with consequent reduction in glomerular filtration and urine output. The renin–angiotensin mechanism is activated with further vasoconstriction and aldosterone release, causing salt and water retention. Release of antidiuretic hormone (ADH) decreases the volume and increases the concentration of urine. However, in early sepsis the patient, although hypovolaemic, may produce inappropriately large amounts of dilute urine (see below).

As cardiac output falls, the hypotension and tachycardia cause poor perfusion of the coronary arteries, and this, in conjunction with hypoxia, metabolic acidosis and the release of specific cardiac depressants (endotoxaemia or pancreatitis), causes yet further cardiac depression and pump failure.

The cells become starved of oxygen, and anaerobic metabolism leads to lactic acidosis. Eventually, the cell membranes cannot pump sodium out of the cells; sodium enters the cells and potassium leaks out (an old axion, 'sodium stays, potassium flees'). Thus, the serum potassium is elevated. Calcium, however, leaks into the cells lowering the serum calcium. Furthermore, the intracellular lysosomes break down and release powerful enzymes causing further damage – *'the sick cell syndrome'*.

The platelets are activated in shock owing to the stagnation of blood in the capillaries. Blood sludging with red cell aggregation may progress to the formation of small clots and, indeed, to DIC. Several coagulation factors are consumed (platelets, fibrinogen, Factor V, Factor VIII, prothrombin), and troublesome bleeding may occur from needle puncture sites, wound edges and mucosal surfaces.

Diagnosis

The prognosis of a shocked patient is related to the *duration* and *degree* of the shocked state, therefore prompt diagnosis of the type of shock is essential. It should be remembered that a thready and irregular pulse can make the measurement of blood pressure inaccurate and misleading. Intra-arterial pressure monitoring should be used. The ECG should be monitored to detect any arrhythmias that may occur. A chest X-ray may reveal mediastinal trauma or cardiac tamponade.

Central venous pressure

The measurement of central venous pressure (CVP) and its response to a small fluid challenge (200 ml of crystalloid or colloid) may assist in distinguishing between cardiogenic shock and hypovolaemic shock, but it must be emphasised that, in the seriously ill patient, the CVP is not a reliable indicator of left ventricular function because of the wide disparity that can exist between the left and the right ventricular functions.

Pulmonary capillary wedge pressure

The pulmonary capillary wedge pressure (PCWP) is a better indicator of both circulating blood volume and left ventricular function. PCWP is obtained by a pulmonary artery flotation balloon catheter (Swan–Ganz). This can be used to differentiate between left and right ventricular failure, pulmonary embolus, septic shock and ruptured mitral valve, and can also be an accurate guide to therapy with fluids, inotropic agents and vasodilators. It may also be used to measure cardiac output by a thermodilution technique simply at the bedside.

H.J.C. Swan. Professor of Medicine, UCLA School of Medicine, Director of Cardiology, Cedars Sinai Medical Center, Los Angeles, California, USA.

William Ganz. Professor of Medicine, UCLA School of Medicine, Senior Research Scientist, Cedars Sinai Medical Center, Los Angeles, California, USA.

Measurement of pulmonary capillary wedge pressure

This specialised procedure requires supervised training, practice, patience and experience in interpreting the values measured and waveforms indicated. Complications include arrhythmias, pulmonary infarction, pulmonary artery rupture, balloon rupture and catheter knotting, in addition to the complication from central venous cannulation. The catheter should not be left *in situ* for more than 72 hours; if further haemodynamic monitoring is required, a new catheter should be inserted.

Method. Strict aseptic central venous cannulation should be performed (e.g. via right internal jugular vein) and using the appropriate introducers, cannula and guidewire, the catheter, flushed and wiped with heparin saline, introduced into the right atrium. The balloon, inflated with 1.5 ml of air, should be advanced slowly via the right ventricle into the pulmonary artery, checked by z-ray and monitored by pressure tracing, which becomes characteristically flat when the balloon wedges in a small branch to give the capillary pressure (indicating left atrial pressure). When the balloon is deflated, the pulmonary artery pressure is obtained. The balloon must *never* be reinflated in the absence of a normal pulmonary artery waveform as this means that the tip alone is wedged and reinflation might therefore rupture the pulmonary artery. Withdrawal of 2–3 cm is mandatory until the waveform reappears and reinflation can be permitted.

The transducer should be placed at the midaxillary point (zero reference point); the normal PCWP is between 8 and 12 mmHg (10.5 and 15.5 cmH_2O), and normal pulmonary artery pressure is 25 mmHg systolic and 10 mmHg diastolic.

Clinical monitoring

In summary, patient monitoring in shock should include:

- pulse;
- blood pressure (recording systolic and diastolic pressure, the pulse pressure, using an intra-arterial line if necessary);
- heart rate and rhythm (cardioscope);
- respiratory rate and depth;
- CVP;
- PCWP in severe shock when the diagnosis is in doubt;
- urine output;
- serial blood gases and serum electrolyte measurements.

Method of central venous catheter insertion (the Seldinger technique)

A commercially available intravenous catheter, made to proper standards and of requisite length (20 cm), is passed into the right, or left, internal jugular vein. A line is drawn between the mastoid process and the sternoclavicular joint. The carotid artery is palpated on this line and the internal jugular vein lies immediately lateral to it at the midpoint of this line. The head-down position is used to prevent air being sucked in (air embolus) and to distend the vein.

Using full aseptic technique, a 7-cm needle, mounted on a syringe, is inserted caudally at 45° to the vertical into the internal jugular vein, the syringe removed and the soft end of the Seldinger wire passed through the needle into the vein. The needle is removed over the wire, and the catheter, placed over the wire, is passed into the vein. The wire is removed, and the catheter sutured into position and covered with a sterile, transparent, self-adherent dressing (e.g. Opsite 2000).

The catheter tip should be positioned in the superior vena cava or right atrium (confirmed radiologically at the first opportunity). Preceding every measurement, the patency of the catheter is confirmed by checking for a swinging movement of the saline column level in time with the patient's respiration. The patency of the catheter may be confirmed by lowering the saline reservoir briefly to check the free reflux of blood in the connecting tubing. It must be emphasised that the use of this method requires supervised training, skill, practice and patience, also referring to the special manuals, because the complications can be serious, for example pneumothorax, haemothorax, brachial plexus and phrenic nerve damage, and carotid artery perforation. The catheter must be removed when not required for CVP measurement, and should not be kept in position as a matter of convenience for electrolyte or parenteral infusions (the latter entering the pleural cavity or the mediastinum can be lethal).

The alternative, subclavian (infraclavicular) approach can be used, but has a higher incidence of complications (e.g. pneumothorax or haemothorax). The catheter may be tunnelled subcutaneously to improve fixation for a long duration and to reduce the incidence of septic complications.

A third approach is the insertion of a longer (60 cm) catheter into the median basilic vein in the antecubital fossa; the tip often does not reach the superior vena cava or right atrium, and therefore may not give an accurate CVP measurement; however, it is useful for a central infusion of fluids or drugs.

Central venous pressure measurement

A saline manometer for measuring central venous pressure should be used. This has a sterile glass or plastic tube manometer against a centimetre scale; a spirit level is used to set zero (0) to the midaxillary point or the manubriosternal angle. A three-way stopcock allows isotonic saline: (1) to run into the vein from the reservoir; (2) to fill the manometer; and (3) to exclude the reservoir and to allow the fluid in the manometer to fall to the level of the CVP.

The catheter is connected to the saline manometer, and readings are taken of the saline level with the *zero reference point at the midaxillary level.* The normal is 5–8 cm; if the CVP is low, the venous return should be supplemented by intravenous infusion, but not if the pressure is high. Readings with the zero reference point at the midaxillary level should

S.I. Seldinger, b. 1921. Swedish radiologist and physician.

never exceed 10; if the readings are taken at the manubriosternal angle (angle of Louis), as they may have to be in a surgically draped patient, the range is 3–4 cm lower than midaxillary readings.

Treatment of shock

The management of all types of shock should be vigorous and dedicated. The objectives are to increase the cardiac output and to improve tissue perfusion, especially in the coronary, cerebral, renal and mesenteric vascular beds. The plan of action should be based on: (1) the primary problem – arrest of haemorrhage, draining pus, etc.; (2) improving ventricular filling by giving adequate fluid replacement, for example human albumin solution or fresh frozen plasma, in sepsis and burns; (3) improving myocardial contractility with inotropic agents – dopamine, dobutamine, adrenaline infusions; and (4) correcting acid–base disturbances, using molar sodium bicarbonate when the pH of arterial blood is less than 7.2, and electrolyte abnormalities, especially potassium and calcium levels.

In endotoxic shock, once the haemodynamic status has been improved, full doses of the appropriate antibiotics are given to treat the causal infection. The circulation may be deluged with bacterial membrane debris which may intensify the endotoxic insult to the patient. This may be ameliorated by giving specific gamma-globulins to bind the endotoxin; the antibiotic polymixin E may also adsorb some of the endotoxins. This will reduce systemic inflammatory effects, diminish capillary leakage and improve organ perfusion.

Diabetic patients in endotoxic shock are in a precarious position. Careful monitoring and control of their nutrition and insulin requirements are necessary under the instruction of a clinician with a special interest in diabetes.

Vasodilators (hydralazine, phentolamine, glyceryl trinitrate infusions and chlorpromazine boluses) may be given provided the blood volume has been corrected and cardiac depression treated such that the systolic blood pressure is 90 mmHg or more. The indication is persistent vasoconstriction with oliguria, high CVP or PCWP and pulmonary oedema. Such therapy will improve cardiac output and tissue perfusion, and reduce the work done by the heart. *It must be emphasised that vasodilators can only be used with extreme caution and full haemodynamic monitoring*, because the sudden production of vasodilation in a hypovolaemic or dehydrated patient can be followed by a catastrophic fall in arterial blood pressure. These drugs should be given only in small intravenous doses or infusions and only until the extremities become warm and pink, and the veins are dilated and well filled.

Parenteral fluid therapy

The rational administration of parenteral fluids is one of the most significant advances in the care of acutely ill patients in the twentieth century. However, despite advances in the monitoring of cardiovascular variables, the questions of what? when? and how much? remain areas of enormous controversy.

In the 1930s Blalock suggested that it was the loss of blood rather than the '*release of evil humors*' that led to death after major trauma and recommended treatment by the administration of intravenous fluids. It was not until the 1940s and World War II that blood and plasma were widely used for the treatment of blood loss. Ironically, the same period highlighted the problems of inducing anaesthesia in vasoconstricted hypovolaemic casualties. When thiopentone was used as a sole intravenous anaesthetic agent at Pearl Harbour on 9 December 1941 there were numerous deaths as a result of vasodilatation and cardiovascular collapse. In the 1940s and 1950s descriptions of postoperative retention of salt and water as part of the *metabolic response to surgery* led to a widespread reluctance amongst surgeons and anaesthetists to administer crystalloids to their patients. The 1960s brought a swing back the other way when Shires and others demonstrated an increased survival in experimental animals that were bled and then reinfused blood plus additional crystalloid. The ensuing enthusiasm for the infusion of crystalloids led to the publication of Moore and Shires' now famous article calling for 'moderation'.

Colloids or crystalloids?

The colloid–crystalloid argument rages to this day: if one was clearly better than the other there would not be a controversy. The common link in the majority of articles on this subject is the final conclusion that it is dose not choice of fluid that is the real issue – and '*the proper dose of any drug is enough*' (Dr J.H. Drysedale). Certainly if the aim is to restore the circulating blood volume this will be achieved with a smaller volume and thus more rapidly by using a colloid.

Diagnosing hypovolaemia

Hypovolaemia can occur as a consequence of a wide variety of pathological processes. The nature of the fluid lost should dictate the choice of replacement fluid. Clinical history, whether first or second hand, in combination with appropriate laboratory investigations, should be the most useful guides to a rational fluid regimen. However, hypovolaemia from whatever cause is an acute medical emergency. Any degree of hypovolaemia jeopardises oxygen transport and increases the risk of tissue hypoxia and the development of organ failure. The greater the degree and duration of hypo-

A. Blalock. Late Professor of Surgery, Johns Hopkins Hospital, Baltimore, Maryland, USA.

G.T. Shires. Professor of Surgery, Cornell University, New York, USA.

F.D. Moore. Late Professor of Surgery, Peter Bent Brigham Hospital, Boston, Massachusetts, USA.

volaemia the greater the risk. Therefore, the initial treatment is to restore the circulating volume as quickly and effectively as possible.

Hypovolaemia may be divided into three categories: covert compensated hypovolaemia, overt compensated hypovolaemia and decompensated hypovolaemia.

Covert compensated hypovolaemia

This is the commonest yet least often diagnosed form of hypovolaemia. It refers to the presence of a reduced circulating blood volume without very obvious associated physical signs. Price found that healthy volunteers could have 10–15 per cent of their blood volume removed with no significant change in heart rate, blood pressure, cardiac output or blood *flow* to the splanchnic bed (gut, etc.). However, splanchnic blood *volume* was reduced by 40 per cent. The subjects in his study had essentially autotransfused and were maintaining the systemic circulating volume at the expense of the splanchnic circulating volume. This same process happens when we donate a unit of blood with no obvious adverse effects. Over the course of the next few hours we feel thirsty and therefore drink more, we also ingest salt and at the same time reduce urine output of salt and water. We make new proteins and blood cells, and very soon everything has returned to normal with no sequelae. In sick patients, however, many of the natural compensating mechanisms malfunction and this, coupled with the fact that fluid intake is being determined by a second party, namely the physician, makes hypovolaemia common.

Covert compensated hypovolaemia is extremely difficult to diagnose. In the conscious patient central nervous system (CNS) symptoms are the best guide. In the experiments performed above, all of the subjects developed CNS symptoms ranging from drowsiness and nausea to hiccoughs. Any thirsty patient should be assumed to be hypovolaemic until proven otherwise. Urinalysis showing an increased urinary osmolality and decreased sodium concentration is the most useful laboratory investigation.

Although covert compensated hypovolaemia is common and probably contributes significantly to morbidity, the majority of patients withstands the insult. If the hypovolaemia persists consequent end-organ hypoperfusion may be present for many days before it manifests itself as organ dysfunction. By this time the patient is usually in a state of overt compensated hypovolaemia.

Overt compensated hypovolaemia

Here there is hypovolaemia to an extent that the reflex mechanisms required to maintain perfusion to *vital* organs are obvious on clinical examination but the blood pressure is maintained. As before, clinical history is essential. On examination the patient will demonstrate the manifestations of an increased sympathetic drive with tachycardia, a wide arterial pulse pressure, and typically increased systolic blood pressure and cool clammy skin, particularly at the hands and feet. There may be other evidence of an inadequate cardiac output such as drowsiness, confusion and an increased respiratory rate. If the diagnosis is uncertain additional dynamic bedside tests can be performed such as gentle head-down bed tilting, leg raising or the administration of a bolus of intravenous fluid. If the diagnosis of hypovolaemia is correct then the increase in venous return may result in a reduction in heart rate, narrowing of pulse pressure, reduction in respiratory rate and overall improvement in well-being. If the diagnosis remains uncertain, or coincidental medical problems such as heart or lung disease make performing or interpreting such tests difficult, then more complex investigations may be required.

With the exception of electrolyte and blood gas analysis the majority of laboratory investigations is of little use in the acute phase. Arterial blood gas analysis can be performed rapidly; hypovolaemic patients are commonly hypoxaemic and may have a metabolic acidosis as a consequence of an inadequate cardiac output. Urinalysis, as described above, may support the diagnosis of hypovolaemia but no single test is diagnostic. Rapid determinations of total blood volume are not yet available.

Except for extreme cases the clinical interpretation of CVP by examination of the jugular venous waveform is unreliable and has no place in the management of hypovolaemic patients. If there is any doubt about the diagnosis, particularly in patients with cardiorespiratory disease, the patient needs a CVP catheter. The insertion and, indeed, interpretation of the information available from central venous catheters carries a significant morbidity and mortality so they should only be inserted and managed by experienced clinicians. For a more detailed account of central venous catheterisation readers are referred to Rosen *et al.* As a general rule the right internal jugular approach is favoured. The subclavian vein may be particularly difficult to locate in the hypovolaemic patient and the risk of arterial cannulation, haemorrhage and pneumothorax is then greatly increased. If during insertion steep head-down tilt produces no adverse effects and it is difficult to visualise or palpate neck veins, the judicious administration of at least 500 ml of colloid by a peripheral route before proceeding is sensible and safe. In the unlikely event that fluid administration produces a deleterious effect the infusion can be stopped easily, the head-down tilt corrected and the patient sat up.

In cases of ventricular dysfunction and/or severe pulmonary disease there will be a misleading discrepancy between right and left atrial filling pressures. If the information obtained from the CVP catheter is confusing, it may be necessary to insert a pulmonary artery flotation (Swan-Ganz) catheter. The pulmonary artery occlusion pressure (PAOP) provides an index of left ventricular filling pressure and may help to clarify the situation. It is important to realise that right atrial pressure and PAOP are influenced not only by the circulating volume but also by the degree to which the circulation is constricted, the compliance of the right and left heart, as well as pain, agitation, etc., causing increases in sympathetic tone. Low values are sensitive indicators of hypovolaemia, but high values do not necessarily mean the patient is well filled. Dynamic tests using fluid challenges give much more information and should always be tried in patients with evidence of an inadequate circulation. The administration of 200–500 ml of colloid over 5–10 minutes and comparison of the CVP or stroke volume (not the cardiac output) before the challenge and 5–10 minutes after the infusion has finished is the most useful guide. A sustained rise in CVP or PAOP of 3 mmHg and failure of the stroke volume to increase suggest the circulation is well filled.

Decompensated hypovolaemia

This is what many people refer to as shock. The degree of hypovolaemia is such that reflex redistribution of blood flow is insufficient to compensate and *vital* organs are no longer adequately perfused. The mean arterial blood pressure falls and may be difficult to record as peripheral pulses are often impalpable. The blood supply to the heart and lungs is compromised, which further reduces cardiac output, causes ventilation/perfusion (V/Q) mismatching and compounds the problem. Tachycardia changes to bradycardia as myocardial oxygenation becomes critical and the conscious level is severely obtunded. If untreated this clinical state rapidly progresses to total circulatory arrest. No special equipment or investigations are needed to make the diagnosis of decompensated hypovolaemia and to start aggressive volume replacement therapy. Misdiagnosis and inappropriate over-transfusion is an overrated problem. Delay in the treatment of hypovolaemic shock greatly reduces the chances of successful resuscitation. Most causes of hypovolaemic shock carry a far better prognosis than any condition that presents in a similar fashion but would be made worse by a fluid challenge.

The consequences of hypovolaemia

Decompensated hypovolaemia will result in end-organ damage and death if it is not treated rapidly and completely. Probably a far more common and insidious source of morbidity and mortality is the compensated hypovolaemias. As described above, a small reduction in circulating blood volume rapidly results in a far more significant reduction in splanchnic blood volume and in particular the supply to the innermost layer of the gut lumen, the mucosa. It is becoming increasingly clear that hypoperfusion of the gut mucosa is of fundamental importance in the pathogenesis of multiple organ dysfunction (see below).

Therefore, hypovolaemia is a potential killer in any disease process. The manifestations of persistent covert compensated hypovolaemia may not be seen for many days. Once a patient has overt hypovolaemia the chances of successful treatment are already significantly reduced with the exception of simple acute haemorrhage. Most patients are referred to intensive care units once they have progressed to decompensated shock with established organ failure. By that stage it is probably too late to make a significant difference to outcome. The early recognition and treatment of hypovolaemia is essential in any disease process.

Treatment of hypovolaemia

Very few patients benefit from fluid restriction; if there is evidence of hypovolaemia it should be treated. Inotropes should be used only when the circulating volume has been corrected.

Occult hypovolaemia is very difficult to diagnose. Therefore, in conscious patients who can drink the most rational approach is to be generous with fluids. Access is important, as is strength and volition. The patient with a full water jug and a raging thirst is commonplace. The aim should be an asymptomatic patient (i.e. no thirst) with good urine volumes (in excess of 0.5 ml/kg/hour) and normal urinalysis. The overriding principle is that fluid overload is easy to treat, whereas fully established organ failure is incurable.

Overt hypovolaemia should be considered a medical emergency and treatment is required urgently. The intravascular space must be resuscitated in minutes to hours *not* hours to days, as is currently common practice. Restoration of total body water and electrolytes will be slower. Treatment should be started following a presumptive diagnosis of hypovolaemia; by all means send laboratory investigations but do not wait for the results before starting treatment.

High-flow oxygen therapy should be given to all hypovolaemic patients until arterial blood gas analysis confirms normoxia. A pulse oximeter is useful if available. Venous access should be secured with short, large-bore cannulae, allowing large volumes to be infused rapidly. Ideally a 14G cannula in an arm vein should be used. These allow flow rates twice those of a 16G cannula. CVP catheters are of very limited use in the early phase of resuscitation, and are difficult and hence more dangerous to place. They should only be used if the diagnosis of hypovolaemia is in doubt or if no other access is available.

The initial choice of fluid in overt hypovolaemia should be a colloid for the reasons stated above. The need for blood (see below) should not delay initial resuscitation. Cardiac arrest due to a low haemoglobin concentration is very unusual; cardiac arrest due to hypovolaemia is relatively common. Resuscitation should be a continuous process with the doctor at the bedside re-evaluating the patient. Failure of a fluid challenge to secure improvement requires the use of more invasive monitoring. Each fluid challenge must be seen to produce a definite improvement. Precharted fluid regimens and remote management cost lives.

Just as patients compensate for volume loss in the early stages of hypovolaemia, so an apparently resuscitated patient may still have a significant volume deficit. The aim for immediate resuscitation should be normal measures of pulse, blood pressure and CVP, urine output > 0.5 ml/kg/hour with normal urinary osmolality and sodium concentration. Any metabolic acidosis should be seen to be correcting. Thereafter, one must try to maintain normovolaemia. This is a continuous process. Critically ill patients may have capillary leak and will therefore have a continuing colloid requirement. Gelatins, being small molecules, are poorly retained and can be replaced by hydroxyethyl starch, plasma or blood at this stage. In sepsis this requirement may be very large (see below).

The importance of blood in immediate resuscitation, the threshold at which one should transfuse urgently (i.e. consider using group-compatible, uncross-matched blood or even Group O blood) and even the target haemoglobin level are controversial. Resuscitation should not be delayed whilst waiting for blood to be grouped; if acute anaemia is secondary to the bleeding resuscitation should be with Group O blood or group-compatible blood as it becomes available. Otherwise colloid should be used initially and cross-matched blood and relevant blood products should be used when they are ready. Packed cells are not colloid and have little plasma expanding effect; transfusions with large amounts of packed cells will require supplementation with colloid. The age of the blood is important (old blood is acidic, with decreased oxygen-carrying capacity and poor red cell deformability) – use the youngest possible blood and whole blood if it is available.

Hypovolaemia and the surgical patient

Hypovolaemia is extremely common among patients undergoing surgery. It remains standard practice in the UK to deny patients food or drink for a minimum of 6 hours prior to elective surgery in an attempt to reduce the risk of pulmonary acid aspiration syndrome. It is not uncommon for this to extend to 10 or even 20 hours due to unforeseen delays. Preoperative fluid restriction is currently a matter of debate. Indeed, there is evidence suggesting that the administration of oral fluids to patients until 2 hours prior to elective surgery has produced a more favourable effect on gastric contents than total starvation. Yet no attempt is routinely made to maintain normal hydration in preparation for surgery, despite numerous previous studies demonstrating the benefits of fluid administration for even the most minor surgical procedures. Recently a study on fit young patients having elective laparoscopic sterilisation under general anaesthesia demonstrated a reduced morbidity by the administration of crystalloid during the operation. It is commonly taught that as part of the stress response to surgery patients have increased levels of ADH and aldosterone postoperatively and thus retain salt and water. As a result of this the overzealous administration of intravenous fluids is feared. Whilst it is probably true that ADH levels do rise in all postoperative patients, the presence of hypovolaemia per se may be responsible for much of the increase. A reduction in urine output in the first 24 hours after surgery may be acceptable, but a fall to oliguric levels (<0.5 ml/kg/hour) is not. Using the gastric tonometer, reduced splanchnic perfusion as a consequence of hypovolaemia has been demonstrated to be common during major surgery and associated with the development of postoperative organ failure. It is difficult to find any objective evidence to support the hypothesis that peripheral oedema or the accumulation of extravascular lung water, as opposed to pulmonary oedema due to left ventricular failure, has any significant adverse effects. On the contrary, the evidence supporting the prophylactic administration of intravenous fluids to patients having major surgery is impressive.

Hypovolaemia and cardiogenic shock

Conventional management of the patient with acute pulmonary oedema is still all too often based on diuretics. Unlike congestive cardiac failure, the usual problem in acute left ventricular failure is not an excess of total body salt and water but an acute redistribution of a normal quantity. This leads to an effectively hypovolaemic patient, particularly if they have been treated enthusiastically with diuretics. The most appropriate treatment is to reduce pre- and after-load with infused vasodilators such as GTN to encourage redistribution of fluid in a more normal fashion and to consider using inotropes and even judicious colloid challenges guided by a pulmonary artery catheter if vasodilators do not produce a rapid improvement. This is particularly important in right ventricular infarction, where the effect of hypovolaemia and poor right ventricular function is to underfill the left ventricle which in itself is usually underperforming.

The treatment of patients with congestive cardiac failure is more difficult. The basic principle should remain the maintenance of an adequate circulation with the use of vasodilators to improve overall haemodynamics supplemented with diuretics as necessary. The fact that so many patients tolerate diuretic-based regimens so well reflects the inherent robustness of the average human being!

Therapeutic interventions aimed at preventing organ failure

The widespread use of blood and plasma for the first time during World War II resulted in the recognition of a new phenomenon – 'irreversible shock'. It became apparent that numerous hypovolaemic casualties could have their vital signs restored with the administration of intravenous blood and plasma only to develop 'secondary shock', often days after the original insult, which rapidly became resistant to any form of treatment. Fifty years later the main thing that seems to have changed is the terminology used to identify the same condition. The terms multiple organ failure syndrome (MOFS), multiple systems organ failure (MSOF) and, most recently, multiple organ dysfunction syndrome (MODS) have all been used to describe 'irreversible shock' and organ failure. Rather like the elephant, it seems that we have difficulty describing it but we all know one when we see one.

In 1943 Blalock summarised the causes of irreversible shock seen in the Armed Forces as:

> ... (1) haemorrhage uncomplicated by gross trauma; (2) burns; (3) trauma to large masses of muscle; and (4) the re-establishment of circulation in a damaged ischaemic area.

In the same dissertation he suggests that:

> ... the initial phases (of shock) are certainly associated with and probably dependent upon a reduction in the volume of effective circulating blood ... Investigations have indicated that at some time in the development of irreversible shock there appear effects that may be ascribed either to toxic substances elaborated in areas of tissue damage or to a derangement of metabolism produced by a circulation which, either locally or generally, has been compromised over a long time.

The currently proposed theories of the pathogenesis of organ failure differ mainly in the fine detail, in particular many of the 'toxic substances' or mediators have been identified. Currently, we recognise and have tried to define more clearly the clinical conditions of the systemic inflammatory response syndrome (SIRS) and MODS.

It is postulated that, as a result of an insult, uncontrolled activation of inflammatory pathways may result in tissue destruction and subsequent organ failure. Inflammation is an essential component of the healing process. From a wide variety of stimuli (e.g. trauma, burns, infection) the final common pathway results in vasodilation, increased endothelial permeability, thrombosis, and leucocyte migration and activation. The systemic inflammatory response syndrome is the latest term proposed to describe a failure of localisation. MODS, due to tissue damage in organs distant to the site of the original injury, is the clinical manifestation of SIRS. Irrespective of the initiating stimulus (e.g. surgery, bacterial infection, pancreatitis), the morphology of necropsy specimens in both animal models and patients is remarkably constant. There is microvascular occlusion, endothelial destruction, interstitial oedema, leucostasis and thrombosis. Therefore, there would seem to be a dichotomy. Inflammation is essential for successful recovery from infection or injury, yet an excessive and uncontrolled inflammatory response can result in organ dysfunction or failure. One hypothesis is that there is a level of stimulation that, once exceeded, leads to uncontrolled activation of inflammatory pathways. There would appear to be a critical balance between activation and modulation (Fig. 4.1).

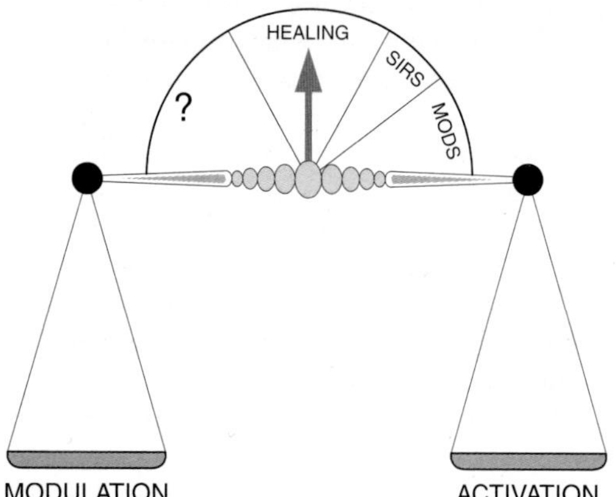

Fig. 4.1 The fine balance between activation and modulation of inflammatory pathways in the pathogenesis of postoperative organ dysfunction.

1. **Primary insult**
   - Infection
   - Trauma (e.g. surgery)
   - Pancreatitis
   - Burns
2. **Compounding insult**
   - Hypoxia
   - Hypovolaemia
   - Nosocomial infection
   - Bacterial and endotoxin leakage from GI tract
   - Malnutrition
3. **SIRS**
   - Increased cytokine production
   - Failure to localise cytokines
   - Abnormal nitric oxide synthesis
   - Contact, coagulation and complement activation
   - Abnormal arachadonic acid metabolism
   - Neutrophil sequestration and degranulation
   - Free radical production
4. **MODS**
   - Established microvascular occlusion
   - Tissue hypoxia
   - Cellular dysfunction

Fig. 4.2 The stages in the development of multiple organ dysfunction syndrome (MODS).

Fully established multiple organ failure is almost always fatal. A greater understanding of the pathogenesis of MODS has provided the basis for treatment regimens currently being used clinically or tested experimentally for the prevention of organ damage. Figure 4.2 summarises the various stages that are thought to lead to the development of MODS and therefore are targets for intervention. The rationale behind the apparent success, or failure, of a cross-section of these regimens is discussed below.

The primary insult

As always, the earliest treatment is most effective and prevention is better than cure. If we assume that the primary insult is unavoidable, has been correctly diagnosed and treated, then all subsequent forms of treatment are aimed at limiting the degree of tissue damage.

Compounding insults

Avoiding tissue hypoxia – simple resuscitation with intravenous fluids

The commonest compounding insult is probably tissue hypoxia as a result of inadequate basic resuscitation. Treating the primary insult is almost a waste of time without restoration of an adequate circulating blood volume. The majority of patients will respond to the administration of intravenous fluids and supplementary oxygen via a face mask. There is little doubt that if the aim is to restore the intravascular volume then this can be done most efficiently using a colloid. As one of the central abnormalities in SIRS is thought to be endothelial leak, one might hope that a colloid with a larger molecular weight than albumin might be more effectively retained within the vascular compartment and therefore more likely to maintain microvascular flow and organ perfusion. However, there are no human data that demonstrate that any particular solution (colloid or crystalloid) is better than another in terms of outcome, even though there is approximately a 100-fold price difference between the cheapest and most expensive alternatives. There are, however, good data to suggest that to avoid tissue hypoperfusion you need to give enough of whatever you choose and you need to give it promptly with the appropriate level of monitoring. For rapid restoration of haemodynamic function a colloid does the job more efficiently than a crystalloid. Albumin has no demonstrable advantages over cheaper alternatives such as the modified gelatins.

Treating tissue hypoxia – the global approach

The rationale here is that patients with SIRS are thought to have an occult tissue oxygen debt in spite of apparently normal global cardiovascular variables such as blood pressure and urine output, and that by increasing total body oxygen delivery, commonly by the administration of inotropes, this debt will be repaid and hypoxic tissue damage will be avoided. In patients undergoing high-risk major surgery and critically ill patients on the intensive therapy unit (ITU) there appears to be a positive correlation between a high oxygen delivery and survival. In patients undergoing high-risk major surgery prophylactically increasing cardiac output and oxygen delivery to predetermined *supranormal* levels has been associated with a decrease in subsequent organ dysfunction and mortality. However, the same principles when applied to established critically ill patients on the ITU has met with very limited success. Once a critical degree of tissue hypoperfusion is established then the situation is apparently irreversible.

There is an ever increasing list of *designer* vasoactive drugs (e.g. dobutamine, dopexamine, enoximone, piroximone, milrinone, amrinone) that can be used to manipulate global haemodynamics in sepsis. They have attractive hypothetical advantages in terms of their effects on global oxygen flow variables that can be confirmed in animal models and humans. However, there is no evidence to suggest that they are any more effective than the cheaper alternatives such as adrenaline and noradrenaline in terms of outcome.

Treating tissue hypoxia – the regional approach

As a result of the enormous amounts of research that have focused on global oxygen delivery in SIRS and MODS, it has become evident that regional perfusion may be compromised in patients who have apparently adequate global oxygen delivery and consumption. Probably the most commonly monitored end organ in the ITU has been the kidney, as urine output is easy to measure and relates crudely to function. The production of 0.5 ml/kg/hour of urine is accepted as an indicator of adequate regional perfusion. Unfortunately, although anuria carries a very poor prognosis the converse is not true. Many reno-protective agents have failed to modify outcome in humans. In animal models the use of mannitol, frusemide and low-dose renal dopamine infusions has been shown to protect the kidney, but this has not been demonstrated in the clinical environment. This may be because the infusion of a *renal dose* of dopamine, for example, may well produce a diuresis but cannot be expected to protect the kidney from coexisting hypoxia and hypovolaemia unless it is used as just a part of a total patient management regimen. Many believe that such agents used in isolation do more harm than good as they maintain an adequate urine output in the face of tissue hypoperfusion and also increase myocardial work.

More recently much attention has focused on the splanchnic region. In particular, the measurement of gastrointestinal luminal PCO_2, using a gastric or sigmoid tonometer, and calculation of gastrointestinal mucosal pH have become fashionable as indices of splanchnic perfusion. Splanchnic perfusion and, in particular, that to the gut mucosa is compromised early and preferentially in shocked states. There is also a hypothesis that gut mucosal hypoperfusion may result in leakage of gut luminal contents into the bloodstream and that this may be a proinflammatory factor tipping the balance in favour of SIRS and MODS. In support of this hypothesis gut mucosal hypoperfusion, as determined by the presence of a mural acidosis measured with a tonometer, has been shown to be the most sensitive predictor of MODS and death in patients undergoing major surgery and on the ITU. Certain therapeutic manoeuvres have been demonstrated to improve gut mucosal perfusion both in animal models and in humans. These include the administration of intravenous fluids, dobutamine, dopexamine and donor blood.

Avoiding nosocomial infections

Once a patient has some degree of organ dysfunction on an ITU they are thought to be at greater risk from nosocomial infection. In the prevention of secondary infection good handwashing and the avoidance of cross-infection carried by staff probably have the greatest impact. Assuming that such cross-infection is avoided then the patient is his or her own enemy and bacteria carried in the gastrointestinal tract provide the commonest source of secondary infection. Nosocomial pneumonia is thought to occur commonly as a result of spillage from the upper gastrointestinal tract into the lungs. It has been demonstrated that the administration of H_2-receptor antagonists with the intention of reducing gastric acidity and avoiding stress ulceration also encouraged the growth of bacteria in the stomach and an increased incidence of nosocomial pneumonias. The use of sucralfate as stress ulcer prophylaxis has the advantage of also being bacteriostatic and has been associated with a decreased incidence of nosocomial pneumonia. Another approach to the problem of secondary infection from the gastrointestinal tract is selective decontamination of the digestive tract (SDD) with the aim of reducing the incidence of secondary infection, from both overspill and translocation. SDD involves the use of a variety of topical and intravenous antimicrobial agents with the aim of removing the pathogenic gut flora but maintaining the commensal anaerobes. Numerous studies have demonstrated that SDD and/or modifying the gastric intraluminal pH reduces the incidence of nosocomial pneumonia. However, reducing the incidence of nosocomial pneumonias has had a far lesser effect on outcome than one might anticipate for a true cause and effect relationship.

Treating endotoxaemia

Endotoxin is a recognised potent activator of various cellular and humoral pathways involved in the generalised inflammatory response. Endotoxins are mostly comprised of lipopolysaccharide, and most of their biological activity resides in the lipopolysaccharide section. The core region of lipopolysaccharide is nearly identical for most strains of Gram-negative bacterial endotoxins. Supranormal levels of naturally occuring endotoxin core antibodies have been associated with a reduction in organ failure in patients following high-risk surgery and on the ITU. However, in two large multicentre trials of patients with presumed Gram-negative infection, the results of giving donor antibodies against the core region of endotoxin have been inconclusive. Active immunisation would be an attractive alternative for patients scheduled for major surgery, and evidence from animal experiments has been encouraging. However, there is no currently available antiendotoxin vaccine. Other potential antiendotoxin strategies undergoing human testing include bacteriocidal/permeability-increasing protein (BPI), endotoxin-neutralising protein and dextran–polymixin B conjugate, all of which have the ability to protect animals from endotoxin-mediated toxicity.

Systemic inflammatory response syndrome

The organo-protective therapeutic regimens cited above seem to work if used prophylactically, as is the case in major surgery. However, the results of adopting similar regimens in established MODS are rather disappointing. This would suggest that once a systemic inflammatory response is unresponsive to cardiovascular manipulations and antimicrobials then if the progression to MODS is to be avoided organ protection must come from a different line of attack. An increased understanding of the host-derived mediators of the tissue destruction seen in MODS has opened up a whole new field of therapeutic agents directed against them. It is hoped that specific manipulation of key mediators will at least halt the tissue damage in its tracks and hopefully be curative.

Cytokines

Protein cytokines play an important part in the mobilisation, localisation and subsequent activity of leucocytes in the inflammatory reaction. Tumour necrosis factor alpha (TNF-α) and the interleukins (IL) have emerged as prime targets for experimental manipulation. In animal models of septic shock, treatment with monoclonal antibodies to TNF-α and various interleukins (e.g. IL-1) have improved survival. There are ongoing trials of inhibitors of both TNF-α and IL in human sepsis. Unfortunately, the early reports have been inconclusive.

Decreasing cytokine synthesis and secretion

Corticosteroids reduce TNF-α mRNA translation in response to a stimulus and thus reduce secretion. Numerous studies have demonstrated the protective effects of corticosteroids in animal models of septic and haemorrhagic shock. The use of low-dose dexamethasone has been shown to improve outcome in paediatric patients with meningitis. From a purely hypothetical viewpoint, steroids should be the answer to the treatment of SIRS. However, two large multicentre, randomised trials of high-dose dexamethasone used in the treatment of septic shock failed to demonstrate any improvement in survival.

Nitric oxide

In 1987 it was reported that the endothelium-derived relaxant factor was identical to the free radical nitric oxide (NO). NO is synthesised from L-arginine by a constitutive enzyme present in the endothelium, which has a physiological role in the control of blood pressure, and by an inducible nitric oxide synthase, which is expressed in vessel walls and phagocytic cells in response to endotoxin or cytokines. NO has a myriad of actions but is predominantly a vasodilator and can modify the neutrophil–platelet interactions that may result in the microvascular occlusion seen in MODS. These effects create a therapeutic dilemma. Should you give NO in an attempt to restore microvascular flow or block its effects to restore the blood pressure in septic shock? In patients with severe acute respiratory distress syndrome inhaled NO has been demonstrated to reduce pulmonary artery pressure and improve pulmonary oxygenation without affecting systemic vascular resistance. However, it has also been demonstrated that blocking the production of NO from its precursor L-arginine is possible by the administration of arginine analogues such as N^G-monomethyl-L-arginine (L-NMMA). In animal studies the administration of NO antagonists has been shown to restore the vascular response to catecholamines and improve survival.

Arachadonic acid metabolites

There is a multitude of animal and human evidence to suggest that metabolites of arachadonic acid play key roles in the pathogenesis of MODS, both protective (e.g. prostaglandin E_2) and deleterious ones (e.g. leukotrienes and thromboxane). Cyclooxygenase inhibitors such as ibuprofen or indomethacin, which are nonsteroidal anti-inflammatory drugs, have been shown to reduce tissue damage and improve survival in animal models of sepsis.

Neutrophils

Degranulating neutrophils as part of a systemic inflammatory response are said to cause microvascular injury and promote organ dysfunction by the release of destructive enzymes and the generation of oxygen free radicals. Free radical scavengers such as superoxide dismutase, allopurinol and even vitamin C are universally successful in reducing the tissue damage seen in septic and haemorrhagic shock models. Provisional reports from at least two human studies claim success from free radical scavenging.

Contact, coagulation and complement activation

A common clinical feature of SIRS is a coagulopathy. Histologically the microvascular abnormality seen in MODS is not unlike clot. This has led to the assumption that there is a disturbance of the balance between procoagulant and anticoagulant pathways in SIRS that can manifest itself most vividly in the disseminated intravascular coagulation seen in meningococcal meningitis. There are preliminary results suggesting that the administration of clinical concentrates of inhibitors of the contact system such as antithrombin III and C1-esterase inhibitor may modify the outcome in established SIRS.

Endogenous anti-inflammatory agents

It is now recognised that most proinflammatory acute-phase reactants are balanced by the production of endogenous anti-inflammatory acute-phase reactants. For example, antagonists to soluble IL-1 and TNF-α are produced by hepatocytes and released into the circulation, thereby reducing the inflammatory response. The anti-inflammatory cytokine IL-10 is a potent macrophage-deactivating factor, and injection of recombinant IL-10 has been shown to protect mice from endotoxic shock. IL-10 is thought to regulate the effects of other cytokines (e.g. TNF-α), rather than block them completely, and therefore has the potential for maintaining optimal balance in the inflammatory system.

Multiple organ dysfunction syndrome

There are no animal or human data to suggest that fully established MODS is treatable. This does not mean that all patients who have MODS die. However, the small percentage who survive have probably done so because supportive care has given them a chance to get better.

Conclusion

Prevention of MODS by the prompt diagnosis and treatment of the primary insult coupled with cardiovascular resuscitation and supportive care has an extremely high success rate in patients who have some hope of long-term survival. However, once the same group of patients has established organ failure the outlook is extremely gloomy.

Further reading

American College of Surgeons' Committee on Trauma. *Advanced Trauma Life Support, Student Manual*, American College of Surgeons, Chicago, IL (only available as part of the ATLS course).

Blalock, A. (1930) Experimental shock: the cause of low blood pressure produced by muscle injury. *Archives of Surgery*, **20**, 959–96.

Blalock, A. (1943) A consideration of the present status of the shock problem. *Surgery*, **14**, 487–508.

Dobb, G.J. and Donovan, K.D. (1992) Bedside catheterization. In *Care of the Critically Ill Patient* (eds J. Tinker and W.M. Zapol), Springer, London, pp. 1205–19.

European Resuscitation Council (1990) *Guidelines for Advanced Life Support*, A statement by the Advanced Life Support Working Party of the European Resuscitation Council.

Halford, F. (1943) A critique of intravenous anesthesia in war surgery. *Anesthesiology*, **4**, 67–9.

Moore, F.D. and Shires, G.T. (1967) Moderation. *Annals of Surgery*, **166**, 300–1.

Price, H.L., Deutsch, S., Marshall, B.E., Stephen, G.W., Behar, M.G. and Neufeld, G.R. (1966) Haemodynamic and metabolic effects of haemorrhage in man with particular reference to the splanchnic circulation. *Circulation Research*, **18**, 469–74.

Rosen, M., Lotte, P. and Ng, S. (1992) *Handbook of Central Venous Catheterisation*, W.B. Saunders, London.

Salmon, J.B. and Mythen, M.G. (1993) Pharmacology and physiology of colloids. *Blood Reviews*, **7**, 114–20.

Shires, T., Coln, D., Carrico, J. and Lightfoot, S. (1964) Fluid therapy in hemorrhagic shock. *Archives of Surgery*, **88**, 688–93.

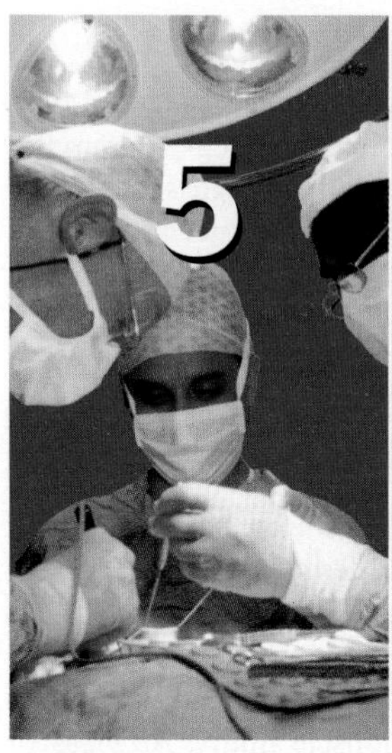

5 Nutritional support and rehabilitation

Nutrition

Malnutrition

In surgical practice malnutrition is common, being present before, or occurring after, operations in about 50 per cent of patients, possibly more in some parts of the world.

Preoperative malnutrition may be due to starvation or to a failure of digestion. Starvation is caused by:

- difficulty in obtaining food (poverty);
- difficulty in swallowing food (dysphagia);
- difficulty in retaining swallowed food (vomiting);
- self-neglect, e.g. in the elderly and in alcoholics.

Failure of proper digestion may, for example, be due to pancreatic or biliary disease (carcinoma or jaundice due to stones), and duodenal and jejunal conditions (fistula or blind-loop syndrome).

Postoperative (post-traumatic) malnutrition is, in most cases, of a transient nature consequent upon a short period of starvation and the stress reaction to trauma. Recovery from any nitrogen deficit (Table 5.1) due to protein catabolism will follow on return to normal feeding. Any delay in return to a normal diet, such as may be imposed by the dictates of the operation (oesophagectomy), or a complication (paralytic ileus from peritonitis), means that severe malnourishment is likely to occur.

Bailey & Love's Short Practice of Surgery, 23rd edition. Edited by R.C.G. Russell, N.S. Williams and C.J.K. Bulstrode. Published in 2000 by Arnold Publishers.

Table 5.1 Typical daily postoperative nitrogen loss

	Nitrogen loss (g)	*Muscle loss (g)*
Herniotomy	3	80
Appendicectomy	6	200
Cholecystectomy	12	320
Fractured femur	15	400
Oesophagectomy	90	2500
Peritonitis	18	570
Sepsis	23	730

Hypercatabolic state. Severe sepsis (subphrenic abscess), severe trauma (burns) and other severe disturbances of major viscera (pancreatitis) are accompanied by an accelerated and profound breakdown of tissue proteins.

In starvation, the metabolic changes are directed to minimising tissue loss and, in some circumstances, humans can survive for about 120 days. Glucose reserves are available only for 24 hours and thereafter are derived principally from muscle, so that catabolism begins almost immediately after food deprivation. In the first 72 hours, there is a rapid weight loss due to loss of sodium and water, then the resting metabolic expenditure falls and daily nitrogen losses over 2 weeks fall from about 10 g to 3–4 g. Progressively fat provides most of the energy requirements yielding 38 kJ/g while carbohydrate derived by gluconeogenesis in the liver from amino acids is utilised by the brain, adrenal glands and red cells – all obligatory glucose users. After about 21 days, the central nervous system adapts to using ketones derived from fat. The gluconeogenesis and ketosis of starvation may be easily inhibited by glucose intake.

Protein in lean tissue is constantly turned over and renewed. Normally the processes of protein synthesis and breakdown act in equal and opposite directions to keep the muscle mass in an adult constant – at about 40 per cent of total body weight. It seems likely that under normal circumstances the provision of an adequate nutrient supply of amino acids allows protein synthesis to exceed breakdown during and after meals, whereas between meals the opposite pertains, thus maintaining a balance over a 24-hour period. Insulin and amino acids appear to stimulate muscle protein synthesis and insulin inhibits protein breakdown. Lean tissue may be lost by a variety of methods. In starvation, chronic illness and immobilisation, muscle protein synthesis is depressed below the level of protein breakdown. Such a pattern is found in patients suffering from heart failure, carcinoma, emphysema, hypothyroidism and cirrhosis, whereas a patient confined to bed will suffer an exacerbation of the process causing muscle wasting.

In sepsis, inflammation, trauma and burns, the muscle wasting results from a massive loss of amino acids from muscle tissue with depressed muscle protein synthesis and enhanced muscle breakdown. The mechanism is uncertain but injury and sepsis trigger a co-ordinated series of inflammatory and immune responses and the stimulation of macrophages to produce cytokines such as tumour necrosis factor and interleukin-1. These cytokines are associated with proteolysis, particularly the breakdown of myofibrillar proteins but only in the presence of elevated corticosteroid concentrations.

After injury or surgical operation

There is an increased oxygen and calorie consumption and a negative nitrogen balance (Cuthbertson). The increase in resting metabolic expenditure ranges from minimal after uncomplicated surgery to 30 per cent with multiple fractures, 45 per cent in peritonitis and up to 100 per cent in burns. An increase in metabolic rate and protein catabolism of more than 25 per cent is regarded as a hypercatabolic state.

The endocrine profile, activated by fear, apprehension and nervous stimuli from damaged tissues, is altered after stress with an increase in secretion of most hormones, in turn resulting in changes in substrate handling by the body.

Glycogen breakdown in muscle and liver is accelerated principally by adrenaline and glucagon, leading to increased blood glucose levels, while increased cortisol and glucagon induces gluconeogenesis from amino acids. Lipolysis – fat breakdown – is increased by growth hormone, glucagon and noradrenaline. Thus control of glucose levels is impaired and, together with depressed peripheral clearance, results in 'the diabetes of injury'.

The stimulated protein breakdown in the postoperative period is associated with a change in synthesis rate in the body cell mass, and this results in a negative nitrogen balance indicating loss of protein derived from muscle and viscera. Larger losses are seen in muscular athletic men and the smallest losses in wasted patients. Epidural anaesthesia inhibits the normal postoperative increases in cortisol, adrenaline, aldosterone and growth hormone, and so may reduce the negative nitrogen balance. Nitrogen balance may be improved during enteral or parenteral feeding if the patient can be mobilised.

Studies following patients for up to 1 year following uncomplicated surgery suggest that the maximum weight loss occurs after 2 weeks and that normal body composition is restored after 6 months.

A particularly unpleasant effect of surgery is the period of mental and physical tiredness that follows it. It is not a particular problem in patients who feel well before surgery, but in those with preoperative tiredness, it is worst postoperatively at the end of the first week; at 4 weeks it is similar to the initial preoperative level, and it usually disappears after 3 months. Voluntary muscle functions deteriorate in a similar pattern to fatigue but postoperative nutrition, which restores muscle mass, does not influence postoperative fatigue, leading to speculation that the symptoms of fatigue have both a physiological and psychological basis.

Uncomplicated, minimally invasive surgery is believed to be associated with minimal postoperative fatigue and a shortened convalescence. Initial studies suggest that the neuroendocrine response is similar to a comparable open operation, and further studies are required to resolve this paradox.

Severe sepsis is characterised by an increased rate of whole body protein catabolism, and when prolonged the depletion of visceral protein results in multiple organ failure. In patients with sepsis, both protein synthesis and catabolism are increased with a much greater increase in catabolism resulting in protein loss. The increase in protein synthesis may be the result of increased hepatic protein synthesis of acute-phase proteins. Intermediate metabolism in sepsis is directed at increasing substrate availability by lipolysis, glycogenolysis, protein catabolism and hepatic glucose production. Studies in septic patients have provided evidence that the myofibrillar proteins, retin and myosin, are particularly catabolised in sepsis. The principal mediators are tumour necrosis factor, interleukin-1 and glucocorticoids.

Fat oxidation increases with sepsis and is the principal source of energy in the patient with sepsis, while hepatic glucose production occurs despite hyperglycaemia and a low respiratory quotient. The increased substrate turnover is accompanied by an increase in resting energy expenditure.

The effects of malnutrition include poor wound healing manifesting as wound dehiscence (Chapter 3) and leaking anastomoses of bowel, delayed callus formation, disordered coagulation, reduced enzyme synthesis, impaired oxidative metabolism of drugs by the liver, immunological depression with increasing susceptibility to infection, decreased tolerance to radiotherapy and cytotoxic chemotherapy, all with the severe mental apathy and physical exhaustion of the patient.

Some clinical indications for nutritional support are:

- preoperative nutritional depletion;
- postoperative complications:
  - ileus more than 4 days,
  - sepsis,
  - fistula formation;
- intestinal fistula;
- massive bowel resection;
- management of:
  - pancreatitis,
  - malabsorption syndromes,
  - ulcerative colitis,
  - radiation enteritis,
  - pyloric stenosis;
- anorexia nervosa;
- intractable vomiting;
- maxillofacial trauma;
- traumatic coma;
- multiple trauma;
- burns;
- malignant disease;
- renal failure;
- liver disease;
- cardiac valve disease.

Sir David Cuthbertson, CBE, 1900–1989. Glasgow Royal Infirmary, Scotland.

Assessment and management

It is essential for the clinician to be aware of the need to assess the state of nutrition of a patient and, if malnutrition is present or threatens, to consider the nutritional requirements, and then to use methods of sustaining normality or rectifying any deficiency. Between 1 and 2 per cent of elderly patients have serious subnutrition as a consequence of inadequate dietary intake.

Assessment

A malnourished patient has a characteristic appearance, lean and hungry in most cases of starvation, lean and apathetic in post-traumatic depletion, with a superimposed hectic flush around sunken cheeks and pinched nose in a hypercatabolic state. The clinician, when placing a comforting hand on the patient's shoulder, discerns the bony scapula bereft of almost all its muscle. However, these clinical observations only detect gross malnutrition and therefore measurement of the nutritional status is essential (Goode). The following parameters are included.

1. *Body weight*. Careful weighing on a bed weighing machine is the obvious way of detecting the progress or otherwise of the patient. The desirable weight of the patient can be checked by reference to the appropriate tables, or by applying the body mass index (BMI) = weight (kg)/height^2 (m). A woman should have an index of 20, 21 or 23, and a man 20.5, 22 or 23.5 according to size of frame (small, medium or large).
2. **Upper arm circumference.** Feeding is indicated if the circumference is less than 23 cm in females and 25 cm in males.
3. **Triceps skinfold thickness.** Using a skinfold caliper, the minimum is 13 mm in females and 10 mm in males.
4. **Serum albumin** should not be less than 35 g/litre.
5. **Lymphocyte count.** Less than 1500/mm^3 indicates an impaired cellular defence mechanism.
6. ***Candida* skin test.** A negative reaction also means defective cell-mediated immunity.
7. **Nitrogen balance studies.** The total nitrogen intake is compared with the loss from all sources, such as urine, fistula drainage and nasogastric aspirate (1 litre = 1 g nitrogen). A greater loss than intake indicates a negative balance and tissue breakdown. A positive balance means anabolism–tissue synthesis.

Other measurements include those determining the rate of muscle breakdown, such as urinary creatinine excretion, or 3-methylhistidine excretion. Body potassium and nitrogen are used to assess the absolute size of the body cell mass. [^{14}C] Leucine incorporation is a measure of the synthesis rate, while serum transferrin is used as a measure of visceral protein synthesis (needs to be more than 1.5 g/litre).

Anthony William Goode. Professor of Endocrine and Metabolic Surgery, University of London, The Royal London Hospital, London, England.

Nutritional requirements

These include carbohydrate, fat, protein, vitamins, minerals and trace elements (Table 5.2).

Energy is provided by carbohydrate and fat. A healthy adult at rest requires 6300–8400 nonprotein kilojoules per day for energy (1500–2000 calories). Carbohydrate provides 16.8 kJ/g (4.1 kcal/g) and fat 37.8 kJ/g (9.1 kcal/g). The number of nonprotein kilojoules given should bear a definite relationship to the nitrogen intake. A typical regime would feature 8400 kJ (2000 kcal) to 13 g N (about 150 to 1).

Nitrogen requirements. The minimum for dynamic tissue turnover, and so to keep a healthy adult in positive nitrogen balance, is about 35–40 g of protein or 5.5–6.5 g of nitrogen per day. The hypercatabolic patient requiring hyperalimentation may need three or four times this amount of protein. A daily negative nitrogen balance of 10 g is not unusual and is equivalent to a loss of 62.5 g of protein or 300 g of muscle tissue.

Vitamins. Whatever the method of feeding, vitamins are necessary as supplements, as they are essential for the maintenance of normal metabolic function.

The water-soluble vitamins B and C act as coenzymes in collagen formation and wound healing. Postoperatively, the vitamin C requirement increases to 60–80 mg/day. Preoperative depletion is exacerbated by anorexia, smoking, aspirin and barbiturate therapy. Vitamin B_{12} is given 500 µg intramuscularly (i.m.) weekly, particularly to those with initial low levels (coeliac disease, Crohn's disease, ileal resection or bypass, blind-loop syndrome, tapeworm infestation, reduced pancreatic secretion, tropical sprue, excess alcohol intake, anticonvulsant therapy and after gastric surgery). As the serum folate falls, especially in those on parenteral nutrition, folinic acid is required daily in doses of 3–6 mg i.m.

The fat-soluble vitamins A, D, E and K are reduced in steatorrhoea and the absence of bile. Vitamin A, 5000 units per week, is required after surgery and, when appropriate, it enhances the antitumour effect of cyclophosphamide. Vitamin K 5–10 mg i.m. weekly reduces any bleeding tendency. If commercially available vitamin additives are put into an infusion, the container should be protected from the light.

Table 5.2 Daily calorie and nitrogen requirements (*after* Johnston)

	Postoperative	*Hypercatabolic states*
Water (ml/kg)	35	40–45
Energy [kJ (kcal)/g]	147 (35)	1890–2310 (40–55)
Nitrogen [kJ (kcal)/g]	756 (180)	840–1176 (200–280)
Nitrogen (g/kg)	0.2	0.25–0.30

Ivan David Alexander Johnston. Emeritus Professor of Surgery, University of Newcastle upon Tyne, England.

Minerals and trace elements

Sodium, potassium, iron, calcium and magnesium deficiencies must be identified and made good (Chapter 4). Zinc deficiency is manifest as a rash on the face and perineum which does not respond to antifungal therapy, stomatitis which causes disturbance of taste (dysgeusia) and alopecia. Copper deficiency results in leucopenia and anaemia, while lack of chromium may give rise to glucose intolerance. The 14 trace elements that are considered essential for normal enzyme activities include manganese, cobalt, molybdenum and vanadium. It is to be remembered that long-term parenteral nutrition can result in depletion.

Methods of feeding. These are predominantly enteral and less commonly parenteral.

Enteral nutrition

By mouth

Obviously, as this is the natural way, it should always be attempted. Only when it is known that this route cannot be used or is ineffective are other methods considered.

Feeding by mouth demands *common sense, cleanliness and compassion* on the part of the medical attendants. It is *common sense* to ensure that an adequate, palatable and varied diet, including all the nutritional requirements, is provided at regular intervals, more frequently than regular meal times if necessary. It is common sense to begin with a liquid diet as soon as bowel sounds return after an abdominal operation, and not, for example, to allow a plate of fish and chips to be put in front of a patient the day after a gangrenous appendix has been removed. Promotion to semisolid (light) and then to more solid food (full diet) follows in steps of 3–7 days according to progress. *Cleanliness* in the preparation and serving of food and of the utensils used is of paramount importance in avoiding gastrointestinal infection causing vomiting and diarrhoea. A salmonella infection among elderly patients and children may be a mortal blow. *Compassion* is needed to ensure that the patient actually receives and ingests the proffered food. Food must be placed within reach of an enfeebled patient. Assistance is often required and should be freely given. Dental care may be necessary to facilitate oral intake and false teeth may need consideration. Table 5.3 shows a representative range of the enteral diets available. Dieticians and pharmacists should be involved in the prescribing of enteral feeding regimes in much the same way as they are involved in parenteral feeding.

Table 5.3 Examples of enteral diets

	Nitrogen (g)	*Fat (g)*	*Carbohydrate (g)*	*Energy (kJ/kcal)*	*Osmolality (mmol)*
Liquids [constituents per litre (as applied)]					
Clinifeed favour	6.0	33.1	140.0	4200/1003	335
Isocal	5.1	42.0	126.0	4240/1013	290
Powders (constituents per 100 g)					
Ensure	2.2	31.5	54.5	1831/437	N/A
Flexical	1.6	15.0	66.9	1856/443	N/A

Suppliers: Clinifeed – Roussel Laboratories Ltd, Uxbridge, Middx, UK; Isocal and Flexical – Mead-Johnson (Squibb) Pharmaceuticals, Slough, Bucks, UK; Ensure – Abbott Laboratories Ltd, Maidenhead, Berks, UK. N/A = Not applicable.

By nasogastric tube

A nasogastric tube which has been passed to allow regular gastric aspiration to be performed may also be used for feeding liquidised diets. Fine-bore tubing can be used instead, being favourably received by most patients as less irritating than the larger tube. It is invaluable when passed with the aid of an endoscope through an oesophageal stricture into the stomach, enabling the effects of starvation to be reversed. In some patients, the tube can be sited in the duodenum, especially if there are problems of gastric stasis or oesophagogastric reflux.

Technique of fine-bore tube insertion and usage

The patient may be sitting or lying, preferably the former. The introducer wire is lubricated with water and inserted into the fine-bore tube. Pass the tube through the nose via the nasopharynx and oesophagus into the stomach. Withdraw the wire and tape the tube to the patient. Check the position of the tube by radiography as passage into a bronchus can occur quite easily. Alternatively, a quick check can be made by injecting 5 ml of air down the tube and listening through a stethoscope for its bubbling entry into the stomach.

Administration of the feeds is either by gravity or by means of an infusion pump.

Problems of tube feeding

Gastric emptying should be normal. In ill patients ensure that the stomach empties by injecting 60 ml water down a nasogastric tube and aspirate 4-hourly. If after 24 hours fluid is passing through the stomach, commence feeding for the first day and aspirate intermittently to ensure that the stomach empties. Then remove the tube and introduce the fine-bore tube.

Blockage of a 1-mm bore tube is cleared by flushing through with 2 ml water – do not add effervescent potassium to the feed as curdling will follow.

Most fine-bore tubes incorporate a male 'luer' lock connector making the nasogastric drip system incompatible with intravenous lines.

Check the drip rate hourly.

All feeds should be stored at 4°C until use, not exposed to room temperature for more than 8 hours and discarded if not used after 12 hours. As diet kitchens may be a source of *Klebsiella* infection, the bacteriological monitoring of feeds is desirable.

Unwanted effects. Nausea, vomiting and pulmonary aspiration are avoided by regulation of the infusion rate and ensuring initial gastric emptying. Diabetes and hyperosmolar states are related to high carbohydrate intake with particular hazard for the established diabetic. Diarrhoea is common and the pathogenesis is not fully understood, but fluid and electrolytes are secreted into the bowel in response to a high osmotic load. The use of broad-spectrum antibiotics is also associated with diarrhoea. Recent studies suggest that osmolality, electrolyte content and volume of the feed are not implicated in the onset of diarrhoea. It is now probable that the bypassing of the cephalic phase of feeding when a tube is *in situ* results in suppression of distal colonic motor activity with the onset of diarrhoea. Commence with half strength feed and increase slowly to standard concentration over days given at a slow, constant rate, avoiding milk because of possible lactose intolerance and a high fat content giving steatorrhoea. Mild disturbances of liver function can be associated with both enteral and parenteral feeding, due to intrahepatic cholestasis. Metronidazole 500 mg twice daily may prevent overgrowth of the anaerobic bacteria responsible.

By tube enterostomy

Tube enterostomy is the operative placement of a tube or catheter into the gastrointestinal tract. It is indicated when the passage of a fine-bore nasogastric tube is not possible or when more than 4 weeks of enteral feeding is anticipated. The common contraindications include complete or partial gastric or intestinal obstruction. The tube is usually placed as a specific surgical procedure or as an adjunct to intra-abdominal surgery.

A choice of procedure is to fashion either a gastrostomy or jejunostomy. The contraindications to the former are:

- gastric disease;
- impaired gastric emptying;
- significant gastro-oesophageal reflux;
- loss of the gag reflex.

Jejunostomy is the procedure of choice for the ease of placement of the tube, the initiation of early postoperative feeding, and the avoidance of the risk of pulmonary aspiration.

By gastrostomy (Figs 5.1 and 5.2)

There are two long-term types of gastrostomy: Stamm and Janeway. An upper abdominal (midline) incision is optimal for giving the best exposure and the catheter can be placed laterally away from the incision. The Stamm gastrostomy is the simplest to perform and is particularly valuable as a temporary procedure or in the patient who is a poor postoperative

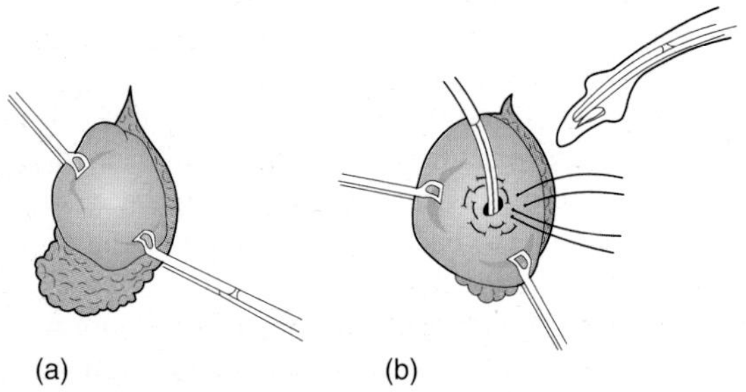

Fig. 5.1 Stamm temporary gastrostomy. Tube inserted into the gastric fundus. Whenever possible, the appropriate portion of stomach for insertion is brought through or surrounded by omentum (a) to act as a seal; (b) tube (usually a Foley catheter of large size) inserted into the stomach through a double row of purse-string sutures in the gastric wall.

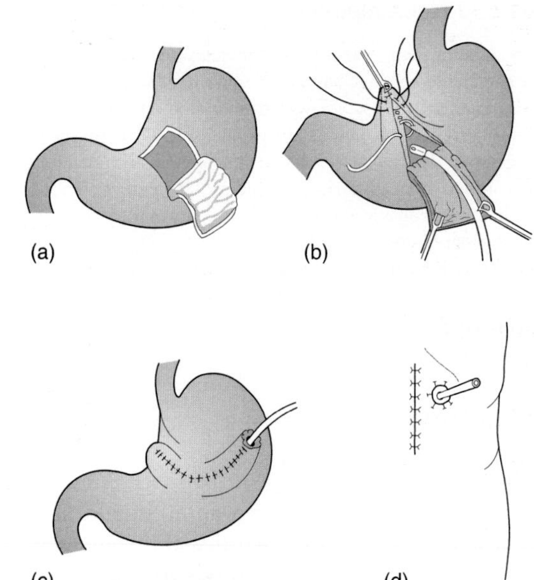

Fig. 5.2 Janeway permanent gastrostomy. (a) A rectangular flap is taken from the anterior gastric wall; (b) a gastric tube is fashioned around an indwelling gastrostomy tube; (c) the gastric tube is brought through the abdominal wall lateral to the incision and the orifice sewn to the skin by direct mucocutaneous suture; (d) final position.

risk. Inadvertent removal of the tube is followed by rapid shrinkage of the cutaneous orifice. To preserve the established gastrostomy a tube must be promptly reinserted. Caution must be exercised to ensure that the new tube is *in situ* before feeding is recommenced. A Janeway gastrostomy is preferred if there is a need for permanent tube feeding.

When a quick temporary measure is necessary, the ink-well (Kader–Senn) technique is valuable. The tube should be large and, as in all gastrostomies, the end of the tube should be directed towards the fundus.

Complication rates as high as 30 per cent have been associated with gastrostomy procedures, reflecting poor nutritional status, impaired wound healing and pulmonary complications because of immobility. Leakage around the tube can be controlled by inserting a larger catheter with a balloon and taping the tube with gentle traction.

The endoscopic placement of gastrostomy tubes in therapeutic endoscopy is an innovation during the last decade (Figs 5.3 and 5.4). Percutaneous endoscopic gastrostomy has reduced the need for the surgical fashioning of a feeding gastrostomy under general or local anaesthesia. Thus, whenever a surgical gastrostomy is indicated, a percutaneous endoscopic technique may be used. As the gastroscope must be passed into the stomach, a complete oesophageal obstruction will be an absolute contraindication, as are ascites, sepsis, abnormal clotting and peritoneal dialysis. The patient should have no intake for 8 hours before the procedure. The basic gastrostomy is fashioned in a retrograde manner from within the stomach. A suture is placed through the anterior abdominal and gastric wall and brought out through the mouth. A catheter with a tapered tip is then fixed to the oral end of the suture from the abdominal wall. The catheter is then delivered through the abdominal wall. The holding sutures are removed from the abdominal wall after 1 week.

There is a 3 per cent incidence of major complications, sepsis, puncture of another viscus such as the colon or the need for a laparotomy. Minor complications in 7 per cent of cases include wound infection and circumstomal drainage.

Edward Gamaliel Janeway, 1841–1911. American physician.
Frederic E.B. Foley, 1891–1966. American urologist.

Bronislaw Kader, 1863–1937. Surgeon, Poland.
Nicholas Senn, 1844–1908. Surgeon, USA.

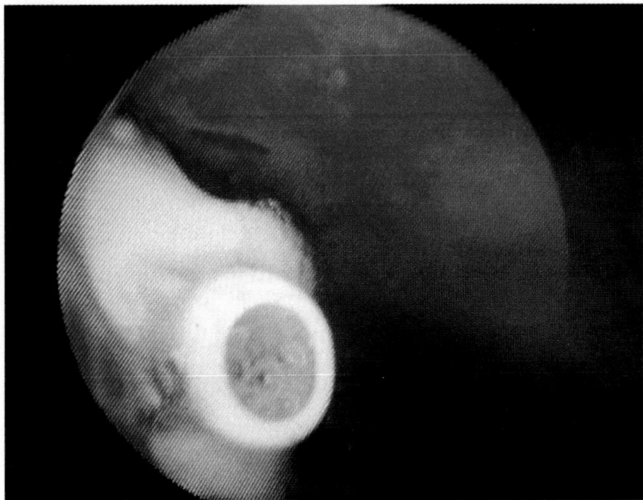

Fig. 5.3 Endoscopic view of gastrostomy fashioned from within the stomach.

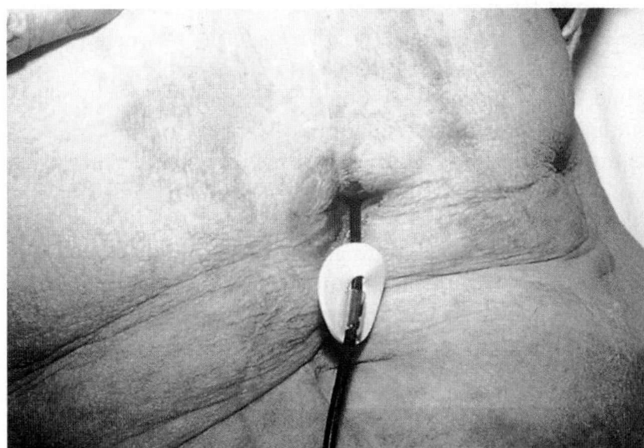

Fig. 5.4 External view of gastrostomy tube *in situ* at the end of the placement procedure.

A tract forms within 2 weeks and, if the catheter is removed, another of similar size may be inserted within a few hours.

By jejunostomy (Figs 5.5 and 5.6)

There are two types of feeding jejunostomy: a Witzel jejunostomy with formation of a serosal tunnel, and a needle jejunostomy using a catheter of a small gauge. The ease of jejunostomy as an adjunct to an intra-abdominal surgical procedure has increased in popularity.

It is of importance to control infusion rates of nutrients, particularly with a jejunal feed. The perceived benefits of an enteral pump infusion system include:

- more efficient nutrient delivery;
- reduced abdominal discomfort;
- decreased incidence of osmotic diarrhoea.

A particular advantage is the pump alarm system indicating an empty bag, line occlusion or a failing pump battery system. This safety mechanism promotes mobility for the patient, a more continuous energy

Friedrich Oskar Witzel, 1856–1925. Surgeon, Bonn, Germany.

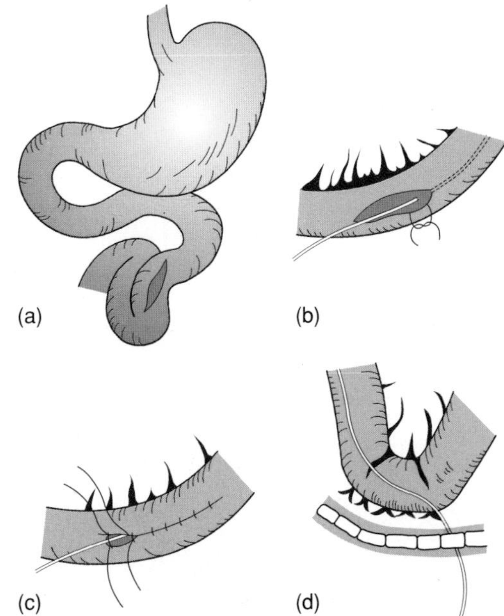

Fig. 5.5 Witzel jejunostomy. (a) The site of election for insertion of a catheter into the jejunum is 30 cm below the ligament of Treitz; (b) a fine-bore catheter is inserted through the seromuscular tunnel (groove) in the jejunal wall and fastened at the point of the mucosal penetration by an anchor stitch; (c) the incision is closed over the fine catheter in the tunnel of the jejunal wall; (d) the jejunum is sutured to the anterior abdominal wall.

intake than an intermittent feeding regimen and a mechanism providing security and confidence for the patient, and nursing and medical staff.

Parenteral nutrition

Parenteral nutrition by intravenous feeding is used in less than 4–5 per cent of all hospital admissions, either when enteral feeding is not possible, or to supplement deficient enteral feeding. It has been suggested that although the incidence of serious, noninfectious complications is lower in patients receiving total parenteral nutrition, the incidence of septic complications is substantially higher and only in severely malnourished patients do the benefits outweigh the risks.

Total parenteral nutrition is particularly complicated by displacement of the catheter, sepsis, mechanical problems and metabolic derangements – which occur in up to 10 per cent of postoperative patients.

Intravenous (i.v.) fat has many immunosuppressive effects: i.v. long-chain triglycerides reduce the functions of the reticuloendothelial system and neutrophils and the ratio of T-helper to T-suppressor cells. Contraindications include cardiac failure, severe liver disease, disorders of fat metabolism, uncontrolled diabetes, shock and severe blood dyscrasias. It must be remembered that total parenteral nutrition is not to be undertaken lightly. It is potentially hazardous and can be dangerous in inexperienced hands. The formation of multidisciplinary nutritional care teams

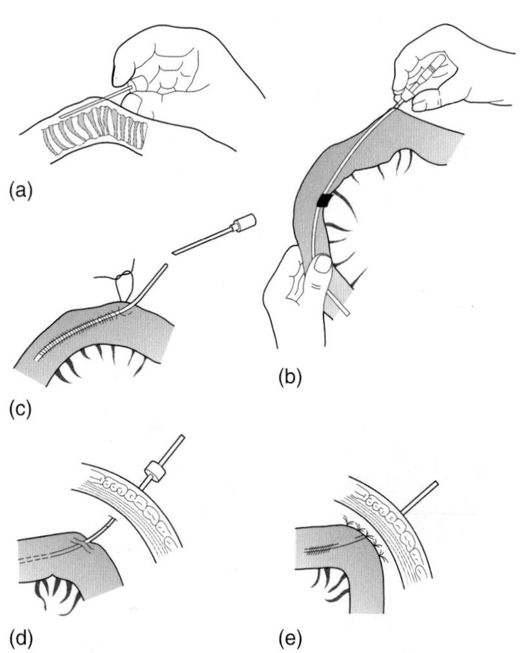

Fig. 5.6 Fine-needle jejunostomy. (a) A large-bore needle is inserted obliquely through the wall of the jejunum into the bowel lumen; (b) a catheter with a stylet is then passed through the needle into the surrounding anchor stitch after removal of the stylet; (d) the end of the catheter is brought out through the large-bore needle inserted through the abdominal wall; (e) the jejunum is secured to the anterior abdominal wall. On elective removal of the tube, the jejunostomy stoma is self-closing.

including dieticians and pharmacists is a major advance and their advice should be sought.

When planning an intravenous feeding regimen, first weigh the patient and calculate the fluid needs for the next 24 hours. Energy and nitrogen intake should be calculated on a body weight basis, remembering that daily needs may change. Daily biochemical patient monitoring is essential (Table 5.4).

Most feeding teams decide on the nitrogen and energy requirements of their patients, and tailor-make the feeds

Table 5.4 Monitoring feeding regimens

Daily	Body weight Fluid balance Full blood count, urea and electrolytes Blood glucose Urine and plasma osmolality Electrolyte and nitrogen analysis of urine and gastrointestinal losses Acid–base status
Thrice weekly	Serum calcium, magnesium and phosphate Plasma proteins Liver function tests Clotting studies
Ten days	Serum B_{12}, folate, iron, lactate and triglycerides Trace elements

Table 5.5 Some available solutions for i.v. feeding

	Nonprotein energy [kJ (kcal)/litre]	*N (g/litre)*	*Na (mmol/litre)*	*K*
Vamin 9 Glucose	1680 (400)	9.4	50	20
Synthamin 14	N/A	14.3	73	60
Aminoplex 14	N/A	13.4	35	30
Intralipid 20 per cent	8400 (2000)	N/A	N/A	N/A
		Mg	*PO_4*	*Ca*
Vamin 9 Glucose		1.5	N/A	2.5
Synthamin 14		5	30	N/A
Aminoplex 14		N/A	N/A	N/A
Intralipid 20 per cent		N/A	15	N/A

N/A = Not applicable.

from the wide variety of amino acid solutions with and without electrolytes, and the various concentrations of dextrose and fat available (Table 5.5). Typically, these are mixed under laminar flow sterile conditions in the pharmacy into 3-litre bags giving sufficient for 24 hours or, better still, supplied to specifications by one of the companies involved in the manufacture of i.v. solutions. Twenty per cent glucose is equivalent to 3200 kJ/litre (770 kcal/litre) and Intralipid 20 per cent (KabiVitrum) is equivalent to 8400 kJ/litre (2000 kcal).

As most glucose solutions are hypertonic and irritant, they are usually given through central veins, the cannulation of which requires technical finesse. In the short term, the nutritional requirements in aseptic patients can be adequately met with mixtures of amino acids, fat and glucose given peripherally. Fat buffers the vein wall and sometimes subtherapeutic doses of heparin and hydrocortisone are given to act locally in the prevention of thrombophlebitis. The energy requirements of surgical patients have often been overestimated; few will require more than 8400 kJ (2000 kcal) per day (Macfie).

Technique for central venous catheter insertion with a skin tunnel (Fig. 5.7)

Percutaneous catheter insertion requires expertise to prevent the *complications* which may occur in one in five attempts. These are air embolism, pneumothorax and injury to the subclavian artery or brachial plexus because of significant variation in relationship of the subclavian vein to the clavicle and first rib. A subclavian vein cutdown technique may be employed to allow cannulation of the vein under direct vision. A silicone rubber catheter of 1 mm diameter (Vygon, Vygon UK Ltd, Uxbridge, UK) is inserted by intraclavicular approach, the introducer inserted under local anaesthetic through a 1-cm skin incision (A) 2 cm below the midclavicular point. The position of the catheter is checked radiologically, ensuring the tip is in the superior vena cava or right atrium. The catheter hub is removed and the introducer withdrawn. The introducer is now inserted through the skin puncture at (B) about 7 cm below and medial to (A); it is passed through the subcutaneous tissue to

J. Macfie. Consultant surgeon, Scarborough, England.

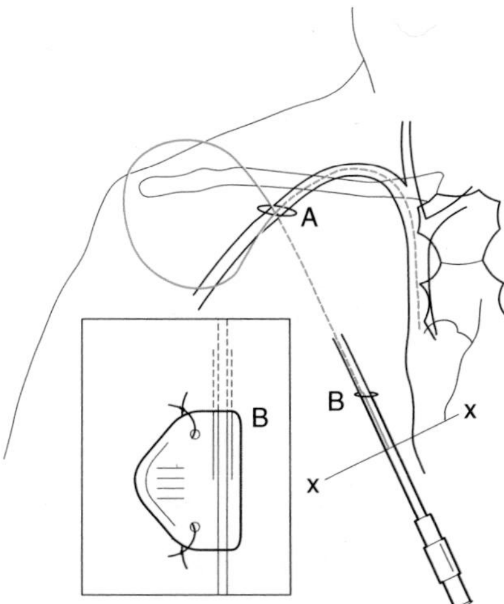

Fig. 5.7 Subclavian catheterisation with a skin tunnel. NB. The sedated patient is placed in the head-down position. The procedure is carried out in a clean room using strict aseptic technique. Insert: the plastic clip, which grips the emerging catheter at B, and sleeve are suitably anchored with sutures (after J. Powell-Tuck).

emerge at (A) and the catheter threaded through the introducer at (A) until it is seen within the transparent introducer at (B). The introducer is partially withdrawn and cut at X–X so that 2 cm remains in the tunnel and 2 cm protrudes, and the catheter pushed fully through the 4-cm sleeve, avoiding kinks at (A). (A) and (B) are cleaned with chlorhexidine in alcohol and sprayed with povidone iodine powder. Incision (A) is closed with a stitch and covered with a sterile dressing. *Caution:* it is possible for the catheter tip to perforate the vein wall. If this occurs in the pleural cavity a pneumothorax can be caused. Before the infusion is started, it is essential to confirm by a free backflow of blood that the catheter remains in the lumen of the vessel.

Commence feeding using half-strength solution and increase to the desired daily intake over days. Additives to solutions should be avoided and given through a separate line, although central mixing in pharmacy allows addition under sterile conditions into a 3-litre bag delivery system.

Catheter-related sepsis may occur in up to a third of patients fed parenterally. Skin flora are important in the pathogenesis of this sepsis and the skin at the site of the catheter insertion should be swabbed on alternate days. Bacteriological skin culture shows a strong association between microbial growth, usually *Staphylococcus epidermidis,* and the development of catheter-related infection. Factors known to increase the risk of infection include variation from the strict nursing protocol for care of the catheter, the age of the patient and the duration of hospital stay before the institution of parenteral nutrition.

Home parenteral nutrition

Chronic intestinal failure results in a failure of adequate nutrient absorption from the gut to maintain body weight. This may follow extensive bowel resection, multiple high output fistulas, motility disorders and extensive Crohn's disease. Such patients require prolonged nutritional management by a skilled and experienced team. Long-term home parenteral nutrition depends upon suitable case selection and extensive patient training by experienced nurses, together with a comprehensive hospital pharmaceutical service: the patient will live at home and manage his or her own parenteral feeding. With successful treatment, many patients are able to return to work or care for the home and family unaided or with minimum help.

Notes on solutions. Fructose, sorbitol or alcohol solutions are potentially disadvantageous owing to an associated lactic acidosis or hepatocellular damage. Fat, isotonic preparations of vegetable oils in water with an emulsification agent or purified egg phospholipid in Intralipid (to stabilise the mixture) should not be used 12 hours before blood sampling as they interfere with analysis. The rate of clearance of intravenous fat is increased after surgery or when energy demands are high (Feggetter).

The nitrogen sources are either casein hydrolysates, or laevorotatory isomers of amino acids. In such solutions, all essential amino acids should be present with a broad spectrum of the nonessential amino acids. No single amino acid should predominate since, if its use is inefficient, this will interfere with the use of the others (Tweedle). In sepsis, renal failure and hepatic failure, the use of solutions containing only essential amino acids, isoleucine, leucine, valine, phenylalanine, lysine and tyrosine is under investigation.

Complications. The initial complications of parenteral feeding arise from *malposition of the catheter tip* and radiographic confirmation of the site of the catheter tip is mandatory before infusion. *Infection,* particularly septicaemia, arises from continuous direct vascular access and immune depression in malnourished patients, together with the solutions being ideal bacterial and fungal culture media. Catheter insertion with strict asepsis, daily care of the entry site cleaned with 1–2 per cent tincture of iodine and alcohol solutions, and the strict use of the line only for nutrient solutions all contribute to prevention. However, if a patient develops an unexplained fever, hypotension, vomiting, diarrhoea, confusion or seizures, a full clinical examination with appropriate radiology and bacteriological culture of blood, sputum, urine and swabs of the catheter site are indicated. If a source of infection is discovered it is treated, but if no source is found and the fever persists for 24 hours, remove the catheter and send the tip for bacteriological and fungal culture, *Candida albicans,* staphylococci or *Klebsiella* frequently being isolated. Recommence the parenteral regimen using a new catheter at a fresh site.

Prolonged use of amino acids and glucose alone will result in essential fatty acid deficiency, with *dermatitis, anaemia and increased capillary permeability,* a complication avoided by the use of intravenous fat solutions or essential fatty acids rubbed into the skin weekly. Similarly, *hypophosphataemia* is seen with such regimens and accentuated by the use of insulin, resulting in enzyme defects, adenosine-5′-triphosphate (ATP) deficiency and a shift to the left in the oxygen dissociation curve. This is prevented by a daily intake of 13 mmol of potassium dihydrogen phosphate. Table 5.6 lists some clinical syndromes and biochemical disorders resulting from drug–nutrient interactions and Table 5.7 lists other biochemical complications. *Jaundice* occurring during parenteral nutrition is cholestatic, perhaps the result of sepsis, malnutrition and hypoxia.

Severe hepatic *steatosis* is rare during total parenteral nutrition. However, transient hepatic abnormalities are so common that some authorities regard it as the most frequent metabolic complication. A cholestatic picture tends to predominate with increases in alkaline phosphatase and bilirubin. Elevations of serum transaminases may also be found. Hepatic biopsy performed in the jaundice phase shows histological evidence of fatty infiltration, periportal lymphocytic infiltration with bile duct proliferation and intrahepatic cholestasis or biliary sludging resulting in extrahepatic obstruction.

Jeremy Powell-Tuck. Physician, The Royal London Hospital, London, England.

Jeremy George Weightman Feggetter. Surgeon, Ashington and Freeman Hospitals, Newcastle-upon-Tyne, England.
David Ernest Frederick Tweedle. Surgeon, University of South Manchester, England.

Table 5.6 Some clinical syndromes and biochemical disorders resulting from drug–nutrient interactions

Drug	*Nutrient*	*Syndrome*
Alcohol	Thiamine (B_1)	Wernicke's encephalopathy
Antacids	Phosphate	
	Hypophosphataemia	
	Aluminium-containing	
Anticonvulsants	Folate	Anaemia
Primidone	Vitamin K	Hypoprothrombinaemia
Antifolates	Folate	Stomatitis
	Methotrexate	
	Pyrimethamine	
	Trimethoprim	
Anti-infectives		
Amphotericin	Magnesium	Hypomagnesaemia
	Potassium	Hypokalaemia
Isoniazid	Pyridoxine (B_6)	Peripheral neuropathy
	Niacin	Pellagra
Tetracyclines	Calcium	Depressed bone growth
	Magnesium	Disturbed mitochondrial enzyme functions
Beta-blockers	Glycogen	Hypoglycaemia
Corticosteroids	Glucose	Hyperglycaemia and glycosuria
	Water	Fluid retention
	Sodium	Sodium retention
	Potassium	Hypokalaemia
	Calcium	Osteoporosis
Diuretics	Magnesium	Hypomagnesaemia
	Potassium	Hypokalaemia
Diuretics–thiazide	Glucose	Hyperglycaemia

Table 5.7 Biochemical complications during parenteral nutrition and their correction

Complication	*Clinical presentation*	*Cause*	*Correction*
Hyponatraemia	Confusion	Water intoxication	Reduce water intake
	Apathy	GI or renal loss	Increase Na^+ intake
Hypokalaemia	Apathy	Inadequate K^+ intake	Increase K^+ intake
	Cardiac irregularity	GI or renal loss	
Hypomagnesaemia	Weakness	Inadequate Mg^{2+} intake	Increase Mg^{2+} intake
	Vertigo	GI or renal loss	
	Convulsions		
Hypophosphataemia	Apathy, confusion, paraesthesias, red blood cell (RBC) oxygen dissociation	Inadequate inorganic phosphate intake	Increase PO_4 intake
Azotaemia	Apathy	Dehydration	Increase water intake
		Energy:nitrogen imbalance	Increase energy:nitrogen ratio to 185:1
Hyperammonaemia	Apathy, seizures, coma	Hepatic dysfunction	Reduce infusion rate or stop altogether
		Amino acid deficiency	
Hyperglycaemia	Increased blood sugar	Unsuspected diabetes	Treat underlying cause
		Underlying sepsis	Treat underlying cause
		Excess infusion of carbohydrate	Reduce infusion rate
Hypoglycaemia	Lethargy	Interrupted infusion	Give dextrose
	Vasoconstriction		
Hyperosmolar dehydration	Hyperglycaemia	Hyperglycaemia	Correct hyperglycaemia and give half-strength saline
	Dehydration		
	Increased serum sodium and osmolality		
	Apathy		
	Coma		

The syndrome differs somewhat between infants and adults. In the former, typical morphological changes and jaundice, fatty metamorphosis and even cirrhotic transformation are described, whereas older patients predominantly have enzyme derangements.

The pathophysiology of hepatic dysfunction is not entirely understood.

Up to 40 per cent of surgical patients have an elevation of alkaline phosphatase, particularly if the feeding solution contains more than 214 kJ/kg daily, while it has been suggested that reduction in carbohydrate intake by increased use of a fat solution reduces liver dysfunction. In the vast majority of patients, hepatic function disturbance is both mild and self-limiting and spontaneous recovery is invariable after cessation of total parenteral nutrition.

In the patient with jaundice, it is proposed that cyclical nocturnal total parenteral nutrition reverses abnormalities when replacing continuous parenteral nutrition. *Metabolic acidosis,* much less common if fructose and alcohol are avoided, may arise from infusion of available hydrogen ions in amino acid solutions and is simply corrected with sodium bicarbonate solution.

Steroids. Anabolic steroids (e.g. Durabolin 25 mg i.m. weekly) may be used to improve nitrogen balance, but the effect may not be observed for some days.

Rehabilitation

It is not enough to save the patient's life or to carry out a successful operation for a benign condition: whenever possible, the patient should be restored to full social and work capacity. This aim demands more than surgical 'cure': rehabilitation will be required in many cases. The importance of this can be judged by the well-documented fact that a patient who suffers a severe and incapacitating injury or accident that keeps him or her from returning to work for 12 months is unlikely ever to return to full employment, however good his or her recovery from the injury appears to be. While orthopaedic and neurosurgical centres provide the bulk of surgical patients requiring a programme of active physical rehabilitation, such centres should be equipped to assist patients recovering from medical disorders as well, e.g. cardiac and 'stroke' patients. With the steadily enlarging proportion of elderly patients surviving, there is an increasing demand for facilities for vascular patients (amputees) and patients with gastrointestinal diseases, principally cancer of the lower bowel (colostomised cases).

Motivation is an important element in rehabilitation. In the USA, a company employee or union-supported victim of trauma takes five times longer to resume his or her normal work than a self-employed person. Therefore, rehabilitation should include a programme of psychological and emotional readjustment in which the family should play an active supportive role. Although rehabilitation can involve the surgeon, pastor, marriage counsellor, occupational therapist, physiotherapist, vocational training assistance scheme, prosthetic counsellor, psychiatrist, health visitor and the family doctor, in many cases practical guidance and effective support should emanate from the surgeon who carried out the primary care. Nothing is more important than the timely recall by the surgeon at the time of the initial surgical procedure that his or her patient will require appropriate rehabilitation to achieve the best result.

While maintaining a caring and human approach, the surgeon must be prepared to be firm with patients who play for sympathy as they try to avoid achieving independent status during their rehabilitation programme.

Further reading

Benyon, S. (1998) *Metabolism and Nutrition.* Mosby, London.

Little, R.A. and Wenierman, J. (eds) (1998) *Energy Metabolism in Trauma.* Ballière Tindall, London.

Garrow, J.S. and James, W.P.T. (eds) (1999) *Human Nutrition and Dietetics.* Churchill Livingstone, London.

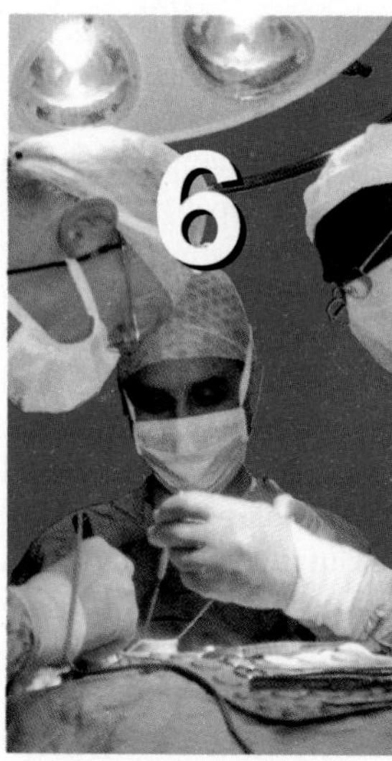

6 Anaesthesia and pain relief

General principles

Effective general anaesthesia for surgery began in 1846 when W.T.G. Morton gave ether for dental extraction in Massachusetts General Hospital, shortly to be followed by the successful use of ether for amputation of the leg in University College Hospital, London. Anaesthesia gained good public repute when Queen Victoria accepted *chloroform à la reine* from Dr John Snow during the birth of Prince Leopold in 1857. Local anaesthesia originated with the use of topical ophthalmic cocaine in Vienna in 1884 (*by Koller, a friend of Freud*), to be followed by the gradual development of local infiltration, nerve blocks, intrathecal (colloquially termed spinal anaesthesia) and, eventually, epidural anaesthesia.

In the UK, training and standards in anaesthetic practice have been led predominantly by the Association of Anaesthetists of Great Britain and Ireland and the Faculty of Anaesthetists of the Royal College of Surgeons. The latter achieved autonomy as the College of Anaesthetists, and in 1993 gained its charter as a Royal College.

Together with the specialist societies, they have fostered advances and developments in anaesthesia for all of the surgical subspecialities, and for obstetric and paediatric anaesthesia, intensive care, trauma and resuscitation, and acute and chronic pain relief. Many advances in anaesthesia have facilitated or are driven by changes in surgical practice. Optimal patient care results from the surgeon and anaesthetist working as a team, and requires a working knowledge of each other's craft. This is especially true in the presence of complex medical and surgical problems, demanding a joint approach to risk–benefit assessment and preoperative medical optimisation.

The importance of multidisciplinary collaborations at national level for successful audit, analysis of performance, and drafting of practice recommendations and policy is exemplified by the Confidential Enquiries into Maternal Deaths (Triennial Reports) and into Perioperative Deaths (CEPOD) in the UK. Surgical and anaesthetic joint working parties have resulted in influential documents such as *Pain after Surgery*.

Intraoperatively, the anaesthetist should provide the general anaesthetic triad of unconsciousness, pain relief and muscular relaxation, while ensuring maintenance of tissue perfusion and oxygenation. Monitoring of vital functions is mandatory, and must include electrocardiography, blood pressure and oxygen saturation.

Throughout, the anaesthetist's prime duty is to the patient's safety and welfare, but it is also important to

William Thomas Green Morton, 1819–1968. Massachusetts, USA. In 1886 he gave ether for dental extraction and by this success spread the use of anaesthesia.

John Snow, 1813–58. English physician. Introduced the use of ether as anaesthetic into English surgical practice (1846/7).

Carl Koller, 1857–1944. American ophthalmologist. Associate of Sigmund Freud at Vienna General Hospital. Introduced cocaine as a local anaesthetic in eye operations (1884) and thus inaugurated the use of local anaesthesia in other types of surgery.

Sigmund Freud, 1856–1939. Austrian neurologist and founder of psychoanalysis. Professor of Neuropathology (1902–38), University of Vienna, Austria.

Bailey & Love's Short Practice of Surgery, 23rd edition. Edited by R.C.G. Russell, N.S. Williams and C.J.K. Bulstrode. Published in 2000 by Arnold Publishers.

optimise the operative conditions. A collective duty of care exists to prevent injuries such as cutaneous burns or to vulnerable structures such as nerves and eyes.

An anaesthetist's care extends into the postoperative period, at least until it has been clearly delegated to another person on the surgical ward or intensive care unit. Indeed, the modern anaesthetist is developing a more defined role as 'perioperative physician', with recognition of the continuing care beyond the immediate recovery period. Organisational and individual conduct has been recently outlined in the *Guide to Good Practice*, published jointly in the UK by the Association of Anaesthetists of Great Britain and Ireland, and the Royal College of Anaesthetists.

Preparation for anaesthesia

Recognition of general medical and specific anaesthetic risk factors facilitates the implementation of pre-emptive measures and improves patient safety. Early assessment, liaison with the anaesthetist and appropriate investigations avoid unnecessary delays. In any case, the anaesthetist who is to be present during the operation should assess the patient preoperatively and participate in the preparation for surgery.

Preoperative evaluation and management

Investigation of the general condition of the patient before surgery should be specific according to the general history and clinical signs. Investigations in fit people are unnecessary and uneconomic, but indicated tests should be performed as early as possible, preferably before admission. Routine haematological and biochemical screens, with electrocardiography and chest radiography, are prudent investigations in elderly people receiving general anaesthesia for all but minor surgery. The saving of a serum sample for transfusion cross-match, a check for hepatitis antigen and a sickle-cell screen, if indicated, should not be forgotten.

Cardiovascular disease

Uncontrolled hypertension and angina, dysrhythmias and cardiac failure are common reasons for postponement of elective procedures. Correction of hypertension and ischaemic heart disease is essential and needs to be continued through the operative period, even though the patient may be unable to take oral drugs. Fast atrial fibrillation needs to be controlled before anaesthesia. Symptomatic disorders of sino-atrial conduction require pacemaker insertion before anaesthesia, as do all cases of either Mobitz type 2 second-degree block or third-degree heart block. In an emergency, transvenous temporary pacing wires or external pacing can be used. Modern variable-rate demand pacemakers may require resetting to fixed-rate mode, but are generally stable during anaesthesia. However, a cardiological opinion should be sought, bipolar diathermy employed if possible and the diathermy plate should be positioned so that the current does not cross the heart or pacemaker wires.

Recent myocardial infarction is a strong contraindication to elective anaesthesia. There is a significant mortality from anaesthesia within 3 months of infarction, and elective procedures should ideally be delayed until at least 6 months have elapsed.

Patients with valvular disease will need corrective treatment of any preoperative infections, and appropriate perioperative prophylactic antibiotic cover, to avoid subacute bacterial endocarditis.

Patients with cardiac disease need careful preoperative evaluation. Much can be derived from a detailed history including exercise tolerance and drug history. Echocardiography has enabled noninvasive assessment of cardiac function. Any electrolyte abnormality (especially hypokalaemia) or anaemia should be corrected and the circulatory volume should be maintained at normal level. Perioperatively, the presence of an adequate urine output is a useful indicator of adequacy of the circulating volume.

Operative procedures create an increased demand for oxygen due to pain, surgical stress and temperature loss. Patients with cardiac disease may need a period of elective postoperative mechanical pulmonary ventilation after surgery, until the period of raised oxygen consumption has passed. The careful anaesthetist and surgeon plan such care before surgery.

Respiratory disease

Thoracic surgical procedures demand specific preoperative tests of respiratory function including spirometry and blood gas analysis. In general surgical practice, respiratory infection and asthma are the common problems needing treatment before anaesthesia. In chronic respiratory failure, careful attention should be given to perioperative physiotherapy, early mobilisation and treatment of infection. Measurement of oxygen saturation and blood gas tensions preoperatively give a very useful guide to future values on recovery. The need for postoperative ventilatory support should be anticipated. Regional anaesthesia as appropriate is advantageous in respiratory disease. Upper abdominal and thoracic procedures are unsuited to regional anaesthesia alone, as positive pressure ventilation under general anesthesia is necessary.

Gastrointestinal disease

Aspiration of gastric contents carries a high risk of acid pneumonitis, pneumonia and death. Regurgitation in the presence of a hiatus hernia, or from 'the full stomach', may result from emergency (nonstarved) cases, bowel obstruction or paralytic ileus and indicates mandatory precautions during anaesthesia. A rapid sequence induction is conducted, in which the patient is 'preoxygenated' and cricoid pressure is applied from loss of consciousness until the lungs are protected by tracheal intubation. Bowel obstruction requires preoperative nasogastric aspiration and careful correction of fluid and electrolyte balance before anaesthesia is induced.

Woldemar Mobitz, b. 1889. German physician.

H_2-receptor blocking agents such as ranitidine are administered if there is an increased risk of regurgitation, ideally at least 2 hours preoperatively.

Anaesthesia in the presence of jaundice carries a high risk of renal damage. The anaesthetist should ensure that no hypovolaemia occurs and that a good urine output is present before induction, by the preoperative infusion of intravenous crystalloid solutions. A diuretic agent should only be used if the circulating volume is first assessed to be adequate.

Metabolic disorders

Familial porphyria and hyperpyrexia are hereditary metabolic disorders associated with high anaesthetic risks. Phaeochromocytoma is also associated with severe anaesthetic complications. The presence of these disorders requires highly specific preanaesthetic planning. Diabetes and adrenal suppression from steroid therapy are also common metabolic disorders which complicate anaesthesia.

Noninsulin-dependent diabetic patients on diet and oral hypoglycaemic agents will need blood sugar measurement during anaesthesia. An intravenous infusion of glucose may be required if the long-acting hypoglycaemic effects persist even if the agent was omitted on the day of surgery.

Except for minor surgery, an intravenous infusion of glucose with soluble insulin is likely to be necessary with close monitoring and control of blood sugar levels. Insulin-dependent diabetes always needs preoperative conversion to control with rapidly acting soluble insulin by intravenous infusion on the operative day, and this is continued until the patient has recovered from the operation. In practice, for maintenance of blood sugar levels, it is best to keep a constant infusion of 5–10 per cent glucose with potassium supplementation through a separate intravenous channel at about 2 litres/24 hours. Soluble short-acting insulin is given continuously by intravenous syringe pump, with the rate indicated by frequent (1–4-hourly) measurement of blood glucose concentration. The plasma potassium level needs careful control. The circulating volume should be manipulated independently via a separate infusion of normal saline, blood or colloid. In this way a steady control of blood glucose concentration can be easily achieved by an experienced nurse.

Patients who are receiving corticosteroids or who have received them in the past 2 months require supplemention with hydrocortisone during and after surgery to avoid adrenal insufficiency (Addisonian crisis).

Coagulation disorders

Whether iatrogenic (including therapeutic) or pathological in origin, coagulation disorders need careful assessment before surgery with a coagulation screen, or clotting factor and platelet measurements. In acquired disorders, such as disseminated intravascular coagulation, fresh frozen plasma or cryoprecipitate and platelets may be given to the patient by the anaesthetist perioperatively to control haemorrhage. Patients receiving therapeutic warfarin need to cease treatment several days preoperatively and have prothrombin time (PT) measurement until the International Normalised Ratio (INR) falls to about 1.5 from the therapeutic range of 2.0–4.2. At an INR of 1.5, surgical haemostasis should be achieved. Vitamin K can be used to hasten the reversal of warfarin but it is a long-acting agent and can cause weeks of resistance to warfarin after surgery, so it is better to avoid it. When the risk of thrombosis and embolism is high, an intravenous infusion of heparin can be used to replace warfarin. The heparin can be stopped or reversed with protamine for the period of surgery. Rapid control of heparin activity is easy, but it is not so with warfarin.

Neurological disease

In cerebral disease and trauma, hypoxia, hypercarbia and respiratory obstruction raise intracranial pressure and can cause cerebral damage. In the presence of deteriorating consciousness, management of the airway and ventilation is of prime importance, and especially so in traumatic injury in which early endotracheal intubation and pulmonary ventilation should precede supine positioning for computed tomography (CT) of the brain. Particular care of the neck during intubation is necessary if a cervical fracture is suspected. Skull traction and awake intubation under local anaesthesia are sometimes used.

Anticonvulsant drugs must be continued during surgery on epileptic patients, and this may necessitate using intravenous administration.

In peripheral neuropathies and myopathies, the need for prolonged periods of postoperative ventilation should be anticipated.

Anaesthesia and psychiatric disease

General, rather than regional, anaesthesia is usually necessary. Tricyclic antidepressants and monoamine oxidase inhibitor drugs potentiate sympathomimetic agents so adrenaline and cocaine must be avoided. Pethidine can also cause hypertension with these drugs. Other narcotic analgesic agents can be used but caution is necessary as their side effects can be potentiated, especially with monoamine oxidase inhibitors.

Starvation before surgery

Standard practice for many years has been 6 hours' abstinence from food and 4 hours' abstinence from fluids. Recently, there has been a shift to permit clear, nonfizzy fluids up to 2 hours preoperatively. These rules apply whenever loss of protective laryngeal reflexes may pertain, as during regional anaesthesia and sedation. Small children are usually given a glucose drink about 4 hours preoperatively to prevent perioperative hypoglycaemia.

Thomas Addison, 1793–1860. Physician, Guy's Hospital, London, England.

Consent for surgery and anaesthesia

Informed consent should be obtained by the surgical team, preferably the operating surgeon, before any sedation is given, but the anaesthetist should still explain anaesthetic procedures, especially regional and spinal techniques, and discuss potential sequelae.

Preoperative drugs and treatment

Preoperative sedative and analgesic medication is becoming much less common. Heavy sedative, antiemetic, antitussive, amnesic medication was previously used for the relatively unpleasant inductions of anaesthesia with pungent inhalational agents. Except for patients who are already in pain, opioid analgesic agents are generally first given during induction of anaesthesia, administered intravenously for rapid onset of action prior to surgery. For reduction of anxiety, oral short-acting benzodiazepines are now more commonly used 1–2 hours preoperatively, especially for children. Oral trimeprazine is also still popular for children.

For the increasing numbers of day-case procedures, preoperative sedation is avoided so as to promote rapid emergence from anaesthesia and mobilisation.

The anticholinergic agents, atropine, glycopyrronium and hyoscine, are used to reduce respiratory and oral secretions. They are not essential with modern anaesthetic agents, but still useful for airway surgery and endoscopy. Atropine and glycopyrronium also protect against vagal dysrhythmias, for which administration at induction is just as effective, and can cause alertness and tachycardia. Hyoscine is pleasantly sedative without the cardiac effects of atropine, but it can cause excessive sedation in infants or the elderly.

Antithrombotic prophylaxis is usually initiated preoperatively in major surgery, commonly by subcutaneous heparin injection. Particular attention must be given to higher risk patients such as women taking contraceptive and hormone-replacement drugs, and those undergoing pelvic, hip, knee and cancer surgery. Low-dose progesterone preparations may be effectively covered by subcutaneous heparin, but other less commonly prescribed forms of contraceptive hormone treatment may need to be stopped 1 month before major surgery.

Preoperative chest physiotherapy, possibly with bronchodilator treatment, may be indicated.

If indicated, prophylactic antibiotic agents are given by the anaesthetist in concert with the surgeon, either with the premedication or intravenously at induction of anaesthesia.

General anaesthesia

Induction of anaesthesia

Intravenous injection is most common in contemporary practice, although the recent introduction of nonpungent sevoflurane has led to renewed use of inhalational induction. Inhalational induction is useful in young children, or 'needle phobic' adults, and may also be used in patients who are at risk of airway obstruction or pulmonary aspiration (of, for example, blood) when the patient is put into the lateral position with head-down tilt to drain the fluid away from the trachea. For intravenous induction, propofol with its rapid recovery is replacing the long-standing barbiturate agent, thiopentone. Analgesic agents are frequently also injected at the time of anaesthetic induction.

Maintenance of anaesthesia

Following the induction of anaesthesia, inhalational volatile or intravenous anaesthetic agents are continuously administered to maintain an adequate depth of anaesthesia. Adding nitrous oxide contributes analgesic and weak anaesthetic effects, which reduce the concentration of volatile anaesthetic agent required for maintenance. To provide a safety margin, at least 30 per cent oxygen is added to the inspired mixture. Although still employed in some parts of the world, ether has generally been replaced by halothane, enflurane and isoflurane. Desflurane and sevoflurane are the most recently introduced agents, conferring the advantages of fewer side effects and more rapid recovery.

The use of nitrous oxide is slowly waning, as oxygen-enriched air with volatile or intravenous maintenance gains popularity.

If compressed sources of oxygen, nitrous oxide or air are scarce, then air may be drawn into the anaesthetic circuit, either by the (unparalysed) patient's own respiratory effort or by a mechanical ventilator.

Total intravenous anaesthesia, a technique undergoing contemporary resurgence, avoids the use of inhalational anaesthetic agents and is claimed to provide enhanced quality and rapidity of recovery. It is also used when inhalational anaesthesia may be impractical, such as during airway laser surgery or endoscopy, and is popular for cardiopulmonary bypass. It is also indicated in spinal surgery during neurophysiological monitoring of cord integrity, as evoked potential signals are suppressed by inhalational anaesthesia. Intravenous anaesthesia avoids atmospheric pollution, and is usually conducted by infusing propofol and a short-acting opioid analgesic agent, such as fentanyl or alfentanil, in combination with neuromuscular block and pulmonary ventilation with a mixture of air and oxygen.

Management of the airway during anaesthesia

General anaesthesia reduces the tone of the muscles required to preserve airway patency, and hence the need for manual methods (e.g. jaw thrust), or devices such as the Guedel or laryngeal mask airways, or endotracheal tubes.

Sir Ivan Magill developed the endotracheal tube during World War I to facilitate plastic surgery around the mouth

---

Arthue E. Guedel, b. 1883. American anaesthesiologist.

Sir Ivan Magill, KCVO, 1888–1986. Anaesthetist, Westminster, Brompton and Dreadnought Hospitals, London, England. Pioneered nasotracheal intubation, direct laryngoscopy and endobronchial intubation.

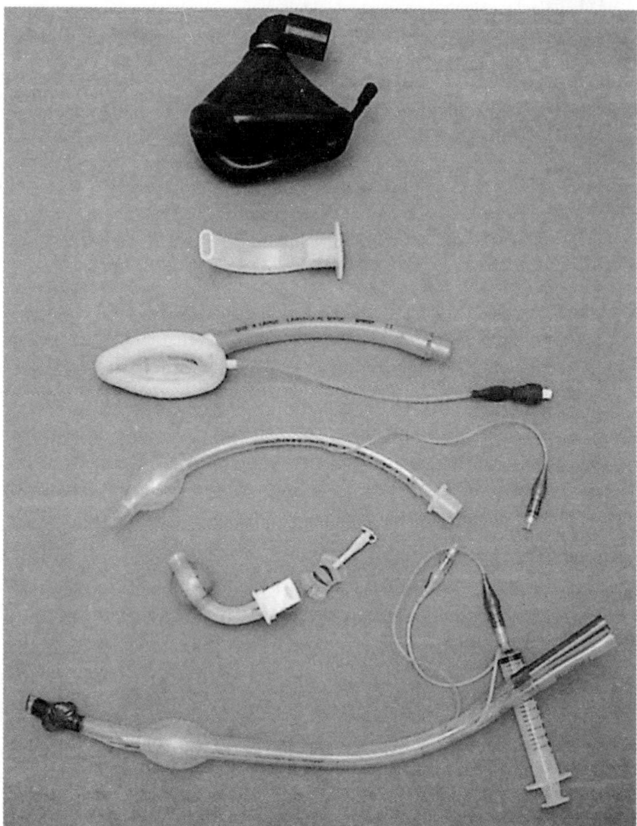

Fig. 6.1 Instruments for control of the airway. Descending from the mouth to the bronchus: face mask and oropharyngeal airway; laryngeal mask; oro- or nasotracheal tube (cuff inflated); cuffed tracheostomy tube; double-lumen right endobronchial tube (tracheal and bronchial cuffs) (*courtesy of R.M. Bowen-Wright*).

without a face mask. The addition of a cuff to the tube allowed a seal of the trachea to protect the lungs from aspiration of blood or secretions, and later mechanical positive pressure pulmonary ventilation.

The following means of airway control in the anaesthetised or unconscious patient are used (Fig. 6.1).

Positioning of the tongue and jaw

The anaesthetist thrusts the jaw forward, from behind the temporomandibular joints, thereby elevating the tongue off the posterior pharyngeal wall, which may also be achieved by inserting an artificial oropharyngeal airway such as the 'Guedel'. The anaesthetic gases are given through a face mask.

The *laryngeal mask airway* (LMA) (developed by Archie Brain) is also inserted via the mouth, and is positioned with the mask over the larynx, sealed by an inflatable cuff. It frees the anaesthetist's hands from holding the patient's jaw or face mask. Its placement is less stimulating than endotracheal intubation. It has proved to be a reliable means of maintaining a patent airway, and is a technique readily taught to nonanaesthetists for emergency airway management. It is likely to replace the face mask for immediate care prior to endotracheal intubation.

The *endotracheal tube* may be passed into the trachea via either the mouth or the nose. It is usually placed by direct laryngoscopy, using a laryngoscope, but it is occasionally impossible to visualise the larynx. A fibre-optic technique may be used in which the tracheal tube is 'rail-roaded' over the flexible laryngoscope, once the tip has been steered into the trachea.

A cuffed endotracheal tube is used to facilitate artificial ventilation or surgery around the face or airway, and to protect the lungs if there is a risk of pulmonary aspiration. If fluid may collect in the mouth from above (as in nasal surgery), a throat pack is placed in the oropharynx.

Although endotracheal intubation is generally straightforward, complications do occur:

- accidental and unrecognised oesophageal intubation;
- accidental intubation of a main bronchus;
- trauma to larynx, trachea or teeth;
- aspiration of vomitus during neuromuscular blockade for intubation;
- failure to intubate and loss of airway control;
- disconnection or blockage of the tube;
- delayed tracheal stenosis, in children or after prolonged intubation.

Careful observation of physical signs and constant vigilance, aided by pulse oximetry, capnography of the expiratory gases, inspiratory oxygen concentration measurement and ventilator disconnection alarms are mandatory to minimise these risks.

Tracheostomy tube

Anaesthesia can safely be conducted through a tracheostomy tube but it should have an inflatable cuff for airway control. Silver or fenestrated tracheostomy tubes should therefore be replaced by plastic cuffed tubes at induction of anaesthesia.

Endobronchial tube

In pulmonary and open oesophageal surgery, selective intubation of either bronchus is usual to facilitate deflation of the lung on the operated side. Its use is essential to protect the normal lung in the presence of a bronchopleural fistula.

Ventilation through a bronchoscope

The lungs can be ventilated during bronchoscopy by intermittent jets of oxygen down a cannula within the bronchoscope. The oxygen entrains air by the Venturi effect to generate enough pressure and flow to inflate the lungs.

The technique demands constant observation of the patient's chest movement.

Dr Archie Brain invented the LMA in a development effort spanning 1981–88.

Giovanni B. Venturi, b. 1746. Italian physicist.

Neuromuscular blockade during surgery

Pharmacological blockade of neuromuscular transmission provides relaxation of muscles to facilitate surgery and mechanical positive pressure ventilation. Muscle tone may also be reduced by very deep anaesthesia, but may compromise the circulation. Neuromuscular blockade demands complete control of the airway and ventilation by the anaesthetist. The depolarising muscle relaxant, suxamethonium, rapidly provides excellent intubating conditions of brief duration, but commonly causes postoperative diffuse muscle pains, and rarely may cause a prolonged block if the patient is deficient in plasma pseudocholinesterase.

The competitive neuromuscular blocking agents such as curare and its modern successors produce a prolonged effect which may persist into the postoperative period. Atracurium, cisatracurium, vecuronium and rocuronium share more predictable activity profiles and are less dependent on hepatorenal function. A peripheral nerve stimulator is also used to check for adequate depth of blockade during surgery, and to confirm satisfactory recovery of neuromuscular function prior to extubation of the trachea. The advent of neuromuscular blockade in the 1940s facilitated many advances in abdominal and thoracic surgery, but introduced the risk of accidental patient awareness during surgery.

Haemostasis and blood pressure control

Although the dangers of profound hypotension are nowadays well accepted, a 20–30 per cent reduction of mean arterial blood pressure from the awake preoperative level in fit patients is still deemed acceptable, and can greatly improve the quality of the operative field and reduce total blood loss. Reduction of venous pressure at the wound by correct patient positioning and avoidance of any causes of venous obstruction (Fig. 6.2), and maintenance of satisfactorily deep anaesthesia and slightly reduced arterial carbon dioxide tension, further contribute to providing a dry surgical field.

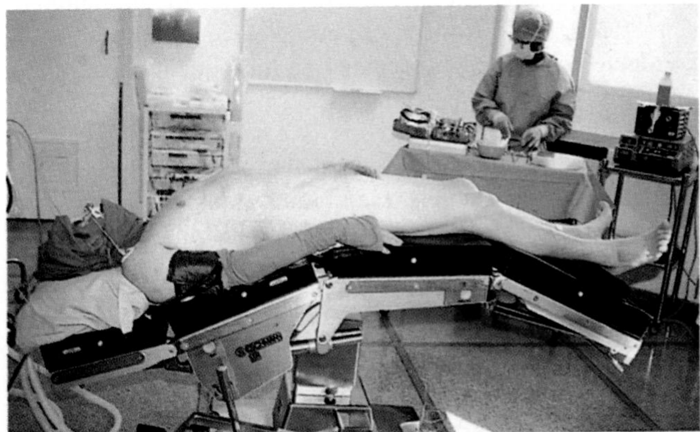

Fig. 6.2 Position for retropubic prostatectomy. A good operative field with controlled hypotension is obtained by positioning the operative site at the apex of the body – a principle for all surgery (*courtesy of R.T. Turner-Warwick, CBE*).

Hypotensive drugs may be used to produce deliberate controlled hypotension if there is a clear surgical benefit to be obtained, although preservation of cerebral perfusion and oxygenation remains paramount. The surgeon must be aware of the prevailing blood pressure, particularly at the time of ensuring satisfactory haemostasis prior to wound closure. Usually, the anaesthetist will attempt to bring the blood pressure back to the normal level at this stage of the procedure.

Management of temperature during anaesthesia

Hypothermia develops quickly during anaesthesia and surgery due to vasodilation, cold infusions of fluid, and loss of body heat by radiation and fluid evaporation from open body cavities. It is a particular hazard in children because of the high ratio of body surface area to body mass. The elderly are also at particular risk as hypothermia and shivering increase oxygen consumption and vascular resistance, predisposing to myocardial infarction. In high-risk patients and for long operations, warm air blowers and warming blankets should be used, and fluids for intravenous infusion, or irrigation of body cavities or organs (such as the bladder and renal pelvis), should be warmed to body temperature. Careful intraoperative temperature control greatly reduces postoperative morbidity.

Monitoring during anaesthesia

Accurate monitoring of vital functions during anaesthesia is now regarded as obligatory in all parts of the world. Surgery should not be practised where proper facilities for monitoring and cardiopulmonary resuscitation are not available. The basic parameters monitored are inspiratory oxygen concentration, oxygen saturation by pulse oximetry, expiratory carbon dioxide tension measurement, blood pressure and the electrocardiogram. For major surgery, invasive, direct monitoring of the circulation is used, but the potential value of information gained must be weighed against the possible dangers of placing intra-arterial or central venous or pulmonary artery catheters. Hourly observation of urine output via a urinary catheter is most helpful in assessing renal perfusion. Ventilators should all have airway pressure monitors and disconnection alarms.

In the UK, the Association of Anaesthetists recommends the following standards of routine monitoring in the anaesthetised patient (Fig. 6.3):

- the continuous presence of an adequately trained anaesthetist;
- regular blood pressure and heart rate measurements (recorded);
- continuous monitoring of the electrocardiography (ECG) throughout anaesthesia;
- continuous analysis of the oxygen content in the inspiratory gas mixture;
- oxygen supply failure alarm;
- ventilator disconnection alarm;

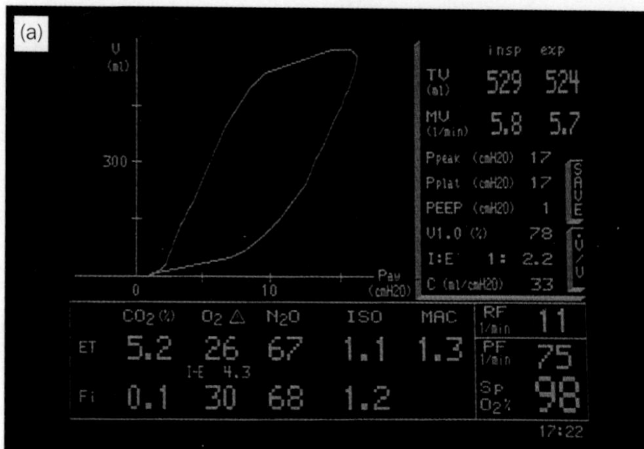

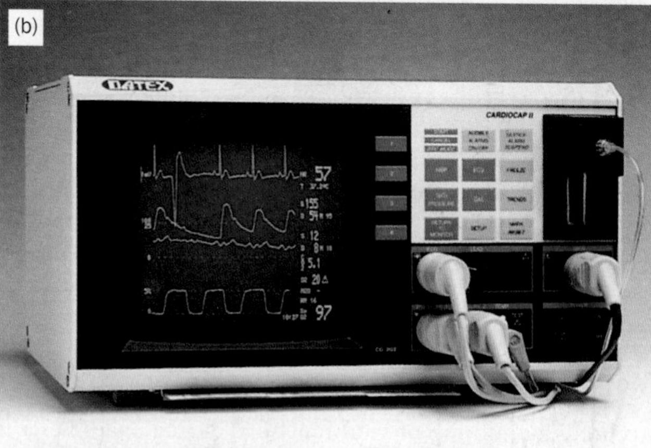

Fig. 6.3 Anaesthetic monitoring devices. (a) Respiratory parameters, including spirograph and volatile agent concentration (International Standards Organisation); (b) cardiac monitoring (electrocardiography, heart rate, arterial and central venous pressures, pulse oximetry and body temperature) (*courtesy of Datex*).

- pulse oximeter;
- capnography (measurement of end-tidal carbon dioxide content);
- temperature measurement availability;
- neuromuscular monitoring availability.

In the USA, spirometry during anaesthesia is regarded as necessary.

Recovery from general anaesthesia

Recovery from general anaesthesia should be closely supervised by trained nursing staff in an area equipped with the means of resuscitation and with adequate monitoring devices. An anaesthetist should be readily available. For the seriously ill patient, a high dependency unit or intensive care unit may be necessary until the patient's condition is satisfactory and stable. The transition from tracheal intubation with ventilatory support to spontaneous breathing with an unprotected airway is a time of increased risk, when respiratory arrest or obstruction may occur.

The common causes of failure to breathe after general anaesthesia are:

- obstruction of the airway;
- central sedation from opioid drugs or anaesthetic agents;
- hypoxia or hypercarbia of any cause;
- hypocarbia from mechanical overventilation;
- persistent neuromuscular blockade;
- pneumothorax from pleural damage during anaesthesia or surgery;
- circulatory failure leading to respiratory arrest.

Management of blood pressure in the recovery room

Hypotension

This may be due to hypovolaemia, prolonged vasodilation or myocardial depressant effects of anaesthetic drugs, cardiac dysrhythmia or hypoxaemia. Management is by treatment of the cause.

Hypertension

Hypertension is common postoperatively, usually of brief duration and associated with peripheral vasoconstriction due to pain, fear, cold or shivering, or pre-existing hypertensive disease. Hypertension predisposes to cerebral and myocardial damage, and needs active management. If it persists in the presence of adequate pain relief, sublingual nifedipine and intravenous labetalol or hydralazine are useful. Rarely, control with more powerful intravenous drugs such as sodium nitroprusside or glyceryl trinitrate is necessary, in conjunction with direct intra-arterial blood pressure monitoring.

General anaesthesia for day-case surgery

Day-case management already accounts for about 40 per cent of procedures in UK hospitals and is intended to reach over 60 per cent. While the principles remain the same, it is even more necessary for the day-case patient to recover rapidly from general anaesthesia and mobilise with the minimum of side-effects. Longer and more complex operations are now conducted as day cases, demanding high-quality anaesthesia and effective analgesic strategies.

Careful selection of patients is essential with regard to coexisting diseases, the nature of the proposed surgery, the availability of a suitable escort and transport home, and domiciliary care. Well-controlled nondebilitating chronic diseases do not preclude day care, but may require a longer period of postoperative supervision before permitting discharge home.

General anaesthesia combined with regional anaesthesia, as for inguinal hernia repair, is often suitable. Anaesthetics which promote rapid recovery such as propofol, sevoflurane and desflurane are used. Drugs with prolonged depressant central action, including premedicant drugs, are avoided and, where possible, analgesics should act peripherally or be of short duration if centrally acting. Where possible, patients are managed with a laryngeal mask or face mask, although endotracheal intubation is the necessary airway control for many day cases such as oral or ear, nose and throat (ENT) procedures, and is generally uncomplicated.

With the patient relatively isolated from immediate medical supervision and advice, postoperative analgesia must be carefully tailored to the procedure, especially in the case of the more painful procedures (such as hernia repair, haemorrhoidectomy, tubal surgery, meniscectomy) for which stronger analgesics and combinations should be provided. Regular postoperative dosing is recommended to avoid breakthrough pain, as may particularly occur following the initial benefits of local anaesthetic.

General anaesthesia and cardiopulmonary bypass

The technique is discussed in Chapter 48 of this book.

Anaesthetic agents and oxygen cannot be delivered to the circulation through the lungs when the lungs are bypassed, so all drugs are given directly into a vein or into the blood while it passes through the oxygenator.

Local anaesthesia

Choice of a local anaesthetic technique depends upon its feasibility for a particular procedure and the patient's willingness and ability to co-operate, as well the surgeon's and anaesthetist's preference. Local anaesthesia may be the reliable and traditional method for some minor surgical procedures which do not warrant general anaesthesia. One of the main advantages is the continuation of pain relief into the postoperative period, by either drugs with a prolonged duration of action or delivery of further local anaesthetic increments via a catheter.

However, local anaesthesia is not infallible, and may be contraindicated by allergy or local infection. Epidural and intrathecal anaesthesia includes sympathetic blockade which may result in vasodilatation and systemic hypotension, and may confer greater intraoperative risk than a carefully managed general anaesthetic.

Complications may be local, such as infection or haematoma, or systemic if overdosage or accidental intravascular injection leads to toxic blood levels. The latter may manifest as depressed conscious level, convulsions and/or cardiac arrest (particularly bupivacaine), and may be heralded by circum-oral paraesthesia and light-headedness. Addition of adrenaline to the local anaesthetic solution increases the risk of cardiac arrhythmia associated with accidental intravascular injection. Prilocaine overdosage causes methaemoglobinaemia. Recently introduced local anaesthetics such as ropivicaine and laevo-bupivacaine are claimed to have enhanced safety profiles.

Addition of adrenaline (commonly 1:200 000–1:125 000 concentration) to the local anaesthetic solution hastens the onset and prolongs the duration of action, and permits a higher dose of drug to be used as it is more slowly absorbed into the circulation. Adrenaline should not be used in hypertensive patients, or for patients taking either monoamine oxidase inhibitor or tricyclic antidepressant drugs, as its cardiovascular effects are potentiated. It should not be used in end-arterial locations, where there is no collateral circulation, such as fingers and toes, or around the retinal artery.

The potential risk of life-threatening sequelae mandates the availability of appropriately skilled personnel and resuscitation equipment including oxygen, as prerequisites if local anaesthesia is practised.

The following exemplify sensible upper dose limits suitable for a 70 kg adult.

- Lignocaine 200 mg (10 ml of 2 per cent) or lignocaine with adrenaline (1:200 000) 500 mg. Lignocaine 1 per cent is effective for most sensory blocks and addition of adrenaline enables a greater volume to be used. Thus, up to 50 ml of lignocaine 1 per cent with adrenaline (1:200 000) can be infiltrated into the tissues.
- Bupivacaine 150 mg (30 ml of 0.5 per cent). Addition of adrenaline would enhance the safety of this high dose. Bupivacaine is more cardiotoxic than lignocaine. Bupivacaine 0.25 per cent is effective for sensory block against moderate stimulus. Bupivacaine must never be injected into a vein, and is absolutely contraindicated from use for intravenous regional anaesthesia. (Bier's block is commonly used for procedures such as reduction of Colle's fracture and carpal tunnel decompression.) Bupivacaine is a long-acting drug lasting for about 6 hours.
- Prilocaine 400 mg (40 ml of 1 per cent). The presence of blue–brown skin colour indicates methaemoglobin toxicity.

Topical anaesthesia

Topical anaesthetic agents are used on the skin, the urethral mucosa, nasal mucosa and the cornea. The agents used are amethocaine, because it is well absorbed by mucosa, cocaine for its vasoconstrictive properties, lignocaine and prilocaine. A lignocaine and prilocaine eutectic mixture ('EMLA' cream) is commonly used on the skin of children before venepuncture.

Local infiltration

This is the method most commonly used by both surgeons and physicians. It is not necessary to starve the patient preoperatively unless the procedure carries a high risk of intravascular or intrathecal injection. Infiltration of local anaesthetic drug may be into or around a wound, ideally with particular attention to neuroanatomical territories and boundaries. Contraindications are local infection

August Karl Gustav Bier, 1861–92. Berlin surgeon.

Abraham Colles, 1777–1843. Professor of Surgery, Royal College of Surgeons in Ireland (1804–36) and Surgeon Doctor, Steven's Hospital, Dublin, Ireland.

and clotting disorder. Not only will local infiltration spread the infection, but local anaesthetic drugs are ineffective in conditions of acidity as produced by infection. Local infiltration in the presence of a clotting disorder may result in haemorrhage, or may produce haematoma, potentially fatal in the airway, as in dentistry.

Regional anaesthesia (without general anaesthesia)

Regional anaesthesia involves blockade of major nerve trunks which innervate the site of surgery. It is usually performed by an anaesthetist with the necessary skills. However, both intrathecal (spinal) and epidural anaesthesia should only be conducted by experienced practitioners using full aseptic techniques.

It is in any case required that a doctor other than the operator is present to monitor continuously and resuscitate the patient if necessary. If regional anaesthesia fails, general anaesthesia may be necessary. Compensation for an inadequate regional block by heavy sedation carries great dangers including airway obstruction and pulmonary aspiration of gastric contents. These may easily go unrecognised by a single-handed operator. All patients should be starved preoperatively and monitored. In emergency surgery, regional anaesthesia carries the advantage of preservation of the protective laryngeal reflexes, particularly in emergency obstetric anaesthesia, for which epidural or spinal regional anaesthesia is commonly the method of choice. The reduction in blood pressure with spinal and epidural anaesthesia can be advantageous in reducing intraoperative blood loss, but only if the surgeon strives to achieve haemostasis prior to wound closure and restoration of normal blood pressure.

When sedation has been used for surgery under regional anaesthesia, respiratory obstruction may occur postoperatively when the surgical stimulus has ceased. Oxygen saturation measurement by pulse oximetry is required monitoring during regional anaesthesia.

Regional anaesthesia had a very clear advantage over general anaesthesia when general anaesthetic agents carried high morbidity and mortality rates. In contemporary practice this advantage is less pronounced or even reversed. However, regional anaesthesia may be advantageous for patients who have debilitating respiratory disease. In cardiovascular disease, general anaesthesia with support of the circulation and pulmonary ventilation is often more advantageous than risking hypotension and tachyarrhythmias exacerbating ischaemic heart disease and resultant angina, which may occur with regional anaesthesia. Regional anaesthesia does provide excellent analgesia into the postoperative period, reducing the need for centrally acting analgesic agents.

The most clear indications for spinal and epidural anaesthesia are in obstetric practice to spare the mother from the risk of pulmonary aspiration because of the full stomach usually present in labour, and also to spare the newborn from the depressant action of the general anaesthetic and analgesic drugs.

General and regional anaesthesia combined

Combining the two methods of anaesthesia in well-balanced measure enables a patient to receive a lighter general anaesthetic and to have the advantage of good postoperative analgesia. At its simplest, the infiltration of an abdominal wound with local anaesthetic agent will facilitate comfortable breathing in the recovery room.

Regional local anaesthetic techniques

Spinal, plexus and major nerve local anaesthetic blockade may be employed alone or in combination with sedation or general anaesthesia. It is most commonly used for limb, abdominal and thoracic surgery, and obstetric analgesia and surgery.

It is imperative that a second medical practitioner, and not the surgical operator, is responsible for supervision and monitoring of the patient during the procedure.

Preoperative patient preparation for elective regional anaesthesia includes that required for general anaesthesia, with explanation of the local anaesthetic procedure. In emergency, it is safer to use regional anaesthesia on an unstarved patient rather than general anaesthesia, for the risk of aspiration of gastric contents is much reduced although not absent. Some forms of regional anaesthesia with long-acting drugs, such as epidural bupivacaine anaesthesia, result in prolonged motor block and may be unsuitable if the patient is expected to be an ambulant day case.

The recently introduced subcutaneous low-molecular-weight heparins (LMWH) for prophylaxis for deep venous thrombosis are longer acting than heparin, and appear to have increased the risk of intraspinal haematoma. Epidural and spinal injections (and catheter insertion or removal) should only be performed at least 12 hours after a LMWH dose, and the next LMWH dose delayed for at least 2 hours. The LMWH doses must therefore be timed appropriately. As with many perioperative management issues, optimal care depends upon close liaison between anaesthetist and surgeon.

Electrocardiogram, pulse oximetry and blood pressure measurements should be performed during regional anaesthesia. Oxygen by face mask should be given to frail or sedated patients during surgery.

Common local anaesthetic techniques

In awake patients the nerve blocks must provide comprehensive numbness throughout the surgical field. The following field blocks are commonly used.

- Brachial plexus block for surgery on the arm or hand.
- Field block for inguinal hernia repair. The iliohypogastric and ilioinguinal nerves are blocked immediately inferomedial to the anterior superior iliac spine. The genitofemoral nerve is infiltrated at the midinguinal point and at the pubic tubercle. If a large volume of local anaesthetic is used, the peritoneal sac can be anaesthetised before the incision, but care must be taken to avoid drug toxicity.

Local anaesthetic with 1:200 000 adrenaline prolongs the duration of action and reduces toxicity by producing vasoconstriction. The line of the skin incision should be infiltrated with the mixture.

- Regional block of the ankle. This can be used for surgery on the toes and minor surgery of the foot.

Intravenous regional anaesthesia

The arm to be operated on is exsanguinated by elevation and/or compression, and then isolated from the general circulation by the application of a tourniquet inflated to a pressure well in excess of the systolic arterial pressure. The venous system is then filled with local anaesthetic agent, injected via a previously placed indwelling venous cannula. The drug diffuses from the bloodstream into the nerves to produce an effective block. The arm is more suitable for this procedure (Bier's block) than the leg because the large volume of drug required for the latter can easily lead to toxicity. The tourniquet must only be deflated after adequate time has elapsed (at least 20 minutes) to allow for the residual venous drug load to fall to a safe level, before it is washed back into the general circulation. Cardiac arrest or convulsions may well occur if the tourniquet is accidentally released before the drug is fixed; this was particularly noted with bupivacaine, which has been banned from use in this procedure after reports both of a number of deaths and of directly toxic effects on the heart. Prilocaine 0.5 per cent up to 50 ml is recommended as the safest agent to use. As above, a separate medical practitioner should supervise the block and monitor the patient, while the surgeon operates.

Intrathecal anaesthesia

Spinal anaesthesia in the awake patient is useful for some forms of surgery in the pelvis or lower limbs. Hyperbaric solutions of bupivacaine are injected as a 'single shot' into the cerebrospinal fluid, to produce rapidly an intense blockade, usually within 5 minutes. Autonomic sympathetic blockade results in hypotension, necessitating prior intravenous fluid loading and titration of vasoconstrictor drugs. If the hyperbaric solution is allowed to ascend too high, severe hypotension and ventilatory failure occur. This factor limits the use of spinal anaesthesia to surgery below the segmental level of T10.

Postoperative headache, due to cerebrospinal fluid leakage through the dural perforation, is nowadays much less common as a result of modern needles (very fine with a round or pencil point tip and side aperture) designed to split rather than cut the dural fibres.

Spinal anaesthesia is much used for Caesarean section, prostatectomy and lower limb surgery. Intrathecal opioid drugs are used to produce postoperative analgesia but there is a significant risk of respiratory depression.

Epidural anaesthesia

Epidural anaesthesia is slower in onset than intrathecal anaesthesia, but has the advantage of multiple dosing and hence prolonged use, as an indwelling catheter may be threaded into the epidural space. Hence, epidural anaesthesia can provide good pain relief extending into the postoperative period. Urinary retention is common, necessitating catheterisation of the bladder. Epidural anaesthesia also includes sympathetic blockade, but it is of slower onset, as is the resulting hypotension, which may be easier to control and can be used to advantage for the surgery, in reduction of blood loss. If a weak solution of bupivacaine or the newer ropivicaine is chosen, epidural anaesthesia can be used to produce a predominantly sensory block for analgesia after upper abdominal or thoracic surgery. The contemporary trend is to combine weak solutions of local anaesthetic with opioid agents such as the lipid-soluble diamorphine or fentanyl, the latter producing analgesia by their action on the opioid receptors in the spinal cord. However, the potential complication of epidural opioid analgesia is delayed respiratory arrest from rostral spread and central depression, as late as 24 hours after the last dose. Hence, regular monitoring of conscious level and respiratory rate, and facility to immediately reverse the opioid with intravenous naloxone or to resuscitate, are essential prerequisites.

Epidural anaesthesia (with bupivacaine or ropivicaine) remains the standard method of anaesthesia during labour and interventional delivery. In contrast to local anaesthetic agents, epidural opioid agents alone do not produce hypotension, so they are preferable for patients who are mobile. There is a current trend towards their use in labour for this reason, but alone they would not produce adequate analgesia for surgical intervention.

Caudal epidural anaesthesia is produced by injection of local anaesthetic agent through the sacrococcygeal membrane. Its main uses are to supplement general anaesthesia and for very effective postoperative pain relief. This analgesic technique is much used in paediatric surgery.

Perioperative pain relief (acute pain management)

Optimal management of acute postoperative pain requires planning, patient and staff education, and tailoring to the type of surgery and the needs of the individual patient. Patients vary greatly (up to eight-fold) in their requirement for analgesia, even after identical surgical procedures. Undertreatment results in unacceptable levels of pain with tachycardia, hypertension, vasoconstriction and 'splinting' of the affected part. Painful abdominal and thoracic wounds restrict inspiration, leading to tachypnoea, small tidal volumes, and inhibition of the patient from effective coughing and mobilisation. This predisposes to chest infection, delayed mobilisation, deep venous thrombosis, muscle wasting and pressure sores.

However, analgesic administration above the patient's requirement increases the risks of side effects such as nausea, vomiting, somnolence and dizziness or, if greatly in excess, severe central effects including depressed consciousness and respiration. This is fortunately rare, and can be avoided by sensible initial dosing followed by titration until the patient is comfortable. Exaggerated fears of opioid-induced central depression and addiction have led all too commonly to inhibition amongst staff from prescribing and administering adequate doses of opioids. Intermittent intramuscular dosing also leads to delays in administration of the 'controlled' opioids compounded by the time to onset of action of action.

As a result of these common deficiencies, a Joint Working Party of the Royal Colleges of Anaesthetists and Surgeons was convened, which published the report *Pain after Surgery* in 1990. It recommended the establishment of acute pain teams, comprising medical and nursing specialists, to oversee the implementation of guidelines for practice including routine recording of pain levels, and educating both staff and patients. Combinations of analgesic methods [local anaesthesia and nonsteroidal anti-inflammatory drugs (NSAIDs) with opioid drugs] were advocated, as were the more sophisticated methods of pain management such as 'patient-controlled analgesia'.

The Working Party report also encouraged further use of combined treatments (termed balanced analgesia) such as with:

- local anaesthetic blocks – excellent short-term analgesia, but requires skill and has a small failure rate. Continuous catheter techniques prolong pain relief but are only appropriate for inpatients;
- spinal opioids – generally very useful for appropriate types of surgery, but again requires skill, and is limited by concerns over severe respiratory depression;
- NSAIDs – in combination reduce requirement for opioids and alone are useful for moderate pain, but are limited by concerns over side effects, such as renal impairment, peptic ulceration and inducing acute bronchospasm in asthmatics. They are not adequate as sole analgesic therapy after major surgery.

The report called for further research and, amongst other aims, hoped for the advent of a powerful analgesic on a par with morphine, but without marked respiratory depressant activity. While the development of tailor-made opioid agonists with differential receptor activity has not yet solved this problem, attention turned more to finding alternative pathways at which to attenuate the afferent pain impulses. For example, clonidine has been administered epidurally to stimulate the spinal cord adrenergic inhibitory mechanisms.

Severe acute pain increases morbidity after trauma or surgery.

Appreciation of pain pathways and the three main classes of pain – nociceptive, neuropathic/sympathetic and that of mainly psychological origin – together with enhanced awareness of pain, has led to new and multimodal treatment strategies.

The methods of prevention are:

- adequate analgesia by intravenous narcotic drugs at the time of surgery;
- regional anaesthesia alone or supplementing general anaesthesia during surgery to prevent excitation of central pathways;
- the use of prostaglandin inhibitory drugs during surgery. Diclofenac suppositories are effective in reducing the pain from tissue damage in bone and muscle, and are used at the time of operation.

These three approaches used together are good at preventing the cycle of pain and muscle spasm from becoming established in the recovery period.

The same methods can be used for managing the pain of acute trauma.

Postoperative pain management

Severe pain from a large incision in a frail patient may require high doses of intravenous opiate drugs leading to elective postoperative endotracheal intubation and ventilation until the patient is stable. This approach should be used if the patient is likely to become hypoxic through struggling in pain if other methods of pain relief are not effective. Other methods of pain relief, properly used, can usually prevent the need for mechanical ventilation even in very major thoracic and abdominal surgery. Acute pain relief teams, using continuous methods of pain relief in high dependency areas well equipped with monitoring, are becoming a routine feature of the postoperative care in both the USA and the UK. Regular intramuscular morphine injection, supplemented by anti-inflammatory analgesic drugs and, possibly, a regional anaesthetic block, are effective treatment for the majority of surgical patients. Each patient should have a pain relief measurement chart for regular assessment with other routine nursing observations. Special methods of pain relief used under close supervision are:

- continuous epidural anaesthesia with opiate or local anaesthetic drugs;
- continuous intravenous opiate analgesia;
- patient-controlled analgesia by injection intravenously or epidurally of opioid analgesia. The patient is trained to give a bolus dose of drug by pressing a control button on a machine whose functions have been regulated by the medical staff. The strength, frequency and total dose of drug in a given time are all limited by computer.

Effective postoperative pain relief encourages early mobilisation and hospital discharge.

Simple analgesic agents

In minor surgery, and when the patient is able to eat after major surgery, aspirin and paracetamol are often the only drugs necessary to control pain. Fear of metabolic acidosis and Reye's syndrome of hepatotoxicity in children have

Douglas Reye, 1912–77. Australian pathologist and physician. First described Reye's syndrome in 1963.

made paracetamol a preferable drug to aspirin in the younger age group. Codeine phosphate is the analgesic favoured after intracranial surgery because it does not have a powerful respiratory depressant effect; it may never be given intravenously as it causes profound hypotension on intravenous injection. Patients with a tendency to peptic ulceration may need cover with omeprazole or misoprostol during analgesic treatment with anti-inflammatory agents.

Chronic pain relief

In surgical practice, the patient with chronic pain may present for treatment of the cause (e.g. pancreatitis) or have concomitant pathology. Surgery itself may have been the cause of the now chronic symptom, as acute pain may progress to chronic pain. There is a developing belief that inadequate treatment of acute pain may make this more likely.

Chronic, intractable pain may be of malignant or benign origin and of several types.

- Nociceptive pain – pain may result from musculoskeletal disorders or cancer activating cutaneous nociceptors. Prolonged ischaemic or inflammatory processes results in sensitisation of peripheral nociceptors and altered activity in the central nervous system leading to exaggerated responses in the dorsal horn of the spinal cord. The widened area of hyperalgesia and increased sensitivity (allodynia) has been attributed to increased transmission of afferent pain impulses consequent upon this spinal cord dynamic plasticity.
- Neuropathic (or neurogenic) pain – dysfunction in peripheral or central nerves (excluding the physiological pain due to noxious stimulation of the nerve terminals). Neuropathic pain is classically 'burning', 'shooting' or 'stabbing', and may be associated with allodynia, numbness and diminished thermal sensation. It is poorly responsive to opioids. Examples include trigeminal neuralgia, metatarsalgia, postherpetic and diabetic neuropathy. Monoaminergic, tricyclic and anticonvulsant drugs are the mainstay of treatment.
- Psychogenic pain – psychological factors play a greater or lesser role in many chronic pain syndromes. Whichever the primary cause may have been, depressive illness and chronic pain may exacerbate each other.

The treatment of pain of malignant origin differs from that of pain of a benign cause, and may be the more difficult to overcome. Drugs, preferably, should be taken by mouth, but the patient must be regularly reassessed to ensure that analgesia remains adequate as the disease process changes.

Malignant disease

In intractable pain, the underlying principle of treatment is to encourage independence of the patient and an active life in spite of the symptoms. The main guide to the management of cancer pain is the World Health Organisation Booklet (now in its second edition), which portrays three levels of treatment. The 'pain stepladder' includes the following treatments:

- first rung: simple analgesics – aspirin, paracetamol, NSAIDs, tricyclic drugs or anticonvulsant drugs;
- second rung: intermediate strength opioids – codeine, tramadol or dextropropoxyphene;
- third rung: strong opioids – morphine. (Pethidine has been withdrawn from the second edition.)

Oral opiate analgesia is necessary when the less powerful analgesic agents no longer control pain on movement, or enable the patient to sleep. Fear that the patient may develop an addiction to opiates is usually not justified in malignant disease.

Oral morphine can be prescribed in short-acting liquid or tablet form and should be administered regularly every 4 hours until an adequate dose of drug has been titrated to control the pain over 24 hours. Once this is established, the daily dose can be divided into two separate administrations of enteric-coated, slow-release morphine tablets (MST morphine) every 12 hours. Additional short-acting morphine can then be used to cover episodes of 'breakthrough pain'. Nausea is a problem early in the use of morphine treatment and may need control by antiemetic agents, e.g. haloperidol, methotrimeprazine, metoclopramide or ondansetron. Nausea does not usually persist, but constipation is frequently a persistent complication requiring regular prevention by laxatives.

Infusion of subcutaneous, intravenous, intrathecal or epidural opiate drugs

The infusion of opiate is necessary if a patient is unable to take oral drugs. Subcutaneous infusion of diamorphine is simple and effective to administer. Epidural infusions of diamorphine can be used on mobile patients with an external pump. Intrathecal infusions are prone to infection, but implantable reservoirs with pumps programmed by external computer are being used for long-term intrathecal analgesia. Intravenous narcotic agents may then be reserved for acute crises, such as pathological fractures.

Neurolytic techniques in cancer pain

These should only be used if the life expectancy is limited and the diagnosis is certain. The useful procedures are:

- subcostal phenol injection for a rib metastasis;
- coeliac plexus neurolytic block with alcohol for pain of pancreatic, gastric or hepatic cancer. Image intensifier control is essential;
- intrathecal neurolytic injection of hyperbaric phenol – this technique is useful only if facilities for percutaneous cordotomy are not available as it can damage motor pathways;
- percutaneous anterolateral cordotomy divides the spinothalamic ascending pain pathway – this is a highly effective technique in experienced hands, selectively eliminating pain and temperature sensation in a specific limited area.

Alternative strategies include:

- the development of hormone analogues, such as tamoxifen and cyproterone, enables effective pharmacological therapy for the pain of widespread metastases instead of pituitary ablation surgery;
- palliative radiotherapy can be most beneficial for the relief of pain in metastatic disease;
- adjuvant drugs such as corticosteroids to reduce cerebral oedema or inflammation around a tumour may be useful in symptom control. Tricyclic antidepressants, anticonvulsants and, occasionally, flecainide are also used to reduce the pain of nerve injury.

Pain control in benign disease

Surgical patients may have persistent pain from a variety of disorders including chronic inflammatory disease, recurrent infection, degenerative bone or joint disease, nerve injury and sympathetic dystrophy. Chronic pain may result from persistent excitation of the nociceptive pathways in the central nervous system, invoking mechanisms such as spontaneous firing of pain signals at *N*-methyl-D-aspartate receptors in the ascending pathways. Such activity is poorly responsive to opiates; neuroablative surgery is unlikely to produce prolonged benefit and may make the pain worse.

As is well known, amputation of limbs may result in phantom limb pain, the likelihood being further increased if the limb was painful before surgery. Continuous regional local anaesthetic blockade (epidural or brachial plexus), established before operation and continued postoperatively for a few days, is believed to reduce effectively the establishment of phantom pain.

The following are treatments for chronic pain of benign origin.

- Local anaesthetic and steroid injections – these can be effective around an inflamed nerve and they reduce the cycle of constant pain transmission with consequent muscle spasm. Epidural injections are used for the pain of nerve root irritation associated with minor disc prolapse. This treatment should be in association with active physiotherapy to promote mobility.
- Nerve stimulation procedures – acupuncture, transcutaneous nerve stimulation and the neurosurgical implantation of dorsal column electrodes aim to increase the endorphin production in the central nervous system altering pain transmission.
- Nerve decompression – decompression of the trigeminal nerve at craniotomy is now performed for trigeminal neuralgia, rather than percutaneous coagulation of the trigeminal ganglion, in patients who are fit for craniotomy.

Treatment of pain is dependent on sympathetic nervous system activity. Even minor trauma and surgery (often of a limb) can provoke chronic burning pain, allodynia, trophic changes and resultant disuse. The syndrome has been attributed to excessive sympathetic adrenergic activity inducing vasconstriction and abnormal nociceptive transmission. Management may include:

- test response to systemic α-adrenergic blockade using intravenous phentolamine;
- intravenous regional sympathetic blockade using guanethidine, under tourniquet;
- local anaesthetic injection of stellate ganglion or lumbar sympathetic chain.

Percutaneous chemical lumbar sympathectomy with phenol under radiographic control is practised by both surgeons and anaesthetists for relief of rest pain in advanced ischaemic disease of the legs. It can also promote the healing of ischaemic ulcers by improving peripheral blood flow.

Drugs in chronic benign pain

Escalating doses of opioid analgesic drugs are to be avoided, and certainly the patient must not become dependent on analgesic injections. However, for debilitating levels of chronic pain, opioid drugs are indicated. Combinations of drugs often prove useful to achieve the optimal combination of efficacy with minimal side-effects.

Paracetamol and NSAIDs are the mainstay of musculoskeletal pain treatment, but NSAIDs are handicapped by gastrointestinal intolerance and peptic ulceration. These carry significant levels of noncompliance, contraindication and morbidity. Specific cyclo-oxygenase 2 inhibition, with preservation of protective cyclo-oxygenase 1 activity, promises to improve tolerability and safety in nonsteroidal anti-inflammatory treatment.

The tricyclic antidepressant drugs and anticonvulsant agents are often useful for diminishing the pain of nerve injury, although side-effects can prove troublesome and reduce compliance.

In the management of chronic pain of benign cause, a multidisciplinary approach by a team using psychologists, physiotherapists and occupational therapists under medical supervision can often achieve much more benefit than the use of powerful drugs. To help the chronic benign pain patients who do not respond to conventional means, 'pain management programmes' have been devised, comprising a multidisciplinary approach of pain specialists, psychologists, phyisiotherapists and occupational therapists. They help a number of the patients to cope with the pain and resume a higher quality life.

Further reading

Rawal, N. (ed.) (1998) *Management of Acute and Chronic Pain*, BMJ Books, London.

Wildsmith, I. and Armitage, E.N. (eds) (1990) *Principles and Practice of Regional Anaesthesia*, Churchill Livingstone, Edinburgh.

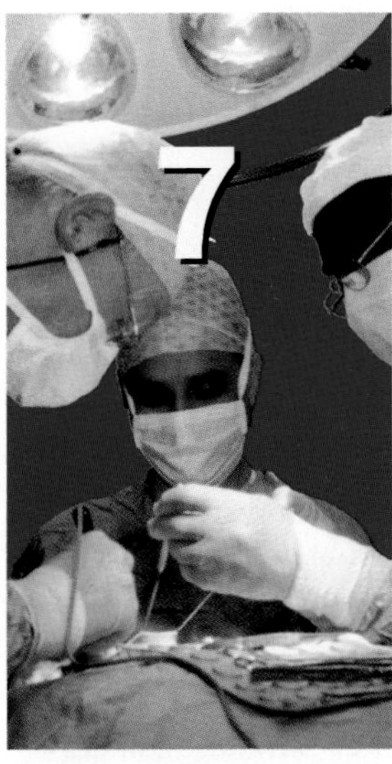

7 Wound infection

Physiology and manifestation

Background. It is clear that the Egyptians knew about infection. They certainly were able to prevent putrefaction which is testified in their skills of mummification. Their medical papyruses also describe the use of salves and antiseptics to prevent wound infections. This had also been known, although less well documented, by the Assyrians and the Greeks, particularly in Hippocratic teachings, which had refined the use of antimicrobial practice. The use of wine and vinegar to irrigate open infected wounds before successful secondary closure was practised widely. Common to all these cultures, and the later Roman practitioners, was a dictum that whenever pus developed in an infected wound it needed to be drained.

Galen recognised that localisation of infection (suppuration) in wounds inflicted in the gladiatorial arena often heralded recovery, particularly after drainage of the pus (*pus bonum et laudabile*). Sadly, this dictum was misinterpreted by many until well into the Renaissance; many practitioners actually promoted suppuration in wounds by application of many noxious substances, including faeces, in the misbelief that healing could not occur without pus formation. There was occasional light in this long, dark tunnel: Theodoric of Cervia, Ambroise Paré and Guy de Chauliac all realised that clean wounds, closed primarily, could heal without infection or suppuration.

The understanding of the causes of infection came in the nineteenth century. Microbes had been seen under the microscope, but Koch laid down the first definition of infective disease (Koch's postulates). These were basically that a particular microbe could be considered responsible for an infection when it was found in adequate numbers in a septic focus, could be cultured in pure form from specimens taken from the focus and could cause similar lesions when injected into another host.

The Austrian obstetrician, Ignac Semmelweis, showed that maternal mortality caused by puerperal sepsis could be reduced from over 10 per cent to under 2 per cent by the simple act of hand washing between postmortem examinations and the delivery suite.

Louis Pasteur recognised that microorganisms spoilt wine and Joseph Lister applied this knowledge to the reduction of organisms in compound fractures allowing surgery without infection. However, his toxic phenol spray and principles of antiseptic surgery soon gave way to aseptic surgery at the turn of the century – a technique still employed in modern operating theatres.

Hippocrates, 460–377 BC. Greek physician and surgeon. The 'father of medicine'.
Galen, 130–200. Roman gladiatorial surgeon, pathologist and philosopher.
Theodoric of Cervia, 1205–96. Surgeon of Bologna, Italy.

Bailey & Love's Short Practice of Surgery, 23rd edition. Edited by R.C.G. Russell, N.S. Williams and C.J.K. Bulstrode. Published in 2000 by Arnold Publishers.

Ambroise Paré, 1510–90. French military surgeon.
Guy de Chauliac. Thirteenth-century French surgeon.
Robert Koch, 1843–1910. Professor of Hygiene and Microbiology, Berlin, Germany.
Ignac Semmelweis, 1818–65. Austrian obstetrician. Died of a septic illness in his home country of Hungary.
Louis Pasteur, 1822–95. French chemist and bacteriologist. Founder of Pasteur Institute, Paris, France.

The concept of a 'magic bullet' which could kill microbes but not their host led to early sulphonamide chemotherapy. The antibiotic penicillin, the discovery of which is ascribed to Alexander Fleming, was isolated by Florey and Chain. The first patient to receive penicillin was Police Constable Alexander, who had a severe staphylococcal illness. He made a partial recovery before the penicillin ran out but later relapsed and died. Since then there has been a huge increase in antibiotic groups with improved antibacterial spectra. Few staphylococci are now sensitive to penicillin but streptococcal illnesses respond, although they are seen increasingly rarely in surgical practice. Many bacteria develop resistance through the acquisition of β-lactamases which can break up the β-lactam ring, common in the formula of many antibiotics. In general surgery, the synergy of aerobic Gram-negative bacilli with anaerobic *Bacteroides* spp. presents the most challenging infection. Wide-spectrum antibiotics can be given empirically to treat such infections, or more specific, narrow-range antibiotics given based on culture and sensitivity. The range of surgery now practised owes much to rational antibiotic use – faecal peritonitis may not be considered to be lethal, and wounds made in the presence of such contamination can heal primarily without infection in 80–90 per cent of patients. Patients undergoing prosthetic surgery or who are immunosuppressed can be spared infection in their wounds by the appropriate use of prophylactic antibiotics.

Physiology

Bacteria are normally prevented from causing infection in tissues by intact epithelial surfaces, but these are broken down by surgery. In addition to this mechanical barrier, there are other protective mechanisms, i.e. chemical (such as the low gastric pH), humoral (antibodies, complement and opsonins) and cellular (phagocytic cells, macrophages, polymorphonuclear cells and killer lymphocytes).

Host response is weakened by malnutrition which may present as obesity as well as recent rapid weight loss (Table 7.1). Metabolic diseases, diabetes mellitus, uraemia and jaundice may weaken defences, and disseminated cancer may also be included together with immunosuppression caused by radiotherapy, chemotherapy, steroids and acquired immunodeficiency syndrome (AIDS) (Figs 7.1 and 7.2).

When enteral feeding is suspended in the perioperative period, the gut rapidly becomes colonised and bacteria, particularly Gram-negative bacilli, translocate to mesenteric nodes. Release of endotoxin may follow, which further increases susceptibility to infection. In these circumstances, nonpathogens become important (opportunism).

Table 7.1 Risk factors for increased risk of wound infection

- Malnutrition (obesity, weight loss)
- Metabolic disease (diabetes, uraemia, jaundice)
- Immunosuppression (cancer, AIDS, steroids, chemotherapy and radiotherapy)
- Colonisation and translocation in the gastrointestinal tract
- Poor perfusion (systemic shock or local ischaemia)
- Foreign body material
- Poor surgical technique (dead space, haematoma)

The pathogenicity and size of bacterial inoculum also relates to the chance of developing an established wound infection after surgery. Poor surgical technique that leaves devitalised tissue, excessive dead space or haematoma may increase this risk. Foreign materials of any kind, including sutures and drains, promote infection. A logarithm reduction in the number of organisms is needed to cause a wound infection in the presence of a silk suture. These factors need consideration in prosthetic orthopaedic and vascular surgery.

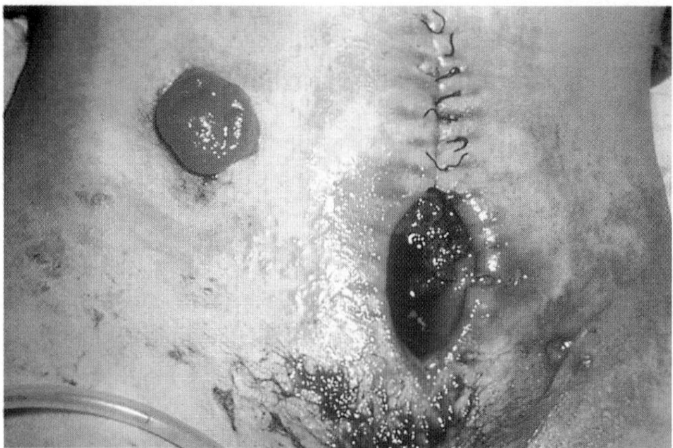

Fig. 7.1 Major wound infection and delayed healing presenting as a faecal fistula in a patient with Crohn's disease.

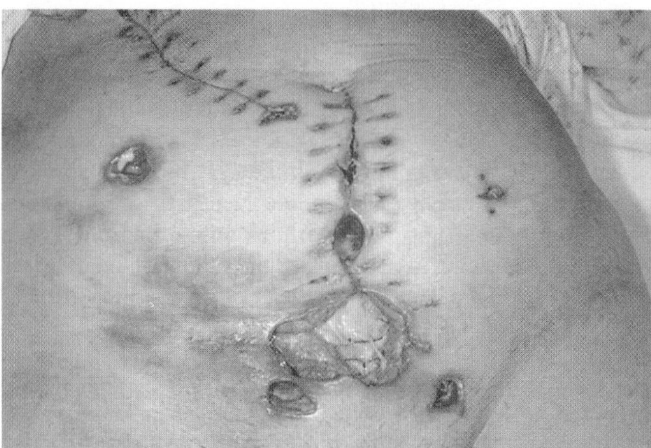

Fig. 7.2 Delayed healing relating to infection in a patient on high-dose steroids.

Lord Joseph Lister, 1827–1912. Professor of Surgery, Glasgow, Edinburgh and King's College Hospital, London, England.

Alexander Fleming, 1881–1955. Discoverer of Penicillium notatum. *Microbiologist, St Mary's Hospital, London, England.*

Lord Howard Walter Florry, 1878–1968. Professor of Pathology, Oxford, England.

Sir Ernst Boris Chain, 1960–78. Professor of Biochemistry, Imperial College, London University, England.

Hans Christian Joachim Gram, 1853–1938. Professor of Pharmacology and Medicine, Copenhagen, Denmark.

In the first 4 hours after a breach in an epithelial surface and underlying connective tissues made during surgery or trauma, there is a delay before host defences can become mobilised through acute inflammatory, humoral and cellular processes. This period is called the 'decisive period' and it is during these first 4 hours after incision that bacterial colonisation and established infection can begin. It is logical that prophylactic antibiotics will be most effective during this time.

Local and systemic manifestation

Infection of a wound can be defined as the invasion of organisms through tissues following a breakdown of local and systemic host defences. Sepsis is the systemic manifestation of a documented infection, the signs and symptoms of which may also be caused by multiple trauma, burns or pancreatitis. Bacteraemia should not be confused with this systemic inflammatory response syndrome (SIRS) although the two may coexist (see Table 7.2). Septic manifestations are mediated by release of cytokines [such as interleukins (IL) and tumour necrosis factor (TNF)] and other modules from polymorphonuclear and phagocytic cells and, in its most severe form, presents as multiple system organ failure (MSOF). Infection may cause SIRS through the release of lipopolysaccharide endotoxin from the walls of dying Gram-negative bacilli (mainly *Escherichia coli*) and other toxins, which in turn causes release of cytokines (Fig. 7.3). A reduced defence to wound infection follows.

Pathogens resist host defences by release of toxins, particularly in unfavourable anaerobic conditions, which favours their spread in wound infections. *Clostridium perfringens,* which is responsible for gas gangrene, releases many spreading proteases such as hyaluronidase, lecithinase and haemolysin. Many resistant pathogens can produce β-lactamases which destroy the β-lactam ring of antibiotics. This resistance can be acquired and passed on through plasmids.

The human body harbours approximately 10^{14} organisms. They are released into tissues by surgery, contamination

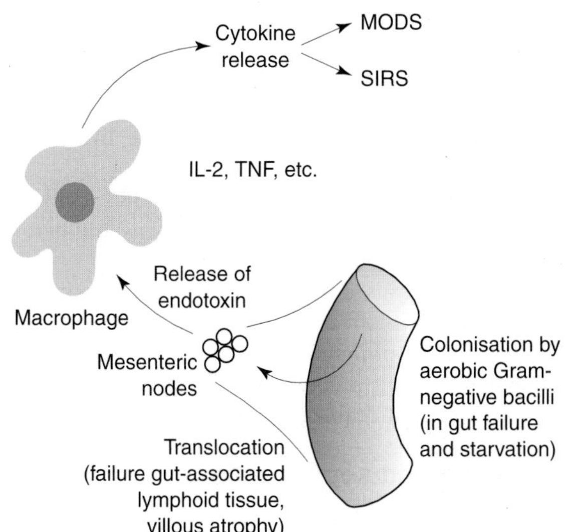

Fig. 7.3 Gut failure, colonisation and translocation related to the development of multiple organ dysfunction syndrome (MODS) and systemic inflammatory response syndrome (SIRS).

Table 7.2 Definitions in sepsis

- Systemic inflammatory response syndrome (SIRS); two of:
  - Hyperthermia (>38°C) or hypothermia (<36°C)
  - Tachycardia (>90/min no β-blockers) or tachypnoea (>20/min)
  - White cell count $>12 \times 10^9$/litre or $<4 \times 10^9$/litre
- Sepsis is SIRS with a documented infection
- Severe sepsis or sepsis syndrome is sepsis with evidence of one or more organ failure [respiratory (acute respiratory distress syndrome), cardiovascular, renal (usually acute tubular necrosis) or central nervous system]

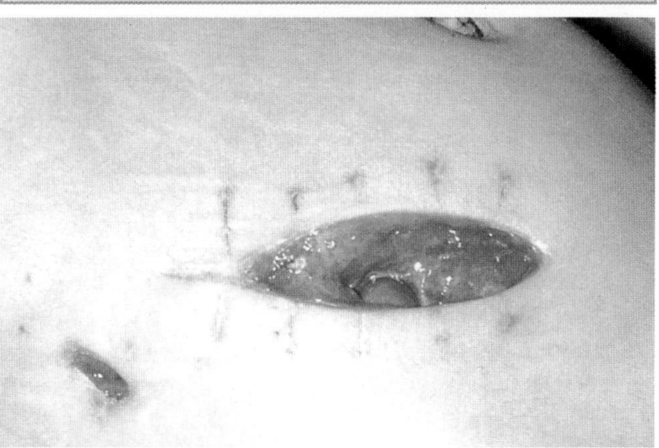

Fig. 7.4 Major wound infection with superficial skin dehiscence.

being most severe when a hollow viscus is opened (e.g. colorectal surgery). Any infection which follows may be termed primary, community acquired or endogenous. Exogenous infections are usually hospital acquired (nosocomial) and are secondary, being introduced into the tissues after surgery not during it, unless introduced via inadequately filtered air in the operating theatre.

A major wound infection is defined as a wound which discharges pus and may need a secondary procedure to be sure of adequate drainage (Fig. 7.4). There may be systemic signs of tachycardia pyrexia and a raised white count (SIRS). The patient may be delayed in returning home beyond the planned day. Minor wound infections may discharge pus or infected serous fluid but should not be associated with excessive discomfort, systemic signs or delay in return home (Fig. 7.5). The differentiation of major and minor wound infection is important in audit trials of antibiotic prophylaxis and is of relevance to 'league tables' of hospital infection as major wound infections must be accounted for.

Types of infection

Wound abscess

A wound abscess presents all the Celsian clinical features of acute inflammation: *calor* (heat), *rubor* (redness), *dolor* (pain)

Aurellas Cornelius Celsus, c. *30* AD. *Roman surgeon. Author of* De Re Medica Libri Octo.

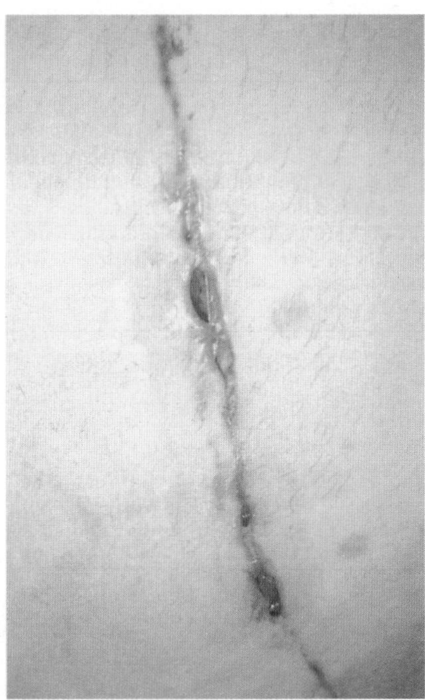

Fig. 7.5 Minor wound infection which settled spontaneously without antibiotics.

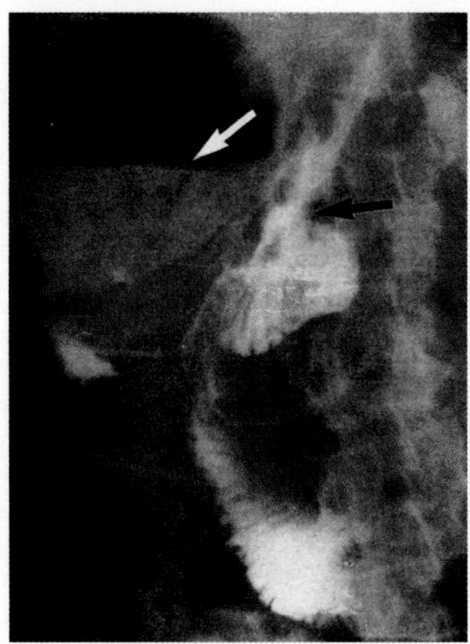

Fig. 7.6 Plain radiograph showing a subphrenic abscess with a gas/fluid level (white arrow). Gastrografin is seen leaking from the oesophago-jejunal anastomosis (after total gastrectomy) towards the abscess (red arrow).

and *tumor* (swelling), to which can be added *functio laesa* (loss of function – if it hurts the infected part is not used). Pyogenic organisms, predominantly *Staphylococcus aureus,* cause tissue necrosis and suppuration. Pus is also composed of dead and dying white blood cells which release damaging cytokines, oxygen-free radicals and other molecules. An abscess is surrounded by an acute inflammatory response, and a pyogenic membrane composed of fibrinous exudate and oedema, and the cells of acute inflammation. Granulation tissue (macrophages, angiogenesis and fibroblasts) forms later around the suppuration and leads to collagen deposition. If excessive or partly sterilised by antibiotics (antibioma), a chronic abscess may result. Abscesses usually track along planes of least resistance and point towards the skin. Wound abscesses may spontaneously discharge through a surgical incision but most take 7–9 days to form after surgery. Many infections may present after the patient has left hospital.

Abscesses may need débridement and curettage with an exploration to break down all loculi before resolution can occur. Persistent chronic abscesses may lead to sinus or fistula formation. In a chronic abscess, lymphocytes and plasma cells are seen with sequestration and later calcification. Certain organisms are related to chronicity, sinus and fistula formation, e.g. mycobacteria and actinomyces, and should not be forgotten.

Perianastomotic abscesses may be the cause or result of anastomotic leakage. Deep cavity abscess (pleura or peritoneum) may be difficult to diagnose or locate even when there is strong clinical suspicion (Fig. 7.6). Plain or contrast radiographs may not be helpful, whereas ultrasonography, computerised tomography, magnetic resonance imaging and isotope scans are usually accurate and may allow guided aspiration without the need for surgical intervention.

The role of antibiotics in the treatment of wound abscesses is controversial unless there are signs of spreading infection (cellulitis or lymphangitis). Surgical decompression and curettage must be adequate and may allow resuture without antibiotics but this is also controversial. Delayed primary or secondary suture is safer.

Cellulitis and lymphangitis

This is the nonsuppurative invasive infection of tissues. In addition to the cardinal signs of inflammation, there is poor localisation. Spreading infection is typical of organisms such as β-haemolytic streptococci (Fig. 7.7), staphylococci (Fig. 7.8) and *C. perfringens.* Tissue destruction and ulceration may follow, caused by release of streptokinase, hyaluronidase and other proteases.

Systemic signs (toxaemia) are common: SIRS, chills, fever and rigors. These follow release of exotoxins and cytokines but blood cultures are often negative.

Lymphangitis is caused by similar processes but presents as painful red streaks in affected lymphatics. Cellulitis is usually located at the point of injury and subsequent tissue infection. Lymphangitis is often accompanied by painful lymph node groups in the related drainage area.

Bacteraemia and septicaemia

These are unusual in superficial wound infections but common after anastomotic breakdown. They are usually transient and follow procedures undertaken through infected tissues (particularly instrumentation in infected bile or urine).

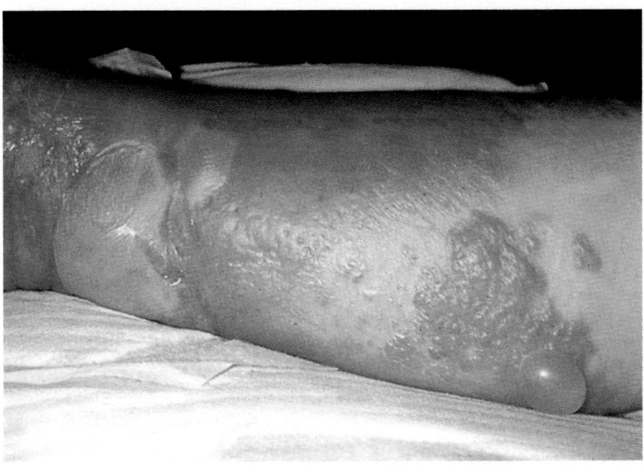

Fig. 7.7 Streptococcal cellulitis of the leg following a minor puncture wound.

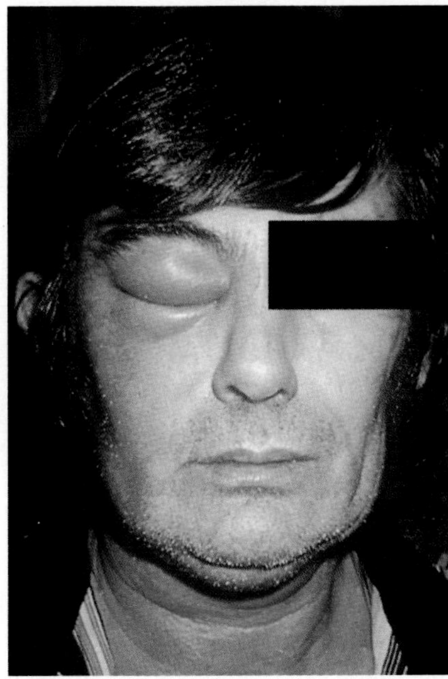

Fig. 7.8 Staphylococcal cellulitis of face and orbit following severe infection of an epidermoid cyst of scalp.

Bacteraemia is important when prosthetics have been implanted, particularly cardiac valves. Septicaemia commonly relates to colonisation and translocation in the gastrointestinal tract and may follow anastomotic breakdown accompanied by MSOF (Fig. 7.3). Aerobic Gram-negative bacilli are mainly responsible but *S. aureus* and fungi may be involved, particularly after the use of broad-spectrum antibiotics.

Specific wound infections

Gas gangrene is caused by *C. perfringens*. The Gram-positive, spore-bearing bacilli are widely found in nature, particularly soil and faeces, which is relevant to military and traumatic surgery, and colorectal operations. Patients who are immunocompromised, diabetic or have malignant disease are at risk, particularly when anaerobic wound conditions are present with necrotic or foreign material. Wound infections are associated with severe local wound pain and crepitus (gas in the tissues which may also be noted on plain radiographs). The wound presents a thin, brown, sweet-smelling exudate, from which bacteria can be recognised on Gram staining. Oedema and spreading gangrene follow the release of collagenase, hyaluronidase, other proteases and α-toxin. Systemic complications with circulatory collapse and MSOF supersede without appropriate intervention.

Prophylaxis in patients at risk should always be considered, particularly amputation for peripheral vascular disease. Once established, large doses of intravenous penicillin and aggressive débridement of affected tissues are required. The use of hyperbaric oxygen is controversial.

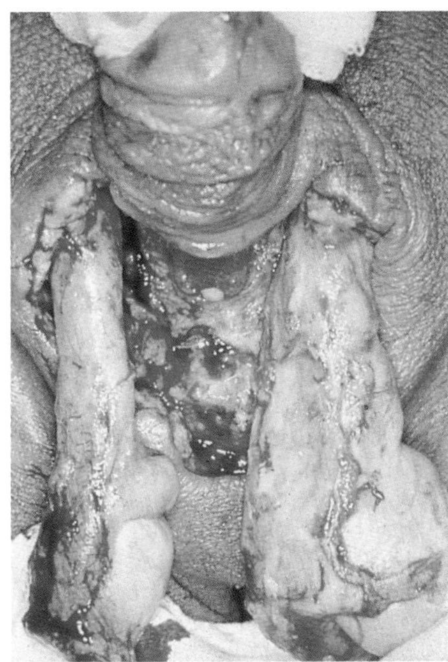

Fig. 7.9 A classic presentation of Fournier's gangrene of the scrotum with 'shameful exposure of the testes' following excision of the gangrenous skin.

Synergistic spreading gangrene (necrotising fasciitis) is not caused by clostridia. A mixed pattern of organisms is responsible – coliforms, staphylococci, *Bacteroides* spp., anaerobic streptococci and pepto-streptococci have been implicated. Synonyms have been associated with abdominal wall infections (Meleney's synergistic hospital gangrene) and scrotal infection (Fournier's gangrene, Fig. 7.9). Patients are almost always immunocompromised (such as diabetes mellitus). The initial wound may have been minor, but severely

Frank Lamont Meleney, 1889–1963. Professor of Clinical Surgery, Columbia University, New York, USA.

Jean Alfred Fournier, 1832–1914. Founder of the Venereal and Dermatological Clinic, St Louis, Paris, France.

contaminated wounds are more likely to be the cause. Severe wound pain, signs of spreading inflammation with crepitus and smell lead on to widespread gangrene. The extent of subdermal spread of gangrene is always much more extensive than at first is apparent. Wide-spectrum antibiotic therapy must be combined with aggressive circulatory support and wide excision and laying open of affected tissue. Débridement may need to be extensive. Patients who survive need large areas of skin grafting.

Treatment

Following the trend to discharge patients earlier, many wound infections may be missed by surgeons unless they undertake a prolonged and carefully audited follow-up with family doctors. Suppurative wound infections take 7–10 days to develop, whereas cellulitis around wounds caused by invasive organisms (such as the β-haemolytic streptococcus) appears in 3–4 days. Major wound infections with systemic signs (Fig. 7.10) or evidence of cellulitis justify the use of appropriate antibiotics. The choice may be empirical or based on culture

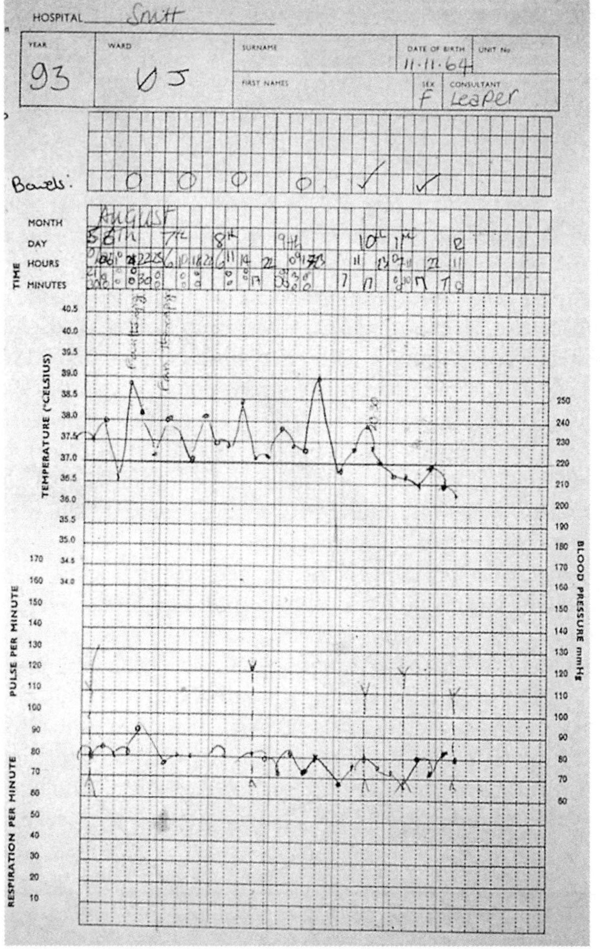

Fig. 7.10 Classic swinging pyrexia related to a perianastomotic wound abscess which settled spontaneously on antibiotic therapy.

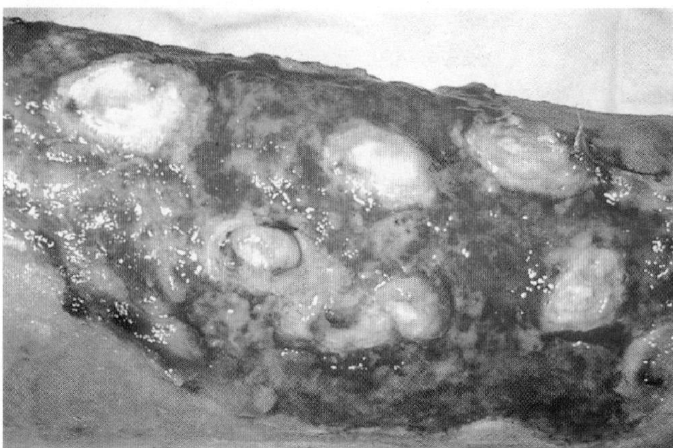

Fig. 7.11 Mixed streptococcal and staphylococcal infection of a skin graft with very poor 'take'.

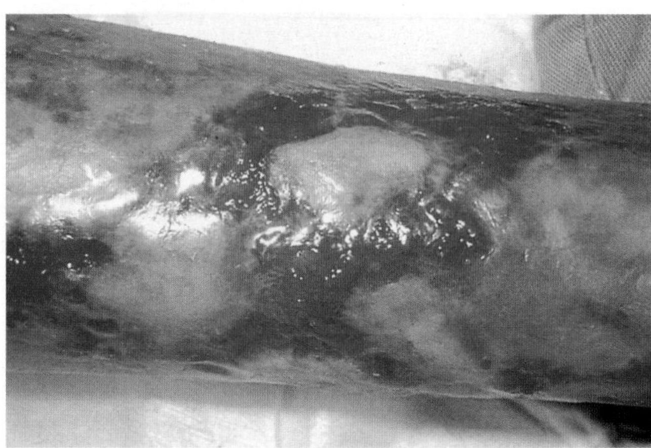

Fig. 7.12 After 5–6 days of antibiotic, the infection in Fig. 7.11 is under control and the skin grafts are clearly viable.

and sensitivities of isolates harvested at surgery. Although the identification of organisms in wound infections is necessary for audit and wound surveillance purposes, it is usually 2–3 days before sensitivities are known (Figs 7.11 and 7.12). It is illogical to withhold antibiotics but if clinical response is poor by the time sensitivities are known then antibiotics can be changed. This is unusual if the empirical choice of antibiotics is sensible – change of antibiotics promotes resistance and risks complications, such as *Clostridium difficile* enteritis.

When the wound is under tension or there is clear evidence of suppuration removal of sutures aids evacuation of pus. There is no evidence that subcuticular continuous skin closure enhances or worsens the effect of suppuration. In severely contaminated wounds, e.g. laparotomy for faecal peritonitis, or incisions made for drainage of an abscess, it is logical to leave the skin layer open. Delayed primary or secondary suture is undertaken when the wound is clean and granulating (Figs 7.13 and 7.14). Leaving wounds open after dirty operations is not practised as widely in the UK as in the USA or mainland Europe.

When taking pus from infected wounds, specimens should be sent fresh for microbiological culture. Swabs should be

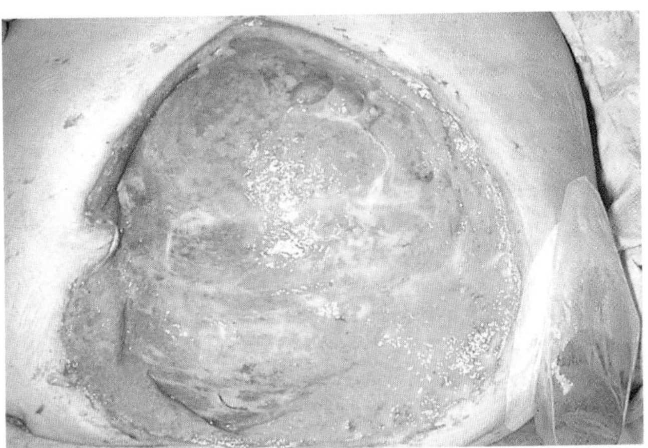

Fig. 7.13 Skin layers left open to granulate after laparotomy for faecal peritonitis. Wound clean and ready for closure.

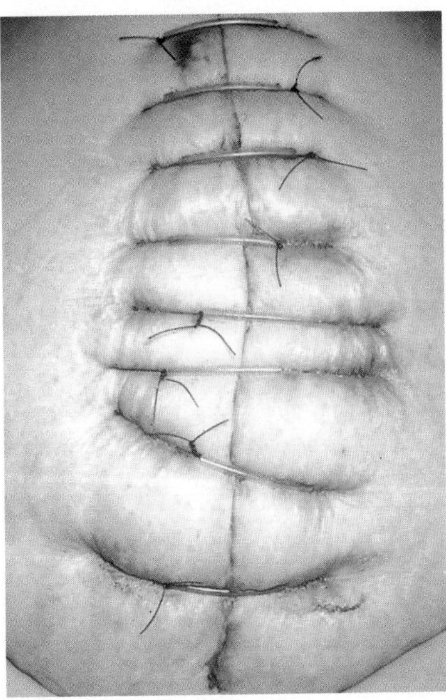

Fig. 7.14 Secondary closure of wound.

placed in transport medium but as large a volume of pus as possible is likely to yield more accurate results. Communication with microbiologists is essential for the most meaningful results. If bacteraemia is suspected, repeat specimens may be needed to exclude negative results.

Reports on infective material can be based rapidly on an immediate Gram stain. Aerobic and anaerobic culture on conventional media allows sensitivities to be assessed by disc diffusion. The measurements of minimum inhibitory antibiotic concentrations (M1C90 in mg/litre), together with measurements of endotoxin and cytokine levels, are usually only used in research.

Many dressings are now available for use in wound care. These are listed in Table 7.3. Polymeric films are used as incise drapes and also to cover sutured wounds but are not indicated for use in wound infections. Agents that can be used to help débride open infected wounds, others to absorb excessive exudate or to encourage epithelialisation and formation of granulation tissue are also listed (Fig. 7.15).

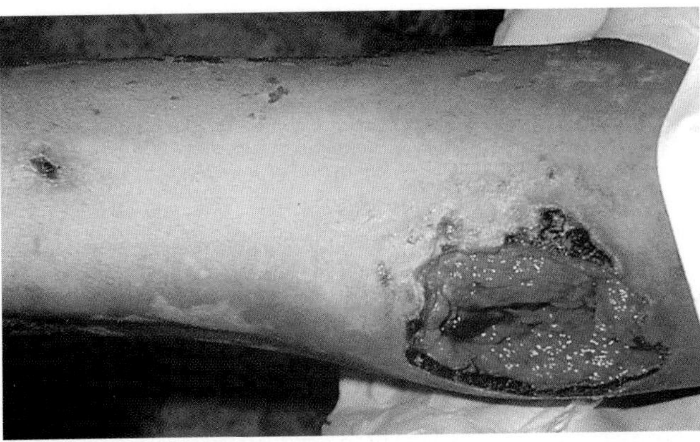

Fig. 7.15 Infected animal bite/wound of the upper thigh treated by open therapy following virulent staphylococcal infection. Deep cavity wounds such as this can be débrided and kept moist by many of the modern dressings listed in Table 7.3.

Prophylaxis

Prophylactic antibiotics. If antibiotics are given empirically they must exert their action when local wound defences are at their least (the decisive period). Ideally, maximal blood and tissue levels should be achieved at incision before contamination occurs. Intravenous administration at induction of anaesthesia is optimal. In long or prosthetic operations, or unexpected contamination, antibiotics may be repeated 8 and 16 hours later. The empiric choice of an antibiotic depends on the expected spectrum of organisms likely to be encountered, the cost and local policies, which are based on experience of local resistance trends. The use of the newer, wide-spectrum antibiotics for prophylaxis should be avoided. Table 7.4 gives some examples of prophylaxis which can be used in elective surgical operations.

Lower limb amputation should be covered against *C. perfringens* using 1.2 g of benzyl penicillin intravenously at induction or anaesthesia and 6-hourly thereafter for 48 hours.

Patients with known valvular disease of the heart (or with any implanted vascular or orthopaedic prosthesis) ought to have prophylaxis during dental, urological or open viscus surgery. Single doses of wide-spectrum penicillin, e.g. amoxycillin, orally or intravenously administered, are sufficient for dental surgery. In urological instrumentation a second generation of cephalosporin, such as cefuroxime, is sufficient but, in open viscus surgery, addition of metronidazole should be considered.

Preoperative preparation. Short preoperative hospital stay lowers the risk of acquisition of methicillin-resistant *S. aureus* (MRSA) and multiply resistant, coagulase-negative staphylococci (MRCNS). The value of personal hygiene is obvious (both patient and surgeon). Open, infected skin lesions should preclude admission to the operating theatres.

Table 7.3 Surgical dressings

Type	*Name (example)*	*Indications and comments*
Débriding agents	Benoxyl-benzoic acid Aserbine-benzoic and salacyclic acid Variclene-lactic acid	Used only in necrotic sloughing skin ulcers. Provide acidic environment. Claimed to enhance healing with débriding action
Enzymatic agents	Varidase-streptokinase/streptodornase	Activate fibrinolysis and liquiefy pus on chronic skin ulcers
Bead dressings	Debrisan Iodosorb Other paste dressings	Remove bacteria and excess moisture by capillary action in deep granulating wounds. Antimicrobials may be added but with questionable topical benefit
Polymeric films	Opsite Bioclusive Tegaderm	Primary adhesive transparent dressing for sutured wounds or donor sites
Foams	Silastic (elastomer) Lyofoam Allevyn	Elastomeric dressing can be shaped to fit deep cavities and granulating wounds. Absorbent and nonadherent
Hydrogels	Geliperm Intrasite	Maintain moist environment. Polymers can absorb exudate or antiseptics (but adding antiseptics is of doubtful benefit). Semipermeable, allow gas exchange
Hydrocolloids	Comfeel Granuflex	Complete occlusion. Promote epithelialisation and granulation tissue. Maintain moisture without gaseous exchange across them
Fibrous polymers	Kaltostat Sorbsan	Absorptive alginate dressings. Derived from natural (seaweed) source. Like polymeric hydrocolloids and hydrogels can pack deep wounds
Biological membranes	Porcine skin, amnion	Used for superficial chronic skin ulcers. No proven advantage
Simple miscellaneous	Gauzes: viscose/cotton with nonadherent coating (Melolin). Tulles: nonadherent paraffin impregnation	Simple absorptive dressings only used as secondary dressings to absorb exudate. Added antimicrobials probably confer no benefit. Added charcoal absorbents may reduce swelling. Relatively cheap but of questionable effectiveness

Table 7.4 Suggested prophylactic regimens for operations at risk

Types of surgery	*Organisms encountered*	*Prophylactic regimen suggested*
Vascular	*Staphylococcus epidermidis* (or MRCNS) *Staphylococcus aureus* (or MRSA) Aerobic Gram-negative bacilli (AGNB)	3 Dose flucloxacillin ± gentamicin, vancomycin or rifampicin if MRCNS/MRSA a risk
Orthopaedic	*Staphylococcus epidermidis/aureus*	1–3 Dose wide-spectrum cephalosporin (with antistaphylococcal action). Gentamicin beads
Oesophagogastric	Enterobacteriaceae Enterococci (including anaerobic/ viridans streptococci)	1–3 Dose second-generation cephalosporin and metronidazole in severe contamination
Biliary	Enterobacteriaceae (mainly *E. coli*) Enterococci (including *Streptococcus faecalis*)	1 Dose second-generation cephalosporin
Small bowel	Enterobacteriaceae Anaerobes (mainly *Bacteroides*)	1–3 Dose second-generation cephalosporin ± metronidazole
Appendix/colorectal	Enterobacteriaceae Anaerobes (*Bacteroides* streptococci)	3 Dose second-generation cephalosporin (alternatively gentamicin) with metronidazole. (Oral, poorly absorbed antibiotics controversial)

All regimens are intravenous and should start preoperatively. In elective operations, antibiotics can be given at induction of anaesthesia. In emergency operations (or in contamination during elective surgery) antibiotics should be given at diagnosis and prolonged as therapy for 3–5 days if necessary.

The value of antiseptic bathing (usually chlorhexidine) is popular in Europe but there is no hard evidence for its efficacy in reducing wound infections. Preoperative shaving should be avoided except for aesthetic reasons or to prevent adherence of dressings. Shaving should be undertaken immediately before surgery but poses a higher infection rate (over 5 per cent) when performed the night before because minor skin injury enhances superficial bacterial colonisation. Cream depilation is messy but clipping is best, with least infection (reportedly under 2 per cent in clean wounds).

Scrubbing of operators' hands with aqueous antiseptics should be confined to nails for the first operation of the day (repeated extensive scrubbing releases more organisms), with washing to the elbows, repeated alone for subsequent operations. Skin preparation of the operative site is adequate with one application of an alcoholic antiseptic (over 95 per cent reduction in flora and fauna). Antiseptics in common use are listed in Table 7.5.

Theatre technique and disciplines also contribute. Only careful surveillance can ensure the quality of theatre ventilation, instrument sterilisation and aseptic technique. Operator skill in gentle manipulation and dissection of tissues is much more difficult to measure but avoidance of dead space, excessive use of diathermy and haematomas surely contribute. There is no evidence that drains, incise drapes or wound guards help to reduce wound infection.

Similar wound surveillance is needed in postoperative care. Secondary (exogenous) nosocomial infections are related to poor hospital wound care. Outbreaks of MRSA are rare but serious. This organism also acts as a marker of adequacy of postoperative wound care but can be very difficult and expensive to eradicate.

Careful audit should lead to changes in practice and follow-up should ensure that loops are closed. It is critical that surgeons manage their own audit – league tables kept by nonmedical or related personnel must be accurate but are to be deprecated. Scoring systems are useful in audit but, in general, have only been used in wound infection research.

Classification of wounds

Potential for infection

The best measure of wound contamination at the end of an operation, and the risk of developing infection, is to sample tissue in the wound edge. Bacteria will already be affected if antibiotic prophylaxis has been given, but the theoretical degree of contamination relates well to infection rates (Table 7.6). When wounds are heavily contaminated or an incision is made into an abscess, continuing prophylaxis as therapy is justified. Infection rates after nonprosthetic clean surgery may be higher if looked for. Antibiotic prophylaxis is controversial.

Bacteria involved in wound infection

Streptococci form chains and are Gram positive on staining (Fig. 7.16). The most important is the β-haemolytic streptococcus which resides in the pharynx of 5–10 per cent of the population. It is in group A of the Lancefield A–G carbohydrate antigens. The alternative name of *Streptococcus pyogenes* is deserved because of its tendency to spread (cellulitis) and to cause tissue destruction through release of

Table 7.5 Classification of antiseptics commonly used in general surgical practice

Name	*Presentation*	*Uses*	*Comments*
Chlorhexidine (Hibiscrub)	Alcoholic 0.5% Aqueous 4%	Skin preparation Skin preparation. Surgical scrub in dilute solutions in open wounds	Has cumulative effect. Effective against Gram-positive organisms and relatively stable in presence of pus and body fluids
Povidone-iodine (Betadine)	Alcoholic 10% Aqueous 7.5%	Skin preparation Skin preparation. Surgical scrub in dilute solutions in open wounds	Safe, fast-acting broad spectrum. Some sporicidal activity. Antifungal. Iodine is not free but combined with polyvinylpyrrolidone (povidone)
Cetrimide (Savlon)	Aqueous	Hand washing Instrument and surface cleaning	*Pseudomonas* spp. may grow in stored contaminated solutions. Ammonium compounds have good detergent action (surface active agent)
Alcohols Hypochlorites	70% ethyl, isopropyl Aqueous preparations (Eusol, Milton, Chloramine T)	Skin preparation Instrument and surface cleaning. (Débriding agent in open wounds?)	Should be reserved for use as disinfectant
Hexachlorophane	Aqueous bisphenol	Skin preparation Hand washing	Has action against Gram-negative organisms

Table 7.6 Wound infection rates currently seen after general surgical operations

Type of surgery	*Infection rare (%)*	*Rate before prophylaxis*
Clean (no viscus opened)	1–2	The same
Clean–contaminated (viscus opened, minimal spillage)	<10	Gastric surgery up to 30% Biliary surgery up to 20%
Contaminated (open viscus with spillage or inflammatory disease)	15–20	Variable but up to 60%
Dirty (pus or perforation, or incision through an abscess)	<40	Up to 60% or more

streptolysin, streptokinase and streptodornase. *Strepococcus faecalis* is the enterococcus in Lancefield group D (often found in synergy with other organisms) and the γ-haemolytic (no haemolysis on blood agar) peptostreptococcus is an anaerobe. Both may be involved in wound infection after large bowel surgery. The α-haemolytic *Streptococcus viridans* is not related to wound infections. The streptococci are still sensitive to penicillin; erythromycin and cephalosporins are alternatives in case of allergy.

Staphylococci form clumps and are Gram positive (Fig. 7.17). *Staphylococcus aureus* is the most important pathogen in this group and resides in the nasopharynx of up to 15 per cent of the population. It can cause exogenous suppuration in wounds (and implanted prosthetics), and MRSA can be involved in epidemics. Doctors and nurses may need to be swabbed and carriers identified and treated in an epidemic. Infections are usually localised (see Wound abscess above). Most hospital *S. aureus* strains are now β-lactamase producers and are resistant to penicillin. Sensitivity to flucloxacillin, vancomycin, aminoglycosides, some cephalosporins and fusidic acid (used in osteomyelitis) is still high.

Staphylococcus epidermidis (syn. *albus* and most conventionally coagulase-negative *Staphylococcus*) was regarded as a commensal but is now recognised as a major threat in prosthetic (vascular and orthopaedic) surgery. It exists in hospitals as a nosocomially acquired organism MRCNS and is resistant to many antibiotics.

Clostridial organisms are Gram-positive, obligate anaerobes which produce resistant spores (Fig. 7.18). *Clostridium perfringens* is the cause of gas gangrene (Specific wound infections above). *Clostridium tetani* causes tetanus following implantation in the tissues or a wound by release of the exotoxin tetanospasmin. A short prodromal period is related to development of severe spasms including opsithotonus, respiratory arrest and death. A longer prodromal period of 4–5 weeks is associated with a much milder form of the disease. Prophylaxis with toxoid is the best preventative treatment but, once established, minor débridement with benzyl penicillin and relaxants (even with ventilation) may be required. The use of antitoxin is controversial.

Clostridium difficile is the cause of pseudomembranous colitis but is not involved in wound infection.

Aerobic Gram-negative bacilli (AGNB) are normal inhabitants of large bowel. *Escherichia coli* and *Klebsiella* spp. are lactose fermenting; *Proteus* is nonlactose fermenting. Most organisms in this group act in synergy with *Bacteroides* to cause wound infections after bowel operations (in particular appendicitis, diverticulitis and peritonitis). The pseudomonads tend to colonise burns and tracheostomy wounds, as well as the urinary tract (all members of this group are a cause of urinary tract infection). Pseudomonads may be regarded as markers and colonise wards and intensive care units from which they may be difficult to eradicate. Surveillance of cross-infection is important in outbreaks. Hospital strains become resistant to β-lactamase which can be transferred by plasmids and individual sensitivity testing may be needed. Wound infections only need antibiotic therapy when there is progressive or spreading

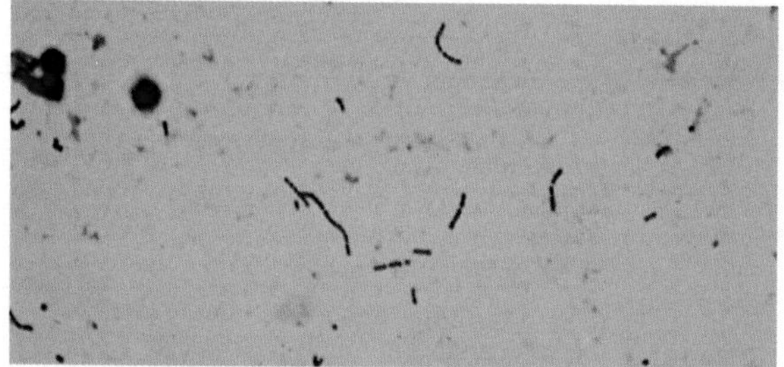

Fig. 7.16 Streptococci.

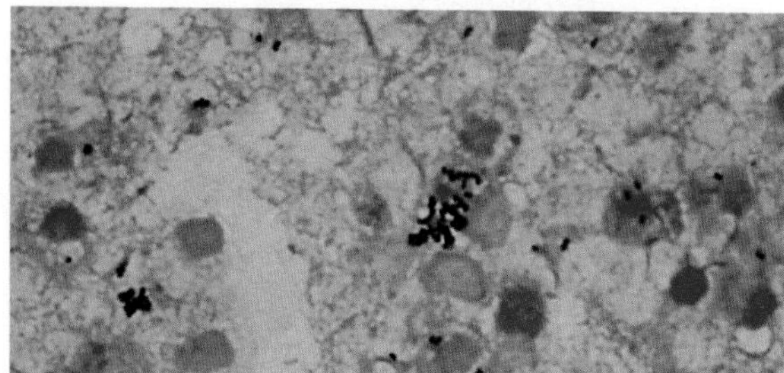

Fig. 7.17 Staphylococcal pus.

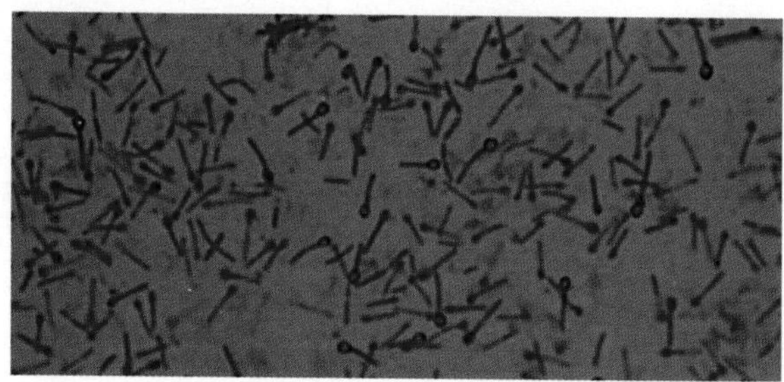

Fig. 7.18 *Clostridium tetani* (drumstick spores).

infection with systemic signs. The aminoglycosides are effective but some cephalosporins and penicillin may not be. Many of the new quinolones, e.g. ciprofloxacin, or carbapenems, e.g. meropenem, are useful in severe infections.

Bacteroides are nonspore-bearing, strict anaerobes which colonise the large bowel, vagina and oropharynx. *Bacteroides fragilis* is the principal organism which acts in synergy with AGNB to cause wound infection after colorectal or gynaecological surgery. They are sensitive to the imidazoles, e.g. metronidazole, and some cephalosporins, e.g. cefotaxime.

Principles of antimicrobial treatment

Antimicrobials may be used to prevent (Prophylaxis above) or treat established wound infection. The use of antibiotics for established infection in wounds ideally requires the isolation of the bacterium and a determination of its sensitivity; this is the overriding first requirement, for after antibiotics are administered, the clinical picture may be confused, the patient no better, and the opportunity to make a precise diagnosis has been lost. However, it is unusual to have to treat wound infections with antibiotics. Only spreading infection or signs of systemic sepsis really justify them. Appropriate treatment must include drainage of pus and débridement if necessary.

Presented with pus, or other material draining from a wound, the microbiologist can isolate the causative organisms and this may guide therapy. There are two approaches to treatment:

- the use of a narrow-spectrum antibiotic to treat a known sensitive infection, e.g. an MRSA sensitive to flucloxacillin (or if not, vancomycin), isolated from pus;
- the use of broad-spectrum antibiotic combinations where the organism is not known or where it is suspected that there may be one, two or more, usually gut-derived bacteria responsible for the infection acting in synergy. Thus, during and following emergency surgery within the abdomen, or requiring the opening of bowel where any of the gut organisms may be responsible for subsequent peritoneal or bacteraemic infection, a combination of broad-spectrum penicillin, such as ampicillin or mezlocillin with an aminoglycoside, e.g. gentamicin, and metronidazole may be used postoperatively to support the patient's own body defences.

Alternatives are a cephalosporin, e.g. cefuroxime, with metronidazole (increasingly popular as gentamicin toxicity and monitoring of levels are avoided), or monotherapy using a carbapenem or quinolone.

In surgical units with multiple resistant *Pseudomonas* or other Gram-negative species (such as *Klebsiella*) which have become 'resident opportunists', there may become a need for a rotation of antipseudomonal and anti-Gram-negative chemotherapy between the broad-spectrum penicillins, e.g. azlocillin 2 g i.v. 8-hourly and cephalosporins, e.g. ceftazidime 50–100 mg/kg per day, or cefotaxime 2 g 8-hourly. The use of these routines, the monitoring of subsequent wound infection and the alternation of combinations of chemotherapy should be monitored by the infection control team. It should not be forgotten, in treating postoperative pyrexial infection, that a failure to respond to a very broad spectrum of these combined antibiotics requires a critical bedside review to exclude collections of pus and other causes of a raised temperature.

New antibiotics should be used with caution and, wherever possible, sensitivities should have been obtained. There are certain general rules from which the choice of antibiotics may be based originally; thus it is unusual for *Pseudomonas aeruginosa* to be found as a primary infecting organism unless the patient has had surgical or hospital treatment. Local antibiotic sensitivity patterns vary from centre to centre and from country to country, and the sensitivity patterns of common pathogens will be known to the hospital microbiologist.

Antibiotics used in treatment and prophylaxis of wound infection

Antimicrobials may be produced by living organisms (antibiotics) or by synthetic methods. Some are bactericidal, e.g. penicillins and aminoglycosides, and others bacteriostatic, e.g. tetracycline and erythromycin. In general, penicillins act upon the cell wall and are most effective against bacteria that are multiplying and synthesising new cell wall materials. The aminoglycosides act at ribosomal level, preventing or distorting the production of proteins required to maintain the integrity of the enzymes in the bacterial cell.

Penicillin. Florey and Chain produced the first therapeutic preparation in 1941, benzylpenicillin, which has proved most effective against Gram-positive pathogens including most streptococci, the clostridia and some of the staphylococci which do not produce β-lactamase. It is still effective against actinomycosis, which rarely is a cause of wound infection, and may be used to treat spreading streptococcal infections specifically, even if other antibiotics are required as part of therapy of a mixed infection. All serious infections, e.g. gas gangrene, require high-dose intravenous benzylpenicillin, e.g. 1.2 g 4-hourly.

Flucloxacillin and methicillin. These are β-lactamase-resistant penicillins and are therefore of use in treating staphylococcal β-lactamase-producing organisms. This is the only reason for using them; and flucloxacillin has poor activity against other pathogens.

Ampicillin and amoxycillin. These β-lactam penicillins are absorbed orally or may be given parenterally. Pharmacodynamically, amoxycillin is superior. Both are effective against enterobacteriaceae, against *E. faecalis* and the majority of group D streptococci, but not species of *Klebsiella* or *Pseudomonas*.

Mezlocillin and azlocillin. These are ureidopenicillins with good activity against species of *Enterobacter* and *Klebsiella*. Azlocillin is particularly effective against *Pseudomonas*. Each has some activity against *Bacteroides* and enterococci, but each is susceptible to β-lactamase. Combined with an aminoglycoside, mezlocillin is a valuable treatment for severe mixed infections, particularly Gram-negative organisms in the immunocompromised patient. *Klebsiella* strains are best treated with mezlocillin, *Pseudomonas* strains with azlocillin.

Clavulanic acid is available combined with amoxycillin for oral treatment. This anti-β-lactamase protects the amoxycillin from inactivation by β-lactamase-producing bacteria. It is of considerable value for treating *Klebsiella* strains and β-lactamase-producing *E. coli* infections, but of no value against *Pseudomonas* strains. Sometimes it is used for localised cellulitis or superficial staphylococcal infection and should be used for infected human and animal bites. It is available for oral or intravenous therapy.

Cephalosporins. There are many β-lactamase-susceptible (not further considered here) and β-lactamase-stable cephalosporins available. There are three that find a place in surgical practice: cefuroxime, cefotaxime and ceftazidime. The first two are most effective in intra-abdominal skin and soft tissue infections, being active against *S. aureus*, and most enterobacteria. As a group, the enterococci (*S. faecalis*) are not sensitive to any of the cephalosporins. Ceftazidime, although being active against the Gram-negative organisms and, to a lesser extent, *S. aureus*, is most effective against *P. aeruginosa*. These cephalosporins may be combined with an aminoglycoside, such as gentamicin, or an imidazole, such as metronidazole, if guaranteed anaerobic cover is needed.

Aminoglycosides. Gentamicin and tobramycin have similar activity and are particularly effective against the Gram-negative enterobacteriaceae. Gentamicin is effective against many strains of *Pseudomonas*, although resistance develops rapidly, but all aminoglycosides are inactive against anaerobes and streptococci. Serum levels immediately before and 1 hour after intramuscular injection must be taken 48 hours after the start of therapy, and dosage should be modified such that the trough level remains at or below 2.5 mg/litre and the peak level should not rise above 10 mg/litre. Ototoxicity and nephrotoxicity may follow sustained high toxic levels. They have a marked postantibiotic effect and single large doses are effective and may be safer.

Vancomycin is most active against Gram-positive bacteria. It is ototoxic and nephrotoxic. Serum levels should be monitored but this antibiotic has proved most effective against multiresistant staphylococcal infection and, when given orally, it is effective against *C. difficile* in cases of pseudomembranous colitis.

Metronidazole is the most widely used member of the imidazole group and is active against all anaerobic bacteria. It is particularly safe and may be administered orally (up to 600 mg 8-hourly), rectally (up to 1 g suppository 8-hourly) or intravenously (500 mg 8-hourly). Infections with anaerobic cocci and strains of *Bacteroides* and *Clostridia* are effectively treated – or prevented – by its use. Metronidazole is responsible for the reduction of anaerobic infections after abdominal, colorectal and pelvic surgery.

Mention has been made of meropenem which, together with imipenem, is a member of the carbopenems, which are stable to β-lactamase. They have useful broad-spectrum anaerobic as well as Gram-positive activity but are expensive.

The quinolones are potent microbicidal agents with action against *Pseudomonas* spp., e.g. ciprofloxacin. Their clinical role in managing wound infection has not been defined.

Further reading

Cohen, I.K., Diegelmann, R.F. and Lindblad, W.J. (1992) *Wound Healing. Biochemical and Chemical Aspects*, W.B. Saunders, Philadelphia, PA.

Davis, J.M. and Shires, G.T. (1991) *Principles and Management of Surgical Infections*, J.B. Lippincott Co., Philadelphia, PA.

Howard, R.J. and Simmons, R.L. (1988) *Surgical Infectious Diseases*, 2nd edn, Appleton and Lange, Norwalk, CT.

Leaper, D.J. and Harding, K.G. (1998) *Wounds: Biology and Management*, Oxford Medical, Oxford.

Majno, G. (1977) *The Healing Hand. Man and Wound in the Ancient World*, Harvard University Press, Cambridge, MA.

Taylor, E.W. (1992) *Infection in Surgical Practice*, Oxford Medical, Oxford.

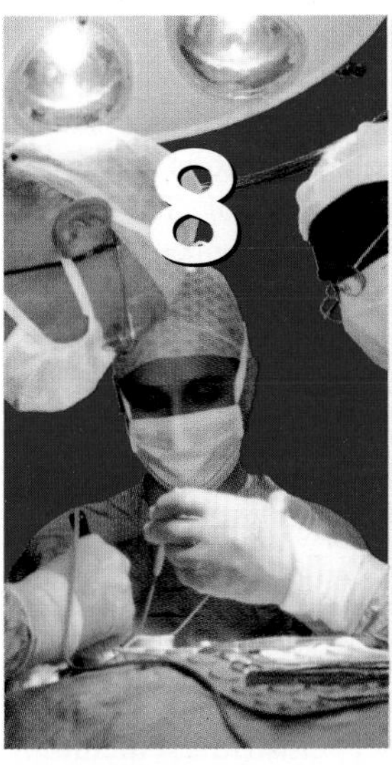

8 Special infections

Clostridia

Tetanus

It has been estimated that, every year, between 300 000 and 500 000 cases of tetanus occur world-wide with an overall mortality of 40–45 per cent. In the UK, 200 cases occur annually, and the condition is also relatively uncommon elsewhere in Europe, in the former Soviet Union and in North America. The burden of this agonising infection falls on those in the other countries of the world, particularly on the children, the neonates (*tetanus neonatorum*) and the elderly. An education programme to have universal active immunisation can and will lead to a reduction in the number of cases and, significantly, the mortality. Tetanus toxoid (now known as tetanus vaccine) practically eliminated tetanus in the armies during World War II. Today, if active immunity is properly initiated and maintained in an individual, death is unlikely even in the presence of clinical tetanus.

Clostridium tetani, the causal organism, is a Gram-positive anaerobic rod with terminal spores (drumstick appearance, Fig. 7.18). Found in manure and soil (notably in market garden areas), it will invade any wound. It multiplies and produces a powerful toxin in any deep, contused wound in the presence of dead tissue, foreign bodies and other bacteria. Penetrating injury from the hoof of an animal can be associated with this infection, while the prick from a rose thorn in a well-manured rose garden can be the sting of death to an elderly assiduous horticulturalist. The exotoxin produced in the inoculation site inhibits the cholinesterase at the motor endplates, resulting in an excess of acetylcholine locally and, therefore, a sustained state of tonic muscle spasm. The exotoxin also travels along the nerves to the central nervous system and causes extreme hyperexcitability of motor neurons in the anterior horn cells, thereby evoking explosive and widespread reflex spasms of muscle in response to sensory stimuli. Once fixed in the nerve tissue, the toxin can no longer be neutralised by antitoxin.

Hans Christian Joachim Gram, 1853–1938. Professor of Medicine, Copenhagen, Denmark.

Bailey & Love's Short Practice of Surgery, 23rd edition. Edited by R.C.G. Russell, N.S. Williams and C.J.K. Bulstrode. Published in 2000 by Arnold Publishers.

Period of onset

The shorter the interval between the first symptom and the first reflex spasm the poorer is the prognosis. (Hippocrates, *circa* 46–77 BC, is believed to have been the first to recognise this fact.) If the interval is less than 48 hours, death is likely. It should be remembered that wounds containing tetanus organisms may have healed and been forgotten for months or years before some (unknown) change produces the right conditions for the organism to multiply and produce toxin (*latent tetanus*).

Symptoms and signs

Dysphagia, jaw stiffness and severe pains in the neck, back and abdomen precede the tonic muscle spasms. The sardonic smile of tetanus (*risus sardonicus*) is evidence of the onset of tonic muscle spasm. Respiration and swallowing become progressively more difficult, and reflex convulsions occur affecting all muscles and causing great pain, opisthotonus (spasm of the extensors of the neck, back and legs to form a

Hippocrates, by common consent the father of medicine, was born on the Greek Island of Cos, off Turkey, in about 460 BC and died in 375 BC.

backward curvature) and even muscle rupture. The spasms are spontaneous, but can be induced by trivial stimuli such as noise or movement and, when severe, will prevent respiration and produce cyanosis. Between the reflex convulsions, the tonic muscular spasm remains, thus distinguishing tetanus from strychnine poisoning. The temperature is elevated, the pulse is rapid, and respiratory failure and death during a cyanotic attack will usually follow if treatment is not initiated.

At an early stage, the symptoms and signs of tetanus might be mistaken for tonsillitis, flu, backstrain or an acute upper abdominal condition. Therefore, careful examination of the patient for a wound is of paramount importance.

Treatment

Isolation, quietness and comfort, drainage of pus and wound toilet will be needed. Human anti-tetanus globulin (e.g. Humotet) is given intramuscularly (i.m.) to limit the effects of free toxins and should be used in doses of 25–500 units to give cover throughout the period of establishing active immunity by giving toxoid (tetanus vaccine, adsorbed) i.m. Equine tetanus antiserum has been used but about 20 per cent of patients develop serum sickness and occasional anaphylactic reactions occur. Antibiotics, including penicillin and metronidazole, are indicated along with measures to protect the lungs.

Stage 1. A mild case, where there is tonic rigidity alone, will require initial sedation, relaxation by drugs such as promazine up to 200 mg i.m. and a barbiturate or diazepam [~50 mg intravenously (i.v.)]. These drugs will be needed approximately four times during any 24-hour period.

Stage 2. A seriously ill patient, with dysphagia and reflex spasm, will need to have a nasogastric tube passed and sedation continued. The diet, the need for intravenous nutrition, the maintenance of balanced protein intake, and of renal function and cardiac function will be priorities. A tracheostomy should be considered if the patient has any difficulty in breathing. The meticulous care of the tracheostomy tube includes suction and humidification (Chapter 43).

Stage 3. In dangerously ill patients, a major cyanotic convulsion will require curarisation, e.g. up to 40 mg tubocurarine i.v. initially and afterwards i.m. to maintain relaxation. It should be remembered that the curarised patient, although unresponsive, is conscious and sensitive and can hear everything that is being said. Intermittent positive-pressure respiration should be provided, and intensive nursing care with increasing sedation would be needed because it has been estimated that a patient at this stage will require at least 350 individual acts of nursing each day. The objective is to reduce the risk of death from spasms or pneumonia wherever possible, while realising that a lethal amount of toxin has already caused severe damage to the motor neurons and the brain with concomitant myocarditis and vascular failure. If recovery takes place, the patient can be weaned from the ventilator (after about 14 days as long as convulsions do not recur when the effects of the relaxants wear off).

Results. With the proper attention to nursing care, prophylactic antibiotic therapy, active and passive immunisation against tetanus and, where indicated, tracheostomy, curarisation and assisted respiration, the death rate can be reduced to approximately 15 per cent. The results in the very young and very old nevertheless are still poor. The tetanospasmin produced by the infection is insufficient to generate an immune response so a course of immunisation is recommended on recovery.

Gas gangrene

Wounds allowing the patient's own faecal flora, or clostridial spores in the soil, to enter the tissues can give rise to anaerobic gas-producing infections. Surgery around the hip joint and leg amputations are at high risk from this postoperative complication, as are the wounds of warfare (Chapter 19). *Clostridium perfringens (welchii)* is usually the cause in about 80 per cent, but other clostridia, including *Clostridium novyi* (*Clostridium oedematiens*), *Clostridium histolyticum*, *Clostridiumbifermentans* and *Clostridium septicum* may be causal. *Clestridium welchii* is found in the stools and therefore is also found on the perineum and, occasionally, as normal flora in the vagina. The clostridia produce numerous toxins, including an α-toxin believed to be important in the pathogenesis of gas gangrene.

Clostridial invasion of a traumatised muscle affects the whole of that muscle from origin to insertion, producing a foul-smelling necrosis of the bundles which lose contractibility and become dull red, green or black in appearance. If septicaemia occurs, gas is produced in many organs, notably the liver (which at necropsy drips with frothy blood – the 'foaming liver').

Subcutaneous tissues alone can be infected; the foul-smelling necrosis, often spreading extensively, can begin in the margin of an abdominal or a thoracic wound.

Clinical features

The wound is under tension and between the sutures the pouting edges exude a brownish and foul-smelling fluid. The skin becomes discoloured – a khaki colour – owing to associated haemolysis. Crepitus can usually be detected. (Crepitus, to the examining hand, feels like an old hair mattress.) A radiograph will show the gas in the muscles or under the skin. The patient, although toxic and pale, with raised pulse, misleadingly appears mentally clear.

Treatment

Treatment, to be effective, requires immediate action:

1. maximum doses of penicillin (up to 2.4 g 4-hourly) – traditionally the treatment of choice, although recent work suggests a better outcome with clindamycin and metronidazole;

William Henry Welch, 1850–1934. Professor of Pathology, Johns Hopkins University, Baltimore, Maryland, USA. Discovered the causative organism of gas gangrene in 1892.

2. blood transfusion;
3. either exposure of all the affected muscle groups by long incisions or, in the subcutaneous infections, multiple subcutaneous drainage and slough extraction by incisions into the subcutaneous tissue;
4. hyperbaric oxygen where this is available. It is said to be helpful in the postoperative period.

The use of antiserum used to be recommended, but clinical experience was variable, stocks are now depleted and there has been little interest in resuming production.

Clostridial pseudomembranous colitis

This is an acute, profuse, antibiotic-associated diarrhoea which produces characteristic changes of the colon, recognisable sigmoidoscopically by a pseudomembrane and subsequently by sloughing of the colonic mucosa. The organism responsible, *C. difficile*, produces a toxin which cross-reacts with *Clostridium sordellii* antitoxin to produce a serious, sometimes fatal, colitis. The toxin can be demonstrated by its cytopathic effect in cell culture as well as by a number of commercial enzyme-linked immunosorbent assay (ELISA) kits. The organism can be cultured from stool but this does not necessarily indicate a pathogenic role. A spectrum of disease is recognised, ranging from antibiotic-associated diarrhoea (AAD) to antibiotic-associated colitis (AAC) to pseudomembranous colitis (PMC). The incidence is high among older patients, especially where broad-spectrum antibiotics (penicillins and cephalosporins) or clindamycin have been used, although almost every antibiotic has been implicated.

Treatment involves stopping antibiotic therapy where possible, general supportive measures and oral metronidazole or vancomycin. Relapse is well documented and further courses of therapy may be required. Being a sporing organism, it survives well in the hospital environment and in some centres is a considerable problem. It is readily transmitted by hand contact.

The salmonellas

Salmonella typhi, paratyphi. These are enteric pathogens which cause enteric fevers with bacteraemia, osteomyelitis and sometimes perforation of ileal ulcers. Persistence of the bacteria in the gallbladder may lead to the carrier state and subsequently person-to-person spread in the community (see Chapter 54). The use of ciprofloxacin 500 mg twice daily for 10 days is recommended for *S. typhi* infections although resistance has now been demonstrated in the Indian subcontinent. It is useful as it prevents or cures long-term carriage, and resistance to the more commonly used drugs (ampicillin, chloramphenicol) has reached very high levels in some parts of the world.

The other salmonellas are associated with food poisoning, diarrhoea and, therefore, dehydration. Control of the symptoms only is usually required, and the use of antimicrobials is not usually helpful for thereby resistant strains are encouraged, excretion can be prolonged, and in any case the intestinal symptoms are self-limiting. In the unusual event of systemic spread and bacteraemia, it will be necessary to use the antibiotics to which the isolate is sensitive. If treatment is started before the organism is isolated, a broad-spectrum penicillin combined with an aminoglycoside may then be required. The commonest nontyphoid salmonellas are *S. typhimurium, S. enteritidis* and *S. virchow.* They are found in cattle, calves, poultry, turkeys and domestic animals, and infection in humans is by direct spread from contaminated food. These organisms can spread within a hospital if patients (or staff) with diarrhoea are not recognised as a risk; close contacts of excreta must be properly protected by apron and gloves to reduce the likelihood of the infection being spread by unwashed hands which have become contaminated with faeces.

Daniel Elmer Salmon, 1850–1914. American pathologist.

Mycobacteria

Tuberculosis

Mycobacterium tuberculosis was discovered by Robert Koch in 1882, while he was working in the Imperial Health Office, Berlin, Germany. This acid-fast bacillus is spread by airborne infection (or from infected cows in the case of bovine tuberculosis). There are three routes of primary infection:

- direct spread to lungs;
- from tonsils to the lymph nodes of the neck where an abscess may form and track round the edge of the sternomastoid muscle, producing a collar-stud abscess;
- from lower ileal infection to the lymph nodes of the ileocaecal angle.

The bacterium, which produces no pigment, grows well at 37°C and may be seen, if there are very many organisms, in the Ziehl–Neelsen stained smear. Growth of the bacteria takes 6 weeks; thus sensitivities to the antituberculous drugs will be delayed. Recently, new techniques – including the polymerase chain reaction (PCR) – have given hope that more rapid diagnosis will soon be possible.

For the accounts of the manifestations of this disease in various organs as applied to the practice of surgery, the reader is referred to the appropriate chapters of this book.

Guidelines for treatment

Nutrition and hygienic living conditions are still crucially important in preventing the spread of this infection.

Treatment with triple therapy consisting of rifampicin 600 mg, isoniazid 300 mg and pyrazinamide 1500–2000 mg per day given orally for at least 2–3 months is the standard chemotherapy at present, followed by 6 months of double therapy (rifampicin plus isoniazid). Sensitivity testing is usually available at the end of the first period of triple therapy and, if the source of the infection is with an organism that is resistant to one of these drugs, appropriate changes can then be made. Ethambutol may be of use in resistant cases. In cases of pulmonary tuberculosis, the sputum should be examined to assess progress every month until the smears are negative, but should the number of acid-fast bacilli increase or the cultures remain positive, the development of resistance or noncompliance of the patient with treatment should be considered.

Robert Koch, 1843–1910. Professor of Hygiene and Bacterial Pathology, Berlin, Germany (1855–1910).
F. Ziehl, 1859–1926. German bacteriologist.
F.K.A. Neelsen, 1854–94. German pathologist.

Genitourinary and orthopaedic tuberculosis is usually effectively treated by the standard 9-month course but the use of pyrazinamide with rifampicin and isoniazid may be required. All of these antituberculous drugs have side effects which may require repeated careful assessment and control; isoniazid causes a peripheral neuritis, ethambutol produces visual impairment and rifampicin is hepatotoxic. Pyrazinamide should be avoided in patients with gout.

It should be remembered that it is nigh impossible to eradicate every tubercle bacillus from the body. Lying dormant and enveloped in fibrous tissue, any remaining bacilli are still able to cause a flare-up of the disease, particularly after trauma, after gastrointestinal operations resulting in nutritional deficiency, and in old age, immune deficiency or long-term use of steroids. Of great concern recently is the appearance of multidrug-resistant tuberculosis (MDRTB). This has arisen as a result of poor compliance with treatment. Although there are some drugs available to treat these strains, patients with underlying immunosuppression often fail to respond and this means that the disease is now a serious threat among patients with human immunodeficiency virus (HIV) infection. Several outbreaks have been described among acquired immunodeficiency syndrome (AIDS) sufferers and a number of healthcare workers has also been infected. Drugs that may be useful in the treatment of MDRTB include ethionamide, ofloxacin, capreomycin and cycloserine.

Opportunist mycobacteria

'Slow-growing' opportunist mycobacteria may be found producing lesions similar to *M. tulerculosis* in susceptible patients. Thus, *M. kansaslii* is a slow-growing opportunist mycobacterium which may cause pulmonary lesions. *Mycobacterium chelonael* and *M. fortuitum* occasionally cause subcutaneous abscesses following skin trauma. This group should always be remembered in the differential diagnosis of subcutaneous abscesses associated with skin traumas or injections (e.g. tetanus immunisation). Skin granulomas in swimmers may be caused by *M. marinum,* while the surgically important Buruli ulcer occurring in East Africa, which affects the exposed surface of the limbs, is caused by *M. ulcerans,* and presents as a spreading granulomatous nodule which subsequently breaks down and forms an ulcer. Incision of the nodule at an early stage and treatment with rifampicin may prevent an ulcer forming, but secondary infection of a Buruli ulcer may result in fibrosis and considerable deformities of a limb as a result. *Mycobacterium avium-intracellulare* is becoming increasingly recognised as a pathogen in patients with AIDS. All of the opportunist mycobacteria should be cultured to assess their sensitivity to the antimycobacterial drugs.

Leprosy (Hansen's disease)

Gerhard Hansen first showed that leprosy was a bacterial infection caused by *M. leprae*. Because of the stigma attached to leprosy, Dr R.G. Cochrane and others recommended that it should be referred to as Hansen's disease. There are probably from 10 to 15 million leprosy sufferers in the world today.

Leprosy is an infectious disease widely spread throughout the tropical and subtropical areas of the world. It is caused by *M. leprae*, an acid-fast bacillus morphologically like the tubercle bacillus. It is mainly, but not entirely, contracted in childhood and late adolescence. While the mode of transmission regarding the portal of entry of *M. leprae* is not known, the source of infection is mainly from the nasal secretions of patients with lepromatous leprosy and not from their skin. Leprosy is no longer endemic in northern Europe, as it was in the Middle Ages, and in Norway until the late nineteenth century; neither is it now spread by immigrants in Europe. These facts suggest that leprosy requires for its transmission some factors associated with poverty or lack of hygiene that are common in the areas where it is still endemic. A vast change in the outlook for this disease has occurred in the last 30 years. The condition was formerly regarded as hopeless, but in spite of the fact that it is now curable, only 25 per cent of the cases of this widely spread disease are under treatment. It is probably true to say that leprosy causes more paralysis, deformity and misery than any other disease, but that, in many cases, these could now be prevented by modern therapy, given an adequate service for early diagnosis.

Although leprosy is a systemic infection, it presents predominantly as an infection of the skin, upper respiratory tract and dermal and peripheral nerves. Leprosy must always be considered in a patient presenting with a combination of skin *and* neural disorder, particularly because of the variation in the preponderance of these two manifestations and the tremendous variation in the appearance and histopathology of the dermal lesions among individual patients with leprosy. These diverse manifestations led to a plethora of classification systems until Ridley and Jopling found that there was a spectrum of disease in leprosy determined by the resistance of the host (Fig. 8.1). The spectrum ranges from polar lepromatous (LL) to polar tuberculoid (TT) leprosy, denoting patients with minimal and maximal irreversible capacities to mount an immunological response against *M. leprae*. The majority of patients is more labile in having some residual immunological capacity against *M. leprae,* and thus are represented as borderline (BB), or borderline lepromatous (BL) or borderline tuberculoid (BT), if they veer more

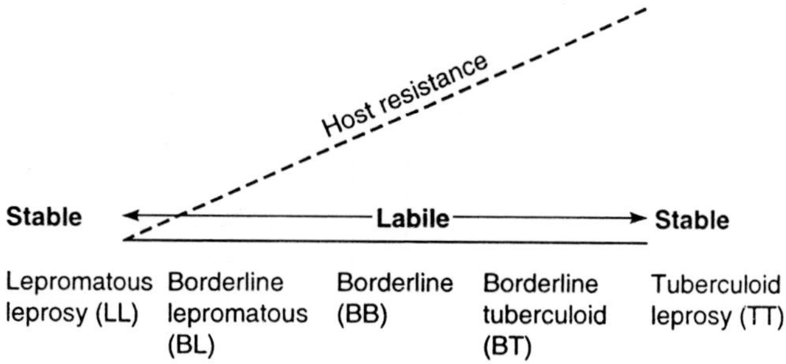

Fig. 8.1 Ridley–Jopling classification of leprosy based on immunity of host.

Gerhard Henrik Armauer Hansen, 1841–1922. Physician in Charge of a Leper Hospital near Bergen, Norway.
Robert Greenhill Cochrane. Former Medical Superintendent, Kola Ndoto Leprosarium, Shinyange, Tanzania.
Dennis Snow Ridley. Consultant pathologist, Hospital for Tropical Diseases, London, England.
William Henry Jopling. Former consultant leprologist, Hospital for Tropical Diseases, London, England.

towards lepromatous or tuberculoid leprosy. If left untreated, patients anywhere within the borderline spectrum can deteriorate towards lepromatous leprosy, whereas under treatment they will shift towards polar tuberculoid leprosy.

Lepromatous leprosy

There is little or no resistance, the bacilli multiply with little cellular response, until the subcutaneous tissues may be loaded with masses of bacilli, many of them distending macrophages as large 'globi'. The cellular infiltrate is mainly of macrophages with a few lymphocytes.

Tuberculoid leprosy

There is a strong tissue response, the bacilli are not numerous and are seldom seen except by special concentration methods. The histology consists of an epitheloid granuloma, many lymphocytes and a few giant cells.

Characteristically, *tuberculoid* leprosy causes sharply localised lesions often affecting only one part of the body, while *lepromatous* leprosy is symmetrical and extensive. Since the damage in leprosy is mainly due to the response of the host cells, tuberculoid leprosy causes early, severe but localised deformity, while lepromatous leprosy causes deformity late, and more mildly and widely spread. The most severely deformed patients are those affected by some of the borderline forms where the disease may be both widespread through the body and also rather violent in its reactions.

A unique feature of the disease is its predilection not only for the surface of the body, but also for the cool part of the surface. Warm areas such as the axilla and gluteal cleft are spared, while the parts of the upper respiratory tract, such as the lining of the nose, are severely involved. The testis is affected, while the ovary, and other deeply placed glands and organs, are unaffected. Since leprosy does not affect the vital organs of the body, it rarely causes death, and patients do not even feel ill for most of the time they have the disease.

During treatment, many patients manifest acute episodes, which are referred to as 'reactions', of which there are two distinct types.

1. The 'lepra or type 1 reaction' occurs in the borderline form of leprosy (BT, BB and BL), in which the skin lesions become erythematous, warm to touch and may break down, and the nerves swell and become painful and tender to touch. It is usually caused by a rapid increase in cell-mediated immunity by the host with an outpouring of lymphocytes into the lesions giving rise to acute inflammation with associated oedema. For this reason, the lesions have been referred to as 'reversal reactions', advantageous by resulting in destruction of *M. leprae,* but causing irreversible destruction of axons when the inflammation and oedema occur in nerves.
2. The other type of reaction is referred to as erythema nodosum leprosum (ENL or type 2 reaction), usually occurring during treatment, but confined to patients with lepromatous type leprosy (BL, LL). Here there are no changes in the established leprosy lesions, but new crops of very small erythematous lesions in the skin appear associated with systemic symptoms such as malaise, fever and nerve and joint pain. Occasionally, rhinitis, acute iridocyclitis, swollen and tender lymph glands, acute epididymo-orchitis and proteinuria occur. This is an Arthus-type reaction, due to the deposition of immune complexes in and around blood vessels, locally or generalised throughout the body, and more akin to chronic serum sickness. This reaction may come and go or be persistent, and can in its most severe form be fatal.

One of the most characteristic features of leprosy is its effect on nerves (Fig. 8.2). Histologically, the cellular infiltrate may be seen localised around nerve fibres in and under the skin and, on clinical examination, superficial nerves such as the ulnar and posterior auricular may be observed to be swollen and tender. The anaesthesia that results from nerve involvement is an important point in diagnosis, and is also a cause of secondary damage and deformity. Much of the loss and disfigurement of hands and feet which has always been associated with leprosy is now known to be due not to leprosy itself, but to the damage and misuse which follow loss of pain sensation.

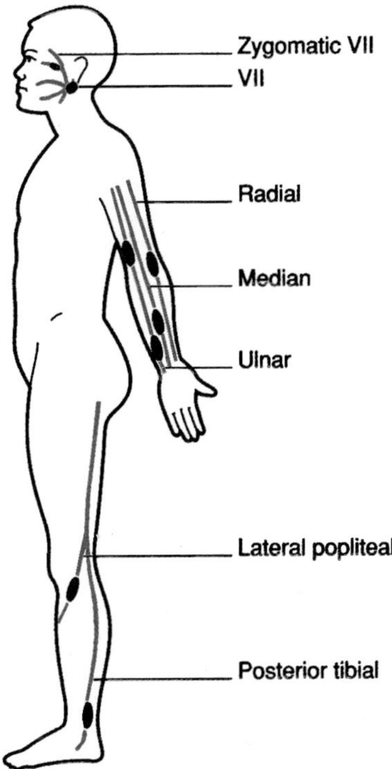

Fig. 8.2 Sites of motor paralysis in leprosy: ulnar nerve just below joint or wrist joint; median nerve just above wrist joint; lateral popliteal at knee joint; posterior tibial above ankle joint; facial nerve in the bony canal or the zygomatic branch; radial nerve at the elbow (rarely) (*after Paul Brand*).

Medical treatment

Until 1980, dapsone (diaminodiphenyl sulphone, DDS) was the standard treatment for leprosy. The problems of DDS resistance and the inordinately long duration of therapy have led to today's standard treatment – multidrug therapy (MDT). For multibacillary cases (which include LL, BL, BB and some BT cases), the treatment duration is 2 years or until negativity is achieved, whereas for paucibacillary leprosy (which indudes all tuberculoid cases and many BT cases) the treatment duration is 6 months or until the lesions become inactive. Rifampicin, the first bactericidal drug against *M. leprae,* is given in a dose of 600 mg a day for 2 days at the beginning of each month, while DDS is given in a dose of 100 mg daily. This two-drug regimen is adequate for paucibacillary cases. For multibacillary leprosy clofazimine at 50 mg daily is added as the third drug. Recently, clarithromycin, ofloxacin and minocycline have been shown to be effective.

For reactions, symptomatic treatment, including analgesics, is given for milder cases. Evidence of nerve damage indicates a necessity to start steroid therapy. For the more severe reactions, reversal and ENL, it is absolutely essential to treat with steroids to protect the nerves and to keep the patient going. In ENL reactions, but only in LL cases, thalidomide has proved to be very beneficial and is also useful in the treatment of steroid dependency. Thalidomide, if available, is used to treat only male patients, or females outside the childbearing years, because of its known teratogenic effects. Psychotropic drugs, e.g. chlorpromazine and amitriptyline, are often needed in cases of severe reaction to treat associated psychological disturbances.

Decompression of nerves

The relief of compression caused by the thickened nerve sheath and by the fibrous roofs of tunnels at entrapment sites (cubital, carpal and tarsal tunnels) is an important supplementary procedure to prevent further damage to the involved peripheral nerve trunks. Intractable pain is a definite indication, while increasing paralysis, in spite of treatment with steroids, is a further indication for nerve decompression.

Surgery

The deformities of leprosy are divided into *primary* – those which are caused directly by leprosy and its reactions and *secondary* – those which result from anaesthesia and consequent misuse. The stigma of leprosy is the stigma of deformity, and a wide-open field awaits the plastic surgeon in this disease.

The face. ***Primary deformity.*** The skin of the face becomes thickened and sometimes nodular in lepromatous leprosy (Fig. 8.3); the forehead, cheeks, nose and ears are especially affected. The result in the acute phase is referred to as 'leonine facies'. This infiltration subsides under medical treatment, but may leave the skin wrinkled and without its normal support, producing, in a younger person, a caricature of old age. The hair of the eyebrows falls out and the lateral cartilages and septum of the nose may be destroyed, leaving collapse of the centre of the nose and lifting of the tip towards the bridge (Fig. 8.4). The upper branches of the facial nerve may be paralysed, giving rise to lagophthalmos; the lower branches are sometimes partially paralysed.

Patients with the above deformities usually find it quite impossible to return to normal social relationships even though their leprosy may be cured. Plastic surgery can completely transform such faces using a postnasal inlay to the nose (Fig. 8.4) and an 'island flap' for the eyebrows. A temporalis muscle segment reactivates the eyelids and a facelift may restore more normal contours to the skin.

Eyes. Some of the blindness of leprosy is simply due to exposure following paralysis of the eyelids. This is correctable by plastic surgery. Other causes of loss of vision are lepromatous infiltration of the anterior segment of the eye and acute allergic changes of the tissues associated with reaction. Acute iridocyclitis is one of the commonest manifestations of this allergic reaction. Any redness of the eye or loss of visual acuity in leprosy demands full examination and prompt treatment if the sight is to be saved. Treatment should include atropine and hydrocortisone eyedrops as well as oral steroids.

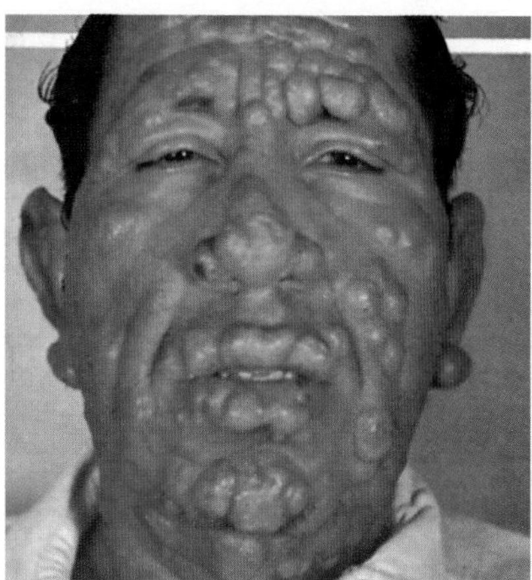

Fig. 8.3 Nodular lepromatous leprosy.

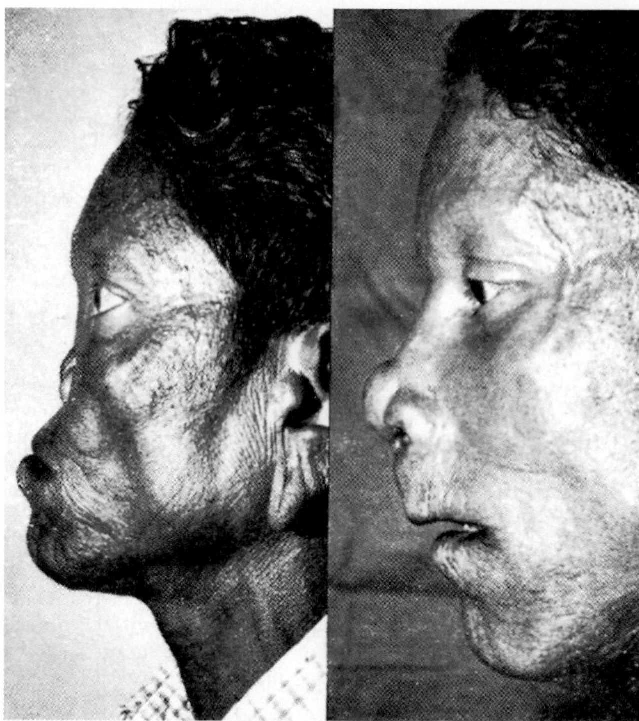

Fig. 8.4 Extreme case of nasal collapse (left). After postnasal epithelial inlay (right) (*courtesy of N.H. Antia, from the Annals of the Royal College of Surgeons of England, with permission*).

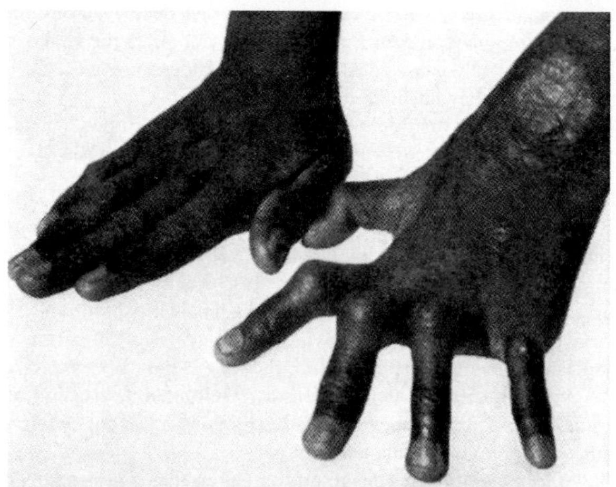

Fig. 8.5 Clawed left hand in leprosy. The patient commonly loses the use of all the small muscles of the hand, but few forearm muscles. The fingers are clawed and the thumb lies completely unopposed (*courtesy of Dr R.G. Cochrane, London, England*).

Hands (Fig. 8.5). The work on reconstruction of the hand in Hansen's disease was started by Professor Paul Brand.

Primary deformity. In the upper limbs, leprosy causes paralysis, frequently in the ulnar nerve at the elbow and in the median nerve at the wrist (Fig. 8.2) but rarely in the motor part of the radial nerve (1 per cent).

Treatment. The extensor carpi radialis brevis muscle is extended into the hand with free grafts which run along the lines of the lumbrical

Paul Wilson Brand. Chief of the Rehabilitation Branch, US Public Health Service Hospital, Carville, Louisiana, USA.

tendons to correct the clawing of the fingers. The flexor sublimis tendon to the ring finger is withdrawn in the forearm and rerouted to oppose the thumb along the line of the abductor brevis. In this way the fingers and thumb may be balanced and function almost normally. Before attempting operation it is important to make sure that the fingers are made mobile by massage and exercise.

Secondary deformity. Since the hand is often totally anaesthetic, patients frequently burn or damage themselves by the uninhibited strength which they use through their fingertips. Their hands become scarred and progressively absorbed until only stumps remain. It takes patience and perseverance to teach patients that their hands can be preserved only by constant alertness to foresee possible dangers, and constant gentleness to their own tissues which are not protected by pain. Once they are convinced that it is not leprosy that is destroying their fingers, they may be willing to accept the discipline of caring for themselves.

Feet. *Primary deformity.* In the lower limbs, the posterior tibial nerve is often involved at the ankle, giving rise to 'clawing' of the toes and anaesthesia of the sole of the foot. The lateral popliteal nerve may also be destroyed, giving rise to footdrop. The medial popliteal nerve is never involved, so the tibialis posterior muscle can be safely used to correct footdrop.

Secondary deformity. The anaesthesia of the sole of the foot is very serious because almost every patient with insensitive feet sooner or later develops trophic ulceration. If patients then continue to walk on their ulcers, the condition progresses and the infection spreads until, after a few years, the foot is contracted and distorted, and destroyed to the point where amputation must be advised.

It is important for patients to understand the pathology of their ulcers and to realise that they are not due directly to leprosy. These ulcers heal readily with rest in a plaster cast and their recurrence can be prevented by the regular use of special footwear designed to spread the weight evenly over the whole foot.

Treponemas

Syphilis derives its name from a poem by a physician, Girolamo Fracastoro (1478–1553), published in Venice in 1530. The poem tells of the shepherd, Syphilus, who was struck down by the disease as a punishment for insulting Apollo.

On his return from Haiti in 1493, Christopher Columbus (1451–1506) brought back syphilis, parrots and rare plants. The King and Queen of Spain received him with highest honours.

For a detailed description of venereal syphilis, reference should be made to a textbook on sexually transmitted disease (STD).

Acquired syphilis

Acquired syphilis is an STD infection caused by *Treponema pallidum*, a delicate spiral organism (spirochaete), 6–15 m in length. A dramatic decline in incidence after the introduction of penicillin has been followed by a gradual but significant increase throughout the world.

Transmission is by direct contact with a surface lesion containing treponemes, which penetrate the skin or mucosa at the point of contact. Since treponemes are present only in the surface lesions of *early* syphilis, i.e. primary, secondary and the first 2 years of latency, syphilis is only infective during that period. After 2 years, acquired syphilis is rarely communicable and the ulcerative cutaneous lesions of tertiary syphilis are not infective as they contain few, if any, treponemes. The organism dies rapidly on drying, hence infective early lesions are predominantly sited on moist areas, e.g. genitals, mouth and anus, so that infection almost always occurs during intercourse including orogenital contact and – of great importance now – homosexual practices involving the anus and rectum.

Girolamo Fracastoro, 1478–1553. Italian physician, astronomer and poet. Professor of Philosophy at the University of Padua, 1502. Demonstrated the specific character of fevers and discovered typhus.

Clinical features

The disease is divided into four stages: primary, secondary, latent and late.

Primary syphilis. A primary sore or chancre (Figs 8.6 and 8.7) develops at the site of entry of the treponemes in about 3–4 weeks. It may resolve at any stage of its development and thus be quite atypical. It may simulate other penile or vulval lesions, traumatic lesions such as splits or tears,

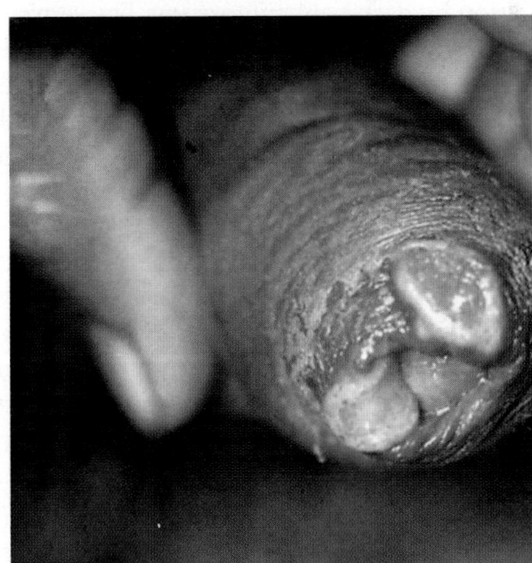

Fig. 8.6 Penile primary chancres.

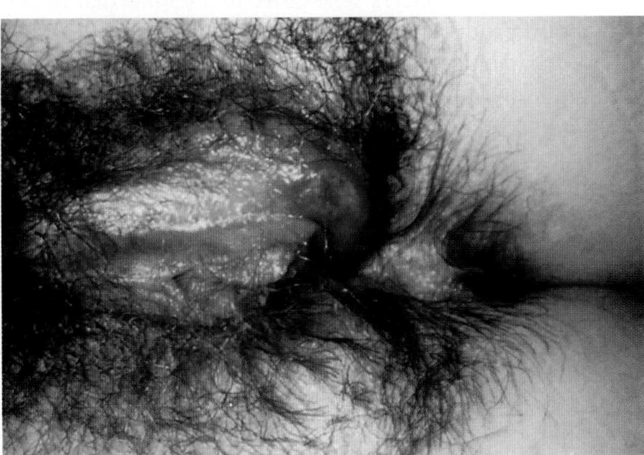

Fig. 8.7 Vulval chancre.

chancroid, herpes genitalis, burns, furuncles and carcinoma, as well as balanoposthitis and lymphogranuloma venereum (Chapter 67).

Starting as an indurated papule, it becomes eroded and when fully developed will present the following signs of a classic Hunterian chancre: a shallow, indurated, painless, nonbleeding ulcer, usually single, oval or round, with a raised hyperaemic margin, often extending into a dusky red oedema. A painless, discrete and 'shotty' enlargement of the associated lymph nodes occurs which has a rubbery consistency. The prepuce of the penis *must* always be fully retracted as otherwise tiny sores in the coronal sulcus may be missed. As there are no constitutional symptoms, a female patient will be unaware of the presence of a cervical chancre, a lesion which accounts for about 45 per cent of all sores in that sex. Extragenital chancres of the lip[1], tongue, nipple, etc., are now rare, but rectal and perianal primaries are common in homosexuals and are usually atypical, frequently resembling painful anal fissures which occasionally get excised in error. Spasm of the anal sphincter is usually less with true sores and a typical (lateral) inguinal lymphadenitis may be present.

Diagnosis is by finding *T. pallidum* in the clear exudate from the lesion by dark-field microscopy. The serum tests do not become positive for 10–90 days (usually 3–5 weeks) after the appearance of the chancre, hence initial negative results must never be interpreted as excluding primary syphilis. This is because the tests identify a gradually developing antibody response. The tests should be repeated for up to 3 months where doubt persists.

Secondary syphilis. Signs usually appear in 6–12 weeks, extremes being 3 weeks to 6 months. The commonest sign is a dull red or coppery rash, which is generalised, symmetrical, indolent and nonirritant. Often inconspicuous, sometimes absent (in 25 per cent of cases), the rash is characteristically pleomorphic, being roseolar or macular at first, with papular, papulosquamous or other elements appearing later. Papules on contiguous moist sites, e.g. vulva and perineum, may enlarge to form condylomata lata, fleshy, wart-like growths teeming with treponemes. Small, round, superficial erosions may occur in the mouth where they may coalesce to form the so-called snail-track ulcers. The rash can resemble that of any known rash-producing condition in the whole of medicine. A generalised, painless lymphadenopathy often occurs, and less common symptoms include sore throat, hoarseness, 'moth-eaten' alopecia, hepatitis, iritis, and bone and joint pains. Bone pains may be severe and prolonged for several weeks without any other supporting signs, and the diagnosis is often missed. Acute meningitis or cranial nerve or spinal root palsies due to an irregular pachymeningitis occur. Constitutional effects, malaise, headache, backache and pyrexia, normally mild, are occasionally of prostrating severity. Secondary syphilis is also a cause of pyrexia of unascertained origin (PUO).

Full spontaneous recovery always occurs.

Latent syphilis. This follows the untreated secondary stage and lasts from 2 years to a lifetime. There are no signs, but the serum tests are positive.

Late syphilis (syn. tertiary syphilis). Syphilis in all its stages is essentially a vascular disease. In each stage, treponemes cause inflammatory reactions in the perivascular lymphatics with plasma cell cuffing of terminal vessels. In the tertiary stage only there is subsequent obliterative endarteritis, tissue necrosis and fibrosis. Since almost any structure may be involved, the signs can be extraordinarily variable, and will be referable to the site or system involved. Only about 35 per cent of untreated syphilitics will develop tertiary syphilis. About 5–15 years after infection, 10 per cent will develop neurosyphilis, 10–12 per cent cardiovascular syphilis and after 6 months up to many years later, 10–15 per cent will develop late benign syphilis involving less vital structures. The three types are not mutually exclusive. The typical lesion of late benign syphilis is the localised gumma (Fig. 8.8) or diffuse gummatous infiltration. The gumma is a syphilitic hypersensitivity reaction consisting of granulation tissue with central necrosis. Sloughing of a subcutaneous gumma may produce the typical, painless, punched-out gummatous ulcer with a 'wash-leather' base (Fig. 8.9). On healing, it leaves a silvery 'tissue-paper' scar. Alter-

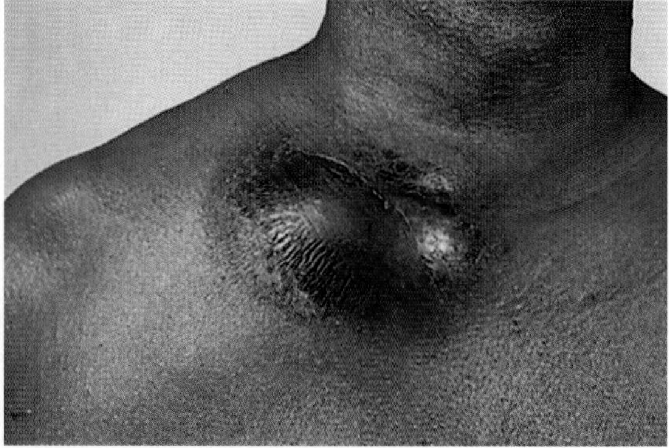

Fig. 8.8 Gumma overlying the sternoclavicular joint. A classic site.

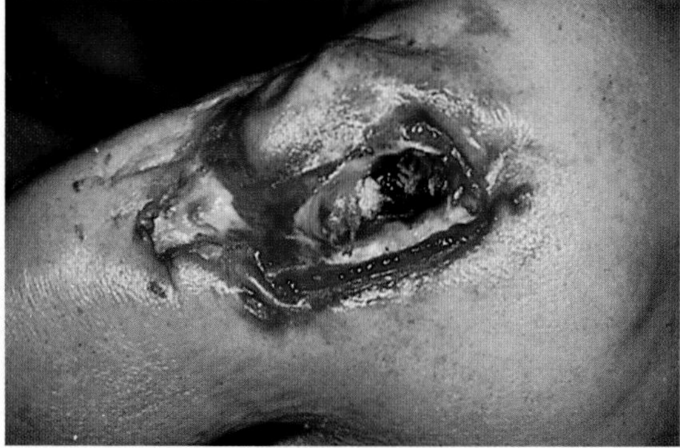

Fig. 8.9 Punched-out gumma of the shoulder. This lesion was characteristically painless.

John Hunter, 1728–93. Surgeon, St George's Hospital, London, England. To further his knowledge of venereal disease he inoculated either himself or another with syphilis in 1767.

[1]*Primary sores on the lips usually result from kissing, and a case is recorded in which a gentleman with secondary ulceration of the mouth infected five young ladies at a dance, each of whom developed a chancre on the lip.*

natively, the gummatous process may be nodular or infiltrative without ulceration, and slow peripheral spread occurs with central healing. The individual lesions are round and indurated, and grouped lesions are circinate in outline with sharply defined, hyperpigmented margins.

Diagnosis. *Dark-field microscopy.* This is performed on aspirates from skin or mucous membrane lesions and is the quickest method of diagnosis in early acquired syphilis.

Serological tests for treponemal diseases are of two types.

1. *Nonspecific (syn. reagin, nontreponemal, lipoidal antigen tests).* Examples are the cardiolipin Wasserman (WR), Kahn, Meinicke, and Venereal Disease Research Laboratory (VDRL) slide test. The last is the best. These test the presence of any antibody reagin in the serum of patients with treponemal infections, but biological false positives (BFP) arise from reagin present in nontreponemal conditions, e.g. malaria, vaccinia, glandular fever, and also after any kind of vaccination. Stronger and persistent reactions may occur in leprosy, sarcoidosis, collagen diseases and chronic liver disorders. A diagnosis of syphilis requires confirmation from one or more of the specific tests.
2. *Group-specific tests (treponemal antigen tests).* Examples are: Reiter's protein complement fixation test (RPCF), *Treponema pallidum* haemagglutination assay (TPHA), absorbed fluorescent antibody test (FTA Abs) and *Treponema pallidum* immobilisation test (TPI).

The first is obsolescent (in the UK) and the last rarely required. The routine practice is to perform the VDRL and TPHA adding the FTA if either is positive or the clinical findings justify it. In primary syphilis, the usual order of conversion is FTA, VDRL with rising titre and TPHA, although this sequence is not invariable. After treatment, the VDRL usually reverts to negative in up to 6 months, the FTA in 70 per cent, but the TPHA hardly ever, of which facts the patients must be told – 'a little scar in the blood' is usually adequate. Persistence of treponemal antibodies, if it is known that adequate treatment has been given, is not a cause for concern but if there is any doubt, confirmed reactions on repetition should be treated as for latent infection.

Treatment

No local treatment except isotonic saline should be applied to a suspected chancre until dark-field examinations have proved negative on 3 successive days. No treponemicidal antibiotics should be prescribed until syphilis is confirmed or excluded, but if there is secondary infection a course of sulphonamides may help. Penicillin has supplanted all other forms of treatment. A high cure rate is achieved in early syphilis with intramuscular procaine penicillin G 1.2 g daily for 15 days. This dosage is prolonged to 21–30 days for late syphilis. Clinical and serological observation should be continued for 2 years after treatment. In penicillin-allergic patients, tetracycline and erythromycin are alternatives. The best treatment is doxycycline 100 mg twice daily for the equivalent period.

Jarisch–Herxheimer reaction. About 6 hours after the first injection, 60 per cent of early syphilitics will develop pyrexia, malaise and possible rigors lasting for a few hours only. Patients must be warned about this. The reaction is infrequent in late syphilis, but may be more serious. In late cases only, prednisone 10 mg four times daily for 3 days before the main treatment should prevent it.

Prognosis is excellent after standard treatment for early syphilis. In late syphilis, particularly of the cardiovascular system, cure of the underlying disease may not significantly improve the condition of the patient.

Congenital syphilis

Transmission. Infection occurs when treponemes from an infected expectant mother cross the placental barrier to the foetal circulation. The more recent the mother's infection, the more likely is this to occur and the more serious the effects on the child. The results of foetal infection vary from death in late foetal life or early infancy, or the birth and normal development of an apparently healthy child who, nevertheless, has latent congenital syphilis.

Early congenital syphilis. Signs in the newborn, which may be delayed for a few weeks, include a generalised rash, mucous erosions as in secondary syphilis and the 'snuffles', a syphilitic rhinitis with nasal discharge which interferes with suckling causing loss of weight, epiphysitis, periostitis, osteochondritis, hepatosplenomegaly and basal meningitis. Signs may be so slight as to escape notice or so severe as to cause death in early infancy, usually due to syphilitic 'pneumonia alba'.

Late congenital syphilis. The extraordinary variety of clinical manifestations which can occur in acquired tertiary syphilis can also occur in childhood or puberty in late congenital syphilis, e.g. congenital neurosyphilis, cutaneous, visceral or skeletal gummata, but congenital cardiovascular syphilis is practically unknown. In addition, some manifestations, the stigmata, occur in congenital, but never in acquired, syphilis.

The stigmata of late congenital syphilis (Hutchinson's classic triad) consist of the following:

1. interstitial keratitis: the most frequent of the stigmata is a syphilitic hypersensitivity reaction with onset between 5 and 15 years. The cornea becomes inflamed causing pain, lacrimation and photophobia. It tends to be bilateral and recurrent. Prolonged severe recurrent attacks result in a hazy 'ground glass' appearance of the cornea, with yellowish-red corneal patches in severe cases (salmon patches, not to be confused with the salmon-patch birthmark). It is uninfluenced by antisyphilitic treatment but can be controlled by local cortisone treatment;
2. eighth nerve deafness: a progressive, bilateral, perceptive deafness, onset about puberty, but occasionally delayed until later and uninfluenced by treatment;
3. Hutchinson's teeth: a peg or band-shaped deformity of the upper central incisors, second dentition. Moon's molars (mulberry molars): the 6-year molars erupt with dwarfed cusps. Other classic signs include nasal deformities, e.g. saddle nose (Fig. 8.10), collapsed nasal septum (Fig. 8.11), perforation of the palate (Fig. 8.12), sabre tibia, Clutton's joints (painless effusions, commonly in the knee joint) and parietal bossing.

A.P. von Wasserman, 1866–1925. German physician.

R.L. Kahn, b. 1887. American bacteriologist who developed a test for syphilis.

H.C. Reiter, 1881–1969. German physician.

A. Jarisch, 1850–1902. Austrian dermatologist.

Karl Herxheimer, 1861–1944. Dermatologist, Frankfurt, Germany.

Sir Jonathan Hutchinson, 1828–1913. Surgeon, The London Hospital, London, England (1859–83). Described Hutchinson's teeth and the triad in 1858.

Henry Moon, 1845–92. Dental Surgeon, Guy's Hospital, London, England (1870–87). Described Moon's molars in 1876.

Henry Hugh Clutton, 1850–1909. Surgeon, St Thomas's Hospital, London, England. Described these joints in 1886.

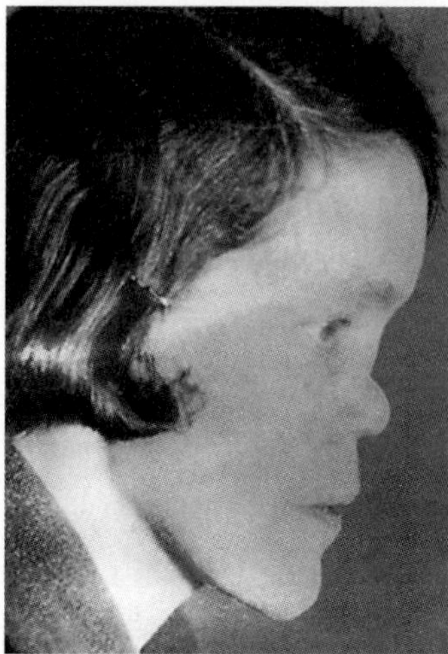

Fig. 8.10 Saddle nose of congenital syphylis.

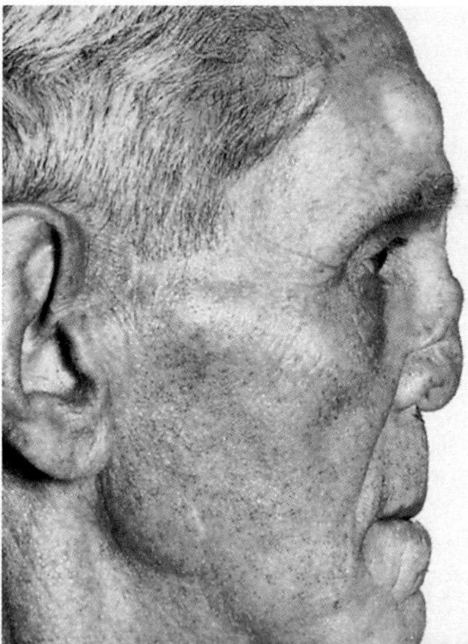

Fig. 8.11 Collapsed nasal septum of congenital syphylis.

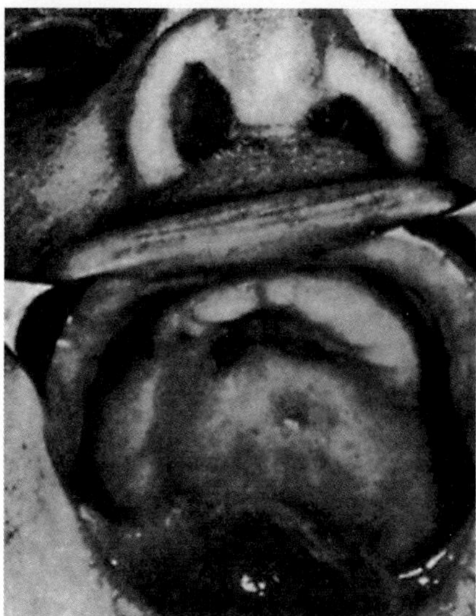

Fig. 8.12 Perforation of palate.

Prevention and treatment. A dosage of 1.2 million units of procaine penicillin G given to the mother for 15 days as early as possible in pregnancy not only will protect her from the ravages of late syphilis, but will prevent infection of the foetus, or may even cure it *in utero*, if already infected. An infected neonate, whose mother received no treatment during pregnancy, should be treated as for late acquired syphilis with the dosage adjusted to weight.

Neonatal serology. An expectant mother who has received no treatment during pregnancy, or who is an untreated latent syphilitic, may produce a child free from syphilis but seropositive owing to passive transfer of maternal antibodies. This serological problem can be solved by performing tests on the immunoglobulin G (IgG) and IgM fractions of the infant's serum but not on the cord blood. In the case of passive transfer, the IgG tests will be positive and the IgM tests negative. Positive IgM tests indicate active disease in the child since the IgM fraction of the maternal serum proteins does not cross the barrier of the normal placenta. Exceptions occur if the placenta has been damaged from other causes. In all cases, careful clinical and serological follow-up of mother and child is essential. The virtual disappearance of congenital syphilis from the UK and similar countries is one of the great triumphs of modern medicine.

Syphilis contacts. At all stages of the disease, the known contacts must be followed up. This applies to late and congenital cases when other members of the patient's family are often found to have untreated latent syphilis.

Yaws[2] (framboesia[3])

Yaws is an endemic disease of rural areas in tropical countries of high humidity. The causative organism, *Treponema pertenue*, appears indistinguishable from *T. pallidum* and produces identical serological reactions. Direct contact with an early lesion is the usual mode of transmission. It is not sexually transmitted. The primary lesion is most frequently seen on the legs of children. About a month after infection, a papule appears at the site of entry of the treponeme; this ulcerates giving the lesion a pink, raised, raspberry-like (framboesia[2]) appearance. Secondary lesions, usually papillomatous, appear some weeks later. After 5 or more years of latency, a minority of patients develops late gummatous-like lesions of soft tissue or bone similar to those of tertiary syphilis. The cardiovascular and nervous systems are not involved and congenital yaws does not occur. Treat as for syphilis.

Other infections (nonviral)

Candidiasis

Candida albicans (formerly called *Monilia*) is a yeast, frequently present in small numbers in the healthy bowel and mouth. It may cause primary infection in the newborn or superinfection when flora are disturbed by antibiotic treatment. In thrush (candidal stomatitis) white patches are seen in the mouth; it may occur in infants, in postoperative patients, and with ill-fitting dental plates. Vaginitis is common in pregnancy and diabetes. *Candida* may infect moist skin under breasts and the nailfolds, and cause severe intertrigo.

[2] *The possible answer to 'What's yaws?' is 'Syphilis'.*

[3] *Framboise (Fr.) = raspberry.*

Administration of broad-spectrum antibiotics often results in proliferation of *Candida* in the respiratory tract and bowel, and may be responsible for digestive upsets. Systemic candidiasis with invasion of lung and bloodstream is a complication of immunosuppression in transplantation surgery, and in the chemotherapy of malignant disease. Oral thrush also occurs in AIDS.

Candida infections are treated by the topical antibiotic nystatin or by gentian violet. Treatments for vaginal candidiasis include pessary treatment with clotrimazole (Canesten), miconazole nitrate (Gynodaktarin), econazole (Ecostatin) or isoconazole nitrate (Travogyn) from 1 to 6 days or nystatin for 14 days. Ketoconazole 200 mg twice daily for 5 days and fluconazole 150 mg (single dose) are more recent oral treatments. In all cases of treatment failure, the male partner should be investigated for balanoposthitis, easily cured with clotrimazole or nystatin ointments locally.

Aspergillus

Aspergillus species can cause a variety of clinical syndromes.

Asthma

A type I hypersensitivity reaction.

Allergic bronchopulmonary aspergillosis

May be due to a type I and type III hypersensitivity reaction. Asthma and a chronic cough with sputum production occur and bronchiectasis may result.

Aspergilloma

A chronic infection in a previously damaged area of lung, e.g. an old tuberculous cavity, producing a characteristic radiographic appearance. Haemoptysis may result and surgical removal may be necessary.

Disseminated aspergillosis

Usually found in immunocompromised patients such as those undergoing chemotherapy for leukaemia. Treatment involves the use of amphotericin B.

Chancroid (soft sore)

This infection is rare in Western countries. It is caused by the Gram-negative bacillus Ducrey (*Haemophilus ducreyi*). Two to 5 days after infection, sores, often multiple, appear on the genitals. They become pustular and ulcerate, forming rounded, painful, soft, readily bleeding ulcers with undermined edges. Inguinal adenitis follows, the swollen nodes being hard and tender causing a feeling of stiffness in the groin. Resolution may occur at this stage, but suppuration may follow, the nodes becoming matted together forming a fluctuant unilocular abscess (bubo) with red overlying skin, in one or both groins. The bubo should never be incised since healing is very slow. Aspiration is correct. Phagedaena (a rapidly destructive ulceration) sometimes occurs.

Treatment. Any antibiotic which may prevent the identification of *T. pallidum* in a case of concomitant syphilitic infection, or when the aetiology of the lesion is in doubt, is contraindicated. The mainstay of treatment has been co-trimoxazole 960 mg twice daily or erythromycin 500 mg four times daily for 1 week. However, resistance to co-trimoxazole is now appearing. Ciprofloxacin 500 mg twice daily for 3 days is an alternative. Regular daily cleaning of ulcers with isotonic saline is recommended.

Gonorrhoea

This venereal disease is discussed in relation to the genito-urinary system in Chapters 67 and 68.

Lymphogranuloma venereum

This is described in Chapter 67.

Granuloma inguinale

This is described in Chapter 67.

Erysipelas

Erysipelas is a spreading inflammation of the skin and subcutaneous tissues due to an infection by *Streptococcus pyogenes* (β-haemolytic streptococcus Lancefield group A). Poor hygienic living conditions, recurrent upper respiratory tract infections, debilitating illness and extremes of life are predisposing causes, and the lesion develops around a scratch or abrasion which is the site of inoculation of the streptococcus. A rapid toxaemia associated with the local infection and a rose-pink rash extending over the adjacent skin rapidly develops. The rash has a very clear edge and considerable oedema occurs (Fig. 8.13) over some tissues when infected, e.g. orbit or scrotum. Following the fading of the rash, a brown discoloration of the skin remains. The *S. pyogenes* remains fully sensitive to penicillin (see also 'Antimicrobial chemotherapy').

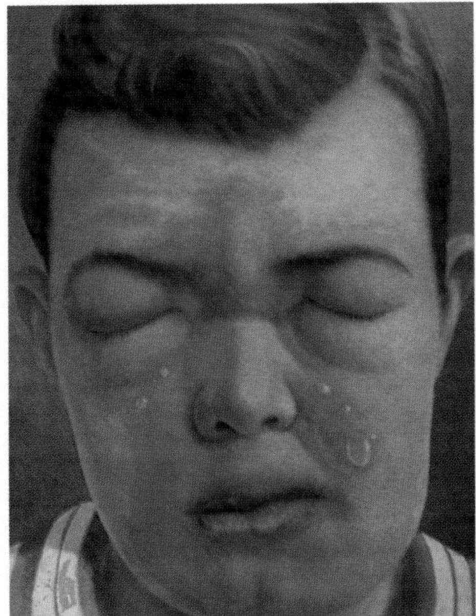

Fig. 8.13 Erysipelas with lymphatic oedema of face and eyelids. The patient was unable to open his eyes.

Augusto Ducrey, 1860–1940. Professor of Dermatology, Pisa, Italy. Described the causative organism of chancroid in 1889.

Rebecca Craighill Lancefield, 1895–1981. American bacteriologist. She developed a streptococci classification system.

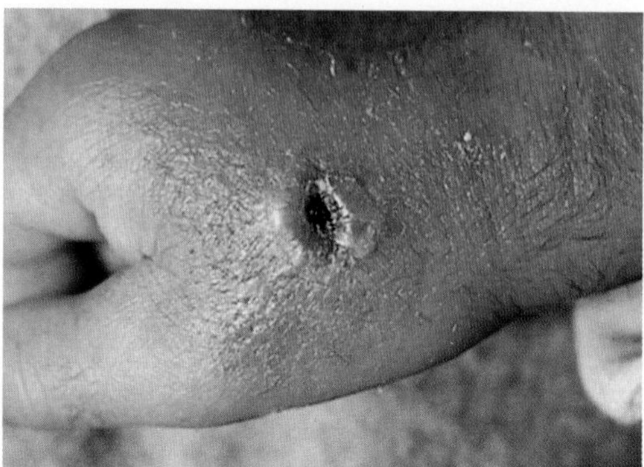

Fig. 8.14 Anthrax pustule (*courtesy of Dr W.D. Paterson, Carlisle, England*).

Anthrax

Bacillus anthracis is a large, Gram-positive, aerobic, spore-forming rod. It is very resistant to heat and antiseptics. The disease is found in cattle and is likely to appear in people who handle carcasses, wool, hides, hair and bone meal.

The cutaneous type is the commonest human variety; the incubation period is from 3 to 4 days. The lesion usually commences on an exposed portion of the body, such as the hands, forearms or face. An itching papule (Fig. 8.14) occurs, around which a patch of induration soon becomes evident. The papule suppurates and is replaced by a black slough, and a ring of vesicles appears on the surrounding indurated area. This stage comprises the typical 'malignant pustule'. A brawny, congested area of induration develops around the site of infection. The regional lymph nodes are involved. Toxaemia is always in evidence. A smear of vesicle fluid is used to confirm the diagnosis by culture and animal inoculation.

Treatment. Penicillin is the treatment of choice.

Prevention. This must include precautions to sterilise potentially infected animal products and wool from countries where the disease is endemic. A vaccine is available for those at special risk of exposure.

Differential diagnosis. The condition is easily mistaken for a severe furuncle (Chapter 37).

Other forms of anthrax are rarely, if ever, now seen, e.g. wool-sorter's disease, a pneumonia due to inhalation of spores, and an alimentary type, following ingestion of spores.

Actinomycosis

This disease is caused by *Actinomyces israelli*, an anaerobic, Gram-positive, branching, filamentous organism which sometimes lives as a harmless parasite in the tonsillar crypts and dental cavities of the otherwise normal mouth. It is popularly supposed that it occurs in corn and grasses, but the pathogenic bacillus does not. If the organism invades tissue, it causes a subacute pyogenic inflammation with considerable induration and sinus formation. Trauma and the presence of carious teeth are important predisposing factors in the development of lesions in the mouth.

Diagnosis depends on finding the organism in pus or in tissue section. Pus should be collected in a sterile tube (a swab is usually insufficient) and inspected in a good light for the presence of pinhead-sized 'sulphur granules'. On microscopy, the granules are seen to consist of Gram-positive branching bacilli. The peripheral filaments radiate[4] from the central part of the granule and may be surrounded by Gram-negative tissue clubs.

James Israel, 1848–1926. Urologist, Germany. Discovered Actinomyces bovis *in humans in 1878.*

[4]Actinomyces = *ray fungus.*

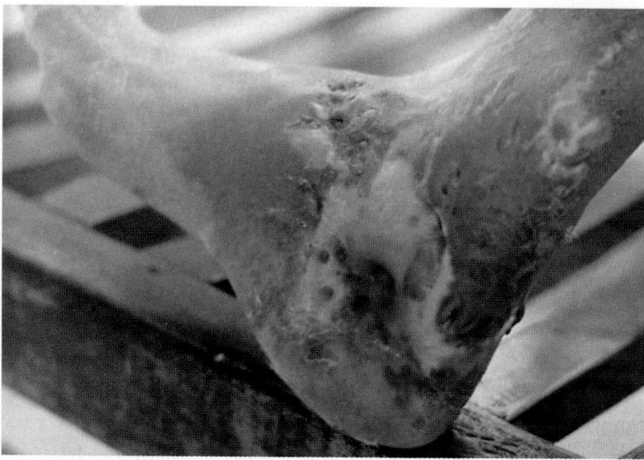

Fig. 8.15 Madura foot. Note the deep surface of the ulcer, sloping epithelialised margin and multiple sinsuses (*courtesy of Dr Sami-Ur-Rahman Khan, Aligarh, India*).

Culture. The presence of secondary organisms often makes this difficult.

The lesions are characterised by the formation of a firm, indurated mass, the edges of which are indefinite. Lymph nodes are not affected, but if a vein is invaded, pyaemia is likely.

There are four main clinical forms of actinomycosis.

- Faciocervical is the commonest. The lower jaw is more frequently affected, often adjacent to a carious tooth. The gum becomes so indurated that it simulates a bony swelling. Nodules appear, which soften and burst; the overlying skin of the face and neck becomes indurated and bluish in colour, softening occurs in patches. Abscesses burst through the skin and sinuses follow.
- Thorax. The lungs and pleura are infected, either by aspiration of the bacillus or by direct spread from the pharynx or neck, or even upwards through the diaphragm. The chest wall, in the late stages, becomes riddled with sinuses. An empyema is not uncommon, and the infection can easily spread through the diaphragm to the liver and the subphrenic spaces.
- Right iliac fossa (see Chapter 57).
- Liver (see Chapter 52).

Treatment. *Actinomyces* is usually sensitive to penicillin, tet racycline and some other antibiotics, e.g. lincomycin, but the sensitivity should be checked in the laboratory. A prolonged intensive course of penicillin (10 megaunits reducing to 4 megaunits daily) is usually the best treatment until all signs of the disease have disappeared.

Madura foot (and hand). See Fig. 8.15 and Chapters 30 and 31.

Parasitic diseases

- **Filariasis.** See Chapter 17.
- **Hydatid disease.** See Chapter 52.
- **Bilharziasis.** See Chapter 65.
- **Amoebiasis.** See Chapter 57.
- **Dracunculus medinensis.** See Chapter 12.

Viruses

Hepatitis A virus (HAV)

This is described in Chapter 52.

Hepatitis B virus (HBV)

This may follow blood transfusion, plasma infusion and, rarely, the administration of sera, infection resembling infective hepatitis except that the incubation period is about 12 weeks. Transmission by plasma has been reduced by avoiding the pooling of plasma from a large number of donors. Transmission by syringes is prevented if all syringes are disposable. It occurs amongst those who are drug addicts and possibly after tattooing or ear piercing. There is an extremely high rate among certain homosexual communities. In certain centres more than 50 per cent of male homosexual patients have antibody indicating exposure and about 5 per cent have active disease. In Athens, a group of prostitutes was found to have a rate 20 times that of married pregnant women, possibly due to more frequent coitus near the period or to other sexually transmitted diseases, producing bleeding that transmits the infection.

Infection with hepatitis B virus is associated with the appearance in the blood of one or more antigens, *viz.* hepatitis B surface antigen (HBsAg), hepatitis Be antigen (HBeAg), the Dane particle (probably the complete virus) and DNA polymerase activity. Under electron microscopy, particles can be seen in the sera of these patients and are associated with the virus. These particles are antigenic. Such patients usually suffer the severest form of hepatitis. The antigen is the scourge of renal dialysis and transplantation units, and hospital staff must avoid contact with blood from such patients.

A genetically engineered vaccine is now available (Engerix B). Three doses produce a good antibody response in most recipients, although poor responders may need a booster. Good antibody levels usually persist for about 5 years and a booster is recommended at this time. It is important that the injection is given intramuscularly in the deltoid as this produces a higher response rate than the buttock. All surgeons are strenuously recommended to have a course of this vaccine.

Hepatitis nonA nonB is a variant, with an incubation period similar to HBV, but with milder clinical features. Several causative agents have been described, one of which is **hepatitis** C. Detection of antibodies to hepatitis C indicates exposure to the disease and the presence of viral ribonucleic acid (RNA) in the blood indicates chronic infection. There is a number of serotypes with varying responses to therapy with a combination of interferon and ribavirin. Sadly, a large number of patients relapses after treatment and the development of new and more effective antiviral agents is awaited.

Further reading

Benenson, A.S. (ed.) (1995) *Control of Communicable Disease Manual*, 16th edn, American Public Health Association, Washington, DC.

Mandel, G.L., Douglas, R.G. and Bennett, J.E. (1989) *Principles and Practice of Infectious Diseases*, 3rd edn, Churchill Livingstone, Edinburgh.

Manson-Bahr, P.E.C. (1996) *Manson's Tropical Diseases*, 20th edn, W.B. Saunders, London.

Shanson, D.C. (1988) *Microbiology in Clinical Practice*, 2nd edn, Wright, London.

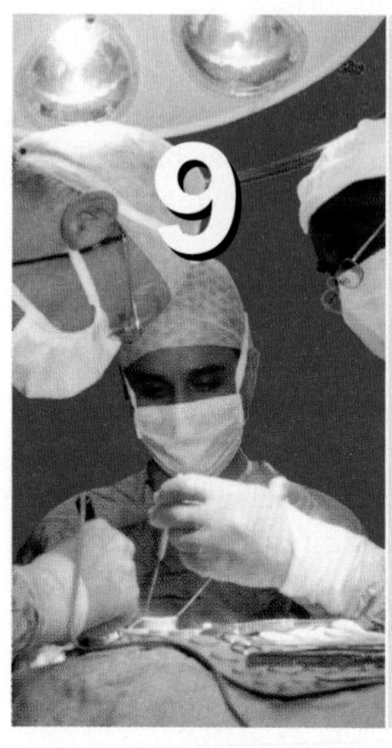

9

Acquired immunodeficiency syndrome (AIDS)

Introduction

The human immunodeficiency virus type 1 (HIV-1) is a member of the slow virus (lentovirus) family of retroviruses. It is a distant relative of the human T-cell lymphocytotrophic virus (HTLV)-1 and HTLV-2 viruses which produce some human leukaemia, but is more closely related to nonhuman retroviruses which produce degenerative disease in animals, such as the simian immune deficiency syndrome which occurs in monkeys.

Retroviruses are ribonucleic acid (RNA)-coded viruses that contain reverse transcriptase which transcribes viral RNA into deoxyribonucleic acid (DNA) within the host genome (Fig. 9.1). Viral infection of the host cell may be either latent, where the DNA is integrated but viral replication does not occur, or productive, where RNA and virus assembly occurs. One reason that the host immune system is ineffective at clearing HIV-infected cells is that the proportion of latently infected cells is high in relation to productively infected cells.

HIV-1 has a cell-surface protein (gp 120) which recognises and binds to receptors on several types of human cells. In particular, HIV binds to the CD4 receptor which is carried in high density on the surface of the CD4+ lymphocyte (helper T-lymphocyte). Other reservoirs of HIV infection are macrophages, neural, renal and perhaps epithelial cells.

Bailey & Love's Short Practice of Surgery, 23rd edition. Edited by R.C.G. Russell, N.S. Williams and C.J.K. Bulstrode. Published in 2000 by Arnold Publishers.

Effect of immune dysfunction

The extent of depletion in immune function correlates with the loss of CD4+ helper T-cells. However, there is also destruction of dendritic cells, damage to the thymus and immune dysregulation associated with production of autoantibodies and of immune complexes with persistent complement activation. Functional impairment of CD4+ lymphocytes

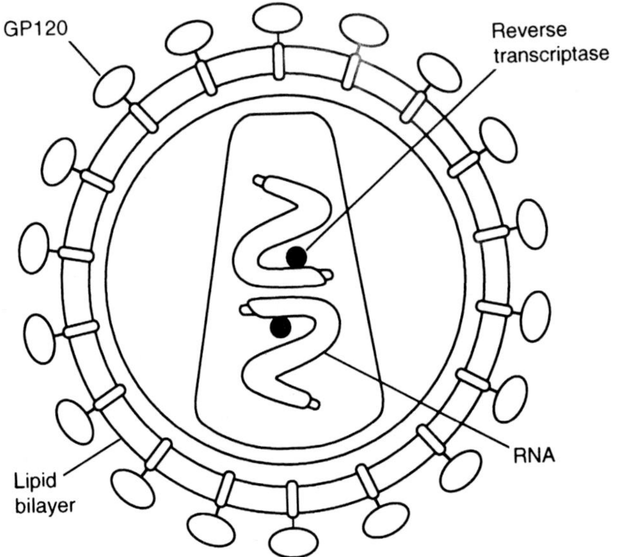

Fig. 9.1 HIV consists of an RNA core adjacent to an enzyme (reverse transcriptase) which produces RNA-coded DNA production in the host cell. The cell surface receptor (gp 120) recognises CD4 helper T-lymphocytes.

results in disorders of antibody production, delayed hypersensitivity and macrophage function. In addition, secretory immune deficiency occurs in the gut with depletion of immunoglobin A (IgA)-containing jejeunal and rectal plasma cells. This results in a vulnerability to many opportunistic infections, an increased risk of cancer development, and malnutrition due to a reduction in nutrient absorption and metabolism.

Natural history of HIV disease

Following infection by the HIV-1 virus into the blood, there is a brief **seroconversion** illness which is characterised by flu-like symptoms and lymphadenopathy. There then follows a latent period when the infected subject remains well but which is associated with a progressive fall in CD4+ lymphocyte count (Fig. 9.2). The progress of the disease has been classified by the US Centers for Disease Control (Table 9.1). It is expected that 25–35 per cent of those infected will develop acquired immunodeficiency syndrome (AIDS) within 2 years of infection if left untreated. The mortality from AIDS is thought to be 100 per cent. HIV-l viral titres are at their highest during the initial 'seroconversion' and the late-AIDS phases of the illness (Fig. 9.2).

Table 9.1 The Centers for Disease Control (CDC) classification of HIV disease

Group	*Description*
I	Acute infection
II	Asymptomatic infection
III	Persistent generalised lymphadenopathy
IV	Other disease
Subgroup A	Constitutional disease
Subgroup B	Neurological disease
Subgroup C	Secondary infectious diseases
Category C-1	Specified secondary infectious diseases listed in the CDC surveillance definition for AIDS
Category C-2	Other specified secondary infectious diseases
Subgroup D	Secondary cancers, including those within the CDC surveillance definition for AIDS
Subgroup E	Other conditions

It can be seen that AIDS is defined as CDC group IV.

The likely period of survival of an HIV-seropositive patient is important in assessment for both emergency and elective surgery. There are three important factors: CD4 (T-helper cell) count, HIV plasma load, and the ability of the patient to receive antiretroviral therapy (HAART).

HIV-seropositive patients die as a result of a wide variety of opportunistic infections caused by the CD4 count falling below a critical level. A low CD4 count is often the best guide to likely clinical events or death within the near future, whereas the plasma viral load (a surrogate for extent of viral production) is the best long-term guide to prognosis – in part because it predicts the rate at which the CD4 count is likely to fall. The likelihood of developing AIDS has been reduced by HAART therapy. This normally consists of at least two nucleoside analogues plus a non-nucleoside reverse transcriptase inhibitor or a proteinase inhibitor. Such therapy is capable of inhibiting all detectable viral replication and clearing the virus from both plasma and lymph nodes. The CD4 count also usually rises dramatically. While the long-term prognosis associated with such therapy is unknown, a pragmatic view would be that the immediate prognosis is likely to be related to whether the patient has further antiviral treatment options available. If so, then even in the face of a low CD4 count and a high plasma load, the patient might live for a considerable period. However, if no further antiviral treatment is feasible, the prognosis is poor and relates predominantly to the current CD4 count level.

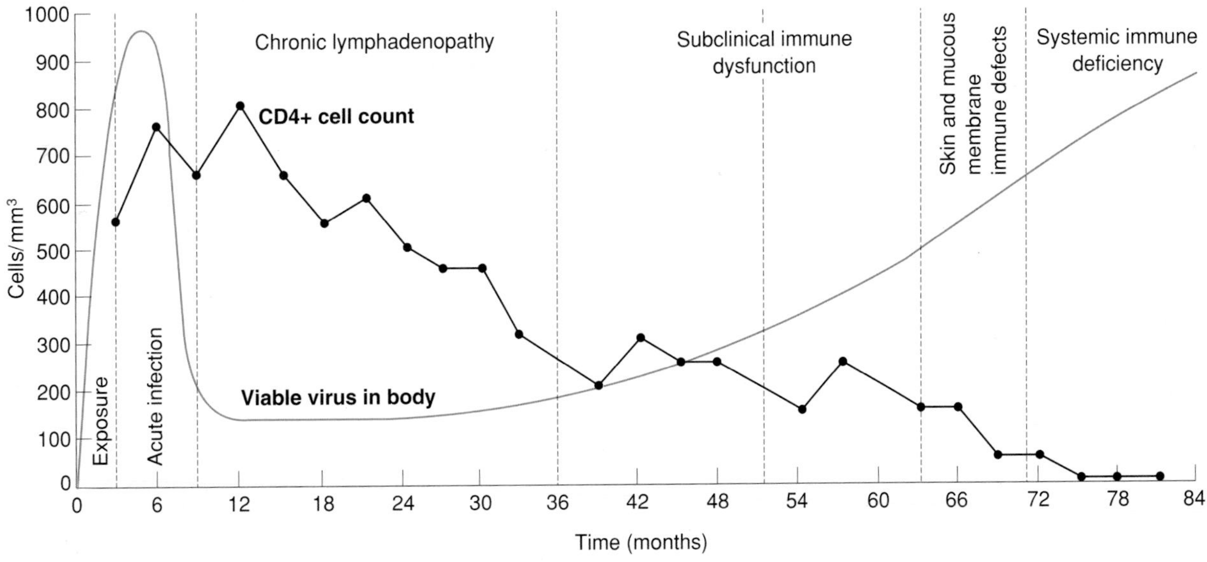

Fig. 9.2 After infection with HIV there is an initial acute rise in viable virus in the circulation which is followed by a fall in viral levels and a later decrease during the AIDS phase of the illness. These changes are associated with a progressive fall in CD4+ cell count.

Transmission

The most certain mode of transmission is by transfer of infected blood. The HIV-1 virus is considerably less infective than hepatitis B, and 1 ml of infected blood contains approximately 50 HIV-1 compared with 10^9 hepatitis B particles. Groups at high risk for acquisition of HIV-1 infection are:

- homosexuals and heterosexuals who indulge in anoreceptive intercourse. The risk of infection increases with the number of partners, associated infections such as gonorrhoea and a history of hepatitis B. Infection may be via traumatic breaches in the anorectal mucosa;
- drug addicts who become infected by using a contaminated needle from an HIV-1 positive source;
- haemophiliacs who receive factor VIII prepared from HIV-infected blood;
- sub-Saharan Africans. In Africa, heterosexual transmission and HIV enteropathy (diarrhoea-wasting syndrome, 'slim' disease) are more frequent than in the West. It is not clear whether this is because of different social patterns of heterosexual sex compared with the West or a difference in the infectivity rate of heterosexual intercourse among Africans compared with non-Africans.

Prevalence

More than 250 000 Americans had developed AIDS and a further 1–2 million worldwide were thought to be infected with HIV-1 by 1991. The highest incidence in South America is in Brazil where homosexual transmission, as in the West, is the most significant factor. In the UK over 150 000 persons are thought to be HIV positive, of whom over 5000 have developed AIDS.

Presentation to the surgeon

HIV-positive patients may develop any of the diseases which present to surgeons, and these are normally managed in the same way as in the non-HIV patient while taking special precautions to prevent cross-infection of HIV disease (see below). However, there are some specific conditions which are associated with the HIV disease syndrome and which occasionally require surgical intervention. Areas in which the surgeon may become involved are:

- the management of colorectal and anal disorders including infections and cancer;
- lymph node excision biopsy where there is diagnostic uncertainty;
- the provision of chronic venous access to facilitate chemotherapy for infections (particularly cytomegalovirus retinitis) or neoplasms.

Anal diseases

Warts

These are usually sexually transmitted, although anoreceptive intercourse is probably not necessary for the development of anal canal warts (Fig. 9.3). The treatment of these warts requires local scissor excision or destruction by some other local method, for example diathermy or laser. Less extensive wart infection can be controlled by application of podophyllin. The wart virus (human papilloma virus) is able to incorporate in the human genome and some types promote cancer development. In the presence of reduced immune surveillance, this can result in early neoplastic change within the anal epithelium which is termed anal intraepithelial neoplasia (AIN). The risk of progression of this intraepithelial neoplasia to invasive anal malignancy is small, although a precise figure is unknown. The finding of AIN in HIV disease is probably of little clinical significance since progression to invasive malignancy is unlikely within the prognosis of the HIV disease. The objective of anal wart treatment in these patients should be to control the local discomfort or leakage associated with the warts. AIN may also occur in the absence of warts (Fig. 9.4), although these patients are probably infected with human papilloma virus.

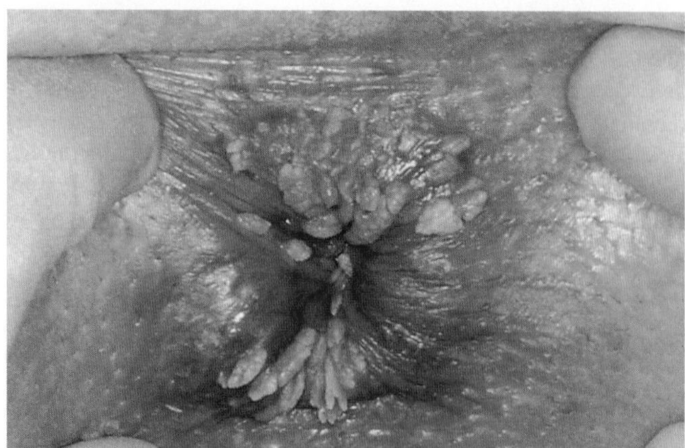

Fig. 9.3 Typical anal canal warts in an HIV-positive male.

Perianal sepsis

The usual varieties of anal fistula can develop in HIV-positive patients. The combination of local anal trauma resulting from anoreceptive sex with reduced immunity probably results in an increased risk of perianal sepsis. Perineal healing is reduced in patients with advanced HIV disease associated with a low CD4+ lymphocyte count. In those patients who do not have a CD4+ count of less than 100, conventional management of perianal sepsis is appropriate.

For patients with severe reduction in CD4+ count who are likely to have AIDS, a more conservative approach to control sepsis, for example, with the use of a seton, is probably more appropriate. It was initially believed that perianal sepsis was more complex in the HIV than in the non-HIV patient population. However, subsequent experience does not suggest that HIV-positive patients are more likely to have difficult or complicated high fistulas.

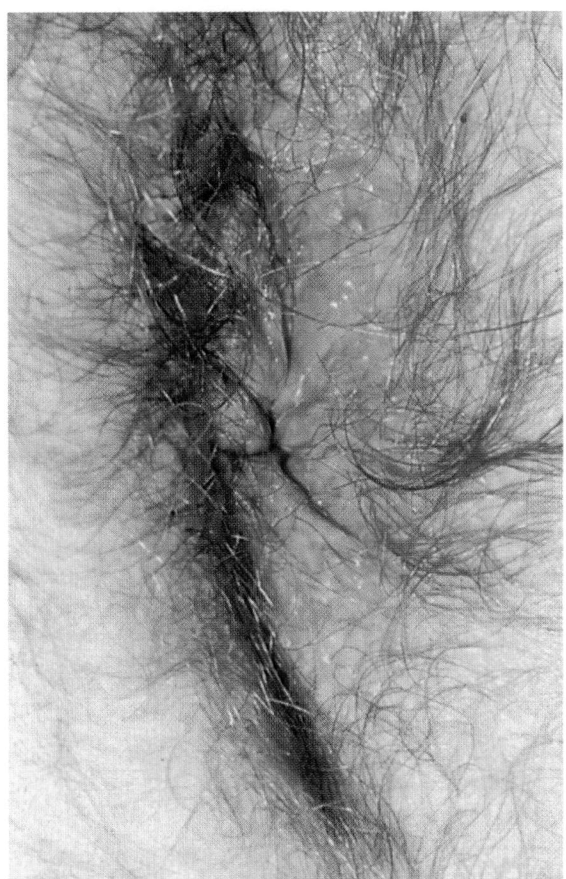

Fig. 9.4 A small area of skin irregularity can be seen adjacent to the anal sphincter. This was an area of anal intraepithelial neoplasia in a patient with AIDS who did not have anal warts.

Anorectal ulceration

Ulcers may occur in any part of the anal canal (Fig. 9.5) or lower rectum, and are usually associated with AIDS. In some cases they can be shown to be due to herpes simplex virus infection, but in other cases no organism has been demonstrated, although infection remains the most likely cause. Treatment for herpes simplex virus with acyclovir should be tried first. Occasionally, excision of the ulcerated area with a gentle anal stretch can be helpful. In some cases it is not possible to achieve healing of the ulcer.

Anal neoplasia

The probability of an HIV-positive patient with anal symptoms having anal neoplasia is much higher than in the non-HIV population. The commonest anal neoplasms are squamous carcinoma of the anal canal (Fig. 9.6), Kaposi's sarcoma involving the anal canal, and perirectal or perianal non-Hodgkin's lymphoma. Lymphoma can produce a tense painful swelling in the ischiorectal fossa which is easily mistaken for perianal sepsis. Thus needle aspiration is helpful before incision and drainage of suspected ischiorectal abscesses in the HIV-positive patient since this may avoid a breach in the skin overlying the lymphoma with subsequent risk of ulceration. The majority of patients with anal neoplasia has advanced HIV disease.

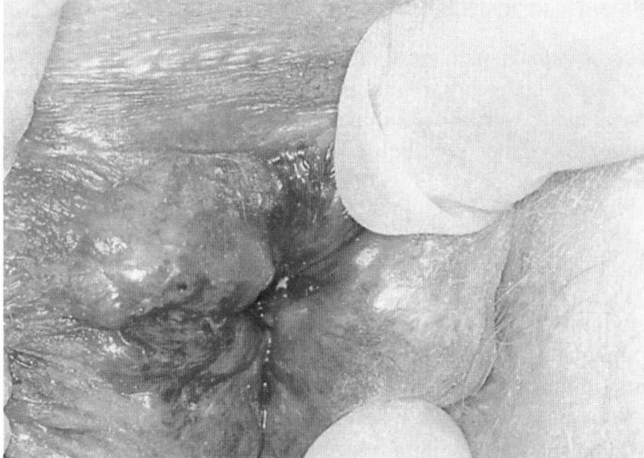

Fig. 9.5 Oedamatous anal canal with mucosal ulceration in an AIDS patient.

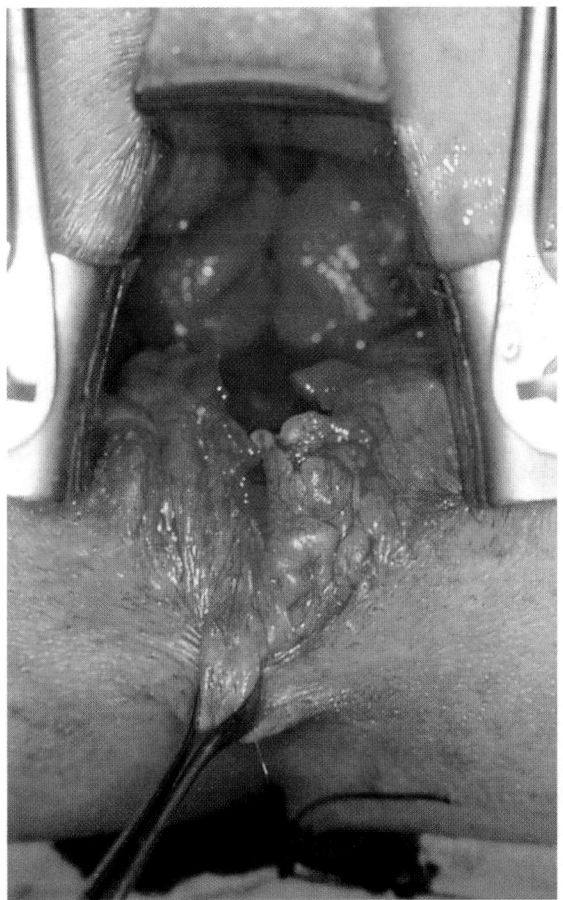

Fig. 9.6 Squamous carcinoma arising posteriorly in the anal canal in association with anal warts.

Moritz K. Kaposi, 1837–1902. Dermatologist, Vienna, Austria.
Thomas Hodgkin, 1798–1866. British physician.

Faecal incontinence

Homosexuals who undergo repeated anorectal intercourse weaken the internal anal sphincter. The association of a weakened internal anal sphincter with some degree of infective proctitis (see below) can produce minor faecal incontinence.

The acute abdomen in AIDS

Abdominal pain occurs in over 10 per cent of all AIDS patients. However, only 5 per cent of AIDS patients with abdominal pain require surgery, and this includes a small group of patients who develop acute abdominal symptoms where emergency laparotomy is necessary. The principal indications for emergency laparotomy in the AIDS patient are as follows.

Appendicitis

This presents as in the normal population. Where the signs and symptoms suggest a diagnosis of appendicitis in an HIV-positive patient, then appendicectomy should be carried out and the postoperative course is similar to the non-HIV patient.

Infective colitis

This arises from infection with cytomegalovirus and a variety of other organisms, and can result in severe bloody colitis (Fig. 9.7), toxic megacolon or colonic perforation which may be life threatening.

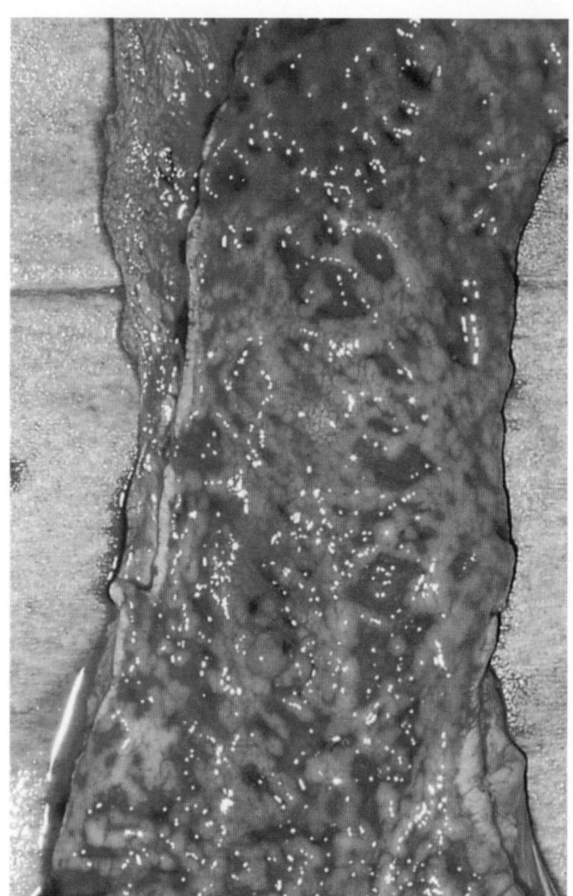

Fig. 9.7 Colitis in an HIV-positive male with cytomegalovirus infection. It is not clear whether the colitis is produced by the cytomegalovirus or by other associated infections.

Mycobacterium avium intracellulare infection

This produces an illness in which generalised symptoms are more prominent with vague abdominal pain associated with fever and marrow suppression. Laparotomy is better avoided in these patients if possible. The diagnosis can be made by marrow aspirate or needle biopsy of enlarged lymph nodes.

Non-Hodgkin's lymphoma (Fig. 9.8)

Diagnostic laparotomy to obtain lymph node tissue for histological examination should be avoided where possible. Occasionally, patients undergoing chemotherapy treatment for non-Hodgkin's lymphoma develop acute abdominal symptoms, for example, due to small bowel perforation at the site of tumour necrosis. The general experience with emergency laparotomy in the HIV-positive individual in this situation has been disappointing, and it is probably better avoided.

Overall, where conventional clinical criteria indicate the need for emergency laparotomy, the results in the HIV-positive patient suggest a 10 per cent perioperative mortality with a median survival of about 6 months following emergency surgery. Thus, this policy does seem to offer some additional life to these unfortunate patients.

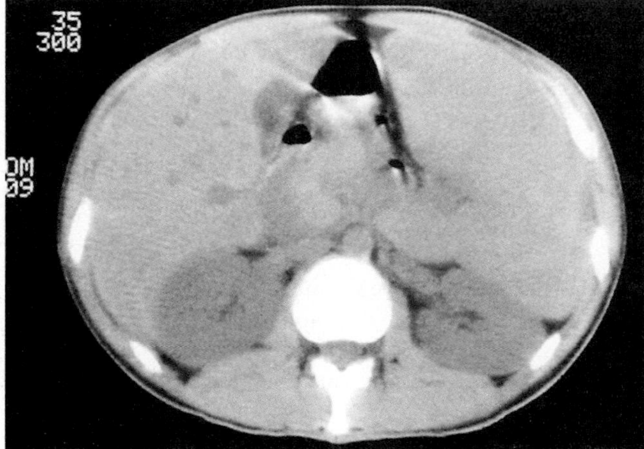

Fig. 9.8 Upper abdominal computerised tomography scan showing periaortic lymphatic enlargement and splenomegaly in an HIV-positive patient with lymphoma (*courtesy of Dr Brian Gazzard, Chelsea and Westminster Hospital, London, England*).

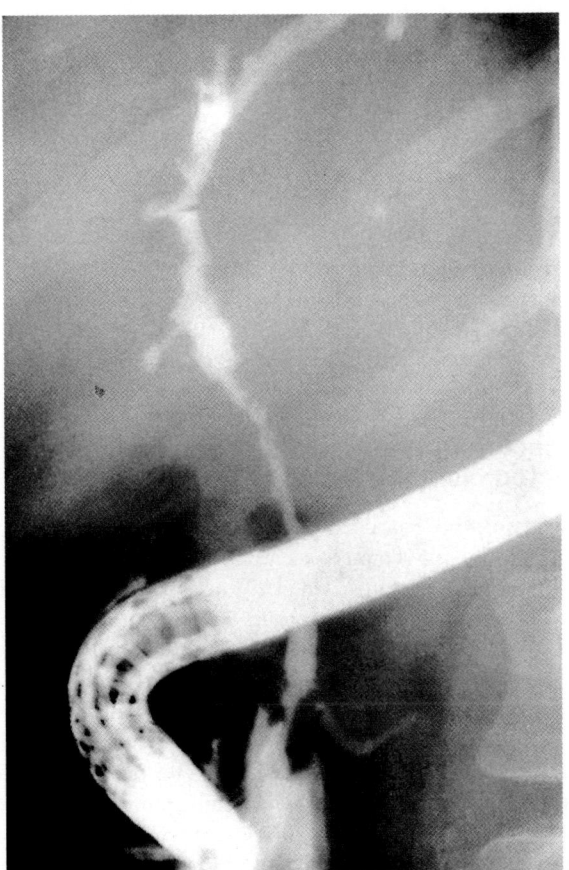

Fig. 9.9 Endoscopic retrograde cholangiopancreatogram showing AIDS-related sclerosing cholangitis (*courtesy of Dr Brian Gazzard, Chelsea and Westminster Hospital, London, England*).

Cholangitis

Some patients with advanced HIV disease develop liver function test abnormalities consistent with cholangitis. Endoscopic retrograde cholangiopancreatography in these patients reveals changes which are similar to sclerosing cholangitis (Fig. 9.9). The aetiology of this condition is not clearly established but it is thought that the inflammation has an infective basis, perhaps cytomegalovirus. Surgical treatment is not required.

Lymphoma

In addition to abdominal non-Hodgkin's lymphoma (see above) lymphomatous swellings can occur in other areas of the body, particularly the parotid and in the mediastinum. Tissue biopsy is occasionally helpful where there is uncertainty about whether the lymph node enlargement is due to lymphoma or to infection. However, major surgical excision biopsy is unhelpful.

Splenectomy

Splenectomy is occasionally indicated to correct an HIV-related form of autoimmune thrombocytopenia.

Risk of transmission of HIV disease from patient to surgeon

The surgeon is regularly exposed to blood, which is the most infective medium for HIV transmission. The risk must be greater where there are more HIV particles in the blood and this occurs during the earliest and later stages of the disease (Fig. 9.2). Thus, patients undergoing surgery who have had a recent seroconversion illness and who may be unaware that they are HIV positive are infectious, as well as patients who are known to be HIV positive. The extent of risk to the surgeon depends on the prevalence of HIV in the patient population, the number of procedures carried out by the surgeon, and the length of the period of risk. It is estimated that the risk to a surgeon working in a high-prevalence American or European inner city area over a 30-year career is roughly a one in 800 chance of acquiring HIV infection. In Africa, where the prevalence of HIV disease is thought to be much higher and the risk of HIV infection in blood products is also higher, a similar career risk has been estimated to be as high as one in four.

Sources of infection

The principal route of occupationally acquired HIV infection in healthcare workers is by skin perforation with a hollow needle containing HIV-infected blood. Although infection has been reported after solid needle skin perforation, the risk seems to be about 10-fold less than with hollow needle perforation where more blood may be injected. Extensive splashing of mucous membranes and skin, as occurred with spillage of a pack of blood over a nurse, has also been reported to produce HIV infection.

Precautions

Although screening of all patients for HIV infection before routine surgery would identify a substantial proportion of patients who might infect the surgeon, this has not been accepted because of political and social constraints in most countries. The risk of contamination to the surgical team can be reduced by the use of 'universal precautions' involving wearing either safety spectacles or a face mask (Fig. 9.10), and a gown which provides waterproof protection to the surgeon's anterior trunk and arms. In addition, boots rather than open-toed shoes should be worn to improve protection to the feet should something sharp be dropped. Needle-stick injuries to the hands most frequently occur on the index finger and palm adjacent to the thumb of the nondominant hand. This is presumably a result of passing the needle through tissue with a needle holder held by the dominant hand and attempting to locate the tip of the needle with the nondominant hand which is also used to retract tissue. Skin contamination from glove perforation can be reduced approximately fivefold by wearing two pairs of gloves. It is usually more comfortable if the larger-sized glove is worn on the inside next to the skin and a half-size, smaller glove is worn as the outer second layer.

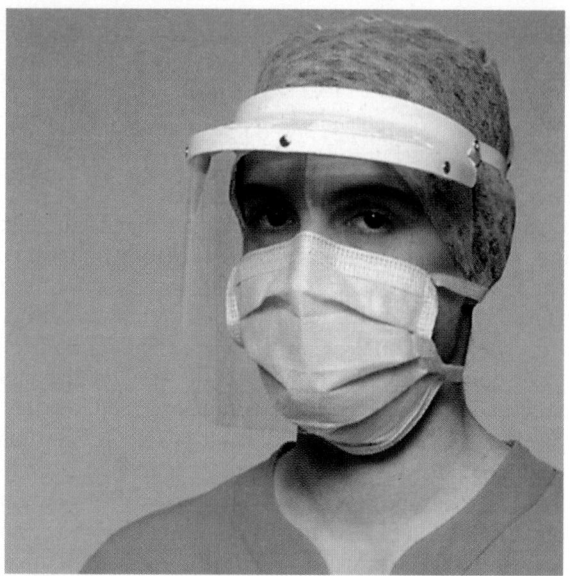

Fig. 9.10 Lightweight mask which can be used for protection of the eyes when operating on patients at high risk for HIV infection.

The most important operative precaution is to carry out the procedure in an orderly manner. Surgical assistants should be kept to a minimum and should be instructed not to move while the operation is proceeding. If the assistants' position is to be adjusted then the operating surgeon should stop operating while changes are being made. This should avoid the risk of the operating surgeon injuring an assistant's hand while it is being moved across the operative field. The operation should proceed in a slow and methodical manner with meticulous attention to haemostasis, taking care to avoid unexpected rapid bleeding which changes the tempo of the procedure and increases the risk of inadvertent injury to the operators. No sharp instruments or scalpels should be passed across the operative field from hand to hand. All instruments are passed from the scrub nurse to the surgeon and back to the scrub nurse in a dish (Fig. 9.11), thereby reducing the risk of injury while passing instruments.

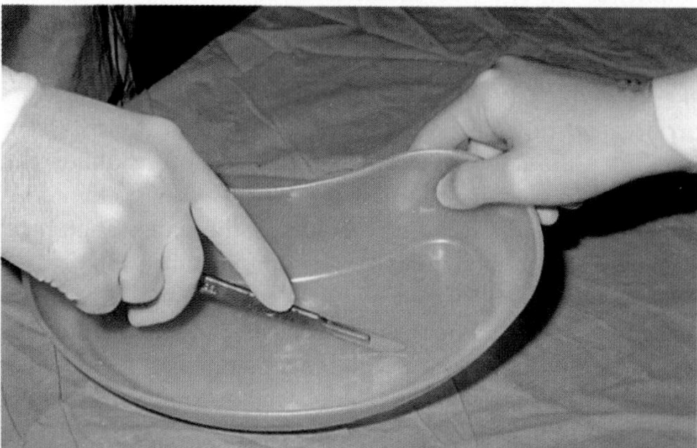

Fig. 9.11 Sharp instruments should be passed between scrub nurse and surgeon in a kidney dish to reduce the risk of sharps injury when operating on patients at high risk for HIV infection.

It is not practicable to adopt universal precautions in all patients, although the precautions related to operative technique should be carried out with all cases regardless of HIV status. It may be helpful to screen patients for factors in the history which are known to predict a higher risk of HIV positivity. These factors are:

- homosexual lifestyle;
- a history of intravenous drug abuse;
- a history of haemophilia treated with factor VIII;
- residents of sub-Saharan Africa;
- the partners of the above, higher risk groups.

Procedure in the event of contamination with infected blood

A surgeon who has been contaminated with HIV-infected blood should immediately clean the contaminated area by washing under running water. Where the source patient comes from a high-risk group and the HIV status is unknown, it is important that postexposure prophylaxis to HIV should be offered. This should be started within 1 hour of the injury where possible, so it is inappropriate to await the result of an HIV antibody test in a high-risk patient before commencing the prophylaxis. The prophylaxis consists of: zidovudine 250 mg twice daily, lamivudine 150 mg twice daily and indinavir 800 mg three times daily for 1 month. The surgeon should then be given hepatitis prophylaxis since the risk of developing hepatitis after contamination with blood from a high-risk patient is greater than the risk of HIV infection. A baseline HIV test should be carried out immediately since seroconversion will not have occurred immediately after injury. The HIV test should then be repeated approximately 12 weeks after contamination to determine whether seroconversion has occurred. This is obviously a period of great anxiety, and advice about domestic relations and procedures at work should be obtained from an HIV counsellor.

Where a medical practitioner discovers that he or she is HIV positive, the requirement of the UK General Medical Council is that 'if their duties involve performing or assisting in surgical or invasive procedures, they must seek and act upon occupational advice on any modifications or limitations to their duties which may be necessary for the protection of patients'.

Infection of the patient by the surgeon

Patient infection from an HIV-positive dentist while undergoing a dental procedure has occurred. Patient cross-infection may also have occurred from an HIV-positive to an HIV-negative patient undergoing a minor surgical procedure on the same operating list. There is no reported case of a patient undergoing a general surgical procedure acquiring HIV infection from the surgeon.

Further reading

Albaran, R.G., Webber, J. and Steffes, C.P. (1998) CD4 cell counts as a prognostic factor of major abdominal surgery in patients infected with the human immunodeficiency virus. *Archives of Surgery*, **133**, 626–31.

Harris, H.W. and Schecter, W.P. (1997) Surgical risk assessment and management in patients with HIV disease. *Gastroenterology Clinics of North America*, **26**, 377–91.

Lord, R.V. (1997) Anorectal surgery in patients infected with human immunodeficiency virus: factors associated with wound healing. *Annals of Surgery*, **226**, 92–9.

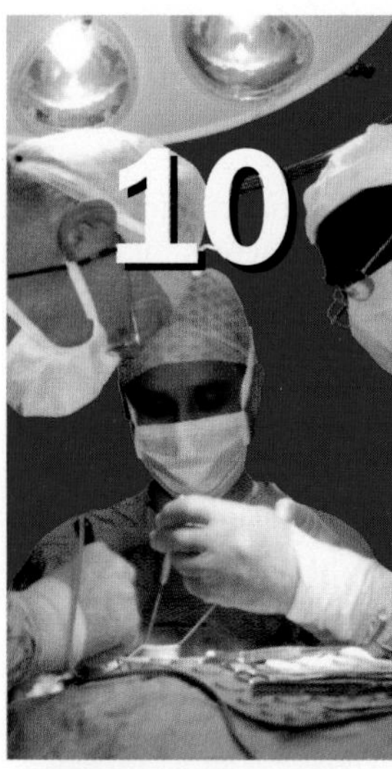

Sterile precautions

Introduction

Surgical infection still causes considerable morbidity and high costs to the health-care systems, and is becoming increasingly important in medicolegal aspects. Although antibiotic prophylaxis, utilising single high-dose broad-spectrum antibiotics, is important, it has unfortunately tended to lull surgeons into a state of unjustified security where too little attention to sterile precautions, and particularly surgical technique, is paid.

Wound infection results from bacterial contamination of the wound. Infection rate is proportionate to:

- number of bacteria;
- type of bacteria;
- incisions involving mucus surfaces;
- sites of existing infection in the body;
- the use of prosthetic implants.

An appreciation of the sources of bacteria is important and in abdominal surgery these may be summarised as:

1. endogenous from the patient's viscera (98 per cent);
2. endogenous from the patient's skin;
3. contamination from the air in the operating theatre – rare (by comparison, in 98 per cent of orthopaedic infections the contaminating organisms are ultimately derived from the air with 30 per cent of these sedimenting directly into the wound and the remainder on to drapes and then become dislodged into the wound);
4. direct contamination, such as punctured gloves – very uncommon.

Bailey & Love's Short Practice of Surgery, 23rd edition. Edited by R.C.G. Russell, N.S. Williams and C.J.K. Bulstrode. Published in 2000 by Arnold Publishers.

The theatre

The siting of the theatre, by contrast to its design, is not of major importance from a bacteriological point of view, although obviously it should not be adjacent to an incinerator or refuse. Clean and dirty areas should be separated and well demarcated with trafficking of personnel kept to a minimum through the sterile area. The dirty corridor should have an independent exit for contaminated materials.

The scrub room

Design of the scrub room should incorporate:

- two doors leading to the corridor and into the theatre;
- sinks with taps that can be manipulated with the elbows and soap holders that can be manipulated by foot pedals or the elbows. Good drainage and suitable panels incorporated in the sink to prevent splashing of clothes;
- anti-slip floors;
- easily cleaned shelves for gownpacks and gloves;
- adequate facilities for separate disposal of linen and paper;
- brushes for cleaning finger nails.

The operating room

The operating room should have a double-door entrance from the anaesthetic room and a double-door exit into the clean corridor. There will also be two small door entrances from the clean store room where sutures, dressings and needles are kept (this is a subsidiary of the main store in the theatre area) and an opening from the scrub room. There is also a single exit door to the dirty corridor for removal of drapes, instruments and waste products at the end of the procedure. All the doors should be well sealed in order to comply with the air ventilation system.

The operating table should be adjustable with all working parts sealed. The cushions should be easy to clean and in good repair. The lights should be adjustable, sealed and easily cleaned with facilities for attachment of light handles so that the surgeon and scrub team can adjust them. The plaster work and floor should be well sealed and any defects must be repaired as a matter of urgency as disturbance of plaster or the soaking through of leaking water will cause an increase in the bacterial content in the theatre environment.

- Fixed surfaces in the operating theatre should be avoided and reliance placed on steel trolleys. X-ray viewers should be inset into the wall and kept in good repair, as should electric sockets.

Control of air quality

Because the nonvisceral bacteriological contamination of wounds is predominantly from the air in theatre, it is essential that modern theatres are fitted with controlled ventilation and filters. For a general surgical theatre the maximum benefits can be obtained from 20 air changes per hour using a 5-mm pore size filter. In an unventilated operating theatre the bacteria present in air can be as high as 3000 colony forming units (CFU) per m^3. With appropriate ventilation and air changes this can be reduced to 200 CFU/m^3.

In general surgery there is conflicting evidence as to whether improvement in ventilation has reduced postoperative infection, but in orthopaedic surgery there is no such ambiguity as air is a significant factor in the development of postoperative infection and modern orthopaedic operating theatres utilise ultra-clean air where the bacterial count is kept below 10 CFU/m^3. The principle includes the provision of a rapid high-volume flow of air over the operating theatre with high-efficiency particulate filters. Essential measures, in addition to efficient air ventilation and filtration, include:

- reduction in the number of individuals in the theatre;
- avoidance of excess movement of individuals in the theatre;
- ensuring that the air vents are not obstructed and that the doors are closed.

Instruments

- Cleaning is a process which removes contamination but does not necessarily destroy microorganisms. It is an essential prerequisite of decontaminating equipment before sterilisation or disinfection is undertaken.
- Sterilisation results in the complete destruction or removal of all viable microorganisms including spores and viruses. In practice it may be difficult to establish. The term is usually applied to solid objects, such as instruments and equipment, but not to skin.
- Disinfection reduces the number of viable microorganisms but will not necessarily inactivate viruses and bacterial spores. It may be classified into:
  (a) high level – which is cidal to spores, bacteria and viruses;
  (b) medium – which is cidal to bacteria and viruses;
  (c) low – which is cidal to only bacteria and viruses of low resistance.

It is applicable to delicate instruments that will be damaged by sterilisation.

Sterilisation

Sterilisation by steam

Instruments can be sterilised by steam under pressure using autoclaves. Vegetative bacteria, including tuberculosis, and viruses such as hepatitis B, hepatitis C and human immunodeficiency virus (HIV) and heat-resistant spores, including *Clostridium tetani* and *Clostridium perfringens*, are killed. The combination of pressure, temperature and time with the moist heat is important:

- 134°C (30 lb/in.^{2}) for a hold time of 3 minutes;
- 121°C (15 lb/in.^{2}) for a hold time of 15 minutes;
- prepacked materials and instruments are processed through a porous load autoclave which incorporates a prevacuum cycle necessary to extract air. If this is not achieved then the dried saturated steam cannot penetrate efficiently. Unwrapped instruments can be sterilised in a small autoclave within the theatre precinct, which is convenient when instruments are dropped.

Monitoring

All autoclaves must be regularly maintained according to the manufacturer's instructions, and a record should be kept of the cycle time, the prevacuum phase, the pressure and temperature. In addition, the steam penetration test (Bowie–Dick test) and chemical indicators, for example Brownes tubes or impregnated tapes, are used to ensure that such errors as poor packing do not prejudice the efficiency of the process. Biological indicators are not appropriate.

Sterilisation by ethylene oxide

Ethylene oxide is a highly penetrative noncorrosive gas which has a broad-spectrum cidal action. It is utilised for heat-sensitive materials including electrical equipment. It is not recommended for ventilator respiratory equipment or soiled instruments because organic debris, including serum, has a marked adverse effect.

Sterilisation by hot air

This is inefficient compared with moist steam sterilisation, but it has the advantage in the ability to treat solid

George Frederick Dick, 1881–1967. Physician, Professor and Head of Medicine, University of Chicago, USA.

nonaqueous liquids grease/ointments and to process closed (airtight) containers. Lack of corrosion may be important, particularly with instruments with fine cutting edges such as ophthalmic instruments. It cannot be used for substances such as rubber, plastics and intravenous fluids which are denatured.

Sterilisation by low-temperature steam and formaldehyde

This uses a combination of dried saturated steam and formaldehyde, with the main advantage being that sterilisation is achieved at a low temperature (73°C) and the method is therefore suitable for heat-sensitive materials and items of equipment with integral plastic components. It is not recommended for sealed, oily items or those with retained air. Some plastics and fabrics absorb formaldehyde, releasing this in a delayed manner which may cause hypersensitivity to the users.

Sterilisation by irradiation

This technique employs gamma rays or accelerated electrons. It is an industrial process and is particularly appropriate to the sterilisation of large batches of similar products, such as syringes, catheters and intravenous cannulas. The delivery of an irradiation dose in excess of 25 kGy is accepted as providing adequate sterility assurance.

Disinfection

Cleaning of items is essential before disinfection is undertaken and the efficiency also depends on:

1. the nature of microorganisms;
2. the load of microorganisms;
3. the duration of exposure to the agent;
4. the temperature.

Disinfection with low-temperature steam

Typical conditions include exposure to dry saturated steam at a temperature of 73°C for a period of 20 minutes at a pressure below atmospheric. This is a useful process for dealing with dirty returns from the operating theatre or clinics which may be contaminated with protein from bodily secretions and microorganisms. Following this method of disinfection the instruments must be cleaned.

Disinfection with boiling water

This utilises soft water at 100°C at normal pressure for 5 minutes. Instruments must be thoroughly cleaned before being utilised.

Disinfection with formaldehyde

Formaldehyde gas is a broad-spectrum antimicrobial agent. This process utilises a cabinet which is airtight and circulates gaseous formaldehyde up to 50°C.

Disinfection with glutaraldehyde

A 2 per cent solution of glutaraldehyde is effective against most bacterial viruses, including hepatitis B and C and HIV, and is particularly useful for the decontamination of flexible endoscopes.

- Thorough cleansing is essential.
- The degree of decontamination is proportional to the time of immersion.
- It is a toxic substance and causes irritant, allergic reactions to the staff, particularly skin reactions, which limits its use.

Safeguards for equipment during sterilisation

Safeguards during sterilisation must include:

- thorough cleaning;
- appropriate packing for the sterilisation of disinfection process in order to avoid reduced penetration of the active agent. This is particularly important in the packing in the autoclave;
- arrangements of articles so that all surfaces are directly exposed to the agent. This includes opening or unlocking jointed instruments and disassembling instruments;
- the use of chemical indicators routinely;
- the interval monitoring of sterilisation process with chemical, thermal and, sometimes, biological indicators;
- the utilisation of flash sterilisation, where a temperature of 147°C is used at a pressure of 40 lb/in.^{2}, is now rare and should only be considered in an emergency situation;
- a careful maintenance plan for all sterilisation processes.

Theatre staff

Bacterial infection

The presence of an infected skin lesion, such as a boil, paronychia or carbuncle, known carrier state, particularly in the nares and the presence of an acute bacterial infection, particularly an upper respiratory tract infection, must lead to the exclusion of such a person from the team. There is good microbiological evidence to show that failure to do so will lead to an increasing number of infections.

Showering

Showering is preferable to bathing and the utilisation of a 4 per cent chlorhexidine gluconate soap by the surgical team is of benefit before the start of an operating list, and has been recommended for the operating surgeon between cases when the procedure is long.

Clothing and gowning

Desquamation principally occurs from the lower half of the body and the changing from normal clothes to clean linen reduces the bacterial count; cotton pores are 100 μm in size whereas skin scales are 5–60 μm, and thus cotton clothing will not serve as a barrier. Cotton suits worn below cotton gowns results in a decrease in bacterial count in air by 30 per cent. The newer bacterial impermeable fabrics further reduce the count but are of no value when worn over cotton pyjamas because the desquamation process continues and bacteria still escape, particularly at the ankles but also at the neck. The wearing of elastic anklets on trousers will reduce bacterial counts by 47 per cent. The most effective reduction of airborne bacteria is obtained by using the Charnley exhaust gowns – this is particularly important in orthopaedic procedures, but probably not significant in general surgery.

Caps are usually worn, although the amount of pathogenic bacteria dispersed is unlikely to be of any significance in general surgery, but may again be significant in implant surgery.

- Pyjamas with elasticated ankles and wraparound breathable membrane fabrics will reduce the bacterial count.
- In orthopaedic surgery, use of the Charnley exhaust gown is optimal.

Masks

The oropharynx is a low-level source of bacteria (36 bacteria per 100 words spoken are generated), the number of bacteria that settle on culture plates is not affected by wearing a mask and several studies exist to show that the wearing of masks in general surgery does not affect the wound infection rate, although the wearing of masks in implant surgery is appropriate as their use has been shown to decrease the number of bacteria detected at the operating site.

- Their use is indicated in implant and orthopaedic surgery.
- They offer protection to the wearer.
- Reduction of speech at the operating table is important.

Gloving

Although gloving or double gloving is widely practised there is little evidence that wound infection is related to glove puncture. This would suggest that disinfection of the hands is important in keeping the incidences of wound infection low.

Scrubbing up

Brushes should only be used for cleaning finger nails. A scrub-up time of 3–5 minutes with chlorhexidine soap or povidone iodine soap is utilised; the former is a broad-spectrum rapidly active agent with persistent activity, whereas the latter has a relatively short duration. The technique should include thorough washing of the hands to the elbows, with removal of the soap in the direction hand to elbow.

Excess soap is not required but a steady and methodical method of massage is important, and adequate drying is again essential, the preferred technique using paper towels in the direction hand to elbow. Jewellery should be removed.

The operation

Preoperative preparation of patient

Factors to be taken into account include the following.

- Preoperative showering with hexachlorophane is widely used in Sweden but not elsewhere; subjects shower twice on the day before and once on the day of surgery. This has been shown to reduce the incidence of wound infection. The former practice of wrapping limbs, before vascular surgery, in povidone–iodine dressings has not been shown to reduce infection rates.
- A short preoperative hospital stay is important; this reduces both the presence of pathogenic bacteria on the skin and the incidence of nasal carrier state (*Staphylococcus aureus*) among patients on the ward.
- Preoperative screening with swabbing of the skin and nose is expensive, and has not been shown to have been of value in altering outcome in terms of infection.
- Shaving – the trauma of shaving undoubtedly results in lacerations to the skin, which can increase infection rate; it is preferable to use either clippers or, ideally, depilation cream but the latter is expensive.
- Transport – the value of trolleys as opposed to transportation in the bed has not been shown to alter infection rates; similarly, the value of transfer trolleys, i.e. keeping one trolley for outside theatre use and one for inside theatre use, and the use of a sticky mat at the theatre entrance have been shown to be ineffective measures.

Skin preparation

Before arrival in theatres the skin of the operation site should be washed with detergent-impregnated soap. This both cleans and degreases the skin. In the operating theatre antiseptic solutions, usually of an alcohol-based detergent such as chlorhexidine or povidone–iodine, give optimal disinfection. The solution should be allowed to dry to maximise the reduction of bacteria, and pools of residual alcoholic solution, such as occur at the umbilicus or in the perineum, must be dried off completely, otherwise there is a danger of burning with the use of diathermy. The vagina and perineum should be cleaned with aqueous chlorhexidine and cetrimide solution. Adhesive plastic drapes are widely used and have the advantage of keeping either cotton or fabric drapes in place, but there is no evidence that they reduce the incidence of wound infection.

The procedure

High standards of asepsis in the operating theatre demand clear protocols or guidelines with regard to the conduct of surgery, and must be monitored by the theatre manager. The proper performance of surgery ensures safety for the patient, surgeon and staff.

Instruments must be handled in such a way as to avoid injury to the patient and staff.

- Sharps should be kept in receivers and disposed of safely using sealed containers.
- Instruments should not be left on drapes where they can directly injure the patient or damage the drapes, breaching asepsis.
- Disposable instruments, particularly those with contaminated blood, should be discarded securely in labelled containers.
- Instruments should be well maintained so that no body fluid remains on the instruments after washing.
- When the preliminary count is done at the start of an operation, instruments should be checked so that all joints, nuts, screws and surfaces that slide over each other are clean with no detritus present, and move freely.
- Swabs should be counted carefully and stored in the special plastic racks containing individual 'swab pockets'.

High-risk infection procedures

Again, there should be careful protocols for the handling of blood and body fluids in order to reduce the risk of auto-infection and cross-infection, for hepatitis B and C viruses, HIV and cytomegalovirus; such precautions are of particular importance in patients who have pre-existing infection or who are immunosuppressed.

General measures include:

- education of staff so that they are fully aware that there is a full vaccination programme for hepatitis B;
- the availability of advice for staff in the event of injury.

practical measures include:

- identifying high-risk patients on the operating list;
- reduction of the number of staff in the theatres to cover essential roles only;
- removal of all extraneous equipment from the theatre;
- Staff should avoid contact with contaminated body fluids, especially blood, and in this respect abrasions should be covered. If the member suffers from eczema, he or she should be excluded from the theatres and if contamination does occur rapid washing should be undertaken.
- When handling potentially contaminated blood or body fluids, scrub staff should use nonpermeable gowns and masks with eye protection and should double glove. Circulating personnel should use plastic aprons and wear gloves.
- Spills should be dealt with by staff wearing gloves and using absorbent disposable clothes; hypochlorite 1 per cent solution may be applied to blood spilt on the floor.
- Particular care should be taken with the handling of sharps, which should always be kept in receivers.
- Swabs should be counted but not left exposed, as for routine operations on a spike rack, they should be placed in deep 'swab pockets' on plastic racks.
- Disposable equipment should be placed in yellow bags at the earliest possible time, then sealed and double bagged with a hazard label attached.
- Soiled linen should be placed in special alginate bags and sent to the laundry clearly marked. At the end of the case all surfaces should be cleaned with detergents and the Domestic Officer informed.

Conclusion

Antibiotics, both prophylactic and therapeutic, have not reduced the essential role of asepsis and sterile precautions. Protocols with regard to instrument sterilisation, equipment maintenance, air filtration and ventilation, and staff behaviour are essential. Regular staff education is imperative.

Further reading

Emmerson, A.M. (1996) Asepsis and antisepsis. In *Clinical Surgery in General*, 2nd edn (eds R.M. Kirk, A.O. Mansfield and J.P.S. Cochrane), Churchill Livingstone, Edinburgh, pp. 179–186.

Holton, J. (1994) Infection control: facts and fantasy in the operating theatre. *Surgical Infection*, **6**(2), 39–42.

Peel, A.L.G. (1999) Adjuncts to surgery. In *Clinical Surgery in General*, 3rd edn (eds R.M. Kirk, A.O. Mansfield and J.P.S. Cochrane), Churchill Livingstone, Edinburgh, pp. 204–210.

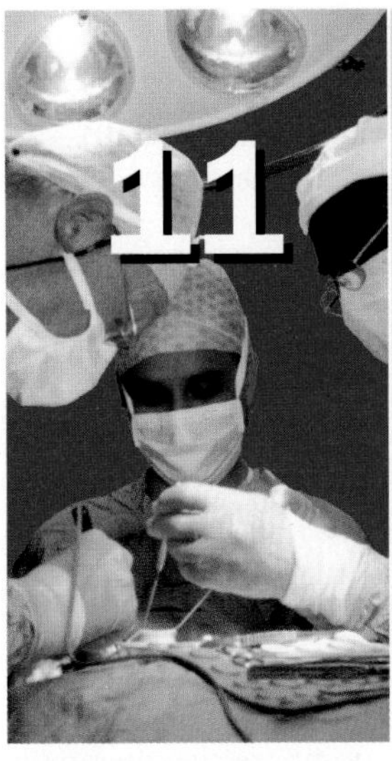

11 Transplantation

Historical perspective

Since early times the idea of tissue and organ transplantation has captured the imagination of successive generations, and over the centuries numerous fanciful descriptions of successful transplants have been recorded. One of the most widely cited early examples is that of the Christian Arab saints Cosmas and Damien. They were reputed, around 300 AD, to have successfully replaced the diseased leg of a patient with that from a black man who had died several days earlier (Fig. 11.1). The modern era of transplantation began in the 1950s and relied on surgical techniques for anastomosing blood vessels which had been developed at the beginning of the twentieth century by Mathieu Jaboulay and Alexis Carrel. The first successful kidney transplant was a living donor transplant performed between identical twins in 1954 at the Brigham Hospital in Boston by Joseph Murray and colleagues. This and other kidney transplants between identical twins demonstrated the technical feasibility of kidney transplantation, but attempts to perform renal transplanta-

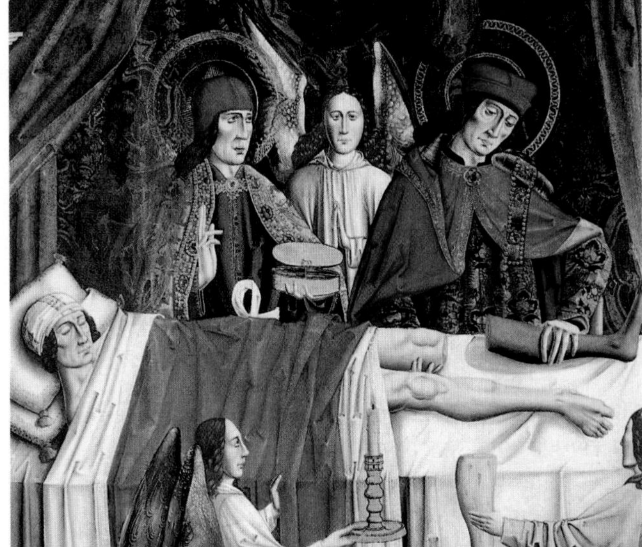

Fig. 11.1 Depiction of Saints Cosmas and Damian performing a miraculous transplantation of the leg. Oil painting attributed to the Master of Los Balbases (Wellcome Institute Library, London).

Cosmas and Damien, third century. Cosmas and Damien were the patron saints of physicians and apothecaries.

Mathieu Jaboulay, 1860–1913. Surgeon, Lyon, France.

Alexis Carrel, 1875–1944. Surgeon, Lyon, Paris, France. Awarded the Nobel Prize for Medicine in 1912 for work on vascular anastomosis and transplantation.

Joseph E. Murray. Professor Emeritus of Plastic Surgery at Harvard Medical School. Awarded the Nobel Prize for Medicine and Physiology in 1990 for work on kidney transplantation.

Bailey & Love's Short Practice of Surgery, 23rd edition. Edited by R.C.G. Russell, N.S. Williams and C.J.K. Bulstrode. Published in 2000 by Arnold Publishers.

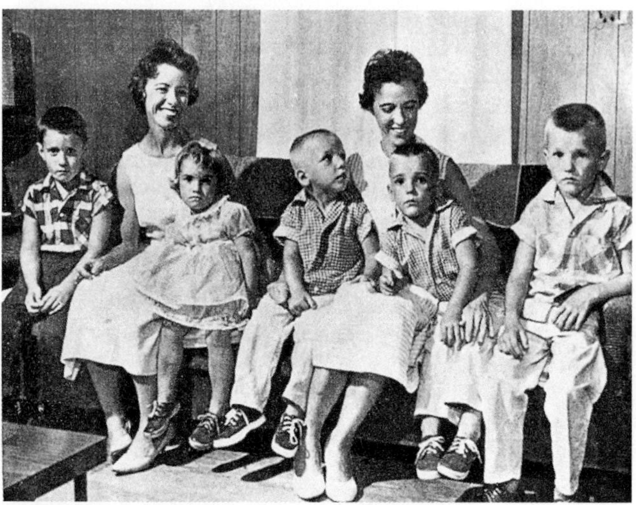

Fig. 11.2 One of the early Boston recipients of a kidney transplant from an identical twin shown here with her twin sister and their children.

tion when the donor and recipient were not genetically identical failed because no effective immunosuppressive therapy was available (Fig. 11.2). Then, in 1959, Schwartz and Dameshek discovered that 6-mercaptopurine had immunosuppressive properties, and Roy Calne showed that azathioprine, a derivative of 6-mercaptopurine, prevented rejection of canine kidney transplants. From the early 1960s, a combination of azathioprine and corticosteroids was used with success in the clinic to prevent graft rejection after kidney transplantation. These chemical agents were sometimes supplemented with a polyclonal antilymphocyte antibody given at the time of transplantation as immunoprophylaxis or used to treat an episode of graft rejection. The cyclosporin era began in the late 1970s following the discovery of the new agent by Borel at the Sandoz laboratories in Basle and the demonstration, by Calne, of its potent immunosuppressive properties in clinical studies. The introduction of cyclosporin was a major advance and cyclosporin (usually given together with azathioprine and steroids) not only improved the results of renal transplantation but also allowed transplantation of the heart and liver to be undertaken with acceptable results. Organ transplantation is now well established as an effective treatment for selected patients with end-stage organ failure. Transplantation of the kidney, liver, pancreas, heart and lungs are all routine procedures, and transplantation of the small intestine is becoming more widely practised. Today, transplant activity is limited only by the shortage of cadaveric organs.

Definitions

- Allograft (synonymous with the old term homograft) – an organ or tissue transplanted from one individual to another.
- Syngeneic graft (isograft) – a transplant between identical twins.
- Orthotopic graft – a transplant placed in its normal anatomical site.
- Heterotopic graft – a transplant placed in a site different to that where the organ is normally located.
- Xenograft – a graft performed between different species.

Graft rejection

Allografts provoke a powerful immune response that results in rapid graft rejection unless immunosuppressive therapy is given. The pioneering studies of Medawar in the 1940s and 1950s firmly established that allograft rejection was due to an immune response and not a nonspecific inflammatory response. Later studies demonstrated that T-lymphocytes play an essential role in orchestrating the graft rejection response. The immunological effector mechanisms responsible for graft rejection are those that have evolved to provide protection from pathogens – in other words there are no unique immunological mechanisms causing graft rejection. Cytotoxic T-cells, delayed-type hypersensitivity and antibody-dependent effector mechanisms all play a role.

The allograft rejection response is directed against a group of cell-surface molecules called the 'human leucocyte antigens' (HLAs) which were first described by Dausset in 1958. HLAs are highly polymorphic (i.e. the amino acid sequence is very variable between individuals) and play a special role in immune recognition. Their normal physiological function is to display antigenic peptides derived from foreign pathogens so that they can be recognised by T-lymphocytes.

There are two types of HLA molecule – HLA class I and HLA class II. HLA class I molecules comprise a polymorphic α-chain which is associated with a smaller nonpolymorphic chain known as a β_2-microglobulin. HLA class II molecules comprise two polymorphic polypeptide chains designated α and β. The tertiary structure of HLA class I and HLA class II is similar. In both classes of HLA molecule, the extracellular domains form a cleft, the purpose of which is to bind and display foreign peptides for surveillance by T-lymphocytes (Fig. 11.3). Each individual HLA molecule only binds one peptide at a time but can bind a wide range of different

Robert S. Schwartz. Professor of Medicine, Tufts University School of Medicine, USA.

Jean-Francois Borel. Research scientist, Switzerland.

Sir Roy York Calne. Emeritus Professor of Surgery, Cambridge University, England.

Sir Peter Brian Medawar, 1915–87. Zoologist and immunologist, London, England. Awarded the Nobel Prize for Medicine in 1960 for work on immunological tolerance.

Jean Dausset. Immunologist, Paris, France. Awarded the Nobel Prize for Medicine in 1980 for his discovery of human leucocyte antigens.

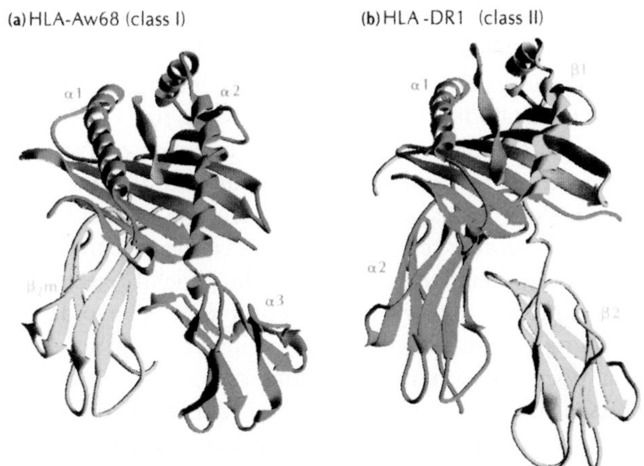

Fig. 11.3 The three-dimensional structure of the extracellular domains of HLA class I and II. The α_1- and α_2-domains of class I and the α_1- and β_1-domains of class II form a cleft which is floored by a β-pleated sheet and walled by two α-helices. The cleft binds an antigenic peptide and displays it for recognition by a T-lymphocyte. (Redrawn with permission from Stern and Wiley, *Structure*, **2**, 245–52, 1994.)

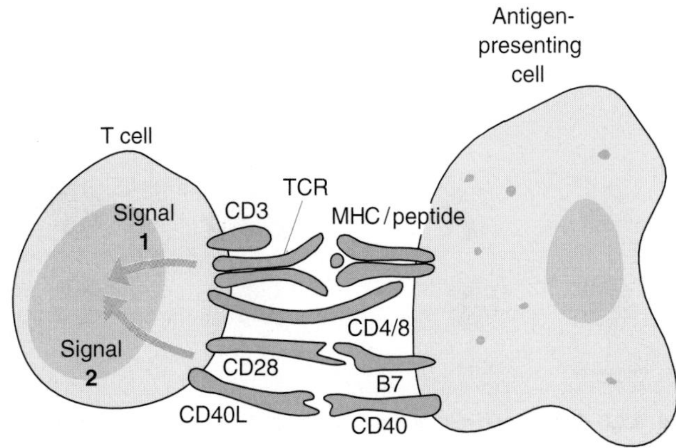

Fig. 11.4 Molecular events involved in T-cell activation.

peptides. The two classes of HLA molecule differ with respect to the source of the peptides they bind. HLA class I molecules present antigenic peptides derived from within the cell, for example antigenic peptides derived from intracellular viruses. HLA class II molecules, in contrast, present peptides derived from the extracellular environment. In the context of organ transplantation it is important to note that the peptide-binding grooves of HLA molecules never lie empty. When they are not occupied by an antigenic peptide derived from an invading microorganism they are occupied by nonantigenic peptides derived from intracellular proteins, including peptides derived from HLA molecules themselves.

HLA class I antigens are present on all nucleated cells, while HLA class II antigens have a more restricted distribution and are expressed stongly on antigen-presenting cells such as dendritic cells, macrophages and B-lymphocytes. However, HLA class II expression is readily inducible on all cell types by cytokines such as interferon-γ. HLA molecules expressed on donor tissues trigger a strong graft rejection response in the recipient by virtue of their special role in T-cell recognition and the fact that they are so polymorphic. It is rare for two unrelated individuals to have a completely identical set of HLA molecules. The high degree of HLA polymorphism between individuals is clearly unfortunate from the viewpoint of organ transplantation because it ensures immunological incompatibility between unrelated individuals. However, transplantation of organs is nonphysiological and it is reassuring to remember that the existence of extensive HLA polymorphism provides a survival advantage for the human species by maximising the chance that a given population will be able to recognise and mount an effective immune response to new pathogens.

T-lymphocytes recognise peptide antigens bound to HLA molecules through their T-cell receptor (TCR), and each T-cell expresses a unique TCR that binds to a particular HLA–peptide complex. During their development, T-cells that recognise self-derived peptides displayed by self HLA are normally deleted as they mature in the thymus gland, thereby eliminating self-reactive T-cells and avoiding autoimmunity.

The TCR is a heterodimer comprising an α- and β-chain. It associates at the surface of the T-cell with the CD3 complex, which is involved in intracellular signalling after the TCR is activated by engaging antigen. Mature T-cells bear either CD4 or CD8 coreceptors and these bind to nonpolymorphic regions of class II and class I HLA, respectively, on antigen-presenting cells. Activation of a T-cell by an antigen-presenting cell requires the delivery of two distinct signals (Fig. 11.4). The first signal (signal 1) is delivered after ligation of the T-cell receptor with an HLA–antigen complex. The second signal (signal 2) is delivered following the interaction of additional nonpolymorphic ligand–receptor molecules or costimulatory molecules on the surface of the antigen-presenting cell and T-cell.

In the context of organ transplantation, allogeneic HLA molecules are exceptionally strong antigens because they are able to stimulate T-cells directly without the need to be broken down into short peptides and presented in the cleft of an HLA molecule. This pathway of antigen recognition is unique to transplantation and is called *direct allorecognition*. All of the commonly transplanted organs have large numbers of dendritic cells distributed throughout their parenchyma. These professional antigen-presenting cells are richly endowed with class I and class II antigens and possess all of the necessary costimulatory molecules to trigger activation of recipient T-cells. Allogeneic molecules can also be processed like other types of antigen and displayed as antigenic peptides associated with HLA molecules on recipient antigen-presenting cells – this is termed *indirect allorecognition* and makes an important contribution to graft rejection.

After encountering alloantigens, activated T-cells undergo a period of clonal expansion which is dependent on IL-2 and other T-cell growth factors. CD4 T-cells, through release of cytokines, play a central role in orchestrating the various effector mechanisms which are responsible for graft rejection (Fig. 11.5). The cellular effectors of graft rejection include

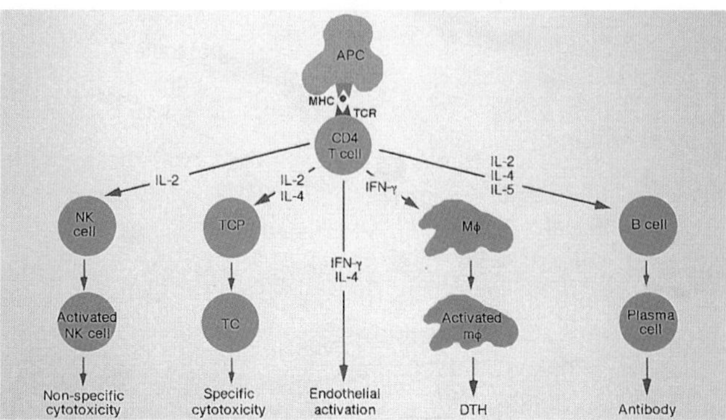

Fig. 11.5 The central role of the CD4 T-cell in orchestrating the effector mechanisms of allograft rejection.

cytotoxic CD8 T-cells that recognise donor HLA class I antigens expressed by the graft and cause target cell death by releasing lytic molecules such as perforin and granzyme. Graft-infiltrating CD4 T-cells that recognise donor HLA class II mediate direct target cell damage and are also able, by releasing cytokines such as interferon-γ, to recruit and activate macrophages which act as nonspecific effector cells. Finally, CD4 T-cells provide essential T-cell help for B-lymphocytes that produce alloantibodies which bind to graft antigen and induce target-cell injury directly or through antibody-dependent cell-mediated cytotoxicity.

Types of allograft rejection

Allograft rejection can be divided into three distinct types on the basis of timescale and underlying pathophysiology:

- hyperacute rejection (occurs immediately);
- acute rejection (occurs in the first 6 months);
- chronic rejection (occurs months and years after transplantation).

Hyperacute rejection is avoidable and acute rejection, although common, can usually be reversed by immunosuppressive therapy. Chronic rejection occurs after all types of organ transplantation and, because it is largely resistant to currently available immunosuppressive therapy, is a major cause of graft failure. Allograft rejection manifests itself as functional failure of the transplant and is confirmed by histological examination. Biopsy material is obtained from renal and pancreas grafts by needle biopsy, and from hepatic grafts by percutaneous or transjugular liver biopsy. Cardiac grafts are biopsied by transjugular endomyocardial biopsy, and lung grafts by transbronchial biopsy. After small intestinal transplantation, mucosal biopsies are obtained from the graft stoma or more proximally by endoscopy. A standardised histological grading system, termed the Banff classification (named after the Canadian town where the initial scientific workshop was held) defines the presence and severity of allograft rejection after solid organ transplantation.

Hyperacute rejection is due to the presence in the recipient of preformed cytotoxic antibodies against HLA class I antigens expressed by the donor. These may arise from blood transfusion, a failed transplant or previous pregnancy. This type of rejection also occurs if an ABO blood group-incompatible organ graft is performed. After revascularisation of the graft, antibodies bind immediately to the vasculature, activate the complement system, and cause extensive intravascular thrombosis and graft destruction within minutes and hours. Kidney transplants are particularly vulnerable to hyperacute graft rejection, whereas heart and liver transplants are relatively resistant to this type of rejection. In clinical practice, hyperacute rejection can be avoided by performing a cross-match test on recipient serum to ensure that it does not contain antibodies directed against HLAs expressed by a prospective kidney donor. Even in the presence of a strongly positive cytotoxic cross-match test, liver transplants rarely undergo hyperacute rejection, although their long-term survival is inferior. It is not clear why the liver is so resistant to hyperacute rejection, but one factor may be that that it is less susceptible to ischaemia than the kidney by virtue of its dual blood supply: 60 per cent of the hepatic blood supply derives from the portal vein and 40 per cent from the hepatic artery.

Acute allograft rejection usually occurs during the first 6 months of transplantation but may occur later. It is mediated predominantly by T-lymphocytes, but alloantibody may also play an important role. Acute rejection is characterised by mononuclear cell infiltration of the graft (Fig. 11.6). The mononuclear cell infiltrate is heterogeneous and includes cytotoxic T-cells, B-cells, natural killer (NK) cells and activated macrophages. Antibody deposition may also be present. All types of organ allograft are susceptible to this form of rejection and it occurs in 25–50 per cent of cases. Fortunately, the majority of acute rejection episodes can be reversed by appropriate immunosuppressive therapy.

Chronic allograft rejection occurs after the first 6 months, and is due to antibody- and cell-mediated effector mechanisms All types of transplant are susceptible to chronic rejection and it is the major cause of allograft failure. Interestingly, however, the liver appears more resistant than other solid organs to the

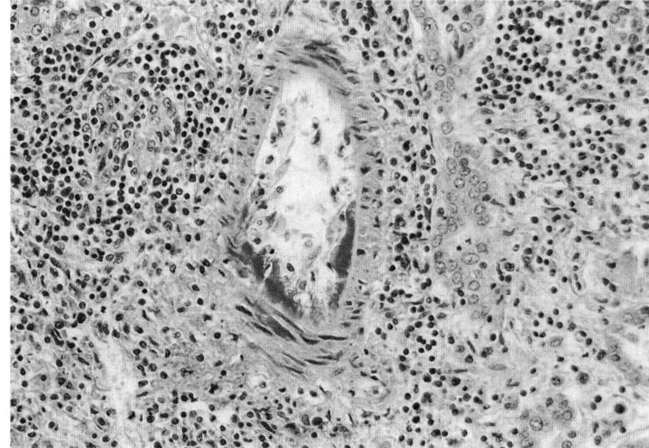

Fig. 11.6 Severe acute renal allograft rejection with a heavy mononuclear cell infiltrate and intimal arteritis.

destructive effects of chronic rejection. The pathophysiology of chronic allograft rejection is not completely understood. The underlying mechanisms are immunological, and both alloantibodies and cellular effector mechanisms appear to contribute. However, it is now clear that alloantigen-independent factors also play a role in the pathogenesis. A number of risk factors for chronic rejection has been identified in the context of renal allograft rejection. These are:

- previous episodes of acute rejection;
- degree of HLA mismatch;
- long cold ischaemia time;
- cytomegalovirus (CMV) infection;
- raised blood lipids;
- inadequate immunosuppression (poor compliance).

The single most important risk factor for chronic rejection is acute rejection. After kidney transplantation, acute rejection with vascular inflammation and recurrent episodes of acute rejection are strongly predictive of subsequent graft failure from chronic rejection.

The histological picture of chronic rejection is dominated by vascular changes with arterial myointimal proliferation which results in ischaemia and fibrosis (Fig. 11.7). In addition to vasculopathy, there are organ-specific features of chronic graft rejection. These are:

- kidney – glomerular sclerosis and tubular atrophy;
- pancreas – acinar loss and islet destruction;
- heart – accelerated coronary artery disease (cardiac allograft vasculopathy);
- liver – vanishing bile duct syndrome;
- lungs – obliterative bronchiolitis.

Chronic rejection causes functional deterioration in the graft resulting after months or years in graft failure. Unfortunately, currently available immunosuppressive therapy has had little effect in preventing chronic rejection.

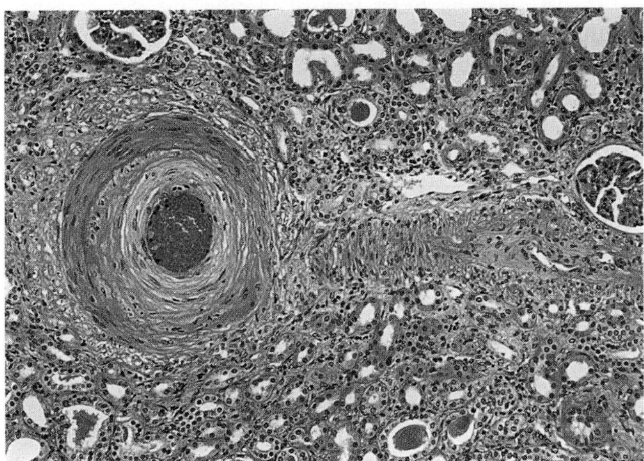

Fig. 11.7 Chronic renal allograft rejection. The small artery shows severe myointimal proliferation and luminal narrowing resulting in ischaemic fibrosis.

Histocompatibility testing and screening for presensitisation

HLA molecules are encoded by the major histocompatibility complex (MHC), a cluster of genes situated on the short arm of chromosome 6 (Fig. 11.8). The HLA class I antigens comprise HLA-A, -B and -C, and the HLA class II antigens comprise HLA-DR, -DP, and -DQ. Expression of MHC genes is codominant, i.e. the genes on both the maternally derived and the paternally derived chromosomes are expressed. Consequently, an individual may express between six and 12 different HLAs, depending on the degree of homozygosity (shared genes) at individual loci. Determination of the HLA or tissue type of an individual was traditionally performed on T- and B-lymphocytes by serological methods using a panel of antisera directed against the different HLA specificities in a microcytotoxicity assay, as described by Terasaki in 1965. However, increasing reliance is now placed on DNA-typing techniques to determine tissue type. These include techniques such as polymerase chain reaction (PCR) analysis using HLA sequence-specific primers.

In renal transplantation, attempts are made to match the donor and recipient histocompatibility antigens for as many of the relevant HLAs as possible. In addition to reducing the risk of graft loss from rejection, a well-matched kidney allograft that subsequently fails is less likely to cause sensitisation to the HLAs that it expresses. It is particularly important in children and young adults to avoid, where possible, grafts that are mismatched for common HLAs because, if retransplantation is required subsequently, it may be difficult to find an organ donor that does not express the antigens to which the recipient has become sensitised. In terms of organ transplantation, HLA-A, -B and -DR are the most important antigens to take into account when attempting to match donor and recipient in an attempt to reduce the risk of graft rejection (Fig. 11.9). HLA matching has a relatively small but definite beneficial effect on renal allograft survival (HLA-DR

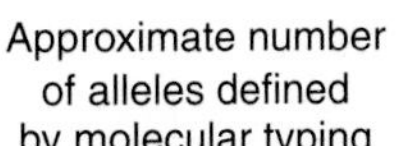

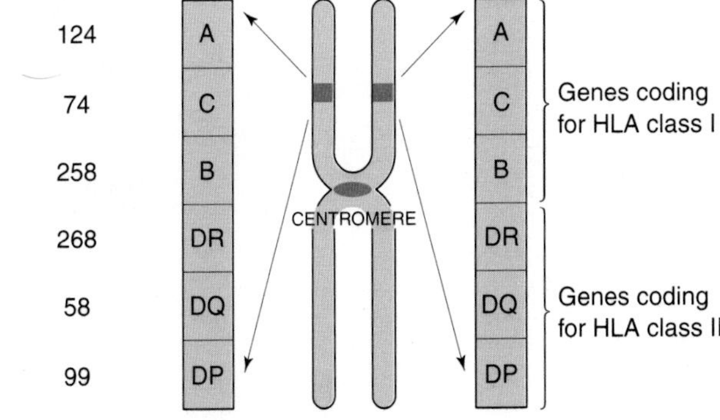

Fig. 11.8 The HLA system on the short arm of chromosome 6.

Paul Terasaki. Scientist, Los Angeles, California, USA.

> HLA-B > HLA-A). Recipients who receive well-matched renal allografts may require less intensive immunosuppression and also have less trouble from rejection episodes. It is common practice to express the degree of HLA matching between the donor and recipient in terms of whether or not there are mismatches at each locus for HLA-A, -B and -DR. A '000 mismatch' is a full-house or complete match, whereas a '012 mismatch' is matched at the HLA-A locus, has one mismatched HLA-B antigen and is mismatched for both DR antigens. Cadaveric kidneys are allocated in some countries, including the UK, by a points system which optimises HLA matching but also takes into account other factors, such as time on the waiting list and the relationship between the donor and recipient age. Allocation of organs for transplantation must also take into account the relative size of donor and recipient. This is not an issue in renal transplantation as adult kidneys can be readily used for paediatric recipients (and vice versa). However, for heart, lung, liver and small bowel transplantation, it is important to consider size compatibility between the donor and recipient.

HLA matching does not appear to confer an advantage for liver transplants and, although it is beneficial in cardiac transplantation, it is not practicable because of the relatively small size of the recipient pool and the short permissible cold ischaemic time.

As already noted, however, it is essential for all types of organ graft to ensure blood group compatibility. Permissible transplants are:

- group O donor to group O, A, B or AB recipient;
- group A donor to group A or AB recipient;
- group B donor to group B or AB recipient;
- group AB donor to group AB recipient.

There is no need to take account of rhesus (Rh) antigen compatibility in organ transplantation. Interestingly, after an

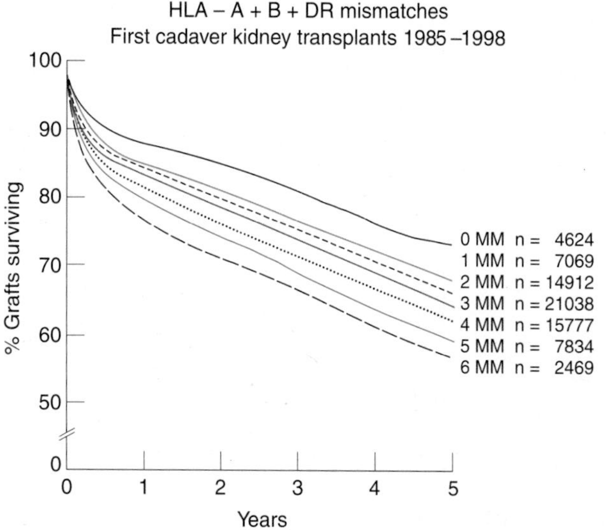

Fig. 11.9 Beneficial effect of HLA matching on renal allograft survival (*courtesy of Gerhard Opelz, Collaborative Transplant Study*).

ABO mismatched but permissible liver transplant (O donor into non-O recipient and A or B liver into an AB recipient) about 50 per cent of recipients develop an early and transient episode of haemolysis due to antibodies produced by donor lymphocytes in the transplanted liver.

In contrast to HLA matching, which is very desirable but not vital to success, the detection of sensitisation to HLA antigens in prospective renal allograft recipients is absolutely essential in order to avoid hyperacute rejection. Immediately before renal transplantation, a cross-match is performed by testing recipient sera against donor T-cells (which express HLA class I but not class II). When the cross-match test is positive transplantation should not proceed as anti-HLA class I antibodies cause hyperacute rejection. An additional cross-match test using donor B cells (which express both HLA class I and class II antigens) is also performed to detect antibodies directed against HLA class II antigens. A negative T-cell but positive B-cell cross-match may indicate the presence of HLA-specific anti-class II antibodies, and these are associated with an increased likelihood of acute rejection and a poor clinical outcome. Patients on the renal transplant waiting list should be screened for the development of HLA antibodies on a regular basis and especially after potential priming to HLAs by blood transfusion. Sensitisation is particularly common after blood transfusion in women who have been previously primed to paternal HLAs during pregnancy. Recipient sera are screened against an HLA-typed panel representing a broad range of HLA types found within the general population so that the specificity of recipient HLA antibodies can be determined. Highly sensitised recipients are arbitrarily defined as those whose sera contain immunoglobin G (IgG) HLA-specific antibodies reacting with > 85 per cent of the donor cell panel. Traditionally, cross-matching is performed by complement-dependent lymphocytotoxity, but flow cytometric cross-matching is becoming more widespread. Flow cytometric cross-matching is more sensitive than cytotoxicity, and is particularly valuable for screening highly sensitised recipients and patients undergoing retransplantation.

Patients awaiting heart transplantation are also screened for the presence of panel-reactive antibodies. Relatively few patients are highly sensitised (< 10 per cent) but in those who are, a prospective cross-match using donor lymphocytes should be performed. Although heart allografts rarely undergo hyperacute rejection, cardiac transplantation in the presence of a positive cross-match is associated with a high incidence of graft loss from accelerated acute rejection. In practice, highly sensitised heart transplant recipients are difficult to transplant because prospective cross-matching is problematic owing to the time constraints imposed by the short donor cold ischaemia time.

Immunosuppressive therapy

Evolution of immunosuppressive therapy

In tracing the development of clinical immunosuppression, three different eras can be identified:

- the early or precyclosporin era (from the early 1960s to the late 1970s);
- the cyclosporin era (from the early 1980s);
- the modern era (the 1990s).

Until the discovery of cyclosporin in the late 1970s, steroids and azathioprine were used for immunoprophylaxis. During the cyclosporin era the monoclonal antibody OKT3, directed against the CD3 molecule expressed on T-lymphocytes, also became available and was sometimes used along with cyclosporin-based regimens as immunoprophylaxis (especially in North American centres) or to treat steroid-resistant graft rejection. The 1990s can be regarded as the modern era of immunosuppression. Although cyclosporin is still the mainstay of many immunosuppressive regimens, several new agents have now been introduced. The place of cyclosporin has been challenged by tacrolimus and other important immunosuppressive agents have recently become available, including mycophenolate mofetil, rapamycin and monoclonal antibodies directed against the interleukin-2 (IL-2) receptor (CD25). When considering immunosuppressive therapy for organ transplantation, the transplant surgeon is now faced with an increasing range of different agents from which to choose (Table 11.1).

Calcineurin blockers

Cyclosporin and tacrolimus, although structurally distinct, exert their principal immunosuppressive effect through the same pathway. Each of the two agents binds within the T-cell to a particular cytoplasmic protein or immunophilin (cyclosporin binds to cyclophilin and tacrolimus to FK binding protein). The resulting immunophilin–drug complex then blocks the activity of calcineurin (a phosphatase) within the cytoplasm of the T-cell. Calcineurin plays a critical role in facilitating the transcription of IL-2, the main T-cell growth factor, and other cytokines after T-cell activation. By blocking cytokine synthesis, cyclosporin and tacrolimus exert a potent immunosuppressive effect. The two agents share a number of side effects, the most notable of which is nephrotoxicity (Table 11.2). Cosmetic side effects may be particularly distressing for the patient (Fig. 11.10). The calcineurin blockers have a relatively small therapeutic window, and monitoring of whole blood drug levels is an important guide to optimal therapy. If, after renal transplantation, the graft fails to function immediately because of acute tubular necrosis, calcineurin blockers may be withheld temporarily to avoid the risk of drug-induced nephrotoxicity. The relative efficacy of cyclosporin and tacrolimus in preventing graft rejection is broadly comparable, and the choice between the two agents is dependent on the preference of the transplant unit and on individual patient tolerance to the different side effects of the two agents.

Table 11.1 Immunosuppressive agents and their mode of action

Agent	*Principal mode of action*
Azathioprine	Prevents lymphocyte proliferation
Mycophenolate mofetil	Prevents lymphocyte proliferation
Cyclosporine	Blocks IL-2 gene transcription
Tacrolimus	Blocks IL-2 gene transcription
Rapamycin	Blocks IL-2 receptor signal transduction
OKT3 monoclonal antibody	Depletion and blockade of T-cells
ALG/ALS	Depletion and blockade of lymphocytes
Anti-CD25 monoclonal antibody	Targets activated T-cells
Corticosteroids	Widespread anti-inflammatory effects

Table 11.2 Side effects of immunosuppressive agents used in organ transplantation

Agent	*Side effect*
Corticosteroids	Hypertension, dyslipidaemia, diabetes, osteoporosis, avascular necrosis, Cushingoid appearance
Azathioprine	Leucopenia, thrombocytopenia, hepatotoxicity, gastrointestinal symptoms
Cyclosporin	Nephrotoxicity, hypertension, dyslipidaemia, hirsuitism, gingival hyperplasia
Tacrolimus	Nephrotoxicity, hypertension, dyslipidaemia, neurotoxicity, diabetes
Mycophenolate mofetil	Leucopenia, thrombocytopenia, gastrointestinal symptoms
Sirolimus	Thrombocytopenia, dyslipidaemia
Antilymphocyte globulin	Leucopenia, thrombocytopenia
OKT3	Cytokine release syndrome, pulmonary oedema, leucopenia
Anti-CD25	None described

Antiproliferative agents

Lymphocytes are among the most rapidly proliferating cells in the body, and lymphocyte proliferation and clonal expansion is an integral part of the immune response to an allograft. The antiproliferative agents available for immunoprophylaxis are azathioprine and mycophenolate. Azathioprine is converted

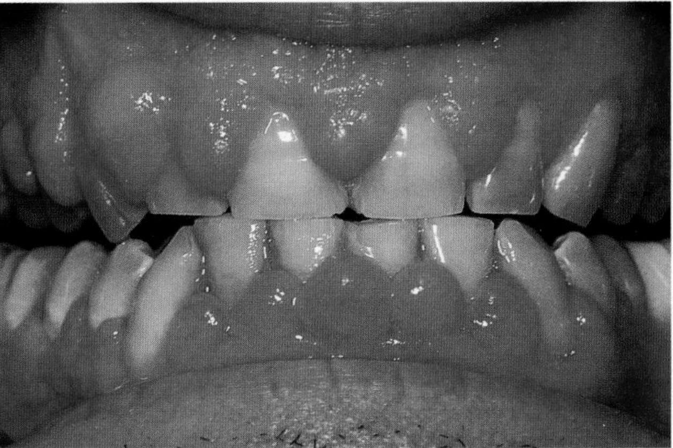

Fig. 11.10 Gingival hyperplasia as a result of cyclosporin treatment.

in the liver to its active metabolite 6-mercaptopurine which blocks purine metabolism and thereby inhibits cellular proliferation. Mycophenolate is a recently introduced antiproliferative agent that, after ingestion, is converted to its active metabolite, mycophenolic acid. It inhibits the enzyme inosine monophosphate dehydrogenase that is the rate-limiting enzyme in the *de novo* pathway of purine nucleotide synthesis. Because lymphocytes do not have a salvage pathway for purine synthesis, their ability to proliferate is selectively impaired.

Steroids

Steroids have always been an important component of immunoprophylactic regimens. Glucocorticoids are potent anti-inflammatory agents and have wide-ranging effects on the immune response. Because of their numerous and well-known side effects, many centres attempt to withdraw gradually steroids from patients who have stable graft function at around 1 year after transplantation, but this sometimes precipitates a rejection episode and necessitates continued treatment with steroids.

Antibody therapies

Many North American transplant units also include antilymphocyte antibody preparations as part of their immunoprophylaxis – so-called 'quadruple therapy'. A polyclonal antilymphocyte preparation (ALG or ALS) may be used or, alternatively, a monoclonal antibody directed against CD3 or CD25 (IL-2 receptor) on T-cells may be given. In Europe, the use of antibody preparations is more common after heart transplantation, where irreversible rejection is usually synonymous with death of the patient. Antibody therapy is often used in renal transplantation for patients who are thought to be at particular risk from graft rejection, for example highly sensitised and second- or third-time graft recipients.

Rapamycin

Rapamycin is a newly discovered immunosuppressive agent that was isolated from a fungus found on Easter Island. Like tacrolimus, it is a macrolide which binds within the T-cell to FK binding protein. However, the mode of action of rapamycin is completely different to that of both cyclosporin and tacrolimus. It acts by interfering with intracellular signalling from the IL-2 receptor and arrests T-cell division in the G1 phase. Rapamycin and cyclosporin therefore act at different stages in T-cell activation and their immunosuppressive effects are synergistic.

Immunosuppressive regimens

When selecting an immunosuppressive regimen some of the important points to bear in mind are as follows.

- The challenge is to provide levels of immunosuppression that are sufficient to protect the graft from rejection without exposing the recipient to excessive risk from infection and malignancy as a result of nonspecific immunosuppression.
- Immunoprophylaxis is started at the time of transplantation and continued indefinitely (as maintenance therapy), although the requirement for immunosuppression is highest in the first few weeks after transplantation when the risk of acute rejection is greatest.
- Individual immunosuppressive protocols vary somewhat but almost all use a combination of immunosuppressive agents. All include a calcineurin blocker (cyclosporin or tacrolimus) as the main agent and this is most often given along with an antiproliferative agent (azathioprine or mycophenolate mofetil) and steroids – so-called 'triple therapy'. Less often, a calcineurin blocker is used with an antiproliferative agent alone or with steroids alone (dual therapy).
- A few renal transplant units use monotherapy with a calcineurin blocker and then add other agents only if needed to treat rejection. At the other end of the spectrum, some units, particularly those in North America, advocate the use of antibody induction therapy (monoclonal or polyclonal preparations) followed by a calcineurin blocker, an antiproliferative agent and steroids (quadruple therapy).
- Many renal transplant units reserve the more intensive antibody induction protocols for recipients judged to be at increased risk of graft rejection (e.g. highly sensitised recipients and grafts with a poor HLA match).
- The principles of immunoprophylaxis are similar for all types of organ transplantation. However, after thoracic organ transplantation there is a tendency to use more intensive immunosuppression than for kidney transplantation, in part because loss of a heart or lung graft from rejection almost inevitably culminates in death. Interestingly, liver grafts seem less susceptible to graft rejection, for reasons that are still unclear.
- The place of the newer immunosuppressive agents, such as rapamycin and anti-CD25 monoclonal antibodies, still remains to be established but recent trials have shown promising results.

Acute rejection during the first 6 months of transplantation occurs in around 20–40 per cent of transplant recipients. Fortunately, the majority of acute rejection episodes responds to a short course of high-dose steroid therapy. This can be given as three daily intravenous doses of methylprednisolone (0.5–1 g/dose) or a several-day course of oral prednisolone (e.g. 200 mg tapering to 20 mg). If the response to treatment is inadequate or if acute rejection recurs it can often be treated successfully by recourse to antilymphocyte antibody therapy and/or switching from cyclosporin to tacrolimus (or vice versa).

Complications of immunosuppression

All immunosuppressive regimens used in organ transplantation increase the risk of infection and malignancy.

Infection

Transplant recipients receiving immunosuppressive therapy are at high risk from opportunistic infection, especially by viruses. Opportunistic infection is a potential problem in all transplant recipients, but those receiving aggressive immunosuppressive therapy after liver, heart, lung and small bowel transplantation are most at risk. Chemoprophylaxis is important in high-risk recipients.

Bacterial infection

The risk of bacterial infection is highest during the first month after transplantation. Transplant recipients are, like all patients undergoing major surgery, at risk of bacterial infections in the wound, respiratory tract and urinary tract. It is standard practice to give a broad-spectrum antibiotic to cover the perioperative period as prophylaxis against wound infection and possible bacterial contamination of the donor organ. The risk of bacterial infection is greatest in transplant recipients who are critically ill before or after surgery and are in the intensive care unit with indwelling catheters and lines. After recovery from surgery, the risk of bacterial infection is much reduced. Tuberculosis is a concern in patients who have previously had mycobacterial infection and in patients from the Indian subcontinent, and it is usual to give immunochemo-prophylaxis to these individuals for a period of 6–12 months after transplantation.

Viral infection

The risk of viral infection is highest during the first 6 months after transplantation and the most common problem is CMV infection. Most adults (> 80 per cent) develop CMV infection when they are children and have acquired immunity, as evidenced by the presence of IgG antibodies to CMV. Following organ transplantation, CMV disease may arise because of reactivation of latent infection or because of primary infection that can be transmitted by an organ from a CMV-positive donor. The recipients at most risk from CMV infection are those who are CMV seronegative and receive an organ from a CMV-seropositive donor. Matching seronegative donors with seronegative recipients is an effective strategy for reducing the risk of CMV infection but is not very practicable. CMV disease typically presents with a high swinging fever, lethargy and leucopenia. The severity of the disease is variable and the clinical picture depends on the organ system most affected. It may present as:

- pneumonia;
- gastrointestinal disease;
- hepatitis;
- retinitis;
- encephalitis.

Severe CMV disease is potentially fatal. Prophylaxis for CMV consists of passive immunisation using hyperimmune immunoglobulin or, more commonly now, administration of antiviral agents in the form of aciclovir or ganciclovir. A diagnosis of active CMV infection can be confirmed by serology, detection of CMV antigenaemia, CMV culture, PCR to detect viral DNA and histological examination of biopsy material. Treatment is with ganciclovir and is more effective when given pre-emptively on the basis of increased viral load as judged, for example, by quantitative PCR analysis for CMV.

Herpes simplex virus (HSV) infection is common after transplantation and is usually due to reactivation of latent infection. It causes mucocutaneus lesions around the mouth and sometimes the genitalia. These usually respond to topical treatment with acyclovir, but in severe cases systemic antiviral therapy is needed. Disseminated HSV infection is rare. Varicella zoster infection occurs more frequently in transplant patients and should be treated with systemic antiviral therapy.

Protozoal infection

Pneumocystis carinii is the most important protozoal infection after transplantation. It occurs during the first few months and presents with respiratory symptoms. The diagnosis is made by examination of bronchoalveolar lavage fluid or lung biopsy material for evidence of parasite infection. Prophylaxis with co-trimoxazole is highly effective and is usually continued for 6 months after transplantation.

Fungal infection

Invasive fungal infections are uncommon in renal transplant recipients but infection with *Candida* or *Aspergillus* is more common after other types of solid organ transplantation. Fungal infection usually occurs in the first 3 months after transplantation, and early diagnosis and aggressive treatment are essential to avoid fatal infection.

Malignancy

After transplantation there is an increased risk of developing certain types of malignant disease, especially those tumours where viral infection plays an aetiological role. The increased risk of malignancy is particularly high for skin cancer and non-Hodgkin's lymphoma. Most of the skin cancers seen are squamous cell carcinomas, but basal cell carcinoma and malignant melanoma are also more common (Fig. 11.11). The risk of skin cancer after transplantation rises with age and with exposure to sunlight, and it has been predicted that 50 per cent of transplant patients will develop a skin malignancy by 20 years. Patients must be warned of this risk before they undergo transplantation and advised to use an effective sun-screen. They should undergo regular review of their skin to detect malignancy and when such lesions occur they must be treated promptly and aggressively.

The risk of developing non-Hodgkin's lymphoma is significantly increased after transplantation. This type of malignancy is classified as post-transplant lymphoproliferative disease (PTLD). Most of them are Epstein–Barr virus-induced B-cell tumours. The overall risk of PTLD is around 1 per cent per

Thomas Hodgkin, b. 1798. English physician.
Y.M. Barr, b. 1932. English pathologist, Bristol, England.

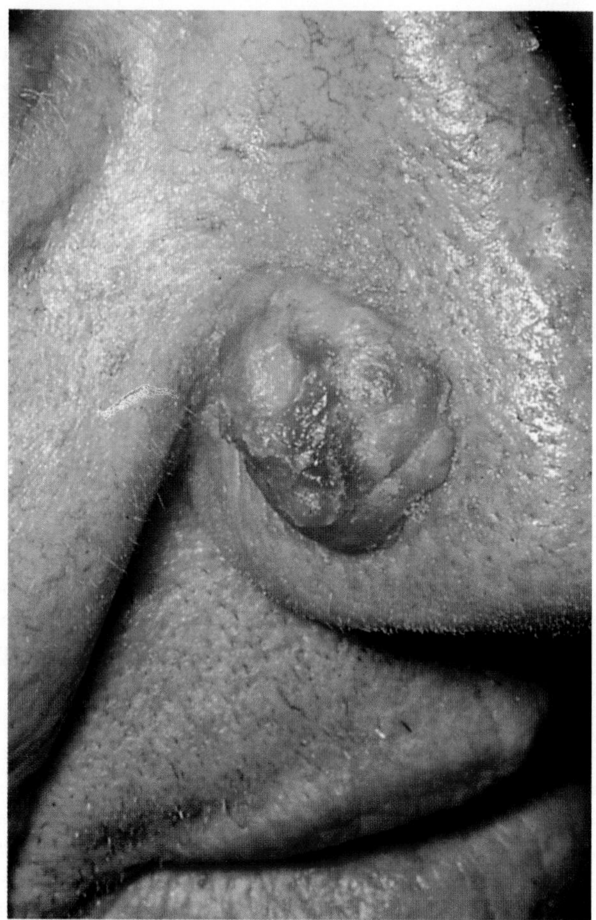

Fig. 11.11 Squamous cell carcinoma on the nose of a transplant recipient following long-term immunosuppression.

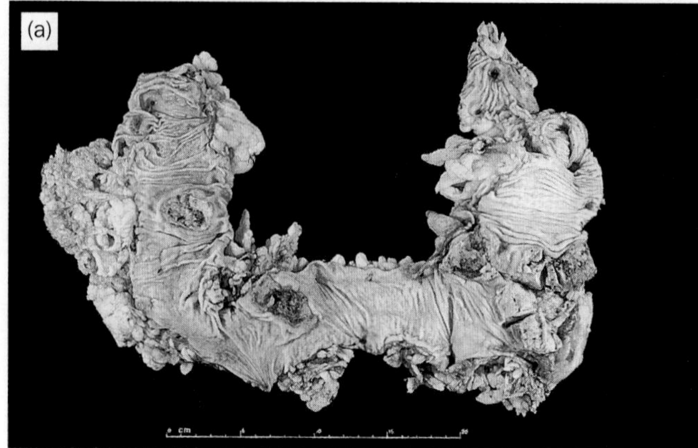

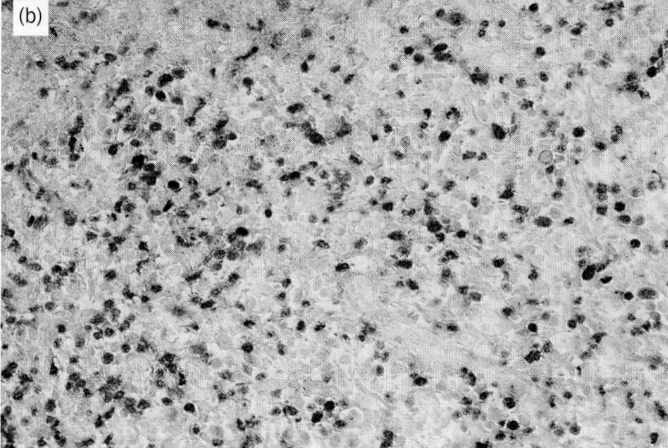

Fig. 11.12 (a) Intestinal post-transplant lymphoproliferative disease (PTLD). Note multiple lesions in terminal ileum and colon. (b) Atypical B-lymphocytes stained positive with a probe for EBV-DNA (*courtesy of C. Watson, R. Chavez-Cartaya and D. Wight*).

annum and is highest in patients who have received aggressive immunosuppression. PTLD may occur in lymph nodes or at extranodal sites such as the gastrointestinal tract, lung, liver or in the transplanted organ (Fig. 11.12). If PTLD is identified at an early stage reduction or cessation of immunosuppressive therapy may cause disease regression and result in a cure. When advanced it is usually fatal. Both disseminated disease and central nervous system (CNS) involvement have a very poor prognosis.

Transplant patients also have a 300-fold increased risk of developing Kaposi's sarcoma, although this malignancy is still very uncommon after transplantation.

Organ donation

Most of the organs used for transplantation are obtained from brainstem-dead, heart-beating cadaveric donors and in the majority of cases multiple organs are procured. However, the number of organs required to satisfy the needs of transplantation far exceeds the number of cadaveric organs available. This has prompted a relaxation in the organ-specific donor selection criteria and the use of organs from so-called 'marginal donors'. In the case of kidney transplantation there is a trend towards increased living donor transplantation and the use of kidneys from nonheart-beating cadaver donors.

Determination of brainstem death

Brain death occurs when severe brain injury causes irreversible loss of the capacity for consciousness combined with the irreversible loss of the capacity for breathing. In most countries, it is accepted that the condition of brain death equates in medical, legal and religious terms with death of the patient. The concept of brain death arose through necessity in the management of patients with irreversible brain damage on life support where there was no prospect for recovery. It was not in the interest of such patients, their relatives or the hospital in which they were being treated to delay their inevitable demise by continuing with futile life support. Acceptance of the concept of brain-death had major implications for organ transplantation as it allowed the possibility for removal of viable organs from brain-dead patients before their circulation failed.

Moritz K. Kaposi, 1837–1902. Dermatologist, Vienna, Austria.

In the UK, and many other countries, brain death is defined in terms of permanent functional death of the brainstem as neither consciousness nor spontaneous respiration is possible in the absence of a functional brainstem. A diagnosis of brainstem death should only be considered when certain preconditions have been met. The patient must have suffered major brain damage of known aetiology, be deeply unconscious and require artificial ventilation. Traumatic head injury and sudden intracranial haemorrhage are the most common causes of brainstem death. Particular care must be taken to ensure that muscle-relaxant agents and drugs with known CNS-depressant effects are not contributing to the clinical picture. Hypothermia, profound hypotension and metabolic or hormonal conditions that may contribute to CNS depression and confound the diagnosis of brainstem death must also be excluded. When the necessary preconditions have been satisfied formal clinical assessment of the brainstem reflexes can be undertaken (Table 11.3). The UK guidelines state that the tests should be performed on two separate occasions by two clinicians experienced in this area. At least one of the two clinicians should be a consultant and neither should be connected with the transplant team. The time that must elapse between the two sets of brainstem tests is not specified in the guidelines and is determined on the basis of clinical judgement. In the UK there is no requirement to perform electrophysiological or brain perfusion studies to aid the diagnosis of brainstem death. Particular care is required in the diagnosis of brainstem death in neonates and infants.

Evaluation of the cadaveric donor

After a brainstem-dead donor has been referred to the transplant team with a view to organ donation the general suitability of the potential organ donor must be carefully assessed. Particular care must be taken to assess the donor from the point of view of transmissible infectious agents and malignancy. The medical history should be carefully scrutinised and evidence of risk factors for human immunodeficiency virus (HIV), such as intravenous drug abuse, sought. The presence of HIV infection is an absolute contraindication to organ donation, as is hepatitis B infection (in most countries) and active systemic sepsis, for example major abdominal infection. The presence of malignancy within the past 5 years is also an absolute contraindication to organ donation, with the exceptions of low-grade primary tumours of the CNS, nonmelanotic tumours of the skin and carcinoma *in situ* of the uterine cervix. If there are no general contraindications to organ donation consideration is then given to organ-specific selection criteria.

Table 11.3 Clinical testing for brainstem death

- **Absence of cranial nerve reflexes:**
  - Pupillary reflex
  - Corneal reflex
  - Pharyngeal (gag) and tracheal (cough) reflex
  - Oculovestibular (caloric) reflex
- **Absence of motor response** to painful stimuli applied to head/face and absence of motor response within the cranial nerve distribution to adequate stimulation of any somatic area. The presence of spinal reflexes does not preclude brainstem death
- **Absence of spontaneous respiration** – after preventilation with 100 per cent oxygen for at least 5 minutes the patient is disconnected from the ventilator for 10 minutes to confirm absence of respiratory effort, during which the arterial CO_2 tension should be $\geq$ 6.65 kPa to ensure adequate respiratory stimulation. To prevent hypoxia during the apnoeic period, oxygen (6 litres/minute) is delivered via an endotracheal catheter

The demand for cadaveric organs for transplantation far exceeds the supply and, consequently, there has been a progressive relaxation in the organ-specific selection criteria. The chronological age of the donor is less important than the physiological function of the organs under consideration for transplantation. As a rough guide acceptable donor age ranges for each of the commonly transplanted organs are as follows:

- kidney – 2–74 years;
- liver – 0–75 years;
- heart – 0–65 years;
- lung – 0–60 years;
- pancreas – 10–50 years.

The organs to be donated should generally be free from primary disease. Kidney donors should not have evidence of primary renal disease. They should have a reasonable urine output and normal serum urea and creatinine, although acute terminal elevations are acceptable. Liver donors should not have hepatic disease, although impaired liver function tests are common in cadaver donors and do not necessarily preclude donation. Heart donors should not have a history of pre-existing heart disease. They should have a normal electrocardiogram (ECG); in doubtful cases an echocardiogram may also be necessary. Lung donors should have no history of primary lung disease. The chest X-ray and gas exchange should be satisfactory, and bronchial aspirates should be free from fungal and bacterial infection. Pancreas donors should not have a history of diabetes mellitus, but elevations of blood glucose and serum amylase are not uncommon in cadaveric donors and do not preclude transplantation.

Organ procurement

When brainstem death has been confirmed, management of the donor is aimed at preserving the functional integrity of the organs to be procured. Brainstem death produces profound metabolic and neuroendocrine disturbances leading to cardiovascular instability. Careful monitoring and management of fluid balance is essential. Inotropic support is given and there may be a role for the use of tri-iodothyronine (T3) and argipressin.

Procurement of multiple organs from a cadaveric donor requires co-operation between the thoracic and abdominal surgical teams. A midline abdominal incision and median sternotomy are used to obtain access. After dissection of the organs to be procured, they are perfused *in situ*. The heart is perfused with cold cardioplegia solution via a cannula in the ascending aorta, and the lungs are perfused via a cannula in the pulmonary artery. The abdominal organs are perfused with chilled organ preservation solution via an aortic and portal cannula. Blood and perfusate are vented from the left atrial appendage and the inferior vena cava. This produces rapid cooling of the organs, reduces their metabolic activity and preserves their viability. Additional surface cooling of the abdominal organs may be achieved by application of saline ice slush. The heart and lungs are excised followed by the liver and pancreas and then the kidneys, either *en bloc* or separately. The extent to which the abdominal organs are dissected prior to cold flush depends on the preference of the surgical team. Some surgeons perform minimal dissection prior to cold perfusion and complete the dissection of the abdominal organs *in situ* or on the back table after the organs have been removed *en bloc*. During procurement of the liver care is taken to ensure that, if there is an aberrant hepatic artery arising from the superior mesenteric artery, it is included in the aortic patch. Similarly, care is taken to ensure that any polar renal arteries are included on an arterial patch with the renal artery. A length of the donor iliac artery is excised for use in reconstructing the arterial supply of the pancreas.

After removal from the donor the organs may undergo a further flush with chilled preservation solution and are then each placed in two sterile plastic bags and stored at 0–4°C by immersion in ice while they are transported to the recipient centre to await implantation. After the donor organs have been excised, samples of donor spleen and mesenteric lymph nodes are obtained for determination of tissue type and for the cross-match test.

Various organ-preservation solutions are available for flushing organs before simple cold storage. They all contain impermeants to limit cell swelling, buffers to counter acidosis and electrolytes, the composition of which reflects that of intracellular rather than extracellular fluid. Commonly used preservation solutions include University of Wisconsin (UW) solution and Eurocollins solution, but there are many others.

Table 11.4 Composition of UW solution

Potassium lactobionate (mmol/litre)	100
Sodium phosphate (mmol)	25
Magnesium sulphate (mmol)	5
Adenosine (mmol/litre)	5
Allopurinol (mmol/litre)	1
Gluthione (mmol/litre)	3
Raffinose (mmol/litre)	30
Hydroxethyl starch (g/litre)	50
Insulin (U/litre)	100
Dexamethasone (mg/litre)	8
Potassium (mmol/litre)	135
Sodium (mmol/litre)	35
Osmolality (mOsm/litre)	320
pH	7.4

Table 11.5 Maximum and ideal cold storage times (approximate)*

Organ	*Optimum (hours)*	*Safe maximum (hours)*
Kidney	< 24	48
Liver	< 12	24
Pancreas	< 10	24
Small intestine	< 4	8
Heart	< 3	6
Lung	< 3	8

*Assuming zero warm ischaemic time and that the organs are obtained from a nonmarginal donor.

The use of UW solution (Table 11.4) (developed by Belzer and colleagues) is particularly effective for liver grafts and, after perfusion with UW, the liver can be stored safely for up to 24 hours. The length of time for which an organ can be stored before transplantation varies depending on the type of organ (Table 11.5). After arriving at the recipient transplant centre any necessary bench surgery is undertaken prior to implantation.

Nonheart-beating (asystolic) donors

There is renewed interest in the use of kidneys from nonheart-beating or asystolic donors in an attempt to address the shortage of organs for transplantation. Kidneys may be procured from patients who are dead on arrival at the hospital or who have died in hospital after withdrawal of support or following unsuccessful resuscitation. In order to minimise the warm ischaemic time, a double-balloon catheter is introduced into the aorta via a femoral cut-down and used to cool the kidneys *in situ* by chilled perfusate, preferably within 30 minutes of circulatory arrest. Kidneys obtained from nonheart-beating donors invariably suffer from delayed function and this approach is not suitable for organs other than the kidney.

Living kidney donors

Currently, living donor renal transplants account for around 20 per cent of the total renal transplant activity. The justification for living donor renal transplantation is based on the shortage of cadaveric transplants and the superior results obtained. Most living donor transplants are between genetically related individuals. However, living donor kidney transplants performed between genetically unrelated individuals also fare better than even well-matched cadaveric grafts, and this observation has given rise to an increase in living unrelated kidney transplantation activity, usually between spouses or partners. It is essential to ensure in all cases of living donation that the prospective donor is fully informed and is free from coercion to donate and that the risk to the donor is small.

Folkert O. Belzer. Surgeon, Madison, Wisconsin, USA.

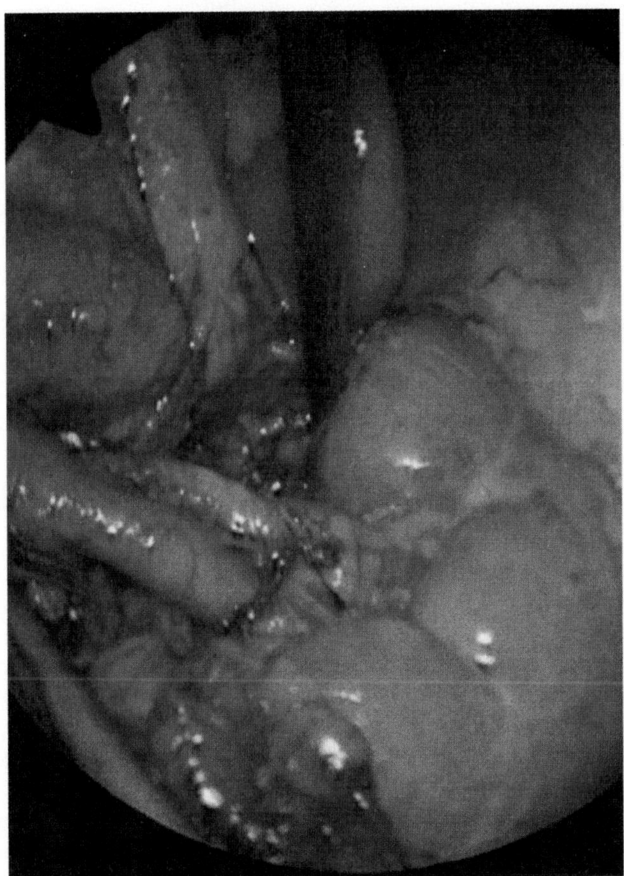

Fig. 11.13 Laparoscopic living donor nephrectomy. The left kidney has been mobilised on its vascular pedicle. After staple/transection of the renal vessels the kidney will be removed via a small midline incision and flushed with chilled organ preservation solution before implantation (courtesy of P. Veitch and M. Nicholson).

Live donation should proceed only after the prospective donor has undergone rigorous assessment to ensure that they are suitable. Before the donation it is essential to perform renal imaging (commonly a selective renal angiogram) to delineate the anatomy of the arterial supply to the kidneys. If the left kidney has a single renal artery it is usually chosen for transplantation because it has a longer renal vein which simplifies the transplant operation. Donor nephrectomy is undertaken either through a loin incision and retroperitoneal approach or through a midline abdominal incision and transperitoneal approach. Laparoscopic donor nephrectomy has recently attracted interest but its role in living donation is not established (Fig. 11.13). The mortality rate for live donation is less than 0.05 per cent and the major complication rate is around 5 per cent. In the long term, a slight elevation in proteinurea and a small rise in blood pressure accompany unilateral nephrectomy.

Living donors: extrarenal organs

Living donors have occasionally been used to provide segments of liver, pancreas, small bowel and lung for transplantation but this is more controversial. Several hundred living related liver transplants have been performed worldwide, predominantly in countries where cadaveric donation is not practised. The left lateral segment or left lobe from an adult is transplanted into a paediatric recipient. In countries where heart-beating cadaver donation is undertaken, live donor liver transplantation has been superceded by the techniques of liver reduction or liver splitting. The latter approach allows the liver from a cadaver donor to be split in two, so that the right lobe can go to an adult and the left lobe to a paediatric recipient (Fig. 11.14). In North America, living donor combined kidney and segmental pancreas transplantation has been undertaken to treat insulin-dependent diabetics with end-stage renal disease. In occasional patients living donor small bowel transplantation has been performed using a small bowel graft which comprises a length of around 1.5 m of ileum. Finally, a small number of living donor segmental lung transplants has been performed. To provide sufficient pulmonary tissue without compromising the donor it is necessary to use segments from two different donors for each recipient. The ethical issues raised by living donation for extrarenal organs are understandably complex.

Resumption of function following organ transplantation

It is crucial that following heart, lung or liver transplantation, the transplanted organ resumes satisfactory function immediately. If primary nonfunction occurs the only option is rapid re-transplantation. After kidney, pancreas or small bowel transplantation immediate graft function is desirable but not vital. The factors that influence the functional integrity of a transplanted organ are shown in Table 11.6.

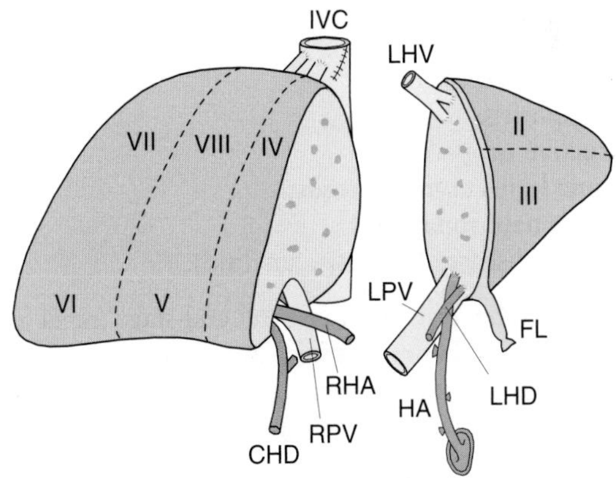

RHD – Right hepatic duct
FL – Falciform ligament
IVC – Inferior vena cava
PV – Portal vein
HA – Hepatic artery (on aortic patch)
LHV – Left hepatic vein
CHD – Common hepatic duct

Fig. 11.14 An adult liver may be split, according to Couinard's segments, so that the left lateral segment (segments II and III) can be transplanted into a child and the right lobe (together with segment IV) can be transplanted into an adult.

Table 11.6 Factors influencing organ function after transplantation

- Donor characteristics:
  - Extremes of age
  - Presence of pre-existing disease in the transplanted organ
  - Haemodynamic and metabolic instability
- Procurement-related factors:
  - Warm ischaemic time
  - Type of preservation solution
  - Cold ischaemic time
- Recipient-related factors:
  - Technical factors relating to implantation
  - Haemodynamic and metabolic stability
  - Immunological factors, e.g. sensitisation status
  - Presence of drugs which impair function

Kidney transplantation

Patient selection

Renal transplantation is the preferred treatment for many patients with end-stage renal disease because it provides a better quality of life for them than dialysis. Transplantation releases patients from the dietary and fluid restrictions of dialysis and the physical constraints imposed by the need to dialyse. It is also more cost-effective than dialysis.

In the UK, around 80–100 people per million population develop end-stage renal disease and the incidence increases with age. The causes of end-stage renal disease are numerous and include the following:

- glomerulonephritis;
- diabetic nephropathy;
- hypertensive nephrosclerosis;
- renal vascular disease;
- polycystic disease;
- pyelonephritis;
- obstructive uropathy;
- systemic lupus erythematosus;
- analgesic nephropathy;
- metabolic diseases (oxalosis, amyloid).

Frequently, the primary cause of end-stage renal disease remains uncertain. For renal transplantation, as for other types of organ transplantation, careful patient selection is essential. Before acceptance as suitable candidates on the transplant waiting list, a transplant surgeon and nephrologist should formally assess all patients. A significant number of patients is likely to be considered unsuitable for renal transplantation because of major comorbid disease, especially cardiovascular disease. In the UK around half of the dialysis population are currently on the waiting list for renal transplantation.

The nature of the primary renal disease does not generally affect the decision to proceed to transplantation. Some of the glomerulonephritides (notably focal segmental glomerulosclerosis) may subsequently affect a transplanted kidney but this only occasionally results in failure of the graft in the first 5 years. In the case of primary oxalosis, combined kidney and hepatic transplantation is usually undertaken to eliminate the metabolic defect and thereby prevent early graft failure from the formation of further oxalate stones.

The age of patients with end-stage renal failure accepted for dialysis has gradually risen over the last two decades and in the UK the mean age of patients starting dialysis is around 70 years. There is no absolute upper age limit to renal transplantation but inevitably older patients (over the age of 65 years) are less likely to be considered suitable candidates because of major cardiovascular and other comorbid disease.

A careful assessment of comorbid disease that might significantly reduce the chances of successful outcome after transplantation is essential. Rigorous evaluation of the cardiovascular system is particularly important. Cardiovascular disease is very common in the dialysis population, especially those with diabetes, and is the major cause of death after transplantation. Before listing patients for transplantation it is important to ensure that their urinary tract is functional and that there is no need for corrective urological surgery. Only when there is long-standing renal sepsis, or in the case of very large polycystic kidneys which intrude into both iliac fossae, is native nephrectomy required before transplantation can be undertaken. Finally, the prospective transplant recipient must be judged likely to comply with immunosuppressive therapy.

Immunosuppressive therapy increases the risk of infection and malignancy. Consequently, pre-existing malignancy is an absolute contraindication, and even after curative treatment transplantation should not be considered for at least 3 years. Similarly, the presence of active infection is an absolute contraindication to transplantation.

Technique of renal transplantation

The transplant kidney is placed in the iliac fossa, in the retroperitoneal position, leaving the native kidneys *in situ*. After induction of general anaesthesia a central venous line and a urinary catheter are inserted. It is helpful to distend the bladder with saline containing methylene blue to allow it to be identified with certainty prior to ureteric implantation. A curved incision is made in the lower abdomen and after dividing the muscles of the abdominal wall, the peritoneum is swept upwards to expose the iliac vessels. These are dissected free so that they can be controlled with vascular clamps. The kidney is then removed from ice and the donor renal vein is anastomosed end-to-side to the external iliac vein. The donor renal artery on a Carrel patch of donor aorta is then anastomosed end-to-side to the external iliac artery (Fig. 11.15a). If the donor renal artery lacks an aortic patch, as in the case of a living donor transplant, it is usually preferable to anastomose the donor artery end-to-end to the recipient internal iliac artery (Fig. 11.15b). While the vascular anastomoses are being undertaken the kidney is kept cold by application of ice. Following completion of the venous and arterial anastomoses the vascular clamps are removed and the kidney is allowed to reperfuse with blood.

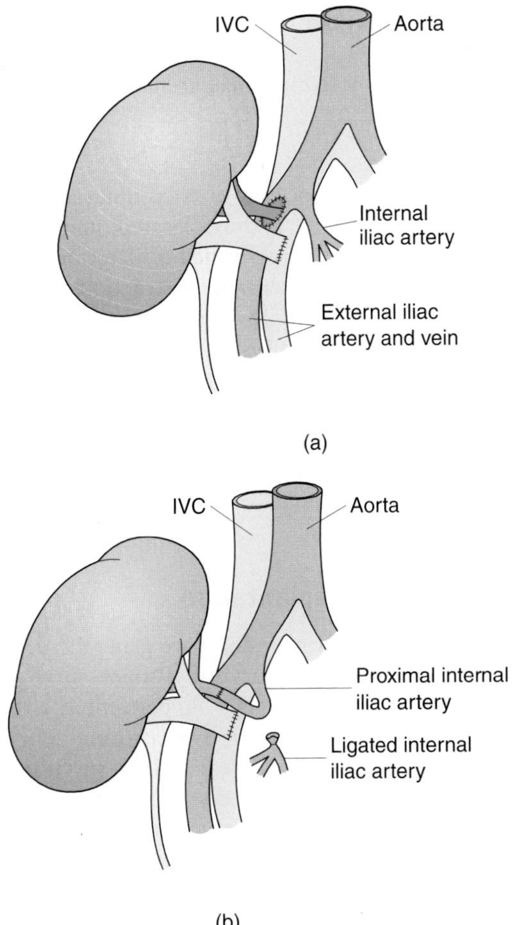

Fig. 11.15 Implantation of renal allograft. (a) The renal artery on a Carrel patch is anastomosed to the external iliac artery. (b) The renal artery is anastomosed end-to-end to the internal iliac artery.

The ureter, which is kept reasonably short to avoid the risk of distal ischaemia, is then anastomosed to the bladder (Fig. 11.16). This is most often achieved by direct implantation of the ureter into the dome of the bladder with a mucosa to mucosal anastomosis followed by closure of the muscular wall of the bladder over the ureter to create a short tunnel – the Lich–Gregoire technique. A double-J ureteric stent is often left *in situ*, especially if there are technical difficulties, and removed after several weeks during cystoscopy. Alternatively, the ureter may be implanted by the Leadbetter–Politano technique where the bladder is opened to allow the creation of a submucosal antireflux tunnel. Before closing the transplant wound it is important to ensure that the kidney is lying in a satisfactory position without kinking or torsion of the vessels. In small children receiving an adult donor kidney the abdomen is opened through a midline incision and the graft is placed intra-abdominally with anastomosis of the renal vessels to the aorta and vena cava.

Willy Gregoire. Chef du Clinique Urologique, Brussels, 1962–87.
Robert Lich Jr. Urologist, Louisville, Kentucky, USA.

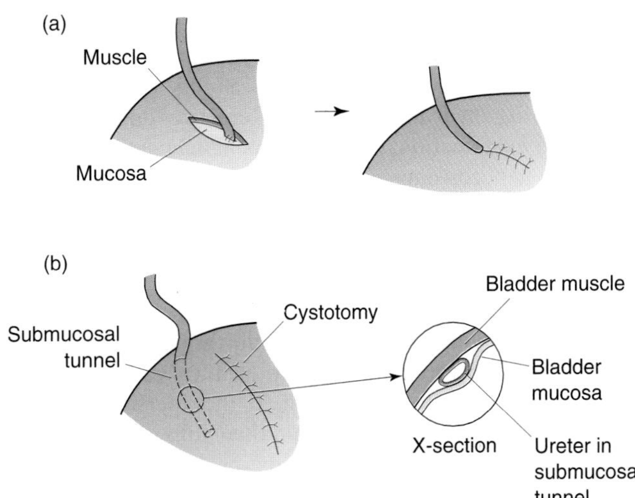

Fig. 11.16 Ureteric implantation. (a) Gregoire–Lich technique. (b) Leadbetter–Politano (pull-through) technique.

Technical complications

Vascular complications

The incidence of vascular complications after renal transplantation is quite low. Renal artery thrombosis occurs in approximately 1 per cent of cases. Renal vein thrombosis is more common (up to 5 per cent of cases), and although sometimes owing to technical error, the aetiology is uncertain. It presents as sudden pain and swelling at the site of the transplant and the diagnosis is confirmed by Doppler ultrasound. Urgent surgical exploration is indicated and in most cases transplant nephrectomy is required. The incidence of renal vein thrombosis can be minimised by giving low-dose heparin or aspirin prophylaxis. Renal artery stenosis presents late (often years) after transplantation with increasing hypertension and decreasing renal function. It may occur in up to 10 per cent of grafts, is diagnosed by angiography and is best treated by angioplasty rather than open surgery.

Urological complications

Urological complications occur in up to 10 per cent of patients in the early post-transplant period, but their incidence can be reduced by leaving a temporary ureteric stent *in situ*. Urinary leaks result from technical errors at the ureteric anastomosis or because of ureteric ischaemia. They present with discomfort and leakage of urine from the wound and usually require surgical intervention and reimplantation of the ureter into the bladder or anastomosis of the transplant ureter to the native ureter. Obstruction of the transplant ureter may occur early or late. Causes of obstruction include

Wyland F. Leadbetter. Urologist, Massachussets General Hospital, USA.
Victor A. Politano. Urologist, Massachusetts General Hospital (now at University of Miami), USA.
Christian Johann Doppler, 1803–53. Austrian physicist.

technical error, external pressure from a haematoma or lymphocele and ischaemic stricture. It presents with painless deterioration in transplant function and is confirmed by demonstrating hydronephrosis and ureteric dilatation on ultrasound examination. Initial treatment is by percutaneous antegrade nephrostomy and insertion of a stent. Surgical intervention may be needed to treat strictures that are not amenable to correction by ballon dilatation.

Lymphocele

Peritransplant lymphoceles are usually asymptomatic, but occasionally they become large enough to cause ureteric obstruction or oedema of the leg. If they persist, surgical intervention may be needed to drain them into the peritoneal cavity. This can often be achieved by an ultrasound-guided laparoscopic approach.

Investigation of graft dysfunction

Graft dysfunction during the early postoperative period is a common problem. Possible causes are:

- acute tubular necrosis;
- arterial/venous thrombosis;
- urinary leak/obstruction;
- calcineurin blocker toxicity;
- hyperacute/accelerated acute rejection.

Delayed graft function as a result of acute tubular necrosis occurs in up to 50 per cent of cadaveric kidney transplants but is uncommon following living donor transplantation. Often the recipient produces significant volumes of urine from their native kidneys, making the diagnosis of delayed function more difficult. The incidence of delayed function can be minimised by optimising donor management before kidney procurement and by reducing the cold ischaemia time by avoiding unnecessary delay before implantation. As a first step in the management of early graft dysfunction, the urinary catheter should be irrigated in case it is occluded by a blood clot. Hypovolaemia, if present, should be corrected with the aid of central venous pressure (CVP) monitoring. A Doppler ultrasound examination of the graft is the single most important investigation as it allows exclusion of vascular thrombosis and urinary obstruction as causes of graft dysfunction. In addition, a renal radionucleotide scan is often performed and provides information on renal perfusion and excretion. If graft dysfunction is still present after several days it is usual to perform an ultrasound-guided needle biopsy of the kidney to ensure that graft rejection is not present. To avoid the risk of nephrotoxicity, calcineurin blockers are often withheld or given in reduced doses until graft function is established. If calcineurin blockers are not withheld, it is important to monitor their blood levels carefully to avoid nephrotoxicity. Acute tubular necrosis usually resolves within the first 4 weeks of transplantation but a small number of grafts suffers primary nonfunction.

Allograft dysfunction developing late (> 1 month after transplant) may be due to:

- acute/chronic rejection;
- drug toxicity;
- ureteric obstruction (lympocoele/ureteric stricture);
- recurrent disease;
- infection.

Blood levels of cyclosporine or tacrolimus are assessed to ensure that they are not unduly elevated, and ultrasound examination of the graft is performed to determine whether ureteric obstruction is present. If obstruction is detected, it is further investigated by percutaneous antegrade pyelography. Ureteric stenosis may be amenable to balloon dilatation but a long stricture may require reimplantation of the transplant ureter (or renal pelvis) into the bladder or into the native ureter. If there is uncertainty about the cause of graft dysfunction, transplant biopsy should be performed to establish whether allograft rejection is present.

Outcome after transplantation

The results of organ transplantation are generally defined in terms of patient and graft survival. Patient survival after cadaveric renal transplantation is > 90 per cent at 1 year and > 80 per cent at 5 years. Graft survival is around 85 per cent at 1 year and 65 per cent at 5 years. Graft survival after a second transplant is only marginally worse than after a first graft. After living related kidney transplantation, overall graft survival is > 90 per cent at 1 year and > 80 per cent at 5 years. Graft survival after transplantation can also be expressed in terms of the half-life of the graft. The half-life for grafts obtained from living donors is substantially longer than for cadaveric grafts:

- cadaveric grafts – 7 years;
- living unrelated – 9 years;
- living haploidentical – 12 years;
- living identical – 24 years.

If a kidney transplant fails late after transplantation, transplant nephrectomy may be indicated, especially if the graft is causing symptoms. The operation is undertaken via the original wound but the kidney is dissected free from the renal capsule and delivered into the wound. The renal vessels are then ligated and divided, leaving behind the original vascular anastomosis.

In addition to graft survival, it is important to consider the extent to which transplantation improves the physical and mental well-being of the patient, and allows them to lead a satisfactory social life. As other types of solid organ transport, successful kidney transplantation undoubtedly leads to a substantial improvement in quality of life. However, whereas some recipients return to a normal or near-normal life, others fare much less well, and for the group overall the quality of life after transplantation falls short of that seen in normal healthy individuals. Organ transplantation is best regarded, therefore, as an effective form of therapy rather than a complete cure.

Pancreas transplantation

Successful pancreas transplantation restores normal control of glucose metabolism and obviates the need for insulin therapy in patients with diabetes mellitus. Improved control of blood glucose levels in diabetes undoubtedly reduces the risk of secondary complications such as retinopathy, peripheral vascular disease and nephropathy. However, in considering the indications for pancreas transplantation, these advantages have to be weighed carefully against the risks posed both by the transplant procedure itself and by the immunosuppressive therapy required to prevent graft rejection. For most patients with diabetes, the additional risks associated with pancreas transplantation and immunosuppression are such that the operation can only be justified when kidney transplantation for diabetic nephropathy is also being undertaken. The only additional risks of pancreas transplantation in such patients relate to the transplant operation itself. In the USA, around half of all diabetic patients undergoing kidney transplantation also receive a pancreas transplant. In most cases, the kidney and pancreas are obtained from the same donor, so-called 'simultaneous pancreas and kidney transplantation' (SPKT). Sometimes pancreas transplantation is performed in patients who have already undergone successful kidney transplantation – 'pancreas after kidney transplantation' (PAKT). Occasionally, pancreas transplantation alone (PTA) can be justified, for example to treat labile diabetes or hypoglycaemic unawareness.

Careful patient selection is essential to avoid excessive mortality and morbidity. The procedure is usually reserved for those patients with type I diabetes who are relatively young (under the age of 50 years) and do not have advanced coronary artery disease or peripheral vascular disease. Echocardiography and coronary angiography are mandatory during assessment of recipient suitability for transplantation.

Surgical technique

Most centres now perform transplantation of the whole pancreas together with a segment of duodenum, essentially as pioneered by Lillehei in1966. Segmental pancreas transplantation is still performed occasionally, especially in France. SPKT is usually performed through a midline incision (Fig. 11.17). The pancreas graft is placed intraperitoneally in the pelvis, usually on the right, and the kidney graft is placed either intraperitoneally or extraperitoneally on the left side. The donor vessels of the pancreas graft are anastomosed to the recipient iliac vessels and the exocrine secretions are dealt with by anastomosing the graft duodenum to either the bladder (urinary drainage) or the small bowel (enteric drainage). The pancreas graft functions immediately after revascularisation, although supplementary insulin may be required for a few days. Technical complications usually occur early and include vascular thrombosis of the graft (5–10 per cent) and anastomotic leaks. Wound infection occurs in around 10 per cent of patients and intra-abdominal infection is

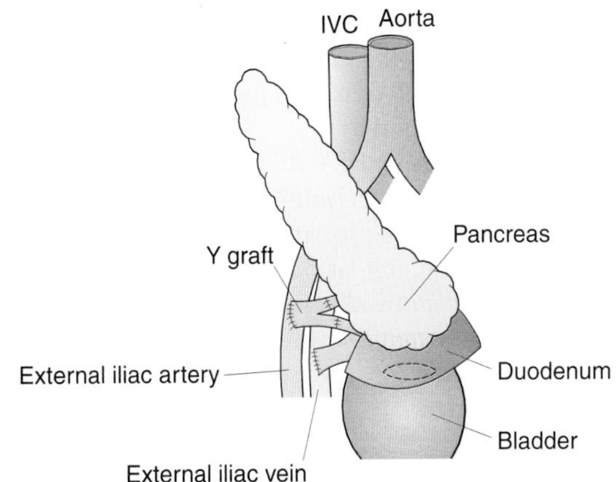

Fig. 11.17 Pancreas transplant operation with urinary drainage of the exocrine secretion via a duodenocystostomy. A 'Y' graft using donor iliac artery is often used to reconstruct the divided splenic and superior mesenteric arteries of the graft prior to implantation.

relatively common. The specific complications of enteric drainage include intra-abdominal sepsis and gastrointestinal haemorrhage (anastomotic). Bladder drainage of the exocrine pancreas may result in the following complications:

- bladder/duodenal anastomotic leaks;
- cystitis (due to effect of pancreatic enzymes);
- urethritis/urethral stricture;
- reflux pancreatitis;
- urinary tract infection;
- haematuria;
- metabolic acidosis (due to loss of bicarbonate in the urine).

Urinary drainage of the pancreas has the advantage that urinary amylase levels can be used to monitor for graft rejection. However, after bladder drainage, urinary complications are common and, in around 20 per cent of cases, are severe enough to require conversion to enteric drainage. Many centres now prefer primary enteric drainage after SPKT. Acute rejection after SPKT usually involves both the kidney and pancreas graft and serum creatinine can be used, therefore, as a surrogate marker for pancreas graft rejection. Urinary drainage is still preferable after PTA and PAKT because it allows pancreas graft rejection to be monitored by serial measurement of urinary amylase. A fall in urinary amylase is indicative of acute rejection. Measurement of blood glucose levels are less useful as an early indicator of rejection. Acute graft rejection is common but usually responds to treatment with steroids.

Results of pancreas transplantation

The results of pancreas transplantation have improved significantly over the last decade. After SKPT, the 1-year patient survival rate is greater than 90 per cent, and the 1-year graft survival rate for pancreas and kidney grafts, respectively, is

Richard Lillehei. Surgeon, University of Minnesota, USA.

80 and 90 per cent. Most deaths are due to cardiovascular complications or overwhelming infection. Patient and kidney graft survival after SKPT in patients with diabetic nephropathy are at least as good as after kidney transplant alone in this group. The results of PTA are not as good as after SKPT (1-year pancreas graft survival 70 per cent) because acute rejection is more difficult to monitor in the absence of a kidney allograft. The aim of pancreas transplantation is to provide freedom from insulin treatment and to improve the quality of life. The extent to which pancreas transplantation halts the progression of the secondary complications of diabetes is still unclear.

Transplantation of isolated pancreatic islets

Treatment of diabetes by transplantation of isolated islets of Langerhans is a more attractive concept than vascularised pancreas transplantation because major surgery and the potential complications of transplanting exocrine pancreas are avoided. Pancreatic islets for transplantation are obtained by mechanically disrupting the pancreas after injection of collagenase into the pancreatic duct. The islets are then purified from the dispersed tissue by density gradient centrifugation and can be delivered into the recipient liver (the optimal site for transplantation) by injection into the portal vein. Islet transplantation has been performed in diabetics receiving immunosuppression because of a kidney transplant. Although some degree of islet cell function occurs initially this is not sustained. Obtaining a critical mass of islet tissue for transplantation is problematic and isolated pancreatic islets are particularly susceptible to graft rejection. Attempts have been made to protect isolated islet cells from rejection by encapsulating them inside semipermeable membranes. The protective membranes are designed with a pore size that allows insulin to pass through but prevents antibodies and leucocytes from reaching the islets, thereby avoiding the need for immunosuppressive therapy. A major attraction of this approach is that islets isolated from animals can be used, and bioartificial pancreas grafts containing xenogeneic islets are currently under evaluation.

Liver transplantation

Starzl first attempted liver transplantation in 1963, and by 1967 had obtained prolonged survival. The first liver transplant performed outside the USA was undertaken in Cambridge by Calne in 1968. Throughout the 1970s liver transplantation remained a hazardous procedure that frequently failed, but the introduction of a number of changes led to improved results. These included improved immunosuppression, in the form of cyclosporin, together with improved patient selection and refinements in organ preservation and attention to technical aspects of the transplant operation. Liver transplantation is now a routine operation in specialist centres.

Indications and patient selection

The indications for liver transplantation fall into four groups:

- chronic cirrhosis;
- acute fulminant liver failure;
- metabolic liver disease;
- primary hepatic malignancy.

The most common indication for transplantation is chronic liver failure. In adults the causes include primary biliary cirrhosis, viral liver disease, alcoholic liver disease and sclerosing cholangitis. In children, who account for around 10–15 per cent of all liver transplants, biliary atresia is the most common indication for transplantation. Acute fulminant liver failure requiring transplantation on an urgent basis accounts for approximately 10 per cent of liver transplant activity and is viral or drug (e.g. paracetamol) induced. There is a variety of metabolic diseases for which transplantation offers the prospect of cure. These include Wilson's disease, oxalosis and α_1-antitrypsin deficiency. Hepatic malignancy is only occasionally treated by liver transplantation because of the high risk of tumour recurrence. Hepatomas, when they occur in a cirrhotic liver, may be best treated by transplantation and some centres consider transplantation for cholangiocarcinoma, although there is a high risk of recurrent disease.

Technique of liver transplantation

A transverse abdominal incision with a midline extension is made and the diseased liver mobilised (Fig. 11.18). Because of portal hypertension the recipient hepatectomy is often the most difficult part of the operation, especially if there has been previous surgery in the region. The common bile duct is divided, as are the right and left hepatic arteries. The inferior vena cava is clamped and divided above and below the liver, and the portal vein is clamped and divided allowing the recipient liver to be removed. Occlusion of the vena cava and portal vein results in a reduction in cardiac output and may necessitate the use of veno-venous bypass. The bypass circuit delivers blood from the portal vein and inferior vena cava back to the heart via a cannula inserted into the axillary vein or the internal jugular veins. After placing the donor liver in position, the supra- and infrahepatic caval anastomoses are performed The portal vein and the hepatic arterial anastomosis are then completed and the graft is reperfused. Finally, biliary drainage is re-established, usually by a duct-to-duct anastomosis (without the use of a T-tube). It may be necessary, for example in recipients with biliary atresia or sclerosing cholangitis, to reconstruct the biliary drainage by a bile duct to Roux loop anastomosis. An alternative 'piggy-back' technique of liver transplantation is sometimes preferred in which the diseased native liver is dissected from the intact inferior vena cava and the suprahepatic vena cava of the donor is anastomosed end-to-side to the anterior wall of the recipient cava.

Many patients undergoing liver transplantation are extremely ill and the surgery involved can be very technically demanding. Optimal perioperative management is crucial to a successful outcome and presents a major challenge. Blood loss

Paul Langerhans, b. 1847. German pathologist.

Thomas E. Starzl. Professor of Surgery, Pittsburgh, USA.
Samuel A.K. Wilson, b. 1877. English neurologist.

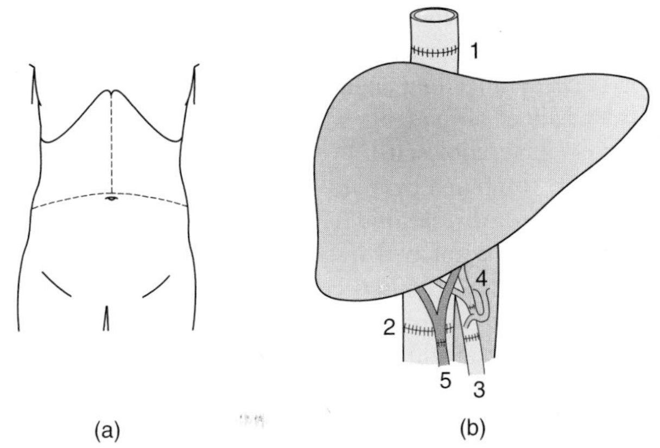

Fig. 11.18 (a) Incision used for liver transplantation. (b) Completed implantation. The anastomoses, in order of performance are: (1) suprahepatic cava; (2) infrahepatic cava; (3) portal vein; (4) hepatic artery; (5) bile duct.

during and after the transplant procedure can be very considerable and management of coagulopathy is particularly important. Coagulation is assessed repeatedly throughout the peritransplant period. Many centres use a thromboelastogram to supplement the information from standard coagulation screening (Fig. 11.19). The thromboelastogram comprises an oscillating cuvette into which a small blood sample is placed and into which a piston suspended by a torsion wire is then lowered. As the sample clots, fibrin strands transmit elastic forces to the piston and are recorded to provide an index of coagulation.

Technical complications

Haemorrhage

Meticulous homeostasis during the transplant operation is important in order to minimise the risk of early haemorrhage. It may occasionally be necessary to pack the peritransplant area for 2–3 days to achieve adequate haemostasis when there is diffuse oozing despite correction of coagulopathy. Evacuation of extensive perihepatic haematoma may be required to avoid secondary infection.

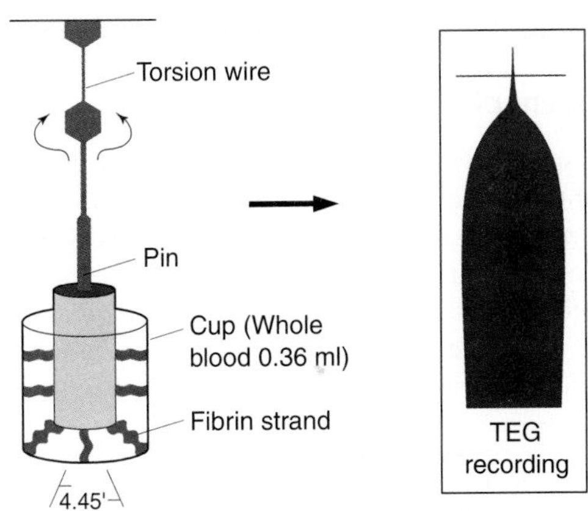

Fig. 11.19 Thromboelastogram. (Reproduced with permission from Mallet, S.V. and Cox, D.J.A. *British Journal of Anaesthesia*, **69**, 307–31, 1992.)

Vascular complications

Hepatic artery thrombosis may occur spontaneously or as a result of acute rejection, and is more common in paediatric recipients. It may present as a rise in serum transaminase levels, unexplained fever or bile leak. Doppler ultrasound or angiography are used to confirm the diagnosis and urgent retransplantation is usually required. Portal vein thrombosis presents more insidiously and does not usually require retransplantation.

Biliary complications

Biliary leaks are now relatively uncommon and biliary stenosis is a more common problem. It usually occurs late after transplantation and is managed by endoscopic dilatation and stenting, and less often by surgical correction.

Paediatric liver transplantation

Until recently, the major factor limiting paediatric liver transplantation was the lack of suitably sized donor livers. However, as noted earlier, the development of techniques for using adult livers that have been reduced in size by cut-down techniques has greatly alleviated the problem. For small children, the lateral segment of the left lobe is often used but the entire left lobe or the right lobe may also be used in this way.

Outcome after liver transplantation

The outcome after liver transplantation depends on the underlying liver disease and the best results are seen in patients with chronic liver disease (Fig. 11.20). Patients undergoing transplantation as a result of acute liver failure have a higher mortality in the early post-transplant period because of multiorgan failure, but those who make a satisfactory recovery have very good long-term liver allograft survival. Conversely, patients transplanted for tumour have a very good early outcome but ultimately fare much less well because of recurrent malignancy. Patients receiving a liver transplant following hepatitis B or hepatitis C infection often develop graft failure as a result of recurrent viral disease.

Small bowel transplantation

Progress in small bowel transplantation has lagged well behind that of other types of solid organ transplantation. Intestinal transplants stimulate a particularly strong graft rejection response, probably because the small intestine contains very large amounts of lymphoid tissue. Moreover, ischaemia and rejection increase intestinal permeability and allow translocaton of bacteria from the lumen of the bowel. Added to this, the operation is often complex and made technically difficult because of repeated previous abdominal surgery. Consequently, graft rejection and infection remain a major problem after small bowel transplantation and the results obtained are inferior to those seen after other types of

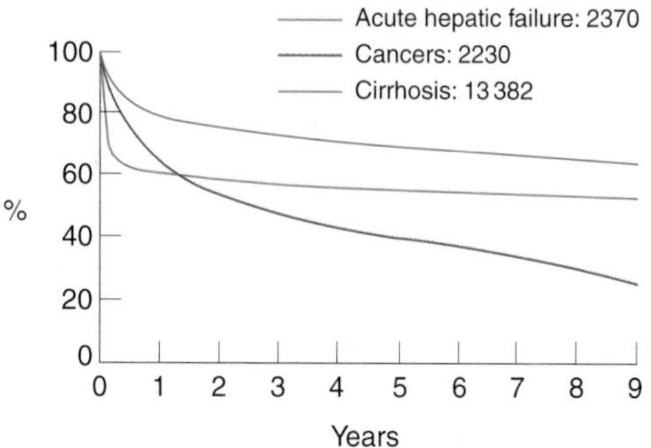

Fig. 11.20 Outcome after liver transplantation (data from European Liver Transplant Registry).

organ transplantation. Small bowel transplantation is a treatment option for patients with intestinal failure as defined by the loss of intestinal function to the extent that long-term parenteral nutrition is required. Intestinal failure may result from short bowel syndrome after resection of the intestine or from intestinal dysfunction. The conditions that may give rise to intestinal failure include the following:

- intestinal atresia;
- necrotising enterocolitis;
- volvulus;
- disorders of motility;
- mesenteric infarction;
- Crohn's disease;
- trauma;
- desmoid tumours.

Because of the substantial risks associated with small bowel transplantation, the procedure should be considered only for those patients where long-term total parenteral nutrition (TPN) has failed, usually because venous access has become impracticable or because of frequent life-threatening line sepsis. The need for small bowel transplantation is estimated at around 0.5–1.0 patients per million population and around 50 per cent of cases are children.

Small bowel transplantation may be carried out as an isolated procedure, performed together with a liver transplant or undertaken as a component of a multivisceral transplant. Around half of all small bowel transplants are performed in children. Where possible, isolated small bowel transplantation is undertaken because patient survival is higher.

A small bowel transplant from a cadaveric donor comprises the entire small bowel but it is no longer considered advisable to include the ascending colon in the graft. The superior mesenteric artery of the graft (with an aortic patch) is anastomosed to the recipient aorta and the superior mesenteric vein is anastomosed to the inferior vena cava or to the side of the portal vein. The proximal end of the small bowel graft is anastomosed to the recipient jejunum or duodenum. The distal end of the graft is anastomosed to the side of the colon (with a loop ileostomy) or is fashioned as an end ileostomy. A gastrostomy tube (to overcome delayed gastric emptying) and a feeding jejunostomy tube are inserted.

About half of all patients who require small bowel transplantation have cholestatic liver disease secondary to TPN and require combined liver and small bowel transplantation. Cholestatic liver disease due to TPN is especially common in children. When combined liver and small bowel transplantation is carried out the two grafts are transplanted *en bloc*. The donor aorta is fashioned into a conduit including the superior mesenteric and coeliac arteries, and anastomosed to the recipient aorta. The portal vein anastomosis is as for isolated liver transplantation.

Multivisceral or 'cluster' transplants may be necessary in the case of large desmoid tumours where excision of both the small bowel and adjacent organs is required, when there has been extensive thrombosis of the splanchnic vessels and for generalised disorders of gastrointestinal motility.

The 1-year graft survival rate after small bowel transplantation is about 60 per cent for both isolated small bowel transplantation and combined liver and small bowel transplantation. After 3 years the graft survival rate is around 40 per cent. As already noted, however, patient survival is better after isolated small bowel transplantation than after combined liver and small bowel transplantation, where loss of the graft usually equates with death of the recipient. Most of the mortality after small bowel transplantation is due to sepsis and multiorgan failure. The risk of infection after small bowel transplantation is heightened by the additional requirements for immunosuppression in order to control graft rejection. This accounts for the relatively high incidence of lymphoproliferative disease (around 10 per cent) observed in patients who have undergone small bowel transplantation. Because of the large amount of donor lymphoid tissue transplanted graft-versus-host disease (GVHD) may occasionally be an added complication. Despite the hazards, small bowel transplantation offers patients with intestinal failure a chance to lead an active life free from the constraints of long-term nutritional support.

Thoracic organ transplantation

Heart transplantation

Dr Christiaan Barnard performed the first human heart transplant in Cape Town, South Africa, in 1967. The operation was based on the experimental work of Richard Lower and Norman Shumway in Stanford, and Shumway subsequently went on to pioneer successful cardiac transplantation in the clinic. Heart transplantation is now considered an effective treatment for selected patients with end-stage

Burrill Bernard Crohn, b. 1884. Gastroenterologist, Mount Sinai Hospital, New York, USA.

Christiaan Neethling Barnard. Surgeon, Cape Town, South Africa.
Richard Lower. Surgeon, Richmond, Virginia, USA.
Norman E. Shumway. Professor Emeritus, Stanford University, USA; Surgeon, Stanford University, USA.

cardiac failure. The most common indications for heart transplantation are idiopathic cardiomyopathy and ischaemic heart disease, but other indications include valvular heart disease, myocarditis and congenital heart disease.

Transplantation is considered only in patients with end-stage heart disease which has failed to respond to all other conventional therapy and where predicted survival without transplantation is only 6–12 months. Suitable candidates are New York Heart Association (NYHA) class III (symptoms on mild exertion) or class IV (unable to perform any physical activity without discomfort, which may occur at rest). Transplantation is usually limited to patients under the age of 65 years who do not have irreversible damage to other organ systems. The preoperative assessment is rigorous and measurement of pulmonary vascular resistance is mandatory because when it is raised the perioperative mortality is high.

Technique of heart transplantation

A median sternotomy is performed and the patient is given systemic heparin, placed on cardiopulmonary bypass and cooled to 28°C. After cross-clamping the aorta, the recipient heart is excised at the mid-atrial level. The donor heart is then removed from ice and the left atrium is then opened by making incisions (Fig. 11.21) in the posterior wall between the orifices of the pulmonary veins to create an atrial cuff. The left and then right atrial anastomoses are performed and the aortic and pulmonary arterial anastomoses are then completed (Fig. 11.22). The patient is then re-warmed and weaned from cardiopulmonary bypass. Total orthotopic cardiac transplantation is an alternative but rarely used procedure in which the entire recipient heart is excised and the donor heart is implanted by caval (superior and inferior), pulmonary vein (right and left), aorta and pulmonary arterial anastomosis. Occasionally, heterotopic cardiac transplantation is undertaken where the donor heart is placed adjacent to and augments the recipient's own heart.

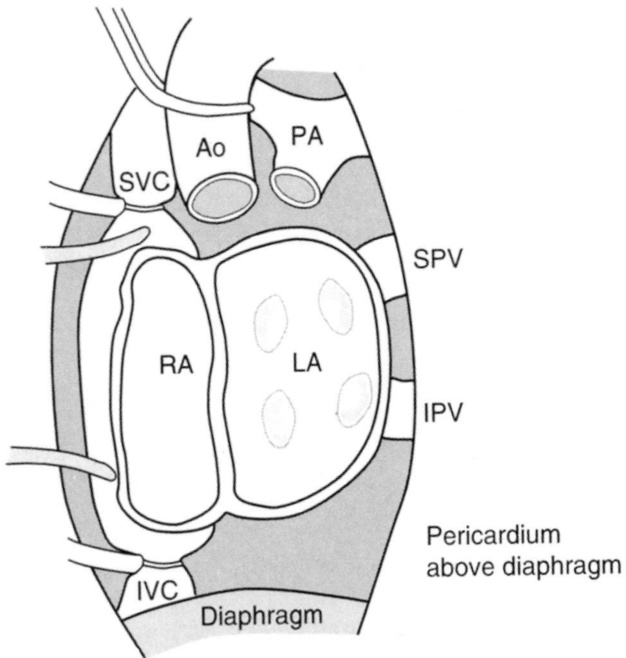

Fig. 11.21 Recipient cardiectomy. After median sternotomy, the recipient is placed on cardiopulmonary bypass. Venous cannulas for bypass are sited in the superior vena cava (SVC) and inferior vena cava (SVC) via punctures in the right atrium, and oxygenated blood is returned via a cannula in the ascending aorta (Ao). The diseased recipient heart is excised leaving behind cuffs of right and left atria. PA, pulmonary artery; IPV, SVP, inferior and superior pulmonary veins; LA, left atrium (*courtesy of J. Dunning*).

Heart–lung, single-lung and double-lung transplantation

Pulmonary transplantation became a clinical reality when Dr Bruce Reitz performed the first successful combined heart–lung transplant in 1981. Combined heart–lung transplantation is still sometimes used, especially for patients with pulmonary vascular disease where there is cardiac dysfunction due to congenital (e.g. Eisenmenger's syndrome) or acquired cardiac dysfunction. For most patients with end-stage pulmonary disease, however, single- or double-lung transplantation has now replaced heart–lung transplantation. Lung transplantation is more economical in terms of organ usage, although if heart–lung transplantation is undertaken for isolated respiratory disease, the healthy native heart can be used for transplantation – the so-called 'domino

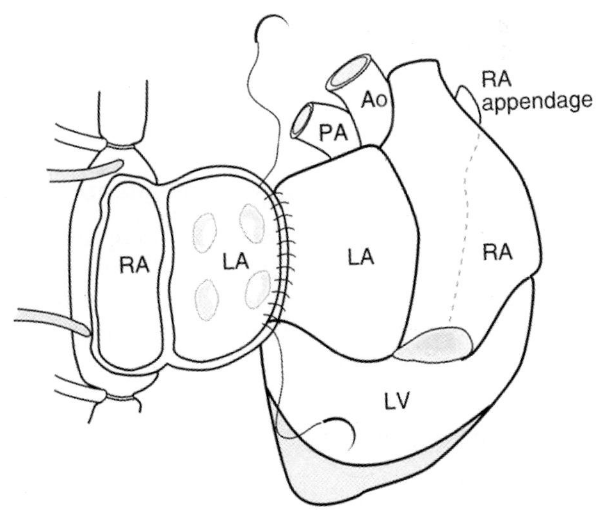

Fig. 11.22 Implantation of the donor heart. The donor left atrium is opened by an incision connecting the four pulmonary veins, excising the central portion. The left atrial anastomosis is performed, starting at the lateral wall of the donor and continuing inferiorly and superiorly, concluding with the interatrial septum. The right atrial anastomosis is performed matching the recipient atrium by an incision towards the donor right atrial appendage (dotted line), which avoids the sinus node at the cavoatrial junction. Finally, the pulmonary artery and aortic anastomoses are completed. Abbreviations as for Fig. 11.21.

Bruce Reitz. Surgeon. Stanford, USA.
Victor Eisenmenger, 1822–1909. German physician.

procedure'. Heart–lung transplantation is performed through a median sternotomy taking particular care to avoid injury of the phrenic and vagus and recurrent laryngeal nerves during excision of the recipient heart and lungs. The recipient right atrium and aorta are divided as for orthotopic cardiac transplantation and the donor heart–lung block is readied for implantation, incising the right atrium from the divided inferior vena cava. An end-to-end tracheal anastomosis is performed, and the right atrial and aortic anastomoses are performed as for cardiac transplantation.

Single- and double-lung transplantation is an effective therapy for selected patients with end-stage chronic lung disease where declining lung function limits life expectancy. Suitable candidates typically have NYHA class III or IV symptoms and a life expectancy of less than 2 years despite optimal medical therapy. Common indications are pulmonary fibrosis, pulmonary hypertension and cystic fibrosis. Single-lung transplantation is performed for pulmonary fibrosis. Patients with cystic fibrosis and other forms of septic lung disease require excision of both native lungs and bilateral or *en bloc* double-lung transplantation, because single-lung transplantation results in soiling of the transplant from the native diseased lung. Single-lung transplantation is performed through a posterolateral thoracotomy, and double-lung transplantation through bilateral thoracotomy or median sternotomy. During lung transplantation the donor pulmonary veins on a left atrial cuff are anastomosed to the recipient left atrium. Next, the bronchial anastomosis and the pulmonary arterial anastomosis are completed. Cardiopulmonary bypass is usually required if pulmonary hypertension is present. Dehiscence of the airway anastomosis used to be common after heart–lung and lung transplantation but improvements in organ preservation and surgical technique have dramatically reduced the incidence of this often fatal complication to < 5 per cent. Late airway stenosis at the bronchial anastomosis due to ischaemia occurs in around 10 per cent of bronchial anastomoses and is treated by dilatation.

Outcome after thoracic organ transplantation

One- and 5-year graft survival after heart transplantation is around 85 and 70 per cent, respectively. The results after heart–lung and lung transplantation are less good with 1-year graft survival rates of around 75 per cent and 5-year survival rates of around 40 per cent.

Future prospects

The two major problems in organ transplantation are:

- chronic graft rejection and the side effects of nonspecific immunosuppression;
- the shortage of organs for transplantation.

A long-standing goal in organ transplantation has been the development of strategies for inducing specific immunological tolerance. Transplantation tolerance would eliminate the need for long-term nonspecific immunosuppressive agents, leaving the immune system intact for defence against infection. It has long been possible to induce transplant tolerance in experimental animals by a variety of preconditioning regimens that often involve antigen pretreatment schedules. So far, however, there is no clinically applicable strategy for inducing transplant tolerance.

The demand for human organs for transplantation is so great that cadaveric donors cannot ever satisfy it. Many consider that the solution is to perfect xenotransplantation, and there is general agreement that the pig is the most suitable source of xenogeneic organs. However, all humans have preformed antibodies directed against carbohydrate antigens expressed by pig organs and these result in hyperacute rejection. The dominant carbohydrate antigen responsible is galα-1,3-gal. Progress has been made towards circumventing hyperacute xenograft rejection, for example by using organs from pigs that have been made transgenic for human complement regulatory proteins. However, such organs are still rejected within a few weeks by primates, despite the use of potent immunosuppressive agents. In addition to the complex immunological problems posed by xenotransplantation, there is a risk that pig organs may transmit infectious agents, and there is particular concern about the risks posed by porcine endogenous retrovirus (PERV). Finally, there are unanswered questions regarding the extent to which pig organs are able to fulfil the physiological demands required of them after transplantation into a human.

Further reading

Busuttil, R.M. and Klintmalm, G.B. (eds) (1996) *Transplantation of the Liver*, W.B. Saunders, Philadelphia, PA.

Collins, G.M., Dubernard, J.M., Land, W. and Persjin, G.G. (eds) (1997) *Procurement, Preservation and Allocation of Vascularised Organs*, Kluwer, Dordrecht.

Klinck, J.R. and Lindop, M.J. (eds) (1998) *Anesthesia and Intensive Care for Organ Transplantation*, Chapman and Hall, London.

Morris, P.J. (ed.) (1994) *Kidney Transplantation: Principles and Practices*, 4th edn, W.B. Saunders, Philadelphia, PA.

Schofield, P.M. and Corris, P.A. (1998) *Management of Heart and Lung Transplantation Patients*, W.B. Saunders, Philadelphia, PA.

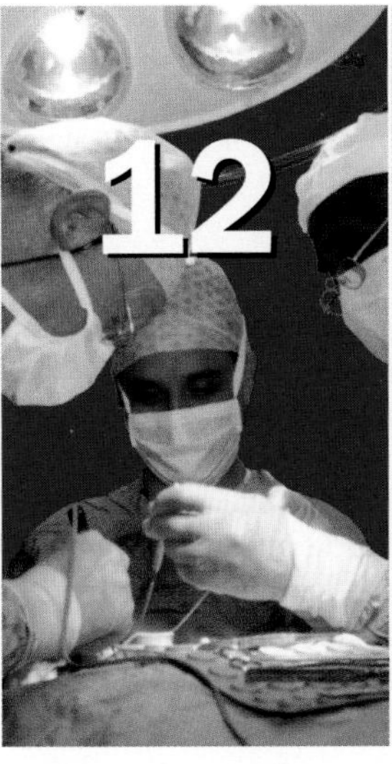

Tumours. Cysts. Ulcers. Sinuses

Tumours

A tumour is a new growth of tissue (a mass) which can refer to an inflammatory swelling such as Pott's puffy tumour (Chapter 35) or to a neoplastic growth. A neoplastic tumour is an uncontrolled proliferation of a clone of cells without useful function.

Causation

Cancer is a disease of genes. The cell is the basic unit of organisation and control. The genetic code is contained within the deoxyribonucleic acid (DNA) molecule present within the cell nucleus. Genes make proteins which govern the function and structure of a cell. There are around 100 000 genes (human genome) representing approximately 10 per cent of the DNA; each cell expresses 5–150 000 genes. Since all genes are present in each cell nucleus, any gene may be expressed if the gene promoter is switched on, as occurs in neoplasia. Cancer is caused by disease of genes which control production of daughter cells from stem cells, cell proliferation, terminal differentiation and programmed cell death (apoptosis); from the Greek – shedding of autumn leaves. There are three important classes of genes involved in cancer:

- tumour suppressor genes, which control the cell cycle by slowing down the cycle or triggering apoptosis (TP53, P16, APC, RB1);
- oncogenes, which promote cell proliferation by increasing signalling activity from the cell surface to the transcription apparatus on gene promoters (KRAS, ERBB2, C-MYC);
- growth factors and their receptors which are switched on by oncogenes or switched off by tumour suppressor genes (EGF, TGFa, IGF, FGF).

Percival Pott, 1914–88. Surgeon, St Bartholomew's Hospital, London, England. Described this fracture-dislocation of the ankle in 1975.

Bailey & Love's Short Practice of Surgery, 23rd edition. Edited by R.C.G. Russell, N.S. Williams and C.J.K. Bulstrode. Published in 2000 by Arnold Publishers.

A benign tumour grows by expansion without invasion of the extracellular matrix. A malignant tumour (cancer) grows by invasion into the extracellular matrix; most solid tumours also invade the basement membrane of endothelium and metastasise. The unit of cancer is the altered malignant cell which proliferates (clone). Different clones usually arise with different characteristics, such as the ability to metastasise via blood vessels or lymphatics. Cancer is a disease of genes which may be inherited or acquired (Table 12.1). Inherited cancers are caused by a specific DNA

Table 12.1 Causes of cancer

Cause	*Examples*
1. Inherited	Familial adenomatous polyposis (FAP), hereditary nonpolyposis colon cancer (HNPCC), familial breast cancer, familial breast–ovarian cancer, familial retinoblastoma, familial atypical multiple mole and melanoma (FAMMM), neurofibromatosis
2. Chemical carcinogenesis	Lung cancer (tobacco-associated nitrosamines), bladder cancer (aromatic amines), mesothelioma (asbestos); other common cancers (carcinogens suspected but not identified)
3. Ultraviolet irradiation	Malignant melanoma, basal cell carcinoma, squamous cell carcinoma
4. Ionising radiation	Thyroid cancer, bone marrow cancer, skin cancers
5. Viruses	Nasopharyngeal cancer, endemic Burkitt's lymphoma, Hodgkin's disease (40 per cent), post-transplant lymphomatous proliferative disease (PTLPD), Kaposi's sarcoma, cervical cancer, adult T-cell leukaemia lymphoma (ATLL), liver cancer
6. Cellular instability and senescence	Marjolin's ulcer, osteosarcoma; other common cancers occurring in older patients

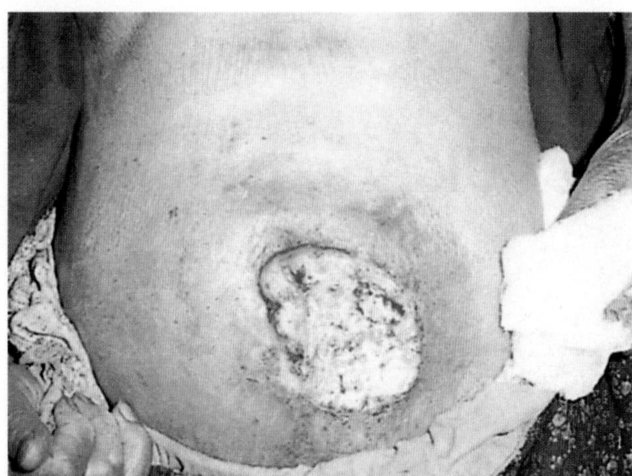

Fig. 12.1 Kangri cancer (*courtesy of Dr Omar J. Shah, Brinagar, Kashmir, India*).

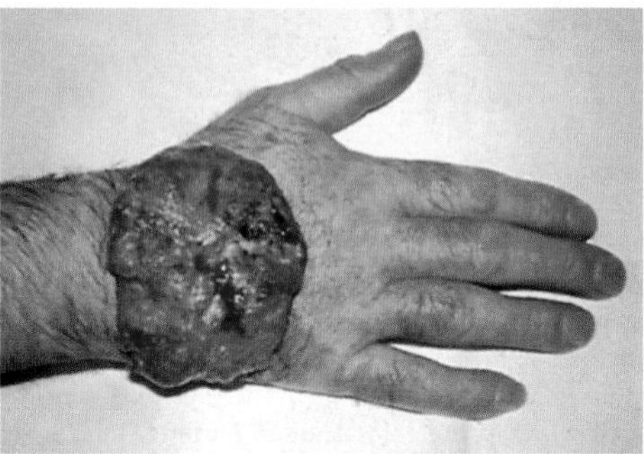

Fig. 12.2 Squamous cell carcinoma on the back of the hand of a tar worker.

mutation of a tumour suppresser gene inherited in all cells. In cells of the organ affected, the (second) homologous gene is lost, initiating a sequence of genetic mutations culminating in cancer. Chemical carcinogens probably account for the majority of sporadic (acquired) cancers. Natives of Kashmir are prone to cancer of the skin of the thighs and lower abdomen. This is due to their habit of keeping warm by squatting and hugging earthenware pots containing glowing charcoal [the pot being termed a *fangri* (Fig. 12.1)], with the result that the adjacent skin is irritated by heat and fumes. 'Chimney-sweep's' cancer' (Chapter 68), 'countryman's lip', and 'tar workers' cancer' (Fig. 12.2) are other examples of carcinoma due to chemical carcinogens. DNA strand breaks are induced by ultraviolet and ionising radiation which, if not repaired, lead to cancer. Cellular instability from ageing of stem cell-lines (many common cancers) or chronic inflammation leads to increased cell proliferation and reduced apoptosis. This results in malignant transformation. Squamous cell carcinoma occasionally occurs in a chronic ulcer (Fig. 12.3) or in a scar (Chapter 13, 'Marjolin's ulcer'). A fibrosarcoma also may arise in a scar. At least 20 per cent of cancers world-wide are caused by oncogenic viruses.

Environmental cofactors are also important. *Helicobacter pylori* is linked to the development of gastric cancer by an unknown mechanism. A diet high in calories and rich in saturated fats (from red meat) is implicated in many cancers including those of the colorectum and pancreas. In viral carcinogenesis there are specific cofactors for different cancers: malaria (Burkitt's lymphoma), immunosuppression (post-transport lymphomatous proliferative disease – PTLPD), human immunodeficiency virus (Kaposi's sarcoma – see Chapter 13), smoking (cervical cancer) and aflatoxins (liver cancer).

Jean Nicolas Marjolin, 1780–1850. Surgeon, Paris, France. Described the develpoment of carcinomatous ulcers in scars in 1828.

Definitions

- Hypertrophy is an increase in the size of an organ without an increase in cell numbers.
- Hyperplasia is an increase in the size of an organ due to an increase in cell numbers.
- Metaplasia. The epithelium from which the tumour grows has already changed its characteristics: bladder transitional epithelium to squamous epithelium, gallbladder columnar to squamous epithelium, bronchial columnar to squamous epithelium, gastric columnar epithelial pattern to intestinal epithelial pattern and oesophageal squamous to columnar epithelium (Barrett's oesophagus).
- Dysplasia. This represents the earliest changes of neoplastic transformation than can be detected at the microstructural level (e.g. by light microscopy). In fact, genetic mutations are detectable at an earlier stage. Alterations in intracellular organisation, the individual size and shape of the nucleus, cellular size and shape and intercellular three-dimensional organisation indicate dysplasia. These changes may be classified as mild, moderate or severe dysplasia. Any grade of dysplasia may revert to normal due to elimination of the neoplastic clone, but is least likely with severe dysplasia.

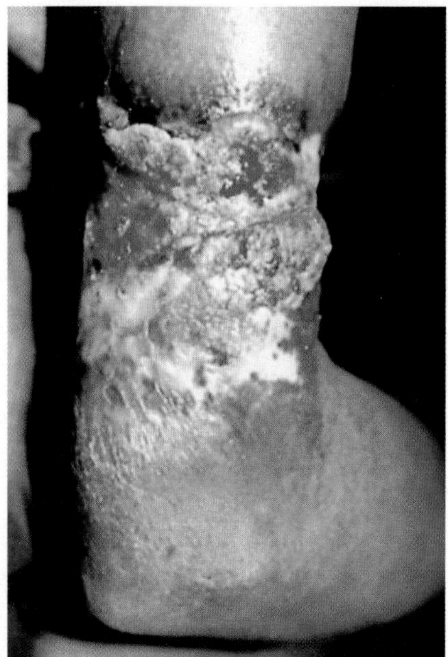

Fig. 12.3 Squamous cell carcinoma in a varicose ulcer (Marjolin's ulcer).

Denis P. Burkitt, b. 1911. Ugandan physician.
Moritz K. Kaposi, 1837–1902. Dermatologist, Vienna, Austria.
Norman Barrett, 1903–79. Surgeon, St Thomas's Hospital, London, England.

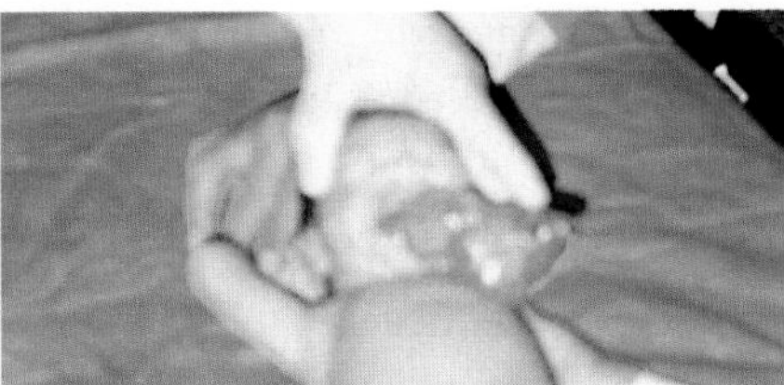

Fig. 12.4 An 8-cm teratomatous tumour arising in the buccal cavity of a neonate: the tumour contained cartilage and muscle (mesoderm), neural elements (ectoderm) and epithelium resembling gut (endoderm). The tumour was removed successfully (*courtesy of Drs D. Pratap and R. Saha, Department of Surgery, M.L.B Medical College, Jhans, India*).

- Carcinoma *in situ*. Severe dysplasia may progress to carcinoma *in situ*: the cellular, nuclear and three-dimensional architecture resemble cancer but without invasion into the extracellular matrix.
- Genotype. This is the molecular structure of any cell. A malignant genotype will have losses and mutations of tumour suppresser genes and the presence of oncogenes.
- Phenotype. This is the appearance of a cell at a microstructural level (microscopic phenotype) and its functional state (biological phenotype). A changed genotype will always precede a particular phenotype: for a time the cell may appear to be normal even though it has already acquired a malignant genotype.

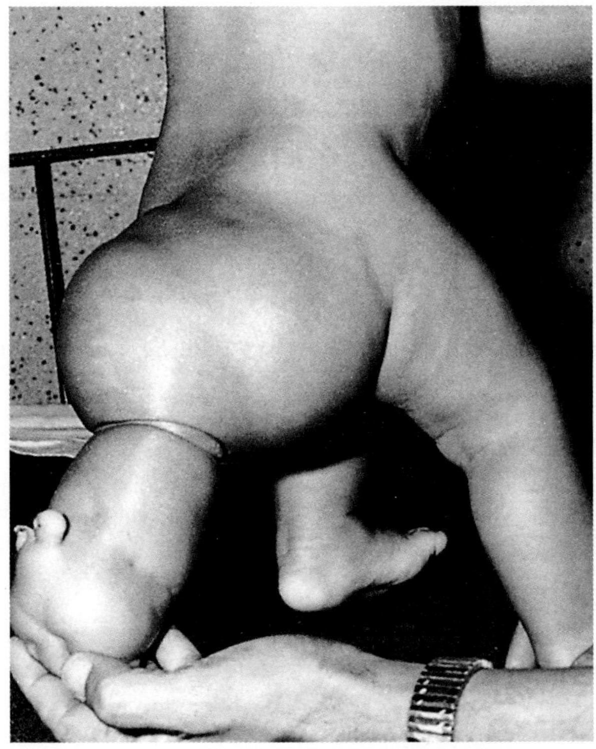

Fig. 12.5 This sacrococcygeal teratoma had taken the shape of a leg (a third leg!). It had rudimentary toes and nails. It was successfully operated on [*courtesy of A.C. Bose, MS, FACS, Senior Consultant (Surgery) Armed Forces, India*].

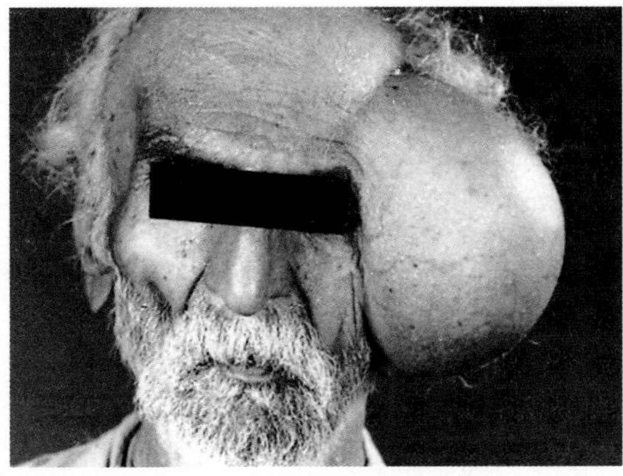

Fig. 12.6 Typical external angular dermoid cyst (very large).

- Differentiation. Depending on the degree to which the cells and organisation (morphology) of tumours resemble the parent tissue they are divided into well-differentiated, moderately differentiated and poorly differentiated forms.
- Anaplasia. Tumours are usually composed of cells which resemble those of the tissue from which they arise. Complete loss of differentiation (anaplasia) is associated with an aggressive cancer.
- Teratomas arise from embryonic stem cells containing representative cells from all three embryonic layers: ectoderm, endoderm, mesoderm (Fig. 12.4). Teratomatous dermoids contain hair and teeth, muscle and gland tissue. An unusual type is the sacrococcygeal teratoma (Fig. 12.5), which can be considered as *foetus in foeto* (an 'included' foetus).
- Blastomas develop from 'unipotent' cells, and arise from any one of the three embryonic layers (e.g. neuroblastoma).
- Dermoid cysts. 'Dermoid' is a loose term given to cysts lined by squamous epithelium occurring in various parts of the body. Sebaceous cysts are lined by superficial squamous cells and should more accurately be called 'epidermoid'.
  - *Teratomatous dermoids* (see above) are found in the ovary, testis retroperitoneum, superior mediastinum and the presacral area. Malignant change (carcinomatous or sarcomatous) can occur.
  - *Sequestration dermoids* (see Cysts, below) are not new growths, but are formed by the inclusion of epithelial 'nests' beneath the surface at places where lines of developing skin meet and join: midline, external angular process (Fig. 12.6), root of nose (Chapter 37), branchial cysts (Chapter 43).
  - *Implantation dermoids* (see Cysts, below) may follow puncture wounds, commonly of the fingers, when living epithelial cells are implanted beneath the surface.
- Benign tumour. A benign tumour is usually encapsulated, and does not disseminate or recur after complete removal. Symptoms and effects, which can be harmful, are due to its size, position, and pressure. Certain adenomas secrete a

hormone which may affect bodily functions. Benign tumours are often multiple.

- Malignant tumour. The characteristics of malignancy are:
  - invasion of surrounding tissues;
  - pleomorphism (variable shapes) of cells and nuclei;
  - rapid growth;
  - the tendency to spread to other parts of the body (metastasis) by the lymphatics, the bloodstream, along nerve sheaths and across body cavities;
  - general weight loss (cachexia in advanced disease).

At an early stage, evidence of invasion is the most important sign of malignancy. Many cells of a malignant tumour have an abnormal number of chromosomes which is not a multiple of the usual haploid number (= 'aneuploidy').

It has been suggested that the division of tumours into these two major groups imposes a concept which is too rigid (Walter). A third group of intermediate tumours exists which includes some carcinoid tumours, adenoma of the bronchus, 'mixed' salivary tumours and basal-cell carcinoma. These intermediate types invade locally, but are much less inclined to lymphatic or especially vascular dissemination.

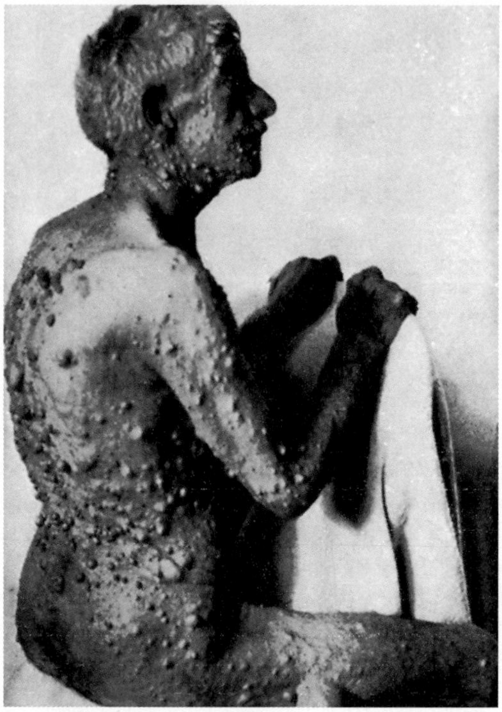

Fig. 12.7 Neurofibromatosis.

Benign tumours

Adenoma

Adenomas arise in secretory glands, and resemble the structure from which they arise. They are encapsulated, and sometimes they secrete hormones which profoundly influence metabolism, as in the case of the thyroid, parathyroid and pancreas. Occasionally an adenoma contains a large proportion of fibrous tissue, e.g. the hard fibro-adenoma in the breast, while in other situations, notably the pancreas and thyroid gland, cystic degeneration is common. Those arising from superficial glands of mucous membrane are liable to pedunculation, as in the case of a rectal 'polyp'.

Papilloma

A papilloma consists of a central axis of connective tissue, blood vessels and lymphatics; the surface is covered by epithelium, either squamous, transitional, cuboidal or columnar, according to the site of the tumour. The surface may be merely roughened, or composed of innumerable delicate villous processes, as in the case of those occurring in the kidney, bladder and rectum. In these situations, papillomas resemble malignant tumours, as secondary growths arise by implantation and, sooner or later, the tumour becomes frankly malignant (Chapter 65). Other common sites for papillomas are the skin, the colon, the tongue and lip, the vocal cords and the walls of cysts (particularly those in the breast and ovary).

Friedrich Daniel von Recklinghausen, 1833–1910. Professor of Pathology, Strasbourg, France (1872–1906). Described generalised neurofibromatosis in 1882.

John B. Walter. Associate Professor of Pathology, University of Toronto, Toronto, Ontario, Canada.

Fibroma

A true fibroma (containing only fibrous connective tissue) is rare. Most fibromas are combined with other mesodermal tissues such as muscle (fibromyoma), fat (fibrolipoma) and nerve sheaths (neurofibroma). Multiple tumours are not uncommon as, for example, in neurofibromatosis (von Recklinghausen's disease, Fig. 12.7).

Fibromas are either *hard* or *soft*, depending on the proportion of fibrous to the other cellular tissue. Soft fibromas are common in the subcutaneous tissue of the face, and appear as soft, brown swellings.

Desmoid

This unusual type of fibroma occurs in the abdominal wall (see Chapter 62). An intraperitoneal form is associated with familial adenomatous polyposis (see Chapter 57).

Keloid

This overgrowth of fibrous tissue commonly occurs in scars, especially of black people.

Lipoma

A lipoma is a slowly growing tumour composed of fat cells of adult type. Lipomas may be encapsulated or diffuse. They occur anywhere in the body where fat is found and earn the

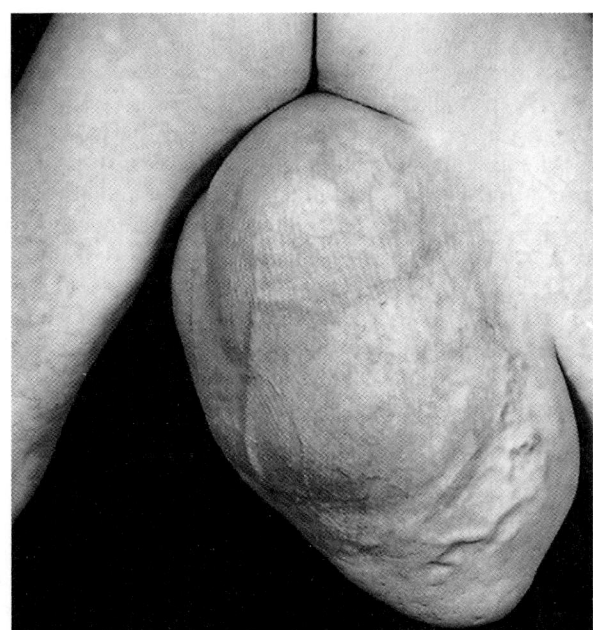

Fig. 12.8 Giant lipoma of the thigh.

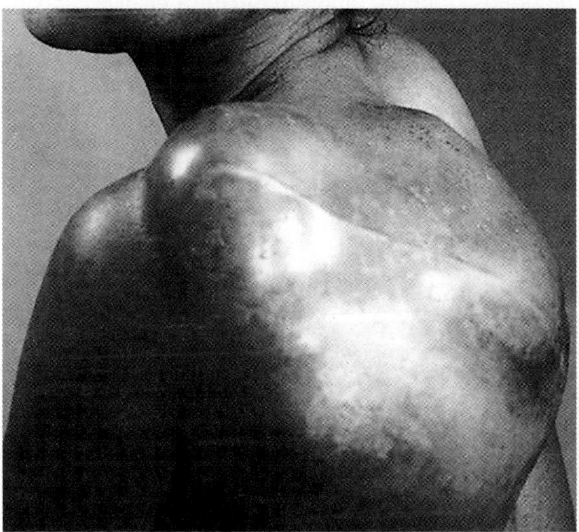

Fig. 12.9 Liposarcoma. Note incision of previous operation (*courtesy of Dr R.S. Naik, Durg, India*).

titles of the 'universal tumour' or the 'ubiquitous tumour'. The head and neck area, abdominal wall and thighs are particularly favoured sites.

Encapsulated lipomas are among the commonest of tumours. The characteristic features are the presence of a definite edge and lobulation. A sense of fluctuation may be obtained. As would be expected, a lipoma deeply situated is liable to be mistaken for other swellings. Most lipomas are painless, but some give rise to an aching sensation which may radiate.

Multiple lipomas are not uncommon. The tumours remain small or moderate in size, and are sometimes painful, in which case the condition is probably one of *neurolipomatosis. Dercum's disease (adiposis dolorosa),* characterised by tender deposits of fat, especially on the trunk, is an associated condition.

Should the lipoma contain an excessive amount of fibrous tissue, it is termed a *fibrolipoma.* In other cases, considerable vascularity is present, often with telangiectasis of the overlying skin, in which case the tumour is a *naevolipoma.* Large lipomas of the thigh (Fig. 12.8), the shoulder (Fig. 12.9) and the retroperitoneum occasionally undergo *sarcomatous* changes. *Myxomatous degeneration, saponification* and *calcification* sometimes occur in lipomas of long duration.

Clinically, circumscribed lipomas are classified according to their situation.

- *Subcutaneous.* Commonly found on the shoulders or the back, although no part of the body is immune. A lipoma may be present over the site of a spina bifida. Subcutaneous lipomas occasionally become pedunculated (lipoma arborescens).
- *Subfascial.* Occurring under the palmar or plantar fascia, they are liable to be mistaken for tuberculous tenosynovitis, as the tough, overlying fascia masks the definite edge and lobulation of the tumour. Difficulty is encountered in complete removal as pressure encourages the tumour to ramify. Subfascial lipomas also occur in the areolar layer under the epicranial aponeurosis and, if of long duration, they erode the underlying bone, so that a depression is palpable on pushing the tumour to one side.
- *Subsynovial.* From the fatty padding around joints, especially the knee. In the knee, they are apt to be mistaken for Baker's cysts but are easily distinguished as, in distinction to a cyst or bursa, their consistency is constant whether the joint is in extension or flexion.
- *Intra-articular.*
- *Intermuscular.* Mainly in the thigh or around the shoulder. Owing to transmitted pressure, the tumour becomes firmer when the adjacent muscles are contracted. Weakness or aching results, owing to mechanical interference with muscular action. The condition is often difficult to distinguish from a fibrosarcoma.
- *Parosteal* occasionally occur under the periosteum of a bone.
- *Subserous* are sometimes found beneath the pleura, where they constitute one variety of innocent thoracic tumour. A retroperitoneal lipoma may grow to enormous dimensions, and simulate a hydronephrosis or pancreatic cyst.
- *Submucous* occur under the mucous membrane of the respiratory or alimentary tracts. Rarely a submucous lipoma in the larynx causes respiratory obstruction. A submucous lipoma can occur in the tongue. One situated in the intestine is likely to cause an intussusception, which may be the first indication of its presence.
- *Central nervous system.* Lipomas may occur anywhere within the extradural spaces, the spinal cord and brain; they usually arise from the pia mater, within the central subarachnoid spaces (especially the quadrigeminal cisterns); a lipoma of the corpus callosum may be accompanied by calcification on the convex margins.
- *Intraglandular.* Lipomas have been found occasionally in the pancreas, under the renal capsule and in the breast (Chapter 46).
- *Retroperitoneal.* Large lipomas are seen not infrequently in the retroperitoneal tissues. Some of them turn out to be liposarcomas.

William Baker, 1839–96. British surgeon.
Francis Xavier Dercum, 1856–1931. Neurologist, Jefferson Medical College, Philadelphia, Pennsylvania, USA. Described adiposis dolorosa in 1888.

Treatment

If a lipoma is causing trouble on account of its site, size, appearance or the presence of pain, removal is indicated.

During operation, any finger-like projections of the tumour into the surrounding tissue should also be removed. Although the tumour is relatively avascular, care is needed to obtain complete haemostasis in the resulting cavity otherwise a haematoma is common, which may be followed by infection and delay in wound healing; drainage is often necessary.

Diffuse lipoma occasionally occurs in the subcutaneous tissue of the neck, from which it spreads on to the preauricular region of the face. The tumour is not obviously encapsulated, and gives rise to no trouble, beyond being unsightly.

Neuroma

True neuromas are rare tumours, and occur in connection with the sympathetic system. They comprise the following types:

- *Ganglioneuroma,* which consist of ganglion cells and nerve fibres. It arises in connection with the sympathetic ganglia, and therefore is found in the retroperitoneal tissue, or in the neck or thorax.
- *Neuroblastoma,* which is less differentiated than the ganglioneuroma, the cells being of an embryonic type. The tumour somewhat resembles a round-celled sarcoma, and disseminates by the bloodstream. It occurs in infants and young children. It may occasionally undergo spontaneous remission.
- *Myelinic neuroma* is very rare, being composed only of nerve fibres, as the ganglion cells are absent. They arise in connection with the spinal cord or pia mater.

Neurilemmoma (syn. Schwannoma)

These lobulated and encapsulated tumours arise from the neurilemmal cells. They are soft and whitish in appearance. They displace the nerve from which they arise and can be removed (Fig. 12.10).

Neurofibroma

Neurofibroma arise from the connective tissue of the nerve sheath. The following varieties are described.

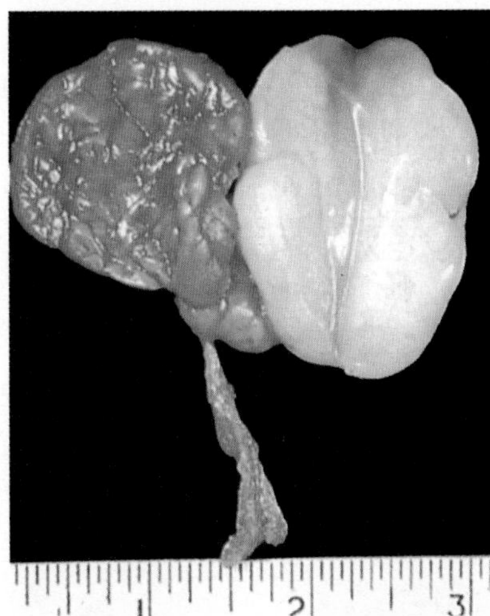

Fig. 12.10 Neurilemmoma of the lingual nerve attached to submandibular salivary gland.

Theodor Schwann, 1810–82. Professor of Anatomy, Louvain and Liège, Belgium.

Local

A single neurofibroma is usually found in the subcutaneous tissue. The 'painful subcutaneous nodule' forms a smooth firm swelling which may be moved in a lateral direction, but is otherwise fixed by the nerve from which it arises. Paraesthesia or pain is likely to occur from the pressure of the tumour on the nerve fibres which are spread over its surface. Cystic degeneration or sarcomatous changes occur occasionally.

Neurofibromas may also grow from the sheath of a peripheral nerve or a cranial nerve, e.g. the acoustic tumour (Chapter 35). As the nerve fibres are 'part and parcel' of the tumour they are difficult to remove without removal of the nerve itself. In major nerves recurrence is a problem, as is malignant (sarcomatous) change.

Generalised neurofibromatosis (syn. von Rechlinghausen's disease of nerves)

In this inherited (autosomal-dominant) disease, any cranial, spinal or peripheral nerve may be diffusely or modularly thickened (Fig. 12.7). The overgrowth occurs in connection with the endoneurium. Associated pigmentation *(café au lait)* of the skin is common, and sarcomatous changes may occur.

Plexiform neurofibromatosis

This rare condition usually occurs in connection with branches of the fifth cranial nerve (Fig. 12.11), although it may occur in the extremities (Fig. 12.12). The affected nerves become enormously thickened as a result of myxofibromatous degeneration of the endoneurium.

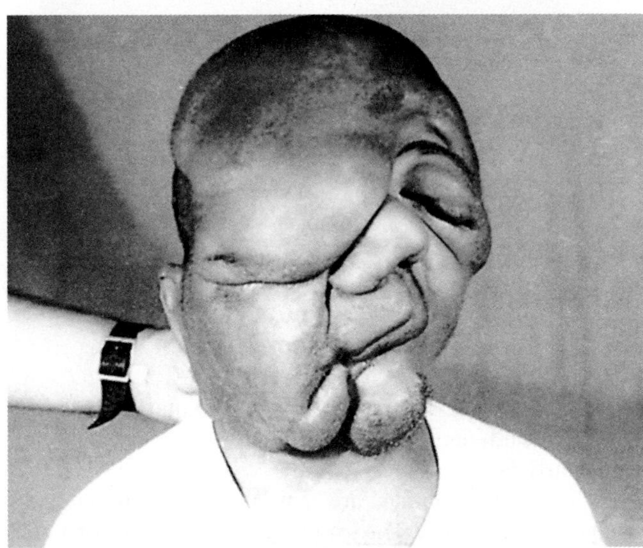

Fig. 12.11 Plexiform neurofibromatosis of the fifth cranial nerve. If occurring in the scalp, the underlying skull may be eroded, and in other situations the involved skin sometimes hangs down in pendulous folds with grotesque effects (cf. Treves' Elephant Man) (*courtesy of Dr P. Nayak, MS, Bombay, India*).

Sir Frederick Treves, 1853–1923. Surgeon, The London Hospital, London, England.

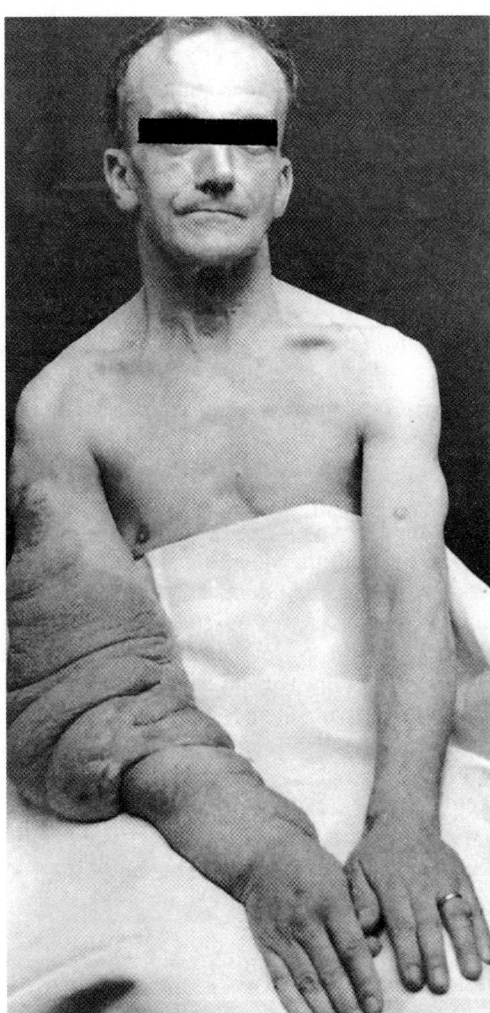

Fig. 12.12 Plexiform neurofibromatosis affecting the right arm.

Elephantiasis neuromatosa

Elephantiasis neuromatosa is a rare variant congenital condition. The skin is coarse, dry and thickened, resembling an elephant's hide, and the subcutaneous tissues become greatly thickened. If a leg is affected, the patient finds walking increasingly difficult. A famous patient of the London Hospital with this condition (the 'Elephant Man') was befriended by his surgeon, Sir Frederick Treves (see also Figs 12.11 and 12.12).

False neuroma

Arises from the connective tissue of the nerve sheath after injury to a nerve (lacerations or amputation). These swellings consist of fibrous tissue and coiled nerve fibres.

Haemangiomas

Haemangiomas are described in Chapter 13. They are represented in various forms, capillary, cavernous and plexiform being common.

Philip Michael Peters, 1916–77. Pathologist, Royal Northern Hospital, London, England.

Glomangioma (syn. glomus tumour)

These tumours arise from a cutaneous glomus composed of a tortuous arteriole which communicates directly with a venule, the vessels being surrounded with a network of small nerves. These specialised organs regulate the temperature of the skin, and are found in the limbs, especially the nail beds. The tumour is compressible. The associated pain is out of all proportion to the size of the tumour, which may be only a few millimetres in diameter. The pain is burning in nature and radiates peripherally, and is more often noticeable when the limb is exposed to sudden changes in temperature.

On section the tumour consists of a mixture of blood spaces, nerve tissue and muscle fibres derived from the wall of the arteriole (angiomyoneuroma). Large cuboidal cells are frequently seen (glomal cells). Cutaneous glomus tumours grow very slowly, and do not become malignant. They should be excised.

Hamartoma

The term hamartoma is roughly translated from the Greek as a 'fault', and its original meaning was 'missing the mark in spear throwing'. It is a developmental malformation consisting of overgrowth of tissue or tissues proper to the part. The possible range therefore is very wide and the lesions are often multiple. Common lesions that are hamartomas are benign pigmented moles, and the majority of angiomas and neurofibromas. On rare occasions a malignant change occurs in a hamartoma, but for practical purposes the lesion is benign (Peters).

Malignant tumours

Carcinomas arise from cells which are ectodermal or endodermal in origin, and they are classified squamous, basal-celled or glandular (adenocarcinomas). Sarcomas occur in connection with structures of mesoblastic origin, hence fibrosarcoma, osteosarcoma. Germ cell tumours arise from germ cells (teratoma, seminoma, thecoma). Ovarian cancer is an adenocarcinoma: it does not arise from oocytes.

Carcinoma

Squamous cancer arises from surfaces covered by squamous epithelium, particularly as a result of ultraviolet or ionising radiation and chronic irritation. Chronic irritation of transitional cells (e.g. by a stone in the renal pelvis) or columnar cells (e.g. the gall bladder) will cause a change in these cells to a squamous type (*squamous metaplasia*), which may lead on to carcinoma. The regional lymph nodes are likely to be invaded, and may also be infected from the sepsis attendant upon the primary growth. Blood-borne metastases occur, but uncommonly from skin squamous cell carcinoma.

Macroscopically, squamous cell carcinomas are either proliferative or ulcerative. On section solid masses of polyhedral cells are seen, which invade the deeper structures. 'Cell-nests' are usually apparent in slowly growing cases, and are due to deeper cells becoming flattened and undergoing keratinisation. 'Prickle' (acanthotic) cells are characteristic, and resemble those present in the epidermis.

Basal-celled (syn. rodent ulcer)

See Chapter 36.

Glandular

Glandular carcinoma commonly occurs in the alimentary tract, breast and uterus, and less frequently in the kidney, prostate, gall bladder and thyroid. Three types of glandular carcinoma may be recognised:

- *carcinoma simplex,* in which the cells are arranged in circumscribed groups, no glandular structure being recognisable. This type commonly occurs in the breast, and the majority of cells are spheroidal or polygonal in shape;
- *adenocarcinoma,* so called from the tendency of the cells to form acini, which resemble those of the gland from which they are derived. The alveoli are ductless, and the walls are composed of layers of cells which invade the surrounding tissues. The cells of the primary growth, and even of the metastases, sometimes retain secretory powers; bronchial adenocarcinomas are well known for this;
- *colloid* (mucoid) is a degenerative process which develops in tumours arising from mucin-secreting cells. The mucin permeates the stroma of the growth, which appears as a gelatinous mass and is typically seen in the colon and stomach.

Glandular carcinoma is also subdivided into various types, e.g. encephaloid (soft), scirrhous (hard) and atrophic scirrhous (stony-hard). These distinctions depend clinically on their rate of growth, and pathologically on the relative proportions of fibrous tissue and gland elements. Examples occur in the breast (Chapter 46). All these glandular types of cancer are best regarded as adenocarcinomas.

Methods of spread

Direct spread (local extension). Invasion takes place readily along connective tissue planes, but no structures are resistant. Veins are invaded commonly. Arteries are rarely invaded. Muscle is less susceptible to invasion or metastatic deposits than other tissues. Fascia also limits direct extension, e.g. Denonvillier's fascia for rectal carcinoma.

Lymphatics by invasion and by embolism.

- *Invasion.* The malignant cells grow along the lymphatic vessels from the primary growth (permeation). This may even occur in a retrograde direction. The cancer cells stimulate perilymphatic fibrosis, but this does not stop the advance of the disease. In some instances, notably malignant melanoma (Chapter 13), groups of cells may so overcome the surrounding fibrosis that they give rise to intermediate deposits between the primary growth and the lymph nodes.
- *Embolism.* Cancer cells which invade a lymphatic vessel can break away and are carried by the lymph circulation to a regional node, so that nodes comparatively distant from the tumour may be involved in the early stages.

Blood stream. Cancer cells may be detected in the venous blood draining an organ involved in carcinoma. A carcinoma of the kidney may invade the renal vein and grow inside the lumen into the vena cava. Malignant emboli may be arrested in the lungs, liver and bone marrow (secondary deposits – metastases). Thyroid, breast and bronchial cancers also commonly disseminate via the blood stream.

Implantation. Implantation of carcinoma has been observed in situations where skin or mucous membrane is in close contact with a primary growth. Examples of this *'kiss cancer'* are carcinoma of the lower lip affecting the upper, and carcinoma of the labium majus giving rise to a similar growth on the opposite side of the vulva. Recurrence after operation is occasionally due to *implantation* of malignant cells in the wound. Examples of this mischance are the appearance of a malignant deposit in the scar after suprapubic removal of a primary carcinoma of the bladder, and nodules of carcinoma in the scar of the incision after mastectomy for a carcinoma of the breast. When a cavity is involved, free-floating cells from a carcinoma may spread like snowflakes all over its serous surface. For the abdomen, *transcoelomic spread* is specially notable when cells from a colloid carcinoma of the stomach gravitate on to an active ovary and give rise to malignant ovarian tumours (Krukenberg's tumour, Chapter 51); intracavitary dissemination can also take place within the pleura and cerebrospinal spaces.

Nerve sheaths. Adenocarcinomas, especially pancreas, may disseminate along nerve sheaths.

Grading and staging

Grading and staging are used to assess the degree of malignancy of the tumour as an indication of the prognosis, and may be used as a guide to determine the type and the extent of the treatment which is required. Advanced staging and grading may indicate the need for adjuvant methods of treatment, e.g. by chemotherapy or irradiation.

Grading. Grading predicts the aggressiveness of a malignant neoplasm by characterising its microscopic appearance taking into account the degree of differentiation, nuclear and cellular appearance, architectural integrity and the proportion of active mitoses.

- Grade 1: well differentiated;
- Grade 2: moderately well differentiated;
- Grade 3: poorly differentiated.

Staging. (i) TNM classification. This has been adopted by the International Union against Cancer (UICC) and has been extended to many sites of cancer. This is a detailed clinical staging which is arrived at simply by the clinician ascertaining the following points. What is the

Charles Denonvillier, 1808–72. Parisian surgeon.

Friedrich Ernst Krukenberg, 1870–1946. Ophthalmologist, Halle, Germany Wrote a classic paper on malignant tumours of the ovary in 1896.

extent of the primary Tumour? Are any lymph Nodes affected? Are there any Metastases? The information so obtained is scored, e.g. in carcinoma of the breast, as follows:

Tumour	*Nodes*	*Metastasis*
T_1 2 cm or less. No skin fixation	N_0 No nodes	M_0 No metastasis
T_2 More than 2 cm, but less than 5 cm. Skin tethered or dimpled. No pectoral fixation	N_1 Axillary nodes movable (a) not significant, (b) significant	M_1 Metastases are present including involvement of skin beyond breast, and contralateral nodes
T_3 More than 5 cm, but less than 10 cm. Skin infiltrated or ulcerated. Pectoral fixation	N_2 Axillary nodes fixed	
T_4 More than 10 cm. Skin involved but not beyond breast. Chest-wall fixation	N_3 Supraclavicular nodes. Oedema of arm	

(i) Thus, for example, one patient may have an early carcinoma which is $T_1N_0M_0$, while in another late case the extent of the disease may be $T_2N_2M_1$.
(ii) **Manchester staging**. This is a method of staging clinical spread of carcinoma of the breast (see Chapter 46).
(iii) **Dukes' staging**. This is a method of classifying the spread of carcinoma of the rectum and colon and is described in Chapter 60.

Sarcomas

Sarcomas differ from carcinomas, not only in their derivation, but in their earlier age incidence, as they are most common during the first and second decades. Sarcomas often grow rapidly and dissemination occurs early via the bloodstream (e.g. 'cannon-ball' secondary deposits in the lung from an osteogenic sarcoma).

The macroscopic appearance of a sarcoma varies considerably. As the word implies, most tumours appear as a fleshy mass, but their consistency depends on the relative proportion of fibrous and vascular tissue. Haemorrhage commonly occurs owing to the very thin walls of the veins, which in some places are represented merely by venous spaces.

Sarcomatous cells may reproduce tissue similar to that from which the tumour originated, e.g. osteosarcoma or chondrosarcoma. Sometimes a sarcoma develops in pre-existing benign tumours, such as fibroma or a uterine fibroid, and also in bones which are affected by osteitis deformans (Chapter 26).

Fibrosarcoma

Fibrosarcoma is composed of spindle cells of varying lengths (the rounder they are the more malignant they are), and occurs in muscle sheaths, scars and as a fibrous epulis. A fibrosarcoma of a muscle sheath presents as an elastic or firm and slowly growing swelling. Dilated veins over the tumour suggest malignancy, and if not obvious they may be demonstrated by infrared photography. On palpation the tumour often feels warm and pulsation may even be detected. Fibrosarcomas not uncommonly arise in scar tissue, sometimes many years after the scar developed. Sir James Paget described this as a 'recurrent fibroid'.

Treatment of sarcoma

The spread of a fibrosarcoma is hastened by incomplete removal. *The moral is that wide excision with surrounding healthy tissues should be practised in all cases.* This may mean amputation in the case of a limb. If untreated or if wide local excision is unsuccessful, a fibrosarcoma eventually fungates through the skin. Metastases are widely scattered and, unfortunately, radiotherapy has but little effect on either the primary growth or the secondary deposits. Sarcomas are often susceptible to anticancer drugs, but fibrosarcomas are more resistant than other types. Sarcoma of bone is sensitive to radiotherapy, which is used in some cases as an alternative to amputation (Chapter 25).

Lymphomas

Lymphomas arise in lymph nodes, tonsils, Peyer's patches or lymph nodules in the intestines. Lymph nodes of the neck or mediastinum are most commonly affected (Chapter 17). They have a bad prognosis.

Synovioma

This rather uncommon tumour may arise in any synovial joint or tendon sheath, especially those of the hand. It appears as a soft, painless swelling, and sarcomatous changes can occur. The diagnosis can only be established by excision and biopsy of the tumour.

Naevus and melanoma

Naevus and melanoma are described in Chapter 13.

Endothelioma; mesothelioma

The endothelial linings of blood vessels, lymphatic spaces and serous membranes occasionally give rise to neoplasms. They can be malignant. They arise from the pleura (Chapter 47) and rarely from the pericardium or peritoneum. Asbestos inhalation may provoke their development. 'Blue' asbestos fibres especially have been shown to be a cause. The original cells are flattened, but they become spheroidal or cuboidal when neoplastic changes occur. The 'endothelioma' (meningioma) of the dura mater is thought to arise from the arachnoid membrane, which is *not* an endothelial structure (Chapter 35).

Peritheliomas

Peritheliomas are tumours arising in the endothelial lining of small blood vessels or lymphatics. Carotid body tumours are probably of this nature (Chapter 43).

Sir James Paget, 1814–99. Surgeon, St Bartholomew's Hospital, London, England.
Johann Conrad Peyer, 1653–1712. Swiss anatomist.
Cuthbert Esquire Dukes, 1890–1977. Consulting pathologist, St Mark's Hospital, London, England.

Benign to malignant transformation

Certain benign neoplasms are prone to undergo malignant changes, and it is important, for both treatment and prognosis, to realise when this occurs. Some or all of the following changes may be recognised:

- **increase in size:** comparatively rapid enlargement is always suspicious, e.g. a neurofibroma which is becoming sarcomatous;
- **increased vascularity:** dilated cutaneous veins, ulceration and bleeding in the case of a superficial growth (e.g. melanoma);
- **fixity:** due to invasion of surrounding structures;
- **involvement of adjacent structures:** e.g. facial palsy suggests malignant change in an otherwise longstanding parotid pleomorphic adenoma;
- **dissemination:** discovery of secondary deposits.

Cysts

The word cyst is derived from the Greek word meaning 'bladder'. The pathological term 'cyst' means a swelling consisting of a collection of fluid in a sac which is lined by epithelium or endothelium.

True cysts

True cysts are lined by epithelium or endothelium. If infection supervenes, the true lining may be destroyed and replaced by granulation tissue. The fluid is usually serous or mucoid and varies from brown-staining by altered blood to almost colourless. In epidermoid, dermoid and branchial cysts the contents are like porridge or toothpaste, as a result of the shedding of desquamated cells. Cholesterol crystals are often found in the fluid of branchial cysts.

False cysts (pseudocysts)

Walled-off collections of fluid not lined by epithelium are not regarded as true cysts. A pseudocyst of the pancreas is an encysted collection of pancreatic enzyme-rich fluid lined by granulation tissue or fibrous tissue. Pancreatic pseudocysts are often in the retroperitoneum deep to but bulging into the lesser sac; they may occur anywhere in the abdominal cavity and even track into the mediastinum and pleural cavities. In tuberculous peritonitis, fluid may be walled off in cystic form by adherent coils of intestine. Fluid may collect in the centre of a tumour (cystic degeneration), due to haemorrhage or necrosis. This can also happen in the brain as a result of ischaemia, and an 'apoplectic cyst' is formed. In acute pancreatitis fluid collections loculated by viscera and fibrin are called 'acute fluid collections'; these often occur in the lesser sac but are neither cysts nor pseudocysts as they are not lined by either epithelium, granulation tissue or fibrous tissue.

A classification of cysts

Congenital	Sequestration dermoids
	Tubuloembryonic (tubulodermoid)
	Cyst of embryonic remnants
Acquired	Retention
	Distention
	Exudation
	Cystic tumours
	Implantation dermoids
	Trauma
	Degeneration
Parasitic	Hydatid, trichniasis, cysticercosis

Congenital cysts

The sequestration dermoid is due to dermal cells being buried along the lines of closure of embryonic clefts and sinuses by skin fusion. The cyst therefore is lined by epidermis and contains paste-like desquamated material. The usual sites are:

- the midline of the body – especially in the neck;
- above the outer canthus (external angular dermoid, Chapter 35);
- in the anterior triangle of the neck (branchial cyst, Chapter 43).

Tubuloembryonic (tubulodermoid) cysts occur in the track of an ectodermal tube used in development, e.g. a thyroglossal cyst from the thyroglossal duct or a postanal dermoid from the postanal gut. In the brain, ependymal cysts arise from the sequestration of cells of the enfolding neurectoderm.

Cysts of embryonic remnants. These arise from embryonic tubules and ducts which normally disappear or are only present as remnants. They should not be confused with teratomatous cysts, e.g. dermoid. There are many examples in the urogenital system, e.g. in the male from remnants of the paramesonephric duct (Müllerian) – the hydatid of Morgagni, or from the mesonephric body and duct (Wolffian) (Chapter 64). Cysts of the urachus and the vitellointestinal duct are other examples of cysts of embryonic remnants (Chapter 65).

Acquired cysts

Retention cysts are due to the accumulated secretion of a gland behind an obstruction of a duct. Examples are seen in the pancreas, the parotid, the breast, the epididymis and Bartholin's gland. A sebaceous cyst starts with the obstruc-

Johannes Peter Müller, 1801–58. Professor of Anatomy and Physiology, Berlin, Germany.
Giovanni Battista Morgagni, 1682–1771. Professor of Anatomy, Padua, Italy.
Faspar Friedrich Wolff, 1733–94. Professor of Anatomy and Physiology, St Petersburg, Russia.
Caspar Bartholin, Secundus, 1655–1738. Professor of Medicine, Anatomy, and Physics, Copenhagen, Denmark.

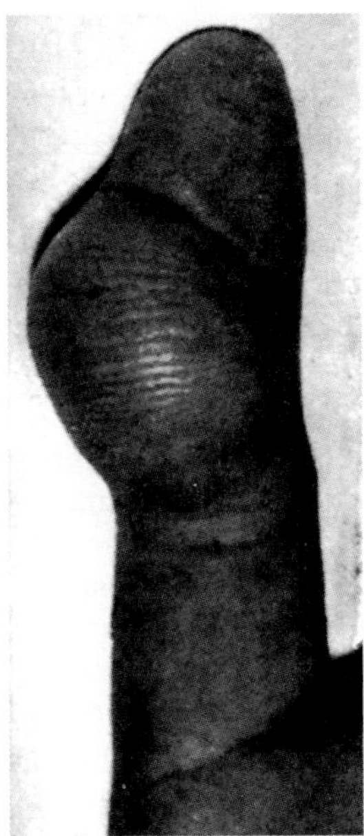

Fig. 12.13 Implantation dermoid. The contents are desquamated cell debris, which may undergo mucoid degeneration.

tion of a sebaceous gland, but this is followed by the downgrowth and the accumulation of desquamated epidermal cells, thus turning it into an epidermoid cyst. In the epididymis, if the retention cyst contains sperms, it is known as a 'spermatocele'.

Distension cysts occur in the thyroid from dilatation of the acini, or in the ovary from a follicle. Lymphatic cysts and cystic hygromas are distension cysts. **Exudation cysts** occur when fluid exudes into an anatomical space already lined by endothelium, e.g. hydrocele, a bursa, or when a collection of exudate becomes encrusted.

Cystic tumours. Examples are cystic teratomas (dermoid cyst of the ovary) and cystadenomas (pseudomucinous and serous cystadenoma of the ovary).

Ganglia. See Chapter 29.

Implantation dermoids arise from squamous epithelium which has been driven beneath the skin by a penetrating wound. They are classically found in the fingers of women who sew assiduously and metal workers (Fig. 12.13).

Trauma

A haematoma may resolve into a cyst. This sometimes happens to haematomas of muscle masses in the loin and anterolateral aspects of the thigh or the skin. They are located between muscle, facial or subcutaneous planes and contain straw- or brown-coloured fluid containing cholesterol crystals. They become lined by endothelium and calcium salts may be laid down. Aspiration is only of temporary value, and a cure depends upon complete excision of the lining. Within the cranium, a haematogenous cyst can cause the same problems as any expanding, space-occupying lesion.

Degeneration cysts

These have already been discussed under false cysts.

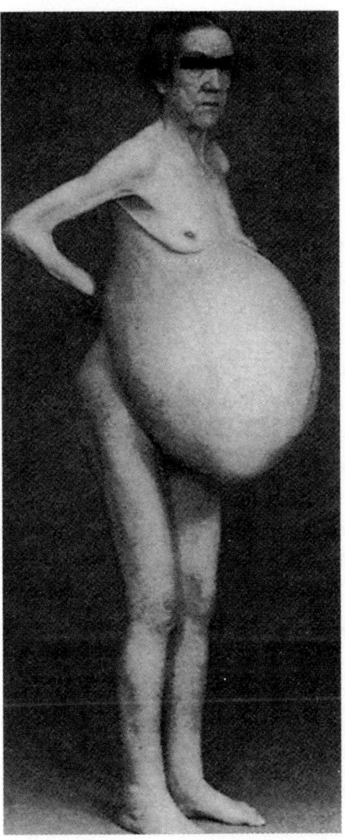

Fig. 12.14 Cachexia ovarica. The patient successfully underwent an operation for a giant ovarian cyst containing 15 litres of fluid. The site, size and weight of the cyst combined to cause the classical appearance of cachexia, lordosis, oedema of the legs and an anxious expression which are generally associated with an advanced cancer.

Parasitic cysts

These are encrusted forms in the life cycle of various worms:

- *Hydatid cyst of* Taenia echinococcus. This is described later according to the organ involved, e.g. liver, Chapter 52; lung, Chapter 47.
- *Trichiniasis.* Cysts of *Trichina spiralis,* affecting muscle.
- *Cysticercosis.* Cysts of *Taenia solium.* A disease of the pig, humans being rarely affected. Eosinophilla is present. The cysts occur in any organ. They calcify and may cause clinical effects according to their situation, especially in the brain. Only those cysts which are actually causing symptoms should be excised.

Clinical features

The swelling usually has a smooth, spherical appearance. *Fluctuation* depends upon the pressure of fluid within: a tense cyst feels like a solid tumour, although careful palpation between two fingers may elicit a characteristic elasticity. *In addition, a solid tumour is most hard at the centre; a cyst is least hard at the centre.* If fluctuation is present, a cyst may be confused with a cold abscess or a lipoma. A cold abscess usually has a peculiar rim of thickening surrounding the soft centre. A lipoma may well test clinical acumen. *Transillumination,* while brilliantly clear in cysts containing serous fluid, does not really distinguish between a lipoma and a dermoid or branchial cyst. There is even an old axiom that 'when in doubt, hedge on fat'. According to circumstances, ultrasonography, computerised tomography (CT) or magnetic resonance imaging (MRI), a test aspiration or excision reveals the true nature of the swelling.

Cysts may be painful, especially when infection or haemorrhage causes a sudden increase in intracystic tension. Sometimes they change in size for no apparent reason. Occasionally, they diminish owing to rupture through a facial plane.

Effects are according to site and size. As with benign tumours, a cyst may compress ducts and blood vessels, e.g. the main bile duct may be obstructed by a choledochal cyst, a renal cyst or a hydatid cyst. The pelvic veins may be obstructed by an ovarian cyst, the patient presenting for treatment of her varicose veins. The sheer size of an ovarian cyst (Fig. 12.14) may so increase intra-abdominal tension as to bring the patient to hospital with symptoms of a hiatus hernia.

Complications

Infection

The cyst becomes tense and painful, and adherent to surrounding tissues. An abscess may form and discharge on the surface and result in an ulcer or a sinus (viz. Cock's peculiar tumour, Chapter 13). Healing will not occur until the whole lining of the cyst or the embryonic track is excised.

Haemorrhage

Sudden haemorrhage, as may occur in a thyroid cyst, causes a painful increase in size. In this particular case, breathing may be difficult because of pressure on the trachea.

Torsion

Torsion may occur in cysts which are attached to neighbouring structures by a vascular pedicle. Ovarian dermoids are sometimes brought to notice in this way as acute abdominal emergencies. The cyst (or cysts – they may be bilateral) turns to a purple or black colour as the venous and then the arterial supply is cut off.

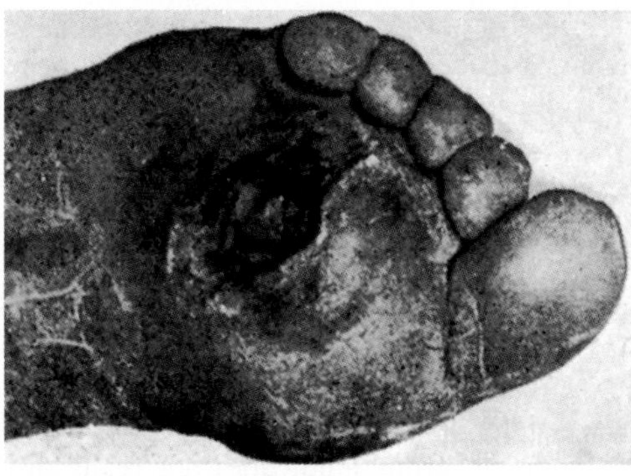

Fig. 12.15 Perforating ulcer in a diabetic.

Calcification

Calcification follows haemorrhage, or infection, and may be the result of reaction to a parasite, e.g. hydatid cyst.

Cachexia ovarica

Enormous cysts are rarely seen nowadays (Fig. 12.14).

Ulcers

An ulcer is a discontinuity of an epithelial surface. There is usually progressive destruction of surface tissue, cell by cell, as distinct from death of macroscopic portions, e.g. gangrene or necrosis. Ulcers are classified as *nonspecific, specific* (e.g. tuberculous or syphilitic) or *malignant*.

Nonspecific ulcers are due to infection of wounds, or physical or chemical agents. Local irritation, as in the case of a dental ulcer, or interference with the circulation, e.g. varicose veins, are predisposing causes.

Trophic ulcers [*trophe* (Greek) = nutrition] are due to an impairment of the nutrition of the tissues, which depends upon an adequate blood supply and a properly functioning nerve supply. Ischaemia and anaesthesia therefore will cause these ulcers. Thus, in the arm, chronic vasospasm and syringomyelia will cause ulceration of the tips of the fingers (respectively painful and painless). In the leg, painful ischaemic ulcers occur around the ankle or on the dorsum of the foot. *Neuropathic* ulcers due to anaesthesia (diabetic neuritis, spina bifida, tabes dorsalis, leprosy or a peripheral nerve injury) are often called *perforating ulcers* (Fig. 12.15). Starting in a corn or bunion, they penetrate the foot, and the suppuration may involve the bones and joints and spread along fascial planes upwards, even involving the calf.

The life history of an ulcer consists of three phases.

Extension

During the stage of extension the floor is covered with exudate and sloughs, while the base is indurated. The discharge is purulent and even blood stained.

Transition

The transition stage prepares for healing. The floor becomes cleaner, the sloughs separate, induration of the base diminishes and the discharge becomes more serous. Small, reddish areas of granulation tissue appear on the floor and these link up until the whole surface is covered.

Repair

The stage of repair consists of the transformation of granulation to fibrous tissue, which gradually contracts to form a scar. The epithelium gradually extends from the now shelving edge to cover the floor (at a rate of 1 mm per day).

Edward Cock, 1805–92. Surgeon, Guy's Hospital, London, England.

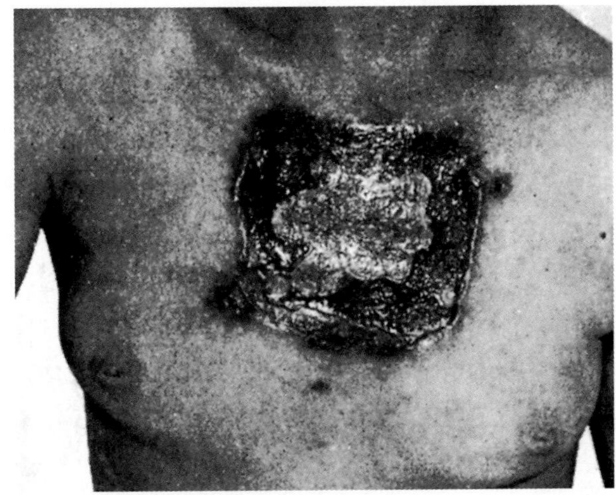

Fig. 12.16 Dermatitis artefacta. This condition is due to self-mutilation, e.g by the application of irritants, such as corrosives. The patient usually has a hysterical temperament, or litigation may be involved.

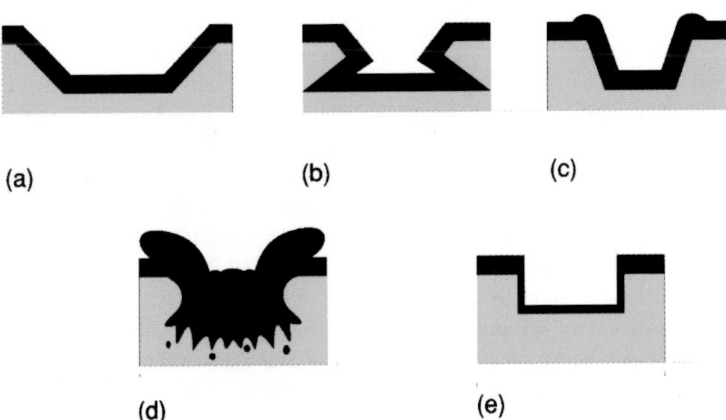

Fig. 12.17 Some characteristic shapes of the edges of ulcers. (a) Nonspecific ulcer: note shelving edge; (b) tuberculous ulcer: note undermined edge; (c) basal-cell carcinoma (rodent ulcer): note rolled edge, which may exhibit small blood vessels; (d) epithelioma: note heaped-up, everted edge (and irregular thickened base); (e) syphilis: note punched-out edge (and thin base which may be covered by a 'wash-leather' slough).

This healing edge consists of three zones – an outer of epithelium, which appears white, a middle one, bluish in colour (where granulation tissue is covered by a few layers of epithelium), and an inner reddish zone of granulation tissue covered by a single layer of epithelial cells. The red colour of granulation tissue is due to the high density of new capillaries (neo-angiogenesis).

Clinical examination of an ulcer

This should be conducted in a systematic manner. The following are, with brief examples, the points which should be noted.

- **Site**, e.g. 95 per cent of rodent ulcers occur on the upper part of the face. Carcinoma typically affects the lower lip, while a primary chancre of syphilis is usually on the upper lip.
- **Size**, particularly in relation to the length of history, e.g. a carcinoma extends more rapidly than a rodent ulcer, but more slowly than an inflammatory ulcer.
- **Shape**, e.g. a rodent ulcer is usually circular. A gummatous ulcer is typically circular, or serpiginous due to the fusion of multiple circles. An ulcer with a square area or straight edge is suggestive of 'dermatitis artefacta' (Fig. 12.16).
- **Edge** (Fig. 12.17). A healing, nonspecific ulcer has a shelving edge. It is pearly, rolled or rampant if a rodent ulcer, and raised and everted if an epithelioma, undermined and often bluish if tuberculous, vertically punched out if syphilitic.
- **Floor**. The floor is that which is seen by an observer, e.g. watery or apple-jelly granulations in a tuberculous ulcer, a wash-leather slough in a gummatous ulcer.
- **Base**. The base is what can be palpated. It may be indurated as in a carcinoma or attached to deep structures, e.g. a varicose ulcer to the tibia.
- **Discharge**. A purulent discharge indicates active infection. A blue–green coloration suggests infection with *Pseudomonas pyocyaneus*. A watery discharge is typical of tuberculosis. It is bloodstained in the extension phase of a nonspecific ulcer. *Bacteriological examination* may reveal colonisation by coagulase-positive staphylococci. Spirochaetes are found in a primary chancre (Chapter 8).
- **Lymph nodes** are not enlarged in the case of a rodent ulcer, unless due to secondary infection. In the case of carcinoma, they may be enlarged, hard and even fixed. The inguinal nodes draining a syphilitic chancre of the penis are firm and 'shotty', but contrarily the submandibular nodes draining a chancre of the lip are greatly enlarged.
- **Pain**. Nonspecific ulcers in the extension and transition stages are painful (except for the anaesthetic trophic type). Tuberculous ulcers vary, that of the tongue being very painful. Syphilitic ulcers are usually painless, but an anal chancre (of a homosexual) may be painful (cf. anal fissure, Chapter 61).
- **General examination**. Evidence of debility, cardiac failure, all types of anaemia, including sickle-cell anaemia, or diabetes must be sought.
- **Pathological examinations**, e.g. biopsy, will confirm carcinoma. The serological and Mantoux tests may be of value for syphilis and tuberculosis, respectively.
- **Marjolin's ulcer**. See Chapter 13.

Local (topical) treatment of nonspecific ulcers

Any underlying cause is treated, e.g. varicose veins (Chapter 16), diabetes, arterial disease. Many lotions and nonadhesive applications are used to aid the separation of sloughs, hasten granulation and stimulate epithelialisation. The basic requirements of an ideal dressing are that should:

Charles Mantoux, 1877–1947. Physician, Le Cannet, France.

- maintain a high humidity between the wound and the dressing;
- remove excess exudate and toxic compounds;
- permit gaseous exchange of oxygen, carbon dioxide and water vapour;
- provide thermal insulation to the wound surface and be impermeable to microorganisms;
- be free from particles and toxic wound contaminants;
- allow easy removal with no trauma at dressing change;
- be safe to use and be acceptable to the patient;
- be cost-effective.

Antiseptics and topical antibiotics

Antiseptics can do more harm than good when used inappropriately. They can interfere with the normal healing process, are toxic to fibroblasts and may permit more virulent organisms to dominate. The routine use of antiseptic and hypochlorite solutions should be avoided. If a wound needs cleaning, this can be achieved safely and more economically with normal saline warmed to body temperature prior to use. If a topical antiseptic is necessary, aqueous chlorhexidine 1 in 5000 solution is effective against a wide range of Gram-positive and -negative organisms and some fungi, but not spores. Povidine iodine has a broad spectrum of activity but its antibacterial effect is reduced by contact with pus or exudate. It should not be used on patients who are sensitive to iodine. Topical antibiotics are not recommended routinely as resistance and sensitisation following application may arise. Flamazine is a hydrophilic cream containing silver suphadiazine 1%, which is a broad-spectrum antibacterial agent and very effective against *Pseudomonas*, useful for the prevention of Gram-negative sepsis in patients with severe burns.

Wound dressings

Hydrocolloid dressings such as Granuflex or Comfeel consist of a thin polyurethane foam sheet bonded on to a semipermeable polyurethane film, which is impermeable to exudate and microorganisms. When the dressing comes into contact with wound exudate it interacts to form a gel which expands into the wound. The moist conditions produced under the dressing promote angiogenesis and wound healing without causing maceration. They can be used in the treatment of leg ulcers, pressure sores, minor burns and many types of granulating wound. A hydrocolloid dressing can be applied to small wounds containing dry slough or necrosis: the dressing prevents the loss of water vapour from the surface of the skin, and this effectively rehydrates the dead tissue, which is then removed by autolysis.

Hydrogel (Intrasite gel) is a pale yellow/colourless transparent aqueous gel. When it comes into contact with a wound, the dressing absorbs excess exudate and produces a moist environment at the surface of the wound without causing tissue maceration. It may be applied to many different wounds including leg ulcers, pressure sores, surgical wounds and granulating tissue. It is particularly useful in the treatment of dry, sloughy or necrotic wounds, promoting rapid débridement by facilitating rehydration and autolysis of dead tissue. It reduces the feeling of pain and can be used as a carrier of other medicines, e.g. metronidazole, for the control of odour caused by infection with sensitive organisms. (It is useful in fungating tumours where the aim is not to heal the wound but to manage the distressing symptoms caused by it.) Intrasite should be secured with a secondary dressing such as an absorbent pad or Tegaderm depending on the wound.

Alginates (Kaltostat) consist of an absorbent fibrous fleece composed of the mixed sodium and calcium salts of alginic acid. In the presence of exudate or other body fluids containing sodium ions, the fibres absorb liquid and swell, calcium ions present in the fibre are partially replaced by sodium, causing the dressing to take on a gel-like appearance which promotes healing. The fibres are held in place with a secondary dressing such as an absorbent pad or Tegaderm depending on the amount of exudate. Alginate dressings can be used for the management of bleeding wounds including cuts and lacerations and also for a wide range of exuding lesions including leg ulcers, pressure sores and most other granulating wounds. Most suitable for heavy to moderately exudating wounds. In the presence of low exudate the Kaltostat must be moistened with saline before application to avoid adherence. The alginates are biodegradable so it is not necessary to remove every fibre if it will damage the healing tissue.

Lyofoam is a low-adherent comformable polyurethane foam sheet. The side of the dressing that is to be placed in contact with the skin has been heat treated to render it hydrophilic, whilst the outer surface remains hydrophobic. The dressing is freely permeable to gases and water vapour but resists the penetration of aqueous solutions and exudate. The dressing absorbs blood and any other tissue fluids but the aqueous component is lost by evaporation through the back of the dressing. Strike-through occurs laterally and not at the top of the dressing. The dressing maintains a moist warm environment at the surface of the wound, which is conducive to granulation and epithelialisation. Foam sheet dressings may be used on a variety of exudating wounds including leg ulcers, pressure sores, sutured wounds, burns and donor sites.

Tegaderm consists of a thin polyurethane membrane coated with a layer of an acrylic adhesive. The dressing allows for a moist environment at the surface of the wound by reducing water vapour loss from the exposed tissue. It is permeable to both water vapour and oxygen and impermeable to microorganisms, providing an effective barrier to external contamination. Scab formation is prevented and epidermal regeneration takes place at an enhanced rate, compared with that which occurs in wounds treated with traditional dry dressings. Tegaderm may be used in the treatment of minor burns, pressure areas, donor sites, post-operative wounds and a variety of minor injuries. It is also effectively used as a protective cover to prevent skin breakdown due to friction or continuous exposure to moisture.

Alleyvn cavity wound dressing is a highly comformable absorbent dressing consisting of a soft, polymeric outer membrane with a three-dimensional honeycomb-like structure containing a mass of hydrophilic polyurethane chips. The outer membrane is perforated to allow exudate to be drawn into the interior of the dressing where it is absorbed and retained by the 'chips'. This type of dressing is used for heavily exudating, full-thickness sloughy wounds, usually combined with Intrasite gel; it can be used alone with clean, deep, exudating wounds.

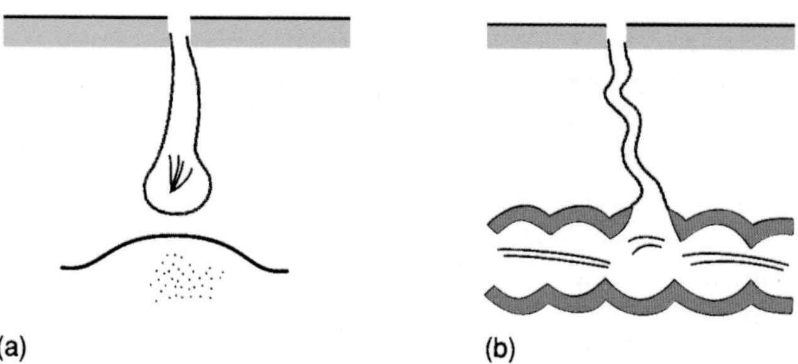

Fig. 12.18 (a) A sinus, and (b) a fistula. Both usually arise from a preceding abscess. (a) This shows that a sinus is a blind track, in this case a pilonidal sinus with its hairs; (b) this shows that a fistula is a track connecting two (epithelial) lined surfaces, in this case a colocutaneous fistula.

Sir William Leishmann, 1865–1926. Professor of Pathology, Royal Army Medical College, London, England.

Most of the above dressings are also available with added properties which improve their basic function, such as Kaltocarb. This is Kaltostat with a layer of activated charcoal cloth attached. This is effective as a primary dressing in the management of infected malodorous wounds.

As the wound heals if granulation tissue continues to grow past the epidermal layer, the dressing used to stimulate granulation should be discontinued and a Lyofoam dressing should be applied. If after 1 week there is no improvement Terra-cortil ointment containing hydrocortisone and oxytetracycline applied sparingly to the wound may be effective. This should be covered with a Lyofoam dressing and should be used for no longer than 5 days. Silver nitrate may be used with heavy overgranulating tissue but it is not recommended, usually because of its toxicity and the risk of sensitivity and staining.

Oriental sore (syn. Delhi boil, Baghdad sore, etc.)

This disease is due to infection by a protozoal parasite, *Leishmania tropica,* and is a common condition in Eastern countries which is occasionally imported to Western zones. An indurated papule appears on an exposed surface, usually the face. If untreated, this breaks down to form an indolent ulcer, which eventually leaves an ugly, pigmented scar. The condition readily responds to intravenous injections of antimony tartrate, but very small lesions can be treated by carbon dioxide snow, and also curettage.

Bazin's disease (syn. erythema induratum) is due to localised areas of fat necrosis and particularly affects adolescent girls. Symmetrical purplish nodules appear, especially on the calves, and gradually break down to form indolent ulcers, which leave in their wake pigmented scars. Tuberculosis may be a cause in many instances, the ulcers responding to antituberculous drugs (Fig. 12.17) (Chapter 8).

Sinuses and fistulas

A sinus (Latin = a hollow; a bay or gulf) is a blind track (usually lined with granulation tissue) leading from an epithelial surface into the surrounding tissues. Pathological sinuses must be distinguished from normal anatomical sinuses (e.g. the frontal and nasal sinuses). A fistula (Latin = a pipe or tube) is an abnormal communication between the lumen or surface of one organ and the lumen or surface of another, or between vessels. Most fistulas connect epithelial-lined surfaces (Fig. 12.18). Sinuses and fistulas may be *congenital* or *acquired.* Forms which have a congenital origin include preauricular sinuses (Chapter 37), branchial fistulas (Chapter 43), tracheo-oesophageal fistulas (Chapter 50) and arteriovenous fistulas (Chapter 15). The acquired forms often follow inadequate drainage of an abscess. Thus, a perianal abscess may burst on the surface and lead to a sinus (erroneously termed a blind external 'fistula'). In other cases, the abscess opens both into the anal canal and on to the surface of the perineal stem resulting in a true fistula-in-ano (Chapter 61). Acquired arteriovenous fistulas are caused by trauma or operation (for renal dialysis).

Persistence of a sinus or fistula

The reason for this will be found among the following:

Pierre Antoine Ernest Bazin, 1867–78. Dermatologist, Hôpital St Louis, Paris, France.

- a foreign body or necrotic tissue is present, e.g. a suture, hairs, a sequestrum, a faecolith or even a worm (see below);
- inefficient or nondependent drainage: long, narrow, tortuous track predisposes to inefficient drainage;
- unrelieved obstruction of the lumen of a viscus or tube distal to the fistula;
- high pressure, such as occurs in fistula-in-ano due to the normal contractions of the sphincter which force faecal material through the fistula;
- the walls have become lined with epithelium or endothelium (arteriovenous fistula);
- dense fibrosis prevents contraction and healing;
- type of infection, e.g. tuberculosis or actinomycosis;
- the presence of malignant disease;
- ischaemia;
- drugs, e.g. steroids, cytotoxics;
- malnutrition;
- interference, e.g. artefacta;
- irradiation, e.g. rectovaginal fistula after treatment for a carcinoma of the cervix;
- Crohn's disease;
- high-output fistula, e.g. duodeno-cutaneous fistula.

Treatment

The remedy depends upon the removal or specific treatment of the cause (see appropriate pages).

Guinea worm (syn. dragon worm, *Dracunculus medinensis*) (Fig. 12.19)

This is a cause of a persisting sinus on the lower leg. The larval form enters through the wall of the stomach

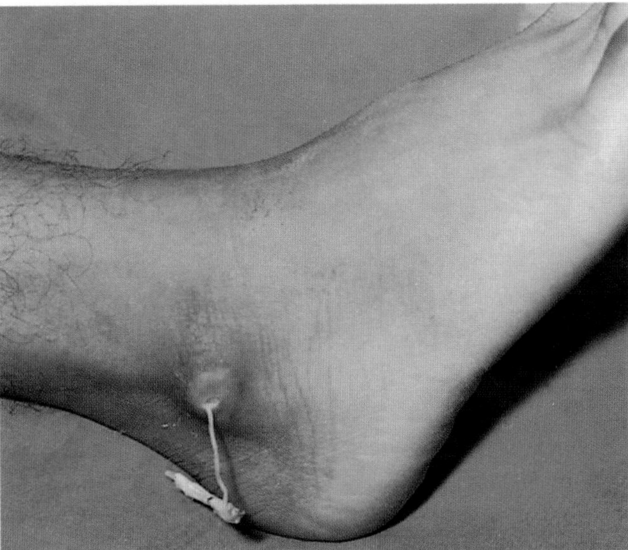

Fig. 12.19 Sinus?, Ulcer? – presenting in a UK outpatient department. The 30-cm female guinea worm is carefully extricated by being wound on a matchstick, a few turns a day to prevent breakage and retraction.

or duodenum in drinking water contaminated by a tiny cyclops crustacean which has consumed the larvae. Settling in the abdominal connective tissue, the male and female mate, the pregnancy lasting about a year, and the female wanders in the subcutaneous tissues to select for egg laying a part of the anatomy likely to be submerged in water (containing the cyclops), usually the lower leg. Cellulitis, abscesses, ulcers and sinuses follow, through which the embryos are discharged, hopefully to be eaten by the cyclops. Baid travelled the interior of India and in 500 cases discerned a syndrome of the infestation, presenting with conjunctivitis (allergic) in 11 per cent, fibrous contracture of joints in 19 per cent, periostitis with osteomyelitis in 21 per cent and acute arthritis in 65 per cent.

J.C. Baid. Surgeon, Jodhpur, India.

Acknowledgement

The sections on Tropical treatment, Antisepsis and Wound dressings were written by Sister Lorraine Bosonnet, Senior Sister, Professional Surgical Unit, Royal Liverpool University Hospital.

Further reading

Ellis, H.A. (1994) *Spot Diagnosis in Surgery,* 2nd edn, Blackwell Scientific, Oxford.

Moschella, S.L. and Hurley, H.J. (eds) (1992) *Dermatology,* 3rd edn, W.B. Saunders, London.

Walter, J.B. and Israel, M.S. (eds) (1987) *General Pathology,* 6th edn, Churchill Livingstone, Edinburgh.

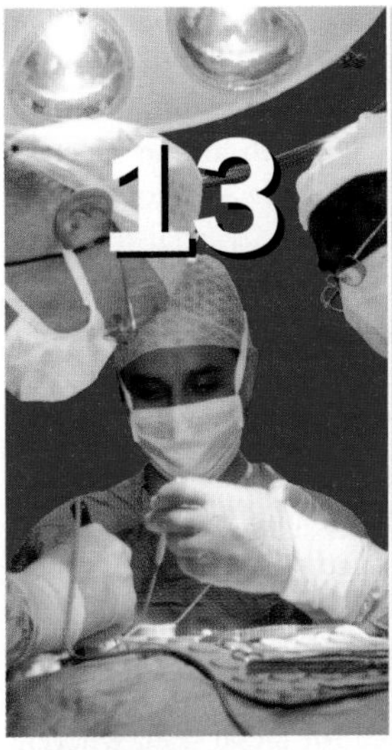

13 Plastic and reconstructive surgery, skin lesions

Plastic surgery

Plastic surgery is defined as 'repair or reconstruction of lost, injured or deformed parts of the body chiefly by transfer of tissue'. The term plastic concerns moulding and reshaping of tissues and comes from the Greek *plastikos* ('that may be moulded'). When tissues are moved or reshaped the most important principle governing this process is respect for their blood supply. The two fundamental methods by which tissues are moved are grafts or flaps. A graft is a piece of tissue that is moved without its blood supply and relies on its recipient bed to re-establish a blood supply. A flap is a piece of tissue that is moved maintaining its blood supply and is not reliant on the recipient site for its vascularity. Historically reconstruction was complex and multistage, with ample opportunity for vascular complications to arise. In the last 30 years there has been a revolution in our understanding of the blood supply of the skin and of other tissues[1]. Flaps can now be reliably designed on single named blood vessels, greatly increasing their power and versatility. Plastic surgical techniques are used in a wide variety of surgical procedures in all parts of the body, and in the treatment of a wide variety of pathologies. These techniques can be learnt and used by other specialists, but most plastic surgeons would feel that optimal care is provided where the plastic surgeon works together with a surgeon from another discipline to each bring their own expertise to bear on the problem.

Priorities in reconstruction

When presented with any defect it is important to recognise that the most important priority is to achieve primary healing. The purpose of reconstructive procedures is to avoid the adverse consequences of healing by second intention in terms of delay and poor function. If one can achieve quiet primary healing and thereby restore the patient to function a superior result in terms of appearance will usually result. It is essential, however, that these three priorities are observed in the correct order: first healing, then function and lastly appearance. Where these aims cannot be achieved by direct closure of a wound a more complex technique is selected from the reconstructive toolbox. Planning and selection are central to the practice of plastic surgery. In any one patient

[1]*In part this has been a rediscovery since much work was done by Manchot in the nineteenth century by means of cadaver dissections and Salmon in the 1930s and 1940s by means of meticulous radiographs of injected cadaver skin.*

Bailey & Love's Short Practice of Surgery, 23rd edition. Edited by R.C.G. Russell, N.S. Williams and C.J.K. Bulstrode. Published in 2000 by Arnold Publishers.

Carl Manchot, 1866–1932. Physician in Hamburg. Published 'Die Hautarterien des Menschlichen Körpers (The Cutaneous Arteries of the Human Body)' in 1889 when still a medical student in what is now Strasbourg, France.

Michel-Marie Salmon, 1903–73. Professor of Anatomy and then Professor of Paediatric and Orthopaedic Surgery in Marseille, France. Published 'Artères de la Peau (Arteries of the Skin)' in 1936.

there is a number of reconstructive options. The reliability and quality of the reconstruction must be balanced against the donor site morbidity.

Priorities in plastic surgery
1. Healing
2. Function
3. Cosmetic

Skin grafts

Skin grafts are harvested from a donor site and transferred to a recipient site on which they must survive, a process known as take. All skin grafts initially adhere to the recipient bed by the formation of fibrin. Oxygen and nutrients diffuse through by a process known as plasmatic imbibition to keep the graft alive. New blood vessels then grow from the recipient site and link up with dermal capillaries to re-establish a blood supply, a process known as inosculation. Thin skin grafts are more likely to survive by imbibition and will revascularise readily and are therefore more likely to take than thicker grafts. Thicker grafts, however, will have more dermis, more sebaceous glands, greater structural integrity and a lesser tendency to contract.

Partial-thickness skin grafts

Partial-thickness skin grafts consist of epidermis and a variable thickness of dermis. There remains some dermis on the donor site that heals by epithelialisation from the cut ends of hair follicles and sweat glands in a manner similar to the healing of a graze or a superficial burn. The thigh is most frequently used as a donor site, but almost anywhere else can be used. Grafts are harvested using a skin graft knife or a power dermatome. These consist of a blade and a guard that can be adjusted to determine the thickness of the graft. Hand knives require practice to use and the graft obtained remains dependent on the tension in the donor site skin, the pressure that the surgeon applies, the speed and length of the strokes used and the angle of application of the blade (Fig. 13.1). With air- or electric-powered dermatomes these factors become less important and more consistent results can be obtained. Partial-thickness grafts are used to resurface relatively large areas of skin defect and are particularly useful in burns (Fig. 13.2a and b).

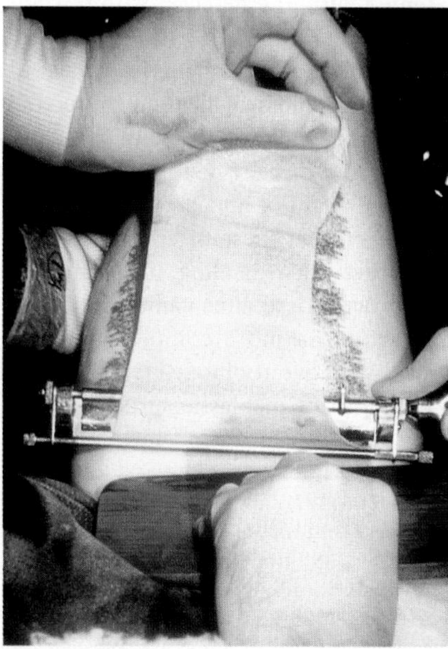

Fig. 13.1 Cutting a partial-thickness skin graft.

Full-thickness grafts

Full-thickness grafts consist of epidermis and all of the dermis; the donor site will not epithelialise and must be closed, usually directly. Suitable donor sites are postauricular, supraclavicular and groin. Full-thickness grafts are most commonly used in repairing defects on the face (Fig. 13.3a–c). Grafts taken from above the clavicles retain the ability to blush and can provide a very good colour match for facial skin, whereas grafts from below the clavicles will tend to look pale. Full-thickness grafts are harvested using a scalpel and forceps, dissecting at a level just below the dermis. As they are thick special care is needed to ensure good apposition to a well-vascularised bed to ensure good take.

Composite grafts

Composite grafts consist of skin and some underlying tissue such as fat and cartilage. Again, donor sites must be closed directly. Composite grafts carry the highest risk of failure yet potentially can repair complex defects. These grafts have to be carefully designed to be as thin as possible and have a large area of inset in order to survive. Their maximum thickness can only be a few millimetres; it is futile to replace larger portions of composite tissues – for larger defects flap repairs are needed. Portions of ear, skin and cartilage can be used to reconstruct nasal defects. Amputated fingertip pulp in children will sometimes survive if carefully replaced as a composite graft.

Other tissues

Other tissues can also be transferred as grafts. Cartilage grafts are commonly used in nasal and ear reconstruction. Cartilage is an avascular tissue; survival of transplanted chondrocytes depends entirely on diffusion of nutrients. Bone grafts are widely used for skeletal reconstruction. Nerve, tendon, vein, fascia and cornea are also all in common use.

Technical aspects

Graft take is only possible at well-vascularised recipient sites. Grafts will not take on bare bone, bare tendon or cartilage, but can survive on periosteum, paratenon and perichondrium. The graft must remain adherent to the bed until it revascularises; shearing forces must be eliminated. Meticulous care with suturing and dressings is essential. Where grafts are applied over mobile areas appropriate splintage must be used. Limbs that have been grafted should be elevated to reduce venous pressure during the process of

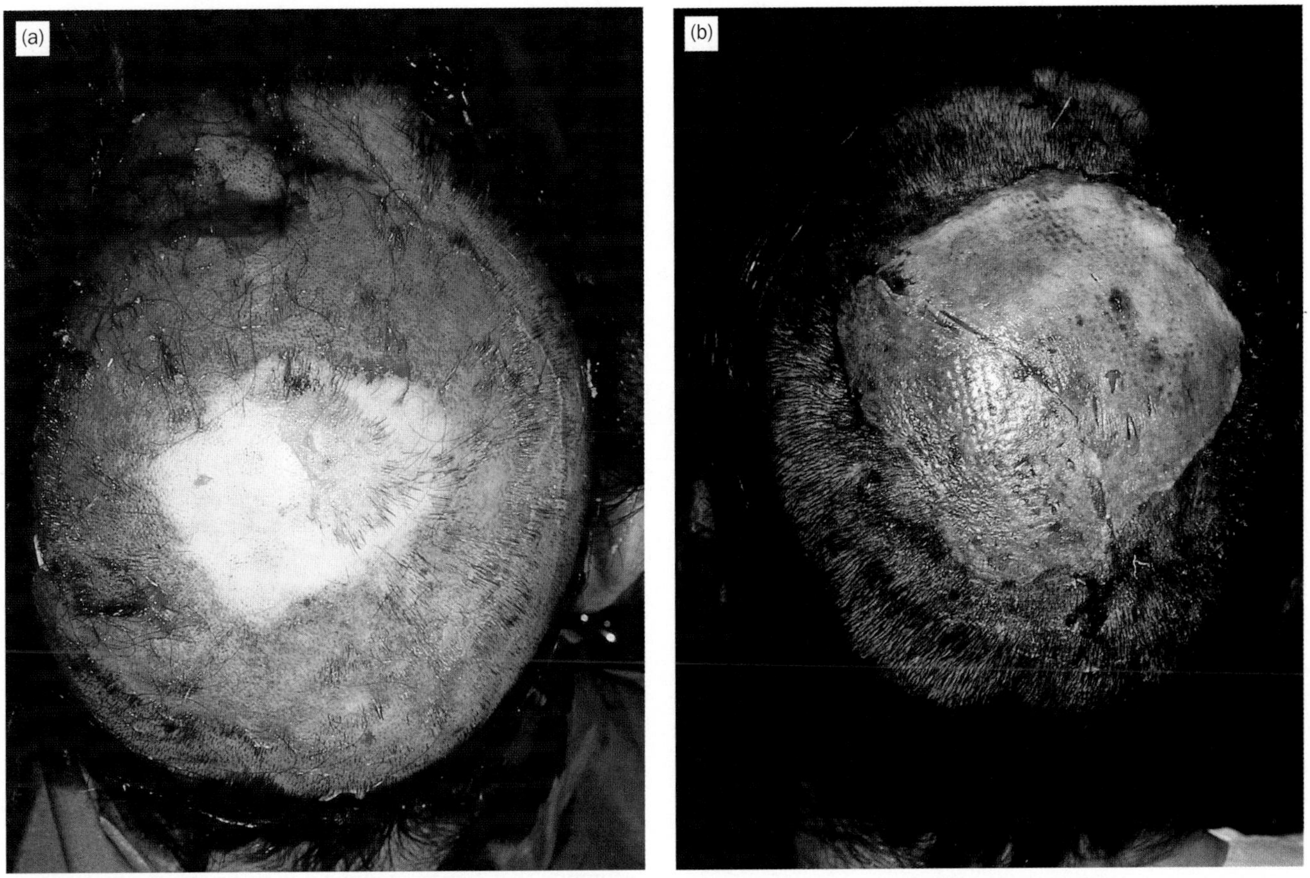

Fig. 13.2 (a) A deep burn of the scalp that requires excision and skin graft. (b) At 14 days complete skin graft take is evident. The wound is healed, but since he has lost all the hair follicles in the scalp he will have alopoecia. Delayed reconstruction of this may be needed.

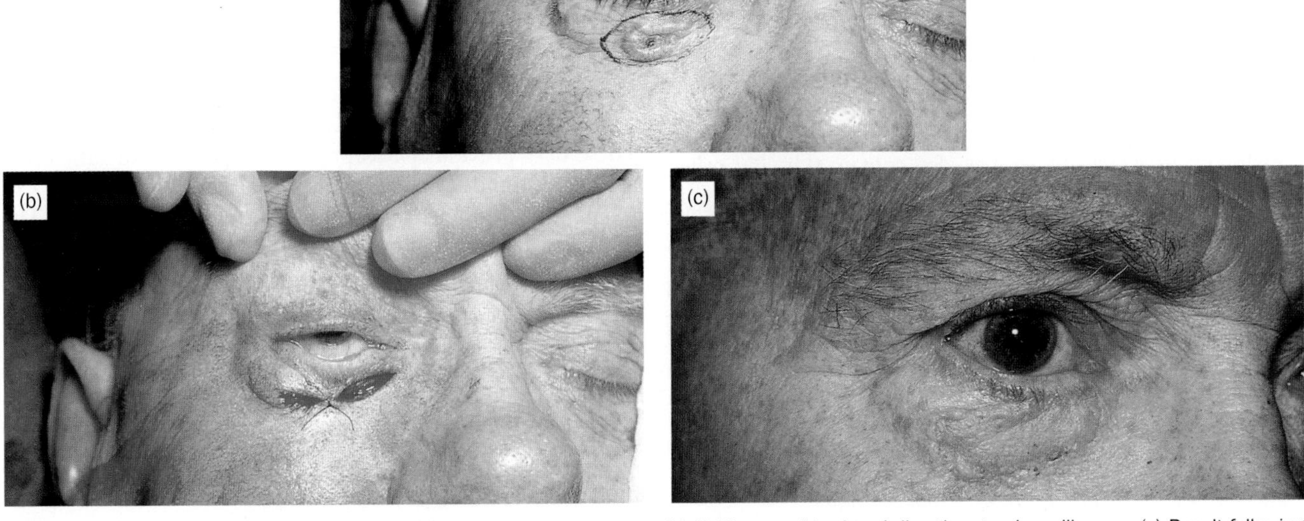

Fig. 13.3 (a) A basal cell carcinoma of the lower eyelid requiring excision. (b) If this wound is closed directly ectropion will occur. (c) Result following repair using a postauricular full-thickness skin graft – there is no ectropion.

revascularisation. Haemostasis at the recipient site must be good to prevent bleeding beneath the graft resulting in its elevation by clot and failure of take. Skin grafts can be stored in a refrigerator at 4°C for 2 weeks for delayed application. Grafts take well on granulation tissue, but excessive contamination with bacteria will prevent take. Streptococci at levels above 10^5 microorganisms per gram of tissue will result in graft loss. Preparation of the bed with dressings may help; it may be necessary to excise the granulation tissue.

Terminology

The definitions of flaps and grafts used above describe the vascular basis of the tissue transfer and the constituents of the transferred tissue. Most tissue transfer is from one place to another in the same person. However, there are other forms of transfer and further terminology is needed to explain the genetic basis of these transfers. An autograft is tissue transferred from one location to another on the same patient. An isograft is tissue transferred between two genetically identical individuals, such as the first successful renal transplant that was between identical twins. An allograft is tissue transferred between genetically different members of the same species. Most solid organ tissue transplantation involves this type of transfer. Rejection of the transplanted tissue will occur unless immunosuppressant drugs are used. A xenograft is tissue transferred from a donor of one species to a recipient of another species. Xenografts are usually small amounts of tissue rendered acellular before implantation to prevent rejection.

Flaps

More complex defects and avascular defects require flap cover. Flaps can consist of skin only, or be complex composites of skin, muscle, bone or other tissues. As their complexity increases so do their power and ability to reconstruct more complex defects. Flaps can be classified according to the geometry of their transfer such as rotation, advancement or transposition. A more useful classification is provided by their vascular basis. The vascular supply of a flap is known as its vascular pedicle; some flaps have more than one vascular pedicle. The term pedicle is also used to describe the base or attachment of a flap, which may also contain skin and other tissues as well as the vascular pedicle. Where the skin is divided all the way around a flap it is called an island flap.

[2]*Flaps from the cheek and forehead were used in India as early as 1000* BC *for nasal reconstruction. Tagliacozzi in 1597 published his method using flaps from the arm. Multitudes of flaps were utilised in the nineteenth century. Tansini in 1896 described the latissimus dorsi flap for breast reconstruction. The significance of the vascular basis of these flaps was not appreciated during the development of modern plastic surgery after World War I and World War II.*

Gaspar Tagliacozzi, 1546–99. Surgeon in Bologna, Italy.

Iginio Tansini, 1855–1926. Professor of Surgery Modena, then Palermo, then Pavia, Italy.

The development of flap surgery

Flaps have been used since ancient times, often to repair complex defects[2]. In the first half of the twentieth century, however, the only flaps that were considered possible were skin flaps consisting of rectangular portions of skin and subcutaneous tissue with length to breath ratio of 2 to 1.5:1. Such flaps were of limited arc of transfer and their use to reconstruct distant defects involved multistage surgery. Bipedicled flaps were tubed to form tubed pedicle flaps that were attached to an arm carrier and then transferred in several stages using multiple delays to a recipient site. It was possible to perform complex reconstructions using these methods, but each stage risked vascular compromise and flap loss, and donor site scarring was considerable. This all took a long time and such flaps, when the transfer was completed, depended on the local vascularity of the recipient site and did not bring in an independent blood supply of their own. Modern flap practice has developed since the discovery of the vascular anatomy of potential flap territories and the vascular patterns of skin blood supply.

Random pattern flaps

The vascular basis of random pattern flaps is the subdermal plexus of blood vessels. These flaps are widely used for local repair of adjacent defects, particularly on the face. Many geometric designs are possible. A particularly useful pattern is a rhomboid flap (Fig. 13.4a–d). The Z-plasty is a local flap technique that can be employed in a variety of situations, in particular treatment of contractures and scar revision. A Z-plasty or a combination of Z-plasties can lengthen a contracture, change the direction of a scar, alter tension, reposition specialised structures and improve the appearance of a scar (Fig. 13.5a and b). It involves the transposition of triangular flaps. The maximum lengthening is achieved by using 60° angles of flap design. Lengthening depends on laxity at right angles to the contracture since it occurs at the expense of shortening in a perpendicular direction.

Axial pattern flaps

Skin flaps with a known direct superficial vascular pedicle passing along their long axis are known as axial pattern flaps. These defy previously accepted length-to-breadth ratios that applied to random pattern flaps and thereby long flaps can reliably be designed with longer axes of rotation[3]. The forehead flap, the deltopectoral flap and groin flap all share this vascular pattern.

[3]*In a series of experiments in the 1960s raising flaps in pigs, Milton discovered that flaps made under similar conditions survive to the same length regardless of width. He realised that the most important factor was including a dominant vessel in the pedicle. He further discovered that islanded flaps with a segmental vessel in their base survived to a greater length than random skin flaps. Thus, he predicted the flap revolution that was about to occur.*

Stuart Harry Milton, 1935–71. Physiologist, Nuffield Department of Surgery, Oxford, England.

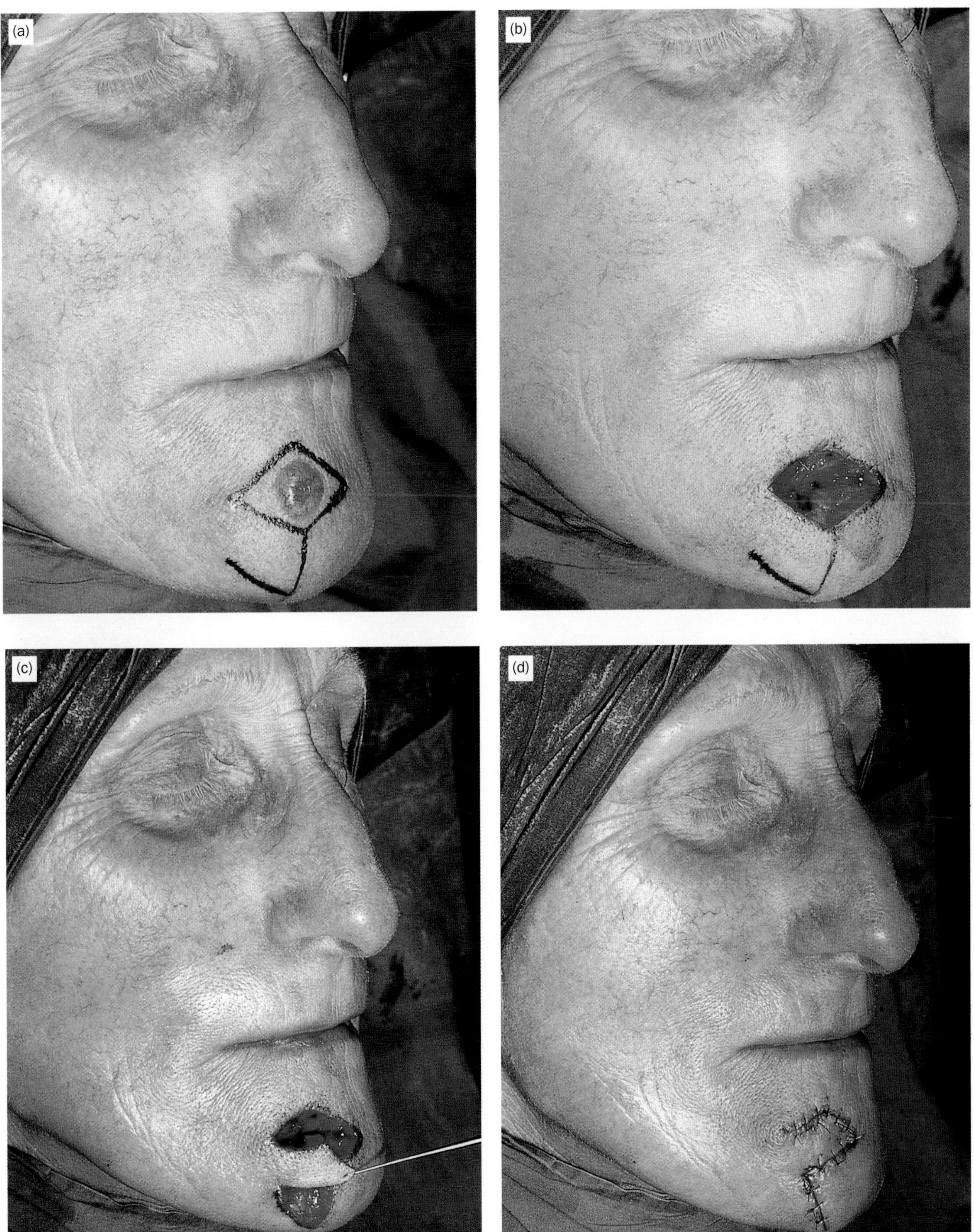

Fig. 13.4 (a) A basal cell carcinoma on the chin. Excision margins and the proposed rhomboid flap repair have been drawn. (b) The basal cell carcinoma has been excised. (c) The rhomboid flap has been raised and is being transposed. (d) The flap has been sutured in place.

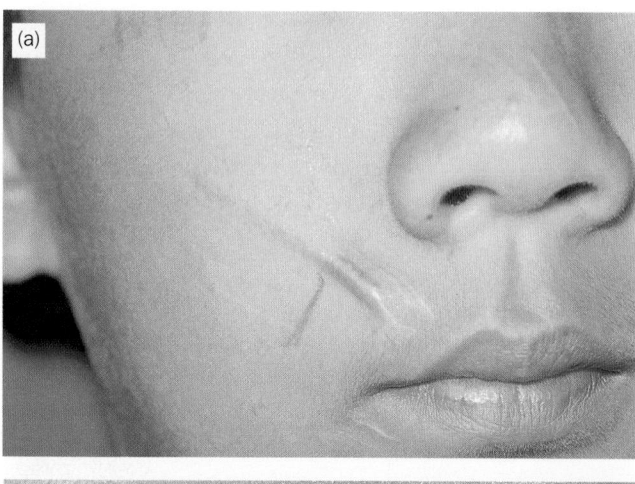

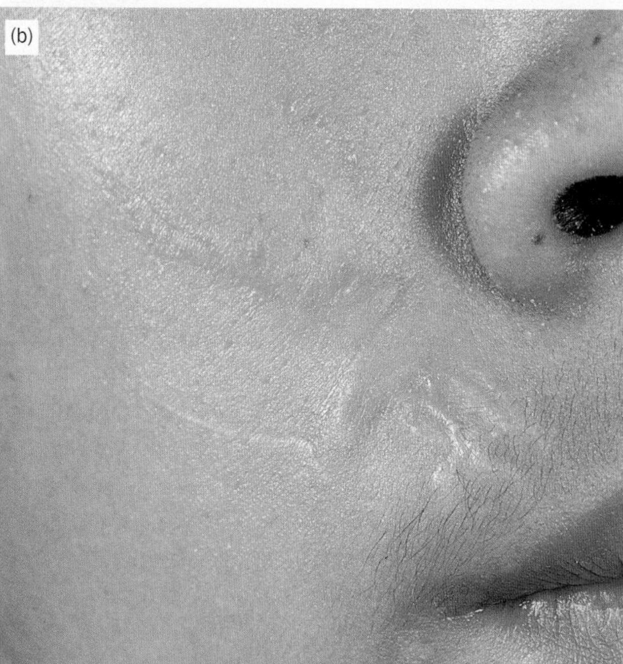

Fig. 13.5 (a) A hypertrophic scar on the cheek that runs across the relaxed skin tension lines. (b) Result after Z-plasty scar revision with resolution of the hypertrophy and a scar with its central limb running along a line of election.

Fasciocutaneous flaps

In many parts of the body blood vessels pass along the deep fascia or, in association with intermuscular septae, pass perforating vessels to supply the overlying skin. These flaps are raised along with the vascular pedicle by dissecting along the relevant fascial plane. Long vascular pedicles can be created, often with quite large vessels at their base. Fasciocutaneous flaps can be transferred loco-regionally, or the vascular pedicle divided, the flap transferred to a distant site and the flap revascularised by microsurgical anastomosis to recipient vessels adjacent to the defect. This technique of free tissue transfer has further extended the versatility of flap reconstruction. Fasciocutaneous flaps can be skin only or can include associated tissue to provide vascularised bone or

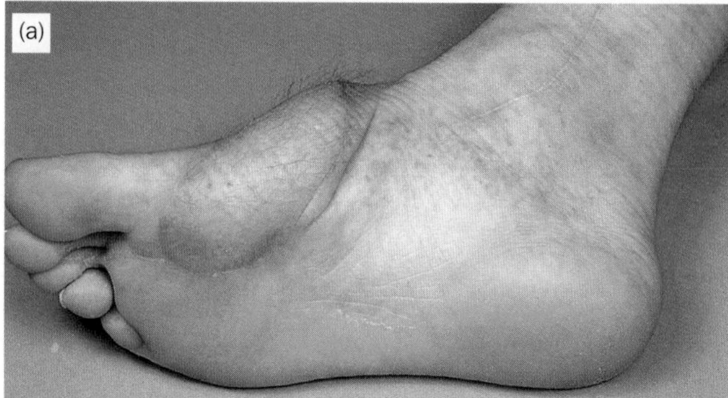

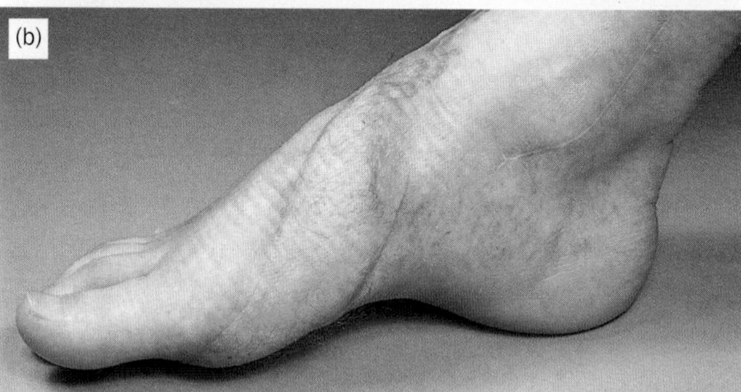

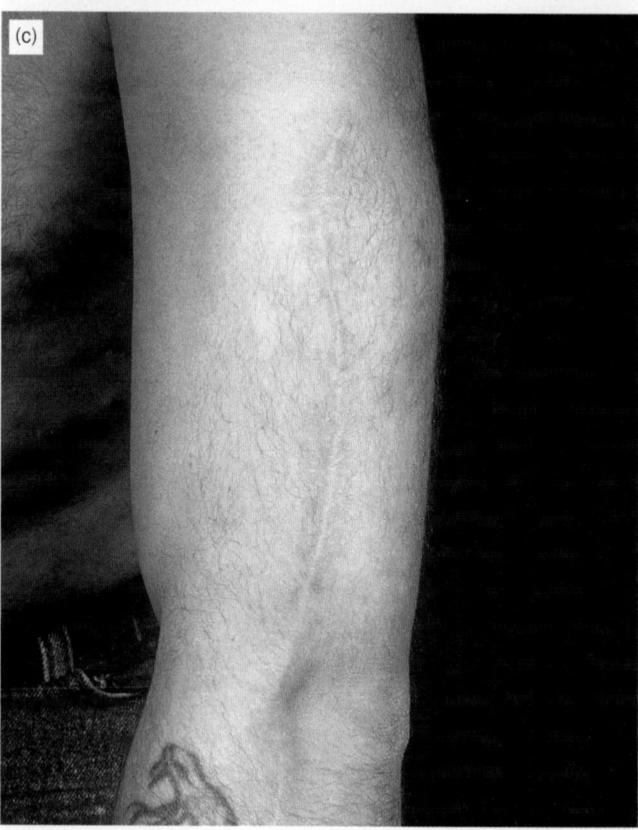

Fig. 13.6 (a) A free lateral arm flap has been used to resurface a post-traumatic plantar defect beneath the first metatarsal head. (b) An extension of the skin paddle passes around the medial aspect of the foot to allow the vascular pedicle to reach the dorsalis pedis vessels. The cutaneous nerve to the skin flap has been joined to a branch of the superficial peroneal nerve to restore some sensation to the flap. (c) The donor site on the arm has been closed directly.

nerve. Examples include the radial forearm flap, the scapular flap and the lateral arm flap (Fig. 13.6a–c). Almost any perforating blood vessel can be used as the vascular basis for a flap if carefully identified and dissected out. These so-called perforator flaps are the latest extension of flap design.

Muscle and musculocutaneous flaps

Muscles have predictable patterns of vascular anatomy that permit the elevation of a muscle on one or more of its vascular pedicles for use as a muscle flap, either locally or as a free tissue transfer. Many muscles also have perforating vessels passing from their substance into the overlying skin enabling musculocutaneous flaps to be designed. Musculocutaneous flaps based on the latissimus dorsi and rectus abdominis muscles are particularly useful in breast reconstruction (Fig. 13.7a and b). These same muscles are widely used as free muscle flaps to repair defects in the lower limb associated with open tibial fractures (Fig. 13.8a–c). Gluteus maximus and tensor fascia lata flaps are used for pressure-sore closure. Muscle flaps can be used as functional transfers where their nerve supply is left intact or re-established at the recipient site. Such techniques are applied

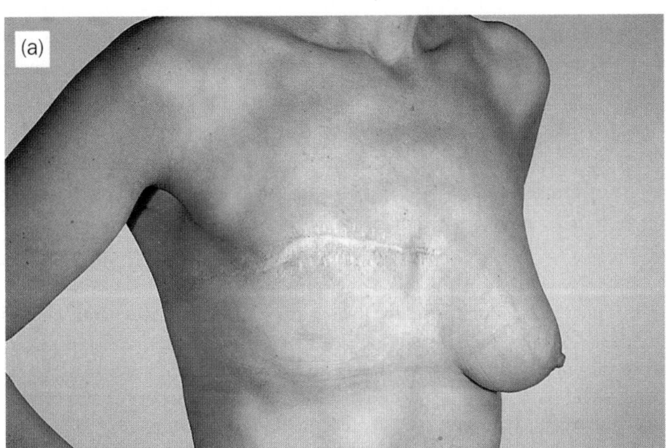

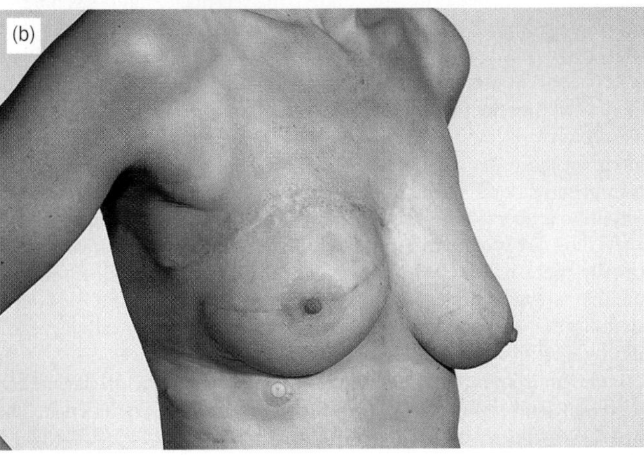

Fig. 13.7 (a) A patient has requested reconstruction after a right mastectomy. (b) Result following latissimus dorsi flap and a submuscular expander prosthesis. A custom-made nipple areola prosthesis has also been used.

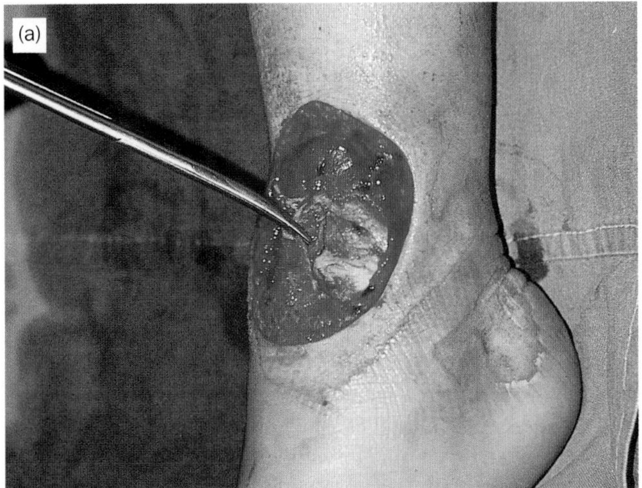

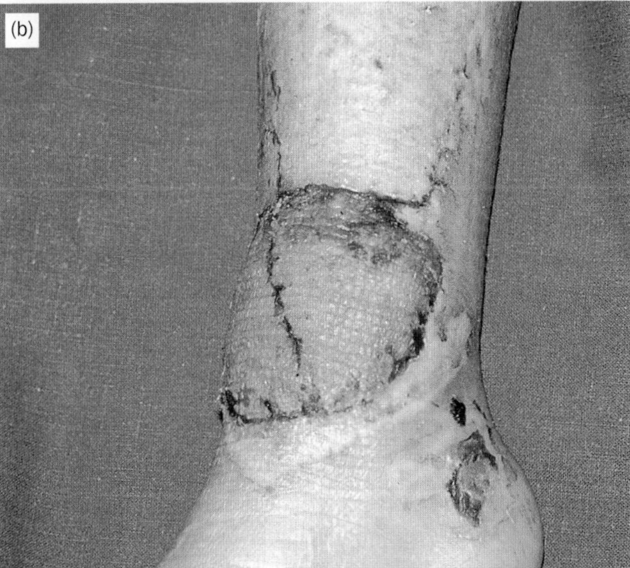

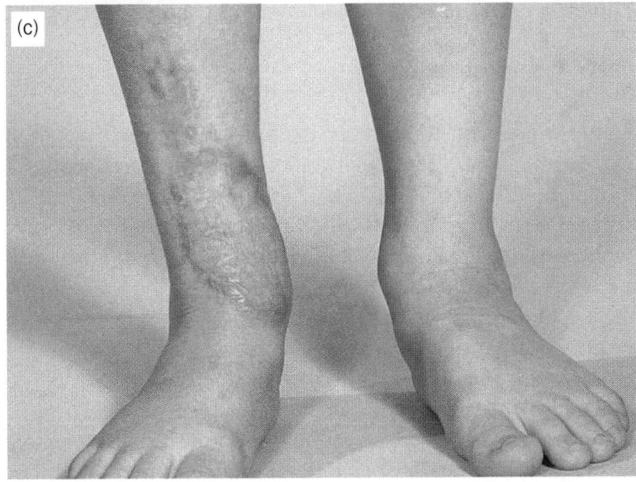

Fig. 13.8 (a) A 7-year-old boy has had his right ankle run over. He has an area of skin loss and an epiphyseal fracture. The exposed epiphysis requires urgent flap cover. (b) Early result from latissimus dorsi free muscle flap repair and skin graft. (c) Late result showing stable flap coverage and acceptable contour. The fracture has united. There was no growth disturbance as a result of the epiphyseal injury.

to the rehabilitation of brachial plexus injury, anal incontinence and facial palsy.

Free tissue transfer

The development of high-quality binocular operating microscopes, swaged microsutures and microsurgical instrumentation has, along with advances in the understanding of flap vascular anatomy, enabled reliable free flap surgery. The first successful microsurgical free tissue transfer was a toe transfer to reconstruct the thumb. Microsurgical transfer of toes or portions of toes to reconstruct hand defects has now become a routine procedure in hand surgery. Most of the other types of flaps described above can be reliably transferred microsurgically. Free tissue transfer allows the design of customised composite flaps without the constraints of loco-regional flap transfers. Successful free flap transfer requires careful planning of the most appropriate flap to reconstruct the defect. Of prime importance is selection of the recipient vascular axis; the operation is designed to ensure the microvascular anastomosis is done to the largest available vessels, thus maximising blood flow. Other factors such as keeping the patient warm, ensuring the patient has a good circulating volume, providing perioperative and postoperative analgesia where possible with regional anaesthesia are also important. Technical issues such as ensuring atraumatic dissection and vessel handling, avoiding tension and kinking of vascular pedicles and gentle irrigation of the vessel lumen with heparinised solutions are essential.

Experienced teams can expect success rates in excess of 95 per cent for most free tissue transfers, placing it amongst the most reliable of techniques. Flap failure is best detected by regular observation of the flap by experienced individuals. If there is any doubt the patient must be rapidly returned to theatre and the microvascular anastomoses inspected. Prompt re-exploration will usually salvage a failing flap.

Tissue expansion

A recent addition to the reconstructive surgeon's options is tissue expansion. Here, a silicone balloon is placed beneath the planned donor site. The balloon is then inflated by percutaneous injections of saline over several weeks in order to increase the area of the expanded flap. It is then possible at a second operation to remove the silicone balloon and utilise the expanded tissue. Tissue expansion has the advantage of creating large flaps of tissue at sites where this might otherwise be impossible. Where expansion is done adjacent to a defect, the flap will often have ideal properties to reconstruct that defect. It can often be transferred by simple techniques, and sensation can be preserved. Often the donor site can be closed directly if sufficient tissue has been created.

Skin lesions

The skin is the largest organ of the body, with a surface area of between 10 000 and 18 000 cm^2 in the average adult, accounting for approximately 15 per cent of the total body weight. The multiple functions of the skin allow humans to adapt to a wide variety of environmental conditions. An important aspect of the function of skin is that of protecting deeper structures. It also has an important role in thermoregulation, metabolism (vitamin D production), immunological defence, a sensory interface with our surroundings and a psychological expression of an individual to their surroundings. The skin as an organ is vulnerable to a wide variety of diseases and conditions. Ageing is accompanied by a loss of elasticity and wrinkling. Degenerative changes result from excessive exposure to ultraviolet radiation and environmental factors. Reactions to chemicals and drugs are also common, and the skin is probably susceptible to more different types of tumours than any other organ. Lesions arise from any of the structures that are present in the skin.

Skin infections

Staphylococcal infections

Most skin infections are staphylococcal and relatively minor. They will settle with no specific treatment; topical antiseptics may be used or systemic antibiotics if the infection does not settle or spreads. Patients with unexplained infections should be checked for diabetes mellitus. The sensitivity of the organisms is determined so that the appropriate antibiotic can be chosen should the need arise. Incision and drainage are indicated when pus is present. If severe, lymphangitis or cellulitis can develop. Various clinical presentations exist.

Boil (syn. furuncle) is an infection of a pilosebaceous unit with perifolliculitis, which usually proceeds to suppuration and central necrosis. A 'blind boil' is one that subsides without suppuration. Boils are common on the face, head and neck. Boils are frequently associated with overwork, worry, debility or other undermining influences. They may be the presenting symptom of diabetes mellitus.

Furunculosis of the external auditory meatus is extremely painful, as the skin is attached to the underlying cartilage, and swelling is accompanied by considerable tension.

Stye (syn. hordeolum) is due to infection of an eyelash follicle. Should softening occur around a hair follicle, particularly an eyelash, removal of the hair allows the pus to escape.

Carbuncle[4] is an infective gangrene of the subcutaneous tissues, which often occurs in the nape of the neck. The subcutaneous tissues become painful and indurated, and the overlying skin is red (Fig. 13.9). Unless the condition is aborted by prompt treatment, extension will occur and, after a few days, areas of softening appear, the skin sloughs and discharges pus. Usually there is one central large slough, surrounded by a 'rosette' of smaller areas of necrosis. The general treatment and organism identification are similar to those described for boils. Many carbuncles are aborted if antibiotics are used adequately in the early stages.

Impetigo is an intradermal infection (Fig. 13.10). The primary lesion is bullous, and soon ruptures to form an erosion and then a crust. The

[4] *'Carbunculus' in Latin, 'anthrax' in Greek, is the word for charcoal. The ancients saw in these conditions burning sores upon the skin – hence they likened them to glowing coal.*

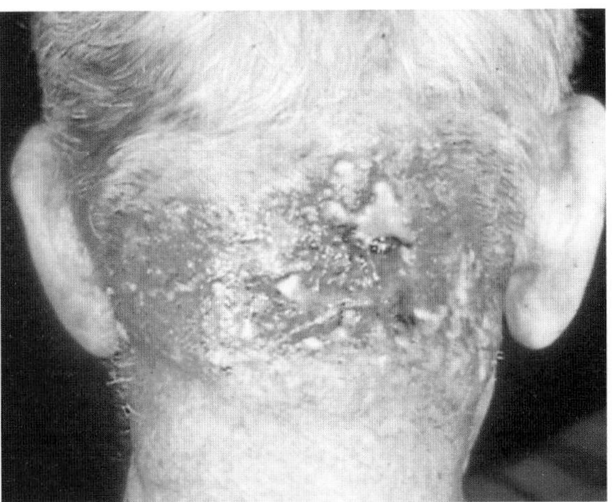

Fig. 13.9 Carbuncle of the neck (*courtesy of Herbert Bourns, Bristol*).

infection is contagious, and in rugby football one player so infected can spread the disease among team mates and the opposing side (the condition being known as scrumpox). Treatment is by careful washing of the face to remove crusts using chlorhexidine soap and lotion (1 per cent); systemic antibiotics are used in those cases that are resistant to local treatment.

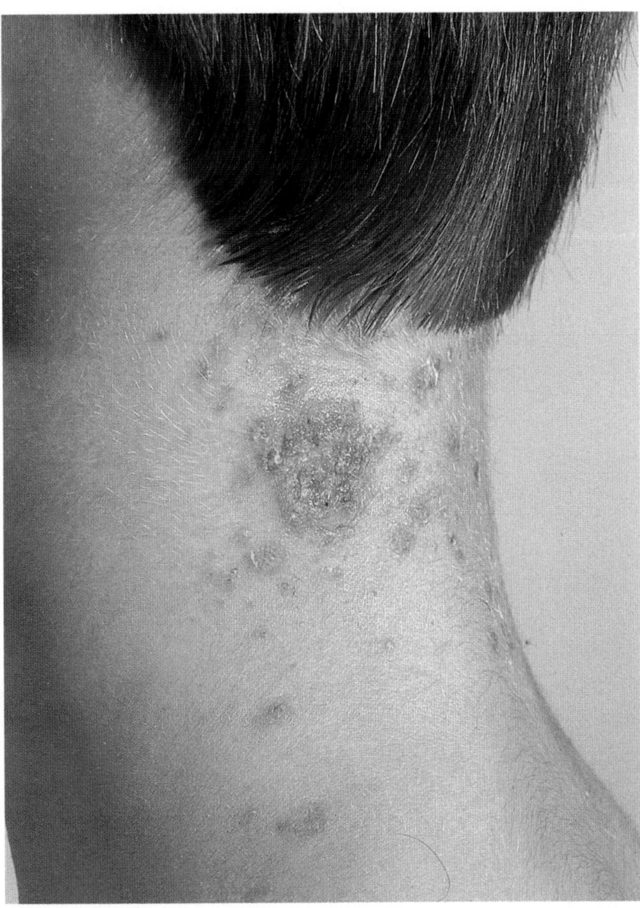

Fig. 13.10 Impetigo on the neck of a 9-year-old boy (*courtesy of Edward Coleman, Oxford*).

Necrotising fasciitis (syn. Meleney's streptococcal gangrene, Fournier's gangrene)

Necrotising fasciitis is a destructive invasive infection of skin, subcutaneous tissue and deep fascia, with relative sparing of muscle. Bacteriology can be *polymicrobial* involving a synergistic combination of anaerobes and facultative species such as coliforms or nongroup A streptococci; or *monomicrobial* due to group A beta-haemolytic streptococci. Common sites are the genitalia, groins and lower abdomen (Fig. 13.11a), although necrotising fasciitis has been reported at almost any site. Patients are unwell, febrile, with areas of subcutaneous induration and erythema; surgical emphysema is palpable if gas-forming organisms are involved; necrotic patches of skin develop. Treatment is by wide surgical excision of all affected soft tissues; very large defects can be

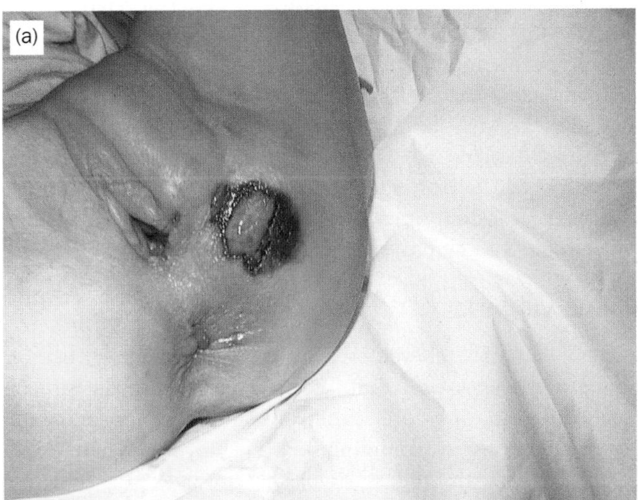

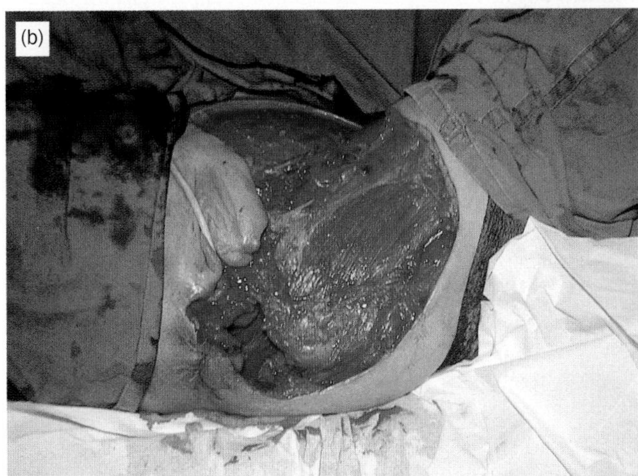

Fig. 13.11 (a) Necrotising fasciitis of the buttock arising in association with a rectal carcinoma that had perforated into the ischiorectal fossa. There was widespread surgical emphysema. (b) Following excision of all affected soft tissues a large defect was created.

Frank Lamont Meleney, 1889–1963. Professor of Clinical Surgery, Columbia University, New York, USA.

Jean Alfred Fournier, 1832–1914. Dermatologist in Paris, France.

created (Fig. 13.11b). Antibiotics and supportive therapy are also administered. Mortality is high and is increased if surgical treatment is delayed or insufficiently radical. Necrotising fasciitis can arise without any history of injury, but can also follow operations or more localised infections. Risk factors for the development of this condition include diabetes mellitus, malnutrition, obesity, corticosteroid drugs and immune deficiency.

Hydradenitis suppurativa

Hydradenitis suppurativa (apocrinitis) is a chronic cicatrising suppurative process caused by apocrine gland hyperplasia (Fig. 13.12). It is common in the second and third decades of life and three times more common in women than men. It occurs most commonly in the axilla, but can also affect the groins and perineum. Locally, duct obstruction from keratin plugging occurs leading to rupture of apocrine glands into the dermis and subdermal tissues with subsequent superimposed infection. Pain can be severe. A course of metronidazole has been found to be useful owing to the fact that *Bacteroides* is a common causative organism; a prolonged course of erythromycin can be curative. If the condition does not respond, then surgical excision is necessary. If a wide area of skin needs to be removed, the wound needs to be covered by a split-skin graft.

Lupus vulgaris

Lupus vulgaris (tuberculosis of the skin) usually occurs between the ages of 10 and 25, the face being the site of election. One or more cutaneous nodules appear, with congestion of the surrounding skin (Fig. 13.13). When blood is expressed with a glass slide, the brownish (apple-jelly) nodules of individual tubercles can be seen. Extension occurs very slowly, but ulceration is likely to follow sooner or later. The resulting ulcer tends to heal in one situation as it extends to another. The mucous membranes of the mouth and nose are sometimes attacked, either primarily or by extension from the face. Oedema occurs if the fibrosis caused by the lupus obstructs the normal lymphatic drainage. Infection in the nasal cavity may be followed by necrosis of underlying cartilage. Treatment is with anti-tuberculous chemotherapy; the lesion should be excised if healing is slow. Squamous cell carcinoma is prone to occur in a lupus scar (Fig. 13.14).

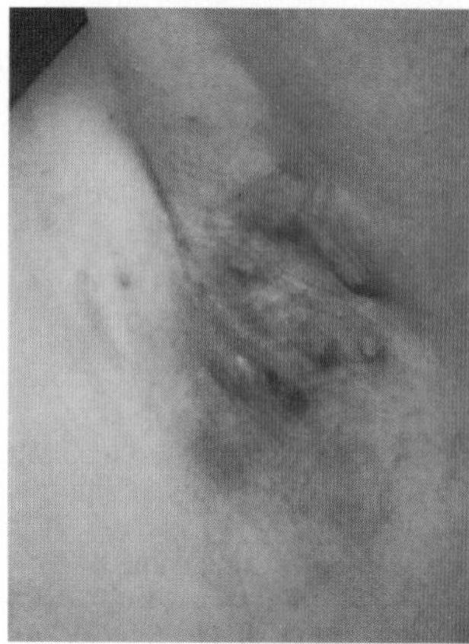

Fig. 13.12 Hydradenitis infection of axillary sweat glands and hair follicles.

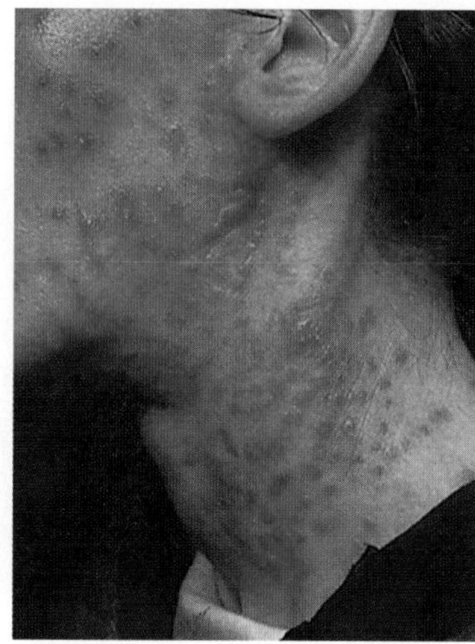

Fig. 13.13 Lupus vulgaris.

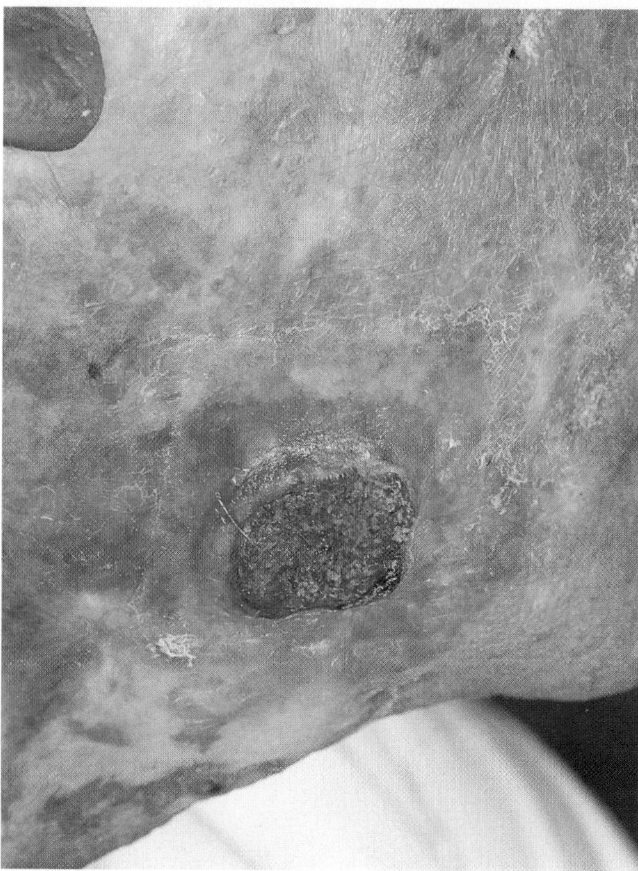

Fig. 13.14 Squamous cell carcinoma arising in scarred skin following lupus vulgaris.

Cysts

Epidermoid cyst[5] (syn. sebaceous cyst, wen)

These cysts contain keratin and its breakdown products, surrounded by a wall of stratified squamous keratinising epithelium (the commonly used term *sebaceous cyst* is incorrect – these cysts only rarely have associated sebaceous glands and do not contain sebum). Epidermoid cysts often have a punctum. They are inherited in an autosomal dominant fashion. The common sites are the face, neck, shoulders and chest, areas favoured by acne vulgaris. Lesions may be solitary but are commonly multiple. They enlarge slowly and may become inflamed and tender from time to time. Suppuration may occur. The contents of an infected cyst become semi-liquid and usually very foetid. Recurrent infective episodes cause the cyst wall to become adherent to surrounding subcutaneous tissue, and consequently more difficult to remove. If ulceration occurs it can resemble squamous cell carcinoma to which the term 'Cock's peculiar tumour' may be applied (Fig. 13.15). The contents of a cyst sometimes escape slowly from the duct orifice and dry in successive layers on the skin, forming a 'sebaceous horn' (Fig. 13.16). Treatment is by surgical excision (except if inflamed, when it is better incised and drained). This can be performed under local anaesthesia; an ellipse of skin including the punctum is removed with the cyst. Unless the wall is completely removed, recurrence is likely.

Pilar cysts

Pilar cysts are usually multiple and occur on the scalp, and they have no punctum. Histologically, their lining is similar to the external root sheath of the hair follicle.

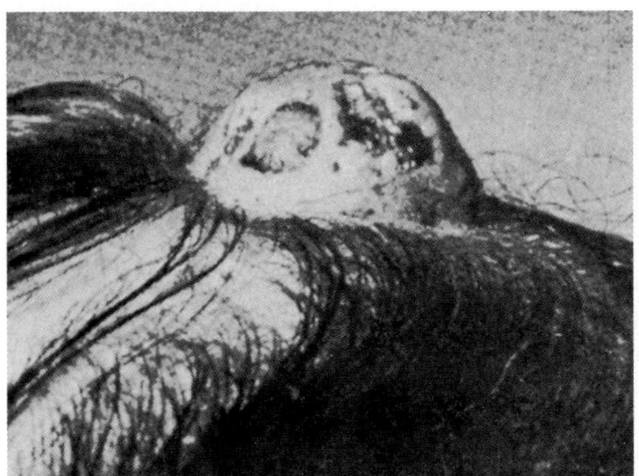

Fig. 13.15 Cock's 'peculiar tumour' (an infected, ulcerated sebaceous cyst).

[5]*Sir Astley Paston Cooper, 1768–1841. Surgeon, Guy's Hospital, London, England (1800–25). In 1821 he received a Baronetcy and one thousand guineas for successfully removing an infected sebaceous cyst from the head of King George IV.*
Edward Cock, 1805–92. Surgeon, Guy's Hospital, London, England.

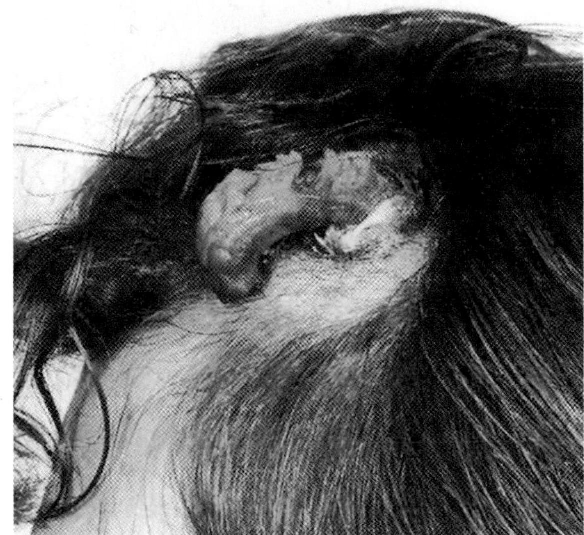

Fig. 13.16 Sebaceous horn of the scalp.

Implantation dermoids

Implantation dermoids may result from deep implantation of a fragment of epidermis by a penetrating injury. Traumatic inclusion cysts usually appear on the palmar or plantar surfaces of the hands, or on the buttocks or knees.

Callosities, corns and warts

Callosity (French: 'callosite') is a localised thickened or hardened part of skin which is an acquired, superficial, circumscribed, yellow–white, flat, thickened patch of hyperkeratotic material. They occur at the regions of pressure or friction on the hands and feet and they are usually not painful. They are commonly occupational, occurring, for instance, on a gardener's hands. There is no need for treatment, although paring may be necessary and should be carried out by a fully trained chiropodist.

Corn (Old French: *corn* = grain) is a horny induration of the cuticle with a hard centre, caused by undue pressure, chiefly affecting toes and feet. They are circumscribed, horny thickenings, cone-like in shape with their apex pointing inwards and their base on the surface. They occur at sites of frictional pressure and usually will spontaneously disappear when the aetiological factor is removed. Skilled treatment is important in patients with diabetes or with a poor peripheral circulation when a secondary infection may precipitate gangrene.

Wart (Old English: *wearte*) is a dry, rough excrescence on the skin (Fig. 13.17). It is a virus-induced tumour that undergoes spontaneous resolution. Transmission is by direct or intimate contact, the virus material usually being inoculated through an abrasion. It is well recognised that patients with immune deficiencies develop widespread resistant warts. They tend to occur on sites of trauma, such as the beard area, hands, genital region and feet. All warts first appear as small, smooth nodules often more easily palpable than seen. Warts are more common in children and young adults, but can be present at any age, causing pain and even difficulty in mobility. Plantar warts occur on the sole and are usually multiple. They may be so tender as to render standing or walking exceedingly uncomfortable. Treatment ranges from folk remedies to sophisticated modern techniques, but the important factor remains that there is no 100 per cent cure. Surgical removal is contraindicated as it leads to scarring

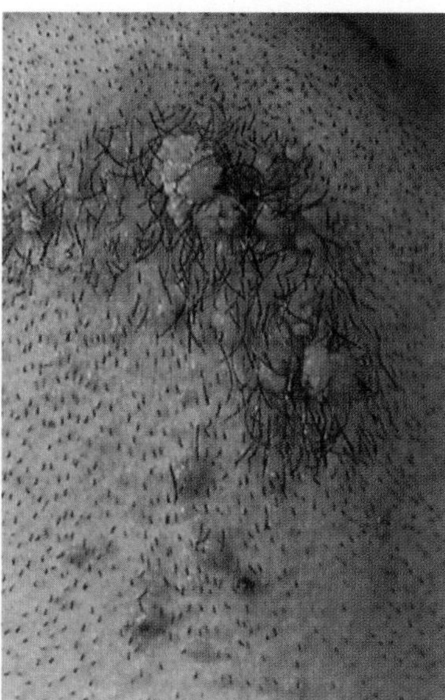

Fig. 13.17 Cutaneous warts.

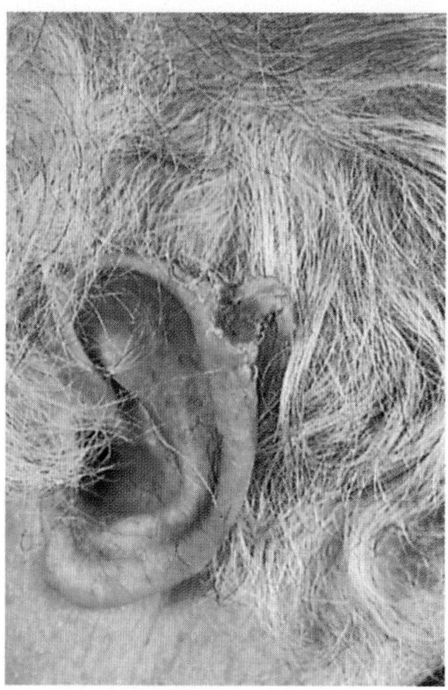

Fig. 13.18 Keratin horn of the ear.

and recurrences are frequent. Curettage and diathermy give excellent results, as does cryotherapy, but the latter is often accompanied by pain. The irritant 50 per cent podophyllin in liquid paraffin gives good results. Use of liquid nitrogen is probably easier and is more effective. Recalcitrant lesions may respond to 585-nm pulsed dye laser irradiation.

Venereal warts and moist warts (papillomata acuminata) occur in the genital region.

Herpes simplex is a viral skin infection that is recurrent in about 1 per cent of the population. An immunosuppressed patient may show dissemination with viraemia and may become seriously ill, requiring treatment with acyclovir infusions. Topical or oral acyclovir is available for the treatment of localised disease.

Orf is caused by the virus that produces pustular dermatitis in sheep. Those infected will have been in contact with sheep in one form or another. The lesions are usually single but may be multiple. The initial lesion is a dusky red papule that enlarges to 1–2 cm in diameter and then resembles a large domed pustule. This is a self-limiting condition that resolves in 5–8 weeks.

Benign growths

Congenital naevi

Congenital (verrucous, epidermal) naevi[6] are common entities which may be single or multiple, and appear at birth or in early childhood. They are warty growths of brownish colour, but large horny excrescences may be present.

Keratin horn (Fig. 13.18)

This is also seen in old people and is a papilloma with excess keratin formation.

[6]*Naevus (Latin) = a birthmark but often used to mean simply a mark or blemish on the skin.*

Seborrhoeic keratosis (basal cell papilloma, seborrhoeic wart or senile wart)

This is a benign tumour caused by overgrowth of epidermal keratinocytes. They are frequently pigmented and often develop in large numbers on the trunk, face and arms of persons in or past middle life and are most common in the elderly. Seborrhoeic keratoses are very common in Caucasians and often are not mentioned by the patient, being accepted as harmless and part of the inevitable ageing process. Both sexes are equally affected. Usually they look like a verrucous plaque stuck on the epidermis, varying from dirty yellow to black and have loosely adherent, greasy keratin on the surface. They are usually ovoid, measuring from 1 mm to several centimetres. An eruption of seborrhoeic warts may be preceded by an inflammatory dermatosis. The superficial type has to be distinguished from simple and malignant lentigo. The domed pigmented variety may resemble a melanoma, especially if it is inflamed. However, with local antibacterial treatment and protection from injury, it returns to its normal state after a few days. If the lesions are asymptomatic removal is not required. Where treatment is indicated shave excision or curettage and diathermy leaves a flat surface that covers with normal epithelium in 1 week. Cryosurgery is also successful.

Dermatofibroma (sclerosing angioma, histiocytoma, fibroma simplex, subepidermal nodular fibrosis)

This occurs in skin as firm, indolent, single or multiple nodules. Some follow minor trauma or insect bites, which may have acted as a trigger to this tissue reaction. It may possibly be a tumour of the dermal dendrocyte. In adults, the nodules are situated most commonly on the extremities, occurring in both sexes of all age groups after puberty (Fig.

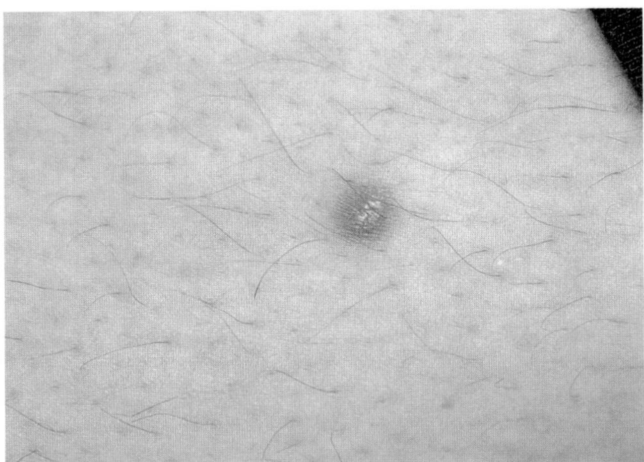

Fig. 13.19 Dermatofibroma on the lower limb.

13.19). They usually present as a small, well-defined nodule that may or may not be elevated above the surface of the skin. It is hard, button-like and freely mobile over the underlying tissues that touch the epidermis. They often itch, vary in size and are frequently pigmented. Excision is only recommended for symptomatic nodules.

Molluscum fibrosum

Molluscum[7] fibrosum are polypoid or filiform soft fleshy skin tags that occur on the neck, trunk and face. They are frequently found together with seborrhoeic warts. They are always pedunculated and frequently constricted at their base. They are round, soft, elastic and frequently pigmented. Treatment is by excision or cautery.

Pilomatrixoma

Pilomatrixoma (calcifying epithelioma of Malherbe) is a benign hair-follicle-derived tumour. These are solitary, hard tumours that appear to be growing from the deep surface of the skin. They occur mostly on the face (Fig. 13.20), neck and arms. The size usually varies between 0.5 and 3 cm in diameter. The tumour may arise at any age but 60–80 per cent occur in the first two decades. Clinically, it resembles a rather hard epidermoid cyst.

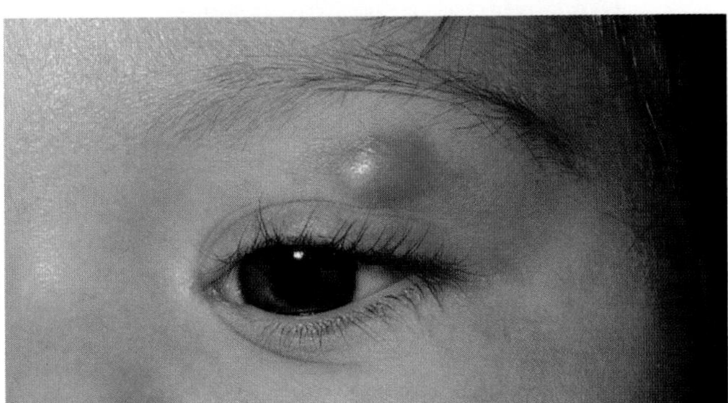

Fig. 13.20 Pilomatrixoma on left upper lid of a child.

Sebaceous adenoma

Isolated lesions are very rare. Multiple sebaceous adenomas occur in association with epilepsy in the condition tuberose sclerosis.

Cylindroma

Cylindroma (syn. 'turban' tumour) is so called from the arrangement of the stroma in peculiar transparent cylinders, which are thought to be of apocrine origin. The tumour gradually forms an extensive, turban-like swelling extending over the scalp (Fig. 13.21). Ulceration is uncommon and the tumour is relatively benign. Cryotherapy may control the progression of this condition.

Rhinophyma (syn. potato nose) (Fig. 13.22)

This is a glandular form of acne rosacea. The skin of the nose, particularly the distal part, becomes immensely thickened and the openings of the sebaceous follicles are easily seen. The capillaries become dilated and the nose assumes a bluish-red colour. Surgical treatment, by paring away the excess tissue, gives a great improvement. Rarely, basal cell carcinomas are associated with this lesion.

Sarcoid (Boecks)

This is a generalised disease that may affect skin. In the skin it occurs as reddish-brown nodules which are soft and rarely ulcerate. Giant cells are found, but tubercule bacilli can never be isolated.

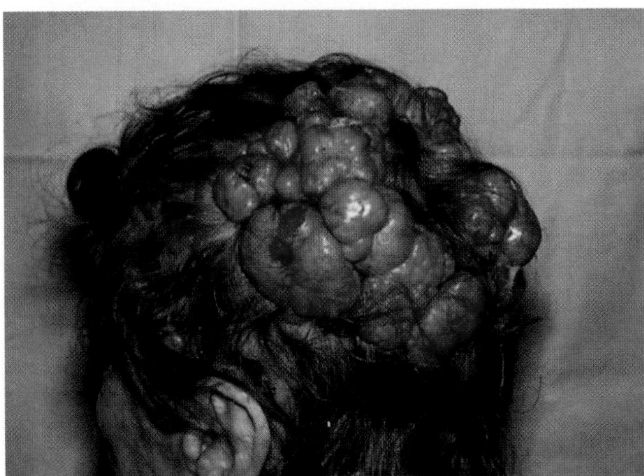

Fig. 13.21 Cylindroma (turban tumour).

[7]*Mollusc (Latin:* molluscus *= soft) = a soft protuberance on the skin.*

Albert Malherbe, 1845–1915. Professor of Pathological Anatomy and Histology, Nantes, France.

Caesar Boeck, 1845–1917. Norwegian dermatologist.

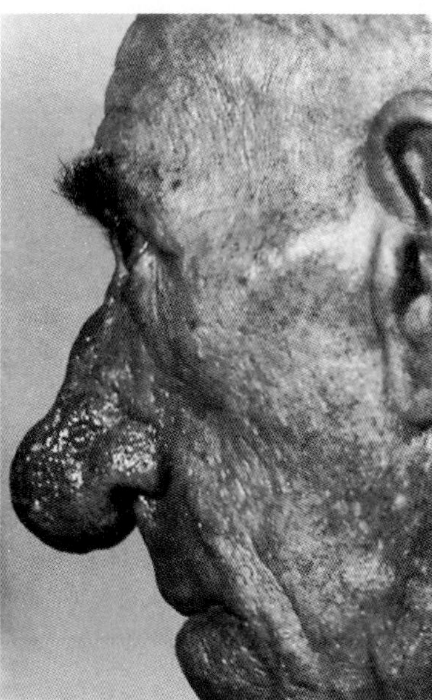

Fig. 13.22 Rhinophyma.

Cutaneous horns (Bland-Sutton)

These may be sebaceous horns (Fig. 13.16), wart or corn horns (Fig. 13.23), cicatrix horns (Fig. 13.24) or nail horns.

Vascular anomalies

Many different and confusing terms have been used to describe vascular lesions. Mulliken and Glowacki's classification based on endothelial characteristics, helps in diagnosis, planning, management and predicting the course of these lesions. This classification has three major categories:

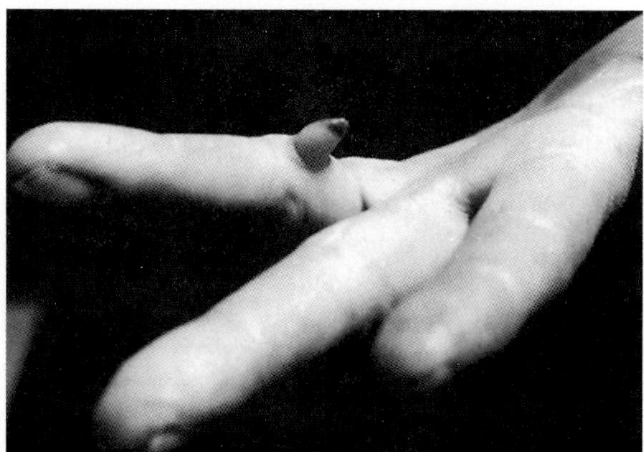

Fig. 13.23 Horn of a corn (*courtesy of Dr Sheetal Singh, Srinagar, Kashmir, India*).

Sir John Bland-Sutton, 1855–1936. Surgeon, The Middlesex Hospital, London, England, and President of the Royal College of Surgeons, classified horns in 1911.

Professor John B. Mulliken. The Children's Hospital, Harvard Medical School, Boston, Massachusetts, USA

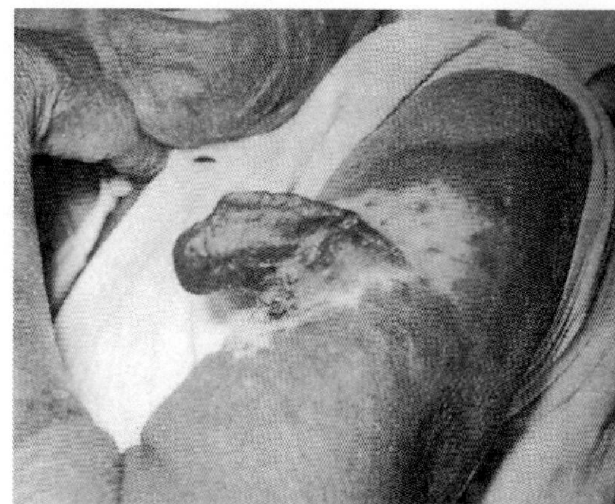

Fig. 13.24 A cicatrix horn in a burn scar (*courtesy of R.R. Deskmukh, Dhautoli, Nagpur, India*).

- haemangiomas: show endothelial hyperplasia;
- malformations: have normal endothelial turnover;
- ectasias: have normal endothelial turnover, but also have vascular dilatation.

Haemangioma (Fig. 13.25)

These are the most common tumours of infancy and have a typical history. The baby is normal at birth and at the age of 1–3 weeks is noted to have a red mark. This increases rapidly for some weeks or even up to 3 months, until the typical 'strawberry' or raspberry-like swelling is present. Clinically, the sign of emptying may be demonstrable. The lesion is composed of immature vasoformative tissue. The subcutaneous tissue as well as the skin is often involved, and

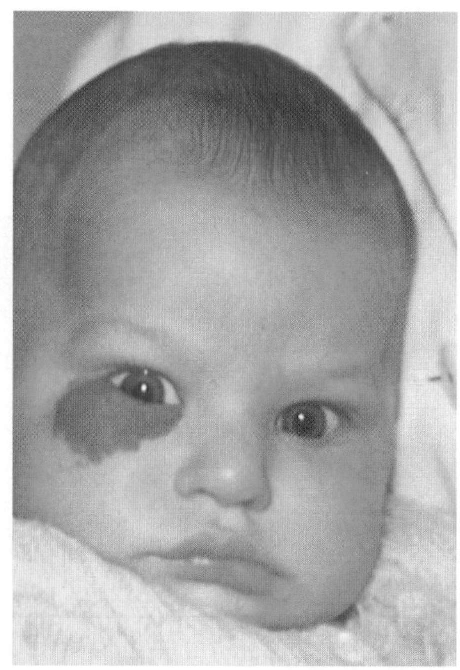

Fig. 13.25 Haemangioma.

in severe cases the muscles may be affected. From the age of 3 months to 1 year the haemangioma grows with the child, and then it ceases to grow. Eventually the colour fades and flattening occurs so that at the age of 9 years 90 per cent demonstrate complete involution. Bleeding is rarely a problem and responds to local pressure. Ulceration occurs in about 5 per cent of the cases, particularly in those areas that are commonly abraded, e.g. lips and perineum. Wound care will prevent infection and promote re-epithelialisation. Pulsed dye laser therapy has also been used to promote the involution of the superficial vessels. Visual obstruction from periorbital haemangiomas (Fig. 13.26) can result in amblyopia or anismetropia if total visual obstruction occurs for more than a week in the first year. Nasopharyngeal obstruction may cause obstruction in infants who are obligate nose breathers. Auditory canal obstruction is seen occasionally with lesions affecting the parotid gland. Intervention should be considered in bilateral conditions which last beyond 1 year of age.

Kasabach–Merritt syndrome occurs owing to platelet trapping within the lesions. Congestive cardiac failure with multiple cutaneous haemangiomas or large visceral haemangiomas results from dilated vessels and arteriovenous shunting. Skeletal distortion and cosmetic deformities in the form of telangectasias, hypopigmentation and contour abnormalities have been observed. The final result (Fig. 13.27) is better if natural involution is allowed to occur rather than if an attempt is made to hasten regression by any operative or physical methods. Many interventions are possible and should be considered only in special circumstances. Intralesional and oral steroids have been demonstrated to produce involution of these lesions. Surgical debulking and laser photocoagulation – both superficially and intralesionally – have also been used. Radiation therapy carries a high risk of disturbance of growth and is dangerous.

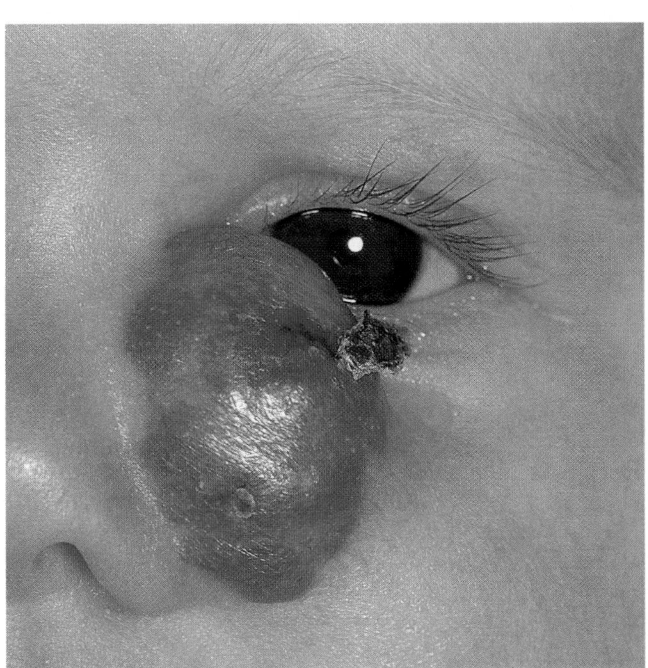

Fig. 13.26 Periorbital haemangioma beginning to encroach on the visual field.

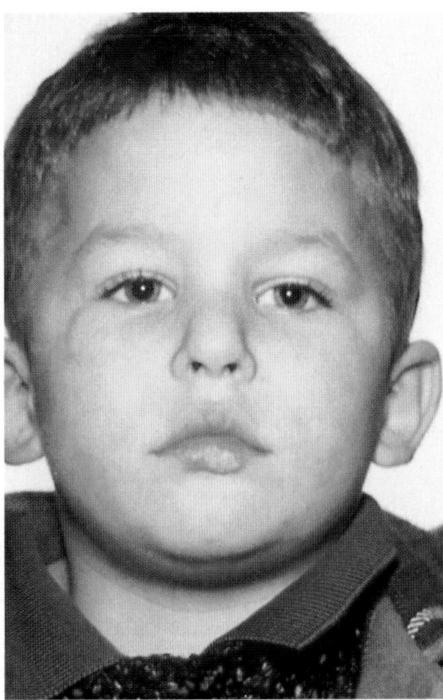

Fig. 13.27 Haemangioma, same case as Fig. 13.25 with conservative treatment after 7 years.

Vascular malformations

These are structural and morphological anomalies due to faulty embryological morphogenesis. The lesions are present at birth, grow commensurate with the child and do not regress. They can lead to underlying soft tissue or bony hypertrophy, nodular development and discoloration as a consequence of blood vessel ectasia with age. The natural history of these lesions is determined by their haemodynamic and lymphodynamic characteristics.

- High-flow lesions include arterial malformations and arteriovenous malformations (arterial plexiform angiomas, cirsoid aneurysm).
- Low-flow lesions include lymphatic (LM) venous (VM) and capillary (CM – port-wine stain). Frequently these lesions combine arterial, venous and lymphatic elements.

Port-wine stains

Port-wine stains (Fig. 13.28) are intradermal capillary malformations that change very little throughout life, although the colour may alter a little and they may become nodular in some areas. Treatment is for reason of appearance. Treatment of choice for these lesions is the use of the pulsed tunable dye laser.

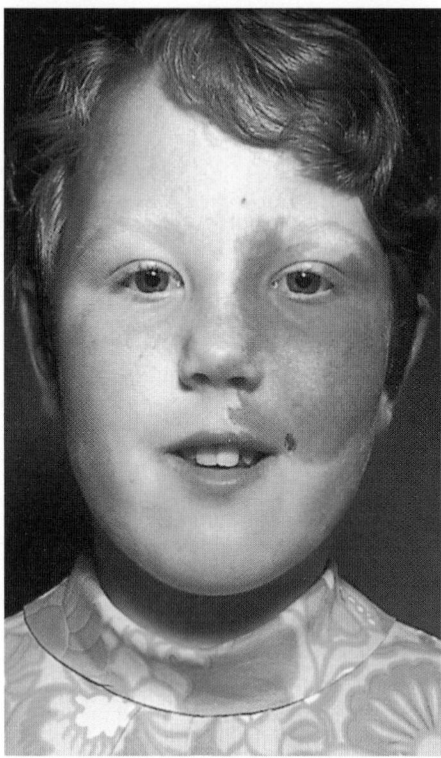

Fig. 13.28 Port-wine stain.

Glomus tumours

Glomus tumours, frequently in the subungal regions, represent arteriovenous anastomoses (Suquet–Hoyer canals). They are frequently removed because of the pain and to obtain a diagnosis.

Ectasias

These represent acquired lesions such as telangectasias (spider naevus). Lesions on the lower extremities are venular (thread veins); however, facial telangiectasia is mostly due to arteriolar vasodilatation. Lower extremity lesions respond to either microsclerotherapy or laser photocoagulation. Those on the face can be treated by photothermolysis using a pulsed dye laser.

Miscellaneous vascular lesions

Pyogenic granuloma

Pyogenic granulomas (Fig. 13.29) are common acquired, reactive, proliferative vascular lesions of the skin and mucous membranes, arising after minor trauma. The lesion looks like a haemangioma, but has a typical natural history. Usually single, it consists of a red, soft or moderately firm, more or less pedunculated nodule that grows rapidly to a size varying from 0.5 to 2.0 cm in diameter. Most commonly it is seen on the face, the fingers and toes. Treatment is excision.

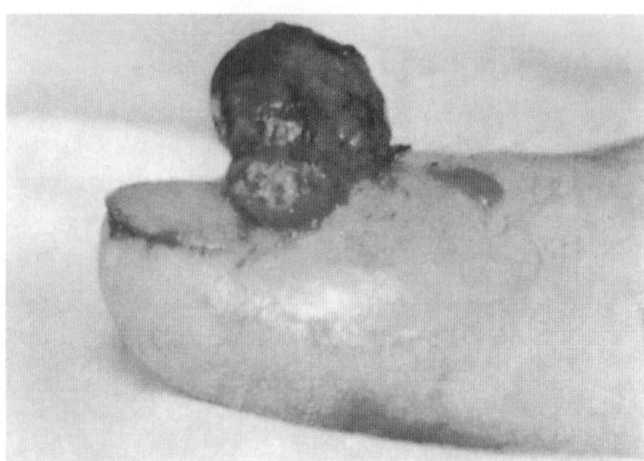

Fig. 13.29 Pyogenic granuloma. The surface shows atrophic epidermis, but often has crusts.

Macular stains

Macular stains (salmon patch, also called 'stork bites'; not to be confused with the 'patch' in syphilis) are present at birth over the forehead in the midline, and over the occiput. They disappear by the age of 1 year and so may represent a physiological process rather than a pathological lesion.

Benign pigmented lesions

Simple melanocytic tumours

The melanocyte is generally believed to be derived from the neural crest. In normal skin, melanocytes appear as clear cells in the basal layer of the epidermis. They may become increased in number in the layers of the skin to form benign pigmented naevi (moles) which include:

- lentigo, which are present within the basal layer of the epidermis;
- junctional naevi, which occur as localised aggregations projecting into the dermis;
- dermal naevi, which occur entirely within the dermis;
- compound naevi, which show the features of both the junctional and dermal naevi.

These simple melanocytic tumours may arise anywhere in the skin including the nail bed. They are seen occasionally in the conjunctiva of the eye, but are rare in other mucous membranes. Pigmented naevi may occur at any age but commonly appear in childhood and adolescence as small, brown, flat or slightly raised lesions in the skin. These are usually of junctional or compound type, but with increasing age they either atrophy or mature into dermal naevi. One or more melanocytic naevi are present in over 95 per cent of white adults. Naevi on the palms, soles and genitalia have an evil reputation as they were thought at one time to be especially prone to become malignant but, in fact, site is not a risk factor.

The **blue naevus** (Fig. 13.30) is a tumour of dermal melanocytes and occurs most commonly on the face, on the

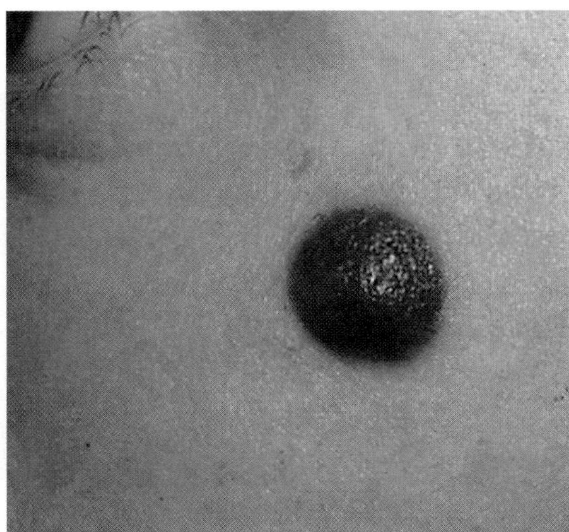

Fig. 13.30 Blue naevus of the face.

dorsum of the hands and feet, and over the sacrum in certain races (Mongolian blue spot). It is very darkly pigmented and because of its overlying layer of normal, although sometimes thinned, epidermis, looks shiny and blue or slate-grey in colour. Malignant change is exceptionally rare. Congenital naevi are rare. They are often darkly pigmented and may be hairy and papillary in appearance (Fig. 13.31). Occasionally, they cover extensive areas of skin, up to 25 per cent or more of the body surface. They may undergo malignant change even during childhood. With this exception, naevi are virtually always benign before puberty. Treatment may be indicated for cosmetic reasons, if by reason of its position the lesion is subject to the nuisance of repeated trauma, e.g. cut when shaving or rubbed by clothing. Although there is no evidence that trauma causes malignant change, if the history suggests that malignant change has occurred (see below under Malignant melanoma), surgical excision is the only acceptable treatment; all lesions must be sent for histological examination.

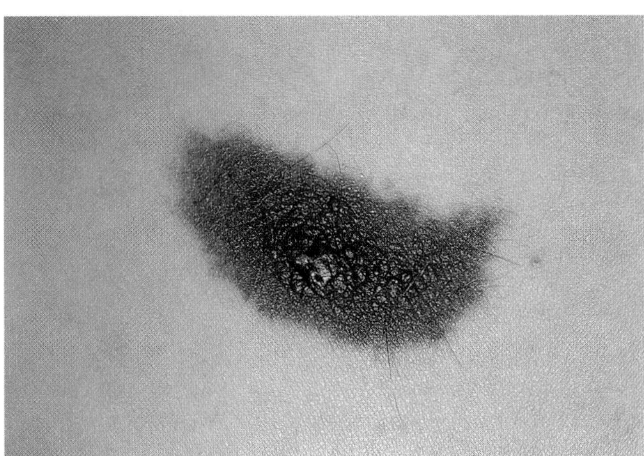

Fig. 13.31 Congenital naevus.

Café-au-lait macules are light-brown flat macules that are often apparent at birth. They are present as solitary lesions, or in increased numbers in syndromes such as neurofibromatosis and Albright's syndrome.

Premalignant lesions

Actinic keratoses

Actinic keratoses (senile keratoses, solar keratoses) are areas of epidermal dysplasia giving rise to cutaneous scaling, usually observed in sun-exposed fair skin. These lesions are potentially malignant. Superficial lesions are best removed by rapid and even freezing with carbon dioxide or liquid nitrogen on a cotton wool bud. Diathermy preceded by curettage of horny lesions is equally effective, but more likely to leave superficial scarring. Indurated lesions are best excised. Multiple lesions may clear with topical 5-fluorouracil cream. An effective sunscreen is important as improvement follows avoidance of sunlight, which is also important prophylactically. Radiotherapy should not be used for solar keratoses.

Bowen's disease

Bowen's disease is an intraepidermal squamous cell carcinoma that is potentially malignant and appears as a persistent, progressive, usually flat, red, scaly or crusted plaque (Fig. 13.32). It is more frequently seen in the elderly. It is triggered mainly by solar radiation, but if those keratoses with Bowen's features are separated off, the cause most frequently found is arsenic ingestion. Most patients are

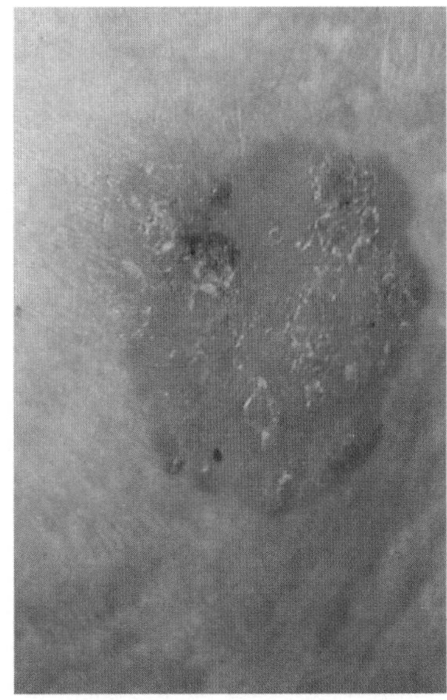

Fig. 13.32 Bowen's disease.

John Templeton Bowen, 1857–1940. Professor of Dermatology, Harvard Medical School, Boston, Massachusetts, USA. Described precancerous dermatosis in 1912.

unaware of having been exposed to arsenic as its presence in a mixture taken medically may have been concealed from them or forgotten. The rate of transformation of Bowen's disease to invasive squamous cell carcinoma is still disputed. Untreated, 3–5 per cent of patients will develop an invasive squamous cell carcinoma. The possibility of a viral cause of Bowen's disease has been postulated. The lesions most likely to be mistaken for Bowen's disease are solar keratoses, psoriasis, multifocal (superficial) basal cell carcinoma and squamous cell carcinoma. If the diagnosis is uncertain on the first examination, the lack of improvement when steroids are applied is suggestive of Bowen's disease. Distinction from the flat type of solar keratosis may be impossible clinically. A biopsy may be necessary to establish a diagnosis. Locally destructive therapy such as cryotherapy or curettage and cauterisation is often used. Recurrence may be due to inadequate treatment of the superficial tumour or failure to destroy deeper extensions down appendage structures such as hair follicles. Radiotherapy, if used, has to be in full tumour doses. Chemotherapy with local cytotoxic agents such as 5-fluorouracil can be applied to small lesions with good effect. Surgical excision is the best treatment if the lesion is not too large.

Erythroplasia of Querat

Erythroplasia of Querat describes Bowen's of the glans penis. It occurs most commonly in uncircumcised males.

Radiodermatitis

This is an area of skin damaged by excessive exposure to X-irradiation. Early erythema occurs which goes on to desquamation and pigmentation. If the dose is very great ulceration may occur. Later atrophy, irregular hyperpigmentation, telangiectasia and hair loss occur. Eventually, squamous cell carcinoma may develop.

Chronic scars

A carcinoma which develops in a scar (Marjolin's ulcer) (Fig. 13.33) presents the following characteristics. It grows slowly, as the scar is relatively avascular. It is painless, as scar tissue contains no nerves. Secondary deposits do not occur in the regional lymph nodes as lymphatic vessels have been destroyed. If the ulcer invades normal tissue surrounding the scar, it extends at a normal rate, and lymph nodes are then liable to be involved.

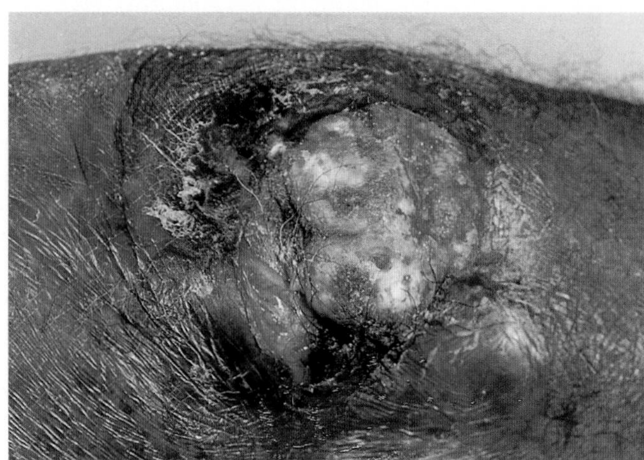

Fig. 13.33 Marjolin's ulcer. Malignant change 36 years after burns to the elbow.

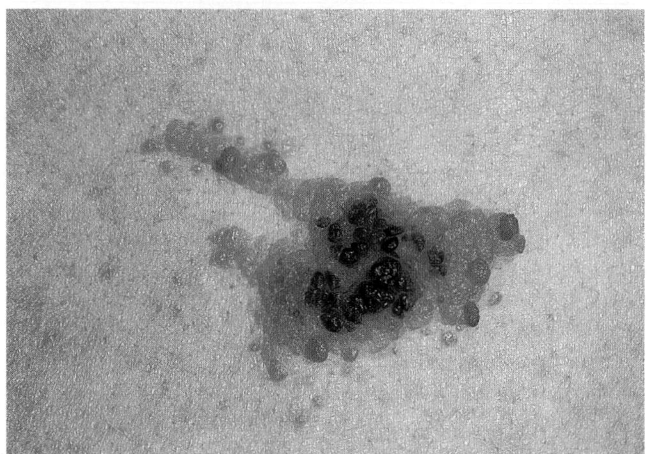

Fig. 13.34 Sebaceous naevus (of Jadassohn) on the back of a young female.

Sebaceous epidermal naevus

Sebaceous epidermal naevus (of Jadassohn, organoid naevus) (Fig. 13.34) is a common condition, frequently affecting the scalp. It initially appears as a raised papular yellow area, developing into a papillomatous area as the child matures. Up to 10 per cent of these may develop into basal cell carcinomas. Very rarely these develop into syringocystadenoma papilliferum – an anomaly of the apocrine gland. Treatment consists of complete excision.

Jean Nicolas Marjolin, 1780–1850. Surgeon, Paris, France. Described the development of carcinomatous ulcers in scars in 1828.

Porokeratosis

Porokeratosis (of Mibelli) is characterised by annular plaques with horny borders. About 13 per cent may transform into basal cell or squamous cell carcinomas.

Malignant lesions

Basal cell carcinoma

Basal cell carcinoma (BCC, rodent ulcer) is the commonest form of skin cancer and typically affects individuals between the ages of 40 and 79 years; more than 50 per cent are male and more than 85 per cent of these lesions occur in the head and neck region. These tumours are thought to originate

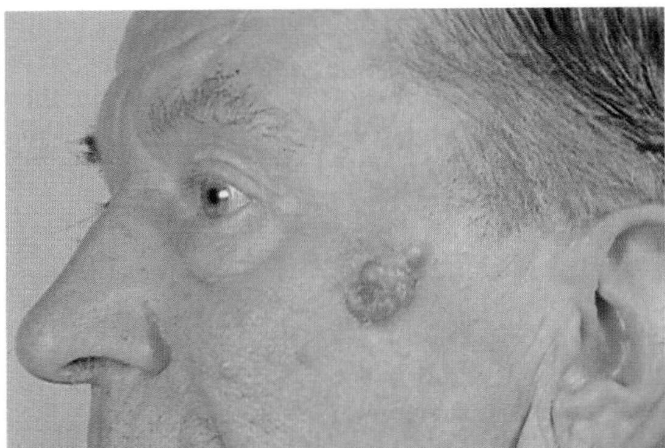

Fig. 13.35 Typical basal cell carcinoma.

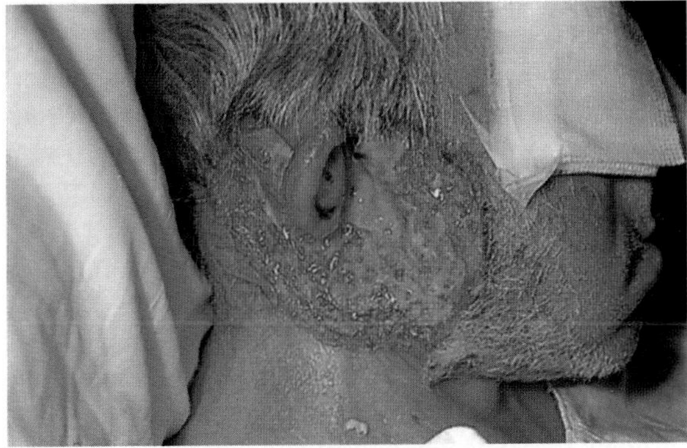

Fig. 13.36 Advanced BCC with massive local destruction.

from pluripotential epithelial cells of the epidermis and hair follicles. BCCs grow slowly, but become locally invasive and penetrate deeper tissues – hence the term rodent ulcer (Figs 13.35 and 13.36). Metastasis is rare. The patient gives a history of a 'spot' that fails to heal. Typically these tumours have a nodular appearance with a pearly rolled edge (which is apparent on stretching the skin) and telangiectatic vessels. Histologically, 26 different varieties of BCC have been described. However, clinically the following are recognised, in order of frequency:

- nodular: 50–54 per cent;
- superficial: 9–11 per cent;
- cystic: 4–8 per cent;
- pigmented: 6 per cent;
- morpheic: 2 per cent.

Several treatments are possible, as follows.

- Surgical excision – the treatment of choice with cure rates between 85 and 95 per cent.
- Electrodessication and curettage commonly used for small superficial lesions (2–5 mm in diameter) gives cure rates between 85 and 100 per cent.
- Radiotherapy. BCC is very radiosensitive and has an overall response of 92 per cent in selected patients. This is reserved for elderly patients who are not suitable for surgery or for specialised anatomical sites.
- Moh's micrographic surgery (chemosurgery) involving serial horizontal excision and mapping of the tumour. Usually reserved for recurrent lesions, tumours in difficult areas or those with indistinct borders (morpeaform).

Following complete excision it is unnecessary routinely to follow-up these patients unless they have a familial disposition for BCC formation (Gorlin's syndrome).

Squamous cell carcinoma

Squamous cell carcinoma (SCC) is a malignant tumour that arises in an area that has had some premalignant change. These tumours appear more inflammatory, feel more indurated and ulcerate sooner compared with BCC. The malphigian or squamous cell layer of the skin is implicated in the development of this cancer. There is a strong correlation with damage to the skin by the sun (Fig. 13.37a and b), and can be experimentally produced by ultraviolet light. Occasionally it arises as a complication of long-standing chronic granolas, such as syphilis, lupus vulgaris and leprosy, chronic ulcers, osteomyelitis, hidradenitis suppurativa, long-standing venous ulcers or old burn scars. Histologically, these tumours are characterised by invasive nests of cells showing variable central keratinisation and horn cell formation. There is no

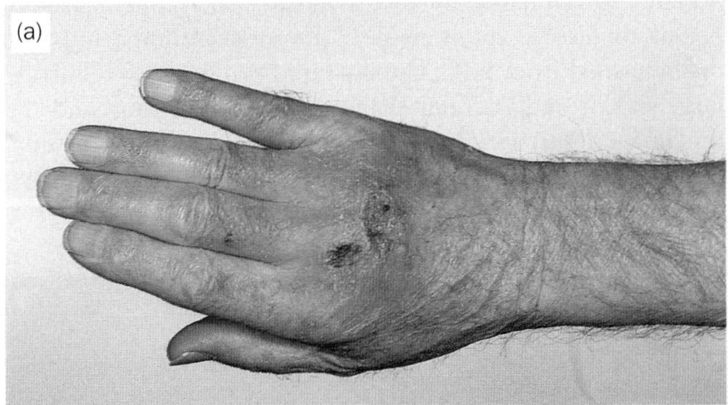

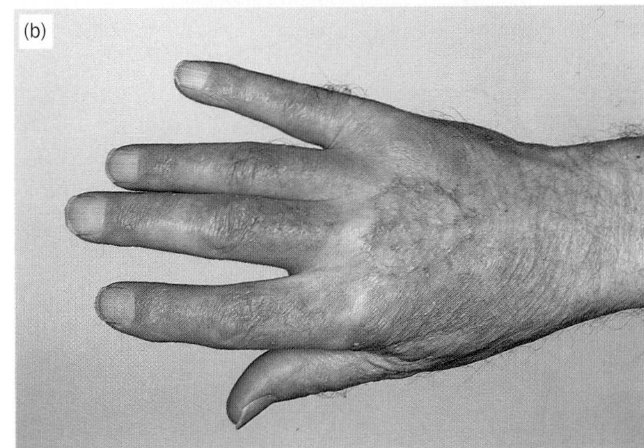

Fig. 13.37 (a) Squamous cell carcinoma on the dorsum of the hand (note actinic damage to surrounding skin). (b) Result following excision and reconstruction with a split thickness graft.

peripheral palisading as occurs in BCC. The cells vary from large, well-differentiated cells to completely anaplastic cells. Lesions of the ear and lip metastasise much earlier even when they are relatively well differentiated. Regional nodes may become enlarged, either as a result of infection of the ulcer or from metastases. Treatment should primarily involve complete eradication of the tumour by the following methods.

- Surgical excision is the most appropriate treatment for SCC of the skin, with the surgical margin being dependent on the tumour diameter and on the site of the lesion.
- Radiotherapy should be used for massive unresectable tumours in critical anatomical sites. Postoperatively it may be used for persisting tumour or where clearance is doubtful.

Verrucous carcinoma

Verrucous carcinoma are well-differentiated SCC which invade locally but rarely metastasise. These commonly occur on the palm and soles; here they are known as carcinoma ciniculatum.

Keratoacanthoma

Keratoacanthoma (molluscum sebaceum) (Fig. 13.38) arises as a rapid proliferation of squamous epidermal cells. The nodule grows rapidly for 6–8 weeks at which time it usually begins to resolve spontaneously. Keratoacanthoma must be distinguished from SCC. Usually rapid evolution to relatively large size, irregular crater shape and keratotic plug, and the undamaged surrounding skin make a distinction possible. Spontaneous healing further confirms the diagnosis. Histologically, it is difficult to differentiate between a keratoacanthoma and SCC. There is also a possibility of a highly anaplastic SCC behaving like a keratoacanthoma. Excision biopsy is mandatory if the diagnosis is in doubt as curetted specimens yield poor sections.

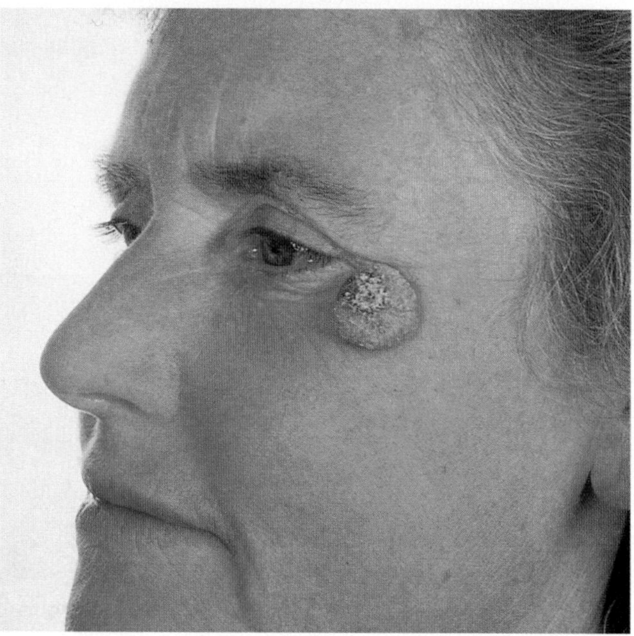

Fig. 13.38 Keratoacanthoma.

Melanoma

Cutaneous melanoma is a malignant neoplasm arising from epidermal melanocytes. The earliest description is in the writings of Hippocrates in the fifth century BC. John Hunter described a 'cancerous fungous excrescence' in 1787, which has subsequently been diagnosed as a melanoma. It has been considered a rare tumour with unpredictable behaviour. It varies from spontaneous regression to rapid progression and death. However, the disease is no longer rare. The rate of increase in the incidence of melanoma is greater than for any other cancer in Caucasians with the exception of bronchogenic carcinoma. Its incidence has doubled every 10 years in countries close to the equator and every 10–15 years in more temperate zones. Incidence has quadrupled in Australasia and doubled in Norway, Britain, America and Canada in the last 30 years. This increase in incidence is not observed in other skin cancers. The incidence is 40 per 100 000 in Queensland, Australia, but only 4 per 100 000 in Scotland. It accounts for almost all the deaths from skin cancer.

It is likely that between a third and a half of all melanomas develop in a benign naevus of many years' standing. Melanoma does not exhibit any overall sex predilection. The commonest site for females is the lower leg and in males the front or back of the trunk. In the Bantu, the sole of the foot is the most frequent site; they can also occur on the palms and other depigmented areas, but do not arise in the black skin of the remainder of the body for a reason that is not understood. Rarely, melanoma arises in the eye, in the meninges or at the mucocutaneous junction zones, e.g. anus and mouth. There is now strong evidence that the increase in exposure to sunlight is mainly responsible for the rapid increase in this skin cancer. It is well known that solar irradiation, which is now much more dangerous as a result of the decreasing ozone layer, is associated with all skin cancers. Ethnic origin, climate, socioeconomic status and lifestyle are all risk factors interacting with sun exposure. The other evidence with reference to sun exposure is that patients with pathological conditions, such as albinism and xeroderma pigmentosa, are susceptible to forming melanomas. A proportion will arise in a Hutchinson's freckle (see below). Clark *et al.* in 1975 produced a concept of a 'radial growth phase' to describe the atypical proliferation of intraepidermal melanocytes which precedes the development of dermal invasion (vertical growth phase) in all except nodular melanoma.

Sir Jonathan Hutchinson, 1828–1913. Surgeon, The London Hospital, London, England. He described the melanotic freckle in 1892.
W.H. Clark. Pathologist, USA.

Four parameters of histological grading are used, as follows.

1. The most important parameter is the depth of invasion as measured by the thickness (Fig. 13.39). The thickness is measured by an optical micrometer from the top of the granular layer of the epidermis to the deepest melanoma cells in the dermis (Breslow, 1975). There is good evidence that tumour thickness is a better measure of prognosis than level of invasion, and also more reproducible by different observers. Lesions less than 0.76 mm in thickness have a very favourable prognosis.
2. Ulceration, and
3. a high mitotic rate carry a poor prognosis.
4. Regression, if present, for some thin melanomas may have an appreciable risk of metastases, presumably because the lesion at some point in the past had been of a sufficient thickness to have metastasised.

Clinical features

Clinically, five types are recognised:

- lentigo maligna;
- superficial spreading;
- nodular;
- acral-lentiginous;
- amelanotic.

Superficial spreading melanomas are the most common (64 per cent). They occur on any part of the body and are usually greater than 0.5 mm in diameter. A variegated coloured pattern and an irregular edge are characteristic. The lesion is usually palpable.

Nodular melanoma. This is the most malignant, occurring in about 12–25 per cent of cases and found in the younger age groups. It may occur on any part of the body, and is always palpable and usually convex in shape. The colour is commonly uniform and is usually blue, grey or black. It sharply delineates from the surrounding tissue, and has a smooth surface and an irregular outline. Ulceration may occur earlier, leading to weeping or bleeding.

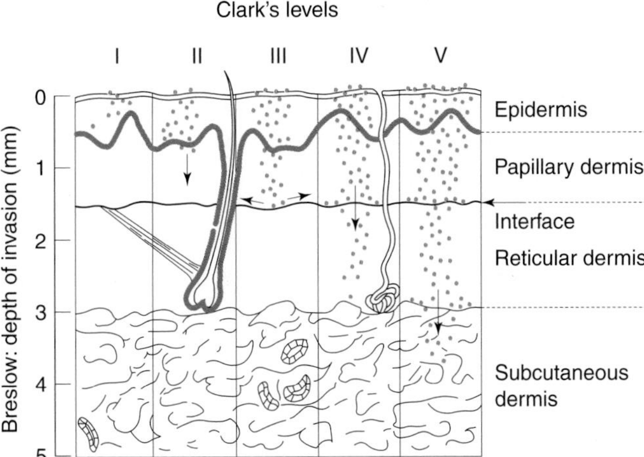

Fig. 13.39 Depth of invasion of melanoma – Clark's level and Breslow's thickness.

A. Breslow. Pathologist, USA.

Lentigo maligna melanoma (Hutchinson's melanotic freckle) is the least common (7–15 per cent) and least malignant. It occurs most frequently on the face in people aged over 60 years. It may occur on any part of the body habitually exposed to the sun. It begins as an irregularly pigmented, flat, brown macule which grows very slowly over a period of 1–15 years, advancing and regressing in various areas. There is a great variation in colour from brown to tanned black within the tumour itself. Malignant change is recognised by thickening and the development of discrete tumour nodules. They may ultimately grow to 5 cm and a very irregular outline is also characteristic (Fig. 13.40a and b).

Acral-lentiginous melanoma. These occur on the palms and soles and also include subungual melanomas (Fig. 13.41). They are the most common type of melanoma found in Japan. They carry a poor prognosis similar to nodular melanoma.

Amelanotic. In this form, the lesion may be pink but usually close inspection will reveal some pigmentation at the base (Fig. 13.42). Amelanotic melanoma seem to carry an even worse prognosis than nodular pigmented melanoma. They may often present with regional lymph node metastases.

Clinical recognition

Malignant melanoma is almost unknown before puberty. The development of a malignancy in a mole should be suspected if any of the following changes occur:

Major signs	*Minor signs*
Change in size	Inflammation
Change in shape	Crusting or bleeding
Change in colour	Sensory change, e.g. itch
	Diameter 5 mm or more

Suspicious lesions should be removed completely with a 2 mm margin; use of incision or punch biopsies is deprecated since accurate histological staging is impossible, and the treatment is dependent on the histology.

Spread

Malignant melanoma may spread by local extension, by the lymphatics or by the bloodstream. Tumour cells may reach the regional lymph nodes by embolism but spread by lymphatic permeation is also seen, producing local satellite (Fig. 13.43a) and/or 'in-transit' deposits between the primary growth and the regional nodes (Fig. 13.43b) resulting in secondary lymphoedema. Blood-borne metastases are seen in the lungs, liver, brain, skin and rarely in the bones. They may also involve unusual sites, e.g. the small intestine, heart and breasts. Secondary deposits are typically black, but

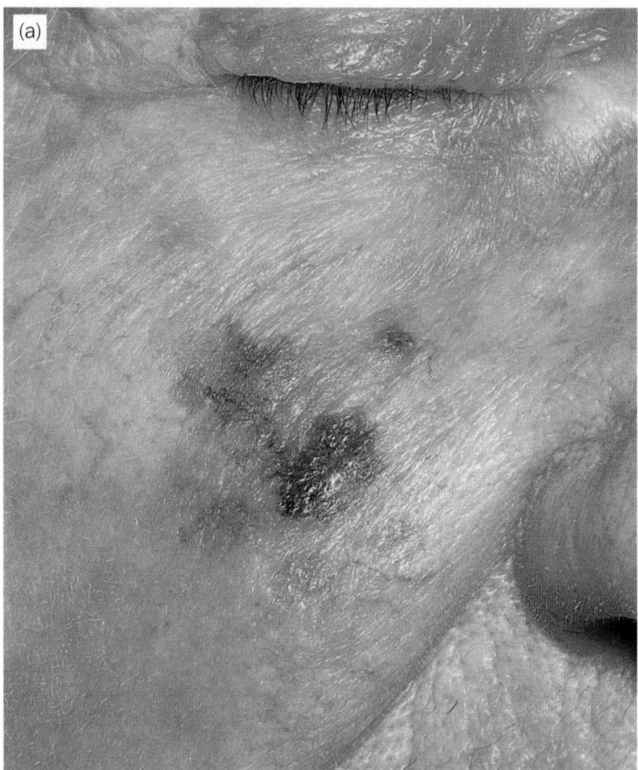

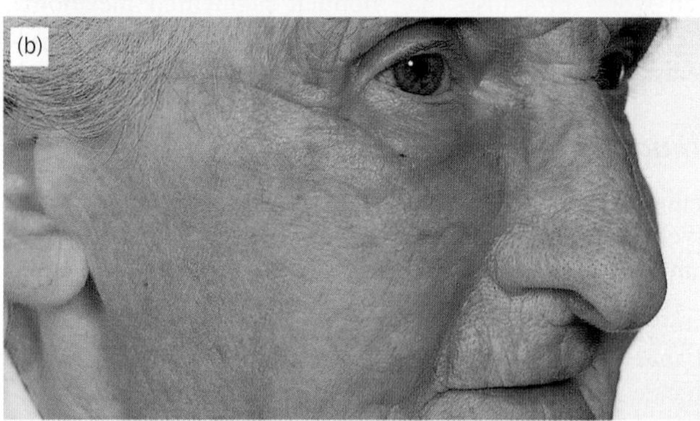

Fig. 13.40 (a) Lentigo maligna melanoma showing irregular margin. (b) Result following excision and reconstruction with a local cheek advancement flap.

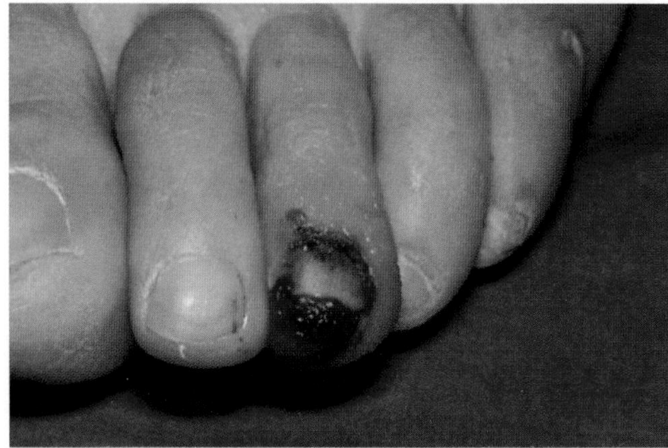

Fig. 13.41 Subungual malignant melanoma.

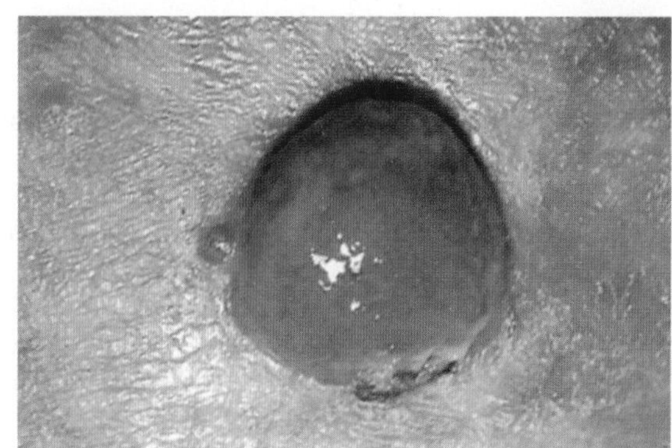

Fig. 13.42 Amelanotic melanoma: note the minimal pigmentation at the base of the tumour.

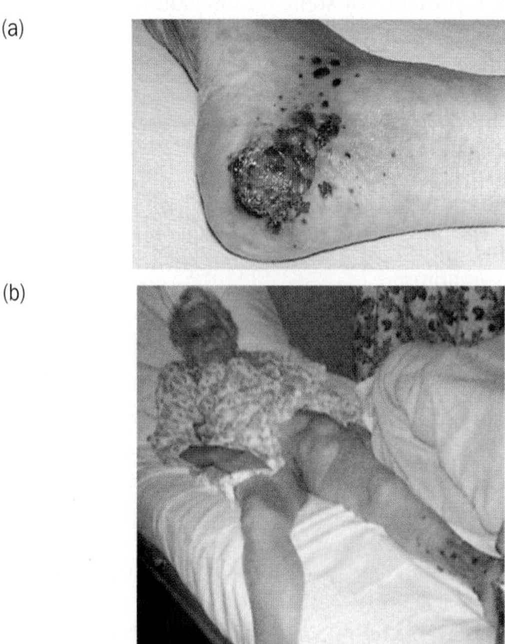

Fig. 13.43 Malignant melanoma. (a) Typical satellite nodules; (b) enormously enlarged regional lymph nodes (of groin).

sometimes contain little or no melanin, even when the primary tumour is heavily pigmented. Extensive visceral involvement may cause melanuria.

Staging

Using the American Joint Committee on Cancer/International Union Against Cancer (AJCC/UICC) staging system is recommended (Table 13.1).

Treatment

This is primarily surgical.

- There should be complete surgical excision.
- Minimum margin of 1.0 cm and a maximum of 2.0 cm should be made. This represents the clinical margins at surgery and not histopathological margins.

Table 13.1 AJCC/UICC staging system for malignant melanoma

Stage	*Primary tumour (pT)*	*Lymph node (N)*	*Distant metastases (M)*
IA	pT1	N0	M0
IB	pT2	N0	M0
IIA	pT3	N0	M0
IIB	pT4	N0	M0
IIIA	Any pT	N1	M0
IIIB	Any pT	N2	M0
IV	Any pT	Any N	M1
Primary	*Breslow thickness*	*Clark's level*	
pTis	Melanoma *in situ*	I	
pT1	Melanoma <0.75 mm	II	
pT2	Melanoma 0.76–1.5 mm	III	
pT3	Melanoma 1.51–4.0 mm	and/or IV	
pT4	Melanoma 4.0 and/or satellites within 2 cm of primary	and/or V	
Nodes			
N0	No nodes involved		
N1	No node >3 cm in diameter		
N2	Any node >3 cm in diameter or 3 or more in transit metastases		

- Wide excision was advocated first by Handley in 1907 based on his pathological studies of the frequency of centrifugal dermal lymphatic permeation into the surrounding skin. Surgeons recommended a 5-cm margin of excision around primary malignant melanomas; this is no longer advocated.
- Do not excise beyond the deep fascia.
- Margins may have to be altered for cosmetic or functional reasons, e.g. periorbital region.

Survival from primary melanoma management falls with increasing tumour thickness (Table 13.2).

Treatment of lymph nodes

Lymph node biopsy. Fine-needle aspiration cytology (FNAC) is preferable to excision biopsy. Open biopsy may increase risk of tumour spillage, but if needed the incision should be placed so that it can be excised in continuity with the lymph node field.

Elective node dissection. This is not recommended for the large majority of patients. A report of satellitosis or lymphatic invasion should warrant consideration of node dissection. Clinically involved nodes require therapeutic node dissection.

Therapeutic dissection for clinically positive nodes requires radical clearance by those with expertise in the surgery of this condition. Limited dissection or 'node picking' is not acceptable. Adequate clearance gives a good prognosis with a 10-year survival of 50 per cent when one node is involved. However, with more nodes involved or extranodal spread the survival rates decrease and radiotherapy may be considered. Groin dissections may be complicated by the development of lymphoedema.

Lymphatic mapping and sentinel node biopsy is a technique initially described by Cabannas in 1974 for penile carcinoma and popularised by Morton in 1994 for melanoma. This may provide an approach to identify those patients who may be appropriate for elective lymph node dissection by detecting the presence of micrometastases in the sentinel node. This technique identifies the first echelon nodes ('sentinel node') using lymphoscintography following an intradermal injection of radioactive colloid around the primary site. The position of these nodes is marked on the skin and identified intraoperatively by injecting patent blue dye around the site of the primary and using a hand-held gamma probe to help to identify the position of these nodes. This accurately indicates the presence or absence of micrometastases in a nodal field.

Loco-regional recurrent melanoma

Loco-regional recurrent melanoma involving skin and soft tissues when isolated should be treated surgically. Patients with multiple local or in-transit recurrences should be considered for specialist treatment with isolation perfusion with high-dose cytotoxic agents (Fig. 13.44). Carbon dioxide laser ablation may be used for multiple small cutaneous lesions; or surgical resection for isolated pulmonary, cerebral, intestinal and intraperitoneal recurrences. In some patients it is advisable not to resect subsequent cutaneous metastases as they can be used as an indicator of response to systemic therapies or monitoring that of new local treatments.

Melanoma in childhood

Melanoma in childhood is rare; however, the clinical behaviour is similar to that in adults. The differential diagnosis is of the pigmented Spitz naevus (juvenile melanoma) which has previously been confused as a melanoma. This is a variant of the compound naevus in childhood. In cases of malignant melanoma in childhood the treatment is exactly the same as that for melanoma in adults.

Table 13.2 Ten-year survival rates from South Australian Cancer Registry 1996

pTis	Melanoma *in situ*	100 per cent
pT1	Melanoma <0.75 mm	97.9 per cent
pT2	Melanoma 0.76–1.5 mm	90.7 per cent
pT3a	Melanoma 1.51–3.0 mm	75.4 per cent
pT3b-pT4	Melanoma >3.0 mm	55.0 per cent

W.S. Handley. Surgeon, Middlesex Hospital, London, England.

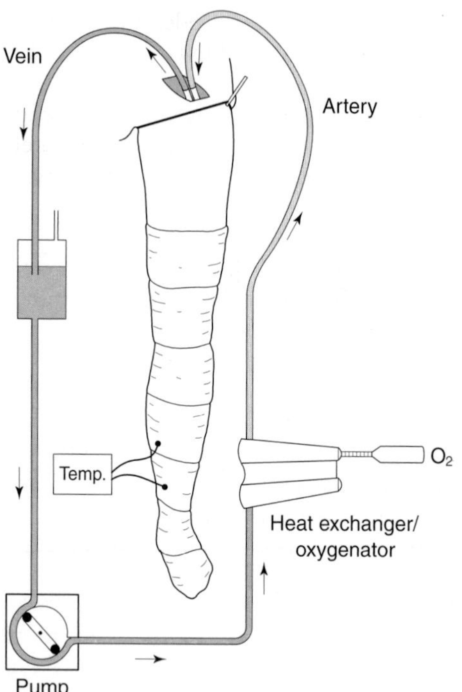

Fig. 13.44 Method for performing isolated limb perfusion using a tourniquet.

Other malignancies

Dermatofibrosarcoma protuberans (Fig. 13.45)

This is a locally malignant tumour arising in the dermis and composed of more or less mature fibroblasts. It is usually situated on the trunk, particularly in the flexural regions, and in its early stages can look very similar to a histiocytoma. Treatment is by wide excision with a margin of 3 cm. Local recurrence invariably follows inadequate surgery.

Kaposi's sarcoma

This is a neoplasm of multifocal origin derived from proliferating capillary vessels and perivascular connective tissue cells. In Europeans, it is a disease of late adult life, running an indolent course affecting the legs of elderly men. Amongst the immunocompromised population it appears much earlier. There is an endemic form in various parts of Africa. The tumour also occurs in association with acquired immuno deficiency syndrome (AIDS). The AIDS-related form runs a rapid course with painful lesions at multiple sites and metastatic spread. The lesions have a dark blue or purplish colour. At first they are macular, and when they become tumid, pressure may produce blanching to reveal a brown tinge. The process usually begins on the extremities, most commonly on the feet, but occasionally on the hands, ears or nose. Treatment is by radiotherapy.

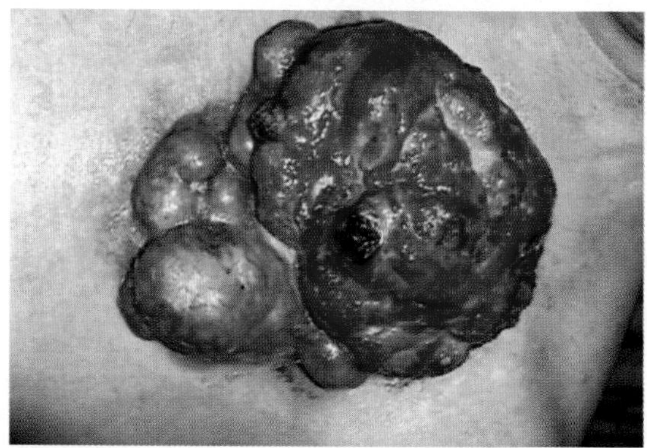

Fig. 13.45 Dermatofibrosarcoma protuberans.

Moritz K. Kaposi, 1837–1902. Dermatologist, Vienna, Austria.

Angiosarcoma

This is a rare tumour largely seen in elderly males. The lesions occur most commonly on the scalp or face and may present either as a subcutaneous plaque in the skin, as a nodule, particularly on the scalp, or as a single or multiple bluish-purple discoloration of the skin. Metastatic disease is largely to the cervical lymph nodes and lungs.

Lymphangiosarcoma

This is a long-standing complication of lymphoedema and it occurs on the brawny oedematous arm of the postradical mastectomy patient or in a lower limb following groin dissection. Conservative breast surgery and the use of special elastic compression stockings have made this condition much less common. It is usually fatal.

Primary cutaneous malignant lymphoma

This is rare and can be divided broadly into three types:

- mycosis fungoides and Sezary syndrome (a rare and fatal reticulosis with unusual giant cells in the blood and skin);
- primary cutaneous non-Hodgkin's lymphoma;
- primary cutaneous Hodgkin's lymphoma.

Mycosis fungoides is a term given to a condition characterised by initial infiltration of the skin by malignant lymphocytes with subsequent involvement of lymph nodes, spleen, liver, bone marrow and other organs. Patients usually present between the ages of 40 and 60 years with a long-standing history of dermatitis, exfoliative erythroderma or a papular rash, which in time progresses to plaque and then tumour formation. The diagnosis of lymphoma of the skin should be made by a biopsy and treatment is by radiotherapy and/or chemotherapy.

Merkel cell tumour

Merkel cell tumour (trabecular cell carcinoma, primary neuroendocrine carcinoma) arises from Merkel cells as an

The Merkel cell was first identified in 1875 on the mole's snout. Merkel, F. (1876). Arch Mikrosk Anat, **11**, *636–52.*

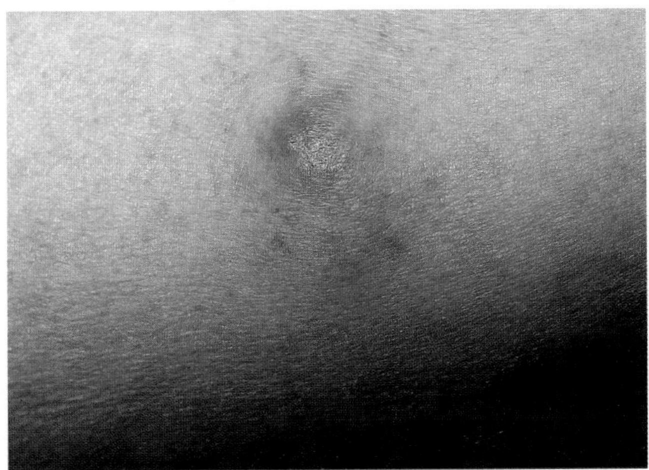

Fig. 13.46 A Merkel cell tumour.

enlarging blue–red nodule (Fig. 13.46). Local metastases occur in 75 per cent and distant spread in 25 per cent of cases. Treatment is by surgical excision of the primary with a 2–5-cm margin followed by radiotherapy to the site of the primary and the regional nodal basin.

Metastatic malignant tumours

These are tumours formed by malignant cells originating from another site, and frequently from another tissue, conveyed to the skin by the blood and lymphatic circulation. The skin is not uncommonly secondarily involved by malignant lymphoma and leukaemia as a manifestation of generalised disease. Most malignant tumours can produce cutaneous metastases, but some seed to the skin more than others. Hypernephroma, an uncommon malignancy, accounts for 9 per cent of skin metastases. The most frequent primary sites are breast, stomach, lung, uterus, large intestine, kidney, prostate gland, ovary, liver and bone.

Further reading

Aston, S.J., Beasley, R.W. and Thorne, C.H.M. (1997) *Grabb and Smith's Plastic Surgery*, Lippincott-Raven, Philadelphia, PA.

Cormack, G.C. and Lamberty, B.G.H. (1994) *Arterial Anatomy of Skin Flaps*, Churchill Livingstone, Edinburgh.

MacKie, R.M. (1996) *Skin Cancer*, 2nd edn, Martin Dunitz, London.

Mathes, S.J. and Nahai, F. (1997) *Reconstructive Surgery Principles, Anatomy and Technique*, Churchill Livingstone, Edinburgh.

McGregor, I.A. and McGregor, A. (1995) *Fundamental Techniques of Plastic Surgery*, Churchill Livingstone, Edinburgh.

Taylor, G.I. and Palmer, J.H. (1987) The vascular territories (angiosomes) of the body: experimental study and clinical applications. *British Journal of Plastic Surgery*, **40**, 113–41.

Venkataswami, R. (1992) Microsurgery in a developing country. In *Recent Advances in Plastic Surgery 4* (eds I.T. Jackson and B.C. Sommerlad), Churchill Livingstone, Edinburgh.

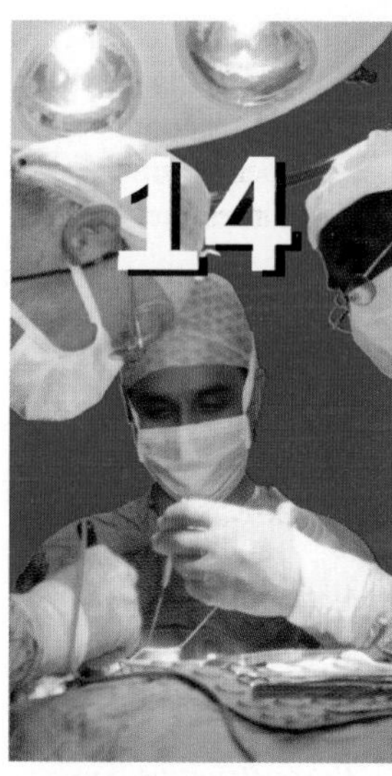

14 Burns

Introduction

The arrival of the victim of a burning accident at the emergency department is one of the most dramatic events in surgical practice. The suddenness of the accident, the visibility of the damage, the pain, fear and the reactions of onlookers all combine to create an atmosphere of tension. The immediate needs of the patient for resuscitation and pain relief may temporarily interfere with the usual assessment of the patient by history and examination. However, the history of the mechanism of burning is of major importance in assessing its likely severity. Detailed inquiry must be made as soon as the patient's condition allows, information being gained from either the patient or a third party. Clinically, the severity of the burn is estimated from the area of the burned surface and the depth of the burn wound.

On arrival a burns case should be treated like any other trauma case. There may be problems with the airway, a broken cervical spine and internal injuries. ABC (airway, breathing, circulation) applies as usual. If there is soot or charring around the mouth and nose, the possibility of smoke or even flame inhalation must be considered. Laryngeal oedema can develop rapidly and lung function can deteriorate. Endotracheal intubation should be considered early, but this should only be attempted by a highly experienced anaesthetist. A needle cricothyroidotomy set should be assembled and ready for use. There will only be one chance at endotracheal intubation and if that fails because of laryngeal oedema a surgical airway will be needed immediately. If laryngeal oedema is possible early intubation is prudent, and mandatory if a transfer to another unit is required. The airway must be secure before transfer.

Assessment of the burn area

An approximate clinical rule in wide use is the 'rule of nines' which acts as a rough guide to body surface area (Fig. 14.1). The examining doctor should assess the total area involved and how much of the area is partial thickness and how much full thickness. As a general rule, an adult with more than 20 per cent of the body surface involved or a child with more than 10 per cent of body surface area involved will require intravenous fluid replacement. However, an intravenous access line may be necessary for adequate analgesia for much smaller areas of burn and many children in particular will require fluid replacement because of vomiting. For smaller percentages than the above, it is necessary to maintain an adequate oral intake of fluid. The prognosis depends upon the percentage body surface area burned. A rough guide is that if the age and percentage add together to a score of 100 then the burn is likely to be fatal. A child may therefore survive a large burn, but even a small burn in an elderly patient is potentially fatal.

Intravenous access in a burnt child may be difficult. Both rectal and intraosseous infusion (into the upper third of the tibia) offer useful alternatives.

Bailey & Love's Short Practice of Surgery, 23rd edition. Edited by R.C.G. Russell, N.S. Williams and C.J.K. Bulstrode. Published in 2000 by Arnold Publishers.

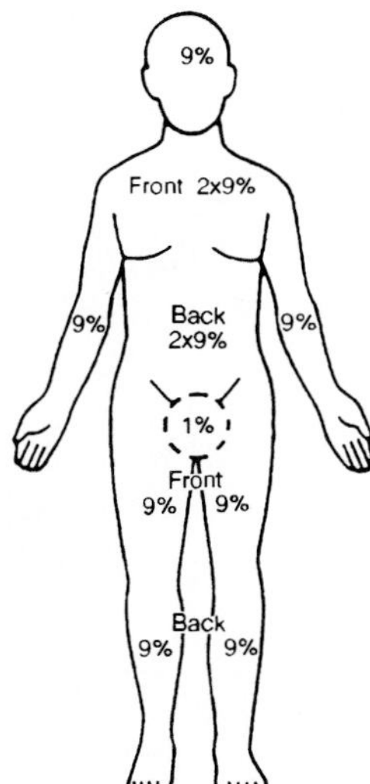

Fig. 14.1 The 'rule of nines' may be used to estimate the total body surface area burnt (%TBSA) of adults. By adding together the affected areas the percentage of the total body surface that is burnt can be calculated quickly. This rule does not apply strictly to infants and children. In a child aged 1 year the head and neck area is 18 per cent and each leg is 14 per cent. A useful aide-memoire is that the patient's hand (fingers and palm) is 1 per cent body surface area (*after Wallace*).

Assessment of burn depth

Burn depth depends, in thermal injury, upon:

- the temperature of the burning agent;
- the mode of transmission of heat;
- the duration of the contact.

Much of this information can be obtained from taking a good history of the injury. Clinical examination of the burn wound may also show characteristic features.

Skin anatomy

The epidermis is the most superficial layer of the skin and provides the waterproofing layer. It is constantly replaced from the basal layer. The dermis is the thicker underlying area that supplies the strength and integrity of the skin. It has a rich blood supply from the subdermal capillary network. It contains the adnexal structures – hair follicles, sebaceous glands and sweat glands. These adnexal structures contain epithelial cells that can proliferate and heal a partial-thickness wound by epithelialisation.

Superficial burns

These have the ability to heal themselves by epithelialisation alone. Epidermal burns look red, are painful, blisters are not present, and they heal rapidly without sequelae. Superficial dermal burns are blistered and painful; they should heal by epithelialisation within 14 days without scarring, but sometimes leave long-term pigmentation changes.

Deep burns

These have lost all adnexal structures and if left can only heal by second intention with scarring. Deep dermal burns may be blistered and have a blotchy red appearance with no capillary return on pressure and absent sensation to pinprick. Full-thickness burns have a white or charred appearance; again sensation is absent. This charred layer consists of denatured, contracted dermis and is called an *eschar*.

In practice most burns contain areas of differing burn depth. Decision making is easy where burns are obviously superficial or obviously deep, with difficulties arising in the distinction between the deeper superficial burns and deep dermal burns.

Mechanisms of injury

A burn is a tissue injury from thermal (heat or cold) application, or from the absorption of physical energy or chemical contact (Table 14.1). Each has its own distinctive features and management problems.

Scalds

Hot water produces a particularly well-defined type of skin damage (Fig. 14.2). The temperature of boiling water (100°C) or steam is constant and the major determinant of the severity of injury is the duration of contact. In the home, spills from kettles or cooking pots are common injuries of childhood. As with all burning accidents, those least able to protect themselves (the very young, the very old and the very drunk) are particularly vulnerable. Children reaching up to grasp the flex of an electric kettle, or a pot handle, can drench themselves in boiling water, and the larger the volume, the more severe the injury in terms of area and depth. Even a cup of tea or coffee can cause considerable scalding. In predicting the outcome, it is worthwhile knowing whether milk has been added, thus lowering the temperature, although this question may seem frivolous to an anxious parent. Common areas involved are the face, neck and upper trunk or limbs. Although spills cool rapidly, limiting the duration of damage, the worst injuries of this type may leave permanent scarring. Immersion in boiling water, or prolonged steam exposure as in some industrial accidents (where superheated steam may have a temperature above 100°C), are particularly dangerous and likely to cause deeper burns.

Table 14.1 Classification of burns

Type of burn	*Tissue injury*
Scalds	Partial-thickness/deep dermal skin loss
Fat burns	Usually full-thickness skin loss
Flame burns	Patches of partial and full thickness
Electrical burns	Full thickness with deep extensions
Cold injury	Ice formation, tissue freezing, vasospasm
Friction burns	Heat plus abrasion
Ionising radiation	Early tissue necrosis, later tissue dysplastic changes
Chemical burn	Inflammation, tissue necrosis, systemic effects

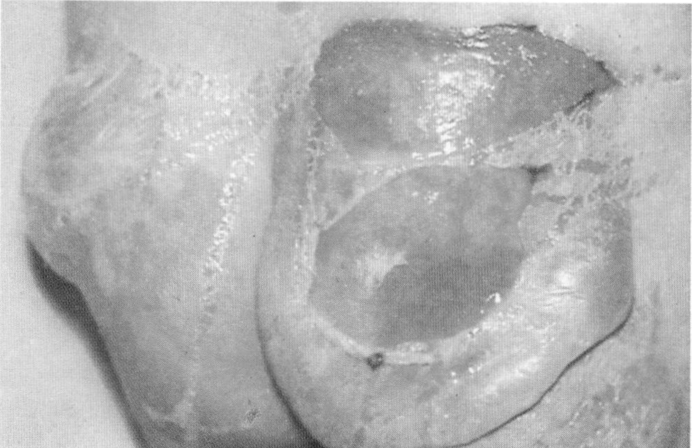

Fig. 14.2 Burnt (scalded) buttocks in a child, said to have sat down in a bucket of hot water.

Fat burns

Cooking fat or oil has a much higher temperature (180°C) than boiling water and hot fat cools slowly on the skin surface. Spills therefore cause deep burns (Fig. 14.3).

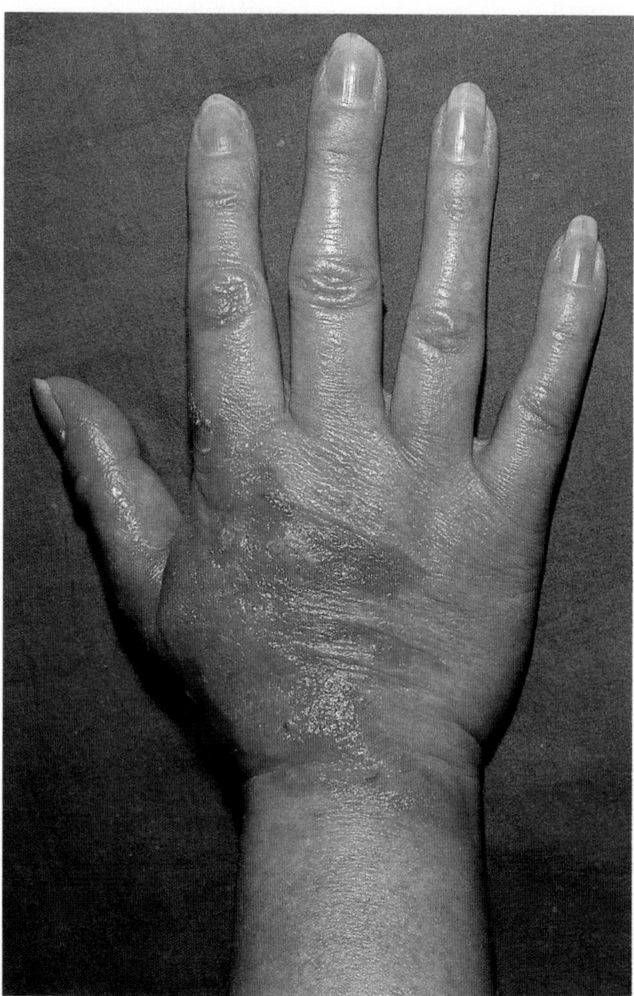

Fig. 14.3 Typical hot fat burns of the hand. These are usually deep dermal and often require excision and grafting.

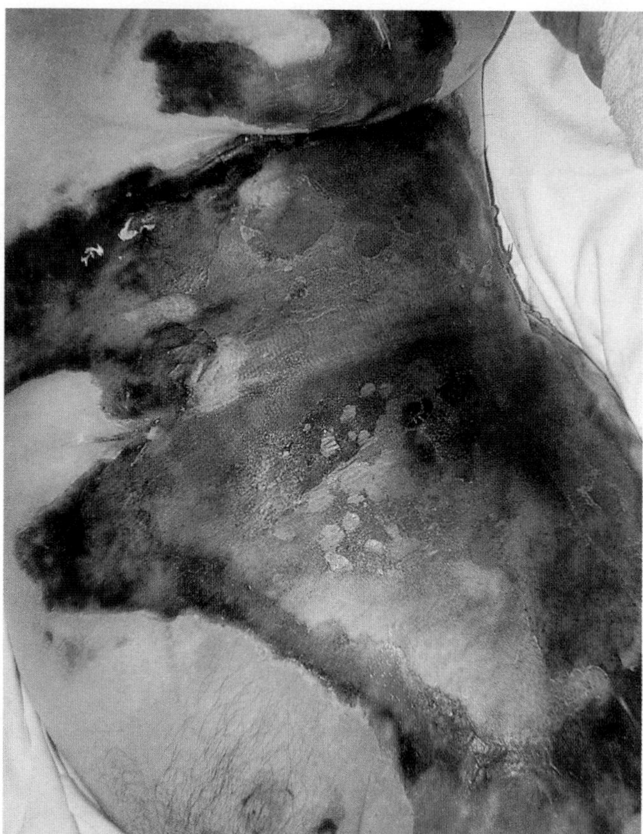

Fig. 14.4 Full-thickness flame burns; this patient's clothes caught fire.

Flame burns

Flame burns have a varied aetiology: house fires, clothing fires, spills of petrol on the skin, butane gas fires. They often occur in confined spaces and may be associated with inhalation injury (Fig. 14.4). It is important to know whether the clothing ignited and how the flames were extinguished (did clothing burn away?). Generally, deep burns will result. Some garments may protect, but if clothing ignites there is a prolonged flame contact with the skin. Flame-retardant clothing may burn under extreme conditions.

Electrical burns

The passage of electric current through the tissues causes heating that results in cellular damage. Heat produced is a function of resistance of the tissue, the duration of contact and the square of the current. Bone is a poor conductor of electrical current, whereas blood vessels, nerves and muscles are good conductors. Bone can therefore become very hot and cause secondary damage to tissues near to the bone. Low voltage (<1000 V) such as from a domestic supply (240 V, 50 Hz) causes significant contact wounds and may induce cardiac arrest, but no deep tissue damage (Fig. 14.5). High-voltage burns (>1000 V) cause damage by two mechanisms: flash and current transmission. The flash from an arc may cause a cutaneous burn and ignite clothing, but will not result

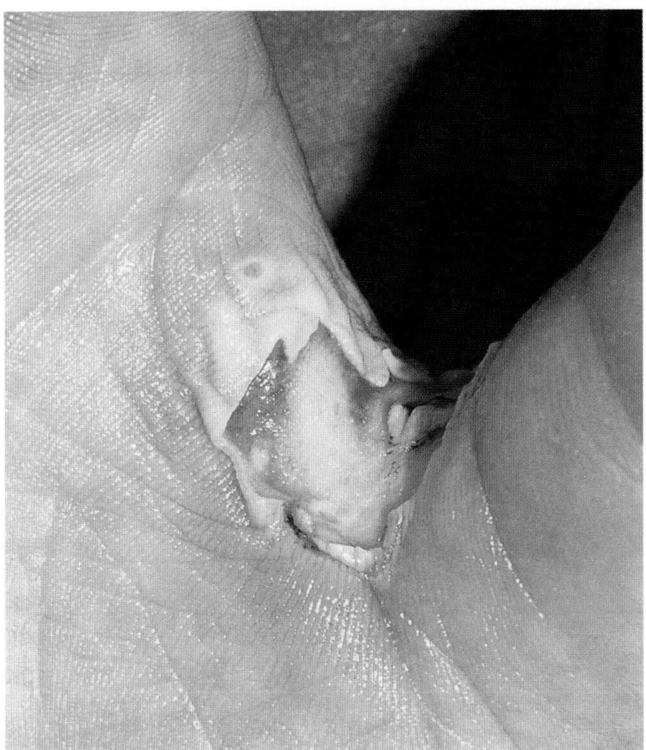

Fig. 14.5 Low-voltage electrical contact burn to the first web space. This is a deep burn requiring surgical treatment (see Figs 14.9 and 14.10).

in deep damage. High-voltage current transmission will result in cutaneous entrance and exit wounds and deep damage. Lightning strikes cause very high-voltage, very short -duration discharge. A direct strike has a high mortality. A side strike may cause superficial burns to the skin and deep exit burns to the feet. Internal damage is not common, but respiratory and then cardiac arrest occur. Some 'electrical' injuries are not associated with the passage of current through the tissues, such as bar-fire burns, where a child grasps a heated and unguarded element of an electric fire and the damage is due to heat alone.

Cold injury

Tissue damage from cold can occur from industrial accidents due to spills of liquid nitrogen or similar substances. The injuries cause acute cellular damage with the possibility of either a partial-thickness or full-thickness burn. Severe cooling can freeze tissues and ice formation is particularly likely to cause cellular disruption. Freezing injuries, however, seem to be less damaging to the connective tissue matrix than heat injuries. Frostbite is due to prolonged exposure to cold and there is often an element of ischaemic damage. Vasoconstriction reduces the resistance of the tissue to cold exposure as the warming effect of the circulation is reduced. There is therefore combined tissue damage from freezing, together with vasospasm. Such injuries occur after exposure to severe cold such as that encountered in mountain regions or arctic conditions. It is a rare injury in the UK.

Friction burns

The tissue damage in friction burns is due to a combination of heat and abrasion.

There is generally a superficial open wound that may progress to full-thickness skin loss. Friction burns may be associated with degloving injuries where the damage is judged to be deep. Early surgical excision and skin cover is the best means of management.

Ionising radiation

X-irradiation may lead to tissue necrosis. Such injuries are exceedingly rare if industrial and medical safety precautions are working. The tissue necrosis may not develop immediately. These injuries are generally limited in area and surgical excision, and flap reconstruction may be appropriate management. Of greater significance is the long-term cumulative effect of ionising radiation in the induction of skin cancers and other tumours.

Chemical burns

Numerous chemicals in industrial and domestic situations can cause burns. Tissue damage depends on the strength and quantity of the agent and the duration of contact. Some agents penetrate deeply or may have specific toxic effects. Chemicals cause local coagulation of proteins and necrosis, and some also have systemic effects (e.g. liver and kidney damage with tannic, formic and picric acids). The harmful effect will continue until the chemical is diluted or neutralised. The most important initial treatment is dilution with running water. Some specific agents cause particular problems or have specific remedies (Table 14.2).

Effects of burn injury

The effects of the burn upon the patient can be considered as:

- local;
- regional;
- systemic.

Local effects

Tissue damage

Heating of tissue results in direct cell rupture or cell necrosis. At the periphery the cells may be viable, but injured. In addition, collagen is denatured and damage to the peripheral microcirculation occurs. The capillaries are either thrombosed where the damage is severe or in less damaged areas there is increased capillary permeability such that the tissues become oedematous and there is external leakage of serous fluid. The essential difference between a partial-thickness and full-thickness skin loss is the depth of injury, but it is possible that the former may progress to the latter.

Table 14.2 Specific problems and remedies for chemical burns

Agent	*Problem*	*Remedy*
Acids	Very painful	Irrigation Sodium bicarbonate
Hydrofluoric acid	Corrosive Penetrates deeply Hypocalcaemia Arrythmias	Irrigation Calcium gluconate 10% gel Calcium gluconate 10% injections Early excision
Alkali	Penetrates slowly and deeply	Prolonged irrigation >1 hour Excision
Cement	Alkali burns Symptoms develop late	Prolonged irrigation
Bitumen	Hot liquid burns 150°C	Cooling Irrigation Remove bitumen using vegetable oil
Phosphorus	Particles burn into skin Systemic effects	Irrigation Removal of particles

Inflammation

There is a marked and immediate inflammatory response. In the areas least damaged by burning, this is manifest simply as erythema. The precise cause of this immediate vasodilation may represent a neurovascular response similar to Lewis's triple response. Mild areas of erythema resolve within a few hours. More severely damaged tissue may develop a more prolonged inflammatory response. Macrophages produce inflammatory mediators or cytokines (e.g. transforming growth factor-p) and phagocytose necrotic cells. Neutrophils and later lymphocytes provide protection against infection.

Damaged tissue separates by an active cellular process described as desloughing, generally complete by 3 weeks.

Infection

The damaged tissue represents a nidus for infection. Burn wounds will almost inevitably be colonised by microorganisms within 24–48 hours and this may remain as a local wound or regional infection. There may in addition be a bacteraemia or septicaemia and metastatic infections may develop at other sites. Bacteraemia is a common cause of fatality in a severe burn and may occur at any time from the first day until the point when all the wounds have entirely healed. Beta-haemolytic streptococci and pseudomonas produce protease enzymes that prevent skin graft adhesion.

Regional problems in burns

Circulation

Limb circulation may be compromised. Direct damage to a main limb vessel is unlikely, although it may occur from high-tension electrical burns. If there is gross oedema in a limb following burning, the swelling and tissue tension may lead to venous obstruction. This is particularly likely where there is circumferential burn tissue (eschar) which is incapable of distending. There is also the possibility of a muscle compartment syndrome affecting the flexors and/or extensor compartments of the upper limb or any compartment of the lower limb. The circulation of the intrinsic muscles of the hand may be compromised by oedema alone and this may lead on to ischaemic fibrosis and contractures. The accumulation of large quantities of interstitial fluid in the hand will inflate the elastic tissues of the hand, tending to drive it into a claw posture (metacarpal–phalangeal joint extension, proximal interphalangeal joint flexion).

Systemic effects from burning

Fluid loss

Fluid may be lost from damaged capillaries either by visible external loss or internally into the tissues from oedema in the region of the burn. In addition, there may be more extensive oedema of the region or even of the entire body. It is likely that this is mediated by cytokines acting on the microcirculation. Prevention of hypovolaemia is the most important function in early burn resuscitation. Effective fluid replacement will minimise the risk of other systemic complications.

Multiple organ failure

There may be progressive failure of renal or hepatic function or heart failure. The precise cause of these complications is uncertain and has often been attributed to fluid loss, 'toxaemia' from infection, or uncontrolled overreaction of the inflammatory response to sepsis. Multiple organ failure may, however, occur without obvious systemic infection.

Thomas Lewis. Physician, University College London, England.

Inhalation injury

These occur in those trapped in enclosed spaces. They are particularly common in association with burns of the head and neck. Various parts of the respiratory tract may be injured. The inhalation of hot gases causes a thermal burn to the upper airway. This is manifest early on by stridor, hoarseness, cough and respiratory obstruction. Inhalation of the products of combustion causes a chemical burn to the bronchial tree and lungs. This is manifest by hypoxia, acute respiratory distress syndrome and respiratory failure; it may be of delayed onset. Systemic absorption of, in particular, carbon monoxide (but also hydrogen cyanide from burning plastics) causes poisoning. Carbon monoxide displaces oxygen from haemoglobin to form carboxyhaemoglobin, reducing the oxygen-carrying capacity of the blood. It also has intracellular effects. Patients who survive the original incident may arrive confused or unconscious. Inhalation injury has an additive effect on mortality in all burns.

Systemic complications

There are well-documented systemic complications in association with burns such as Curling's (gastric or duodenal) ulcer that may result in acute haematemesis. Immunosuppression increases the risk of septic complications. Later, there is a catabolic response to trauma with severe weight loss. Nonspecific complications include urinary tract infection from catheterisation, deep vein thrombosis and pulmonary embolism.

Clinical features of burn injuries

Pain

Pain is immediate, acute and intense with superficial burns. It is likely to persist until strong analgesia is administered. With deep burns there may be surprisingly little pain.

Acute anxiety

The patient is often severely distressed at the time of injury. It is frequent for patients to run about in pain or in an attempt to escape, and secondary injury may result.

Fluid loss and dehydration

Fluid loss commences immediately and, if replacement is delayed or inadequate, the patient may be clinically dehydrated. There may initially be tachycardia from anxiety and later a tachycardia from fluid loss.

Local tissue oedema

Superficial burns will blister and deeper burns develop oedema in the subcutaneous spaces. This may be marked in the head and neck, with severe swelling which may obstruct the airway. Limb oedema may compromise the circulation.

Thomas Blizard Curling, 1811–88. Surgeon, London, England.

Special sites

Burns of the eyes are uncommon in house fires as the eyes are tightly shut and relatively protected. The eyes, however, may be involved in explosion injuries or chemical burns. Burns of the nasal airways, the mouth and upper airway may occur in inhalation injuries.

Coma

Following house fires, the patient may be unconscious and the reason for this must be ascertained. Asphyxiation or head injury must be excluded. Burning furniture is particularly toxic and the patient may suffer from carbon monoxide or cyanide poisoning.

Management of the burned patient

First aid

Stop the burning process

Flames from burning clothing or from burning inflammable substances on the skin surface should be extinguished by wrapping the patient in a fire blanket or any other readily available garment such as the bystander's own clothing. Some fire extinguishers are suitable for extinguishing flames on the skin surface. With electrical burns it is important that any live current is switched off, and with chemical burns the first-aid worker must avoid contact with the chemical. Burned or water-soaked clothing should be removed.

Cool the burn surface

Immediate cooling of the part is beneficial and should continue for 20 minutes. With scalds, irrigation with cold water under a tap is best and many a child has had scald damage successfully limited by pouring a readily available jug of cold water or milk immediately over the scalded area. Irrigation in cold water is particularly valuable for chemical burns. Hypothermia must be avoided. Do not use ice or iced water. The ideal temperature of cooling water is 15°C, but 8–25°C is effective. The burn should then be wrapped in any clean linen or plastic 'cling film' and the patient transported immediately to hospital.

Emergency examination and treatment

The order of priorities in the management of a major burn injury is:

- A: airway maintenance;
- B: breathing and ventilation;
- C: circulation;
- D: disability – neurological status;
- E: exposure and environment control – keep warm;
- F: fluid resuscitation.

Many of these observations and manoeuvres are shared with those considered good practices in any trauma situation. In severe facial and neck burns early endotracheal intubation or tracheostomy should be considered. Early escharotomy may be needed in circumferential chest or limb burns where respiratory or circulatory disturbance is observed. An altered conscious level may be caused by carbon monoxide poisoning.

Fluid resuscitation

It is important at an early stage to secure large-bore intravenous lines. Samples are taken for haemoglobin, urea and electrolytes, and blood cross-matching. Blood gases and blood analysis for carbon monoxide or cyanide poisoning are required in the unconscious patient. Having estimated the percentage burned surface area and measured the body weight, initial fluid resuscitation can be planned. The simplest formula (for adults) is:

3–4 ml/kg body weight/% burn/in the first 24 hours.

Half of this volume is given in the first 8 hours and the rest in the next 16 hours. Timings begin from the time of the burn, not the start of resuscitation. Hartmann solution is preferred, but other isotonic fluids may be used. Metabolic fluid requirements are also needed. Formulae are only a guide and the adequacy of fluid resuscitation is monitored by regular clinical assessment. A urinary catheter is essential. Urine output is the best guide to adequate tissue perfusion; in an adult one should aim for 30–50 ml/hour.

Further management

It is important to complete a detailed history of pre-existing problems and of the burn injury. A detailed physical examination and examination of the burned area is carried out. Adequate pain relief must be provided, usually by means of intravenous morphine. Good notes and a drawing of the burn area are needed. Smaller burns may be managed satisfactorily on an outpatient basis with arrangements for further dressing either at a hospital follow-up clinic or by the general practitioner. Patients with major burns should ideally be treated in a specialised burns unit. Indications for referral include:

- burns requiring fluid resuscitation;
- burns of special areas (face, hands, feet, perineum, genitalia);
- full-thickness burns >5 per cent body surface area;
- circumferential limb or chest burns;
- electrical burns;
- chemical burns;
- burns in children or the elderly;
- where nonaccidental injury is suspected in the case of a child;
- associated medical conditions or pregnancy;
- associated other trauma.

Adequate assessment, resuscitation and fluid administration should be secured before transfer of the patient. The trend towards early surgical excision and closure of the wound dictates that any patient with a wound which is unlikely to heal spontaneously should have the benefit of a plastic or burns surgical opinion at the earliest possible stage. A burns unit is often the most convenient place to undertake regular dressings. Dressing changes in an appropriate area are likely to minimise cross-infection, although formal isolation is rarely used unless a patient is shown to have an antibiotic-resistant organism, such as methicillin-resistant *Staphylococcus aureus*. The burns unit provides facilities for immediate physiotherapy and occupational therapy to minimise limb stiffness. Nutritional support is available. Early establishment of normal feeding appears to protect the small bowel mucosa and prevent translocation of Gram-negative bacteria. Inhalation injuries often require ventilation and monitoring by blood gases and bronchoscopy. These are best managed in a respiratory intensive care unit with appropriate surgical support for the management of the burn wound.

Dressings

Epidermal burns with erythema and no blisters do not need dressings. Analgesia and moisturising cream are used. Burns the face are generally treated by exposure, largely because of

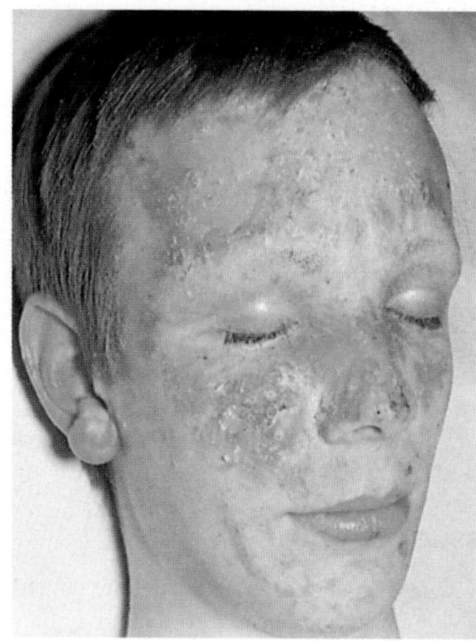

Fig. 14.6 Flash burns to the face, a firework injury.

Henri Albert Charles Antoine Hartmann, 1860–1952. Professor of Surgery, Paris, France.

Hans Christian Joachim Gram, 1853–1938. Professor of Medicine, Copenhagen, Denmark.

the difficulty of dressing (Fig. 14.6). Where there is much crusting it may be necessary to apply an ointment such as petroleum jelly, particularly around the eyes, and frequent toilet of the eyes and orifices may be needed. Burns of the trunk and limbs are usually dressed. Where possible the burns should be inspected by an experienced doctor to check on the assessment of area and depth before the application of dressings, as appearances may subsequently be difficult to interpret. Superficial dermal burns with blistering are usually dressed to absorb exudate, prevent desiccation, provide pain relief, encourage epithelialisation and prevent infection. Appropriate dressings are plastic films, hydrocolloids, preserved cadaver or pig skin, alginates or paraffin gauze. A thick layer of gauze may then be placed on top to allow transudation of any fluid and layers of wool or padding are applied over this to act as a sump for exudate. Dressing changes are painful and should not be performed more than necessary. Partial-thickness skin injuries heal within 2–3 weeks. Any wound that remains unhealed or granulating at 3 weeks will not heal satisfactorily without surgical intervention. Plastic surgical advice should certainly be sought by 3 weeks or at an earlier stage if the wound is extensive or showing evidence of considerable slough formation. Enzyme preparations may be used to facilitate sloughing. Where deep burns are being managed with dressings a topical antimicrobial agent such as silver sulphadiazine cream is used.

Infections

There is controversy about the use of routine antibiotic administration. It is almost inevitable that a burned surface will become colonised by microorganisms. The administration of broad-spectrum antibiotics on a routine basis is likely to encourage the emergence of resistant organisms. Children suffering from burn wounds are often given routine antibiotics to limit the possibility of metastatic infection. Almost any organism may colonise a wound. Beta-haemolytic streptococci are likely to delay healing and should be treated. *Staphylococcus aureus* is a frequent pathogen and *Pseudomonas* particularly grows on raw surfaces. These organisms may be best treated by local antiseptic preparations, although where there is any evidence of cellulitis, antibiotics should be administered. Frequent wound swabs should be cultured and where there is any rise in temperature, blood cultures should be taken.

Whether to administer an antibiotic before an organism is cultured from the blood is an individual clinical decision that depends on the severity of the patient's condition.

Monitoring for the onset or progress of infection should consist of:

- routine temperature measurement;
- frequent wound swab cultures;
- wound inspection by an experienced doctor or nurse at the time of dressing change;
- blood cultures.

Toxic shock syndrome

Toxic shock syndrome (TSS) is a life-threatening, exotoxin-mediated disease caused by *S. aureus*. It can occur in children who often have small body surface area burns. It presents with fever, a rash, myalgia, diarrhoea and vomiting and can progress rapidly to hypotension and multiorgan failure. Treatment is by dressing change, fluid resuscitation, antibiotics and immunoglobulin. Mortality can be high, but prompt active intervention appears to be effective. It is important to have a high index of suspicion regarding this condition when treating burned children.

Surgical treatment

Partial-thickness burns should heal without surgical intervention, but full-thickness burns require surgical management. There are two alternative policies for deep burns. One can await spontaneous desloughing and apply split-skin grafts at 3 weeks. This policy has the advantage that early operation can be avoided, but has the disadvantage of slow healing and greater scarring that follows a granulating wound. Alternatively, early excision of the burn is carried out with the application of skin cover, usually a skin graft, but where indicated a flap. This has the advantage of obtaining rapid healing and early restoration of function, and minimises the risk of adverse scarring. Where facilities allow, a policy of early operation for deep burns is preferred. Early tangential excision of skin grafting is a technique used for deep dermal burns, usually performed within 48 hours. Successive layers of the burned tissue are shaved with a split-skin grafting knife until a healthy bleeding dermal bed is reached upon which the skin grafts are applied. The rationale of this treatment is that deep dermal burns will heal slowly with considerable scarring. The healing process can be expedited by this method. It is a technique that requires considerable experience in the interpretation of the wound bed. Any surgery of this type is associated with considerable blood loss and limbs should be operated on with the assistance of a tourniquet. On the trunk it may be necessary to use a dilute infusion of adrenaline subcutaneously. Following excision of burned

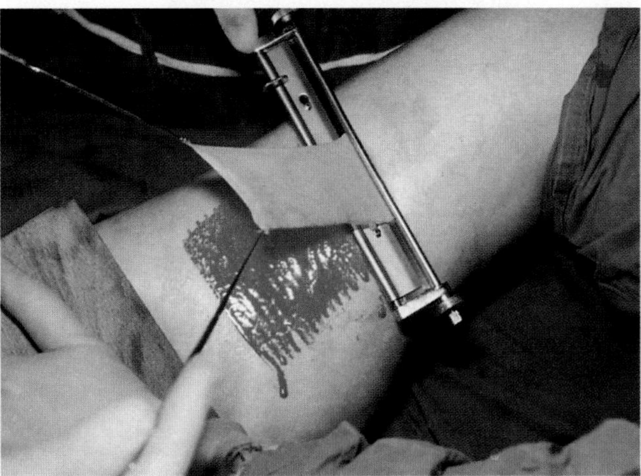

Fig. 14.7 Cutting a split-skin graft (*courtesy of P.L. Levick, Birmingham*). The graft is taken from normal thigh skin held tense by an assistant. This graft is elevated with skin hooks for demonstration purposes.

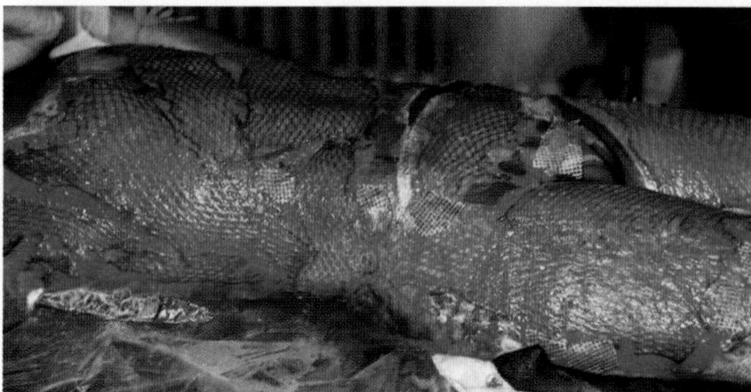

Fig. 14.8 Full-thickness burn wounds covered by mesh grafts (*courtesy of J.P. Gowar, Birmingham*). Meshing increases the area of the skin grafts and allows blood and exudate to escape, thus minimising haematoma.

tissue, skin cover is by split-skin autograft cover (Fig. 14.7). This is harvested from a donor site on an unburned area of skin. Care should be taken in selecting the donor site to produce the least possible cosmetic deficit. All grafts in children should be harvested from the buttocks. With extensive burns, the thighs are the first choice and other sites on the limbs and trunks may be necessary in addition. The skin graft can be meshed to expand its area. This is a system by which the graft is expanded by passing it through a machine that places multiple cuts in the skin. The skin can then be stretched and the cuts open out into small, diamond-shaped wounds. In this way the skin can be expanded 1/2–3 times depending on the expansion of the diamonds. Meshed skin also has the advantage that it allows free drainage of fluid from beneath the graft area (Fig. 14.8). Cadaveric allografts may be used for temporary cover.

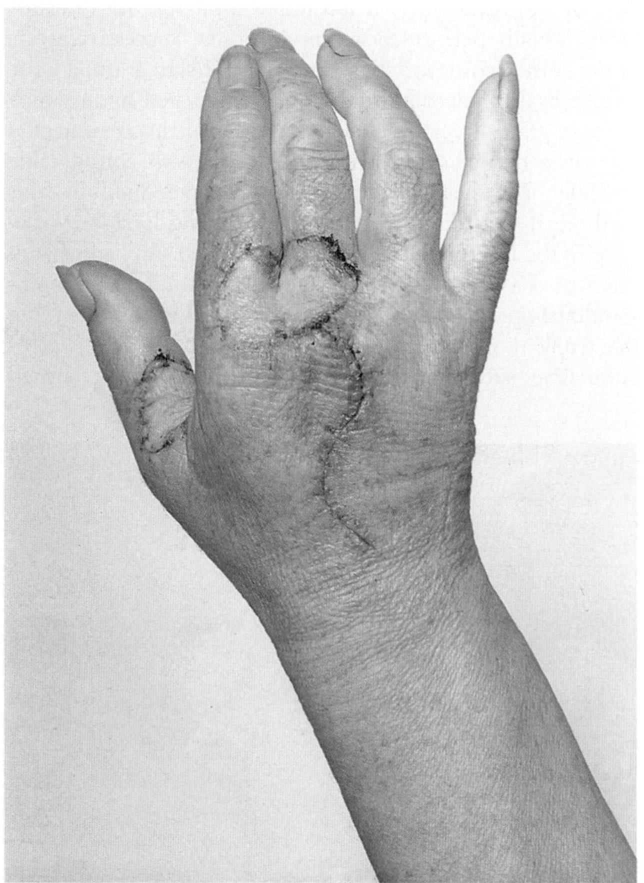

Fig. 14.9 The deep electrical burn of the first web space (Fig. 14.5) has been excised and closed using a second dorsal metacarpal artery flap, transferring a flap from the second web to reconstruct the first web. The flap donor site is covered by a full-thickness skin graft from the groin.

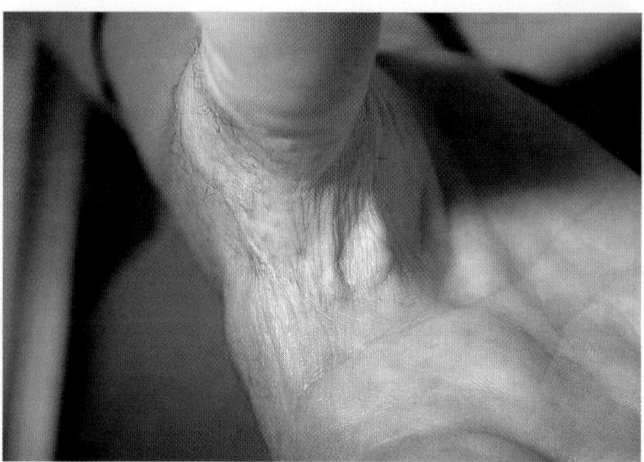

Fig. 14.10 Late result showing a mobile web space reconstruction. Skin grafts contract during the process of take, whereas flaps retain their size and mobility and are essential for reconstruction in mobile areas.

Cadaveric dermis has also been used as definitive cover with the addition of cultured autografts of keratinocytes. Keratinocyte grafting may have a larger role in establishing skin cover in the future. It is possible to grow large areas of keratinocyte autografts that facilitate healing, although the long-term future of the grafted skin cells remains uncertain. In deep burns, those with exposed structures (nerves, tendons, and vessels) or those overlying joints primary flap cover may be needed (Figs 14.9 and 14.10). Localised burns can usually be excised and closed in a single episode. Patients with extensive burn injuries may need repeated operations over many weeks to achieve healing. Once healed the process of rehabilitation can be more actively pursued.

Mobilisation and rehabilitation

The move towards earlier excision and skin cover and early mobilisation of the patient succeeds in reducing the incidence of complications such as infection and deep vein thrombosis. Most burns units have an intensive programme of physiotherapy and mobilisation without which limb oedema would progress to joint contractures.

Surgical reconstruction of the burn injury

The major complication of burn injury is scarring (Fig. 14.11). Lumpy hypertrophic or keloid scars can be limited by the

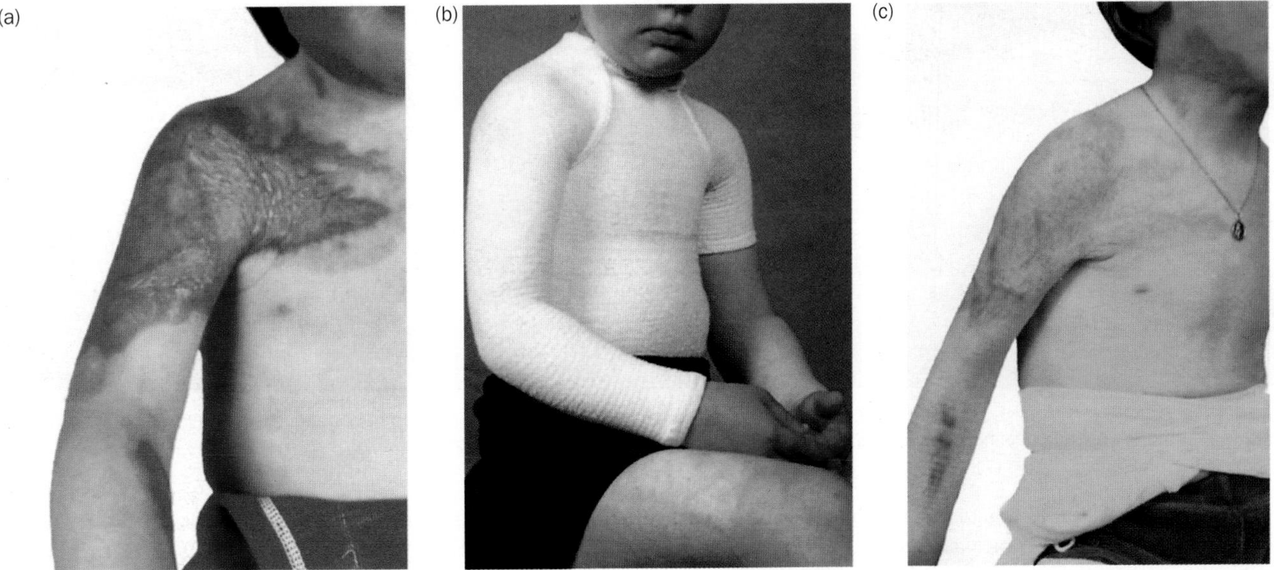

Fig. 14.11 The treatment of hypertrophic scars with pressure garments. (a) A typical example of active hypertrophic scarring following a full-thickness scald from a spilt cup of tea; (b) pressure garments were worn continuously for 14 months; and (c) the scar matured.

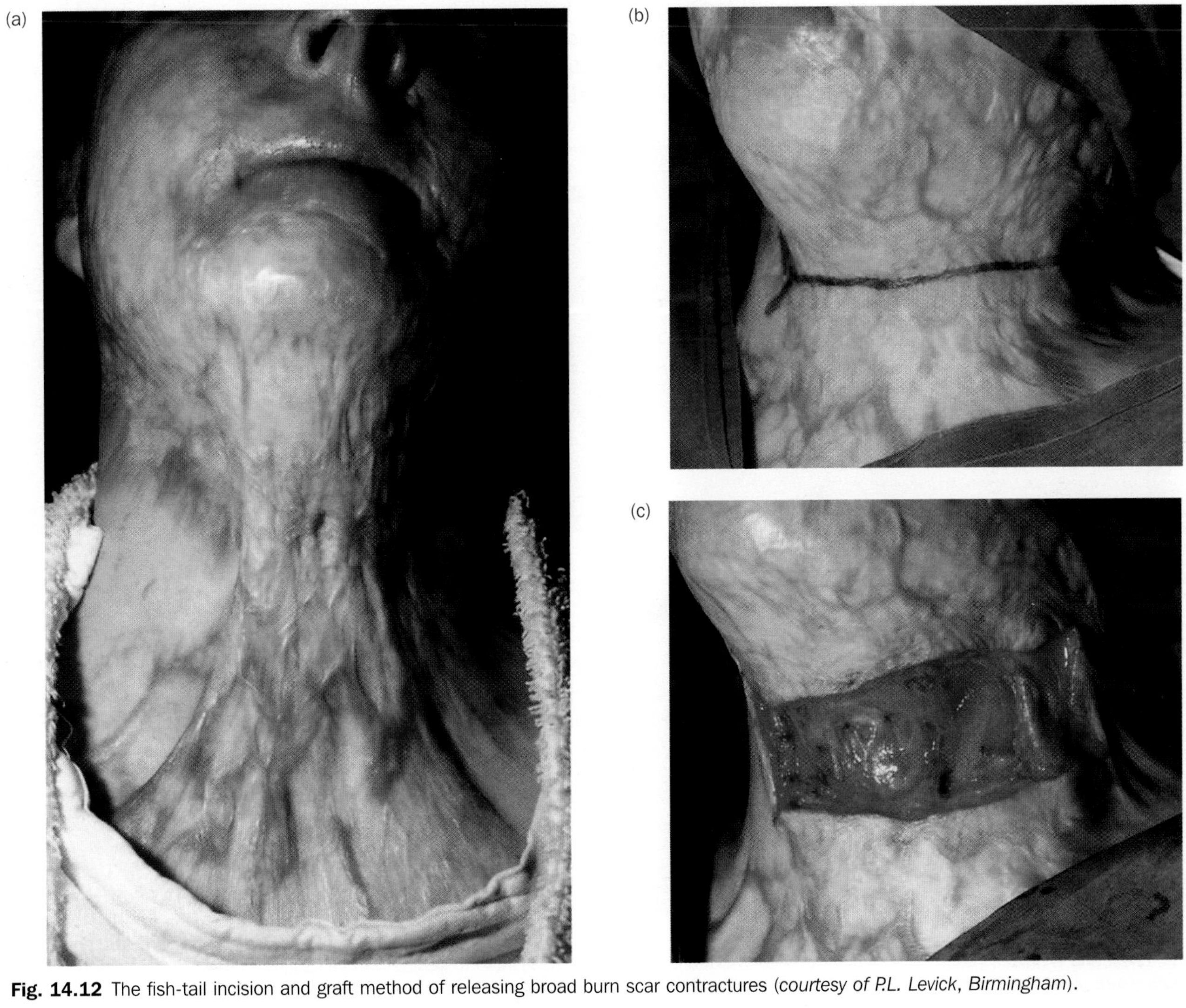

(a) (b) (c)

Fig. 14.12 The fish-tail incision and graft method of releasing broad burn scar contractures (*courtesy of P.L. Levick, Birmingham*).

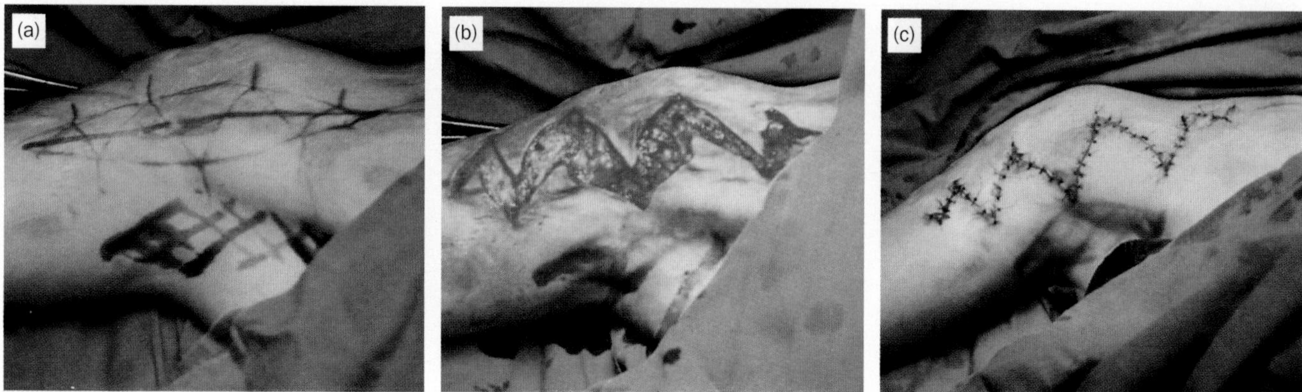

Fig. 14.13 (a, b, c) The Y–V plasty; (d) method of releasing burn scar contractures, the skin flaps are not undermined (unlike those of the Z plasty) and note that the axillary hair-bearing skin remains undisturbed (*courtesy of P.L. Levick, Birmingham*).

application of pressure, and patients are routinely fitted with Lycra pressure garments. Topical silicone sheeting may also be beneficial in limiting scar hypertrophy. Surgery is usually inappropriate for hypertrophic scars since they gradually improve with time (Chapter 3). Where burn scars cross surfaces near-joint scar contractures may occur. Late surgical reconstruction may be needed to release these contractures (Fig. 14.12). Broad contractures require releaser and insertion of skin grafts; such operations are particularly valuable in restoring the range of motion of a joint, but often leave a less than pleasing aesthetic result. Where there is a localised linear contracture a better technique may be Y–V plasty (Fig. 14.13). In some circumstances contractures can be released and burn scar area reduced by means of tissue expansion. This technique allows gradual stretching of marginal skin by implanting expander balloons under the adjacent normal skin. These are serially injected with saline through a port, thereby enlarging the expander and

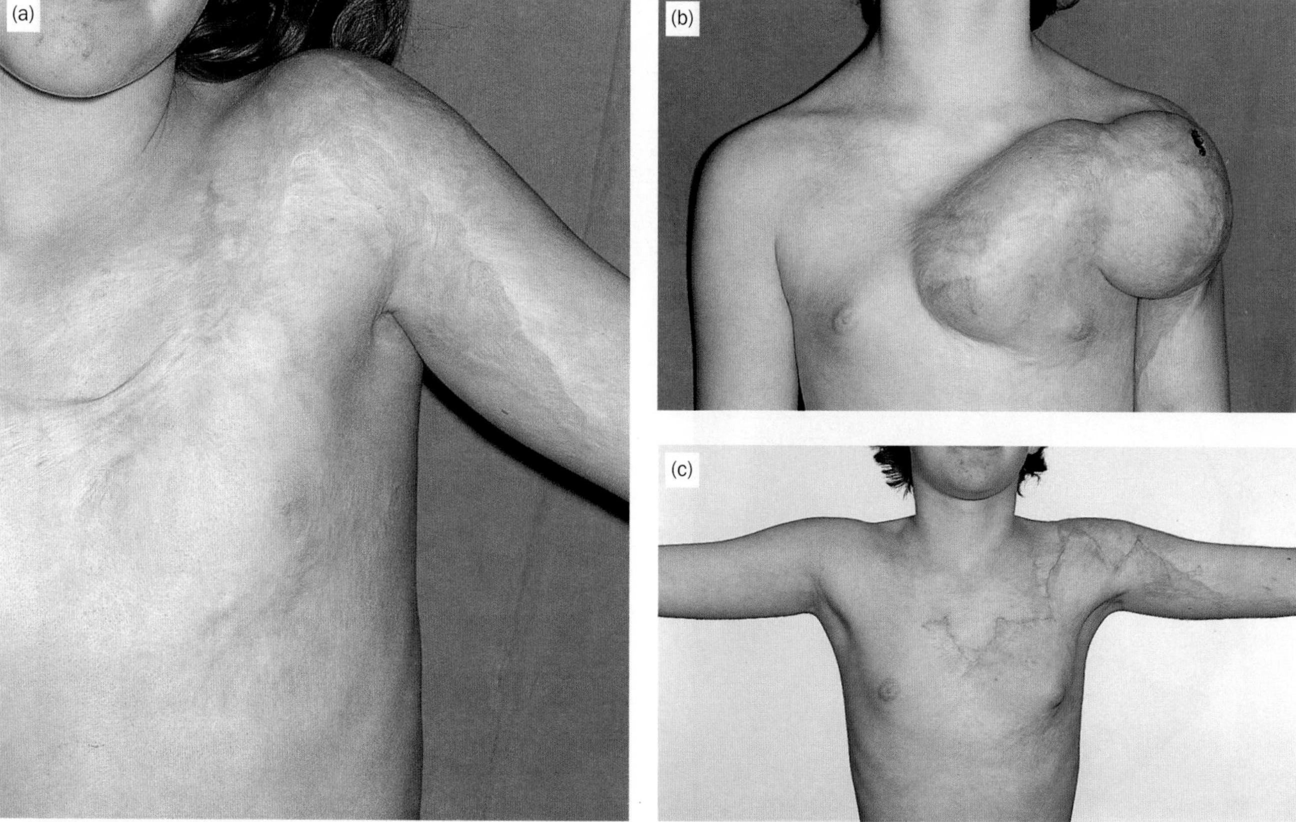

Fig. 14.14 (a) Burn scarring on the anterior chest in a teenage girl resulting from a scald in infancy. (b) There is a degree of contracture across the anterior chest and shoulder. Tissue expanders have been inserted and progressively inflated to generate more tissue. (c) It is now possible to release the contracture using the expanded flaps; a Y–V plasty was used. Late result showing good release without elevation of the nipple.

stretching the overlying skin. At a second operation the expander is removed and the excess skin stretched over the grafted area to aid reconstruction (Fig. 14.14). Tissue expansion is particularly useful in reconstruction of burn alopoecia. Missing eyebrows can be reconstructed by hair-bearing grafts or flaps. Extensive procedures may be necessary to reconstruct facial features such as the eyelids, lips and nose. In the long term, areas healed by skin grafting may be unstable and chronic ulceration in a grafted area may rarely lead on to a squamous carcinoma.

Further reading

Settle, J.A.D. (1986) *Burns – The First Five Days*, Smith and Nephew Pharmaceuticals, Romford.

Settle, J.A.D. (1996) *Principles and Practice of Burns Management*, Churchill Livingstone, Edinburgh.

The Australia and New Zealand Burn Association (1996) *Emergency Management of Severe Burns (EMSB) Course Manual*, ANZBA.

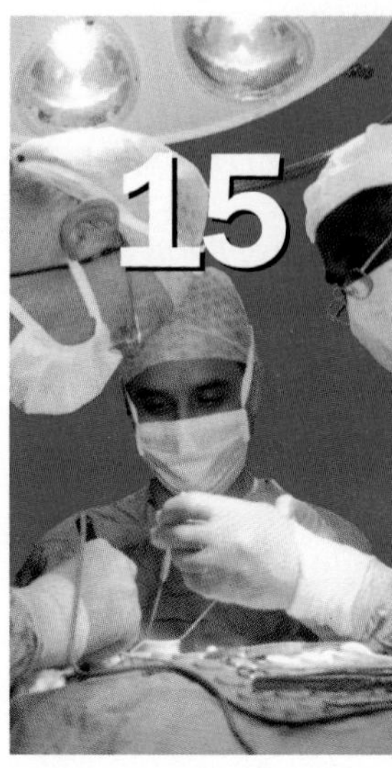

15 Arterial disorders

Conditions encountered in arteries include: stenosis or occlusion, dilatations (aneurysms), arteritis and small-vessel abnormalities.

Arterial stenosis or occlusion

Cause and effect

Arterial stenosis or occlusion is commonly caused by atherosclerosis, but can occur acutely as a result of emboli or trauma. Stenosis or occlusion produces symptoms related to the organ which is supplied by the artery: e.g. lower limb – claudication, rest pain and gangrene; brain – transient ischaemic attacks and hemiplegia; myocardium – angina and myocardial infarction; kidney – hypertension or infarction (Fig. 15.1); intestine – abdominal pain and infarction. The severity of the symptoms is related to the size of the vessel occluded and the alternative routes (collaterals)[1] available (Fig. 15.2).

Symptoms and signs of lower limb arterial stenosis or occlusion

Intermittent claudication[2]

Intermittent claudication is a cramp-like pain felt in the muscles that:

- is brought on by walking;
- is not present on taking the first step (contrast osteoarthrosis, Chapter 26);
- is relieved by standing still (contrast lumbar intervertebral disc nerve compression, Chapter 33).

The distance walked is called the **claudication distance.** It is a very subjective distance which varies only slightly from day to day in the same patient. It is altered by walking up hill or

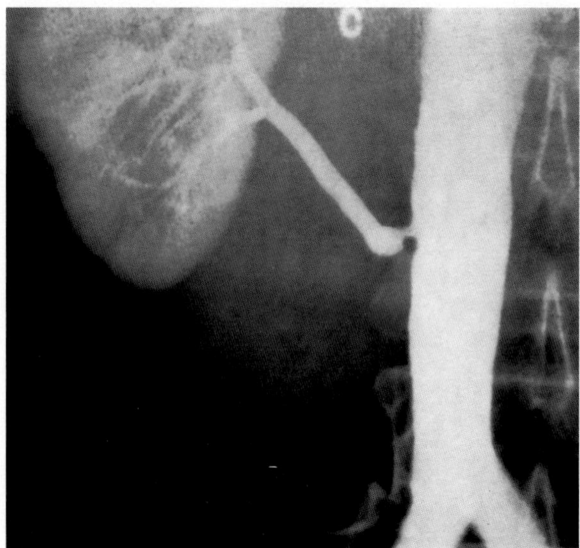

Fig. 15.1 Renal artery stenosis. Arteriogram by retrograde femoral catheterisation. Note the poststenotic dilatation.

[1]*Collateral circulation was demonstrated first by John Hunter, 1728–93. Surgeon, St George's Hospital, London, England.*

[2]*Claudication, from the Latin claudicatio – to limp. The Roman emperor Claudius 10* BC *to 54* AD *walked with a limp, possibly due to poliomyelitis.*

Bailey & Love's Short Practice of Surgery, 23rd edition. Edited by R.C.G. Russell, N.S. Williams and C.J.K. Bulstrode. Published in 2000 by Arnold Publishers.

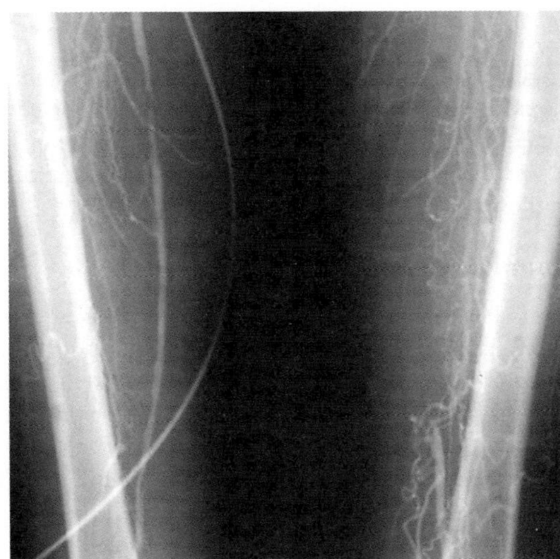

Fig. 15.2 Right superficial femoral stenosis. Left superficial femoral occlusion (causing claudication). Note collateral vessels.

against a wind, the speed of walking, or by changes in general health such as anaemia or heart failure.

The pain of claudication is most commonly felt in the calf, but can affect the thigh or buttock. Pain in the buttock occurring on exercise (walking) and associated sexual impotence, which result from arterial ischaemia, are given the eponymous title 'Leriche syndrome'. Claudication less commonly occurs in the upper limb in subclavian, axillary or brachial artery obstruction, the pain being brought on by such activities as writing or manual labour.

Rest pain

Rest pain is severe pain felt in the foot at rest, made worse by lying down or elevation of the foot. Characteristically, the pain is worse at night; it may be somewhat relieved by hanging the foot out of bed or by sleeping in a chair. Night cramps, which are short, severe muscle cramps of unknown origin, should not be confused with rest pain.

Coldness, numbness and paraesthesia

Coldness, numbness and paraesthesia are common in moderate as well as severe ischaemia but, in the absence of colour changes, it is essential to exclude a neurological cause.

Colour changes (Fig. 15.3)

Moderate or severely ischaemic limbs become blanched on elevation and develop a purple discoloration on dependency. Any bright red speckling is due to the extravasation of red cells through capillary walls. The angle of elevation at which blanching first occurs gives a rough guide to the degree of ischaemia.

Rene Leriche, 1879–1955. Surgeon, Strasbourg, France. First described the syndrome that bears his name in 1940.

(a)

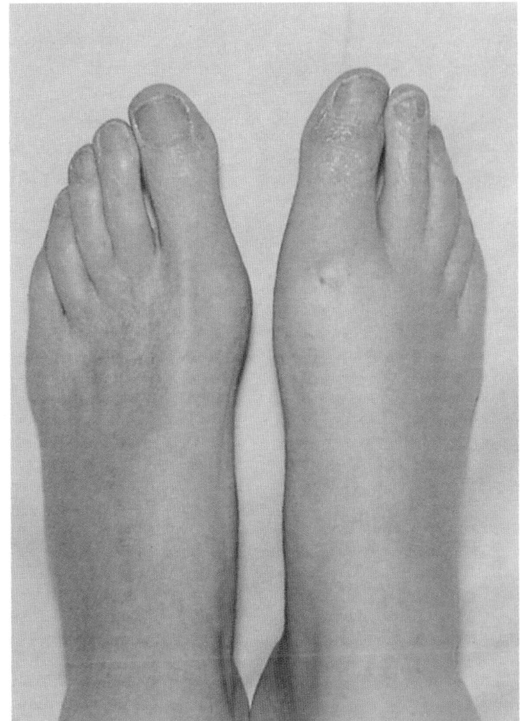

(b)

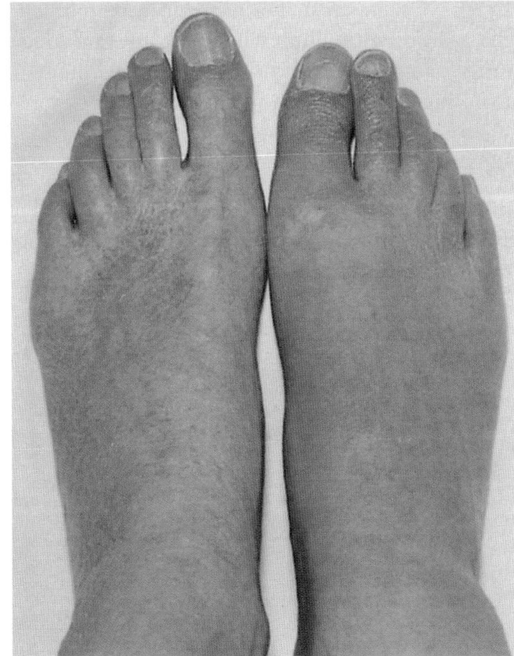

Fig. 15.3 Colour changes with (a) elevation and (b) dependency.

Ulceration and gangrene

Ulceration occurs with severe arterial insufficiency and often presents as a painful, superficial erosion between toes. Alternatively, small, shallow, indolent nonhealing ulcers may occur on the dorsum of the feet, on the shins and especially around the malleoli. The blackened mummified skin and

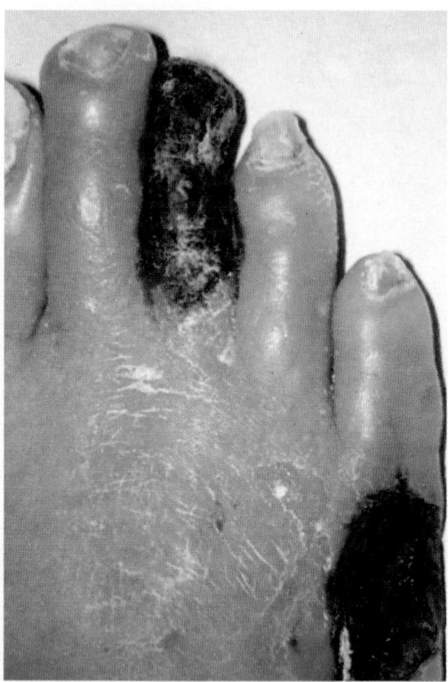

Fig. 15.4 Severe chronic ischaemia with dry gangrene.

tissues of frank gangrene are unmistakable to the observer (Fig. 15.4), but it must be remembered that in acute ischaemia a dead, white limb which becomes mottled means impending gangrene and not an improvement in the circulation. Fig. 15.5 shows a typical case.

Pregangrene

The combination of rest pain, colour changes, oedema and hyperaesthesia, with or without ischaemic ulceration, is frequently referred to as pregangrene.

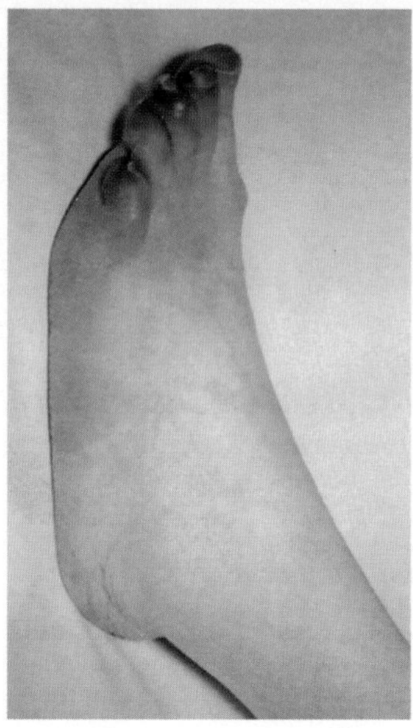

Fig. 15.5 Severe acute ischaemia (embolism – too late for embolectomy).

Temperature

A severely ischaemic foot is usually cold but sometimes paradoxically may feel warmer than the noninvolved foot. The acutely ischaemic limb tends to take on the temperature of its surroundings and may feel quite warm under the bedclothes.

Sensation and movement

Acutely ischaemic limbs are frequently paralysed and without sensation. These are ominous physical signs and such a limb has a poor prognosis in the absence of active treatment. Severe chronic ischaemia does not produce paralysis, but hyperaesthesia is common, especially in those areas of skin on the borderline of gangrene. Gentle handling of such limbs is essential.

Arterial pulsations

Arterial pulsations below an occlusion in a main artery are usually absent or, in the presence of good collaterals, diminished. In patients with vascular symptoms, it is standard practice to feel the pulsations in the radial arteries, the carotid arteries, the abdominal aorta, the femoral arteries in the groins, the popliteal arteries behind the knees (an easily palpable popliteal artery may be aneurysmal), the posterior tibial arteries behind the medial malleoli and the dorsalis pedis arteries on the dorsum of the feet. Diminution of a pulse can best be appreciated by comparing it with the pulse in the other limb, provided that the latter is normal. Expansile arterial pulsation with a mass may indicate an aneurysm. In arterial occlusion with a highly developed collateral circulation, or in main artery stenosis, the distal pulses may be normal to palpation. The following physical sign is then useful.

The 'disappearing pulse'

Where peripheral pulses are apparently normal, exercising the patient to the point of claudication may unmask the effect of an arterial obstruction by causing the previously palpable pulse to disappear. After a minute or two of rest the disappearing pulse reappears. The explanation is that exercise produces vasodilatation below the obstructing lesion and the arterial inflow, reduced by the lesion, cannot keep pace with the increasing vascular space; arterial pressure falls and the pulse disappears.

Arterial bruits

A vascular examination should include auscultation of the subclavian arteries in the supraclavicular fossas, the carotid arteries behind the angle of the mandibles, the abdominal aorta and the femoral arteries in the groins and over the adductor (subsartorial) canals. A systolic bruit over an artery is due to turbulence and indicates a stenosis of the artery.

Systolic bruits

Systolic bruits are conducted distally. Thus a bruit in the neck at the level of the angle of the mandible without any supraclavicular bruit frequently means a carotid artery stenosis. Where, however, a bruit is heard at both sites, its origin may be more proximal, e.g. aortic valve, aortic arch, brachiocephalic or subclavian arteries. Under these circumstances the carotid artery may prove quite normal. The patient with renal artery stenosis shown in Fig. 15.1 had a bruit over the renal artery. A continuous 'machinery' murmur over an artery usually indicates the presence of an arteriovenous fistula.

Venous refilling

The limb should be elevated for 30 s and then laid flat on the bed. Normal refilling occurs within seconds. Reduced venous filling is often present in the severer forms of arterial insufficiency, but is also common in vasospastic disease and in cold weather.

Harvey's sign

If the two index fingers are placed firmly side by side on a vein and the finger nearer the heart is moved so as to empty a short length of vein, the release of the distal finger will allow the speed of venous refilling to be observed. Increased venous return and varicosities of veins are associated with arteriovenous fistulas.

Impotence

Impotence from failure to achieve an erection is often a feature in male patients with an occlusion in the region of the bifurcation of the aorta and the internal iliac arteries (Leriche's syndrome).

Relationship of clinical findings to the site of disease

By associating the symptoms and signs found in a case of arterial disease, the site of the major arterial obstruction can be determined (Table 15.1).

Table 15.1 Relationship of clinical findings to site of disease

Aortoiliac obstruction	Claudication in both buttocks, thighs and calves Femoral and distal pulses absent in both limbs. Bruit over aortoiliac region. Impotence common (Leriche)
Iliac obstruction	Unilateral claudication in thigh and calf and sometimes buttock Bruit over iliac region Unilateral absence of femoral and distal pulses
Femoropopliteal obstruction	Unilateral claudication in calf Femoral pulse palpable with absent unilateral distal pulses
Distal obstruction	Femoral and popliteal pulses palpable
Ankle pulses absent	Claudication in calf and foot

The best results from surgery are obtained by operation on the larger vessels which allow a high volume of blood flow through bypass grafts. For instance, aortoiliac bypass is longer lasting than femorotibial bypass.

William Harvey, 1578–1657. Physician, St Bartholomew's Hospital, London, England. First described circulation of the blood in his course of lectures at the Royal College of Physicians of London in 1615.

Double blocks

The presence of another (secondary) obstruction can usually be inferred. For example, a patient with signs of iliac artery obstruction, but with rest pain and pregangrene of the foot, must have a secondary obstruction as collateral circulation around an isolated iliac artery obstruction is usually excellent. The severe symptoms indicate a secondary obstruction, probably in the femoral or popliteal arteries.

Investigation of arterial stenosis or occlusion

Many patients with symptoms due to arterial disease without stenosis or occlusion do not need active treatment. This decision can often be made without submitting the patient to a series of special investigations. Active treatment includes angioplasty and surgical reconstruction.

General

Patients with arterial disease tend to be elderly and atherosclerosis is a generalised disease. If surgery is indicated, a full assessment is essential.

Investigations

Investigations relevant to diabetes, abnormalities of lipid metabolism, anaemia, conditions causing high blood viscosity, e.g. polycythaemia and thrombocythaemia (in small-vessel disease), include a full blood count (including erythrocyte sedimentation rate and platelets), plasma fibrinogen, protein

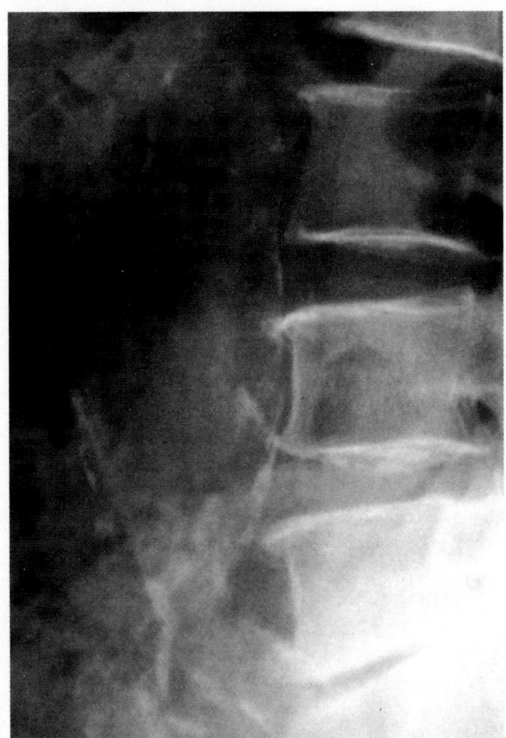

Fig. 15.6 Plain lateral radiograph of the abdomen reveals an abdominal aortic aneurysm outlined by calcium flecks.

electrophoresis, blood and urine glucose and blood lipid profile. A plain radiograph of the abdomen will show the presence of arterial calcification and flecks of calcium may outline an aneurysm (Fig. 15.6). Heart failure, myocardial ischaemia, hypertension and age-related diseases such as bronchial problems and neoplasia should also be excluded.

Electrocardiography (ECG)

Although a normal ECG does not exclude severe coronary artery disease, a grossly abnormal ECG may influence the decision for surgery in patients with lower limb disease.

Exercise ECG gives a more accurate cardiac assessment, although many of the patients are severely limited in their ability to exercise.

Radioisotope ventriculography

This is an isotope technique measuring left ventricular ejection fraction which correlates well with cardiac function.

Echocardiography

This noninvasive technique is often useful in assessing left ventricular function.

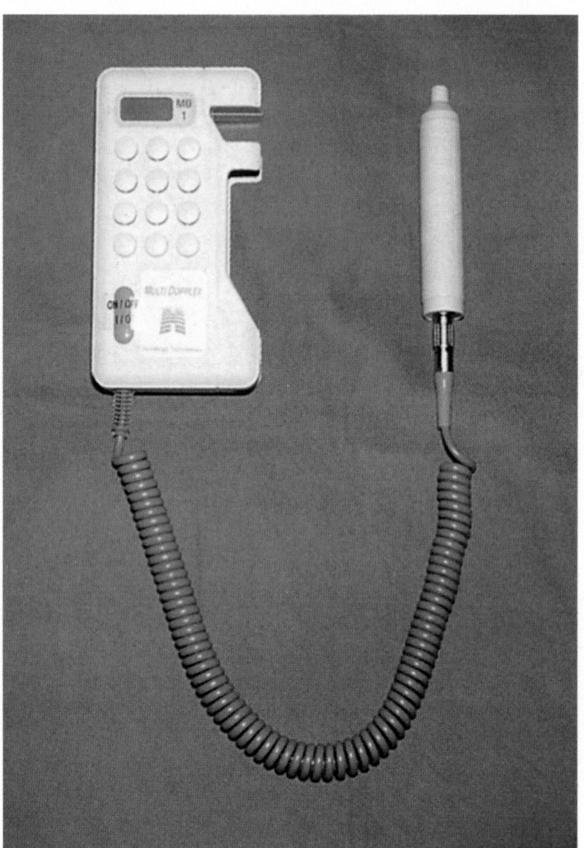

Fig. 15.7 Simple hand-held Doppler ultrasound probe.

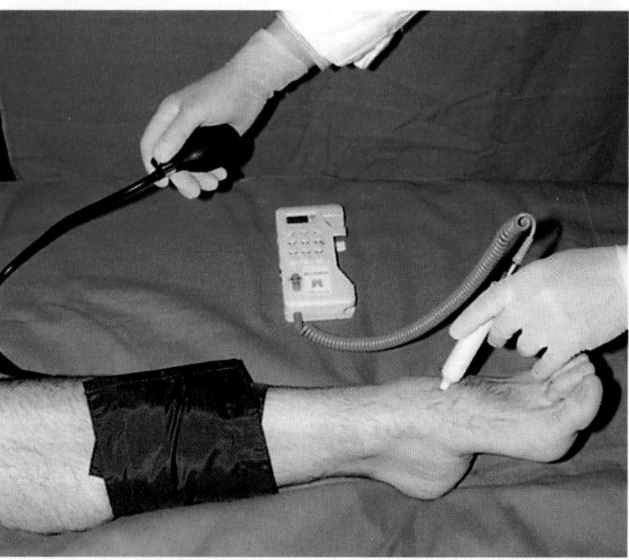

Fig. 15.8 Hand-held Doppler probe and sphygmomanometer used to determine systolic pressure in the dorsalis pedis artery, as part of assessing the ankle:brachial pressure index.

Doppler ultrasound blood flow detection (Figs 15.7 and 15.8)

A continuous wave ultrasound signal is beamed at an artery and the reflected beam picked up by a receiver. The change in frequency in the reflected beam compared with that of the transmitted beam is due to the Doppler shift, resulting from the reflection of the beam by moving blood cells. The frequency change may be converted into an audio signal and, in arteries, a pulsatile sound typically results. Doppler ultrasound equipment can, therefore, be used as a very sensitive type of stethoscope in conjunction with a sphygmomanometer to assess the systolic pressure in relatively small vessels. This is often possible even at sites where the arterial pulse cannot be palpated.

The ankle:brachial pressure index (ABPI) is the ratio of systolic pressure at the ankle to that in the arm. Generally, the higher of the recordings of pressure in the dorsalis pedis and posterior tibial arteries serves as the numerator, with the higher systolic pressure between the brachials serving as the denominator. The resting ABPI is normally about 1.0; values below 0.9 indicate some degree of arterial obstruction. A value of less than 0.3 suggests imminent necrosis. It must be appreciated, however, that values approaching normality at rest may still be associated with intermittent claudication. Retesting after exercise is useful in this context: in normality ABPI will rise while occlusive disease may result in a depression of ABPI.

A Doppler ultrasound probe can also be used to assess differences in arterial blood pressure between segments of a limb, thereby giving an indication of the site of a stenosis. In the leg, the cuff is commonly placed above the ankle, at midcalf and midthigh, to provide 'segmental pressures'. Artefacts are due especially to calcified arteries, which may be incompressible and lead to a falsely high limb pressure or ABPI result. This is particularly the case in diabetics.

Christian Johann Doppler, 1803–53. Austrian physicist.

Duplex imaging

This is an investigative technique of major importance in vascular disease. A duplex scanner uses B-mode ultrasound to provide an image of vessels (Figs 15.9 and 15.10). This image is created through the different ability of different tissues to reflect the ultrasound beam. A second type of ultrasound, namely Doppler ultrasound, is then used to insonate the imaged vessels and the Doppler shift obtained is analysed by a dedicated computer in the duplex scanner. Such shifts can give detailed knowledge of vessel blood flow, turbulence, etc. Some scanners have the added sophistication of colour coding which allows visualisation of blood flow on the image. The various colours indicate change in direction and velocity of flow; points of high flow generally indicate a stenosis. It should be appreciated that modern duplex scanning is at least as accurate as angiography in certain circumstances. In terms of cost-effectiveness and safety, duplex scanning is generally to be preferred to angiography if they are considered to be equally useful in any given clinical context.

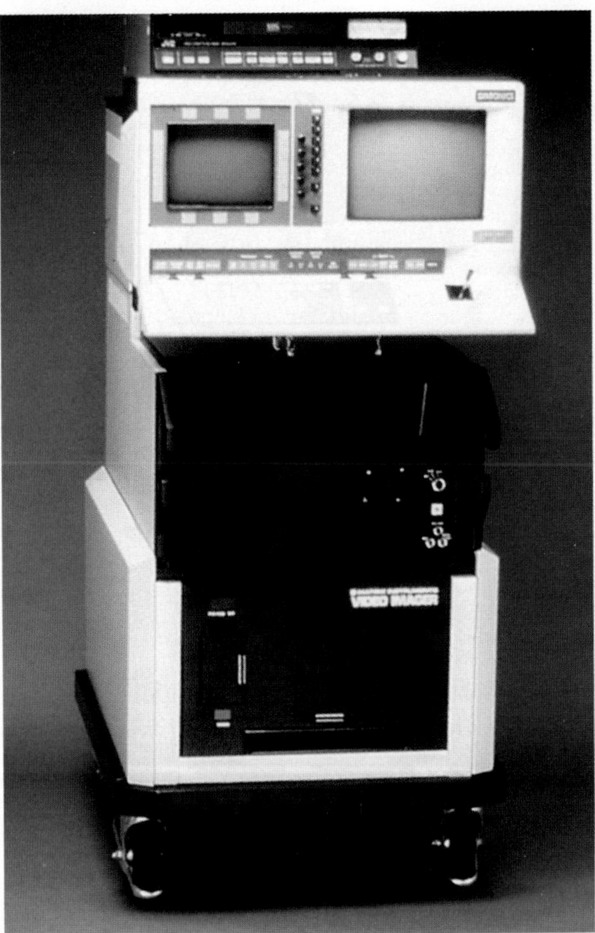

Fig. 15.9 Duplex scanner.

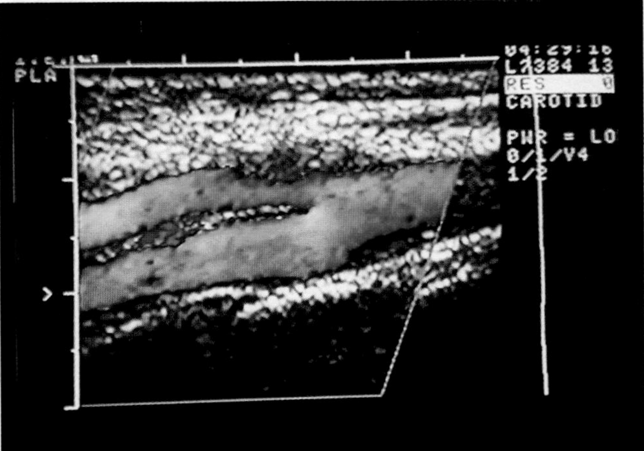

Fig. 15.10 Colour duplex scan of carotid vessels in neck showing stenosis at common carotid bifurcation (*courtesy of Dr Paul Allan, Royal Infirmary, Edinburgh, Scotland*).

Plethysmography

Plethysmography assesses changes in volume of a limb or digit over the cardiac cycle. Air-filled cuffs or mercury in rubber strain gauges have typically been used. For most clinical purposes the test has been superseded by duplex scanning, although plethysmography may still have certain research uses.

Oculoplethysmography

Oculoplethysmography (OPG) uses fluid- or air-filled cups attached to the eye by suction to investigate carotid artery disease. Once again, the technique has largely been superseded by duplex scanning.

Treadmill

A treadmill with a slight incline is a useful diagnostic apparatus in the assessment of walking distance in claudicants. Patients are known to be very poor assessors of walking ability in terms of distance; objective measurement using the treadmill is recommended.

Arteriography (syn. angiography)

In lower limb disease it is symptoms and their severity which decide whether intervention is needed. An arteriogram is done only after a decision has been taken that intervention is appropriate. Even then, it may be advisable in some circumstances to precede the arteriogram with a duplex scan. This is so especially in the field of carotid artery disease where arteriography is associated with a stroke rate of between 1 and 2 per cent. Many surgeons are content to operate on carotid artery disease solely on the results of a duplex scan without arteriography.

Arteriography involves the injection of a radio-opaque solution into the arterial tree, generally by a retrograde percutaneous method usually involving the femoral (occasionally the brachial or axillary) artery. This retrograde method is known as the Seldinger technique (Figs 15.11 and 15.12). Direct arteriography, by puncturing, for example, the carotid artery or aorta, is more hazardous; it is outdated and no longer in use. Hazards include thrombosis, arterial dissection, haematoma, neurological dysfunction and anaphylaxis. Anaphylactic reactions can occur even with a trial injection and informed consent should always be obtained for this form of imaging.

S.I. Seldinger, b. 1921. Swedish radiologist.

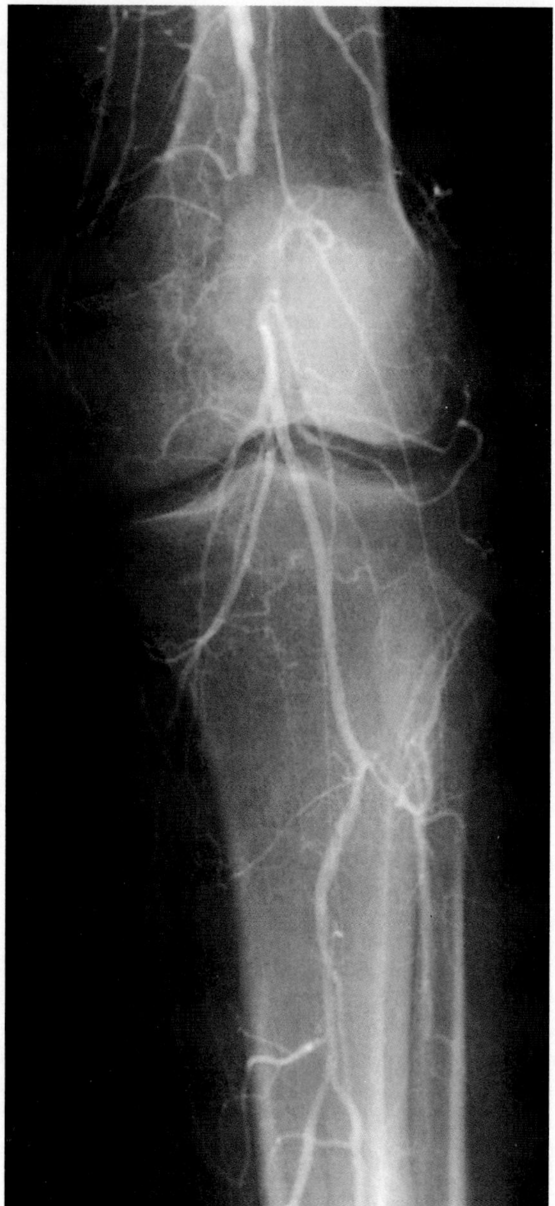

Fig. 15.11 Arterial occlusion just above the knee causing claudication of the calf, good collateral circulation (arteriogram by Seldinger technique).

Digital subtraction angiography (DSA)

This technique, which is in widespread use, employs a computer system to digitise the angiographic information (Fig 15.13). It allows the image before contrast injection to be subtracted from the contrast image, yielding great clarity. DSA may be carried out by arterial or venous injection. The former allows the use of finer catheters and less contrast agent than conventional angiography.

The latter avoids the need for arterial puncture completely, although rather high volumes of contrast agent must be injected into a large vein.

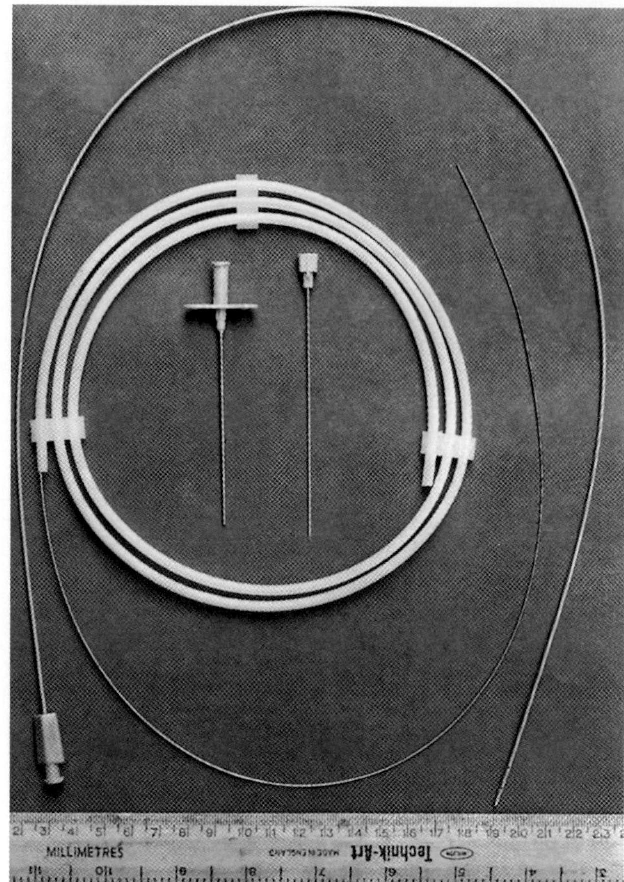

Fig. 15.12 Seldinger needle and guidewire for introducing an arterial catheter.

Management of arterial stenosis or occlusion

Explanation and advice

Patients are worried by the presence of pain on walking. Once told that walking is not doing harm, many are content to live within the limitations imposed by their claudication. Spontaneous improvement occurs in some patients over the first 6 months after an occlusive episode as collateral vessels are developed.

Adjustment of lifestyle

Adjustments to everyday habits of transport can increase mobility within the claudication distance, e.g. the use of a bicycle or a car.

Stopping smoking

Particularly for patients with Buerger's disease (see later in this chapter). Progression of the disease and graft failure after surgery are more common in any patient who continues to smoke.

Leo Buerger, 1879–1943. Professor of Urologic Surgery, New York Polyclinic Medical School, New York, USA. Described thromboangiitis obliterans in 1908.

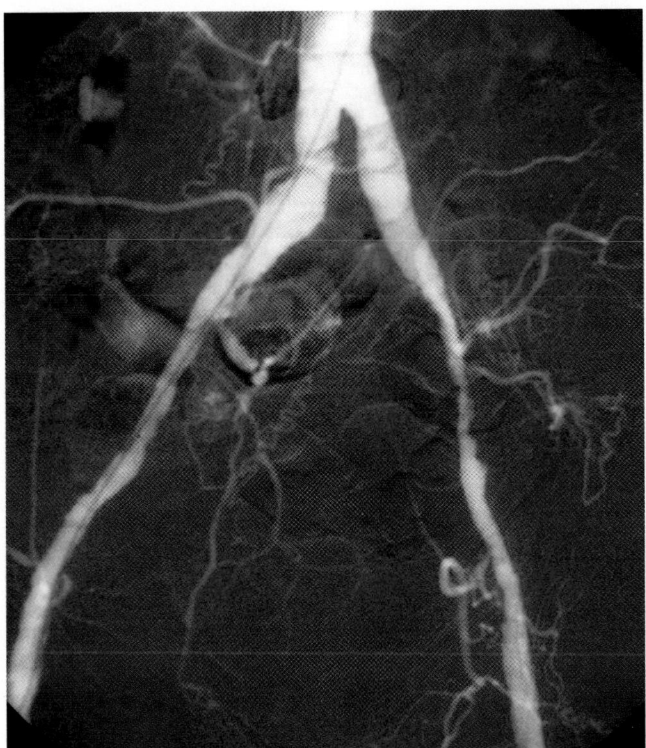

Fig. 15.13 Digital subtraction aortography by intra-arterial injection. Note the retrograde Seldinger catheter within the right iliac artery. The proximal left external iliac artery is stenosed.

Taking regular exercise

Within the limits of the pain.

Diet

To reduce weight in the obese and, more specifically, in the treatment of hyperlipidaemia.

Drugs

Vasodilator drugs are ineffective in the management of arteriosclerotic disease.

- Praxilene (naftidrofuryl oxalate) may alter tissue metabolism, increasing the claudicating distance by allowing a greater oxygen debt to be incurred.
- Trental (oxpentifylline) has some effect on whole blood viscosity.
- Prostacyclin is currently being evaluated and may have a role in the management of the critically ischaemic limb.

Lipid abnormalities

The first line of treatment is dietary to reduce weight (if necessary) and to reduce fat intake. Patients who have no primary metabolic disease and who achieve an ideal weight but remain lipaemic should be considered for drug treatment.

Diabetes and hypertension

These should be treated by standard methods. In hypertension, the overzealous reduction of blood pressure by the use of beta-adrenoceptor blocking drugs can worsen claudication.

Care of the feet

This includes avoiding socks with holes and amateur chiropody, which can spark off gangrene in the toes and heels, particularly in diabetic patients.

Heel raise

Claudication distance may be increased by raising the heels of shoes by 1 cm. The work of the calf muscles is reduced thereby.

Analgesics and position

Rest pain can be relieved to some extent in some patients by the use of analgesics and elevation of the head of the bed (Buerger's position).

Aspirin

In dispersible form this may be prescribed for its anti-adhesive effect on platelets. A dose of 150 mg/day is usual.

Sympathectomy

Sympathectomy is not effective in claudication but occasionally it may relieve ischaemic rest pain and ulceration. However, it must be recognised that the results of sympathectomy are very much poorer than those of bypass surgery or percutaneous transluminal angioplasty. Sympathectomy can only be justified when it is not technically possible to operate or employ balloon angioplasty. The details of lumbar sympathectomy (operative and chemical) are given at the end of this chapter.

Transluminal angioplasty (Figs 15.14 and 15.15)

Arterial occlusive disease may be treated by inserting a balloon catheter into an artery and inflating it within a narrowed area. This may be done

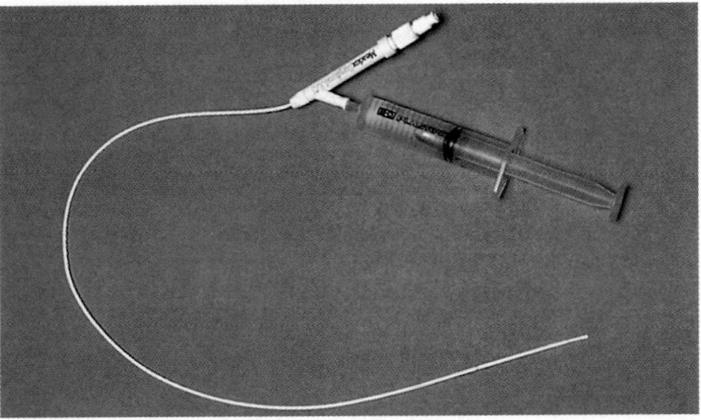

Fig. 15.14 Balloon catheter for percutaneous transluminal angioplasty.

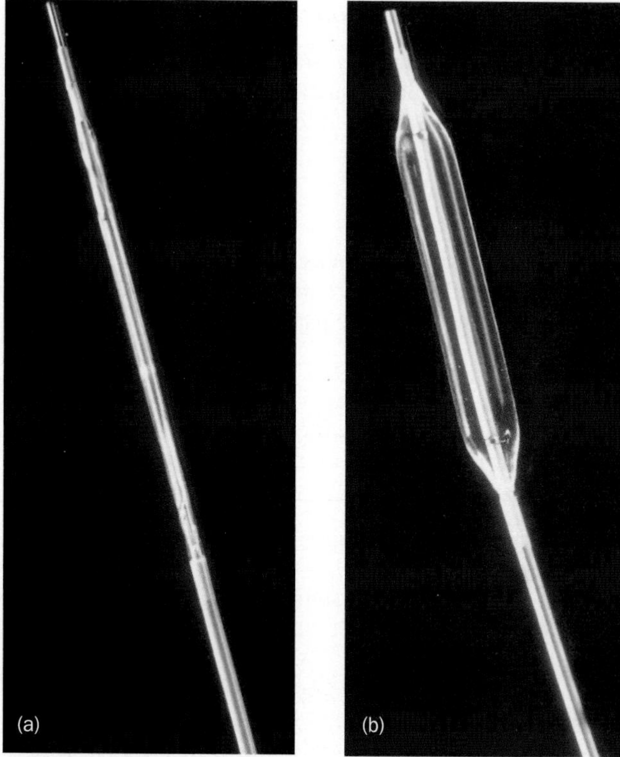

Fig. 15.15 (a) Catheter balloon deflated; (b) balloon inflated.

at the same time as an operation but, more usually, it is carried out percutaneously in the radiology department (Figs 15.16 and 15.17). Percutaneous transluminal angioplasty (PTA) may be used for stenoses or short occlusions; in the latter case the occlusion must first be traversed by a guidewire. Balloon angioplasty has had its major success in dilating the iliac vessels. To a lesser extent the vessels of the leg itself may be dilated with a good outcome.

Technique. A femoral arteriogram is performed and a guidewire inserted through any stenosis to be treated. The balloon catheter is then inserted over the guidewire. The balloon is positioned within the stenosis (confirmed by angiography). The balloon is then inflated for approximately 1 minute and then deflated. This is repeated before withdrawal of the catheter.

Atherectomy

A variety of new devices is available to allow the percutaneous removal of atheroma from within the vessel in the radiology department. These cutting catheters have several styles and their use in certain circumstances, e.g. eccentric plaque, may be efficacious.

Intraluminal stents (Figs 15.18 and 15.19)

In certain circumstances after balloon dilatation, the vessel fails to stay adequately dilated and it may then be possible to hold the lumen open using a metal stent. Such a device may be introduced on a balloon catheter; the balloon itself when inflated expanding the stent, which acts as a rigid skeleton for the vessel, keeping it widely patent. The catheter balloon is deflated and the catheter removed. An alternative type of self-expanding stent is held compressed by a sheath of plastic in a delivery system. When the stent has been positioned at the appropriate arterial site the sheath is withdrawn and the stent self-expands to hold the lumen open. The results of stenting have not been fully assessed but early results suggest that the technique has considerable promise.

Operations for arterial stenosis or occlusion

Site of disease and type of operation

Aortoiliac occlusion with good calibre vessels below the site of disease responds well to aortofemoral bypass (Fig. 15.20a). If the disease is limited in extent, an iliac endarterectomy might be considered, but PTA with or without a stent is probably a better alternative if technically possible. In the patient who is unable to withstand major abdominal surgery and who has pronounced ischaemia due to aortoiliac occlusion, a femoro–femoral or ilio–femoral crossover bypass may be considered (if only one iliac system is involved with disease) or an axillo–bifemoral bypass may be done (if both iliac segments are diseased).

Superficial femoral and profunda femoris artery occlusive disease often produce unilateral symptoms. For long-distance claudication, conservative treatment is usually suitable. For more severe disease a supervised exercise programme may be appropriate. In certain circumstances, when the occlusive appearance on angiography is favourable and the patient fully understands the risks and benefits of intervention, angioplasty or bypass may be considered. A femoropopliteal bypass graft (Fig. 15.20b) is the most usual operation (to overcome a blocked superficial femoral artery). Long-term graft patency is related to the inflow and outflow from the graft. It is also related to the material used for the bypass. The patient's own saphenous vein gives the best results when used either as a reversed conduit or *in situ* after valve disruption. In some patients a profunda femoris origin stenosis is noted and this situation can be helped by a small patch angioplasty to relieve the diseased site.

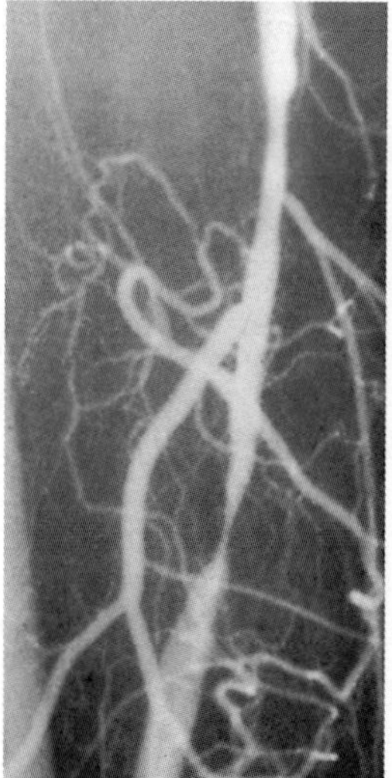
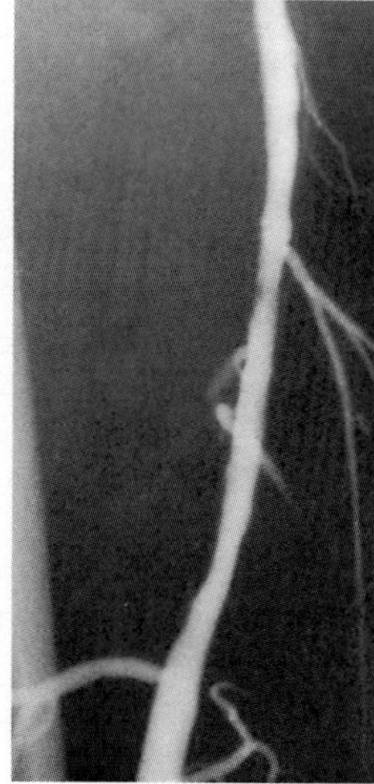

Fig. 15.16 Narrowed superficial femoral artery before and after transluminal angioplasty (*courtesy of J. McIvor, FRCR, London*). An advantage of this technique is that it can be done under local anaesthesia using the Seldinger technique (Fig. 15.12) of percutaneous arterial puncture, and therefore useful in the treatment of those patients who are medically unfit for major surgery.

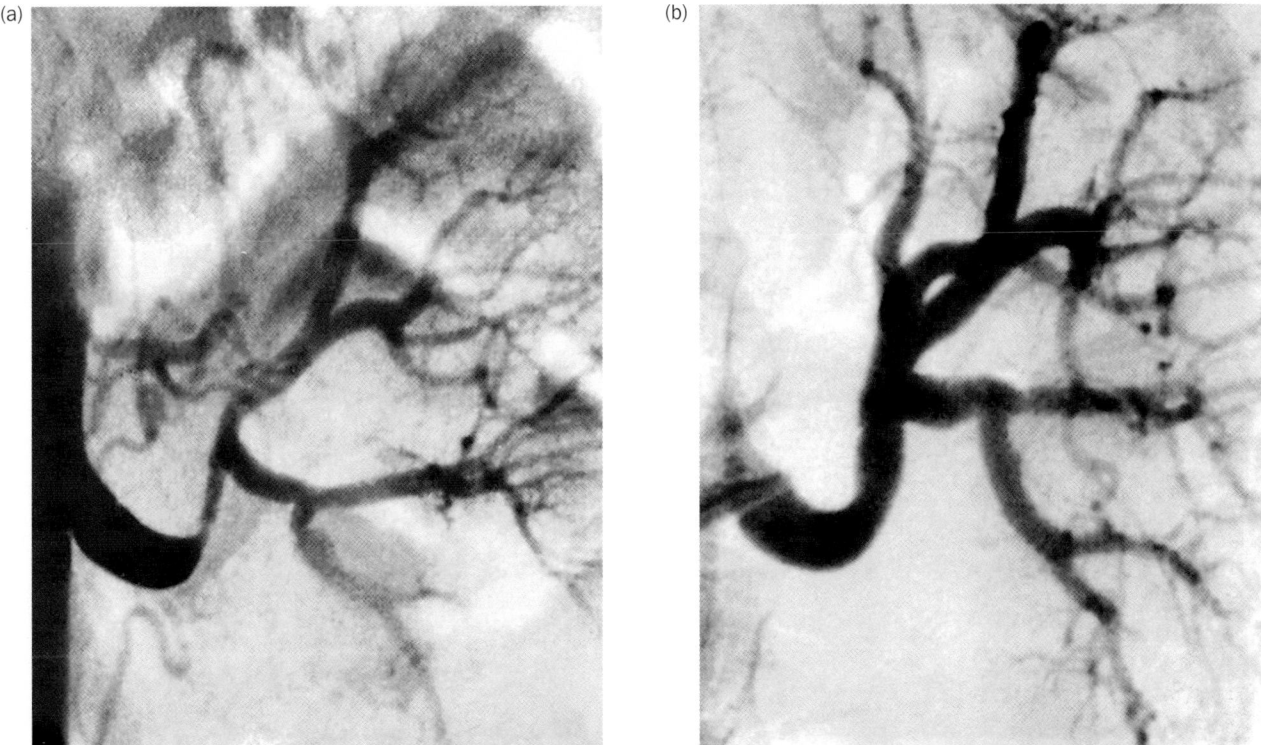

Fig. 15.17 (a) Before and (b) after balloon dilatation of a severely stenosed left renal artery in a 20-year-old woman with uncontrollable hypertension. The blood pressure fell to normal after the procedure. The stenosis was probably due to fibromuscular hyperplasia but there was no tissue available for histological diagnosis.

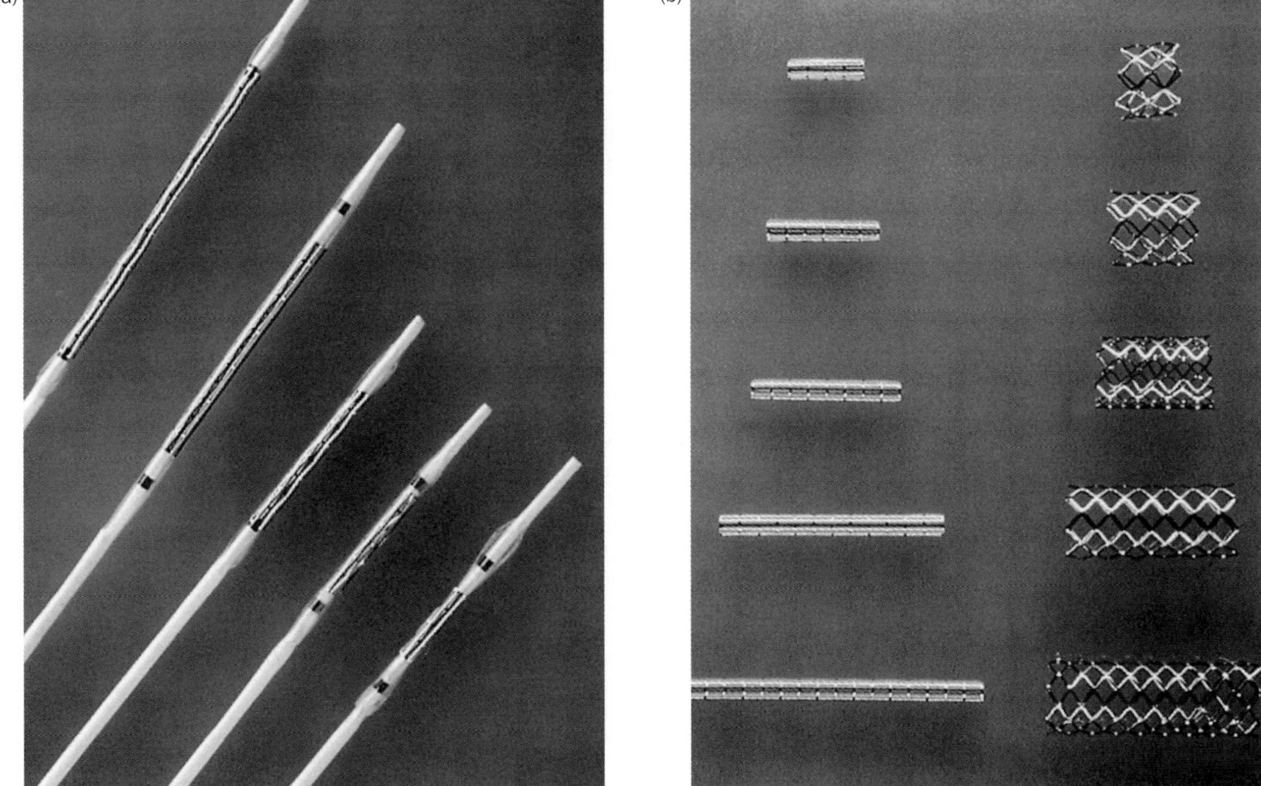

Fig. 15.18 (a) Balloon catheters carrying stents; (b) nonexpanded (left) and expanded stents (right) (*courtesy of Johnson and Johnson Interventional Systems, Bracknell, Berks, England*).

(a)

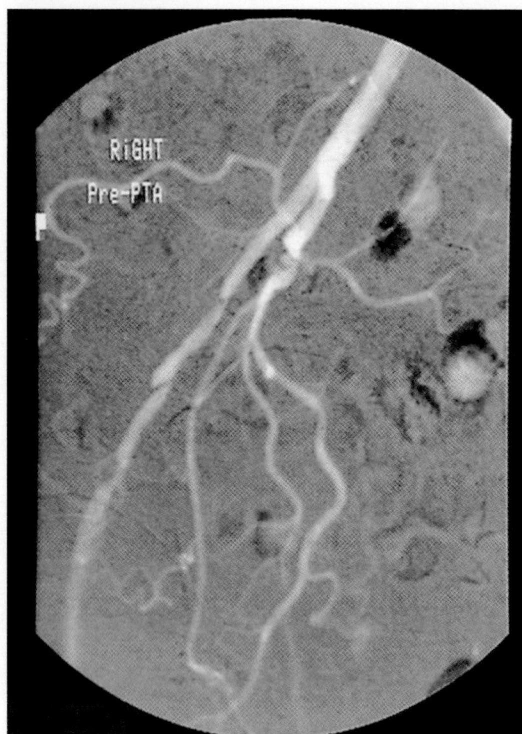

(b)

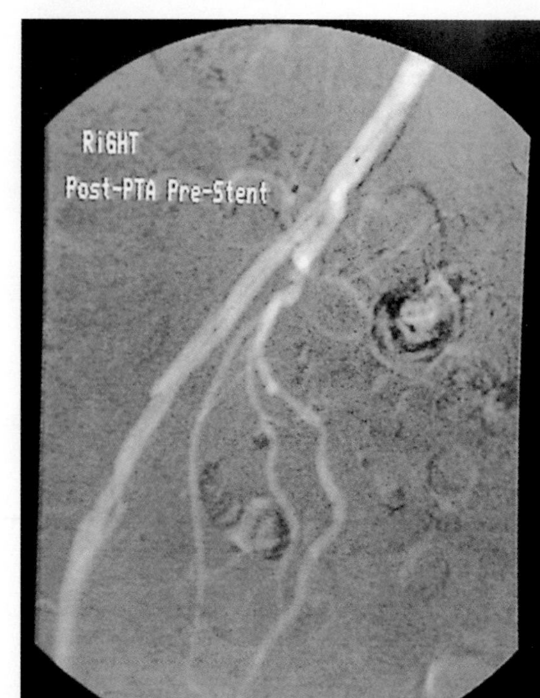

(c)

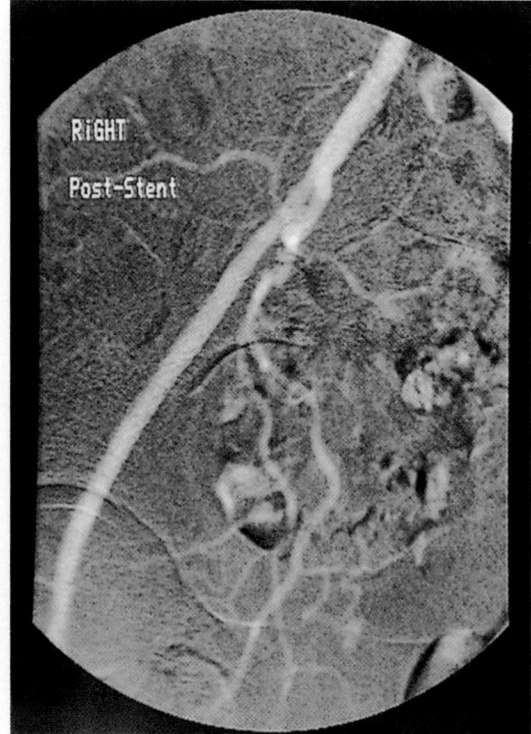

Fig. 15.19 (a) External iliac artery stenosis before dilatation; (b) after dilatation by percutaneous transluminal angioplasty; (c) dilated artery patency assured by stent (*courtesy of Johnson and Johnson Interventional Systems, Bracknell, Berks, and Dr W. Shaw, Ninewells Hospital, Dundee, Scotland*).

Occlusive disease below the popliteal artery used to be widely regarded as unreconstructable but it is increasingly recognised that bypass to the tibial vessels, even down to ankle level, can be met with reasonable success. The most usual and successful conduit is the long saphenous vein used in the *in situ* fashion after disrupting the valves with a valvulotome. If the saphenous vein is not available from either leg, it may still be realistic to carry out the surgery with a polytetrafluoroethylene (PTFE) graft; many surgeons construct the lower anastomosis using a small collar of vein between the PTFE and the recipient artery. This technique (Miller cuff) may give prolonged patency.

Prosthetic materials

For bypass of the aortoiliac segment the favoured material is Dacron (Fig. 15.21a). Prostheses come in two types: woven and knitted. Woven grafts tend to leak less when first exposed to blood flow during surgery, but newer knitted prostheses may be sealed with gelatin or collagen by the manufacturer and may leak even less than their woven counterparts. In the final analysis, there is probably little to choose between any of the styles of Dacron graft; all achieve satisfactory results. For bypass in the femoropopliteal region, if autogenous long saphenous vein (or other veins such as the short saphenous or arm vein) is not available, PTFE (Fig. 15.21b) or glutaraldehyde-tanned, Dacron-supported, human umbilical vein (Fig. 15.21c) may be employed. In general, any vein used requires a diameter of at least 3.5 mm. For profundaplasty, a small piece of vein may be used or, alternatively, PTFE or Dacron.

Suture materials for vascular surgery are usually monofilament in nature; polypropylene has been particularly popular. In the aorta it is

---

Justin H. Miller. Australian Surgeon.

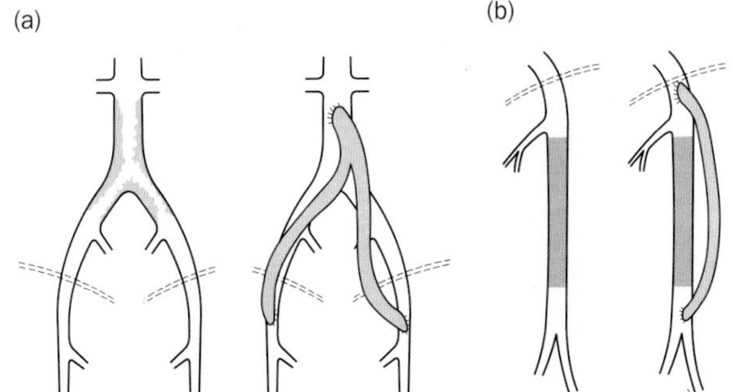

Fig. 15.20 (a) Atherosclerotic narrowing of the aortic bifurcation. Aorto-bi-femoral graft to bypass stenosis. (b) Superficial femoral artery occlusion with profunda femoris stenosis providing poor collateral circulation. Femoropopliteal graft used to bypass the occluded area into good 'runoff' below.

usual to use 2/0 or 3/0 polypropylene. In the femoral artery at the groin it is usual to use 4/0 or 5/0 polypropylene. Finer sutures, up to 7/0, may be needed further down the limb. PTFE may (alternatively) be stitched using a suture of the same material. PTFE sutures tend to cause less bleeding through stitch holes in the graft substance.

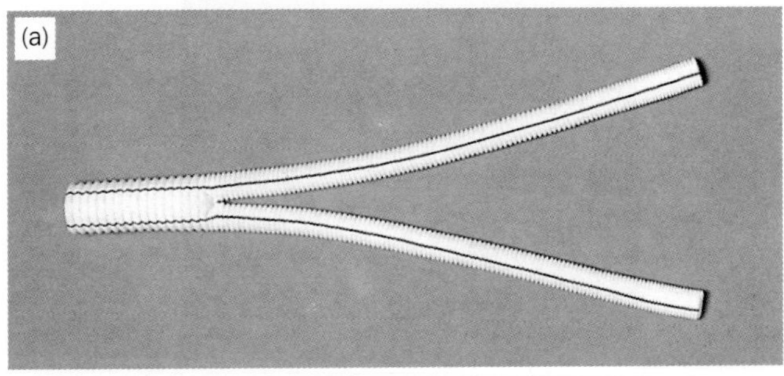

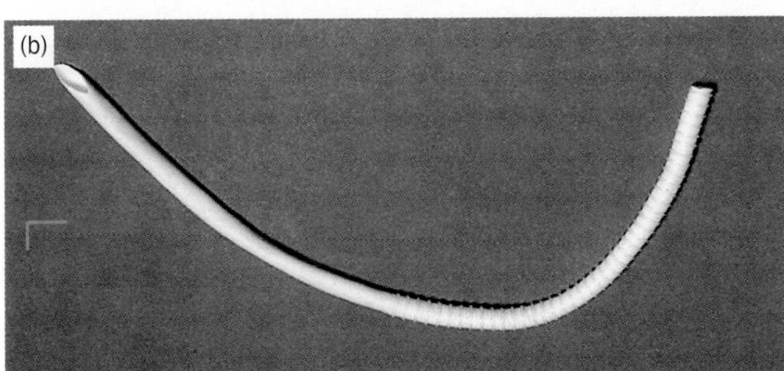

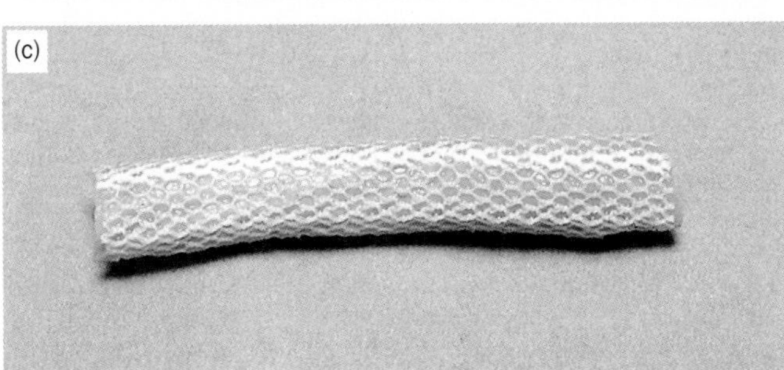

Fig. 15.21 (a) Dacron bifurcation graft; (b) polytetrafluoroethylene graft; (c) human umbilical vein graft.

Operative details

Aortofemoral bypass graft. The aorta is approached through a midline or transverse abdominal incision. The common femoral arteries and their branches are exposed through vertical groin incisions. The small bowel is retracted to the right and the posterior peritoneum opened. Retroperitoneal tunnels are made from the aorta to the groins. Heparin (5000 units) is given intravenously and the vessels are clamped. A vertical incision is made in the anterior aspect of the aorta to which an obliquely cut, bifurcated Dacron graft is sutured. The graft limbs are then fed down to the groins where they are in turn anastomosed to the common femoral arteries or, if there is evidence of profunda stenosis, to an arteriotomy running from the common femoral vessel down into the profunda. The posterior peritoneum is closed carefully over the Dacron to prevent adhesion of the graft to bowel. The abdomen and groin wounds are closed without drainage.

Femoropopliteal bypass. The popliteal artery above or below the knee is exposed through a medial incision. The femoral artery is exposed at groin level. The long saphenous vein may be treated in two different ways. First, it may be excised, its tributaries tied, reversed and sutured into the limb as a bypass. Second, it may be left in place (*in situ*) and the valves disrupted with a valvulotome, either blindly or using an angioscope. The graft is then sutured to the femoral artery proximally and to the popliteal vessel distally. Suction drains are rarely necessary.

Femorodistal bypass. This surgery is usually carried out using long saphenous vein in the *in situ* mode. Great care must be taken at the conclusion of the procedure to assess the conduit and the lower anastomosis. This may be done using completion angiography or angioscopy (Figs 15.22 and 15.23).

Profundaplasty. The common femoral artery and its branches are exposed through a vertical incision. After giving intravenous heparin and clamping the vessels, an incision is made into the common femoral artery and carried down into the profunda, effectively dividing the stenotic profunda origin. The arteriotomy is then closed with a vein, Dacron or PTFE patch to widen the narrowed segment.

Other arterial operations and salvage procedures

Femorofemoral crossover graft is useful for relieving an iliac artery occlusion when the other iliac artery is patent with a strong femoral pulse. An 8-mm Dacron or PTFE graft is tunnelled subcutaneously above the pubis and anastomosed end-to-side to the common femoral arteries on each side. Blood from the patent iliac system is then carried through this graft to vascularise the ischaemic limb.

Axillofemoral graft is useful for salvaging a pregangrenous limb in a poor-risk patient with bilateral iliac obstruction. A long 8-mm PTFE graft is tunnelled subcutaneously, from an end-to-side anastomosis with the axillary artery proximally, to reach the femoral artery of the involved limb in the groin where the distal anastomosis is made. The axillary artery will carry a sufficient volume of blood to maintain the circulation in the arm and revascularise the lower limb. The short-term results are usually good and in these patients with their poor general condition, the poorer, long-term result is usually less important. An axillobifemoral bypass carries twice as much bloodflow through its long limb as does an axillo(uni)femoral bypass; the former has a correspondingly improved patency rate. Salvage operations should not be performed for intermittent claudication alone. Gangrene and loss of limb may result if the operation should fail.

Adjuncts to direct arterial surgery. Blood-flow estimations (by Doppler ultrasonography or electromagnetic flowmeter) or on-table arteriography at the completion of the operation are useful techniques for ensuring that there have been no errors of surgical technique before the wound is closed.

(a)

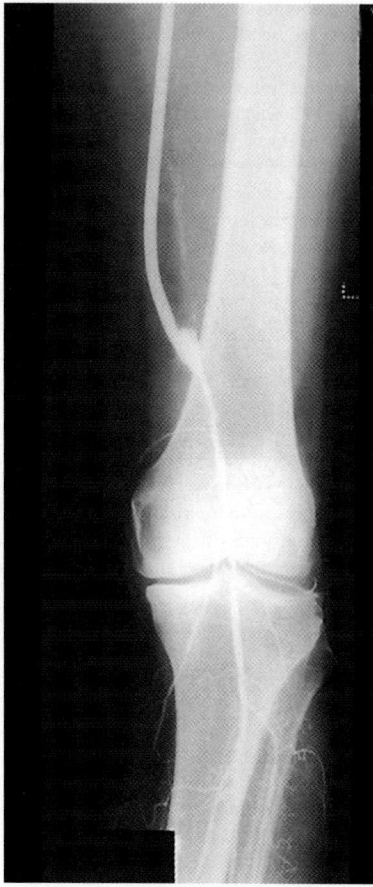

(b)

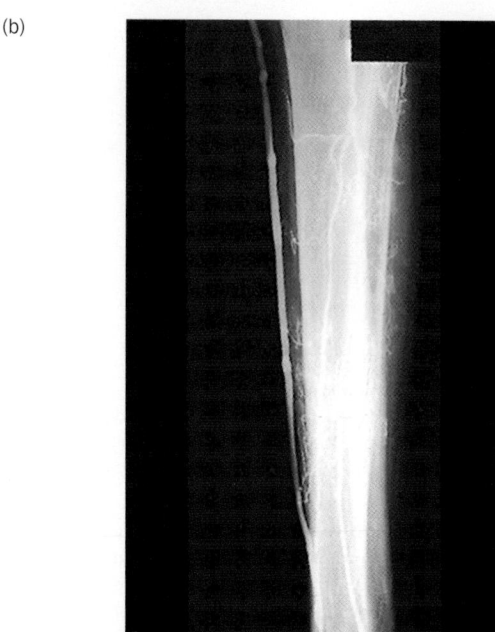

Fig. 15.22 (a) Completion angiogram of femoropopliteal bypass graft (with Miller cuff); (b) completion angiogram of femorodistal bypass graft *in situ*.

Results of operation

The long-term results of aortoiliac reconstructive surgery are good; they are usually only marred by progressive disease producing femoropopliteal occlusions at a later date. Femoropopliteal surgery is less successful. The immediate postoperative success rate for vein bypass exceeds 90 per cent but many cases fail in the first 18 months after operation and, at the end of 5 years, the success rate is usually only between 50 and 60 per cent. The results of femoropopliteal endarterectomy are less good in both the short and long term. Dacron or PTFE bypass also gives a poorer result than vein, with 5-year success rates of less than 50 per cent. The rather poor long-term results of femoropopliteal surgery emphasise that these operations should only be used for clear indications.

Other sites of atherosclerotic obstruction

The principles of arterial surgery as stated above can be applied to other arteries which are stenosed by the disease.

Carotid stenosis may cause transient ischaemic attacks (TIAs). These are recurrent and, by definition, short-lived mini-strokes. Resolution occurs within 24 hours (usually within a few minutes) but TIAs are a warning of impending major stroke. Patients with TIAs should have a duplex scan (not an angiogram) in the first instance. If the scan confirms carotid occlusive disease at an appropriate site, then formal angiography may be considered desirable. Some surgeons operate frequently on duplex scan evidence alone, without angiographic confirmation of disease.

Carotid atheroma classically affects the internal carotid artery origin (Fig. 15.24). The usual procedure is a carotid endarterectomy which involves clamping the vessels, an arteriotomy in the common carotid artery continued up into the internal carotid artery through the diseased segment, removal of the occlusive disease (endarterectomy) and closure of the arteriotomy, often with a patch (vein, PTFE or Dacron). During clamping, some patients will have inadequate cerebral blood flow (especially if the contralateral carotid vessels are compromised). Such a situation may be recognised by recording a low pressure in the distal internal carotid artery above the level of the clamp. It may be necessary in such circumstances to insert a temporary silicone shunt over the arterial field being worked upon.

Subclavian artery stenosis may cause claudication and (rarely) frank ischaemia of an arm. The subclavian lesion may also have an effect by causing artery-to-artery embolisation. This may lead to loss of digits. The condition may be treated by endarterectomy or bypass but nowadays percutaneous transluminal balloon angioplasty is the treatment of choice. It must be noted, however, that some

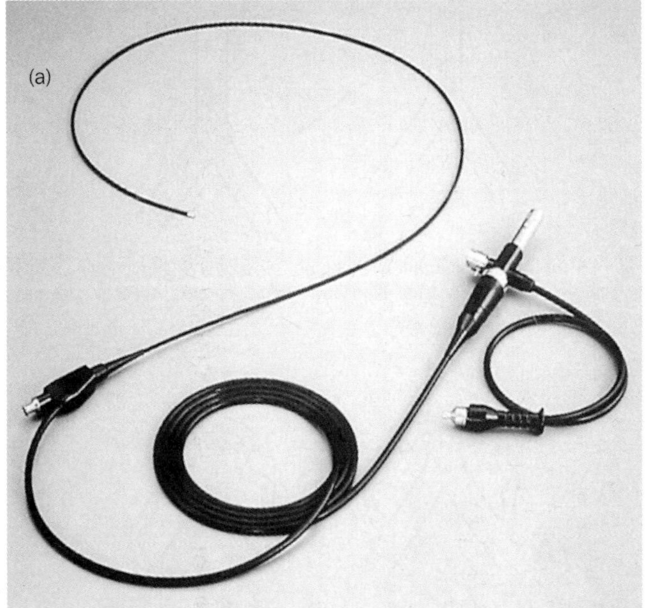

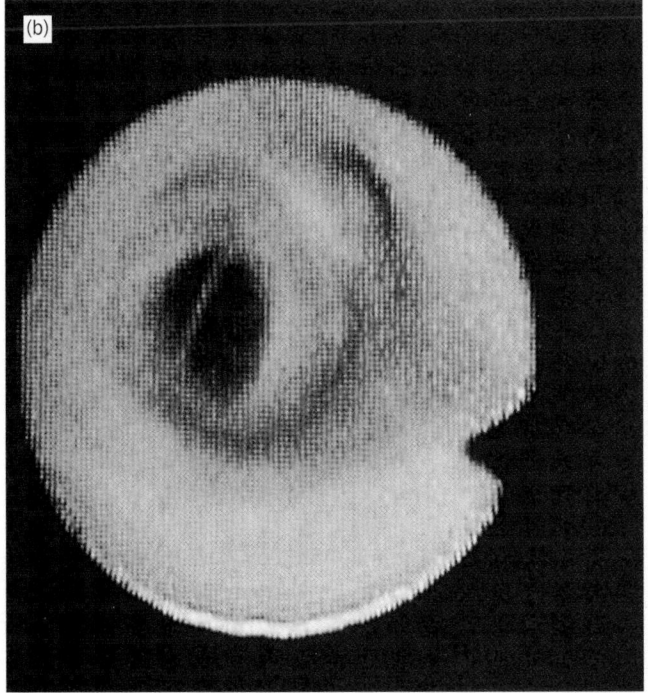

Fig. 15.23 (a) Olympus angioscope – in practice this is connected to a light source and television monitor; (b) angioscopic view of uncut valve cusp in a vein graft *in situ* (*courtesy of Key Med Ltd, Southend-on-Sea, England*).

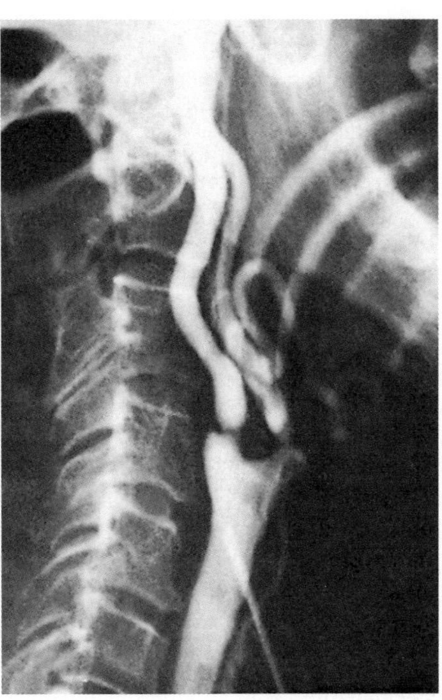

Fig. 15.24 Carotid stenosis. A unilateral localised stenosis suitable for operation. Also some narrowing of the external carotid. Note: a rather similar double narrowing is seen in some carotid body tumours (Chapter 43).

subclavian artery lesions are associated with neck pathology such as cervical rib. Any underlying pathology must be corrected at the time of arterial repair.

Subclavian steal syndrome. If the first part of the subclavian artery is obstructed, the vertebral artery may provide a collateral circulation into the arm by reversing its direction of flow. This may cause periods of cerebral ischaemia. The classic syndrome of syncopal attack and visual disturbance associated with arm exercise and a diminished blood pressure in the affected limb is rather rare. Asymptomatic reversal of flow in the vertebral artery, recognised by either duplex scanning or angiography, is much commoner. In symptomatic patients, percutaneous transluminal angioplasty may relieve the problem, or the situation may be corrected by endarterectomy or a bypass from the ipsilateral common carotid artery to the third part of the subclavian artery.

Enteric artery occlusive disease. Pain after eating that has no obvious diagnosis in a patient with known atheromatous disease and weight loss may be due to enteric artery occlusion. In general, two of the three enteric vessels (coeliac axis, superior mesenteric artery, inferior mesenteric artery) must be occluded to produce 'intestinal claudication'. Great care must be taken to exclude all other diagnoses before contemplating surgical endarterectomy or bypass.

Renal artery stenosis may be responsible for hypertension and, eventually, loss of renal function. In general it is possible to control hypertension using drugs. When this pathology is associated with loss of renal tissue, however, arterial intervention is indicated. Both percutaneous transluminal angioplasty and arterial surgery have their specific place in this disease. A variety of operations is available ranging from endarterectomy, aortorenal bypass, renal artery revascularisation using another vessel (such as the splenic artery), to renal autotransplantation.

Coronary artery disease. See Chapter 48.

Acute arterial occlusion

Sudden occlusion of an artery is commonly due to either emboli or trauma.

Embolic occlusion

An embolus is a body which is foreign to the bloodstream and which may become lodged in a vessel and cause obstruction.

Simple emboli

Simple emboli are due to blood thrombus. The sources are most commonly mural thrombus following a myocardial infarct (a third of cases), mitral stenosis, cardiac arrhythmias (particularly atrial fibrillation) and aneurysms. Emboli may lodge in any organ with resultant ischaemia and symptoms:

- **brain**: the middle cerebral artery (or its branches) is most commonly affected, resulting in hemiplegia, permanent or temporary (transient ischaemic attacks);
- **retina**: amaurosis fugax is fleeting blindness caused by the passage into the central retinal artery of a minute thrombus emanating from an atheromatous plaque in the carotid artery. Complete obstruction causes total and permanent blindness;
- **mesenteric vessels**: causing engorgement and possible gangrene of the corresponding loop of intestine;
- **spleen**: commonly affected with local pain and enlargement;
- **kidneys**: resulting in loin pain and haematuria;
- **lungs**: pulmonary embolism (Chapter 47) is a catastrophe which may fatally interrupt convalescence after operation. Haemoptysis and dyspnoea are usual in survivors;

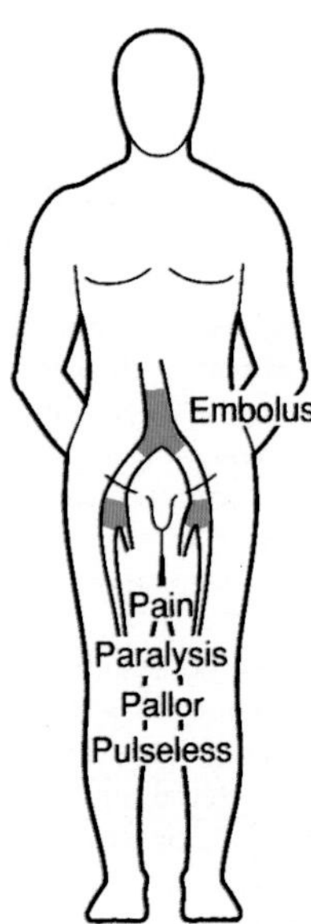

Fig. 15.25 The symptoms and signs of embolism 'four Ps'. The fifth feature, anaesthesia, is often stated to be paraesthesia (the fifth P) but, in truth, complete loss of sensation in the toes and feet is characteristic.

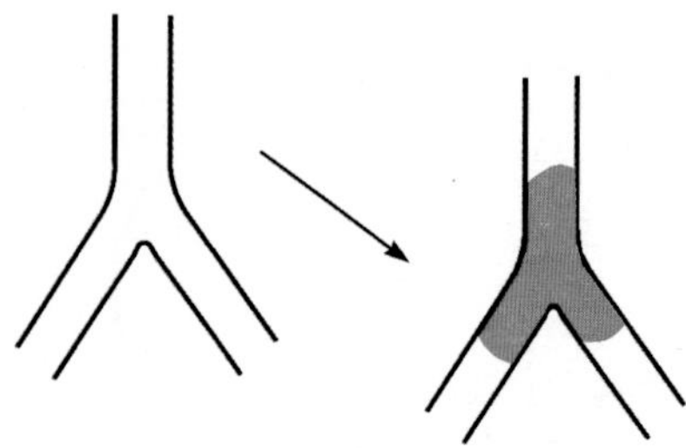

Fig. 15.26 Aortic bifurcation embolus. Source for embolus – recent myocardial infarct or atrial fibrillation. This causes severe, dramatic symptoms.

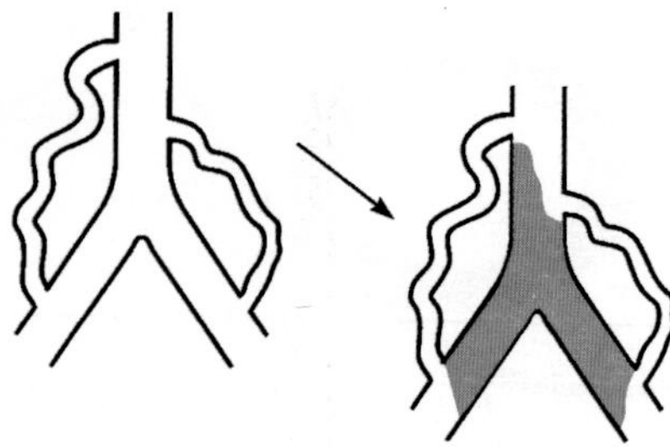

Fig. 15.27 Aortic bifurcation thrombosis. No source of embolus but previous claudication. Claudication worse but no dramatic event.

- **lower limbs**: pain, pallor, paresis, pulselessness and paraesthesia (more correctly anaesthesia) (Fig. 15.25). Acute arterial occlusion due to an embolus differs from atherosclerotic occlusion in that the occlusion is sudden. Indeed, the clinical differences between these two causes of occlusion in the lower limb are as set out in Figs 15.26 and 15.27. It is essential to differentiate between these two causes of occlusion, because they may require different forms of treatment.

Embolic arterial occlusion is an emergency, generally requiring treatment immediately the diagnosis is made.

Clinical features

In the legs, the dramatic symptoms which occur when major vessels are occluded deserve re-emphasis – pain, pallor, paresis, loss of pulsation and anaesthesia (Fig. 15.25). The limb is cold and almost immediately the toes cannot be moved (contrast with venous occlusion when muscle function is not affected). The diagnosis can be made clinically in the majority of cases. The patient, who has no previous symptoms of claudication or limb pain and has a source of emboli, suddenly develops severe pain or numbness of the limb which becomes cold with mottled blue and white discoloration. Movement of the toes becomes progressively more difficult and sensation to touch is lost. Pulses are absent distally, but the femoral pulse may be palpable (even thrusting) if the clot is lodged in a low bifurcation of the femoral artery. This is because distal occlusion results in forceful expansion of the artery with each pressure wave, despite the lack of flow.

Treatment

Because of the ensuing stasis, thrombus can extend distally and proximally to the embolus. The immediate administration of heparin 5000 units intravenously can reduce this extension and maintain patency of the surrounding (particularly the distal) vessels until the embolus can be treated. The relief of pain is essential because it is severe and constant. Embolectomy or thrombolysis are the treatments available for patients with limb emboli.

Embolectomy (and thrombectomy)

Local or general anaesthesia is used, depending upon the patient's general condition and the scope of the proposed operation. The artery, bulging with clot, is exposed and held up by slings or fine rubber tubing. Through a longitudinal or transverse incision the clot begins to extrude and is removed, together with the embolus (Fig. 15.28). Arterial clamps are applied as bleeding occurs, special note being made of the degree of retrograde bleeding (back bleeding).

Fogarty catheterisation. This is the most effective method of removing proximal and distal extension thrombus and also allows an embolus or thrombus to be removed from a vessel remote from the arteriotomy. The Fogarty catheter is like a ureteric catheter, with a balloon tip, and is introduced until it is deemed to have passed the limit of the thrombus. The balloon is inflated and the catheter withdrawn slowly, together with the clot. The procedure is repeated until bleeding occurs. The method is valuable in patients with an aortic bifurcation embolus, since the clot and embolus can be extracted by insertion of balloon catheters via the common femoral arteries in the groin and the patient is saved from a laparotomy. Postoperatively, anticoagulant therapy is continued.

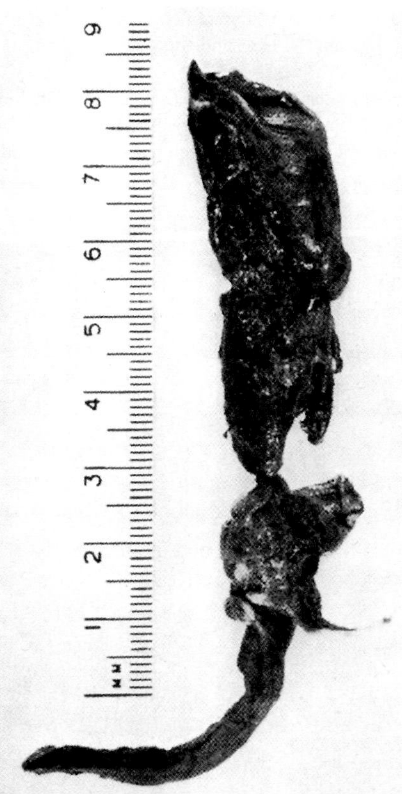

Fig. 15.28 Aortic embolectomy. The extension thrombosis extended proximally up to the renal, and distally into the iliac, arteries.

Thomas J. Fogarty. Surgeon, University of Oregon Medical School, Portland, Oregon, USA.

Prevention of further emboli is achieved by treatment of the cause, whenever possible, and by reducing the chance of further thrombus formation by using long-term anticoagulation with warfarin.

Intra-arterial thrombolysis (Fig. 15.29)

If ischaemia is not so severe that immediate operation is mandatory, it may be possible to treat either embolus or thrombosis by intra-arterial thrombolysis. Because of the nature of thrombosis as opposed to embolism, thrombolysis is more useful in the former condition. Indeed, it may well be the treatment of choice on many occasions.

Arteriography of the ischaemic limb is carried out (usually via the common femoral artery) in the radiology department and at the conclusion of the procedure a narrow catheter (5 French gauge) is passed into the occluded vessel and left embedded within the clot. Into this catheter a thrombolytic agent is infused over a period of several hours. In addition, heparin 250 units per hour is added to the infusate. Intra-arterial thrombolysis may be carried out in a well-staffed ward, but some workers prefer the safety of either a high dependency unit or an intensive care unit.

The common thrombolytic agents are streptokinase, urokinase and tissue plasminogen activator (TPA). In the UK, the most frequently used agent is now TPA, streptokinase having fallen into some disfavour owing to allergy. TPA also has a more rapid action which may be clinically useful. The speed of thrombus dissolution can be further improved by replacing the infusion technique by a pulse-spray method; this requires a special catheter and delivery system.

Whichever drug is used, regular angiograms are carried out to check on the extent of lysis. Using streptokinase, lysis was usually complete within 48 hours. TPA may achieve lysis within 24 hours and pulse-spray TPA may take less than 6 hours. Lysis should be abandoned if there is no progression of dissolution of clot with time. There are several contraindications to the technique, the most important of which are recent stroke, bleeding diathesis and pregnancy.

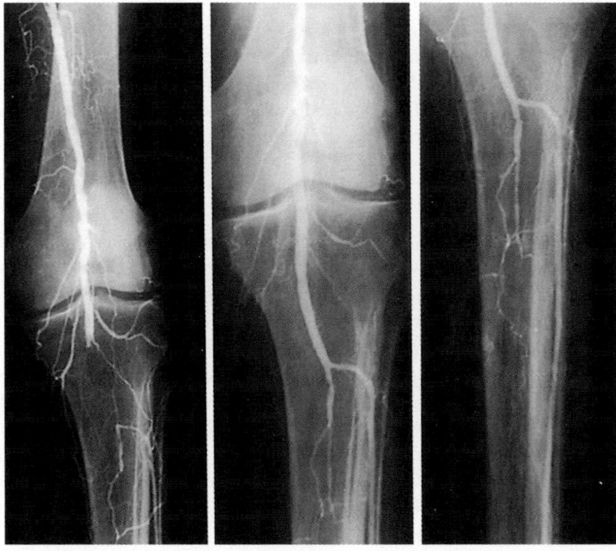

Fig. 15.29 Angiogram of occluded popliteal artery (left) before thrombolysis and at 12 hours (middle) and 18 hours (right) after lysis.

Mesenteric artery occlusion

Acute mesenteric occlusion can be either thrombotic (following atherosclerotic narrowing) or embolic.

Thrombotic occlusion follows progressive narrowing and so the symptoms also tend to be progressive with weight loss, abdominal pain (usually postprandial) and leucocytosis. Once the abdominal pain becomes severe, diarrhoea, systemic hypovolaemia and haemoconcentration occur. By this stage, the patient is ill out of proportion to the physical signs. Treatment is arteriography followed by percutaneous transluminal angioplasty or surgical bypass if the bowel has not already infarcted.

Embolic occlusion results in sudden, severe abdominal pain, with bowel emptying (vomiting and diarrhoea), and a source of emboli present (usually cardiac). Arteriography and embolectomy or bypass surgery can reduce the otherwise high mortality in these patients.

Air embolism

Air may be accidentally injected into the venous circulation, e.g. artificial pneumothorax, or sucked into an open vein. Thus venous air embolism occasionally complicates operations on the neck or axilla if a large vein is inadvertently opened, or it may be an accessory cause of death following a cut throat. The risks associated with intravenous infusion are reduced by the use of a drip chamber containing a spherical plastic float which plugs the exit when the fluid falls to a dangerous level. When air enters the right atrium it is churned up; the foam then enters the right ventricle and causes an air-lock in the pulmonary artery, which may end in right-sided heart failure.

Treatment. Trendelenburg's position encourages air to pass into the veins of the lower half of the body and the patient is placed on the left side so that air will float into the apex of the ventricle, away from the pulmonary artery. Oxygen is administered to counteract hypoxaemia and to assist in the excretion of nitrogen. In serious cases the right ventricle should be aspirated by a needle passed upwards and backwards from below the left costal margin. If this fails, the heart is rapidly exposed for aspiration under direct vision.

Air may occasionally enter the left side of the heart, e.g. at open heart surgery, following puncture of a pulmonary vein during artificial pneumothorax or through a patent foramen ovale (paradoxical embolism). It may from there embolise coronary or cerebral arteries. Treatment is along similar lines to venous air embolism. Air embolism is also a risk following fallopian tube insufflation and following illegal abortion. The air may travel to the brain via the paravertebral veins.

Fat embolism

This condition, which is more common than generally supposed, usually follows severe injuries with multiple or major fractures. Cases have also been recorded following electroconvulsive therapy. The fat may be derived from bone marrow or adipose tissue, but recent work suggests that it is metabolic in origin, perhaps by aggregation of chylomicrons. Symptoms are evident a day or so after injury and two more-or-less distinct types, cerebral and pulmonary, are recognised. In the cerebral type, the patient becomes drowsy, restless and disorientated (delirium tremens may be suspected). Subsequently, the patient is comatose, the pupils become small and pyrexia ensues. The pulmonary type is ushered in with cyanosis, which increases in intensity, and signs of right heart failure. White froth may occur at the mouth and nostrils. It may be mistaken for bronchopneumonia or left ventricular failure. One of the earliest signs may be emboli in the retinal arteries, which cause striate haemorrhages and 'fluffy' patches of exudate. The sputum should be examined for fat droplets and fat may be excreted in the urine. A fall in the haemoglobin value of the blood is a constant sign. Petechial haemorrhages often occur.

Treatment consists of oxygen, early heparinisation and intravenous low molecular weight dextran.

Other forms of emboli include infective emboli of masses of bacteria or infected clot, which may cause mycotic aneurysms, pyaemia or infected infarcts; parasitic emboli due to the ova of *Taenia echinococcus* – and *Pilaria sanguinis hominis* (see Chapter 17) and emboli of malignant cells (e.g. hypernephroma, see Chapter 64).

Fredrich Trendelenburg, 1844–1924. Described this sign in 1895.

Therapeutic embolisation

This is used to arrest haemorrhage from the gastrointestinal, urinary (Fig. 15.30) and respiratory tracts, to treat arteriovenous malformations by blocking their arterial supply and to control the growth of unresectable tumours. Arterial embolisation requires accurate selective catheterisation using the Seldinger technique.

Examples. The left gastric or gastroduodenal artery may be occluded to treat a bleeding ulcer. Occlusion of the hepatic artery often relieves the pain of primary and secondary liver tumours and will usually control the endocrine effects of hormone-secreting tumours, such as metastatic carcinoid (Fig. 15.31). Renal artery embolisation has been used to devascularise a renal tumour prior to surgery and to arrest persistent haemorrhage from an unresectable tumour. In patients with bleeding oesophageal varices, the portal system can be entered by percutaneous catheterisation through the liver and the veins supplying the varices can be embolised.

A wide range of materials have been used and they include blood clot, gel foam sponge, human dura, plastic microspheres, balloons, ethyl alcohol, quick-setting plastics and mechanical devices made of stainless

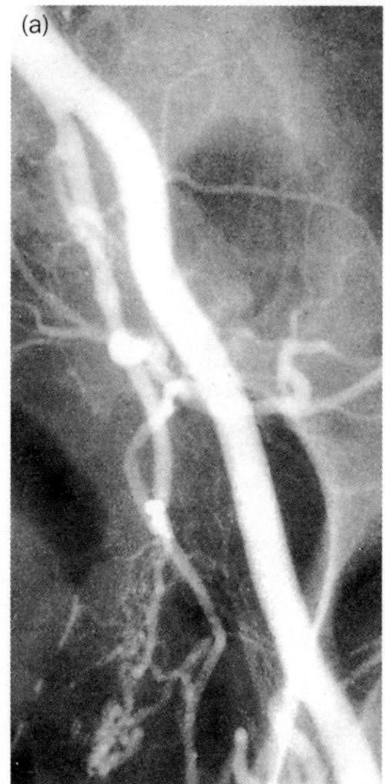

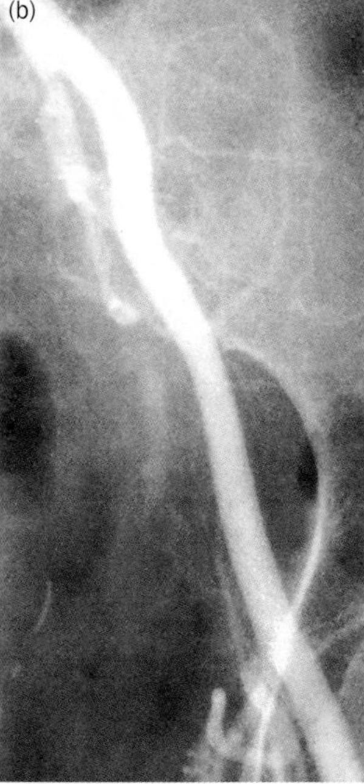

Fig. 15.30 (a) Before and (b) after therapeutic embolisation of the internal iliac artery in a patient with gross haematuria from an ulcerating bladder carcinoma (*courtesy of F. McIvor, FRCR, London, England*).

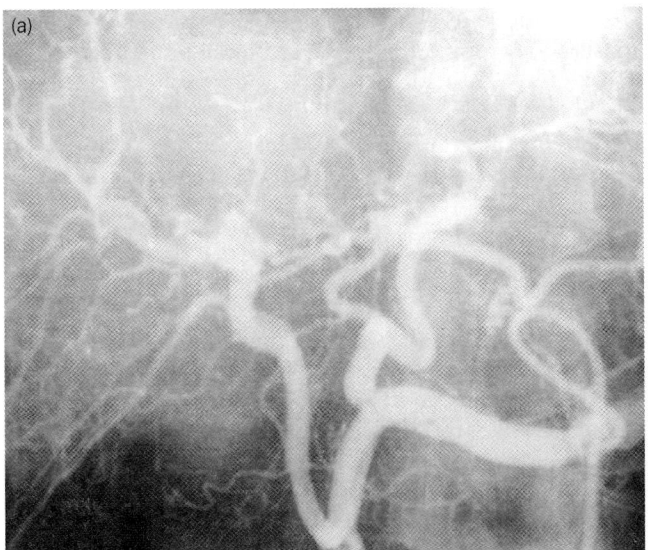

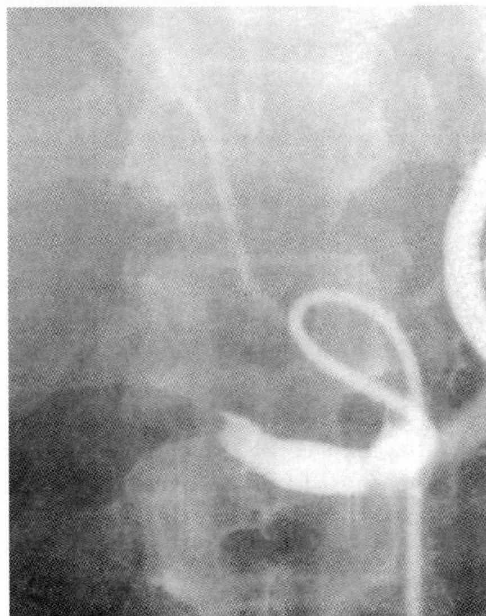

Fig. 15.31 (a) Before and (b) after embolisation of common hepatic artery bifurcation in a patient with the carcinoid syndrome.

steel coils and wool. Therapeutic embolisation is usually carried out under local anaesthesia and has a low morbidity. This is particularly useful for patients with advanced malignant disease where palliation is the aim of the procedure.

Caisson and decompression disease

These similar conditions may affect divers and those who work in compressed air chambers or who ascend in unpressurised aircraft to above 8000 m. If decompression is too rapid, bubbles of nitrogen are set free in the tissues and bloodstream, and occlude small vessels. Symptoms include pain in the muscles or joints, which may be excruciating (the 'bends'), and neurological disturbances; if the spinal cord is affected the patient suffers from weakness of the legs and sphincters. In severe cases, the lungs may be affected, and the patient complains of tightness of the chest and a dry cough (the 'chokes'). Caisson disease requires recompression followed by gradual decompression. The high-altitude flyer is relieved by gradual descent. Inhalation of oxygen assists the excretion of nitrogen. If the spinal cord is not permanently damaged the prognosis is good, but hypertrophic changes may persist in the ends of long bones.

Acute arterial occlusion due to trauma

Arteries (like all tubes) can be occluded as a result of changes:

- in the lumen, e.g. thrombosis;
- in the wall, e.g. subintimal haematoma;
- in the surrounding tissues, e.g. compartment syndrome.

The history of trauma should alert the clinician to check the pulses in the affected limb. There may be obvious injury, for example 'butcher's thigh', when the boning knife slips and enters the groin, but sometimes in blunt injury the lack of surface changes may be misleading. Absent pulses with rest pain, or skin colour and temperature change, suggest arterial occlusion. In many Western nations, the commonest cause of arterial trauma is iatrogenic. In this group, the commonest event is femoral or brachial artery damage at cardiac catheterisation; the latter vessel is much more prone to iatrogenic complications and should be avoided if possible by those using catheter techniques.

Preoperative assessment

Preoperative assessment including arteriography is valuable. It is also useful to recognise pre-existing atherosclerotic disease.

Operative procedure

On exposing a damaged artery, an obvious laceration may be found – remember to look for a puncture wound in the back of an artery in a stabbing. If this is very small, e.g. from a needle puncture, a single suture may suffice to repair a leak. If damage is more widespread and if thrombosis forms part of the picture, it may be necessary to resect a damaged segment (Fig. 15.32). If the resection is very limited, it may be possible to reconstitute the vessel by direct anastomosis of the cut

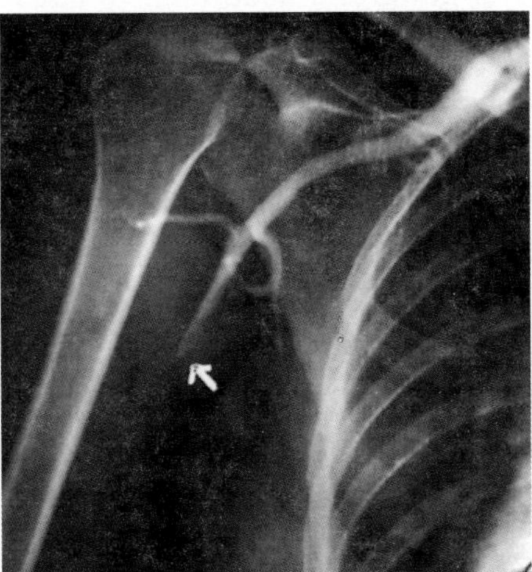

Fig. 15.32 Arteriogram showing axillary artery thrombosis in a woman following trauma to the axilla over the headboard of a bed during the second stage of labour.

ends. In general, however, a short interposition graft (vein is best) is to be preferred. The vein should not be taken from the damaged limb because concomitant deep venous trauma may be present and superficial veins may be required to return blood centrally.

It should first be appreciated that occlusion due to trauma should never be casually ascribed to arterial spasm; ischaemia after trauma demands urgent action. Second, the results of operating on traumatised arteries are, in general, good. The outflow is not compromised by atheromatous disease in most cases. If the return of blood supply to the limb after arterial declamping is not very obvious, preoperative angiography is mandatory. Not only may there be a problem with the local arterial reconstruction but also thrombosis (from stasis) or embolism at a distal site may be present and may require separate attention.

Fractures of bone occur frequently alongside arterial injuries and require stabilisation, both in their own right and to protect the vascular repair. Stabilisation may be carried out before or after the vascular reconstruction (depending on how acute is the ischaemia) and fixation (often external) is greatly to be preferred to traction, for obvious reasons.

Compartment syndrome (Chapter 21)

It must also be remembered that in the lower limb the additional problem of compression of the main artery due to haematoma or oedema in the fixed fascial compartments of the calf, especially the anterior tibial compartment, can cause distal ischaemia (and crush syndrome renal effects). The treatment is urgent fasciotomy to release the external compression on the artery.

Gangrene

Gangrene implies death with putrefaction of macroscopic portions of tissue. It is commonly seen affecting the distal part of a limb, the appendix or a loop of small intestine, and sometimes organs such as the gallbladder, the pancreas or the testis. Note that the term necrosis applies mainly to the death of groups of cells, although it is extended to include bone, i.e. a **sequestrum**. A **slough** is a piece of dead, soft tissue, e.g. skin, fascia or tendon.

Varieties of gangrene according to cause

Secondary to arterial obstruction from disease, for example:

- thrombosis of an atherosclerotic artery;
- embolus from the heart in atrial fibrillation or after coronary thrombosis;
- arteritis with neuropathy in diabetes;
- Buerger's disease;
- arterial shutdown in Raynaud's disease or ergotism;
- effect of intra-arterial injections – thiopentone and cytotoxic substances.

Infective: boils and carbuncles, gas gangrene, gangrene of the scrotum (Fournier's gangrene).

Maurice Raynaud, 1834–81. Physician, Hopital Lariboisiere, and Professor Agrege, Paris, France. Published his thesis De L'Asphye Locale et La Gangrene Symetrique des Extremites *in 1862.*

Jean Alfred Fournier, 1832–1914. Dermatologist in Paris, France.

Traumatic: direct, such as crushes, pressure sores and the constriction groove of strangulated bowel; or indirect, due to injury of vessels at some distance from the site of gangrene, e.g. pressure on the popliteal artery by the lower end of a fractured femur.

Physical, e.g. burns, scalds, frostbite, chemicals, irradiation and electricity.

Venous gangrene: see Chapter 16.

Clinical features of gangrene (Figs 15.4 and 15.5)

A gangrenous part lacks arterial pulsation, venous return, capillary response to pressure (colour return), sensation, warmth and function. The colour of the part changes through a variety of shades according to circumstances (pallor, dusky grey, mottled, purple) until finally taking on the characteristic dark brown, greenish black or black appearance, which is due to the disintegration of haemoglobin and the formation of iron sulphide.

Clinical types

Dry gangrene occurs when the tissues are desiccated by gradual slowing of the bloodstream; it is typically the result of atherosclerosis. The affected part becomes dry and wrinkled, discoloured from disintegration of haemoglobin and greasy to the touch.

Moist gangrene occurs when venous as well as arterial obstruction is present, when the artery is suddenly occluded, as by a ligature or embolus, and in diabetes. Infection and putrefaction are always present, the affected part becomes swollen and discoloured, and the epidermis may be raised in blebs. Crepitus may be palpated, owing to infection by gas-forming organisms. Moist gangrene is manifest also in such conditions as acute appendicitis and strangulated bowel.

Separation of gangrene

Separation by demarcation

A zone of demarcation between the truly viable and the dead or dying tissue appears first. It is indicated on the surface by a band of hyperaemia and hyperaesthesia. Separation is achieved by the development of a layer of granulation tissue which forms between the dead and the living parts. These granulations extend into the dead tissue until those which have penetrated farthest are unable to derive adequate nourishment. Ulceration follows and thus a final line of demarcation (separation) forms which separates the gangrenous mass from healthy tissue.

In dry gangrene, if the blood supply of the proximal tissues is adequate, the final line of demarcation appears in a matter of days and separation begins to take place neatly and with the minimum of infection (so-called separation by aseptic ulceration). Where bone is involved, complete separation takes longer than when soft tissues alone are affected, and the stump tends to be conical as the bone has a better blood supply than its coverings.

In moist gangrene, there is more infection and suppuration extends into the neighbouring living tissue, thereby causing the final line of demarcation to be more proximal than in dry gangrene (separation by septic ulceration). This is why dry gangrene must be kept as dry and aseptic as possible, and why every effort should be made to convert moist gangrene into the dry type.

Vague demarcation; spread of gangrene; skipping and die-back. In many cases of gangrene from atherosclerosis and embolism, the line of final demarcation is very slow to form or does not develop. Unless the arterial supply to the living tissues can be improved forthwith, the gangrene will spread to adjacent tissues or toes, or will suddenly appear as 'skip' areas further up the limb. Signs of skipping should always be carefully looked for. Black patches suddenly appear, perhaps on the other side of the foot, on the heel, on the dorsum of the foot or even in the calf. Infection, another cause of the spread of gangrene, may spread upwards beyond the line of separation along the lymphatic vessels or cellular tissue into healthy parts; extensive inflammation then results. Except in diabetic gangrene without concomitant atherosclerotic obstruction, these forms of spread do not usually respond to efforts to save the limb and an above-knee amputation becomes necessary. To attempt local amputation in the phase of vague demarcation is to court failure, as gangrene reappears in the skin-flaps ('die-back').

Treatment of gangrene

General principles

A limb-saving attitude is needed in most cases of symptomatic gangrene affecting hands and feet. The surgeon is concerned with how much can be preserved or salvaged[3]. With arterial disease all depends upon there being a good blood supply to the limb above the gangrene, or whether a poor blood supply can be improved by such measures as percutaneous transluminal angioplasty or direct arterial surgery. A good or an improved blood supply indicates that a conservative excision is likely to be successful and a major amputation may be avoided. A life-saving amputation is required for a badly crushed limb, rapidly spreading symptomatic gangrene and gas gangrene.

General treatment includes that of cardiac failure, atrial fibrillation and anaemia, to improve the tissue oxygenation. A nutritious diet, essential in all forms of gangrene, and the control of diabetes, when present, are additional items of care. Pain, especially night pain, may be difficult to relieve. Nonaddictive drugs should be used whenever possible.

[3]*Sir William Fergusson, 1808–77. Surgeon, Royal Infirmary, Edinburgh, later Professor of Surgery, King's College Hospital, London, England, said that amputation is 'one of the meanest, and yet one of the greatest operations in surgery: mean, when resorted to where better may be done – great, as the only step to give comfort and prolong life'.*

Local treatment

Care of the affected part includes keeping it absolutely dry. Exposure and the use of a fan may assist in the desiccation and may relieve pain. The limb must not be heated. Protection of local pressure areas, e.g. the skin of the heel or the malleoli, is required otherwise fresh patches of gangrene are likely to occur in these places. A bed-cradle, padded rings, foam blocks and air beds are useful preventive aids. Careful observation of a gangrenous part will show whether the lifting of a crust, or the removal of hard or desiccated skin, will assist in demarcation, the release of pus and the relief of pain.

Varieties of gangrene

Diabetic gangrene

Diabetic gangrene is due to three factors. These are:

- trophic changes resulting from peripheral neuritis;
- atheroma of the arteries resulting in ischaemia;
- excess of sugar in the tissues which lowers their resistance to infection (Fig. 15.33), including fungal infection.

The neuropathic factor impairs sensation and thus favours the neglect of minor injuries and infections, so that inflammation and damage to tissues are ignored. Muscular involvement is frequently accompanied by loss of reflexes and deformities. In some cases, the feet are splayed and deformed (neuropathic joints). Thick callosities develop on the sole and are the means whereby infection gains entry, often following amateur chiropody. Infection involving fascia, tendon and bone can spread proximally with speed via subfascial planes.

Clinical examination and investigations include those on the urine and blood for diabetes. Palpable dorsalis pedis and posterior tibial pulses, and the absence of rest pain and intermittent claudication, imply that there is no associated major arterial disease. A bacteriological examination is made of any pus. A radiograph may help to reveal the extent of any osteomyelitis.

Treatment. The diabetes must be brought under control by diet and appropriate drugs. The gangrene is treated along the

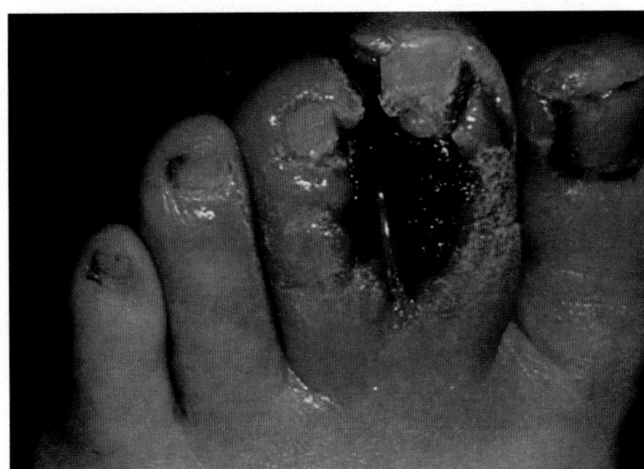

Fig. 15.33 Diabetic gangrene.

lines already described, the accent being on conservatism if there is no major arterial obstruction. A rapid spread of infection requires drainage of the area by incision and the removal of any obviously dead tissue. This may often involve free and extensive laying open of infected tissue planes. Adequate surgical drainage of pus and the control of infection due to bacteria and fungi may then be followed by rapid healing. After healing, protection of the affected part is essential.

Direct traumatic gangrene

Direct traumatic gangrene is due to local injury and may arise as a result of crushes, pressure (as in the case of splints or plasters) or bedsores. Gangrene following severe injury, e.g. a street accident in which a vehicle passes over a limb, is of the moist variety and excision without delay is usually indicated. Amputation may be performed as close to the damaged part as will leave the most useful limb.

Bedsores

Bedsores (syn. decubitus ulcers) are predisposed to by five factors – pressure, injury, anaemia, malnutrition and moisture. They can appear and extend with alarming rapidity in patients with disease or injury of the spinal cord and other patients with debilitating illness. It is important to recognise patients at risk and take adequate prophylactic measures. These measures include the avoidance of pressure over the bony prominences, regular turning of patients and nursing on specially designed beds, which reduces the pressure to the skin. These beds include the high air loss Clinitron bed, low air loss Mediscus bed and the very low air loss OSA 1000. There are advantages in not blowing large quantities of air around the ward, and also advantages in being able to articulate the patient, yet removing the increased pressure and sheer forces produced by such articulation (Chapter 33). Preventive measures are of the utmost importance. Thus pressure over bony prominences is counteracted by a 2-hourly change of posture and protection by foam blocks. A water bed or a ripple bed is sometimes desirable. Injury due to wrinkled draw-sheets and maceration of the skin by sweat, urine or pus is combated by skilled nursing and the use of an adhesive film such as Opsite (Fig. 15.34).

A bedsore is to be expected if erythema appears which does not change colour on pressure. The part must be kept dry. An aerosol silicone spray may be used. Actual bedsores may be treated either by lotions or by exposure to keep them as dry as possible. Once pressure sores develop, they are extremely difficult to heal. They should be kept clean and débrided, and the use of rotation flaps should also be considered. The haemoglobin of the patient should be maintained at a normal level by transfusions of packed cells if needed. If the patient is young and otherwise healthy, excision of the dead tissue and flap pedicle skin grafting is often successful.

Indirect traumatic gangrene

Indirect traumatic gangrene is due to interference with blood vessels:

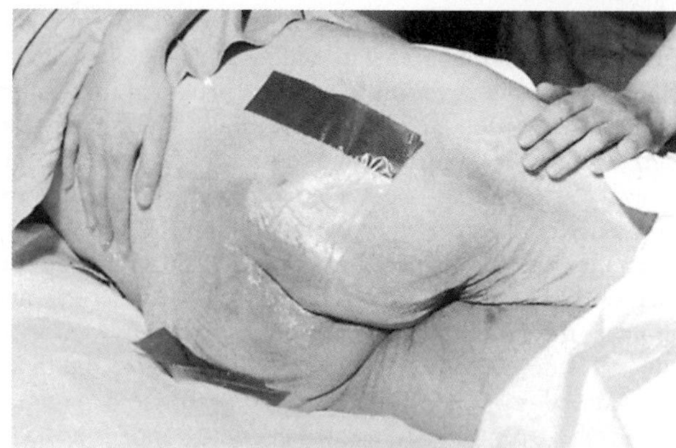

Fig. 15.34 Opsite being applied to combat an incipient bedsore.

- from pressure by a fractured bone in a limb or by strangulation (Fig. 15.35) (strangulated hernia, Chapter 62);
- thrombosis of a large artery following injury;
- ligation of the main artery of a limb, as after division by injury;
- poor technique for local digital anaesthesia. The combination of a tourniquet and an adrenaline-containing local anaesthetic solution can lead to permanent occlusion of all the arteries (Chapter 30).

The likelihood of gangrene depends upon the sufficiency of the collateral circulation.

Treatment directed to the cause, e.g. closed or open reduction of a fracture together with direct arterial surgery for the damaged vessel, will usually prevent the onset of gangrene. The limb must be kept cool, so as to reduce metabolism to the minimum. When gangrene is slow to develop, a line of demarcation will indicate the level of vitality. If moist gangrene occurs and spreads rapidly, amputation may be needed to save the patient's life.

Ergot

Ergot, a cause of gangrene among dwellers on the shores of the Mediterranean Sea and the Russian steppes who eat rye bread infected with *Claviceps purpurea*, also occurs in migraine sufferers who, for

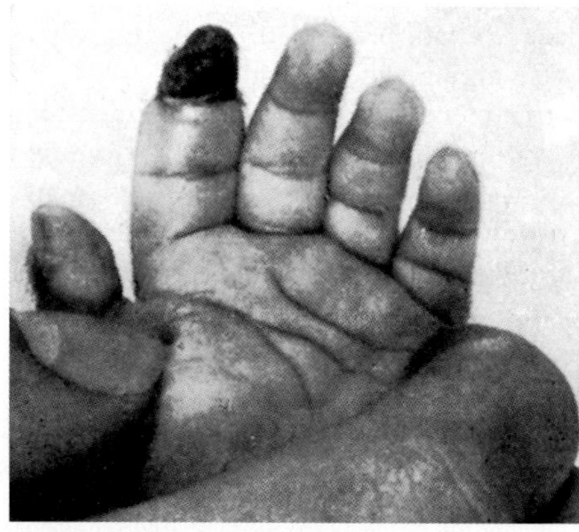

Fig. 15.35 Indirect traumatic gangrene of a newborn infant's finger, accidentally caused by a thread of cotton.

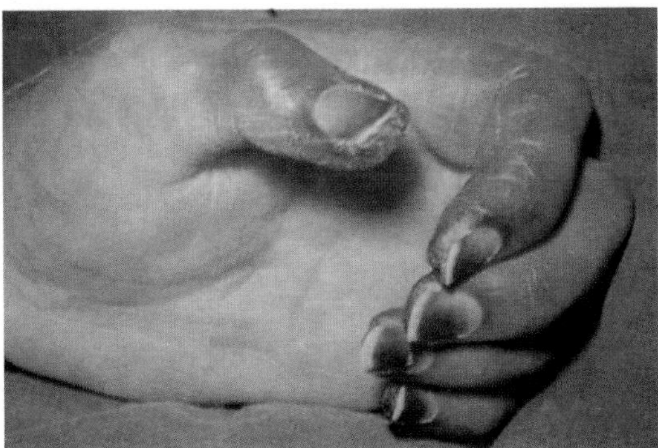

Fig. 15.36 Gangrene due to ergot. The patient had taken repeated doses of ergotamine tartrate for 'migraine' while on a transatlantic flight (*courtesy of Professor Dame Sheila Sherlock, London, England*).

prophylactic reasons, unwittingly take ergot preparations over a long period. The fingers, nose and ears may be affected (Fig. 15.36).

Physical and chemical causes of gangrene

Frostbite is due to exposure to cold, especially if accompanied by wind or high altitude (e.g. climbers and explorers). It is also encountered in the elderly or the vagrant during cold spells (Fig. 15.37). Pathologically, there is damage to the vessel walls, which is followed by transudation and oedema. The sufferer notices severe burning pain in the affected part, after which it assumes a waxy appearance and is painless. Blistering and then gangrene follow.

Treatment. Frostbitten parts must be warmed very gradually. Any temperature higher than that of the body is detrimental. The part should be wrapped in cottonwool and kept at rest. Friction, e.g. rubbing with snow, may damage the already devitalised tissues. Warm drinks and clothing are provided and powerful analgesics are required to relieve the pain which heralds the return of circulation. Paravertebral injection of the sympathetic chain may be helpful in relieving associated vasospasm. Amputations should be conservative. Hyperbaric oxygen (Chapter 4) may help.

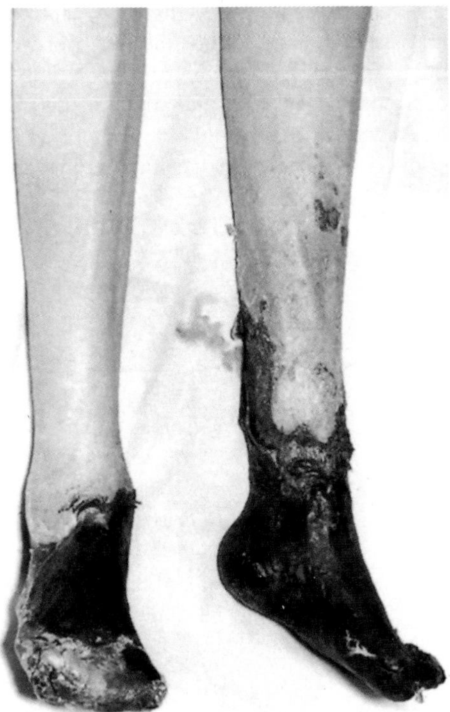

Fig. 15.37 Frostbite in Fulham, London, England. An elderly lady, living with insufficient food or heating. Conservative amputations were successful.

Trench foot is due to cold, damp and muscular inactivity; it is predisposed to by tight clothing, such as garters, puttees and ill-fitting boots. Prophylaxis is of paramount importance. Numbness is followed by pain, which is excruciating when boots are removed. The skin is mottled like marble and, in severe cases, blisters containing blood-stained serum develop; moist gangrene follows. The pathology is similar to that of frostbite and the treatment is essentially the same.

Inadvertent intra-arterial injection of thiopentone can happen when a high division of the brachial artery results in one of its two terminal branches, usually the ulnar, passing superficially downwards in the antecubital fossa. The appreciation by palpation of pulsation of the vessel and of the withdrawal of bright red blood prior to injection should prevent this calamity. Injection causes immediate and severe burning pain, with blanching of the hand. The needle should be left in position, and 5 ml of 1 per cent procaine and/or 2 per cent papaverine sulphate injected to reduce vascular spasm. Dilute heparin solution may also be given intra-arterially if the needle is in position. Intra-arterial thrombolysis and intravenous low molecular weight dextran may be employed. Brachial block should also be performed and repeated as necessary. Even so, gangrene of one or more fingers may occur.

Drug abuse. Inadvertent arterial injection of drugs is becoming common in many countries with significant numbers of drug addicts. Usually the femoral artery in the groin is involved, and presentation is with pain and mottling distally in the leg. Often all pulses down to ankle level are retained. If pulses have been lost, angiography and intra-arterial thrombolysis may be considered (possibly with dextran and heparin in addition). If pulses are retained, dextran and heparin may be given but there is no firm evidence of their efficacy in this condition. Many cases are self-limiting and resolve spontaneously. It should be remembered that many of these patients carry the human immunodeficiency virus (HIV) or have frank acquired immunodeficiency syndrome (AIDS).

Chemical gangrene. Carbolic acid (phenol) is the most dangerous, as anaesthesia masks the pain which occurs before the onset of gangrene. *Carbolic compresses should never be used*, for fingers have been lost by application of compresses even as dilute as 1:80. The gangrene is due to local arterial spasm. In addition, there is danger of severe systemic effects from absorption of phenol. Local bicarbonate soaks should be applied. Later, excision of the slough and skin grafting are necessary.

Ainhum (Fig. 15.38), a disease of unknown aetiology, usually affects black males (but some females) who have run barefoot in childhood.

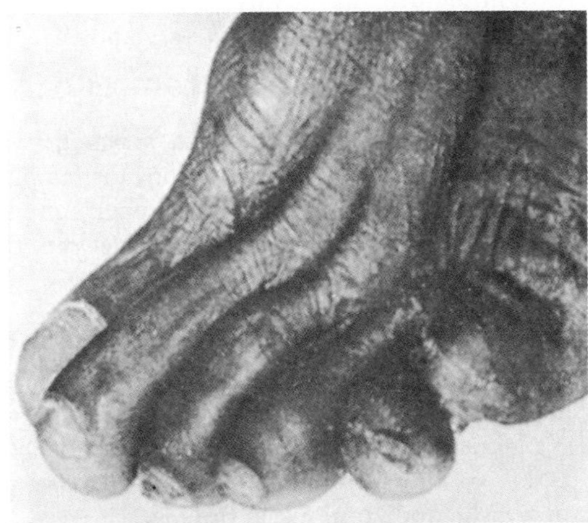

Fig. 15.38 Ainhum (*courtesy of Dennis Morrissey, FRCS, Birmingham*).

Besides Central Africa, there are reports from Central America and the East. A fissure appears at the level of the interphalangeal joint of a toe, usually the fifth. This fissure becomes a fibrous band, which encircles the digit and causes necrosis. The treatment is either early Z-plasty or, later, amputation.

Venous gangrene is discussed in Chapter 16.

Amputation

Amputation should be considered when part of a limb is dead, deadly or a dead loss.

Dead

Arterial occlusion or stenosis, if sufficiently severe, will lead to tissue infarction with putrefaction of macroscopic portions of tissue (gangrene). The occlusion may be in major vessels (atherosclerotic or embolic occlusions) or in small peripheral vessels (diabetes, Buerger's disease, Raynaud's disease, inadvertent intra-arterial injection, ergotism). If the obstruction cannot be reversed and the symptoms are severe, amputation is indicated.

Deadly

Moist gangrene with its accompanying putrefaction and infection is dangerous, for the infection spreads to surrounding viable tissues, and cellulitis with severe toxaemia and overwhelming systemic infection can occur. Amputation is indicated as a life-saving operation. Antibiotic cover should be broad and massive. Other life-threatening situations for which amputation may be required include gas gangrene (as opposed to simple gas infection, Chapter 8), neoplasm (such as osteogenic sarcoma) and arteriovenous fistula.

Dead loss

This applies to the following:

- severe laceration and fracture with partial amputation due to the trauma of road accident or bomb-blast injury (e.g. mines) (Chapter 19);
- severe contracture or paralysis, e.g. poliomyelitis, may make the limb impossible to use, and may hinder walking or any movement. Amputation can improve mobility;
- severe rest pain without gangrene in a patient with an ischaemic foot may be an indication for amputation because of the relentless severity of the pain. Amputation under those circumstances can improve the quality of life.

Distal amputation

In patients with small-vessel disease (diabetes and Buerger's disease), gangrene of the toes occurs with relatively good blood supply to the surrounding tissues. Therefore, local amputation of the toe can result in healing.

In diabetic patients:

- infection tends to track up the tendon sheath;
- infection tends to recur if the wound is closed;
- neuropathy often makes early mobility possible because of lack of pain.

For these reasons, when the metatarsophalangeal joint region is involved in diabetes, 'ray' excision is recommended, taking part of the metatarsal and cutting tendons back (Fig. 15.39). The wound should not be sutured but loosely packed with gauze soaked in an antiseptic solution such as proflavine. Early mobility aids drainage provided cellulitis is not present. For less extensive gangrene, if amputation is taken through a joint, healing is improved by removing the cartilage from the joint surface.

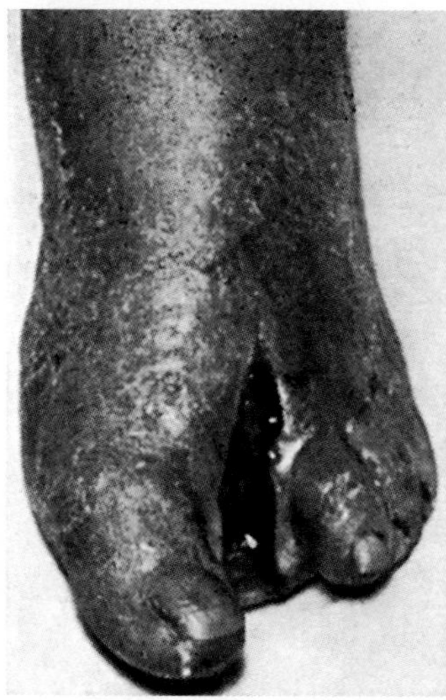

Fig. 15.39 Conservative amputation for diabetic gangrene ('ray' excision).

Transmetatarsal amputation

Transmetatarsal amputation can be used in similar circumstances, where several toes are affected and irreversible ischaemia has extended to the forefoot, as in Buerger's disease; a viable long plantar flap is essential for this operation to heal successfully (Fig. 15.40).

Major amputation

Preoperative preparation/informed consent

The patient should, whenever possible, be given time to come to terms with the inevitability of amputation and, ideally, once the alternatives between a painful useless limb or a painless useful (artificial) one are explained, the patient will make the final decision. This approach to the matter prevents the patient feeling that the loss of the limb is being imposed, possibly making him or her less positive in attitude to retraining. In gangrene of the foot, especially with 'skip' areas, this is the time for explanation of, and consent for, above-knee amputation should an attempt at below-knee section prove inadvisable on account of inadequate blood

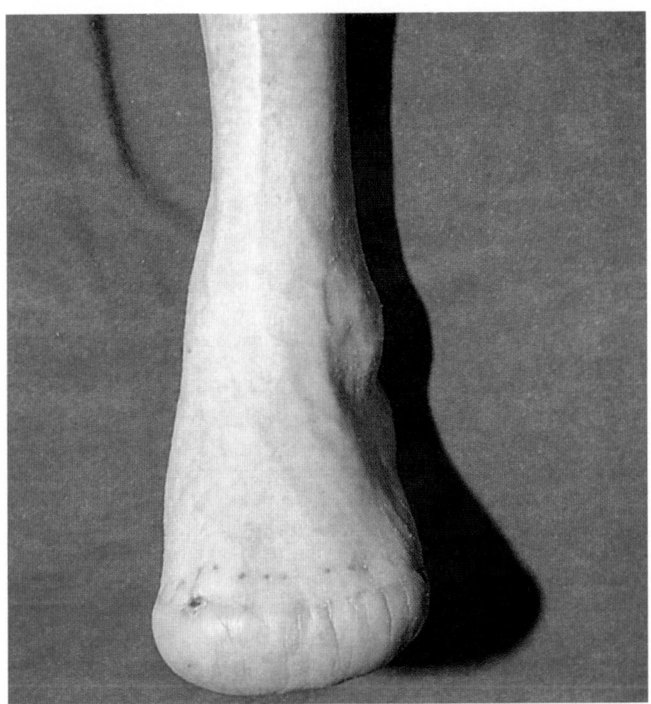

Fig. 15.40 Transmetatarsal amputation for diabetic gangrene of the toes.

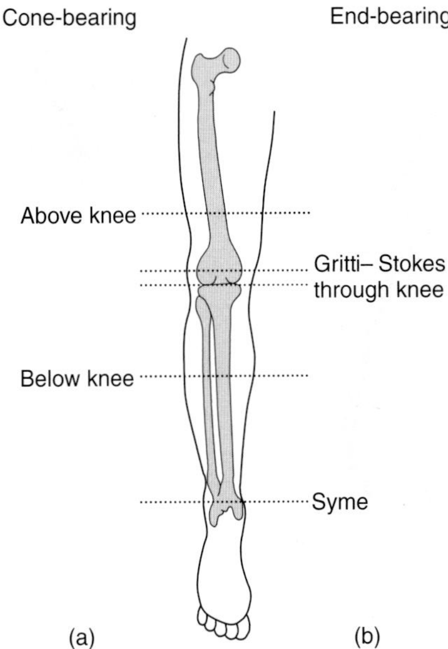

Fig. 15.41 Choice of site: (a) cone-bearing and (b) end-bearing amputations.

supply to the flaps. The general condition of the patient needs to be maintained and/or improved, e.g. anaemia corrected and pain controlled.

Physiotherapy before the operation enables the patient to get used to the exercises that will prevent muscle wasting and flexion deformity of the hip.

Antibiotics should be given with the premedication to prevent clostridial infection (Chapter 8), particularly in above-knee amputations.

Analgesia. The appropriate level of analgesia should be maintained up to the time of operation (and see Postoperative analgesia in Chapter 6).

Assessment of joints. Flexion contracture or severe arthritis may influence the level of amputation and/or the final degree of mobility.

Choice of operation (Fig. 15.41)

Where good limb-fitting facilities exist, above- or below-knee amputations are preferable because the best cosmetic and functional results can be obtained by the cone-bearing amputation stumps. [Note the words 'cone-bearing'. The term conical stump is reserved for an entirely different pathological entity – that which occurs when the growing humerus (or tibia), following amputation in a child, stretches the stump tissues and skin into an unsightly cone. (Main growth occurs in the epiphyses located 'toward the knee and away from the elbow'.)] If limb-fitting facilities are limited, end-bearing amputation may be preferable (Syme's, through-knee, Gritti–Stokes) so that simple prostheses (peg leg or simple boot) can be used. Syme's amputations are not suitable for severely ischaemic atherosclerotic limbs because of the poor healing of the heel flap.

Cone-bearing amputations. For above- or below-knee amputations, with good stump shape and limb-fitting facilities, it is possible to have a prosthesis held in place simply by suction, without any cumbersome and unsightly straps.

- The stump must be of sufficient length to give the required leverage: below the knee – not less than 8 cm (preferably 10–12 cm); above the knee – not less than 20 cm.
- There must be room for the artificial joint (the stump must not be too long); above the knee ideally 12 cm proximal to the knee joint and below the knee 8 cm proximal to the ankle joint are needed for the mechanism.

A below-knee amputation is much better than an above-knee (or Gritti–Stokes) amputation in terms of eventual mobility. Every attempt should be made to preserve the knee joint if the extent of ischaemia or trauma allows this.

Below-knee amputations

Two types of skin flap are commonly used: long posterior flap and skew flap. Skew flaps were described by K.P. Robinson. Whatever method is chosen it is wise to remember the old rule that the total length of flap or flaps need to be at least one and a half times the diameter of the leg at the point of bone section.

James Syme, 1799–1871. Professor of Clinical Surgery, University of Edinburgh, Scotland.
Rocco Gritti, 1828–1920. Surgeon, Milan, Italy.
Sir William Stokes, 1839–1900. Dublin surgeon.
K.P. Robinson. Emeritus Consultant Surgeon, Roehampton Hospital, England.

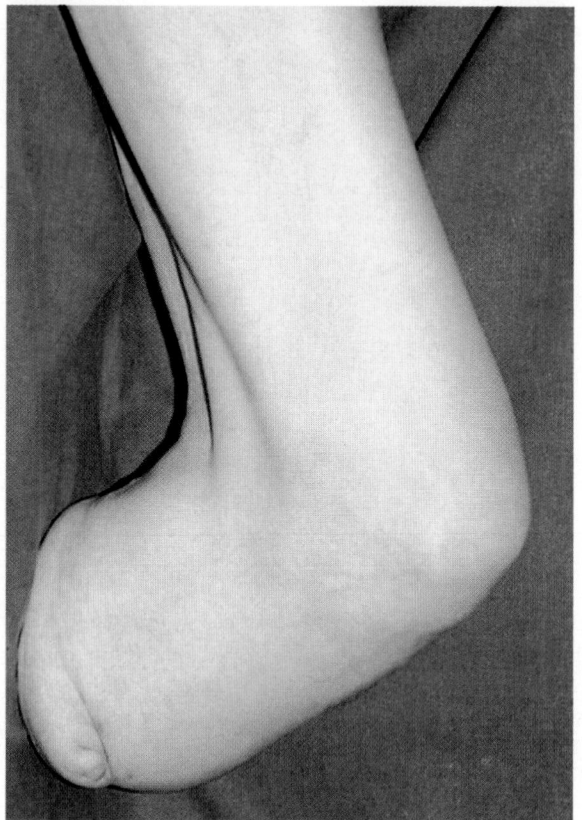

Fig. 15.42 Classic long posterior flap type of below-knee amputation.

Long posterior flap below-knee amputation (Fig. 15.42). In cases of trauma a tourniquet is applied at the thigh, but not in cases of ischaemia. Anteriorly, the incision is deepened to bone and the lateral and posterior incisions are fashioned to leave the bulk of the gastrocnemius muscle attached to the flap, muscle and flap being transected together at the same level. If bleeding is inadequate, the amputation is refashioned at a higher level. Blood vessels are identified and ligated. Nerves are not clamped but pulled down gently and transected as high as possible. Vessels in nerves are ligated. The fibula is divided 2 cm proximal to the level of tibial division using bone cutters, the skin and muscle being retracted to avoid damage. The tibia is cleared and transected at the desired level, the anterior aspect of the bone being sawn obliquely before the cross-cut is made. This, with filing, gives an anterior smooth bevel which prevents pressure necrosis of the flap. The long muscle/skin flap is tapered after removing the bulk of soleus muscle (most of the gastrocnemius may be left), the area is washed with saline to remove bone fragments and the muscle and fascia are sutured with catgut or Dexon to bring the flap over the bone ends. A suction drain is placed deep to the muscle and brought out through a stab incision in the skin. The skin flap should lie in place with all tension taken by the deep sutures. Interrupted skin sutures are inserted. The drain can be attached to the skin by adhesive tape instead of sutures, allowing its removal without the need to take down the stump dressing. Gauze, wool and crêpe bandages make up the stump dressing.

Skew flaps. This form of below-knee amputation seeks to make use of anatomical knowledge of the skin blood supply. Equally long flaps are developed; they join anteriorly 2.5 cm from the tibial crest, overlying the anterior tibial compartment, and posteriorly at the exact opposite point on the circumference of the leg. After division of bone and muscle in a fashion similar to that above, the gastrocnemius flap is sutured over the cut bone end to the anterior tibial periosteum with catgut or Dexon. Finally, drainage and skin sutures are inserted and the limb is dressed as in the long posterior flap operation.

Above-knee amputations

The site is chosen as indicated above, but may need to be higher if bleeding is poor on incision of the skin. Curved equal anterior and posterior skin flaps are made of sufficient total length (one and a half times the anterior/posterior diameter of the thigh). Skin, deep fascia and muscle are transected in the same line. Vessels are ligated. The sciatic nerve is pulled down and transected cleanly as high as possible and the accompanying artery ligated. Muscle and skin are retracted, and the bone is cleared and sawn at the point chosen. Haemostasis is achieved. The muscle ends are grouped together over the bone by means of catgut or Dexon sutures incorporating the fascia. A suction drain deep to the muscle is brought out through the skin clear of the wound and affixed with tape so that removal can takes place without disturbing the stump dressing. The fascia and subcutanous tissues are further brought together so that the skin can be apposed by interrupted sutures without tension. Gauze, wool and crêpe bandages form the stump dressing.

Gritti–Stokes and through-knee amputations

Gritti–Stokes and through-knee amputations are rarely done nowadays. In the Gritti–Stokes type, the section is transcondylar.

Syme's amputation

It is essential to preserve the blood supply to the heel flap by meticulous clean dissection of the calcaneum. The tibia and fibula are sectioned as low as possible to the top of the mortice joint. This type of procedure is rarely applicable in patients with occlusive vascular disease.

Postoperative care of an amputation

Pain relief

Diamorphine or other opiates should be given regularly (Chapter 6).

Care of the good limb

Attention is focused on the amputation, but a pressure ulcer on the good foot will delay mobilisation, despite satisfactory healing of the stump. The use of a cradle to keep the weight of bed clothes off the foot and pressure area care are adjuncts to good nursing care.

Exercises and mobilisation

Immediately, the prevention of flexion deformity can be achieved by the use of a cloth placed over the stump with sand bags on each side to weight it down. Once the drain has been removed, exercises are started to build up muscle power and co-ordination. A stump bandage is applied each day to mould the shape of the stump. Mobility is progressively increased with walking between bars and the use of an inflatable artificial limb which allows weight-bearing to be started before a pylon or temporary artificial limb is ready

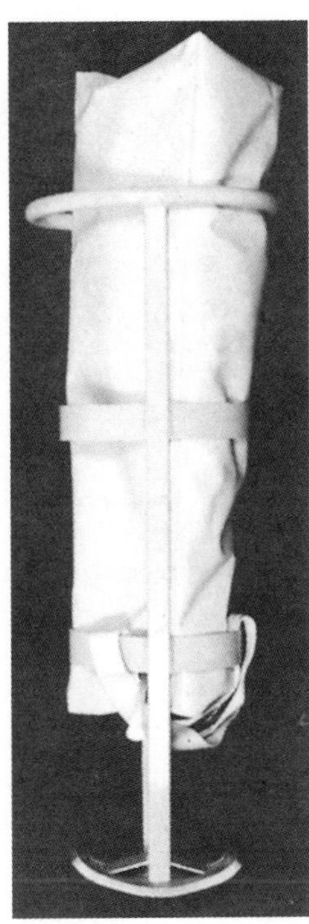

Fig. 15.43 Inflatable artificial limb.

(Fig. 15.43). It is emphasised that the whole episode in the patient's life should be conducted in an attitude of promotion through the stages towards full independence. Early assessment of the home (part of the whole programme) allows time for minor alterations, such as the addition of stair rails, movement of furniture to give support near doors, and clearance in confined passages.

Complications

Early complications include the following: reactionary haemorrhage, which requires return to the theatre for operative haemostasis; a haematoma, which requires evacuation; and infection, usually from a haematoma. Any abscess must be drained. Depending upon the sensitivity reactions of the organisms cultured, the appropriate antibiotics are given. Gas gangrene can occur in a midthigh stump, the organisms coming from contamination by the patient's faeces. Wound dehiscence and gangrene of the flaps are due to ischaemia; a higher amputation may well be necessary. Amputees are at risk of deep vein thrombosis and pulmonary embolism in the early postoperative period. Prophylaxis with subcutaneous heparin 5000 units twice daily is advised for several weeks after operation.

Late. Pain is sometimes a problem due to unresolved infection (sinus, osteitis, sequestrum), a bone spur, a scar adherent to bone, an amputation neuroma from the outgrowth of nerve fibrils which become attached to skin, muscle or fibrous tissue, or a phantom limb.

Phantom pain. Patients frequently remark that they can feel the amputated limb and sometimes that it is painful. The surgeon's attitude should be one of firm reassurance that this sensation will disappear. Other late complications include ulceration of the stump due to pressure effects of the prosthesis or increased ischaemia. Rarely, an ulcer is artefactual (Fig. 12.16). Some patients are troubled by cold and discoloured stumps, especially during the winter.

Arterial dilatation (aneurysm)

Dilatations of localised segments of the arterial system are called aneurysms. They can either be true aneurysms, containing the three layers of the arterial wall in the aneurysm sac, or false aneurysms, having a single layer of fibrous tissue as the wall of the sac, e.g. aneurysm following trauma (Fig. 15.44). Aneurysms can also be grouped according to their shape [fusiform, saccular (Fig. 15.45), dissecting], or to their aetiology [atherosclerotic, traumatic, syphilitic, collagen disease (Marfan's syndrome), mycotic]. The term mycotic is a misnomer because, while it indicates infection as a causal element in the formation of the aneurysm, this is hardly ever due to a fungus. In general, mycotic aneurysms are due to bacteria. Aneurysms occur all over the body in major vessels such as the aorta, femoral, popliteal, subclavian and carotid arteries, or in smaller vessels, such as the cerebral, mesenteric, splenic and renal arteries. The majority is true fusiform atherosclerotic aneurysms.

(a)

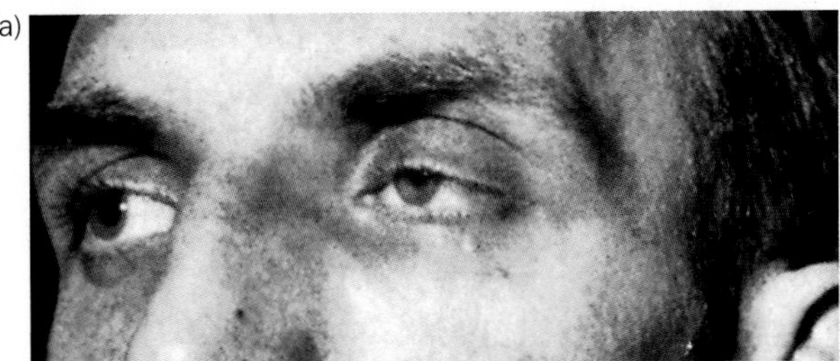

(b)

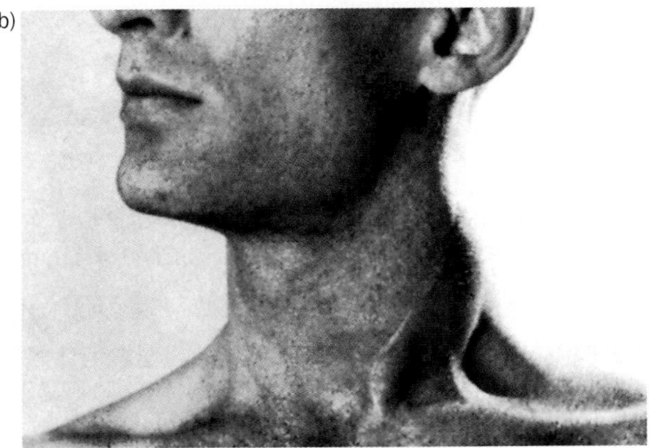

Fig. 15.44 (a) The ptosis, myosis, and enophthalmos of a Horner's syndrome, due to concomitant severance of the cervical sympathetic nerve. (b) A false, and rapidly extending, aneurysm of the common carotid caused by a stab wound.

Antonin Bernard Jean Marfan, 1858–1942. Professor of Paediatrics, Hopital des Enfants-Malades, Paris, France. Described this syndrome in 1896.

Johann Freidrich Horner, 1831–86. Professor of Ophthalmology, Zurich, Switzerland. Described the syndrome which bears his name in 1869.

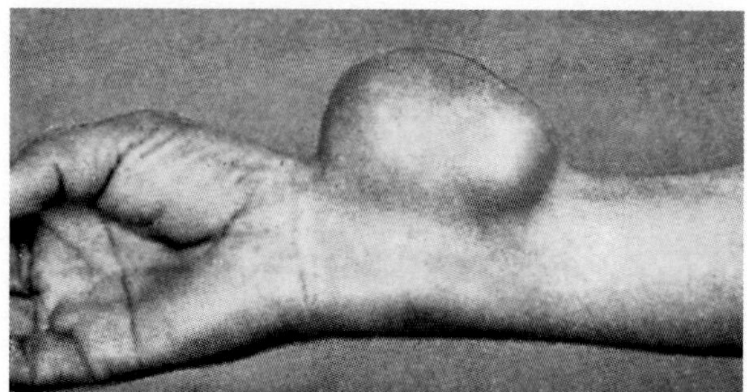

Fig. 15.45 Saccular aneurysm of the radial artery (*courtesy of Professor A.K. Toufeeq, Lahore, Pakistan*).

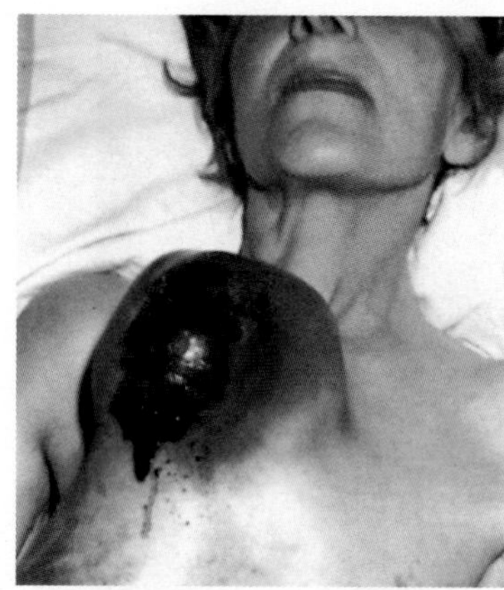

Fig. 15.46 An aortic aneurysm has eroded the sternum and is about to rupture (*the late Raymond Heisby, FRCS, Liverpool, England*).

Symptoms

All aneurysms can cause symptoms due to expansion, thrombosis, rupture or the release of emboli. The symptoms relate to the vessel affected, the site supplied or the tissues compressed by the aneurysm. Emboli from an aortic aneurysm can occasionally cause ischaemia of the toes and thrombotic occlusion of a popliteal aneurysm is a well-recognised cause of gangrene of the foot.

Clinical features of an aneurysm

Intrinsic

A swelling exhibiting expansile pulsation is present in the course of an artery. The pulsation diminishes if proximal pressure can be applied; the sac itself is compressible (although large aneurysms are frequently full of mural thrombus and may not be compressible), filling again in two or three beats if proximal pressure is released. A thrill may be palpable and auscultation sometimes reveals a bruit.

Extrinsic

Neighbouring or distal structures are affected. Thus pressure on veins or nerves causes distal oedema or altered sensation. Bones, joints or tubes, such as the trachea or oesophagus, are sometimes affected, but structures which are resilient, such as the intervertebral discs, often withstand prolonged pressure.

Differential diagnosis

Swelling under an artery

An artery may be pushed forwards, e.g. the subclavian by a cervical rib, and thus rendered prominent. Careful palpation distinguishes this condition.

Swelling over an artery

Transmitted pulsation is liable to be mistaken for that caused by expansion. However, posture may diminish pulsation; thus a pancreatic cyst examined in the genupectoral position falls away from the aorta, and consequently pulsation is less definite.

Pulsating tumours

Pulsating tumours include bone sarcoma, osteoclastoma and metastasis, especially from a hypernephroma.

An abscess

Before making an incision into a swelling believed to be an abscess, e.g. of the chest wall (Fig. 15.46), in the groin, in the axilla or in the popliteal fossa, it is essential to make sure that it does not pulsate. This mistake has been made many times.

A serpentine artery

A serpentine artery, e.g. innominate, carotid.

Abdominal aortic aneurysm

Abdominal aortic aneurysm is the commonest type of aortic aneurysm and is found in 2 per cent of the population at autopsy; 95 per cent are due to atherosclerosis and 95 per cent occur below the renal arteries.

Symptomatic aneurysms cause either minor symptoms, such as back pain and abdominal pain, or sudden, severe symptoms when they expand and rupture.

Asymptomatic aneurysms are found incidentally on physical examination, radiography or ultrasound investigation.

Ruptured abdominal aneurysm

Abdominal aortic aneurysms can rupture anteriorly into the peritoneal cavity (20 per cent) or posteriorly into the retroperitoneal space (80 per cent). Less than 50 per cent of patients with rupture survive to reach hospital.

Anterior rupture results in free bleeding into the peritoneal cavity. Very few of these patients reach hospital alive. Those who do have had a prolonged period of hypotension and shock, and consequently the results of surgery are poor.

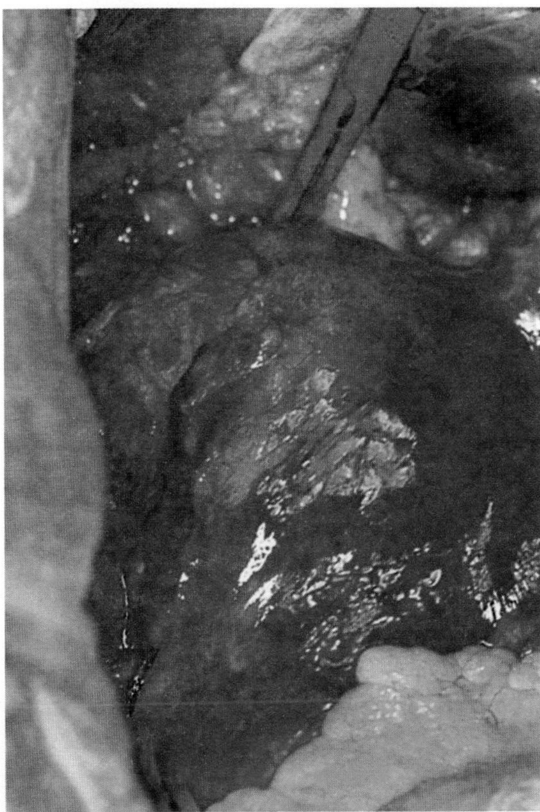

Fig. 15.47 The retroperitoneal haematoma of a ruptured aortic aneurysm. The patient is anaesthetised (on the operation table after towels have been placed – if in severe shock). Through a full-length midline or transverse incision the small bowel is lifted to the patient's right side to expose the aorta and the haematoma lying behind the posterior peritoneum. The aortic pulsation is palpated through the haematoma at its upper limit and fingers are insinuated on each side of the aorta. With finger and thumb control the upper clamp is positioned and closed on the aorta. The procedure is then as for a planned case. In this illustration the clamp is at the proximal end of the aneurysm; the haematoma has spread from the left paracolic gutter to encircle the aneurysm and the aortic bifurcation.

Posterior rupture produces a retroperitoneal haematoma (Fig. 15.47). There is a brief period in many of these patients when a combination of moderate hypotension and the resistance of the retroperitoneal tissues stops the haemorrhage. The patient remains conscious, but in severe pain. If no operation is performed, the mortality is 100 per cent. Operation results in a better than 50 per cent survival.

To achieve the best results, the diagnosis must be made early. The clinical features include sudden, severe back pain, accompanied in some cases by a brief loss of consciousness. The femoral pulses in one or both groins may be diminished or absent. A pulsatile mass is palpable in the abdomen and there are signs of shock. The procedure is as follows.

- Two good intravenous infusion lines and a central venous pressure line must be inserted as soon as the patient arrives in hospital or the diagnosis made once admitted.
- Blood is sent for immediate cross-match of 8 units.
- Infusion of saline, or volume-expanding fluids (Chapter 4), is given to raise the systolic blood pressure to approx. 100 mmHg. *On no account should the blood pressure be allowed to rise unduly as further uncontrolled haemorrhage may be stimulated.*
- A urinary catheter is passed.
- If the patient appears to be stable, although in pain, the operation may be delayed until cross-matched blood is ready but the patient should still be *transferred immediately to the operating room* so that surgery may be commenced immediately if haemodynamic problems develop.

It should always be remembered that the definitive treatment of burst aneurysm is operation, not monitoring and resuscitation.

Abdominal aneurysm without rupture

Patients most commonly present without symptoms although they may have pain, usually felt in the back in the lumbar region and in the upper abdomen. In addition, pain can occur in the thigh and groin due to nerve compression. Gastrointestinal, urinary and venous symptoms can also be caused by abdominal aneurysm. As a general rule, in the presence of a pulsatile mass if symptoms cannot be reasonably explained by another lesion, they must be assumed to be due to the aneurysm (until proved otherwise) and the aneurysm placed in the symptomatic group.

Indication for surgery

Symptomatic aneurysm

Without surgery, 80 per cent with a symptomatic aneurysm will be dead in a year. With surgery, 80 per cent will be alive in a year. Surgery is indicated, therefore, in patients who are otherwise medically fit. The risk of operation is increased particularly in the presence of hypertension, chronic airway disease, recent myocardial infarction and impaired renal function. Chronological age is not a bar to surgery, but few patients are fit enough for this type of procedure once over the age of 80.

Asymptomatic aneurysm

Aneurysm found incidentally on examination, radiography or ultrasound in an otherwise fit patient needs repair if over 5.5 cm in diameter on ultrasound. The annual incidence of rupture rises from 1 per cent in aneurysms that are 5.5 cm in diameter to over 20 per cent in those that are 7 cm in diameter. As elective surgery carries a 2–5 per cent mortality, the balance is in favour of surgery once the diameter is above 5.5 cm, provided there are no medical contraindications to surgery.

Investigations

After taking a careful history and examining the patient, the following investigations are performed: urine analysis to exclude diabetes, in particular, haemoglobin estimation, full blood count, erythrocyte sedimentation rate (ESR), blood group and cross-match if surgery is contemplated within a few days; electrocardiogram (ECG); liver function tests; blood lipids; electrolytes and urea; chest radiography and ultrasonography of the abdomen to assess aneurysm diameter (Fig. 15.48).

An aortogram may be useful in delineating the proximal and distal extent of the aneurysm before surgery; it does not permit assessment of diameter because the sac is usually filled with circumferential clot leading to a falsely narrow angiographic appearance. Involvement of the renal arteries by the aneurysm should be suspected if it is not possible to palpate the upper limit of the aneurysm below the xiphisternum with the patient lying flat (only 5 per cent of cases). In such circumstances aortography, computerised tomography (CT) and/or magnetic resonance imaging are essential (Figs 15.49–15.51).

(a)

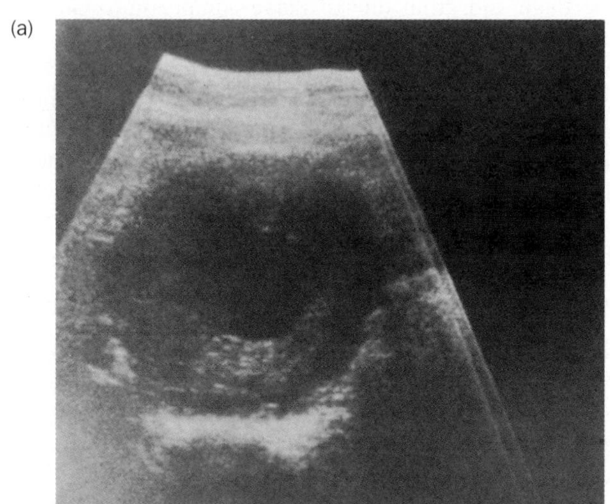

(b)

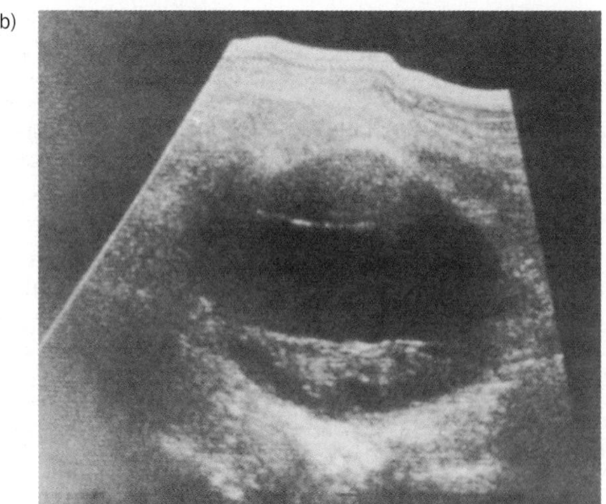

Fig. 15.48 Ultrasound of an aortic aneurysm showing the large clot-filled sac with a small central lumen (transverse (a) and longitudinal (b) scans).

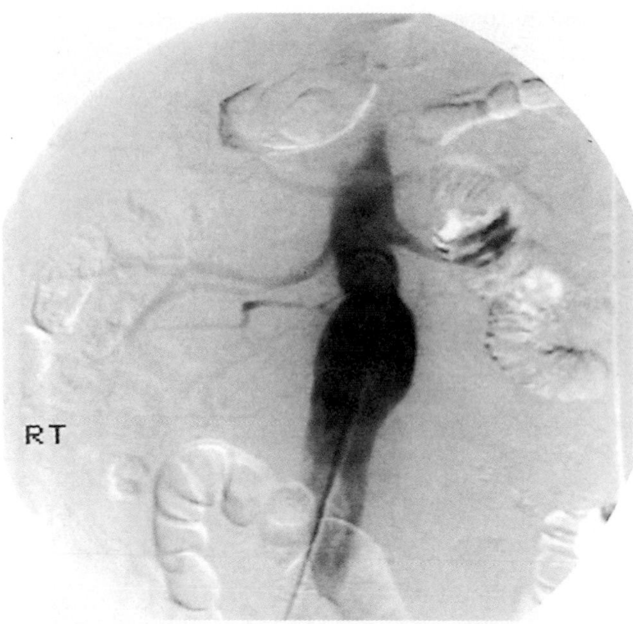

Fig. 15.49 Angiogram of abdominal aortic aneurysm. The neck of the aneurysm is inferior to the renal arteries.

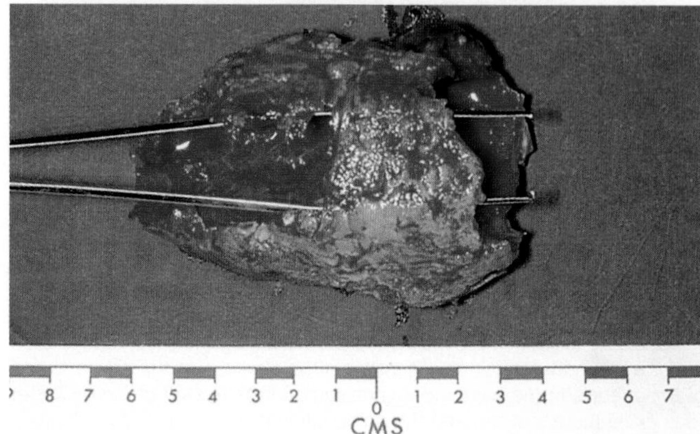

Fig. 15.50 Thrombus removed from an abdominal aortic aneurysm; this thrombus is the reason an angiogram may give a false impression of aneurysm diameter.

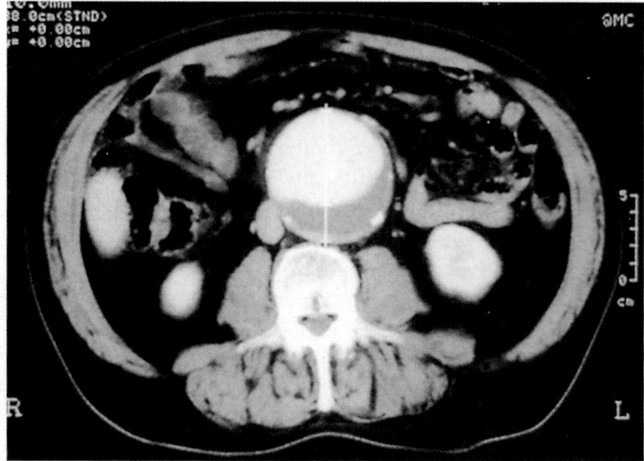

Fig. 15.51 Computerised tomogram of abdomen showing an aortic aneurysm. Blood flowing through the thrombus-containing sac is enhanced with contrast agent and appears white.

(a) (b)

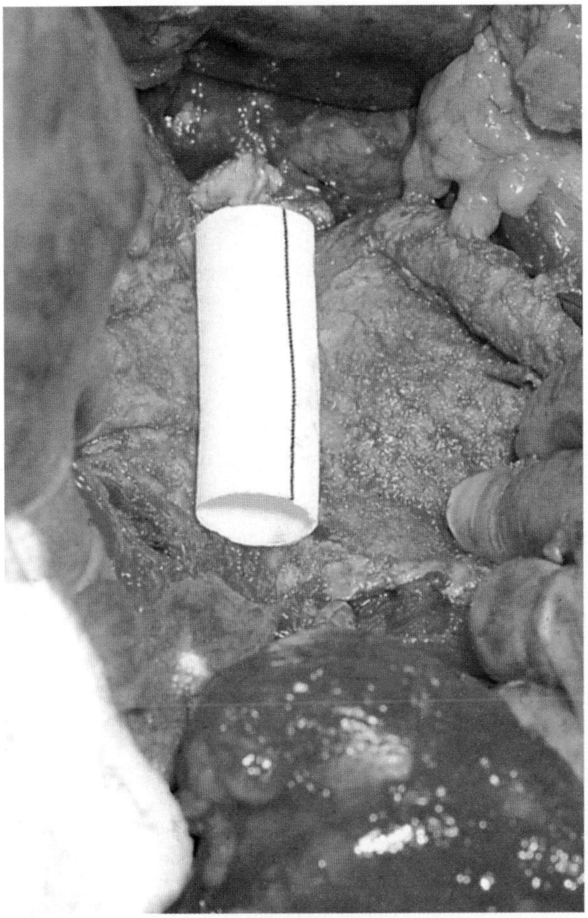

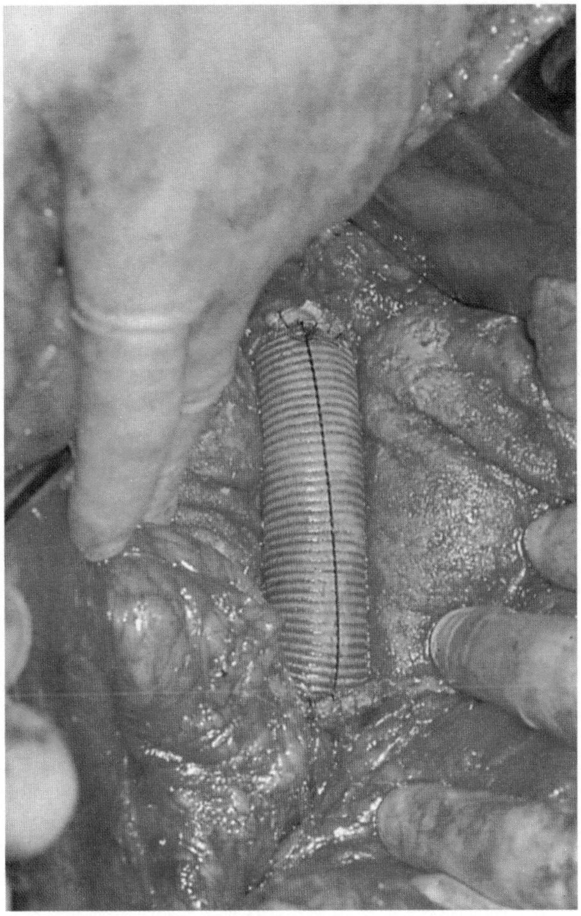

Fig. 15.52 (a) Aneurysm sac opened. Note that the posterior wall of the aorta immediately above and below the sac is not divided. A Dacron tube graft is laid in place within the sac ready for suture; (b) graft sutured in place and vascular clamps removed.

Open surgical procedure (Figs 15.52 and 15.53)

Under general anaesthesia, with the patient lying supine with a urinary catheter and central venous line *in situ*, a full-length midline or upper transverse incision is made. The small bowel is lifted to the patient's right and the aorta identified. The posterior peritoneum overlying the aorta is opened and the upper limit of the aneurysm is identified. A plane is sought between the aorta and vena cava below the left renal vein. The iliac arteries are then dissected free from surrounding structures, heparin is given, and clamps are applied above and below the aneurysm. The aneurysm is opened longitudinally to the right of the inferior mesenteric artery, and back-bleeding from lumbar and mesenteric vessels controlled by sutures placed from within the aneurysm sac. The graft is then sutured end to end inside the aneurysm sac (2/0 or 3/0 Prolene). The upper clamp is released and haemostasis achieved. The lower end is then sutured to the aortic bifurcation in a similar manner. Clamps are released carefully, to one leg at a time, because hypotension and arrhythmias can occur if release is too rapid. The aneurysm sac is then closed round the graft (Fig. 15.54) and the posterior peritoneum closed to exclude the graft and suture lines from the intestine (to reduce the risk of fistula formation). The abdomen is then closed in layers. Occasionally, when the iliac vessels are also involved with dilatation or severe atheroma, it is necessary to construct an aorto-bi-iliac or aorto-bifemoral bypass, rather than use a simple aorto-aortic tube graft.

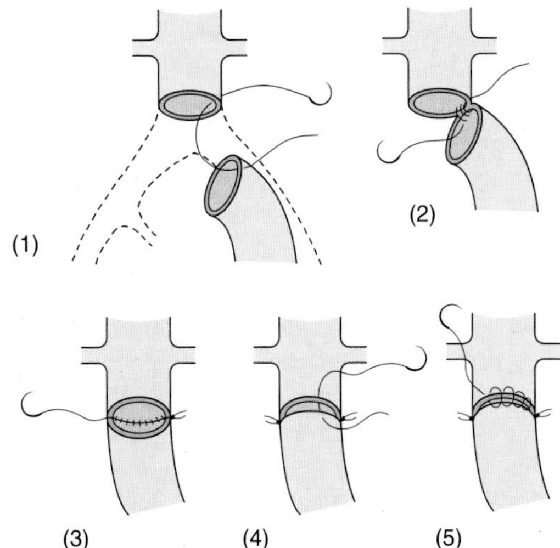

Fig. 15.53 Aortic aneurysm repair (end-to-end within aneurysmal sac). The initial stitch is placed at '2 o'clock', leaving two-thirds of the diameter posteriorly (1). The posterior continuous sutures are placed (2) and completed (3). The anterior suture line started at the initial stitch (4) and the anterior suture line completed (5).

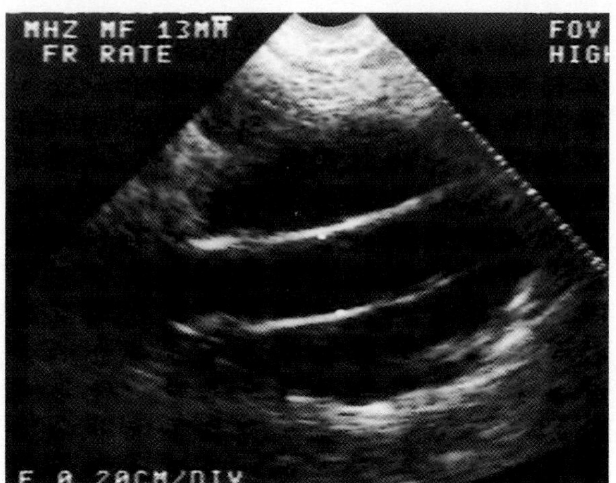

Fig. 15.54 Aortic graft. Transverse scan showing the graft in the dilated aortic bed.

Endoluminal stent-graft procedure

Many major vascular surgical centres are now able to offer this minimally invasive treatment for certain aortic aneurysms, generally on an elective or a semi-elective basis. The aorta is accessed via the common femoral arteries, which are exposed surgically. Under radiological control, a delivery system is guided up into the aorta and a stent-graft placed within the aortic sac; this usually comprises aortic body and one iliac, the opposite iliac being replaced by a separate single iliac stent-graft introduced from the opposite common femoral artery. The stent system must be able to produce a blood-tight seal at the uppermost (infrarenal aortic) level of the graft, at both iliac levels distally, and at the junction between the aorto-uni-iliac stent-graft and its contralateral iliac partner. The technique has been carried out successfully so far in a few thousand patients world-wide but concerns remain about stent-graft fragmentation with the passage of time, and leakage (endoleak) at the interface of vessel and stent-graft or from patent lumbar arteries.

Postoperative complications

The commonest complications following open repair of abdominal aortic aneurysms are respiratory (lower lobe consolidation, atelectasis and 'shock lung'). Haemorrhage occurs in relatively few cases provided anticoagulation is not continued beyond the immediate operative period and haemostasis is satisfactory at the end of the procedure. A degree of colonic ischaemia due to lack of collateral blood supply occurs in 10 per cent of all cases; fortunately this severe complication usually resolves spontaneously. Renal failure and infection of the graft are rarely seen following nonurgent procedures, but can complicate procedures for repair of ruptured aneurysm. Other complications are sexual dysfunction, fistula formation and spinal cord ischaemia.

Aortoduodenal fistula

Aortoduodenal fistula is an uncommon but treatable complication of abdominal aortic replacement surgery. It should be suspected whenever haematemesis or melaena occurs in the months or years after operation. A successful outcome may be achieved by prompt operation, separating aorta from duodenum, closing the holes and interposing some omentum.

Peripheral aneurysm

Popliteal aneurysm accounts for 70 per cent of all peripheral aneurysms. Two-thirds of them are bilateral. Three-quarters develop complications within 5 years if treated conservatively. Careful examination of the abdominal aorta is indicated if a popliteal aneurysm is found because one-third are accompanied by aortic aneurysms. Popliteal aneurysms present as a swelling behind the knee, or with symptoms due to complications, such as severe ischaemia of sudden onset following thrombosis, or ischaemic ulceration of the toes due to emboli. Surgery, possibly preceded by intra-arterial thrombolysis, is indicated urgently in the presence of complications to prevent amputation, and in asymptomatic cases, to prevent complications. Diagnosis can be difficult and relies on palpation of a pulsatile mass behind the knee. As a general guide, if the popliteal pulse is easily felt in a patient who is not thin, the presence of an aneurysm should be considered. Ultrasound and CT scan can be helpful in confirming the diagnosis. Treatment is either a bypass graft with ligation of the aneurysm or an inlay graft.

Femoral aneurysm. ***True*** aneurysm of the femoral artery is uncommon. Complications occur in less than 3 per cent and so conservative treatment is indicated initially. Look for aneurysms elsewhere: more than half are associated with abdominal or popliteal aneurysms.

False aneurysm of the femoral artery occurs in 2 per cent of patients after arterial surgery at this site. Many are infective in origin and rupture is possible, making surgical treatment indicated. Local repair with reanastomosis at the groin under suitable antibiotic cover may be successful, but bypass, clear of the infected area, with subsequent excision of the infected graft is often the only way of preventing further problems.

Iliac aneurysm (Fig. 15.55) usually occurs in conjunction with aortic aneurysm and rarely occurs on its own. On its own, it is difficult to diagnose clinically and so 50 per cent present already ruptured. Surgical treatment is indicated, with bypass, and exclusion of the aneurysm by ligation above and below the dilatation.

Aneurysms of the ascending aorta and arch require cardiopulmonary bypass for reconstruction to be undertaken. These, together with dissecting aneurysms of the thoracic aorta and traumatic false aneurysms in that situation, are considered in Chapter 48.

Arteriovenous fistula (AVF)

Communication between an artery and a vein (or veins) may be either a congenital malformation, or acquired by the trauma of a penetrating wound or a sharp blow. Arteriovenous fistulas are also created surgically in the arms or legs of

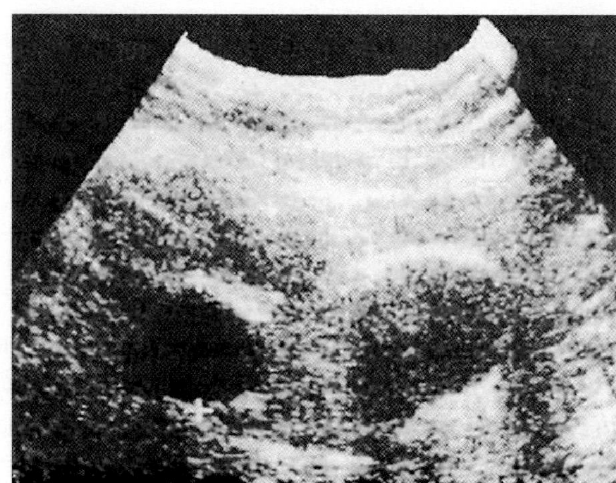

Fig. 15.55 Ultrasound revealing bilateral iliac aneurysms.

patients undergoing renal dialysis (Chapter 64). All arteriovenous communications have a structural and a physiological effect.

Structural effect

The structural effect of arterial blood flow on the veins is characteristic as they become dilated, tortuous and thick walled (arterialised) (Fig. 15.56). It also makes the lesions diffuse and so renders surgical procedures difficult.

Physiological effect

The combination of an uncontrolled leak from the high-pressure arterial system and an enhanced venous return and venous pressure results in an increase in pulse rate and cardiac output. The pulse pressure is high if there is a large and persistent shunt. Left ventricular enlargement and, later, cardiac failure occur. A congenital fistula in the young may cause overgrowth of a limb. In the leg, indolent ulcers may result from relative ischaemia below the short circuit.

Clinical signs

Clinically, a pulsatile swelling may be present if the lesion is relatively superficial. On palpation, a thrill is detected and auscultation reveals a buzzing continuous bruit. Dilated veins may be seen, in which there is a rapid blood flow. Pressure on the artery proximal to the fistula causes the swelling to diminish in size, the thrill and bruit to cease, the pulse rate to fall [known variously as Nicoladoni's (1875) or Branham's (1890) sign] and the pulse pressure to return to normal.

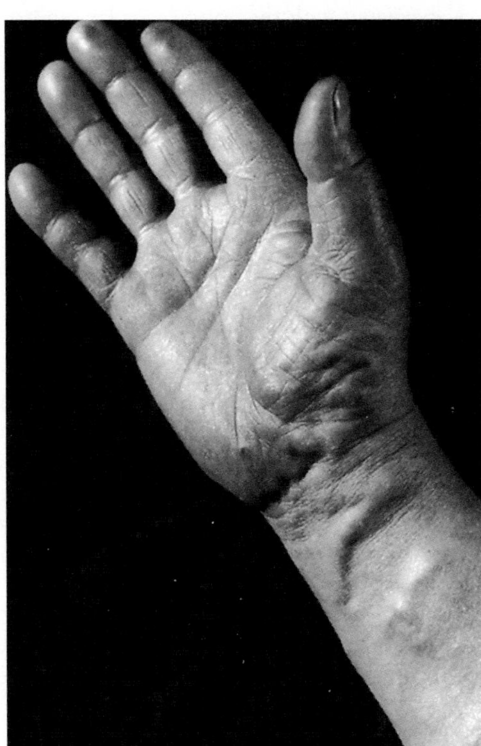

Fig. 15.56 Post-traumatic arteriovenous aneurysm at the wrist. Note the prominent (varicose) arterialised veins.

Arteriography

Arteriography confirms the lesion, which is noteworthy for the speed with which venous filling occurs. It is often difficult to pinpoint the actual site of the fistula.

Treatment

Embolisation by the radiologist or excision is advocated only for severe deformity or recurrent haemorrhage. It is often wise to enlist the aid of a plastic surgeon so that proper ablation and reconstruction can be effected. Ligation of a 'feeding' artery is of no lasting value and is likely to be detrimental as it may preclude treatment by embolisation.

The **acquired** lesions especially tend to be progressive and embolisation or operation is indicated if feasible and safe. At operation the vessels are separated and, if possible, repaired by suture, any intervening sac being excised. Failing this, ligation of the involved artery and vein is required both above and below the lesion (quadruple ligation). Bypass grafts may be required.

Arteritis

Thromboangiitis obliterans (Buerger's disease)

This is a condition characterised by occlusive disease of the small and medium-sized arteries (plantars, tibials, radial, etc.), thrombophiebitis of superficial or deep veins, and Raynaud's syndrome occurring in male patients in a young age group (usually under the age of 30 years). Usually one or two of the three manifestations are present and occasionally all three. The condition does not occur in women or nonsmokers. It is not, as used to be stated, more common in Russian Jews; cases are seen in different races all over the world. Histologically, localised inflammatory changes occur in the walls of arteries and veins leading to thrombosis. The usual symptoms and signs of arterial occlusive disease are present. Gangrene of the toes and fingers is common and progressive. Arteriography sometimes shows a characteristic 'corrugation' of the fermoral arteries as well as the distal arterial occlusions and helps to distinguish the condition from presenile atherosclerosis. Other forms of arteritis, e.g. polyarteritis nodosa, must be excluded.

Investigations

A formal vascular assessment should be undertaken, e.g. ESR, autoantibodies, coagulation screening and lipid profile.

Carl Nicoladoni. Nineteenth-century surgeon, Vienna, Austria.
H.H. Branham. Nineteenth-century surgeon, USA.

Treatment

The treatment is total abstinence from smoking. While this will arrest the disease it will not reverse established arterial occlusions. A mere reduction in smoking is not sufficient to prevent the relentless progression of this devastating condition. Established arterial occlusions may be treated along the usual lines and sympathectomy may be a useful adjunctive procedure. Nevertheless, amputations, conservative if possible, may eventually be required.

Other types of arteritis

Other types of arteritis are encountered in rheumatoid arthritis, diffuse lupus erythematosus and polyarteritis. Treatment is similar. Diabetes was discussed earlier.

Temporal, occipital and ophthalmic arteritis

Localised infiltration with inflammatory and giant cells leads to arterial occlusion, ischaemic headache and tender, palpable, pulseless (thrombosed) arteries in the scalp. The major catastrophe of irreversible blindness occurs when the ophthalmic artery is occluded. A raised ESR and a positive temporal artery biopsy call for immediate prednisolone therapy to arrest and reverse the process before the ophthalmic artery is involved. The dose must be reduced as soon as possible, in line with clinical improvement and a fall in the ESR, to a maintenance dose which is controlled under long-term surveillance.

Takayasu's arteriopathy

Takayasu's arteriopathy (syn. obliterative arteritis of females, pulseless disease) causes narrowing and obstruction of major arteries. It usually pursues a relentless course (Fig. 15.57).

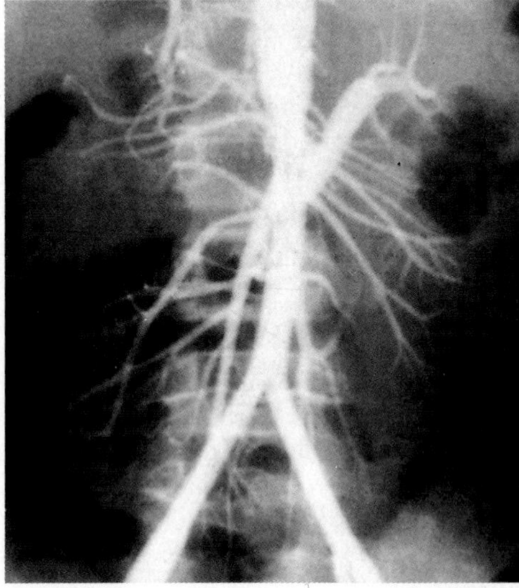

Fig. 15.57 A bypass vein graft from the aorta to the left renal artery in a young girl with bilateral renal artery stenosis causing hypertension. The subclavian and other arteries were also occluded by Takayasu's arteriopathy.

U. Takayasu, b. 1871. Japanese ophthalmologist who studied in Tokyo, St Thomas's Hospital, London, and Breslau. Published a paper on Takayasu's disease in 1908.

Cystic myxomatous degeneration

An accumulation of clear jelly (like a synovial ganglion) in the outer layers of a main artery may occasionally be encountered, especially in the popliteal artery. The lesion so stiffens the artery that pulsation disappears and claudication occurs when the limb is flexed (as on walking up stairs). Arteriography shows a smooth narrowing of an otherwise normal artery and a sharp kink or buckling when the knee is flexed. Decompression, by removal of the myxomatous material, is all that is required, but the 'ganglion' may recur and require excision of part of the artery with interposition vein graft repair.

Vasospastic conditions

Raynaud's syndrome

Raynaud's syndrome may be primary or secondary. The primary idiopathic form usually occurs in young women and affects the upper extremities more than the lower. The peripheral pulses are normal. The condition is attributable to abnormal sensitivity in the direct response of the arterioles to cold. When cooled, these vessels constrict and, as a result, the part (usually the fingers) becomes blanched and incapable of finer movements. The capillaries then dilate and fill with slowly flowing deoxygenated blood, the digits therefore becoming swollen and dusky. As the attack passes off, the arterioles relax, oxygenated blood returns into the dilated capillaries and the digits become red. Thus the condition is recognised by the characteristic sequence of blanching, dusky cyanosis and red engorgement, often accompanied by pain. In the idiopathic form, superficial necrosis is very uncommon. Early cases must be distinguished from chilblains and vascular disturbances sometimes associated with the costoclavicular syndrome, and from the other causes of secondary Raynaud's syndrome.

Conservative treatment

Protection from cold and avoidance of pulp and nail-bed infections are part of the conservative regimen that is advised for mild cases. The use of calcium antagonists, such as nifedipine, may also have a role to play and electrically heated gloves can be useful in winter. Sympathectomy has been discredited in this condition.

Secondary Raynaud's syndrome

This was previously called Raynaud's disease (a term to be avoided). Although peripheral vasospasm may be noted in atherosclerosis, thoracic outlet syndrome, carpal tunnel, etc., the term secondary Raynaud's syndrome is most often used for a peripheral arterial manifestation of the collagen diseases, especially progressive systemic sclerosis (scleroderma) and systemic lupus erythromatosis. It may also follow the use of vibrating tools (when it is commonly known as 'vibration white finger'), e.g. pneumatic road drills, mining borers and chain saws, which vibrate at certain frequencies.

Treatment

Treatment is directed primarily at the underlying condition, although the conservative measures outlined above are often helpful. The syndrome when secondary to the collagenoses leads frequently to necrosis of digits and multiple amputations. Sympathectomy yields disappointing results and is rarely used. Nifedipine, steroids and vasospastic antagonists may all have a place. Patients with vibration white finger should avoid vibrating tools.

Acrocyanosis

Acrocyanosis, *crurum puellarum frigidum*[4], may be confused with Raynaud's disease, but it is painless and is not paroxysmal. Affecting young females, the cyanosis of the fingers and, especially, the legs may be accompanied by paraesthesia and chilblains. In severe cases, sympathectomy may be tried. If merely affecting the calves, a differential diagnosis is Bazin's disease.

Preganglionic cervicodorsal sympathectomy

Supraclavicular method. Through a supraclavicular incision, the clavicular part of the sternomastoid, the posterior belly of the omohyoid and the scalenus anterior muscles are divided, the phrenic nerve being displaced medially. The subclavian artery is exposed and depressed; the suprapleural fascia is divided so that the dome of the pleura can be displaced downwards. The stellate ganglion is identified as it lies on the first rib (Fig. 15.58). The sympathetic trunk is traced downwards and divided below the third thoracic ganglion. All rami communicantes associated with the second and third ganglia and the nerve of Kuntz, a grey ramus running upwards from the second thoracic ganglion to the first thoracic nerve, are meticulously divided. Occasionally, the approach is *under* a high arching subclavian artery.

Transthoracic method. This gives a greater exposure and facilitates the removal of the sympathetic chain from the fifth ganglion up to the lower fringe of the stellate ganglion. It tends to give better results than the supraclavicular method and can be employed when that has failed. In women where cosmetic effects are a consideration, the approach can be made via an axillary incision through the third space (Hedley Atkins). The sympathetic chain is easily seen and after dividing the pleura, it is dissected out, care being taken to avoid damage to the intercostal vessels, which may cause tedious haemorrhage. Care should also be taken, when making and suturing the approach wound, to avoid damage to the nerve to serratus anterior, giving rise to 'winging' of the scapula.

Endoscopic method. This seeks to achieve a sympathectomy via the transthoracic route using a suitable endoscope, e.g. a cystoscope or laparoscope. A Verres needle is passed via the axilla to induce a CO_2 pneumothorax. A trochar and cannula are then employed to introduce the endoscope. The sympathetic chain is visualised and a coagulating electrode used to disrupt the ganglia. Some surgeons carry out the procedure without using CO_2, the lung being simply deflated by the anaesthetist using a double-lumen endotracheal tube. The endoscopic method is now the procedure of choice for cervicodorsal sympathectomy.

Lumbar sympathectomy

Operative method. Using a transverse loin incision, an extraperitoneal approach is used in which the colon and peritoneum, to which the ureter clings, are stripped medially so as to expose the inner border of the psoas muscle (Fig. 15.59). The sympathetic trunk lies on the sides of the bodies of the lumbar vertebrae; on the right side it is overlapped by the vena cava. Lumbar veins are apt to cross the trunk superficially. The sympathetic trunk is divided on the side of the body of the fourth lumbar vertebra. It is then traced upwards to be divided above the large second lumbar ganglion, which is easily recognised by the number of white rami which join it. Care should be taken not to mistake small lymph nodes,

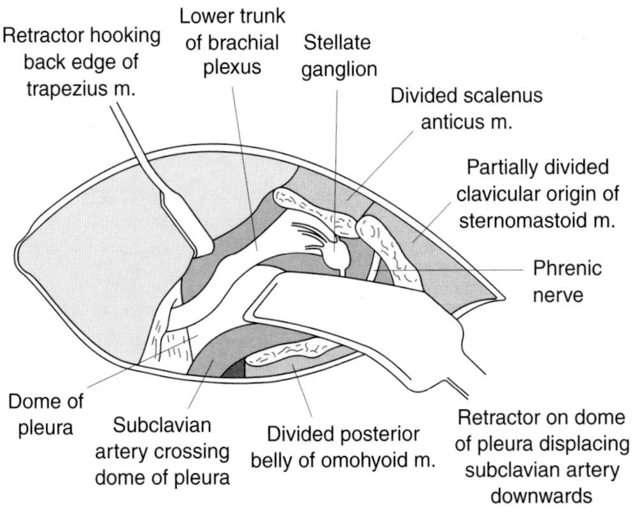

Retractor hooking back edge of trapezius m.
Lower trunk of brachial plexus
Stellate ganglion
Divided scalenus anticus m.
Partially divided clavicular origin of sternomastoid m.
Phrenic nerve
Dome of pleura
Subclavian artery crossing dome of pleura
Divided posterior belly of omohyoid m.
Retractor on dome of pleura displacing subclavian artery downwards

Fig. 15.58 Cervical sympathectomy: exposure of the superior ganglion of the sympathetic chain through a supraclavicular approach.

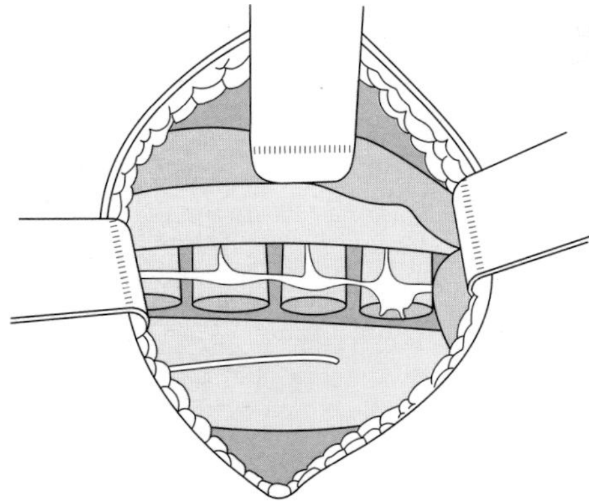

Fig. 15.59 Left lumbar sympathectomy. The central retractor is holding back the peritoneum and ureter to expose the aorta and the psoas muscle, between which lies the sympathetic chain. Note that the second lumbar ganglion, adjacent to the lower pole of the kidney, has connecting rami to the spinal cord. The genitofemoral nerve is seen emerging through the fibres of the psoas.

[4]*Puellarum = of girls, frigidum = cold.*

Pierre Antoine Ernest Bazin, 1807–78. Dermatologist, Hopital St Louis, Paris, France.

Albert Kuntz, 1879–1957. Professor of Anatomy, St Louis, Missouri, USA.

Sir Hedley John Barnard Atkins, 1905–83. Past President, The Royal College of Surgeons of England. Emeritus Professor of Surgery, Guy's Hospital, London, England.

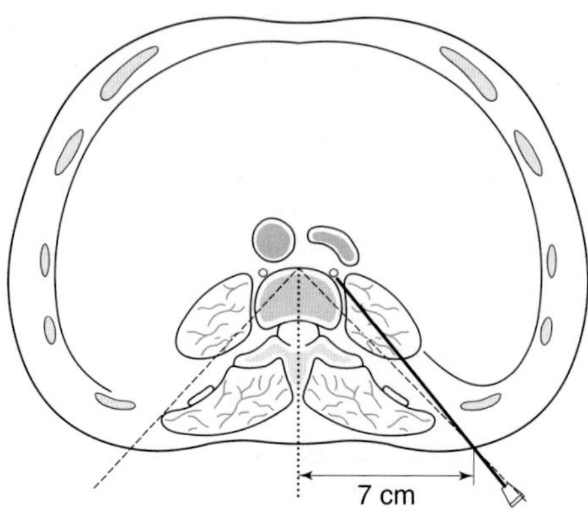

Fig. 15.60 Lumbar paravertebral injection.

lymphatics, the genitofemoral nerve or the occasional tendinous strip of the psoas minor for the sympathetic chain. It is possible to perform the operation via an endoscope after the creation of a suitably expanded retroperitoneal tissue plane. Along with a decline in the recognised indications for sympathectomy there has been a move away from the operative approach in favour of the less hazardous chemical (phenol) sympathectomy.

Chemical method. This is contraindicated in patients taking anticoagulants. Under radiographic fluoroscopic control, with the patient in the lateral position, local anaesthetic is injected. A long spinal needle is then inserted (Fig. 15.60) to seek the side of the vertebral body and to pass alongside it to reach the lumbar sympathetic chain. After confirming the needle position by injection of contrast agent, approximately 5 ml of phenol in water (1:16) is injected. This is usually done at two sites: beside the bodies of the second and fourth lumbar vertebrae. Great care is needed to avoid penetrating the aorta, cava or ureter; the plunger of the syringe must always be drawn back before injection to exclude the presence of blood.

Further reading

Bell, P.R.F., Jamieson, C.W. and Ruckley, C.V. (eds) (1992) *The Surgical Management of Vascular Disease*, W.B. Saunders, London.

Jamieson, C.W. and Yao, J.S.T. (eds) (1997) *Rob and Smith's Concise Vascular Surgery*, Chapman & Hall, London.

Moore, W.S. (ed.) (1998) *Vascular Surgery: A Comprehensive Review*, 5th edn, W.B. Saunders, Philadelphia, PA.

Rutherford, R.B. (ed.) (1995) *Vascular Surgery*, 4th edn, W.B. Saunders, Philadelphia, PA.

Veith, F.J., Hobson, R.W., Williams, R.A. and Wilson, S.E. (eds) (1994) *Vascular Surgery: Principles and Practice*, 2nd edn, McGraw-Hill, New York.

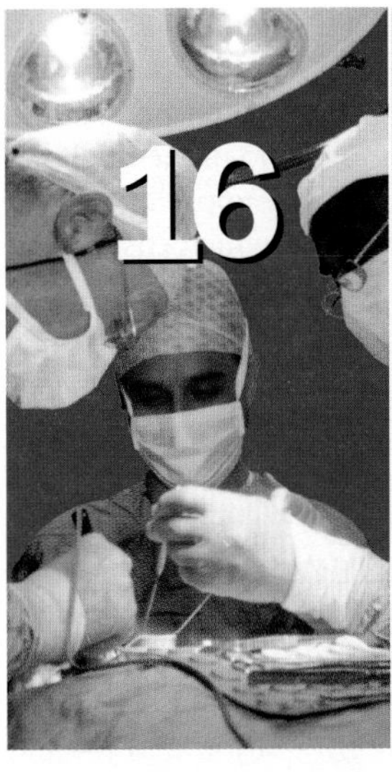

16 Venous disorders

Introduction

Venous disorders are very common and especially affect the lower limb. Twenty per cent of the population suffer with varicose veins and 2 per cent have skin changes which may precede venous ulceration. At any one time 200 000 people in the UK have active venous ulceration. The provision of wound care and bandaging costs the National Health Service £600 million per annum.

Anatomy of the venous system in the limbs

Arterial blood flows through the main axial arteries to the upper and lower limbs. It returns via the deep and superficial veins. In the upper limb the superficial veins are more important in carrying blood back to the heart. In the lower limb, the superficial veins carry only about 10 per cent of the blood, while the remainder passes via the deep veins. The superficial veins lie superficial to the muscle fascia of the limb. The principal superficial veins in the leg are the long and short saphenous veins (Fig. 16.1). In the arm, the cephalic and basilic veins are the principal superficial veins.

Interestingly, venous diseases occur much more frequently in the lower limb than in the upper limb, and most often in the superficial veins. The deep veins of the lower limb may be

Fig. 16.1 The superficial veins of the lower limb.

Bailey & Love's Short Practice of Surgery, 23rd edition. Edited by R.C.G. Russell, N.S. Williams and C.J.K. Bulstrode. Published in 2000 by Arnold Publishers.

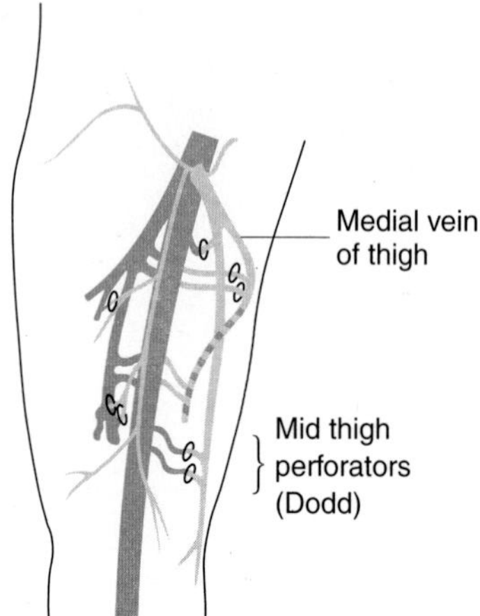

Fig. 16.2 The main deep veins of the lower limb.

the site of life-threatening venous thrombosis or venous valvular incompetence resulting in leg ulceration. Each major axial artery has at least one and often a pair of accompanying veins named after the artery (Fig. 16.2). The superficial and deep veins join at a number of points. The short saphenous vein terminates at the saphenopopliteal junction (SPJ) and the long saphenous vein at the saphenofemoral junction (SFJ) in the groin. Here the flow in the superficial veins joins that in the deep veins. There is, in addition, a number of places in the calf and thigh where flow in the superficial veins may also join that in the deep veins. These is the ankle, calf and thigh communicating or perforating veins (Fig. 16.3). The names of these veins come from their course from the superficial to the deep venous system in which they perforate the deep fascia of the leg. Near the ankle are the Cockett perforating veins, near the knee the Boyd perforators and in the thigh the Hunterian perforating vein. All veins in the upper and lower limbs contain valves every few centimetres which ensure that blood flows towards the heart.

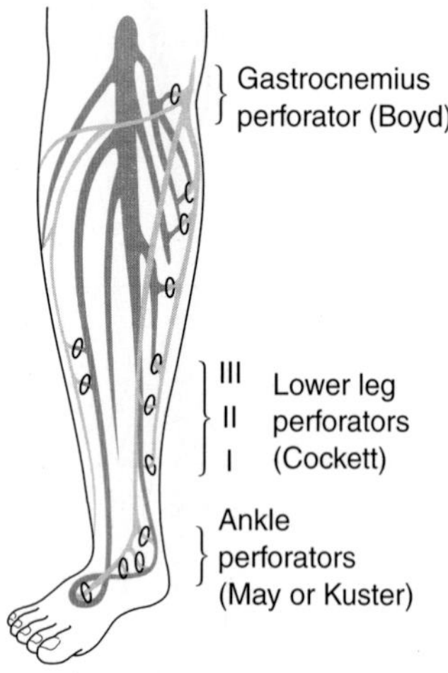

Fig. 16.3 Lower limb perforating veins – points at which blood should flow from the superficial to the deep veins.

Frank Bernard Cockett. Emeritus Surgeon, St Thomas' Hospital, London, England.

John Hunter, 1728–93. Scottish anatomist, physiologist and pathologist. Surgeon, St George's Hospital, London, England.

Venous pathophysiology

Blood flows into the leg because it is pumped by the heart along the arteries. By the time it emerges from the capillaries it is at a low pressure (about 20 mmHg), but this is enough for the blood to return to the heart. Blood from the muscles of the leg returns through the deep veins. Blood from the skin and superficial tissues, external to the deep fascia, drains via the long and short saphenous veins – SFJ and SPJ – and communicating veins into the deep veins. Valves prevent the flow of blood from the deep to the superficial system.

The venous pressure in the foot vein on standing is equivalent to the height of a column of blood, extending from the heart to the foot. However, the same is true of the arterial system so that on standing the arterial blood pressure at the ankle rises by 80–100 mmHg, depending on the height of the person. So the blood continues to circulate, even in the absence of muscle activity. However, we also have a sophisticated series of muscle pumps that act as peripheral hearts in the venous system (Fig. 16.4). These are made up of the deep veins of the calf and thigh which are surrounded by muscle. In addition, there is a foot pump which ejects blood from the plantar veins as pressure is placed on the foot during walking. On exercise the calf and thigh muscles contract compressing the veins and ejecting blood towards the heart. The direction of venous blood flow is controlled by the venous valves. The pressure within the calf compartment rises to 200–300 mmHg during walking and this is more than enough to propel the blood in the direction of the heart (Fig. 16.5). During the muscle relaxation phase, the pressure within the calf falls to a low level and blood from the superficial veins flows through the perforating veins into the deep veins. The consequence of this is that the pressure in the superficial veins falls during walking. This can be monitored by a cannula placed in a superficial vein of the foot and connected to a pressure transducer. Normally the pressure in

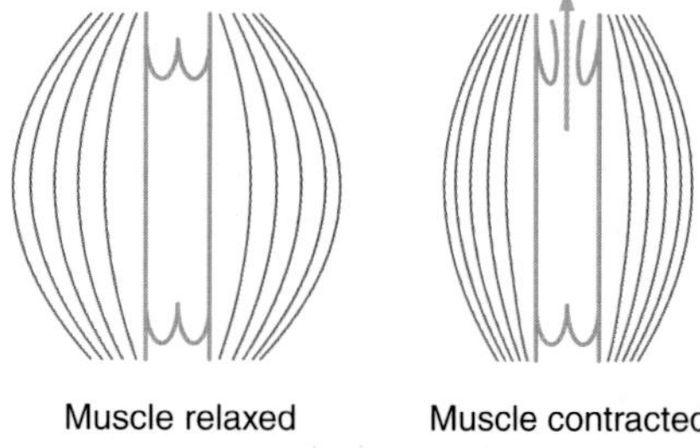

Fig. 16.4 Diagram to show a muscle venous pump such as that present in the calf.

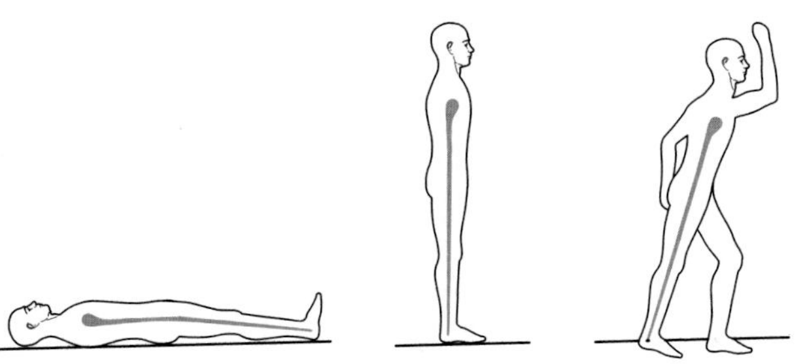

Fig. 16.5 Effect of exercise on the superficial venous pressure in health and disease.

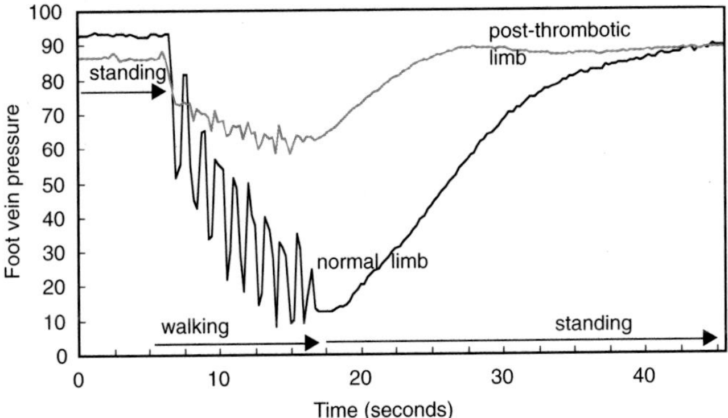

Fig. 16.6 Physiology of the calf muscle pump – pressure traces.

the superficial veins of the foot and ankle falls from a resting level of 80–100 mmHg to about 20 mmHg (Fig. 16.6).

This ability to reduce the pressure in the superficial venous system is crucial to the health of the lower limb. Patients with damage to the veins in whom the superficial venous pressure does not fall during exercise may develop varicose eczema, skin damage and, eventually, leg ulceration.

Venous incompetence – varicose veins

One of the most common problems with the veins of the leg is failure of their valves. This occurs frequently in the superficial venous system resulting in varicose veins, which affect 10–20 per cent of the adult population in Westernised countries. In developing countries, where a primitive way of life is maintained, there is a very low incidence of varicose veins. The reasons for this difference are unclear but are probably related to differences in diet. A further major factor is inheritance: women in whom neither parent has varicose veins have a 10 per cent risk of developing varices, but when both parents are affected there is an 80 per cent chance. Men are affected less frequently than women.

The mechanisms that cause the superficial vein valves to fail have not been fully established. What appears to happen is that first a small gap appears between the valve cusps at the commisure (where the valve leaflets join the vein wall). This gap widens and more reverse flow (venous reflux) is allowed. The valve cusps degenerate and holes develop in them. Eventually they disappear completely (Fig. 16.7). The vein below the valve responds by dilating. Varicose veins may eventually reach five times their usual size if left to develop for long enough.

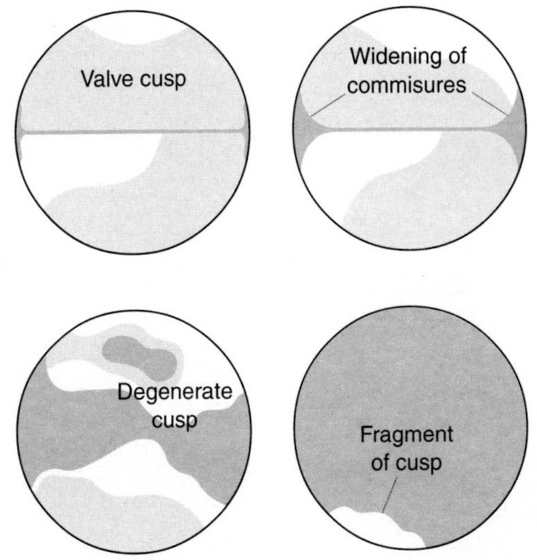

Fig. 16.7 Stages of development of venous valvular incompetence.

In the past it was thought that varicose veins were caused by anatomical abnormalities in the deep vein valves. It is now clear that this is not true. Varicose veins often develop in the calf when the veins above are normal. This seems to be a process where congenital and environmental factors accumulate to cause valve failure.

Varicose veins are thought to develop more often in people who stand during their work. People who sit or walk are at less risk of developing varices. They often develop during pregnancy under the influence of oestrogen and progesterone which cause the smooth muscle in the vein wall to relax.

Clinical features

Varicose veins are very common; they may either give no symptoms or cause aching and discomfort in the legs. Varices are recognised as tortuous dilated veins in the leg, but physiologically speaking *a varicose vein is one which permits reverse flow through its faulty valves.* Varices of the major tributaries of the saphenous veins or the saphenous veins themselves are large (5–15 mm diameter) and usually start in the calf (Fig. 16.8). Later varices of the long saphenous system may also appear in the thigh. Patients may develop much smaller varices. These range from 0.5-mm diameter vessels in the skin, which are commonly referred to as *thread veins* or dermal flares, and are usually purple or red in colour. Slightly larger veins (1–3 mm diameter) lying immediately beneath the skin may also present as small varicosities. These are usually referred to as *reticular varices.* The association of thread veins and reticular varices is frequently seen, and these probably reflect a type of varicose veins which is confined to the smallest size of vein. These tiny veins are associated with superficial venous incompetence in about 30 per cent of

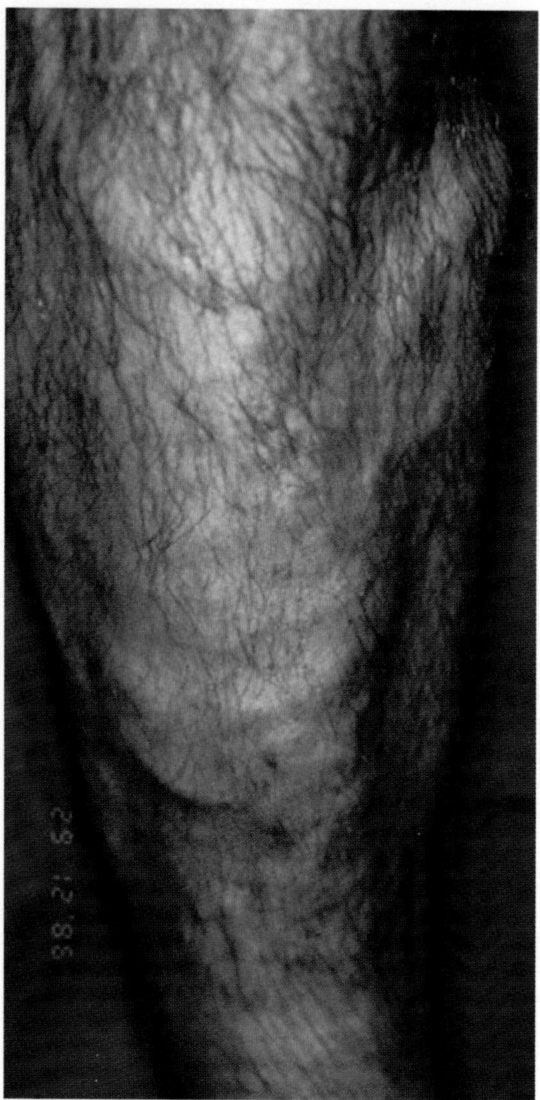

Fig. 16.8 Varicose veins.

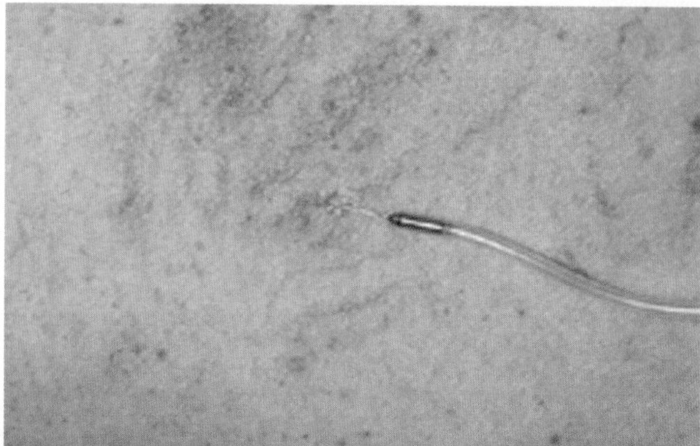

Fig. 16.9 Dermal flares, commonly called 'thread veins'.

cases. They require different treatment from large varices (Fig. 16.9). The combination of small varicosities and much larger truncal and tributary varices is often seen, but each type may occur on its own. The symptoms reported by patients affected by either type of varices are very numerous. Often there are no specific symptoms but the cosmetic appearance is unsatisfactory. Patients may also report aching especially on standing, itching, 'restless legs' and ankle swelling. The severity of the symptoms is unrelated to the size of the veins, and is often more severe during the early stages of development of varices.

Complications of varicose veins

Occasionally complications of varicose veins may develop. These include *thrombosis*, which is referred to as superficial thrombophlebitis. Usually this remains in the superficial veins and may cause considerable discomfort. Sometimes thrombosis extends into the deep venous system to cause deep vein thrombosis, although this is infrequent. Spectacular *haemorrhage* can occur when large superficial varices are damaged. This is easily controlled by lying the patient down, elevating the leg and applying a compression bandage. The most serious problem is venous *ulceration* which complicates varicose veins in less than 5 per cent of patients. However, it is a troublesome and painful condition which requires careful management if the ulcer is to heal.

Venous incompetence – deep vein incompetence

Valvular incompetence of the deep veins may develop in the same way as in the superficial venous system, with the degeneration of the valve cusps resulting in reverse flow in these veins. In other patients it may develop following a deep vein thrombosis. When the deep veins fill with thrombus a new channel appears (recanalisation) after a number of weeks or months. However, the deep vein valves are destroyed by this process and, although the veins carry blood, the valves no longer work and reverse flow is allowed. Some veins are severely scarred by the recanalisation process so that they also become very narrow and ineffective at carrying blood. Occasionally veins fail to recanalise at all. This is sometimes seen following a venous thrombosis in the iliac veins. Under these conditions the blood must find an alternative way round the blockage and collateral veins develop. In the leg the long and short saphenous veins may act as collateral channels and may double in size to accommodate the additional blood flow. In patients with chronic iliac vein occlusion large suprapubic or abdominal varices may be seen carrying the collateral flow.

Clinical features of deep vein incompetence

A number of patients with severe deep vein damage has little to show for their problems. In patients with venous valvular incompetence the calf muscle increases in size, apparently in response to the greater work in returning blood from the leg. There may be some *ankle oedema*, especially in those patients who have persistent venous obstruction. A proportion of patients develops skin complications. These may range from mild eczema to severe ulceration. An early sign of skin injury is *brown pigmentation* due to haemosiderin deposition in the skin. This occurs because the high venous pressures which result from damage to the muscle pumping mechanism cause red blood cells to be forced out of capillaries in the skin where their haemoglobin breaks down to form haemosiderin. A later and more serious stage is *lipodermatosclerosis* in which palpable induration develops in the skin and subcutaneous tissues. This particularly affects the gaiter area of the leg, just above the malleoli, and may be the precursor of leg ulceration. Contraction of the skin and subcutaneous tissues is seen and the ankle becomes narrower. The combination of a narrow ankle and prominent calf is often referred to as a 'champagne bottle leg' (Fig. 16.10). *Atrophie blanche* may also develop. In this condition the superficial blood vessels are lost from the skin and white patches develop. These indicate that the skin has been severely damaged by the venous valvular incompetence. Venous ulceration may develop in these areas.

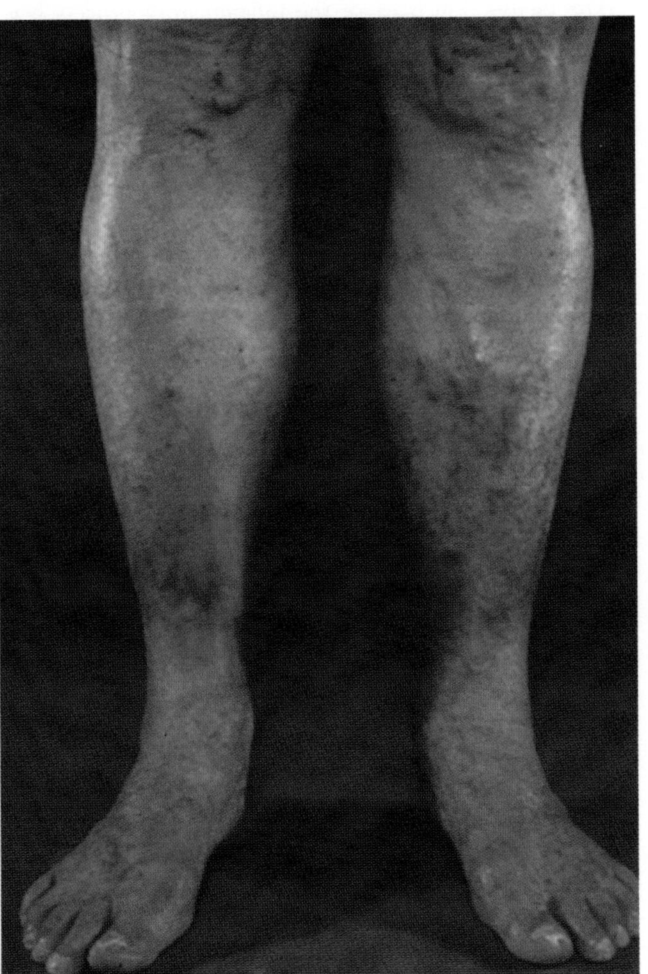

Fig. 16.10 Lipodermatosclerosis (scaring) and haemosiderosis (brown pigmentation of the skin) in a patient with venous disease.

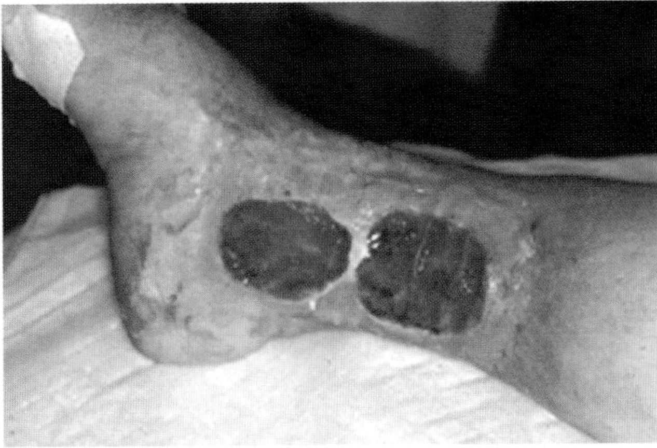

Fig. 16.11 Venous ulceration.

Patients may remain untroubled by many of these symptoms and may not seek medical advice until venous ulceration develops. Even then, it is thought that less than half of the patients with venous leg ulcers are known to their general practitioners (Fig. 16.11).

Effects of deep and superficial venous incompetence on the vascular physiology of the leg

When the venous valves fail, the ability of the muscle pumps to reduce the pressure in the leg is decreased. Following muscle contraction blood may return to the leg rapidly by flowing in the reverse direction along deep or superficial veins. Incompetence of the deep veins usually has a more severe effect on the venous physiology than does superficial venous incompetence as the deep veins are much larger than the superficial veins. The effect of reverse flow in the deep or superficial veins is to prevent the superficial venous pressure from falling during exercise. This is referred to as 'ambulatory venous hypertension' and is the main cause of venous leg ulceration. Persistently raised venous pressure tracks back to the microcirculation of the skin and causes skin damage that eventually may result in venous ulceration.

In some patients veins remain permanently blocked following a deep vein thrombosis leading to the blood experiencing difficulty leaving the leg. This usually causes worse symptoms than venous valvular incompetence alone. Swelling of the leg, especially ankle oedema, is often a feature in patients with persistent venous obstruction. In many cases the passage of time allows deep veins to recanalise and the ankle oedema may then become less severe. However, the recanalised veins are likely to be incompetent and the features of venous hypertension may then predominate.

How does ambulatory venous hypertension cause leg ulceration?

The damage caused by venous hypertension in patients with venous disease is confined to the skin and subcutaneous tissues. The main focus of the damage is in the capillaries in the skin. These increase in size and length, and become very convoluted and are described as 'glomerulus like' (Fig. 16.12). The amount of capillary endothelium is increased in the skin and many more capillary loops are cut on histological sections of damaged skin. This results in the development of a fibrotic process affecting the skin and subcutaneous fat which comprise the condition of lipodermatosclerosis. Around the capillaries are many inflammatory cells, especially macrophages. The combination of capillary proliferation and inflammation accounts for the appearance of liposclerotic skin, which looks inflamed. A perivascular cuff is present around the capillaries, which is made up of many connective tissue proteins including fibrin, collagen IV and fibronectin. This perivascular cuff is probably the result of chronic inflammation and occurs in many other types of inflammatory processes. It was originally thought that the fibrin cuff acted as a barrier to diffusion preventing nutrient exchange between the capillaries and the tissues. The *'fibrin cuff' hypothesis* was accepted for many years as the explanation for venous ulceration. Research and theoretical calculations have shown that there is no physical barrier to the diffusion of nutrients to the tissues in this condition.

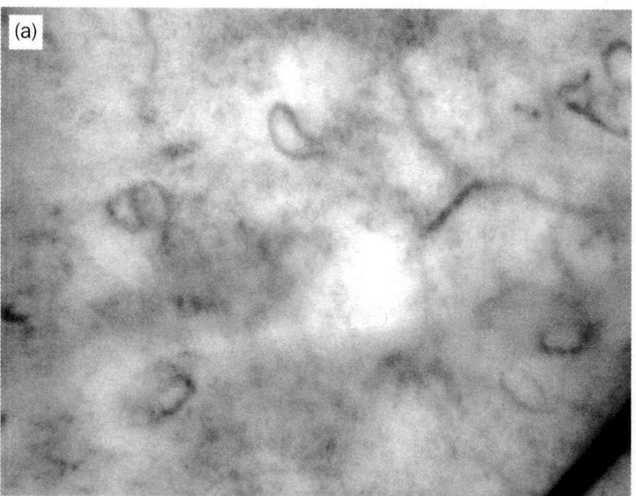

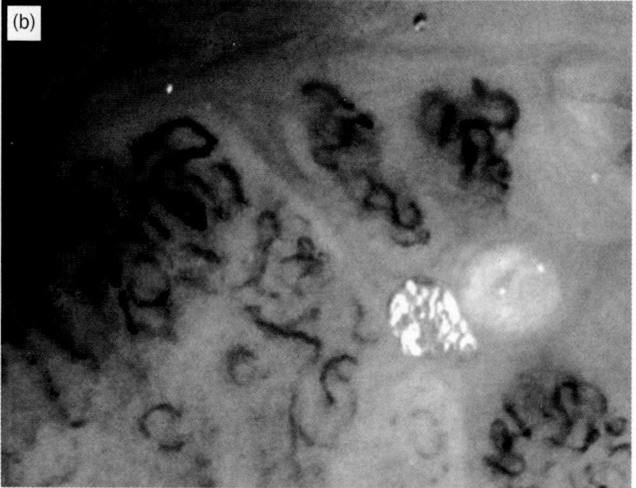

Fig. 16.12 The skin capillaries in health and disease – the appearance of the skin capillaries in patients with lipodermatosclerosis is sometimes said to be 'glomerulus like'.

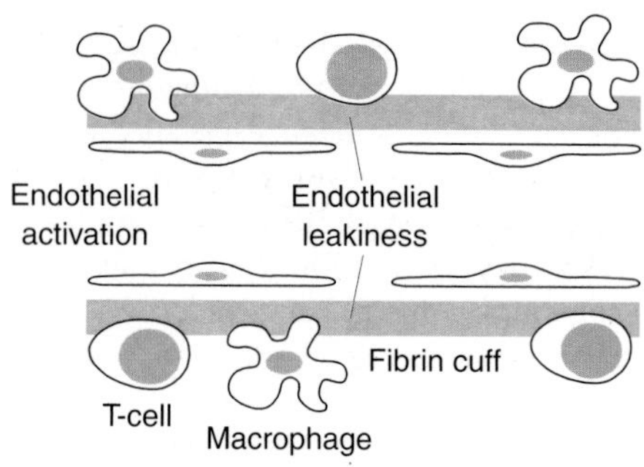

Fig. 16.13 Diagram of a diseased capillary from the skin of a patient with chronic venous disease showing the fibrin cuff and possible mechanisms of leucocyte injury.

The factors which cause the inflammatory process have been sought. It has been shown that venous hypertension causes leucocyte sequestration in the microcirculation of the leg. Patients with chronic venous disease resulting in lipodermatosclerosis and venous ulceration trap more leucocytes than do subjects with normal limbs. It has been shown that these 'trapped' leucocytes become activated and release the proteolytic enzymes that are normally used in defence against infection. This, in turn, causes injury to the capillary endothelium. It seems likely that inappropriate activation of leucocytes instigates the series of events that results in leg ulceration. The frill mechanism is incompletely understood and further investigation of the processes involved may eventually lead to the development of better treatments for venous ulceration. This mechanism is referred to as the *'white cell trapping hypothesis'* and was first proposed in 1988 (Fig. 16.13).

Investigation of venous disease

A full history should always be taken, enquiring about any injury to the leg or swelling which may suggest a previous episode of deep vein thrombosis. Patients report a wide range of symptoms associated with venous disease. These include *tiredness, aching, tingling* and *ankle swelling* which get progressively worse towards the end of the day and are relieved by elevating the leg. Sometimes patients report cramps in the legs, which are usually worse at night. Patients with more severe venous disease may notice the skin changes that occur. Pain in the calf on walking is usually attributable to lower limb arterial disease, referred to as intermittent claudication. Patients with severe deep vein obstruction may also develop bursting pain in the calf on walking, due to the very high venous pressures that may occur under these conditions.

A clinical examination carried out with the patient standing will reveal the extent of any varicose veins and whether they are associated with the long or short saphenous systems. Further information may be gained by using a tourniquet test (Brodie, 1846; Trendelenburg, 1890) to determine the source of varices. The tourniquet is often replaced by the hand of the examiner used to compress the long or short saphenous vein. The patient lies and the leg is elevated to empty the veins. The tourniquet is applied high on the thigh and the patient stands again. The speed at which the varices fill is observed. In the case of varices from the long saphenous vein these fill within a few seconds without a tourniquet, but with the trunk of the long saphenous vein compressed in the thigh much slower filling takes place over 15 or 20 seconds. If filling is not controlled by an above-knee tourniquet, then a tourniquet is applied to compress the short saphenous vein, just below the knee. If the varices now fill slowly then the source of venous reflux is from the SPJ. If the varices continue to fill rapidly some further source must be the cause. The patient may have incompetent deep veins or a calf perforating vein. The success of tourniquet tests lies in the ability of the examiner to assess the varices and their rate of filling. This may be easy in the case of large varices, but can be vary difficult with smaller varices. Considerable practice is required for successful application of these tests (Fig. 16.14).

The clinical examination should continue by noting the presence and extent of any skin changes or ulceration at the ankle. An examination of the peripheral pulses should be carried out. Venous and arterial disease of the lower limb often coexist, especially in more elderly patients. An abdominal examination completes the clinical examination in patients presenting with lower limb varices, as these may occasionally be the result of an abdominal neoplasm causing venous obstruction.

More detailed information than can be obtained from clinical examination is useful in the management of patients with primary varicose veins and essential in the management of patients with recurrent varices, a history of lower limb venous thrombosis or venous leg ulcers.

Doppler ultrasound

A Doppler assessment is now the minimum level of investigation required before treating somebody with venous disease. A Doppler flow probe can be used to exclude arterial disease and to determine the patency of a vein, and a bidirectional flow probe used to detect venous reflux. This investigation is carried out with the patient standing. The Doppler probe is first placed over the SPJ and the blood flow assessed to locate the venous flow in the common femoral vein. With one hand the examiner gently squeezes the calf to produce an acceleration of blood flow in the veins. This is heard as a 'whoosh' from the loudspeaker of the Doppler machine. The calf compression is released and any reverse flow in the veins sought. With practice it is possible reliably to identify venous reflux in the SFJ. The examination may be repeated with the probe held over the long saphenous vein in the mid-thigh region, to confirm that the venous reflux lies in the superficial vessels. Some surgeons use a tourniquet to occlude the superficial veins, in the same way as when performing a Trendelenburg test. The probe may also be held over the SPJ while the calf is compressed and released to test the competence of veins in this region. In the popliteal fossa it is more difficult to distinguish between deep and superficial venous incompetence (Fig. 16.15).

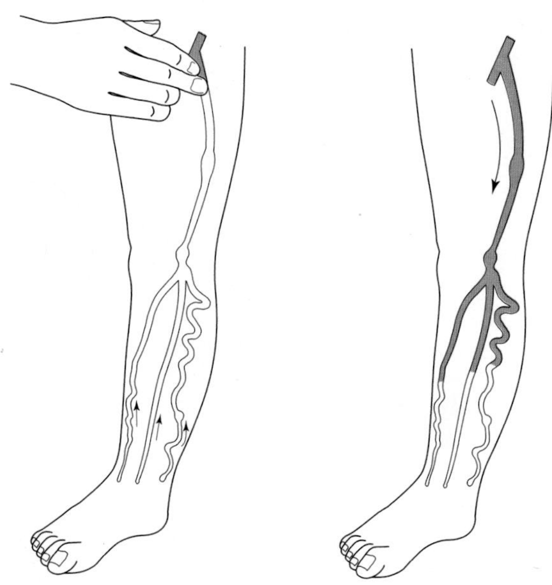

Fig. 16.14 Tourniquet tests used in the diagnosis of superficial venous incompetence.

This method is very useful when examining patients with primary varicose veins, especially those which are thought to result from SFJ incompetence. The popliteal fossa contains many veins and if venous reflux is heard it is difficult to be certain from which veins it arises. However, in patients with primary varices saphenopopliteal incompetence is usually readily identified. All surgeons who regularly treat patients with varicose veins should be competent at this type of investigation. Where the source of recurrent varices or a leg ulcer is sought, duplex ultrasonography is usually more reliable.

Photoplethysmography and other plethysmographic techniques

In this investigation a probe is attached to the skin to assess venous filling of the surface venules by measuring light transmission of the skin. The filling of these vessels reflects the pressure in the superficial veins of the leg. The patient sits

Sir Benjamin Collins Brodie, 1783–1862. Surgeon, St George's Hospital, London, England.

Fredrich Trendelenburg, 1844–1924. Professor of Surgery, Rostock 1875–82; Bonn 1882–95 and Leipzig 1895–1911.

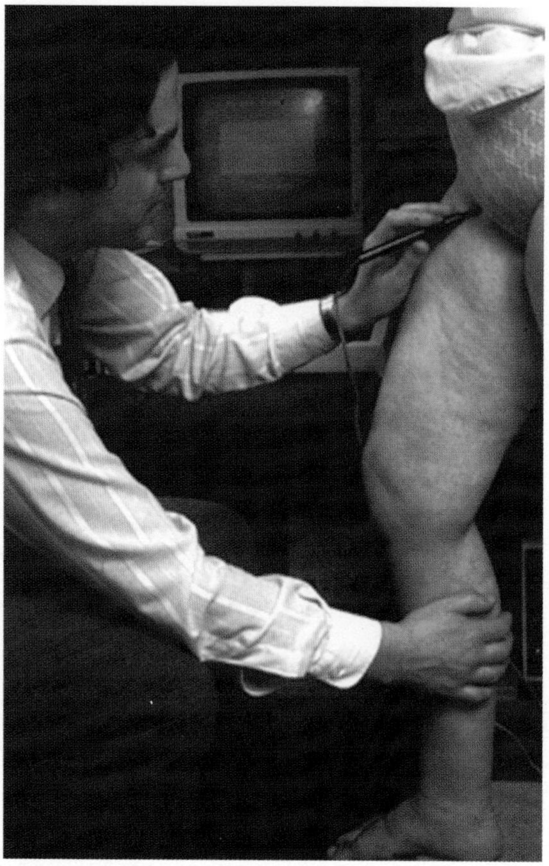

Fig. 16.15 Doppler ultrasound examination of the venous system of the lower limbs.

quietly until the trace stabilises. Then he or she performs a series of 10 dorsiflexions at the ankle. The venous pressure falls in the superficial veins of the leg and the skin venules empty, so the photoplethysmography (PPG) trace falls. The patient then sits and the veins refill. Under normal conditions venous refilling occurs through arterial inflow alone, a slow process taking 20 or 30 seconds when the limb is at rest. In patients with venous incompetence the veins also fill via venous reflux, which speeds the refilling process. Fast refilling times mean that one or more veins in the leg are incompetent. The test can be repeated after the application of a tourniquet above the knee to occlude the long saphenous vein, and then below the knee to occlude both the long and short saphenous veins. This helps to establish which set of superficial veins is incompetent (Fig. 16.16).

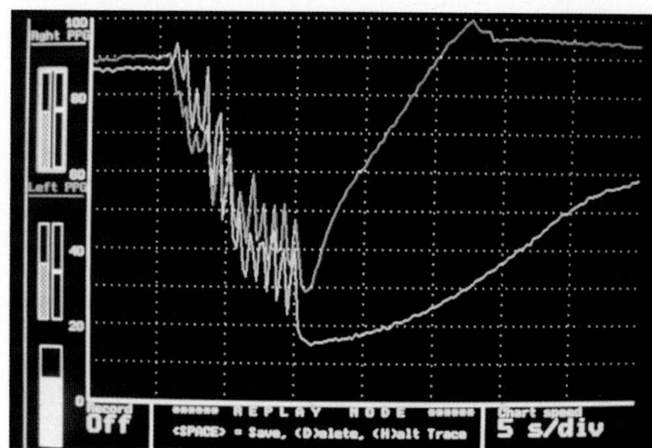

Fig. 16.16 Photoplethysmography traces demonstrating normal refilling. Lower trace: abnormal refilling in a patient with superficial venous insufficiency.

A number of other plethysmographic tests is used to evaluate the venous system physiology including the air plethysmograph, light reflex rheography and strain gauge plethysmograph. These are usually used by vascular surgeons in vascular laboratories or by specialists in venous diseases. All are used to quantify the impairment of venous function caused by obstructed or incompetent venous valves.

Duplex ultrasound imaging

This technique involves the use of high-resolution B-mode ultrasound imaging and Doppler ultrasound to obtain images of veins and simultaneously measure flow in these vessels. It allows direct visualisation of the veins and provides functional, as well as anatomical, information. Modern duplex ultrasound machines represent blood flow as a colour map which is superimposed on the greyscale image of the vessel. This technique is highly reliable in the investigation of arteries and veins, and is the most appropriate investigation to use when detailed analysis of the anatomy and physiology of the venous system is required.

The examination is performed with the patient standing. In this position the veins are filled and easily seen on the ultrasound image. The flow in the veins is assessed in exactly the same way as when using a hand-held Doppler probe. The examiner images the vein that he or she wishes to study and compresses the calf with his/her hand to produce forward flow. This results in upward flow towards the heart in a normal vein, and is shown as blue in the colour flow map. The calf is then released to test the competence of the valves. Competent veins show no flow, but incompetent veins allow reverse flow which is represented as red in the colour flow map. All lower limb veins may be imaged with ease using modern ultrasound machines, and therefore the patency and competence of all lower limb veins may be tested. The examiner steadily works his/her way from the groin to the ankle testing each major deep and superficial vein along the limb. This allows a comprehensive map of the

Christian Johann Doppler, 1803–53. Austrian physicist.

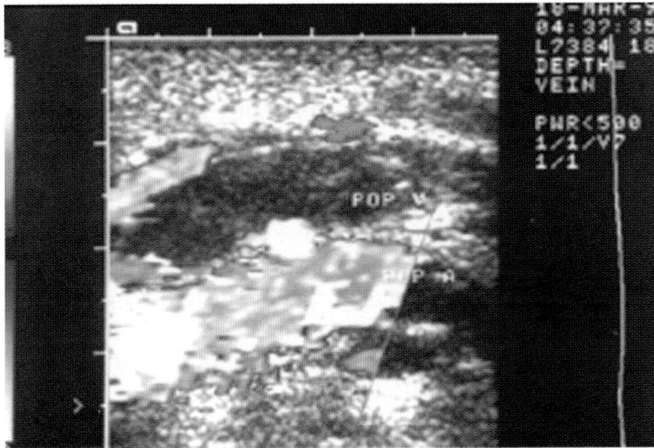

Fig. 16.17 Deep vein thrombosis in the popliteal vein. Blood attempting to flow round the thrombus, seen here as a filling defect.

veins to the leg to be constructed. Blocked or incompetent veins can be readily identified by a skilled vascular technologist. The origin of varicose veins and venous ulceration can be identified, and in patients with suspected deep vein thrombosis the presence of thrombus can be seen (Figs 16.17–16.19).

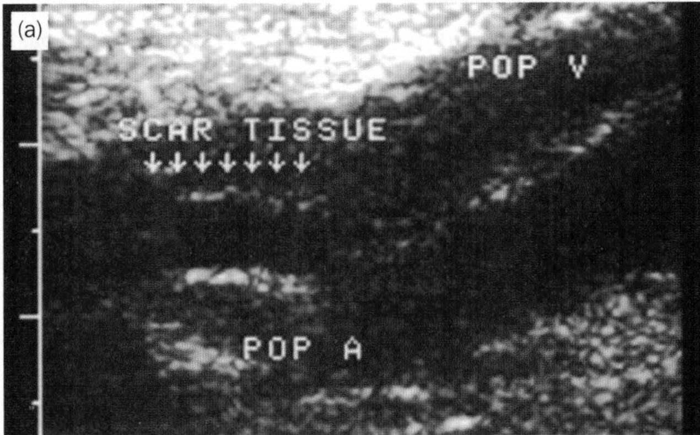

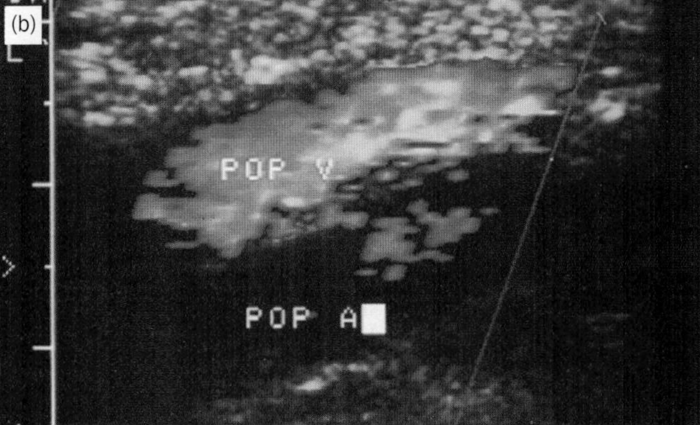

Fig. 16.18 Flow through the popliteal vein. Forward flow is demonstrated on the left. On release of the calf compression reverse flow is seen on the right indicating venous reflux.

Venography

This investigation is the X-ray equivalent of duplex ultrasonography. Historically it preceded ultrasonography and has been widely used in the past for the assessment of patients with vein problems. An ascending venogram is performed by canulating a vein in the foot in order to inject X-ray contrast medium. A narrow tourniquet is applied just above the malleoli to direct blood flow into the deep veins and an injection of nonionic contrast material given to outline the veins. The technique provides excellent anatomical information but gives much less information about the veins where the valves have failed. It is a useful examination for suspected deep vein thrombosis where ultrasonography is not available.

Incompetent veins can be shown by descending venography. Here a cannula is inserted in the femoral vein and contrast material injected with the patient standing. The contrast material is heavier than blood and flows down the limb though incompetent valves. Both ascending and descending phlebography is required to establish as much information as is provided by duplex ultrasonography.

The source of recurrent varicose veins may be identified by a varicogram. Contrast material is injected into one of the varicosities and followed to identify its source. Again, duplex ultrasonography has largely replaced this investigation (Fig. 16.20).

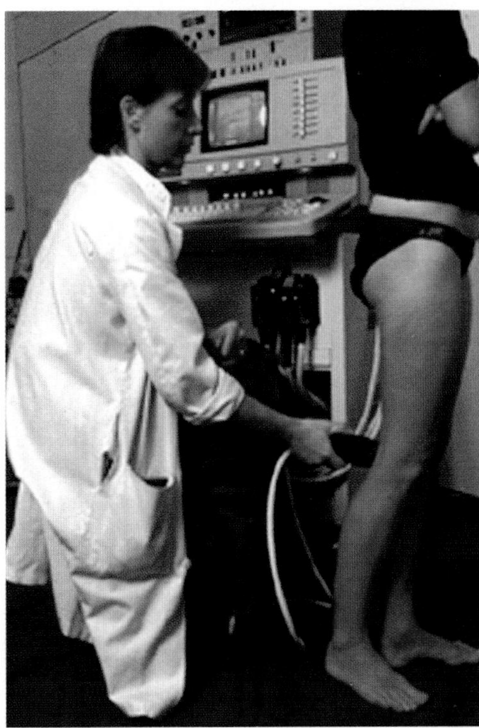

Fig. 16.19 Duplex imaging. A patient with varicose veins being assessed by Duplex ultrasound machine.

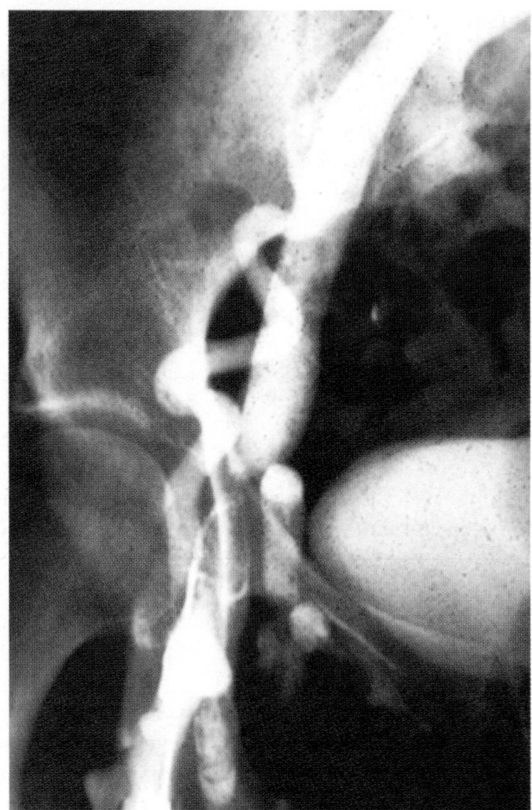

Fig. 16.20 Example of a venogram.

Management of patients with varicose veins

A history should be taken from the patient to find out how long the varices have been present and if any event seemed to cause them. A history of previous lower limb deep vein thrombosis should be sought. Venous thrombosis may follow lower limb fractures, so this also should be asked about. Superficial varices which develop after a venous thrombosis may be the only route of venous drainage in the lower limb and should not be removed until the patency of the deep veins of the limb has been shown. Patients may also have received previous surgical or other treatment for their varices. Any previous treatment may greatly alter the surgical management of the patient. When the SFJ has been ligated previously, a further operation here is technically much more demanding for the surgeon and should not be performed unless recurrence at the previous operation site has been conclusively demonstrated. Unfortunately, patients often have only a vague recollection of their previous vein operations and therefore diagnostic ultrasound imaging or venography is essential to establish the anatomy and source of varices in patients with recurrent varicose veins.

Clinical examination should establish the extent and size of varices, as well as the presence of any associated skin changes. Tourniquet tests should be used to decide the location of venous incompetence. All patients considered for surgical treatment of their varices should be examined using a hand-held Doppler ultrasound device to confirm the source of the varices.

Patients with recurrent varices or a history suggestive of previous venous thrombosis and any patient with skin changes should be fully investigated using duplex ultrasonography or venography. The presence of ankle pulses should be confirmed by palpation or, if necessary, by measuring the ankle blood pressure using Doppler ultrasound.

The treatment of varicose veins following a proper assessment may include reassurance, the use of elastic compression stockings, injection sclerotherapy or surgical treatment. The treatment of choice depends on the size of the varices, their extent and the symptoms that they produce.

Compression stockings

The symptoms of varicose veins may be relieved by the use of compression stockings. These are available for the treatment of venous disease in three grades of compression, classes 1–3. Light compression stockings may be helpful in the early stages of varicose veins but do not prevent the development of more varices or result in the disappearance of veins.

Injection sclerotherapy

This treatment is best used in the management of small varices and those where the main long and short saphenous veins, and their major tributaries, are competent. This type of treatment is also effective where the larger varices have been removed surgically and only small varices remain. In the past, sclerotherapy has been used in the management of incompetence of the main saphenous trunks. Evidence suggests that varicose veins managed in this way recur much more rapidly than following surgical treatment.

The basis of sclerotherapy is that a solution which destroys the endothelial lining of the veins is injected. In the UK the most widely employed drug is sodium tetradecyl (STD), which chemically is a soap. To be effective, the sclerosant has to be given into an empty vein that is compressed immediately after the injection has been given to avoid the development of thrombosis within the vein. It is easy to produce thrombophlebitis which can recanalise and result in the recurrence of the varices. The aim is to produce sclerosis with the vein being replaced by a fibrous cord, incapable of recanalisation and recurrence (Fig. 16.21).

Technique

The limb is examined with the patient standing and the position of the varices that should be injected marked on the skin. The needle is inserted into the vein with the patient sitting down and the leg in a horizontal position. A 23G or 25G needle is usually used for this. The position of the needle in the vein is confirmed by drawing back on the syringe. Injection of the sclerosant outside the vein causes tissue necrosis and ulceration, and must be avoided. The leg is elevated to empty the veins and a small volume of sclerosant (0.5 ml) is injected into the vein. Compression is

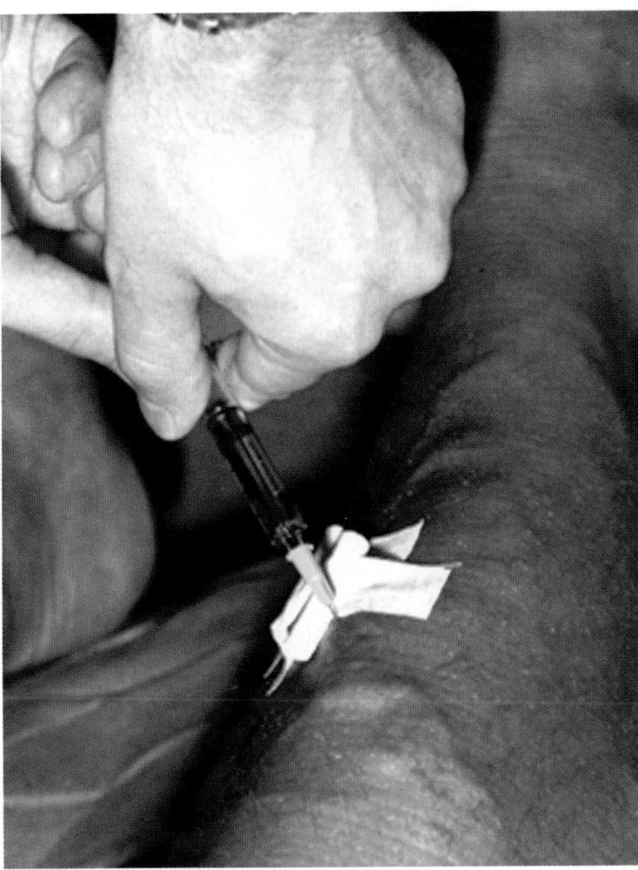

Fig. 16.21 Sclerotherapy for varicose veins.

immediately applied to the vein being treated with the fingers and a firm bandage applied. Treatment is usually commenced at the ankle so that the bandage can be applied progressively from the ankle to the groin as treatment progresses along the limb. A latex foam pad is put over the sites of the injection and incorporated within the bandage. Skin sensitivity to rubber may lead to allergic reactions if the latex pads come into direct contact with the skin. Immediately after the bandage has been completed, the patient is asked to walk to encourage the blood to circulate reducing the risk of venous thrombosis in the limb and also reducing the venous pressure in the varices of the calf.

Further sessions of sclerotherapy continue at weekly intervals until all lower limb varices have been treated. The patient should wear a compression bandage or stocking for 3–6 weeks after the completion of a course of sclerotherapy This ensures that the veins which have been treated do not suffer thrombosis and are converted into a fibrous cord, achieving sclerosis of the vein.

Complications

The complications of this treatment include skin pigmentation and ulceration if the sclerosant is not injected within a vein. Small regions of thrombophlebitis are often seen during a course of sclerotherapy. Deep vein thrombosis develops only rarely.

Microsclerotherapy

Thread veins and reticular varices may be treated by injection through a very fine needle, a treatment referred to as 'microsclerotherapy'. Very dilute sclerosing solutions are used. The most frequently employed drugs used for this are STD and polidocanol. A skilled practitioner can insert a 30G needle into dermal flares and successfully eradicate these tiny veins. Compression bandaging is usually applied after this treatment for 1–5 days. Treatment of these veins is normally regarded as a cosmetic procedure.

Surgical treatment of varicose veins

Surgical treatment of varicose veins is widely used and is effective in removing varicose veins of the main saphenous trunks, as well as their tributaries, down to a size of about 3 mm. Veins smaller than this are best treated by sclerotherapy. Surgical removal of varices is inappropriate where these form a major part of the venous drainage of the limb, for example where a deep vein thrombosis has destroyed the main axial limb veins and the patient relies on the superficial veins. This possibility may be suggested by the patient's medical history and can be confirmed by duplex ultrasonography or venography.

The main principles of surgical treatment are to ligate the source of the venous reflux (usually the SFJ or the SPJ) and to remove the incompetent saphenous trunks and the associated varices. Sapheno-femoral ligation alone, sometimes referred to as a 'Trendelenburg procedure', is associated with a high rate of recurrence of varices. Recent research has shown that it is necessary to remove the long saphenous vein to ensure that as much venous reflux as possible is eliminated. Similarly, communications between the many deep veins in the popliteal fossa and the short saphenous vein mean that some patients develop recurrences in the short saphenous vein due to the re-establishment of reflux from these veins. This problem may be eliminated by removing the short saphenous vein. Removal of the saphenous veins has the disadvantage that both veins are accompanied by a nerve that may be damaged in the vein stripping operation. To avoid nerve injury the long saphenous vein should not be removed below mid-calf level and great care should be exercised in removing the short saphenous vein.

Venous anatomy is particularly variable, and for some veins preoperative vein localisation is very helpful. The termination of the short saphenous vein may lie from 2 cm below the knee to 15 cm above the knee. Its course and termination can be readily identified by ultrasound imaging and marked on the skin with an indelible pen before the operation, reducing the risk of damage to nerves and arteries in the popliteal fossa. Perforating veins in the calf and thigh, and residual segments of the saphenous veins left after previous venous surgery, can also be localised in this way (Fig. 16.22).

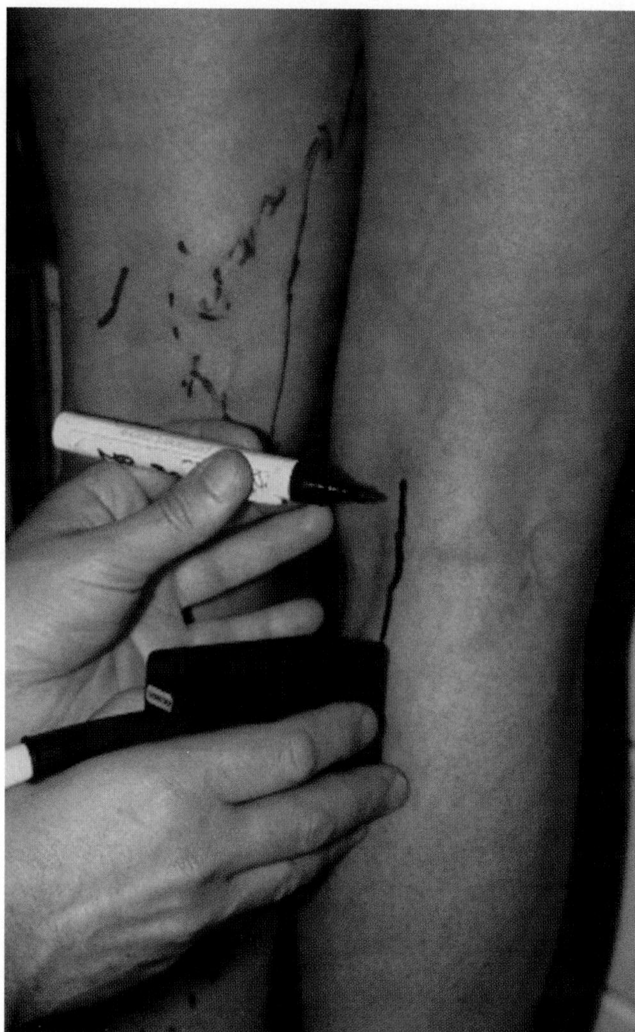

Fig. 16.22 Preoperative ultrasound localisation of the saphenopopliteal junction.

Technique of saphenofemoral junction ligation

An oblique incision is made in the groin commencing over the femoral artery and extending 4 cm medially. The long saphenous vein is exposed and the common femoral and superficial femoral veins are identified before dividing the long saphenous vein. Having divided the long saphenous vein, all branches should then be isolated and divided. The SFJ should be tied flush with the femoral vein. Any tributary of the saphenous vein or femoral vein left in this operation may be the source of a future recurrence, so it is important that all are ligated and divided. It is important that the femoral vein is inspected carefully for at least 1 cm above and below the SFJ, and any tributaries ligated and divided.

The conventional way of removing the saphenous vein is with a Babcock stripper. This consists of a flexible wire which is passed down the long saphenous vein. The end is identified in the upper third of the calf and a 2-mm incision is made to retrieve the stripper. An olive about 8 mm in diameter is attached to the upper end and the saphenous vein is removed by firm traction on the wire in the calf.

More recently 'inverting' or 'invaginating' stripping has become popular. The aim here is to reduce the damage to the tissues around the vein leading to less bleeding and post-operative pain. This may be done in a number of different ways. A rigid metal 'pin-stripper' has recently been developed (Fig. 16.23). This is passed down the inside of the saphenous vein and recovered through a small incision in the upper part of the calf. A strong suture is attached to the end of the stripper and firmly ligated to the proximal end of the vein (Fig. 16.24). Pulling gently on the stripper, the long saphenous vein will invert and can be delivered through a 2-mm incision in the mid-calf region (Fig. 16.25). No olive is used and the technique relies on the strength of the vein. Should the vein break, an instrument with a small olive on one end is used to recover the remaining saphenous vein.

Technique of saphenopopliteal junction ligation

Accurate preoperative ultrasound localisation of this junction makes the operation easy, as the position of the SPJ is

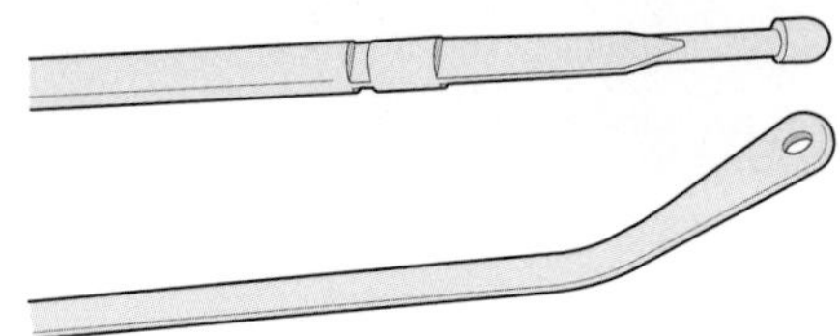

Fig. 16.23 Oesch pin-stripper. A small notch at the back (above) indicates the direction of the small tip (below).

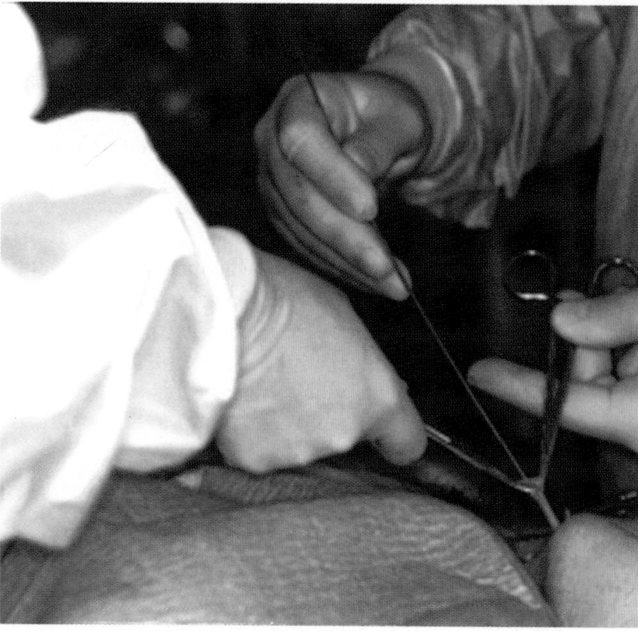

Fig. 16.24 The vein does not directly attach to the end of stripper and this allows the vein to be inverted.

William Wayne Babcock, 1872–1963. American surgeon.

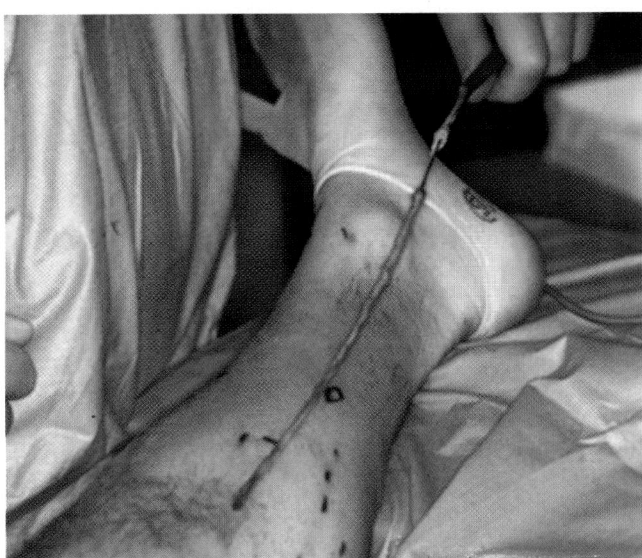

Fig. 16.25 This figure illustrates recovery of the metal stripper through a small 1.5-mm incision.

notoriously variable. A skin incision is made over the junction and the deep fascia incised to reveal the short saphenous vein beneath. The vein is followed to the SPJ, where the short saphenous vein enters the side of the popliteal vein. The vein can then be ligated and divided close to the popliteal vein. This operation may not be enough to eliminate venous reflux in the short saphenous vein because communication with the gastrocnemius (muscle) veins in the calf is often present and may lead to further varicosities arising from the short saphenous vein. Many surgeons now routinely strip the short saphenous vein to prevent this problem. This is best done using an inverting technique as the sural nerve lies close to the vein and may be damaged if a large olive is used.

A pin-stripper (Oesch) is passed down the short saphenous vein as described above for the long saphenous vein. This is recovered through a 2-mm incision made at the mid-calf level. A heavy suture is used to attach the vein to the upper end of the stripper and gentle traction applied to the stripper. The inverted vein appears in the calf incision.

Removing superficial varices

Varicose veins do not disappear following saphenous vein stripping and should be removed through small incisions. It was standard practice to insert artery forceps through the incision in order to remove varices. However, this necessitates long incisions in the leg which require suturing and are unsightly. European phlebologists have developed instruments to minimise the size of incision required for this procedure. The technique is referred to as 'hook phlebectomy' and uses small hooks which may be inserted through incisions of only 1–2 mm (Fig. 16.26). The hook is used to capture a small section of a varicosity and bring it to the surface where is may be grasped using a large artery forceps; the remaining vein is then teased through the tiny incision. The aim is to remove all the varicosities through incisions that require no suture. Closure of the incisions is achieved using adhesive strips or dressings. The cosmetic outcome from this procedure is excellent.

The results of varicose vein surgery depend on the care taken with the preoperative assessment, the preoperative marking and the determination of the surgeon to remove all the superficial varicosities. Patients may complain of symptoms of varicose veins, but most remain unsatisfied until they achieve a good cosmetic result following treatment!

Postoperative management

Compression bandaging is applied to the limb at the end of the operation to prevent excessive bruising. In fact, some surgeons apply compression to the limb before stripping the long saphenous vein. After 1 or 2 days the bandages may be replaced by a thigh-length high compression stocking (class 2 compression is appropriate). This can usually be removed easily to allow the patient to take a shower and can then be reapplied.

Complications of varicose vein surgery

Bruising and discomfort are common following removal of varices, especially where the veins were of very large diameter. However, the pain usually requires only mild analgesics.

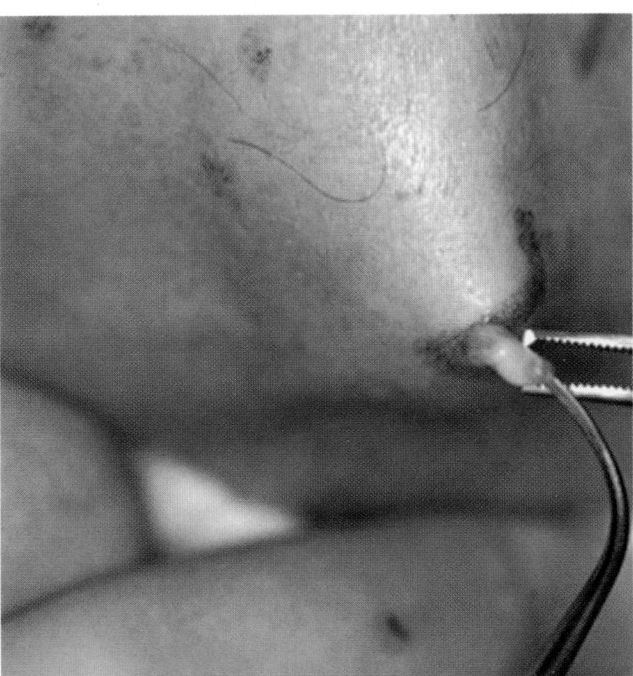

Fig. 16.26 Hook phlebectomy – varicose veins may be removed through very small incisions in the leg.

Sensory nerve injury is seen occasionally after removal of varicose veins. The saphenous nerve and its branches accompany the long saphenous vein in the calf, the sural nerve accompanies the short saphenous vein. Damage to the main part of these nerves occurs in about 1 per cent of operations, but small areas of anaesthesia may occur more frequently (in up to 10 per cent of patients). The adoption of inverting stripping techniques and avoidance of stripping the long saphenous vein below mid-calf level have reduced the risk of damage to these nerves. All patients should be warned before surgery that they may experience small areas of numbness and tingling after the operation. These changes are usually reversible but can be quite persistent.

Motor nerve injury is an uncommon complication of varicose vein surgery and may occur during exploration of the popliteal fossa if care is not taken to protect the nerves in this region. Preoperative ultrasound localisation of the short saphenous vein helps in limiting the extent of the dissection in this region and risk to the nerves during dissection. Venous thrombosis is often seen in residual varices following varicose vein surgery and resolves without the need for specific treatment. The risk of this is reduced if all visible varices are removed at the time of surgery. Deep vein thrombosis occurs in about one operation per 1000 following varicose vein surgery. The factors which result in increased risk are described below. Patients who have previously suffered a deep vein thrombosis seem to be particularly at risk and should receive full prophylactic measures, usually low-dose subcutaneous heparin in addition to compression stockings. Patients receiving oestrogen treatment may also be at increased risk of venous thrombosis, and heparin prophylaxis should be considered.

Venous reconstructive surgery

Surgery to the deep veins is limited by the absence of suitable prosthetic grafts or any satisfactory way of creating a venous valve. Surgery may be carried out for venous occlusion and for deep venous insufficiency. Patients who might be considered for these procedures include those who have persisting swelling of the lower limb after a previous venous thrombosis, even when a number of years has passed and collateral veins have had the opportunity to develop. The presence of a functional obstruction must be confirmed using direct venous pressure measurements. In the case of suspected iliac vein obstruction, the pressure in the femoral vein is measured with the patient lying supine. If there is a substantial rise in venous pressure during exercise then venous obstruction is confirmed. An alternative method is to measure the venous pressure in the hand and foot veins with the patient lying supine (the Raju test). Normally the foot venous pressure is the same as the hand venous pressure or no more than 5 mmHg greater. If venous obstruction is present the pressure difference is greater, with pressure differences of 10–15 mmHg indicating significant venous obstruction.

Venous obstruction

In patients with venous obstruction venous bypass procedures can be performed. Simple bypass with vein or prosthetic material may be used in the larger vessels, such as the iliac veins and vena cava. One problem is to find a vein of large enough calibre to insert in this region. These are sometimes constructed from opened out sections of saphenous vein reconstructed as a spiral graft (Fig. 16.27). Alternatively a Palma operation can be carried out. This involves mobilising the long saphenous vein in the opposite leg, tunnelling the distal end of the long saphenous vein across suprapubically and inserting it into the femoral vein below the obstruction. Blood then drains from the affected leg via the long saphenous vein into the femoral vein in the opposite leg (Fig. 16.28).

In patients who have obstruction of the superficial femoral vein, the long saphenous vein may be connected to the popliteal vein in the same limb, allowing blood to flow along the superficial veins more easily (May–Husni procedure). However, in the majority of patients with chronic superficial femoral vein obstruction, the blood flows along the long saphenous vein to reach the groin and therefore this operation is not required.

Venous incompetence

The surgical treatment of deep venous insufficiency remains a difficult problem that is dealt with in a few centres. Venous valves in the deep veins may be repaired if their incompetence is a consequence of primary valve failure. Kistner has described two methods of repairing incompetent valves, and successful completion of this operation may lead to long-term maintenance of leg ulcer healing. However, the operations are technically difficult and there is a risk of thrombosis which may destroy the reconstructed valve (Fig. 16.29). In patients who have previously suffered a deep vein thrombosis, transplantation of a segment of axillary vein has been carried out. This is usually attempted in patients who have damage to the deep veins following a previous venous thrombosis. The risk of further episodes of venous thrombosis makes the likely success of such operations as low as 50 per cent.

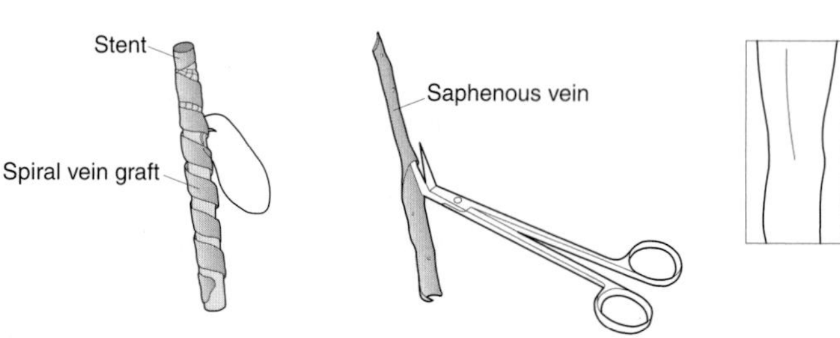

Fig. 16.27 Deep vein reconstruction using a spiral graft of saphenous vein.

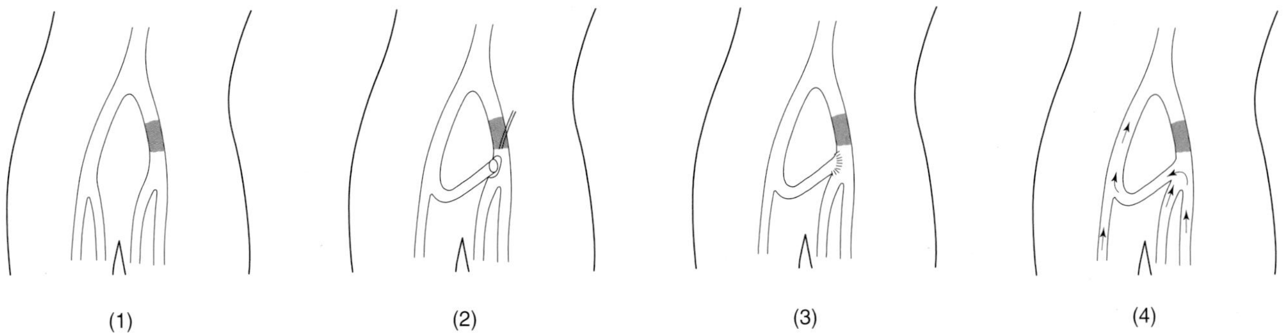

Fig. 16.28 Palma procedure – a femorofemoral vein graft constructed from the saphenous vein.

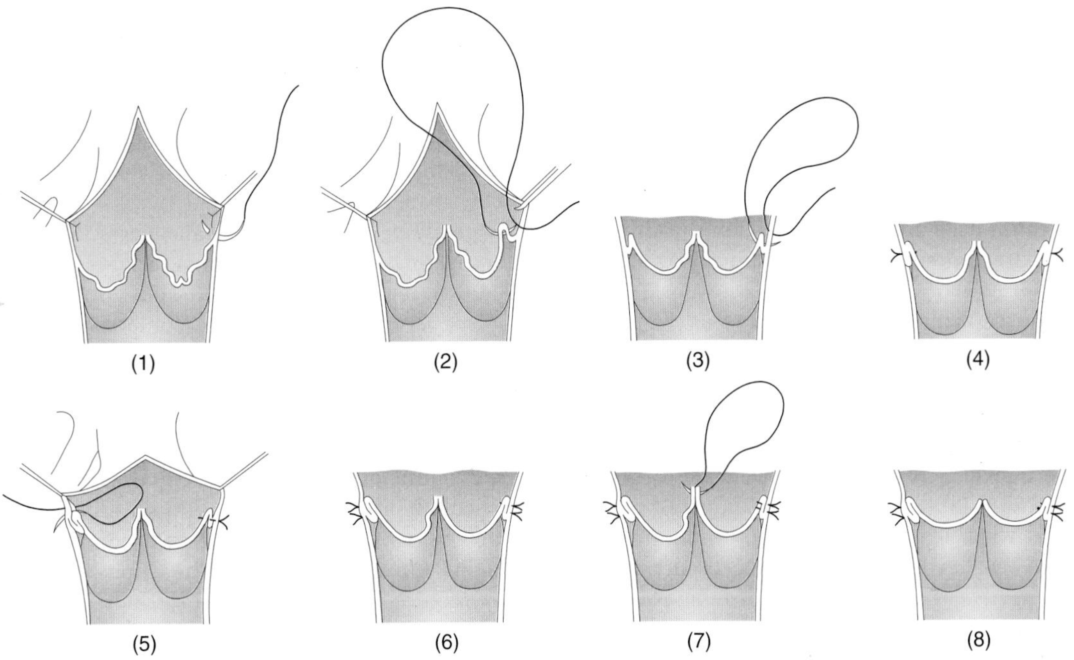

Fig. 16.29 Kistner-type valve repair for deep vein incompetence.

Leg ulcers

The most common cause of leg ulceration in Western countries is venous disease of the lower limb. However, many patients have other causes for their leg ulcer. The most frequent associated cause is peripheral arterial disease, which may be the sole cause for ulceration or may occur with venous disease. Because of this common association with arterial disease, patients presenting with leg ulceration should be investigated for arterial disease as well as for vein problems. In addition, a number of other common conditions may cause leg ulceration. A brief list of the causes of leg ulcers is given in Table 16.1.

Examination and investigation

Clinical examination should be performed carefully. The ulcer itself should be examined to establish its location. Venous ulcers usually lie just proximal to the medial or lateral malleolus, although they may extend to the ankle and dorsum of the foot. Venous ulcers are accompanied by lipodermatosclerosis and haemosiderosis. If these are not present then the ulcer is probably not of venous origin. The presence of obvious varicose veins should be recorded, although these are often not present or not visible in patients with venous ulcers. The peripheral pulses should be palpated to assess the peripheral arteries. The presence of loss of sensation in the foot or area of ulceration should be assessed, especially in a diabetic patient. Diabetic leg ulceration usually affects the foot and is almost always associated with peripheral neuropathy.

In patients suspected of suffering lower limb venous or arterial disease as the cause of the ulceration, complete examination of the venous system by duplex ultrasonography combined with measurement of Doppler ankle blood pressures is the most appropriate investigation in the first

Table 16.1 Some common causes of leg ulcers

- Venous disease of the lower limb
- Peripheral arterial disease
- Diabetes
- Neuropathy
- Rheumatoid disease
- Autoimmune disease (systemic sclerosis, systemic lupus erythematosus)
- Trauma
- Malignant ulcers (basal cell carcinoma, squamous cell carcinoma, malignant melanoma)
- Infective

instance. This investigation is highly effective in establishing the location of incompetent veins and assessing the extent of post-thrombotic vein damage. In those patients with venous ulceration, between 40 and 50 per cent have ulceration due to superficial venous insufficiency alone. Simple noninvasive tests can exclude those patients with arterial occlusion and identify those with deep and superficial venous insufficiency. Patients with pure superficial venous insufficiency, i.e. varicose ulcers – ulcers due entirely to varicose veins, respond well to surgical treatment of their varicose veins (Fig. 16.30). Where severe arterial disease is found it may be necessary to undertake detailed duplex ultrasound or angiographic examination of the arteries. Should the vascular system prove to be normal, blood tests may be done to test for systemic inflammatory disorders [e.g. rheumatoid disease, systemic lupus erythematosus (SLE)]. In addition, a biopsy of the ulcer may be helpful when it is not clearly due to an arterial or venous cause. A small proportion of leg ulcers is of malignant origin and any persistent ulcer, especially in an unusual place, should be biopsied to detect malignancy. Squamous cell and basal cell carcinomas are the most frequent cause of leg ulceration due to neoplasms, although occasionally malignant melanomas are found. In addition, malignant change may complicate a long-standing venous ulcer (Marjolin's ulcer). This should be suspected where part of an ulcer shows evidence of proliferation. This type of tumour is usually a squamous cell carcinoma.

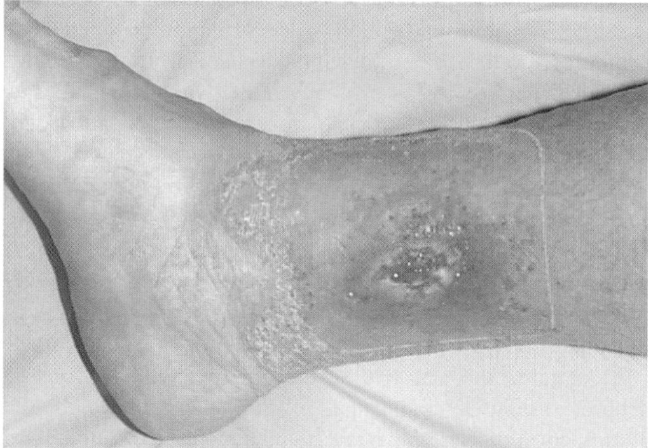

Fig. 16.30 Extensive venous ulceration entirely due to missed superficial venous insufficiency.

Management of venous leg ulcers

In patients who have venous ulceration due to superficial venous incompetence alone, varicose vein surgery is effective in producing ulcer healing in those patients who are fit enough to undergo this treatment. In the authors' experience it is not necessary to delay surgery until the ulcer has healed. The ulcer is covered by a dressing during surgery and prophylactic antibiotics are given to prevent infection of the surgical wounds with any bacteria present in the ulcer. Ulcers managed in this way usually heal rapidly (within 4 weeks) following surgery.

In those patients with deep venous insufficiency or who are unfit or unwilling to undergo surgery, standard ulcer management should be used. The mainstay of this is local ulcer management combined with the application of compression. The ulcer is cleaned by soaking in tap water (the use of sterile water is unnecessary) and débriding the ulcer to remove any slough. The skin of the leg often becomes very scaly beneath compression dressings and should be treated with emulsifying ointment. No topical application has been shown to speed the healing of a venous leg ulcer, and patients with venous disease of the lower limb are very likely to become allergic to dressing materials. Topical antibiotics are ineffective in healing leg ulcers and are particularly likely to produce skin sensitisation. They should never be used in the management of venous ulceration. Patients who have eczematous reactions around their ulcers may require the use of topical steroids to treat the allergic response. The dressing material should follow standard guidelines – see Chapter 3 on 'Wounds, tissue repair and scars'.

The most important factor in achieving healing is the use of high levels of compression. The use of dressings alone leads to a very slow rate of ulcer healing. It has been found that pressures of 30–45 mmHg applied to the ulcer are much more effective than lower levels of compression. These can be achieved by the use of compression stockings or by bandaging. Class 3 stockings exert about 30 mmHg compression at the ankle but require the patient to have sufficient strength in their hands to apply these. They are useful in younger patients who wish to manage their own ulcer. Frail patients often cannot manage this type of stocking, but may be able to apply two stockings of lower compression to the limb or use a stocking with a zip fastener in the seam. The compression need only be applied to the ulcer region, so patients with venous leg ulcers should wear below the knee

Jean Nicolas Marjolin, 1780–1850. Surgeon, Paris, France. Described the development of carcinomatous ulcers in scars in 1828.

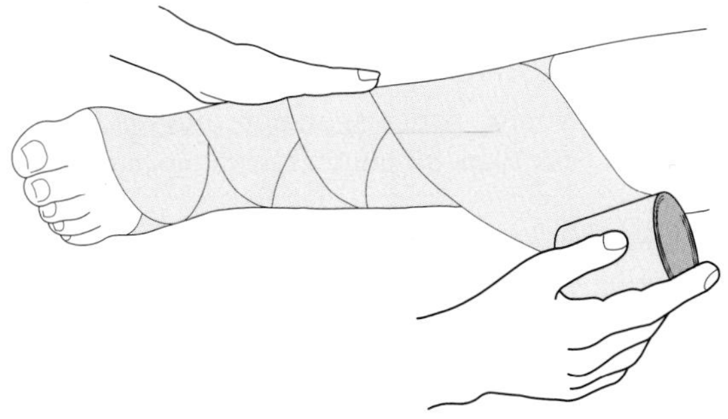

Fig. 16.31 Four-layer bandaging technique for venous ulceration.

stockings. Patients who are unable to manage with stockings are treated using multilayer bandaging regimes. These must be applied by a person trained in the procedure, as the use of lower pressures leads to slow ulcer healing and too high a pressure may cause injury to the leg. The best known of these techniques is the 'four-layer bandage' developed at Charing Cross Hospital in London. This method achieves pressures of 45 mmHg at the ankle and has been shown to produce healing of 70 per cent of venous ulcers within 12 weeks. The bandage must be changed once or twice per week (Fig. 16.31). The requirement that, for leg dressings, a nurse must change the dressing leads to a great deal of investment in the provision of community nursing services. Community nurses spend about 30 per cent of their time attending to leg ulcers and this leads to enormous expenditure by the National Health Service on this problem. It has been estimated that in the UK between £600 million and £800 million per annum is spent in the management of leg ulcers.

Prevention of recurrence

Even when healing has been achieved there is a risk that further ulcers may develop. Patients with healed ulcers should be encouraged to wear support stockings and rest with their feet elevated whenever possible. Recurrence rates of 25 per cent per year are accepted as the norm for such patients. In those who have been treated surgically for superficial venous incompetence the risk of reulceration is about 2–3 per cent per year.

Drug treatment for leg ulcers

No drugs have been found which are more effective than compression bandaging in the management of venous leg ulceration. Antibiotics have no effect on ulcer healing but are required if infection develops around an ulcer. This usually takes the form of cellulitis but, surprisingly, only occurs occasionally. A few drugs have been investigated to assess their efficacy in venous ulcer healing. These have included aspirin, oxpentifylline (Trental, Hoechst), prostaglandin E1 analogue and diosmin (Daflon 500 mg, Servier). All of these have an effect on leg ulcer healing but none is currently in widespread use. Future developments in understanding of the pathology of leg ulcers may lead to improvements in drug treatment for this condition.

Venous thrombosis

Venous thrombosis of the deep veins is a serious life-threatening condition which may lead to sudden death in the short term or to long-term morbidity due to the development of a post-thrombotic limb and venous ulceration. The most frequent location of deep vein thrombosis is in the lower limb. This condition may arise spontaneously or after injury to the limb. In modern medical practice the most common cause of lower limb venous thrombosis is following hospital admission for treatment of medical or surgical conditions. In 10 per cent of patients who die in hospital, the cause of death is pulmonary embolism following a lower limb deep vein thrombosis (Fig. 16.32).

Factors which lead to venous thrombosis

These were originally described by Virchow over a century ago. He suggested that the following factors may lead to clotting in the veins.

1. Changes in the vessel wall with damage to the endothelium due to injury or inflammation. This is known to happen following previous deep vein thrombosis.
2. Diminished rate of blood flow in the veins. In modern medical practice this occurs during and after operations, and in debilitating conditions such as strokes and myocardial infarction.
3. Increased coagulability of the blood. This also occurs following surgery and in the presence of infection or systemic malignancy.

Much more is now understood about the clotting cascade that results in the deposition of thrombus, as well as the fibrinolytic system that removes thrombus. Congenital deficiencies in either of these systems may result in increased susceptibility to thrombosis in that individual (Table 16.2).

Thrombophilia

Severe deficiencies of antithrombin III, protein C or protein S lead to severe or fatal episodes of venous thrombosis at an

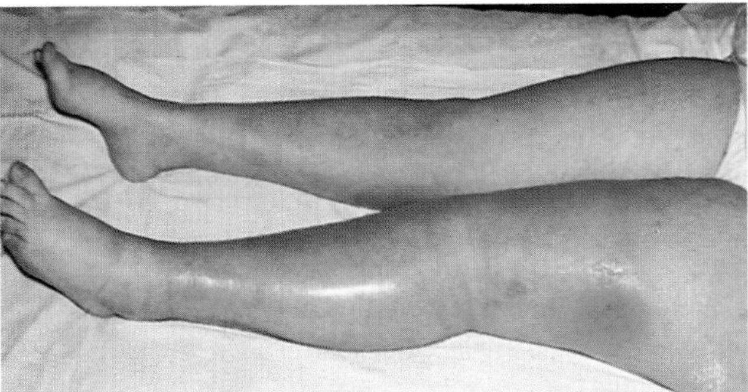

Fig. 16.32 Clinical deep vein thrombosis. Other conditions can simulate these signs.

Rudolf Carl Virchow, 1821–1902. German pathologist.

Table 16.2 Abnormalities of thrombosis and fibrinolysis which lead to increased risk of venous thrombosis

Congenital:
- Deficiency of antithrombin III, protein C or protein S
- Antiphospholipid antibody or lupus anticoagulant
- Factor V Leiden gene defect or activated protein C resistance
- Dysfibrinogenaemias

Acquired:
- Antiphospholipid antibody or lupus anticoagulant

early age. More mild deficiencies may present as recurrent episodes of venous thrombosis in later life. Activated protein C resistance results in only a modest increase in the risk of venous thrombosis, perhaps presenting as deep vein thrombosis in the lower limb following hospital treatment for some other condition. However, this abnormality is fairly common, occurring in 6–7 per cent of Caucasian people. In any patient presenting with an episode of venous thrombosis a family history of thrombotic episodes should be sought.

Spontaneous venous thrombosis may occur following injury to the leg such as a severely sprained ankle, as the consequence of an infection or following a period of immobility. Long-haul air travel is recognised as the cause for venous thrombosis in a number of people who are obliged to spend long periods in conditions permitting little movement of the legs. Long car journeys may also cause venous thrombosis in the lower limbs in susceptible individuals. In a proportion of patients an underlying malignancy appears to be the precipitating factor. In a patient who develops venous thrombosis in the absence of any identifiable cause clinical examination and special investigations should be arranged to detect common malignancies (leg, lung, stomach, large bowel).

Patients receiving treatment in hospital are at increased risk of venous thrombosis. This includes patients being treated surgically or for medical conditions. The factors which result in increased risk of venous thrombosis include advancing age and greater complexity of surgical treatment. Orthopaedic operations on the lower limbs (hip and knee replacements) are especially likely to result in venous thrombosis. The risk of venous thrombosis associated with particular surgical procedures is summarised in Table 16.3. However, medical patients are also at risk, particularly those being treated for strokes and other neurological conditions. Any patient with myocardial infarction or any serious illness runs the risk of venous thrombosis of the lower limb. Should this thrombus detach and become a pulmonary embolism, the result may be fatal. A large number of medical conditions, in addition to those mentioned above, may lead to venous thrombosis. These are listed in Table 16.4.

Prevention of deep vein thrombosis

All patients admitted to hospital or being treated for a serious illness should be assessed for the risk of deep vein thrombosis. These patients may be considered at low risk, moderate risk or high risk:

- low risk – young patients, minor illnesses, operations lasting for less than 30 minutes with no additional risk factors;
- moderate risk – patients over the age of 40 years with debilitating illnesses, undergoing major surgery but no additional risk factors;
- high risk – patients over the age of 40 years with serious medical conditions, such as stroke and myocardial infarction, and undergoing major surgery with additional risk factor, such as a past history of venous thromboembolism, extensive malignant disease or obesity.

Both mechanical and pharmacological methods are effective in preventing deep vein thrombosis. Graduated compression stockings (TED stockings) have been shown in clinical trials to reduce the incidence of deep vein thrombosis. Sequential pneumatic compression devices have also been shown to reduce the incidence of deep vein thrombosis in patients (Fig. 16.33). Their efficacy is enhanced if graduated compression stockings are worn as well.

Pharmacological methods evaluated include: low-dose heparin, low-molecular-weight heparin, dextran and adjusted dose warfarin. There is now good scientific evidence that low-dose heparin is effective in reducing the incidence of deep vein thrombosis and pulmonary embolism. Most studies suggest that the use of 5000 units of heparin, given subcutaneously two or three times a day, is effective. This should be continued for at least 5 days. The risk of developing a deep vein thrombosis following hospital discharge has now been recognised, and deep vein thrombosis prophylaxis probably ought to be extended into the postdischarge period. Low-molecular-weight heparin is effective in reducing the incidence of deep vein thrombosis. It has been shown to be more effective than low-dose heparin in orthopaedic patients and as effective in patients undergoing general surgical procedures. The advantages of low-molecular-weight heparin over standard heparin include once a day administration and a lower risk of bleeding complications, making it more suitable for out of hospital use.

Pulmonary embolism

Pulmonary embolism is a potentially fatal complication of lower limb deep vein thrombosis. A clot from the lower limb veins becomes detached from its site of formation and passes via the inferior vena cava and right heart to the pulmonary arteries. Here it may totally occlude the perfusion to part or all of one or both lungs. This leads to collapse or sudden death in some patients and is a medical emergency. Treatment includes full, immediate anticoagulation with intravenous heparin combined with standard methods of resuscitation. Large emboli may be treated by infusion of fibrinolytic drugs into the pulmonary arteries via catheters inserted via arm or leg veins.

Table 16.3 Risk factors for deep vein thrombosis

Risk category	*Risk of venous thromboembolism (assessed by objective tests)* Calf vein thrombosis (per cent)	Proximal vein thrombosis (per cent)	Fatal pulmonary embolism (per cent)
High risk: • General and urological surgery in patients aged over 40 years with recent history of deep vein thrombosis or pulmonary embolism • Extensive pelvic or abdominal surgery for malignant disease • Major orthopaedic surgery of lower limbs	40–80	10–30	1–5
Moderate risk: • General surgery in patients aged over 40 years lasting for 30 minutes or more and in patients aged below 40 years on oral contraceptives	0–40	2–10	0.1–0.7
Low risk: • Uncomplicated surgery in patients aged under 40 years without additional risk factors • Minor surgery (i.e. less than 30 minutes) in patients aged over 40 years without additional risk factors	< 10	< 1	< 0.01

Diagnosis of deep vein thrombosis

The symptoms and clinical features of a lower limb deep vein thrombosis are listed in Table 16.5. The most significant findings are tenderness in the calf and oedema at the ankle. However, these may also be attributable to other conditions. Pain in the calf on dorsiflexion of the ankle (Homan's sign) has been described in many textbooks. However, this is a very misleading clinical sign and provides no useful information about the presence or otherwise of a lower limb venous thrombosis. *It should no longer be used.* Some patients with deep vein thrombosis of the lower limb may have no symptoms in the leg, but present with severe dyspnoea due to pulmonary embolism.

Signs and symptoms of deep vein thrombosis

The clinical features a lower limb deep vein thrombosis are given in Table 16.5.

Objective diagnosis of deep vein thrombosis

The only reliable way to detect venous thrombosis is using an imaging investigation. The test of choice is duplex ultrasonography because it is a noninvasive, hazard-free method of investigation. If this is not available, then ascending phlebography should be undertaken. For diagnosis of pulmonary embolism, enhanced helical computerised tomography (CT) scanning is considered the standard test and is replacing isotope imaging studies. Treatment with anticoagulants is potentially hazardous and should not be commenced until a definite diagnosis has been made.

John Homans, 1877–1954. American surgeon. He described his sign, which is pain in the calf experienced on dorsiflexion of the foot, in cases of thrombosis of the calf veins, in 1941.

Table 16.4 Risk factors for venous thromboembolism

Patient's factors	*Disease or surgical procedure*
Age	Trauma or surgery, especially of pelvis, hip, lower limb
Obesity	Malignancy, especially pelvic, abdominal metastatic
Varicose veins	Heart failure
Immobility (bed rest > 4 days)	Recent myocardial infarction
Pregnancy	Paralysis of lower limb(s)
Puerperium	Infection
High-dose oestrogen therapy	Inflammatory bowel disease
Previous deep vein thrombosis or pulmonary embolism	Nephrotic syndrome
Thrombophilia	Polycythaemia
Deficiency of antithrombin III, protein C or protein S	Paraproteinaemia
Antiphospholipid	Paroxysmal nocturnal haemoglobinuria antibody or lupus anticoagulant
	Behçet's disease
	Homocystinaemia

Table 16.5 The clinical features of deep vein thrombosis

Swelling
Pain
Redness or no apparent signs and symptoms
Dilated superficial veins
Calf tenderness
Low-grade pyrexia

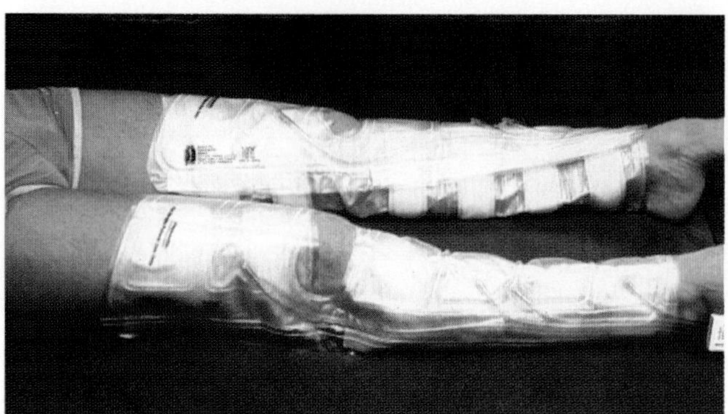

Fig. 16.33 Intermittent pneumatic compression device commonly used for the prevention of deep vein thrombosis.

Treatment of deep vein thrombosis

In treating an established deep vein thrombosis it is important to make the correct diagnosis. Twenty per cent of patients with clinical signs and symptoms of a deep vein thrombosis have normal deep veins. The differential diagnosis includes ruptured Baker's cyst, superficial thrombophlebitis, calf muscle haematomas and a ruptured plantaris tendon. All of these diagnoses can be demonstrated on ultrasonography, which has the advantage of allowing the examination of the soft tissues, something which venography is unable to do.

Having made the diagnosis of a deep vein thrombosis and confirmed it by duplex ultrasound imaging or venography, treatment should be instituted. Standard treatment involves intravenous heparin with the dose adjusted according to the weight of the patient and controlled by the activated partial thromboplastin time (APTT). The duration of heparin treatment should be at least 5 days. The aim is to minimise the risk of pulmonary embolism and encourage the thrombus to resolve. At the same time, the patient should be commenced on warfarin. The aim here is to reduce the risk of a further recurrence of venous thrombosis. Warfarin does not remove the clot from blocked veins and the duration of treatment (usually 3–6 months) is selected to prevent further episodes of venous thrombosis. Warfarin dosage is controlled by measuring the international normalised ratio (INR) by regular blood tests. The INR should be prolonged to between 2.5 and 3.5 times the control value. Patients with recurrent venous thromboembolic problems should be anticoagulated for life.

The use of subcutaneous injections of low-molecular-weight heparin for the treatment of deep vein thrombosis is an alternative method of anticoagulation. The dose is based on the patient's weight and treatment given without blood tests to control the dose. This has been found to produce reliable anticoagulation without the risk of haemorrhage. This may in future become a very convenient way to manage patients with acute deep vein thrombosis, either in hospital or at home. Warfarin treatment is commenced at the same time and controlled using the INR in the same way as for the intravenous heparin regime.

Venous thrombectomy

Occasionally massive venous thrombosis in the lower limb leads to severe impairment in the blood supply to the limb, leading to ischaemia and, eventually, gangrene. This is a surgical emergency and requires rapid relief of the venous obstruction. This can be achieved surgically by opening the femoral vein via an incision in the groin and removing all clot from the deep veins of the leg and pelvis. This operation used to be more widely performed on the assumption that it would reduce the severity of post-thrombotic vein damage following a deep vein thrombosis. However, very few surgeons now perform this operation. The more modern treatment of thrombolysis, achieved by passing a catheter into the affected vein and infusing a fibrinolytic drug such as streptokinase or tissue plasminogen activator (TPA), is reducing the need for this operation (Fig. 16.34).

Prevention of pulmonary embolism

In some patients the risk of pulmonary embolism is very great, e.g. a large venous thrombosis in the lower limb where anticoagulation is contraindicated (e.g. following a haemorrhagic stroke). In others, pulmonary embolism occurs despite full anticoagulation with warfarin. Pulmonary embolism may be prevented by the insertion of an inferior vena cava filter which traps large thrombi in its wires and prevents them from occluding the pulmonary arteries. These filters are usually placed by a radiologist via the femoral or jugular vein under X-ray control without the need for an open surgical procedure (Fig. 16.35).

Superficial vein thrombosis

Venous thrombosis (thrombophlebitis) often occurs in superficial veins. This is a frequent complication of varicose veins and may follow cannulation of a vein for an intravenous infusion. Spontaneous superficial thrombophlebitis may occur in the presence of polycythaemia, polyarthritis and Buerger's disease and may also herald the

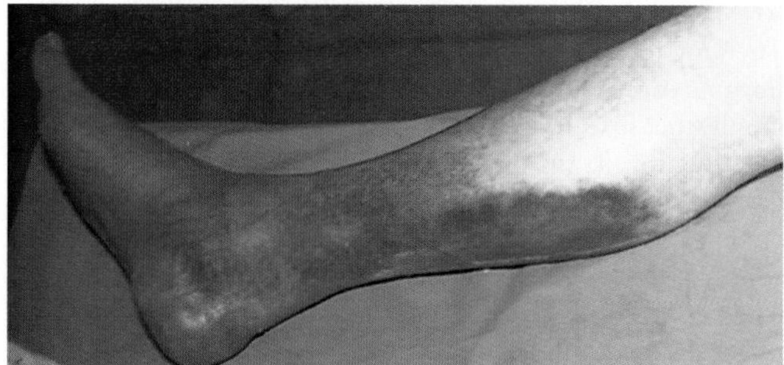

Fig. 16.34 Venous gangrene. Deep vein thrombosis.

William Morrant Baker, 1838–96. Surgeon, St Bartholomew's Hospital, London, England. Described these cysts in 1877.

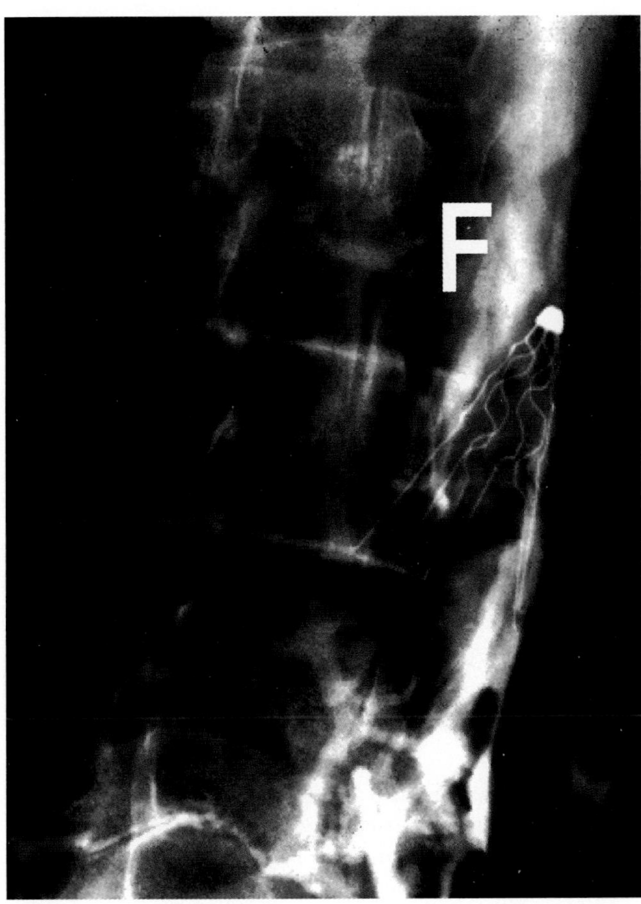

Fig. 16.35 Greenfield inferior vena cava filter, used to prevent pulmonary embolism from the lower limb veins.

presence of a visceral cancer. This condition does not carry the severe risks of deep venous thrombosis and is normally treated symptomatically. Patients benefit from simple analgesics and anti-inflammatory drugs. Occasionally deep

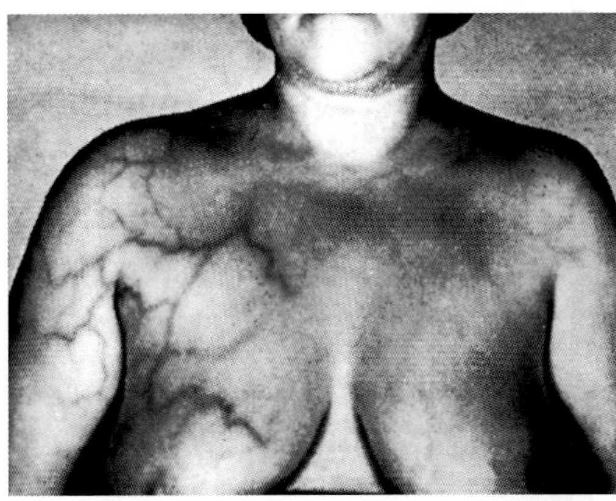

Fig. 16.36 Collateral venous circulation following thrombosis of axillary vein infrared photograph.

vein thrombosis may complicate superficial venous thrombosis and should be investigated where there is a clinical suspicion that thrombosis may have reached the deep veins. Patients with varicose veins should be advised to undergo surgical treatment for their varices as further episodes are likely in these patients.

Axillary vein thrombosis

Thrombosis of the axillary vein may occur following excessive exercise or as a complication of thoracic outlet syndrome. It is occasionally associated with a cervical rib. The arm becomes swollen and the superficial veins are distended. Early treatment with anticoagulants may result in rapid resolution. In severe cases the use of fibrinolytic therapy, streptokinase or TPA may be considered. Definitive treatment of the thoracic outlet syndrome by surgical decompression of the subclavian vein may be needed, for example by resection of the first rib (Fig. 16.36).

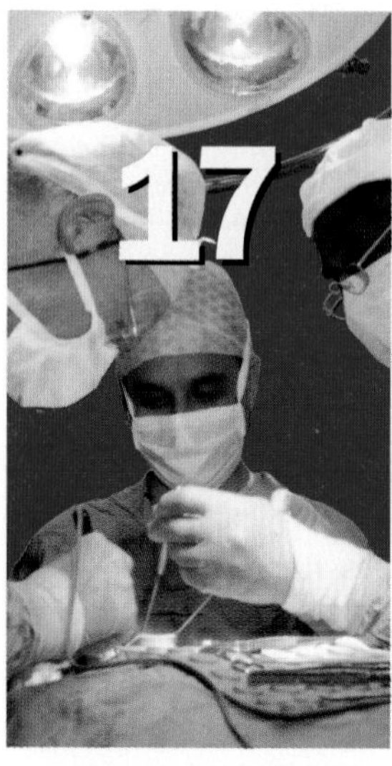

Lymphatic system

Introduction

The lymphatic system was first described by Erasistratus in Alexandria more than 2000 years ago. However, the anatomy was not described in detail until the seventeenth century and William Hunter, in the late eighteenth century, was the first to describe the function of the lymphatic system as we now understand it. Starling's pioneering work on the hydrostatic and haemodynamic forces controlling the movement of fluid across the capillary provided further insights into the function of the lymphatics. In the past two decades this knowledge has been further refined through the application of advanced *in vivo* microscopic techniques and the advances in molecular biology. Nevertheless, there is much about the lymphatic system that is not yet understood and debate continues over the precise aetiology of the commonest abnormality of the system; namely, lymphoedema.

Anatomy and physiology of the lymphatic system

Functions

1. Removes water, electrolytes, low-molecular-weight moieties (polypeptides, cytokines, growth factors) and macromolecules (fibrinogen, albumen, globulins, coagulation and fibrinolytic factors) from the interstitial space and returns them to the circulation.
2. Permits the circulation of lymphocytes and other immune cells.
3. Intestinal lymph (chyle) transports cholesterol, long-chain fatty acids, triglycerides and the fat-soluble vitamins (A, D, E and K) directly to the circulation, bypassing the liver.

Development and macroanatomy

In the embryo, the lymphatic system develops from four cystic spaces, located one on either side of the neck and one in each groin. These cisterns enlarge and develop communications (lymphatic vessels) that permit lymph from the lower limbs and abdomen to drain via the cisterna chyli, lying between the aorta and azygos vein, into the thoracic duct. This duct is a major lymph channel which passes cephalad on the left of the bodies of the thoracic vertebrae to enter the left side of the neck, where it drains into the left internal jugular vein at its confluence with the left subclavian vein. Lymph from the head and right arm drains via a separate lymphatic trunk, the right lymphatic duct, into the right internal jugular vein. Lymph nodes develop as condensations along the course of these lymphatic highways.

Lymphatics accompany veins everywhere in the body except in the cortical bony skeleton and central nervous system, although the brain and retina possess analogous systems (cerebrospinal fluid and aqueous humour, respectively). The lymphatic system comprises lymphatic channels,

Erasistratus of Chios c. *304* BC–c. *250* BC. *Greek anatomist and physician.*
William Hunter, 1718–83. British anatomist and obstetrician.
Ernst Henry Starling, 1866–1927. Physiologist, University College Hospital, London, England.

Bailey & Love's Short Practice of Surgery, 23rd edition. Edited by R.C.G. Russell, N.S. Williams and C.J.K. Bulstrode. Published in 2000 by Arnold Publishers.

lymphoid organs (lymph nodes, spleen, Peyer's patches, thymus, tonsils) and circulating elements (lymphocytes and other mononuclear immune cells).

Microanatomy and physiology

Lymphatic capillaries

Lymphatics originate within the interstitial space either from specialised endothelialised capillaries (initial lymphatics) or from nonendothelialised precapillary channels such as in the liver (spaces of Disse). Initial lymphatics capillaries are unlike arteriovenous capillaries in that they:

- are blind-ended;
- are much larger (50 μm);
- allow the entry of molecules up to 1000 kDa in size because the basement membrane is fenestrated, tenuous or even absent and the endothelium itself possesses intra- and intercellular pores.
- The abluminal surface of the endothelium is intimately related to the interstitial matrix through anchoring collagen and elastic filaments. In the resting state initial lymphatic capillaries are collapsed. When interstitial fluid volume and pressure increase, the space expands and the lymphatic capillaries and their pores are held open by these filaments to facilitate increased lymphatic drainage.

Terminal lymphatics

Lymphatic capillaries drain into terminal (collecting) lymphatics which possess bicuspid valves and endothelial cells rich in the contractile protein actin. Larger collecting lymphatics are innervated and surrounded by smooth muscle. Valves partition the lymphatic into segments termed lymphangions which are believed to contract sequentially in order to propel lymph into the lymph trunks. The area of skin drained by a single terminal lymphatic is termed an areola. Although there is some overlap between adjacent areolata, there are lymphatic watersheds and there is limited capacity for bypass flow when a main collecting duct or lymph trunk is blocked.

Lymph trunks

Terminal lymphatics lead to lymph trunks which have a structure that is similar to veins: a single layer of endothelial cells, lying on a basement membrane overlying a media comprised of smooth muscle cells that are innervated with sympathetic, parasympathetic and sensory nerve endings. About 10 per cent of lymph arising from a limb is transported in deep lymphatic ducts that accompany the main neurovascular bundles. The majority of lymph, however, is conducted, in epifascial lymph ducts, against venous flow from the core of the limb to the surface. Superficial ducts form lymph bundles of various sizes which are located within strips of adipose tissue and tend to follow the course of the major superficial veins.

Johann Konrad Peyer, 1653–1712. Swiss anatomist.

Starling's forces

The distribution of fluid and protein between the vascular and interstitial spaces depends on the balance of hydrostatic and oncotic pressures between the two compartments (Starling's forces), together with the relative impermeability of the blood capillary membrane to molecules over 70 kDa. In health there is net capillary filtration into the interstitial space of 2–4 litres per 24 hours which is removed by the lymphatic system. Disease processes which disturb Starling's forces lead primarily to oedema that is low in protein, whereas diseases which primarily impair lymphatic drainage lead to high-protein oedema (lymphoedema).

Transport of particles

Particles enter the initial lymphatics through interendothelial openings and vesicular transport through intraendothelial pores. In contradistinction to arteriovenous capillaries, the larger the particles the greater the lymphatic uptake. Large particles are actively phagocytosed by macrophages and transported through the lymphatic system intracellularly.

Mechanisms of lymph transport

Whereas resting pressures in the interstitial fluid compartments of the skin and subcutaneous tissues are negative (–2 to –6 mmH_2O) pressures within lymphatics are positive, indicating that lymph flows against a small pressure gradient. It is believed that prograde lymphatic flow depends on two mechanisms:

- transient increases in interstitial pressure secondary to muscular contraction and external compression;
- the generation of alternating suction and propulsive forces through the sequential contraction and relaxation of lymphangions separated by valves that prevent retrograde flow.

Lymphangions respond to increased lymph flow in much the same way as the heart responds to increased venous return, in that they increase their contractility and stroke volume. Contractility is also enhanced by noradrenaline, serotonin, certain prostaglandins and thromboxanes, and endothelin-1. Pressures of up to 30–50 mmHg have been recorded in normal lymph trunks and up to 200 mmHg in severe lymphoedema. Lymphatics modulate their own contractility through the production of nitric oxide. Contractility appears to be inhibited by haemoglobin, haem-containing proteins and oxygen-derived free radicals.

Transport in the thoracic and right lymph ducts is also dependent on the changes in intrathoracic pressure that occur with respiration, as well as changes in central venous pressures through the cardiac cycle. Cardiac and respiratory disease may, therefore, have an adverse effect on lymphatic function.

Lymphovenous communications were first observed on lymphangiography and were thought to act as safety valves that would allow decompression of a hypertensive lymphatic system. While lymphscintigraphy may reveal lymphovenous communications in normal limbs, they have been reported to be absent in some cases of lymphoedema, for example post-mastectomy. The pathophysiological importance of this observation remains uncertain.

In summary, in the normal limb, lymph flow is largely due to intrinsic lymphatic contractility, although exercise, limb movement and external compression do increase lymphatic return. However, in lymphoedema, where the lymphatics are constantly distended with lymph, these forces assume a much more important functional role and this explains the success of physical therapy.

Acute inflammation of the lymphatics

Acute lymphangitis occurs when a deep or superficial infection, often due to *Streptococcus pyogenes* or *Staphylococcus aureus*, spreads to the draining lymphatics and lymph nodes (lymphadenitis) where an abscess may form. Eventually this may progress to bacteraemia or septicaemia. The normal signs of infection (rubor, calor, dolor) are present and a red streak is seen in the skin along the line of the inflamed lymphatic (Fig. 17.1). The part should be rested to reduce lymphatic drainage, elevated to reduce swelling and the patient treated with intravenous antibiotics based upon actual or suspected sensitivities. Failure to improve within 48 hours suggests inappropriate antibiotic therapy, the presence of undrained pus either in the lymph nodes or at the site of primary infection, or the presence of an underlying systemic disorder (malignancy, immunodeficiency). The lymphatic damage caused by acute lymphangitis may lead to recurrent attacks of infection and lymphoedema.

Lymphoedema

Definition

Oedema is due primarily to defective lymphatic drainage in the presence of (near) normal net capillary filtration.

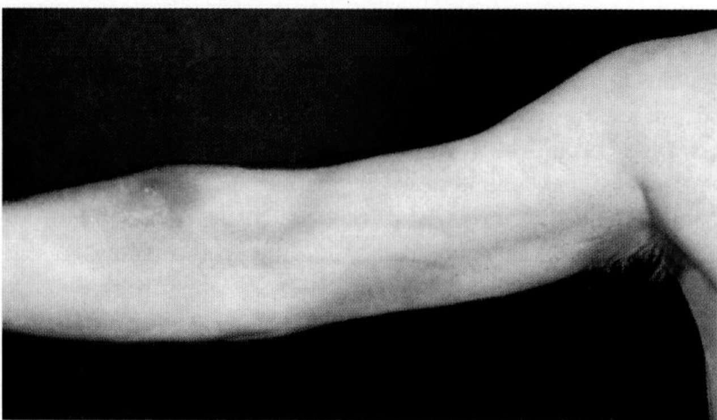

Fig. 17.1 Acute lymphangitis of the arm. Erythematous streaks extend from the site of primary infection on the volar aspect of the forearm to epicondylar nodes at the elbow and thence to enlarged and tender axillary lymph nodes.

Pathophysiology

Lymphoedema is the end result of insufficient lymphatic outflow due to aplasia, hypoplasia, primary decreased lymphatic contractility (with or without valvular insufficiency) or inflammatory obliteration. Lymphatic hypertension occurs and leads to distension with secondary impairment of contractility and valvular competence. Lymphostasis leads to the accumulation of fluid, proteins, growth factors and other active peptide moieties, glycosaminoglycans and particulate matter, including bacteria. As a consequence, there is increased collagen production by fibroblasts, an accumulation of inflammatory cells (predominantly macrophages and lymphocytes) and activation of keratinocytes. The end result is protein-rich oedema fluid, increased deposition of ground substance, subdermal fibrosis, and dermal thickening and proliferation.

Cross-sectional imaging of the affected limb by means of computerised tomography (CT) or magnetic resonance imaging clearly indicates that lymphoedema, unlike all other causes of oedema, is confined to the epifascial space comprising the skin and subcutaneous tissues. Although muscle compartments may be hypertrophied as a result of the increased work involved in limb movement, they are characteristically free of oedema.

Classification

Lymphoedema was originally classified by Allen in 1934 who subdivided it into primary lymphoedema, in which the cause is unknown (or at least unproved), and secondary lymphoedema, in which there is a clear aetiology (Table 17.1). Primary lymphoedema is usually further subdivided on the

Table 17.1 Aetiological classification of lymphoedema

Primary lymphoedema	Congenital (onset < 1 year old) – sporadic
	Congenital (onset < 1 year old) – familial – (Milroy's disease*)
	Praecox (onset 1–35 years of age) – sporadic
	Praecox (onset 1–35 years of age) – familial (Meige's disease*)
	Tarda (onset after 35 years of age)
Secondary lymphoedema	Bacterial infection
	Parasitic infection (filariasis)
	Fungal infection (tinea pedis)
	Exposure to foreign body material (silica particles)
	Primary lymphatic malignancy
	Metastatic spread to lymph nodes
	Radiotherapy to lymph nodes
	Surgical excision of lymph nodes
	Trauma (particularly degloving injuries)
	Superficial thrombophlebitis
	Deep venous thrombosis

*These terms are used variably.

James Alfred Van Allen, b. 1914. American physicist. Inventor of Van Allen belts, also known as radiation belts.

Table 17.2 Clinical classification of lymphoedema (Brunner)

Grade	*Clinical features*
Subclinical (latent)	There is excess interstitial fluid and histological abnormalities in lymphatics and lymph nodes but no clinically apparent lymphoedema
I	Oedema pits on pressure and swelling largely or completely disappears on elevation and bed rest
II	Oedema does not pit and does not significantly reduce upon elevation
III	Oedema is associated with irreversible skin changes: fibrosis, papillae

basis of age of onset and the presence of a family history. Lymphoedema may also be classified on the basis of lymphangiographic findings (see below) and clinical severity regardless of the underlying cause (Table 17.2).

History

The age of onset of painless swelling, together with the presence or absence of a family history or coexistent pathology, will allow differentiation of primary from secondary lymphoedema to be made in most cases. It is important to remember that in developed countries lymphoedema is a relatively uncommon cause of limb swelling (Table 17.3).

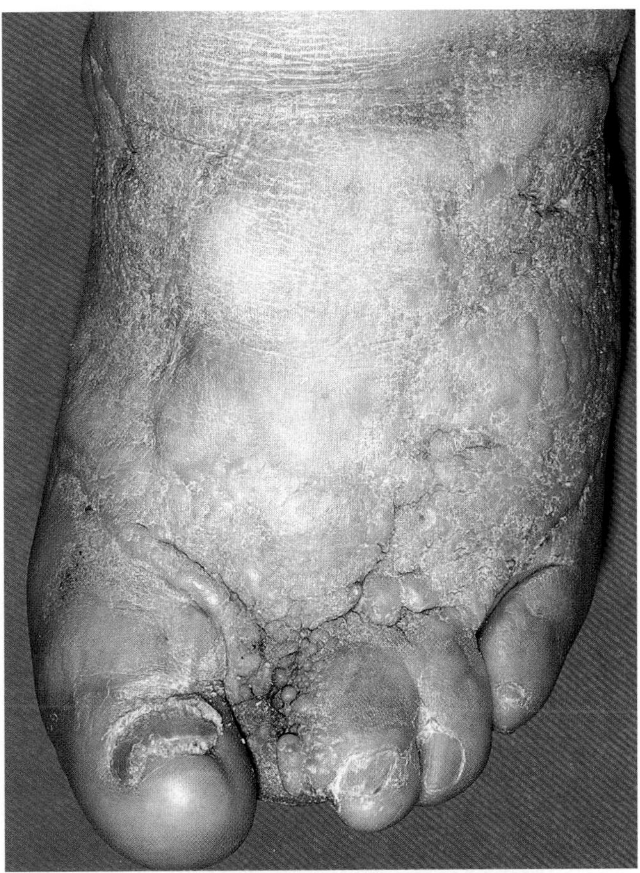

Fig. 17.2 The foot of a patient with typical lymphoedema.

Table 17.3 Differential diagnosis of the swollen limb

Nonvascular or lymphatic	General disease states	Cardiac failure from any cause. Liver failure. Hypoproteinaemia due to nephrotic syndrome, malabsorption, protein losing enteropathy. Hyperthyroidism (myxoedema). Allergic disorders including angioedema and idiopathic cyclic oedema. Prolonged immobility and lower limb dependency
	Local disease processes	Ruptured Baker's cyst. Myositis ossificans. Bony or soft tissue tumours. Arthritis. Haemarthrosis. Calf muscle haematoma. Achilles tendon rupture
	Retroperitoneal fibrosis	May lead to arterial, venous and lymphatic abnormalities
	Gigantism	Rare. All tissues are uniformly enlarged
	Drugs	Corticosteroids, oestrogens, progestagens; monoamine oxidase inhibitors; phenylbutazone; methyldopa; hydralazine; nifedipine
	Trauma	Painful swelling due to reflex sympathetic dystrophy
	Obesity	Lipodystrophy, lipoidosis
Venous	Deep venous thrombosis	There may be an obvious predisposing factor such as recent surgery. The classical signs of pain and redness may be absent
	Post-thrombotic syndrome	Swelling, usually of the whole leg, due to iliofemoral venous obstruction. Venous skin changes, secondary varicose veins on the leg and collateral veins on the lower abdominal wall. Venous claudication may be present
	Varicose veins	Simple primary varicose veins are not usually associated with significant leg swelling
	Klippel–Trenaunay syndrome and other malformations	Rare. Present at birth or develops in early childhood. Comprises an abnormal lateral venous complex, capillary naevus, bony abnormalities, hypo(a)plasia of deep veins and limb lengthening. Lymphatic abnormalities often coexist
	External venous compression	Pelvic or abdominal tumour including the gravid uterus. Retroperitoneal fibrosis
Arterial	Ischaemia reperfusion	Following lower limb revascularisation for acute and chronic ischaemia
	Arteriovenous malformation	May be associated with local or generalised swelling
	Aneurysm	Popliteal. Femoral. False aneurysm following (iatrogenic) trauma

Johann Conrad von Brunner, 1653–1727. Swiss anatomist.

William Morrant Baker, 1838–96. Surgeon, St Bartholomew's Hospital, London, England.

Maurice Klippel, 1858–1942, and André Feil, b. 1884, both neurologists in Paris, France, described this condition in a joint paper in 1912.

Signs

Unlike other types of oedema, lymphoedema characteristically involves the foot (Fig. 17.2). The contour of the ankle is lost through infilling of the submalleolar depressions, a 'buffalo hump' forms on the dorsum of the foot, the toes appear 'square' owing to confinement of footwear and the skin on the dorsum of the toes cannot be pinched because of subcutaneous fibrosis (Stemmer's sign). Lymphoedema usually spreads proximally to knee level and less commonly affects the whole leg (Fig. 17.3). Lymphoedema will pit easily at first but, with time, fibrosis and dermal thickening prevent pitting except following prolonged pressure. Chronic eczema, fungal infection of the skin (dermatophytosis) and nails (onychomycosis), fissuring, verrucae and papillae are frequently seen in advanced conditions. Frank ulceration is rare except in the presence of chronic venous insufficiency, but the two conditions not infrequently coexist and chronic venous insufficiency may actually lead to lymphatic insufficiency (Fig. 17.4). Ulceration can also develop after minor trauma and be slow to heal (Fig. 17.5). Protein-losing diarrhoea, chylous ascites, chylothorax, chyluria and discharge of lymph from skin vesicles (lymphorrhoea, chylorrhoea) suggest lymphangectasia (megalymphatics) and chylous reflux, but this is rare. Ulceration, nonhealing bruises and raised purple-red nodules should lead to suspicion of malignancy. Lymphangiosarcoma was originally described arising in postmastectomy oedema (Stewart–Treves syndrome) but can

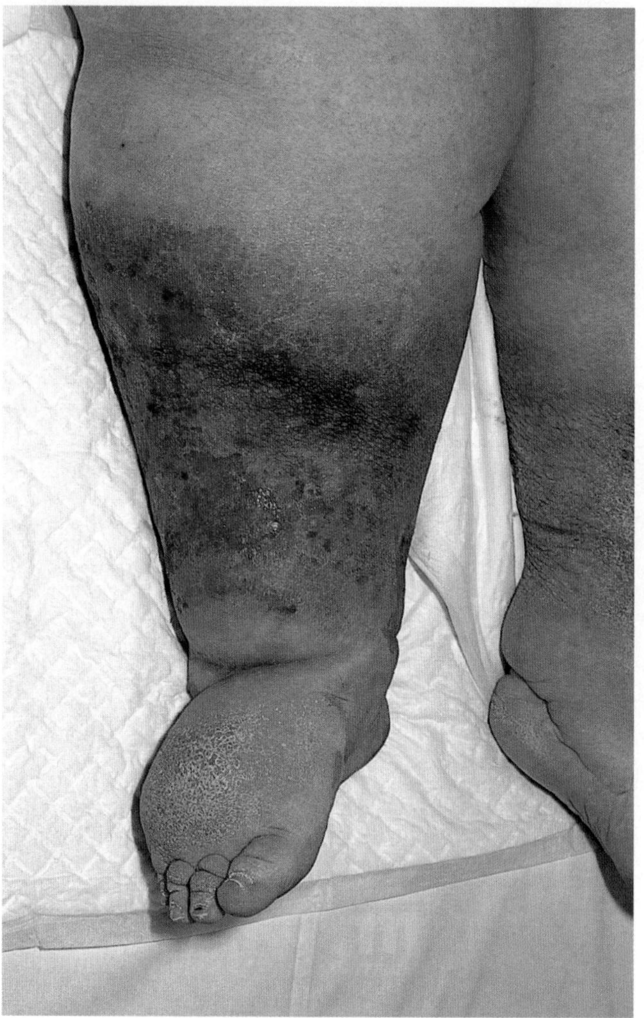

Fig. 17.3 The lower leg of patient with typical lymphoedema.

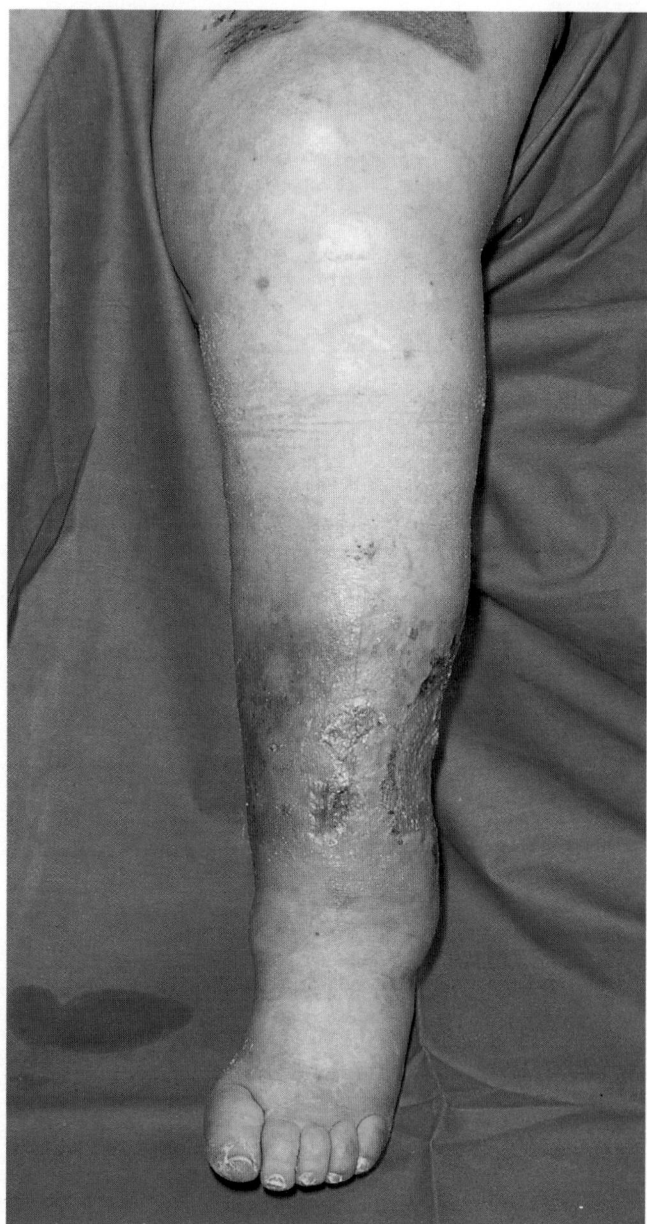

Fig. 17.4 A patient with lymphoedema who also had a previous deep venous thrombosis. Note the presence of skin changes typical of chronic venous insufficiency, including a laterally placed 'venous' ulcer.

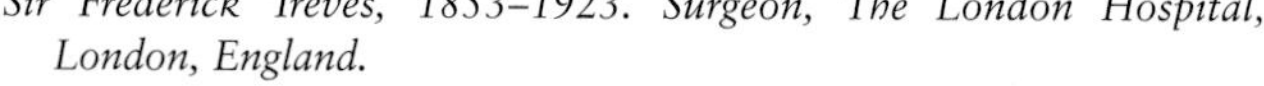

Sir Frederick Treves, 1853–1923. Surgeon, The London Hospital, London, England.

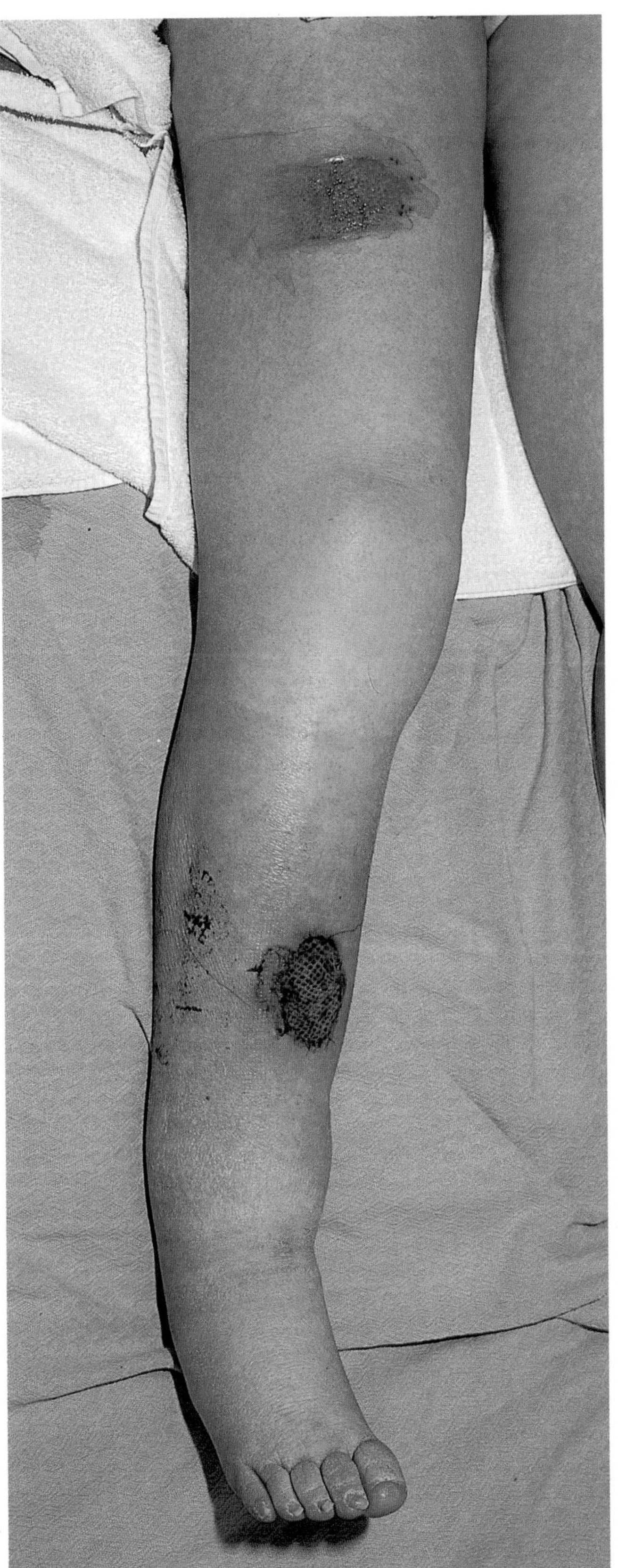
Fig. 17.5 Traumatic ulcer in a patient with lymphoedema praecox treated successfully with a split skin graft.

arise in any in long-standing lymphoedema. It is rare, aggressive, usually diagnosed late and frequently leads to loss of limb or life.

Primary lymphoedema

Pathophysiology

Primary lymphoedema affects only one or two people per 100 000 under 20 years of age. Approximately 10 per cent have a positive family history.

Nonfamilial primary lymphoedema

It has been proposed that all cases of primary lymphoedema are due to an inherited abnormality of the lymphatic system, sometimes termed 'dysplasia *in utero*'. However, it is more likely that many sporadic cases occur in the presence of a (near) normal lymphatic system and are, in reality, examples of secondary lymphoedema for which the triggering event has gone unrecognised. In animal models, simple excision of lymph nodes and/or trunks leads to acute lymphoedema that resolves within a few weeks, presumably due to collateralisation. The human condition can only be achieved by inducing extensive lymphatic obliteration and fibrosis, for example by injecting silica particles; even then there may be considerable delay between the injury and the onset of oedema. It is likely that most nonfamilial primary lymphoedema is due to chronic injury over many years due to seemingly trivial (but repeated) bacterial and/or fungal infections, insect bites, barefoot walking (silica), deep venous thrombosis or episodes of superficial thrombophlebitis. Primary lymphoedema is much more common in the legs than the arms. This may be due to gravity and a bipedal posture, the fact that the lymphatic system of the leg is less well developed than that of the arm in terms of the volume of tissue drained, or the increased susceptibility of the lower extremity to trauma and/or infection.

Familial primary lymphoedema

In familial cases it is assumed that there must be some, as yet undefined, genetic susceptibility of the lymphatic system to such injury. This may be:

- a structural problem such as aplasia or hypoplasia;
- a functional problem such as defective lymphatic contractility;
- an immune deficiency.

However, at the present time, the exact mechanisms causing familial primary lymphoedema remain speculative.

Lymphoedema congenita

Congenital lymphoedema (onset at or within a year of birth) is more common in males, more likely to be bilateral and to involve the whole leg, and accounts for less than 5 per cent

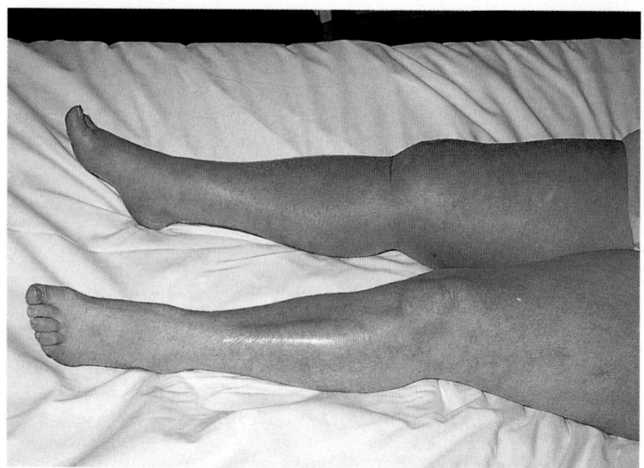

Fig. 17.6 This woman, in her sixth decade, presented with rapid onset of lymphoedema of the right leg. On further investigation she was found to have locally advanced bladder carcinoma. Note that, unlike most cases of lymphoedema, the swelling is greater proximally than distally.

of primary lymphoedema. Milroy's disease describes familial lymphoedema that is present at birth or is noticed shortly thereafter. Congenital lymphoedema is also associated with other disorders, such as yellow nail and Pierre–Robin syndrome (micrognathia).

Lymphoedema praecox

Lymphoedema praecox (onset from 1 to 35 years of age) is three times more common in females than males, has a peak incidence shortly after menarche, is three times more likely to be unilateral than bilateral, usually only extends to the knee and accounts for about 20 per cent of primary lymphoedema. The familial form is referred to as Meige's disease and represents about one-third of all cases.

Lymphoedema tarda

Lymphoedema tarda develops, by definition, after the age of 35 years but, in practice, is a disease of middle age. It is often associated with obesity and, histologically, lymph nodes are replaced with fatty and fibrous tissue. The cause is unknown. Lymphoedema developing for the first time in later life should prompt a thorough search for underlying malignancy, particularly of the pelvic organs, prostate and external genitalia; such malignancy may be found in up to 10 per cent of patients. It is worth noting that in such patients lymphoedema often commences proximally in the thigh rather than distally (Fig. 17.6).

Lymphangiographic classification

Browse has classified primary lymphoedema on the basis of lymphangiographic findings (Table 17.4, Figs 17.7 and 17.8). These findings are related to the clinical presentations described above.

Megalymphatics

Some patients with lymphatic hyperplasia possess megalymphatics in which lymph or chyle refluxes freely under the effects of gravity against the physiological direction of flow. The megalymphatics usually end in thin-walled vesicles on the skin surface causing excoriation, secondary infection, fluid electrolyte and protein depletion; serous surfaces of

Table 17.4 Lymphangiographic classification of primary lymphoedema

	Congenital hyperplasia (10 per cent)	*Distal obliteration (80 per cent)*	*Proximal obliteration (10 per cent)*
Age of onset	Congenital	Puberty (praecox)	Any age
Sex distribution	Male > female	Female > male	Male = female
Extent	Whole leg	Ankle, calf	Whole leg, thigh only
Laterality	Unilateral = bilateral	Often bilateral	Usually unilateral
Family history	Often positive	Often positive	No
Progression	Progressive	Slow	Rapid
Response to compression therapy	Variable	Good	Poor
Comments	Lymphatics are increased in number although functionally defective, there is usually an increased number of lymph nodes. May have chylous ascites, chylothorax and protein-losing enteropathy	Absent or reduced distal superficial lymphatics. Also termed aplasia or hypoplasia	There is obstruction at the level of the aortoiliac or inguinal nodes. If associated with distal dilatation the patient may benefit from a lymphatic bypass operation. Other patients have distal obliteration as well

William Forsyth Milroy, 1855–1942. Professor of Clinical Medicine, University of Nebraska, Omaha, Nebraska, USA. Described hereditary oedema of the legs in 1892.

Pierre Robin, 1867–1950. French histologist and stomatologist.

Joe Vincent Meige, 1892–1964. Gynaecological Surgeon, Massachusetts General Hospital, Boston, Massachusetts, USA.

Norman Browse, President of Royal College of Surgeons, 1992–95.

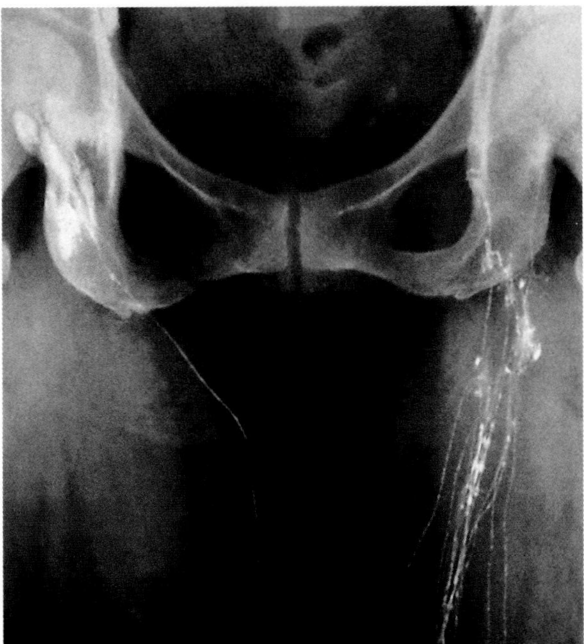

Fig. 17.7 This patient presented with congenital lymphoedema of the right leg. The lymphangiogram shows lymphatic hypoplasia.

peritoneal (chylous ascites) or pleural (hydrothorax, chylothorax) cavities; or mucosal surfaces of the intestine (protein losing enteropathy), kidney or bladder (chyluria) (Fig. 17.9).

Secondary lymphoedema

This is the most common form of lymphoedema. There are several well-recognised causes.

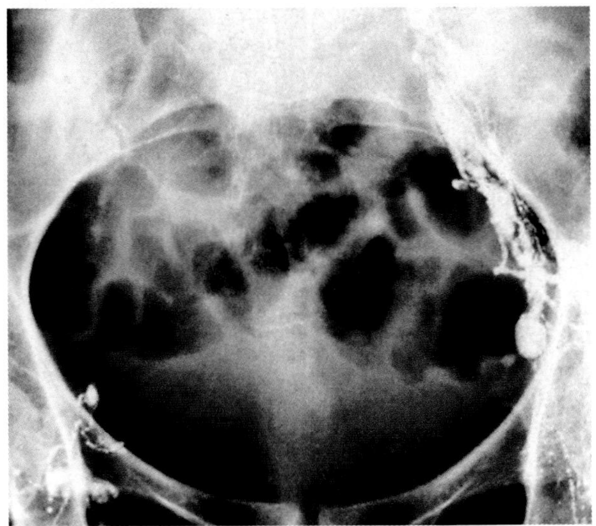

Fig. 17.8 This patient presented with lymphoedema of the right leg. Bipedal lymphangiogram demonstrated normal lymphatics in the right leg up to the inguinal nodes but no progression of contrast above the inguinal ligament; a case of proximal obstruction.

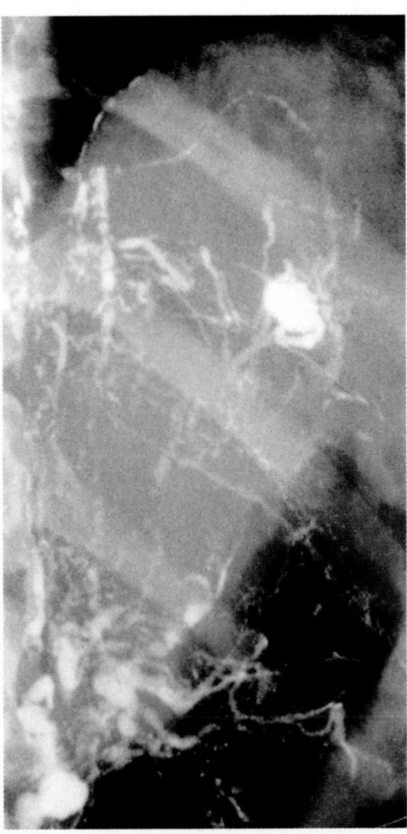

Fig. 17.9 Lymphangiogram demonstrating reflux from dilated para-aortic vessels into the left kidney in a patient with filariasis who presented with chyluria.

Filariasis

This is the commonest cause of lymphoedema worldwide, affecting up to 100 million individuals. It is particularly prevalent in Africa, India and South America where 5–10 per cent of the population may be affected. The viviparous nematode *Wucheria bancrofti*, whose only host is humans, is responsible for 90 per cent of cases and is spread by the mosquito. The disease is associated with poor sanitation. The parasite enters lymphatics from the blood and lodges in lymph nodes where it causes fibrosis and obstruction, due partly to direct physical damage and partly to the immune response of the host. Proximal lymphatics become grossly dilated with adult parasites. The degree of oedema is often massive, in which case it is termed 'elephantiasis' (Fig. 17.10). Immature parasites (microfilariae) enter the blood at night and can be identified on a blood smear, a centrifuged specimen of urine or in lymph itself. A complement fixation test is also available and is positive in present or past infection. Eosinophilia is usually present. Diethylcarbamazine destroys the parasites but does not reverse the lymphatic changes; although there may be some regression over time. Once the infection has been cleared treatment is as for primary lymphoedema. Public health measures to reduce mosquito breeding, protective clothing and mosquito netting may be usefully employed to combat the condition.

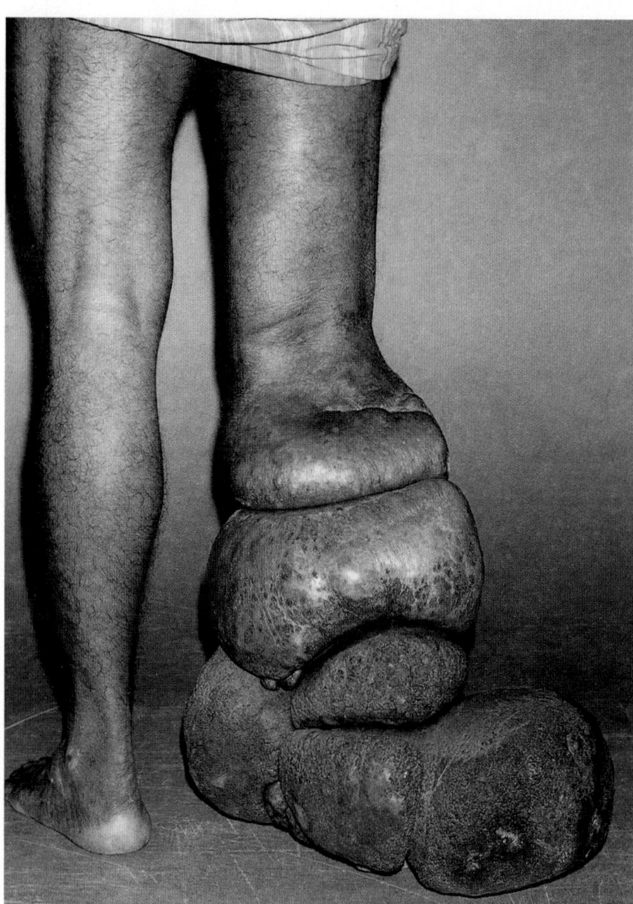

Fig. 17.10 Elephantiasis due to filariasis. (*Photograph reproduced with permission from Mr R. Kaje, Jipher, India.*)

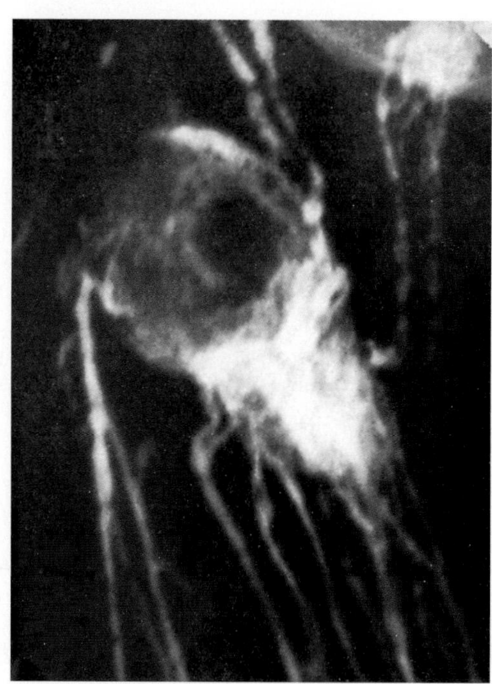

Fig. 17.11 Lymphangiogram showing a filling defect in an inguinal affected by metastatic malignant melanoma.

Malignancy and its treatment

This is the most common cause of lymphoedema in developed countries. Hodgkin's and non-Hodgkin's lymphoma may present with lymphoedema, as may malignant melanoma which has metastasised to regional lymph nodes (Fig. 17.11) and malignancy of the pelvic organs (ovary, uterus, bladder), anus, prostate, testes, penis and breast (*peau d'orange*). More often lymphoedema is a result of treatment, either surgical excision of draining lymph nodes and/or radiotherapy. Lymphoedema following treatment for breast carcinoma is the commonest example, but fortunately this is decreasing in incidence as surgery for the condition has become more conservative (Fig. 17.12). Lymphoedema may occur after radical mastectomy (up to 60 per cent), modified radical mastectomy (up to 20 per cent), local excision with either axillary node clearance *or* radiotherapy (less than 5 per cent), and local excision with axillary node clearance *and* radiotherapy (up to 40 per cent).

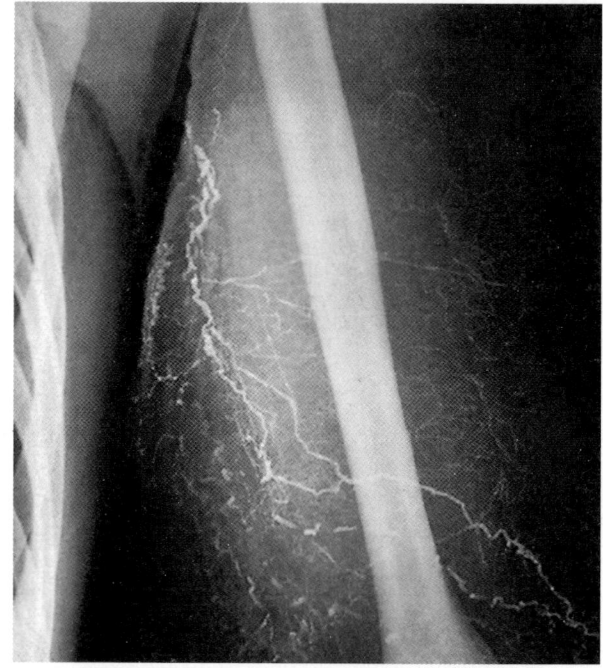

Fig. 17.12 Obstructive lymphoedema of the left arm secondary to radical mastectomy and radiotherapy for breast carcinoma.

Trauma

This is an unusual cause of lymphoedema but is especially seen after degloving injuries of the extremities.

Acute cellulitis

As described above, acute bacterial lymphangitis is a frequently observed triggering event for secondary lymphoedema.

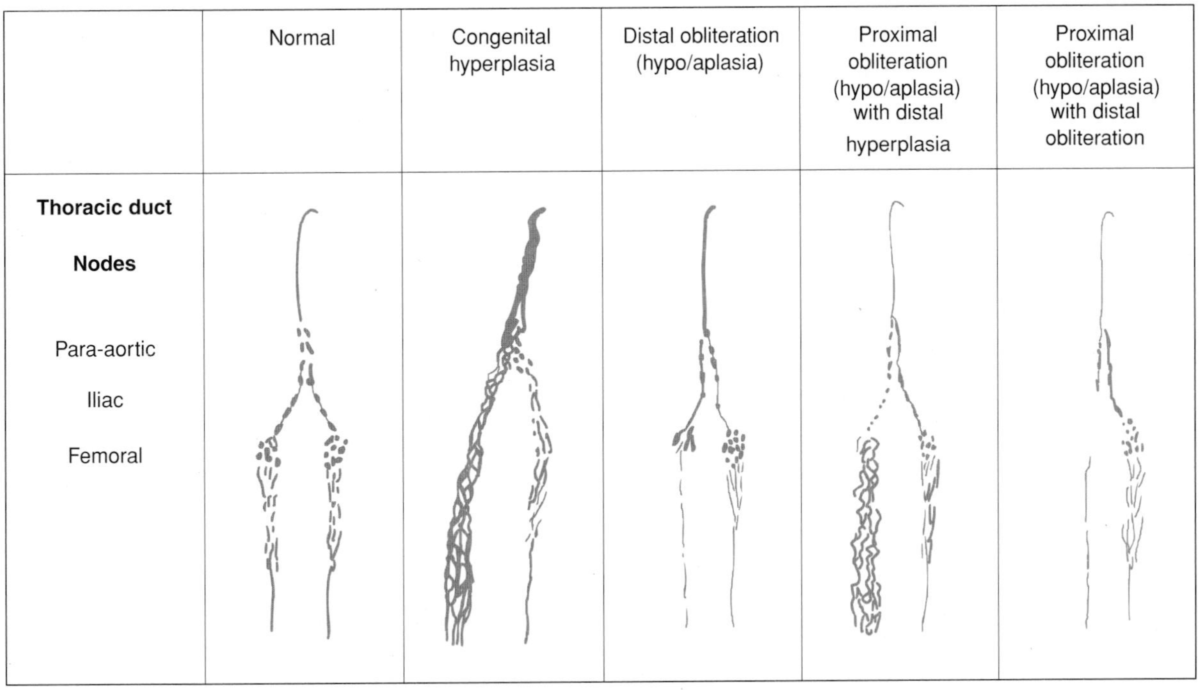

	Normal	Congenital hyperplasia	Distal obliteration (hypo/aplasia)	Proximal obliteration (hypo/aplasia) with distal hyperplasia	Proximal obliteration (hypo/aplasia) with distal obliteration
Thoracic duct					
Nodes					
Para-aortic					
Iliac					
Femoral					

Fig. 17.13 Lymphangiographic patterns of primary lymphoedema.

Other causes

Other rare, but well-documented, causes of secondary lymphoedema include tuberculosis, rheumatoid arthritis (chronic inflammation and lymph node fibrosis), and snake and insect bites. It is likely that deep venous thrombosis, chronic venous insufficiency and superficial thrombophlebitis can lead to lymphoedema. Indeed, lymphatic abnormalities are frequently observed in patients who have the skin changes of chronic venous insufficiency and venous ulceration.

Factitious lymphoedema

This may be caused by application of a tourniquet (a rut and sharp cut-off is seen on examination) or 'hysterical' misuse.

Investigation of lymphoedema

Are investigations necessary? Many clinicians diagnose lymphoedema purely on the basis of history and examination, especially when the swelling is mild and there are no apparent complicating features. Severe swelling, with unusual features, or where there may be more than one pathology contributing to the clinical picture usually warrants further investigation. Not only will this allow the diagnosis to be confirmed, but it may also provide useful prognostic information and guide management decisions.

Investigation techniques

Listed are several procedures used in the investigation of lymphoedema.

'Routine' tests. A full blood count, plasma urea and electrolytes, creatinine, liver function tests, chest radiograph and midnight blood smear for microfilariae may be indicated.

Contrast lymphangiography. Although few centres now perform this technique, it remains the standard by which all other lymphatic imaging is judged and provides precise information about the anatomy of the lymphatic system. It is now generally reserved for preoperative evaluation of patients with megalymphatics who are being considered for bypass or fistula ligation.

Technique (Kinmonth, Browse, Wolfe). The patient is admitted for limb elevation to reduce swelling and facilitate lymphatic cannulation. Originally a vital dye such as patent blue was injected and its ascent in the lymphatics to the regional nodes (in about 5–10 minutes) simply observed with the naked eye (visual lymphangiography). In patients with obliterated lymphatics dermal backflow could be observed soon after injection and the appearance of dye at the groin was delayed. This technique was soon replaced with direct contrast lymphangiography. Under local anaesthesia, a small transverse incision is made in the dorsum of the foot after 1 ml of isosulphan blue has been injected subcutaneously to identify the lymphatics. Lymphatics are dissected out under loupe magnification and a 30G needle used to infuse lipid-soluble contrast at a rate of 1 ml in 8 minutes to a maximum of 7 ml (taking about 1 hour) into each limb. Serial radiographs are taken during injection and at intervals up to 24 hours. As the procedure is uncomfortable and patients are often unable to lie still, it is frequently performed under general anaesthesia. In a normal limb the injection will usually fill between five and 15 superficial valved medial lymphatic vessels in the thigh as well as most of the inguinal lymph nodes; iliac nodes fill at between 30 and 45 minutes. Deep lymphatics, which are frequently paired and follow the deep vessels, as well as the lateral superficial lymphatics are not usually seen except in disease. Four main anatomic patterns of lymphatic disease are identified by

John Bernard Kinmonth, 1916–82. Professor of Surgery, St Thomas' Hospital, London, England.

John R. Wolfe. Surgeon, St Mary's Hospital, London.

lymphangiography; namely congenital hyperplasia, distal obliteration (hypo/aplasia), proximal obliteration with distal hyperplasia and proximal obliteration with distal obliteration (Table 17.4 and Fig. 17.13).

Isotope lymphoscintigraphy. This has largely replaced contrast lymphangiography and is used in most centres as the primary diagnostic technique.

Technique. The patient lies supine. Radioactive technetium-labelled antimony sulphide colloid particles (10 nm diameter) are injected into the web space between the second and third toes (or fingers) with a 27G needle bilaterally. This is associated with 5–10 seconds of stinging, about which the patient must be warned. The particles are specifically taken up by lymphatics and about 30 per cent of the tracer is absorbed in 3 hours. Immediately after injection a gamma camera is positioned to include the inguinal region in its upper field. During the first hour, 12 5-minute dynamic anterior exposures are taken. The patient is requested to exercise with a foot ergometer (to permit reproducible exercise and tracer clearance) for 5 minutes initially and then for 1 minute out of every subsequent 5 minutes. At 1 and 3 hours, and in selected patients at 6 and 24 hours, 20-minute whole body exposures are taken. Between exposures the patient is ambulant.

Interpretation. In a normal leg activity ascends the anteromedial aspect of the limb. Several lymph channels are seen in the calf but in the thigh they cannot usually be distinguished. Normally, radioactivity first appears in the inguinal (axillary) nodes at between 15 and 60 minutes and is symmetrical; individual nodes cannot usually be distinguished. At 60 minutes there is only faint uptake in the liver and bladder. At 3 hours there is intense activity over the liver and good symmetrical uptake in inguinal, pelvic and abdominal lymph nodes; the thoracic duct may also be seen. Most groups interpret lymphoscintigraphy qualitatively as attempts to perform quantitative assessment have produced inconsistent results. It is not possible to distinguish primary from secondary lymphoedema with certainty. However, lymphoscintigraphic patterns can be correlated to some extent with lymphangiographic findings.

- Distal obliteration is also known as aplasia or hypoplasia and is associated with little or no removal of tracer from the injection site, little or no activity in the regional nodes at 1 or 3 hours, and a cutaneous pattern of tracer distribution (dermal backflow). Although the time taken for radioactivity to reach the groin is prolonged, onward passage from there is usually normal.
- Proximal obliteration is associated with normal uptake from the injection site and appearance of tracer in inguinal nodes. However, there is a failure of tracer to progress from the inguinal lymph nodes and collaterals crossing over to other side are present.
- Lymphangectasia is associated with abnormal collections of tracer activity indicating extravasation into the peritoneal or pleural cavities or into viscera. Lymphocoeles and dilated lymph channels (megalymphatics) are also seen.

Computerised tomography. The main role of CT is to exclude pelvic or abdominal mass lesions. Although lymphoedema itself can be visualised on CT, it is of little diagnostic value in this respect.

Magnetic resonance imaging. Magnetic resonance imaging can provide clear images of lymphatic channels and lymph nodes, and can also distinguish venous and lymphatic disease as the cause of a swollen limb. However, it cannot at present provide the information available from lymphoscintigraphy, and as a cross-sectional imaging technique it appears to have little advantage over CT.

Pathological examination. In cases where malignancy is suspected, samples of lymph nodes may be obtained by fine needle aspiration, needle core biopsy or surgical excision.

Management of lymphoedema

Physical methods

The patient should elevate the foot above the level of the hip when sitting, elevate the foot of the bed when sleeping and avoid prolonged standing. Various forms of massage are effective at reducing oedema. Single- and multiple-chamber intermittent pneumatic compression devices are also useful. In most clinics the mainstay of therapy is correctly fitted graduated compression hosiery. Pressures exceeding 50 mmHg at the ankle may be required to control oedema. Below-knee stockings are usually sufficient. The patient should put the stocking on first thing in the morning when the leg is at its least swollen. General advice regarding exercise and weight reduction, if necessary, is sensible.

Drugs

Diuretics are of no value in pure lymphoedema. Their use is associated with side effects including electrolyte disturbance. The hydroxyrutosides are reported to be beneficial, as are the coumadins, but there are no scientifically robust data to support their use. Antibiotics should be prescribed promptly for cellulitis; penicillin V 500 mg four times daily for streptococcal infection and flucloxacillin 250 mg four times daily for staphylococcal infection are suitable. In severe cases there should be no hesitation in admitting the patient to hospital, elevating the limb and administering antibiotics intravenously. Antibiotics should be continued for at least 7 days or until all signs and symptoms have abated. Erythromycin is a reasonable alternative for those who are allergic to penicillin. In patients who suffer recurrent spontaneous episodes of cellulitis, long-term prophylactic antibiotic therapy may be indicated. Fungal infection (tinea pedis) must be treated aggressively; topical clotrimazole 1 per cent or miconazole 2 per cent used regularly is sufficient in most cases, but in refractory situations systemic griseofulvin 250–1000 mg daily may be required. The feet must be dried after washing and the skin kept clean and supple with water-based emollients to prevent entry of bacteria.

Surgery

Only a small minority of patients with lymphoedema benefits from surgery. Operations fall into two categories: bypass procedures and reduction procedures.

Bypass procedures

In less than 2 per cent of patients with primary lymphoedema, lymphangiography will demonstrate proximal lymphatic obstruction in the ilio-inguinal region with essentially normal distal lymphatic channels. In theory at least, such patients might benefit from lymphatic bypass. A number of methods has been described, including the omental pedicle, the skin bridge (Gillies), anastomosing lymph nodes to veins (Neibulowitz), the ileal mucosal patch (Kinmonth) and, more recently, direct lymphovenous anastomosis with the aid of the operating microscope. Although the last two techniques do appear to lead to significant improvement in about 50 per cent of patients, it is not possible to predict which patients will benefit. The procedures are technically demanding, not without morbidity and there is no controlled evidence to suggest that these procedures produce a superior outcome to best medical management alone.

Limb reduction procedures

These are indicated when a limb is so swollen that it interferes with mobility and livelihood. These operations are not 'cosmetic' in the sense that they do not create a normally shaped leg and are usually associated with significant scarring. Four operations have been described.

Sistrunk. A wedge of skin and subcutaneous tissue is excised and the wound closed primarily. This is most commonly employed to reduce the girth of the thigh.

Homan. Skin flaps are elevated and subcutaneous tissue is excised from beneath the flaps, which are then trimmed to size to accommodate the reduced girth of the limb and closed primarily. This is the most satisfactory operation for the calf (Figs 17.14 and 17.15). The main complication is skin flap necrosis. There must be at least 6 months between operations on the medial and lateral sides of the limb and the flaps must not pass the midline. This procedure has also been used on the upper limb but is contraindicated in the presence of venous obstruction or active malignancy.

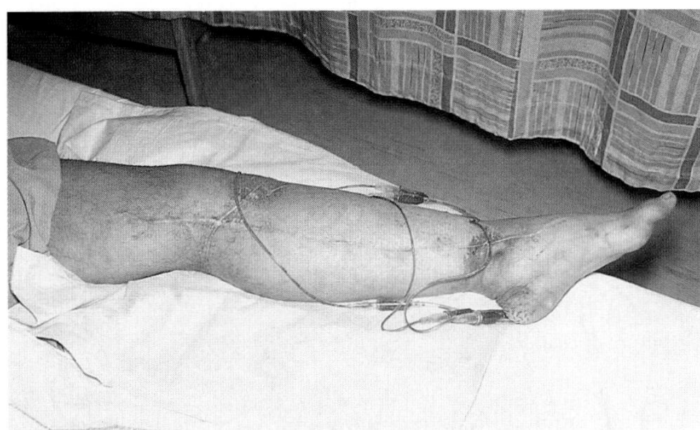

Fig. 17.15 This patient underwent a Homan's reduction procedure on the medial aspect of his left calf 5 days previously. Note the presence of suction drains removing lymphatic fluid. Postoperatively, the patient was also placed in a multichamber sequential compression device to prevent reaccumulation of lymphoedema. Once the wounds are satisfactorily healed the patient is fitted with compression hosiery which should be worn indefinitely.

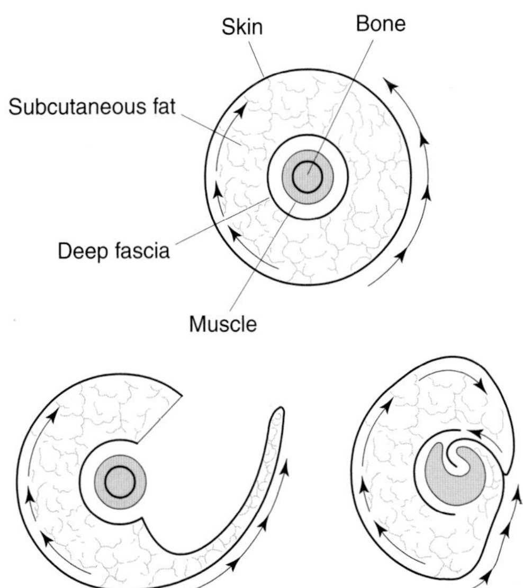

Fig. 17.16 A cross-sectional representation of Thompson's reduction operation; the buried dermal flap.

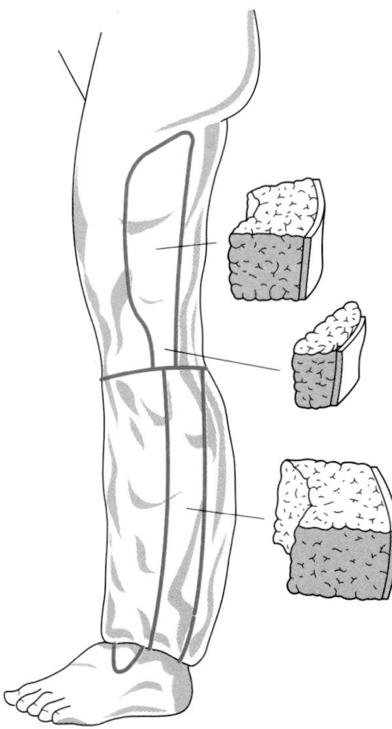

Fig. 17.14 Homan's procedure involves raising skin flaps to allow the excision of a wedge of skin and a larger volume of subcutaneous tissue down to the deep fascia. Surgery to the medial and lateral aspects of the leg must be separated by at least 6 months to avoid skin flap necrosis.

Walter Ellis Sistrunk Jr, 1880–1933. Professor of Clinical Surgery, Baylor University College of Medicine, Dallas, Texas, USA.

John Homans, 1817–1954. American surgeon. He described his sign, which is a pain in the calf experienced on dorsiflexion of the foot, in cases of thrombosis of the calf veins, in 1941.

Fredrick Thompson. 1910–75. Plastic Surgeon, Mount Vernon Hospital, London.

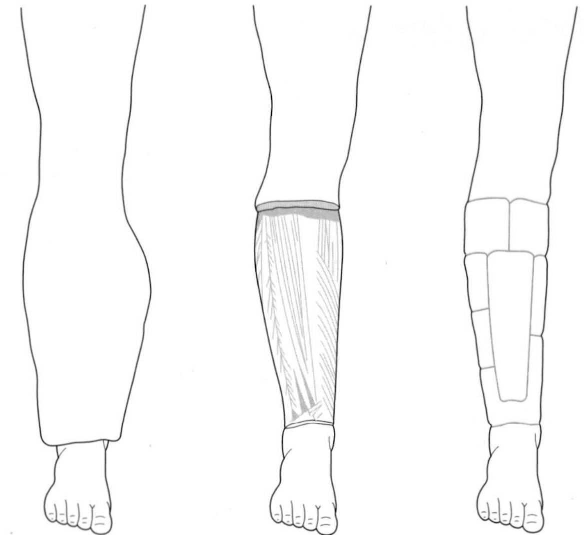

Fig. 17.17 Charles' procedure involves circumferential excision of lymphoedematous tissue down to and including the deep fascia followed by split skin grafting. This procedure gives a very poor cosmetic result but does allow the surgeon to remove very large amounts of tissue and is particularly useful in patients with severe skin changes.

Thompson. One denuded skin flap is sutured to the deep fascia and buried beneath the second skin flap (the so-called buried dermal flap) (Fig. 17.16). This procedure has become less popular as pilonidal sinus formation is common, the cosmetic result is no better than that obtained with Homan's procedure and there is no evidence that the buried flap establishes any new lymphatic connection with the deep tissues.

Charles. This operation was initially designed for filariasis and involved excision of all the skin and subcutaneous tissues down to deep fascia with coverage using split skin grafts (Fig. 17.17). This leaves a very unsatisfactory cosmetic result and graft failure is not uncommon. However, it does enable the surgeon to reduce greatly the girth of a massively swollen limb.

Other excisional surgery

Scrotal, penile and labial lymphoedema may be highly symptomatic causing embarrassment, preventing intercourse and impeding micturition. Minor swelling may be treated with support hosiery but severe swelling is best treated with excisional surgery. Lymphoedema of the eyelid may be treated by lid reduction.

Chylous ascites and chylothorax

The diagnosis may be obvious if accompanied by lymphoedema of an extremity, especially if the latter is associated with vesicles. However, some patients develop chylous ascites and/or chylothorax in isolation, in which case the diagnosis can be confirmed by aspiration and the identification of chylomicrons in the aspirate. Cytology for malignant cells should also be carried out. CT scan may show enlarged lymph nodes, and CT with guided biopsy, laparoscopy or even laparotomy and biopsy may be necessary to exclude lymphoma or other malignancy. Lymphangiography may indicate the site of a lymphatic fistula which can be surgically ligated. Even if no localised lesion is identified, it may be possible to control leakage at laparotomy or even remove a segment of affected bowel. If the problem is too diffuse to be corrected surgically, a peritoneal venous shunt may be inserted, although occlusion and infection are important complications. Medical treatment comprising the avoidance of fat in the diet and the prescription of medium-chain triglycerides (which are absorbed directly into the blood rather than via the lymphatics) may reduce swelling. Chylothorax is best treated by pleurodesis with either bleomycin, talc, pleural stripping or tetracycline. In some cases this leads to death from lymph-logged lungs as the excess lymph has nowhere to drain.

Chyluria

Filariasis is the most common cause, with chyluria occurring in 1–2 per cent of cases 10–20 years after initial infestation. It usually presents as painless passage of milky white urine, particularly after a fatty meal. The chyle may clot leading to renal colic and hypoproteinaemia may result. A clot forms in the urine on standing which does not dissolve on shaking with an equal amount of ether. The urine contains chylomicrons, and oral ingestion of fat with Sudan Red turns the urine pink. Chyluria may also be caused by ascariasis, malaria, tumour and tuberculosis, and the differential diagnosis includes gross pyuria, phosphaturia and caseous material from tuberculosis. Intravenous urography and/or lymphangiography will often demonstrate the lymphourinary fistula. Treatment includes a low-fat and high-protein diet, increased oral fluids to prevent clot colic, and laparotomy and ligation of the dilated lymphatics. Attempts have also been made to sclerose the lymphatics either directly or via instrumentation of the bladder, ureter and renal pelvis.

Lymphangiomas

Lymphangioma circumscriptum

This involves superficial proliferation of capillary sized lymphatic vessels which comprise fluid-filled vesicles on the surface and larger cisternae in the subcutaneous tissues and even adjacent muscles. These clear or slightly haemorrhagic skin vesicles have been considered either as hamartomas or as a localised deficiency in skin lymphatic drainage. Affected skin and a generous amount of subcutaneous tissue containing the vessels may be excised if they cause symptoms, but even with generous margins recurrence is common.

Cystic hygroma

Cystic hygroma is an abnormal lymph-filled, often multilocular, space which usually presents in childhood as a soft, brilliantly transluminable swelling in the base of the neck. It is also found in the head and inguinal regions as they develop from primitive lymph cisterns. It behaves like a benign tumour and grows gradually in size, leading to cosmetic problems and compression of surrounding structures. Recurrence is common after simple aspiration and injection of sclerosant. Excision is technically challenging due to the large number of vital structures in the vicinity.

Mesenteric lymph cysts

These cysts present as well-defined mobile lumps within the abdomen, the nature of which can be confirmed by either ultrasound or CT. They may be resected together with the overlying segment of small bowel if they cause symptoms.

Further reading

Browse, N. (1986) *Reducing Operations for Lymphoedema of the Lower Limb*, Wolfe, London.

Gloviczki, P. (1994) Direct operations on the lymphatics. In *Rob and Smith's Operative Surgery: Vascular Surgery* (eds C.W. Jamieson and J.S.T. Yao), Chapman & Hall, London, pp. 624–35.

O'Donnell, T.F. and Howrigan, P. (1992) Diagnosis and management of lymphoedema. In *Surgical Management of Vascular Disease* (eds P.R.F. Bell, C.W. Jamieson and C.V. Ruckley), W.B. Saunders, London, pp. 1305–28.

Szuba, A. and Rockson, S.G. (1997) Lymphedema: anatomy, physiology and pathogenesis. *Vascular Medicine*, 2, 321–6.

Wolfe, J.H.N. (1994) Lymphography. In *Rob and Smith's Operative Surgery: Vascular Surgery* (eds C.W. Jamieson and J.S.T. Yao), Chapman & Hall, London, pp. 615–24.

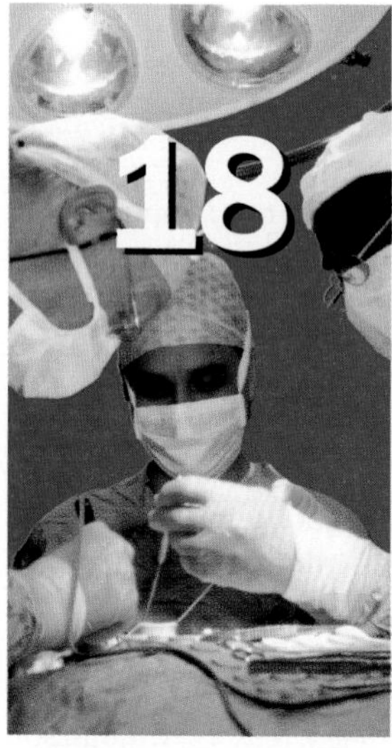

18 Accident and emergency surgery

Introduction and epidemiology

Injury is the leading cause of death and disability in the first four decades of life and is the third most common cause of death overall. This holds true even in acquired immunodeficiency syndrome (AIDS)-prevalent areas of the world. Yet, the National Academy of Science in the United States has labelled injury as the 'neglected disease of modern society'. A similar view prevails in the UK, where a leading emergency surgeon has referred to 'trauma as the neglected stepchild of modern medicine'. Public health officials world-wide concede that there is a global epidemic of violence with an increasing trend towards penetrating injury caused by knives, guns and terrorist devices. This has led to injury as a subject of study undergoing a renaissance over the last 10 years.

In the UK accidental and deliberate injury results in more than 18 000 deaths annually, with 60 000 hospital admissions costing £2.2 billion, which represents 1 per cent of gross national product (GNP). For every injury-related death there are 10 other survivors with serious injury, two of whom will have permanent disabilities. A staggering 120 000 people die from trauma each year in the USA. Ballistic trauma accounts for more than 30 000 of these, most of them in the prime of life. The cost to the USA is between $75 and $100 billion – more than the cost of the Gulf war in 1990.

Bailey & Love's Short Practice of Surgery, 23rd edition. Edited by R.C.G. Russell, N.S. Williams and C.J.K. Bulstrode. Published in 2000 by Arnold Publishers.

Mechanisms of injury

By convention, injury is classified into several categories – these are listed below.

> Types of injury
>
> - Penetrating
> - Nonpenetrating blunt
> - Blast overpressure
> - Thermal
> - Chemical
> - Other, including crush and barotrauma

In this chapter discussion centres on blunt, penetrating and blast injury only.

Impact between the body and an external object may result in tissue compression, stretching, tearing and other deformation ranging in severity from trivial to tissue injury beyond recoverable limits. The severity of damage is related to many factors, the most important of which are the amount of energy transferred and the nature and extent of the tissues over which it is applied.

In penetrating injury of low velocity and low available energy, tissue damage is focused over a small area, for example injuries caused by low-energy handguns, knives, sharp instruments, spikes of glass, wood or metal. Injury severity and outcome is related to the tissues involved. While low-velocity and low-energy injury to the soft tissue in the forearm will be slight, a similar injury involving the mediastinum might be lethal. In this case debates concerning velocity and energy transfer become academic. In high-velocity injury, associated with the potential for high-energy transfer, damage to structures may extend over a wide area remote from the wound track (see later).

In blunt injuries mechanisms may be multiple and tissue damage of complex aetiology. Mechanisms are listed below.

> Mechanisms of blunt injuries
>
> - Acceleration
> - Deceleration
> - Rotational
> - Stretch and shear

Victims of motor vehicle accidents may be injured either by rapid deceleration or by deformation with intrusion of vehicle components into the interior of the vehicle. In a crash, as deceleration occurs, the occupant's body is thrown against the interior of the vehicle, often referred to as the 'second collision'. There is also a 'third collision' between soft tissues and skeletal structures. All may contribute to injury, the extent of which will depend on the body region involved, degree of restraint and severity of the impact. Deformation and intrusion may result in blunt, penetrating or crush injury. Prolonged entrapment may exacerbate matters. Ejection of an occupant may occur, in which case rapid deceleration of the body occurs when it strikes the ground or another vehicle. Ejection is associated with increased likelihood of serious injury and death. When a pedestrian is struck by a moving vehicle there is often an acceleration injury in addition to the direct trauma at the sites of impact (Fig. 18.1). In an adult, injury is commonly due to bumper (fender) impact to the limbs; in children, such an impact is over a wider area often involving the chest and abdomen, and is associated with multiple injuries and high mortality.

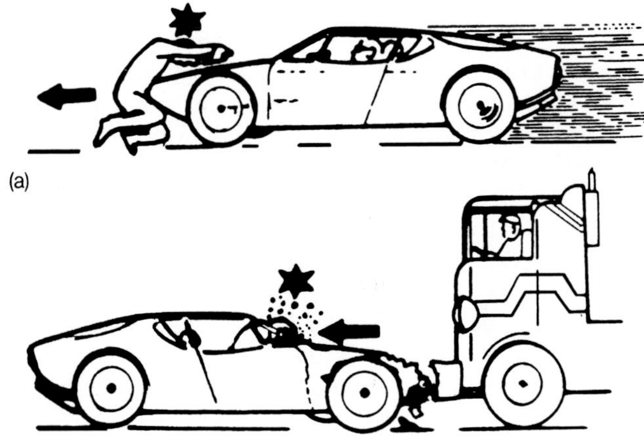

Fig. 18.1 (a) A victim struck by a fast-moving vehicle suffers blunt trauma (*) and acceleration injuries. (b) In head-on impaction-type injuries, the victim suffers blunt trauma (*) and deceleration injuries.

Patterns of injuries in road traffic accidents

Although the variety of injuries that may occur in a road traffic accident is vast, consistent patterns of injury are observed. The following are typical combinations:

- head, face and cervical spine injuries;
- cervical whiplash and sternal injuries;
- sternal fracture and dorsal spine injury;
- lower rib fractures with injury to kidneys, liver or spleen;
- intra-abdominal and diaphragmatic injuries;
- pelvic fracture with lower urinary tract injury;
- lower limb fracture with hip dislocation or spinal fracture.

Seat-belt injuries

While the wearing of automobile seat belts has undoubtedly saved many lives and has also reduced the incidence and severity of injuries to passengers, there are instances in which significant injury may be produced by their use. These lesions are secondary to restraint caused by the seat belt, whereby the occupant is forced by inertia against the straps as the vehicle rapidly decelerates. Injury may also be attributed to incorrect seat belt usage resulting in 'submarining' below the lap section of the belt on impact. While injuries to the head, face, lung, heart, aorta and liver/spleen are rarer since the introduction of seat belts, an increased incidence of injuries to stomach, duodenum, pancreas, small bowel and mesentery has been noted. Major intra-abdominal vessels may also be traumatised and fractures of the lumbar spine can occur.

Airbags

There is considerable interest in the use of airbags for drivers and front seat passengers. Evidence of their effectiveness and safety is gradually emerging with increased use. While they have saved lives, deaths, particularly in front-seat child passengers, have been reported. These were related to inadvertent inflation in slow-speed impacts with inflation velocity sufficient in some cases to decapitate. More evidence is required.

Death following injury

Dr Donald Trunkey has pointed out that deaths following injury fall broadly into three groups giving a distinct trimodal pattern (Fig. 18.2).

- Immediate deaths (50 per cent) – those occurring immediately or within the first few minutes of injury and usually due to widespread damage to the brain or upper spinal cord, the heart or major vessels, or multiple injuries. This first peak is due to injuries which are generally lethal so that little can be done in their management that is likely to affect outcome. Reduction of this peak can only be achieved by preventive measures such as wearing of

Donald D. Trunkey. Chairman, Department of Surgery, Portland, Oregon, USA.

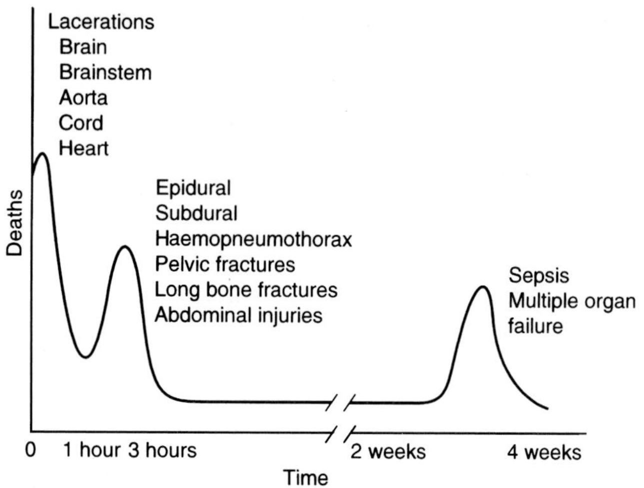

Fig. 18.2 Trimodal distribution of death following trauma based on 1500 autopsies. (adapted with permission from *Trauma* by D. Trunkey, published by *Scientific American*, 1983.)

appropriate seat belts in automobiles, head protection on bicycles and motorcycles, road safety legislation and education for pedestrians.

- Early deaths (30 per cent) – those occurring within the first few hours after injury [called by some the 'golden hour(s)' of trauma]. These deaths are deemed preventable and are due to facial injuries with developing *airway* obstruction, lethal disruption of the *breathing* mechanism, massive blood loss into body cavities or from multiple long bone fractures leading to collapse of the *circulation,* and *dysfunction* of the central nervous system due to space-occupying collections of blood within the skull. This became the basis of the ABCDE approach to initial assessment of the severely injured (see later).
- Late deaths (20 per cent) – those occurring days or weeks after injury, generally due to sepsis and multiple organ failure. Organ failure may involve the heart, kidney, liver, lung, brain and haemopoietic systems.

It is among those cases represented by the second and third peaks that potentially preventable deaths occur.

Modern management of the injured

Before turning to retrieval, hospital reception and care of the injured it is necessary to outline the fundamental changes in the management of the injured that have taken place in recent decades. The 1988 Royal College of Surgeons of England report on the management of the multiply injured highlighted that at least one in five, and possibly as many as one in three, trauma deaths in hospital were avoidable. They further concluded that death in such cases was due to medical mismanagement at every level and throughout all specialties. Later that year the Advanced Trauma Life Support Course (ATLS®) was introduced, followed by the Advanced Trauma Nursing Course (ATNC). More recently the Pre-Hospital Trauma Life Support Course (PHTLS) was introduced for those working in the prehospital setting. These training courses have radically altered the way in which the injured patient is perceived and managed throughout the chain of care from point of injury onwards. In this chapter concern is focused on management by surgeons in hospital. Nevertheless, readers must be aware that recovery following injury is dependent upon a collaborative approach involving health professionals throughout the chain of care. A break in the chain at any point is likely to affect outcome adversely. ATLS and its derived variants such as ATNC and PHTLS provide a framework and a common language throughout the chain.

The Advanced Trauma Life Support approach

Following the death of his wife and serious injury to his three children in an air crash in the 1970s, an American orthopaedic surgeon, Dr James Styner, introduced a structured trauma management training programme which was soon adopted by the American College of Surgeons and developed into the ATLS educational package now in widespread use in the UK and in 23 other countries. To date, over 200 000 doctors have been trained and the approach is now regarded as the gold standard in early trauma initial assessment and resuscitation.

The philosophy

ATLS management is based on a 'treat lethal injury first, then reassess and treat again' strategy. The steps in management are given below.

> ATLS component steps
>
> - Primary survey – identify what is killing the patient
> - Resuscitation – treat what is killing the patient
> - Secondary survey – proceed to identify all other injuries
> - Definitive care – develop a definitive management plan
>
> NB. Primary survey and resuscitation must be concurrent.

The philosophy is based on the urgency and crisis surrounding early management of a multiply injured patient whose life is in danger. Underpinning this approach is the quite recent realisation that death following injury is a function of time and occurs in a predictable and measurable way.

Dr Donald Trunkey's demonstration of the trimodal distribution of death has already been alluded to in Fig. 18.2. The ATLS approach focuses on the second or early death group where death is preventable. Within this so-called preventable group, death will follow if treatment is withheld or delayed and will do so in a predictable way. Early and effective treatment during the period when the second group of deaths occurs also reduces the number of deaths during the third phase of the trimodal distribution.

An obstructed airway in a victim with head injury will kill in 3–4 minutes, well before death might occur from the effects of injury to the brain. Equally, a life-threatening injury within the thorax will kill before a life-threatening bleed within the abdomen. Finally, major haemorrhage in the limbs, chest or abdomen will kill before a life-threatening space-occupying lesion. While these are generalisations and exceptions do occur, they support the 'primary survey and resuscitation' management doctrine. The elements of this ABCDE approach are listed below and will be explained in more detail later.

Elements of the primary survey

- **A**irway with cervical spine control
- **B**reathing and ventilation
- **C**irculation with control of haemorrhage
- **D**ysfunction of the central nervous system
- **E**xposure in a controlled environment

Prehospital retrieval and management

The aim should be for rapid and smooth transfer of patients from the scene of the accident to a hospital that is well equipped and adequately staffed, with trained personnel to deal quickly and efficiently with all of the injuries encountered.

A 'scoop and run' policy is best where transfer time to hospital is short. A 'stay and play' policy may be required in the face of entrapment but prehospital personnel must be properly trained and equipped (to PHTLS standards, for example). In all cases, attention is first paid to securing an adequate airway. Gloves are worn and a two-finger 'sweep' is used to clear solid material from the mouth and pharynx combined with good suction under direct vision to remove fluid and debris. Airway patency is then maintained by chin lift or jaw thrust manoeuvres, lifting the mandible forwards and, if appropriate, inserting an airway device (oropharyngeal/nasopharyngeal or endotracheal according to clinical judgement and expertise available). If unable to open the airway by the above, a surgical cricothyroidotomy may be performed in patients over the age of 12 years by inserting a 6-mm paediatric cuffed tracheostomy tube through the cricothyroid membrane (Fig. 18.3). Under the age of 12 years the cricoid membrane is very narrow and the cricoid cartilage is the only complete ring preventing airway collapse. Under these circumstances, a needle cricothyroidotomy may buy some time (20 minutes) provided that a means of jet-insufflating oxygen through the needle is available. Proprietary mini-tracheostomy sets should not to be used. These have a very narrow internal diameter and do not allow spontaneous ventilation. They are indicated only in critical care environments for bronchial toilet. Finally, access to the trachea should not be attempted under these conditions – tracheostomy is time-consuming and fraught with danger.

Meanwhile, attention is paid to protecting the cervical spine by the use of a well-fitting semirigid neck brace, sandbags and forehead strapping. Modern spine boards incorporate neck restraint pads and straps, and may be used in lieu of sandbags and forehead strapping (Fig. 18.4).

Other measures include ensuring adequate ventilation and oxygenation, covering and sealing open 'sucking' chest wounds, controlling external bleeding by direct pressure and monitoring the neurological status. The 'AVPU' method is recommended in the prehospital setting.

Prehospital mini-neurological examination

- **A** – **A**lert
- **V** – Responds to **V**oice
- **P** – Responds to **P**ain
- **U** – **U**nresponsive
- Pupils – Size and reaction

If there is any obvious long bone fracture of an extremity with gross deformity, the limb should be gently drawn into alignment and a traction splint applied.

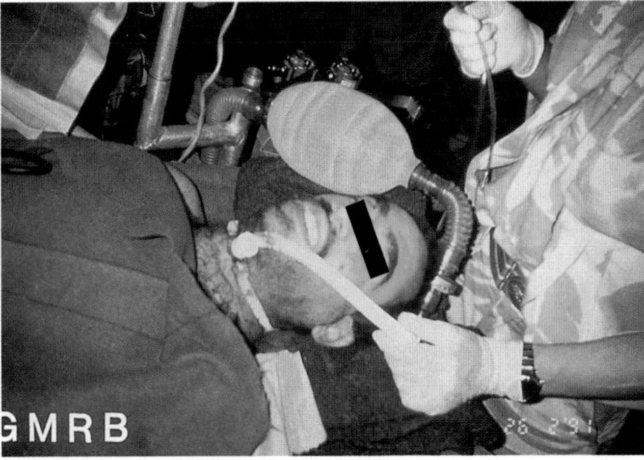

Fig. 18.3 A wounded solider during the Gulf war. Impending airway obstruction necessitated the insertion of a 6-mm paediatric tracheostomy tube through the cricothyroid membrane. The casualty, while able to ventilate spontaneously, is being assisted with a bag–valve–mask device entraining oxygen (*courtesy of The BATLS training team, Chester*).

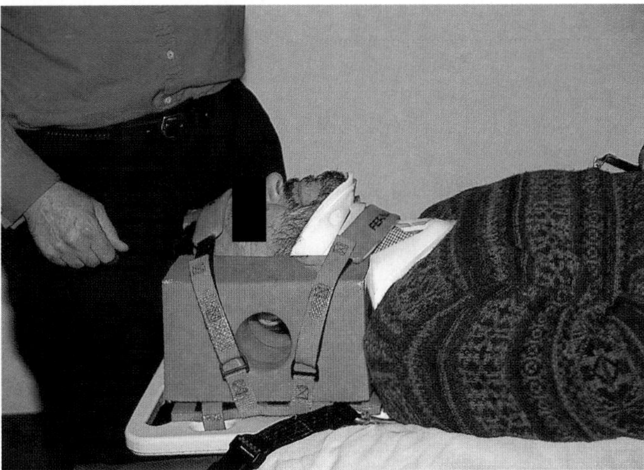

Fig. 18.4 An injured patient on a long spine board with cervical spine immobilisation.

Controversy exists regarding the prehospital role in resuscitation by intravenous fluid infusion. Vascular access in a cold, shocked injury victim is often difficult and time-consuming, and there is emerging evidence that a degree of hypotension (systolic blood pressure 80–85 mmHg) may be safely tolerated (see later). If circumstances dictate that transfer time will be prolonged, or when entrapment and difficulty in extrication is encountered, then more sophisticated and advanced life-support measures may be instituted with the caveat made at the beginning of this section.

Management in hospital

Reception in hospital

Planning and preparation

Accident departments dealing with the injured must have purpose-built and well-equipped resuscitation rooms. Medical staff should ideally be trained in a trauma system – ATLS provides an ideal framework within which to work and certification will soon be compulsory in the UK. Certification is already compulsory in North America. Nursing and other professional staff should also be trained within the system. Another advantage of a structured approach relates to equipment and layout. Working within a system removes debate concerning intravenous fluid type and amounts, techniques and investigations to be performed, and the summoning of appropriate specialists. Agreement in these areas is laid down in advance and allows medical teams to work within a common language and sequence.

The trauma team

While a suitably trained doctor can successfully assess and resuscitate an injured patient while working to a system, it is obvious that a team approach is more efficient and is quicker. This is the vertical (alone) versus the horizontal (team) argument. Dr Peter Driscoll in Salford has shown clearly the benefits of a team in improving outcome. The team should initially comprise four doctors, five nurses and a radiographer. Roles should be paired and tasks allocated on a pre-agreed basis. To avoid chaos, there should be no more than six people physically attending to the patient at any one time. Others should stand back until called to perform specific tasks such as vascular access, radiographic assessment or assisting in log rolling. The team should have a leader responsible for co-ordination and at least one member should be a trained general surgeon. Injury is a surgical disease and surgical consultation is required throughout.

Controversy once surrounded the mobilisation of the trauma team, with accusations of inappropriate call-out resulting in time wasted from clinics and operating lists. This has now been resolved by widespread acceptance of trauma team call-out criteria. Agreed factors indicating high risk of multiple injuries and justifying trauma team mobilisation are (after Champion):

- penetrating injury to the chest, abdomen, head, neck or groin;
- two or more proximal long bone fractures;
- flail chest and pulmonary contusion;
- evidence of high-energy impact:
  - falls of 2 m (6 feet) or more;
  - changes in velocity in an road traffic accident of 32 km/hour (20 miles/hour) or more estimated from outward deformity of car;
  - rearward displacement of front axle;
  - sideward intrusion of 35 cm or more on the patient's side of the car;
  - ejection of the patient;
  - rollover;
  - death of another person in the same car;
  - pedestrian hit at more than 32 km/hour.

Initial assessment and resuscitation

The objectives in this phase are to seek and manage immediately life-threatening conditions. In ATLS language this is the 'primary survey and resuscitation', following an ABCDE sequence in every circumstance. The description that follows holds good for vertical (alone) or horizontal (team) management. The only radiographs permitted during this phase are:

- cross-table lateral cervical spine;
- antero-posterior supine chest X-ray;
- antero-posterior plain pelvic film.

A – Airway management and cervical spine control

Injury to the cervical spine is assumed in the presence of injury above the clavicle, loss or alteration of conscious level, involvement in high-speed collisions or where there is a history of neck pain. Airway assessment and management is performed with the cervical spine immobilised in the neutral position by manual in-line immobilisation or by a well-fitting neck brace, sandbags and forehead tape. Many injured patients arrive in the accident department with neck protection already *in situ*. In a conscious patient, speaking in a normal voice, the airway is patent and the brain is being adequately perfused. If the patient does not reply to a simple question, the airway is opened and dealt with as described for prehospital personnel. If there is any doubt concerning the integrity of the airway, skilled anaesthetic help should be summoned if not already present as part of an attending trauma team. All injured patients require supplemental oxygen at 15 litres/minute via a mask with a rebreathing bag.

Peter Driscoll. Senior Lecturer in Emergency Medicine and Critical Care, The Hope Hospital, Salford, England.

Howard Champion. Professor of Surgery and Trauma, Department of Surgery, Uniformed Services University for the Health Sciences, Bethesda, Maryland, USA.

B – Breathing and ventilation

The neck and chest are exposed. Examination involves inspection, palpation, percussion and auscultation. The examination starts in the neck with inspection for wounds, condition of neck veins, wounds and evidence of tracheal injury. The respiratory rate is counted and recorded, with the time noted. Chest symmetry and respiratory effort are assessed. Wounds and bruising are noted. Palpation, particularly to include the sides and back (without spinal movement), is performed gently followed by percussion and auscultation. A dull percussion note and absent breath sounds over a hemithorax in the presence of shock are indicative of massive haemothorax (see Box 18.6). The objective is to hunt out and treat the six life-threatening thoracic conditions listed below.

Immediately life-threatening thoracic conditions

- Airway obstruction (dealt with under 'A')
- Tension pneumothorax
- Massive pneumothorax (> 1500 ml blood in a hemithorax)
- Open pneumothorax ('sucking wound')
- Flail segment with pulmonary contusion
- Cardiac tamponade (almost always penetrating injury)

Tension pneumothorax requires immediate needle thoracocentesis in the second intercostal space in the midclavicular line on the affected side, followed by tube thoracostomy through the fifth intercostal space just anterior to the midaxillary line. Massive haemothorax is a combined breathing (B) and circulation (C) problem with death likely from hypovolaemic shock and impaired ventilation. Management is therefore by vigorous support of the circulation followed by tube thoracostomy. Open pneumothorax is managed by sealing the wound with a dressing secured on three sides followed by tube thoracostomy. Following insertion of the tube, the dressing is sealed on the fourth side. Flail segment with underlying contusion (always present) requires consultation with anaesthetic colleagues as endotracheal intubation and mechanical ventilation may be required to maintain adequate arterial oxygen saturation. Diagnosis of cardiac tamponade requires a high index of suspicion, particularly if a penetrating wound is noted medial to the nipples anteriorly or medial to the scapulae posteriorly. Needle pericardiocentesis may be life-saving in the short term; thoracotomy and repair are required for definitive management.

C – Circulation and haemorrhage control

This begins with assessment for signs of shock (see Chapter 4). Tachycardia in a cold patient indicates shock. Equally, shock associated with injury is hypovolaemic until ruled out. Causes of shock are listed below.

Causes of shock following injury

- Hypovolaemic – haemorrhagic (most common)
- Cardiogenic or pump failure (cardiac tamponade, tension pneumothorax or myocardial contusion)
- Neurogenic (often combined with hypovolaemic shock and masked)
- Septic (a late event > 24 hours and associated with missed faecal spillage)

An early attempt should be made to assess the degree of blood loss. Table 18.1 lists four classes based on volume loss expressed as actual amounts and percentages (to be used for adults only).

Blood loss may be external and obvious, or internal and covert, or combinations of both. External bleeding sites are dealt with by direct pressure at this stage. A hunt must be undertaken for signs of covert bleeding. Bleeding in the chest will have been noted already. The abdomen and pelvis must be rapidly assessed for signs of injury. A good aide-mémoire is 'blood on the floor and four more':

- blood on floor or environment, including clothing;
- blood in the chest (dull percussion note);
- abdomen (wounds, abrasions, tenderness but may be silent);
- pelvis (usually associated with obvious pelvic disruption);
- limbs (should be obvious).

The presence of shock demands the presence of a surgeon, appropriate to the region injured if this is obvious. Whereas intravenous fluid administration has a vital role, the emphasis must be on stopping the bleeding by surgical means. Vascular access for resuscitation is by cannulation of peripheral veins – if this fails, venous cut-down at the ankle or elbow is recommended. Once a cannula is in position, 20 ml of blood should be withdrawn for group, type or full cross-match depending on the degree of urgency. Central access will be required later for monitoring but is not a good route for initial resuscitation owing to slow flow rates, technical difficulty and uncertainty concerning position of the catheter

Table 18.1 Classification of shock (hypovolaemic)

	Class 1	*Class 2*	*Class 3*	*Class 4*
Blood loss	< 15 per cent (750 ml)	15–30 per cent (0.8–1 litre)	30–40 per cent (1.5–2 litres)	> 40 per cent (> 2 litres)
Systolic blood pressure	No change	No change	Reduced	Reduced markedly
Pulse rate	Slight increase	100–120 beats/minute	> 120 beats/minute, weak	> 120 beats/minute, thready
Respiratory rate	Normal	Increased	> 20 breaths/minute	20–30 breaths/minute
Urinary output	30 ml/hour	20–30 ml/hour	> 20 ml/hour	Negligible
Capillary refill	Normal (2 seconds)	Delayed (> 2 seconds)	Delayed (> 2 seconds)	Very delayed
Colour	Normal	Pale and cold	Pale and cold	Grey–ashen
Mental state	Alert	Anxious	Anxious and aggressive	Drowsy, confused, unconscious

tip. There is revival of interest in interosseous access for adults. It is too early to comment on its utility for general use. Its place is well established for children under the age of 6 years and should be resorted to without hesitation if peripheral access fails on two attempts. Special paediatric interosseous needles are available commercially.

In adults, 1–2 litres of warmed Hartmann's (Ringer's) solution is recommended as an initial fluid challenge. The initial volume in children is calculated according to weight and is by convention 20 ml/kg body weight. This bolus may be repeated once.

The patient should now be reassessed. The three responses that may be seen are given below.

Responses to initial fluid challenge

- Immediate and sustained return to normal vital signs
- Transient response with later deterioration
- No improvement

Immediate responders are likely to have less than 20 per cent blood loss and bleeding will have ceased spontaneously or by direct pressure – an open fracture of tibia, for example. Transient responders may have intra-abdominal or thoracic bleeding, and surgical intervention will be required. Non-responders are bleeding actively, usually in a body cavity, or shock is nonhaemorrhagic in nature. Hypovolaemic patients have lost over 40 per cent of their blood volume, demanding immediate surgical intervention. Continuing intravenous fluid administration may actually be detrimental.

D – Dysfunction of the central nervous system

The AVPU and pupillary assessment carried out by pre-hospital personnel is repeated (see Box 18.5). In addition, a rapid assessment of motor and sensory function is performed looking only for gross and obvious signs. A more detailed assessment will be carried out during the secondary survey (see later).

E – Exposure and environment

Any remaining clothing should now be removed. The environment must be considered. If too cold, hypothermia will ensue. Blankets or air heaters should be used if available.

Critical decisions

The response of the injured patient to the primary survey and resuscitation phase will influence decision making. A patient in whom no life-threatening condition was found, or one whose condition responded well and in a sustained way, is now fit for a full secondary assessment which may be carried out in the resuscitation room or in a ward area following admission. Some patients will have failed to respond and require immediate removal to the operating theatre. Examples include disruptive pelvic injury, major liver laceration or injuries to multiple body systems requiring immediate control of blood loss – these are relatively rare. Initial surgery in this instance is part of the primary survey and a secondary survey, although deferred, must not be forgotten. Good note-keeping and records are vital. A significant number of patients will respond transiently and is best taken to a critical care environment where more advanced resuscitation techniques and assessments are possible. Such patients will require surgery but it is usually possible to investigate and plan in advance. Examples include splenic laceration, bowel injury, diaphragmatic disruption, or multiple fractures and soft-tissue wounds. In summary, the patient may be taken to the ward, critical care unit or to theatre.

Secondary survey

This phase comprises a head-to-toe examination of the undressed and stable patient. It is lengthy and includes a detailed history if this is feasible. The examination may be conducted in any order. The description here starts with the head and works distally. At this time check that vital signs monitoring devices are *in situ*. These should include a pulse oximeter and an oesophageal or a rectal thermometer. During this phase detailed radiographic procedures including computerised tomography (CT) and dye studies may be performed. Patients should be stable and can therefore travel safely for CT, ultrasound or even magnetic resonance imaging (MRI) investigations if these are indicated.

Head and Glasgow Coma Scale (GCS)

A thorough check is undertaken for signs of external injury such as bruising, laceration or bony deformity. Depressed skull fractures may or may not be palpable.

Table 18.2 Glasgow Coma Scale (GCS)

Eye opening	
Spontaneous	4
To voice	3
To pain	2
None	1
Verbal reponse	
Orientated	5
Confused	4
Inappropriate words	3
Incomprehensible sounds	2
None	1
Motor response	
Obeys command	6
Localises pain	5
Withdraws (pain)	4
Flexion (pain)	3
Extension (pain)	2
None	1
Total	3–15

Henri Charles Antoine Hartmann, 1860–1952. Professor of Surgery, Paris, France.
Sydney Ringer, 1834–1910. British physician.

At this stage, the patient's conscious level is determined by applying the GCS, which measures eye opening, best verbal response and best motor response. The coding for each is given in Table 18.2.

The use of this coding system is detailed fully in Chapter 35 on 'Cranium and head injury'. Neurological deterioration may indicate a haemorrhagic space-occupying lesion or rising intracranial pressure, or it may be due to hypoxia and hypoperfusion. Hypercarbia and hypoxia are the commonest causes of the preventable 'second injury' in head-injured patients. Hypotension in a head-injured adult should lead to a further search for evidence of blood loss elsewhere.

The nostrils and external auditory meatus are examined for rhinorrhoea or otorrhoea. *Cerebrospinal fluid from these orifices mixed with blood produces a double ring if dropped on a hospital sheet or pillowcase.*

Face

Maxillofacial injuries are discussed in Chapter 38. In summary, the eyes are checked for foreign bodies, perforation, subconjunctival haemorrhage, visual acuity, and pupillary and corneal reflexes. The mandible is checked for fracture and stability. Maxillary stability is also assessed – fractures of the middle third of the face may be displaced with risk to the airway, either immediately or late as a result of expanding haematoma. The mouth is checked again for broken teeth, loose dentures and foreign bodies. Check also for retropharnygeal haematoma. This may be associated with previously undetected cervical spine injury.

Neck

Look for subcutaneous emphysema. Palpate (gently) the cervical spine. A lateral radiograph showing all seven cervical vertebrae and the upper border of the first thoracic is essential in all multisystem injury patients. Particular care should be taken not to miss lesions at C1, C2 and C7 levels – fractures and dislocations at these levels are notoriously unstable. Downward traction on the arms while the film is being taken will enhance the demonstration of the lower cervical and T1 vertebrae. In some cases a 'swimmer's view' may be necessary – see also Chapter 33 on the spine.

Thorax

Start by repeating the steps on thoracic assessment performed in the primary survey. The search is now for potentially life-threatening and less serious injuries. These are listed below. Remember, penetrating and blunt injury below the nipples (male patient) raises the likelihood of injury to intra-abdominal structures, in particular the liver, spleen, stomach and transverse colon. Simple haemothorax and pneumothorax may be picked up on an anteroposterior (AP) supine chest radiograph. Tube thoracostomy will suffice in most instances. Check also for the integrity of diaphragm, particularly on the left.

Secondary survey – potentially life-threatening injuries

- Pulmonary contusion
- Myocardial contusion
- Aortic tear
- Diaphragmatic tear
- Oesophageal tear
- Tracheobronchial tear

Abdomen

The secondary survey is the phase of 'fingers and tubes' in every orifice. This particularly applies to the abdomen. Nasogastric and urinary catheters are inserted for diagnostic and assessment purposes. The abdomen is now fully examined in the usual way. A rectal examination and inspection of the perineum is mandatory. At this time please read the relevant sections on specific injuries in Chapters 50–61 inclusive. Wounds should be covered with sterile dressings or towels. Eviscerated bowel should be covered in warm wet packs and must not be returned to the peritoneum at this stage. Assessment of the abdomen in cases of penetrating trauma is relatively easy. In most instances the abdomen will need to be explored. In some large centres, protocols may permit local exploration of stab wounds in stable patients. Difficulty arises in cases of blunt injury, all the more when multiple injuries are present or where the conscious level is altered. Diagnostic peritoneal lavage, ultrasound examination or, in some specialist centres, laparoscopy may be required to detect covert intra-abdominal injury. The retroperitoneum is notoriously silent. All of the foregoing remarks refer to stable patients. Any deterioration should lead to consideration of rapid surgical exploration.

Pelvis

The pelvis is gently compressed and distracted manually to check for pain enhancement and pelvic stability. If not already to hand, an AP radiograph of the pelvic ring should be obtained. Blood at the urinary meatus may indicate urethral injury. If injury is suspected, get expert help. If not available, do not catheterise; instead, place a suprapubic catheter. Please also read the sections on specific injuries in Chapters 63–68 inclusive.

Spinal injuries

Please read the relevant sections in Chapter 33. Tests are made for peripheral sensory and motor defects. In spinal injuries with unstable fractures, further neurological damage can be caused by moving the patient inappropriately. Full examination will require the patient to be log rolled when sufficient personnel are present. At least five people are needed. The team leader should control the neck and coordinate. Three others are needed to effect rolling the torso and limbs, and a doctor to examine the back and perineum. A rectal examination is performed if not done before. In large urban centres, severely injured patients may be transported to hospital on a long spine board. Removal from the board on to a hospital trolley requires the same care as for a log roll.

Extremities

The limbs should be fully assessed for evidence of injury. This should include a complete neurovascular examination. Appropriate radiographs may be obtained at this stage. Readers are also referred to Chapters 21–23 for more detailed discussions on specific injuries.

Drug administration

As part of the early management of the injured patient, consideration should be given to administration of analgesics. Opiates are best, given in small intravenous increments. Antibiotics and tetanus prophylaxis may also be appropriate.

Definitive care plan

A position should now have been reached where a daily management and definitive plan is initiated. Patients with multiple injuries may require the attention of a number of specialists. A decision on 'ownership' must be made but with arrangements for all involved to have access. The patient should not 'fall between two stools', without anyone in overall charge. The most appropriate person to take primary responsibility in such cases is usually the general or orthopaedic surgeon.

Emerging concepts and techniques

Permissive hypotension

Also called hypotensive resuscitation, this concept is of increasing interest to trauma surgeons faced with intra-abdominal or intrathoracic haemorrhage. The important question is whether the systolic blood pressure needs to be returned to premorbid levels utilising fluid resuscitation. In nontrauma patients, vascular patients for example, controlled preoperative hypotension is well established in certain situations. Further, recent research in the USA seems to deprecate the use of rapid infusion systems (RIS), with evidence emerging that large volume fluid resuscitation to achieve normal systolic blood pressures is associated with increased mortality compared with injured patients resuscitated with small fluid volumes prior to surgery. An increasingly accepted view holds that moderate hypotension – systolic blood pressure of 85–90 mmHg – is sufficient to maintain vital organ perfusion and avoids a hypertensive overshoot with the risk of precipitating further haemorrhage. The concept is still new in the care of the injured and further trials on optimal fluids, levels of permissive hypotension and the effects of delay before surgery are needed before it can be safely assimilated. *The most important message to retain is that the best treatment for ongoing haemorrhage is to turn off the tap and not to continue infusion of fluids, including blood products.*

Damage control – staged or abbreviated laparotomy

The concept of staged operative procedures for the severely injured patient is not new. The earliest uses of the approach concerned perihepatic packing for extensive liver injury. While the commonest indication remains catastrophic intra-abdominal haemorrhage, the technique now has wider application. The technique should usually be considered as part of the primary survey and resuscitation phases in patients who fail to respond to nonoperative resuscitation methods. The indications suggested by Dr Gene Moore and his colleagues in Denver are listed in Table 18.3.

Table 18.3 Indications for staged or abbreviated laparotomy (damage control)

- Inability to achieve control of haemorrhage in the face of worsening coagulopathy
- Inaccessible major venous injury
- Time-consuming procedure in a poorly resuscitated patient
- Management of extra-abdominal life-threatening injury (e.g. active pelvic haemorrhage)
- Inability to close abdominal wall due to reperfusion splanchnic oedema
- Re-assessment of intra-abdominal contents required (e.g. compromised intestinal blood supply due to extensive mesenteric injury)

The technical aspects of the procedure are dictated by the pattern of injuries. The objectives are listed below.

Objectives of staged or abbreviated laparotomy

- Arrest haemorrhage
- Control or limit coagulopathy
- Limit cavity contamination
- Protect viscera and limit fluid/protein loss

Having achieved the objectives, the patient is returned to a critical care environment for continuing monitoring, resuscitation and in-depth investigation prior to a second definitive procedure. Moore terms this 'physiological restoration in a surgical intensive care unit'. Timing for the definitive procedure varies but is usually within 24 hours of the damage-control procedure.

Focused abdominal sonogram for trauma (FAST)

Portable, hand-held ultrasound is now being used by trauma surgeons in the USA in the evaluation of patients with blunt thoracoabdominal trauma, and is the preferred initial technological assessment of the patient. It belongs early on in the secondary survey, although some centres advocate its use during the 'C' component of the primary survey to localise intra-abdominal haemorrhage and to rule out cardiac tamponade in overtly shocked patients where no haemorrhage source is evident. The technique is rapid, with only four areas being scanned at the initial investigation (Fig. 18.5). One of the greatest challenges will be to train trauma surgeons in the use of the technology.

Ernest E. Moore. Chief, Department of Surgery, Denver Health Medical Center and the University of Colorado Health Sciences Center, USA.

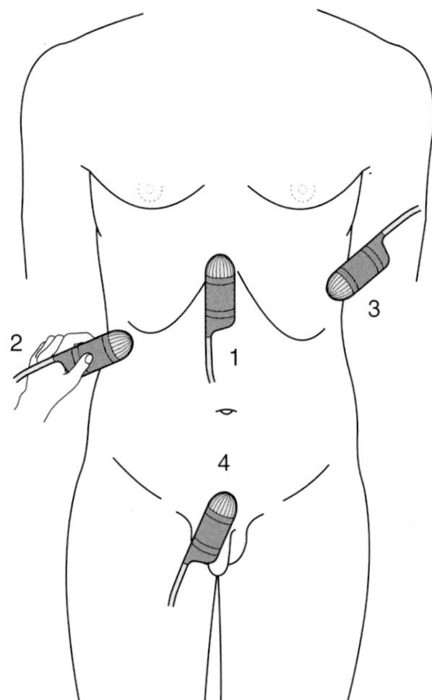

Fig. 18.5 The four areas to be scanned during focused abdominal sonogram for trauma (FAST). The aim is to rule out cardiac tamponade, the presence of free blood and solid organ disruption.

Multiple and mass casualties

In both major civil disasters and war, patient numbers may for a time exceed the capacity of medical teams to render normal care. Under these circumstances, it is necessary to sort casualties on the basis of need so that available resources and personnel can render the 'most for the most', to quote an American military surgeon. This is 'triage' and it is outlined below. Triage assessments and categorisation should be delegated to a senior, experienced and trained doctor. Failure to perform correct triage will disrupt optimal management for those most at need and divert scarce resources, often to those who can wait. Triage is a dynamic process and needs to be repeated at each level of care from point of injury until arrival in hospital. In general, field triage is for evacuation to hospital. Once in hospital, triage is for access to resuscitation and to operating rooms. The concept is at the heart of major incident planning and is outlined below.

Triage

Triage (from the French 'trier') means to sift or to sort and refers to the allocation of injured patients into certain categories for action by emergency teams. A common scheme of assessment is presented below.

- *Triage sieve* – a quick survey is made to separate the dead and the walking from the injured.
- *Triage sort* – remaining casualties are now assessed and allocated to three or four groups according to local protocols:
  - category 1 – critical and cannot wait. Airway obstruction and catastrophic haemorrhage are examples;
  - category 2 – urgent. Serious injury but can wait a short time, 30 minutes in most systems;
  - category 3 – less serious injuries. Not endangered by delay;
  - category 4 – expectant. Severe multisystem injury. Survival not likely;
  - (optional) – heavy manpower demands.

The system outlined above is only one of many. Readers should familiarise themselves with local custom and policy. The ABCDE of ATLS is now used increasingly as a means of assessment for grading.

Audit and quality assurance

Injury severity scoring systems

Statistical analysis of injury severity and the most effective means of managing injured patients is relatively recent and is slowly replacing anecdote and unfounded assumptions. An example is the GCS, to which reference has already been made. The most widely applied is the Revised Trauma Score (RTS). Data combined from vital signs and level of consciousness are mathematically combined into a single variable that correlates with outcome (Table 18.4). There is a myriad of others. Readers are referred to Professor Yates' paper in the publication *ABC of Major Trauma*.

Major trauma outcome study (MTOS)

First developed in the USA, MTOS is an ongoing audit of the effectiveness of injury management and is now in widespread use in the UK. Utilising the TRISS (combination of the RTS and Injury Severity Score weighted for age and premorbidity) method with additional input on prehospital events, initial management including time to resuscitative interventions and the grading of medical staff, MTOS is applied to patients with severe injury and to those who die or are transferred to specialist units. The benefits are summarised in Box 18.11.

Box 18.11 Benefits of MTOS

- Measures injury severity
- Records management and outcome
- Provides a database for audit
- Allows comparison of performance

Table 18.4 Revised Trauma Score (RTS)

Glasgow Coma Scale	*Systolic blood pressure (mmHg)*	*Respiratory rate (breaths/minute)*	*Points*
13–15	> 89	10–19	4
9–12	76–89	> 29	3
6–8	50–75	6–9	2
4–5	1–49	1–5	1
3	0	0	0

David W. Yates. Professor of Accident and Emergency Medicine, Hope Hospital, Salford, England.

Further reading

Driscoll, P. (1996) Initial assessment and management – I: primary survey. In *ABC of Major Trauma* (eds D. Skinner, P. Driscoll and R. Earlam), BMJ Publishing Group, London, pp. 1–5.

Driscoll, P. and Skinner, D. (1996) Initial assessment and management – II: secondary survey. In *ABC of Major Trauma* (eds D. Skinner, P. Driscoll and R. Earlam), BMJ Publishing Group, London, pp. 6–10.

Hyde, J.A.J., Rooney, S.J. and Graham, T.R. (1998) Hypotensive resuscitation. In *Trauma* (eds I. Greaves, J.M. Ryan and K.M. Porter), Arnold, London, pp. 177–85.

Walters, M. and Yates, D.W. (1997) Epidemiology of road traffic accidents. In *Scientific Foundations of Trauma* (eds G.J. Cooper, H.A. Dudley, D.S. Gann, R.A. Little and R.L. Maynard), Butterworth-Heinemann, Oxford, pp. 151–64.

Westaby, S. (1989) *Trauma Pathogenesis and Treatment*, Heinemann Medical Books, Oxford.

Yates, D.W. (1996) Scoring systems. In *ABC of Major Trauma* (eds D. Skinner, P. Driscoll and R. Earlam), BMJ Publishing Group, London, pp. 83–7.

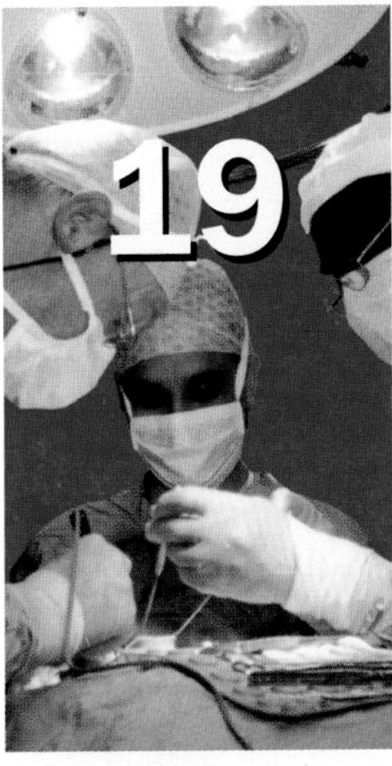

19 Warfare injuries

Introduction and epidemiology

Penetrating missile wounds, injuries from blast phenomena and burns are the typical features of modern conventional war. This chapter is concerned only with missile wounds and blast injury. Burn injury is covered in Chapter 14. Missile wounds are caused by bullets or by fragments from exploding shells, mines or bombs. Exposure to blast phenomena may result in unique and complex injury patterns, and these will be described.

There is a wealth of data on the cause and distribution of wounds in wars over the last 30 years. Care is needed in interpretation as the number of wounded varies greatly in each series. For example, Vietnam data cover over 17 000 casualties. In contrast, Gulf war data are restricted to 63 casualties. Inclusion criteria are also very variable and many fail to record multiple injuries to different body systems in single casualties – the hallmark of modern war injury. Tables 19.1–19.3 summarise the available data.

Table 19.1 Cause of war wounds 1966–1991

War zone and date	*Fragments (per cent)*	*Bullet (per cent)*	*Mine (per cent)*	*Other (per cent)*
Vietnam 1966–1967	37	26	11	26
Vietnam 1970	45	30	3	22
Falklands 1982	45	32	11	12
Lebanon 1982	32	20	4	44
Afghanistan 1985	50	38	10	2
Gulf 1991	72	20	8	–

While care is needed in interpreting the available data, some broad statements concerning war injury can be made. The most common wounding agent in surviving casualties is a fragment wound, not a bullet wound as many erroneously believe. Limb injuries predominate, pointing to the high lethality of hits to the trunk and head. The most startling revelation is the emerging incidence of multiple hits to multiple body regions in survivors. This is a deliberate policy – the aim in modern war is to incapacitate, not kill. The reason is clear: large numbers of surviving casualties are a major financial and logistic burden on a nation engaged in total war.

In conclusion, the factors that govern the nature, severity and outcome of a war wound are many and include the weapon systems deployed, the environment in which the weapon systems are deployed, and the quality and timing of medical management. In short, there is no single entity that merits the description 'the war wound'.

Wound ballistics and mechanisms of injury

As a missile traverses the body it causes injury by transferring some or all of its available energy, and this is manifested by lacerating and crushing tissues in its path and, in some cases, injury remote from the missile path (see below). The amount of energy transferred may be expressed by the formula:

Bailey & Love's Short Practice of Surgery, 23rd edition. Edited by R.C.G. Russell, N.S. Williams and C.J.K. Bulstrode. Published in 2000 by Arnold Publishers.

Table 19.2 Distribution of war wounds 1966–1991

War zone and date	*Head and neck (per cent)*	*Thorax (per cent)*	*Abdomen (per cent)*	*Upper limb (per cent)*	*Lower limb (per cent)*
Vietnam 1966–1967	24	20	14	40	50
Middle East 1973	15	8	6	29	27
Falklands 1982	14	7	12	27	41
Afghanistan 1985	12	3	12	26	43
Gulf 1991	6	12	11	44	75

Table 19.3 Gulf war 1991 – missile wounds and body areas involved (*n* = 51)

	Patients	
Number of body areas	*Number*	*Percentage*
1	19	37
2	10	20
3	10	20
4	9	17
> 5*	3	6

*One surviving casualty had 47 wounds across three body systems.

$$KE = \frac{1}{2}M\left(V_1^2 - V_2^2\right)$$

where KE is the available energy, M is the mass, and V_1 and V_2 are the velocities at entry and at exit, respectively. In general, bullets fired from handguns and most modern fragment munitions are propelled at low velocity, have low available energy (100–500 J) and result in *low-energy transfer wounds*. Missiles with high available energy (2000–3000 J) include high-velocity assault rifle bullets (> 900 m/second) and some large fragments, and have potential to cause *high-energy transfer wounds* (Figs 19.1 and 19.2). Some modern high-performance handguns are now capable of firing high-velocity bullets with high available energy.

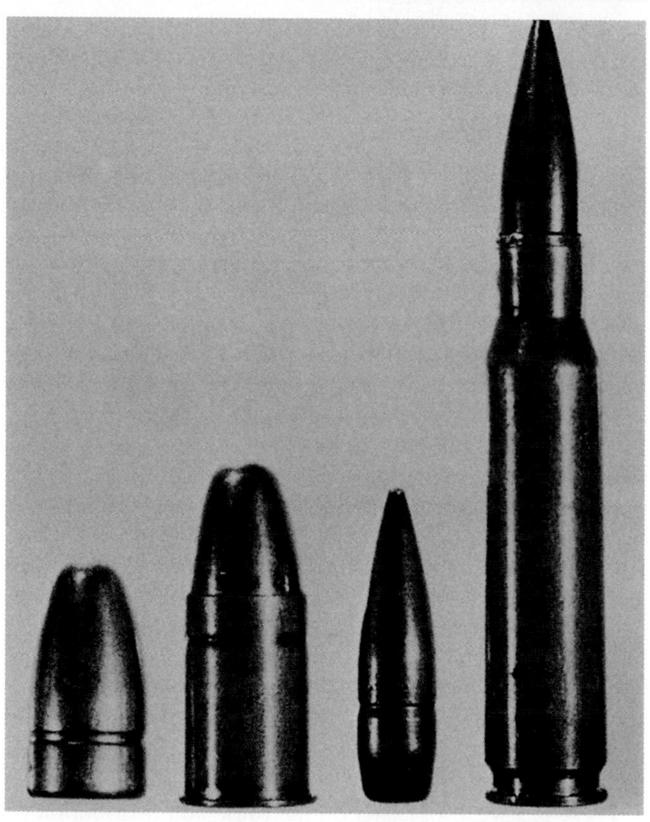

Fig. 19.1 Two bullets shown with and without their casings. A low-velocity type of bullet is shown on the left and a high-velocity bullet on the right (*courtesy of Professor T.G. Parks, Belfast*).

By convention, missile wounds are now described in terms of energy transfer, not velocity as was the custom, recognising that velocity is merely one factor determining energy available and its transfer to tissues. *Low-energy transfer* wounds are characterised by injury confined to the wound track. *High-energy transfer* wounds also cause local laceration and crush injury but have, in addition, the potential to cause injury remote from the wound track associated with a phenomenon known as temporary cavitation (Fig. 19.3).

The extent of cavitation depends upon the density and elasticity of the target organ or structure, and in certain circumstances is associated with injury many centimetres away from the missile wound track.

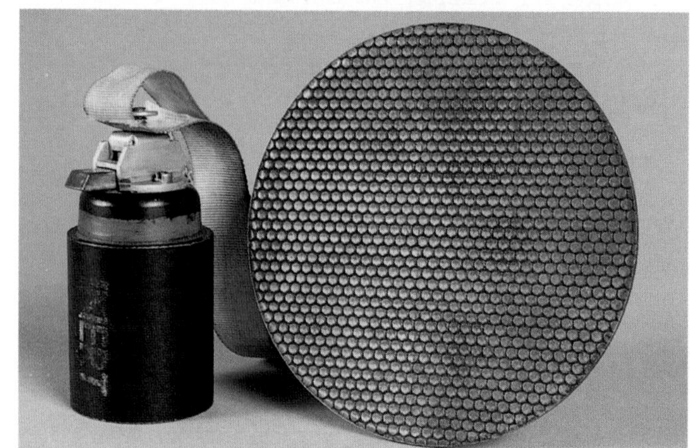

Fig. 19.2 Bomblet pressed from a patterned plate to create partially preformed fragments. (Reproduced with permission from *Ballistic Trauma*, edited by J.M. Ryan *et al*., published by Arnold, London, 1997.)

Cavitation within solid organs such as the liver, spleen and kidney results in shattering with high morbidity and mortality. The extent of injury to bowel is variable. In general, the small bowel fares better than the colon, particularly if the latter is loaded with faeces. A similar event in an elastic tissue

(a)

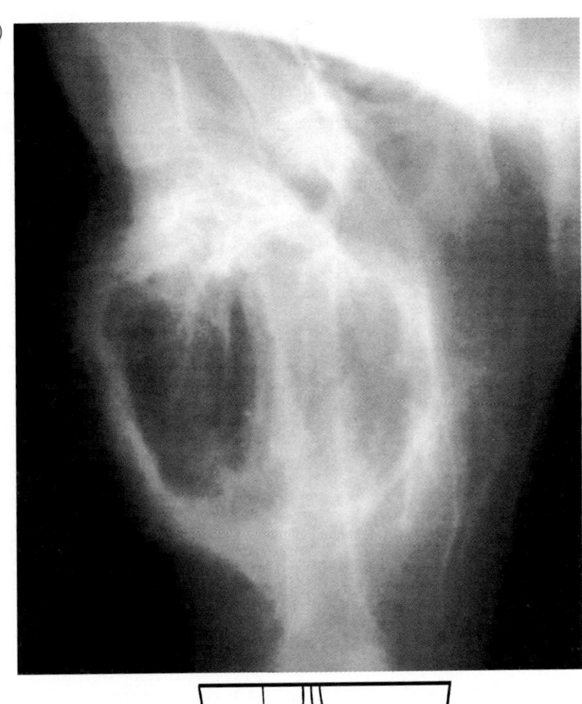

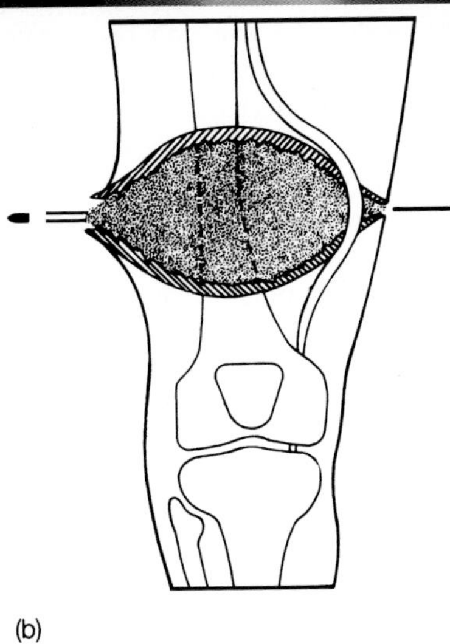

(b)

Fig. 19.3 High-velocity (high available energy) energy missile (experimental). (a) Radiograph taken 30 milliseconds after the bullet traversed the limb; (b) cavitational extent due to energy transfer of the high-velocity missile. The arteries and nerves are often temporarily displaced by such an insult.

such as the lung may result in quite modest injury. In the limb the position is more complex and controversial. While voluntary muscle may merely stretch if injured in isolation, bone fares badly. As a rule, bone involvement results in severe injury due to high-energy transfer with disruption of the missile and involved bone, with generation of secondary missiles. Extensive devitalisation of muscle is a typical finding. Devitalised muscle in the depths of a missile wound provides the perfect culture medium for the growth of pathogenic bacteria, a fact recognised by military surgeons for centuries. Nerves and blood vessels respond unpredictably with injury, ranging from minimal bruising to complete disruption. Within the closed skull there is, in addition, a rapid, high-pressure shock wave causing widespread disruption and injury at a distance. Thus, vital centres at the base of the brain may be injured by a wound of the cranium.

Management of missile injuries

Missile wounds of soft tissue

Management of the soft tissue wound is a formal procedure consisting of clearly defined stages. This is the part of early management most frequently neglected by surgeons with limited or no experience of war surgery. The entrance and exit wounds do not indicate the considerable damage that may have occurred to deeper structures (Fig. 19.4).

This can only be detected by full exploration. In limb wounds, exploration is followed by thorough wound excision, after which, with very few exceptions, the wound should be left open. Delayed primary closure should follow within 4–7 days after injury. Having followed the Advanced Trauma Life Support (ATLS®) guidelines, the patient will have been completely undressed prior to surgery, but it is wise to retain any pressure dressings over a wound until the operation is due to begin. The operation should consist of the following stages.

1. After photographing the wound and cleaning it with an antiseptic, generous longitudinal incisions are made through the skin to allow visualisation and access to the deeper structures and to facilitate subsequent extension of the exposure, should this be required. A minimal amount of skin edge (i.e. only that which has been contaminated)

(a)

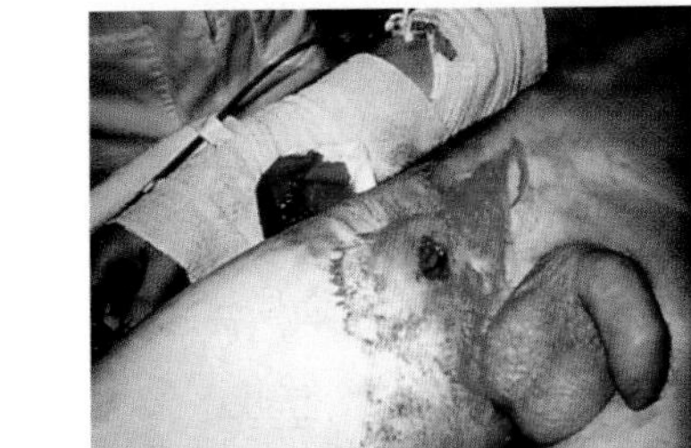

(b)

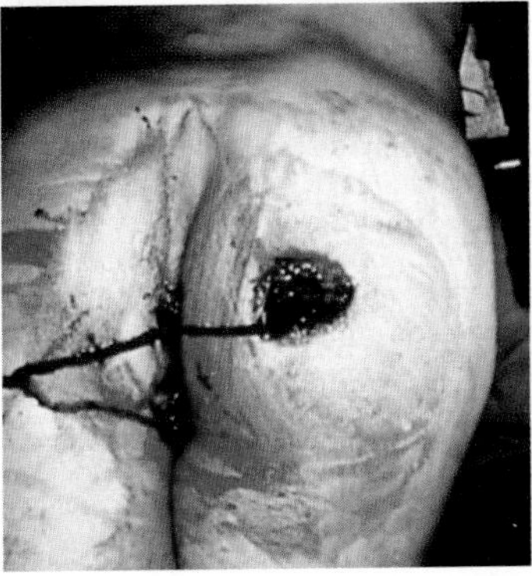

Fig. 19.4 High-energy transfer wound caused by a high-velocity assault rifle bullet. (a) Entrance wound and (b) exit wound. Note that in this instance the exit wound is larger than the entrance wound, indicating that temporary cavitation took place closer to the exit wound.

should be excised around the entrance and exit wounds. Skin is remarkably resistant to injury – scrubbing with a nail brush will remove most contaminants and indriven debris, allowing skin excision to be kept to a minimum.

2. The deep fascia is exposed over the length of the skin incisions, and must be incised in a longitudinal direction to allow full inspection of the area damaged by the wounding missile and to decompress the underlying muscle which will swell subsequently. This is the true meaning of the much misused term *débridement*[1] (Fig. 19.5).
3. Neurovascular bundles in the wound track must be identified and examined, but nerves should not be dissected out at the initial exploration. Nerves considered to be injured and warranting later exploration may have their position marked with a nonabsorbable suture marker to ease subsequent identification. It is important to examine the patient for nerve injury before the operation if this is possible and to record in the operation notes the nature of the nerve injury. The majority of nerve injuries is neuropraxias which do recover.

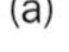
(a)

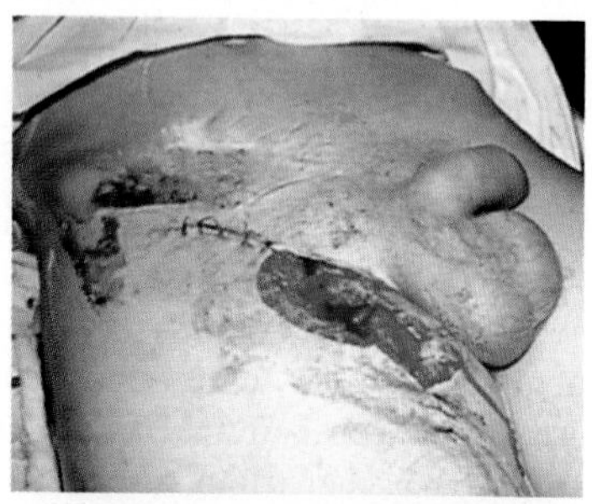

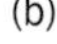
(b)

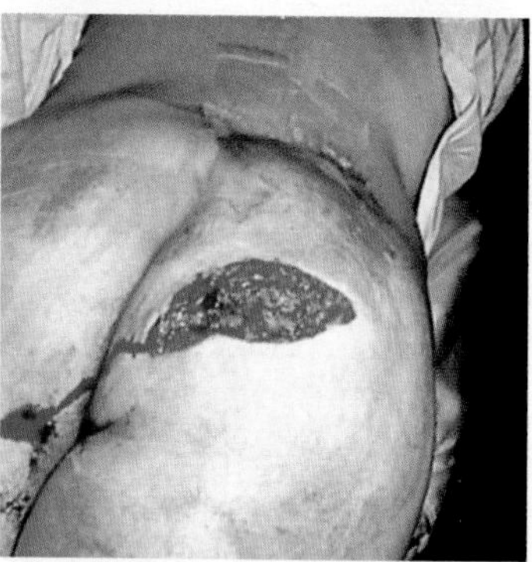

Fig. 19.5 High-energy transfer wound. (a) Extensive exploration of the entrance wound in the groin was required to complete adequately wound débridement and excision, and gain control of the damaged femoral artery. The extent of skin incision is clearly demonstrated; this was partially restored at initial operation after exploration and repair of the large vessels. (b) The exit wound over the right buttock is shown here on completion of wound excision and before delayed primary closure some days later.

[1]*Débridement (unbridling or unleashing). The term was introduced by Baron Dominique Jean Larrey, 1766–1842, Surgeon to Napoleon's Imperial Guard. He used it to describe the process of laying a wound open to facilitate removal of bullets, bits of loose cloth, detached pieces of bone and soft tissue. He and his contemporaries did not excise tissue in the modern sense and his procedure was much less extensive than the formal wound excision practised today.*

4. Foreign matter should be removed from the wound. Pieces of clothing are especially sought, both in the missile track and in the tissue planes on either side. It is not necessary to remove every piece of metal seen on a radiograph. Multiple, very small metal fragments from modern munitions may, in any case, be very difficult to locate and remove.
5. Dead muscle that does not bleed or contract, is mushy in consistency or has an unhealthy colour must be excised. These criteria comprise is the '4 Cs' for muscle excision.

The '4 Cs'

- Colour
- Contractility
- Consistency
- Capillary bleeding

6. Tendon repair should not be performed at this initial procedure. Tattered ends should be trimmed.
7. Major artery and vein damage must be noted. Where possible, the ends should be trimmed and sutured. If any tension is likely to develop, a reversed vein graft may be inserted to bridge the gap and the repair covered by healthy muscle. The rest of the wound should be left open for delayed primary closure. Synthetic grafts must not be used. A plastic shunt inserted into an injured artery can be used to revitalise tissue distal to the site of injury prior to definitive repair. In combined arterial and venous injury, concomitant shunting of both vessels may be undertaken. Temporary shunting has a vital role where major vascular damage is associated with fractures of long bones. In this instance, blood flow is established via the shunt(s), and the fracture is reduced and immobilised using an external fixator, after which definitive vascular repair is undertaken.
8. Bone shattered by high-energy transfer will in many instances still have attachment to periosteum or muscle. Such fragments must not be discarded. Loss of bone may result in malunion (e.g. shortening) or nonunion. Contaminated bone may be cleaned by using that useful instrument of military surgery, the Volkmann's spoon or curette.
9. Injured joints need thorough inspection and cleaning by copious irrigation with saline to remove organic matter. Any exposed articular cartilage should be covered by at least one layer of healthy tissue, preferably synovium, otherwise muscle or skin should be used.
10. At the end of the operation the wound should be irrigated thoroughly with saline to remove any remaining debris. Haemostasis should be secured with the aid of hot packs and the wound left open without closure of either fascial layer or skin, even in the presence of exposed bone. A lightly fluffed gauze dressing should be placed over the wound to allow free drainage. Packing must be avoided.

Richard von Volkmann, 1830–89. Professor of Surgery, Halle, Germany.

11. Immobilisation in a well-padded splint allows the soft tissues to recover, a principle expounded by Hugh Owen Thomas at the turn of the century. Split plaster of Paris splints are ideal even in the absence of a fracture. Femoral shaft fractures should be immobilised in a traction splint.
12. Antibiotic cover is advised for all wounds; third-generation cephalosporins or agents with an equivalent spectrum being ideal. In all abdominal, pelvic and perineal wounds, metranidazole is given in addition (see Chapter 7).

Delayed primary closure

All wounds treated by wound excision and left open should be inspected about 4–6 days after injury. Provided the wound looks healthy, delayed primary closure is indicated. This should be by interrupted suture, split skin graft or a combination of both.

Traumatic amputations

Traumatic amputations should be surgically tidied, completed at the lowest level possible and the skin left open for delayed primary closure. If there is much skin loss or if a limb is very swollen, split skin grafting may be used to effect wound closure in order to avoid skin tension. If, at the time of delayed primary closure, dead muscle is found, which is not uncommon in traumatic amputation due to antipersonnel mines, the muscle is excised and the wound left open for a further period before closure.

Missile wounds of the abdomen

Every penetrating and perforating missile wound of the abdomen should be explored by laparotomy. Before surgery, a nasogastric tube should be passed into the stomach and a urinary catheter into the bladder. Bladder catheterisation must be preceded by a digital rectal examination. Timing of exploration will vary. In some cases, operation will be undertaken as part of resuscitation leaving little or no time for planning (see the section on 'Damage control' in Chapter 18). In others, preoperative stabilisation is possible and time is available for investigation, including haematology, biochemistry and radiology. In all cases blood in realistic quantities must be available.

A full midline incision from xiphisternum to pubis is recommended. It has the advantage of facilitating rapid access and extension laterally or into the chest where required. The commonest source of bleeding in survivors is from the small bowel mesentery, but major haemorrhage may come from the solid organs, such as liver or spleen, or from the major vessels. Haemorrhage must be controlled and careful examination is then made of all the abdominal contents.

In all wounds of the stomach, the lesser sac must be opened to inspect the posterior gastric wall. Retroperitoneal haematoma in the region of the duodenum requires inspection of its posterior wall by Kocher's method (Chapter 51). Haematoma surrounding the retroperitoneal parts of the ascending and descending colon may also necessitate exploration, but nonexpanding retroperitoneal haematomas over the kidneys are best left undisturbed.

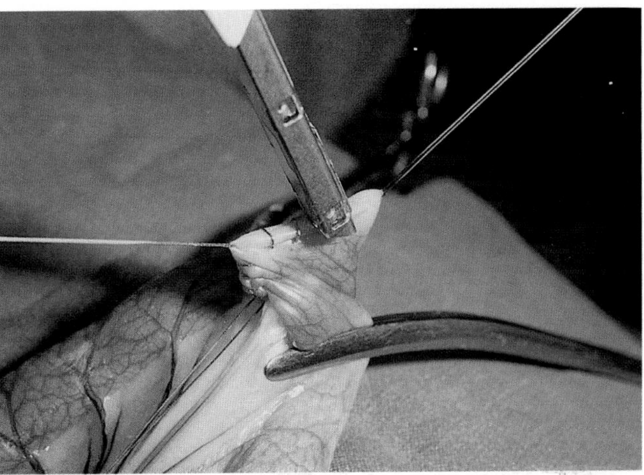

Fig. 19.6 A proprietary skin stapler (Autosuture Premium 35) being used to construct an end-to-end small bowel anastomosis. This technique is fast, easily taught and is particularly useful in war when faced with multiple procedures in large numbers of casualties. (Reproduced with permission from *Ballistic Trauma*, edited by J.M. Ryan *et al.*, published by Arnold, London, 1997.)

Small intestinal perforations are either excised and closed transversely, or the damaged section is resected if there are multiple holes in a short length (Fig. 19.6) Mesenteric tears may also require bowel resection (see Chapter 56).

Colon and rectal wounds (see also Chapter 57)

For most injuries of the *right side of the colon*, primary repair or primary resection is satisfactory. Occasionally, where severe wounding with extensive contamination has occurred, a vented ileotransverse anastomosis is warranted. Rarely, the two ends are brought to the surface as proximal ileostomy and distal mucous fistula, respectively.

On the left side a one-stage procedure may be undertaken if favourable circumstances pertain, i.e. minimal peritoneal contamination, limited blood loss, and a time interval between injury and operation of less than 8 hours. However, if injury is associated with high-risk factors, the injured colon is resected and the proximal end brought out as a colostomy and the distal end as a mucous fistula. If the distal end cannot be brought to the surface, as in low sigmoid or rectal injuries, it may be closed off as in a Hartmann procedure (Chapter 60). Subsequent restoration of bowel continuity will be required.

Extraperitoneal rectal injuries are repaired if feasible and defunctioned by establishing a sigmoid end colostomy. Good

Hugh Owen Thomas, 1834–91. Surgeon, Liverpool, England. He introduced the Thomas splint in 1875.

Emil Theodor Kocher, 1841–1917. Professor of Surgery, Berne, Switzerland.
Henri Charles Antoine Hartmann, 1860–1952. Professor of Surgery, Paris, France.

dependent drainage is best achieved by a presacral, retrorectal drain brought out between the tip of the coccyx and the anus. *The control of haemorrhage in pelvic injuries can be difficult and may require ligature of the internal iliac artery.*

Rectal injury

Renal injury is best treated conservatively if this is possible. Fortunately, immediate nephrectomy is rarely indicated. A divided ureter may be brought to the surface or may be repaired over a 'pigtail' stent.

Bladder and urethral injuries

Bladder and urethral injuries are treated by suprapubic cystostomy with placement of a suprapubic drain after wound excision.

Liver injuries

In 50 per cent of cases of hepatic injury surviving to reach a surgical centre, bleeding has stopped and is not a problem at laparotomy, a reassuring statistic for the youthful surgeons usually faced with such cases. Where bleeding is still occurring, damage control techniques are particularly appropriate in a warfare setting (see section on 'Damage control' in Chapter 18). Manual compression and perihepatic packing are recommended, and may allow a patient to survive to reach a more sophisticated surgical facility in the rear of the fighting area. If these simple measures do not work, and provided that the operator is experienced, finger fracture with exposure of bleeding points followed by individual ligation, or more formal resection procedures, will be needed (see also Chapter 52). These are rare eventualities. In all cases, generous drainage of the spaces surrounding the liver is important.

Damage to the spleen and pancreas

Damage to the spleen and tail of pancreas may require resection, although in some cases splenorrhaphy may be feasible. Missile injury of the head of the pancreas is seldom seen in the operating room because injury to it and surrounding structures is usually fatal. In a very few cases it may be possible to apply a Roux loop of jejenum to create an internal fistula.

Peritoneal toilet

Using warm saline, it is important to assist the removal of all spilled bowel contents and blood clot.

Closure

The laparotomy wound is closed using the mass closure technique. The missile entrance and exit wounds should be excised as described earlier and left open initially with a view to delayed primary closure at 4–6 days.

Missile wounds of the chest

(See also Chapter 47.) Penetrating missile wounds of the chest are common in war and are associated with a high mortality if simple life-saving measures are neglected. It is important to secure an airtight seal of open wounds of the chest to prevent a potentially fatal open pneumothorax. This is immediately followed by tube thoracostomy. This should been done during the primary survey. Failure to do so will result in collapse of the lung on the affected side with alteration of the ventilation/perfusion ratio and, in addition, will progressively decrease the quantity and quality of air entering the affected lung. As dyspnoea increases due to anoxia, the mediastinum shifts on respiration and decreases venous return to the heart – the clinical picture in the later stages is identical to a tension pneumothorax.

All penetrating wounds of the chest require adequate venting of the pleura by formal tube thoracostomy. This simple procedure will prevent the accumulation of blood or air under tension. The position of the tube should be confirmed by chest radiography. Once pulmonary function has been stabilised, missile entry and exit wounds are excised. During the excision of a large chest wall wound, the pleural cavity is often entered; this need not cause concern. The opportunity should be taken to remove any retained foreign material, arrest haemorrhage (usually from an intercostal or internal mammary vessel) and to oversew or staple holes in the adjacent lung. On completion the pleural opening must be sealed either by direct pleural closure (often difficult) or by utilising overlying healthy soft tissue, and the wound(s) left open for subsequent delayed primary closure.

These simple measures will suffice for more than 80 per cent of chest wounds. The remainder will require formal thoracotomy, often urgently. The usual indications are listed below.

Indications for formal thoracotomy

- More than 1.5 litres initial blood loss
- Continuing loss of > 200 ml/hour
- Cardiac tamponade
- Other mediastinal injuries
- Persistent air leak
- Retained foreign bodies > 1.5 cm in diameter

Even in cases where thoracotomy is indicated, considerable delay can often be tolerated provided adequate resuscitation is initiated quickly. Thoracotomy for retained foreign bodies is often a late and planned procedure.

In thoracoabdominal injuries, the thoracic component is treated by tube thoracostomy and the abdominal component by laparotomy through a midline incision. Formal thoracoabdominal incisions risk contamination of the chest cavity by faeces and should be avoided.

Missile wounds of the head

The penetrating high-energy transfer missile wound of the head is usually lethal. The management of penetrating low-energy transfer and tangential wounds depends initially on measures described in the primary survey and resuscitation phases (see Chapter 18). These will ensure a protected airway, adequate ventilation, and maintenance of blood pressure and perfusion pressure to permit oxygenation of the brain. Good radiographs are mandatory to localise foreign bodies and bone fragments. Computerised tomography (CT) images are invaluable in planning surgical exploration. Wound excision should be carried out using gentle irrigation and suction to remove devitalised brain and bony fragments. Every effort, including the use of temporalis fascia or fascia lata, should be made to close overlying dura. The skin overlying the head and face is an exception to the delayed primary closure rule. Blood supply is excellent, allowing primary closure which also serves to control blood loss from the scalp.

Intermittent positive pressure ventilation (IPPV) assists in the reduction of intracranial pressure by reducing brain swelling. Intracranial pressure transducers inserted through burr holes may be employed to monitor intracranial pressure in the postoperative phase.

Shotgun injuries

Accidents from large-bore shotguns are common and often lethal when injury is sustained at close range. It is never possible to retrieve all the shot and, indeed, to do so would result in unacceptable damage to uninjured soft tissues. Wound excision should be carried out on the major wound, particularly looking for indriven wadding and plugs of clothing. Laparotomy is essential if it is thought that any of the shot has traversed an abdominal viscus. The retention of lead shot in the body can result in a dangerously high lead concentration, which should be monitored. After a time, this concentration will fall as a result of encapsulation of the lead pellets by fibrous tissue.

Summary: dos and don'ts of missile injuries

Do:

- incise skin generously;
- incise fascia widely;
- identify neurovascular bundles;
- excise all devitalised tissue;
- remove all indriven clothing;
- leave wound open at end of surgery;
- dress wounds with fluffed gauze;
- record all injuries in the notes.

Don't:

- excise too much skin;
- practise keyhole surgery;
- repair tendons or nerves;
- remove attached pieces of bone;
- close the deep fascia;
- insert synthetic prostheses;
- pack the wound;
- close the skin.

Blast injuries

Mechanism of explosive blast injury

The explosive pressure that accompanies the bursting of bombs or shells ruptures their casing and imparts a high velocity to the resulting fragments. These fragments have the potential to cause even more devastating injury to the tissues than bullets. They are unstable in flight and may tear through tissue at high speed in a tumbling fashion. These statements are particularly true of old artillery shells and terrorist bombs where the casing fragments naturally into pieces of variable size. However, the trend in conventional war is towards carefully engineered weapons which carry preformed munitions, such as notched wire or ball bearings, or have their casing etched to allow predictable fragmentation patterns resulting in a multitude of small, relatively low-energy fragments (Fig. 19.2). The aim is to incapacitate, not kill, by inflicting multiple low-energy transfer wounds to two or more body systems.

In addition, all explosives are accompanied by a complex blast wave. The two main components of this wave are a blast pressure wave (known as dynamic overpressure), with a positive and negative phase, and the mass movement of air (known as blast wind) (Fig. 19.7).

The positive pressure phase of the blast wave lasts for only a few milliseconds, but close to an explosion it may rise to over 7000 kN/m^2. As the healthy tympanic membrane ruptures at about 150 kN/m^2, it is evident that the effects on the human body of such an explosion can be devastating, especially in confined areas. Like sound waves, the blast pressure waves flow over and around an obstruction and affect anyone sheltering behind a wall or in a trench. The pressure affecting such a person is known as the *incident pressure* (defined as the pressure level at 90° to the direction of travel of the blast shock front). Also, any person standing in front of a wall or other vertical surface facing an explosion is subjected to the added effect of a *reflected pressure*. The negative effect of a pressure wave is of low amplitude, lasts longer than the positive wave and is of doubtful clinical significance.

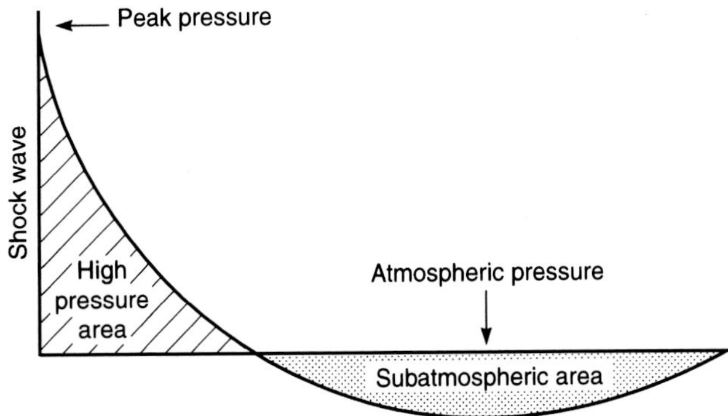

Fig. 19.7 Pressure changes that occur as a result of a bomb explosion. A blast produces two pressure changes: a high-pressure shock wave, followed by a subatmospheric (suction) phase. Injuries are mainly due to the initial shock wave but are aggravated by the subatmospheric phase.

A mass movement of air or dynamic pressure results from the rapidly expanding gases at the centre of the explosion which displaces air at supersonic (greater than the speed of sound in air) speed. This has been described by an eminent blast scientist as 'fresh air moving very fast'. The mass movement of air results in what is colloquially known as *blast wind* and disrupts the environment, hurling debris and people. This phenomenon results in injury patterns ranging from traumatic amputation to total body disruption. The mass movement of air may disrupt buildings, causing entrapment and crush injuries.

Blast pressure waves travel at the speed of sound in the medium being traversed. In water, velocity and distance are greater and injuries tend to be more complex and severe. For example, blast pressure waves in air rarely affect the gastrointestinal tract to any clinically significant extent in survivors; however, in water, the blast wave exerts a 'water hammer' effect with significant rates of gastrointestinal perforation.

When the body is impacted by a blast pressure wave, it *couples* into the body and sets up a series of stress waves which are capable of injury, particularly at air–fluid interfaces. Thus, injury to the ear, lungs, heart and, to a lesser extent, the gastrointestinal tract (see above) is notable. The exact mechanisms of injury at each specific tissue are still the subject of controversy but need not unduly worry readers as this topic is debated well by Cripps and Guy in *Trauma* and by Ryan *et al.* in *Ballistic Trauma*, as listed in the 'Further reading' section of this chapter.

General management of blast injuries

The structures injured by the primary blast wave, in order of prevalence, are the middle ear, the lungs and the bowel. However, the most common urgent clinical problem in survivors is usually penetrating injury caused by blast-energised debris and fragments from the casing of the exploding device (see below). Many of those exposed will have blunt, blast and thermal injuries in addition to more obvious penetrating wounds (the clinical picture is usually referred to as *combined injury*). The deafness of the victims of blast, due to disruption of the tympanic membrane, makes communication with them difficult and may complicate early assessment and management. Here, the primary survey and resuscitation phases of a system such as ATLS are particularly apt. The management of penetrating wounds differs little from that of missile wounds referred to earlier. The soft-tissue wounds are usually heavily contaminated with dirt, clothing and secondary missiles such as wood, masonry and other materials from the environment. Such contaminants may be driven deeply into adjacent tissue planes opened up by the force of the explosion. The propensity for wound infection in these cases is considerable and is often underestimated. Some cases are associated with multiple wounds of varying severity affecting a limb (Fig. 19.8).

It may not always be practical to explore every wound at first surgery. The larger and deeper wounds should have priority of management due to the more serious consequences of infection. In many blast injuries one cannot be sure of complete wound excision and, therefore, it is imperative that all blast wounds should be left open at the end of the initial operation and delayed primary closure performed 4–6 days later.

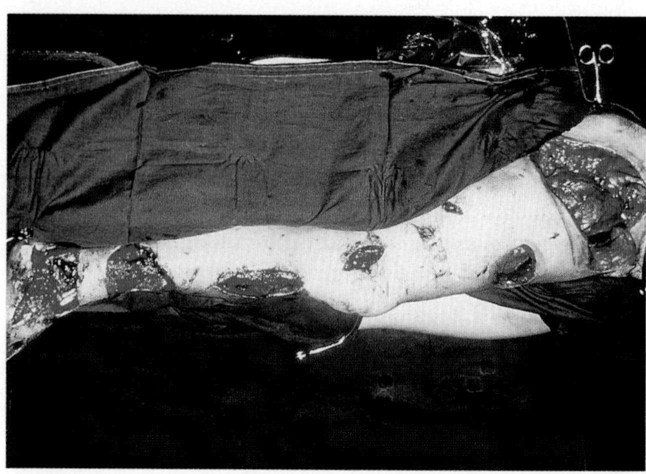

Fig. 19.8 A civilian victim of a terrorist bombing in London. Note the multiplicity of limb wounds, all of which are heavily contaminated. (Reproduced with permission from *Ballistic Trauma*, edited by J.M. Ryan *et al.*, published by Arnold, London, 1997.)

Regional management of blast injuries

Here one is particularly concerned with identifying specific injuries caused by the primary blast wave.

Auditory system

Blast damages the hearing in three ways. There may be rupture of the tympanic membrane, dislocation of the ossicles or widespread disruption of the inner ear. The latter is sometimes accompanied by permanent deafness. It should be remembered that the likelihood of ear damage depends on the angle between the incident blast wave and the external auditory meatus. Although deafness is a certain indicator of exposure to significant blast loading, its absence does not imply the absence of blast injury to other systems.

Respiratory system

Injury to the lung parenchyma is complex and the exact mechanisms are still the subject of debate. Undoubtedly, the impacting primary blast wave may cause a rapid inward movement of the chest wall and result in underlying pulmonary contusion, but this is not the principal mechanism in the severe and progressive acute lung injury picture seen in small numbers of survivors. In these casualties it is probable that the initial blast wave couples into the chest resulting in stress waves which spread out, reflect and reinforce at tissue interfaces. At air–fluid interfaces they may result in considerable disruption. This is particularly notable at the alveolar–capillary membrane and leads to capillary leakage resulting in a spreading haemorrhagic alveolar contamination (Fig. 19.9).

An inflammatory cascade now ensues resulting in a post-blast respiratory insufficiency (PBRI), which is virtually indistinguishable from adult respiratory distress syndrome (ARDS) following generalised sepsis or fat embolism syn-

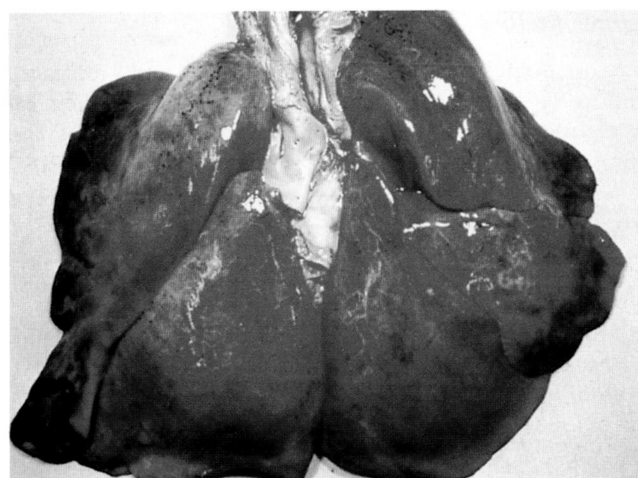

Fig. 19.9 Blast lung showing extensive haemorrhage of both lobes due to blast (*courtesy of Professor T.G. Parks, Belfast*).

drome (FES), and posing a difficult clinical problem in critical care units. PBRI varies from a mild and localised area of pulmonary contusion injury to a fulminating and rapidly fatal condition involving both lungs. This rapid and progressive condition is relatively rare, as casualties sufficiently close to suffer extreme blast loading to the chest wall are usually killed by multiple penetrating wounds or are dismembered by blast winds. In severe cases, respiratory insufficiency may be further precipitated by overtransfusion with electrolyte solutions. The clinical picture is typical – patients develop a cough with frothy blood-stained sputum, dyspnoea and a feeling of apprehension, bordering on a foreboding of impending doom – they are often right. A pulse oximeter will show a resistant low saturation, with values well below 90 per cent. Blood gas analysis confirms arterial hypoxia and a raised carbon dioxide partial pressure (PCO_2). Chest radiographs in the initial stages may show localised contusion injury but, as the inflammatory cascade builds, radiographic evidence becomes generalised with bilateral fluffy infiltrates spreading out from the hilum of both lungs (Fig. 19.10).

Specific clinical management of an established case remains controversial. There is still little hard evidence to guide clinicians. However, most agree with the guidelines listed in below.

Postblast respiratory insufficiency (PBRI) – clinical guidelines

- Work within the ABCDE system of the ATLS system
- Avoid overhydration while maintaining vital organ perfusion
- Administer high-flow oxygen (12 litres/minute) with mask and rebreathing bag
- Carry out arterial blood analysis to assess need for further measures
- Resort to mechanical ventilation early to ensure adequate oxygenation
- Use positive end-expiratory pressure (PEEP) carefully while avoiding excessive peak and plateau pressures
- Corticosteroids should be avoided

(a)

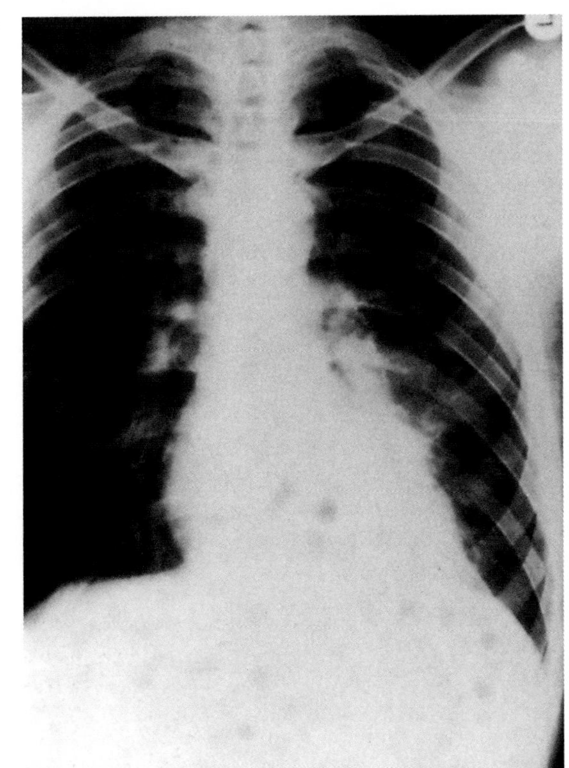

(b)

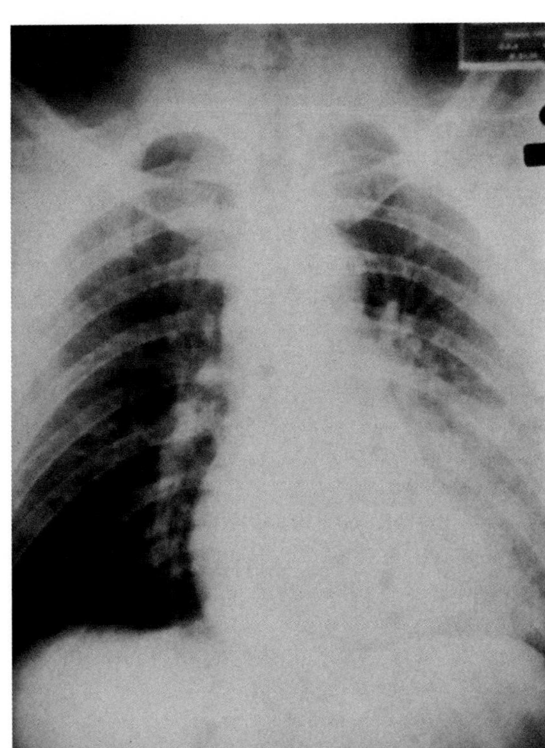

Fig. 19.10 (a) Chest radiograph of a soldier admitted immediately after sustaining minor burns, lacerations and bruises from a terrorist booby-trap bomb. (b) Chest radiograph 3 hours later showing pulmonary contusion. No treatment was required; there was spontaneous resolution. (Royal Army Medical College.)

Gastrointestinal tract

Injury to gas-filled viscera is more common in underwater explosions than air blasts. Perforation of the stomach, small intestine and caecum is most common. The clinical presentation is one of increasing abdominal pain accompanied by signs of peritonism and often gas under the diaphragm. In the presence of clear physical signs urgent laparotomy is indicated. In cases where signs are few but the risks are high, ultrasonography, CT, diagnostic peritoneal lavage and laparoscopy should be considered. There is no single modality agreed by all. Serological assessment of gut-associated enzymes is still an experimental tool and no reliable serum marker of intestinal injury is available.

The eye

The eye should be examined in both the primary and secondary surveys, yet injury is easily missed. Conjunctival haemorrhage following blast exposure may herald a more serious underlying problem of penetration of the globe by blast-energised debris or fragments. The pupil must be carefully examined and any abnormality, distortion of the iris or the presence of a hyphema, for example, should be investigated by an ophthalmologist.

Other factors

Factors that increase the morbidity and mortality following bomb blast injuries are associated chemical and thermal burns, and the inhalation of toxic gases and smoke.

Further reading

Coupland, R.M. (1993) *War Wounds of Limbs – Surgical Management*, Butterworth-Heinmann, Oxford.

Dufour, D., Viroman Jensen, S., Owen-Smith, M. *et al.* (1988) *Surgery for Victims of War, ICRC Publications*, Geneva.

Cripps, N.P.C. and Guy, R.J. (1998) Primary blast injuries: mechanisms, pathophysiology and treatment. In *Trauma* (eds I. Greaves, J.M. Ryan and K.M. Porter), Arnold, London, pp. 314–34.

Kirkby, G. and Blackburn, G. (1981) *Field Surgery Pocket Book*, HMSO, London.

Ryan, J.M., Rich, N.M., Dale, R.F., Morgans, B.T. and Cooper, G.J. (eds) (1997) *Ballistic Trauma – Clinical Relevance in Peace and War*, Arnold, London.

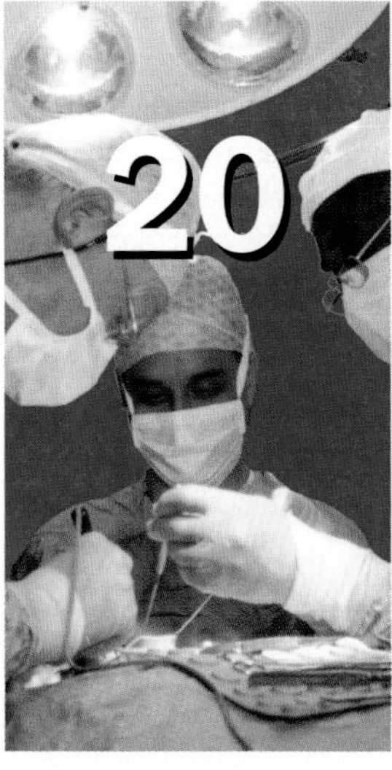

20 History taking and examination in musculoskeletal disorder

The history

Learning objectives

1. To understand the three key types of history, their function and the different way in which they are obtained.
2. To understand the three zones of abnormality that a history should address.

Introduction

The importance of taking a history in musculoskeletal disorders is threefold (Table 20.1).

- Its first function is to allow the patient to list the problems that they are experiencing and to define what it is that they are hoping to gain from this consultation. This part of the history should be used to 'set the agenda' for the consultation.
- The second task is to draw out from the patient a full description of those symptoms which confirm one diagnosis, or which exclude others. This is the 'diagnostic phase'.
- The final phase is only needed if surgery is a possible option. The questions here are directed at determining the patient's 'fitness for surgery'.

Table 20.1 Phases of taking a history

Setting the agenda	*Making a diagnosis*	*Fitness for surgery*
Open questions	Directed questions	Specific questions
Patient lists his/her problems and expectations	Clinician explores the details of symptoms	Clinician checks for risk factors and that the patient is in optimal condition

Bailey & Love's Short Practice of Surgery, 23rd edition. Edited by R.C.G. Russell, N.S. Williams and C.J.K. Bulstrode. Published in 2000 by Arnold Publishers.

Setting the agenda

In this phase the patient should be encouraged with open questions to do most of the talking. As they talk it should be possible to divide the patient's problems into three main areas: pain, dysfunction and deformity (Table 20.2).

Pain

Patients should be asked to define in what way the pain troubles them, as the answer may give the clue to how this can best be managed if it cannot be cured. For example, if it is pain at night stopping sleep, then a combination of pain killers and sleeping tablets might offer the best solution if no other is available. If, however, the pain occurs in a joint on weight-bearing a splint might stabilise the joint and make the pain manageable.

Table 20.2 Areas of musculoskeletal problems

- Pain
- Dysfunction
- Deformity

Dysfunction

A patient may complain of loss of function as a result of pain, stiffness, weakness, instability or even locking. In the first instance the patient should be allowed to describe in their own words what it is they can no longer do. This may be something like inability to reach up to hang clothes on the washing line. This problem will later be translated into a clinical diagnosis, but at this stage should be reported in the patient's own words.

Deformity

This may be much more of a concern to the patient than might seem reasonable to you. Patients may want bunions corrected not because they are painful (although they may initially claim this), but because they are unsightly. It is crucial to be clear about the patient's real reasons for seeking treatment, and what it is they hope you will be able to do about it before embarking on the next stage of the interview.

Summary

This part of the interview should be summarised and recorded as the patient's problems and expectations.

History for diagnosis

The 'history for diagnosis' leads directly on from taking a 'history for agenda' but the structure of the interview changes. Instead of open questions aimed at getting the patient to talk about how they see their problems, each question is now carefully designed to confirm or exclude a differential diagnosis derived from the initial part of the interview. The same categories are used as before – pain, dysfunction and deformity – but this time the characteristics of each are explored in detail, searching for clues to causation, association and alleviating factors. The main areas to be covered are as follows.

Onset

A careful history of how the problem was first noticed is diagnostically useful. In sports medicine it is usual to divide onset into three categories: acute extrinsic, acute intrinsic and chronic (Table 20.3).

Acute extrinsic. This is associated with external trauma. A limb which is deformed, after being hit with a stick, is likely to be broken. If it is painful but not deformed then it is likely to be bruised.

Acute intrinsic. This occurs when the human body is under load and fails. In young people this may be a ligament (e.g. anterior cruciate ligament in a footballer, who twists at speed on a fixed foot). In older people it might be a broken bone (e.g. a fractured neck of femur in an elderly osteoporotic patient who tripped).

Chronic. These problems are those where the onset is not clearly associated with any traumatic event, but just gradually appears. An example is osteoarthritis of the shoulder.

Table 20.3 Types of onset

Acute extrinsic	*Acute intrinsic*	*Chronic*
For example, a patient hit with a stick	For example, an elderly osteoporotic patient trips and falls	For example, an elderly patient with gradual onset of pain in the shoulder
Butterfly fracture of the ulna	Fractured neck of femur	Osteoarthritis of the shoulder

Association

The human brain is programmed to seek patterns, and may do so even when there is no pattern to see. Just because a patient feels that there is an association between an event and onset of an illness does not mean that this is correct. Conversely, you may need to seek associations which had not occurred to the patient.

Development

The natural history of the problem may also give clues to diagnosis causation and even treatment. If the condition spontaneously resolves, then returns, the cause for recurrence needs to be sought. For example, being compelled to sit for a long period in one place may exacerbate pain from a prolapsed intervertebral disc.

Nature

The type of pain in particular may give you a clue as to the origin.

Throbbing pain associated with sweats and chills may be an infection.

Deep boring pain, which wakes the patient from sleep, may be caused by a tumour.

Similarly, dysfunction needs to be explored carefully to see whether it is caused by weakness, pain, instability, locking or even lack of confidence.

History for surgery

If surgery is a possibility you need to know whether it would be safe before you offer it as a treatment option. This can be divided into two sections. The first is identification of conditions, which increase the risk of anaesthesia and of surgery morbidity. The second involves determining whether

Table 20.4 History for surgery – co-morbidity

- Does the patient have a condition which might pose a risk to surgery?
- Are these conditions under good control, so that risks are minimised?

those conditions have been brought into the best possible control to minimise the risk. Orthopaedic surgery is rarely life-saving, but can be very useful for improving quality of life. It is quite acceptable to take a known risk and operate on a high-risk patient provided that you and the patient are aware of what you are doing. It is quite unacceptable to operate on a patient when either you and/or the patient are not aware of the increased risk, or when the condition has not been brought under the best control possible, and so the patient is being exposed to an unnecessary risk Table 20.4).

Factors in the history which point to high-risk patients are:

- patients who have had problems with previous anaesthetics;
- a history of cardiac or circulatory problems – previous myocardial infarcts, angina, cardiac arrhythmias, high blood pressure, peripheral vascular disease, previous strokes or transient ischaemic attacks;
- breathing problems – chronic breathing problems such as asthma or chronic bronchitis. Acute problems such as chest infection;
- metabolic problems – diabetes and steroid treatment;
- urinary tract problems – benign prostatic hypertrophy which has not been treated.

Musculoskeletal examination

Learning objectives

1. To understand a simple system for examining the musculoskeletal system.
2. To learn the specific features to be sought in each area of the body.

Musculoskeletal examination works on a simple system originally designed by Apley. It consists of four-letter words divided into threes.

The first stem is:

- look;
- feel;
- move.

The second stem branching off from each of these first two stems is:

- skin;
- soft (tissue);
- bone.

Finally, 'move' is divided into:

- active;
- passive;
- stability.

Alan Apley. Rowley Bristow Hospital, Pyrford, died c. 1995.

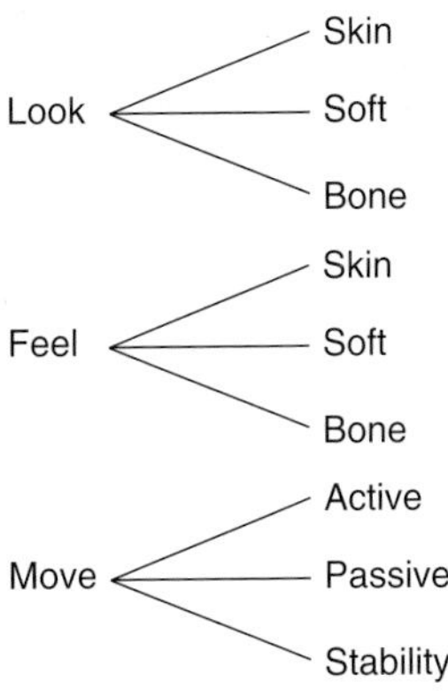

Look

You cannot look with your hands. Once you let your hands on to the patient, your ability to notice things with your eyes seems to be lost. While looking, it may be better to put your hands behind your back to remind you to look first, and to show the examiner what you are doing.

Make sure that you can see enough of the patient's body. This means exposing at least one joint above and one below the area in question. It also means exposing the opposite side. It is said by some that the human body was made bilaterally symmetrical to help orthopaedic surgeons distinguish abnormal from normal. Do not spurn such ready-made help.

It is not always necessary to lay the patient down for an orthopaedic examination. It may be easier if the patient remains standing, provided that they are comfortable to do this. In this position it is easier to look at the patient's back as well as their front. It is important to inspect all sides of the patient to make sure that no lesion is missed.

Skin

Look once at the skin for:

- bruising and wounds – evidence of recent injury;
- redness – signs of inflammation;
- scars – the archaeology of injury;
- sweating – loss of sweating may indicate nerve damage.

Soft tissues

Look a second time at the soft tissues. Now you are looking for:

- swelling – a cardinal sign of injury and inflammation;
- wasting – signs of disuse and nerve damage, the archaeology of injury.

Bones

Look a third time at the bones (shape of the skeleton). Look for:

- deformity – unusual angles or joints held in unusual positions.

Summarise

You have now looked at three zones. Summarise these in your mind and make a record of what you have found.

Feel

Once again you will test in three zones: skin, soft tissue and bone.

Skin (temperature, sensation)

- Temperature – stroke the patient's limbs with the back of your hand. It is more sensitive than the front. Use the patient's other side for comparison. Warmth may indicate inflammation. A cold limb may indicate nerve or vascular damage.
- Sensation – if you ask the patient to shut their eyes and then test whether their feeling is normal, you are in danger of missing nerve damage. Patients do not always close their eyes when asked (especially if they are drunk). The question 'Is that normal?' is a closed question which invites the answer 'Yes'. A better system is to leave the patient with their eyes open and then stroke first the normal limb then the other limb lightly. Ask if the touch on the two limbs feels the same. By comparing the two sides the patient should be able to detect any change in sensation, however slight.

Soft tissue (tenderness, lumps and circulation)

When you feel the soft tissues, you must be very careful to avoid hurting the patient. The best way to do this is to place your hands on the area under examination, then look up and watch the patient's face as you palpate. This way you will be certain to spot immediately that you are causing discomfort or even pain. You will then be able to stop what you are doing immediately to prevent further suffering. If you fail to do this in an examination and then cause pain to a patient, the examiner will regard this as a serious transgression.

Feel for:

- tenderness – as you press with your fingers try to describe to yourself the actual anatomical structure that you are palpating: subcutaneous fat, bursae, muscle bodies, tendons, nerves, arteries and ligaments;
- lumps and effusions – each time you feel an abnormality under the skin you should be able to run through a checklist of features of a lump. A simple system is shown in Table 20.5.
- distal circulation – feel for peripheral pulses and check capillary filling. When checking pulses, take the patient's pulse elsewhere at the same time. This should ensure that it is the patient's pulse you are feeling, not your own.

For capillary filling, simply press in on the tip of a digit and say under your breath 'capillary filling'. If the blanching has not disappeared by then, there is diminished capillary filling. Before diagnosing local vascular damage, check whether the circulation is reduced generally (as it might be in shock).

Table 20.5 History and examination of a lump or swelling

The steps needed to diagnose a lump in the musculoskeletal system are given by the acronym SWELLING:

- **S**tart – did it appear gradually or after trauma? A lump which appears immediately after trauma may be a haematoma. Does it hurt (all the time or just on movement)? One which appears spontaneously and is very painful is more likely to be infection
- **W**here – does it lie in the skin, fat, muscle, tendon, nerve, capsule or bone? Which of these tissues is it attached to? You will need to try to move the skin over it. If it is attached to skin and there is a punctum it is probably a sebaceous cyst. If it is attached to muscle it will be mobile until the muscle is contracted. If it is attached to a nerve, it may move freely in one direction (across the line of the nerve), but resist movement at right angles to this (along the line of the nerve)
- **E**xternal features – size, surface, separation. The size needs to be carefully defined so that future examinations can decide whether it has increased in size or not. Swellings with lumpy surfaces may be loculated as in lipomas. Lumps with ill-defined margins may be malignant, those with smooth well-defined margins are more likely to be benign
- **L**ymph nodes – are the local lymph nodes enlarged? Both infection and malignancy can cause enlargement of the local lymph nodes
- **L**iquid – is it fluctuant? Tests for fluctuance are described under examination of the knee where this test is commonly needed to determine whether there is an effusion in the joint
- **I**nternal features – is it tender? How hard is it? Lumps which are tender are more likely to be infection, especially if they are hot and red. Hardness defines whether the lump is likely to be made of bone/cartilage (hard), muscle/fat (softer) or fluid (fluctuant)
- **N**oise – bruit and thrill. The cardinal signs of a vascular lump
- **G**eneral – examination of whole patient. Are there any other lumps, or signs of generalised disease?

Bone (bone outlines and joint margins)

Watch the patient's face, feel the bone and joint margins gently for areas of tenderness, steps and lumps. Again, try to work out what anatomical structure your fingers are touching as you palpate.

Summary

Review your findings. Try to decide what structures are tender, what structures are swollen, wasted or displaced, and whether the circulation and sensation to the distal limb is normal. If not, where is the likely damage?

Move

Once again there are three phases of the examination, but this time they are active, passive and stability.

Active

The patient should move their own joints within the limits of pain. Use simple language to explain what you want them to do, and if necessary demonstrate the movement.

Passive

Don't take the range of movement beyond the active range without watching the patient's face.

Stability

There are two types of stability: dynamic and static. Dynamic stability is provided by muscle power; static stability by ligaments and intact joint surfaces.

Dynamic stability. Measure the force that the patient can develop by showing them the movement, then asking them to repeat it while you try to stop them. For each movement, try to work out which muscles are the drivers of that movement, which nerves supply them and the nerve root values.

Static stability. Static stability tests the integrity of the ligaments and the joint surface. The joint should be gently stressed in each direction controlled by a ligament, while watching the patient's face to make sure that you don't hurt the patient. You do not need to use any force. Indeed, the tests will not work if you do, as the patient's muscles will go into spasm and hide the underlying static instability.

General principles of lower limb examination

Before you put the patient on the couch, ask them to walk up and down and look at their gait. See if they are limping.

Types of limp

The limp caused by any specific diagnosis is usually a complex mixture of several pathological processes, which can be divided simply into the following groups to produce an easily remembered (if ill-spelt) mnemonic:

- Long;
- Incoordinated;
- Muscle weakness;
- Pain;
- Stiff.

Long. If one limb is short then the other is long in relation to it. The patient bobs up and down when walking, when looked at from the front. However, the cadence (rhythm) of the gait is normal. There is equal time spent on each limb.

Incoordinated. The uncoordinated gait – walking has been described as controlled falling (McNeil, Alexander). In patients with neuromuscular disorders the falling is less controlled and so the patient's limp is similar to a normal person who has tripped or who is drunk. The arms are swung around to act as counterbalances. The legs frequently scissor across each other and the gait has no rhythm to it.

Muscle weakness. ***Hip (Trendelenberg gait).*** The patient's body sways sideways to and fro when looked at from the front. The patient uses the trunk muscles to lift the pelvis high enough to swing the leg through, as they cannot lift the pelvis alone.

Knee. Patients with weak quadriceps (often seen after polio) use a trick manoeuvre to lock the knee as they take weight on the leg. As they swing the leg forward, they flick the lower leg forward so that the knee extends fully well before the heel strikes the ground. They then hold the knee locked straight by keeping their hand in their pocket and pushing back on the front of the thigh as the foot comes down to heel strike. If they do not do this then the knee may buckle into flexion as they start to take weight on the leg.

Alexander McNeil. Professor of Anatomy, Loughborough, England.
Friedrich Trendelenburg, 1844–1924. Professor of Surgery, Rostock (1875–82), Bonn (1882–95) and Leipzig (1895–1911).

Ankle. With a weak ankle the patient lifts the foot very high in order to swing the leg through without catching their toes. The foot also lands with a slap on the ground because there is no control over it.

The painful limp (antalgic gait). The patient spends less time on the painful limb than the painless one. They also bob up and down when looked at from the front, dropping down as they take weight on the bad limb, and rising back up again as they take weight on the good limb. This gait can be confused with the 'long' leg gait, but there is a major difference. The cadence is abnormal. The gait is dot–dash–dot–dash because so much less time is spent on the painful limb than on the painless one.

The stiff limp. *Hip.* The patient tends to sway forwards and backwards when looked at from the side. They also hoist the pelvis up as they bring the hip through to stop it dragging on the ground.

Knee. Patients with a stiff knee often swing the leg out to the side as they walk. This is because you need to be able to lift the knee to avoid catching your toe on the ground as you bring the leg forward for the next stride.

Ankle. Patients with a stiff ankle walk with a foot that rocks forward from heel to toe in a very pronounced way.

The foot and ankle

In this chapter the examination starts with the foot and ankle. On a live patient the examination should first be directed to the part of the body with the problem (see the section on 'The history' in this chapter).

Look

Watch the patient walking, both with their shoes on and barefooted.

Look at the shoes for signs of abnormal wear.

The wear on the shoe tells you about rubbing not pressure. The normal wear pattern is for a corner to be worn off the posterolateral side of the heel (the normal point for heel strike). There may then be a circular wear pattern under the ball of the big toe (where toe off occurs as the foot provides its final drive and then lifts off). These two areas of wear may be linked in a very old shoe by a line of wear along the lateral side of the sole where most of the weight is taken during the stance phase of the stride.

Skin

Look for calluses, corns, bunions and scars, particularly in the following.

- At the base of the big toe for a bunion.

A bunion is a red swelling on the medial side of the metatarsophalangeal joint consisting of inflamed skin, a subcutaneous bursa and an osteophyste on the joint margin of the medial side of the metatarsal head (Fig. 20.1). In gout the whole metatarsal phalangeal joint will be red and swollen.

- Under the metatarsal heads.

In rheumatoid arthritis the fat pad under the metatarsal heads thins, and the heads become prominent and tender immediately beneath the skin of the sole of the foot. The patient complains of pain in the sole of the foot when walking as if walking barefoot on pebbles. Areas of thickened callous skin form over the metatarsal heads.

- Over the dorsum of interphalangeal joints and over the tips of the toes in patients with claw toes.

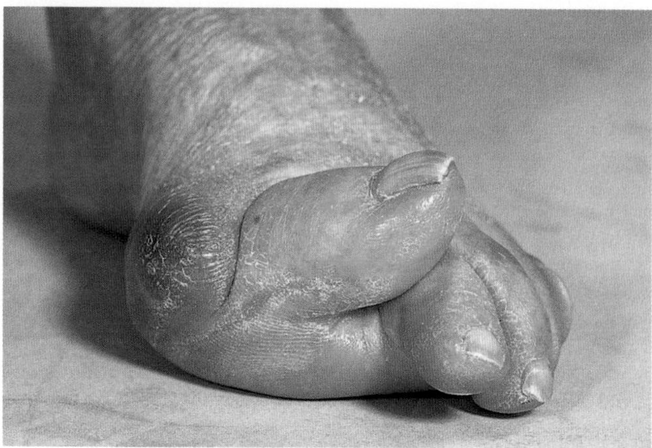

Fig. 20.1 A bunion.

Feet do not fit easily into most shoes, even when they are normal. If the toes have started to claw then the pulp of the toe will be driven into the floor of the shoe, while the dorsum of the interphalangeal joints will be driven into the top of the shoe (a sort of contracoup injury) (Fig. 20.2).

- Over the base of the fifth metatarsal if the patient is walking on the outside of the foot.

A bunion can form on the outside of the foot at the base of the fifth metatarsal. This is sometimes called a bunionnette.

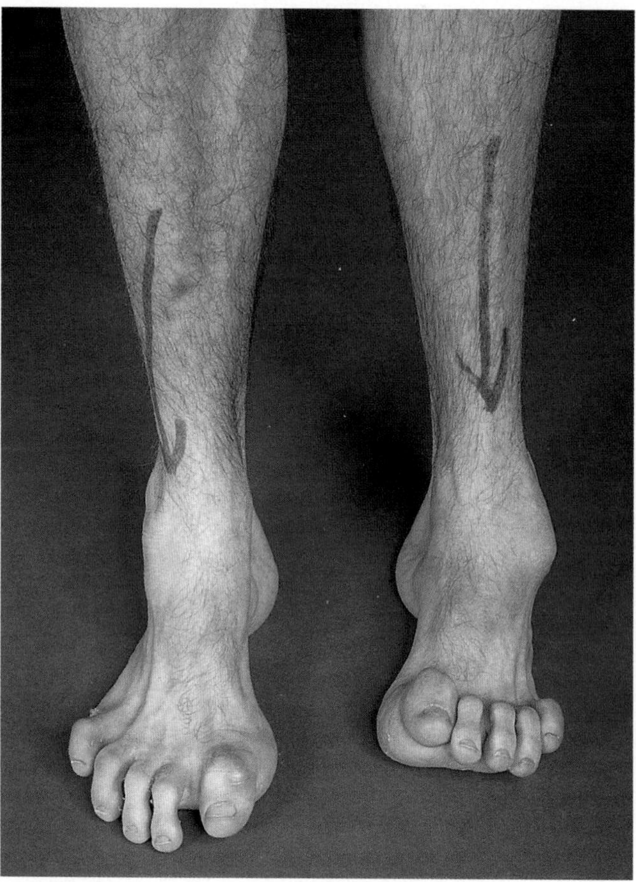

Fig. 20.2 Claw toes and wasting of intrinsic muscles of the foot.

- Over the heel.

The counter of shoes (the part that wraps around the heel) can rub on the calcaneum producing a bunion on the insertion of the achilles tendon into the bone.

- Check also for scars, cuts and redness everywhere on the foot including the sole of the foot.

Soft tissues (swelling and wasting)

Swelling in the foot is commonly seen on the dorsum only. In the ankle joint it is commonly seen at the front of the ankle.

Wasting is in seen in neurological conditions, and there may be wasting in the clefts between the metatarsals. Wasting may be associated with clawing of the toes (see Fig. 20.2).

Bone

With the patient standing, the heel should be in very slight valgus. The medial side of the foot (the arch) does not normally quite touch the ground, but is not raised so high that you can put a finger between it and the ground. The heel pad, the lateral side of the foot, all the metatarsal heads and the pulps of all the toes are on the ground when the patient is standing erect and relaxed. The toes should be relatively straight, not clawed (flexed at the interphalangeal joints and extended at the metatarsal phalangeal joint) or hammered (extended at the distal interphalangeal, and metatarsal phalangeal joint, flexed at the proximal interphalangeal joint) (Fig. 20.3).

Feel

Skin

Inflammation. Feel for heat. ***Sensation.*** In neuropathies, such as that caused by diabetes, the distal sensation may be lost, and the toes may be numb. In nerve compression in the spine (e.g. prolapsed intervertebral disc) it should only be necessary to compare the two sides by testing the sole, the medial side and lateral side, each of which is supplied by a different nerve root.

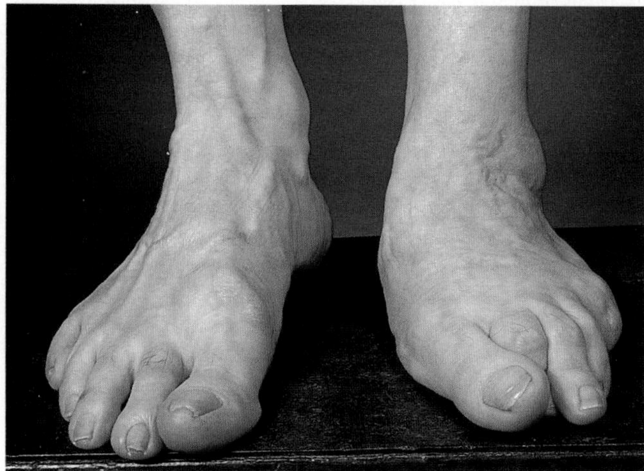

Fig. 20.3 Hammer toe – second toe to the left.

Soft tissue

Pulses. The easiest foot pulses to feel are the posterior tibial behind the medial malleolus, and the dorsal pedis between the proximal ends of the first and second metatarsals (Fig. 20.4). The toes should also be tested for capillary fillings.

Swelling. Feel the ankle joint for an effusion. It may even be possible to feel cross-fluctuation if there is a tense effusion in the ankle joint.

Wasting and gaps. Feel the tendoachilles passing up from the heel into the calf muscle. If it is ruptured it may be possible to feel a gap in the tendon.

However, an acute rupture is usually so bruised and tender that the gap is not as easy to feel as it should be. The site of tenderness will give you a clue as to whether the rupture is mid-substance or is at the musculotendinous junction (much higher in the calf). It is important to distinguish between these two as the management and prognosis are very different.

Tenderness. The extensor tendons of the toes in the dorsum of the foot and up the front of the tibia will be very tender and may even produce crepitus if there is tenosynovitis. If they are tender, ask the patient to move the tendons and you may feel crepitus under your fingers.

Bone

Tenderness. In injuries around the ankle, start feeling at the proximal fibula head, just below the knee. The Maisonneuve fracture is a sprain of the ankle with a spiral fracture of the fibula proximally. Palpate for tenderness down the length of the fibula to its tip (the lateral malleolus), and then over the lateral collateral ligament as it passes from there to the calcaneum. Then palpate down the medial side of the leg, down the tibia, to the tip of the medial malleolus and on to the medial deltoid ligament. Feel the talus and navicular, on the dorsomedial side of the forefoot. Feel the fifth metatarsal head on the lateral side of the midfoot (a common site for a fracture after an inversion injury).

After a fall from a height check for tenderness in the calcaneum, as this may be fractured. If the forefoot has been trapped (frequently behind the pedals of a car in a head-on crash) then check for tenderness in the bones of the forefoot. These may be both fractured and dislocated if the forefoot is twisted.

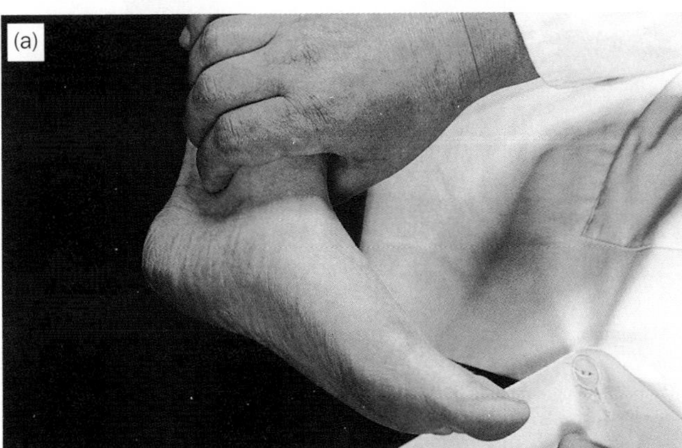

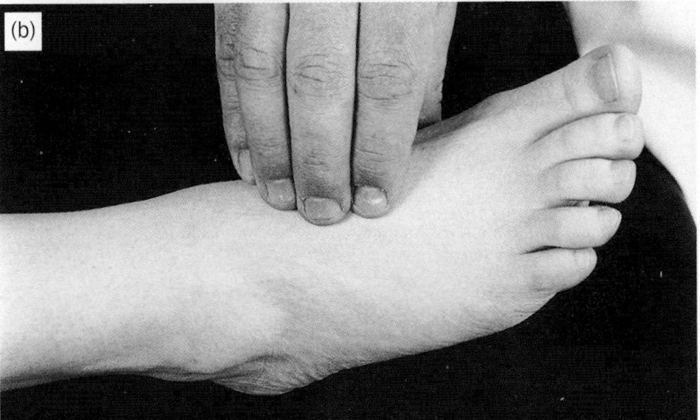

Fig. 20.4 Feeling dorsalis pedis and posterior tibial pulses.

Move

Active

Ask the patient to walk towards you then away from you. Look for limps.

The Windlass test. Make the patient stand on their toes while you look from in front and from behind. Some patients' feet look very flat when at rest. This can simply be a physiological flat foot. As soon as these patients stand on their toes, the arch forms (Fig. 20.5). In pathological flat foot the arch does not form.

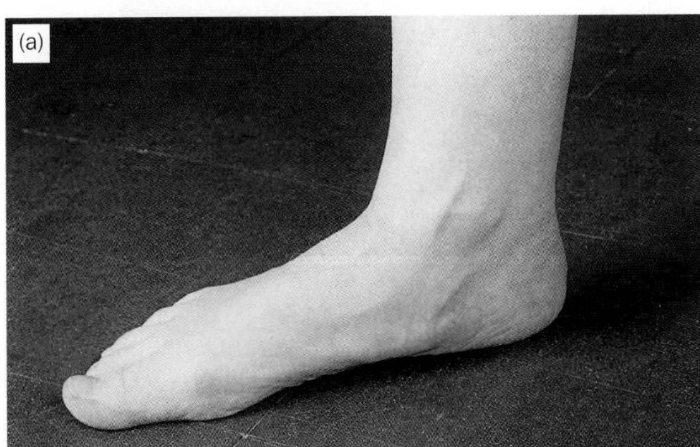

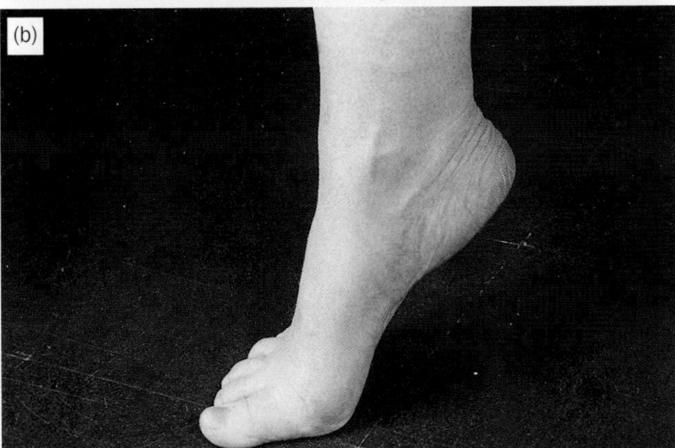

Fig. 20.5 The Windlass test. (a) At rest, the arch of the foot may be obvious. (b) As the patient rises on to their toes the arch of the foot increases. The test is normal. If the arch does not crease the patient has a pathological flat foot.

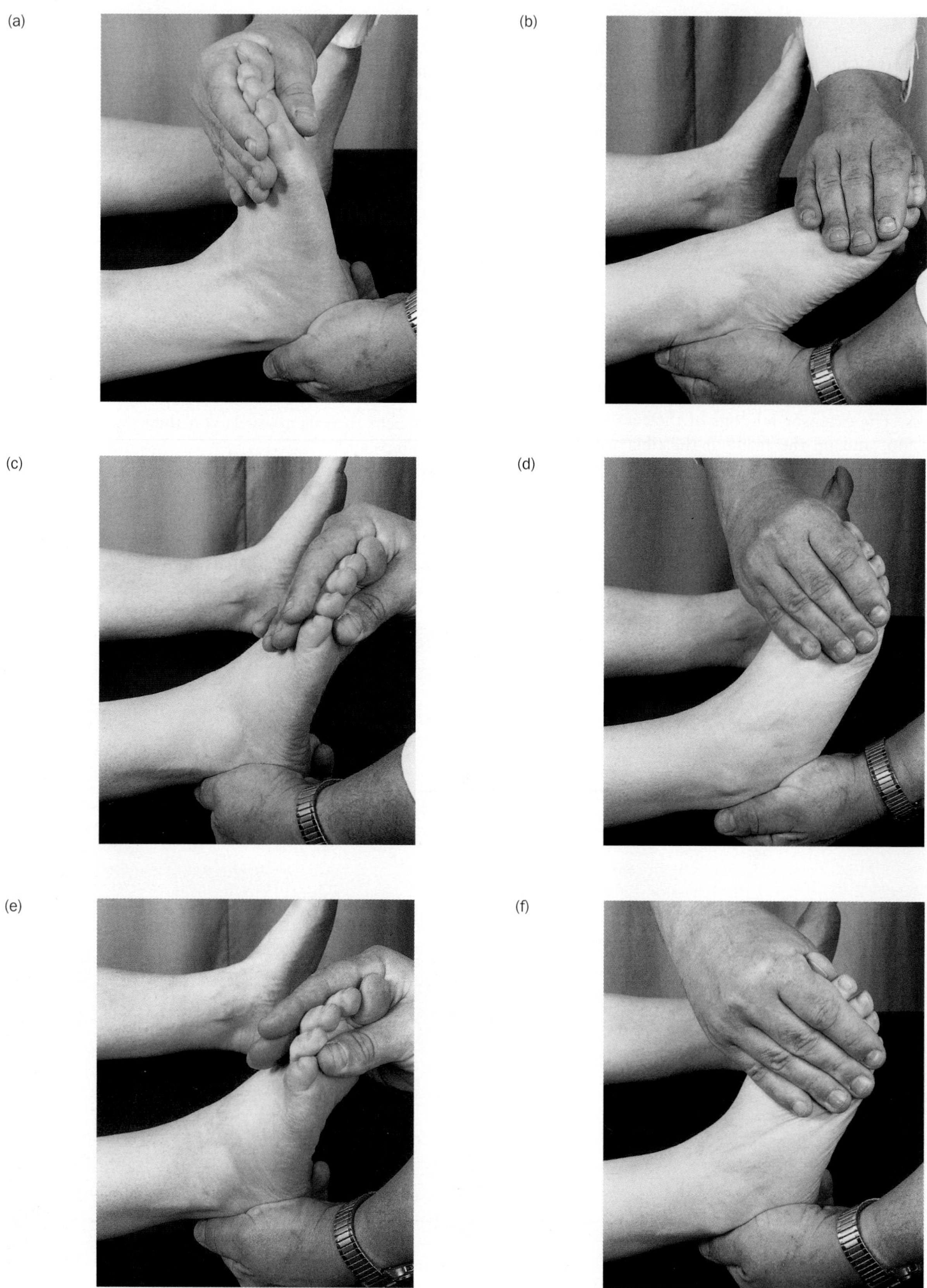

Fig. 20.6 The Apley test for movement of the ankle, the subtalar and the midfoot. The hands remain in the same position throughout testing first dorsiflexion and plantarflexion then subtalar movements (inversion and eversion) and, finally, forefoot movement (pronation and supination). (a) Dorsiflexion. (b) Plantarflexion. (c) Eversion. (d) Inversion. (e) Pronation. (f) Supination.

Other movements. You should also ask them to move their toes, and move the ankle through a full range of movement (flexion, extension, inversion and eversion).

Passive

The Apley test. If you hold the heel in one hand and the forefoot in the other, the ankle, subtalar and metatarsal mobility can be tested one after the other without moving your hands. Rocking the ankle by moving your hands in opposite directions, like a see-saw, tests ankle mobility. Tilting the foot outwards and inwards using both hands together tests subtalar movement. Twisting the forefoot while holding the hindfoot still tests midtarsal mobility (Fig. 20.6).

Hallux rigidus and claw toes. The metatarsal phalangeal joint of the big toe is stiff in hallux rigidus.

In claw toes the metatarsophalangeal joint is commonly dislocated with the phalanx riding dorsally over the metatarsal head (Fig. 20.2). Check for passive correction of the metatarsal phalangeal joint and proximal phalangeal joints.

Stability

Stability of the ankle and foot joints is not easy to test, especially after acute trauma.

If the ankle is dislocated the talus will be visible pressing hard against the skin anterior and lateral to the foot. It should be reduced at once both to save the skin (which may otherwise become necrotic) and to make the patient more comfortable.

Resisted

Test for power of extensor hallucis longus (Fig. 20.7). Remember, this muscle is specifically served only by the L5 nerve root, and is a key test for damage to this nerve in a prolapsed intervertebral disc.

In polio and other neurological disorders, each muscle will need to be tested in turn. One way to do this is to put the tips of your fingers over the muscle body, or its tendon, while holding the limb still with the other hand. The patient is asked to try to move the limb against the resistance that you have created. Your fingertips will detect whether there is any activity in the muscle, as the movement itself might be produced by alternative muscles, the so-called 'trick manoeuvres'. The power of each muscle can be graded using the Medical Research Council (MRC) power scale (Table 20.6).

Simmonds' test. The patient lies face down, feet over the end of the bed. Squeeze the calf and the foot should passively dorsiflex (Fig. 20.8). If it does not, the tendoachilles is likely to be ruptured.

Table 20.6 MRC muscle power scale

Grade	*Description*
1	Flicker of movement
2	Moves but not against gravity
3	Moves just against gravity
4	Not quite full power
5	Full power

Morris Simmonds, 1855–1925. German pathologist.

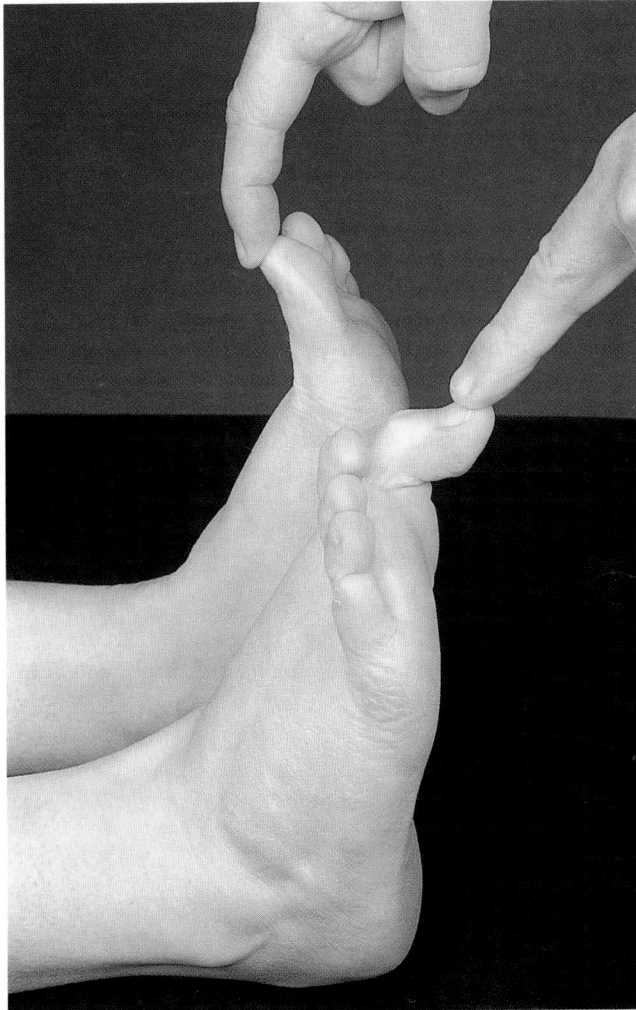

Fig. 20.7 Testing the power of the extensor hallucis longus.

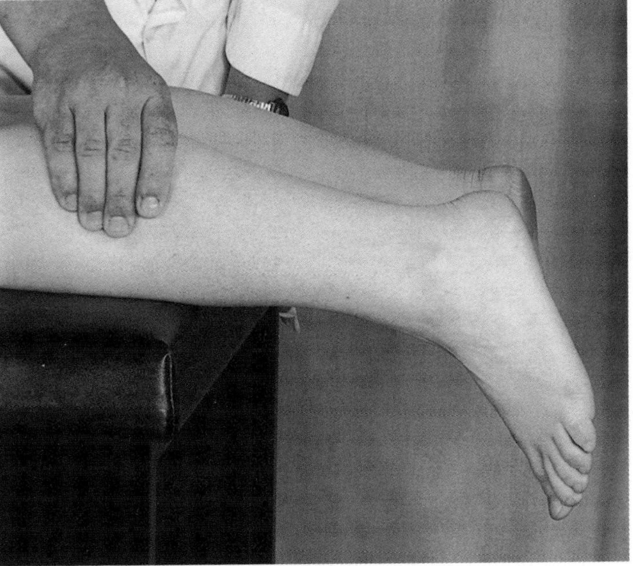

Fig. 20.8 Simmonds' test. If the foot plantarflexes when the calf is squeezed the tendoachilles is intact.

The knee

General

Watch a patient walking first before starting examination of the lower limb.

Look also from in front or behind to see whether the knees are aligned in the sagittal plane. Varus knees (or bow legs) have clear space visible between the knees when the ankles are together. It is not uncommon to see slight varus in males, a normal variant. Severe varus is commonly seen in osteoarthritis which commonly attacks the medial compartment of the knee first, as the arthritis destroys the joint which then collapses.

Valgus knees tend to brush together as the patient walks even though the ankles may be wide apart. This deformity is commonly seen in rheumatoid arthritis, which attacks the lateral side of the knee first and leads to collapse there.

Look

Expose the legs fully including thighs (rolled up trousers is not enough).

Skin

Check for redness, scars and lacerations. (Do not forget the back of the knee.)

Soft tissue

Swelling. Look for an effusion in the knee. The dimple on the medial side of the knee will be lost compared with the other side if there is an effusion.

Wasting. Vastus medialis can be clearly seen if the patient is asked to force their knees into hyperextension. This muscle wastes within days of a knee injury, and will fail to bulge when contracted, compared with the other side.

Bone

Check for knock-knee, bow legs, fixed flexion and for the position of patella (Fig. 20.9).

Fixed flexion is the position of comfort in the knee and tends to develop secondary to any acute infection or inflammation.

The patella almost always dislocates laterally (Fig. 20.10). If not reduced it may remain jammed outside the lateral femoral condyle.

Feel

Skin

Temperature. Inflammation of the knee will produce a knee hot to the touch compared with the other side.

Sensation. Damage to nerves at or around the knee will produce disturbance of sensation distally. The same examination as described in the section on 'The foot and ankle' should therefore be performed.

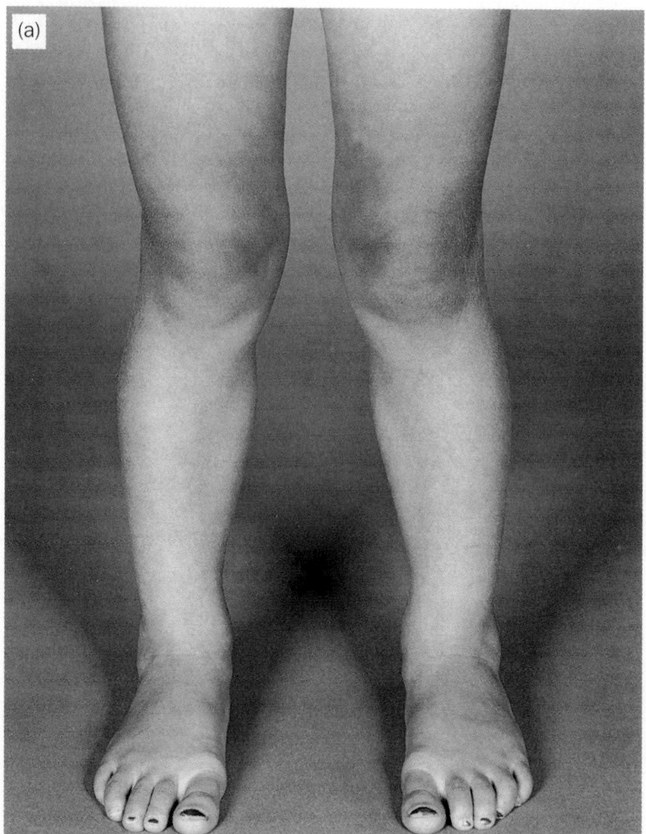

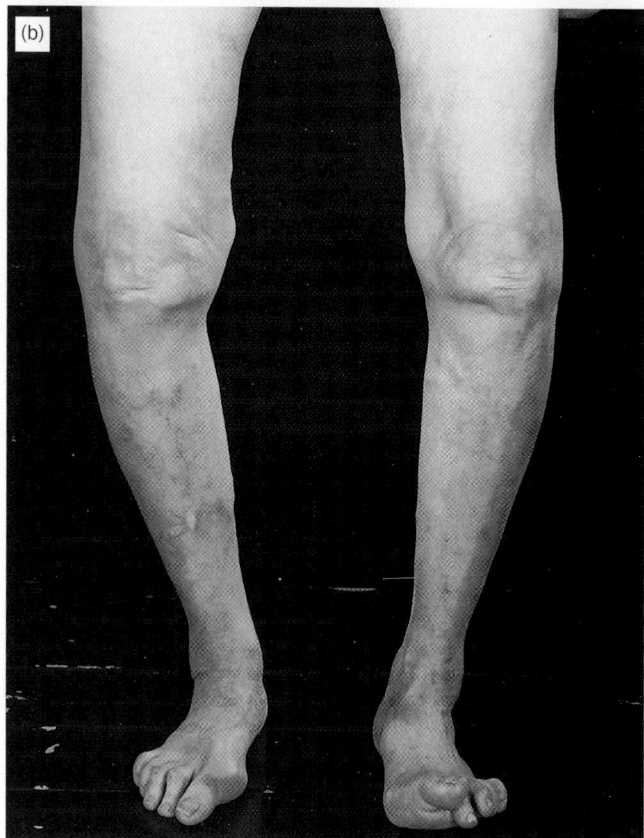

Fig. 20.9 Knock-knee and bow legs.

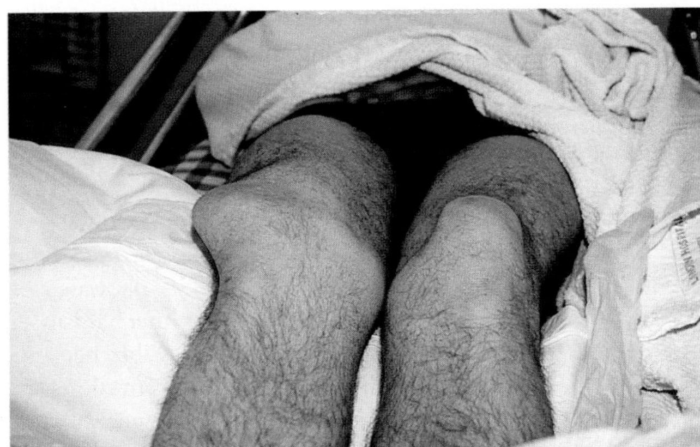

Fig. 20.10 Dislocated patella.

Soft tissue

Swelling. Check for a knee effusion, using either a patella tap, cross fluctuation or a stroke test.

Stroke test. With the patient lying supine, empty the medial side of the knee joint by stroking any fluid up into the suprapatella pouch. Then watching the medial side of the knee carefully, stroke down the front of the thigh squeezing any fluid lying in the suprapatella pouch back into the medial side of the knee. As the fluid returns the dimple on the medial side of the knee pops out (Fig. 20.11).

The margin of the synovium can most easily be felt on the medial side above the patella. It can be rolled under your fingers, but is only palpable if the synovium is thickened.

Baker's cyst. This is an outpouching of the synovium through a defect in the capsule posteriorly. It can be difficult to feel. As soon as the knee is flexed the cyst disappears, but reappears in full extension. It is associated with osteoarthritis of the knee. The patient will guide your fingers to the lump if you are having difficulty finding it.

Wasting. Atrophy of the vastus medialis is more easily seen than felt.

Circulation. The distal pulses and capillary filling should be checked in the same way as examination of the foot.

Bone

The margins of the patella, the femoral condyles and the margins of the tibial plateau are all easy to feel as they are subcutaneous. The underside of the patella may be tender if there is synovitis of the knee when the inflammed synovium is compressed against the bone.

The inferior pole of the patella is tender if there is tendonitis of the patella tendon origin (jumper's knee).

The fat pad beneath the patella tendon is tender in Hoffa's syndrome, an inflammation commonly brought on by sudden forced hyperextension of the knee.

William Morrant Baker, 1838–96. Surgeon, St Bartholomew's Hospital, London, England.

The tibial tubercle is enlarged and tender when the insertion of the patella tendon is inflammed (Osgood–Schlatter's syndrome), a common condition in athletic adolescents.

A tear in the meniscus may produce tenderness at the joint line margin over the area of the tear.

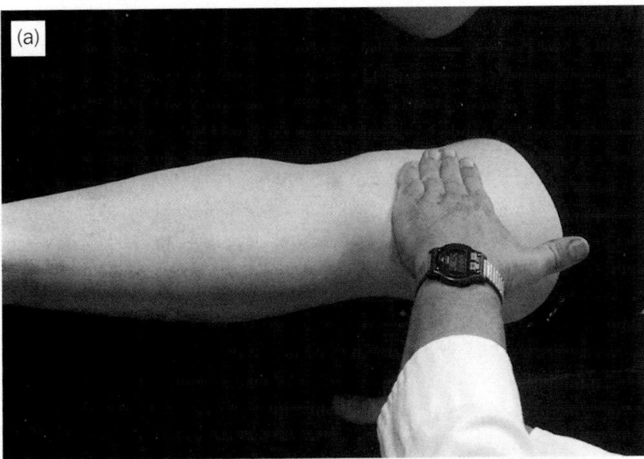

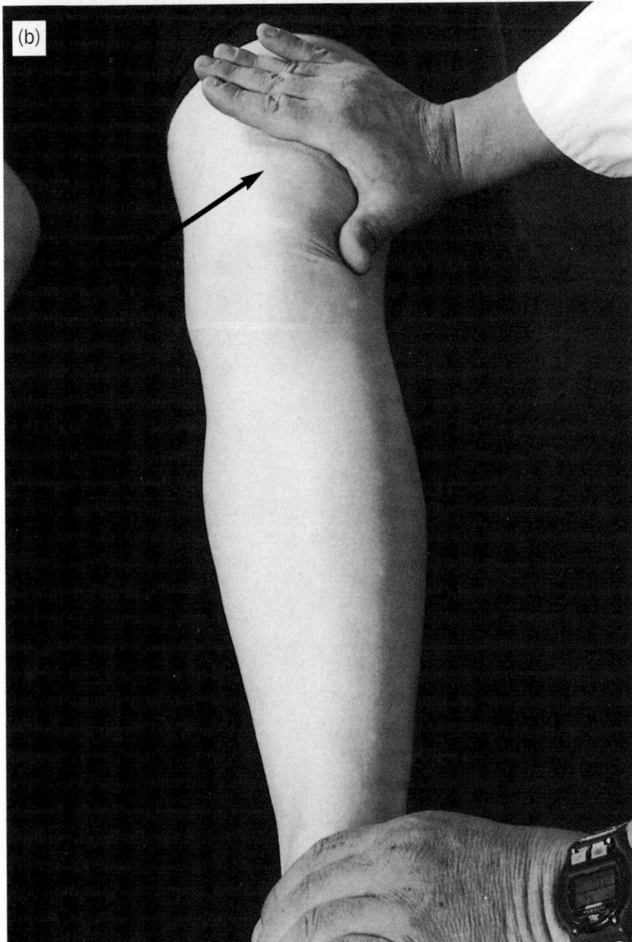

Fig. 20.11 Stroke test for fluid in the knee. (a) Any fluid in the knee is stroked up into the suprapatella pouch. (b) The fluid is forced back down and a watch kept for a pouting of the dimple on the medial side of the patella (see arrow).

The medial collateral ligament extends from two finger's breadth above the knee joint to four fingers breadth below the joint. Tenderness over the ligament may indicate traumatic damage to the ligament.

Move

Active

Flexion. The knee should be able to flex until the heel touches the buttock. Loss of flexion can be measured by the number of centimetres that the heel stops short of the buttock, rather than by actually measuring the angle of the knee. Comparison with the other side gives a sensitive guide to loss of range of movement.

Extension. The patient should be asked to force their knee into the bed. Most knees hyperextend at least by a few degrees.

Passive

Flexion. The knee can be bent up passively, but be sure to watch the patient's face, especially if you push the knee beyond the active range of flexion. It may be limited because of pain.

Extension. With the patient lying supine and relaxed the feet can be raised off the bed by lifting under the heels. Any loss of extension will be visible because one knee will remain higher (in fixed flexion) than the other.

In posterior ligamentous damage to the knee (as may occur in a hyperextension injury) the knee may hyperextend excessively. In this case the abnormal limb will be lower than the other.

Lag test. A subtle test for quadriceps weakness is to ask the patient to lift their leg 10 cm off the bed. Most patients can do this and, indeed, even if the quadriceps mechanism is completely ruptured this manoeuvre is still possible because the patient uses the lateral retinaculum to lock the knee in extension. The patient is then asked to bend the knee 20° and straighten it, again with the leg still in the air (Fig. 20.12). The patient will not be able to return the knee to its original extension if the quadriceps muscle is weak. This loss of flexion is not a fixed flexion deformity (they have already demonstrated that the knee will extend); it is caused by weakness in the quadriceps and is known a 'quads lag'.

Stability

Collateral ligaments. The integrity of the collateral ligaments can only be tested when the knee is slightly flexed. In full

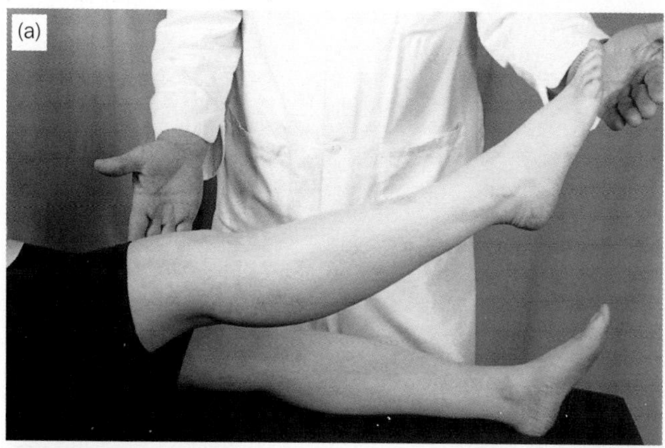

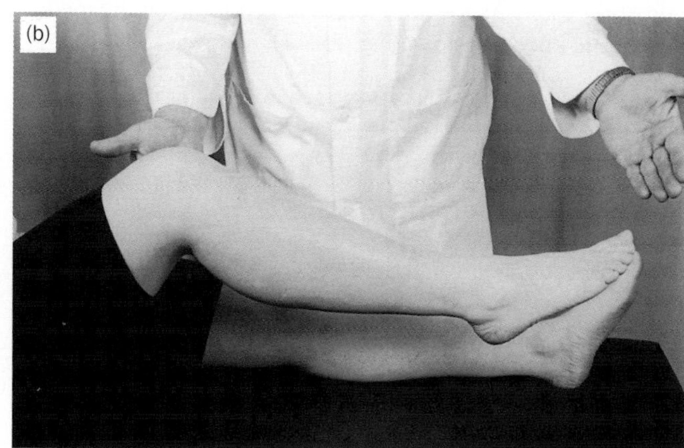

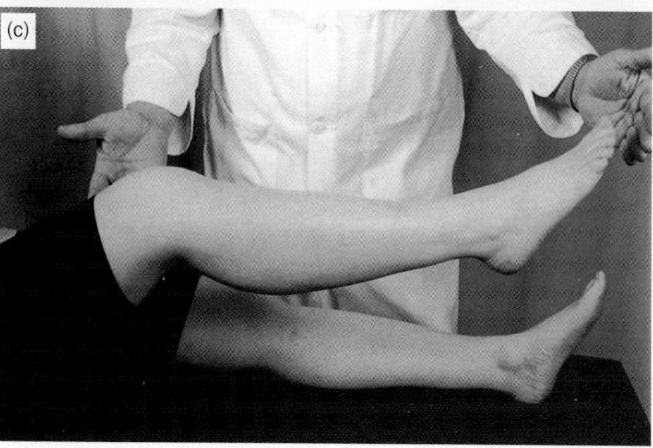

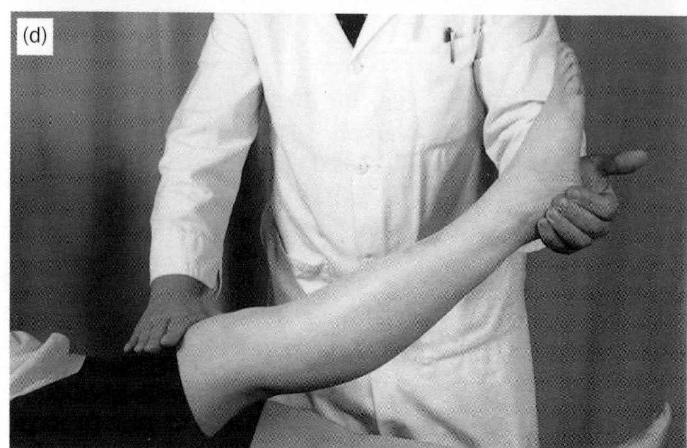

Fig. 20.12 The lag test. (a) Step 1 – the patient lifts the leg with the knee straight. (b) Step 2 – the patient flexes their knee. (c) Step 3 – the patient is now asked to try to extend the knee again without support. If they are not able to extend it fully there is a 'flexion deformity'. (d) Step 4 – the patient is helped to extend their knee. If it will not extend further there is a 'fixed flexion deformity'. If it will, there is a 'quadriceps lag'.

extension the stability of the posterior capsule masks any collateral ligament instability. However, if the knee is flexed more than a few degrees, the knee rotates when stress is put on the knee to test medial and lateral stability, and it is not possible to check integrity of the ligaments. The leg should be rested on the bed with the patient supine. One of your hands should be put behind the knee to lift it slightly into flexion, hold it stable and feel with thumb and fingers over the joint line. Your other hand should grasp the patient's ankle, and gently stress the lower leg into varus (putting load on the lateral collateral ligament) then into valgus (stressing the medial collateral ligament) while still holding the knee with your other hand (Fig. 20.13). Knee ligaments vary in their laxity between patients, and it is a difference between the two sides which once again gives a clue to instability. Pain over the ligament on stressing without instability suggests a partial tear.

Cruciate ligaments. The anterior is the cruciate ligament most commonly injured.

History. The patient is commonly twisting on a flexed knee and the foot jams on the ground. There is often a loud crack and the knee swells immediately (with blood). If the injury occurs during sport the patient cannot play on and is usually carried off. The injury may be accompanied by a torn meniscus or, indeed, the instability may subsequently cause a torn meniscus. If the quadriceps are allowed to waste (as they will without treatment) the knee will be unstable giving way on turns and swelling up each time this occurs. If the meniscus is also torn the knee may lock intermittently (become jammed in flexion).

The posterior cruciate has a completely different mechanism of injury. It can occur either as a result of a hyperextension injury, or if the tibia is driven backwards with the knee in flexion (the dashboard injury).

There are several tests for cruciate disruption but one simple method is as follows. The patient lies supine with both knees bent up to a right angle and the feet resting on the bed. The examiner looks from the side to see whether one tibial tubercle is lying further back than the other. If the tubercle on the injured side is lying further back then the knee has a posterior sag (suggestive of a posterior cruciate ligament injury). The examiner then grasps the uninjured knee with fingers meeting in the popliteal fossa and thumbs side by side over the tibial tubercle. Sit on the patient's foot to keep it still and then rock the upper tibia gently backwards and forwards against the femur, feeling for the amount of laxity in the joint. Now repeat the manoeuvre with the injured limb, comparing the amount of 'play' in the injured knee with the normal one. If there is more play and the injured knee had a posterior sag then the posterior cruciate is ruptured. If there was no sag then the problem is rupture of the anterior cruciate (Fig. 20.14).

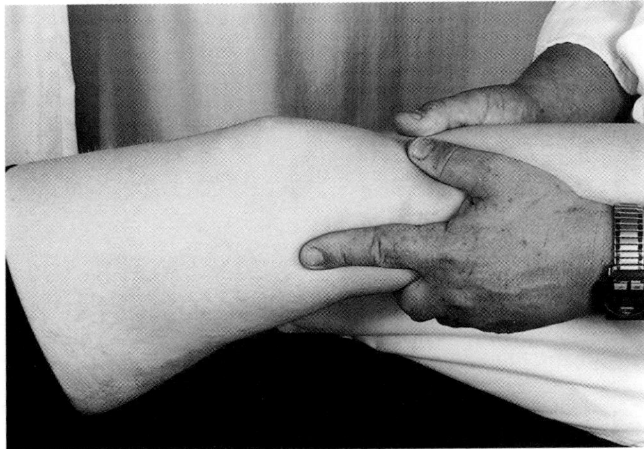

Fig. 20.13 Hand position for testing of collateral ligament stability in the knee.

The pivot shift test. This test relies on the fact that an anterior cruciate deficient knee frequently has some rotatory instability in extension. In this position the femoral condyles rolling on the tibia do not control rotation well. With the patient lying supine and the examiner sitting at the patient's foot facing up the bed, one hand is used to lift the leg off the bed by the ankle and to rotate the tibia inwards on the femur. The examiner's other hand presses against the lateral side of the knee pushing it into valgus, so that the lateral femoral condyle is engaged firmly with the tibial plateau. This hand now gently pushes the knee into flexion (Fig. 20.15). If there is anterior cruciate instability the knee starts to

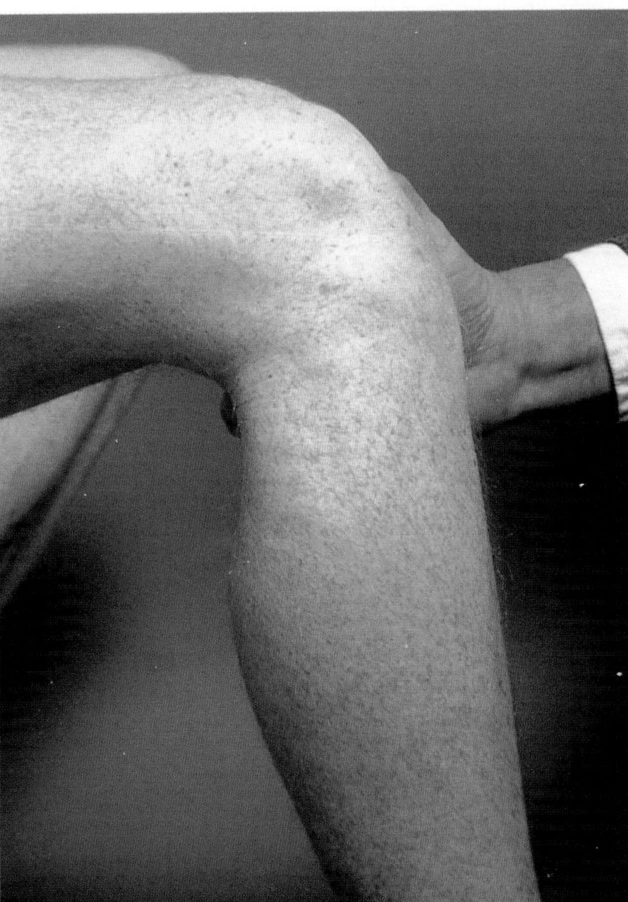

Fig. 20.14 Anterior draw. The tibia is unstable on the femur and has fallen forward. The anterior cruciate ligament is disrupted.

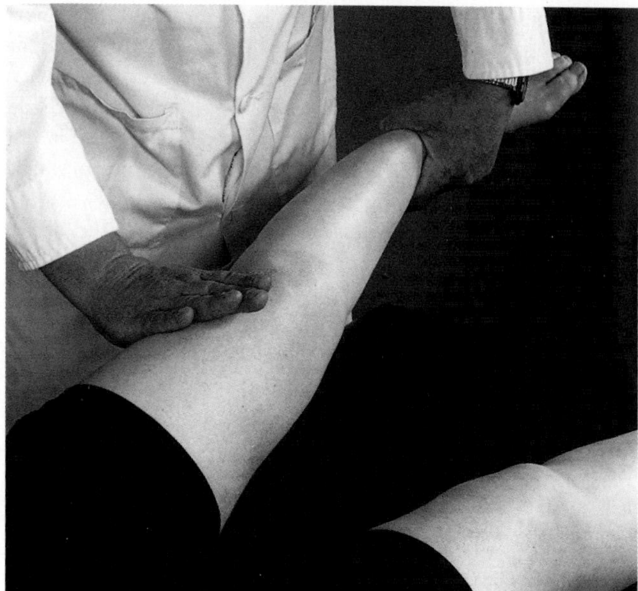

Fig. 20.15 Position of hands for the pivot shift test.

bend under the guidance of the examiner's hand, but then jams at about 10° of flexion. The tibia has rotated so much on the femur (because of the absent anterior cruciate ligament) that the knee will no longer work as a hinge, but jams as soon as it tries to do so. As the examiner's hand pushes the knee on into flexion, the knee has to come out of internal rotation so that the jammed joint can continue to flex. The jolt as the tibia derotates under the examiner's hand is clearly palpable to the examiner and to the patient. It is even easier to feel if the examiner's thumb lies tucked behind the fibula head. It is then forced smartly back when the derotation occurs. This test should be done very gently. If it is not the patient will be hurt and the test will be inconclusive because muscle spasm will mask the pivot shift.

Patella apprehension.

History. Patients who have lax ligaments (are double-jointed) are much more susceptible to dislocation of the patella. The dislocation commonly occurs during a twisting manoeuvre on a flexed knee and if the knee cap relocates immediately the injury can closely mimic the history of an anterior cruciate rupture. The knee swells at once (with blood) and the patient is unable to walk on it. If the patella stays out the patient may claim that they saw a lump on the medial side of the knee. This is in fact the medial femoral condyle (the patient assumes that the patella indicates the position of the knee). Examination of a knee which has recently had a dislocated patella is very difficult as the knee is stiff, swollen and very painful. However, patients who dislocate a patella have frequently previously dislocated the other patella and the patella apprehension test can be performed on the opposite knee.

The test. If patients have ever dislocated their patella they will be anxious about dislocating it again. If the knee is placed in extension and the patella pushed laterally, flexing the knee will encourage the patella to dislocate over the lateral femoral condyle (Fig. 20.16). As soon as this starts to happen the patient will become very apprehensive. Do not continue – just note the apprehension; you do not want to actually dislocate the patella.

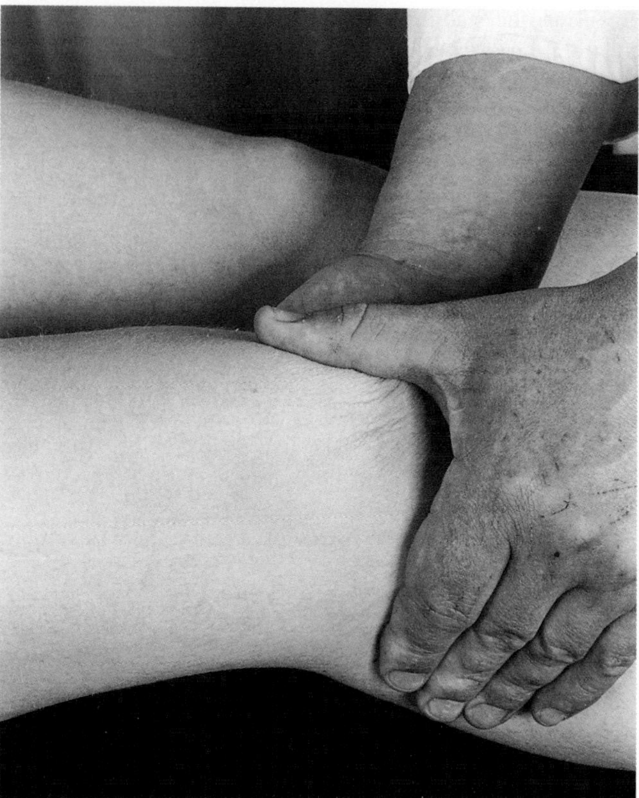

Fig. 20.16 Patella apprehension test. The patella is formed laterally as the knee is passively flexed with the examiner's other hand.

The hip

The hip is rarely involved in extrinsic trauma but is commonly affected by intrinsic trauma (fractured neck of femur) and by chronic conditions (osteoarthritis). The examination of the joint is made more difficult by the fact that it is covered by muscles. It is also likely to present with pain referred to the knee, and can be the site of pain referred from the spine.

Look

Limp

Watch the patient walk, and look for a limp. The limp of a stiff hip is difficult to spot as the patient rocks their pelvis with the femur on the affected side, but fixed flexion deformity is common and leads to the patient walking with a characteristic stooped gait.

Skin

The scars from surgery on the hip are usually on the lateral side of the hip.

Soft tissue

Gluteal wasting can occur if the superior gluteal nerve was damaged after hip surgery, but beware of confusing gluteal wasting with loss of lumbar lordosis caused by back problems. The tilt of the pelvis may make it look as if there is bilateral gluteal wasting.

Bone

There is little to see because the hip is so deeply buried, but a limp may give a clue to underlying bony deformity.

Feel

Skin

As the joint is so deeply buried the only item that needs checking is distal sensation. Damage to the femoral nerve produces numbness over the front of the thigh. Damage to the sciatic nerve will produce numbness in the lower leg.

Soft tissues

Peripheral pulses can, again, be tested in the foot.

Bone

The hip can be palpated anteriorly in the groin beneath the femoral pulse, but the hip is deep and difficult to feel. Tenderness on the lateral side of the hip arises from the greater trochanter or is referred from the spine. Pain posteriorly is usually the sciatic nerve or, once again, has been referred from the spine.

Leg length discrepancy

Leg length discrepancy can be caused by bones in the two limbs being of unequal length, such as might occur after a fracture. It can also be caused by deformity such as a fixed flexion deformity of the hip. Leg length discrepancy caused solely by short bones is known by convention as 'true' leg length discrepancy. That caused by joint deformity is known as 'apparent' shortening. Most leg length discrepancy is caused by a mixture of the two.

True leg length discrepancy. It is usual to measure the 'true' leg length discrepancy first by putting both legs as straight as possible, and then measuring the leg which cannot be put straight. The other leg is then put into an identical position, so that the deformity has no effect on leg length discrepancy. If the end of the tape measure is held firmly between the pulp of the thumb and the side of the index finger the tip of the thumb can be used to trace the inguinal ligament upwards until it catches in the notch immediately below the anterior superior iliac crest. A similar manoeuvre can be used at the lower end of the leg. The tip of the examiner's other thumb is traced up the calcaneus, until it jams in the notch immediately below the medial malleolus. The measure is repeated on the other limb which is first put in the identical position.

In order to decide which bone(s) are responsible for the shortening, the patient should lie supine and the knees should be bent up to a right angle. The examiner should then look at the knees from the side. If the femur on the short side lies lower then the shortening is below the knee. If the tibia lies further back then the shortening lies above the knee. If the shortening is above the knee then palpation of the greater trochanters will reveal whether the shortening is in the femoral neck or in the femoral shaft. If the shortening is below the knee then palpation of the medial and lateral malleolus will reveal whether the shortening is above or below the ankle.

Apparent leg length discrepancy. Apparent leg discrepancy is that caused by joint deformity and is best calculated from the difference in true leg length, as measured above, and the difference in leg length when both legs are put as straight as possible.

Leg length discrepancy is very difficult to measure accurately using clinical methods, but can be measured very precisely, when necessary, using X-rays with grids superimposed. An alternative method clinically is to give the patient raised blocks to walk over. The height of the blocks is raised under the sole of the shorter leg until the patient feels that the short leg is now too long. Reduction of the height by 5 mm usually produces a measure which can be used as a shoe raise to correct leg length inequality. Discrepancies of 1 cm or less can usually be hidden inside the shoe. Raises of up to 2–3 cm can be put on the heel only, so keeping the shoe light. Raises of more than this usually require a raise of the sole and the heel.

Move

Active and passive

In the hip active and passive movements are measured together in the modified Thomas's test, which will be described below.

Modified Thomas's test. The patient bends up both their knees and hips actively, rolling themselves into a ball. The examiner can then carefully (watching the patient's face) push the hips into further flexion (passive flexion). The flexion of the two hips can now be checked and compared. The patient is now asked to hold the affected hip flexed by holding their shin in their hands. This fixes the pelvis in full flexion. The other leg is now carefully extended as far as comfortable and a note made of the angle that the femur makes to the couch in full extension. The normal leg is now flexed back up again as far as possible, and held there by the patient. The abnormal hip is now allowed to extend (carefully watching the patient's face) until it too will extend no further (Fig. 20.17). Again, the angle that the femur makes with the couch is noted and compared with the recording made on the other side. Both legs are now lowered on to the bed and a note is made of the range of flexion and extension of both hips, noting that the examination was performed with the pelvis in full flexion.

Abduction. Lay your forearm across the patient's pelvis with the tips of your fingers resting on one anterior superior iliac spine and your forearm resting on the other one nearer

Hugh Owen Thomas, 1834–91. Surgeon, Liverpool, England. Regarded as founder of orthopaedic surgery. He introduced his splint in 1875.

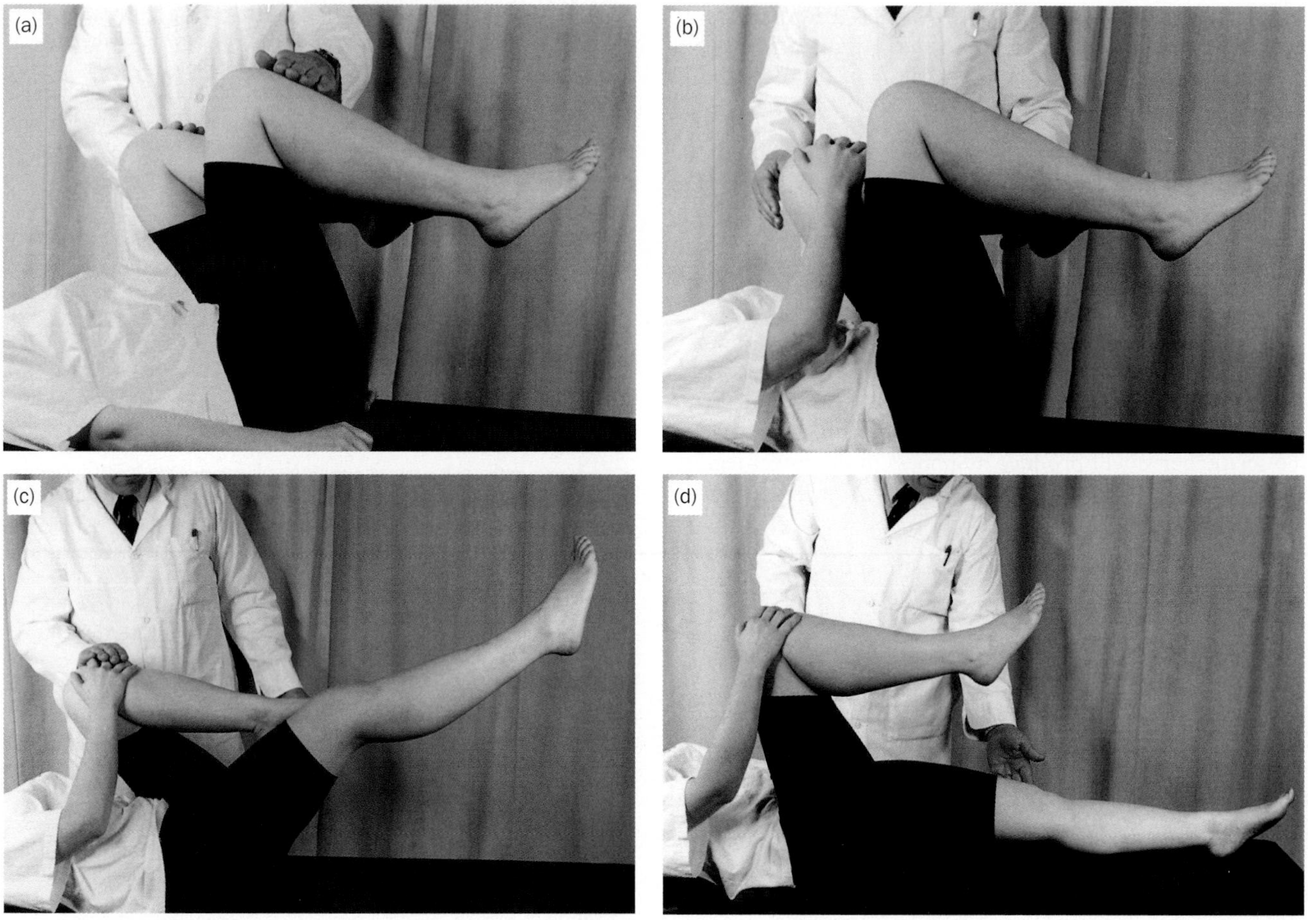

Fig. 20.17 Modified Thomas's test. (a) The patient actively flexes both hips fully. (b) Grasping the good leg to keep it flexed. (c) Drop the bad leg into extension. The loss of extension is fixed flexion deformity. (d) They then flex fully the bad leg, grasp it and extend the other leg to feel for its fixed flexion.

to you. Abduct first one hip and note the angle when you feel the pelvis starting to move under your hands. Return that leg to its original position and repeat the manoeuvre with the other leg.

Abduction. Still leaving one hip abducted, adduct the other hip across until the pelvis starts to move. Put that hip back in abduction and adduct the other hip, noting the range of movement of abduction and adduction on both sides (Fig. 20.18).

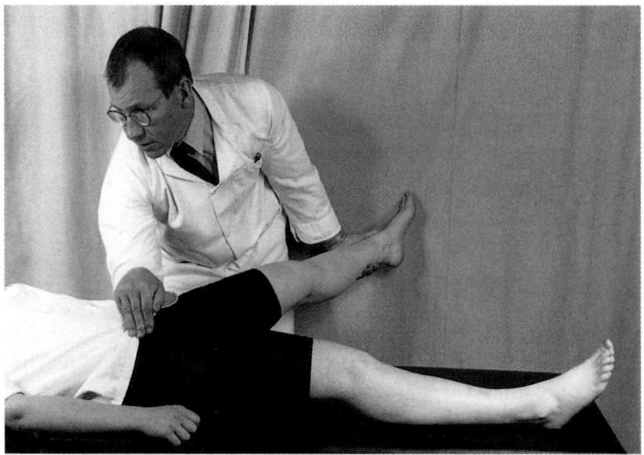

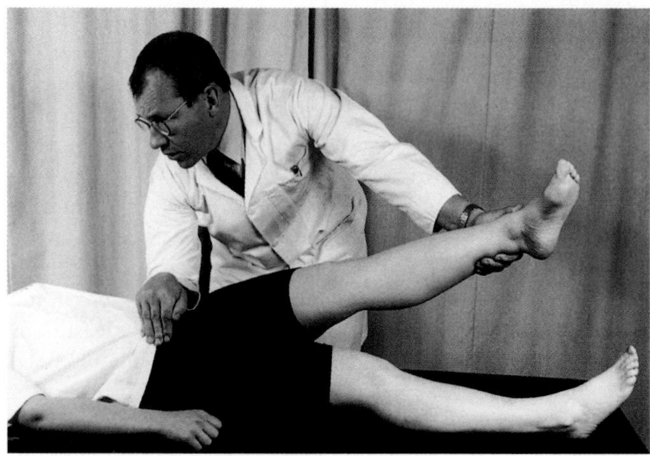

Fig. 20.18 Making sure the pelvis remains still while testing abduction and adduction. The examiner must watch the patient's face to be sure they do not cause any pain.

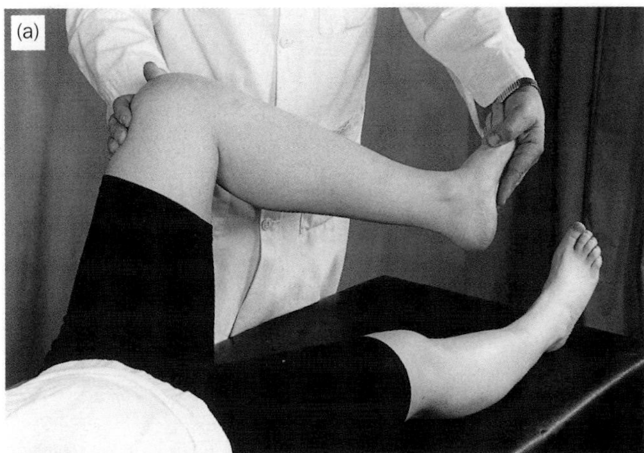

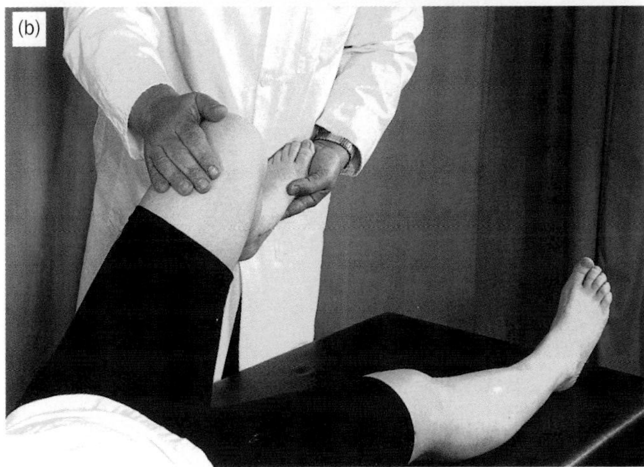

Fig. 20.19 Testing rotation of the hip joint with the hip flexed to 45° and the knee flexed at 90°.

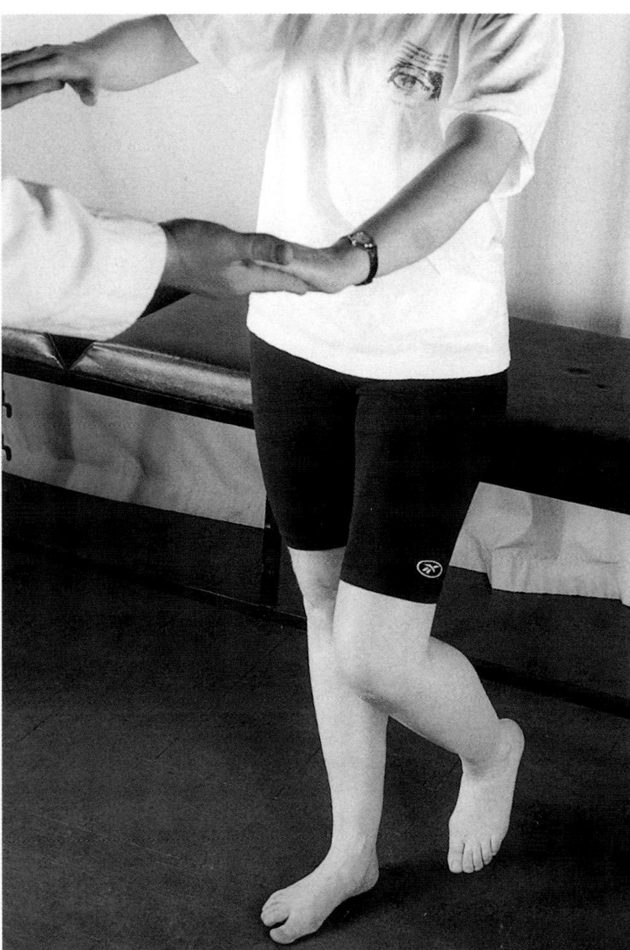

Fig. 20.20 Trendelenburg test. As the patient stands on the right leg with weak abductors they push down with their left hand to save themselves from falling.

Rotation. Rotation of the hip will always be limited in extremes of extension and flexion, as the capsule of the hip is already tight. It is therefore important to test the range of movement of the hip in the mid-range with the thigh flexed at 45°. If the knee is flexed to 90° the tibia can be used as a lever and a protractor. Watch the patient's face, and test internal and external rotation, comparing the two sides. Note that when the foot comes across the body you are testing external rotation, and when the foot comes out to the side you are testing internal rotation (Fig. 20.19).

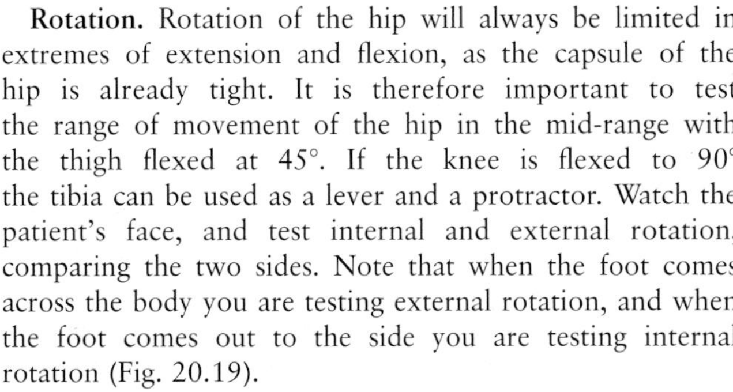

Stability

The Trendelenburg test. This is a test of stability of the hip joint or of weakness of the gluteal muscles, such that the patient has great difficulty taking all of their weight on the affected leg. The most sensitive way of performing this test is to ask the patient to stand on both legs facing you, and to place their hands palm downwards on your hands held palm upwards. The patient is asked first to stand on their healthy leg, then repeat the manoeuvre on the affected leg. If the test is positive the examiner will feel a firm push downwards from the patient's hand on the affected side as the patient tries to transfer their weight on to the affected limb (Fig. 20.20).

Tests for referred pain

Pain in the hip can be referred down from the spine, while pathology in the hip can produce pain in the knee. A simple test which can help distinguish pathology in the hip from pathology elsewhere is the 'pastry rolling test'. With the patient lying supine on the couch start with the unaffected side. Place the palm of one of your hands on the patient's shin, and the other on their thigh. Keep your hands flat with the fingers straight, and roll the leg as one to and fro under your hands as if you were rolling pastry. If there is no problem in the hip, the patient will relax completely after a couple of rolls, and their foot will flop to and fro at the end of the leg (Fig. 20.21). Repeat the test on the affected side. If there is pain and/or stiffness in the hip joint the patient will not relax, the foot will not flop to and fro, and there will be a distinct resistance to movement at the end of internal and external rotation. Pathology in the knee does not do this because the knee joint is being rolled as one. Similarly, the sciatic nerve is not irritated by internal and external rotation of the hip, so pathology in the spine has no effect on this test.

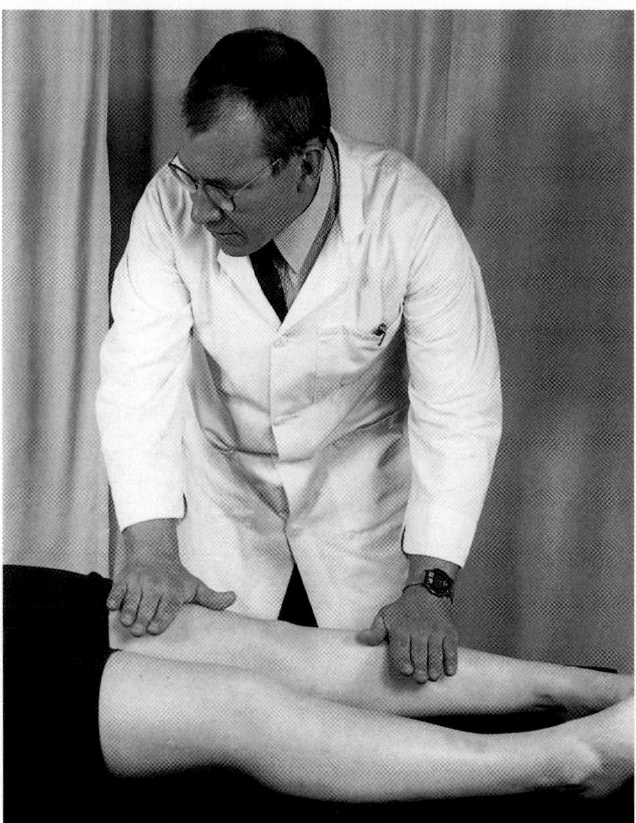

Fig. 20.21 Pastry roll test for pain in the hip and from pain (?) to the hip.

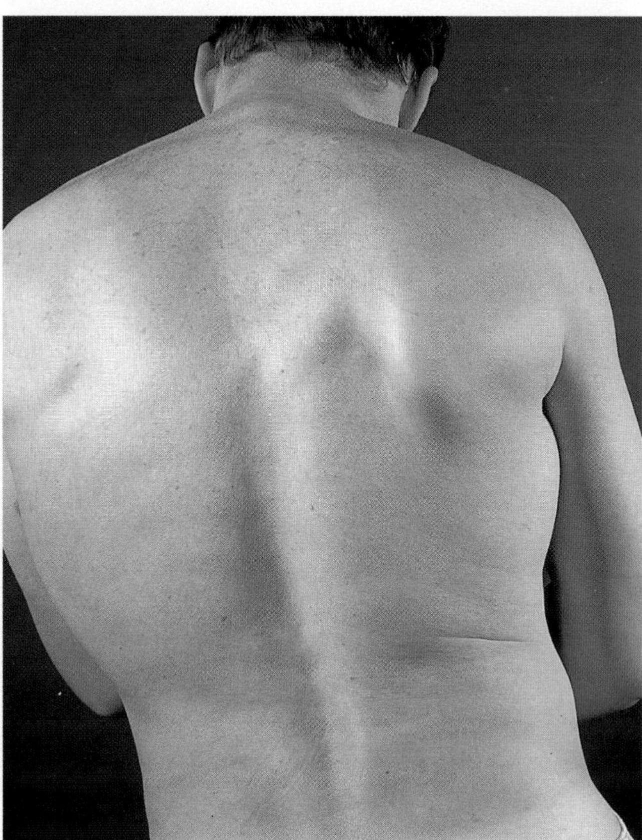

Fig. 20.22 Loss of lumbar lordosis and paraspinal muscle spasm caused by prolapsed intervertebral disc.

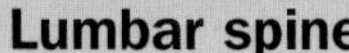

Lumbar spine

The lumbar spine is another part of the anatomy which can be best examined initially with the patient standing up. Exposure is important and the back must be visible as far down as the natal cleft. The key to the examination of the lumbar spine is a full examination of the lower limbs. Irritation of nerves in the spine can mimic problems in the lower limb. Whenever you see a patient with problems in the lower limb, keep in the back of your mind that this problem could be referred from the spine.

Look

Skin

Look for hairy tufts and dimples at the base of the spine which may indicate an underlying spina bifida.

Soft tissue

Look at the muscles on each side of the spine. If they are very prominent they may be in spasm.

Bone

The lumbar spine should have a smooth concavity (lumbar lordosis). Loss of lordosis and flattening of the buttocks go with muscle spasm (Fig. 20.22).

If the spine is curved laterally (scotiosis) then there are three common causes. The legs may be unequal in length (postural scoliosis). This scoliosis will disappear when the patient sits down. Secondly, there may be a fixed scoliosis in the thoracic spine, with a compensatory scoliosis in the lumbar region below it. Thirdly, there may be spasm in the muscles around the lumbar spine caused by pain.

Feel

Skin

Sensation. Test sensation in both legs. Sensory loss is most likely to be detectable distally, so simply compare touch on the lateral and medial side of both feet. If this is abnormal, then continue to a full neurological examination. Test for any loss of sensation in the perineal area if the patient complains of sudden onset of pain and numbness in both legs (cauda equina syndrome).

Soft tissue

Feel the muscles on each side of the spine for spasm.

Bone

Trace the line of the spine with your fingers, checking for scoliosis.

Feel the spine of the L5 and the S1 vertebrae. A step between the two may indicate a spondylolisthesis.

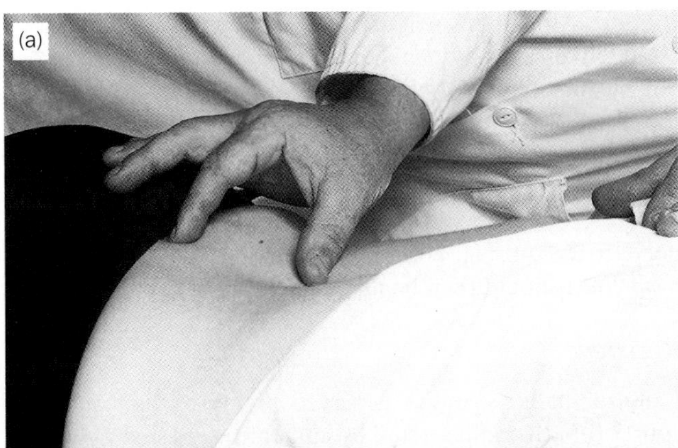

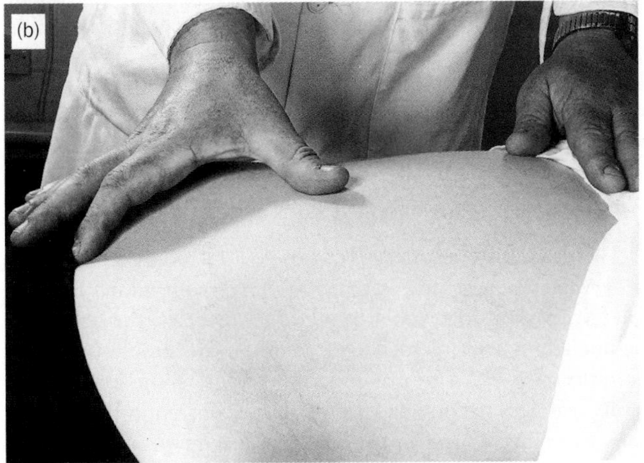

Fig. 20.23 Testing mobility in the lumbar spine. (a) Index finger over the lumbar–sacral junction, thumb over thoracolumbar junction. (b) Index finger and thumb separate as lumbar spine flexes.

Move

Active

Flexion/extension. Place the tip of your thumb over the T12–L1 junction, and the tip of your index finger of the same hand over the lumbosacral junction. Ask the patient to reach forward to try to touch their toes. Note the distance that your thumb and tip of finger separate as the patient bends forward (Fig. 20.23). This distance is a measure of lumbar flexibility.

Note also how far the tips of the patient's fingers can reach down their legs when they bend forwards. The distance that they can reach is an indication of total spinal flexibility combined with hip flexibility.

Most patients cannot touch their toes, but some hypermobile patients can put the palms of their hands on the floor. Flexibility depends on fitness, age, gender and overall body mobility, and varies enormously between individuals.

Lateral deviation. Ask the patient to slide first one hand and then the other down the side of their thigh, bending laterally. The spine should bend smoothly from top to bottom. Total mobility can be recorded by noting the distance that each hand can move down the side of that thigh (Fig. 20.24).

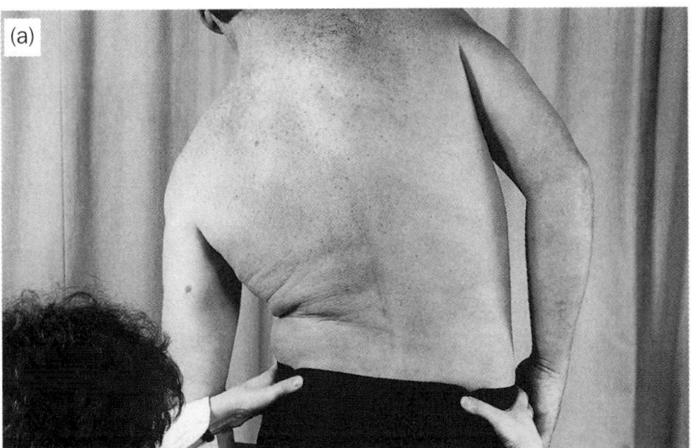

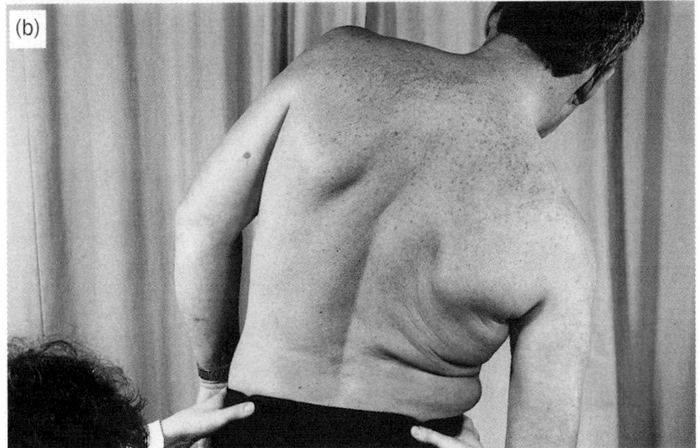

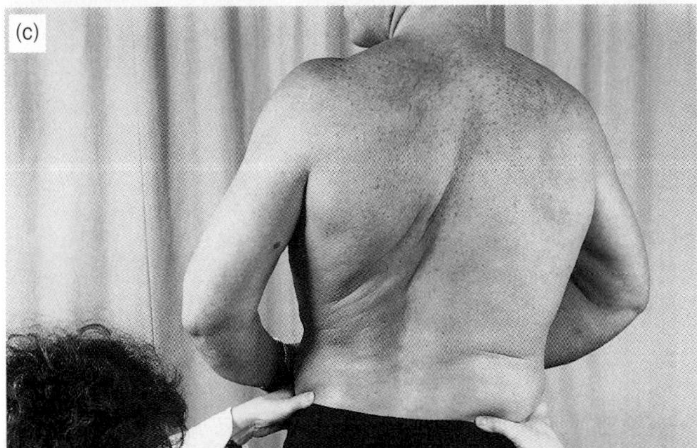

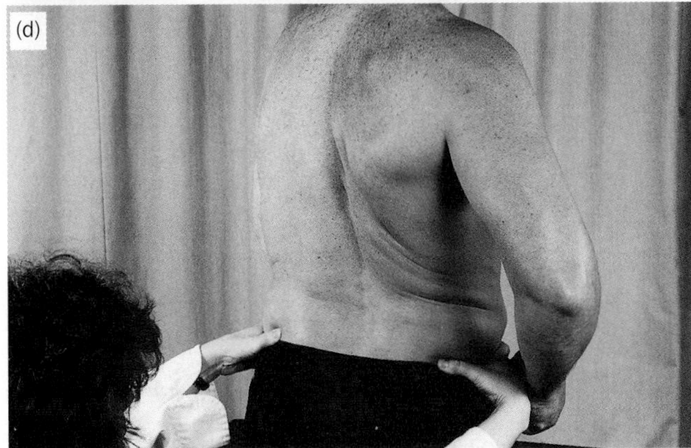

Fig. 20.24 Testing lateral deviation and rotation of the spine.

Rotation. Stand behind the patient and hold their pelvis still with both hands. Ask the patient to twist round and look over their shoulder, first in one direction and then the other. Note the angle that the shoulder girdle can form with the pelvis (Fig. 20.24).

For these last three tests record whether any of the manoeuvres are limited by pain, and if so where.

Passive

The Lasegue or straight leg raise test. This test can be painful and so should only be performed slowly while watching the patient's face at all times. The test should be abandoned if pain becomes severe. It is a test of sciatic nerve irritability and relies on the fact that when the straight leg is flexed fully at the hip the roots of the sciatic nerve move as much as 2 cm through the vertebral foraminae. If the nerve is compressed and/or inflamed this movement will cause pain.

Pick up the leg least affected by the pain and gently bend the hip and the knee until both joints are fully flexed. Note the range of movement of both hip and knee.

Gradually straighten the knee, while allowing the hip to extend only as much as the patient feels is necessary for comfort. All patients will get some discomfort in the back of the thigh during this manoeuvre as the hamstring muscles are put on full stretch. While keeping the knee straight, let the hip drop 10° into extension so that any pain from tight hamstrings is relieved. Then take the foot and dorsiflex the ankle fully. This stretches the sciatic nerve. Pain in the back radiating down the full length of the leg indicates sciatic nerve irritation (Fig. 20.25).

The test should then be repeated with the opposite leg.

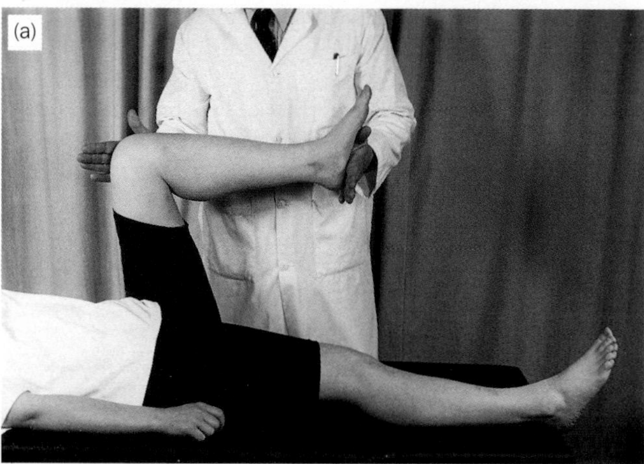

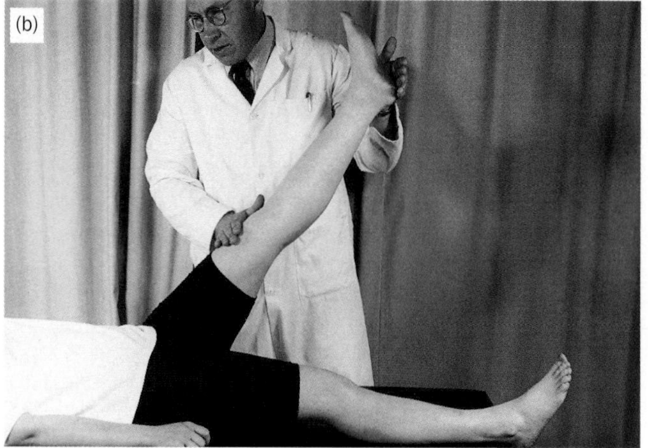

Fig. 20.25 The Lasegue test. (a) The hip is flexed to check for limitation. (b) The knee is straightened and the hip extended until pain from tight hamstrings is released. (c) The foot is dorsiflexed to stretch the sciatic nerve.

Resisted

Extensor hallucis longus is served purely by lumbar nerve root 5 (L5). It can be tested by comparing resisted extension of the tip of the big toes. Stand at the feet of the patient and press down on the big toenails of each patient while asking them to resist this pressure. If one distal phalanx drops into flexion easily compared with the other toe despite the best efforts of the patient, there is likely to be an L5 lesion (Fig. 20.7).

Testing for motor weakness

L5 is the commonest nerve root to be affected by a prolapsed intervertebral disc and is the only nerve root which is completely responsible for serving one muscle (the extensor hallucis longus) and so is easy to test. The simplest test for compromise of L4 motor function is loss of the knee reflex and weakness in the quadriceps (demonstrated in the section on 'The knee'). The ankle reflex is lost in S1 damage, but beware; it is commonly missing in elderly patients even without nerve root damage.

Thoracic spine

Look

Skin and soft tissues

There are no common lesions in the thoracic spine which can be seen in the skin or soft tissues.

Bone

The thoracic spine is normally convex, and straight in the sagittal plane.

If it is very convex and painful the patient may have Scheuermann's disease, a condition of unequal growth of the front and back of the spine which presents in adolescence.

Lateral curvature of thoracic spine accompanied by rotation is called scoliosis. As the patient bends forward to touch their toes the associated rib hump increases in size. This is diagnostic of scoliosis.

Holger Werfel Scheuermann, 1877–1960. Radiologist, Municipal Hospital, Sundby, Copenhagen, Denmark. Described juvenile kyphosis in 1920.

Lasegue did not describe this test. His student Forst did in 1881, but gave the credit to his boss – an early example of currying favour.

Feel

Skin, soft tissues and bone

In cases of possible trauma to the thoracic spine the patient should be immobilised on a spine board. A full check of distal neurology should be performed if the patient is alert enough to co-operate. When the time comes to examine the thoracic spine, the patient should be log-rolled using at least three trained staff working as a team. The whole length of the spine should be palpated for tenderness and steps. If any are found the patient should be kept on a spine board until all the necessary investigations have been performed. The spinal cord lies in the thoracic spine so neurological damage may appear as an upper motor neuron lesion in the lower limbs and/or a lower motor neuron lesion in nerve roots originating from the thoracic spine. Any sensory loss may spread progressively (the apparent level of the lesion rises) in the hours after the injury. A very careful examination of perineal sensation should be performed. Preservation of function in these sacral roots (central sparing) is a good prognostic sign that some recovery may occur over the next months.

Move

Active, passive and stability

There are no simple tests for mobility or stability of the thoracic spine and, indeed, if stability is in doubt the thoracic spine should be not be moved. It should be immobilised while investigations are performed to avoid the risk of causing further neurological damage.

A full neurological examination of the lower limbs will be needed if neurological damage in the thoracic spine is possible. Immediately after the injury there may be spinal shock with reduced power and tone. This will mimic a lower motor-neuron lesion. Later, the picture of an upper motor-neuron lesion will appear with hyper-reflexia and clonus. Clonus is tested by smartly dorsiflexing the ankle. If the gastrocnemius contracts more than once or twice, then clonus is present.

Cervical spine

The cervical spine can be difficult to see, particularly in women. It is important to get the hair up out of the way, but patients should not use their own arms to do this. A theatre nurse's cap may be helpful. Just as the key to examination of the lumbar spine is a neurological examination of the lower limb, the key to the examination of the cervical spine is a neurological examination of the upper limbs.

Look

Skin

Look for scars and sinuses, particularly around the cervical lymph node area and over the thyroid. Surgical approach to the neck can be made from the front, the side or the back.

Soft tissue

Look for spasm of the trapezius muscles and the sternomastoid muscles.

Bone

The cervical spine normally has a lordosis like the lumbar spine. If this is lost there is probably muscle spasm caused by pain.

Feel

Skin

Test for sensory loss in hands and feet.

Soft tissue

Feel for spasm in the trapezius muscles.

Bone

Palpate down the contour of the cervical spine feeling for gaps or for tender areas.

Move

Active

Flexion/extension. The patient should be asked to bend their neck forward and put their chin on their chest. Look to see whether the cervical lordosis is lost. They should then extend their neck by looking up at the ceiling. Note the angle that the face makes with the ceiling as a measure of extension.

Lateral rotation. Ask the patient to look over their shoulder on each side keeping their shoulders still. Note the angle that the chin makes with the shoulders on each side.

Lateral deviation. Ask the patient to lay one ear on that shoulder, then the opposite ear on the other shoulder. Note how close they can bring each ear to its shoulder without shrugging the shoulder upwards. Note whether any of these manoeuvres are painful in extreme.

Neurological testing

The neurology of both upper and lower limbs should be tested. Lesions in the lower limbs are likely to be upper motor neuron; those in the upper limb are likely to be lower motor neuron. For testing motor power in the upper limb it is probably only necessary to test grip and the power to spread the fingers apart. Grip tests power of the finger flexors as well as the wrist extensors, so covering most of the middle cervical nerve roots. Abduction of the fingers is supplied by the lower cervical roots including T1, so testing these two manoeuvres covers most of the motor roots from the cervical spine apart from the uppermost ones.

Passive and stability

These do not contribute much to diagnosis of problems in the cervical spine.

The shoulder

The examination of the shoulder is most easily performed if the patient is standing with their shirt and vest removed. It is not necessary to remove the brassiere.

Look

Look at the patient standing both from in front and from behind.

Skin

Look for scars. Check in the axilla for sinuses.

Soft tissue

Check for wasting of the deltoid (increased angularity of the shoulder) (Fig. 20.26). This is commonly caused by damage to the axillary nerve during an anterior dislocation of the shoulder.

Wasting of the supraspinatus and infraspinatus (hollows above and below the spine of the scapular) occurs with a tear of the rotator cuff. Check for a bulge low in the upper arm which is especially prominent when the patient flexes their elbows. When the long head of the biceps ruptures the body of the muscle retracts back down the arm.

Use the other side of the patient's body for comparison.

Bone

The commonest deformity is a subluxed acromioclavicular joint, which appears as a prominent lump on the distal end of the clavicle (Fig. 20.27). An anterior dislocation of the shoulder itself is first noticeable because of the loss of the rounded contour of the shoulder. The bulge in front of the shoulder (the humeral head lying anteriorly) is easier to see when you start looking for it. Otherwise, it can easily be masked by the swelling of the acute injury.

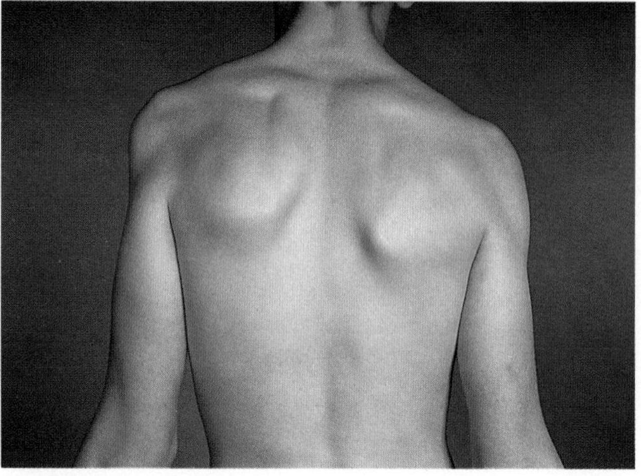

Fig. 20.26 Deltoid wasting. Secondary to axillary nerve damage after dislocation of the shoulder.

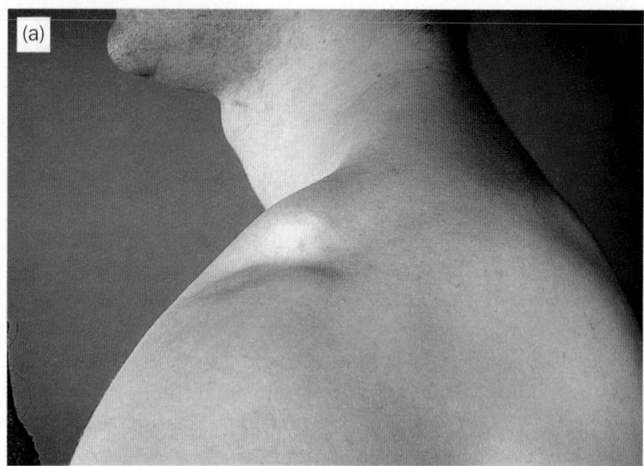

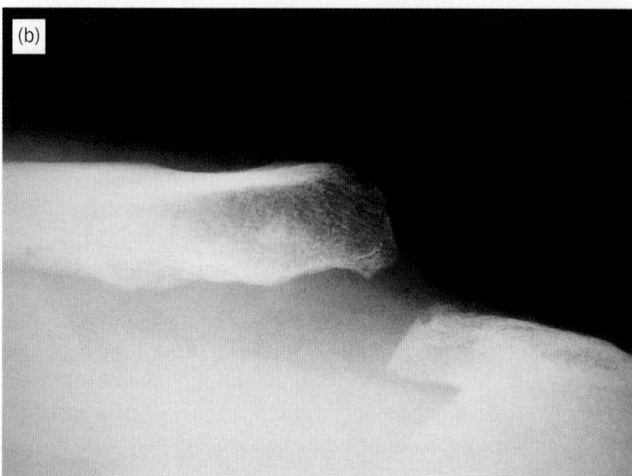

Fig. 20.27 Acromioclavicular subluxation.

Feel

Problems in the shoulder can be referred from the neck or arise from the shoulder complex itself.

The epaulette sign

Before starting the examination, ask the patient to show you where they are feeling pain. If they are able to localise the pain with the tip of one finger then the pathology is probably in the shoulder. If, however, they rub the whole hand over the top of the shoulder then the pain is likely to be referred from a lesion in the neck. The patient rubs their hand over the position of epaulettes on a soldier's uniform, hence the name of the test.

Localisation in the shoulder

Within the shoulder complex problems commonly arise either from the acromioclavicular joint, from problems in the rotator cuff including the subacromial bursa or from the glenohumeral joint itself. The examination should be designed to distinguish between these possibilities.

Skin

Feel for heat. Test distally for loss of sensation, comparing soft touch on both sides. Test the outer and inner side of the upper and lower arm, then the medial and lateral side of the hand.

Soft tissue

Feel the trapezius muscle for tenderness (common in referred pain from the neck). Tenderness under the margin of the acromion suggests problems with the rotator cuff complex.

Bone

Feel along the clavicle starting at the sternoclavicular joint palpating for tenderness, particularly at the junction of the clavicle with the acromion. Palpate the outlines of the acromion and feel for tenderness immediately beneath the acromion in the subacromial bursa starting anteriorally, moving laterally and finishing posteriorally. Note any tender sites.

Move

Active

Ask the patient to put their hands first behind their head, and then behind their back. These two movements effectively test the functional range of movement in the shoulder. Record how far they can reach towards the back of their heads and up their backs.

Stand behind the patient and ask them to raise both arms from their sides out laterally and 30° forward (in the plane of the scapula) vertically up above their heads. Watch the movement of the scapula in relation to the humerus. There should be a scapulohumeral rhythm. In the first part of abduction the scapula moves very little, perhaps only 1° for every 2° that the humerus moves. In the second part of movement the scapula and humerus tend to move almost together. That is a normal rhythm. Note if there is a catch in this movement, and ask them to point where they experience pain if they get a catch. Pain under the lower margin of the acromion suggests an impingement.

Passive

With their arms at their sides, flex their forearms to 90° pointing their hands straight forward. Put one hand on the shoulder joint and use the other hand gently to turn the forearm outwards externally rotating the shoulder. Crepitus in the shoulder suggests arthritis in the glenohumeral joint. Pain and complete stiffness is associated with adhesive capsulitis (frozen shoulder).

Stability

Thumb-down test. This test is specific for problems of impingement and inflammation in the subacromial bursa.

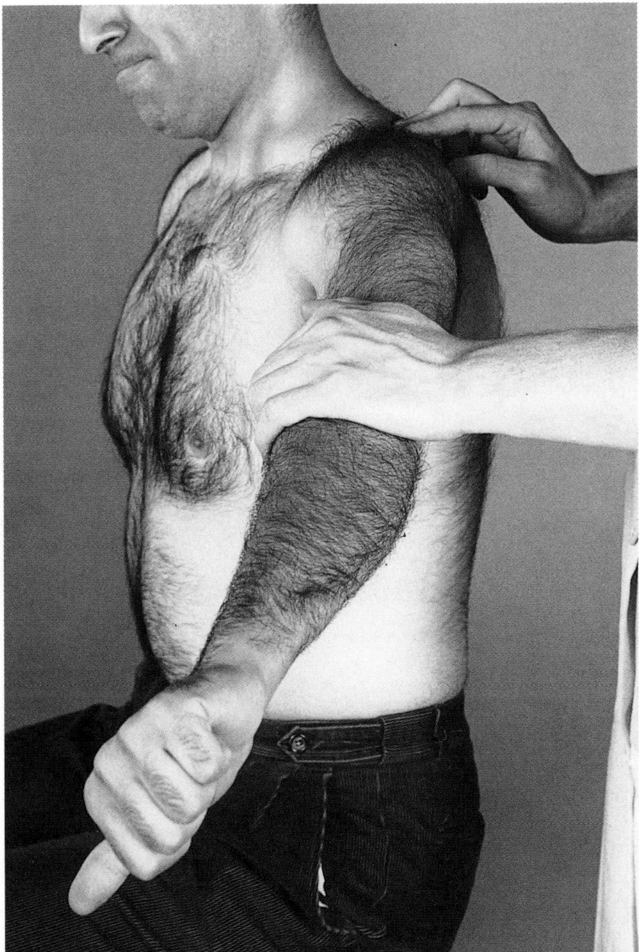

Fig. 20.28 Thumb-down test for acromial impingement.

The patient is asked to flex the shoulder to just under 90° in the plane of the scapula (laterally and 30° forward). With the patient holding their arm straight out in this position, push down gently on the arm so that they have to maintain the position against resistance (Fig. 20.28). If they experience sharp pain in the subacromial area they have an impingement problem.

Apprehension sign. The shoulder commonly dislocates anteriorly when the arm is above the head and externally rotated. If the patient has ever experienced a previous dislocation, putting the patient in that position makes them feel as if the shoulder is about to dislocate (Fig. 20.29). Only do this test gently, and watch the patient's face. You do not want to dislocate the shoulder.

Sulcus test. In patients who have had a previous dislocation the shoulder joint tends to be lax. Drawing down on the patient's arm when they are relaxed allows the humerus to drop away from the acromion, producing a sulcus (groove) in the unstable shoulder which is more prominent than on the normal side (Fig. 20.30).

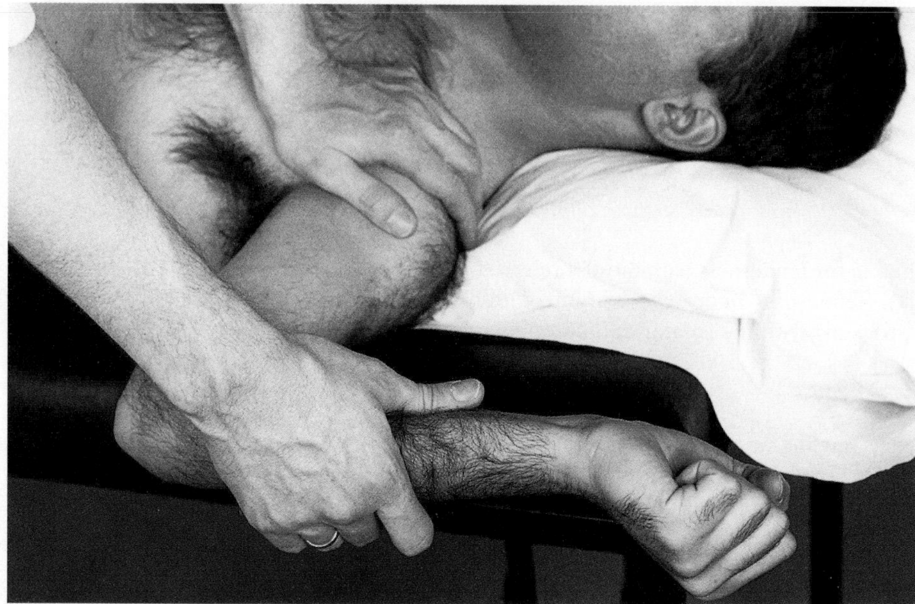

Fig. 20.29 Apprehension test for previous anterior dislocation of the shoulder.

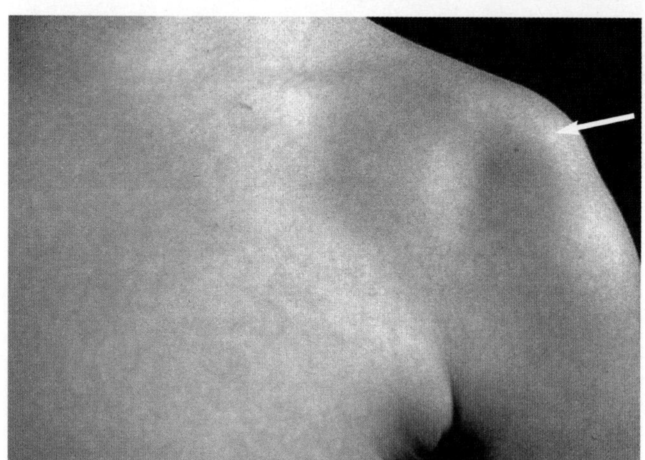

Fig. 20.30 Sulcus test (arrow points to sulcus).

The elbow

The elbow is a subcutaneous joint, which is quite simple to examine. Exposure should include the whole of both arms. It is not sufficient just to roll up the sleeves.

Look

Skin

Look for scars and for redness, especially over the olecranon.

Soft tissue

Swelling can be seen mainly in the dimples either side of the olecranon. Wasting as a result of a lesion around the elbow is commonly the result of an ulna nerve palsy. There will therefore be wasting in the hypothenar eminence and of the intrinsic muscles in the hand.

Bone

Look at the carrying angle of the elbow, the angle that the forearm makes with the upper arm as the arm lies by the patient's side with the hands facing forward (Fig. 20.31). Fixed flexion can be seen in comparison with the other arm if the arms are held out horizontally in front with the palms upwards.

Feel

Skin

If the elbow joint is inflamed it will feel hot as it is a subcutaneous joint.

Sensation. The sensation in the hand should be checked. The ulna nerve is the one most likely to be injured around the elbow. Its sensory distribution is the lateral one and a half fingers of the hand.

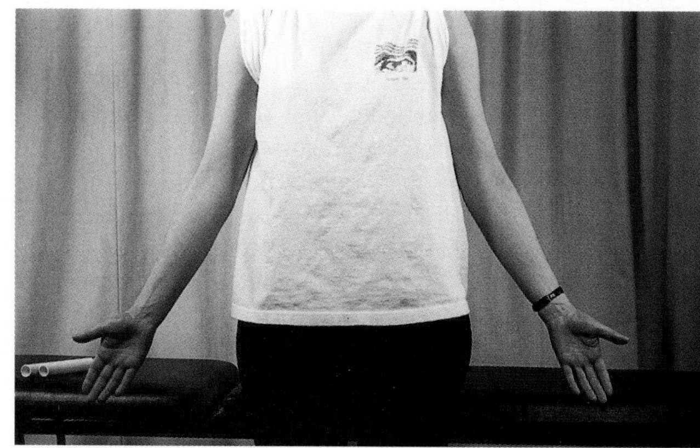

Fig. 20.31 Carrying angle of the elbow.

Soft tissue

Cross fluctuation in the elbow joint between the posteromedial and posterolateral pouches can be elicited if there is an effusion in the elbow. The ulna nerve can be felt by rolling it under your fingers between the medial epicondyle and the olecranon. If it is tender it is probably inflamed.

Bone

Tenderness over the lateral epicondyle is found in tennis elbow.

The radial head can be felt best by passively pronating and supinating the forearm while feeling for the radial head. It is slightly lumpy and can be felt under the tip of your finger as it rotates. Tenderness indicates a fracture if it is acute, or arthritis if it is chronic.

Move

Active

Flexion/extension. The range of movement of elbows can be compared by moving both elbows together with the shoulders forward flexed 90° (Fig. 20.32). The normal elbow hyperextends slightly, but the variation is large.

Pronation and supination. This is tested with the elbows at a right angle and with the fingers out straight or with a pencil gripped in the fist to act as a protractor (Fig. 20.33).

Passive

Repeat the above movements holding the patient's wrist in one hand and the elbow clasped between the thumb and index finger on the epicondyles. Watch the patient's face to avoid causing pain.

Stability

The stability of the elbow can be tested in extension, stressing the collateral ligaments.

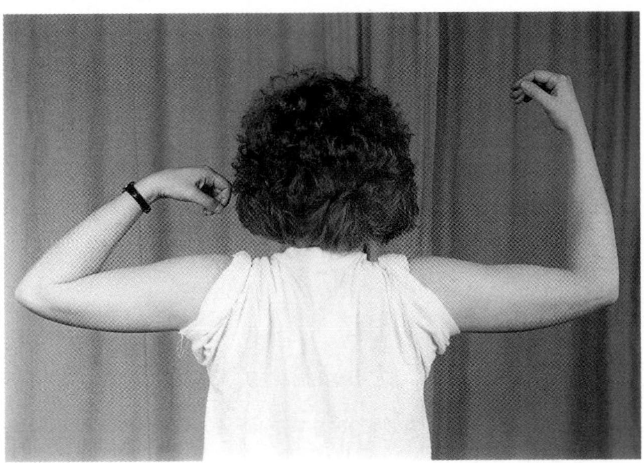

Fig. 20.32 Measuring flexion of the elbow.

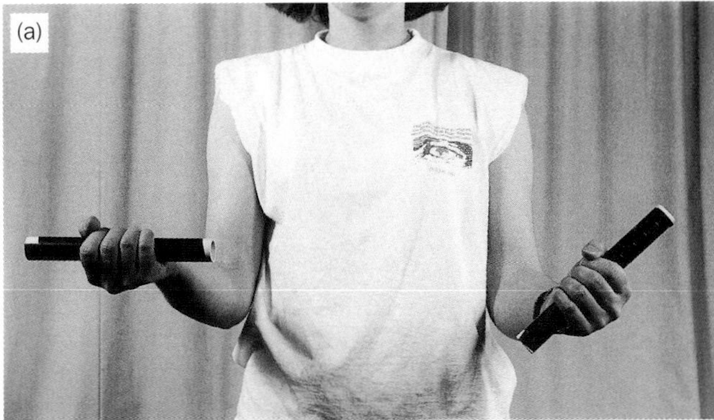

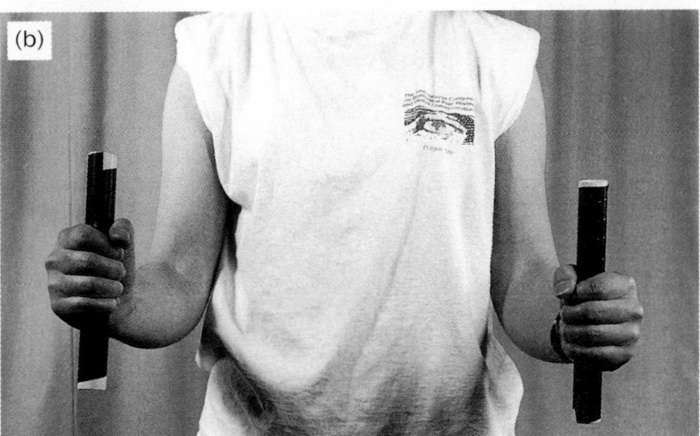

Fig. 20.33 Measuring pronation and supination of the forearm.

The wrist

Look

Skin

Look for scars, particularly over the palmar side of the wrist. The thin scar of a carpal tunnel release may be almost invisible unless carefully looked for.

Soft tissue

Swelling and wasting. Swelling is visible mainly on the dorsal side, or over the radial styloid (De Quervain's tenosynovitis). Wasting can occur in the thenar or hypothenar eminence. It can also be seen between the metacarpals in the dorsum of the hand. Thenar eminence wasting can best be seen by putting the two hands side by side, thumb upwards, and looking down at the thumbs from above. Any slight difference in shape can then be clearly seen (Fig. 20.34).

Bone

Look for prominence of the ulna styloid and for radial drift of the wrist characteristic of rheumatoid arthritis.

Fritz De Quervain, 1868–1940. Professor of Surgery, Berne, Switzerland.

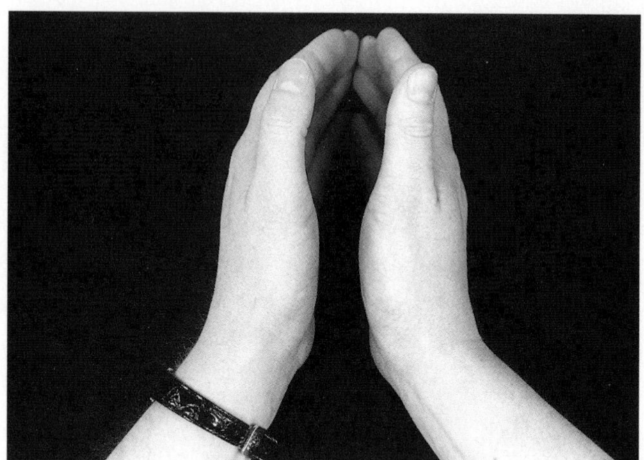

Fig. 20.34 Checking for thenar wasting.

Feel

Skin

Test sensation in the hand by comparing the sides. The median nerve can be tested over the palmar surface of the thumb and the index finger, the ulna nerve over the little finger. The sensory distribution of the radial nerve is a patch over the dorsum of the base of the thumb.

Soft tissue

Feel for the radial pulse and capillary filling at the fingertips.

Synovial thickening can be felt in the wrist either dorsally or on the palmar side.

Tinel's test. This is a test for inflammation in the median nerve. This is usually caused by compression in the carpal tunnel. Lay the patient's hand on the table, palm upwards, and tap with the tip of your index finger over the median nerve at the wrist crease. Tingling or lightning pains into the fingers suggest that the median nerve is being compressed.

De Quervain's tenosynovitis. The extensor tendons to the thumb can become inflamed from overuse. The tendon sheath is tender and it is sometimes possible to feel crepitus in the tendon if it is moved gently while palpating over it.

Bone

Scaphoid fracture. The waist of the scaphoid can be felt in the anatomical snuff box and the proximal pole can be felt anteriorly at the front of the base of the thumb.

Carpal instability. Trauma to the wrist can produce tears in the carpal ligaments. Chronic tears can be tender to palpation.

Jules Tinel, 1879–1952. French neurologist.

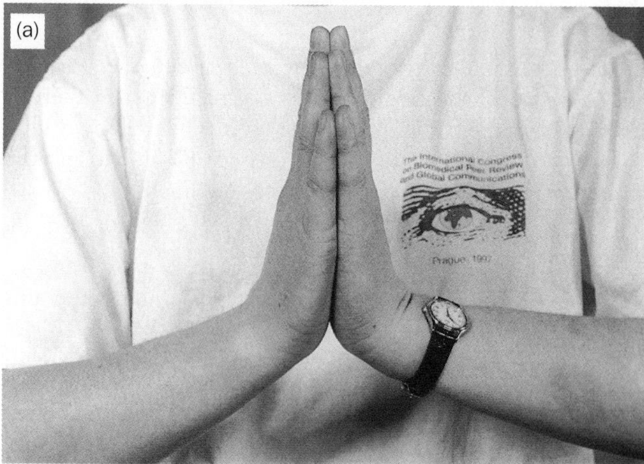

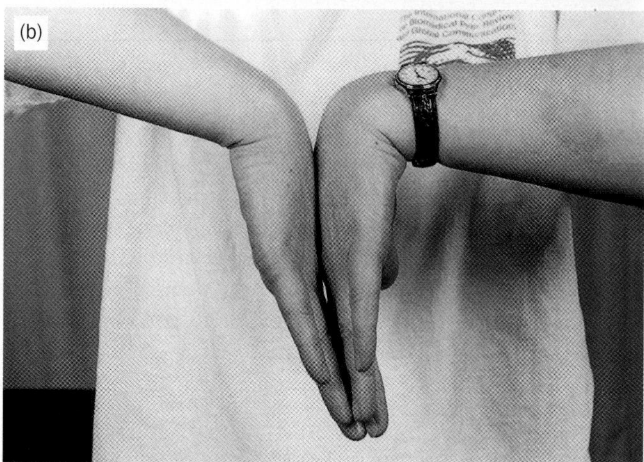

Fig. 20.35 The prayer test for measuring flexion and extension of the wrist.

Move

Active

Extension is tested by the patient pushing their two hands together into a 'prayer' position but with the elbows raised so that the forearms are in line with each other (Fig. 20.35). If there is loss of extension the palms will not be able to meet together and/or one forearm will tend to be dropped. Palmar flexion is performed in the same way, but with the hands pointing down and the backs of the hands in contact.

Passive

Ulna and radial deviation are tested by taking the patient's hand in your own and forcing the hand into these positions, comparing the two sides.

Stability and resisted movement

The stability of the wrist is not easy to test, but checking power grip tests the power of the finger flexors, the wrist extensors and the stability of the wrist.

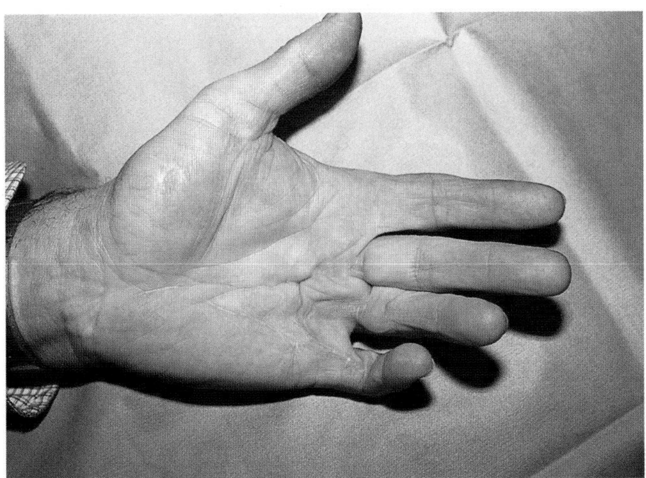

Fig. 20.36 Dupuytren's contracture.

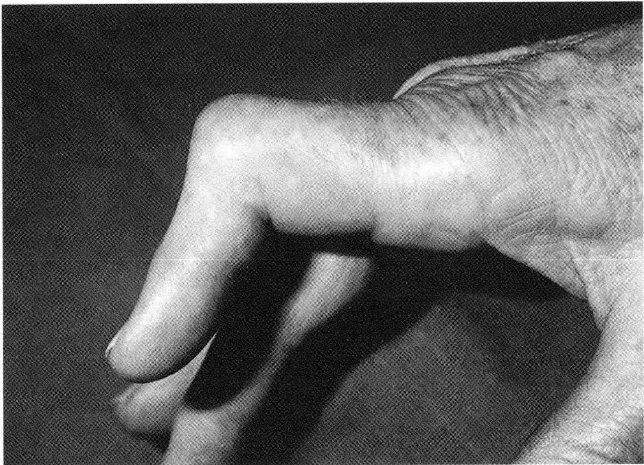

Fig. 20.38 Swan neck and boutonnière deformities in a hand affected by rheumatoid arthritis.

The hand

Look

Skin

Look for tight bands in the palm leading up to the fingers or even thumb (Dupuytren's contracture) (Fig. 20.36).

Soft tissue

Check for thenar and hypothenar wasting (see previous section on 'The wrist') but also check for wasting in the clefts between the fingers dorsally (damage to the ulna nerve or T1).

Bone

Look for Heberden's nodes (Fig. 20.37) over the distal interphalangeal joints dorsally (associated with osteoarthritis). Look for swan neck and boutonnière (Fig. 20.38) deformities. Swan neck deformities have an extension at the middle interphalangeal joint with flexion at the distal interphalangeal joint. Boutonnière deformity is extension at the distal interphalangeal joint with flexion at the middle interphalangeal joint.

Both of these are associated with rheumatoid arthritis. Look also for dropped fingers. If one finger lies lower than the others when the hands are held out, test for rupture of the extensor tendon by asking the patient to extend the finger against resistance. Look for subluxation of the metacarpal phalangeal joints and for ulna drift of the fingers (also associated with rheumatoid arthritis) (Fig. 20.39).

Feel

Skin

Feel for loss of sensation in the tips of the fingers. Review the sensory distribution of the median, ulna and radial nerves. If there is any doubt about the sensation then proceed to test two-point discrimination.

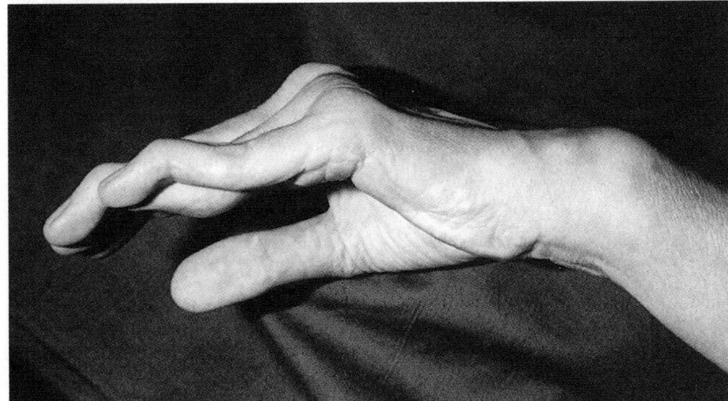

Fig. 20.37 Heberden's nodes.

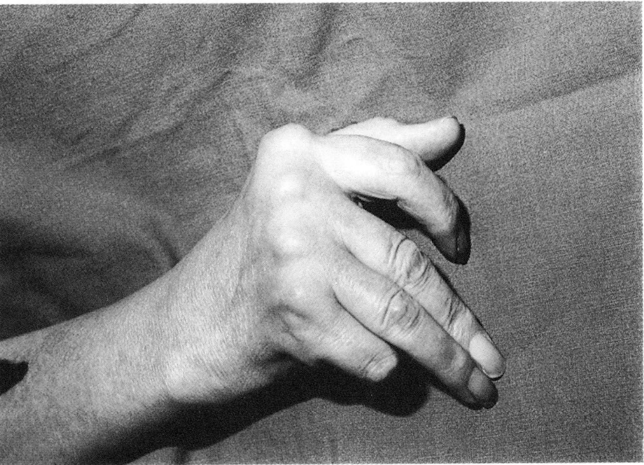

Fig. 20.39 Deformities associated with rheumatoid arthritis. Swelling of metacarpophalangeal joint and ulna deviation.

William Heberden, 1710–1801. Physician, London, England.

Baron Guillaume Dupuytren, 1777–1835. Surgeon, Hôtel Dieu, Paris, France.

Soft tissues

Check for capillary filling in the fingertips.

Feel for wasting in the first dorsal interosseous on the radial side of the first metacarpal. This muscle is plump and easily palpable. Damage to the ulna nerve or to the T1 nerve root can be detected from wasting in this muscle.

Bone

Feel for swelling and tenderness over the metacarpal phalangeal and interphalangeal joints.

Move

Active

Test roll-up of the fingers from full extension to full flexion. Test flexion of the metacarpal phalangeal joints in isolation while keeping the proximal and distal interphalangeal joints extended. This tests the patient's control of the intrinsic muscles. Test abduction of the fingers (a further test of small muscles in the hand).

Passive, stability and resisted

Test the power of the extensors, individually pushing down on each finger.

Superficialis tendon test. Flexor digitorum profundus usually has only one muscle belly supplying the tendons to all of the fingers. Profundus can therefore be immobilised by holding all the fingers bar the one being tested in full extension, grasping them in your hand. If the test finger is still able to flex, then superficialis to that finger is active (Fig. 20.40).

Profundus test. Flexor digitorum profundus is the only tendon that inserts in the distal phalanx. If the finger is held by the middle phalanx, the power of the profundus tendon can be tested (Fig. 20.41).

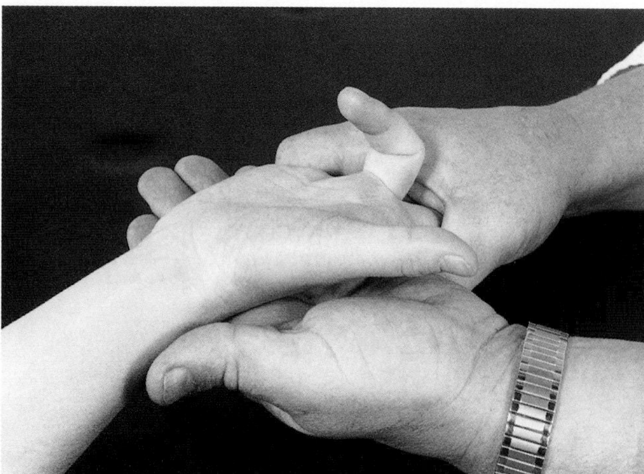

Fig. 20.40 Testing power in the flexor digitorum superficialis having immobilised profundus by holding the other fingers extended.

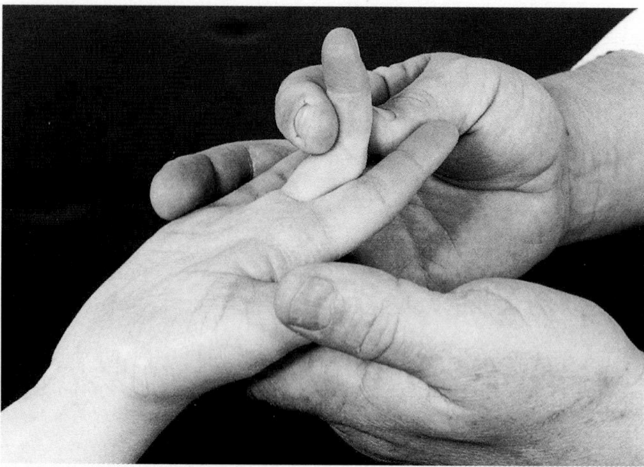

Fig. 20.41 Testing power of the flexor digitorum profundus.

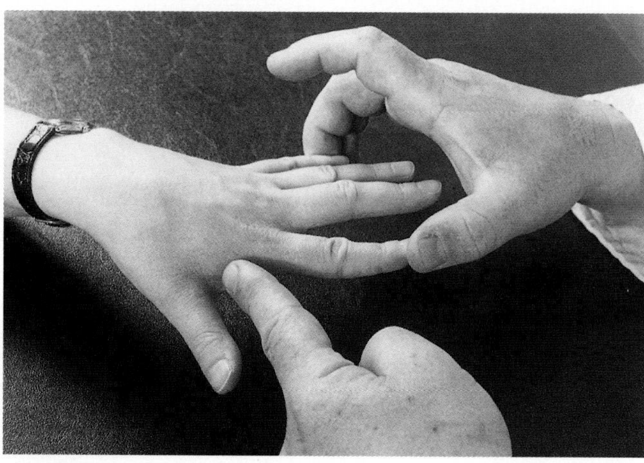

Fig. 20.42 Testing for weakness in the first dorsal interosseous muscle, characteristic of damage to the ulna nerve.

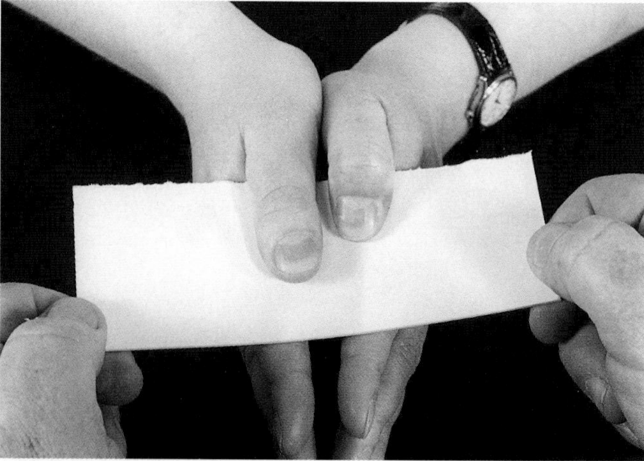

Fig. 20.43 Froment's test. As the patient resists the card being dragged out of their fingers, the thumb bends up on the side with intrinsic muscle weakness.

Jules Froment, 1878–1946. Professor of Clinical Medicine, Lyons, France.

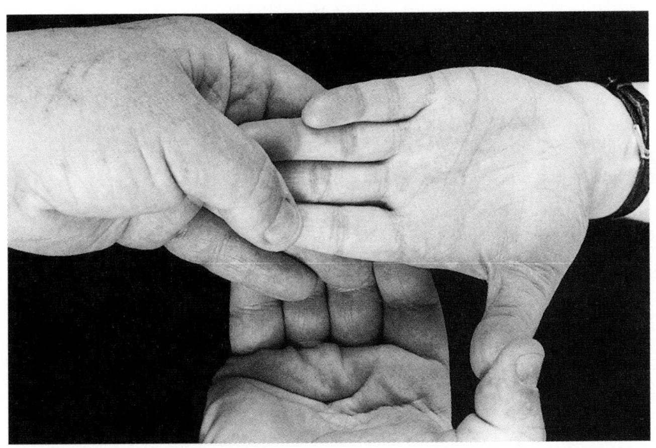

Fig. 20.44 Testing abductor power of the thumb. Weakness is characteristic of damage to the median nerve.

Intrinsics. The power of the intrinsic muscles of the hand is tested by asking the patient to abduct the fingers against resistance, and feeling for contraction in the first dorsal interosseous muscle on the index finger side of the web space (Fig. 20.42).

Froment's test. The patient is asked to grip a sheet of paper between the index finger and thumb of both hands. If the intrinsic muscles of the hand are normal the patient can grip firmly with the thumb in extension. However, if there is weakness, particularly of the adductor pollicis, the thumb cannot remain straight while flexor hallucis longus contracts hard, so the thumb flexes (Fig. 20.43).

Abductors of thumb. The abductors of the thumb are supplied by the median nerve. Power is tested by asking the patient to raise the thumb from the palm against resistance (Fig. 20.44).

Summary

The examination of the musculoskeletal system follows a standard pattern whichever part of the body is being examined. The system is quick and simple, and ensures that no critical physical signs are missed.

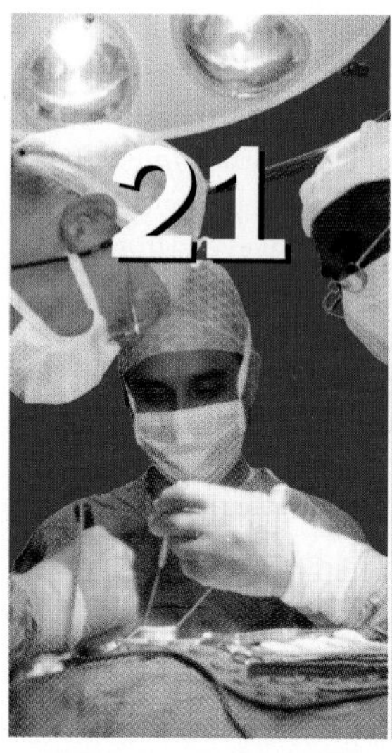

21

Fractures and dislocations

Learning objectives

- To know how to investigate a patient who may have a fracture or dislocation.
- To be able to describe a fracture or dislocation concisely and correctly.
- To understand the principles of reduction and holding a fracture or dislocation.
- To know the common complications of fractures and dislocations, and how to check for them.
- To understand the basic pathophysiology of fracture healing.

Significance of fractures and dislocations

Fractures (breaks) and dislocations are failures of the skeleton to cope with the loads put upon it. When they do occur there are other structures which can also fail which may not be so obvious but which may have much more serious consequences. After the initial trauma, tissues tend to spring back into place. Nerves and blood vessels may also have been stretched far beyond their physiological limit at the time of trauma. If the nerve has been disrupted and the ends have separated, surgery may improve the prognosis dramatically. If the blood supply to that limb has been disrupted, then it is a surgical emergency to restore that circulation (Fig. 21.1).

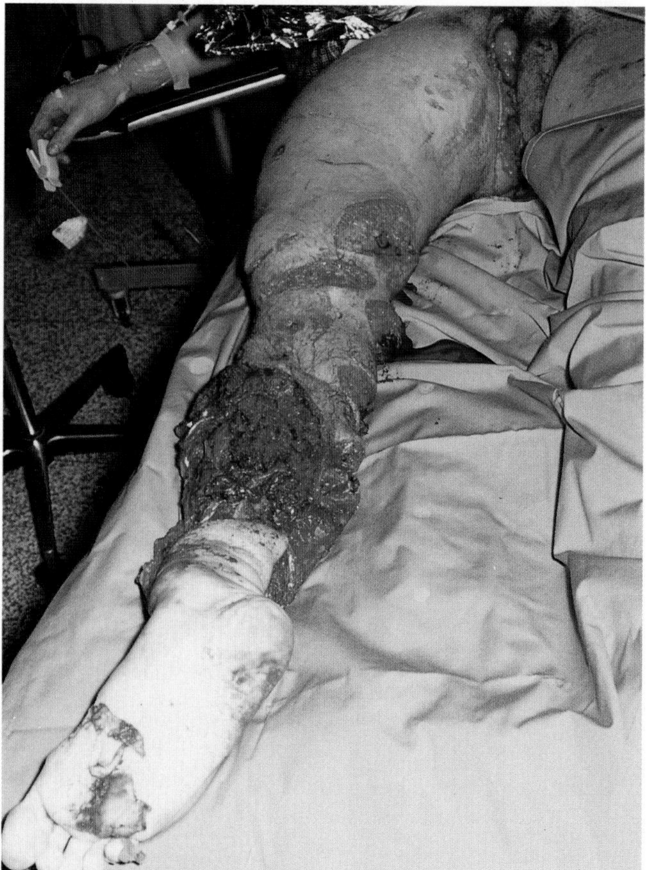

Fig. 21.1 A high-velocity motor cycle accident. The tibia is broken but the real problem is that the blood supply to the foot is disrupted.

Bailey & Love's Short Practice of Surgery, 23rd edition. Edited by R.C.G. Russell, N.S. Williams and C.J.K. Bulstrode. Published in 2000 by Arnold Publishers.

The check for neurovascular damage in a traumatised limb is, if anything, more important than the diagnosis of the fracture or dislocation.

Importance of the history

The history gives important clues to the type of trauma likely. The energy of trauma is related to the mass and the square of the velocity. The direction of the trauma will also affect the injury that you should be seeking. The important thing to remember is that if the trauma was severe enough to fracture or dislocate the skeleton, then it is highly likely that there was enough energy to cause a second or even a third dislocation or a fracture.

Do not relax once you have found the fracture or dislocation – start looking for more.

Patterns of injury

The history of the injury will give a clue to the pattern of the injury. A fall from a height with the casualty landing on their feet will produce a characteristic pattern of injury. This might include bilateral fractures of the calcaneum, pilon fractures of the ankle (the talus is driven up into the lower tibia), depressed fractures of the tibial plateau, central dislocation of the acetabulum and crush fractures of the vertebrae (Fig. 21.2).

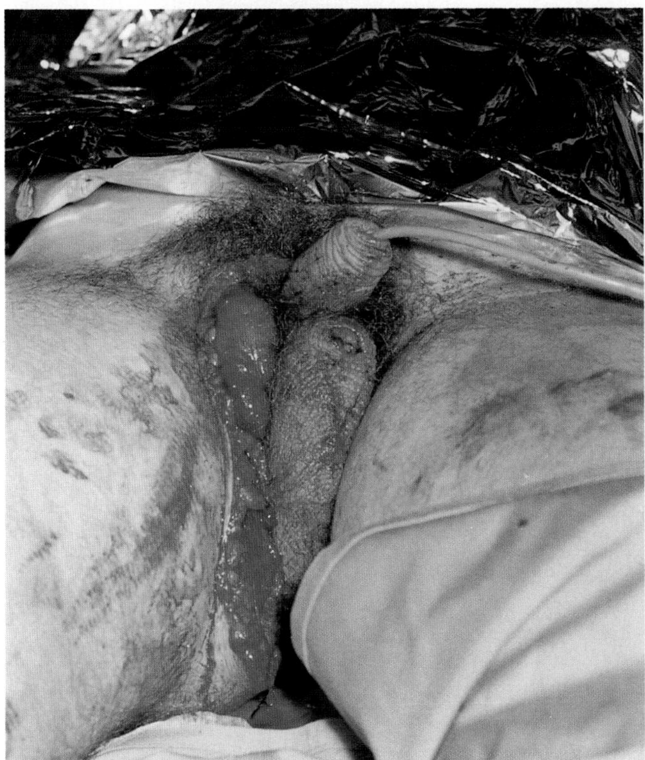

Fig. 21.2 A second image of the same patient in Fig. 21.1. Not only is the tibia broken, but the pelvis has a vertical shear fracture, the urethra is damaged and the testicle extravascated.

Examination

The musculoskeletal examination is described in Chapter 20. The key features are to make sure that the patient's overall condition is stable by checking their airway, breathing and circulation before concentrating on the musculoskeletal injuries. The examination should then be systematic from top to bottom of the body, with complete exposure and care taken to check the patient's back as well as their front. For each limb, be sure to check the distal circulation and neurogy. Finally, it is important to record these findings.

Describing a dislocation or fracture

Dislocations and subluxations

A dislocation is a complete disruption of a joint. The articular surfaces are no longer in contact. A subluxation is a partial dislocation. Some of the articular surface is in contact, but the congruence of the two joints has been lost. For either a dislocation or subluxation the joint needs to be named, and the direction of the disruption should be described (e.g. an inferior glenohumeral dislocation).

Fractures

Classification by quality of bone in relation to load

Fractures occur when the load to which they are subjected exceeds their intrinsic strength. A simple *traumatic fracture* occurs when an excessive load is applied to normal bone. A *pathological fracture* is produced when the strength of the bone is reduced by disease. In this case a force which is within normal limits leads to a fracture. The disease could be generalised osteoporosis, or a localised lytic lesion from a metastasis (Table 21.1).

If bones are subjected to a very large number of loads, none of which alone would be enough to break the bone, then the mechanical structure of the bone can gradually fatigue and the bone will then break. This is particularly a problem for people playing high-level sport and produces a *stress fracture*.

Partial or greenstick fracture. Bones in young people are very flexible. They bend and then may buckle or partially break, instead of breaking cleanly when overloaded (as bones in adults do). One characteristic of a greenstick fracture is that there may be a discontinuity in one cortex of the bone, but not in the other (Fig. 21.3).

Table 21.1 Types of fracture

Fracture type	*Bone strength*	*Load*
Traumatic	Normal	Abnormal
Pathological	Abnormal	Normal
Stress	Weakened with time	Normal but repeated
Greenstick	Abnormal (child)	Abnormal

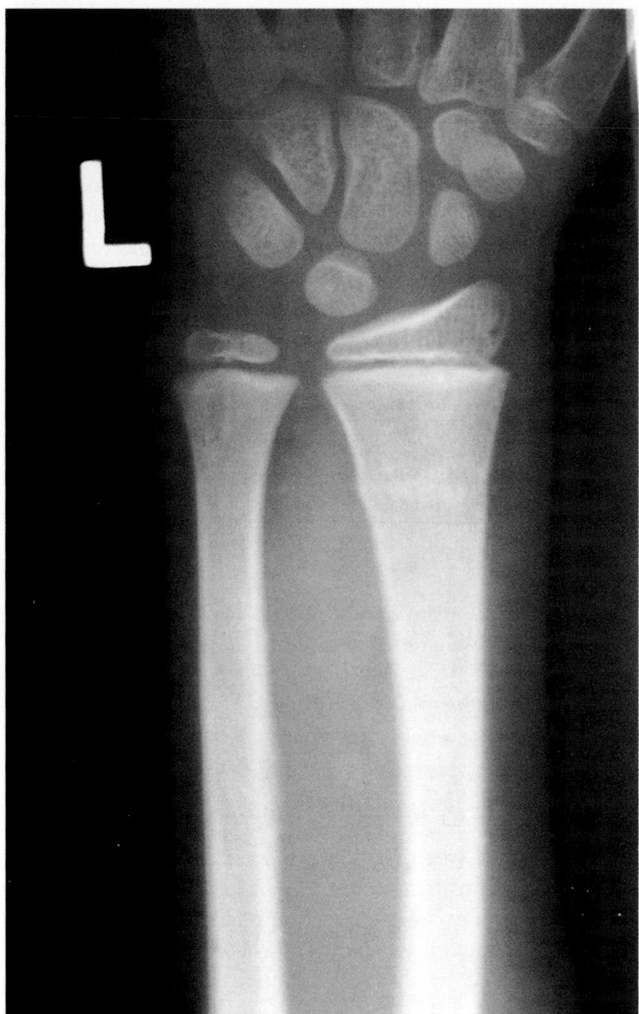

Fig. 21.3 Greenstick fracture in a young child with deformable bones. The distal radius has buckled 1 cm proximal to the epiphyseal plate.

Classification by direction of force

Compression fractures. If the load applied along the length of a bone exceeds that of its strength then it may collapse into itself. This is especially common in the elderly if the bones are osteoporotic, and so are less able to resist a heavy load. The fracture may be difficult to see. There may only be a small overlap of the cortical margins of the fracture, while the medulla may look diffusely radio-opaque (white) because the trabeculae have collapsed into each other. Overall, the bone will be shortened and may also be angulated.

Avulsion or distraction fracture. Here the two fragments of bone are pulled apart. In young patients a ligament or tendon may be stronger in tension than the bone into which it inserts. If the load is excessive the bone tears apart. These fractures are particularly common where strong muscles insert into small bones. Examples are the patella (the quadriceps muscle), the olecranon (triceps) and the fifth metatarsal head (peroneus tertius).

Spiral fractures. If a long bone is twisted along its axis a spiral fracture may result. The length of the spiral is easy to underestimate. It is especially important to see whether there is any extension into the articular surface of the bone. The tibia is particularly susceptible to spiral fractures when the foot is firmly fixed to the ground (by studs or another player's foot) and the player's body continues to twist.

Transverse fractures. If a long bone is bent along its long axis then a transverse fracture may result.

Butterfly fractures. If a bone is struck a direct blow, it is common for a more complex fracture to result where two break lines spread out obliquely from the point of contact of the blow, producing a free-floating 'butterfly' fragment between the two fractures.

Comminuted fractures. Comminuted fractures occur when a large amount of energy is dissipated into a bone. The bone breaks into fragments which may *impact* into each other or separate and become *displaced* (Fig. 21.4).

Classification by anatomical site

A long bone is divided into three main zones. The *diaphysis* is the narrow part of the main shaft. It usually has a thick cortex and a medulla filled with trabecular bone. The

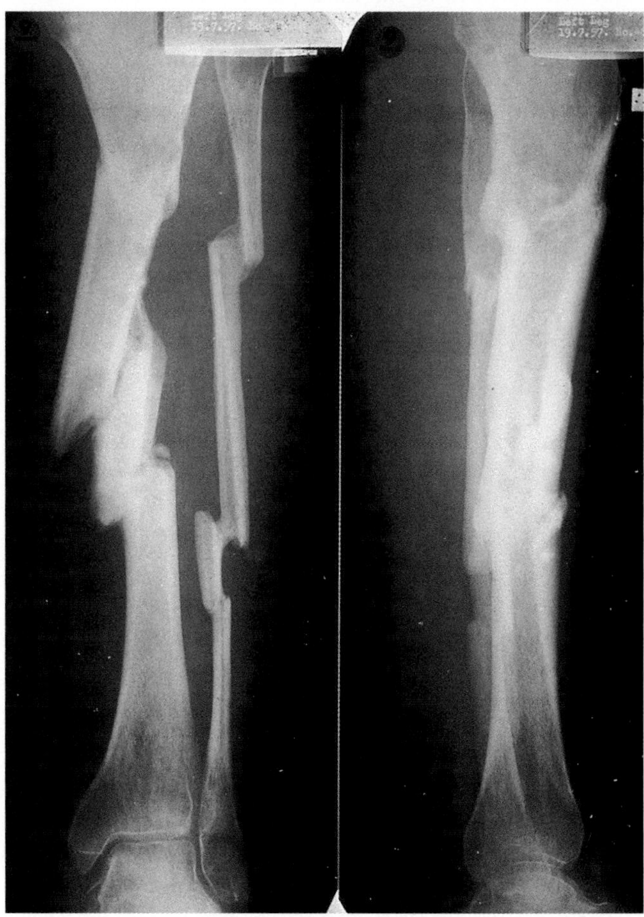

Fig. 21.4 Comminuted fractures.

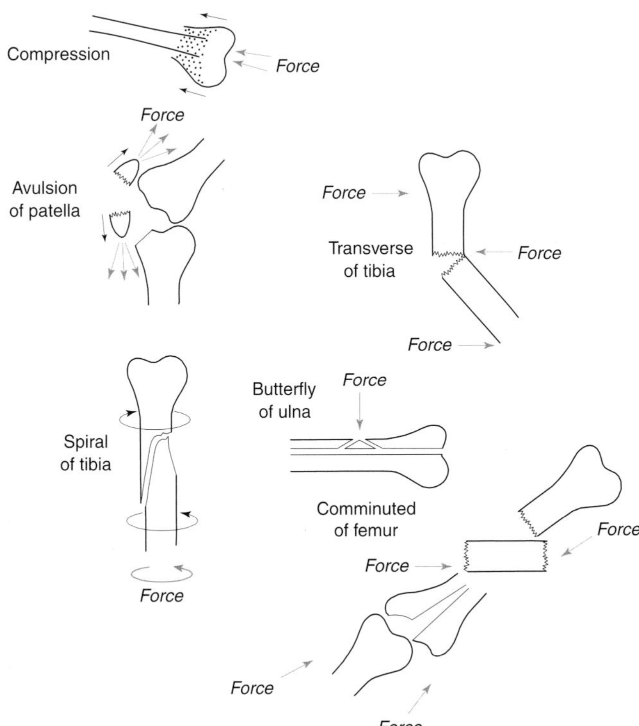

Fig. 21.5 Classification of fractures by shape.

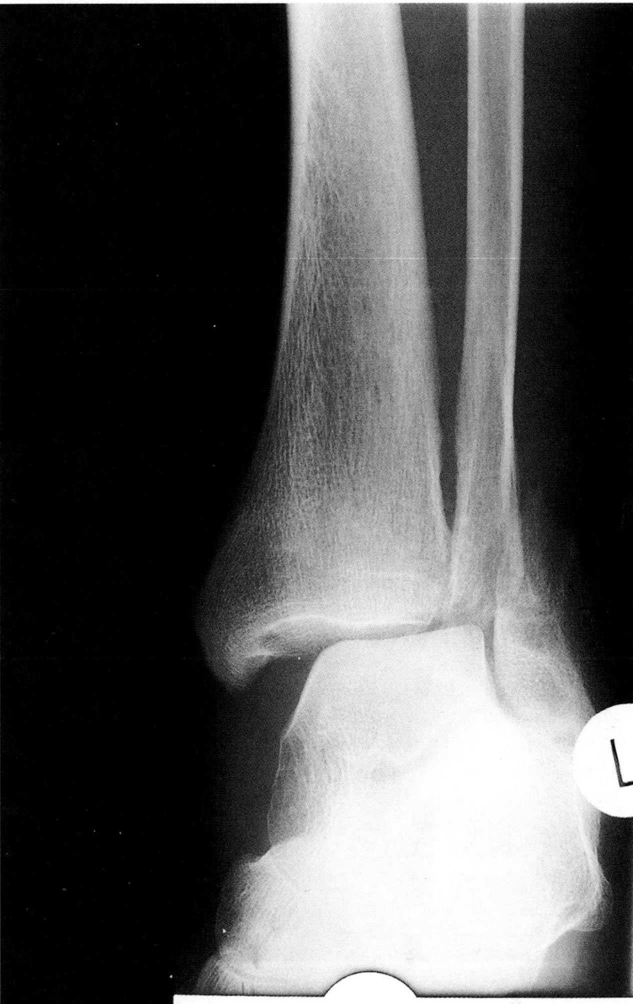

Fig. 21.6 Intra-articular ankle fracture. This will produce early aggressive osteoarthritis if not anatomically reduced.

metaphysis is the flare at each end between the diaphysis and the epiphyseal (growth) plate. It has thinner cortical bone and its medulla is, again, filled with trabecular bone. The ends of a long bone beyond the epiphyseal plate are called the *epiphyses* (singular epiphysis). They are covered mainly by articular cartilage but may have a cuff of thin cortical bone. In infants and children, in whom the bones are still growing, the epiphyseal plate will be open. The plate is weaker than the bone around and so fractures tend to track along it or even across it. *Epiphyseal fractures* are important because they can have a poor prognosis. Fractures into the joint (*articular fractures*) are also important because they carry a very poor prognosis if they are not anatomically reduced (Fig. 21.6).

Classification of epiphyseal fractures

The Salter Harris classification of epiphyseal fractures is the simplest and the commonest used (Table 21.2 and Fig. 21.7).

Grade 1. In this case there is a small crack along the metaphyseal side of the epiphyseal plate. This side is made up of dying chondrocytes and ossifying cartilage. The fracture does not affect the blood supply to the epiphyseal plate nor does it affect the anatomy of the germinal layer. It therefore heals quickly and without long-term problems, like children's bone elsewhere.

Grade 2. Here the fracture line again travels along the metaphyseal side of the plate but, before reaching the far cortex, it breaks out and tracks down into the metaphysis. This is by far the most common epiphyseal fracture, and for the same reason as given above has a good prognosis. Even if the fracture is markedly displaced the prognosis remains good. In children the bone will remodel and grow straight over the next year, especially if no rotatory abnormality is involved. In fact, one of the greatest risks in a grade 2 fracture is causing growth arrest by damaging the growth plate while reducing the fracture, especially if this is attempted after a few days when the fracture may already be uniting.

Robert Salter. Professor of Surgery, Children's Hospital, Toronto, Canada.
W.R. Harris. Orthopaedic Surgeon, Toronto, Canada.

Table 21.2 The Salter Harris classification of fractures involving the epiphyseal plate

Fracture type	*Anatomy*	*Frequency*	*Prognosis*
1	Runs along epiphyseal plate	Rare	Good
2	Metaphyseal fragment	Very common	Good
3	Extends into epiphysis	Rare	Poor if not reduced
4	Crosses epiphyseal plate	Rare	Poor if not reduced
5	Crushes epiphyseal plate	Very rare	Very poor

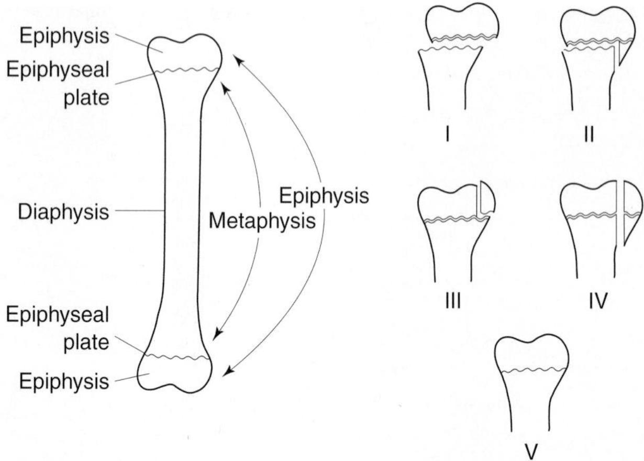

Fig. 21.7 Anatomy of the growing bone in relation to the Salter Harris classification of epiphyseal plate fracture.

Grade 3. In this case the fracture line does not run along the epiphyseal plate at all. It crosses from the metaphysis to the epiphysis. If it is displaced then it may heal with a step in the epiphyseal plate. Bony union may occur across the epiphyseal plate and block further growth, causing a most disfiguring progressive deformity of the limb if it is not promptly released. The key to the management of this type of fracture is anatomical reduction if it is displaced. This type of epiphyseal plate fracture is rare.

Grade 4. Here the fracture line travels along the distal (epiphyseal) side of the growth plate affecting both the blood supply and the anatomical integrity of the germinal cells. The fracture line does not travel the whole length of the epiphyseal plate but deviates off into the epiphysis itself and out on the articular suface. This is a second reason why this fracture has a poor prognosis. Not only is the growth plate likely to be damaged, but the articular surface may be incongruent. This predisposes the joint to early arthritis. The key to successful management of this type of fracture is anatomical reduction. This will be best performed by open surgery. Once again, this type of fracture is rare.

Grade 5. This is a rare and difficult fracture to diagnose. The injury is a severe crush of the epiphyseal plate. The X-ray may only look abnormal in retrospect, and this is indeed how this type of fracture is usually diagnosed. The consequence of complete disruption of the growth plate is complete growth arrest. There is little that can be done to prevent this, or indeed deal with it, once it has occurred.

Open fractures. At the time of a fracture the soft tissues over the bone will also be damaged. If the skin is broken there is a high probability that at some time during the accident the fracturing bone came into contact with the outside world, and so could be contaminated with bacteria. If there is no broken skin anywhere near a fracture, the fracture can be assumed to be *closed* and will initially be free of infection. If, however, there is any break in the skin anywhere near the fracture it is important that the fracture is classified as open and treated as such. The bone will need exposing and a careful search made to allow all dead or contaminated tissue to be removed. The wound will also need washing out and should be left open. It is always best to err on the safe side, and if there is any doubt whatsoever to treat the fracture as 'open'.

Classification by position

Bones have a very strong covering (the periosteum) which is invisible on X-ray. When a bone breaks the periosteum is torn, but it is unusual for the periosteum to be completely disrupted. This is very important for othopaedic surgeons because the periosteum can be used to obtain a good position when reducing a fracture. It can even act before that. Its elasticity may serve to reduce the fracture after the trauma. If a fracture is seen to be undisplaced on X-ray, that does not mean that it was never displaced, it just means that much of the periosteum is intact. Even *displaced fractures* usually have at least part of the sleeve of periosteum intact (on the side of concave curvature), but once again the displacement at the time of trauma was always greater than that seen afterwards. This is why apparently innocuous looking minimally displaced fractures with a small puncture wound over them should be assumed to be open.

Deciding whether a fracture is stable or unstable is yet another type of classification, 'classification by management'.

Classification by management

Stable fractures are those which are unlikely to move further. *Unstable fractures* are those which will continue to displace if action is not taken to hold the fracture secure. There is a gradation of stability which depends on the following factors.

Site. Fractures in weight-bearing bones are more likely to be displaced by 'normal' loads than those in bones which can easily be protected from load, such as the long bones of the arm.

Shape. Spiral fractures tend to be unstable, while impacted fractures tend to be very stable. The more displaced the fracture, the more unstable it is likely to be.

Displacement. Undisplaced fractures may have the periosteum intact and are therefore stable. The more displaced the fracture, the more unstable it is likely to be.

Behaviour of the patient. Patients who are prepared to be careful can maintain the position of a fracture which would become displaced in a young hard-drinking male, who is not prepared to take any advice.

International classifications

The AO classification is an internationally agreed classification of fractures using a simple alphanumeric code. The first number relates to the bone (humerus is 1, radius and ulna are 2, etc.). The second number relates to the position of the fracture on the bone (1 is proximal, 2 diaphyseal and 3 is distal). The position number is followed by a letter which defines the severity of the fracture. For proximal and distal fractures (types 1 and 3) 'A' is extra-articular, 'B' is partial articular and 'C' is intra-articular. For diaphyseal fractures (type 2) 'A' is a simple fracture, 'B' is a wedge or butterfly type and 'C' is comminuted or complex. This letter is followed by a further number which classifies the fracture still further.

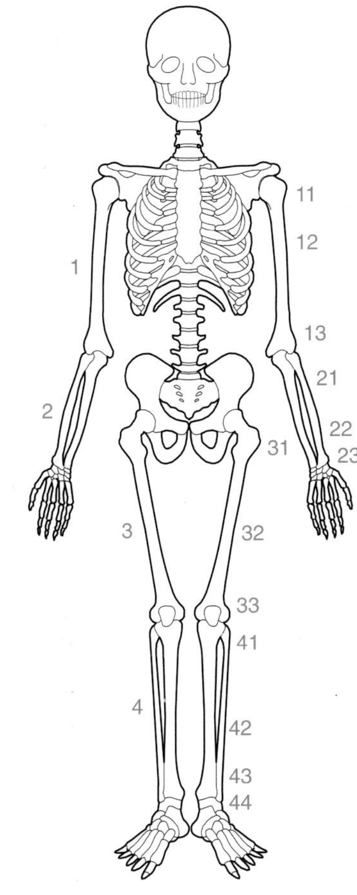

Charts are available to help you to decide the exact classification of each fracture (see Fig. 21.8)

The advantage of this classification is that it is international and has been carefully validated to make sure that, as far as possible, everyone looking at the same fracture would classify it in the same way. The disadvantage is that a string of numbers is not very memorable. If you say to most trauma surgeons that a fracture is a 32B3.2, it is unlikely that they would immediately know that you were talking about a distal third comminuted fracture of the femur.

A second problem is that for a classification to be useful it should point to both treatment and prognosis. One of the key features which determines treatment and indeed prognosis in a fracture is soft-tissue damage (especially whether the fracture is open or not). A second major feature is whether a fracture is displaced or not, as this may make a big difference to any decision on management. Neither of these two important prognosticators is covered in the AO classification.

Principles of management

Early treatment (neurovascular problems)

The principle of management of fractures is to deal with life- and limb-saving problems first. This means paying attention to ABC (airway, breathing and circulation) and to the neurovascular status of the limb before dealing with the fracture itself. If there is vascular compromise and the limb is distorted, it is always worth straightening the limb as far as possible in case it is simply the pressure of the displaced bone which is causing the problem.

Reduction of fractures and dislocations

Some fractures may not need reduction, especially if the minimal malunion which results will cause no cosmetic or

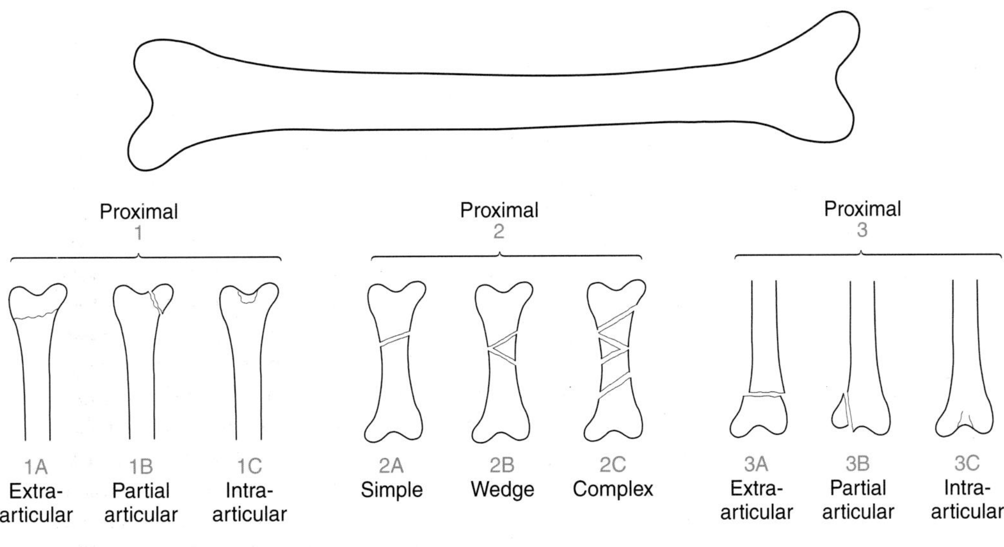

Fig. 21.8 The international AO classification of fractures.

Table 21.3 Stages of management of a fracture

Reduce	*Hold*	*Rehabilitate*
Only if displaced and malunion will compromise function	For comfort To prevent redisplacement	Build muscle power Reduce stiffness
	Allow early return to function for patient	Rebuild propioception

functional problem. An impacted stable fracture, which is only slightly displaced, may actually be made worse by reduction. The position may be improved but the fracture will become unstable. This may make future management much more difficult.

Holding a fracture

Once a fracture has been *reduced* it needs to be *held* until it has *united* (the bone ends have joined together).

Rehabilitation

Once the fracture is stabilised, the patient may need help with *rehabilitation* so that they can return to as full and as independent a life as possible (Table 21.3).

Indications for reduction

If a fracture is allowed to heal in a displaced position the fracture will unite, but it may go on to *malunion*. This may be unacceptable either because it is ugly (deformity) or because it interferes with the function of the limb. Malunion is not usually painful.

Remodelling in children

Fractures in children remodel as the skeleton grows. Some deformity can therefore be accepted because this will correct itself over the following months. Grade 2 epiphyseal fractures in children are easy to reduce but may then slip back out of a satisfactory position. Re-reduction carries a risk of causing growth plate damage (especially if it is performed more than 2 or 3 days after the fracture). Under these circumstances it may be better to accept the malunion resulting from a slip rather than risk an epiphyseal arrest while trying to produce a perfect reduction.

Stable impacted fractures

If the fracture is stable and impacted then it will heal quickly with a minimum need for protection. *Disimpaction* (separation of the fragments) and reduction will automatically make the fracture unstable. The fracture will then need more sophisticated methods for holding it. In the elderly, a rapid return to independent existence may be more important than cosmesis. A stable distal radius (Colles) fracture in an elderly patient who is only just managing to cope with independent existence may be best left unreduced and managed in a removable splint for comfort. Within 2 weeks it will be almost painless and can be used for everyday activities. Reduction would require a plaster for at least 4 weeks, during which time bathing and cooking might prove impossible.

Reduction

Reducing a fracture involves trying to return the bones to as near to their original position as possible (Fig. 21.9). Reduction can be performed *open*, in which case the fracture is exposed surgically so that the fragments can be reduced under direct vision. If a fracture is reduced *closed*, then the accuracy of the reduction can only be checked on an X-ray. An advantage of closed reduction is that the soft tissues and blood supply should not be disrupted any further than occurred at the time of the trauma.

If a fracture is closed and can be reduced closed it should be. If it is already open, then the opportunity should be used when cleaning the wound to make sure that reduction is anatomical by performing an open reduction.

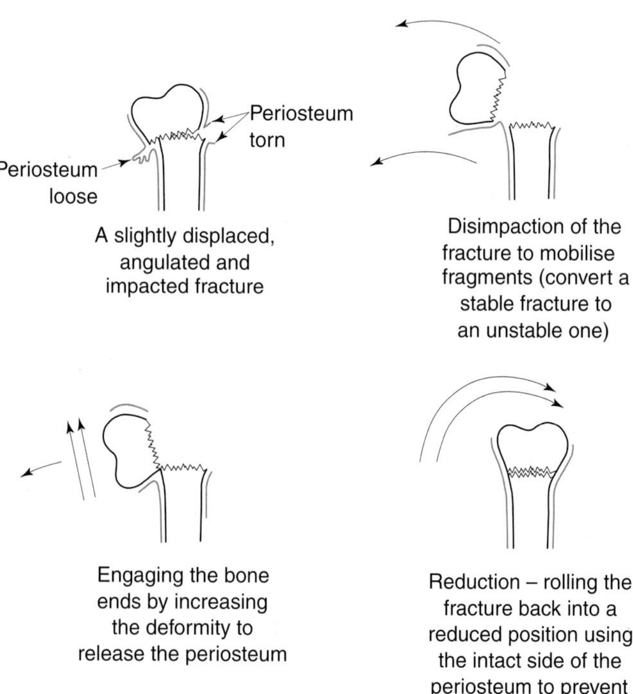

Fig. 21.9 Four stages of reduction of a fracture.

Abraham Colles, 1777–1843. Professor of Surgery, Royal College of Surgeons in Ireland (1804–36) and Surgeon Doctor, Steven's Hospital, Dublin, Ireland. Described this fracture in 1814.

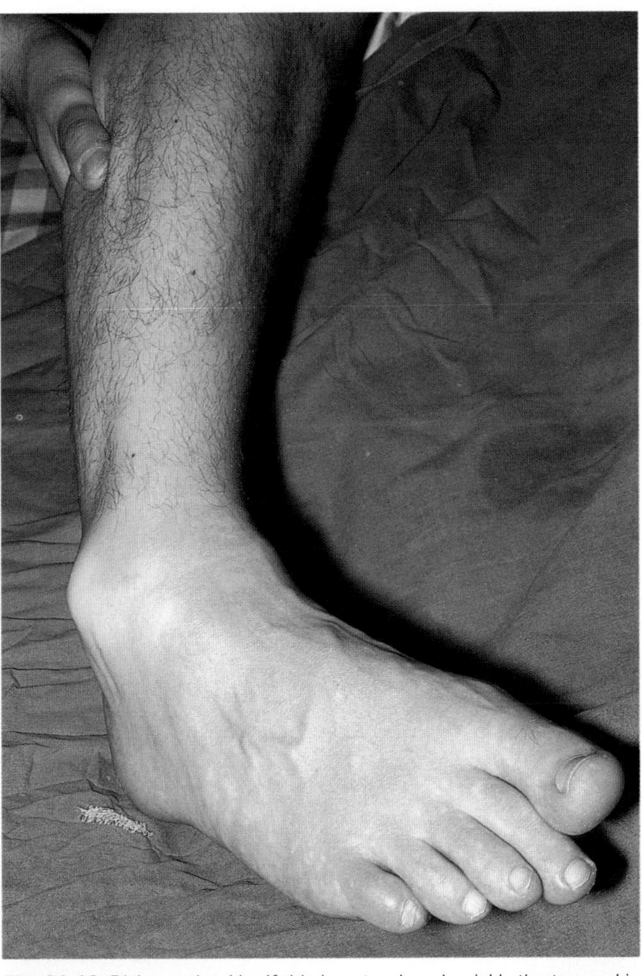

Fig. 21.10 Dislocated ankle. If this is not reduced quickly the tense skin over the ankle will necrose and create an open fracture dislocation. This is an indication for emergency reduction.

Emergency reduction

Emergency reduction should be undertaken immediately and without analgesia if the circulation or the skin of a limb is compromised (Fig. 21.10).

Principles of closed reduction

Closed reduction is always preferable to open reduction provided that a comparable reduction can be obtained and held. Closed reduction relies on the attachments of the bone to soft tissues (periosteum and/or ligaments) to obtain and to hold reduction. Intra-articular fractures, where fragments may not have any soft-tissue attachments, cannot usually be reduced closed. These fractures also need accurate reduction if traumatic secondary arthritis is to be avoided and so are best performed open to make sure that reduction is anatomical. In children the bones may not be clearly visible on X-ray because they have not yet fully ossified, especially around the elbow. Open reduction may be needed to be certain that reduction has been achieved (Table 21.4).

Table 21.4 Indications for open reduction

Open fractures	The wound needs opening up and washing out
Fractures which cannot be reduced closed	Closed reduction has failed or will obviously be impossible
Displaced intra-articular fractures	Important to achieve perfect reduction to avoid arthritis
Grossly unstable	Internal fixation provides stability allowing the patient to mobilise
Displaced children's intra-articular fractures	Lack of ossification makes checking closed reduction impossible

Pain relief

Patients need to be free of pain when reducing fractures, so a general anaesthetic will be required if a regional block is not possible. If there is no neurovascular compromise this is not an urgent operation, so time should be allowed for the patient's stomach to empty before a general anaesthetic is administered. It may be best to send the patient home with a splint and analgesia so that the procedure can be performed as a semi-planned procedure on a fully staffed list the following morning. If there is any chance that the reduction will not be successful, and that the fracture will need to be opened, then this should be planned in advance (another good reason to leave the case over until the following morning). You will also need to plan how you are going to check that the fracture has indeed reduced satisfactorily, so you will need to book either an image intensifier or plain X-rays, and the patient will need to be positioned so that imaging in two planes is possible. You will also need to plan how to hold the fracture and what facilities (such as plaster or traction pins and frames) you will need.

Value of the periosteum

When a bone fractures the periosteum remains largely intact, especially on the concave side of the fracture. This strong membrane is not visible on the X-ray and so its value in guiding the fracture to a stable reduction may not always be fully appreciated. Impacted fractures which are also partially displaced will need *disimpacting* before the displacement can be corrected. Disimpaction is carried out by applying steady distraction to the fracture until you feel the bone ends separate. The force applied should be no more than 4 or 5 kg as otherwise there is a danger (especially in the elderly) of *degloving* the limb (pulling off the skin and soft tissues). If the fracture does not initially disimpact, then the fracture should be bent further than it is already angulated, 'exaggerating the deformity'. This manoeuvre should disengage the jammed ends. The limb will lengthen slightly, and the fracture will become floppy. Traction should be continued for another couple of minutes to drive oedema out of the tissues around the fracture. This will allow the soft tissues to extend to their normal length and make the reduction easier.

Engaging the bone ends

The intact periosteum on the concave side of the fracture can now block reduction unless the tension is taken off it. This is done by angulating the fracture even further than before, and sliding the fractured end of the distal fragment up the cortex of the proximal fragment until it slips over the broken edge of the proximal fragment. As soon as this occurs the fracture can be rolled into place with the jagged ends of the fracture interdigitating like gear wheels. When the fracture comes to anatomical alignment, the intact periosteum on what was the concave side will become tight and prevent *overcorrection* of the fracture. Providing that any lateral pressure exerted on the fracture is in the direction of overcorrection the fracture will remain stable, splinted by the periosteum.

Open reduction of fractures

Exposure of a fracture should allow adequate access to see as much of the fracture as necessary while minimising damage to soft tissues. It should also minimise damage to the periosteum, which will be providing the bulk of the blood supply to the broken bone fragments. If that blood supply is lost then the fracture cannot unite. The incision will have to take into account any wounds already present and should be *extensile* (able to be extended if necessary). If a plate is to be put on the bone the incision should be planned to enable the plate to be put on the side of the bone which will be in tension. If there is skin and soft-tissue loss then incisions should be planned with a plastic surgeon to ensure that *skin and soft-tissue cover* of the bone and fixation can be obtained at the end of the operation. Fractures which are contaminated and those which are open (which must be treated as contaminated) are an emergency, but not a life-threatening one. Every hour that goes by increases the risk of the fracture becoming infected, so surgery needs to be performed as soon as the anaesthetist feels that it is safe.

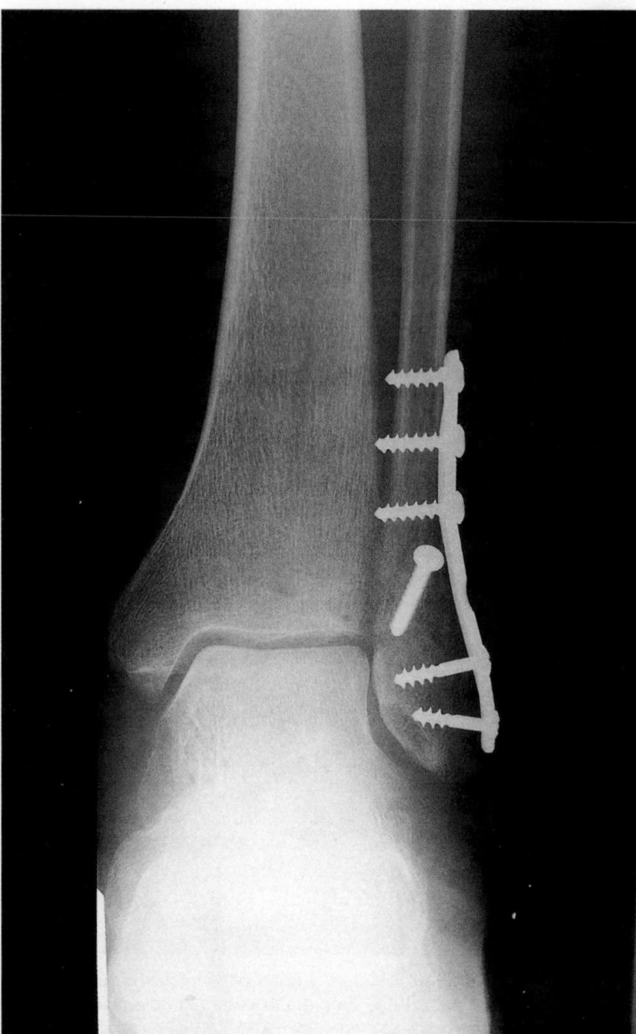

Fig. 21.11 Open reduction and internal fixation (ORIF) of an ankle fracture allows arthritis to be avoided, as well as allowing early weight bearing.

Principles of holding fractures

There are two main ways in which a fracture can be held which make a profound difference to the way in which the fracture heals. *Rigid fixation* blocks the normal callus formation of bone healing. The bone appears to be unaware that there is a fracture if there is no movement at the fracture site. As the bone undergoes normal physiological remodelling, the fracture cleft is gradually obliterated by new bone. This takes about a year. During that time the fixation must share the loads normally taken by the bone. Most implants fatigue under the repetitive load imposed by the human body, and will soon fail if the bone does not heal and take over its original function. Fracture healing is therefore a race against time: the bone must unite before the implant fails or the construct will collapse. Nonrigid fixation (such as plaster of Paris) allows limited movement and loading of the fracture site. The aim is to allow movement and load to stimulate callus formation without allowing the fracture to re-displace. This delicate balancing act depends on the quality of the fixation, the type of fracture and the compliance of the patient (Fig. 21.11).

Pathophysiology of fracture healing

When a bone breaks there is disruption of periosteum, cortical bone, trabecular bone and the blood vessels which run in the periosteum and the medulla. There is haemorrhage and immediate release of cytokines. This signals to cells locally that damage has occurred. These cytokines attract macrophages which start the cleaning-up process. They also attract undifferentiated stem cells which migrate in and start differentiating into fibroblasts and bone-producing cells. These stem cells probably come from the periosteum and the endosteum, and normally lie latent.

The haematoma around the fracture is invaded with small capillaries while the macrophages remove the haematoma itself. At the same time connective tissue is laid down. The connective tissue slowly organises.

This pattern of layers of organised tissue appears first as a collar arising from the periosteum close to the end of each broken bone. The collars appear to grow towards the collar on the other bone. Eventually, the spurs of callus meet and bridge the fracture site. They become increasingly thick and strong fibrocartilage stabilises the fracture. This period, which in the adult occurs over the first few weeks after the fracture, is described as the fracture becoming sticky. It may still be possible to angulate the fracture but it is no longer possible to translate the fracture (move it from side to side). Meanwhile, in the fracture cleft itself, osteoclasts continue to resorb haematoma and other dead tissue and to eat away the broken bone ends. This can result in the fracture becoming more obvious on X-ray over the first few weeks and can indeed make fractures visible which were initially invisible (e.g. the scaphoid). The callus of fibrous cartilage around the fracture cleft becomes calcified and then ossified (so that it is visible on X-ray). Ossification starts at the bone ends but in the centre of the fracture cleft, where oxygen levels may be very low, cartilage may be laid down initially rather than bone. This cartilage is then replaced by bone (*endochondral ossification*). It is not clear whether the callus is derived from the haematoma or from the periosteum, but it is clear that movement stimulates the production of a callus.

When the fracture can no longer be angulated with normal loads, and it is not painful to try, the fracture is said to be *clinically united*. On X-ray, when the strands of ossified callus can be seen to be stretching continuously from one bone end to another, the fracture is said to be *radiologically united*. In neither case is the fracture at full strength yet, but at this stage limited activity can be undertaken safely. Finally, the callus forms a fat cuff of woven bone from one bone end to the other. This callus is at least as strong as the bone around it because biomechanically it has widened the diameter of the tube and this confers extra strength. This stage is called consolidation.

Over the next months the woven bone is replaced by Haversian cortical bone which remodels over the following years.

Rigid immobilisation. If the fracture is rigidly immobilised with a plate there is no stimulus for callus formation. Macrophages remove the haematoma and the dead bone ends. The normal process of remodelling produced by osteoclasts tunnelling through the bone and osteoblasts laying down new bone in their wake gradually obliterates the fracture cleft and reconstitutes normal bone. This process is slow and even in a young patient may take up to a year. If the fixation of the fracture is not completely rigid then some callus will form rapidly, but the patient may be able to resume near-normal function because the fracture is held stable if not immobile by the fixation. This partial rigidity therefore offers the best of both worlds, with rapid biological healing combined with the benefits of early mobilisation of the patient.

Types of fixation

Fixation can be divided into external and internal. Implants which are fitted directly on to or put down the inside of the bone and are then covered with soft tissues and skin are classified as *internal fixation*. Those where the mechanical strength of the construct is outside the skin are defined as *external fixation*.

Types of internal fixation

Screws can be used to hold plates on to bone or can be used in their own right to hold bone fragments together. In orthopaedics, screws have been standardised to an agreed set of diameters. The threads of the screws also come in two standard forms, one for cortical and the other for cancellous bone. The size of these threads and their pitch (the distance between each thread) is specifically designed to give the best possible grip in healthy human bone. The drills, which create the holes for these screws, are also standardised to allow as snug a fit of the screws as possible without putting undue load on the bone. 'Taps' are also supplied which cut the grooves in the bone to take the threads of the screws. Tables are available in every orthopaedic theatre to show which drill should be used for which screw.

Clopton Havers, 1650–1702. Anatomist and physician, London, England.

Lagging

If a screw is to be used to compress two bone fragments together it is important that the thread of the screw should only grip the distal fragment in which the tip of the screw is embedded. As the screw is tightened the shoulder of the screw (the part that tapers in under the head) presses down on the proximal fragment and compresses the two fragments together. If the thread of the screw engages with the proximal fragment the screw can actually hold the fragments apart. There are techniques used to ensure that the fragments are drawn together as the screw is tightened. First, a screw can be used which has no proximal thread, just a smooth shaft. This is known as a 'lag' screw. An alternative strategy is to use

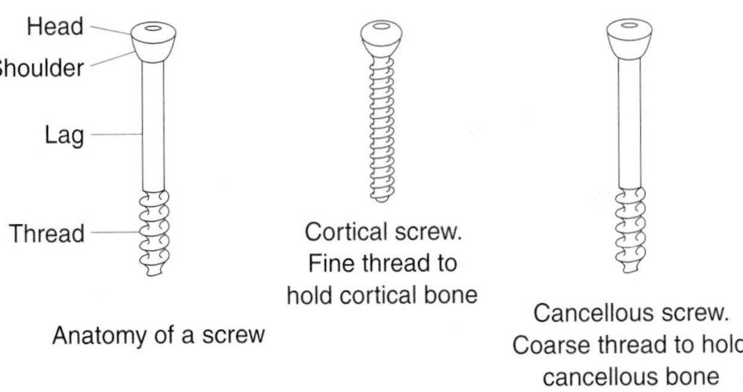

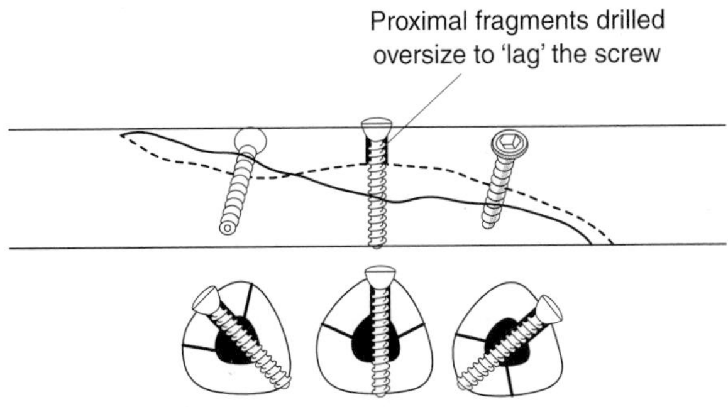

Fig. 21.12 Types of AO screws and the techniques used for 'lagging' to compress the fragments together.

a fully threaded screw, but to drill the hole in the proximal fragment to a slightly larger size so that the screw threads cannot engage with the wall of the hole. This is called lagging the drill hole and serves the same purpose as using a lag screw (Fig. 21.12).

Plates

The plates come in several sizes, each designed to be used with a standard set of screws. They are designed to fit on to the curved surface of bone and to be held there by screws. The plates can be used for several purposes and there are specific plates designed for each function (Fig. 21.14).

Buttress plates. Buttress plates prevent one fragment of bone slipping on another. They are especially useful in oblique fractures in load-bearing bones where they will stabilise what is a very unstable fracture configuration.

Dynamic compression plates (DCP). Dynamic compression plates have oval screw holes in them with tapered walls. If the screw holes are drilled into the bone at one end of these holes (there are drill guides to assist in doing this) then the plate slides along the bone as the screw is tightened home. If the plate has already been firmly fixed to the other fragment then the slip can be used to compress the fragments of bone tightly together. This has the benefit of stabilising the construct by increasing the area of contact. It also appears to stimulate healing by putting the bone edges in close apposition.

Neutralisation plates. Neutralisation plates are used to prevent bone ends from being distracted. They can therefore be used to resist angular forces by being placed on the side of a bone which goes into tension when load is applied (the side that opens when the fracture bends). Plates with screws are excellent at resisting tension and this is how they are used in neutralisation. Plates have very little resistance to bending and so should never be put on the side of the bone which is in compression and which will go into concave angulation when load is applied.

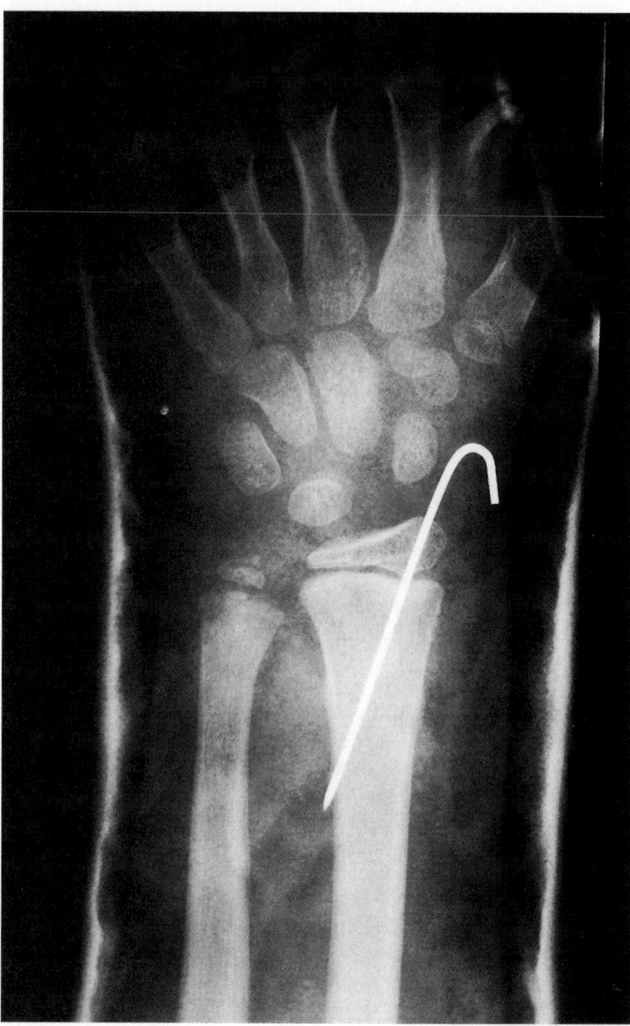

Fig. 21.13 An unstable epiphyseal plate fracture held with percutaneous Kapanji wire.

Wires

Wires are much less traumatic than plates and screws. They can be used temporarily to hold fragments reduced while plates and screws are applied. They can also be used to resist shear where loads are not great. They are especially useful in children's fractures where plates and screws could damage the epiphyseal plate (Fig. 21.13). Wires can cross the growth plate without causing long-term effects, and if left protruding from the skin can be removed when the fracture is secure without the need for a further anaesthetic.

Kapanji wires are a technique which can be used in fractures where impaction may have left a defect which leaves the fracture unstable when reduced. After the fracture has been disimpacted and reduced, wires are introduced into the fracture cleft on the side of the defect. As soon as the tip of the wire is in the medulla the wire is tilted so that its tip travels proximally and embeds on the inside of the far cortex. One or more wires placed in this way substitute for the missing cortex and work with the intact periosteum on the other side to create a stable reduction.

Figure of eight wiring allows a strong wire suture to be woven over the cortex of bone which is in tension. The construct is not prominent and so fits well subcutaneously and is commonly used on the olecranon and on the patella (Fig. 21.14).

Nails

Intramedullary nails. Implants driven down the medulla of a long bone suffer from a significant mechanical disadvantage because they must be narrower than the bone into which they are introduced. Nevertheless, the medulla can provide a natural guide for the implant and introducing the nail into one end of the bone (under image intensifier control) minimises the risk of infection from opening the fracture, and preserves the periosteal blood supply. In recent years the scope of intramedullary nails has been increased enormously

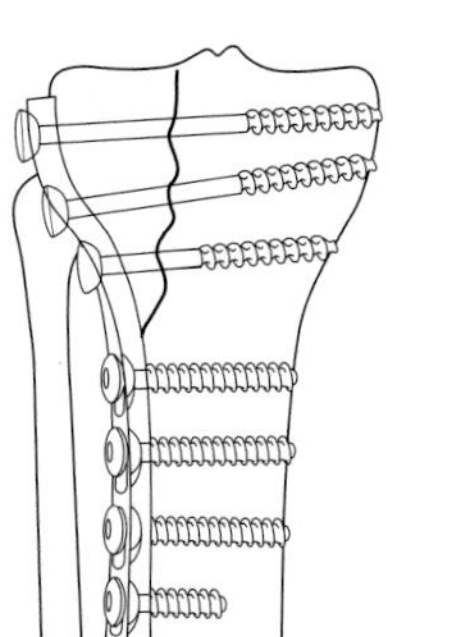

A buttress plate prevents the slip of one fragment over the other

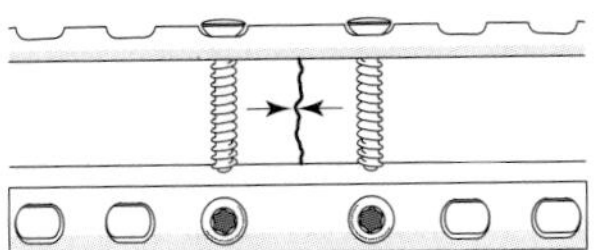

Dynamic compression plate (DCP). The oval holes allow compression to be applied to the fracture site as the screws are tightened

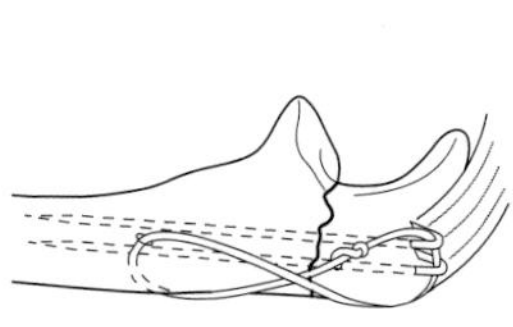

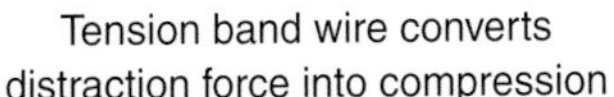

Tension band wire converts distraction force into compression

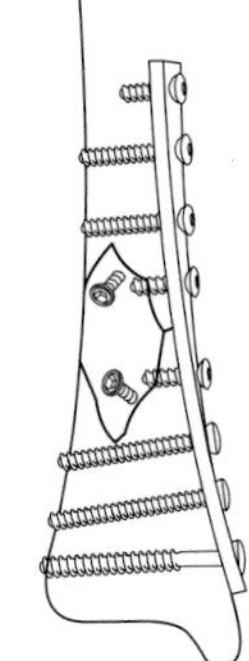

Neutralisation plate. Pre-bent to the shape of the bone held with 7 cortical screws and one cancellous screw

Fig. 21.14 Types of internal fixation with plates and wires.

by the introduction of the *locking nail*. This system has holes through the nail at each end. Using jigs or an image intensifier, screws can be passed through the bone, the hole in the nail and out through the opposite cortex of the bone. This produces a construct which holds the bone rigidly and is especially resistant to twisting. It allows an intramedullary nail to be used for a far greater range of long-bone fractures. Some of the newer nails can now be passed down the medulla without requiring any reaming in advance, the *unreamed nails*. This makes the operation quicker and reduces the trauma to the patient.

In summary, internal fixation can allow very accurate reduction of fractures under direct vision, and allows strong and stable fixation so that the patient can rapidly return to everyday activities with the minimum of inconvenience. The disadvantage is that the patient requires carefully planned and complex surgery which carries a risk of infection if sterile technique is not strictly adhered to.

Disadvantages and complications of internal fixation

The disadvantages of internal fixation are those of damage to soft tissues, especially blood supply. The rigidity of fixation slows the natural healing process, even though it allows earlier mobilisation of the patient. Internal fixation is technically demanding, requires a large range of implants and instruments, and is best performed in ultraclean theatres as infection is a disaster. Internal fixation requires careful preplanning and the best surgery is performed if the fractures are drawn out on stencils first, and the problems of reduction and obtaining mechanical stability planned in advance. This includes size and type of plates, and position of screws. Only in this way can the operation be performed quickly and cleanly (minimising the risk of tissue damage and infection) so that the strongest fixation is obtained.

Internal fixation is best performed under a tourniquet, if possible, in order to obtain a blood-free view. There are complications inherent in using a tourniquet such as cuff damage to nerves as a result of inflation to an excessive pressure, and problems of reperfusion injury if the cuff is left up too long.

Exposure of the fracture may damage the soft-tissue attachments to the bone and produce avascular fragments, which will delay or even prevent fracture union. Soft-tissue dissection should therefore be kept to a minimum, but must be adequate to obtain a clear view and access. All incisions should be designed so that they can be extended safely if necessary – *extensile exposure*.

The risk of infection can be minimised by cleaning out open fractures and leaving them open, with the fractures stabilised until it is certain that all dead and contaminated tissue has been removed. Only when they are clean should they be closed (*delayed primary closure*). When internal fixation is used infection is minimised by performing quick, tidy and well-planned surgery, and by adhering to strict theatre discipline on theatre sterility. Surgery should be covered by three doses of a broad-spectrum antibiotic which has good activity against *Staphylococcus* (the commonest infective organism) and *Streptococcus* (the second most common).

Internal fixation can also leave unsightly scars, and these should be planned to minimise cosmetic deformity without compromising access.

Drills and screws can damage nerves and vessels. Drill guards should always be used to prevent soft tissues being inadvertently dragged into a spinning drill. When the drill is cutting into the far cortex the hand that the surgeon is using to hold the drill should have a straight finger resting on the limb through which the drill is passing, and only light pressure should be applied to the drill so that when the drill then comes out through the far cortex it will not suddenly penetrate deep into the soft tissues on the far side of the bone, where it might perforate a nerve or vessel.

Removal of internal fixation

Implants for internal fixation are made of surgical-grade stainless steel and should not corrode. Nevertheless, the alloys contain transitional metals such as chromium and vanadium whose salts are allergenic, toxic and may even be carcinogenic. Despite this, there is little evidence that metalware left in patients for long periods causes any chemical or even allergic problems. Children should have metalware removed if it is likely to compromise growth. It should be removed as early as possible because periosteal bone grows rapidly over the plates and makes their removal difficult. Internal fixation also shields the bone around it from load, and so may cause local osteoporosis. The load passing down the bone may then peak at the end of a plate (a *stress raiser*) and cause a fracture. Internal fixation of a fracture next to an old plate already embedded in the bone is very difficult to manage. Despite this, it is now normal practice to leave plates and even intramedullary nails in the patient unless there is a specific reason why they should be given another anaesthetic and be subjected to a further operation to remove them.

External fixators

An alternative way to holding a fracture is to insert pins and wires into the bone on each side of the fracture, and to attach these to an external frame which provides the structural integrity. Fixators can be as simple as a set of pins incorporated into a plaster through single- and double-bar fixators, to ring fixators holding the bone through tensioned wires (Fig. 21.15). There is a trade-off between cost, ease of fitting, adjustability, rigidity and convenience to the patient (Table 21.5). The choice of fixator will depend on what is available and the use to which it is to be put.

Uses of an external fixator

Emergency use of the external fixator

Fixators are used for two main reasons in an emergency.

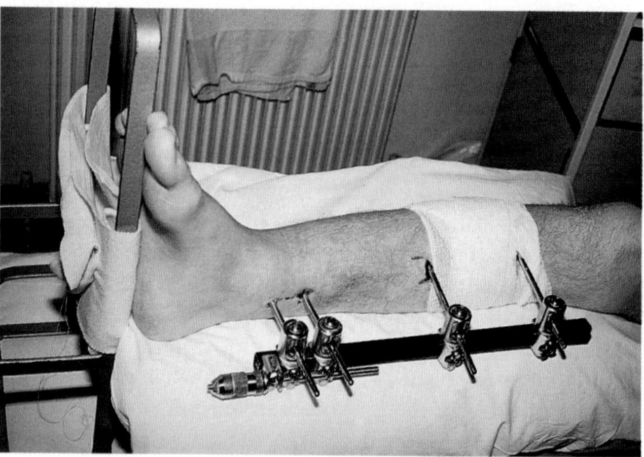

Fig. 21.15 External fixators.

Table 21.5 Choice criteria of external fixators

Fixator type	*Low cost*	*Easy to fit*	*Easy to adjust*	*Rigid*	*Versatile*	*Convenience to patient*
Pins in plaster	Yes	Yes	No	No	No	Fair
One-bar fixator	Fair	Fair	Fair	Fair	Yes	Good
Two-bar fixator	Fair	Fair	Fair	Yes	Yes	Fair
Rings	No	No	No	Yes	Fair	No

Pelvis. They can be used to stabilise an unstable pelvic fracture to try to reduce life-threatening haemorrhage from the pelvic veins. Closing and stabilising an open pelvis fracture may reduce bleeding by reducing movement of the pelvic veins. This may stabilise clots and reduce haemorrhage. Closing the pelvis may increase the intrapelvic pressure and tamponade the veins to reduce bleeding. A bar fixator attached to pins inserted into the pelvic wings will need to be used. The bar should be set as low as possible to give enough room over the abdomen should a laparotomy be needed.

Neurovascular compromise. If a limb has an unstable fracture and has lost its blood supply the skeleton needs to be stabilised before the vascular repair can be performed. One option is to insert a *stent* and provide a temporary blood supply to the limb while a definitive orthopaedic fixation is performed. An alternative is to use an external fixator which can be applied quickly to stabilise the fracture so that the vascular surgeon can start work with the minimum of delay. The disadvantage of this approach is that an external fixator may not be the optimal way of stabilising that particular fracture, but once it has been applied the risk of infection from the pin tracks makes a conversion to a plate or an intramedullary nail potentially risky.

Nonemergency use of the external fixator

Soft tissue damage. If there is extensive damage to the soft tissues then it may not be possible to achieve good cover of the bone. If bone is contaminated and/or exposed internal fixation may not be advisable. Under these circumstances an external fixator may offer the best option. The position of the pins can be planned with the plastic surgeons to enable them to rotate flaps without the fixator or the pins getting in the way.

Leg lengthening and correction of deformity. Over the last decade one of the great advances in orthopaedics has been the discovery that bones can be lengthened gradually – *callostasis*. Segments of bone can be moved across defects and, if the periosteum is left as intact as possible, new bone will be laid down in the defect – *bone transport*.

In order for the pins of the fixator to be able to move through the soft tissues as the bones move they need to be very thin, and it is now routine to use wires which gain their rigidity by being tensioned on a ring (the *Ilizarov* technique). The key to the technique is to move the bone so slowly that new bone can be laid down in its track, but not so slowly that the bone unites and prevents any further distraction. The fixation pins must be positioned to avoid damaging vital structures as they carve through the soft tissues. Care must also be taken to avoid overstretching nerves and vessels, and to avoid contractures caused by ligaments, tendons and muscles failing to extend in concert with the bone.

Gavriil Ilizarov, 1921–92. Orthopaedic surgeon, Kurgan, Russia.

Determining union

Clinical union

A bone is clinically united when putting load on the fracture produces no detectable movement and no pain. The fracture site will not yet be as strong as the bone around it, but it is united.

Radiological union

This is not the same as clinical union. It occurs when the callus around the fracture can be seen to pass from one broken bone end to the other without a gap between. The fracture across the medulla of the bone may still be visible, but the callus around the bone is continuous. The bone should now be able to cope with normal loads, but will not be as strong as the bone around it. From a management point of view, it is the time when movement and loading of the limb should be increased to build up muscle power, mobility and proprioception. If the patient plays sport or works in a job involving heavy labour they should not return to this unless the bone is protected, or until the fracture has consolidated (Fig. 21.16).

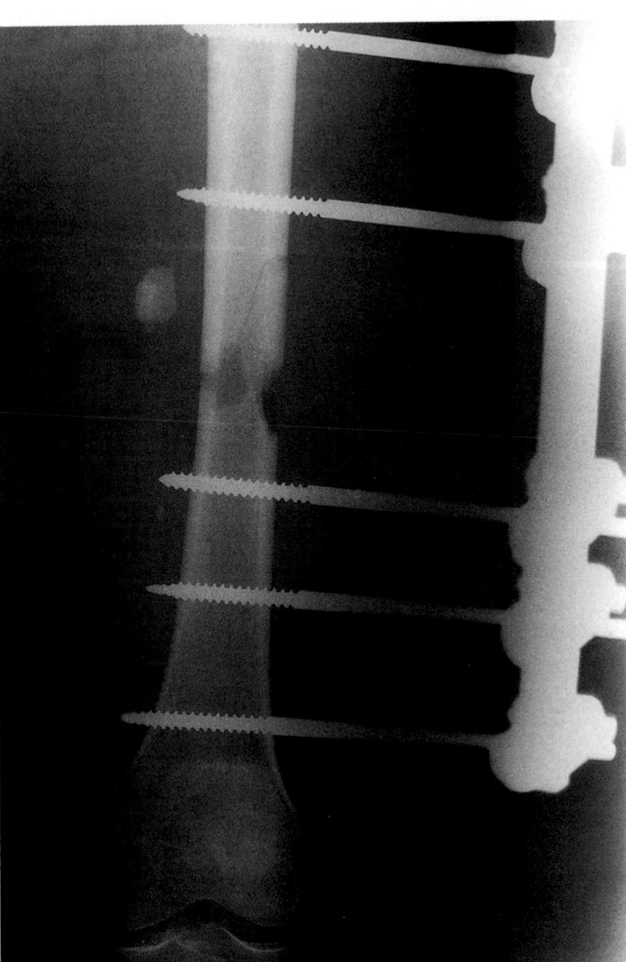

Fig. 21.16 This tibial fracture has radiologically united but has not yet consolidated.

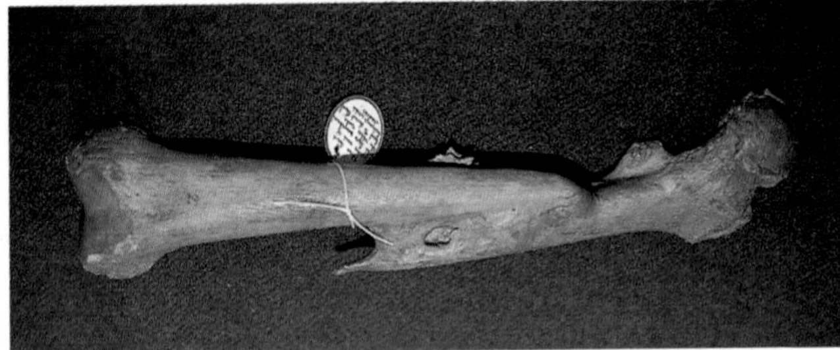

Fig. 21.17 This bone is malunited but the fracture has consolidated.

Consolidation

Consolidation takes much longer than union, and is defined as the time when the process of fracture healing is complete and the strength of the bone has risen to normal levels or even beyond. The formation of callus around a fracture creates a strong cuff. The diameter of this cuff is greater than the diameter of the bone itself, and so a consolidated fracture can be stronger than the original bone (Fig. 21.17).

Restoring function

When a fracture occurs, there will be damage to soft tissues. Muscles may be bruised or torn. Ligaments may be ruptured, joints filled with blood, and nerves and blood vessels damaged. The original philosophy in orthopaedics was that the key to management of fractures was immobilisation, and of injury was rest. This has now all changed. Fractures are stabilised to allow mobilisation of the limb and the patient. Rigid fixation of the fractures actually inhibits callus formation and slows healing. However, stabilisation of the fractures allows the patient to start moving the soft tissues to promote healing and reduce stiffness. It also allows the patient to return to a normal independent life sooner. Physiotherapy is a key element in the rehabilitation of trauma cases. It:

- allows early mobilisation of the limb while ensuring that loads are not so excessive that the fixation will fail;
- provides instruction and advice to the patient on their own rehabilitation;
- builds the patient's confidence;
- re-trains proprioception so that the feedback loops between sensors of joint position and tendon load start to co-ordinate with motor nerves serving the muscles.

Table 21.6 Complications of limb injuries

	Early	*Late*
Local	Neurovascular loss, compartment syndrome, degloving, pain, fracture blisters	Nonunion (hypertrophic, atrophic), malunion, stiffness, wasting, infection, osteoarthritis
Systemic	Hypovolaemic shock, shocked lung, other injuries	Myoglobinuria, multiorgan failure, depression

Complications of limb injury

The complications of injuries can be divided into early and late, local and systemic, and those specific to certain methods of fixation (Table 21.6).

Early local

The key complication is the loss of circulation distal to the injury. A second commonly missed problem is degloving of the skin and subcutaneous fat, which lose their blood supply as they are torn from the deeper tissues. This injury is easy to miss, but if a careful check is made for loss of sensation and capillary filling, and there is a high coefficient of suspicion from the history, then appropriate action can be taken as all of the dead tissue needs to be removed and skin cover is urgently needed. Compartment syndrome is a condition which develops if an injured muscle swells inside a compartment bounded by an inelastic fascia. The most common sites for this problem are the forearm and the muscle compartments surrounding the tibia and fibula. As the muscle swells the pressure within the compartment rises until it becomes so high that it actually cuts off the blood supply to the limb. If urgent action is not taken the muscle dies and scars up, producing *Volkmann's contracture* (Fig. 21.18). An identical situation can be created if a dressing is put on too tight or if a complete plaster is applied to a limb without adequate padding, and before the limb has finished swelling. For the first few hours after trauma it is wise to put on only well-padded back-slab plasters and only complete them on the following day. If the fracture cannot be held without a close-fitting plaster it may be better to wait before carrying out the definitive reduction as the patient needs to be admitted to hospital and to be put under very close observation. The simplest test for developing compartment syndrome is severe pain on extending the digits distal to the injury. Loss of pulses and/or loss of sensation can be late and unreliable signs which should not be relied on. Measuring intracompartmental pressures with a wick catheter is also unreliable and should only be relied on if the patient is unconscious and no other technique is possible. If there is any suspicion that a compartment syndrome might be developing then all dressings should be removed, even if this means losing the fracture position. If this does not lead to an immediate improvement then the patient should be taken to theatre and a fasciotomy performed. The compartment should be opened from end to end and left open until the swelling has settled.

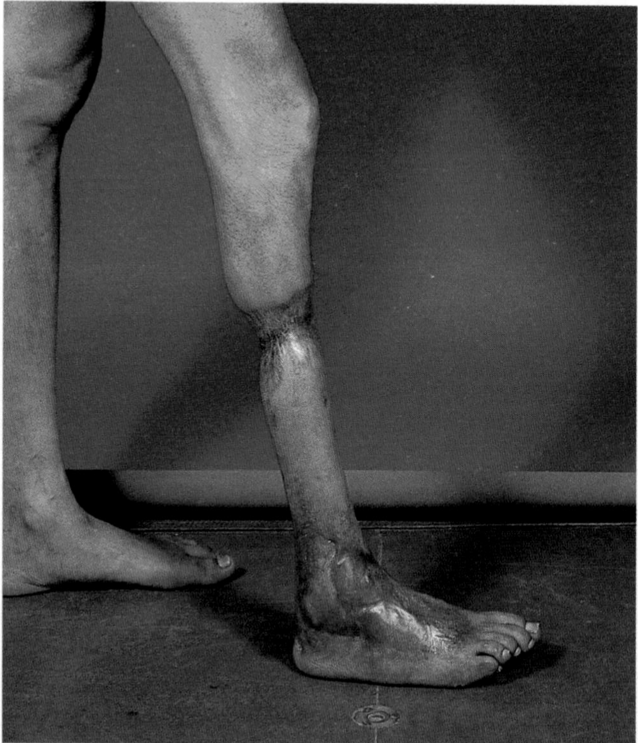

Fig. 21.18 Volkmann's ischaemia caused by a plaster which was too tight.

Richard W. Volkmann, 1800–77. German surgeon.

Fracture blisters

These are a side effect of the soft tissue trauma (Fig. 21.19). They are fragile and quickly burst, creating an open wound which is contaminated. They are a contraindication to internal fixation because of the risk of infection.

Swelling

Soft-tissue swelling is commonly association with fractures. If it severe it is a hindrance to open reduction and internal fixation (ORIF) because the swelling may make it impossible to close the wound at the end of operation. If severe swelling is expected (it is very common with ankle fractures) there is a short window within hours of the accident when surgery may be feasible; after that there may be a period of several days when surgery is impossible. During that time every effort should be made to reduce the swelling as quickly as

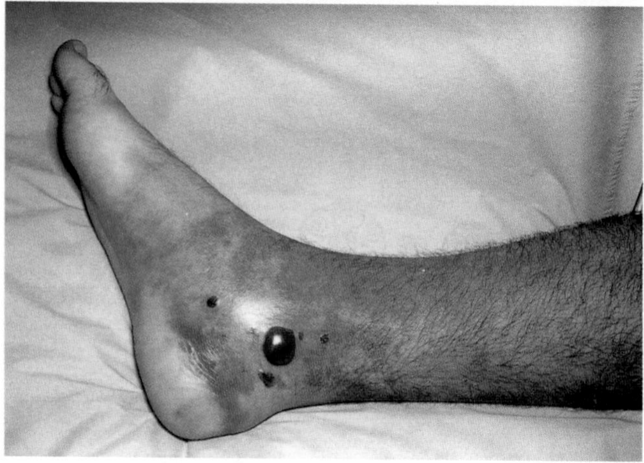

Fig. 21.19 Fracture blisters over an ankle fracture.

possible. The techniques for reducing swelling are given by the acronym RICE: Rest, Ice, Compression and Elevation. Pneumatic stockings can pump away the swelling by intermittent compression. Elevation should be used with care if the circulation to the limb is already compromised.

Early systemic

The main complications arise secondary to hypovolaemic shock. The second problem is that injuries come in clusters, and so a careful search must be made for other injuries to the patient, including those to soft tissues and vital organs, such as the lungs.

Late local

Limbs that are injured tend not to be moved. In limbs that are not moved the joints become stiff, the muscles waste and the circulation deteriorates, so that the healing of the limb may be compromised.

Osteomyelits

If wounds were not cleaned properly or surgery became contaminated the fracture may become infected. Once infection is established it can be very difficult to eradicate, in fact some would say that chronic osteomyelitis is never cured as it can break out again at any time.

The principles of management are to remove all dead and infected bone, then to try to achieve union with strong bone and adequate soft-tissue cover. The amount of bone that needs to be removed is always difficult to estimate and more than you had originally hoped.

Nonunion

Fractured bones which have lost their blood supply, either because of the energy involved at the time of injury or because of the handling of soft tissues at the time of surgery, may go on to *atrophic nonunion*. The bone ends become thin and pointed, and there is no sign of any attempt at union.

If the fracture moves too much then a *hypertrophic nonunion* may result (overabundant callus), but with a persisting fracture cleft held open by excessive movement at the fracture site. If the fracture unites in a bad position (*malunion*) the limb may look very ugly, but may also not work properly. If the radius and ulna unite in a poor position the forearm will lose all ability to pronate and supinate (Fig. 21.20). A common cause for malunion is a failure to supervise the healing of a fracture adequately. If protection is removed too soon, or the patient is not seen often enough, then the fracture may slip and then unite in a poor position. Avoid calling a patient back as an outpatient more than absolutely necessary, but while the fracture is still uniting be sure that the next appointment occurs before union has occurred, so that if there is a slip there is time for a correction of reduction and to secure fixation. Intra-articular fractures which are not anatomically reduced will lead to rapid onset of osteoarthritis. Accurate reduction can be difficult to obtain, especially if there is bone loss, and can be even more difficult to maintain until union has occurred if early movement of the limb is also a priority.

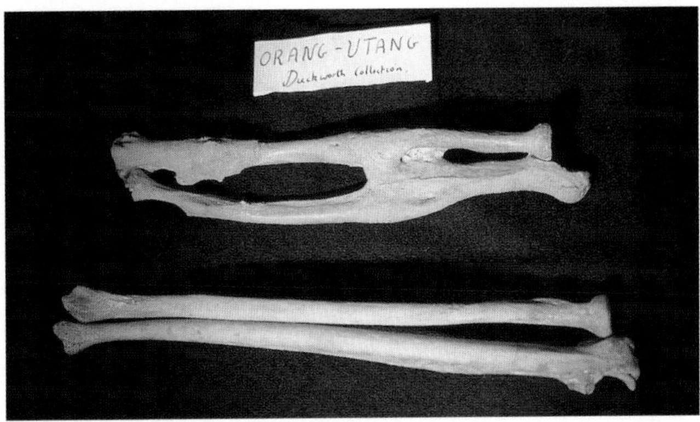

Fig. 21.20 Cross-union in the radius and ulna of an orang-utan.

Late systemic

The late systemic complications can be divided into organic and psychiatric. The initial period of hypovolaemia, and even hypoxia, in polytrauma can lead to irreversible damage locally and systemically. The key to the management of these conditions is prevention. Early aggressive management of the trauma with oxygen and fluids should minimise the time and severity of the insult. If there has been a significant injury then there is a high risk of multiorgan failure which is best managed on an intensive care unit. If there is an open wound with muscle necrosis and this dead tissue is not excised, there is a risk of infection including gas gangrene. Even if the dead tissue does not become infected, there will be a release of muscle degradation products into the bloodstream as the tissue revascularises. These products include myoglobin, which darkens the urine to a dark-brown colour, but also clogs the glomeruli, causing renal failure. The treatment once again is prevention. First, where possible, tissues should not be allowed to become ischaemic. Trapped limbs should be released as quickly as possible, and patients should be kept well oxygenated and well perfused. Dead muscle should be excised and wounds left open for further inspection and excision until cleared of all dead and contaminated tissues. The patient should be given plenty of fluids to maintain diuresis. It is thought that rapid flow of fluids through the kidneys may reduce the build-up of myoglobin and reduce the risk of renal failure.

Shocked lung

This condition develops in patients who have been involved in major trauma. Over the days after the trauma the patient's oxygenation deteriorates despite adequate ventilation and perfusion. The lungs become stiffer and more difficult to ventilate, and chest X-ray shows diffuse clouding. The condition appears to be more likely to occur if the patient is severely hypovolaemic for long periods. This is yet another reason to aim for early aggressive rehydration.

Psychiatric disorders

Patients who survive a suicide attempt may remain deeply psychiatrically disturbed. As soon as they are conscious a pychiatric opinion needs to be sought. If when they start to be mobile they continue to want to take their lives special measures may need to be taken, especially if the orthopaedic wards are not on the ground floor.

Patients who were not psychiatrically disturbed at the time of the accident may become depressed afterwards. This is especially true if the patient lost a close relative or friend in the accident, or if there are awkward questions over who was to blame. It can also occur if treatment takes some time, or the patient is severely scarred, requires an amputation or is left in continuous pain. The modern limb reconstruction techniques, involving multiple plastic and orthopaedic operations which are so time-consuming and technically demanding, can leave a patient physically capable but a mental invalid. You should give careful consideration to the possibility that early amputation with rapid return to normal life in a well-fitting prosthesis could give a better result for a patient with a mangled limb than many months spent reconstructing a limb which could end up useless, painful and ugly.

Further reading

Browner, B.P., Jupiter, J.B. and Levine, A.M. (eds) (1992) *Skeletal Trauma: Fractures, Dislocations, Ligamentous Injuries*, W.B. Saunders, London.

Canale, S.T. (ed.) (1998) *Campbell's Operative Orthopaedics*, 9th edn, Mosby, London.

Gregg, P.J., Stevens, J.G. and Worlock, P.H. (1995) *Fractures and Dislocations: Principles of Management*, Blackwell Science, Oxford.

Rockwood, C.A., Green, D.P. and Bucholz, R.W. *et al.* (1996) Fractures, Vols I–III, *Fractures in Adults, Fractures in Children*, Lippincott Williams & Wilkins, London.

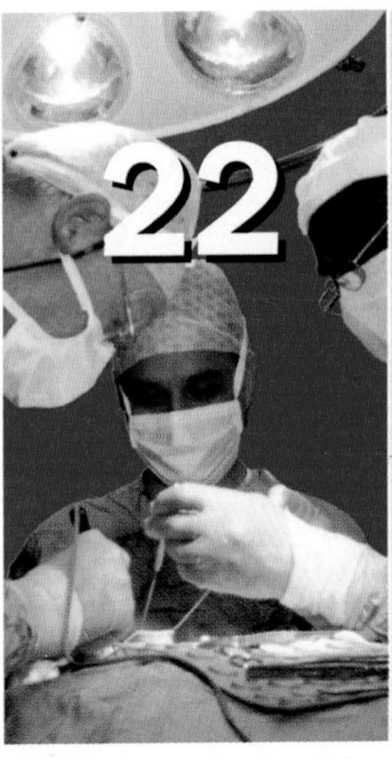

22 Problems in the shoulder and elbow

Congenital abnormalities

Sprengel's deformity

This is the most common congenital abnormality around the shoulder, and results from a failure of normal descent of the scapula. In the embryo, the scapula forms in the midcervical region, and then descends to its midthoracic position. With the Sprengel deformity, the scapula is high, small and rotated, and in approximately 50 per cent of cases the scapula is connected to the cervical spine by the omovertebral body, a fibrous or bony bar. In addition there may be other congenital deformities, which include rib abnormalities, scoliosis of the thoracic spine, or cervical spine abnormalities including the Klippel–Feil syndrome (congenital fusion of the cervical vertebrae) (Fig. 22.1).

Treatment

The major problem is usually cosmetic rather than functional, and this is particularly true for unilateral deformities. In these cases excision of the omovertebral body or superior angle is performed. Surgery is occasionally required to improve function, and in these circumstances more complex reconstructive procedures are carried out.

Otto Sprengel, 1852–1915. Surgeon, Brunswick, Germany.
Maurice Klippel, 1858–1942. Neurologist in Paris, France. Described this condition in a joint paper with Feil in 1912.
André Feil, b. 1884. Neurologist in Paris, France. Described this condition in a joint paper with Klippel in 1912.

Bailey & Love's Short Practice of Surgery, 23rd edition. Edited by R.C.G. Russell, N.S. Williams and C.J.K. Bulstrode. Published in 2000 by Arnold Publishers.

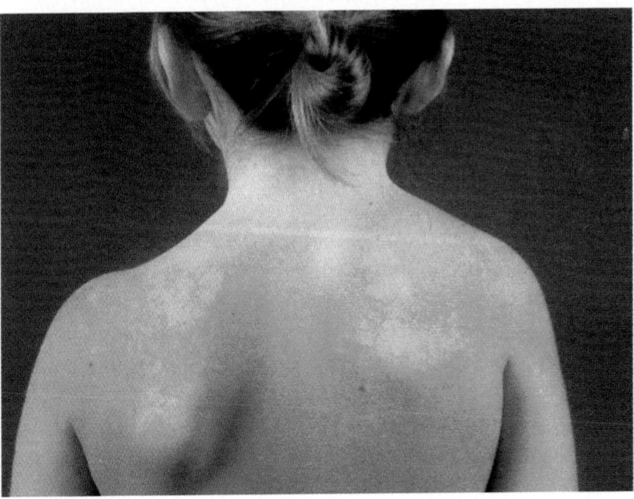

Fig. 22.1 Demonstrating Sprengel's shoulder. The right shoulder of a 4-year-old girl. The scapula is riding high and the shoulders are at uneven levels.

Acquired conditions

The painful shoulder

After back pain, shoulder pain is the second most common musculoskeletal problem seen by primary care physicians. The commonest causes of the painful shoulder in adults are disorders of the rotator cuff, particularly the supraspinatus tendon. Although conditions such as the painful arc syndrome, impingement, rotator cuff tears and cuff tear arthritis are often considered as separate conditions, in reality they are part of a spectrum of disorders of the supraspinatus tendon. Other causes of shoulder pain include calcific tendonitis, frozen shoulder and degenerative disease.

Disorders of the rotator cuff

In common with some other tendons of the body, the supraspinatus tendon has a relatively poor blood supply, and this can predispose to both degenerative changes and tearing of the tendon. The anterolateral portion of the tendon is initially affected and swelling of this portion may lead to impingement between the greater tuberosity of the humerus and the anterior acromion with its attached coraco-acromial (CA) ligament. This leads to pain, particularly on active abduction or flexion, and initially leads to a painful arc between 60–120°.

Abnormalities of the bone occur, with hooking of the anterior acromion. These are probably secondary changes, rather than the primary cause of the pain, but surgical treatment is often directed against the acromion and the CA ligament.

History and examination

The patient is usually middle aged, and the initial symptoms may be due to a specific traumatic incident or a period of overuse of the arm, or there may be no precipitating events. The pain is activity related, particularly on overhead activities, such as reaching up to shelves or hair washing. Gardening and household activities often produce symptoms. Some patients complain of significant weakness, and this may indicate the presence of a rotator cuff tear.

On examination, there is often no local tenderness. Active movements may be limited, and usually reproduce the symptoms, which occur between 60–120° of abduction and flexion (Fig. 22.2). There is usually much less pain on passive movements, and this confirms the mechanical nature of the pain. Weakness of both supraspinatus and infraspinatus may be demonstrated, and suggest the possibility of a tear in the cuff. Specific impingement tests have been described and help to confirm the diagnosis (Figs 22.3 and 22.4). Radiographs may be normal, but usually there are signs of subacromial sclerosis.

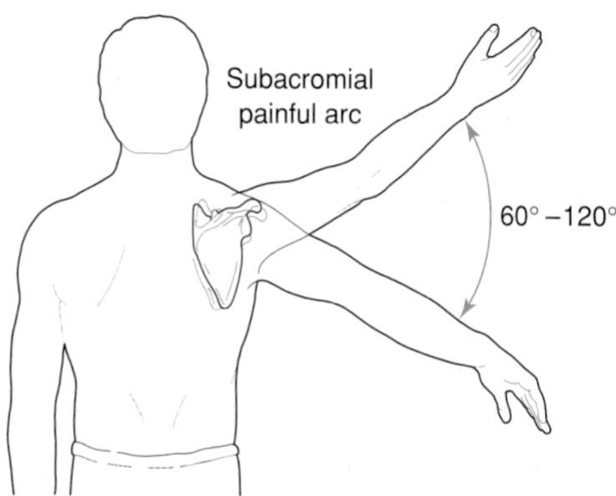

Fig. 22.2 Demonstrating impingement pain in the arc of abduction between 60° and 120°.

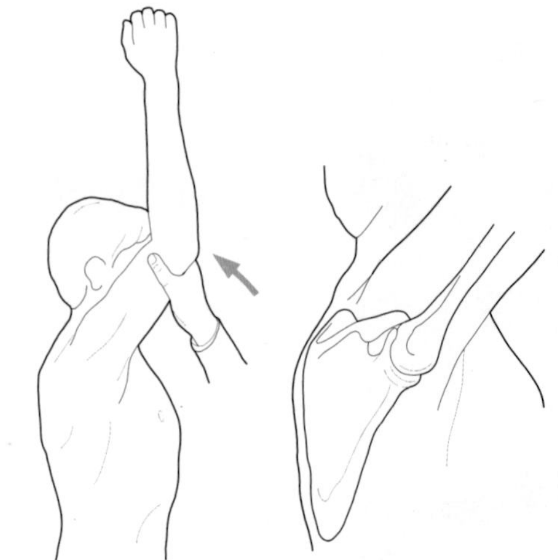

Fig. 22.3 Neer's test producing impingement pain on full flexion.

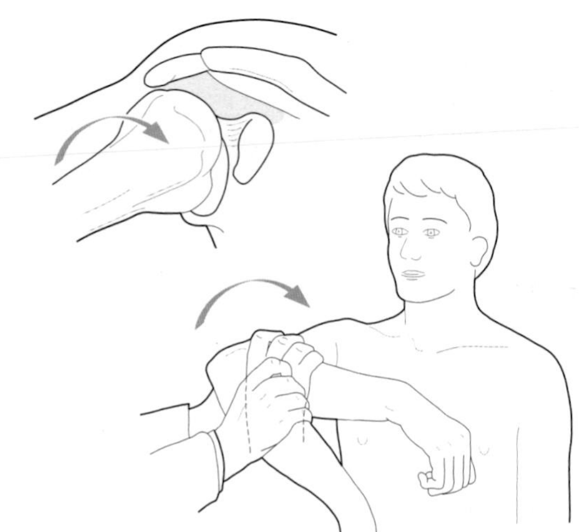

Fig. 22.4 Hawkin's test for impingement. Impingement pain is produced by abducting and flexing to 90° and then by internally rotating the humerus thus moving the greater tuberosity on the under surface of the acromion.

Subacromial injection of local anaesthetic and cortisone often leads to improvements in the symptoms and they are used for both diagnostic and therapeutic purposes. If the diagnosis is correct, the symptoms are usually improved. The benefit may only be short lived, but this is a valuable diagnostic aid. Improvement in symptoms occurs for a few weeks after the injection, but subsequent relapse commonly occurs.

Further investigations

A subacromial injection is the most useful diagnostic test, and this is easily performed in the out-patient clinic. Further investigations such as ultrasound and magnetic resonance imaging (MRI) are used to determine the presence of a tear of the rotator cuff if surgery is contemplated; they have little place in the diagnosis of impingement (Fig. 22.5).

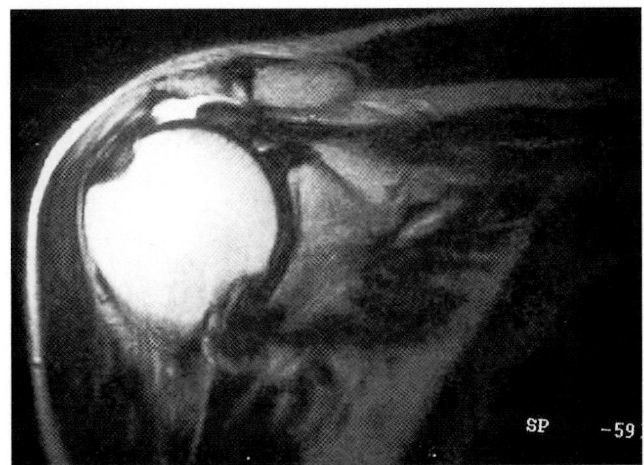

Fig. 22.5 An MRI scan of a shoulder demonstrating a full-thickness tear of the supraspinatus tendon.

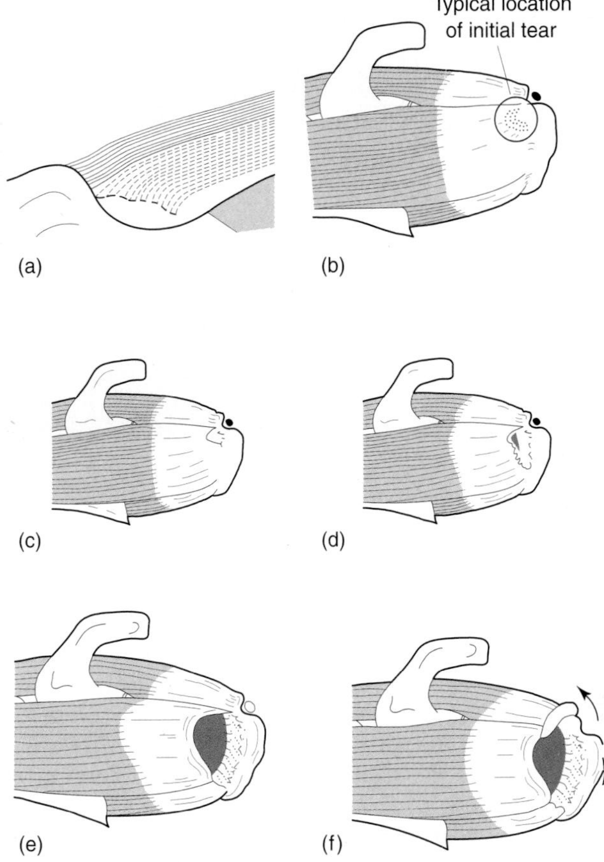

Fig. 22.6 (a) Rotator cuff tears usually begin on the under surface of the rotator cuff (the joint side). (b) The typical tear begins in the anterior part of the supraspinatus just behind the rotator interval and the long head of biceps. (c) The tear then develops as a horseshoe shape. (d) The tear usually extends along the attachment of the greater tuberosity developing an 'L' shape. (e) Usually gradually, but sometimes suddenly, after a fall the tear may extend to involve the whole of the supraspinatus. (f) This tear may extend further to involve the infraspinatus posteriorly and anteriorly to affect the upper part of subscapularis and may be associated with a dislocation of the long head of the biceps tendon. The long head of the biceps tendon may also rupture.

Treatment

It is likely that most patients will settle with conservative treatment. The initial treatment is by cortisone injection, and this is repeated up to three times if there is prolonged relief of symptoms. Specific physiotherapy has a role, particularly in the early stages, but most patients who present to specialist clinics will only have a limited response. Surgery is eventually required in 50 per cent of these patients, and is indicated when symptoms, sufficient to limit activities, have been present for over a year. Decompression of the rotator cuff is carried out, either arthroscopically, or by an open procedure, with removal of the anterior overhang and division of the CA ligament. In addition, repair of a rotator cuff tear may be required. In the absence of a rotator cuff tear, the prognosis is good.

Rotator cuff tears

Patients with rotator cuff tears are usually slightly older than patients with impingement. Tearing of the supraspinatus muscles also starts at the front lateral edge of the tendon, and can progress posteriorly along the tendon, detaching it from the greater tuberosity. The tendon retracts medially leading to a U-shaped tear. The patient is usually unaware of the rotator cuff tearing, and large tears of several years' duration may be present before the patient seeks medical attention (Fig. 22.6).

Small tears of the supraspinatus

These are very common and may be found in up to 20 per cent of the normal population, in the absence of any specific shoulder symptoms. The tear is usually less than 1 cm in length and, in the absence of significant pain, is not of a sufficient size to cause weakness of the shoulder.

Treatment of small tears. Treatment is dependent on the presence and severity of impingement symptoms. In the absence of symptoms, the tear can be left unrepaired, and the patient kept under review. Progression of the tear is an indication for repair. If impingement is a significant problem, decompression is carried out, and the tear can be repaired if appropriate.

Intermediate tears

Tears of 2–3 cm (as measured on ultrasound) are usually associated with symptoms of impingement or weakness of the shoulder, and these will often require decompression and repair of the supraspinatus. This can be carried out through a lateral sabre-type incision. The tendon is mobilised, and then sutured into a bony trough created on the edge of the greater tuberosity, using osseous sutures. Results of repair are good for intermediate tears, but full recovery will take several months.

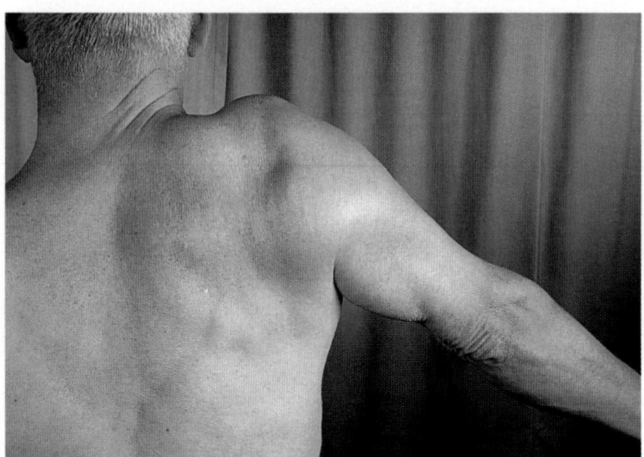

Fig. 22.7 A full-thickness tear of the rotator cuff produces failure of abduction. The shoulder is characteristically hunched up. There is wasting of the infraspinatus and supraspinatus.

Large tears of the supraspinatus

These are often 5 cm or greater, and may extend into infraspinatus. They are usually associated with weakness of the shoulder, and abduction may be limited to 60°, often with a characteristic hunching of the shoulder (Fig. 22.7). With massive tears of the rotator cuff, superior migration of the humeral head can occur, and this further impairs function. In addition, secondary osteoarthritis of the glenohumeral head may occur due to the resulting incongruity of the joint.

Treatment of large tears. If symptoms of impingement or weakness are sufficient, decompression and repair should be considered. Unfortunately repair is not always possible as the medial edge of the tendon retracts, and it may be impossible to mobilise this to close the defect. Tendon grafts and synthetic meshes have been used to close this defect but the results are less than satisfactory. This is due to degeneration and disuse atrophy of the supraspinatus associated with a chronic tear, and although the gap may have been closed there is poor function from the repaired tissue.

In many patients with large tears, the predominant symptom is still pain rather than weakness and in these patients if the tear is irreparable by direct suture, simple decompression is carried out. Up to 80 per cent of these patients will have good relief of symptoms and improved function, despite the unrepaired rotator cuff tear.

Acute tears of the rotator cuff

Most tears of the supraspinatus are due to degeneration and, as discussed above, will be associated with impingement symptoms. Occasionally a large tear of the rotator cuff can result from trauma, in the absence of any previous shoulder symptoms. These patients present soon after the event with profound weakness and loss of function but minimal pain. On examination, there is marked restriction of abduction, usually to less than 90°, with a characteristic hunching of the shoulder. This is due to elevation and rotation of the scapula to attempt to aid abduction. Diagnosis is confirmed by ultrasound or MRI, and early exploration and repair is indicated. Unlike the large degenerate cuff tears the acute tear is usually repairable if surgery is carried out early. Often no decompression is necessary, as the front edge of the acromion is normal with no evidence of overhang. In middle-aged and elderly patients an acute cuff tear can occur after shoulder dislocation.

Frozen shoulder

This is a painful shoulder condition of unknown aetiology that affects the capsule of the shoulder. The rotator interval between supraspinatus and subscapularis is affected predominantly. The disease most commonly affects females in their 50s, and is more common in diabetics and patients with heart or thyroid disease.

History and examination

The pain is often of sudden onset and may follow minor trauma. It is severe and often disturbs sleep, and fractures or joint infection may be considered in the differential diagnosis. In the early stages, the shoulder is difficult to examine owing to the pain, but as the disease progresses the range of motion is reduced, both actively and passively. Local tenderness is often felt anteriorly over the rotator interval. The pathognomonic sign of frozen shoulder is loss of external rotation and this differentiates it from rotator cuff disease. Plain X-rays exclude other intra-articular pathology.

Clinical course

The clinical course of frozen shoulder can be divided into three stages as follows.

- Stage 1 – a *painful phase* – can last for 2–9 months. The shoulder becomes increasingly painful, especially at night, and the patient uses the arm less and less. The pain is often very severe, and may be unrelieved by simple analgesics.
- Stage 2 – a *stiffening phase* – can last for 4–12 months and is associated with a gradual reduction in the range of movement of the shoulder. The pain usually resolves during this period, although there is commonly still an ache, especially at the extremes of the reduced range of movement.
- Stage 3 – the *thawing phase* – lasts for a further 4–12 months and is associated with a gradual improvement in the range of motion.

The clinical course runs over a period of 1–3 years and usually resolves without any long-term sequelae.

Treatment

Often no treatment is required and the condition will usually resolve as described above. The range of motion may be slightly reduced compared with the unaffected side, but the vast majority of patients has no functional problems.

Treatment in the acute stage is pain relief. Corticosteroids may be tried but have variable effects. Active and passive mobilisation can be carried out if comfort allows but aggressive physiotherapy should be discouraged.

Surgery is usually reserved for prolonged stiffness affecting function but can also produce good pain relief in the acute stage. Surgical treatment has a limited place in management. Manipulation under anaesthetic may produce an increased range of motion. Arthroscopic distension of the joint with saline allows inspection of the shoulder before treatment. If these measures fail to produce any benefit, open release of the rotator interval can be carried out through an anterior approach.

Calcific tendonitis

This is a common disorder of unknown aetiology which results in an acutely painful shoulder. Calcium is deposited within the supraspinatus, and it is thought that this may be part of a degenerative process. The differential diagnosis includes frozen shoulder, with both conditions occurring most commonly in middle-aged women.

History and examination

This pain is usually of rapid onset, often with no precipitating cause. In common with impingement, the pain is felt on the anterolateral aspect of the shoulder and is worse with activities, particularly overhead activities. The pain can be very severe and usually disturbs sleep. On examination, the shoulder is tender anterolaterally, and there is often some restriction of active and commonly passive motion. External rotation will be possible and this differentiates the condition from frozen shoulder.

The calcific deposits can be seen on plain radiographs, lying within the supraspinatus tendon, inferior to the acromion and just medial to the tuberosity of the humerus. They can also be seen on ultrasound (Fig. 22.8).

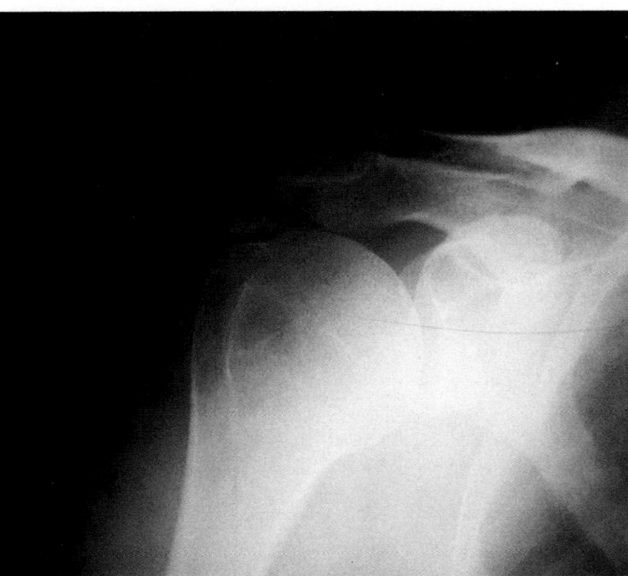

Fig. 22.8 Demonstrating calcification of the supraspinatus tendon.

Treatment

Simple analgesia should be tried together with physiotherapy, although specialist referral is commonly indicated. Calcific tendonitis usually responds to subacromial injection of corticosteroid, although a course of several injections may be necessary. The condition is often self-limiting with resolution of the symptoms and resorption of the calcium.

Surgery

Resistant cases of calcific tendonitis are an indication for surgical treatment. Open excision of the calcific deposits can be carried out through a sabre incision but arthroscopy of the shoulder with subacromial decompression is an alternative. The cuff can be debrided and, if the deposits are prominent, they can be removed through a smaller incision.

The prognosis for calcific tendonitis is generally good.

Arthritis of the shoulder

Rheumatoid arthritis

The glenohumeral joint is commonly involved in inflammatory arthritis, particularly rheumatoid arthritis (RA), with up to one-third of these patients developing severe problems. Initially the pain is related to synovitis and this responds to medical management, including intra-articular steroid injection.

Impingement symptoms can also occur, either with or without a rotator cuff tear. These will respond to subacromial injection but decompression may be indicated. Arthroscopic synovectomy can be carried out at the same time but, in general, open synovectomy is not indicated in the management of RA of the shoulder. Chemical synovectomy may be indicated for symptoms that are resistant to medical treatment but this is not commonly performed for RA.

For advanced disease, glenohumeral arthroplasty is indicated, with very good relief of pain, but there is often little improvement in the preoperative stiffness.

Osteoarthritis

Osteoarthritis of the glenohumeral joint is either primary or more commonly secondary. Secondary arthritis is usually due to previous trauma or to end-stage rotator cuff disease, in association with a massive tear of the cuff and superior migration of the humeral head.

Treatment. As with osteoarthritis of other joints, medical measures are initially tried. Failure of medical management is an indication for surgery. Débridement of the joint and osteotomy have little if any place in the management of glenohumeral osteoarthritis, and joint replacement is the treatment of choice. Both total shoulder replacement and hemiarthroplasty, without glenoid replacement, can be carried out (Fig. 22.9). Total shoulder replacement should only be carried out if the rotator cuff is intact. In most patients with RA, and all patients with cuff tear arthritis, the cuff is deficient and hemiarthroplasty is therefore the most common replacement performed; this can be carried out through an anterior deltopectoral approach. Shoulder

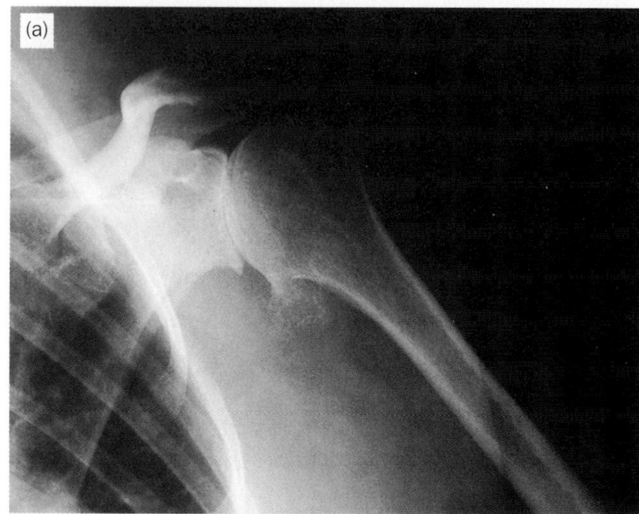

replacement is a very good pain-relieving procedure but, in general, will not restore movement to a stiff shoulder.

Arthrodesis of the joint is an alternative in the younger patient, especially if there is a history of sepsis or any neurological problem that would affect the stability of a joint replacement. The perioperative morbidity is higher, however, and 3–4 months of immobilisation are required. The patient retains a surprisingly good range of movement at the shoulder and can function well owing to scapulothoracic movement (Fig. 22.10).

Arthritis of the acromioclavicular (AC) joint

Degenerative changes of the AC joint on plain radiographs are relatively common and are usually age related. Symptomatic disease, however, usually affects males in their 20–40s and is commonly due to a previous injury. It is often seen in individuals who play sport or are involved in an occupation that stresses the upper limbs. If inferior osteophytes are present, impingement on the underlying rotator cuff can occur.

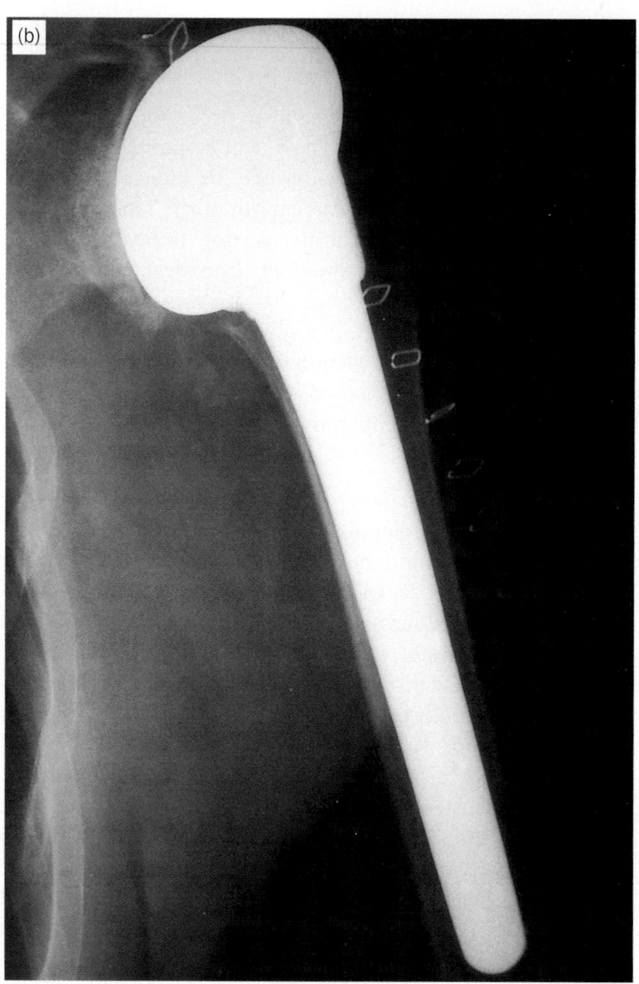

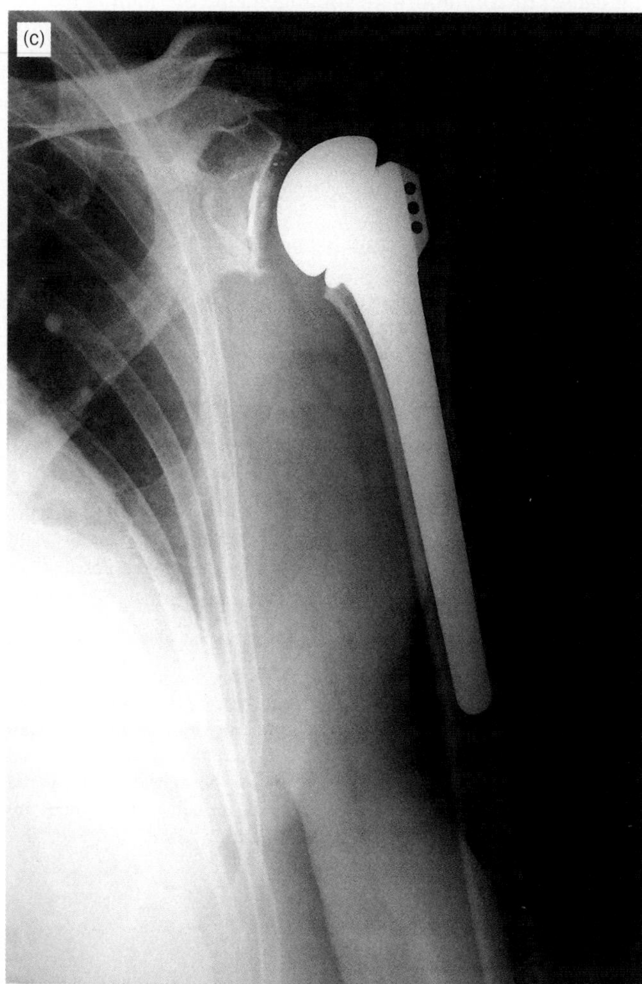

Fig. 22.9 (a) X-ray demonstrating typical appearances of a shoulder in advanced osteoarthritis with subchondral sclerosis and osteophyte formation. (b) If the rotator cuff is torn then a hemiarthroplasty may be performed. (c) If the rotator cuff is intact and there is not excessive glenoid erosion then a total shoulder replacement is indicated.

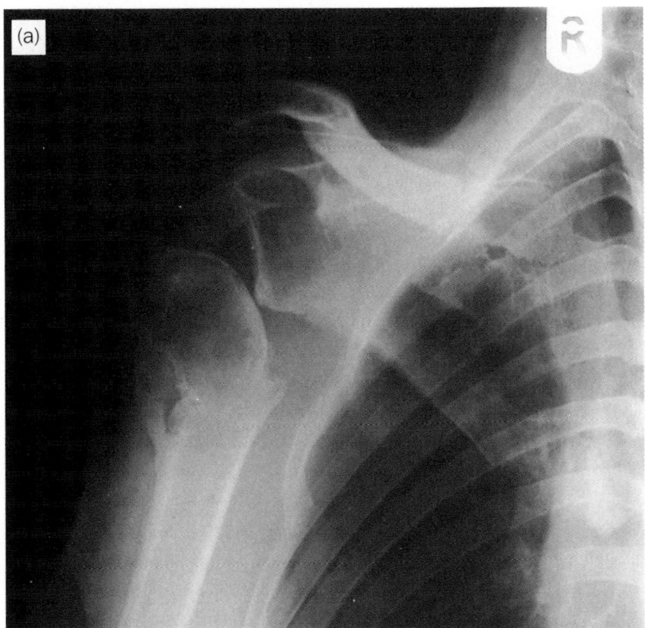

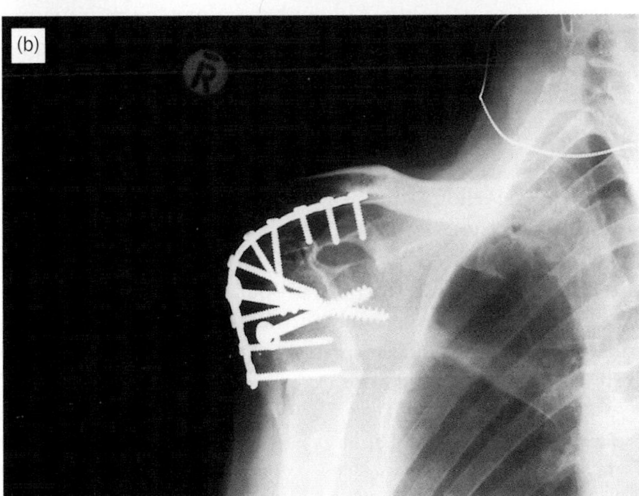

Fig. 22.10 (a) Post-traumatic osteoarthritis of the shoulder with considerable deformity and subluxation of the humeral head. (b) This is managed with arthrodesis by single lag screws and a 3.5-mm reconstruction plate. The plate is screwed to the spine of the scapula and to the humeral shaft.

History and examination. The pain is activity related and, unlike most causes of shoulder pain, it is well localised, with the patient pointing to the AC joint as the source of the pain. On examination, there is usually a bony abnormality, with prominence of the distal end of the clavicle. This may be tender and movement of the joint by depressing the clavicle whilst pushing up the humerus will reproduce the pain. Flexing and adducting the arm to place the hand behind the opposite shoulder will also produce pain. An intra-articular injection of local anaesthetic will confirm the joint as the site of the pain. If the symptoms are related to the inferior osteophytes, the pain is less well localised, and impingement signs and symptoms are present.

Treatment. Intra-articular injection of corticosteroids will usually produce some benefit and a course of three injections may be tried. If medical management fails, then surgery may be appropriate. The distal 1/2 to 1 cm of the clavicle is excised by a direct approach, with good relief of pain and no functional difficulties. In patients with predominately impingement symptoms, arthroscopic debridement of the osteophytes can be carried out.

Rupture of the biceps tendon

Rupture of the long head of biceps is a relatively common condition, occurring in middle age and in the elderly. The condition is closely related to rotator cuff disease and the tendon usually ruptures owing to chronic attrition. Although many patients present acutely, an asymptomatic biceps rupture is a relatively common finding during arthroscopy for rotator cuff surgery.

History and examination

The patient usually complains of something giving, often when they are lifting. The arm is often bruised and when the patient flexes the elbow a lump is evident in the middle of the biceps. The lump is initially tender and power is diminished (Fig. 22.11).

Treatment

This condition is treated conservatively, and the patient can be reassured that the pain will ease and the power return, although this may take several months.

Rupture of the distal insertion of biceps is an uncommon condition that usually occurs in younger patients, particularly after a sporting injury. Again pain and weakness are present but, unlike rupture of the long head, the weakness will not improve. Surgical repair is indicated.

Instability of the glenohumeral joint

Traumatic dislocation of the shoulder will be considered in the next section but recurrent instability is a common sequela

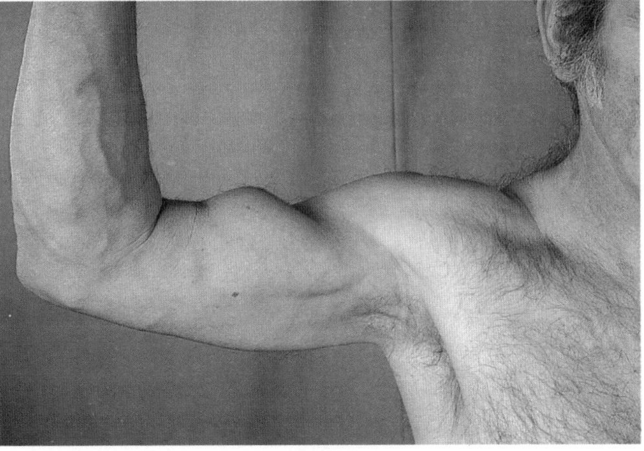

Fig. 22.11 Long head of biceps rupture.

of dislocation. Recurrent traumatic instability is age related, with over half of shoulder dislocations becoming recurrent in the under 25 year olds. In some patients, the shoulder may dislocate after relatively little force, and a further group of patients with shoulder instability may be able to dislocate the shoulder at will. The diagnosis is based on an accurate history and further investigations, other than plain radiographs, are not usually required.

Classification

There are many ways of classifying shoulder instability, based on direction, the degree of violence required as well as considering subluxations and true dislocations. There is a spectrum of instability but, in general, three groups of patients can be considered as follows (Fig. 22.12).

Recurrent traumatic instability. This is predominately in one direction, most commonly anteroinferiorly. There is a definite traumatic event initially, although less violence is required subsequently. The patient is aware of apprehension on certain activities and sport may be made difficult. The shoulder may sublux or dislocate and often the dislocation has to be reduced in a medical facility. On examination, there is a full painless range of motion but apprehension on forced abduction and external rotation (Fig. 22.13). Other joints are usually normal. As discussed in the section on trauma, there is usually a Bankart defect with detachment of the anteroinferior glenoid labrum and damage to the humeral head (Fig. 22.14).

Treatment. Conservative treatment has little place and, if the instability causes functional difficulties, surgery is indicated. For anterior instability, repair of the Bankart defect, in addition to some tightening of the capsule, will produce good results in 90–95 per cent of patients. This is carried out through an anterior deltopectoral approach (Fig. 22.13). For recurrent posterior instability (uncommon) tightening of the posterior capsule through a posterior approach is carried out.

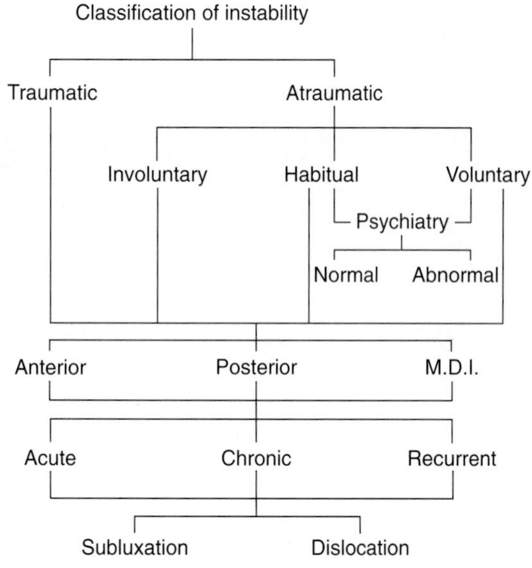

Fig. 22.12 Classification of instability of the shoulder.

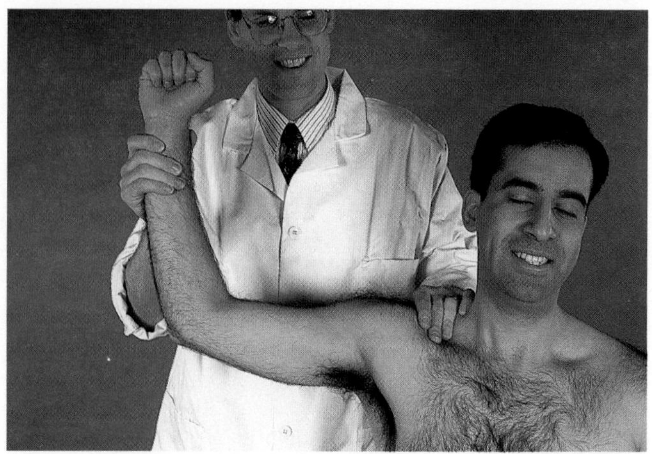

Fig. 22.13 Demonstrating the anterior apprehension test.

Atraumatic instability. Although there may be an initiating event, this is often less traumatic, for example a fall climbing stairs rather than a sporting injury. In many cases there is no initial injury and the instability may occur in more than one direction. The shoulder usually subluxes rather than dislocates and the patient can often reduce the shoulder themself. The subluxation is painful and the patient will not dislocate the shoulder at will. On examination, generalised ligament laxity is commonly present and the shoulder can often be subluxed inferiorly to produce a sulcus sign, with a lateral sulcus appearing beneath the acromion as the arm is pulled down. Apprehension tests are again positive but often in more than one direction.

Treatment. Physiotherapy, by an experienced therapist, should be tried first in these patients. As well as muscle strengthening re-education of the patient and shoulder is necessary, and specific muscle groups may need to be targeted.

Approximately half of the patients will require surgery and a capsular tightening procedure is carried out through an anterior approach. This is a successful procedure but there is a higher failure rate than with patients found to have a Bankart defect. Arthroscopic shrinkage of the capsule may have a place in these patients, and this is currently being evaluated.

Habitual dislocation. This is a much smaller group of patients, but one which does not respond well to surgical treatment. The patient is able to sublux the shoulder at will and this is usually not painful (Fig. 22.15). There is underlying joint laxity, which is usually generalised, and there is rarely a significant traumatic event. The patient may sublux the shoulder as a 'party trick', or for emotional or psychological reasons.

A.S. Blundell Bankart, 1879–1951. Consulting surgeon, Royal National Orthopaedic Hospital, London, England.

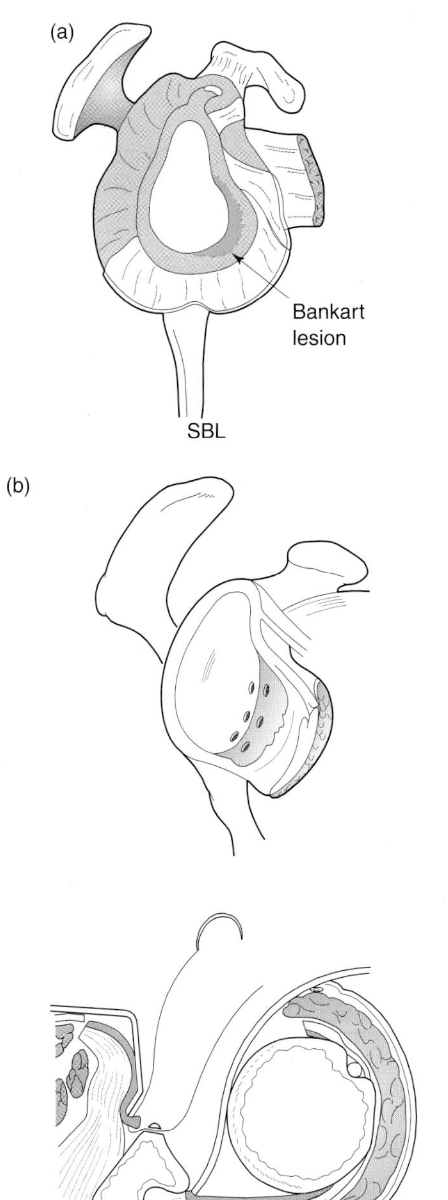

Fig. 22.14 (a) Demonstrating the Bankart lesion of the anteroinferior capsule and labrum of the shoulder. (b) The Bankart repair involves reattachment of the labrum and capsule to the anterior part of the glenoid using sutures through bone.

Treatment. It is vital that these patients are assessed and managed by an experienced therapist. The patient must be educated to avoid subluxing the shoulder and shown exercises as appropriate. Surgery is associated with a high failure rate and should be avoided.

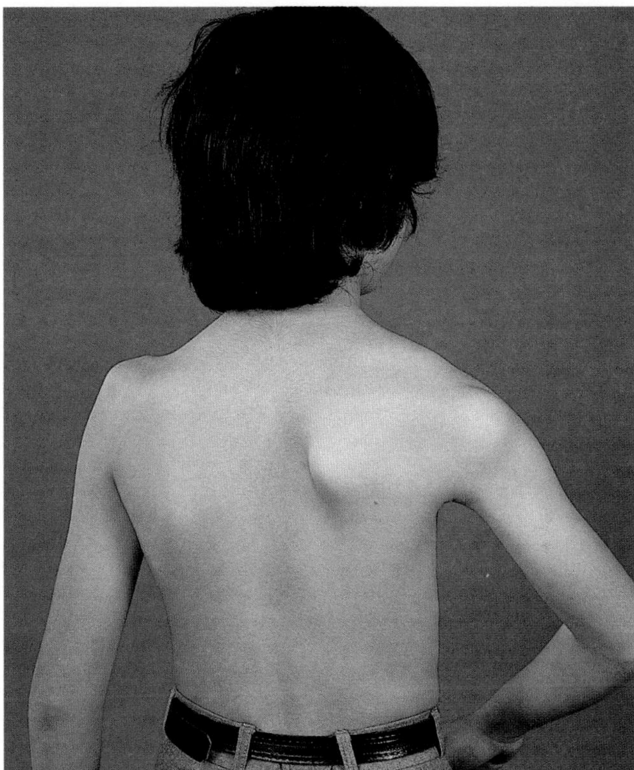

Fig. 22.15 Multidirectional voluntary dislocation of the shoulder. This 9-year-old boy can voluntarily dislocate his shoulder posteriorly.

Disorders of the elbow

Tennis elbow

Excluding traumatic conditions, this is the most common cause of pain around the elbow, and usually occurs in patients in their 30–50s. The exact cause is unknown but the condition commonly follows a period of overactivity, particularly an unaccustomed activity that involves active extension and suppination of the wrist. The tendon of extensor carpi radialis brevis is most commonly involved and, at exploration, a partial tear and chronic inflammatory tissue have been described.

History and examination

The patient complains of pain around the lateral epicondyle and in the back of the forearm. This is activity related and often a particular activity is implicated. There is not usually a history of trauma, but the patient may relate the onset to a period of unusual activity. On examination, the patient is locally tender, which is commonly just distal and anterior to the lateral epicondyle rather than the epicondyle itself. Forced palmar flexion and pronation against resistance reproduces the pain. The diagnosis is essentially a clinical one, although ultrasound and MRI may be indicated if there is any doubt.

Treatment

The prognosis is generally good. Many cases probably resolve without the need for any medical input, particularly if the precipitating activity can be avoided. Simple analgesia may be sufficient, but often a local injection of hydrocortisone is required. This can be repeated if there is some response, but repeated injections should be avoided. Physiotherapy, particularly local measures including ultrasound, can help, as can a tennis elbow splint, which is designed to alter the pull of the muscle. Surgery may be occasionally indicated and local excision of the abnormal tissue will produce good results in 70–80 per cent of patients.

Golfer's elbow

This is less common and involves the flexor origin around the medial epicondyle. Ulnar nerve entrapment should be considered in the differential diagnosis and treatment is on similar lines. If medical treatment fails and surgery is being considered, further imaging such as ultrasound or MRI is appropriate to localise any abnormal tissue.

Arthritis of the elbow

Rheumatoid arthritis

The elbow is commonly involved in rheumatoid arthritis and can be a source of considerable discomfort and functional limitation. Medical management is initially tried but surgery is commonly required. If the elbow has good preservation of joint surfaces, then chemical synovectomy may be indicated, but again this is not commonly carried out in RA. If there is considerable pain and restriction of pronation and suppination, rather than flexion and extension, radial head excision and synovectomy is appropriate. This produces good short-term improvement but there is a high relapse rate.

With end-stage disease, particularly with gross joint destruction, elbow arthroplasty is indicated. This is becoming more commonly performed and good results with 80–90 per cent of patients problem-free at 10 years (Fig. 22.16).

Osteoarthritis

Primary osteoarthritis of the elbow is rare and most cases of degenerative disease are due to previous trauma, osteochondritis dissecans or congenital problems such as epiphyseal dysplasia or radial head abnormalities. The patient is usually male, in their 40–60s and often works in a profession that requires heavy use of the upper limb. Pain is the chief complaint, although on examination there will usually be a 20–30° fixed flexion deformity and limited suppination. The history and examination should concentrate on differentiating the pain of a degenerate joint, which is activity related and predictable, from that of sudden unexpected pain and locking, which suggests loose bodies within the elbow (see below). In addition, ulnar nerve symptoms are more common in the arthritic elbow.

Treatment. Often no treatment is required other than reassurance about the nature of the condition. Osteoarthritic elbows seldom deteriorate rapidly and often the symptoms will improve after retirement. For the patient who is unable to carry out his normal activity, early retirement or a change of work is the best solution, as there is no satisfactory surgical procedure that will guarantee a return to a heavy manual job. Débridement is practised in the USA and will increase the range of motion; however, lack of movement is seldom a major complaint by the patient. Resurfacing arthroplasty using tendon or fascia has been tried but, in general, gives a less than satisfactory outcome. Joint replacement should not be carried out in a patient who wishes to return to heavy work but is indicated for severe pain and functional problems in a more sedentary patient. Arthrodesis of the elbow is rarely carried out.

In general, the results of elbow replacement for osteoarthritis are not as good as for RA. This may be related to the different lifestyles of the patients.

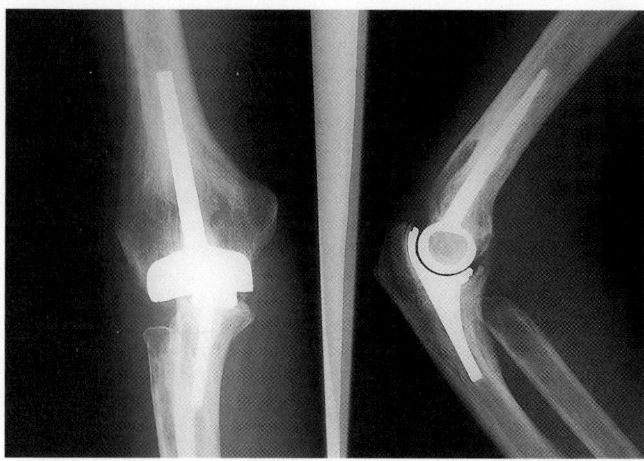

Fig. 22.16 A Kudo unlinked semiconstrained total elbow replacement.

Loose bodies

After the knee, the elbow is the second most common site of symptomatic loose bodies. The most common cause is osteoarthritis but in the younger patient osteochondritis dissecans is the usual cause. Most patients complain of sudden unexpected pain and locking of the elbow, and often they have to shake or manipulate the elbow to relieve it. Plain radiographs will confirm the diagnosis in 90 per cent of cases and further investigation is not necessary. Arthroscopic removal is indicated and, in the presence of mechanical symptoms, good results can be expected in most patients. In the absence of an appropriate history simple removal of loose bodies from a degenerate elbow will not result in any lasting benefit.

Osteochondritis dissecans

Osteochondritis dissecans is much less common in the elbow than the knee, and usually affects the capitellum. Teenage boys are usually affected and the condition is often related to sporting activities. The main symptoms are pain and swelling, and on examination there is a loss of full extension. Treatment is normally conservative with a rest from sport, but arthroscopy may be required if the fragment detaches and the patient develops mechanical symptoms suggestive of a loose body.

Olecranon bursitis

Inflammation of the olecranon bursa is relatively common. The elbow is often very red, warm, swollen and painful, and a septic arthritis may initially be suspected. The signs and symptoms are, however, confined to the back of the elbow (Fig. 22.17) and movement within an arc of 30–130° is usually possible. The bursitis is usually chemical rather than infective, and management consists of rest, ice, anti-inflammatories and a compression dressing. If there is any suspicion of a penetrating wound, antibiotics should be administered but formal drainage of the bursa should be avoided, unless purulent material is present.

Chronic bursitis can occur and may be associated with small calcific nodules. In general these should not be removed and surgical excision of the bursa should be avoided if possible.

Ulnar nerve compression

This is the second commonest nerve entrapment after carpal tunnel syndrome. The most common sites of compression are around the elbow and there is a number of possible sites:

- the arcade of Struthers and the medial intermuscular septum – as the nerve passes into the posterior compartment of the distal humerus;
- medial epicondyle – particularly if osteophytes are present;
- cubital tunnel – as the nerve passes between the two heads of flexor carpi ulnaris (Fig. 22.18).

A nerve palsy may also be due to a flexion or a valgus deformity of the elbow.

History and examination

Unlike carpal tunnel syndrome, compression of the ulnar nerve may not be painful and the patient may present with weakness of the hand in association with paraesthesia. On examination a positive Tinnel's sign is usually present, particularly at the site of compression, and wasting and weakness of the intrinsic muscles of the hand are evident. Nerve conduction studies are usually carried out, unless the site of compression is obvious. In addition, plain radiographs of the elbow should be obtained, particularly if any deformity is present.

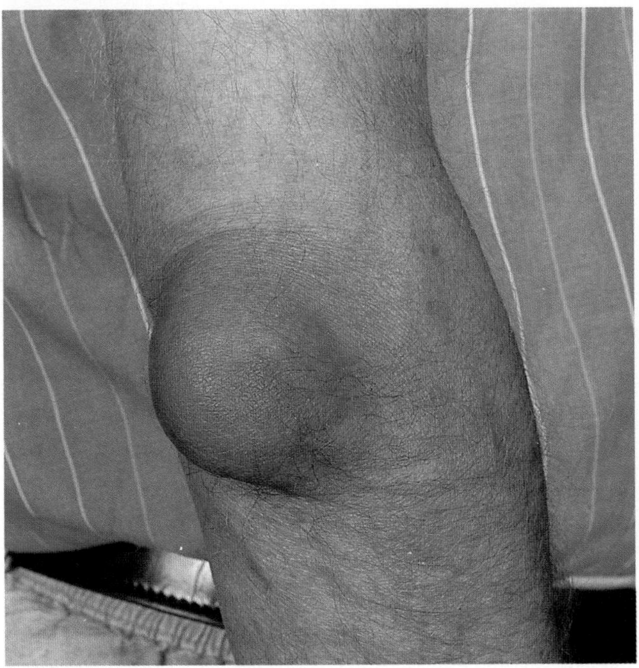

Fig. 22.17 Olecranon bursitis.

Treatment

Despite the absence of pain, decompression of the nerve should be carried out. The nerve can be explored through a medial or posterior approach. Opinion is divided on whether simple decompression is sufficient or whether there is a need for formal anterior transposition of the nerve. Transposition is usually necessary in cases of deformity, or if the nerve is unstable after decompression. For most other situations decompression without transposition is sufficient, provided all sites of possible compression have been explored.

Any paraesthesia should resolve but the prognosis for the return of hand power should be guarded as the recovery is unpredictable.

Compression of both the radial and median nerves at the elbow occurs but this is much less common than ulnar nerve compression (Fig. 22.19).

Infections of the upper limb

Osteomyelitis

Osteomyelitis of the upper limb is very uncommon in adults, unless there are specific predisposing factors such as penetrating wounds. As with other sites, staphylococci and streptococci are commonly implicated, although in the immunocompromised patient other organisms may be encountered. The treatment of osteomyelitis of the upper limb does not differ from other sites.

In children, osteomyelitis of the proximal humeral metaphysis can occur but this is much less common than osteomyelitis of the proximal femur or around the knee.

Septic arthritis

In both adults and children, septic arthritis of the shoulder or elbow is uncommon. Arthroscopy is preferred to formal

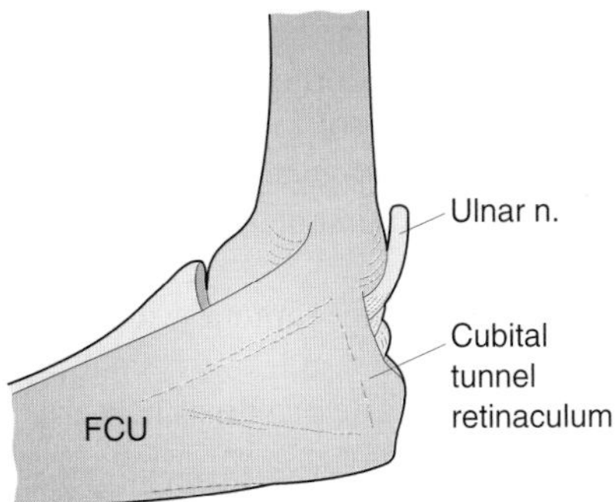

Fig. 22.18 One site of ulnar nerve compression is as the ulnar nerve passes through the cubital tunnel retinaculum.

MEDIAN AND ULNAR NERVES: SENSORY SUPPLY TO THE HAND

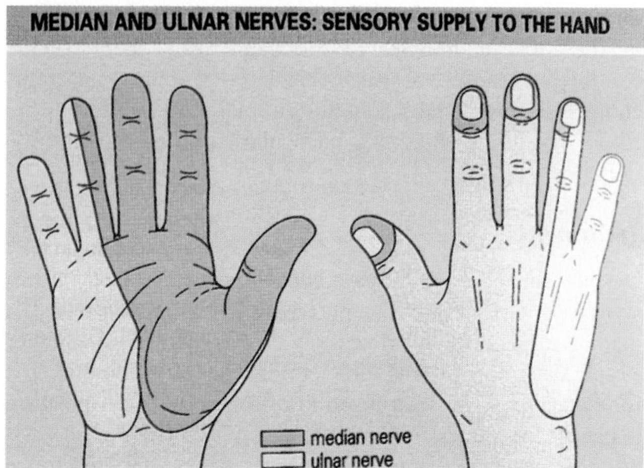

Fig. 22.19 Describing the cutaneous distribution of the median and ulnar nerves in the hand.

arthrotomy for washing out the shoulder. The elbow may be washed out arthroscopically or via a lateral Kocher-type approach.

Tuberculosis

The shoulder and elbow are relatively uncommon sites for tuberculosis (TB) and treatment is along conventional lines. Secondary degeneration can occur and may be difficult to manage. A previously infected joint is one of the few indications for shoulder arthrodesis but the elbow presents a dilemma. Arthrodesis of the elbow is not a good procedure and there is little information on the outcome of other methods of treatment after previous TB.

Tumours of the upper limb

Tumours are unusual around the elbow but the proximal humerus is a relatively common site. It is the third most common site for both osteosarcomas and fibrosarcomas, after the distal femur and proximal tibia. Treatment is on conventional lines. The shoulder is the second most common peripheral site after the proximal femur for chondrosarcomas, and the scapula body is also a common site. The principal method of treatment for chondrosarcomas is surgical excision and this may be technically difficult around the shoulder. Subtotal excision of the scapula can be carried out with good preservation of function if the glenoid can be left. The humerus is also a relatively common site for lymphomas and Ewing's tumour. Treatment is, again, along conventional lines.

Benign and intermediate tumours such as osteochondromas, giant cell tumours and aneurysmal bone cysts are also relatively common. The proximal humerus is the most common site for unicameral bone cysts, which are thought to represent an abnormality of cells of the growth plate. They commonly present as pathological fractures in children around the age of 10 and affect boys more commonly than girls. The lesion may resolve after fracturing but local medical treatment is often required (Fig. 22.20).

The humeral shaft is a common site for secondary deposits and intramedullary nailing may be required for pathological fracture or impending fracture. The majority of primary tumours is found in the breast or prostate, but secondary spread from the thyroid, lung, kidney and bowel can also occur.

Fractures of the upper limb in adults

Introduction

Fractures of the upper limb are very common injuries in all age groups. In adults, between the ages of 15–49, these injuries are more common in males and are usually due to

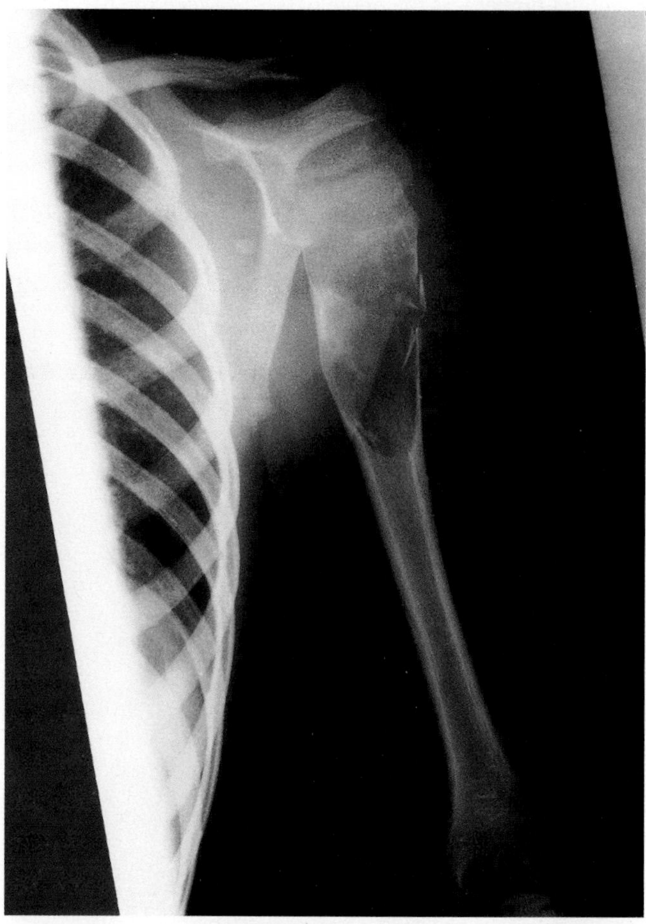

Fig. 22.20 Fracture through a benign cyst of the proximal humerus.

Emil Theodor Kocher, 1841–1917. Swiss surgeon and professor at Bern. Known especially for work on the thyroid gland.

James Ewing, 1866–1943. Professor of Oncology, Cornell University, Medical College, New York, USA.

high-energy mechanisms such as road traffic accidents. Between the ages of 65 and 89 there is a considerable increase in the incidence of fractures, particularly in females. These are associated with osteoporosis and may follow minor trauma such as a fall from a standing height. Many of these injuries are relatively minor, for example clavicle fractures, which usually require no more than symptomatic treatment. Some injuries, such as displaced forearm fractures, require internal fixation but the final result is usually good. Some of the injuries, however, particularly complex fractures of the proximal humerus, often result in poor results despite aggressive management including primary joint replacement.

Specific injuries

Fractures of the clavicle

Fractures of the clavicle are very common, accounting for 5–10 per cent of all fractures. Males are more commonly affected than females (2.5:1) and, in males, the most common age group is the under 20s. The fracture is usually due to sporting injuries or road traffic accidents. In females the elderly are commonly affected, often following a simple fall. The fracture may be caused by direct trauma or indirectly such as a fall on the outstretched hand. The majority of fractures is closed injuries.

Most fractures occur in the midshaft of the bone and are often associated with overlap of the fragments. Fractures of the lateral end of the clavicle may result in superior displacement of bone if the coracoclavicular ligaments are involved. Fractures of the medial end of the clavicle are uncommon.

Treatment. The vast majority of clavicle fractures is treated conservatively with the limb rested in a broad arm sling. Mobilisation can be commenced as comfort allows, with a return to full activities within 3–6 weeks. Attempts at reduction, including bracing back the shoulders with a figure-of-eight bandage, are rarely necessary. Malunion is common but is not usually a functional problem. Nonunion may occur in up to 5 per cent of fractures and is more common after high-energy mechanisms such as road traffic accidents (Fig. 22.21).

Surgery. Open reduction and plate fixation are occasionally required and may be indicated for open fractures associated neurovascular injuries or fractures of the lateral end of the clavicle with significant displacement of the fragments. Internal fixation and bone grafting are indicated for symptomatic nonunions.

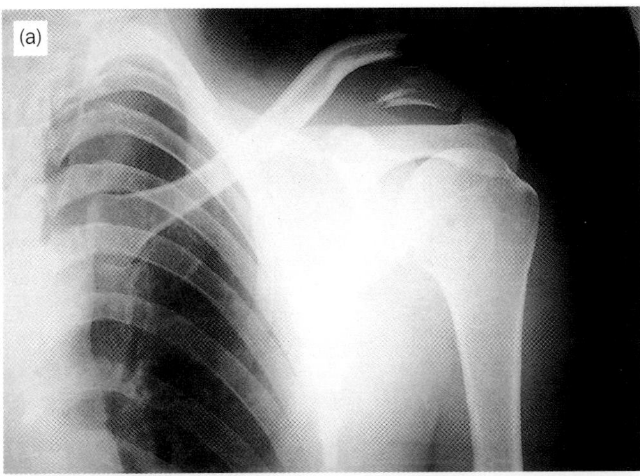

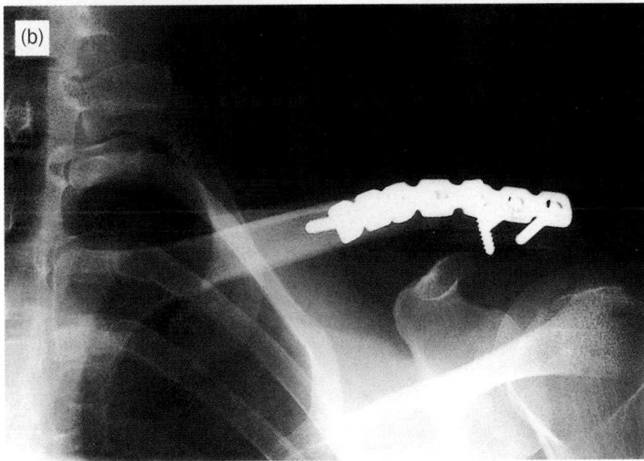

Fig. 22.21 (a) Fracture of the distal third of the clavicle with wide separation of fragments. (b) The fracture has been reduced and secured with a 3.5-mm reconstruction plate.

Acromioclavicular joint injuries

Disruption of the AC joint is a relatively common injury and is typically seen in young males. It is usually caused by trauma, commonly sporting injuries, and is associated with superior subluxation or dislocation of the lateral end of the clavicle (Fig. 22.22).

Classification.

- Type 1 – the capsule and coracoclavicular ligaments are damaged but not ruptured, and no subluxation of the joints occurs.
- Type 2 – the joint is subluxed, with some superior displacement of the clavicle; this is associated with increased damage to, but not rupture of, the ligaments.
- Type 3 – the ligaments are ruptured and the clavicle dislocates superiorly.
- Type 4 – the lateral end of the clavicle dislocates and lies subcutaneously due to severe soft tissue injury.
- Type 5 – the clavicle dislocates and lies posterior to the acromion (rare).
- Type 6 – the clavicle dislocates and lies inferior to the acromion (rare).

Treatment. Most injuries can be treated conservatively, with good results expected. A broad arm sling can be used, with mobilisation as comfort allows. In certain circumstances, early surgery may be indicated, especially for the less common type 4–6 injuries. Late reconstruction of the AC joint is occasionally required for persistent displacement of the clavicle associated with pain and functional impairment.

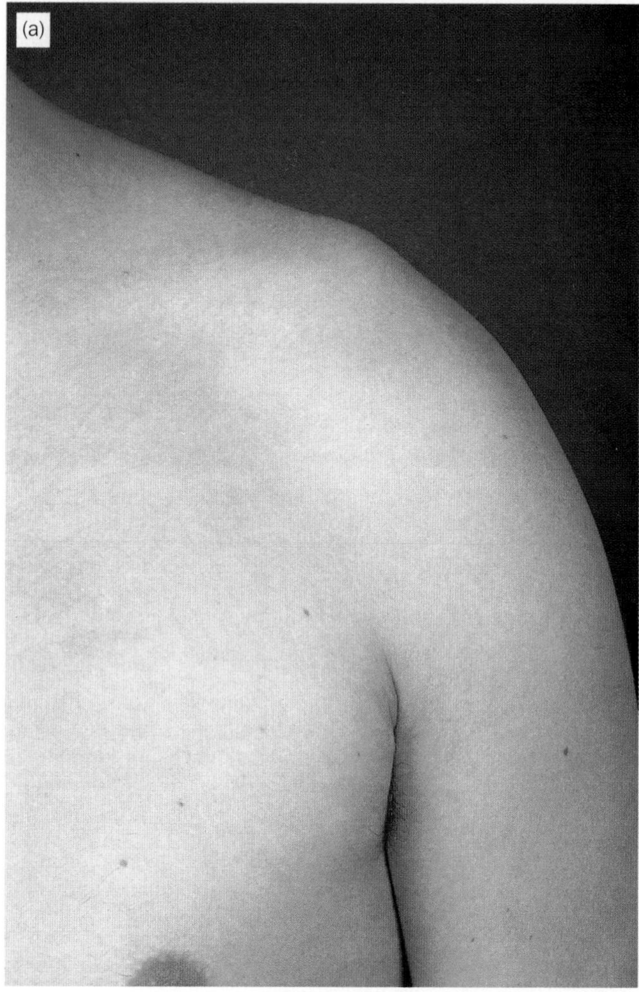

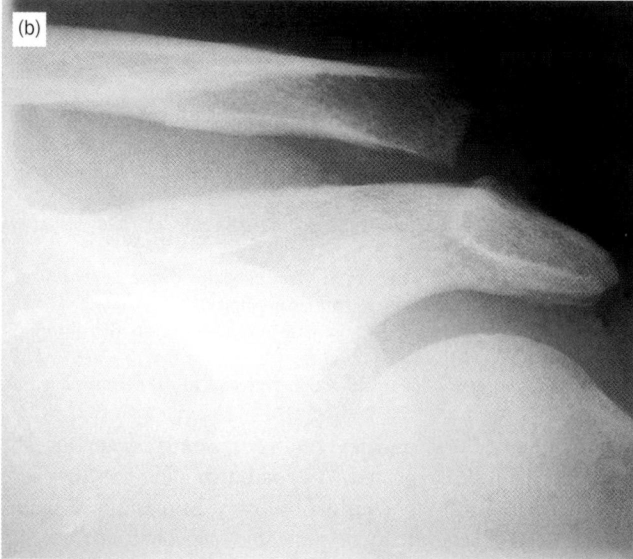

Fig. 22.22 (a) Cosmetic deformity of an acromioclavicular joint dislocation. (b) Radiograph demonstrating complete dislocation of the acromioclavicular joint.

Scapular fractures

These are uncommon injuries and are usually caused by direct trauma, often due to road traffic accidents. Most can be treated conservatively. Internal fixation is indicated for some articular fractures of the glenoid.

A glenoid fracture usually represents a fracture dislocation of the shoulder. The size and displacement of the fragment must be assessed and this can be done by computerised tomography. Conservative treatment with immobilisation will be required for minimally displaced fractures, although rarely for more than 3 weeks. Indications for internal fixation, usually by a lag screw technique, include large displaced fragments and an unstable shoulder. Operative approach, method of fixation and postoperative mobilisation will be determined by the fracture pattern and fixation achieved at surgery.

Dislocation of the glenohumeral joint

Approximately 45 per cent of all joint dislocations in adults occur at the glenohumeral joint. Most dislocations occur anteriorly and result from a forced abduction/external rotation mechanism, often due to sporting injuries. The injury is therefore more common in males in the age group 21–30, although glenohumeral dislocation does occur in elderly females. In this age group rotator cuff damage may occur in association with the dislocation.

Dislocation is frequently associated with damage to the glenoid labrum and detachment of the anteroinferior segment, the Bankart lesion. In addition, damage to the back of the humeral head can occur as a Hill–Sachs lesion (Fig. 22.14). Both of these abnormalities predispose to recurrent dislocation. Less than 5 per cent of primary dislocations are posterior.

Treatment. The dislocation should be reduced as early as possible and this can usually be accomplished under sedation. There are three common methods of reduction dislocations. Following reduction, the arm is rested in a sling for approximately 1 week and mobilisation commenced. Prolonged immobilisation, as previously recommended, does not seem to influence the recurrent dislocation rate.

Hippocratic method. The patient lies supine on a bed, although classically the patient lies on the ground. Traction is applied to the arm with the elbow extended and the arm is flexed and abducted at the shoulder. As traction is continuously applied, the humeral head is eased back into the joint by the surgeon's stockinged foot.

Kocher's method. Traction is applied to the arm, with the elbow flexed to 90°. The arm is slowly externally rotated, and then internally rotated and flexed across the body to reduce the shoulder. This may be modified by abducting as well as externally rotating the arm, and a collar and cuff bandage can be used to provide counter-traction over the humeral head. All these manoeuvres should be carried out gradually as spiral fractures of the humerus and brachial plexus injuries have been reported.

Lucius Hill. Surgeon, Mason Clinic, Seattle, Washington, USA.

Hanging-arm method. This method may be tried without sedation. The patient is placed face down on a bed or bent over a chair. The arm is allowed to hang free, with the elbow extended; an intravenous fluid bag can be tied to the arm to provide traction.

Complications. *Nerve palsy.* Neurological dysfunction is common after shoulder dislocation and electrophysiological tests have revealed abnormalities in over half of the patients. Significant problems occur in approximately 5 per cent of patients, with the axillary nerve, or occasionally the suprascapular nerve, involved. The majority of palsies recovers with conservative treatment.

Recurrent dislocation. This is age related and is usually due to the presence of a Bankart lesion. In the under 25s approximately 60 per cent will have further instability and approximately half of these will require surgery. Only 25 per cent of the over 34 age group will have further problems. Instability of the glenohumeral joint is considered in more detail in the previous section.

Posterior dislocation of the glenohumeral joint is much less common and has been associated with epilepsy and electrocution. The humeral head appears light-bulb shaped on anteroposterior radiographs, an appearance that is normally seen on a lateral or an axillary view. Reduction is achieved by applying traction to the abducted arm and then gently externally rotating the arm.

Proximal humeral fractures

Fractures of the proximal metaphysis of the humerus are one of the most common fractures in the elderly with a dramatic increase in incidence after the age of 60. They account for approximately 5–7 per cent of adult fractures and are most common in elderly females.

Classification of fractures. Proximal humeral fractures were classified by Neer in 1970 and this is still an accepted classification. Minimally displaced fractures are ignored, and the fractures are classified by anatomical location and the number of main fragments. The more severe injuries consist of four main parts: the shaft, the articular surface, together with separate, displaced greater and lesser tuberosities (Fig. 22.23).

Treatment. Treatment of these injuries is dependent on the severity and displacement of the fractures. The majority of fractures is minimally displaced and treated conserva-tively with good results expected. Two to three weeks of immobilisation in a sling is recommended. Displaced fractures, particularly in the younger patient, are treated by internal fixation with a plate and screws, multiple pins or an intramedullary device; again good results can be anticipated.

The treatment of four-part fractures in the elderly osteoporotic patient is still unresolved owing to the unsatisfactory results with all methods of treatment. Conservative treatment can result in a stiff painful shoulder but operative treatment often results in the same outcome. A number of methods of fixation have been described including plates and screws, multiple wires, tension band wiring and intramedullary devices. Insecure fixation in the osteoporotic bone, together with difficulties in reattaching the tuberosities and subsequent rotator cuff problems, will produce poor results. Primary replacement of the humeral head, with a metal prosthesis, is frequently performed and was originally recommended by Neer for severe injuries. Unfortunately hemiarthoplasty is also frequently complicated by stiffness or rotator cuff problems.

Avulsion of the greater tuberosity

This fracture is included in the classification described by Neer but should also be considered separately. The injury is often associated with dislocation of the glenohumeral joint and represents a rotator cuff injury. The fracture may appear to be minimally displaced after reduction of the dislocation.

Treatment. Displaced fractures should be anatomically fixed with screws through a lateral approach. Undisplaced fractures may be treated conservatively but regular review, initially with weekly radiographs, is required. Malunited fractures will lead to impingement symptoms which do not respond as well to later decompression.

Humeral shaft fractures

These injuries account for approximately 3 per cent of adult fractures and are most common in patients in their 70s, usually as a result of a simple fall; approximately 80 per cent of the patients are female. A second, slightly smaller peak in incidence occurs in patients in their 20s. In this group 80 per cent of the patients are male and the injury is due to a road traffic accident or sport. The majority of humeral shaft fractures is closed injuries, with open fractures and associated injuries being more common in the younger age group (Fig. 22.24).

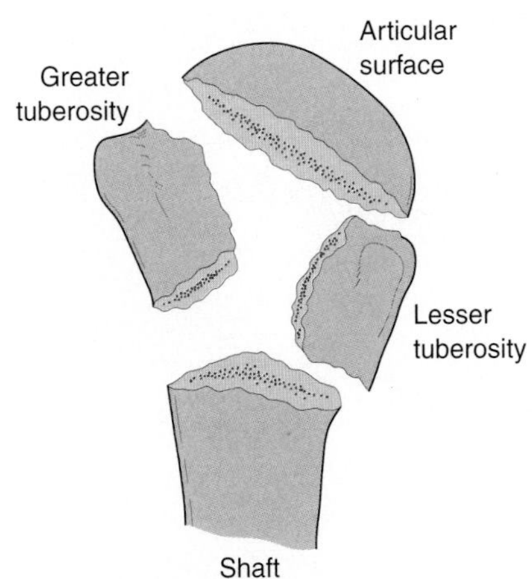

Fig. 22.23 Neer's classification of four-part fracture of the proximal humerus divides the humerus into the articular surface, the greater tuberosity, the lesser tuberosity and the shaft.

Charles Summer Neer II. Orthopaedic surgeon, Columbia-Presbyterian Medical Center, New York, USA.

Treatment. The majority of humeral fractures can be treated conservatively, particularly in the elderly, with good return of function anticipated. A sling or splintage is employed for 2–3 weeks, at which time mobilisation can be commenced. Hanging casts have been recommended, but can result in distraction of the fracture site and increased risk of nonunion.

Surgery. Operative treatment is indicated in patients with open fractures, associated vascular injuries and particularly in patients with multiple injuries. Open reduction and plate fixation is the most common method of stabilisation, although intramedullary nailing from either a proximal or distal entry point is commonly used. External fixation is occasionally indicated for associated severe soft tissue problems.

Complications. ***Nonunion.*** Up to 10 per cent of humeral fractures will be complicated by nonunion, particularly transverse fractures of the midshaft of the bone. Treatment is usually internal fixation and bone grafting of the nonunion site with subsequent healing in most cases.

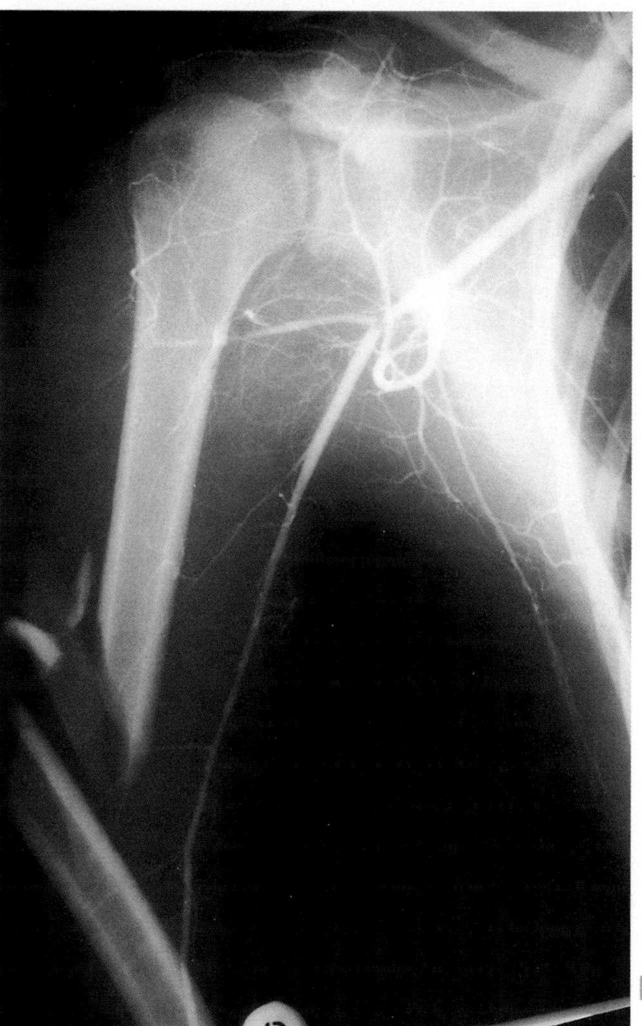

Fig. 22.24 High-energy injury of the humerus producing a fracture of the shaft of the humerus with associated vascular injury showing on the arteriogram.

Nerve palsy. Radial nerve palsy can also occur in up to 10 per cent of patients, with a wrist drop and loss of extension of the fingers. The majority will recover and therefore the injury is treated conservatively, with the patient managed with physiotherapy and a radial nerve splint. Up to 10 per cent of these patients will have no recovery of function and may require exploration of the nerve at about 3 months after the injury. Early exploration is indicated if the nerve is initially intact but dysfunction occurs after closed or open management.

Distal humeral fractures

These are the least common of the metaphyseal fractures of the upper limb, and commonly require internal fixation and early mobilisation to produce good results. As with clavicle fractures, the injury is more common in young males and is usually due to moderate to severe trauma. In the elderly distal humeral fractures are more common in females and again are usually due to mild or moderate trauma.

Anatomy and classification of fractures. The elbow consists of a medial and lateral column, with an articular surface at the distal end. The trochlea at the end of the medial column articulates with the ulna and contributes to flexion and extension at the elbow. The capitellum, the articular surface of the lateral column, articulates with the radial head and contributes to pronation and supination at the elbow.

Anatomically the fractures may involve the medial or the lateral column in isolation, with separation of the condyle from the rest of the humerus. These are relatively uncommon, accounting for only 5 per cent of elbow fractures in adults. The more complex injuries involve both columns, with complete separation of the articular surface from the diaphysis, together with a fracture through the articular surface. It is these T- or Y-shaped fractures that can be particularly difficult to treat.

Treatment. Minimally displaced fractures can be treated conservatively with splintage followed by gentle mobilisation as comfort allows. In adults immobilisation of the elbow for longer than 2–3 weeks should be avoided as stiffness and functional restriction can occur. This is particularly true for complex injuries, or following operative management of the fractures.

For displaced fractures internal fixation is recommended for all age groups; stable fixation with plates and/or screws should be used to allow early mobilisation. Single column fractures can usually be stabilised through a limited approach but the complex T- or Y-fractures require a wide exposure of the joint to ensure accurate reduction, and usually two plates are necessary for stable fixation to the humeral shaft. In order to gain the necessary access, osteotomy of the ulna is usually required and these injuries require surgical skill and experience to achieve good results.

In the elderly osteoporotic patient, especially with very distal fractures, stable internal fixation is not possible. In these patients primary elbow replacement has been carried out with good results. This avoids the need for an osteotomy, with its risk of nonunion and implant problems, and allows immediate mobilisation of the elbow.

Radial head fractures

These are relatively common fractures; the majority occurs in females, in the age group 20–50, after a fall on the outstretched hand.

Approximately 40 per cent of fractures are undisplaced, involving only part of the articular surface. In a further 40 per cent a fragment of the radial head is displaced, with depression of the articular surface. The remainder of the fractures involves all of the articular surface, either as a single fragment with a fracture of the radial neck or as a comminuted fracture of the radial head.

Some fractures are not visible on plain radiographs, although evidence of an effusion can often be seen. This injury should be suspected in patients with a typical history, pain over the radial head and restricted movement of the elbow.

Classification. A number of classifications has been described but one of the most commonly used is that described by Mason (Fig. 22.25):

- type 1 – undisplaced partial articular (marginal) fractures;
- type 2 – displaced marginal fractures;
- type 3 – comminuted fractures of the radial head.

Treatment. Undisplaced fractures are treated by a temporary collar and cuff support, followed by early mobilisation. If the elbow is particularly painful, aspiration of the haemarthrosis can be carried out followed by intra-articular injection of local anaesthetic. Aspiration can be safely carried out through the centre of the triangle formed by the lateral epicondyle, radial head and the olecranon.

The treatment of displaced, partial articular fractures is dependent on the size and displacement of the fragment. Small fragments (<25 per cent of the articular surface) are treated conservatively, unless the range of motion is significantly restricted. In these circumstances aspiration of the joint and injection of local anaesthetic is carried out. If there is still a block to extension, and particularly full supination, exploration of the elbow via a lateral incision is indicated. Large fragments are treated by open reduction and internal fixation with small screws if possible; smaller fragments can be excised.

More complex injuries are treated by internal fixation, although this may not be possible if significant comminution is present. In these circumstances excision of the radial head can be carried out. If, however, there is any damage to the collateral ligaments of the elbow or the interosseous membrane of the forearm, prosthetic replacement may be indicated. This is seen in patients sustaining high-energy injuries, such as road traffic accidents or falls from a height. In these patients radiographs of the entire forearm including wrist should be obtained, and the distal examined carefully, both clinically and radiologically.

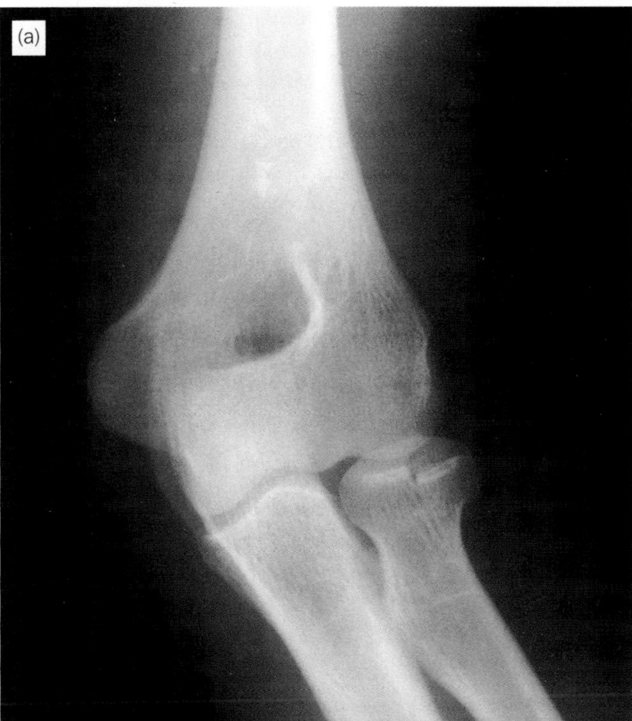

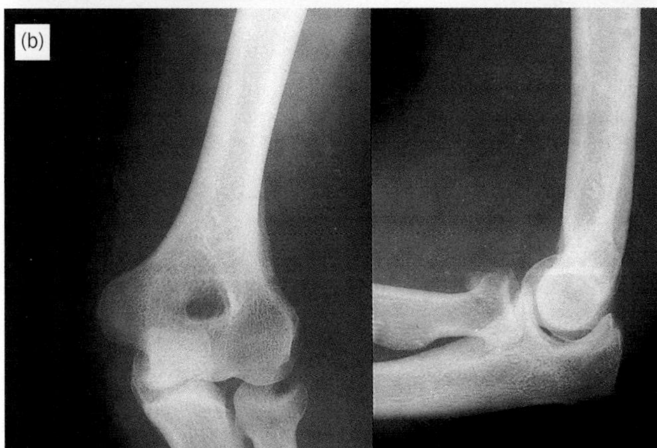

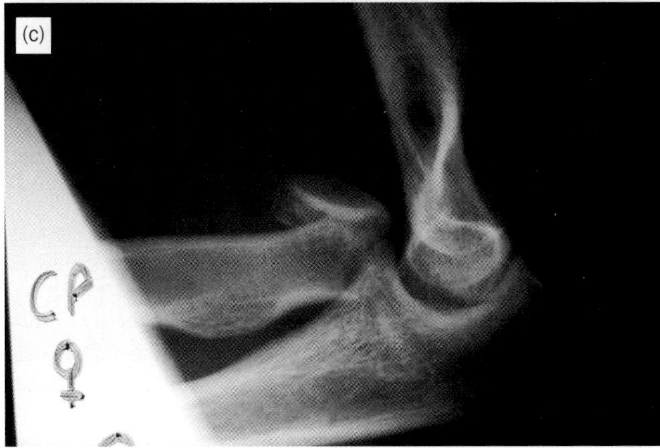

Fig. 22.25 (a) A minimally displaced fracture of the radial head. (b) A moderately displaced fracture of the radial head involving more than 25 per cent of the joint surface. (c) A grossly displaced fracture of the radial head and neck.

Olecranon fractures

These are common injuries and are usually due to indirect trauma such as a fall on the outstretched hand. The injury is essentially an avulsion fracture due to the pull of the triceps muscle. Most fractures are intra-articular, although extra-articular fractures do occur with a small bony fragment avulsed (Fig. 22.26).

Classification. A number of classifications has been described but the main factors that determine the treatment are the location and displacement of the fracture, and the number of fragments.

Treatment. Undisplaced fractures can be treated conservatively, but late displacement can occur and regular review is necessary. Most fractures are displaced and internal fixation is indicated. Extra-articular and two-part intra-articular fractures can be treated with a tension band wiring system, using a figure-of-eight wire and intramedullary wires or screws. Stable internal fixation should be achieved to allow early mobilisation of the elbow. A tension band wire is not suitable for comminuted articular fractures or more distal fractures, and plate fixation is recommended.

The prognosis for this injury is good, with a full functional recovery expected. The metal is often prominent and can be troublesome. It can be removed, if necessary, after the fracture has healed.

Elbow dislocation

Approximately 20 per cent of all dislocations occur at the elbow and most occur in children and young adults. The elbow usually dislocates posteriorly and is due to axial loading on a slightly flexed elbow. Fractures of the distal humerus, radial head and coronoid may be associated with the injury (Fig. 22.27).

Treatment. The elbow should be reduced as soon as possible and this is usually accomplished by closed means. Traction is applied with the arm slightly flexed and the olecranon can usually be pushed over the distal humerus, reducing with a definite clunk. Postoperatively the arm is immobilised in a collar and cuff, and mobilisation commenced after 1 week. Prolonged immobilisation should be avoided as the elbow often becomes stiff.

Complications. ***Instability***. In most cases the elbow is stable after reduction but occasionally there is a tendency for the elbow to redislocate in extension. In these circumstances, after reduction, the elbow is managed in a cast brace preventing full extension initially. The extension block can be gradually reduced over 2–3 weeks. Late instability is rarely a problem after simple dislocation and is more usually associated with complex fracture dislocations.

Stiffness. Some loss of extension is not uncommon after elbow dislocation but is rarely a functional problem unless the arm has been immobilised for long periods.

Forearm fractures

These account for approximately 5 per cent of adult fractures and the majority occur in young adults as a result of moderate to severe trauma. In contrast to many other fractures, these are unusual in the more elderly osteoporotic patient.

Most of these fractures involve both bones and result from indirect trauma. Single bone injuries can occur and are usually caused by direct violence, such as a blow with a stick. Single bone fractures can also occur in association with a joint injury of the other forearm bone,

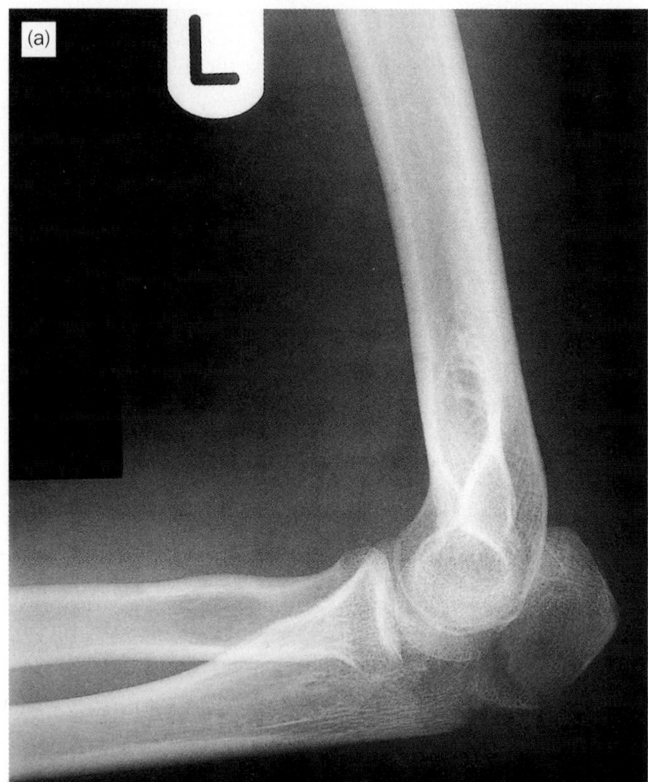

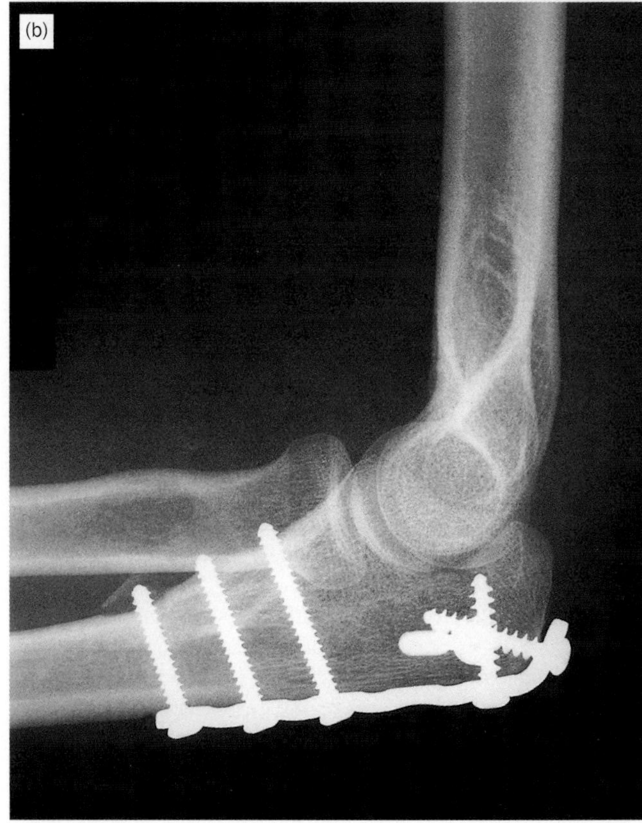

Fig. 22.26 (a) A fracture of the olecranon with considerable comminution at the joint surface. (b) Because of comminution of the joint surface this fracture has been fixed with a plate and screws rather than tension band wire.

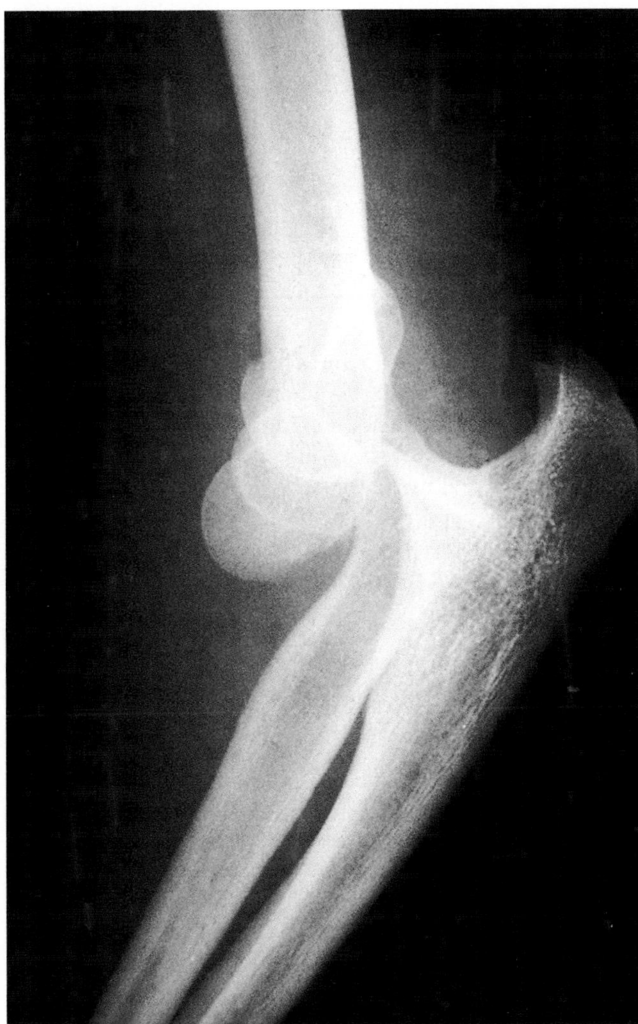

Fig. 22.27 Dislocation of the elbow.

and this injury must be considered. Radiographs of the elbow and wrist joints should be obtained in all forearm fractures.

Treatment. The vast majority of these fractures is displaced, and open reduction and internal fixation with plates is indicated. Both bones are usually plated, through separate incisions, with early postoperative mobilisation. Conservative treatment is not usually recommended as rotation at the fracture site is difficult to correct or control in plaster. Full functional recovery can be expected in these patients. The forearm plates, particularly the radial, should not be removed unless there are specific indications, as a high complication rate has been reported.

Specific injuries. *Monteggia fractures.* Proximal ulna fractures may be associated with dislocation of the radial head but these account for only 1 per cent of forearm fractures. If the ulna fracture is reduced accurately, the radial head usually reduces and no specific treatment is necessary (Fig. 22.28).

Galeazzi fractures. Again these are relatively uncommon and consist of a distal radial fracture with disruption of the distal radio-ulnar joint.

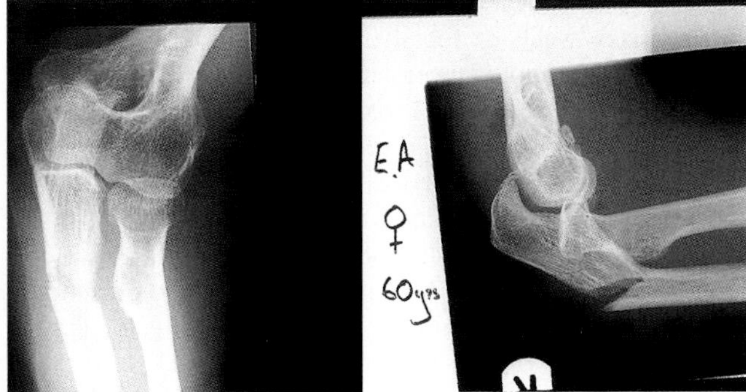

Fig. 22.28 A reversed Monteggia fracture in an adult. The ulna is fractured and the radial head is dislocated posteriorly.

Open reduction of the distal radius is carried out and the reduction of the distal ulna confirmed. If this is unstable, immobilisation in suppination or even cross pinning to the radius is carried out.

Fractures and dislocations of the upper limb in children

Introduction

It must be realised that children are not merely small adults, and this is particularly true with fractures and dislocation of the upper limb. Although superficially the injuries may appear to be the same, the pattern and prognosis of the injuries are often very different. Fractures of the proximal humerus in adults are a major problem; they are often complicated by nonunion, avascular necrosis and a poor functional outcome, and the patient may require joint replacement. In children the fracture usually represents an epiphyseal injury and the prognosis is very good, often without treatment, despite significant angulation at the fracture site. Shoulder dislocation, a common adult condition, is very uncommon in children. Apparent dislocations in children are often due to epiphyseal fractures and again may not require treatment. It is therefore necessary to be aware of the ossification centres of the upper limb when dealing with these injuries.

Ossification

A large part of the body of the scapula is ossified at birth. A secondary ossification centre appears in the coracoid during the first year and fuses by about the 15th year. The acromion usually develops two ossification centres, with all ossification centres fused by about the age of 20. These may be confused with fractures on radiographs or predispose to epiphyseal separation. Failure of fusion of the acromion resulting in an os acromiale occurs in about 5 per cent of the population, although there is a number of different reports of the incidence in the literature.

Giovanni Battista Monteggia, 1762–1815. Professor of Anatomy and Surgery, Milan, Italy.
Ricardo Galeazzi, 1866–1952. Orthopaedic Surgeon, Milan, Italy.

The clavicle develops two ossification centres around the fifth to sixth week of foetal life. These fuse within a few weeks of their appearance; failure of this may produce a congenital pseudoarthrosis of the clavicle. A secondary ossification centre appears in the medial end of the clavicle in the late teens. An epiphyseal injury may occur before the appearance of this ossification centre giving the appearance of a sternoclavicular dislocation. This epiphysis fuses by about the age of 25. The lateral end occasionally develops a secondary ossification centre at the age of 18–20. This is usually small and rapidly fuses to the shaft.

The shaft of the humerus is evident at birth, with the head appearing by about 6 months. The greater and lesser tuberosities appear around the age of 2 and 5 years, and fuse by the age of about 6 to produce a conical growth plate. In children under the age of 6 fracture through this growth plate is usually a Salter and Harris type I injury, as before the tuberosities fuse the growth plate is more transverse. In the older child a Salter and Harris type II fracture occurs through the conical growth plate. The proximal growth plate accounts for 80 per cent of the humeral growth.

There are six ossification centres around the elbow and the usual order of appearance is shown below in Table 22.1, together with the approximate time of appearance. In general ossification centres appear earlier in females than males.

The shafts of both the radius and ulna are evident at birth.

Table 22.1 Ossification centres and the approximate age of appearance

Ossification centre	*Approximate age of appearance*
Capitellum	By 2 years
Proximal radial epiphysis	4–6 years
Medial epicondyle	5–9 years
Trochlea	7–11 years
Olecranon	8–10 years
Lateral epicondyle	8–13 years

General principles

With any childhood injury the possibility of child abuse must always be considered. In general this does not apply to injuries around the shoulder, as most of these injuries occur in those over 5 years old, an age at which child abuse resulting in fractures is uncommon. In the under 5 year old a proximal humerus fracture is rarely due to child abuse, although clavicle fractures especially in those under 18 months should be viewed with suspicion. Spiral fractures of the humerus in young children should also be considered as nonaccidental injuries, although distal humeral fractures and elbow fractures in general are usually not due to child abuse. If, however, the mechanism of injury does not fit the history given or there was a significant delay in presentation, then nonaccidental injury should be considered.

In a child of any age, an open fracture must be treated by operative débridement and stabilisation of the fracture site. In children, as in adults, polytrauma is a relative indication for surgical treatment.

Epidemiology

The risk of at least one fracture up to the age of 16 in a boy has been reported to be 42 per cent. In girls the quoted figure is 27 per cent. Of these, fractures of the distal forearm are the most common, accounting for about 20 per cent of the total. Fractures of the clavicle accounted for 8 per cent, the fourth most common site of fracture in children, with the midshaft of the forearm and the supracondylar region of the humerus both causing about 3 per cent of the fractures. The proximal humerus accounted for 2 per cent, and other fractures around the shoulder accounted for less than 1 per cent of all childhood fractures.

Specific injuries

Sternoclavicular joint

Dislocations of this joint are rare in children and most apparent dislocations, even in adults up to the age of about 25, represent epiphyseal separations. True dislocations and epiphyseal injuries can be manipulated and are often stable, even if unstable fixation of these injuries should be avoided. Internal fixation may damage nearby structures with disastrous results, and wires should be avoided as migration into the chest has been reported. Rapid healing and remodelling will occur. Posterior displacement may be a surgical emergency if vital structures are compromised.

Fractures of the clavicle

Fractures of the medial end of the clavicle are considered above.

Fractures of the shaft of the clavicle account for the majority of clavicle fractures. Many are caused by a fall on the outstretched hand; a bicycle, climbing frame, or bunk bed is commonly involved. Green-stick fractures commonly occur and may be missed on initial radiographs. Temporary rest in a sling for a short period is all that is required for most of these fractures. Displaced fractures of the clavicle are very common but rarely require reduction. In many countries, including many American centres, attempts are made to reduce the displacement with a figure-of-eight bandage to retract the scapula. To be effective this has to be tight, often uncomfortably tight, and needs constant adjustment. A broad arm sling for 2–3 weeks until comfortable is all that is required. Malunion is very common but rarely a functional problem; nonunion is very uncommon in children. Relatives can be reassured that the prominent callus will usually resolve over the subsequent months.

Open reduction and fixation with wires or a plate may be occasionally required. The indications are similar to

W.R. Harris. Orthopaedic surgeon, Toronto, Canada.
Robert Salter. Professor of Surgery, Children's Hospital, Toronto, Canada.

those in the adult; open fracture, skin compromise, vascular injury, etc.

Fractures of the lateral end of the clavicle may also be confused with joint dislocations, as discussed below.

Acromioclavicular joint

True dislocations of this joint are unusual in children, especially in the younger child. The ligaments around the joint are very strong and often the lateral end of the clavicle will fracture, although this may not be apparent on radiographs if unossified. Even with true dislocations the inferior periosteum may be left behind with the conoid and trapeziod ligaments intact. These will heal and remodel with conservative treatment, with a sling for comfort followed by early mobilisation.

Scapular fractures

In children as in adults fractures of the body of the scapula are uncommon injuries and usually represent direct violence. The significance of this injury is the likely injury to the chest wall and possible pulmonary contusion rather than the scapula fracture itself. These injuries will almost always be treated conservatively with analgesia and a sling for comfort. The arm should be mobilised as comfort allows.

Fractures of the glenoid are also very uncommon injuries in children.

Dislocation of the glenohumeral joint

Shoulder dislocation in children is unusual except in the adolescent as the ligaments are stronger than the epiphysis; usually a Salter and Harris fracture of the proximal humerus will occur. In adolescents as in adults, glenohumeral dislocation is commonly due to a sporting injury and is nearly always an anterior dislocation. Treatment is along adult lines with early closed reduction using standard techniques. The redislocation rate is age related and is higher in the child or adolescent, with a recurrent dislocation rate of 70–80 per cent reported in the age group 12–16. Approximately 50 per cent of these patients require a stabilisation procedure. Atraumatic dislocations can occur in children with joint laxity or connective tissue disorders.

Proximal humerus

Fractures of the proximal humerus usually occur in the older child or adolescent. Not only are accidents more common at this age but the perichondral ring may be weaker just before skeletal maturity. The majority of injuries occurs through the growth plate; Salter and Harris type II in the older child and type I in the younger child. In the younger child, child abuse should be considered, although humeral shaft fractures are more common in child abuse. Salter and Harris type III and IV are very uncommon injuries of the proximal humerus.

Fracture displacement is common and is due to the pull of the pectoralis major attaching to the distal fragment which tends to pull it anteriorly and medially. Although residual shortening is common, the majority of patients will have satisfactory functional results. It has also been reported that manipulation of a displaced fresh fracture did not improve the final outcome when humeral growth or function was assessed.

Treatment. Treatment therefore is generally conservative; not only because of the remodelling potential but also because of the malalignment that can be accepted around the shoulder generally. Forty-five degrees of angulation and 50 per cent of displacement can be accepted. In the younger child 70 per cent angulation and any bony contact should heal with good functional results. The fracture is usually treated in a collar and cuff sling, although rarely a hanging cast may be used in the older child with significant shortening or angulation.

If the position is unacceptable closed reduction is attempted and the fracture held with two or three wires. These wires can be removed after 3 weeks.

Open reduction may occasionally be required for soft tissue interposition often the biceps tendon and this can be achieved through a standard deltopectoral approach. Fracture stabilisation is carried out as described as above.

Metaphyseal fractures

This may occur with direct trauma or may occur as a pathological fracture, classically through a unicameral bone cyst. Displacement is not usually significant; angulation may occur but rarely produces a functional problem. The fractures usually heal rapidly with conservative treatment in a sling. The proximal humerus is the only common site for pathological fractures around the shoulder.

Humeral shaft fractures

These injuries are less common in children than in adults. The fracture is usually transverse or short oblique in pattern, and is due to direct violence; an appropriate history should be available. Nonaccidental injury should always be considered with this injury, particularly in the younger child or with spiral fractures which are due to a twisting force.

Treatment. The vast majority of fracture can be treated conservatively with either a simple collar and cuff or a plaster U-slab. Union is usually rapid, particularly in the younger child, considerable remodelling can occur and so malunion rarely results in a functional problem. Nonunion is uncommon in children.

Internal fixation is occasionally required for open fractures, associated vascular injuries and the polytrauma patient.

Supracondylar fractures of the humerus

This is the most common fracture around the elbow in children and usually occurs in children under the age of 10. The injury is usually due to a fall on the outstretched hand with an extended elbow and this results in a hyperextension injury with posterior angulation, with or without posterior displacement of the distal fracture. Between 1 and 5 per cent of supracondylar fractures are caused by a flexion injury and associated with an anterior deformity.

Radiological diagnosis. Displaced fractures are readily diagnosed by plain radiographs but angulated fractures may be difficult to assess. Comparison views of the other elbow can be taken but a number of radiographic lines can be assessed on the injured elbow, as follows.

- Capitellum angle. The capitellum is normally angulated and displaced anteriorly to the humeral shaft. In the normal elbow, a line drawn through the centre of the capitellum joins a line drawn down the humeral shaft at an angle of 30°.
- Anterior humeral line. A line drawn along the anterior cortex should pass through the central portion of the capitellum.
- Anterior coronoid line. A line drawn along the coronoid process of the ulna should just pass through the anterior portion of the capitellum.

All of the above lines are drawn on true lateral radiographs. In addition, on a true anteroposterior view, Bauman's angle can be assessed. This is the angle formed between the growth plate of the capitellum and a line perpendicular to the humeral shaft. The normal angle is approximately 30° and can be used to assess the adequacy of reduction of a fracture (Fig. 22.29).

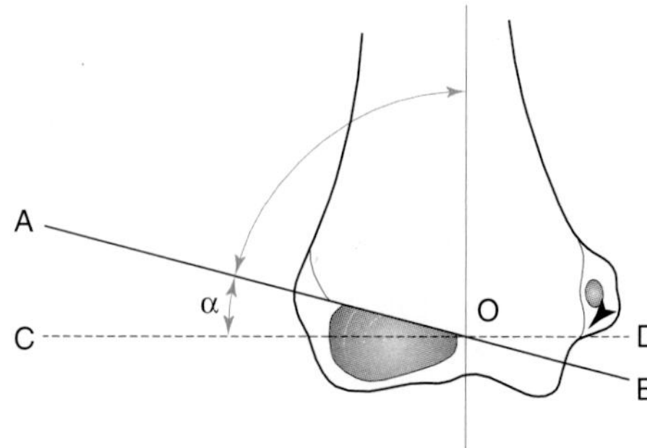

Fig. 22.29 Calculation of Bauman's angle. This angle is formed between the growth plate of the capitellum and a line drawn perpendicular to the humeral shaft. The normal angle is 30°.

Classification. As noted above supracondylar fractures can be divided into extension types and the much less common flexion types. Extension types are further subdivided into three types dependent on the angulation and displacement (Fig. 22.30).

- Type 1. The fractures are undisplaced but the radiographic lines should be carefully assessed to confirm this.
- Type 2. The fractures are angulated posteriorly, but the posterior periosteum remains intact, and prevent displacement and overlap of the fracture fragments.
- Type 3. The fractures are completely displaced with shortening and overlap of the fragments.

Treatment. Type 1 fractures can be treated conservatively in a collar and cuff, with 90° of flexion at the elbow. This is maintained for 2–3 weeks, with a check radiograph taken after 1 week. As with the initial film, the undisplaced nature of the fracture should be confirmed by plotting the appropriate lines.

Type 2 fractures should be treated by closed reduction if the position is unacceptable. Thirty degrees of extension can be accepted due to the remodelling that will occur in the younger child. Bauman's angle should be corrected if there is any varus or valgus deformity as this will not remodel. Significant rotational deformity is uncommon with this type of fracture. Reduction is usually straightforward and the position can be maintained with the elbow at 90°. Rarely wires may be required to hold an unstable reduction (Fig. 22.31).

Type 3 fractures usually require reduction but this is often difficult and the fracture site is commonly unstable after reduction, with a significant rotational element. Under general anaesthetic traction is applied to the suppinated forearm. The mediolateral displacement of the distal fragment is reduced by direct finger pressure and the carrying angle restored by comparison with the uninjured side. The extension element of the fracture is the last thing to be corrected by flexing the elbow maximally while applying posterior pressure to the distal fragment. The reduction should be confirmed radiographically, however the X-ray source rather than the arm should be moved to obtain the views. This avoids the risk of fracture displacement if the arm is rotated.

If the reduction is satisfactory, the position can be maintained by maximum flexion but this may cause vascular compromise, and loss of reduction may occur if the elbow extends. It has been recommended by a number of authors that the reduction should be held by two wires. Cross wires through both condyles may be used but care must be taken to avoid an ulnar nerve palsy, as the nerve may be difficult to locate in the swollen elbow. An open technique may be used on the medial side, or the wire may be inserted through an anterior starting point. Alternatively, two wires may be inserted from the lateral side but biomechanically this is not as strong a fixation.

Failure to obtain a reduction is an indication for open reduction but in the very swollen elbow, traction is a better option. This may be temporary, until the swelling reduces, but can be used as a definitive method of treatment. Traction may be applied using a bone crew inserted into the ulna, or by longitudinal skin traction. Surprisingly, the patient becomes relatively pain free very quickly (Fig. 22.32).

Complications. ***Vascular injury.*** Occlusion of the brachial artery is an uncommon but serious complication. Despite the absence of a radial pulse, the arm has a good collateral supply and will not necessarily become ischaemic. Both skin temperature and colour should be assessed, together with Doppler investigation of the pulse.

The treatment of vascular compromise is early reduction of the fracture under general anaesthetic. If the pulse returns the arm should be monitored carefully. Failure of circulatory return is an indication for exploration of the artery and fracture site, with open reduction and internal fixation with wires. An arteriogram may be obtained but should not be allowed to delay exploration.

Neurological injury. Transient neurological problems are relatively common after supracondylar fractures. The radial nerve is reported to be the most commonly affected, followed by the median nerve. Treatment is conservative for 3 months initially with good recovery expected.

Volkmann's ischaemic contracture. Flexion contractures of the fingers and wrist are caused by fibrosis of the anterior compartment of the forearm due to a missed compartment

Christian Johann Doppler, 1803–53. Austrian physicist.
Richard von Volkmann, 1830–89. Professor of Surgery, Halle, Germany.

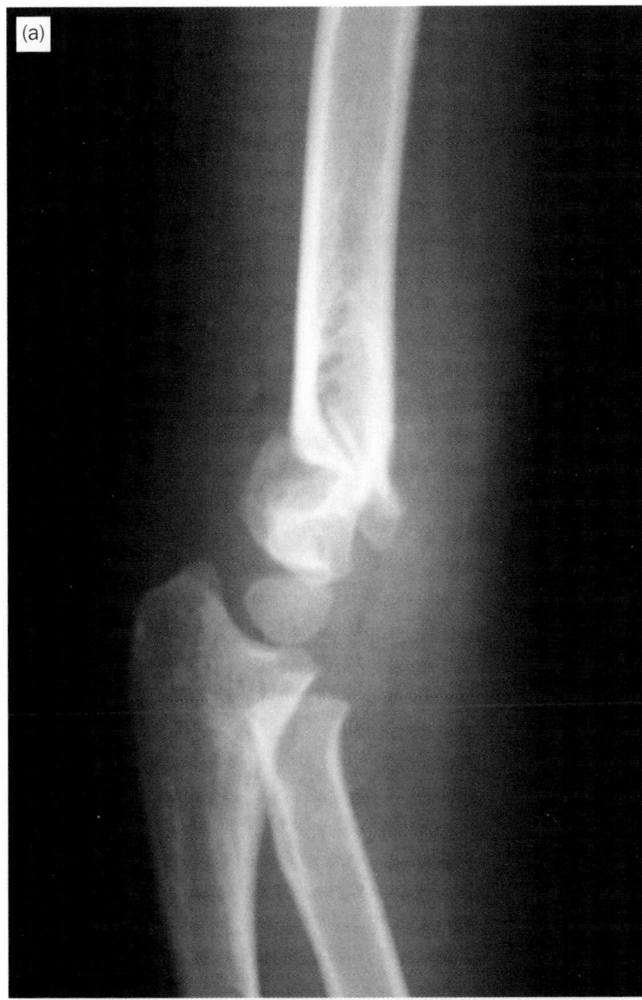

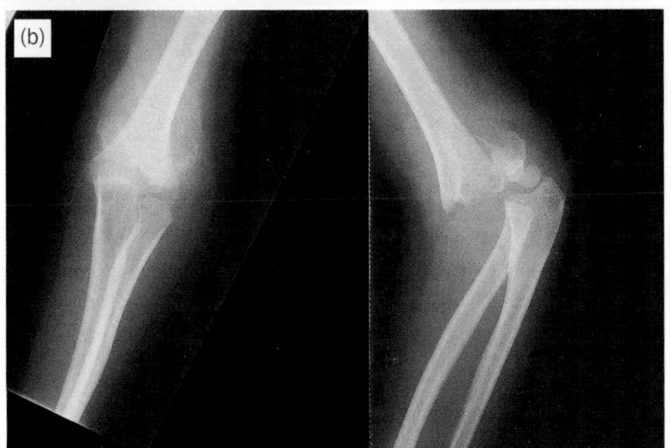

Fig. 22.30 (a) A type II fracture of the supracondylar region of the humerus with posterior tilt but an intact posterior periosteum. (b) A type III fracture with complete displacement of the distal fragment.

syndrome. It can usually be prevented by avoiding immobilisation in excessive flexion of the elbow. If greater than 90° of flexion is required to maintain a reduction, the reduction should be held by wires and the elbow extended.

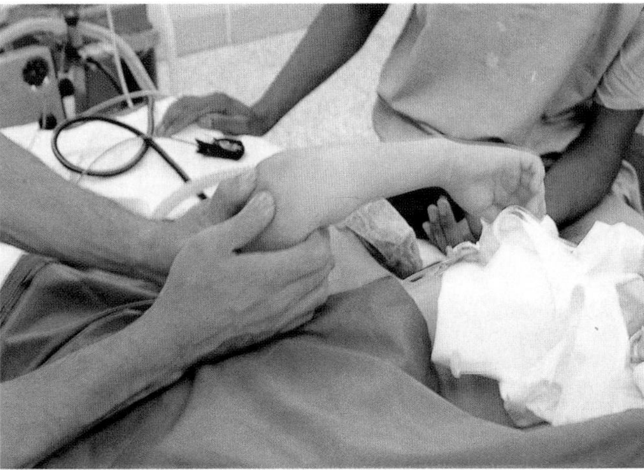

Fig. 22.31 Reduction of type II supracondylar fractures is achieved in elbow flexion using digital or thumb pressure.

Disproportionate pain in the forearm, paticularly on passive extension of the fingers, should be treated by immediate release of all dressings, even if this compromises the reduction. If pain persists fasciotomy is indicated.

Malunion. Some degree of malunion is relatively common after supracondylar fracture. A flexion or extension deformity will remodel and observation is indicated. Varus malunion, with a gunstock deformity, is unsightly but is usually not a functional problem. Corrective osteotomies, if necessary, should probably be delayed until skeletal maturity. Valgus deformity may be associated with a tardy ulnar nerve palsy and may require treatment.

Condylar and epicondylar fractures

Lateral condyle. This is a relatively common injury and, after supracondylar fractures, is the second most common elbow fracture in children. It is usually due to a fall on the outstretched hand. Although this injury can occur in younger children the diagnosis is usually apparent on plain radiographs due to the early appearance of the ossification centre of the capitellum (see above) (Fig. 22.33).

Classification. Milch has classified this injury based on the location of the articular fracture. A type I fracture either passes through the ossification centre of the capitellum or just passes through the aspect of the trochlea. In either case the majority of the trochlea is intact and the elbow does not dislocate. In type II fractures the fracture line passes at or medial to the trochlear groove and the elbow joint may dislocate if the fracture displaces.

Treatment. Undisplaced fractures can be treated by immobilisation for approximately 3 weeks, but check radiographs are required. Most fractures are, however, displaced, and open reduction and internal fixation is required as closed reduction is seldom possible. Anatomical reduction is required and wires or screws can be used.

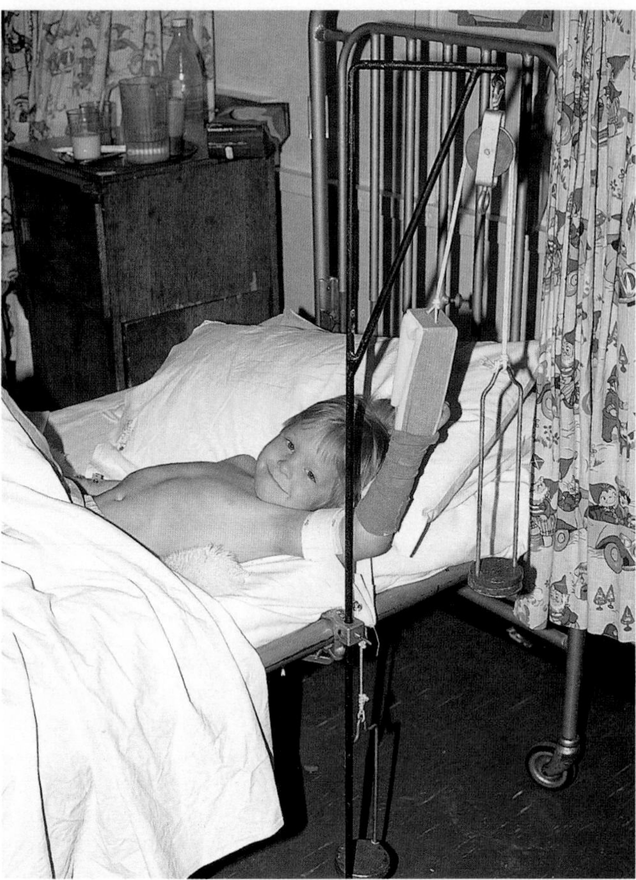

Fig. 22.32 A supracondylar fracture may be managed postreduction in longitudinal skin traction.

Complications. Nonunion occasionally occurs, often as a result of missed fractures or inadequate fixation. This may lead to a valgus deformity and tardy ulnar nerve palsy. Internal fixation and bone grafting can be utilised, either at presentation or at skeletal maturity.

Medial epicondyle. This is the third most common fracture around the elbow and is usually seen in older children. It is due to an avulsion injury and, despite the proximity of the ulnar nerve, it is rarely affected. Diagnosis can usually be made on plain radiographs, although, as with all children's fractures, comparison views of the other side can be taken if there is any doubt (Fig. 22.34).

Treatment. Undisplaced fractures can be treated conservatively, with early mobilisation as comfort allows. Displaced fractures are usually internally fixed, especially if instability of the elbow is present.

Other elbow fractures

Fractures of the medial condyle, lateral epicondyle and T-intercondylar fractures are rare in children; treatment depends on displacement.

Elbow dislocation

This is an uncommon injury in children. As with adults the elbow usually dislocates posteriorly and radiographs should be studied carefully for associated fractures. Treatment is early reduction; instability is rarely a subsequent problem.

Proximal radius fractures

These are the fourth most common of the fractures around the elbow in children. They differ from the intra-articular radial head fractures seen in adults as, with children, the injury usually occurs through the epiphysis of the radial neck,

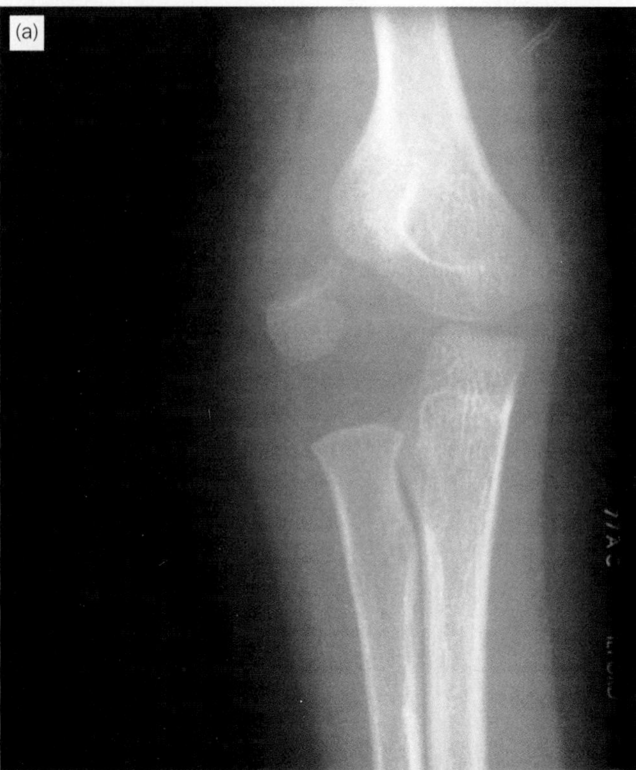

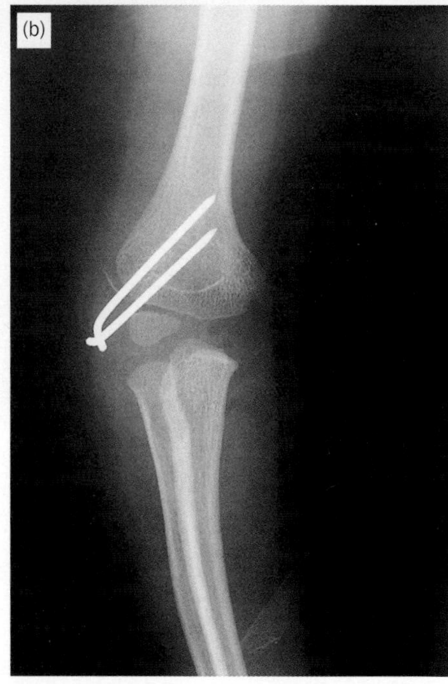

Fig. 22.33 (a) A Milch I lateral condylar fracture of the humerus. (b) The fracture has been reduced and held with K-wires.

and the articular surface displaces as a single piece. The injury usually results from a fall on the outstretched hand, although it can occur in association with a posterior dislocation of the elbow. This fracture usually occurs after the ossification centre of the proximal radius appears and so the diagnosis is readily made on plain radiographs.

Treatment. In common with many children's fractures there is considerable potential for remodelling. Up to 30° of angulation can be accepted, provided there is growth remaining. These injuries can be treated with a simple sling followed by early mobilisation.

If angulation exceeds 30°, manipulation under anaesthetic is carried out, which can be aided by the use of a percutaneous lever to push the radial head. For irreducible or completely displaced fractures (commonly seen after elbow dislocation) open reduction is carried out. This is usually supplemented by wire fixation, but wires should not be placed across the radiocapitate joint. These are removed after 2–3 weeks followed by mobilisation.

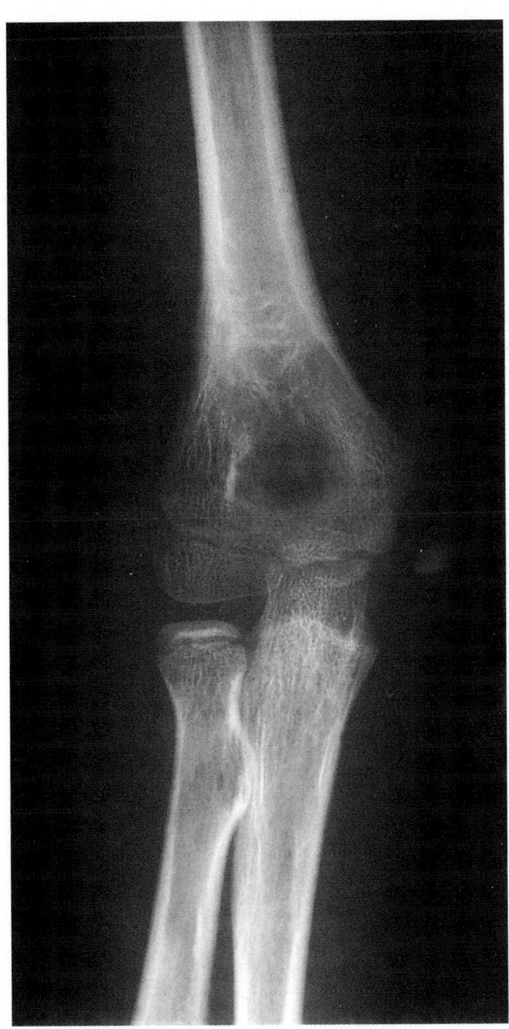

Fig. 22.34 A medial epicondylar fracture of the distal humerus.

Olecranon fractures

These are uncommon injuries and are often minimally displaced. For the occasional injury with significant displacement, open reaction and tension band wiring along adult lines is recommended.

Fractures of the forearm bones

Fractures of the radius and ulna are the most common fractures in children. The distal third of the bones is most commonly involved and the injury can occur in all age groups after the age of walking. Many injuries are green-stick fractures, often with angulation at the fracture site. Completely displaced fractures do occur and can be difficult to manage by closed means. The combination of a completely displaced distal radius fractures with a green-stick fracture of the distal ulna is also common and can be difficult to control in plaster.

Aetiology. In common with many injuries of the upper limb, forearm fractures are usually due to a fall on the outstretched hand. It is believed there is also a rotational element with forced suppination. Diagnosis is readily made on plain radiographs, although a fracture line may not always be evident; in this situation the cortical bulge of the torus or buckle fracture can be seen.

Treatment. Many of these fractures are minimally displaced and can be treated conservatively with 2–4 weeks in plaster, depending on the age of the child. Fractures of the distal sixth of the forearm can be managed in a below-elbow plaster; more proximal fractures require the elbow to be immobilised.

Manipulation under anaesthetic should be considered if angulation of the fracture site exceeds 20°. The age of the child and the potential for remodelling should be considered, as correction of up to 10° per year is possible. Although remodelling of an angulation of 30–40° is possible in the younger child, parental pressure to correct the obvious deformity may be an indication for manipulation.

Displaced fractures can also be managed by manipulation, as a periosteal hinge often remains intact and can be used to hold the reduction. Failure to reduce the fracture is an indication for open reduction and internal fixation, usually with a plate; small two- to four-hole plates can be used in younger children. Instability of the fracture site after a satisfactory reduction, either at the original operation or at subsequent out-patient review, is an indication of a temporary thin wire to maintain reduction. Thin wires can be safely passed across the distal radial epiphysis, provided care is taken and repeated attempts are avoided. The wire is removed after 2–4 weeks.

One fracture pattern which is notorious for loss of reduction is a completely displaced fracture of the distal radius with an intact or green-stick fracture of the ulna; wiring of the radius at the initial operation should be considered.

Complications. *Malunion.* This is relatively common after closed reduction of a displaced fracture. Often, by the time the malreduction is diagnosed, the fracture is too sticky to allow remanipulation and the position has to be accepted. For

(a)

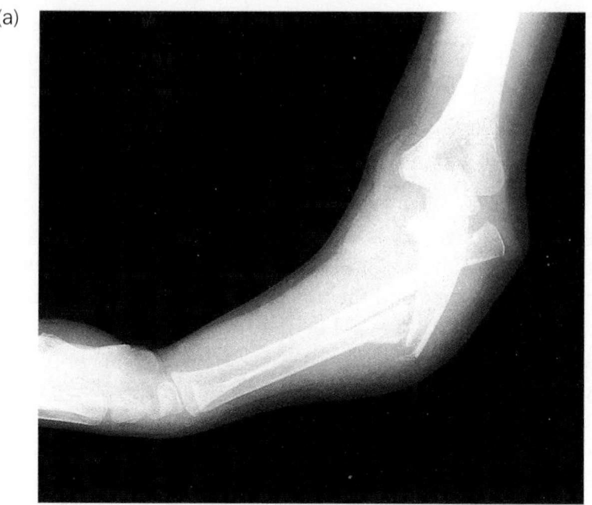

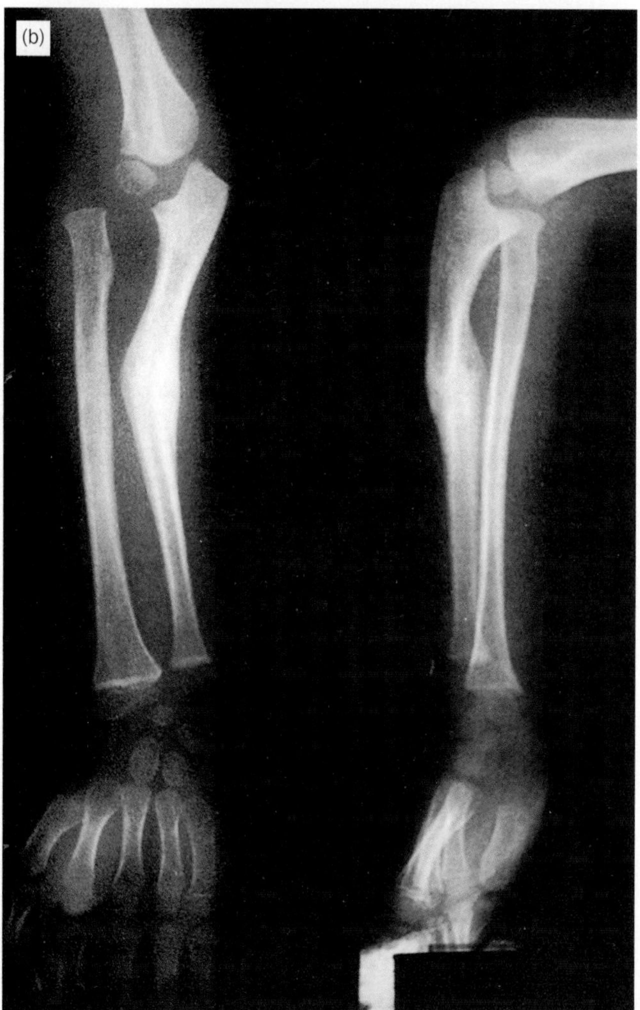

Fig. 22.35 (a) A Monteggia fracture involving fracture of the ulna and anterior dislocation of the radius. (b) If this fracture is not reduced and held with plate or K-wires then the radial head will remain dislocated and the ulna will malunite. Considerable restriction of elbow movement can occur.

fractures of the distal forearm with volar or dorsal angulation, considerable remodelling, as described above, can occur and the patient can be reassured. For malunions involving a rotation element, particularly with shortening of one bone, take down of the fracture site or osteotomy has to be considered.

Refracture. This is not an uncommon complication and usually occurs in the first few weeks after the plaster is removed. Although it may be due to inadequate immobilisation, the usual cause is a return to the original cause of the injury. Although a pathological process should considered it is not usually present and treatment should follow similar lines to a first-time injury.

Compartment syndrome. This is uncommon after a simple forearm fracture and severe pain is usually due to a tight dressing. All patients requiring a general anaesthetic for manipulation should be admitted overnight and the limb elevated. Severe pain should be treated by immediate splitting of the plaster and all dressings down to the skin. In the vast majority of cases this will provide immediate relief but a compartment syndrome should be considered if pain persists, particularly in patients with complicated injuries. Compartment syndrome is treated by fasciotomy, irrespective of the age of the child.

Monteggia fracture

This injury, characterised by a dislocation of the radial head at the elbow together with a (usually proximal) ulna fracture, is uncommon in children, accounting for less than 1 per cent of all forearm fractures. As in adults it is imperative that the joint above and the joint below a fracture should be visualised radiographically. With the forearm, if a fracture of only one bone is evident, the wrist and elbow joints must be examined and radiographs obtained (Fig. 22.35).

In children this injury can often be managed by manipulation and immobilisation in an above-elbow plaster. Follow-up radiographs must be obtained as redisplacement can occur. If a reduction cannot be achieved open reduction and internal fixation is indicated.

Galeazzi fracture

In children this injury is also uncommon and often consists of a distal radius fracture with separation of the distal ulna epiphysis, rather than a true joint disruption. It often occurs in the older child and, as with proximal humeral fractures, may be due to a weakness of the perichondral ring. Closed reduction is usually possible with this injury.

Further reading

Morrey, B.F. (1993) *The Elbow and Its Disorders*, W.B. Saunders, London.

Rockwood, C.A. Jr, Green, D.P., Heckman, J.D. *et al.* (1997) *Fractures*, Lippincott Williams & Wilkins, London.

Rockwood, C.A. Jr, and Matsen, F.A. III (1998) *The Shoulder*, W.B. Saunders, London.

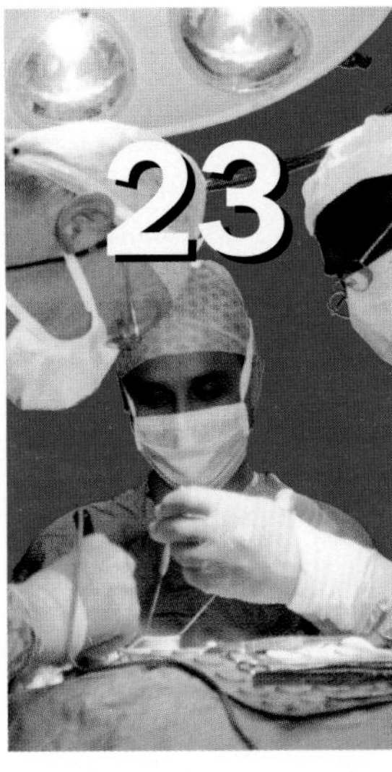

The pelvis and lower limb

Fractures of the pelvis

Fractures of the pelvis are relatively common in osteoporotic elderly patients. In this age group they are low-energy injuries and may, in fact, be pathological fractures. A careful check should be made for abnormalities which might suggest a benign lytic lesion or a metastatic tumour. In young patients, a pelvic fracture is associated with very high-energy accidents and carry a mortality of up to 20 per cent. This is because of the associated injuries. The pelvis is a stable ring, made up of bones and ligaments. If there is a displaced fracture of the pelvis then it must be broken in at least two places, and the ring is likely to be unstable. Unstable pelvic fractures carry a very poor prognosis because they are associated with torrential retroperitoneal bleeding from the pelvic veins. Immediate temporary stabilisation of the pelvic ring may be life-saving by helping the pelvic veins to clot off through tamponade, and by reducing the chance of movement displacing the clot. Pelvic fractures are also associated with damage to the rectum, the vagina and the urethra (especially in the male). A careful examination of all these structures should be performed in any patient with a significant pelvic fracture.

Bailey & Love's Short Practice of Surgery, 23rd edition. Edited by R.C.G. Russell, N.S. Williams and C.J.K. Bulstrode. Published in 2000 by Arnold Publishers.

Classification of pelvic fractures

Fractures outside the ring

These fractures do not disrupt the structure of the ring and occur either following a direct blow or as a traction injury of an epiphysis. In fractures of the sacrum a careful check should be made for nerve damage as the sacral nerves are likely to be involved.

Fractures of the coccyx can occur when the patient falls on to their backside. The fracture is very painful but usually settles after a few weeks. If it does not, then treatment is very difficult as coccydynia (pain in the coccyx) seems to be associated with a neurotic personality. Neither injection of the fracture site with local anaesthetic and steriods nor excision of the coccyx reliably relieves the pain.

Traction injuries

The origin of rectus femoris can be avulsed when, for example, a patient kicks a heavy wet football. Similarly, in Fig. 23.1 the adductor tubercle can be avulsed if the leg is forcibly abducted. Both of these fractures settle with rest.

Fracture of the iliac wing

The iliac wing can be broken following direct trauma, or indeed when harvesting bone graft (Fig. 23.1). No active treatment is necessary.

Single fractures of the ring

These fractures are by definition undisplaced and commonly

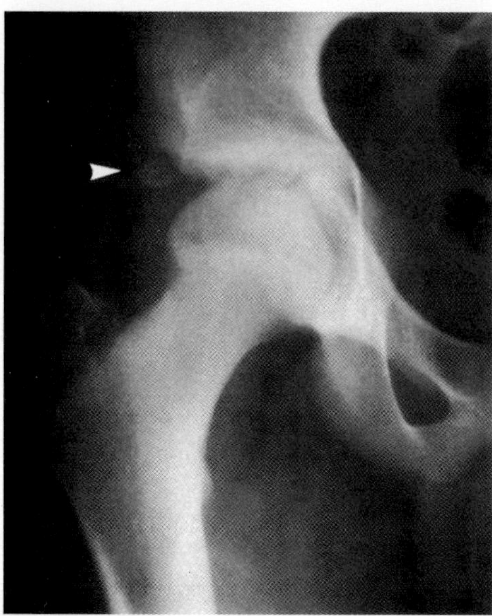

Fig. 23.1 Avulsion of the anterior inferior iliac spine.

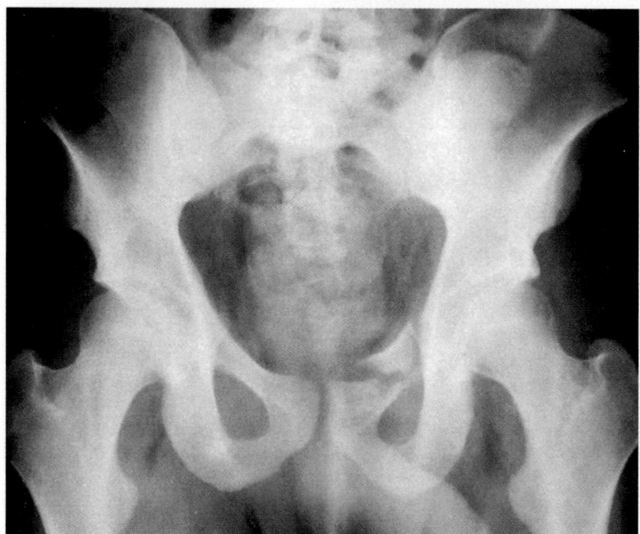

Fig. 23.2 Fracture of the pubic ramus (single fracture of the ring) (*courtesy of Keith Willett*).

occur either through the pubic or ischial ramus (Fig. 23.2). They are common in the elderly following a fall and may be pathological, through a metastasis or even a lytic lesion created by hyperparathyroidism (Brown tumour).

Fractures in or around the acetabulum

A fall from a great height on to the feet or a direct blow to the greater trochanter can fracture the pelvis around the acetabulum. The femoral head can be driven centrally through the floor of the acetabulum into the pelvis (the central acetabular fracture) (Fig. 23.3). Alternatively, either the front wall (the anterior pillar) or the back wall (the posterior pillar) of the acetabulum can be fractured. In extreme cases a combination of these injuries occurs. A simple anteroposterior (AP) and lateral view of the pelvis does not reveal the true nature of the injury, and it is usual to take oblique X-rays which show more clearly the extent of the injury to the anterior and posterior pillar. Computerised

Francis Robert Brown, 1889–1967. Surgeon, Royal Infirmary, Dundee, Scotland.

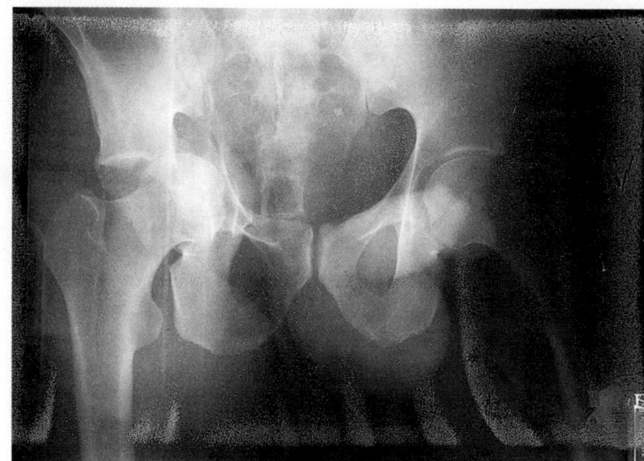

Fig. 23.3 A central acetabular fracture. Failure to reduce will inevitably lead to arthritis (*courtesy of Keith Willett*).

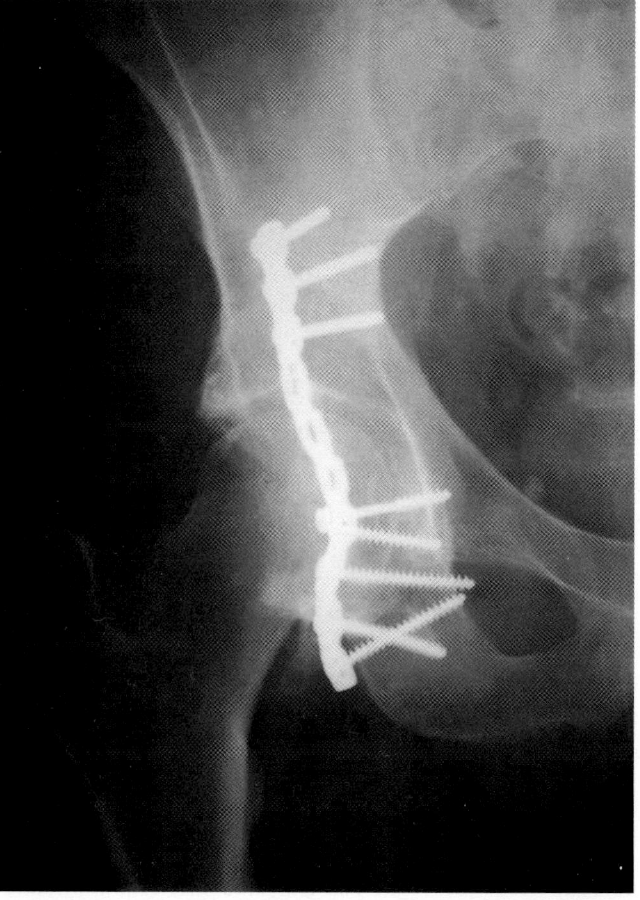

Fig. 23.4 Reconstruction of a posterior pillar fracture (*courtesy of Keith Willett*).

tomography (CT) scans with three-dimensional reconstruction can give even further information about the nature and extent of the fracture, and the number and extent of displacement of the fragments. This information is important for planning the treatment. If there is damage to the posterior pillar of the acetabulum then a careful check must be made for damage to the sciatic nerve which runs close to the posterior pillar (Fig. 23.4).

Treatment. Fractures around the acetabulum can be treated nonoperatively with skeletal traction for 6–8 weeks. Although this method of treatment is uncomplicated and safe, the results are poor if there is a displaced intra-articular fracture.

Traumatic osteoarthritis of the hip is inevitable, and subsequent treatment with an arthrodesis or even a joint replacement will be required within a few years. This may, however, be the only option if the patient's overall condition is so poor that major surgery is dangerous, or if the relevant surgical expertise is not available. The alternative is surgical reconstruction of the pelvis using plates bent to the contour of the surface of the pelvis and screws to stabilise fractures. This type of surgery is both difficult and complex, and carries a significant morbidity and mortality to the patient through blood loss and damage to the nerves around the pelvis. If, however, a stable congruent surface to the acetabulum can be recreated the prognosis to the patient is very good indeed.

Double fractures of the ring

Displaced fractures of the pelvis must by definition involve a fracture through two parts of the pelvic ring. It is not always possible to see the second fracture line as it may pass through the sacral iliac joint. These fractures are very high energy and are intrinsically unstable (Fig. 23.5). They are associated with a high mortality because of associated injuries and the massive retroperitoneal haemorrhage involved. Therefore, for the reasons described above, they may need stabilising immediately with an external fixator to reduce haemorrhage when the patient is turned (Fig. 23.6).

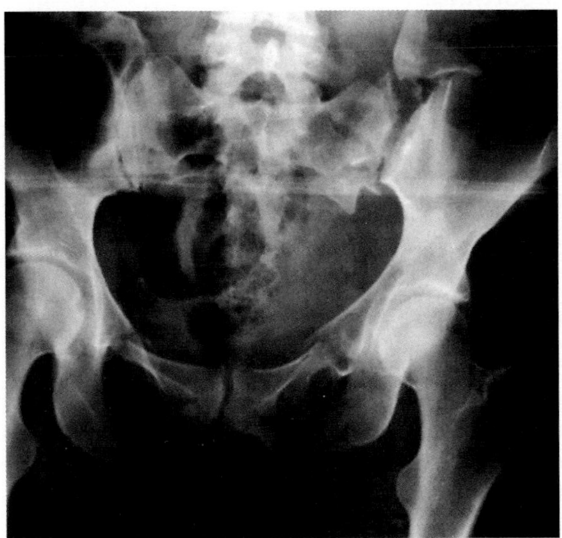

Fig. 23.5 Double fracture of the pelvic ring with disruption of the left sacroiliac joint (*courtesy of Keith Willett*).

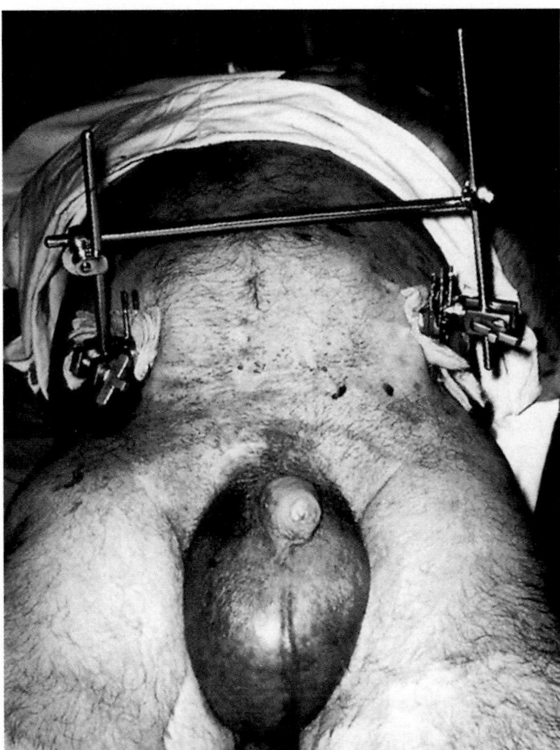

Fig. 23.6 Fractured pelvis held by an external fixator. Note bruising of the scrotum, which is characteristic of pubic rami fractures.

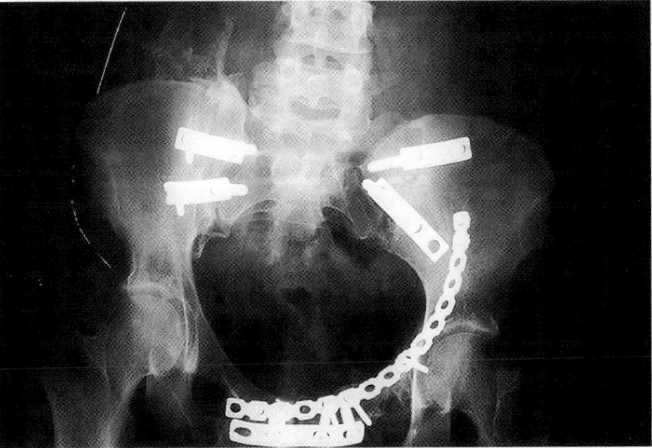

Fig. 23.7 Reconstruction of an unstable pelvic fracture using screws and reconstruction plates (*courtesy of Keith Willett*).

They are also associated with damage to the nerves of the sacral plexus as well as injuries to the pelvic organs, particularly the male urethra.

Treatment. Initially these patients may be too sick to embark on a formal reduction and stabilisation of the pelvic ring (Fig. 23.7). The operation therefore may have to be delayed for up to 10 days. Beyond that the operation becomes difficult because callous formation prevents fracture reduction.

Table 23.1 Problems in the hip by age group

At birth	*Newborn*	*Child*	*Adolescent*	*Adult*	*Elderly*	*Senile*
Congenital dislocation of the hip	Septic arthritis	Perthes' disease	Slipped upper femoral epiphysis	Secondary arthritis	Osteoarthritis	Fractured neck of femur

Table 23.2 Causes of arthritis of the hip

Congenital dislocation of the hip	*Septic arthritis*	*Perthes' disease*	*Slipped upper femoral epiphysis*	*Inflammatory arthritis*	*Trauma*	*Primary osteoarthritis*
Hip does not form normally. Incongruent and abnormal cartilage	Articular cartilage damaged	Avascular necrosis leads to collapse of head	Abnormal growth plate leads to deformed hip	Pannus destroys articular cartilage	Incongruent joint	Cause unknown

The hip

The hip is one of the 'bread-and-butter' joints in orthopaedics, and provides a very substantial proportion of the total workload of an orthopaedic surgeon. In infants the problem of congenital dislocation of the hip is important because it is treatable if diagnosed early. The hip is also susceptible to septic arthritis, especially in the newborn (Table 23.1). In children, Perthes' disease, an avascular necrosis of the hip, poses a major therapeutic challenge. In the young adolescent slipped upper femoral epiphysis needs early diagnosis if problems are to be avoided for the rest of the child's life. In the young adult hip dysplasia may start to cause problems which will eventually go on to arthritis of the hip and which will pose severe problems for future hip replacement. In the elderly primary osteoarthritis of the hip is so common that, in Britain alone, over 50 000 total hip replacements are performed each year. Osteoporosis and problems of balance in the elderly also brings about a rapid rise in the incidence of fractured neck of femur. This, too, requires surgical treatment, providing the majority of major operations needed in trauma services.

Principles of history and examination of the hip

Pain – localisation and radiation

Patients find pain originating from the hip very difficult to localise. Children presenting at the clinic with a limp, a painful knee and a normal knee X-ray (King's triad) will usually be found to have a problem in the hip not the knee. Similar problems occur in the elderly, who may complain of pain down the front of the thigh and into the knee, when the diagnosis is osteoarthritis of the hip. However, pain originating from the back can radiate down into the buttocks into the greater trochanter. Examination of a patient complaining of pain in the hip needs to concentrate on determining whether this pain is arising from the spine, the knee or the hip itself.

Disability – activities of daily living

Patients with a stiff hip complain primarily of difficulty getting in and out of the bath and low chairs, as well as problems with getting socks and shoes on. The combination of pain and stiffness from osteoarthritis may also limit their walking distance.

Deformity

Problems in the hip lead to flexion and adduction of the joint. This leads to a tilt of the pelvis and a leg which appears to be shortened. The patient will therefore stoop and limp because of pain, weakness and deformity.

Osteoarthritis

Most osteoarthritis is called primary because there is no known preceding cause. There is a genetic effect, but the reason why some joints apparently last the lifetime of a patient while others disintegrate is not well understood. Secondary arthritis can occur following congenital subluxation of the hip, Perthes' disease secondary to trauma or an inflammatory arthritis such as rheumatoid (see Table 23.2).

Prevention

There is some evidence that young people involved in high-intensity sport and/or heavy-duty work are more susceptible to osteoarthritis later in life, but the affect is surprisingly small. Secondary osteoarthritis may be prevented by minimising the damage to the joints caused by the primary disease. In trauma articular fractures should be anatomically reduced. In inflammatory joint disease every effort should be made to reduce the level of inflammation.

George Clemens Perthes, 1868–1927. Professor of Surgery, Tübingen, Germany.

John King. Consultant orthopaedic surgeon, London Hospital, England.

Treatment

In the early stages osteoarthritis affects the patient in all three main areas of orthopaedic endeavour. It causes pain, disability and some deformity. It may also cause high levels of anxiety in the patient who may be worried that the condition is going to rapidly deteriorate and spread to other joints, destroying their quality of life. Many patients are resistant to taking tablets of any sort. There is no evidence that pain killers or anti-inflammatory drugs do anything but relieve the symptoms, and they may even accelerate the pathological changes. The key issue at this early stage for the quality of life of the patient is to maintain mobility and to avoid deformity. Physiotherapy should be used to show the patient how to keep joints mobile and muscles in good condition. The psychological benefit of this is also almost certainly important.

More severe osteoarthritis

As the condition becomes more severe regular analgesia may be needed. The use of centrally acting pain killers, such as paracetamol, combined with nonsteroidal anti-inflammatory drugs appears to provide a synergistic effect in terms of pain relief, but care must be taken to avoid gastric irritation and ulceration.

Indications for joint replacement

Indications for joint replacement are:

- pain;
- stiffness;
- loss of independence.

In the elderly, loss of independence through disability is a crucial issue. A painful stiff and deformed hip may prevent a person from sleeping, from doing up their shoes, from going out to do their shopping and even from using a car or a bus. This combined with chronic pain may convert a cheerful outgoing involved member of society into a depressed and isolated individual reliant on others for their needs. The cost to the individual and to society is out of all proportion to the pathological effect of the disease itself. A total hip replacement reverses this cycle. Combined with the judicious use of physiotherapy and occupational therapy, this gives the patient the confidence to return to an active independent life. In the patient over 65 years with a life expectancy of around 20 years, total hip replacement is the treatment of choice for osteoarthritis. In the younger patient the likelihood is that the joint replacement will not last the lifetime of the patient. They can be replaced (a revision operation) but this is technically difficult and the next operation does not last as long as the first. In younger patients secondary osteoarthritis is more common than primary and in these patients fitting the hip replacement securely in the abnormal anatomy may be much more difficult than in a simple elderly patient. The patient may also put greater loads on the hip. If a patient has a normal life expectancy, the younger the patient the more carefully alternatives to total hip replacement must be considered.

Rheumatoid arthritis

Total hip replacement in patients with rheumatoid arthritis is a successful operation. Perhaps this is because the patient has put very little load on the hip, but the relief of pain and the increase in mobility can have a dramatic effect on the quality of life of the patient.

Alternatives to total hip replacement

Juvenile chronic arthritis

In these patients the disability in other joints and the lack of demand that they make on the hip replacement makes it the treatment of choice despite their young age. Nevertheless, there are considerable technical difficulties; these patients have all the complications of long-term steroid therapy and the hip joint may be too small for normal implants because it was damaged with arthritis before it had fully developed.

Hip dysplasia

Patients with hip dysplasia may start to develop arthritis in their teens or early 20s. X-rays will show subluxation of the hip joint which rides up the deficient acetabular wall and there may already be signs of point loading on the edge of the acetabulum with osteoarthritis starting to form. The treatment of this condition is contentious but most surgeons would recommend some form of osteotomy to try to obtain better cover for the femoral head. The purpose is to spread the load of the hip joint over a larger articular surface, and so an osteotomy on the acetabular side is the preferred technique. The whole acetabulum can be detached from the rest of the pelvic ring and rotated so that an adequate roof is produced. The operation is technically very difficult to perform and there is a risk of causing complete avascular necrosis and chondrolysis of the acetabular cartilage.

An alternative is to cut through the ileum immediately above the acetabulum and to displace the acetabulum inwards under this shelf, so creating a new roof for the acetabulum. This operation too is difficult to perform and, given the rarity of the cases and the problems of finding matched controls, there is no evidence that this operation or any other for that matter makes any difference to the outcome of the hip. A third operation is to lift a wedge of bone on a proximally based cortical pedicle and create a roof by packing bone graft inside the wedge. This is the simplest of the operations but the least attractive from a biomechanical point of view. If these operations are successful and a new roof is created for the acetabulum in one way or another the secondary advantage of this type of surgery is that it makes total hip replacement in the future much easier. Otherwise there are great difficulties in setting the cup in the pelvis because there is no bony roof to provide support for it.

> Hip dysplasia
>
> - Pelvic osteotomy spreads the load and may make total hip replacement easier

Osteoarthritis secondary to trauma in the young adult

Young, fit adults put a great load on the total hip replacement and will also have a life expectancy in excess of 30–40 years. They may be in severe pain and will push hard for a total hip replacement having heard of the marvellous results which can be obtained in the elderly. It is important to explain to them that the lifetime of the hip may be as little as 5 years in a young patient and that subsequent revisions are likely to have an even shorter life. The better option in the young fit patient is a hip arthrodesis. The operation, if successfully performed, will completely remove pain and produce a strong, stable hip. This should last their lifetime without further problems. It is even possible to unpick an arthrodesis and replace it with a total hip replacement if problems start in the other hip or in the knee below the arthrodesis. The disability of a successful hip arthrodesis is slight. The patient can walk and run, but can usually only climb ladders one step at a time. The stiff hip does not apparently interfere with the ability to have sexual intercourse or to have children, and the only time when it is particularly a problem is when sitting in a chair. Because the hip is only fused in slight flexion the patient may have to slump in a chair with the leg sticking out in front. This posture can appear very irritating to fellow passengers in a bus if they are not aware of the reason for it. Technically, the arthrodesis can be difficult to perform, but with the advent of modern techniques (using cobra plates) and bone graft a secure arthrodesis should be obtainable. It is important to make sure that the hip is arthrodesed in a good position. The ideal is neutral or slight abduction with some 20–30° of flexion. It is all too easy to let the hip slip into adduction when there will be unnecessary relative shortening. If the hip is fixed in too much abduction then the leg is too long and it may be difficult to obtain adequate swing through. However, there will be some shortening from fixing the hip in a little flexion (to allow sitting) so a little abduction may compensate for that.

Hip arthrodesis

- Produces a painless hip
- Does not wear out
- Can be replaced with a total hip replacement later
- Ideal for a young active patient

Secondary osteoarthritis in the older patient or in a patient who has a disease in other joints

Arthrodesis should not be considered in patients who already have back problems or who have arthritis in other joints. In these cases it increases the patient's disability and may exacerbate the pain from osteoarthritis in the other joints. An alternative in the older patient who is still too young for a total hip replacement is the femoral osteotomy.

The femur is divided in the intertrochanteric region and then fixed securely using a dynamic hip screw or a plate. It has been suggested that the cause of the deep pain in osteoarthritis is venous hypertension, and that the osteotomy relieves this hypertension. This cannot be the only explanation as, radiologically, there may be a dramatic improvement in the joint surface with apparent regrowth of articular cartilage. One element of the osteotomy is to change the angle of the femoral head so that a new area of little worn articular cartilage can be brought to bear on the acetabulum. If the osteotomy also shortens the femur slightly then the pelvis will dip down in compensation and in effect the acetabulum will give more cover to the femoral head and it too will bring a new area of articular cartilage into the load-bearing zone. Femoral osteotomy gives a variable relief of pain from osteoarthritis, but it is reasonable to offer the patient up to 5 years of pain relief, and it may be much longer. There is nothing to stop a total hip replacement being performed after an osteotomy, so the advantage of using an osteotomy to buy time in a patient who is a little too young for a total hip replacement makes this a very attractive option. The operation needs to be planned carefully in advance with tracings made from the X-rays to decide exactly what type of wedge, if any, is to be taken out of the femur. If the femur is to be rotated as well then it is advisable to put pins into the femur either side of the osteotomy so that the angle of rotation can be carefully measured. The osteotomy is fixed with either a blade plate or with a dynamic hip screw. If the fixation is secure then the patient should be able to weight-bear partially using crutches immediately after surgery and can start full weight-bearing at 3 months.

Indications for osteotomy in hip arthritis

- Young patients not suitable for total hip replacement
- Problems in more than one joint not suitable for arthrodesis

Total hip replacement

Total hip replacement is the mainstay of treatment for osteoarthritis and rheumatoid arthritis of the hip, and for patients over the age of 65 years is the operation of first choice. In patients between the age of 55 and 65 years the pros and cons should be weighed up carefully against osteotomy. Below the age of 55 years total hip replacement should only be undertaken in exceptional circumstances and arthrodesis should be the treatment of choice.

Management of hip arthritis

- > 65 years – total hip replacement
- 55–65 years – osteotomy
- < 55 years – arthrodesis

Indications for surgery

The indications for an operation are primarily pain when it can no longer can be controlled by using pain killers. A secondary indication is interference with mobility and quality of life.

Types of total hip replacement

There are nearly 100 different designs of total hip replacements currently on the market and in almost none of them is there an adequate long-term follow-up which a surgeon could use to decide which design to use (Fig. 23.8). Designs can be classified into some simple categories which are given in Table 23.3 (see also Fig. 23.9).

Table 23.3 Classification of types of joint replacement

Categorisation	*Type*		*Comments*
Fixation to bone	Cemented	Uncemented	Cementless are more expensive; the methods of fixation are unproven
Articular surfaces	Femoral head – stainless steel, colbalt chrome, titanium, ceramic	Acetabulum, high-density polyethylene, ceramic, metal	Metal on polyethylene is well proven but produces wear particles. Ceramic on ceramic is expensive and, as yet, only better in theory
Head size	22 mm head	28–32 mm heads	Small heads have low friction but put high loads on the polyethylene and may wear rapidly. Large heads increase the friction, reduce the loading, increase stability but reduce the amount of polyethylene available for the acetabulum

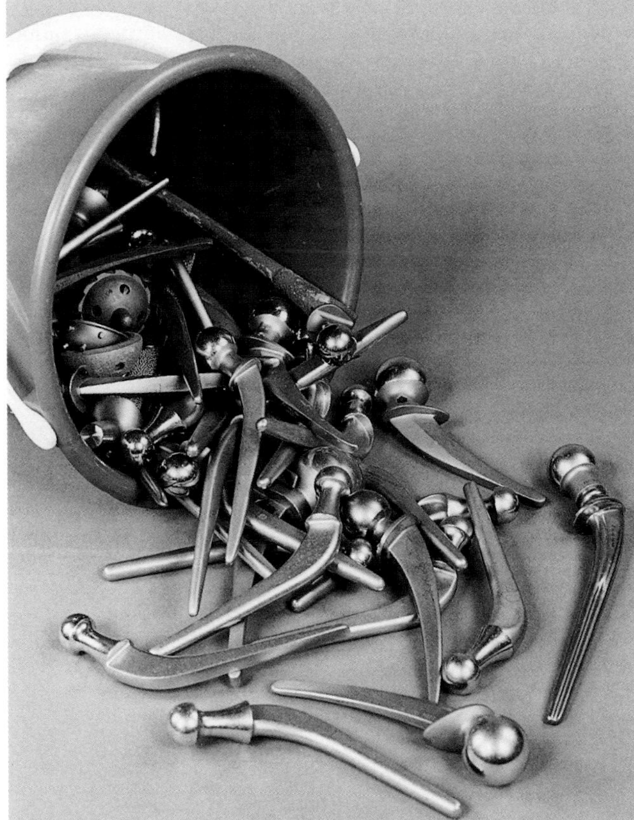

Fig. 23.8 Variety of joint replacement types removed at revision surgery.

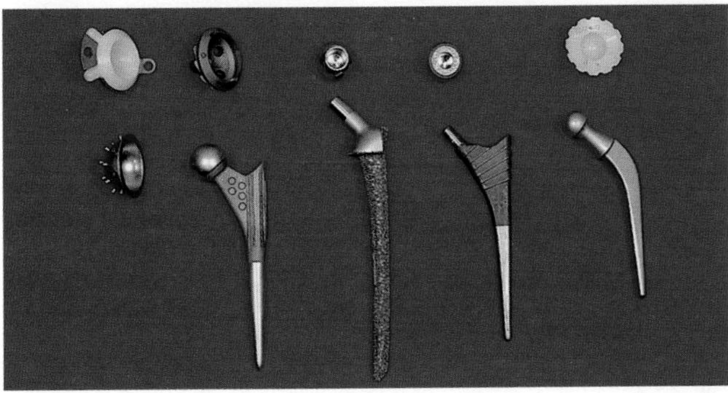

Fig. 23.9 Some varieties of materials shape and fixation methods in total joint replacement.

Methods of fixation

Traditionally, hip replacements were fixed into a bed of polymethyl methacrylate (PMMA) cement. The cement is a grouting agent, in other words it acts as a spacer between the implant and the irregularly shaped cavity into which it is being put. A powder of PMMA cement is mixed with the monomer which is itself quite toxic to both patient and staff. The two are mixed together until an exothermic reaction starts and the cement begins to set. This takes 5–7 minutes. The cement is then put into the cavity and the implant pushed in on top of the cement until it is properly bedded in. Over the next 10 minutes the cement sets, becoming quite hot as it does so. The cup is cemented into place first. The process is then repeated with the femoral component. As the cement sets, some of the methyl methacrylate polymer is released into the patients blood stream and can cause a drop in the patient's blood pressure. The heat produced by the cement setting may cause a layer of bone necrosis around the cement and it has been suggested that this may lead to early loosening. If fragments of the cement break away and get into the joint they will act as an abrasive and cause third-body wear. This destroys the artificial joint surface and releases a large amount of debris, which then sets up an inflammatory reaction. If the cement around the implant breaks or becomes loose it too will release particles which stimulate an inflammatory response. This too can lead to resorption of bone around the implant. This is called aseptic loosening as there is no evidence that infection has any role in this type of loosening. In response to these findings surgeons have attempted to design implants which can be fixed into the bone without the use of PMMA cement. In dentistry there has been considerable success with bone bonding to implants made of titanium for osseous integration and those which are coated in a layer of hydroxyapatite ceramic. Unfortunately, in joint replacement surgery this success has not been reproduced. Implants designed for cementless implantation are much more expensive to manufacture and need to be fitted much more carefully is there is to be any chance of good binding between the bone and the implant. Once they have been implanted the load on the interface should be kept to a minimum until osseous integration has had a chance to take place. Unfortunately, if this ever occurs it is likely to take many months, and even if a patient does not weight-bear during that time the micromovement between implant and bone may prevent osseous integration. This is because the hip joint is a fulcrum to powerful muscles around the hip. Even lifting the leg up off the bed may produce loads through the hip joint of three or four times body weight. One further practical advantage of cementless joint replacement is that when these implants do come loose, they should be easier to change as there is no need to remove all the cement from inside the femoral canal. Unfortunately, this too is only a theoretical advantage. Cementless hip replacements which start loosening and become painful may, nevertheless, have small areas where osseous integration has occurred. This can make them quite as difficult to remove as a cemented implant. There is currently no evidence whatsoever to support the use of the more expensive and difficult to implant cementless implants, although hydroxyapatite coating looks promising.

Joint surfaces

The original total hip replacements designed by Charnley eventually used a joint surface of metal on high-density polyethylene. The coefficient friction between these two surfaces is far higher than articular cartilage, but because a small head size was used the actual force on the implants remained low. High-density polyethylene has good shock-absorbing properties but does wear slowly over the years producing small particles which can stimulate an inflammatory response in the joint. It is felt that this inflammatory response can, once again, be responsible for aseptic loosening. The macrophages actually start to resorb bone and may stimulate osteoclasts to do the same. There has therefore been a move towards using joints which do not produce wear particles. Ceramic femoral heads bearing on polythene cups have far lower friction, but ceramic femoral heads on ceramic acetabular cups have the lowest friction of all. They are, however, very difficult and very expensive to manufacture. Metal-on-metal implants should also have a low coefficient of friction and produce very few wear particles. These implants were frequently used in the early days of joint replacement but had a bad reputation for loosening. It is currently claimed that this was because they were not manufactured to a high enough tolerance, and that the surfaces were binding together, loosening the implant. There is as yet, however, no evidence that the newer metal-on-metal implants offer anything but theoretical advantages.

Head size

The original implants used a small head size of 22 mm to reduce friction (Fig. 23.10). This has the added advantage of allowing plenty of room inside the acetabulum for a thick polythene cup which has plenty of room for wear and which should have good shock-absorbing capabilities. The small head, however, does carry a theoretical higher risk of dislocation, because the diameter of the head is so small that a relatively small displacement of the hip out of the socket allows it to dislocate. Biomechanical calculations show that the load on the polythene cup produced by a small head is close to the limits which can be tolerated by the polythene, and therefore recently manufacturers have been moving towards a larger size of femoral head. The disadvantage of this increased head size is that the friction increases and so the force on the interface between the acetabular cup and the bone will be increased. Theoretically, this will increase the chance of loosening.

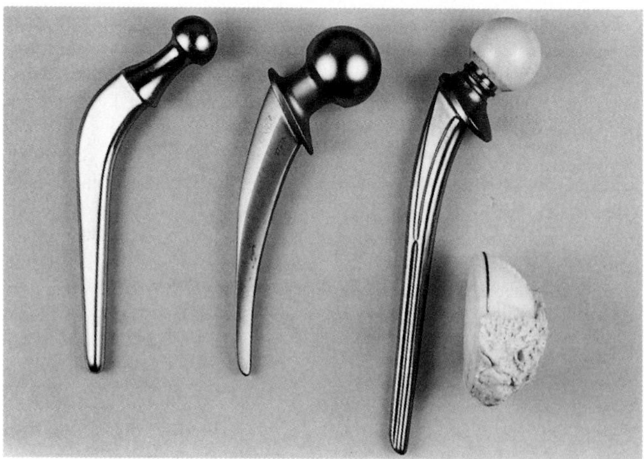

Fig. 23.10 Different head sizes: 22 mm on the left; 32 mm in the middle. The right-hand implant has a ceramic head aimed at reducing friction, despite the larger size.

Sir John Charnley, 1911–82. Professor of Orthopaedic Surgery, University of Manchester, England.

Choice of implant

Currently, the best long-term results have been obtained with some of the older and cheaper cemented implants. In good hands these implants should give over 50 per cent of the patients a trouble-free joint for over 10 years. In younger patients the figures are not so good, and once a joint has been revised the lifetime of the second implant appears to be shorter. New designs (Fig. 23.11) should not be introduced on to the market without proper trials being performed. Surgeons should be able to explain to their patients who will be performing the operation, the published results of the design that they are using and the ongoing results of the design in their own hands.

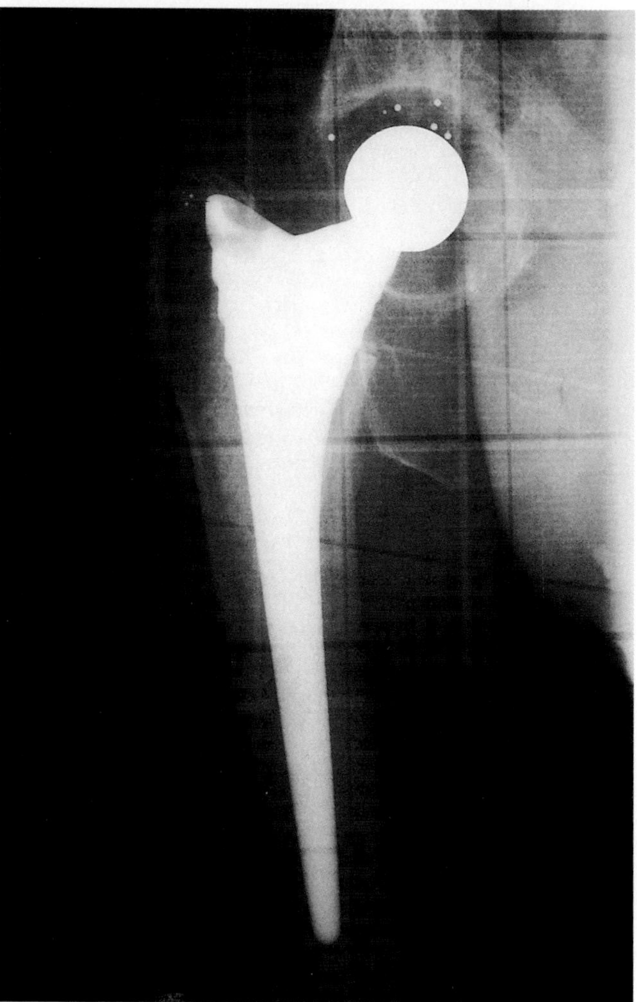

Fig. 23.11 X-ray of a newer type of joint replacement using a research technique designed to predict failure in clinical trials – stereoradiogrammetry (RSA).

Surgical technique

There are three commonly used approaches to total hip replacement. The fact that there are three suggests that there are advantages and disadvantages to each.

The anterolateral approach

The anterolateral approach has been popularised by many surgeons, particularly Hardinge. The patient can be positioned on the table either in the lateral position or supine with a sandbag under the buttock to raise it clear from the table. If the supine position is used then the patient needs to be placed as close to the edge of the table as possible as otherwise access is restricted. A 15-cm incision is centred over the greater trochanter curving 45° backwards above the greater trochanter and running straight down the line of the femur below the greater trochanter. Tensor fascia lata is divided over the greater trochanter and held apart with a self-retaining retractor. Gluteus medius is divided off the front of the greater trochanter, until the capsule is exposed. The fibres of gluteus medius are gently divided above the greater trochanter for a few centimetres (no further or the neurovascular bundle may be damaged). A sharp retractor can now be introduced over the capsule and the front of the femoral head into the anterior wall of the acetabulum, taking care not to damage the femoral nerve. The anterior capsule is divided removing as large an ellipse as possible but taking care, particularly inferiorly, not to cut blind into veins running in the soft tissue just outside the hip joint. The assistant now takes the patient's leg, bending the knee at right angles, and dislocates the hip by external rotation. Great care should be taken not to use too much force during this manoeuvre as otherwise the femur will be fractured. If the hip cannot be dislocated safely then the femoral neck should be cut and then the femoral head removed using a bone screw in the same way as the femoral head is removed during surgery for a subcapital fractured neck of femur.

The trochanteric approach

This is an important approach because it gives excellent access to the hip, and is also a very useful approach for reconstruction of the pelvis after pelvic fracture. However, in all but expert hands reattachment of the greater trochanter after surgery has given significant complications. Nonunion of the greater trochanter can be painful and weakens the hip considerably. The approach should only be used after careful training.

The patient can be placed supine on the table and a straight or curved incision made centred over the greater trochanter. Tensor fascia lata is divided along the lines of its fibres and the soft tissue cleaned off the lateral side of the femur and the greater trochanter. A Gigli saw is passed over the top of the femoral neck beneath the insertion of the abductors and the greater trochanter taken off with an oblique osteotomy continuing the line of the femoral neck across the femur. Some people insert a Steinmann pin into the lateral cortex of the femur to tent the Gigli saw so that an oblique chevron-type osteotomy is performed. The hip can now be dislocated anteriorly. Before the femoral component is cemented into place wires are laid in place ready for reattachment of the greater trochanter.

The posterior approach to the hip

This approach is quick and easy. Access is good but there is an increased risk of posterior dislocation after surgery.

The patient is placed in the full lateral position and an incision is made centred over the greater trochanter with the upper arm curving backwards at 45° and the lower arm passing straight down the femur. Tensor fascia lata is divided along the line of its fibres and retracted. The hip is internally rotated by the assistant holding the lower leg. This exposes the short external rotators of the hip. The sciatic nerve runs over these muscles and should be identified and carefully retracted. The short external rotators are then divided on stay sutures and are folded back over the sciatic nerve to protect it. The capsule is now divided; a wide ellipse may be needed to be taken before the hip can be dislocated. Alternatively, an H-shaped incision can be made so that the capsule can be repaired once the hip replacement has been performed.

Performing the total hip replacement

The knee should be bent to 90° and the tibia placed either horizontal or vertical in relation to the floor, so that you can be sure of the orientation of the femoral shaft. If the femoral neck has not already been cut it should now be cut at the correct level allowing 10–20° of anteversion if it is a posterior approach, slightly less anteversion if it is antrochanteric or anterolateral approach. The level of the cut on the femoral neck can be determined by laying a trial prosthesis against the femur and marking where the neck of the implant lies when the centre of the head is level with the centre of the old femoral head. The femur now needs to be retracted out of the way of the acetabulum taking care not to damage the sciatic nerve or the femoral nerve with the retractor. Further excision of the capsule may be necessary before the femur is released adequately to do this. The ligamentum teres and any other soft tissue is excised from the acetabulum.

The acetabulum is now reamed with a strawberry reamer pushed in along the line that the acetabular cup will occupy when it is placed in the acetabulum. Reaming should continue until the osteophytes around the central fovea have been removed. The size of the strawberry reamer should be increased until it is just gripping the edges of the old acetabulum. Reaming should be continued until all the articular cartilage has been removed and subchondral bone is exposed. Keyholes need to be drilled in the subchondral bone to provide extra support for the cement, avoiding the weight-bearing superolateral area. The keyholes do not need to be more than a couple of millimetres deep and should not broach the medial wall. They are therefore best placed into the anterior and posterior pillars. Choose the correct size of acetabular cup for the reamer that has been used so that a thin mantle of cement will lie all the way around the implant. Check that the acetabular cup when inserted will lie comfortably just inside the acetabulum and that its superolateral margin is bearing on the superolateral margin of the acetabulum when it is placed with 30–45° of cover and 10–20° of anteversion. The acetabulum should then be packed with a dry swab and the retractors removed.

The femur should now be rotated to expose the cancellous bone in the femoral neck and to deliver the femur up and out of the wound so that rasps can be inserted without touching the gluteal muscles or the skin. A sharp lever may need to be inserted under the greater trochanter to help this. Spoon out the medullary contents of the femur keeping the convex side of the spoon always facing the dorsum of the femur. This will prevent the spoon inadvertently being driven out through the lateral cortex of the femur. Clear out the cancellous bone, particularly in the greater trochanter, until the spoon can be inserted straight down the

Kevin Hardinge. Orthopaedic surgeon, Wrightington.

Leonardo Gigli, 1863–1908. Obstetrician and Director, Santa Maria Nuova Hospital, Florence, Italy. Introduced his saw for pubiotomy in 1894 and adapted it for craniotomy in 1898.

Fritz Steinmann, 1872–1932. Surgeon, Berne, Switzerland. Described a pin for skeletal traction in 1907.

femoral canal. Insert rasps into the femoral canal, always applying pressure so that the shoulder of the rasp is pressing back against the greater trochanter and the tip is pressing towards the medial cortex of the femur. Once again, this will avoid the all too common complication of the rasp penetrating the lateral cortex of the femur. Continue rasping until a trial prosthesis can be inserted into the femur and lies comfortably with the tip resting against the medial cortex of the femur. Wrap a swab around the neck of the trial component and carry out a trial reduction with a trial acetabulum in place.

The purpose of the trial reduction is to check the orientation of the femur and the acetabulum, and to check that tension in the soft tissues is adequate to stabilise the components but not so great that reduction will prove impossible once cementing has been performed. If the reduction is satisfactory mix the first batch of cement and, when it is no longer sticky but wrinkles when compressed, change gloves and insert the cement into a clean, dry acetabulum. Insert the chosen cup, apply pressure directly up the line of the cup allowing for adequate cover and anteversion. Remove excess cement from around the cup, particularly posteriorly. When the cement has set, check that all extraneous cement has been removed and cover the acetabular component with a swab. Insert a cement restrictor into the femoral canal. Wash out the femoral canal with copious volumes of saline and then pack the canal with dry swabs and start mixing the cement for the femoral canal using a cement gun. When the cement is ready, remove the swabs and inject the cement into the femoral canal from the bottom up. Insert the femoral component, ensuring that the rotation does not change as the implant is inserted and that the tip of the femoral component runs down the centre of the canal, or even slightly medially. Continue to apply pressure to the femoral component once it has bedded down, and remove all extra cement.

When the cement has set check that all extra cement has been removed and that there are no fragments lying loose in the wound. Reduce the implant and test stability in full internal and external rotation in both full extension and full flexion. Make a note if stability is compromised in any way so that postoperative care can make allowance for this. Wash out the wound with copious volumes of saline. If the sciatic nerve was visualised, check once again that it is intact and undamaged. Close the muscles in layers over two drains, one deep and one superficial.

Postoperatively, the patient should be managed in troughs or with an abduction pillow to keep the legs slightly abducted. If there is gross instability then a plaster spica may need to be applied, including the feet if rotation needs to be controlled. After an uneventful total hip replacement the patient can be mobilised as soon as resources are available. If the patient has already been taught how to use crutches before surgery then mobilisation will be much easier. The patient should avoid sitting on a low seat or on a lavatory seat which has not been raised for at least 6 weeks after surgery as this position invites dislocation. If social circumstances are satisfactory the patient can be discharged home between day 7 and day 10. An annual review should be performed for the rest of the life of the patient in order to gain information about the natural history of total hip replacement and to identify aseptic loosening early before there is too much damage to the bone. The results of this annual review should be used to build up a bank of information on a unit's success with joint replacement. It should also be made available to any national register so that long-term results on large numbers can be used to see how the successful joint replacement process may be improved.

Prophylactic antibiotics

There is good evidence that at least three doses of a broad-spectrum antibiotic should be used to cover total hip replacement. If this is combined with the use of laminar flow operating theatres, the chance of a total hip replacement becoming infected should be less than 2 per cent. One dose of the antibiotics should be given at induction and the other two doses to cover the next 24 hours. There is no evidence that giving antibiotics for any longer than this confers any added benefit.

Thromboprophylaxis

The total death rate after total hip replacement is around nine deaths per 1000 patients in the first 90 days. Three of those deaths would have occurred in the normal population even if they had not had a total hip replacement. Therefore the excess number of deaths is six people per 1000, i.e. less than 1 per cent. Only a small proportion of those deaths is caused by pulmonary embolus, the major cause of death being myocardial infarct and stroke. There is no evidence that thrombopropylaxis affects the overall death rate or, more particularly, the very low death rate for pulmonary embolus. There is clear evidence that thromboprophylaxis reduces the rate of deep vein thrombosis, but it is not clear whether this translates into a reduction in pulmonary embolus or even postphlebitic limb. There has been little research into the complications of thromboprophylaxis. Haematoma formation is associated with an increased rate of infection but no studies have been performed to determine whether thromboprophylaxis affects the infection rate or, indeed, loosening of total hip replacements. There is also no evidence that mechanical methods such as stockings or even foot pumps affect the death rate after total hip replacement. There is some evidence that compression stockings can, in fact, increase the instance of deep vein thrombosis. Despite the prodigious efforts by the pharmaceutical industry to prove the efficacy of thromboprophylaxis, there is as yet no evidence to support its use or, indeed, to show that it does more harm than good. Therefore, under the present circumstances there is no merit in using any form of thromboprophylaxis.

Consent for total hip replacement

Consent for total hip replacement should involve, like any other consent, checking what the patient knows about the operation after introductions have been made. You should then explain to the patient exactly what the operation involves. It is very helpful here to have a model of a hip replacement for the patient to look at and to feel. Patients also like to be told where they will be when they wake up, when they can first have visitors and when they are likely to go home. You should then deal with the outcome of the operation in terms of pain relief and mobility. The patient also needs a clear explanation of the alternatives to the operation. In other words, what is the likely natural history of their disease if they do not have surgery, as it is only if they have the knowledge of the choices available to them that they can make an informed decision. There are unlikely to be any variations to the operation under anaesthetic and therefore these do not have to be described as they do in some other operations, but the patient does need to have described to them the common complications and the serious ones (Table

Table 23.4 Check sheet – consent

Introduction – give your own name and competence to consent; check patient's name; explain what you are doing	
Background – check what they know and explore how much they want to know	
E	**what is wrong with the patient** – diagnosis
X	**what you are proposing to do** – defence to 'battery'
P	**the expected outcome** – short and long term
L	**choices of treatment** – including doing nothing
A	**variations** – alternatives that may be necessary while under anaesthetic (if sedation used)
I	**complications and risks** – of procedure: specific conditions, clear description and what action will be taken
N	**right of refusal** – the patient needs to know that the decision is theirs. They can also have time to think about it
Check understanding – ask the patient to review what has been discussed	
Open question to finish – e.g. Is there anything else you would like to discuss?	
Record – what was discussed and what was agreed	

23.4). In British law it is usually accepted that any complication more common than 1 per cent needs to be described to the patient. In the case of total hip replacement the risks are: dislocation (2–5 per cent), damage to the sciatic or femoral nerve (1–2 per cent), infection (1–2 per cent), fracture or penetration of the femur (1–2 per cent), death from any causes (< 1 per cent). The patient also needs to be warned that they may have an inequality of leg length after surgery.

The patient needs to be warned that they are likely to receive a blood transfusion during the operation.

Postoperative care

Most patients, especially males, are prone to urinary retention. If they are not catheterised at surgery then they should be carefully observed postoperatively. Nerve damage is one of the commoner complications. As soon as the patient awakes a check should be made that there is no damage to the nerves around the hip, especially the sciatic nerve. A simple test is to ask the patient to dorsiflex the foot. The patient should be carefully nursed to avoid flexion or adduction of the hip joint.

Revision of total hip replacment

A significant number of total hip replacements now coming to operation is revisions of primary total hip replacements which are loose. There are two main causes for loosening. The first is sepsis and the second is aseptic loosening (Fig. 23.12), possibly due to an inflammatory response secondary to particle wear. A hip replacement, which is becoming loose develops increasing pain. Septic loosening usually starts within months of the operation and the history may give a clue to the problem. The patient may have had a persistent discharge after surgery and pain relief may not have been complete. The organism involved is usually a low-grade pathogen such as *Staphylococcus epididymis*. The infection cannot be eradicated using antibiotics, but the symptoms may improve if adequate doses of the correct antibiotics are used. A needle aspiration of the synovial fluid may give a positive culture, but normally it is only at the time of surgery that the diagnosis can be made. It is now normal to send tissue for frozen section histology at the time of surgery. If signs of infection are seen in the histology then the implant is assumed to be loose because of infection.

Revision of the infected total hip replacement

If it has been decided from preoperative aspiration or from frozen section at surgery that the hip replacement is infected then further specimens of the membrane surrounding the hip need to be sent for formal culture. Then, and only then, should the patient be given the first dose of antibiotics. The infective organism is likely to be a *Staphylococcus* and so it is normal to give an antibiotic with good cover for this organism. Both femoral and acetabular components are removed with all the cement. The acetabulum and femoral canal are irrigated with saline and a further check is made that all foreign material and fibrous membrane have been removed. A decision must be made as to whether to insert gentamycin-inpregnated beads and to leave the patient on traction for 6 weeks without a hip joint to allow any infection to settle before inserting a new implant (a so-called 'two-stage revision'). The alternative is to replace the joint at the same operation (a 'one-stage' revision). Either way there is good evidence that the new implant should be put in using antibiotic-inpregnated cement as this reduces the likelihood of a recurrence of infection. A special revision implant may need to be used which may have a longer stem (Fig. 23.13).

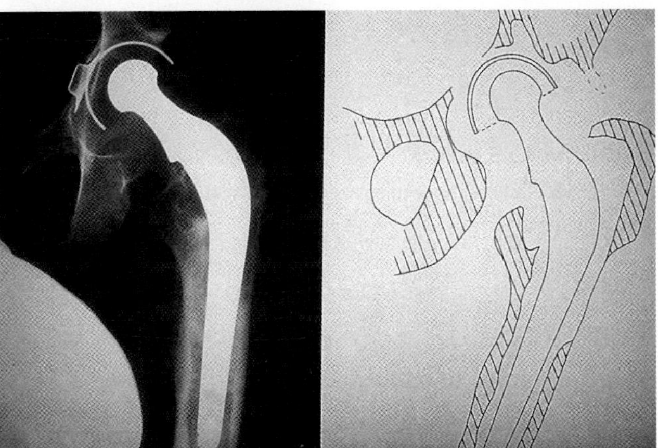

Fig. 23.12 Aseptic loosening of a total hip replacement. Diagram shows the extent of bone resorption.

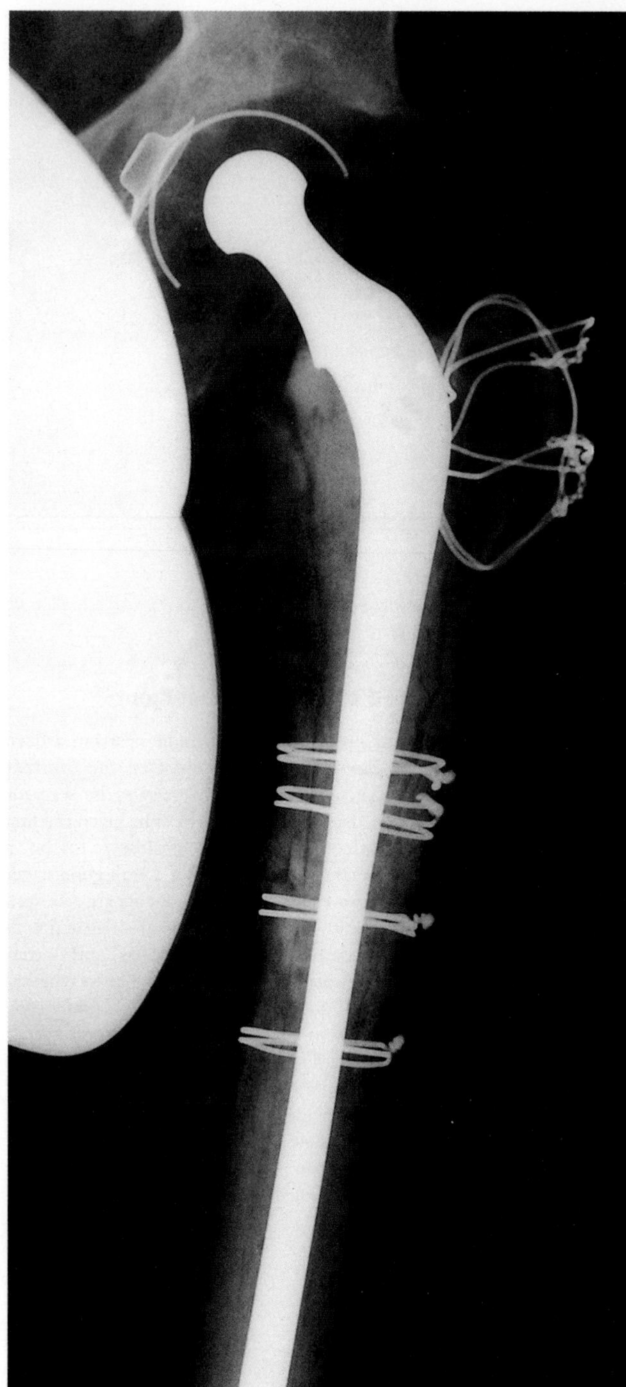

Fig. 23.13 Revision hip replacement using a very long stem to bridge a lytic area at the tip of the primary stem. Despite removal of the greater trochanter to improve access (wired back afterwards), the femur fractured at surgery and was fixed with cerclage wires during cementing.

Management of aseptic loosening

In this case a one-stage revision is performed. Some people would, nevertheless, use an antibiotic-inpregnated cement in case an occult infection had been missed. It is wise to take multiple bacteriological swabs of the membrane around the hip before prophylactic antibiotics are given. Postoperatively, there is a much higher risk of dislocation and it is normal to keep the patient in bed for several days and then to mobilise with great care. Before embarking on this operation patients need to be consented for the possibility that they may wake up without a hip replacement (the Girdlestone operation).

Fractures of the upper femur

Epidemiology

Fractures of the upper end of the femur are both common and serious. In children a slipped upper femoral epiphysis (a fracture of the epiphyseal plate) will lead to a lifetime of pain and disability. In adults a fracture of the upper end of the femur is a very high-velocity injury which is difficult to treat. In the elderly fractured neck of femur is the 'bread-and-butter' of orthopaedic trauma practice, with over 100 000 cases of fractured neck of femur each year in Britain alone.

Subcapital fractured neck of femur

This is a very common fracture in the elderly osteoporotic patient. The sclerosis produced by osteoarthritis tends to protect the patient from this fracture so the hip joint itself is usually healthy at the time of the accident. The problem with this fracture is that the majority of the blood supply to the femoral head travels up the femoral neck. A subcapital fractured neck of femur (Fig. 23.14) may destroy the blood supply to the femoral head. The older the patient, and the more displaced the fracture, the less likely the head is to recover its blood supply.

History

Some patients actually give a history of feeling the femur break and then falling as a result of this, while others appear to break the femur as a result of the fall. Either way, they complain of severe pain in the hip and are usually unable to walk.

Examination

The leg may appear shortened and externally rotated.

Investigation

On an AP X-ray the fracture may be difficult to see, but it will be shown more clearly on the lateral view as the head may displace posteriorly. On the AP X-ray the only clue to the presence of a fracture may be a discontinuity in the trabecular lines running up the femoral neck into the head.

Garthorne Robert Girdlestone, 1881–1950. Nuffield Professor of Orthopaedic Surgery, Oxford, England.

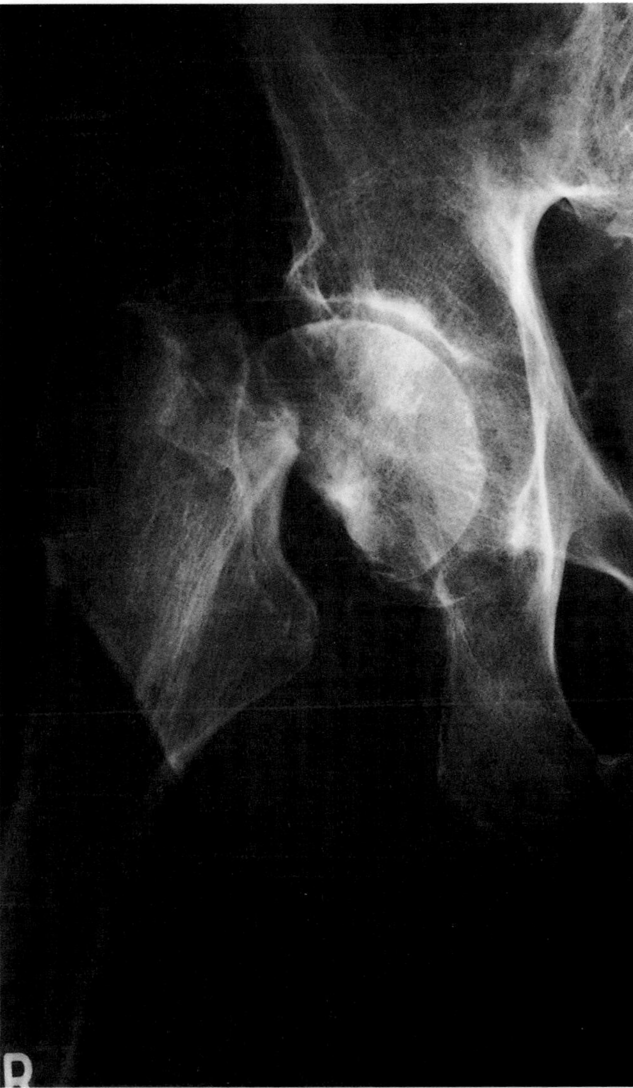

Fig. 23.14 Subcapital fractured neck of femur. Garden grade 3 – grossly displaced but not completely off-ended.

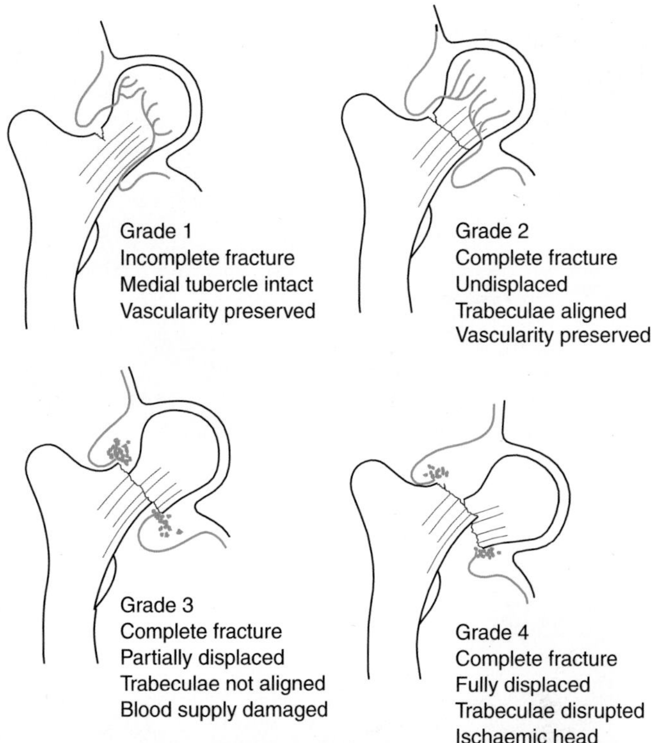

Fig. 23.15 Garden grading of subcapital fractured neck of femur.

Table 23.5 Treatment of grades of subcapital fractured neck of femur by approximate age

Age (years)	*Grade 1*	*Grade 2*	*Grade 3*	*Grade 4*
< 50	Pin *in situ*	Pin *in situ*	Reduce and pin	Total hip replacement or reduce with pin
50–70	Pin *in situ*	Pin *in situ*	Reduce and pin	Hemiarthroplasty
70–80	Pin *in situ*	Pin *in situ* or hemiarthroplasty	Hemiarthroplasty	Hemiarthroplasty
> 80	Hemiarthroplasty or pin *in situ*	Hemiarthroplasty or pin *in situ*	Hemiarthroplasty	Hemiarthroplasty

Treatment

The Garden classification divides these fractures into four grades (see Fig. 23.15 and Table 23.5):

- grade 1 is an incomplete fracture of the neck;
- grade 2 is a complete fracture of the neck without displacement;
- grade 3 has moderate displacement of less than half the diameter of the femoral neck;
- grade 4 is a complete off-ended femoral head as seen in the AP or lateral X-ray.

R.S. Garden. Former orthopaedic surgeon, Preston Royal Infirmary, England. Described his classification in the Journal of Bone and Joint Surgery *in 1961.*

If grade 1 or 2 fractures are left untreated they may rapidly displace and become grade 3 or 4.

In grade 1 fractures it is generally agreed, whatever the age group, that the treatment of choice is AO screws or other pins introduced up the femoral neck to hold the femoral head in position. In grade 4 fractures, whatever the age group, it is unlikely that the femoral head will survive. In patients under 50 years of age they should be taken to theatre as quickly as possible to reduce and pin the head as quickly as possible, and fix with screws (Fig. 23.16). The hope is that the femoral head will revascularise before it collapses. In patients older than this, the chance of survival of the femoral

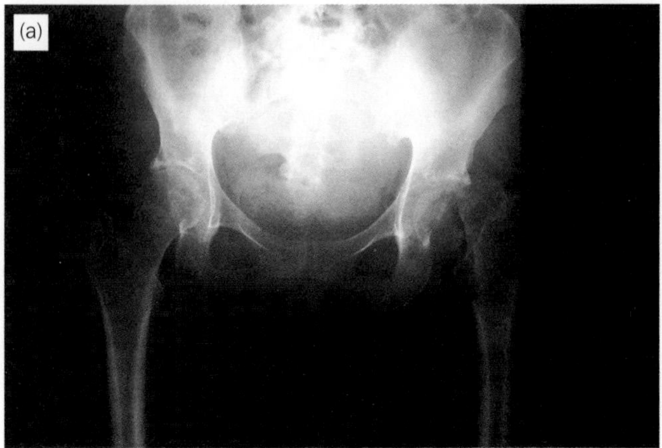

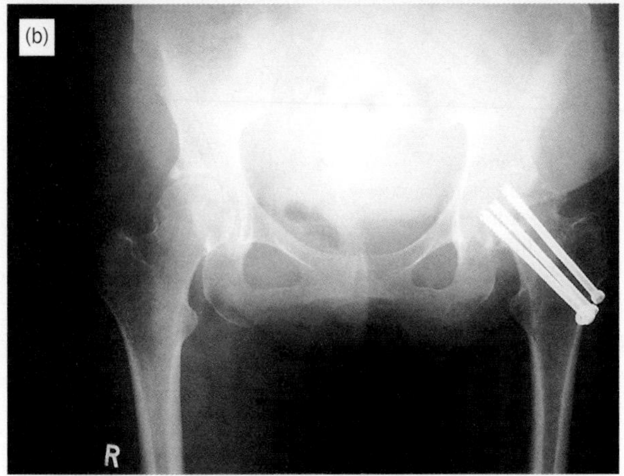

Fig. 23.16 Screws for undisplaced subcapital fractured neck of femur (*courtesy of Keith Willett*).

head is so low that it is best to replace it straight away. In young patients (under 65), a total hip replacement should be performed, but in older patients a hemiarthroplasty can be used. In the hemiarthroplasty the acetabulum with its normal articular cartilage is left alone but the patient's femoral head is replaced by an implant whose head has the same diameter as the head being removed. This articulates with the patient's normal acetabulum. The cemented variety of this implant is usually known as a 'Thompson' prosthesis; the uncemented variety is known as an 'Austin Moore' (Fig. 23.17). There is good evidence that the cemented hemiarthroplasty does better than the uncemented in the long term. In the older patient (with a life expectancy of 5 years or less) it is normal to go ahead and perform a hemiarthroplasty on patients with a Garden 2, 3 or 4 fracture. The risk of avascular necrosis is so high and the destruction of quality of life when this occurs so great, that it is simpler to sort out the problem in one go. The chance of the hemiarthroplasty giving the patient good function to the end of their days is high and so this is the operation of choice.

Frederick Roeck Thompson. Professor of Orthopaedic Surgery, New York Polyclinic Medical School, New York, USA.

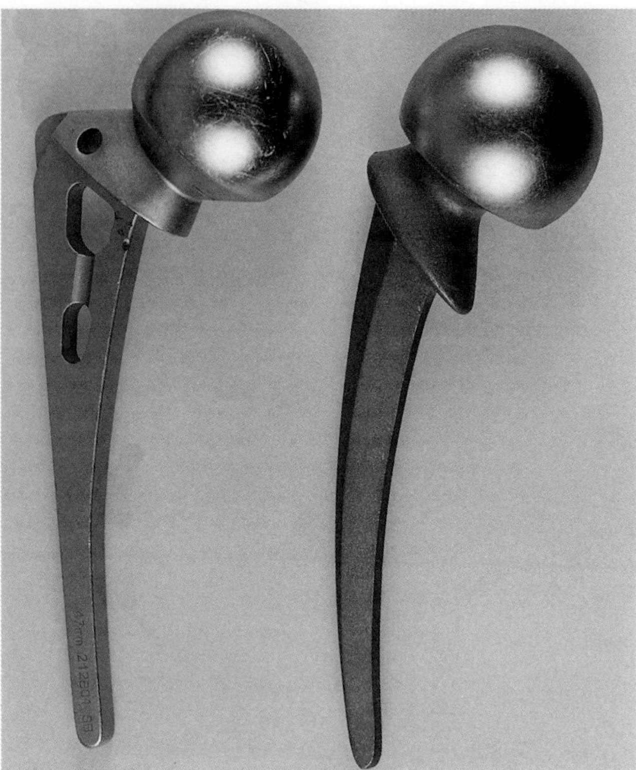

Fig. 23.17 Hemiarthroplasty for displaced subcapital fractured neck of femur. On the left is an Austin Moore (used uncemented), on the right the Thompson (cemented) prosthesis.

Problems

If the femoral head is retained reduction can be difficult to achieve and if pins are used they may displace into the acetabulum. Avascular necrosis is then a risk depending on the age of the patient, the degree of displacement and the time to reduction. If the head is replaced then dislocation, bleeding and infection are early complications, as well as damage to the nerves around the hip when replacing the joint. Late complications are loosening of the replacement, and sometimes the acetabulum can be eroded away by the implant, creating a protrusio-type arthritis (Figs 23.18 and 23.19).

Subcapital fractured neck of femur

- Common in osteoporosis
- Treatment depends on displacement and age
- Complication – avascular necrosis

Avascular necrosis of the hip

Epidemiology

Avascular necrosis is a rare but important problem in all age groups (Table 23.6). In the infant it may follow as a complication of septic arthritis, the pressure of the effusion denying the head of the femur its blood supply. In children, spontaneous avascular necrosis is called Perthes' disease. In adults it may be caused by steroids or heavy alcohol intake, and can occur in people who work in an environment which is at high pressure (divers or people who work in tunnels). It is also found

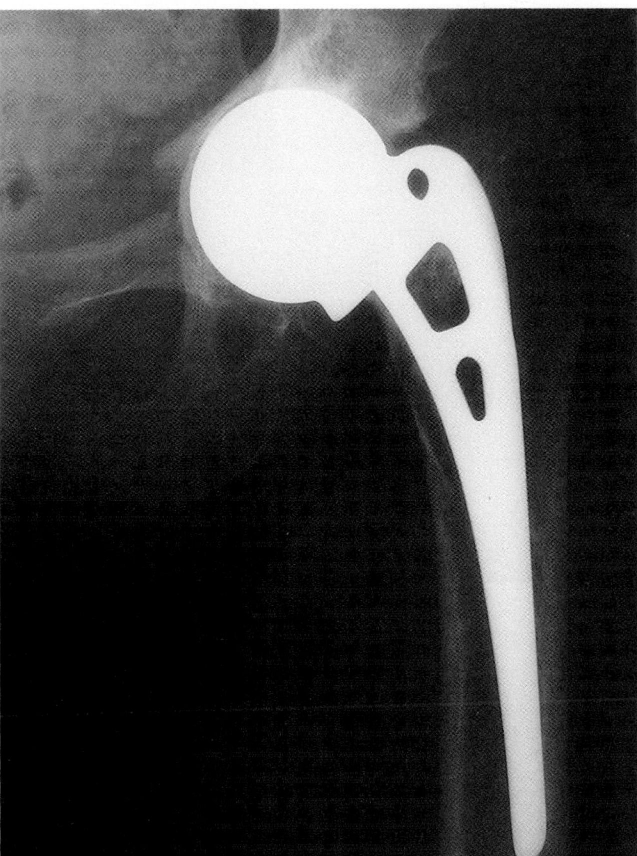

Fig. 23.18 Protrusion of a Thompson hemiarthroplasty in a patient with soft bone.

occurring spontaneously in patients with blood abnormalities such as sickle cell anaemia and thalassaemia. It is a very common problem in the elderly following a displaced subcapital fractured neck of femur. These are managed by replacing the dead femoral head with a hemiarthroplasty before the sequelae of avascular necrosis can develop.

Pathophysiology

The head of the femur is one of the areas of the body most susceptible to avascular necrosis. The underlying pathophysiology of the condition is not known but it is believed that the blood supply to the femoral head is lost either through thrombosis of the vessels entering the head or because of interosseous hypertension. The marrow of the femoral head becomes replaced with fat and the bone dies. Subsequently, there will be a zone of revascularisation which will be incomplete if the avascular area is large. Finally, there is a zone of reossification. During this period the joint is at risk of collapse. Once collapse has occurred full recovery is not possible and secondary arthritis sets in.

History

The patient may complain of sudden onset of pain in the hip or gradually increasing joint pain.

A careful family history will be needed to exclude sickle cell and thalassaemia. A social history should carefully cover alcohol intake, and a history of having worked underground or under water using high pressure. This exposure might have taken place some years before the onset of symptoms in the joint.

Medical history should specifically cover treatment with steroids.

Examination

On examination there may be nothing to find, except for a painful limitation of range of movement.

Investigation

Ultrasound may reveal a small effusion around the hip but X-rays are normal unless the avascular necrosis has been caused by a fracture. A radioisotope scan will show a dead area of the femoral head later surrounded by a hyperaemic area of revascularisation. Magnetic resonance imaging (MRI) may also show one or more avascular areas. If

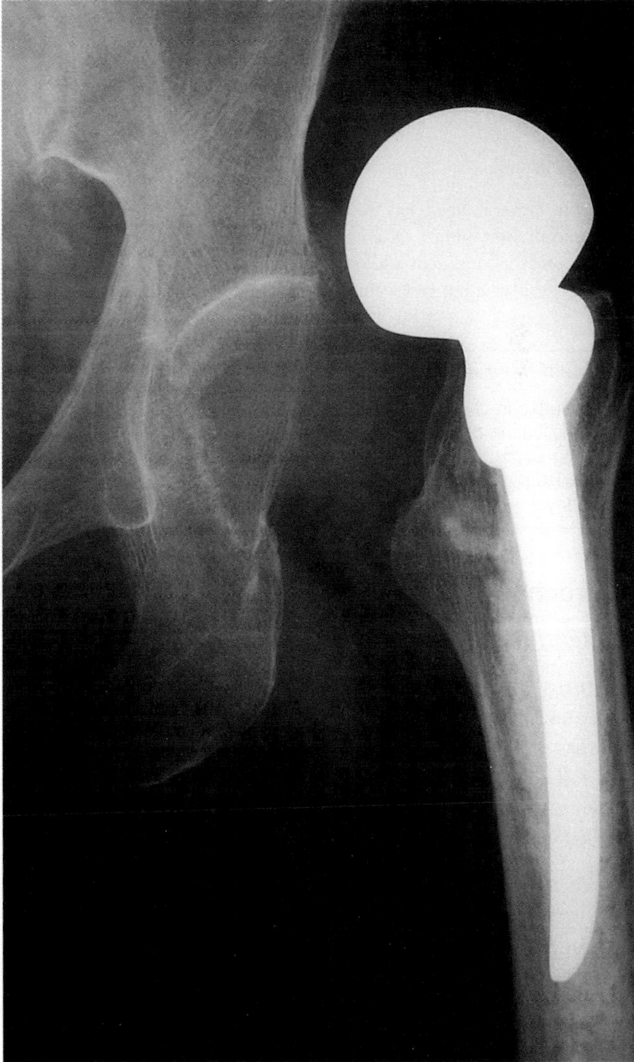

Fig. 23.19 Dislocated Thompson hemiarthroplasty (*courtesy of Keith Willett*).

Table 23.6 Causes of avascular necrosis

Congenital	Sickle cell anaemia, thalassaemia
Drug induced	Steroids, alcohol
Environmental	Caisson's disease (diving)
Trauma	Previous subcapital fracture
Infectious	Previous septic arthritis

any of these areas are in the weight-bearing part of the femoral head then there is a risk that the femoral head will collapse before revascularisation occurs. If this does occur, secondary osteoarthritis of the hip starts and a total hip replacement may be needed. If the diagnosis can be made early before the femoral head has collapsed, there is a chance of protecting the femoral head until it revascularises. This may prevent collapse.

Treatment

If the femoral head has not collapsed a 'forage' operation (where a core of bone is removed from the femoral neck and femoral head through a window in the lateral femoral cortex) can be used to decompress the femoral head. There is no clear evidence that this operation makes any difference to the natural history of avascular necrosis. If the avascular area is in the main weight-bearing area of the femoral head a further option is to perform an osteotomy. The head is rotated to bring a healthier part of the head into the main weight-bearing area of the hip joint to prevent collapse.

Problems

Once the femoral head has collapsed osteoarthritis is inevitable, with pronounced shortening as the hip collapses followed by stiffness as the joint becomes incongruent and osteoarthritis sets in. The options then are an arthrodesis or a hip replacement. Osteotomy is unlikely to help at this stage.

Avascular necrosis

- Idiopathic in children = Perthes' disease
- Complication of alcohol and steroids in adults
- Complication of sickle cell and thalassaemia in all ages
- Avoided by hemiarthroplasty following subcapital fracture in the elderly

Pertrochanteric fractured neck of femur

Epidemiology

Fractures through the trochanters of the femur are as common as subcapital fractured neck of femur. They can occur in patients with osteoarthritis of the hip and are caused by a trip or a fall on to the hip.

Pathophysiology

Unlike subcapital fractures these can occur in association with arthritis of the hip. In the younger adult they can occur with high-velocity trauma.

History

The patient complains of sudden severe onset of pain in the hip and is unable to weight-bear.

Examination

On examination the leg is often short and internally rotated.

Treatment

The fracture is highly unstable (Fig. 23.20) and the patient cannot mobilise until it has been stabilised. This fracture can be managed on traction but it is very difficult to reduce the

(a)

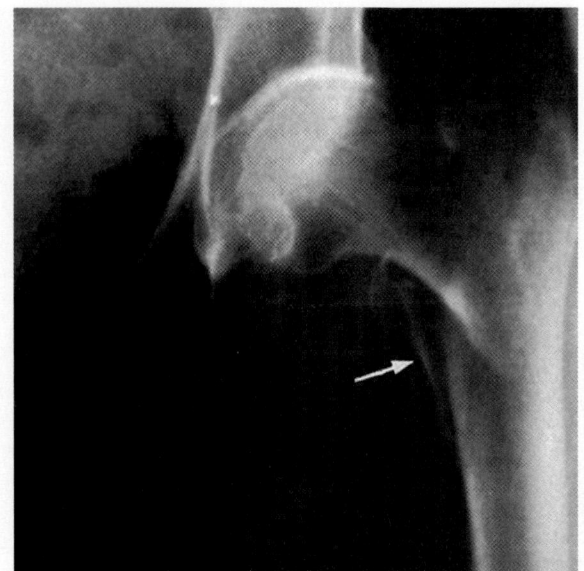

(b)

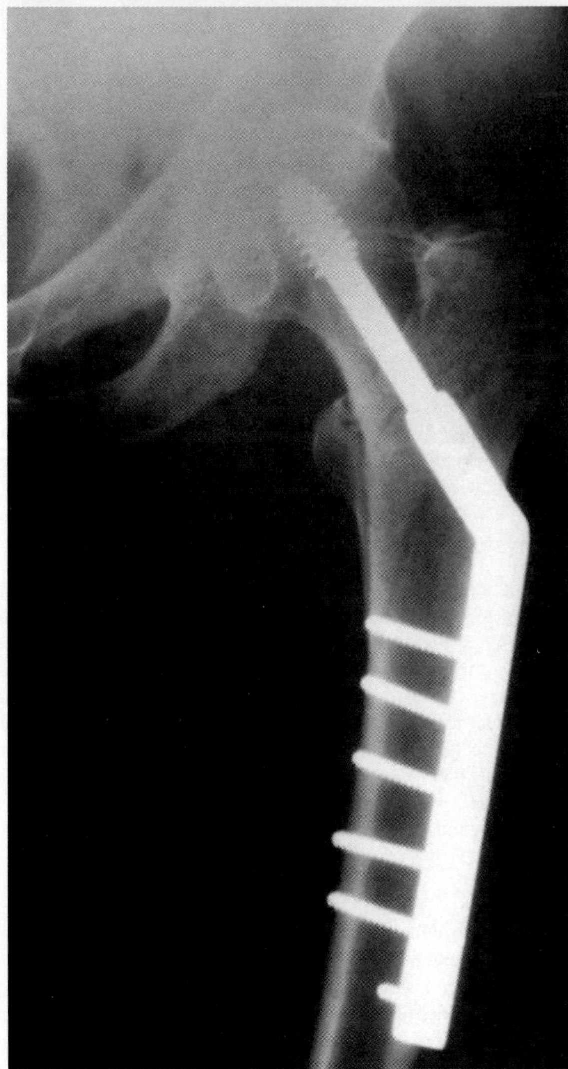

Fig. 23.20 (a) Pertrochanteric fractured neck of femur. (b) Dynamic hip screw for treatment.

fragments and the patient would need to in bed for a minimum of 12–18 weeks.

The patient is usually very elderly and this length of time in bed would destroy their sense of independence and put them at risk for developing hypostatic pneumonia, urinary tract infection and bed sores. The blood supply of the femoral head is not affected by this fracture and therefore avascular necrosis is not a problem. However, the fracture requires a very strong fixation because of the enormous forces which go through the hip. The dynamic hip screw (DHS) is made up of two parts which can slide in relation to each other but do not allow binding (Fig. 23.20). The first part is a heavy-duty plate which is fixed to the lateral cortex of the femur with cortical screws. The second part is a rod which passes up through a slot in the plate into the femoral neck. Its threaded end crosses the fracture line to engage and hold the femoral head. As the patient weight-bears on the healing fracture the broken ends of the bone collapse into each other and compress the fracture. The sliding-rod mechanism of the DHS allows this to happen without allowing the hip to fall into varus. This prevents the plate breaking at the fracture, or indeed the rod penetrating through into the femoral head and acetabulum.

Problems

Some fractures are difficult to reduce and can result in poor placement of the DHS. If this happens the fixation will fail, and the fracture collapses into a painful nonunion which is difficult to reconstruct.

> Pertrochanteric fractured neck of femur
>
> - Common in the elderly
> - Does not cause avascular necrosis
> - Nonoperative treatment is slow and difficult
> - A dynamic hip screw (DHS) allows compression while providing a secure fix allowing immediate mobilisation

Operative procedure. Dynamic hip screw for intertrochanteric fracture

The patient is anaesthetised and then carefully placed on a well-padded orthopaedic table with the leg to be operated on extended on traction applied to the foot by a boot (Fig. 23.21). Countertraction comes from a post in the patient's groin. The opposite leg is bent up and abducted as far as possible to allow an image intensifier to be placed in between the patient's legs. This allows the operator to see AP and lateral pictures of the hip. The patient must be firmly anchored to the operating table as it easy for the patient to roll off. The operation must not begin until both the surgeon and the anaesthetist are satisfied that the patient is secure, and the radiographer is satisfied that she or he can obtain clear pictures AP and lateral of the femoral head and the upper femur. Under image intensifier control the fracture is reduced using the traction boot to control the rotation and traction on the lower leg. Ideally, the fracture is fully reduced and the femoral neck set horizontal by slight internal rotation of the lower leg to correct for femoral neck anteversion. In very unstable fractures closed reduction is not possible and further reduction will be needed once the hip has been exposed. Through a small lateral incision over the greater trochanter a guide wire is introduced through the lateral femoral cortex, up the femoral neck and into the femoral head. The wire is introduced on a jig at a fixed angle of 135° to the femoral shaft. It is crucial to get this wire properly positioned by checking both AP and lateral views. The wire should be central or, if that is not achievable, it should err on the side of being in the lower and anterior quadrant of the hip where the bone is strongest. Once the wire is properly positioned, a measuring device is used to determine the length of screw which will need to be used. The cannulated drill is set to produce a drill hole of the correct length. Using the prepositioned wire as a guide, and under image intensifier control, the drill is passed up across the fracture and close to but not through the subchondral bone. The hole is measured again and then tapped (a thread cut into it), and a DHS is inserted until its tip lies just beneath subchondral bone of the femoral head. It is important that this screw lies in the centre of the femoral head. A blade is then fitted on to the back of the screw where it protrudes out to the lateral femoral cortex. This plate is then fixed on to the distal femur using cortical screws. A check X-ray is taken at the end of the operation to show that the plate and sliding screw are correctly positioned. The patient is mobilised the following day and encouraged to put weight through the hip so that the fracture ends are driven together.

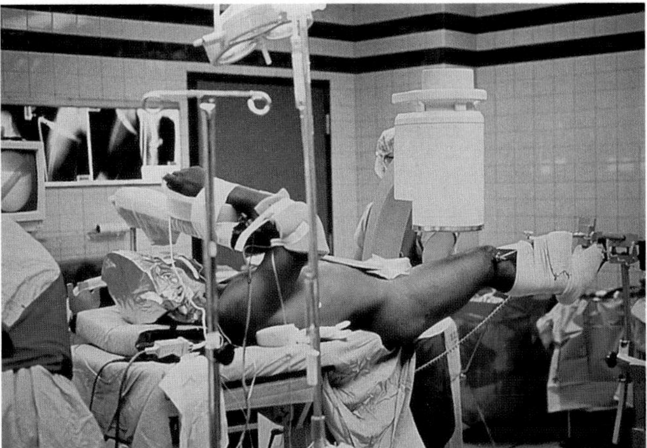
Fig. 23.21 Patient on the orthopaedic table prior to draping.

The commonest errors in this operation are to fail to obtain good views on the X-ray before starting, and to insert the screw before the fracture is properly reduced.

Prognosis. The mortality after hemiarthroplasty for subcapital fractured neck of femur and DHS for trochanteric fractures in the elderly is high, with as many as 25 per cent of the patients dead within 6 months. This is in part because these fractures occur in a very elderly age group but is also because the fractures may be one part of a terminal illness. There are also likely to be difficulties in getting these patients out of hospital unless there is a very active team in the community whose task it is to provide suitable accommodation for these patients. For many of them the fracture is the straw that breaks the camel's back, so that those who were living alone now need to move to sheltered accommodation while those who are in sheltered accommodation may need to move into a home. The chance of a patient surviving and of returning to their previous accommodation is most strongly affected not by their physical state but by their mental state. Demented patients carry a bad prognosis.

Subtrochanteric fracture of the femur

Epidemiology

This is a rare fracture and a difficult one to manage (Fig. 23.22).

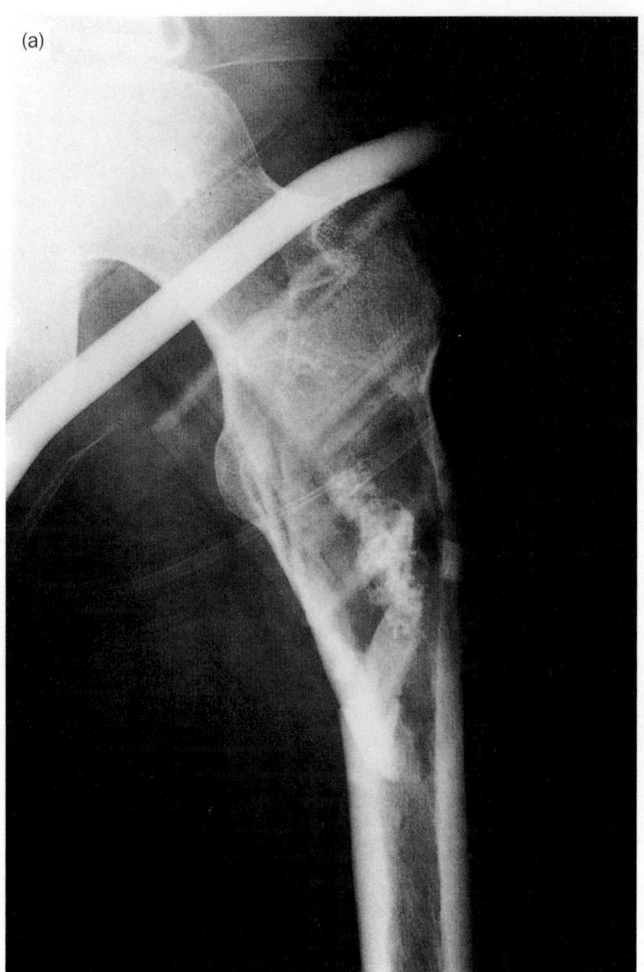

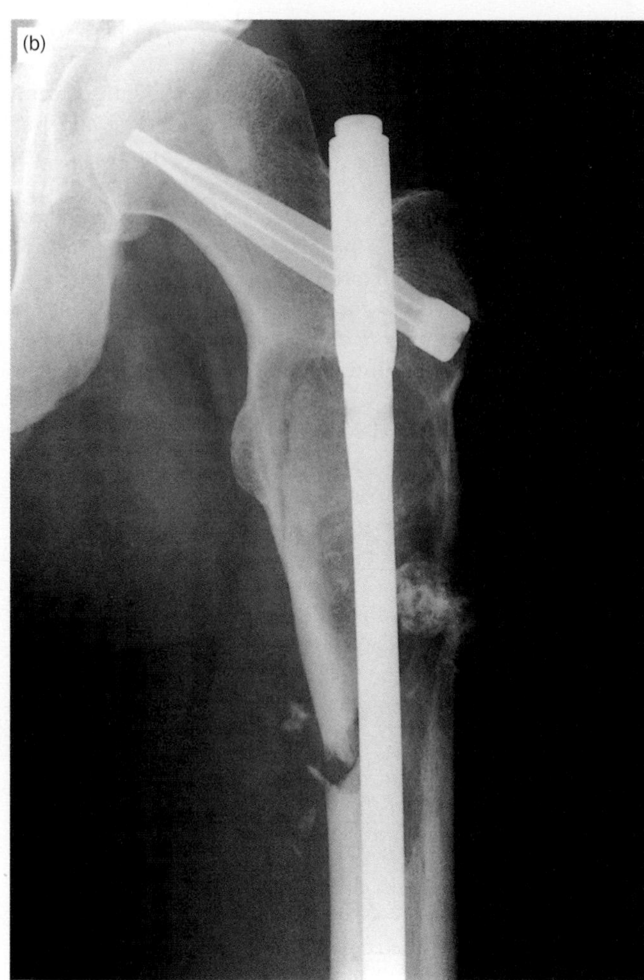

Fig. 23.22 Subtrochanteric fractured neck of femur (a) before and (b) after nail fixation (*courtesy of Keith Willett*).

Pathophysiology

This fracture tends to be a high-velocity fracture or a pathological fracture through a lytic lesion.

History

Because of its pathophysiology it is important to check for other injuries or a history of pain elsewhere.

Examination

The presentation is similar to a fractured neck of femur with pain in the upper thigh and shortening. The leg is short and may be rotated. A careful check should be made for distal neurovascular status.

Investigation

X-rays will be needed of the fracture and the whole length of the femur in case there are any other fractures. In pathological fractures a bone scan will help to identify silent lesions which may profoundly affect the treatment. Many surgeons routinely X-ray the opposite femur. If there are lytic lesions in one femur there are probably some in the other too.

Treatment

The proximal fragment tends to be drawn into flexion by the powerful muscles around the hip and there is no form of traction or plaster which can stabilise the fragments or bring them into good alignment. The thick layer of soft tissue covering the bones in this area also makes an external fixator difficult to use. A plate with a blade inserted into the femoral neck to provide proximal stability can be used, but if the medial cortex is deficient, as it usually is, then the plate may bend and break before the fracture unites (Fig. 23.23). If an intramedullary nail is to be used, the nail needs to be very strong and to have an attachment device which serves to fix it to the proximal femur and femoral neck. It will also need to be locked distally. Nails as strong as this also tend to be stiff so are difficult to insert without causing further damage to the femur. The trauma to the patient is also considerable and, in the case of patients with pathological fractures secondary to malignant disease, there is a high risk of pulmonary embolus on the operating table. Anticoagulation will need to be used with care as blood loss is another major complication of this surgery.

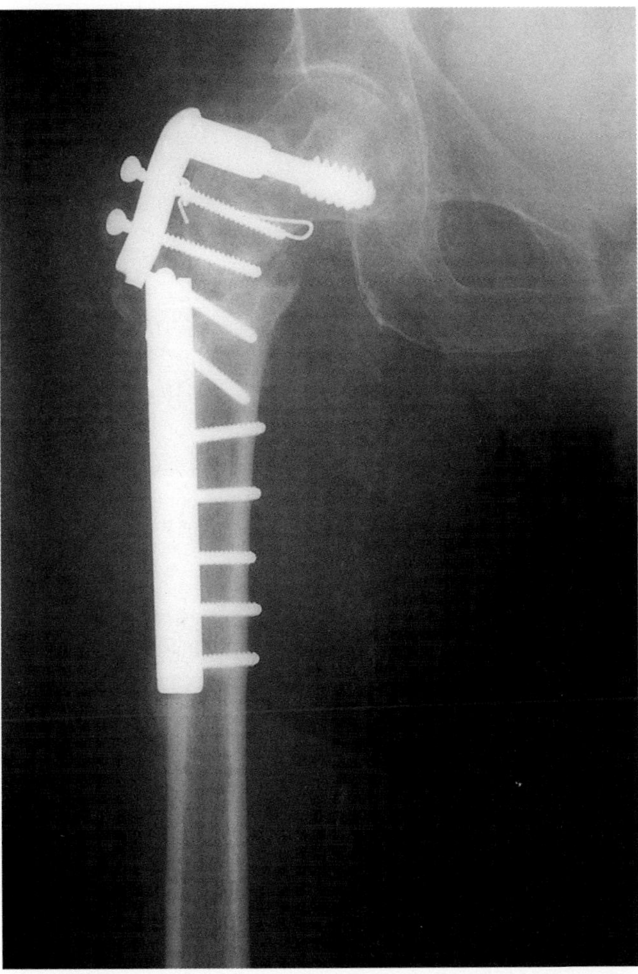

Fig. 23.23 Failed fixation of the fracture. The plate fatigued before the fracture could unite.

Problems

This is a difficult fracture in which to obtain stable fixation. A long-plated DHS may be difficult to apply, while a heavy-duty reconstruction nail carries a high risk of exploding the femur in inexperienced hands. Nerve damage may also result if the fracture is distracted when driving the nail.

> Subtrochanteric fracture of the femur
>
> - High-velocity or pathological fracture
> - Nonoperative treatment commonly leads to malunion
> - A reconstruction nail is the best treatment but is difficult to use safely

Fractures of the shaft of the femur

Fractures of the shaft of the femur can occur in any age group. In young children the spiral fracture of the femur is one of the fractures which occurs commonly in nonaccidental injury but rarely at any other time. The force required to cause a spiral fracture of a child's femur is so great that it is unlikely that the child can exert this force by falling. In the adult a shaft fracture of femur is usually associated with a high-energy injury such as a motorcycle crash. In the elderly this fracture is again associated with pathological fractures secondary to a lytic lesion. It is unusual for this fracture to be associated with neurovascular damage, but in a high-velocity accident in a young adult this must always be born in mind.

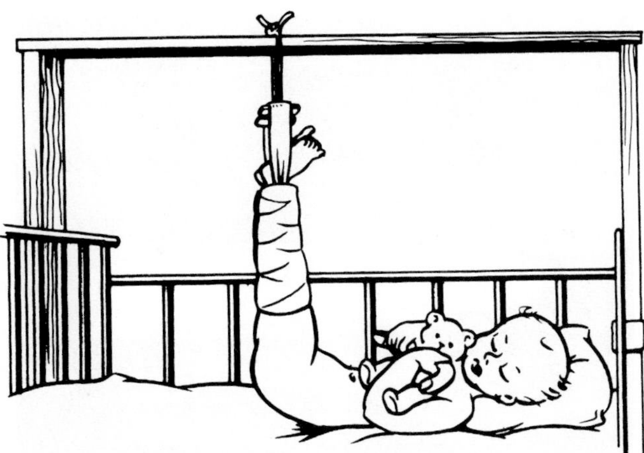

Fig. 23.24 A 'gallows' splint. Traction is applied by means of strapping, and the legs are slung up to the cross-piece so that the pelvis is just lifted from the mattress (a position which is very convenient for nursing purposes). The child's weight acts as countertraction. Alternatively, children of this age can be treated in a plaster spica.

> Causes of fractures of the shaft of the femur
>
> - In children, may be nonaccidental injury
> - In adolescents, usually high-velocity injury
> - In the elderly, may be pathological

Treatment in children

This fracture heals very quickly in children and the fracture can be stabilised with nonoperative means (Fig. 23.24). In children under the age of 2 years, vertical skin traction can be used to hang the legs off the bed. Static traction can be used and the legs raised until the child's bottom is floating just off the bed. Surprisingly, the children do not find this traction uncomfortable and nursing is easy. It is easy to tell when the fracture has united as the child starts spinning around and hanging off the bed by its legs. In the young child the femur is capable of considerable remodelling, so a perfect reduction is not necessary.

> Treatment of fractured shaft of femur
>
> - In infants – gallows traction
> - In children and adolescents – balanced traction
> - In adults and the elderly – locked nail

Treatment of the fractured shaft of femur in the child before epiphyseal closure

If there is still growth potential in the femur then internal fixation should be avoided as this may cause damage to the epiphyseal growth plate. The

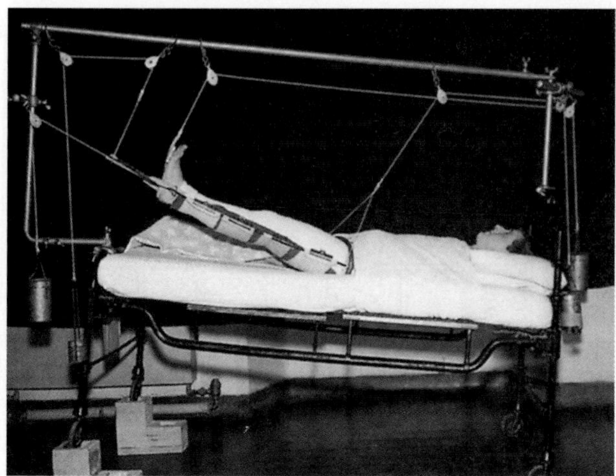

Fig. 23.25 Fixed traction applied with a Thomas splint and adhesive strapping to the skin. Hinges at the knee convert a Thomas splint into a Fisk and allow early mobilisation of the knee joint.

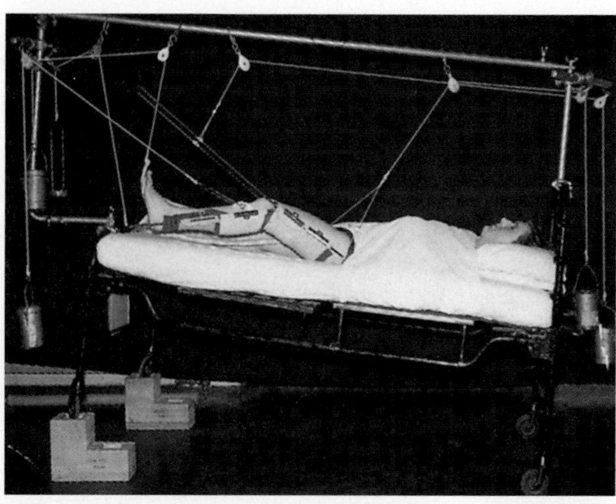

Fig. 23.26 The principal elements of sliding traction: traction and countertraction. Hamilton Russell dynamic traction means that the patient can move around in the bed.

majority of growth in the femur occurs in the distal epiphysis, but nevertheless both should be protected if at all possible. A fractured femur in an adolescent can be managed on Hamilton Russell balanced traction or on static traction using a Thomas splint, but in this case it is wise to use a Fisk hinged knee piece to allow early mobilisation of the knee joint to prevent stiffness in the knee (Fig. 23.25). If traction is applied through a tibial pin, care must be taken not to apply the traction for too long as there is a risk of causing stretching of the ligaments around the knee. This produces a permanently lax and unstable knee (a frame knee). As soon as the fracture is sticky, there may be place for taking the child off traction and putting the leg into a cast brace with knee hinges so that they can start mobilising. Great care must be taken to watch that the femur does not fall into varus at this stage. Initially, weekly check X-rays will be needed.

Treatment of fractured femur in the adult

Traction for fractured mid-shaft femur can also be used in the adult but requires that the patient stay in bed for 12–16 weeks. Once the fracture has been settled into a satisfactory position there is no reason why the last weeks of this traction should not be carried on at home where the patient can be nursed by his or her family (Fig. 23.26). Traction may also offer some advantages when the fracture is open and the femur heavily contaminated. There will inevitably be an increased risk of infection if plating or an intramedullary nail is used, and it may be advisible to leave the patient on traction at least for a few days until the wound has settled down. However, this is not an excuse for failing to be aggressive about removing all contaminated tissue from the wound at the time of the accident (débridement). The wound should be left open, and re-exploring and clearing away of dead or contaminated tissue should continue until the wound is clean. An external fixator can be applied to the lateral side of the femur to stabilise the fracture but the thick muscles overlying the bone can produce problems with pin tract infections. Internal fixation of the femur can be performed either with a plate or with an intramedullary nail.

If a plate is to be used then it should be very heavy duty and the exposure will need to be extensive, as there will need to be at least four holes for fixation of the plate above the fracture and four holes below the fracture. If the fracture is spiral then lag screws will need to be placed to draw the fragments together, either through or separate from the plate. If the medial cortex is deficient then this will need to be buttressed with bone graft and great care will need to be taken when mobilising the femur as the plate will be vulnerable to bending loads. The femoral shaft is ideally suited to an intramedullary nail which, if the equipment and expertise is available, can be introduced closed from the proximal end and then locked both proximally and distally. This will give adequate stability to both bending and rotation forces to allow the patient to weight-bear immediately (partial weight-bearing if it is an unreamed nail) and to leave hospital as soon as they have recovered from the surgery and are able to walk safely. The operation must be performed with great care as the complication rate even in the best hands is high. The common complications are listed in Table 23.7.

Table 23.7 Common complications of femoral nailing

- Nerve damage due to overdistraction of the fracture when driving down the nail
- Breakage of the flexible reamers
- Problems with the guidewire being driven down into the knee
- Nails being put in the driver too long or too short
- Breakage of the femur while inserting the nail
- Getting the nail jammed in the femur
- Failure to get the locking screws through the holes in the nail
- Malrotation of the femur
- Infection

Hugh Owen Thomas, 1834–91. Surgeon, Liverpool, England. Although he never held a hospital appointment, preferring to attend patients in their homes, he is regarded as the founder of orthopaedic surgery. He introduced his splint in 1875.

Alternatives to intramedullary nailing

A simpler alternative to intramedullary nailing is the use of rush pins introduced through the lateral and/or medial condyles of the femur. Rush pins are flexible rods which can be passed into the femur through a small skin incision at the knee and which are slightly curved so that by twisting them they can be used to cross the fracture site and pass up into the femoral neck. The femur can be stacked with rush nails until a relatively tight fixation is obtained. Four or five rush nails passed up the femur are not as strong as an intramedullary nail and are particularly poor at controlling rotation. They do, however, prevent translation at the fracture site but do not prevent impaction. Although they are relatively simple to insert they do tend to back out, and a patient should certainly not be encouraged to more than toe touch with the leg until the fracture has started to unite.

Metastases in the femur which have not yet fractured

Wherever possible, secondaries in the femur or any other long bone should be referred to an orthopaedic department before the pathological fracture occurs. They are much easier to manage at this stage than they are after the fracture has occurred through the lytic lesion. It is said that the femur is at imminent risk of pathological fracture if a lytic lesion has eroded more than half the thickness of the cortex or there is erosion over more than 2 cm of the cortex. If either of these signs is present then immediate action needs to be taken to stabilise the femur before it breaks. Before embarking on surgery X-rays should be taken of the whole length of both femurs as there is likely to be more than one metastatic lesion and this may affect the choice of surgery. The purpose of the surgery is to fix the bones so that they do not break, so that the last weeks or months of the patient's life are not spent in pain and disabled. However, the patient must be warned of the risks of the surgery which are high (particularly death from pulmonary embolus). As soon as the bones are fixed the patient can be transferred back to medical care for radiotherapy or cytotoxic drugs, depending on the most appropriate management.

Indications for prophylactic fixing of lytic lesions in the femur

- 50 per cent of the cortex eroded
- > 2 cm invaded
- Check for other lesions

Supracondylar fractures of the femur

Supracondylar fractures occur in young adults involved in very high-energy accidents or in the elderly who fall awkwardly. There are many different patterns of fracture, but not uncommonly a fracture line enters the knee joint through the intercondylar notch creating an unstable Y-shaped fracture. The X-rays may be difficult to interpret because the fracture line down into the knee joint may be hidden behind the patella but a careful check must be made for this as it alters the surgery required. In the elderly neurovascular compromise is unusual, but in the young high-velocity accident the popliteal vessels and nerves lie close to the fracture and may easily be damaged.

The nonoperative management of the supracondylar fracture of the femur

This fracture is normally unstable. It is too close to the knee joint to manage in plaster and even in traction the distal fragment tends to flex. If it is not possible to move the knee early the gastrocnemius tends to become tethered down to the fracture site and permanent stiffness in the knee results. The nonoperative management of the supracondylar fracture therefore tends to end with a malunion and a stiff knee.

Operative management of supracondylar fractures

Special plates have been designed for the management of supracondylar fractures, and it is a fracture where preoperative planning, of drawing out of the fragments on tracing paper and then fitting templates to the reduced fragments allows a logical operation to be designed.

If there is an intercondylar fracture this may need to be fixed first with large lag screws and then a blade plate introduced to attach the distal fragment to the proximal. Bone grafting may be needed on the medial side if there is a defect. Internal fixation allows early mobilisation of the knee but weight-bearing may need to be protected with a cast brace until union has been achieved.

Supracondylar and intracondylar fractures of femur

- Check carefully for extra fracture lines
- Nonoperative treatments lead to malunion and stiffness
- Plan surgery with templates drawn on to tracings of X-rays
- Mobilise early

The knee

The knee does not feature prominently in children's orthopaedics, but commonly poses problems in adolescents with anterior knee pain otherwise known as chondromalacia patellae. Subluxation and dislocation of the patella may also start to cause problems at this age. In the young adult problems with the knee are exceptionally important. All contact sports and high demand sports, such as skiing, produce a rich crop of sports injuries. Rheumatoid arthritis affects the knee in the later stages just as it affects the hip, and in the elderly osteoarthritis of the knee is as common as osteoarthritis of the hip, and within the next few years total knee replacement may become as common an operation as total hip replacement. Certainly, it is already quite as successful.

History of knee injury

The history of an accident can be divided into three types: acute extrinsic, the patient was struck on the knee; acute intrinsic, something snapped or gave way in the knee; and chronic, where the onset was gradual and not related to any specific event. Each of these kinds of history is related to a completely different diagnosis (Table 23.8).

Table 23.8 Differential diagnosis according to type of history

Type of history	*Differential diagnosis*
Acute extrinsic	Tibial plateau fracture
Acute intrinsic	Torn mensiscus, dislocated patella, torn ligaments
Chronic	Anterior knee pain, Osgood–Schlatter disease, jumper's knee, plica, arthritis

Robert B. Osgood, b. 1873. American surgeon.
Carl Schlatter, b. 1864. Swiss surgeon.

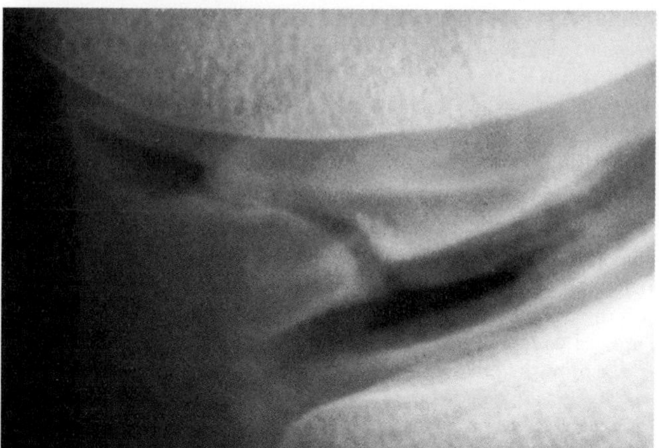

Fig. 23.27 Arthrogram of torn meniscus using contrast showing a clear split in the meniscus.

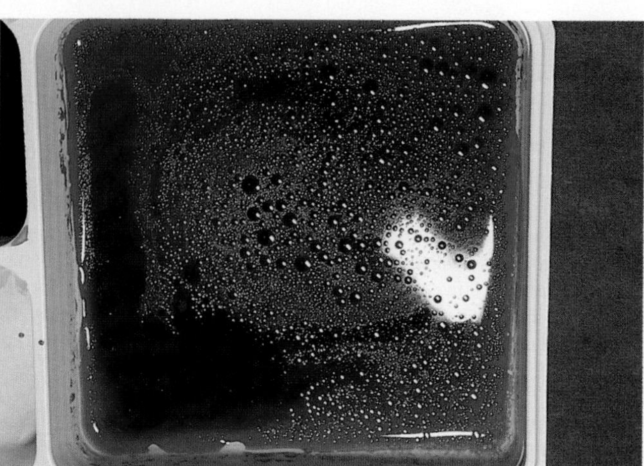

Fig. 23.28 Fat in aspirate from a haemarthrosis of the knee indicates that an intra-articular fracture has occurred.

Investigation for torn meniscus

A torn meniscus only shows up on X-ray if dye is used (an arthrogram – see Fig. 23.27). It also shows up very well on MRI. The investigation of choice is therefore MRI. If, however, the history is absolutely clear of mechanical locking, then arthroscopy is the investigation of choice, as it is going to be necessary anyway and it allows treatment to be undertaken at the same time. If, however, the diagnosis is in doubt than a noninvasive investigation such as MRI is the first line of investigation, the only problem being that interpretation of the MRI can be difficult and there is an incidence of false positives.

Osteochrondritis of the knee

A small flake fracture of the articular surface of the knee is also possible after a twisting injury. The presentation is very similar to a torn meniscus and plain X-rays may miss the diagnosis unless the defect is silhouetted in one of the views. Both MRI and CT scan are used in making the diagnosis, but arthroscopy can miss it because unless the whole of the articular surface is carefully probed the actual defect may be invisible from the surface and systematic probing of the whole articular surface will be needed to find the actual defect. If the fragment is small and breaks away into the joint it may cause mechanical locking and needs to be removed. If it is large then an attempt should be made to replace it using a recessed screw, buried pins or some kind of bone glue. If it is not felt to be possible to replace the fragment some people drill the base of the defect to stimulate healing by providing a blood supply to the damaged area, but the cartilage will only be replaced by fibrocartilage which has poor wear properties.

Ruptured anterior cruciate ligament

This is an epidemic in modern sport. It occurs when a very high twisting force is applied to the bent knee. If contact sports did not allow the use of studs on boots the injury would probably almost disappear. It is only when the foot is fixed firmly to the ground and the body continues to twist fast on it that the injury is inevitable. The patient often hears a loud crack in the knee and collapses. They cannot play on both because the pain is severe and because the knee swells rapidly and is unstable. The other common cause for an acute haemarthrosis following an acute intrinsic injury to the knee is dislocation of the patella. A careful history and examination will distinguish the two conditions. In patella dislocation the patient may have noticed something out of place immediately after the accident or have had the problem before. Sometimes the patella remains dislocated.

Aspiration of the joint will produce a dramatic reduction of pain. If there are fat globules in the aspirate then a fracture must be suspected as marrow has escaped into the joint (Fig. 23.28).

Treatment of the ruptured anterior cruciate ligament

In the child the anterior cruciate avulses with a fragment of bone. It is relatively simple to fix this fragment back into the tibia either with a bone screw or with sutures passed through to the front of the tibia. In the adult the anterior cruciate tears its central part, where there is no capacity to heal. This does not necessarily mean that surgery to substitute the ligament is required. In a significant number of patients intense physiotherapy rebuilds the control of the knee to levels where the absence of an anterior cruciate does not hamper performance. In other patients whose performance is compromised by an anterior cruciate-deficient knee it is a perfectly valid option for the patient decide to modify their lifestyle to cope with their disability. For example, they may decide that the time has come to give up contact sport. It is only after these first two options have been exhausted that the possibility of performing surgery to substitute for the anterior cruciate ligament should even be considered. Even then the surgery is complex, the rehabilitation is difficult and there is no evidence in the long term that functionally the knee maintains any greater stability, or that reconstruction protects the knee from osteoarthritis. There is also now good evidence that some of the synthetic ligaments used are not strong enough for the loads exerted on them and break up in the knee. If they do so the debris may cause an inflammatory arthritis. Finally, it is very difficult to make sure that the substitute ligament has the right biomechanical properties and is correctly positioned to give a stable knee without causing stiffness. A substitute ligament cannot have a proprioceptive function in the knee, a role that some people feel is one important facet of the anterior cruciate ligament's role.

As the ligament does not heal, the alternatives are either to realign the structures outside the knee to prevent the instability caused by anterior cruciate deficiency or a second possibility is to take a ligament from elsewhere in the patient and route it through the track of the anterior cruciate to re-create the function of the ligament. A third option is to put in a synthetic ligament. A ligamentous augmentation device (LAD) is a synthetic ligament which in itself is not strong or elastic enough to undertake the function of an anterior cruciate but combined with tendon material from the patient is supposed to perform this function.

Extra-articular repair

The Macintosh operation involves reefing the lateral dynamic structures of the knee. It pulls back on the lateral tibial plateau in flexion in an attempt to stop it sliding forward in a uncontrolled way (the pivot shift), which makes the knee so unstable in twisting and turning.

Intra-articular repair

Intra-articular repairs can be performed either through the arthroscope or open. The Jone's repair involves freeing the proximal end of the middle third of the patella tendon and rerouting this tendon through the knee along the line of the anterior cruciate. Semitendinosus tendon can be used in a similar way or a synthetic tendon can be inserted. The key issue surgically is to make sure that the origin and insertion of this new ligament are in the correct place to allow free movement of the knee without undue laxity.

Posterior cruciate

A posterior cruciate tear is commonly associated with a hyperextension injury and disruption of the posterior structures of the knee (Fig. 23.29). Treatment of the knee in a plaster usually allows the posterior capsule to heal up. There is then little functional disability despite the fact that the posterior cruciate does not heal.

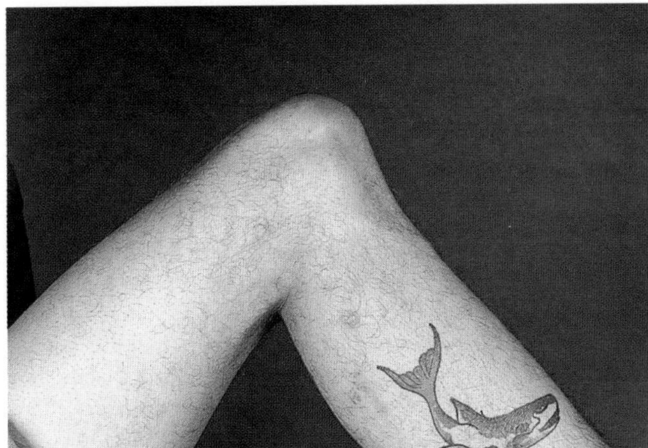

Fig. 23.29 Ruptured posterior cruciate ligament. The tibia lies back on the femur and can be drawn forward from there (a paradoxical anterior draw test).

Rupture of the medial collateral ligament

Ruptures of the medial collateral ligament occur when the leg is forced into valgus usually by a blow on the outside of the leg. With moderate trauma there is usually only a tear of the short cruciate ligament. If the force is greater then the medial collateral ligament disrupts. The knee is grossly unstable when stressed into valgus. If on X-ray a flake of bone can be seen avulsed from the femur then reattachment using a screw is relatively straightforward. The medial collateral ligament inserts into the tibia well below the knee joint and avulsion in this area can also be repaired surgically by suturing the tendon back. Midsubstance tears at the level of a joint are more difficult to repair, and surgery is not necessary. A cast brace for 6 weeks allowing for flexion of the knee but protecting it from valgus forces will encourage good healing.

Anterior knee pain – chondromalacia patellae

This condition tends to start in the teens and is more common in girls than in boys. It may follow an injury to the knee, particularly a dislocation of the kneecap. The patient gives a history that they have pain on stairs, particularly going down stairs when the knee may actually feel unsafe. They also experience severe pain when sitting for any length of time. When they try to move after the knee has been still for a while the pain may be so severe that the knee feels locked. This is not true mechanical locking. It seems to be more to do with synovial inflammation. On examination, there may be some quadriceps wasting, there is not usually an effusion but there is tenderness if the synovium around the patella is pressed against the patella itself. This is sometimes confused with tenderness beneath the patella; it is the synovium caught between your finger and the patella that is causing the pain as there are no nerve fibres under the patella itself.

Management

There is no proven treatment for this condition, but because its severity fluctuates it is a diagnosis which has attracted all sorts of unusual therapies. There is little doubt that pain killers and nonsteroidal anti-inflammatory drugs make little or no difference to the pain. Strapping and tubigrip can actually make the pain worse, and there is no evidence that avoiding activities which make the pain worse makes any difference to the natural history of the condition. The use of crutches, plaster cylinders and even wheelchairs merely seems to confirm the child in the role of an invalid. There is always quadriceps inhibition and eventually wasting, so exercises to build up the quadriceps, particularly the vastus medialis, should be encouraged. Unfortunately, these exercises can be quite painful, but if the child is encouraged to contract the muscles isometrically (without moving the knee) the pain can be minimised. There are several surgical operations described for this condition but there is no evidence that any of them do any good and some of them certainly make the condition worse, so they should be avoided.

Dislocating kneecap

It is most common to see a patient who has had a previous dislocation. The kneecap normally relocates itself, but if it has not the patient can be given nitrous oxide. When the knee is straightened the patella will relocate. Immediately after a dislocation the patient will have a quadriceps lag and should therefore be protected with a back slab and crutches. Physiotherapy should be started at once. If there have been recurrent dislocations, then swelling may be minimal but quadriceps wasting may be marked. It is then even more important to arrange physiotherapy to build up the muscles around the knee if further dislocations are to be avoided.

Surgery for the dislocated patella (Fig. 23.30) should only be undertaken as a last resort. If the patient has built up the quadriceps well but the kneecap is still unstable then initially a soft-tissue realignment of the patella should be considered by performing a lateral release. This involves dividing the lateral retinaculum of the patella so that the pull on the patella is more medial.

Dislocation of the knee

In high-energy accidents the knee can be dislocated. The tibia is driven backwards and dislocates posteriorly. The key feature in this injury is that there is a high risk of neurovascular injury. The pulses to the foot must be intact before and after relocation, and even if they return great care must be taken that a compartment syndrome does not develop. The knee can then be treated in a plaster for 6 weeks with active quadriceps exercises.

Fractured patella

There are two types of fractured patella. The first is a direct blow to the patella, which tends to shatter the patella into many fragments which do not displace as the patella tendon and the fibres which run over the patella itself are usually intact. The second type of fracture is an avulsion fracture where the patella snaps in half under the load of the quadricep muscle trying to prevent the knee from being forcibly flexed. In the latter case the fracture is usually transverse and displaced.

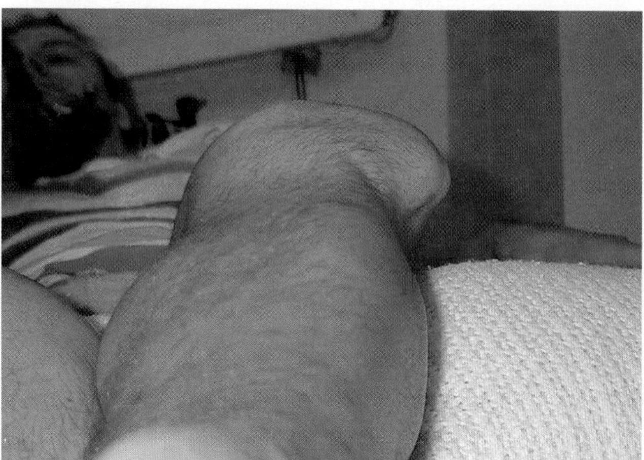

Fig. 23.30 Dislocated patella.

Management of the communited undisplaced fracture

There is often an open wound over the patella and this needs cleaning. If it is contaminated it should be left open for delayed primary closure. It is unlikely that the patella can be reconstructed when it is in a large number of fragments, and therefore the choice is either to treat the patella as a 'bag of bones' (simply mobilised without any attempt at reduction) or to excise it. The patella acts as a fulcrum for the quadriceps tendon and a stabiliser, so if it is excised the knee may subsequently be weaker and less stable. However, if it is moblised early as a 'bag of bones' the articular surface may be smoothed but will never be truly congruent and early oesteoarthritis in the patellofemoral joint is inevitable.

Management of the displaced transverse fracture of the patella (avulsion)

The fracture can be managed in exactly the same way as an olecranon fracture with wires passed through the patella and a figure-of-eight tension band passed around the outside of the patella. The load of the quadriceps passing through the patella and down the patella tendon into the tibial tubercle serves to compress the fracture provided that the outer cortex is held together with a tension band (Fig. 23.31). The patient is mobilised with partial weight-bearing until the fracture is healed. The pins and wires are then removed as otherwise they cause skin irritation.

Tibial plateau fractures

Tibial plateau fractures occur in the elderly when the knee is forced into varus or valgus and the osteoporotic bone fails before the ligaments. Fracture can also occur in the young adult but are then associated with very high-energy injuries which may also have damaged the ligaments and caused fractures elsewhere. The pattern of fracture of the plateau depends on the direction of the force exerted. If the knee was forced into valgus then there tends to be a depressed fracture of the lateral plateau; if the knee is forced into varus then, similarly, the medial plateau will be fractured. If there is an axial force then both plateaux may be damaged. A check should always be made on the contralateral side of the fracture for ligamentous disruption as the compressed side will have acted as a fulcrum for the load to come on to the opposite ligament. There are two main types of tibial plateau fracture. The first is a vertical cleft fracture where a whole

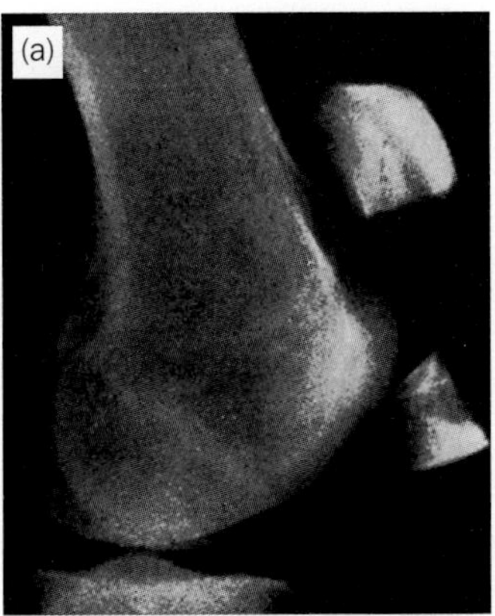

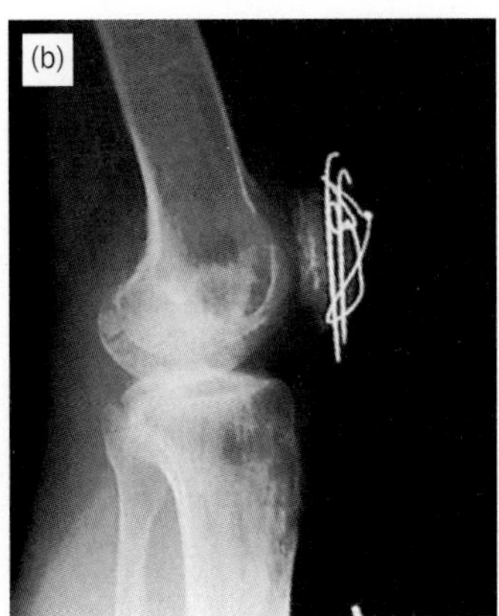

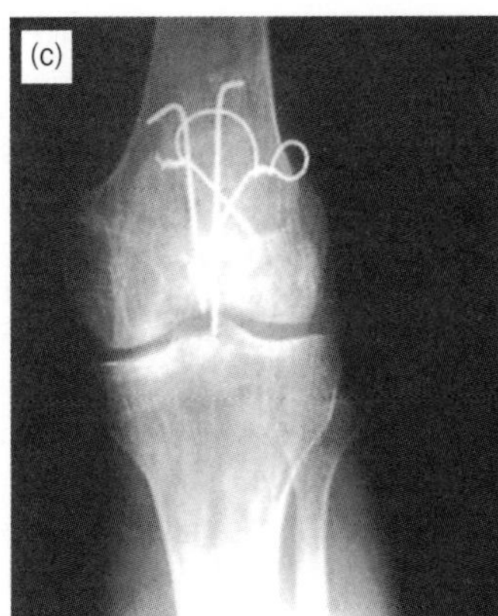

Fig. 23.31 Transverse fractures of the patella (a), fixed internally by means of two wires and a figure-of-eight tension band (b and c). (*courtesy of Keith Willett*).

fragment is displaced downwards. The second is an egg-shell-type fracture where the plateau is buckled in by the femoral condyle. Most fractures are a mixture of these two types. The buckle 'egg-shell' fracture can be quite difficult to see on an X-ray, as it is often only part of the plateau (usually the posterior part) that is depressed. Unless a careful check is made the intact part of the plateau will give the appearance that the knee is normal in both the AP and the lateral directions. Fractures in which there is more than 2 mm displacement in the articular surface or in which the joint is unstable need open reduction and internal fixation in all but the most elderly and frail patient. The investigation of choice is therefore tomography or a CT with reconstruction of the tibial plateau in the vertical axis to show the size and depth of the depressed section. The final decision on whether the knee needs reconstructing may have to made under anaesthetic when the stability can be tested.

Management of vertical shear fractures

If the fracture is a pure vertical shear fracture with displacement of more than 2 mm then the fragment needs to be exposed, elevated, and fixed back with a buttress plate and lag screws across the knee. Early partial weight-bearing and mobilisation can then be started.

Management of depressed fractures

In these cases the joint may need to be opened so that the fragments can be elevated under direct vision. The incision should be extended down beside the tibia and a small window opened in the cortex into which a punch can be introduced. The fragments can then be elevated from inside the bone and the cavity packed with bone graft. If there is combined vertical shear fracture then this can be fixed with a buttress plate (Fig. 23.32). Most of the load to the knee goes through the medial side so a fracture of the lateral plateau may only need protecting with a cast brace to prevent the knee going into valgus, but a fracture of the medial plateau should be nonweight-bearing for some weeks.

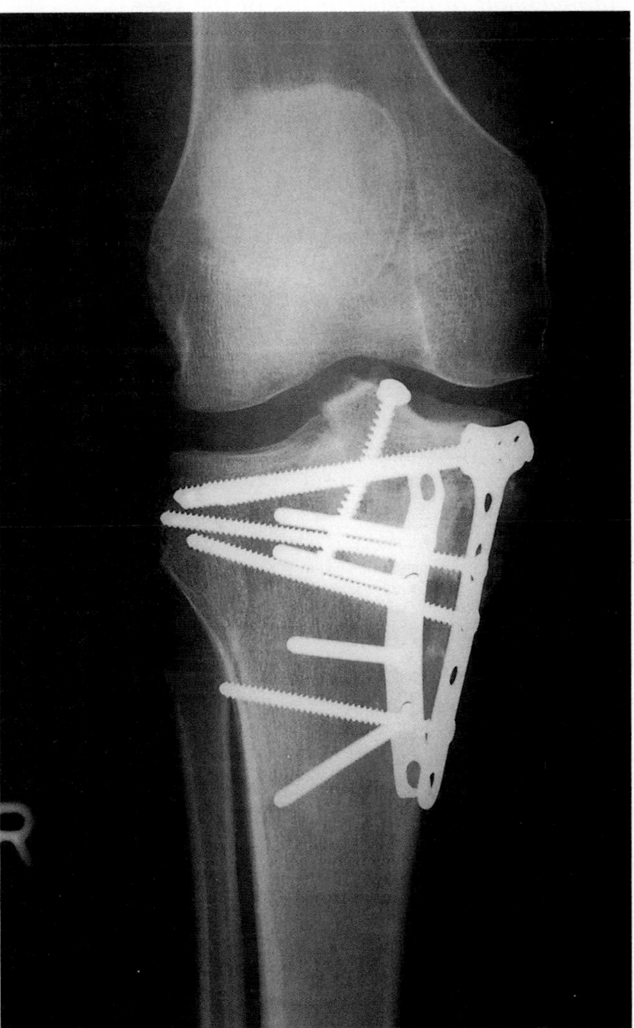

Fig. 23.32 Reconstruction of a tibial plateau fracture (*courtesy of Keith Willett*).

Rheumatoid arthritis of the knee

Rheumatoid arthritis commonly affects the knee, but the diagnosis is simple as it is one of the later joints to be affected. In the first instance the problem is pain and swelling secondary to an aggressive synovitis. At this stage medical treatment, nonsteroidal anti-inflammatory drugs, pain killers, splints and physiotherapy are the best choice. Synovectomy can be performed chemically using short-acting radioisotopes. Surgical synovectomy can also be performed through an arthroscope. This is technically difficult because of the florid synovitis and should only be undertaken if there is still a good range of movement and the articular surfaces are well preserved. In the later stages of rheumatoid arthritis there is severe arthritis in the lateral compartment with a contracture of the lateral structures of the knee, producing external rotation of the tibia and a fixed flexion deformity. Total knee replacement is now the operation of choice but this may need to be combined with a careful soft-tissue release to obtain a stable straight knee.

Management of osteoarthritis of the knee

Osteoarthritis of the knee may be idiopathic or secondary to trauma. The disease may affect all three compartments of the knee: the patellofemoral joint as well as both the medial and lateral compartments of the knee, but its main effect appears to be on the medial compartment. Initially the patient may present with pain on walking. Weight-bearing X-rays may show slight narrowing of the medial joint space. If medical treatment and physiotherapy are no longer controlling the symptoms and there appears to be a major inflammatory element to the disease then an arthroscopic washout should be considered. It is not known how this operation works but it can give considerable relief of pain in the short term. A valgus osteotomy may help to transfer the weight-bearing away from the medial compartment and more equally into the medial lateral compartment. This is only suitable if the lateral compartment shows no sign of arthritis on X-ray, the knee is stable and there is a good range of movement (at least 90°).

Operative technique for high tibial osteotomy for osteoarthritis

The degree of varus (Fig. 23.33) should be measured carefully on long leg X-rays. The size of wedge which needs to be removed from the tibia should then be calculated with the aim of putting the knee in neutral or very slightly into valgus. At operation a laterally based wedge is removed from tibia just below the joint surface leaving the medial cortex intact to stabilise the osteotomy. An alternative procedure is the 'dome osteotomy', where a series of drill holes in the shape of an arch is drilled through from the front of the tibia to the back and then joined using a sharp osteotome. The distal tibia can then be rotated in the dome to correct the alignment of the knee. As with the wedge osteotomy, the new position can then be held using a long leg plaster. Care must be taken in either operation to avoid damaging the vessels immediately behind the knee, which lie very close to the bone especially if the knee is extended. These procedures are therefore best all performed with the knee well flexed.

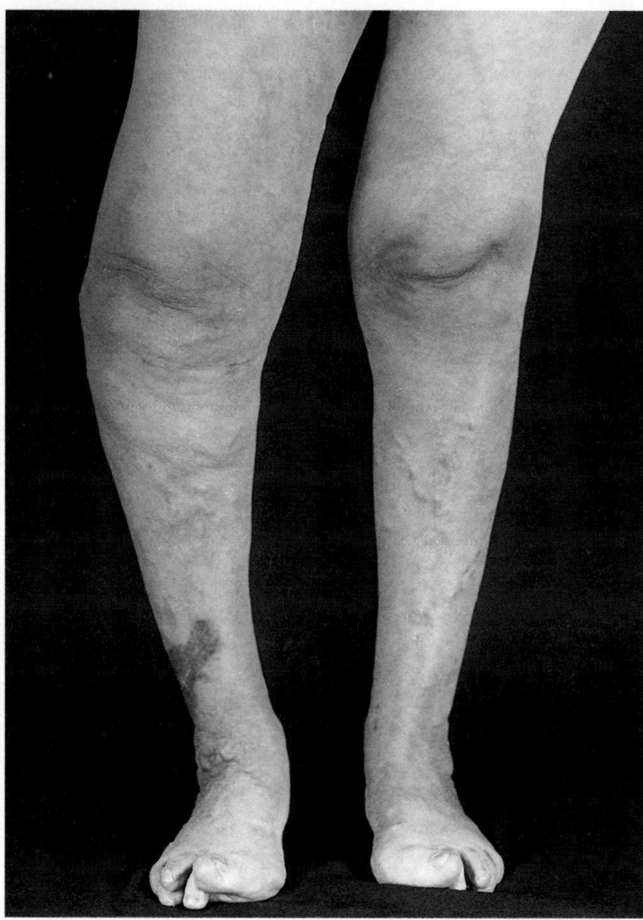

Fig. 23.33 Osteoarthritis of the knee with marked varus deformity.

Knee replacement

Most knee replacements are total condylar knee replacements (Fig. 23.34). The femoral component replaces both femoral condyles and there is a tibial plateau component which covers the tibia. An optional extra is a resurfacing component for the back of the patella. Unicompartmental knee replacements are available, but unicompartmental arthritis is not that common, and technically these implants can be difficult to insert.

Operative technique for total condylar knee replacement

The patient is placed supine on the table. It is not necessary to use a tourniquet although many people do. The risk of causing vascular damage, especially in the elderly, outweighs any possible advantages in obtaining a blood-free field. A long midline anterior incision should be made from 10 cm above the patella to 3 cm below the tibial tubercle. This incision can be curved slightly medially. The incision is carried down to the patella and patella tendon without undercutting the edges. The medial margin of the patella tendon and of the patella is now exposed and the incision carried on through this tissue to the knee joint. Above the patella the incision is brought round to the midline of the patella and then extended vertically up the quadriceps muscle in the midline for 10 cm above the knee. The patella is turned upside down and dislocated laterally and the knee flexed up to 90°. Any bleeding in

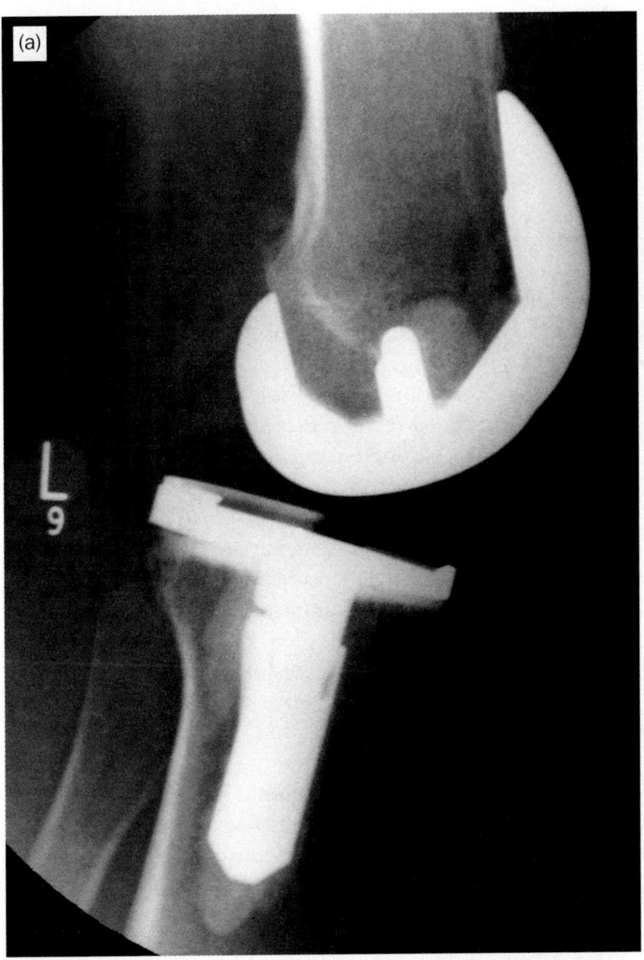

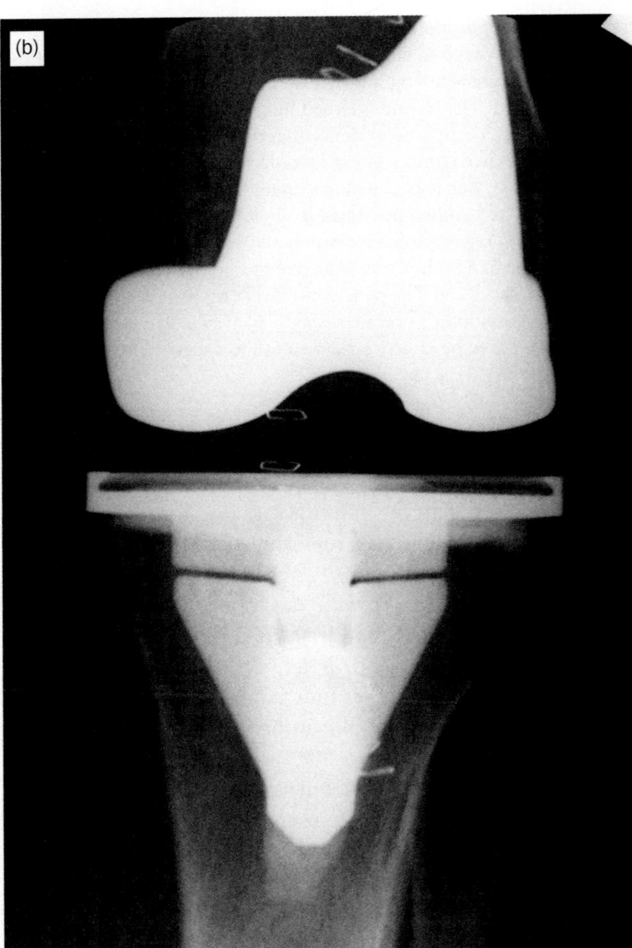

Fig. 23.34 X-rays of total condylar knee replacement.

the wound edges should now stop so that a tourniquet would now serve no further useful function. The fat pad and menisci are excised and a jig is placed on the femur. The jig should be sized so that the femoral component will be the same size as the condyles it is replacing.

Having checked that rotation is correct the anterior and posterior cuts should then be made on the femur. Very little of the anterior condyles should be removed. Each fragment of the posterior condyle should be about the size of a thumb nail and no thicker than the thickness of the replacement metal component. The tibial jig should now be applied. Two types of jig are available. One is fitted on a rod passed down the medulla of the tibia and relies on the tibial shaft anatomy being normal and the entry hole being in the centre of the tibia. The second type of jig (extramedullary jigging) relies on the surgeon clipping the jig to the tibia and achieving the correct alignment by eye. This second system relies more on the surgeon's skill and expertise, and tends to be used more by experienced knee surgeons who may wish to make allowances for abnormal anatomy. The cut on the tibia should only remove as much tibia as is needed to make room for the thickness of the thinnest of the tibial components. If there is a defect in either the medial or the lateral plateau no attempt should be made to remove the defect by cutting lower, as the defect can be filled with cement or, indeed, with special components that can be fitted to the implant. The gap between the cut top of the tibia and the posterior cut of the femur should be measured with the knee in 90° of flexion using the spacers provided on the instrument tray. This gap measured will include the thickness of the tibial component and of the femoral component.

With the knee now extended, and using the same spacer, a mark should be made on the femur so that the distal cut of the femur is made at a height that will keep the components in the same amount of tension through flexion and extension. If, however, it is found that it is difficult to get the distal tibia in the correct alignment to the femur in extension (7° of valgus) then a soft-tissue release may need to be carried out on either the medial or lateral collateral ligaments. The lateral ligament is best released from the femur; the medial side can be released from both femur and tibia until the knee is in correct alignment in extension. A similar amount of bone should then be cut from the femoral condyles as the thickness of the metal of the components, allowing for any defects in the femur caused by osteoarthritis. The distal cut in the femur should now be carried out using a jig to ensure that it is at the correct angle to the anterior and posterior cuts. The corners are trimmed where necessary, and a trial femoral component can be fitted to test against a trial tibial component. It is now possible to see whether the cuts have been put in the right place and whether the tension of the knee in both flexion and extension is correct. On good designs the tension in flexion should be slightly less than in extension to allow rotation of the tibia on the femur in flexion. If the alignment and tension are good then the components can be cemented into place. There is no evidence that resurfacing the back of the patella makes any difference to the long-term outcome, and the complications of this thin implant are well described. Nevertheless, the patellofemoral joint is clearly a potential source of pain and some surgeons argue that it should be replaced.

The patella is reduced and a single tacking suture put in to hold the medial retinaculum to the patella. A check is then made that the patella tracks normally in the new intercondylar groove. If it does not, osteophytes may need to be trimmed from the edge of the patella. If the lateral retinaculum is too tight then a lateral retinacular release may need to be performed. The wound is closed in layers and the knee placed in a back slab splint. There is no evidence that continuous passive movement after surgery either reduces blood loss, decreases pain or improves the overall outcome, but it is commonly used. The key to success is good postoperative physiotherapy aimed at building up the power of the quadriceps then regaining full extension and at least 90° of flexion. Total knee replacement does not give immediate pain relief in the same way as a total hip replacement. The patient also needs to do a great deal of work over the next 6 months to regain strength and range of movement in the knee. This needs to be clearly explained to the patient before embarking on the surgery.

Complications of total knee replacement

Total knee replacement is subject to wound breakdown if care is not taken with the anterior incision. If the wound does break down then the knee replacement is likely to become infected.

Tourniquet damage is well described, especially in the elderly. The tourniquet may fracture atherosclerotic plaques in the femoral vessels and, if left on too long, may cause nerve damage. If tourniquet time is more than 1 hour in the elderly, the tourniquet should probably be released and then reinflated after 10 minutes.

Tourniquets can also cause burns if alcohol-based skin preparation solution is allowed to seep down into the tourniquet padding (Fig. 23.35).

Damage to the vessels behind the knee can be avoided by making the cuts on the tibia with the knee flexed and being very careful not to let the saw cut too deep.

The retractor on the lateral side of the knee must be used with care if damage to the lateral popliteal nerve is to be avoided.

If the knee is put in too loose it may be unstable and require bracing.

The infection risk of total knee replacements is around the same as total hip replacements, somewhere below 2 per cent. The risk of infection can be reduced using three doses of prophylactic antibiotics specifically to cover *Staphylococcus*.

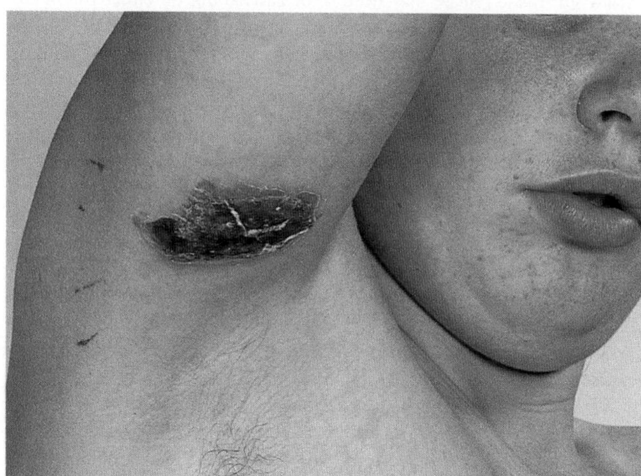

Fig. 23.35 Tourniquet burn of the upper arm in a young man where the preparation solution was allowed to seep under the tourniquet.

The incidence of deep vein thrombosis after total knee replacement appears to be high, but few of these cases produce any clinical symptoms. The overall death rate after total knee replacement is low (less than 1 per cent, and the death rate from pulmonary embolus even lower). There is, therefore, no evidence to support the use of thromboprophylaxis in total knee replacement, either chemical or mechanical.

Some total knee replacements fail to mobilise quickly particularly if physiotherapy resources are not good or the patient lacks motivation. After 2 weeks a manipulation under anaesthetic may need to be performed to release any adhesions. This must be done with great care to avoid breaking the femur.

Total knee replacement does not produce immediate relief of pain but if severe pain persists the possibility of aseptic or septic loosening must be considered. The joint should be aspirated and fluid sent for culture. If a trial of antibiotics does produce relief of pain then the diagnosis of septic loosening is most likely and a revision should be considered.

Aseptic loosening of total knee replacements probably occurs in a similar way to the hip, with particulate wear stimulating an inflammatory response. Special implants are available for revision but tissue should be sent at the time of surgery for histology and bacteriology. The problems of wound healing after a revision are considerably increased, as is the risk of infection and stiffness.

The tibia

Fractures of the tibial shaft can occur after repetitive loading (stress fractures) or following a single major traumatic event. The tibia is a subcutaneous bone on its anteromedial margin and so any significant displacement of the fracture is likely to result in an open injury. This skin over the tibia is also a notoriously poor healer, and therefore the open fracture of the tibia is an especially challenging problem for the trauma surgeon.

Mechanism of injury

The mechanism of injury is particularly important with respect to the energy involved, likely contamination of the wound and subsequent problems with healing.

Stress fractures

Stress fractures are particularly common in the tibia, particularly in runners. The patient initially complains of pain during exercise, then pain during and after exercise, and finally pain at all times. On examination there may be little to find except for the fact that the tibia may be tender to percussion. Initially the X-ray may be normal but after some weeks a faint haze of callous may form locally over the site of the invisible fracture. This X-ray, if combined with a history of continuous pain, is also characteristic for osteosarcoma. Careful imaging with MRI or CT scan should be able to distinguish these two diagnoses.

Management of stress fractures. This condition can prove very difficult to manage. It may occur at a crucial phase in an athlete's training programme and at some stage, preferably sooner rather than later, it is going to become clear that training for the next few months, or indeed that season, is over. This can be very difficult for an athlete to accept, but until it is the condition is unlikely to settle. One problem may be the boredom that sets in if the significant proportion of the day, which was previously devoted to sport, is now to be spent resting. The alternative is to devise forms of exercise which are as strenuous and as time-consuming as the original activity, but which do not stress the tibia. For runners the nearest sport is cycling, a more remote possibility swimming. As the fracture is incomplete, it should not require any extra protection.

Low-energy direct blow fractures to the tibia

The tibia may be broken by a direct blow such as a bumper injury to a pedestrian. Despite the low-energy nature of the injury the skin and soft tissues may be damaged over the fracture, so the fracture may be technically open. If the fracture is a simple transverse fracture or a small butterfly fragment the fracture may be stable to axial compression. In this case nonoperative treatment will be best. If, however, there is a large butterfly fragment the fracture is likely to be unstable and treatment in plaster may lead to unacceptable shortening. Because of its subcutaneous position the tibia is ideally suited to the use of an external fixator (Fig. 23.36), except that the tibia is slow-healing bone and external fixators on the whole delay healing rather than stimulate it. Nevertheless, an external fixator offers a viable option where facilities for internal fixation are limited, or where it is felt that the damage to the skin and soft tissues over the bone makes the risk of internal fixation too high.

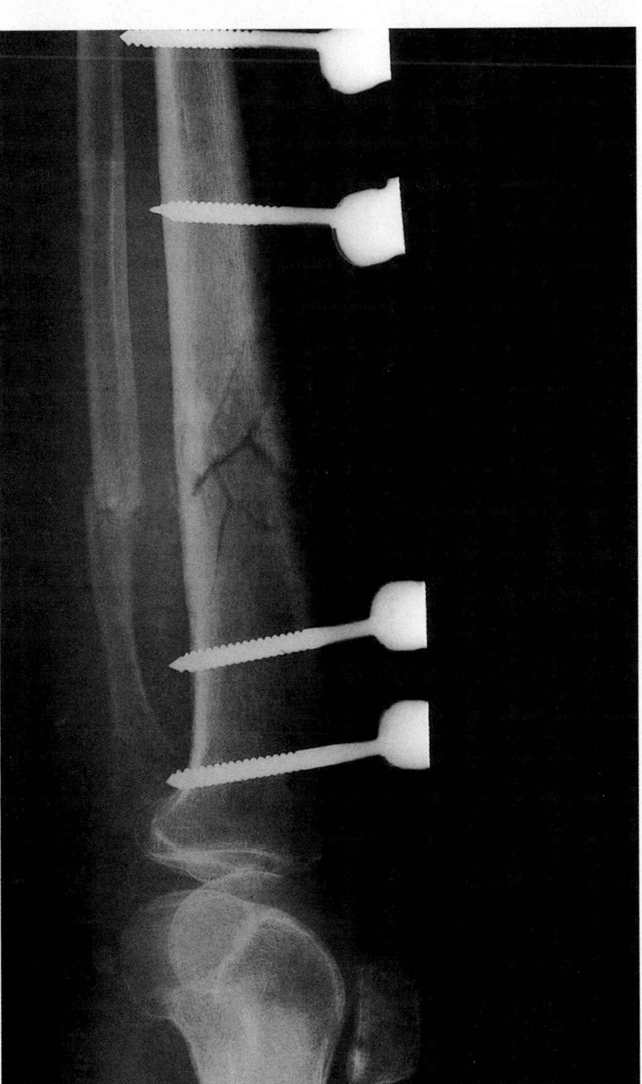

Fig. 23.36 Tibial fracture managed with an external fixator.

Internal fixation can be performed using either a plate or an intramedullary nail. A plate cannot be fixed on the anteromedial border of the tibia because it is subcutaneous. If there is any soft-tissue defect then a careful plan will need to be made with the plastic surgeons to ensure that cover of the fracture and plate can be obtained. This may mean rotating a musculocutaneous flap. A plate cannot be applied if cover cannot be obtained. Some surgeons apply bone graft to all tibial shaft fractures which are plated because of their reputation for poor healing.

The tibia is well suited to intramedullary nailing (Fig. 23.37), especially using the newer type of unreamed nail. Fixation can be obtained without unduly disturbing the fracture. Proximal and distal locking provides control of axial

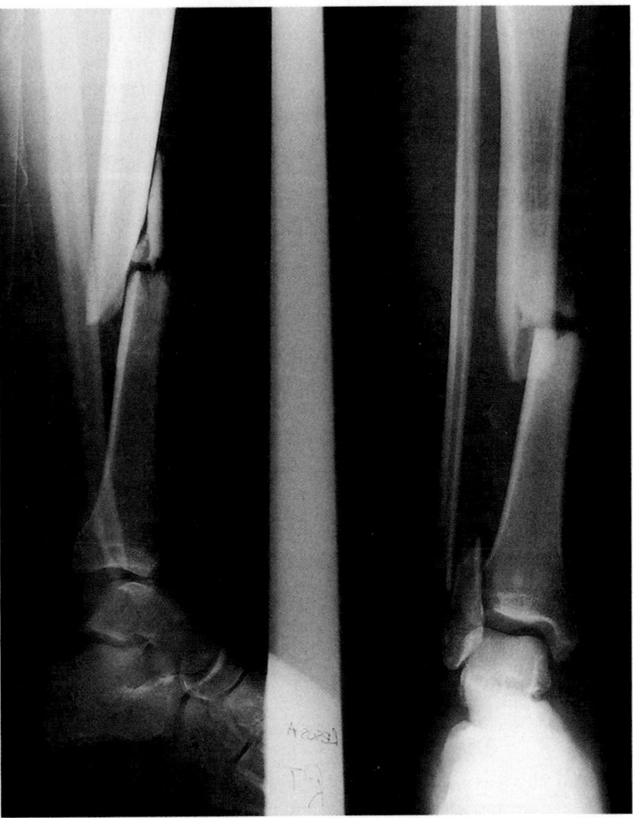

Fig. 23.37 Spiral midshaft fracture of the tibia. This is suitable for intramedullary nailing if the equipment facilities and skills of the surgeon are adequate. It could also be managed on traction followed by cast bracing or even with an external fixator.

compression and gives rotational stability. A nail allows immediate mobilisation of the patient, although with the unreamed nail they should probably remain partial weight-bearing on crutches for the first 6–8 weeks. The technique can apparently be used without undue risk of infection even in open fractures provided that there is no significant contamination or major soft-tissue damage. The operation should only be performed by an experienced team with excellent X-ray image intensifier facilities as the complication rate of this operation is high even in experienced hands.

Operative technique for unreamed intramedullary nailing

The patient is placed supine on a fracture operating table and the tibia set either vertically with the femur horizontal or horizontally with the femur vertical with the tibia above the rest of the table. Either way, the opposite leg must be put in a different position so that the image intensifier can get a clear AP and lateral view of the whole length of the tibia. The knee must be bent up to the right angle to obtain access to the front of the tibia. A Steinmann pin may be inserted into the calcaneum to provide the traction needed to hold the tibia straight. If the tibia is allowed to hang vertical then the weight of the tibia will provide that traction, but access from the image intensifier may be more difficult. A small incision is made over the medial margin of the patella tendon and the entry area on the extra-articular superior surface of the tibia is identified by pushing back the fat pad with a periosteal elevator. An entry hole is made into the tibia in the midline 2 cm back from the anterior margin. A guide pin is inserted and a check made on the image intensifier that the pin is indeed central and can be induced to pass down the tibia, not out of the posterior cortex. This is only possible if the knee is flexed at least 90° so that the roll back of the knee joint moves the femoral condyles and patella back out of the way. It also relies on the entry point being made well enough forward to allow the pin to pass vertically down the tibia without impinging initially on the anterior cortex and further down on the posterior cortex.

Leaving the guide pin in place a circular cutter should be introduced over this pin to open up a entry hole in the top of the tibia. A guidewire should then be introduced and passed beyond the fracture down to the sclerotic remains of the growth plate immediately above the ankle joint. Its length should be measured and an unreamed nail mounted on its introducer, checking that the proximal screw guides are on the medial side and that the nail's curve is concave anteriorly. The nail should be gently driven down, taking great care that initially it does not penetrate the posterior cortex. When it reaches the fracture site the nail should be driven slowly across the fracture site under direct image intensifier control until the tip is just above the ankle joint. The image intensifier should then be centred over the distal holes making sure that the image of each hole is round and not oval, and is exactly in the centre of the image intensifier screen. Through a small skin incision the drill should then be passed through the bone and through the locking hole. The length of screw needed is measured with a depth gauge, and the two distal screws are introduced from the medial side. The traction should then be removed and the nail at the proximal end hammered back a little to draw the two fragments together, as they may be slightly distracted when the nail is driven down. The jig is used to put locking screws in the proximal end after once again checking that rotation is correct.

A final check is made using the image intensifier to ensure that all screws are passing through the nail and engaged on both cortices (Fig. 23.38). A check is also made of the distal circulation. Postoperatively, sensation should be checked and the patient put under observation to ensure that circulation to the foot is maintained and that a compartment syndrome is not developing. The operation and immediate postoperative period should be covered with prophylactic antibiotics. The patient can start mobilising the next day but should remain on crutches until the fracture starts to unite. If the patient cannot be trusted to be careful then it may be wise to put on a plaster gaiter to protect the nail.

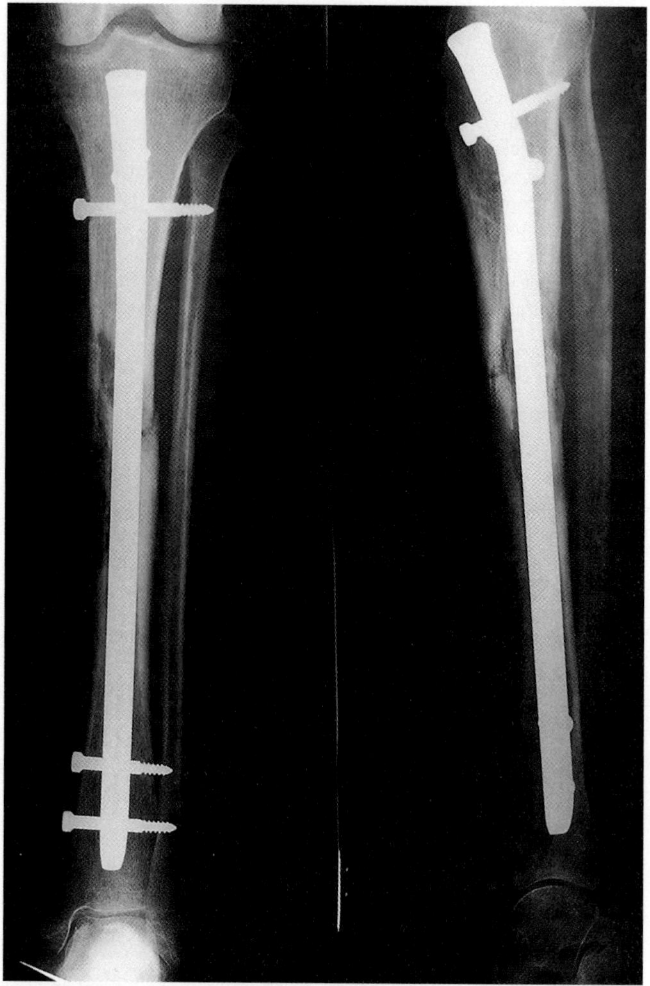

Fig. 23.38 X-rays of a tibia fixed with a locked intramedullary nail (courtesy of Keith Willett).

Management of the severely crushed tibia

In the high-energy injury to the tibia or where there are has been severe crushing, the fracture may be highly unstable, contaminated and surrounded by damaged soft tissues which cannot cover the fractures (Fig. 23.39). The patient will need resuscitating and a check made for other injuries. The neurovascular status of the foot distal to the fracture will also need to be checked. Where possible, polaroid photographs should be taken and then the fracture site wrapped in sterile saline swabs. The management of this fracture is going to be by a team approach but the continuous re-exposure of the fracture for each member of the team to inspect should be avoided as this will increase the overall risk of infection. The first decision which will need to be made is whether the limb is salvageable at all or whether an early amputation will

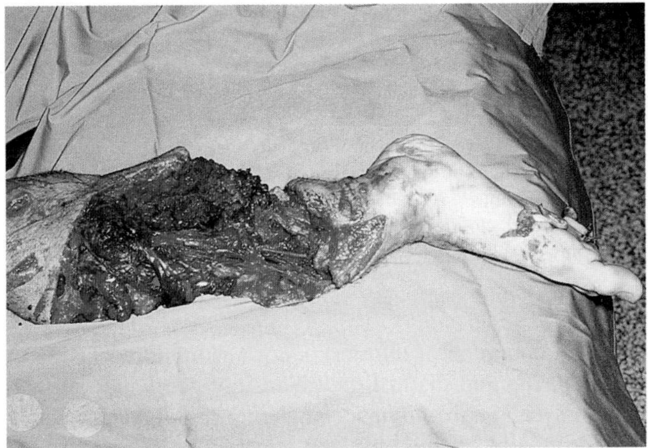

Fig. 23.39 Mangled limb. Although the foot is relatively uninjured it has no circulation or nerve supply. Amputation is indicated.

provide the quickest return of the patient to active life. In the case of land mine injuries, the damage appears to be more severe the further distal one goes and the decision on amputation can be a simple one. In isolated injuries of the tibia, however, the decision will depend on the age of the patient and the function of the distal limb. If the patient is elderly or the distal limb's sensational vascular supply is compromised then serious consideration must be given to whether the unit has the expertise to provide this patient with a sensate and functional foot and union of the tibia. The worst possible scenario is to find that the limb is not salvageable after a year of heroic effort. By then the patient's morale will be sapped and amputation is unlikely to lead to a rapid return to independent living. In contrast, an early amputation followed by rapid rehabilitation through a limb-fitting unit might have allowed return to work within 6–8 weeks.

Complications of tibial fracture and their management

Loss of circulation to the foot

This is the most important complication and treatment must be started immediately. If the limb is angulated it should be put straight immediately in case the cause is merely kinking vessels to the foot. If this does not produce an immediate improvement in circulation and the patient is young enough for a repair of the vessels distal to the trifurcation to be a possiblity, then arrangements need to be made immediately for surgery with an arteriogram on the table. In some units a temporary stent is inserted to start reperfusion of the foot before stabilisation of the fracture is attempted. In other units the fracture is first stabilised. Otherwise there is a risk of disrupting the vascular repair when stabilising the fracture. However, stabilising the fracture significantly prolongs the warm ischaemic time of the foot so if it is decided to stabilise the fracture first then this must be done as quickly as possible. When circulation returns to the lower limb there is a high probability of developing a compartment syndrome. Fasciotomies will usually be required.

Neurological damage to the lower limb

If the soft-tissue damage around the fracture is so extensive that the nerves cannot be repaired then primary amputation should be considered. An insensate limb is unlikely to be of any use to the patient. If the nerves are damaged in continuity, then some recovery can be expected and salvage of the limb should be attempted. In closed injuries it is likely that damaged nerve is in continuity and reasonable recovery can be expected provided that the blood supply to the foot is restored as quickly as possible.

Infection

Infection of closed tibial fractures should be rare but of open tibial fractures is common. All fractures with a puncture wound over them, however small, should be treated as open fractures with contamination. They are all treated in the same way. The skin edges of the wound should be excised and the wound extended so that a clear view of all damaged tissue can be obtained. Any dead and necrotic tissue should be removed and the wound should be washed out with several litres of saline. The wound should be left open and re-inspected at 24 hours. Again, any necrotic or contaminated tissues should be excised and the wound washed out. This process should be repeated until the wound is clean. When this occur delayed primary close can be performed. Throughout this time high levels of intravenous broad-spectrum antibiotics should be used aimed at covering *Staphylococcus*, *Streptococcus* and *Clostridium*. If infection develops when internal fixation is in place then the surgeon is caught on the horns of a dilemma. Stabilisation of the fracture is needed to bring infection under control but foreign material may be acting as a focus for the infection. If a nail is in place then exchange nailing may need to be performed under intravenous antibiotic cover. If a plate has been used then this too may need to be replaced and all infected tissue excised and the wound washed out. An alternative is to change fixation to an external fixator while removing all internal metalware.

Compartment syndrome

A compartment syndrome may develop at any time in the first 48 hours after the accident or after surgery. The patient usually complains of severe unremitting pain with some numbness in the foot. The foot may be cold but there may still be pulses even though a compartment syndrome is developing. Passive dorsiflexion of the toes produces severe pain in the leg. There are no reliable investigations for compartment syndrome and if the condition is suspected then the suspicion should be acted on.

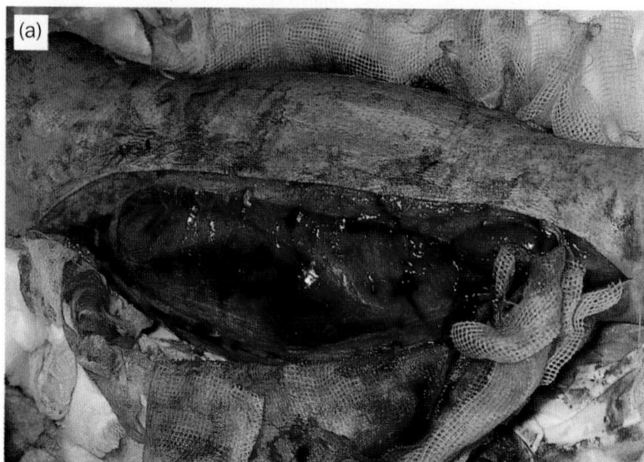

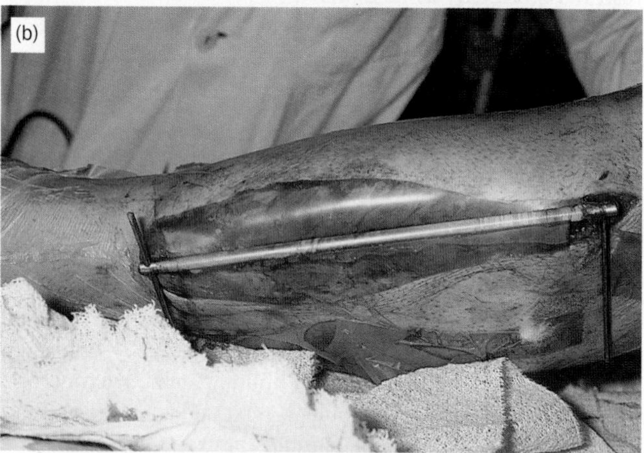

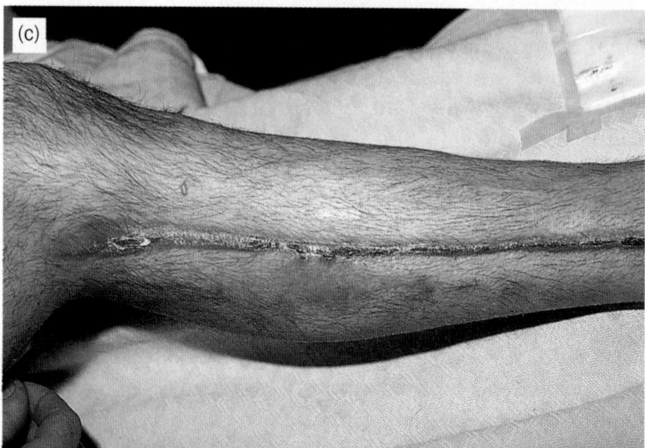

Fig. 23.40 Fasciotomy closure device being used to close a large fasciotomy over a period of 1 week: (a) immediately postfasciotomy; (b) 4 days later; and (c) after healing.

Operation note for fasciotomies

The Mubarek fasciotomy is probably the most reliable form as it ensures that all four compartments are decompressed. An anterolateral incision allows the anterior and perineal compartment to be entered through one incision. Care is taken not to damage any nerves running in the fascia. The fascia is divided, first with a sharp knife and then with a pair of scissors, under direct vision. If a compartment syndrome is present the muscle will pout out a deep purple in colour, and if the fasciotomy was performed soon enough the muscle will then pink up. A second incision is then made posteromedially allowing decompression of the superficial and deep posterior compartments. The deep posterior compartment is the most likely site for a compartment syndrome. If any dead muscle is found it should be excised. Even if no dead muscle is found the wound should be left open and reinspected at 24–48 hours when it will be easier to see whether muscle is dead or viable. At that stage all dead muscle can be excised and closure performed with a split skin graft or with a fasciotomy closure device (Fig. 23.40).

Nonunion

Atrophic nonunion of the tibia is not uncommon. The blood supply to the mid shaft of the tibia is not good and the soft-tissue cover is also minimal. High-energy trauma may strip the periosteum off the tibia and infection may further compromise healing ability. If after 8–12 weeks the tibia is showing no radiological signs of union then delayed union is occurring and may go on to nonunion. If a plate or nail has been used there is a risk that the metalwork will fatigue before the fracture unites. Bone grafting can be used to stimulate callus formation. If an intramedullary nail is already in place then exchange nailing may need to be considered to stabilise the fracture with a new nail which has not yet started to fatigue. Hypertrophic nonunion usually develops if there is too much movement at the fracture site. This is unlikely to occur if internal fixation or an external fixator is used but might occur if a plaster is used to hold the fracture.

Treatment. The fracture site should be opened and the cleft of the fracture cleaned of all fibrous tissue. Consideration should then be given to inserting a reamed nail or putting on a carefully moulded plate to compress the fracture ends and stabilise them. Bone graft should then be put around the fracture site. The patient should only be mobilised under careful supervision of a physiotherapist.

Injuries around the ankle

Minor injuries around the ankle must be one of the commonest presenting conditions in a casualty department. Most of these are minor sprains which only require RICE (Rest, Ice, Compression, Elevation). Nonsteroidal anti-inflammatory drugs may help the pain, reduce swelling and speed rehabilitation. A simple sprained ankle is usually the result of a patient going over on their ankle (an inversion and internal rotation of the foot on the tibia). On examination tenderness is confined to the lateral side of the ankle and is localised over the ligament. The bone itself is not tender. More serious injuries to the ankle have a pattern characterised by the way in which the injury occurred. The injuries caused by inversion and external rotation of the foot on the tibia occur in a sequence. First, the posterior part of the distal fibula fractures off (Fig. 23.41). If the injury is more serious then the foot continues to rotate and the medial collateral ligament fails or the tip of the medial malleolus is pulled off. At this stage the ankle becomes unstable. Finally, if the force continues further, the posterior capsule fails by ripping off the posterior

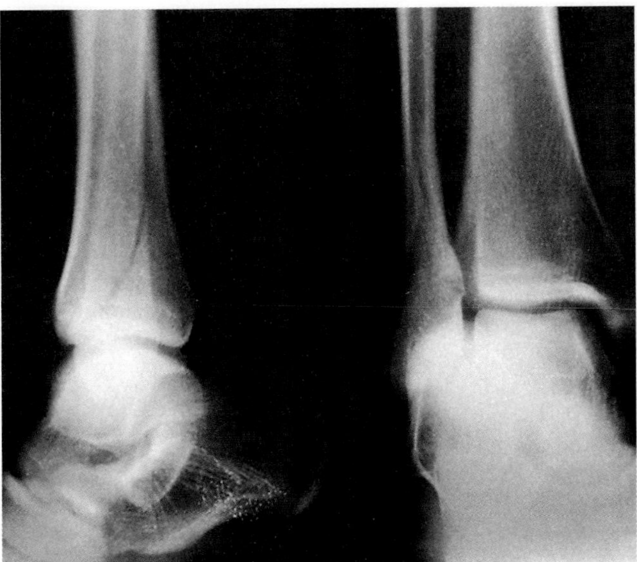

Fig. 23.41 Ankle fracture, first degree. The characteristic line of the fracture of the fibula is seen on the lateral view.

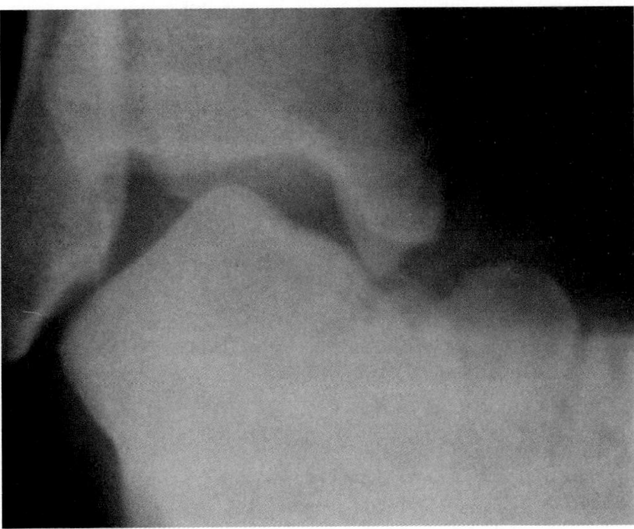

Fig. 23.43 Inversion stress radiograph of an ankle with rupture of the lateral ligament. An anteroposterior view showing gross talar tilt indicating a complete rupture of the lateral ligament. A routine anteroposterior radiograph of the ankle revealed no abnormality.

malleolus of the tibia, completely disrupting the ankle joint (see Fig. 23.42).

If the deforming force on the foot is pure inversion then it is usual for the lateral structures to fail first. There is either a rupture of the lateral ligament or avulsion of the tip of the fibula. If, however, only the ligament is ruptured the X-ray may look normal as there will be no fracture visible and the ankle at rest will lie in its normal anatomical position. If the ankle is stressed while the X-ray is taken, by holding the foot inverted using lead-protective gloves, the full extent of the injury will be immediately apparent on the X-ray (see Fig. 23.43). If the injury is more serious, and especially if there is a medial compression element to the fracture, then a vertical shear fracture may develop separating off the medial malleolus (see Fig. 23.44). Some of the standard forms of fracture pattern are shown in Fig. 23.45.

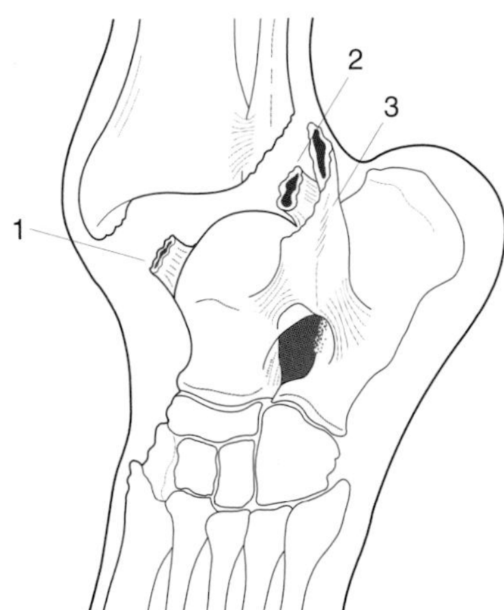

Fig. 23.42 The morbid anatomy of a third-degree external rotation injury of the ankle. Note that the medial malleolus (1), the third malleolus (2) and the lateral malleolus (3) are all attached directly or indirectly by ligaments to the talus or os calcis and, hence, that they move with the foot. (For clarity, the talus is shown in this figure as lying distal to the tibia. In fact, it lies behind the lower end of the tibia.)

Value of the history

The history may be helpful in defining what type of ankle injury is likely. Remember that the fracture may have occurred because the ankle was held stationary while the body continued to move. The patient's description of the injury may need translating into the actual movements of the foot on the tibia and fibula.

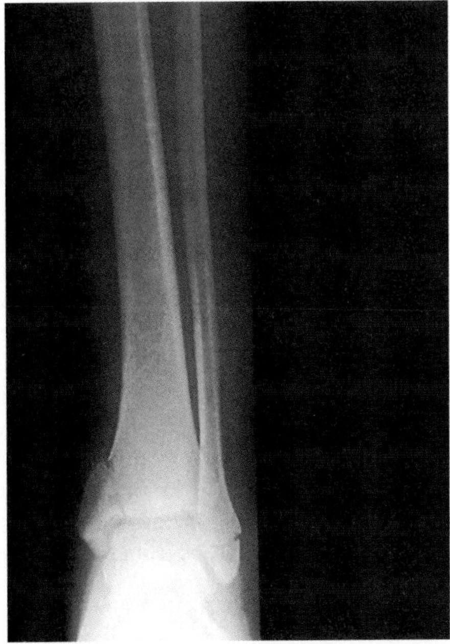

Fig. 23.44 Ankle fracture. Medial compression failure results in a near vertical fracture line because it is 'pushed off'.

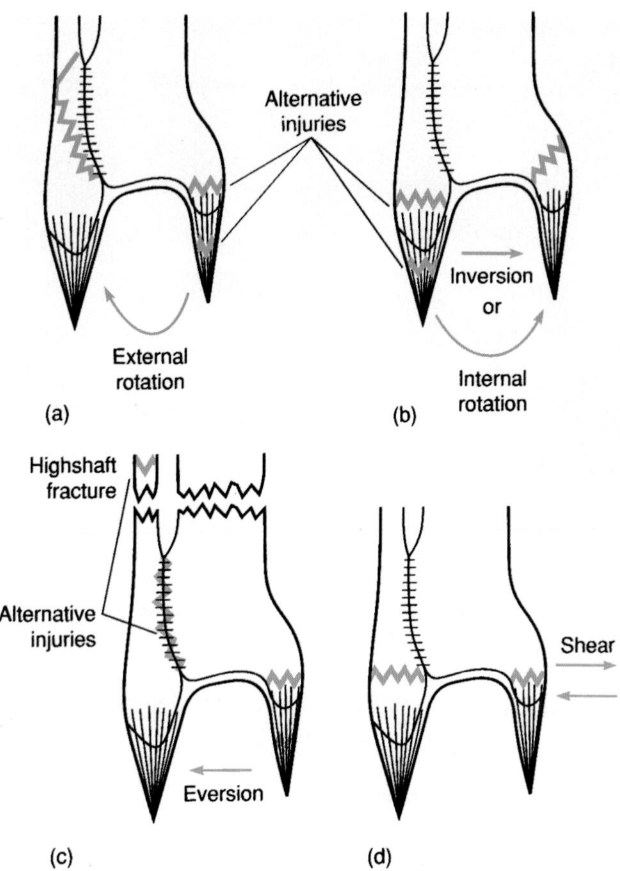

Fig. 23.45 Varieties of ankle fracture.

Examination

The neurovascular status of the foot should always be tested first. In an ankle dislocation, the circulation to the foot may be compromised, as is the viability of the skin over the extruded talus. Reduction of the fracture is an emergency, if skin necrosis is to be avoided (see Fig. 23.46).

Palpation should start at the proximal fibular head. The Maisonneuve-type fracture is an external rotation of the foot on the ankle. The fibula rotates with the talus, avulsing the anterior diastasis but fracturing just below the knee at the fibula neck. The fracture is not normally noticed on an X-ray centred on the ankle, and therefore only clinical examination will reveal the tenderness which warns you to look for this fracture. Careful palpation down the full length of the fibula and on to the lateral collateral ligament will reveal whether there is likely to be a fracture of the fibula or a tear of the ligament. Similar palpation of the medial malleolus and deltoid ligament will give information about the medial side of the ankle. It is always worth including the fifth metatarsal head in this examination, as an inversion of the ankle can result in an avulsion fracture of peroneus tertius from the metatarsal head.

Investigation

Two X-ray views of the ankle will be needed. Most fractures are much better seen in one view than another. The posterior malleolar fracture is very difficult to see in the AP X-ray because it is obscured by the talus and the rest of the tibia. The posterior spiral fracture of the fibula is also difficult to see in the AP X-ray as it is hidden by the silhouette of the intact fibula. A very careful check should be made on the AP X-ray to make sure that the talus has not shifted in the mortice (the socket created by the fibula and the medial malleolus). If the joint space between the talus and the medial malleolus is wider than the joint space between the talus and the plafond of the tibia, then the diastasis ligament between the tibia and the fibula is likely to be disrupted or there is an unstable fracture pattern. If this state of affairs is left untreated then early aggressive arthritis of the ankle will result.

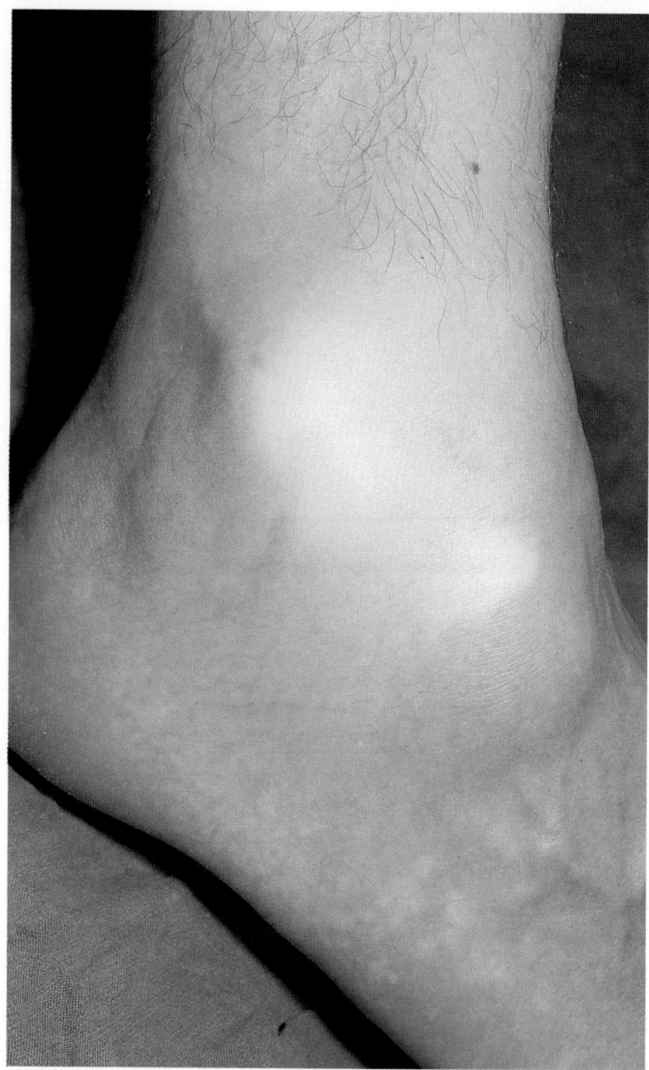

Fig. 23.46 Dislocated ankle. The talus is pressing on the skin. Reduction is urgent if skin necrosis is to be avoided.

Unusual fractures of the ankle

A direct compression force, such as caused by landing on the feet from a height, can drive the talus up into the tibia, destroying the tibial plafond. The principle of management is

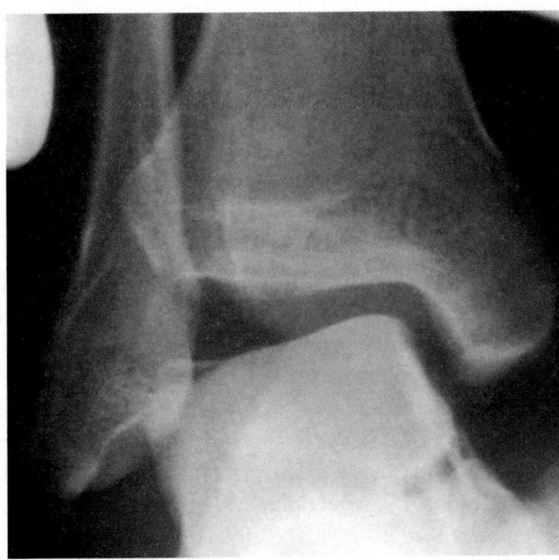

Fig. 23.47 Inversion stress radiograph of an ankle with rupture of the lateral ligament. There is a less marked tilt than in Fig. 23.43, but note the transchondral fracture of the dome of the talus where the talus strikes the fibula. A routine anteroposterior radiograph of the ankle revealed no abnormality (*courtesy of Keith Willett*).

the same as for any other fracture, reconstruction of a congruent joint surface. However, this can be very difficult to achieve.

Twisting injuries to the ankle in unusual positions such as full plantar flexion may produce a chip fracture of the talus (see Fig. 23.47). These fractures can be difficult to see as they can be very posterior and lie hidden behind the rest of the talus in a normal X-ray. A shoot-through view of the ankle joint in full plantar flexion should reveal the injury.

Footballers who use the front of the foot for kicking a ball can develop a prominent osteophyte on the front of the tibia, which can then fracture. The appearance of the ankle joint even before a fracture has occurred can be quite unusual because of the prominent osteophyte.

Management

If the injury to the ankle joint is stable with the foot plantigrade then the fracture can be treated in a simple plaster. This should be split for the first 24 hours to allow for swelling, but can then be closed. A very careful check should be made that the talus is stable within the mortice. If you are dealing with an unstable fracture pattern, then the plaster will need changing regularly to maintain a close fit as the swelling goes down. Regular checks using X-rays will also be necessary to make sure that displacement has not occurred.

It is important to keep the foot dorsiflexed in plaster, otherwise a fixed flexion deformity of the ankle may develop within a few weeks. If the fracture pattern is stable then weight-bearing can be allowed, but the plaster will need to be reinforced with a foot piece or an external shoe to protect against wear. If the fracture is unstable then weight-bearing must not be allowed. If you feel that the patient is unlikely to understand or co-operate with this instruction, then a simple solution is to incorporate the knee in plaster flexed to 90°. This effectively prevents them getting the foot to the ground, and increases the overall stability of the plaster.

If the injury is of such severity that the ankle joint is unstable and cannot be held in a stable configuration with plaster alone, then open reduction and internal fixation must be considered. Avulsion of the medial malleolus can be reduced and held with a lagged screw, while a vertical shear fracture may require lag screws and a buttress plate. The oblique fracture of the fibula is both more difficult to reduce and more difficult to fix and will require a third tubular plate applied anteriorly or posteriorly with lag screws across. Plates applied directly to the lateral side of the fibula are too bulky and prevent closure of the wound.

Timing of surgery

Unstable ankle injuries produce enormous swelling. If surgery is attempted when swelling is excessive then it will be impossible to close the wounds at the end of surgery, and a simple closed fracture will be converted into a complex open fracture. Surgery should therefore be undertaken within a few hours of the injury before the swelling has become too great. Otherwise the ankle should be elevated and a pneumatic splint used, if available, until the swelling has gone down enough for surgery to be possible. A simple test is to see whether the skin over the ankle is slack enough to create a small pucker with pressure between the fingertip and the thumb. If it is not, then it is too tight for surgery and the wound will not close (Fig. 23.48).

Postoperative care

The normal aim of internal fixation is to create a stable skeleton so that full mobilisation can be undertaken. This is unlikely to be achieved in ankle fractures. The purpose of internal fixation is to create a congruent ankle joint so that

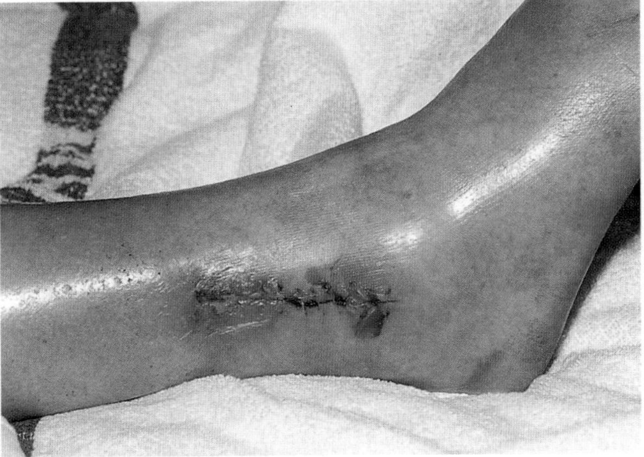

Fig. 23.48 Wound breakdown after surgery – surgery was attempted when there was still too much swelling for closure without tension.

early arthritis is avoided. The ankle will still need protecting with plaster, and the patient will need to remain nonweight-bearing for at least 2 weeks and then partial weight-bearing until union has occurred. If a removable plaster is used then early active mobilisation of the ankle joint can be started under the supervision of a physiotherapist, so that stiffness is avoided and swelling is brought down as quickly as possible. Once bone union has occurred and ligaments are felt to be healed an intensive programme of physiotherapy is needed to restore full range of movement in the ankle, and to build up proprioception in the ankle joint. This is carried out using a wobble board (a small platform with a half-ball underneath which requires considerable skill to balance on). Patients should only be allowed to return to contact sport once they have regained full control of the ankle joint as otherwise they will simply repeat the injury.

Ruptured tendoachilles

This injury occurs most commonly in the middle aged. It occurs without warning and is often associated with strenuous exercise such as playing a game of squash. The patient describes hearing a sharp crack behind the heel, and may look around to see if she or he has been struck. There is immediate pain and weakness in the ankle. However, the patient may still be able to plantar flex the foot quite forcibly using the flexor digitorum and flexor hallucis longus. The diagnosis is therefore not as easy to make as might first appear. In a true rupture of the tendon there is swelling and tenderness over the tendoachilles about 3 cm above the heel. If it is possible to palpate deeply, a clear step can be felt in the tendoachilles, especially when compared with the other side. Sometimes the swelling is so great and the patient is in so much pain that it is not possible to feel this step. An alternative injury is a tear at the musculotendinous junction of gastroenerimus much higher up in the calf. Here the tenderness is much less well localised, some 10 cm above the heel and overall the calf is much more swollen. This injury has a completely different treatment and prognosis, and it is therefore important to distinguish between the two. If the patient is laid prone on the examination couch with their feet hanging over the edge, squeezing of the calf produces severe pain in a rupture of the musculotendinous junction, but in a true rupture of the tendoachilles there is little pain but the foot fails to plantar flex on pressure (see Chapter 20 on examination of joints).

Treatment

Treatment of the tear of the musculotendinous junction is immobilisation with the foot in full plantar flexion and non-steroidal anti-inflammatory drugs. As the pain and swelling go down, gentle mobilisation can be started. Healing is quick as there is a good blood supply.

Treatment of the ruptured tendoachilles is a completely different matter. There is a very poor blood supply, and if the ends are not brought into close apposition the tendon will either fail to heal or heal elongated. Either way, there will be a severe weakness of plantar flexion of the ankle. Non-operative treatment consists of putting the leg in plaster with the foot fully plantar flexed and the knee flexed to 90° initially to bring the tendon ends together. After 2 weeks the plaster is reduced to a below-the-knee plaster and the patient is allowed to mobilise on crutches. Over the next weeks, serial plasters are applied gradually bringing the foot up to a normal plantar grade position over a period of 6 weeks. The patient is then allowed to mobilise gently, but full activity is not allowed for a minimum of 3 months. There is a significant rate of re-rupture. Healing the second time is even slower and the likelihood of a fixed plantar flexion deformity even greater. Surgical treatment can be performed either percutaneously or under direct vision. The tendon ends are sutured together using strong nylon sutures. The stitches are very difficult to insert as the tendon is macerated and stitches tend to cut out unless they are placed very carefully. If the sutures are pulled too tight the tendon tends to bunch up and then it is impossible to close the wound. There is a significant incidence of wound breakdown and some people would question whether wound healing is any faster or the rate of re-rupture any lower in surgical repair compared with nonoperative treatment.

Injuries to the foot

The foot is very susceptible to crush injuries. Even if there are no fractures, the damage to the soft tissues causes swelling and stiffness, and is very slow to heal. Prevention is always better than cure, and in Britain all workers are obliged to wear steel-tipped toe-capped boots if there is a possibility of a heavy object landing on or running over their feet. Degloving injuries occur where there is a shearing force on the foot, such as occurs when a wheel of a vehicle runs over the foot. The injury may appear trivial with no fractures on X-ray and merely a blotchy area of skin over the dorsum of the foot. If this skin is insensate, then it is almost certainly been stripped from its underlying blood and nerve supply. Over the next few days the area will demarcate and necrose. In some cases the degloving is complete at the time of the accident (see Fig. 23.49), and it is clear that amputation is

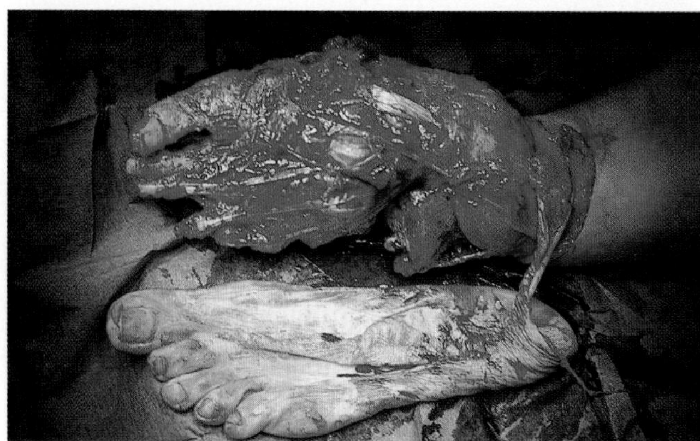

Fig. 23.49 A foot degloved by a road-laying machine running over a worker's foot.

the only option. Minor degloving injuries require excision of all dead tissue and immediate grafting if the foot is salvageable.

Frostbite

The toes are particularly susceptible to frostbite, which may be quite painless initially and may not be noticed by the patient. Once again, prevention is far better than cure, and experienced climbers go to great lengths to make sure that frostbite is not setting in. Once it has occurred demarcation occurs over a period of days and, provided that the tissues do not become infected, simple excision of the necrotic areas can be performed when the boundary between dead and living tissue is clear (Fig. 23.50).

Fractures of the hindfoot

The talus

Most of the surface of the talus is intra-articular, and so any fracture needs to be perfectly reduced if osteoarthritis is to be avoided. An extra complication is that the blood supply to the proximal half of the talus travels up the neck of this bone. A fracture across the neck leads to avascular necrosis in the same way as a fracture across the waist of the scaphoid bone. These fractures need early reduction and careful monitoring for the onset of avascular necrosis.

The calcaneum

Patients landing on their heels from a great height are likely to suffer a series of fractures passing through the body, including fractures of one or both heel bones. The bone tends to split and to crush. If the fracture is not reduced then the hind foot is greatly widened when it heals, making shoe fit difficult. The fracture lines commonly extend into the subtalar joint, and lead to pain and stiffness in the subtalar joint (Fig. 23.51). This makes walking difficult, especially on rough ground such as building sites. Open reduction and internal fixation of these fractures are extremely difficult because the anatomy of the fracture is difficult to see on X-ray and there is commonly massive bone loss in the body of the calcaneum (Fig. 23.52). Wounds in the hind foot are slow to heal and swelling may make closure of the wound difficult

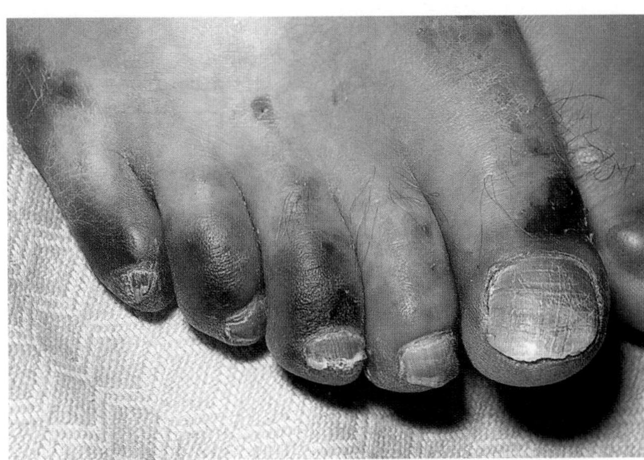

Fig. 23.50 Frostbite of the toes which has started to demarcate.

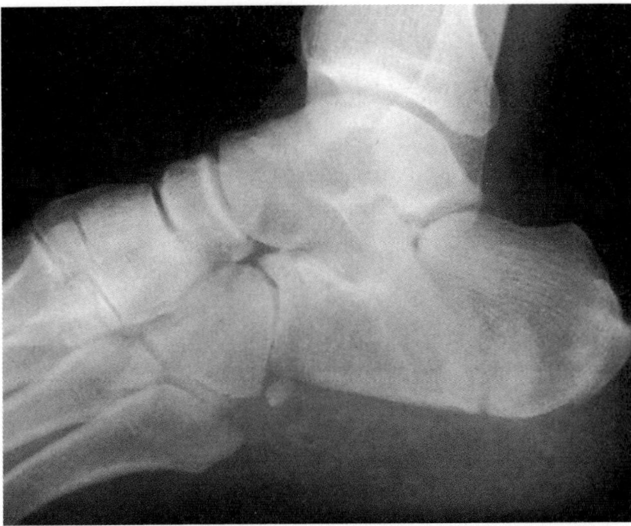

Fig. 23.51 Fracture of the os calcis involving the subtalar joint (*courtesy of Keith Willett*).

(a)

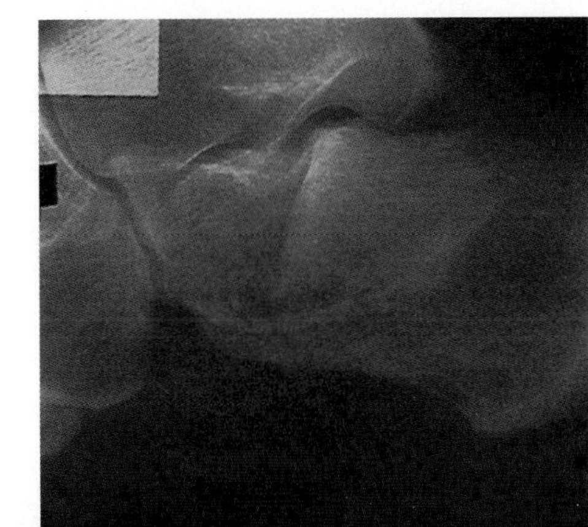

(b)

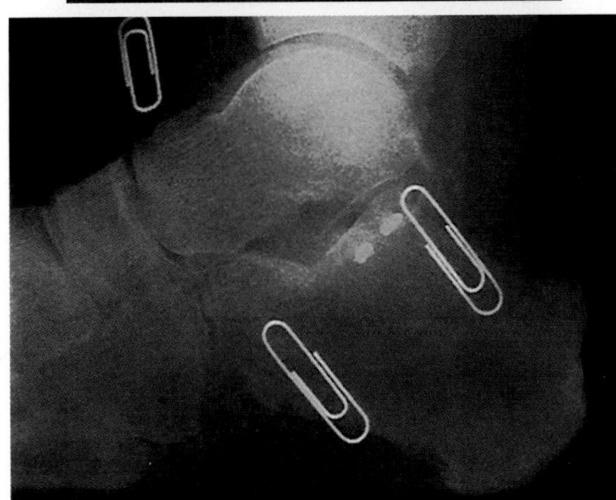

Fig. 23.52 Fracture of the os calcis with displacement of the posterior facet: (a) preoperation; (b) following elevation and internal wire fixation (seen between 'marker' paper clips) (*courtesy of Keith Willett*).

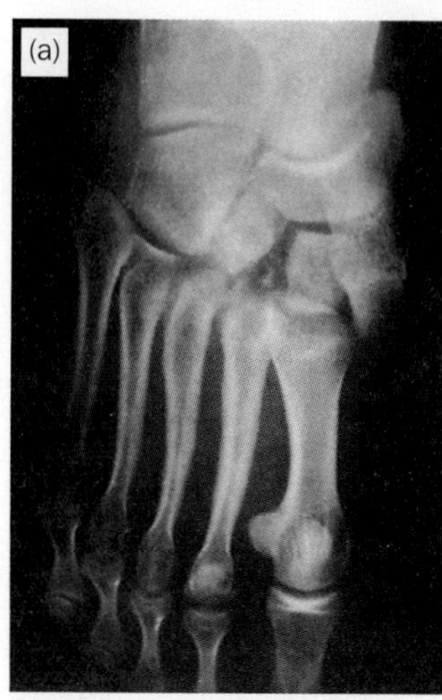

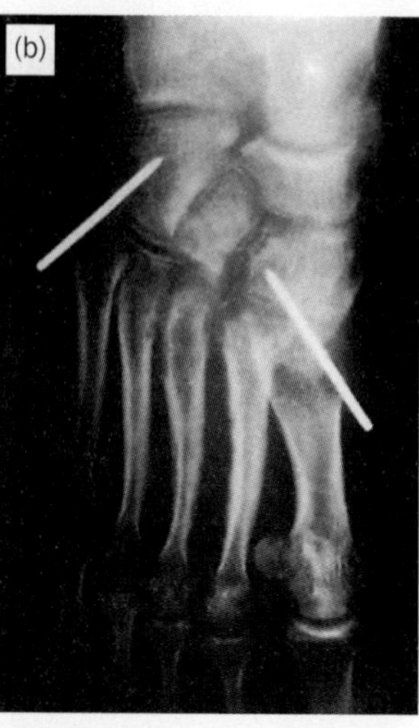

Fig. 23.53 (a) Tarsometatarsal (Lisfranc) dislocation. (b) Treated by open reduction and fixation by wire (*courtesy of Keith Willett*).

anyway. The technique should only be attempted in units with considerable experience and with special equipment for reduction and holding of fractures.

Fractures and dislocations of the midfoot

This injury, sometimes named a Lisfranc fractive, is commonly seen following head-on road traffic accidents where the feet are jammed between the pedals of the car. These injuries are a blend of fractures and dislocations combined with massive soft-tissue swelling. If they are not reduced the arch of the foot is lost and the foot becomes stiff and painful. Reduction is best performed under an image intensifier and Kirschner wires are used to transfix the midfoot to hold fractures and dislocations reduced (Fig. 23.53).

Jacques Lisfranc, 1790–1847. French surgeon. He described the joint but not the dislocation.

Fractures and dislocations of the toes

These injuries are common, and if they are stable when reduced can be treated symptomatically or with a buddy strapping (tapping the injured toe to the adjacent toe). If the fracture or dislocation is unstable then the toe can be held by transfixing it with a wire driven through from the distal phalanx into the metatarsal head.

Further reading

Browner, B.P., Jupiter, J.B. and Levine, A.M. (eds) (1992) *Skeletal Trauma: Fractures, Dislocations, Ligamentous Injuries*, W.B. Saunders, London.

Canale, S.T. (ed.) (1998) *Campbell's Operative Orthopaedics*, 9th edn, Mosby, London.

Gregg, P.J., Stevens, J.G. and Worlock, P.H. (1995) *Fractures and Dislocations: Principles of Management*, Blackwell Science, Oxford.

Rockwood, C.A., Green, D.P. and Bucholz, R.W. *et al.* (1996) Fractures, Vols I–III, *Fractures in Adults, Fractures in Children*, Lippincott Williams & Wilkins, London.

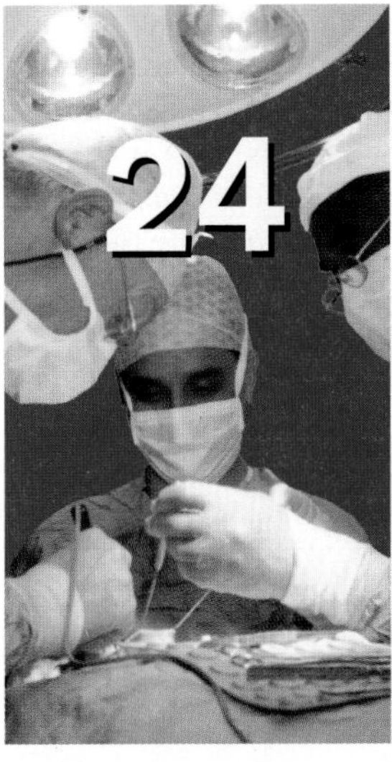

Diseases of bones and joints: infections

Education goal

To understand the importance of early diagnosis and aggressive treatment of osteomyelitis and septic arthritis so as to prevent the formation of chronic osteomyelitis and secondary osteoarthritis.

Learning objectives

- To know the importance of having a high index of suspicion for osteomyelitis and septic arthritis in the neonate.
- To recognise the value of blood cultures to isolate an organism before starting antibiotics.
- To learn the importance in giving high-dose intravenous antibiotics.
- To understand the importance of early drainage and washout of joints in preventing secondary arthritis.
- To recognise the common forms of crystal arthropathy.

Acute osteomyelitis

Pathogenesis

Acute osteomyelitis now commonly occurs in three different groups.

Bailey & Love's Short Practice of Surgery, 23rd edition. Edited by R.C.G. Russell, N.S. Williams and C.J.K. Bulstrode. Published in 2000 by Arnold Publishers.

1. It can occur in the premature baby, possibly as a result of blood-borne spread of infection from intravenous cannulae or other portals.
2. Secondary to open fractures where there has been inadequate cleaning of a wound or it has been closed before it is clean.
3. Following joint replacement or open reduction in internal fixation of fractures where contamination of the bone has occurred.

Osteomyelitis of the neonate

An infant with acute osteomyelitis will be fretful and pyrexial and will not feed. The only clue to the underlying diagnosis may be the child failing to move one limb. Premature babies on intensive care are particularly susceptible, especially as they will have drips and arterial lines, all of which can act as a source for septicaemia. The infection may be remote from the source as the infection spreads through the bloodstream. Unlike osteomyelitis in older patients, the pathogen need not be *Staphylococcus aureus*. It may be *Streptococcus*, *Pneumococcus*, *Haemophilus influenzae* or even *Escherichia coli*. The key to successful treatment is a high index of suspicion leading to early diagnosis by blood culture. High-dose intravenous antibiotics should be started as soon as possible but not before blood cultures have been taken. If the diagnosis and treatment are delayed, pus may collect either under the periosteum or within the medulla of the bone. The epiphyseal plate may be damaged and it will not be possible to bring the infection under control until the abscess has been drained.

Osteomyelitis in the neonate

- Premature are babies susceptible
- The baby may not move the limb
- Organism may not be *Staphylococcus*
- Antibiotics should be started as soon as cultures have been taken

Antibiotics must be started blind after blood cultures have been taken because if the disease can be sterilised within the first 48 hours of onset, complete resolution can be guaranteed. If, however, the diagnosis is reached more than 48 hours after the onset of symptoms, it should be assumed that there is a collection of pus and therefore surgery to drain this pus should be considered. Flucloxacillin should be given at a daily dose of 250 mg/kg in the very young child. Ampicillin 150 mg/kg should also be considered because it has a better spectrum against *H. influenzae*. If the child fails to settle rapidly, it must be assumed either that the organism is not sensitive to the antibiotic being used or that there is a collection of pus present which requires drainage.

Operation

Drainage of pus

Under general anaesthetic, the skin is opened over the most tender red area. The incision is carried down to the periosteum and when this is opened it is usual to find pus expressed at high pressure. This pus should be sent for culture. If no pus is found it is probably worth drilling through the cortex to make sure that there is no pus in the medullary cavity (Fig. 24.1).

Osteomyelitis in open fractures

Any fracture which connects to a wound in the skin must be managed as an open fracture. The haematoma around the fracture acts as a perfect culture medium if any organisms succeed in colonising it. The key to avoiding this situation is to open the wound, fully wash out the haematoma and remove any dead or contaminated tissue. The fracture should then be stabilised and the wound left open. The wound should then be checked every 24–48 hours until it is clear that all dead and contaminated tissue has been removed and clean granulation tissue is forming. Then, and only then, can delayed primary closure (DPC) be attempted.

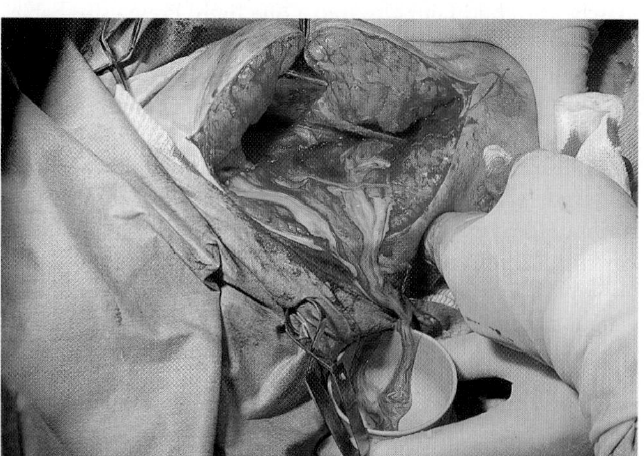

Fig. 24.1 Draining an infected total hip replacement in a patient who was immunocompromised.

Osteomyelitis in open fractures

- All open fractures are contaminated
- Wash out and remove dead tissue
- Leave wound open
- Only close once wound is clean

Osteomyelitis in association with orthopaedic implants

Orthopaedic procedures should always be performed in sterile conditions, preferably in an operating theatre with laminar flow. At least three doses of prophylactic antibiotics should be used, the first given 1 hour before the procedure starts, the second 8 hours later and the third 8 hours after that. There is no evidence that continuing antibiotics beyond this reduces the risk of infection. There is, however, good evidence that prolonged use of antibiotics increases the risk of producing multiple antibiotic-resistant staphylococci (MARS). Any organism introduced into the operative field effectively turns the exposed bone into an open fracture. The most likely organism will be *S. aureus* and therefore an antibiotic with good activity against this organism should be used. Flucloxacillin has excellent activity against *Staphylococcus*. If *Streptococcus* is a possibility, then penicillin should be added.

Preventing infection of orthopaedic implants

- Strict operative discipline with laminar flow
- Three doses of antibiotics starting 1 hour before surgery
- Reopen and wash out suspicious wounds and persisting haematomas

Features which suggest that an orthopaedic operation has become infected

Postoperatively, many patients have a pyrexia in the first 24 hours but it rarely goes above 38°C. If this pyrexia persists or the temperature goes above 38°C then a careful check should be made for a source of infection. This may be the lungs, urine or the wound itself. If a wound is infected it may appear red and swollen, and may start discharging old blood (Fig. 24.2). A persistently discharging haematoma is infection until otherwise proven. The patient should be taken back to theatre, the wound opened and deep samples taken for histology and bacteriology before any antibiotics are given. The wound should be carefully washed out and all dead tissue excised. Infection is more likely to occur in patients who are immunocompromised. The most common cause for this is diabetes or steroids.

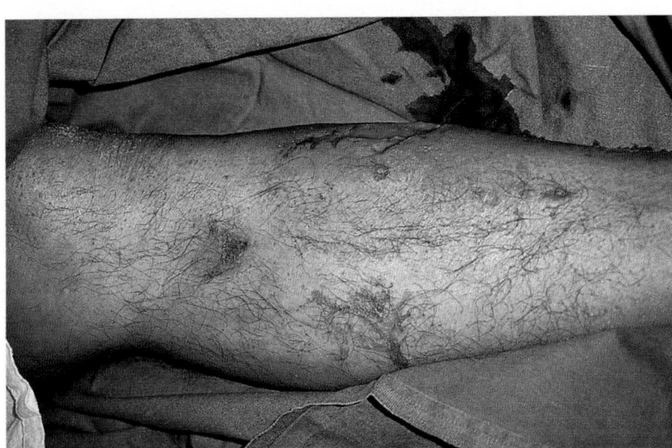

Fig. 24.2 Infected wound. This shin laceration was closed primarily without adequate cleaning. Gas gangrene has developed and the patient died 10 days later.

Chronic osteomyelitis

Once osteomyelitis is established it is almost impossible to eradicate. The intraosseus blood vessels thrombose and the bone infarcts. Pus lifts the periosteum. If the process continues the pus ruptures through the periosteum, tracks into the soft tissues and may even discharge through the skin remote from the initial site of infection. The bone may die and form a sequestrum. The new bone formed by the periosteum which has been lifted is known as an involucrum. Once there is dead bone the infecting organisms have a permanent site where they can survive beyond the reach of the body's immune system or of antibiotics. Any time that the patient's resistance to infection is reduced, the infection can break out again and produce a septicaemia. Brodie's abscess is a chronic abscess walled off in sclerotic bone. This can remain dormant for many years.

Treatment of chronic osteomyelitis

All dead tissue needs to be removed. If there is a fracture, this will need to be stabilised. If there was previous fixation which has become infected then this will need replacing. The dead bone is very sclerotic and extremely difficult to remove without causing a new fracture. It is also very difficult to be certain that all dead bone has been removed. If it is not, then the infection will recur. The introduction of the Ilizarov fixator and modern distraction techniques allow much more radical excision with a real prospect of reconstructing a functioning limb.

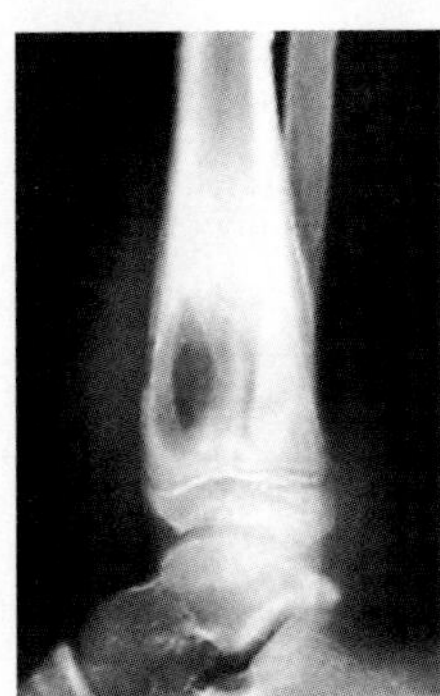

Fig. 24.3 Brodie's abscess of the lower end of the tibia, revealing a band of sclerosis surrounding a central lucent area.

Sir Benjamin Brodie, 1783–1862. Surgeon, St George's Hospital, London, England.

Chronic osteomyelitis

- Excise all dead tissue
- Take deep cultures
- Give appropriate antibiotics
- Reconstruct limb

Discitis of the spine

In the elderly, infection of the invertebral disc can occur spontaneously. It may arise from haematogenous spread from a urinary tract infection through the lumbar plexus and commonly involves Gram-negative organisms. The infection is low grade and insidious in onset. The patient complains of increasingly severe back pain which is also present during the night, not just in the day during activity. The patient may have a low-grade fever and the white cell count and erythrocyte sedimentation rate (ESR) may be raised. The diagnosis can be difficult to make on X-ray because degenerative changes present in the elderly spine may make the characteristic signs of collapse of the disc space difficult to spot. However, if the diagnosis is considered, careful scrutiny of the X-rays may show a soft-tissue shadow swelling in the prevertebral space with destruction of the adjacent vertebral body endplates. Needle aspiration under image intensifier will allow the organism to be identified and its sensitivity determined. Treatment with the appropriate antibiotic, initially intravenously and then orally, should cure the condition.

Tuberculous osteomyelitis

Tuberculous osteomyelitis is rare and occurs following haematogenous spread from the primary focus in the lung or in the gut. In the spine it is usual for two adjacent vertebral bodies to be involved (Pott's disease). The vertebrae collapse but the posterior structures remain intact, so the spine angulates into a kyphos. An abscess forms, which may put pressure on to the spinal cord or the nerve roots, but which also tracks forward in the prevertebral space. From there it follows fascia, and in the case of low thoracic or lumbar tuberculosis may follow the psoas muscle from its original origin to its insertion in the lesser trochanter of the femur. There

Gavriil Ilizarov, 1921–92. Orthopaedic Surgeon, Kurgan, Russia.
Hans C. J. Gram, 1853–1938. Danish Physician.
Percival Pott, 1714–88. Surgeon, St Bartholomew's Hospital, London, England. Described this fracture dislocation of the ankle in 1765.

the pus may track through the subcutaneous fat and discharge through the skin. There is little inflammation because the abscess cavity is remote from the point of discharge so it is a 'cold' abscess.

In the developed world, tuberculosis is again on the increase in patients who are immunocompromised either because of diseases such as acquired immunnodeficiency syndrome (AIDS) or because they have been immunosuppressed. The organism is becoming increasingly resistant to standard antibiotics such as rifampicin. The failure of some patients, such as drug addicts, to comply fully with the treatment regime, further increases the risk of spread of antibiotic-resistant tuberculosis.

Septic arthritis

Arthritis caused by sepsis is a rare but important surgical emergency. Some organisms such as *S. aureus* may have a collagenase, which actually dissolves the articular surface. If the joint is not sterilised within 24–48 hours, irreversible damage will occur to the articular surface, which will inevitably lead to aggressive arthritis and even ankylosis (fusion) of the joint. Pus in the joint may interfere with the nutrition of the articular cartilage, which has no blood supply itself but derives nutrients from the synovial fluid. In acute arthritis the rapid accumulation of pus leads to a sharp rise in intra-articular pressure. This is extremely painful for the patient, but also tamponades the blood vessels in the capsule. This is the main blood supply to both the femoral head and the humeral head, and so avascular necrosis will occur if the pressure is not quickly relieved.

Epidemiology

Septic arthritis occurs most commonly in children but can also occur in adults whose resistance to infection has been reduced, such as diabetics, and can also occur after surgical intervention, such as arthroscopy. The onset is sudden with extreme pain in the joint. The patient may have rigors and will certainly feel shivery and generally unwell.

Examination

The joint may be red, hot and swollen, and held in the position of comfort (see Table 24.1). However, the most characteristic feature is the quite extraordinary amount of pain experienced by the patient when any attempt whatsoever is made to move the joint. If the joint moves even 1° the patient cries out with pain. If this sign is present, then both diagnosis and treatment run hand in hand. The pressure in the joint needs to be relieved without delay and the organism needs to be identified. Needle aspiration of the joint will provide fluid for microscopy and culture and start the decompression of the hip. In the child this will need to be done under a general anaesthetic, and is most easily performed using an image

(a)

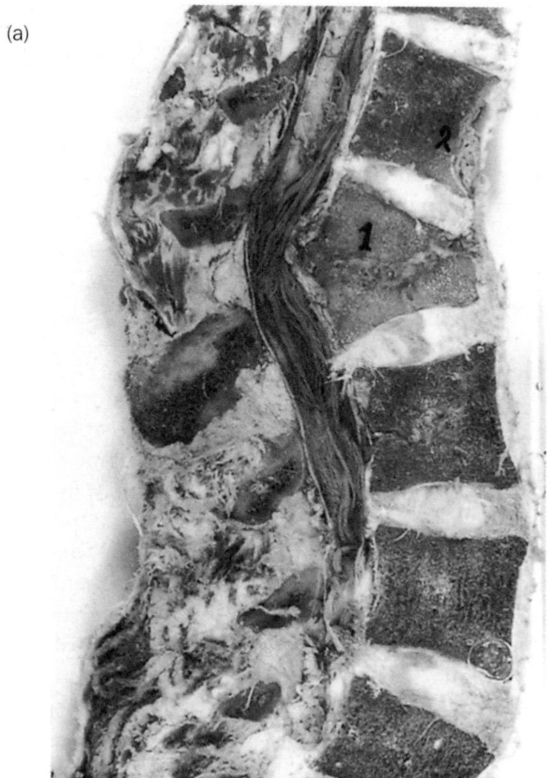

(b)

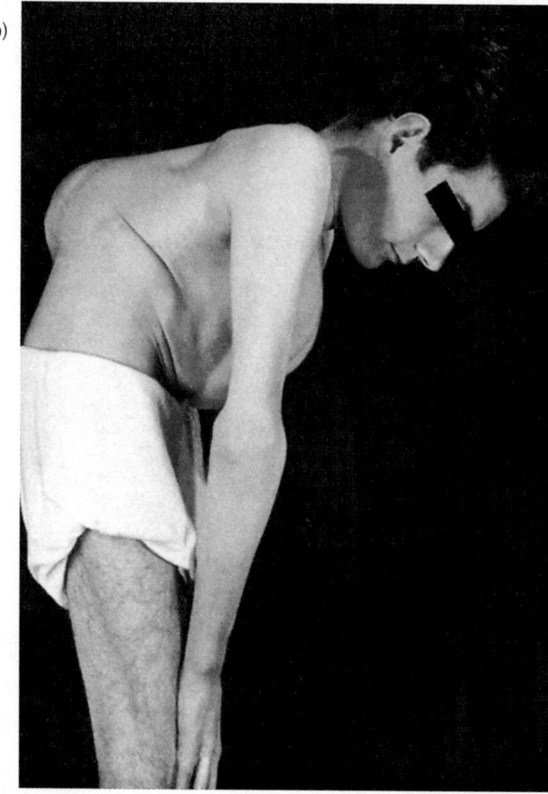

Fig. 24.4 (a) Tuberculosis of the spine. L1 and L2 (1) have collapsed to produce wedging (and hence kyphos). A further tuberculosis lesion is present in D12; (b) the clinical appearance of kyphos due to tuberculosis of the spine (*courtesy of the London Hospital Museum, London, England*).

Table 24.1 Suppurative arthritis: physical signs and optimum positions for joint ankylosis

Joint	*Position*	*Site of maximum swelling*
Shoulder	Adducted	Under the deltoid along the tendon of the biceps and in the axilla
Elbow	Flexed at a right angle and pronated	On either side of the triceps tendon
Wrist	Slight flexion	Under extensor and flexor tendons
Hip	Flexed, adducted and externally rotated	Upper part of Scarpa's triangle
Knee	Flexed	Suprapatellar bursa and either side of patellar tendon
Ankle	Slightly plantarflexed (and inverted at the subtalar joint)	Anteriorly and on either side of the Achilles' tendon

intensifier. If pus is found in the joint then the best treatment is to proceed immediately to a complete decompression of the joint and wash out either through the arthroscope or by open arthrotomy. It is important that organisms are washed out of the joint as quickly as possible to prevent collagenase from damaging the articular surface. It is equally important that the pressure within the joint is reduced to normal to prevent avascular necrosis and to allow normal nutrition of the articular cartilage. Intravenous antibiotics should also be given as the patient is likely to be septicaemic (Fig. 24.5). The initial antibiotic should be chosen according to whether the organism identified at microscopy is Gram-negative or Gram-positive. The antibiotic can be changed later when the sensitivity is known.

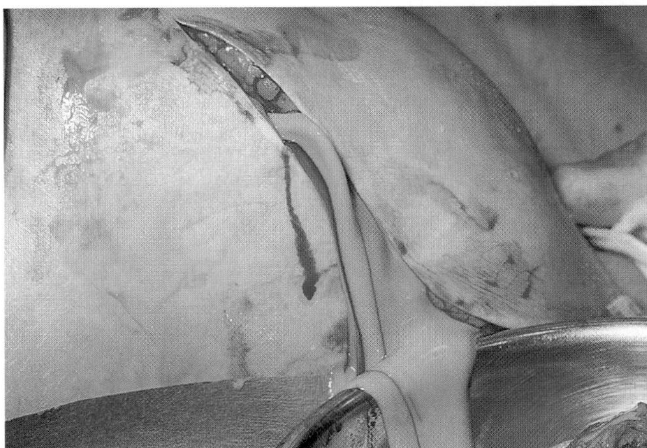

Fig. 24.5 Drainage of a septic joint.

Antonio Scarpa, b. 1747. Italian anatomist and surgeon.

Achilles, the Greek hero, was the son of Peleus and Thetis. When he was a child his mother dipped him in the River Styx, so that he should be invunerable in battle. The heel by which she held him did not get wet and was therefore unprotected. Achilles died from a wound in the heel, received at the siege of Troy.

Late diagnosis of septic arthritis

In immunocompromised patients the symptoms of septic arthritis may not be so florid, and initially the diagnosis may not be suspected. If it is likely that septic arthritis has been present for several days, then it is unlikely that the infection can be brought under control without a synovectomy, and the prognosis for the joint is poor. It should be splinted in a position of best function, as a painless arthrodesis will be the best outcome that can be hoped for. The position of function is not the same as the position of comfort, and therefore the joint will need careful splintage. After acute septic arthritis there is usually bony ankylosis. This provides a stable painless limb, but if the ankylosis is not solid, or if the joint has fused in a poor position, a formal arthrodesis may need to be performed once the infection has been brought under control. This operation will need to be covered with antibiotics, as it may produce a further recurrence of septicaemia.

Tuberculous arthritis

Tuberculous arthritis can be of slightly more insidious onset than acute septic arthritis, but nevertheless the pressure within the joint causes severe pain. The joint is held in the position of comfort but the redness and swelling may not be so pronounced. However, there is marked wasting of the muscles around the joint. The child will be very unwilling to move the joint, and the muscles around the joint may be in tight spasm, preventing it moving. This leads to the characteristic feature of 'night cries'. When the child finally falls asleep the muscle spasm decreases and the joint moves. The child awakes with a characteristic cry of pain.

The treatment once again is decompression of the joint and identification of the organism as soon as possible, then treatment with the appropriate antibiotics. Synovectomy may well be useful, especially if the diagnosis is delayed (as is usual). In tuberculosis the ankylosis is usually fibrous and therefore unstable. Once the infection is brought under control there may then be a place for carrying out a formal bony arthrodesis with the limb in the position of function.

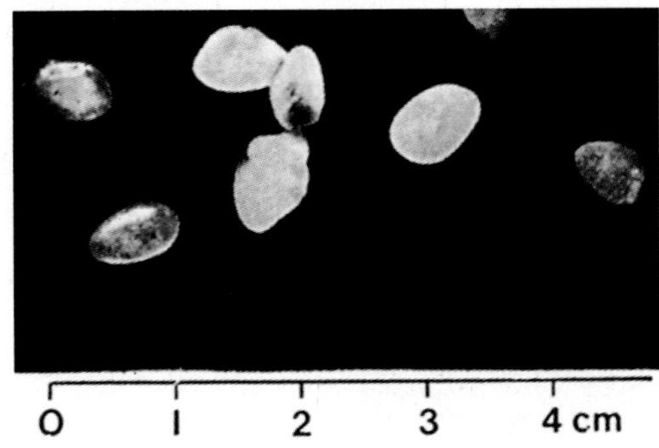

Fig. 24.6 'Melon-seed' bodies from tuberculous synovitis at the wrist.

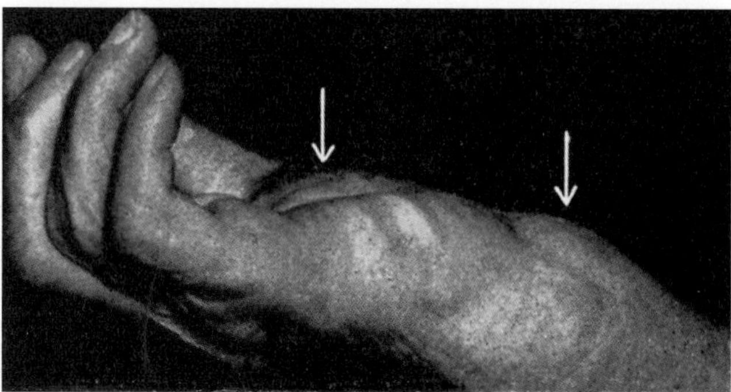

Fig. 24.7 A compound palmar ganglion (tuberculous flexor synovitis at the wrist). The swelling in the palm communicates with the swelling above the wrist and cross-fluctuation can be demonstrated.

Tuberculous tenosynovitis

This is a rare condition. If it occurs in the hand a soft ganglion appears which seems to be multilobulated (the compound palmar ganglion). If this is drained surgically the characteristic finding will be of a synovitis with a synovial effusion full of fibrinous 'melon-seeds'. The treatment is as for tuberculous septic arthritis.

Crystal deposition disorders

Gout, pseudogout and hydroxyapatite deposition are three types of crystal deposition in joints and around joints, and can cause pain and inflammation. In the long term they may actually cause destruction of the joint. They can be confused with infection.

Crystal deposition disorders

Type:	Crystal deposited:
• Gout	• Monosodium urate crystals
• Pseudogout	• Calcium pyrophosphate
• Chondrocalinosis	• Hydroxyapatite

Gout. Normally the patient is unable to metabolise purine normally. This leads to hyperuricaemia and urate crystal deposition in the joints. The condition is very common in men but may be seen in women after the menopause. Most cases are congenital. Secondary causes can be divided into those resulting from overproduction of uric acid or failure of excretion. Myloproliferative disorders may lead to tissue breakdown and overproduction. Any form of renal failure may prevent excretion.

Presentation. The patient suffers sudden attacks of acute arthritis and/or tendonitis as a result of monosodium urate crystals being deposited in the joint in tendon sheaths or in tophi. The patients may also be prone to renal calculi. Any minor trauma or a bout of drinking alcohol may precipitate an attack. This normally occurs in the first metatarsal phalangeal joint of the big toe, the ankle, the finger joints and the olecranon bursa. The joint becomes hot and extremely tender. The skin over it is tense and glassy. If the joint is aspirated birefringent crystals can be seen under polarised light. These confirm the diagnosis. Chronic gout leads to degenerative changes in the joints. Tophi may form on the extensor surfaces of joints and in the ears.

Diagnosis of gout

- History – previous attacks, acute-onset arthritis
- Examination – hot, red, painful site
- Investigation – birefringement crystals in joint aspirate
- Differential diagnosis – septic arthritis

The differential diagnosis is septic arthritis. The patient will usually have had an attack before and will therefore know the diagnosis, but otherwise aspiration of the joint and the finding of crystals rather than pus will give the diagnosis. The X-rays are compatible with an erosive arthritis.

Treatment. The treatment is resting the joint and anti-inflammatories. Allopurinol can be used as a prophylactic agent but must not be started during an acute attack When it is started, a anti-inflammatory should be given at the same time, as otherwise it may actually cause an acute attack.

Pseudogout. Pseudogout involves the deposition of calcium pyrophosphate crystals. It is part of the normal ageing process of a joint. However, patients can develop an acute arthritis resembling gout. It normally occurs in large joints such as the knee. On X-ray the articular cartilage and menisci can be seen to be calcified. Once again, the diagnosis is made by finding birefingent crystals in the synovial fluid. An attack can be treated by aspirating the joint and injecting corticosteroid.

Hydroxyapatite deposition. Hydroxyapatite crystals can also be deposited in a joint, in a bursa or in a tendon sheath. They most commonly give problems in the shoulder, where they can be seen on X-ray as a small area of radio-opacity.

Treatment. The treatment of gout can be divided into the management of an acute attack and the prevention of future acute attacks in patients with an underlying metabolic disorder which predisposes them to further acute attacks.

Treatment of an acute attack of gout

- Analgesia
- Nonsteroidal anti-inflammatories
- Rest
- NOT alloprinol

Hyperuricaemia which is leading to acute attacks.

- Treatment. Allopurinol.

Management of an acute attack. The treatment is symptomatic with analgesia, nonsteroidal anti-inflammatories and rest. Check that any predisposing factors such as diuretics are stopped if possible.

Prevention of further attacks. Regular treatment with allopurinol should bring down the levels of uric acid in the blood and so reduce the chance of further attacks. However, allopurinol should not be started during an acute attack as in the short term it may exacerbate the condition rather than improve it. For the same reason patients need to be warned, when starting antimetabolism drugs, that an acute attack may be precipitated.

Further reading

Browner, B.P., Jupiter, J.B. and Levine, A.M. (eds) (1992) *Skeletal Trauma: Fractures, Dislocations, Ligamentous Injuries*, W.B. Saunders, London.

Canale, S.T. (ed.) (1998) *Campbell's Operative Orthopaedics*, 9th edn, Mosby, London.

Gregg, P.J., Stevens, J.G. and Worlock, P.H. (1995) *Fractures and Dislocations: Principles of Management*, Blackwell Science, Oxford.

Rockwood, C.A., Green, D.P. and Bucholz, R.W. *et al.* (1996) Fractures, Vols I–III, *Fractures in Adults, Fractures in Children*, Lippincott Williams & Wilkins, London.

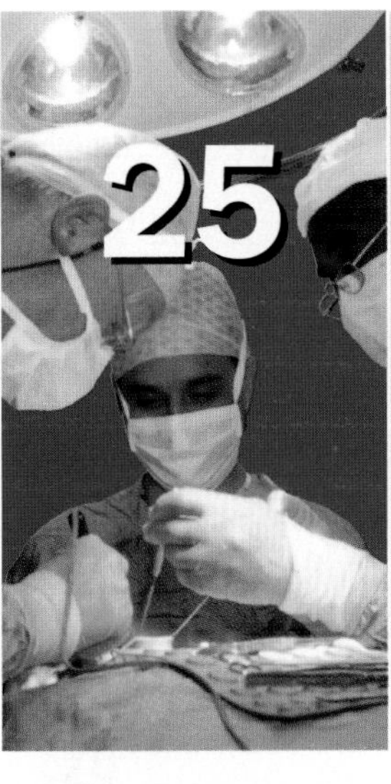

25 Diseases of bones and joints: tumours

Education goal

- To understand that the majority of malignant tumours in bone is secondaries, and that a significant part of their management is palliative.

Learning objectives

- To understand the nomenclature of tumours in the musculoskeletal system.
- To learn the cardinal features of the history, examination and investigations which distinguish benign tumours from malignant ones.
- To learn the importance of making sure that the approach for the biopsy does not compromise further management of the tumour.

Introduction

Benign tumours of the musculoskeletal system are common and frequently show up as an incidental finding on an X-ray taken for other reasons. Metastases in the skeleton are also common, particularly from carcinoma of the breast, the prostate and the kidney. Primary malignant tumours of the musculoskeletal system are rare, apart from those arising from the marrow such as multiple myeloma and lymphoma.

Tumours are named after the tissue from which they have arisen. They can be identified from their shape and their staining. Benign tumours are give the suffix 'oma' and malignant tumours 'sarcoma' (see Table 25.1).

Benign tumours

Many of the benign tumours appear to have been present from birth and to grow with the child. They may be multiple, suggesting a problem in development, and if they are truly benign they stop growing when the child stops growing.

Table 25.1 Classification of bone tumours

Origin	*Benign*	*Malignant*
Cartilage	Osteochondroma Chondroma Chondroblastoma Chondromyxoid fibroma	Chondrosarcoma
Bone	Osteoid osteoma Osteoblastoma	Osteosarcoma
Bone marrow		Multiple myeloma Malignant lymphoma
Fibrous tissue	Desmoplastic fibroma Fibroma	Fibrosarcoma
Unknown origin	Giant cell tumour Fibrous histiocytoma	Malignant giant cell tumour Ewing's tumour Adamantinoma
Vascular tissue	Aneurysmal bone cyst Haemangioma	
Synovium	Synovioma	Synovial sarcoma

Bailey & Love's Short Practice of Surgery, 23rd edition. Edited by R.C.G. Russell, N.S. Williams and C.J.K. Bulstrode. Published in 2000 by Arnold Publishers.

James Ewing, 1866–1943. Professor of Oncology, Cornell University Medical Colege, New York, USA.

Osteochondromas are outgrowths of the bone, which may look much smaller on X-ray than they feel on clinical examination. This is because the outgrowth of bone has a large cartilage cap over it. Growths within the bones such as enchondromas may weaken the bone so that it fractures. The benign tumour is then diagnosed on X-ray with a pathological fracture running across it (Fig. 25.1).

Where possible, benign tumours should be left alone. There are, however, three indications for surgical intervention in a benign tumour (Table 25.2).

1. If there is doubt about diagnosis and a biopsy is needed to determine whether the tumour is, indeed, benign or malignant. In this case surgery should be planned as if the tumour is malignant, and an approach made which allows either complete excision of the tumour or an incision which will not interfere with further surgery later, if a massive implant or amputation is required.
2. If the bone is so weakened that a pathological fracture has occurred or is likely to occur. In this case the contents of the tumour can be curetted out and the cavity filled with chips of bone harvested from elsewhere in the patient.
3. If the bony protuberance is so prominent that it creates a cosmetic deformity or interferes with muscles or joints, so that the limb cannot function normally.

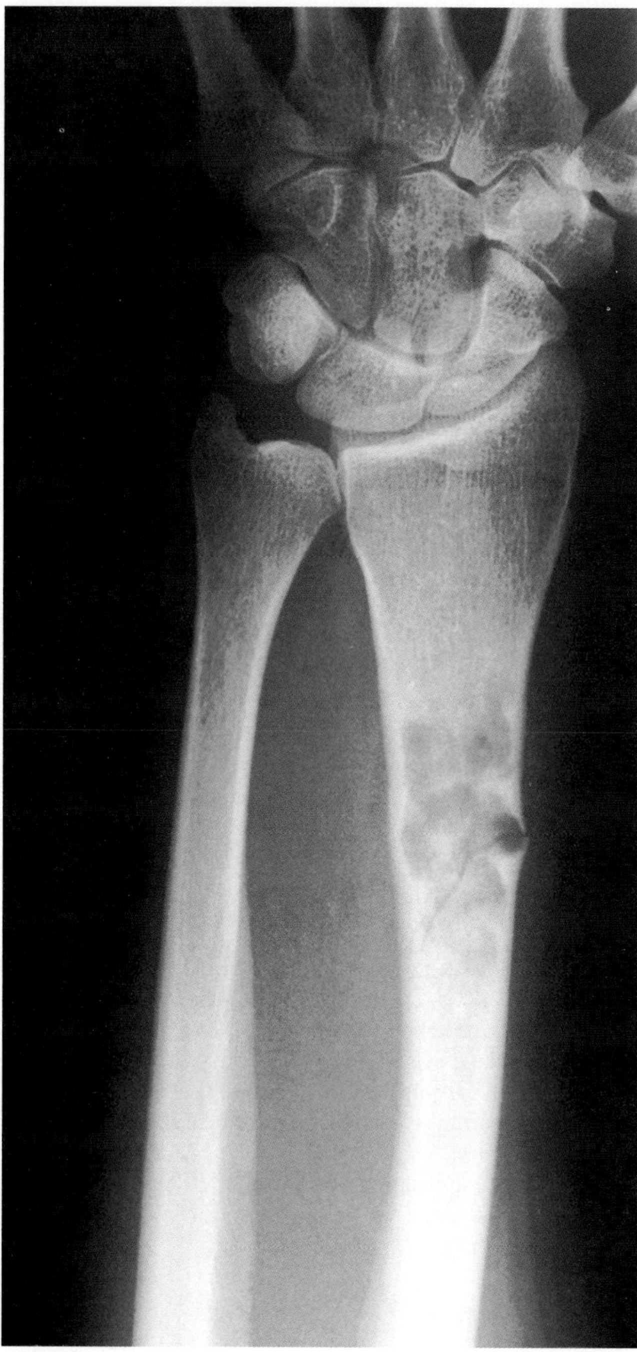

Fig. 25.1 Enchondroma of the distal radius. This was symptomless until a relatively trivial trauma produced a pathological fracture.

Distinguishing between benign and malignant tumours

This can be very difficult in the growing child, and is best handled with a team approach among the surgeon, radiologist and pathologist.

History

Malignant tumours are usually painful. Benign tumours are not. The pain of malignant tumours is very characteristic. It is most noticeable at rest, particularly at night. The site and the age of the patient will also give clues to the likely pathology.

Examination

A lump which has been present for a long time is unlikely to be malignant. Unfortunately, some benign tumours can turn malignant, so a sudden change in size or increase in tenderness in what was previously thought to be a benign tumour should raise suspicions.

Investigations

X-rays

Benign tumours have well-circumscribed margins and may even have a thin rim of sclerosis around a lytic lesion. Malignant lesions do not have clear margins. A subtle, but important, sign is periosteal lifting over the site of the lesion (Fig. 25.2). This indicates inflammation and can be a clear sign of malignancy.

Table 25.2 Indications for surgery in benign bone tumours

Indications for surgery	*Problem*	*Action*
1	Doubt about diagnosis	Plan surgery as if it is malignant
2	Bone weak	Curette and graft
3	Interferes with movement	Excise but send for histology

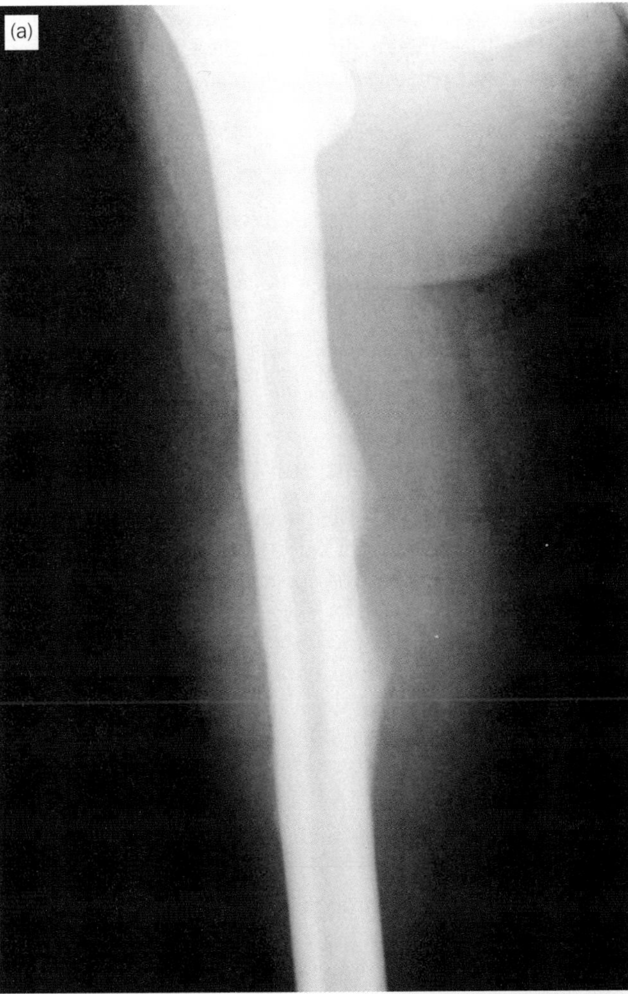

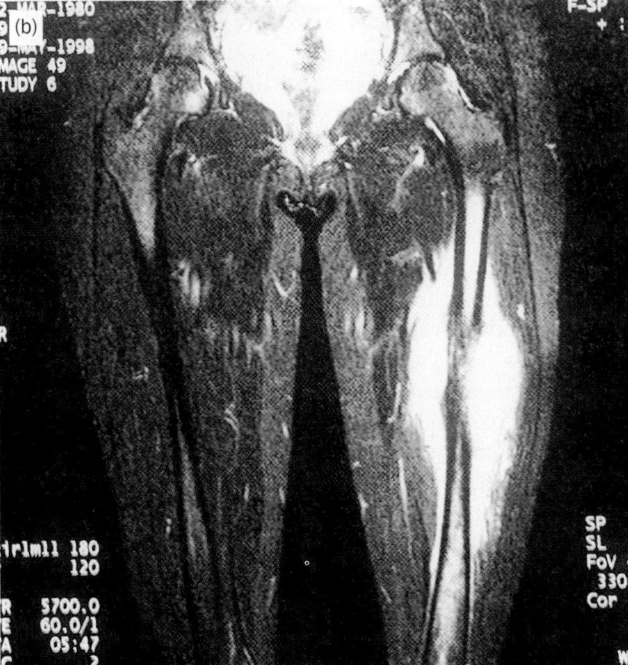

Fig. 25.2 Ewing's sarcoma of the femur. The X-ray shows periosteal lifting. The MRI shows the extent of the lesion.

Periosteal lifting can also occur over a stress fracture and if there is underlying infection, so both these possibilities must be borne in mind when making a differential diagnosis.

Osteochondroma

These benign tumours are common and frequently multiple. The commonest site is in the femur or the tibia around the knee. There are commonly on a bony pedicle which grows away from the epiphyseal plate and which is covered in a large cartilage cap (Fig. 25.3). If they are large they can interfere with the function of the knee. Occasionally they become malignant and if they become painful the possibility of malignant change should be considered.

Osteoid osteoma

These benign tumours occur in children, adolescents and young adults. They are commonest in the femur and tibia but can occur elsewhere, even in the spine. They are unusual as benign tumours in that they produce a constant aching pain,

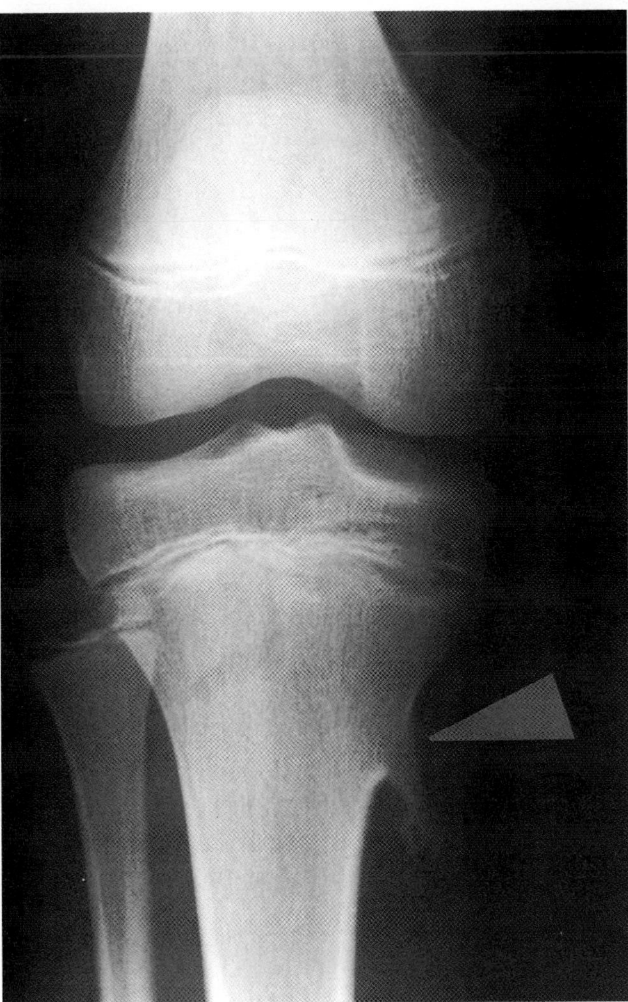

Fig. 25.3 Osteochondroma – the arrow points at the base of the lesion. Note that the stalk grows away from the epiphysis. The cartilage cap is much larger than the X-ray might suggest as it is radiolucent.

which is most noticeable at night and is sometimes relieved by aspirin. They can be very difficult to see on plain X-ray where they may look like an area of slight sclerosis (Fig. 25.4). However, on tomography it may be possible to see the characteristic radiolucent centre. Osteoid osteomas also show up very hot on radioisotope scans. Surgical excision relieves the pain but they can be difficult to find at surgery so careful preparation is needed.

Chondromas

As their name suggests, these tumours are made up mainly of cartilage and are common in the hands and the feet. The medulla of the bone may be scalloped out (enchondroma) and there may be cortical thinning which may produce a pathological fracture. The condition of multiple enchondroma is called Ollier's disease. Malignant change is not common but when many chondromata are present this risk is increased.

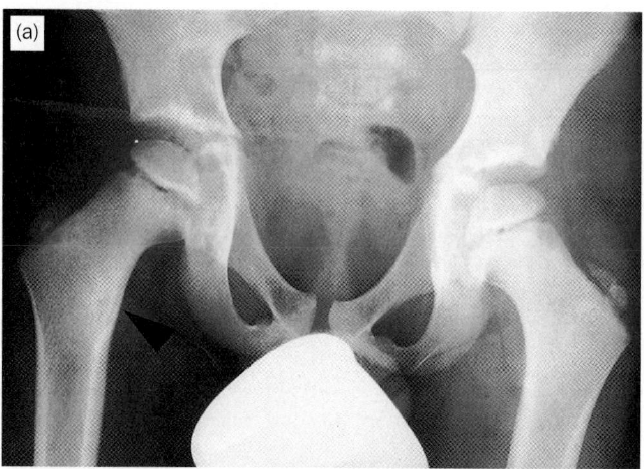

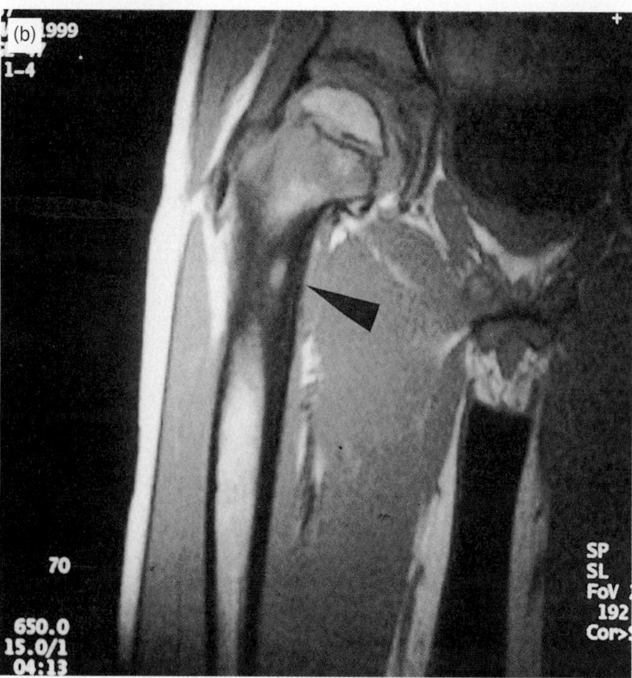

Fig. 25.4 Osteoid osteoma of the right femoral neck. (a) X-ray. (b) MRI. The arrows point to the lesion.

Fibroma

These appear as well-circumscribed lytic lesions in the cortex of bone. They can be difficult to distinguish from fibrous dysplasia, which usually has new bone within the lytic lesion. Another dysplasia, which can cause confusion with a tumour, is the aneurysmal bone cyst. This is an expanding lytic lesion most commonly found in the ends of growing long bones.

Osteoclastoma or giant cell tumour

These benign tumours are filled with undifferentiated spindle cells and multinucleate giant cells (Fig. 25.5). They are commonly found in the epiphysis of a bone, lying close to the epiphyseal plate. The cortex over the tumour may be destroyed and there may be periosteal elevation. They can be treated by block excision but, unfortunately, they are commonly closely associated with a joint. If they are rapidly growing or recur after excision they may be malignant and require more aggressive treatment.

Metastatic tumours

A pathological fracture through a metastatic tumour may be the first clue that a patient has malignant disease. Indeed, the primary may never be found. In other cases metastatic bone disease occurs some time after treatment of the primary tumour. The commonest source of metastases in bone is tumours of the breast, the prostate and the kidney. In patients who are suspected of having metastases, a radioisotope bone scan may show up lesions which are not yet symptomatic, and which may not even be visible on X-ray (Fig. 25.6).

The management of metastases is excision, where these are isolated and relatively slow growing. In the majority of cases radiotherapy and/or chemotherapy can be used to slow the rate of growth of the lesion. If more than 50 per cent of the cortex is eroded over more than 2 cm then it is considered that the long bones are liable to imminent pathological fracture. Under these circumstances it is best to stabilise the bone before it breaks. In the femur, the tibia or the humerus, a prophylactic intramedullary nail can be used to support the bone. Even where a fracture has already occurred, stabilisation and radiotherapy will relieve the patient's pain, allow them to remain mobile and may even allow the fracture to heal.

Before embarking on stabilisation of a metastatic lesion, it is always worth taking an X-ray of the whole bone and of the

Louis Ollier, 1830–1900. Professor of Surgery, Lyons, France.

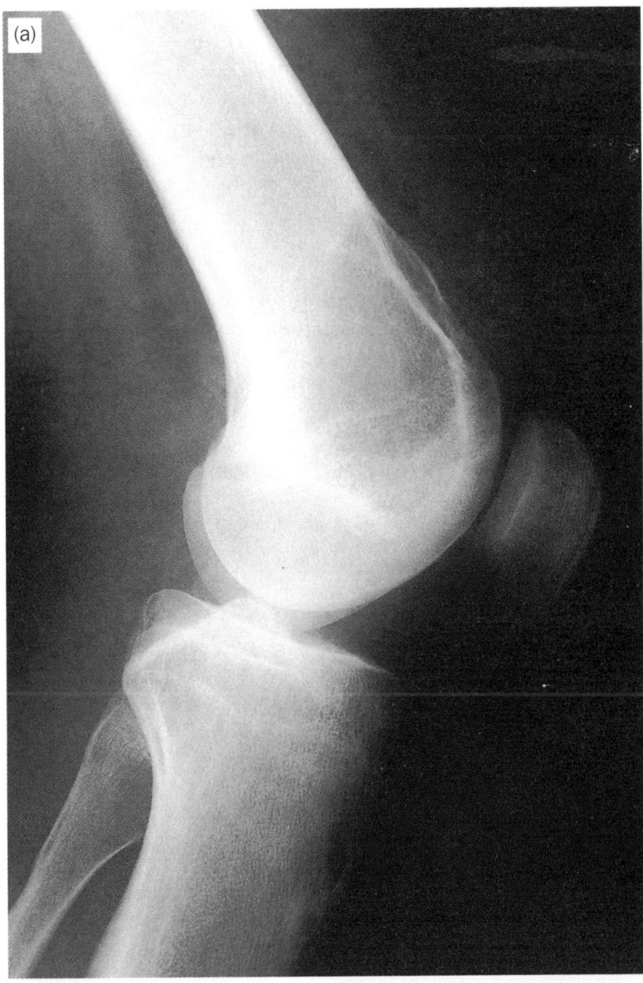

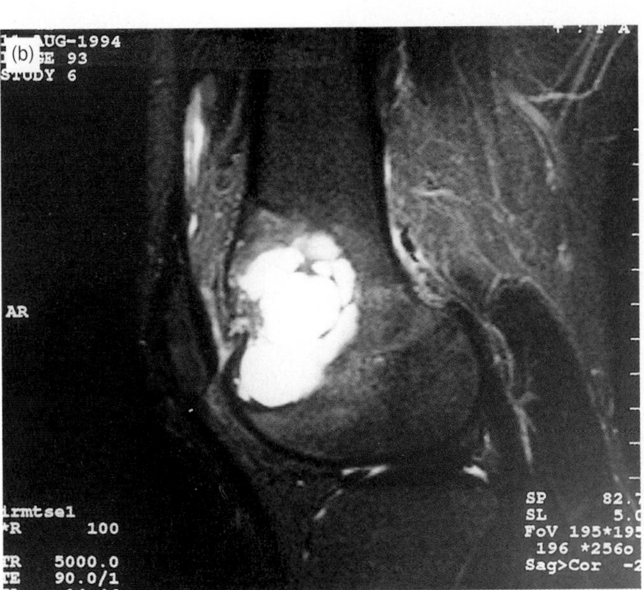

Fig. 25.5 Giant cell tumour of the distal femur. (a) The X-ray shows a lystic lesion. (b) MRI shows fluid in the lesion.

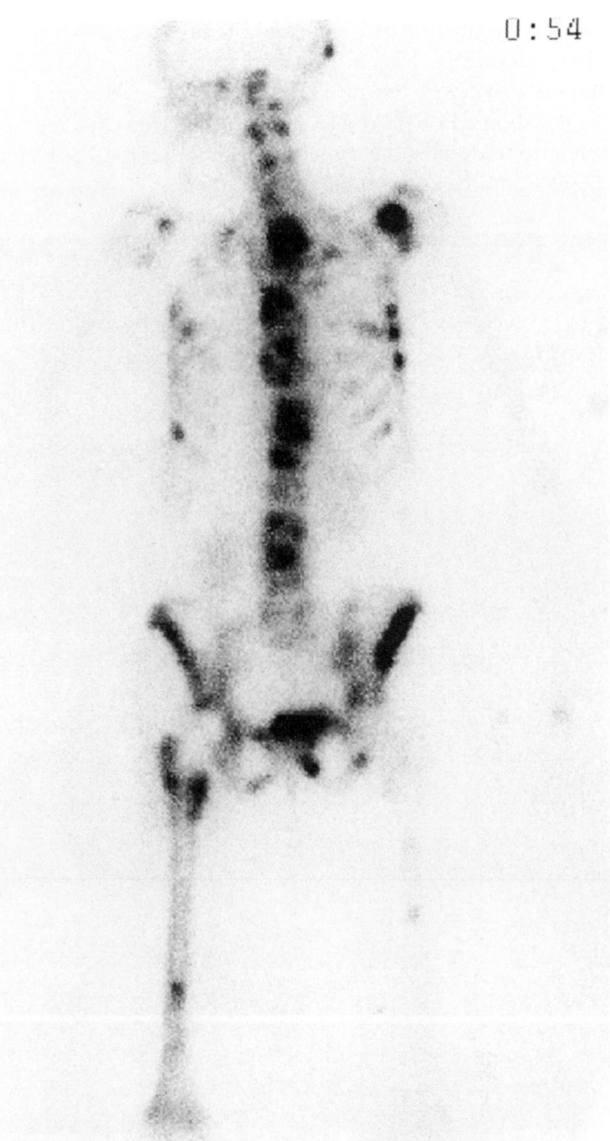

Fig. 25.6 Radioisotope scan showing multiple metastases in the skeleton.

other long bones. It may be that other bones need fixing at the same sitting or that there are so many metastases that stabilisation of one will make no difference to the patient's quality of life. Patients with multiple metastases may have a high serum calcium and this will need checking before embarking on a general anaesthetic. The risk of pulmonary embolus is also high, and patients need to be warned of this when giving their consent for surgery.

Primary malignant bone tumours

These are very rare indeed. The commonest of this rare group is the osteosarcoma. These tumours have very variable histology and occur either in adolescents or in the elderly secondary to Paget's disease. The tumour is metaphyseal

Sir James Paget, 1814–99. Surgeon, St Bartholomew's Hospital, London, England.

(usually the tibia or the femur) and is easy to confuse with a stress fracture or with an infected haematoma. If the diagnosis is suspected, the tumour should not be biopsied. The patient should be referred to a team of doctors who are competent to undertake the surgery, the radiotherapy, the chemotherapy and the counselling of the patient.

Imaging

Characteristically, there is periosteal lifting (Codman's triangle) and 'sun-ray' spicules of new bone within the tumour. Magnetic resonance imaging (MRI) and computerised tomography (CT) scan may be helpful in determining the true extent of the tumour within the medulla (Fig. 25.7).

Treatment

The choice of treatment depends on the histological grading of the tumour, the age of the patient, the presence or absence of secondaries and the wishes of the patient.

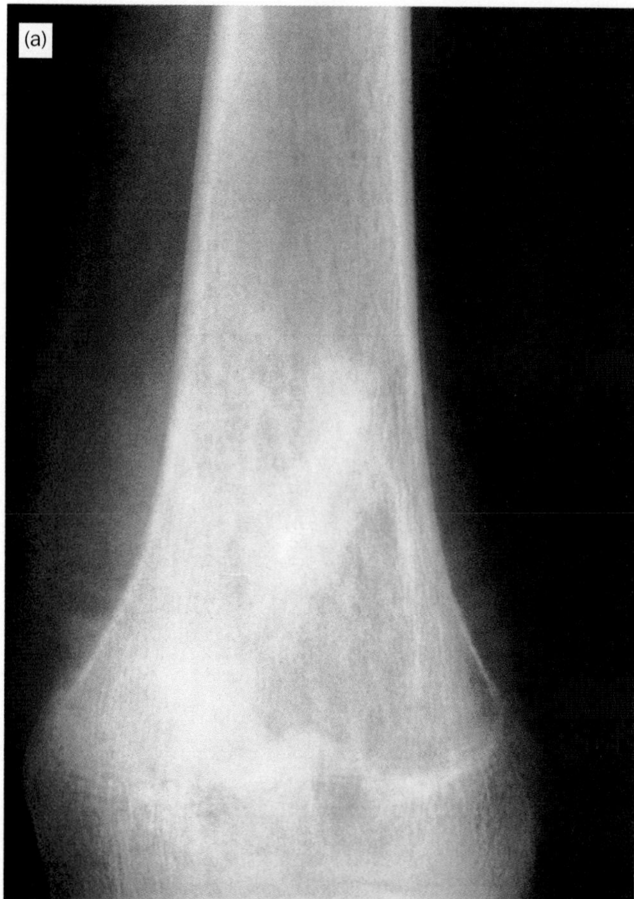

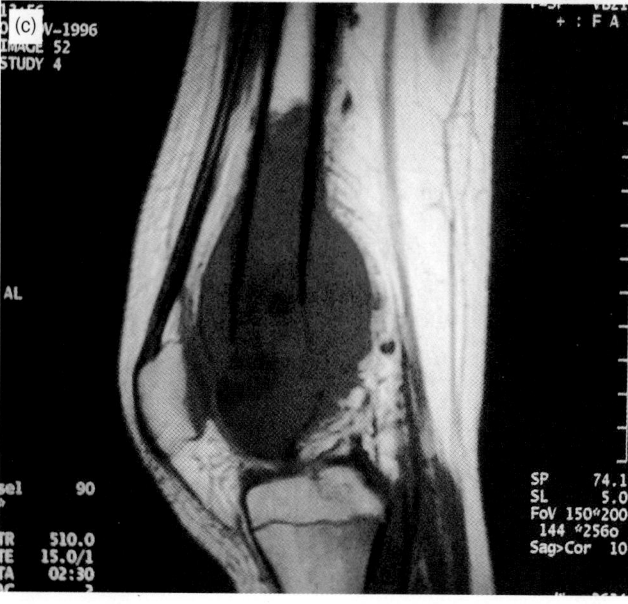

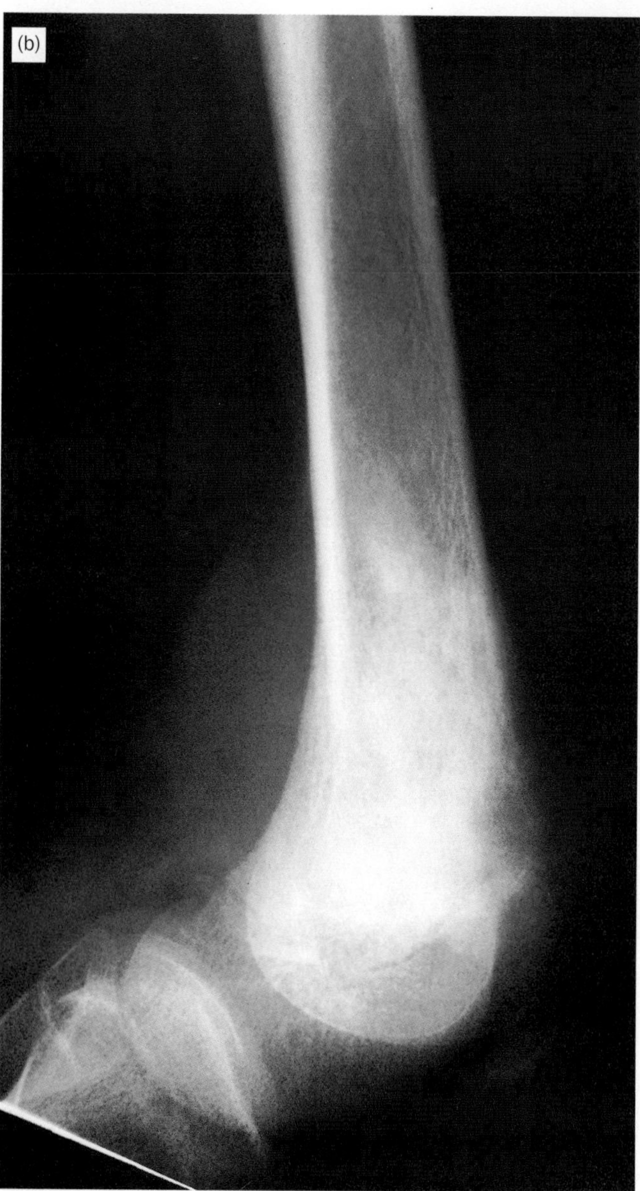

Fig. 25.7 Osteosarcoma of the distal femur. (a) anteroposterior X-ray. (b) Lateral X-ray. (c) MRI of the lesion showing the extent of soft-tissue involvement.

If there is no evidence of secondaries, and it is technically possible, an amputation may be the treatment of choice with chemotherapy used to destroy micrometastases. Alternatively, radiotherapy and chemotherapy to shrink the lesion followed by a massive joint replacement may carry a higher risk of recurrence but may be cosmetically and functionally much more acceptable. If massive joint replacements are to be used in growing children, then designs need to be used which allow for lengthening of the limb as the child grows. Massive allografts using bones and joints from cadaver donors have limited long-term success, and have problems with rejection and the possibility of transmission of infection.

Prognosis

Survival is dependent on the histological grading and the degree of spread, but in cure rates of around 50 per cent can be achieved.

Chondrosarcoma

This tumour commonly occurs in the pelvis, ribs or proximal long bones in middle-aged people. The tumour is lytic with ill-defined boundaries and has speckled calcification within its substance (Fig. 25.8). The grade of malignancy is very variable and is closely linked to the prognosis. Low-grade tumours have a survival rate of 75 per cent at 5 years, while high-grade tumours have a survival rate of less than 10 per cent over the same period.

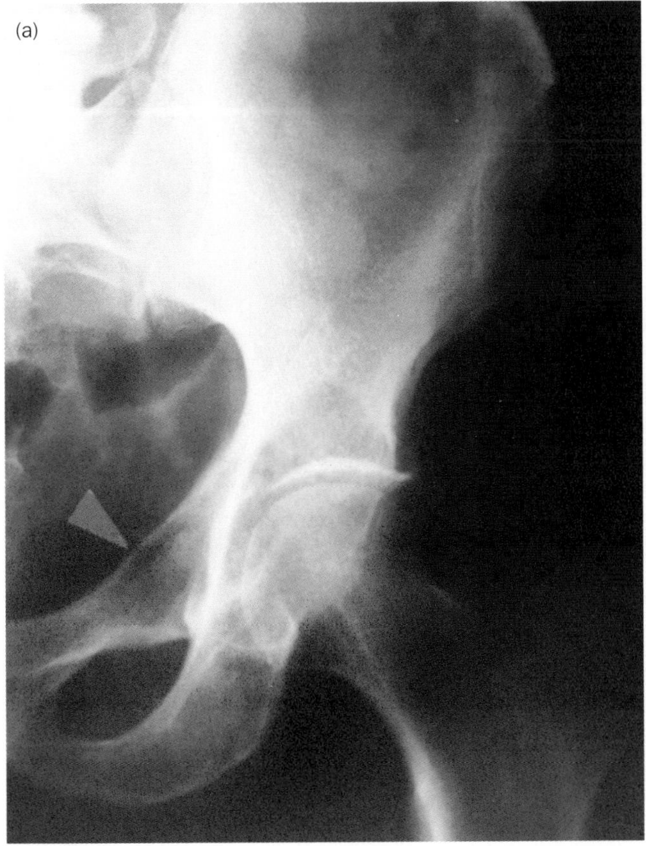

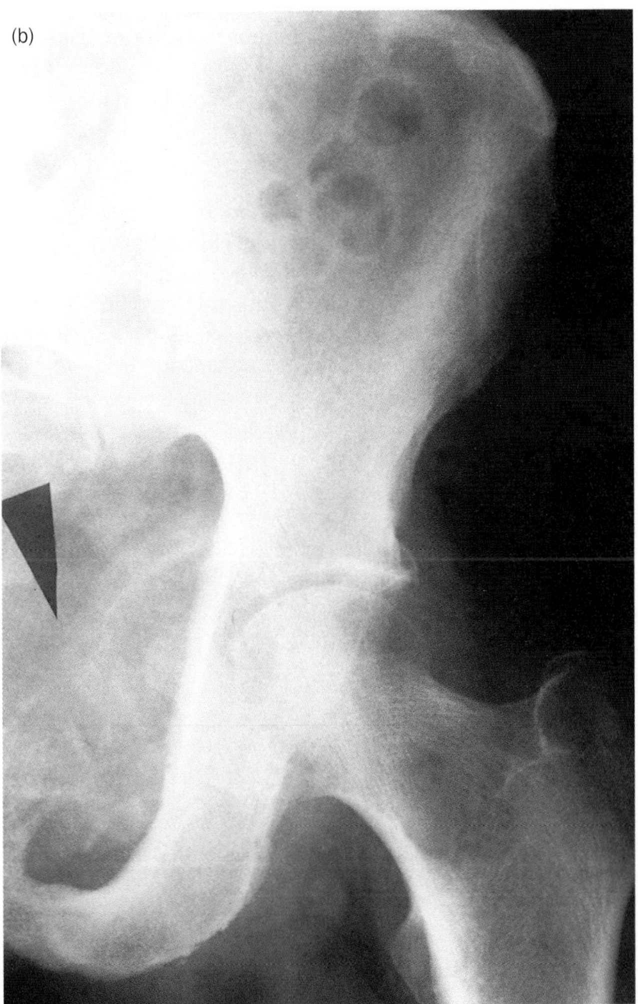

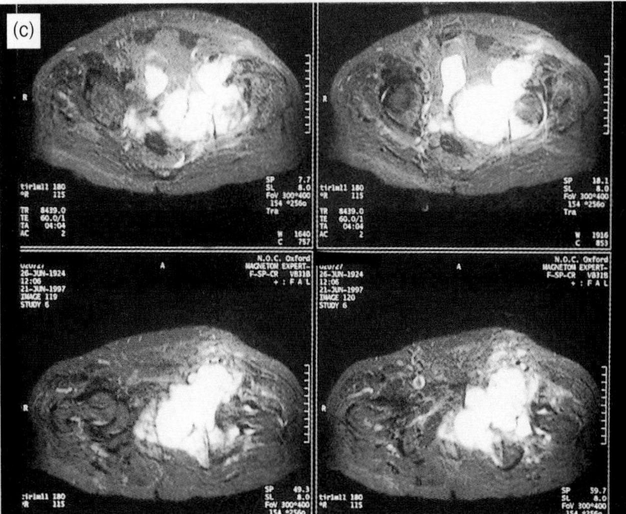

Fig. 25.8 Chondrosarcoma of the pelvis. (a) At first presentation and (b) 21 months later. (c) MRI showing the pelvis filled with tumour.

Fibrosarcoma

These tumours occur most commonly in the metaphysis or diaphysis of the tibia or femur, but may also arise in soft tissue. They metastasise to the lungs and the 5-year survival rate is around 30 per cent.

Synovial sarcoma

This is a highly malignant tumour which metastasises through the blood supply, bloodstream and lymphatics. Five-year survival rate is low whatever treatment is attempted.

Ewing's tumour

This tumour is commonest in childhood and arises in the midshaft or metaphysis of long bones. The child may present with pyrexia and have a high erythrocyte sedimentation rate, so the condition can be confused with osteomyelitis. Radiologically, there may be multiple layers of subperiosteal new bone producing an 'onion skin' arrangement. Although the tumour is highly malignant, aggressive treatment with chemotherapy and radiotherapy has started to produce some survivors (see Fig. 25.2).

Summary

Bone tumours are rare. Most of them are secondaries. Tumours which appear to be primary bone tumours should only be investigated and treated at specialist centres. The quality of life of patients with bone secondaries can be improved dramatically with internal fixation followed by radiotherapy. Pain will be reduced and mobility maintained.

Further reading

Enneking, W.F. (1983) *Musculoskeletal Tumor Surgery*, Churchill Livingstone, London.

Enzinger, F.M. and Weiss, S.W. (1983) *Soft Tissue Tumors*, Mosby, London.

Jaffe, H.L. (1972) *Metabolic, Degenerative and Inflammatory Diseases of Bones and Joints*, Lea and Febiger, Malvern, PA.

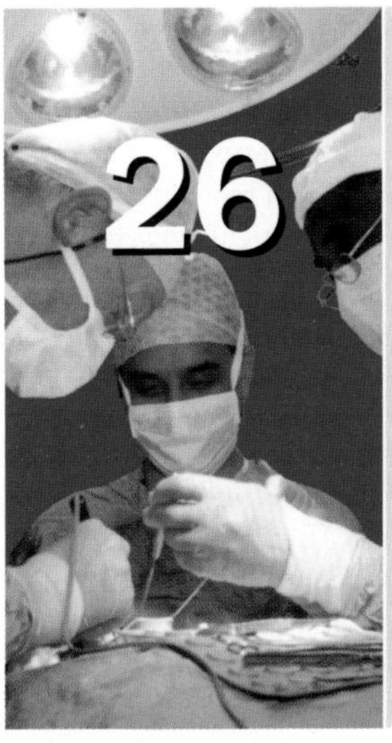

26 Diseases of bones and joints: generalised disease and chronic joint disorders

Educational goal

To understand the presentation and underlying pathological process of the common metabolic and degenerative disorders affecting bone and articular cartilage.

Introduction

Bone is a living structure. It is continuously being broken down by osteoclasts and built up again by osteoblasts. It has a blood supply and a nerve supply, and is therefore subject to diseases and problems just like the rest of the body. Perhaps because of its relatively low rate of turnover it is unusual for a primary bone tumour to occur, but bone is a common site for secondaries. Similarly, bone infection is rare but when it does occur it is very difficult to eradicate.

Articular cartilage has no blood supply at all. It receives its nutrition from synovial fluid. Its powers of healing are therefore very limited. Once damage occurs, repair is difficult if not impossible. Further breakdown is inevitable, slowly at first, then more rapidly.

Disorders of joints

As mentioned above, the articular cartilage has no blood supply. It is nourished by the synovial fluid, the nutrients being produced by the synovial membrane. The nutrients diffuse through the joint, speeded by the movement of that joint.

Bailey & Love's Short Practice of Surgery, 23rd edition. Edited by R.C.G. Russell, N.S. Williams and C.J.K. Bulstrode. Published in 2000 by Arnold Publishers.

Osteoarthritis (Fig. 26.1)

This is the common pathway for all diseases which damage the articular cartilage. The patient complains initially of pain on movement, and over a period the joint becomes stiffer and stiffer, gradually fixing in the position of maximum comfort. The muscles around the joint tend to waste and weakness sets in, further hampering the patient's mobility.

Eventually the joint may actually collapse, the limb shortens and the joint may lose its normal alignment.

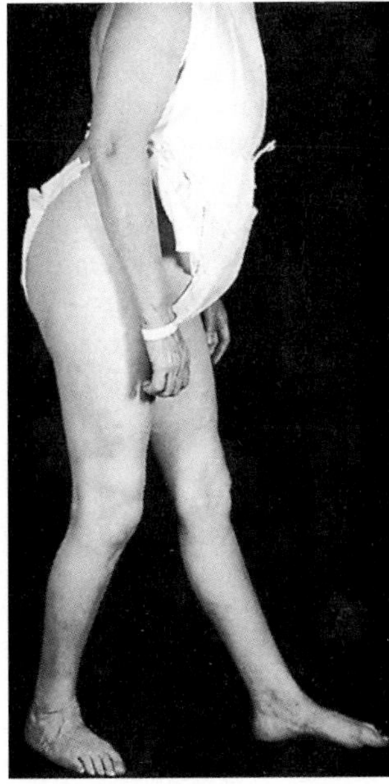

Fig. 26.1 Osteoarthritis of the hip. The patient has fixed flexion and has difficulty standing straight.

Examination

On inspection the joint may be slightly red and there may be swelling of the soft tissues, combined with muscle wasting. The limb is held in the position of comfort and may even be deformed. There may be some heat over the joint, and careful examination usually reveals at least a small effusion (although it can be very large). The osteophytes around the joint may be palpable and the joint line itself is often tender to palpation. Movement will be markedly limited and crepitus may be both palpable and audible. In osteoarthritis, the knee tends to fall into varus (bow legs), while in rheumatoid arthritis the knee falls into valgus (knock knees). The hip tends to flex into internal rotation, and the limb may actually shorten if there is bone loss.

Treatment

The early treatment of osteoarthritis is aimed at treating the pain and disability. Nonsteroidal anti-inflammatories may help with the pain. Physiotherapy should help to maintain mobility. It is said by some that weight loss improves symptoms. Walking sticks and household aids including a seat in the shower and handles around bathroom fittings may help the patient to maintain independent existence.

Once these nonoperative measures are no longer adequate, joint replacement should be considered in the hip, knee and the shoulder, as replacement in these joints now has good long-term results. Even so, in a young active patient, an arthrodesis should always be considered as an alternative. It is strong. It should give complete pain relief and can always be taken down and replaced with an artificial joint if necessary. Arthrodesis should only be considered when a single joint is affected, otherwise it transfers extra load on to already compromised joints.

Aetiology

Primary osteoarthritis develops spontaneously without any apparent predisposing cause.

Secondary osteoarthritis. This is the final common pathway after damage to the joint from some other cause. This may be traumatic, sepsis or inflammatory arthritis. Even repeated bleeds into a joint (as occurs in haemophilia) will cause breakdown of the articular cartilage, and multiple attacks of gout or pseudogout will have the same effect.

Underlying pathology of osteoarthritis

Articular cartilage is a complex structure made up of collagen and proteoglycan molecules which are highly hydrophilic and create the turgor pressure of the articular cartilage which gives it its strength and resilience. The joint surface itself is lubricated by a film of fluid squeezed out of the articular cartilage by the pressure applied. The first signs of osteoarthritis appear to be some softening of the articular cartilage (or at least loss of this turgor pressure) followed by a breakdown in the smooth surface. Microcracks appear in the articular surface (fibrillation) and pieces of the articular cartilage start to break off. These small fragments are mopped up by the macrophages in the synovium but this produces an inflammatory response. At the same time it appears that some form of repair mechanism is going on. This repair mechanism does not seem able to replace the articular cartilage in the load-bearing area of the joint. Instead, there is new bone formation and fibrocartilage laid down around the edge of the joint. This ring of new bone may be visible on the X-ray as osteophytes. The bone arcades lying immediately beneath the articular cartilage and which supported it now become more sclerotic, perhaps because of the increasing load coming on to the bone. The synovial fluid appears to break through the cartilage to create cysts in the subchondral bone. Finally the articular cartilage is completely worn away (eburnation) and there is direct articulation bone to bone. Pain may serve a protective function because in those joints lacking pain perception (Charcot's joints) the disintegration of the joint is both more rapid and more severe. Eventually the bone itself breaks down and the joint collapses completely.

Cardinal features of osteoarthritis on X-ray

These include:

- loss of joint space;
- subchondral sclerosis;
- osteophytes;
- cysts.

Radiological features of osteoarthritis (Fig. 26.2)

These include:

- joint narrowing;
- osteophyte formation;
- subchrondral sclerosis;
- cyst formation.

Rheumatoid arthritis

This is much rarer than osteoarthritis and occurs in a younger age group. Indeed, it can occur in children, when it is called Still's disease. The disease is usually symmetrical and starts in the small joints of the hands and feet. Women are more commonly affected than men. As each joint becomes involved, it becomes red, stiff and painful. After a time the disease burns out in an individual joint, but the damage is done and secondary osteoarthritis now sets in.

History

Characteristically the patient complains of feeling generally unwell and the painful joints are most painful and stiff early in the morning when the patient first gets up. This is in contrast to osteoarthritis where the joint is usually most painful in the evening after a long day's activity.

Jean-Martin Charcot, 1825–93. French neurologist.

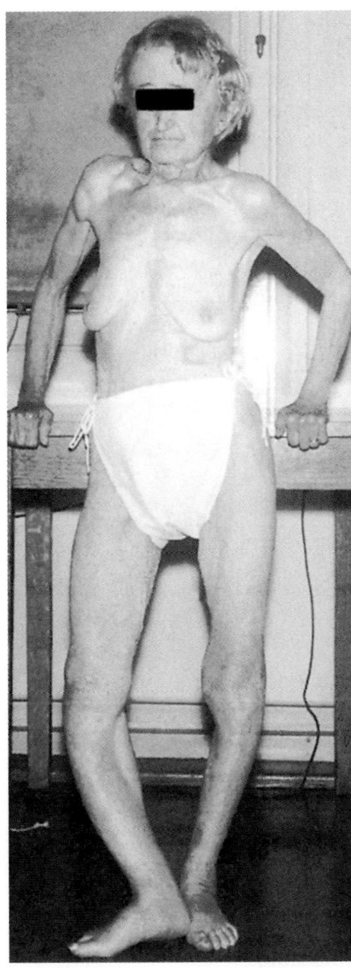

Fig. 26.2 Paget's disease affecting the skull, which is large, and the legs (especially the right tibia) where the bones are thickened and bowed.

Examination

The skin over the joints is red and glassy. The soft tissues are swollen and in the late stages the joints may be subluxed or even dislocated. The skin may be hot to touch and the swelling of the soft tissues is often as much synovial thickening as a synovial effusion. The joint therefore feels doughy rather than having a simple effusion. The bones do not usually have palpable osteophytes. Normal movement is markedly diminished but the joint may be grossly unstable as the ligaments around the joint may have stretched, or the joint surface itself may have collapsed.

Treatment

The bulk of treatment for rheumatoid arthritis is nonoperative. Nonsteroidal anti-inflammatories, analgesics and immunosuppressants, including steroids, are routinely used, combined with splints and with physiotherapy. If these measures fail then surgery needs to be considered. In the early stages where there is massive synovitis but relatively little damage to the articular cartilage as yet, a synovectomy may slow the course of the disease and reduce damage to ligaments and tendons. However, the procedure is not easy to perform and the results are not impressive. Once the joint surface has been destroyed then joint replacement may be the only option. Arthrodesis does not work well in rheumatoid arthritis as the bone is soft and other local joints are involved by disease. Paradoxically, joint replacement works well in rheumatoid arthritis and can be used in the hip, knee, shoulder, elbow and even the metatarsal phalangeal joints. However, fusion of the wrist remains the best solution for severe rheumatoid arthritis of this joint.

Pathology

A pannus of inflammatory tissue spreads from the margin of the joint, across the articular cartilage, creating inflammation in the joint and destroying the articular cartilage. The bone around the joint becomes osteoporotic, possibly because of hyperaemia, and because of disuse. In the late stages the joint may collapse completely.

Charcot's joints – neuropathic joints

Any joint which has lost its nerve supply seems to be susceptible to a particularly aggressive form of arthritis. The condition was originally described with tertiary syphilis but can in fact occur whenever the sensory supply to a joint is affected. There is massive joint destruction combined with new bone formation producing a very disorganised joint in a patient who is complaining of surprising little pain. Once seen it is never forgotten.

Nonspecific seronegative arthritis

Not all arthritis is either osteoarthritis or rheumatoid arthritis. Acute onset of pain in joints can occur secondary to a viral infection or indeed for no known cause. The treatment is symptomatic with anti-inflammatories, splints and physiotherapy.

Chondromalacia patellae – anterior knee pain

This condition occurs in adolescents, particularly girls, and may initially be brought on by a blow to the knee. The patient complains of severe pain in the knee which is worse going down stairs and if they are obliged to sit still for any length of time. After this period of rest any attempt to move the knee is extremely painful and may cause them to collapse. On examination there is surprisingly little to see. There is no redness or swelling and there may be very little thickening of the synovium and no effusion. Range of movement is good but there may be crepitus from the patella. The synovium around the patella is tender to palpation.

Sir George Frederick Still, 1868–1941. Professor of Diseases of Children, King's College Hospital, London, England.

Sir James Paget, 1814–99. Surgeon, St Bartholomew's Hospital, London, England.

This condition can also be caused by maltracking of the patella but in the majority of cases there is no obvious cause to be found.

Luckily, the condition is usually self-limiting and treatment is symptomatic using nonsteroidal anti-inflammatories, splints and physiotherapy and trying to keep the patient as mobile as possible within the limits of pain.

Diseases affecting bone

Paget's disease

This condition seems to involve a dramatic increase in both osteoclasts and osteoblasts in the bone. The bone starts to remodel far too rapidly. The patient complains of bone pain, and over a period of years the bone may gradually change shape, producing a characteristic bowed tibia and an enlarged skull. One bone may be involved in isolation, or several bones can be involved at the same time. The condition becomes increasingly common with age, affecting as much as 10 per cent of the very elderly. The X-ray findings of the bone are quite characteristic. The bone looks larger then it should and there is loss of the clear margin between the cortex and the medulla. The trabecular pattern of the medulla becomes coarse, tangled and confused. The plasma alkaline phosphatase may be markedly raised because of the increased osteoclast activity. The abnormal bone may suffer a pathological fracture. This fracture can be difficult to manage because the bone is deformed and because any attempt to pass a nail down the medulla may produce significant loss of blood. The cortical bone is also extremely hard and it can be very difficult to make drill holes for screws. Surgery on pagetic bone should be approached with great caution by both surgeon and anaesthetist (Figs 26.2 and 26.3).

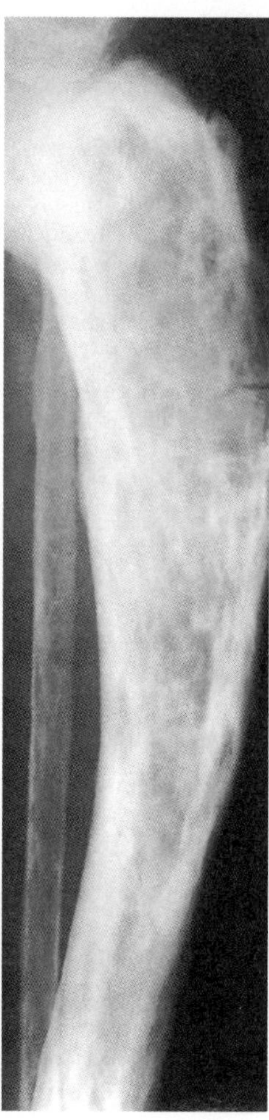

Fig. 26.3 Paget's disease involving the tibia showing the thickening of the bone, bowing, a pathological fracture anteriorly and mottled sclerosis.

Osteoporosis

This condition is becoming increasingly common in the Western world in the elderly but especially in postmenopausal women. It is believed to be related to a fall in oestrogen. The remodelling activity of the bone appears to fall away but osteoblastic activity falls more rapidly than osteoclastic, so there is a gradual thinning of the cortex and trabecular pattern of the bone. The bone gradually weakens until trivial trauma leads to a fracture. The common sites for a fracture are the neck of the femur, a crush fracture of the lumbar or thoracic spine, the head of the humerus and the distal radius. The fractures heal normally but can be difficult to hold with internal fixation because the bone is so soft and spongy.

Rickets/osteomalacia

The failure of bone osteoid to mineralise is called osteomalacia. In children, the disease is called rickets. The cause is a deficiency in vitamin D or in its metabolism. Vitamin D is produced in the skin when exposed to sunlight. It is also absorbed in the diet and is fat soluble. If the patient has a malabsorption syndrome, then vitamin D deficiency may occur. In the body vitamin D is converted to 25-hydroxycholecalciferone in the liver, then to 1,25-dihydroxycholecalciferone in the kidney. In children who lack vitamin D, either because of diet or because of an inbuilt error in metabolism, the costochondral junctions enlarge to form the 'rickety rosary'. The skull develops frontal bosses and the long bones bend, especially the lower third of the tibia. The child is also small. Serum calcium and phosphate are normal but alkaline phosphatase is usually raised. In adults bone deformity is not so marked but the patient may complain of marked muscle weakness. Lytic lesions may appear in the bone called Looser's zones. These are particularly common in the pelvis and may cause a pathological fracture.

Hyperparathyroidism

If for any reason there is excessive production of parathormone there is increased osteoclast activity which leads to lytic lesions in the bone, similar to those seen in osteomalacia. These are called 'Brown tumours', and fractures may occur through these. The osteolytic lesions are partic-

Emil Looser, 1877–1936. Swiss physician.

Francis Robert Brown, 1889–1967. Surgeon, Royal Infirmary, Dundee, Scotland.

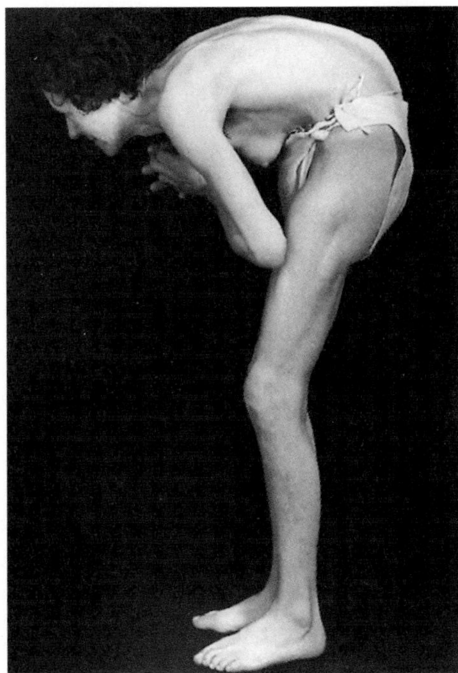

Fig. 26.4 Ankylosing spondylitis.

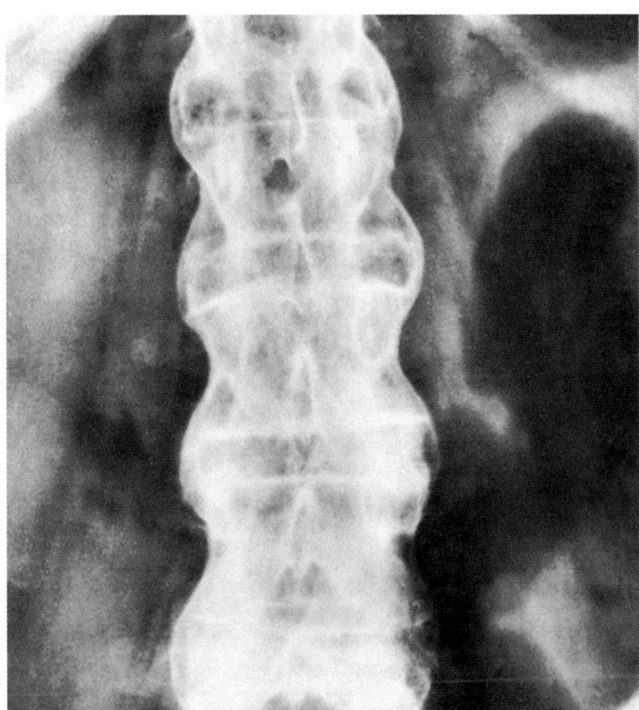

Fig. 26.5 Ossification of the lumbar spine ('bamboo spine').

ularly characteristic in the terminal phalanges and the alveolar margins of the jaws. The patient's serum calcium is raised and serum phosphorus is lowered with the alkaline phosphatase slightly raised. The treatment is to manage the underlying endocrine condition but fractures should be treated as normal and will heal well.

Ankylosing spondylitis

This progressive disorder has some features in common with rheumatoid arthritis. It is much more common in men than women and starts with the central joints of the body. The ligaments around the joints calcify and then ossify, freezing the patient into their deformed position (Fig. 26.4). The tissue antigen HLA-B27 is very common in patients who have ankylosing spondylitis but is rarely found in the normal population. It is therefore diagnostic.

History

The condition starts in early adult life, and starts with painful stiff joints.

Examininination

Reduction of chest expansion is an early physical sign.

Investigation

As mentioned, the HLA-B27 antigen will be positive. The erythrocyte sedimentation rate may be slightly raised and X-rays of the sacroiliac joints show early obliteration with ankylosis. An X-ray of the spine may show ossification of the spinal ligaments (bamboo spine; Fig. 26.5).

Treatment

Early treatment with anti-inflammatories and physiotherapy can reduce the disability. In cases where gross flexion of the spine has occurred an osteotomy can be performed but this is not without risk of causing paraplegia. If the disease includes the hip joints then total hip replacement will help.

Further reading

Scrivenier, C.R., Beandet, A.L., Sly, W.S. and Valle, D. (1960) *The Metabolic Basis of Intented Disease*, 6th edn, McGraw-Hill, London.

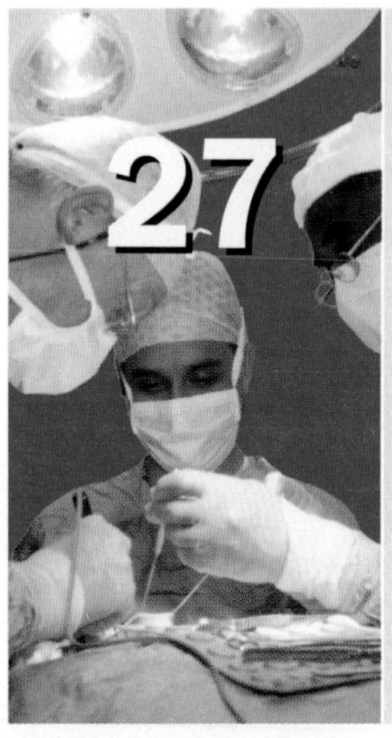

Children's orthopaedics: normal development and congenital disorders

Introduction

Children's orthopaedics is different from its adult counterpart because growth is still taking place. This can work for or against the child and surgeon. On the positive side there are great powers of remodelling and recovery (Fig. 27.1). Conversely, a growth plate injury or congenital shortening of a limb will produce progressive deformity (Fig. 27.2).

The understanding of children's orthopaedics is helped by a knowledge of its terminology (Table 27.1 gives examples).

Many orthopaedic conditions are congenital, i.e. present at birth. Some are immediately obvious, for example the absence of a limb; others such as cerebral palsy or developmental dysplasia of the hip may not be clinically detectable at birth but declare themselves later. In addition, some acquired conditions arise against a background of genetic susceptibility, for example immune deficiency predisposing to infection. Finally, children present great variation within the spectrum of normality (e.g. gait pattern), while others have conditions such as postural abnormalities which are self-limiting. These may cause great concern to a family. Clinical assessment and explanation must be just as thorough as for a child with an obviously severe condition.

Figure 27.3 presents a helpful system for treating orthopaedic conditions in childhood.

The term 'orthopaedics' (straight child) originally referred to correction of deformity in children. The speciality generally has expanded beyond all recognition and this includes

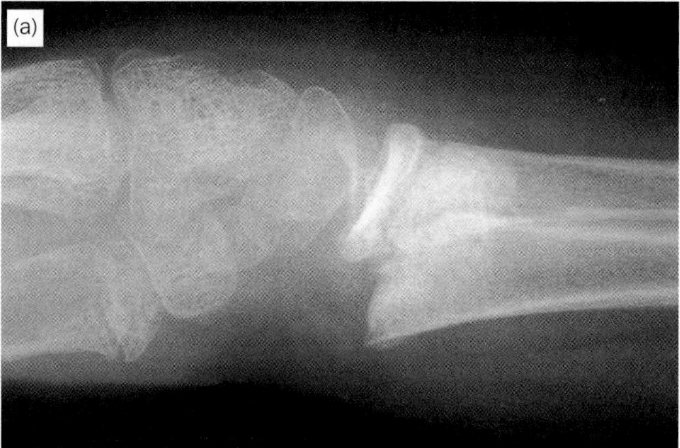

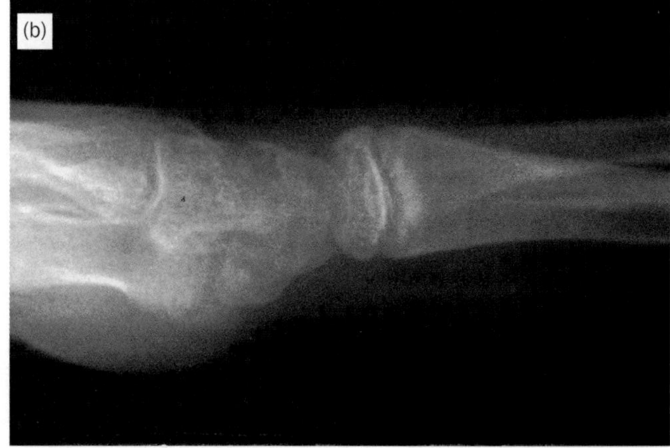

Fig. 27.1 (a) A 2-week-old displaced fracture of the lower radius. The decision was made, wisely, not to manipulate and risk damage to the growth plate. (b) The same wrist 18 months later. Remodelling has corrected the deformity.

Bailey & Love's Short Practice of Surgery, 23rd edition. Edited by R.C.G. Russell, N.S. Williams and C.J.K. Bulstrode. Published in 2000 by Arnold Publishers.

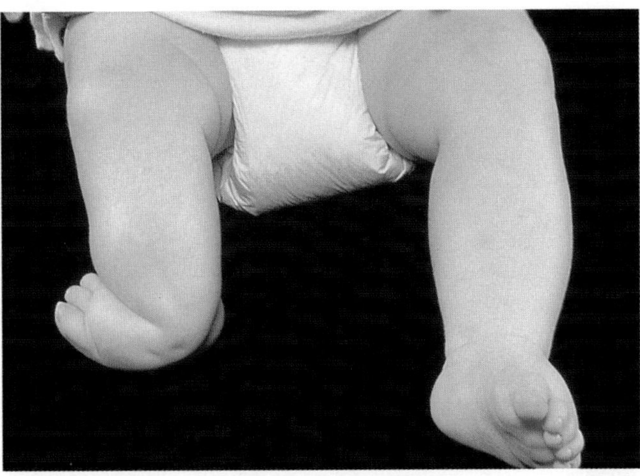

Fig. 27.2 Fibular deficiency. A cause of deformity, mainly shortening.

Table 27.1 Glossary of orthopaedic terms

Term	*Definition*	*Examples*
Varus	Towards the mid line	Genu varum (bow legs) Coxa vara
Valgus	Away from the mid line	Knock knees Coxa valga (cerebral palsy)
Calcaneus	Heel points upwards	Calcaneo valgus
Equinus	Heel points down	Talipes equino varus
Cavus	Arched foot, concave ↓	Pes cavus
Rocker bottom foot	Foot concave ↑	Congenital vertical talus
Anteversion	Femoral neck angled forwards in relation to the shaft	Common in developmental dysplasia of the hip
Recurvatum	Joint can be hyperextended	General joint laxity Congenital dislocation of knee
Foot progression angle	Angles of foot in relation to direction of gait	Intoeing or out-toeing
Foot/thigh angle	Angle between line of foot and thigh (child prone, with knee and ankle at right angle)	External or internal tibial torsion

children's orthopaedics. Not only has deformity to be addressed, often with sophisticated technology for investigation and treatment, but the children's orthopaedic surgeon is concerned with a much wider range of musculoskeletal disease, along with closer involvement in the general care of the child in the community. The role of the orthopaedic surgeon may be primary or secondary, according to the overall needs of the child.

Normal variants and self-limiting conditions

The range of normality in the development of the musculoskeletal system is wide (Table 27.2). At all ages the appearance of a child's limbs or spine includes the components of rotation, angulation and joint laxity. When these are added to the natural clumsiness of a developing youngster it is not

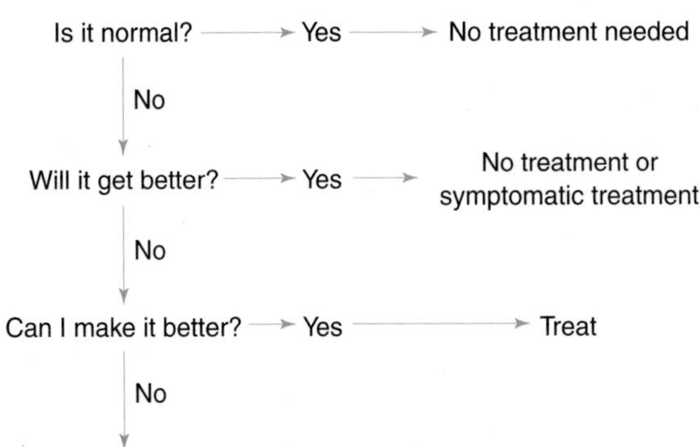

Fig. 27.3 A scheme for treatment of orthopaedic conditions in childhood.

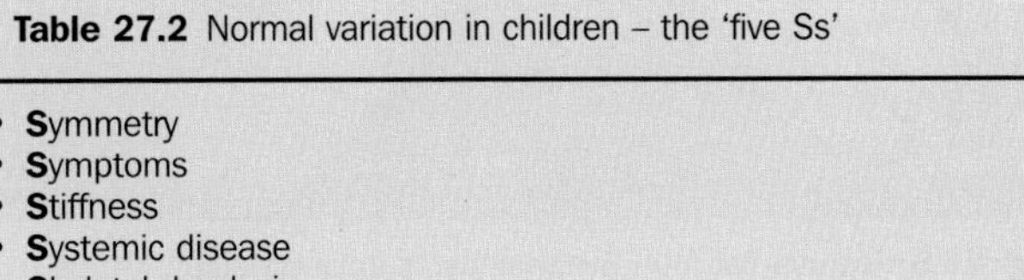

Table 27.2 Normal variation in children – the 'five Ss'

- **S**ymmetry
- **S**ymptoms
- **S**tiffness
- **S**ystemic disease
- **S**keletal dysplasia

surprising that parents may be concerned whether their offspring is normal. Therefore, all consultations must be thorough and sympathetic.

Common reasons for referral are intoeing, bow legs (Fig. 27.4), knock-knees and flat feet (Fig. 27.5). None can be judged in isolation. For example, intoeing (foot progression angle) is the result of the various torsional and angulation components within the femur, tibia and foot.

For example, the child in Fig. 27.6 is normal. The condition is symmetrical and symptomless, the joints are supple and there is no evidence of skeletal dysplasia or systemic disease such as neurological or metabolic condition.

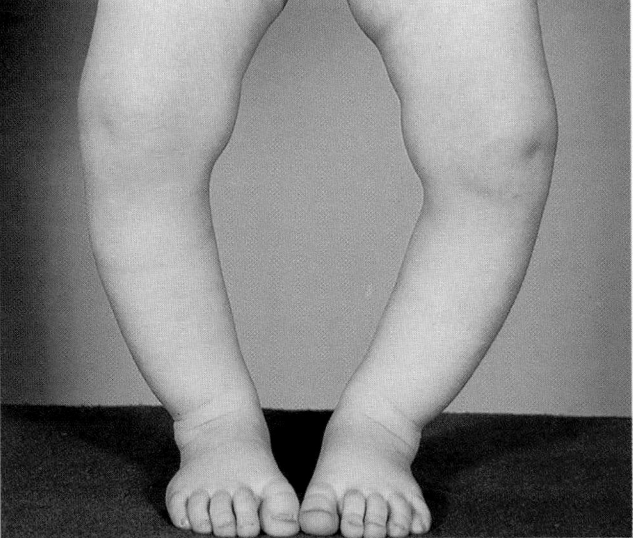

Fig. 27.4 Genu varum. Normal variant. Although dramatic, the condition is symmetrical, the joints move normally, the child is asymptomatic and there is no evidence of systemic disorder (e.g. rickets, neurological disease or skeletal dysplasia).

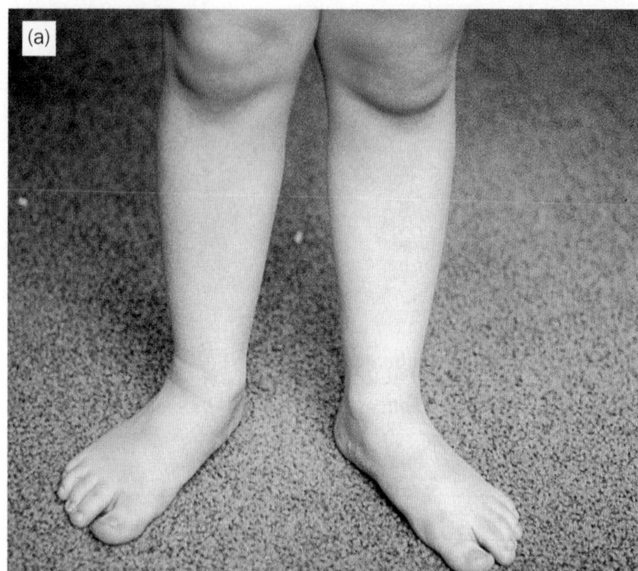

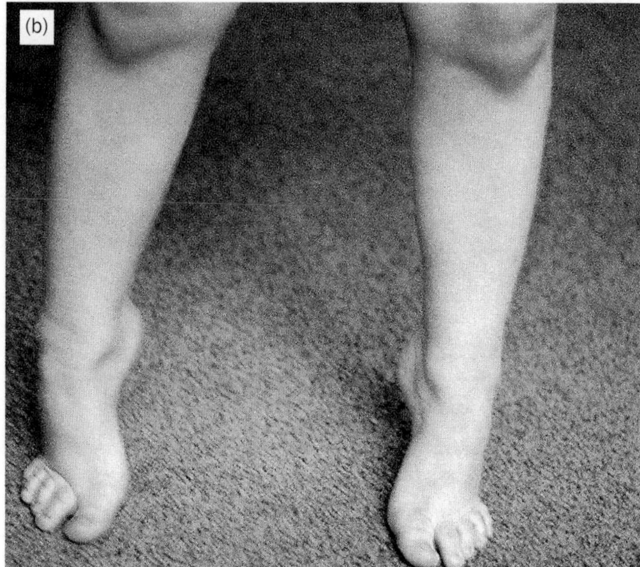

Fig. 27.5 Postural flat foot. Symmetrical, supple condition. On tip-toes there is a normal arch to the foot.

Conversely, the child in Fig. 27.7 is abnormal. There is asymmetry and evidence of a systemic disorder (rickets).

Self-limiting conditions (Table 27.3) are outside the definition of normal variance because they do not fulfil the 'five Ss' rule. They include postural deformities such as calcaneo valgus (Fig. 27.8), moulded baby syndrome (plagiocephaly, infantile scoliosis, tight hip adductors), metatarsus varus (Fig. 27.9) and 'growing pains'. Asymmetry, stiffness and symptoms may be present. The conditions usually correct spontaneously or with minimal treatment such as stretching exercises.

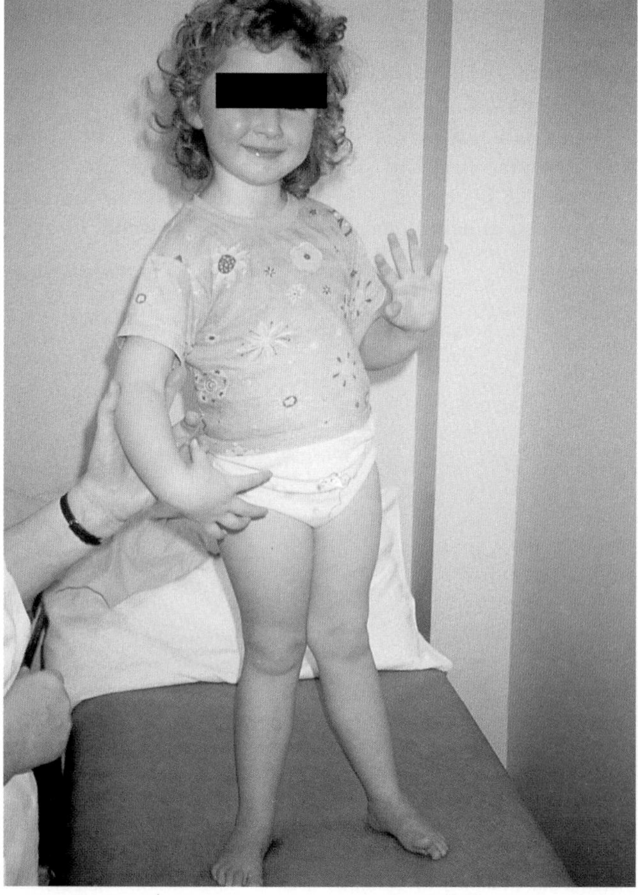

Fig. 27.6 Symmetrical genu valgum, supple joints, normal variant.

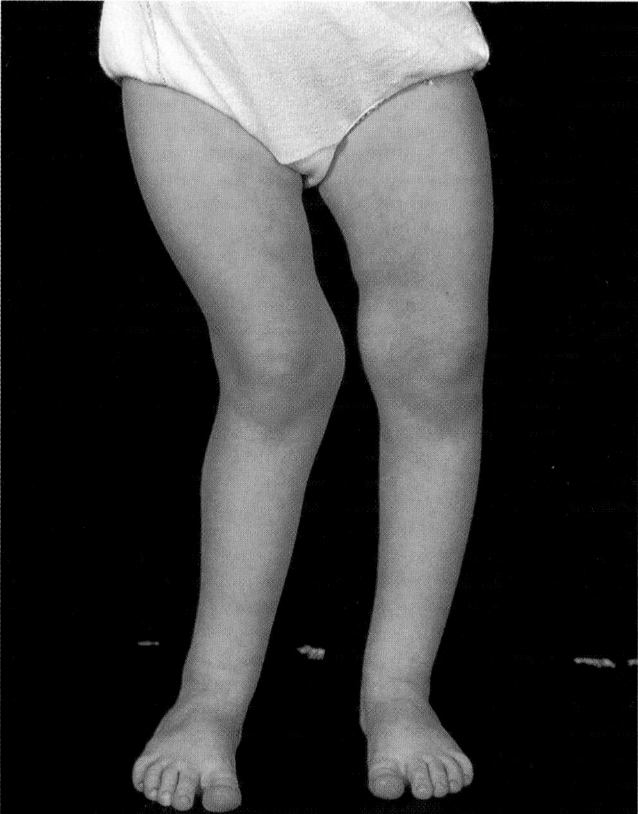

Fig. 27.7 Asymmetrical limb posture. The underlying cause is rickets.

Table 27.3 Self-limiting conditions

- Calcaneo valgus metatarsus varus
- 'Moulded baby' (plagiocephaly, limited abduction of hip and infantile scoliosis)
- External rotation of lower limb
- Hallux erectus
- 'Growing pains'
- Habitual toe walker

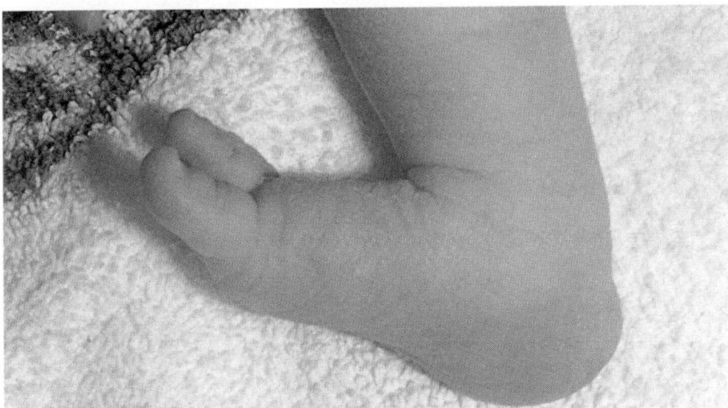

Fig. 27.8 Calcaneo valgus. This will correct spontaneously but is an indicator of possible hip dysplasia.

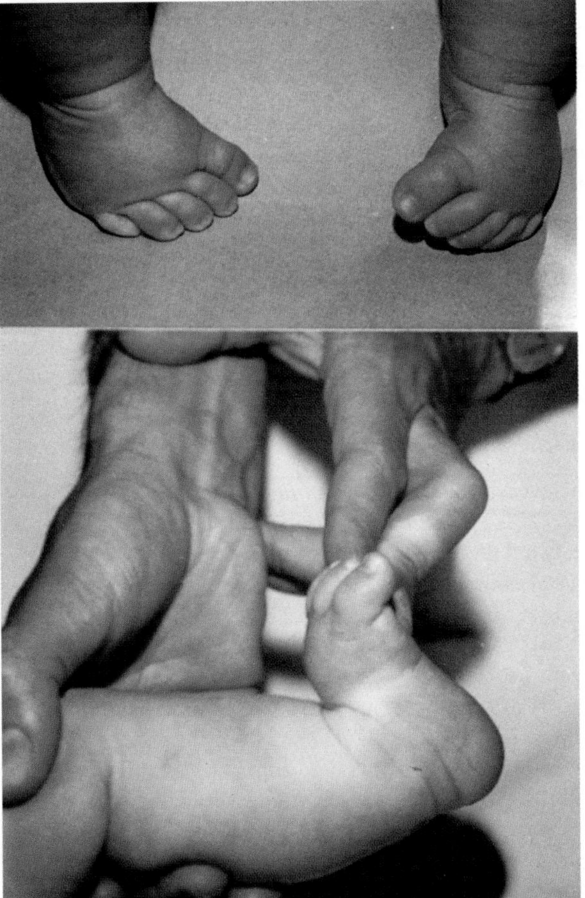

Fig. 27.9 Metatarsus varus. The hindfoot is normal. The forefoot will correct spontaneously in the vast majority of cases.

Congenital disorders

These may be intrinsic malformations within a developing structure (e.g. limb deficiency) (Fig. 27.2), or the result of extrinsic influences, for example postural (Fig. 27.8), neuromuscular (Fig. 27.10) or a malformation elsewhere (Fig. 27.11). Regularly, however, we do not know why a congenital abnormality (e.g. talipes equino varus) has occurred.

Nowadays, diagnostic ultrasound can detect musculoskeletal abnormalities *in utero*. This technology is creating both opportunities and difficulties in the management of an unborn child. Whatever the cause, a significant abnormality diagnosed prenatally or at birth can be devastating to a family. Support and advice from a wide range of experts may be required.

Malformations of the limbs and spine

Musculoskeletal structures develop alongside other body systems. By the 12th week of intrauterine life the spine and limbs are formed, the upper limbs slightly ahead of the lower. Examples of how embryological structures can stray from the path of normal development are shown in Table 27.4.

Because the various organs are developing concurrently, the causes of malformation may affect more than one system. Therefore, when presented with a limb anomaly one should

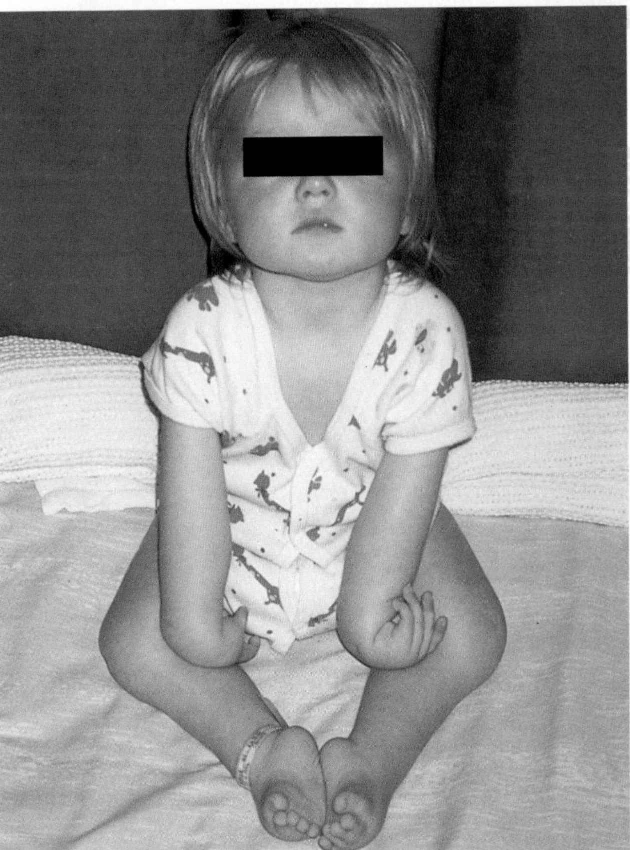

Fig. 27.10 Arthrogryposis. A neuromuscular disorder causing weakness and deformity.

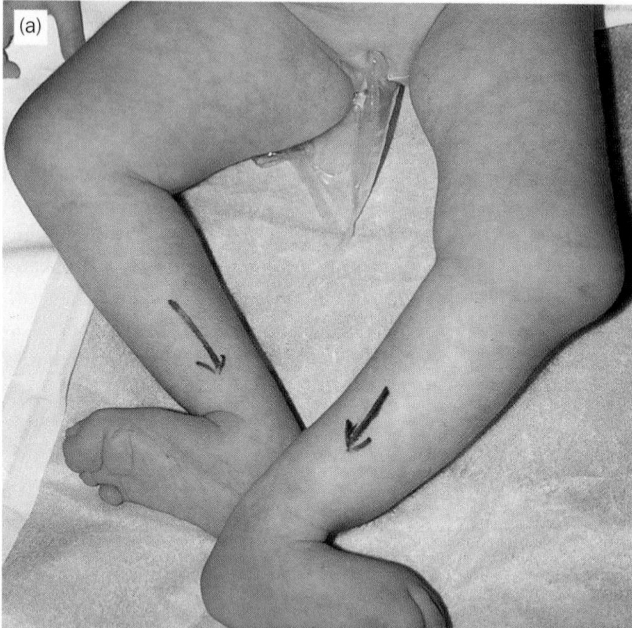

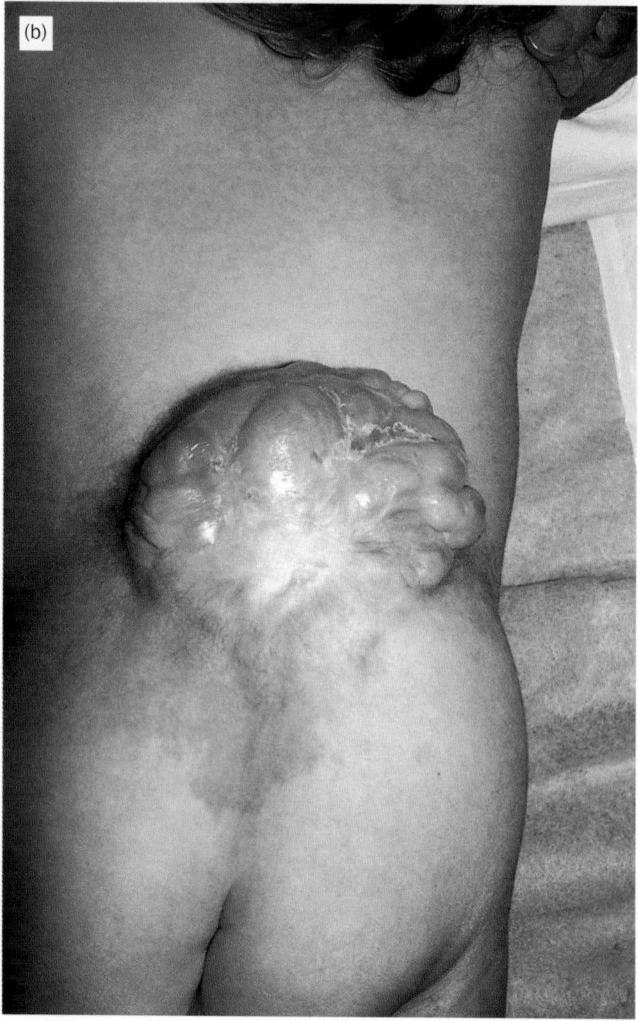

Fig. 27.11 An example of how lower limb deformity (a) can be produced by spina bifida (b).

Table 27.4 Classification of anomalies of the developing limbs and spine

Type	*Examples*
Failure of formation	Femoral deficiency (Fig. 27.12) Fibular deficiency (Figs 27.2, 27.17 and 27.19) Sacral agenesis Hemivertebra Radial club hand (Fig. 27.14) Tibial dysplasia (Fig. 27.15)
Failure of separation	Syndactyly (Fig. 27.20) Radioulnar synostosis Klippel–Feil syndrome Sprengel shoulder (Fig. 27.22) Tarsal coalition
Extra parts	Polydactyly (Fig. 27.25)
Gigantism	Macrodactyly (Fig. 27.24)
Hypoplasia	Short femur
Constriction ring syndrome	Congenital amputation Constriction rings on limbs
Skeletal dysplasia	Achondroplasia (Fig. 27.29) Metaphyseal dysplasia (Fig. 27.28) Osteogenesis imperfecta (Fig. 27.26) Hereditary multiple exostosis (Fig. 27.27)

consider associated abnormalities in, for example, the cardiovascular, urogenital or nervous system.

However, in most cases the children are usually otherwise normal and develop and function well. They are regularly well motivated and do not admit to any disability in spite of obvious physical abnormality. These aspects have to be understood when considering treatment.

In the majority of cases there is no obvious cause, such as thalidomide. Occasionally a genetic (especially in skeletal dysplasia) or syndromic association [e.g. thrombocytopenia, absent radius (TAR syndrome)] is possible.

Congenital malformations

Failure of formation

These cases may present as multiple complex abnormalities (Fig. 27.12) or fit recognisable patterns of deformity (Fig. 27.13). The defects may be classified as transverse [e.g. congenital amputation through a limb) or longitudinal (e.g. femoral deficiency (Fig. 27.13) or radial club hand (Fig. 27.14)]. A longitudinal deficiency may be florid [e.g. tibial dysplasia (Fig. 27.15)] or subtle [e.g. congenital pseudarthrosis of the tibia (Fig. 27.16)]. The limb beyond the defect may be normal (Fig. 27.17) or abnormal (Fig. 27.2).

Femoral deficiency. This ranges in severity from a short femur to total absence. Treatment varies accordingly.

A short femur may be amenable to lengthening. The commonly associated coxa vara may require correction beforehand by valgus osteotomy.

More profound degrees are beyond the limits of surgical leg equalisation. However, children usually function well in

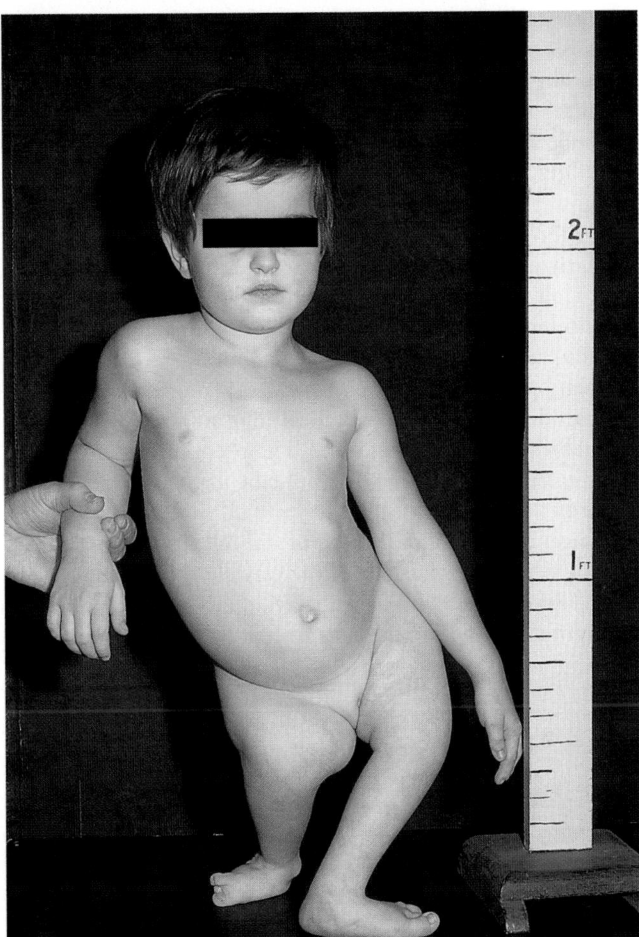

Fig. 27.12 A complex pattern of failure of function in an otherwise normal child.

an extension prosthesis (Fig. 27.18). Indeed, there is a debate whether a child with a congenitally short limb is better served by complex leg equalisation surgery with its regular complications and joint stiffness or by early mobilisation in an extension prosthesis.

Fibular deficiency (Figs 27.2 and 27.17). In this condition the tibia is short and bowed anteriorly, often with an overlying skin dimple. The fibula is wholly or partly absent. The foot is in equino valgus and commonly shows deficiency of the outer rays. The condition also affects the whole limb. There is mild femoral shortening and genu valgum and often the cruciate ligaments are absent.

Treatment is dominated by the overall predicted shortening and the state of the foot. A child with marked shortening and a deformed residual foot is best served by a Syme's amputation at about 1 year. If the foot is normal, it is reasonable to consider correction of the equino valgus deformity and equalisation of leg lengths. This may require a com-

James Syme, 1799–1870. British surgeon. He described the amputation in a medical communication in 1843. He became Professor of Surgery to the University of Edinburgh, Scotland.

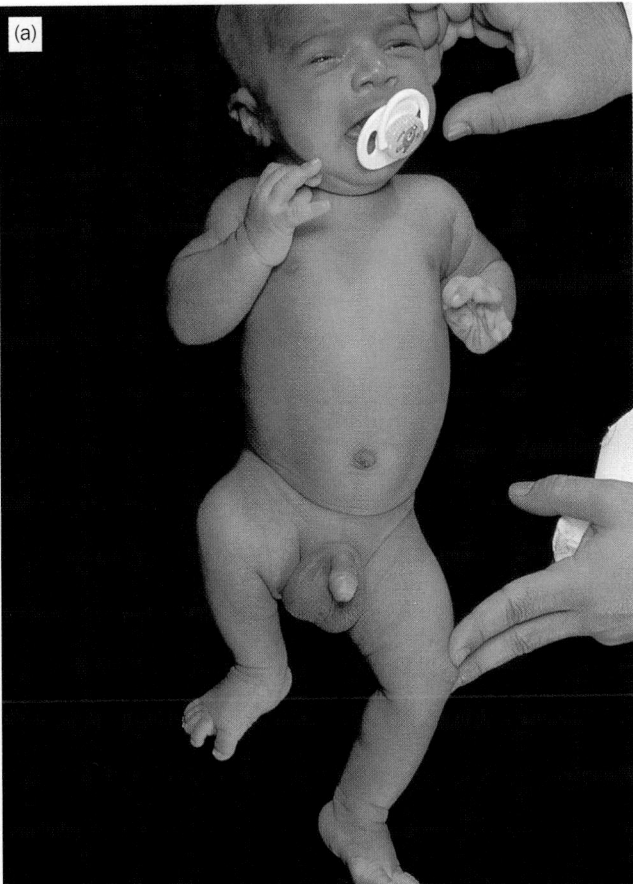

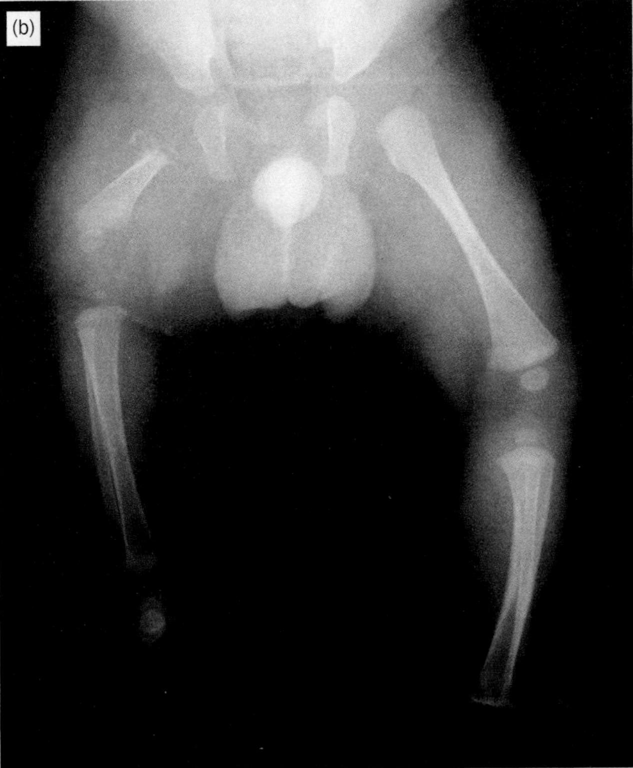

Fig. 27.13 Typical case of femoral deficiency. The limb beyond is normal.

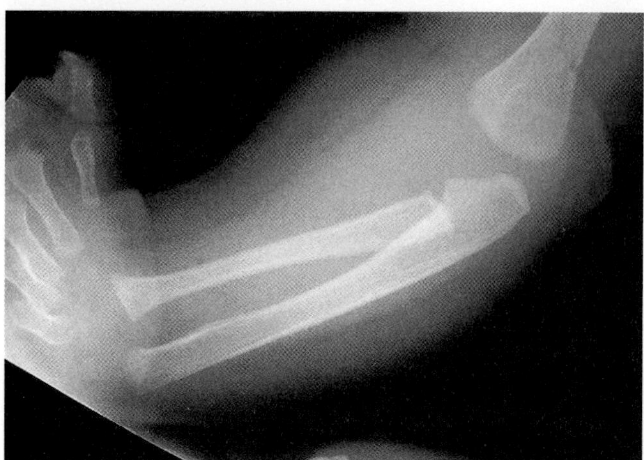

Fig. 27.14 Radial club hand. A longitudinal deficiency. In this case the radial side of the limb is affected and the thumb is deficient.

bination of lengthening of the affected tibia and a shortening procedure, for example epiphysiodesis on the normal side.

Tibial deficiency (Fig. 27.15). The tibia is wholly or partially absent. The foot is in equino varus and, in contrast to fibular deficiency, may be augmented (e.g. polydactyly or diplopodia).

Reconstruction of the foot is usually unsuccessful except in mild cases. If the tibia is absent a 'through the knee' amputation is indicated. If there is a tibial remnant a good option is to fuse the fibula with this and fit the child with an extension prosthesis. It is thereafter usually preferable to amputate the foot to allow better fitting of the prosthesis.

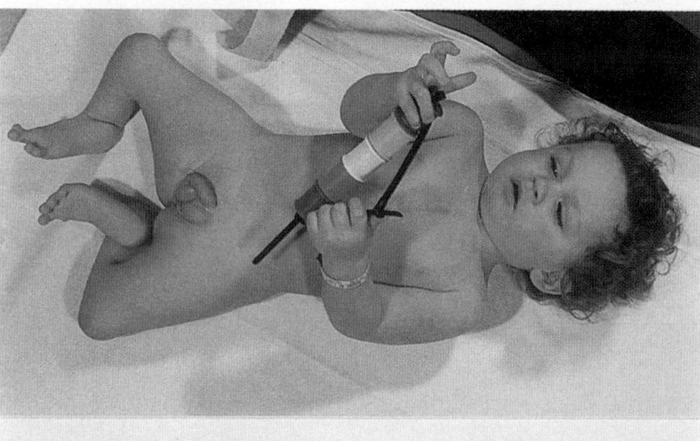

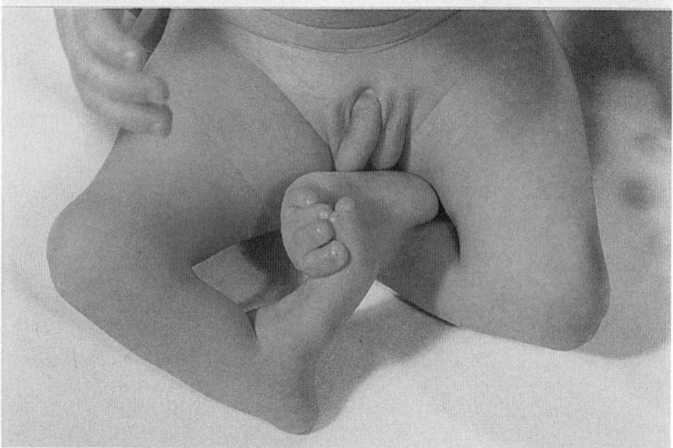

Fig. 27.15 Congenital tibial deficiency. In this case there were no vestigial tibial elements to allow useful reconstruction and the child is now active and mobile following through the knee amputation and prosthesis.

Congenital pseudoarthrosis of the tibia (Fig. 27.16). This is a subtle longitudinal defect causing anterolateral bowing in the lower tibia. The condition may be associated with neurofibromatosis or fibrous dysplasia. The deformity regularly progresses to a beastly fracture for which treatment is difficult and prolonged. The whole armamentarium of the fracture surgeon can be involved including intramedullary fixation, traditional and advanced grafting techniques (e.g. vascularised fibular graft and the Ilizarov method). Even then the pseudoarthrosis may not heal and amputation becomes inevitable in a minority of cases. The prepseudoarthrosis and the treated pseudoarthosis should be braced until skeletal maturity.

Congenital pseudoarthrosis of the clavicle (Fig. 27.19). This defect of the midshaft of the clavicle is probably related to the development of the subclavian artery as it occurs on the right side unless there is dextrocardia.

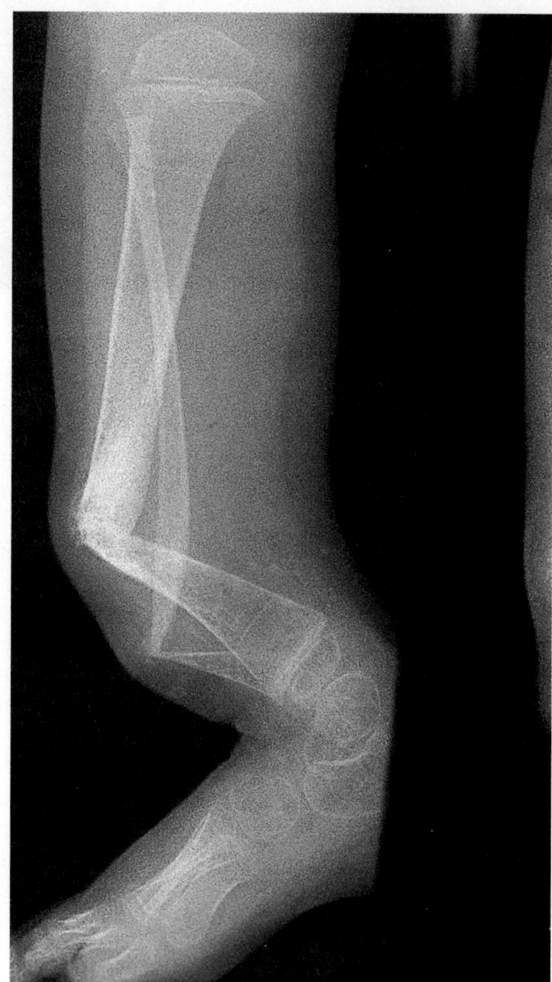

Fig. 27.16 Congenital pseudoarthrosis of the tibia.

Gaveriil A Ilizarov. 1921–92. Orthopaedic surgeon, Kurgan, Russia.

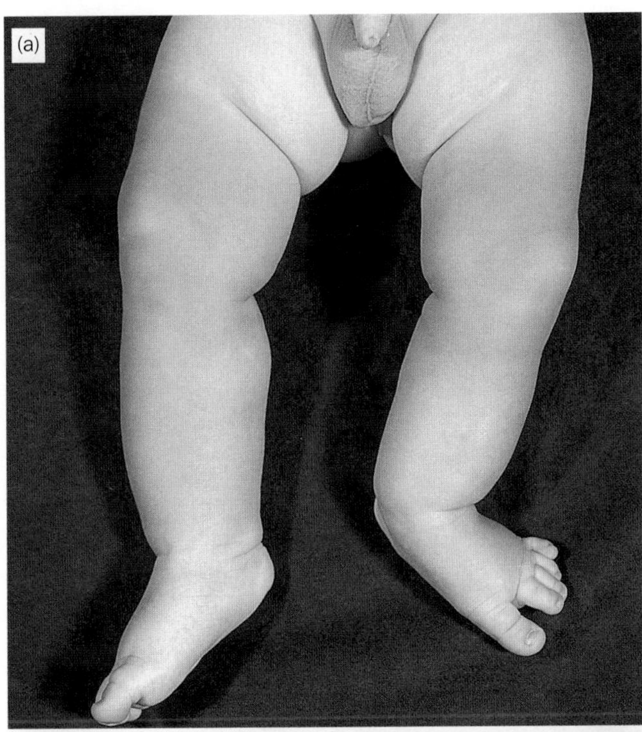

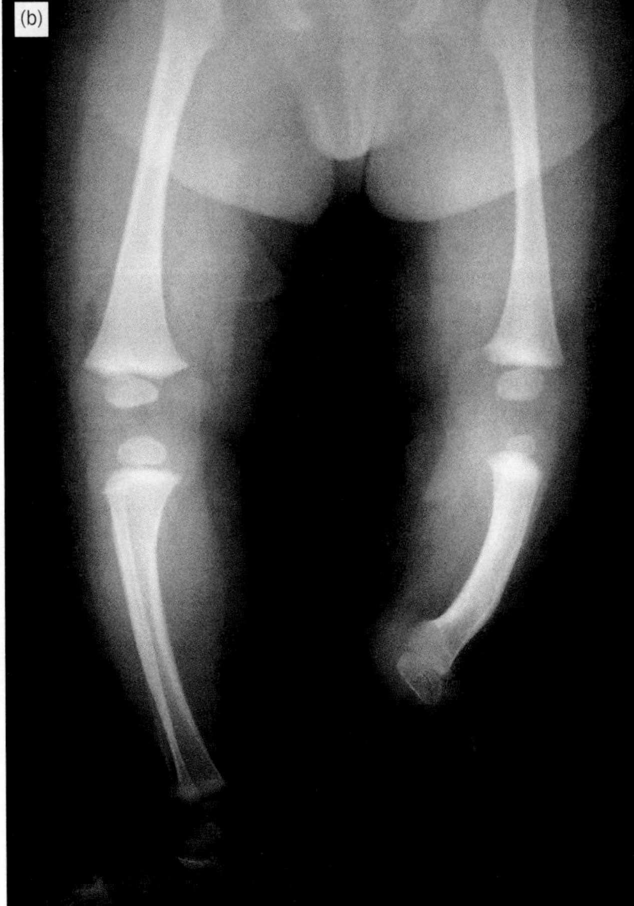

Fig. 27.17 Congenital fibular deficiency. Note that there is femoral as well as tibial shortening.

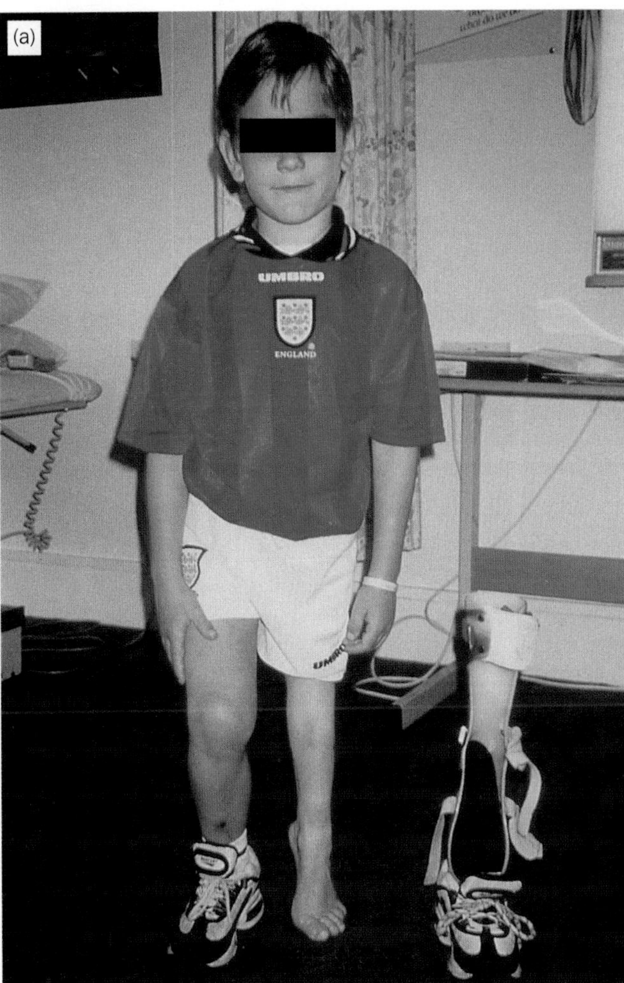

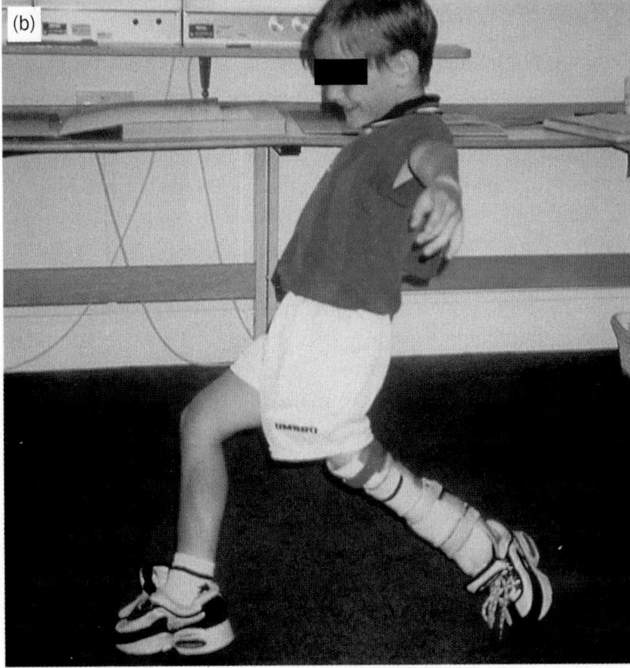

Fig. 27.18 A child with femoral deficiency showing excellent function using an extension prosthesis.

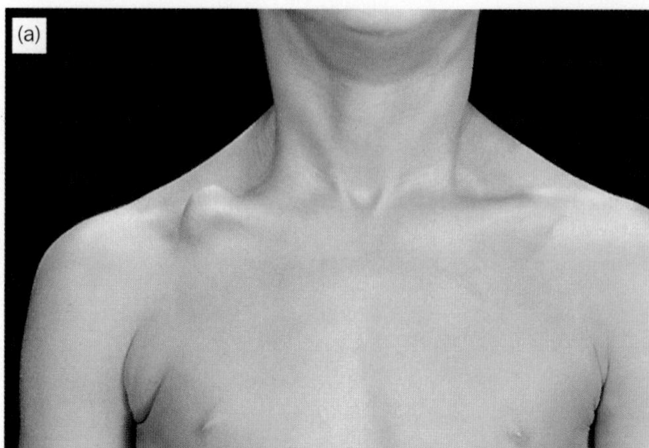

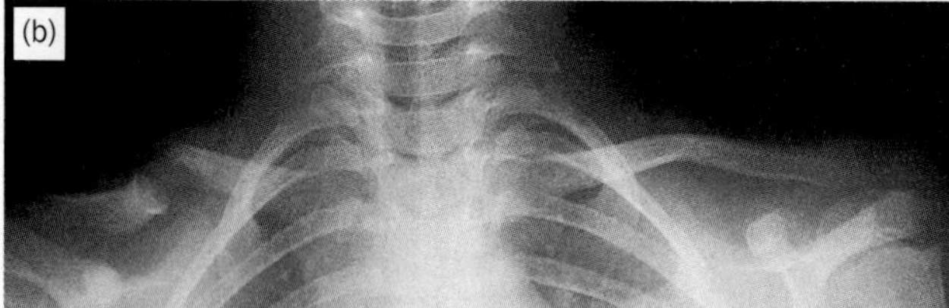

Fig. 27.19 Congenital pseudoarthrosis of the clavicle.

The main problem is cosmetic, although there may be discomfort. If treatment is undertaken the options include excision of the defect with repair of its periostial sleeve or fixation and grafting.

Infantile coxa vara. There is a defect of ossification in the femoral neck, leading to a varus deformity usually requiring corrective osteotomy.

Failure of separation

Syndactyly (fingers and toes) (Fig. 27.20). Three types are described, simple (soft tissue only), complex (bones involved) and acrosyndactyly (digits joined at their tips). Syndactyly as a regular component of syndromic conditions (e.g. Apert's syndrome, constriction ring). Where possible fingers should be separated, although the techniques are demanding and involve flaps and skin grafting. Separation of toes is rarely indicated.

Radioulnar synostosis. The fused radius and ulna are shorter than their counterparts. Abduction of the shoulder effectively mimics pronation. Therefore, a forearm fixed in neutral rotation or slight supination can be compensated by the shoulder and this allows virtually normal hand function. A forearm fixed in pronation cannot be thus compensated and in such cases a rotation osteotomy to bring the hand to the neutral or slightly supinated position may be indicated.

Tarsal coalition. The usual patterns are calcaneonavicular (Fig. 27.21) or talocalcaneal fusions by cartilaginous or bony bars. There may be pain as well as stiffness, particularly in eversion, and the condition is also known as peroneal spastic

Eugene Apert, b. 1868. French paediatrician.

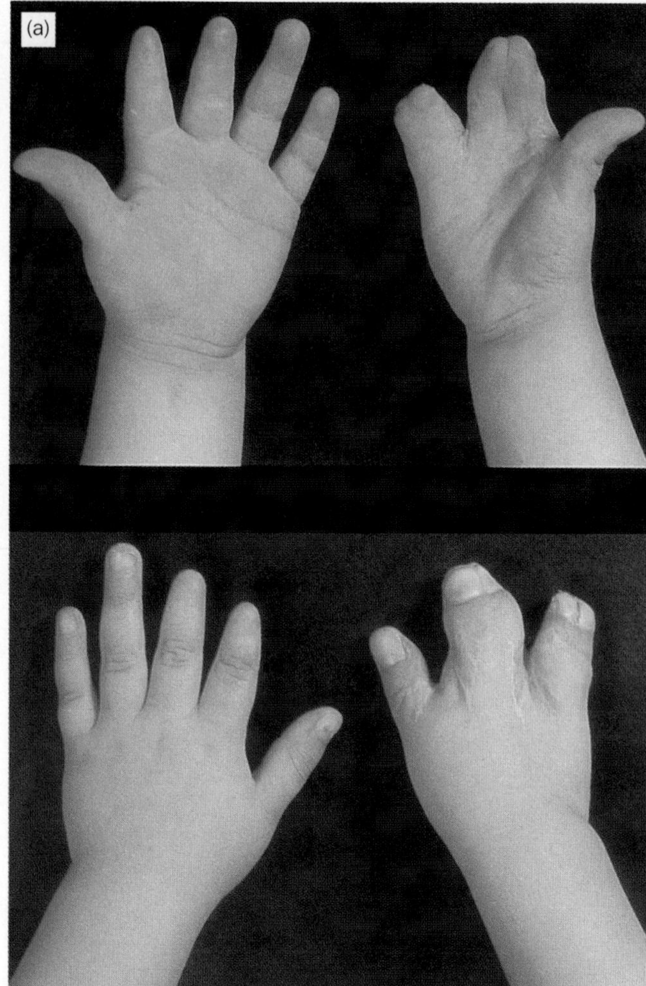

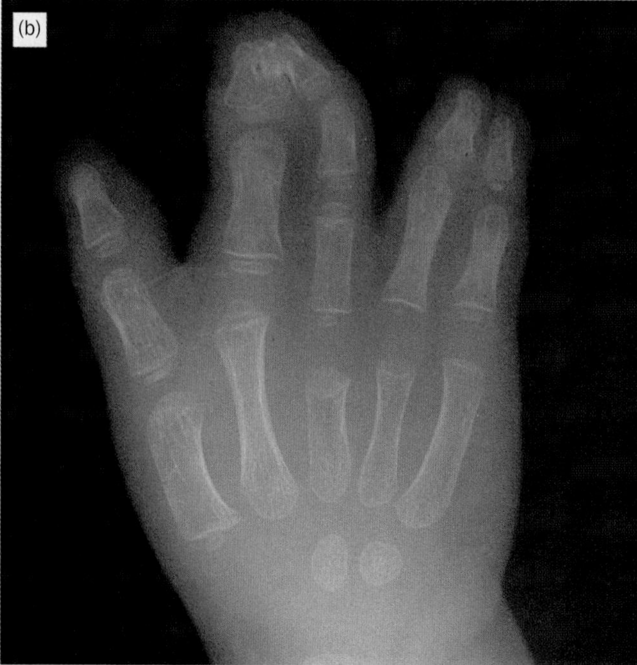

Fig. 27.20 Syndactyly. This patient had constriction ring syndrome and demonstrated the different types of syndactyly.

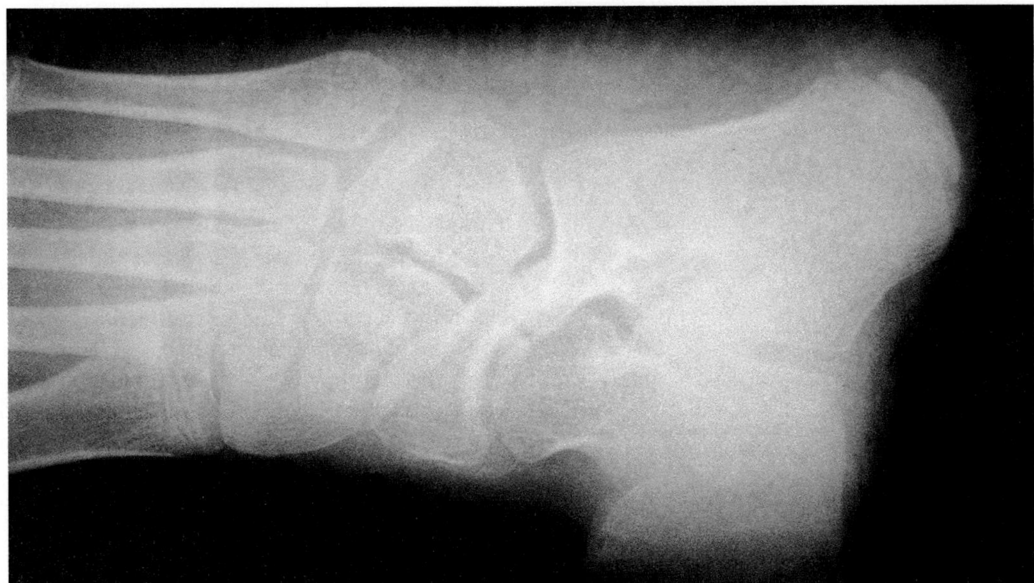

Fig. 27.21 Calcaneonavicular fusion.

flat foot. There may be an associated ball and socket ankle joint. The calcaneonavicular bar can be demonstrated by plain radiographs, whereas computerised tomography (CT) best visualises the talocalcaneal bar. If conservative measures (e.g. analgesics, orthotics) fail, excision of the bar may be indicated. If degenerative changes ensue, arthiodesis may ultimately be required.

Vertebral and scapular anomalies. Vertebrae and ribs may be fused with resultant scoliosis and/or chest wall deformity. Regularly, there are associated abnormalities within the spinal column (e.g. diastomatomyelia) and elsewhere (e.g. urogenital and cardiac systems).

Klippel–Feil syndrome. This comprises multiple congenital abnormalities in the cervical spine leading to a characteristic short, stiff neck and a low hairline. Torticollis, facial asymmetry and webbing of the neck may be apparent.

Sprengel shoulder. This is due to a failure of normal descent of the scapula which remains high and small (Fig. 27.22). There may be a bony tether, the omovertebral bar, between scapula and spine, which is also prone to anomalies.

Treatment is largely for cosmetic reasons. Excision of the superomedial portion or displacement osteotomy of the scapula is a better option than attempts to reposition the whole bone.

Gigantism

A whole limb (Fig. 27.23) or part (Fig. 27.24) can be affected. The condition may be idiopathic or associated with neurofibromatous or a vascular malformation. The gigantic part is distressing for the child and family. Procedures such as debulking and growth arrest are usually unsuccessful. The best results are from amputation, where this is a realistic option.

Maurice Klippel, 1858–1942. Neurologist, Paris, France. Described this condition in a joint paper in 1912.

Andre Feil, b. 1884. Neurologist, Paris, France. Described this condition in a joint paper in 1912.

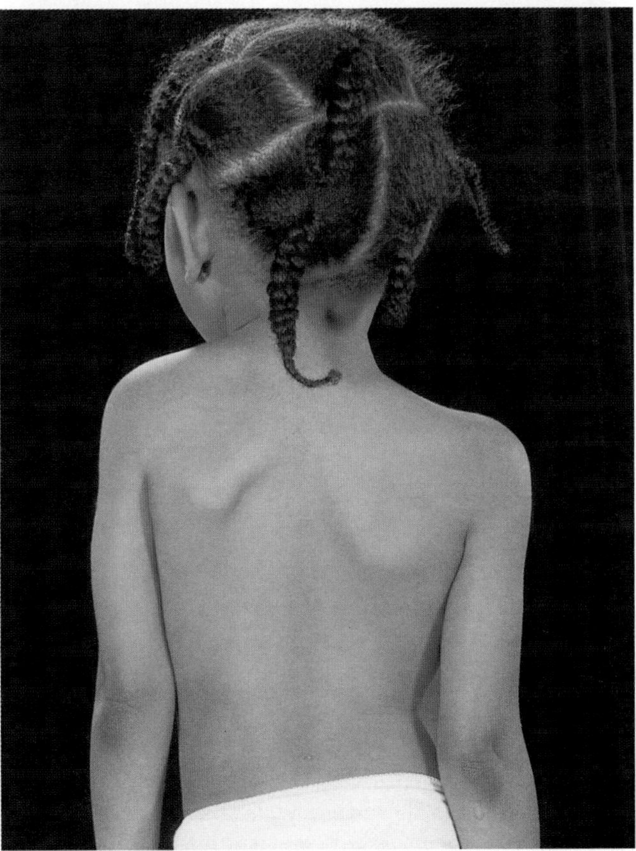

Fig. 27.22 Sprengel shoulder.

Otto Sprengel, 1852–1915. Surgeon, Brunswick, Germany.

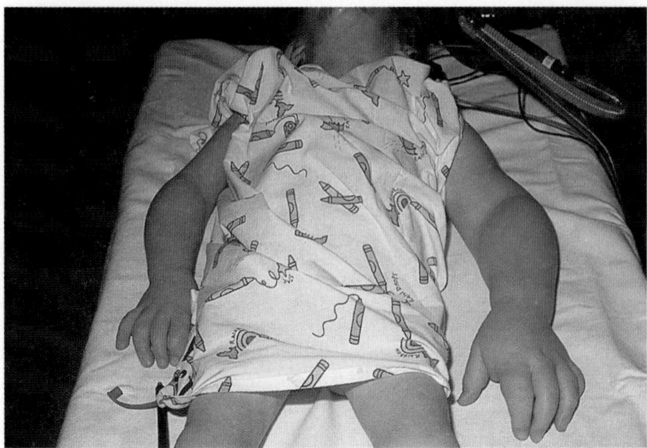

Fig. 27.23 A gigantic left upper limb in a case of Proteus syndrome.

Polydactyly

Extra digits can be an isolated abnormality, part of a pattern of limb malformation (e.g. tibial deficiency with diplopodia) or syndromic, as in chondroectodermal dysplasia (Ellis–van Creveld syndrome) which consists of short-limbed dwarfism, dysplastic nails, hair and teeth, polydactyly and congenital heart disease.

Extra digits usually require removal. It is sometimes difficult to know which digit to sacrifice (Fig. 27.25).

Skeletal dysplasias

These generalised disorders of the skeleton are often genetically determined. They may affect the whole or part of a bone. In some, for example osteogenesis imperfecta, the condition is a generalised disorder affecting connective tissue.

They characteristically produce skeletal deformities and abnormal stature. Although uncommon, they pose complicated problems in management. Their detailed description is outwith the scope of this book but it is possible to summarise them along with suitable examples.

They can be categorised into major groups shown in Table 27.5.

The diagnosis is from clinical data, especially comparing the patient's measurements with standard growth charts, radiographs (typically a skeletal survey) and further tests (e.g. biochemical). In some cases the diagnosis can be made by ultrasound.

(a)

(b)

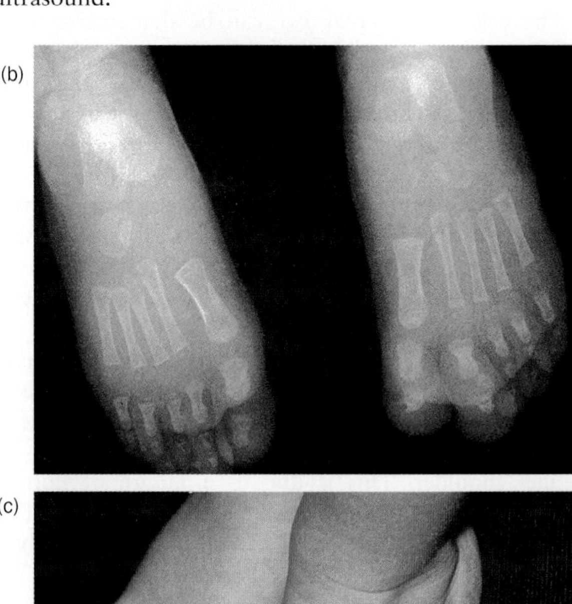

(c)

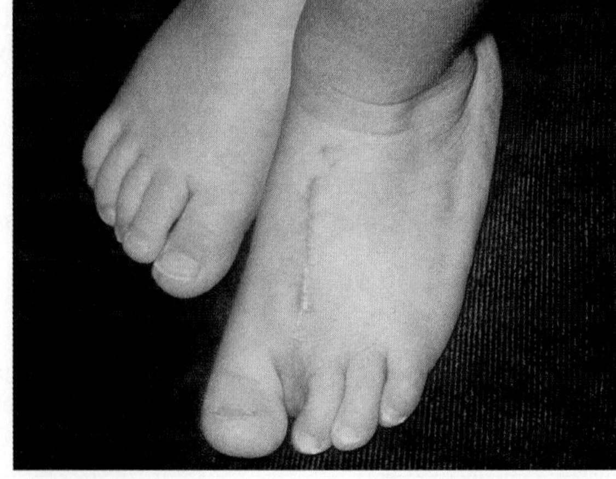

Fig. 27.24 A gigantic second toe, successfully treated by ray amputation.

Richard Ellis. Twentieth-century British physician.
Simon van Creveld, b. 1894. Dutch physician.

Table 27.5 Major groups of skeletal dysplasias

Type	*Examples*
Epiphyseal or spondylo epiphyseal	Multiple epiphyseal dysplasia
Metaphyseal or (includes some metabolic disorders)	Metaphyseal spondylometaphyseal chondrodysplasia
Mesomelic and other forms of short stature (includes some storage disease)	Achondroplasia
Lethal forms of dwarfism	Thanantropic dwarfism
Increased limb length	Marfan's syndrome
Storage diseases	Hurler's syndrome
Metabolic bone disease	Hypophosphataemic rickets
Decreased bone density	Osteogenesis imperfecta
Sclerosing bone dysplasias	Osteopetrosis
Tumour-like bone dysplasias	Hereditary multiple exostosis (diaphyseal aclasis)
Fibrous disorders of bone growth	Neurofibromatosis
Malformation syndromes	Cleidocranial dysostosis

Osteogenesis imperfecta (OI). This relatively common dysplasia (incidence 1:20 000 births) is caused generally by an abnormality of collagen type I and thereby all connective tissues are involved. The joints are loose, bones bend and break, teeth can be abnormal (dentinogenesis imperfecta, DI) and there may be neurological and gastrointestinal problems. The care of these children as with many other dysplasias becomes multidisciplinary. In severe types the children are unable to walk through weakness and deformity. Other methods of locomotion must be used (e.g. bottom shuffling, crutches, wheelchairs).

Four broad types of OI are described but it is not always possible to thus classify a patient.

- Type I(a) – the classic form; blue sclerae, autosomal dominant inheritance and the mildest clinically. Children and adults can be reasonably active with precautions. A neurological problem is premature deafness.

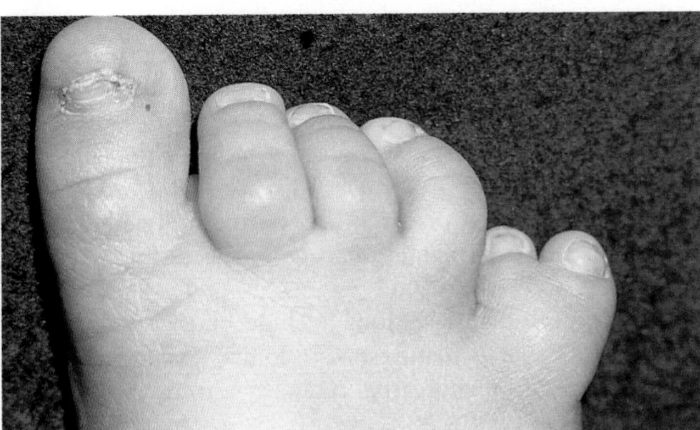

Fig. 27.25 Polydactyly. In this case it was thought better to sacrifice the fifth of the six toes.

- Type II – lethal perinatal form.
- Type III (Fig. 27.26) – severe deforming type. Autosomal recessive. Multiple fractures. The children rarely achieve walking. DI is common.
- Type IV – as for type I but the children are less active and the sclerae are normal. DI is common.

The diagnosis of OI is usually possible from clinical data and radiographs. These can show classical appearances in the limbs, spine and skull (osteopenia, deformities, vertebral collapse and Wormian bones in the skull). However, there are borderline cases which pose great difficulties, especially if the differential diagnosis includes nonaccidental injury. There is yet no test which will unequivocally confirm the diagnosis of OI.

Treatment depends on the individual and the severity of the condition. Any advice must be given within the context of what goals are achievable.

Much can be done through occupational therapy, orthotics, seating and general paediatric care.

The orthopaedic surgeon can help with deformity correction and intramedullary stabilisation of long bones using rods or wires. These can prevent recurrent fractures and help those children who are strong enough to stand and walk.

The value of treatments to increase bone strength (e.g. bisphosphonates) remains unproven.

Osteopetrosis. The bones are dense, hard and brittle. The milder tarda form is autosomal dominant; the severe congenital type is recessive.

Death may occur from lack of bone marrow. Distortion of the orbits may cause blindness. Bone marrow transplantation can be successful.

Bernard-Jean A. Marfan, b. 1858. French paediatrician.

Gertrud Hurler. Twentieth-century paediatrician, Munich, Germany. Described this condition in 1919.

Ole Worm, 1588–1654. Professor of Medicine, University of Copenhagen and personal physician to King Christian V. He described these bones in 1634.

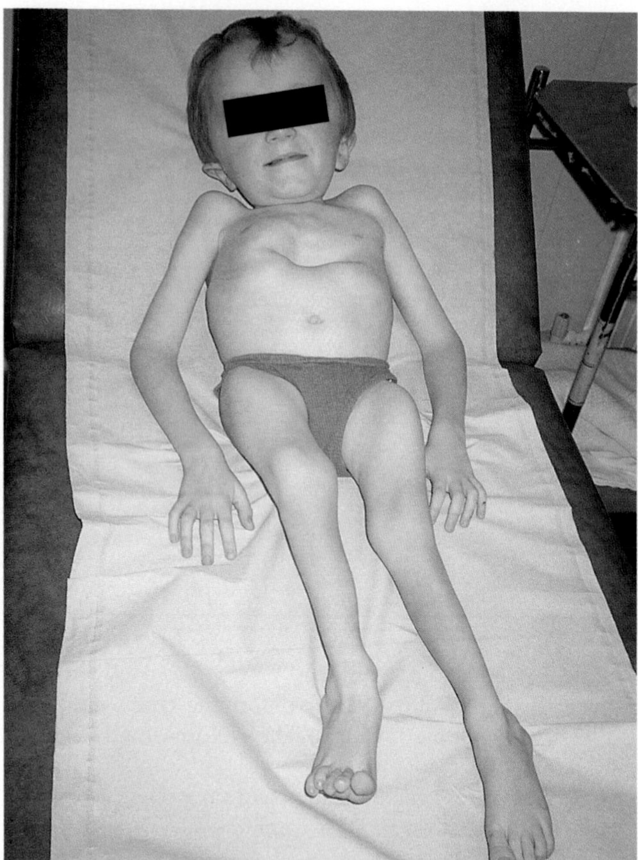

Fig. 27.26 Osteogenesis imperfecta type III. The child shows severe generalised deformities and is unable to stand or walk.

If fractures need fixation, special instruments are needed to overcome the hard bone.

Hereditary multiple exostoses (diaphyseal aclasis) (Fig. 27.27). This is a relatively common, autosomal dominant dysplasia. Cartilaginous-capped exostoses occur at the metaphyses and the osteochondromas grow with the child and stop growing at maturity. The lumps may cause mechanical or cosmetic problems which justify their removal. There may be differential growth disturbances in the forearm or leg leading to ankle, wrist and elbow deformities. Distortion of growth plates may cause, for example, genum valgum. All of these deformities may require surgical correction.

Malignant change in an osteochondroma (chondrosarcoma) is possible, usually after skeletal maturity. The combination of pain and/or enlargement is an indication for further investigation.

Disorders of the epiphyses. Multiple epiphyseal dysplasia can be autosomal dominant. It causes irregular epiphyses which, in the hip can be confused with bilateral Perthes' disease. The hips and knees are prone to early degenerative change.

In spondyloepiphyseal dysplasia the vertebrae are also affected and there may be instability of the atlantoaxial joint.

Disorders of the metaphyses. These result in short stature and deformities such as genum varum which require correction (Fig. 27.28).

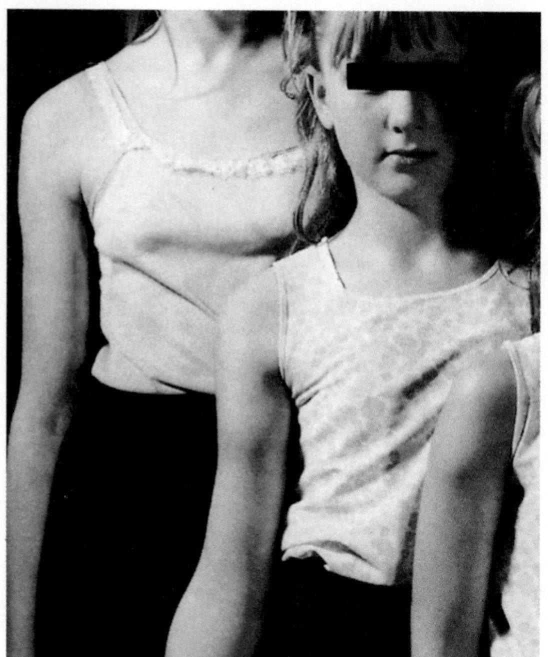

Fig. 27.27 Exostoses of the humerus in three sisters.

Achondroplasia. This is the commonest cause of short-limbed dwarfism (Fig. 27.29). The inheritance trait is autosomal dominant, although many cases arise as new mutations.

The limbs are short with wide metaphyses, there is lumbar lordosis, the forearm bulges and the nasal bridge is low. Trunk height is maintained but spinal stenosis is common.

Cleidocranial dysostosis. This generalised dysplasia includes partial or complete absence of clavicles, ossification defects in the skull, abnormal dentition and a wide symphysis pubis. The absence of clavicles allows the shoulders to be brought together in front of the chest (Fig. 27.30).

Storage diseases. In the mucopolysaccharidoses, the intermediate metabolites of the partial degradation of glycosaminoglycans are stored in various tissues including bone marrow and connective tissues.

The specific enzyme defects responsible for the various types of storage disease (e.g. Hunter's disease, Morquio's disease) are becoming well known. Bone marrow transplantation can be successful in certain types.

The clinical manifestations include short stature, limb deformities, coarse features, stiff joints, expanded bones, mental retardation and carpal tunnel syndrome.

George Clemens Perthes, 1868–1927. Professor of Surgery, Tübingen, Germany.

Charles Hunter, 1872–1955. Canadian physician. Described this condition in 1817.

Luis Morquio, 1867–1935. Professor of Medicine, Montevideo, Uruguay.

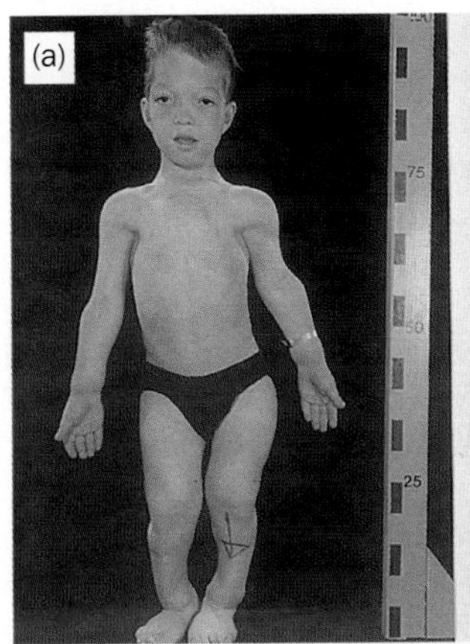

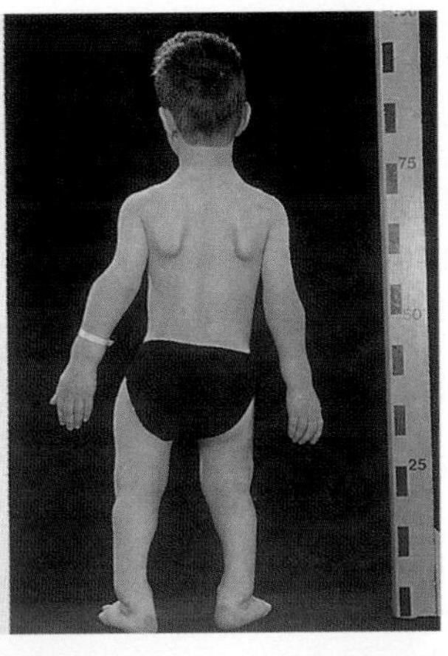

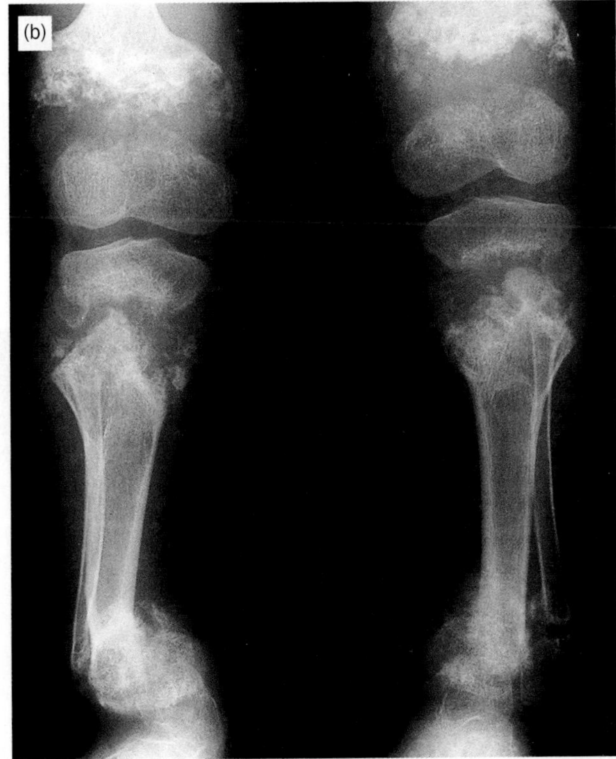

Fig. 27.28 Chondrometaphyseal dysplasia. This child was treated by corrective osteotomies.

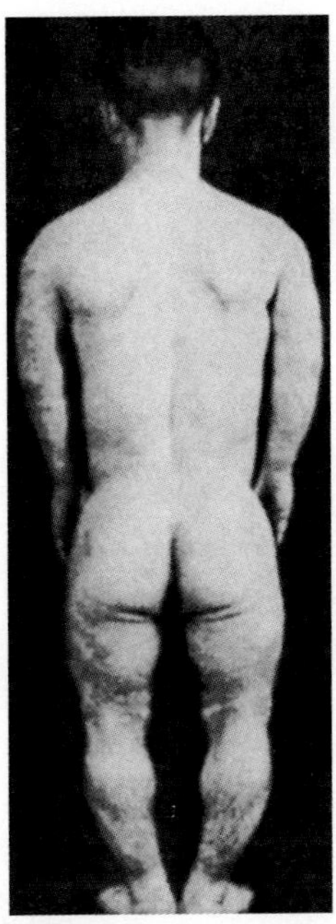

Fig. 27.29 Achondroplasia.

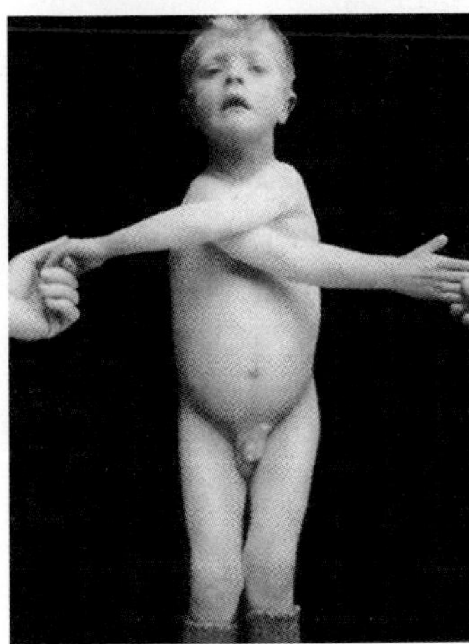

Fig. 27.30 Cleidocranial dysostosis.

Congenital deformities

Developmental dysplasia of the hip (DDH)

This term is more accurate than the older congenital dislocation of the hip (CDH) because it includes dislocation along with other less severe forms, all of which have in common a dysplasia or natural shallowness of the acetabulum. The femoral neck is usually anteverted.

There is a wide spectrum of presentation of DDH from birth to adult life. The condition can manifest as a neonate with clinical hip instability (Fig. 27.31), an infant with limited abduction (Fig. 27.32), a limping toddler (Fig. 27.33), a child or adolescent with dysplasia (Fig. 27.34), or an adult with established degenerative change (Fig. 27.35).

Incidence

This is highest in the neonate where environmental factors such as breech presentation, transient ligamentous laxity and the skills of examiners can influence the rate of detection of instability.

The incidence depends on the criteria by which the diagnosis is made. The rates of detection of neonatal instability in some series approach 20 per 1000 births, whereas the incidence of late presenting dislocations (after the age of 3 months) is generally in the order of 0.5–1 per 1000. The inference is that many cases will stabilise spontaneously and this creates a dilemma for the surgeon as to which cases should be treated.

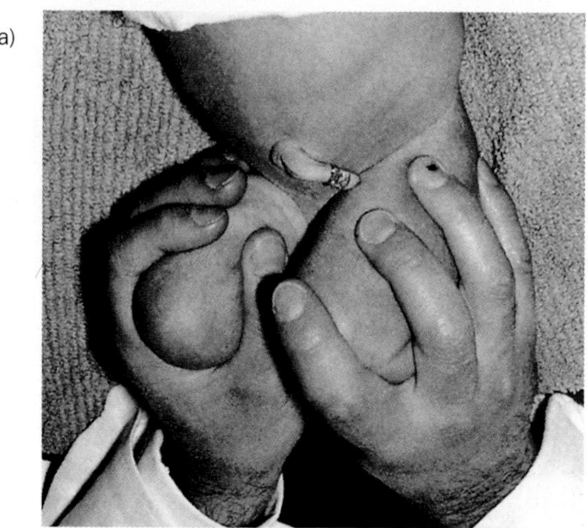

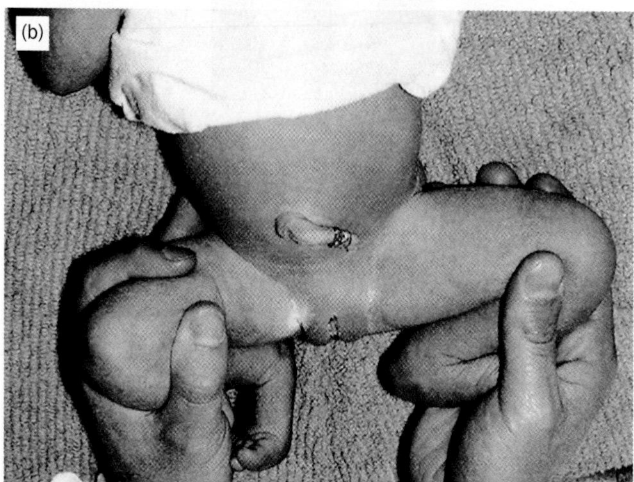

Fig. 27.31 Congenital dislocation of the hip. (a) Barlow test. (b) Ortolani test.

Aetiology

Many factors are related to DDH (Table 27.6). A *family history* of DDH increases the risk up to 30 times. The condition is five times more common in *girls*, possibly related to hormonal factors producing joint laxity. The *left side* is affected more commonly than the right.

Breech presentation, especially the extended position, *first-born children* and *caesarean* section are associated with increased neonatal instability, possibly through restricted foetal movement.

A *foot deformity* or *torticollis* should also alert the examiner to possible associated DDH. Finally, there may be hip dislocation or dysplasia in association with neuromuscular disease syndromic conditions and skeletal dysplasia.

Diagnosis

Neonate. The clinical examination is only part of the general examination. All newborn babies should be screened for hip instability by a skilled examiner using the Barlow and Ortolani tests (Fig. 27.31). The baby should be relaxed and the hips flexed to 90°. It is possible to reduce a dislocated hip by abduction and gentle forward pressure (Ortolani) or dislocate an unstable hip by adduction and gentle backward pressure (Barlow). In both cases a soft clunk is felt as the hip reduces or dislocates.

The specificity of clinical neonatal examination is 100 per cent (no false positives). However, its sensitivity is much lower; even skilled examiners are unable to eliminate late diagnosed cases.

Ultrasonography is a valuable test. It is more sensitive than clinical examination and can detect not only displacement of the femoral head but also varying degrees of dysplasia. Therein lies its weakness for it tends to overdiagnose the condition and thus subject babies to unnecessary treatment. Also, it is very difficult to deliver universal ultrasound screening to communities where the population is mobile, the time in hospital is short, and obstetric and imaging services may be geographically separated.

Radiography can be helpful in the neonate provided care is taken in positioning the patient. However, X-rays are not generally reliable until approximately the age of 3 months (Fig. 27.36).

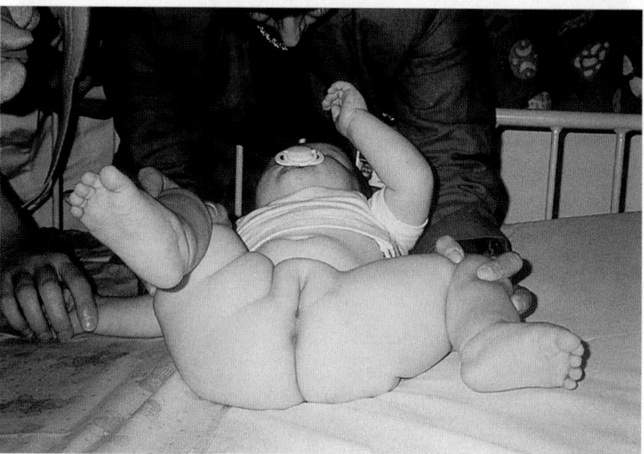

Fig. 27.32 Infant with limited abduction. A sign of possible DDH.

Table 27.6 Factors associated with developmental dysplasia of the hip (DDH)

- Family history
- Sex
- Birth history (e.g. breech presentation)
- Foot deformity
- Torticollis
- Neuromuscular disease
- Syndromic conditions
- Skeletal dysplasia

Marius Ortolani. Twentieth-century Italian orthopaedic surgeon.
Thomas Geoffrey Barlow, 1915–75. Orthopaedic surgeon, Salford Royal Infirmary, Salford, England.

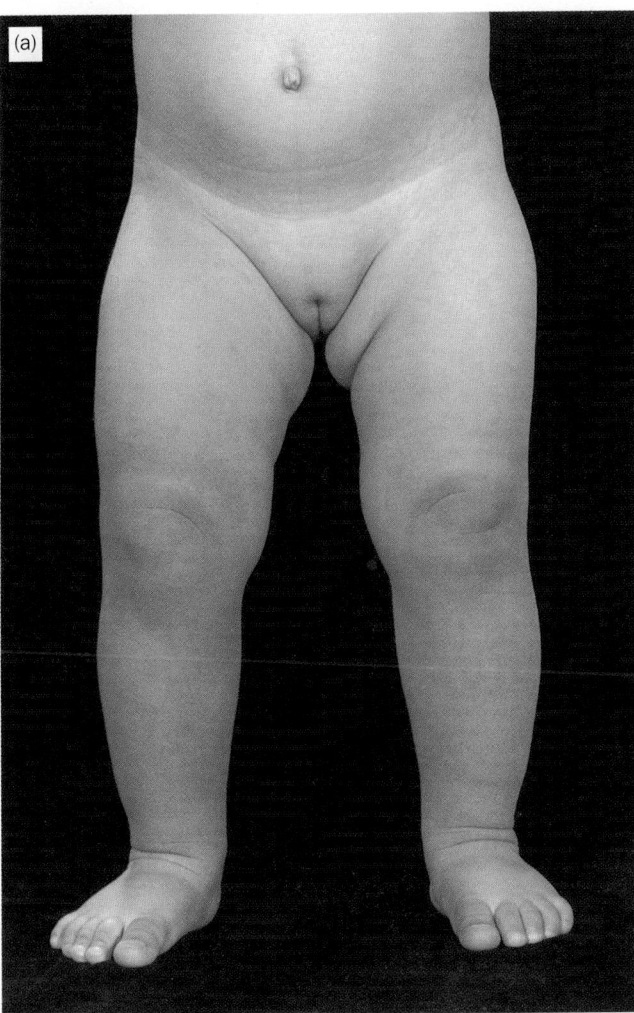

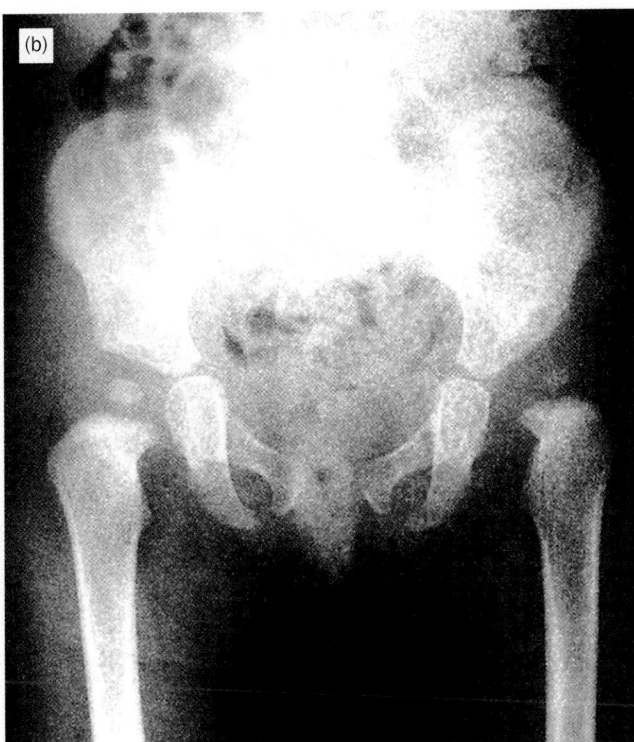

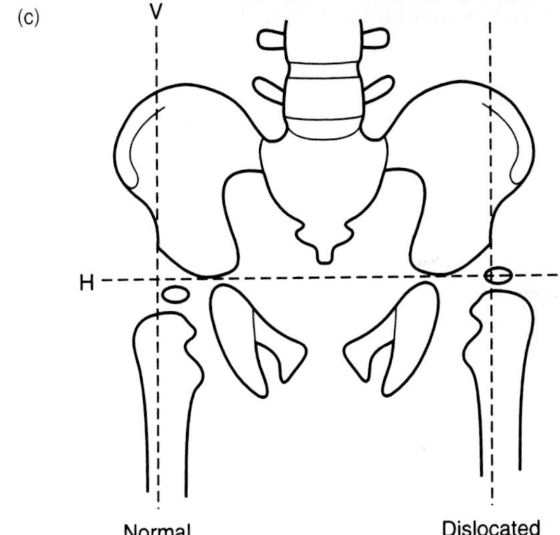

Fig. 27.33 (a) A toddler with a dislocated left hip. The signs can be subtle. (b) and (c) Congenital dislocation of the hip. (b) Radiography; (c) diagrammatic representation of (b). On the normal side, the capital epiphysis lies within the lower medial quadrant formed by the intersection of a vertical line (V), passing through the edge of the acetabulum, with a horizontal line (H), passing across the triradiate cartiliage. On the dislocated side (left), the epiphysis is displaced laterally and superiorly.

Infant. The hips should be examined as part of routine developmental checks, looking in particular for asymmetry, such as an extra thigh crease, shortening of a limb or limitation of abduction (Fig. 27.32).

Child. The child limps, the affected leg is externally rotated, there is an increased lumbar lordosis, and there is regularly an extra thigh crease and limited abduction. However, the signs may be subtle (Fig. 27.33) and easily misinterpreted as part of normal development in an unsteady toddler. A bilateral case is more difficult to diagnose because the gait is symmetrical. Indeed, the condition may be missed until late in childhood.

Adolescent. Pain is the usual feature and an X-ray will reveal dysplasia and possible subluxation.

Adult. Pain is again the usual complaint and X-rays may now show degenerative change as well as dysplasia (Fig. 27.35).

Treatment

Although the details of treatment vary at different ages the principles are the same (Table 27.7) and should all be considered before deciding which one is appropriate for an individual case. The objective is a stable congruous reduction through gentle methods so that the fragile growth plate is not damaged. Such an event (avascular necrosis) is a major complication and usually results in shortening, coxa vara and a greater trochanter, which is high because its growth plate is not affected.

Infant. Traction and surgery are not indicated. The hips can usually be reduced (Ortolani) and should then be held in a harness or splint (Fig. 27.37) for about 8 weeks. A harness

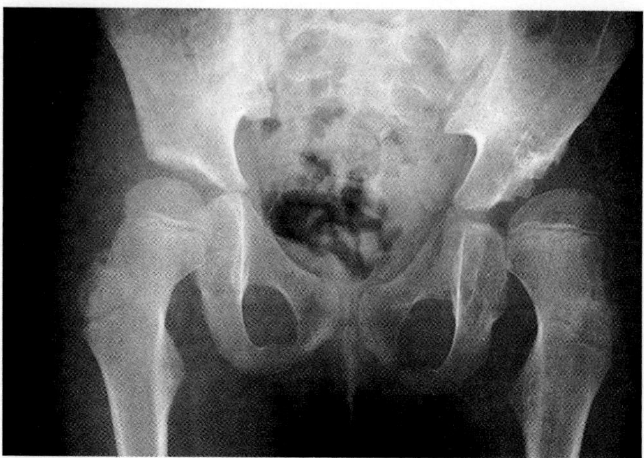

Fig. 27.34 A child with a dysplastic left hip.

allows movement but requires more supervision, and out of expert hands carries a significant failure rate. A splint contains the hips better but thereby carries a risk of avascular necrosis.

A baby, for example, aged 6 months would usually require preliminary traction followed by closed reduction augmented by soft-tissue release (psoas and/or adductor).

An arthrogram is often helpful to define the abnormal soft tissues and confirm a satisfactory reduction.

Toddler and young child. Although it is still possible to achieve reduction by closed methods it becomes more likely that, with age, open reduction along with femoral or innominate osteotomy will be required.

Open reduction. This is usually undertaken through the anterior approach. The iliac apophysis is split. The psoas is divided near its insertion. The capsule is opened and excess trimmed. The ligamentum teres and soft tissues in the acetabular floor are removed. The transverse ligament is divided. The inturned labrum (limbus) may also need to be cut in a radial fashion to allow entry of the femoral head. Reduction can then usually be achieved. However, in the majority of cases it is necessary to complement the reduction with a realignment femoral or innominate (Salter) osteotomy. If reduction is impossible because of a high dislocation, femoral shortening along with realignment is necessary. Postoperatively, the child is held in a cast for 6–8 weeks and then mobilised.

In later childhood, dislocations can still be treated by the combination of open reduction, femoral osteotomy and acetabuloplasty. However, the older the child the more difficult and unrewarding the surgery becomes, especially in bilateral cases.

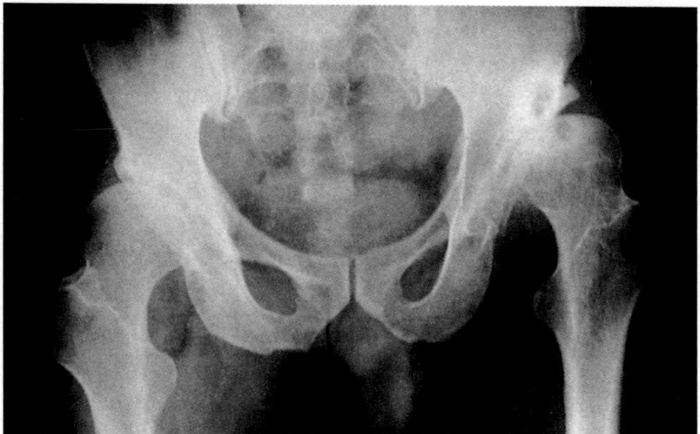

Fig. 27.35 Degenerative change in a dysplastic subluxated left hip.

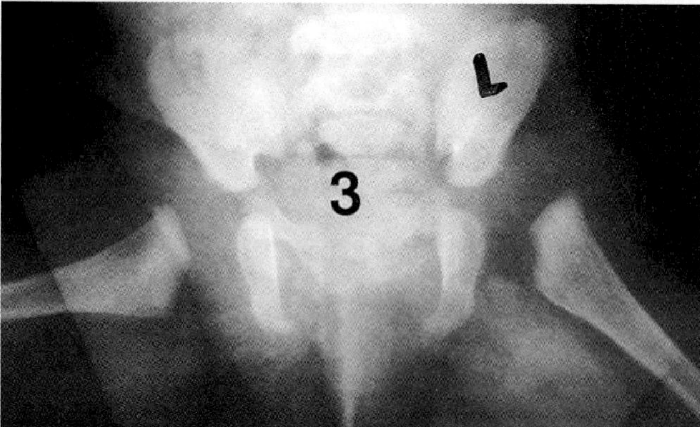

Fig. 27.36 Dislocated left hip in a 3-month-old baby. X-rays may not be reliable before this time.

Adolescent or young adult. Those presenting with a painful dysplastic hip may require surgery. A realignment of the joint through pelvic or femoral osteotomy is only appropriate if there is a congruous hip joint. Otherwise (i.e. subluxation) the acetabulum has to be augmented by other means, for example shelf arthroplasty.

Special cases. DDH associated with neuromuscular disease, syndromic disorders or skeletal dysplasia requires special thought. In such cases (e.g. arthrogryposis, spina bifida) surgery is likely to fail through redisplacement or stiffness. Therefore, it may well be in the child's overall best interests to leave the hip joint alone and restrict one's surgery by treating major limb malalignment by corrective osteotomy.

Coxa vara

This is a descriptive term that describes a decrease in the angle between the femoral neck and shaft. Many conditions can produce this deformity but three general categories are recognised.

Table 27.7 The stages in treating developmental dysplasia of the hip (DDH)

	– *Options*
1. Get it down	– Traction – Femoral shortening
2. Put it in	– Closed or open reduction
3. Keep it in	– Cast – Soft-tissue release (e.g. adductor psoas) – Femorale osteotomy – Innominate osteotomy – Acetabuloplasty
4. Monitor development	

Robert Salter. Professor of Orthopaedic Surgery, University of Toronto, Canada.

- Congenital – this is present at birth and results in shortening of the leg. It is often associated with femoral deficiency.
- Developmental (infantile) – coxa vara develops in early childhood and progresses with growth. The cause is likely to be related to defective enchondral ossification in the metaphysis. Corrective osteotomy may be required.
- Acquired – this group includes cases where the deformity is due to a metabolic disorder (e.g. rickets), trauma (e.g. avascular necrosis in the treatment of DDH) and infection.

Congenital deformities of the feet

Congenital talipes equinus varus (club foot)

If ever there was a condition which exemplified 'Beauty and the Beast' this is it. The deformity can present over a wide spectrum of severity. At one end there are *postural* forms which respond easily to simple treatment; at the other there are severe *fixed* deformities which resist treatment and behave in a beastly fashion.

Incidence. This is generally quoted as one–two cases per 1000 babies.

Aetiology. Although the majority of cases is idiopathic, the condition can regularly be related to factors such as posture, heredity and associated conditions like neuromuscular disease (Table 27.8 and Fig. 27.38).

The risk of club foot is increased 20-fold if a first-degree relative has the condition, and there are examples of racial prevalence, for example among Polynesians. The most difficult club feet tend to be in association with neuromuscular, syndromic or dysplastic conditions.

Clinical features. The baby must be fully examined because of the links between foot deformity, hip disorder and other conditions. The diagnosis of club foot is usually obvious. The hindfoot and forefoot are in equinus and varus (Fig. 27.39). However, the stiffness varies from case to case and it is important to assess whether the deformity is likely to be postural or fixed (Fig. 27.40). Mild postural cases may be corrected above the plantigrade position, whereas a severe fixed deformity falls well short of this.

Pathological anatomy. In fixed deformity the navicular dislocates medially and downwards off the head of the talus, whose neck likewise becomes deformed in the same direction. The front of the os calcis goes medially under the talus, whereas the back of the os calcis is high and lateral, with tethers between it and the fibula. Several tendons are tight (tendo achilles, tibialis posterior, flexor hallucis longus, flexor digitorium longus) and there are contractures of joint capsules and ligaments. Debate continues as to which of the changes in club foot are primary and which are secondary.

Treatment. This depends on stiffness. Mild cases will respond to stretching, whereas fixed deformities will probably need surgery.

Sophus von Rosen. Orthopaedic surgeon, Malmio, Sweden.
Professor Arnold Pavlik. Palacky University, Olmutz, Czechoslavakia. Described the use of his harness in 1957.

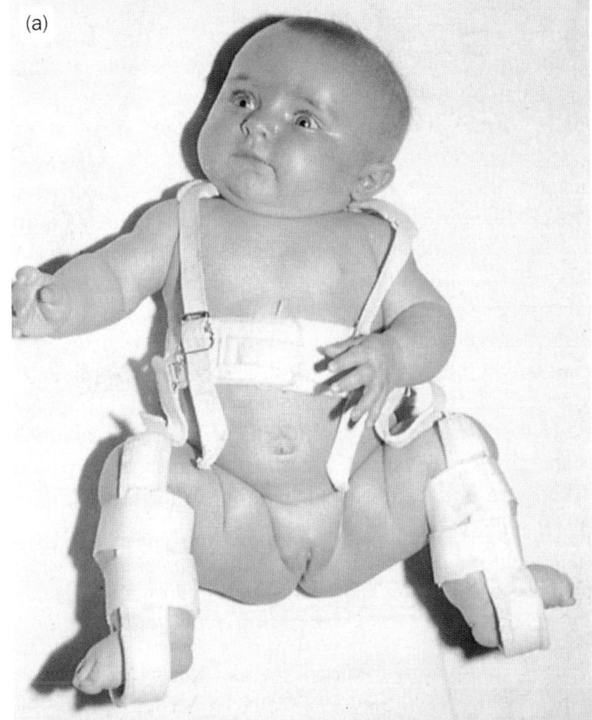

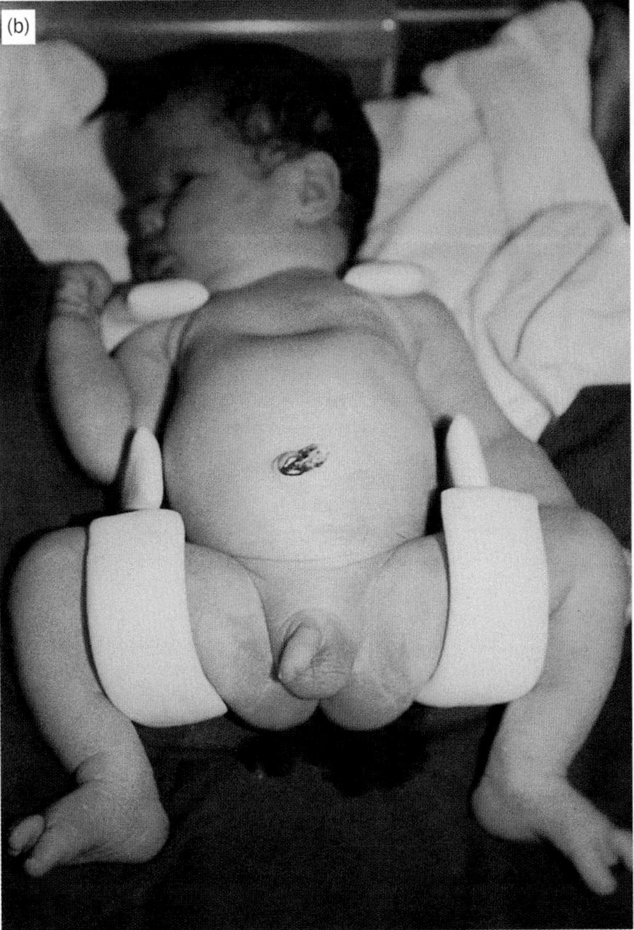

Fig. 27.37 (a) Pavlik harness. (b) von Rosen splint.

The parents must be given careful explanation of the condition. They should understand that club foot alone does not prevent a child walking, and even in the untreated case function can be good (Fig. 27.41). However, the foot cannot be made normal. It usually ends up smaller and stiffer and the calf is thinner. Finally, parents must realise that relapse can occur and, therefore, follow-up until maturity is necessary.

Most babies with significant congenital talipes equinus varus (CTEV) undergo stretching and strapping, usually supervised by a physiotherapist. Alternative methods include serial casts or splints.

Surgeons generally advise nonoperative treatment for 3 months when it is likely to be clear whether soft-tissue surgery is needed. If so, persisting with stretching and splintage is unlikely to remain effective. Indeed, persistent or over-vigorous stretching may cause a breach in the midfoot to produce a rocker bottom deformity which is very difficult to treat.

Primary surgery. This can be undertaken at 3 months, but most surgeons prefer to wait until after 6 months of age. In infants who are handicapped in other ways, and whose prognosis for walking is unclear, it is wiser to wait even longer.

The operation depends on the severity of the condition. The structures to be considered for division or lengthening are tendons (achilles, tibialis posterior, flexor hallucis longus, flexor digitorium longus), joint capsules (ankle, subtalar, calcaneocuboid, talonavicular, naviculocuneiform) and ligaments (talofibular, calcaneofibular, talotibial, peroneal sheath, plantar fascia).

The surgical approach depends on what are to be divided. The posterior route alone will suffice for most cases, whereas a pan-talar release will require a more extensive approach (e.g. Cincinnati). Temporary wires may be used to fix reduced joints, especially the talonavicular. In very severe cases (e.g. arthrogryposis, sacral agenesis) soft-tissue surgery alone will not correct the deformity. In this event, talectomy may be indicated.

Postoperatively, an above-knee cast is applied with the knee at a right angle and the foot as dorsiflexed as the wound and the circulation will allow. The cast is changed at 2–3 weeks when further correction is gained. Difficult cases may need more than one change. Plasters are retained for 8 weeks or so. Thereafter, continuing splintage and supportive footwear may be needed according to severity.

Secondary surgery. Recurrence of deformity (relapse) is, unfortunately, common in severe cases and bony surgery is ultimately necessary. However, most surgeons try to avoid such surgery in patients under the age of 5 years. Meanwhile, repeat soft-tissue release and/or transfer of the tibialis anterior tendon may hold the foot, at least temporarily.

Later on, collateral release (division of medial structures combined with calcaneocuboid fusion), wedge tarsectomy, triple arthrodesis, supramalleolar osteotomy and the Ilizarov technique are possible salvage operations.

Table 27.8 Congenital talipes equino varus

Deformity	*Aetiology*	*Example*
Postural	Intrauterine position	
Fixed	Hereditary and/or racial	Polynesians
	Neuromuscular	Arthrogryposis, spina bifida
	Syndromic	Freeman–Sheldon syndrome (Fig. 27.38)
	Skeletal dysplasia	Diastophic dwarfism
	Idiopathic	

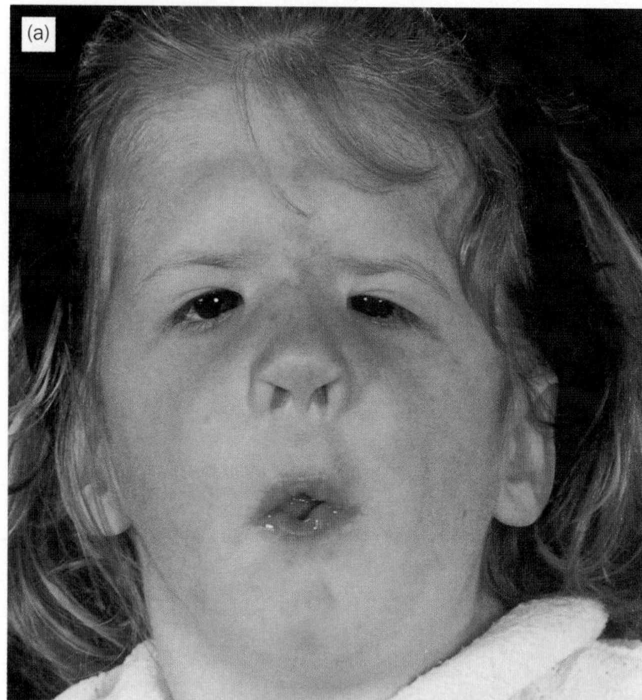

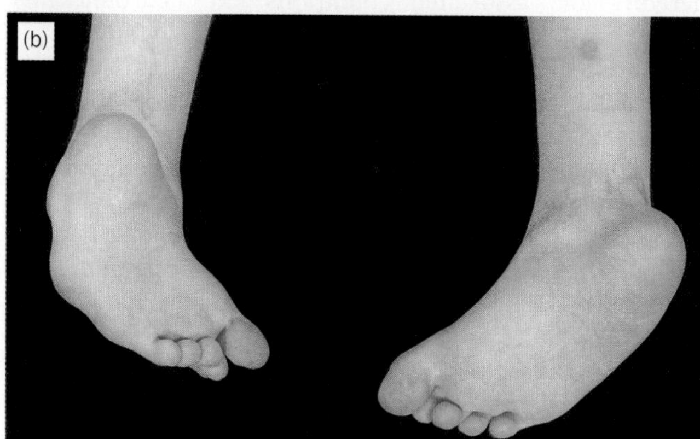

Fig. 27.38 Syndromic cause of congenital talipes equinus varus. In this case Freeman–Sheldon syndrome, which includes: 'whistling faces', severe CTEV and small stature.

Congenital vertical talus

This is a rare condition, 100 times less common than club foot (Fig. 27.42). The hindfoot is in equinus with the talus vertical.

E.A. Freeman, 1900–75. Described the syndrome of cranio-carpo-tarsal dystrophy in a joint paper from the Royal Wolverhampton Hospital, England, in 1938.

J.H. Sheldon, 1920–64. Described the syndrome of cranio-carpo-tarsal dystrophy in a joint paper from the Royal Wolverhampton Hospital, England, in 1938.

Achilles, the Greek hero, son of Peleus and Thetis. As a child his mother dipped him in the River Styx, so that he should be invulnerable in battle. The heel by which she held him did not get wet and was therefore unprotected. Achilles died from a wound to the heel, received at the siege of Troy.

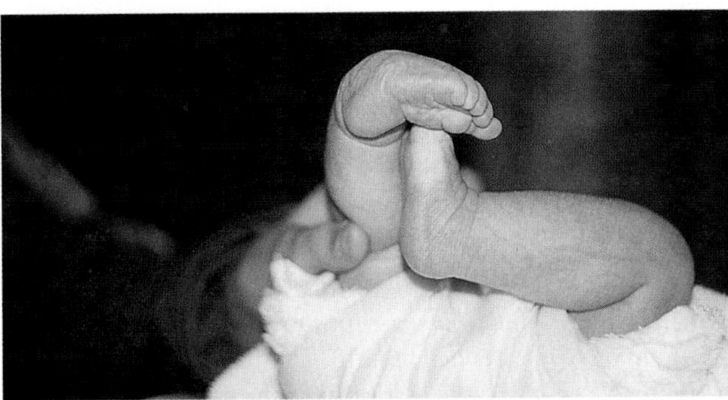

Fig. 27.39 Idiopathic congenital talipes equinus varus. The forefoot and hindfoot are in equinus and varus.

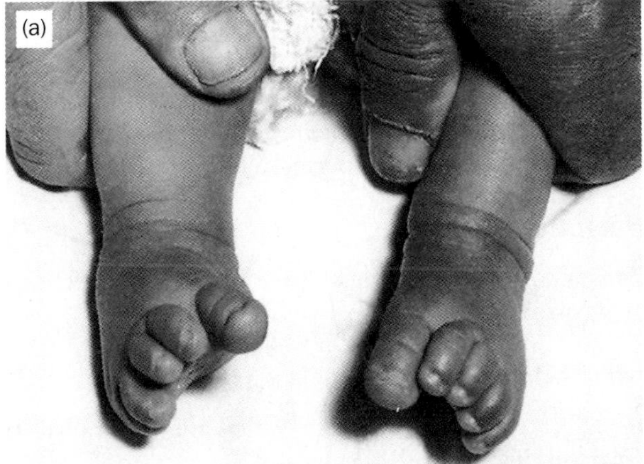

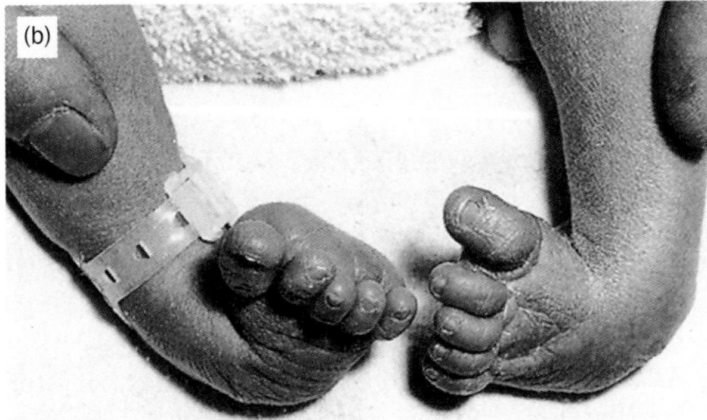

Fig. 27.40 (a) Mild postural congenital talipes equinus varus (CTEV). (b) Severe fixed CTEV.

The navicular is dislocated on to the neck of the talus and the combination gives the appearance of a rocker bottom foot. However, unlike the deformity caused by over-correction of club foot, the talus and os calcis retain a normal relationship.

The condition is regularly associated with neurological disorder. Surgical correction is usually required and involves complex reconstruction of the foot.

Congenital elevation of the fifth toe

The little toe is hypoplastic and sits upon its neighbour. Surgical correction is usually undertaken for cosmetic and/or shoe-fitting problems.

Curly toes

The third and fourth toes are usually affected and flexed at their distal interphalangeal joints. The condition may correct spontaneously and surgery (normally flexor tenotomy) should be delayed until after the age of 3 years, as for symptomatic toes.

Congenital abnormalities of the knee

Patella

There is a number of congenital conditions involving the patella, which may be absent or hypoplastic in association with the nail–patella syndrome. Other features of the syndrome include hypoplasia and splitting of the nails, elbow abnormalities and bony spurs on the ilium. The patella may be bipartite and confused with a fracture; the separate ossicle is usually superolateral. There may be congenital dislocation of the patella, which is small and fixed to the lateral femoral condyle; a fixed flexion deformity of the knee and genu valgum will be noted.

Discoid meniscus

The lateral meniscus is almost always involved, and there is either a complete discoid meniscus of normal mobility or the

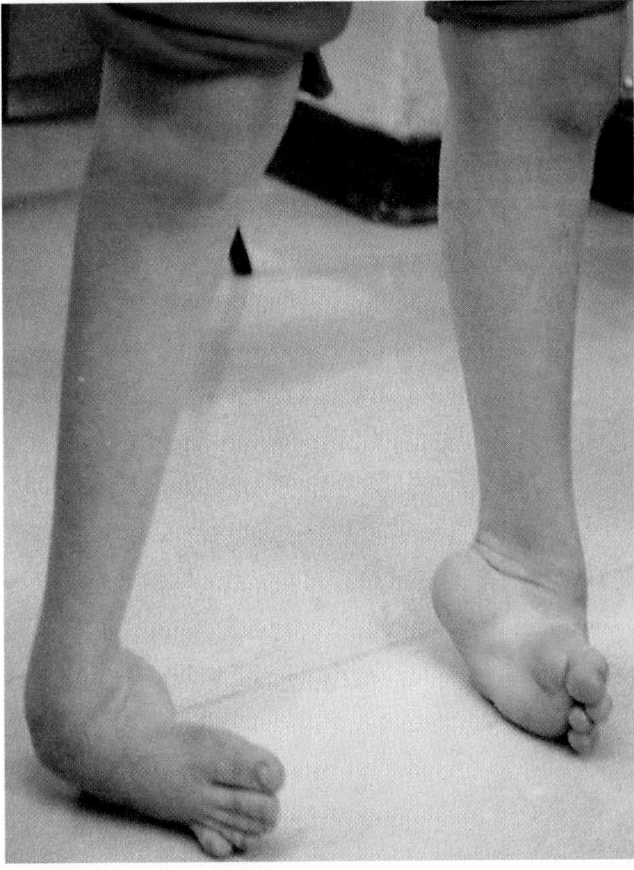

Fig. 27.41 Untreated congenital talipes equinus varus. In spite of severe deformity, function is good.

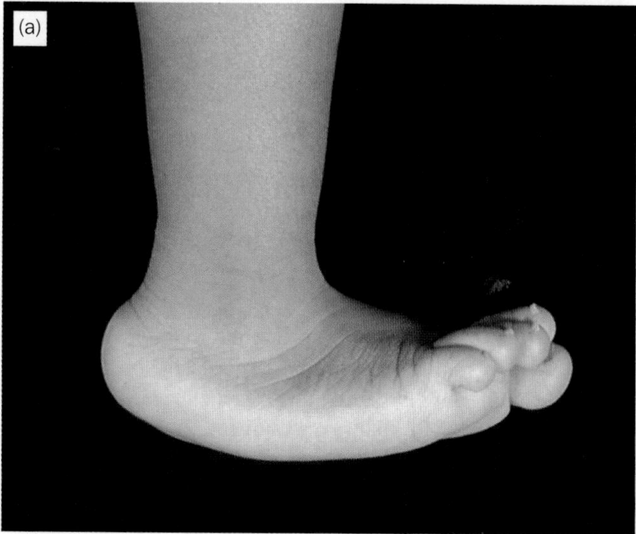

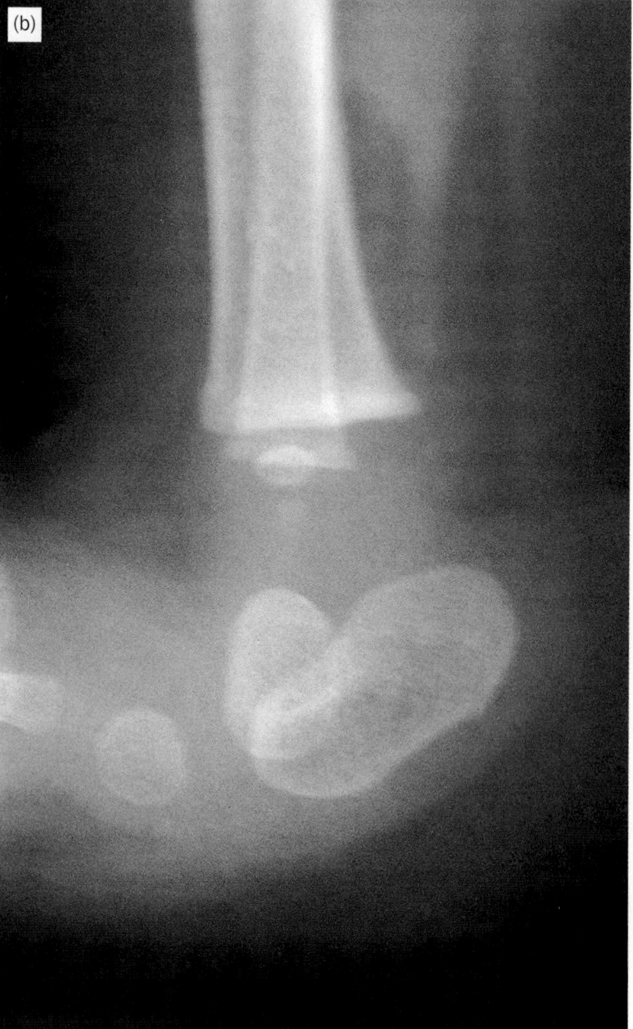

Fig. 27.42 Congenital vertical talus. (a) Clinical. (b) Radiological.

anterior and lateral attachment is deficient resulting in hypermobility. The latter type causes problems of locking and pain. Surgery is often required but where possible meniscal preserving techniques should be used because total menisectomy invariably leads to degenerative change.

Congenital dislocation of the knee

The joint is hypoextended with the tibia displaced forwards on the femur. Mild cases are postural and related to malpresentation (e.g. extended breech). They can be treated by simple splintage or exercises. More severe ones involve quadriceps contractures, which require surgical release (quadricepsplasty).

Congenital deformities of the fingers

Camptodactyly

This is a nontraumatic flexion deformity of the little finger at the proximal interphalangeal joint. Most cases are better left alone as function is usually normal.

Clinodactyly

This is a curvature of a digit in the radioulnar direction. It may be associated with other syndromes.

Kirner's deformity

This affects the little finger in which there is radial and palmar curving of the distal phalanx.

Further reading

Benson, M.K.D., Fixsen, J.A. and Macnicol, M.F. (eds) (1994) *Children's Orthopaedics and Fractures*, Churchill Livingstone, Edinburgh.

Harrold, A.J. and Walker, C.J. (1983) Treatment and prognosis in congenital club foot. *Journal of Bone and Joint Surgery*, **65B**, 8–11.

Wynne-Davies, R., Hall, C.M. and Apley, A.G. (eds) (1985) *Atlas of Skeletal Dysplasias*, Churchill Livingstone, Edinburgh.

J. Kirner. German physician, described this deformity in 1927.

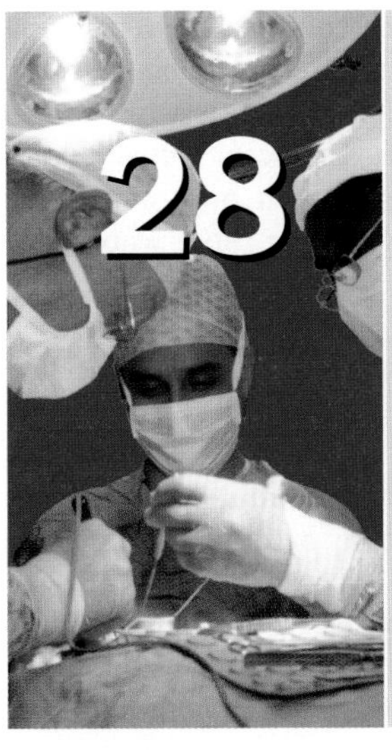

28 Children's orthopaedics: diseases of the growing skeleton

Introduction

Injury or disease affecting the developing skeleton may lead to growth abnormality or deformity. The effects of damage to the growth plate are particularly troublesome. In this chapter, fractures and joint injuries are not discussed. Although most of the conditions described are generally considered to be acquired, they may arise against a background of genetic susceptibility.

Osteochondritis

This loosely defined term embraces three pathological processes involving epiphyses of larger bones or even the whole of a small bone, e.g. in the carpus or tarsus.

The processes are *avascular necrosis* affecting epiphyses normally under compression, *chronic strain injuries* to traction epiphyses and *osteochondritis dissecans,* which is a stress fracture through articular cartilage with or without involvement of subchondral bone. The individual conditions are usually referred to eponymously (Table 28.1).

Avascular necrosis (AVN)

The causes of osteochondritis presenting as AVN are obscure and theories include interruption of arterial supply through trauma, coagulopathy, venous hypertension or disorders of epiphyseal cartilage.

Legg–Calve–Perthes (LCP) disease

This is a mysterious and poorly understood condition. The capital femoral epiphysis undergoes an early stage of infarction, progressing to collapse and fragmentation, followed by healing (Figs 28.1–28.4). The whole process takes several years (Fig. 28.2) and involves part or all of the epiphysis.

Various classifications of the radiological changes have been used, e.g. Catterall, Salter–Thompson, Herring. Unfortunately, they are prone to interobservor error and it is difficult from a single set of X-rays to be sure of the stage or extent of the disease. Moreover, radiological classifications do not reliably relate to the age of the child or the clinical features. For example, a child, especially if young, with whole head involvement may have good movements and very little disability. The condition is relatively benign in the majority of children and does not lead to severe disability or

Arthur Thornton Legg, 1874–1939. Orthopaedic Surgeon, The Children's Hospital, Boston, Massachusetts, USA.

Bailey & Love's Short Practice of Surgery, 23rd edition. Edited by R.C.G. Russell, N.S. Williams and C.J.K. Bulstrode. Published in 2000 by Arnold Publishers.

Jacques Calve, 1875–1954. Orthopaedic surgeon, La Foundation Franco-Americaine, Berck Plage, France.

George Clemens Perthes, 1868–1927. Professor of Surgery, Tubingen, Germany. Legg, Calve and Perthes all described osteochondritis of the head of the femur independently in 1910.

Robert Salter. Professor of Orthopaedic Surgery, Hospital for Sick Children, Toronto, Canada.

George Thompson. Professor of Orthopaedic Surgery, Case Western Reserve University, Cleveland, Ohio, USA.

John Herring. Professor of Orthopaedic Surgery, Dallas, Texas, USA.

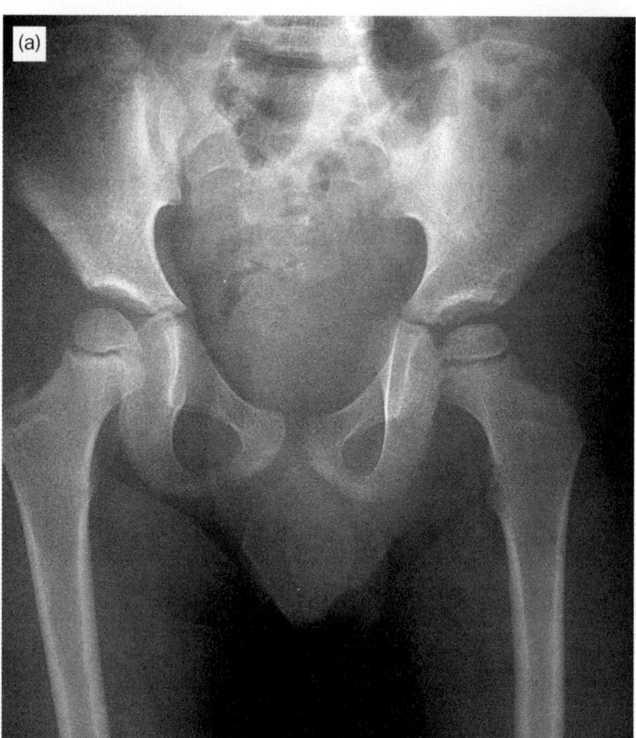

arthritis in adult life. All of these uncertainties make it difficult to select those children who might benefit from treatment in both the short and long term.

Clinical features. The condition can occur between the ages of 3 and 12. It is more common in boys and more frequent in children of low birth weight or those who had a constitutional delay in growth. There is a family history in 12 per cent of cases and the condition may be bilateral in 20 per cent. Synchronous involvement is rare and when seen the diagnosis of multiple epiphyseal dysplasia should be considered.

The usual presentation is pain and a limp. These can be mild and intermittent so the onset may be difficult to define. The pain is usually in the hip region but, like slipped upper femoral epiphysis (SUFE), can be referred to thigh or knee. Therefore children with knee pain should always have their hips examined and X-rayed if there is any suspicion of disease therein.

In LCP disease, flexion is usually maintained but the hips lose abduction and internal rotation. The thigh is usually

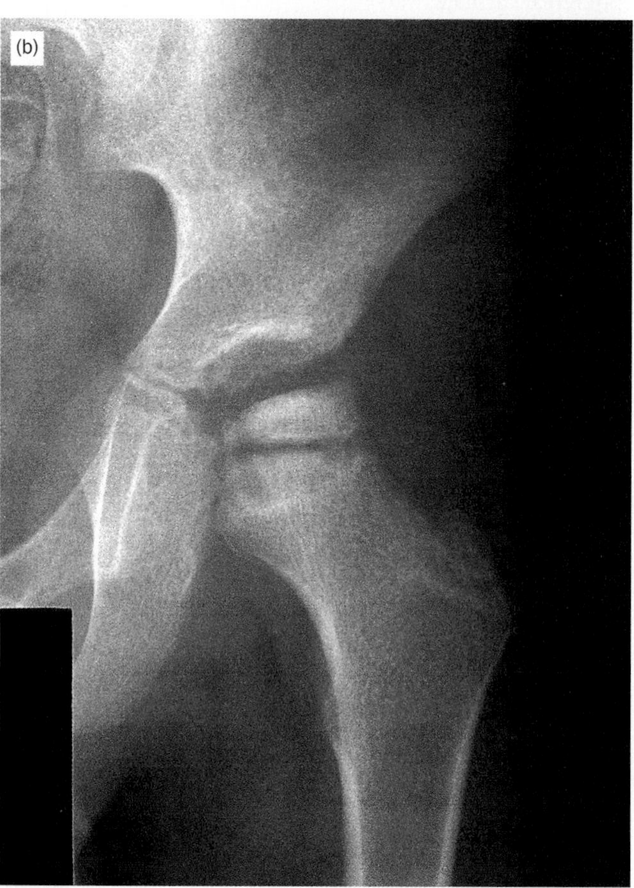

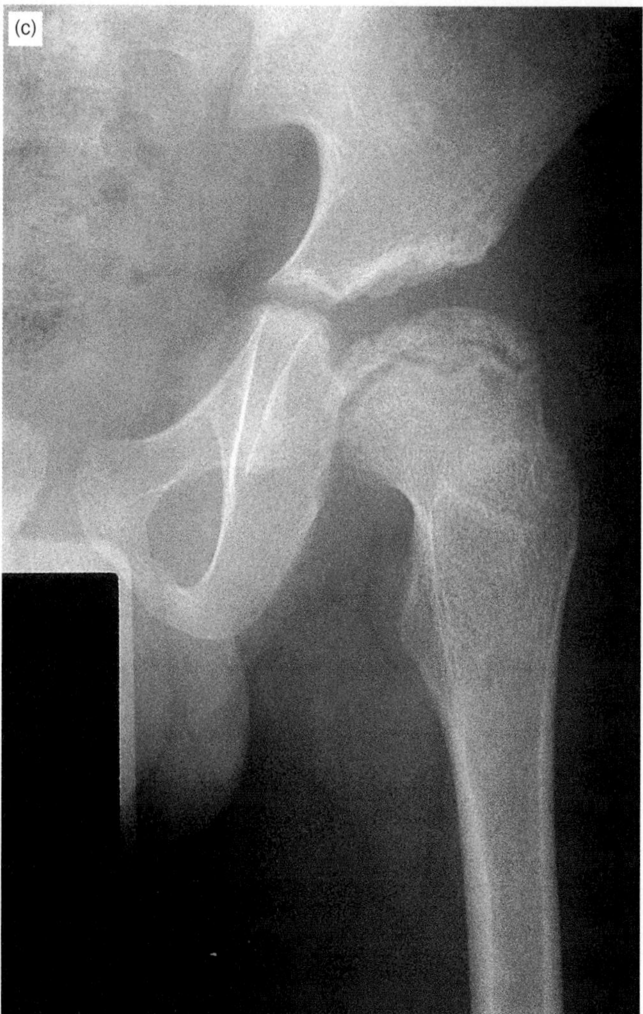

Fig. 28.1 A boy who developed LCP disease aged 5: (a) early stage; (b) fragmentation stage 6 months later; (c) healing stage 2 years after onset. He had no treatment and remained active throughout.

Table 28.1 Classification of osteochondritis

Type	*Examples*
Avascular necrosis	Legg–Calve–Perthes disease Kohler's disease Freiberg's disease Panner's disease Kienbock disease
Chronic strain injuries	Osgood–Schlatter's disease Sinding Larsen disease Sever's disease
Osteochondritis dissecans	Femoral condyle

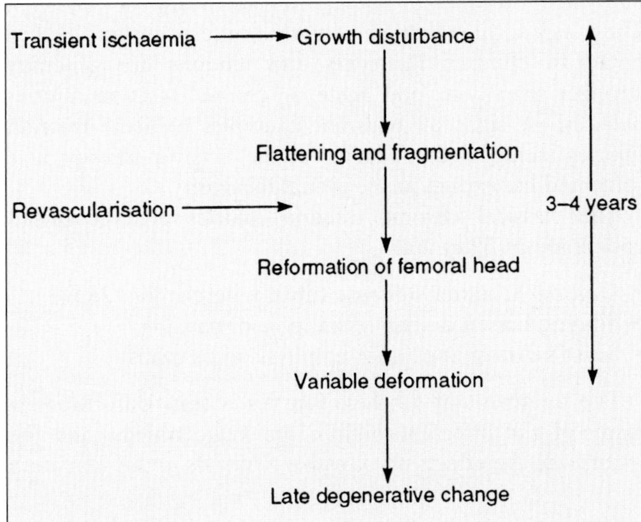

Fig. 28.2 The stages of LCP.

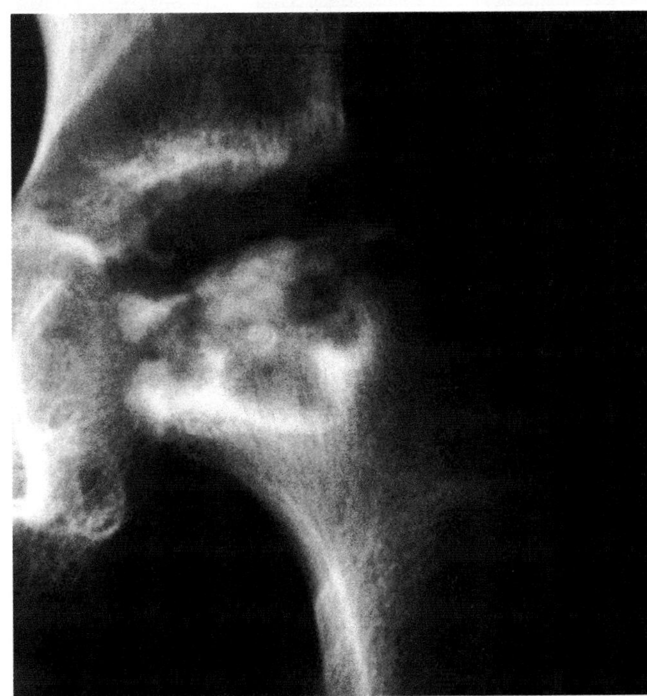

Fig. 28.3 Severe LCP in an older child.

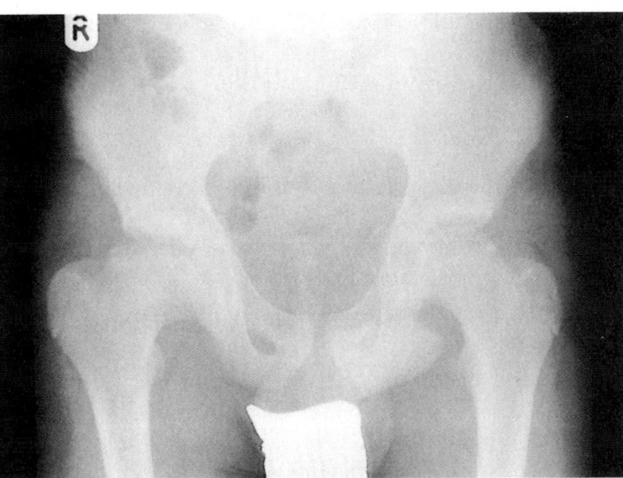

Fig. 28.4 Late changes of LCP disease. Broadening and flattening of the femoral head has healed to aspherical congruity.

thinner than the normal side and the Trendelenburg test frequently positive. In spite of these clinical features the children usually remain active and regularly have to be restrained.

The diagnosis is confirmed by radiographs. Magnetic resonance imaging (MRI) or bone scans may be helpful in the very early stages.

Treatment. The goal is to achieve a congruous joint. The majority of cases will not regain their previous normal shape (spherical congruity) but heal as an oval head (aspherical congruity). However, providing the head matches the socket, the hip is likely to do well in the long term. Where there is a mismatch (aspherical incongruity) the hip does badly.

It is generally agreed that hips should be exercised and kept as mobile as possible, thereby aiming to prevent adduction or flexion deformity and encourage remodelling to a congruous joint. If adduction deformity develops, a period in abduction splintage should be considered.

The role of open surgery, e.g. femoral or innominate osteotomy, is controversial, especially in the younger child. It is difficult to prove that surgery will be beneficial in the long term. In the short term, operations designed to achieve containment of the femoral head may cause damage to the growth plate, usually make a limp worse and may cause incongruity and stiffness. Therefore, if a surgeon cannot feel sure of achieving a congruous joint (an arthrogram may help in the assessment) a better alternative to osteotomy is a shelf-type procedure to augment the acetabulum and thereby give better cover to the femoral head.

In summary, LCP disease is generally benign with a good long-term prognosis. The hip should be kept mobile to avoid deformity and encourage congruous healing. Children who are younger and with partial head involvement do better and

Friedrich Trendelenberg, 1844–1945. Professor of Surgery, Leipzig, Germany.

the role of operations remains controversial. We still do not know how to select accurately those children who will benefit from surgery in the long term.

Freiberg's disease

This affects the distal epiphysis of the second metatarsal and is generally very troublesome. If simple treatment, such as insoles, fails it may be necessary to consider osteotomy or even excision of the metatarsal head.

Kohler's disease

This benign condition affects the tarsal navicular. This normally does not ossify until the fourth year of life and thereby confusion may occur. Kohler's disease presents with pain which is usually not bad enough to warrant more than symptomatic treatment. Radiographs show a flattened navicular (Fig. 28.5) and a comparison view of the other foot is indicated to ensure that one is not dealing with a normal ossification pattern. The children can be advised on activity within the limits of their symptoms and the navicular usually remodels to normality.

Keinbock disease

This affects the carpal lunate and causes troublesome pain and stiffness. It usually affects older teenagers and young adults. The lunate flattens and fragments thereby disturbing the proximal row of the carpus. It is a difficult condition to treat with no reliable surgical option. Various procedures include replacement of the lunate, shortening of the ulna, proximal row carpectomy or even arthrodesis of the wrist.

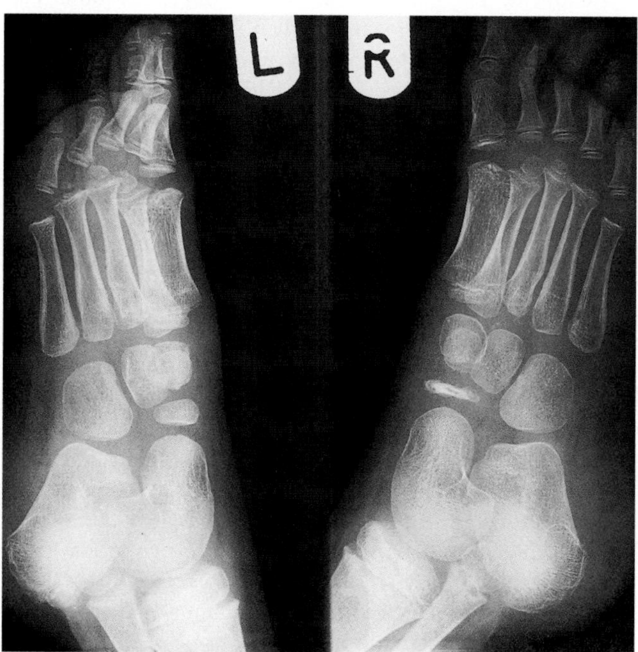

Fig. 28.5 Kohler's disease. Usually benign with the navicular remodelling to normal.

Panner's disease

The capitellum becomes flattened and the elbow stiffens. There is no satisfactory operation for the condition but fortunately good elbow function is usually maintained.

Traction or strain injuries

These can occur wherever powerful muscles are attached to bone. In children ligaments and tendons are generally stronger than bone and acute or chronic traction injuries manifest by signs of avulsion. Examples of acute traction injuries include rectus femoris at the anterior–inferior iliac spine and hamstrings at the ischial tuberosity.

The classical chronic traction injuries are recognised eponymously. They are:

- Osgood–Schlatter's disease (tibial tubercle; Fig. 28.6);
- Sinding Larsen disease (distal pole of patella);
- Sever's disease (posterior epiphysis of os calcis).

The treatment of all these injuries is rest. Unfortunately many of the affected children are keen athletes and the lesions are the effects of excessive demands on an immature

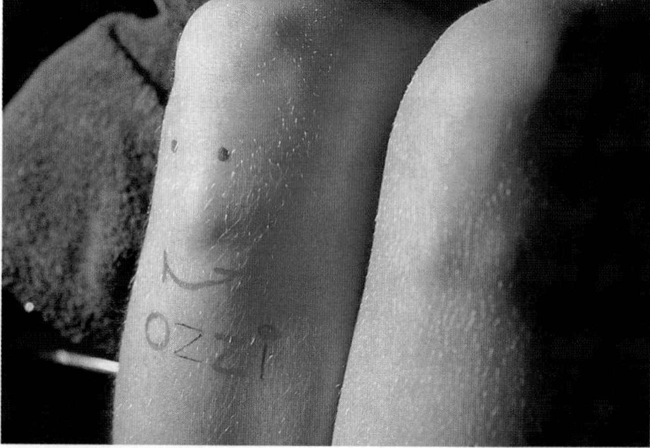

Fig. 28.6 Osgood–Schlatter's disease. The right tibial tubercle is prominent and tender.

Albert Henry Freiberg, 1868–1940. Professor of Orthopaedic Surgery, Cincinatti University, Ohio, USA.

Alban Kohler 1874–1947. Radiologist, Wiesbaden, Germany. Described this condition in 1908.

Robert Keinbock, 1871–1953. Professor of Radiology, Vienna. Described this condition in 1910.

H.J. Panner. Twentieth-century Danish Radiologist. Gave first description of osteochondritis affecting the capitellum humeri.

Robert Bayley Osgood, 1873–1956. Professor Orthopaedic Surgery, Harvard University, Boston, USA.

Carl Schlatter, 1864–1934. Professor of Surgery, Zurich. Osgood and Schlatter described osteochondritis of the tibial tubercle independently in 1903.

Christian Magnus Falsen Sinding Larsen. Norwegian surgeon. Described this disease of the patella in 1921.

James Warren Sever, 1878–1964. Orthopaedic surgeon, Children's Hospital, Boston, USA. Described apophysitis of the os calcis in 1912.

skeleton. It is often unrealistic to impose a total ban on sport; a more practical approach is to advise activity within the limits of the symptoms with the likelihood that the conditions will settle as the skeleton matures.

Osteochondritis dissecans

In this condition, a piece of articular cartilage, with or without the underlying subchondral bone, becomes unstable and may detach into the joint, thereby forming a loose body. The mechanism is acute or chronic trauma.

Common sites include the medial femoral condyle, talus and capitellum. Loose bodies cause pain and locking whereas an unstable fragment may cause discomfort when the joint is stressed.

The lesions may be present on plain X-rays but can also be well demonstrated by MRI.

In general an expectant approach is adopted, unless a troublesome loose body needs removal.

Slipped upper femoral epiphysis

This is a shear failure through the hypertrophic zone of the upper femoral growth plate (physis). The capital epiphysis slips backwards and downwards. SUFE is uncommon. For example, a family doctor in Britain is likely to see only one case in a working lifetime (Table 28.2). Although the condition is classically described in a very overweight (Pickwickian) child, it can occur in a tall or muscular child. Conversely the physis can be weakened by injury or disease, e.g. renal failure, radiotherapy, hyperthyroidism. Thus no type of body build can be considered safe from SUFE (Fig. 28.7).

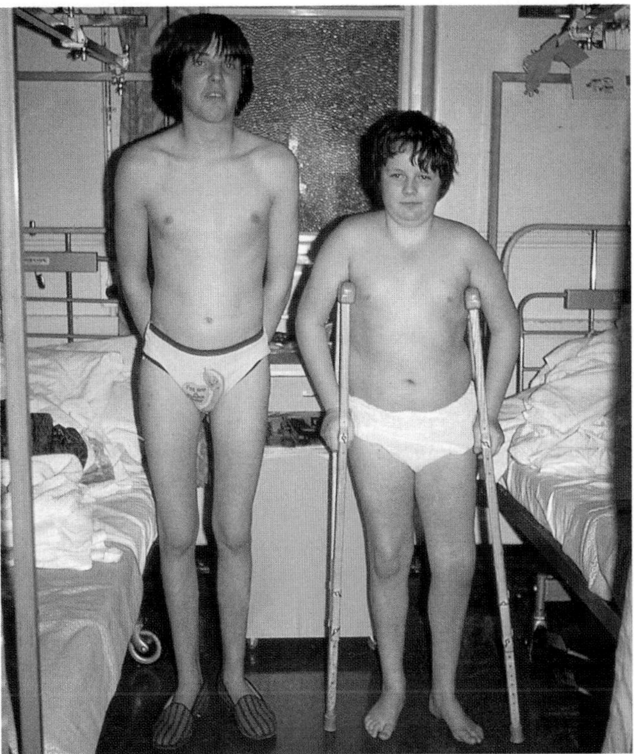

Fig. 28.7 Two boys with SUFE. One preoperative and, the taller, postoperative. Note different body build.

Classification

The condition can be graded according to the degree of slippage as measured in the lateral X-ray. However, such classifications are prone to inconsistencies in measurement owing to differences in positioning and interobserver error. Moreover, they do not relate easily to treatment. There are better classifications, e.g. those of Dunn or Loder (Table 28.3) which complement each other. The former relates presentation to treatment, while the latter usefully defines slips according to whether the child can walk unaided (stable) or requires crutches (unstable). A stable hip would therefore correspond to an early chronic (Fig. 28.8) and an acute on chronic (Fig. 28.9) or late chronic slip with the growth plate open (Fig. 28.10) would be likely to be unstable.

Table 28.2 Hip disorders in childhood

Disorder	*Incidence per general practitioner working lifespan*
SUFE	1
LCP	2
Developmental dysplasia of the hip	3

Dennis Dunn. Consultant orthopaedic surgeon, Black Notley, Essex, England.

Randall Loder. Professor of Orthopaedic Surgery, Philadelphia, Pennsylvania, USA.

Table 28.3 Classification of SUFE

Dunn
Acute
Early chronic (Fig. 28.8)
Acute on chronic (Fig. 28.9)
Late chronic – growth plate open (Fig. 28.10)
– growth plate closed
Osteoarthritis

Loder
Stable (Fig. 28.8)
Unstable (Figs 28.9 and 28.10)

Clinical features

Boys and girls are more or less equally affected but girls tend to get the condition earlier, e.g. ages 9–14 as opposed to 11–16. A girl who has reached menarche is virtually immune. Although the classically overweight picture is commonly seen, no body habitus is exempt.

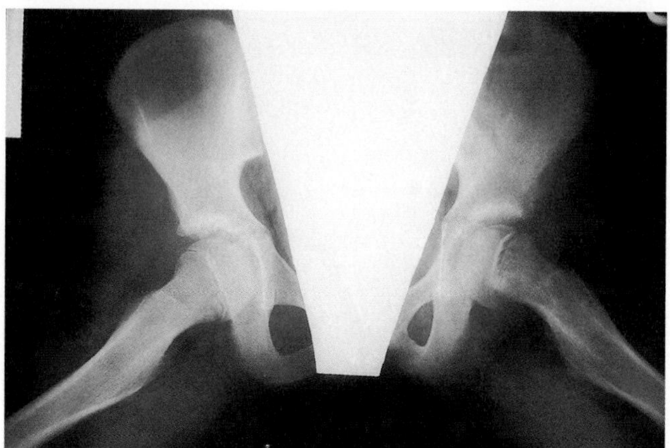

Fig. 28.8 SUFE. Early chronic type (stable). Minor symptoms and a limp.

As the severity and speed of slippage varies, so does the classical presentation. An early chronic (stable) slip may be the cause of mild intermittent pain which is ignored or missed, whereas an unstable acute on chronic or late chronic slip may result in catastrophic loss of function in the limb.

The diagnosis of early slips is usually delayed because this relatively rare condition is not suspected or the symptoms are minor. Pain is classically felt in the groin and thigh but may be referred to the knee. Any child with knee pain should have the hips examined and if necessary X-rayed.

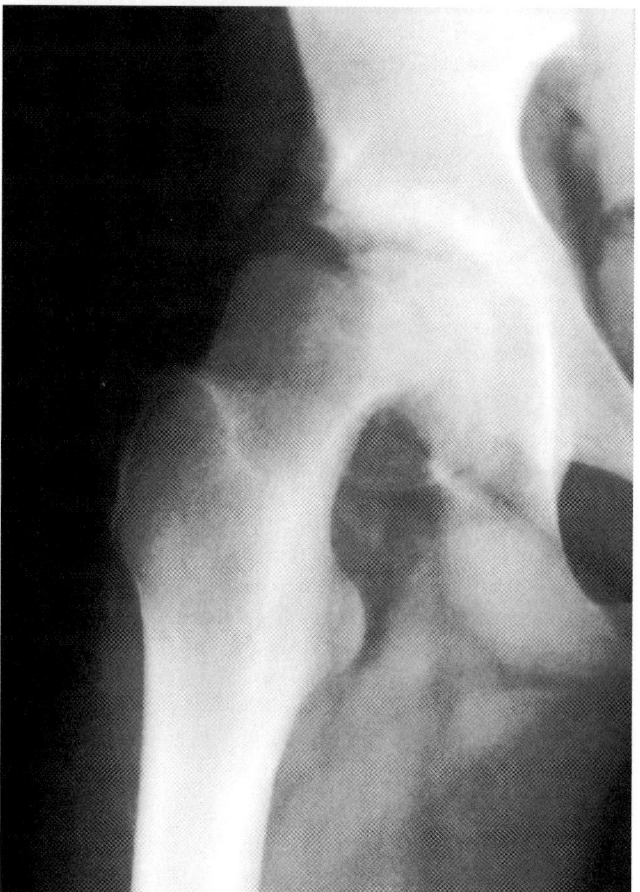

Fig. 28.9 SUFE. Acute on chronic (unstable). The boy had minor symptoms for a few months and then suddenly had severe pain as the epiphysis slipped off the neck.

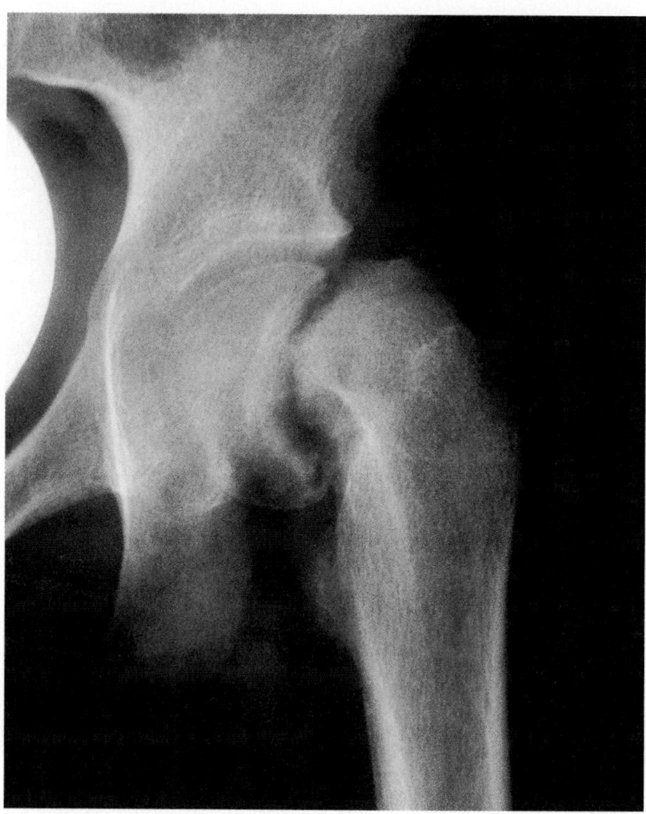

Fig. 28.10 SUFE. Late chronic stage, growth plate open (unstable). The head gradually slipped to this extreme position over a year.

The backward and downward displacement of the epiphysis causes the lower limb to adduct, externally rotate and extend. The hip thereby shows apparent shortening with loss of abduction, internal rotation and flexion.

Investigations

The diagnosis is confirmed on the lateral radiograph but the features are regularly seen on the anterior–posterior view. A computerised tomography (CT) scan can help in defining whether the growth plate is open (Fig. 28.11). Blood tests are usually unhelpful unless there is a suggestion of metabolic or endocrine disorder, e.g. renal failure or hyperthyroidism.

Treatment

The child should be placed on protected weight bearing or even bed rest and traction prior to surgery.

The choices for treatment are fixation *in situ* or realignment, either by reduction of the slip or osteotomy (Table 28.4).

When the growth plate is open one should fix *in situ* if at all possible (Fig. 28.12) because realignment through the growth plate carries a significant risk of AVN. The treatment of unstable slips is thereby controversial. However, an extreme

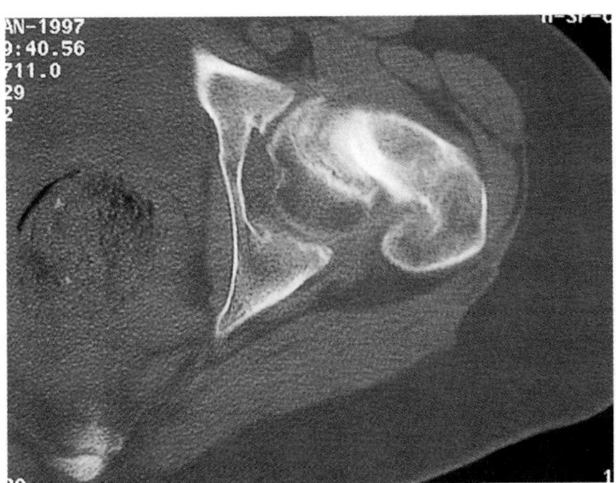

Fig. 28.11 SUFE. In severe slips a CT scan can help to determine whether the growth plate is open.

Table 28.4 Treatment of SUFE

Fixation *in situ*	
Realignment osteotomy	Through growth plate Base of neck Intertrochanteric Subtrochanteric

slip either acute on chronic or late chronic may be impossible to fix *in situ* and reduction before fixation may have to be considered, notwithstanding the risks involved (Fig. 28.13).

Postoperatively the child should be on protected weight bearing for 6 weeks and followed up until both growth plates are fused. The family should be warned of the risk of slippage on the contralateral side (20 per cent). Any evidence of this through symptoms or X-rays demands fixation of that side as well. Routine prophylactic pinning of the opposite side is normally reserved for those children at special risk, e.g. renal failure, hypothyroidism.

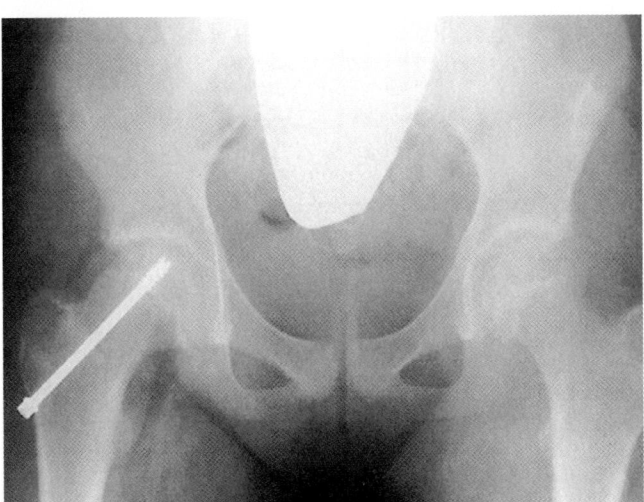

Fig. 28.12 SUFE. Early chronic slip has been fixed *in situ* with a single screw; the optimum treatment where at all possible.

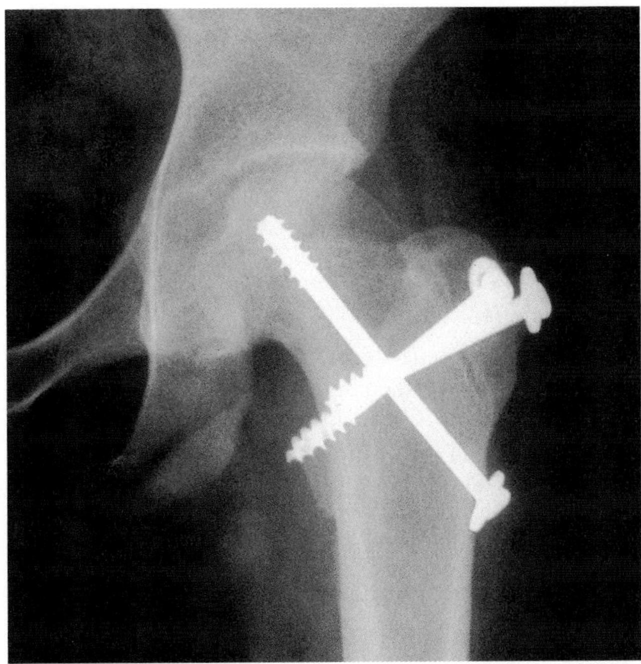

Fig. 28.13 SUFE. Extreme slip (same case as Fig. 28.10) treated by replacement of the head. Significant risk of AVN but in this case successful.

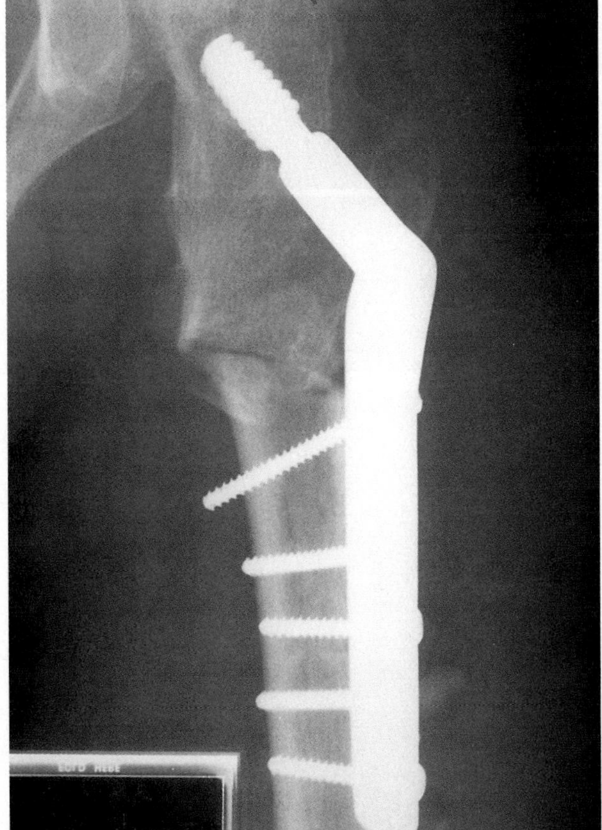

Fig. 28.14 SUFE. Avascular necrosis developed after acute on chronic slip. It was later treated by osteotomy. In spite of severe radiological change the hip is still functioning well.

Complications

Avascular necrosis

This is serious and disabling. It may occur as the result of an acute on chronic slip or may be caused in the course of treating an unstable slip (Fig. 28.14).

Part or all of the head may be involved and the condition does not usually manifest itself radiologically until several months after treatment.

Chondrolysis

This is a poorly understood condition possibly related to autoimmune causes, whereby the hip joint stiffens and narrows. Chondrolysis is not related to the severity of slippage and indeed can occur after prophylactic pinning of the contralateral hip.

Treatment is to prevent contracture and keep the hip mobile while healing occurs.

Osteoarthritis

Although osteoarthritis is a common effect of SUFE, it is generally a forgiving complication. Hips generally function well in the long term and only a minority will require, for example, a hip replacement.

Infection of bone and joint

Osteomyelitis and septic arthritis remain a significant cause of morbidity in paediatric practice. Prompt and adequate treatment is needed to reduce the risk of complications. In some parts of the world tuberculosis is still a serious problem; indeed there are signs it may be on the increase in the Western hemisphere.

Bone and joint infection is usually described in terms of *acute*, *subacute* or *chronic*. No age is exempt from any type. Although there are classical forms of presentation at different ages, skeletal infection can pose great problems in terms of differential diagnosis. For example, trauma or sickle cell crisis can be confused with acute osteomyelitis, benign or malignant bone tumours can mimic subacute or chronic infection (Fig. 28.15) and other causes of inflammatory joint disease, such as juvenile arthritis or irritable hip syndrome, have to be distinguished from septic arthritis (Fig. 28.16).

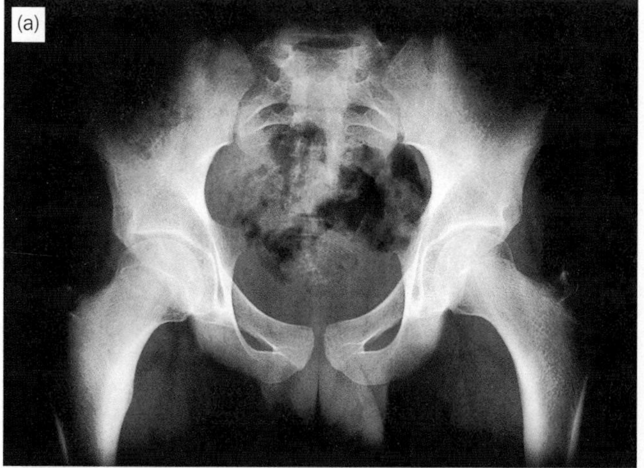

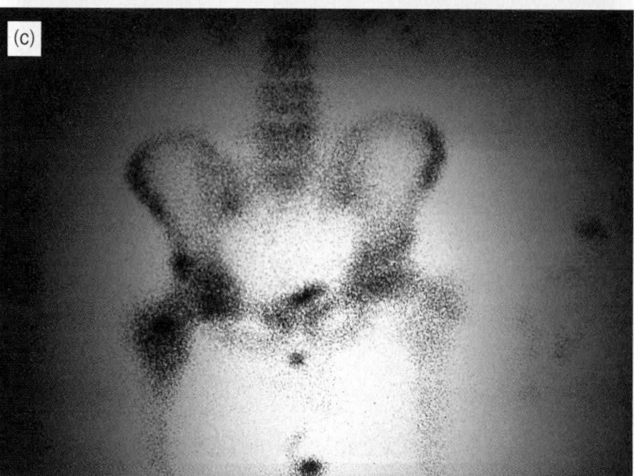

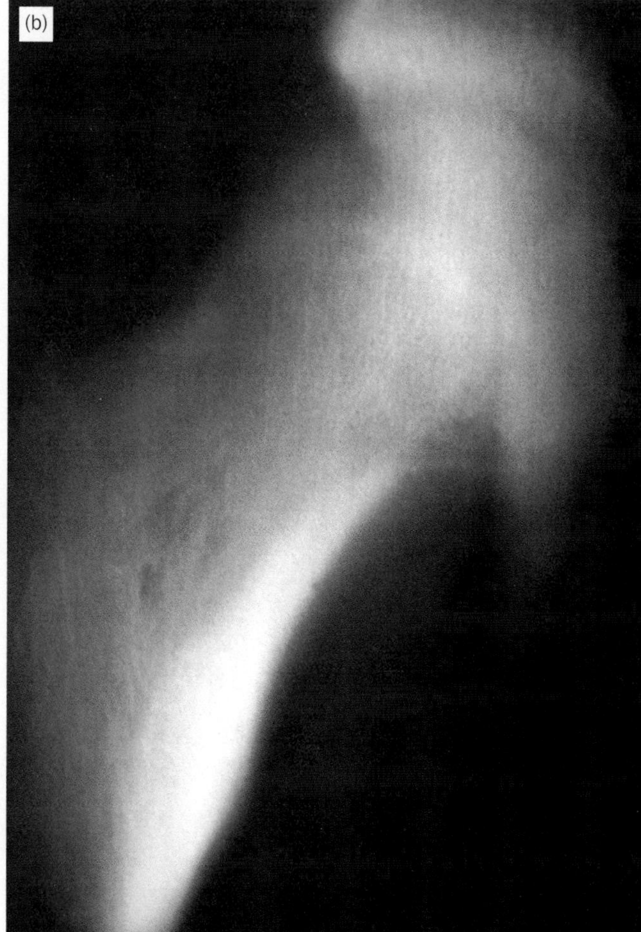

Fig. 28.15 Child aged 12. It was thought that she had chronic infection in her femoral neck but the diagnosis was osteoid osteoma. (a) Plain X-ray; (b) tomogram; (c) bone scan.

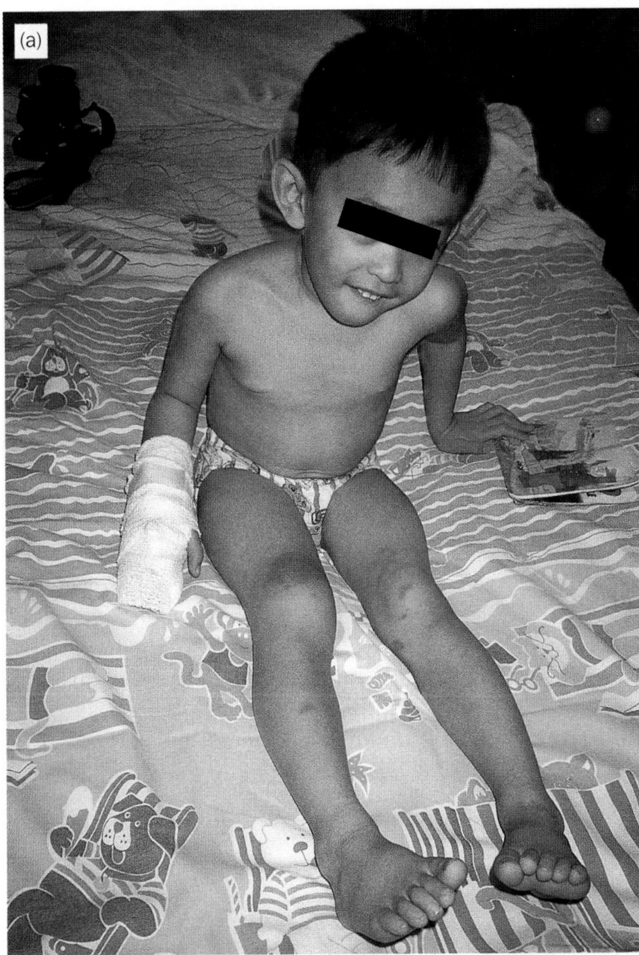

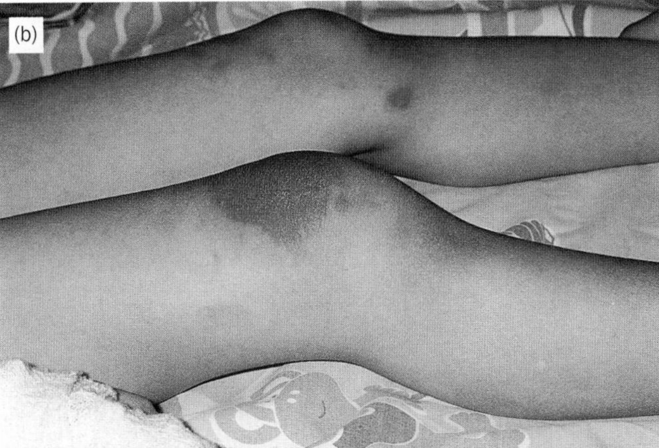

Fig. 28.16 (a) and (b) The appearances resemble septic arthritis but the diagnosis was purpura.

Thus, bone and joint infection my present in many guises, from an acute life-threatening condition to a painless deformity manifesting many years after an unrecognised infection damaged the growth plate.

The treatment of skeletal infection is based on the following principles:

- rest;
- elevation;
- surgical drainage;
- antibiotics;
- nutrition.

In every case, all must be considered although not all may need immediate implementation. For example, an early osteomyelitis may not require surgical drainage or, in another case, antibiotics should be withheld until adequate surgical clearance has removed infected, dead tissue and provided specimens for culture and sensitivity. It is also vital to remember that when surgeons are considering which antibiotic to give or whether a bone should be explored, the importance of resting and elevating a limb, along with correction of nutritional deficiency, including anaemia, must not be forgotten.

The cause of skeletal infection is usually haematogenous spread from without the body or from a septic focus within. In acute osteomyelitis the metaphysis is the common site. Involvement of epiphysis or diaphysis is more often seen in subacute or chronic infections.

Acute infections

Septic arthritis

The hip and knee are the commonest joints affected but the principles of management apply to any joint.

It is difficult to distinguish between septic arthritis of the hip and osteomyelitis of the upper femur. The growth plate and metaphysis are intracapsular and an early osteomyelitis can rapidly progress across the metaphysis directly into the joint. In practice, especially in the neonate, osteomyelitis and septic arthritis of the hip should be considered a single entity.

The usual cause of septic arthritis in any joint is haematogenous spread but direct inoculation can occur, e.g. penetration of the hip during femoral venepuncture. Neonates, the immunosuppressed and children with sickle cell disease are more susceptible.

Bones and joints can be involved as part of septicaemia, e.g. meningococcal. Diagnosis is often delayed in the seriously ill child where attention is directed towards the septicaemia.

Clinical features. The diagnosis is straightforward when there are typical signs such as tenderness, reluctance to move a limb (pseudoparalysis) and fever. In superficial joints an effusion can be demonstrated and the joint is warm. In the hip, ultrasonography is useful to show an effusion. Plain X-rays show this as widening of the joint space (Fig. 28.17) and in severe cases there may be a septic dislocation of the hip.

Treatment. Blood should be taken for blood count, erythrocyte sedimentation rate (ESR) and C-reactive protein. The joint should be aspirated. If pus is obtained or there is any doubt, open surgical drainage and decompression of the joint is indicated. In the hip, this is most easily done through an anterior approach. A section of capsule is excised to ensure free drainage and the joint copiously irrigated. Once

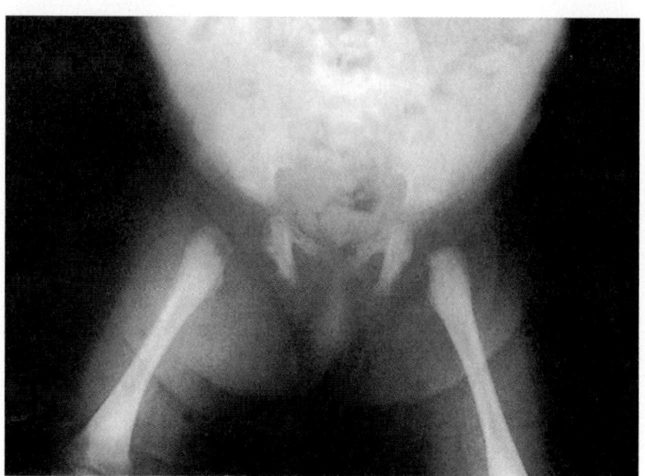

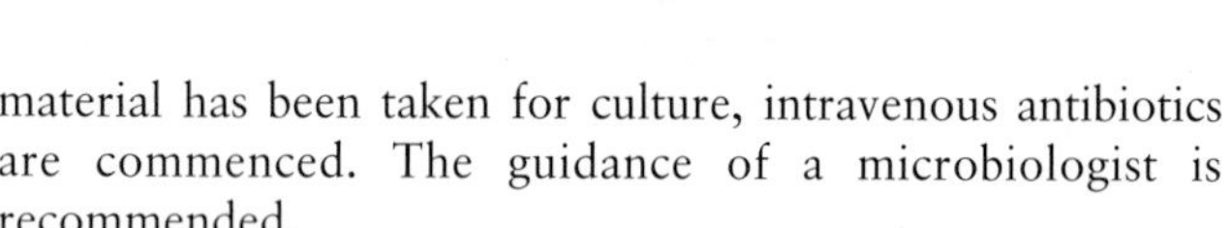

Fig. 28.17 Septic arthritis of the right hip. There is joint space widening and a periosteal reaction in the femoral metaphysis.

material has been taken for culture, intravenous antibiotics are commenced. The guidance of a microbiologist is recommended.

The most common organisms are staphylococci and streptococci. In children under 4, *Haemophilus influenzae* may be found.

If the hip was subluxated or dislocated a hip spica should be applied to keep it reduced. Otherwise bed rest is appropriate until the signs of infection, combined with blood tests, are seen to be settling. In this regard it is easier to monitor and treat a superficial joint, e.g. knee. Pus in a joint is destructive. If treatment is delayed chondrolysis occurs. In the hip, this is followed by avascular necrosis of the femoral head and ultimately limb shortening due to dislocation (Fig. 28.18). A hip thus affected may come to arthrodesis or trochanteric arthroplasty in which the unaffected greater trochanter is placed in the acetabulum to stabilise the hip. Minor damage to the growth plate may not show until late after the infection (Fig. 28.19).

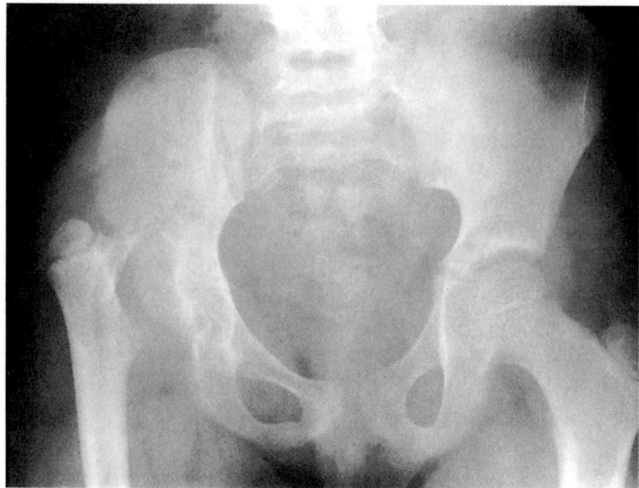

Fig. 28.18 Old septic dislocation of the right hip. The femoral head is destroyed with only a stump of neck remaining.

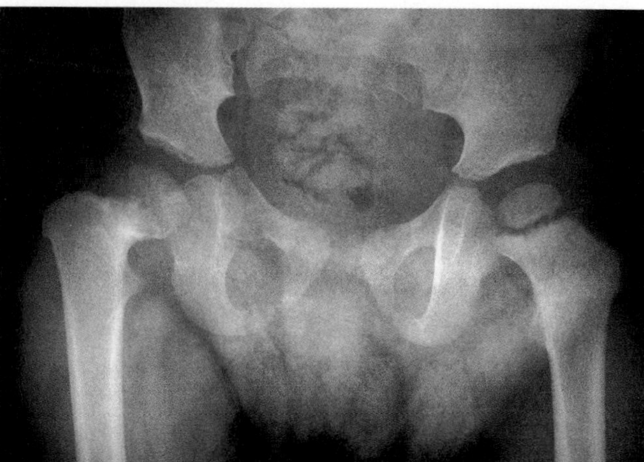

Fig. 28.19 Old septic arthritis of right hip. Late presentation as shortening due to growth disturbance of the femoral neck.

Osteomyelitis

As with septic arthritis, the usual cause is haematogenous spread to the metaphysis and most frequently involves the most rapidly growing ends of long bones. There is often a history of antecedent trauma and osteomyelitis may follow a

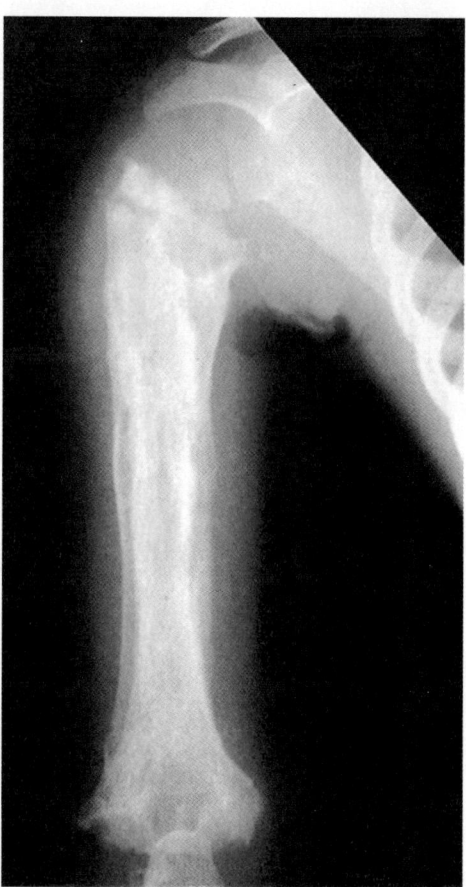

Fig. 28.20 Osteomyelitis of the humerus showing new bone formation (involucrum) around the sequestrum of the original shaft.

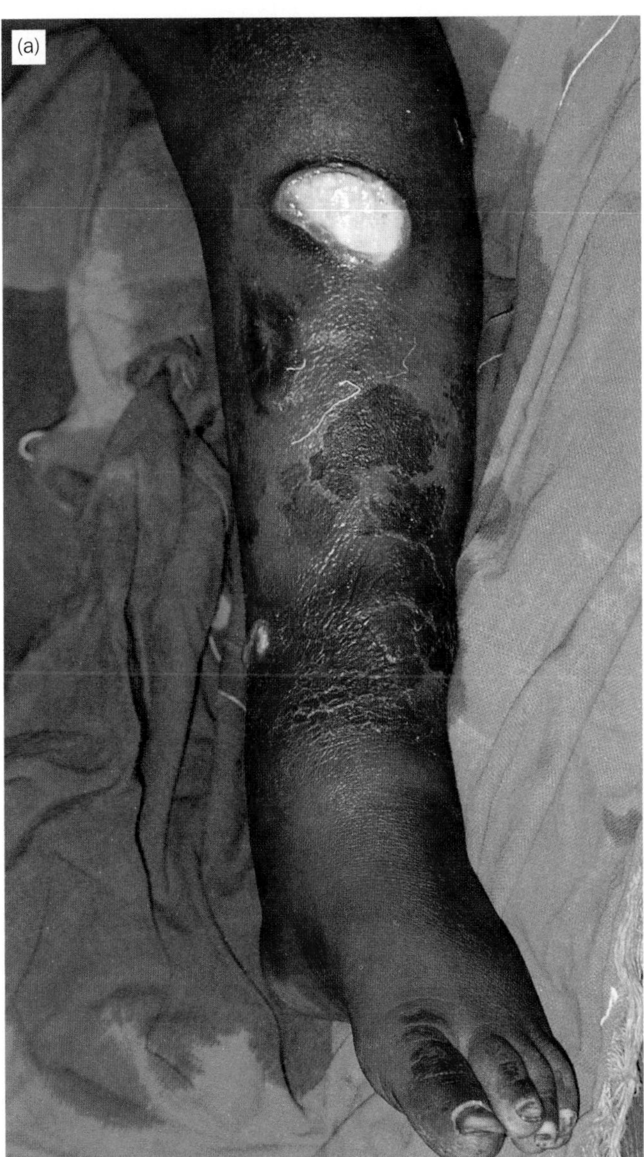

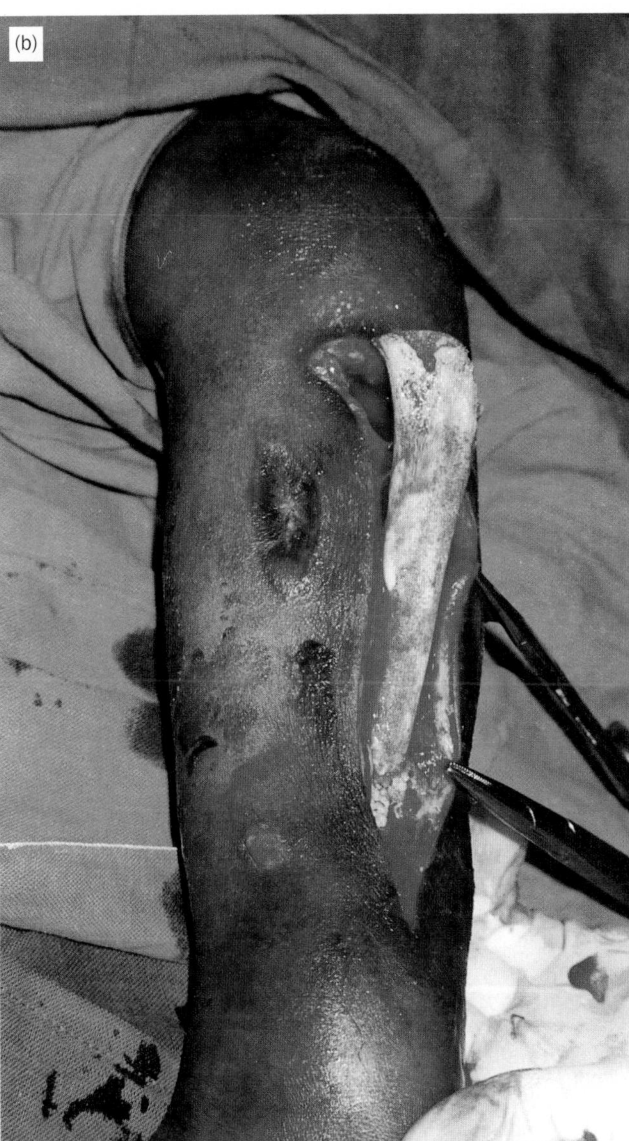

Fig. 28.21 (a) and (b) Neglected osteomyelitis of the tibia. Pus has burst through to the skin. The sequestrum was virtually the whole of the shaft of the tibia which fell out when the leg was drained.

subperiosteal haematoma. The initial inflammatory reaction is followed by an abscess which tracks laterally to lift the periosteum. This deprives the cortex of its blood supply and it may die; a sequestrium. Subperiosteal new bone produces the involucrum (Fig. 28.20). Pus may continue to rupture through the involucrum via cloacae and reach the skin (Fig. 28.21a and b).

Clinical features. Classically, the child is ill with signs of septicaemia. There is local tenderness erythema and increase in local temperature. In severe cases the whole limb is swollen, tender and hot, making localisation difficult. Radiological appearances in osteomyelitis are normal in the early stages, although a bone scan may be helpful.

Treatment. Once pus is formed it must be surgically released. In the genuinely early case (history less than 24 hours) treatment with antibiotics can be started after blood cultures are taken. Provided there is a prompt response (24–48 hours) surgery may be avoided. This approach may also be justified in early severe cases where generalised swelling and tenderness of the whole limb makes localisation difficult. In such cases it is advisable to take blood cultures, commence resuscitation and intravenous antibiotics, and wait 24–48 hours when localising features will develop to direct the surgical approach.

When surgery is required the periosteum is incised and any subperiosteal abscess drained. If there is no subperiosteal abscess, the bone should be drilled to drain any intraosseous pus. Postoperatively the limb should be rested in a cast. Prolonged antibiotic therapy is necessary (at least 6 weeks) because it can be very difficult to eradicate the

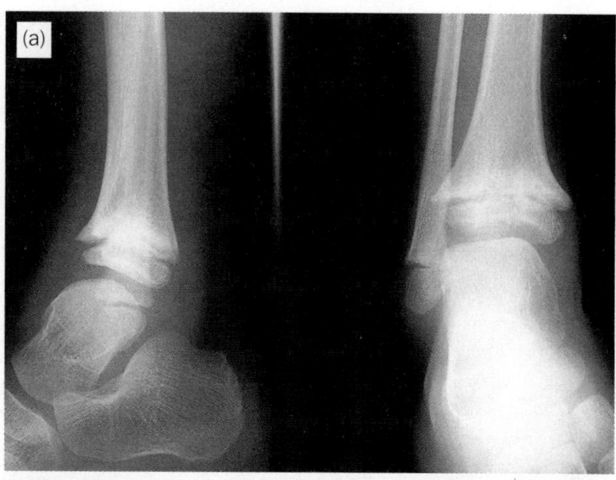

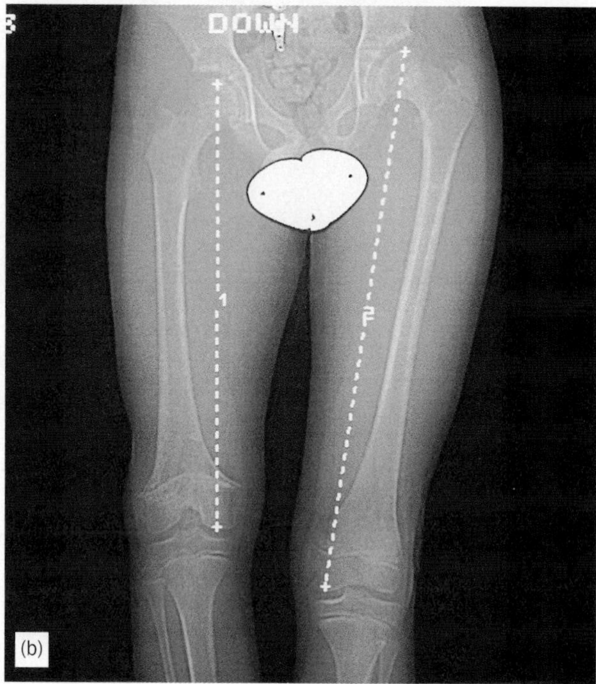

Fig. 28.22 A child who had neonatal septicaemia with multifocal osteomyelitis which damaged several growth plates. He later presented with deformity and shortening at (a) the ankle and (b) femur.

condition permanently: 'once an osteomyelitis, always an osteomyelitis'.

Apart from chronicity, other possible late effects of osteomyelitis include overgrowth of the limb due to stimulation of the growth plate or deformity due to growth plate damage (Fig. 28.22a and b).

Acute infection can affect the spine in childhood. It is often not suspected in a toddler or child who may be generally well; backache, stiffness and a limp are alerting signs. X-rays show disc space narrowing and an MRI scan will highlight the inflamed area. A CT-guided biopsy will probably show infected tissue but it is common that culture is negative or inconclusive. Rather than exploring and draining the spine it is usually worthwhile to treat these children with a spinal brace and broad-spectrum antibiotics whereupon the infection usually subsides, with or without spontaneous fusion between affected vertebrae.

Subacute and chronic infections

The epiphysis is a relatively common site. The diaphysis can also be affected. The clinical features are much less marked than with acute infections and diagnosis is often delayed. Radiographs may show a sclerotic wall around a cyst or in many cases sclerosis may be the only feature. A bone scan may be helpful to distinguish from quiescent harmless bone lesions. In cases where sampling a lesion may be difficult because of its anatomical location or lack of clear definition on radiographs a conservative approach with antibiotics may be indicated. If there is no response, biopsy is indicated to exclude a tumour.

Irritable hip

This is also known as transient synovitis or observation hip. It is essentially a diagnosis of exclusion – most importantly from septic arthritis. It is a common condition in which the child, usually between 4 and 8 years old, presents with pain in the hip of variable severity, reluctance to weight bear and a limp. The cause is usually unknown but there may be a history of preceding trauma or a viral infection. The clinical features vary from a well child with minor loss of movement to the unwell child with a low-grade fever and marked stiffness.

Systemic examination may reveal lymphadenopathy or other evidence of a viral infection, such as a rash. Radiographs are normal or may show slight widening of the joint space. The blood count is normal and the ESR may be minimally raised. The presence of fever, effusion and marked stiffness would be an indication to investigate as a septic arthritis. This would only apply to a minority of cases. The great majority settles with bed rest followed by mobilisation as the hip becomes comfortable

Skeletal tuberculosis

This may present as chronic arthritis (Fig. 28.23) or osteomyelitis.

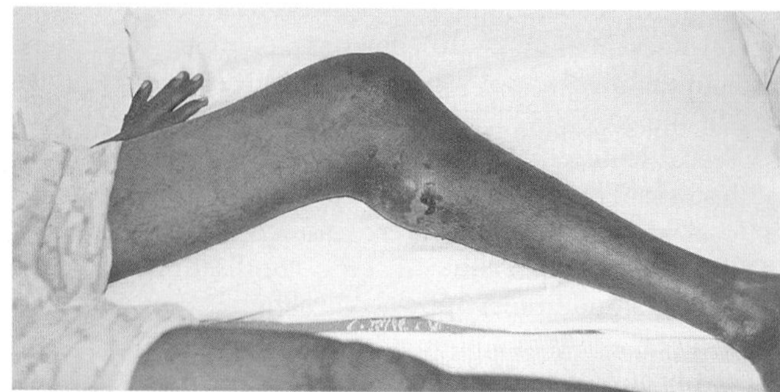

Fig. 28.23 Tuberculous arthritis of the knee.

In the spine it usually involves the adjacent parts of the bodies of two vertebrae. The disc is relatively resistant to tuberculosis but eventually undergoes avascular necrosis although it may sequestrate. Abscesses can spread in various directions by stripping the vertebral ligaments. In the lumbar region, a paravertebral abscess may enter the psoas sheath to appear in the femoral triangle. Clinical features include general malaise, backache and stiffness. The principal complications of spinal tuberculosis are paraplegia and deformity. Paraplegia may occur early or late in the disease. Early paraplegia is usually due to mechanical pressure on the cord from granulation tissue, pus, sequestrated disc material or oedema; ischaemia can also be a cause. Late paraplegia is usually associated with stretching of the spinal cord over an angular deformity, resulting in ischaemia. The usual deformity in spinal tuberculosis is a kyphosis due to collapse of the vertebral bodies. As with other forms of skeletal tuberculosis, treatment should be with appropriate antibiotics. However, it has been shown that, although conservative treatment is effective, there is a risk of a deterioration in the kyphosis and that this is most likely to occur in children and when several vertebrae are involved. Radical anterior débridement and spinal fusion will usually prevent any progression of the deformity.

Neuromuscular orthopaedics

In neuromuscular conditions such as polio, spina bifida, cerebral palsy and the muscular dystrophies, imbalance of muscles and the effects of gravity can result in deformity. Orthopaedic surgery has a valuable role in properly selected patients. However, it is important to remember that surgery is only an incident in the continuing care of these patients. The support of parents, other medical specialists, therapists, orthotists and teachers is essential for good results. The care of these children should be delivered in a co-ordinated way, usually through a paediatrician or general practitioner.

Poliomyelitis

This is usually due to infection by one of three types of poliomyelitis virus, although other members of the enterovirus group can cause clinically and pathologically indistinguishable disease. Effective vaccination has been present for almost 40 years but the disease has not been eliminated from certain parts of the world. The virus enters the oropharyngeal route, passing via the alimentary lymph nodes to enter the circulation with an incubation period of 6–20 days. One or 2 per cent of patients develop neurological disease as the virus affects the anterior horn cells, particularly in the cervical and lumbar enlargements (as well as parts of the brain including the medulla). Weakness in a muscle is in proportion to the number of motor units destroyed. Up to 60 per cent of units have to be damaged before weakness is clinically detectable. Muscles innervated by the cervical and lumbar enlargements are most commonly affected and paralysis is twice as common in the lower than in the upper limb. Orthopaedic surgery is not indicated in the acute or convalescent stages although careful physiotherapy in the convalescent stage is helpful to work individual muscles to maximum capacity without letting normally working muscles become hypertrophied. Paretic muscles must not be over-exercised and contractures in paralysed muscles must be stretched out before exercising them.

In the chronic stage which can be as much as 2 years after onset of the disease, orthopaedic surgery may be indicated. Joint deformities will largely be dictated by the muscle groups affected, although certain patterns of deformity, such as flexion contracture of the knee and hip and calcaneus of the hindfoot, are common. Patients with a weak quadriceps and a flexion contracture may develop 'knee–hand gait' in which the hand supports the knee which cannot be locked into extension. In severe cases patients have to crawl and the pattern adopted is a guide to the muscle groups affected. When all muscles acting on a joint are paralysed it will become flail and unstable. It is surprising that such joints rarely show degenerative changes. When the paraspinal muscles are affected a scoliosis may develop. A disused lower limb grows shorter than normal and leg-length discrepancy is common.

If surgery is to be undertaken in poliomyelitis, it should be preceded by a full assessment, including muscle charting. If orthoses are being considered, it is important to be certain these will be appropriate in the patient's home environment. The surgical options in polio include:

- tendon transfer to augment or replace weak muscles;
- release of contractures by soft-tissue release and/or corrective osteotomy. The knee–hand gait can often be abolished by extension osteotomy of the distal femur which allows the knee to lock in extension. However, in some cases a contracture may help the patient and the surgeon must be circumspect about releasing it (Fig. 28.24);
- stabilisation of flail joints by arthrodesis;
- spinal fusion and instrumentation for scoliosis;
- leg equalisation surgery.

Cerebral palsy

This is classically a nonprogressive injury to the developing brain that usually occurs in the neonatal period. There are several potential causes such as anoxia, intracerebral haemorrhage and infection. There is a strong association with prematurity. In such cases it is debatable whether the neurological damage is due to a naturally impaired brain or caused during delivery. Severe neurological impairment may also be part of syndromic or genetic conditions. Finally there may not be any obvious cause for a child's neurological condition. On rare occasions such a child presenting as 'cerebral palsy' may respond to dopamine treatment.

Cerebral palsy is often not apparent at birth and may only be suspected as an infant fails to reach milestones or shows

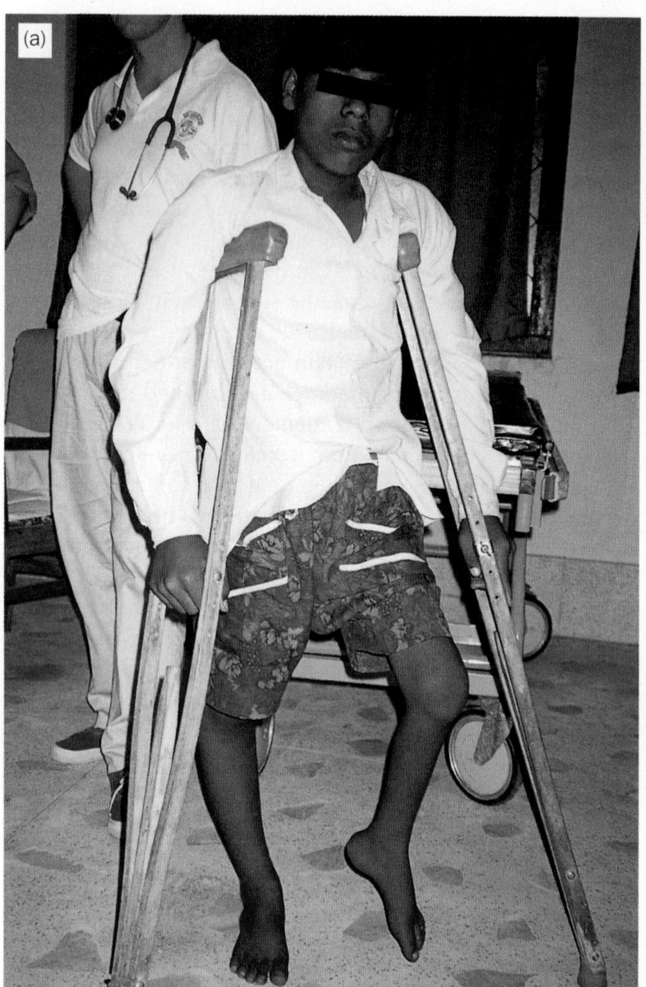

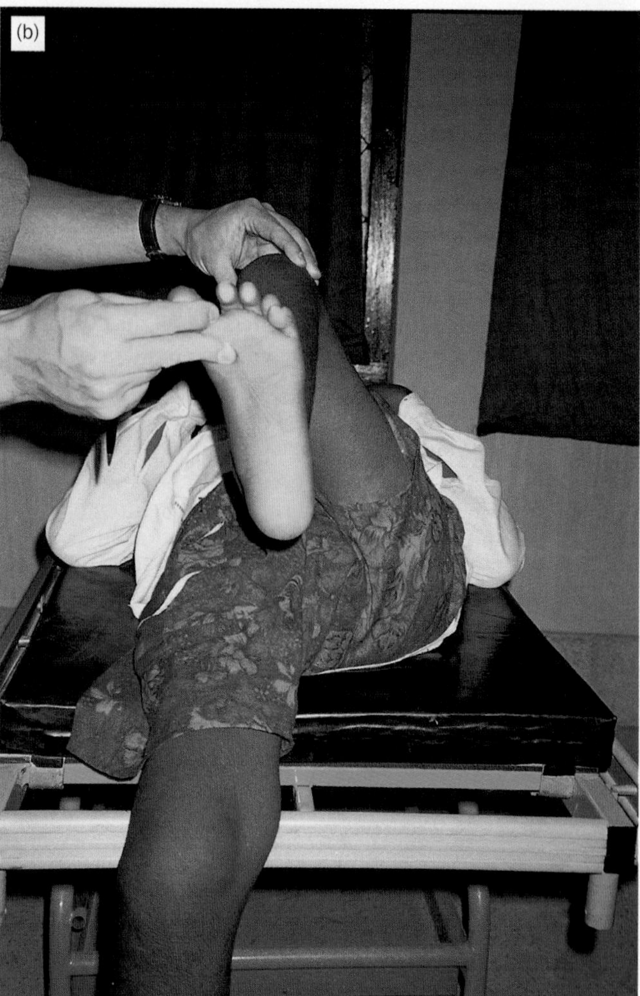

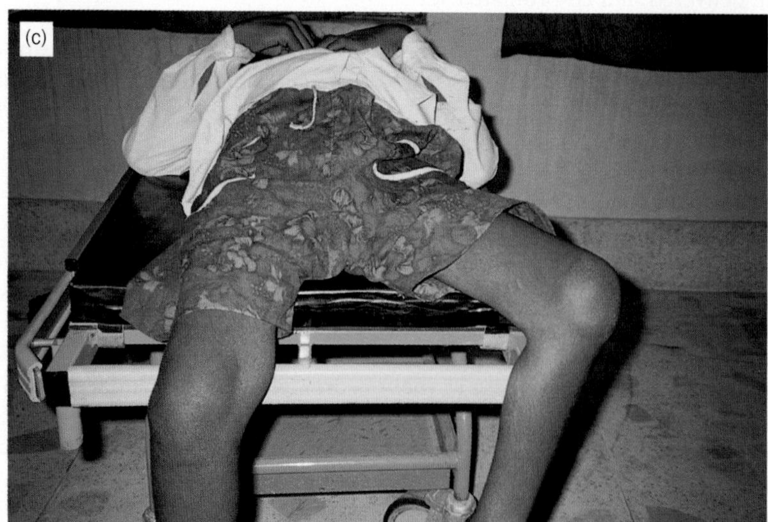

Fig. 28.24 Poliomyelitis with contracture of tensor fascia lata (TFL). (a) With the hip extended the thigh abducts. (b) It can only adduct when the hip and knee are flexed, thereby relaxing TFL. (c) Surgery not indicated because the TFL and knee contractures keep his flail foot clear of ground when using crutches.

evidence of altered muscle tone. For all of these reasons it is important to try and accurately assess the cause and scale of neurological impairment, be it cerebral palsy or otherwise. The skills and armamentarium of the paediatric neurologist are usually required for this.

In cerebral palsy there are various patterns of disability depending on the type and distribution of the motor disturbance (Table 28.5). It is also helpful to grade the condition according to function which should include intellectual ability and whether there is epilepsy (Table 28.6).

The commonest type of disturbance is spasticity which tends to affect flexors rather than extensors. Orthopaedic surgery can only have limited goals in cerebral palsy as it deals with peripheral effects rather than the central problem. Moreover, the orthopaedic surgeon is usually part of a large team involved in the care of the child.

The aim of surgery should be to improve function and facilitate the care of these patients by correcting or preventing deformity. Regular physiotherapy to stretch contractures (Fig. 28.25a and b) and supervise the use of orthoses is essential (Fig. 28.26). Realistic goals must be set. It has to be explained that results can be unpredictable and disappointing especially in dystonic cases. The immediate postoperative care may be hampered by difficulties with nursing and skin problems due to pressure from casts. Rehabilitation is usually prolonged.

The goals and scope of treatment are usually determined by the anatomical distribution and functional ability as follows.

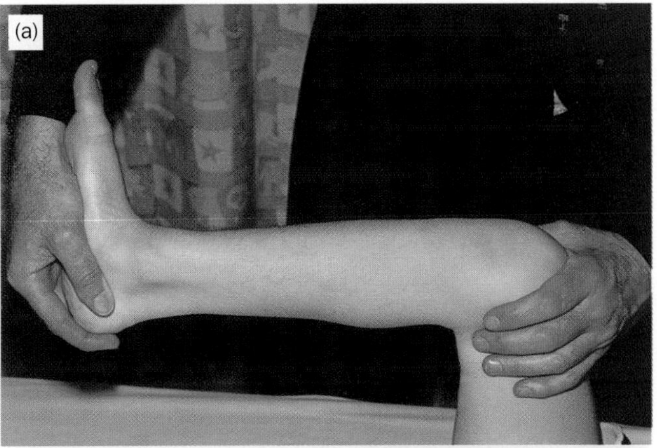

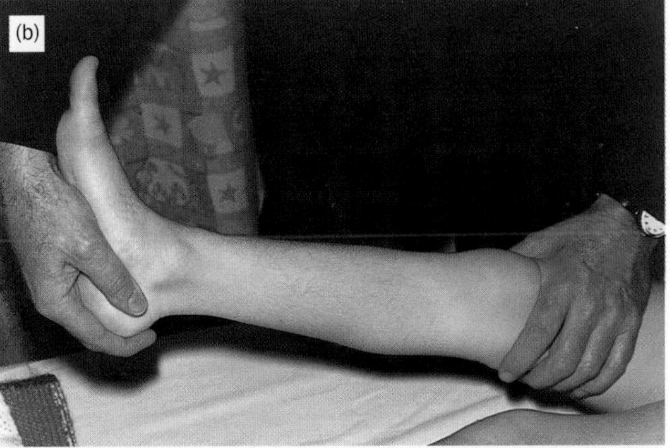

Fig. 28.25 (a) and (b) Cerebral palsy. Stretching a tight calf in knee flexion and extension.

Hemiplegia

The children walk independently and the hip is not at risk. The common problems in the lower limb are equinus or internal rotation. Equinus usually requires physiotherapy, an ankle/foot orthosis (AFO) and frequently elongation of the tendo achilles (ETA). Severe internal rotation can be due to femoral torsion and an external rotation osteotomy may be justified.

The upper limb in hemiplegia is often badly affected. Surgical options to improve function significantly are sadly few but some help can also be given to improve the cosmetic appearance of the hand.

Table 28.5 Classification of cerebral palsy

Neurological type	*Anatomical pattern*
Spastic	Monoplegic (rare)
Dystonic (athetoid)	Hemiplegia
Atonic	Diplegia
Mixed	Quadriplegia (total body involvement)

Table 28.6 Functional grading of cerebral palsy

Walking ability (with or without aids)
Community walker – able to walk in or outside the house
Household walker – walks inside the house only
Therapeutic walker – only able to walk with assistance from another person
Nonwalker
Sitting ability
Independent sitter
Propped sitter
Nonsitter
Intellectual ability, feeding, continence and whether epilepsy

Diplegia

These children can usually walk but in an awkward and difficult fashion (Fig. 28.27). The hips are unlikely to be at risk of displacement. The aim of treatment is to achieve a more energy-efficient gait.

The common deformities are equino valgus, knee flexion and adduction, internal rotation and flexion at the hip. There

Achilles, Greek hero, son of Peleus and Thetis. As a child his mother dipped him in the River Styx, so he should be invulnerable in battle. The heel by which his mother held him did not get wet and so remained unprotected. Achilles died from a wound to the heel, received at the siege of Troy.

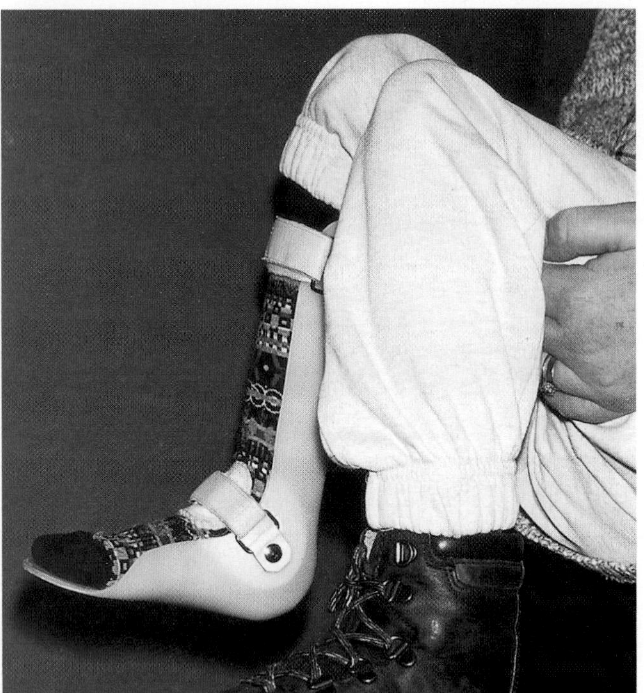

Fig. 28.26 Application of an ankle/foot orthosis to maintain position after stretching (same case as Fig. 28.25).

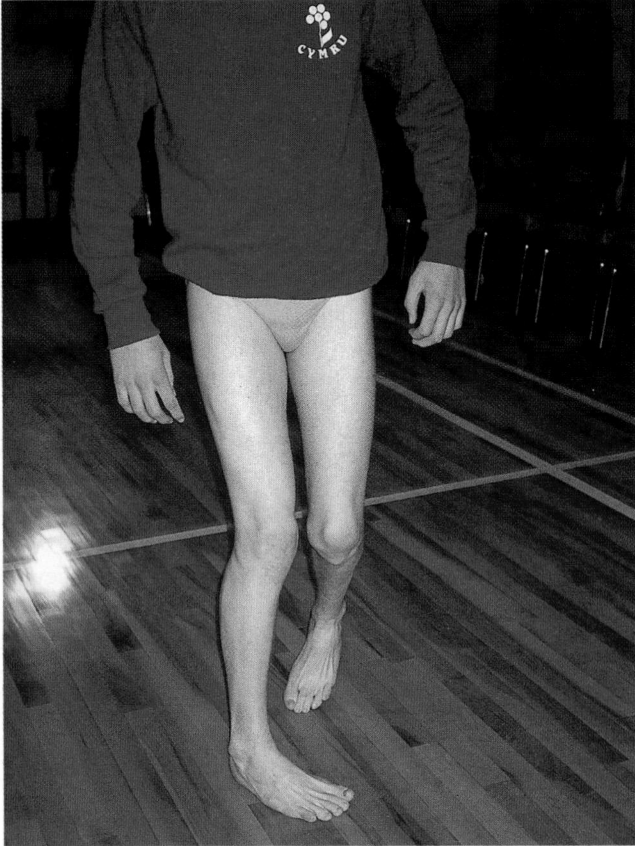

Fig. 28.27 Cerebral palsy. Diplegia. Crouched gait with internal rotation.

may also be rotational deformities of the femur and tibia. Surgery must be carefully planned and gait analysis can be helpful. Whereas operations can be undertaken sequentially, combined multilevel surgery is sometimes preferable. A typical combination would be femoral rotation osteotomies followed by release of adductors, hamstrings and tendo achilles. The rehabilitation after such surgery is prolonged and demanding. It is a year before the final benefits are likely to be felt.

Total body involvement

The children are usually very impaired mentally as well as physically. However, in some, whereas the physical disability may be severe the child can be intellectually bright. There are usually difficulties with incontinence, feeding, nutrition and epilepsy.

The orthopaedic goals in such cases can be summarised as follows.

- **Spine**. Scoliosis is likely and should be anticipated. Early curves can be treated by postural exercises, seating supports and braces. More severe curves require surgical stabilisation to prevent them progressing to unmanageable deformities.
- **Hips**. These are at risk of dislocation because of adductor and psoas spasm. The joints should be monitored clinically and radiologically. Preventive measures include exercises, abduction splints and seating adaptation. If the hip is displacing early surgical options include adductor release of femoral osteotomy (Figs 28.28 and 28.29). In late dislocations which are painful and pose severe nursing or seating problems, the combination of open reduction, femoral osteotomy and acetabular augmentation may be necessary.

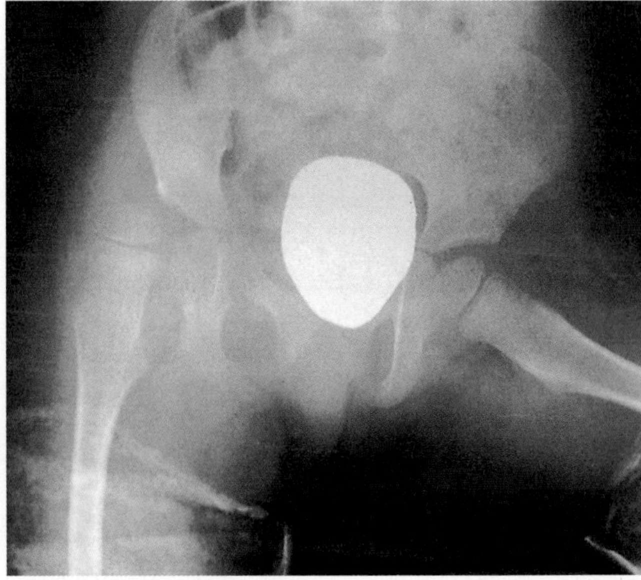

Fig. 28.28 Cerebral palsy. Totally involved child with spastic quadriplegia. Hip is severely subluxated in spite of previous soft tissue release.

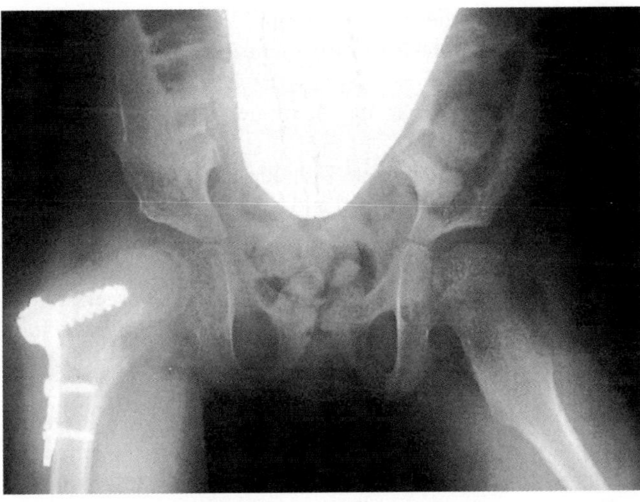

Fig. 28.29 Cerebral palsy. Severely subluxated hip relocated successfully by a varus osteotomy.

- **Seating.** Proper seating is important and is a major factor in maintaining posture and minimising deformity (Fig. 28.30). If hips, knees or ankles pose problems in achieving good seating and transfers usually because of flexion deformities, then soft-tissue releases will have to be considered.
- **Communication skills.** The child should be in the school best suited to his or her particular needs and potential. Computers and electronics can help parents and teachers in this regard.

Spina bifida

Unfortunately, most children with spina bifida have profound lower limb weakness and sensory loss (Fig. 28.31). They regularly need multidisciplinary help from paediatricians, orthopaedic surgeons, neurosurgeons, therapists and orthotists.

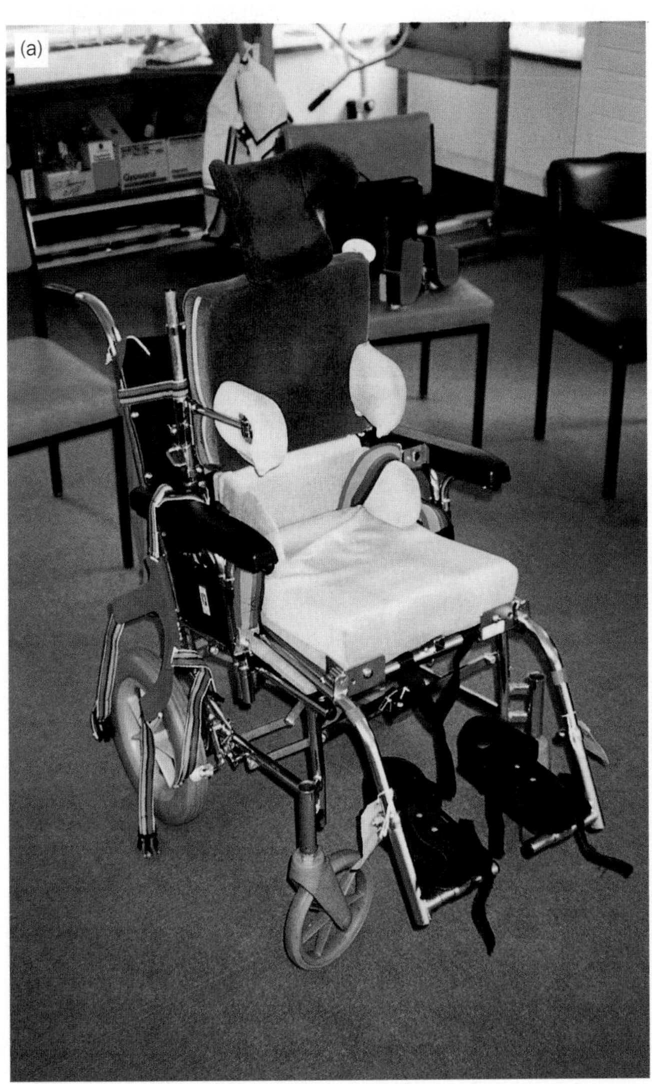

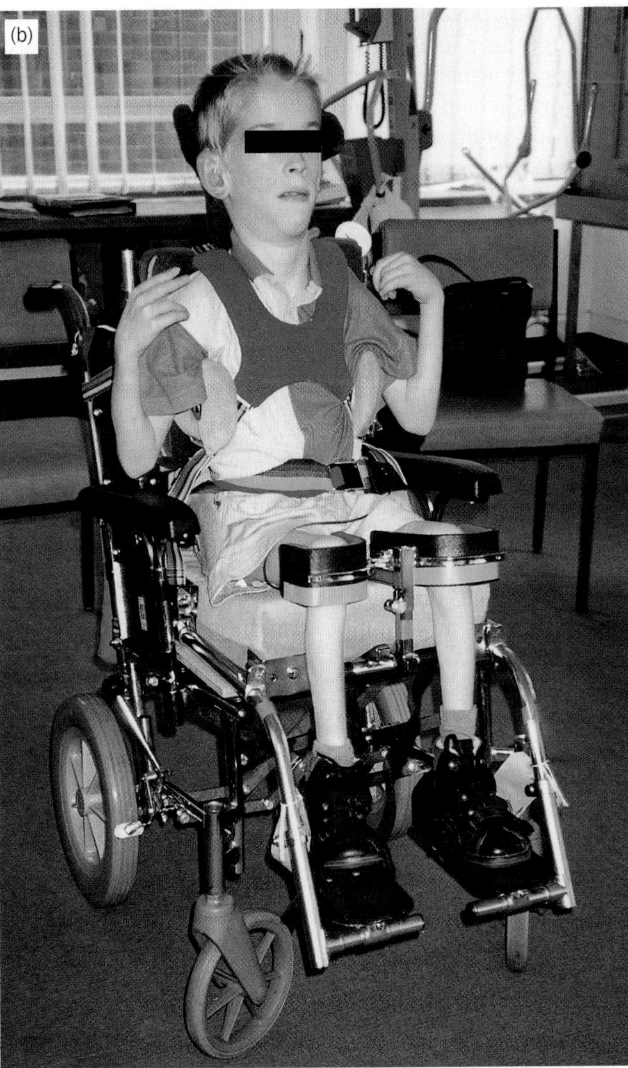

Fig. 28.30 (a) and (b) Cerebral palsy with total body involvement. The importance of good seating to support the head and trunk and prevent deformities at hips and ankles.

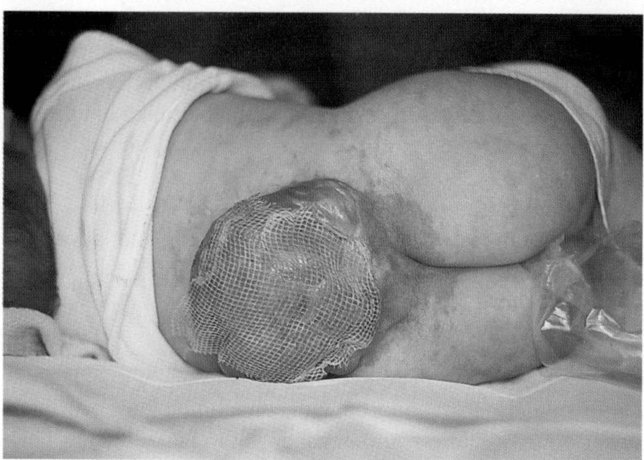

Fig. 28.31 Severe case of spina bifida with paralysis and deformities in the lower limbs.

However, not all spina bifida produces severe disability (Fig. 28.32). Occult forms may cause subtle changes in neurology as a child grows. If a lower limb deformity, weakness or urinary symptoms develop it is advisable to seek neurosurgical help as, with growth, there may be tethering of nerve roots or other pathology such as a syrinx which can be amenable to surgery.

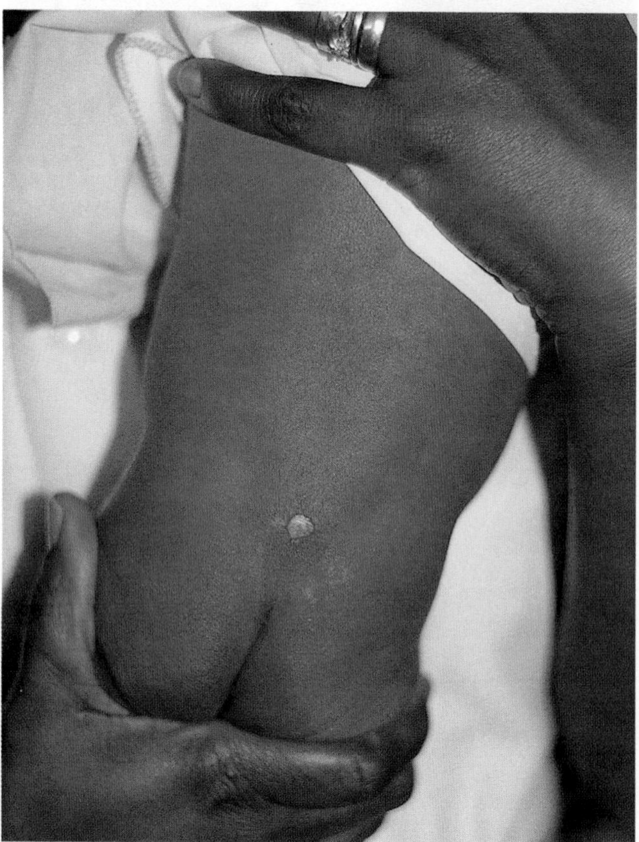

Fig. 28.32 Mild spina bifida. The child was ambulant with no disability or significant deformity.

In severe cases the extent of disability depends on the level of the lesion. In the majority there is some upper motor neuron involvement as well as the classical lower motor neuron lesion. Spasticity may therefore complicate the motor and sensory loss.

The lack of protective sensation means that minor cuts and abrasions may pass unnoticed and lead to infection. Once this involves bone it is extremely difficult to eradicate. Patients and carers must therefore adopt a daily routine of foot inspection and must always try to protect skin. Surgery to the foot in spina bifida is largely to achieve a plantigrade foot which can be fitted with an orthosis and moulded footwear to avoid areas of pressure.

Hip dislocation is common in spina bifida. Most surgeons do not operate for dislocation because of the relatively poor results and prefer to advise it to be left mobile and painless.

Flexion contractures at hip or knee can be treated by soft-tissue release and/or osteotomy. External rotation of the tibia may cause the medial side of the foot to drag along the ground. This can be helped by internal rotation osteotomy of the tibia. Spina deformity is common in higher level lesions and usually takes the form of a kyphosis. This can be controlled with a brace but spinal fusion and instrumentation may be necessary (see Chapter 20).

Muscular dystrophy

The details of the many types of muscular dystrophy which vary in severity and age at presentation are beyond the scope of this book. However, a short discussion of a severe and classical type, namely Duchenne dystrophy, exemplifies the diagnostic and therapeutic approaches, which may be applicable throughout the spectrum of the muscle dystrophies.

Duchenne dystrophy is inherited as a sex-linked condition and only boys are affected. They are not usually diagnosed until after walking, which is delayed. They may present as toe walkers or show difficulties with mobility. For example, when getting up from the floor they use their hands on their thighs to push themselves up into the erect position. They often have thick calves (pseudohypertrophy) and the Achilles tendons are tight. The clinical features plus a raised creatine phosphokinase (CPK) confirm the diagnosis.

The condition is sadly progressive. The children usually come off their feet in late childhood or early teens and die in late adolescence or early adult life. At present there is no cure but gene therapy holds some hope for the future.

Treatment is multidisciplinary and aims to keep the children as mobile as possible and prevent deformity. Immobilisation after any surgery must be for as short a time as possible. Walking can be prolonged by percutaneous lengthening of the Achilles tendons and orthoses.

The spine is particularly liable to deformity. This may be lessened by bracing and seating. However, it regularly progresses beyond these measures whereupon surgical stabilisa-

---

Guillaume B.A. Duchenne, 1806–75. French neurologist.

tion is worthwhile, otherwise the deformity may become very severe and the management difficult and unpleasant for the child during his or her final years. The timing of spinal surgery is important. It should be done before the vital capacity has deteriorated to a dangerous level.

Torticollis (wryneck)

This is frequently related to neurological or muscular conditions. The causes of the abnormal neck posture can be summarised as:

- cervical – congenital and acquired conditions of the cervical spine, painful or otherwise;
- pharyngeal – usually infection, e.g. tonsillitis;
- ocular – squints or visual field defects;
- intracranial – posterior fossa tumours;
- muscular – contracture of the sternomastoid;
- habitual – no obvious organic cause.

The classical type is due to contracture of either or both anatomical heads of the sternomastoid muscle (Fig. 28.33). The cause of contracture is usually unknown. It can follow a sternomastoid tumour, which is probably a traumatic lesion sustained during delivery and usually resolves without long-term effects (Fig. 28.34).

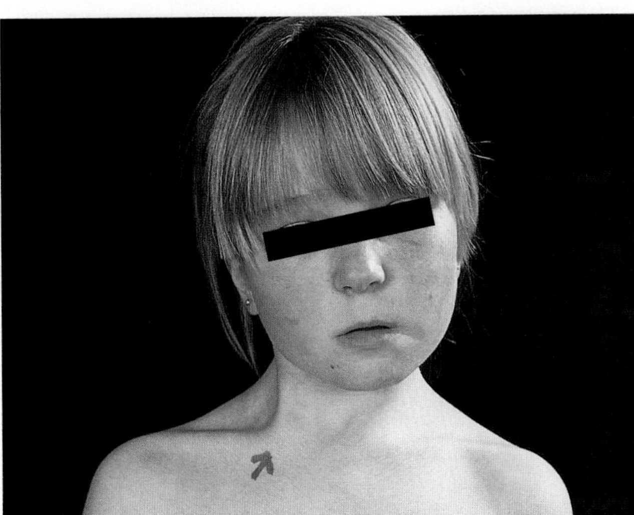

Fig. 28.33 Muscular torticollis. The left sternomastoid is tight, causing the child to look upwards to the opposite side.

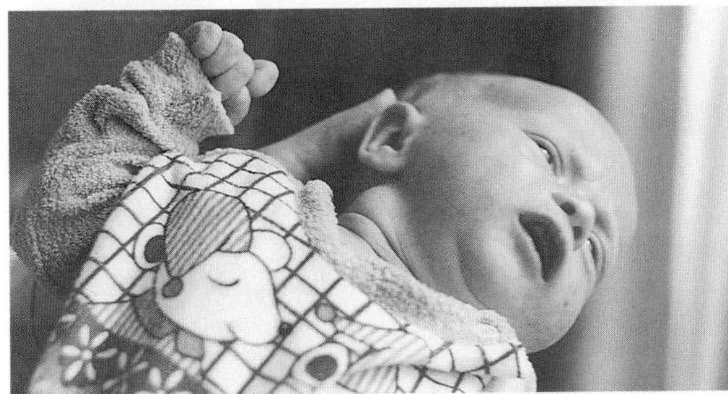

Fig. 28.34 Sternomastoid tumour following precipitate breech delivery. In this case the swelling resolved with no long-term effects.

Treatment is usually by surgical release of the contracture followed by physiotherapy and exercises to re-educate the child back to normal posture and movement.

Spinal deformity

Scoliosis

This is a lateral curvature of the spine but is usually accompanied by a rotational deformity as the spinal column starts to buckle and shorten. In the thoracic region the rotation throws the ribs into prominence producing the cosmetically deforming rib hump (Fig. 28.35a and b) whereas in the lumbar region the same degree of curvature may not be so noticeable. A curve is described as *structural* or *fixed* when there is loss of mobility in the involved segment. This usually occurs because of alterations in the shape of the vertebrae and adaptive changes in soft tissues. A curve is *mobile* when normal flexibility is preserved; such curves are often described as *postural* although strictly speaking the terms are not interchangeable. A postural curve is secondary to the position of the body, one of the commonest causes being leg-length inequality. Curves are also described on the

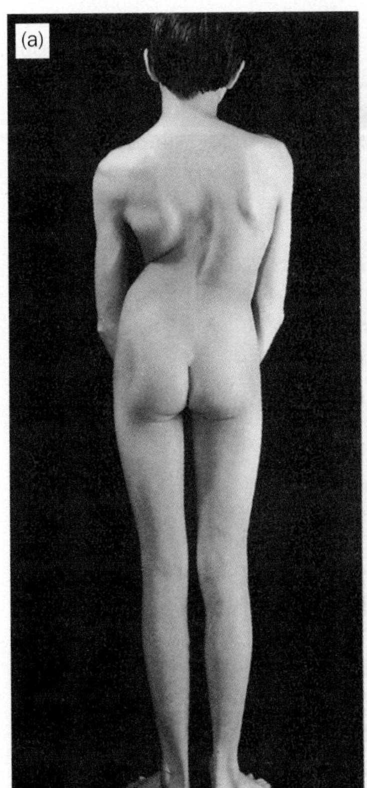

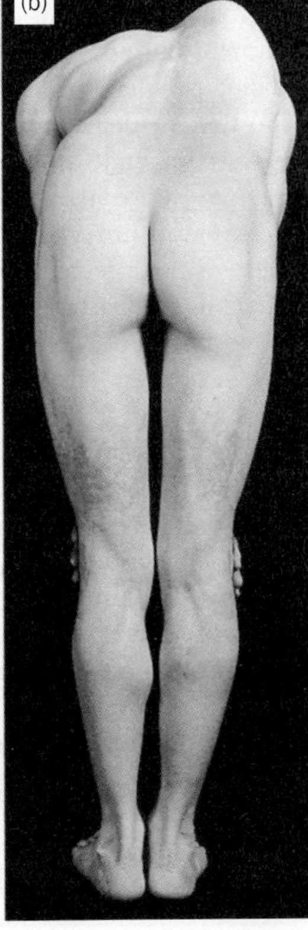

Fig. 28.35 Scoliosis: (a) appearance of the back; (b) 'rib hump' revealed by flexion.

Table 28.7 Causes of scoliosis

	Examples
Congenital	Hemivertebra
Neuromuscular	Cerebral palsy, polio
Thoracogenic	Lung and rib resection
Other conditions	Spinal tumours
	Spinal infection
	Spinal trauma
	Disc prolapse
	Skeletal dysplasias
	Marfan's syndrome
	Neurofibromatosis
	Osteogenesis imperfecta
Idiopathic	

basis of their anatomical site and whether they are *primary* (major) or *secondary* (compensatory) to the primary curve in an attempt to maintain spinal balance.

The causes of scoliosis are summarised in Table 28.7.

Idiopathic scoliosis

Idiopathic scoliosis is the commonest type and is usually considered in three sub groups.

Infantile idiopathic scoliosis may be related to sleeping position. It is usually noted between birth and the age of 1 year. It is often a component of the 'moulded baby syndrome' (plagiocephaly, tight hip adductors, scoliosis, foot deformities). The curves are usually convex to the left and are more common in males. The great majority resolve without treatment but approximately 10 per cent progress and pose difficult problems. Serial examination and radiographs are important to detect progressive cases. Measurement of the rib–vertebra angle difference (Mehta) is helpful in predicting which cases are likely to progress. Treatment is initially by bracing but if unsuccessful there is an indication for anterior release of the affected spinal segments.

Juvenile idiopathic scoliosis. This occurs between the ages of 3 years and puberty. The distinction between juvenile and early adolescent curves is ill defined. However, juvenile curves frequently progress and early bracing is advisable.

Adolescent idiopathic scoliosis is the commonest form and occurs at puberty. It is slightly more common in girls and usually convex to the right. A number of different patterns of curve has been described depending on site and distinguishing between the major and compensatory curves. Appreciation of the patterns is important in assessing the extent and level of spinal fusion. In general, treatment is required for all curves that are progressing. The following are important factors in assessing progression.

- Sex. Progression is more common in girls.
- Age. Progression is more likely when there is potential for skeletal growth. Curves presenting before menarche have more potential for progression. Ossification of the iliac apophysis (Risser's sign) is helpful is assessing skeletal maturity.
- Curve pattern. Double curves are more likely to progress than single thoracic curves which in turn are more likely to progress than lumbar curves.
- Curve magnitude. Progression is more likely with curves over 30°.
- Other factors. Patients with slender spines are more likely to progress.

Clinical features. The above features related to curve progression must be noted. In addition, a history of pain or neurological symptoms makes it important to exclude other causes of scoliosis such as a spinal tumour. On examination, the site, flexibility and cosmetic effects of the curve are noted, as well as spinal balance, i.e. is the head centred over the natal cleft? A neurological examination should be carried out, skin blemishes, e.g. café au lait patches, should be sought and any leg-length discrepancy measured. The curve can only be assessed accurately by radiology (Fig. 28.36).

Treatment. Idiopathic scoliosis can only be treated by bracing and surgery. In general, curves which measure less than 30° should be managed nonoperatively with regular clinical and

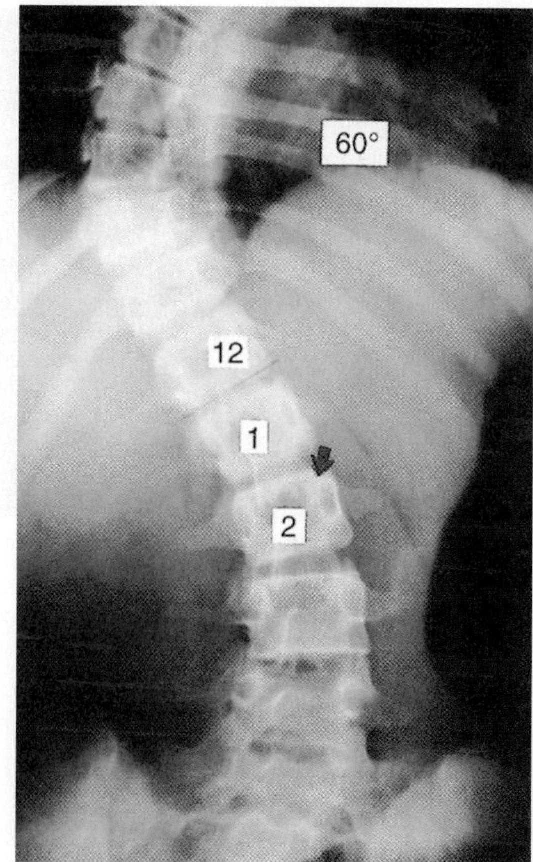

Fig. 28.36 Radiograph of the spine in a case of scoliosis. This curvature measured 60°.

Min Mehta. Orthopaedic Surgeon, Royal National Orthopaedic Hospital, London, England.

Joseph C. Risser. Former Professor of Orthopaedic Surgery, Loma Linda University, Los Angeles, California, USA.

radiological assessment. Earlier intervention should be undertaken in those curves with a worse potential. Once there is clear evidence of progression bracing is used for curves between 30° and 45°. There are two main types of brace. The *Milwaukee* incorporates anterior and posterior struts that support a neck ring and suboccipital pads. The *Boston* brace is an underarm device constructed from a pelvic module fitted with individualised pads to correct lumbar and thoracolumbar curves. Since it can be worn under clothes it is more acceptable than the Milwaukee but is not suitable for high curves.

Surgery is generally indicated when:

- bracing is likely to be ineffective because
  - the curve is too large, i.e. >45°,
  - the site makes it difficult to brace, e.g. high thoracic or true double thoracic curve,
  - the curve is fixed;
- the curve is deteriorating in a young child;
- there is loss of spinal balance;
- the cosmetic appearance needs correction.

The surgical procedures to correct, stabilise and fuse the spine include anterior release, and anterior and posterior instrumentation techniques (Fig. 28.37). Spinal cord monitoring is usually employed during such surgery that aims to produce a balanced, corrected, stable spine with a minimum of fused segments.

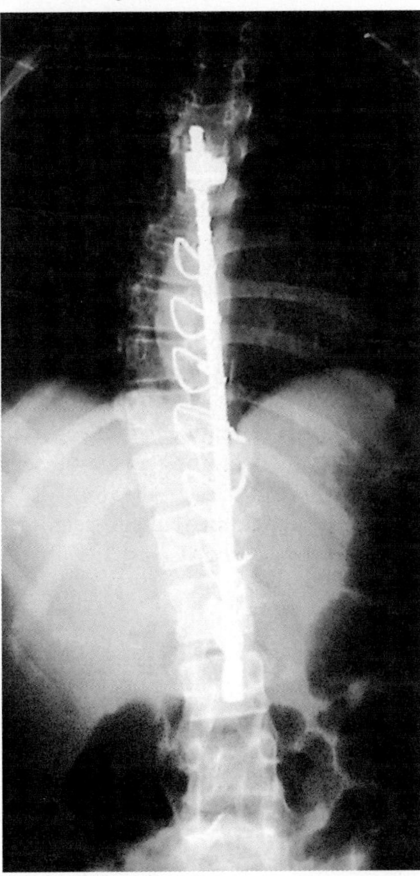

Fig. 28.37 The scoliosis shown in Fig. 28.36 has been corrected by posterior instrumentation (Harrington rod and sublaminar wires).

Congenital scoliosis

This is usually due to a failure of formation, e.g. hemivertebra (Fig. 28.38) or failure of segmentation, e.g. a bar. Mixed patterns can occur and the anomalies may be single or multiple. Associated abnormalities are diastomatomyelia, and cardiac and renal malformations. A unilateral unsegmented bar with a contralateral hemivertebra at the same level along with thoracolumbar anomalies are associated with particularly severe curves. In general, early fusion *in situ* should be undertaken for curves that are progressing or likely to progress. On occasions, other procedures may be appropriate such as hemivertebra excision or growth arrest operations.

Neuromuscular scoliosis

Many neuromuscular conditions such as cerebral palsy, spina bifida, polio and muscular dystrophy can cause a scoliosis. Characteristically a long, C-shaped thoracolumbar curve is found. Left untreated, severe deformities can occur with reduction of respiratory function and great difficulties in nursing. Early bracing is valuable, surgical stabilisation is often necessary and strong internal fixation is necessary to allow early mobilisation.

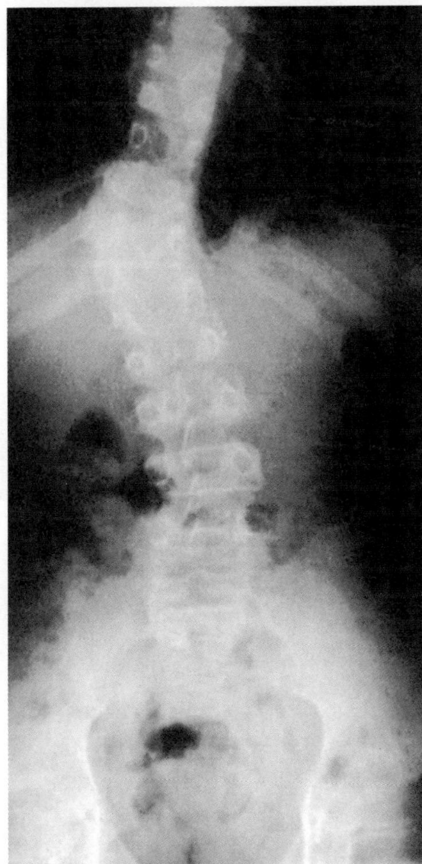

Fig. 28.38 Congenital scoliosis due to hemivertebra at T11.

Paul Harrington, 1911–80. Professor of Orthopaedic Surgery, Baylor College Medicine, Houston, Texas, USA.

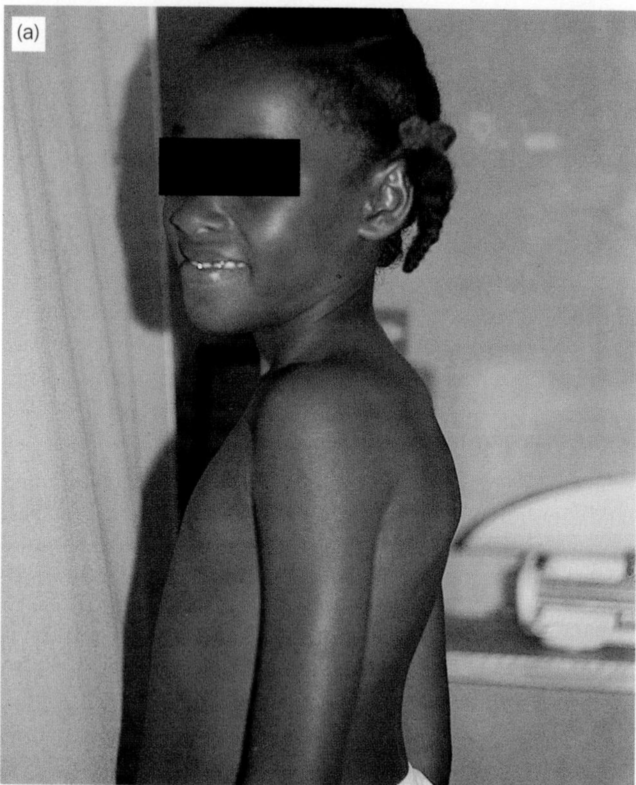

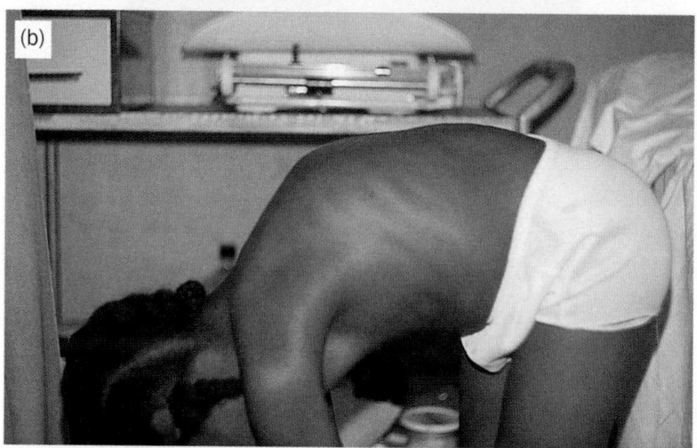

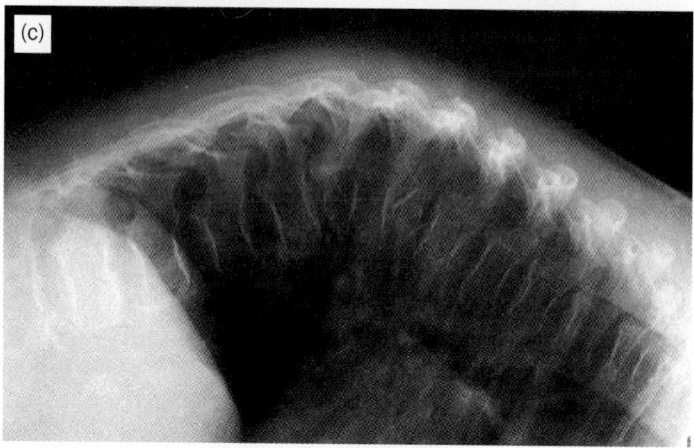

Fig. 28.39 (a), (b) and (c) Child with a thoracic kyphosis, accentuated on forward bending. The cause was sickle cell disease.

Tumours

Tumours involving the vertebrae, e.g. osteoid osteoma or the neural elements, may present as a scoliosis. Any child presenting with significant back pain should be investigated and a bone scan is a useful screening test.

Other conditions

Other conditions associated with scoliosis include infections, disc prolapse, spinal injury and skeletal dysplasias such as neurofibromatosis, Marfan's syndrome and osteogenesis imperfecta.

Kyphosis

A kyphosis is normally present in the thoracic spine but more than 45° is considered to be excessive. The deformity may be idiopathic or occur as a result of:

- congenital abnormalities such as anterior bony bar;
- developmental delay, e.g. cerebral palsy;
- vertebral collapse, e.g. infection, osteoporosis, sickle cell disease (Fig. 28.39a–c).

There is a spectrum of idiopathic scoliosis. In *Scheuermann's disease*, the kyphosis is associated with radiological changes such as irregular vertebral end plates, apparent narrowing of the disc space and wedging of one or more vertebrae. These changes make the kyphosis more rigid than the less severe *postural round back* in which radiographs are normal. Apart from the cosmetic deformity, Scheuermann's disease may be associated with back pain, especially after skeletal maturity and, in severe cases, brace treatment and occasionally fusion may be justified.

Further reading

Benson, M.K.D., Fixsen, J.A. and Macnicol, M.F. (eds) (1994) *Children's Orthopaedics and Fractures*, Churchill Livingstone, Edinburgh.

Herring, J.A. (1994) The treatment of Legg–Calve–Perthes disease. A critical review of the literature. *Journal of Bone and Joint Surgery*, **76a**, 448–58.

Various authors (1996) Slipped upper femoral epiphysis. *Journal of Paediatric Orthopaedics*, **2**, **3**, Part B. Fourteen articles on SUFE.

Bernard-Jean A. Marfan, 1852–1942. Physician, Hopital des Enfants Malades, Paris. Described this syndrome in 1896.

Holger W. Scheuermann, 1877–1960. Radiologist, Municipal Hospital, Copenhagen, Denmark. Described juvenile kyphosis in 1920.

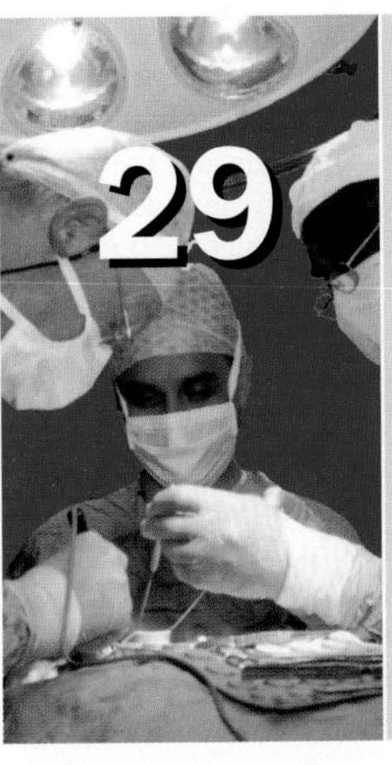

Disorders of muscle, tendons, ligaments; sports medicine

Biomechanics

> Biomechanics is a subject of immense complexity and it is specially difficult for surgeons because graduate engineers often fail to appreciate the abysmal ignorance of mathematics which hampers surgeons in this field. *Sir John Charnley*

Despite this sobering thought from Sir John Charnley, all surgeons who deal with injuries of the musculoskeletal system require a basic understanding of biomechanics. It is the science of the action of forces, internal or external, on the living body and dictates how accidents and overloading produce tissue damage. Effective treatment regimes, surgical or nonsurgical, to restore the mechanical properties of injured structures must be based on knowledge of the fundamentals of biomechanics.

Dynamics

Dynamics is the study of the motion of bodies and forces that produce the motion. There are three subtypes:

- *Kinematics* is the study of motion in terms of displacement, velocity and acceleration without reference to the cause of the motion.
- *Kinetics* relates the action of forces on bodies to their resulting action.
- *Kinesiology* studies human movement and motion.

Sir John Charnley, 1911–82. Professor of Orthopaedic Surgery, University of Manchester, England.

Bailey & Love's Short Practice of Surgery, 23rd edition. Edited by R.C.G. Russell, N.S. Williams and C.J.K. Bulstrode. Published in 2000 by Arnold Publishers.

The guiding principles by which forces act on bodies are encapsulated in Newton's three laws. Statics is the study of the action of forces on bodies at rest and is governed by Newton's first law; if a zero net external force acts on a body, the body will remain at rest or move uniformly. Thus, the sum of the external forces applied to a body at rest equals zero. Newton's second law relates to acceleration. The acceleration (a) of an object of mass (m) is directly proportional to the force applied to the object ($F = ma$). Newton's third law states that for every action there is an equal and opposite reaction. This allows us to analyse the action of forces on the whole body, or limbs, and resolve them.

Biomaterials

The effect of externally applied loads on a particular structure, such as a ligament or tendon, and the resulting internal effects and deformations induced in these structures is the study of biomaterials. The basic terminology is given in Table 29.1.

All materials will eventually fail if sufficient load is placed upon them. If you clamp the medial collateral ligament including its bony attachments and pull it apart (a tensile test) then you would be testing a *structure* whose properties are defined by a load–deformation curve (Fig. 29.1a). If the experiment were modified to include only the ligament then you would be testing it as a *material* resulting in a stress–strain curve (Fig. 29.1b).

Sir Issac Newton, 1642–1727. British scientist and mathematician.

Table 29.1 Common terminology used in the study of biomaterials

Term	*Description*	*Units*
Load	Forces acting on a body (may be compression, tension, bending, shear or torsion)	Newtons
Deformation	Temporary (elastic) or permanent (plastic) change in a dimension of a body under external loading	m
Stress	Load in a specimen divided by its cross-sectional area	N/m^2 (Pascal)
Strain	Proportional measure of the deformation of a body as a result of loading	No units
Stiffness	Ability of a structure to resist deformation (load–deformation)	N/m^2
Young's module of elasticity	Ability of a material to resist deformation (stress–strain)	N/m^2

In Fig. 29.1b the first part of the curve (toe-in) occurs as the natural wavy pattern (crimp) of the fibres is eliminated. As the stress increases the fibres lengthen proportionally, the slope of this line representing Young's modulus (*E*). As the strain increases beyond physiological loads increasing numbers of fibres are injured until the highest stress is recorded immediately prior to failure of the ligament.

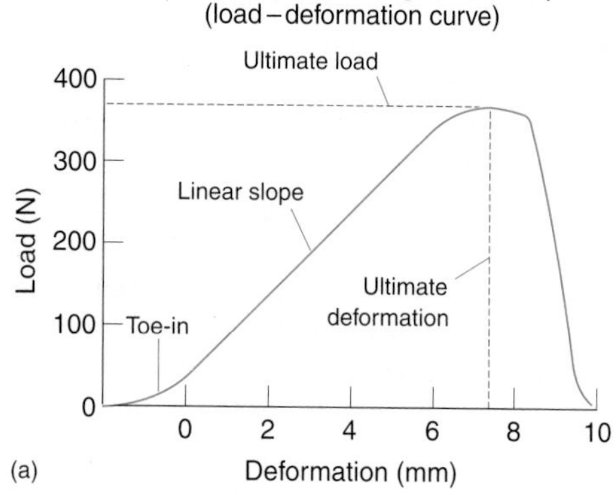

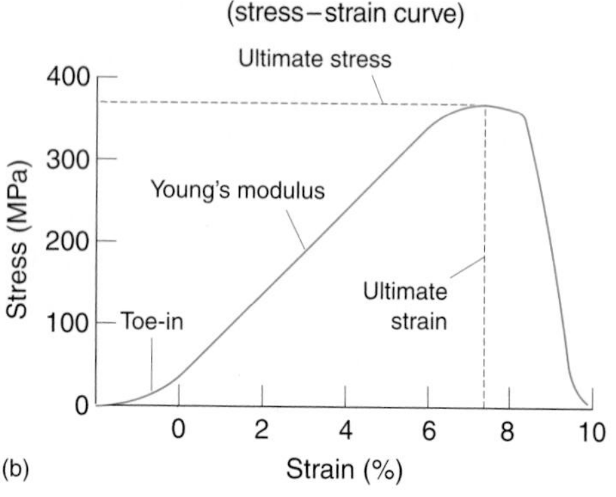

Fig. 29.1 Results of tensile tests on a ligament.

Thomas Young, 1773–1829. British physicist.

It is therefore apparent that if a single load in excess of the ultimate failure load of a structure is applied then it will fail. An example of this occurs when a football player is tackled from the side. The knee is forced into valgus and the medial collateral ligament is loaded in tension. If the load exceeds the ultimate failure load it will rupture completely. If the load is below this then a partial rupture may occur.

If the ligament is partially ruptured and the player manages to continue playing, a second injury of similar magnitude results in complete rupture of the ligament. This brings us to the concept of fatigue failure. Figure 29.2 depicts the relationship between load and the number of stress cycles required to produce failure in a structure. As the applied load diminishes the number of cycles tolerated by the structure increases. Once the load reaches physiological levels then, theoretically, the structure will remain intact however many cycles are applied – the fatigue endurance limit.

The principles outlined in the above example are applicable to all constituents of the musculoskeletal system: bone, tendon, ligament and muscle. Whilst the units will vary between tissue types the patterns will also vary within one tissue depending on the direction of the applied load, and this property is called *anisotropy*. For example, bone has a very high failure load in compression but a relatively low failure load in tension. So far, the principles described could equally well be applied to an inert structure. The challenge of biomechanics is apparent when one considers the multitude of other factors that affect the structural properties of living tissues. Age has a profound influence on both mode of and loads to failure. In growing skeletons the junction between ligaments/tendons and bone is weaker than the ligament itself, and failure typically occurs here. In mature skeletons the failure usually occurs in the midsubstance of the ligament. The failure load of all structures peaks in early adult life and declines thereafter. Ligaments, tendons and muscles are all more compliant (less stiff) at higher temperatures and circulating hormones, particularly sex hormones, can affect the structural properties of soft tissues from one day to the next.

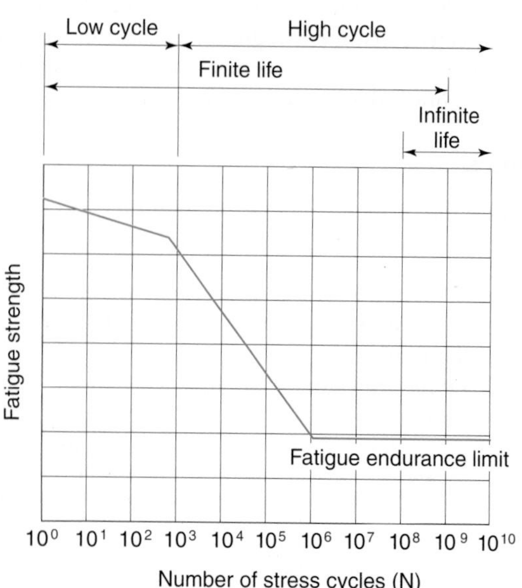

Fig. 29.2 Results of fatigue failure testing.

Diagnosis of sports injuries

The first question that a surgeon must ask himself or herself is whether the extent of the injury is in keeping with the description of the mechanism of injury. In other words, was this normal tissue that was injured because of an abnormal load applied to it, either a single high load or many cycles of low load? In this situation successful resolution of the injury and avoidance of the abnormal load should prevent recurrence. However, if a relatively normal load resulted in injury then the tissue was probably abnormal and the underlying abnormality is the main concern.

All of these points serve to emphasise the importance of good history taking and careful clinical examination. They still form the cornerstone of diagnosis in all branches of medicine but especially with injuries to the soft tissues.

Arthroscopy versus imaging

The principle of using the arthroscope and specialised imaging techniques to diagnose pathology is to be decried. The arthroscope should be used to confirm *and* treat pathology identified by the surgeon from the history and clinical examination. If the signs and symptoms elicited are not sufficient to establish a diagnosis, then an arthroscopy will not advance matters. For example, arthroscopic confirmation of a torn anterior cruciate ligament is a wasted procedure: the knee is either clinically and/or functionally unstable, or it is not; there is nothing to be gained by looking at it.

The careful clinical assessment of the functional stability of an injured ligament is far more valuable than expensive imaging techniques, such as magnetic resonance imaging (MRI) or computerised tomography (CT) scans, which can be very misleading. No one would consider buying a second-hand car from a picture as you cannot tell how well a car goes merely by looking at it. The old rust bucket may look fit for the scrap heap but will drive surprisingly well, whereas the 'top of the range' model with all the extras will not even start! In the same way, tissues that appear to be damaged on scans may 'drive' perfectly well and normal looking tissues may be functionally useless.

Nevertheless, in some situations when a diagnosis is in doubt or there is an unusual presentation of pathology, then arthroscopy and MRI have their place. Identification of meniscal and ligament damage in the knee is 85 per cent accurate using both these techniques and is invaluable in selected cases.

Skeletal muscle

The contractile elements of skeletal muscle are derived from myoblasts. Each muscle is composed of several muscle bundles which in turn contain muscles fibres, the basic unit of contraction. A muscle fibre is an elongated cell and is composed of myofibrils (1–3 μm in diameter and 1–2 cm long) which are collections of sarcomeres. Each sarcomere is composed of thick filaments (myosin) and thin filaments (actin) arranged in an overlapping pattern that allows the filaments to slide past each other. The force generated by a muscle is proportional to its functional cross-sectional area. A muscle contraction is *concentric* when the muscle fibres shorten and the tension within the muscle is proportional to the externally applied load. During an *eccentric* contraction the muscle lengthens (pays out) and the internal force is less than the external force. The latter have the greatest potential for high muscle tension and injury. During an *isometric* contraction tension is generated but the muscle does not shorten.

Muscle fibres are divided into two types: fast twitch and slow twitch. Slow twitch fibres are highly vascularised, and contract slowly and aerobically. They are used in endurance (low-load, high-frequency) activities. Fast twitch fibres contract more quickly and powerfully but they do so at the expense of efficiency and are anaerobic such that they fatigue quickly. The distribution of fast and slow twitch fibres is genetically determined but may be influenced by selective training. Endurance training typically increases the aerobic capacity of the slow twitch fibres by increasing the number of mitochondria and capillary density. Strength training involves using higher loads at lower repetitions and leads to an increased number of myofibrils as well as hypertrophy of fast twitch fibres.

Muscle injury

During physical activity up to 70 per cent of the cardiac output may be diverted to muscle blood flow. It is easy to see that whenever a muscle is injured significant bleeding is an inevitable complication. The injury may be direct, from a blow compressing the muscle against the underlying bone, or it may be indirect due to excessive distraction of the muscle ends. The latter may result in partial or complete rupture of the muscle.

When bleeding occurs within a muscle the clinician must distinguish between intramuscular bleeding, i.e. contained within a muscle sheath, and intermuscular bleeding. Intramuscular haematoma is a more serious injury and the resultant swelling usually persists beyond the first 48 hours, and is accompanied by significant tenderness, pain and impaired muscle function. If the swelling reaches a critical level then an acute compartment syndrome may result (*vide infra*).

With an intermuscular haematoma the dispersal of blood within the facial plains means that after an initial period of increased pressure there is a relatively rapid reduction in pressure and swelling with return of muscle function. Typically, superficial bruising may be visible some distance from the site of injury 24–48 hours later.

A number of factors predisposes muscles to rupture:

- inadequate warm-up prior to exercise;
- fatigue;
- previous injury, resulting in:
  - incomplete recovery of muscle strength,
  - inelastic scar tissue impeding muscle elongation and joint motion,
  - loss of muscle proprioceptive feedback;
- eccentric loading;
- muscle spanning two joints.

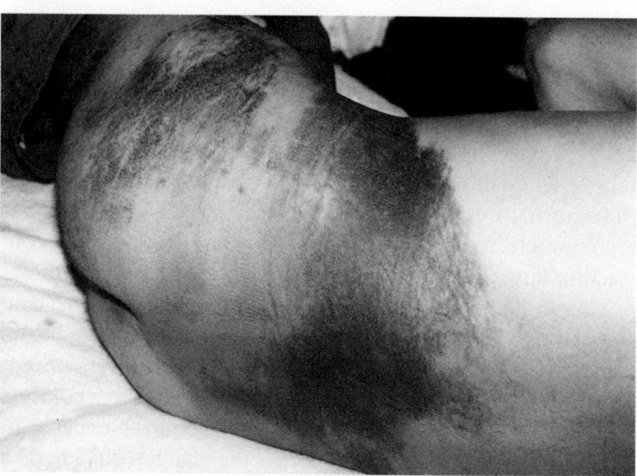

Fig. 29.3 Extensive intermuscular haematoma.

The principles of treatment for any soft-tissue injury, and particularly for muscle injuries, can be remembered using the acronym RICE.

- **R**est
- **I**ce
- **C**ompression
- **E**levation

Treatment should minimise the amount of bleeding within the tissues, and cessation of activity as soon as possible after the injury will allow the fibrin scaffold to develop on the damaged capillaries. A sportsman injured during the course of a game presents the surgeon with a delicate judgement. The injured player may be able to continue playing but the importance of the current match must be weighed against the increasing damage that is being done with every minute that he or she continues to play. However, players in the heat of battle often require a little persuasion to see that curtailing the present game by 20 minutes can save them 2–3 weeks of rehabilitation in the future!

The application of ice and compression vasoconstricts and tamponades the blood vessels, whilst elevation of the limb hampers the player's activity and improves venous drainage.

After 48 hours of this regime a more accurate assessment of the extent and nature of the injury can be made. Inspection and palpation of damaged muscle is usually sufficient to diagnose the majority of injuries. In cases of complete muscle rupture the surgeon must decide whether exploration and apposition of the muscle ends is required. If some continuity of the musculotendinous unit can be demonstrated, for example active extension of the knee when a quadriceps rupture is suspected, then surgery is not required.

Complications of muscle injury

A small proportion of large muscle haematomas will fail to be reabsorbed. The walls of the cyst become endothelialised and aspiration is of no benefit. Resection of the cyst is then required with particular attention to haemostasis to prevent recurrence.

Healing deep intramuscular haematomas, most commonly of brachialis and vastus intermedialis, may lead to the formation of bone rather than fibrous tissue, a process known as myositis ossificans (MO). This condition should be suspected if pain, swelling and restricted motion persist despite adequate rehabilitation. Over-vigorous passive stretching of the muscle in the early phase of rehabilitation may precipitate MO and should be avoided. Plain radiographs demonstrating hazy callus formation confirm the diagnosis. Surgery for symptomatic cases must not be performed until maturation of the ossified area is complete. Radiotherapy or non-steroidals should be given postoperatively to prevent recurrence.

Compartment syndrome

Compartment syndrome is a condition in which high pressure within a closed space bounded by fascia and/or bone reduces capillary blood perfusion below a level necessary for tissue viability with subsequent neuromuscular dysfunction. Acute compartment syndrome is a surgical emergency and is dealt with more comprehensively elsewhere in this book. Chronic compartment syndrome affects athletes and results from the vascular engorgement of muscles during exercise superimposed on muscles hypertrophied by prolonged training. The anterior and deep posterior compartments of the tibia are must commonly affected, but the lateral compartment of the thigh and forearm compartments may also be affected. The symptoms of a rapidly worsening ache or cramping pain felt in the affected compartment characteristically occur at the same time after the start of training. In the same way that a patient with vascular insufficiency will describe cessation of symptoms upon ceasing the activity, so will the symptoms recur if activity is resumed, usually after a shorter interval. Clinical examination with the patient at rest is usually unhelpful, and examination after the patient has exercised may be equally uninformative if a deep muscle compartment is involved. The diagnosis can be made by using intracompartmental pressure monitoring whilst the patient exercises. The resting pressure is often 15–20 mmHg (normal 0–5 mmHg) and may rise with exercise to >100 mmHg. This abnormal elevation will often persist for 15 minutes or more after stopping the exercise. Treatment should aim to correct any abnormalities in the patient's gait or training methods, but subcutaneous fasciotomy of the involved compartments has a good success rate.

Assessment of muscle function

The inability of a patient to perform a satisfactory voluntary muscle contraction should lead the surgeon to consider a potential site of injury anywhere from the cerebral cortex to the muscle. All too often the focus is on the muscle itself, forgetting the neural networks that are required to empower the muscle. The patient may voluntarily or involuntarily inhibit the activity of the muscle because of pain; the central or peripheral nervous system may be damaged or diseased or there may be a more generalised hereditary condition such as Duchenne's muscular

Guillame Benjamin Amand Duchenne, 1806–75. Neurologist, Heidelberg, Germany.

dystrophy. Whilst it is important for the surgeon to consider all possible causes of muscle dysfunction, this chapter will confine itself to the assessment of muscle function in athletes. Muscle power is graded on the Medical Research Council scale:

grade 0 – no movement;
grade 1 – only a flicker of movement;
grade 2 – movement with gravity eliminated;
grade 3 – movement against gravity;
grade 4 – movement against resistance;
grade 5 – normal power.

It is useful in diseased states, but almost all sportsmen have muscle function in grade 5 and still complain of weakness! Tests for muscle function in this situation are divided between functional tests that quantify the ability of a muscle to perform a specific task and objective tests of muscle strength. One example of a functional muscle assessment is the single leg hop test. This tests principally the quadriceps power of an injured knee compared with the control knee. From a single leg stance the athlete jumps as far as he or she can and the distance is recorded. This is then expressed as a percentage of the distance achieved by the control leg. Inevitably, this test requires good function in several other muscle groups as well as the joints above and below the knee. It is therefore less applicable in the comparison of results between patients, but is useful as a means of monitoring one patient's recovery following injury or surgery. Objective tests of muscle strength, such as grip strength using a hand-held dynamometer, are readily performed but the results are often subject to great variation. Furthermore, the relationship between results and functional outcome is often not as close as we would wish. Task-specific outcomes such as running figures of eight for assessment of the lower limbs and performing activities of daily living for use with the upper limb are more time-consuming but have the advantage that the task can be tailored to meet the requirements of the individual.

Proprioception

Full recovery after injury to muscles and joints requires not only their anatomy to be restored but also the neuromuscular reflexes that control their motion. The word proprioception is derived from the Latin word '*proprius*' meaning self or own. It describes a process whereby an individual is aware of the position and movement of a joint. However, it is a rather vague term and its components are usefully considered under three headings.

- Static joint position sense (knowing where the limb is held in space), signalled by slow adapting Ruffini receptors found mainly in the superficial layers of the fibrous capsule of joints.
- Kinesthetic sense (detection of displacement and or velocity) detected by fast adapting Pacinian corpuscles located in the deeper layers of the joint fibrous capsule.
- Unconscious closed loop afferent/efferent neural activity required for reflex activity and regulation of muscle stiffness. This component is signalled by Pacinian and Ruffini receptors but also by Golgi tendon organs (slow adapting) and muscle spindle receptors (fast adapting).

These receptors occur at multiple sites in the body and there is a complex, and poorly understood, interplay between their signals in producing functional stability of joints. Joint stability is maintained by the static mechanical restraints such as the articular geometry and ligaments, as well as a dynamic element provided by the muscles. The relative importance of damage to the neuromuscular, or 'proprioceptive', feedback in maintaining stability of an injured joint has only recently received much attention. Damage to anatomical structures and the resultant change in stability of a joint is relatively easy to assess, whereas techniques for measuring the loss of neuromuscular reflexes that provided functional stability were only developed more recently.

It is now well established that injury to a joint can impair the function of all three of the components of proprioception. This impairment may be improved by rehabilitation programmes that specifically address the restoration of sensory feedback from injured joints. Reconstructive surgery, which one would expect to address only the static mechanical restraints of an injured joint, also improves the proprioception of the joints. Rehabilitation programmes that aim to improve neuromuscular control begin by re-establishing joint position sense and kinesthesia followed by dynamic joint stabilisation by using activities that produce sudden alterations in joint position necessitating reflex neuromuscular control. The final phase of these programmes addresses functionally specific activities for return to the chosen sport.

Whilst the importance of neuromuscular components in maintaining functional stability of joints is universally accepted, the exact role of each of the components is poorly understood and the relationship between loss of neuromuscular reflexes and functional instability is not absolute.

Tendon

Tendons attach muscle to bone and are composed of dense, regularly arranged fascicles, or groups of collagen bundles. The fascicles are surrounded by an epitenon and are closed within the paratendon (tendon sheath). The predominant cells are fibroblasts producing mostly type I collagen (85 per cent dry weight of tendon). Tendons transmit load from muscles to the bone and the collagen fibres tend to orientate themselves along stress lines. The collagen laid down in a healing tendon initially has a haphazard arrangement but when subjected to physiological strains the orientation returns to normal, with restoration of the mechanical properties of the tendon. Tendon pathology may be divided into three types:

- paratendinitis;
- paratendinitis with tendinosis;
- pure tendinosis.

Paratendinitis is inflammation of the investing paratenon and may be diagnosed by eliciting tenderness around the full circumference of the tendon, the site of which does not move with the underlying tendon (Fig. 29.4). It is an extremely painful condition. Paratendinitis usually responds well to anti-inflammatory medication, local physical therapies such as friction massage and ultrasound, and occasionally an injection of local anaesthetic and corticosteroid into the paratenon (*not* into the tendon itself). If the paratendinitis becomes chronic it may be necessary to strip surgically the injured paratenon from the tendon.

Angelo Ruffini, 1864–1929. Italian anatomist.
Falippo Pacini, 1812–83. Italian anatomist.
Camillo Golgi, 1843–1926. Italian pathologist.

Tendinosis is a more sinister condition both to diagnose and to treat. It is usually asymptomatic and is present in an increasing proportion of all tendons with advancing age. The term covers a wide variety of pathological processes: hyaline degeneration, a decrease in the normal cell population and alterations in the matrix.

Treatment for tendinosus is difficult and patients should be warned against the likelihood of a 'quick fix'. Physical therapies aimed at improving the blood supply to the degenerate areas are only moderately successful. Rehabilitation programmes should start with complete rest and only progress within the limits of pain. More recently the emphasis has been on eccentric loading and enhanced proprioceptive feedback to improve tendon healing. Surgical treatment for tendinosis is controversial but a distinction should be made between surgery to remove aggravating mechanical factors, for example subacromial decompression of the rotator cuff tendon, which has a good success rate, and surgery to the tendon itself which is less rewarding. However, encouraging results have been obtained after percutaneous, longitudinal tenorrhaphy of the Achilles tendon, although the risk of precipitating tendon rupture is always present.

Tendon rupture

Rupture is the end point of tendinosis in that there is histological evidence of degeneration present within every tendon that has ruptured. It seems that closed injury cannot rupture a *normal* tendon, failure always occurring at the musculotendinous junction in this instance.

The principles of treatment of a ruptured tendon are similar to those for treating fractures, namely to restore anatomy and maintain it whilst healing occurs. Tendon ends need to be apposed in order to minimise the gap that must be bridged by fibrous tissue. The larger the gap the greater the volume of scar tissue which has inferior biomechanical properties. A large tendon gap also decreases muscle strength by lengthening the musculotendinous unit and reducing the efficiency of its contractions.

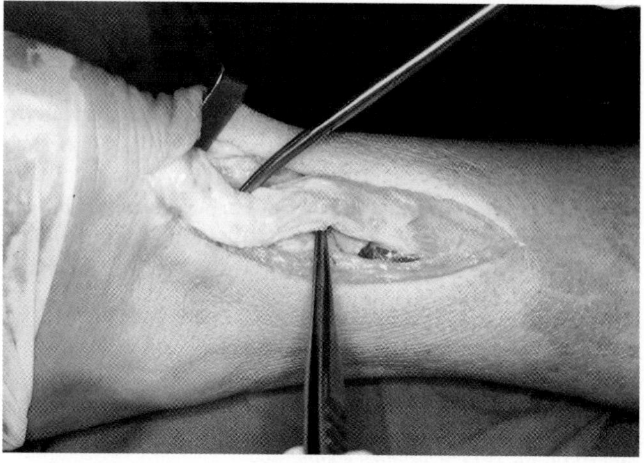

Fig. 29.4 Degenerate Achilles tendon.

All tendons will heal, and indeed this healing may to some extent be impaired by surgery. The surgeon must therefore be clear that benefit will ensue from his or her surgical intervention. The next point to remember is that the strength of any type of surgical repair will only ever be a small fraction of the strength of the intact tendon. Whilst the initial biomechanical properties of a repair may be improved by placing multiple sutures into the tendon ends, this apparent advantage is outweighed by the adverse effect on the vascular regeneration required to produce tendon healing.

Plantarflexing the ankle usually brings the tendon ends together after rupture of the Achilles tendon. Failure to produce tendon apposition may account for the relatively high rate of tendon re-rupture and weakness of calf muscle power in nonoperatively treated patients. In several instances the tendon ends can never be apposed by closed means; examples of this include rupture of the distal insertion of the biceps tendon on to the radial tuberosity and tears of the rotator cuff tendon. Surgery is then required to restore the anatomy whilst preserving the blood supply wherever possible. One advantage of surgical repair of a ruptured tendon is that a graduated rehabilitation programme to maintain muscle function and joint range of motion can be started within a week of surgery.

Ligaments

Ligaments transmit tensile forces across the joint, define the motion limits of the bones with respect to each other and guide the relative movements of bones within the motion limits. Their ultrastructure is similar to that of tendons, the principal difference being that they have a higher elastin content which ensures that joint stability is not entirely rigid. The principles of examination of an injured ligament can be applied to any joint that is readily palpable by direct comparison with the uninjured limb:

grade 0 – normal ligament, normal joint stability;
grade 1 – tenderness at the site of ligament injury, no detectable increase in joint laxity whilst loading the ligament;
grade 2 – increase in joint laxity but with a solid end point;
grade 3 – significant increase in joint laxity with no end point.

Arthometers have been developed to quantify the amount of joint laxity and are most commonly used after cruciate ligament injury in the knee. However, as they only measure the static stability and do not take into account the dynamic stabilisers of a joint, the correlation between arthrometric estimation of joint stability and the functional instability remains poor.

Achilles, the Greek hero, was the son of Peleus and Thetis. When he was a child his mother dipped him in the River Styx, so that he should be invulnerable in battle. The heel by which she held him did not get wet and was therefore unprotected. Achilles died from a wound in the heel, received at the siege of Troy.

The stability of joints varies enormously from one individual to the next. Women's joints tend to be more lax than men's and all joints become stiffer as we grow older. Connective tissue disorders such as Ehlers–Danlos syndrome or Marfan's syndrome should be excluded in patients with hyperlaxity. A patient should be assessed for generalised ligamentous laxity using the criteria of Wynne-Davies:

- elbow hyperextension;
- knee hyperextension;
- foot dorsiflexion of more than 45°;
- thumb can be bent back to touch volar forearm surface;
- fingers can be hyperextended to parallel forearm.

The principles of treatment for ligament injuries are as for tendon injuries. However, ligament injuries are quite commonly multiple, and because of their close proximity to joints the effect on joint motion is more pronounced.

Bursae

Sandwiched between tissues that slide past each other, bursae decrease the frictional forces present. They are endothelial-lined cushions and normally contain little fluid. If they are overloaded they can become inflamed, swollen and very painful. Although the appearances can mimic sepsis, a pathogenic organism is rarely isolated in cases of closed injury. Common sites for bursitis to develop are:

- olecranon;
- psoas tendon;
- greater trochanter;
- iliotibial band;
- prepatellar;
- infrapatellar;
- retrocalcaneal.

Avoidance of the aggravating mechanical factors and a short course of anti-inflammatories is usually sufficient to control symptoms. Intractable cases require aspiration and steroid injections and, more rarely, excision of the indurated bursal wall.

Stress fractures

Bone is a dynamic structure and, unlike the scaffolding of a building, it adapts to the stresses placed upon it according to Wolff's law. Plain radiographs will chart the activity of a limb, the osteopenia of a nonweight-bearing foot or the thickened metatarsal shafts of an army recruit. Fractures of bone may be due to a single high load or cyclical low loads leading to a stress fracture.

Henri Alexander Danlos, 1844–1912. French dermatologist.
Bernard-Jean Antonin Marfan, 1858–1942. French daediatrician.
Ruth Wynne-Davies, an international authority on genetic patterns in orthopaedic conditions. (Scoliosis, congenital dislocation of the hip, foot disorders. Did most of her early work in Edinburgh. She continues her studies in Oxford.)

Any repetitious activity, particularly endurance training, is a risk factor for the development of stress fractures. Diagnosis should be suspected from the patient's history, particularly if there has been a recent change in the training pattern, different footwear, a new playing surface or a sudden increase in intensity. Pain and tenderness are often poorly localised and radiographs may be normal in the early phase. Bone scintigraphy, or MRI if it is available, is the investigation of choice to demonstrate the earliest changes of marrow hypervascularity and trabecular microfracture (Fig. 29.5).

A common theme for treating these conditions is the necessity for a reduction in weight-bearing, particularly high-impact activity, for healing to occur. This disruption to the athlete's training regime requires counselling but, more importantly, a satisfactory replacement activity must be found to keep up the athlete's supply of endorphins! Cycling, with the pedal held under the heel, is the ideal substitute for runners, whilst swimming is less well tolerated.

Two patient subgroups should be identified: children and women. Children often present late with vague symptoms and the radiological changes to the growth plate may be difficult to interpret. The contralateral limb should be X-rayed to provide a control. Female athletes appear to be at increased risk of developing stress fractures. There appears to be a complex interplay between dysmenorrhea, exercise and decreased bone density, particularly if an eating disorder is superimposed.

The distribution of stress fractures amongst runners is: tibia 49 per cent, tarsals 25 per cent, metatarsals 9 per cent, femur 7 per cent and fibula 7 per cent.

The majority of fractures can be treated nonoperatively without great risk, but femoral neck stress fractures must be carefully assessed. There are two types: a tension fracture, which begins as a cortical defect on the superior aspect of the femoral neck, and the compression type, which appears as a haze of callus around the inferior cortex. Failure to recognise these fractures may result in displacement of the fragments with the subsequent risk of osteonecrosis, malunion and nonunion. Internal fixation with multiple screws should be considered in cases where symptoms are not controlled by reduction in weight-bearing.

Stress fractures of the pelvis occur about the ischium, but the ilium and sacrum may be involved. The tarsal navicular and metatarsal stress fractures are the bane of the armed forces owing to marching, but particular care must be taken of the base of fifth metatarsal fracture as it has a high rate of delayed union or nonunion. Stress fractures are not confined to the lower limb and may occur in the ribs, clavicle, acromion, olecranon and metacarpals (Fig. 29.6).

Kasper Fredrich Wolff, 1733–94. Professor of Anatomy and Physiology, St Petersburg, Russia.

Lower leg pain

Lower leg pain is a common complaint in athletes who have recently changed their footware or have increased the intensity of their training. The main diagnoses to be considered are stress fracture of the tibia, chronic compartment syndrome, medial tibial periostitis and tibialis anterior syndrome. The term 'shin splints' is unhelpful and should be avoided.

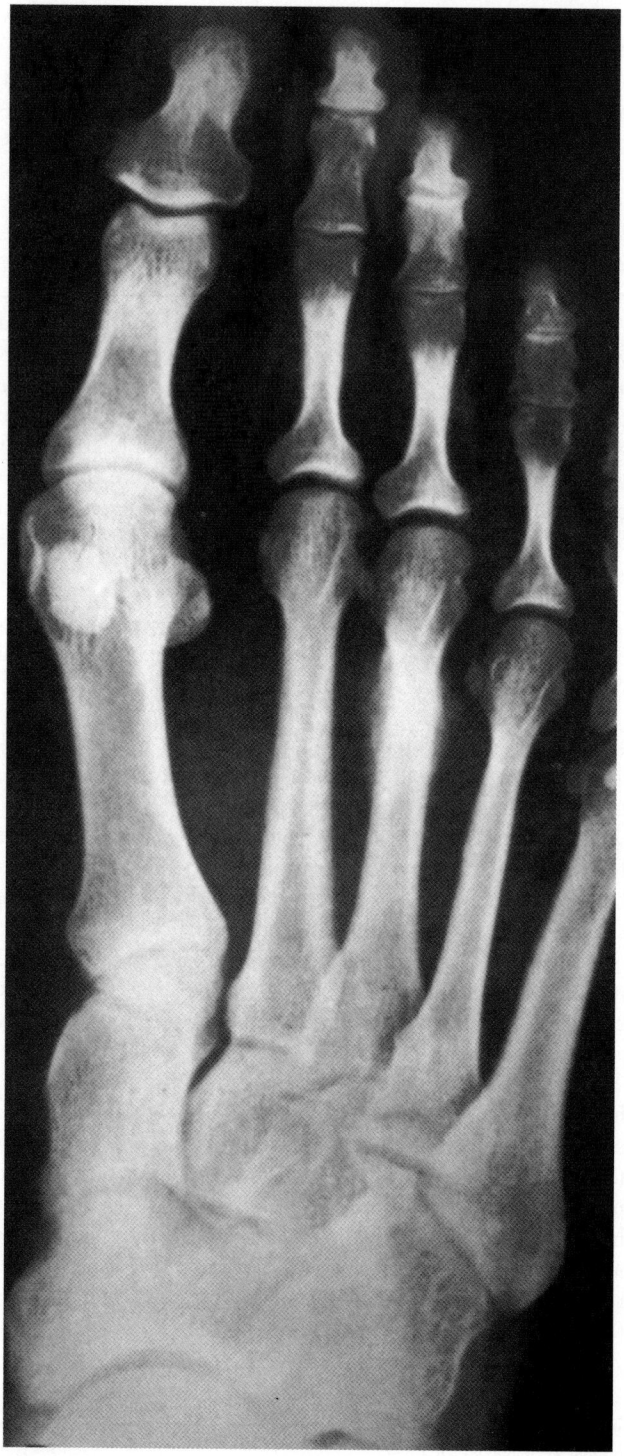

Fig. 29.5 Stress fracture of the third metatarsal.

Stress fracture of the tibia

Stress fractures are not uncommon in the tibia, particularly in long-distance runners. The patient initially complains of pain during exercise, then pain during and after exercise, and finally pain at all times. On examination there may be little to find except that the tibia may be tender to percussion. Initially the X-ray may be normal but after some weeks a faint haze of callous may form locally over the site of the invisible fracture. This X-ray picture, if combined with a history of continuous pain, is also characteristic for osteosarcoma. Careful imaging with MRI or CT scan should be able to distinguish between these two diagnoses.

This condition can prove very difficult to manage. It may occur at a crucial phase in an athlete's training programme and at some stage, preferably sooner rather than later, it is going to become clear that training for the next few months

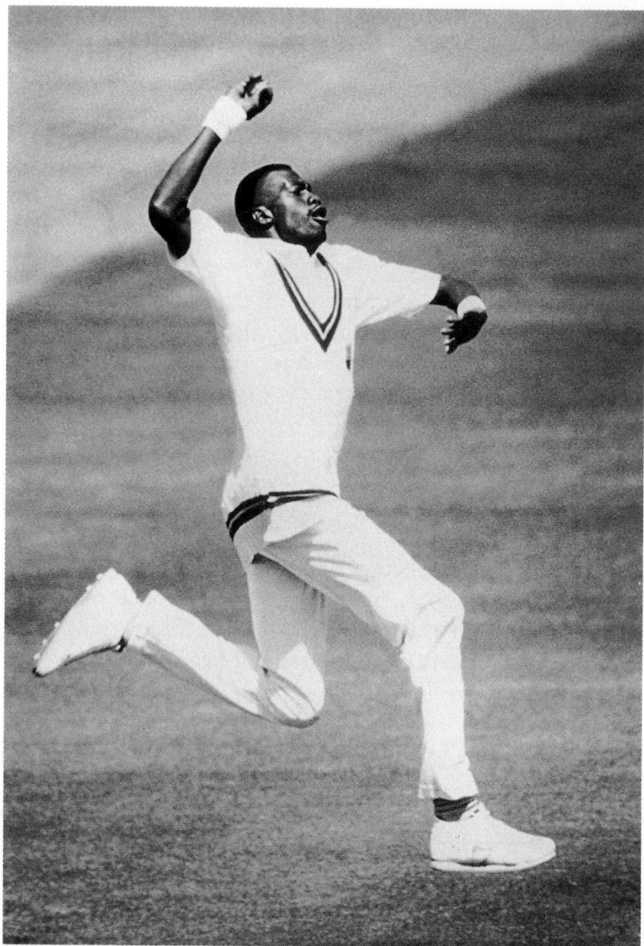

Fig. 29.6 Fast bowlers are at risk of stress fractures of the lower limb and lumbar spine.

or indeed that season is over. This can be very difficult for an athlete to accept, but until it is the condition is unlikely to settle. As the fracture is incomplete it should not require any extra protection, and a modification of activity is usually all that is required for healing.

Chronic compartment syndrome

The anterior and deep posterior compartment is most commonly involved. Physicial examination is generally unhelpful and a diagnosis is made from the history and intracompartmental pressure monitoring whilst the athlete exercises. Subcutaneous fasciotomies of the affected compartment provides good relief of symptoms.

Tibialis anterior syndrome

Acute inflammation in the tendon sheath of the tibialis anterior muscle often arises from over-use of the ankle joint, especially running and jumping on hard surfaces. Tenderness is localised to the tibialis anterior tendon with pain on resisted dorsiflexion of the ankle. Increased temperature, swelling and crepitus may be palpated over the tendon sheath. Resolution is usually swift with a short period of nonweight-bearing and rest.

Medial tibial periostitis

The attachment of the investing muscle fascia into the periosteum of the posteromedial order of the tibia may become inflamed. The pain is often poorly localised by the athlete but tenderness is well localised over the distal medial margin of the tibia, particularly over the lower half of the bone. Resisted plantar flexion aggravates the pain and radiographs should be performed to exclude a stress fracture.

Groin pain

A wide variety of pathologies can present with pain in the groin. The surgeon requires a systematic and methodical approach to the diagnosis based on a sound knowledge of the complex anatomy in the region. The history of pain should give clues as to whether the origin is visceral (more constant) or somatic (exercise related). Each surgeon will develop their own system but it is reasonable to separate the pathologies on the basis of the tissue involved.

Muscles

A large number of muscles takes their origin from or traverse the region of the groin. Inflammation of these musculotendinous origins or partial tears will produce activity-related pain. The principles of assessment are carefully to localise the point of maximal tenderness and then test the muscles in that area with an isometric contraction. Muscles that frequently cause problems are the proximal insertion of rectus femoris just distal to the anterosuperior iliac spine, the adductor musculature inserting into the inferior aspect of the pubic bone and psoas tendon as it courses over the anterior aspect of the hip joint to the lesser trochanter.

Visceral organs

Visceral pain from pelvic organs may produce groin pain and a careful history will have elicited symptoms of systemic upset. Appendicitis, prostatitis, urinary tract infection and gynaecological disorders should always be borne in mind and dealt with appropriately.

Nerve entrapment

Lumbar spine disease causing entrapment of the higher lumbar nerve roots may produce pain radiating round the buttock to the groin. Less commonly the ilio-inguinal (in the inguinal canal) and lateral cutaneous nerve of the thigh (distal to the anterosuperior iliac spine) may be trapped as they pass through the deep fascia.

Hernia

Male athletes who play sports that involve a lot of twisting and turning are prone to developing the 'sportsman's hernia'. This is really a direct 'prehernia' in that no bulge can be demonstrated either clinically or even with specialist scanning techniques. The hernia is a fatigue failure of the transversalis fascia which only becomes symptomatic because of the repeated stresses placed on it by the athlete. The diagnosis is based on the history and tenderness at the deep inguinal ring. This sign is elicited by invaginating the scrotum with the little finger until the tip can be placed directly over the deep inguinal ring. The examination is uncomfortable and so comparison with the normal side is required. Repair is performed in the standard manner either using a mesh or by reefing the conjoined tendon to the inguinal ligament.

Bone and joint

Osteoarthritis of the hip classically presents with groin pain, and the diagnosis should not be excluded because of normal radiographs. Plain radiographs will usually demonstrate a stress fracture of the femoral neck but if there is still doubt then bone scintigraphy or an MRI will establish the diagnosis.

Osteitis pubis is a well-recognised but poorly understood condition. Pain and tenderness are vaguely localised to the anterior pubic bones and intervening symphysis. Plain radiographs may demonstrate changes of fragmentation of the margin of the pubic bones and patchy sclerosis within the symphysis. The aetiology of this condition is unknown; certainly no pathogenic organisms have ever been demonstrated within biopsies. Treatment is frustrating for both surgeon and athlete as it may require a prolonged period of nonweight-bearing activity. Fusion of the pubic symphysis should be avoided as the results are very poor.

Knee

Ligament injuries of the knee

The four major ligaments of the knee (anterior and posterior cruciate, medial and lateral collateral) maintain its stability and guide its motion. The anterior cruciate ligament (ACL) provides the major restraint to anterior translation of the tibia on the femur, and the posterior cruciate ligament (PCL) to posterior translation. The medial collateral ligament (MCL) resists valgus deformation but the lateral collateral ligament (LCL) is the weakest of the four and does little to prevent varus deformity, the majority of restraint coming from the dynamic input of the iliotibial band. All four ligaments work in close harmony and injury to one affects the function of the others. The following combination of injuries is roughly in their frequency of occurrence:

- MCL;
- ACL;
- ACL and MCL;
- PCL;
- PCL and posterolateral structures;
- ACL, MCL, PCL (knee dislocation, rare).

MCL injury

These occur after a valgus injury, commonly during snow skiing. There is pain and tenderness localised to the site of injury, usually the midsubstance or proximal insertion and valgus instability may be elicited. Grade I injuries may be treated symptomatically; grade II–III should be braced with knee motion restricted from 10° to 90° for 3–4 weeks. Athletes should be warned of 'tweaking' pains that persist for up to a year following MCL injury.

ACL and ACL–MCL injury

The history of a noncontact injury when the athlete was running and tried to change direction, felt the knee 'jump', heard a pop and developed immediate swelling is almost diagnostic of ACL injury. If the knee took 2–3 weeks to settle down and the athlete is left with a feeling of, or experiences, instability then any lingering doubts over the diagnosis can be dispelled. Clinical confirmation comes from increased anterior tibial translation with the knee held in 30° of flexion (positive Lachmann test) and abnormal anterior subluxation of the lateral tibial plateau (positive Pivot shift test). The main indication for surgery is the recurrent episodes of instability that patients experience when changing direction or landing from a jump.

ACL rupture is commonly associated with injury to other structures in the knee. Meniscal tears are present 80 per cent of the time and unstable meniscal tears should be repaired at the time of ACL reconstruction. 'Bone bruises' visible on MRI scans represent subchondral oedema and are evidence of impact damage sustained at the time of injury.

All patients with ACL injury should undergo an intensive rehabilitation programme, with special emphasis on hamstring proprioception. The decision making concerning the need for, and technique of, surgical reconstruction is not straightforward. There is a massive body of literature, but very little science. At present, the major determining factors are the degree of knee laxity and the level of sport to which the athlete wishes to return. The decision is relatively easy at each end of the spectrum; the high-demand athlete with a loose knee probably (but *still* by no means certainly) requires reconstruction, whereas the nonsporting office worker with a fairly stable knee does not need a reconstruction. With patients in the middle ground, who may or may not wish to adapt their sporting lifestyle to accommodate their knee, it is reasonable to adopt a wait-and-see policy, and if functional instability develops then reconstruction can be offered at a later date.

Surgery should be delayed until the swelling and range of motion have improved in order to avoid a painful stiff knee postoperatively (arthrofibrosis). Combination ACL–MCL injuries should be braced for 3–6 weeks to allow the MCL to heal and then have the ACL reconstructed.

Techniques of ACL reconstruction

The child's ACL usually avulses with a fragment of bone from the tibia. It is relatively simple to fix this fragment back into the tibia either with a bone screw or with sutures passed through to the front of the tibia. The adult ACL tears midsubstance or at the femoral insertion but rarely heals.

Extra-articular reconstructions

These prevent the abnormal anterior subluxation of the lateral tibial plateau by re-routing the iliotibial band around the LCL. Whilst they abolish the pivot shift phenomenon they do not restore normal knee kinematics and the majority of surgeons no longer uses them routinely.

Intra-articular reconstruction

Suturing the ends of the ACL back together is only possible in the acute injury, but the long-term stability of the knee is poor and the technique has largely been abandoned. The ACL is therefore replaced with a graft placed through bone tunnels which enter the joint at the sites of attachment. Graft positioning is critical to the success of ACL reconstruction, and ideally the graft should not lengthen or shorten by more than 2 mm when the knee is put through its full range of motion, i.e. it is isometric. Prosthetic grafts are very attractive because of the lack of donor morbidity and their high initial strength. However, the early optimism with their use has been dampened as problems have developed due to particulate debris when the grafts fail. They are usually only used if a viable alternative is not available.

Allografts have no donor morbidity but all methods of sterilisation (to prevent disease transmission) significantly reduce the biomechanical properties and delay the revascularisation of the graft.

Autografts are the most widely employed at present, the two most common ones being the middle third of the patellar tendon with patellar and tibial bone blocks at either end, and the quadrupled semitendinosus and gracilis tendon graft. These may be secured with interference screws within the bone tunnels or via sutures to screws/posts on the external cortex (Fig. 29.7). The surgery may be performed open or with the arthroscope, drilling the tunnels from within the joint. The modern trend for accelerated rehabilitation permits early weight-bearing without braces, and athletes can return to contact sport 6 months after reconstruction.

PCL injury

Commonly sustained during road traffic accidents from a direct blow to the front of the tibia, PCL injuries are much less common than ACL injuries (occurring in a ratio of about 1:10). Examine the patient with both knees flexed to 90° and you will see the tibia sagging back on the side of PCL injury. The knee of patients who have a femoral shaft fracture should always be examined to exclude injury to the PCL.

Isolated PCL injuries probably do very well if rehabilitated and, as the surgery to reconstruct them is not as well developed as ACL surgery, nonoperative treatment is recommended.

PCL and posterolateral structures

These are significant injuries but diagnosis is often difficult, and the loss of posterolateral structures (posterior capsule, popliteus tendon and the popliteofibular ligaments) in addition to the PCL can render the knee unstable. In an athletic individual acute reconstruction is probably to be recommended, but the surgery is complex and the results are not yet convincing.

Knee dislocation (combination of three or more ligament injuries)

Thankfully rare and a result of high-energy trauma, knee dislocation is a surgical emergency. Neurovascular injury may occur in 50 per cent of cases despite a normal-looking radiograph, and vigilance must be maintained at all times with these injuries to avoid catastrophe. Reconstruction of all of the damaged structures is difficult surgery but in experienced hands can lead to a reasonable outcome.

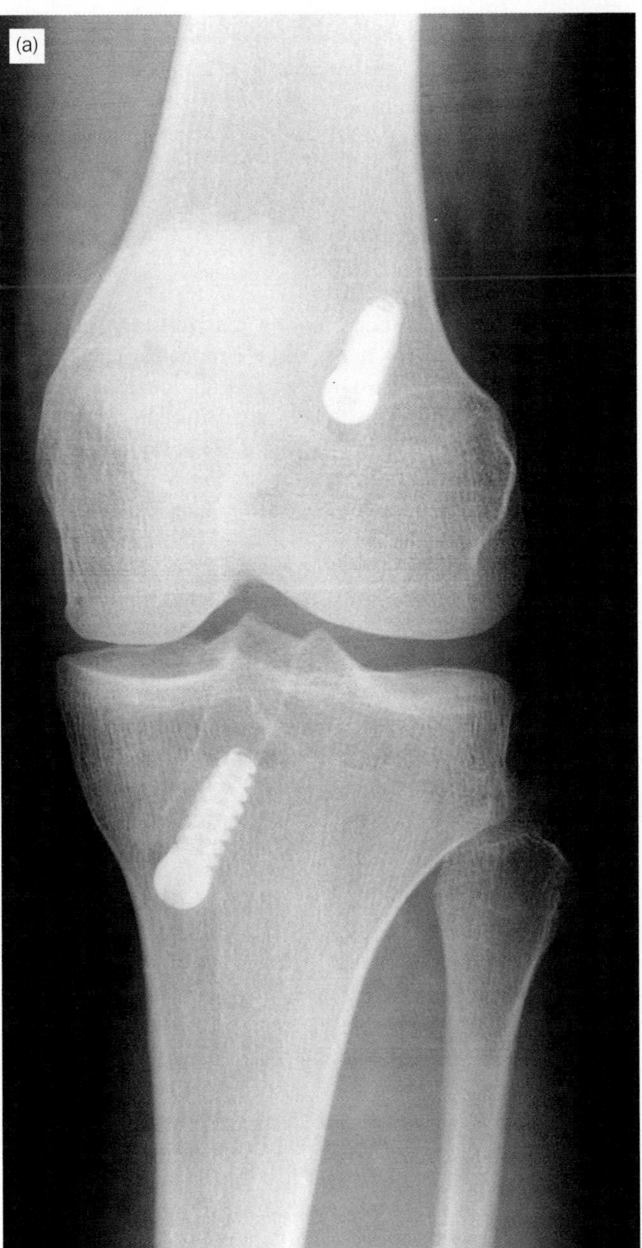

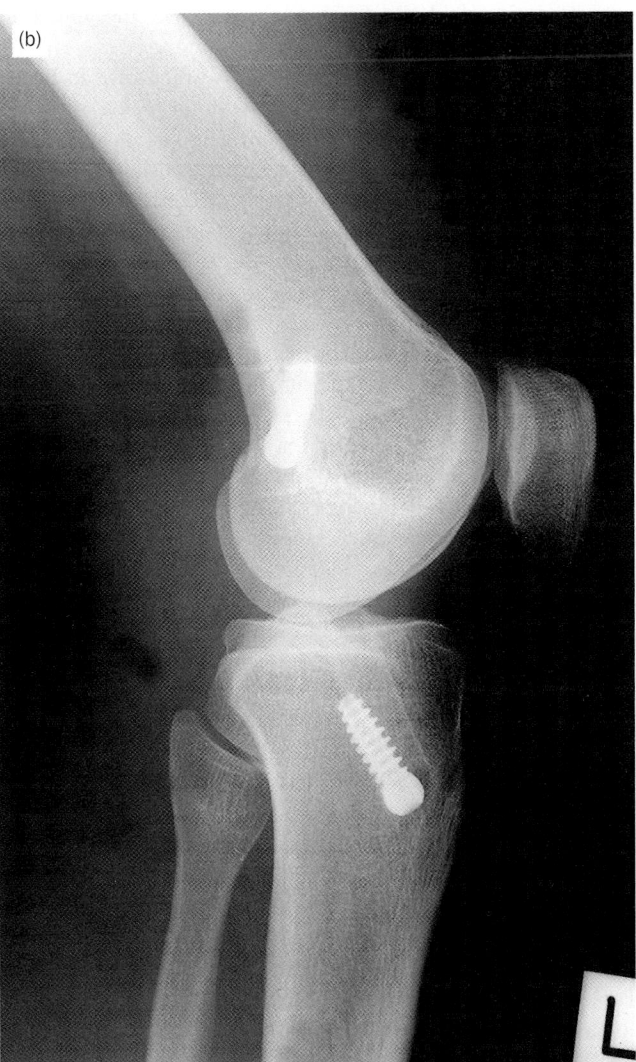

Fig. 29.7 Radiographs of ACL reconstruction demonstrating interference screw positions.

Ankle

Ankle sprains are one of the most common sporting injuries requiring treatment. The mechanism is usually inversion damaging the anterior talofibular (ATF) and subsequently the calcaneofibular (CF) ligaments (Fig. 29.8). Surgery to repair the ligaments is rarely required; functional bracing with early weight-bearing allows the ligaments to heal whilst maintaining ankle motion.

If the recovery after ankle sprain is slow then chondral damage to the talar dome should be suspected. Bone scintigraphy is the most sensitive investigation and lesions can be treated with arthroscopic débridement.

Recurrent lateral instability of the ankle requires a rehabilitation programme concentrating on restoration of proprioception but if this fails then repair is indicated. A direct repair of the ligament ends is usually possible, otherwise the use of a periosteal flap from the fibula or a free hamstring autograft may be used to reconstruct both the ATF and the CF ligaments. The use of some or all of the peroneal tendons for reconstruction is best avoided as they are the dynamic stabilisers to inversion.

Posterior impingement of the ankle is practically an occupational hazard in ballet dancers. With the ankle in point (forced plantar flexion) the posterior malleolus, the talus and the calcaneum compress the soft tissues causing inflammation. An os trigonum may or may not be present, but the diagnosis is made by reproducing the pain of impingement. With the patient prone, plantarflex the ankle and compress the heel whilst moving the forefoot from side to side. Treatment is surgical resection of the soft tissue, or os trigonum if present, via a short medial approach.

Repeated trauma to the anterior joint capsule causes anterior osteophytes ('footballer's ankle') which limit dorsiflexion. These may be resected via the arthroscope.

Forced eversion of the ankle may disrupt the sheath surrounding the peroneal tendons allowing them to sublux anteriorly. The athlete reports a 'snapping' sensation with activity and resisted eversion demonstrates the abnormality. Splints are ineffective at keeping the tendons in place so surgery is required to repair the defect in the sheath, supplementing it with a periosteal flap.

Ruptured tendo achilles

Rupture of the tendo achilles (TA) most commonly occurs in patients in their 40s who experience a sharp snap while running or jumping. Over 80 per cent occur during sport, and the athlete describes a feeling of being struck in the back of the heel. On examination there is tenderness and swelling over the TA and careful palpation may reveal a dent in the TA, especially if it is compared with the other side. Paradoxically the patient may still be able to stand using their long toe flexors, although it may be painful. Simmons' test involves lying the patient face down on the couch with their feet hanging over the edge of the bed. If the calves are squeezed the foot on the normal side plantar flexes but if the TA is ruptured there is no movement. This test is pathognomic of ruptured TA.

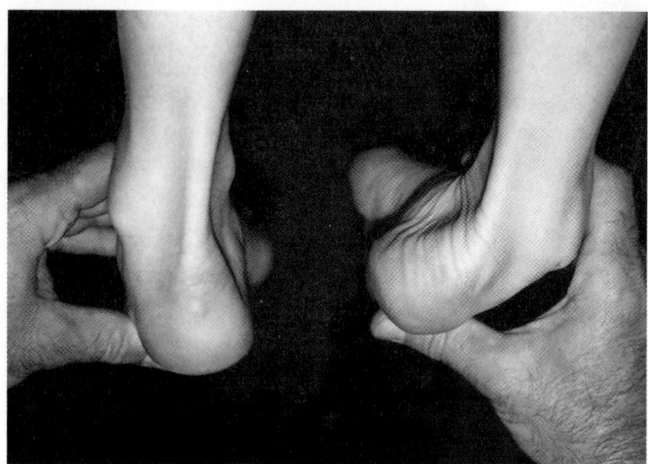

Fig. 29.8 Chronic lateral ligament instability of the ankle.

Management

If the tear is at the musculotendon junction high up in the calf then treatment only needs to be symptomatic, but if it is in the middle of the substance of the tendon then the two ends must be brought into close apposition for healing to occur. This can be done by managing the patient in a below-knee plaster with the ankle in full equinus. Serial plasters are may be used to bring the foot up into neutral. After a total of 6–8 weeks the leg is taken out of plaster and mobilisation of the ankle is started. Surgery to appose the tendon ends may be performed through a longitudinal medial incision (open) or via stab wounds (percutaneous) (Fig. 29.9). Accelerated rehabilitation regimes with functional braces are now commonly used. Ankle mobilisation starting 7 days after repair and 3–4 weeks after nonsurgical treatment lowers the re-rupture rate and maintains better muscle function.

Nonsurgical treatment has a re-rupture rate of 6–10 per cent, open repair risks wound breakdown (1–2 per cent) which is a disaster, and percutaneous repair may lead to sural nerve injury. The results of the few prospective randomised trials have unfortunately been inconclusive, so surgeons should stick to what works best for them.

Shoulder

Instability

Glenohumeral dislocation is not difficult to diagnose but athletes are prone to subtle instability due to stretching of the anterior capsular structures. Abducting the shoulder and using the arm above shoulder height are painful. A diagnosis of subacromial impingement is often made because of a failure to elicit a positive apprehension test. Standing behind the athlete, abduct their shoulder to 90° and then try to pull their elbow posteriorly: if the test is positive they will ask you to stop, not because of pain, but apprehension. In subtle cases of instability you may need to stress the joint by pushing the humeral head forwards with your thumb to reproduce the symptoms.

Treatment should start with a rehabilitation programme to improve proprioception and rotator cuff muscle strength. If there is no improvement after 3 months then a stabilisation is performed by double-breasting the anterior capsule (inferior capsular shift procedure). Athletes with multidirectional instability due to ligamentous laxity should be identified and treated nonoperatively as surgery in these cases is complex and less proven.

Throwing injuries

Throwing involves a number of distinct phases, each with characteristic injuries (Table 29.2). Skeletally immature athletes, despite the same mechanisms of injury, sustain avulsion fractures of the ligament insertions rather than rupture the ligament.

Table 29.2 Different phases of throwing and their injuries

Phase	*Motion*	*Site of injury*
Wind-up	Shoulder hyperextended, externally rotated and abducted	Anterior capsule, long head of biceps
Acceleration (early)	Elbow into valgus	Elbow ulnar collateral ligament rupture, capitellar fractures
Acceleration (late)	Shoulder internal rotation	Latissimus dorsi and pectoralis major rupture, spiral fracture of humerus (rare)
Follow through	Elbow pronation and extension	Posterior elbow impingement

Elbow

Soft-tissue injuries

Rupture of the triceps near its insertion into the olecranon is caused by resisted elbow extension or a fall. The diagnosis is quite often missed as the defect is not readily palpable because of swelling and as gravity can extend the elbow the loss of active extension may not be recognised by the patient immediately. Surgical repair of the avulsion is required for good function.

Avulsion of the biceps tendon from its insertion into the radial tuberosity occurs after violent trauma in young athletes and due to degeneration in older patients. Early reattachment using a small antecubital incision to retrieve the tendon end and a posterior approach to identify the tuberosity usually restores full function.

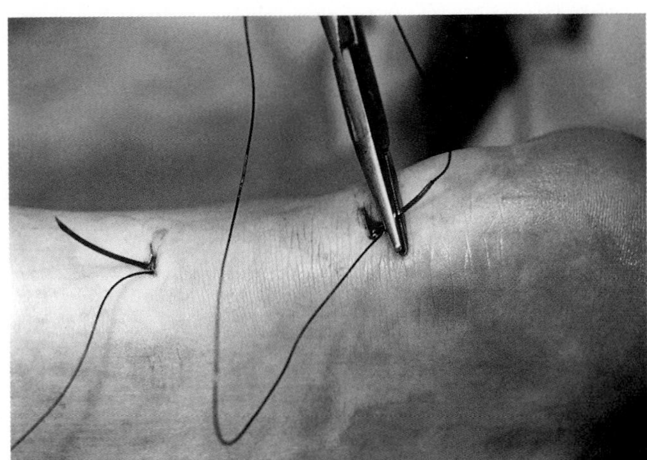

Fig. 29.9 A percutaneous repair of a ruptured Achilles tendon.

Nerve entrapments occur at the elbow, commonly the ulna nerve in the cubital tunnel and occasionally the anterior interosseus nerve within pronator teres. Electrophysiology should be used to confirm the diagnosis before surgical release.

Loose bodies

Throwing sports can lead to repeated minor trauma of the elbow which can manifest in loose bodies. The history of intermittent locking is diagnostic and arthroscopic removal is very satisfying for both surgeon and patient.

Epicondylitis

Medial ('golfer's elbow') and lateral ('tennis elbow') epicondylitis are in fact misnomers as inflammation is secondary to the primary pathology, tendon degeneration. The common flexor origin and the extensor carpi radialis brevis are the respective culprits. Anti-inflammatories, oral and locally injected, are usually ineffective and attention should focus on correcting playing style, grip size (tennis racquet) and equipment (light, graphite racquet) before reducing the frequency of playing. Local physical therapies are beneficial but if these measures fail, the degenerate area is excised and the tendon repaired.

Further reading

Daniel, D., Akeson, W. and O'Connor, J.J. (1990) *Knee Ligaments. Structure, Function, Injury and Repair*, Lippincott Raven, New York.

McLatchie, G.R. and Lennox, C.M.E. (1993) *The Soft Tissues. Trauma and Sports Injuries*, Butterworth-Heinemann, Oxford.

Mow, V.C. and Hayes, W.C. (1997) *Basic Orthopaedic Biomechanics*, Lippincott Raven, New York.

Reid, D.C. (1992) *Sports Injury. Assessment and Rehabilitation*, Churchill Livingstone, London.

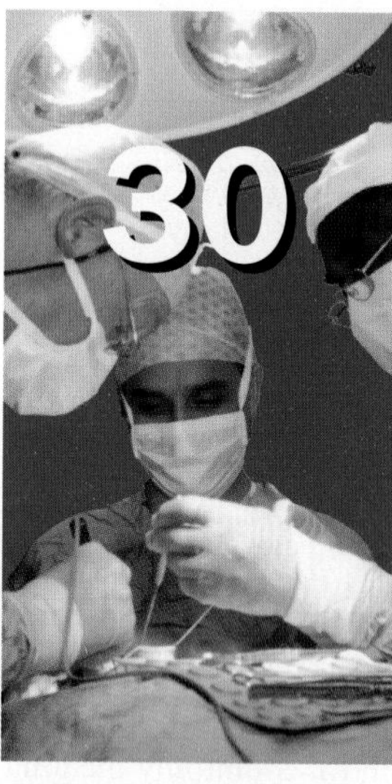

30 Wrist and hand

Function

Wrist

The wrist connects the radius and ulna to the metacarpals. It should provide a stable, mobile, pain-free platform on which the hand can function. It comprises eight bones – scaphoid, trapezium, trapezioid, capitate, hamate, triquetral, pisiform and lunate. A complex system of intrinsic and extrinsic ligaments maintains the alignment of these bones and co-ordinates their movement, whilst the long flexor and extensor tendons contract across them.

Hand

The hand is a very intricate tool with which the individual can receive information from the outside world and then act upon it. It must be supple, sensate, pain-free and co-ordinated. There are several types of grip. The thumb acts as a post against which the index finger moves for *fine pinch* (picking up a pin). The little and ring fingers curl into the palm to provide *power grip* (holding a hammer). The thumb moves to the side of the index finger for *key grip* and to the tips of the index and middle fingers for *chuck grip* (holding a pen). All of the fingers curl for *hook grip* (holding a suitcase).

Bailey & Love's Short Practice of Surgery, 23rd edition. Edited by R.C.G. Russell, N.S. Williams and C.J.K. Bulstrode. Published in 2000 by Arnold Publishers.

Assessment

A careful history and examination is as important for the wrist and hand as anywhere else.

History

- General – Is the patient left- or right-handed? Occupation, hobbies and ambitions? How do the symptoms interfere with these?
- Pain – What is the site of the pain, what makes it better or worse, how long has it been present, does it fluctuate?
- Function – Is the grip weak? Are there problems with fine motor tasks, such as doing up buttons, or coarse tasks, such as opening a jar? Are there clicks or clunks?
- Sensation – Loss of sensation? Tingling? Which part of the hand?
- Injury – The exact nature of the injury: a cut (sharp, blunt, dirty?), a crush, a fall (how far?), a bite, a punch, an avulsion?
- General health – Diabetes? Smoking? Steroids? Cardiac or respiritory problems which may influence the choice of anaesthetic?

Examination

- In the injured patient, are there Airway, Breathing or Circulation problems which should take priority?
- Skin – Are there cuts or bruises? Is there skin loss, and if so are tendons or bone exposed? Are there previous surgical or traumatic scars? Are there signs of infection?

- Bones – Is there deformity or tenderness? The precise of tenderness can be diagnostic, for example a tender lunate with Kienbock's disease or a tender anatomical snuffbox with a scaphoid fracture.
- Joints – Is there deformity or tenderness? *Ligament stability* should be tested by stabilising the proximal bone and gently stressing the distal. The *active and passive range of movement* in each joint should be established. A similar restriction in both active and passive movement may be caused by pain or joint stiffness. A discrepancy may be due to tendon rupture, tendon adhesions or a nerve palsy.
- Tendons – *Passive tenodesis* is a useful screening test: the hand is relaxed and the wrist is moved into flexion and then extension by the examiner. As the wrist extends, the fingers should curl into a neat cascade, and as the wrist is flexed the fingers should open. The function of each individual tendon is established. *Flexor digitorum profundus* is tested in each finger by supporting the proximal interphalangeal joint and middle phalanx then asking the patient to flex the distal interphalangeal joint. *Flexor digitorum superficialis* is tested with the examiner holding the other three fingers straight and asking the patient to flex the proximal interphalangeal joint of the remaining finger. *Extensor digitorum communis* is tested by asking the patient to fully extend the metacarpophalangeal joints (interphalangeal joint extension is a function of the intrinsic muscles).
- Nerves – The nerves supplying the hand can be quickly checked. If there is a cut in the palm or finger, the digital nerves should be tested by checking sensation on each side of the finger tip. *Two-point discrimination* is useful in partial nerve lesions or recovering nerves; two prongs of a paper clip are spread and the patient asked to say whether one or two points can be felt. Normal discrimination in the finger tips is about 6 mm. *Tinel's percussion sign* – tapping on a nerve and causing 'tingling'– is present at the site of nerve compression, a neuroma or at the advancing tip of a recovering nerve. In the unconscious patient or young child, the *plastic pen test* is helpful. If the nerve is normal then the side of a pen brushed gently across the skin will stick because of the intact supply to sweat glands; if the nerve is divided, the pen will brush off smoothly.

Examining the nerves of the hand

Nerve	*Altered sensation*	*Weakness, wasting*
Anterior interosseous	Nil	Flexor pollicis longus, flexor digitorum profundus (FDP) to index
Posterior interosseous	Nil	Extensors of wrist and metacarpophalangeal joint
Median	Thenar eminence, palmar side of thumb, index, middle and radial half of ring finger	Flexor carpi radialis, pronator teres, long finger flexors (except FDP to ring and little), abductor pollicis brevis, opponens pollicis
Ulnar	Ulnar side of hand, palmar side of little finger and ulnar half of ring finger	Flexorcarpi ulnaris, FDP to ring and little finger, adductor pollicis, interossei, hypothenar eminence, Froment's sign
Superficial radial	Anatomical snuffbox	Nil

- Circulation – A white or blue fingertip suggests circulation problems. If the finger nail is compressed and then released, the circulation should return in less than 2 seconds. If not, this suggests either systemic hypotension or loss of the local blood supply. With the *Allen test*, one can tell whether both radial and ulnar arteries are intact. Both are compressed by the examiner's fingers, the patient squeezes his or her hand to express the blood and then relaxes. The hand will be white. The examiner then releases one artery; if the hand does not 'pink up', that artery is occluded or divided. The test is repeated for the other side.

Investigation

- Plain radiographs – The standard views are a *posteroanterior* and *true lateral*. *Oblique views* are helpful particularly for intra-articular fractures and scaphoid fractures. *Special views*, for example stress views for ulnar collateral ligament injuries of the thumb or a clenched fist view for carpal instability, are sometimes needed.
- Magnetic resonance imaging (MRI) – This can detect, for example, Kienböck's disease before it is apparent on plain radiographs and gives some indication of the vascularity of a scaphoid fracture.
- Isotope bone scanning – In difficult cases this helps by disclosing the inflammation that accompanies undisclosed fractures or bone lesions such as osteoid osteoma.
- Wrist arthroscopy – This can diagnose tears of the triangular fibrocartilage complex (TFCC), carpal instability and arthritis. Some TFCC tears are treatable arthroscopically.
- Electrophysiology – For a clinically obvious carpal tunnel syndrome these may not be required; for less clear neurological symptoms these tests detect if and where there is nerve compression.

Basic principles of treatment

Certain principles must be followed when treating conditions of the hand and wrist.

Avoiding swelling and stiffness

The hand swells following injury, surgery or infection (Fig. 30.1); as it swells it tends to fall into a position with the wrist flexed, the metacarpophalangeal joints extended and the interphalangeal joints flexed. This position becomes permanent as the collateral ligaments shrink and the oedematous tissues fibrose. The hand then cannot function properly. To avoid this, one must obey the following three principles.

Robert Kienböck, 1871–1953. Austrian roentgenologist.
Jules Tinel, 1879–1952. French neurologist.
Jules Froment, 1878–1946. Professor of Clinical Medicine, Lyons, France.
Edgar Allen, 1892–1943. Anatomist. Researched reproduction and hormones with Doisy and discovered oestrogen.

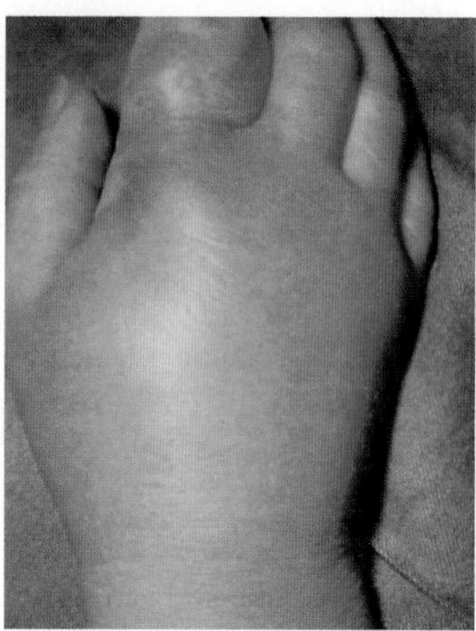

Fig. 30.1 Swelling of the hand is common and must be prevented as much as possible.

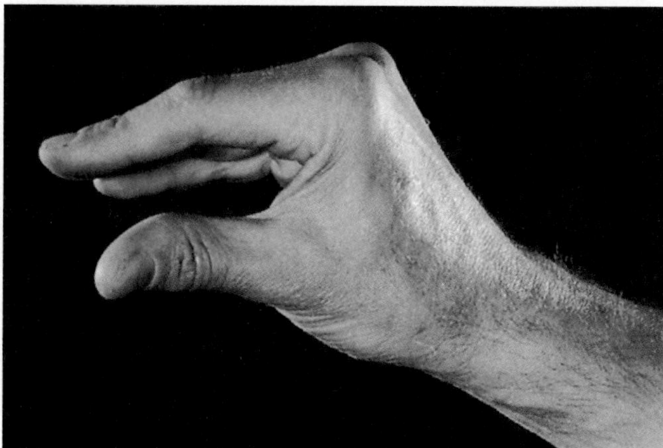

Fig. 30.3 The safe position for splintage is with the wrist extended to 30°, the metacarpophalangeal joints flexed to 90°, interphalangeal joints straight and the thumb abducted forwards from the palm.

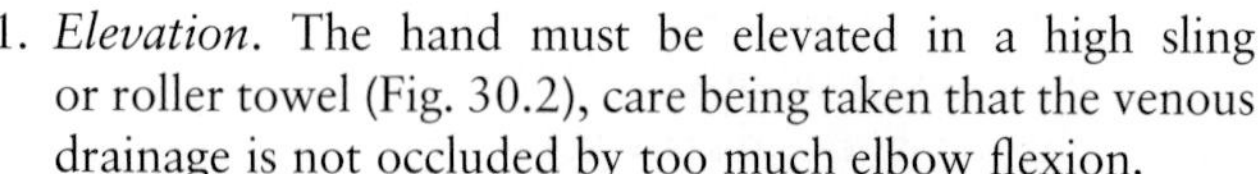

1. *Elevation.* The hand must be elevated in a high sling or roller towel (Fig. 30.2), care being taken that the venous drainage is not occluded by too much elbow flexion.
2. *Splintage.* The wrist should be splinted initially in the position of safety – the 'Edinburgh' position described by James (Fig. 30.3). Dressings must not be too tight.
3. *Movement.* As many joints as possible of the wrist and hand should be moved as early as possible. Rehabilitation should be planned so that the fewest possible joints and tendons are immobilised.

Anaesthesia

Many procedures on the wrist and hand can be performed using local anaesthesia either *proximally* (scalene block, axillary block) or more *distally* (Bier's block, wrist block, digital nerve block or tendon sheath block). In general, if a tourniquet is used for more than about 20 minutes it becomes uncomfortable and so a proximal block or general anaesthetic is preferred.

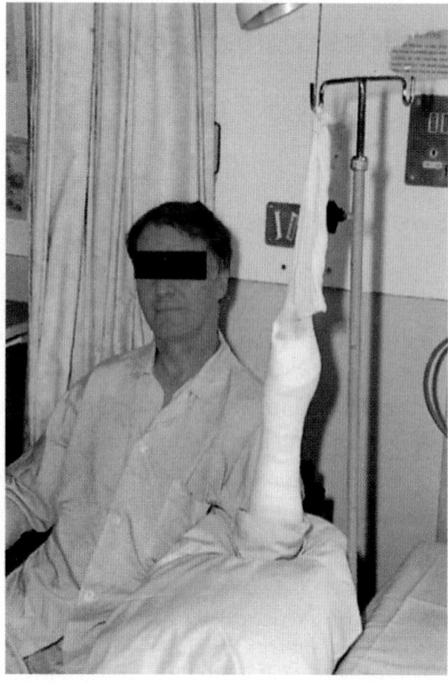

Fig. 30.2 Elevation is important after injury, infection and surgery.

For a digital nerve block, local anaesthetic is introduced into the palm at the level of the distal palmar crease; this is preferable to surrounding the base of the finger with a potentially occlusive 'ring block'. An alternative is to instill about 1 ml of 2 per cent lignocaine beneath the flexor tendon sheath. This takes a little more time to work than a digital nerve block, but lasts for longer and is equally effective.

Tourniquet

A bloodless field is essential for accurate surgery. A well-padded tourniquet above the elbow, inflated to 75 mmHg pressure over the systolic blood pressure, is usually satisfactory. The time should not exceed 2 hours. An Esmarch bandage or a rubber-tube exsanguinator are effective, but should be avoided for tumour or infection cases lest the pathology is spread systemically. In the finger, a tourniquet can be made by placing a sterile glove on the patient, snipping off the tip and then rolling the glove down to the base of the finger.

Incisions

Incisions which cross a flexion crease may produce an uncomfortable and restrictive contracture. Therefore, surgical incisions should be planned to cut across flexor creases at 45° or to lie in neutral areas, such as the midlateral line of the finger. An alternative is to close a straight incision across a flexor crease with a Z-plasty (Fig. 30.4).

August Karl Gustav Bier, 1861–92. Berlin surgeon.
Gip James. Professor of Orthopaedics, Edinburgh.
Esmarch, 1823–1908. German surgeon who devised his bandage during the Franco–Prussian war.

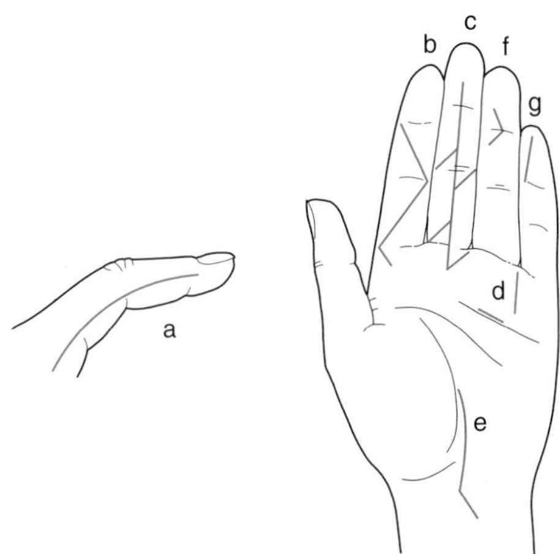

Fig. 30.4 Incisions on the hand: (a) midlateral; (b) Bruner; (c) straight with Z-plasty; (d) web space; (e) carpal tunnel; (f) flexor tendon infection; and (g) pulp space infection.

Splints

Splints can broadly be described as *resting*, *static* or *dynamic* (Fig. 30.5). Resting splints are used to immobilise the hand when there is active inflammation, for example after injury, after surgery or during a flare-up of rheumatoid arthritis or infection. Static splints can be used *continuously* (e.g. for a fracture until healed), *serially* (e.g. gradually changing the angle of a splint to overcome a joint contracture) or *periodically* (e.g. a wrist extension splint at night to reduce symptoms of carpal tunnel syndrome). Dynamic splints allow movement of one group of tendons but not the antagonist, for example to protect either the flexor tendons or extensor tendons after repair.

Injuries

Vascular injuries

Vessel division

A *partial injury* of an artery will not contract and seal itself so it continues to bleed. Bleeding should be controlled with pressure – it is dangerous to use a tourniquet (which can be forgotten) or to clip the vessel blindly (which spoils the chance for repair and can damage the nearby nerve).

Compartment syndrome

Following *crush injuries* and *fractures* of the forearm or hand, or *prolonged ischaemia* from vessel damage, tourniquet or tight dressings, a compartment syndrome can develop. The pressure within the fascial compartments (superficial flexor, deep flexor, extensor, interossei, thenar and hypothenar) rises and occludes the microcirculation which supplies the muscles and nerves. The *symptoms* are pain, tingling, cold; the *signs* are tightness, tenderness and swelling of the muscles, and pain on passive stretching of the muscles in the compartment. The main vessels will not necessarily be occluded as their closing pressure is greater than the pressure required to cut off the microcirculation. Any cast and dressings should be released and, if this does not relieve the ischaemia, then a surgical fasciotomy should be performed. Measurement of the compartment pressures can help in a few cases, but should not delay fasciotomy if the clinical picture is clear.

Julian M. Bruner. Plastic surgeon, Des Moines, Iowa, USA. Described the use of zig-zag incisions in 1967.

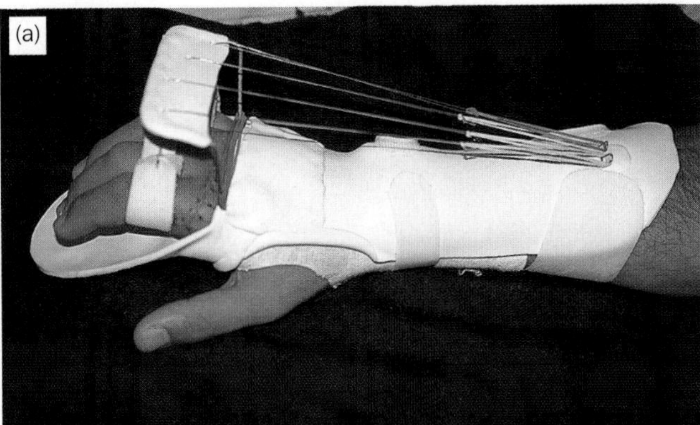

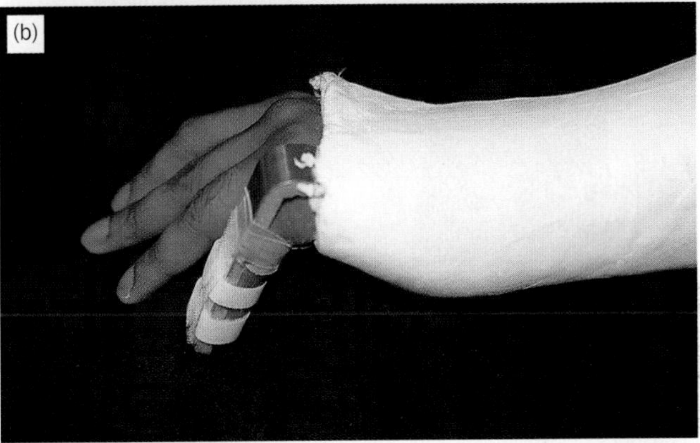

Fig. 30.5 (a) Dynamic splint after repair of the extensor tendons at metacarpophalangeal level, allowing active flexion but passive extension; (b) static splint to protect a fracture of the proximal phalanx fracture.

Fractures

Scaphoid

This bone is fractured by a fall on the outstretched hand. The fracture is easily overlooked – it causes little deformity or pain and does not always show clearly on plain radiographs. However, it is notorious for two reasons – *it may not unite* (particularly in the relatively avascular proximal pole) or *it may present later* with intercarpal collapse and osteoarthritis. If there is doubt about the diagnosis, the wrist is best immobilised and radiographs repeated 2 weeks later. If there is still doubt, isotope bone scanning or MRI scanning will confirm the diagnosis. Plaster immobilisation is needed for at least 8 weeks; delayed union (e.g. if not healed by about 3 months) may merit bone graft and internal fixation (Fig. 30.6). Some unstable displaced fractures probably need early internal fixation.

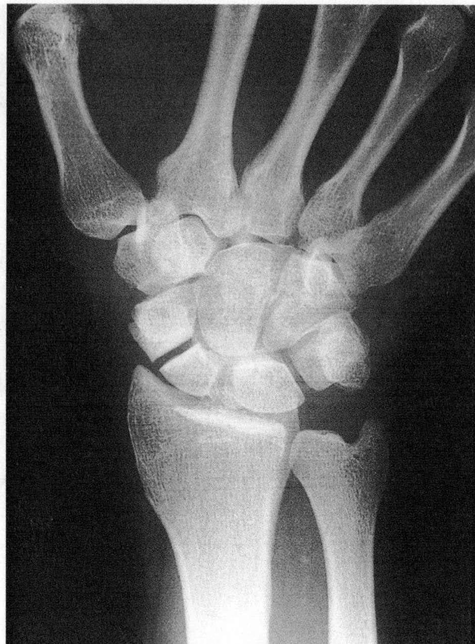

Fig. 30.6 Scaphoid nonunion.

Distal radius

This is commonly injured. There are broadly three groups of fracture.

- *Children*. Usually a Salter Harris type 2 physeal injury, with the distal ulna sometimes fractured as well. Manipulation and plaster fixation for a few weeks is usually adequate. Percutaneous Kirschner wires are sometimes needed for unstable injuries.
- *Young adults*. Usually a high-energy injury, with several intra-articular fragments. Perfect anatomical reduction is most likely to give the best result; this may need a selection of techniques, including bone graft, percutaneous wires, internal fixation and distraction with an external fixator.
- *Older adults*. Typically through osteoporotic bone in a postmenopausal female after a fairly minor fall. This is the classic Colles' fracture. The distal fragment is tilted dorsally and radially; the radius is shortened because of impaction. Reduction is easily achieved by manipulation under regional anaesthesia or haematoma block, but slippage is common and percutaneous wires may be chosen for some.

Metacarpals and phalanges

- Fifth metacarpal neck: usually caused by a punch (hence '*Boxer's fracture*'). Up to 60° of flexion at the fracture site can be accepted because of the spare hyperextension in the fifth metacarpophalangeal joint and because the little finger's function is to flex – a loss of extension is not functionally too important. It is treated with elevation and splintage for a few days and then gentle mobilisation. Surgery is rarely required. The 'dropped knuckle' deformity is permanent.
- Metacarpal shaft fractures: most metacarpal fractures are *stable and undisplaced*, and need a resting splint for 1–2 weeks followed by careful mobilisation. If *spiral*, the finger rotates (no longer points to the scaphoid tubercle along with the other fingers when flexed into the palm); if *angulated* the prominent metacarpal head can be uncomfortable when gripping. Therefore some metacarpal fractures need manipulation and fixation with plates or percutaneous Kirschner wires.
- Phalangeal fractures: whatever the fracture and its management, the fingers must be moved within a few days of injury to avoid stiffness. Most phalangeal fractures are *undisplaced* or can be manipulated under local anaesthetic into a stable, anatomical position. The hand is splinted and elevated for a few days then the fractured finger is strapped to a neighbouring finger and mobilised. If the fracture is *displaced and unstable*, or if the *joint surface is disrupted*, accurate reduction and fixation is needed. Rigid fixation with miniplates and screws allows early mobilisation which prevents stiffness, but unfortunately the soft-tissue dissection required paradoxically can cause stiffness. Therefore, percutaneous wires are generally preferred unless open surgery is needed for reduction.

Robert Salter. Professor of Surgery, Children's Hospital, Toronto, Canada.
W. R. Harris. Orthopaedic Surgeon, Toronto, Canada.
Martin Kirschner, 1879–1942. Professor of Surgery, Heidelberg, Germany. Introduced the use of skeletal wires in 1909.
Abraham Colles, 1773–1843. Professor of Surgery, Royal College of Surgeons in Ireland (1804–36) and Surgeon Doctor, Steven's Hospital, Dublin, Ireland. Described this fracture in 1814.

Ligaments

Carpal instability

No tendons attach to the scaphoid, lunate or triquetrum. These bones are called the 'intercalated segment', and their position and stability are controlled by the stout ligaments interconnecting them. Damage to these ligaments, usually after a fall on the outstretched hand, causes the bones to rotate abnormally in relation to each other (Fig. 30.7). If the scapholunate ligament is ruptured, the lunate tilts dorsally and the scaphoid flexes forward; on the posteroanterior radiograph the flexed scaphoid looks like a 'ring' and the scapholunate gap opens up. Early repair and temporary stabilisation with wires should be considered.

Thumb ulnar collateral ligament

The ulnar collateral ligament of the thumb metacarpophalangeal joint is crucial for stable pinch. It can be torn when the thumb is wrenched radially ('skier's thumb'). A relatively stable sprain is splinted for about 3 weeks; an unstable ligament should be repaired; often the adductor pollicis tendon is trapped between the torn ligament and its insertion. The thumb ulnar collateral ligament can also be stretched with chronic overuse ('gamekeeper's thumb').

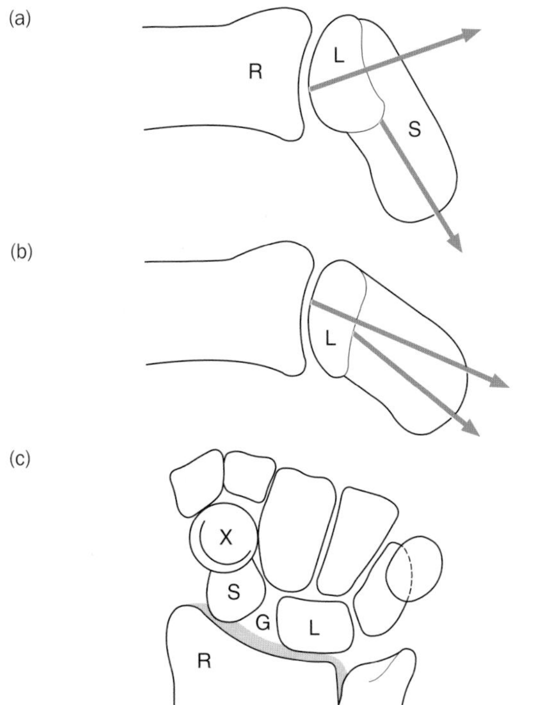

Fig. 30.7 Carpal instability: (a) DISI (dorsal intercalated segment instability) with a flexed scaphoid and extended lunate causing a scapholunate angle greater than 70°; (b) VISI (volar intercalated segment instability) with an extended lunate and scapholunate angle of less than 30°; (c) scapholunate dissociation with a 'ring-shaped' scaphoid and a large gap. R, radius; L, lunate; S, scaphoid; X, ring sign-flexed distal pole of scaphoid; G, scapholunate gap.

Triangular fibrocartilage complex

This important structure attaches the base of the ulnar styloid to the ulnar side of the distal radius. It is continuous with the dorsal and palmar capsule of the ulnar side of the wrist. The TFCC stabilises the distal radioulnar joint. It can be torn, leading to instability of the distal radioulnar joint and ulnar sided wrist pain. The diagnosis is confirmed by arthrography or arthroscopy, and some tears can be repaired.

Dislocations

Perilunate

A fall on the outstretched hand can cause the lunate to dislocate from the surrounding carpus, or for the carpus to dislocate around the lunate. The scaphoid may also be fractured. Median nerve compression may result. The injury is easily missed on radiographs. Prompt reduction should be supplemented by ligament repair and temporary Kirschner wires.

Metacarpophalangeal joints

These can be *simple*, which reduce easily, or *complex*, which usually need open reduction through a dorsal approach because the palmar plate (the thickened palmar capsule) is wedged in the joint.

Bennett's fracture-dislocation

This unstable intra-articular fracture of the thumb carpometacarpal joint is difficult to treat with plaster; closed reduction and percutaneous wire fixation for 5 weeks is more reliable.

Interphalangeal joints

These are usually easy to reduce and are stable. However, an associated fracture of the condyles, tendon avulsion, palmar plate avulsion or collateral ligament tear may need specific treatment.

Tendons

Mallet finger

Forced flexion of the distal interphalangeal joint can rupture the insertion of the long extensor tendon. There may be a bone fragment. Closed reduction and splintage in full extension for 8 weeks is preferable to surgery which has a high complication rate.

Flexor tendons

Flexor tendon injuries have a poor reputation. Surgery is particularly demanding in Bunnell's 'no man's land' – otherwise known as zone II – between the metacarpophalangeal joint and distal interphalangeal joint where both flexor digitorum superficialis and flexor digitorum profundus run in an intricate, tight fibrous sheath (Fig. 30.8). The best outcome is probably with primary repair by an experienced surgeon using special sutures under magnification (Fig. 30.9). Rehabilitation must be meticulous to avoid either *stiffness* or *rupture*. Various splints and mobilisation protocols have been recommended.

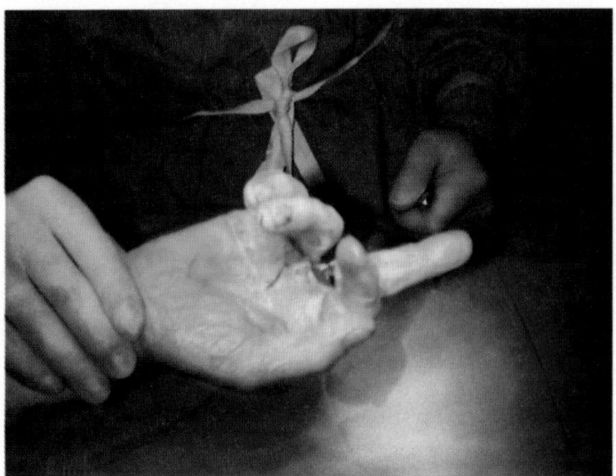

Fig. 30.8 Flexor tendon division – note the alteration of finger posture when the deep and superficial tendons are both divided.

Edward Hallaran Bennett, 1837–1907. Professor of Surgery, Trinity College, Dublin, Ireland.

Sterling Bunnell, 1882–1957. Consultant in hand surgery to the Surgeon General of the United States Army and Navy.

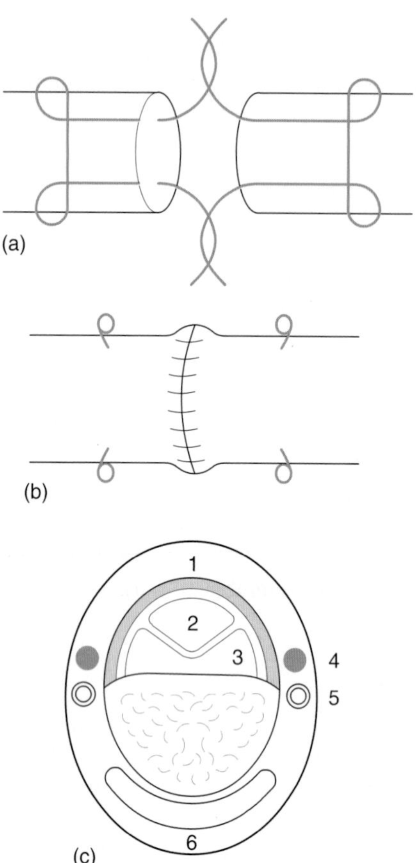

Fig. 30.9 (a) Flexor tendon repair with a core suture supplemented by (b) circumferential suture. (c) The close relationship in 'no man's land' of the: 1, tendon sheath; 2, flexor digitorum profundus; 3, flexor digitorum superficialis. Also: 4, nerve; 5, artery; 6, extensor tendon.

Extensor tendons

Extensor tendon injuries generally have a better outcome than flexor tendon injuries. They usually recover well with careful primary suture and splintage for about 4 weeks. There are two sites where special care must be taken.

- Cuts over the *proximal interphalangeal joint*, if untreated, can lead to a 'boutonnière' (buttonhole) deformity because the central slip no longer extends the proximal joint whilst the remaining extensor mechanism hyperextends the distal joint and flexes the proximal joint. Early repair and splintage is therefore important.
- Cuts over the *metacarpophalangeal joint*, especially following a punch, usually enter the joint and must be thoroughly cleaned.

Fingertip injuries

The choice of treatment depends on the type of injury, as well as the patient's occupation, hobbies and cosmetic demands. Many fingertip injuries will heal when left alone beneath a *semipermeable dressing*. If more than 1 cm^2 of skin is lost, a *skin graft* will speed up the overall time to healing. If the pulp is lost and bone exposed then many techniques are available

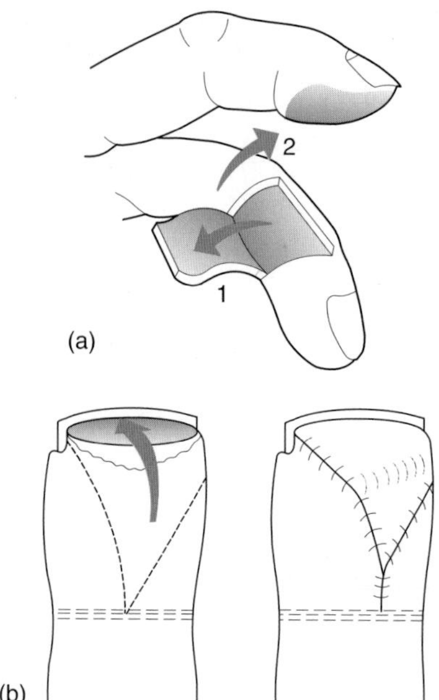

Fig. 30.10 (a) Cross-finger for a palmar oblique fingertip injury with exposed bone. (b) V to Y advancement for a transverse fingertip injury with exposed bone.

to cover the bone and maintain the length of the finger. If early return to manual work is important, then shortening through the distal interphalangeal joint is considered ('*terminalisation*'). Careful attention to detail is important – trimming the condyles, tailoring well-vascularised skin flaps, burying the nerve ends and completely removing the nail bed. If length, sensation and appearance are important (particularly in the thumb and index finger) then a *flap* may be preferred: for example, a cross-finger flap or a V to Y advancement flap (Fig. 30.10).

Replantation

With microsurgical techniques, it is sometimes *both* possible *and* advisable to replant amputated parts (Fig. 30.11).

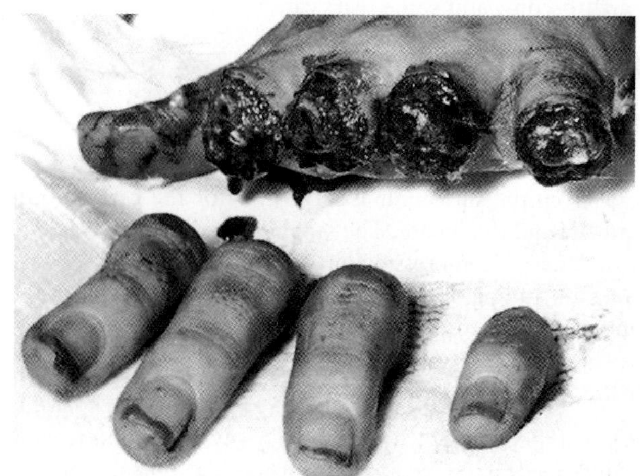

Fig. 30.11 Replantation should be considered for clean-cut amputation of several digits.

Amputated parts should be wrapped in a sterile cloth soaked in sterile saline, and placed in a plastic bag which is placed in water and crushed ice. Replantation is not always advisable. The choice must always be tailored to the individual injury and the individual patient. A single digit replanted proximal to the superficialis insertion is likely to become very stiff, with imperfect sensation and the prospect of a considerable time off work after the first, and often subsequent, surgery. Amputation is often a better option. The thumb, in contrast, functions well enough even if stiff, and replantation should be considered.

> Replantation
>
> Indications:
> - Thumb
> - Single digits in children
> - Single digits at distal interphalangeal joint level
> - Multiple digits
> - Hand, wrist, forearm
>
> Relative contraindications:
> - Single digits in adults
> - Crushed, mangled or avulsed parts
> - Poor general condition of patient
> - Long warm ischaemic time

Infection

Signs include *redness*, *tenderness*, *swelling* (often more apparent on the back of the hand), *lymphangitis* – streaks of red running up the arm – and *lymphadenopathy* (epitrochlear or axillary). Many hand infections will settle within 24–48 hours if elevated, splinted and treated with a best-guess antibiotic. As soon as the signs of inflammation have settled, the hand must be diligently mobilised. If pus appears, it must be drained; the wound should be left open, antibiotics changed according to microbiological advice, and the hand splinted in the Edinburgh position and then mobilised as soon as the inflammation settles.

Acute paronychia

This is the most common infection of the hand, often caused by careless nail trimming or picking the skin around the nail fold (Fig. 30.12). After an initial inflammatory phase, pus is trapped beside the nail. The pus is released by incision on to the nail fold and excision of the outer quarter of the nail.

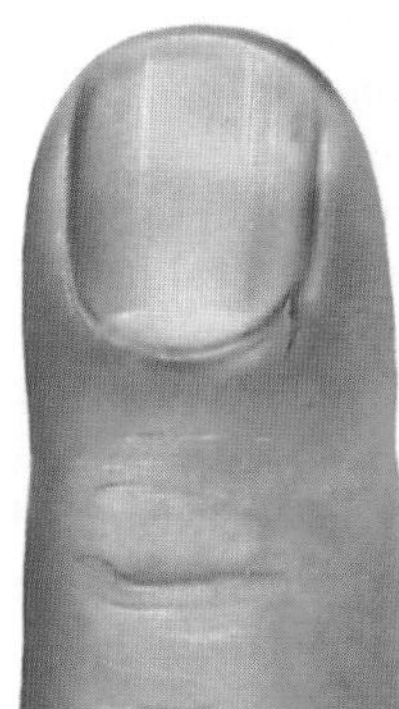

Fig. 30.12 Acute paronychia.

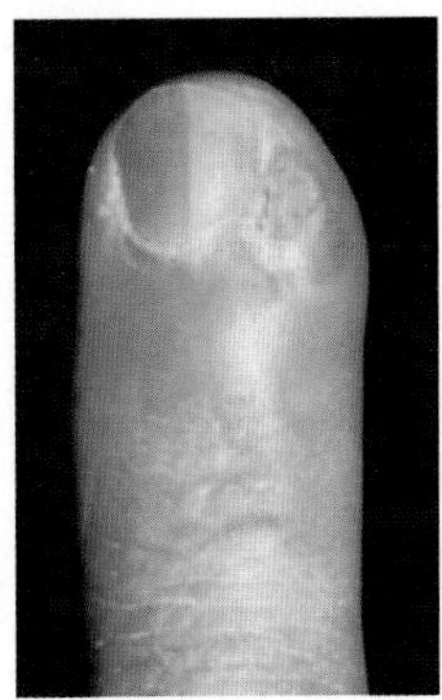

Fig. 30.13 Chronic paronychia.

Chronic paronychia

This appears over several weeks (Fig. 30.13). Rather than a consequence of an acute paronychia, it is usually a chronic fungal infection in those with their hands constantly immersed. Microscopical examination of the scrapings and special fungal cultures will confirm the diagnosis. It may resolve if the hands are kept dry and the nail fold is regularly dressed with antifungal ointment. If this fails, the nail fold is laid open.

Pulp space

Otherwise known as a '*felon*', this causes severe pain in the finger pulp. Pus is trapped between the fibrous septae which bind the specialised fingertip skin to the underlying bone; the bone of the terminal phalanx can also become infected leading to a sequestrum. An abcess should be drained through an oblique incision over the point of greatest tenderness. The differential diagnosis is a *herpetic whitlow*. This is caused by herpes simplex virus and may be found, for example, in dental workers. Small vesicles appear which then become crusty. Surgery should not be performed; it resolves itself over a few weeks.

Flexor tendon sheath infection

There is little spare space within the tendon sheath; an untreated infection rapidly causes adhesions and even tendon necrosis, leading to a stiff, useless finger. The classic signs, described by Kanavel, are a *swollen finger* held in *flexion*, with *exquisite pain on passive extension* and *tenderness precisely* over the flexor sheath. The usual organism is a *Staphylococcus* or a *Streptococcus*. The tendon sheath should be

---

Kanavel, 1874–1938. Professor of Surgery, North Western University, Chicago, Illinois, USA. The fascial spaces were described in his book Infections of the Hand *published in 1933, as well as his sign or point.*

promptly irrigated with normal saline through a fine catheter passed into small incisions over the distal and proximal ends of the sheath. The finger must be moved as soon as the signs of inflammation begin to resolve.

Bites

Serious infection and subsequent loss of function can result from animal or human bites. Human organisms include *Eikenella corridens*; animal bites include *Pasteurella multicodens*. Staphylococci are common in both. These organisms are usually sensitive to broad-spectrum antibiotics such as Augmentin. Wounds should be explored under adequate analgesia and a tourniquet. A common injury is over the knuckle when the opponent's tooth penetrates the metacarpophalangeal joint. The penetration may not be apparent because the four layers (skin, tendon and capsule and synovium) which are injured in *flexion* close over when the knuckle is examined in *extension*. The wound must be excised, the joint thoroughly washed out, and the extensor tendon repaired and splinted.

Other infections

Mycobacterial infections

Tuberculosis in the hand may involve the tenosynovium, joints or bone. The most dramatic is a so-called compound palmar ganglion, with synovial swelling both proximal and distal to the transverse carpal ligament. The diagnosis is confirmed by biopsy. Treatment is by synovectomy and prolonged drug treatment.

Pilonidal sinus

A hair implanted in the palm or web space can cause a cyst with recurrent infection (Fig. 30.14). The cyst should be excised.

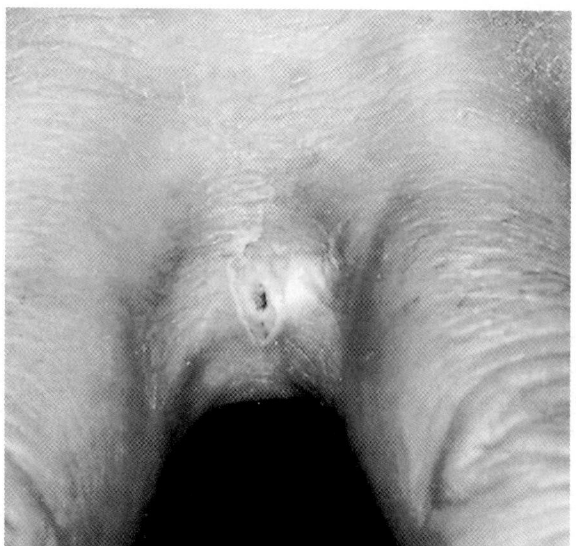

Fig. 30.14 Pilonidal sinus in a barber.

Orf

Transmitted by sheep, this virus causes red papules which become reddish blue and then grey nodules. The condition resolves after a few weeks.

Palmar space infections

Pus can collect deep to the palmar fascia either side of the septum running down to the third metacarpal. The whole hand is swollen and the palm intensely tender. The infection is drained through a longitudinal incision, great care being taken to avoid damage to the tendons, nerves and blood vessels.

Web space infections

Pus can collect in the potential space surrounding the lumbrical muscles as they pass from the palm, across the deep transverse metacarpal ligament into the extensor mechanism. The swelling in the web space tends to spread the adjacent fingers apart. The pus is drained through a longitudinal incision over the web space, taking care not to damage the nearby neurovascular bundles.

Arthritis

Rheumatoid arthritis

Rheumatoid arthritis is a disease which affects many systems and many joints. It can devastate the wrist and hand. The *synovitis* destroys ligaments, tendons and joints, producing pain, deformity and loss of function. *Zig-zag collapse* is typical of rheumatoid arthritis – as one joint deforms in one direction, the next deforms in the opposite (e.g. boutonnière, swan neck, ulnar drift of metacarpophalangeal joints with radial drift of wrist). As the joints deform, the tendons overlying them gain a greater mechanical advantage, leading to greater deformity. Simple *activities of daily living*, such as thumb pinch and opening jars, stress the weakened ligaments and produce worsening deformity (particularly ulnar drift at the metacarpophalangeal joints).

Assessment

For the hand to function well, it must be placed accurately and firmly in place – the elbow, shoulder and wrist must be carefully assessed as well.

History. What are the patient's social circumstance, mobility, occupation and general health? These all influence the treatment that is offered. Which particular joints concern the patient? What is the patient's problem with these joints – pain, instability, weakness, stiffness, appearance? Are there symptoms elsewhere, particularly the shoulder and elbow? What specific functional problems are there?

Examination. Does the patient have a typical pattern of deformity? Are the joints stable or unstable? Is there synovitis in the joints or tendons? What is the active and passive range of movement of each joint? Are these movements painful? Are the tendons intact? Are the muscles weak? Is there a median nerve palsy (from synovitis in the carpal tunnel) or a radial or ulnar nerve palsy (much rarer, from synovitis around the elbow)? Pinch grip and power grip?

Deformities in rheumatoid arthritis

Wrist:
- Radial deviation
- Carpal supination
- Prominent, unstable ulnar head
- Extensor tenosynovitis

Metacarpophalangeal joints:
- Flexion
- Ulnar deviation
- Subluxation, dislocation

Fingers:
- Swan neck
- Boutonniere
- Extensor tendon rupture
- Flexor tendon rupture
- Flexor synovitis
- Congenital deformities

Type	*Example*
Failure of formation	Longitudinal absence-radial (radial club hand), longitudinal absence-ulnar (ulnar club hand), longitudinal absence-central (lobster claw hand)
Failure of differentiation	Syndactyly (fingers joined by skin and sometimes bone)
Duplication	Thumb duplication
Overgrowth	Macrodactyly
Undergrowth	Thumb hypoplasia
Constriction ring syndrome	Simple rings
Generalised skeletal abnormalities	Marfan's, Turner's, Down's, etc.

Nonoperative treatment

Rheumatoid arthritis is best managed with a *team* comprising the patient, physician, physiotherapist, occupational therapist, social worker and surgeon. *Drugs* can reduce symptoms and slow progression. *Resting splints* are helpful during flare-ups. *Appliances* can help with tasks such as turning on taps or opening jars, which would otherwise strain and damage the lax ligaments. *Static splints* stabilise and protect lax joints and improve function.

Surgery

The hand can never be made normal but many patients benefit from carefully planned surgery. Surgery must be tailored for each patient. In general, the shoulders, elbow and wrist should be treated before the hand, and reliable operations (e.g. thumb or wrist fusion) should be undertaken before more uncertain operations (e.g. soft-tissue reconstruction).

There are four indications for surgery:

- pain;
- prevention of progression;
- improving function;
- improving appearance.

Synovectomy of the wrist joint, metacarpophalangeal joints and interphalangeal joints should be considered if medical treatment has failed to control pain, with minimal joint damage on radiographs. Synovectomy of the flexor tendons may be needed if the patient has flexor tendon rupture, poor active finger flexion, trigger finger or carpal tunnel syndrome. Synovectomy of the extensor tendons (often with excision of the distal ulna) removes unsightly swelling and reduces the risk of rupture.

Excision of the distal end of the ulna, often with reconstruction of the associated extensor tendon ruptures, reliably improves pain and function, and prevents extensor tendon rupture.

Replacement of the wrist with silicone or metal–polyethylene implants carries a high risk of failure. Replacement of the metacarpophalangeal joints helps pain and appearance, and the implants can last for a considerable time; the extensor tendons, collateral ligaments and intrinsic tendons all need careful reconstruction to overcome ulnar deviation. Replacement of the proximal interphalangeal joint can maintain some movement but there is an appreciable failure rate.

Fusion of the radiocarpal joint gives a pain-free, stable platform for the hand. An intramedullary pin with bone graft usually suffices. Fusion of the thumb metacarpophalangeal joint and the finger distal interphalangeal joints can considerably improve function by providing stability and removing pain.

Tendon reconstruction is sometimes necessary. A ruptured extensor pollicis longus is treated effectively with an extensor indicis transfer. A ruptured flexor pollicis longus is most reliably treated, if the patient's symptoms need it, by thumb interphalangeal joint fusion. Multiple tendon ruptures on the dorsum of the wrist are managed with side-to-side suture to intact tendons, tendon transfer or a tendon graft.

Swan neck deformity (Fig. 30.15) is caused by imbalance of the flexor and extensor tendons over the finger, subluxation of the metacarpophalangeal joint, tightness of the intrinsic

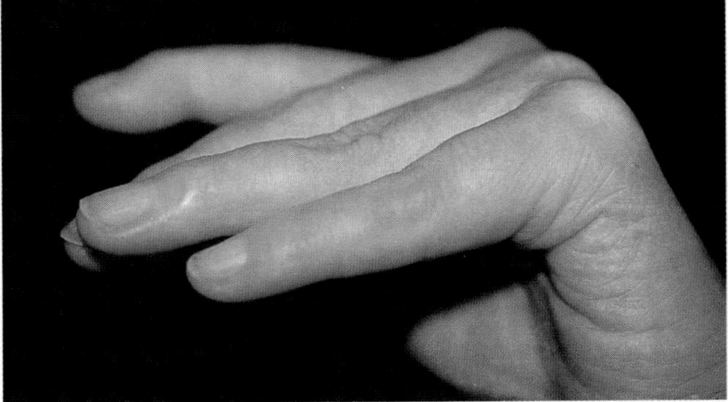

Fig. 30.15 Swan neck deformity.

Bernard-Jean Antonin Marfan, 1858–1942. French paediatrician.
Henry Hubert Turner, b. 1892. American endocrinologist.
John Langdon Down, 1828–96. English physician.

muscles and failure of the palmar plate of the proximal interphalangeal joint. It may need splintage, manipulation, tenodesis, intrinsic muscle release, lateral band release or even fusion depending on the cause and severity.

Osteoarthritis

Wrist

The *radiocarpal joint* may develop osteoarthritis after an intra-articular fracture or infection; it can develop without an obvious cause. If splintage, analgesics and modification of activity fail, then fusion of the wrist at about 20° extension with a dorsal plate and bone graft will give a stable, pain-free wrist. Arthritis may develop around the *scaphoid* after a scaphoid fracture or a scapholunate ligament rupture. If simple measures fail, then bone excision, a limited fusion or total wrist fusion may be needed. The *pisotriquetral joint* can develop osteoarthritis. There is focal tenderness over the joint and 30° supination radiographs show the pathology (Fig. 30.16). If rest, splintage and a steroid injection fail, pisiform excision is helpful.

Hand

Osteoarthritis of the hand is most commonly part of a predisposition to generalised osteoarthritis, particularly in late middle-aged females. Infrequently it follows joint injury or infection. The proximal interphalangeal joints may be involved (Bouchard's nodes), the distal interphalangeal joints (Heberden's nodes) or the carpometacarpal joint of the thumb. The metacarpophalangeal joints and finger carpometacarpal joints are rarely involved. The symptoms do not correlate well with the radiographs. Occasionally surgery is needed. Fusion of the distal interphalangeal joint removes pain and gives good function. The proximal interphalangeal joint can be fused, but the loss of flexion is a significant hindrance; the alternative of replacement with silastic is unreliable. The basal joint of the thumb usually responds to analgesics, steroid injections and splintage. Excision of the trapezium helps the pain but the thumb is weakened. Filling the space with a rolled-up length of palmaris longus, or suspending the base of the first metacarpal with a sling made from part of the flexor carpi radialis tendon, may improve stability of the thumb.

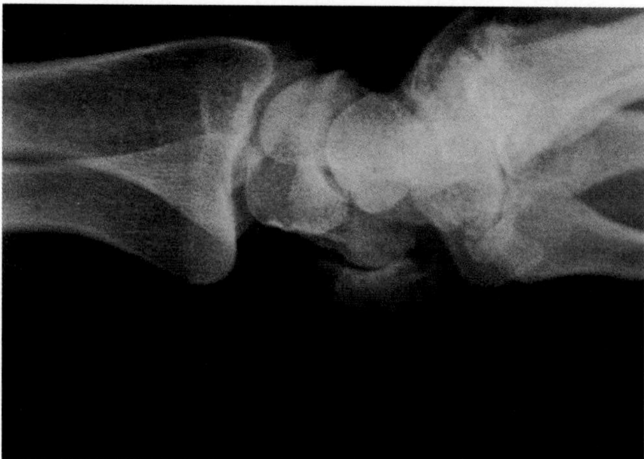

Fig. 30.16 Pisotriquetral arthritis.

William Heberden, 1710–1801. Physician, London, England.

Other forms of arthritis

Gout can easily be mistaken for a septic arthritis in the wrist or finger joints. The diagnosis is confirmed by measuring the serum urate and examining the joint aspirate under a microscope. In more chronic forms, tophi are seen beneath the skin and bone can be eroded. Gout can also cause tenosynovitis leading to trigger finger or carpal tunnel syndrome. *Psoriasis* often involves the joints of the hand and wrist. The nails are pitted and bone may resorb.

Dupuytren's contracture

The condition is inherited as an autosomal dominant trait and is more common in males, with age, smoking, pulmonary tuberculosis, epilepsy, acquired immunodeficiency syndrome (AIDS) and alcoholic cirrhosis. It is usually found in those of Anglo-Saxon descent. Myofibroblasts in the palmar fascia proliferate and contract. Initially, there is a nodular swelling in the palm. The overlying skin then puckers. Cords running into the fingers contract causing a flexion deformity of the metacarpophalangeal and proximal interphalangeal joints. The skin over the back of the proximal interphalangeal joints may thicken (Garrod's knuckle pads – Fig. 30.17) and a few patients may have thickening in the penis (Peyronie's disease) or on the sole of the foot (Ledderhose's disease).

Surgery is advised if the deformity is a nuisance or if the deformity is rapidly progressing, especially at the proximal interphalangeal joint where it soon becomes irreversible.

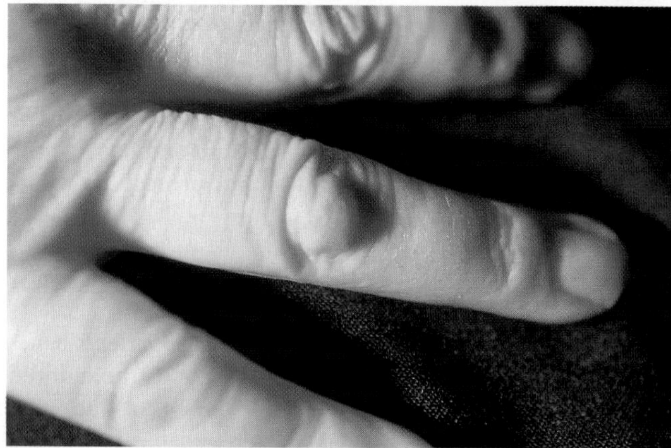

Fig. 30.17 Garrod's knuckle pads.

Sir Alfred Baring Garrod, 1819–1907. British physician. Professor of Medicine, University College of London and then King's College Hospital, London, England.

Francois de la Peyronie, 1678–1747. Surgeon to Louis XIV and founder of the Royal Academy of Surgery, Paris, France.

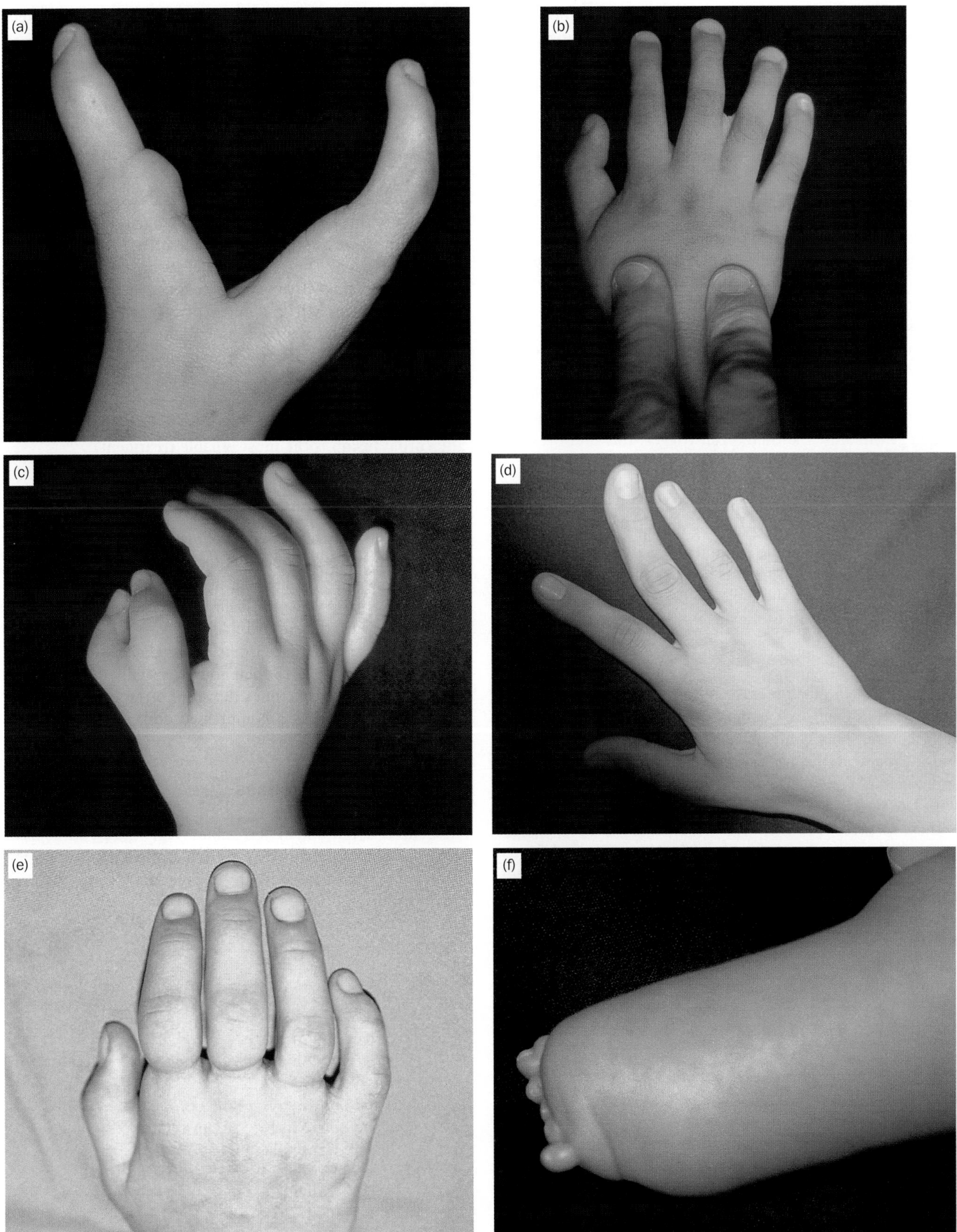

Fig. 30.18 Congenital differences: (a) cleft hand; (b) syndactyly; (c) thumb duplication; (d) macrodactyly; (e) constriction rings; (f) transverse deficiency.

During surgery, care must be taken to avoid the neurovascular bundles. Z-plasties can provide extra skin but occasionally full-thickness skin grafts are needed. The palm wound can be left open – it will heal rapidly with dressings. Surgery is not curative and recurrence is very common.

Tendon disorders

Trigger finger

For reasons which are often obscure, the opening of the flexor tendon sheath (the A1 pulley) thickens and snares the tendon which may secondarily develop a small nodule. When the proximal interphalangeal joint is flexed it locks and then snaps into extension. This often starts only on awakening, and then gradually occurs more frequently during the day. If it does not resolve with a steroid injection into the sheath, then release of the pulley at the level of the metacarpophalangeal joint (distal palmar crease) is successful, watching for the neurovascular bundle. In infants, the thumb can trigger; this often resolves spontaneously by the age of 1 year, but if not surgery is needed, being aware that in the thumb the digital nerves run close to the midline (not the midlateral line as they run in the fingers). In *rheumatoid arthritis*, the triggering is caused either by synovitis or by a nodule in the tendon. Synovectomy, and if necessary excision of a slip of flexor digitorum superficialis, is safer than division of the pulley – the latter can worsen the tendency to ulnar drift of the metacarpophalangeal joints.

De Quervain's disease

The extensor pollicis brevis tendon and abductor pollicis longus tendon run in a compartment beneath the extensor retinaculum. This compartment can constrict the tendons, causing pain at the base of the thumb. Usually occurring spontaneously in middle-aged women, it is also associated with late pregnancy and overuse. Finkelstein's test is positive – there is pain over the radial side of the wrist when the patient's thumb is grasped and the hand is quickly abducted ulnarward. Splintage, nonsteroidal anti-inflammatory medication, steroid injection and ultrasound may help. Surgical decompression is often required, avoiding the superficial radial nerve (lest a very troublesome neuroma occurs) and remembering that there are often extra septae and slips of tendon – the condition will persist if these are overlooked.

Carpal tunnel syndrome

This is common. The typical patient awakens with painful tingling over the radial side of the hand; there is often loss of fine dexterity because of weakness of the abductor pollicis brevis muscle and altered sensation over the thumb, index and middle fingertips. On examination, Tinel's percussion sign is positive over the carpal tunnel and Phalen's test may be positive (tingling in the hand when the wrist is fully flexed). In advanced cases, the thenar eminence is wasted. The diagnosis, if not certain clinically, is confirmed with electrophysiology. Treatment includes splinting the wrist in extension at night, injecting steroid into the carpal canal and surgical release of the transverse carpal ligament.

Fritz De Quervain, 1868–1940. Professor of Surgery, Berne, Switzerland.

Kienbock's disease

The aetiology is unclear, but probably involves both ischaemia and microtrauma in the lunate, causing sclerosis initially, then collapse and finally arthritis. Many patients have a relatively short ulna ('negative ulnar variance'). Patients complain of pain and weakness in the wrist. Very early, bone scan or MRI can detect disease before it shows on plain radiographs. Treatment is initially conservative, with splintage, avoidance of activity and simple analgesics. Surgical shortening of the radius reduces the compressive forces across the lunate and may help those with early disease. In advanced cases with painful osteoarthritis around the lunate, radiocarpal fusion is the most reliable treatment.

Ganglion cysts

These are the most common swellings in the hand. Patients present with concern about the lump and occasionally with pain. The swelling is smooth, well defined, fluctuant and transilluminable. A few resolve with aspiration or compression ('hitting with the family bible'). Surgery should be meticulous otherwise recurrence is likely. Ganglia around the wrist should be traced down to their source, usually the scapholunate ligament and sometimes the scapho-trapezio-trapezioid joint. Histology shows a compressed collagen sheath filled with a mucoid substance.

Congenital differences

These affect about one in 500 babies (Fig. 30.18). Some have a clear genetic cause, while others may follow an intrauterine insult during the second month of pregnancy when the limb buds are forming. These need careful management of both child and parent; surgery is challenging and the patients are best referred to a specialist.

Further reading

American Society for Surgery of the Hand (1996) *Hand Surgery Update*, American Academy of Orthopaedic Surgeons, Rosemount IL.

Brand, P.W. and Hollister, A. (1993) *Clinical Mechanics of the Hand*, 2nd edn, Mosby, St Louis, MO.

Flatt, A.E. (1995) *The Care of the Arthritic Hand*, 5th edn, QMP, St Louis.

Green, D.P. (ed.) (1998) *Operative Hand Surgery*, 3rd edn, Churchill Livingstone, New York.

Lister, G.D. (1993) *The Hand – Diagnosis and Indications*, 3rd edn, Churchill Livingstone, Edinburgh.

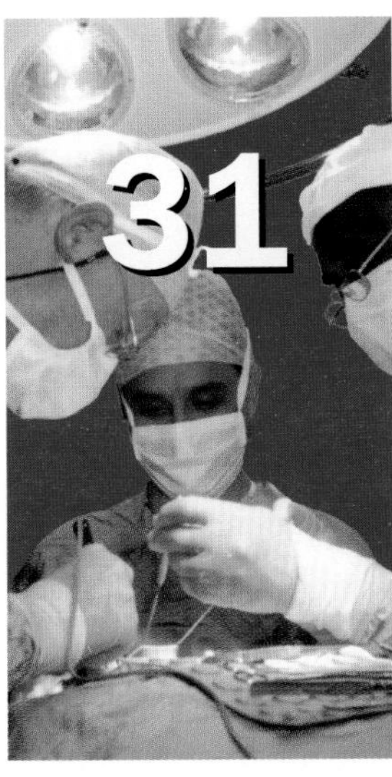

31 The foot

Congenital abnormalities

Congenital abnormalities in the foot can be divided into minor and major abnormalities. Minor congenital abnormalities include many conditions which are inherited. These abnormalities rarely cause significant problems. They largely constitute toe abnormalities such as syndactyly or curly toes; these variations are not uncommon and rarely need any treatment. Congenital hallux varus is not common but can require surgery if severe or progressive. Hallux valgus is surprisingly rare considering its incidence in the adult population. Major abnormalities include genetic disorders, major chromosomal malformations, and failure of formation or differentiation. In addition, there are several conditions which, although present in the newborn child, do not fit into these headings. They can be described as either structural or postural deformities.

Of the major deformities clubfoot or talipes equinovarus is the commonest (Fig. 31.1). It has a familial incidence (one in 1000 live births reduces to one in 35 live births if one sibling is affected) and it has a varied incidence with different ethnic groups (Maoris having the highest incidence). Although this suggests a genetic propensity it seems likely there is a multifactorial mode of inheritance. The exact mechanism of the production of the deformity is unknown; it seems likely that a number of different conditions produces the same deformity. This should be taken into account when planning treatment.

Treatment

Treatment of talipes equinovarus needs to commence within 24 hours of birth. Various techniques for strapping or taping

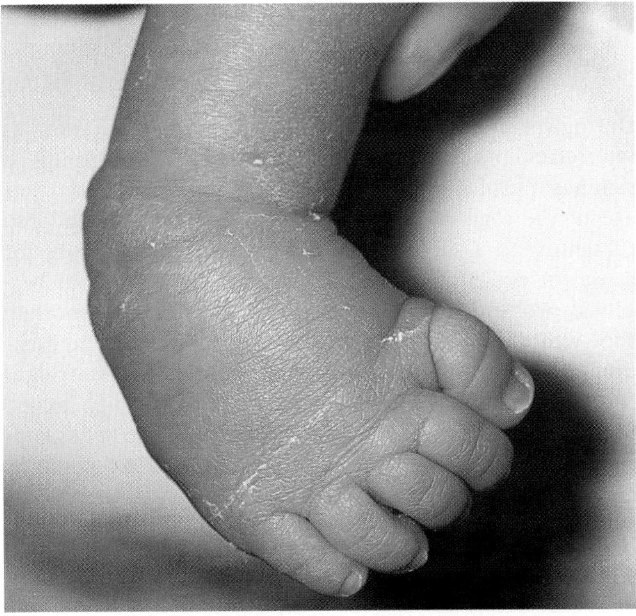

Fig. 31.1 Unilateral talipes equinovarus showing the typical features of equinus, varus, midfoot adduction and forefoot supination.

Bailey & Love's Short Practice of Surgery, 23rd edition. Edited by R.C.G. Russell, N.S. Williams and C.J.K. Bulstrode. Published in 2000 by Arnold Publishers.

the foot or the use of plaster of Paris or special splints have been advocated. What is common to all of these techniques is the need for early treatment and the careful attention to detail. This form of treatment should go on for at least 3 months and, no matter what, should be followed by a period of stretching undertaken by the parents and a suitable therapist. At this stage care should be taken to avoid stretching the midfoot into a rocker bottom foot position in an attempt to correct tight posterior structures. If early treatment is instigated then between 30 and 40 per cent of feet will correct sufficiently not to require surgery.

The remainder of the feet will require surgical correction. Although there is a great deal of controversy about the exact timing of surgery, the extent of surgery and the expected functional result, most authors would advocate that it is undertaken during the first year of life. The aim of surgery is to achieve the best functional result. By ensuring that the foot can be placed in plantigrade (or flat to the floor) position this is likely to be associated with the most satisfactory result. This will require an adequate posterior release to allow the foot to dorsiflex actively at the ankle. The subtalar and midtarsal joints need to be released to allow the primary rotational deformity to be reduced. In many cases this will involve both medial and lateral releases. Continued therapy and splintage should then back up the surgery, having achieved adequate correction, during the first years of life. In particular, the weakness of the peroneal tendons seen in many cases will not improve until at least 18 months of age. Children with this condition should be monitored throughout the period of growth. The genetic propensity for the deformity is likely to continue to be expressed throughout the growing period.

Other major congenital deformities need treatment on their merits with the aim of achieving the best functional result for the child.

Developmental problems

During the period in which the foot is growing a variety of interrelated problems can arise. These fall into two groups of significant problems but represent a relatively small percentage of the total population. The vast majority of children presenting to a surgeon will in fact be normal. The major cause for presentation will be parental concern about perceived problems about the shape of the foot or abnormal shoe wear. The two groups of disorder, foot shape and function, are the conditions leading to a progressive planovalgus (or flat) foot and those that lead to pes cavus or a high arched foot. Some of the toe conditions start to become symptomatic in the childhood years but only in adolescence does the condition of hallux valgus appear as a significant developmental abnormality.

Planovalgus foot

The flat foot is normal providing that the longitudinal arch rises and falls dynamically. In activities such as standing on tiptoes the longitudinal arch rises. This is the basis of the clinical test of great toe dorsiflexion (Fig. 31.2). It is this that allows the body to store energy in the foot during walking. This in turn allows efficient, low-energy-cost locomotion.

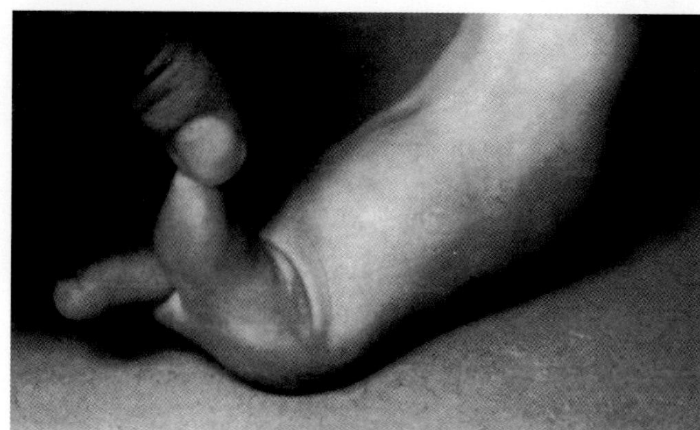

Fig. 31.2 Great-toe extension test to tighten plantar fascia and show the normal arch mechanism.

The flat foot becomes pathological when one of three things happens. First, anything which stops movement in one of the joints of the hindfoot will simply prevent the normal behaviour of this mechanism. The condition of tarsal coalition is the most obvious example of this. This is where there is an abnormal join (fibrous or bony) between two or more tarsal bones.

Second, conditions which affect the integrity of the primary restraints of the various joints involved will result in instability. This leads to the foot deforming into a valgus heel position and into an abducted (and supinated) forefoot position. Conditions such as Marfan's syndrome are examples of this form of problem. Commoner is familial hypermobility, but only a few of these patients exhibit pathological foot function.

Third, imbalance between the secondary restraints can cause progressive deformity. The best example of this is in neurological conditions such as cerebral palsy. Here the spasm in the peroneal muscle groups overcomes the action of the inverters of the foot. The hindfoot is gradually pulled into valgus. This in turn leads to stretching of primary restraints. If the deforming force is unresisted for long enough, the effect is to produce bony deformity; this fixes the deformity. Although this pattern of developing deformity can be applied to the adolescent foot, it also underlies the pattern of development of a progressive planovalgus foot in any age group. In the elderly rupture of the tibialis posterior tendon will cause imbalance of the secondary restraints.

Bernard-Jean Antonin Marfan, 1858–1942. French paediatrician.

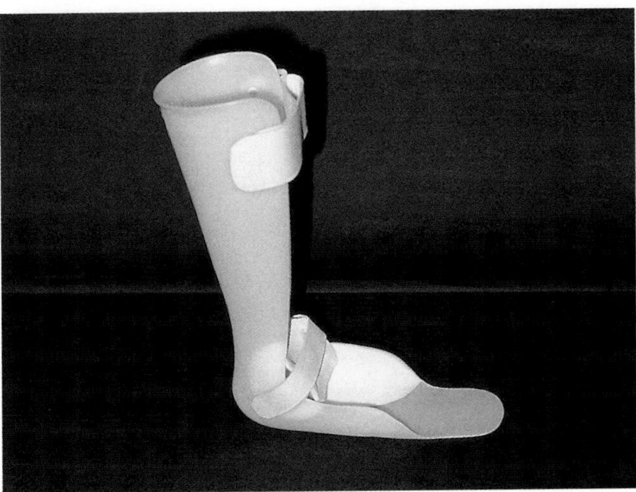

Fig. 31.3 A standard ankle foot orthosis (AFO).

Treatment

This will obviously be dependent on the underlying cause of the progressive deformity.

Primary treatment should always be conservative in nature. In the foot with increased mobility the use of orthoses will control the foot position while a shoe is worn. This diminishes the pressure on the foot created by the shoe; thus the symptoms due to pressure effects are reduced. The shoe itself is less likely to deform and produce abnormal wear contributing to the pressure on the foot. There is no evidence that such devices influence the long-term outcome for the foot. Corrective orthoses in conditions where the deformity is fixed, as in a coalition, do not work. In these circumstances orthoses should be used to increase the cushioning available in the foot. This can reduce symptoms by reducing the forces passing through the foot. Rest and modification of activity can have a profound effect on the symptoms that the patient experiences. This can mean that despite the rigidity of the foot the patient is pain free and has reasonable function. If the joints involved are irritable and painful an injection of a local anaesthetic agent with an intra-articular steroid injection can reduce symptoms until the child is older.

In the neurological conditions such as cerebral palsy, physiotherapy including stretching exercises has a role to play. This allows the imbalance to be corrected passively. The use of ankle foot orthoses to maintain the position of the foot is helpful (Fig. 31.3). If the increased tone in the peroneal and calf muscles is a particular problem then botulinum toxin injections into the muscle bellies can be useful. The effect wears off within days but during the period of reduced spasm the benefit of surgical treatment can be assessed in the knowledge that the paralysis will wear off in the fullness of time. During the period when the toxin is active physiotherapy may overcome the deformity further providing a longer-term benefit.

The principle of surgical treatment is first to balance the forces acting on the foot to remove the deforming forces; second, to correct any deformity that has already developed; third, to stabilise the foot in order to prevent deformity from recurring.

- Release of fixed deformity. This could be soft tissue (as in lengthening the peroneal tendons) or bony (as in the excision of a tarsal coalition).
- Correcting bony deformity. This can be achieved by lengthening the lateral border of the foot using a modified distraction osteotomy originally described by Dillwyn Evans (Fig. 31.4) or by an osteotomy of the os calcis designed to transfer the contact point of the calcaneum medially.
- Balancing the secondary restraints. This may involve tightening of the inverters of the foot. This may include formal reconstruction of the tibialis posterior tendon.
- Reconstructing the primary medial restraints such as the talonavicular joint capsule.

If these principles cannot be achieved then fusion of some or all of the joints of the hindfoot (as in a triple arthrodesis) will allow correction of foot position, reduce pain from damaged joints and prevent recurrence of the deformity.

Pes cavus

The mechanism of the generation of the deformity of the high arch foot is less easy to understand. This is partly because a number of conditions leads to similar although not identical deformity. The common feature of the condition is some element of neurological dysfunction. This leads to the problem of muscle imbalance. The intrinsic muscles are weak leading to a mismatch between the intrinsic and extrinsic muscle power. With equinus deformity the Achilles tendon is tight. This is not an invariable feature of pes cavus and in conditions where the calf muscles are weak there is a calcaneus deformity. In addition there is a group of patients who have a relatively higher inverter power than everter power. This will lead to the foot rotating so that the lateral border is mainly in contact with the floor.

The clinical presentation of patients with pes cavus most commonly occurs in late childhood or early adolescence when the presence of the deformity becomes more obvious. The deformity is obviously influenced by growth but can progress after growth has ceased. Symptoms which are usually present are increased pressure on the forefoot due to clawing of the toes and equinuus, pain on the lateral border of the foot due to a varus heel position and finally feelings of

Dillwyn Evans, 1910–74. Orthopaedic surgeon, Cardiff, Wales.

Achilles, the Greek hero, son of Peleus and Thetis. As a child his mother dipped him in the River Styx, so that he should be invulnerable in battle. The heel by which she held him did not get wet and was therefore unprotected. Achilles died from a wound in the heel, received at the siege of Troy.

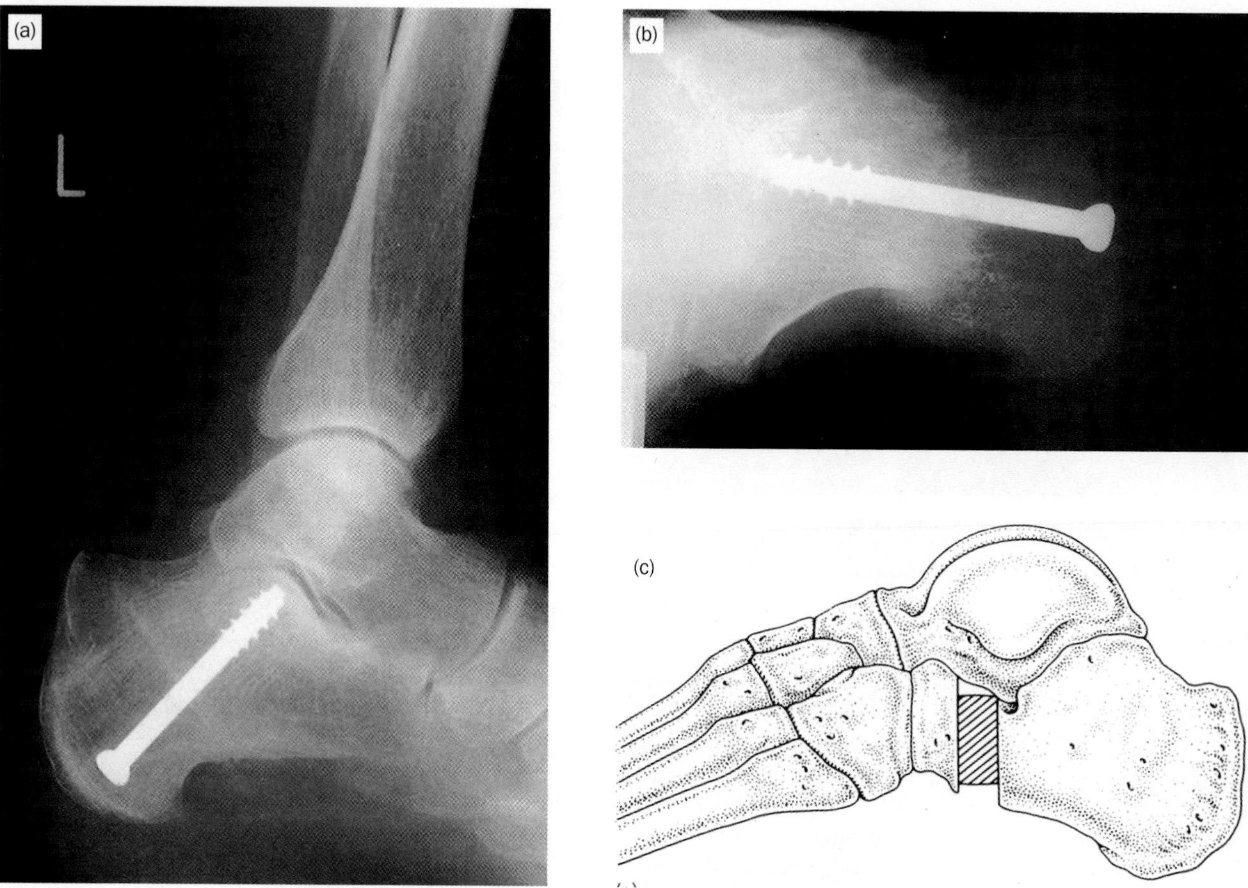

Fig. 31.4 Medial displacement osteotomy. (a) Lateral view; (b) axial view of medial displacement osteotomy; (c) insertion of bone graft in lateral border of foot to lengthen it (Dillwyn Evan's procedure).

insecurity and weakness. Where there is an associated sensory neuropathy, patients can suffer with ulceration. Patients generally need to be monitored to analyse the rate and nature of progressive change.

Because of the variations in specific aetiology, and the progression and nature of the deformity, various management options need to be considered. The use of conservative treatment is important and largely revolves round the use of appropriate shoeware. Shoes need to have extra depth to accommodate toe deformities. The sole needs to be cushioned to absorb the excess pressure. Adjustments can be made to the sole of the shoe with outside wedges to create a corrective force on the outer border of the foot. The same effect can be achieved with insoles. If conservative treatment fails then surgical options need to be considered. With any part of the deformity the first thing to consider is

Table 31.1 Management options in pes cavus

	Mobile	*Fixed*
Claw toes with metatarsalgia	Flexor to extensor transfer and Jones extensor Transfer for great toe	IP joint fusion Extensor to neck of metatarsal Basal dorsiflexion osteotomy of the metatarsals
Plantaris	Extensors to metatarsal necks	Basal dorsiflexion osteotomy Or midfoot wedge osteotomy
Plantaris with hindfoot varus	Extensors to metatarsal necks and tibialis anterior transfer	Jappas type osteotomy + or − tendon transfers
Equinus with plantaris	Tendo–Achilles (TA) lengthening	TA lengthening and midfoot osteotomy
Equinus with varus	TA lengthening plus calcaneal and tibialis posterior transfer	Triple arthrodesis

Sir Robert Jones, 1853–1933. Orthopaedic surgeon, Royal Southern Hospital, England, and nephew of Hugh Owen Thomas.

whether it is mobile or fixed. In general terms mobile deformities can be corrected by soft tissue surgery. Fixed deformity requires bony or joint surgery. An algorithm for the management of pes cavus has to be based on the type of deformity and the nature of the clinical complaint (Table 31.1).

Although this guide gives a concept of the procedures that have to be considered when treating the cavus foot, there is a great variation in the pattern of deformity with different aetiologies. The deformity can progress throughout life. This again has to be taken into account in planning the management of each individual case (Figure 31.5).

Acquired foot problems

Injury

The foot is one of the commonest sites of injury in the body. Because of its relatively rigid structure a great deal of force is necessary to injure the hindfoot. The forefoot including the toes is relatively exposed and therefore susceptible to injury. Also, the high forces going through the foot mean that it is a common site for stress fractures. The principles of fracture management are discussed elsewhere. The foot does present particular difficulties in diagnosis because of the complexity of local bony and joint anatomy. This means that the importance of careful history taking, examination and investigation cannot be emphasised enough. The commonest missed injury is a tarsometatarsal dislocation.

In all foot injuries the full extent of the injury needs to be appreciated, with soft-tissue injuries often being associated with bony injuries. Postinjury rehabilitation is important to treat these elements of the injury.

Infection

Infections in the foot can be considered to be minor and common, or major and fortunately rarer. With a significant proportion of the world's population remaining barefoot, minor skin trauma is a frequent cause of local infection. In the shod population poor shoe fitting has the same effect. The increased incidence of diabetes means that this is now a potent cause of major infections. With the combination of vascular insufficiency, neuropathy and poor cellular function, infection due to diabetes can be extremely difficult to treat. This has considerable implications for the patient. It is also part of why diabetes and its complications represent the greatest single cost drain on many health services in the world.

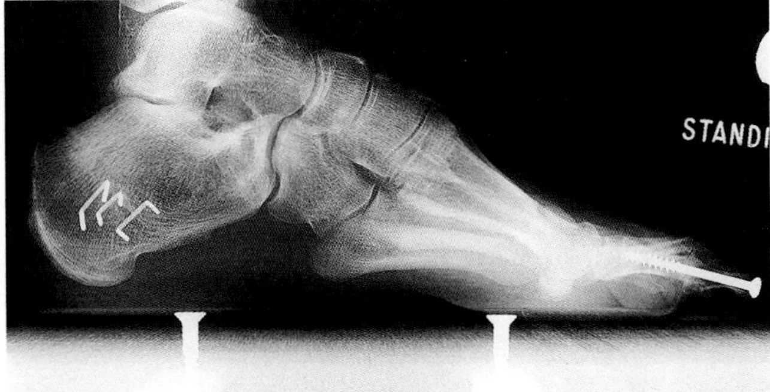

Fig. 31.5 Surgery for pes cavus may have to involve both forefoot and hindfoot procedures to balance the foot, here an os calcis osteotomy in combination with a Jones procedures to correct the position of the great toe.

A careful history and examination must be aimed at elucidating predisposing factors, assessing the extent of the infection, including evidence of more generalised spread. Even with relatively minor bacterial infections lymphatic spread is not uncommon. This leads to lymphangitis and involvement of regional lymph nodes. Investigations must be aimed at establishing the extent of the infection, the nature of the organism involved and any increased risk factors such as poor peripheral blood supply or diabetes. Wound swabs, culture of discharged material and skin scrapings or nail clippings can be helpful in identifying the organism. A full blood count, plasma viscosity, blood sugar and blood cultures can be helpful in determining the exact diagnosis and monitoring the benefit of treatment. Plain X-rays remain the baseline investigation of deeper infection, but newer investigation modalities such as magnetic resonance imaging (MRI) can give extremely helpful information on the deeper spread of infection and particularly address the issue of soft-tissue spread.

Basic principles of management involve rest, elevation, antibiotics and, where necessary, surgical débridement. Regular dressings are needed. Desloughing agents and dressings which keep the recovering granulation tissue moist are important.

Minor infections

These include a variety of extremely common conditions including fungal infections, varrucas, infected blisters, infected bursitis and ingrowing toenails. Associated with ingrowing toenails are paronychia, which need formal surgical drainage. Infections created by chronic or repetitive trauma need the underlying cause treating in order to prevent their recurrence. A good example of this is the ingrowing toenail. This will usually need surgical treatment to get it to settle once infection has been established for any length of time. If the infection is severe simple nail removal maybe sufficient to settle the infection but recurrence is relatively common. Wedge resection of the border of the nail and the associated nail bed is the treatment of choice in most cases; this can be aided by phenolisation. It is important to neutralise the phenol on the nail after application. In some cases complete resection of the nail and nail bed (Zadik's procedure) may be necessary.

Fungal infections are relatively common and can be important as they can cause generalised discomfort that can

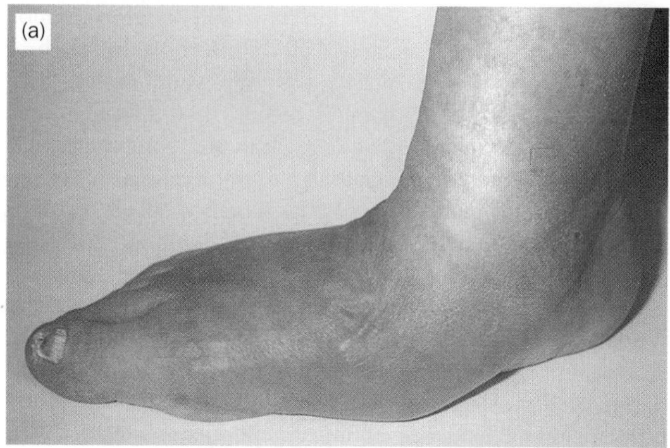

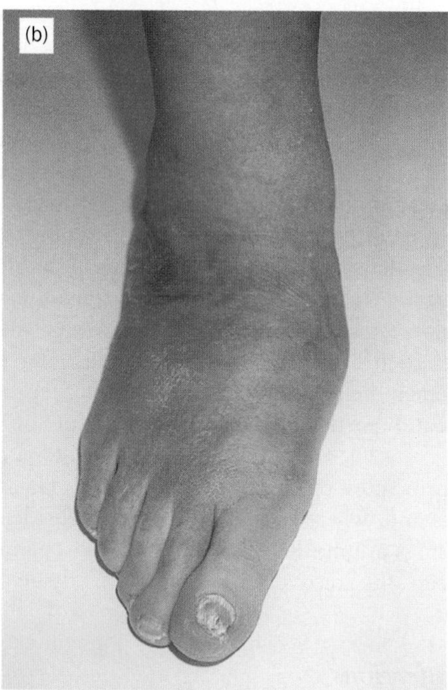

Fig. 31.6 Severe deformity resulting from Charcot changes in the midfoot.

be mistaken for mechanical causes of pain. In addition they commonly affect the nails leading to nail thickening and distortion (onychogryphosis) which in itself can lead to mechanical symptoms.

Major infections

Diabetes accounts for a substantial number of the major foot infections seen. These may be superficial, often associated with ulceration. Deeper infection may involve soft tissues only with abscess formation or can involve bones (osteitis or osteomyelitis). This type of infection can also involve local joints (pyogenic arthritis). The presence of poor vascularity and neuropathy further complicates both diagnosis and management. Neuropathy can lead to Charcot changes in the foot, disrupting joint stability and foot architecture (Fig. 31.6). This leads to increased pressure under the sole of the foot due to the loss of the normal capacity of the foot to absorb load. In addition the bony disruption produces a high incidence of prominence under the sole. This then leads to ulceration. There is a progression from this superficial form of infection through deep infection and abscess formation to osteomyelitis. If not brought under rapid control this will go on to gangrene.

Treatment

If ulceration is present without the presence of deeper infection the clear aim is to heal the skin. After desloughing the ulcer and removing hyperkeratotic skin the ulcer can be dressed locally. The application of a skin-tight plaster of Paris changed on a weekly basis will allow the vast majority of ulcers to heal. It also allows the patient to be mobile. Deep infection without abscess formation can be treated by strict rest, elevation, soft-tissue support and antibiotics. Any form of abscess needs to be drained urgently and the deeper tissues thoroughly débrided. Ulcers which are deeply penetrating in certain sites are more of a problem than elsewhere. The heel is a particular problem in that ulcers lead to a permanent loss of the heel pad. Once an ulcer is healed the use of appropriate insoles and shoes can prevent further ulceration this is much more difficult to achieve when the ulcer has been in the heel.

When fixed deformity occurs as a consequence of neuropathy or Charcot changes due consideration should be given to corrective surgery. The stage of development of the Charcot changes has to be considered. The changes progress through three stages. Stage 1 involves generalised inflammation and fragmentation of bone. In stage 2 the inflammation starts to settle and the bone starts to show signs of

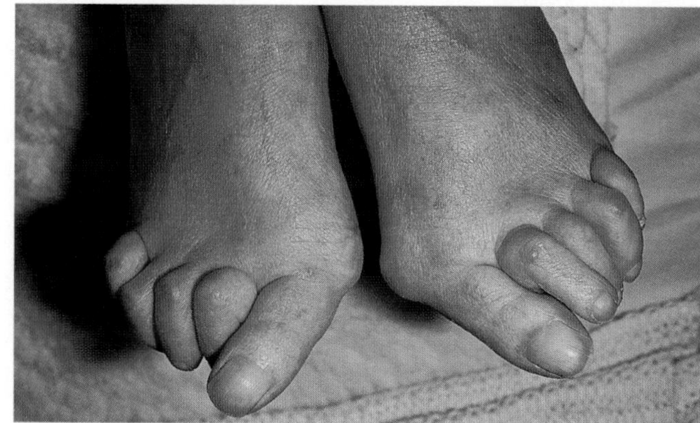

Fig. 31.7 The forefoot is often severely involved in rheumatoid arthritis.

Frank Raphael Zadik, b. 1914. Former orthopaedic surgeon, Wigan Health Authority, England.

Jean-Martin Charcot, 1825–93. French neurologist.

healing. In stage 3 the bone consolidates. Once the changes become stable, surgery to correct deformity, produce stability and reduce any high pressure points can be undertaken.

Ultimately if tissues are clearly not viable then an appropriate amputation should be planned. This should be undertaken at a level where there is a realistic chance of the wound healing.

Other serious infections

Probably the commonest serious 'primary' infection is seen in the madura foot. The causative organism of this is *Nocardia madurae*; this is a filamentous organism similar to actinomyces. World-wide its incidence is still high, affecting particularly populations in the Asian subcontinent and in Africa who go barefoot. It is also has an increased incidence in other areas of the world including southern USA, the South American states and the West Indies. The organism almost certainly gains access to the foot through minor penetrating injuries or splits in the skin. Subsequently the foot forms multiple painless nodules, which ultimately form vesicular eruptions. These ulcerate and form sinuses. These then become secondarily infected. Treatment involves rest, elevation, and antibiotics for the secondary infection and protracted treatment with dapsone or similar agents. Ultimately if the infection persists and leads to disability then amputation can be considered.

Other types of major infection include tuberculosis, bacterial osteomyelitis and/or arthritis, and finally infections such as guinea worm.

Arthritis

Arthritis affecting the foot is a common event in an ageing population. The vast majority will be osteoarthritis.

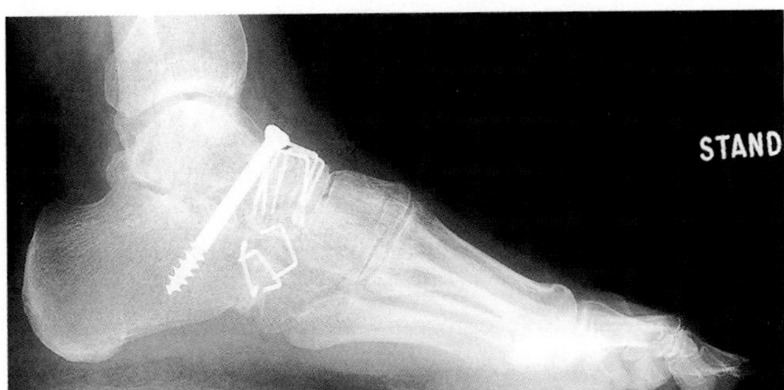

Fig. 31.8 The pain arising from hindfoot deformity can often only by controlled by fusing the subtalar and midtarsal joints, a triple arthrodesis.

The most common joint affected is the first metatarsophalangeal joint.

Inflammatory arthropathies frequently produce foot problems. In rheumatoid arthritis the forefoot is the first part affected. Up to 40 per cent of patients suffering with rheumatoid arthritis regard their feet as being their most troublesome area. Other forms of inflammatory arthritis are also seen in the foot. Of particular note is psoariatic arthritis, which is commonly missed. It is a particular cause of symptoms following minor trauma. Gout is also a cause of a sudden acute arthritis.

Rheumatoid changes

Rheumatoid arthritis creates symptoms in three ways. In the early stages of the disease, pain may be caused by the presence of inflamed synovium, usually in the forefoot and the subtalar joint. It can also affect the tendon sheaths. If the synovitis persists the ligaments and tendons can be damaged and rupture. This means that the joints become unstable, and deform. The toes dislocate at the metatarsophalangeal joints

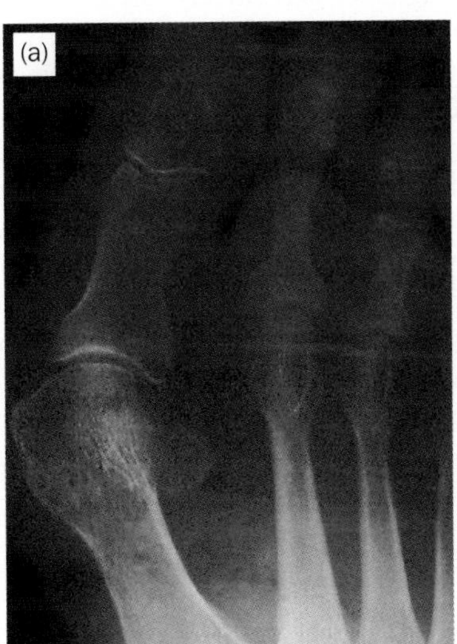

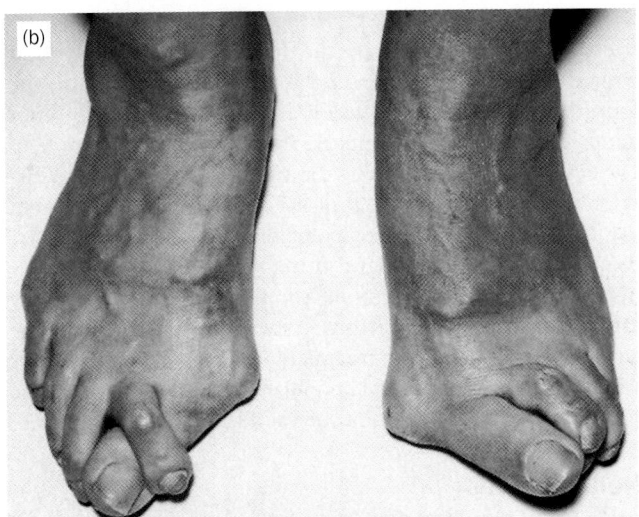

Fig. 31.9 (a) Radiograph of the foot with hallux valgus and metatarsus primus varus. (b) Appearance of the feet with hallux valgus. A bunion is present in both feet, and bunionette is over the head of the fifth right metatarsal. Note the variation of over-riding of the second toes – in both there is a callosity over the proximal interphalangeal joint;

(Fig. 31.7). This produces fixed clawing, with the metatarsal heads being prominent in the sole of the foot. In the hindfoot a combination of instability of the subtalar joint and rupture of the tibialis posterior tendon will produce a progressive planovalgus foot. The synovitis also damages the joint surface.

Patients suffering from an inflammatory arthropathy will complain of pain and swelling in the affected joints. Subsequently, progressive deformity and arthritic change result in metatarsalgia. Pain over the medial side of the foot due to the progressive lateral tilt of the foot is common. Impingement between the calcaneum and the lateral malleolus produces pain on the lateral side. Stress fractures of the lateral malleolus can occur. The secondary osteoarthritis will cause pain in its own right.

Treatment

During the early stages the aim of treatment is to reduce the synovitis and to manage associated pain. Nonsteroidal anti-inflammatory agents are the first-line drugs. Additional pain relief can be obtained from well-cushioned shoes. If drugs do not bring swelling under control, synovectomy should be considered. Once deformity has occurred the treatment is aimed at controlling symptoms. Shoes with cushion insoles and extra depth to allow for toe deformities should be used. If forefoot symptoms persist, surgical correction of the toe deformities should be undertaken, aimed at reducing the symptoms of metatarsalgia. The exact technique used for correcting the forefoot remains controversial. The principles of surgery are to correct the alignment of the toes over the end of the metatarsals. This provides cover for the ends of the prominent metatarsals. The most common technique practised is to excise the metatarsal heads through either a plantar or dorsal approach. At the same time, the first metatarsophalangeal joint is fused to restore the position of the great toe and allow it to take weight.

Progressive deformity of the hindfoot is probably best treated by surgery to correct the position and stabilise the foot; this usually involves fusion of one or the more hindfoot joints (Fig. 31.8). Bone grafts are frequently necessary to help correct the deformity. Reduction of deformity has to be directed towards keeping the foot flat to the floor. Involvement of the ankle can further complicate matters, the ankle frequently tilting into valgus. If the ankle is symptomatically involved then consideration should be given to either arthrodesis or possible arthroplasty of that joint also. The choice between surgical treatments under these conditions will depend on the general and local state of the patient, the position of the patient's hindfoot and their expectation.

Hallux rigidus

This is the most common arthritic condition affecting the foot. The symptoms are those of limitation of movement and pain. It can arise as early as the adolescent years. It is associated with various systemic causes of arthritis such as gout and psoriasis. Most commonly it arises *de novo*. Pathologically it is typified by the presence of dorsal osteophytes and by damage to the articular surface centrally and dorsally. The vast majority of patients presents with severe joint involvement.

Treatment

The first line of treatment is conservative. Education about the nature of the condition is helpful. Advice about footware and stiffening of the sole of the shoe under the first ray can be helpful.

Operative treatment falls into three groups depending on the severity of the condition. In mild or moderate disease dorsal wedge osteotomy of the proximal phalanx can help to reduce pressure over the dorsum of the great toe. If there are mild to moderate changes on the joint surface but a significant dorsal osteophyte a cheilectomy procedure, where the dorsal osteophyte and approximately the dorsal third of the metatarsal head is excised, can be undertaken. If there are severe changes two procedures can be considered. The first is to fuse the first metatarsal to the proximal phalanx. This produces the most reliable result but by definition there is a loss of the range of movement. Approximately 90 per cent of patients who undergo this procedure ultimately find it satisfactory. The second option is to undertake an arthroplasty. A variety of prostheses has been tried without consistent success.

Tumours

Like elsewhere in the body tumours may be benign or malignant, which may be primary or secondary. The foot shows three types of benign tumour: those that are latent or active, and finally those which are locally invasive but do not metastasise.

Primary malignancy is relatively rare but can arise in any of the tissues which go to make up the structure of the foot. They are usually graded on the basis of their differentiation, whether they cross anatomical barriers and obviously whether they have metastasised. More common are metastases from the common malignant tumours: lung, breast and prostate.

Plain X-rays can be helpful, but for thorough preoperative analysis of a tumour, investigations such as computerised tomography (CT) scans, technetium bone scans, MRI scans and high-resolution ultrasound for the vascular tumours may be necessary. Serological studies and investigations such as chest X-rays looking for evidence of distant spread may be required.

Treatment

This may involve simple local excision through to amputation, depending on the nature and extent of the tumour. In the foot it is particularly important to take into account the local anatomy when planning tumour excision.

Ageing in the forefoot

As the foot ages it undergoes a number of changes that relate to original shape of the foot and to changes which occur in the ligaments of the foot. There is a general tendency for the foot to become flatter and broader. The forefoot tends to abduct and the toes deform. The hallux gradually goes into increasing valgus and lesser toes become relatively crowded and longer. The consequence is increasing deformity of the lesser toes (Fig. 31.9). The hindfoot deformities that occur are largely covered by the sections on developmental and arthritic conditions.

Hallux valgus

This is probably the commonest condition seen affecting the forefoot. A wide variety of factors is involved in its aetiology. These include:

- wearing shoes – hallux valgus is commoner in shod populations;
- hereditary predisposition;
- metatarsus primus varus;
- increased length of the first metatarsal; and
- hypermobility of the first ray.

Although all of these factors come into play the pathology of the progressing deformity is essentially the same, there are only two structures which prevent the toe going into valgus, the medial collateral ligament and the abductor muscle of the great toe. If the toe starts to deviate into valgus because of any of the above factors, then the medial capsule stretches and the abductor moves under the metatarsal head by virtue of its attachment to the medial sesamoid. The first metatarsal displaces medially in relation to the great toe and its associated seamoids. Their position is maintained in relationship to the rest of the foot by both primary restraints (the plantar fascia and the transverse tarsal ligament) and the secondary restraints (the intrinsic and extrinsic muscles). The valgus displacement of the great toe exposes the metatarsal head creating a bony prominence, and an adventitious bursa can then form. In some patients the increasing deformity damages the joint producing a secondary osteoarthritis. As the great toe deviates futher it impinges on the second toe producing hammering and ultimately dislocation of the second metatarsophalangeal joint. A cascade of increasing deformity then ensues. Associated with the increasing width of the foot a bunionette may form over the fifth metatarsal.

Treatment

Conservative treatment always has to be considered first. Advice about ill-fitting or tight shoes may relieve symptoms or prevent episodes of infection or minor ulceration. There is a perception that this advice will not be tolerated by women who wish to wear fashion shoes. This is incorrect. If properly advised about the potential risks and complications of surgery many patients will modify their expectations and their footwear. The relationship of the forefoot to the hindfoot has to be considered and can be improved while wearing suitable footware by the use of suitable insoles.

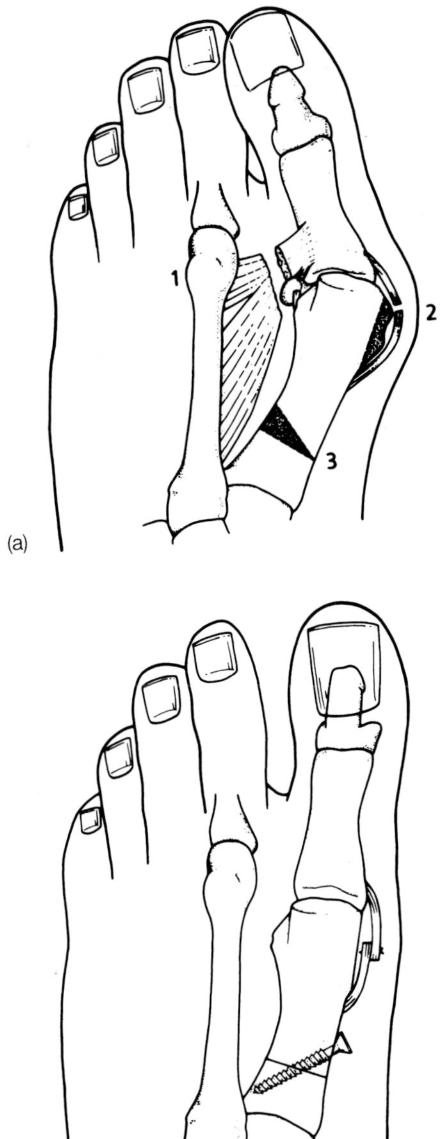

Fig. 31.10 Operation for hallux valgus. (a) The essential steps of the procedure in addition to shaving off the excess bone. 1: Division of tendon of contracted adductors in first web space; 2: tightening of stretched medial collateral ligament; 3: lateral wedge osteotomy at base of first metatarsal. (b) After operation.

Surgical treatment should be considered for persistent symptoms, recurrent ulceration or infection, or increasing deformity leading to increasing symptoms in the lateral part of the foot (Fig. 31.10).

No one operation is the answer to all cases of hallux valgus and a protocol of management should be assumed if results are going to be consistent (Table 31.2). Factors such as age, sex, hallux valgus angle, the angle between the first and

Table 31.2 Hallux valgus (HV) surgical planning (the number of plus signs represent the suitabity of the operation)

	Distal osteotomy	*Proximal osteotomy*	*Phalangeal osteotomy*	*Fusion*	*Arthroplasty*
<30 years	+++++	+++++	+++++	–	–
30–50 years	+++++	+++++	+++++	++	–
50–65 years	+++	++++	+++	+++	++
>65 years	+	++	+	++++	+++
Man	+++	+++	+++	+++++	–
Woman	+++	++++	++++	++	+++
Arthritis	++	–	++	+++++	+++
<25° HV angle	+++++	–	+++	–	–
25°–45°	+	+++++	++	++	++
>45°	–	++	–	++++	+++++
Congruent	++++	+++	+++++	–	–

second metatarsal, hypermobility of the first tarsometatarsal joint and degenerative changes in the first metatarsophalangeal joint have to be taken into account.

Lesser toe deformities

These include:

- hammer toe;
- mallet toe;
- claw toe;
- curly toe;
- metatarsalgia;
- Morton's neuritis and neuroma.

Further reading

Mann, R.A. and Coughlin M.J. (1993) *Surgery of the Foot and Ankle*, 6th edn, Mosby, London.

Wülker, N., Stephens, M. and Cracchiolo A. (eds) (1998) *An Atlas of Foot and Ankle Surgery*, Martin Dunitz, London.

Thomas George Morton, 1835–1903. Surgeon, The Pennsylvania Hospital, Philadelphia, Pennsylvania, USA.

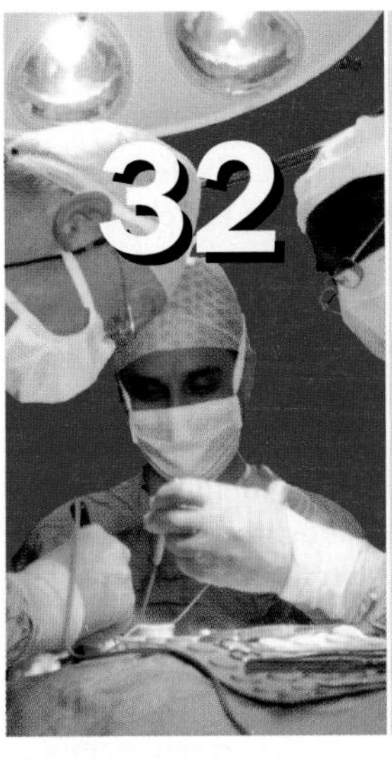

32 Neurological disorders affecting the musculoskeletal system

Introduction

Neurological conditions are not common but they occupy a great deal of time and effort for orthopaedic surgeons. Polio and spina bifida are becoming increasingly rare in the developed world, as is cerebral palsy. Genetic counselling has reduced the incidence of the genetic disorders. In the developing world many of these conditions remain common but simple public health measures should reduce these dramatically in the future.

Classification of neurological disorders

Static, e.g. polio	**Progressive**, e.g. Huntington's	
Sensory, e.g. leprosy	**Mixed**, e.g. disseminated sclerosis	**Motor**, e.g. polio
Flaccid, e.g. peripheral nerve section	**Spastic**, e.g. disseminated sclerosis	**Abnormal movements**, e.g. Huntington's

Static versus progressive

From an orthopaedic point of view, neurological disorders are classified into those which are static and those which are progressive. Static disorders can in fact appear progressive. As an adult gets older and heavier, actions that were previously possible become impossible despite the fact that there has been no deterioration in neurological function. Nevertheless, some conditions such as cerebral palsy and polio tend to be static while other conditions, such as Duchenne muscular dystrophy, are progressive and require a different approach.

Sensory versus motor

Sensory loss such as that caused by traumatic nerve lesions, leprosy and multiple sclerosis may create a limb which cannot be protected from injury, but which is also functionless because the patient does not know where the limb is (loss of proprioception). Other conditions, particularly polio, are pure motor loss. Indeed if there is any associated sensory loss a diagnosis other than polio should be considered. In this case disability and deformity will be a result of loss of muscle power not loss of sensation.

Flaccid versus spastic versus abnormal movements

Flaccid paralysis occurs when a peripheral motor nerve is transected or in the early stages after an upper motor neuron lesion. The limb is flail, and ligaments are susceptible to damage, simply because there is no muscle power protecting them. Spastic paralysis is loss of cortical control of muscles despite the fact that they are contracted in spasm and hyperreflexia. The conversion of an upper motor neuron lesion from flaccid paralysis to spastic paralysis some days after the original lesion may raise false hopes in the patient that recovery is imminent. Spastic paralysis will lead to contractures

Bailey & Love's Short Practice of Surgery, 23rd edition. Edited by R.C.G. Russell, N.S. Williams and C.J.K. Bulstrode. Published in 2000 by Arnold Publishers.

Guillaume Benjamin Armand Duchenne, 1806–75. Neurologist, Heidelberg, Germany.

and gross deformity if great care is not taken to maintain limb mobility. Abnormal movements are a characteristic of other neurological conditions. In Parkinson's disease there is a tremor and a repetitive pill-rolling manoeuvre of the thumb and index finger. In athetoid cerebral palsy, the limbs may writhe and wave around in an uncontrollable manner.

Making a diagnosis

A careful history needs to be taken which includes family history, problems during pregnancy or at birth. If the problem is of recent onset, contact, ingestion or inhalation of heavy metals, pesticides and other toxins should be covered. On examination a careful check needs to be made of the spine for signs of spina bifida. All modalities of sensation need to be carefully checked. Muscle power should be graded according to the Medical Research Council (MRC) Scale and a careful check made for signs of wasting, fasciculation and hyper-reflexia.

Investigations

Electrolytes should be checked routinely as imbalances in both calcium and magnesium can cause neurological problems. Electromyelographs (EMGs) and even muscle biopsies may be needed to determine the diagnosis. Imaging of the spinal cord and of the brain may also be required.

Management

Sensory loss

If the sensory loss is likely to be temporary (such as caused by transected sensory nerve) then the limb should be carefully protected to avoid injuries such as burns. Splints and plaster should also be applied with great caution as the patient will be unaware when they are developing sores at pressure points.

Temporary flaccid paralysis

This can be managed with splints to prevent overloading of ligaments and to maintain function of joints. Physiotherapy will be needed to maintain joint mobility, and to build up muscle power as the nerve supply returns. Lively splints are fitted with springs so that the weak muscle does not have to function but nevertheless the limb can be kept moving by the opposing muscle whose function remains normal.

Spastic paralysis

This is much more difficult to manage and requires regular gentle physiotherapy to try and put joints through a full range of movement without creating spasm. Regular physiotherapy should prevent the development of contractures which may make the deformity very difficult to manage. As a general rule, splints do not work well in spastic paralysis as they can stimulate spasm. The result is then either sores or a broken splint. Deformity as a result of spasticity can only really be treated by weakening the spastic muscle. There are various ways in which this can be done:

(a) the muscle can be divided;
(b) the tendinous insertion of the muscle can be lengthened;
(c) the insertion of the muscle into bone can be released and allowed to slide along the bone reducing the mechanical lever arm;
(d) the muscle can be injected with either a temporary or permanent paralytic agent such as botulin toxin;
(e) the nerve supply to the muscle can be divided.

In children many of these actions causing defunction of the muscle are reversed by the natural healing powers of a child. Transected muscles heal. Divided nerves regenerate. The procedures may therefore need repeating.

In athetosis, paralysis of the muscle with botulin or by transection of the nerve is a possibility but there is usually considerable function available despite the irregular movements of the limb and this loss of function must be balanced against the improvement in abnormal movements.

Trick manoeuvres

Patients with paralysed muscles develop a set of trick manoeuvres aimed to overcome their disability. For example, paralysis of the quadriceps muscle makes it difficult to lock the knee when walking. Patients with this problem frequently walk with their hand in the trouser pocket pressing firmly on the front of the knee and heel strike. This serves to lock the knee for normal locomotion. Patients with paralysis of the shoulder girdle may develop trick manoeuvres with their trunk which enable them to throw their arm high above their head.

Cerebral palsy

Children with cerebral palsy are usually floppy babies at birth. It is some months before the spasticity starts to develop. Even if the cerebral palsy is severe, intelligence is usually normal. It is a grave mistake to underestimate the intelligence or comprehension of these children.

Nonoperative treatment

These children will need assessment of their special needs in terms of walking aids, wheelchairs, etc. They will also need intensive physiotherapy to avoid deformity during growth. The imbalance of muscles across joints and growth plates during the growing period can lead to abnormal growth of bone which can then be very difficult to correct later in life. This is especially true of the spine where a particularly vicious form of scoliosis may develop which is very resistant to treatment. Although every effort should be made to help the child walk, this goal should not become the only goal to the exclusion of everything else. If a child with severe cerebral palsy of the lower limbs does succeed in walking, this is likely to be a temporary triumph. As they get older they are likely to go off their feet again and return to a wheelchair. If all of the parents' and the child's efforts are devoted to

James Parkinson, 1755–1824. British surgeon and palaeontologist.

walking to the exclusion of overall development the child's interest will not be served in the long term.

Surgery for cerebral palsy in the lower limb

Toe walking

Children with cerebral palsy frequently walk on their toes and appear unable to bring the heel to the floor. There can be several reasons for this. If they have a fixed flexion deformity to the hip and a flexion deformity at the knee, the only way in which the foot can get to the ground is by toe walking. Under these circumstances attention should be directed to the hip and/or the knee. If however, correction of the flexion deformity of the hip will not get the foot plantigrade because the tendo achilles is tight, then there may be a place for releasing the tendo achilles at the same time. The old cerebral palsy philosophy was to release one joint at a time, and to review the situation. This was because the release of one muscle group appears to have profound effects on the others. The problem with this was that the child was subject to multiple admissions to hospital before any correction was obtained. A newer approach is to do a global approach to the whole limb releasing hip flexors and adductors as necessary, lengthening the hamstrings behind the knee and lengthening the tendo achilles at the heel. The problem with this one-stage global correction is that the muscles affected by cerebral palsy may already be weak. They will be further weakened by surgery and there may not be adequate strength to hold the leg straight when walking. Some deformities actually help other deformities. For example, if the child is walking with bent knees and weak quadriceps, a fixed plantar flexion of the foot may bring the centre of gravity forwards and provide sufficient power to help the quadriceps to extend the knee and allow the child to walk. Release of the tendo achilles may improve cosmesis but remove the support to the quadriceps so that the child can no longer walk.

In the upper limb spasticity tends to flex the wrist, claw the fingers and draw the thumb into the palm, making the hand functionless and cosmetically unattractive. Fusion of the wrist in slight extension with release of the finger and thumb extensors may improve cosmesis but is unlikely to improve function unless some active flexion of the thumb and fingers is maintained. On the whole tendon transfers in the upper limb for cerebral palsy do not work as muscles lose power when transferred and lose range of movement.

Release of tendo achilles

The tendo achilles can be released with a triple cut through three percutaneous stab incisions. Each incision enters the tendo-achilles vertically. This scalpel blade is then turned to the right angle and half of the tendon is cut through. The superior cut and inferior cut are medial, the middle cut is lateral. Stretch applied to the tendo achilles then results in a sliding release of the tendo achilles which will heal quickly in the lengthened position. The child is put in a plaster with the foot fully dorsiflexed and mobilisation started as soon as possible.

Release of the hamstrings

Hamstring release should allow the knee to come straight but in the older patient it may be necessary to release the posterior capsule of the knee as well. This is a very major undertaking and risks damage to the neurovascular bundle behind the knee. It is particularly difficult if the flexion deformity is very severe because access to the back of the knee becomes very difficult.

Adductor tenotomy of hip

The adductors of the hip can be released through a subcutaneous incision. If the femur is held firmly by the assistant applying steady pressure into abduction, the tendons can be felt tight as bow strings and divided as they insert into the ischial tuberosity. Adductor tenotomy dramatically improves the ability of a child to sit in a chair and makes perineal toilet much easier.

Scoliosis

This can be severe and aggressive in a child with cerebral palsy. Surgery will prevent any further growth of the spine but correction may have to be undertaken early because pulmonary function is being compromised by the deformity of the spine.

Polio and other flaccid paralysis

After the initial acute phase of polio, there should be a rapid improvement in motor function to a steady state. During this time it is important that joints are kept mobile and morale is kept up. In children, compensatory development of other unaffected muscles may allow the child to lead an almost normal life despite quite marked paralysis of some muscle groups. However, tendon transfers can prove very useful in any form of flaccid paralysis, especially if the following rules are adhered to.

- Muscles should only be transferred which are of normal power.
- It must be expected that muscles will drop at least one grade of power when transferred.
- Where possible, muscles should be transferred which operate in the same way or in the same phase of normal movement as the muscle that they are supposed to replace.
- Tendon transfers should not go round sharp corners where they will lose their efficiency.

In children it is important to try and balance muscle power around joints so that deformity does not arise.

Specific tendon transfers

Long thoracic nerve, weakness of thoratis anterior and winging of the scapula can be treated by transferring the pectoralis minor into the inferiomedial aspect of the scapula musculocutaneous nerve. The brachioradialis is spared in an injury to the musculocutaneous nerve and remains as the only weak flexor of the elbow joint. If its insertion is advanced proximally up the humerus to obtain better leverage its power increases.

Radial nerve palsy

This is a common injury after a fracture of the humerus and if there is no prospect of return of function, then transfers of flexor tendons to the extensor side will stabilise the wrist and allow extension of the fingers. The classic transfer is the Robert Jones. Pronator teres is inserted into extensor radialis longus to restore wrist extension. Flexor carpi ulnar is inserted into extensor digitorum to restore finger extension. Palmaris longus when present is inserted into extensor polices longus to restore thumb extension.

Median nerve

There is a number of tendon transfers to improve function of the thumb depending on the level of the median nerve palsy. In distal median nerve palsy, flexor digitorum superfascialis of the ring finger can be passed across to the thumb to help with opposition.

Lateral popliteal nerve

This leads to a foot drop which can be treated by transfer of the tibialis posterior tendon to take the place of tibialis anterior by routing through the interosseous membrane.

Bone operations for flaccid weakness

Athrodesis is especially useful where flaccid weakness is proximal with a normally functioning distal limb. Fusion at the wrist dramatically improves the function of the hand while fusion of the shoulder can make a flail limb functional again. The arthrodesis may also release active muscles for use elsewhere in tendon transfers. Arthrodesis does not work well in cerebral palsy where the spasticity tends to deform the arthrodesis. However, if spastic tendons have been released and there is a persistent fixed flexion deformity, an osteotomy may be simpler than a radical release of capsule. This is particularly true around the knee.

Splintage

Modern splints can be very lightweight and cosmetically not prominent. Splints can be built with springs and locks to improve function. Great care must be taken if there is any sensory loss in the limb to make certain that the splints fit well. Splintage may need to be combined with tendon release and with osteotomy, especially in the severe cavus foot of the child with cerebral palsy, where both a soft-tissue release and bony fusion will be needed to prevent recurrence of the deformity.

Leg length discrepancy

This can be corrected with a shoe raise and in some cases with stapling of epiphyses on the opposite side to reduce growth. Modern techniques of leg lengthening using external fixators offer the opportunity of restoring the patient to normal height, but take time and have severe complications.

Limbs with both sensory and motor loss

A flail limb without sensation may be more of a hazard than a help to the patient and may be better amputated. This is particularly true if the limb is scarred and deformed.

Inherited disorders

Friedreich's ataxia

This is hereditary autosomal recessive. The child presents in early childhood with both a motor and a sensory loss presenting as clumsiness and difficulty walking. From an orthopaedic point of view the main problem is a cavovarus deformity of the foot, which in the young child can be corrected with soft-tissue release but in the older adolescent may require a wedge osteotomy.

Duchenne muscular dystrophy

This is cross-link recessive and again presents in early childhood with difficulty walking and classically with difficulty rising from a sitting position and climbing stairs. There are high levels of serum creatinine kinase and the muscle biopsy is diagnostic. In their early teens patients are wheelchair bound and they normally die in their early twenties. The main input from orthopaedics is correction of scoliosis to improve breathing.

Multiple sclerosis

This is a patchy demyelination of the central nervous system which develops later in life. The patient develops spasticity in the lower limbs with gross deformities. Splintage should avoid these causing too much trouble but tenomities are frequently required round the hip and knee to help the patient to sit.

Progression of static neurological disorders

As patients go into middle age, they put on weight and their muscles may weaken as does their motivation. Patients who were previously able to walk now find themselves confined to a wheelchair. It may be that this situation should be gracefully accepted, as static neurological disorders become an increasing disability to patients as they grow older.

Further reading

Sutherland, S. (1968) *Nerves and Nerve Injuries*, 2nd edn, Livingstone.

Walton, J.N. (ed.) *Brains' Diseases of the Nervous System*, 10th edn, Oxford University Press, Oxford.

Sir Robert Jones, 1858–1933. Orthopaedic surgeon, Royal Southern Hospital, England, and nephew of Hugh Owen Thomas.

Nikolaus Friedrich, 1825–82. German neurologist.

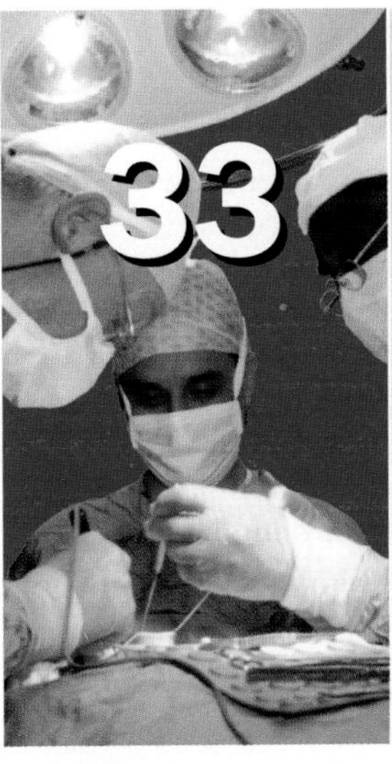

33 The spine, vertebral column and spinal cord

Anatomy of the spine and spinal cord

Vertebral column

This provides a mobile yet protective midline dorsal scaffold housing the spinal cord and cauda equina. Comprising a series of interlocking vertebrae the spinal nerves emerge via intervertebral foramina, the cord joining the brain stem at the foramen magnum (Fig. 33.1a and b).

Developed from the union of adjacent mesenchymal blocks, the basic pattern of anterior body and posterior arch exists throughout. These surround the central canal through which passes the spinal cord, a derivation of the neural plate, and lower down the nerves of the cauda equina. Between each vertebra – which are linked by anterior intervertebral disc and lateral facet joints – runs a series of connecting ligaments to provide significant stability to the spine. These include particularly the anterior and posterior longitudinal ligaments running the full length of the vertebral column from the foramen magnum, attached to the periosteum of each vertebral body by an annulus of each disc. The interspinous ligaments link each spinous process and the supraspinous ligaments skip between the tips of each spinous process along the full length of the spine (Fig. 33.2).

Cervical spine

This comprises seven vertebrae with areas of specialisation. The C1 and C2 vertebrae join to form the atlantoaxial complex, the body of Cl being incorporated into the body of C2 to form the odontoid peg or dens. The Cl or atlas vertebra, therefore, becomes a ring between the occipital condyles of the skull and the C2 or axis vertebra. The posterior arch of Cl has no spinous process and may be incomplete.

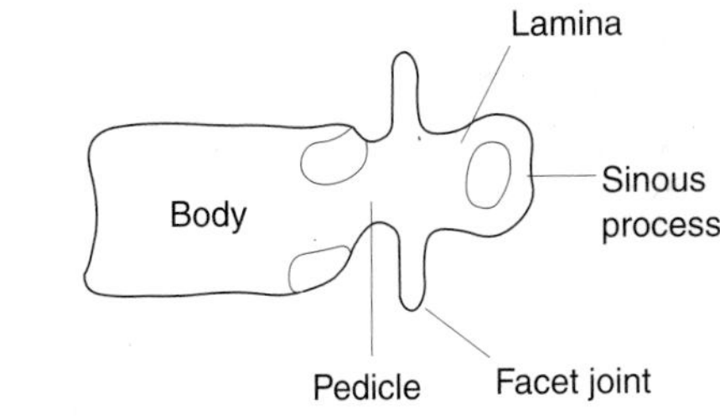

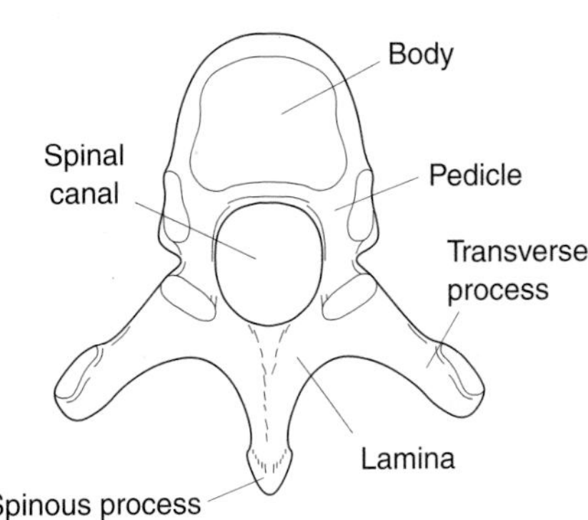

Fig. 33.1 Basic anatomy of a vertebra: (a) lateral view; (b) axial view.

Bailey & Love's Short Practice of Surgery, 23rd edition. Edited by R.C.G. Russell, N.S. Williams and C.J.K. Bulstrode. Published in 2000 by Arnold Publishers.

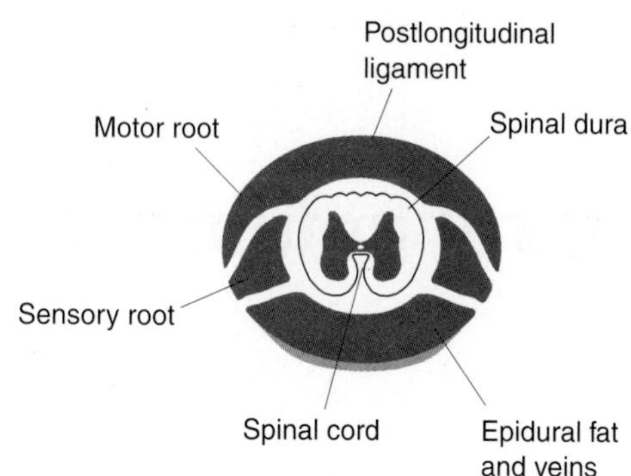

Fig. 33.2 The contents of the spinal canal.

The axis or C2 vertebra forms an easily radiologically visible structure with the dens anteriorly and a large bifid spine posteriorly.

The remaining cervical vertebrae (C3 to C7) also have identifying features. Running in the lateral mass is the foramen transversarium through which passes the vertebral artery from its point of origin at the subclavian artery to where it loops over the lamina of C2 to gain access to the cranial cavity via the foramen magnum. The spinous process of these vertebrae (except C7) are usually bifid. The vertebral artery does not traverse the C7 vertebra and this also has a prominent spinous process which can be palpated, giving rise to its name, the vertebra prominens.

Thoracic spine

Uniform in shape, the heads of the ribs articulate with adjacent bodies of these 12 vertebrae. Gradually the size of the vertebral body and the articular processes increases down towards the more solid lumbar vertebrae.

Lumbar vertebrae

These represent a more mobile part of the spine and yet represent an area of great strength. Formed of five vertebrae the lateral mass, pedicles and laminae are thicker and the spinous processes shorter and more vertical. The last mobile joint between L5 and S1 (lumbosacral junction) joins the spine to the rigid pelvis via the sacrum.

Sacrum

Situated between the iliac bones and joined by the sacroiliac joint, the bones of the sacrum are fused into one triangular shape through which traverse the terminal sacral nerve roots – S2, S3 and S4.

The basic vertebral structure of each component of the sacrum is maintained, but the bones blend into one another to form a smooth anterior and posterior surface.

Coccyx

These very small vertebrae do not transmit any neural structure and are attached to the sacrum.

The spinal canal

This contains the spinal cord and cauda equina enclosed in layers of meninges.

The spinal cord extends from the foramen magnum at the cervicomedullary junction to the conus medullaris – an area of expansion of the cord at the L1/L2 junction.

From that point there is no spinal cord, the nerves continuing as the cauda equina. Surrounding the cord and the cauda equina is arachnoid mater, defining the cerebrospinal fluid (CSF) containing subarachnoid space, and the spinal dura or theca which is continuous with the cranial dura at the foramen magnum and forms a sleeve around each emerging nerve root. It is via this root sleeve that the sequential blood supply gains access to the spinal cord. The epidural space between the spinal theca and the bone of the spinal canal is filled with epidural fat and the epidural venous plexus.

The spinal cord

The cord itself is part of the central nervous system but arising from it are pairs of spinal nerves, each one composing a dorsal sensory root and a ventral motor root to form a numbered mixed spinal nerve (Fig. 33.3).

These emerge via the intervertebral foramenae and are numbered Cl to C8, T1 to T12, L1 to L5 and S1 to S4.

The spinal cord is uniform in appearance with two areas of expansion – in the cervical region corresponding to the origin of the nerve roots to the arm and in the lumbar region at the conus medullaris.

The blood supply to the spinal cord is formed from the descending anterior and spinal arteries, from the vertebral arteries and from the segmental spinal arteries which form an anastomosis up and down the spine. Some of these segmental arteries are significantly enlarged, for example the artery of Adamkewitz at D10.

Assessment of the spine

Trauma

> Always assume that the patient has a spinal column injury until you have proved otherwise

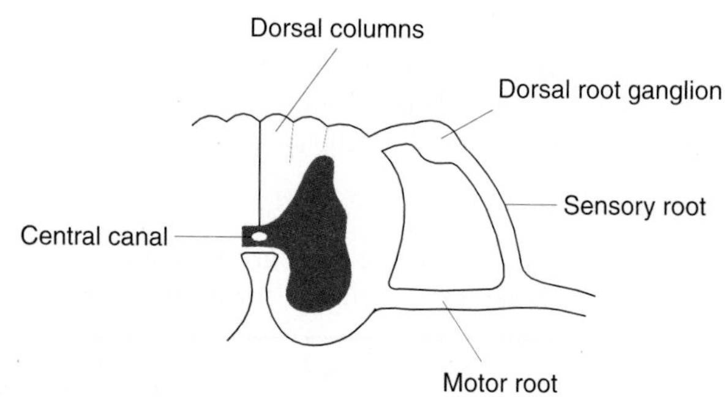

Fig. 33.3 The anatomy of the spinal cord.

It is of great importance to recognise the presence of a spinal injury as early as possible after the injury has occurred. This will prevent further injury to the spinal cord and nerve roots, and give the patient the best chance of a good long-term outcome. Throughout assessment and resuscitation the spine must be suitably immobilised. Initially this can be done with simple in-line immobilisation. Advanced trauma and life support (ATLS) protocols can then be used to resuscitate the patient in the normal way (see Chapter 4).

The patient should be suitably immobilised at the site of the injury on a spine board with a hard collar and with the whole of the spine immobilised. The head should be attached to the board with tape and steadied with sand bags or some similar device (see Fig. 33.4). The patient can then be safely transported to a suitable hospital for further treatment.

There are certain features in an injured patient which should alert the doctor that there may be a spinal injury of some sort:

- evidence of neurological injury;
- multiple injury;
- head injury;
- facial injury;
- high-energy injury (e.g. fall from a height);
- seat-belt abdominal marking (may suggest lumbar injury).

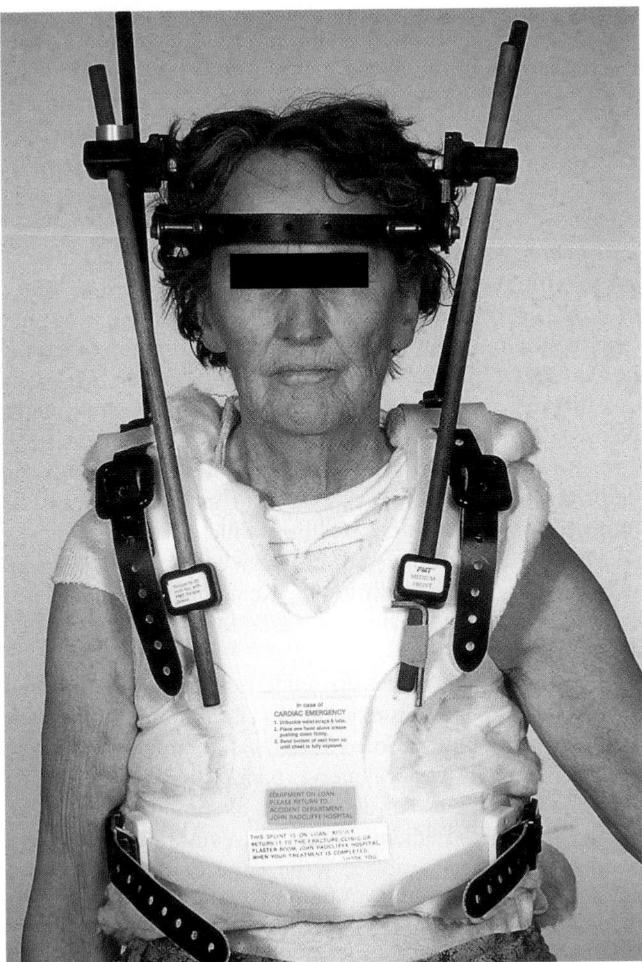

Fig. 33.4 Patient immobilisation.

Assessment of the spine in the unconscious patient with multiple injuries is probably the most difficult. If there are associated life-threatening injuries, it is probably best to carry on and treat these first before the spine is fully assessed. For example, a patient with severe intra-abdominal bleeding may require urgent surgery. It is still mandatory that the spine is protected throughout management, for example moving the patient on to the operating table. Further spinal assessment can then be carried out later.

The spine must always be examined clinically as part of the secondary survey. This can be done easily when the back of the patient is examined. If this is not done, severe injuries such as an open spinal injury may be overlooked for some hours.

In the conscious patient without other severe injuries spinal injury can usually be excluded by the combination of absent pain and a normal clinical examination of the spinal column with a normal neurological examination.

In the conscious patient biplanar X-rays of the symptomatic part of the spine are adequate, and in the cervical spine open mouth view of the odontoid peg should be included. In the unconscious patient assessment of the spinal column is much more difficult because clinical signs are often absent. In the thoracic and lumbar spine full anteroposterior (AP) and lateral X-rays of the spine are required to exclude an injury to the spinal column. In the cervical spine unstable injuries of the neck are easily overlooked, and full AP lateral and odontoid peg views will still overlook about 5 per cent of injuries. One option is to carry out real-time flexion and extension X-rays of the cervical spine using an image intensifier. If there is any evidence of instability at any point the investigation is stopped. An alternative is to carry out magnetic resonance imaging (MRI) scans on all these patients but this is time consuming and difficult in the patient with multiple injuries.

The extent of an injury may not be apparent initially, and further imaging in the form of computerised tomography (CT) or MRI scanning may be required. For example, in the unconscious the upper and lower cervical spine may be very difficult to assess. Most of these patients will require a CT scan of the brain to exclude a space-occupying lesion, and it is convenient to carry out a few CT cuts at the occipitocervical junction and at the cervicothoracic junction to exclude a significant injury, particularly if the cervicothoracic junction has not been visualised on plain films. Similarly, the upper thoracic spine is a very difficult area to visualise on plain films and if there is suspicion of injury, CT scan should be used to assess the area. CT scan will show any disruption of the ring of the vertebra suggesting an unstable injury, and will allow assessment of canal compromise and of subluxation or dislocation of the vertebrae.

MRI scanning is very sensitive, but is better for assessment of soft-tissue injury and less sensitive for assessing bone injury. Where there is no fracture it can be useful for establishing the presence of a soft-tissue injury, it is useful for assessing spinal cord and nerve root compression as well as the extent of spinal cord injury, and it can be helpful in making a long-term prognosis about spinal cord recovery.

If an unstable injury is demonstrated, spinal immobilisation should continue until such time as the spine can be stabilised, or until healing has occurred.

Nontrauma

As in assessment of any part of the skeleton first principles should be followed, or clinical signs will be missed.

- Take a history – 90 per cent of diagnoses can be made at this point.
- Look at the spine standing and lying.
- Palpate the spine.
- Examine the neurological system.
- Examine the peripheral vascular system.
- Watch the spine moving.

The history should include past medical history of importance (e.g. injury or previous similar symptoms) and family history (e.g. for scoliosis). Important parts of the history are:

- pain (site, nature, duration, pain scale, effects);
- disability (sitting, standing, walking, lifting, dressing, travel, social activities, sleep, sex life);
- physical impairment;
- work loss.

Many of these parameters are very difficult to assess in the spine. Pain is a very subjective sensation, and it is difficult to grade the amount of pain which a patient is experiencing. Methods of assessing the amount and quality of the pain include the anatomical pattern of the pain, the use of pain scales such as the visual analogue scale, and pain descriptions such as the short-form McGill pain questionnaire.

In assessing the pain and disability which a patient is experiencing it is important to include an assessment of how **much distress and illness behaviour** the patient is experiencing. This is because the type of treatment chosen may be very different for the patient with significant distress, and because the outcomes of treatment are very different. For example, the outcome of surgery for back pain in those with distress is very much worse than in those who are not distressed. Physical signs which suggest that the patient may be exhibiting abnormal illness behaviour include the following.

Symptoms include:

- whole leg pain;
- tailbone pain;
- whole leg numbness;
- whole leg giving way;
- never free of pain;
- intolerance of treatments;
- emergency admission to hospital.

Signs include:

- superficial widespread nonanatomical tenderness;
- lumbar pain on axial loading of the spine;
- lumbar pain on simulated rotation of the spine;
- straight leg raising which improves with distraction;
- regional sensory disturbance;
- regional motor weakness;
- jerky movements on motor assessment with giving way.

Litigation is an important confounding factor in the treatment of individuals with spinal pain. There is no doubt that the response to treatment is less good in those who are litigating, perhaps because there is little incentive for them to recover. However, there is also good evidence that few patients experience a significant improvement in their symptoms after settlement of the claim.

Physical impairment can be measured and lumbar spine measurements of impairment include those of the American Medical Association and the American Academy of Orthopaedic Surgeons. We have more experience with the use of the Oswestry Disability Index, a 10-question self-administered score of back pain and associated disability which is reliable and reproducible. This combined with a pain score is in regular use in our institutions and allows easy scoring of pain and disability and comparison of pretreatment and post-treatment pain and disability.

Examination technique

Make the patient feel relaxed. Watch how the patient moves and walks, and watch how the patient dresses and undresses. Look at the spine. Is there a deformity or muscle spasm, does the patient have a scoliosis? Are there any associated features such as birth marks or a leg length discrepancy which might suggest a congenital disorder? Examine the range of movement of the spine in the cervical, thoracic and lumbar spine with the patient standing up if possible. The range of spinal movement is difficult to assess accurately, but flexion and extension can be measured with a goniometer if necessary. Deformities should also be assessed for their mobility. It is usually easiest to have the patient lie prone to palpate the spine. This avoids putting the patient off balance, and also allows the muscles to relax. Look to see whether the deformity corrects, for example with a sciatic scoliois, as opposed to a structural scoliosis which will not correct completely. Palpate the spine to see whether there is a step suggesting a spondylolithesis. Remember to look for evidence of inappropriate signs (axial loading and simulated rotation).

With the patient prone the ankle reflexes can be assessed and posterior sensation examined. The femoral stretch test (hip extension with the knee flexed) can be carried out to see whether there is femoral nerve pain. The patient is then asked to lie supine. An assessment of muscle bulk can be made, and measurements made as required. A thorough neurological examination can be carried out including a sciatic stretch test (see Fig. 33.5 and Table 33.1).

Remember to examine the abdominal reflexes where there is any possibility of an upper motor neuron lesion. Hip and knee pathology frequently mimics back pain and these joints

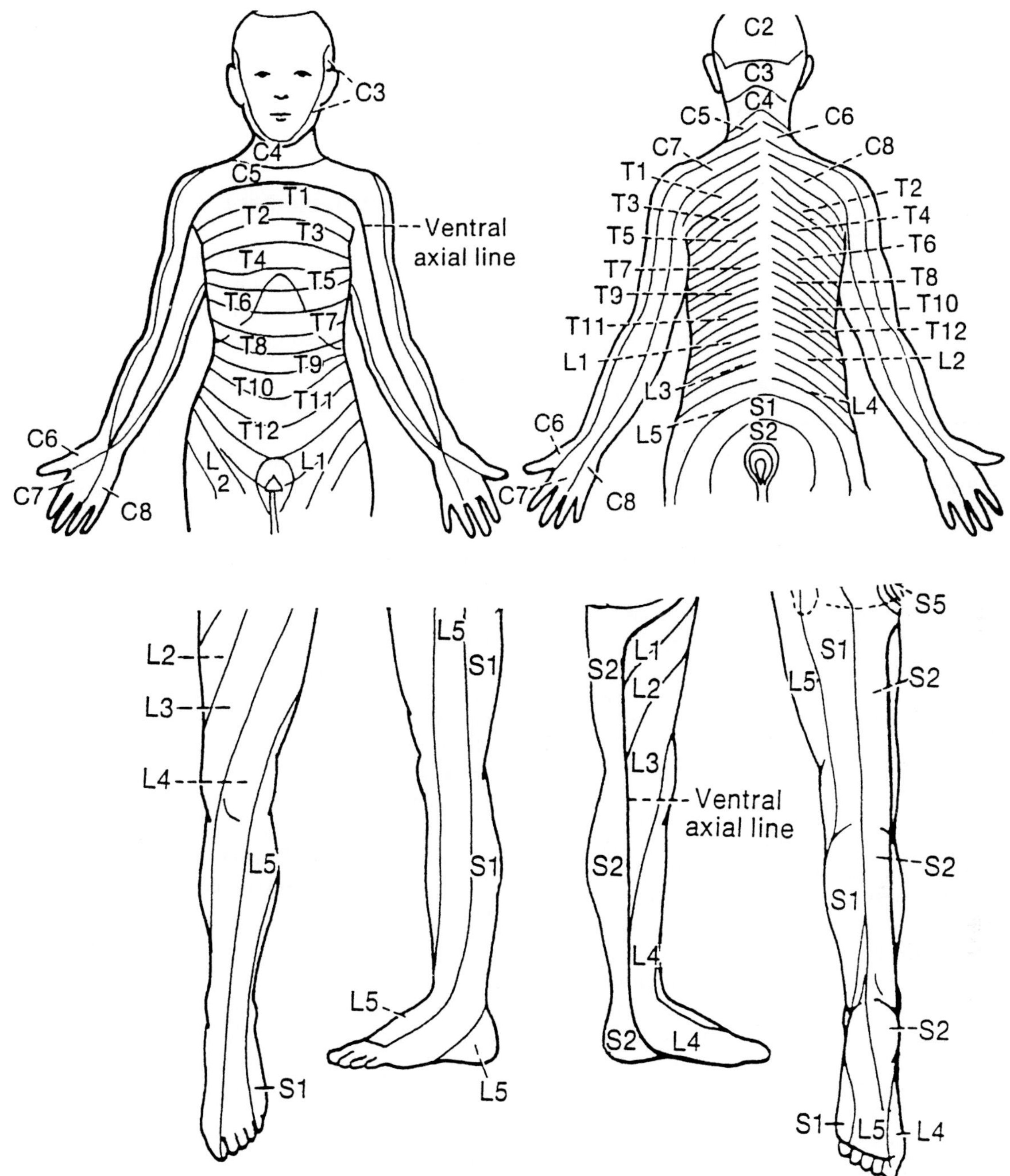

Fig. 33.5 The typical distribution of sensory nerves into 'dermatomal' areas.

should be examined. Remember that spinal stenosis is often contused with intermittent claudication, and the peripheral pulses must be examined. Finally abdominal examination should exclude intra-abdominal pathology as a cause of back pain (e.g. aneurysm) (Table 33.2).

This sounds like a lengthy examination, but with plenty of practice it should be possible to carry out the examination reasonably rapidly (e.g. 5–10 minutes). Does the patient have back pain as the primary problem, does the patient have nerve root pain, or is there a combination? Are there inappropriate signs suggesting illness behaviour?

Investigations

Where malignancy or infection is a possibility haematological investigation is useful [full blood count (FBC), erythrocyte sedimentation rate (ESR), C-reactive protein (CRP), bone biochemistry].

MRI scanning has revolutionised the diagnosis and

Table 33.1 Muscle chart myotomes

Diaphragm	C3/4/5	
Biceps	C5/C6	Biceps reflex
Wrist extension	C6	
Triceps and wrist extensors reflex	C7	Triceps
Finger flexion	C8	Finger jerk
Intrinsics	T1	
Intercostals	T2–T9	
Abdominals	T10–T12	
Cremaster	T12–L1	
Iliopsoas	L3	
Tibialis anterior/quads	L4	Knee reflex
Extensor hallucis	L5	
Gastrocnemius	51	Ankle reflex
Bladder sphincter	S2	
Anal sphincter	S3	

Table 33.2 The features of upper motor neuron lesions due to spinal cord compression or lower motor neuron lesion due to nerve root compression

	LMN lesion	*UMN lesion*
Power	Myotomal loss	Pyramidal loss
Tone	Reduced/normal	Increased
Reflex	Reduced	Brisk
Wasting	Present	Absent
Due to:	Nerve root compression	Spinal cord compression

treatment of patients with spinal problems. Plain X-rays still have their place, for example in the assessment of deformity or trauma, but for most other conditions MRI scanning is a very sensitive investigation. In some respects it is oversensitive and has to be used carefully. MRI scanning does not replace clinical assessment and should be used either to confirm a diagnosis in order to plan treatment or to exclude a lesion, for example spinal dysraphism in a patient with scoliosis. The false-positive rate for abnormalities is very high, especially for conditions such as disc degeneration but even, for example, for disc prolapse. MRI scanning allows assessment of the discs and spinal column, the spinal cord and nerve roots, as well as the structures immediately adjacent to the spine such as the psoas muscles. It allows assessment of neurological compression and of other abnormalities within the spinal canal.

In many parts of the world MRI scanning is not readily available. Plain X-rays will have more use in screening for conditions such as tumours or infection. Compressive lesions can be investigated with CT scanning and, if necessary, CT myelography can be carried out. Myelography alone may still have its place, for example in a compressive lesion in a patient with a metal implant in the spine. Bone scanning is a useful screening test where, for example, a bone tumour is suspected, but MRI scanning has largely replaced this as an investigation.

For assessment of back pain and nerve root pain provocative tests are widely used. Discography can help to assess whether spinal pain arises from a disc, and facet blocks can be used to assess pain in the facets, but also to treat facet pain. Nerve root blocks with local anaesthetic can help to assess whether a particular nerve root is responsible for pain, for example in a patient with multiple-level stenosis.

Trauma management

Most spinal injuries are the result of high-energy trauma. Road accidents and falls are the commonest causes of injury, but in the USA gunshot injuries cause spinal injury relatively frequently. Associated injuries are common.

- Spinal injury at another level 10–15 per cent.
- Head and face injury 26 per cent.
- Major chest injury 16 per cent.
- Major abdominal injury 10 per cent.
- Long bone/pelvic fracture 8 per cent.

Ninety per cent of fractures are simple compression fractures and the majority of these will go on to heal with little consequence. They are best treated symptomatically, initially with rest and then with mobilisation and splinting as necessary.

Seventy-five per cent of patients with an unstable spinal injury will have some sort of neurological injury. The assessment of spinal stability is difficult, especially in the patient who is unconscious, and especially in the cervical spine. Look for general alignment of the spine and for soft-tissue shadows. Is there widening of the anterior cervical soft tissue shadow, for example? Is there subluxation or rotation of one vertebra on another? Flexion extension views can be useful (see above) but should only be done with care by suitably qualified staff.

A scoring system has been devised for assessing cervical stability.

- Anterior element disruption 2
- Posterior element disruption 2
- Sagittal translation >3.5 mm 2
- Sagittal plane rotation >11° 2
- Positive stretch test 2
- Cervical cord injury 2
- Cervical root damage 1
- Abnormal disc narrowing 1
- Dangerous spinal loading in the future 1

If more than five points are scored, then the cervical spine should be considered unstable. In the thoracic and lumbar spine plain X-rays should alert the clinician to possible instability, but this may only be confirmed by CT scan in some cases. Remember that 10 per cent of all injuries are at multiple levels, so always search for the other injury.

Unstable cervical spine injuries

Adequate immobilisation of patients with unstable cervical injuries is mandatory. The patient should have a hard collar, with sandbags at either side of the head and the head should be taped to the bed until adequate treatment is started. Dislocations and fracture dislocations should be reduced as soon as possible. Delay in reduction makes it more likely that neurological injury will occur, and the longer the delay, the more difficult the reduction. However, **beware of the possibility of disc prolapse in the presence of a dislocation.** It is not uncommon for the intervertebral disc to prolapse posteriorly at the time of dislocation. When the dislocation is reduced, this can cause paraplegia as the spinal cord is compressed against the disc. This occurs in about 1 per cent of all these injuries. Therefore MRI scanning is mandatory before closed reduction of these fractures. If MRI scanning is not available, and not likely to be available over the following few hours, then it may be safer to carry out open anterior discectomy with fusion and instrumentation, in order to try to avoid this severe complication occurring.

Closed reduction can be best achieved either with halo traction or with Gardner Wells tongs. These are best applied under local anaesthetic which avoids any risk to the spinal cord with anaesthesia and intubation. Gardner Wells tongs are easier to apply, but do not allow correction of flexion or extension of the head once applied. The other advantage of halo traction is that the halo can then be used together with a jacket for immobilisation of the cervical spine if required (Figs 33.6 and 33.7).

Neurological injury and its management

Some patients with unstable spinal column injuries will sustain damage to either the spinal cord or nerve roots. Further

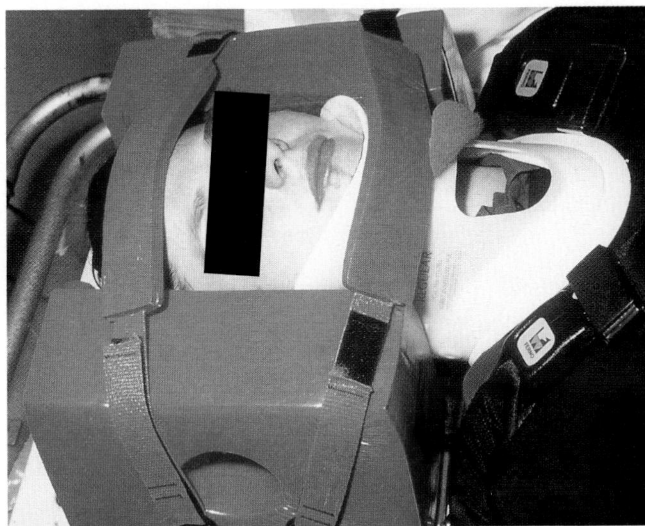

Fig. 33.6 Immobilisation with pads, tapes and a hard collar for transporting all patients in whom a clinical spinal injury is a possibility.

Eldon J. Gardner, b. 1909. American geneticist.
Samuel A. Wells, Jr. Brixby Professor of Surgery and Chairman, Department of Surgery, Washington University School of Medicine, St Louis, Missouri, USA.

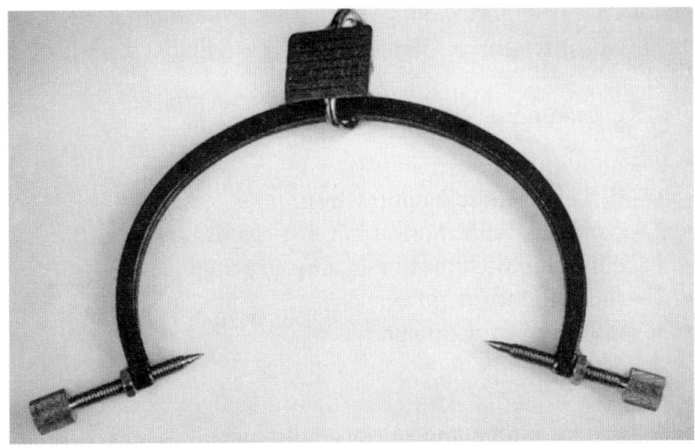

Fig. 33.7 Gardner Wells tongs.

damage may be prevented by suitable immobilisation of the spinal column, although in a small number of patients remorseless deterioration in neurological dysfunction may occur. This is usually due to persistent compression on the spinal cord interfering with the blood supply to the neurological tissues, but may be due to extension of haematoma or oedema in the area of the injury. Deterioration of neurological function following initial assessment is an indication for urgent treatment. Surgery should be considered to stabilise the spine and to decompress the spinal cord and nerve roots.

A randomised controlled study of a large group of patients has suggested that high-dose steroids may improve recovery after spinal cord injury. The suggested regimen is:

- 30 mg per kilogram of body weight bolus of methylprednisolone;
- 5.4 per kilogram of body weight per hour of methylprednisolone for the first 23 hours.

There is some debate in the literature about the real efficacy of this regimen, but serious side effects are rare, and until there is evidence to the contrary it seems reasonable to offer patients high-dose steroids on presentation. If the steroids cannot be given within 8 hours, they are not effective and should be avoided.

It is important to establish as soon as possible whether the injury is incomplete or complete. Often the sacral nerve roots are the least affected in spinal injury probably because they are protected to some extent from the vascular effects of injury. Sacral sensation is best assessed at the same time as the patient is log rolled to examine the spine. If sacral sensation is intact, then the injury is incomplete. If spinal shock has developed, it will not be possible to assess function below the injury until the spinal shock has resolved. Reflex arcs can function below the level of the injury without higher functions. The anal wink and the bulbocavernosus reflexes are examples of these. If they are present, one can assume that the patient is not in spinal shock. During the period of spinal shock these reflexes will be absent and it is not possible to assess whether the spinal cord injury is complete or incomplete. Spinal shock will usually resolve within 24 hours.

Assessment of neurological injury is best carried out using

various scoring techniques. For grading individual muscles the Medical Research Council (MRC) grading system is best used.

MRC grading:

- 0 – no contraction;
- 1 – flicker of muscle contraction;
- 2 – contracts with motion but not against gravity;
- 3 – contracts with motion against gravity;
- 4 – reduced motor power;
- 5 – normal motor power.

Frankel grading:

- A – absent motor and sensory function;
- B – sensation present motor absent;
- C – sensation present, motor present but not useful (MRC grade 2/3);
- D – sensation present, motor useful (MRC grade 4/5);
- E – normal function.

With this information available it is possible to define a neurological injury, to assess improvement or deterioration, and to communicate with others in a meaningful way about the injury.

Cervical spine injuries

Upper cervical spine injuries

Severe neurological injury is rarely seen in practice because it is not usually compatible with life.

Occipital condyle injuries. These are unusual injuries which are difficult to diagnose on plain films. If this type of injury is suspected, CT scanning is the best method of investigation. Some of these injuries are unstable, and if so occipitocervical fusion should be considered.

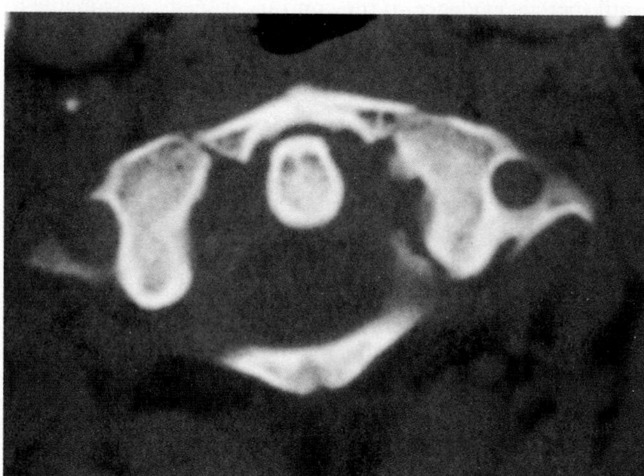

Fig. 33.8 Jefferson fracture CT scan showing three-part fracture through the ring of the atlas.

Sir Geoffrey Jefferson, 1886–1961. Professor of Neurosurgery, University of Manchester, England.

Jefferson fractures. This is a fracture of the ring of C1 and is usually caused by axial loading (Fig. 33.8). The ring can be split in two, three or four places. The amount of displacement can be assessed on the open mouth view, and if there is more than 6.9 mm of displacement, one can assume that the transverse ligament is ruptured, which suggests that the fracture is very unstable. Although the fracture can usually be seen on plain films, CT scan is useful to define the fracture pattern and to be sure that there is no associated injury at adjacent levels.

If the transverse ligament is divided a period of traction may be advisable. We usually treat these fractures in a halo jacket for 3 months; CT scan followed by supervised flexion extension radiographs is advisable at that point to be sure that healing has occurred and that there is no residual instability. Occasionally one part of the ring may fail to heal but the spine may still be stable. Persistent instability or failure to heal requires posterior occipitocervical fusion.

Odontoid fracture. This is the most commonly missed fracture in the cervical spine and comprises 10 per cent of cervical injuries. Failure to diagnose these fractures can result in spinal cord damage and death. Three types of fracture are described (see Fig. 33.9). Type 1 fractures are rare and are usually stable and can be treated symptomatically. Type II fractures (Fig. 33.10) cause the most problems because there is a high incidence of nonunion, especially in displaced fractures (up to 70 per cent). Undisplaced fractures can be treated with halo-jacket immobilisation, although it is also possible primarily to internally fix the fracture with one or two screws through an anterior approach. Displaced fractures can also be treated with anterior fixation which is quite

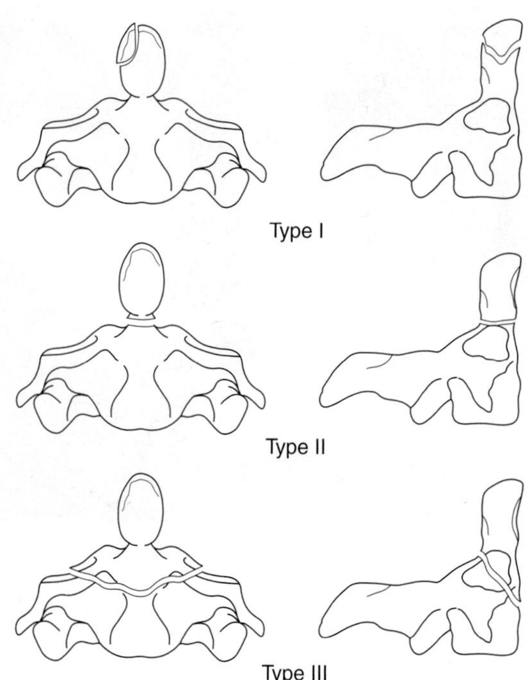

Fig. 33.9 Types of odontoid fracture.

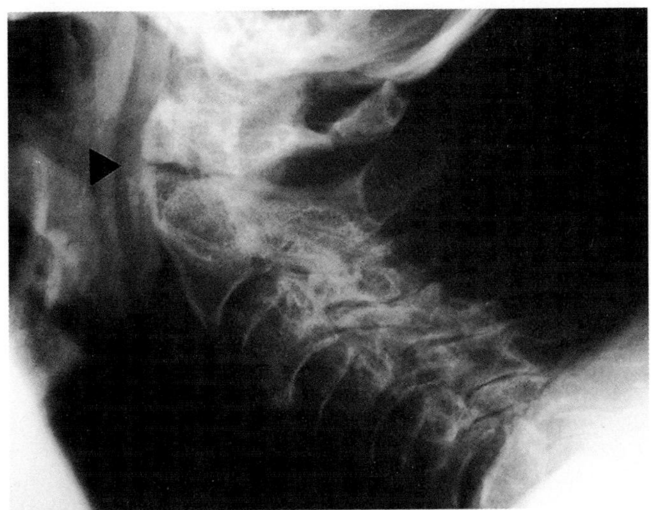

Fig. 33.10 Type II odontoid fracture.

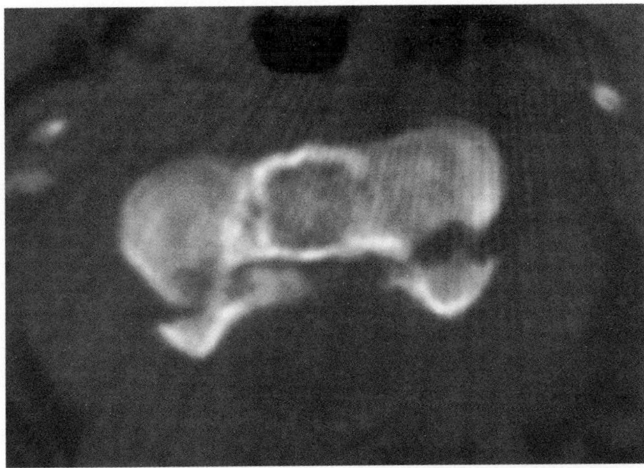

Fig. 33.11 Hangman's fracture CT scan showing fracture passing through the pedicles of C2.

a difficult technique, or with the more traditional technique of posterior C1–C2 fusion. In older individuals a period of immobilisation in a halo or even a sterno-occipitomandibular immobilizer (SOMI) collar may be considered, because they may heal in a stable position, even though the fracture itself does not unite. They are likely to put less demand on their neck, but stability should be assessed at the end of treatment with supervised flexion extension radiographs.

Type III fractures have a much better ability to heal and immobilisation in a halo jacket for 3 months will usually allow the fracture to heal. Again in the very old immobilisation in a SOMI brace or even in a Philadelphia collar may be adequate to allow healing. During treatment the position of the fracture should be monitored, and adjustments made to the position of the head as required to hold the fracture reasonably reduced.

Atlantoaxial instability. This is a common presentation in children and usually presents as inability to straighten the head, which tends to look right or left and slightly up, the so-called cock-robin position. The rotation may be fixed and often follows minor trauma, although it can present spontaneously, or occasionally as a result of local infection in the neck or oropharynx, so a careful examination of the head and neck is required. The diagnosis is made with radiographs and CT scans with the patient looking right and left. If the position of the axis is fixed in relation to the atlas on the two views, then fixed atlantoaxial rotation can be diagnosed. The subluxation can usually be corrected by a short period of halter traction, but occasionally surgery in the form of fusion is required.

Hangman's fracture (Fig. 33.11). This is really a fracture of the pedicle of C2. It comprises 5–10 per cent of cervical injuries, and is caused by hyperextension of the spine. There are three types, type I being the most stable, and type III the most unstable. Type I fractures can be immobilised for 3 months in a halo jacket or in a suitable brace, and they will usually heal. The more unstable the fracture the more likely that spinal fusion will be required as primary treatment. If conservative treatment is chosen for unstable fractures, it is important that the fracture is reduced and held reduced until fracture healing has occurred. This can be established with supervised flexion extension radiographs to check for stability and with CT scans to look for bridging of the fracture.

Lower cervical spine injuries

Wedge fractures. These are the commonest fractures, and are caused by hyperflexion of the spine, but they must be differentiated from burst fractures (see below). This can be done with CT scan. Symptomatic treatment is the rule, and surgery is rarely indicated.

Burst fractures and teardrop fractures. Burst fractures are caused by hyperflexion of the spine with or without axial compression. Fragments of bone are pushed circumferentially, whereas in wedge fractures the bone is simply compressed. Thus, the spinal cord or nerve roots may be compromised, and the majority of these fractures should be considered unstable. They should be treated either with immobilisation or with surgery in the form of fusion and instrumentation.

Teardrop fractures (Fig. 33.12) are really fracture dislocations where part of the injury goes through the lower part of the vertebra and part of the injury is ligamentous. These fractures often look quite benign on radiographs, but they are very unstable and should be treated with respect. Stabilisation is often necessary.

Facet dislocation. These injuries are caused by flexion or flexion and rotation. Either one or both facets may be dislocated (and this can usually be decided on plain films, where if there is less than 25 per cent displacement of one vertebra on the other it is probably one facet, whereas if there is more displacement it is probably both facets). About two-thirds of these patients have some sort of neurological injury, and a third have a complete cord injury. These dislocations should be reduced as soon as possible, provided an anterior disc

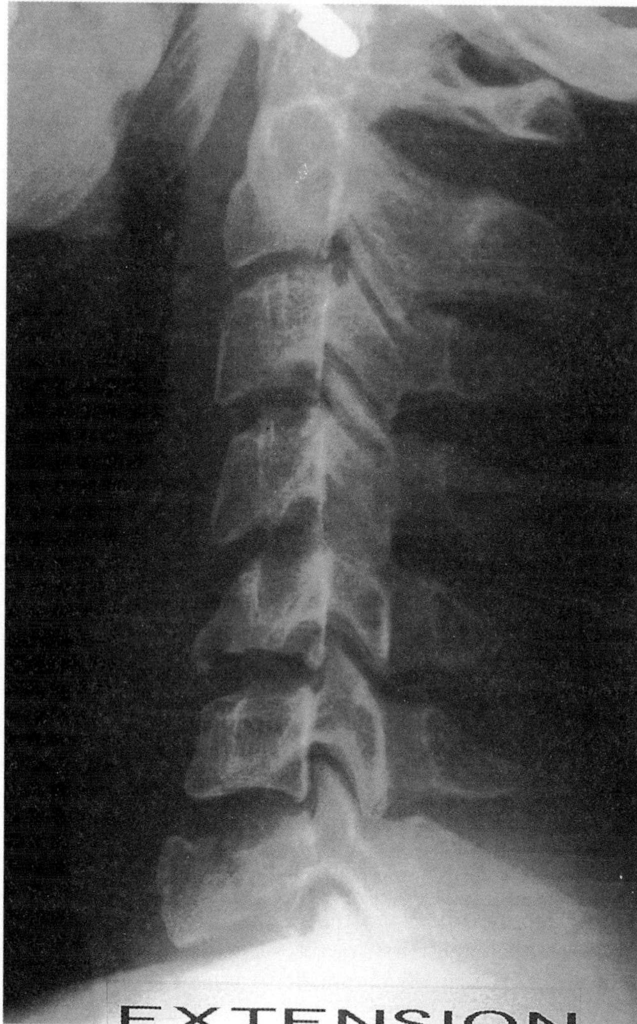

Fig. 33.12 Tear-drop fracture (C5) and burst fracture (C7) in the same patient.

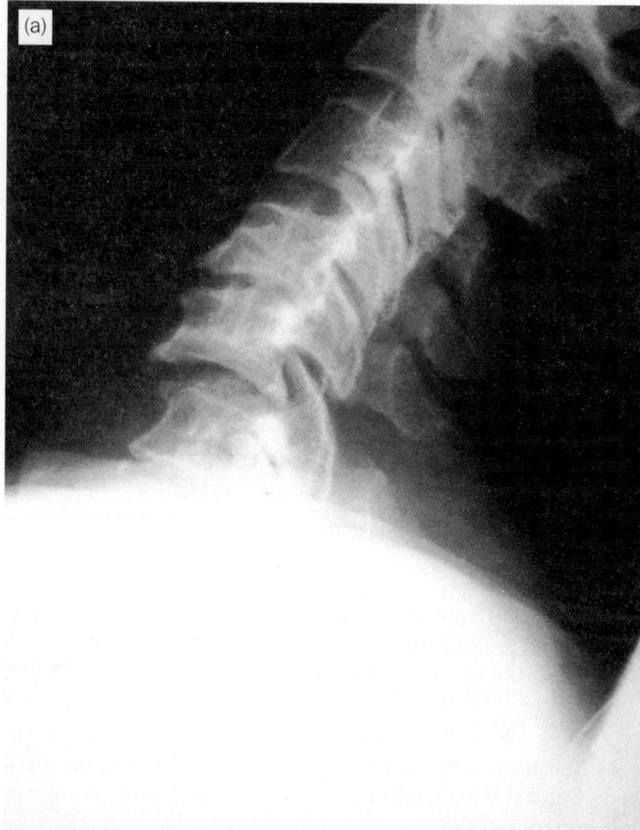

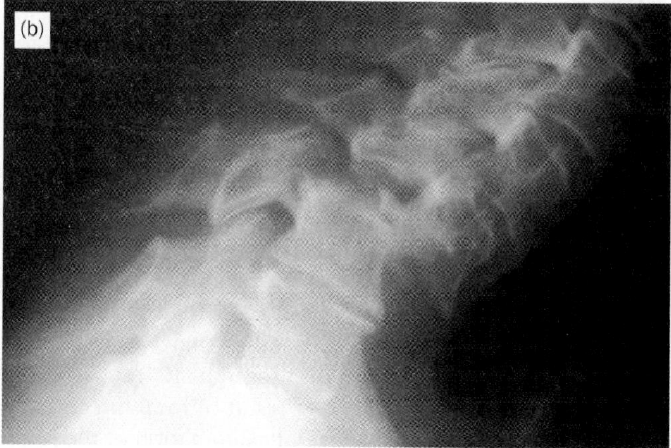

Fig. 33.13 (a) Unifacet dislocation, with less than 25 per cent displacement of C5 on C6. (b) Bifacet dislocation with almost complete dislocation between C5 and C6.

prolapse has been excluded (see assessment above). If the patient has a complete cord injury, the dislocation can simply be reduced on traction (see Fig. 33.13).

Facet dislocations are unstable and once reduced, internal fixation and bone grafting is recommended.

Thoracic and thoracolumbar fractures

These fractures can be classified according to the mechanism of injury or according to the classification method developed by the AO. This classification corresponds with an increasing degree of injury and increasing incidence of neurological injury. It is helpful for communication and for classification in research.

Thoracic fractures (T1–T9)

As in other areas of the spine the commonest fractures are wedge fractures, in the elderly often associated with osteoporosis. These stable fractures can be safely managed with pain relief and mobilisation. Occasionally bracing can be helpful for pain relief.

The spine is splinted by the ribs. Other patterns of fracture are often caused by high-energy injuries, and multiple injuries are not uncommon in these patients. Thoracic fractures and sternal fractures are often associated with aortic rupture, and a high index of suspicion is recommended in the patients. CT scanning will help to make the diagnosis.

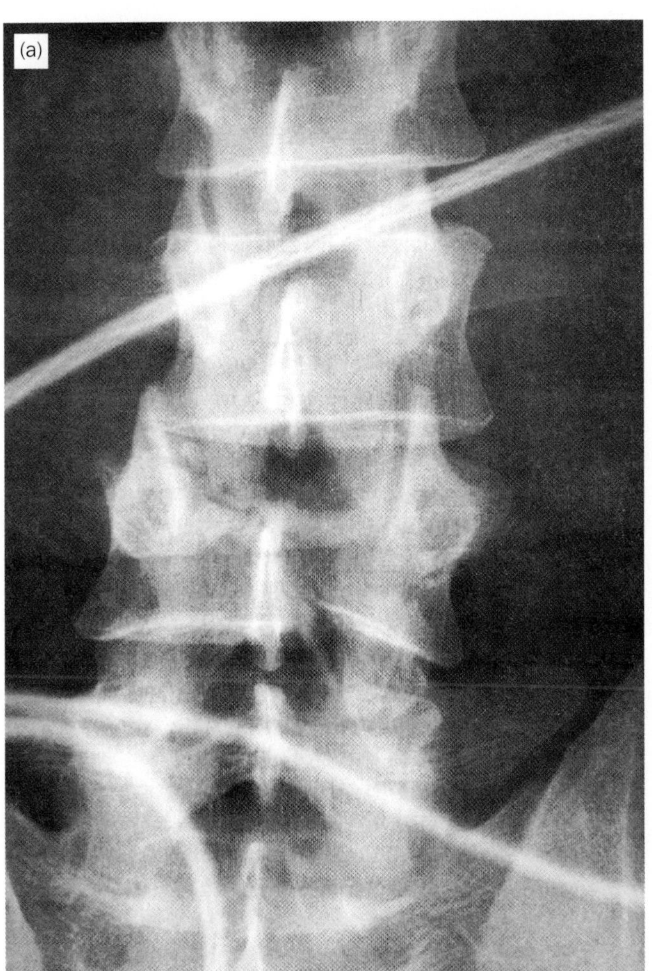

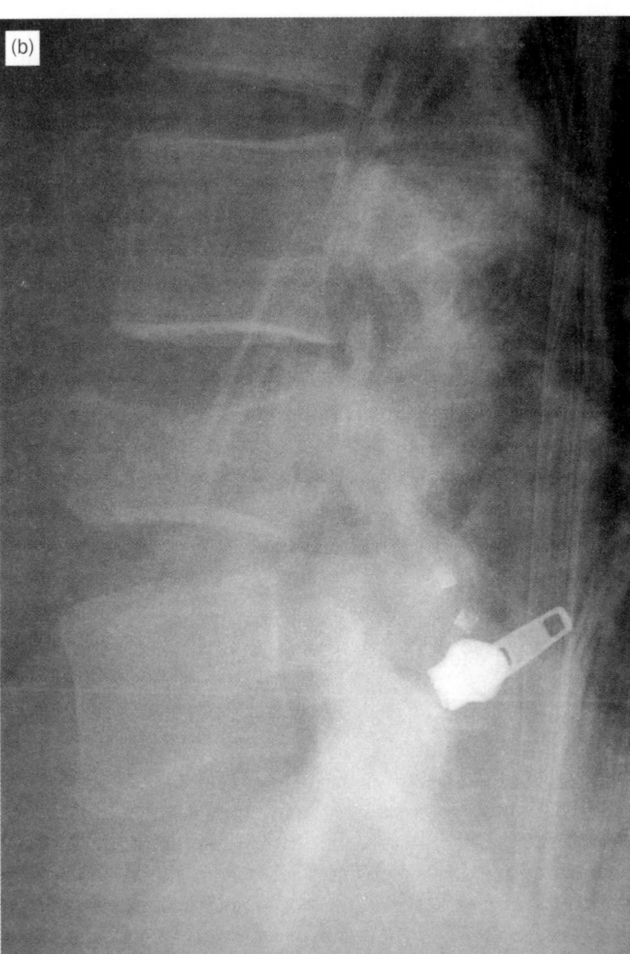

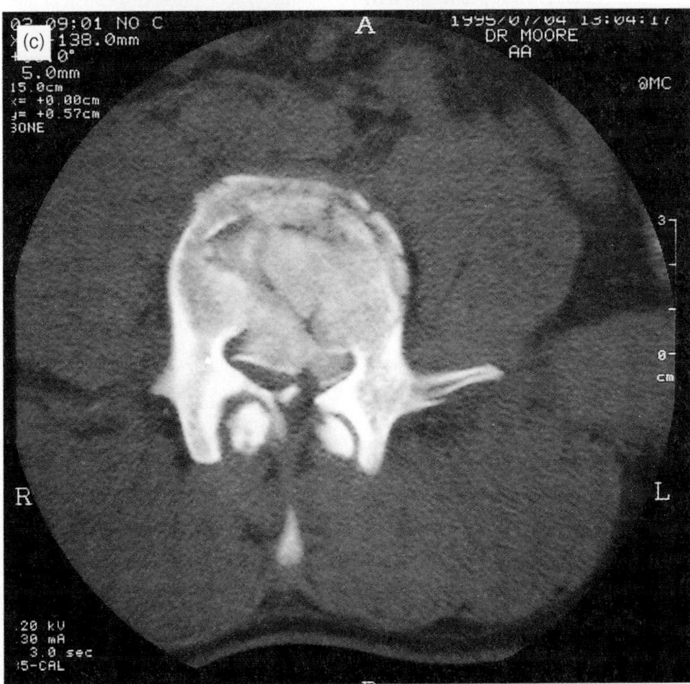

Fig. 33.14 Thoracolumbar burst fracture. Plain films: (a) and (b) show disruption of L4; (c) CT scan shows almost complete occlusion of the spinal canal. Patients had partial injury to the cauda equina.

Some thoracic fractures can be very difficult to diagnose, particularly in the upper part of the thoracic spine. Careful clinical examination should exclude these fractures in the conscious patient, but in the unconscious patients radiographs of the spine must be carefully examined, with a low threshold for carrying out CT scans.

Unstable thoracic fractures can easily displace in the first few hours after a fracture and great care must be taken when moving the patient. Early posterior stabilisation of these fractures is recommended.

Thoracolumbar fractures (T10–L5)

These fractures are more common than thoracic fractures because this part of the spine is not splinted by the ribs. The most common fractures are T12 and L1 because these are at the junction between the stiff thoracic spine and the mobile lumbar spine.

Stable wedge fractures are commonest and can be treated either with mobilisation alone or with bracing initially for pain.

Unstable fractures may cause spinal cord injury or nerve root injury depending on the level of the injury.

Burst fractures may be stable or unstable. If the posterior elements are intact, then the fracture can be considered stable. Unstable fractures can usually be diagnosed on the plain radiographs, with what may appear to be a fracture similar to a wedge fracture, but with widening of the distance between the pedicles (see Fig. 33.14). This implies a fracture of the anterior structures (the body) and the posterior structures (the pedicles). It may however be necessary to carry out a CT scan to see whether the posterior elements are fractured. Clinical examination in the conscious patient will allow some assessment of the posterior structures. If there is no pain and no palpable defect, then the injury is probably stable. In the unconscious patient this may be more difficult and occasionally MRI scans are necessary to assess the whether posterior elements adequately to see if there is ligamentous damage.

Distraction injuries are more commonly associated with neurological injury and are usually unstable injuries. Most of these injuries are a combination of bone and soft-tissue injury, but some pass through the bone alone, so-called chance fractures. Many of these fractures are associated with intra-abdominal injury and careful examination of the abdomen is important.

Rotational injuries are the most common and are usually caused by a combination of forces. They are associated with the highest incidence of neurological injury and are best treated with reduction and internal fixation.

Unstable fractures are best treated with posterior stabilisation of the spine but if there is associated neurological injury, particularly at the level of the conus (T12/L1), anterior vertebrectomy and stabilisation is probably best in order to decompress the spinal cord adequately. In the lumbar spine it is important that fixation is limited to the minimum number of levels in order to maintain lumbar mobility.

Degenerative disease of the spine

Introduction

Pain due to degenerative disease of the cervical and lumbar spine is very common in the general population. A wide variety of terms is used describing this, including lumbago, wear and tear, spondylosis and a slipped disc. What is clear is that parts of the spine are subject to a series of changes in both the intervertebral disc and the adjacent vertebrae. They are associated with local pain and may be associated with the compression of the spinal cord or nerve root. It is also apparent that these changes occur with age. MRI scanning has provided excellent evidence of this disc degeneration, with loss of water content, these changing often without associated pain (see Fig. 33.15). Thinning of the annulus and the appearance of radial slits allow the nucleus to bulge – and may eventually rupture through causing disc prolapse.

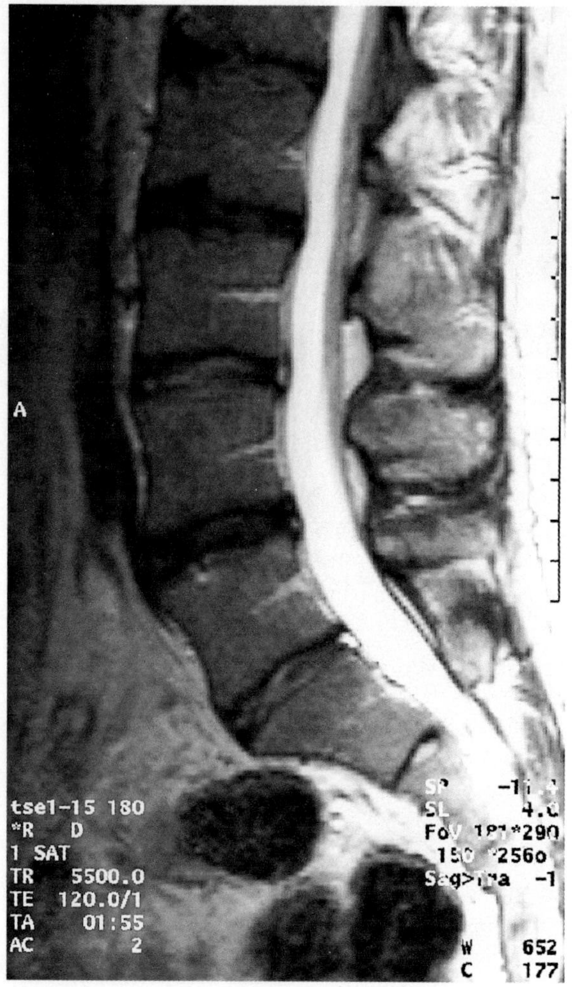

Fig. 33.15 MRI (T2 sagittal) showing changes of dehydration and disc bulging in the lumbar spine of a patient without symptoms.

Progressive collapse of the disc space may allow additional movement, putting extra strain on the apophyseal joints, in which secondary degenerative changes occur with associated ligamentous hypertrophy. Osteophyte formation, due to calcification of the bulging peripheral fibres of the annulus, leads to further narrowing of the spinal, or root exit, canal.

Neurological involvement can therefore occur due to cord, cauda equina or root compression by soft disc, ligamentous hypertrophy or osteophyte formation.

Cervical degenerative disease

Two patterns emerge.

1. **Cervical radiculopathy**. Neck and radicular pain in the arm with, on examination, signs of a lower motor neuron lesion usually affecting C6 or C7. Functional changes and pins and needles may be apparent, the arm pain being the predominant symptom (see Fig. 33.16).
2. **Cervical myelopathy**. Pain and stiffness in the neck with a gritty feeling in the tips of the fingers. Patients will complain of stiffness and a loss of dexterity, with unsteadiness of gait.

The symptoms are usually slowly progressive with, on examination, signs of an upper motor neuron lesion with a glove and stocking distribution sensory loss. The neck pain may not be a major feature. Examination will usually reveal a restricted range of cervical spine movement (see Fig. 33.17).

Commonly seen in the midcervical region, signs of radiculopathy at the affected level may be superimposed. Presence of the deltoid jerk suggests compression above the C4/5 level.

Investigation

Following a careful history and examination to define the pattern of neurological compromise and the clinically

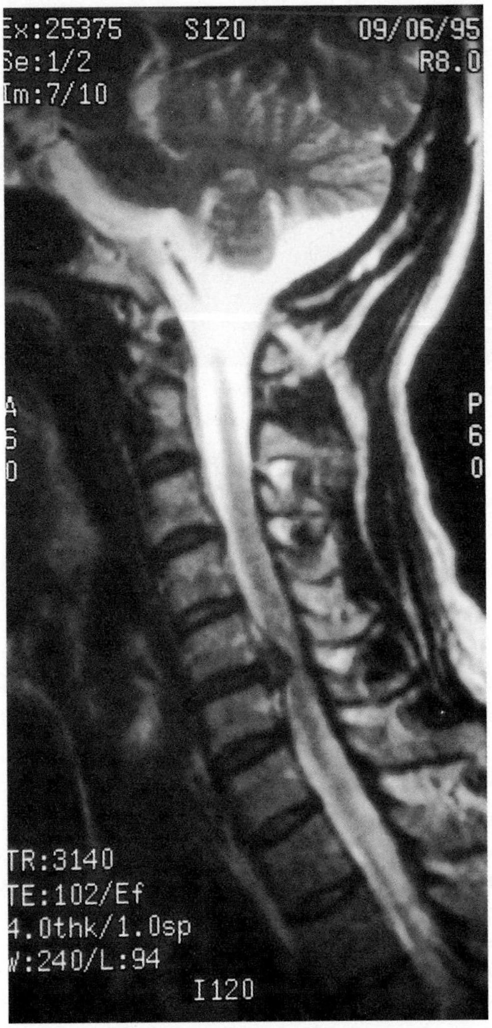

Fig. 33.16 MRI scan (T2 sagittal) showing acute cervical 5/6 soft disc prolapse.

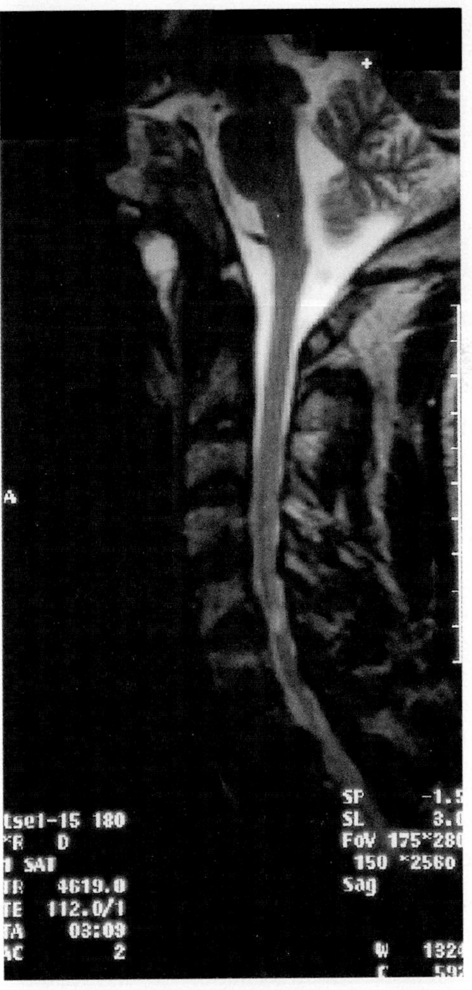

Fig. 33.17 MRI scan (T2 sagittal) showing a narrow spinal canal due to cervical spondylosis with an area of myelomalacia within the spinal cord.

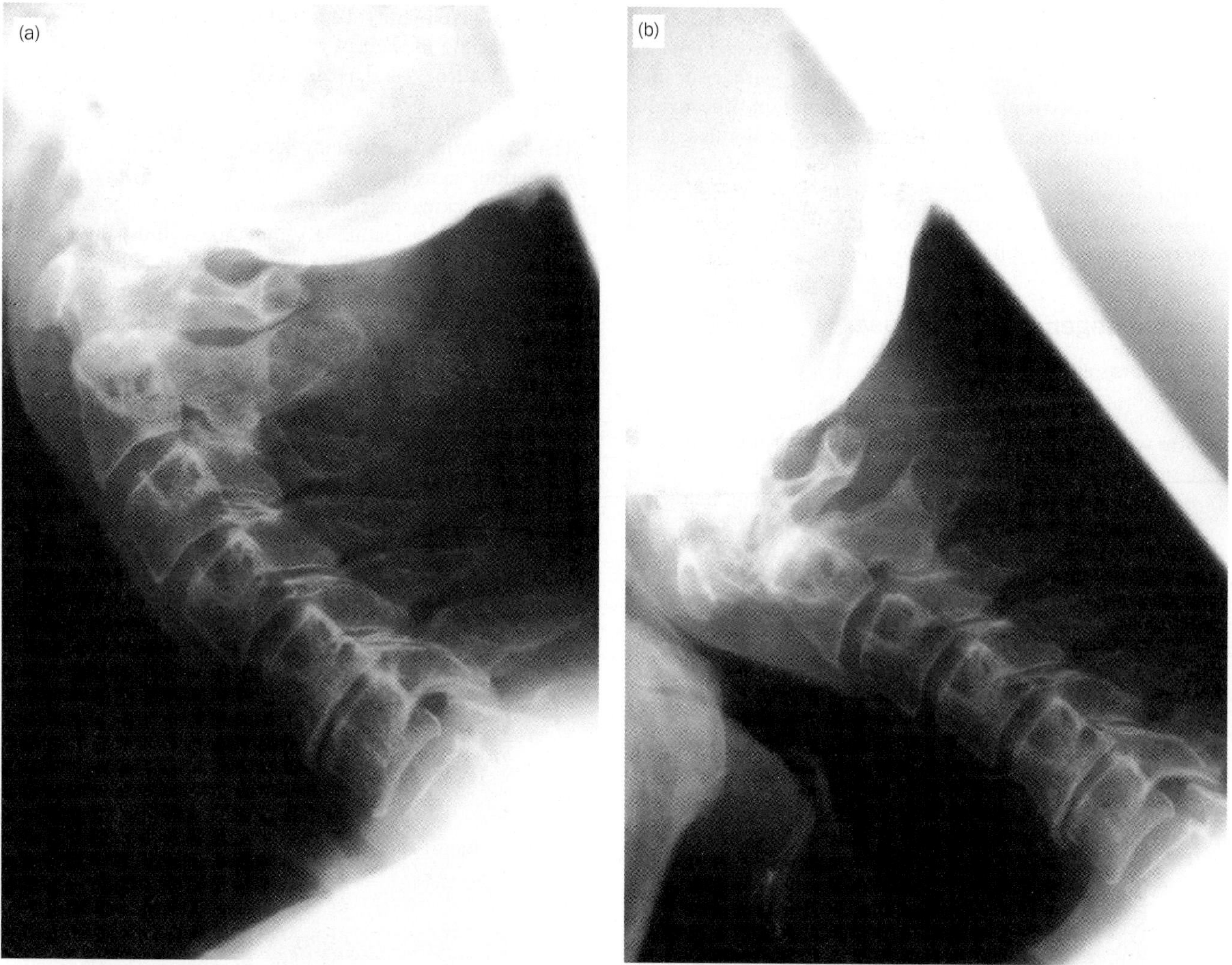

Fig. 33.18 Lateral cervical spine X-rays showing early osteophyte formation: (a) extension; (b) flexion.

affected level, plain X-rays in flexion and extension with an MRI represent the investigations of choice. Cervical myelography is rarely performed, but CT myelography may be helpful if MRI is not available.

Plain X-rays provide details of the bony architecture and evidence of osteophyte formation. Instability can be seen and measured (see Fig. 33.18). MRI in sagittal and axial views allows detailed study of the spinal cord – including changes within the cord itself – together with views of the exiting nerve roots and root canals. MRI does not provide 'dynamic' information about the cervical spine and should be used in conjunction with plain X-rays in flexion and extension (see Fig. 33.19).

Differential diagnosis

For cervical radiculopathy the diagnosis is usually apparent. The differential includes cervical rib, producing a T1 syndrome, ulnar or median nerve entrapment syndromes, metastatic disease in the cervical spine, or even direct brachial plexus involvement via an apical lung tumour (Pancoast syndrome).

For patients with a myelopathy, clearly other causes of spinal cord compromise rarely occur, but should be considered. These include an intraspinal tumour, infection or instability associated with conditions such as rheumatoid arthritis. Beware the tumour at the level of the foramen magnum leading to wasting of the small hand muscles.

Management

Radiculopathy. In over 75 per cent of patients the symptoms will resolve with conservative measures, including rest, analgesia, the use of a cervical collar and physiotherapy by an experienced therapist. Physical therapies are becoming increasingly specialised and appropriately timed treatments will usually produce good results.

Care should be taken with cervical collars. A short-term support can become a long-term crutch. Their length of use should be avoided.

Henry Khurrath Pancoast, b. 1875. Radiologist, Philadelphia, Pennsylvania, USA.

(a)

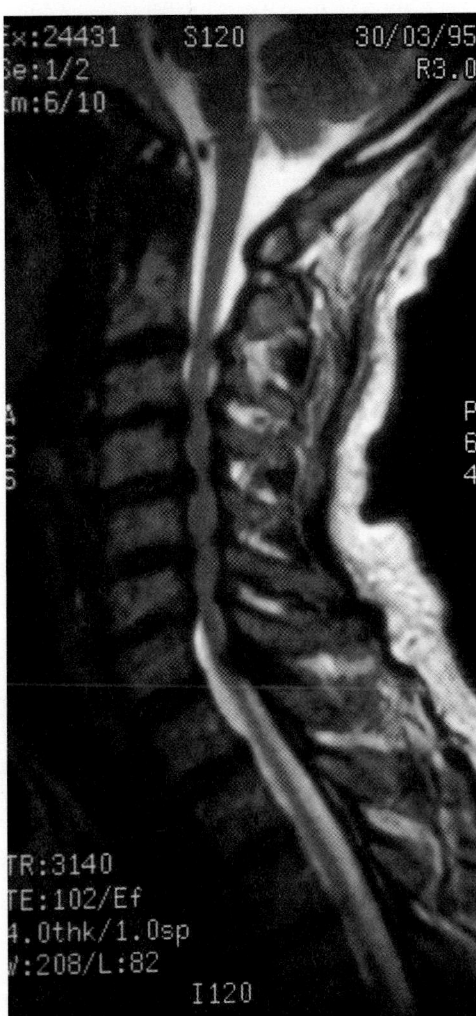

(b)

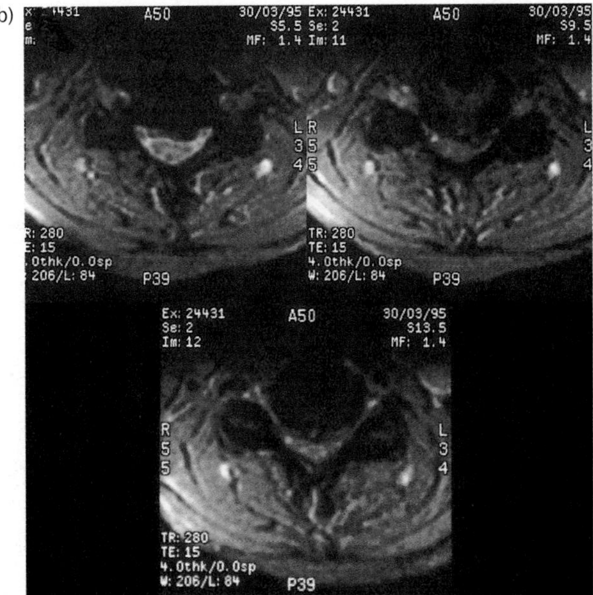

Fig. 33.19 MRI scan (sagittal and axial T2) showing severe cervical cord compression due to cervical spondylosis at multiple levels: (a) sagittal view; (b) axial views.

Surgery is indicated according to the duration and severity of the pain, physical signs, the radiological appearances and – most importantly – the patient's wishes. A good history with physical signs and corresponding radiological changes, and providing a good decompression is achieved, will produce good results.

To effect decompression of the nerve root, either an anterior cervical discectomy approach can be used, or posterior foraminotomy. For soft disc prolapse causing nerve root compression, an anterior approach is most frequently used.

Myelopathy. There is much debate about how and when to proceed to surgery. The aim of the operation is *to prevent further deterioration*. If there is improvement, then this is to some extent a bonus and it is important that the patient and their family are advised of this. Despite decompression, in 30 per cent of patients there will be further deterioration, probably due to vascular changes within the cord itself.

Surgical decompression is, therefore, appropriate for those who are deteriorating, whose symptoms interfere with normal activity, and are accepting of the risks of the procedure.

The aim is to decompress the spinal cord and maintain or establish stability. This can be done by an anterior or a posterior approach to the spine. Anterior approach requires removal of soft disc, osteophytes and hypertrophied ligaments, often over multiple levels. Fusion, intervertebral grafts or onlay plates can then be achieved.

A posterior cervical laminectomy provides easy access to decompress the spine over multiple levels and great care must be taken to avoid spinal cord injury. The decision between anterior and posterior approaches depends again on the pathology, the presence of instability and the experience of the surgeon.

The advantages and disadvantages of the two approaches are considered in Table 33.3.

Table 33.3 The advantages and disadvantages of anterior and posterior approaches to the cervical spine

	Anterior	*Posterior*
Advantages	Easy access to disc	Access to multiple levels
	Evacuate disc	Good root compression
	Fusion by plate/graft	Direct visualisation of root
	Little pain	Fusion not usually required
Disadvantages	Multiple levels difficult	Risk of instability
	May require fusion if unstable	Poor access to disc space
	Loss of mobility	Poor access to osteophytes
	Risk of injury to adjacent structures	Higher risk of cord injury
		Painful procedure

Inflammatory disorders involving the cervical spine

Rheumatoid arthritis

This commonly affects the spine and particularly the cervical spine. Patients often present with stiffness and pain in the neck, and some patients present with neurological symptoms due to compressive myelopathy in the neck. Diseases in the joints in turn lead to soft-tissue destruction and then instability. The three common abnormalities are:

- atlantoaxial subluxation;
- proximal migration of the odontoid with basilar impression;
- lower cervical spine subluxations.

Investigation with flexion and extension radiographs of the neck and MRI scan allow assessment of stability and cord compression. A certain number of patients may require decompression of the spinal cord and appropriate stabilisation. Anterior decompression (transoral), fusion and instrumentation may be appropriate with localised disease. This may be necessary in either the lower or the upper cervical spine (see Fig. 33.20a–c).

Ankylosing spondylitis

This is relatively uncommon, but can present with painful stiffness of the spine. It is more common in males, most of whom will be human leucocyte antigen (HLA) B27 positive. Other inflammatory markers will be raised. In general physiotherapy combined with anti-inflammatory drugs will control symptoms adequately. However, severe deformities will occasionally be seen and these may require major surgery to the spine to effect correction. Occasionally patients with ankylosing spondylitis will present after minor trauma with unstable fractures. These patients should be assumed to have an unstable injury until this has been excluded. Surgical stabilisation leads to satisfactory results in most cases.

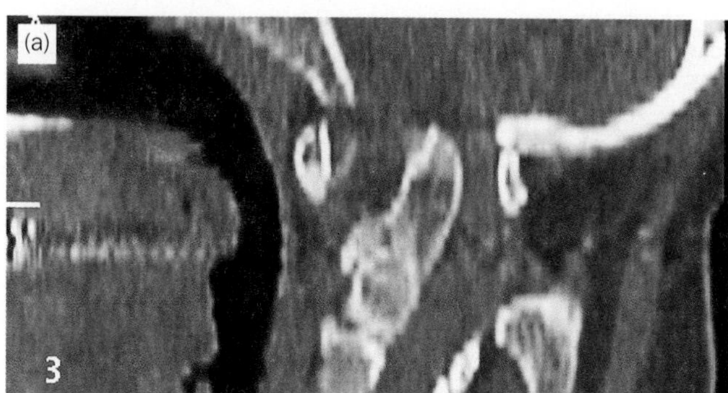

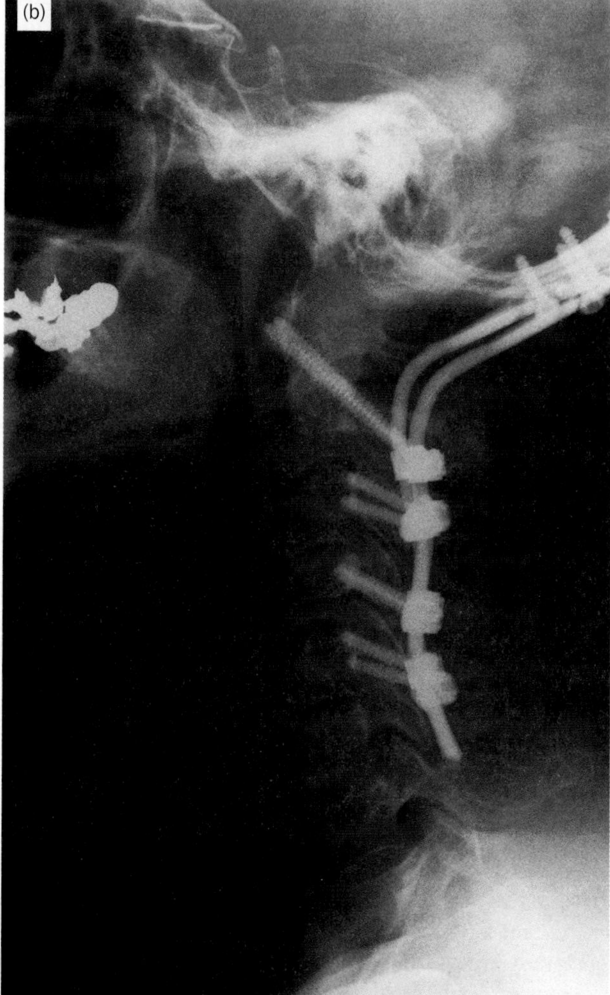

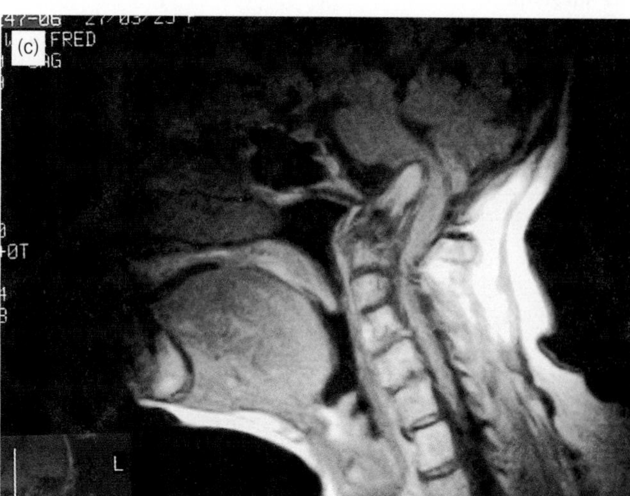

Fig. 33.20 The rheumatoid spine. (a) CT reconstruction showing atlantoaxial instability with basilar invagination of the odontoid peg. (b) MRI scan (sagittal T1) showing severe medullary compression due to atlantoaxial instability with erosion of the odontoid, pannus formation and basilar invagination. (c) Plain lateral cervical spine X-ray after reduction and stabilisation with cervifix on-lay plates.

Thoracic spinal degenerative disease

This is rare. Thoracic disc is the commonest form of degenerative thoracic disease that requires surgery.

Presentation

More common in males (5:3 ratio) and usually in the lower thoracic spine, the patients may present with a history of injury but this usually occurs spontaneously.

Pain may not be a major feature. The symptoms will progress very rapidly over a few days, or may occur insidiously over years. The presenting features are those of progressive spinal cord compression with, initially, often dissociating signs, but if undiagnosed will finally progress to a paraplegia with a sensory level, to loss of sphincter function.

Investigation

Plain X-ray may reveal calcification in the disc at the affected level, with calcification of the protruding disc visible.

CT scan. As part of a CT myelogram, this will confirm the epidural compression at the level of the disc prolapse.

MRI scan remains the investigation of choice. Be aware of the level of the disease and whether it is lateral or central (see Fig. 33.21a and b).

Management

Removal of a thoracic disc represents a very different operation to that of cervical or lumbar disc. The prolapse can be hard and calcified or occasionally soft and liquid, appearing like pus. The dura may even be eroded.

A standard laminectomy is dangerous and a lateral or anterior transthoracic approach is required to excise these lesions.

If truly central, a transthoracic route, with drilling out of the vertebral body above and below the level of the disc prolapse, will allow piecemeal removal of the disc and decompression of the spine.

For the laterally placed discs a costotransversectomy with division of the paravertebral muscles and excision of the rib head provides good access, again drilling away the vertebral bodies above and below the disc to allow its removal. Check the levels very carefully by preoperative and/or peroperative imaging and warn the patient, especially about the risks of paralysis due to surgery.

Lumbar spine

Degenerative disease of the lumbar spine is almost universal with increasing age. The disc ages owing to deterioration of the proteoglycan within the disc, which becomes dehydrated as a result. Therefore the disc becomes narrower and this in turn narrows the nerve root canals where the lumbar nerve roots exit from the spinal canal. Secondary changes also occur in the facet joints with loss of joint space, sclerosis and osteophyte formation.

(a)

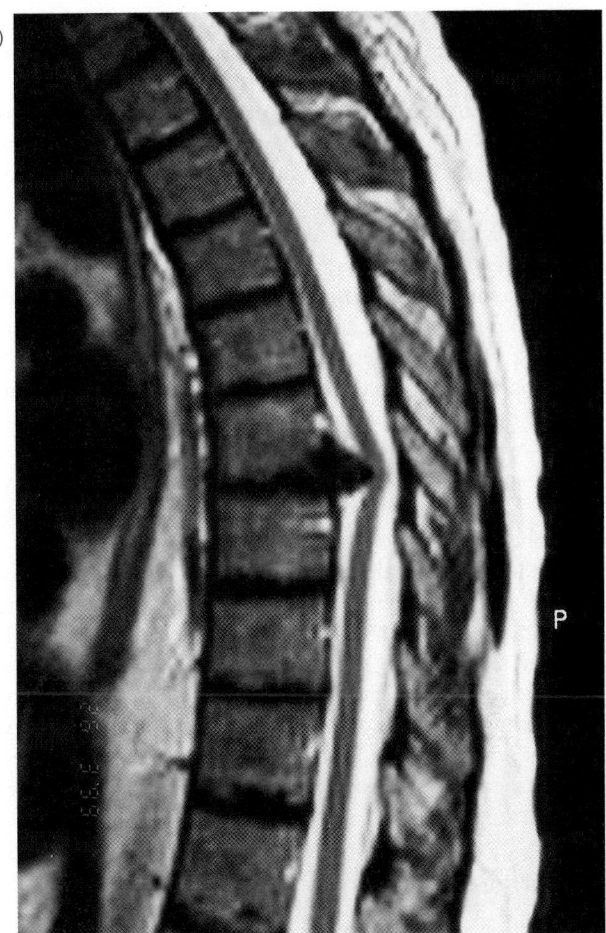

(b)

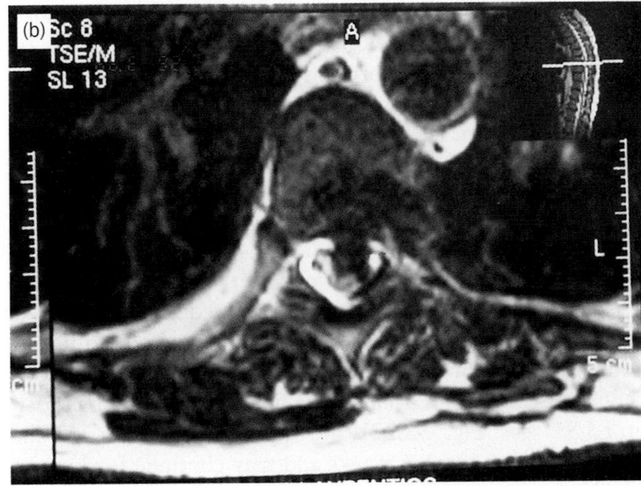

Fig. 33.21 MRI scan (sagittal and axial T2) showing severe thoracic cord compression due to a thoracic disc: (a) sagittal view of thoracic disc; (b) axial views showing that the disc is paracentral towards the left.

Between 70 and 90 per cent of individuals will experience back pain at some point in their lives. The commonest site of pain in the spine is the intervertebral disc. Although the central part of the disc has no nerve supply, the annulus is very sensitive and is often a source of pain. Degeneration tears often occur in the annulus and these can be a source of pain.

Neurological symptoms can also occur as a result of degenerative disease in the spine. Tears of the annulus can allow part of the nucleus pulposus to herniate through the annulus. The weakest part of the annulus is the postero-lateral corner, and as a result the nerve root is often compressed in the lateral part of the spinal canal. More central disc protrusions can also occur and this can result in compression of the cauda equina which lies in the midline throughout most of the lumbar spine. This can cause cauda equina compression with loss of bowel and bladder function. If this occurs, urgent surgical decompression is indicated.

Another effect of degeneration is that spinal stenosis can occur due to a combination of narrowing of the disc, osteophyte formation from the joints and thickening of the ligamentum flavum. The stenosis can either be central, lateral around the exiting nerve roots or a combination of the two. Most patients with spinal stenosis are elderly but some patients present young, and the majority of these has developmental spinal stenosis where the spinal canal is narrow from birth.

Presenting symptoms

Back pain is usually felt in the lumbar area and may radiate to the buttocks and the back of the thighs. If the pain is coming from the upper lumbar region, it may radiate to the front of the thigh. Pure back pain very seldom radiates below the knees. Patients will often complain of spinal stiffness and of difficulty in the activities of daily living such as picking things up, shopping, sitting, walking, running and so on. Back pain can occur in any age group, but beware of the child with back pain because it is likely that there is some more serious underlying condition (see above). Other features of back pain which are worrying include night pain which prevents sleep or unremitting pain which cannot be controlled with pain relief. Spinal tumour or spinal infection must be excluded in these patients.

Disc prolapse

Disc prolapse occurs most commonly in middle age although it can occur in adolescence and in the elderly. The typical history is of an episode of back pain either related to lifting and/or twisting or which occurs spontaneously. Eighty per cent of disc prolapses occur in the lumbar spine, the majority at L5/S1 (see Fig. 33.22) and at L4/L5. The back pain commonly lasts for 2–6 weeks and may continue for longer. The back pain will often improve then but is followed almost immediately by sciatica or nerve root pain. The pain will usually follow one or more dermatomes, and is often associated with neurological symptoms, altered sensation and weakness in the muscles innervated by the compressed nerve roots. Serious neurological symptoms may be an indication for urgent surgery to decompress the nerve roots, but in general a period of waiting is best because 90 per cent of patients will have relief of their pain within 6 weeks. Minor degrees of weakness and numbness will usually improve with time and may resolve completely. Motor weakness is more likely to recover than sensory change.

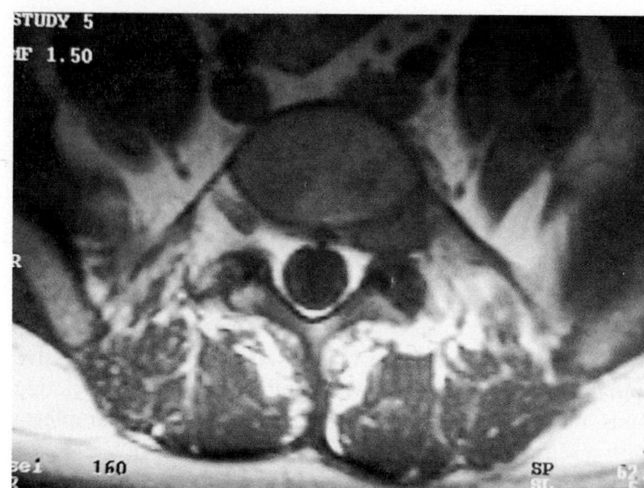

Fig. 33.22 Lateral disc prolapse L5/S1 compressing the exiting L5 nerve root.

Spinal stenosis

Spinal stenosis presents typically in the elderly patient and tends to develop gradually (Fig. 33.23). The patient may develop back pain, especially standing and walking, which is associated with neurological symptoms in the legs. Patients report pain, weakness and numbness in the legs on standing or walking, and their walking distance is usually limited. They may complain that their legs go rubbery or tend to give way. Their symptoms usually resolve with rest, especially sitting down for 5–10 minutes, and then they can continue. They often report fewer symptoms going up hill or walking using a rollator or a shopping trolley. The reason for this is that the spinal canal is made wider with spinal flexion. This helps to differentiate these patients from those with vascular claudication who find it worse uphill. Usually the symptoms of vascular claudication will be relieved more rapidly.

Treatment

The majority of patients with *back pain* can be treated with physical treatments such as physiotherapy, chiropractic, or the various other treatments available. Explaining to the patient that they have a nonprogressive condition which is very common will help them to cope with the symptoms. Medications such as analgaesics and anti-inflammatories can also be used. Adjustments to work situations (e.g. seating) and to day-to-day life (e.g. less driving, more physical

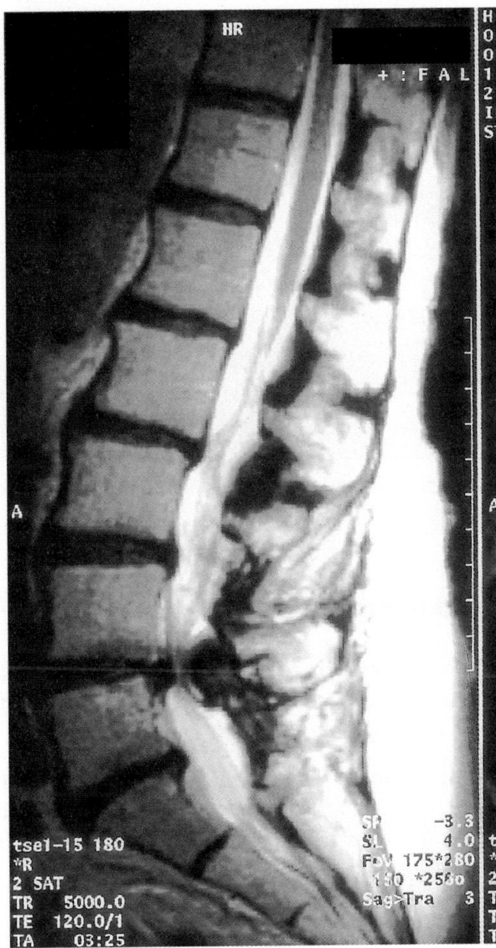

Fig. 33.23 Spinal stenosis at L4/L5.

activity, weight loss) are often much more effective that other measures. A small proportion of patients will develop more severe symptoms which require more intensive physical treatments such as rehabilitation. Surgery to fuse or stabilise the spine is a last resort, and should only be used in selected patients where less invasive methods have been used. Combined anterior–posterior surgery probably has the best results in these patients.

Disc prolapse

Disc prolapse usually resolves within 6 weeks, and simple pain relief may be all that is required in these patients. Longitudinal studies have demonstrated that most of these disc prolapses will resolve with time.

Patients with evidence of cauda equina compression must be managed as an emergency. Symptoms suggestive of this are:

- very restricted straight leg raising bilaterally;
- numbness in the perineum;
- inability to void or difficulty voiding urine;
- inability to have or difficulty in having bowels open;
- lax anal sphincter;
- severe pain.

Not all of these signs are necessarily present in each patient. Emergency MRI scanning or, if not available, CT scan or myelogram will confirm the diagnosis, and treatment is surgical decompression and partial discectomy.

In the patient with simple sciatica various options are available.

- Epidural steroid injection – about 30 per cent success rate, low complication rate, day-case procedure.
- Chemonucleolysis (injection of chymopapain into the disc itself) – about 70 per cent success rate, day case or overnight stay. Often causes back pain in the early stages. May take some weeks to be effective. Low complication rate, occasional anaphylactic reaction to the chymopapain.
- Laser discectomy (laser coagulation of the disc) – success rate 50–70 per cent, less back pain than chemonucleolysis, day-case procedure, low complication rate.
- Microdiscectomy – success rate 80–90 per cent. Three per cent long-term complication rate (e.g. nerve damage, infection, long-term back pain). Requires hospital admission for a few days. Longer convalescence.
- Standard discectomy – as for microdiscectomy, but longer scar, longer in hospital, longer recovery.

There is no reason in most cases why closed techniques cannot be used initially and then open surgery used if other methods fail. In older individuals associated spinal stenosis is common and open techniques are more likely to be effective.

Many patients with *spinal stenosis* are elderly, and nonsurgical methods of treatment may be better for some. Various treatments have been used with fairly low success rates such as lumbar corset, epidural injection of steroids and traction. Physiotherapy with flexion exercises can be helpful in a minority of patients. Calcitonin has been used with some success for treating spinal stenosis, particularly in the elderly who may not be fit for surgery. One-hundred international units of calcitonin are given by intramuscular (i.m.) injection 4 days a week for 4 weeks. Success rates of 20–30 per cent have been reported, but to date there has not been a randomised trial to assess the treatment.

Surgery is effective in about 70 per cent of patients with spinal stenosis. Decompression of symptomatic nerve roots and central stenosis can give very effective relief.

Spondylolisthesis

Spondylolisthesis is a common condition and is usually caused either by spondylolysis or by degenerative change (Fig. 33.24). Spondylolysis is a defect in the bone in the pars

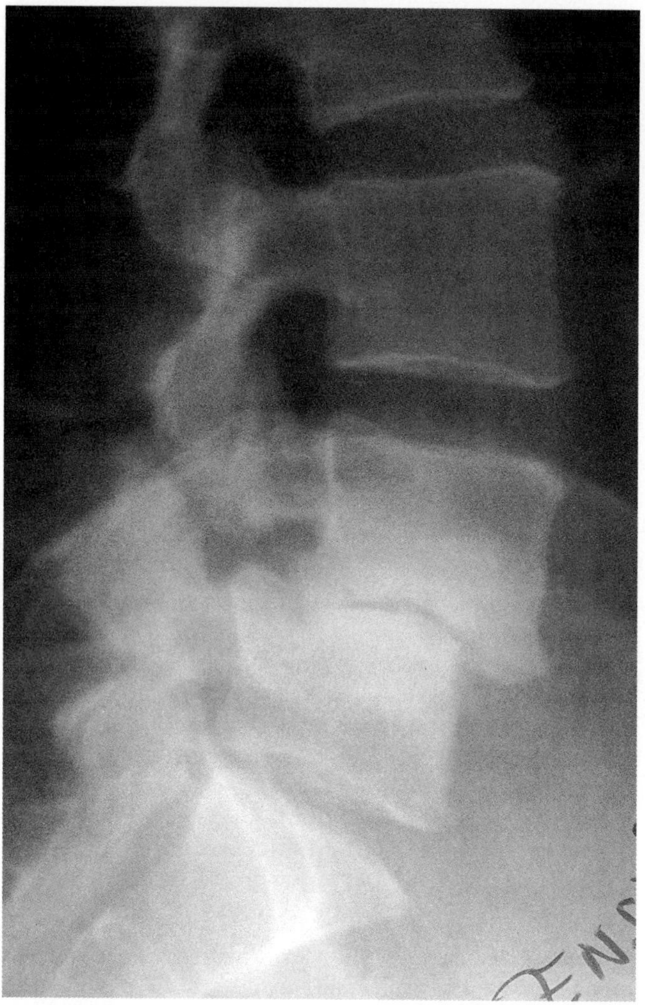

Fig. 33.24 Spondylolisthesis at L4/L5 with narrowing of the intervertebral disc.

interarticularis, and causes a slip between one vertebra and another in some cases. It is present in about 6 per cent of the normal population, is usually asymptomatic and is a common incidental finding. In young individuals presenting with back pain nonoperative measures such as physiotherapy are usually successful in resolving pain, and occasionally a plaster jacket can resolve symptoms. Indications for surgery include nonresolving and serious pain or progressive slip between the two vertebrae. If the spondylolysis is undisplaced and the intervertbral disc at that level is normal, direct repair by bone grafting and internal fixation can be carried out. Otherwise fusion of the motion segment is required. In children internal fixation is seldom required but in adults most surgeons use fixation with interpedicular screws.

Degenerative spondylolithesis is common in the elderly and occurs owing to degeneration of the disc and the associated facet joints. It can be associated with spinal stenosis, and if decompressive surgery is contemplated, it is usually best to carry out an uninstrumented fusion to prevent progression of the slip.

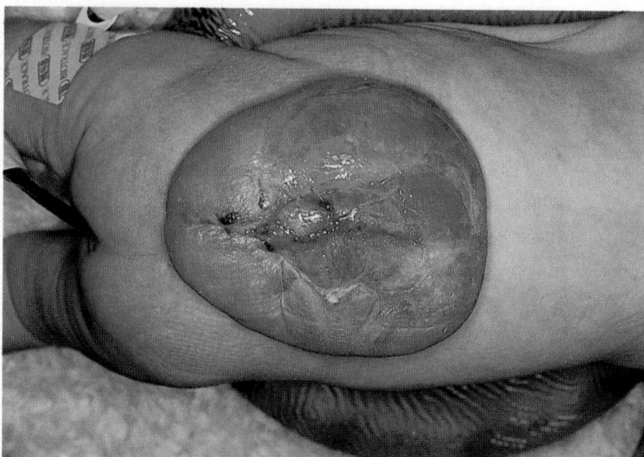

Fig. 33.25 Spina bifida aperta with an open neural tube defect leaking CSF.

Developmental anomalies

The commonest problem to affect the spinal column is failure of the neural tube to close fully, producing one of many patterns of neurospinal dysraphism or spina bifida.

- Spina bifida aperta. The neural tube is open with no skin coverage, through a defect in the posterior vertebral arch. CSF leakage usually occurs with an associated risk of infection (see Fig. 33.25).
- Spina bifida cystica. In this situation there is skin covering the defect which may contain just CSF, so forming a meningocele, or may have neural tissue within the sac, a myelomeningocele.
- Spina bifida occulta. The posterior vertebral arch has a defect within it, but there is no herniation of the neural tube. This defect may be found within 10 per cent of the population. On the skin over the defect various skin changes may be seen, for example a hairy patch (see Fig. 33.26), an area of pigmentation, a fatty lump or

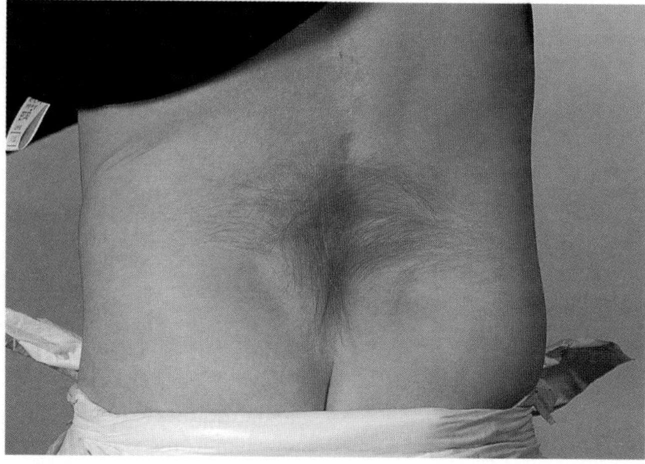

Fig. 33.26 A hairy naevus associated with spina bifida occulta.

dermal sinus. There may also be associated intradural lesions, including lipomas, dermoids, epidermoid tumours and tethering of the cord with thickening of the filum terminale.

Management

Any discussion regarding the treatment of children with this condition should include inheritance. Whilst the majority (90 per cent) of cases occurs sporadically, with an incidence ranging from one to eight per 1000 of the population, children of parents with spina bifida have a 5 per cent risk of having the condition as well.

Prenatal screening to detect alpha-fetoprotein in blood or amniotic fluid, obtained by amniocentesis, together with the use of ultrasound allows the detection of such defects in over 80 per cent with an open neural tube.

Problems of development tend to occur in the lumbo-sacral area and are especially associated with changes in bladder and bowel function. These changes may not become apparent for the first few years of life and can be associated with a totally normal neurological examination.

The higher the lesion the more severe the defect and the worse the neurological condition. In severe cases it can be associated with a complete failure of development of the legs with a complete paraplegia and loss of bladder and bowel function.

If the lesion is open then there are attendant risks of meningitis as well.

Other associated disorders include Arnold–Chiari malformations and, in up to 80 per cent, hydrocephalus.

Investigations

The investigations include:

- complete neurological examination;
- head circumference measurements;
- plain X-rays of the spine (see Fig. 33.27);
- MRI scan of brain and whole spine.

Treatment

For the majority of cases of open dysraphism, closure should be carried out as soon as possible with treatment of the hydrocephalus. Often this is the first of many procedures best provided by a team of surgeons, paediatricians, therapists and nurses.

As regards the patients with closed lesions at birth, they may require surgery at a later stage should progressive neurological signs develop. It should be noted, however, that any procedure may be associated with neurological deterioration.

Julius Arnold, 1835–1915. German pathologist.
Hans Chiari, 1851–1916. German pathologist.

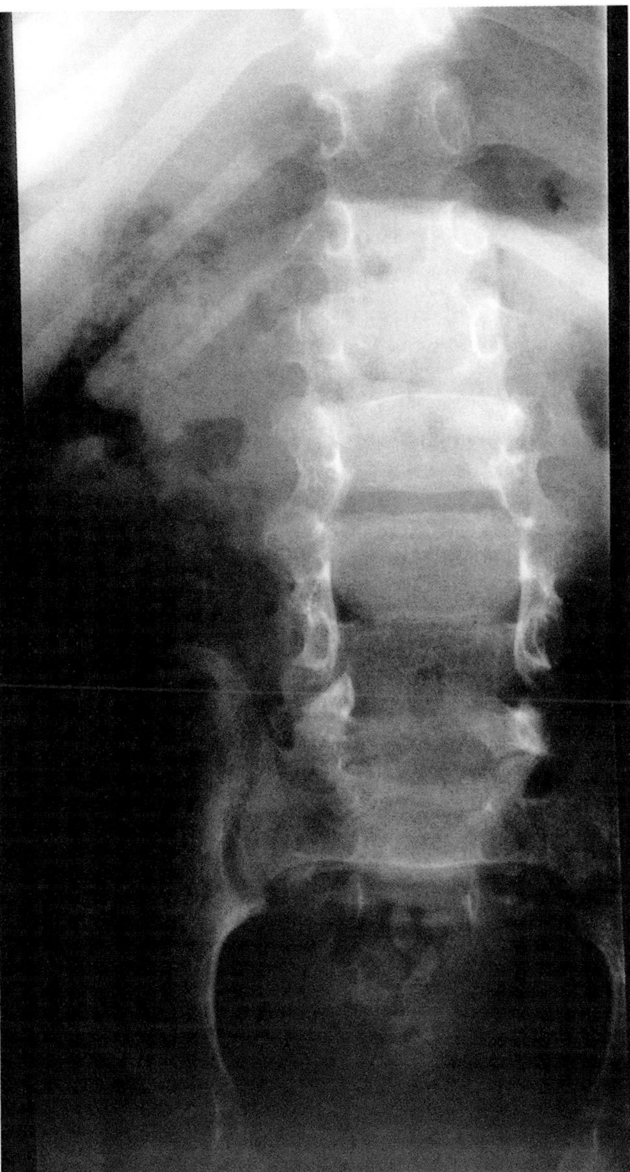

Fig. 33.27 Plain lumbar spine X-ray in a patient with myelomeningocele.

Spinal tumours

These have been divided into:

- tumour of the vertebral column;
- intraspinal tumours.

Tumours of the vertebral column

Between 90 and 95 per cent of spinal tumours are secondary tumours, and occur mostly in older individuals. Although almost any tumour can metastasise to bone the six most common are:

- thyroid;
- breast;

- lung;
- GI tract;
- renal;
- prostate.

The most common among these are breast, lung and prostate. Pain is the commonest cause of presentation and only 10 per cent of individuals present with neurological symptoms alone. Patients may present with pain in the spine itself due to collapse or instability of the spine, or with radicular pain in the distribution of a nerve root. Features of pain which should alert the clinician are night pain and uncontrollable pain which is not relieved by rest. Patients will usually have a history of weight loss and may have a history of previous tumour.

Careful examination of patients presenting with spinal pain may pick up the primary site of the tumour, although in many cases the primary site is not evident.

Plain radiographs of the site of the pain may show vertebral collapse, loss of a pedicle on the AP radiograph, loss of bone substance or occasionally sclerosis of bone (prostate). Bone scans may show tumours, although they are unreliable in myeloma and plasmacytoma. An MRI scan is the most sensitive and reliable way of diagnosing spinal tumours, and allows assessment of the size and invasiveness of the tumour. CT scans can also be used for better definition of bone and bone destruction. Myelography is seldom required now unless MRI scans are impossible (e.g. pacemaker) or difficult technically (e.g. previous metallic implant).

Primary bone tumours do occur in the spine. The most common are:

- benign:
  - haemangioma (10 per cent of autopsies),
  - osteoid osteoma,
  - osteoblastoma,
  - aneurysmal bone cyst,
  - giant cell tumour;
- malignant:
  - myeloma,
  - lymphoma.

Biopsy is indicated in most cases either to confirm the diagnosis or to make the diagnosis. In the terminal patient with a known primary diagnosis biopsy is sometimes not necessary. Diagnosis of the tumour allows planning of appropriate treatment. For example, some tumours are radiosensitive (e.g. lymphoma), whereas others are relatively radioresistant (e.g. lung secondaries).

Three types of biopsy are possible: excisional, incisional and needle biopsy. Occasionally a posteriorly sited tumour will be suitable for excisional biopsy but this is unusual. In most cases a needle biopsy will provide enough material for a diagnosis to be made histologically, but in more complex lesions where there is a subtle differential diagnosis incisional biopsy is probably best. Frozen section can be used so that the whole procedure can be done under one anaesthetic, as long as appropriate staging of the tumour has been carried out beforehand. The needle biopsy should be sited so that the entry point can be excised at the time of definitive surgery.

Excision of the tumour is most commonly carried out for benign tumours in younger individuals where there is a real possibility of cure and where recurrence is possible, for example giant cell tumour. This may require simultaneous anterior and posterior *en bloc* excision of the affected vertebra with a cuff of normal tissue, and then reconstruction of the spine. Osteoid osteoma, in contrast, on the other hand usually requires simple excision of the affected part of the vertebra.

Total excision of malignant tumours may be carried out where the tumour is an isolated tumour and cure of the patient is possible (e.g. some plasmacytomas), but in many cases the tumour cannot be cured either because there is widespread infiltration of the tumour, the tumour has metastasised, or most commonly because the tumour is a distant metastasis of a primary tumour and cure is not possible. In these cases decompression of the neurological structures and stabilisation of the spine are most appropriate.

Intraspinal tumours

'Lumps' within the spinal canal can be classified anatomically or pathologically. Anatomically they may be intradureal or extradural. Pathologically they may be benign or malignant (primary or secondary). Thus a combined classification can be devised (see Table 33.4).

Occurring in one per 100 000 of the population, meningiomas are the commonest intradural lesion accounting for 23 per cent of those visualised, whilst metastatic tumour forms the commonest extradural lesion.

Presenting features

Pain. Usually localised to the anatomical location of the tumour, the pain is progressive over weeks or months, although it may fluctuate in intensity. Characteristically the pain is nocturnal and will often wake the patient at 3 a.m. to 4 a.m. causing them to get up, walk around and maybe try to sleep in a chair. Local tenderness may be present but this is more common with extraspinal tumours.

Radicular signs. Owing to the root irritation this may result in pain in a radicular distribution with associated pins and needles in the corresponding dermatomal area.

Clearly if the root involved is cervical or lumbar in origin the symptoms may mimic cervical brachalgia or sciatica. If the tumour is in the thoracic region the pain will radiate around the chest wall in a dermatomal distribution. Clinical examination may reveal signs of a radiculopathy – indicated by a lower motor neuron lesion of the affected nerves.

Spinal cord/cauda equina signs. Here the signs and symptoms are dependent upon the level of the tumour. If it is above the L1/L2 junction leading to compression of the spinal cord, the patient will develop a progressive spastic paraparesis/quadriparesis with an ascending sensory level, although this may be suspended. Pain due to pressure on the spinal cored is rare. The patient will usually present with a progressive loss of function with pins and needles in the feet (and hands) with, on examination, signs of an upper motor neuron lesion with increased tone, pyramidal distribution weakness, brisk reflexes and extensor plantar responses. Although there is an ascending sensory level, perianal and pericoccygeal sensation may be spared.

Cauda equina compression (below L1/L2 junction) results in symptoms and signs of a lower motor neuron lesion with radicular pain, dermatomal sensory loss and myeotomal loss of power. The reflexes will be reduced with normal or absent plantar responses. Pericoccygeal sensory loss should specifically be examined for, having also made enquiry for changes in bladder, bowel and sexual function. A lack of awareness of the bladder filling, an inability to distinguish the passage of flatus or faeces, and in men erectile dysfunction, all indicate neurological compromise. It should be noted that the neurological picture may be incomplete in the early stages of compression. For example a Brown-Séquard syndrome or contralateral pain and temperature loss with equilateral loss of light touch is occasionally found.

Investigations

Magnetic resonance imaging. With and without gadolinium enhancement, this now forms an investigation of choice. Careful clinical examination with a knowledge of spinal cord anatomy will direct where the imaging is done. A differential diagnosis, according to the classification seen in Table 33.4, can then be made. It should be noted that some tumours can spread throughout the CSF pathways including into the brain, and thus whole neuraxis imaging may be required (Fig. 33.29a and b).

Plain X-rays/CT scan. When dealing with extradural malignant disease the anatomy of the surrounding bone is vital when considering the stability of the spine. This clearly influences the management options. Plain films may show enlargement of the intervertebral canal with a dumb-bell neurofibroma, or scalloping of the vertebral body. In the absence of MRI a CT myelography will provide details of the level of disease, but not the extent, and some information about the relationship to the cord, but not the internal features. CT scan is particularly helpful, however, in performing CT-guided biopsies for extradural tumours (Fig. 33.30a and b).

Other investigations. It should be noted that intraspinal tumours may form part of a systemic disease, for example metastatic tumour, and thus general examination with chest X-ray and routine laboratory tests should always be done.

Francis Robert Brown, 1889–1967. Surgeon, Royal Infirmary, Dundee, Scotland.

Charles Edouard Brown-Séquard, 1817–94. Physician, Natural Hospital for Nervous Diseases, London, England; Professor of Medicine, Harvard University, Boston, Masachussetts, USA, and College de France, Paris, France. Described syndrome in 1851.

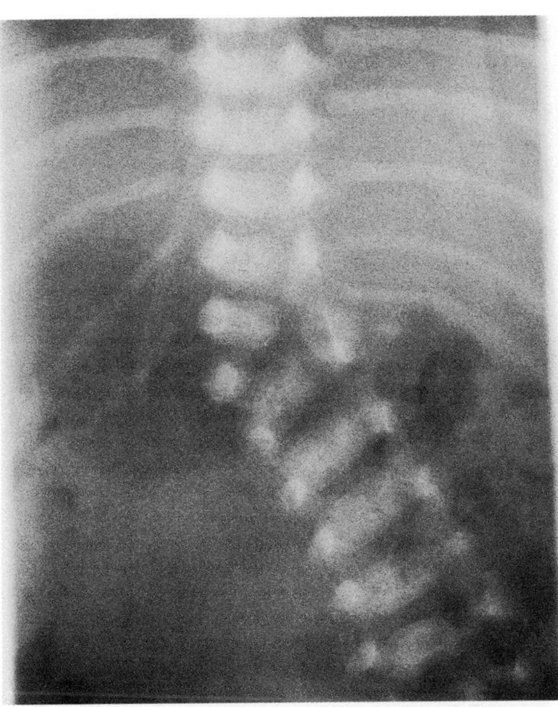

Fig. 33.28 Congenital scoliosis with hemivertebra at the thoracolumbar junction.

Management

Only after a careful history and examination have been performed with review of the radiology and other tests can the course of management be decided. In principle, symptomatic intraspinal tumours should be excised as completely as possible using microneurosurgical techniques and, furthermore, this may have to be done urgently if there is progressive neurological dysfunction. The aims of treatment are:

1. relief of pain;
2. to achieve a histological diagnosis;
3. excision of benign tumours;
4. prevention of further neurological deterioration.

Pain relief. Decompression of the spine with removal of the tumour will usually provide immediate pain relief, even if

Table 33.4 Intraspinal tumours

Extradural	*Intradural*
Benign	Extramedullary
Neurofibroma	Meningioma
Lipoma	Neurofibroma
Meningioma	Intramedullary
Chordoma	Glioma
Malignant	Ependymoma
Metastatic tumour	Haemangioblastoma
Sarcoma	Dermoid
	Lipoma
	Teratoma

(a)

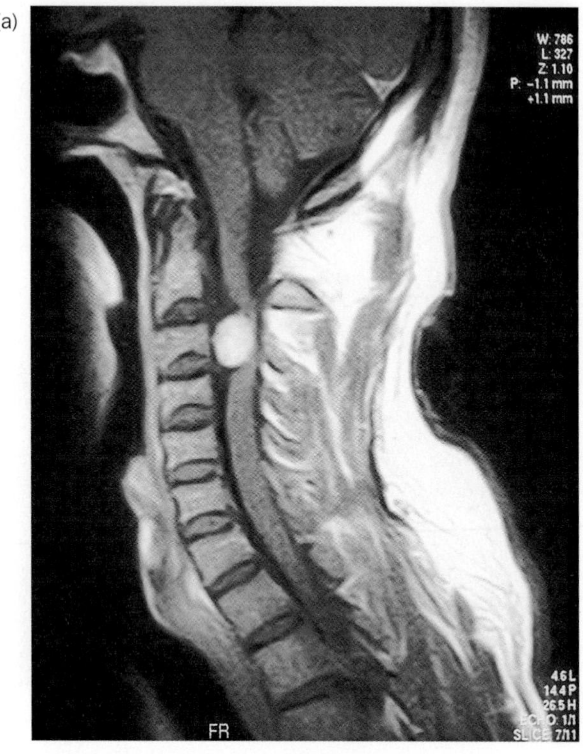

(b)

Fig. 33.29 MRI scan (sagittal T1) showing intraspinal tumours: (a) extramedullary, intradural neurofibroma; (b) intramedullary, cervical cord glioma.

this is incomplete. Radiotherapy of malignant tumours will provide some pain relief but not immediately. Clearly, the patient will suffer postoperative pain, but the severe nocturnal, often interscapular pain will immediately be relieved once the dura is decompressed and the tumour removed.

Achieve histological diagnosis. Clearly this is important when deciding whether further adjunctive therapy will be required. For extradural tumours when surgery is not feasible, a CT-guided needle biopsy can be carried out with a good chance of achieving a histological diagnosis and minimal risk of morbidity.

Excision of benign tumours. Irrespective of whether the tumour is inside or outside the spinal cord, surgery represents the mainstay of treatment using microneurosurgical techniques. Careful definition of the anatomy, debulking of tumour, teasing it away from the surrounding tissues will allow removal with minimum risk of morbidity.

Prevention of further deterioration. Decompression of the spinal cord or cauda equina with either malignant or benign disease will prevent further deterioration and may allow some neurological improvement.

Surgical technique

Patients and their families should be carefully consented prior to operation. A back marker will help with localisation, although advances in technology using the optical tracking systems will not only allow help with location but also help to define the extent of the dissection, especially with intramedullary disease.

A posterior or dorsal approach is usual via a midline incision through a laminectomy. The full cephalocaudal extent of the tumour should be exposed and, if extradural, the dural tissue above and below should be identified to allow gentle excision of the tumour.

Care should be taken to keep the dura intact if at all possible and to avoid injury to the emerging spinal nerves. Surrounding the extradural tumour is often a plexus of veins that will bleed quite profusely as the tumour is decompressed. These should be controlled using bipolar coagulation. The lateral extension of a neurofibroma will often require a second approach at a later stage.

It an intradural tumour is the dura should be opened above and below the tumour and, if required, the dural opening should be done using the microscope. Retaining sutures will retract the dura and all dissection thereafter should be carried out using microinstruments with the help of a microscope. Excision of a neurofibroma will require isolation of the root of origin and its subsequent division. Meningiomas require careful debulking and excision of their origin, whilst keeping the arachnoid planes intact to preserve and protect the spinal cord itself. Care should be taken to avoid any additional compression or distortion of the spinal cord.

If an intramedullary tumour is visible on the surface of the cord then this can be used as a portal of entry to the tumour. If not, a midline myelotomy can be used with tiny pial retraction sutures. This will then allow access to the tumour itself.

For ependymoma or haemangioblastoma a plane intersection can usually be identified, which will allow the tumour to be gently teased away using any cystic component of the tumour to assist with that dissection. Astrocytomas, however, may not have such a well-defined plane and their removal, therefore, is more difficult.

For tumours within the cauda equina, again careful definition of the anatomy – especially the arachnoid planes – is vital. To fully excise a cauda equina ependymoma requires division of the filum terminale. Beware of the sacral roots, which are often closely attached.

Dural closure follows careful haemostasis. This should be watertight to prevent postoperative CSF leakage. Spinal cord monitoring should be carried out where possible.

Spinal artereovenous malformations

First successfully operated on in 1914 by Ellsburg, the classification of these rare lesions has changed as understanding of the aetiology and anatomy has developed.

The revised classification of spinal vascular malformations is as follows.

Dural AV fistulas. This represents a low-flow shunt in the dural sleeve supplied by a dural branch of intervertebral artery. Drainage to superficial intradural veins produces local venous hypertension with venous congestion and an associated myelopathy.

Intradural AVM's. (a) Juvenile – fed by multiple feeders, these high flow lesions may involve the vertebral column. (b) The glomus type – this has a tightly packed nidus usually supplied by one vessel. It may be associated with the arterial aneurysm.

Intradural. This is a direct fistula between the intradural spinal artery and vein. It is defined by an absence of the nidus and associated with haemorrhage from aneurysm or venous varix.

Cavernous angiomas. These are angiographically occult, with normal vascular anatomy. They appear as small blackberry-like lesions, with low flow and are demarcated on MRI scan.

Management

This is usually with progressive symptoms with an ascending myelopathy; it may occasionally present with subarachnoid haemorrhage.

Diagnosis

Depends upon a high index of suspicion, often with the identification of a draining vein on MRI scan. Confirmation should be via the spinal angiography (Fig. 33.31).

Treatment

The aim is to eradicate the fistula and the nidus without compromising the blood supply to the spinal cord. Depending on the vascular anatomy and the type of lesion, this can be achieved either by intravascular therapy, using particle embolisation, or by surgical exposure of the lesion with identification and closure of the fistula (Fig. 33.32).

Spinal infection

Spinal column infection

Spinal column infection is not common and 30 per cent of cases have a significant delay in diagnosis, the average being 3

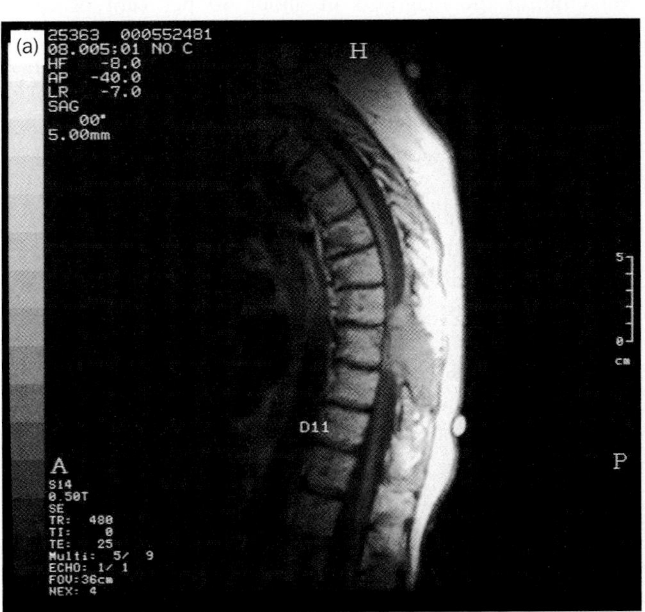

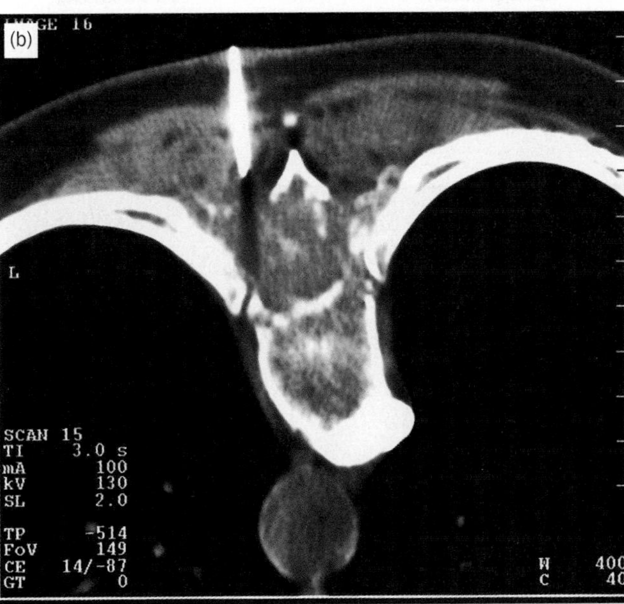

Fig. 33.30 Metastatic deposit causing spinal cord compression. (a) MRI scan (sagittal T1) showing severe thoracic cord compression with both intraspinal and extraspinal disease. (b) CT-guided percutaneous needle biopsy of metastatic deposit.

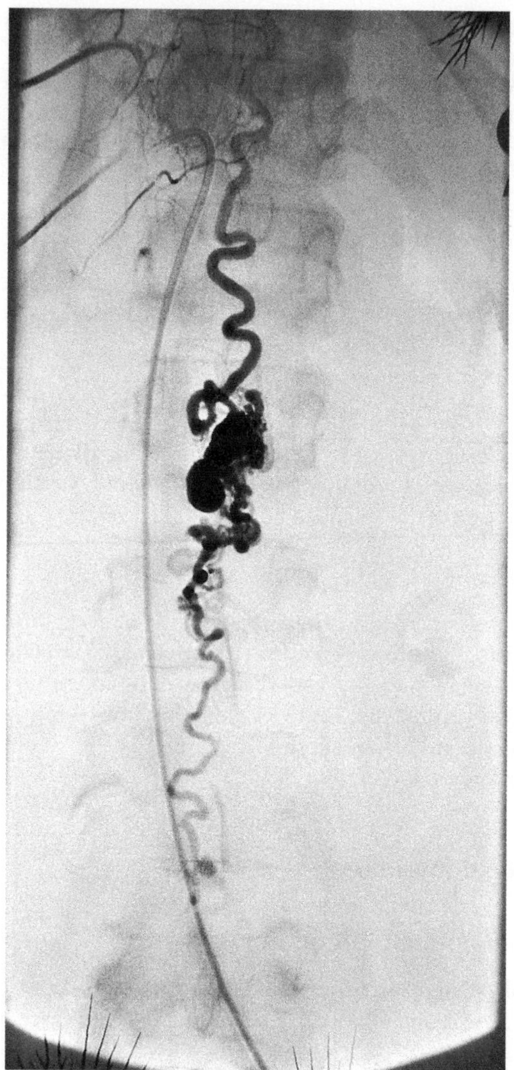

Fig. 33.31 Spinal angiogram demonstrating extensive intradural glomus type arteriovenous malformation.

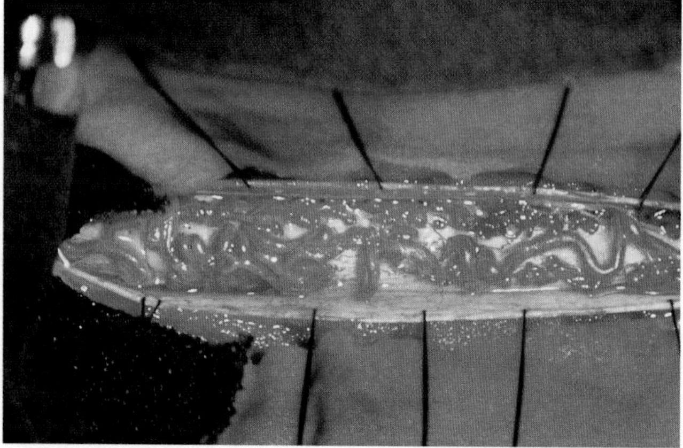

Fig. 33.32 Surgical exposure of the surface of the spinal cord to show the arteriovenous malformation.

months. The common presenting symptoms are fever and unremitting pain especially at night. The distribution is bimodal, occurring in the very young and the very old. In children the infection is frequently sterile and may simply be a discitis. Very young children may present simply with malaise and inability to walk. There may be a scoliosis. The infection is usually centred on the disc, and in the early stages there may be no X-ray changes although MRI will show the typical changes of oedema in the end plates and disc, with changes in the surrounding soft tissues. After 2 weeks narrowing of the disc space usually occurs. Needle biopsy of the disc only grows bacteria in about 40 per cent of cases. Unless the child is septicaemic, expectant treatment can be tried. Established infection or failure to improve requires treatment with broad-spectrum antibiotics. A plaster jacket may be helpful in controlling pain and accelerating resolution of symptoms. In the long term the disc may reconstitute, or occasionally spontaneous fusion of the disc may occur.

Infection of the spinal column is usually more serious in adults. As in children it is usually centred on the disc, and by the time of presentation X-ray changes are usually present in the form of disc space narrowing with destruction of the end plates. The patient may be generally unwell and septicaemic. Many patients have reduced immunity to infection due to conditions such as diabetes or carcinoma, and recent urinary catheterisation or surgery is not uncommon. It is important to establish the bacterium causing the infection if possible before starting treatment. The most common bacterium is *Staphylococcus aureus*, but almost any bacterium can cause the infection and tuberculosis must always be considered as a possibility (see below). Blood cultures should always be carried out and in many cases this will establish the type of bacteria. Needle biopsy of the disc space is an alternative method of diagnosis. This is done under local anaesthetic with X-ray control, and will confirm the diagnosis in about 60 per cent of cases. Surgery tends to be used for patients where there is considerable bone destruction or deformity, neurological compromise due to compression on the spinal cord or failure to eradicate the infection with antibiotics. Simple stabilisation of the infected area combined with antibiotics may be adequate in older individuals, but otherwise débridement of the disc space, bone grafting and stabilisation are most likely to result in cure. Surprisingly internal fixation in these patients rarely seems to cause problems of persistent infection, although it may be advisable to remove the fixation once the bone has healed. Antibiotic treatment is usually continued for some months.

Some cases of disc space infection will progress to epidural abscess. This will present with neurological symptoms and signs and should be drained as a surgical emergency (see below).

Tuberculosis

Tuberculosis is more frequently seen in the Third World than in the developed world but it is becoming more common, and should always be considered as a possible diagnosis in those with spinal infection.

Treatment with multiple antibiotics over long periods has proven very effective in treating spinal tuberculosis, and has been shown to be effective in managing some patients with paraplegia. Eventual fusion of the infected area can be expected in around 80 per cent of patients without surgery. Surgery combined with antibiotics is used where there is a large abscess which requires draining or considerable deformity of the spine. Failure of antibiotic treatment may also be a surgical indication. In general the best surgical results are with anterior débridement and bone grafting of the infected area.

Spinal epidural abscess

Infection within the epidural space is a rare but potentially disastrous condition. Usually due to haematogenous spread from remote sites or associated with intravenous drug usage, pus can collect and spread within the epidural space and cause compression of the spinal cord or cauda equina. Infection may spread from local sites (discitis/vertebral osteomyelitis or paravertebral infection) (see Fig. 33.33) and may present as a postoperative complication.

Staphylococcus aureus represents the commonest causative organism. A variety of other organisms including bacteroides, aerobic and anaerobic streptococci may be found. Consider unusual organisms in association with immune compromise, including fungal infections.

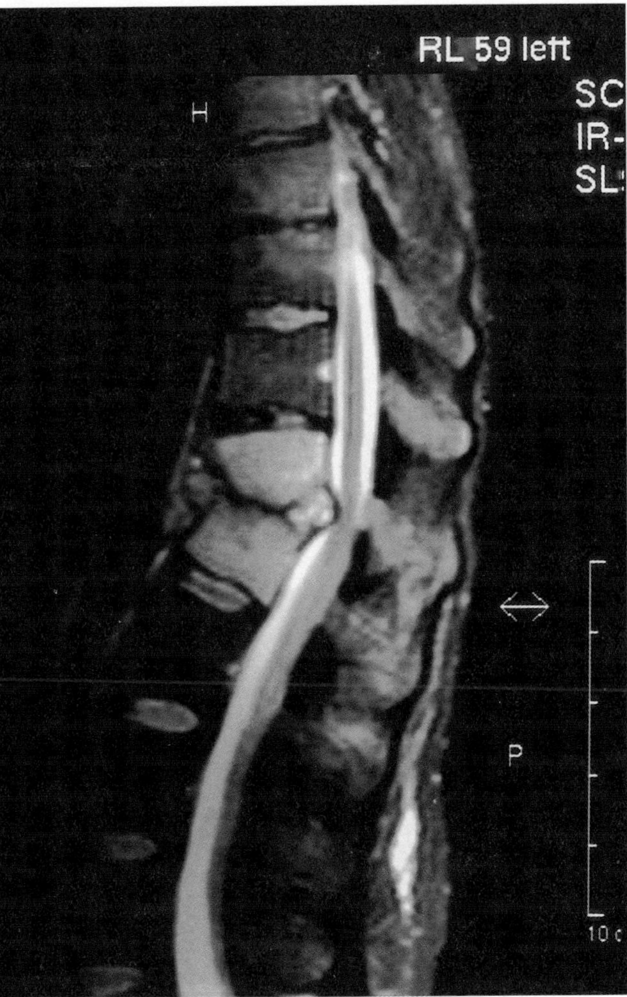

Fig. 33.33 MRI (sagittal T2) of spinal epidural abscess associated with osteomyelitis and discitis.

Presentation

Presentation includes:

- severe local pain;
- systemic signs of infection;
- radicular signs;
- onset of symptoms and signs of cord and cauda equina compression.

Progression of symptoms can be very rapid and therefore early recognition is vital to allow a good outcome. A high index of suspicion to achieve diagnosis before the onset of complete paralysis is very important. If the diagnosis is delayed to this point, vascular thrombosis may result in irreversible paralysis.

Diagnosis

Diagnosis includes:

- clinical awareness of the condition;
- general tests: haemoglobin, white cell count, ESR, CRP, blood cultures, midstream urine;
- plain spinal X-rays, chest X-ray;
- MRI scan.

Plain X-rays may show evidence of osteomyelitis and should be performed, but MRI is the investigation of choice (see Fig. 33.34). The precise location of the abscess and its extent and position in relation to the cord can all be identified. If suspected the investigation must be carried out as an emergency.

In the absence of MRI, myelography and CT myelography would enable the diagnosis of an epidural mass, but it is harder to define the full extent of the lesion. Care must be taken to avoid carrying infection into the intradural compartment at the time of lumbar puncture. If a cervical abscess is suspected, a lumbar spinal puncture can be used, the contrast being run up to the cervical region. However, if the abscess is thought to be in the thoracolumbar region, a cervical puncture must be made. CT myclography will help to define the extent of the lesion and will also provide important anatomical information about adjacent vertebral bodies.

CSF examination shows a mild leucocytosis with elevation of the neutrophil or lymphocyte counts. Protein levels will be increased.

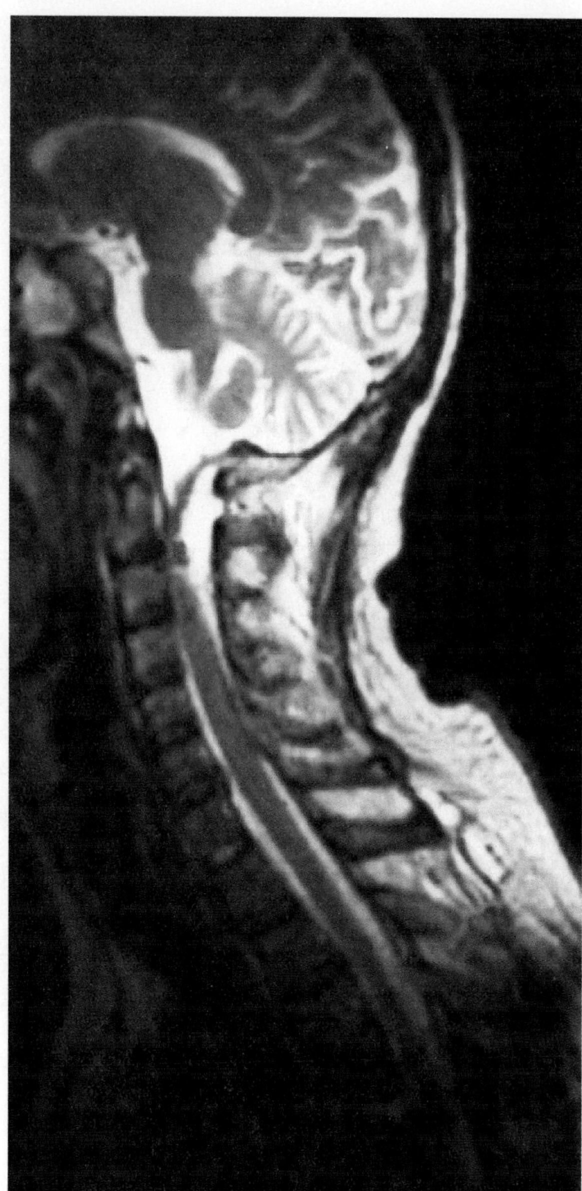

Fig. 33.34 An extensive craniocervical junction epidural abscess visualised on MRI (sagittal T2).

Management

Management of this condition includes:

- surgical drainage of the abscess;
- antibiotic therapy;
- treatment of source of infection/paravertebral infection;
- management of neurological disability.

Patients with an epidural abscess showing signs of severe systemic infection require full supportive therapy.

Drainage of the pus via a posterior or anterior approach should be carried out as an emergency once a diagnosis is suspected. For anteriorly placed lesions, usually in the cervical region, an anterior cervical discectomy with opening of the posterior longitudinal ligament reveals the pus. Samples should be sent for microscopy and Gram stain, set up for culture and antibiotics started. Avoid instrumentation or insertion of bone grafts.

Dorsally placed collections can be drained via a laminectomy.

If available, the advice of a bone infection unit should be taken. Certainly, advice from a medical microbiologist will help in the choice of antibiotic and the duration of treatment. In principle, intravenous therapy via a long intravenous line, and modified according to culture results, should be continued for at least 2 weeks. Be prepared to repeat the MRI scans to ensure that the abscess has been fully drained.

Any residual neurological deficit will require input from physiotherapists and occupational therapists, directed by a rehabilitation facility. Recovery, however, may be slow and protracted over many months.

Finally, any other site of infection should be dealt with as indicated.

Further reading

Kerr, R.S.C., Cadoux-Hudson, T.A. and Adams, C.B.T. (1988) The value of accurate clinical assessment in the surgical management of lumbar disc protrusion. *Journal of Neurology, Neurosurgery and Psychology*, **51**, 169–73.

Tarlov, E.C. (1991) Thoracic disc herniation. In *Neurosurgical Treatment of Disorders of the Thoracic Spine*, American Association of Neurological Surgeons, Park Ridge, IL, pp. 53–8.

Whitecloud, T.S. and Dunsker, S.B. (1994) Anterior cervical spine surgery. In *Principles and Techniques in Spinal Surgery*, Raven Press, New York.

Hans Christian Joachim Gram, 1858–1938. Professor of Medicine, Copenhagen, Denmark.

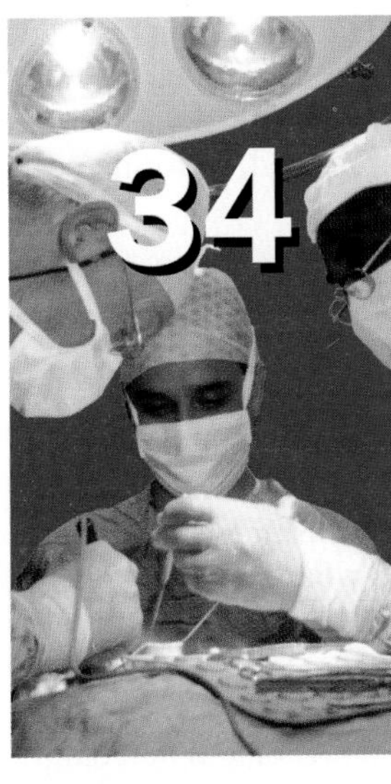

34 Nerves

Introduction

The nervous system is divided into the central nervous system (CNS) and the peripheral nervous system (PNS). The CNS consists of the brain, spinal cord and the first two cranial nerves, while the remaining cranial nerves and the spinal nerves constitute the PNS. The CNS and PNS have fundamentally different responses to injury, the CNS having little ability to regenerate, while the PNS has considerable potential for recovery if conditions are favourable. This chapter deals mainly with surgical disorders of the PNS. Injuries to peripheral nerves have a major effect on the functional outcome after trauma, and therefore careful management from an early stage is important to obtain the best results possible.

Principles of peripheral nerve surgery

Structure of the peripheral nerve trunk

The anatomy of a peripheral nerve trunk is shown in Fig. 34.1. Nerve impulses are conducted by axons. The nerve contains many axons which are supported by connective tissue structures. Neurons consist of a cell body, associated dendrites and usually one axon. In order to remain viable an axon must be connected to its cell body. All axons are surrounded by Schwann cells. In myelinated fibres the Schwann cells form an insulating sheath, each Schwann cell being associated with only one axon. Integrity of the myelin sheath is necessary for conduction of nerve impulses in myelinated fibres. Unmyelinated fibres are composed of several axons wrapped by a single Schwann cell. The Schwann cell basement membrane, together with endoneurial collagen fibres, forms the *endoneurial tube*. Large numbers of nerve fibres are gathered in fascicles surrounded by a connective tissue

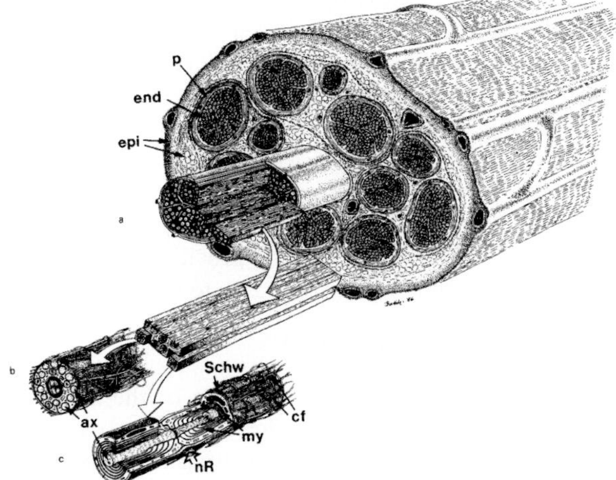

Fig. 34.1 Microanatomy of a peripheral nerve trunk and its components. (a) Fascicles surrounded by a multilaminated perineurium (p) are embedded in a loose connective tissue, the epineurium (epi). The outer layers of the epineurium are condensed into a sheath. (b) and (c) illustrate the appearance of unmyelinated and myelinated fibres, respectively. Schw, Schwann cell; my, myelin sheath; ax, axon; nR, node of Ranvier. (Reproduced with permission from *Nerve Injury and Repair*, by G. Lundborg, 1988, Churchill Livingstone, Edinburgh.)

Bailey & Love's Short Practice of Surgery, 23rd edition. Edited by R.C.G. Russell, N.S. Williams and C.J.K. Bulstrode. Published in 2000 by Arnold Publishers.

Theodor Schwann, 1810–82, French histologist and pathologist.
Louis Antoine Ranvier, 1835–1922. French histologist and pathologist.

sheath called the *perineurium*. The fascicles are bound together and the whole trunk ensheathed by a further connective tissue layer called the *epineurium*.

Response of a nerve to injury

If trauma to a nerve is sufficient to disrupt axons then the distal part of the nerve undergoes Wallerian degeneration. In this process there is lysis of the axoplasm and fragmentation of myelin sheaths leaving an endoneurial tube containing Schwann cells. The axons in the proximal part of the nerve have the potential to regenerate into the endoneurial tubes of the distal segment and subsequently make connections with target organs. The regeneration proceeds slowly with axons growing at only 1–2 mm/day in humans. The extent of damage to the supporting connective tissue layers influences the quality of recovery and is, hence, the basis of the classification of nerve injuries.

Classification of nerve injuries

The most widely used classification of nerve injuries in the UK was described by Seddon (1942) after study of a large number of battle casualties during World War II. There are three types of injury of increasing severity:

- neuropraxia;
- axonotmesis;
- neurotmesis.

Neuropraxia (nerve not working)

This is a local block to conduction of nerve impulses at a discrete area along the course of a nerve. The axons are in continuity and therefore Wallerian degeneration does not occur. Nerve conduction distal to the site of injury remains normal. Experimental work suggests that the conduction block results from localised demyelination of fibres in the damaged segment of nerve. Neuropraxia is a relatively mild injury typically caused by moderate compression such as that caused by a tourniquet, slight stretching or the passage of a missile close to a nerve. Recovery is complete providing the cause is removed, but the time varies from days to several weeks.

Axonotmesis (axons divided)

This represents an anatomical disruption of the axons and their myelin sheaths. However, the supporting connective tissue structures including the endoneurial tubes, perineurium and epineurium are still intact. Wallerian degeneration occurs distal to the site of injury and, hence, distal conduction is lost. Axonotmesis results from a more severe blow or stretch injury to a nerve. For example, radial nerve palsy associated with fracture of the humerus is usually an axonotmesis. Recovery occurs by axon regeneration proceeding at a rate of 1–2 mm/day. Axons regenerate along the same endoneurial tube and therefore connect with the same end organ as before injury. The prognosis is good, restoring near-normal sensory and motor function.

Neurotmesis (whole nerve divided)

This is the state where the nerve has been completely severed or is so seriously disorganised that spontaneous recovery is not possible. The axons and the supporting connective tissue structures are disrupted, and Wallerian degeneration occurs distal to the site of injury. Typically neurotmesis occurs as a result of an open injury such as a stab wound but high-energy traction, injection of noxious drugs and ischaemia can also destroy a nerve in this way.

If appropriate surgical repair is carried out then recovery may occur by axonal regeneration at a rate of 1–2 mm/day. In contrast to axonotmesis, the quality of recovery is never perfect after neurotmesis. This is probably the result of the failure of correct 'rewiring'. Because the endoneurial tubes and other connective tissue structures have been disrupted, even with the best repair, regenerated nerve fibres connect with muscles or sensory organs which they did not previously innervate.

Sunderland's classification

In 1951 Sunderland defined five degrees of nerve injury on the basis of increasing anatomical disruption of the nerve trunk (see Table 34.1). Although Seddon's classification is simpler and more widely used in the UK, Sunderland's classification is useful in its distinction between third- and fourth-degree injuries when exploring a damaged nerve. If the fascicles are in continuity (not worse than third-degree injury) then spontaneous recovery is possible, whereas if the fascicles are disrupted (fourth-degree injury) then spontaneous recovery will not occur and immediate nerve grafting may be considered.

Injection injuries

Injection of toxic substances directly into a nerve leads to a very intense fibrotic reaction in the nerve. Immediate exploration, incision of the epineurium and irrigation of the nerve trunk is recommended, but the outcome is poor.

Table 34.1 Anatomical basis of Sunderland's and Seddon's classifications of nerve injuries (+, intact; , severed)

Sunderland	*Endoneurial*				*Seddon*
Grade	*Axon*	*Tube*	*Perineurium*	*Epineurium*	*Group*
First-degree	+	+	+	+	Neurapraxia
Second-degree		+	+	+	Axonotmesis
Third-degree			+	+	
Fourth-degree				+	Neurotmesis
Fifth-degree					Neurotmesis

Augustus Volney Waller, 1816–70. General practitioner, Kensington, London, 1842–51. Subsequently worked as a physiologist at Bonn, Paris, Birmingham and Geneva.

Sir Herbert John Seddon, 1903–77. Professor of Orthopaedic Surgery, Royal National Orthopaedic Hospital, London, England.

Sydney Sunderland, b. 1910. Melbourne, published the 'bible' of peripheral nerve injuries in 1978.

Clinical features of nerve disorders

As with other medical and surgical problems, diagnosis of conditions affecting nerves is based upon history, examination and special investigations. In the case of trauma it is particularly important to establish the mechanism. High-velocity and open injuries produce more severe nerve injuries.

The clinical findings on examination of patients with nerve injury include motor and sensory dysfunction but depend, in part, upon the grade of injury. With neurapraxia there is usually complete paralysis of the appropriate muscle groups but some sensation and autonomic function is preserved. In the case of axonotmesis and neurotmesis there is complete loss of muscle power, sensation and autonomic function. The latter is most easily shown by lack of sweating in the distribution of the nerve. This is a useful objective sign as it does not require a co-operative patient. The nerve injured and the level at which the injury has occurred can be worked out from a careful physical examination and knowledge of the anatomical distribution of the nerves. Nonetheless, there is significant crossover in sensory function and also in some motor function, particularly when considering nerve roots (Table 34.2 and Fig. 34.2).

It is useful to *grade* the level of dysfunction of nerves, particularly in the assessment of recovery and the results of treatment. The system widely used is the 1975 update of the 1954 Medical Research Council (MRC) classification (Tables 34.3 and 34.4). This grading system is good, and widely used, but is still a rather coarse measure of muscle function and sensation.

Table 34.2 Myotomes

Arm:	
• Shoulder abduction	C5
• Elbow flexion	C5/6
• Elbow extension	C7/8
• Finger flexion	C8
• Small muscles of hand	T1
Leg:	
• Hip flexion	L2/3
• Hip extension	L5/S1
• Knee flexion	L5/S1
• Knee extension	L3/4
• Ankle inversion	L4
• Ankle eversion	L5/S1
• Plantar flexion	S1/2
• Dorsiflexion of foot and toes	L4/5

Table 34.3 MRC classification of motor nerve dysfunction

Grade	*Clinical features*
M0	Complete paralysis
M1	Flicker of muscle activity
M2	Power insufficient to overcome gravity
M3	Movement against gravity
M4	Movement against resistance
M4+	Strong movement, but not normal
M5	Normal, full power

(a)

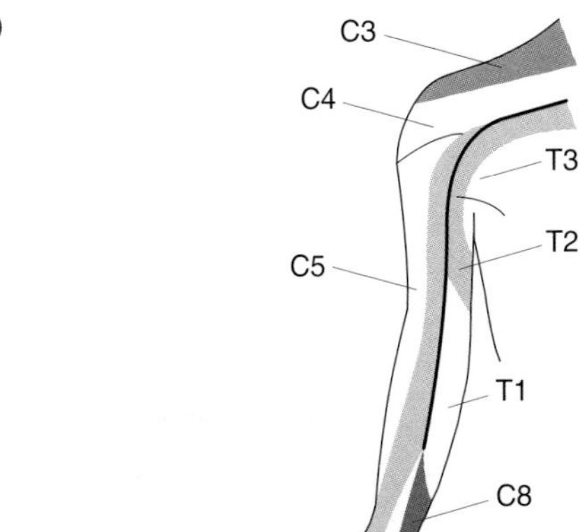

(b)

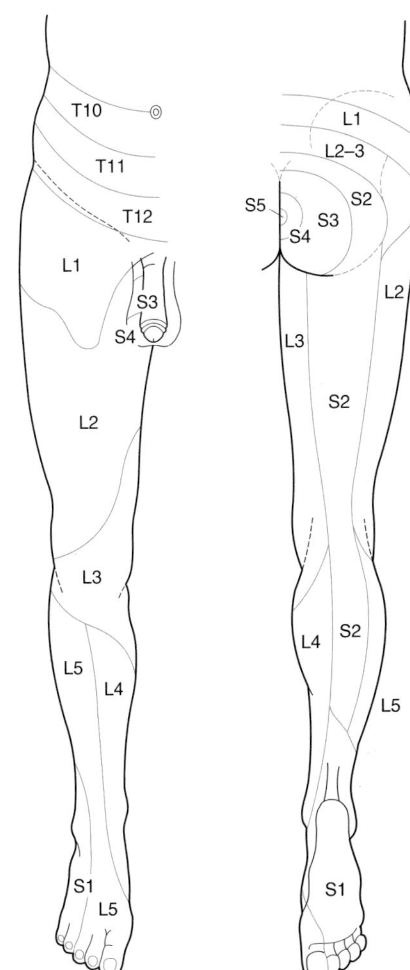

Fig. 34.2 Diagrams showing the dermatomes in the (a) upper limb and (b) lower limb. (Crown Copyright, reproduced with permission of the Controller of Her Majesty's Stationery Office from Medical Research Council, Nerve Injuries Committee, *Aids to Examination of the Peripheral Nervous System* (1976))

Table 34.4 MRC classification of sensory nerve dysfunction

Grade	Clinical features
S0	No sensation
S1	Deep pain sensation
S2	Skin touch, pain and thermal sensation, i.e. protective sensation
S3	S2 also with accurate localisation but deficient stereognosis. Cold sensitivity and hypersensitivity are often present
S3+	Object and texture recognition, but not normal sensation. Good but not normal, two-point discrimination
S4	Normal sensation

Clinical examination needs to be conducted with care, particularly with those patients who may have difficulty co-operating. The findings should be accurately documented. Two-point discrimination is particularly useful for assessing sensation in the hand as it is an objective measurement and normality (approximately 4 mm on the finger pulps) excludes significant nerve injury. If there is any doubt initial first aid should be carried out and the patient re-examined within 48 hours. Diagnosis can be difficult and severe nerve injuries are regularly missed.

Investigation

While the most important assessment of nerve pathology is undoubtedly clinical, useful additional information can sometimes be obtained from neurophysiological studies or imaging.

Neurophysiological investigations require complex stimulation and recording apparatus. Interpretation of the results requires experience and is reliant upon the skill of the neurophysiologist. There are two types of test available.

- Nerve conduction studies – these involve recording sensory or motor nerve action potentials and calculating the conduction velocity for given anatomical segments. Compression neuropathy can be identified by slowing of conduction.
- Electromyography (EMG) – in this test muscle action potentials are recorded in response to voluntary activity. Denervation can be diagnosed and distinguished from reinnervation.

Using these tests it is possible to distinguish between a nerve injury where axons have not degenerated distal to the lesion (neurapraxia) and one were Wallerian degeneration has occurred (axonotmesis or neurotmesis). Axonotmesis and neurotmesis cannot be distinguished.

Magnetic resonance imaging (MRI) is showing some promise in displaying peripheral nerve pathology and is likely to be used routinely in the future. Currently, its main application is in imaging cervical nerve roots after brachial plexus injuries.

Treatment

Open injuries

If there is clinical evidence of a nerve injury associated with a wound, then it should be assumed that the nerve is divided until proven otherwise.

Surgical exploration of the nerves is advisable, once life-threatening haemorrhage has been controlled and providing the general condition of the patient allows operation. In addition, wounds in areas where important nerves are vulnerable to damage should be routinely explored even in the absence of obvious neurological deficit, for example the flexor compartment of the forearm. Early repair of any divided nerves should be performed if possible. Exploration should therefore be undertaken by a surgeon with appropriate experience to carry out repair of nerves if necessary. If a vascular repair is required then nerve repair should normally be carried out at the same time. If the injury is in a site which is difficult to expose surgically, for example the brachial plexus, then transfer to a specialist unit should be arranged as soon as possible.

Closed injuries

Management of closed injuries where nerves have been subjected to stretch or compression is more difficult because the severity of nerve injury may not be clear. Neurapraxia and axonotmesis will recover spontaneously providing the cause, for example compression, is removed. However, surgical repair of the nerve is necessary for there to be any chance of recovery after neurotmesis. Results are markedly better if this repair is carried out early after injury.

Exploration and repair of nerves may be combined with fixation of any associated skeletal injury. In cases of low-energy injury it is reasonable to observe the nerve injury initially, unless operation is being carried for fracture fixation in which case the opportunity should not be missed to confirm nerve continuity. Cases managed nonoperatively should be followed up carefully. If there is clear evidence of recovery after 2–3 months then nonoperative management can continue. If not, then surgical exploration should be considered without further delay. Neurophysiology may be helpful in making the decision in some cases as the tests may detect early recovery which is not evident clinically.

Surgical repair

The essence of a good surgical repair of a nerve is accurate coaptation of the nerve ends without tension in a healthy bed of tissue. At operation the nerve ends are exposed, carefully avoiding further injury. If there has been a clean division of a nerve, then little dissection is usually required and direct suture can be carried out. However, if the nerve ends are ragged or the disruption has been caused by blunt trauma, it is necessary to trim the nerve back to healthy tissue with bulging nerve bundles. In delayed repairs significant scarring and retraction of the nerve ends may have occurred and it is, again, important to trim the nerve back to normal tissue. In these circumstances there will be a gap between the nerve ends. In the past extensive mobilisation of some nerves was recommended to allow direct suture. However, it is seldom possible to get much length by this manoeuvre and the repair is invariably under tension. Therefore, if there a significant gap is present it is usually better to perform nerve grafting. Occasionally, when a nerve injury is combined with a fracture, bone shortening may be justified to allow direct nerve suture.

Timing of nerve repair

Early nerve repair provides the best chance of satisfactory recovery and should be carried out provided that a well-trained surgeon and suitable equipment are available. Occasionally, if a wound is very contaminated then primary nerve repair may not be appropriate. In most circumstances it is possible to carry out early repair if sufficient wound débridement is carried out and plastic surgical expertise is available to provide flap cover of soft-tissue defects. If primary repair is not carried out then it is useful to apply one or two nonabsorbable sutures, either to hold nerve ends together or to suture a nerve end to local soft tissue, thereby minimising retraction and aiding identification at later surgery.

Direct nerve suture

When repairing a nerve, a microscope should be used to aid accurate alignment of the nerve and placement of sutures, which range in the order of 6-0 for large nerves (such as the sciatic nerve), 8-0 for the median nerve in the forearm, and 9- or 10-0 for digital nerves. It is important to orientate the nerve ends with the correct rotation in order to minimise crossover during recovery. The pattern of nerve fascicles and surface blood vessels can be used as guides for alignment. Sutures are usually placed in the epineurium (*epineurial repair*). There is probably no advantage in performing interfascicular repair except at distal sites where the nerve is dividing into terminal branches. Sufficient sutures are inserted to provide epineurial cover for all nerve bundles (Fig. 34.3).

Nerve grafting

When direct nerve suture is not possible an interpositional nerve graft is necessary. This involves harvesting a length of

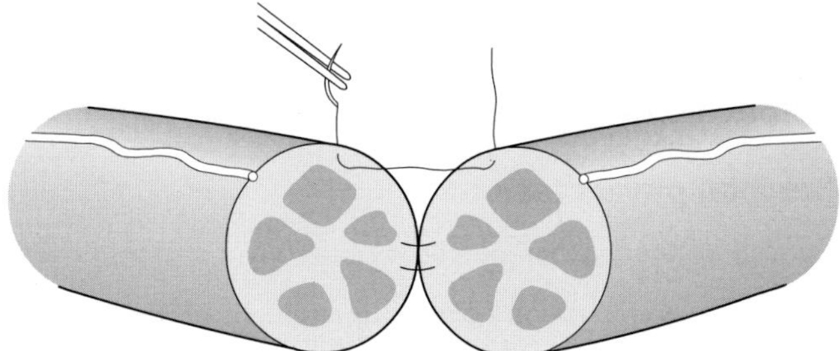

Fig. 34.3 Illustration of direct epineurial suture of a nerve.

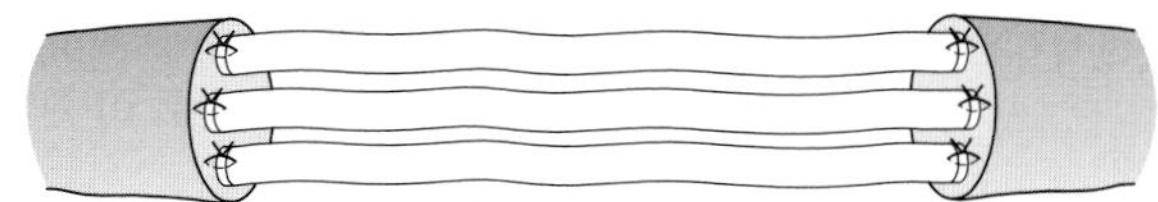

Fig. 34.4 Illustration of cable grafting a large nerve trunk. The strands of nerve graft should connect matching groups of fascicles in the proximal and distal stumps if these can be identified.

an 'expendable' nerve trunk, such as the sural nerve or the medial cutaneous nerve of the forearm. These are long slender nerves which supply only small areas of sensation. The nerve graft is usually cut up so that a number of strands can be used to build up a similar thickness to that of the nerve trunk being repaired (*cable grafting*; Fig. 34.4).

Postoperative management

After wound closure, the limb is immobilised to minimise any tension on the suture line with appropriate flexion of proximal and distal joints. These are held in a cast for a minimum of 3 weeks. It may then be appropriate progressively to extend the proximal and distal joints, thus gradually restoring normal tension to the nerves. After 6 weeks, free mobilisation is permitted, assisted by appropriate physiotherapy.

Follow-up management

After nerve repair patients should have regular physiotherapy to maintain the passive range of movement in all joints prior to muscle recovery. In addition, patients should be monitored clinically to check that nerve recovery is occurring at the expected rate. Tinel's sign is useful in monitoring axon regeneration and should advance at about 1 mm/day. (Elicited by percussing over the course of the nerve, the patient feels tingling in the distribution of the nerve.) In the event of nerve recovery not progressing, then re-exploration of the nerve may be justified.

General factors affecting prognosis

The factors governing the prognosis of nerve repair are both general to all nerves and specific to certain nerves.

Age

Children recover much better than adults and this is probably the most important prognostic factor. Nonetheless, the secondary consequences of paralysis in children may be worse because of the associated growth abnormalities. Age over 50 years is a particularly poor prognostic factor for proximal nerve injuries.

The severity of injury to the nerve

Seddon's classification of nerve injuries relates the severity of injury to the prognosis. However, there are varying grades of neurotmesis which affect the chance of recovery after repair. A clean-cut nerve injury has the best prognosis, whereas

Jules Tinel, 1879–1952. French neurologist.

high-energy injuries, such as high-velocity gunshot wounds or severe traction injuries, damage a greater length of nerve and have a much worse prognosis.

The level of injury

In general, proximal lesions do worse than distal lesions although there do appear to be some exceptions to this rule.

The type of nerve

The classic teaching is that nerves with both sensory and motor fibres fare worse than pure sensory or motor nerves. The latter do not truly exist, as all motor nerves have some afferents from muscle spindles. However, it is certainly true that motor nerves to large muscle groups not requiring fine control have a better prognosis than motor nerves supplying the small muscles of the hand.

Associated injuries

Nerve repairs with associated vascular injuries, soft-tissue damage and fractures are less likely to heal with a satisfactory result. It is important that associated vessels and other structures are repaired as far as possible.

Delay

Early repair of nerves, that is within a few days of injury, gives the best results and is one of the main factors which the surgeon can influence.

Special types of nerve injury

Compression neuropathy

This is the term used to describe chronic dysfunction of a nerve as a result of local compression at some point along its course. Compression neuropathy is one of the most frequent single conditions presenting to orthopaedic and hand clinics. The most common sites of compression are the median nerve at the carpal tunnel and the ulnar nerve at the cubital tunnel or Guyon's canal. These are anatomical sites where the nerve is surrounded by unyielding bone and ligaments. Sometimes there is an identifiable cause such as tenosynovitis within the carpal tunnel, but in many cases there is no obvious cause. Compression of a nerve has a direct effect on the myelin sheaths, as well as causing ischaemia of the nerve with consequent fibrosis. It also appears that damage results from loss of mobility of the nerve at the point of entrapment. The patient initially complains of pain and altered sensation in the distribution of the affected nerve. In more advanced cases there is loss of sensory and motor function. Most compression neuropathies respond to surgical decompression of the affected nerve.

Felix J.C. Guyon, 1831–1920. French surgeon.

Irradiation

Radiation neuritis can occur up to 20 years after the radiation, the classic site being the infraclavicular brachial plexus following radiation for breast cancer. Fortunately, this is rare. Characteristically, there is severe pain with some motor and sensory changes. The pain is very difficult to treat. Surgical exploration and release of nerves has been beneficial in some patients.

Pain

The pain following nerve injuries or other nerve pathology can be of the most severe intractable type, leading to requests for amputation and even depression and suicide. The cause of this pain is poorly understood. Local nonoperative treatment includes encouraging use and movement of the limb, and transcutaneous electrical nerve stimulation (TENS). This works as a counter-stimulus to the pain. In addition to simple systemic analgesics, medication to suppress nerve excitability, such as carbamazepine, and antidepressants, such as amitryptilline, can be useful. There are certain occasions where pain of nerve origin may be influenced by surgical intervention.

Causalgia is pain as a result of an injury (often partial) to a major nerve. The pain typically has an intense burning character. This pain tends to improve with nerve recovery and therefore any surgical measures should be aimed at facilitating this. Sympathectomy may be helpful in resistant cases.

Nerve compression may cause severe pain (neurostenalgia).

Avulsion of spinal nerve roots from the spinal cord, for example with traction injuries to the brachial plexus. This is a complex pain syndrome involving damage to the spinal cord and loss of the normal afferent signals from the limb. Re-establishment of some neurological input is by nerve transfer. In the case of the brachial plexus intercostal nerve transfer may prove useful.

Neuroma – if a nerve is wholly or partially divided and not repaired, for example at amputation, then axons attempting to regenerate form a neuroma on the nerve end. The neuroma may be exquisitely sensitive to any pressure, particularly if it is tethered in scar tissue or situated at a prominent point. Surgery may be helpful to restore continuity of the nerve by repair or grafting, if possible, or to move a neuroma to a less prominent position.

Reflex sympathetic dystrophy (algodystrophy) – this is a specific syndrome which can occur after trauma or surgery where a cycle of pain and dysfunction is set up and leads to a chronic state associated with sympathetic over-activity. The limb involved becomes painful and tender to normal stimuli. This leads to disuse, stiffness and trophic changes. It is important to recognise the condition as early as possible and to break the vicious cycle. In addition to standard analgesics, guanathedine blockade to suppress sympathetic activity is useful to facilitate vigorous physiotherapy.

Specific nerve injuries

Brachial plexus lesions

Damage to the brachial plexus is caused by:

- traction as a result of violent displacement of the shoulder girdle and cervical spine;
- open, penetrating injuries by knife or missile;

- operation in the area (for example, for removal of lymph nodes);
- malignant infiltration at the base of the neck, for example Pancoast syndrome.

Traction injury is particularly associated with road traffic accidents to motorcyclists. Any component of the plexus (Fig. 34.5) can sustain any grade of injury (neurapraxia, axonotmesis, neurotmesis). In addition, nerve roots may be avulsed from the spinal cord (preganglionic injury). According to the degree of injury the paralysis varies from a completely flail and useless arm and hand to paralysis of groups of muscles and anaesthesia according to the roots affected. Injuries are usually divided into:

- supraclavicular;
- infraclavicular,

although it is possible for there to be damage both above and below the clavicle.

The most common pattern of injury to the supraclavicular plexus is a lesion of the C5 and C6 roots and upper trunk (Erb–Duchenne palsy). There is loss of shoulder abduction and external rotation, elbow flexion and forearm supination. Sensation is absent on the outer aspect of the arm and hand. Klumpke described a lesion of the lower roots, but this is rare on its own. Injuries to all of the roots are more common.

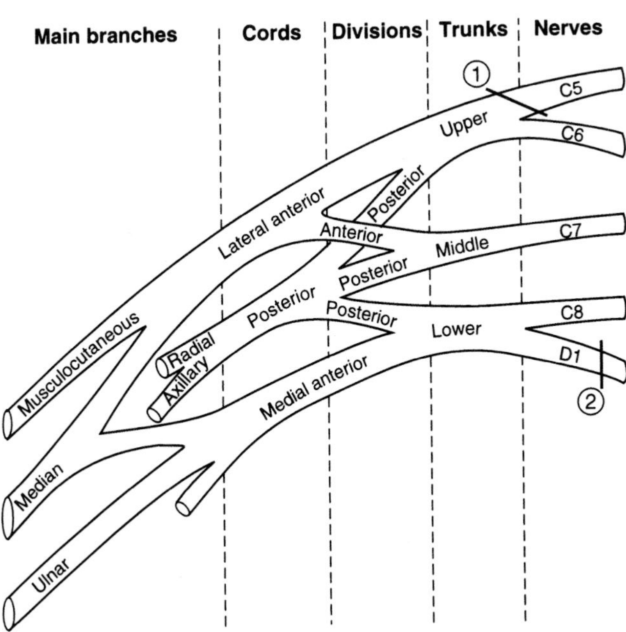

Fig. 34.5 The brachial plexus, showing two classic sites for injury.

Henry Khurrath Pancoast, b. 1875. Radiologist, Philadelphia, USA.
Wilhelm Erb, 1840–1921. Professor of Medicine, Heidelberg, Germany.
Guillaume Benjamine Amand Duchenne (Duchenne de Boulogne), 1806–75. Neurologist, successively in Boulogne and Paris, but never held a hospital appointment.
Madame Augusta Marie Dejerine-Klumpke, 1859–1927. Neurologist, Paris, France.

Management of traction injuries

It is important to establish the mechanism of injury as nerve ruptures are more likely after high-energy trauma. The nerves affected can largely be deduced from careful clinical examination. Signs of preganglionic injury include:

- Horner's syndrome;
- paralysis of the thoracoscapular muscles (innervated by branches near the roots);
- swelling in the posterior triangle of the neck;
- severe pain in the anaesthetic arm.

Investigation includes radiographs of the chest and cervical spine to look for vertebral or rib fractures and to assess phrenic nerve function. In cases of supraclavicular injury myelography, preferably combined with computerised tomographic (CT) scanning, or MRI gives useful additional information on the integrity of the roots before surgery (Fig. 34.6). Neurophysiological assessment is not usually helpful until 2–3 weeks after injury.

Severe traction injuries to the brachial plexus have a devastating effect on the limb and the outlook is often poor. Careful management is therefore important to maximise recovery. If clinical examination reveals complete absence of function of any part of the plexus and the injury was caused by high-energy trauma, then exploration of the brachial plexus is indicated as soon as the general condition of the patient allows. Therefore, transfer to a specialist unit should be arranged as soon as possible. If early surgery is not possible then every effort should be made to operate by 3 months from injury, as the results of repair are undoubtedly worse with increasing delay. At operation the damage to the plexus is carefully documented and nerve grafting is carried out for nerve ruptures. Until recently, repair of avulsed roots was not thought to be possible, but some recovery has now been obtained after repair of ventral (motor) roots within the spinal canal. Alternatively, nerve transfers are performed to restore the most important functions of avulsed roots as far as possible.

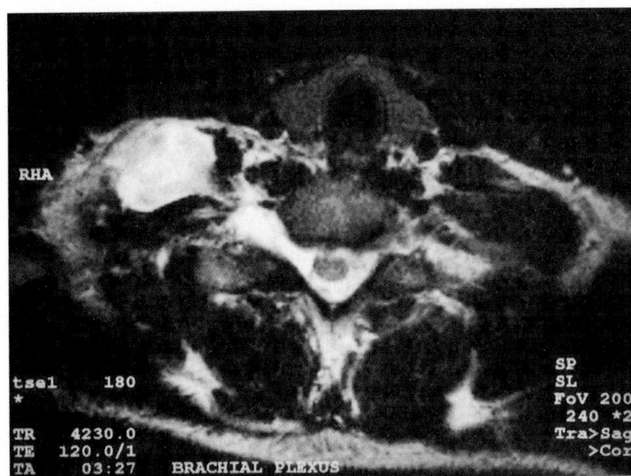

Fig. 34.6 Magnetic resonance image (axial, T2 weighting) showing a right-sided pseudomeningocoele resulting from traumatic avulsion of one of the roots of the brachial plexus.

Friedrich Horner, 1831–86. Professor of Ophthalmology, Zürich, Switzerland. Described his syndrome in 1869.

Stab wounds

Any sharp injury to the brachial plexus should be explored as soon as possible and repaired using nerve grafts.

Obstetric brachial plexus palsy

Injury to the brachial plexus can result from traction on the shoulder girdle during birth. The upper roots are most commonly affected (Erb–Duchenne palsy). The prognosis is good with conservative management in most cases. Physiotherapy is necessary to prevent joint contractures, particularly of the shoulder. The prognosis is improved by surgery to the brachial plexus in approximately 10 per cent of cases. Indications for operation are:

- failure to regain elbow flexion by 3–6 months;
- complete paralysis of the limb.

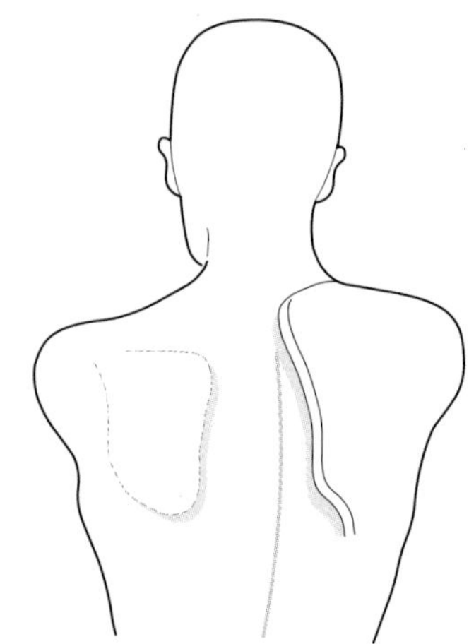

Fig. 34.7 'Winging' of the scapula; the patient is pushing against a wall.

Branches of the brachial plexus

Axillary or circumflex nerve

This is most commonly injured in association with dislocation of the shoulder joint. The deltoid muscle is paralysed and there is a patch of anaesthesia over the outer side of the arm. The majority of cases recovers spontaneously, but rupture of the nerve does sometimes occur and then recovery is only possible if nerve grafting is carried out.

The long thoracic nerve

The long thoracic nerve to serratus anterior (nerve of Bell) may be injured by operations on the breast or chest wall, or is occasionally involved in neuropathies. Paralysis of serratus anterior results in 'winging' of the scapula and difficulty in elevating the arm above a right angle (Fig. 34.7).

Radial nerve

This nerve is most commonly injured in the radial groove in association with fracture of the shaft of the humerus or as a result of pressure, as in 'Saturday night' palsy due to falling into a heavy sleep with the arm over the sharp back of a chair. Clinical features include:

- *motor* – paralysis of brachioradialis, the wrist extensors and extensor digitorum. It should be remembered that extension of the interphalangeal joints will still be present if the hand is supported because of the action of the lumbricals and interossei, which are inserted into the extensor expansions. In higher lesions the triceps will also be affected;
- *sensory* – loss of sensation over the dorsum of the thumb and the first web space. In higher lesions sensation is also lost on the dorsum of the forearm (Fig. 34.8).

Sir Charles Bell, 1774–1842. Surgeon, Middlesex Hospital, London, England (1812–35), Professor of Surgery, Edinburgh, Scotland (1836–42).

Recovery of the radial nerve is usually good either after conservative management or repair, if appropriate.If not, then good results can be obtained by tendon transfer.

Median nerve

The median nerve is classically injured at the elbow or wrist. Injuries at the elbow are due to fractures of the distal humerus or dislocation of the elbow joint. Clinical features include:

- *motor* – paralysis of the pronators of the forearm and flexors of the wrist and fingers, with the exception of the flexor carpi ulnaris and the medial part of the flexor digitorum profundus. The index finger and thumb cannot be flexed at the interphalangeal joints, but flexion of the other fingers is performed by the portion of the flexor digitorum profundus which is supplied by the ulnar nerve. The thenar muscles are paralysed with resulting loss of abduction and opposition of the thumb;
- *sensory* – sensation is lost over the palmar aspect of the thumb, index, middle and the radial half of the ring fingers, as well as part of the palm.

Damage to the median nerve at the wrist is comparatively common as a result of lacerations, fractures of the distal radius or compression in the carpal canal. Clinical features

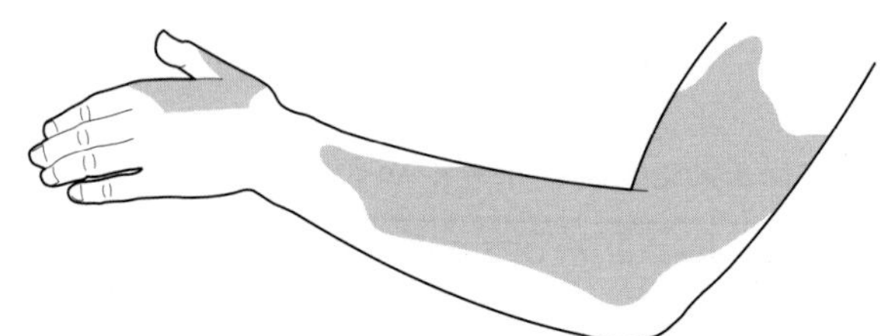

Fig. 34.8 Areas of anaesthesia after a high complete lesion of the radial nerve. If damage is below the origin of posterior cutaneous nerve of the forearm then the sensory loss is limited to the dorsum of the first web space.

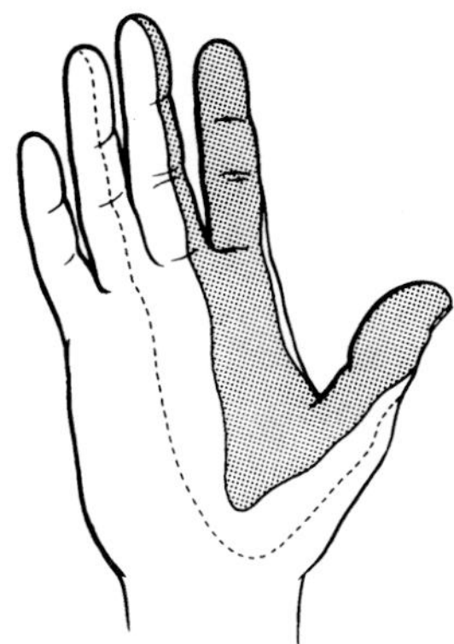

Fig. 34.9 The area of sensory loss in the hand involving the radial three and a half digits after damage to the median nerve proximal to the wrist.

include paralysis of the thenar muscles and loss of sensation on the palmar aspect of the radial three and a half fingers (Fig. 34.9).

Ulnar nerve

The ulnar nerve is most commonly damaged by lacerations in the forearm or entrapment as it passes behind the medial epicondyle of the humerus, in which case decompression or anterior transposition may be indicated.

Clinical features include:

- *motor* – paralysis of the small muscles of the hand, with the exception of the thenar muscles and lateral two lumbricals. The patient is unable to abduct and adduct the fingers, or indeed grip a piece of paper between them (Fig. 34.10). Weakness of flexion of the metacarpophalangeal joints and extension of the interphalangeal joints result in a claw-type deformity. If the patient pinches a piece of paper between the thumb and the index finger the distal phalanx of the thumb assumes a flexed position, as weakness of the adductor pollicis permits over-action of flexor pollicis longus (Froment's sign, Fig. 34.11). In longer standing cases, muscle wasting will be evident in the interosseus spaces and along the medial border of the hand. Lesions proximal to the elbow also cause paralysis of the flexor carpi ulnaris and medial half of the flexor digitorum profundus;
- *sensory* – sensation is lost on the medial one and a half fingers (Fig. 34.12).

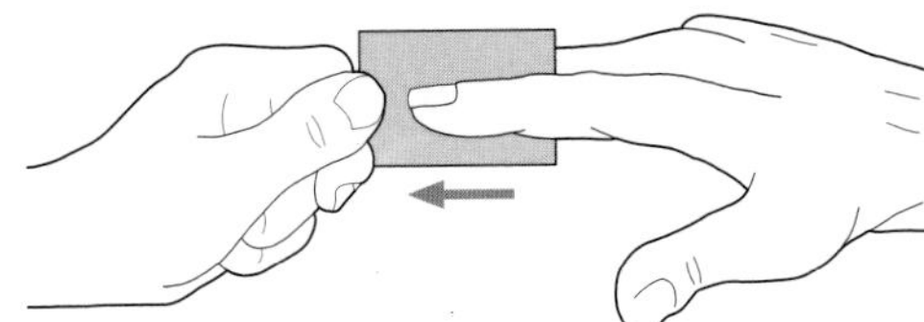

Fig. 34.10 Ulnar nerve injury. Test for weakness of the interosseus muscles.

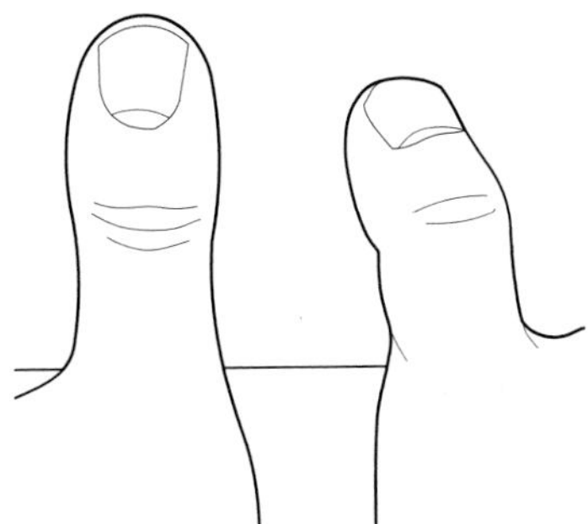

Fig. 34.11 Froment's sign for right ulnar nerve paresis.

Lower limb nerves

Sciatic nerve

The sciatic nerve is occasionally injured by wounds, fractures of the pelvis, posterior dislocation of the hip, operation for hip replacement or tumours. The prognosis for recovery is poor, particularly in proximal injuries. If the lesion is above the origin of branches to the hamstrings, the following features will be present:

- *motor* – the flexors of the knee are paralysed, but some degree of flexion is possible owing to the action of the sartorius and gracilis muscles. Complete paralysis exists below the knee, and the pull of gravity therefore causes foot drop;
- *sensory* – complete loss below the knee, with the exception of the skin supplied by the saphenous nerve, i.e. the medial border of the foot;
- causalgia may complicate partial lesions.

Common peroneal (lateral popliteal) nerve

Partial lesions of the sciatic nerve affect the peroneal division much more frequently than the tibial division. The common peroneal nerve itself is quite sensitive to injury by fractures or dislocations around the knee, pressure from plasters or

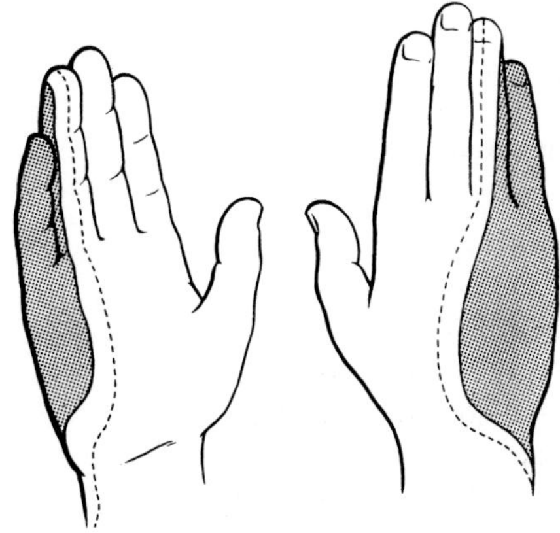

Fig. 34.12 Ulnar nerve injury. The area of sensory loss affecting the ulnar one and a half digits.

Jules Froment, 1878–1946. Professor of Clinical Medicine, Lyons, France.

splints and operations around the knee. Complete lesions will cause:

- *motor* – complete paralysis of the extensor muscles of the ankle and toes and the peroneal muscles, with resulting foot drop and tendency to inversion of the ankle;
- *sensory* – anaesthesia of the dorsum of the foot and toes.

The prognosis depends on the severity of injury, but is poor even after repair for neurotmesis. Function may be improved by tendon transfer at the ankle.

Femoral nerve

The femoral nerve is occasionally injured by stab wounds or operations on the groin. Paralysis of the quadriceps results. The prognosis is good if a laceration of the nerve is repaired early.

Cranial nerves

I. Olfactory nerve

The fine olfactory filaments pass through the cribiform plate to join the olfactory bulb that runs on the undersurface of the frontal lobe. Damage can result from acceleration/deceleration injuries causing shifts in the position of the brain, fractures of the ethmoid bone and meningioma arising from the floor of the anterior cranial fossa. The sense of smell is impaired, and because of the strong relationship between smell and taste this can considerably affect the enjoyment of food and drink.

II. Optic nerve

The optic nerve is an outgrowth from the cerebrum and has an investing nerve sheath, enclosing cerebrospinal fluid, which allows intracranial hydrostatic pressure to be transmitted to the optic fundus. A rise in intracranial pressure may be manifest by swelling of the optic disc (papilloedema). The optic nerve may be damaged as it leaves the skull and glial tumours may arise within the substance of the optic nerve, particularly in children. By testing the visual field, it may be possible to infer the site of intrinsic or extrinsic lesions affecting the optic pathways.

III. Oculomotor nerve

A complete lesion of this cranial nerve causes total paralysis of the levator palperae superioris, resulting in ptosis. A proptosis will occur because of loss of tone of the extraocular muscles which normally exert traction on the globe. Owing to the unopposed action of the sixth and seventh cranial nerves, the eye is deviated downwards and outward and, when the lid is lifted, diplopia will occur. Because of the unopposed action of sympathetic fibres there is dilatation of the pupil, which is unresponsive to both light and accommodation. The length of the intracranial course of the third cranial nerve exposes the nerve to damage either intracranially, as it leaves the skull, or within the orbit. In circumstances of raised intracranial pressure, herniation of the uncus of the temporal lobe through the tentorial notch leads to pressure on the third cranial nerve and a dilated pupil. This is a late and serious sign of raised intracranial pressure.

IV. Trochlear nerve

The fourth cranial nerve supplies the superior oblique muscle and is rarely involved by itself. It is associated with mild diplopia.

V. Trigeminal nerve

This nerve has a sensory portion, conveying sensation from the face and a motor root, supplying the muscles of mastication. There are three divisions of the sensory part of the nerve: the ophthalmic, the maxillary and the mandibular (Fig. 34.13). Large tumours in the cerebellar pontine angle may affect the trigeminal nerve. However, the commonest clinical manifestation of trigeminal nerve dysfunction is trigeminal neuralgia. This condition occurs predominantly in the middle aged and elderly, with a female predominance. It is characterised by severe, dagger-like pain within one or more divisions of the trigeminal nerve. Frequently the pain is triggered by any movement or stimulus to the face. It is becoming increasingly recognised that ectatic vascular loops may cause compression of the fifth nerve, producing these symptoms. Management of trigeminal neuralgia is, in the first instance, with carbamazepine. However, if this fails surgery may be considered to relieve vascular compression in the posterior fossa or to disrupt the trigeminal ganglion using percutaneous thermocoagulation.

VI. Abducens nerve

This nerve supplies the lateral rectus muscle and, when it occurs in isolation, results in diplopia due to the unopposed action of the medial rectus muscle. Because of its long intracranial course, the sixth nerve may be affected by fractures of

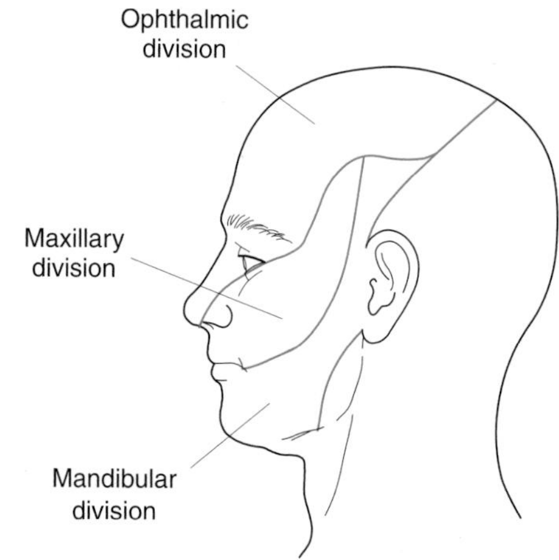

Fig. 34.13 Diagram showing the areas of skin innervated by the sensory divisions of the trigeminal nerve.

the skull base or, alternatively, a supratentorial mass lesion may result in traction of the nerve as it passes over the petrous tip.

VII. Facial nerve

The seventh cranial nerve gives a motor supply to the muscles of facial expression and its sensory branch, the chorda tympani, carries taste from the anterior two-thirds of the tongue.

In clinical practice the motor supply is of most importance. Paralysis of the facial muscles may result from upper or lower motor neuron lesions. Because of bilateral cortical representation of motor supply to the upper half of the face, upper motor neuron lesions, such as those caused by cerebrovascular events, will result in weakness of the face with preservation of eye closure and forehead movement. In a lower motor neuron lesion, all muscles innervated by the facial nerve will be affected and this results in complete facial weakness with loss of resting tone and of facial expression (Fig. 34.14).

The causes of facial nerve damage include:

- cerebellar pontine angle lesions, such as an acoustic neuroma;
- Bell's palsy, a mononeuritis may be related to viral infection;
- trauma to the nerve during surgery on the parotid gland.

Damage to the nerve in the face should be repaired as with other peripheral nerves. If damage or a defect occurs during the course of a cerebellar pontine angle operation, such as removal of an acoustic neuroma, then the facial nerve may be reconstituted using either a nerve graft or a piece of freeze–thawed skeletal muscle. When repair is not possible a nerve transfer of the hypoglossal to the facial nerve or cross face transfer may be carried out. Alternatively, plastic surgical procedures may be used to improve the resting state of the face.

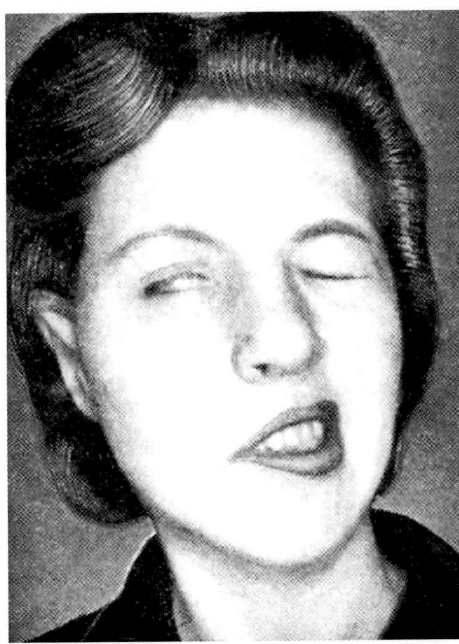

Fig. 34.14 Right-sided facial paralysis as a result of a lower motor neuron lesion.

VIII. Vestibulocochlear nerve

The eighth cranial nerve carries information from the vestibular apparatus and organ of Corti (hearing). The surgical significance of the eighth nerve is that it may be involved in fractures of the middle cranial fossa or be affected by tumours such as an acoustic neuroma.

IX. Glossopharyngeal nerve

The motor supply of the ninth cranial nerve is to the stylopharyngeus muscle, which cannot be tested clinically. Therefore, for the purposes of examination, the ninth cranial nerve carries sensation from the soft palate and the posterior third of the tongue. It mediates the sensory component to the gag reflex. It may be affected by fractures of the skull base or by pathology involving the lower cranial nerve roots as they leave the brainstem.

X. Vagus nerve

This nerve has a small sensory supply to the ear canal, with motor innervation to the palate and vocal cords. Although the nerve may be affected throughout its course, damage to the recurrent laryngeal nerve, which may occur during a thyroid operation as a result of intraoperative traction, division or postoperative haematoma formation, is of particular note. A complete recurrent laryngeal nerve palsy results in paralysis of both abductors and adductors of the corresponding vocal cord, which therefore adopts a halfway position, the so-called cadaveric position. The opposite vocal cord can compensate, closing the glottis, but the range of the voice is impaired. Partial recurrent laryngeal nerve involvement has a predilection to the muscles of abduction leading to adduction of the vocal cord on the affected side. If this is bilateral, stridor can result, which rarely may require tracheostomy.

XI. Accessory nerve

This is the nerve to the sternocleidomastoid and trapezius. It may be damaged by base-of-skull fractures, but it is more commonly affected in its cervical course. It is particularly at risk during operations on the posterior triangle, for example biopsy of lymph nodes. Division of the nerve in the anterior triangle will produce paralysis of the sternocleidomastoid and trapezius muscles (Fig. 34.15). Damage in the posterior triangle will affect only the trapezius, resulting in a drooping shoulder with wasting of the trapezius and often a considerable amount of pain. If the injury is recognised early then direct repair or nerve grafting will usually allow some recovery.

Marquis Alfonso Corti, 1822–88. Italian anatomist.

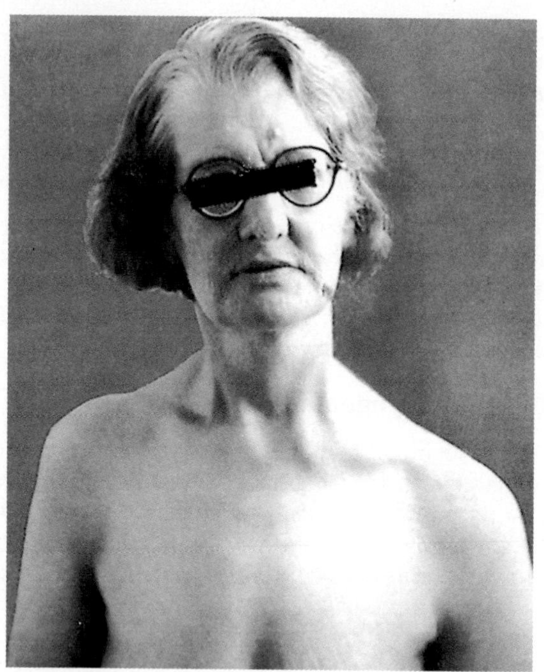

Fig. 34.15 Drooping of the left shoulder and wasting of the trapezius muscle following division of the spinal accessory nerve.

XII. Hypoglossal nerve

This is the motor nerve to the tongue, and damage results in wasting, weakness and fasciculation on the affected side. On protrusion of the tongue, deviation occurs towards the side of the lesion. The twelfth nerve may be involved with intracranial pathology but is more often injured distally, particularly during operations such as those on the submandibular gland.

Further reading

Birch, R., Bonney, G. and Wynn Parry, C.B. (1998) *Surgical Disorders of the Peripheral Nerves*, Churchill Livingstone, Edinburgh.

Gelberman, R.H. (ed.) (1991) *Operative Nerve Repair and Reconstruction*, J.B. Lippincott, Philadelphia, PA.

Green, D.P. (ed.) (1993). *Operative Hand Surgery*, 3rd edn, Churchill Livingstone, New York.

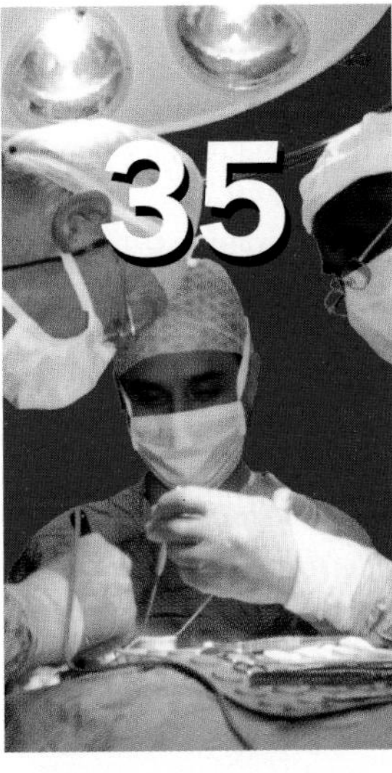

35 The cranium (scalp, skull, brain)

The scalp

There are five layers to the scalp: skin, dense connective tissue, galea aponeutotica, loose connective tissue and pericranium (Fig. 35.1). The scalp receives a rich vascular supply. This arises from both the external and internal carotid arteries with the vessels lying in the dense connective tissue layer. The anterior scalp is supplied by the supratrochlear and supraorbital arteries, and branches of the internal carotid via the ophthalmic artery. The lateral and posterior scalp is supplied by the superficial temporal, posterior auricular and occipital arteries, and branches of the external carotid. The sensory nerves run with the arteries and are derived from the trigeminal nerve at the front and sides. The posterior aspect is supplied by the greater and lesser occipital nerves with motor supply to the occipitofrontalis muscle by the facial nerve. Venous drainage of the face and anterior scalp is via the facial vein. The lateral and posterior aspects are drained by the external jugular vein and the vertebral venous plexus, respectively. The veins of the scalp and face communicate directly with the intracranial venous sinuses via emissary veins, hence infections in the nasal region have the potential to cause cavernous sinus thrombosis. Lymph drainage from the scalp is to the preauricular and occipital lymph nodes.

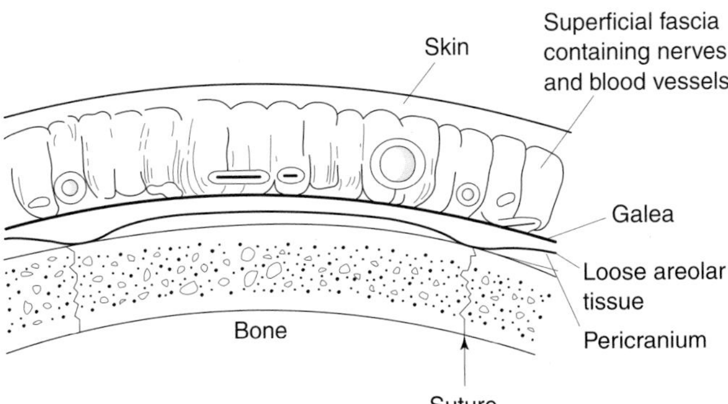

Fig. 35.1 Layers of the scalp: skin, dense connective tissue, galea aponeurotica, loose connective tissue and pericranium.

Bailey & Love's Short Practice of Surgery, 23rd edition. Edited by R.C.G. Russell, N.S. Williams and C.J.K. Bulstrode. Published in 2000 by Arnold Publishers.

The walls of the vessels in the dense connective layer are bound, preventing ready retraction when divided. Wounds to the scalp therefore bleed copiously. When the underlying cranium is intact, it is a safe and simple measure to arrest haemorrhage by compression against bone until haemostasis is achieved by suturing the wound. In the presence of a penetrating wound to the scalp, it is mandatory to exclude a fracture radiologically. If no fracture is present, it is safe to explore the wound, so that foreign bodies and debris may be removed, the wound débrided and the scalp closed. This is done in layers with a resorbable suture to the galea and a nonabsorbable suture to the skin.

The scalp heals readily and therefore it is often possible for skin of questionable viability to be left in place without becoming necrotic. When a scalp wound results in loss of tissue the limiting factor to closure is often the inflexibility of the galea. By performing release incisions in the galea, a moderate-sized defect may be closed. However, when large areas of scalp are missing, more extensive rotational flaps are required. Skin grafts will only take on a layer of intact pericranium.

The loose areolar tissue under the galea aponeurotica is a dangerous zone for infections. Pus can spread freely in this layer and reach the intracranial sinuses through the emissary veins. Abscesses and haematomas under the pericranium are limited to the area of one bone because the pericranium is firmly adherent to the sutures between the skull bones. In infants, blood loss into this layer can often be underestimated leading to cardiovascular decompensation. Osteomyelitis of the skull is associated with a subperiosteal swelling and oedema of the scalp referred to as Pott's puffy tumour (Fig. 35.27). This is now a rare condition but because of the possibility of intracranial sepsis, should be aggressively investigated and treated.

Lesions that occur on the head may be identical to those occurring in the skin elsewhere (Fig. 35.2a and b). Therefore any mobile lesion occurring within the skin should be inspected, investigated and treated using the usual diagnostic criteria. However, when lesions occur in the midline or appear to be more deeply connected within the layers of the scalp, then it is mandatory that more extensive radiological investigations [ideally computerised tomography (CT) or magnetic resonance imaging (MRI)] be performed to exclude any intracranial extension.

The skull

The skull consists of several bones which are fused by means of sutures to form the cranium which encases the

(a)

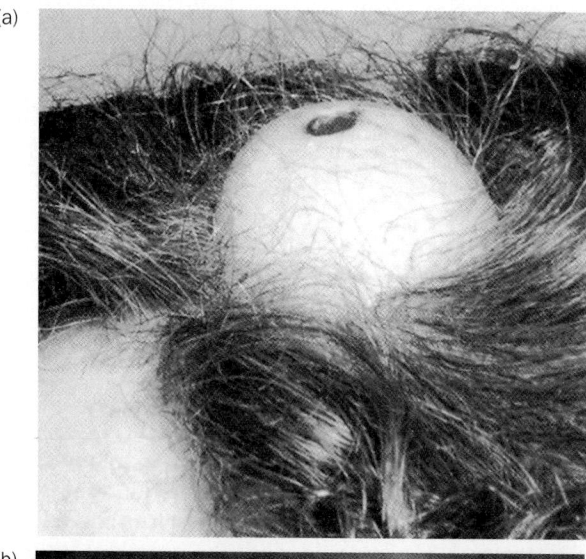

(b)

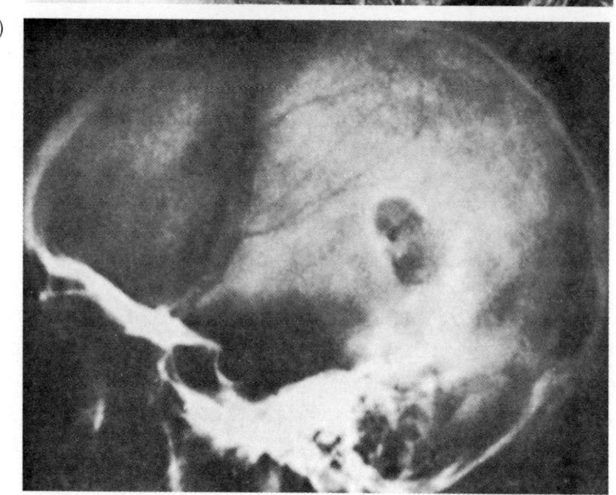

Fig. 35.2 Sebaceous cyst of the scalp.

Percival Pott, 1914–88. Surgeon, St Bartholomew's Hospital, London, England. Described this fracture – dislocation of the ankle – in 1975.

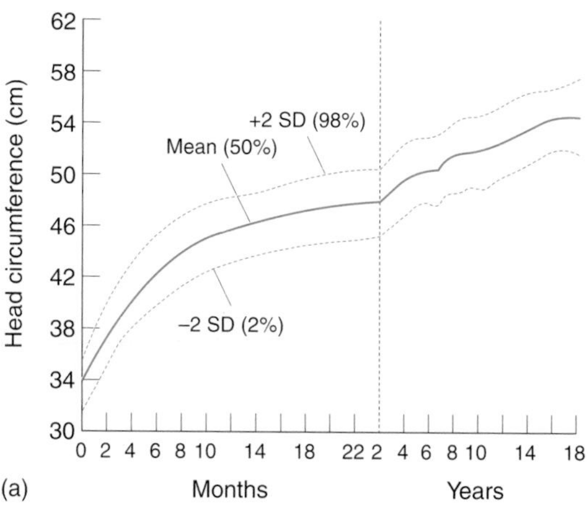

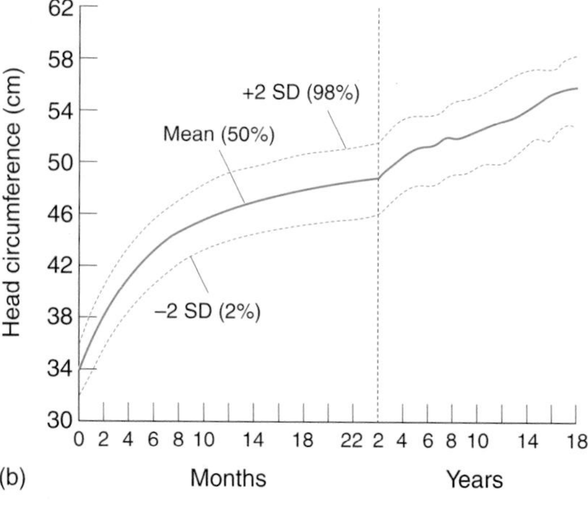

Fig. 35.3 Head circumference in (a) girls and (b) boys from birth to 18 years with the 2 per cent and 98 per cent centiles plotted.

brain and from which the face hangs. The normal skull has a remarkable degree of symmetry about the midline. There is rapid growth of the skull during the first few years of life, a growth which is driven and shaped by the underlying developing brain and the development of the sphenoid bone. If the development of the brain is abnormal, then this can be reflected in the overall skull size. Therefore, macrocephaly may occur as a result of hydrocephalus (Fig. 35.3).

If premature closure of any of the cranial sutures occurs, this may result in loss of midline symmetry and associated developmental abnormalities of the face. The most common type of synostosis is that of the sagittal suture, which results in the characteristic keel-shaped head or scaphocephaly (Fig. 35.4a–c).

Trigonocephaly is caused by premature fusion of the metopic suture (Fig. 35.5), whereas plagiocephaly will result from unilateral coronal or lambdoid synostosis. When more than one suture is involved in the synostotic process, this may result in elevation of the intracranial pressure. This may be as a result of not only restriction of calvarial growth but also obstruction to venous drainage at the base of the skull and respiratory problems. These are commonly associated with syndromic craniosynostosis, such as Crouzon's and Apert's syndrome. Surgery for craniosynostosis is undertaken in specialised units and because of the associated otolaryngological, dental and ophthalmological implications, the approach should be multidisciplinary. Surgery is directed towards increasing the volume of the skull, improving the cosmetic deformity and overcoming airway problems that may contribute to morbidity.

Congenital defects of the skull may occur at any point in the midline from the nasion to the foramen magnum as a result of incomplete fusion. Meningeal prolapses that occur with these defects may contain cerebral tissue and likewise be associated with a degree of structural abnormality of the underlying brain (Fig. 35.6). These lesions are usually situated in the frontonasal region and are not commonly associated with derangement of the cerebral architecture, whereas those occurring more towards the occipital region characteristically have more severe anatomical problems with consequent mental and physical handicaps. Frontonasal encephalocoeles are more common in Asiatic races and may be associated with a degree of hypertelorism. Smooth swellings seen in the roof of the mouth or in the nose in infants and dermal sinuses should be approached cautiously, as these might harbour underlying skull defects with herniation of the intracranial contents. Investigation with CT and often MRI is required to exclude intracranial communication. If this is confirmed, neurosurgical exploration may be required to prevent the risk of future ascending infection.

Octave Crouzon, 1874–1938. French physician.
Eugène Apert, 1868–1940. French paediatrician.

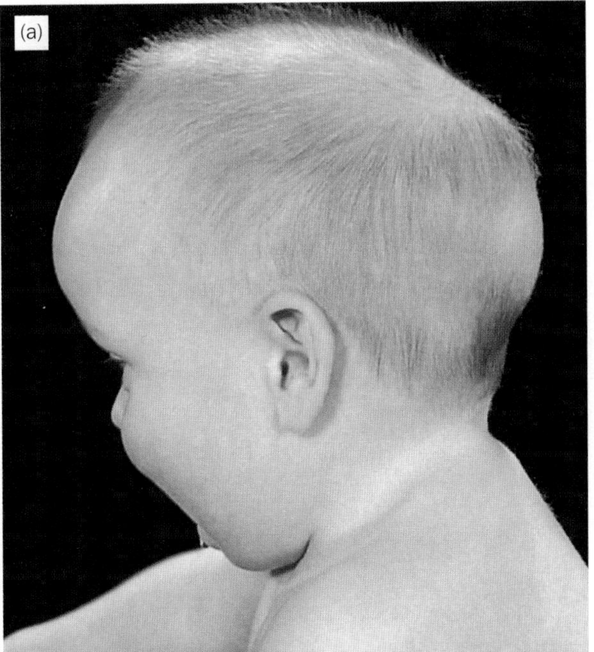

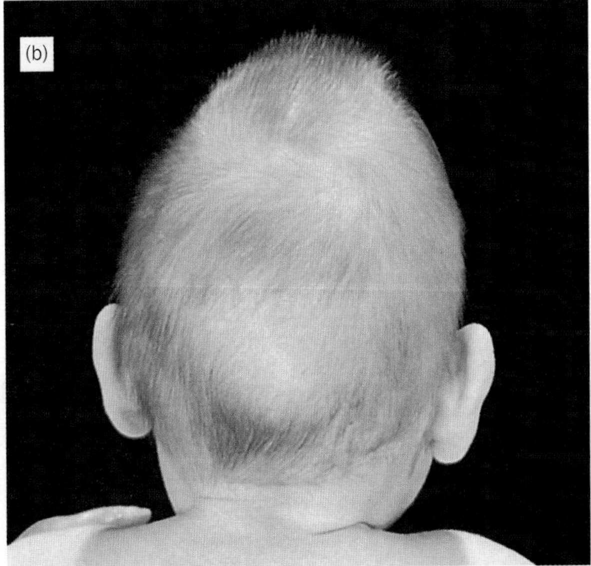

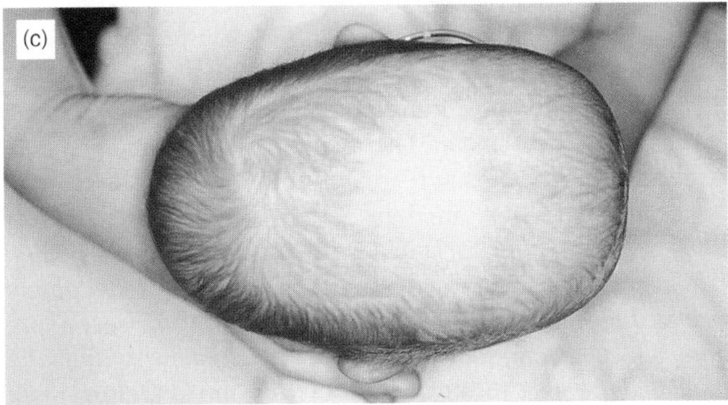

Fig. 35.4 Characteristic appearances of scaphocephaly due to premature fusion of the sagittal suture.

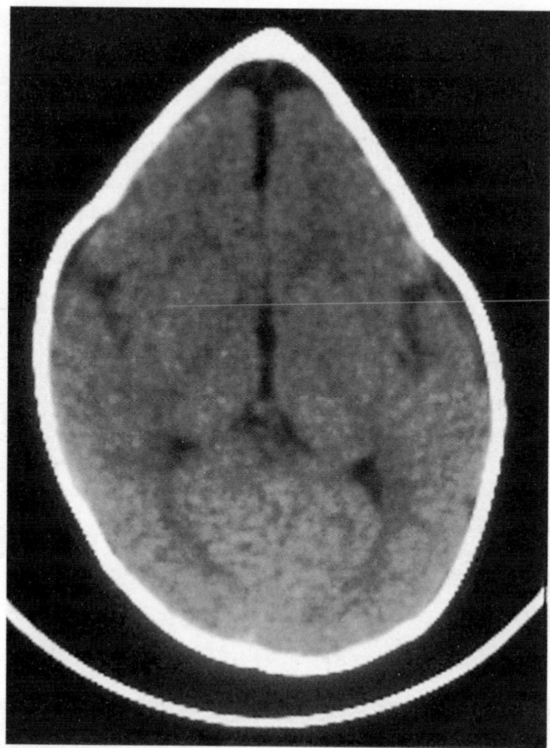

Fig. 35.5 Axial CT showing severe trigonocephaly due to premature fusion of the metopic suture.

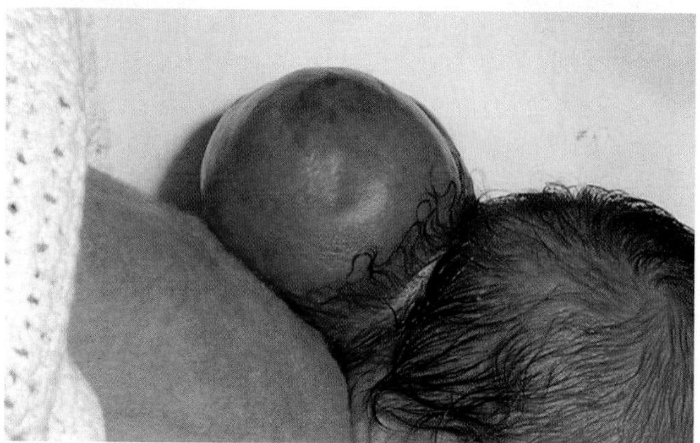

Fig. 35.6 An occipital encephalocoele.

Bony tumours are unusual and may present because of cosmetic deformity. The benign ivory osteoma may be either drilled down or simply excised with the defect being reconstituted by either a split cavarial graft from adjacent bone or filled with an acrylic cranioplasty. Primary malignant growths of the skull are exceedingly rare and more often these lesions are found to be secondary (Fig. 35.7). In childhood, however, lytic lesions within the skull may be as a result of histiocytosis and therefore open biopsy with or without excision or curettage may be indicated.

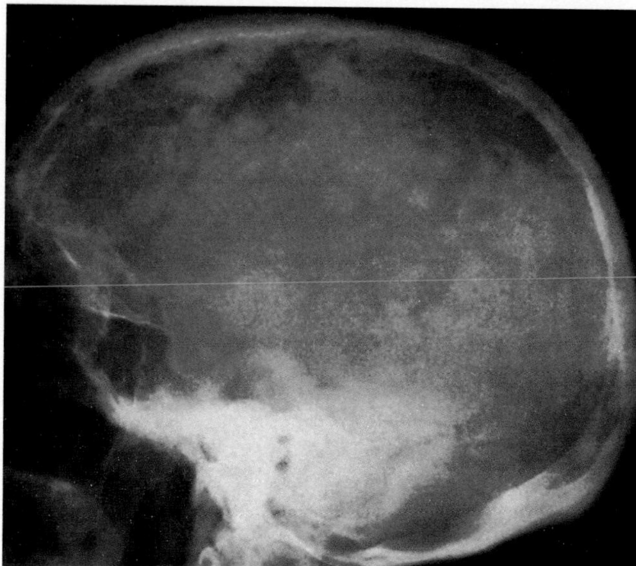

Fig. 35.7 Multiple secondary deposits due to breast carcinoma.

Intracranial disorders

Pathophysiology of raised intracranial pressure

Introduction

The adult skull may be regarded as a rigid unyielding box containing brain, cerebrospinal fluid (CSF) and blood. At normal supine pressures of 5–15 mmHg (6–18 cmH_2O), measured from the level of the foramen of Munroe, these three components maintain volumetric equilibrium. An increase in the volume of any one of the components will result in an increase in intracranial pressure (ICP) unless there is a proportionate decrease in the volume of one of the other components. These observations were first reported by Alexander Munro (Professor of Anatomy, Edinburgh, 1783) and 40 years later confirmed by Kellie – becoming known as the Munro–Kellie doctrine.

Owing to compensatory volumetric changes having physical and physiological limits, the ability to maintain a constant ICP can be exceeded by a change in volume that is too fast or too great. This intracranial pressure–volume relationship is illustrated in the curve (Fig. 35.8). Initially quite large increases in volume produce only small changes in pressure. During this phase the brain adapts by shifting CSF and moving blood from venous structures. A critical point is reached however when small changes in volume cause exponential increases in ICP.

The relationship of volume to pressure is described in terms of compliance or elastance of the intracranial space. Compliance is expressed as dV/dP and is the amount of 'give' available within the intracranial compartment. Elastance is

Alexander Monro, 1733–1817. Professor of Anatomy, Edinburgh, Scotland.

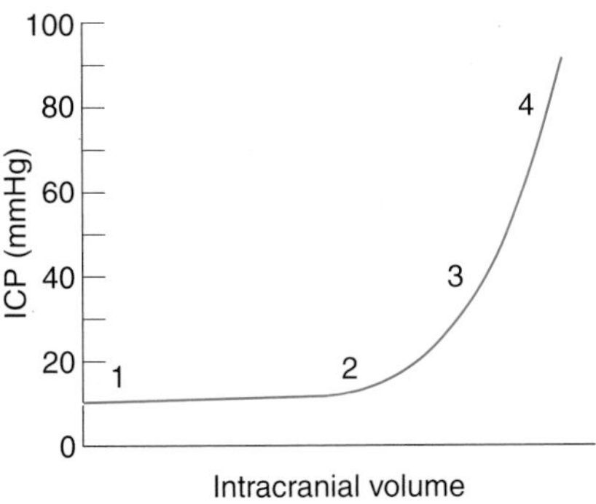

Fig. 35.8 Intracranial pressure volume relationships. At elevated intracranial pressures, a small increase in volume will result in a large increase in pressure.

the inverse and is the resistance offered to the expansion of a mass or the brain itself. When patients initially present with symptoms of raised ICP it is invariably when brain compliance has been reduced and small volume changes have the potential to cause precipitous increases in ICP and a reduced level of consciousness.

Between physiological ranges of blood pressure, the brain is able to maintain a constant cerebral blood flow. This is achieved by a process called autoregulation (Fig. 35.9), whereby the brain adjusts the intracranial vascular resistance. With hypovolaemic shock, malignant hypertension, subarachnoid haemorrhage or diffuse severe head injuries, this ability is compromised and the cerebral perfusion pressure becomes virtually dependent on the mean arterial pressure.

Normal cerebral blood flow (CBF) is about 800 ml/min or 20% of the total cardiac output. The blood flow is a function of the cerebral perfusion pressure (CPP) and the cerebral vascular resistance (CVR).

$$CBF = CPP/CVR$$

The cerebral perfusion pressure is a function of the systemic mean arterial pressure (MAP) and the ICP.

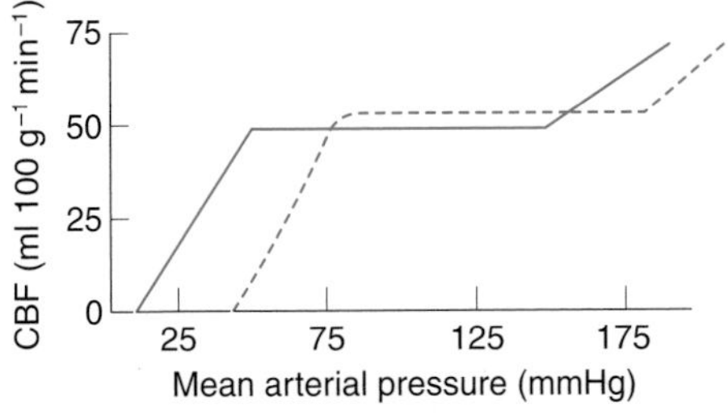

Fig. 35.9 Autoregulation of cerebral blood flow. Cerebral blood flow remains constant over a mean arterial pressure range 50–150 mmHg. The curve is shifted to the left in patients with chronic hypertension.

Harvey Cushing, 1869–1939. Professor of Surgery, Harvard University, Boston, Massachusetts, USA. Described his syndrome in 1932.

$$CPP = MAP - ICP$$

As intracranial pressure increases, in order to maintain a constant CPP, there has to be a compensatory rise in the MAP. A hypertensive response is therefore elicited which classically is associated with a bradycardia. This is termed the Cushing reflex after the eminent American neurosurgeon.

Clinical features

These are largely determined by the underlying cause. However, some of the clinical symptoms and signs will be the same:

- headache;
- nausea and vomiting;
- drowsiness;
- papilloedema.

These headaches are usually worse in the morning owing to vasodilatation caused by hypoventilation and consequent CO_2 retention during sleep. They are typically progressive but relieved by an upright position and are frequently associated with nausea and vomiting. As the brain has no sensation they are caused by traction and distortion of the pain-sensitive blood vessels and dura. Compression of the reticular activating system in the brainstem results in drowsiness. In an infant, raised ICP will cause a tense bulging fontanelle.

As the eyes are extensions of the forebrain, the optic nerves carry with them the meningeal coverings. The ICP is thus transmitted directly to the optic nerve head via the CSF. This results in obstruction to axoplasmic flow in the retinal neurons causing swelling. This is seen on funduscopy as blurring of the disc margins (Fig. 35.10), eventually retinal haemorrhages and if prolonged, optic atrophy. Traction on the abducent (sixth) nerves by caudal displacement of the brainstem may cause nerve palsies – the false localising sign.

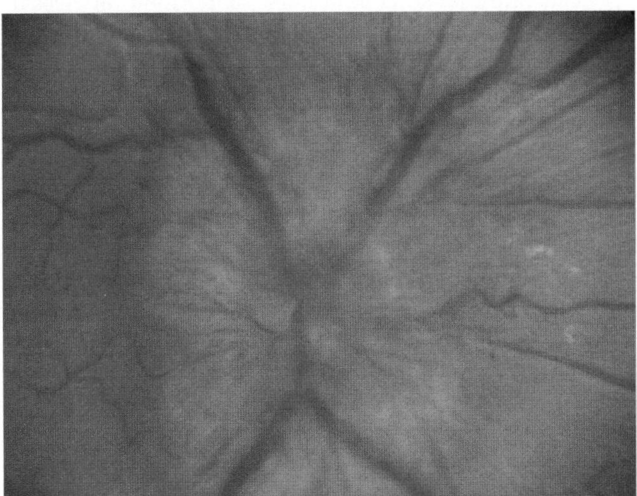

Fig. 35.10 Papilloedema showing a swollen optic disc with blurred margins.

Continuous monitoring of ICP reveals stereotyped variations superimposed upon baseline fluctuations. 'A' waves are transient plateaux of increased pressure to greater than 50 mmHg which last for 5–10 minutes. They are abnormal and indicate low compliance within the intracranial cavity. Skull X-rays may demonstrate sutural separation in children, pronounced 'copper-beating' marking of the cranial vault and thinning of the dorsum sellae with erosion of the posterior clinoid processes.

Treatment

This should primarily be directed at removing the cause for the increased ICP. Intracranial volume can be mechanically decreased by removing an intracranial mass or haematoma, reducing intracranial venous blood volume by facilitating venous outflow via the jugular veins, ventilated to bring the carbon dioxide toxin (PCO_2) down to 4–4.5 (avoiding vasoconstriction in patients with ischaemic disease) or by draining CSF through a ventriculostomy.

Steroids seem most effective in decreasing ICP resulting from vasogenic oedema associated with brain tumours or surgical manipulation (dexamethasone 4 mg 6 hourly). They work by stabilising the blood–brain barrier and reducing oxygen radical injury.

Mannitol, an osmotic dehydrating agent (1 g/kg 4–6 hourly), works by drawing water from parts of the brain with an intact blood–brain barrier. If this is disrupted as in a cerebral contusion, Mannitol can leach out into the brain and potentiate the mass effect. In head injuries it should therefore only be administered after consultation with a neurosurgeon. It becomes ineffective when brain osmolarity becomes iso-osmolar with that of the serum.

Barbiturates given as a bolus (thiopentone 3–5 mg/kg) can reduce ICP, although the exact mechanism remains obscure. Subsequent doses are titrated to give a level of 2.5–3.5 mg per cent. Infusions to control burst suppression on electroencephalogram (EEG) have been postulated to diminish ICP by reducing cerebral metabolism. The initial response is due to vasoconstriction but it is possible to reduce CPP by causing hypotension.

Frusemide reduces ICP by reducing cerebral oedema and CSF production. It may act synergistically with mannitol. Hypothermia down to 34°C is currently undergoing assessment as a brain protection agent.

Although no randomised clinical study has ever been performed conclusively proving the value of ICP monitoring in reducing morbidity following brain injury, there is a clear relationship between raised pressure and morbidity and mortality. The vital physiological parameter in severely head-injured patients is the CPP. This is a function of the mean arterial blood pressure and the ICP and, to optimise outcome, should be maintained above 65 mmHg. This requires a close working relationship between the intensivist and the neurosurgeon.

Head injury

It has been estimated that in the UK, between 200 and 300 per 100 000 of the population are admitted to hospital each year with a head injury, making it one of the most common causes for attending accident and emergency departments. Trauma, in which severe head injury often plays a major role, is also the leading cause of death in the population below 45 years of age. Craniocerebral trauma is consequently a source of major disability and a huge financial and psychological burden upon society.

Despite being encased in a rigid protective skull and cushioned by CSF, the brain is still very vulnerable to trauma, having only the consistency of a well-set jelly. This trauma can take the form of translational acceleration/deceleration forces, rotational forces or direct local sharp penetrating or blunt trauma to the cranium and can involve the scalp, skull or brain, in any combination.

Scalp

Scalp lacerations are common and can give rise to exanguinating haemorrhage if not controlled. This is due to the vessels in the dense fibrous layer being held open. Scalp hair plays an important protective role and by matting into wounds can effectively assist haemostasis but likewise mask significant scalp lacerations. The scalp's rich vascular supply plays an important role in healing, making it a very resilient structure.

Skull

Different types of skull injury may follow blunt trauma.

Simple linear fractures

These require no specific neurosurgical management but are usually markers of the force to which the head was subjected. Patients are usually CT scanned but should also be admitted for at least 48 hours' observation.

Depressed skull fracture

These fractures are a result of blunt trauma, usually to the left frontal region. If the pericranium has been breached the fractures are technically compound. The integrity of the dura is however more important. The dura and brain may be lacerated by the depressed fragment.

The damage done at the time of impact with subsequent risk of epilepsy is irreversible. Surgery is usually undertaken to prevent the risk of infection, to alleviate mass effect and for cosmetic purposes. Contaminated wounds require extensive débridement, a duraplasty and irrigation before closure. A full course of intravenous antibiotics should be administered.

Base of skull fracture

These are relatively frequent fractures, usually diagnosed on clinical grounds. They often result in CSF fistula which may

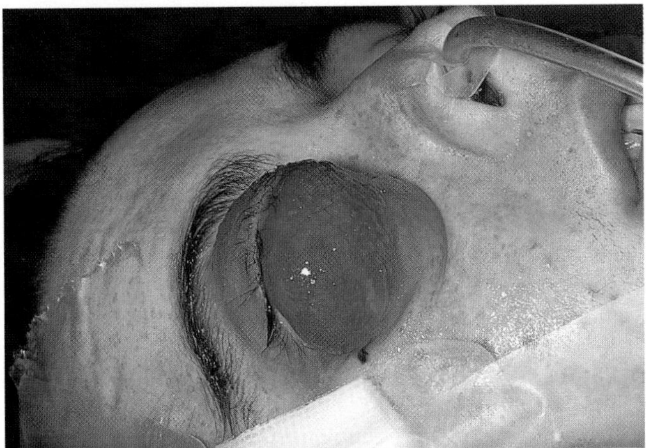

Fig. 35.11 Caroticocavernous fistula, a complication developing following a fracture of the petrous temporal bone and rupture of the internal carotid into the cavernous sinus. The pulsating proptosis and conjunctival oedema are visible and a bruit is audible on auscultation.

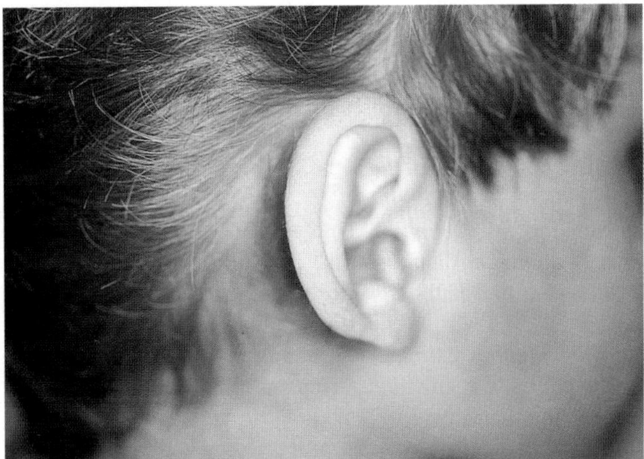

Fig. 35.13 'Battle sign', bruising behind the ear occurring 36 hours after a head injury with petrous temporal base of skull fracture.

persist but usually seal off after a few days. Anterior fossa fractures present with subconjunctival haematomas, anosmia, epistaxis and CSF rhinorrhoea and may occasionally be associated with caroticocavernous fistulae (Fig. 35.11). Periorbital haematomas or 'racoon eyes' indicate subgaleal haemorrhage and not necessarily base of skull fracturing as do subconjuntival haemorrhages extending beyond the conjunctival reflections (Fig. 35.12). Middle fossa fractures present with CSF otorrhoea or rhinorrhoea via the eustachian tube, heamotympanum, ossicular disruption, 'battle sign' (Fig. 35.13) or VII and VIII cranial nerve palsies.

There is no evidence that prophylactic antibiotics diminish the incidence of meningitis. Administering them may just select out more virulent organisms in those that become infected, increasing morbidity and mortality. If one suspects a CSF fistula, the fluid should be screened for beta-transferrin to confirm that it is in fact CSF. Before repair of CSF fistula, it is mandatory to exclude the presence of hydrocephalus. The

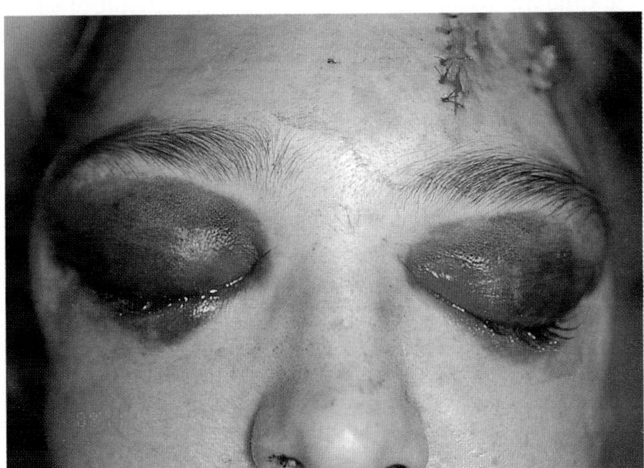

Fig. 35.12 Periorbital ecchymoses ('racoon eyes') due to subgaleal bleeding from frontal trauma.

dura should then be sealed with autologous, vascularised grafts and fibrin glue after cranialisation of the frontal sinuses.

Ping-pong fracture

This is a smooth depression of the cranial vault usually seen in children. Also known as a 'pond' fracture.

Blow-out fracture

These are caused by fracturing of the orbital walls with herniation of orbital contents and subsequent tethering of the globe, resulting in pain and diplopia.

Brain injury

For both treatment and medicolegal purposes, it is important to have an understanding of the mechanisms as to how brain injuries evolve. Abrupt deceleration of a moving head is characterised by a relatively minor injury at the site of impact (coup injury) and an extensive contusion of the brain opposite the point of impact [contre-coup injury (French-'counter-blow')]. Contusions are most likely along the undersurface of the frontal lobes, the tips of the temporal lobes and along the falx.

Abrupt acceleration of an unsupported head occurs when the head is struck by a moving object. The skull accelerates against the brain causing an extensive coup injury of the brain. The remainder of the brain may remain unchanged. When a well-supported head is struck by a moving object, there is little movement of the skull and brain. Most of the force is absorbed by the skull, which will fracture. Damage to the underlying brain results from direct perforation or laceration by skull fragments.

It is thus easy to understand why most cerebral contusions occur without skull fracture and why patients with spectacular fractures are often awake with only minor neurological dysfunction.

Primary brain injury is caused at the time of impact and is irreversible (Fig. 35.14). Secondary brain injury develops subsequent to the impact damage (Table 35.1). The management of head injuries focuses on reducing secondary injuries.

Primary brain injury

Cerebral concussion

This is a clinical diagnosis and is manifested by temporary dysfunction that is most severe immediately after injury and resolves after a variable period. It may be accompanied by autonomic abnormalities including bradycardia, hypotension and sweating. Loss of consciousness often, but not invariably, accompanies concussion. Amnesia for the event is common and varying degrees of temporary lethargy, irritability and memory dysfunction are hallmarks.

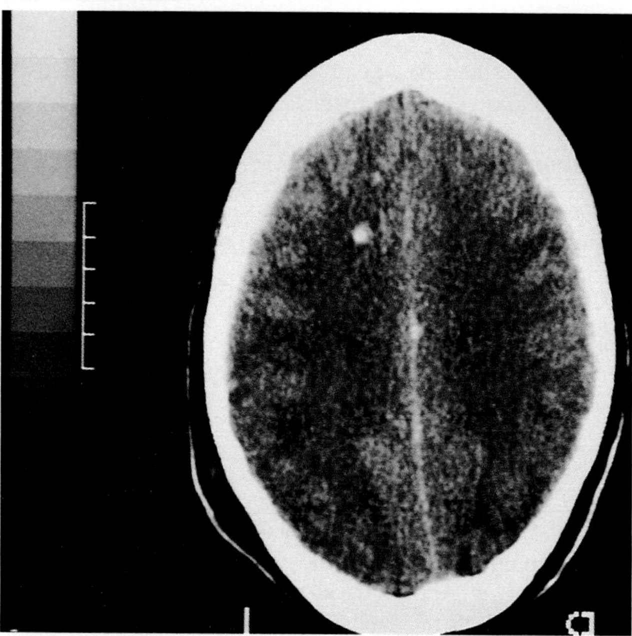

Fig. 35.14 Axial CT showing a diffuse axonal head injury. This demonstrates all three radiological criteria: subarachnoid bleeding, brain swelling and scattered punctate haemorrhages.

Table 35.1 Brain injury

Primary brain injury
Concussion
Cortical contusions/lacerations
Bone fragmentation
Diffuse axonal injury
Brainstem contusions
Secondary brain injury
Intracranial haematomas
Cerebral oedema
Hypoxaemia
Ischaemia
Infection
Epilepsy
Metabolic/endocrine disturbances

Postconcussion syndrome can accompany head trauma and consists of headaches, irritability, depression, lassitude and vertigo. It is more frequent after minor head trauma due to people trying to return to work too quickly.

Cerebral contusion and laceration

This can be demonstrated by CT as small areas of haemorrhage in the cerebral parenchyma. They usually produce neurological deficits that persist for longer than 24 hours. Contusions may resolve together with the accompanying deficit or they may persist. Blood–brain barrier defects and cerebral oedema are common and these lesions enlarge or coalesce with time.

Even without a skull fracture, if sufficient force is delivered to the skull the brain might become lacerated as a result of rapid movement and shearing of brain tissue. The pia and arachnoid may be torn and intracerebral haemorrhage may accompany this lesion. Focal deficits are the rule.

Diffuse axonal head injury

This type of brain damage occurs as a result of mechanical shearing following deceleration, causing disruption and tearing of axons, especially at the grey/white matter interface. Severity can vary from mild confusion to coma and even death. Macroscopically, punctate haemorrhages are visible, especially in the corpus callosum and superior cerebellar peduncle. Microscopically, retraction balls reflecting axonal damage and microglial clusters (hypertrophied microglia) are found diffusely in the white matter.

Secondary brain damage

Intracranial haematomas

Intracerebral haematoma. These appear as hyperdense lesions on CT with associated mass effect and midline shift. They are due to areas of contusion coalescing into a contusional haematoma. They may appear to have a mixed density.

Extradural haematoma occurs usually as a result of squamous temporal bone fractures with laceration of the middle meningeal artery. They can also arise from fractured bone edges or rarely from the dural venous sinuses. The potential space between the dura and bone is developed by the expanding haematoma allowing it to take on the familiar convex configuration due to the adherence of the dura to the inside of the calvarium (Fig. 35.15). The degree of trauma might not be severe and there is typically a lucid interval following the trauma. Frequently, patients present in coma and require urgent evacuation via a burr hole prior to formal craniotomy (Fig. 35.16). Patients do well if delay is minimised.

Subdural haematomas. They are the most common intracranial mass lesions resulting from head injury. Most result from torn bridging veins draining blood from the cortex to the dura. They can also arise from cortical lacerations or bleeding from the dural venous sinuses. They are usually associated with more severe, high-velocity trauma with a

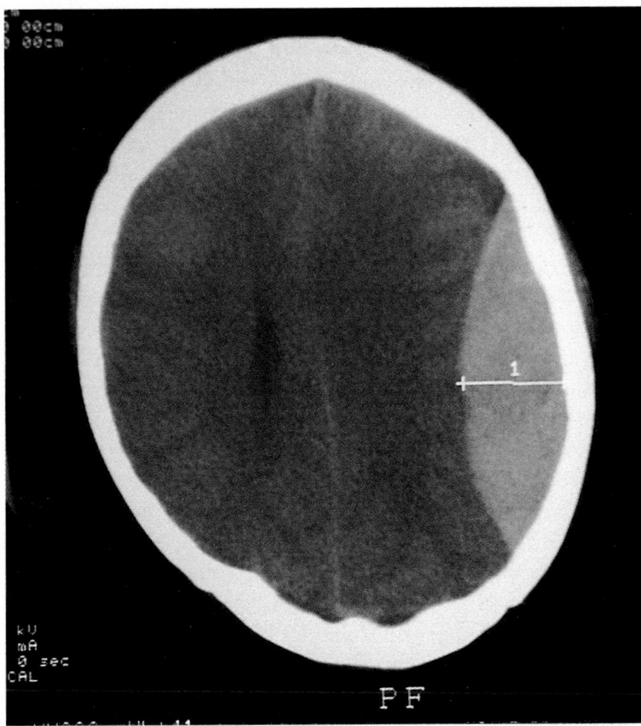

Fig. 35.15 Axial CT showing an acute right frontoparietal extradural haematoma due to a squamous temporal fracture not visible on CT.

poorer outcome, usually in older patients. The blood follows the subdural space over the convexity of the brain and appears as a concave hyperdense lesion. Acute subdural haematomas are more rapidly evolving lesions and early evacuation is mandatory (Fig. 35.17).

Chronic subdural haematomas. These haematomas are most common in infants and in adults over 60 years of age. They present with progressive neurological deficits more than 2 weeks after the trauma. Often the initial head injury has been completely forgotten and the pathology has been attributed to either dementia or a brain tumour until patients are scanned (Fig. 35.18). The initial haemorrhage may be relatively small or may occur in elderly patients with large ventricles or a dilated subarachnoid space. Membranes deriving from the dura and arachnoid mater encapsulate the haematoma which remains clotted for 2–3 weeks then liquefies. The acute clotted blood initially appears white on a CT scan. As it liquefies it slowly becomes black. There is therefore a point in time where it appears isodense with brain and all that can be seen is apparent inexplicable midline shift on an otherwise normal CT. These collections can be removed by drilling burr holes and washing them out with warmed saline.

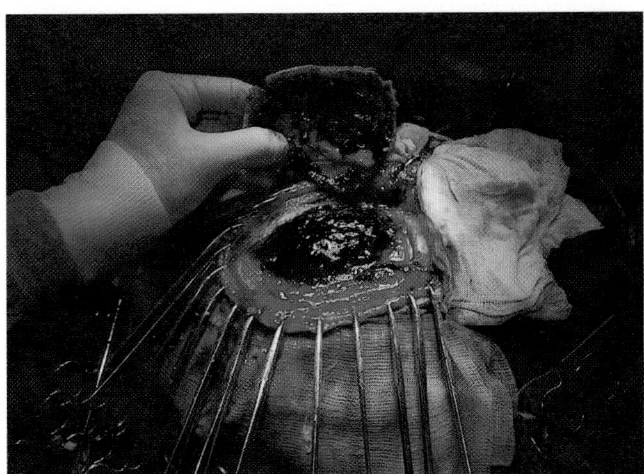

Fig. 35.16 Removal by craniotomy of an acute extradural haematoma.

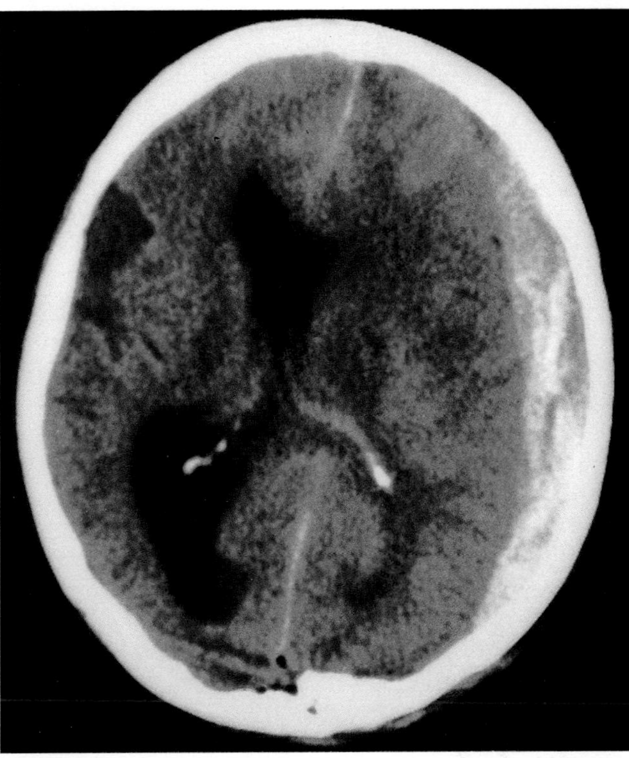

Fig. 35.17 Axial CT showing a right-sided acute subdural haematoma with midline shift.

Cerebral swelling

This results from vascular engorgement, probably due to a loss of autoregulation and an increase in extracellular and intracellular fluid. The exact causative mechanisms are unclear.

Cerebral ischaemia

This is common after severe head trauma and is caused by a combination of either hypoxia or impaired cerebral perfusion. The brain is unable to autoregulate its blood supply with a decrease in blood pressure. Glutamate excess and free radical accumulation lead to neuronal damage.

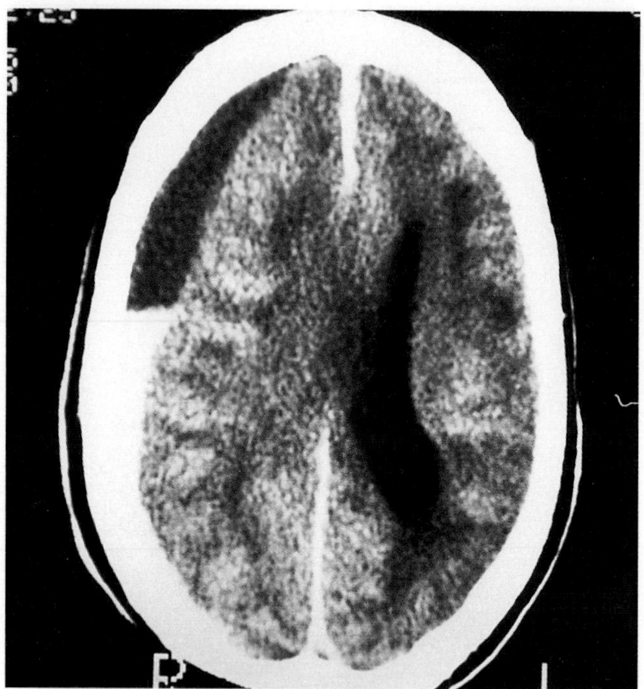

Fig. 35.18 Axial CT showing an acute on chronic subdural haematoma. The fresh clotted blood appears white while the older altered liquid blood appears black.

Infection

Compound depressed fractures or base of skull fractures can lead to either meningitis or cerebral abscess.

Epilepsy

Seizures can increase brain metabolism and blood flow, thereby increasing ICP. Prophylactic anticonvulsants given acutely for the first 2 weeks are said to be of benefit. No benefit from long-term treatment has been demonstrated.

Management

Initial assessment of head injuries must follow Advanced Trauma and Life Support (ATLS®) guidelines with an initial primary survey, then resuscitation, followed by a secondary survey then definitive management or, more simply: airway, breathing, circulation, disability and exposure. Securing an adequate airway preventing obstructive breathing or hypoventilation is critical in unconscious head-injured patients, as is maintaining a decent blood pressure. Care must be taken to secure the neck and spine. When an intracranial haematoma is suspected, an early CT scan is essential.

In the assessment of a head injury points to determine from the history are:

- period of loss of consciousness;
- period of post-traumatic amnesia;
- cause and circumstances of the injury;
- presence of headache and vomiting.

The patient should be examined for evidence of injury (e.g. lacerations and grazes) and the findings clearly documented. Base of skull fracturing should be excluded and the conscious level determined on the Glasgow Coma Scale and monitored (Table 35.2). The pupillary response should be elicited to determine whether there is incipient transtentorial herniation with oculomotor palsy, limb movements and responses recorded.

Once any intracranial haematoma has been evacuated patients should then be admitted to an intensive care unit and ventilated to a PCO_2 of 4–4.5 kPa. A central line, arterial line and a urinary catheter should be inserted. The head of the bed should be positioned 40° up and the patient given analgesia (fentanyl), sedated using propofol or midazolam and paralysed (atracurium). Intravenous fluids administered should be isotonic until nasogastric feeding can be commenced. An ICP monitor (Codman or Camino) should be inserted intraparenchymally and the ICP and CPP monitored. Ideally the ICP should be maintained below 25 mmHg and the CPP above 70 mmHg. If necessary, ionotropes can be used to support the blood pressure and CPP.

Dexamethasone has no benefit. Diuretics such as mannitol and frusemide can be used to lower ICP further but the former must be used with caution in patients with large areas of blood–brain barrier breakdown for fear of potentiating the mass effect. If ICP cannot be controlled by these means alone then steps such as introducing EEG burst suppression therapy with a barbiturate (thiopentone), ventricular or lumbar CSF drainage or polar lobectomies have to be considered.

Repeat CT scan should be considered if there is a delayed deterioration in the mental state, a maintained rise in intracranial pressure or a failure to improve over 24 hours.

Table 35.2 Glasgow Coma Scale

Eye opening	
Spontaneous	4
To speech	3
To pain	2
Nil	1
Best motor response	
Obeys	6
Localises	5
Withdraws	4
Abnormal flexion	3
Extension response	2
Nil	1
Verbal response	
Orientated	5
Confused conversation	4
Inappropriate words	3
Incomprehensible sounds	2
Nil	1

Hydrocephalus

Hydrocephalus is defined as a disproportionate increase in the amount of CSF within the cranium, usually in association with a rise in ICP.

Physiology and circulation of cerebrospinal fluid

The normal volume of circulating CSF is in the region of 140 ml. The fluid both protects and supports the brain and spinal cord, as well as maintaining homeostasis by acting as a transport medium for transmitters and as a method of removing the end products of metabolism. CSF is produced by an active process, 80 per cent of it being derived from the choroid plexus and the rest from the parenchyma. The rate of production is between 0.2 and 0.4 ml/minute, with a daily production rate of approximately 480 ml. This means that the turnover of CSF is approximately three times daily. Production of CSF is regulated, not only by the homeostatic environment, but also neurogenically and in response to alterations in CSF pressure. Resorption of CSF is almost entirely pressure dependent as a result of a hydrostatic gradient existing between the CSF in the subarachnoid space and the arachnoid villi, the point of reabsorption of the CSF into the venous system. There is also some absorption of CSF via the sleeves of the nerve roots.

Most fluid is produced in the lateral ventricles. Normal flow is then down through the foramina of Monro into the third ventricle and subsequently the aqueduct of Sylvius into the fourth ventricle, to pass laterally and inferiorly out of the fourth ventricle via the foramina of Luschka and Magendie, to circulate over the surface of the cortex for reabsorption at the arachnoid villi (Fig. 35.19).

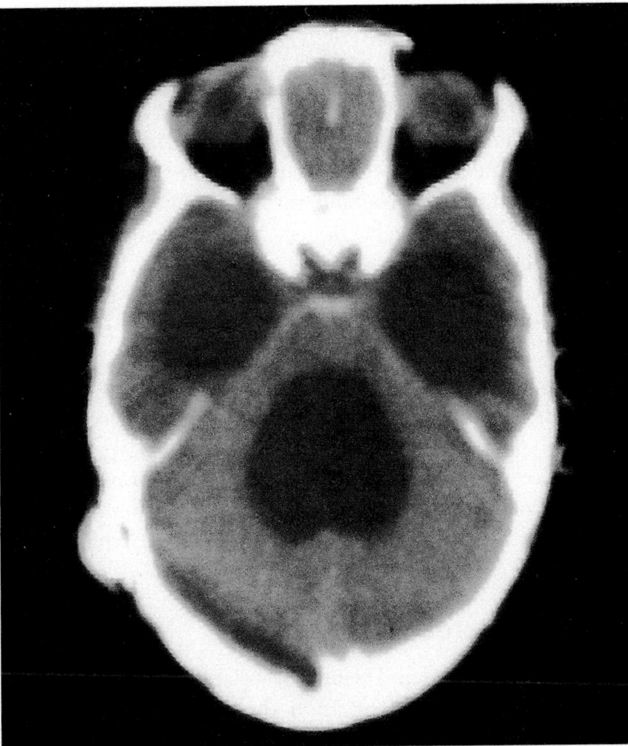

Fig. 35.19 Axial CT showing a neonate with communicating hydrocephalus and markedly dilated ventricles, the temporal horns, specifically which are normally just visible.

Hydrocephalus means an imbalance between the ratio of the CSF to cerebral tissue within the cranium. The first condition to be excluded immediately from a physiological point of view is hydrocephalus *ex vacuo*. This occurs when the ratio is altered as a result of atrophy of the cerebrum with an increase in CSF, purely as a compensatory mechanism. This condition does not have treatment implications, other than being part of the differential diagnosis in a patient with suspected hydrocephalus (Fig. 35.20).

Aetiology

In those patients with the pathophysiological condition of hydrocephalus, an imbalance has occurred between the normal physiological production of CSF and its absorption. This imbalance can be as a result of overproduction of CSF or impaired absorption. Conditions in which CSF is overproduced are uncommon. Typically the choroid plexus papilloma is cited as the most common cause of overproduction and, in most cases, there is no doubt that this does occur. However, in these cases there are compounding problems, such as obstruction of CSF flow, haemorrhage and change in the protein level of the CSF, which may exacerbate the hydrocephalus. As regards conditions where CSF resorption is impaired, there is a rare congenital condition wherein there is a congenital absence of the arachnoid villi. Failure of absorption is usually as a result of alterations in the hydrostatic gradient responsible for CSF absorption or failure of the CSF to circulate adequately to allow absorption to take place.

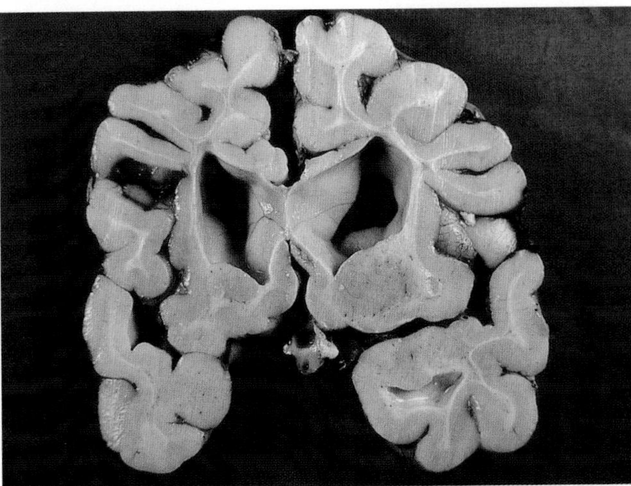

Fig. 35.20 Pathological specimen of a hydrocephalic brain.

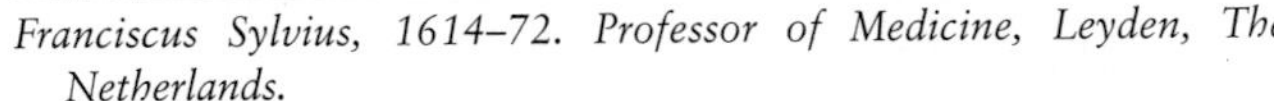

Franciscus Sylvius, 1614–72. Professor of Medicine, Leyden, The Netherlands.
Hubert Luschka, 1820–75. Anatomist, Tübingen, Germany.
François Magendie, 1783–1855. Physician and physiologist, Paris, France.

There is a further concept of obstructive or communicating hydrocephalus. Obstructive hydrocephalus is seen where the normal pathways of CSF flow are for some reason occluded. This may be as a result of conditions such as aqueduct stenosis or as a result of local compression from a tumour. In communicating hydrocephalus no obvious obstruction to CSF flow can be observed and all of the ventricles appear to be communicating freely. In fact, these so-called cases of communicating hydrocephalus usually do have some obstructive element underlying them, the level usually being in the basal system, the subarachnoid space or at the arachnoid villi.

Hydrocephalus may be congential and occur in conjunction with other abnormalities of the central nervous system, such as spina bifida, as a result of congenital aqueduct stenosis or as a result of intrauterine infections. Hydrocephalus acquired postnatally is commonly secondary either to intraventricular and intraparenchymal haemorrhage or to meningitis.

Clinical features

The presenting signs and symptoms related to hydrocephalus are very much dependent upon the age of the patient at presentation. In the neonatal period an increasing head circumference, tense fontanelle and failure to thrive may be the only initial signs, although feeding problems and 'sunsetting' (early down-turning of the eyes) associated with bradycardias may become apparent in the extreme cases (Fig. 35.21).

In older children and adults, hydrocephalus may be manifest principally by gradual development of symptoms of raised ICP, so that headache, nausea and vomiting occur, ultimately followed by a deterioration in the level of consciousness. There may also be associated ataxia and visual disturbance. With increasing age, hydrocephalus secondary to tumours becomes increasingly common and therefore in the older age group the symptoms of hydrocephalus may be combined with those symptoms attributable to the neoplasm itself.

Investigation

Records of the head circumference and its comparison with body weight and length are an integral part of the postnatal follow-up of any child. While this is an essentially somewhat crude method of determining the onset of hydrocephalus, it is nonetheless an easy and noninvasive sequential investigation with an excellent rate of diagnosis. On clinical examination, disproportion of the head to the rest of the body may immediately be evident and palpation of the head will reveal a tense fontanelle and separation of the sutures. Percussion of the head may produce the so-called 'crack-pot sign', while in severe cases it may be possible to transilluminate the head.

In older children and adults, the effects of chronic raised intracranial pressure may be evident on a skull radiograph with separation of the sutures and 'copper beating' of the skull, as well as erosion of the pituitary fossa (Fig. 35.22).

When the anterior fontanelle is patent it is possible to carry out ultrasonography to visualise the ventricular system, and this is also the way in which hydrocephalus is picked up antenatally. In older or younger children where further information is required, CT may be performed to aid in diagnosis. If a tumour is suspected then both enhanced and unenhanced tomography should be performed. The use of MRI to follow patients with hydrocephalus is attractive as no radiation dose is involved. However, accessibility, cost and time preclude this from being a routine investigation. MRI may be required when a tumour is seen to determine the surgical strategy, and when aqueduct stenosis occurs, to rule out a tectal plate tumour.

Management

Medical

Treatment of hydrocephalus is primarily directed towards methods of reducing CSF production. This can be achieved

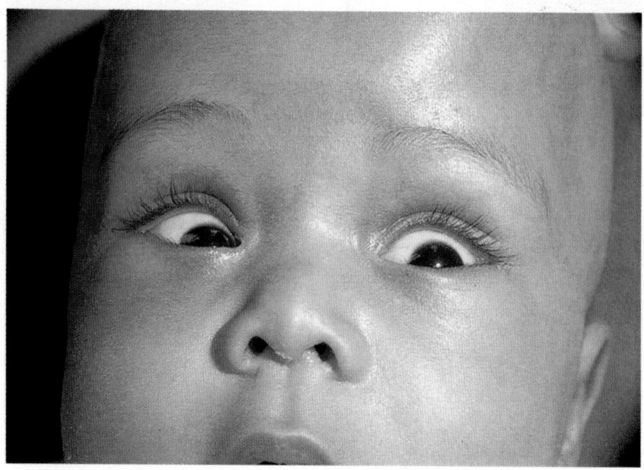

Fig. 35.21 Child with 'setting sun sign' due to hydrocephalus.

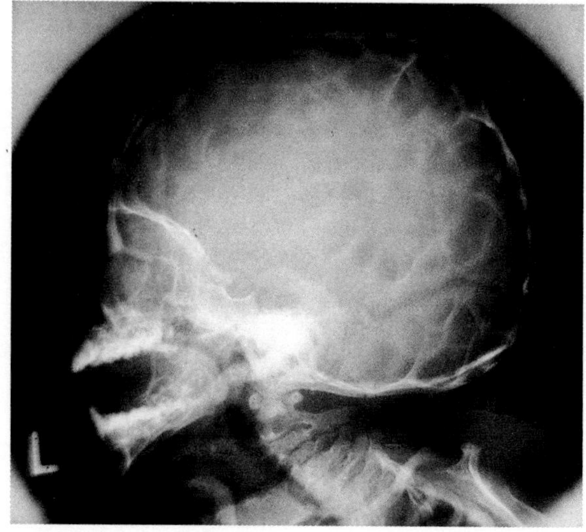

Fig. 35.22 Copper-beaten sign indicative of chronic raised ICP.

by using acetazolamide, which is a carbonic anhydrase inhibitor and may reduce CSF production by as much as 60 per cent. Frusemide also has an effect on CSF production and both drugs, therefore, may be used in the short term. In the long term the effect of these medications appears to be relatively limited and therefore surgical intervention is required.

Surgical

Where an obstruction to the flow of CSF is present, removal of that obstruction, particularly if it is neoplastic in origin, should be the primary goal of surgery. In most patients with obstructive hydrocephalus secondary to tumours, removal of the tumour will result in resolution of the hydrocephalus.

In others with long-standing hydrocephalus and the chronic changes as a result of this, long-term CSF diversion will be required. Surgical management of the hydrocephalus may be directed towards reducing CSF production, bypassing a blockage to normal CSF flow, drainage of CSF externally or finally drainage of CSF in another absorptive viscus. While obliteration of the choroid plexus was first described by Dandy it has failed for several reasons to act as a cure for hydrocephalus. First, the surgical procedure is directed towards the choroid plexus at the lateral ventricles and, as described above, 20 per cent of the CSF is produced by the nonchoroidal surface of the ventricles. Ablation of the intraventricular choroid plexus possibly has a role in the reduction in incidence of shunt obstructions. Bypassing obstruction to CSF flow may be achieved by a variety of means, such as cannulation of the aqueduct of Sylvius or third ventriculostomy, which may be performed endoscopically or at open operation. The first described bypass technique was that described by Torkildsen, where aqueduct stenosis was overcome by passing a catheter from the lateral ventricle into the cisternal magna, thereby reconstituting the normal circulatory pathway. External drainage of CSF may help in the temporary management of acute hydrocephalus but the risk of infection precludes this as a means of long-term management.

The final and most common form of surgical management of hydrocephalus is by an internal diversion. Methods of CSF diversion were first tried in the nineteenth century when attempts were made to divert the CSF by the use of silver wires into the lumbar vertebral bodies. The modern era of internal CSF diversion began in the 1950s when implantable devices with regulatory valves were developed (Fig. 35.23). The proximal site of CSF diversion is usually the lateral ventricle and, while many distal sites have been attempted, the current favoured distal site of CSF absorption is the peritoneum. Two main complications can occur following shunt insertion. The first is infection and the second is shunt malfunction. Infection occurs in about 5 per cent of adult cases and approximately 10 per cent of paediatric cases depending on age mix, as the rate of infection in neonates is much higher than that in older children.

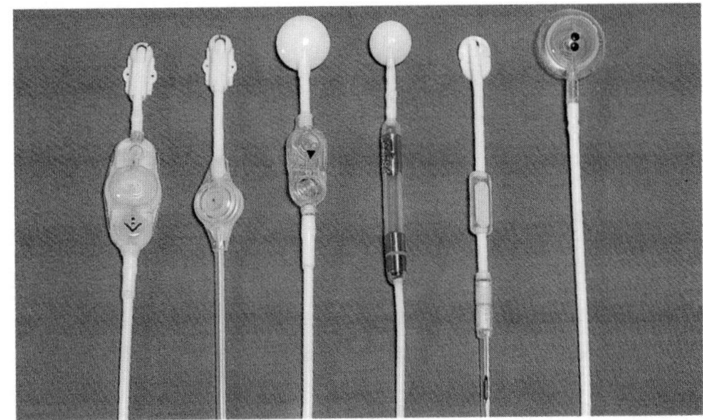

Fig. 35.23 Various types of CSF shunt.

Manifestations of infection usually become apparent within the first few weeks or months following implantation, and treatment of choice is to remove the infected system and treat the patient with intrathecal and intravenous antibiotics. Because infection is often with low-grade organisms, infection may take some time to diagnose. It is for this reason that the previously favoured distal shunting site at the right atrium was abandoned, as chronic bacteraemia was associated with the development of immune complexes leading to renal and pulmonary damage.

Shunt obstruction may occur at any time following shunt insertion and may be due to either ventricular catheter obstruction, valve malfunction or a distal obstruction at the peritoneal catheter. Regrettably, no ideal valve mechanism for CSF diversion has been developed and together with occlusion of the system, the system may also malfunction by overdraining. This is a result of the siphoning effect of the catheter into the peritoneal cavity and can lead to symptoms of headache as a result of the low intracranial pressure and the appearances on tomography of small, slitlike ventricles.

Intracranial infection

Infections involving the central nervous system (CNS) present in a variety of ways and unless diagnosed and treated promptly can result in serious morbidity and mortality. Intracranial infections encountered in neurosurgical practice include bacterial meningitis, brain abscess and subdural empyema.

Meningitis

Bacterial meningitis, although potentially a life-threatening infection, seldom requires neurosurgical intervention. Treat-

Walter Edward Dandy, 1886–1946. Neurosurgeon, Johns Hopkins Hospital, Baltimore, Maryland, USA.
Arne Torkildsen. Neurosurgeon, Norway.

ment involves confirming the diagnosis and identifying the organism by obtaining a CSF sample, usually via lumbar puncture (LP). Broad-spectrum intravenous (i.v.) antibiotics with good CSF penetration should then be commenced without delay (ceftriaxone 2 g 12 hourly and metronidazole 400 mg 8 hourly) and adjusted as cultures and sensitivities become available. In situations where lumbar puncture is deemed impossible or unsafe, unless CSF can be obtained by other means, treatment might have to be empirical. Studies have demonstrated that steroids, commenced early and in combination with antibiotics, can improve outcome by reducing oxygen free radical attack on the brain. Complications are more likely to occur if treatment is not commenced early and may require neurosurgical intervention. The major complications are: cerebral oedema, seizures, hydrocephalus (communicating), subdural effusion, subdural empyema, brain abscess and ventriculitis.

Brain abscess

The treatment of brain abscess has been revolutionised by the availability of CT scanning, metronidazole and stereotaxis. Prior to these modalities, the mortality for brain abscesses ranged between 15 and 40 per cent. Pyogenic inflammation of the brain leading to cerebral abscess may result from: haematogenous spread from a known septic site or occult focus (particularly in patients with right to left cardiac shunts) (Fig. 35.24); contiguous spread from an adjacent infected sinus presumably via retrograde thrombophlebitis; and direct inoculation from trauma. In 20 per cent of patients no cause can be identified (Figs 35.25–35.27).

The organisms most commonly responsible vary depending on the aetiology. With otitis media anaerobic streptococci, *Haemophilus* and Gram-negative anaerobes are involved; with sinusitis *Streptococcus milleri* and *Staphy-*

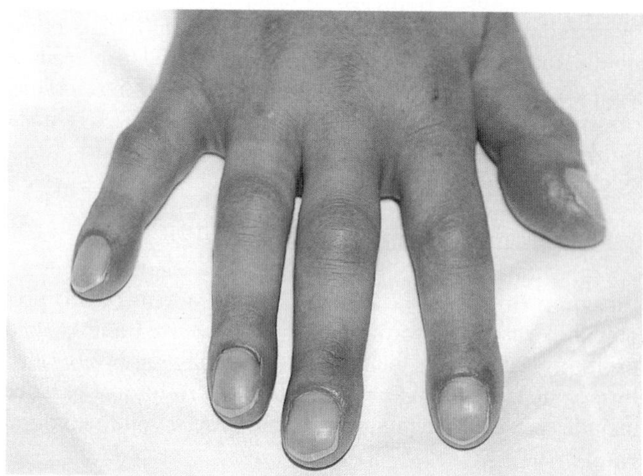

Fig. 35.24 Congenital cyanotic heart disease patient with clubbing.

Hans Christian Joachim Gram, 1858–1938. Professor of Medicine, Copenhagen, Denmark.

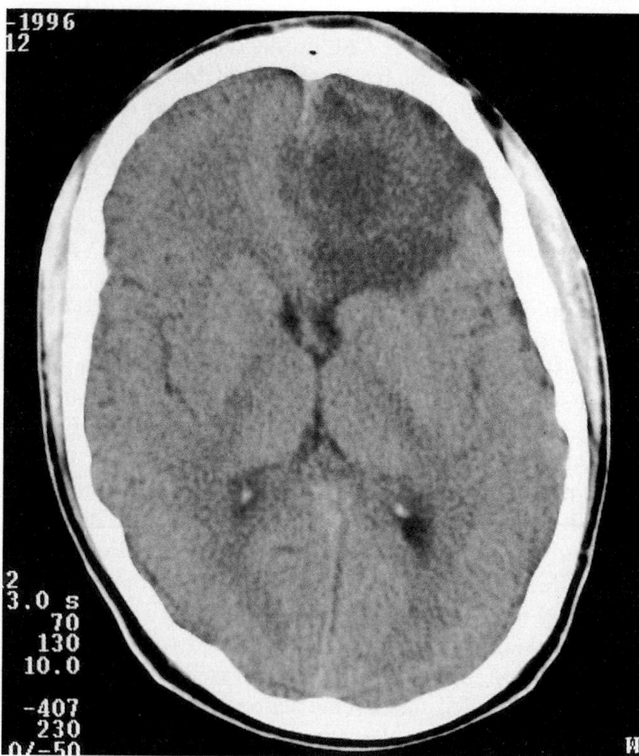

Fig. 35.25 Axial CT with contrast of patient with frontal sinusitus presenting with epilepsy and a hypodense area of cerebritis in the left frontal region.

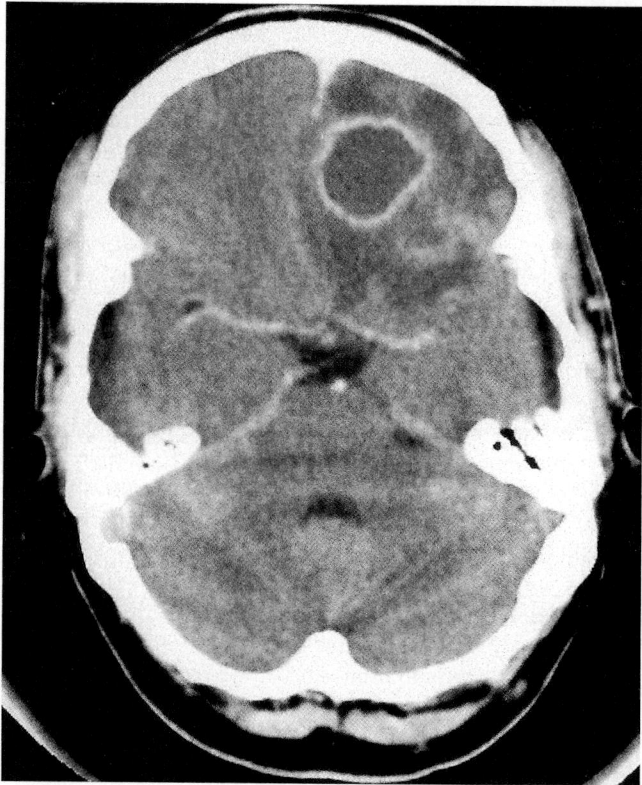

Fig. 35.26 Axial CT with contrast of same patient 2 weeks later. A round ring-enhancing lesion with a hypodense centre has developed – typical of a pyogenic intracerebral abscess.

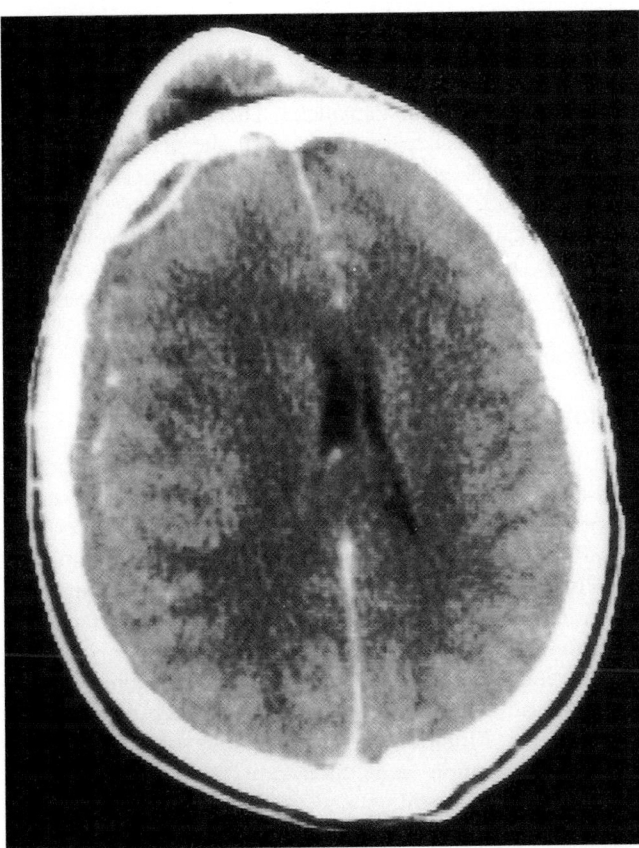

Fig. 35.27 Axial CT of patient with contrast and presenting with chronic frontal sinusitus, seizures and pyrexia. This demonstrates a right hemisphere subdural empyema and a right frontal Pott's puffy tumour.

lococcus; with traumatic inoculation *Staphylococcus*; and with haematogenous spread various organisms are involved.

Clinical features

Patients can present with either features of raised pressure, seizures, meningeal irritation or focal signs, each of which occurs in 50 per cent of patients. Systemic features of infection including pyrexia are frequently absent but the history is usually short with rapid clinical progression. Diagnosis is confirmed by demonstrating a single or multiple low attenuation and smooth, symmetric, ring-enhancing mass lesions with variable oedema on CT. MRI with enhancement will demonstrate similar findings including high signal on T2-weighted images from the surrounding oedema. These lesions arise in an area of cerebritis and can often be multiloculated. Opacification of the sinuses or mastoids can be recognised on both CT and skull X-ray (SxR). Infection markers will demonstrate a leucocytosis and a raised erythocyte sedimentation rate (ESR) and C-reactive protein (CRP), but may initially be normal.

Treatment

The principles of treatment are to identify the bacterial organism, institute intravenous antibiotic therapy (see above), drain or excise the abscess, and aggressively pursue and treat the cause. During the stage of acute cerebritis, prior to abscess formation, surgical treatment is seldom indicated. Steroids reduce oedema around these lesions and are thus invaluable in reducing intracranial pressure but can inhibit formation of the abscess capsule.

Unless very small, intracranial abscesses require surgical management. This is performed by either aspiration through a burr hole, with or without stereotaxis (repeated as necessary) or formal excision. The latter is undertaken if there is persistent reaccumulation of pus despite serial aspirations. Excision may also be considered if the abscess is superficial and easily accessible, and if there is a well-formed capsule which fails to collapse despite repeated aspirations. Patients should have regular follow-up CT scans with contrast until the abscess stops reaccumulating. Anticonvulsant therapy is routinely instituted.

Subdural empyemas

Subdural empyemas, although uncommon, may develop from sinusitus or mastoiditis. The infective agent is frequently *S. milleri*, although other anaerobic or aerobic streptococci, other anaerobes and *Staphylococcus aureus* may also be responsible. These patients are systemically unwell with rapidly progressive neurological signs, a depressed level of consciousness and hemiparesis. Epilepsy occurs in most patients and can often progress to status epilepticus.

Despite this being a surgical emergency, diagnosis is often delayed as the collection on CT scanning is usually subtle to the untrained eye and frequently missed. Treatment is as for an intracranial abscess but the collection requires a formal craniotomy for drainage with exploration of the interhemispheric fissure. The combination of fever and seizures with a background of sinusitus is usually diagnostic of this lesion. Complications include refractory status epilepticus and cortical vein/venous sinus thrombosis.

Human immunodeficiency virus (HIV) infection

Surgical management

The neurological complications of HIV infection have implications for both surgeon and patient. Although transmission of HIV from patients to healthcare workers is extremely rare, the surgeon is at risk from needle stick injury and thus extra care should be taken when dealing with a population at risk. In the acquired immunodeficiency syndrome (AIDS), single or multiple lesions within the brain may develop and patients may present with focal neurological signs, symptoms of raised intracranial pressure or seizures. In the early days of AIDS management, stereotactic biopsies of these lesions were routinely carried out. However, in view of the high proportion of infective lesions, particularly toxoplasmosis, it has now become routine to treat the patient first with a full course of antitoxoplasma treatment. Should this fail or the patient's clinical condition deteriorate, or both, then a stereotactic biopsy should be considered. The differential diagnosis is then between infection with an organism thus far not covered with the therapy given, or tumour, principally lymphomas, or the condition of progressive multifocal leucoencephalopathy (CML). The current clinical course is one of rapid and relentless deterioration and, indeed, when a stereotactic biopsy is required for diagnostic purposes in AIDS, then the overall prognosis is poor. However, biopsy and histological diagnosis allow patients, their partners and families to be counselled as regards prognosis. Furthermore, a histological diagnosis also allows a prospective study of new therapies for AIDS which, it is hoped, will lead to improved long-term prognosis.

Intracranial tumours

Introduction

Although either benign or malignant, almost all brain tumours are malignant in the sense that they may lead eventually to death if not treated. Brain tumours are responsible for 2 per cent of all cancer deaths. The annual incidence of newly diagnosed brain tumours in the USA is approximately 18 per 100 000 persons of which 30 per cent are primary. At autopsy the prevalence is 1–2 per cent. The incidence varies with age. In children tumours of the CNS comprise 20 per cent of all childhood malignancies. There is a peak at 2 years followed by a decline for the rest of the first decade. The incidence then slowly increases, peaking at 20 per 100 000 in late adulthood. The mortality rate averages 5 per 100 000. The classification of brain tumours is determined by their cell of origin. Over 50 per cent are neuroepithelial in origin, 15 per cent metastatic, 15 per cent meningiomas and 8 per cent pituitary tumours. The World Health Organization (WHO) classification is outlined in Table 35.3.

Table 35.3 WHO classification of brain tumours

Neuroepithelial tumours
Gliomas
Astrocytomas
Oligodendrogliomas
Ependymoma
Choroid plexus tumour
Pineal tumours
Neuronal tumours
Ganglioglioma
Gangliocytoma
Neuroblastoma
Medulloblastoma
Nerve sheath tumour
Acoustic neuroma
Meningeal tumours
Meningioma
Pituitary tumours
Germ cell tumours
Germinoma
Teratoma
Lymphomas
Tumour-like malformations
Cranipharyngioma
Epidermoid tumour
Dermoid tumour
Colloid cyst
Metastatic tumours
Contiguous extension from regional tumours, e.g. glomus tumour

Aetiology

The aetiology of brain tumours is still not clearly understood. Although there is no genetic predisposition, chromosome abnormalities have been noted in many CNS tumours (e.g. von Recklinghausen's). Some chemicals show carcinogenic activity in animals producing CNS tumours. Immunosuppression can markedly increase the incidence of primary CNS lymphoma. The current molecular understanding of oncogenesis involves both the addition of oncogenes to the genome and the loss of normally occurring tumour suppresser genes. Mutation in the *p53* tumour suppresser gene is the most common gene alteration and found in both astrocytomas and meningiomas.

Clinical features

The clinical presentation of intracranial neoplasms will be as a result of one or a combination of raised ICP, focal neurological signs, organic mental changes and seizures.

The ability of the intracranial contents to adapt to an increase in volume is limited and ultimately an increase in pressure will occur. This will manifest itself initially as a result of headache due to stretching of the dura. In the initial phase this headache is characteristically worse first thing in the morning and progressive. Nausea and vomiting may occur, followed by disturbance of vision as a result of papilloedema. Finally, a deterioration will occur in the level of consciousness as a serious and late consequence of raised ICP (Fig. 35.28).

Late-onset epilepsy, particularly over the age of 30, should prompt investigations to exclude an intracranial neoplasm. Forty per cent of patients with supratentorial glial tumours will have experienced a seizure by the time they come to surgery. Benign tumours may also be an underlying cause of long-standing epilepsy and may render the seizures surgically remediable. Focal neurological signs associated with intracranial neoplasms are related to the area of cortex involved. Contralateral signs are associated with lesions in the posterior frontal area (motor) or anterior parietal (sensory)

Friedrich Daniel von Recklinghausen, 1833–1910. Professor of Pathology, Strasbourg, France (1872–1906). Described generalised neurofibromatosis in 1882.

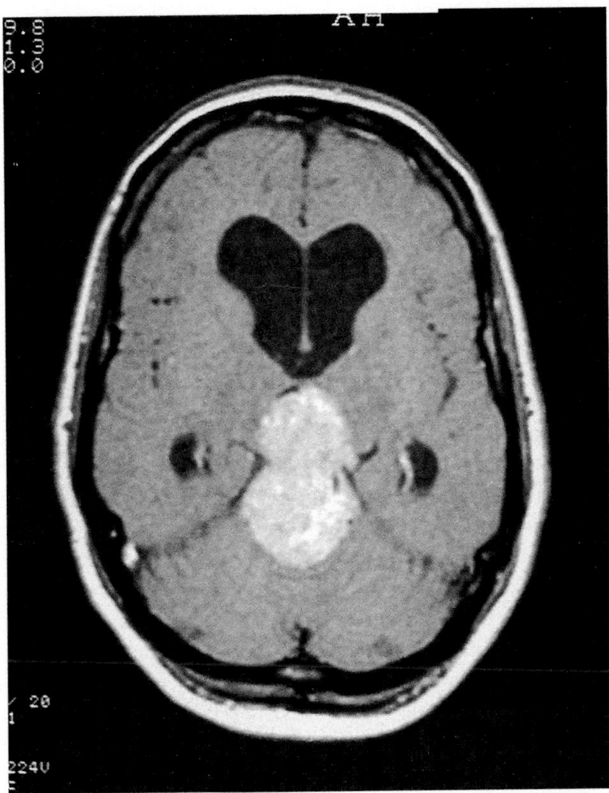

Fig. 35.28 Pineal region tumour causing obstructive hydrocephalus.

lobe. Tumours in the dominant hemisphere may cause problems with language (aphasia) and in the nondominant hemisphere apraxia. The optic pathway may be involved producing various visual symptoms, usually a contralateral homonymous hemianopia. Temporal lobe lesions frequently cause focal seizures with auras and visual field defects. Tumours in the frontal lobes can grow to considerable sizes before producing altered cognitive functioning and subtle personality changes. Subfrontal lesions may involve the olfactory nerves (anosmia). Sellar and parasellar tumours present with visual field and acuity problems due to compression of the optic chiasm. Tumours in relation to the ventricular system may obstruct CSF drainage and result in hydrocephalus, compounding raised ICP. Tumours of the brainstem and cerebellar–pontine angle may result in cranial nerve palsies and long tract signs. Tumours involving the cerebellar vermis cause ataxia, while tumours in the hemispheres produce appendicular signs such as incoordination and nystagmus.

Gliomas

Gliomas account for 50 per cent of adult intracranial tumours and are usually supratentorial. They are of neuroectodermal origin arising from glial cells of which there are four types: astrocytes, oligodendroglioma, ependymal cells and neuroglial precursors. The most frequent is the astrocytoma. They rarely metastasise (except for medulloblastoma and ependymoma) and spread along axonal pathways.

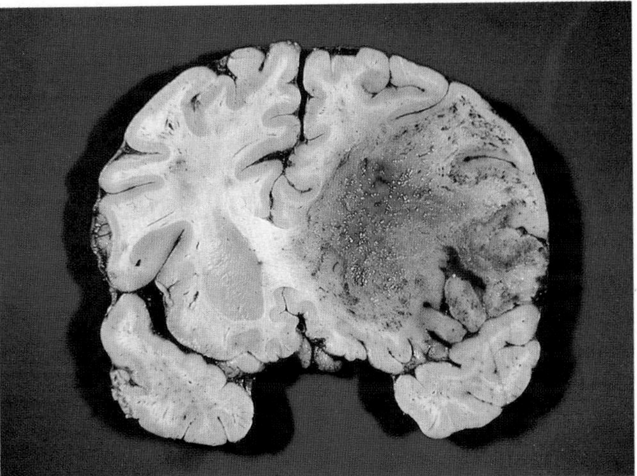

Fig. 35.29 Pathological specimen of a glioblastoma multiform.

Grading is on the basis of histological features, namely the presence of mitoses, necrosis, endothelial proliferation and nuclear atypia. Low-grade tumours have long median survival whereas high-grade tumours (glioblastoma multiforme) have a 20 per cent 2-year survival (Fig. 35.29).

CT scanning before and after contrast is able to localise and confirm the diagnosis in the majority of cases. The enhancement is often irregular around a centre of low density which may represent necrosis. Calcification may be present. MRI is more accurate in defining low-grade lesions. Tissue definition and anatomical localisation of lesions in and adjacent to eloquent areas are also superior, facilitating surgical planning and resection (Fig. 35.30).

The aim of treatment is to obtain a pathological diagnosis and grading and to debulk the tumour, both to alleviate symptoms of raised pressure and as a precursor to adjuvant

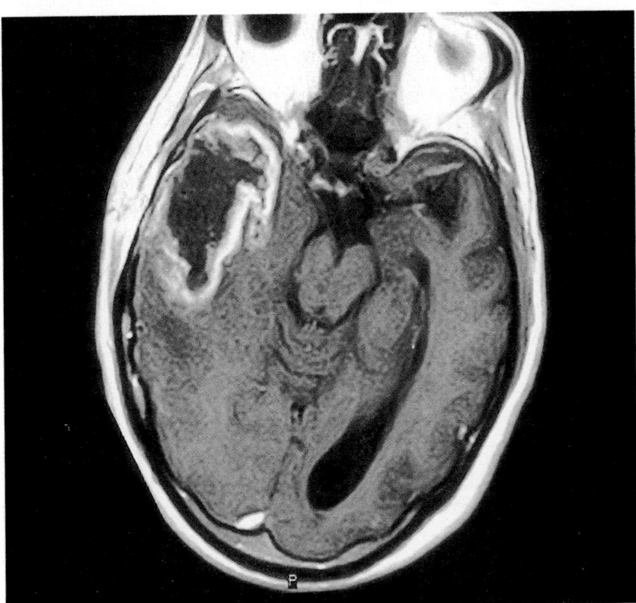

Fig. 35.30 Axial T1-weighted MRI with gadolinium enhancement showing a glioblastoma multiform.

treatments. This usually involves a combination of surgery and radiotherapy and will depend on the size and location of the tumour, as well as the patient's clinical state and age. Patients are started on dexamethasone in order to diminish cerebral oedema prior to surgery. Spread along axons makes total resection impossible unless the lesion is low grade, small and polar. Radiotherapy is usually as an external beam (50–60 Gy fractionated over 30 days), stereotactic focal irradiation using a gamma knife or linear accelerator or brachytherapy (implantation of a radioactive source). Chemotherapy has little role for lesions other than oligodendrogliomas. Photodynamic therapy, immunotherapy and gene therapy are all currently undergoing clinical trials to determine advantages over conventional treatment. In view of the poor prognosis with high-grade lesions, conservative treatment is often appropriate for selected patients.

Metastatic tumours

Metastatic tumours comprise 15 per cent of intracranial tumours. Approximately 30 per cent of deaths are due to cancer and up to 25 per cent of these have intracranial metastatic deposits at autopsy. The common sites of origin are illustrated in Table 35.4. In 15 per cent a primary source is never found. Up to 60 per cent are multiple, with 85 per cent situated above the tentorium. The interval between diagnosis of a primary and cerebral metastasis varies considerably. Melanoma and renal carcinoma may present with haemorrhage.

Metastatic tumours appear isodense on unenhanced CT but enhance vividly after intravenous contrast. Melanoma may appear hyperdense prior to contrast. MRI will frequently reveal lesions not visible on CT. A chest radiograph is essential to exclude a source or other metastic deposits. Steroids should be commenced to reduce peritumour oedema and if surgery is planned an anticonvulsant (phenytoin 300 mg nocte) started. Surgery is appropriate if there is a solitary surgically accessible lesion and no systemic spread, particularly if the primary site is unknown and the histological diagnosis in doubt. This may take the form of either resection or biopsy. Stereotactic or image-guided techniques are often employed. Radiotherapy is used to treat multiple metastases and following resection. More recently focused stereotactic radiosurgery is being used in the treatment of metastases smaller than 2 cm with results comparable to surgery. About 30–50 per cent of patients will survive a year following resection.

Table 35.4 Origin of cerebral metastases

Lung	40 per cent
Melanoma	11 per cent
Kidney	11 per cent
Colon	8 per cent
Unknown	15 per cent

Meningiomas

These account for 15 per cent of intracranial neoplasms and are the most common benign neoplasms. They are uncommon in children, occur more frequently in women than men and their incidence peaks in middle age. They originate from meningothelial cells that occur in the greatest abundance in the arachnoid villi, correlating with their site of occurrence. They are most commonly found along the superior sagittal sinus (parasagittal), over the free convexity and falx, along the sphenoid wing, beneath the frontal lobes (olfactory groove and tuberculum sellae), within the posterior fossa (cerebellopontine angle and foramen magnum), the optic nerve and in the ventricles. They classically arise from a broad base along the dura, may invade bone, and derive their blood supply from the external carotid circulation (Fig. 35.31).

There is a spectrum of histological appearances but malignant meningiomas are relatively rare. Surgical treatment should be, wherever possible, total excision. If this includes the site of dural attachment, the recurrence rate is less than 10 per cent. Incomplete excision of the dural attachment will result in a recurrence rate of between 20 and 30 per cent. Subtotal excision will result in 40 per cent showing progressive growth. The role of radiotherapy is controversial and is usually reserved for tumours with aggressive histological features or recurrent tumours, or where a subtotal resection has been performed.

Nerve sheath tumours

These benign tumours originate from Schwann cells and have a predilection for sensory nerves, especially the eighth nerve

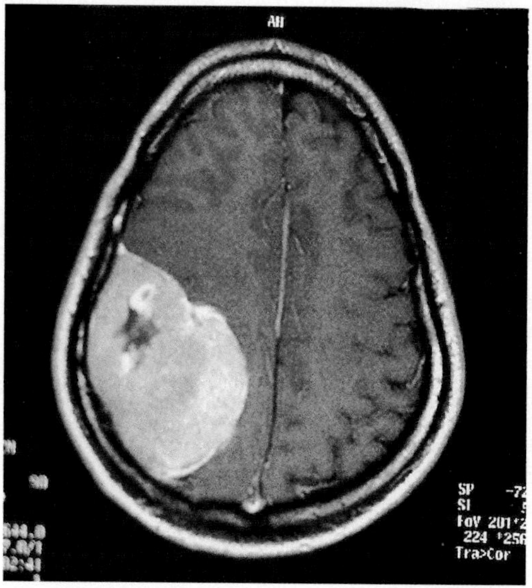

Fig. 35.31 Axial T1-weighted MRI with gadolinium enhancement showing a large dural-based parietal eminence convexity meningioma.

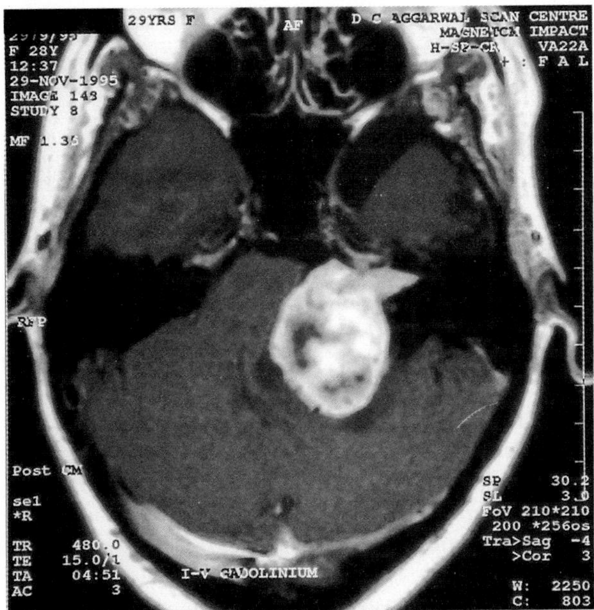

Fig. 35.32 Axial T1-weighted MRI with gadolinium showing a left acoustic neuroma.

(e.g. acoustic neuroma), followed much less frequently by the fifth nerve. Schwannomas of the eighth nerve arise from the superior or inferior vestibular portion in the internal auditory canal. As the tumour grows, it expands the internal auditory canal and extends into the cerebellopontine angle, compressing the pons, cerebellum and cranial nerves (Fig. 35.32). Bilateral Schwannomas of the eighth cranial nerves are diagnostic of type 2 neurofibromatosis. However, the majority of patients harbouring acoustic Schwannomas has no stigmas of this disease. Surgical intervention is aimed at total excision with preservation of neurological function. Patients frequently sustain seventh nerve palsies. More recently 'gamma knife' radiosurgery has been used effectively in the treatment of those tumours with a diameter of less than 30 mm.

Pituitary tumours

Introduction

Pituitary tumours account for 8 per cent of all intracranial tumours. Historically they were classified according to their staining characteristics seen on light microscopy. However, the three types (chromophobe, acidophilic and basophilic) did not correspond closely with the clinical syndromes of pituitary hypersecretion. The subsequent development of immunological staining techniques and electron microscopy provided a more refined classification of pituitary tumours. It is now correct to classify pituitary tumours according to their size (microadenomas, mesoadenomas and macroadenomas) and whether they are endocrine active or inactive (Table 35.5). These features will also determine their presentation.

Clinical features

Pituitary tumours arise in the sella turcica and can expand up into the suprasellar cisterns, compressing the optic chiasm above and resulting in visual failure – classically a bitemporal hemianopia. Careful assessment of the visual fields, visual acuity and optic fundi is therefore essential. They may also invade laterally into the cavernous sinuses on each side, compressing the third to fourth cranial nerves.

Endocrine disturbance is due to either hypopituitarism or excess secretion of a particular pituitary hormone. Prolactin secreting tumours are usually found in younger women and cause loss of libido, infertility, amamenorrhoea and galactorrhoea. Corticotrophin-producing tumours cause Cushing's disease due to cortisol excess. The principal features are moon face, abdominal striae, buffalo hump, hypertension and diabetes mellitus.

Acromegaly is due to an overproduction of growth hormone. The disease is disfiguring, causing prognathism and overgrowth of joints, especially in the hands and feet. Systemic side effects include hypertension, cardiomyopathy, diabetes mellitus, excessive sweating, arthralgias and lassitude. Haemorrhage into a macroadenoma, known as pituitary apoplexy, can precipitate an acute presentation with headache, hypopituitarism and visual failure. Diabetes insipidus, a product of direct hypothalamic involvement, is usually indicative of a craniopharyngioma and rarely caused by pituitary tumours.

Investigation

Diagnosis is confirmed by laboratory assessment of pituitary endocrine function, neuroradiological imaging (Fig. 35.33) and formal visual assessment.

Radioimmunoassay will identify the hormone being secreted. It is important, particularly with acute presentations, to exclude a prolactinoma as the majority of these will respond rapidly to treatment with the dopamine antagonist bromocriptine. Prolactin levels above 200 ng/ml are usually diagnostic. Nonfunctioning macroadenomas may cause hyperprolactinaemia due to distortion of the pituitary stalk or impingement on the hypothalamus. This is because the latter produces prolactin-inhibiting factor, which under normal circumstances suppresses prolactin levels to below 15 ng/ml. Diagnosis of Cushing's disease is made by radioimmunoassay of adrenocorticotrophic hormone (ACTH) in the peripheral blood and petrosal venous sinus sampling.

With the exception of some patients with Cushing's disease, MRI of the sella will confirm diagnosis of an intrasellar mass. The resolution of MRI will also detect all but the smallest (<2 mm) tumours and any extrasellar extension.

Theodor Schwann, 1810–82. Professor of Anatomy, Louvain and Liège, Belgium.

Table 35.5 Classification of pituitary tumours

Secretory product	*Clinical syndrome*	*Endocrine active*
Somatotrophic	Growth hormone (GH) 20 per cent	Acromegaly, giantism
Corticotrophic	Adrenocorticotrophic hormone (ACTH) 15 per cent	Cushing's disease, Nelson's syndrome
Prolactinoma	Prolactin (PRL) 40 per cent	Amenorrhoea, galactorrhoea, impotence
Thyrotrophic	Thyroid-stimulating hormone (TSH) 1 per cent	Hyperthyroidism
Gonadotrophic	Follicle-stimulating hormone (FSH), luteinising hormone (LH) 1–2 per cent	Behaves as endocrine inactive
Endocrine inactive	Alpha subunit 20 per cent	Hypopituitarism

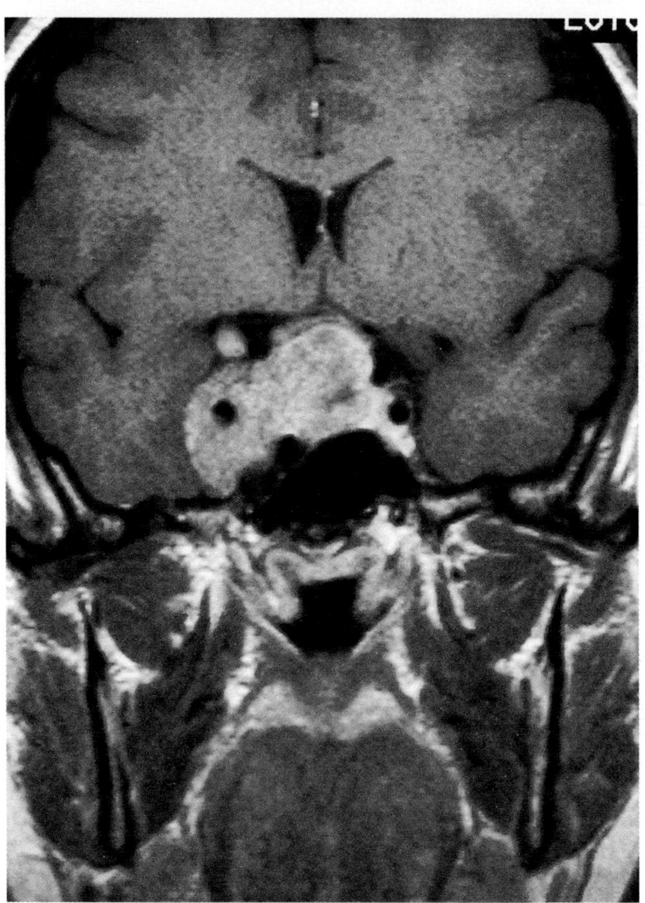

Fig. 35.33 Pituitary nonfunctioning macroadenoma with suprasellar extension and right cavernous sinus invasion.

Treatment

Treatment depends on the endocrine disturbance present and the effect of compression of adjacent neural structures. For prolactinomas, bromocriptine (a dopamine agonist) is commenced. Surgical excision is reserved for macroadenomas compressing the optic chiasm, growth hormone secreting tumours causing acromegaly and ACTH secreting tumours causing Cushing's disease. Occasionally surgery is undertaken in patients with prolactinomas not responding to medical treatment or when unwanted side effects occur. This is usually performed via a transphenoidal route although the transcranial route can be employed. The aim is to preserve normal pituitary function if possible. Surgery should be covered with parenteral hydrocortisone and frequently vasopressin is required.

Radiotherapy is used for subtotal resections and for persistent hypersecretion of pituitary hormones. The long-term follow-up of nonfunctioning pituitary adenomas has shown a recurrence rate approaching 40 per cent at 10 years indicating that there is perhaps a more extensive role for this modality and that postoperative patients should be more closely followed up.

Subarachnoid haemorrhage and aneurysms

Introduction

The blood supply to the brain enters the cranium through the skull base via the paired internal carotid and vertebral arteries. Within the subarachnoid space these vessels communicate to form the circle of Willis and then branch out over the surface of the brain before entering into and supplying the brain parenchyma. Subarachnoid haemorrhage (SAH) occurs when a vessel ruptures into this subarachnoid layer. Patients present with a typical sudden, unusual and severe headache. They may die apoplectically or present with a range of clinical conditions varying from being moribund, to a mild residual headache. The clinical status of these patients is graded according to the World Federation of Neurological Surgeons (WFNS) scale where the Glasgow Coma Scale (GCS) is used to measure consciousness (Table 35.6). This gives a measure of severity and prognosis of the haemorrhage.

Table 35.6 WFNS grading of subarachnoid haemorrhage

	GCS	*Deficit*
0	Unbled	
1	15	
2	13–14	–
3	13–14	+
4	8–12	±
5	3–7	±

Rupert Allan Willis, 1898–1980. Professor of Pathology, Leeds, England.

Table 35.7 Causes of subarachnoid haemorrhage

Aneurysms	70 per cent
Arteriovenous malformations	10 per cent
Idiopathic	5 per cent
Other:	
Spinal AVM	
Tumour	
Coagulopathy	

Epidemiology

The incidence of SAH is 6–16 cases per 100 000 per year representing 2–10 per cent of all cerebrovascular events and can have various causes (Table 35.7). While in some countries SAH is predominantly traumatic in origin, in most, these bleeds arise from thin-walled saccular dilatations or aneurysms situated at the bifurcation of intracranial vessels, particularly upon the circle of Willis (Fig. 35.34a and b). These are usually saccular with a neck and fundus but may be fusiform. They are most likely to be caused by haemodynamic stresses, the result of turbulent blood flow, possibly acting on a weak point in a vessel wall. Such lesions are found in about 7.8 per cent of individuals at post mortem examination. The total prevalence in the general population appears to be in the region of 1.5 per cent and aneurysmal SAH accounts for 0.1 per cent of deaths within the general population. The prevalence increases with each decade reaching a peak at 40–60 years.

Arteriovenous malformations (AVM) are vascular hamartomas. Several groups are recognised. The most common is the true arteriovenous malformation while the other types include cavernous angiomas, venous malformations or capillary telangiectasis. These latter types seldom bleed and are usually incidental findings on MRI. AVMs present with either haemorrhage, epilepsy or a neurological deficit. They may also cause ischaemia by shunting blood away from cerebral tissue ('steal phenomenon') and are graded according to their size, situation and the direction of their venous drainage.

(a)

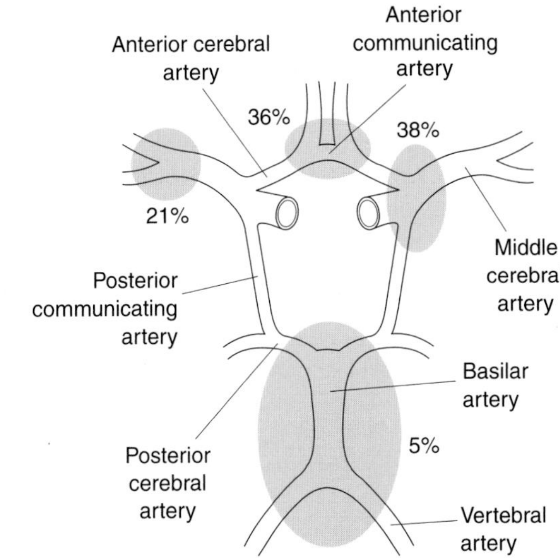

(b)

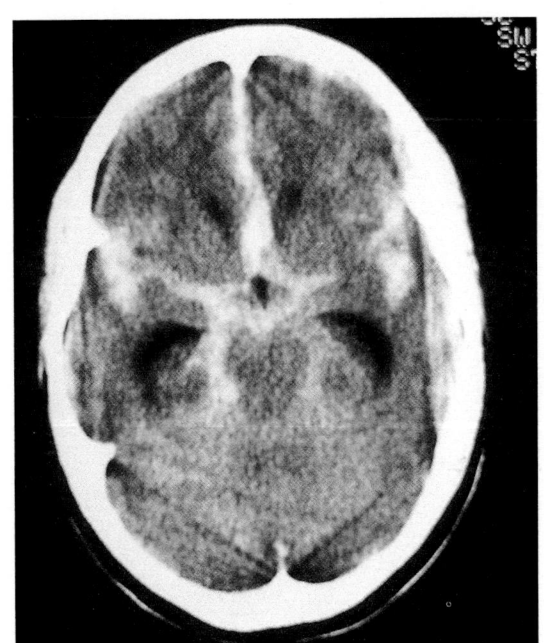

Fig. 35.34 (a) Main sites of intracranial supraclinoid aneurysms. (b) Axial CT demonstrating a diffuse SAH involving the basal cisterns with communicating hydrocephalus.

Clinical features

SAH is typically heralded by a severe, unusual headache of sudden onset, frequently associated with neurological symptoms and often accompanied by nausea and vomiting. This is a result of extravasation of blood under pressure into the CSF space, ventricles or into the brain itself. The accompanying acute rise in ICP causes compromise of the cerebral perfusion pressure and the cerebral blood flow, tamponading the bleed and allowing time for a clot to develop. The patient's level of consciousness may as a consequence be depressed to varying degrees for varied periods of time and there might be concomitant photophobia and neck stiffness from meningeal irritation. Rarely, the patient may develop back and radicular pain as blood accumulates in the spinal canal. Physical examination reveals meningism and a positive Kernig's sign. Fundoscopy can sometimes show globular subhyloid haemorrhages, scattered retinal haemorrhages and occasionally papilloedema. A focal neurological deficit or seizures reveals concomitant parenchymal damage. Fever, leucocytosis and hypertension are not unusual. Although the majority of aneurysms presents with rupture, they can present with symptoms of compression alone resulting in pain, dysfunction (classically a third nerve palsy) or epilepsy.

Investigations

Diagnosis is classically made by LP but all patients should be investigated with CT. This is the investigation of choice and within the first 24 hours of the bleed has a 90 per cent sensitivity, falling to 50 per cent at 3 days. This is able to confirm the diagnosis noninvasively, detect the presence of intracerebral haematomas, exclude hydrocephalus and indicate the likely source of a bleed – directing cerebral angiography. If the CT is normal or equivocal, if the bleed is more than 72 hours old and if no contraindications to LP are present, then the patient should undergo a lumbar puncture looking for uniformly bloodstained CSF, xanthochromia or bilirubin byproducts of haemoglobin breakdown on spectrophotometry (Fig. 35.35a and b). Acute bacterial meningitis can mimic SAH so microbiological analysis should

(a)

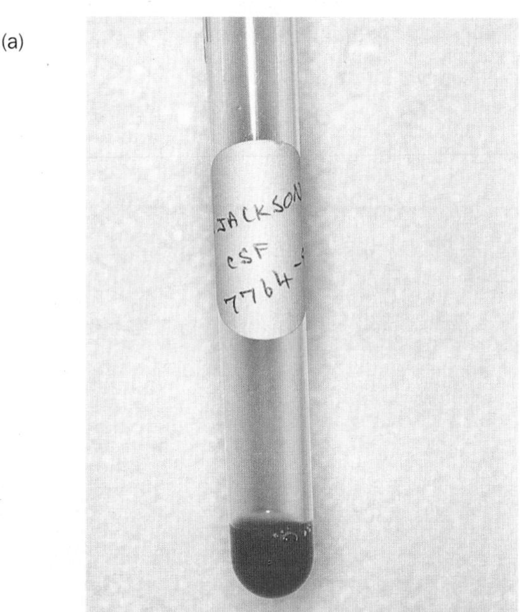

(b)

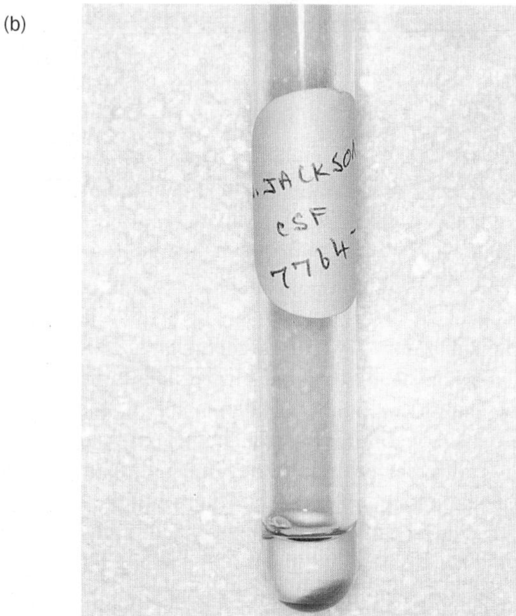

Fig. 35.35 CSF sample from patient presenting with SAH. (a) Test-tube showing uniformly bloodstained CSF. (b) Test-tube showing sample after having been spun down demonstrating xanthochromia in supernatant.

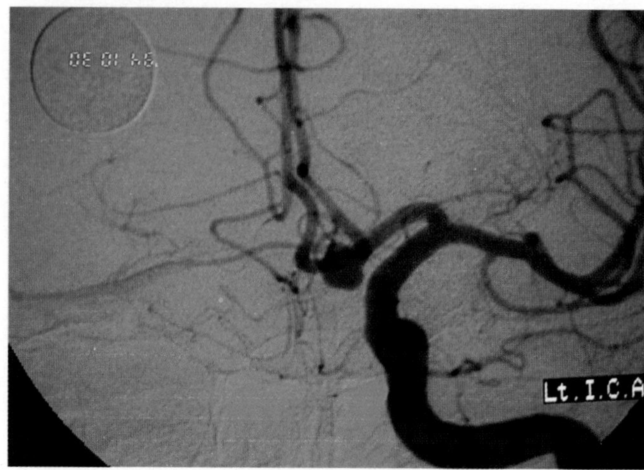

Fig. 35.36 Anteroposterior projection of the internal carotid injection of a cerebral angiogram showing an anterior communicating aneurysm.

also be requested. Confirmation of haemorrhage should be investigated with cerebral angiography to determine the cause (Figs 35.36 and 35.37). This should be considered with some urgency as the potential for a ruptured aneurysm to rebleed within the first 2 weeks is 25 per cent or 60 per cent within 6 months of the initial SAH with a mortality rate of greater than 60 per cent.

Fifteen per cent of aneurysms are multiple and 15 per cent of angiograms will be negative, indicative of an occult source such as a perimesencephalic bleed, a thrombosed aneurysm or a spinal arteriovenous malformation. The first angiogram describing intracranial aneurysms was performed by Moniz in 1933. Bilateral angiography including the internal carotids and vertebral arteries is the gold standard for delineating vascular lesions. With the advent of digitised angiography, it

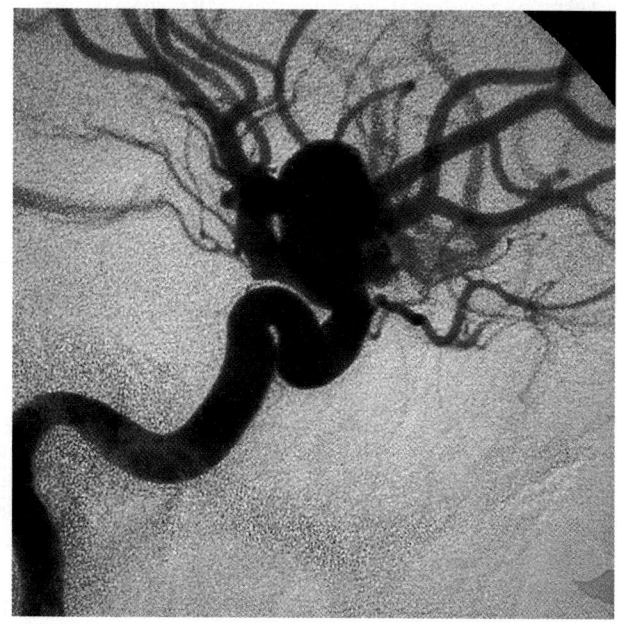

Fig. 35.37 Cerebral angiogram demonstrating a middle cerebral artery aneurysm.

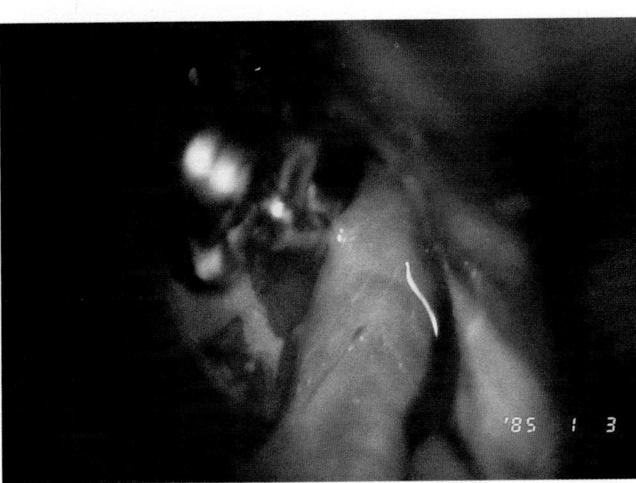

Fig. 35.38 Microscope picture of clipped aneurysm.

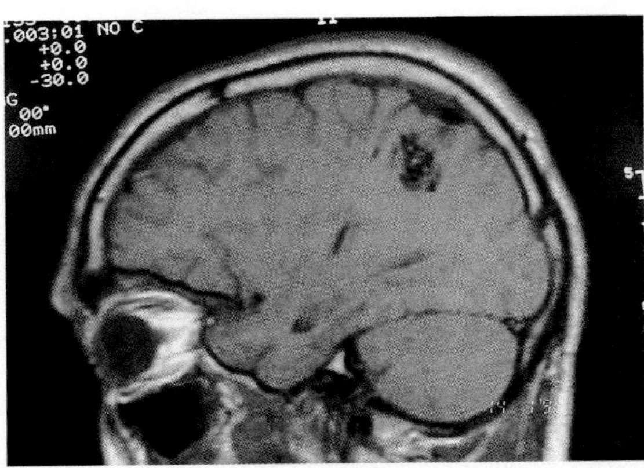

Fig. 35.40 Sagittal T1 MRI sequence of a young male presenting with a seizure. This demonstrates a serpiginous lesion with filling defects of low signal typical of an AVM.

has been possible to reduce significantly the dosage of contrast material given. The increasing sophistication of the noninvasive imaging techniques, magnetic resonance angiographic (MRA) and CT angiography, enables resolution of aneurysms 3 mm in size.

Management

The clinical course of patients with SAH is frequently unpredictable owing to the development of complications. The most severe are rebleeding and delayed ischaemic neurological deficit (DIND) – also known as vasospasm. The risk of rebleeding is 4 per cent in the first 24 hours and 19 per cent in the first 2 weeks, and carries a mortality and morbidity of 60 per cent. Aneurysms are secured by the surgical application of a clip across the neck at craniotomy (Fig. 35.38), isolating it from the circulation. Recently, endovascular techniques have been developed enabling aneurysms to be secured by packing them with platinum coils (Figs 35.38 and 35.39).

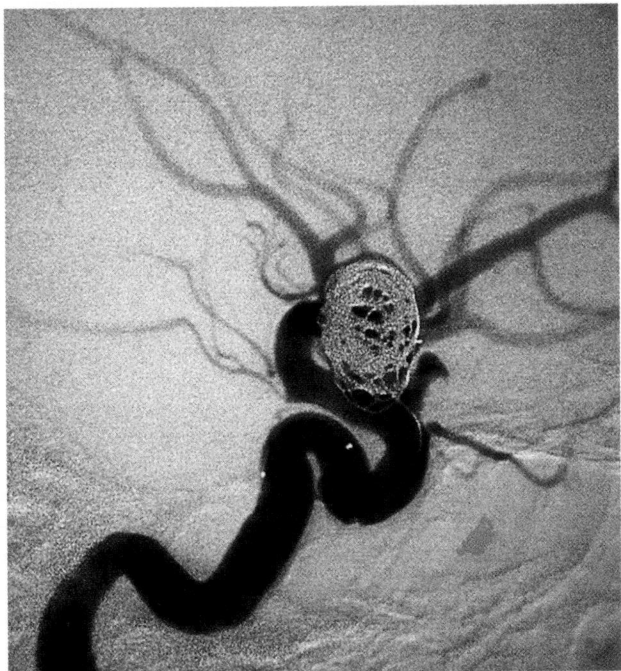

Fig. 35.39 The middle cerebral artery aneurysm undergoing Gugliemi detachable coil (GDC) embolisation.

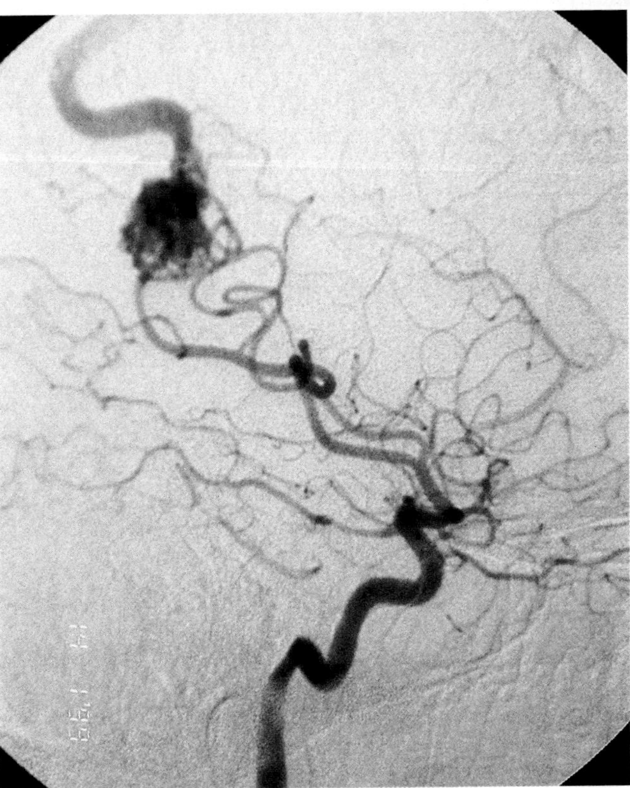

Fig. 35.41 Lateral projection of the internal carotid injection cerebral angiogram on the same patient as in Fig. 35.40. This demonstrates the AVM being fed by middle cerebral vessels and draining into the sagittal sinus.

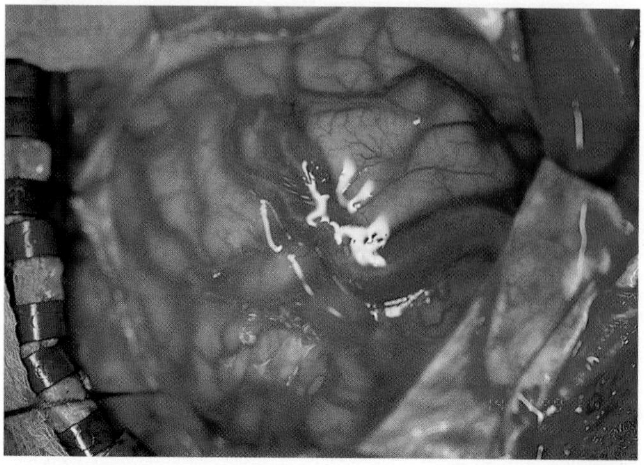

Fig. 35.42 Intraoperative picture of the same patient as in Fig. 35.40 showing the vein pictured in Fig. 35.6 draining into the sagittal sinus.

The cause of vasospasm remains unknown and is a significant cause of morbidity. Overall, 30 per cent of SAH patients will suffer DIND due to vasospasm, with the majority suffering permanent neurological deficits. Treatment of vasospasm relies on maintaining an adequate blood pressure and intravascular volume with intravenous fluids (mixture of 3.5 litres per 24 hours of crystalloid and colloid) since cerebral perfusion is related to arterial pressure and intracranial pressure. Cerebral blood flow is further optimised by decreasing the haematocrit and if necessary using inotropic agents to elevate the blood pressure above physiological levels. All SAH patients develop some degree of hydrocephalus. This usually resolves spontaneously but may require temporary or permanent CSF diversion. Cardiac arrhythmias and hyponatraemia are also frequent complications of this condition.

The potential for rebleeding from an AVM (2–4 per cent per annum) is lower than for an aneurysm and there is therefore less urgency with treatment (Figs 35.40–35.42).

AVMs are treated by either removing the lesion surgically, endovascular embolisation of the nidus, stereotactic radiosurgery or a combination of treatments.

Epilepsy

Introduction

Epilepsy is the commonest neurological condition affecting the general population. In the UK, 300 000 people have active epilepsy, 100 000 of whom are below 15 years of age. Despite the fact that epilepsy is such a common neurological condition, the attention given to the surgical management has been relatively small. Following Horsley's initiative however, great interest was shown in the surgical management of epilepsy but it was for the most part confined to post-traumatic cases and cases with obvious neoplasms (Fig. 35.43). With the invention and development of the EEG in the 1930s, this was integrated into the preoperative evaluation and supplemented by the pioneering work of Jasper and Penfield in Montreal. Their series of patients undergoing surgery for complex partial seizures identified that, where abnormal tissue was found in the resected specimen, the outcome in terms of seizure control was generally good. With the development of effective anticonvulsant medication, epilepsy was generally confined to specialist centres or to those in whom neoplasms could be identified. Indeed, oral anticonvulsant medication is still the first-line management of seizures. However, approximately 20 per cent of patients do not have their seizures adequately controlled on oral anticonvulsants and it is these patients who may benefit from surgery. Surgery is directed towards a focal lesion, the resection of which will abolish seizures. Functional operations may also be carried out to modify seizure spread and therefore ameliorate the patient's condition.

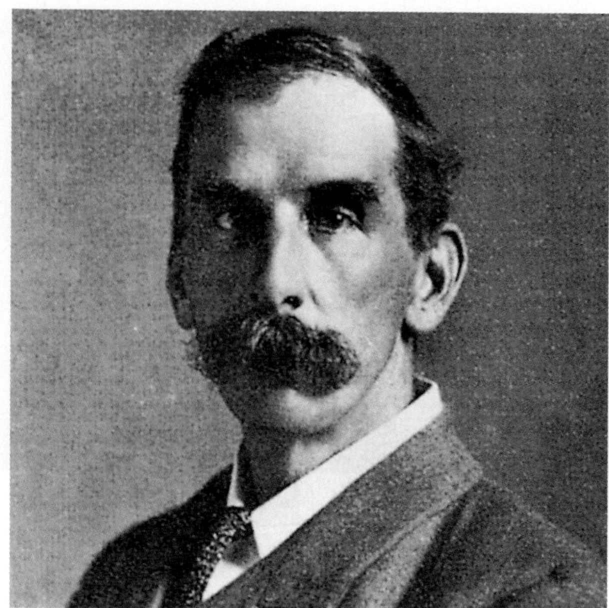

Fig. 35.43 Sir Victor Horsley, Honorary Surgeon, National Hospital, Queen's Square, London, from 1886 to 1916.

Preoperative evaluation

History and examination

A careful history of the onset and nature of the seizures should be made as well as the way that the seizures have changed with time, by either their nature or their frequency. Note should be made of previous medications in addition to current anticonvulsant medication. It is important that the patient should have received an adequate therapeutic trial of the first-choice anticonvulsant drugs before consideration for

Sir Victor Horsley, 1857–1916. Neurosurgeon, National Hospital, London, England. Performed first operation for surgical management of epilepsy in 1886.

Wilder Grove Penfield, 1891–1976. Canadian neurologist. Devised a surgical method for treating epilepsy.

Robert Bentley Todd, 1809–60. Physician, London, England.

surgery. The examination in patients with epilepsy is frequently entirely normal. However, when focal signs do occur, they can be useful in lateralising the seizure focus. Pathology under these circumstances is commonly neoplastic or the result of previous vascular episodes. The history of the circumstances of the patient's birth, particularly whether there were any complications in the antenatal or perinatal period, is important, while the history of a prolonged febrile convulsion in childhood is frequently found in patients who have hippocampal sclerosis and associated complex partial seizures.. Any associated Todd's paralysis with the febrile convulsion may be a very useful lateralising sign. The history should include the impact that the seizures have on the patient's activities of daily living; notably, its effect on education, employment and personal relationships.

Electroencephalography

Interictal scalp recordings may be useful in excluding a patient for surgery on the grounds of widespread abnormal activity or if a recognisable electrographic syndrome can be identified. More commonly the interictal recordings can give broad guidance in terms of lateralisation and localisation of the seizure focus as identified by slow-wave activity or interictal spikes. The information obtained from the scalp recording may be supplemented by more invasive electrodes such as sphenoidal electrodes or alternatively it may be necessary to perform video telemetry and record a seizure on video with a time-locked EEG recording. This allows analysis of the semiology of the seizure as well as the EEG changes associated with the clinical manifestations.

Neuropsychology and neuropsychiatry

Careful neuropsychological testing may reveal fixed functional deficits that lateralise and localise the site of cerebral dysfunction. An evaluation of verbal and performance IQ as well as memory function are also vital parts in preoperative evaluation of seizures arising from the mesial temporal structures. To confirm laterality of language and integrity of memory function on each side, it may be necessary to carry out a Wada test during which sodium amytal is injected under angiographic control into the internal carotid artery, effectively putting the ipsilateral cerebral hemisphere to sleep. Patients are carefully tested before injection, immediately following injection and during the recovery phase to evaluate motor, speech and memory function.

Psychiatric evaluation is an essential part of the preoperative strategy, in that psychiatric morbidity is common both in relation to seizures and in the postoperative period of seizure surgery. Established psychosis is usually deemed a contraindication for surgery for epilepsy, whereas a postictal psychosis is not. Integral to the role of the psychiatrist is the counselling that is necessary before seizure surgery, as often the seizures themselves are only a portion of the patient's morbidity and it is essential that patients and their partners and relatives understand this.

Imaging

Preoperative imaging in patients considered for epilepsy surgery has been revolutionised by the advent of MRI and by an increasing understanding of the necessary sequences and planes of acquisition required to demonstrate the pathological entities responsible for epilepsy. It is becoming increasingly apparent that with more sophisticated imaging techniques, pathology can be demonstrated preoperatively in an ever-increasing proportion of surgical candidates. In patients with seizures emanating from the temporal lobe, the commonest pathological substrate is hippocampal sclerosis. This can be identified on preoperative scans by careful examination of the mesial temporal structures. The volume of the affected hippocampus is reduced while the anatomy may be clearly abnormal, and both the T1 and T2 signals altered. Neoplasms lying within the mesial temporal lobe may also be readily identified and their anatomical boundaries defined, allowing some idea of the feasibility of the extent of tumour resection possible at surgery. In cases of extratemporal epilepsy, tumours may likewise be clearly identified as well as areas of cortical damage or congenital malformations of cortical architecture.

Surgical procedures

Penfield and Falconer clearly identified that, where pathological tissue was found in the resected specimens of patients suffering with epilepsy, then the likelihood of surgical success was high. Further studies have more recently demonstrated that the more complete the resection of pathological tissue, the higher the likelihood of a good surgical outcome. As MRI is now such a powerful investigatory tool, pathology is frequently visualised preoperatively and thus surgery for focal epilepsy is becoming more and more lesional. Thus, when neoplasms are identified, the surgical objective is to excise the lesion in its entirety, with any surrounding abnormal tissue. Where the lesion is small and circumscribed, this may be best achieved using stereotactic or minimally invasive techniques with or without intraoperative EEG.

Approximately 60 per cent of patients being treated for epilepsy suffer from complex partial seizures and their seizure focus is localised to the mesial temporal structures. Therefore resections of the temporal lobe, particularly the amygdala and the hippocampus, are the most frequently performed operations for the surgical management of epilepsy. The extent of the neocortical resection is dependent on whether the lesion is on the dominant or nondominant side and may be further guided by intraoperative EEG. In order that careful dissection of the mesial temporal structures may be safely performed, this part of the procedure requires an operating microscope. Extratemporal resections are dependent on the pathological entity responsible and also upon the eloquence of the brain in which the lesion is situated. Where the lesion is close to or within eloquent areas it may be necessary to carry out the surgery under local anaesthesia with cortical stimulation, so as to minimise the risk of a postoperative neurological deficit.

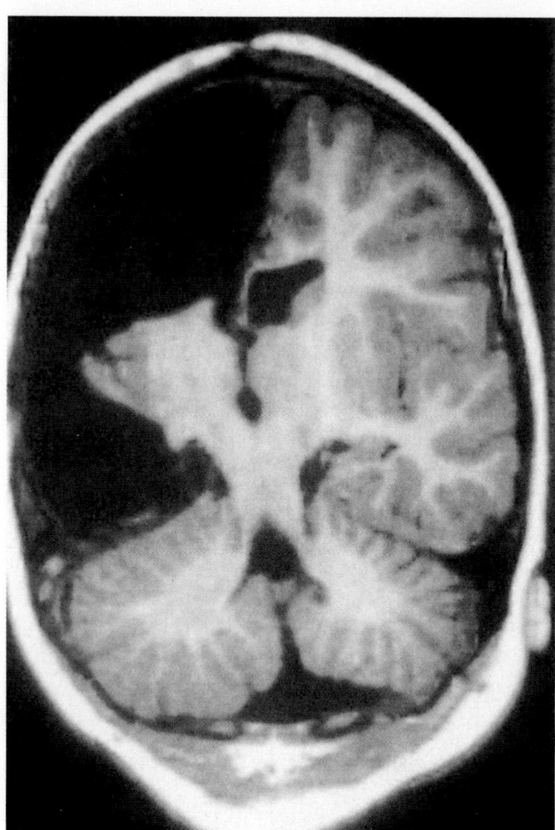

Fig. 35.44 Coronal T2-weighted MRI image following an anatomical right-sided hemispherectomy.

When an extensive area of unilateral hemisphere abnormality exists, as a result of either a congenital or an acquired lesion, consideration may be given to a multilobar or hemisphere resection. Hemispherectomy, or more correctly hemidecortication, is perhaps the most effective operation for treating epilepsy, with a near 80 per cent seizure-free rate postoperatively (Fig. 35.44). However, the inevitable neurological deficits mean that its use is limited and should be considered carefully.

The most commonly performed functional operation is section of the corpus callosum. The aim of surgery is to improve rather than eradicate the seizures. This surgical approach was initially described by Dandy in the management of tumours of the third ventricle but was applied to the management of epilepsy in the 1940s. The indications for callosal resection are far from clear but patients suffering with atonic drop attacks appear to have the best outcome. In the first instance the anterior two-thirds of the corpus callosum are usually divided to minimise the chances of a longstanding disconnection syndrome. If anterior section does not result in improvement in seizures, then the resection may be completed. The rate for extending resection is limited to approximately 10 per cent. More recently, vagal nerve stimulation is being used as an alternative to corpus callosum resection with similar success rates.

Outcome

Surgery for well-circumscribed lesions such as benign tumours and cavernomas produces seizure-free rates as high as 70–80 per cent. In the presence of hippocampal sclerosis, resection of the mesial temporal structures and temporal neocortex will result in an approximately 70 per cent seizure-free rate. Extratemporal resections have a less favourable outcome with a seizure-free rate of between 40 and 50 per cent. This is often the result of a more diffuse pathological process, such as post-traumatic gliosis or neuronal migration defects that underlie the extratemporal epilepsy. Equally important in the postoperative evaluation is an appraisal of neurological, psychological and psychiatric status, which may then be compared with preoperative status to assess the dynamic impact of the seizure surgery.

Movement disorders

Parkinson's syndrome was first described by James Parkinson in 1817. The principal pathological disorder is a depletion of dopamine stores in the cells of the substantia nigra and neostriatum. This produces the classical triad of tremor, rigidity and akinesia. As early as 1820, Parkinson appreciated that stroke ablated contralateral tremor. Over the next century, neurosurgeons lesioned various parts of the central nervous system in an attempt to alleviate this tremor until it was thought that the surgical relief of tremor boiled down to the artificial production of paralysis. The development of stereotactic techniques and a better understanding of the circuitry of the basal ganglia led to the development of the thalamotomy procedure. By 1975, 75 000 thalamotomies had been performed world-wide. However, in 1969, the discovery of levodopa led to the cessation of surgery for Parkinson's disease. The subsequent development of on–off phenomena, dyskinesias and dystonias in patients treated with dopamine led to a revival of interest in movement disorder surgery. New imaging techniques and work on animal models of Parkinson's disease led to the discovery of new targets in the basal ganglia and the procedure as we know it today.

Thalamotomy is used to treat patients with drug-resistant tremor but does little to improve akinesia and rigidity, and has an inconsistent effect on levodopa-induced dyskinesias. Case series have demonstrated that pallidotomy is helpful in reducing levodopa-induced dyskinesias. Underlying parkinsonism also improves but to a lesser degree. Unilateral procedures are usually preferred to bilateral ones as some centres have reported an increase in the risk of complications with the latter such as speech impairment and neuropsychological impairment (Fig. 35.45). More recently, the subthalamic nucleus has been lesioned,

James Parkinson, 1755–1824. Surgeon and palaeontologist.

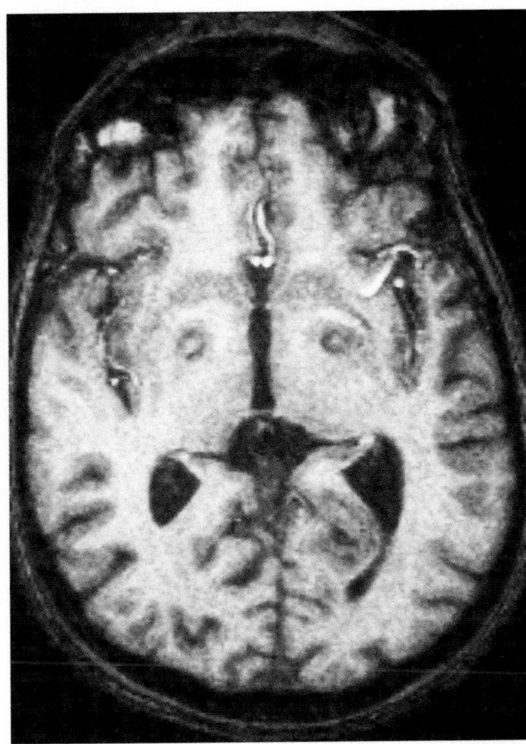

Fig. 35.45 T1-weighted axial MRI showing bilateral stereotactic radiofrequency pallidotomy lesions.

alleviating akinesia in addition to tremor and rigidity. This target does however expose patients to a higher risk of haemorrhage.

Lesions are made either by radiofrequency coagulation after trial stimulation or by deep brain stimulation of any of the sites targeted for lesioning. Although stimulators do not require tissue destruction, they are expensive and prone to technical failures. They can however be turned on and off, programmed as necessary and are reversible.

Neural transplantation of foetal mesencephalon to the neostriatum of humans is a controversial experimental technique which has had variable and questionable success. In addition, the ethics of obtaining foetal tissue and the problems of immunological reactions have led to the call for a moritorium on this procedure until long-term results are available.

Pain

Pain has been described as 'an unpleasant sensory and emotional experience associated with actual or potential tissue damage or described in terms of such damage'. The physician initially confronts pain as the signal of some underlying damage and, as such, an important symptom of numerous diseases. Treatment is aimed at eradicating the disorder responsible for the pain. Occasionally the underlying problem cannot be identified or eradicated. It may even represent damage to the nervous system itself. The above definition also takes account of the emotional aspects of pain which may be all consuming for the patient and suggests the importance of psychological factors in evaluation and treatment.

Table 35.8 Pain treatment continuum

Over-the-counter drugs
Nonsteroidal anti-inflammatory drugs (NSAIDs)
Physiotherapy/manipulation/transcutaneous electrical nerve stimulation (TENS)/acupuncture/muscle relaxation
Oral analgesics/narcotics
Nerve blocks (therapeutic/diagnostic)
Behavioural programmes
Corrective surgery
Long-term oral narcotics
Implantable spinal cord stimulator
Implantable drug delivery
Neuroablation (chemical/surgical)

Patients with pain are usually divided into two groups: those with diseases that limit life expectancy (e.g. malignancies) and those with chronic benign pain. The management of each group is very different. The treatment of pain follows a continuum (Table 35.8) which is determined by the severity of the pain and its response to treatment. It is also essential that chronic pain patients are managed holistically by a pain team including pain-relief specialists and nurses, psychologists, physiotherapists and occupational therapists in conjunction with a neurosurgeon.

Drug therapy is aimed at suppressing pain at points along the pain pathways. Steroids and nonsteroidal anti-inflammatories act directly on chemoreceptors. Afferent pain fibres can be anaesthetised by infiltration with local anaesthetic. Descending pain modulation circuits are influenced by narcotics and antidepressants. Psychotropic and antidepressant drugs (chlorpromazine and haloperidol) are used to treat the affective component of pain.

The optimal surgical treatment for any intractable pain would be to have its effect confined to the painful area, be simple and inexpensive to perform, and be associated with a low mortality and morbidity. In particular it should be associated with a low incidence of neurological deficit.

There are three principal methods of neurosurgical management for pain:

1. operations that interrupt nociceptive pathways by creating lesions in peripheral nerves, roots or ganglia, the spinal cord, various parts of the brain and brainstem, and the sympathetic nervous system;
2. electrical stimulation of pain suppressive systems or blocking pain pathways (peripheral nerve, spinal cord or brain);
3. administration of various drugs to the intraspinal or intraventricular compartments of the CSF pathways.

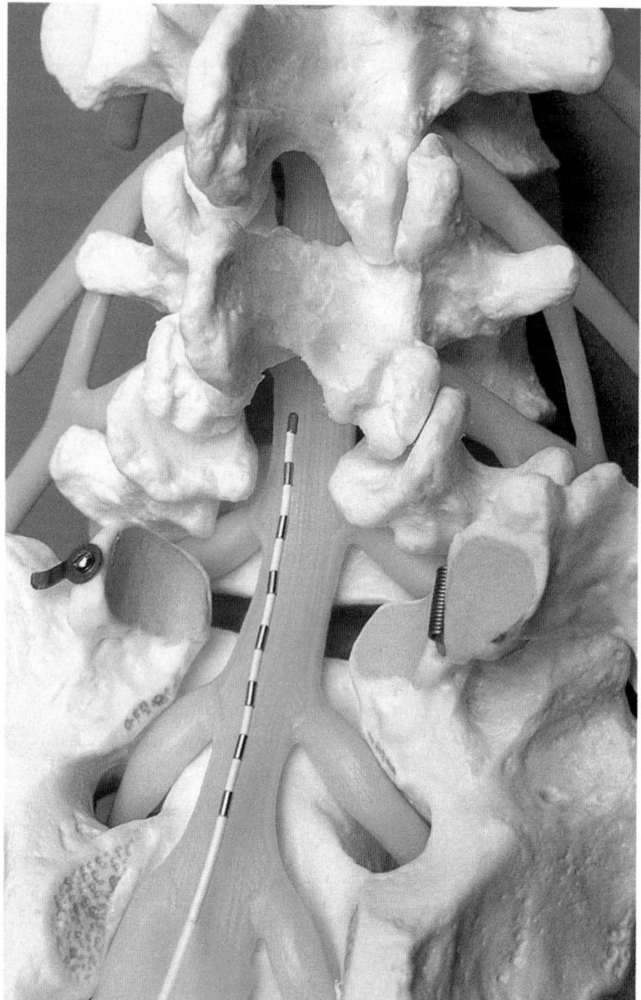

Fig. 35.46 The position of an epidural electrode.

Electrical stimulation of the central nervous system

Epidural stimulation

This is achieved by either totally implanted devices which are powered by a battery with a finite lifespan, or radiofrequency powered devices which have an implanted receiver which is activated by an external stimulator. These are connected to multichannel electrodes. By activating various electrodes and adjusting the pulse width, amplitude and frequency, beneficial stimulation is sought. The electrodes are positioned epidurally over the dorsal columns or more caudally over the cauda equina roots (Fig. 35.46). If paraesthasiae can be induced in the area of pain – significant benefit is virtually assured. This location is most effective for failed back surgery syndrome, arachnoiditis, peripheral vascular disease and angina. Spinal cord stimulation is based on the gate control theory of pain with inhibition of C-fibre conduction. The exact neurochemical and neurophysiolgical mechanisms are poorly understood.

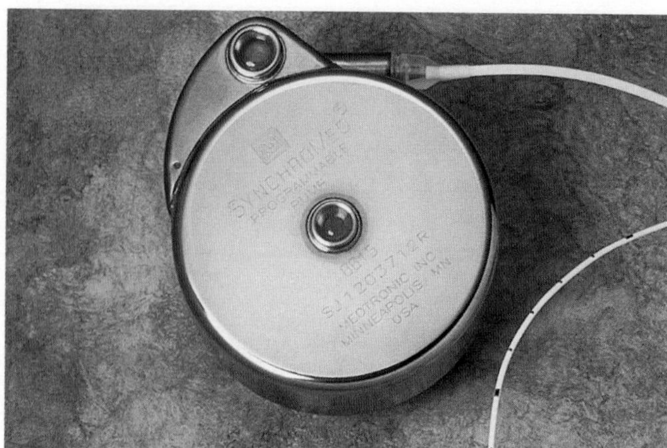

Fig. 35.47 A Medtronic synchronised programmable intrathecal drug-delivery system.

Electrodes can also be positioned epidurally over the motor cortex for more refractory pain syndromes such as thalamic and phantom limb pain. This can be of benefit in 50 per cent of patients.

Deep brain stimulation

Stimulation of the lateral margin of the periaqueductal and periventricular grey matter is thought to affect a pathway running from the midbrain to the dorsal horn, inhibiting nociceptive neurons. The other target area is the ventroposteromedial/ventroposterolateral nuclei of the thalamus which ultimately inhibit spinothalamic tract neurons. These electrodes are implanted stereotactically at specialist centres.

Intrathecal drug delivery

The opiate doses required to maintain patients with chronic pain frequently result in unacceptable side effects such as respiratory depression, drowsiness, urinary retention, nausea and vomiting, and eventually progress towards tolerance. Delivery of opiates into the CSF space via the lumbar or transventricular routes has a potentiated effect directly upon the opiate receptors in the brain and spinal cord at a fraction of the previous dose. This is achieved by implanted drug delivery systems (Fig. 35.47). These can be either manually activated – pressurised systems controlled by capillary resistance utilising different concentrations – or self-activated programmable pumps delivering small aliquots.

Pain associated with spasticity following spinal cord injury can be treated with intrathecal baclofen.

Neuroablative procedures

Ablative procedures have proved effective in relieving certain types of pain but run the risk of producing a neurological deficit without relieving and potentially even exacerbating pain and are hence more suited for patients suffering from pain associated with malignant disease. Sympathectomy is used to treat causalgic and visceral pain. Coeliac ganglion blocks have been especially helpful in treating pain associated with pancreatic disease.

Surgically produced dorsal root entry zone lesions in the spinal cord are especially helpful in treating phantom limb pain, brachial plexus avulsion and discrete spinal cord lesions.

Cordotomy, the surgical interruption of the spinothalamic tract, results in hemianalgesia below the level of the lesion. It is invariably effective in managing unilateral pain associated with metastatic disease but its efficacy diminishes with time. Within 1 year 20 per cent of patients will develop painful dysaesthesias in the anaesthetic area. It is usually performed at C1–2 with the patient awake. Risks include sleep apnoea (Ondine's curse), bladder, bowel and sexual dysfunction. Commissural myelotomy is a longitudinal sectioning of the spinal cord in the sagittal plane to disrupt the crossing fibres of the spinothalamic tract.

Mesencephalotomy reduces the number of functioning ascending fibres in the newer specific and older nonspecific pain pathways. It is effective for pains of the neck, head and upper chest caused by cancer.

Stereotactive cingulotomy is the creation of bilateral medial frontal lesions modifying the patient's response to pain. These central lesions do not remove the painful sensation but alleviate the concomitant suffering.

Alcohol injection, radiofrequency lesioning, balloon compression and avulsion of various components of the trigeminal nerve are all usually effective in the treatment of trigeminal neuralgia but invariably only temporising measures. Intracranial microvascular decompression and partial trigeminal rhizotomy offer long-term relief with lower recurrence rates.

Brain death

Introduction

For as long as medical practice has existed, the layperson has required of medical practitioners that they be knowledgeable about death. For centuries, laypeople and doctors alike have accepted cessation of respiration and heartbeat as the classical signs of death. Advances in cardiopulmonary resuscitation and modern mechanical ventilation have made obsolete the traditional clinical definition of death with a small but significant harvest of irreversibly brain-damaged patients. The worst form of such damage led to the concept of 'coma depasse', first defined by Mollaret and Goulon in 1959. As the number of patients with artificially maintained ventilation and circulation increased, they became to be regarded as a potential source of donor organs. These two developments occurred parallel to but independently of each other, and the diagnosis of brain death did not arise because of the need for donor organs.

The presence of an irreversibly damaged brain in a body in which ventilation and circulation were being maintained by artificial means presented a state in need of a definition. Mollaret and Goulon were the first to investigate this state in their paper 'Le coma depasse'. Many terms for this and other states for which it has been mistaken have been suggested or used, of which the following are the most commonly encountered: cerebral death, brainstem death, brain death, coma depasse, irreversible coma, cortical death, persistent vegetative state and locked-in syndrome.

The high cost of maintaining patients in intensive therapy units (ITUs) and the premium on such limited resources has led significantly to the re-evaluation and management of such states. Nursing and medical staff morale, as well as the emotional toll on relatives, are very real considerations. As these patients may now be potential essential organ donors their care has acquired medicolegal and ethical significance. It is not the primary task of a doctor to provide organs for transplantation but neither is it to deny patients in need of transplant surgery. Before a patient can be considered as having suffered irreversible brain damage, it is mandatory that a positive diagnosis be made of the pathogenesis of this damage. To produce coma, pathological processes must affect the brain diffusely or encroach upon its deep central structures.

Three major groups of lesions can be differentiated:

- supratentorial lesions;
- infratentorial lesions;
- metabolic disorders – which widely depress or interrupt brain function, including anoxia, ischaemia, infections, toxins and essential deficiencies.

The disintegration of function following progressive herniation will end in cessation of spontaneous respiration leading to hypoxic cardiac arrest. If ventilation and circulation are maintained artificially, the heart, kidneys and liver may continue to function for some hours or days but after brainstem death has occurred, cardiac arrest will follow within 2 weeks.

Since Mollaret and Goulon, several committees and reviewers have sought to establish unequivocal and appropriate clinical and EEG criteria for brainstem death based on retrospective analysis of patients who died. The first was the Harvard group who included EEG as part of their criteria. This was later deemed unnecessary by both the Minnesota and British Groups. The latter are as follows.

Before diagnosing brain death several preconditions should be satisfied:

- there should be no doubt that the patient's condition is due to irremediable brain damage of known aetiology (Fig. 35.48);
- the patient should be in a coma on a ventilator because spontaneous respiration has been inadequate or ceased altogether;

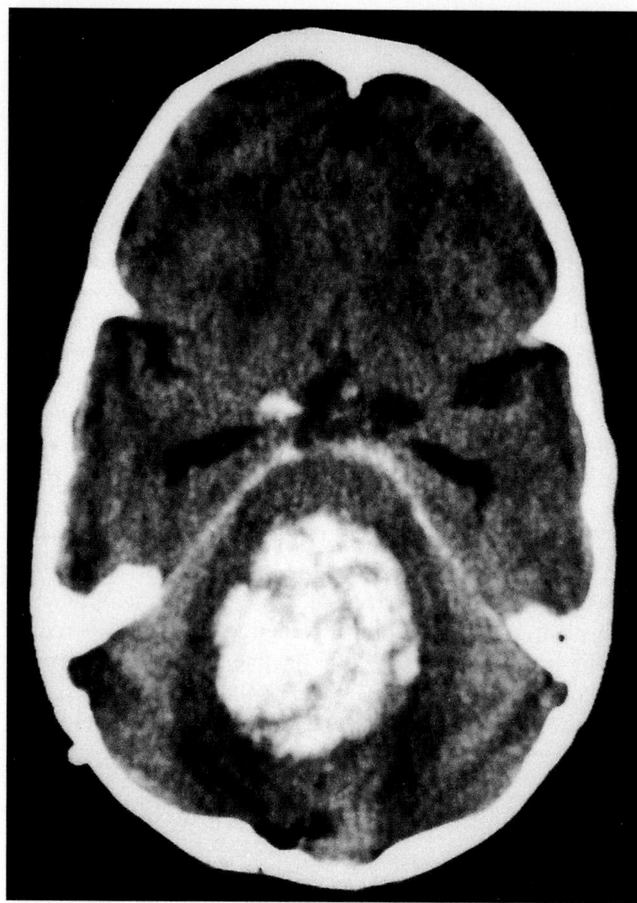

Fig. 35.48 Axial CT through posterior fossa showing fatal brainstem haematoma.

- conditions and drugs which simulate brain death have to be excluded and, if necessary, drug levels measured to ensure that there is no reversible cause for coma. Some drugs (e.g. thiopentone) may take days to be cleared from the system.

Potentially reversible circulatory, metabolic and endocrine disturbances must have been excluded as the cause for the continuation of unconsciousness. It is recognised that circulatory, metabolic and endocrine disturbances are a likely accompaniment of brainstem death (e.g. hypernatraemia and diabetes insipidus) but these are the effect rather than the cause of that condition and do not preclude the diagnosis.

The tests should be performed by two physicians of not less than 5 years' registration, who are not members of a transplant team and at least one of whom is a consultant. The tests are designed to assess brainstem functioning as it is the reticular activating system in the brainstem which is responsible for activating the rest of the cerebrum.

1. The pupils should be fixed and unresponsive to changes in the intensity of incidental light.
2. There should be no corneal reflex.
3. The vestibulo-ocular reflexes should be absent. No eye movements should be observed while at least 50 ml of cold water is infused over each eardrum. Clear access to the membrane must be established by direct inspection.
4. No motor responses within the cranial nerve distribution can be elicited by adequate stimulation of any somatic area. There is no limb response to somatic pressure, bearing in mind that movements mediated at a spinal level might still be possible.
5. There is no gag reflex to bronchial stimulation by a catheter placed down the trachea.
6. No respiratory movements appear when the patient is disconnected from the mechanical ventilator. During this test it is necessary for the arterial CO_2 to exceed the threshold for respiratory stimulation, that is the $PaCO_2$ should reach 6.65 kPa. This should be ensured by measurement of the blood gases. The patient should first be preoxygenated with 100 per cent O_2 for 10 minutes (then with 5 per cent CO_2 in O_2 for 10 minutes – if CO_2 is available). The ventilator should then be disconnected for 10 minutes while 6 litres per minute O_2 via a catheter is infused into the trachea.

If no respiratory effort has been detected and other signs of brainstem dysfunction have been demonstrated the patient may be considered brain dead.

Studies of hundreds of patients in several countries have found that not a single body displaying the criteria of brain death outlined gained any neurological recovery. Despite full and repeated efforts at resuscitation all such reported patients have suffered asystole within days or rarely weeks of the diagnosis. Interestingly in 37 instances the EEG retained at least fragments of electrical activity at a time when the patient was diagnosed as brain dead. In contrast to this, Jennet has shown that of the patients surviving prolonged coma, none ever met the criteria for brainstem death at any stage. Although not all agree, most religious and ethical bodies have expressed themselves in sympathy with the concept that death of the brain signifies death of the person. Pope Pius XII proclaimed in 1958 that the pronouncement of death was the responsibility of the church, stating that when illnesses reached hopeless proportions, death should not be medically opposed by extraordinary measures.

It is imperative that conditions simulating brain death be excluded.

Drug intoxication

CNS-depressant drug poisoning may cause total loss of cerebral function and electrocerebral silence for more than 50 hours followed by complete recovery. Self-induced drug poisoning often involves several drugs, frequently in combination with alcohol. Toxicology screening is not always available and frequently levels do not correlate with the clinical state. Serum concentrations often lag behind brain concentrations.

Hypothermia

The core temperature tends to drop when the brainstem ceases to function. That hypothermia may cause an isoelectric EEG is a theoretical rather than a practical issue. What is important is that hypothermia should be excluded as the cause rather than the result of the coma.

Electrical injury

This may be an important cause of coma, apnoea and fixed pupils.

Brainstem encephalitis

This is a rare form of encephalitis characterised by rapid ophthalmoplegia, ataxia and areflexia with apnoea and coma in severe cases. Although the clinical state may suggest brain death, these patients do not comply with the basic prerequisite of an incontrovertible diagnosis and the physician should be concerned with diagnostic and therapeutic measures rather than speculating about irreversible coma.

Ancillary tests

Ever since the concept of brain death arose, efforts have been made to establish the diagnosis electrophysiologically, the reason being to seek an objective nonclinical mode of diagnosis free of error or bias. These tests are not available in all hospitals and those which have proved to be indisputable indicators of brainstem death have usually occurred in patients in whom the diagnosis was never in doubt. They are listed for completeness and not because they replace clinical testing:

- EEG;
- scalp electromyograms;
- evoked potentials;
- brainstem auditory evoked potentials;
- somatic evoked potentials;
- lower oesophageal contractility;
- arteriovenous O_2 difference;
- cerebral blood flow;
- ocular microtremor.

There is strong evidence that EEG silence for greater than 12 hours in a normothermic patient having had no drugs is not compatible with neurological recovery. Silverman reviewed 2560 isoelectric EEGs lasting for up to 24 hours. Only three patients in this group, all of whom overdosed on CNS antidepressant drugs, recovered cerebral function. Testing in an ITU setting is technically difficult owing to interference. The presence of a few fragments of electrocerebral activity is of dubious significance. Return of EEG activity after silence has also been reported.

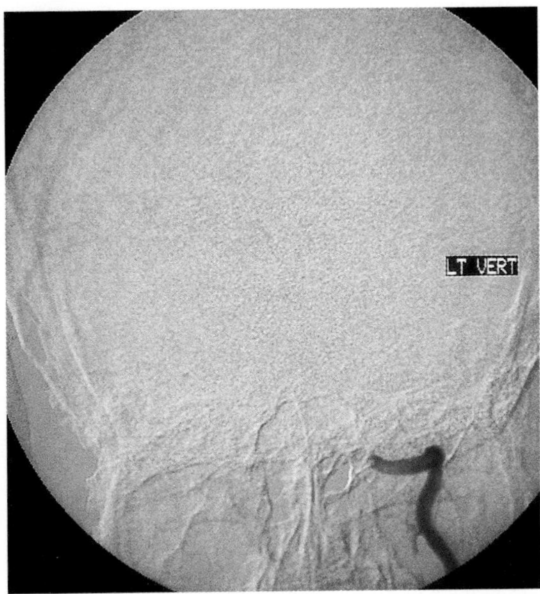

Fig. 35.49 Left vertebral injection of cerebral angiogram demonstrating no filling indicative of brain death.

NB: an EEG does not measure brainstem function. Drugs may cause coma with reversible true electrocerebral silence.

Cessation of cerebral blood flow in patients with raised ICP was first described by Riishede and Ethelberg in 1953. It is a significant indicator of brain death particularly where CT scanning is not available. It is caused by ICP rising above the MAP and by progressive vascular obstruction caused by autolysis in respirator brain (Fig. 35.49).

Ocular microtremor is one of three fixational eye movements measured using the isoelectric strain gauge technique and is an indicator of brainstem activity. Studies by Coakley and Bolger (1999) have shown that this tremor is absent in patients with the diagnosis of brainstem death.

If the viability of certain organs is to be maintained for possible harvesting, mechanical ventilation can be continued and the circulation artificially supported with a clear understanding, however, that these measures are not therapeutic but continued in order to maintain a cadaver in a perfused state. A member of the transplantation team is summoned and all further medical and administrative care of the potential donor should be carried out by them. The request for organ donation must come from the transplant team and not those treating the primary pathology. The staff taking care of the patient declining to brain death have a special responsibility towards the relatives who are going through a very harrowing time. For the layperson it is still a macabre concept to speak of death of a person in whom the heart is still beating.

Further reading

Crockard, A., Hayward, R. and Hoff, J.T. (1992) *Neurosurgery – The Scientific Basis of Clinical Practice*, 2nd edn, Blackwell Scientific, Boston, MA.

Friedman, A.H. and Wilkins, R.H. (1984) *Neurosurgical Management for the House Officer*, Williams & Wilkins, Baltimore, MD.

Jennett, W.B. and Teasdale, G. (1981) *Management of Head Injuries*, Davis, Philadelphia, PA.

Kaye, A. (1997) *Essential Neurosurgery*, 2nd edn, Churchill Livingstone, New York.

Lindsay, K.W. and Bone, I. (1997) *Neurology and Neurosurgery Illustrated*, 3rd edn, Churchill Livingstone, New York.

Morris, P.J. and Malt, R.A. (1994) *Oxford Textbook of Surgery*, Oxford University Press, Oxford.

Plum, F. and Posner, J.B. (1972) *The Diagnosis of Stupor and Coma*, 2nd edn, F.A. Davis, Philadelphia, PA.

Williams, R.H. and Rengachary, S.S. (1996) *Neurosurgery*, 2nd edn, McGraw-Hill, New York.

Working Party for the Department of Health (1998) *A Code of Practice for the Diagnosis of Brainstem Death*, Department of Health, London.

Youman, S. (1990) *Neurological Surgery*, 3rd edn, W.B. Saunders, Philadelphia, PA.

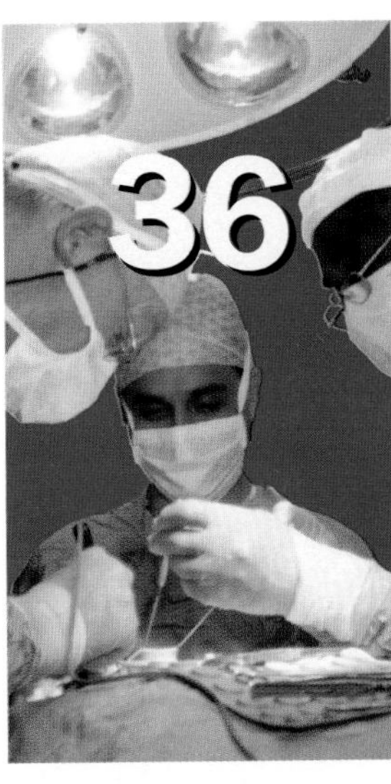

36 The eye and orbit

Periorbital and orbital swellings

Swellings related to the supraorbital margin

Dermoid cysts

Dermoid cysts are usually external angular cysts although they may occur medially (Fig. 36.1). They often cause a bony depression by their pressure, and may have a dumb-bell extension into the orbit. They can also erode the orbital plate of the frontal bone, to become attached to dura, and for this reason it is important to do computerised tomography (CT) of the area before excision.

Neurofibromatosis

Neurofibromatosis may also produce swellings above the eye. The diagnosis can usually be confirmed by an examination of the whole body, as there are often multiple lesions. Proptosis can also result (Fig. 36.2).

Swellings of the lids

Meibomian cysts (chalazion)

These are the most common lid swellings (Fig. 36.3). A meibomian cyst is a chronic granulomatous inflammation of a meibomian gland. It may occur on either upper or lower lids and presents as a smooth painless swelling. It can be felt by rolling the cyst on the tarsal plate. It is distinguished from a stye (hordeolum) which is an infection of a hair follicle, usually painful. Meibomian cysts are treated by incision and curettage from the conjunctival surface. Styes are treated by antibiotics and local heat.

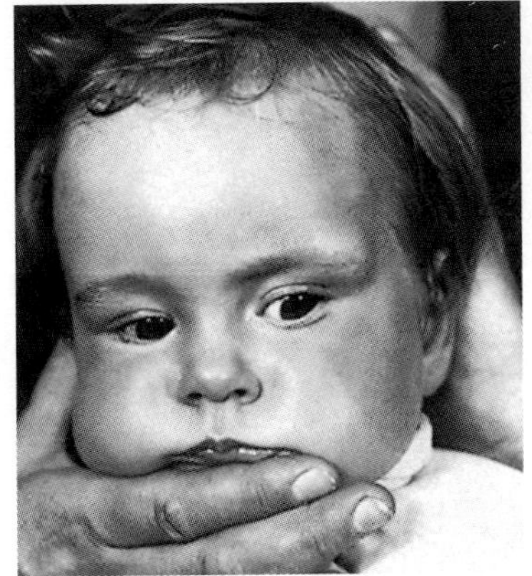

Fig. 36.1 External angular dermoid.

Basal cell carcinomas (rodent ulcers)

This is the most common malignant tumour of the eyelids (Fig. 36.4). It is locally malignant, is more common on the lower lids, and usually starts as a small pimple which ulcerates and has raised edges. It is easily excised in the early stages, and can be treated with local radiotherapy if too big to be excised.

Henrich Meibomian, 1638–1700. German anatomist.

Bailey & Love's Short Practice of Surgery, 23rd edition. Edited by R.C.G. Russell, N.S. Williams and C.J.K. Bulstrode. Published in 2000 by Arnold Publishers.

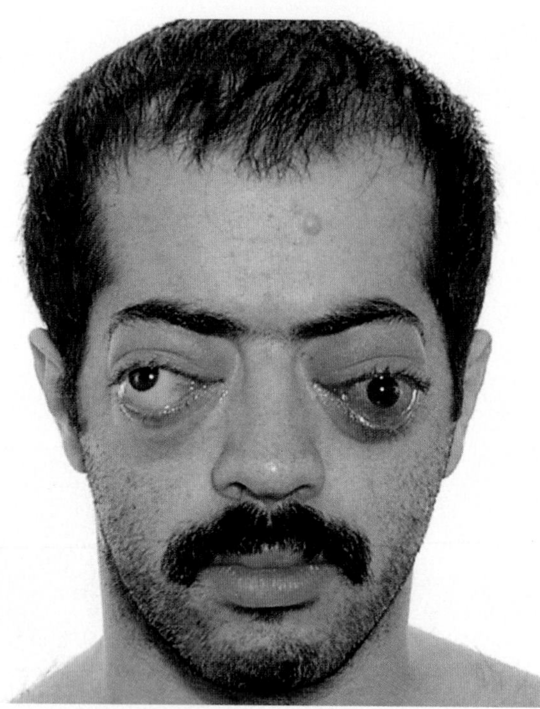

Fig. 36.2 Neurofibroma in the orbit with proptosis and also similar lesion in the forehead.

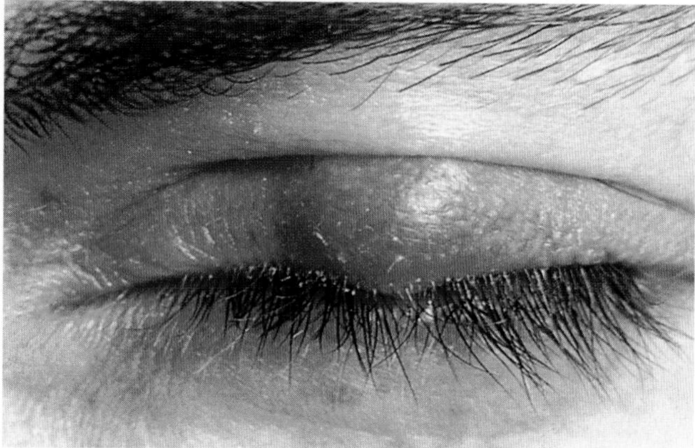

Fig. 36.3 Meibomian cyst (*courtesy of Mr D. Spalton, FRCS*).

Other lid swellings

These can occur, but are less common. These include sebaceous cysts, papillomas, keratoacanthosis, cysts of Moll (Fig. 36.5) (sweat glands) or Zeiss (sebaceous glands) and molluscum contagiosum. When molluscum contagiosum occurs on the lid margin, they can give rise to a mild keratoconjunctivitis and should be curetted.

Carcinoma of the meibomian glands and rhabdomyosarcomas are rare lesions; they need to be treated radically. Meibomian cysts that recur frequently should be submitted to biopsy.

Jacob Anthoni Moll, 1832–1914. Dutch ophthalmologist.

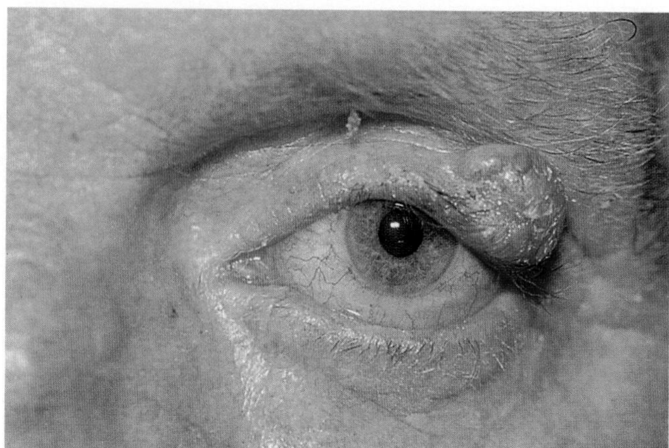

Fig. 36.4 Rodent ulcers (*courtesy of Mr J. Beare, FRCS*).

Swellings of the lacrimal system

Lacrimal sac mucocele

This occurs from obstruction of the lacrimal duct beyond the sac, and results in a fluctuant swelling, which bulges out just below the medial canthus. It can become infected to give rise to a painful tense swelling (acute dacryocystitis). If untreated it may give rise to a fistula. Treatment is by performing a bypass operation between the lacrimal sac and the nose [a dacryocystorrhinostomy (DCR)]. Watering of the eye can occur due to eversion of the lower lid (ectropion), which causes loss of contact between the lower punctum and the tear film, and this must be distinguished from a mucocele.

Lacrimal gland tumours

Pathologically these resemble parotid tumours (Chapter 42). These are swellings of the gland which lie in the upper lateral aspect of the orbit, and eventually they lead to impairment of ocular movements and displacement of the globe forwards, downwards and inwards. They can be pleomorphic adenomas with or without carcinomatous change, carcinomas or mucoepidermoid tumours.

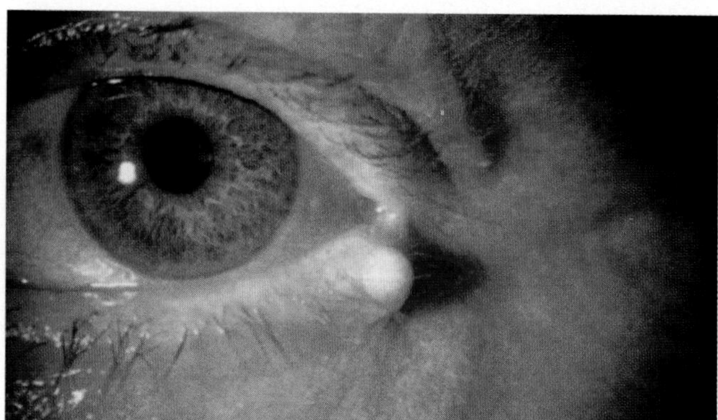

Fig. 36.5 Cyst of Moll.

Orbital swellings

If these reach any size they result in displacement of the globe and limitation of movement. A full description of these is outside the realm of the text, but some of the most common causes include the following.

- *Pseudoproptosis*. This results from a large eyeball, as seen in congenital glaucoma or high myopia.
- ***Orbital inflammatory conditions*** result in orbital cellulitis (Fig. 36.6).
- ***Haemorrhagic lesions*** occur in the orbit, after trauma or retrobulbar injections.
- ***Neoplasia*** affects the lacrimal gland, the optic nerve, the nasal sinuses and glioma (neurofibromatosis) (Fig. 36.6), meningioma and osteoma (Fig. 36.7).
- ***Dysthyroid exophthalmos*** (Figs 36.8, 36.9 and 36.10). Often unrelated to active thyroid disease but can start after thyroidectomy and may need urgent tarsorrhaphy, large doses of steroids or even orbital decompression, if the eyeball is threatened by exposure. This is most easily done into the nasal sinuses (Chapter 44). CT and magnetic resonance imaging (MRI) scans are useful in diagnosis.
- *Pseudotumour*, or malignant lymphoma.
- *Haemangiomas* of the orbit (Fig. 36.11).

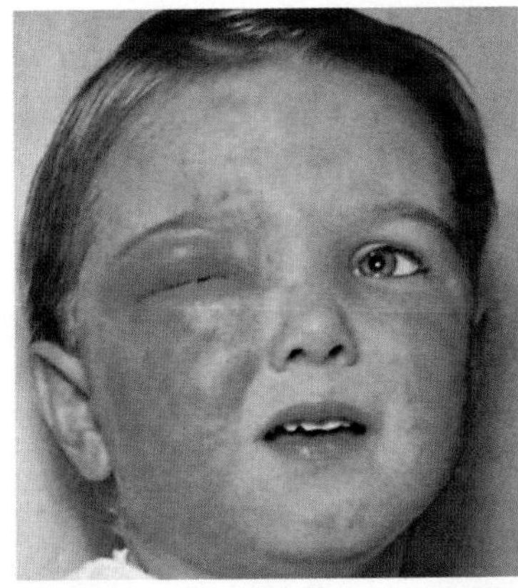

Fig. 36.6 Orbital cellulitis.

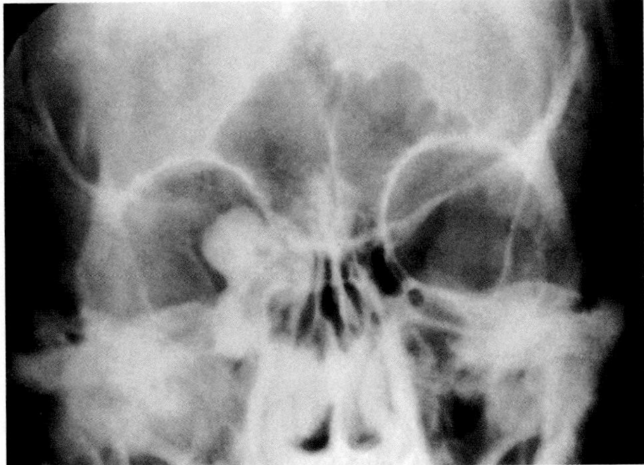

Fig. 36.7 Radiograph showing an osteoma on the nasal side of the orbit giving rise to proptosis.

- *Tumour secondaries or metastases*. These are rare. In children they usually come from neuroblastomas of the adrenal gland, whereas in adults, the oesophagus, stomach, breast and prostate can be sites of primary lesions.

Diagnostic aids

Diagnostic aids include: radiography, tomography, orbital venography, ultrasonography, CT and MRI.

Treatment

Treatment is directed to the cause of the lesion if at all possible, taking care to prevent exposure of the eye and discomfort from diplopia.

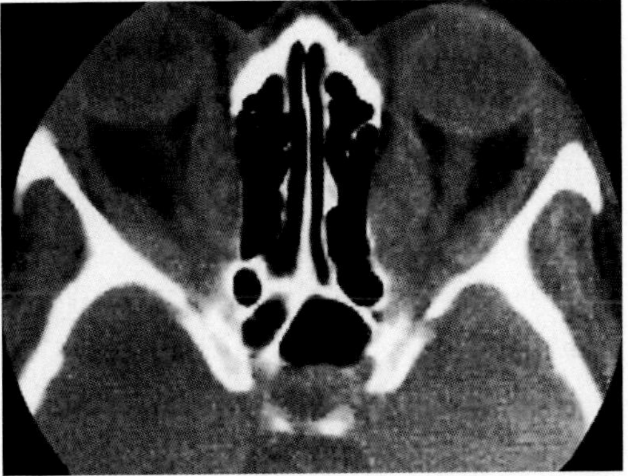

Fig. 36.8 Computerised tomogram of orbit in dysthyroid exophthalmos showing swollen muscles (*courtesy of Dr Glyn Lloyd*).

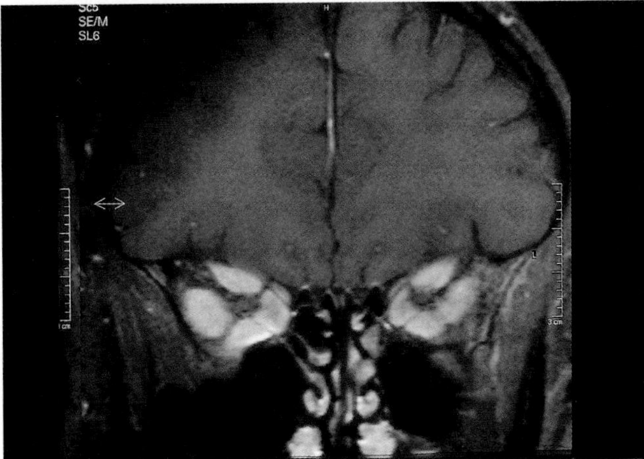

Fig. 36.9 MRI coronal view of orbit showing enlarged ocular muscles in thyroid disease (*courtesy of Dr Juliette Britton*).

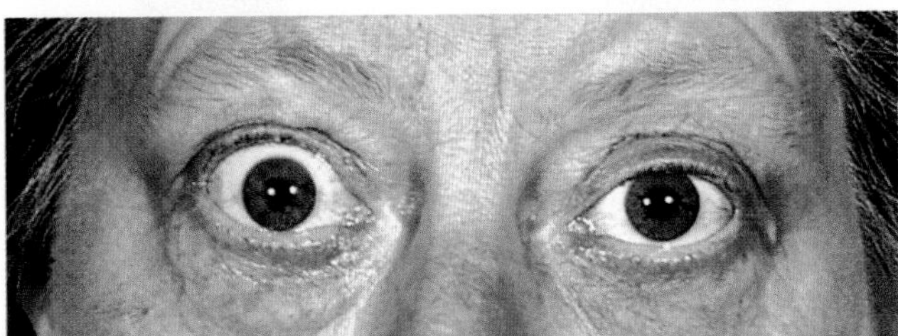

Fig. 36.10 Exophthalmos in dysthyroid eye disease.

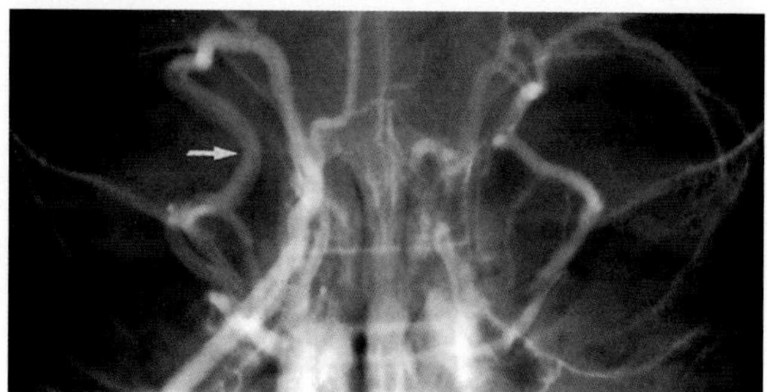

Fig. 36.11 Capillary haemangioma in a child. Orbital venogram demonstrates displacement of the second part of the superior ophthalmic vein (arrow) (*courtesy of Dr Glyn Lloyd*).

Intraocular tumours

Children

Retinoblastoma is a multicentric malignant tumour of the retina, which can be bilateral. Some are sporadic, but many are hereditary. Children with a family history should be carefully monitored from birth. It is often not spotted until the tumour fills the globe and presents as a white reflex in the pupil (Fig. 36.12). Differential diagnosis is from retinopathy of prematurity, primary hyperplastic vitreous and intraocular infections. If the tumour is large, enucleation may be required, but radiotherapy, cryotherapy or laser treatment can cure small lesions.

Adults

Malignant melanoma is the most common tumour, and it originates in the pigment cells of the choroid ciliary body (Figs 36.13 and 36.14) or iris. It can present a reduction in vision, a vitreous haemorrhage or by the chance finding of an elevated pigmented lesion in the eye. Growth can be rapid or fairly slow; as a general rule, the more posterior the lesion the more malignant it is likely to be. Malignancy is ultimately related to the cell type. Spread is often delayed for many years, and often goes to the liver, hence the advice 'beware of the patient with a glass eye, and an enlarged liver'. Treatment is by light or laser coagulation, radioactive plaques, radiotherapy, enucleation and in selected cases it is by local excision using hypotensive anaesthesia. Note: a blind painful eye may hide a malignant melanoma. Diagnosis is made either by direct observation or by ultrasound which shows a solid tumour (Fig. 36.15).

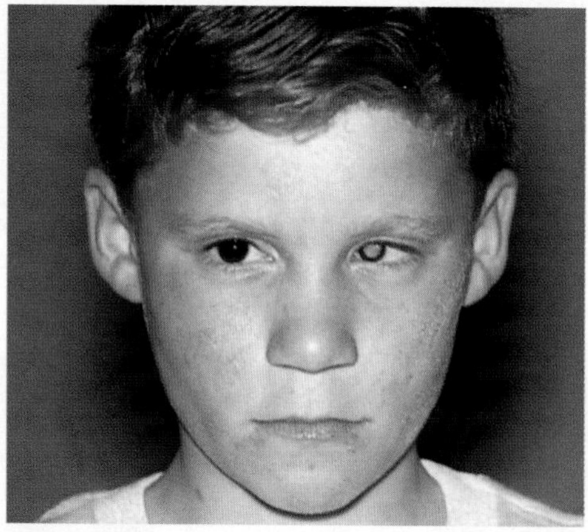

Fig. 36.12 Retinoblastoma giving rise to a white pupillary reflex. This child was first seen with a convergent squint and discharged without a fundus examination. He was next seen many years later with a 'white reflex' and died soon after diagnosis (*courtesy of M.A. Bedford, FRCS*).

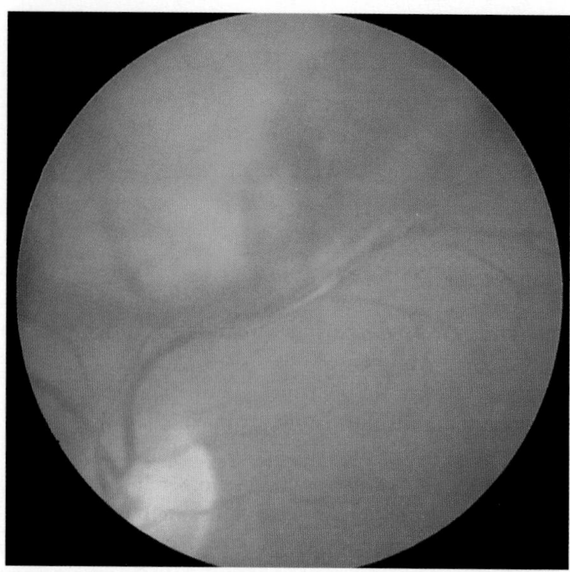

Fig. 36.13 Choroidal melanoma.

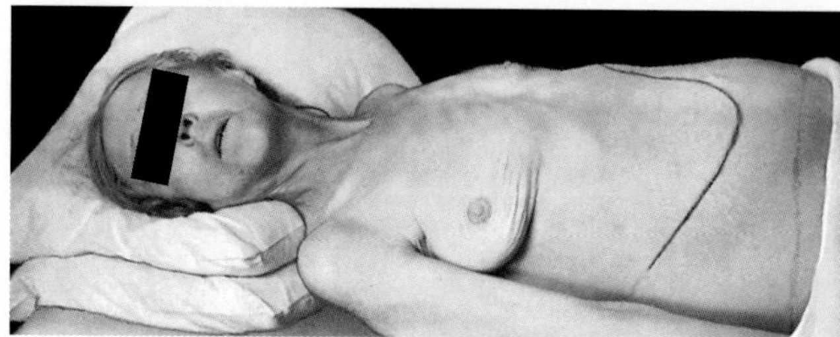

Fig. 36.14 Patient with a greatly enlarged liver who for many years had worn a glass eye after excision of the eyeball for melanoma.

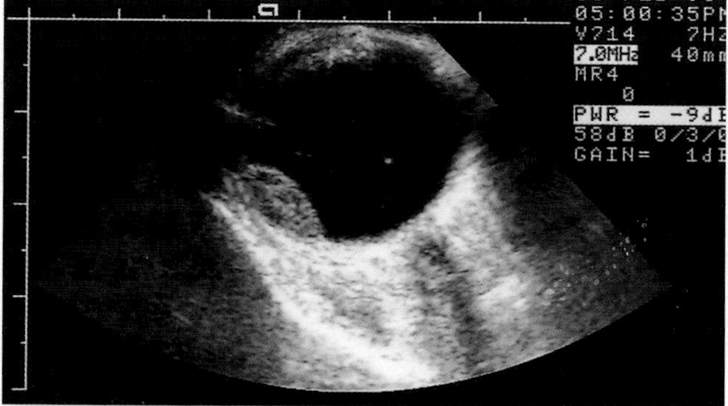

Fig. 36.15 B-scan showing choroidal melanoma (*courtesy of Dr Marie Restori*).

Injuries involving the eye and adjacent structures

Corneal abrasions and ulceration

The cornea is frequently damaged by trauma and foreign bodies (Fig. 36.16). Ulceration can occur with infection or after damage to the facial nerve (Chapter 34). Postherpetic ulceration is common and serious if not treated. Fluorescein instillation can show up corneal ulceration at an early stage. Treatment is by protection (eye pads, tarsorrhaphy or a bandage contact lens), and antibiotics topically and systemically: 0.5 per cent chloramphenicol or ofloxacin eye drops are commonly used. The eye is made more comfortable by the use of mydriatics such as homatropine or cyclopentolate. Herpes simplex ulcers are treated with acyclovir ointment. In countries in the Far and Middle East chronic infection with trachoma can cause corneal opacification and blindness. Corneal grafting is the only cure for an opaque cornea. Osteo–odonto keratoprosthesis can be done in very severe cases of opaque corneas which are not suitable for grafting. Acanthoemeba is a serious cause of corneal infection. This fungal corneal infection usually follows the use of contact lenses. These rare cases need specialist treatment.

Blunt injuries to the eye and orbit

The floor of the orbit is its weakest wall, and in blunt trauma, such as fist injuries, it is often fractured without fractures of the other walls. This is called a blow-out fracture. Clinical signs are enophthalmos, bruising around the orbit and limitation of upward gaze and diplopia. This occurs when the extraocular muscles become trapped in the fracture, and can be identified as a soft tissue mass in the antrum on a radiograph (Fig. 36.17), although tomograms or CT scans may be necessary. Surgical repair of the orbital floor with freeing of the trapped contents may be necessary if troublesome diplopia persists. Large doses of steroids sometimes relieve symptoms in acute cases. If an orbital haemorrhage is too extensive to examine the eye, it may be necessary to examine the eye under anaesthesia because there may be a hidden perforation of the globe. Injuries to the lids and lid margins must be repaired, and if the lacrimal canaliculi are damaged they should be repaired if possible, especially the lower canaliculus, because 95 per cent of tear drainage goes through it.

Blunt injuries can also cause damage to the optic nerve which can result in blindness and a total afferent nerve defect (Figs 36.18 and 36.19).

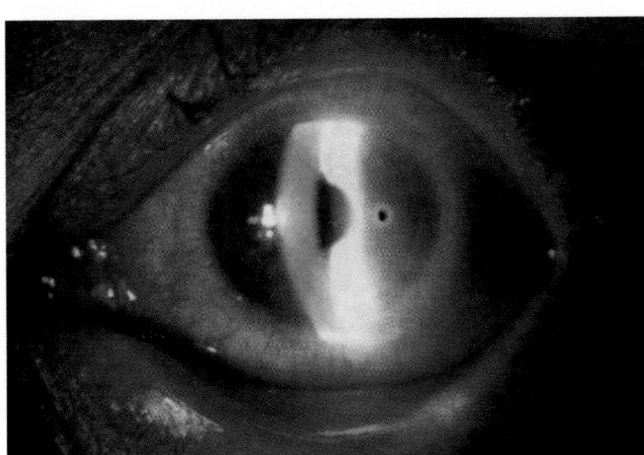

Fig. 36.16 Corneal foreign body.

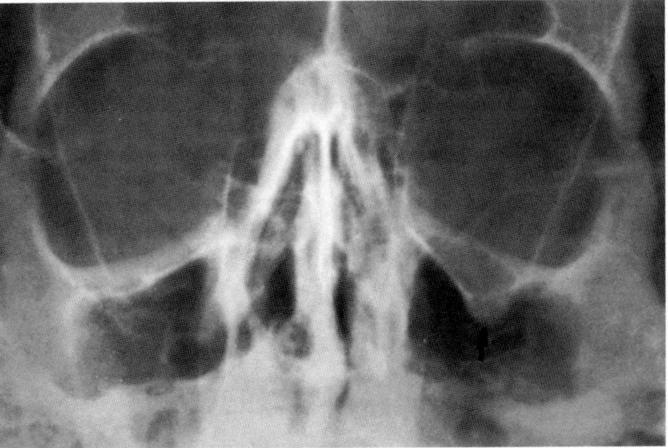

Fig. 36.17 Radiograph showing a blow-out fracture of the orbit (left) with soft tissue in the antrum (*courtesy of Dr Glyn Lloyd*).

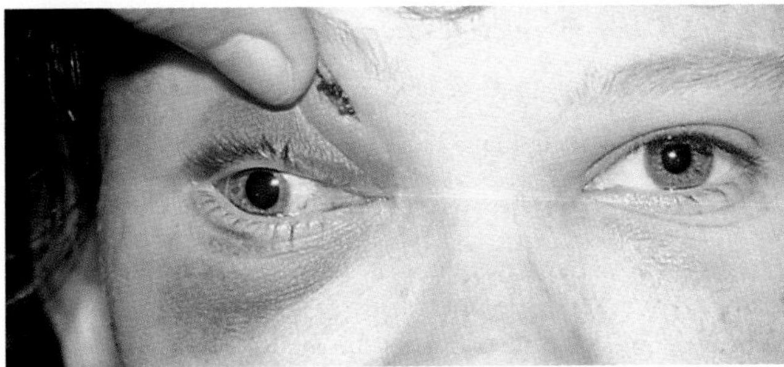

Fig. 36.18 Injury from a ski stick into the right brow. Vision reduced to 'no perception of light' (*courtesy of J. Beare, FRCS*).

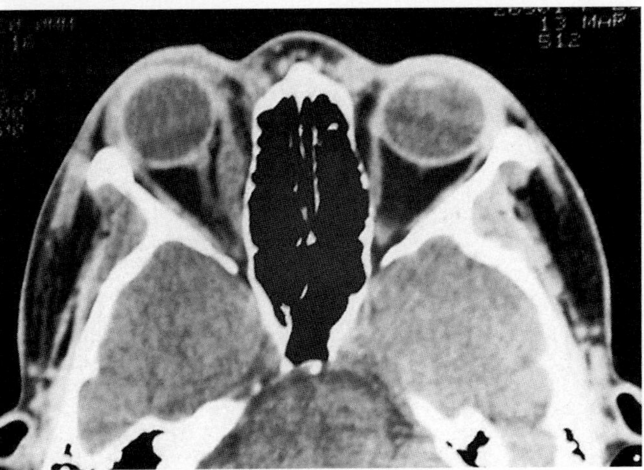

Fig. 36.19 Scan of orbit from Fig. 36.18 showing massive swelling of medial rectus (*courtesy of J. Beare, FRCS*).

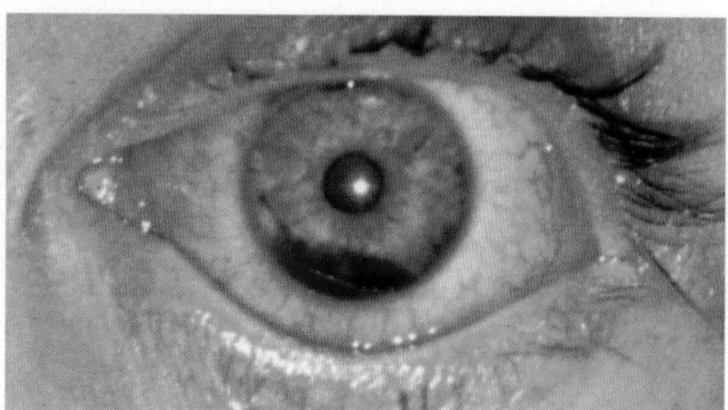

Fig. 36.20 Hyphaema – blood in vitreous chamber after concussional injury.

Concussional injuries

Concussional injuries of the eye can give rise to several problems, which include the following.

- *Hyphaema* (blood in the anterior chamber) (Fig. 36.20). Bed rest and sedation are advised because the main danger in this condition is secondary bleeding, resulting in an acute rise in intraocular pressure and blood staining of the cornea. The use of antifibrinolytic agents (e-aminocaproic acid) has been advocated and, if the pressure rises, surgery to wash out the blood may be necessary.
- *Subluxation of the lens* can be suspected if the iris, or part of the iris, 'wobbles' on movement (iridodonesis).
- *Secondary glaucoma* often associated with recession of the angle.
- *Retinal and macular haemorrhages and choroidal tears* (Fig. 36.21).
- *Retinal dialysis,* which may lead to a retinal detachment and permanent damage to vision (Fig. 36.22).

Penetrating eye injuries

These occur when the globe is penetrated, often in road traffic and other major accidents (Fig. 36.23), and also in injuries from sharp instruments. In the UK, the seat belt law has reduced this type of eye injury by up to 73 per cent in some series. The presence of an irregular pupil suggests prolapse of the iris, and should arouse the suspicion of a penetrating injury. Treatment is immediate surgery to restore the integrity of the globe. If a perforation is suspected, extensive eye examination should not be attempted before anaesthesia because this may lead to further extrusion of the intraocular contents. In severe corneal and intraocular injuries, primary corneal grafting, lensectomy and vitrectomy have considerably improved the visual prognosis; these must be done by an experienced eye surgeon. Injuries to the optic nerves must also be excluded in severe accidents.

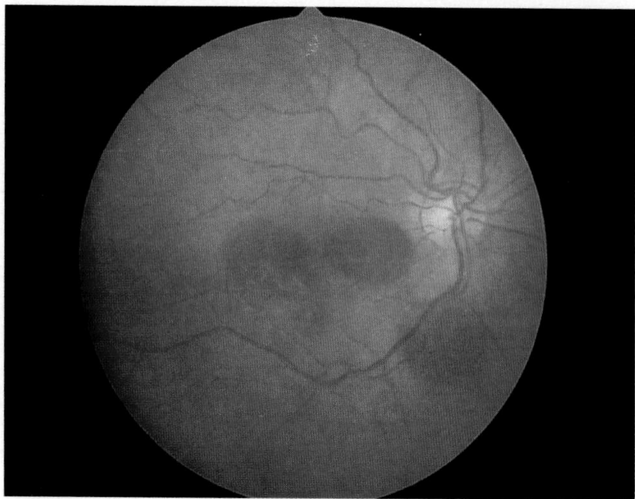

Fig. 36.21 Retinal haemorrhage from a cricket ball injury (*courtesy of J. Beare, FRCS*).

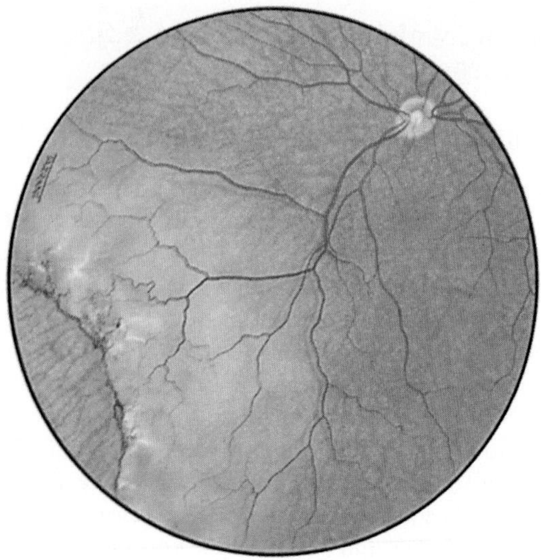

Fig. 36.22 Retinal dialysis after concussional injury.

Intraocular foreign bodies

Intraocular foreign bodies must always be excluded when patients attend the accident and emergency department with a history of working with a hammer and chisel. *Radiography of the orbits should always be performed, and ferrous and copper foreign bodies should always be removed.* Beta-scan ultrasonography can also assist in localising foreign bodies when a vitreous haemorrhage is present. CT can be used, but MRI is contraindicated for orbital lesions.

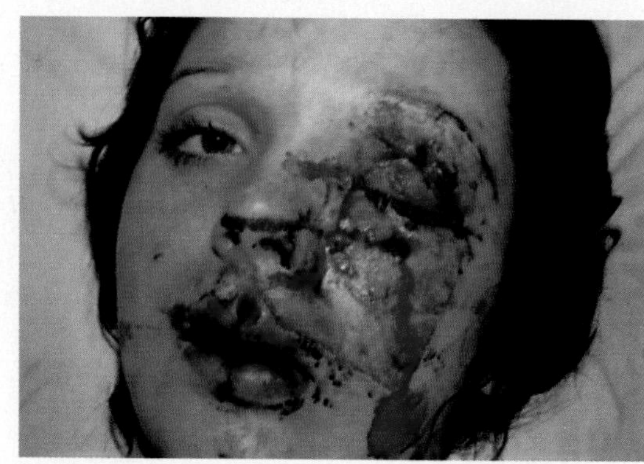

Fig. 36.23 Facial lacerations from windscreen injury: beware of a perforating eye injury.

Burns

Radiation burns

These occur after exposure to ultraviolet radiation after arc welding or excessive sunlight (snow blindness) and sun lamps. Such burns cause intense pain and photophobia due to a keratitis, which may start some hours after exposure. Mydriatic and local steroid drops ease the condition, and healing usually occurs after 24 hours.

Thermal burns

If these involve the full thickness of the lids, corneal scarring may occur, and immediate skin grafting to the lids is necessary. A splash of molten metal may cause marked local necrosis, and may lead to permanent corneal scarring. Treatment is to remove any debris by irrigation, and to instil local atropine, antibiotics and steroids to prevent superadded infection and scarring.

Chemical burns

Chemical burns, and especially alkali burns, can be serious because ocular penetration occurs quickly and ischaemic necrosis can result. Immediate irrigation will ensure that the chemical is diluted as much as possible, and all particles should be removed from the fornices. Treatment can then be continued as with thermal burns. Well-fitting goggles should prevent such injuries (Fig. 36.24).

Differential diagnosis of the acute red eye

The importance of this is in the management of minor ocular complaints, and the recognition of conditions requiring expert attention. Possible causes of the acute red eye can be divided into:

- conjunctivitis;
- keratitis;
- uveitis;
- episcleritis and scleritis;
- acute glaucoma.

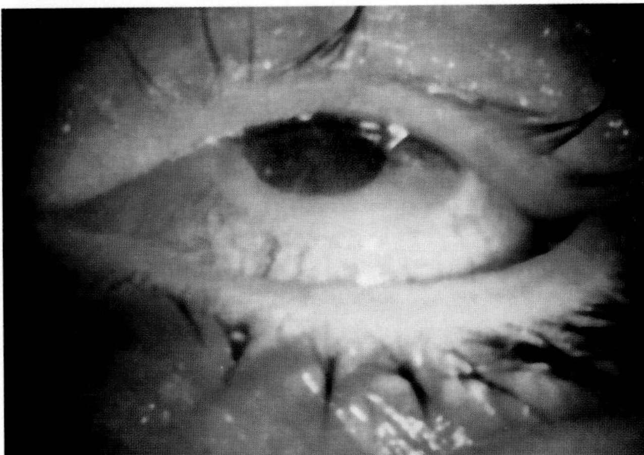

Fig. 36.24 Chemical burn showing conjunctival necrosis.

Conjunctivitis

Symptoms are grittiness, redness and discharge. Causes are infective, viral, traumatic or allergic. In the newborn it can be serious, and gonococcal and chlamydial infection must be excluded. Vernal conjunctivitis (Fig. 36.25) is a form of allergic conjunctivitis, usually worse in the spring and early summer, and often associated with other allergic problems such as hay fever. Clinically, most signs are under the upper lid which may have a cobblestone appearance instead of a smooth surface. Giant pupillary conjunctivitis with large papilli under the upper lid may be seen in soft contact lens wearers. This is usually due to an allergy to the sterilising solutions and may be helped by either using a preservative-free solution or using daily wear disposable lenses where these are applicable. Viral conjunctivitis has become much more common. Chlamydial and adenovirus infections must be considered. Adenoviral infections usually affect one eye

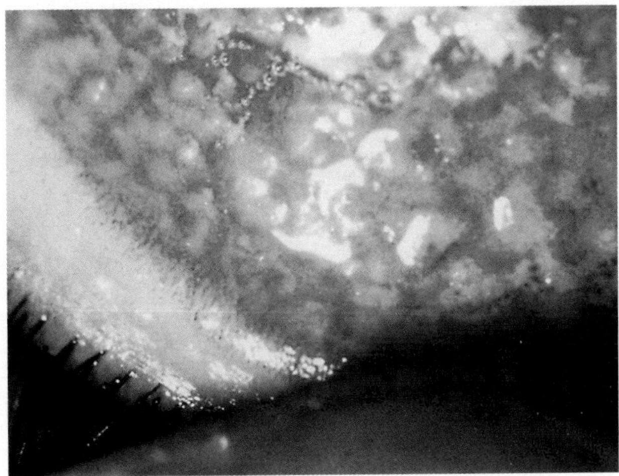

Fig. 36.25 Vernal conjunctivitis (spring catarrh) showing cobblestone appearance under the upper lid.

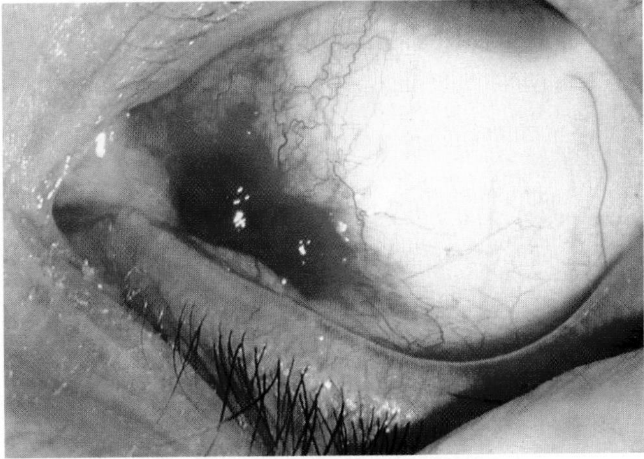

Fig. 36.26 Kaposi's sarcoma of conjunctiva.

much more than the other and are often associated with a palpable preauricular gland. Kaposi's sarcoma can present like a subconjunctival haemorrhage (Fig. 36.26).

Considerable conjunctival irritation can be caused by the lids turning in (entropion) (Fig. 36.27) or turning out (ectropion) (Figs 36.28 and 36.29) and by ingrowing lashes. The lids should be repaired surgically to their normal position.

Vision is not affected in conjunctivitis, but with some virus infections a keratitis may be present, and result in visual loss and pain. All of the other conditions are painful, and usually affect vision.

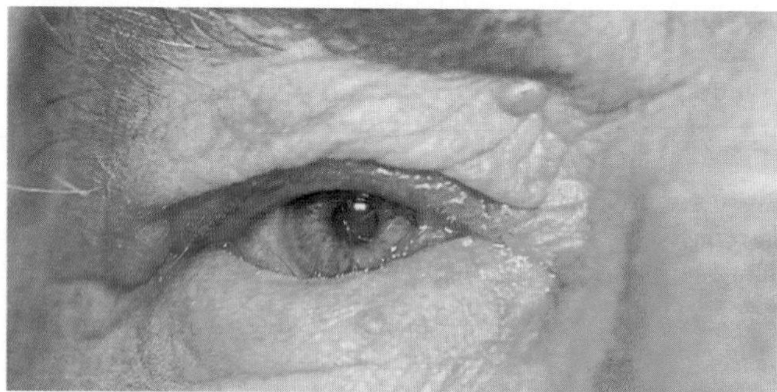

Fig. 36.27 Entropion (*courtesy of J. Beare, FRCS*).

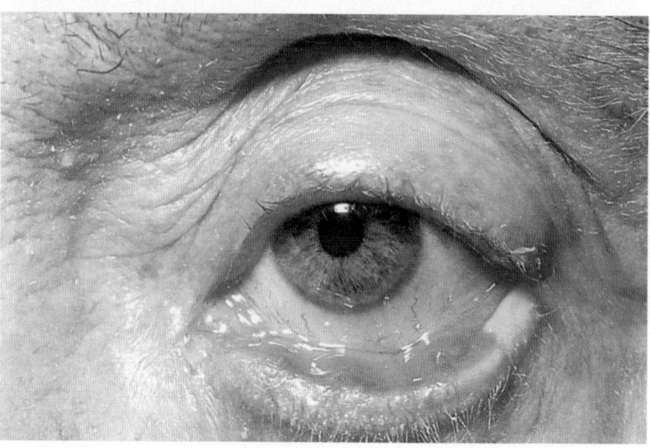

Fig. 36.28 Ectropion, lower lid (*courtesy of J. Beare, FRCS*).

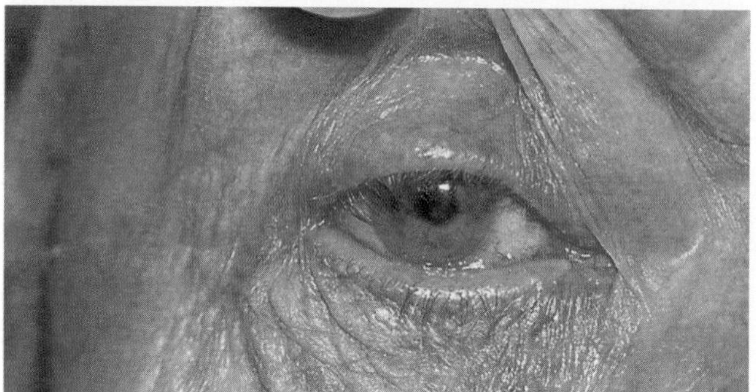

Fig. 36.29 Ectropion, upper lid – chronic staphylococcal infection (*courtesy of J. Beare, FRCS*).

Moritz Kaposi, 1837–1902. Austrian dermatologist.

Keratitis (inflammation of the cornea)

Herpes simplex infection is the most serious, and presents itself as a dendritic (branching) ulcer, shown easily by staining with fluorescein or Bengal rose. It is treated with acyclovir ointment five times a day. The use of steroid drops must be avoided as this can make the condition much worse (Fig. 34.30).

Corneal ulceration may occur due to ingrowing lashes or corneal foreign bodies, marginal ulceration and infected ulcers. Infected ulcers can occur in patients wearing soft contact lenses. **Herpes zoster** (shingles) affects the ophthalmic division of the fifth nerve, and can give rise to a keratitis and uveitis. It is important to exclude the use of steroid drops until a diagnosis has been made. Local anaesthetic drops should also not be given on a regular basis.

Uveitis

This can be anterior (iritis) or posterior. In anterior uveitis the pupil will be small, sometimes irregular, there is circumcorneal injection and there may be keratic precipitates (KPs) present on the posterior surface of the cornea. Pain, photophobia and some visual loss are usually present. Posterior uveitis can present with a white eye and blurred vision. It usually takes a chronic course. Granulomatous diseases, Behçet's disease, toxoplasmosis and cytomegalovirus infection should be excluded. Systemic steroids and cytotoxic drugs are sometimes useful in treating these conditions.

Episcleritis and scleritis

Episcleritis or inflammation of the episcleral tissue often occurs as an allergic reaction following an eye infection (Fig. 36.31).

Scleritis is a more serious condition in which the deeper sclera is involved. There is often an associated uveitis and thinning of the sclera. It may require the use of systemic steroids in order to treat adequately

Scleritis is often associated with severe rheumatoid conditions.

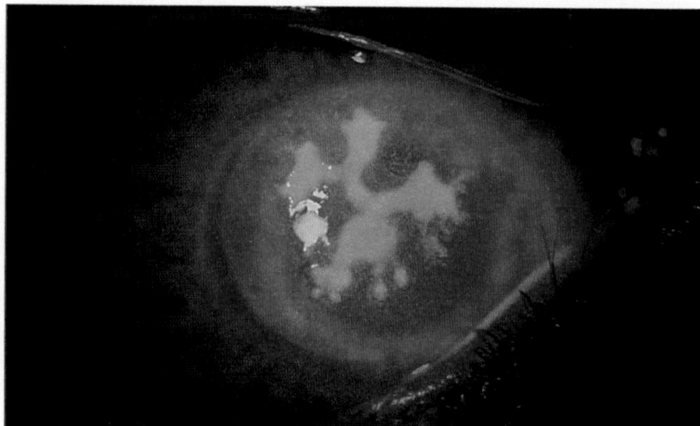

Fig. 36.30 Dendritic staining due to herpes keratitis.

Hulusi Behçet, 1889–1948. Dermatologist, Istanbul, Turkey.

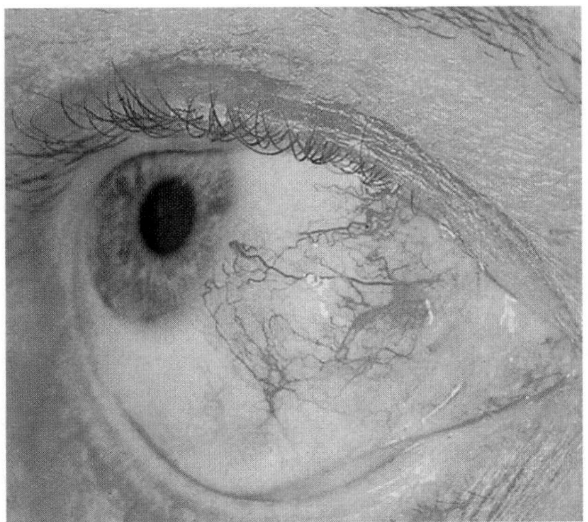

Fig. 36.31 Episcleritis.

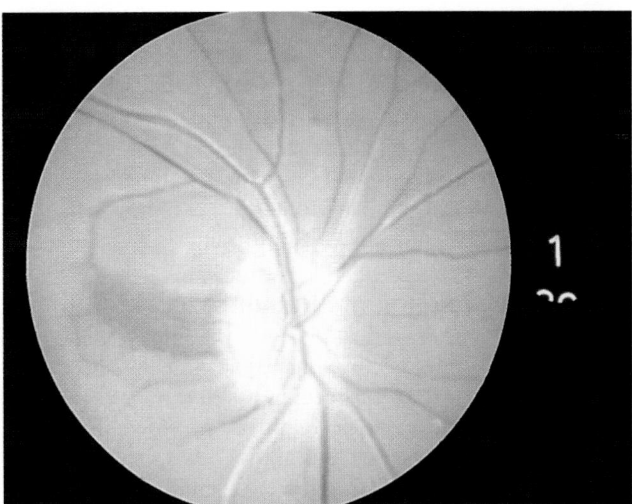

Fig. 36.32 Retinal artery occlusion.

Acute glaucoma

This usually occurs in older, often hypermetropic patients. The cornea becomes hazy, the pupil oval and dilated, the vision very poor and the eye feels rock hard. In severe cases the pain may be accompanied by vomiting, and the pain can be mistaken for one of an acute abdomen. In doubtful cases the use of the tonometer to measure the intraocular pressure is a useful diagnostic procedure. Urgent treatment to reduce the pressure by pilocarpine, acetazolamide and mannitol should be started followed by a surgical iridectomy or laser iridotomy. The condition is usually bilateral, and the second eye usually needs treatment at the same time.

Except for a simple conjunctivitis, which is self-limiting, these conditions require expert treatment and a specialist opinion should be sought.

A painful eye with a third nerve palsy often signifies an intracranial aneurysm and should be investigated immediately.

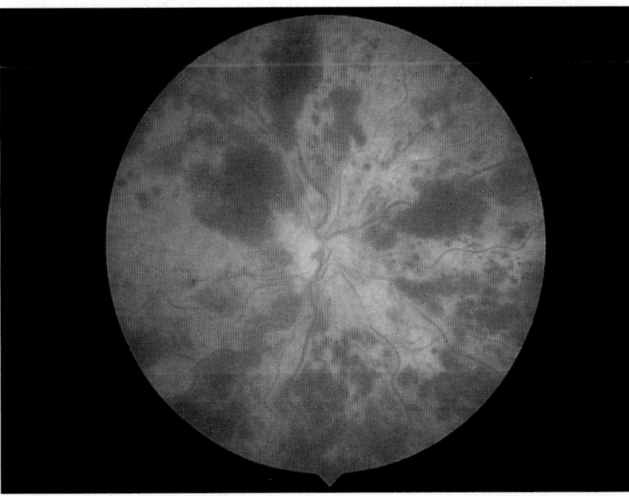

Fig. 36.33 Central retinal vein occlusion.

Painless loss of vision

This may occur in one or both eyes, and the visual loss may be transient or permanent. Possible causes are:

- obstruction of the central retinal artery (Fig. 36.32);
- obstruction of the central retinal vein (Fig. 36.33);
- cranial arteritis;
- ischaemic optic neuropathy;
- migraine and other vascular causes;
- retrobulbar neuritis and papillitis;
- vitreous and retinal haemorrhages;
- retinal detachment (Fig. 36.34);
- macular hole, cyst or haemorrhage;
- cystoid macular oedema often after surgery;
- hysterical blindness.

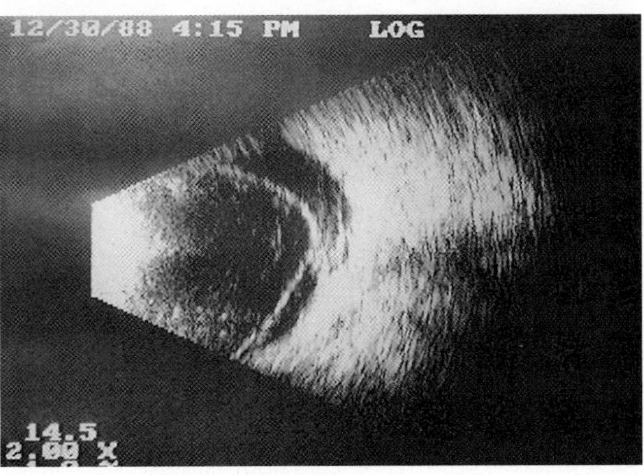

Fig. 36.34 B-scan of a retinal detachment.

Specialist help should be sought in any case of loss of vision. The erythrocyte sedimentation rate and C-reactive protein should be measured immediately if cranial arteritis is suspected, and the carotid system should be examined for bruits and other signs of arteriosclerosis in cases of ischaemic optic neuropathy and central retinal artery occlusion. Glaucoma, hypertension, myeloma and diabetes should be looked for in cases of central vein thrombosis.

Recent developments in eye surgery

In the last two decades, eye surgery has become a microsurgical speciality. Cataract surgery has been transformed by changes in local anaesthesia, implants, phakoemulsification and small incision surgery which allows compressible silicone or acrylic implants to be inserted through a 3-mm incision. The implant power can be more accurately measured by new formulae and the use of A-Scan ultrasonography.

The developments in vitreous surgery have enabled membranes to be peeled off the retina and macular holes to be repaired and have also increased the success rate in retinal detachment surgery with the additional use of gases and silicone oil inserted into the vitreous cavity.

Some paralytic squints can be helped by the use of adjustable sutures or injections of botulinum toxin into the overacting muscles. Refractive error can be treated either by surgery (radial keratometry) or by the excimer laser. This can be combined with LASIK surgery (laser *in situ* keratomeilusis) which involves removing a corneal flap and doing the laser surgery at a deeper level. There have been some concerns about defective contrast sensitivity and problems with night vision after laser correction of myopia. Phakic implants have also been used to correct high refractive errors.

Corneal topography can help in making corneal and refractive surgery more accurate, and the increased use of CT and MRI scans helps to diagnose orbital and intracranial lesions involving the optic pathways (Figs 36.35–36.37). Fluorescein angiography and indocyanine green angiography

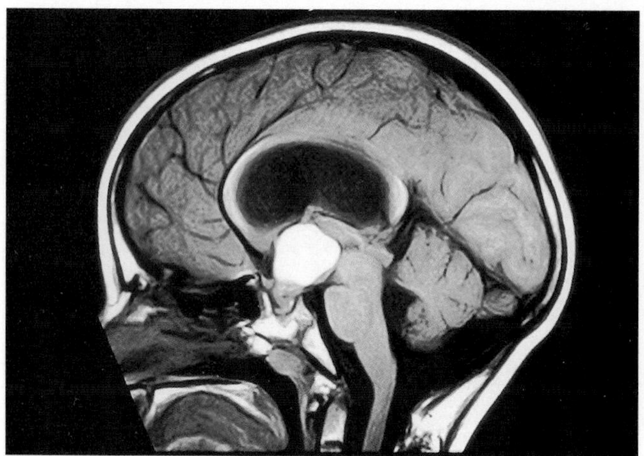

Fig. 36.35 MRI scans, sagittal view. Craniopharyngioma. The mass in the suprasellar cistern is of high signal intensity owing to the proteinaceous fluid that the cyst contains (*courtesy of Dr Juliette Britton*).

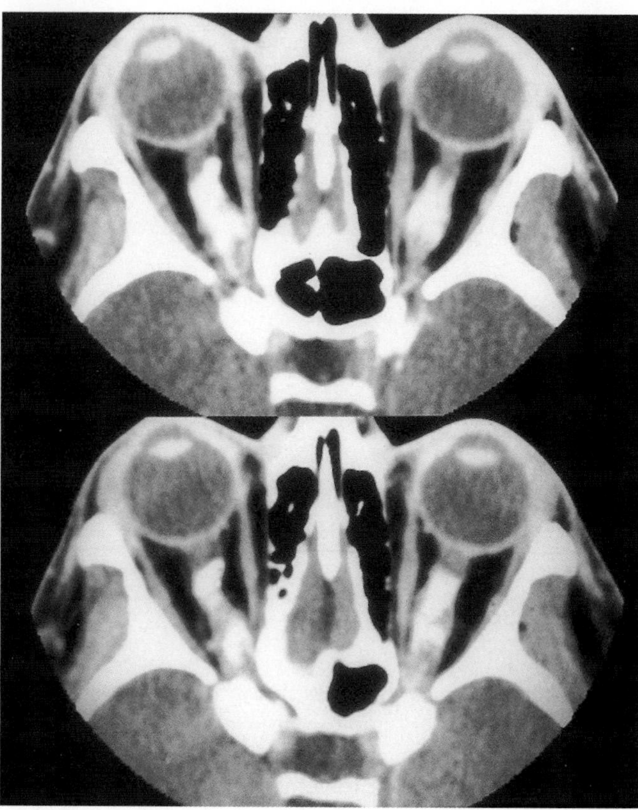

Fig. 36.36 High-resolution CT through orbits showing dense calcification of optic nerve sheaths typical of optic nerve meningioma (*courtesy of Dr Juliette Britton*).

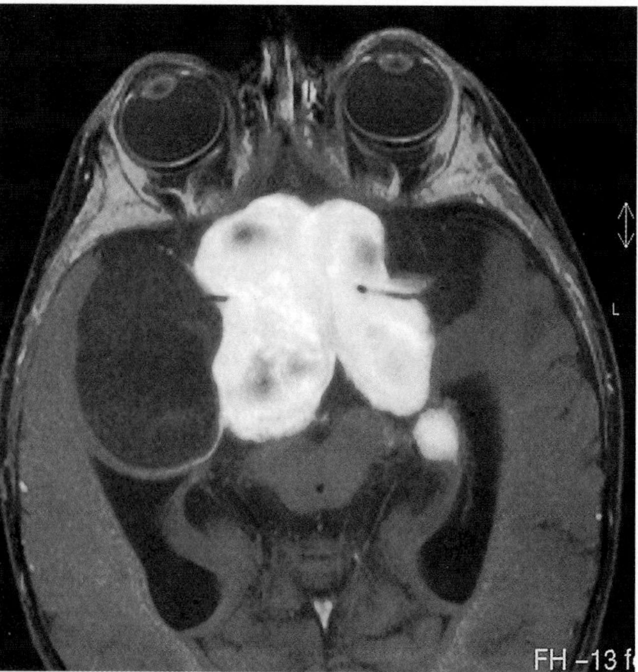

Fig. 36.37 Axial enchanced MRI scans showing a mass involving the optic chasm and extending down the optic nerves and tracts.

help in the diagnosis and occasional treatment of macular lesions. The only advantage of indocyanine green is that the vascularisation of the choroid is much easier to see.

Lasers in ophthalmology

These were originally used as coagulators. The ruby laser was superseded by the argon blue–green laser and then the argon green-only laser, as the blue light was dangerous both to the operator and to the patient's macula. Yellow and red wave lengths are also used and the doubled frequency YAG (yttrium–aluminium–garnet) laser can be used as a coagulator with a frequency of 533. The YAG laser was developed together with extracapsular surgery and is used for capsulotomies, iridotomies and cutting anterior vitreous bands. In its continuous mode it can be used to treat severe glaucomas.

Holmium and erbium lasers have been used to create subconjunctival drainage in glaucoma and the holmium laser can also be used in lacrimal obstruction during a DCR (dacryocystorhinostomy) operation. CO_2 lasers are used to remove external lesion of the eyelids and excimer lasers are used for refractive surgery. The diode laser can be used both as a photocoagulator and for treating the ciliary body in advanced cases of glaucoma. Lasers combined with phakoemulsification to liquefy the human lens are being developed. Laser surgery is making rapid advances and no doubt many new forms of lasers will be developed for use in ophthalmology in the next few years.

Surgical procedures

Excision of an eyeball

Indications include a blind, painful eye, a blind, cosmetically poor eye, intraocular neoplasm and in cadavers for use in corneal grafting.

The operation. The speculum is introduced between the lids and opened. The conjuctiva is picked up with toothed forceps and divided completely all round as near as possible to the cornea, Tenon's capsule is entered, and each of the rectus tendons hooked up on a stabismus hook and divided close to the sclera. The speculum is now pressed backwards and the eyeball projects forwards, blunt scissors, curved on the flat, are insinuated on the inner side of the globe, and these are used to sever the optic nerve. The eyeball can now be drawn forwards with the forceps, and the oblique muscles, together with any other strands of tissue which are still attaching the globe to the orbit, are divided. A swab moistened with hot water and pressed into the orbit will control the haemorrhage. If an orbital implant is inserted to give better eye movement, the muscles are sutured to the implant at the appropriate sites.

Jacques Rene Tenon, 1724–1816. Surgeon, La Salpetière, Paris, France.

Evisceration of an eyeball

As a result of the danger of opening up lymphatic spaces at the back of the globe, and thus favouring meningitis, evisceration is to be preferred to excision in panophthalmitis. The sclera is transfixed with a pointed knife a little behind the corneosclerotic junction, and the cornea is removed entirely by completing the encircling incision in the sclera. The contents of the globe are then removed with a curette, care being exercised to remove all of the uveal tract. At the end of the operation the interior must appear perfectly white.

Incision and curettage of chalazion (meibomian cyst)

The lid margin is everted to allow the application of a meibomian clamp. The ring of the clamp is placed on the palpebral conjunctiva with the granuloma in the centre. An incision is made with a sterile blade in the axis of the gland. The herniating granulomatous tissue is removed with a curette and the gland is scraped clear. Recurrent cysts may have to have the cyst wall dissected away with scissors. A biopsy may be necessary in recurrent cysts to exclude malignant change.

Acquired immunodeficiency syndrome (AIDS) and the eye (See Chapter 9).

Kaposi's sarcomas, purplish or brown nonpruritic nodules or macules, are a frequent early manifestation of AIDS. Commonly affecting the face, especially the tip of the nose, the lesions may involve the eyelids and the conjunctiva.

Fundus lesions are divided into 'noninfective' and 'infective' categories. Noninfective changes consist of cotton-wool spots, haemorrhages and vascular sheathing. These occur in up to 40 per cent of patients with the disease. Infective lesions are usually caused by a cytomegalovirus infection. These lesions may have been described as 'tomato ketchup and salad cream retinopathy', but the pattern is now changing and not so florid. Herpes zoster, toxoplasmosis, pneumocystis and candidiasis lesions can also occur in the retinae. Cytomegalovirus retinitis can be prevented from spreading by treatment with ganciclovir or foscarnet or a combination of the two. These are, however, toxic in the doses required: ganciclovir to the leucocytes, foscarnet to the kidneys.

Intravitreal injections of ganciclovir twice a week until the condition regresses is an alternative if systemic treatment is not tolerated. Intravitreal implants of ganciclovir or foscarnet are now being used.

Neuro-ophthalmological complications in AIDS have been reported, most frequently as nerve palsies associated with intracranial infections with crypotococci and toxoplasmosis, or as a manifestation of an intracranial lymphoma.

Further reading

Blaustein, B.H. (1994) *Ocular Manifestation of Systemic Disease*, Butterworth-Heinemann, Oxford.

Collin, J.R.O. (1989) *A Manual of Systematic Eyelid Surgery*, 2nd edn, Churchill Livingstone, Edinburgh.

Findlay, R.D. and Payne, P.A.G. (1997) *The Eye in General Practice*, Butterworth-Heinemann, Oxford.

Kanski, J. (1995) *Clinical Ophthalmology*, 3rd edn, Butterworth-Heinemann, Oxford.

Roper-Hall, M.J. (ed.) (1989) *Stallard's Eye Surgery*, Wright, Bristol.

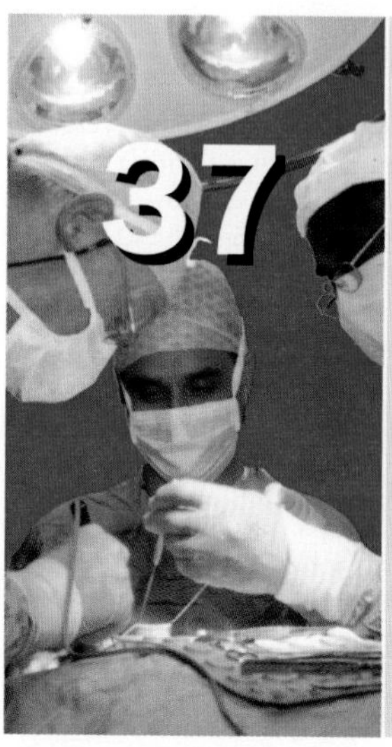

Cleft lip and palate. Developmental abnormalities of the face, palate, jaws and teeth

Cleft lip and palate

Clefts of the lip, alveolus, hard and soft palate are the most common congenital abnormalities of the orofacial structures. They frequently occur as isolated deformities but can be associated with other medical conditions particularly congenital heart disease. They are also an associated feature in over 300 recognized syndromes.

All children born with a cleft lip and palate need thorough paediatric assessment to exclude other congenital abnormalities. In certain circumstances genetic counselling must be sought if a syndrome is suspected.

Incidence

The incidence of cleft lip and palate is one in 600 (1:600) live births, and 1:1000 live births for isolated cleft palate. The incidence increases in Oriental groups (1:500) and decreases in the black population (1:2000). The highest incidence reported for cleft lip and palate occurs in the Native American tribes of Montana, USA (1:276).

Although cleft lip and palate is an extremely diverse and variable congenital abnormality, several distinct subgroups exist, namely cleft lip with/without cleft palate (CL/P), cleft palate alone (CP) and submucous cleft palate (SMCP).

The typical distribution of cleft types is:

- cleft lip alone – 15 per cent;
- cleft lip and palate – 45 per cent;
- isolated cleft palate – 40 per cent.

Cleft lip/palate predominates in males whereas cleft palate alone appears more common in females. In unilateral cleft lip, the deformity affects the left side in 60 per cent of cases.

Aetiology

Contemporary opinion on the aetiology of cleft lip and palate is that cleft lip and palate (CL/P) and isolated cleft palate have a genetic predisposition and a contributory environmental component. A family history of cleft lip and palate in which the first-degree relative is affected increases the risk to one in 25 live births. Genetic influence is more significant in cleft lip/palate than cleft palate alone where environmental factors exert a greater influence.

Environmental factors implicated in clefting include maternal epilepsy and drugs (e.g. steroids, diazepam, phenytoin), although the benefit of antenatal folic acid supplement to prevent cleft lip and palate remains equivocal.

Although most clefts of the lip and palate occur as an isolated deformity, the Pierre Robin sequence remains the most common syndrome. This syndrome comprises isolated cleft palate, retrognathia and a posteriorly displaced tongue (glossoptosis), which is associated with early respiratory and feeding difficulties.

Bailey & Love's Short Practice of Surgery, 23rd edition. Edited by R.C.G. Russell, N.S. Williams and C.J.K. Bulstrode. Published in 2000 by Arnold Publishers.

Pierre Robin, 1867–1950. French histologist and stomatologist.

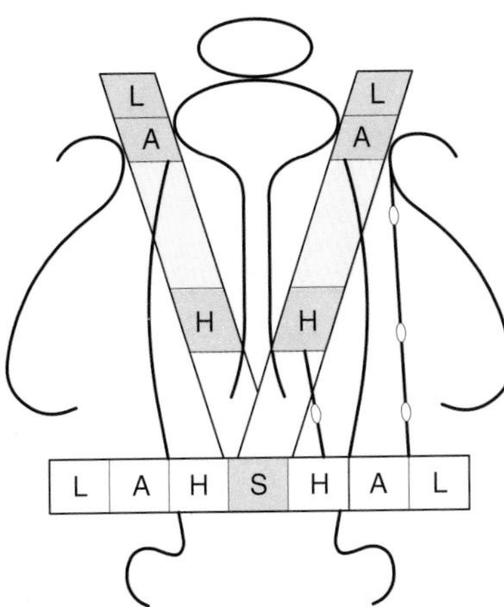

Fig. 37.1 LAHSAL: an anatomical representation of cleft lip (L), alveolus (A), and hard (H) and soft palate (S).

Isolated cleft palate is more commonly associated with a syndrome than cleft lip/palate and cleft lip alone. Over 150 syndromes are associated with cleft lip and palate, although Stickler (ophthalmic and musculoskeletal abnormalities), Shprintzen (cardiac anomalies), Down's, Apert's and Treacher Collins' are most frequently encountered.

Classification

Any classification for such a diverse and varied condition as cleft lip and palate needs to be simple, concise, flexible, exact but graphic. It must be suitable for computerisation but descriptive and morphological. An example of such a classification is the LAHSHAL system which is able to describe site, size, extent as well as type of cleft (Fig. 37.1).

Complete clefts of the lip, alveolus, and hard and soft palate are designated capital L, A, H and S, respectively, whereas incomplete clefts are recorded in small letters; microform clefts are documented with asterisks. Hence, LAHSHAL is the anatomical paraphrase of a complete bilateral cleft lip and palate. Another example, lahSh, represents an incomplete right unilateral cleft lip and alveolus with a complete cleft of soft palate extending partly on to the hard palate.

Primary management

Antenatal diagnosis

An antenatal diagnosis of cleft lip, whether unilateral or bilateral, is possible by ultrasound scan after 18 weeks of gestation. Isolated cleft palate cannot be diagnosed on an antenatal scan. When an antenatal diagnosis is confirmed, referral to a cleft surgeon is appropriate for counselling to allay fears. Photographs of cleft lip shown to parents 'before and after' surgery are invaluable. Introduction to a parent support group and meeting parents of a child with a similar cleft who has undergone surgery may also be extremely helpful.

Feeding

Most babies born with cleft lip and palate feed well and thrive provided appropriate advice is given and support available. Some mothers are successful in breastfeeding, particularly when the cleft is incomplete and confined to the lip. Good feeding patterns can be established with soft bottles (e.g. Mead Johnson) and modified teats (orthodontic, Nuyk). Simple measures, such as enlarging the hole in the teat, often suffice. Feeding plates, constructed from a dental impression of the upper jaw, are rarely necessary to improve feeding. Some babies are provided with an active plate which aims not only to improve feeding but also reduce the width of the cleft lip and palate prior to surgery. The long-term benefit of such a regime remains unproven.

Airway

Major respiratory obstruction is uncommon and occurs exclusively in babies with Pierre Robin sequence. Hypoxic episodes during sleep and feeding can be life threatening. Intermittent airway obstruction is more frequent and managed by nursing the baby prone. More severe and persistent airway compromise can be managed by 'retained nasopharyngeal intubation' to maintain the airway. Surgical adhesion of the tongue to the lower lip (labioglossopexy) in the first few days after birth is an alternative but less commonly practised method of management.

Principles of cleft surgery

The ultimate goal in cleft lip and palate management is a patient with normal appearance of lip, nose and face, whose speech is normal and whose dentition and facial growth fall within the range of normal development.

Surgical techniques are aimed to restore normal anatomy. With the exception of rare conditions such as holoprosencephaly, there is no true hypoplasia of the tissues involved either side of the cleft. There is, however, displacement, deformation and underdevelopment of the muscles and facial skeleton. Emphasis is placed on muscular reconstruction of the lip, nose and face, as well as muscles of the soft palate. Normal or near-normal anatomy promotes normal function, thereby encouraging normal growth and development of lip, nose, palate and facial skeleton. An in-depth understanding of the anatomy of the cleft is invaluable if the surgeon is to achieve normal, or near-normal, anatomical reconstruction.

Anatomy of cleft lip and palate

Cleft lip

The abnormalities in cleft lip are the direct consequence of disruption of the muscles of the upper lip and nasolabial

John L. Down, b. 1828. British physician.
Eugene Apert, 1868–1940. French paediatrician.
Edward Treacher Collins, 1862–1932. Surgeon, Charing Cross and Moorfields Eye Hospital, London, England.

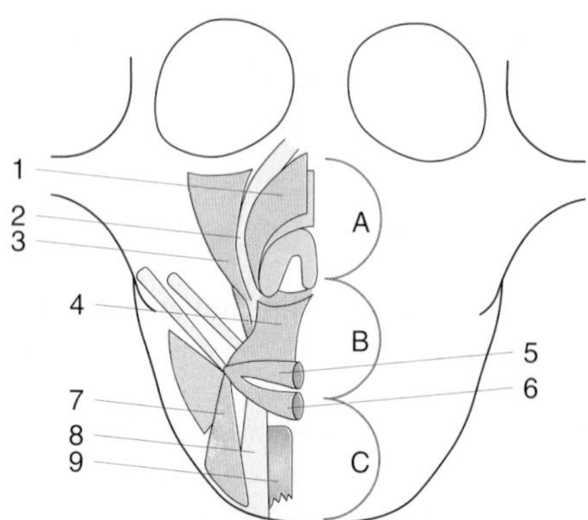

Fig. 37.2 The muscle chains of the face: frontal view. A, Nasolabial (muscles 1–3); B, bilabial (muscles 4–6); C, labiomental (muscles 7–9). Muscles: 1, transverse nasalis; 2, levator labii superioris alaeque nasi; 3, levator labii superioris; 4, orbicularis oris (oblique head) – upper lip; 5, orbicularis oris (horizontal head) – upper lip; 6, orbicularis oris – lower lip; 7, depressor anguli oris; 8, depressor labii inferioris; 9, mentalis.

region. The facial muscles (Fig. 37.2) can be divided into the three muscular rings of Delaire.

Unilateral cleft lip. In the unilateral cleft lip, the nasolabial and bilabial muscle rings are disrupted on one side resulting in an asymmetrical deformity involving the external nasal cartilages, nasal septum and anterior maxilla (premaxilla) (Fig. 37.3). These deformities influence the mucocutaneous tissues causing displacement of nasal skin on to the lip and retraction of labial skin, as well as changes to the vermilion and lip mucosa. All of these changes need to be considered in planning the surgical repair of the unilateral cleft lip.

Bilateral cleft lip. In the bilateral cleft lip, the deformity is more profound but symmetrical. The two superior muscular rings are disrupted on both sides producing a flaring of the nose (due to lack of nasolabial muscle continuity), a protrusive premaxilla and an area of skin in front of the premaxilla, known as the prolabium, devoid of muscle (Fig. 37.4). As in the unilateral cleft lip, the muscular, cartilaginous and skeletal deformities influence the mucocutaneous tissues, which must be respected in planning the repair of the bilateral cleft lip.

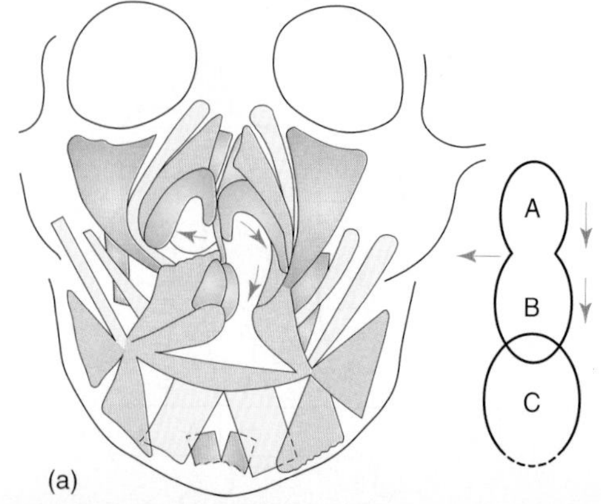

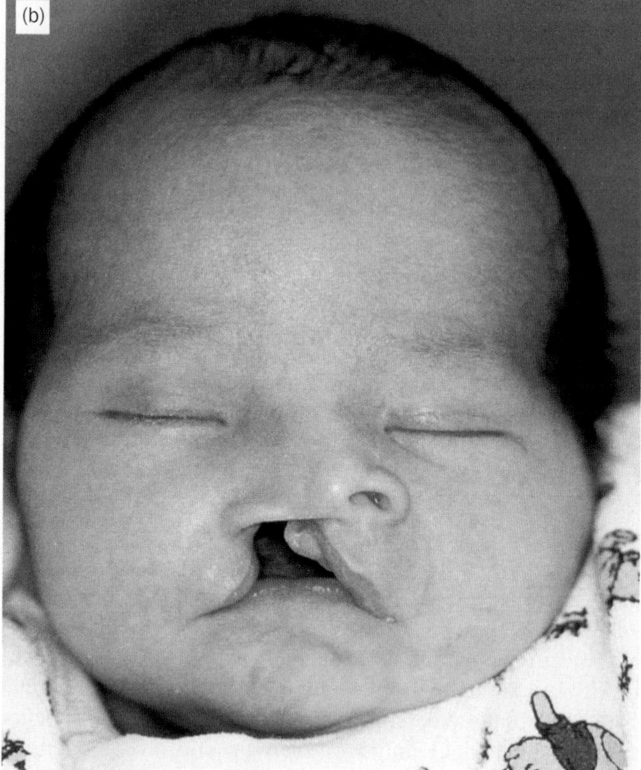

Fig. 37.3 (a) Schematic representation of the disruption of the nasolabial and bilabial muscle chains in unilateral cleft lip. (b) Unilateral cleft lip before muscular reconstruction.

Cleft palate

Embryologically, the *primary* palate consists of all anatomical structures anterior to the incisive foramen, namely the alveolus and upper lip. The *secondary* palate is defined as the remainder of the palate behind the incisive foramen divided into the hard palate and, more posteriorly, the soft palate.

Cleft palate results in failure of fusion of the two palatine shelves. This failure may be confined to the soft palate alone or involve both hard and soft palate. When the cleft of the hard palate remains attached to the nasal septum and vomer, the cleft is termed *incomplete*. When the nasal septum and vomer are completely separated from the palatine processes, the cleft palate is termed *complete*.

Soft palate. In the normal soft palate, closure of the velopharynx, which is essential for normal speech, is achieved by five different muscles functioning in a complete but co-ordinated fashion. In general, the muscle fibres of the soft palate are orientated transversely with no significant attachment to the hard palate.

In a cleft of the soft palate, the muscle fibres are orientated in an anteroposterior direction, inserting into the posterior edge of the hard palate (Fig. 37.5).

Hard palate. The normal hard palate can be divided into three anatomical and physiological zones (Fig. 37.6). The

Jean Delaire. Professor of Stomatology and Maxillofacial Surgery, University of Nantes, France, 1960–91.

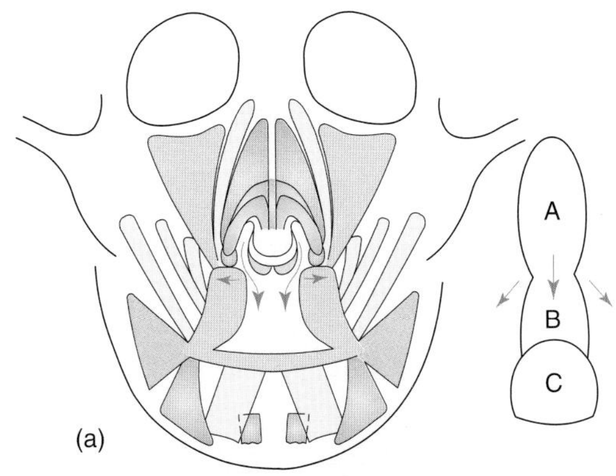

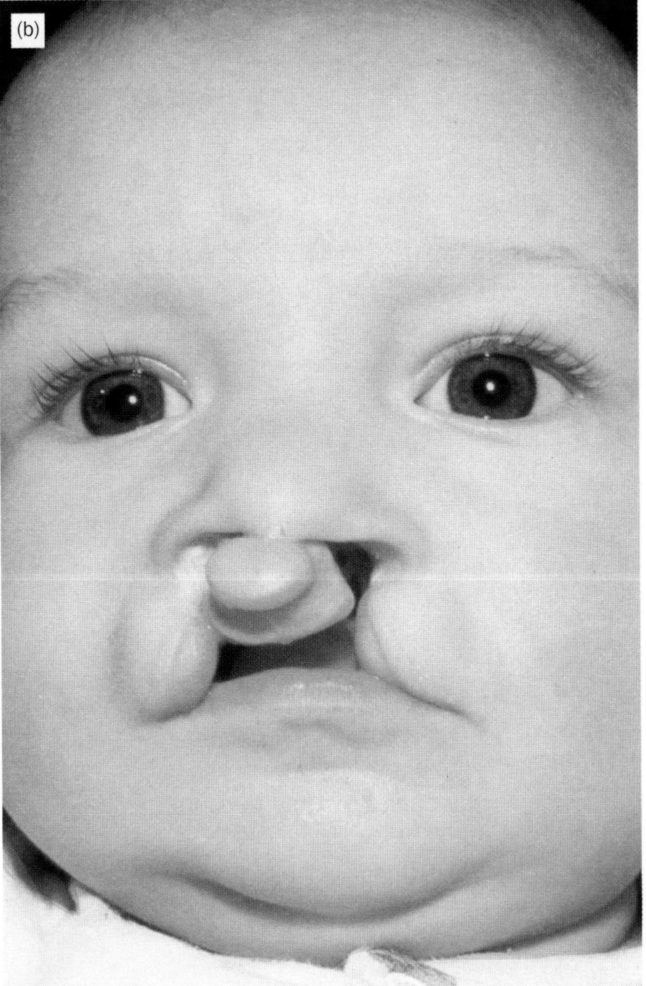

Fig. 37.4 (a) Schematic representation of the disruption of the nasolabial and bilabial muscle chains in bilateral cleft lip. (b) Bilateral cleft lip before muscular reconstruction.

central *palatal fibromucosa* is very thin and lies directly below the floor of nose. The *maxillary fibromucosa* is thick and contains the greater palatine neurovascular bundle. The *gingival fibromucosa* lies more lateral and adjacent to the teeth.

In performing surgical closure of cleft palate the changes associated with the cleft must be understood to obtain an

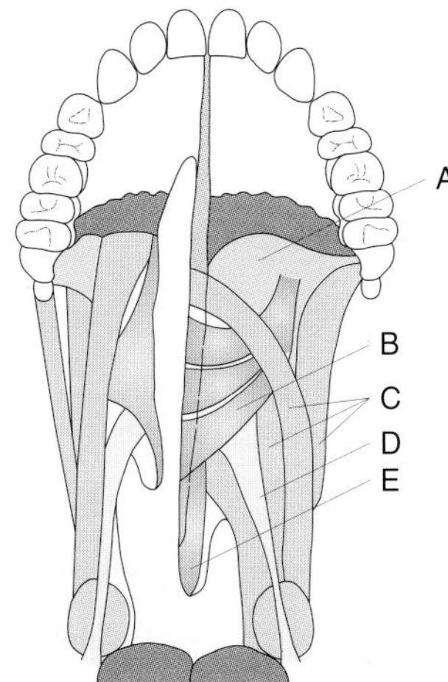

Fig. 37.5 Muscles of the soft palate: (left) cleft palate; (right) normal anatomy. A, Tensor palati; B, levator palati; C, palatopharyngeus; D, palatoglossus; E, musculus uvulae.

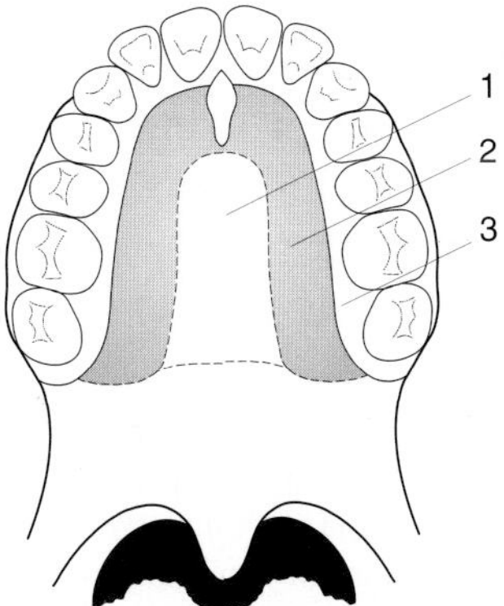

Fig. 37.6 The three mucosal zones of the hard palate: (1) palatal fibromucosa; (2) maxillary fibromucosa; (3) gingival fibromucosa.

anatomical and functional repair. In complete cleft palate the median part of the palatal vault is absent and the palatal fibromucosa is reduced in size. The maxillary and gingival fibromucosa are not modified in thickness, width or position.

Surgical techniques

There have been many different surgical techniques and sequences advocated in cleft lip and palate management. Cleft lip repair is commonly performed between 3 and 6 months of age, whereas cleft palate repair is frequently performed between 6 and 18 months.

The Delaire technique and sequence (Table 37.1) is one of many regimes currently practised.

Cleft lip surgery

Skin incisions (Figs 37.7 and 37.8) are developed to restore displaced tissues including skin and cartilage to their normal position, whilst gaining access to the facial, nasal and lip musculature.

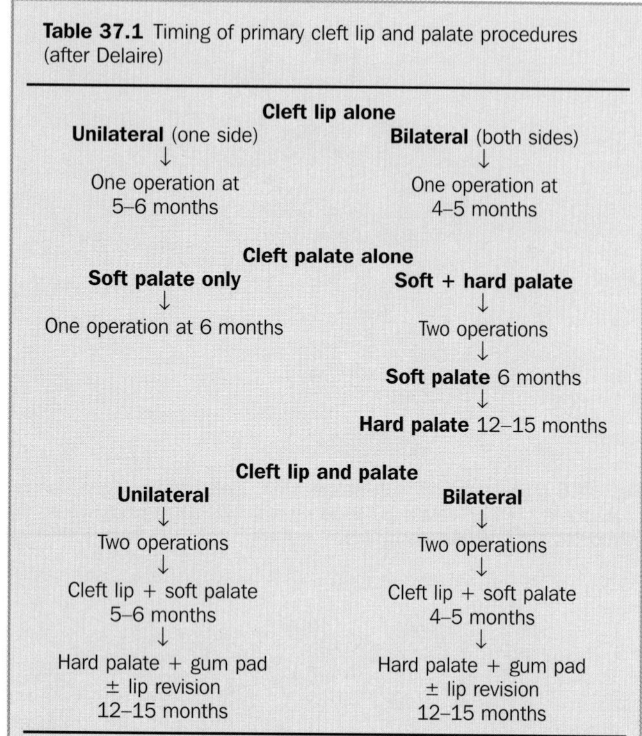

Table 37.1 Timing of primary cleft lip and palate procedures (after Delaire)

Cleft lip alone

Unilateral (one side)	**Bilateral** (both sides)
↓	↓
One operation at 5–6 months	One operation at 4–5 months

Cleft palate alone

Soft palate only	**Soft + hard palate**
↓	↓
One operation at 6 months	Two operations
	↓
	Soft palate 6 months
	↓
	Hard palate 12–15 months

Cleft lip and palate

Unilateral	**Bilateral**
↓	↓
Two operations	Two operations
↓	↓
Cleft lip + soft palate 5–6 months	Cleft lip + soft palate 4–5 months
↓	↓
Hard palate + gum pad ± lip revision 12–15 months	Hard palate + gum pad ± lip revision 12–15 months

Muscular continuity is achieved by subperiosteal undermining over the anterior maxilla. Nasolabial muscles are anchored to the premaxilla with nonresorbable sutures. Oblique muscles of orbicularis oris are sutured to the base of the anterior nasal spine and cartilaginous nasal septum. Closure of the cleft lip is completed by suturing the horizontal fibres of orbicularis oris to achieve a functioning oral sphincter (Figs 37.9 and 37.10).

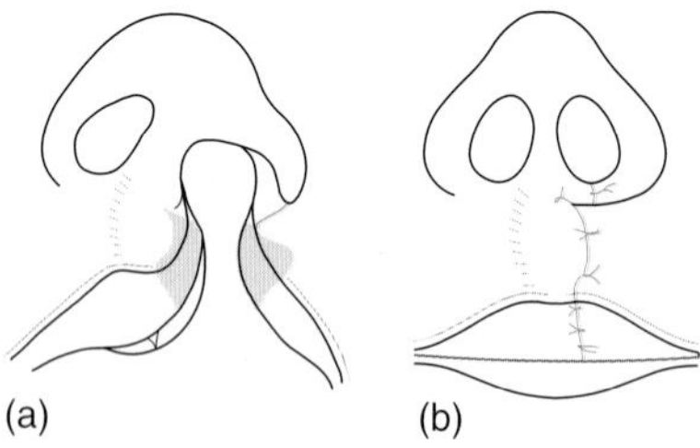

Fig. 37.7 Skin incisions for left unilateral complete cleft lip (*after Delaire*).

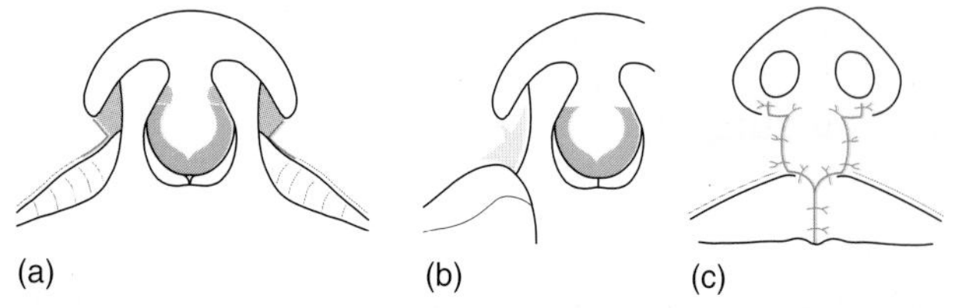

Fig. 37.8 Skin incisions for bilateral complete cleft lip (*after Delaire*).

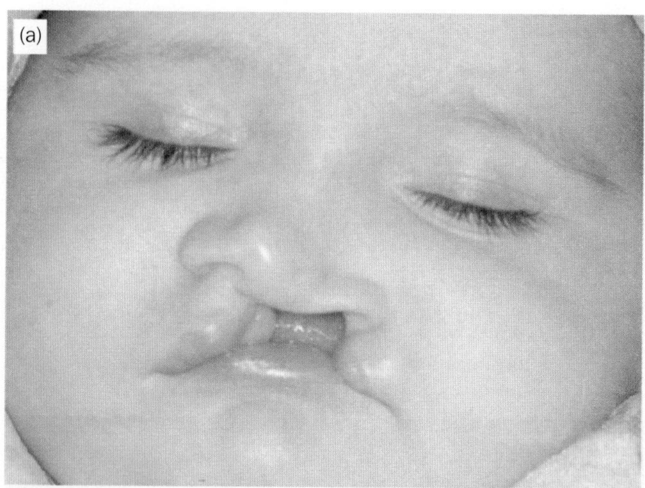

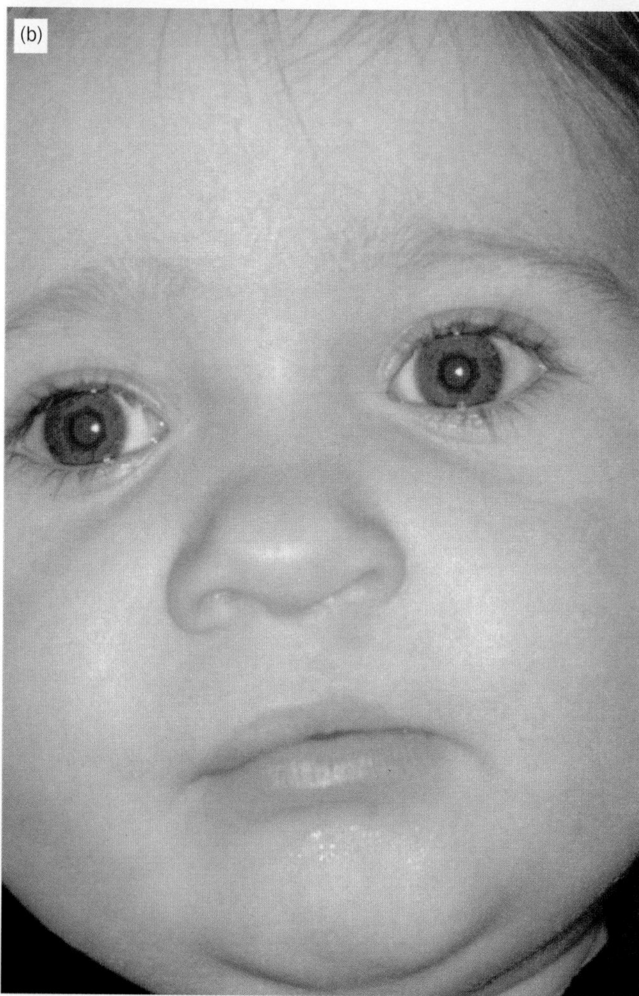

Fig. 37.9 Unilateral cleft lip (a) before and (b) after muscular reconstruction.

Cleft palate surgery

Cleft palate closure can be achieved by one- or two-stage palatoplasty. The surgical principle is mobilization and reconstruction of the aberrant soft palate musculature (Fig. 37.11),

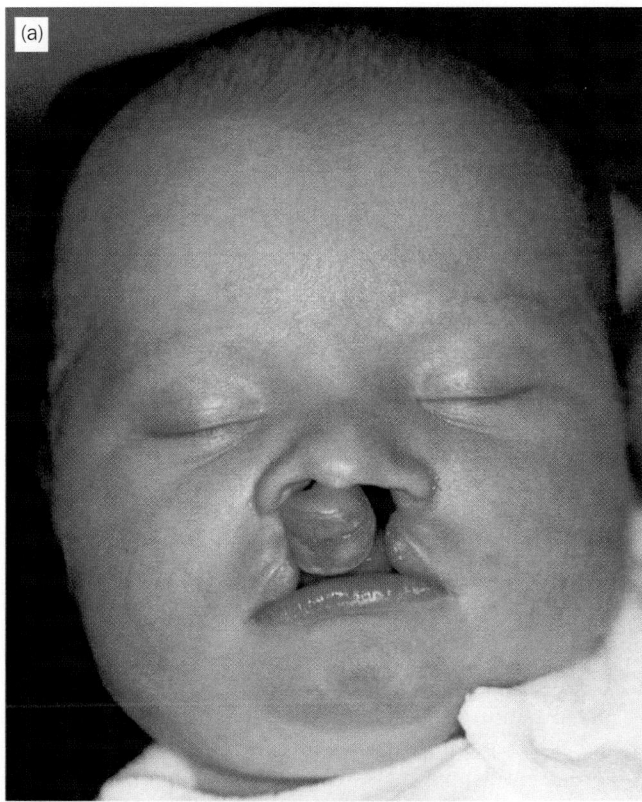

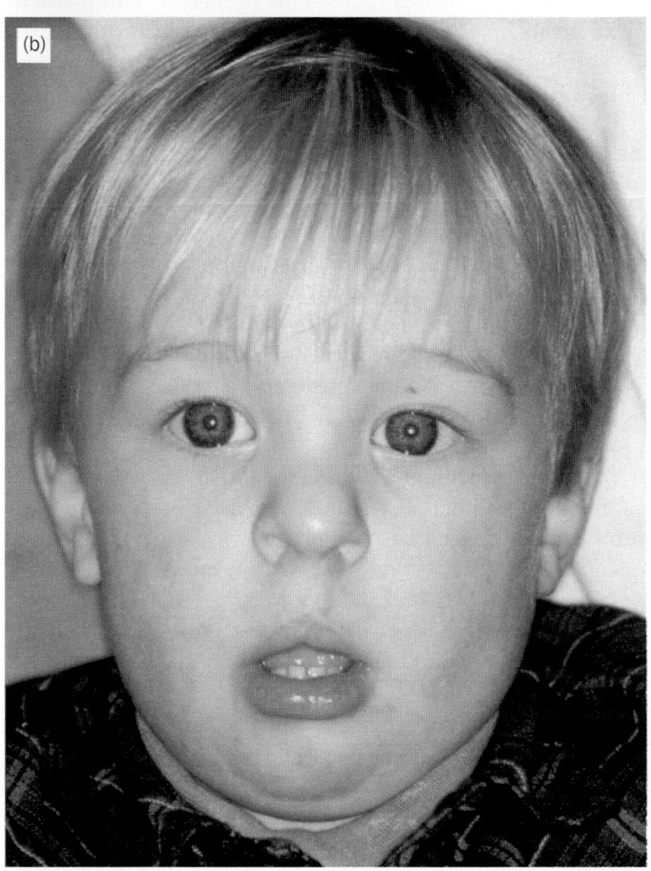

Fig. 37.10 Bilateral cleft lip (a) before and (b) after muscular reconstruction.

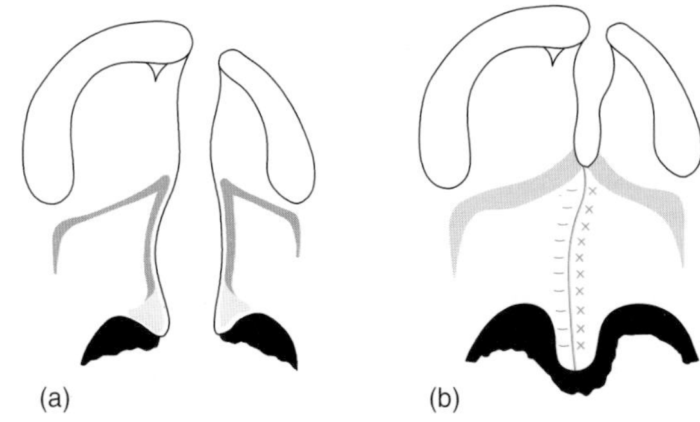

Fig. 37.11 Method of repair of cleft palate. First-stage palatoplasty to reconstruct muscles of the soft palate.

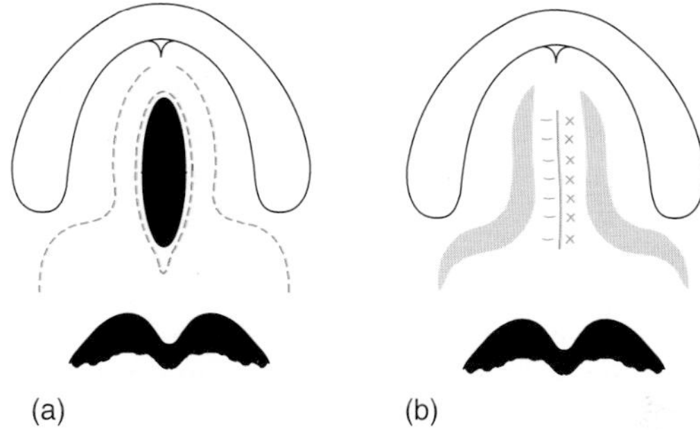

Fig. 37.12 Schematic representation of closure of the hard palate. Second-stage palatoplasty achieved with a two-layered closure.

together with closure of the residual hard palate cleft by minimal dissection and subsequent scar formation (Fig. 37.12). Excess scar formation in the palate adversely affects growth and development of the maxilla. The philosophy of two-stage closure encourages a physiological narrowing of the hard palate cleft to minimize surgical dissection at the time of the second procedure.

Secondary management

Following primary surgery, regular review by a multidisciplinary team is essential. Many aspects of cleft care require long-term review.

Hearing

Eustachian tube dysfunction plays a central role in the pathogenesis of otitis media with effusion in babies and children born with a cleft palate. Children with a cleft lip alone exhibit the same frequency of otitis media as their age-matched noncleft counterparts. It has been recently recognised that a child with a craniofacial anomaly including cleft lip and palate is at increased risk of a sensorineural hearing deficit. All children born with a cleft lip and palate should undergo assessment before 12 months of age for *sensorineural and conductive hearing loss* by auditory brainstem responses (ABR) and tympanometry, respectively.

Bartolomeo Eustachio, b. 1520. Italian anatomist.

Sensorineural hearing loss is managed with a hearing aid, whilst the management of secretory otitis media remains more controversial. Early (6–12 months old) prophylactic myringotomy and grommet temporarily eliminates middle ear effusion. Regular audiological testing may be as appropriate, reserving surgery for established secretory otitis media with infection. No firm evidence is available to support the interventional approach over the conservative regime. Nevertheless, the relationship between hearing loss and potential speech problems remains important. Regular audiological assessment during childhood is of utmost importance.

Speech

Initial speech assessment should be performed early (18 months) and repeated regularly to ensure that problems are identified early and managed appropriately.

Common speech problems associated with cleft lip and palate are:

- Velopharyngeal incompetence – this is associated with increased nasal airflow and resonance producing a nasal or 'hypernasal' quality to speech. It frequently reflects poor function of soft palate associated with inadequate muscle repair.
- Articulation problems – these either arise as a compensatory mechanism to overcome velopharyngeal incompetence or, less commonly, are due to jaw/dental and occlusal abnormalities.

Investigation by:

- videofluoroscopy
- nasal airflow studies (aerophonoscopy)
- nasendoscopy

is helpful in defining the exact mechanism of the problem which aids management.

Speech problems are managed by:

- speech and language therapy;
- secondary palatal surgery:
  - intravelar veloplasty (muscular reconstruction of soft palate);
  - pharyngoplasty;
- speech-training devices.

Dental

Dental anomalies are common findings in children with cleft lip and/or palate. Various phenomena include delayed tooth development and delayed eruption of teeth; morphological abnormalities are also well documented. The number of teeth may be reduced (hypodontia) or increased (hyperdontia), and occurs most commonly in the region of the cleft alveolus involving the maxillary lateral incisor tooth. These abnormalities can occur in both primary and secondary dentition.

Table 37.2 Timing of secondary cleft procedures

Secondary procedure	*Age (years)*
Lip/nose revision	2–adult
Velopharyngeal surgery	3–8
Alveolar bone graft	7–11
Orthognathic surgery	16+
Rhinoplasty	16+

All children with cleft lip and palate should undergo regular dental examination. Dental management should also include preventive measures such as dietary advice, fluoride supplements and fissure sealants.

A well-maintained and disease-free dentition in childhood is an absolute prerequisite for orthodontic treatment.

Orthodontic management

Many children with cleft lip and palate require orthodontic treatment.

Orthodontic treatment is commonly carried out in two phases:

- mixed dentition (8–10 years) – to expand the maxillary arches as a prelude to alveolar bone graft;
- permanent dentition (14–18 years) – to align the dentition and provide a normal functioning occlusion. This phase of treatment may also include surgical correction of a malpositioned/retrusive maxilla by maxillary osteotomy (Fig. 37.13).

Secondary surgery for cleft lip and palate

Good outcome in cleft lip and palate is directly attributable to the quality of primary surgery. Poorly executed primary surgery leads to residual deformity of the lip and nose, together with poor speech. Impaired growth of the midface (maxilla) is now attributed to poor and traumatic primary surgery. Surgical techniques must endeavour to minimize scarring.

Despite adequate primary surgery, residual problems do occur and are managed with appropriate secondary procedures (Table 37.2).

The management of children with cleft lip and palate is complex, requiring the skill of a multidisciplinary team. Each team should include professionals who are appropriately qualified with specialist training, treating an adequate number of patients per year. Meticulous record-keeping of photography, radiology, dental casts and speech recording are indispensable, and permit regular audit and improved outcomes.

Developmental abnormalities of the face, palate, jaws and teeth

Treacher Collins' syndrome (Fig. 37.14)

Treacher Collins' syndrome or mandibular facial dysostosis has a variable presentation. The cardinal features are of an

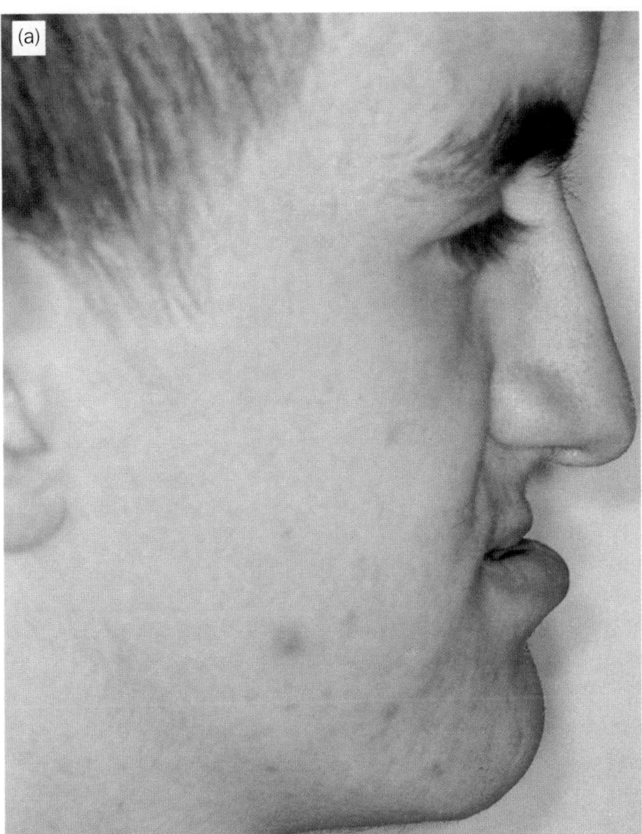

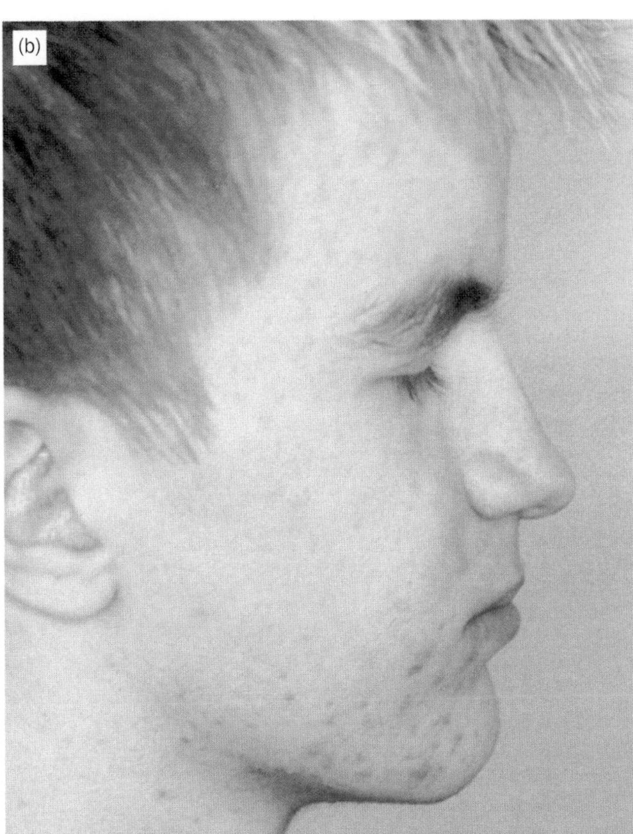

Fig. 37.13 Correction of midface retrusion by maxillary advancement osteotomy (a) before and (b) after surgery.

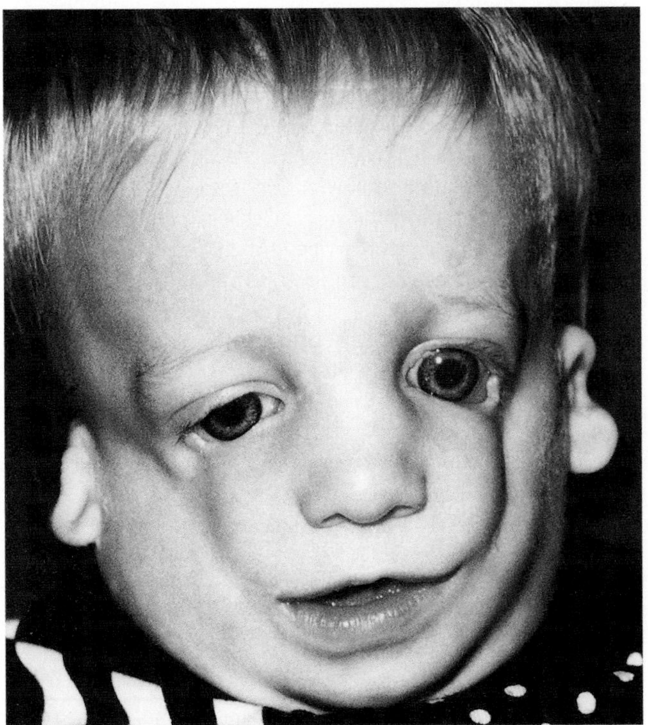

Fig. 37.14 Teacher Collins' syndrome is characterised by antimongoloid palpable fissures and coloboma, with hypoplasia of the midface. (*Reproduced with kind permission of Mr S. Wall.*)

antimongoloid palpable fissure with a coloboma or groove in the outer portion of the lower lids with deficiency of the eyelashes. There is generally hypoplasia of the midface and zygomatic bones, and occasionally of the mandible. There may be malformation of the external ear unilaterally or bilaterally. Macrostomia and facial clefts may accompany this condition.

Crouzon's disease (Fig. 37.15)

This is also known as craniofacial dysostosis and may occur together with syndactyly. This is a genetic disease characterised by protruberant frontal bones, a hypoplastic maxilla with relative mandibular prognathism. The hypoplasia may be so severe that the globes of the eye are protruberant to a degree that corneal ulceration and loss of sight can occur. There may well be a hyperteliorism and divergent strabismus. Most patients have a normal cerebral function.

Pierre Robin's syndrome

This condition is characterised by micrognathia (small lower jaw) and glossoptosis. There is almost always a cleft palate. The overall impression is of bird faces. It does not appear to be an inherited syndrome and it has been thought that extreme flexion of the neck during foetal life may contribute

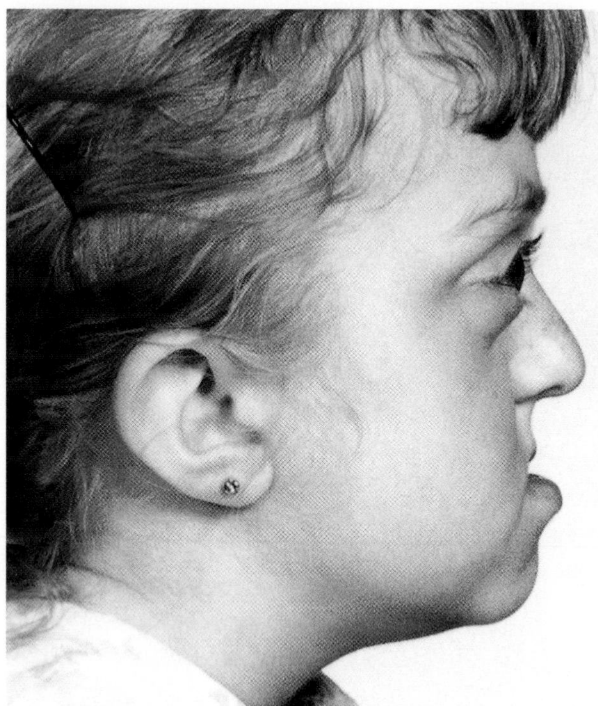

Fig. 37.15 Crouzon's disease is characterised by protruberant frontal bones and hypoplastic maxilla with prominent globes. (*Reproduced with kind permission of Mr S. Wall.*)

to the disorder: the tongue is thrust upwards between the palatal shelves which fail to fuse so causing the cleft palate to develop. Recent work on gene function suggests that deficiencies one of the transformation growth factors (TGFB3) is responsible. Respiratory obstruction due to poor control of the tongue and difficulties with suckling require careful neonatal management.

Hemifacial microsomia (first arch syndrome – Fig. 37.16)

In this condition tissues which seem to have been derived from the first branchial arch are deficient. A better understanding of the embryology, and experimental work by Poswillo, have indicated that there may be haemorrhage from the stapedial artery around the sixth week of intrauterine development. Tissues that were in development at that time are damaged by the haemorrhage and the subsequent reorganisation so that tissues are smaller or fail to develop completely. The expression is variable but there is always hypoplasia or absence of the mandibular condyle and part of the ramus of the mandible. The masticatory muscles are deficient, and the external, middle and inner ear may fail to develop. Thus, there is the appearance of hypoplasia or the affected side of the face and head with the pinna absent and the external auditory meatus rudimentary or absent. Skin tags over the side of the face beneath the ear are common. The child is almost always deaf in the affected ear. As the growth centre at the mandibular condyle is deficient, the deformity progresses throughout early life and particularly at puberty. The patient requires expert craniofacial surgery that is delayed as long as possible but is generally carried out at the age of 8 years. Further surgery is usually required postpuberty.

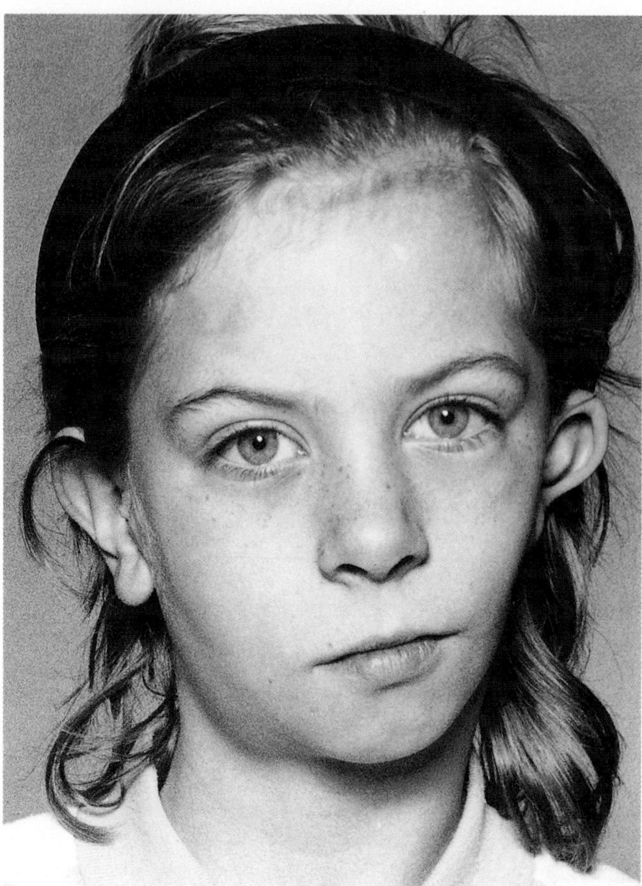

Fig. 37.16 Hemifacial microsomia. The presentation is variable but there is always hypoplasia or absence of the mandibular condyle and part of the ramus of the mandible, with distorted pinna and deformed hearing apparatus. (*Reproduced with kind permission of Mr S. Wall.*)

Maxillomandibular disproportion

Angle, an American orthodontist, put the occlusion of the teeth into three classes:

- class I – normal relationship of the lower to the upper teeth in the molar area;
- class II – the lower molar teeth are placed posterior to the normal position;
- class III – the posterior molar teeth are placed anterior to the normal position.

Octave Crouzon, 1874–1938. French physician.

David E. Poswillo. Formerly Professor of Oral Surgery, The United Medical and Dental Schools (Guy's Hospital Dental School), London, England. Formerly Professor of Teratology, Royal College of Surgeons of England.

This classification has been extended to include the facial skeleton such that:

- skeletal II – small mandible is placed posterior to the normal position in relation to the maxilla;
- skeletal III – mandible is placed anterior to the normal position relative to the maxilla.

It is a helpful description of a facial skeletal deformity, but it only describes the mandible in relation to the maxilla which itself may be hyperplastic or hypoplastic. Thus, the 'Hapsburg jaw' which described the familial features of the royal houses of Europe in the nineteenth century describes a large lower jaw, a hyperplastic mandible, which is frequently associated with a hypoplastic maxilla which accentuates the deformity in the mandible.

The most common deformity of the facial skeleton in the Caucasian is the hypoplastic mandible – skeletal class II – which gives the impression of a hyperplastic maxilla as the upper teeth are very prominent. A hyperplastic maxilla alone is very unusual. Bimaxillary protrusion is a racial characteristic of the African races. Occasionally the mandible may grow large and asymmetric owing to hyperplasia of the mandibular condylar neck. Rarely, a hemimandible may be hypoplastic.

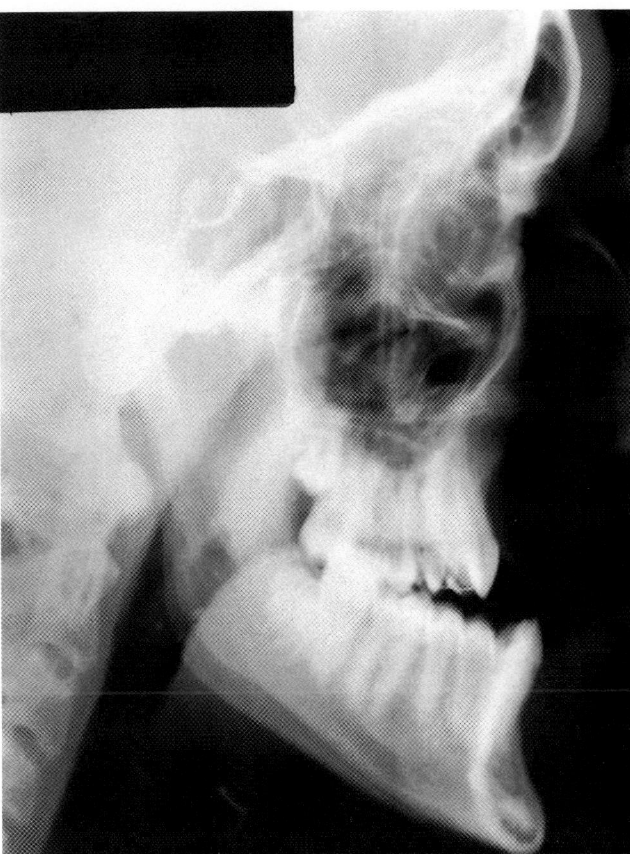

Fig. 37.17 Gross maxillomandibular disproportion before treatment by bimaxillary osteotomies.

Orthognathic surgery

Orthognathic surgery is the term given to the correction of deformities of the teeth and jaws. It should always be undertaken in close co-operation with consultant orthodontists and consultant oral and maxillofacial surgeons. Correction of maxillomandibular disproportion is frequently directed towards changing the position of both the maxilla and the mandible, usually at the end of the growth period. It is essential that there should be a team approach, with treatment planning usually commencing at the age of 12–13 years. Treatment of the syndromes, some of which are described above, may require much earlier treatment (see below). The orthodontist prepares the dental arches for their new position preoperatively, and continues postoperatively with the ultimate goal of a perfect dental occlusion within 6 months of the surgery.

The orthognathic surgery is generally carried out through incisions within the mouth avoiding skin incisions where possible. The upper and lower jaws are mobilised individually and fixed by means of small stainless steel or titanium plates and fixed by means of stainless steel or titanium miniplates. Splinting of the upper and lower teeth by various means is undertaken intraoperatively to achieve an accurate and planned occlusion. Usually it is possible to leave the mandible free for the mouth to be opened at the dangerous times in the first 24 hours postoperatively. An example of maxillomandibular disproportion may be seen in Fig. 37.17, with the effect of bimaxillary surgery in Fig. 37.18.

Craniofacial surgery

Craniofacial surgery is undertaken in a few designated centres in the UK where the team of an orthodontist and a maxillofacial surgeon is augmented to include a craniofacial surgeon (usually with plastic surgery training), neurosurgeons and ear, nose and throat (ENT) surgeons. The whole team includes dedicated nursing staff, both in the ward and in the operating theatre, speech therapists and audiologists. The principles of treatment are to correct deformities from the cranium downwards. Thus, in Crouzon's disease (see above) the craniofacial surgeon with the neurosurgeon will correct the cranial deformity in the first 2–3 years of life, and will return to deal with the midface by the age of 6 or 7 years, often in co-operation with the maxillofacial surgeon. Final correction will be to the mid and lower face with the patient in their mid-teens where they may be treated much like a more straightforward orthognathic case. The surgical principles involve dividing the various bones of the face and skull, inserting bone grafts where appropriate, and maintaining the position of the bones by miniplates or microplates made of stainless steel or titanium. The surgery to the cranium as far forward as the nose and lateral border of the orbits may be carried out through a coronal incision, pulling the scalp downwards and forwards over the face. For access to particular areas, incisions are made through the skin around the orbits at sites where the scarring is barely noticeable.

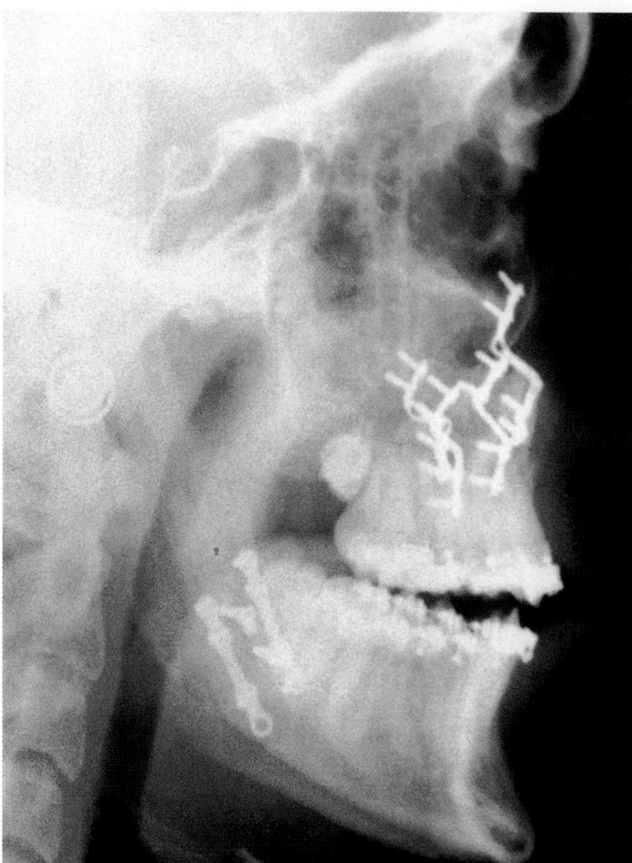

Fig. 37.18 Gross maxillomandibular disproportion shown in Fig. 37.17 after it has been treated by bimaxillary osteotomies.

New developments in osteogenic distraction in the early growth period in the severe abnormalities may greatly change and reduce the major surgery that is currently undertaken on patients with facial deformity.

Other developmental abnormalities in the face and jaws

Failure of fusion, or inclusions of epithelium where various processes meet during development, can lead to cysts and fistulae around the face, the jaws and the neck. Cysts may develop and then become infected, leading to persistent sinuses. Examples are as follows.

- *Pre-auricular cyst* – fusion of the six tubercles around the external auditory canal can lead to formation of one or more narrow, blind pits or, perhaps, a cyst. Infection of the cyst may lead to a persistent discharging sinus which would need to be excised.
- *Periauricular dermoid cyst* – these may develop from under the pinna as a fluctuant swelling, usually posteriorly. They occur in the position where the two adjacent auricular tubicles should merge.
- *Globulomaxillary cyst* – cysts may develop in the alveolus in the position where the globulomaxillary processes should fuse with the frontonasal process. The cyst occurs lateral to a vital second upper incisor and canine. These have to be differentiated from a radicular cyst developing on a nonvital lateral incisor.
- *Nasolabial cyst* – these occur in a similar position to the globulomaxillary cyst, but in the soft tissues of the upper lip. They are extremely rare.
- *Cysts of the incisive canal* – the two palatal shelves fuse with the premaxilla at the site of the exit from the palate of the nerve of the incisive canal. This canal may form a cyst or be patent, leading to recurrent infections in this area. Those that have a patent canal may enjoy the party trick of producing a high-pitched squeaking or whistling sound as they raise the pressure in the mouth, discharging air into the nose.
- *Oral dermoids* – these are derived from embryonic epithelium and can occur anywhere where the facial processes fail to fuse completely. They are rare, but the most common site is the midline of the floor of the mouth. They should not be confused with the ranula, which is a mucous extravasation cyst derived from the lingual gland.
- *Branchial cysts* – these occur in the lateral aspect of the upper neck of young adults as a slow-growing fluctuant swelling. It had been assumed that these occur as a result of failure of fusion branchial arches. They are lined with lymphoid tissue, and the current view is that they are derived from cystic transformation of glandular epithelium included in lymphoid aggregates during embryogenesis. The current nomenclature is lymphoepithelial cyst.
- *Oral tori* (Figs 37.19 and 37.20) – it is uncertain as to whether these are true developmental abnormalities. They occur at two major sites, the most common lies on the medial side of the mandibular alveolus in the region of the premolar teeth. Less frequently midline palatal tori occur, again in line with the premolar teeth. These are dense,

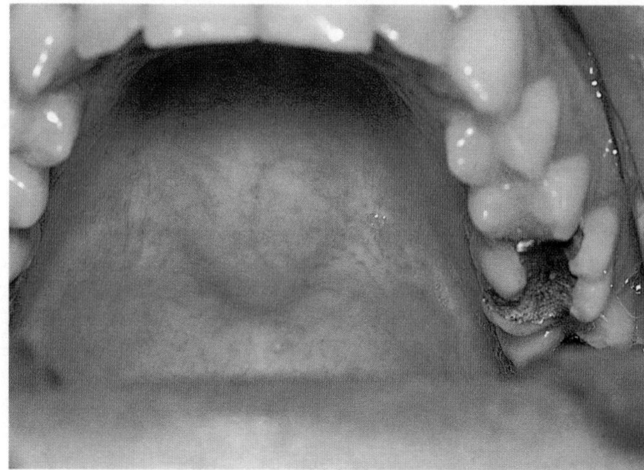

Fig. 37.19 An example of mandibular tori. They grow slowly throughout life and only need removal if lower dentures are to be constructed.

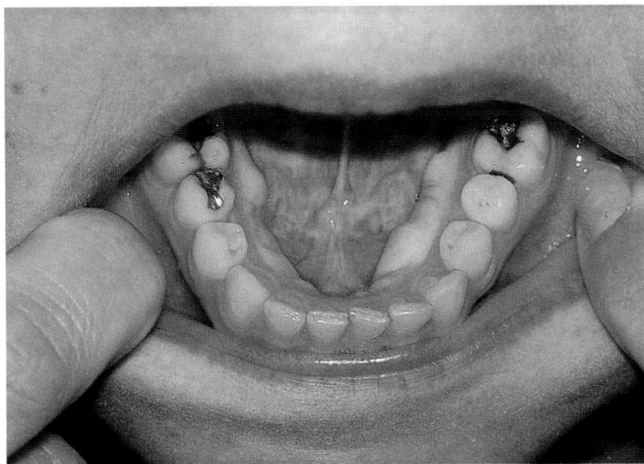

Fig. 37.20 Upper tori are always in the midline. They are bony hard, grow slowly and need treatment only if an upper denture is required.

bony swellings that cause no problem apart from occasional ulceration, particularly if dentures are to be worn. They are only removed if they cause difficulty in the wearing of dentures.

- *Cysts in the thyroglossal tract* – the thyroid gland develops as an evagination of the epithelium at the junction of the anterior two-thirds and the posterior third of the tongue, the foramen caecum. A vestigial epithelial remnant may remain and cysts may occur along the line of this duct. They may be anywhere on a line from the surface of the tongue (Fig. 37.21), down to and behind the hyoid bone or to the isthmus of the thyroid gland. Occasionally thyroid tissue may develop and remain at the site of origin in the base of the tongue.

Surgical treatment

Cysts are, by definition, epithelially lined cavities, and where swellings cause difficulty, embarrassment or recurrent infections the lining has to be removed. Where infection may cause sinus formation, the epithelial track has to be removed. The surgery may be major and complex, or minor, according to site.

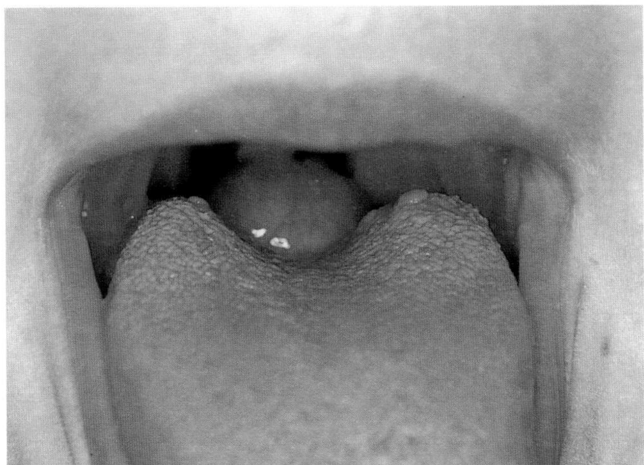

Fig. 37.21 Cysts in the thyroglossal tract.

Congenital and developmental anomalies of the teeth

Dental lamina

Teeth develop from the dental lamina, a strand of epithelium originating from the oral mucosa, which migrates backwards from the incisor region of both mandible and maxilla beginning in the sixth week of intrauterine life. As it migrates backwards tooth buds are formed which eventually develop into the teeth and roots, each with its characteristic shape, according to the position in the jaw. Abnormalities in its migration may lead to abnormalities that are laid out below. The concept of the dental lamina, however, has changed in recent years, as it would seem that the epithelium responsible for developing the teeth is not the dental lamina as such but modifications of the oral mucosa. This invaginates beneath the alveolus progressively posteriorly from the incisor region under the influence of genes and activators, which are specific for each part of the mouth, in a time-window of 2–3 days.

The total number of the secondary dentition is 32. The third molar or wisdom tooth may fail to develop in any of the four quadrants. Lack of space may cause them to impact into the second molars or backwards into the ramus. These may lead to pericoronal infection later in life and the third molars may require removal. The upper lateral incisors may fail to develop or develop as small, peg-shaped teeth. This is normally associated with an impaction of the canines and is thought to be associated with faults in the dental lamina or gene deficiencies during development.

Failure to develop a large number of primary and secondary teeth is known as hypodontia. It may be associated with other forms of ectodermal dysplasia where there is a lack of sebaceous and sweat glands. Considerable problems are encountered in providing a functional dentition, particularly during the growth period.

Supernumerary teeth and odontomes

Supernumerary teeth tend to occur in the same areas where teeth may be absent – the lateral incisor, second premolar and the third molar areas. Generally they are smaller than the normal teeth in the same area and seldom develop little more than a crown and a vestigial root. They may be multiple. In the incisor region they may be responsible for the failure of eruption of adjacent permanent teeth, particularly the central and lateral incisors and canine. They generally lie palatal to their normal counterparts. They have to be removed to allow eruption of the permanent teeth to occur. Rarely, in the third molar region, dentigerous cysts may develop around the crown. These are characterised by a radiographic appearance of a cyst enveloping the crown of the tooth that is displaced.

Odontomes are aggregations of tooth-like material and may take the form of multiple small teeth (denticles, a compound complex odontome) or irregular masses of dentine, cementum and enamel (complex composite odontome). They lie within the alveolus, frequently inhibiting the eruption of the adjacent teeth and are encapsulated. The most common site is the premolar region of the mandible. Odontomes are, in effect, hamartomas. Once formed they do not increase in size. Occasionally they become infected.

Developmental disturbances in the structure of the teeth

The enamel of primary and secondary dentition may be affected by a number of genetic or congenital conditions. There may be effects due to local problems such as trauma during birth or infection. The most notable change affecting all teeth is the result of amelogenesis imperfecta which is genetic and may be dominant or recessive. It is an ectodermal disturbance and the anomalies can range from pits in the teeth to failure of enamel development. It may be associated with osteogenesis imperfecta. By contrast, dentinogenesis imperfecta affects the mesodermal portion of the odontogenic apparatus. The appearance of the teeth is variable with the poorly supported enamel taking on a opalescent tinge. The enamel is readily damaged. Both amelogenesis and dentinogenesis imperfecta result in rapid early tooth loss.

Odontogenic cysts and tumours

Abnormalities in the dental lamina may form benign cysts and odontogenic tumours (keratocyst, odontogenic myxoma). A malignant form, ameloblastoma, is variable between cystic and solid, and is locally invasive. The most common site for these to occur is in the third molar region and ramus of the mandible.

Congenital and developmental abnormalities of the gums

Congenital epulis of the newborn

This uncommon tumour is seen in the anterior mandible and can reach a relatively large size. It is pedunculated and mobile, and can cause extreme concern to parents. It is simple to remove and has no long-term consequences.

Predeciduous teeth

At birth, or shortly afterwards, hard tooth-like structures may be detected in the lower alveolus and can cause the mother considerable discomfort during breastfeeding. These do not represent primary dentition or 'a third set of teeth' as the structures, although calcified, do not take the form of normal teeth. Simple removal is advised where breastfeeding is undertaken.

Further reading

Bergland, O., Semb, G. and Abyhoim, F. (1986) Elimination of the residual alveolar cleft by secondary bone grafting and subsequent orthodontic treatment. *Cleft Palate–Craniofacial Journal*, **23**, 175.

Kriens, O. (1990) Documentation of cleft lip, alveolus and palate. In *Management of Cleft Lip and Palate* (eds J. Bardach and H.L. Morris), W.B. Saunders, Philadelphia, PA, p. 127.

Markus, A.F. and Delaire, J. (1993) Functional primary closure of cleft lip. *British Journal of Oral Maxillofacial Surgery*, **31**, 281.

Markus, A.F., Smith, W.P. and Delaire, J. (1993) Primary closure of cleft palate: a functional approach. *British Journal of Oral Maxillofacial Surgery*, **31**, 71.

Nicolau, P. (1983) The orbicularis oris muscle: a functional approach to its repair in the cleft lip. *British Journal of Plastic Surgery*, **36**, 14.

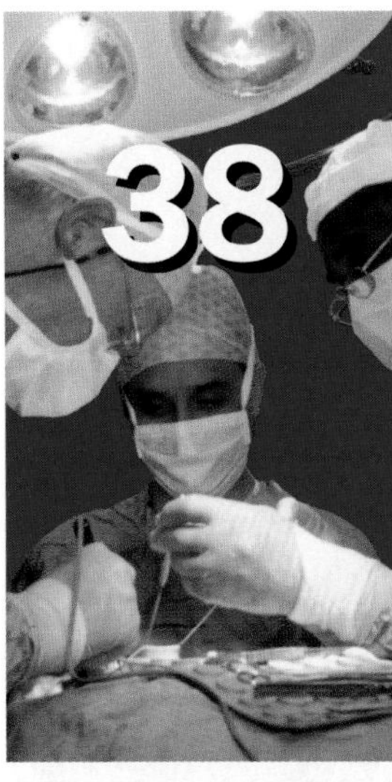

38 Maxillofacial injuries

Introduction

Injuries to the face are common but the majority is relatively minor. A few are major and complex, requiring exacting technique and infinite care in management. It must be remembered always that an intact and unscarred face is important to the well-being of the individual, and thus all injuries, however trivial, should be treated thoughtfully and sympathetically, with every effort always to produce an optimal outcome. In addition, even trivial blows to the face may:

- cause injuries which compromise the airway;
- directly or indirectly cause a head injury (a fall to the ground so banging the head, for instance);
- cause injuries to the cervical spine.

Injuries to the face and facial bones result from both sporting activities and accidents, and intentional violence. The major injuries in the past were as a result of road traffic accidents, but the compulsory wearing of seat belts, car air bags, head restraints and laminated windscreens have reduced all of these greatly. However, the reduction in damage from this source has been almost matched by the increase in deliberate injury from bodily violence where 'putting the boot in' has become a fashion with appalling results.

Clinical effects

The mouth and nasal passages are the upper airway, and lacerations and fractures of the facial skeleton may give rise to immediate or delayed respiratory obstruction. Immediate obstruction may arise from inhalation of tooth fragments, accumulation of blood and secretions, and loss of control of the tongue in the unconscious or semiconscious patient. To avoid this, the patient should always be nursed in the semiprone position (Fig. 38.1) with the head supported on the bent arm, and never lying on their back. Damaged teeth, blood and secretions can then fall out of the mouth and gravity pulls the tongue forward. As the patient is manoeuvred into the correct nursing position, the neck should be supported and held in a neutral position – a protective collar is advisable until a fracture of the cervical spine has been excluded. Under no circumstances should the chin be pulled up to straighten the airway. An intracranial injury should always be considered as a possibility, however minor the injury to the face.

Initial haemorrhage after a facial injury can be dramatic. Sustained bleeding is unusual but emergency surgery to stabilise the facial fractures and control bleeding may be required. The most likely causes of circulatory failure in a bad facial injury are accompanying skeletal injuries or a ruptured viscus, and these should always be actively sought for in the shocked patient.

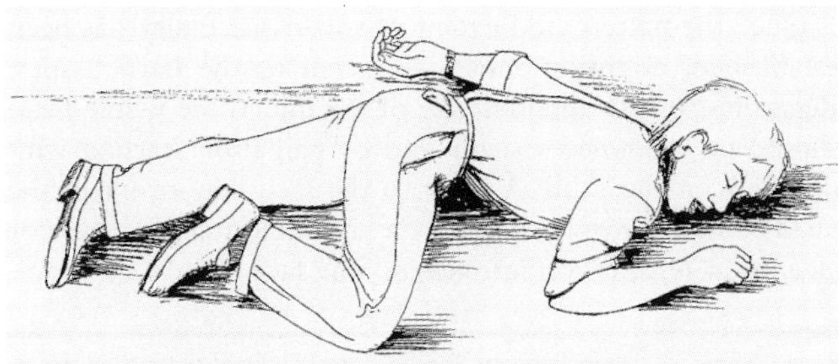

Fig. 38.1 The patient should be nursed in the semiprone position to allow secretions, blood and foreign bodies to fall from the mouth.

Bailey & Love's Short Practice of Surgery, 23rd edition. Edited by R.C.G. Russell, N.S. Williams and C.J.K. Bulstrode. Published in 2000 by Arnold Publishers.

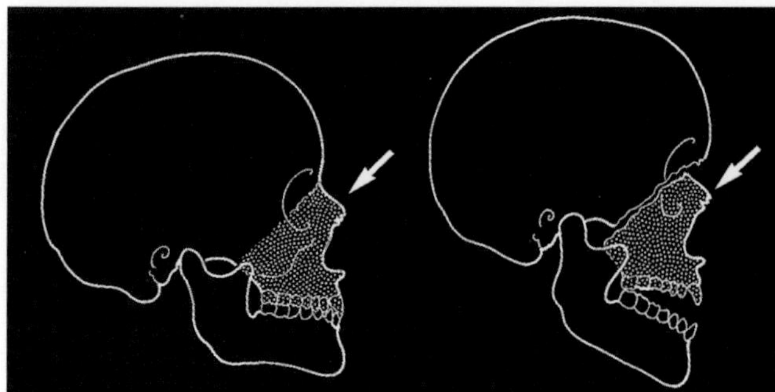

Fig. 38.2 A blow from the front of the face may separate the facial skeleton from the base of the skull and thrust it backwards and downwards.

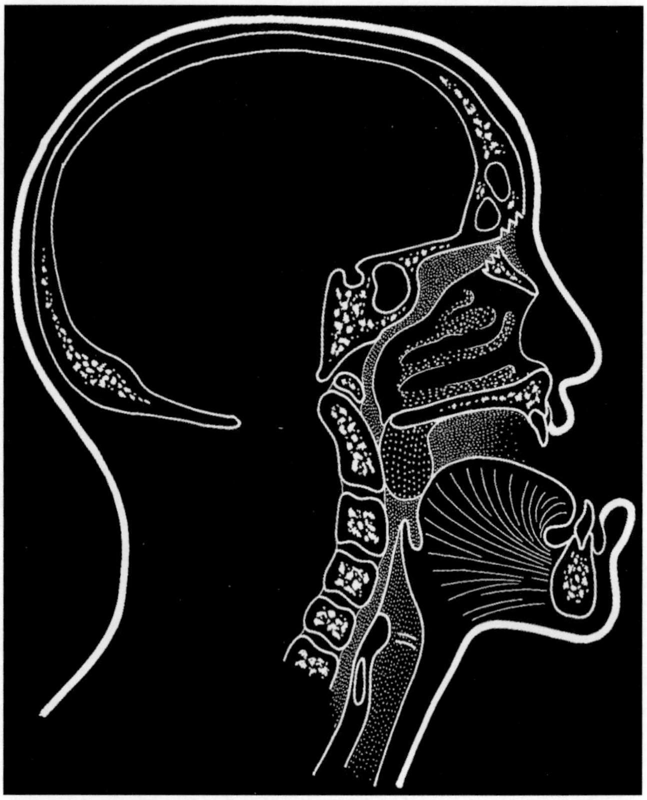

Fig. 38.3 Loss of nasopharangeal space and oedema of the soft palate and tongue may close off the airway in severe maxillofacial injuries, 2–3 hours after the injury.

Oedema is a particular feature of all fractures of the facial skeleton and tends to develop within 60–90 minutes. Thus, a patient with a shattered face may appear to have a good airway immediately after the blow, but that airway may rapidly change and become occluded by swelling of the tongue or facial and pharyngeal tissues. This problem must always be borne in mind when the middle third of the face is involved. In Le Fort III fractures (see below) the facial bones may be thrust downwards and backwards along the base of the skull. As it does so, the posterior teeth of the upper and lower jaw contact first and the mouth is held open giving the impression of a good airway (Fig. 38.2). As swelling supervenes, the soft palate and the tongue may swell to meet, so closing the pharyngeal airway and leading to acute respiratory obstruction (Fig. 38.3). Whenever this is suspected, the 'golden hour' must be used to insert an oropharyngeal airway, even though the patient may appear conscious and unobstructed. If this is not done an emergency tracheostomy may have to be undertaken later with great risk to the patient.

Examination of the injuries

The examination of the patient should be under a good light with consideration of the airway and other collateral injuries always in mind. It is easy to be deviated from examining the whole patient by the dramatic effects of the facial injury. The rapid onset of oedema may make the examination of the face and routine head injury observations difficult – occasionally it is impossible to prise the eyelids apart to examine the pupil, for instance. Lacerations should be explored gently first and, if necessary, cleaned using sterile saline, aqueous antiseptic solution and/or dilute hydrogen peroxide.

Once the pattern and extent of soft-tissue injury has been established, attention should be given to the hard tissues. Regardless of the apparent site of the injury, the whole head should be examined visually and by palpation starting with the vault of the skull. A blow to the face may result in the head being thrown back against a hard object and a bruise or laceration on the occiput missed. The face should be examined from in front. Any asymmetry and displacements should be noted, although oedema may make this difficult. Gentle palpation, using both hands and wearing surgical gloves, gives the most information in searching for step deformities. Tenderness over sites of known weakness and potential for fracture (see below) is a very good guide for the possibility of fracture of the bone beneath. A suitable system is to examine from above downwards – the supraorbital and infraorbital ridges, the nasal bridge, the zygomas, including the zygomatic arch. The mandible should then be examined starting at the condyles bilaterally and then following the posterior and lower border of the mandible as far as the midline. All middle third injuries are accompanied by bleeding from the nose, and Le Fort II and III injuries frequently have a cerebrospinal fluid (CSF) leak with anterior or posterior CSF rhinorrhoea. All fractures of the maxilla lead to mucosal tears with bleeding from the nose. A particularly useful sign in the fractured zygoma is the frequent subconjuctival haemorrhage which will be found to have no posterior border when the patient is asked to look to the opposite side (Fig. 38.4). This gives a positive indication of a fracture of the bone behind.

The patient should then be examined intraorally with good illumination; a pen torch is insufficient. The lips should be parted and the occlusion of the teeth examined. The upper and lower teeth normally 'fit' together even if the occlusion

René Le Fort, b. 1869. Surgeon, Paris, France. Defined these fractures as early as 1901 by macabre research in which he dropped rocks, etc., on the faces of cadavers.

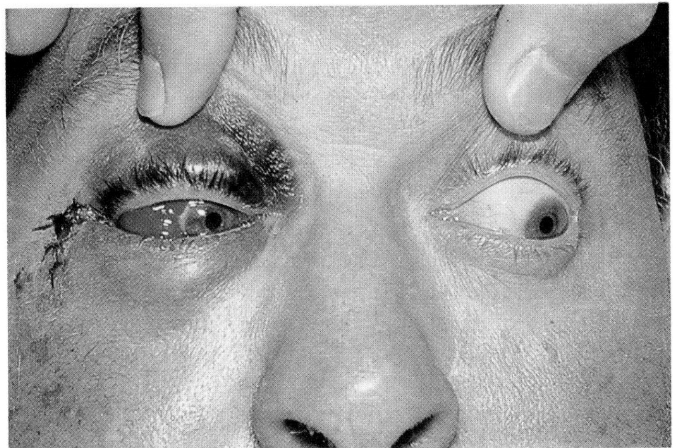

Fig. 38.4 Fractures of the zygoma cause subconjunctival ecchymosis and there is no posterior border to it as the patient looks away from the side of the fracture.

is naturally irregular – if they do not, a fracture of the jaws is likely. All fractures of the alveolus (the bone holding the teeth) tear the gingiva and are compound into the mouth: the examiner should look for sites of bleeding. A haematoma in the floor of the mouth is a good indication of a fracture of the mandible, particularly in the edentulous case. The cheeks, throat and tongue should be examined at the same time. Movement of the jaw should be tested – deviation from the midline at rest or on opening suggests a fracture of the side to which the jaw is deviating.

If a fracture of the maxilla is suspected, the upper dental arch should be grasped between index finger and thumb of one hand in the molar region, while the other is placed on the forehead. A gentle pull on the maxilla forward and backward, or side to side, will reveal movement between the examining hands. With the mandible, gentle manipulation across the suspected site of a fracture will confirm the presence of the fractue if 'spinging' is felt and seen. Confirmation of a fractured zygoma may be made by palpating the fractured antral wall above the upper molar teeth in the buccal sulcus.

The facial examination should be completed by testing for sensation over the face. Anaesthesia or parathesia suggests a fracture proximally along the path of the nerve. Thus, anaesthesia of the cheek and upper lip suggests a fracture going through the infraorbital foramen, while anaesthesia of the lower lip suggests a fracture of the mandibular body. It is important to confirm that the patient has sight in both eyes. This may be difficult in the very oedematous patient with circumorbital haematoma, but a pen torch shone through the lids will confirm that the optic nerve is intact. Where possible, vision should be checked for diplopia by asking the patient to follow the light of the pen torch in both central and extremes of gaze. Diplopia may mean that there is damage to the thin orbital plates of bone, particularly the infraorbital plate.

All findings should be recorded accurately, preferably with diagrams to include measurements of lacerations and displacements. Photographs of the initial injury can be very helpful if litigation is likely to follow.

Investigations

Blood tests

Baseline full blood picture and serum electrolytes should be recorded, and the blood should be grouped when it is thought that much bleeding has occurred and more bleeding is likely.

Radiographs

Posteroanterior occipitomental radiographs taken at 10 and 30° are the best initial radiographs to illustrate the site and displacement of the maxilla; an opaque antrum is a good indication that there may be a fracture of the maxilla. A panoramic oral radiograph (orthopantomogram) is the radiograph of choice for the mandible as it shows the whole bone from condyle to condyle. If the patient cannot be positioned in the machines to achieve these views, radiographs should wait until the patient is fit enough. Poor radiographs can be misleading, and treatment can only be carried out on good ones. The orbital floor may be visualised best by a computerised tomography (CT) scan in the coronal plane, and may also be used to identify the presence and site of other middle third fractures. If a CT scan is to be made, always consider including the upper cervical spine in addition to the face.

Fractures of the facial skeleton

Fractures of the facial skeleton may be divided into those in the upper third (above the eyebrows), the middle third (above the mouth) and the lower third (the mandible). Fractures tend to occur through points of weakness – the sutures and foramina, and in thin unsupported bone.

The upper third

The patterns of fracture of the skull tend to be random but there are points of weakness, mainly involving the frontal sinuses and the supraorbital ridges.

The middle third

Fractures of the middle third of the face have been studied extensively and René Le Fort in 1911 classified fractures according to patterns which he created on cadavers using various degrees of force. The Le Fort classification is used extensively today throughout the world. While Le Fort classified the fractures from superior to inferior, the custom today is that the classification runs inferiorly to superiorly (Fig. 38.5).

The **Le Fort I** fracture effectively separates the alveolus and palate from the facial skeleton above. The fracture line runs through points of weakness from the pyriform aperture, through the lateral and medial wall of the maxillary sinus running posteriorly to include the lower part of the pterygoid plates.

The **Le Fort II** fracture is pyramidal in shape. The fracture involves the orbit, running through the bridge of the nose, and the ethmoids whose cribriform plate may be fractured, leading to a dural tear and CSF leak. It continues to the

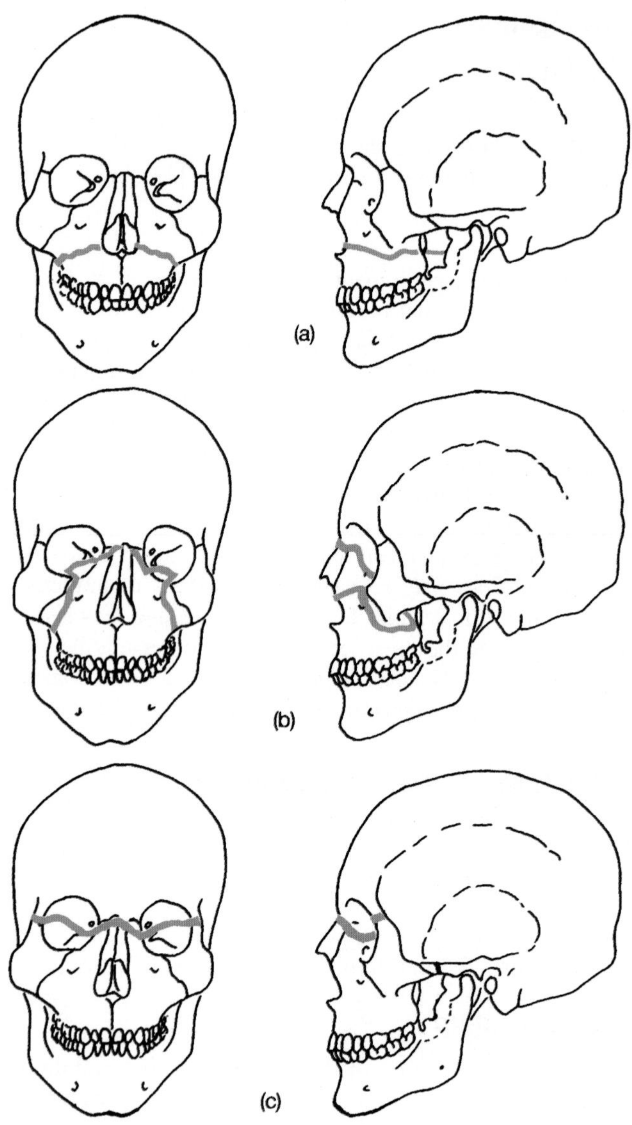

Fig. 38.5 Maxillary fractures as classified by Le Fort. (a) Le Fort I; (b) Le Fort II; (c) Le Fort III.

medial part of the infraorbital rim, through the infraorbital foramen and through the infraorbital fissure. The orbital floor is always involved. It continues posteriorly through the lateral wall of the maxillary antrum at a higher level than the Le Fort I to the pterygoid plates at the back. The nasal septum is displaced and lateral walls of the nose are fractured.

The **Le Fort III** fracture effectively separates the facial skeleton from the base of the skull – the fracture lines run high through the nasal bridge, septum and ethmoids, again with the potential for dural tear and CSF leak, and irregularly through the bones of the orbit to the frontozygomatic suture. The zygomatic arch fractures, and the facial skeleton is separated from the bones above at a high level through the lateral wall of the maxillary sinus and the pterygoid plates. The nasal septum will be fractured and may be displaced.

These fractures are seldom confined exactly to this classification and may be combinations of any of the above.

The zygoma

This is the most common fracture of the middle third of the face apart from the nose, as the patient turns the cheek to approaching danger. The fractures occur though points of weakness – infraorbital margin, the frontozygomatic suture, the zygomatic arch and the anterior and lateral wall of the maxillary sinus. Tears on the mucosa of the antrum lead to bleeding from the nose. The infraorbital plate of bone is always involved to a greater or lesser extent and may cause entrapment of the orbital contents.

Blow-out fractures of the orbit

Direct trauma to the globe of the eye may push it back within the orbit. The globe is a fairly robust structure and as it is thrust backwards, the pressure increases within the orbit and the weaker plates of bone may fracture, without necessarily fracturing the bones of the orbital rim. Such injuries can occur where a pointed object hits the globe of the eye – for example, a bent elbow of a standing man inadvertently being thrust into the orbit of a person sitting. A finger deliberately thrust into the eye may have the same effect. The weakest plate of bone, commonly the infraorbital plate, ruptures and the orbital contents herniate downwards into the maxillary antrum. On rebound, as the pressure within the orbit is reduced, the small fractured pieces of bone may entrap the orbital contents, particularly the inferior oblique and inferior rectus muscles, leading to failure of the eye to rotate upwards. Enophthalmus and profound diplopia can follow although initially both may be concealed by oedema. Anaesthesia over the distribution of the infraorbital nerve may be an important clue to the blow-out fracture. Pain is experienced on movements of the eye as the entrapped muscle is stretched. There may be enophthalmos although this may be masked in the early stages by oedema. Any fracture that may involve the orbital floor (Le Fort II and zygomatic bone) must be considered a potential for orbital content entrapment too.

Fractures of the mandible

These are usually as a result of blows from the side or from the front to the lower third of the face. The condylar neck is the weakest part of the bone and is the most frequent site of fracture (Fig. 38.6) while other fractures tend to occur through unerupted teeth (the impacted wisdom tooth) or where the roots are long (the canine tooth). Blows from the side may fracture at the point of injury but, as the force is transmitted to the base of the skull via the condylar neck, this may fracture first. Blows from the front may cause fracture in the midline and fractures of both condyles. Individual sharp blows with a blunt instrument may fracture a segment away from the mandible. Blows from below may cause the mandible to be thrust upwards fracturing the alveolus and teeth as they hit their fellows in the maxilla. Fractures of the mandibular body may also fracture the teeth in the fracture line.

Much has been made in the past of the 'butterfly' fracture of the mandible. Here a segment of mandible in the midline

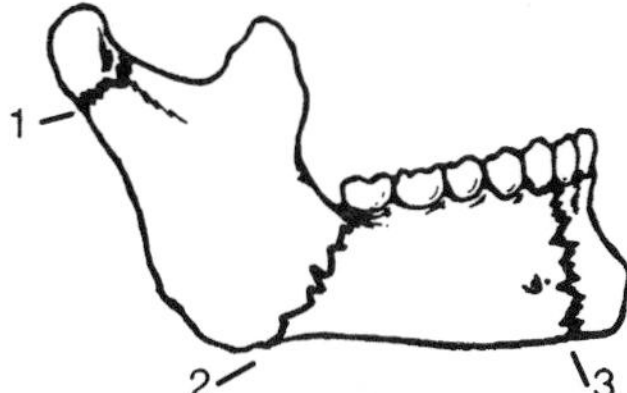

Fig. 38.6 The patterns of fracture of the mandible. (1) The neck of the condyle is the most common site, followed by (2) the angle of the mandible through the last tooth. (3) The third point of weakness is in the region of the canine tooth.

is detached from the rest of the mandible with fractures in the canine regions. The segment of bone takes on the appearance of a butterfly, and this will include the anterior insertion of the tongue (geniohyoid and genioglossus). Conceptually, the tongue may fall back and occlude the airway. First, the fracture is extremely rare, and second, the patient can still control the tongue, if allowed to by a good nursing position (see above).

Treatment

Soft-tissue injuries

Facial soft tissues have an excellent blood supply and heal well. They should be sutured as soon as possible after the injury after careful exploration, débridement and cleaning, particularly where glass or plastic may be embedded. The tissues should be meticulously clean and scrubbed, as retained dirt may cause tattooing and hypertophy of the scar. Many lacerations may be closed using local anaesthesia, injecting into the edges of the wound. If the patient is due to have a general anaesthetic and there is a delay, the wounds should be closed in advance by local anaesthesia. Tissue sufficiently traumatised to have lost its blood supply should be removed with a sharp scalpel, and the edge to which it is to be apposed trimmed to fit as appropriate.

Great care should be taken to replace tissues very accurately, particularly in cosmetically important landmarks such as the vermillion border of the lips, the eyelids and nasal contours. Haemostasis is important. Muscle and underlying layers should be brought together with absorbable sutures so that the edges of the wound lie passively within 2 mm of their final position. Then fine monofilament sutures (5-0 or 6-0) are used to bring the wound edges together (Fig. 38.7). All sutures should be placed so as to avoid compromising the blood supply of the apices of small flaps. Vacuum drains are used where there is concern over dead space beneath the wounds. The lacerations should be covered by antibiotic ointment and this should be replaced two to three times per day. This prevents the sutures causing scarring of the skin. Intravenous dexamethasone 8 mg twice daily for 2 days and broad-spectrum antibiotics should be prescribed. Sutures may be removed from the third day.

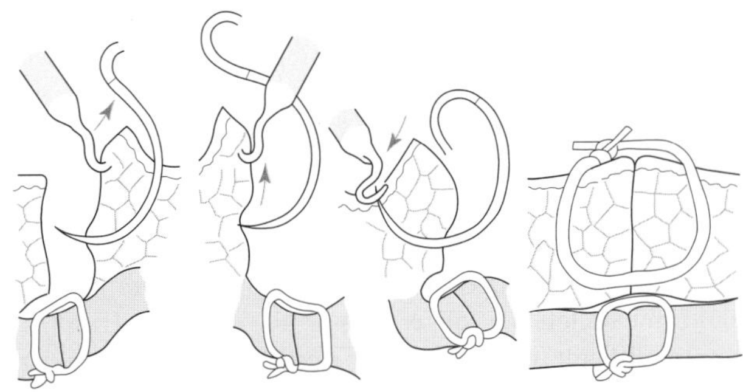

Fig. 38.7 Facial wound. The method of skin closure avoiding inversion of the wound edges. The skin suture has a greater depth of deep tissue than at the surface.

Facial nerve injury

The facial nerve may be severed in the depth of a lateral facial wound. If this is suspected, primary repair should be attempted, particularly where clinical signs suggest that a main division is involved. Locating the divided branches in oedematous and damaged tissue may be extremely difficult. Proximal and distal flaps in relatively normal adjacent tissue may have to be raised to identify the nerve on each side of the laceration. The severed nerve may then be traced towards the laceration and the ends approximated using an operating microscope, and the nerve and laceration sutured. Attempt at primary repair is always worthwhile, although extremely difficult, as secondary repair is generally unsatisfactory.

Parotid duct

Lacerations in the same vicinity as those that transect the facial nerve may also transect the parotid duct. The suggested management is to insert a small cannula in the parotid duct from within the mouth and then pass it distally until it appears in the wound. The position of the duct is identified and the proximal end may be found from the site of the distal end as the tissues are approximated and the cannula runs into it. The laceration of the facial tissues may be sutured in the normal way avoiding any tendency to displacement across the ends of the duct. Some advise that the parotid duct is sutured side to side to avoid stricture. Two days of intravenous dexamethasone (8 mg twice a day) should follow the surgery. Antibiotics are recommended.

The lacrimal apparatus

The lacrimal apparatus may be involved in damage to the eyelids and nasal bones in Le Fort II and III injuries. The tissues are generally grossly oedematous and the manipulation required to reduce the fractures adds to the difficulties of identifying the cannaliculae. Most surgeons do not attempt repair primarily but refer to an appropriate plastic or ophthalmic surgeon if epiphora become a problem later. Surprisingly, few patients suffer epiphora after a year has elapsed from the injury.

Injuries to the facial bones

The fractured nose

This is the most common fracture of the face. Best results are achieved when oedema has been allowed to settle so that accurate reduction can be achieved. Reduction of oedema may be assisted by intravenous or intramuscular dexamethasone 8 mg twice daily preoperatively. However, surgery should not be left for longer than a week, as reduction may become difficult or impossible. Accurate reduction always requires a general anaesthetic and an endotracheal tube. A throat pack should always be inserted. Reduction should be directed first to repositioning the nasal bones, disimpacting with Walshams's forceps with the external blade covered with rubber tubing so as to avoid damage to the skin. The nasal bones are first taken laterally to disimpact them, and then medially to reposition them. It is wise to start on the side opposite to the blow which broke the nose. The septum is then grasped with Asch's forceps, manipulated until it is straight, and then positioned in the groove of the nasal crest and vomer. Asch's forceps may be used to pull the disimpacted nasal bones forward to their previous unfractured position. If there is a suggestion that the insertion of inner canthi has been involved, or the nasal bones have been thrust into the ethmoid sinuses, then open reduction may be required (see treatment of Le Fort III). The nasal bones may need supporting by a pack within the nasal bridge. This is best done using ribbon gauze inserted into the finger(s) of a rubber surgical glove previously placed beneath the reduced nasal bones (to reduce the discomfort of pack removal at 3 days). A protective nasal plaster may be placed and removed at 1 week.

Fractures of the maxilla

Treatment of fractures of the maxilla should be undertaken in a maxillofacial unit. They always require a general anaesthetic given through a cuffed nasotracheal tube. Careful intubation is required ensuring that the tube is directed posteriorly, not superiorly, on insertion. Correctly placed tubes are of no risk to the cranial base however extensive the fracture. Occasionally it may be necessary to begin the operation with an oral tube, and then transfer to a nasal tube once the maxilla is reduced and held. Final positioning of a concomitant fractured nose may be left until the end of the operation, just after the nasal tube has been removed. Conversely, if it is necessary to leave in a nasopharangeal airway, a second airway should be inserted in the other nostril, so as to keep the nares equally distended. A tracheostomy may be required occasionally.

The principle of reducing and stabilising fractures of the frontal and facial bones is that the surgeon starts at the top and works down. Where there are extensive lacerations, these may be used, perhaps with small extensions, to approach the fracture lines. Where there are no convenient lacerations, fractures of the frontal bone and supraorbital ridges and fractures of the nasal root may be approached through a coronal incision at the vault of the skull, high in the hair line. The incision is taken from just in front of each ear across the vault of the skull and reflected forwards until the supraorbital ridges are exposed. The supraorbital nerve is identified and freed and the flap extended as required. The nasal root, the lateral orbital rim and zygomatic arch may be exposed through this route. All of the fractured bones may be reduced and held by stainless steel or titanium miniplates or microplates and wires, under direct vision. Bone deficiencies in this area or in the infraorbital plate may be made up with free cranial cortical bone grafts, with the donor sites available through the coronal incision. Where the nasal bones are spread, leading to an orbital hyperteleorism, the root of the medial canthal ligaments may be identified and sutured to the opposite side to restore canthal width.

When the stabilisation of the upper part of the face is complete, attention may be given to the midface. Incisions in the lower eyelid (blephoroplasty incisions) or lower conjunctival sac are used to explore fractures of the infraorbital margin. These also give access to the orbital floor and are used to treat blow-out fractures. The rim may be fixed using miniplates or microplates or wires as above, and the floor of the orbit reconstituted with bone, titanium or alloplastic material according to choice, held by wires or screws.

The lower part of the maxilla is approach through a gingival sulcus incision above the maxillary teeth as far back as the second molar. Fractures may be identified with ease through this route and fixed with plates or wires. The dental arch is restored to its original shape as far as possible so that it matches the previous occlusion with the lower teeth. To achieve accurate location, dental archwires or eyelet wires (see below) may need to be inserted. Where this is anticipated, the necessary wiring is done before the main part of the operation is commenced.

The principle of treatment is to restore the fragments to their original position. To achieve this, usually it is necessary to reduce the maxilla first with Rowe's disimpaction forceps which grasp the palate between the nasal and palatal mucosa. Considerable force is sometimes required in a series of downward, forward and sideways movement to free it, particularly where the operation has been delayed. After 3 weeks, full disimpaction is often impossible.

With the advent of miniplates and microplates, indirect fixation with pins and halo frame is seldom used. If the fragments are multiple and the whole restored maxilla remains unstable, external fixation may be the only answer. Then the principle is that the mandible is fixed to the cranium, with the maxilla as a sandwich between the two. Cranial fixation is by

William Johnson Walsham, 1847–1903. St Bartholomew's Hospital, London, England.

Morris Joseph Asch, 1833–1902. Surgeon, New York Eye and Ear Hospital, New York, USA.

Norman Lester Rowe. Late Consultant in Oral and Maxillofacial Surgery, Queen Mary's Hospital, Roehampton and Westminster Hospital, London, England.

a halo or supraorbital pins, and mandibular fixation is by pins inserted in the body on each side. All of the pins are connected together with connecting bars secured by universal joints. When the teeth of each jaw are fixed together with intermaxillary fixation (see below) the anteroposterior position of the face is likely to be correct. The vertical dimension is adjusted through the connecting bars fixed by universal joints on to the pins. This means that the jaws are fixed together during recovery, and careful attention should be given to advising the recovery staff on how to release the apparatus in an emergency.

Fractures of the mandible

Fractures of the mandible frequently are reduced and then fixed with intermaxillary fixation (IMF). IMF is a means of splinting the upper and lower arches of teeth together. First, eyelet wires or arch bars are fixed to the upper and lower teeth. Eyelet wires consist of a small loop about 4 mm in diameter twisted in the centre of a length of 0.35-mm stainless steel wire. Each loop is threaded between and around pairs of teeth, and twisted together on the buccal side, with one of the ends going through its own loop. This makes very secure fixation. Four or five eyelets are required for each dental arch. These are most suitable where there is a full, or near full, arch of teeth in each jaw. Where there has been tooth loss with irregular gaps around the mouth, then arch bars may have to be used. These are prefabricated lengths of stainless steel tape or wire, with hooks coming off at 8–10-mm intervals. These are wired to individual teeth so that there are two arch bars opposing one another in each jaw. IMF is applied between the loops of the eyelet wires or the hooks of the arch bars. In the past, custom-made silver cap splints were used, cemented to the opposing jaws. These are rarely used now.

For future comfort of the patient, it is very important to restore the dental occlusion to its original position. With simple minimally displaced fractures, eyelet wiring is all that is required (Fig. 38.8). This may be achieved without general anaesthetic. Undisplaced fractures and fractures of the mandibular condyle may require no active treatment.

Displaced fractures, or fractures which have markedly disturbed the occlusion, will require a general anaesthetic. A cuffed nasotracheal tube is required without a throat pack (a throat pack may make it difficult to achieve the correct occlusion). Fractures of the body of the mandible may be explored through intraoral or extraoral incisions according to the access required, and the fractures reduced and fixed with miniplates and/or wires. Any fractured teeth should be removed and also those previously compromised by extensive caries or infection. It is unnecessary to remove healthy teeth in the fracture line. To be sure of achieving a correct occlusion it is wise to use temporary intraoperative IMF. There are occasions when the best results can be achieved with IMF alone. In this event, it is necessary to remove the IMF during recovery, so as not to risk complications involving the airway. IMF may be inserted after 12 hours when the patient has recovered from the general anaesthetic. It is retained for 3–4 weeks.

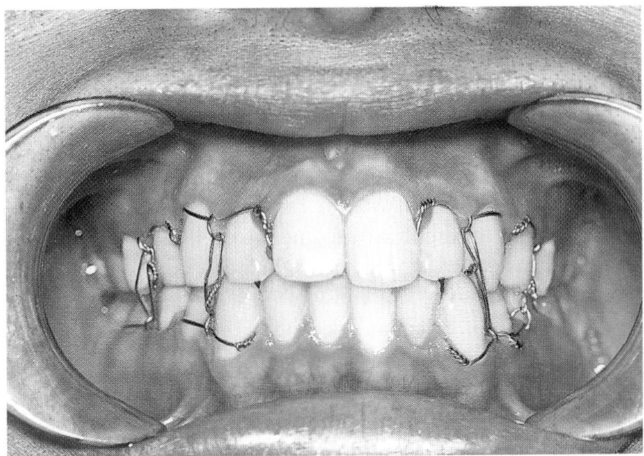

Fig. 38.8 Intermaxillary fixation using eyelet wires.

Fractures of the edentulous mandible generally are plated using miniplates. In the atrophic mandible, the raising of periosteum should be kept to a minimum as the blood supply to the jaw may be compromised. Where there is fear that the blood supply may be seriously disadvantaged by the insertion of plates, Gunning's splints may be constructed. These require dental impressions and are then constructed in the laboratory. In effect, these are like upper and lower dentures, but with the teeth replaced with plastic in which hooks are placed (the patient's dentures may be used). Each splint is wired to the respective jaw – the mandible, with wires going around the mandible (circumferential wires) and the maxilla, with wires going around the zygomatic arches. The circumferential wires around the mandible are sited to stabilise the fracture line. The hooks placed on the buccal surfaces of the plastic arch are used to apply IMF when the patient has recovered from the anaesthetic. The IMF is released after 4–6 weeks.

Fractures of the mandibular condyle may cause disturbance to the occlusion with deviation of the mandible to the side of the fracture. In unilateral fractures, this disturbance may correct spontaneously in a few days. If it is still present at 10 days, or where both condyles are fractured, open surgery may be required to one of the condyles to prevent an anterior open bite developing. The open bite occurs due to the vertical pull of the muscles of mastication shortening the ramus. The posterior teeth contact first and the anterior teeth remain apart. Functionally and cosmetically, this is very undesirable and is almost impossible to counteract by secondary procedures. Simply to fix the mandible in IMF, with or without posterior block to overcome the tendency to open bite, is insufficient. Direct surgical approaches to the condylar neck are difficult owing to the parotid gland and facial nerve lying in close proximity. Preauricular incisions com-

Thomas Brian Gunning, 1813–89. Dentist, New York, USA. Invented a vulcanite jaw splint. Noted for his successful treatment of the fractured jaw of William H. Seward, President Lincoln's Secretary of State.

bined with incisions at the lower border of the mandible do give access but reduction of the bones is difficult through these approaches. A simple and effective approach is via a tangential incision at the angle of the mandible that gives access to the bone beneath, between the facial and cervical branches of the facial nerve. The angle of the mandible is identified and the periosteum raised up both sides of the ramus as far as the fracture line. Access to the displaced condyle is achieved by removing the posterior border of the mandible with a vertical subsigmoid cut, running from the sigmoid notch of the mandible down to the angle of the jaw. The condyle may then be removed and offered up to the excised segment of mandible. The two bone fragments are located and fixed together with miniplates outside the body. The restored bone is then returned to the patient and secured to the distal mandible with a miniplate.

Fractures of the zygoma

Second to the fractured nasal bone, this is the most common fracture of the maxilla. Displacement is usually posteriorly, but it is important to assess the actual displacement by studying the occipitomental radiographs. Most fractures may be reduced by the Gillies approach. This entails an incision in the hairline superficial to the temporal fossa about 15 mm long, at 45° to the vertical. It is deepened down to and through the temporal fascia. A channel is prepared behind the fascia and down to the body of the zygoma and arch. A Bristow's or Rowe's elevator is then inserted beneath the body of the zygoma or arch, according to the site of fracture. Considerable force is applied in the opposite direction to that calculated to have been delivered by the blow which caused the fracture. After reduction, the position of the zygoma can be checked by palpating the bony prominences of the arch, and the lateral and inferior orbital rims. As all fractures of the zygoma involve the orbital floor, it is essential to apply a forced duction test to the globe to ensure that the inferior oblique or inferior rectus muscle is not trapped. For this to be done properly, the lower eyelid should be retracted and the inferior rectus muscle grasped in the lower fornix. The globe can then be rotated upwards and should move freely. Any restriction in movement suggests entrapment of intraorbital tissues and the floor of orbit should be explored as for a blow-out fracture (see below). It is essential to warn the anaesthetist that this manoeuvre is being done, as it can lead to a severe bradycardia.

Should the fracture seem unstable, direct wiring or plating may be necessary. The frontozygomatic suture should be exposed by a small incision just behind the lateral part of the eyebrow and visualised. Displacements may be reduced and generally the fracture becomes stable once this fracture is fixed. Occasionally it is necessary to explore and fix fractures of the infraorbital rim (see above).

Walter Rowley Bristow, 1882–1947. Orthopaedic Surgeon, St Thomas's Hospital, London, England.

If the fragments are very unstable owing to comminution, packing the antrum via a Caldwell–Luc incision in the mouth may be necessary. The antrum should be first examined using a fibre-optic light source, with particular attention given to the orbital floor. Then, with the orbital floor reduced and protected, and the body of the zygoma supported by an assistant, the antrum may be packed from above down with a 2-inch ribbon gauze soaked in Whitehead's varnish. Great care must be exercised not to overpack the antrum and displace the orbital contents. The incision is closed with a tail of ribbon gauze sutured into the wound to allow drainage. The pack is removed at 3 weeks.

All patients who have had operations around the orbit should be observed formally at 15-minute intervals for 9–12 hours. The condition of the eye, the pupil size and the appreciation of light should be recorded. Occasional complications arise, the most serious of which is a developing haematoma in the periorbital tissues or the cone between the ocular muscles. Increasing exophthalmous and loss of vision constitute a postoperative emergency requiring immediate action to reduce the pressure of the haematoma.

Blow-out fractures

The mechanism has been explained above. The floor of the orbit is approached either through a blephoroplasty incision in the lower eyelid or through the inferior fornix. Keeping superficial to the tarsal plate of the lower lid, the infraorbital margin is identified and the periosteum raised, being careful not to displace the delicate fragments of bone constituting the fracture. The periorbital tissues are gently separated from the bones of the fracture and freed so that no trapping remains. The apex of the orbit should not be explored for fear of damage to the optic nerve or spasm of the retinal artery. Defects of the orbital floor may be made up with bone from the cranium (see above) or the opposite antral wall, titanium mesh, or other suitably rigid materials. Reinforced silastic sheet is no longer thought adequate. The materials are fixed with wires, screws or plates and the wound is closed.

General

Fractures of the facial skeleton are almost always compound and prophylactic antibiotics are important. Penicillin and metronidazole singly or in combination are ideal for those patients who are not allergic. The cephalosporins are an alternative. Where there is the possibility of a CSF leak from a dural tear above a fractured cribriform plate of the ethmoid

George Walter Caldwell, 1866–1946. Otolaryngologist in New York, San Francisco and Los Angeles. Described his operation for treating suppuration of the maxillary antrum in 1893.

Henri Luc, 1855–1925. Otolaryngologist, Paris. Described his operation in 1889.

Walter Whitehead, 1849–1913. Surgeon, Manchester Royal Infirmary, Manchester, England.

bone (Le Fort II and III), suitable antibiotics which cross the blood–brain barrier (chloramphenicol, for example) should be given to avoid the risk of meningitis or later intracranial abcess. All patients with fractures of the facial skeleton benefit from intraoperative and postoperative dexamethasone, to reduce swelling.

Intermaxillary fixation makes it impossible to chew. It is important that the patient receives the advice of a dietician so that high calorific value food may be taken through the IMF. It is surprising how patients find a way to take fluid and semi-solids through clenched teeth. In the badly injured, parenteral feeding may be required. It is wise to leave a nasogastric tube in place, inserted at the time of operation, for as long as food cannot be taken normally.

Dislocation of the mandibular condyles

Dislocation of the mandibular condyles is a relatively uncommon condition and occurs usually after a wide opening of the mouth. Occasionally it may accompany a blow to the face, particularly a blow to the jaw with the mouth already open. The patient is unable to close the mouth as the condyles have translated in front of the articular eminence and spasm of the closing muscles traps them there. It may be very painful. An attempt should be made to reduce the dislocation by manual manipulation. This is achieved by standing in front of and above the seated patient and grasping the mandible with gloved hands with the thumbs on the occlusal surfaces of the teeth, and the index and middle fingers below the lower border of the mandible. It is wise to wrap the thumbs each in a gauze square. Sudden downward and backward movement is applied bilaterally with an assistant supporting the head. If this fails, one repeat attempt concentrating on one side at a time may then succeed. Reduction may be assisted by injecting local anaesthetic around both joints. Occasionally it may be necessary to sedate the patient with intravenous midazolam or even resort to a general anaesthetic.

Further reading

Rowen, N.L. and Williams, J.L. (eds) (1985) *Fracture of the Facial Skeleton*, Churchill Livingstone, Edinburgh.

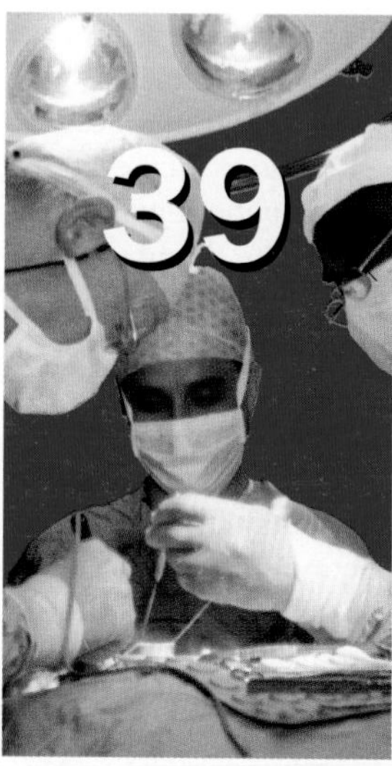

39 The nose and sinuses

Surgical anatomy of the nose

The supporting structures of the nose are shown in Fig. 39.1. The paired nasal bones join in the midline with a suture and are supported by the septum, which consists of the anterior quadrilateral cartilage, the perpendicular plate of the ethmoid and the vomer (Fig. 39.2). In children the length of the nasal bone equals its width, whereas in the adult the length is three times the width. The lateral wall of the nasal cavity contains the superior, middle and inferior turbinates (Fig. 39.3). Opening on to the lateral nasal wall are the ostia of all the nasal sinuses except for the sphenoid sinus (Fig. 39.4). The nasolacrimal duct opens into the inferior meatus beneath the inferior turbinate approximately 3 cm posterior to the external nasal opening. Below the middle turbinate is the middle meatus into which the nasofrontal duct, the anterior ethmoid cells and the maxillary antrum open (Fig. 39.5). The superior meatus between the middle and superior turbinates contains the opening for the posterior ethmoid cells. The sphenoid ostium lies at this level on the anterior wall of the sphenoid sinus. The nasal cavities and sinuses are lined by respiratory epithelium. The olfactory mucosa, innervated by fibres from the olfactory nerve, lines the area of the olfactory cleft and the cribriform

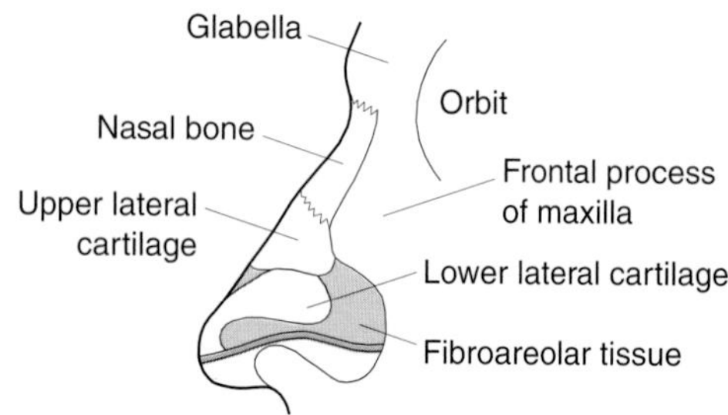

Fig. 39.1 The nasal skeleton.

Bailey & Love's Short Practice of Surgery, 23rd edition. Edited by R.C.G. Russell, N.S. Williams and C.J.K. Bulstrode. Published in 2000 by Arnold Publishers.

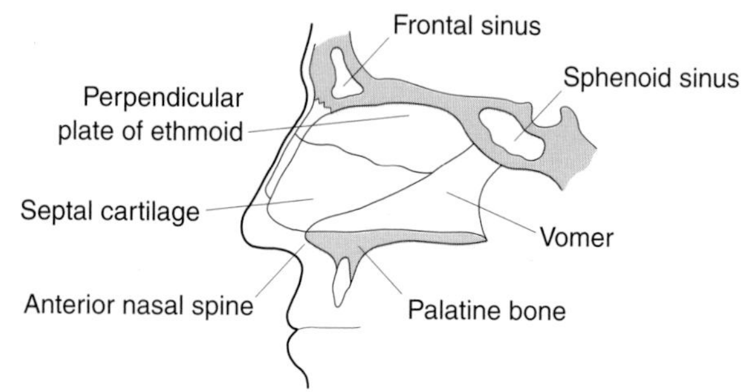

Fig. 39.2 The left side of the nasal septum.

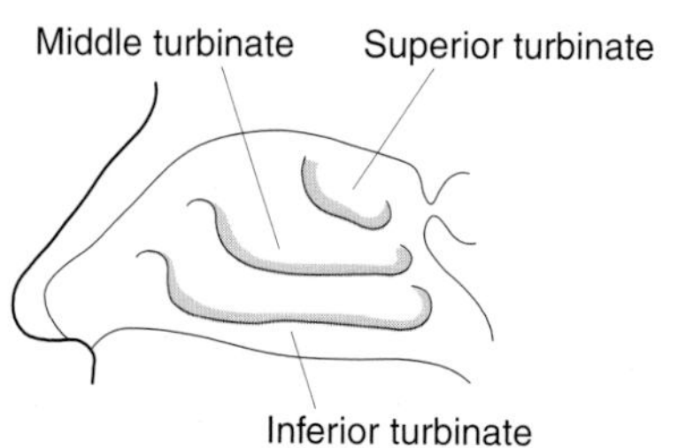

Fig. 39.3 The right lateral nasal wall.

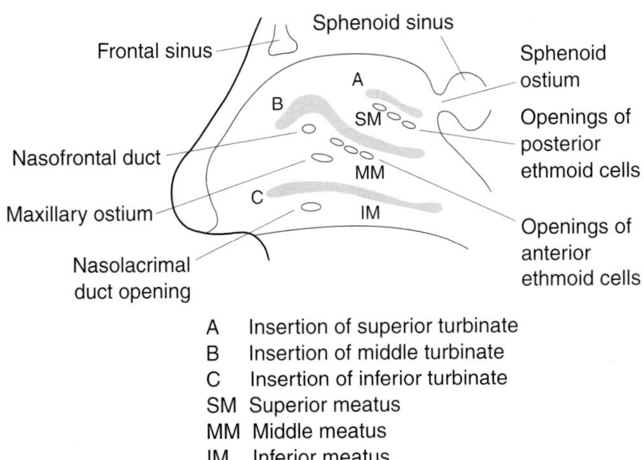

Fig. 39.4 The right lateral nasal wall with turbinates removed to show sinus ostia.

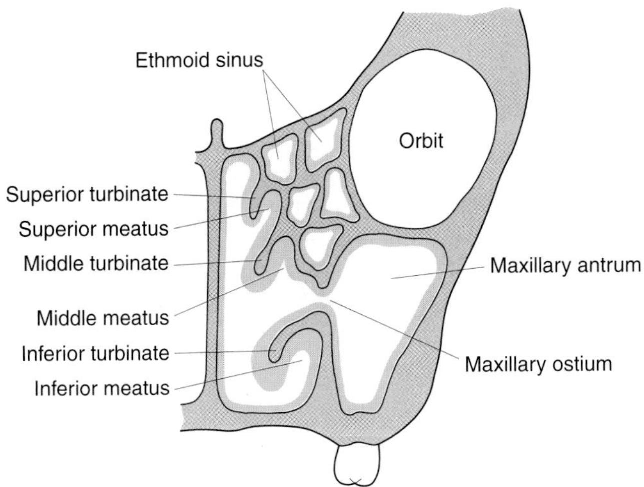

Fig. 39.5 Coronal section through the left maxillary and ethmoid sinuses.

plate. The nasal fossae and sinuses receive their blood supply via the external and internal carotid arteries. The external carotid artery supplies the interior of the nose via the maxillary and sphenopalatine arteries. The greater palatine artery supplies the anteroinferior septum via the incisive canal. The contribution from the internal carotid artery is via the anterior and posterior ethmoidal arteries which are branches of the ophthalmic artery (Fig. 39.6). All of these arteries anastomose

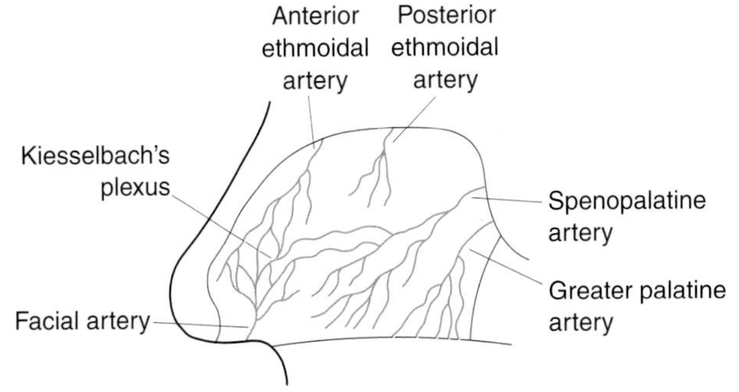

Fig. 39.6 The left side of the nasal septum showing the arterial supply.

to form a plexus of vessels (Kiesselbach's plexus) on the anterior part of the nasal septum. Venous drainage is via the ophthalmic and facial veins and the pterygoid and pharyngeal plexus. Intracranial drainage into the cavernous sinus via the ophthalmic vein is of particular clincial importance because of the potential for intracranial spread of nasal sepsis. The nasal cavity and sinuses have a sensory nerve supply provided by the first and second branches of the trigeminal nerve. The olfactory epithelium is supplied by the olfactory nerve. Autonomic innervation comprises sympathetic fibres to the blood vessels via the cervical and pterygopalatine ganglia. Parasympathetic fibres also synapse in the pterygopalatine ganglion before passing to the mucous glands.

Investigation

Plain X-rays are of limited value in the assessment of sinus disease. A minimum of four views – namely occipitomental, occipitofrontal, submentovertical and lateral views – are required to demonstrate the paranasal sinuses adequately. Computerised tomography (CT) scanning is far superior in demonstrating sinus pathology. Coronal and axial scans are necessary for detailed assessment.

Nasal airway resistance can be assessed by means of rhinomanometry which can be performed by either active or passive techniques. It may be used to quantify pre- and post-medical and surgical treatment for nasal obstruction and for the assessment of response to treatments for rhinitis.

Both rigid and flexible nasoendoscopes can be used for direct visualisation of the nasal fossa and the paranasal sinuses. Endoscopic techiques can be used for diagnosis and treatment.

Trauma to the nose

Injuries to the nose are commonly sustained in fights, sporting injuries and road traffic accidents. A blunt injury of moderate force may lead to springing of the nasal septal cartilage with separation of the overlying mucoperichondrium. Bleeding into this potential space will cause a septal haematoma which may be unilateral or bilateral. The haematoma will give rise to nasal obstruction and can be easily overlooked in the presence of extensive facial injuries. It is, however, an important diagnosis not to miss because untreated, a septal haematoma will progress to abscess formation and ultimately result in necrosis of the septal cartilage. Robbed of this support the tip of the nose will collapse. A septal haematoma should be treated by incision and evacuation of the blood clot. The insertion of a small silicone drain and packing of the nasal fossa will prevent reaccumulation and encourage the mucoperichondrium to readhere to the septal cartilage. A broad-spectrum prophylactic antibiotic should be prescribed.

Wilhelm Kiesselbach, 1839–1902. German laryngologist.

A more violent blunt injury to the nose can fracture the nasal bones. This may be a simple crack of the nasal bones without displacement, but greater force may result in deviation of the bony nasal complex laterally (Fig. 39.7) or depression of the bony pyramid if the blow is directly from the front. Greater impacts from this direction may cause a comminuted fracture and widening of the nasal bones or involve the lacrimal bones causing a nasoethmoidal fracture. Lateral injuries with displacement of the nasal bones may also be associated with a C-shaped fracture of the septal cartilage and the anterior portion of the perpendicular plate of the ethmoid (Jarjavay fracture). Nasal bone fractures can extend into the lacrimal bone tearing the anterior ethmoidal artery to produce catastrophic haemorrhage. This may be delayed, occurring only as the soft-tissue swelling subsides and the torn artery opens up.

Violent trauma to the frontal area of the nose can result in a fracture of the frontal and ethmoid sinuses extending into the anterior cranial fossa. Dural tears and brain injuries are then at risk from ascending infection through the fracture line from the nose or sinuses which may progress to meningitis or a brain abscess.

Cerebrospinal fluid (CSF) rhinorrhoea is a certain sign of a dural tear. There may be associated surgical emphysema, proptosis with or without loss of vision or frontal pneumoencephalocele. Anosmia occurs in 75 per cent of patients with these injuries, and cranial nerves II–VI may be injured. A clear discharge from the nose may be confirmed to be CSF by a simple stix test demonstrating the presence of glucose, which is not present in nasal mucus. Such injuries are managed by neurosurgical exploration to remove bone fragments, repair the skull base and close the dura. Late complications of this injury include CSF fistula, recurrent late meningitis, brain abscess, osteomyelitis and the formation of mucopyoceles.

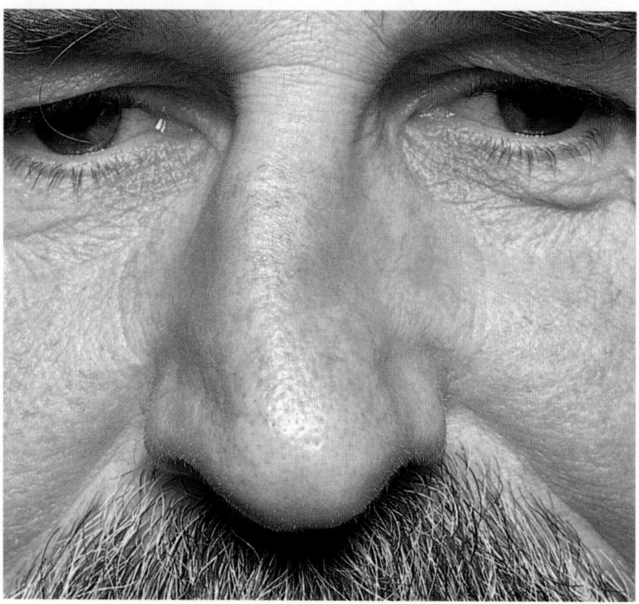

Fig. 39.7 Fracture of the nasal bones with lateral displacement of the bony nasal complex.

Management of fractured nasal bones

Fractured nasal bones are often accompanied by extensive overlying soft-tissue swelling and bruising which may hinder the assessment of the underlying bony deformity. Reviewing the patient 4–5 days later will give time for the soft-tissue swelling to subside and make subsequent assessment of any deformity much easier. If a fracture to the nasal bones has caused a significant degree of nasal deformity then this should be corrected by manipulation of the nasal bones under general anaesthesia. This must be carried out within 10 days of the injury while the bony fragments are still mobile. The deviated nasal bones are repositioned to restore the correct alignment of the nose or, in the case of a depressed fracture, the fragments are elevated and supported if necessary with anterior nasal packing. Often a satisfactory result can be obtained by simple manipulation, but should this fail then a rhinoplasty procedure (see later) may be necessary at a later date to obtain further improvement in the appearance of the nose. Any blow to the nose may cause displacement or fracture of the cartilagenous septum giving rise to post-traumatic nasal obstruction. Unlike the nasal bones, the nasal septum cannot be manipulated back into position and requires a formal septoplasty to restore the anatomy and the patency of the nasal airways (see later).

Nasal trauma – summary

- Do not overlook a septal haematoma
- Displaced nasal bone fractures should be reduced within 10 days of injury
- Severe epistaxis suggests lacrimal bone fracture and anterior ethmoid artery injury
- CSF rhinorrhoea indicates fracture involving frontal or ethmoid sinuses with a dural tear

Epistaxis

Although in the majority of patients this is a relatively easy clinical problem to deal with, this may not always be the case and in certain situations the haemorrhage may be life threatening. The most common site of bleeding is from Kiesselbach's plexus in Little's area of the anterior portion of the septum (Fig. 39.6). The usual cause is microtrauma to these blood vessels sandwiched between the mucosa and the underlying cartilage. In young children, heavy bleeding sometimes occurs from an engorged retro-columellar vein. Less often bleeding arises from the lateral nasal wall. Anterior bleeding is common in children and young adults as a result of nose blowing or picking. In the elderly, arteriosclerosis and hypertension are the underlying causes of arterial bleeding from the posterior part of the nose. The degeneration of the muscle layer of small arteries with age and the gradual replacement with collagen and calcification hinder post-traumatic vasoconstriction and prolong bleeding. Less com-

James Lawrence Little, 1836–85. Professor of Surgery, University of Vermont, Burlington, Vermont, USA.

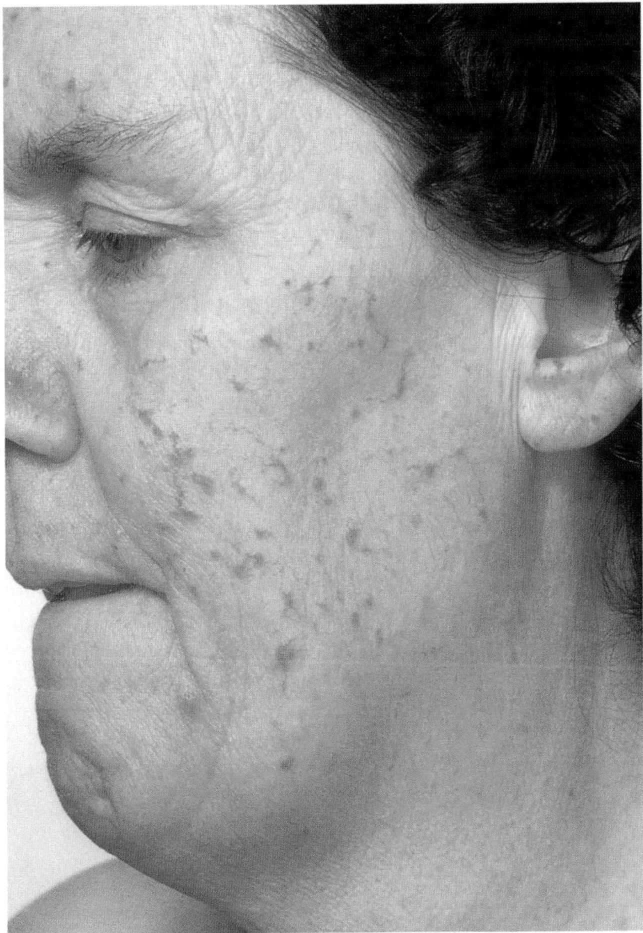

Fig. 39.8 Osler's disease showing multiple telangiectasia.

mon causes are trauma, foreign bodies within the nose, blood diseases, disorders of coagulation and malignant tumours of the nose or sinuses. Nasopharyngeal angiofibroma is a rare condition that affects boys and may lead to massive life-threatening attacks of bleeding. Hereditary haemorrhagic telangiectasia (Osler's disease) gives rise to recurrent multifocal bleeding from thin-walled vessels deficient in muscle and elastic tissue (Fig. 39.8).

Management of epistaxis

Bleeding from Kiesselbach's plexus may be controlled by silver nitrate cautery under local anaesthesia. Bleeding from further back in the nose, as seen in the elderly, may require anterior nasal packing with Vaseline-impregnated ribbon gauze. The packing is inserted in layers starting on the floor of the nasal cavity. Sometimes hypoxia can be induced by nasal packing and may be exacerbated in patients with chronic obstructive airways disese. The packing is usually kept in place for 48 hours and the patient commenced on a broad-spectrum antibiotic. An alternative to anterior packing

Sir William Osler, 1849–1919. Canadian-born physician.

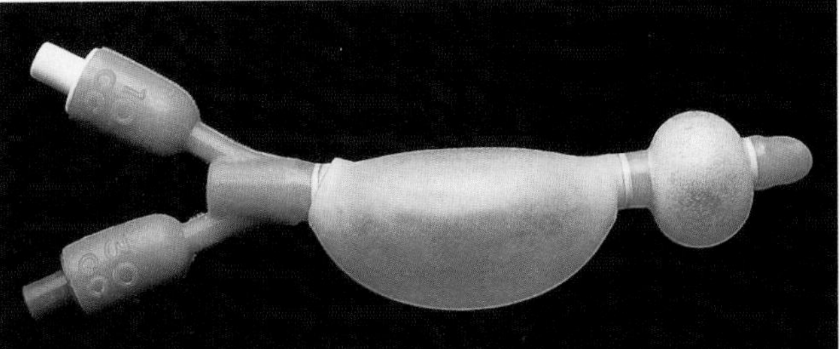

Fig. 39.9 Epistaxis balloon catheter.

is the use of an epistaxis balloon catheter (Fig. 39.9). The catheter is inserted in the nose and the distal balloon is inflated first within the choana to secure the catheter and then the proximal balloon, which is sausage shaped, is inflated within the nasal cavity proper. These catheters are usually effective but can be quite uncomfortable.

Sometimes anterior nasal packing alone is not sufficient to control haemorrhage and posterior nasal packing may be required. This is usually carried out under general anaesthesia inserting a gauze pack into the nasopharynx, which is then secured by tapes passed through each side of the nose and tied together across a protected columella. A third tape is brought out through the mouth and taped to the patient's cheek. The nasal fossae are then packed with anterior nasal packs. All packs are left in for 48 hours and prophylactic antibiotics are given. The tape attached to the cheek is to facilitate removal of the pack usually without a general anaesthetic.

In uncontrolled life-threatening epistaxis where the above methods have proved ineffective, haemostasis is achieved by vascular ligation. Depending on the origin of bleeding it may be necessary to ligate the internal maxillary artery in the pterygopalatine fossa and the anterior and posterior ethmoidal arteries within the orbit. An alternative measure is external carotid artery ligation above the origin of the lingual artery.

In Osler's disease anterior nasal packing is best avoided if at all possible because it is most likely to lead to further mucosal trauma and bleeding. High-dose oestrogen induces squamous metaplasia of the nasal mucosa and has been used effectively in treating this condition. In some cases however, it may be necessary to resort to excision of the diseased nasal mucosa via a lateral rhinotomy and replace it with a split skin graft – a procedure known as septodermoplasty. It is not unknown, however, for the grafted skin to undergo similar abnormal vascular change over time.

Epistaxis – summary

- Young people bleed from the anterior septum – Kiesselbach's plexus
- Older people bleed from the posterior part of the nose
- Silver nitrate cautery is good for controlling anterior septal bleeding
- Moderate bleeding may require anterior nasal packing
- Severe bleeding may require anterior and posterior nasal packing
- Persistent bleeding will probably require arterial ligation

Nasal polyps

Nasal polyps are benign swellings of the ethmoid sinus mucosa. Histologically polyps consist of a water-logged stroma infiltrated with eosinophils. The cause of polyp formation is unknown but it is thought that it may be related to a disorder of arachidonic acid metabolism. Nasal polyps are erroneously linked to allergic rhinitis, but many patients with allergic rhinitis never have polyps and many patients who suffer from nasal polyposis have no evidence of nasal allergy. Approximately a third of patients with nasal polyps also have asthma, while the triad of nasal polyps, aspirin allergy and asthma is not uncommon.

The vast majority of nasal polyps arises from the ethmoid sinuses, each individual ethmoid air cell giving rise to a single polyp as its swollen mucosal lining prolapses out of the air cell to hang down inside the nasal cavity. Polyps can arise from the other nasal sinuses, and a single large polyp arising from the maxillary antrum is referred to as an antrochoanal polyp. This usually fills the nose and eventually prolapses down into the nasopharynx. The diagnosis can often be made by looking into the patient's mouth and observing the fundus of the polyp hanging down beyond the free margin of the soft palate. Ethmoid polyps are usually bilateral but when unilateral in an adult or associated with bleeding then malignancy must be excluded. Nasal polyps are unusual in children and if multiple often occur in conjunction with cystic fibrosis in 10 per cent of cases. A unilateral nasal polyp in a child must be distinguised from a meningocele or encephalocele by high-resolution CT scanning of the anterior cranial fossa.

Clinical features

Polyps cause nasal ostruction associated with watery rhinorrhoea and often anosmia. They are easily identifiable within the nose as pale, semitransparent grey masses which are mobile and insensitive when palpated with a fine probe, allowing them to be distinguished from turbinate hypertrophy. Extensive nasal polyposis often gives rise to secondary pansinusitis, by occluding the ostia and interfering with sinus ventilation. If left untreated they will eventually result in expansion of the nose and prolapse through the nasal vestibule (Fig. 39.10).

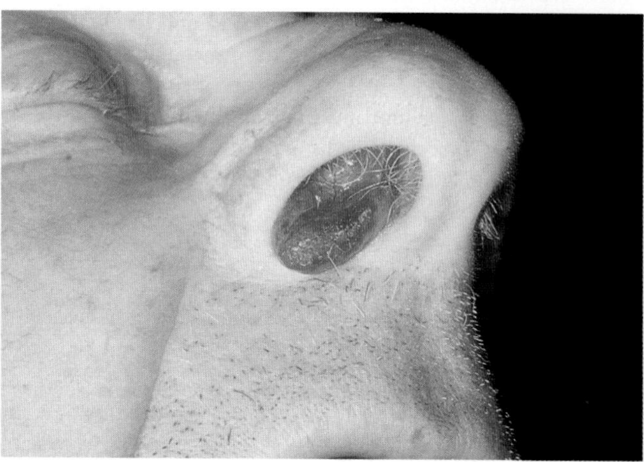

Fig. 39.10 Nasal polyp presenting at the right nasal vestibule.

Management of nasal polyps

Polyps are best treated by surgical removal either by avulsion with a nasal snare or with a powered nasal microresector (Fig. 39.11). Antral lavage should be performed at the same time. Benign transitional cell papilloma (inverted papilloma) can be mistaken for simple nasal polyps (see later) and therefore the polyps should always be submitted for histological examination.

Polyps often recur in a seemingly random and unpredictable way. There is evidence to suggest that long-term treatment with low-dose topical nasal steroids (betamethasone) postoperatively lessens the tendency for polyps to recur. After multiple recurrence external ethmoidectomy should be considered. Although polyp formation may still occur after the procedure, the interval between recurrences will be longer. Polyps usually shrink while a patient is taking oral steroids but recur when treatment is stopped.

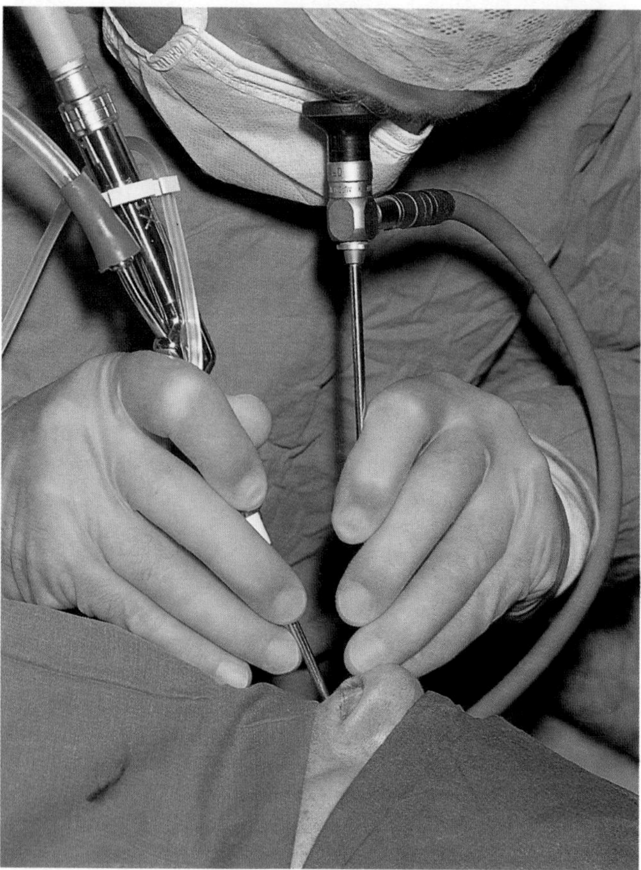

Fig. 39.11 Powered nasal microresector. An oscillating blade within a narrow metal sheath cuts off tissue at the window in the sheath. Continuous irrigation with suction keeps the window and operating field clear.

Nasal polyps – summary

- Polyps are insensitive to touch
- Transitional papilloma may be mistaken for simple polyps
- Polyps can be removed by nasal snare or powered nasal microresector
- Recurrent polyps may require external ethmoidectomy
- Meningocele and encephalocele should be excluded in children with polyps
- Bleeding polyps may indicate malignancy

Nasal septum

The nasal septum consists of the quadrilateral cartilage anteriorly and the bony perpendicular plate of the ethmoid and vomer posteriorly. Few, if any, people are born with an entirely straight septum and symmetrical nasal airways. In some individuals a naturally occurring deviated nasal septum gives rise to significant nasal obstruction. In others minor nasal trauma is responsible for displacement of the septum and restriction of the nasal airway (Fig. 39.12). Further encroachment of the anterior nasal airway can occur if the ventral edge of the septal cartilage is dislocated from the columella and projects into the nasal vestibule. Inferior turbinate hypertrophy is frequently seen on the concave side of a deviated nasal septum. This is particularly likely to occur after nasal injury. The physical obstruction of the nasal airway by a deviated septum is readily apparent on anterior rhinoscopy.

Septal deformity can be corrected by means of a septoplasty procedure or by a submucus resection of the septum (SMR). In the former procedure the septal cartilage is preserved but the anatomical abnormalities giving rise to its deformity such as a twisted maxillary crest or inclination of the bony septum are corrected, permitting the septal cartilage to be repositioned in the midline with the restoration of nasal airway patency. In the SMR procedure the deformed septal cartilage is excised, while preserving a dorsal strut along with the anterior 5 mm of septal cartilage in order to support and maintain the normal shape of the nasal tip. Both operations are performed through a vertical incision of the septal mucosa with elevation of mucoperichondrial flaps.

Postoperatively, the nose is packed for 24–48 hours to prevent haematoma formation. Complications of septal surgery include septal perforation giving rise to excessive crusting within the nose, nasal obstruction and epistaxis. If too much cartilage is excised in the SMR procedure the loss of support to the dorsum of the nose may result in a saddle deformity or drooping of the tip of the nose.

Septal perforation

The causes of septal perforation are listed in Table 39.1. The commonest cause is a complication of septal surgery. Septal perforations seldom heal spontaneously. They give rise to extensive crusting at the margins of the perforation, often with mucosal bleeding. If situated towards the front of the septum embarrassing whistling can occur. Patients also often complain of a sensation of nasal obstruction.

Crusting can be controlled to a degree with nasal douches or the use of topical antiseptic creams to minimise mucosal drying. A great variety of operations has been described to close septal perforations but none of them has met with universal success. A more certain option is to occlude the perforation by inserting a sialastic biflanged prosthesis (Fig. 39.13).

Rhinitis

Rhinitis is inflammation of the nasal mucous membranes and can be of various types (Table 39.2). A clinical diagnosis of rhinitis can be made if a patient has two or more of the following symptoms: anterior rhinorrhoea, postnasal catarrh, nasal obstruction, nasal itch or irritation, and sneezing. The management of these conditions is determined largely by the type of rhinitis and the predominant symptom and lies within

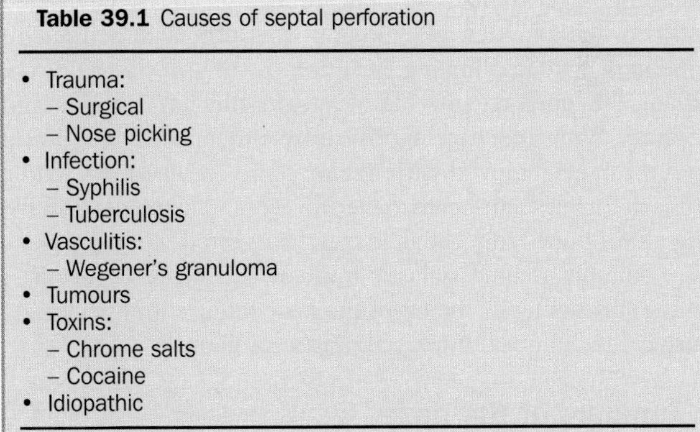

Table 39.1 Causes of septal perforation

- Trauma:
  - Surgical
  - Nose picking
- Infection:
  - Syphilis
  - Tuberculosis
- Vasculitis:
  - Wegener's granuloma
- Tumours
- Toxins:
  - Chrome salts
  - Cocaine
- Idiopathic

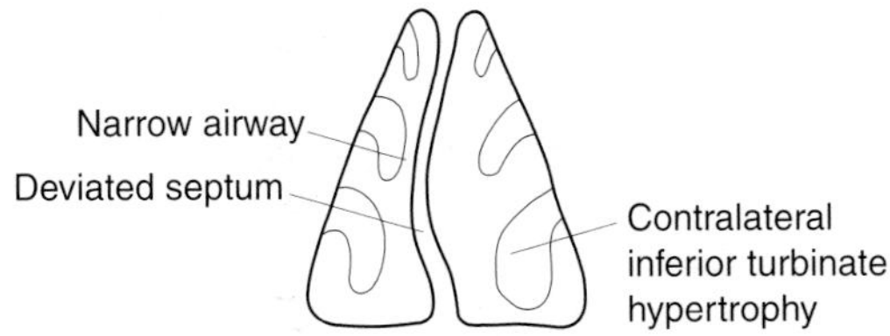

Fig. 39.12 Anterior diagram of nasal fossae. Deviated nasal septum to the patient's right side restricting the nasal airway.

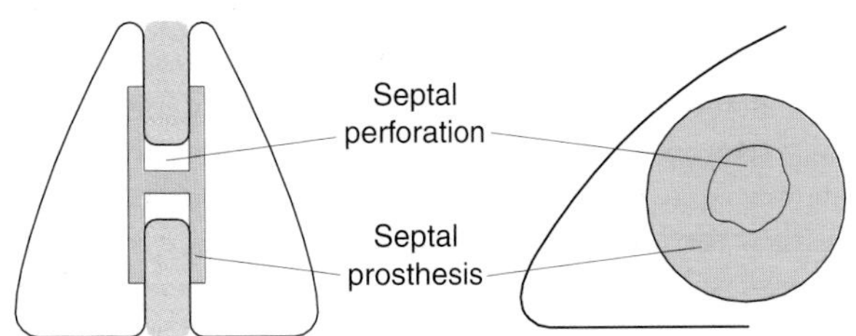

Fig. 39.13 Anterior and lateral diagrams of nasal septal perforation showing occlusion with a prosthesis.

Table 39.2 Classification of rhinitis

- Allergic rhinitis
- Intrinsic rhinitis
- Infective rhinitis
- Unusual types of rhinitis:
  - Atrophic rhinitis
  - Drug-induced rhinitis
  - Hormonal rhinitis
  - Occupational rhinitis
  - Rhinitis medicamentosa
  - Sarcoidosis
  - Wegener's granulomatosis

the province of the otolaryngologist, seldom requiring surgery and therefore not referred to further in this chapter.

External nasal deformity

Anomalies of the shape of the nose may be congenital or acquired. The latter may be the result of trauma, previous nasal surgery or destructive processes such as Wegener's granulomatosis. Correction of a deformity of the bony nasal complex is referred to as a rhinoplasty procedure and if combined with a procedure to correct a deviation of the nasal septum the procedure is known as a septorhinoplasty. In a standard rhinoplasty procedure the nasal bones are approached through an intercartilagenous incision between the upper and lower lateral cartilages within the nasal fossa and the soft tissues covering the nasal skeleton are elevated. Superior and lateral osteotomies are used to mobilise the nasal bones, which are then repositioned to produce a pleasing shape to the nose. This procedure can also be carried out through an external approach where the skin of the columella is divided allowing elevation of the soft tissues of the tip of the nose to provide access to the nasal bones and septum. With adequate exposure by either method a dorsal hump can be removed with hammer and chisel and a saddle nose deformity can be corrected by dorsal augmentation using either bone from the iliac crest, harvested septal cartilage or a suitably shaped sialastic implant. Cosmetic deformities of the soft tissues of the tip of the nose require the specialised surgical techniques of a facial plastic surgeon.

Tumours of the nose

Benign tumours

Osteomas of the nasal skeleton are not uncommon and are usually detected on X-ray as an incidental finding. They are usually seen in the frontal and ethmoid sinuses (Fig. 39.14). Some may produce symptoms such as headache or recurrent sinusitis if the location interferes with the drainage of one of the paranasal sinuses. Plain X-rays demonstrate a calcified, well-demarcated tumour of variable size. In symptomatic individuals the osteoma can be removed via the frontal sinus or an external ethmoidectomy.

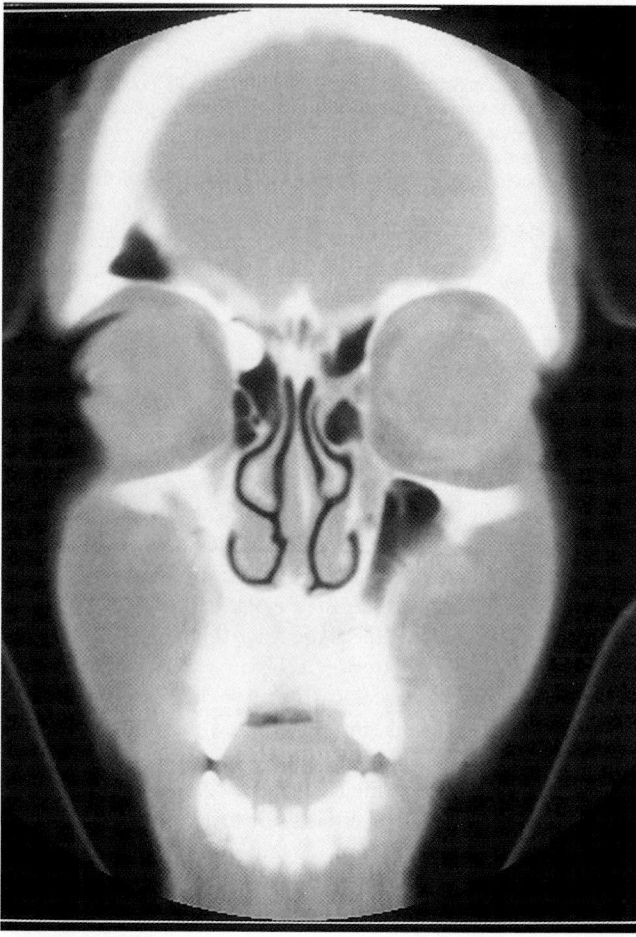

Fig. 39.14 Coronal CT scan showing small osteoma in the right ethmoid sinus adjacent to the orbit.

Transitional cell papilloma (inverted papilloma) can occur in both the nasal cavity and the nasal sinuses. They can be quite extensive (Fig. 39.15) and give rise to nasal obstruction and sometimes epistaxis. Although usually unilateral, red, firm and vascular they can sometimes look like simple nasal polyps, and in 25 per cent of cases the diagnosis is made by the pathologist after a routine nasal polypectomy. When large they can erode the lateral nasal wall and infiltrate the antrum and ethmoid. Calcification within the tumour may be seen on CT scanning along with sclerosis of bone at the margins of the growth. Transitional cell papilloma can undergo malignant change; synchronous lesions occur in 5–10 per cent, while metachronous lesions develop in 1 per cent of cases.

For this reason more radical surgery is employed than for simple polyps to ensure complete removal of all papillomata and will usually involve a partial maxillectomy.

Benign nasal tumours – summary

- Osteomas are frequently asymptomatic
- Transitional papilloma may undergo malignant change

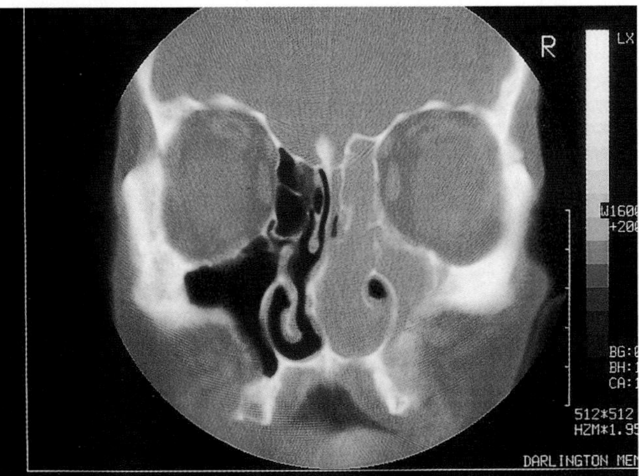

Fig. 39.15 Coronal CT scan showing extensive transitional papilloma involving right maxillary antrum and ethmoid sinuses.

Malignant tumours

Skin tumours involving the nose are not uncommon. Basal cell carcinomas (rodent ulcer) are confined to the head in 86 per cent of cases and of these 26 per cent occur on the nose. Adequate surgical excision may require some form of reconstructive flap procedure to eliminate the resulting defect. Keratinising squamous cell carcinoma is the second most common tumour of the external nose, which should be adequately excised with a generous margin of healthy skin and the defect reconstructed with a local flap. About 10 per cent of all melanomas occur in the head and neck. Wide surgical excision is mandatory, frequently requiring the skills of a plastic surgeon for reconstruction (see Chapter 13 on 'Plastic surgery').

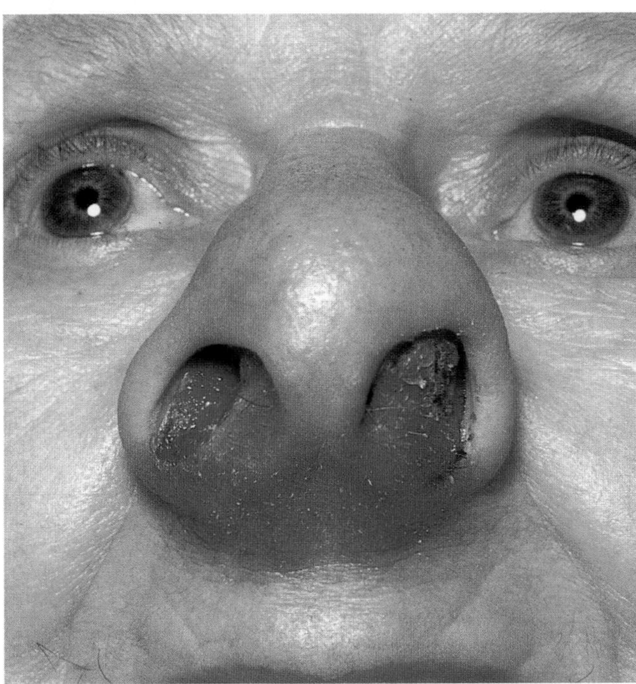

Fig. 39.16 Squamous cell carcinoma of the nasal septum.

The most common tumours to occur within the nasal cavity and paranasal sinuses are squamous cell carcinoma (Fig. 39.16), adenoidcystic carcinoma and adenocarcinoma. (Table 39.3). Presenting symptoms include unilateral nasal obstruction, chronic nasal discharge, which is often haemorrhagic and offensive, and loss of skin sensation on the face (trigeminal nerve). There may be swelling of the cheek, buccal sulcus or the medial canthus of the eye and a feeling of fullness or pressure within the nose or face. Suspicious signs of invasion of neighbouring tissues include diplopia, proptosis, loosening of the teeth (Fig. 39.17), trismus, cranial nerve palsies and regional lymphadenopathy.

Table 39.3 Classification of nasal and sinus tumours

- Benign epithelial tumours:
  - Papillomas
  - Minor salivary gland tumours
  - Dermoids
  - Gliomas
  - Encephaloceles
- Benign osseous tumours:
  - Osteoma
  - Fibrous dysplasia
  - Ossifying fibroma
  - Osteitis fibrosa cystica
  - Giant cell epulis
- Benign connective tissue tumours:
  - Chondroma
  - Meningioma
  - Haemangioma neurofibroma
  - Angiofibroma
  - Eosinophilic granuloma
- Intermediate tumours:
  - Basal cell tumour
  - Transitional cell papilloma
  - Extramedullary plasmacytoma
  - Ameloblastoma
- Malignant epithelial tumours:
  - Squamous cell carcinoma
  - Adenocarcinoma
  - Transitional cell carcinoma
  - Anaplastic carcinoma
  - Malignant melanoma
  - Olfactory neuroblastoma
  - Adenoid cystic carcinoma
  - Metastatic carcinoma
- Malignant osseous tumours:
  - Osteogenic sarcoma
  - Malignant fibrous histiocytoma
  - Ewing's sarcoma
- Malignant connective tissue tumours:
  - Fibrosarcoma
  - Rhabdomyosarcoma
  - Chondrosarcoma
  - Haemangioperiocytoma
  - Lymphoma
  - Midfacial necrotizing lesions

James Ewing, 1866–1943. American pathologist.

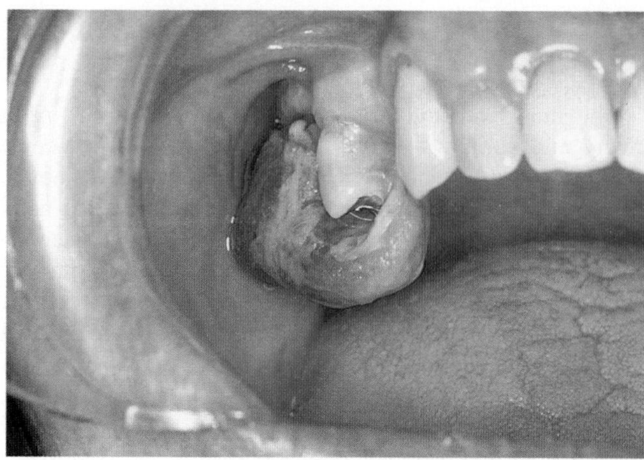

Fig. 39.17 Maxillary antral carcinoma presenting through an oroantral fistula.

Biopsy via nasal endoscopy will permit a tissue diagnosis, while assessment of bone errosion and the extent of the disease can be determined by CT scanning (Fig. 39.18). If invasion of the skull base is suspected then angiography will be required, and distant metastases to lung, bone, brain and liver should be excluded.

Patients with sinus or intranasal malignancy are best managed in a combined clinic where the expertise of ear, nose and throat (ENT) surgeons, maxillofacial surgeons and radiotherapists can be employed. Detailed surgical management is outside the scope of this book, but the adequacy of any surgical resection will need to be confirmed by frozen section control of soft-tissue margins. Inevitably reconstruction will require the use of myocutaneous flaps or free grafts with microvascular anastomosis. Surgery is followed by radiotherapy. At present chemotherapy is reserved for palliation of inoperable tumours.

> Malignant nasal tumours – summary
>
> - Skin cancer of the nose requires wide excision and expert reconstruction
> - May present late with signs of invasion
> - Should be managed by ENT and maxillofacial surgeons with a radiotherapist

Paranasal sinus infection

Patients with paranasal sinusitis will usually only be referred to an ENT surgeon if they have failed to respond to conservative treatment with antibiotics or if complications are developing.

Maxillary sinusitis

Patients with persistent maxillary sinusitis have postnasal discharge, headache which is variable in severity and location, nasal obstruction and usually general malaise. The nasal mucosa is swollen and bathed in mucopurulent secretions. Plain sinus X-rays may show a fluid level in the antrum or complete opacity (Fig. 39.19).

The most likely causative organisms are *Streptococcus pneumoniae* and *H. influenzae*. As the infection becomes chronic the likelihood of anaerobic infection increases. The consideration of a *Branhamella catarrhalis* as a primary pathogen and the possibility of β-lactam-producing

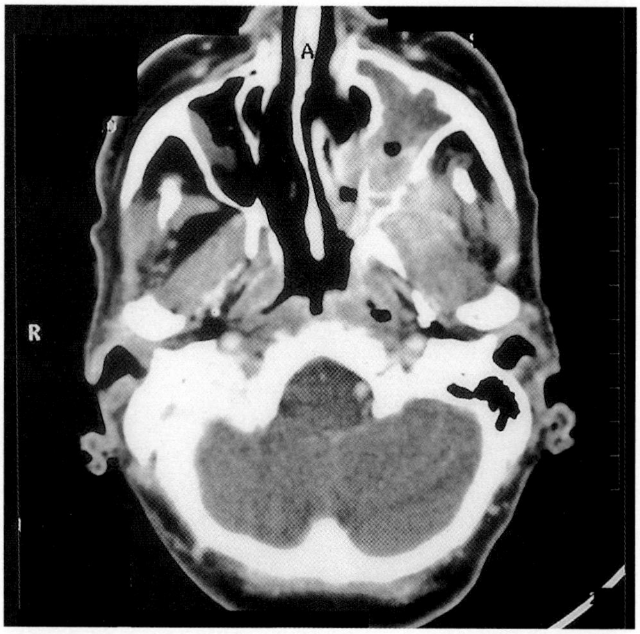

Fig. 39.18 CT scan showing extensive maxillary antral carcinoma invading adjacent structures.

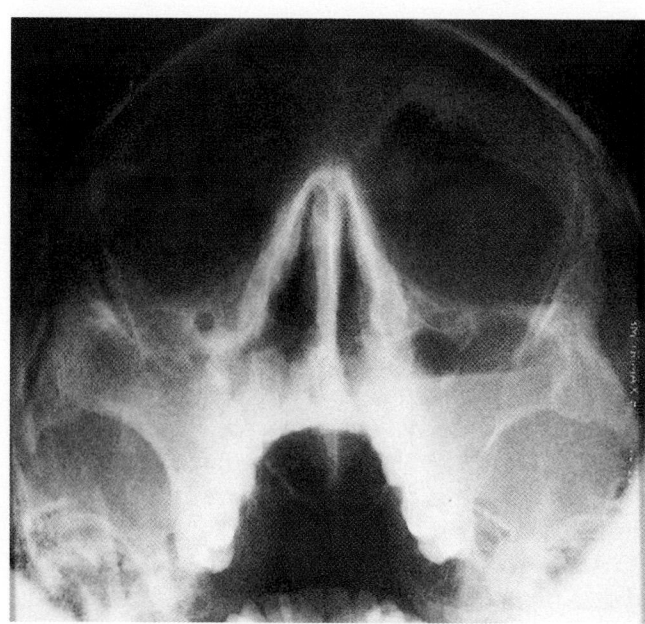

Fig. 39.19 Plain X-ray showing fluid level in the left maxillary antrum and total opacity of the right side.

strains of *H. influenzae* will also influence the choice of antibiotic.

Adequate penetration of antibiotics into chronically inflamed sinus mucosa is doubtful, and therefore treatment may need to be given for several weeks. Topical nasal decongestants such as ephedrine nasal drops will often encourage the sinus to drain. About 10 per cent of infections of the maxillary antrum are due to dental sepsis from anaerobic organisms. The resultant mucopurulent nasal secretion has a foul smell and taste. Maxillary sinusitis from any cause may, through irritation of the superior alveolar nerve, give rise to referred upper toothache.

Antral lavage under local or general anaesthesia allows confirmation of the diagnosis and provides the opportunity to obtain samples for bacteriology. The antrum is entered through the inferior meatus below the inferior turbinate where the bone separating the antrum from the nasal fossa is extremely thin and can be penetrated by a trocar and cannula (Fig 39.20).

If infection has caused a significant degree of inflammation and fibrosis of the lining of the antrum then the natural ostium may be completely obstructed. In this situation an intranasal inferior meatal antrostomy may be fashioned to facilitate drainage from the antrum. Alternatively, intranasal endoscopic techniques may be employed to create a middle meatal antrostomy. The middle turbinate is lifted and the infundibulum is located and enlarged anteriorly, sometimes requiring the excision of the anterior end of the uncinate process under direct endoscopic control. The antrum itself can be inspected through the antrostomy using a combination of 30° and 70° rigid endoscopes (Fig. 39.21). For persisting disease a Caldwell–Luc radical antrostomy may be performed, whereby the entire diseased maxillary sinus mucosa is removed through an opening in the anterior wall of the antrum via an incision in the upper gum. Once the diseased antral mucosa is removed a large window is created in the lateral nasal wall allowing drainage into the inferior meatus.

Endoscopic nasal surgery allows a more functional approach to diseases of the paranasal sinuses and the indications for radical antrostomy are on the decline. Areas of chronically diseased mucosa and infected granulation tissue hinder mucociliary transport and lymphatic drainage leading to retained secretions and the perpetuation of infection. Intranasal endoscopic operations permit the precise removal of diseased mucosa with minimal trauma to adjacent tissues. By removing scar tissue from the narrow recesses within the nose, ventilation and internal drainage can be restored allowing permanent resolution of the chronically inflamed mucosa. In this way precise endoscopic surgery directed towards the middle meatus and the ethmoid system restores the normal physiological function of the paranasal sinuses with minimal mucosal resection (Fig. 39.22).

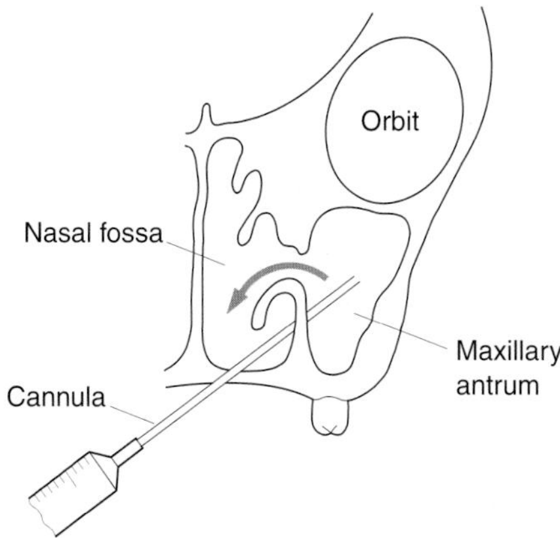

Fig. 39.20 Diagram of maxillary antral lavage.

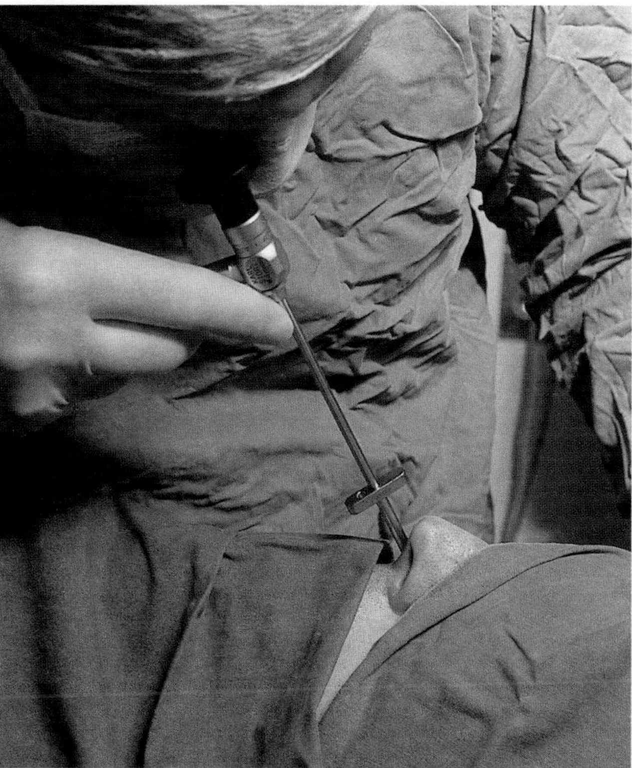

Fig. 39.21 Inspection of the right maxillary antrum using a rigid endoscope.

Complications of maxillary sinusitis

Untreated chronic maxillary sinusitis can lead to acute cellulitis or osteitis and rarely, if there is a breach in the roof of the antrum, infection may spread into the orbit.

> Maxillary sinusitis – summary
>
> - Commonest organisms *S. pneumoniae* and *H. influenzae*
> - May result from dental sepsis
> - Antral lavage is diagnostic and therapeutic
> - Intranasal antrostomy or endoscopic middle meatal antrostomy may be needed

George Walter Caldwell, 1866–1946. Otolaryngologist who practised successively in New York, San Fransisco and Los Angeles. Described his operation for treating suppuration of the maxillary antrum in 1893.

Henri Luc, 1855–1925. Otolaryngologist, Paris. Described his operation in 1889.

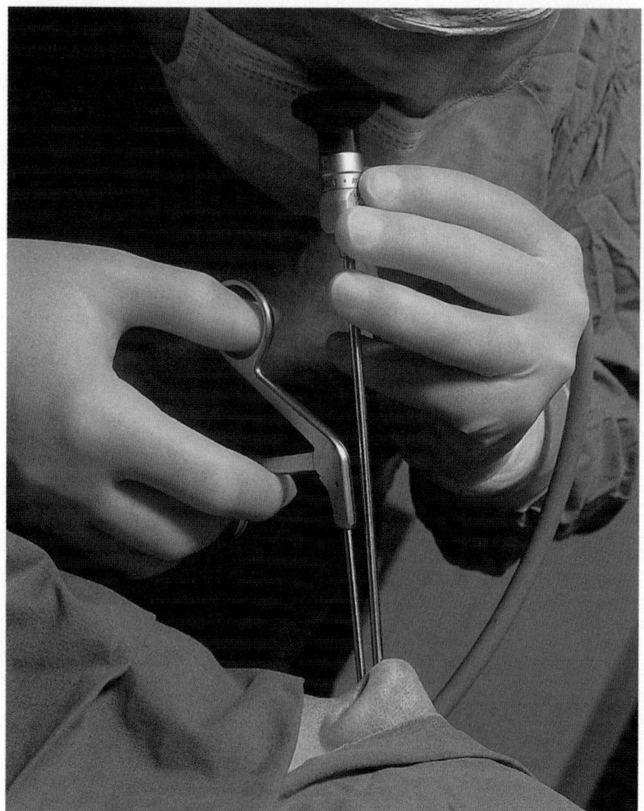

Fig. 39.22 Function endoscopic nasal surgery.

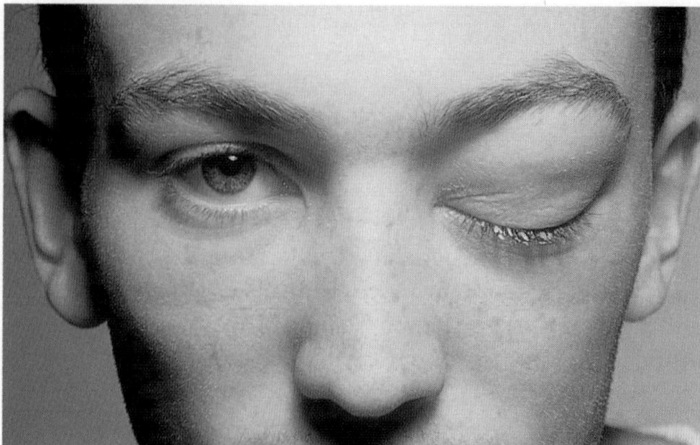

Fig. 39.23 Left periorbital cellulitis complicating left-sided acute ethmoiditis.

Frontoethmoidal sinusitis

If treated promptly with antibiotics and topical nasal decongestants this type of sinus infection is unlikely to be a long-term problem. If allowed to persist chronic frontoethmoiditis gives rise to mucopurulent catarrh, frontal headaches, pressure feeling between the eyes, nasal obstruction and hyposmia. Nasal endoscopy will confirm pus issuing from the middle meatus. The ethmoid sinuses can only be properly assessed radiologically by CT scanning, including coronal as well as axial sections. If frontoethmoiditis fails to settle with conservative treatment then frontal drainage may be required. The frontal sinus is entered through its anterior wall via a small incision below the medial end of the eyebrow. After pus is drained a small sialastic tube is left in the wound to allow regular irrigation of the sinus. Where the disease is more extensive intranasal endoscopic ethmoidectomy may be required. Removal of the uncinate process provides access to the osteomeatal complex, so that if necessary the entire ethmoid complex can be cleared and the frontonasal recess opened. If endoscopic nasal equipment is not available then the tried and tested radical external ethmoidectomy through a Lynch–Howarth incision provides excellent access to the frontal, ethmoid and sphenoid sinuses. Chronic frontal sinus disease can be cleared by means of an osteoplastic flap procedure. Using an X-ray template, the boundaries of the frontal sinus are marked out and a fissure burr is used to cut through the frontal bone along the outline of the sinus. The front wall of the sinus is then prised downwards and forwards to produce an inferiorly based osteoplastic flap. The diseased lining can then be removed and the sinus obliterated with fat taken from the anterior abdominal wall.

Complications of frontoethmoiditis

These are potentially extremely serious. Quite often infection can spread to involve the other sinuses because of the close proximity of their ostia. Orbital cellulitis is not an uncommon complication (Fig. 39.23) and may progress to an extraperiosteal abscess, which typically displaces the eyeball down forwards and laterally. If unrecognised and untreated this can lead to blindness. Treatment consists of intravenous broad-spectrum antibiotic and an orbital decompression by an external approach. Orbital cellulitis may progress to cavernous sinus thrombosis and septicaemia. Spread of infection by direct bone penetration or via the diploic veins can give rise to either extradural, subdural or frontal lobe abscess formation.

Frontoethmoidal sinusitis – summary

- May require open surgical drainage
- Chronic frontal sinusitis may require obliterative osteoplastic flap procedure
- Orbital complications may threaten sight
- Intracranial complications include cerebral abscess and cavernous sinus thrombosis

Further reading

Mackay, I.S. and Bull, T.R. (1988) *Scott Brown's Otolaryngology*, Butterworths, London.

Maran, A.G.D. and Lund, V.J. (1990) *Clinical Rhinology*, Thieme, New York.

Wigand, M.E. (1990) *Endoscopic Surgery of the Paranasal Sinuses and Anterior Skull Base*, Thieme, New York.

Sir Philip Lynch, 1893–1982. Canadian ophthalmologist.
W.G. Howarth, 1879–1962. London otolaryngologist.

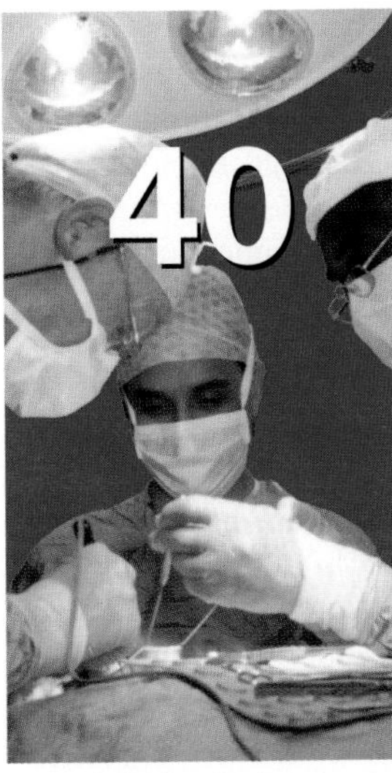

40 The ear

Surgical anatomy of the ear

The *external ear* consists of the pinna and the ear canal. The pinna is made of yellow elastic cartilage covered by tightly adherent skin. The external and middle ear develop from the first two branchial arches. The external ear canal is 3 cm in length, the outer two-thirds is cartilage and the inner third is bony. The skin on the lateral surface of the tympanic membrane and the inner two-thirds of the ear canal is highly specialised. It does not simply shed like the skin from the rest of the body. It migrates outwards from the tympanic membrane and along the ear canal. As a result of this migration most people's ears are self-cleaning. Disorders of skin migration can result in ear disease (e.g. cholesteatoma). The external canal is richly innervated and the skin is tightly bound down to the perichondrium so that oedema in this region results in severe pain.

The lymphatics of the external ear drain to the retroauricular, parotid, retropharyngeal and deep upper cervical lymph nodes.

The *middle ear* contains the ossicles. Laterally it is bounded by the tympanic membrane, medially by the cochlea, anteriorly by the eustachian tube and posteriorly it communicates with the mastoid air cells (Fig. 40.1). Entwined in this tiny space is the facial nerve which pursues a tortuous course through the middle ear and exits the skull base at the stylomastoid foramen. Knowledge of the anatomy of the middle ear is important because infection can spread through it to the cranial cavity which lies millimetres away.

The *tympanic membrane* has three layers: an inner mucosal layer, a dense fibrous middle layer and the outer stratified squamous epithelium (skin). The upper portion that lies above the lateral process of the malleus is called the pars flaccida. The lower portion, making up the majority of the drum, is called the pars tensa (Fig. 40.2).

The tympanic membrane and ossicles act as a transformer system converting vibrations in the air to vibrations within the fluid-filled inner ear (perilymph).

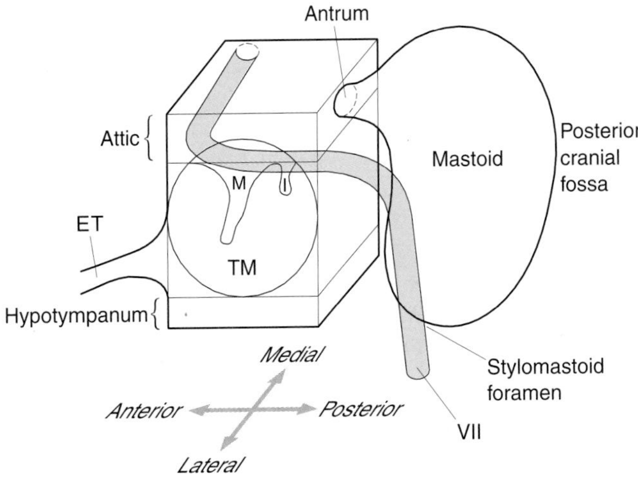

Fig. 40.1 Diagram to show the relations of the middle ear. ET: eustachian tube; TM: tympanic membrane.

Bartolomeo Eustachio, b. 1520. Italian anatomist.

Bailey & Love's Short Practice of Surgery, 23rd edition. Edited by R.C.G. Russell, N.S. Williams and C.J.K. Bulstrode. Published in 2000 by Arnold Publishers.

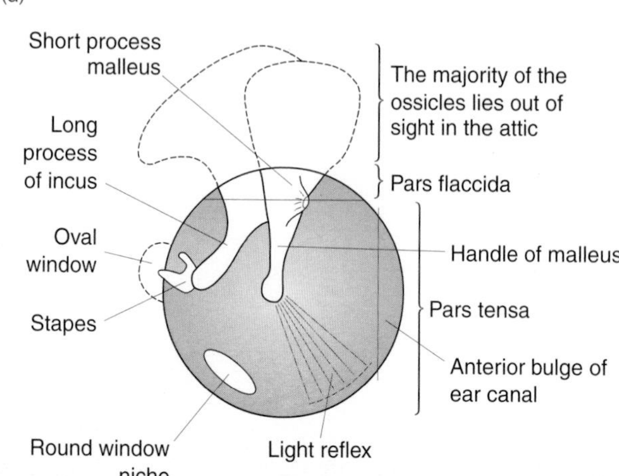

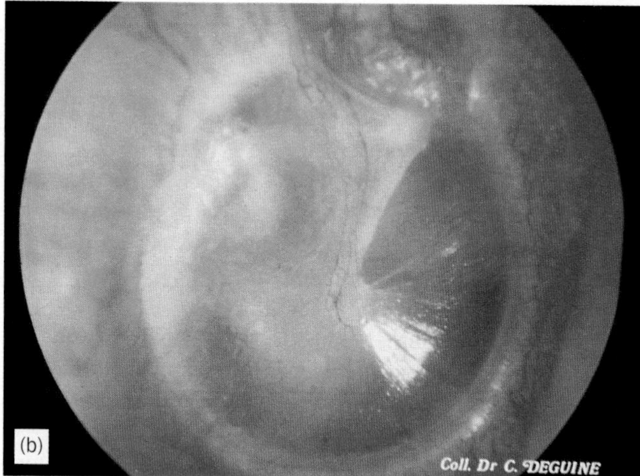

Fig. 40.2 Right tympanic membrane and diagram to illustrate anatomy (*courtesy of Dr Christian Deguine*).

The evolution of the middle ear is interesting. Fish do not have one, whereas amphibians (e.g. salamanders) have a single strut for an ossicle. At an air–water interface there is a 30 decibels loss of sound energy. The mammalian middle ear overcomes virtually all of this potential loss of sound energy.

The *inner ear* comprises the cochlea and vestibular labyrinth (saccule, utricle and semicircular canals). These structures are embedded in dense bone called the otic capsule.

The cochlea is a minute spiral of two and three-quarter turns. Within this spiral, perilymph and endolymph are partitioned by the thinnest of membranes (Reissner's membrane). The endolymph has a high concentration of potassium similar to intracellular fluid, and the perilymph has a high sodium concentration similar to extracellular fluid. Maintenance of the ionic gradients is an active process and is essential for neuronal activity.

There are approximately 15 000 hair cells in the human cochlea. They are arranged in rows of inner and outer hair cells. The inner hair cells act as mechanicoelectric transducers, converting the acoustic signal into an electric impulse. The outer hair cells contain contractile proteins and have an efferent nerve supply from the brain. They serve to tune the basilar membrane on which they are positioned.

Each inner hair cell responds to a particular frequency and when stimulated it depolarises and passes an impulse to the cochlea nuclei in the brainstem.

The vestibular labyrinth consists of the semicircular canals, the utricle and saccule, and their central connections. The three semicircular canals are arranged in the three planes of space at right angles to each other. As in the auditory system, hair cells are present. In the lateral canals the hair cells are embedded in a gelatinous cupula, and shearing forces, caused by angular movements of the head, produce hair cell movements and generate action potentials. In the utricle and saccule the hair cells are embedded in an otoconial membrane which contains particles of calcium carbonate. These respond to changes in linear acceleration and the pull of gravity.

Impulses are carried centrally by the vestibular nerve, and connections are made to the spinal cord, cerebellum and external ocular muscles.

The *sensory nerve supply* of the ear is complex. The external ear is supplied by the auriculotemporal branch of the trigeminal nerve (V), and this supplies most of the anterior half of the pinna and the external auditory meatus. The greater auricular nerve (C2,3), together with branches of the lesser occipital nerve (C2), supply the posterior part of the pinna. The VIIth, IXth and Xth cranial nerves also supply small sensory branches to the external ear; this explains why the vesicles of herpes zoster affecting the VIIth nerve appear in the concha (see Fig. 40.29 later). The middle ear is supplied by the glossopharyngeal nerve (IX).

This complicated and rich sensory innervation means that referred otalgia is common and may originate from the normal area of distribution of any of the above nerves. A classic example is the referred otalgia caused by a malignancy in the pyriform fossa of the pharynx or a cancer of the larynx.

Anatomy of the ear

- Referred otalgia has many causes (e.g. cancer of the larynx)
- Middle ear is intimately related to the cranial cavity
- The VIIth nerve has a tortuous course through the ear

Conditions of the external ear

Congenital anomalies

Congenital anomalies can range from total absence of the ear through to mild cosmetic deformities such as tiny accessory auricles or skin tags. External ear anomalies can be isolated or may be associated with middle ear deformity. The external and middle ear originate from the first and second branchial arches, whereas the cochlea is of neuroectodermal origin. This means that an individual may have no pinna or ear canal but a normal cochlea may well be present. In these circumstances, sound can be transmitted from a hearing aid connected to an osteointegrated peg that is screwed into the mastoid bone.

Table 40.1 Conditions of the external ear

Congenital	Microtia Preauricular sinuses Prominent ears
Trauma	Haematoma of the pinna Foreign bodies
Inflammatory	Otitis externa Necrotising otitis externa Furuncle
Neoplasms	Benign: osteomas, papillomas, adenomas Malignant: basal and squamous cell carcinomas

Children who have a significant deformity of the pinna (microtia) can be helped with osteointegrated implants to which a prosthetic ear is connected (Fig. 40.3). The ear can be unclipped prior to playing violent sport (e.g. rugby) and this unsettles the opposition.

Preauricular sinuses are a common congenital abnormality and occasionally need excising because of recurrent infections and discharge. The sinus usually ends near the external canal but occasionally the track is very extensive and is closely related to the facial nerve, which makes life exciting.

Prominent ears are a common deformity which usually results from the absence of the antihelix curve. Various cartilage scoring methods are available to correct this deformity.

Trauma

Trauma often affects the external ear. A haematoma of the pinna occurs when blood collects between the perichondrium and the cartilage. The cartilage receives its blood supply from the perichondrial layer and will die if the haematoma is not evacuated (cauliflower ear). An extensive excision, under general anaesthetic, with a pressure dressing and antibiotic cover is recommended (see Fig. 40.4).

Foreign bodies in the ear canal need to be treated with the greatest respect. If an object is not simply removed at the first attempt, it is better to do it with the aid of a microscope and general anaesthesia. An active 2-year-old with a bead in the ear can be a formidable opponent (Fig. 40.5).

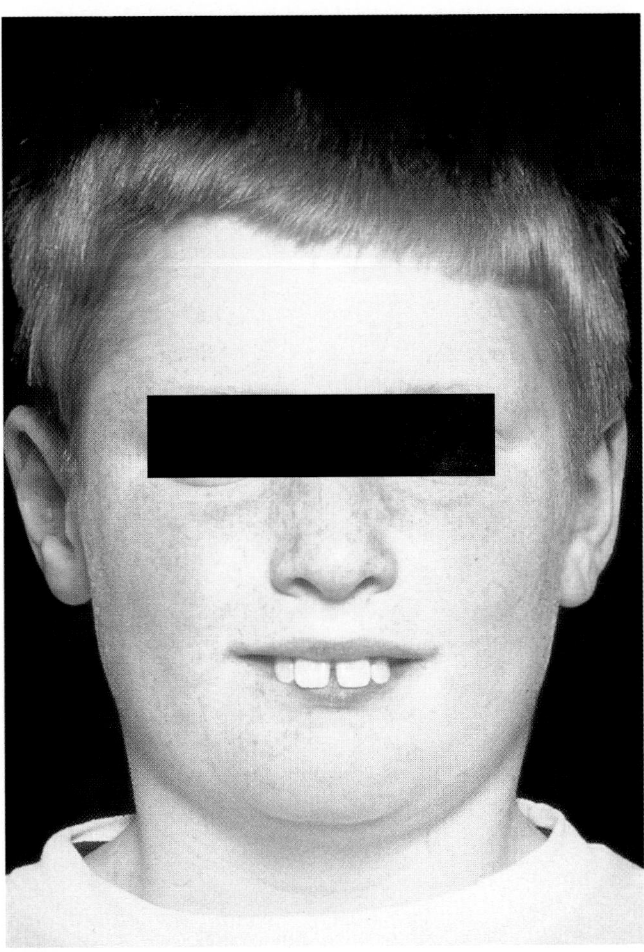

Fig. 40.3 This young man can remove his prosthetic right ear, which is attached to an osteointegrated stud, before playing rugby.

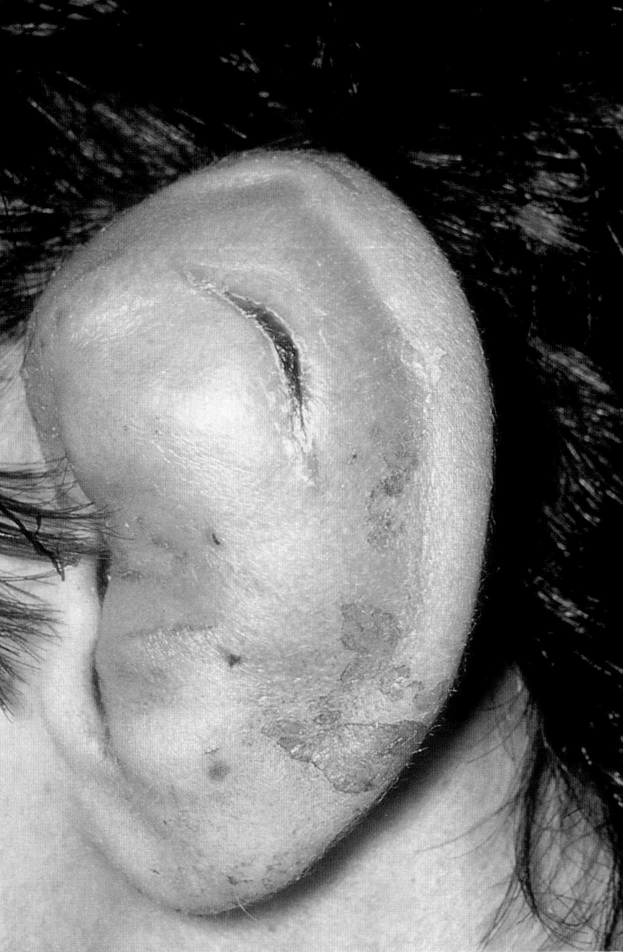

Fig. 40.4 Haematoma of the pinna.

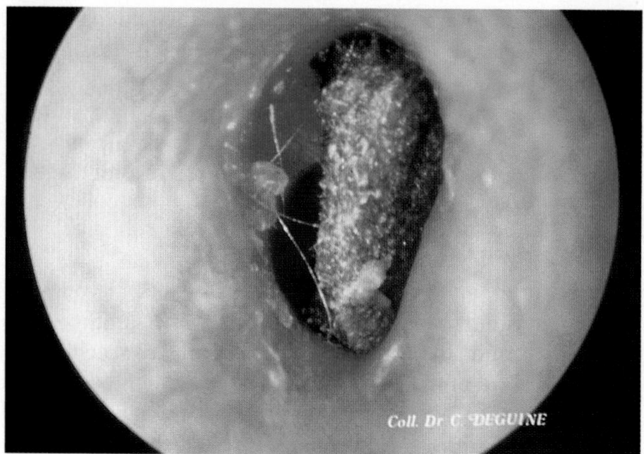

Fig. 40.5 Removal of a foreign body from the ear canal can be a challenge (*courtesy of Dr Christian Deguine*).

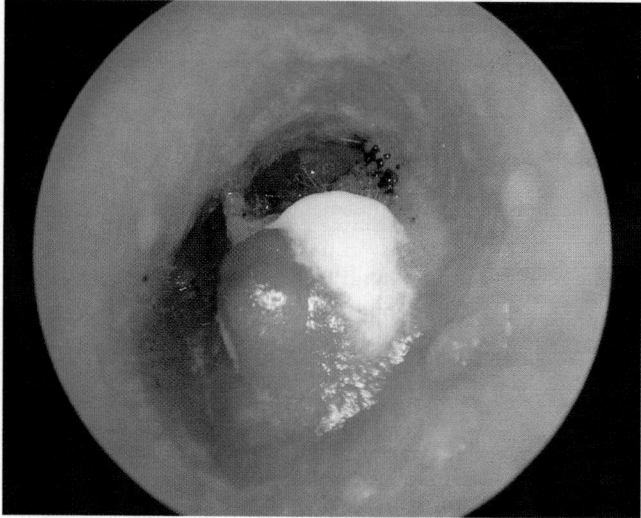

Fig. 40.6 Fungal otitis externa. Note the spores!

Inflammatory disorders

Inflammatory disorders of the external ear are extremely common. Otitis externa frequently presents to general practice and to ear, nose and throat (ENT) surgeons. There is generalised inflammation of the skin of the external auditory meatus. It can occur as an acute episode or can run a more chronic course. The cause is often multifactorial but includes general skin disorders, such as psoriasis and excema, and trauma. Common pathogens are pseudomonas and staphylococcus bacteria, and amongst fungi, candida and aspergillus. Once the skin of the ear canal becomes soggy and oedematous, skin migration stops and debris collects in the ear canal which acts as a substrate for the pathogens. The hallmark of acute otitis externa is severe pain (evidently on a par with childbirth). Unlike otitis media, movement of the pinna elicits pain. The condition is often bilateral.

The initial treatment is with topical antibiotics and steroid ear drops, together with analgesia. If this fails meticulous removal of the debris with the aid of an operating microscope is required. Regular cleaning of the canal, together with topical steroids, needs to be continued until normal skin migration resumes. If fungal infection is present it can easily be recognised by the presence of hyphae and spores within the canal (Fig. 40.6). Fungal infection causes irritation and itch, and the treatment is meticulous removal of the fungus and any debris, as well as stopping any concurrent antibiotics.

Systemic antibiotics are rarely required for otitis externa but should be used if cellulitis of the pinna occurs (Fig. 40.7).

Necrotising otitis externa is a rare but very important condition. It presents as a severe, persistent, unilateral otitis externa in an immunocompromised individual, for example it is important to think of the diagnosis in an elderly diabetic. Osteomyelitis of the skull base occurs and usually the infecting organism is *Pseudomonas aeruginosa*. Several cranial nerves (VII, IX and X) may be destroyed by the progressing infection. Intensive systemic antibiotic treatment is required and the disease process is monitored by high-resolution imaging.

A furuncle of the external ear is an infection of a hair follicle and is due to a staphylococcal infection. Moving the pinna causes extreme pain. Local treatment of the ear canal (oto-wick and steroid drops) together with systemic antibiotic therapy is required.

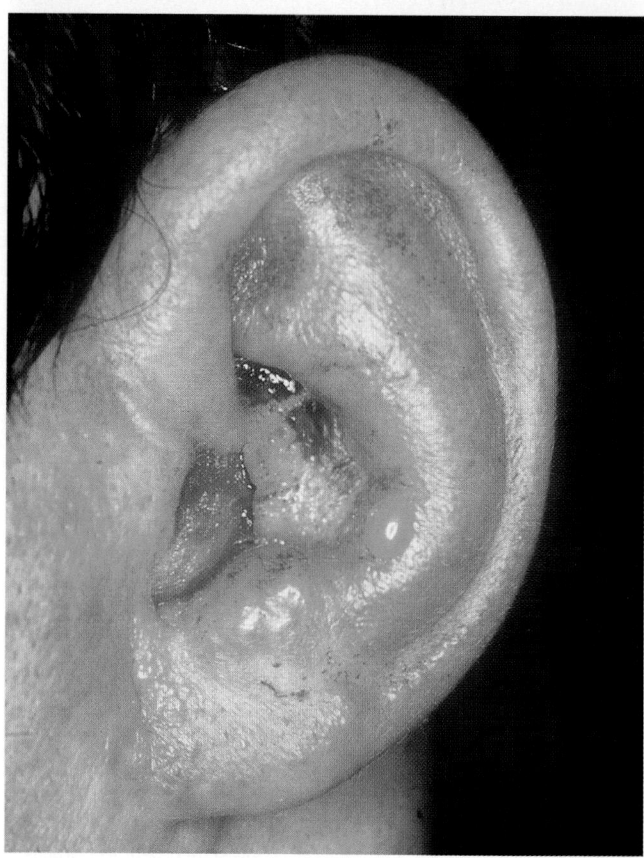

Fig. 40.7 Cellulitis of the pinna.

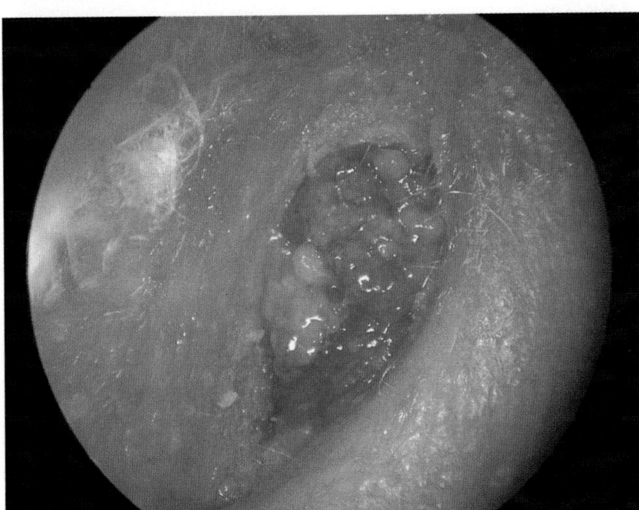

Fig. 40.8 Squamous cell carcinomas of the external ear usually originate from the pinna; in this case the tumour is growing from the canal (*courtesy of Mr N. Beasley*).

Neoplasms

Benign neoplasms

Benign neoplasms of the external ear are common if osteomas are included. These arise from the bone of the ear canal in individuals who have done a lot of swimming in cold water. No treatment is required unless they obstruct the migration of skin out of the canal. Other benign tumours include papillomas and adenomas.

Malignant primary tumours

Malignant primary tumours of the external ear are either basal cell or squamous cell carcinomas (Fig. 40.8). Both may present as ulcerating or crusting lesions which grow slowly and may be ignored by elderly patients. Squamous cell carcinomas may metastasise to the parotid and/or neck nodes and need radical surgical clearance. The ear canal may be invaded by tumours from the parotid and postnasal space carcinoma which 'creep' up the eustachian tube. All resectable malignant tumours of the ear are treated primarily with surgery with or without the addition of radiation therapy.

The external ear

- Otitis externa responds to topical medication
- Unilateral otitis externa in a diabetic may be fatal
- Auricular haematoma needs a robust incision, drainage and pressure dressing
- Think osteointegration for congenital malformations

Table 40.2 Conditions of the middle ear

Congenital	First and second branchial arch deformities
Trauma	Perforations
	Ossicular discontinuity
Inflammatory	Acute otitis media
	Mastoiditis
	Otitis media with effusion (glue ear)
	CSOM: tubotympanic disease; atticoantral disease
	Tuberculous otitis media
	Otosclerosis
Neoplasms	Benign: glomus tumours
	Malignant: squamous cell carcinoma

Conditions of the middle ear

Congenital anomalies

Congenital anomalies of the middle ear may be isolated or may be associated with other ear or general congenital deformities. There is a number of branchial arch syndromes – for example Pierre Robin's syndrome, craniofacial dysostosis, Down's syndrome and Treacher Collins' syndrome. If there is an external ear abnormality, it should raise suspicion of an underlying middle ear deformity. Middle ear deformity can be assessed by high-resolution computerised tomography (CT) scanning and, if the inner ear is normal, reconstructive surgery of the middle ear can be very successful.

Trauma

Trauma to the middle ear can result in a perforated tympanic membrane (Fig. 40.9a). Such perforations usually heal spontaneously (Fig. 40.9b). Trauma can result is ossicular discontinuity and typically it is the incus that is displaced. Various operations termed 'tympanoplasties' are available to reconstruct the damaged ossicular chain and repair the tympanic membrane if necessary.

Inflammatory disorders

The most common inflammatory condition of the middle ear is acute suppurative otitis media. It is extremely common in childhood and is characterised by purulent fluid in the middle ear. Mastoiditis may be associated with otitis media because the mastoid air cells connect freely with the middle ear space. The tympanic membrane is hyperaemic and bulges owing to pressure from the pus in the middle ear (Fig. 40.10). The child suffers extreme pain until the tympanic membrane bursts. The most common infecting organisms are *Streptococcus pneumoniae* and *Haemophilus influenzae*. Appropriate systemic antibiotics should be given for 10 days.

The incidence of acute mastoiditis has diminished with the widespread use of antibiotics for otitis media. Sometimes, however, a child will have had a number of courses of antibiotics, none of which completely resolves the middle ear infection. In such cases the pain and swelling behind the ear may not be quite so apparent as in Fig. 40.11. When mastoiditis is present, if the tympanic membrane can be seen, there is always a sag in the posterior superior part of the drum. (Conversely, a normal tympanic membrane excludes mastoiditis.) Treatment requires hospital admission and

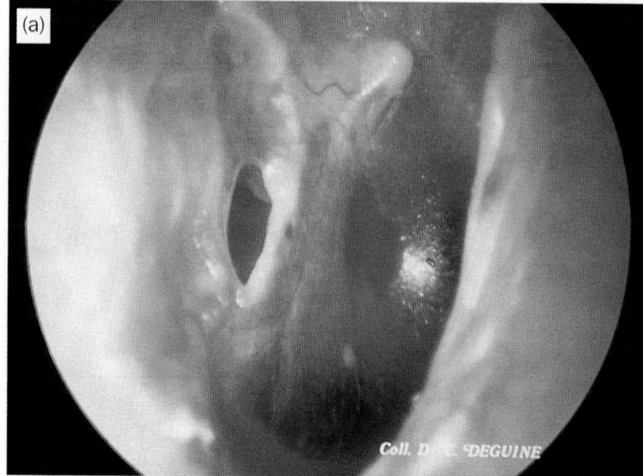

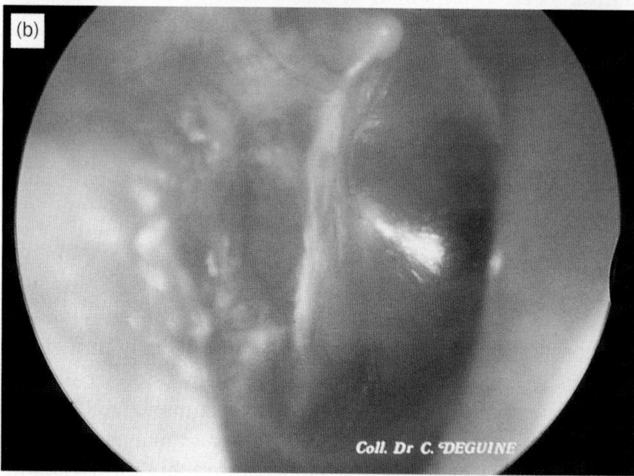

Fig. 40.9 (a) Traumatically perforated tympanic membrane. (b) Same tympanic membrane has healed 2 days later (*courtesy of Dr Christian Deguine*). (Reproduced with permission from by O'Donoghue, G.M., Bates, G.J. and Narula, A. *Clinical ENT*, Oxford University Press, Oxford, 1991.)

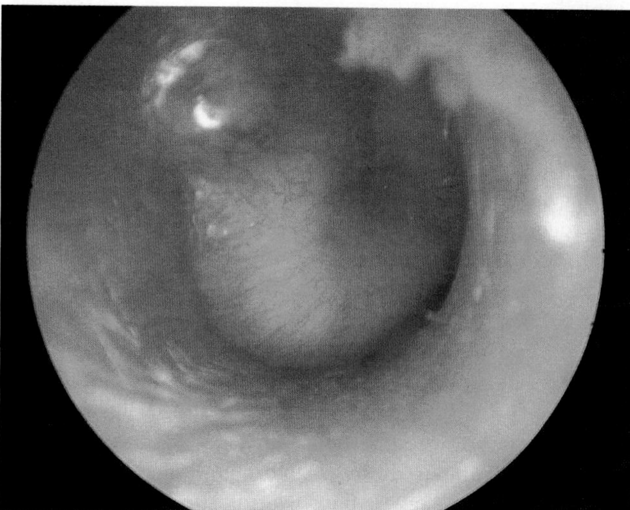

Fig. 40.10 Acute otitis media. Note the bulging tympanic membrane. Left ear.

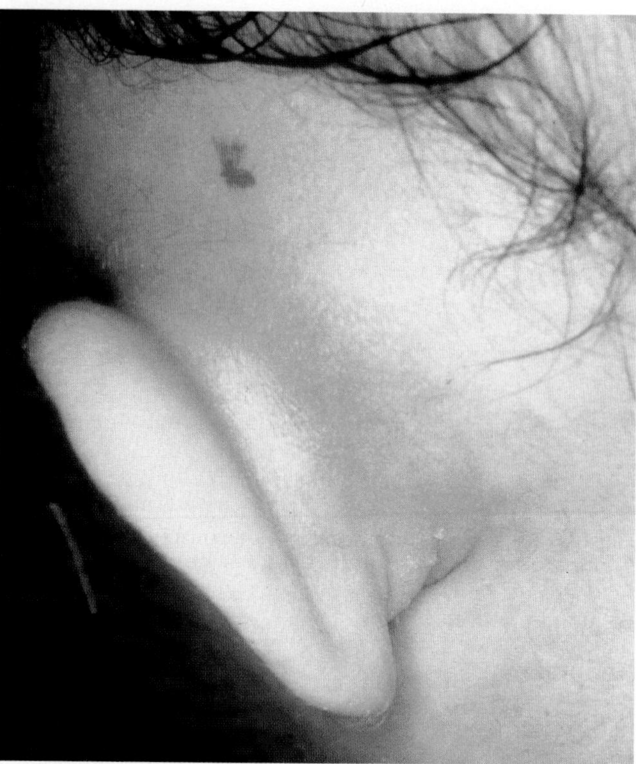

Fig. 40.11 Child with acute mastoiditis whose tympanic membrane is shown in Fig. 40.10.

intensive parenteral antibiotics. If this does not resolve the infection quickly a cortical mastoidectomy is required, together with a myringotomy.

Mastoiditis

- Sequelae of acute otitis media
- May be masked by antibiotics
- Requires intensive antibiotics and/or drainage

Otitis media with effusion (glue ear) is very common with the majority of children experiencing at least one episode of it during development. Many factors have been implicated, although it is primarily thought to be due to poor eustachian tube function. Oxygen is continually being absorbed by the middle ear mucosa and this results in a negative middle ear pressure unless the eustachian tube opens to replenish the air. This negative middle ear pressure initially results in transudation of fluid into the middle ear space (Fig. 40.12). If the hypoxia continues, a mucoid exudate is produced by the glands within the middle ear mucosa. This sticky exudate is referred to as 'glue ear'.

The following symptoms may be associated with glue ear:

- hearing impairment which often fluctuates;
- delayed speech;
- behavioural problems;
- recurrent ear infections – this occurs because the exudate is an ideal culture medium for microorganisms;
- reading and learning difficulties at school.

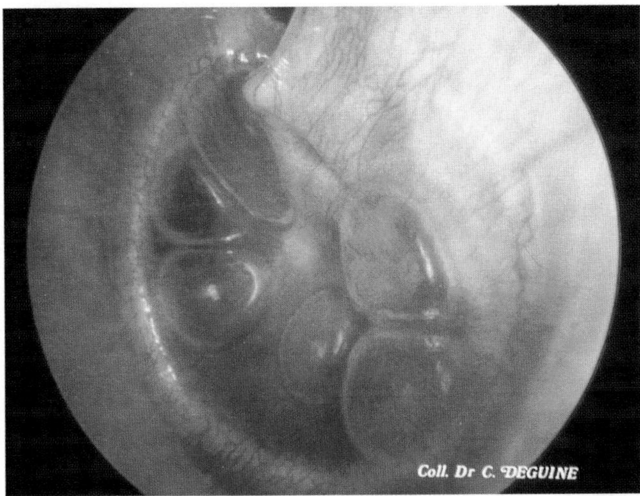

Fig. 40.12 The initial serous transudate of glue ear. Left ear (*courtesy of Dr Christian Deguine*). (Reproduced with permission from O'Donoghue, G.M., Bates, G.J. and Narula, A., *Clinical ENT*, Oxford University Press, Oxford, 1991.)

If these symptoms are present for a short time only, it is likely that no long-term sequelae will develop. However, if symptoms persist, particularly a long-term bilateral conductive hearing loss, the child will miss out on educational opportunities and may not fulfil his or her academic potential. The otoscopic findings of exudative glue ear are of a dull drum that is immobile on pneumatic otoscopy (Fig. 40.13).

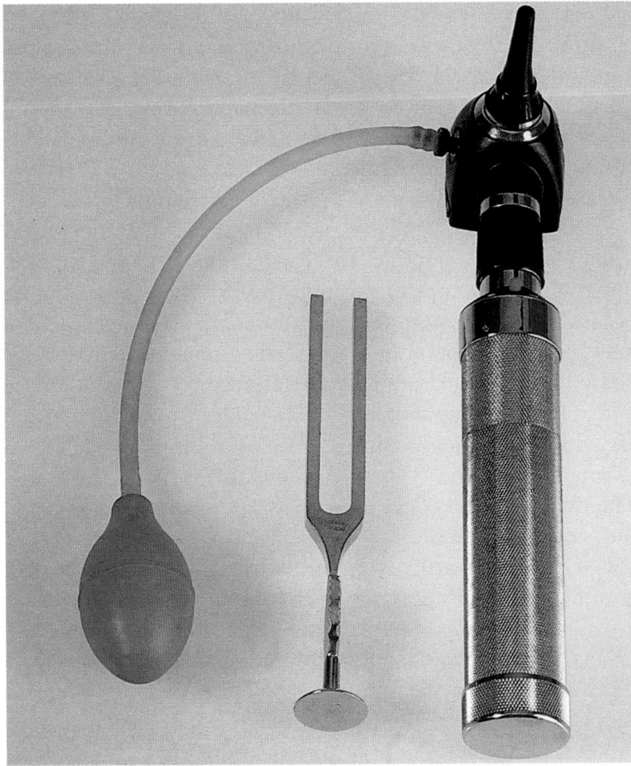

Fig. 40.13 Pneumatic otoscope and tuning fork (essential diagnostic tools).

The tympanic membrane is retracted and radial blood vessels may be present (Fig. 40.14). Of children first presenting with bilateral glue ear, 50 per cent of the effusions will resolve spontaneously within 6 weeks of onset. Initially, a 'wait and watch' policy is therefore appropriate. If the bilateral glue ear persists with a significant hearing loss then treatment is required.

There is no substantial evidence for medical treatment. Use of the Otovent device (Fig. 40.15) may improve eustachian tube function and is worth trying while waiting for resolution of the effusion. However, surgical intervention is the only effective way of curing glue ear. Both ventilation tube (grommets) and adenoidectomy are effective. The controversy is not whether surgery works but when to intervene.

Insertion of ventilation tubes and/or an adenoidectomy require a general anaesthetic. The ventilation tube is placed in the anterior inferior portion of the tympanic membrane because there is no important

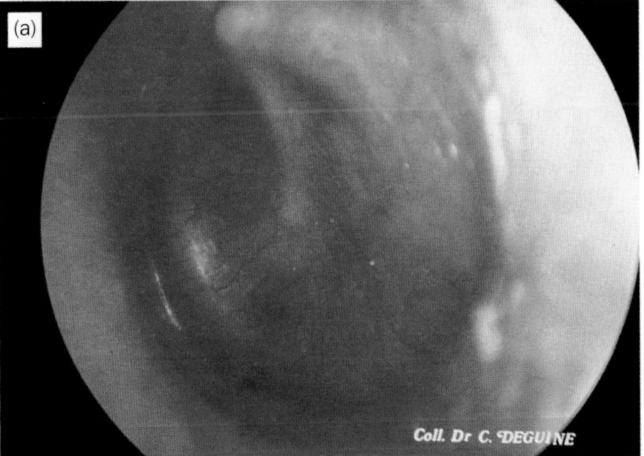

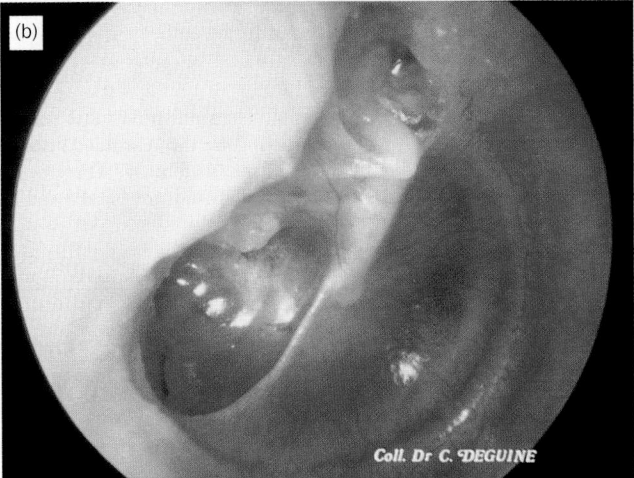

Fig. 40.14 (a) Left exudative glue ear. The tympanic membrane is dull and retracted. The light reflex has gone and there are radial blood vessels. The drum does not move with pneumatic otoscopy. (b) Right ear. Advanced exudative glue ear with retraction pockets (*courtesy of Dr Christian Deguine*). (Reproduced with permission from O'Donoghue, G.M., Bates, G.J. and Narula, A. *Clinical ENT*, Oxford University Press, Oxford, 1991.)

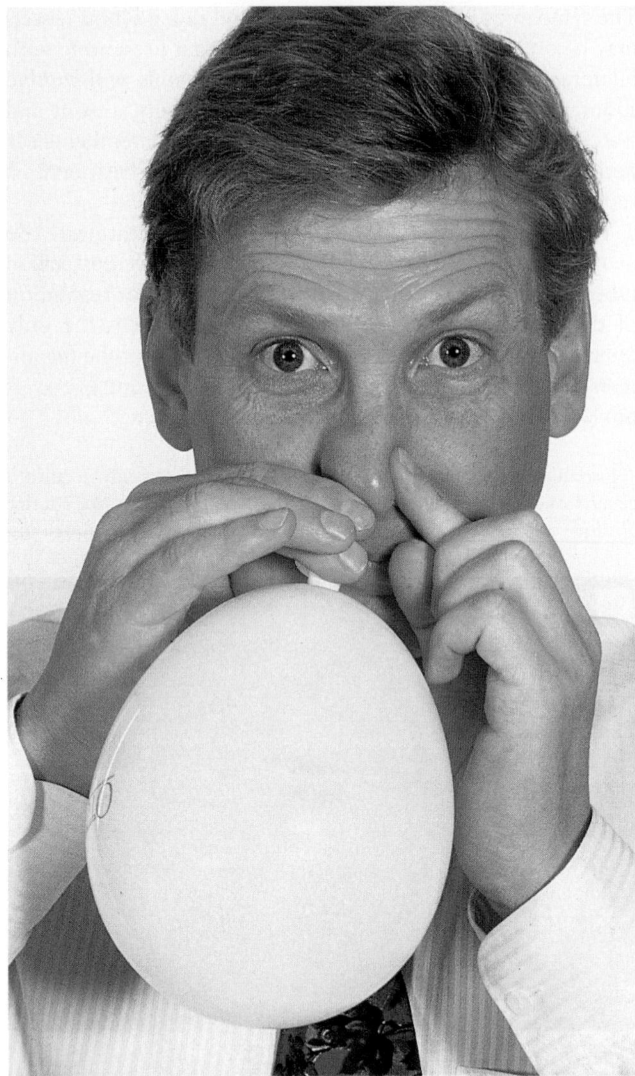

Fig. 40.15 Otovent device demonstrated by the author.

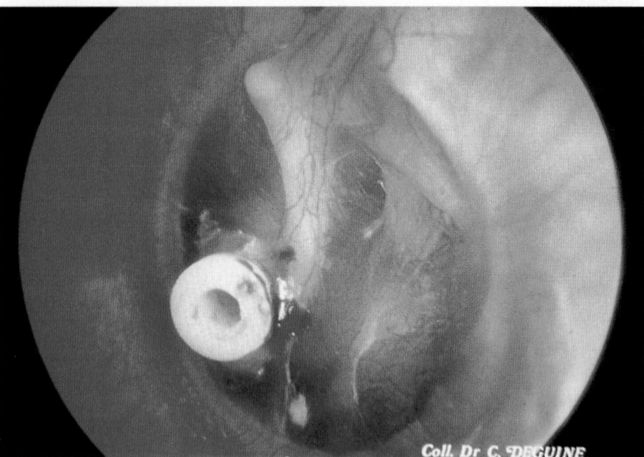

Fig. 40.16 Ventilation tube in tympanic membrane. Left ear (*courtesy of Dr Christian Deguine*).

clockwork behind this part of the drum. The ventilation tubes stay in position for approximately 6–18 months and are then extruded because of the migratory behaviour of the tympanic membrane. There is no reason why children with ventilation tubes should not be allowed to swim (Fig. 40.16).

> Otitis media with effusion (glue ear)
>
> - Very common, peaks at 18 months and 5 years
> - Majority of children need no treatment
> - Prolonged hearing loss treated with ventilation tubes and/or adenoidectomy

A middle effusion in adults is relatively rare and when it occurs does not usually last long. The condition is often associated with an upper respiratory tract infection. A persistent unilateral effusion in an adult should always be viewed with suspicion. A nasopharyngeal carcinoma may cause the effusion by blocking the opening of the eustachian tube in the postnasal space. This is the most common carcinoma in males in southern China.

Chronic suppurative otitis media

Chronic suppurative otitis media (CSOM) is classified into two types: tubotympanic disease, in which there is a perforation of the pars tensa; and atticoantral disease, in which a retraction pocket develops from the pars flaccida.

CSOM of the tubotympanic type. CSOM of the tubotympanic type can result from trauma or infection. When perforated the tympanic membrane usually repairs itself, but occasionally the outer layer of the tympanic membrane fuses with inner mucosa and a chronic perforation results (Fig. 40.17). With this type of disease the patient's main symptoms are of an intermittent or chronic mucoid discharge associated with a mild conductive hearing loss. It is rare for this type of disease to be associated with intracranial complications.

A diagnosis is made on otoscopy and the tuning forks usually suggest a conductive hearing impairment. The first-line treatment is topical antibiotic and steroid drops, and on occasion microsuction. If medical treatment fails, the patient may request an operation to graft the tympanic membrane in order to give a dry ear. This operation is termed a myringoplasty (type I tympanoplasty). The edges of the perforation are freshened and a small piece of temporalis fascia is inserted under the tympanic membrane to graft the drum. The raw epithelial edges then grow across the graft to repair the tympanic membrane.

CSOM of the atticotympanic type. CSOM of the atticoantral type is important because of the complications associated with it. Cholesteatoma is the alternative name and means a cyst or sac of squamous epithelium that is present in the attic part of the middle ear. The exact aetiology of cholesteatoma is not known, although poor eustachian tube function is implicated (e.g. patients with cleft palates have relatively poor eustachian tube function and have a higher incidence of cholesteatoma).

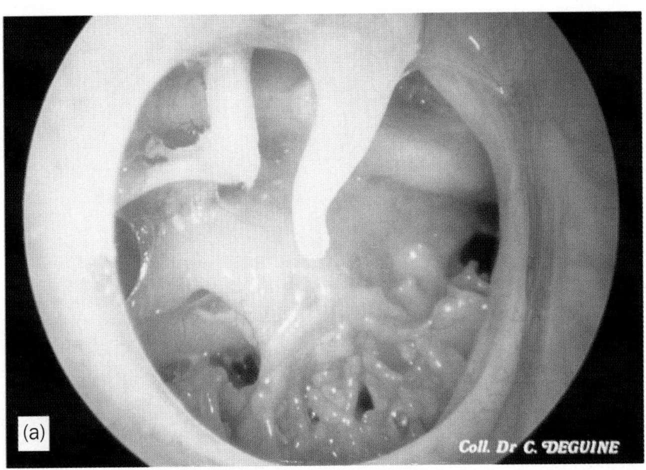

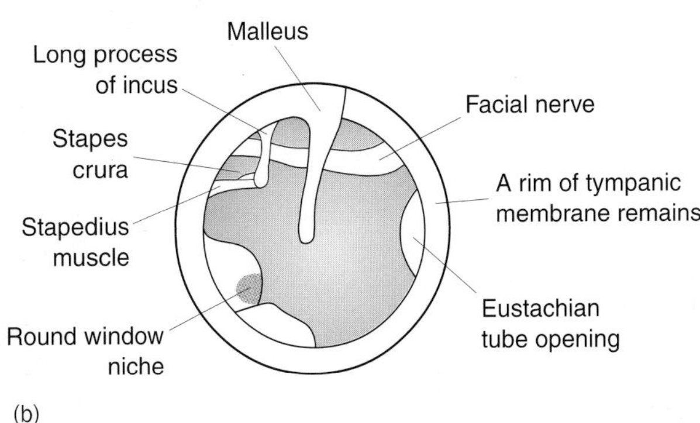

Fig. 40.17 (a) Tubotympanic CSOM showing central perforation. Right ear. (b) Diagram to illustrate anatomy. (*courtesy of Dr Christian Deguine*).

A retraction pocket develops in the pars flaccida and, if the squamous epithelium cannot migrate out of this pocket, a cholesteatoma results. The expanding ball of skin causes a low-grade osteomyelitis which results in the release of fatty acids from the bone. This gives the discharge its characteristic faecal smell. Invariably the discharge is accompanied by hearing loss and mild discomfort. The patient may simply put up with the symptoms until a severe complication occurs.

The hearing loss that is caused by cholesteatoma may be conductive due to erosion of the incus or sensorineural due to direct erosion of the cochlea or migrations of toxins into the inner ear. Vestibular symptoms may occur because of erosion of the semicircular canals or the migration of toxins into the vestibule. Pressure or erosion of the facial nerve is relatively unusual.

The close proximity of the middle ear and mastoid to the middle and posterior cranial fossae means that intracranial sepsis can result from chronic ear disease. The infection spreads to the dura via emissary veins which connect the middle ear mucosa to the dura or by direct extension of the disease through the bone. Meningitis, extradural, subdural or intracerebral abscess, or a combination of these may occur. The main causes of intracranial sepsis in the UK are chronic ear disease and chronic sinus disease.

Diagnosis should be suspected on otoscopy (Fig. 40.18). Pus, crusts, granulations or a whitish debris in the attic are hallmarks of the disease. Examination under the microscope, audiometry and, sometimes, CT scanning are indicated.

The treatment is surgical and follows the principle of exposing the disease, excising the disease and then exteriorising the affected area. Two commonly applied operations for this disease are an atticotomy and a modified radical mastoidectomy.

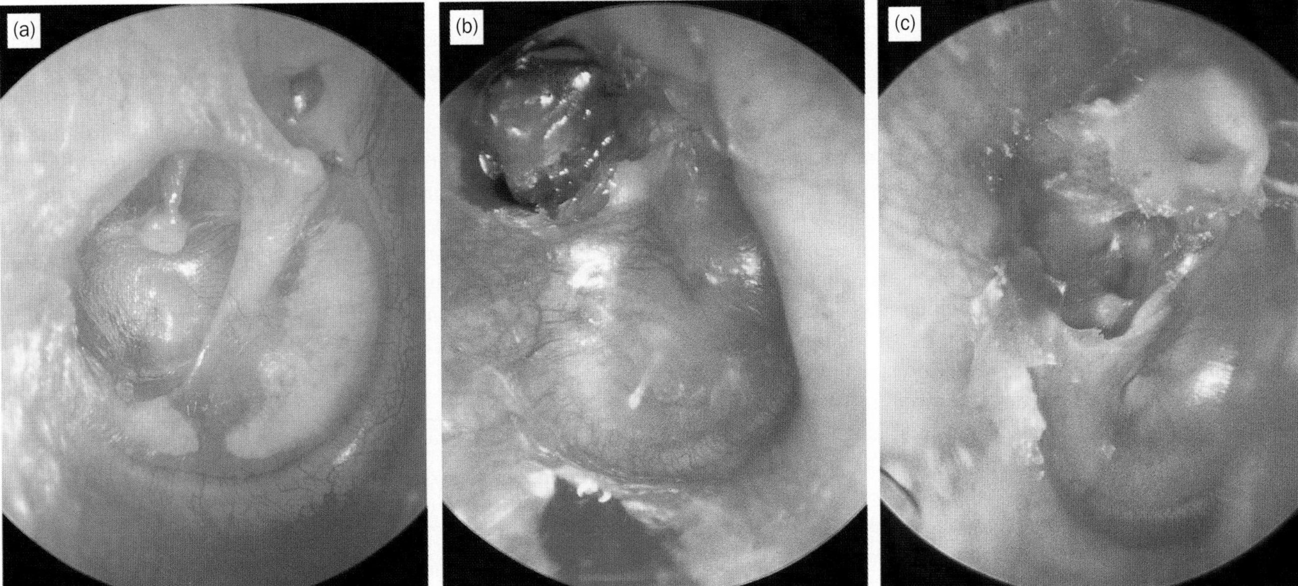

Fig. 40.18 (a) Empty attic retraction pocket, right ear. (b) Attic crust covering cholesteatoma, right ear. (c) Attic erosion with cholesteatoma, right ear.

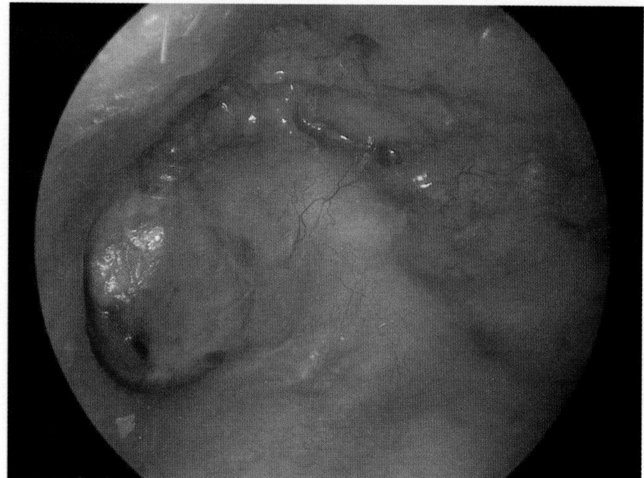

Fig. 40.19 Dry mastoid cavity, left ear. Remnant of tympanic membrane is separated from the mastoid bowl by the facial ridge.

An atticotomy or modified radical mastoidectomy is performed by making an incision behind the ear (postauricular), or between the tragus and the pinna (endaural). The attic part of the bony ear can is drilled away and the retraction pocket is followed back into the mastoid until the end of the disease is found. An attempt is made to excise totally the pocket and then the resulting cavity is usually lined with temporalis fascia. A mastoid cavity heals with normal skin that does not migrate, and for this reason patients with a mastoid cavity need to be seen in an out-patients' clinic on a regular basis. Any skin that collects in the mastoid cavity needs to be removed with the aid of a sucker and a microscope (Fig. 40.19).

Chronic suppurative otitis media (CSOM)

- In tubotympanic CSOM there is a perforated tympanic membrane and frequently a mucoid discharge
- Atticoantral CSOM:
  - Is skin in an attic retraction? = cholesteatoma
  - Presents with hearing loss and smelly discharge
  - Is a common cause of intracranial sepsis

Tuberculous otitis media is an important cause of suppuration in some countries. The diagnosis should always be considered in any ear which fails to respond to standard therapy. A swab for appropriate culture studies, coupled with chest radiography, will usually confirm the diagnosis.

Otosclerosis is a condition in which new abnormal spongy bone is laid down in the dense otic capsule. Of particular importance is the bone that is laid down around the footplate of the stapes which impedes the mobility of the stapes and results in a conductive hearing loss (Fig. 40.20). Toxins released from the new bone formation may also cause a gradual sensorineural hearing loss. Otosclerosis is more common in women, and in 50 per cent of patients there is a family history. The typical presentation is of a conductive hearing loss in a young woman with the condition being exacerbated by the hormonal flux of pregnancy. A similar type of stapes fixation occurs in osteogenesis imperfecta and is known as Van der Hoeve's syndrome. Otosclerosis is often bilateral. A diagnosis should be suspected in any patient with a conductive hearing loss and a normal tympanic membrane.

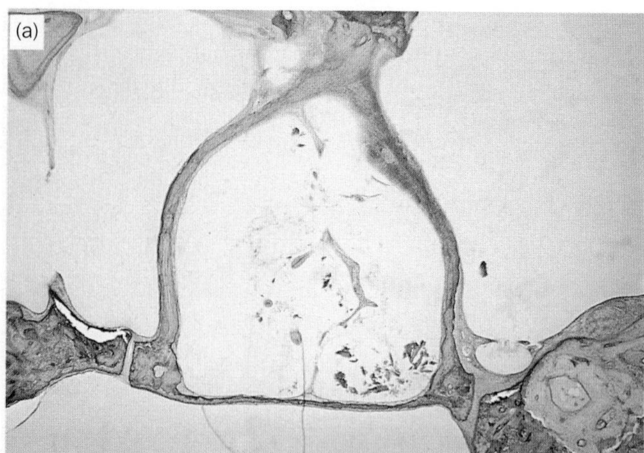

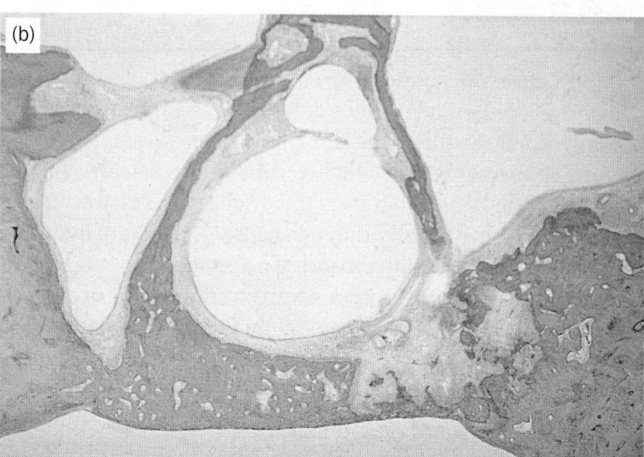

Fig. 40.20 Section of normal stapes (a) and section of stapes affected by otosclerosis (b).

The treatment options are simple reassurance, a hearing aid or a stapedotomy operation. In the stapedotomy operation, the stapes crura are removed and a small hole is drilled in the fixed stapes footplate. A vein graft is then inserted over the hole and a piston linking the incus to the vein graft is delicately placed in position (Fig. 40.21). In 90 per cent of cases the operation is highly successful, but rare complications include severe sensorineural hearing loss and balance disturbance.

Otosclerosis

- New bone formation in otic capsule
- Stapes fixation
- Options:
  - Reassurance;
  - Hearing aid;
  - Stapedotomy

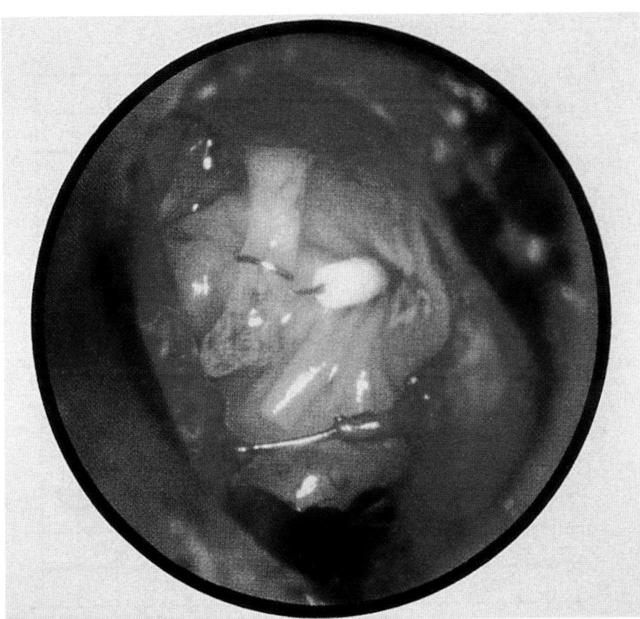

Fig. 40.21 The stapedotomy operation showing piston linking incus to vein graft, left ear.

Neoplasms

Neoplasms of the middle ear are rare, the most common being a glomus tumour (Fig. 40.22). Glomus tumours arise from nonchromaffin paraganglionic tissue. The carotid body tumour arising in the neck is an example of this type of tumour. In the temporal bone three types of glomus tumour are recognised and classification depends on the location: glomus tympanicum (arising in the middle ear), glomus jugularae (arising next to the jugular bulb) and glomus vagali (skull base).

Pulsatile tinnitus is a classic symptom of these tumours. Hearing loss occurs and may be either conductive or sensorineural, and paralysis of the VIIth, IXth, Xth, XIth and/or XIIth nerves may occur. The classic sign is a cherry-red mass lying behind the tympanic membrane. An audible bruit may be heard with a stethoscope over the temporal bone. The treatment of choice is preoperative embolisation followed by surgical excision. Radiotherapy is also effective.

Squamous cell carcinoma may also occur within the middle ear. It usually presents with deep-seated pain and a blood-stained discharge. The facial nerve may be paralysed. Squamous carcinomas usually arise in a chronically discharging ear and can certainly arise in a chronically infected mastoid cavity. Radical surgical excision with or without radiotherapy provides the only chance of cure.

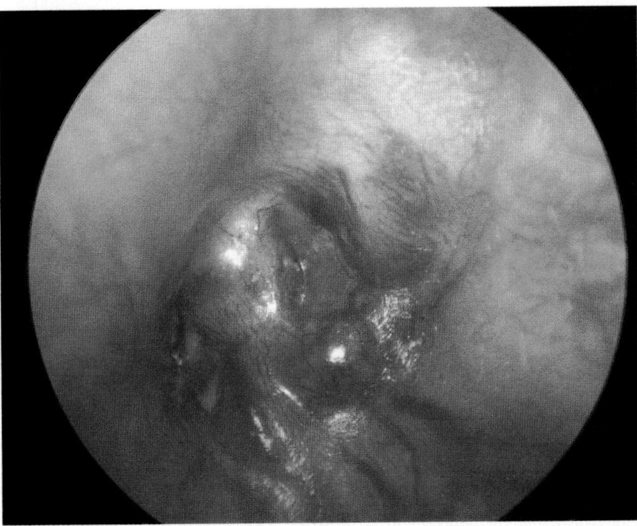

Fig. 40.22 Glomus tumour in the middle ear, left ear.

Conditions of the inner ear

Congenital

Congenital inner ear disorders may be associated with external or middle ear abnormalities or exist on their own. The most common anomaly is dysplasia of the membranous labyrinth, although dysplasia of the bony labyrinth and even total aplasia of the ear may occur. Intrauterine infections, including rubella, toxoplasmosis and cytomegalovirus, can cause inner ear damage. Perinatal hypoxia, jaundice and prematurity are also risk factors for a hearing loss. After birth, meningitis may cause profound sensorineural hearing loss.

If a child's parents suspect a hearing impairment it is important to believe them, especially when glue ear has been excluded. In children in whom there is a suspicion of sensorineural hearing loss, brainstem-evoked audiometry is used to establish hearing thresholds (Fig. 40.23). If some hearing is present, the early fitment of hearing aids can maximise the neural plasticity that is present in the developing brain. If a child has a profound hearing loss, then early intervention with a cochlea implant may be appropriate (Fig. 40.24). Most cases of profound sensorineural hearing loss are due to

Table 40.3 Conditions of the inner ear

Congenital	Dysplasia
	Infections
Degenerative	Presbycusis
	Tinnitus
Trauma	Noise
	Temporal bone fractures
	Barotrauma
	Oto-toxics
	Benign paroxysmal positional vertigo (BPPV)
Vascular occlusion	Sudden sensorineural hearing loss
Inflammatory	Viral labyrinthitis
	Ménière's disease
	Bell's facial palsy
	Herpes zoster (Ramsay Hunt's syndrome)
Metabolic	Diabetes
	Thyroid disease
Neoplasms	Acoustic neuroma
	Meningiomas

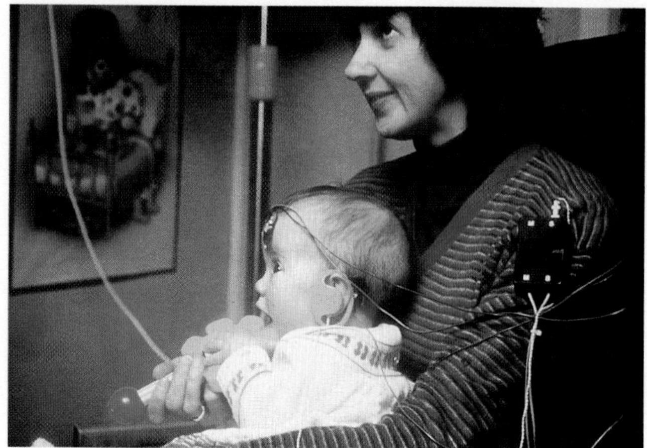

Fig. 40.23 Evoked response audiometry. A simple noninvasive objective test of hearing thresholds. (Reproduced with permission from by O'Donoghue, G.M., Bates, G.J. and Narula, A., *Clinical ENT*, Oxford University Press, Oxford, 1991.)

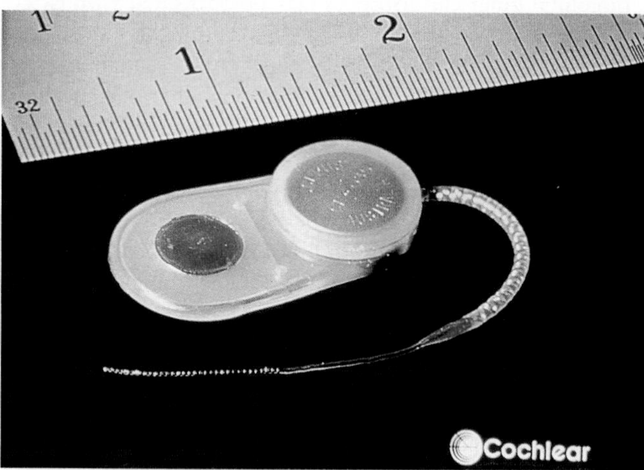

Fig. 40.24 Multichannel cochlear implant. Cochlear Corporation.

loss of cochlear hair cells so that an implant inserted through the round window can selectively stimulate the cochlear neurons which usually remain intact.

Degenerative

Presbyacusis, a degenerative disorder, is a term used to describe the hearing loss of old age. It is characterised by a gradual loss of hearing in both ears, with or without tinnitus. The hearing loss usually affects the higher frequencies and a classical audiogram is shown in Fig. 40.25.

The consonants of speech lie within the high-frequency range which makes speech discrimination difficult. Examination of an elderly person's cochlea shows loss of hair cells, particularly at the basal turn of the cochlea. With ageing the dynamic range of hearing is also reduced so that elderly people often find loud noises uncomfortable. This phenomenon is known as 'recruitment'.

Many patients with presbycusis are concerned that they may lose their hearing completely and need reassurance. Hearing aid technology has improved dramatically and most patients now benefit (Fig. 40.26). Care and attention to detail when fitting the hearing aid are essential, together with monitoring the patient's progress. If this does not occur the hearing aid ends up in the bedroom drawer.

(a)

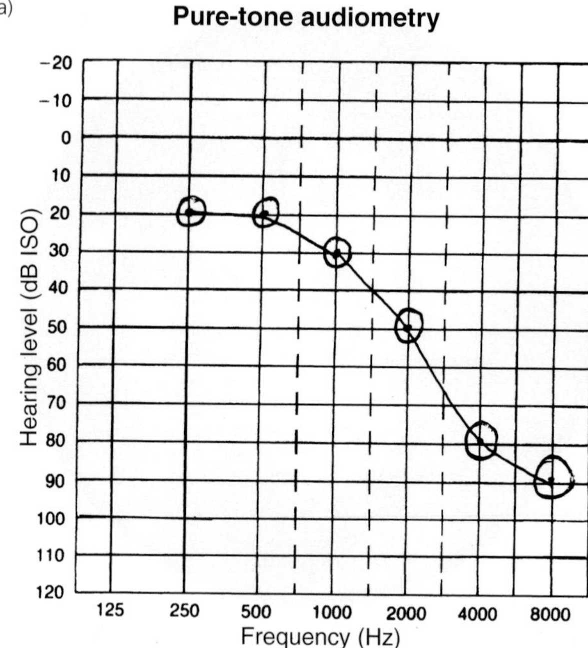

(b)

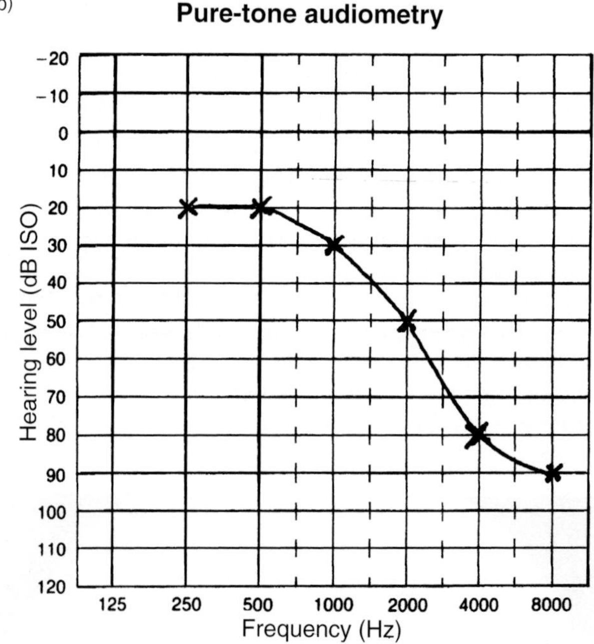

Fig. 40.25 Typical audiogram of presbyacusis.

Tinnitus describes an abnormal noise that appears to come from the ear or within the head. It may have an extrinsic cause, for example the pulsatile tinnitus of a glomus jugularae tumour. Usually, however, the tinnitus is generated within the cochlea, and most people will experience tinnitus at some time in their life.

Tinnitus frequently accompanies presbycusis, as well as any condition that damages the inner ear structures. Most individuals adapt to the presence of tinnitus but in some patients it proves intrusive. Reassurance

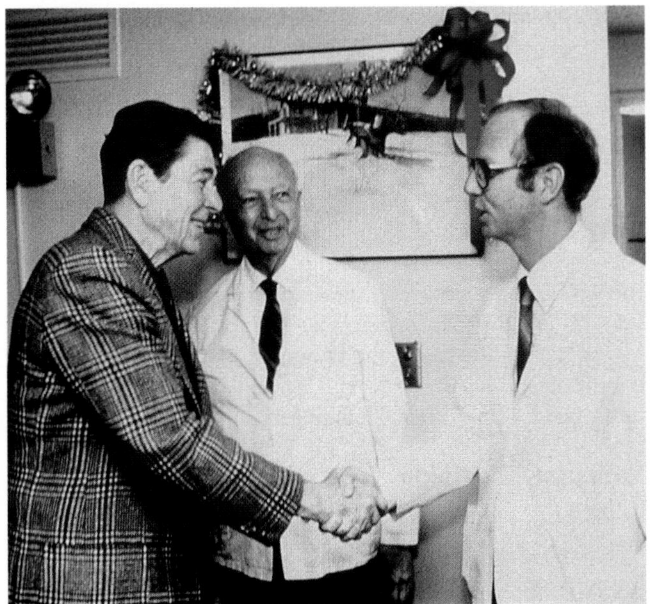

Fig. 40.26 A well-known patient receives his hearing aid.

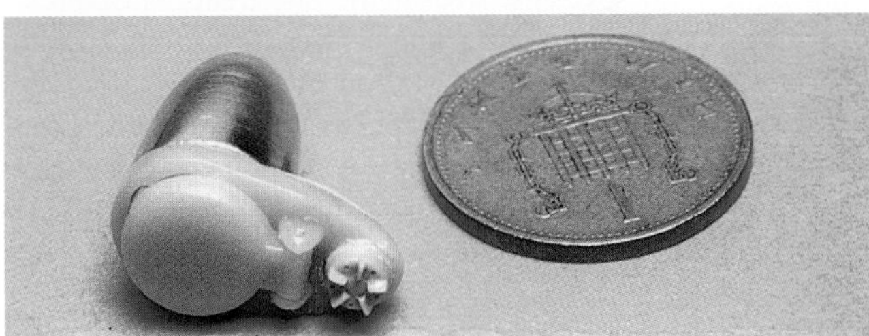

Fig. 40.27 A tinnitus masker (the coin is 20 mm diameter).

and relaxation therapy are highly effective, as is a hearing aid for patients who also have presbycusis. An ENT surgeon who was a keen fisherman found that he could not hear his tinnitus when fishing next to a waterfall. From this observation tinnitus maskers have been developed (Fig. 40.27). A masker provides a similar noise to the tinnitus and 'blanks it out'.

Trauma

Trauma to the inner ear can be caused by noise or direct injury. Hair cells within the cochlea are damaged by sudden acoustic trauma (blast injury or gun fire) or by prolonged exposure to excessive noise. The sensorineural hearing loss that results is greatest at high frequencies (particularly 4000 Hz) and is often accompanied by tinnitus (Fig. 40.28). The law in the UK requires that workers are protected from noise, but in a disco an individual relies on common sense!

The otic capsule is the hardest bone in the body but if trauma to the head is severe temporal bone fractures may occur. These tend to be either longitudinal (80 per cent) or transverse (20 per cent). Transverse fractures usually involve the labyrinth and lead to a sensorineural hearing loss which is permanent. Profound vertigo occurs initially followed by gradual compensation. In about 50 per cent of cases there is an associated facial nerve paralysis.

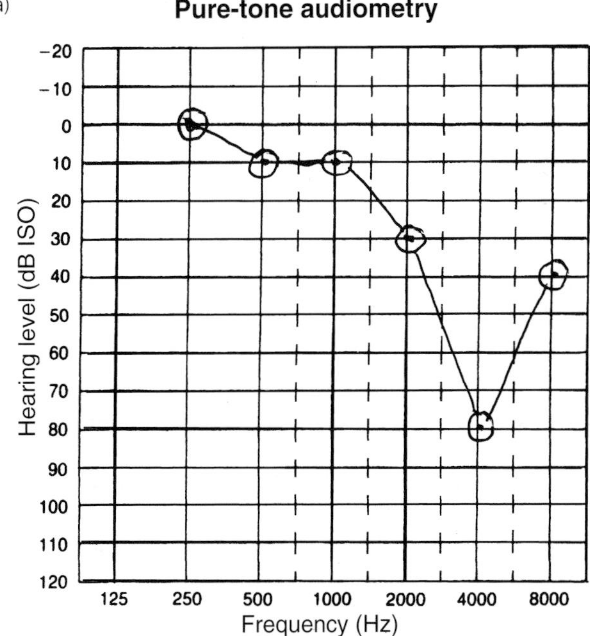

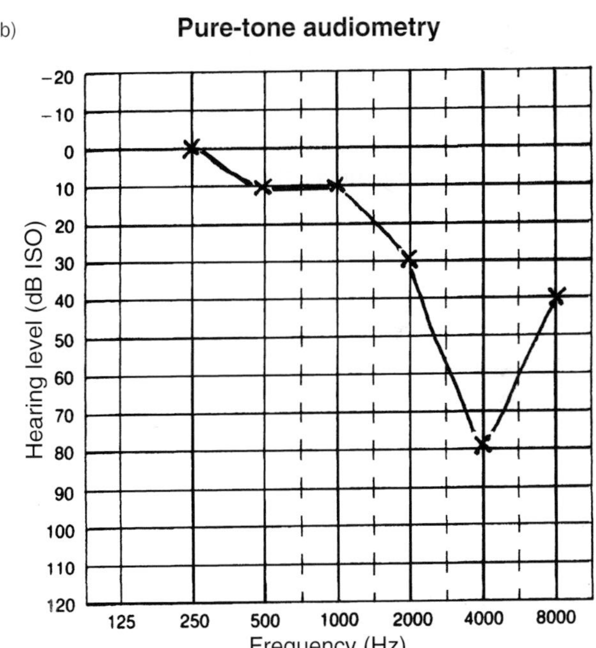

Fig. 40.28 Typical audiogram of noise damage.

When assessing a severely injured patient, it is important to record the facial nerve function and, in particular, whether any facial weakness is partial or total. Total facial paralysis immediately following a head trauma suggests a major injury to the nerve and under certain circumstances exploration of the facial nerve to decompress it or repair it may be appropriate. Longitudinal fractures usually spare the labyrinth but frequently involve the external meatus and roof of the middle ear.

Important physical findings that may accompany a skull base fracture include a haematoma over the mastoid bone (Battle's sign), blood in the external ear or a laceration along the roof of the external canal. Cerebrospinal fluid (CSF) otorrhoea or CSF rhinorrhoea (if the tympanic membrane is intact) may occur. A conductive hearing loss may be present because of fluid in the middle ear or disruption of the ossicular chair. A high-resolution CT scan is required to assess skull base fractures.

> Facial paralysis
>
> - Think complete or partial
> - Protect the eye
> - Otoneurological examination to find cause
> - Early treatment with steroids and/or antiviral therapy dependent on aetiology

Barotrauma is a rare cause of a sudden sensorineural hearing loss (SNHL) or acute vestibular disturbance. Rapid changes in pressure across the labyrinthine membranes may occur with diving or flying and may allow air to be forced into the cochlea. Any individual with a sudden sensorineural hearing loss requires urgent hospital admission, and in those with a history of barotrauma it may be appropriate to raise the tympanic membrane and to search for a leak of perilymph in the region of the oval or round window.

Drug ototoxicity is a form of trauma that may damage the inner ear. Some drugs differentially affect the cochlea causing hearing loss and tinnitus while others pick out the vestibular system causing vertigo. Aminoglycocides are well known to be ototoxic, as is cisplatinum. Recognition of risk factors, such as poor renal function in patients being treated with aminoglycocides, is most important. Although many topical ear drops contain aminoglycocides, there is little evidence that such topical treatment causes sensorineural hearing loss if used for short periods.

Benign paroxysmal positional vertigo (BPPV) may follow head or neck trauma. Vertigo is an illusion of movement and BPPV is characterised by intermittent attacks of vertigo that occur when the head is moved in a certain position. Typically the vertigo only lasts for a few seconds and is not associated with other otological symptoms. Positional testing can evoke nystagmus and helps in the diagnosis of this condition. The condition is usually self-limiting and special manoeuvres described by Epley help the majority of patients (Fig. 40.29).

Vascular occlusion

A reduction in labyrinthine blood flow with associated hypoxia is the most likely cause for most cases of sudden onset of severe sensorineural hearing loss. All patients with a sudden sensorineural hearing loss should be referred immediately for specialist treatment. The treatment consists of bed rest, steroids and, in some centres, the administration of Carbogen (an oxygen and carbon dioxide mixture). Five per cent of acoustic neuromas present with a sudden sensorineural hearing loss and therefore radiological investigation, preferably with magnetic resonace imaging (MRI), is required to exclude this tumour.

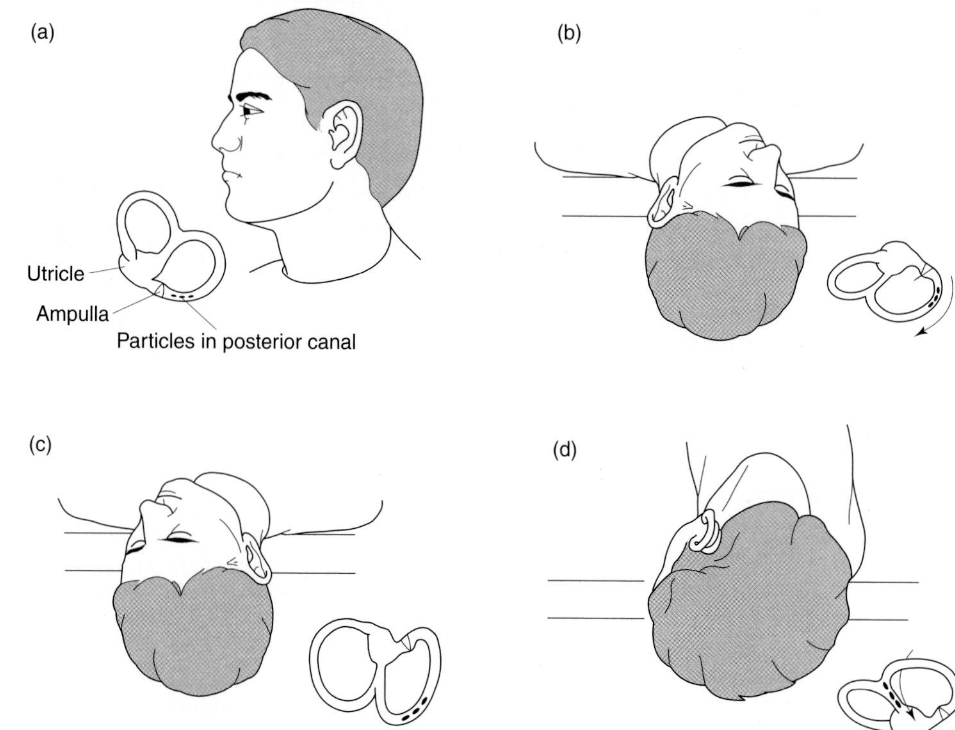

Fig. 40.29 The Epley manoeuvre for benign paroxysmal positional vertigo (BPPV).

Inflammatory disorders

Inflammation caused by a viral infection is thought to account for acute vestibular failure (vestibular neuronitis). This condition is characterised by a sudden onset of vertigo. The vertigo is so severe that the patient often takes to his or her bed for between 2 and 5 days. Central compensation then occurs, although recurring episodes of vertigo for up to 18 months can occur. This is thought to be due to incomplete compensation for the original vestibular damage.

The aetiology of *Ménière's disease* is not known. The condition is characterised by a triad of symptoms. Intermittent attacks of vertigo, a fluctuating sensorineural hearing loss and tinnitus. The patient often has a sensation of pressure in the affected ear before an attack. The hearing loss typically affects the lower frequencies and is virtually the only type of sensorineural hearing loss that fluctuates. The time-course of the vertigo characteristically lasts between 30 minutes and 6 hours. It is often accompanied by nausea and vomiting. Although the cause of the condition is unknown, the pathology is well documented. There is an excessive accumulation of endolymphatic fluid (hydrops) and it is thought that the distension of the endolymphatic compartment may rupture Reissner's membrane which leads to mixing of endolymph and perilymph. This is the basis for the cochlear–vestibular failure which characterises the condition. The investigations include pure-tone audiometry, electrocochleography and MRI scan if available. The latter is required to exclude an acoustic neuroma which may mimic the symptoms of Ménière's disease.

Viral infections that involve the facial nerve are possibly one of the commonest causes of facial weakness (80 per cent). *Bell's palsy* results from a viral infection of the facial nerve. The nerve swells and is compressed in its labyrinthine portion as it passes from the internal auditory meatus towards the middle ear. If the patient presents within the first 48 hours, treatment with high-dose steroids is appropriate. Not all facial nerve palsies are due to viral infection and a thorough otoneurological examination is required. The facial nerve can be damaged within the brainstem at the cerebellopontine angle, within the internal auditory meatus, within the middle ear, at the skull base and within the parotid. It is essential to consider these potential sites of facial nerve damage in any patient with VIIth nerve paralysis.

Ramsey Hunt's syndrome is caused by herpes zoster virus. It is characterised by a facial palsy and is often associated with facial pain and the appearance of vesicles on the ear drum, ear canal and pinna (Fig. 40.30). Vertigo and sensorineural hearing loss (VIIIth nerve) accompany it. Treatment with aciclovir is effective if given early.

Prosper Ménière, b. 1799. French physician.
Charles Bell, b. 1774. Scottish surgeon.
James Ramsay Hunt, b. 1874. American neurologist.

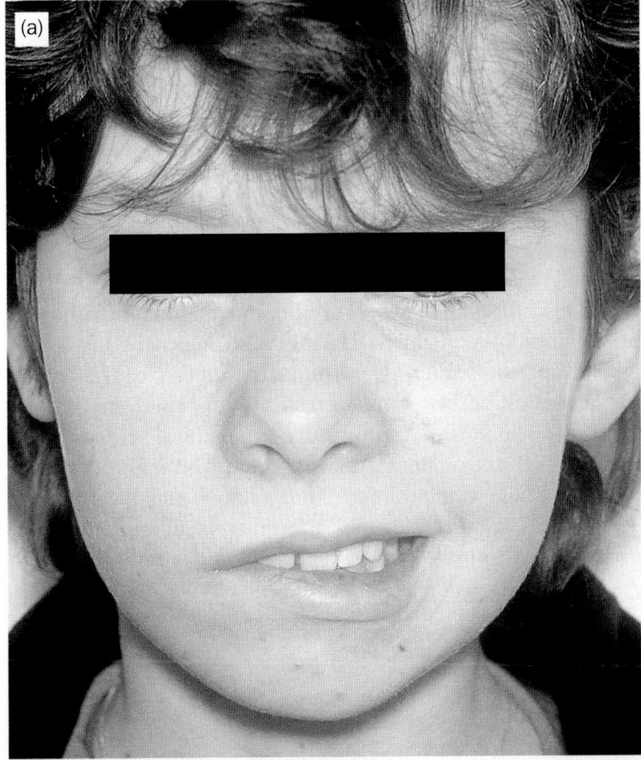

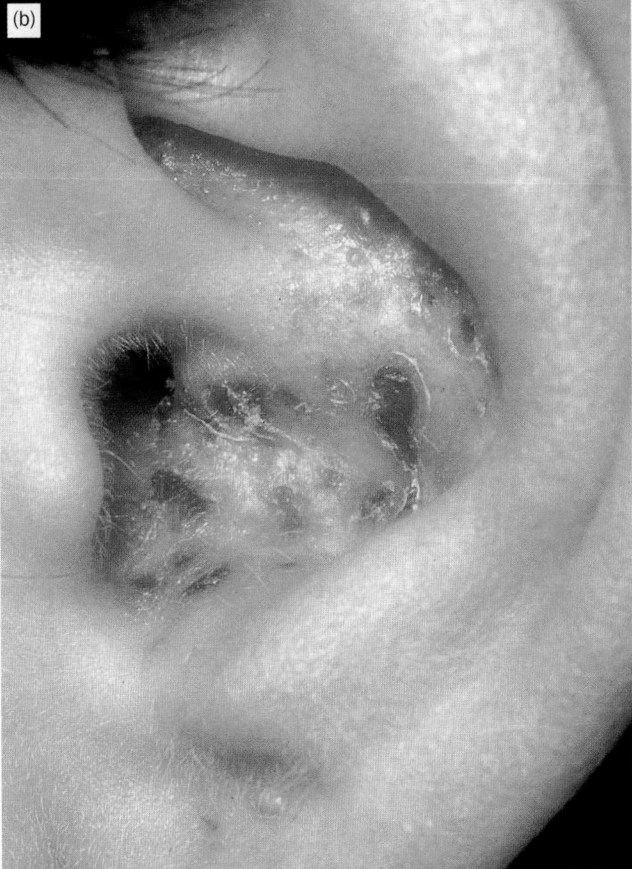

Fig. 40.30 Herpes zoster infection of the VIIth (a) and VIIIth (b) nerves with vesicles on the pinna.

Metabolic causes

The metabolic causes of inner ear damage include diabetes mellitus and thyroid disease, both of which may cause sensorineural hearing loss.

Neoplasms

Tumours of the inner ear are uncommon but can present with sensorineural hearing loss, tinnitus and vertigo. Acoustic neuromas, which are actually Schwannomas of the vestibular division of the VIIIth nerve, are the most common, followed by meningiomas. Acoustic neuromas grow slowly and somewhat unpredictably and as they expand can cause cranial nerve palsies, brainstem compression and raised intracranial pressure. The early symptoms are a unilateral sensorineural hearing loss or unilateral tinnitus, or both. It is important to diagnose these tumours early and remove them when they are small. The morbidity and mortality from surgery is directly related to tumour size. If the tumour is removed when it is small, there is an extremely good chance of preserving facial nerve function.

The investigation of choice for detecting acoustic neuromas is MRI (Fig. 40.31). In many centres patients with any unilateral otological symptoms are screened using MRI. If MRI is not available, CT scanning is the next best diagnostic tool. Occasionally, in an elderly patient, 'a wait and see' policy may be adopted. In such patients repeat MRIs can be used to monitor the tumour.

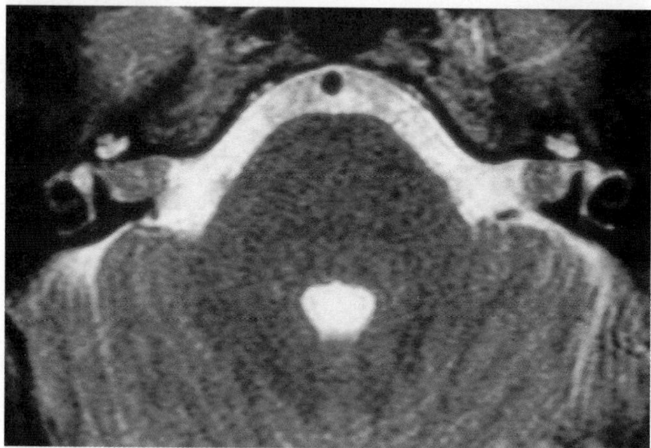

Fig. 40.31 MRI showing bilateral acoustic neuromas; patient had neurofibromatosis.

Friedrich T. Schwann, b. 1810. German anatomist.

There are three main surgical approaches for resecting acoustic neuromas. A *temporal craniotomy and a direct middle fossa* approach is used for small tumours only. The *translabyrinthine* approach is entirely through the ear and does not breach the dura. The neurosurgeon and ENT surgeon work together. There is minimal disturbance to the patient, although the hearing is completely destroyed. A *suboccipital* approach is performed by a neurosurgeon doing a craniotomy with the ENT surgeon removing bone at the internal auditory meatus. Traction on the cerebellum is required. This increases the morbidity. In some cases, however, what remains of the hearing can be preserved using this approach. The physiological monitoring of the facial nerve and auditory nerve during surgery has improved acoustic nerve surgery results.

The inner ear

- Presbycusis: bilateral high-frequency loss
- Unilateral tinnitus or sudden sensory neural hearing loss needs to be investigated for possible acoustic neuroma
- Sudden sensory neural hearing loss needs immediate treatment

Further reading

Booth, J. (ed.) (1997) *Scott-Brown's Otolaryngology*, 6th edn, Vol. 3, Butterworth-Heinemann, Oxford.

Ludman, H. and Wright, A. (eds) (1998) *Mawson's Diseases of the Ear*, 6th edn, Arnold, London.

Van Hassell, A., Milford, C.A. and Bleach, N. (eds) (1997) *Operative Otolaryngology*, Blackwell Scientific, Oxford.

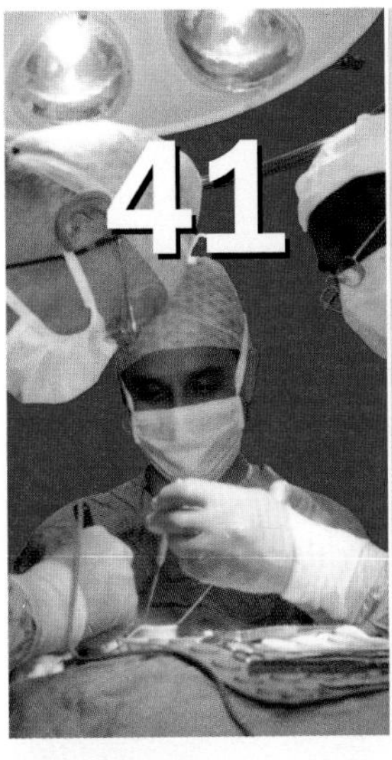

Oral and oropharyngeal cancer and precancer

Oral and oropharyngeal cancer

In global terms, oral–oropharyngeal cancer is the sixth most common malignancy. In the Western world it accounts for only 2–4 per cent of all malignant tumours, although there is now good evidence to show that the incidence is increasing particularly in younger people. By contrast, in Asia oral–oropharyngeal malignancy is the commonest malignant tumour which in parts of India accounts for no less than 40 per cent of all malignancy. It is estimated that globally there are nearly 500 000 new cases annually and that by the year 2000 there will be 1.5 million people alive with oral cancer at any one time.

Oral–oropharyngeal cancer is an almost entirely preventable disease being caused by tobacco either with or without alcohol. In the West this is mostly cigarette smoking combined with alcohol abuse, the risk of both in combination being greater than the summation of the risks of each individually.

In Asia and the Far East the use of Pan and reverse smoking are the major aetiological agents. Epidemiological evidence strongly suggests that again it is the presence of tobacco in the betel quid which is the major agent, although there seems also to be some relationship to the source of slaked lime and the areca nut itself.

The incidence in women appears to be increasing and there is a worrying cohort of young patients, mostly male and particularly with tongue cancer, who show a sharp increase in incidence after a gradual fall earlier in the twentieth century. This recent trend seems not to be related to tobacco and alcohol consumption and has been observed throughout Europe and North America.

Local control of disease at the primary site and the management of neck disease have improved, yet despite this cure rates and survival rates have not improved during the last 40 years remaining at approximately 55 per cent survival at 5 years.

Both recurrence of local disease and failure to control lymphatic metastases in the neck are early events and clearly have a negative effect on 5-year survival figures. There is no doubt, however, that during the past 20 years great advances have been made in the management of oral cancer, and persistence of local disease and lymphatic metastasis are now less common events. Why then have cure rates not improved?

Field changes in the upper aerodigestive tract result in the phenomenon of multiple primary cancers. The longer a patient survives his or her index tumour, the greater the risk of developing a second or third primary tumour either elsewhere in the oral cavity or in the larynx, bronchus or oesophagus.

Even if the patient does not develop a second primary tumour, he or she is then at risk of developing distant metastatic disease. It is probable that although until recently rarely recognised during life, metastasis via the bloodstream is a relatively early event in oral cancer. Currently, 20 per cent of all cancer-related deaths in patients with a tumour in the oral cavity or oropharynx are due to distant metastasis with no evidence of disease in the head or neck. Thus, oral cancer is a 'systemic' disease from an early stage.

Bailey & Love's Short Practice of Surgery, 23rd edition. Edited by R.C.G. Russell, N.S. Williams and C.J.K. Bulstrode. Published in 2000 by Arnold Publishers.

Resection

Surgical advances have been primarily in techniques of access surgery and in reconstruction. The widespread adoption of lip splitting and mandibulotomy has facilitated safe three-dimensional resections of tumours in the tongue and floor of mouth incontinuity with the lymphatics in the neck. A better understanding of the patterns of invasion of the mandible by adjacent tumour has allowed the development of rim resections, avoiding the sacrifice of mandibular continuity in many cases, without risking local recurrence. In recent years there has been the development of skull base access surgery using well-established oral and facial osteotomy techniques which have rendered previously inoperable tumours operable. This is particularly true for tumours extending into the pterygoid, infratemporal and lateral pharyngeal regions.

Reconstruction

Primary reconstruction is now the rule to the great advantage of patients. Previous reconstruction techniques were often unreliable, and when bony reconstruction was involved they were often staged. It was reasonably felt that before embarking on such prolonged and insecure techniques a period of time should be allowed to elapse to demonstrate that local recurrence was unlikely before reconstruction was attempted. With current techniques based largely on muscle flaps – pectoralis major, trapezius and latissimus dorsi – and free tissue transfer, based on microvascular techniques, primary reconstruction is not only reliable but produces acceptable functional and cosmetic results.

Radiotherapy

High-energy beams, computerised planning and simulation have greatly reduced the morbidity of radiotherapy by reducing the dosage to the adjacent tissues. Teeth are no longer routinely extracted prior to radiotherapy regardless of their state, and osteoradionecrosis is now an unusual complication.

Although not a new technique, brachytherapy using iridium wire implants is regaining popularity. For suitable tumours – T1 and early T2 tumours in mobile soft tissues – this technique delivers very high-dose local irradiation continuously with very little irradiation to adjacent tissues (Fig. 41.1). Local control rates are excellent. Currently, considerable interest is being shown in hyperfractionation techniques, whereby a higher total tumour dose can be achieved by giving more but smaller fractions of radiation.

Chemotherapy

Although many single agents or combinations of drugs can result in a response rate around 60 per cent, there is no evidence that this results in an increase in survival time or cure rate. Some centres advocate the use of induction chemotherapy prior to surgery but, again, there is no evidence based upon prospective studies that this improves survival. Palliative chemotherapy using agents such as cisplatin and 5-flurouracil are sometimes helpful for painful or fungating tumours.

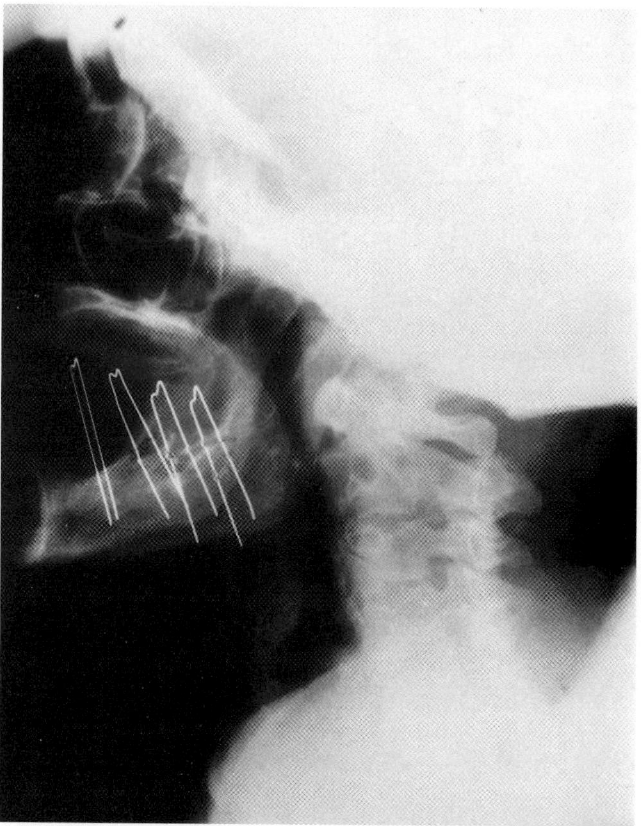

Fig. 41.1 Radiograph of iridium wire hairpins inserted for the treatment of a tongue cancer. Even spacing of the hairpins is essential to achieve a homogeneous tumour dose.

Clinical aspects

Oral cancer has a predeliction for certain sites within the mouth, notably the lateral margins and ventral tongue, floor of mouth, retromolar trigone, buccal mucosa and palate. The majority – more than 85 per cent – is mucosal squamous cell carcinomas. Malignant tumours arising in the minor salivary glands are next in frequency with lymphomas, malignant melanomas, sarcomas and metastatic tumours making up the remainder.

Premalignant lesions

The association of oral carcinoma and other oral mucosal lesions has been recognised for many years. Often these lesions are in the form of white plaques ('leucoplakia') or bright red velvety plaques ('erythroplakia'). They may be present for periods of months to years prior to the onset of malignant change and often they will be present together with the carcinoma at presentation. Because of this association the assumption was made that such lesions led directly to invasive carcinoma and hence were themselves premalignant.

Some white plaques do undoubtedly have a potential to undergo malignant transformation, and an examination of established carcinomas will show many to exist in association with white plaques. However, the majority of oral carcinomas is not preceded by or is associated with leucoplakia.

Although historically oral 'leucoplakia' has been recognised as premalignant, the risk of malignant transformation is not as great as was previously thought. Early literature suggested a 30 per cent or higher incidence of malignant transformation of these lesions whereas more recent authors quote an incidence of between 3 and 6 per cent.

The following oral lesions are now definitely considered to carry a potential for malignant change:

- leucoplakia;
- erythroplakia;
- chronic hyperplastic candidiasis.

A further group of conditions, although not themselves premalignant, are associated with a higher than normal incidence of oral cancer:

- oral submucous fibrosis;
- syphilitic glossitis;
- sideropenic dysphagia.

There remains a further group of oral conditions about which there is still some doubt as to whether their association with oral cancer is causal or casual:

- oral lichen planus;
- discoid lupus erythematosus;
- dyskeratosis congenita.

Leucoplakia

Using the term leucoplakia (Fig. 41.2) either in a histological or clinical context is a matter of defining what one means by the term. The World Health Organisation (WHO) has defined leucoplakia as 'any white patch or plaque that cannot be characterised clinically or pathologically as any other disease'. This definition has no histological connotation.

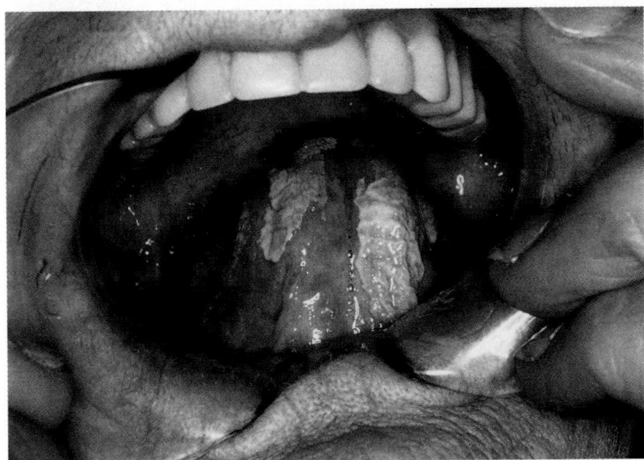

Fig. 41.2 The photograph shows the typical appearance of a homogeneous leucoplakia arising on the ventral aspect of the tongue.

Clinical features

Clinically leucoplakia may vary from a small circumscribed white plaque to an extensive lesion involving wide areas of the oral mucosa. The surface may be smooth or it may be wrinkled, and many lesions are traversed by cracks or fissures. The colour of the lesion may be white, yellowish or grey, with some being homogeneous whilst others are nodular or speckled on an erythematous base. Many lesions are soft whereas other thicker lesions feel crusty. Induration suggests malignant change and is an indication for immediate biopsy. It is important to recognise that it is the speckled or nodular leucoplakias which are the most likely to undergo malignant change.

Potential for malignant change

It has been shown that the incidence of ultimate malignant change in oral leucoplakia increases with the age of the lesion. One study showed a 2.4 per cent malignant transformation rate at 10 years which increased to 4 per cent at 20 years. It also showed that as the age of the patient increased so did the risk of malignant transformation: for patients younger than 50 years it was 1 per cent whereas for those between 70 and 89 years it was 7.5 per cent during a 5-year observation period. Studies have shown that, in southern England, leucoplakia of the floor of the mouth and ventral surface of the tongue has a particularly high incidence of malignant change. This study suggested that this occurrence was due to pooling of soluble carcinogens in the 'sump' of the floor of the mouth.

Aetiology

Tobacco smoking and chewing are undoubtedly important aetiological factors. In Indians who smoke or chew tobacco (often as a component of the betel quid) the incidence of leucoplakia in those of 60 years of age is 20 per cent, whereas in those who neither smoke not chew tobacco the incidence is 1 per cent.

The role of alcohol in the development of oral leucoplakia is difficult to assess. Few studies have been reported, but it has been shown that in patients with leucoplakia the incidence of excessive alcohol consumption is greater than in those free of leucoplakia.

Management

In any patient presenting for the first time with oral leucoplakia a careful history – particularly looking for aetiological factors – and a detailed clinical examination should precede the histological examination of biopsies of any suspicious areas. Suspicion should be aroused by any areas of ulceration or induration or where the underlying tissues are bright red and hyperaemic.

If there is a history of tobacco consumption then the patient should be persuaded to stop immediately. It has been shown that if the patient stops smoking entirely for 1 year the leucoplakia will disappear in 60 per cent of the cases.

Whenever severe epithelial dysplasia or carcinoma *in situ* is present, surgical excision or carbon dioxide laser excision of the lesions is mandatory. Small lesions may be excised, the margins of the adjacent mucosa undermined and the defect closed by advancing the margins. For larger defects the area should be left to epithelialise spontaneously or alternatively the area can be skin grafted. On the tongue the graft is quilted on to the raw area, whereas on the cheek, floor of mouth or palate the graft can be retained in place by suturing a suitable pack overlying it.

When only mild to moderate epithelial dysplasia is present the patient should be followed up at 4-monthly intervals and the lesions recorded in the notes either photographically or diagrammatically.

Erythroplakia

Erythroplakia (Fig. 41.3) is defined as 'any lesion of the oral mucosa that presents as bright red velvety plaques which cannot be characterised clinically or pathologically as any other recognisable condition'. Such lesions are usually irregular in outline, although clearly demarcated from adjacent normal epithelium. The surface may be nodular. In some cases erythroplakia coexists with areas of leucoplakia. The incidence of malignant change in erythroplakias is 17-fold higher than in leucoplakia. In every case of erythroplakia there are areas of epithelial dysplasia, carcinoma *in situ* or invasive carcinoma. Clearly, all erythroplakic areas must be completely excised either surgically or with a carbon dioxide laser, and the specimens submitted for careful pathological examination.

Chronic hyperplastic candidiasis

In chronic hyperplastic candidiasis (Fig. 41.4), dense chalky plaques of keratin are formed, the plaques being thicker and more opaque than in noncandidal leucoplakia. Such lesions are particularly common at the oral commissures extending on to the adjacent skin of the face.

In 1969 Cawson drew attention to the high incidence of malignant transformation in these candidal leucoplakias, suggesting that the invasive candidal infection is the cause of the leucoplakia and not merely a superimposed infection. It has also been suggested that in such patients there may be an immunological defect which allows the *Candida albicans* to invade the epithelium and may render the patient susceptible to malignant change.

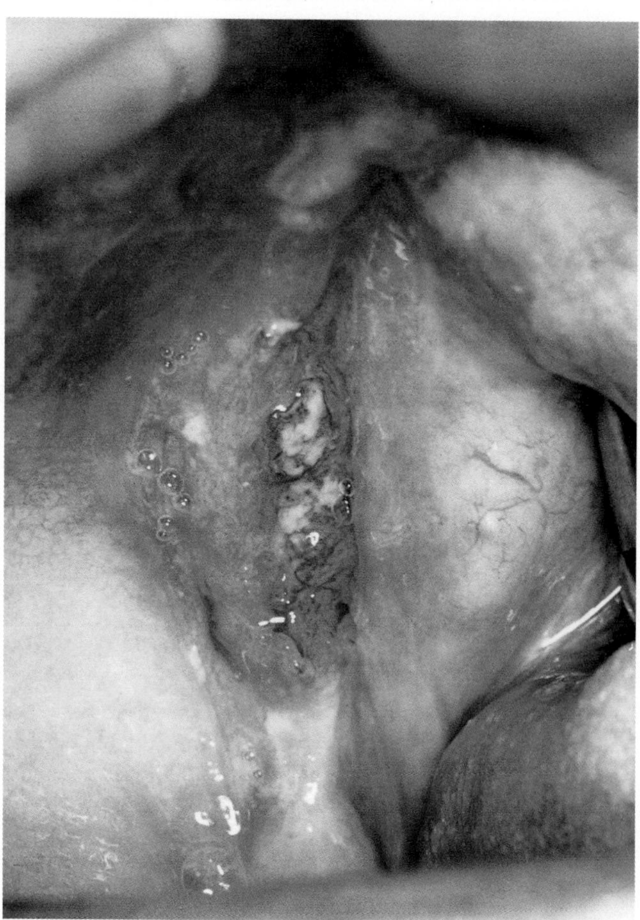

Fig. 41.3 Erythroplakia, in this case arising on the buccal mucosa posteriorly, is always a warning sign that the patient will soon develop an invasive carcinoma.

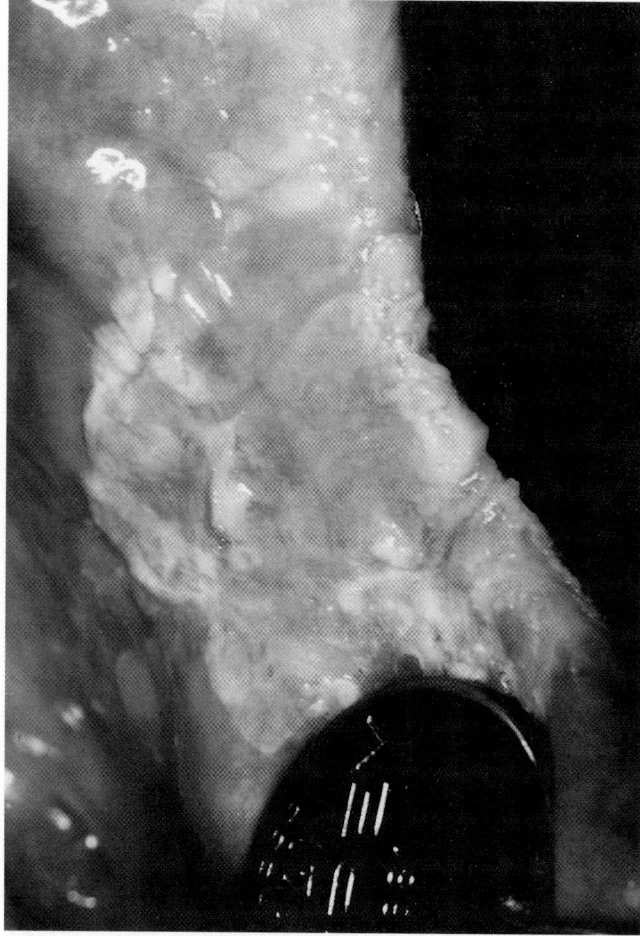

Fig. 41.4 Chronic hyperplastic candidiasis has a greater risk of malignant change than noncandidal leucoplakia. The commissures region as shown here is a typical site.

It is thought that treatment with nystatin, amphotericin or miconazole to eliminate the candidal infection will reduce the risk of malignant change. However, treatment may be necessary for many months to eliminate the organisms and reinfection is a constant problem. Surgical excision is recommended for persistent lesions.

Oral submucous fibrosis

Oral submucous fibrosis (Fig. 41.5) is a progressive disease in which fibrous bands form beneath the oral mucosa. These bands progressively contract so that ultimately opening is severely limited. Tongue movements may also be limited. The condition is almost entirely confined to Asians. Histologically it is characterised by juxta-epithelial fibrosis with atrophy or hyperplasia of the overlying epithelium which also shows areas of epithelial dysplasia. Paymaster in 1956 first discussed the precancerous nature of submucous fibrosis. He noted the onset of a slowly growing squamous cell carcinoma in one-third of such patients. The aetiology is obscure. Hypersensitivity to chilli, betel nut, tobacco and vitamin deficiencies have been implicated. Canniff has investigated the various enzyme components of the constituents of the 'betel quid', and has characterised some alkaloids and collagenases that may be responsible for the connective tissue changes which lead to epithelial atrophy and ultimate malignant degeneration. Tissue culture experiments have shown that alkaloids in the betel nut – particularly arecoline – stimulate collagen synthesis and the proliferation of buccal mucosal fibroblasts. Tannins also present in the betel nut stabilise the collagen fibrils and render them resistant to degradation by collagenase.

The scar bands of submucous fibrosis which result in difficulty in opening can be treated either by intralesional injection of steroids or by surgical excision and grafting, but this has little effect in preventing the onset of squamous cell carcinoma in the generally atrophic oral mucosa. Any aetiological factors should, of course, be eliminated.

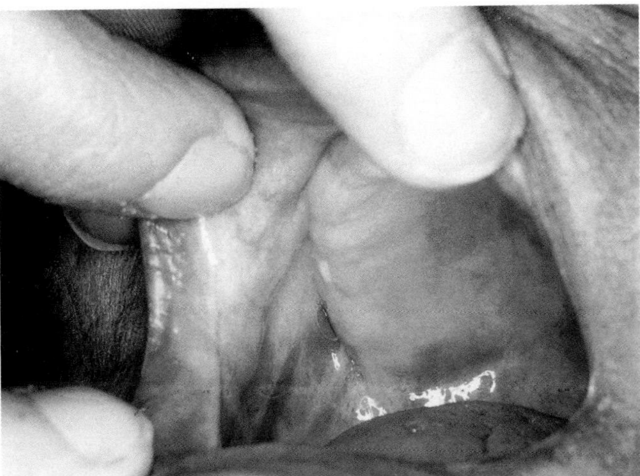

Fig. 41.5 This photograph of a patient with oral submucous fibrosis shows the thin pale atrophic mucosa and vertical scar bands in the buccal tissues.

Syphilitic glossitis

Prior to the antibiotic era, syphilis was an important predisposing factor in the development of oral leucoplakia and oral cancer. The syphilitic infection produces an interstitial glossitis with an endarteritis which results in atrophy of the overlying epithelium. This atrophic epithelium appears to be more vulnerable to those other irritants which cause oral cancer or oral leucoplakia. As these changes are irreversible there is no specific treatment, although active syphilis must be treated. Regular follow-up is essential. It should be noted that squamous cell carcinomas may arise in syphilitic glossitis even in the absence of leucoplakia.

Sideropenic dysphagia (Plummer–Vinson syndrome, Paterson–Kelly syndrome)

In 1936 Ahlbom showed the relation between sideropenic dysphagia and oral cancer. Sideropenic dysphagia (Fig. 41.6) is particularly common in Swedish women, and this accounts for the high incidence of cancer of the upper alimentary tract in this group and the higher incidence of women with oral cancer in Sweden. Of women with oral cancer in Sweden, 25 per cent were sideropenic.

The pathogenesis of oral cancer in such patients may be similar to that of syphilitic glossitis. The sideropenic dysphagia leads to epithelial atrophy, which in itself is excessively vulnerable to carcinogenic irritants. Although the anaemia will respond to treatment with iron supplements, it is not known whether such treatment reduces the risk of subsequent malignant change.

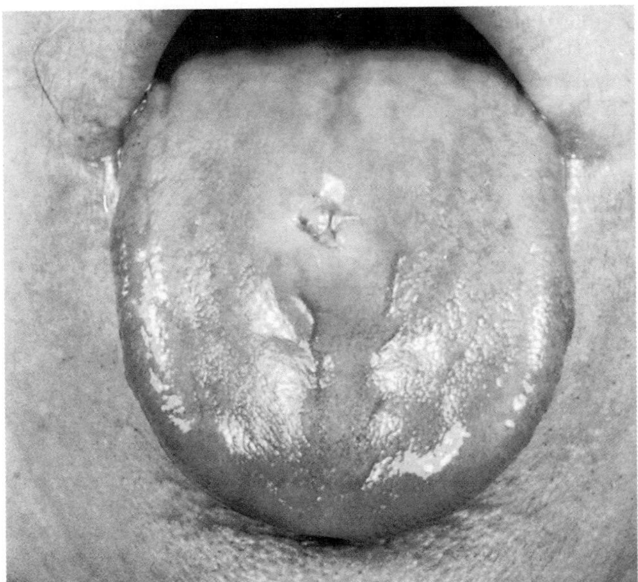

Fig. 41.6 In sideropenic dysphagia the oral mucosa is thin, pale and atrophic as seen in this tongue.

Henry S. Plummer, 1874–1957. Physician, Mayo Clinic, Rochester, Minnesota, USA.
Porter P. Vinson, b. 1890. American physician.
Donald R. Paterson, b. 1863. Welsh physician.
Adam B. Kelly, b. 1865. Scottish physician.

Oral lichen planus

There have been some reports that in erosive or atrophic lichen planus (Fig. 41.7) there is a risk of malignant transformation. If there is an association between lichen planus and oral cancer the relation only exists with atrophic or erosive lichen planus. All patients with erosive or atrophic lichen planus should be carefully reviewed. Erosive lichen planus should be treated with topical steroids and, in severe cases, systemic steroids may be necessary.

Discoid lupus erythematosus

The oral lesions of discoid lupus erythematosus consist of circumscribed, somewhat elevated, white patches usually surrounded by a telangiectatic halo. Epithelial dysplasia may be seen on histological examination and this may lead to malignant transformation. Malignant change usually occurs in those lesions of the labial mucosa adjacent to the vermilion border, and occurs more often in men than in women. Such patients with discoid lupus erythematosus should be advised to avoid bright sunlight and when in the open air to apply an ultraviolet barrier cream to the lips.

Dyskeratosis congenita

This syndrome is characterised by reticular atrophy of the skin with pigmentation, nail dystrophy and oral leucoplakia. Eventually, the oral mucosa becomes atrophic and the tongue loses its papillae. Finally, the mucosa becomes thickened, fissured and white.

Clinical presentation and diagnosis of oral cancer

Early diagnosis of oral cancer should lead to better treatment results and, ideally, the clinical diagnosis of oral cancer should be easy. Oral lesions, unlike those at many other sites, give rise to early symptoms. In general, patients become aware of and usually complain about minute lesions within the mouth and biopsy may be carried out under local analgesia. Yet, despite all the above, between 27 and 50 per cent of patients present for treatment with late lesions. Many of these patients are elderly and frail and, therefore, delay the effort of visiting their doctor or dentist. Many of this group of patients wear dentures and are accustomed to discomfort and ulceration in the mouth and thus see no urgency in seeking treatment. Furthermore, the practitioner is often not suspicious that a lesion may be malignant and the lesion is often treated initially with antifungal therapy, antibiotics, steroids and mouth-washes, thus contributing to further delay in the ultimate diagnosis and treatment. Another factor is that oral cancer is not usually painful until such time as either the ulcer becomes secondarily infected or the tumour invades sensory nerve fibres.

The tongue

The majority of tongue cancers occurs on the middle third of the lateral margins, extending early in the course of the disease on to the ventral aspect and floor of the mouth (Fig. 41.8). Approximately 25 per cent occur on the posterior third of the tongue, 20 per cent on the anterior third and rarely (4 per cent) on the dorsum.

Early tongue cancer may manifest in a variety of ways. Often the growth is exophytic with areas of ulceration. It may occur as an ulcer in the depths of a fissure or as an area of superficial ulceration with unsuspected infiltration into the underlying muscle. Leucoplakic patches may or may not be associated with the primary lesion. A minority of tongue cancers may be asymptomatic, arising in an atrophic depapillated area with an erythroplakic patch with peripheral streaks or areas of leucoplakia.

Later in the course of the disease a more typical malignant ulcer will usually develop, often several centimetres in diameter. The ulcer is hard in consistency with heaped-up and often everted edges. The floor is granular, indurated and bleeds readily. Often there are areas of necrosis. The growth infiltrates the tongue progressively causing increasing pain and difficulty with speech and swallowing. By this stage pain is often severe and constant, radiating to the neck and ears. Lymph node metastases at this stage are common – indeed 50 per cent may have palpable nodes at presentation. Because of

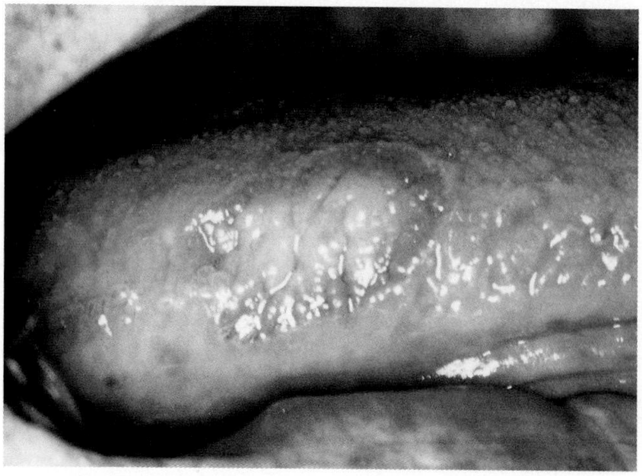

Fig. 41.7 It is now recognised that errosive lichen planus, particularly as shown here on the lateral border of the tongue, carries an increased risk of malignant change.

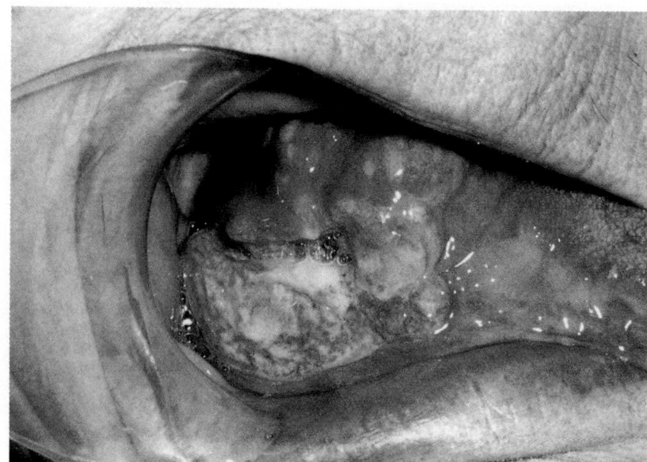

Fig. 41.8 Carcinoma of the tongue often starts as an indolent non-healing exophytic ulcer on the lateral border of the tongue. Pain is a late feature.

the relatively early lymph node metastasis of tongue cancer, 12 per cent of patients may present with no symptoms other than 'a lump in the neck'.

The floor of the mouth

The floor of the mouth is the second most common site for oral cancer (Fig. 41.9). It is defined as the U-shaped area between the lower alveolus and the ventral surface of the tongue; carcinomas arising at this site involve adjacent structures very early in their natural history. Most tumours occur in the anterior segment of the floor of the mouth to one side of the midline.

The lesion usually starts as an indurated mass which soon ulcerates. At an early stage the tongue and lingual aspect of the mandible become involved. This early involvement of the tongue leads to the characteristic slurring of the speech often noted in such patients. The infiltration is deceptive but may extend to reach the gingivae, tongue and genioglossus muscle. Subperiosteal spread is rapid once the mandible is reached. Lymphatic metastasis, although early, is less common than with tongue cancer. Spread is usually to the submandibular and jugulodigastric nodes and may be bilateral.

Cancer in the floor of the mouth cancer is associated with a pre-existing leucoplakia more commonly than at other sites.

The gingiva and alveolar ridge

Carcinoma of the lower alveolar ridge occurs predominantly in the premolar and molar regions (Fig. 41.10).

The patient usually presents with proliferative tissue at the gingival margins or superficial gingival ulceration. Diagnosis is often delayed because there is a wide variety of inflammatory and reactive lesions which occur in this region in association with the teeth or dentures. Indeed, there will often be a history of tooth extraction with subsequent failure of the socket to heal prior to definitive diagnosis. Another common story is that of sudden difficulty in wearing dentures.

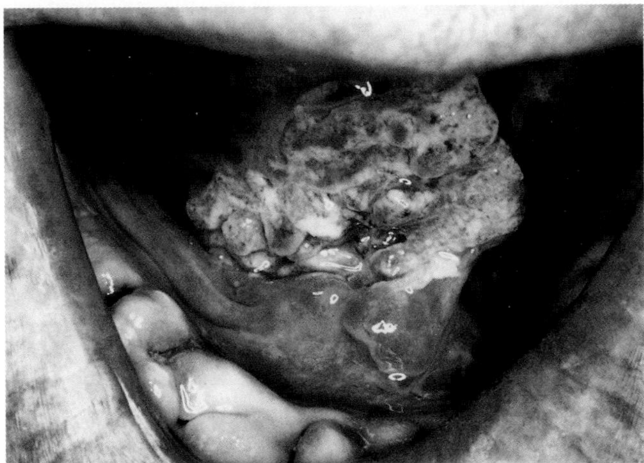

Fig. 41.9 Carcinoma in the floor of the mouth is often associated with a pre-existing leucoplakia.

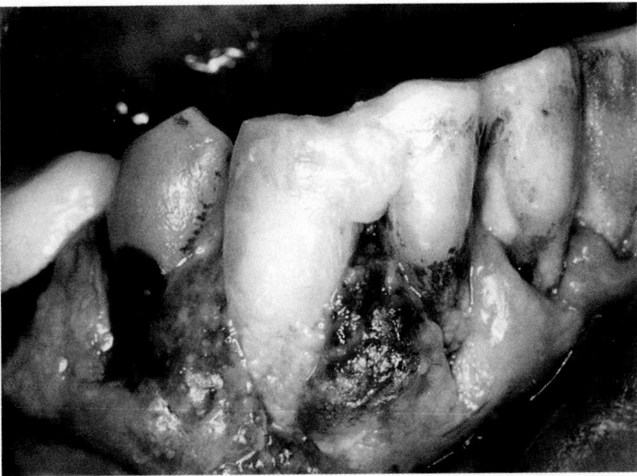

Fig. 41.10 The diagnosis of gingival carcinoma is often delayed as it can mimic chronic gingival infection and presents as loose teeth and bleeding gums.

Regional nodal metastasis is common at presentation, varying from 30 to 84 per cent, although false-positive and false-negative clinical findings are common.

The buccal mucosa

The buccal mucosa extends from the upper alveolar ridge down to the lower alveolar ridge and from the commissure anteriorly to the mandibular ramus and retromolar region posteriorly (Fig. 41.11). Squamous cell carcinomas mostly arise either at the commissure or along the occlusal plane to the retromolar area, the majority being situated posteriorly. Exophytic, ulcero-infiltrative and verrucous types occur. They are subject to occlusal trauma with consequent early ulceration and often become secondarily infected. The onset of the disease may be insidious, the patient sometimes presenting with trismus due to deep neoplastic infiltration into the buccinator muscle. Extension posteriorly involves the anterior pillar of the fauces and soft palate with consequent worsening of the prognosis. Ulcero-infiltrative lesions will often involve the overlying skin of the cheek resulting in multiple sinuses. Lymph node spread is to the submental, submandibular, parotid and lateral pharyngeal nodes.

Verrucous carcinoma occurs as a superficial proliferative exophytic lesion with minimal deep invasion and induration. Often the lesion is densely keratinised and presents as a soft white velvety area mimicking benign hyperplasia. Lymph node metastasis is late and the tumour behaves as a low-grade squamous cell carcinoma.

The hard palate, maxillary alveolar ridge and floor of antrum

These three sites are anatomically distinct, but a carcinoma arising from one site soon involves the others (Fig. 41.12). Consequently, it can be difficult to determine the exact site of origin. Except in countries where reverse smoking is practised, cancer of the plate is relatively uncommon. The

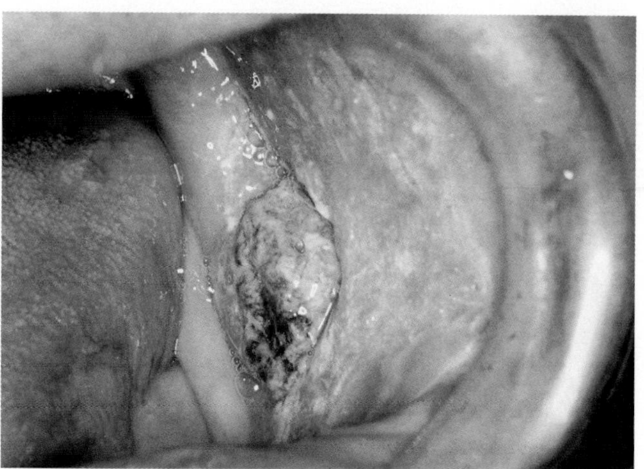

Fig. 41.11 This exophytic buccal carcinoma has arisen in an area of widespread leucoplakia.

majority of squamous cancers arises in the antrum and later ulcerates through to involve the hard palate. The majority of malignant tumours arising from the palatal mucosa is of minor salivary gland origin. Palatal cancers usually present as sessile swellings which ulcerate relatively late. A finding in contrast to mandibular alveolar tumours is that deep infiltration into the underlying bone is uncommon.

Carcinomas arising in the floor of the maxillary antrum often present as palatal tumours. Although the fully established picture of antral carcinoma is difficult to miss, the early symptoms are nonspecific and may mimic chronic sinusitis. Tumours of the lower half of the antrum below Ohngren's line usually present with 'dental' symptoms because of early alveolar invasion. The commonest presenting feature is pain, swelling or numbness of the face. Later symptoms of nasal obstruction, discharge or bleeding, and dental symptoms such as painful or loose teeth, ill-fitting dentures, oro-antral fistula or failure of an extraction socket to heal, soon follow. Lymph node metastasis from carcinomas of the palate and floor of the antrum occurs late but carries a poor prognosis.

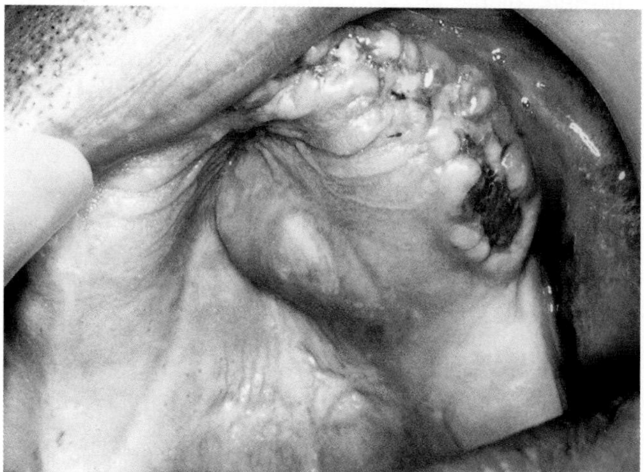

Fig. 41.12 Carcinoma arising in the floor of the maxillary antrum often presents with palatal swelling and nonhealing tooth sockets.

Diagnosis

The diagnosis of intraoral carcinoma is primarily clinical, and a high index of suspicion is necessary for all those clinicians seeing and treating patients with oral symptoms. A careful and detailed history with particular attention to recording the dates of the onset of particular signs and symptoms precedes the clinical examination. All areas of the oral mucosa are carefully inspected and any suspicious lesion is palpated for texture, tethering to adjacent structures and induration of underlying tissue.

Investigation

Surgical biopsy

A clinical diagnosis of oral cancer should always be confirmed histologically. Within the oral cavity a surgical biopsy can nearly always be obtained using local anaesthesia. An incisional biopsy is recommended in all cases. Whenever possible the patient should be seen at a combined clinic by a surgeon and radiotherapist before even the biopsy is carried out, but provided careful records are made an initial incisional biopsy is acceptable and may save time in the planning and execution of subsequent therapy. The biopsy should include the most suspicious area of the lesion and include some normal adjacent mucosa. Areas of necrosis or gross infection should be avoided as they may confuse the diagnosis.

Fine needle aspiration biopsy

This technique is applicable mainly to lumps in the neck, especially suspicious lymph nodes in a patient with a known primary carcinoma. It consists of the percutaneous puncture of the mass with a fine needle and aspiration of material for cytological examination. The method of aspiration needs no specialised equipment and is fast, almost painless and without complications. The node is fixed between finger and thumb and then punctured by a 21G or 23G needle on a 10-ml syringe, the gauge of the needle depending on the size of the node. Important points to note are that the needle is properly pushed on to the syringe to prevent air leaking in when the plunger is withdrawn and that a small amount of air is already in the syringe (about 2 ml) before the node is punctured in order subsequently to expel the aspirate from the needle on to the slide.

Radiography

Plain radiography is of limited value in the investigation of oral cancer. At least 50 per cent of the calcified component of bone must be lost before any radiographic change is apparent. Furthermore, the facial bones are of such a complexity that confusion from overlying structures makes X-ray diagnosis more difficult. However, rotational pantomography of the jaws can be helpful in assessing alveolar and antral involvement, provided that the above limitations are understood.

Computerised tomography

The increasing availability of computerised tomography (CT) scanning has undoubtedly been of great benefit in the investigation of head and neck tumours. However, for intraoral tumours its value is more limited. For the evaluation of antral tumours, particularly assessment of the pterygoid regions, CT has superseded plain radiography and conventional tomography. CT is also of value in the investigation of metastatic disease in the lungs, liver and skeleton.

Radionuclide studies

Technetium (Tc) pertechnetate bone scans of the facial skeleton are of little value in the diagnosis of primary oral cancers. There will be obvious clinical disease long before bone changes are visible on a Tc scan. Furthermore, such scans are not specific and will show increased uptake wherever there is increased metabolic activity in the bone.

Ultrasound

Abdominal ultrasound to detect liver metastases is probably as accurate as CT scanning. As it is noninvasive, readily available and cost effective, it is probably the most appropriate technique for assessing the liver.

Management of the primary tumour

Choice of treatment

The principal treatments available for primary tumours remain surgery and radiotherapy. The basic decision to be made is between radical radiotherapy and elective surgery. If the former is chosen, surgery is reserved for 'salvage', i.e. for biopsy-proven recurrent or residual disease. If surgery is chosen, radiotherapy may be used in an adjuvant manner, either preoperatively or postoperatively, but the operation remains fundamentally the definitive curative procedure. Preferences for one or other policy vary considerably between treatment centres.

Many factors must be considered in deciding the optimum management for each individual patient. These include the site, stage and histology of the tumour, and the medical condition and lifestyle of the patient. Ideally, every patient should be seen at a joint consultation clinic by a surgeon and radiotherapist who assess objectively and agree the optimum strategy of management for the particular individual. The following factors should influence the decision on treatment policy.

Site of origin

The choice of treatment depends on the part of the mouth in which the tumour arises. The management of primary tumours at the various anatomical sites is discussed later. In general, surgery is preferred for those tumours arising on or involving the alveolar processes; for other sites surgery and radiotherapy are alternatives.

Stage of disease

A small lesion which can be excised readily without producing any deformity or disability is, in general, best managed surgically. Surgery is also usually more appropriate for a very large mass or where there is invasion of bone, provided the tumour is operable, because of the low cure rates by radiotherapy in these circumstances. The management of lesions of intermediate stage, i.e. larger T1, most T2 and early exophytic T3 tumours, is more controversial as policies of elective surgery or radical radiotherapy produce generally similar survival rates; hence, discussion centres on the likely functional results and morbidity of either approach.

When there is involvement of cervical lymph nodes the primary and nodes are normally both treated surgically. However, there is no clear evidence that a primary tumour is less likely to be cured by radiotherapy in the presence of lymph node metastases than in their absence.

Previous irradiation

It is not advisable to retreat a tumour arising in previously irradiated tissue. Such a tumour is likely to be relatively radioresistant because of limited blood supply. Re-irradiation of normal tissue is very likely to result in necrosis.

Field change

Where multiple primary tumours are present, or if there is extensive premalignant change, surgery is the preferred treatment. Radiotherapy in these circumstances is unsatisfactory; irradiation of the entire oral cavity causes severe morbidity and may not prevent subsequent new primary tumours arising from areas of premalignant change.

Histology

The histology report on a biopsy specimen has a relatively small influence on choice of treatment. The less common adenocarcinoma and melanoma are relatively radioresistant, and therefore should be treated surgically whenever possible. The grade of malignancy of a squamous carcinoma does not normally influence its management, there being little evidence to suggest that a well-differentiated primary should be treated differently from a poorly differentiated one.

A possible exception is the verrucous carcinoma, which is the subject of much controversy. The observation has been made that where large lesions of this histological type are treated by radiotherapy recurrences appear in some cases which are of a much more anaplastic pattern than the original primary, and it has become widely accepted that radiotherapy induces 'anaplastic transformation'.

It seems probable that some verrucous carcinomas already contain foci of more malignant cells prior to treatment, and that these cells are the ones most likely to survive after radiotherapy and give rise to recurrence. In practice, most verrucous carcinomas present at an early stage as superficial exophytic lesions and are suitable for local excision. When they cannot be excised locally the weight of evidence suggests that they can be dealt with safely in the same way as squamous carcinomas of other types, and either surgery or radiotherapy be chosen as the primary treatment modality according to the site and stage of the lesion and the condition of the patient.

Age

The patient's age is often quoted as an important factor which must be taken into account when deciding on a course of management. With a young patient there is the fear that if radiotherapy is given it may induce a malignancy in years to come; in fact, this risk is very small compared with the mortality of the disease itself. Elderly patients tend to be poor surgical risks, but they also tend to do badly with radiotherapy, especially external radiotherapy, and often deteriorate and may die as a result of the debility and poor nutritional status induced by the irradiation. Chronological age per se should not necessarily be regarded as a contraindication to surgery.

Carcinoma of the lip

Carcinoma of the lip most commonly arises at the vermilion border of the lower lip away from the line of contact with the upper lip. Only 15 per cent arise from the central third and commissure regions, and 5 per cent from the upper lip.

Initially the tumours tend to spread laterally rather than infiltrating deeply; eventually, if uncontrolled, they can spread into the anterior triangle of the neck and invade the mandible. Lymph node metastases occur late. Both surgery and radiotherapy are frequently employed and are highly effective methods of treatment, each giving cure rates of about 90 per cent.

Up to one-third of the lower lip can be removed with a V- or W-shaped excision with primary closure (Fig. 41.13). This method is suitable for tumours up to 2 cm in diameter. The residual defect is reconstructed by approximating and suturing the borders in three layers; mucosa, muscle and skin. Particular attention should be paid to the correct alignment of the vermilion junction. This simple procedure can readily be performed under local anaesthetic on an out-patient basis. Initially the lip will appear tight, but this improves after about 3 months.

If more than one-third of the lip is removed, primary closure results in microstomia. Therefore, for more extensive lip resections it is necessary to utilise local flaps for reconstruction. For large central defects of the lower lip, particularly in patients who do not have ageing wrinkled faces, the 'stepladder' approach of Johanson gives excellent cosmesis as the reconstruction advances symmetrical bilateral flaps from the lower third of the face (Fig. 41.14). This results in a 'mini facelift' and the scars are concealed in the labiomental groove around the chin point. For defects more laterally, in the lower lip, the upper lip and particularly involving the commissure, Fries' 'universal procedure' gives excellent functional results with acceptable cosmesis especially in the ageing face (Fig. 41.15). With this technique, lateral facial flaps are developed following full-thickness incisions in the cheeks parallel to the branches of the facial nerve. These flaps are then advanced into the lip defect with the sacrifice of Burrows' triangles to prevent piling up of the facial tissues.

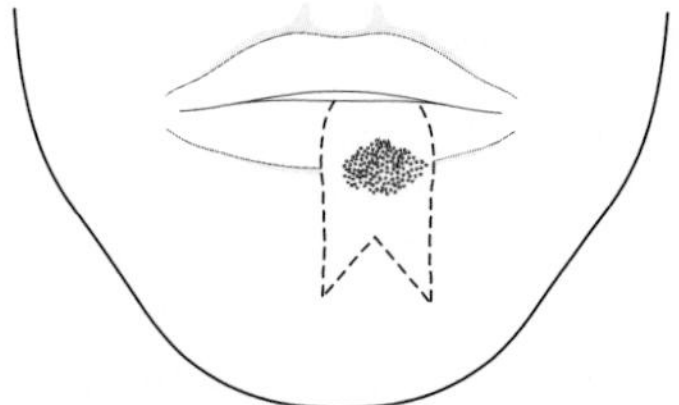

Fig. 41.13 Up to one-third of the lower lip can be excised and reconstructed using a 'W-plasty'.

The majority of lower lip cancers is caused by ultraviolet radiation and often the entire vermilion border will show actinic changes. Whenever these changes are seen a total lip shave would be undertaken in addition to resection of the primary tumour. The resection is reconstructed either by advancing labial or buccal mucosal flaps or, if such tissue is inadequate, by the use of a pedicled anteriorly based tongue flap. After 3 weeks the pedicle is divided and the flap finally set into the lip.

Carcinoma of the tongue

Surgery is the treatment of choice for early lesions suitable for simple intraoral excision, for tumours on the tip of the tongue and for advanced disease when surgery should be combined with postoperative radiotherapy. For intermediate-stage disease surgery and radiotherapy have similar outcomes. When performing surgical excision of less than one-third of the tongue, formal reconstruction is not

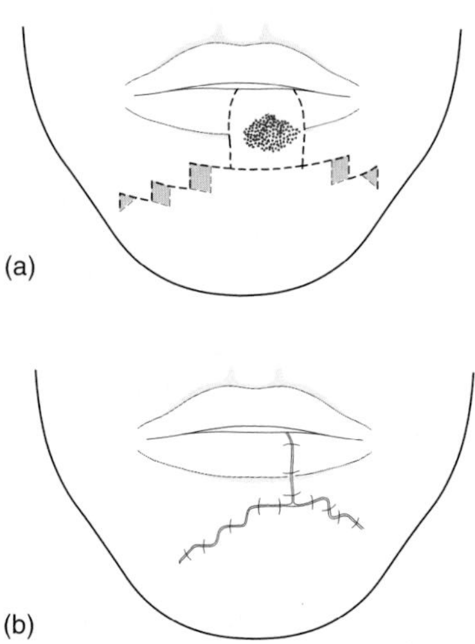

Fig. 41.14 (a) and (b) The Johansen 'stepladder' procedure can be used for more extensive carcinomas of the lower lip. It heals very well leaving an inconspicuous scar.

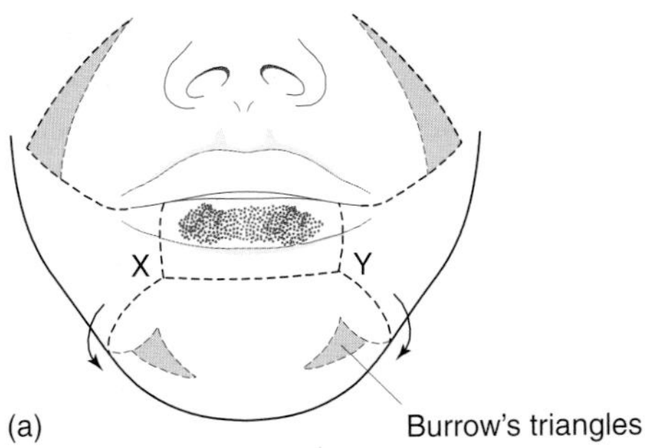

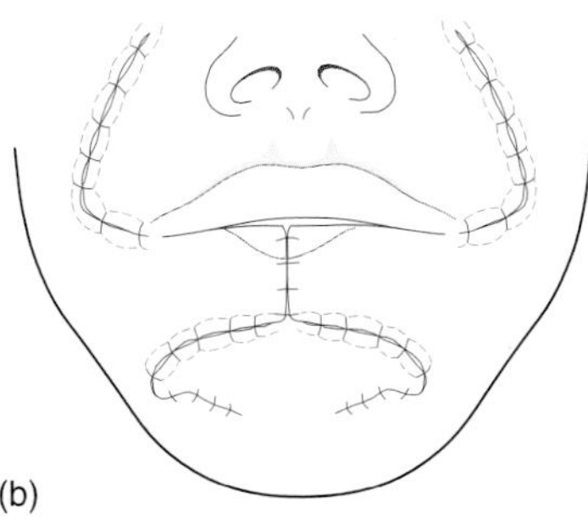

Fig. 41.15 (a) and (b) The Fries modification of the Bernard flap is very versatile and can be used for total lip reconstruction of both upper and lower lips. Burrows' triangles of redundant skin are excised in the nasolabial and submental regions.

necessary. Indeed, the best results are obtained by not attempting to close the defect or to apply a split-skin graft. The base of the residual defect should be fulgurated and then allowed to granulate and epithelialise spontaneously. Such treatment is relatively pain free and results in an undistorted tongue. When available a carbon dioxide laser may be used for the partial glossectomy. The postoperative course is relatively pain free, oedema is minimal and healing occurs with minimal scarring.

Any tongue carcinoma exceeding 2 cm in diameter requires at the very least a hemiglossectomy. Many such tumours will infiltrate deeply between the fibres of the hyoglossus muscle. Extensive tongue lesions often involve the floor of the mouth and alveolus. Under any of these circumstances a major resection is indicated. Access is best via a lip split and mandibulotomy (Fig. 41.16). The pull-through procedure is not recommended as it is very difficult to achieve adequate excision in all three dimensions with a limited access. As the resection opens the submandibular space the resection should include a dissection of the neck on the same side as the tumour. The type of neck dissection will depend upon the node status of the patient. A rim resection of the mandible is indicated if the tumour reaches but does not invade the alveolus. Such extensive defects require reconstruction with distant flaps. If the volume of the tongue defect does not exceed two thirds of the original tongue a radial forearm free flap with microvascular anastomosis gives a good functional result. For very large volume defects, for total glossectomy or for deeply infiltrating tumours, when the resection extends to the hyoid bone, more bulky flaps are required to fill in the dead space and prevent food pooling.

A pectoralis major muscle flap is the best method. Whenever it is possible, without compromising the resection, at least one of the hypoglossal nerves should be preserved. If this is done, most patients will eventually relearn to swallow and will establish reasonable speech.

Carcinoma of the floor of the mouth

Floor of mouth cancers spread to involve the under surface of the tongue and the lower alveolus at a relatively early stage. Therefore, surgical excision will nearly always include partial glossectomy and marginal resection of the mandible. The resultant defect must always be reconstructed with either a local or a distant flap. It is unacceptable to advance the lateral margin of the residual tongue to the buccal mucosa as this causes very severe difficulties with speech and mastication. Small tumours of the floor of the mouth that do not show deep infiltration can be treated by simple excision.

It is important that a 1-cm margin of normal-appearing mucosa be excised around the tumour. The resulting defect can either be left to granulate if a carbon dioxide laser was used for the excision, or fulgurated if diathermy excision was used. Alternatively, if the defect is large it can be repaired using bilateral nasolabial flaps tunnelled into the mouth and interdigitated anteriorly. The submandibular duct should be identified proximally, well clear of the distal margin of the excision and brought out into the floor of the mouth or lingual gutter posteriorly.

For larger lesions and those involving the ventral tongue and/or the alveolus, surgical access is gained via a midline or lateral (anterior to the mental foramen) mandibulotomy and lip split. As these extensive tumours have a high incidence of nodal involvement, the resection is undertaken in continuity with an ipsilateral neck dissection (Fig. 41.17).

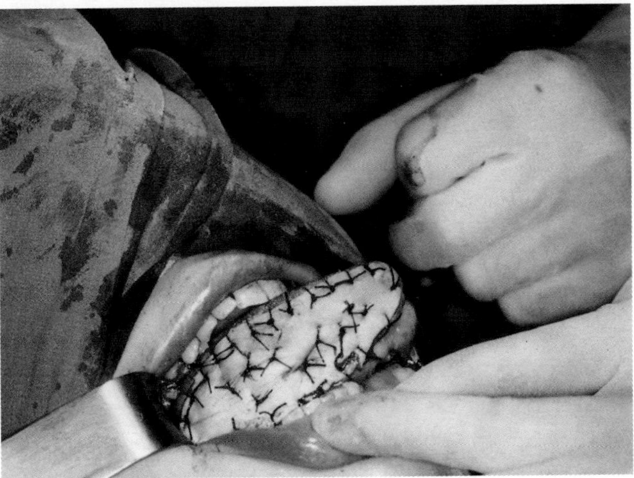

Fig. 41.16 For T1–T2 tongue cancers requiring hemiglossectomy, the resulting defect can be repaired with a simple quilted split-skin graft.

Recent work has demonstrated the pattern of bone invasion by carcinoma of the floor of the mouth. Invasion in the edentulous mandible is almost exclusively via deficiencies in the cortical bone of the alveolar crest. In the dentate mandible invasion is usually via the periodontal ligament and is nearly always above the insertion of the mylohyoid muscle. Once tumour has invaded the mandible it soon enters the inferior dental canal and perineural spread occurs anteriorly and posteriorly. Consequently, in many cases the continuity of the mandible can safely be maintained provided a marginal resection is carried out which includes the inferior dental canal from the lingula to the mental foramen.

When there is evidence of gross tumour invasion of the bone resection of the mandible is mandatory. In order to avoid functional and cosmetic deformity, immediate primary reconstruction is essential. The choice lies between reconstruction with vascularised bone, a free corticocancellous graft or an alloplastic system usually supplemented with cancellous bone mush.

Carcinoma of the buccal mucosa

Lesions strictly confined to the buccal mucosa should be excised widely including the underlying buccinator muscle, followed by a quilted split-skin graft. For more extensive lesions with more complicated three-dimensional shapes, i.e. lesions extending posteriorly to the retromolar area, maxillary tuberosity or tonsillar fossa, reconstruction with a free radial forearm flap is advisable; this adapts very well to such shapes and remains soft and mobile postoperatively (Fig. 41.18).

In situations where a free flap is not appropriate, alternatives are the buccal fat pad or the forehead flap. The buccal fat pad has proved to be a useful local flap for the reconstruction of small intraoral defects up to 3 × 5 cm. This well-vascularised flap can be left raw to epithelialise spontaneously, and is used to reconstruct maxillary defects, hard and soft palate defects, and cheek and retromolar defects. For large defects at these sites its use can be combined with the temporalis muscle flap.

The use of the forehead flap, an axial flap based on the superficial temporal artery, was first described by McGregor in 1963. It is a very reliable flap able to reach most areas within the mouth including the anterior floor of the mouth. However, it is now rarely used because it results in a very obvious cosmetic defect at the donor site; it is a two-stage procedure requiring division of the pedicle at 3 weeks; and it requires the creation of a tunnel, either deep or superficial, to the zygomatic arch when the flap is needed in the oral cavity.

Carcinoma of the lower alveolus

In general, surgery is the treatment modality of choice for all alveolar carcinomas, except for patients unfit for surgery. Access is achieved via a lip-split approach. Now that the patterns of bone invasion are better understood, the continuity of the mandible can often be preserved by performing a marginal resection. If bone invasion is so extensive that the mandible must be resected in continuity, primary reconstruction should always be undertaken as the results are always better than those of delayed reconstruction.

Several techniques are available for immediate reconstruction of the mandible. Historically, free corticocancellous grafts harvested from the iliac crest or rib grafts have been used. Provided there is a good watertight cover to the graft, results can be very satisfactory, although it is difficult to reconstruct the chin prominence with this technique. Boyne and Leake have advocated the use of cancellous bone from

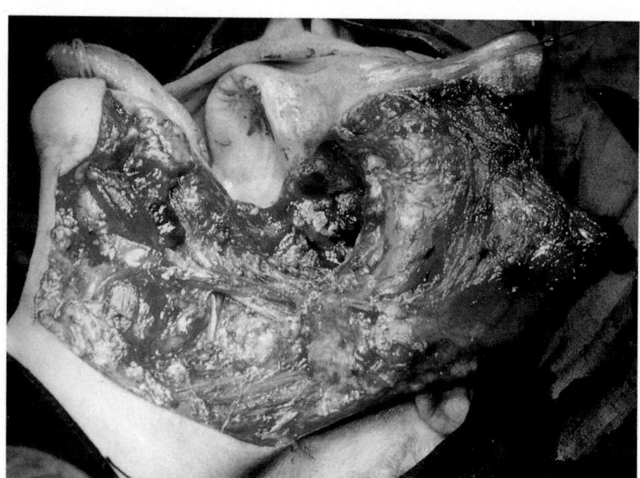

Fig. 41.17 For access to the floor of the mouth, posterior maxilla and oropharynx a lip-splitting procedure with or without a mandibulotomy gives wide exposure enabling a three-dimensional resection of the tumour to be undertaken.

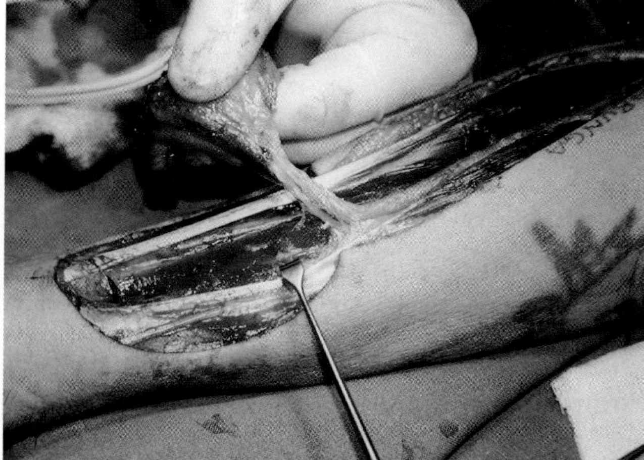

Fig. 41.18 Microvascular free transfer of tissues has allowed much more sophisticated one-stage reconstructions to be undertaken. The radial forearm flap illustrated here is the workhorse of oral reconstruction.

Ian McGregor, d. 1997. Plastic surgeon, Glasgow, Scotland.

the ilium packed into mesh trays preformed to match the resected part of the mandible. The early dacron trays did not prove successful, but the titanium trays currently available have given excellent results (Fig. 41.19).

Microvascular tissue transfer is currently favoured for immediate mandibular reconstruction. The radial forearm flap with a section of the radius, the compound groin flap based on the deep circumflex iliac vessels and free fibula flaps have all been advocated (Fig. 41.20). A problem with the radial flap is that the harvested bone, although restoring mandibular continuity, is barely adequate for prosthetic reconstruction.

Soft-tissue cover for all of these reconstruction techniques is critical. With microvascular free flaps the associated skin is used. For cancellous bone mush in titanium trays, and for corticocancellous grafts, the pectoralis major muscle-only flap is most useful (Fig. 41.21). The pedicle is brought up through the neck and the flap introduced into the floor of the mouth. The flap is then wrapped around the bone graft and sutured back on to itself on the labial aspect. Thus, the bone graft is totally enveloped in well-vascularised soft tissue. The mucosal resection margins are then sutured to the exposed muscle at their appropriate sites and the bare muscle allowed to epithelialise spontaneously. Such flaps withstand immediate postoperative radiotherapy, and the subsequent insertion of osseointegrated implants has not proved to be a problem.

Carcinoma of the retromolar trigone

The retromolar trigone is defined as the anterior surface of the ascending ramus of the mandible. It is roughly triangular in shape with the base being superior behind the third upper molar tooth and the apex inferior behind the third lower molar.

Tumours at this site may invade the ascending ramus of the mandible. They may also spread upwards in soft tissue to involve the pterygomandibular space, which can be difficult to detect clinically or radiologically.

A lip split and mandibulotomy are needed to gain access to the retromolar region. Small defects can often be reconstructed with a masseter or temporalis muscle flap. Larger defects are best reconstructed with a free radial forearm flap which can be made to conform very well to the shape of the defect at this site.

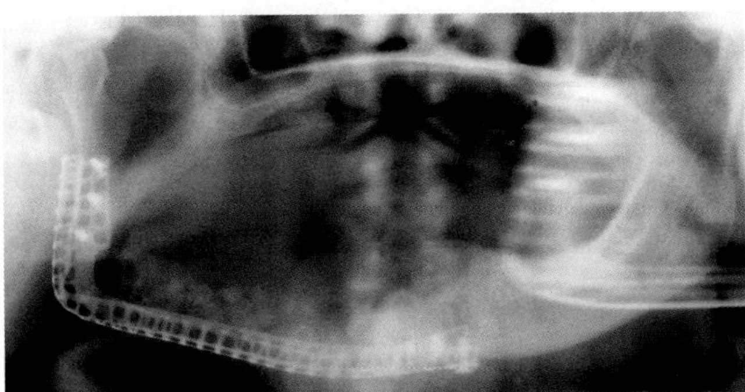

Fig. 41.19 Titanium mesh trays packed with bone-mush harvested from the ilium are useful for mandibular reconstruction when more sophisticated techniques are not available.

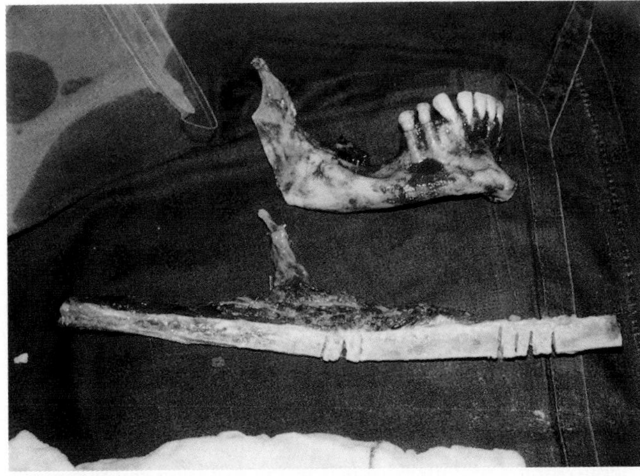

Fig. 41.20 This photograph shows a fibula bone graft harvested with its soft-tissue pedicle. Osteotomy cuts have been made to enable the graft to be shaped to match the resected specimen.

Carcinoma of the hard palate and upper alveolus

These sites are considered together as they are closely adjacent and both are rare sites of origin of primary squamous carcinoma. A squamous carcinoma presenting at either of these sites is more likely to have arisen in the maxillary antrum than in the oral cavity. An exception is on the Indian subcontinent where carcinoma of the hard palate is seen in association with reverse smoking. Tumours of minor salivary

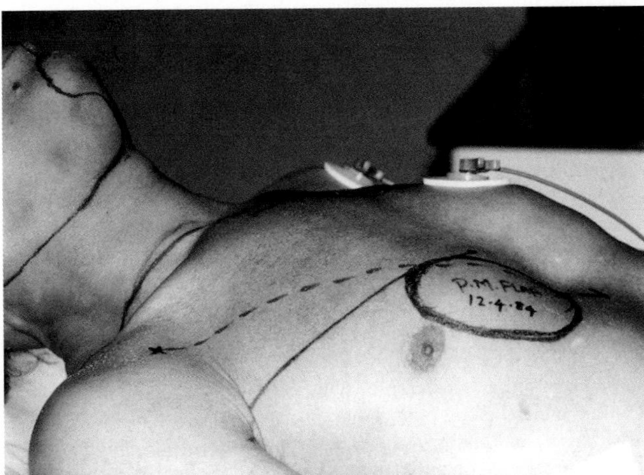

Fig. 41.21 The pectoralis major myocutaneous flap based on the acromiothoracic artery and veins (dotted line) is a very reliable flap and easily reaches the oral cavity. The pedicle is brought up through the neck following neck dissection including removal of the sterno-cleido-mastoid muscle to create space.

glands are much more common than squamous carcinomas on the hard palate. The vast majority of squamous carcinomas which present in the upper gum or hard palate arises from the maxillary antrum.

A tumour confined to the hard palate, upper alveolus and floor of the antrum can be resected by conventional partial maxillectomy. A more extensive tumour confined to the infrastructure of the maxilla requires total maxillectomy. If the preoperative investigations indicate extension of disease into the pterygoid space or infratemporal fossa a more exten-sive procedure is necessary. The chance of obtaining a cure by surgery alone is small, and postoperative radiotherapy is essential. A combined anteroposterior or lateral facial approach is required. If the tumour extends superiorly to involve the dura then a combined neurosurgical procedure will be required.

Following a maxillary resection the resulting cavity should be skin grafted to ensure rapid healing and to prevent contracture of the overlying soft tissues.

The defect created by surgery will require either reconstruction or a prosthesis. Various techniques have been described for reconstruction; Obwegeser described a technique using split ribs. More recently, the temporalis muscle flap has been advocated. The temporalis muscle flap is a simple technique and has the advantage that it carries with it its own blood supply. It must be remembered that if such a reconstruction is to be undertaken subsequently, it is essential that at the time of the original maxillectomy the coronoid process of the mandible is not excised, because if it is resected the blood supply to the mobilised temporalis muscle will have been compromised and the flap will necrose.

Malignant melanoma

Oral melanomas are rare. The peak age incidence is between 40 and 60 years; nearly 50 per cent are on the hard palate and about 25 per cent are on the upper gingivae. About 30 per cent of melanomas are preceded by an area of hyperpigmentation, often by many years. Pigmentation varies from black to brown, while rare nonpigmented melanomas (15 per cent of oral melanomas) are red. Oral melanomas may be flat but are usually raised or nodular, and asymptomatic initially, but may later become ulcerated and painful or bleed. Because of their rapid growth, most oral melanomas are at least 1 cm across, and approximately 50 per cent of patients have metastases at presentation (Fig. 41.22).

Clinically, size and rapid growth, particularly if associated with destruction of underlying bone or presence of metastases, are obvious indicators of a poor outcome.

Microscopically, tumour thickness, measured in millimetres from the granular cell layer to the deepest identifiable melanocyte (the Breslow thickness), is the main guide to prognosis. With cutaneous melanomas the 5-year survival rate is inversely proportional to the Breslow thickness. The poor prognosis of oral melanomas is probably due to their later detection than more conspicuous skin tumours.

Other indicators of poor prognosis are malignant melanocytes in blood vessels and multiple, or atypical, mitoses. The morphology of the melanocytes or the amount of the melanin does not appear to affect the outcome.

Once the diagnosis has been confirmed, the only hope of cure is provided by the widest possible excision followed by radical radiotherapy. There is no evidence that chemotherapy is of signifcant value except for palliation. The over 5-year survival rate appears to be about 5 per cent.

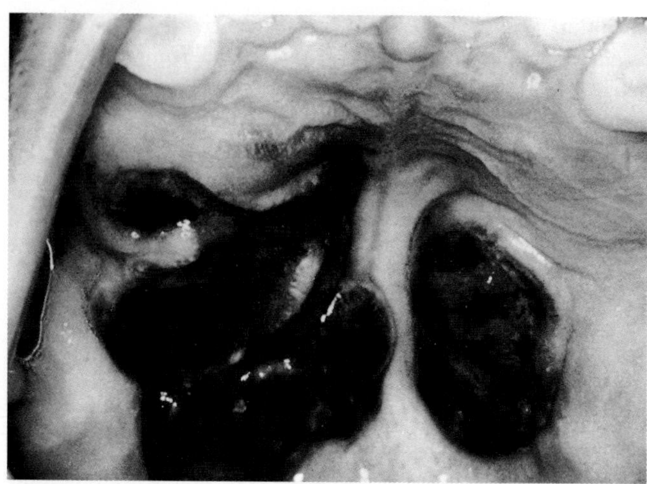

Fig. 41.22 Intraoral malignant melanoma most usually arises as here on the palate.

Management of the neck

Patients staged N0. The regional lymph nodes, although clinically impalpable, sometimes contain occult foci of malignant cells. It seems reasonable to expect, therefore, that removal or treatment of regional lymph nodes, even when clinically clear, would improve cure rates. Alternatively, it can be argued that treatment of the regional nodes in all cases is unnecessary, as only a minority has metastases in the nodes.

The arguments expressed in favour of elective block dissection are:

- the incidence of histologically involved nodes in N0 necks varies from 25 to 65 per cent;
- survival rates are considerably lower in patients who develop node metastases;
- the recurrence rate following block dissection is higher in advanced disease when there is extracapsular spread or multiple nodes;
- by waiting for clinically detectable disease to develop, many patients will have a worse prognosis;
- some patients fail to attend regular follow-up and may not appear again until nodal metastases are extensive;
- block dissection of the neck carries negligible mortality and an acceptable morbidity;
- retrospective reviews confirm that patients undergoing elective neck dissection have higher survival rates;
- failure to control nodal metastases is a frequent cause of death.

The arguments against elective neck dissection are that:

- it is rare for treatment to fail in the neck when the primary is controlled – only 4.5 per cent in one large series;

- the incidence of histologically positive nodes in elective neck dissections exceeds the incidence of subsequent clinical nodal metastases, suggesting that some microscopic foci are destroyed by the body's defences;
- the primary may recur or a second primary develop and metastasise into the dissected neck, making subsequent management very difficult;
- elective neck dissection gives no guarantee against recurrence of the tumour in the neck;
- block dissection has a considerable morbidity;
- removal of regional lymph nodes may remove a barrier to the further spread of disease;
- there is no prospectively controlled trial to support the argument that elective neck dissection does improve the prognosis.

On balance, the weight of these arguments favours prophylactic neck dissection.

As the submandibular triangle often has to be opened as part of the resection of the primary, a function sparing elective neck dissection for tumours in the floor of the mouth and lower alveolar ridge and tongue is advocated. This dissection, in which structures such as the accessory nerve, internal jugular vein and sterno-cleido-mastoid muscle are preserved, can be justified. Further, a survey showed that of 501 cancers of the oral cavity, 34 per cent of nodes were found to be positive after elective radical neck dissections. Over 96 per cent of these histologically postive nodes would have been removed by a supra-omohyoid dissection.

The operation should preferably be seen as a staging procedure on which is based the decision to give radical postoperative radiotherapy. All patients with two or more positive nodes or extracapsular spread should be treated with postoperative radiotherapy.

An alternative approach is elective irradiation of the clinically negative neck, and indeed there is good evidence that this is of some benefit in preventing subsequent nodal disease. Certainly, elective irradiation to 40 Gy carries less morbidity than elective neck dissection.

Patients staged N1/N2a/N2b. At present, evidence suggests that the treatment of choice is radical neck dissection, either alone or combined with postoperative radiotherapy if multiple nodal involvement or extracapsular extension is found in the resected specimen (Fig. 41.23). In those patients unfit for radical surgery, radical external beam irradiation is indicated.

Patients staged N2c. It is uncommon for patients with oral cancer to present with bilateral nodes. When they do so, there is often a large inoperable primary tumour which is best treated by external radiation. It therefore seems logical to treat the neck also by irradiation. Occasionally, particularly in young patients, bilateral neck dissection can be justified. A full radical neck dissection is undertaken on the ipsilateral side and the internal jugular vein is spared if possible on the contralateral side. Most often postoperative radiotherapy will be required for multiple nodal involvement or extracapsular spread. In such situations, severe post-treatment oedema or congestion of the face and tongue may be anticipated.

J. MacFie. Consultant surgeon.

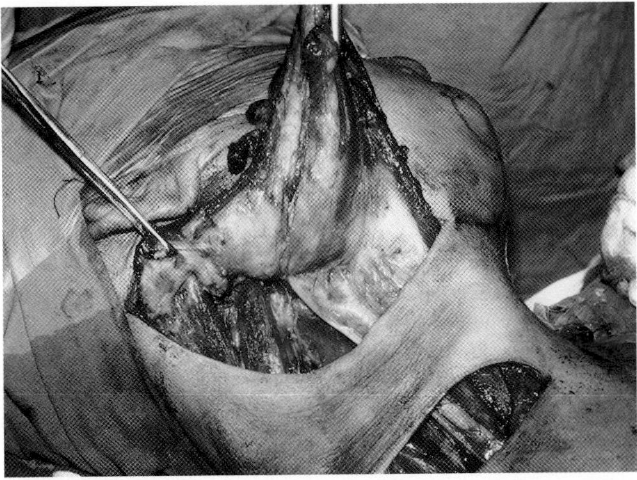

Fig. 41.23 This photograph illustrates a radical neck dissection undertaken via MacFie incisions. The common carotid artery and the carotid bifurcation can be seen. The internal jugular vein, sterno-cleido-mastoid muscle and accessory nerve which are being removed have been lifted upwards.

Patients staged N3. N3 indicates massive involvement, usually with fixation. Large fixed nodes are often associated with advanced primary disease with a poor prognosis. Surgery is not normally advisable: removal of the common or internal carotid artery with replacement, or extensive resection of the base of the skull, although technically feasible, is seldom advisable. Treatment is most often by external radiotherapy. In a few younger patients with resectable primaries, it is worth rendering a fixed mass in the neck operable by preoperative radiotherapy.

Nodal metastases appearing after primary treatment

Provided that follow-up at regular intervals is rigorously maintained, it should be possible to detect a lymph node metastasis while it is still relatively small and therefore operable. Fine needle aspiration cytology is particularly useful in this situation to confirm that the palpable node is a carcinoma rather than reactive. Whenever positive, or if there is any doubt, a radical neck dissection is performed, followed by external irradiation if multiple involved nodes or extracapsular spread are found.

Further reading

Avery, B.S. (1998) Neck dissections. In *Operative Maxillofacial Surgery* (eds J.D. Langdon and M.F. Patel), Chapman & Hall, London, pp. 295–302.

Cawson, R.A., Langdon, J.D. and Eveson, J.W. (1996) *Surgical Pathology of the Mouth and Jaws*, Wright, Oxford.

Langdon, J.D. and Henk, J.M. (eds) (1995) *Malignant Tumours of the Mouth, Jaws and Salivary Glands*, Arnold, London.

McGregor, I.A. and McGregor, F.M. (1986) *Cancer of the Face and Mouth*, Churchill-Livingstone, Edinburgh.

Ord, R.A. (1998) Local resection and local reconstruction of oral carcinomas, and jaw resection. In *Operative Maxillofacial Surgery* (eds J.D. Langdon and M.F. Patel), Chapman & Hall, London, pp. 273–94.

Soutar, D.S. (1993) Free flaps in intra oral reconstruction. In *Microvascular Surgery and Free Tissue Transfer* (ed. D.S. Soutar), Arnold, London.

Vaughan, E.D. (1990) The radial forearm free flap in orofacial reconstruction, personal experience in 120 consecutive cases. *Journal of Cranio-Maxillofacial Surgery*, **18**, 2–7.

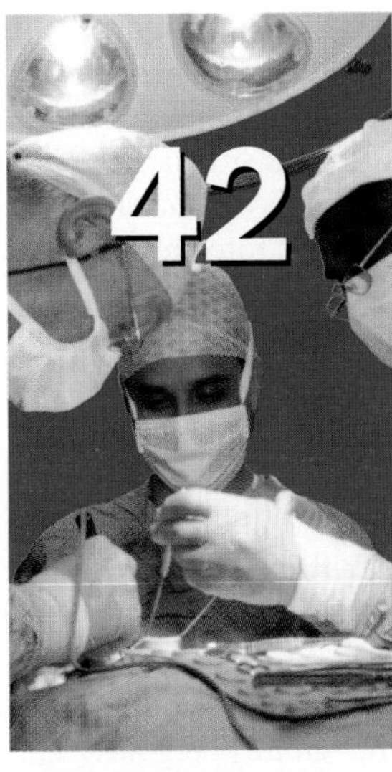

42 Salivary gland disorders

Developmental disorders (Table 42.1)

Aplasia/agenesis

Congenital absence of one or more of the major salivary glands can occur but is very rare. When it does it is usually the parotid gland that is affected.

Duct atresia

Again this disorder is extremely rare. Usually the submandibular duct in the floor of the mouth fails to canulate during embryological development. The newborn infant presents within 2 or 3 days of life with submandibular swelling on the affected side due to a retention cyst in the submandibular salivary gland.

Congenital fistula

Patients with branchial cleft anomalies present usually with unilateral painless swellings in the region of the parotid. Rarely they are bilateral. They form sinus tracts either in the crease behind the pinna or in front of the tragus. They discharge saliva intermittently. Abscess formation due to secondary infection may occur. Complete surgical excision of the sinus tract is essential. The dissection is often very extensive and full dissection of the facial nerve may be required.

Bailey & Love's Short Practice of Surgery, 23rd edition. Edited by R.C.G. Russell, N.S. Williams and C.J.K. Bulstrode. Published in 2000 by Arnold Publishers.

Ectopic and aberrant salivary tissue

Ectopic salivary tissue can develop anywhere within the territory of the first and second branchial arches in the lateral neck, pharynx or middle ear. Salivary tissue is regularly found in lymph nodes within the neck and can be mistaken for metastatic disease when found in a neck dissection specimen.

Although rare, the most commonly recognised ectopic salivary tissue is the Stafne bone cyst. This presents as an asymptomatic clearly demarcated radiolucency at the angle of the mandible below the inferior dental canal. It is formed by an invagination into the bone of the lingual aspect of the mandible by an ectopic lobe of the adjacent submandibular salivary gland.

Accessory lobes

An accessory parotid lobe is the most common developmental anomaly. It occurs in as many as 20 per cent of

Table 42.1 Developmental disorders

Aplasia/agenesis	Rare Usually parotid
Atresia	Rare Usually floor of mouth Retention cysts
Congenital fistula	Associated with branchial clefts
Ectopic/aberrant	Accessory parotid lobe common Enclaved salivary tissue common in cervical nodes Middle ear cleft and mastoid Stafne bone cavity

subjects. Its position is constant arising from the horizontal component of the parotid duct as it crosses the masseter muscle. Its importance lies in the fact that any of the diseases that can affect the salivary glands may involve the accessory lobe and lead to diagnostic confusion as the possibility is not considered. This is because the symptoms and signs are not within the normal anatomical territory of the parotid.

Inflammatory disorders (Table 42.2)

Viral

Mumps

The mumps virus is a paramyxovirus and is the most common cause of acute painful parotid swelling affecting children. The disease starts with a prodromal period of 1 or 2 days during which the child experiences feverishness, chills, nausea, anorexia and headache. This is typically followed by pain and swelling of one or both parotid glands. The parotid pain can be very severe and is exacerbated by eating or drinking. Symptoms resolve spontaneously after 5–10 days.

Table 42.2 Inflammatory disorders

Viral	Mumps is the commonest cause of acute parotitis May be atypical: unilateral or predominantly submandibular Lasting immunity Other viruses may cause identical symptoms/signs
Bacterial	Acute: usually parotid Ascending infection Dehydration Cachexia Obstruction Chronic: usually submandibular Often secondary to obstruction by stones
Recurrent parotitis of childhood	M:F 2:1 Recurrent Resolves at puberty Punctate sialectasis
Specific 'infection'	Mycobacterial Cat-scratch disease Syphilis Toxoplasmosis Deep mycoses Sarcoid Wegener's granulomatosis
Allergic	Foods, drugs and metals Very rare
Radiation	Acute parotitis 24 hours after irradiation Transient rise in salivary amylase Self-limiting
HIV-associated	Similar to Sjögren's syndrome Autoantibodies negative Lymphoma can occur Multiple parotid cysts
Minor glands	Sarcoid Stomatitis nicotina Acute necrotising sialadenitis

In a classical case of mumps the diagnosis is based on the history and clinical examination. However, the presentation may be atypical or sporadic or have predominantly unilateral or even submandibular involvement. In this situation, paired blood specimens taken approximately 10 days apart are used to confirm the diagnosis. One episode of infection confers lifelong immunity.

A number of other viral agents – Coxsackie A and B, para-influenza 1 and 3, enteric cytopathogenic human orphan viruses (ECHO) and lymphocytic choriomeningitis – can all cause identical signs and symptoms.

Bacterial

Acute ascending bacterial sialadenitis affects mostly the parotid glands. Historically it was described in dehydrated, cachectic patients often following major abdominal surgery when the patient was on a 'nil by mouth' regime. The reduced salivary flow and oral sepsis resulted in bacteria colonising the parotid duct and subsequently involving the parotid parenchyma. With current medical practice and improved oral hygiene patients are rarely allowed to become dehydrated and this clinical pattern is uncommon. The typical patient presenting with an acute ascending bacterial parotitis now is an otherwise fit young adult with no obvious predisposing factors (Fig. 42.1).

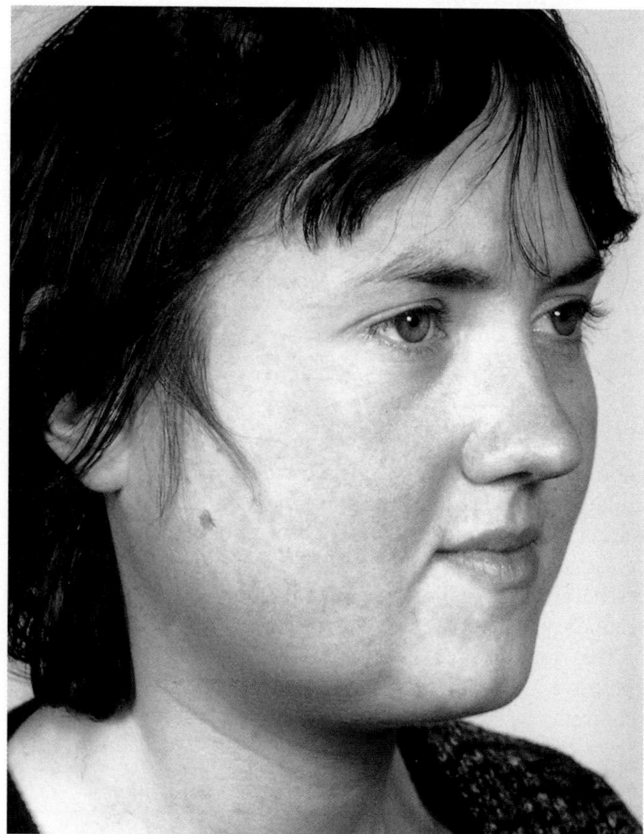

Fig. 42.1 This young nurse presents with acute bacterial parotitis. There are no obvious precipitating factors.

The clinical presentation is of the onset of tender, red, painful parotid swelling over a few hours. There is associated malaise, pyrexia and often regional lymphadenopathy. Pain is exacerbated on attempting to eat or drink. The parotid swelling may be diffuse but often it is localised to the lower pole of the gland presumably because the infection tends to localise under the effect of gravity.

If the gland is gently 'milked' by massaging the cheek, cloudy turbid saliva can be expressed from the parotid duct and this should be cultured. The infecting organism is usually *Staphylococcus aureus* or *Streptococcus viridans*. Sialography must never be undertaken during the acute phase of infection as the retrograde injection of infected material into the duct system will result in bacteraemia. Ultrasound imaging shows the characteristic dilatation of the acinae (Fig. 42.2).

If the patient presents at an early stage before abscess formation, the infection can usually be controlled with antibiotics. In a patient not allergic to penicillin a combination of a broad-spectrum penicillin and a penicillinase-resistant agent is usually effective. If the gland becomes fluctuant indicating abscess formation, the pus must be drained. Occasionally it is possible to drain the abscess by aspirating the pus through a large-bore hypodermic needle but usually it is necessary to undertake formal surgical drainage under general anaesthesia (Table 42.3).

Chronic bacterial sialadenitis is far more common in the submandibular salivary gland and it usually occurs secondary to chronic obstruction. Unfortunately the submandibular gland has a poor capacity for recovery following infection

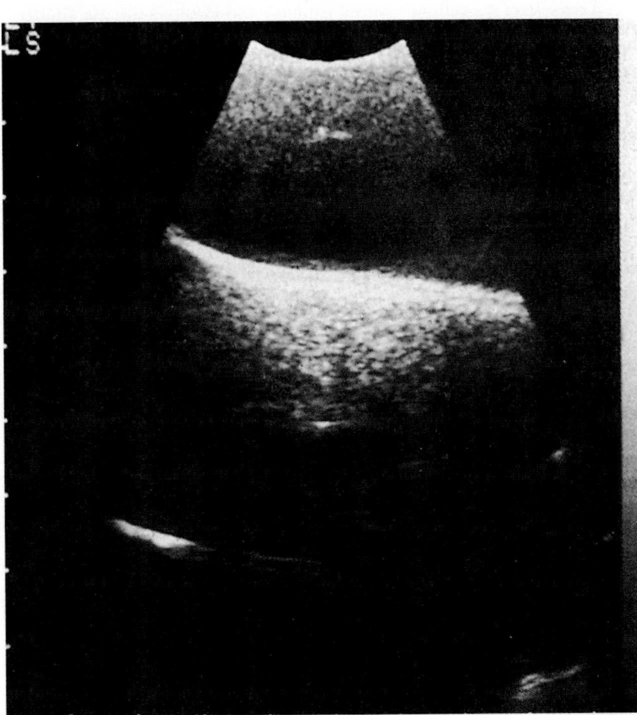

Fig. 42.2 Ultrasound scan of a chronically infected parotid gland demonstrating sialectasis.

Table 42.3 Management of acute bacterial sialadenitis

- Never perform sialography in acute phase
- Culture saliva from duct orifice
- Start broad-spectrum and penicillinase-resistant antibiotics immediately
- Refer for surgical drainage if gland is fluctuant
- Encourage fluids
- Sialography following resolution of symptoms to assess salivary function

and, in most cases following control of any acute symptoms with antibiotics, the gland itself must be removed. During the operation great care must be taken not to damage the mandibular branch of the facial nerve when making the incision, the lingual nerve when mobilising the gland and clamping the duct and the hypoglossal nerve when separating the gland from the floor of the submandibular triangle.

Recurrent sialadenitis of childhood

Recurrent sialadenitis of childhood exists as a distinct clinical entity but little is known regarding its aetiology and prognosis. It is characterised by the rapid swelling of usually one parotid gland accompanied by pain and difficulty in chewing as well as systemic symptoms such as fever and malaise. Although each episode of parotid swelling is normally unilateral the opposite side may be involved in subsequent episodes. Each episode of pain and swelling lasts for 3–7 days and is followed by a quiescent period of a few weeks to several months. Occasionally episodes are so frequent that the child loses a considerable amount of schooling. The onset is usually between 3 and 6 years although it has been reported in infants as young as 4 months. The diagnosis is based on the characteristic history and is confirmed by sialography which shows a very characteristic punctate sialectasis often likened to a snow storm against a dark night sky (Fig. 42.3).

Traditionally the episodes of parotitis have been treated with antibiotic and symptoms settle within 3–5 days on such a regime. Occasionally recurrent episodes are so frequent that prophylactic antibiotics are required for a period of months or years. Spontaneous resolution of symptoms seems to occur at puberty.

Specific 'infections' (*granulomatous sialadenitis*)

Mycobacterial infections

Tuberculosis and nontuberculous parotitis typically presents as a tumour-like swelling of the gland. Symptoms are usually minimal with little pain and no pyrexia. Often the diagnosis is not suspected and the mass is excised by formal parotidectomy.

Cat-scratch disease

Cat-scratch disease is caused by *Bartonella henselae*. It is a common disease in the USA but is not often seen in the UK. Children are usually affected. Symptoms follow a scratch by a cat when a small pustule forms at the site of the scratch. There is an associated lymphadenitis usually affecting the cervical nodes and mild pyrexia and encephalopathy with occasional transient cranial nerve palsies. The parotid glands are swollen in 3 per cent of cases. The condition is self-limiting and resolves without treatment.

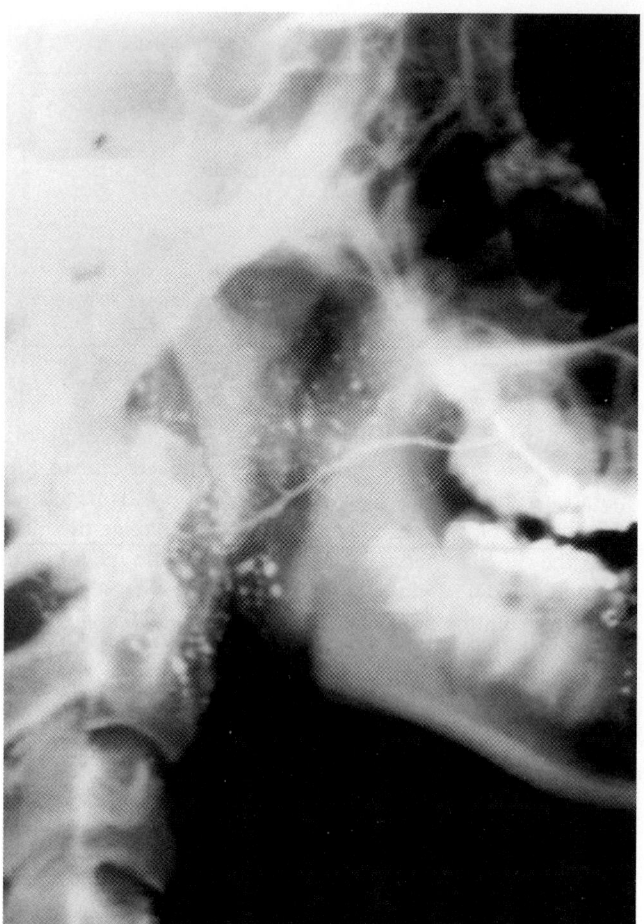

Fig. 42.3 Recurrent parotitis of childhood shows characteristic 'snowstorm' sialectasis on sialography.

Syphilis

Syphilis parotitis is now rare in the UK as the disease itself is uncommon. The glands can be involved in the acute early stages but are more often involved in tertiary syphilis with gumma formation, gland destruction and dense fibrosis.

Toxoplasmosis

Toxoplasmosis is due to the protozoan organism *Toxoplasma gondii*. In most cases infection is not recognised and is asymptomatic. When symptoms do occur the patient usually presents with lymphadenopathy and malaise sometimes accompanied by a headache and sore throat. The enlarged lymph nodes are rubbery and are not tender. On occasion the patient presents with isolated unilateral parotid swelling some weeks before the lymphadenopathy develops. In this situation a parotidectomy is often performed which leads to the diagnosis. Diagnosis is further confirmed by the detection of a positive Sabin–Feldman dye test on the serum. The disease follows a self-limiting course and resolves spontaneously after weeks or months. If symptoms are severe the patient is treated with a 3- or 4-week course of pyrimethamine and sulphadiazine.

Deep mycoses

Fungal infections of the salivary glands occur only in immunocompromised patients and are most commonly seen in human immunodeficiency virus (HIV)-positive patients. Salivary gland involvement is usually just one manifestation of a more generalised infection. The patient presents with a tumour-like swelling of the affected gland. Often there is extensive central necrosis. Fresh material is needed for culture and identification of the organism. Treatment is by appropriate systemic antifungal chemotherapy.

Sarcoid

Sarcoidosis has a predeliction for salivary tissue, but only rarely is salivary swelling the presenting feature. Parotid gland involvement occurs in 10 per cent of cases classically as part of Heerfordt's syndrome which comprises parotid swelling, anterior uveitis, facial palsy and fever. Xerostomia may be a prominent feature. A less usual presentation is with bilateral parotid and submandibular swelling which is one of the causes of Mikulicz' syndrome. In each of these presentations salivary involvement is widespread and representative histology can be obtained from a minor salivary gland biopsy. Rarely the patient will present with a localised tumour-like swelling in one parotid gland – the so-called sarcoid pseudotumour. In the absence of other signs or symptoms the diagnosis is only likely to be made following parotid surgery for a presumed neoplasm.

Wegener's granulomatosis

Although the typical presentation is chronic granulomatous ulceration and destruction in the nasopharynx or sometimes the oral cavity, Wegener's granulomatosis can involve the major salivary glands. Diagnosis is based on the histological finding of necrotising arteritis often associated with numerous giant cells and granulomas. Pulmonary and renal involvement is very common. Treatment is by cytotoxic chemotherapy such as cyclophosphamide or azathioprine. The prognosis is poor.

Granulomatous disease of minor salivary glands

Granulomatous cheilitis, Melkersson–Rosenthal syndrome (recurrent facial palsy/facial swelling/fissured tongue) and Crohn's disease all affect the minor salivary glands of the lips. Cheilitis glandularis is a rare disorder mainly of adult males in whom the lower lip becomes swollen and hard. The labial salivary glands become nodular and their orifices are inflamed and swollen.

Allergic sialadenitis

A variety of potential allergens causing acute parotid swelling has been identified. Some foods, drugs (most frequently chloramphenicol and tetracycline), metals such as nickel and pollens have been incriminated.

Radiation sialadenitis

Following the start of therapeutic irradiation when the parotid glands are within the radiation field the patient develops an acute parotitis usually after 24 hours. The glands are swollen and tender and there is a marked rise in salivary amylase and the salivary flow rate is reduced. The reaction is self-limiting and resolves after 2 or 3 days even though the radiotherapy continues. This reaction is quite distinct from the permanent radiation atrophy that occurs with therapeutic doses above 50 Gy, which develops progressively some weeks after the radiation has been completed.

Albert Bruce Sabin, b. 1906. Polish-born American microbiologist.
C.E. Heerfordt, 1871–1973. Danish ophthalmologist.
Johann von Mikulicz-Radecki, 1850–1905. Polish surgeon. Described his disease in 1892.

Human immunodeficiency virus-associated sialadenitis

Chronic parotitis in children is almost pathognomonic of HIV infection. In adults a sicca syndrome and lymphocytic infiltration of the salivary glands are more usual. The presentation of HIV-associated sialadenitis is very similar to classical Sjögren's syndrome. Dry mouth, dry eyes and swelling of the salivary glands together with lymphadenopathy suggest the diagnosis. Histologically the condition closely resembles Sjögren's syndrome and differentiation may be difficult. However, autoantibodies including antinuclear, rheumatoid factor, SS-A and SS-B are absent unless the patient coincidentally has a connective tissue disorder. Acquired immunodeficiency syndrome (AIDS)-associated lymphoma presenting as salivary gland swelling has also been described.

Another presentation of salivary gland disease in HIV-positive patients is multiple parotid cysts causing gross parotid swelling and significant facial disfigurement. On imaging with computerised tomography (CT) or magnetic resonance imaging (MRI) the parotids have the appearance of Swiss cheese with multiple large cystic lesions. The glands are not painful and there is no reduction in salivary flow rates. Surgery may be indicated to improve the appearance (Fig. 42.4).

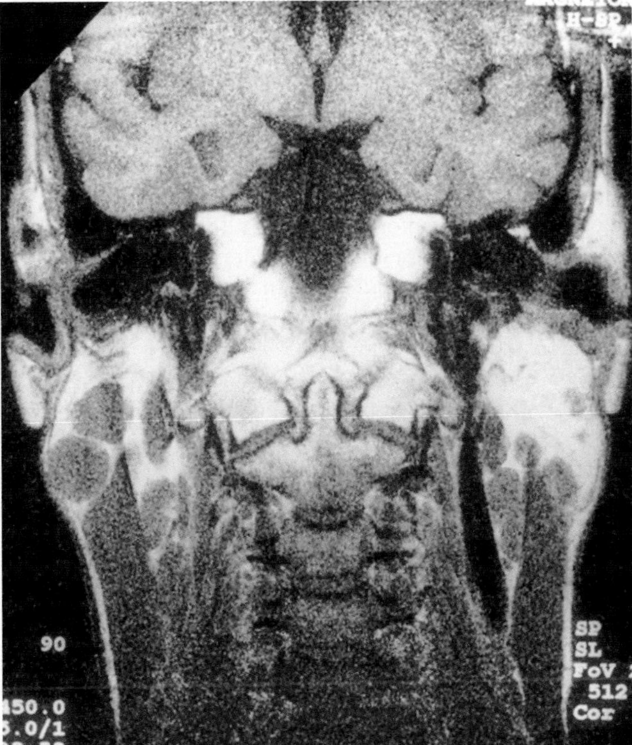

Fig. 42.4 Giant parotid cysts shown here bilaterally on this MRI are increasingly seen in long-term survivors of HIV infection.

Sialadenitis of minor salivary glands

Acute necrotising sialometaplasia is an unusual condition which was first described in 1973. It occurs only on the hard palate in the molar region in the vault of the palate midway between the midline and the gingival margin. It is only seen in heavy smokers. It has a characteristic appearance which resembles a carcinoma with central ulceration and raised erythematous margins. The ulcer may be as much as 3 cm in diameter. As it so closely resembles a carcinoma the diagnosis is often made on the basis of a surgical biopsy. The lesions are self-healing but often take 10–12 weeks to resolve (Fig. 42.5).

Obstruction and trauma (Table 42.4)

Papillary obstruction

Occasionally a rough upper molar tooth or an overextended denture flange will irritate the parotid papilla. If this is sufficient to cause ulceration with consequent inflammation and oedema this may obstruct salivary flow, particularly at meal times when the flow rate is increased. In this situation the patient has classical rapid-onset pain and swelling at meal times.

If the trauma to the parotid papilla continues there will be progressive scarring and fibrosis in the soft tissues and permanent stenosis of the papilla can occur. A papillotomy will be required. This is a simple procedure performed under local anaesthesia. A probe is inserted into the orifice of the papilla and with a scalpel blade the papilla is split open by incising down on to the probe. This lays open the papilla and divides the stenosis allowing free drainage of saliva.

Stone formation (sialolithiasis)

Eighty per cent of all salivary stones occur in the submandibular gland, 10 per cent occur in the parotid, 7 per

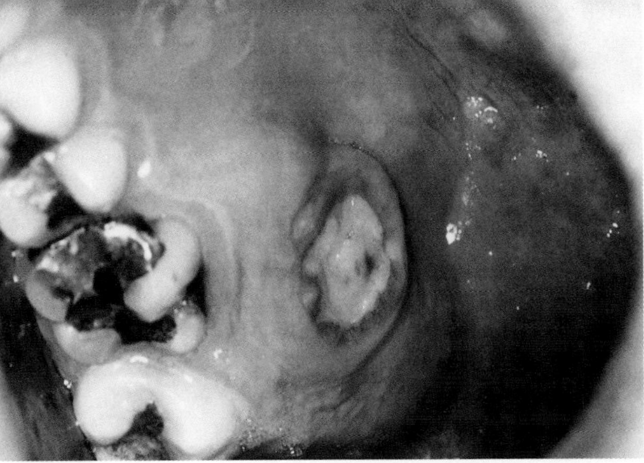

Fig. 42.5 Acute necrotising sialometaplasia occurs exclusively in tobacco smokers. The raised borders of the ulcer mimic carcinoma.

Ernst G. Melkersson, 1898–1932. Swedish physician.
Curt Rosenthal. Twentieth-century German psychiatrist.
Burrill Bernard Crohn, b. 1884. Gastroenterologist, Mount Sinai Hospital, New York, USA.

cent in the sublingual gland and the remainder occurs in the minor salivary glands. It is believed that the majority of stones occurs in the submandibular glands because their secretions contain mucus and the viscosity is higher. Eighty per cent of submandibular stones are radio-opaque and can be identified using plane radiographs. By contrast the majority of parotid stones are radiolucent and cannot be detected on plane radiography (Fig. 42.6).

The classical presentation is of acute pain and swelling at meal times. Onset is rapid – within a minute of starting the meal – and the swelling resolves over a period of about 1 hour after the meal is completed.

However, this classical picture only occurs when the stone causes almost complete obstruction often when it is impacted at the opening of Wharton's duct. More often the stone causes only partial obstruction and is lying either within the hilum of the gland or within the duct in the floor of the mouth. In this situation the patient may complain of occasional swelling often with minimal discomfort or of a chronically enlarged mass in the submandibular triangle with episodes of dull aching pain. This results from chronic bacterial infection arising in an obstructed gland with salivary stasis and poor emptying. Often a salivary stone is totally asymptomatic and is discovered coincidentally during radiography for other reasons. If a stone is identified on plane radiographs, no other investigation is necessary. Parotid stones often impact at the parotid papilla or alternatively take on a 'stag-horn' shape and form at the junction of the two main collecting ducts and the Stenson's duct (Fig. 42.7). If the stone is trapped at the duct papilla it can often be released by gently probing and carrying out dilatation of the papilla. It may be necessary to slit the duct in order to release the stone.

If the stone is lying in the submandibular duct in the floor of the mouth anterior to the point at which the duct crosses the lingual nerve (second molar region) the stone can be released by opening the duct longitudinally (Fig. 42.8). It is important to pass a large suture around the duct proximal to the stone so that during the operative procedure the stone cannot be displaced backwards in the duct. Once the stone has been released the wall of the duct should be sutured to the mucosa of the floor of the mouth to maintain an opening for the free drainage of saliva. No attempt should be made to repair the duct wall as this will lead to stricture formation. A parotid stone located at the confluence of the collecting ducts can be released surgically by raising a preauricular flap, exposing the parotid duct and again incising it longitudinally to release the stone.

Table 42.4 Obstruction and trauma

Papillary obstruction	Check biting Overextended denture flange
Stones	80% submandibular 80% radio-opaque Mostly calcium phosphate and calcium carbonate
Duct wall	Strictures secondary to calculus Direct trauma (e.g. floor of mouth) Parotid duct in masseteric hypertrophy Tumours may obstruct collecting ducts
Mucocele	Lower lip Buccal mucosa posteriorly Mucous extravasation cyst Mucous retention cyst Ranula

Obstruction in and around the duct wall

Scarring and fibrosis in the duct wall stricture formation will also result in obstruction to salivary flow. It often results as a complication of long-standing sialolithiasis but it may occur as a result of trauma particularly to the floor of the mouth. Subsequent healing and scarring can result in a stenosis of the duct. In patients with masseteric hypertrophy the parotid duct may be stretched around the anterior border of the muscle and this may cause obstruction of salivary flow at meal times.

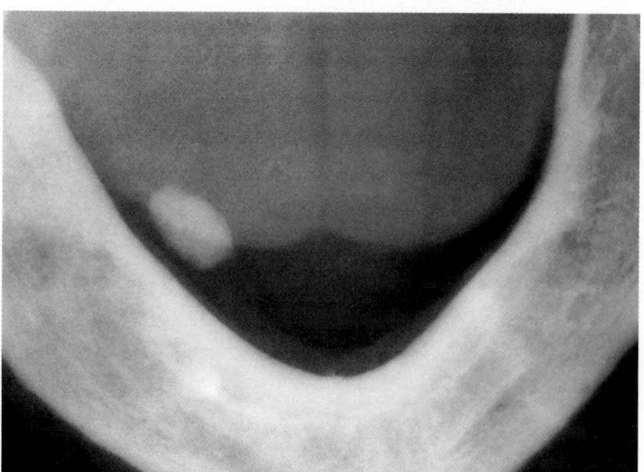

Fig. 42.6 Submandibular salivary stones are best demonstrated on anterior occlusal radiographs.

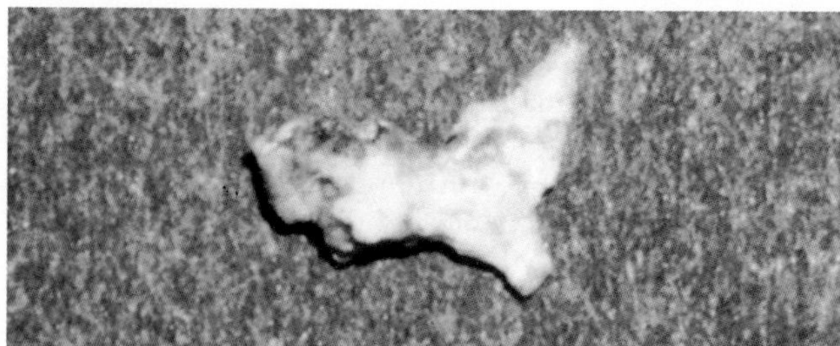

Fig. 42.7 This typical parotid calculus shows the stag-horn appearance of the stone which formed at the junction of the principal collecting ducts and the main duct.

Thomas Wharton, 1616–75. Physician, St Thomas' Hospital, London, England. Said to have remained on duty during the plague.

Niels Stensen, 1638–86. Professor of Anatomy, Copenhagen, Denmark. He abandoned medicine for the church on being appointed Bishop of Titiopolis. He is also regarded as 'The Father of Geology'.

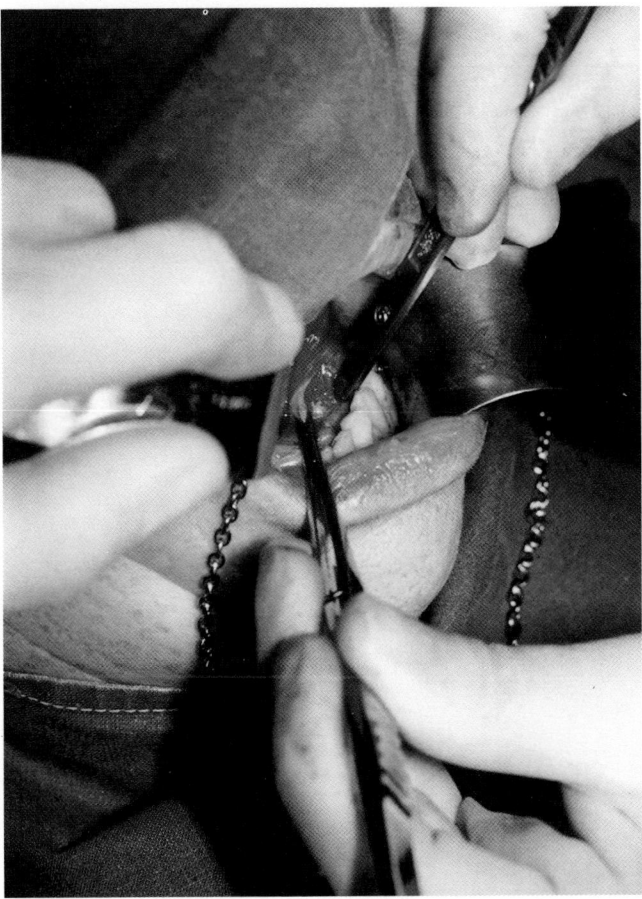

Fig. 42.8 Calculi arising in the anterior two-thirds of the submandibular duct – anterior to the lingual nerve – are readily removed by making a linear incision along the duct.

Mucoceles

Mucus retention cysts and mucus extravasation cysts arise in the minor salivary glands as a result of mechanical damage to the gland or its duct. The common sites are on the mucosal aspect of the lower lip particularly in patients with a deep overbite and in the buccal mucosa posteriorly where an upper wisdom tooth is erupting buccally. Typically the patient presents with a history of recurrent swellings that develop over days or weeks, rupture and then recur after a few weeks. The cysts rarely exceed 1 cm in diameter and are tense bluish sessile swellings. The treatment is not to the cyst itself but to the underlying minor gland which should be excised under local anaesthesia.

A ranula is no more than a large mucocele arising from the sublingual gland. Classically the ranula presents as a large tense bluish swelling in the floor of the mouth anteriorly often displacing the tongue (Fig. 42.9). However, the ranula may push its way though the midline mylohyoid dehiscence in the floor of the mouth and enter the submental space presenting as a midline swelling in the upper neck. This is the 'plunging ranula'. The treatment of a ranula is excision of the sublingual gland.

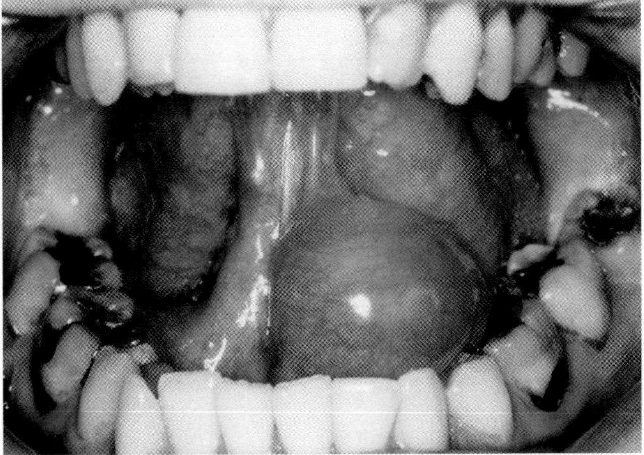

Fig. 42.9 This photograph shows a classical ranula arising from the left sublingual gland.

Salivary neoplasms (Table 42.5)

Salivary neoplasms comprise 1.2 per cent of all neoplastic disease.

Nearly all salivary neoplasms present as slowly growing masses which have often been present for several years. Even malignant salivary tumours usually grow slowly. Unfortunately pain is not a reliable indication of malignancy. Certainly if a malignant salivary neoplasm is invading a sensory nerve pain or paraesthesia can occur but frequently at surgery one sees a nerve macroscopically invaded by tumour but which has been functioning normally preoperatively. Furthermore benign tumours often present with pain and aching in the affected gland presumably due to capsular distension and possibly also due to an element of outflow obstruction. Therefore the only reliable clinical indication of malignancy is facial nerve palsy in the case of the parotid, induration and/or ulceration of the overlying skin or mucosa and regional lymphatic metastasis.

The investigation of salivary neoplasms

For parotid and submandibular tumours CT and MRI scanning are the most helpful imaging techniques (Figs 42.10 and 42.11). They will confirm that the mass being investigated is indeed intrinsic to the gland, they accurately image the borders of the tumour and show whether it is well circumscribed and benign or diffuse, invasive and malignant. In addition they show the relationship of the tumour to other anatomic structures and help with the planning of subsequent surgery.

Open surgical biopsy of intrinsic neoplasms of the major glands is absolutely contraindicated. At least 75 per cent of all parotid tumours and more than 50 per cent of all submandibular gland tumours will prove to be benign pleomorphic adenomas. This tumour which is only poorly encapsulated is very tense and if an incision is made into it the contents of the tumour burst into the surrounding tissue planes and it is impossible to eradicate the microscopic

Table 42.5 Salivary tumours – WHO Classification (1991–simplified)

1. Adenomas	Pleomorphic adenoma	Any age M:F 1:1 75% of all parotid tumours 50% of all submandibular tumours
	Warthin tumour	Over 60 years M:F 4:1 15% of parotid tumours (only occurs in parotid)
2. Carcinomas	Acinic cell carcinoma	Often low grade
	Mucoepidermoid carcinoma	Often low grade More common in USA
	Adenoid cystic carcinoma	Invariably fatal but good 5- and 10-year survival Perineural spread Pulmonary metastases
	Adenocarcinoma Squamous cell carcinoma Undifferentiated carcinoma	All have a poor prognosis
	Carcinoma in pleiomorphic adenoma	Very rare 25% 5-year survival
3. Nonepithelial tumours	Haemangioma	Mostly infants Usually parotid Frequent spontaneous regression
	Lymphangioma Neurofibroma Neurilemoma	Any gland affected
4. Malignant lymphoma		
5. Unclassified and allied conditions		

spillage of tumour cells. If this happens the patient will develop multiple local tumour recurrences over many years unless they are subjected to radical postoperative radiotherapy, which is best avoided in the management of benign disease. Clearly if there is skin infiltration or ulceration an open biopsy is essential to establish a preoperative diagnosis upon which to plan surgery. For tumours of the minor salivary glands particularly in the palate there is a much higher chance of the tumour being malignant and as it is not necessary to open up other tissue planes to gain access to the tumour as open incisional biopsy is important.

Fine needle aspiration (FNA) biopsy is a safe alternative to open biopsy of a major gland. Evidence suggests that provided the needle gauge does not exceed 18 G there is no risk of seeding viable tumour cells. Although advocates of this technique claim high accuracy and specificity, there is inevitably a high risk of sampling error.

Epithelial tumours

Seventy-five per cent of all salivary epithelial tumours arise in the parotid glands and, of these, only 15 per cent are malignant. Just over 10 per cent occur in the submandibular glands and, of these, approximately one-third are malignant. About 15 per cent of tumours occur in the minor salivary glands and nearly half of these will be malignant. Tumours arising in the sublingual glands are rare (0.3 per cent) but nearly all of them will be malignant.

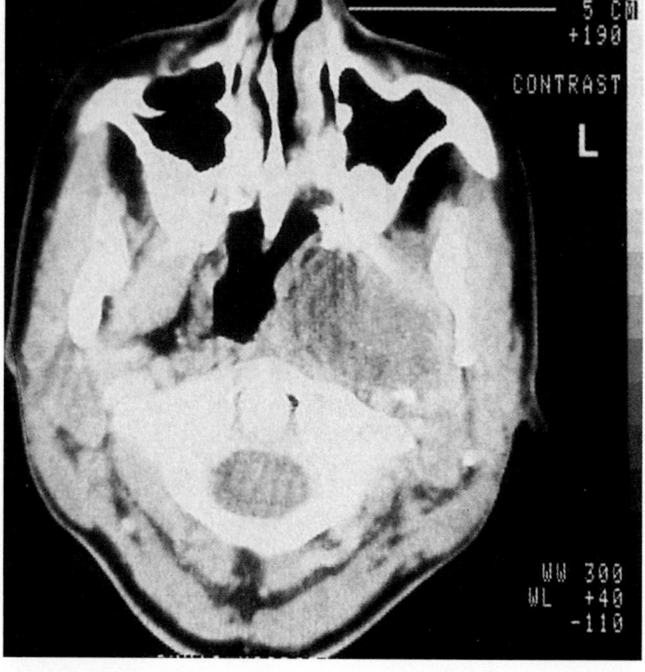

Fig. 42.10 CT scan of a deep lobe parotid tumour showing the attenuated layer of parapharyngeal fat.

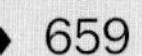

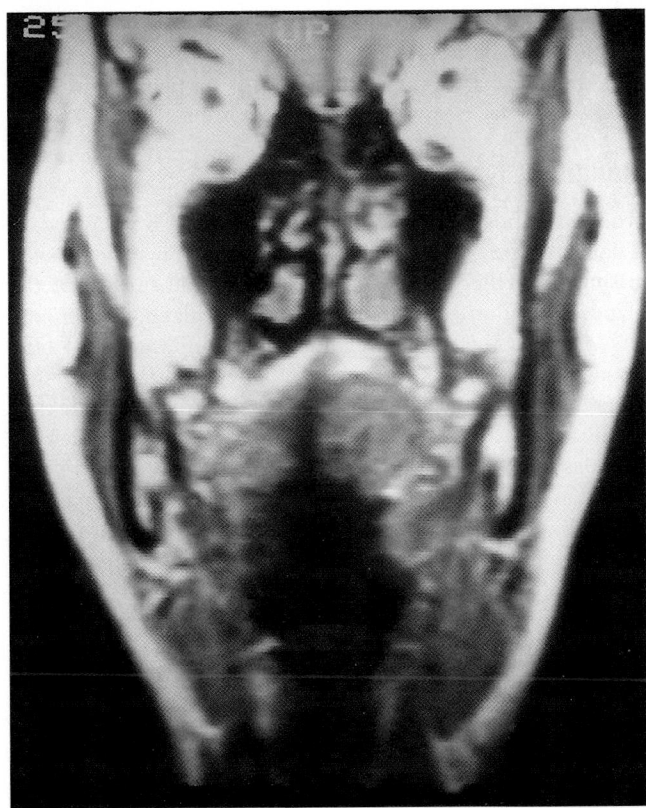

Fig. 42.11 This MRI scan shows a large adenoid-cystic carcinoma arising at the junction of the hard and soft palate.

Both benign tumours – adenomas – and malignant tumours – carcinomas – occur.

Adenomas

Of the variety of benign adenomas that has been described only two – the pleomorphic adenoma and Warthin's tumour – arise with any frequency.

The pleomorphic adenoma occurs at any age (mean 42 years) and has an equal sex incidence. It accounts for at least 75 per cent of parotid tumours and more than 50 per cent of submandibular tumours. It accounts for rather less than 50 per cent of minor gland tumours. Clinically the tumour has the texture of cartilage and has an irregular and bosselated surface. In the palate, the overlying mucosa is rarely ulcerated. Very rarely after a number of years the tumour may undergo malignant change and for this reason all patients presenting with pleomorphic adenomas should be advised to undergo surgical removal of the tumour (Fig. 42.12).

The Warthin's tumour occurs only in the parotid gland where it accounts for approximately 15 per cent of all neoplasms. It is a disease of the elderly with a mean age of presentation of 60 years. Historically it had a male:female ratio of 4:1 but it is now becoming increasingly common in females. Recent evidence suggests that this tumour is related to cigarette smoking. It is also unusual in that in 10 per cent of cases it arises either bilaterally or is multicentric in the one gland. It does not undergo malignant change.

Carcinomas

The acinic cell carcinoma and the mucoepidermoid carcinoma, although undoubtedly malignant tumours with a potential for local invasion and metastatic spread, are frequently very low grade histologically and do not require the radical treatment needed for more aggressive tumours. Together they account for only 5 per cent of all tumours at any site. The mucoepidermoid tumour is much more common in the USA where it forms 10 per cent of all salivary neoplasms.

The adenoid cystic carcinoma, adenocarcinoma, squamous cell carcinoma and undifferentiated carcinoma are all aggressive malignant tumours that carry a poor prognosis regardless of treatment. The adenoid cystic carcinoma is characterised by relentless perineural spread along the cranial nerves and into the brain. However, it grows extremely slowly and

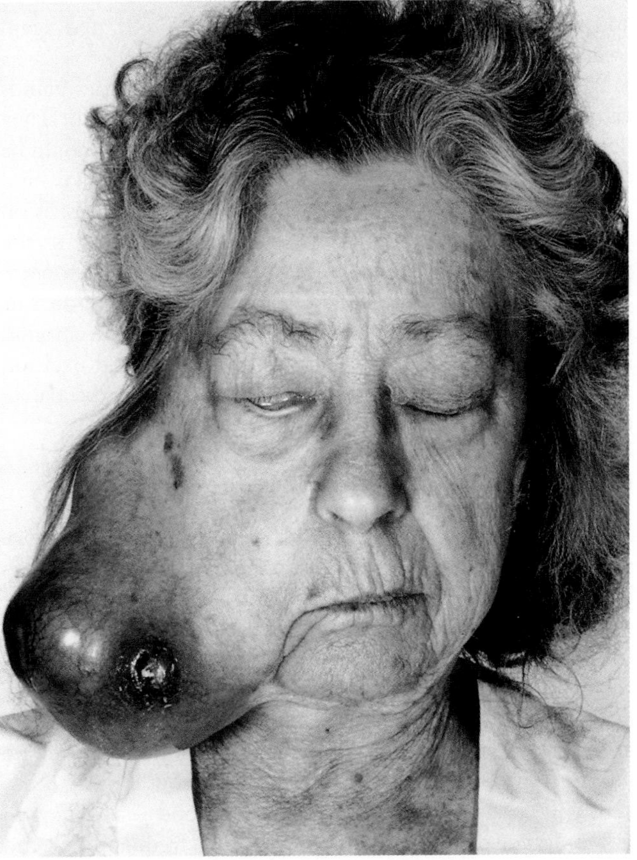

Fig. 42.12 This giant pleomorphic adenoma has been present for many years. It has recently undergone more rapid growth and is ulcerating, indicating malignant degeneration.

Alfred Scott Warthin, 1866–1931. Professor of Pathology, University of Michigan, Ann Arbor, USA.

although inevitably fatal the 5- and 10-year survival figures are 70 per cent and 40 per cent, respectively. It is also unusual in having a predilection for distant metastasis to the lungs where it produces often multiple cannon ball tumours which remain symptomless for many years. The other carcinomas mentioned above have 5-year survival figures of around 25–35 per cent.

Management of epithelial tumours

Both benign and malignant tumours arising in the parotid or submandibular glands are treated surgically by excision with surgical clearance. In the parotid gland this is by either superficial or total parotidectomy according to the location of the tumour. Unless the patient presents with facial nerve palsy (indicating a malignant tumour) the facial nerve is always preserved. In the submandibular gland treatment is always by excision of the gland. If when a definitive pathological diagnosis is received the tumour is malignant then the patient should receive radical postoperative radiotherapy. In those cases when the tumour involves skin or other adjacent structures or where there is lymphatic metastasis the patient should undergo radical excision, including a neck dissection and sacrificing any structures invaded by tumour, and again treated with postoperative radiotherapy.

Pleomorphic adenomas arising in the minor salivary glands can be treated by local excision with a 5-mm margin. They do not invade periosteum and so in the palate they should be excised subperiosteally. Mucoepidermoid carcinomas and acinic cell carcinomas require rather more radical excision with a 10-mm margin and, when they are situated in the palate, palatal fenestration should be undertaken. Postoperative radiotherapy is only indicated for high-grade tumours or if the margins are not clear. For the remaining carcinomas arising in the minor salivary glands radical surgical excision and postoperative radiotherapy are indicated. In the palate this will be by maxillectomy.

Nonepithelial tumours

A variety of nonepithelial tumours can arise in the salivary glands. Haemangiomas and lymphangiomas (cystic hygromas) occur in childhood. Haemangiomas occur mostly in the parotid and appear shortly after birth and grow progressively for several months. The majority undergoes spontaneous regression by 2 years of age. Females are more frequently affected. Lymphangiomas are less common. They may affect any of the salivary glands. They form sponge-like multicystic lesions. Fifty per cent are manifest by 12 months and 90 per cent will be evident by the end of the second year. They do not undergo spontaneous involution. They frequently extend into the neck and mediastinum, and can undergo dramatically rapid growth causing respiratory obstruction. Treatment is by complete surgical excision but this may be technically very difficult.

Neurofibromas and neurilemmomas are the commonest nonepithelial tumours arising in adults. Clinically they are not distinguishable from other salivary tumours and are only diagnosed following surgery for a presumed epithelial tumour. Lipomas occur in the parotids particularly in adult males. They are treated by surgical excision.

Malignant lymphomas

True extranodal lymphoma arising in the salivary glands – usually the parotids – is rare. More common is lymphoma arising from the lymph nodes either on the surface of the glands or within the parenchyma of the gland. Lymphoma also arises in the salivary glands, as a complication of HIV disease, and also in benign lymphoepithelial lesion and Sjögren's syndrome. The peak incidence for nonHodgkin's lymphoma is the sixth and seventh decades and females are twice as likely as males to be affected.

Salivary gland lymphomas usually present as firm painless swellings and more than 90 per cent occur in the parotids. If the lymphoma is confined to the parotid, treatment is by parotidectomy with postoperative radiotherapy. If there is evidence of spread beyond the salivary gland, treatment is by polychemotherapy according to the accepted protocols based on histological characterisation.

Unclassified and allied conditions

Sialosis is an uncommon noninflammatory cause of salivary swelling usually affecting the parotid glands symmetrically. It is usually associated with metabolic and endocrine conditions such as alcohol abuse, diabetes mellitus, pregnancy, malnutrition and some drugs (usually sympathomimetics). It usually affects middle-aged and elderly adults who present with bilateral soft parotid swellings. Biopsy of the glands reveals extensive fatty replacement but otherwise normal tissues. No treatment is known to be effective but sometimes parotidectomy is required to correct the disfigurement.

Necrotising sialometaplasia, benign lymphoepithelial lesion, salivary duct cysts, Kuttner tumour and cystic lymphoid hyperplasia of HIV disease can all mimic salivary gland neoplasia. Similarly, branchial cysts and dermoids can present diagnostic confusion on occasion. As has already been discussed both sarcoid and toxoplasmosis can present as parotid pseudotumours.

Degenerative conditions (Table 42.6)

Sjögren's syndrome

Sjögren's syndrome is an autoimmune condition causing progressive destruction of the salivary and lachrymal glands. In 1933 Sjögren first described the association of keratoconjunctivitis sicca (dry eyes) and xerostomia (dry mouth). Shortly thereafter he noted that these symptoms frequently

---

Thomas Hodgkin, 1798–1866. British physician.

occurred in patients with rheumatoid arthritis (RA). It has since been realised that Sjögren's syndrome can occur in association with any connective tissue disorder. Indeed the association is very much commoner in many connective tissue disorders than it is with rheumatoid arthritis. Only 15 per cent of patients with RA develop Sjögren's syndrome whereas 30 per cent of patients with systemic lupus erythematosis and nearly all patients with primary biliary cirrhosis do so. This combination of dry eyes, dry mouth and a connective tissue disorder – most often RA as this is by far the most frequent connective tissue disorder – is called secondary Sjögren's syndrome. The same combination of dry eyes and dry mouth but without association with a connective tissue disorder is known as Primary Sjögren's syndrome. Primary Sjögren's syndrome also differs from secondary Sjögren's syndrome by virtue of more severe xerostomia and xerophthalmia, more widespread dysfunction of other exocrine glands, a higher incidence of developing lymphoma and a different antibody profile.

Females are affected more often than males in the ratio of 10:1. Typically they are middle aged. The presenting complaint is usually of the underlying connective tissue disorder and only later does the patient become aware of a gritty feeling in the eyes due to dry eyes or of dry mouth. Occasionally there is enlargement of the parotid glands bilaterally and even more rarely the enlarged parotids are painful (Fig. 42.13). Superinfection of the mouth with *Candida albicans* is frequent. Less frequently the patient develops bacterial sialadenitis due to ascending infection from the mouth. The condition does not invariably progress to total xerostomia and for any individual patient it is not possible to predict the outcome. The characteristic features of the condition are progressive lymphocytic infiltration, acinar destruction and proliferation of duct epithelium of all salivary and lachrymal tissue.

The diagnosis is often based on the characteristic history. No laboratory investigation is pathognomonic of either primary or secondary Sjögren's syndrome. However, the following investigations are usually undertaken:

1. Sialography reveals the progressive damage from punctate sialectasis to total parenchymal destruction leaving no more than a grossly dilated duct (Fig. 42.14).
2. Labial salivary gland biopsy can be misleading particularly if only one minor gland is harvested. The characteristic lymphocytic infiltration is focal and a single gland may not show the changes. A minimum of three glands should be submitted to the pathologist.
3. Estimation of salivary flow may be unhelpful as the normal variation in flow rates makes the interpretation of the results difficult.
4. Vital staining of the cornea with rose bengal and examination of the cornea with a slit-lamp is a very sensitive assessment of a dry eye.
5. Autoantibody screen. See Table 42.7.
6. Blood tests usually show a moderately raised erythrocyte sedimentation rate (ESR) and a mild microcytic anaemia (the anaemia of chronic disease).

The management of Sjögren's syndrome must be symptomatic. No known treatment modifies or reverses the xerostomia and keratoconjunctivitis sicca. Artificial tears are essential to protect the cornea. For the dry mouth various artificial saliva preparations are available but often the patient prefers to use frequent drinks and learns to carry a bottle of water with them at all times. If patients are to use

Table 42.6 Degenerative conditions

Primary Sjögren's	More severe xerostomia Widespread exocrine gland dysfunction No underlying connective tissue disorder
Secondary Sjögren's	F:M 10:1 Middle aged Rheumatoid arthritis is commonest underlying connective tissue disorder
Benign lymphoepithelial disorder	Not benign! 20% develop lymphoma Diffuse parotid swelling 20% bilateral

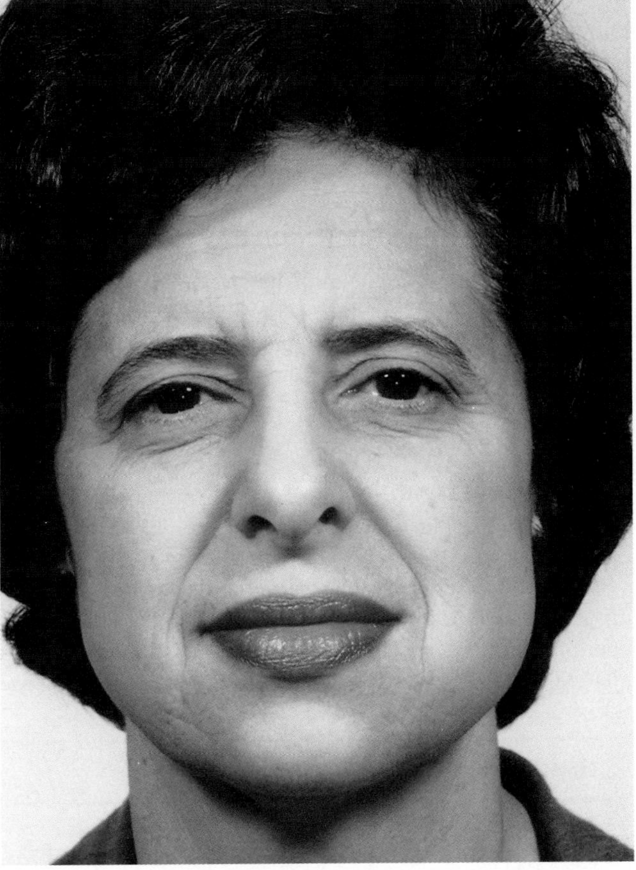

Fig. 42.13 On occasion, Sjögren's syndrome presents with parotid gland enlargement as seen in this 47-year-old female.

Henrik Samuel Sjögren, b. 1899. Stockholm ophthalmologist.

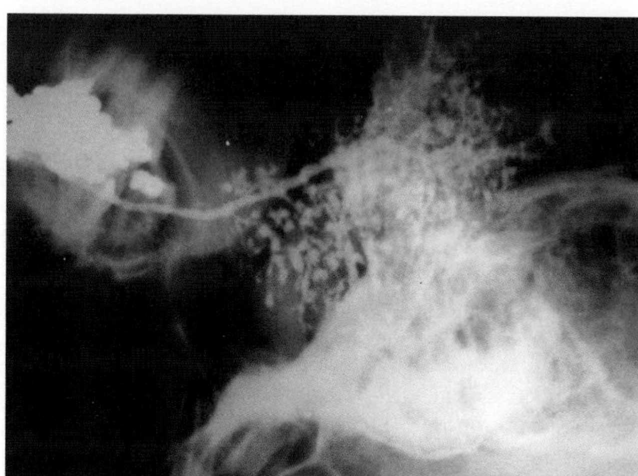

Fig. 42.14 Sialographic changes in Sjögren's syndrome shows punctate (cavitatory) sialectasis.

saliva substitutes it is important that, if they are dentate, the product should not have a low pH and should contain fluoride as rampant dental caries are a frequent complication. There is also increased incidence of developing lymphoma in patients with Sjögren's syndrome. The risk is highest in those with primary Sjögren's syndrome. Monocytoid B-cell lymphoma is the usual complication. Its onset is often heralded by immunological changes (falling immunoglobulin levels, falling titre of rheumatoid factor, rising B_2-microglobulin titre, rising serum macroglobulin titre and the appearance of monoclonal light chains in the serum and urine), lymphadenopathy and weight loss.

'Benign' lymphoepithelial lesion

The term 'benign lymphoepithelial lesion' was coined by Godwin in 1952. Use of the word 'benign' to describe the lesion is misleading as approximately 20 per cent of patients with benign lymhoepithelial lesion or Sjögren's syndrome ultimately develop lymphoma. Histologically it is not possible to distinguish benign epithelial lesions from Sjögren's syndrome. Both are characterised by lymphocytic infiltration, acinar atrophy and ductal epithelial proliferation. Indeed they may well be manifestations of the same condition.

Clinically benign lymphoepithelial lesion presents as diffuse swelling of the parotid. The swelling is firm and often painful. In 20 per cent of cases the parotid swelling is bilateral. Eighty per cent of patients are female and most are over 50 years old at presentation. Often there is an associated connective tissue disorder and the risk of developing lymphoma is particularly high in those with rheumatoid arthritis. Most patients will be treated by parotidectomy in order to establish the diagnosis but if any parotid remnants are left, the swelling may recur again with the risk of lymphomatous change. Prolonged follow-up is essential.

Table 42.7 Autoantibodies in Sjögren's syndrome

Autoantibody	Primary	Secondary
Salivary duct ab	10–36%	67–70%
Rhesus factor	50%	90%
SS-A antibody	5–10%	50–80%
SS-B antibody	50–75%	2–5%

Mikulicz' syndrome

In 1888 Mikulicz described benign, asymptomatic, symmetrical enlargement of the lacrimal and salivary glands. His original publication described a series of patients who clearly had a variety of different conditions. Benign lymphoepithelial lesion, Sjögren's syndrome, lymphoma, lymphocytic leukaemia, sarcoid and sialosis can all present in this way. The term Mikulicz' syndrome is not helpful and should not be used (Fig. 42.15).

Xerostomia

A complaint of dry mouth is common. It seems to be particularly frequent in postmenopausal women who also complain of a burning tongue or mouth. Normal salivary flow decreases with age in both men and women. The situation is further confused as patients with Sjögren's syndrome are frequently unaware of having a dry mouth and patients who complain of dry mouth frequently have normal salivary flow rates. The most common causes of xerostomia in order of frequency are:

- chronic anxiety states and depression;
- dehydration;
- drugs – many drugs have been implicated in causing xerostomia as an undesirable side effect (Table 42.8);
- salivary gland diseases as described earlier.

Xerostomia can be difficult to treat. Treatment is aimed at the relief of symptoms and the avoidance or control of complications. Frequent sips of water help most patients. Artificial salivas are not well accepted but their lubricant properties may be particularly useful at meal times. Cholinergic drugs such as pilocarpine can be tried but their side effects – diarrhoea and pupillary dilatation – often outweigh any benefit.

Rampant caries and destructive periodontal disease are major complications due to oral infection. Meticulous oral hygiene and the weekly use of topical fluoride are essential. There is a high incidence of oral candidosis and antifungal drugs are necessary.

Sialorrhoea (Table 42.9)

Some drugs and painful lesions in the mouth increase salivary flow rates. In normal health this is rarely noticed as the excess saliva is swallowed spontaneously. 'False ptyalism' is more common and is a well-recognised delusional symptom or

Johannes von Mikulicz, 1850–1905. Polish surgeon.

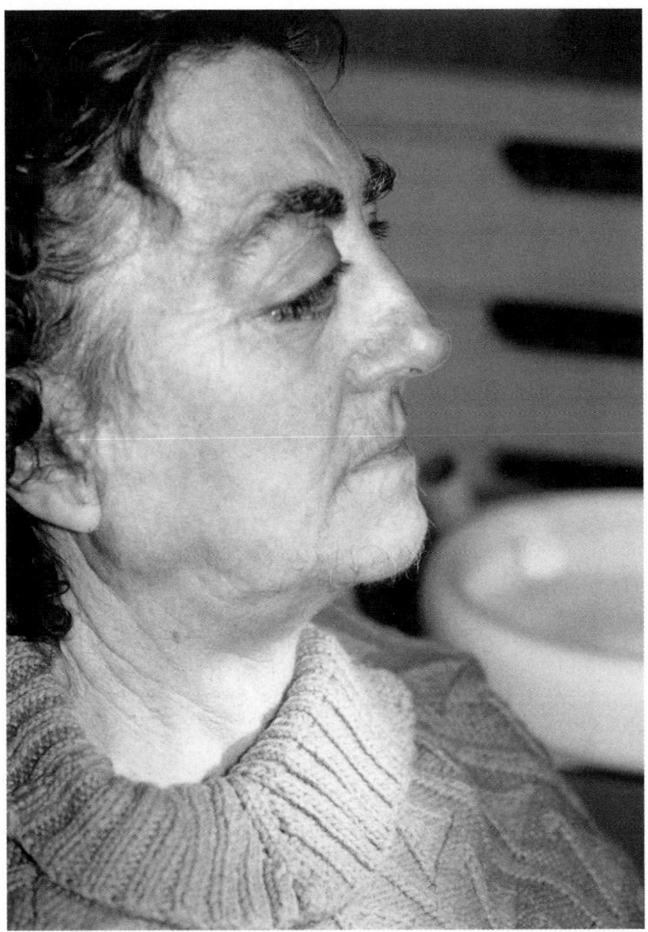

Fig. 42.15 This photograph of a patient with lymphoma presenting with Mikulicz' syndrome shows enlargement of the lachrymal gland with proptosis and enlargement of the parotid and submandibular glands. These changes were bilateral.

occurs due to faulty neuromuscular control leading to drooling despite normal saliva production. Uncontrollable drooling is usually treated surgically. As the submandibular gland contributes most resting saliva, attention is directed at these glands bilaterally. The submandibular ducts can be mobilised and repositioned in the base of the anterior pillars of the fauces. Alternatively the two glands may be excised.

Table 42.8 Drugs which cause xerostomia

Antimuscarinic drugs	Atropine and analogues Tricyclic antidepressants Monoamine oxidase inhibitors Phenothiazines and related drugs Benzhexol and related drugs Antihistamines Ganglion blockers Antiemetics
Sympathomimetic drugs	Ephidrine/phenylpropylamine Isoprenaline and related bronchodilators Amphetamines

Table 42.9 Causes of sialorrhoea

Local	Painful oral ulcers Oral wounds (extractions/surgery) Dentures/appliances
Systemic	Nausea Reflux oesophagitis
Toxic	Iodine Heavy metal poisoning
False ptyalism	Psychogenic Bell's palsy Parkinson's disease Stroke Cerebral palsy

Surgery of salivary gland disease

The most common indication for removal of the sublingual salivary gland is in the management of a ranula, which is a mucous extravasation/retention cyst of the gland. Neoplasms of the sublingual gland occur only rarely but nearly all tumours at this site will be malignant. In this situation surgery is the same as that for any other malignancy in the floor of the mouth – resection with a clear margin often involving the mandible and when necessary *en bloc* with a neck dissection. Before an incision is made it is helpful to infiltrate the floor of the mouth with a local anaesthetic containing a vasoconstrictor. For simple excision of the sublingual gland, a linear incision is made in the floor of the mouth parallel to and just lateral to the submandibular duct, with care taken not to extend the incision more posteriorly than the first molar tooth so as to avoid damage to the lingual nerve (Fig. 42.16). The incision should open the cavity of the ranula and allow the mucinous contents to be aspirated. The submandibular duct is now carefully identified and retracted medially. Stay sutures passed through the margins of the mucosa are helpful to aid retraction. Using blunt dissection with scissors the lingual nerve is identified. The sublingual gland which lies adjacent to the inner cortex of the mandible is then mobilised and its multiple ducts which drain into the submandibular duct are divided carefully in order not to damage the duct itself. The anterolateral part of the sublingual gland may be attached to the periosteum of the mandible by fibrous tissue and this must be divided carefully. Following removal of the gland, the mucosa of the floor of the mouth is loosely closed with two or three plain gut sutures. When sublingual gland excision is necessary for a tumour, it should be removed with a wide margin including a rim resection of the mandible (Fig. 42.17).

Sir Charles Bell, 1774–1842. Scottish physician, The Middlesex Hospital, London, England.
James Parkinson, 1755–1824. English physician.

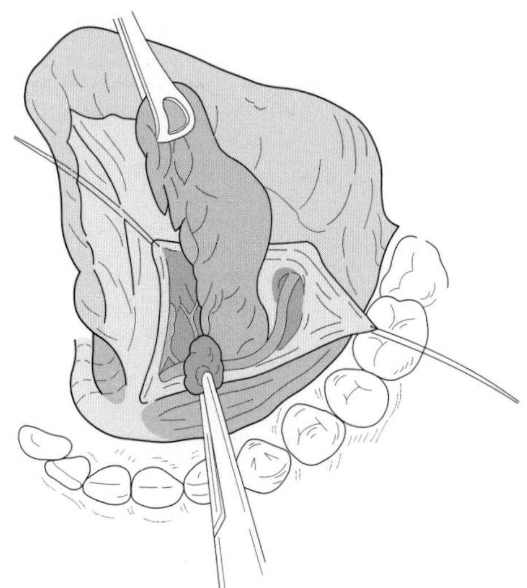

Fig. 42.16 The sublingual gland is removed through an incision in the floor of the mouth just lateral to the submandibular duct.

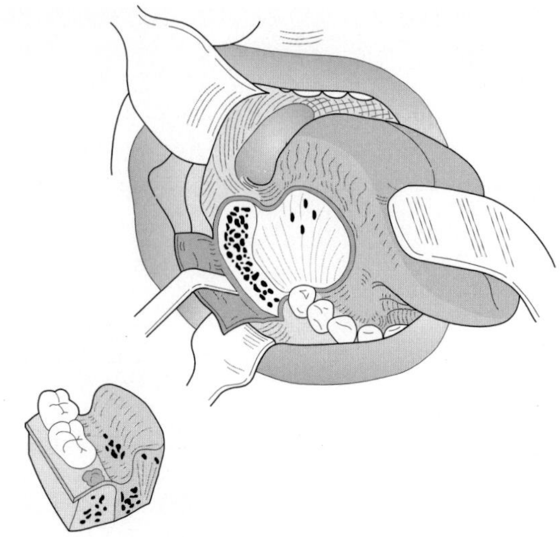

Fig. 42.17 Tumours arising in the sublingual gland are nearly always malignant and require excision with clear margins often including the adjacent bone.

Complications

Damage to the lingual nerve posteriorly or the submandibular duct medially is avoided by careful surgical technique. Meticulous haemostasis is required to avoid a postoperative haematoma in the floor of the mouth.

Submandibular gland excision

The patient is positioned supine on the operating table with moderate neck extension and the chin rotated to the opposite side. It is helpful to have head-up tilt on the operating table as this reduces venous engorgement. Following routine skin preparation and draping the incision is mapped out. The line should run within a skin crease in the neck at least 3 cm below the lower border of the mandible in order to avoid risk of damaging the mandibular branch of the facial nerve as it loops down below the lower border of the mandible. The incision should be approximately 7 cm long. The incision line is then infiltrated with conventional dental local anaesthetic solution containing 2 per cent lignocaine and 1:80 000 adrenaline. This results in some vasoconstriction which limits capillary ooze and helps to define tissue planes.

The incision is made with either a number 15 blade or a fine cutting diathermy whilst the assistant puts tension across the incision line. The incision is made directly down to platysma. The subcutaneous fat is stripped with firm pressure and a swab from the underlying muscle for approximately 1 cm on each side of the incision as this facilitates a layered closure later. The underlying platysma is then incised to the full extent of the skin incision again with either a blade or cutting diathermy. The assistant can now retract the wound margins using 'cat paws' or Allis forceps applied to the cut edge of the platysma muscle (never the skin edges!).

The underlying investing layer of the deep cervical fascia is next divided, preferably with scissors, after the fascia is first tented outwards with toothed forceps. Often the fascia consists of a series of separate laminae like an onion skin but occasionally it is composed of a single thicker sheet. Again the fascia should be divided along the full length of the incision to avoid the operative field becoming ever smaller.

Posteriorly, the fascial incision approaches the angular tract where the deep cervical fascia splits to form the investing layer that has just been incised and the deeper layer that forms the floor of the submandibular triangle containing the submandibular gland.

The mandibular branch of the facial nerve normally runs on the deep aspect of the investing layer of fascia although occasionally it lies between the platysma and the fascia. Great care must be taken to protect the mandibular branch.

The anterior facial vein which lies in the connective tissue overlying the submandibular gland is clamped, divided and tied. The loose connective tissue is separated with scissors to expose the submandibular gland. The dissection from now on continues on the capsular surface of the gland. For chronically infected glands there is frequently extensive fibrosis, and care and patience are required to maintain this plane. For all tumours contained within the submandibular gland capsule, this plane is safe as it forms an effective barrier. For malignant tumours that have infiltrated beyond the capsule, a full submandibular clearance, usually as part of a neck dissection, and often including the periosteum of the lower and inner aspect of the mandible, is needed.

The anterior pole of the superficial lobe of the submandibular gland is first mobilised and retracted upwards with Allis forceps (Fig. 42.18). This reveals the posterior belly of the digastric muscle which is then gently retracted downwards with a small Langenbeck retractor. This exposes the facial artery which emerges from behind the stylohyoid muscle and passes upwards and forwards to enter the deep surface of the

Oscar Huntington Allis, 1836–1921. American surgeon.

submandibular gland. The artery is then clamped, divided and tied. Great care must be taken to secure the proximal ligature. As the vessel is divided it retracts out of sight and, if the ligature slips, the bleeding end of the vessel can be very difficult to identify.

The course of the facial artery is variable. Often it deeply penetrates the substance of the gland to emerge again at its upper border. Sometimes the artery lies in a groove in the deep aspect of the gland. The dissection in the plane of the submandibular gland capsule continues to mobilise the anterior pole of the superficial lobe of the gland, which is then gently retracted posteriorly. During this dissection a number of small arteries and veins will be identified entering the gland. These should be carefully clamped, divided and tied or diathermised according to their size. As the dissection continues posteriorly along the lower border of the mandible, the facial artery and anterior facial vein are encountered as they hook around the mandible. The vessels are again clamped, divided and ligated at this point.

At this stage in the operation, the anterior pole of the superficial lobe of the gland can be retracted posteriorly to reveal the groove between the superficial and deep lobes of the submandibular gland. The posterior border of the mylohyoid muscle lies within this groove. It is gently freed with scissors and then retracted forwards with a Langenbeck retractor. The deep lobe of the submandibular gland can now be mobilised either with a finger or by opening the blades of the scissors applied to the surface of the gland. On the deep aspect of the deep lobe, one or two small veins may be encountered running from the gland through the underlying hyoglossus into the lingual veins. If these veins are not tied or adequately diathermised, troublesome bleeding may be encountered.

The submandibular salivary gland can now be pulled downwards revealing the V-shaped lingual nerve. The apex of the V is the point at which parasympathetic secretomotor fibres tether the lingual nerve to the salivary gland. It is very important to identify carefully the V of the lingual nerve and its parasympathetic fibres as the latter must be transected to free the gland (Fig. 42.19). As these fibres are cut, the lingual nerve springs forwards. Finally the submandibular duct is clamped, divided and tied as far forward as possible with just enough left to drain the major sublingual gland which empties into the duct. A thin layer of loose connective tissue remains in the gland bed overlying the hypoglossal nerve.

The wound is inspected for any bleeding points, a vacuum drain inserted and the wound closed in layers using a subcuticular suture to close the skin. The wound edges are reinforced with skin closure tapes.

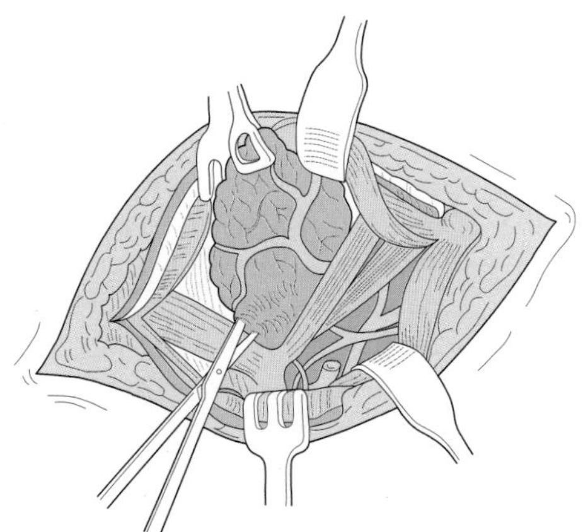

Fig. 42.18 During the excision of the submandibular gland, the anterior pole of the superficial lobe is mobilised and retracted upwards.

Berhard von Langenbeck, 1810–87. German surgeon.

Complications

Three cranial nerves are at risk during removal of the submandibular salivary gland – the mandibular branch of the facial nerve, the lingual nerve (a branch of the third division of the trigeminal nerve) and the hypoglossal nerve.

When chronic infection and subsequent fibrosis have occurred, it is sometimes difficult to identify the lingual nerve and the deep aspect of the deep lobe may be attached to the hypoglossal nerve. At these stages of the operation, the surgeon must be convinced that these structures have been identified before using any sharp dissection.

Meticulous haemostasis is required throughout the operation as many of the vessels entering and leaving the submandibular gland are only apparent when the gland is under traction and as soon as they are divided the vessels retract into the adjacent muscle planes.

Parotidectomy

Treatment of parotid tumours is by superficial parotidectomy for all benign tumours in the superficial lobe and total parotidectomy for all benign deep lobe and dumb-bell tumours. Such tumours including deep lobe tumours should never be approached from the pharyngeal aspect. The facial nerve is preserved in all cases.

The prognosis for malignant parotid tumours is poor. There is little evidence that radical parotidectomy, which includes sacrificing the entire facial nerve, adds significantly

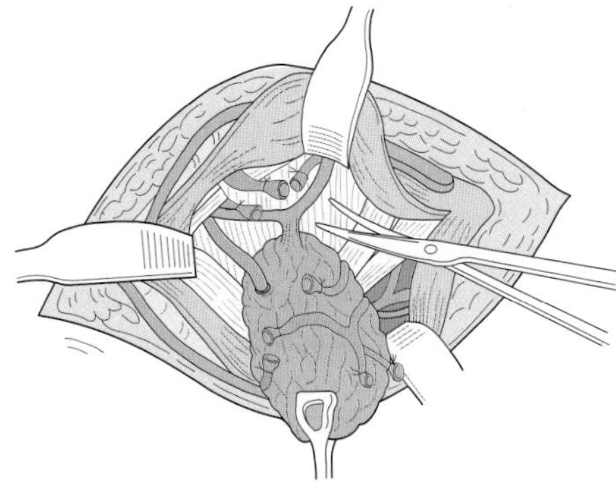

Fig. 42.19 The parasympathetic fibres which anchor the submandibular gland to the lingual nerve must be carefully divided whilst preserving the continuity of the lingual nerve.

to the patient's survival. It does, however, considerably increase the morbidity. For this reason, superficial or total parotidectomy for malignant tumours is undertaken with preservation of those branches of the facial nerve not macroscopically invaded by tumour. This is followed in all cases of malignant parotid tumours by radical radiotherapy.

Similarly, 'supraradical' surgery for adenoid cystic carcinomas is not advocated. This tumour, although probably always fatal in the long term, is compatible with a useful 10-year survival rate. It is difficult, therefore, to justify extensive mutilating surgery without offering a cure. Adenoid cystic carcinomas whose macroscopic margins remain within the parotid are treated by total parotidectomy followed by radical radiotherapy. For more extensive tumours, radical dissection with as wide a margin as is anatomically appropriate whilst being compatible with reasonable rehabilitation followed by radical radiotherapy will ensure excellent local control of tumour. The radiotherapy field should include the skull base in order to control the perineural tumour extensions.

For any malignant parotid tumours with skin involvement, facial nerve weakness, mandibular invasion, extension into the infratemporal fossa or lymph node metastasis, radical resection often in continuity with radical neck dissection must be undertaken with reconstruction with the use of appropriate flaps and followed by radical postoperative radiotheraphy.

Surgical technique

Whenever the facility is available and the patient fit, hypotensive anaesthesia is used, as this considerably reduces oozing and thus makes it easier to trace the facial nerve fibres. The incision line is infiltrated with lignocaine hydrochloride and 1:80 000 adrenaline and the incision made with a knife or fine cutting diathermy. Following a preauricular incision extending downwards to continue in a suitable skin crease in the neck, the skin flap is raised in the plane of the preparotid fascia and then held forward by suturing the margins for the flap to the adjacent towels. The blood-free plane anterior to the external auditory meatus is opened up by blunt dissection and this leads the surgeon down to the base of skull just superficial to the styloid process and the stylomastoid foramen. This plane is then gently opened up in an inferior direction by blunt dissection until the trunk of the facial nerve is seen. With large posterior tumours this plane may be difficult to open up. In this situation it is helpful to identify the posterior belly of the digastric muscle in the cervical extension of the incision. The anterior border of the sternocleidomastoid muscle is mobilised and retracted inferiorly to display the digastric muscle beneath it (Fig. 42.20). This manoeuvre necessitates sectioning the great auricular nerve. The posterior belly of the digastric is traced upwards and backwards to its insertion on to the mastoid, which lies immediately below the stylomastoid foramen, thus leading the operator to the facial nerve from below.

There are four anatomical landmarks leading to the identification of the trunk of the facial nerve as it leaves the stylomastoid foramen (Fig. 42.21).

1. The cartilaginous external auditory meatus forms a 'pointer' at its anterior, inferior border indicating the direction of the nerve trunk.
2. Just deep to the cartilaginous pointer is a reliable bony landmark formed by the curve of the bony external meatus and its abutment with the mastoid process. This forms a palpable groove leading directly to the stylomastoid foramen. Unfortunately this groove is filled with fibrofatty lobules that often mimic the trunk of the facial nerve which can lie as much as 1 cm deep to this landmark.
3. The anterior, superior aspect of the posterior belly of the digastric muscle is inserted just behind the stylomastoid foramen.
4. The styloid process itself can be palpated superficial to the stylomastoid foramen and just superior to it. The nerve is always lateral to this plane and passes obliquely across the styloid process. A branch of the postauricular artery is usually encountered just lateral to the nerve.

Once the facial nerve trunk has been identified the superficial lobe of the parotid can be exteriorised by opening up

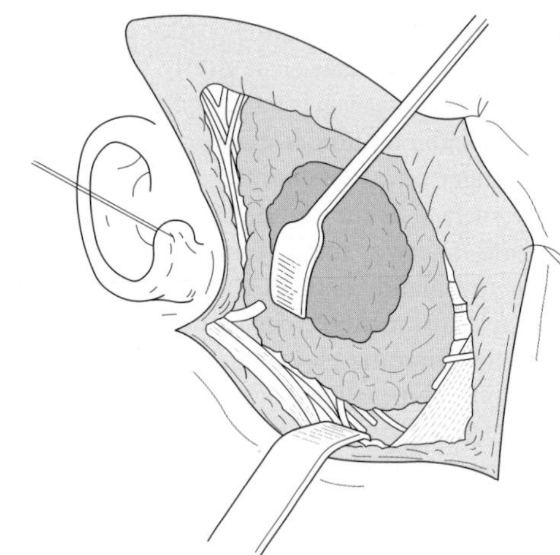

Fig. 42.20 The trunk of the facial nerve may be identified at the insertion of the digastric muscle into the mastoid.

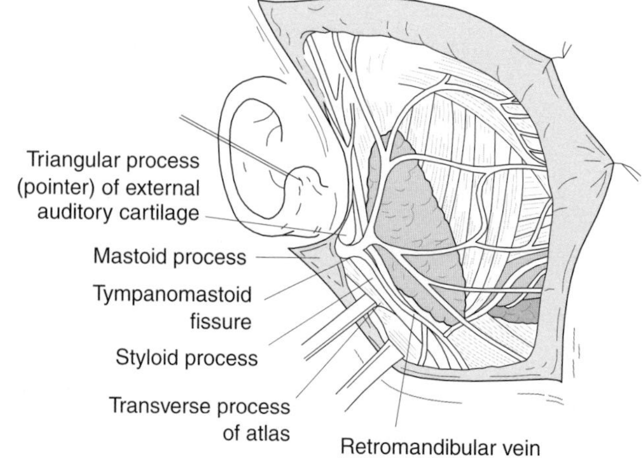

Fig. 42.21 This diagram shows the anatomical landmarks leading to the identification of the trunk of the facial nerve.

the plane in which the branches of the facial nerve run between the two lobes by blunt dissection. Initially, as it leaves the stylomastoid foramen, the trunk of the facial nerve turns abruptly to become more superficial and also divides into the larger zygomaticofacial trunk and smaller cervicofacial trunk. The five main branches of the nerve are then followed peripherally through the parotid until the superficial lobe is completely freed. This part of the operation is performed using fine scissors, opened up in the plane of the facial nerve branches, with care always taken to identify the nerve fibre before dividing parotid tissue (Fig. 42.22).

During the lower part of the dissection, branches of the posterior facial vein will be encountered immediately deep to the marginal mandibular branch. Great care must be taken when vascular clamps are applied to these branches to avoid damaging the facial nerve.

If the superficial parotidectomy is being performed for chronic infection, the duct should be tied off as far forward as possible to prevent recurrent ascending infection from the oral cavity.

If the tumour lies in the deep lobe of the gland a conventional superficial parotidectomy is performed as described. Next, the branches of the facial nerve are mobilised and lifted on nylon tapes to enable the deep lobe to be freed around its margins and removed when the mass is dropped downwards (Fig. 42.23). As this space is wedge shaped with its apex superior, it is almost invariably possible to do this. The deep lobe is covered by a capsule (the deep layer of the deep cervical fascia which splits to envelope the parotid) and is surrounded by the parapharyngeal fat. Thus, it is relatively easy to mobilise the deep lobe by blunt dissection with either scissors or a finger. Only very rarely is it necessary to perform a mandibulotomy to gain access to the deep lobe.

Very rarely – most often after recurrent infection with fibrosis or previous radiotherapy – the trunk of the facial nerve cannot be confidently identified. In this situation the peripheral branches of the nerve are identified at the anterior border of the parotid and traced centrally towards the stylomastoid foramen.

Following removal of the parotid gland the blood pressure is returned to normal, all bleeding points are controlled, a vacuum drain is placed and the wound closed in layers. A pressure dressing is then applied for 48 hours.

Complications

Permanent facial nerve paralysis following superficial or total parotidectomy is rare except when branches of the facial nerve have been deliberately sacrificed. When the facial nerve or its branches are sacrificed as a result of macroscopic tumour involvement, an immediate nerve graft may be undertaken using conventional microneural techniques.

Temporary weakness due to neuropraxia occurs in approximately 30 per cent of operations but recovers rapidly, usually within 6 weeks. Anaesthesia of the skin flap slowly resolves as the sensory nerves regenerate from the periphery.

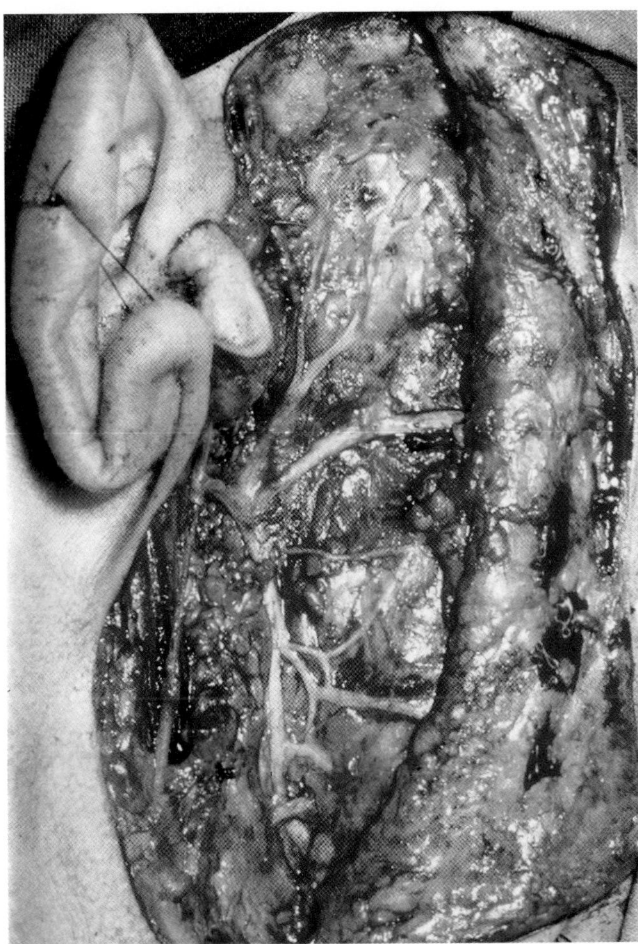

Fig. 42.22 Following removal of the superficial lobe of the parotid, the trunk of the facial nerve and its major branches can be seen.

Anaesthesia of the ear lobe due to sectioning of the great auricular nerve can be troublesome, particularly in females who find it difficult to wear earrings. Recovery can take up to 18 months and sometimes is never complete.

Gustatory sweating (Frey's syndrome) is a regular sequel to parotidectomy occurring in up to 54 per cent of cases. Surgical manoeuvres to treat it once established are not successful and most patients either learn to live with it or alternatively use an antiperspirant containing aluminium chloride.

Spillage of a benign pleomorphic adenoma should not occur if a formal superficial parotidectomy is undertaken. However, there are four circumstances where even with meticulous surgical technique this can happen:

- extremely large pleomorphic adenomas occupying the entire superficial lobe making mobilisation of the gland difficult;
- tumours that are intimately associated with branches of the facial nerve requiring very delicate dissection along the capsule of the tumour to release the nerve;
- tumours with lobular extensions extending beneath the mastoid, zygomatic arch or mandible;
- some tumours that are abnormally friable with even routine retraction of the superficial lobe resulting in rupture.

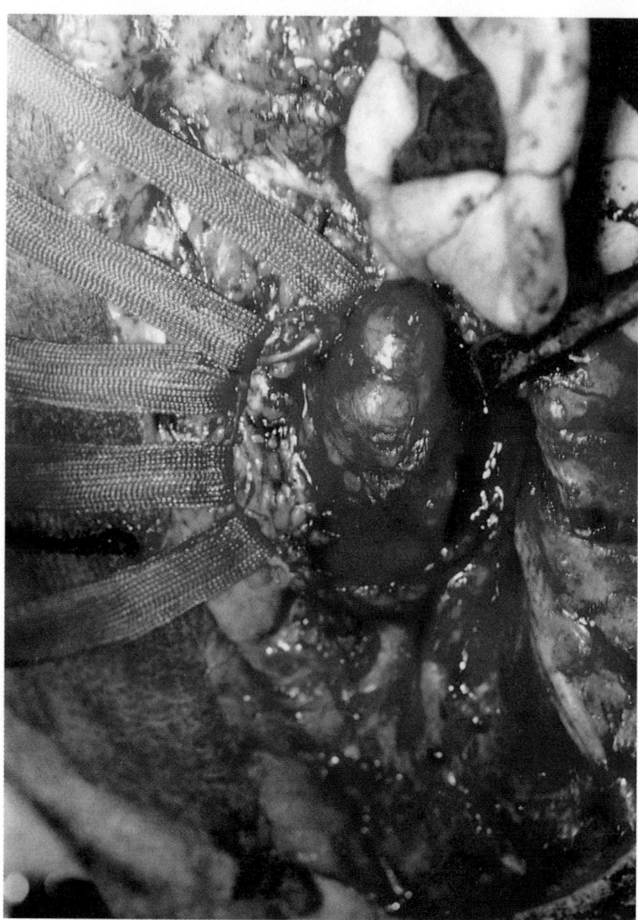

Fig. 42.23 By careful retraction of the branches of the facial nerve access is gained to the tumour in the deep lobe of the parotid gland.

If rupture occurs an extremely careful inspection of the wound must be undertaken and the area thoroughly irrigated. In all such cases postoperative radiotherapy should be undertaken in order to avoid multiple recurrences due to tumour seeding.

Other rare complications such as sialocele or salivary fistula occasionally follow parotidectomy. Both complications are managed conservatively and resolve spontaneously after days or weeks. Very rarely a parotid fistula persists despite attempts at surgical closure. In this situation postoperative radiotherapy will destroy the residual functioning acinar tissue and allow the fistula to close.

Radiotherapy

Parotid tumours are often considered to be 'radioresistant'. This is not true: regression after radiotherapy is usually slow, but this reflects the slow cell turnover time of the majority of these tumours, rather than the inability of radiation to effect a cure. There are many reports of long-term local control of large inoperable tumours by radiotherapy. Nevertheless, the chance of successful radiotherapy does seem lower than in the case of squamous cell carcinoma, and therefore the primary treatment should be surgical wherever possible.

Radiotherapy is of value for the inoperable tumour, and also should be used postoperatively whenever there is a risk of incomplete excision such as rupture of a pleomorphic adenoma. It should also be used prophylactically to radical dosage following excision of any malignant parotid tumour. In cases where reoperation is required for recurrence or where there is gross residual tumour, radiation in high doses increases survival significantly.

Adenoid cystic carcinoma has been reported to be the most consistently radioresponsive tumour type. In view of the propensity of this tumour for later recurrence, it is doubtful whether high local control rates at 3 or 5 years really indicate radiocurability.

A wide volume around the tumour should be irradiated, especially in the case of adenoid cystic carcinoma. A dose close to the limits of normal tissue tolerance is necessary.

Further reading

Cawson, R.A., Gleeson, M.J. and Eveson, J.W. (1997) *Pathology and Surgery of the Salivary Glands*, Isis Medical Media, Oxford.

Hobsley, M. (1983) *A Colour Atlas of Parotidectomy*, Wolfe, London.

Langdon, J.D. (1998) Sublingual and submandibular gland excision and parotid surgery. In *Operative Maxillofacial Surgery* (eds J.D. Langdon and M.F. Patel), Chapman & Hall, London, pp. 375–90.

Norman, J.E., De, B. and McGurk, M. (1995) *Colour Atlas and Text of the Salivary Glands*, Mosby-Wolfe, London.

Rankow, R.M. and Polayes I.M. (1976) *Diseases of the Salivary Glands*, W.B. Saunders, Philadelphia, PA.

Seward, G.R. (1968) Anatomic surgery for salivary calculi. *Oral Surgery, Oral Medicine, Oral Pathology*, **25**, 670–8; **25**, 810–16; **26**, 1–7.

Siefert, G., Miehlke, A., Haubrich, J. and Chilla, R. (1986) *Diseases of the Salivary Glands*, Thieme, Stuttgart.

Luiji Frey, 1889–1944. Physician, Neurologist Clinic, Warsaw, Poland.

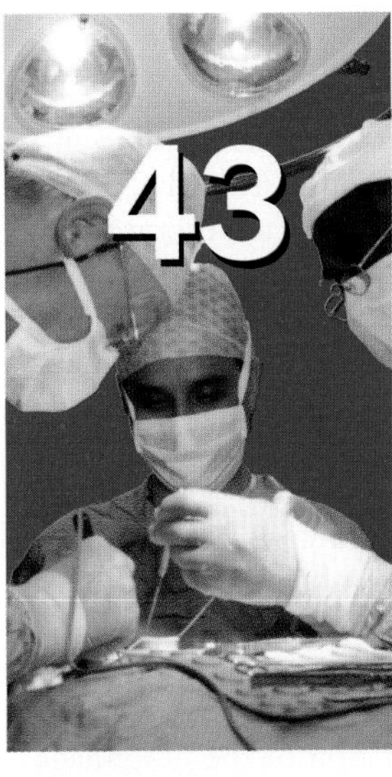

43 Pharynx, larynx and neck

Clinical anatomy and physiology

The pharynx

The pharynx is a fibromuscular tube forming the upper part of the respiratory and digestive passages. It extends from the base of the skull to the level of the sixth cervical vertebra at the lower border of the cricoid cartilage where it becomes continuous with the oesophagus. It opens anteriorly into the nose, mouth and larynx from above downwards, and is therefore divided into three parts, the nasopharynx, oropharynx and hypopharynx (Fig. 43.1).

Nasopharynx

The nasopharynx lies anterior to the first cervical vertebra and has the openings of the eustachian tubes in its lateral wall, behind which lie the pharyngeal recesses, the fossae of Rosenmüller. The adenoids are situated submucosally at the junction of the roof and posterior wall of the nasopharynx. The nasopharynx is closed off from the oropharynx during swallowing by the raising of the soft palate and contraction of the palatopharyngeal sphincter.

Bartolomeo Eustachio, b. 1520. Italian anatomist.
Johann Christian Rosenmüller, 1771–1820. Professor of Anatomy and Surgery, Leipzig, Germany.

Bailey & Love's Short Practice of Surgery, 23rd edition. Edited by R.C.G. Russell, N.S. Williams and C.J.K. Bulstrode. Published in 2000 by Arnold Publishers.

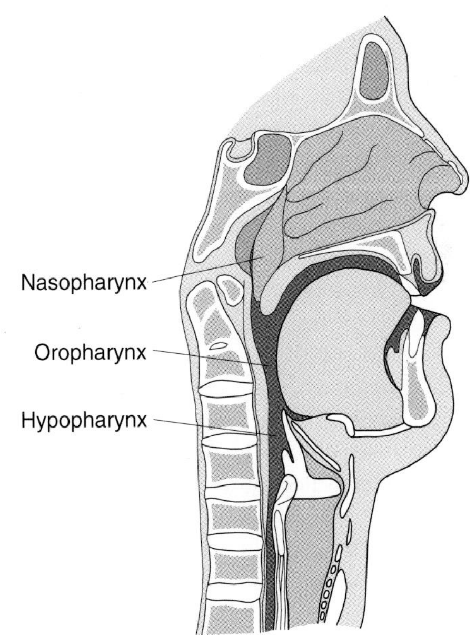

Fig. 43.1 The component parts of the pharynx.

Oropharynx

This is bounded above by the soft palate, below by the upper surface of the epiglottis and anteriorly by the anterior faucial pillar which contains the palatoglossus muscle. The oropharynx therefore contains the palatine tonsils situated in the lateral wall between the anterior and posterior pillars of the fauces and the posterior third of the tongue. These palatine tonsils are

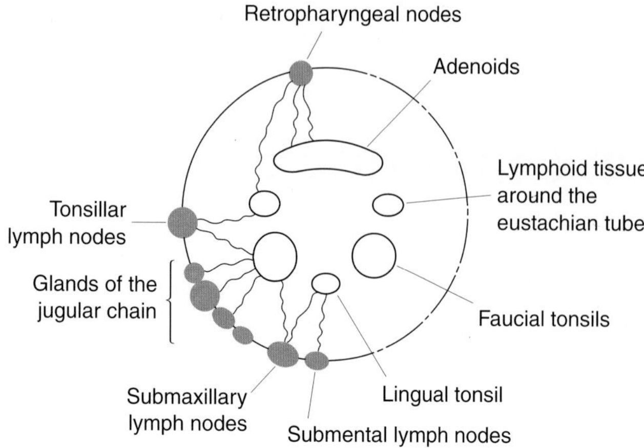

Fig. 43.2 Waldeyer's ring.

part of the complete ring of lymphoid tissue (Waldeyer's ring) which additionally comprises the adenoids and the lingual tonsils on the posterior third of the tongue. This ring of lymphoid tissue occupying the entry of the air and food passages is constantly exposed to new antigenic stimuli. It is an important part of the mucosal-associated lymphoid tissue (MALT) which processes antigen and presents it to T-helper cells and B-cells. The tonsillar tissue produces immunoglobin G (IgG), IgA and a small amount of IgD. These immunoglublins are secreted into the pharynx and their output is increased in response to a wide variety of inflammatory processes (Fig. 43.2).

The tissue of Waldeyer's ring undergoes physiological hypertrophy during early childhood as the child is exposed to increasing amounts of antigenic stimuli; there is often a similar hypertrophy of the cervical lymph nodes and, indeed, the abdominal lymph nodes (the aetiology of mesenteric adenitis). The tonsils contain tortuous crypts which can harbour pus and microorganisms. Clothing the lateral two-thirds of each tonsil is the capsule, a well-defined structure composed of fibrous and elastic tissue, and muscle fibres. The tonsil has an exceptionally good blood supply. It is well to bear in mind that a tortuous facial artery may be closely related to the lower pole. On the lateral aspect of the tonsil is a varying number of paratonsillar veins which may be the source of serious venous bleeding following tonsillectomy. This may particularly occur when the bleeding end retracts into the upper part of the tonsillar fossa, and this must be found and ligated before the patient leaves the operating room.

Hypopharynx

The hypopharynx is bounded above by the upper border of the epiglottis and anteriorly by the sloping laryngeal inlet. Its inferior border is the lower border of the cricoid cartilage where it continues into the oesophagus. The hypopharynx is commonly described anatomically of being composed of three areas: the piriform fossae, the posterior pharyngeal wall and the postcricoid area. The mucosa of these areas is in direct continuity with no distinct barriers, and disease processes, such as malignant neoplasms, can easily involve more than one area.

Swallowing

Swallowing is a complex neuromuscular act. Trauma and disease may result in dysphagia and at times aspiration of food and fluid into the airway. In considering the diseases which involve the pharynx and larynx, it is important to have a basic understanding of swallowing and the functions of the larynx. Swallowing consists of three stages: oral, pharyngeal and oesophageal (Fig. 43.3). Knowledge of the physiology of normal swallowing and the problems as a consequence of disease has been enhanced in the last two decades by use of videofluoroscopic techniques. This is the radiographical evaluation of the passage of a bolus of radio-opaque liquid or solid from the point at which it enters the oral cavity down to its passage within the stomach. This investigation is considerably more accurate than the older-fashioned radiological examination of barium swallow, where the object was to concentrate on the plain X-ray examination of the oesophagus, rather than the new technique which shows a complete video of all stages of swallowing. This can be reviewed on many

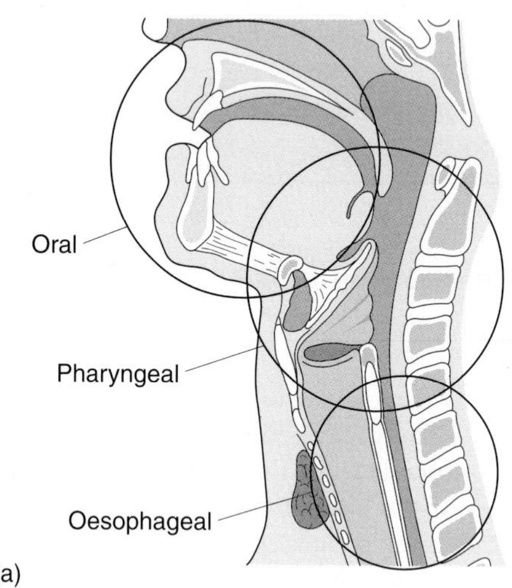

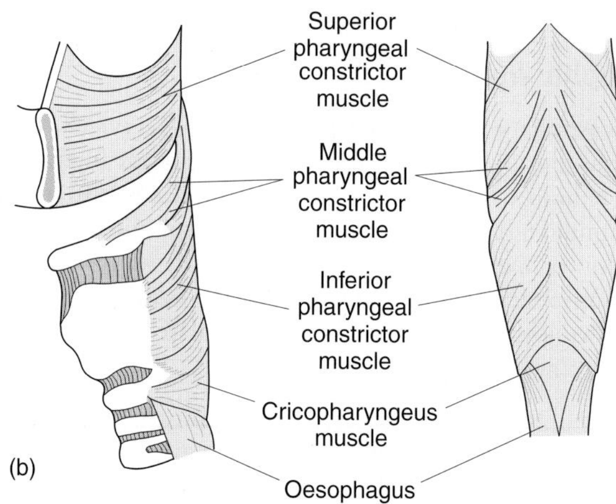

Fig. 43.3 The three phases of swallowing and muscles involved. [Reproduced with permission from McGregor, I.A. and Howard, D.J. (eds), *Rob and Smith's Operative Surgery, Head and Neck Part 2*, Butterworth-Heinemann, Oxford, 1992, p. 440.]

occasions, if necessary, and gives far more detail than plain radiograph films.

Swallowing is mediated via efferent fibres passing to the medulla oblongata through the second division of the trigeminal nerve (V), glossopharyngeal (IX) and vagus nerves (X). The afferent pathway is from the nucleus ambiguous, and is mediated via the glossopharyngeal (IX), vagus (X) and hypoglossal (XII) nerves.

Damage to these major cranial nerves at any point along their pathway, by trauma or disease, may cause dysphagia with or without aspiration.

In the oral voluntary phase of swallowing the lips, cheeks, tongue, floor of mouth, teeth and palate participate in preparing the food. The food is held in the oral cavity, lateralised for mastication and then formed into a bolus. The tongue propels the formed bolus posteriorly into the oropharynx in the second involuntary pharyngeal phase. The soft palate is elevated to prevent nasopharyngeal escape, and the lateral and posterior walls contract to propel the food downwards. The larynx moves upwards and forwards as the posterior tongue moves backwards and downwards.

The main function of the larynx is in fact not the production of voice but the protection of the tracheobroncheal airway and lungs. It is basically a three-tiered sphincter mechanism: the first tier consisting of the epiglottis, aryepiglottic folds and arytenoids; the second the false cords; and the third level the true vocal folds. The whole larynx not only moves upwards and forwards but the three-tier sphincter mechanism closes on every occasion that swallowing occurs.

As the food enters the piriform fossa there is an anticipatory relaxation of the upper oesophageal sphincter and the food enters the oesophagus. Oesophageal peristaltic waves then convey the food down into the stomach. Gravity aids both the involuntary pharyngeal and oesophageal phases of swallowing.

Relations of the pharynx (Fig. 43.4)

- The parapharyngeal space – this potential space lies lateral to the pharynx and is of importance when understanding disease of the pharynx and neck. It is a potential space which extends from the base of the skull above to the superior mediastinum below, and it is occupied by the carotid vessels, internal jugular vein, deep cervical lymph nodes, the last four cranial nerves and the cervical sympathetic trunk. Infection and suppuration of the cervical lymph node in the parapharyngeal space most commonly occurs from infections of the tonsils or teeth (particularly the third lower molar tooth). It may then spread throughout the parapharyngeal space up to the skull base or down to the paraoesophageal region and superior mediastinum.
- Retropharyngeal space – this potential space lies posterior to the pharynx bounded anteriorly by the posterior pharyngeal wall and its covering buccopharyngeal fascia and posteriorly by the cervical vertebrae and their covering muscles and fascia. It contains the retropharyngeal lymph nodes, which are usually paired lateral nodes, but which are separated by a tough median partition which connects the prevertebral with the buccopharyngeal fascia. These nodes are more developed in infancy and young children, and it is at this age that they are most likely to be involved in inflammatory processes which, if severe, may affect swallowing and respiration as a consequence of gross swelling and suppuration of the retropharyngeal space.

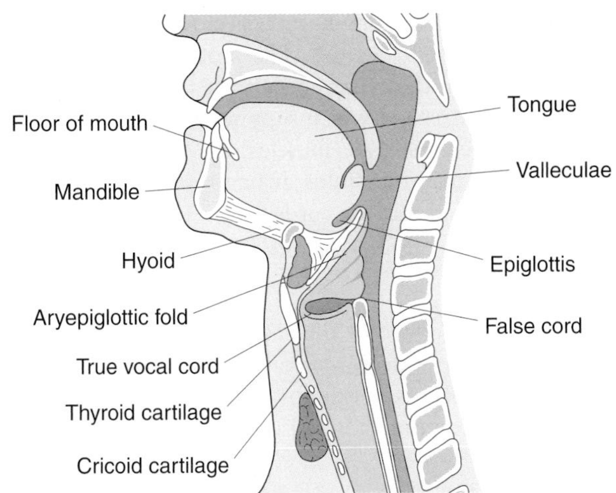

Fig. 43.4 Sagittal diagram of upper aero-digestive tract. [Reproduced with permission from McGregor, I.A. and Howard, D.J. (eds), *Rob and Smith's Operative Surgery, Head and Neck Part 2*, Butterworth-Heinemann, Oxford, 1992, p. 442.]

Larynx

The larynx is the protective sphincter which closes off the airway during swallowing. In humans and some other mammals it is also responsible for the generation of sound, which in humans is modified by the pharynx, oral cavity, nasal passages, sinuses, tongue, lips and teeth to produce speech. The larynx has a mainly cartilaginous framework which may ossify in later life and which consists of the hyoid bone above, the thyroid and cricoid cartilages, and the intricate arytenoid cartilages posteriorly.

The cricoid cartilage is the only complete ring in the entire airway and bounds the subglottis which is the narrowest point of the airway. This is the commonest site for damage from endotracheal tubes, occasionally causing laryngotracheal stenosis.

An anatomical description of the larynx divides it into the supraglottis, glottis and subglottis (Fig. 43.5). The true vocal folds (often incorrectly called the vocal cords) are normally white in contrast to the pink mucosa of the rest of the larynx and airway. The true vocal folds meet anteriorly at the mid-level of the thyroid cartilage, whereas posteriorly they are separate and attached to an arytenoid cartilage. This arrangement produces the 'V' shape of the glottis (Fig. 43.6).

Nerve supply

The sensory nerve supply to the larynx above the vocal folds is from the superior laryngeal nerve and below the vocal folds from the recurrent laryngeal nerve. Both of these nerves are branches of the vagus (X). The motor nerves supply to the larynx is from the recurrent laryngeal nerve, which is a branch of the vagus and which supplies all intrinsic muscles. Only one of these intrinsic muscles, the posterior cricoarytenoid, abducts the vocal folds during respiration. All other intrinsic muscles adduct the cords.

Lymphatics

The lymphatic drainage of the supraglottis above the vocal folds is to the upper deep cervical nodes, whilst in contrast that of the subglottis is to inferior deep cervical nodes and to the paratracheal and mediastinal nodes.

- The vocal folds themselves have a very sparse lymphatic drainage. The commonest form of malignant disease affecting the true vocal folds is squamous cell carcinoma, and tumours confined to the true vocal folds do not metastasise to lymph nodes unless they spread into supraglottic or subglottic tissue.
- All of the intrinsic muscles of the larynx are supplied by the recurrent laryngeal nerve, and therefore damage to this nerve or to the vagus nerve will cause paralysis of the vocal fold on the side of the damage.

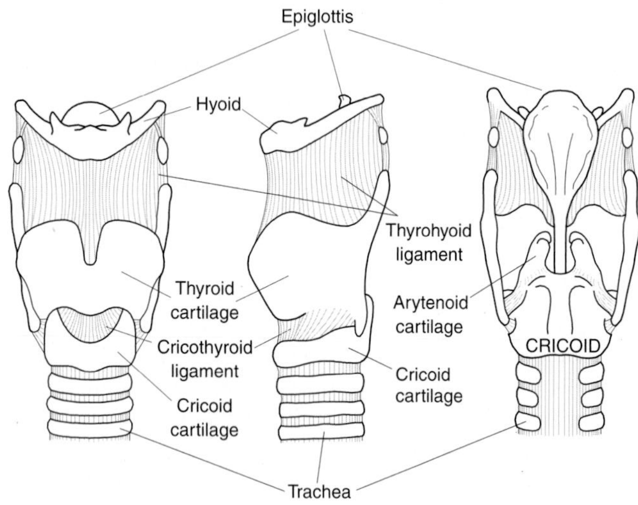

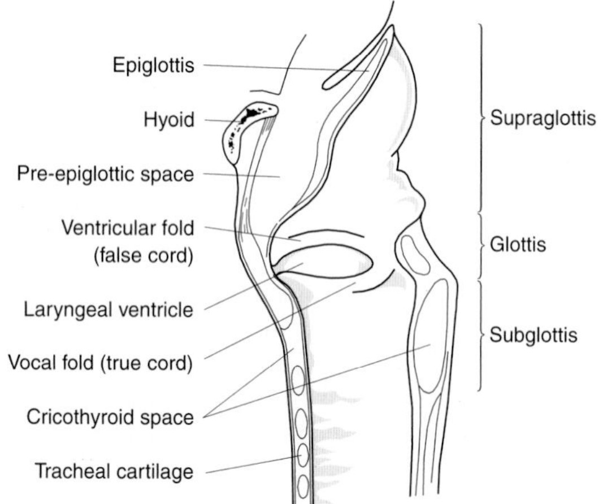

Fig. 43.5 Anatomy of the larynx. [Reproduced with permission from O'Connor, F. and Lund, V.J. (eds), *Aird's Companion in Surgical Studies*, Churchill Livingstone, London, 1998, Fig 20.37.]

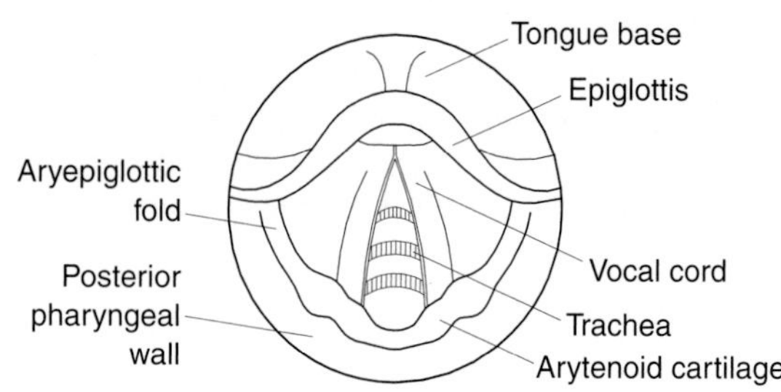

(a) Vocal cords abducted (open)

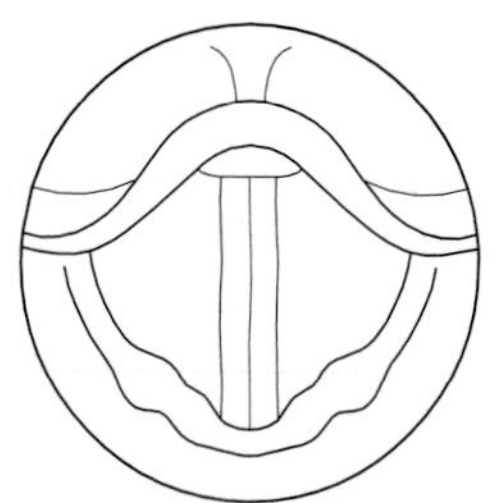

(b) Vocal cords adducted (closed)

Fig. 43.6 Diagram showing a view of the larynx on indirect laryngoscopy: (a) vocal cords abducted; (b) vocal cords adducted. [Reproduced with permission from O'Connor, F. and Lund, V.J. (eds), *Aird's Companion in Surgical Studies*, Churchill Livingstone, London, 1998, Fig 20.38.]

Phonation/speech

During expiration air from the lungs passes out through the larynx under pressure and the vocal folds channel this into a column of high-speed vibrating air, thus producing sound. This sound is converted into intelligible speech by the remainder of the vocal tract, i.e. the pharynx, tongue, lips, teeth and the resonating chambers of the nose and sinuses. The larynx functions by closing the vocal fold against the air being exhaled from the lungs but the rise in subglottic pressure forces the vocal folds apart slightly for an instant with accompanying vibration of the vocal fold epithelium. The opening and closing occurs in rapid sequence to produce a vibrating column of air which is the source of sound. The pitch of the sound is controlled by the frequency of the vocal fold epithelial vibration, which in turn is determined by the thickness, length and tension of the vocal folds controlled by the intrinsic musculature. The loudness or intensity of the sound is governed by the expiratory air pressure and the amplitude of the vocal fold vibrations.

Paralysis or overt disease of the vocal folds or closely associated laryngeal structures will give rise to disturbance of the sound and creation of the symptom of hoarseness (Table 43.1).

Table 43.1 Functions of the larynx

1. Protection of the lower respiratory tract by:
   - closure of the laryngeal inlet;
   - closure of false cords;
   - closure of glottis;
   - cessation of respiration;
   - cough reflex
2. Phonation
3. Respiration – control of pressure
4. Fixation of chest – aids lifting, straining and climbing

The neck

The neck is divided into anterior and posterior triangles by the sternocleidomastoid muscle. The anterior triangle extends from the inferior border of the mandible to the sternum below, and is bounded by the midline and the sternocleidomastoid muscle. The posterior triangle extends backwards to the anterior border of trapezius and inferiorly to the clavicle. The upper part of the anterior triangle is commonly subdivided into the submandibular triangle above the digastric muscle and the submental triangle below. The lymphatic drainage of the head and neck is of considerable clinical importance (Fig. 43.7). The most important chain of nodes is the deep cervical nodes which run adjacent to the internal jugular vein. The other main groups are the submental, submandibular, preauricular and postauricular, occipital and posterior triangle nodes.

The upper deep cervical nodes, which contain the large jugulodigastric node, drain the oropharynx, including the tonsils, posterolateral aspects of the oral cavity, superior aspects of the larynx and piriform fossae, and are the commonest site of enlargement due to disease in these areas.

The upper deep cervical nodes may be palpated along the anterior border of the sternocleidomastoid muscle but when the muscle is well developed or the neck is obese it may be difficult to evaluate their true size and under these circumstances clinical examination may be unreliable.

Metastatic spread of squamous cell carcinoma, which accounts for 80 per cent of malignant disease of the head and neck, most commonly occurs with tumours of the nasopharynx, tongue base, tonsil, piriform fossae and supraglottic larynx. When an enlarged neck node is detected and the possibility of malignant disease suspected, it is these five primary sites which must receive careful investigation.

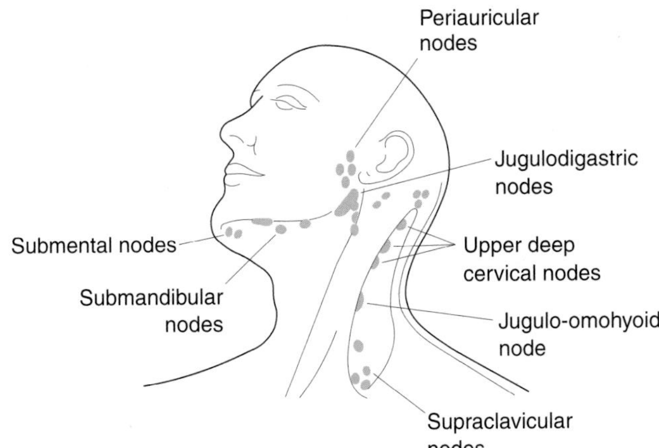

Fig. 43.7 Diagram showing distribution of cervical lymph nodes.

Metastatic spread to regional lymph nodes in the neck is managed surgically in many cases by resection of the neck nodes, and a detailed knowledge of their anatomy is thus required. The parotid and submandibular salivary glands, and the thyroid and parathyroid glands, are additional important neck structures which will be covered separately in their respective chapters.

Clinical examination

Pharynx and larynx

Prior to examination of the pharynx, the oral cavity should be examined with the aid of a good light and tongue depressors (Fig. 43.8).

The ear, nose and throat (ENT) surgeon customarily uses a reflecting mirror on the head or a headband-mounted fibre-optic light source which permits use of both hands to hold instruments. Inspection should include the buccal mucosa and lips, the palate, the tongue and floor of the mouth, all surfaces of the teeth and gums, opening and closing of the mouth, and dental occlusion. Patients should be asked to elevate the tongue to the roof of the mouth and protrude the tongue to both the right and the left. Palpation may be required using one or two fingers gently intraorally to feel any swellings, and this may be combined with extraoral palpation of the submental and submandibular lymph nodes and salivary glands. Simple percussion of the teeth may reveal tenderness indicating adjacent pathology in the maxilla or mandible.

Examination of the mouth without adequate illumination, the use of a tongue depressor, and gentle palpation may fail to reveal common and important pathology.

Following examination of the oral cavity, the oropharynx is inspected with the light and with the tongue depressor placed firmly on to the tongue base to depress it inferiorly.

The anterior and posterior faucial pillars, the tonsil, retromolar trigone and posterior pharyngeal wall should all be inspected for colour changes, ulceration, pus, foreign bodies and swellings.

Even with an experienced examiner, approximately one-third of patients cannot tolerate the depression of the posterior base of tongue without gagging. Pain and trismus as a con-

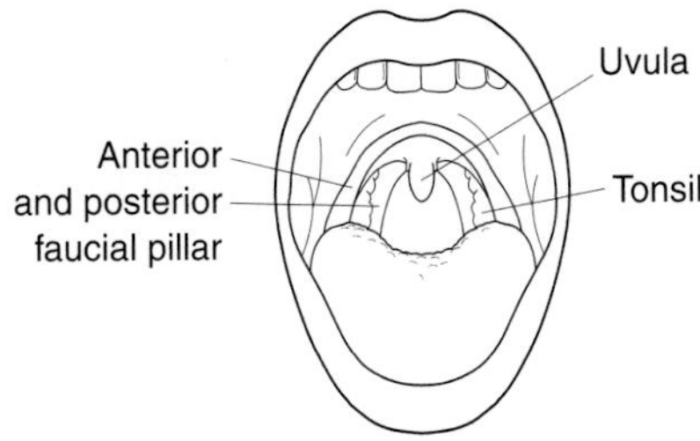

Fig. 43.8 Diagram showing oral cavity and oropharynx.

sequence of pharyngolaryngeal or neck pathology may add to the difficulty of the examination. However, if the patient is co-operative the nasopharynx may be further examined by posterior rhinoscopy using a postnasal mirror introduced along the tongue depressor and moved so that a mirror image is seen of the nasopharynx. Likewise, further examination of the inferior oropharynx, larynx and piriform fossae can be obtained by indirect laryngoscopy using laryngeal mirrors. Both of these mirror examination techniques require the use of a headlight and both of the examiner's hands. Indirect laryngoscopy allows visualisation of the larynx to the level of the vocal folds, and sometimes additional views of the subglottic and tracheal airway. Vocal fold mobility may be assessed.

Fibre-optic pharyngolaryngoscopy

The fibre-optic nasendoscope is passed through the nose under topical anaesthesia, and the entire nasopharynx, oropharynx and larynx can be seen and demonstrated to others. This technique allows high-quality visualisation in over 90 per cent of patients (Fig. 43.9).

Modern fibre-optic nasendoscopes have produced tremendous improvements in examination of the nasal cavities, pharynx and larynx. They are now widely available and should be used whenever possible.

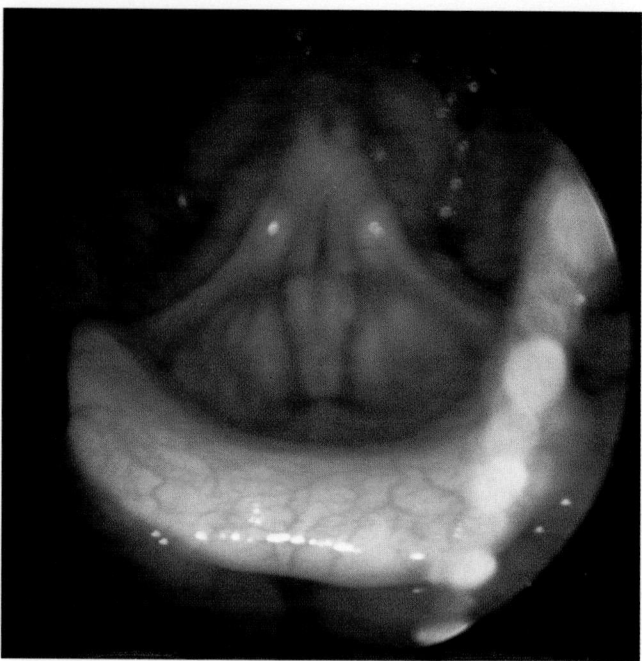

Fig. 43.9 View of larynx with fibre-optic endoscopy.

The neck

With the patient sitting, expose the whole neck so that both clavicles are clearly seen. Inspect the neck from in front and ask the patient to swallow, preferably with the aid of a sip of water. Note the movements of the larynx and any swelling in the neck. Ask the patient to protrude the tongue if there is a midline neck swelling. A thyroglossal cyst will move upwards with the tongue protrusion. Then stand behind the seated patient who should sit with the chin flexed slightly downwards to remove any undue tension in the strap muscles, plastysma and sternocleidomastoids. Palpate the neck bilaterally using the pulps of the fingers, not the tips. It is important to palpate the groups of lymph nodes in a definite manner comparing the two sides of the neck. Begin with the superficial chain around the upper neck and carefully palpate the entire length of the deep cervical nodes around the internal jugular vein.

On examining for a lump in the neck it is often helpful to ask the patient to point to the lump first. Ask them whether the lump is tender. A swelling beneath the sternomastoid muscle may be considerably larger than your evaluation on palpation. If you are suspicious that a neck node is enlarged as a result of malignancy (it may be hard, irregular or fixed to overlying skin or to deep structures) then it is mandatory to inspect the nasopharynx, tonsils, tongue base, piriform fossa and supraglottic larynx (Table 43.2).

Investigation of diseases in the pharynx, larynx and neck

Plain lateral X-rays

Plain lateral radiographs of the neck and cervical spine may show soft-tissue abnormalities; of particular importance is the depth and outline of the prevertebral soft-tissue shadow. The outline of the laryngotracheal airway may be a useful guide to the presence of disease in the pharynx and larynx (Fig. 43.10). Radio-opaque foreign bodies may be visible, impacted in the pharynx, larynx or upper oesophagus.

There should be no air within the upper oesophagus, if this is seen it is indicative of pathology.

Table 43.2 Key points of history and examination

1. Mouth
   Adequate light source and two spatulas to examine the mouth
   - Examine:
     - teeth, gums, gingival sulci
     - buccal mucosa, opening of parotid duct
     - floor of mouth
     - hard and soft palate
     - retromolar trigone region ('coffin corner')
     - anterior and posterior faucial pillars, tonsils
     - posterior pharyngeal wall
     - tongue (observe full movements)
   - Palpate:
     - salivary glands/ducts
2. Larynx, oropharynx and hypopharynx
   Indirect laryngoscopy – mirror and headlight
   Direct flexible fibre-optic pharyngolaryngoscopy
3. Nasopharynx
   Rigid Hopkin's rod endoscopy
   Flexible fibre-optic nasendoscopy
4. Neck
   - Inspect:
     - tongue protusion
     - observe swallowing
   - Palpate:
     - if a mass is palpable, evaluate for size, site, shape, consistency, superficial and deep fixation, fluctuation, transillumination, auscultation

Barium swallow

This X-ray has traditionally been used to assess the pharynx and oesophagus using simple barium liquid and plain X-rays. However, it has now been superseded in many places by the use of videofluoroscopic studies which record the moving images of a small quantity of radio-opaque liquid, enabling evaluation of the oral and pharyngeal phases of swallowing in much more detail (Fig. 43.11).

Manometric analysis and pH recordings within the pharynx and oesophagus are used in specialised units and may be coupled with simultaneous videofluoroscopy to assess changes in luminal pressure and pH to define muscular incoordination and the role of reflux of low-pH gastric contents.

Computerised tomography (CT) scanning

CT scanning is widely used to assess head and neck disorders, and the increasing quality of the images provides much improved demonstration of disease in the pharynx, larynx and neck. Intravenous contrast given at the same time as the CT scan (dynamic scanning) further improves the demonstration of disease in these areas (Fig. 43.12).

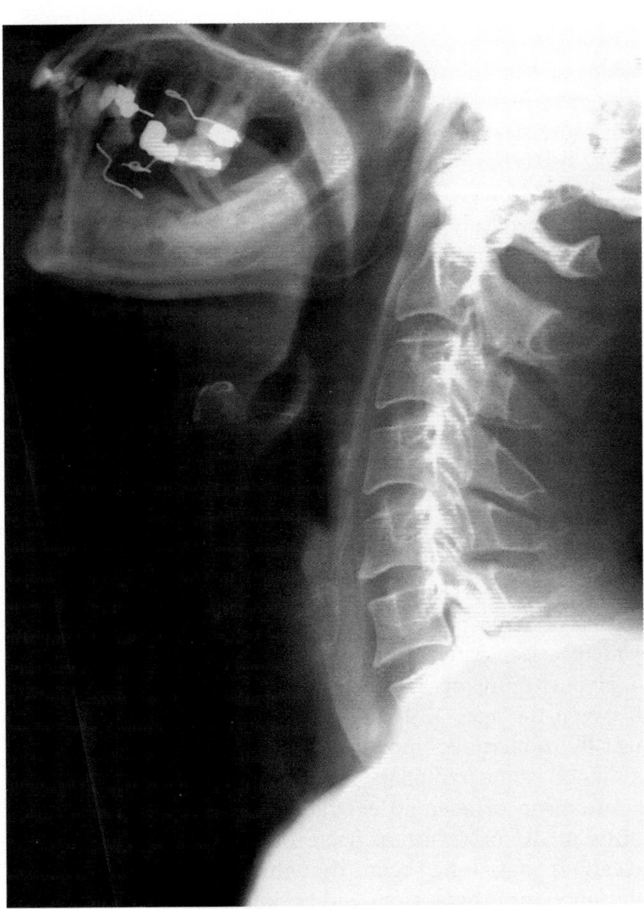

Fig. 43.10 Plain lateral X-ray showing normal anatomy.

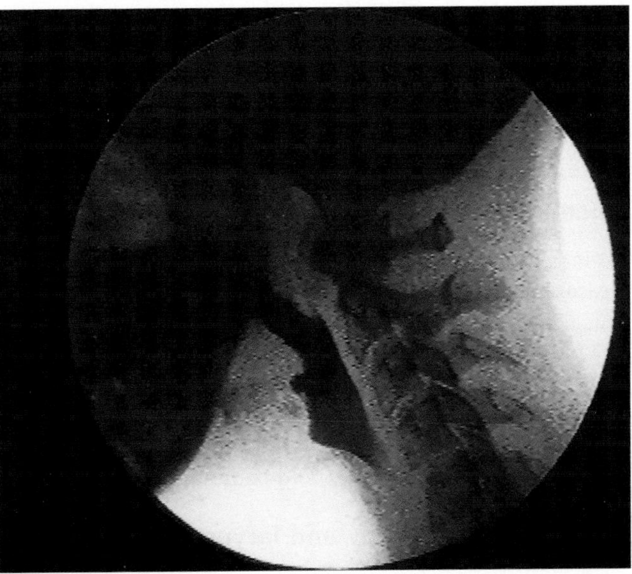

Fig. 43.11 Videofluoroscopy image showing liquid barium in the upper pharynx in normal swallow.

Other techniques

Magnetic resonance imaging (MRI) is being increasingly used and may give better soft-tissue definition of some diseases but poorer definition of bony and cartilaginous structures. Ultrasound scanning can be useful in differentiating solid lesions, e.g. malignant lymph nodes from cystic lesions such as a branchial cyst.

Fine needle aspiration cytology

This technique can be performed under local anaesthesia either in the out-patient department or in a cytology clinic.

Fine needle aspiration cytology is useful particularly if a neck lump is thought to be malignant. Increasingly high rates of accurate histological diagnosis are reported and there is *no* evidence of spread of tumour through the skin track caused by the fine hyperdermic needle used with this technique.

Fine needle aspiration may be further aided by ultrasound or CT guidance.

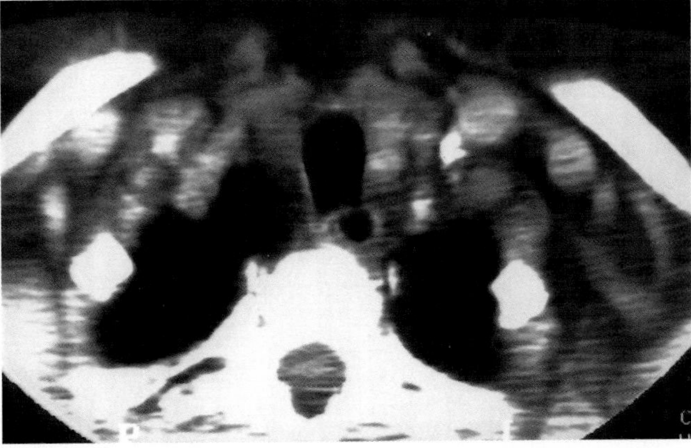

Fig. 43.12 Axial CT scan showing normal larynx and pharynx.

Angiography or digital subtraction vascular imaging

These may be indicated if a vascular lesion such as a carotid body tumour is suspected. Angiography may have a therapeutic role to play by facilitating embolisation of the lesion.

Voice analysis

An increasing variety of techniques is now available for the measurement of vocal function including videostroboscopy. This technique utilises a flexible or rigid endoscope coupled to a video-camera and a stroboscopic light. This allows identification of the fine epithelial movements of the vocal folds and demonstrates this on a monitor to the patient, doctor and speech therapist. This technique allows very sensitive assessment of laryngeal vocal fold pathology.

Direct pharyngoscopy and laryngoscopy

An examination of the pharynx, larynx and neck under general anaesthesia may be required as a result of problems with the routine examination of patients. This may be due to an inadequate view as a consequence of trismus from pain, poor patient compliance, or large obstructive pharyngeal or laryngeal pathology. These examinations may be further aided by the use of an operating microscope, or rigid telescopes (Hopkin's rods) which improve the visualisation of the pharynx and larynx (Fig. 43.13).

Diseases of the pharynx

Nasopharynx

Enlarged adenoid

The most common cause of an enlarged adenoid (there is only one nasopharyngeal adenoid, despite the common use of the term 'adenoids') is physiological hypertrophy (Fig. 43.14). The size of the adenoid alone is not an indication for removal. It is often associated with hypertrophy of the other lymphoid tissues of Waldeyer's ring. If excessive hypertrophy causes blockage of the nasopharynx in association with tonsil hypertrophy, the upper airway may become compromised during sleep causing obstructive sleep apnoea. This condition is becoming increasingly diagnosed, and is important because it can cause sleep deprivation and secondary cardiac complications. It has been implicated in some cases of a sudden infant death syndrome. The most common symptom is snoring, which is typically irregular, with the child actually ceasing respiration (apnoea) and then restarting with a loud inspiratory snort. The child is often restless and may take up strange sleeping positions as he or she tries to improve the pharyngeal airway. Surgical removal of the tonsils and adenoid is curative, but it is important to avoid sedative premedications and opiate analgesics postoperatively because they may further depress the child's respiratory drive. Obstructive sleep apnoea may also occur in adults, where the obstruction may result from nasal deformity, a hypertrophic soft palate associated with an altered nasopharyngeal isthmus, obesity and general narrowing of the pharyngeal airway, or supraglottic laryngeal pathology. Surgery may be indicated following investigation by means of a sleep study, during which measurement of the patient's sleep pattern and arterial oxygenation is undertaken.

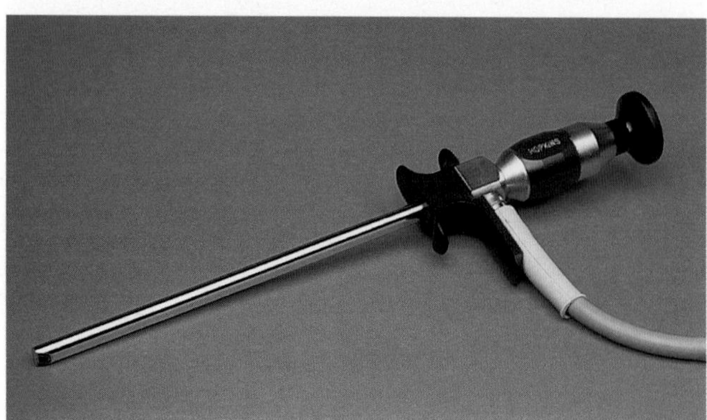

Fig. 43.13 Slide showing a rigid Hopkin's rod or endoscope.

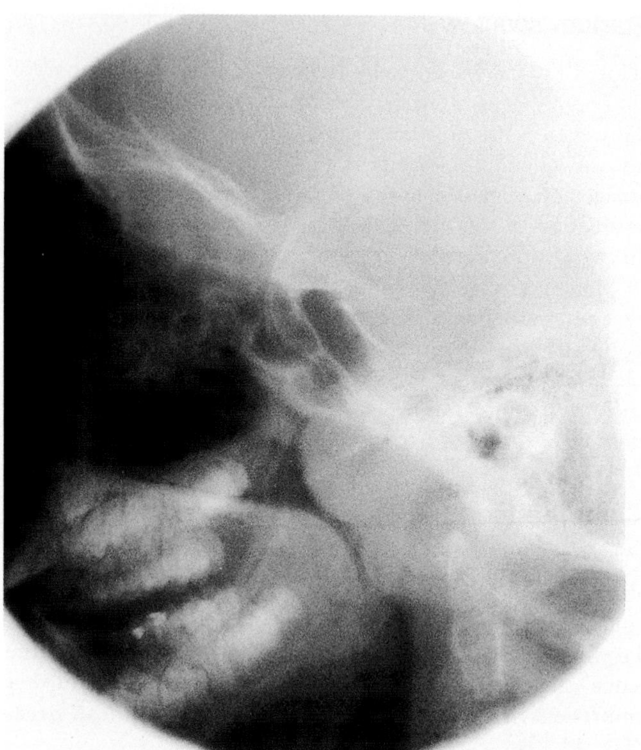

Fig. 43.14 Plain lateral X-ray showing a large pad of adenoid in postnasal space.

Hypertrophy of adenoid tissue most commonly occurs between the ages of 4 and 10 years, but the adenoid tissue usually undergoes spontaneous atrophy during puberty, although some remnants may persist into adult life. The relationship of adenoid enlargement to recurrent secretory otitis media or recurrent acute otitis media is not entirely clear. It has long been thought that eustachian tube dysfunction results from either inflammatory oedema or interference with palatal elevation which opens the eustachian tube. However, the exact relationship has not been determined and many children who have secretory otitis media do not always benefit from adenoid removal.

Adenoidectomy

Adenoid tissue can be removed alone or in conjunction with a tonsillectomy.

Indications are:

- obstructive sleep apnoea associated with postnasal obstruction;
- postnasal discharge;
- recurrent acute otitis media or prolonged serous otitis media usually longer than 3 months' duration;
- recurrent rhinosinusitis.

Operative technique. The adenoid tissue is removed with a guarded curette (Fig. 43.15) pressed against the roof of the nasopharynx and then carried downwards in a moderately firm sweeping movement bringing the excised adenoid into the oropharynx (Fig. 43.16). The guard on the curette secures the adenoid and prevents it from dropping inferiorly into the airway. A postnasal swab is placed into the nasopharynx until all haemorrhage has ceased.

Reactionary or secondary haemorrhage during the recovery period may require the placing of a nasopharyngeal pack under a further anaesthetic. This can occasionally cause respiratory depression in children and adults, and they require strict observation while the pack is in place.

Tumours of the nasopharynx

Benign. There are two main types of benign tumour of the nasopharynx: the angiofibroma and the antrochoanal polyp.

Angiofibroma. This is often termed 'nasopharyngeal angiofibroma', but this is incorrect as the tumour arises in the area of the sphenopalatine foramen in the posterior part of the nasal cavity. However, it readily expands into the nasopharynx and, although the tumour is not malignant in that it never metastasises, it does spread relentlessly over the skull base expanding anteriorly into the nasal cavities displacing the nasal septum, compressing the posterior wall of the maxillary antrum and often entering it by bone erosion. Likewise, it may enter and expand the sphenoid sinus and spread laterally through the pterygopalatine fissure and onwards into the infratemporal fossa occasionally to reach the soft tissues of the cheek and orbit via the inferior orbital fissure. Inferiorly it may fill the nasopharynx, depress the soft palate and eventually appear within the oropharynx (Fig. 43.17).

Macroscopically there is a firm reddish-blue tumour covered with normal mucous membrane, but ulceration may occur if the tumour hangs into the oropharynx or becomes exposed anteriorly at the nostril. Microscopically it is composed of immature fibroblasts and blood vessels, and it remains benign even in its advanced stages. It should probably be regarded as a hamartoma. Clinically the tumour is confined to male patients commonly between the ages of 8 and 20 years, i.e. around puberty. It occasionally occurs in the 20s and 30s.

It rarely regresses and usually causes progressive nasal obstruction, recurrent severe epistaxis, purulent rhinorrhoea and occasionally loss of vision due to compression of the optic nerve. Although the tumour is rare, these symptoms in a young boy should always arouse suspicion.

The tumour occurs in many countries around the world but is most common in northern India. The reasons for this are unknown.

Standard clinical examination may easily reveal the tumour in the nasal cavity or nasopharynx, but CT scanning best demonstrates the extent of the tumour and its accompanying bony erosion. MRI scanning will further define the soft-tissue extent and with these two modern investigations angiographic evaluation is rarely indicated.

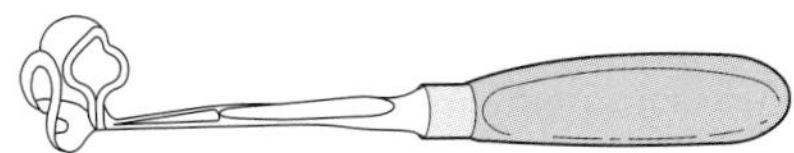

Fig. 43.15 St Clair Thomson's adenoid curette.

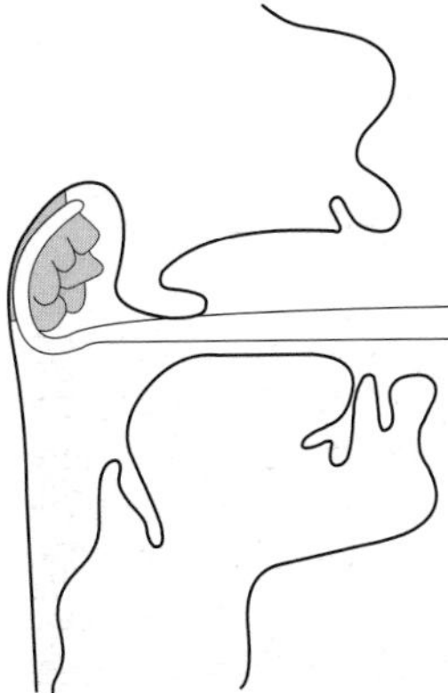

Fig. 43.16 Curettage of the adenoid.

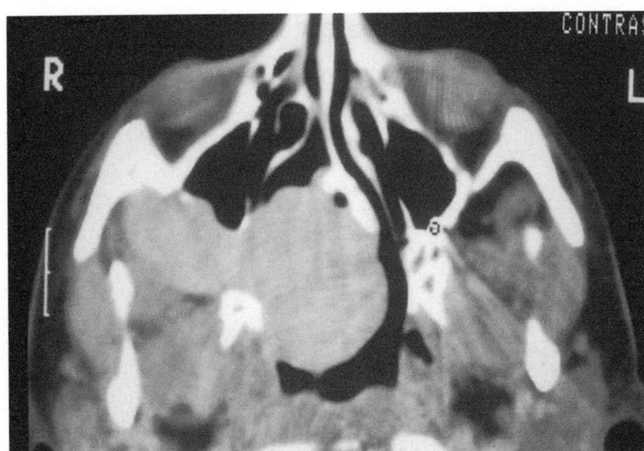

Fig. 43.17 Axial CT scan showing juvenile angiofibroma presenting in the nasopharynx and nasal cavity with erosion of the medial pterygoid plate and extension into infratemporal fossa.

Sir St Clair Thomson, 1859–1943. Surgeon, Ear Nose and Throat Department, King's College Hospital, London, England.

Biopsy should be avoided unless clinical and radiological examination is not clear. There should be definite reasons for undertaking biopsy, and matched blood must be in readiness and the surgeon prepared to deal with the haemorrhage.

Whilst radiotherapy has occasionally been advocated, surgical resection is by the far commonest management worldwide and requires an adequate exposure of the entire region either through a midfacial degloving approach or a lateral rhinotomy (Figs 43.18 and 43.19). Both of these approaches allow ligation of the feeding maxillary artery. A transpalatal approach may be used for the smaller tumours but this does not give full control of any potential bleeding.

Antrochoanal polyp. This relatively uncommon lesion is not a tumour but a simple mucosal polyp. It does not arise in the nasopharynx, but from the maxillary antrum, from which it prolapses into the nasal cavity and thence expands backwards into the nasopharynx and occasionally down into the oropharynx (Figs 43.20 and 43.21). It also commonly occurs in young males, and therefore may mimic a tumour of the nasal cavity or nasopharynx. It is distinguished clinically from an angiofibroma by its avascularity, pale colour, its site of origin on endoscopic examination and imaging, as it is a simple mucosal polyp. Whilst it may be removed intranasally by an avulsion snare, a portion often remains in the antrum producing recurrent symptoms and it requires complete removal via an endoscopic approach through the middle meatus or, occasionally, a Caldwell–Luc procedure to prevent recurrence.

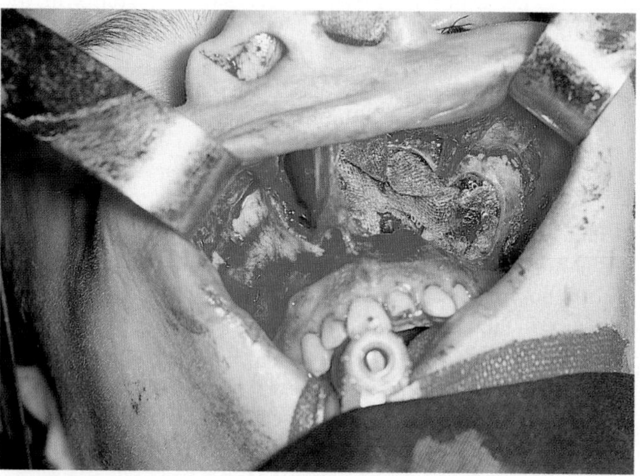

Fig. 43.18 Intraoperative photograph showing exposure during midfacial degloving approach.

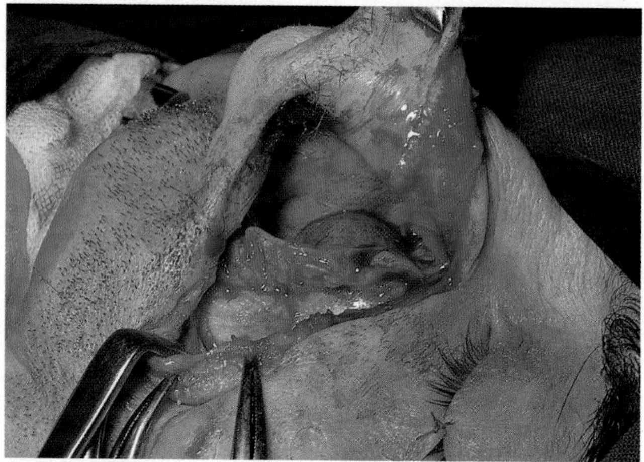

Fig. 43.19 Intraoperative photograph showing an incision in lateral rhinotomy.

Malignant. Nasopharyngeal carcinoma is an interesting squamous cell carcinoma with a very variable incidence. In most parts of the world the tumour is rare with an incidence of less than one person in 100 000 per year. However, it is a common tumour amongst southern Chinese, and this high-risk population has rates of 30–50 people per 100 000 per year. In the rest of China there are substantial variations in the incidence but, in general, the incidence decreases from south to north. Higher frequencies of nasopharyngeal carcinoma are also observed in emigrant southern Chinese populations in south-east Asia and elsewhere around the world, and it is also more common amongst Eskimo, the Kadazans in East Malaysia and parts of northern Africa. It is now well accepted that mechanisms leading to development of a cancer often involve a multistep process, and the aetiology of nasopharyngeal carcinoma is most likely to be multifactorial with no single cause adequately explaining the epidemiology of the disease. However, it is also clear that three well-defined major aetiological factors are involved in its development (Table 43.3). The exact mechanism as to how these factors act is not yet fully understood. The majority of squamous carcinomas of the nasopharynx is undifferentiated and the morphology of this tumour is characteristic. Only a few are well-differentiated squamous carcinomas, and these two lesions make up over 90 per cent of nasopharyngeal malignancy in endemic areas. Other rare epithelial tumours are adenocarcinoma and adenoid cystic carcinoma. B- and T-cell lymphomas also occur in this region and should not be confused with the more common undifferentiated carcinoma.

Nasopharyngeal carcinoma affects a younger age group of the population than almost any other head and neck neoplasm. In endemic regions at least 60 per cent of patients are under 50 years of age and this applies to both sexes.

Clinical features. Symptoms are closely related to the position of the tumour in the nasopharynx and the degree of distant spread which may be present. Early symptoms are often minimal in nature and thus liable to be ignored by both patient and doctor.

- Approximately half the patients will present with a mass in the neck. This percentage is even higher in patients under 21 years of age. It indicates that the tumour has already reached an advanced stage. Fine needle aspirate or a biopsy of a neck node showing undifferentiated carcinoma requires immediate thorough examination of the nasopharynx.
- The nasopharynx may look normal or only minimally asymmetric but contain submucosal nasopharyngeal carcinoma. Nasal complaints occur in one-third of patients and aural symptoms of unilateral deafness, as a consequence of

Table 43.3 Aetiological factors of nasopharyngeal carcinoma

- Genetic, e.g. Cantonese
- Infective, e.g. Epstein–Barr virus
- Environmental, e.g. salted fish

eustachian tube obstruction and secretory otitis media, occur in approximately 20 per cent. Neurological complications with cranial nerve palsies due to disease on the skull base occur relatively late in the disease but are a poor prognostic factor.

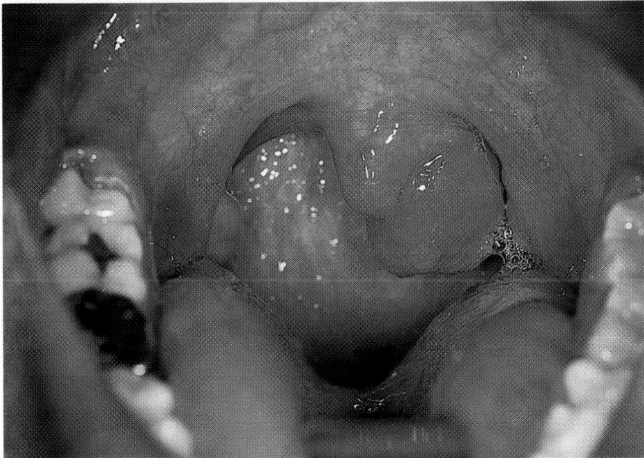

Fig. 43.20 Intraoral view showing a fleshy polyp hanging in the oropharynx.

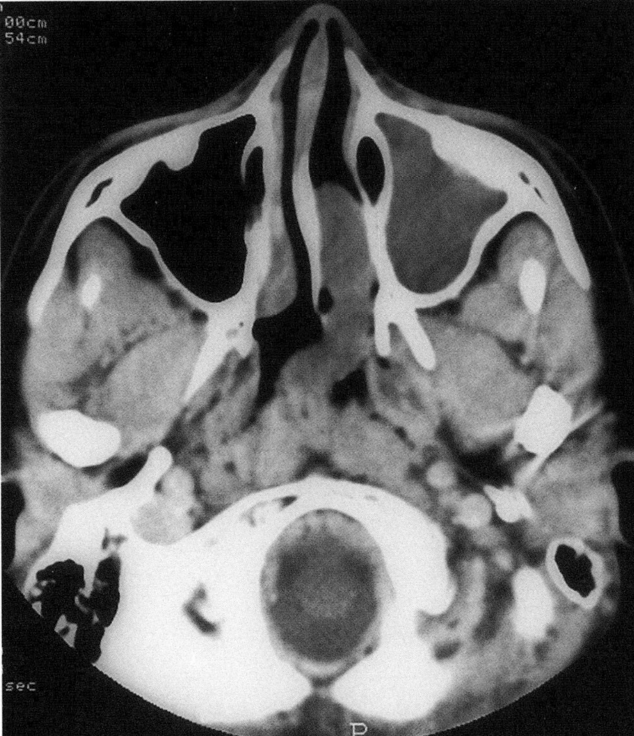

Fig. 43.21 Axial CT of an antrochoanal polyp (as seen in Fig. 43.20) with opaque maxillary antrum, and a mass in the nasal cavity and nasopharynx.

A biopsy of the nasopharynx is mandatory if there is suspicion of nasopharyngeal malignancy.

The traditional method of indirect examination with a mirror, although adequate in some patients, has been superseded by direct inspection carried out by a flexible or rigid nasendoscope. If topical anaesthesia is used, a biopsy may be taken. Serological investigation for Epstein–Barr virus-associated antigenic markers, in combination with the clinical and histological examination, is valuable for the early detection of disease. Highly sensitive assays for antiviral antibodies, together with the newly discovered virus-associated serological markers, are assisting not only in the early detection but in the treatment and control of this disease. IgA antiviral capsid antigen (VCA) antibody has recently been evaluated in mass surveys in southern China and has been found to be an excellent screening method for the early detection of nasopharyngeal carcinoma in high-risk groups.

Imaging. Imaging is essential to determine the extent of the disease and to enable correct staging. In areas where CT and MRI are available plain film radiography of the nasopharynx and other ancillary methods, such as xerography and tomography, have now been superseded. A chest X-ray, however, should still be performed. CT has a major role in determining the size and position of the tumour essential for radiotherapy planning and assessing the response to treatment, diagnosing recurrence and detecting complications.

Treatment. Primary treatment of nasopharyngeal carcinoma is radiotherapy. The majority of the tumours belongs to the radiosensitive undifferentiated squamous cell group. With the advent of CT, precise radiotherapy treatment planning is now possible and brachytherapy (intracavitary and interstitial radiotherapy) and chemotherapy are increasingly added in the management plan. Elective external radiotherapy is given to the neck in all cases, even when no neck nodes are apparent. For early disease, 3-year disease-free survival rates of more than 75 per cent are now common. However, late disease has figures of only 30–50 per cent for 3-year disease-free survival. Although the benefit of modern radiotherapy is beyond doubt, the value of additional chemotherapy remains debated, but it is likely that a combination of chemotherapy and radiotherapy will produce better locoregional control of the tumour. Surgery is reserved for recurrent disease in neck nodes and the occasional removal of recurrent skull base disease which has not responded to additional radiotherapy or chemotherapy.

Oropharynx

Acute tonsillitis

This common condition is characterised by a sore throat, fever, general malaise, dysphagia, enlarged upper cervical nodes and sometimes referred otalgia. Approximately half the cases are bacterial, the most common cause being a

Michael Anthony Epstein, b. 1921. English pathologist, Bristol, England.
Y.M. Barr, b. 1932. English pathologist, Bristol, England.

Table 43.4 Nasopharyngeal carcinoma: main presenting complaints

1. Systemic
   - Cervical lymphadenopathy
2. Local
   - Unilateral serous otitis media, otalgia
   - Nasal obstruction, bloody discharge, epistaxis
   - Cranial nerve palsies, especially III–VI then IX–XII

pyogenic group A streptococcus. The remainder is viral and a wide variety of viruses has been implicated; in particular, infectious mononucleosis may frequently be mistaken for bacterial tonsillitis. On examination the tonsils are swollen and erythematous, and yellow or white pustules may be seen on the palatine tonsils, hence the name 'follicular tonsillitis'. A throat swab should be taken at the time of examination and blood for Paul–Bunnell testing (Fig. 43.22).

Treatment. Paracetamol or similar analgesia may be administered to relieve pain and gargles of glycerol–thymol are soothing. The condition is frequently sensitive to benzyl or phenyoxymethylpenicillin (penicillin V) and these are given until antibiotic sensitivities are known. Ampicillin is avoided as it may exacerbate the situation and precipitate a rash in patients with infectious mononucleosis. Most cases resolve in a few days.

Quinsy

This is the formation of an abscess in the peritonsillar region causing severe pain and trismus, and most usually associated with streptococcal infection (see Fig. 43.23). Trismus caused by spasm induced in the pterygoid muscles from the spreading infection may make examination difficult. This may be overcome by the instillation of local anaesthesia into the posterior nasal cavity (thereby anaesthetising the sphenopalatine ganglion) and directly into the oropharynx. This simple manoeuvre aids subsequent examination which should be carried out with good illumination and suction. A diffuse swelling of the soft palate just superior to the involved tonsil is seen displacing the uvula medially and, in more advanced cases, there may be an area of pus pointing underneath the thin mucosa.

Treatment. In the early stages where no distinct abscess is pointing, intravenous broad-spectrum antibiotics are indicated and may produce resolution. However, if there is frank abscess formation, incision and drainage of the pus can be carried out under local anaesthesia (Fig. 43.24). A small scalpel is best modified by winding a strip of adhesive tape around the blade so that only 1 cm of the blade projects. In teenagers and young adults the patient sits upright and an incision is made in the position shown in Fig. 43.24. This is approximately mid-way between the base of the uvula and

John R. Paul, b. 1893. American physician.
Walls W. Bunnell, b. 1902. American physician.

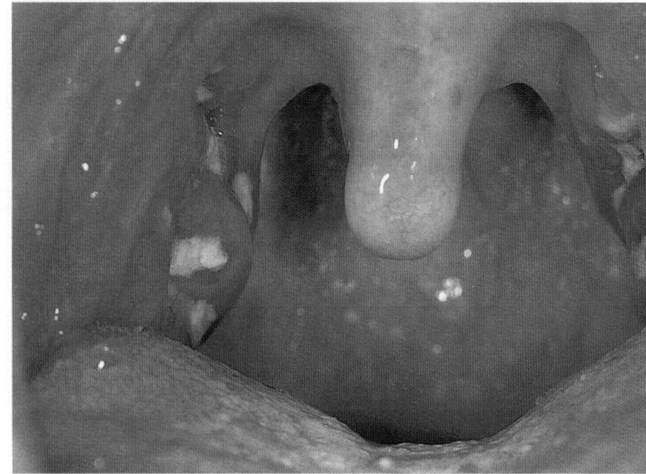

Fig. 43.22 Photograph showing acute follicular tonsillitis.

the third upper molar tooth. This may produce immediate release of pus but, if not, dressing forceps are now pushed firmly through the incision directly backwards and, on opening, pus may then be encountered. In small children general anaesthesia may be required.

Chronic tonsillitis

Chronic tonsillitis usually results from repeat attacks of acute tonsillitis in which the tonsils become progressively damaged and provide a reservoir for infective organisms.

Tonsillectomy. Indications for tonsillectomy may be divided into absolute or relative (Table 43.5). When the size of the tonsils is contributing to airway obstruction or a malignancy of the tonsils is suspected, the decision to perform tonsillectomy is relatively straightforward. Complete tonsillectomy is preferable to wedge biopsies when squamous cell carcinoma is suspected, and bilateral tonsillectomy is performed in the case of suspected lymphoma as part of the staging process.

Considerable interest now focuses on the area of sleep apnoea and related problems. Patients should be admitted for

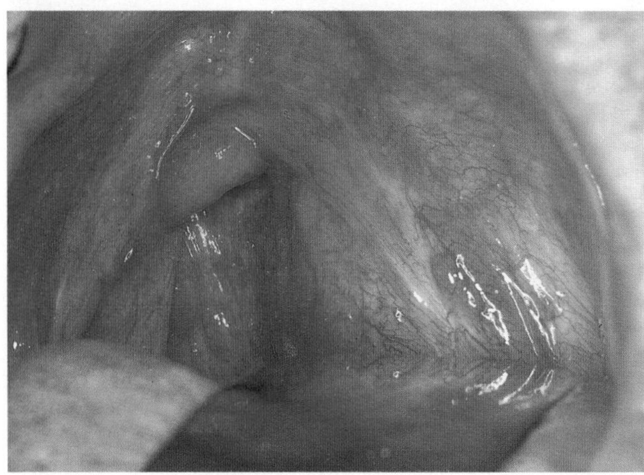

Fig. 43.23 Photograph showing quinsy (peritonsillar abscess).

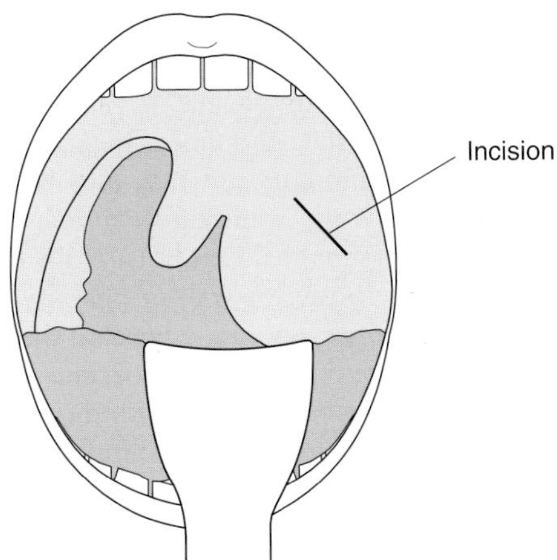

Fig. 43.24 Site of incision in peritonsillar abscess.

formal sleep studies to establish the exact extent and site of the problem following which a variety of medical and surgical treatments may be deemed appropriate, one of which is tonsillectomy.

Recurrent acute tonsillitis is the commonest relative indication for tonsillectomy in children and adolescents, although it is important that these attacks are well documented and do not simply constitute a minor sore throat usually of viral origin and of short duration. Chronic tonsillitis more frequently affects young adults in whom it is important to establish that chronic mouth breathing secondary to nasal obstruction is not the main problem rather than the tonsils themselves.

Ideally, the procedure should be undertaken when the tonsils are not acutely infected, and it is important to discuss factors which may increase the tendency to bleed. Blood transfusion is rarely required but it is normal practice to perform a 'group and save' in children under 15 kg in weight.

Dissection tonsillectomy is carried out under general anaesthesia during which the patient lies supine with the head extended and with the surgeon sitting at the end of the operating table. The mucosa of the anterior faucial pillar is incised and the tonsil capsule identified. Using blunt dissection the surgeon separates the tonsil from its bed until only a small inferior pedicle is left (Fig. 43.25). Usually a snare is used to separate it from the lingual tonsil. Ribbon gauze is placed in the tonsillar bed and pressure applied for some minutes following which bleeding points may be controlled by ligature or by bipolar diathermy. Following surgery, the patient is kept under close observation for any systemic or local evidence of bleeding with regular monitoring of pulse and blood pressure, and observation to see whether the patient is swallowing excessively (Fig. 43.26). The patient is kept nil by mouth for the first few hours in case an immediate (or reactionary) haemorrhage should necessitate a return to theatre. After this period the patient is encouraged to use the mouth and a normal diet rapidly instituted. Paracetamol is preferred to aspirin-containing analgesics. Patients are generally allowed home on the following day and are warned that they may experience otalgia due to referred pain from the glossopharyngeal nerve and that late (or secondary) haemorrhage may occur up to 10 days following the surgery, which would necessitate their immediate return to hospital.

Table 43.5 Indications for tonsillectomy

1. Absolute
   - Sleep apnoea, chronic upper respiratory tract obstruction, cor pulmonale
   - Suspected tonsillar malignancy
2. Relative
   - Documented recurrent acute tonsillitis
   - Chronic tonsillitis
   - Peritonsillar abscess (quinsy)
   - Tonsillitis resulting in febrile convulsions
   - Diphtheria carriers
   - Systemic disease due to β-haemolytic streptococcus (nephritis, rheumatic fever)

Haemorrhage is obviously the most common complication, occurring in the immediate postoperative period (Table 43.6). Local pressure, hydrogen peroxide, gargles and general supportive measures may help in mild cases, but it is generally wisest to return to theatre for definitive treatment particularly in younger patients. Blood loss is replaced with crystalloid whilst a cross-match is performed, and frequent observations of blood pressure, pulse and respiratory rate are made. Adequate analgesia is given without causing respiratory depression. With the patient seated upright in bed the mouth is examined under reasonable illumination to determine the site of bleeding and if possible to suction away clots from the tonsillar fossa. A swab soaked in 1 in 1000 adrenaline may be held against the bleeding area in a co-operative patient, but if this is not possible and/or the bleeding persists theatre should be alerted. Under general anaesthesia it may be possible to identify a bleeding spot, but often a more generalised ooze is observed and suturing of the tonsil bed combined with the

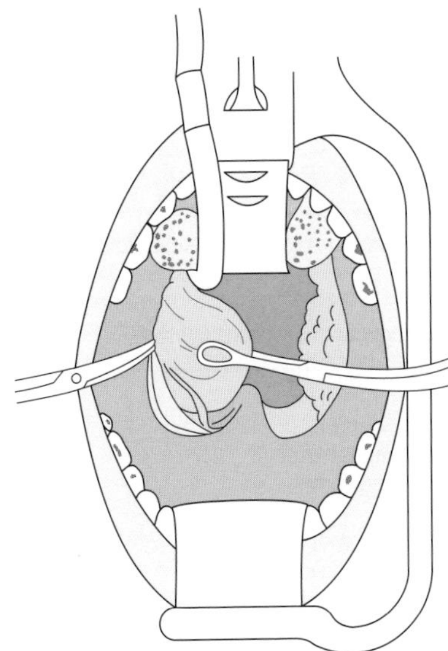

Fig. 43.25 Removal of the tonsils.

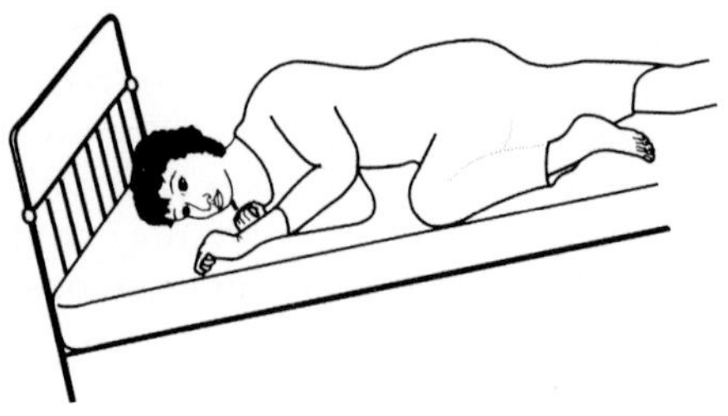

Fig. 43.26 Positioning of the patient after tonsillectomy.

application of Surgicel and bipolar diathermy is often more successful than attempted placement of ligatures.

Late haemorrhage is generally secondary to infection and patients should be immediately commenced on intravenous antibiotics with aerobic and anaerobic cover. Significant or persistent bleeding may require a further general anaesthetic and undersewing of the surgical bed, which by this time will often be covered with slough and granulation tissue. Post-operative tonsillar haemorrhage must still be regarded as a serious and life-threatening complication and should not be underestimated, particularly in the younger patient.

Parapharyngeal and retropharyngeal abscess

Parapharyngeal abscess. The parapharyngeal abscess may be confused with a peritonsillar abscess but the maximal swelling is *behind* the posterior faucial pillar and there may be little oedema of the soft palate. The patient is usually a young child and there may be a severe degree of general malaise. With an obvious abscess pointing into the oropharynx, drainage may be carried out with a blunt instrument or the gloved finger but general anaesthesia is frequently required and the expertise of a senior anaesthetist, good illumination and good suction are absolutely essential. A large parapharyngeal abscess may compromise both the airway and swallowing. In the earlier cases admission to hospital and the institution of fluid replacements coupled with intravenous antibiotics may produce resolution. The advanced cases also require intravenous antibiotics.

Acute retropharyngeal abscess

This is the result of suppuration of the prevertebral lymph nodes and, again, is most commonly seen in children with most of the cases occurring in those under 1 year of age. It is associated with infection of the tonsils, nasopharynx or oropharynx, and is frequently accompanied by severe general malaise, neck rigidity, dysphagia, drooling, a croupy cough, an altered cry and marked dyspnoea. Indeed, dyspnoea may be the prominent symptom, and may also be accompanied by febrile convulsions and vomiting.

Table 43.6 Complications of tonsillectomy

1. Anaesthetic
   - Traumatic intubation
   - Cardiopulmonary arrest
   - Malignant hyperthermia
2. Surgical
   - Haemorrhage (immediate or late)
   - Infection
   - Pain/otalgia
   - Postoperative airway obstruction
   - Velopharyngeal insufficiency

These children should always be carefully examined, and an inspection of the posterior wall of pharynx may show gross swelling and an abscess pointing beneath the thinned mucosa. In countries where diphtheria still occurs, an acute retropharyngeal abscess may be confused with this but the presence of the greyish-green membrane aids differentiation. Occasionally, a foreign body, most commonly a fish bone which has perforated the posterior pharyngeal mucosa, will give rise to an abscess in this situation in older children and young adults.

These patients should be admitted to hospital and intravenous antibiotics instituted immediately. Surgical drainage of the abscess may not be necessary but, if so, requires experienced anaesthesia as on induction care must be taken to avoid rupturing the abscess. The airway is protected by placing the child in a head-down position whilst a pair of dressing forceps guided by the finger may be thrust into an obvious abscess in the posterior wall with the contents being evacuated. On other occasions an approach anterior and medial to the carotid sheath via a cervical incision may be required.

Chronic retropharyngeal abscess

This condition is now rare and most commonly the result of an extension of tuberculosis of the cervical spine which has spread through the anterior longitudinal ligament to reach the retropharyngeal space. In contrast to the acute retropharyngeal abscess, this condition occurs almost solely in adults and radiology usually shows evidence of bone destruction and loss of the normal curvature of the cervical spine. The spine may be quite unstable and undue manipulation may precipitate a neurological event. In addition to the retropharyngeal swelling seen intraorally, there may be fullness behind the sternocleidomastoid muscle on one side. A chronic retropharyngeal abscess must not be opened into the mouth, as such a procedure may lead to secondary infection. Drainage of the abscess may not be necessary if suitable treatment of the underlying tuberculosis disease is instituted. If it is necessary then it should be carried out through a cervical incision anterior to the sternocleidomastoid muscle with an approach anterior and medial to the carotid sheath to the retropharyngeal space. The cavity is opened and suctioned dry after taking biopsy material. Occasionally surgery is required to decompress the spinal cord if there is a progressive neurological deficit.

Glandular fever (infectious mononucleosis)

This systemic condition is usually caused by Epstein–Barr virus but similar features can be due to cytomegalovirus or toxoplasmosis.

Clinical features. The tonsils are typically erythematous with a creamy-grey exudate, and they appear almost confluent and usually symmetrical in contradistinction to a quinsy. In addition to the discomfort and dysphagia, the patient may drool saliva and have respiratory difficulty, particularly on inspiration. They commonly have a high temperature and gross general malaise with other notable cervical or generalised lymphadenopathy. Occasionally an enlarged spleen or liver may be detected. These features most commonly occur in teenagers and young adults, and diagnosis can be confirmed by serological testing showing a positive Paul–Bunnell test, an absolute and relative lymphocytosis, and the presence of atypical monocytes in the peripheral blood.

Treatment. Analgesia and maintenance of fluid intake are important. A small number of patients requires admission to hospital if the airway is compromised and a short course of steroids may be helpful. If this is necessary it should only be carried out as an in-patient where the airway can be constantly monitored. Antibiotics are of little value and, indeed, ampicillin is contraindicated because of the frequent appearance of a widespread skin rash.

Human immunodeficiency virus

The human immunodeficiency virus (HIV) is the causative agent of acquired immunodeficiency syndrome (AIDS) which, although it was initially associated with intravenous drug users and homosexual males, is now spreading in many parts of the world to affect the heterosexual community. It can affect almost all of the head and neck structures at any point during the disease. The initial seroconversion may present with the symptoms of glandular fever which is followed by an asymptomatic period of variable length. In the pre-AIDS period, prior to the full-blown symptoms of the AIDS-related complex, many patients have minor upper respiratory tract symptoms which are often overlooked such as otitis externa, rhinosinusitis and a nonspecific pharyngitis. As the patient moves into the full-blown AIDS-related complex a persistent generalised lymphadenopathy is frequently found affecting the cervical nodes which is usually due to follicular hyperplasia. However, patients may also develop tumours such as Kaposi's sarcoma, sometimes seen in the oral cavity, and high-grade malignant B-cell lymphoma affecting the cervical lymph nodes and nasopharynx. In addition, multiple ulcers may be found in the oral cavity or pharynx associated with herpes infection. Severe candida may affect the oral cavity pharynx or even larynx, and a hairy leucoplakia may affect the tongue (Fig. 43.27). There is also an increased incidence of squamous cell carcinoma of the oral cavity.

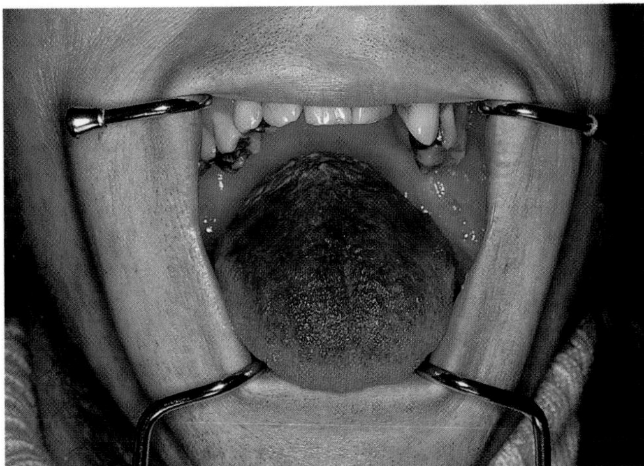

Fig. 43.27 Intraoral view showing hairy tongue in an HIV-positive patient.

The globus syndrome

A wide variety of patients has a predominant symptom of a feeling of a lump in the throat (Latin: globus = lump). The symptom most commonly affects adults between 30 and 60 years of age. This feeling is not true dysphagia as there is no difficulty in swallowing. Most patients notice the symptom more if they swallow their own saliva, i.e. a forced dry swallow, rather than when they eat or drink. The aetiology of this common symptom is unknown but some patients may have gastro-oesophageal reflux or spasm of their cricopharyngeus muscle. The symptom may be associated with the presence of a pharyngeal pouch, or tumours in the oropharynx, hypopharynx or upper oesophagus.

The original name of globus hystericus is unhelpful and although these patients may be anxious and at times introverted, they none the less require full examination to exclude local disease. Radiological and endoscopic investigation may be necessary to exclude an underlying cause.

Pharyngeal pouch

The pouch is a protusion of mucosa through Killian's dehiscence, a weak area of the posterior pharyngeal wall between the oblique fibres of thyropharyngeus and the transverse fibres of cricopharyngeus at the lower end of the inferior constrictor muscle. These fibres, along with the circular fibres of the upper oesophagus, form the physiological upper oesophageal sphincter mechanism. Quite why the pouch forms is not yet clear even with modern videofluoroscopic and manometric studies. Many patients with pharyngeal pouches have been demonstrated to have normal relaxation of the upper oesophageal sphincter mechanism in relation to swallowing, but others have been shown to have incomplete pharyngeal relaxation, early cricopharyngeal contraction and abnormalities of the pharyngeal contraction wave. As the pouch enlarges the resistance of the vertebral column behind usually causes it to turn laterally to the left (Fig. 43.28).

Clinical features. Patients suffering from this condition are commonly more than 60 years of age and it is twice as common in women as in men.

In the initial phases when there is a small diverticulum the patients may present with globus-type symptoms of a feeling of something in the throat or minor difficulties and slight regurgitation on swallowing. A videofluoroscopic or barium swallow study may show abnormalities of the upper

Moritz K. Kaposi, 1837–1902. Dermatologist, Vienna, Austria.

oesophageal sphincter in association with the small pouch. As the diverticulum enlarges patients may experience regurgitation of undigested food sometimes hours after a meal, particularly if they are bending down or turning over in bed at night. They are sometimes awoken at night with a feeling of tightness in the throat and a fit of coughing. Occasionally they may present with recurrent unexplained chest infections as a result of small amounts of liquid and food being aspirated from the pouch. As the pouch increases in size the patients may notice gurgling noises from the neck on swallowing and the pouch may become large enough to form a visible swelling in the neck. This swelling may increase when the patient drinks and, indeed, there may be increasing difficulty with swallowing associated with weight loss and cachexia.

Radiological examination. If a pharyngeal pouch is suspected, this is an extremely useful examination. A thin emulsion of barium is given to the patient as a barium swallow (Fig. 43.29) or, better still, as part of a videofluoroscopic swallowing study. Care should be exercised in patients who cough on swallowing indicating they may have aspiration. Just a few millilitres of barium is sufficient to outline the pharynx pouch and upper oesophagus. The videofluoroscopic study gives additional information about the pharyngeal contraction waves and the performance of the upper oesophageal sphincter. Occasionally there is an associated hiatus hernia at the lower end of the oesophagus and this should be excluded. A chest X-ray is important to exclude aspiration pneumonitis.

Rigid oeosophagoscopy or pharyngoscopy under general anaesthesia is unnecessary for diagnosis and may be dangerous. When the diagnosis is unsuspected, oesophagoscopy performed without realising the pathology may be associated with the tip of the oesophagoscope entering the pouch and perforating the fundus. Subsequent mediastinitis is associated with a high mortality.

Treatment. Surgery is indicated when the pouch is associated with progressive symptoms, and particularly when a prominent cricopharyngeal bar of muscle associated with abnormality of the upper oesophageal sphincter mechanism causes considerable dysphagia. In very elderly patients a decision to operate may be offset by the general condition of the patient. Preoperative physiotherapy and attention to the respiratory, cardiovascular and nutritional aspects of the patient are important. Preoperative chest physiotherapy and perioperative antibiotics are recommended. In the classical operation the opening to the pouch is first identified using a pharyngoscope and a nasogastric tube placed into the oesophageal lumen to allow postoperative nutrition. This initial endoscopy is often difficult because the normal oesophageal opening is small compared with the lumen of the pouch but it may be facilitated by using a Dohlmann' s rigid endoscope which allows better visualisation. The nasogastric tube allows identification of the oesophagus subsequently by palpation and facilitates the myotomy, in addition to allowing postoperative feeding. The pouch may be packed with ribbon gauze soaked in proflavin solution to aid identification of the neck of the pouch.

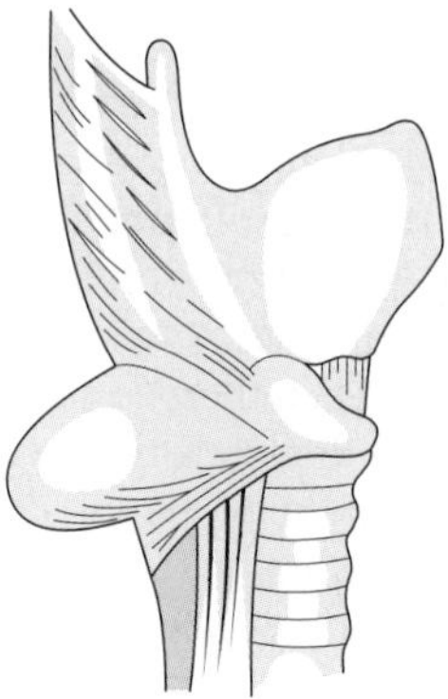

Fig. 43.28 Diagram of a pharyngeal pouch.

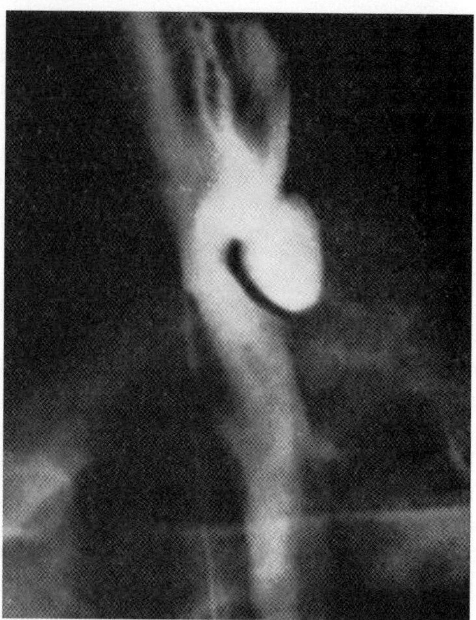

Fig. 43.29 Barium swallow showing a pharyngeal pouch.

A lower neck incision along the anterior border of the left sternocleidomastoid muscle, or a transverse crease incision, is then used and the sternocleidomastoid muscle and carotid sheath are retracted laterally and the trachea and larynx medially. The middle thyroid vein is divided and, if necessary, the inferior thyroid artery is found and ligated well laterally. The retropharyngeal space is entered above the inferior corner of the thyroid cartilage, thereby avoiding risk of damage to the recurrent laryngeal nerve. The pouch is found medially behind the lower pharynx and is carefully isolated and dissected back to its origin at Killian's dehiscence. It may then be excised and the pharynx closed in two layers or, if it is small, it may invaginated into the pharyngeal lumen before closing the muscle layers. In all cases a myotomy dividing the fibres of the cricopharygeus muscle and the upper oesophageal circular muscle fibres must be performed. The wound is usually closed with drainage and the patient fed through the nasogastric tube for 3–7 days.

Complications. This classic operation has been associated with wound infection, mediastinitis, pharyngeal fistula formation and stenosis of the upper oesophagus. Variations have been tried which include simply hitching up the pouch into a superior position without excising it, thus allowing the fundus and body to empty continuously into the oesophagus. This is unsatisfactory with the larger pouches. Endoscopic division of the bar of muscle forming the anterior wall of the pouch and the posterior aspect of the lumen of the oesophagus has been advocated for many years using Dohlmann's instruments and, more recently, a laser applied via a special pharyngoscope. There is increasing evidence that both the open operative intervention and previous endoscopic techniques can be improved by using an endoscopic stapling technique, whereby a specialised staple gun is passed down a modified pharyngoscope which safely divides the anterior wall of the pouch and the posterior wall of the oesophagus. This completes a full myotomy and allows any food and fluid to drain from the pouch directly down the oesophagus. The staples provide an instant two-layer closure at the site of division, and this endoscopic technique is associated with very low morbidity and a high success rate for the relief of the patient's symptoms. Low morbidity is particularly important in this elderly group of patients.

Sideropenic dysphagia

Prolonged iron deficiency anaemia may lead to dysphagia, particularly in middle-aged females. In addition, they may have koilonychia, cheilosis and angular stomatitis, together with lassitude and poor exercise tolerance. The dysphagia is caused by a postcricoid web, and these patients have a higher incidence of postcricoid malignancy. Prognosis of these postcricoid tumours is very poor, requiring radical treatment with radiotherapy and major surgery, and it is therefore important to prevent this problem by recognition and treatment of the anaemia. The syndrome is associated with the names of Plummer and Vinson, and Patterson and Brown Kelly.

Tumours of the oropharynx

Benign

Benign tumours of the oropharynx are rare, papillomas being the most common. These are usually incidental findings and are rarely of any importance.

Malignant

The most important epithelial tumour is squamous cell carcinoma, which constitutes roughly 90 per cent of all epithelial tumours in the upper aerodigestive tract (Figs 43.30 and 43.31). In the oropharynx the proportion is less (70 per cent) because of the higher incidence of lymphoma (25 per cent) and salivary gland tumours (5 per cent).

Aetiology

Squamous carcinomas of the oropharynx have strong associations with cigarette smoking and the consumption of alcohol, and these two factors cause varying incidence throughout the world. In countries where the consumption of tobacco and alcohol is associated with poor oral hygiene these malignancies assume major importance. Due to the rich lymphatic drainage of the oropharynx, cervical node metastatases are common. They may be the only presenting feature with an apparent occult primary often being unsuspected and missed in the tonsil or tongue base.

The majority of lymph node metastases from oropharyngeal squamous carcinomas is to the jugulodigastric node. This is the commonest site for the so-called 'branchial cyst carcinoma', but several studies in recent times have shown that this is probably an extremely rare pathology and that usually the diagnosis represents cystic degeneration in a jugulodigastric node from a small undetected primary squamous carcinoma in the tonsil or tongue base. Squamous cell carcinomas are most common in the sixth and seventh decades and more frequent in men.

Treatment

Treatment patterns vary with facilities, but early tumours may be cured by radiotherapy, laser excision or more conventional excision. Recurrent disease following radiotherapy is managed surgically, and repair of the oropharynx may require regionally based myocutaneous flaps or free flaps with microvascular anastomosis. Neck dissection is required in a large proportion of cases of advanced disease. Postoperative dysphagia with aspiration, as a result of interference in the complex neuromuscular control of the second phase of swallowing, is a particular problem in these patients. More advanced tumours may also require additional resection of the mandible or an associated total laryngectomy, so this type of surgery is best carried out in a centre undertaking this work on a regular basis.

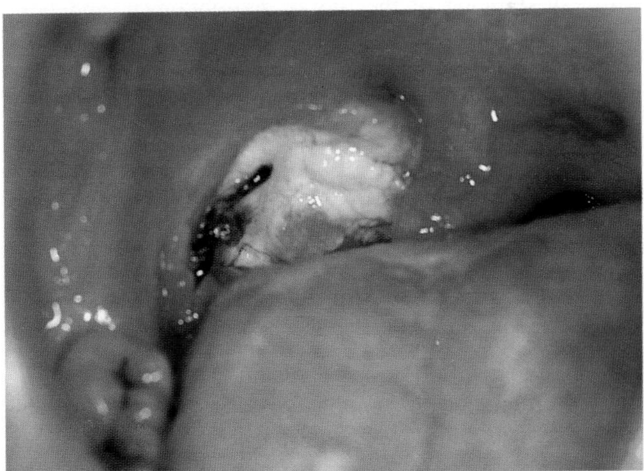

Fig. 43.30 Squamous cell carcinoma of the right tonsil.

Henry S. Plummer, 1874–1957. Physician, Mayo Clinic, Rochester, Minnesota, USA.

Donald Rose Patterson, 1862–1939. Surgeon, Ear, Nose and Throat Department, Royal Infirmary, Cardiff, Wales.

Adam Brown Kelly, 1865–1941. Surgeon, Ear, Nose and Throat Department, Victoria Infirmary, Glasgow, Scotland.

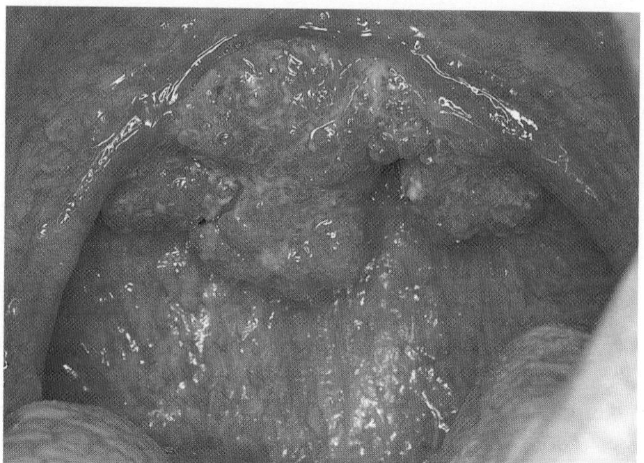

Fig. 43.31 Squamous cell carcinoma of the soft palate.

Lymphoma of the head and neck

Lymphomas of the head and neck may arise in nodal or extranodal sites, and both Hodgkin's disease and nonHodgkin's lymphoma commonly present as lymph node enlargement in the neck. Hodgkin's disease is rare in the oropharynx, but nonHodgkin's lymphoma accounts for 15–20 per cent of tumours at this site in some countries. Most are of the B-cell type and have features in common with other tumours of MALT sites. Many of the lymphomas of the oropharynx have no demonstrable deposit elsewhere in the body when a full lymphoma investigation is carried out. On occasions, however, they may be secondary or coincident with deposits at other sites in the neck, the gastrointestinal tract, lung and the testes. Further evaluation with CT scanning of the thorax and abdomen, and bone marrow evaluation are essential. Radiotherapy is undoubtedly the treatment of choice for localised nonHodgkin's lymphoma and may give control rates as high as 75 per cent at 5 years. For disseminated nonHodgkin's lymphoma the treatment of choice is systemic chemotherapy. Combination chemotherapy is used in patients with an unfavourable histological type.

Tumours of the hypopharynx

Benign

Benign tumours of the hypopharynx are very rare, the most common being the fibroma and the leiomyoma. These are polypoid tumours which usually present with dysphagia and are seen on videofluoroscopy or barium swallow. They show a smooth constant mass lying in the lumen of the hypopharynx or oesophagus.

Thomas Hodgkin, 1798–1866. Physician, Guy's Hospital, London, England.

Malignant

Malignant tumours of the hypopharynx are almost exclusively squamous cell carcinoma with a predominance of moderate and poor differentiation. The tumours are usually classified according to their anatomical site of origin from the piriform fossa, postcricoid region or posterior pharyngeal wall but, as mentioned in the section on pharyngeal anatomy, it can be difficult to determine the site of origin when a tumour has spread to involve one or more of these areas. Even differentiation between laryngeal and hypopharyngeal tumours can be difficult in the advanced disease when the aryepiglottic fold has been replaced or covered by tumours. Marked differences in the incidence of these tumours occur throughout the world in association with factors such as iron deficiency anaemia (see subsection on Sideropenic dysphagia) and they may be associated with marked submucosal spread of 10 mm or more which further complicates their evaluation.

- Tumours arising from the piriform fossa and posterior pharyngeal wall may spread to upper or lower cervical nodes. Tumours arising in the postcricoid area typically metastasise to paratracheal and paraoesophageal nodes which may not be palpable. As with oropharyngeal tumours, alcohol and tobacco are two principal carcinogens implicated in these tumours. Postcricoid carcinoma, although essentially a rare disease, is more common in women than men.
- The diagnosis of hypopharyngeal carcinoma should be considered in all patients presenting with dysphagia or hoarseness, particularly if they have a history of iron deficiency and anaemia, smoking or significant alcohol consumption.

On examination indirect laryngoscopy may show only subtle signs of disease such as oedema or pooling of saliva unilaterally in a piriform fossa, or diminution of vocal fold mobility. All regions of the neck must be assessed in a systematic manner. Fine needle aspirate is advocated for suspicious nodes. A suspected primary may require videofluoroscopy or barium swallow study, endoscopy and biopsy, and CT or MRI scanning if available. A chest X-ray should be taken to detect a second primary or metastasis.

Treatment

Squamous carcinoma of the hyopharynx commonly presents late and carries a poor prognosis. Early lesions may be treated with radiotherapy alone, and surgery is generally used for recurrence after radiotherapy or as primary excision in advanced disease. Total pharyngolaryngectomy is commonly required and, for lesions extending into the upper oesophagus, oesophagectomy and total thyroidectomy may additionally be needed.

Reconstruction of the excised pharynx and/or oesophagus may be undertaken by the use of a myocutaneous flap, free jejunal transfer or gastric transposition. These major surgical techniques require excellent preoperative preparation of the patient and surgical teams with a high standard of expertise as they have a potential mortality and a wide variety of complications. Swallowing and voice rehabilitation are necessary to support patients after this major surgery if they are to adjust themselves and maintain some quality of life.

Cytotoxic drugs have not been found to have significant value as an adjunct to surgery or radiotherapy in the treatment of patients with hypopharyngeal squamous carcinoma. It is to be hoped in the future that they will produce better results so that the major surgery and its associated debility can be avoided. Before deciding to give chemotherapy in any form of squamous carcinoma of the head and neck one has to balance the prognosis of the disease against the expected relief and possible toxic side effects. The most commonly used agents are cisplatin, 5-fluorouracil (5FU) and methotrexate. These drugs are best administered by doctors expert in their use and as part of controlled trials until we can evaluate the most suitable method of administration and the best combination of agents.

Diseases of the larynx

Emergencies

Stridor

Stridor means noisy breathing. It may be inspiratory or expiratory or occurring in both phases of respiration. Inspiratory stridor is usually due to an obstruction at or above the vocal folds and most commonly is a result of an inhaled foreign body or acute infection such as epiglottitis. Expiratory stridor is usually from the lower respiratory tract and gives rise to a prolonged expiratory wheeze. It is most commonly associated with acute asthma or acute infective tracheobronchitis. Biphasic stridor is usually due to obstruction or disease of the tracheobronchial airway and distal lungs.

Stridor in children (Table 43.7)

Infants and children presenting with stridor need assessment with a full history and careful examination if appropriate. If on presentation a child is cyanosed and severely unwell the airway must be secured as soon as possible but it is often possible to obtain a brief history from the parents, with important pointers. A nurse or colleague may be detailed to do this whilst the resuscitation is taking place.

History. In infants in the first year of life it is important to establish whether the stridor is associated with particular activities such as swallowing, crying or movement. These may suggest congenital laryngomalacia or subglottic stenosis. If the stridor is exacerbated by feeding, particularly in the first 4 weeks of life, this suggests a vascular ring or tracheo-oesophageal fistula. If the cry is weak or abnormal this suggests a vocal fold palsy. If the problem only occurs in association with an upper respiratory tract infection and, in particular, is biphasic this would suggest congenital subglottic stenosis. In a young child inspiratory stridor and drooling suggest acute epiglottitis, whereas biphasic stridor without drooling suggests laryngotracheobronchitis or croup.

Examination.

Observe the child carefully at rest; do not attempt to move or handle the child, particularly if the stridulous child is being held by its mother or other family member.

Once a baby starts to cry it may be impossible to study its resting respiratory pattern for some time. Ask the mother, not a nurse or a colleague, to move a baby or young child into different positions such as face down and supine, and watch for changes in its respiratory pattern and level of distress. Observe any drooling and with neonates and infants always try to watch the child being fed, listening to the trachea and chest with a stethoscope if possible. Always examine the whole child, looking for any evidence of congenital abnormalities before attempting any examination of the throat.

If a child is stridulous and drooling and sitting upright in its mother's arms or chair do not attempt to lie it down and do not attempt to look inside the mouth.

These are potentially life-threatening circumstances as the child may aspirate a large quantity of thick saliva contained within its oral cavity. The child does not wish to attempt swallowing in the case of a retropharyngeal abscess, parapharyngeal abscess or acute epiglottitis as these conditions are so painful. It is particularly important in acute epiglottitis as the aspiration of thick saliva may be associated with further laryngeal spasm and a respiratory arrest. Restlessness, increasing tachycardia and cyanosis are important signs of hypoxia. If the child is not distressed and drooling, and not markedly stridulous it may be co-operative enough for it to be possible to look inside the mouth and check the palate, tongue and oropharynx.

In stridulous children, particularly neonates and infants, a transcutaneous oximeter is invaluable if available. It may be placed on the child before any examination and during any subsequent management. A resuscitation trolley with the necessary equipment for emergency intubation or tracheostomy should be close at hand, if at all possible, before commencing examination and investigation of these children.

Investigation. In addition to the oximeter, plain lateral X-rays of the neck and a chest X-ray can be obtained but only if the child's condition permits. If the child is severely stridulous they should *not* be sent to an X-ray department without access to medical staff or resuscitation equipment. The X-rays may confirm the presence of a foreign body or show soft-tissue shadowing consistent with a retropharyngeal or parapharyngeal abscess, acute epiglottitis or chest disease.

Examination under anaesthesia.

Examination under anaesthesia is essential in all children whose diagnosis remains in doubt.

This requires a high level of skill and close co-operation between surgeon and anaesthetist, and appropriate rigid laryngoscopes, bronchoscopes, endoscopic Hopkin's rods and an operating microscope should be made available.

Equipment should be available at all times to undertake an urgent tracheostomy to establish or maintain an airway.

Acute epiglottitis (Table 43.7)

This illness may occur in adults, although fortunately the stridor rarely progresses as rapidly as in children. In children it is of rapid onset and tends to occur in children of 2 years of age or over. Stridor is usually associated with drooling of saliva. The condition is caused by *Haemophilus influenzae* infection which initially causes a severe pharyngitis at the junction of the oropharynx and hypopharynx before progressing to produce inflammation and oedema of the laryngeal inlet. As it progresses it actually involves the whole of the supraglottic larynx, with severe oedema of the ariepiglottic folds and epiglottis being the most notable component; hence the commonly used term 'acute epiglottitis'. Examination and investigation are outlined above, but these children frequently require intensive management with emergency intubation or tracheostomy followed by oxygenation, humidification, continuous oximetry and antibiotics such as ampicillin or chloramphenicol to combat the haemophilus infection. This may be associated with septicaemia and blood cultures should be obtained.

Children with acute epiglottitis may develop airway obstruction rapidly. Insertion of a spatula into the mouth may precipitate a respiratory arrest and is best avoided. Infants and children have small airways and high oxygen demand. It is extremely important to pre-empt any respiratory arrest.

Laryngotracheobronchitis (croup)

This is usually of slower onset in contrast to acute epiglottitis and occurs most commonly in children under 2 years of age. It is usually viral in origin and the cases often occur in clusters. The children have a biphasic astridor and often hoarseness, and a typical barking cough. Airway intervention is required less often but admission to hospital with oxygenation and humidification coupled with antibiotics may be necessary if there are signs of secondary infection.

Table 43.7 Acute paediatric stridor

1. Congenital
   - Laryngomalacia
   - Laryngeal web
   - Subglottic stenosis
2. Acquired
   - Inflammatory – angioneurotic oedema
   - Traumatic – impacted foreign body, laryngeal fracture
   - Infective – epiglottitis, laryngotracheobronchitis
   - Neurological –vocal fold palsy
   - Neoplasia – benign laryngeal papillomatosis

Foreign bodies

Both children and adults may inhale foreign bodies. Young children will attempt to swallow a wide variety of objects, but coins, beads and parts of toys are particularly common. In adults the aspiration is usually of food, particularly inadequately chewed bones and meat. This is more common in elderly edentulous adults and occasionally portions of dentures may be inhaled, particularly in association with road traffic accidents.

Clinical features. The history is often paramount and it is important to always believe the patient, particularly a parent who gives a history of foreign body ingestion or inhalation in a child, even though the pain, dysphagia, coughing, etc., may have settled. Adult patients will, on the whole, have a clear recall and the diagnosis is more easy, but this may not always be the case particularly if the patient is suffering from mental illness. Fish bones may lodge in the tonsils or base of tongue with minimal symptoms but in certain areas of the world, notably Asia, small fish bones may impact in the tonsils, oropharynx or hypopharynx and give rise to parapharyngeal and retropharyngeal abscess formation.

Examination. Examination may be prevented by trismus, pain and anxiety, but the presence of a foreign body may be suspected by a salivary pool within the piriform fossa or adjacent oedema and erythema of the pharyngolaryngeal mucosa.

Radiology.

Radiology may be helpful but is not critical. Fish bones are often not visible on plain X-rays, and a normal plain X-ray does not exclude a foreign body within the pharynx, larynx, oesophagus or lungs.

Specialised studies may help in cases of doubt using tomography of the neck, CT scan or a gastrograffin swallowing study in the case of a suspected oesophageal foreign body.

Treatment. In the case of an inhaled foreign body causing severe stridor in a neonate or infant it may be removed either by hooking it from the pharynx with a finger or by inverting the child carefully by its ankles and slapping its back. In a larger child it may be more appropriate to bend them over your knee with their head hanging down and again strike them firmly between the shoulders. In the case of adults an impacted laryngeal foreign body may be coughed out in association with a Heimlich manoeuvre. This involves standing behind the patient, clasping the arms around the lower thorax such that the knuckles of the clasped hands come into contact with the patient's xiphisternum, and then a brief firm compression of the lower thorax may aid instant expiration of the foreign body.

If none of these immediate emergency measures removes the foreign body and the patient is cyanosed and severely stridulous, an immediate cricothyroidotomy or tracheostomy may be necessary.

In less urgent cases, if the radiography is not useful but a foreign body is strongly suspected, then detailed endoscopy under general anaesthesia may be indicated.

It is important to remember that the symptoms of foreign body ingestion are more reliable than the results of specialist radiology investigations.

Other causes of acute pharyngolaryngeal oedema

Angioneurotic oedema, radiotherapy, laryngeal trauma associated with road traffic accidents, corrosives, scalds and smoke ingestion may all cause significant pharyngolaryngeal oedema, in addition to the acute infective conditions mentioned elsewhere. Hoarseness is the predominate symptom along with dysphagia prior to the increase in dyspnoea. If laryngoscopic examination is possible marked oedema of the supraglottis and pharynx can be seen. Humidified oxygen, adrenaline nebulisers, systemic antihistamines and steroids may be valuable in these cases. Morphine should not be given to these patients to combat their distress as it may cause respiratory depression and respiratory arrest. If the dyspnoea progresses intubation or tracheostomy will be necessary.

Tracheostomy and other emergency airway measures (Table 43.8)

This procedure is to relieve airway obstruction or to protect the airway by fashioning a direct entrance into the trachea through the skin of the neck. Tracheostomy may be done as an emergency when the patient is *in extremis* and the larynx cannot be intubated but it is not always an easy procedure, particularly in the obese patient, and should not be embarked upon unless absolutely necessary. An easier alternative for the inexperienced doctor is the insertion of a large intravenous cannula or, alternatively, a small tube into the cricothyroid membrane which lies in the midline immediately below the thyroid cartilage. Emergency intubation is a further option when the laryngotracheal airway is not obstructed, and tracheostomy may be performed following initial endotracheal intubation.

Choice of operation

- The degree of urgency in establishing tracheostomy will determine the method used, but preference should always be for the elective procedure. One of the most appropriate pieces of advice in surgery is 'the time to do a tracheostomy is when you first think it may be necessary'. All of the potential complications of tracheostomy are markedly decreased if a meticulous elective procedure is performed under controlled circumstances by an experienced team.

If time allows the following should be undertaken:

- inspection and palpation of the neck to assess the laryngotracheal anatomy in the individual patient;
- indirect or direct laryngoscopy;
- tomography of the larynx and upper trachea;

Henry J. Heimlich, b. 1920. American surgeon.

Table 43.8 Indications for tracheostomy

1. Acute upper airway obstruction – e.g. an inhaled foreign body, a large pharyngolaryngeal tumour, or acute pharyngolaryngeal infections in children
2. Potential upper airway obstruction – for example after major surgery involving the oral cavity, pharynx, larynx or neck
3. Protection of the lower airway – for example protection against aspiration of saliva in unconscious patients as a consequence of head injuries, faciomaxillary injuries, comas, bulbar poliomyelitis or tetanus
4. Patients requiring artificial respiration

- assessment of pulmonary function.

- Whenever possible the procedure should be adequately explained to the patient beforehand, with particular emphasis on the inability to speak immediately following the operation and possible difficulties with swallowing.

Emergency tracheostomy. If a skilled anaesthetist is unavailable local anaesthesia is employed, but in desperate cases where the patient is unconscious none is required. The only word of warning would be in those patients who have suffered severe head and neck trauma, and may have an unstable cervical spine fracture. Cricothyroidotomy may be more suitable under these circumstances.

If it is possible the patient should be laid supine with padding placed under the shoulders and the extended neck kept as steady as possible in the midline. This aids palpation of the thyroid and cricoid cartilage between the thumb and index finger of the free hand. The movements of the fingers of the free hand are important in this technique. The operation is more difficult in small children and thick-necked adults as the landmarks are difficult to palpate.

A vertical midline incision should be made from the inferior aspect of the thyroid cartilage to the suprasternal notch and continued down between the infrahyoid muscles (Fig. 43.32). There may be heavy bleeding from the wound at this point, particularly if the neck is congested as a result of the patient's effort to breathe around an acute upper airway obstruction. No steps should be taken to control this haemorrhage, although an assistant and suction apparatus are valuable if available. The operator should feel carefully, and without undue haste, for the cricoid cartilage using the index finger of the free hand whilst retracting the skin edges by pressure applied by the thumb and middle finger. If the situation is one of extreme urgency a further vertical incision straight into the trachea at the level of the second, third and fourth ring should be made immediately without regard to the presence of the thyroid isthmus (Fig. 43.33). The knife blade is rotated through 90° thus opening the trachea. At this point the patient may cough violently as blood enters the airway. The operator should be aware of this possibility and avoid losing the position of the scalpel in the open trachea. Any form of available tube should be inserted into the trachea as soon as possible and blood and secretion sucked out. Once an airway has been established haemostasis is then

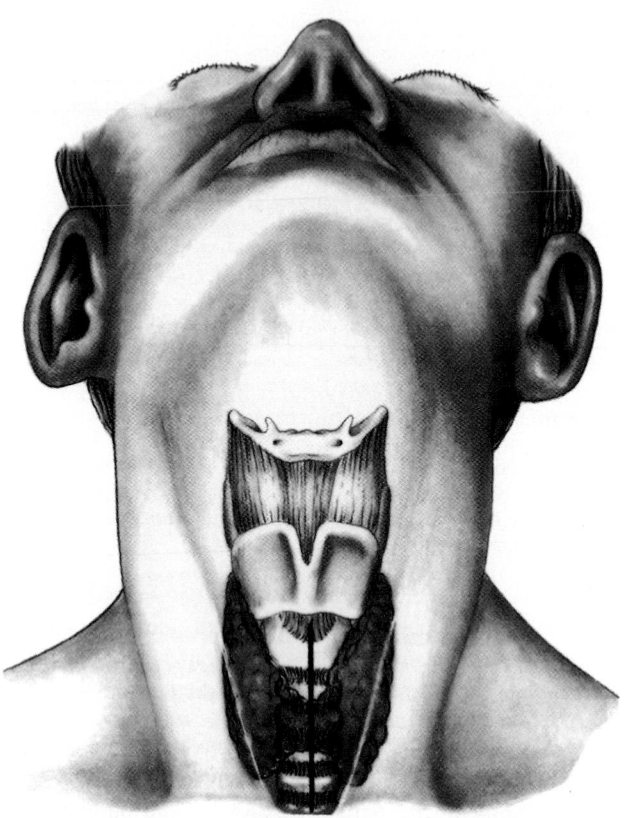

Fig. 43.32 Diagram showing the position of skin incision in an emergency tracheostomy. [Reproduced with permission from McGregor, I.A. and Howard, D.J. (eds), *Rob and Smith's Operative Surgery, Head and Neck Part 1*, Butterworth-Heinemann, Oxford, 1992, p. 29.]

secured. With the emergency under control the tracheostomy should be refashioned as soon as possible.

Should additional equipment and more time be available once the cricoid cartilage has been identified, blunt finger dissection inferiorly can be used to mobilise the thyroid isthmus which should be divided between haemostats, clearing the trachea before making a vertical incision through the second–fourth rings. A tracheal dilator should be inserted through the tracheal incision and the edges of the tracheal wound separated gently. In cases of suspected HIV infection or diphtheria the surgeon should place a swab over the wound so that the violent expiratory efforts which may follow do not contaminate the operator(s) with infected mucus and blood. When respiratory efforts have become less violent a tracheostomy tube should be inserted into the trachea and the dilator removed. It is important that the surgeon keeps a finger on the tube while the assistant ties the attached tapes round the patient's neck.

Elective tracheostomy.

The advantage of an elective procedure is that there is complete airway control at all times, unhurried dissection and careful placement of an appropriate tube.

Close co-operation between the surgeon, anaesthetist and scrub nurse is essential, and attention to the details will markedly reduce possible complications and morbidity from the procedure. Following induction of general anaesthesia and endotracheal intubation, the patient is positioned with a combination of head extension and placement of an appropriate sandbag under the shoulders (Fig. 43.34). There should be no rotation of the head. Children's heads should not be over-extended as it is possible to enter the trachea in the fifth or sixth rings under these circumstances. The inexperienced surgeon may find the insertion of a bronchoscope in the trachea of great help when performing tracheostomy in young children. A transverse incision may be used in the elective situation. The thyroid isthmus is divided carefully and oversewn, and tension sutures are placed either side of the tracheal fenestration in children (Figs 43.34–43.38). A Bjork flap may be used in adults. The advantages of the Björk method far outweigh the potential disadvantages, and the method is particularly useful for those surgeons who undertake occasional tracheostomy or where the level of skill and experience of the nursing staff are limited. Performed correctly it is safe and allows reintroduction of a displaced

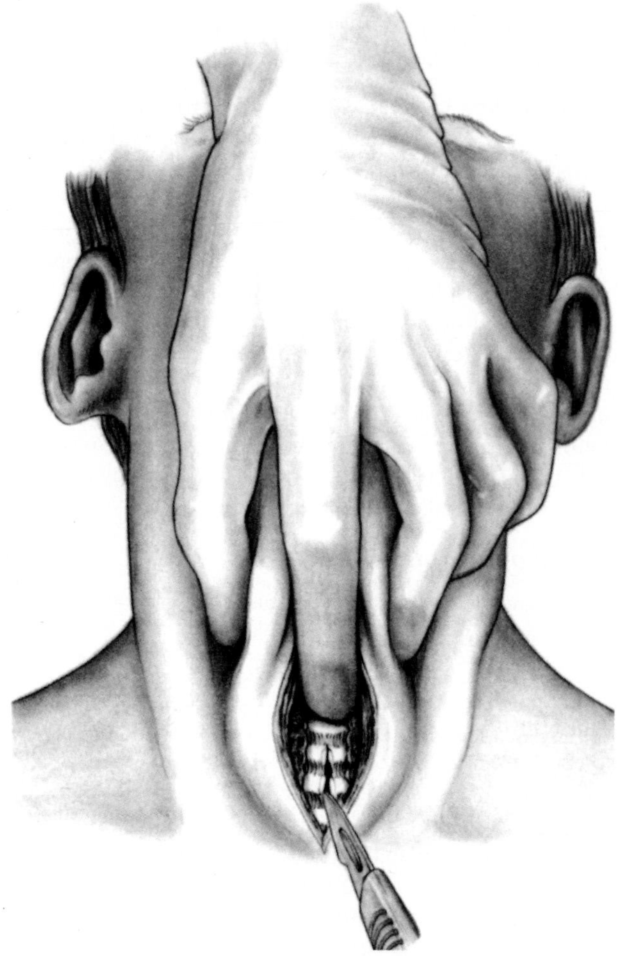

Fig. 43.33 Diagram showing an incision in the trachea in an emergency tracheostomy. [Reproduced with permission from McGregor, I.A. and Howard, D.J. (eds), *Rob and Smith's Operative Surgery, Head and Neck Part 1*, Butterworth-Heinemann, Oxford, 1992, p. 30.]

tube with the minimum of difficulty. The inferiorly based flap is begun at its apex with an incision on the superior aspects of the second ring and extended down either side through the second and third rings. The tip of the flap should be stitched to the inferior edge of the transverse skin incision using horizontal mattress sutures through the structure of the second ring. These sutures should be generous enough so that they will not cut out. The first tracheal ring should not be violated under any circumstances.

Tracheostomy tubes. These are basically made of two materials, silver or plastic (Fig. 43.39). Both materials have been used to make tubes of various sizes with varying curves, angles, cuffs, inner tubes and speaking valves. A cuffed tube is used initially, which may be changed after 3–4 days to a noncuffed plastic or silver tube. The pressure within the tube cuff should be carefully monitored and should be low enough not to occlude circulation in the mucosal capillaries. When in position the tube should be retained by double tapes passed around the patient's neck with a reef knot on either side. It is important that the patient's head is flexed when the tapes are tied otherwise they may become slack when the patient is moved from the position of extension, thereby resulting in a possible displacement of the tube if the patient coughs. Alternatively, the flanges of the plastic tube may be stitched directly to the underlying neck skin.

Knowledge of the physiological changes induced by tracheostomy is an essential requirement for the understanding of postoperative management. All forms of tracheostomy and cricothyroidotomy bypass the upper airway and have the following advantages:

- the anatomical dead space is reduced by approximately 50 per cent;
- the work of breathing is reduced;
- alveolar ventilation is increased;
- the level of sedation needed for patient comfort is decreased and, unlike endotracheal intubation, the patient may be able talk and eat with a tube in place.

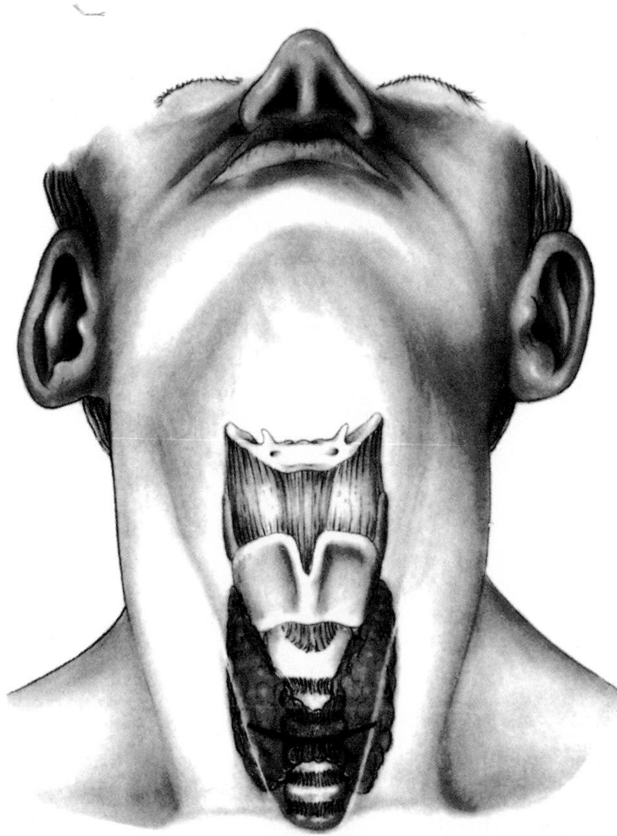

Fig. 43.35 Diagram showing the position of a skin incision in an elective tracheostomy. [Reproduced with permission from McGregor, I.A. and Howard, D.J. (eds), *Rob and Smith's Operative Surgery, Head and Neck Part 1*, Butterworth-Heinemann, Oxford, 1992, p. 33.]

However, there are several disadvantages:

- loss of heat and moisture exchange performed in the upper respiratory tract;
- desiccation of tracheal epithelium, loss of ciliated cells and metaplasia;

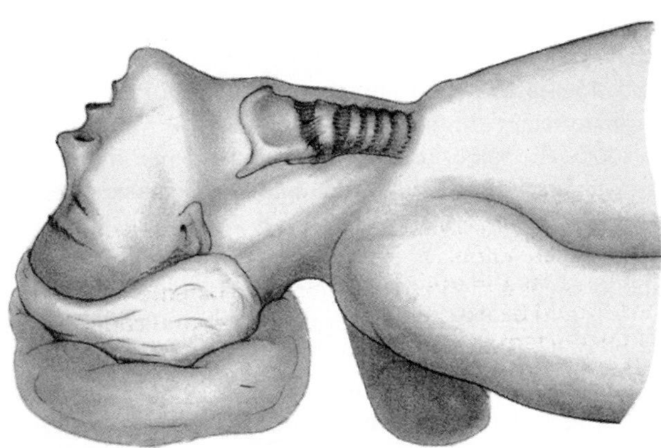

Fig. 43.34 Position of the patient for elective tracheostomy. [Reproduced with permission from McGregor, I.A. and Howard, D.J. (eds), *Rob and Smith's Operative Surgery, Head and Neck Part 1*, Butterworth-Heinemann, Oxford, 1992, p. 32.]

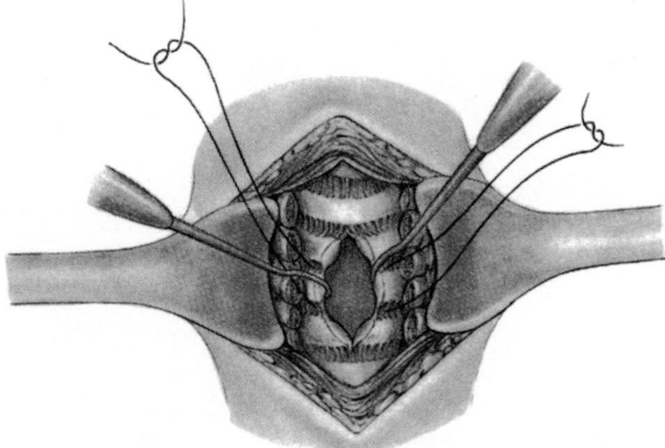

Fig. 43.36 Diagram showing tracheal fenestration in an elective tracheostomy. [Reproduced with permission from McGregor, I.A. and Howard, D.J. (eds), *Rob and Smith's Operative Surgery, Head and Neck Part 1*, Butterworth-Heinemann, Oxford, 1992, p. 35.]

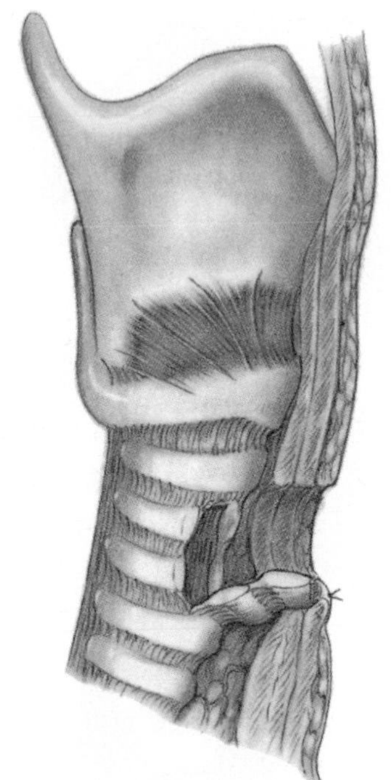

Fig. 43.37 Diagram showing a Bjork flap. [Reproduced with permission from McGregor, I.A. and Howard, D.J. (eds), *Rob and Smith's Operative Surgery, Head and Neck Part 1*, Butterworth-Heinemann, Oxford, 1992, p. 36.]

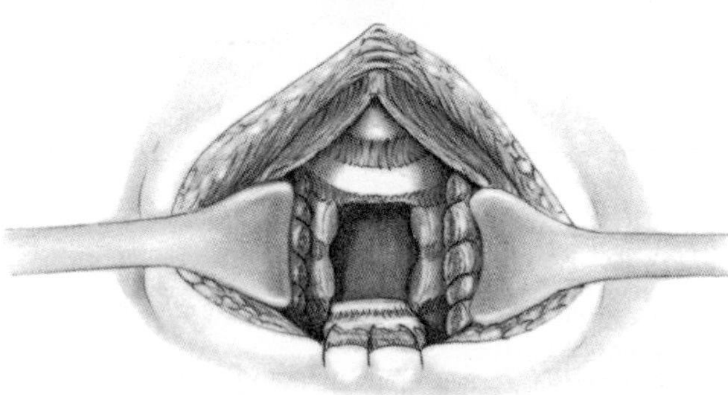

Fig. 43.38 Diagram showing fenestration in a Bjork flap. [Reproduced with permission from McGregor, I.A. and Howard, D.J. (eds), *Rob and Smith's Operative Surgery, Head and Neck Part 1*, Butterworth-Heinemann, Oxford, 1992, p. 36.]

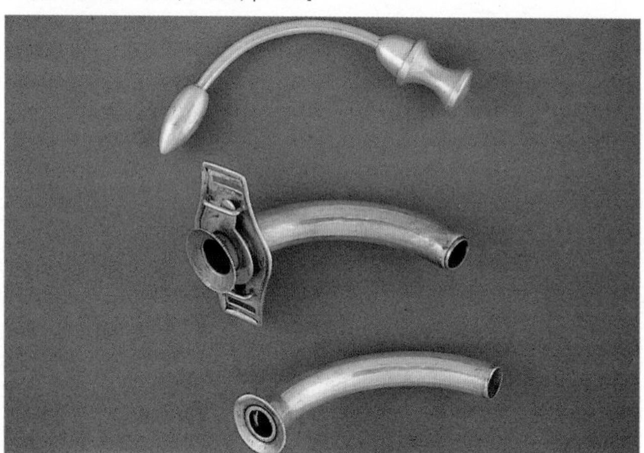

Fig. 43.39 Silver tracheostomy tube; inner, outer tubes and introducer.

Table 43.9 Tracheostomy: postoperative management

- Suction – efficient, sterile as often as required
- Humidification (± oxygen)
- A warm well-ventilated room
- Position of tube and patient
- Spare tube, introducer, tapes, tracheal dilator
- Change of tube, inner tube, possible speaking valve
- Physiotherapy

- the presence of a foreign body in the trachea stimulates mucus production. Where no cilia are present this mucociliary stream is arrested;
- the increased mucus is more viscid, and thick crusts may form and block the tube, particularly in children;
- whilst many patients with a tracheostomy can feed satisfactorily, there is some splinting of the larynx which may prevent normal swallowing and lead to aspiration. This aspiration may be 'silent', i.e. not apparent.

Postoperative treatment is designed to counteract these effects, and frequent suction and humidification are most important (Table 43.9). A trolley must be placed by the bed containing a tracheal dilator, duplicate tubes and introducers, retractors and dressings. Oxygen should be at hand and, in the initial period, a nurse must be in constant attendance. Humidification will render the secretions less viscid; a sucker with a catheter attached should be on hand to keep the tracheobronchial tree free from secretions. The catheter must be kept in a sterile holder and introduced with aseptic precautions by all concerned. When mucus is very tenacious and consequently difficult to aspirate, isotonic saline or a mucolytic agent may be administered through the tracheostomy tube by a fine nebuliser. If there is an inner tube it should be removed and washed in sodium bicarbonate solution every 4 hours or more if necessary. A number of complications is associated with tracheostomy but all can be avoided with care and attention to operative and postoperative detail (Table 43.10).

Other emergency airway procedures. ***Fibre-optic endotracheal intubation.*** In most emergency situations endotracheal intubation is the most direct and satisfactory method of securing the airway. Nasotracheal intubation in expert hands is also a well-established technique and is particularly useful if the patient has trismus, severe mandibular injuries, cervical spine rigidity or an obstructing mass within the oral cavity. Both of these forms of intubation can be aided in difficult patients by passing a modern fibre-optic endoscope through the centre of an entrotracheal tube, hence guiding it into the larynx and trachea under direct vision (Fig. 43.40).

Transtracheal ventilation. This technique has been increasingly advocated in the last decade and, although some specialist equipment is required, the actual technique is simple and effective. It will allow ventilation of the patient for periods in excess of 1 hour and will often give ample time to allow for a more organised elective procedure.

Table 43.10 Tracheostomy: complications

1. Intraoperative complications
   - Haemorrhage
   - Injury to paratracheal structures particularly the carotid artery and recurrent laryngeal nerve and oesophagus
   - Damage to the trachea
2. Early postoperative complications
   - Apnoea caused by a fall in the PCO_2
   - Haemorrhage
   - Subcutaneous emphysema, pneumomediastinium and pneumothorax
   - Accidental extubation, anterior displacement of the tube, obstruction of the tube lumen and tip occlusion against the tracheal wall
   - Infection
   - Swallowing dysfunction
3. Late postoperative complications
   - Difficult decannulation
   - Tracheocutaneous fistula
   - Tracheo-oesophageal fistula, tracheoinnominate artery fistula with severe haemorrhage
   - Tracheal stenosis

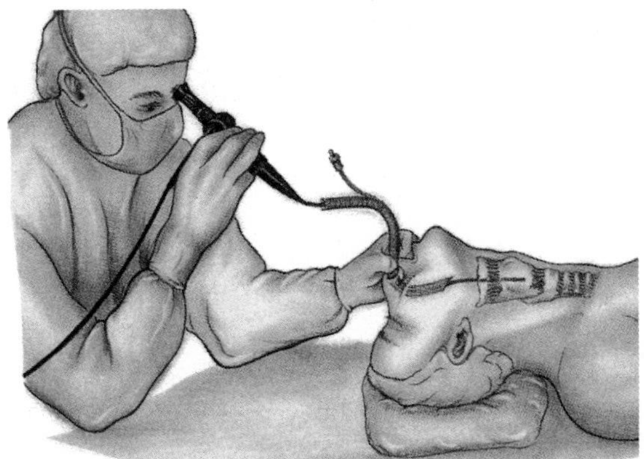

Fig. 43.40 Diagram showing fibre-optic endotracheal intubation. [Reproduced with permission from McGregor, I.A. and Howard, D.J. (eds), *Rob and Smith's Operative Surgery, Head and Neck Part 1*, Butterworth-Heinemann, Oxford, 1992, p. 40.]

The cricothyroid membrane is located by palpation of the neck with the index finger, and a 14G or 16G plastic-sheathed intravascular needle and a 10-ml syringe containing a few millilitres of lignocaine are introduced in the midline and directed downwards and backwards into the tracheal lumen (Fig. 43.41). The needle is advanced steadily and negative pressure is placed on the syringe until bubbles of air are clearly seen. The tissues of the neck may be infiltrated with the anaesthetic if desired and the tracheal mucosa likewise partly anaesthetised by the introduction of 1–2 ml after gaining the lumen. The needle is removed and the plastic-sheath cannula remains in the trachea. It is attached by means of a Luer connection to the high-pressure oxygen supply. Ventilation may be undertaken in a controlled manner with a jetting device with the chest being observed for appropriate movements. If there is severe obstruction of the laryngopharynx by the foreign body or tumour, the exhaled outflow of gases can be aided by placement of one or two further cannulae as exhalation ports. This procedure gains extremely rapid control of ventilation and requires a minimum of technical expertise.

Cricothyroidotomy. Cricothyroidotomy has gained increasing support in some centres and is advocated when endotracheal intubation is not possible. It has the advantages of speed and ease requiring little equipment and surgical expertise. However, its use for all but the briefest access to the airway remains controversial, and there are conflicting reports with regard to the subsequent incidence of complications, particularly those of subglottic stenosis and long-term voice changes.

The patient's neck is extended and the area between the prominence of the thyroid cartilage and the cricoid cartilage below is palpated with the index finger of the free hand. In the emergency situation a vertical skin incision is recommended with dissection rapidly carried down to the criocothyroid membrane. A 1-cm transverse incision is made through the membrane immediately above the cricoid cartilage and the scalpel twisted through a right angle to gain access to the airway (Figs 43.42). If available artery forceps, dilator or tracheal hook will aid improving the aperture and the insertion of an available tube (Figs 43.43).

Depending on the degree of emergency it may be necessary for the surgeon to assess the results of the procedure by direct laryngoscopy, and the authors recommend that careful consideration should be given to conversion of the cricothy-

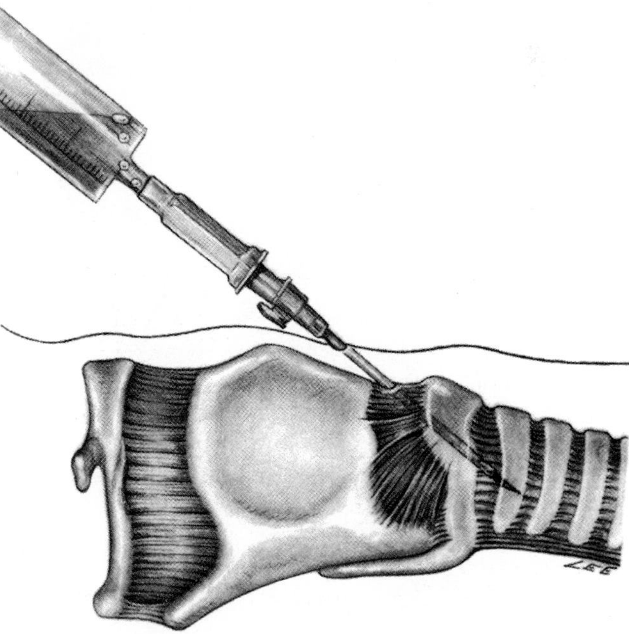

Fig. 43.41 Diagram showing transtracheal needle introduction. [Reproduced with permission from McGregor, I.A. and Howard, D.J. (eds), *Rob and Smith's Operative Surgery, Head and Neck Part 1*, Butterworth-Heinemann, Oxford, 1992, p. 41.]

roidotomy to a tracheostomy. Although there is debate about the frequency of subglottic stenosis following this procedure, there is general agreement that it is much increased if any long-term ventilation is undertaken via even a modest size tracheostomy tube through the cricothyroid membrane.

Laryngeal disease causing voice disorders

Vocal nodules

These are known as singers' nodules in adults and screamers' nodules in children (Fig. 43.44). They are fibrous thickenings of the vocal folds at the junction of the middle and anterior third, and are the result of vocal abuse. Speech therapy is therefore the preferred treatment and the lesions will resolve spontaneously in most cases. Occasionally the nodules will need to be surgically removed using modern microlaryngoscopic dissection or laser techniques. Follow-up by the speech therapist is necessary until all of the underlying errors in voice production are overcome.

Vocal fold polyps

These are usually unilateral and may be associated with an acute infective episode, cigarette smoking and vocal abuse (Fig. 43.45). Speech therapy is again indicated, but the polyps usually require removal by microdissection or laser surgery.

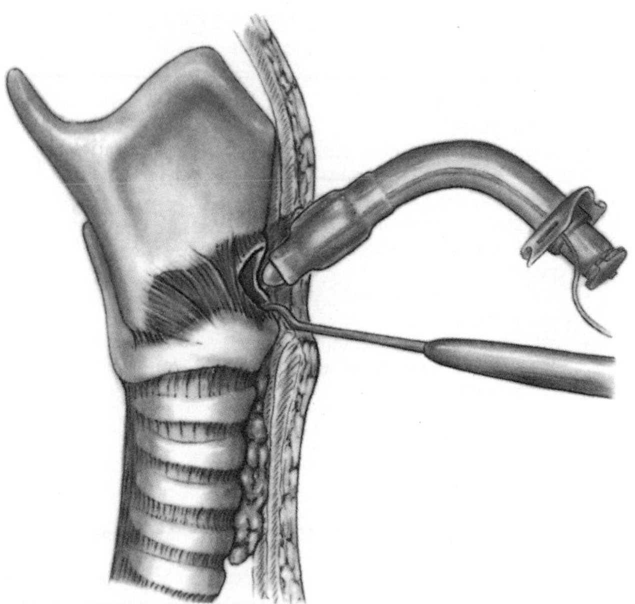

Fig. 43.43 Diagram showing insertion of a tube after cricothyroidotomy. [Reproduced with permission from McGregor, I.A. and Howard, D.J. (eds), *Rob and Smith's Operative Surgery, Head and Neck Part 1*, Butterworth-Heinemann, Oxford, 1992, p. 43.]

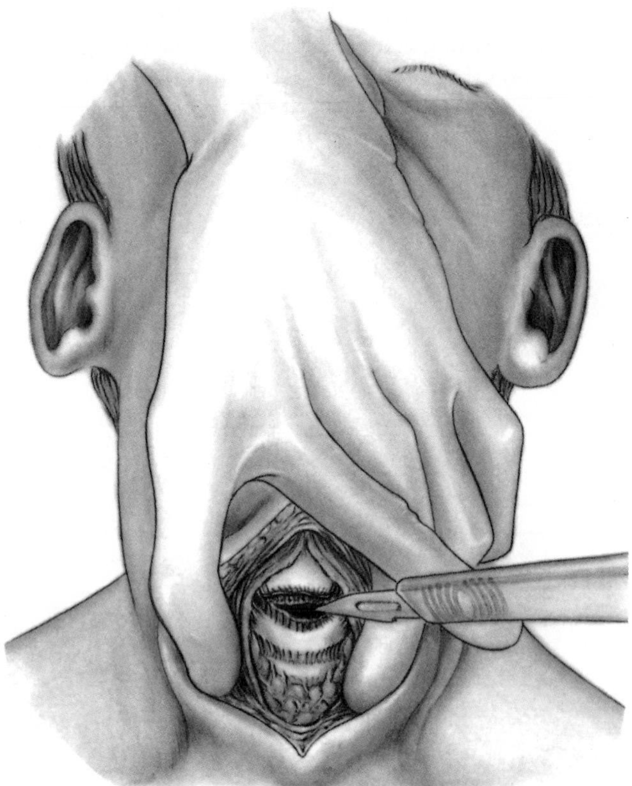

Fig. 43.42 Diagram showing an incision in a cricothyroidotomy. [Reproduced with permission from McGregor, I.A. and Howard, D.J. (eds), *Rob and Smith's Operative Surgery, Head and Neck Part 1*, Butterworth-Heinemann, Oxford, 1992, p. 42.]

Laryngeal papillomata

These occur mainly in children but can also present in adults. They are most commonly found on the vocal folds but may spread throughout the larynx and tracheobronchial airway (Fig. 43.46). They are caused by papilloma viruses and need removal by laser surgery in order to maintain a reasonable voice and airway. Antiviral treatment by such drugs as interferon remains of doubtful value at present. Endoscopic laser surgery is the least traumatic way of removing these lesions and should not produce scarring or cause implantation of the papillomata elsewhere in the airway.

Acute laryngitis

This often occurs in association with upper respiratory tract infections in association with a cough and pharyngitis. It may, however, be localised to the larynx, is usually viral and settles quickly if the patient rests the voice during the active inflammation. Steam inhalations are soothing along with mild anal-

Table 43.11 Causes of hoarseness

- Localised vocal fold pathology, e.g. vocal nodule, polyps or laryngeal papillomatosis. Acute or chronic laryngitis
- Vocal fold palsy
- Laryngeal tumours
- Nonspecific voice disorders, functional dysphonia

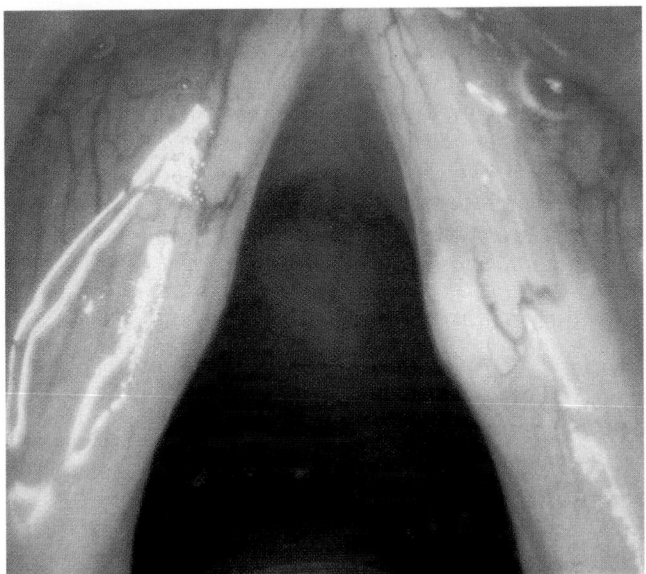

Fig. 43.44 Photograph of vocal cord nodules.

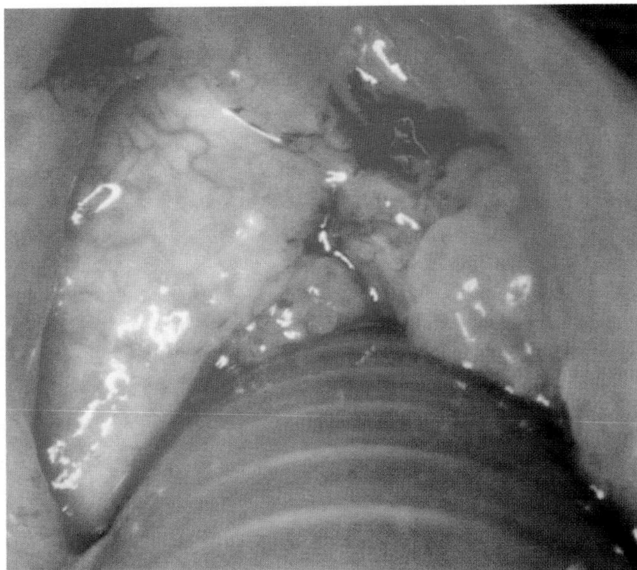

Fig. 43.46 Photograph of laryngeal papillomata.

gesics but antibiotics are unnecessary. The condition should resolve in 2–3 weeks with voice care.

Hoarseness lasting for 3–4 weeks should always be referred for an ENT opinion, particularly in smokers.

Chronic laryngitis

Chronic laryngitis may be specific and can be caused by mycobacteria, syphilis and fungi. Treatment is directed towards the causative organism. Nonspecific laryngitis is common, and the main predisposing factors are smoking, chronic upper and lower respiratory sepsis and voice abuse. In some cases the laryngeal mucosa may become dysplastic, particularly over the true vocal folds, and is a premalignant condition. It may require microlaryngoscopic examination and biopsy. Treatment is by the elimination of any predisposing factors, particularly smoking, and attention to any vocal abuse under the guidance of a speech therapist.

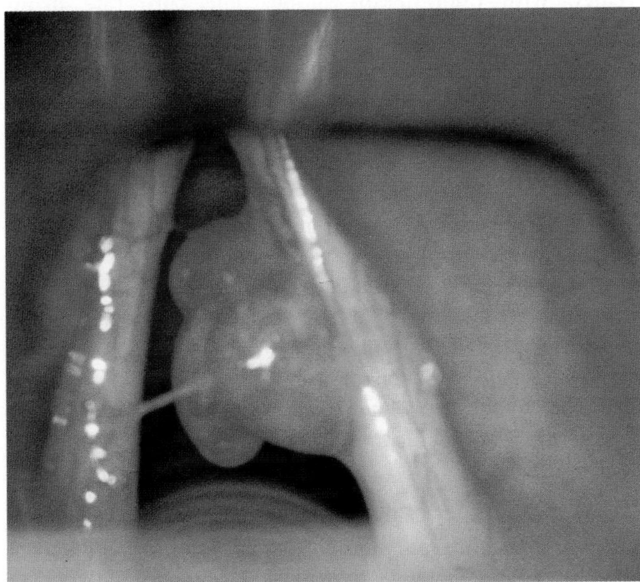

Fig. 43.45 Photograph of a vocal cord polyp.

Diagnosis of chronic laryngitis should not be made unless the larynx has been fully evaluated by a laryngologist.

Vocal fold palsy

This may be unilateral or bilateral, but a unilateral left vocal fold palsy is the commonest as a consequence of the long intrathoracic course of the left recurrent laryngeal nerve which arches around the aorta and may be commonly involved in inflammatory and neoplastic conditions involving the left hilum (Fig. 43.47).

Lung cancer is the commonest single cancer in many parts of the world and a left vocal fold palsy should be considered to be due to a carcinoma of the lung until proved otherwise.

Other malignant lesions can cause a similar effect and may arise in the nasopharynx, thyroid gland or oesophagus. Bilateral vocal fold paralysis is uncommon and tends to occur after thyroid surgery or head injuries (Table 43.12).

Clinical features

Unilateral recurrent laryngeal nerve palsy of sudden onset produces hoarseness which is most notable for lack of volume to the voice and occasionally may be associated with difficulty in swallowing liquids and weakening of the cough. These symptoms may be short lived and the voice may return to normal within a few weeks as the muscles in the opposite vocal fold compensate and move it across the midline to meet the paralysed vocal fold which usually lies in the paramedian position. Owing to this efficient compensation, in slowly progressive lesions the patient may only experience slight weakness of the voice with prolonged use.

Bilateral recurrent laryngeal nerve palsy is an occasional and very serious complication of thyroidectomy. Acute dyspnoea occurs as a result of the paramedian position of both vocal folds which reduce the airway to 2–3 mm and which tend to get sucked together on inspiration. In severe cases tracheostomy or intubation is necessary immediately otherwise death occurs from asphyxia.

Investigation of vocal fold paralysis is most easily encompassed nowadays by a CT scan from skull base to diaphragm. This technique has replaced the multiple previous investigations which were necessary and reveals most of the pathology which may give rise to an undiagnosed vocal fold palsy. Approximately 20–25 per cent of cases of vocal fold paralysis occurs without known pathology and spontaneous recovery may occur. In unilateral vocal fold paralysis, where compensation does not occur, the paralysed fold may be medialised by injecting Teflon paste lateral to the vocal fold and displacing it medially. Alternatively, a small external operation on the thyroid cartilage may be undertaken in order to enter the paraglottic space and displace the fold medially (thyroplasty). These surgical procedures should be performed early if the cause is carcinoma of the bronchus and the outlook of the patient is poor. When the pathology is unknown it may be better to wait for a period of 1 year to see whether spontaneous improvement occurs and to allow further recovery with the help of speech therapy.

In bilateral vocal fold paralysis the patients frequently require tracheostomy, but surgery may be carried out to remove a small portion of the posterior aspect of one vocal fold or a portion of one arytenoid cartilage. These procedures are most easily performed endoscopically with a carbon dioxide laser. They increase the size of the posterior glottic airway allowing the patient to be decannulated or even to avoid a tracheostomy in the first place. Some laryngologists have advocated reinnervation procedures for the paralysed larynx by rotating a nerve muscle combination into the larynx from the neck. However, these techniques have not yet found widespread acceptance.

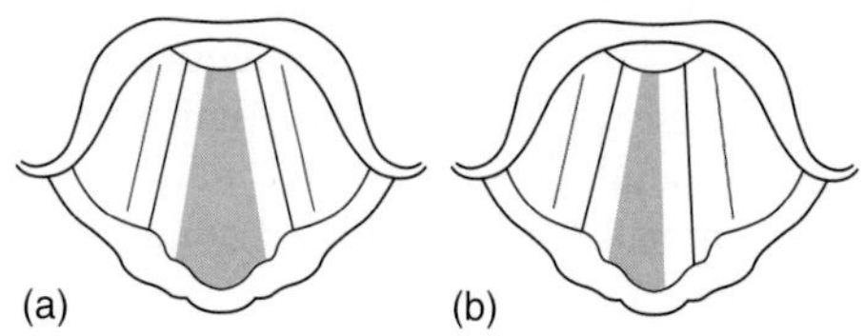

Fig. 43.47 Vocal cord positions (a) Normal; (b) Cord palsy.

Table 43.12 Causes of vocal fold palsy

1. Congenital (infants)
2. Acquired
   - Traumatic:
     - direct to neck
     - postsurgical, e.g. thyroidectomy
   - Infective:
     - viral (rare)
   - Neoplastic:
     - carcinoma of the lung involving left hilum
     - carcinoma of the larynx
     - carcinoma of the thyroid
     - carcinoma of the oesophagus
   - Vascular:
     - aortic aneurysm
   - Neurological:
     - lower motor neuron disease
   - Idiopathic

Tumours of the larynx

Benign tumours of the larynx are extremely rare and squamous carcinoma of the larynx predominates over all others, being responsible for more than 90 per cent of tumours within the larynx. It is the commonest head and neck cancer and almost always occurs in elderly male smokers. However, over the past two decades the sex incidence has changed as a consequence of increasing smoking amongst women, and in some areas they now make up more than 20 per cent of the patients. The squamous epithelium of the vocal folds and the respiratory epithelium of the supraglottis undergo dysplastic change stimulated by cigarette smoking and other factors. The incidence of laryngeal cancer in the three compartments supraglottis, glottis and subglottis varies around the world; the glottis is generally the commonest site followed by the supraglottis (Fig. 43.48). True carcinomas of the subglottis are very rare and most are a consequence of inferior spread from the glottis.

Clinical features

The frequent glottic origin means that patients almost always present with hoarseness. This is of great importance because if a diagnosis can be made while the tumour is in the first stage, i.e. confined only to one vocal fold, these cancers have more than a 90 per cent 5-year disease-free cure rate when treated with radiotherapy alone. The cure rate drops dramatically once the lymphatically rich supraglottis or subglottis is involved, owing to spread to neck nodes. The appearance of more than one neck gland halves the overall prognosis of the patient.

Investigations

Direct laryngoscopy, preferably a microlaryngoscopy, together with Hopkin's rod examination allows precise determination of the extent of the tumour and biopsy confirms an exact histology (Table 43.13). CT and MRI scanning give further details of the extent of larger tumours demonstrating escape of the tumour outside the larynx and suspicious nodal involvement within the neck which may not be determined on clinical examination.

Treatment

Early supraglottic and glottic tumours stages I and II are optimally treated with megavoltage radiotherapy where these facilities exist. Five-year cure rates for stages I and II are

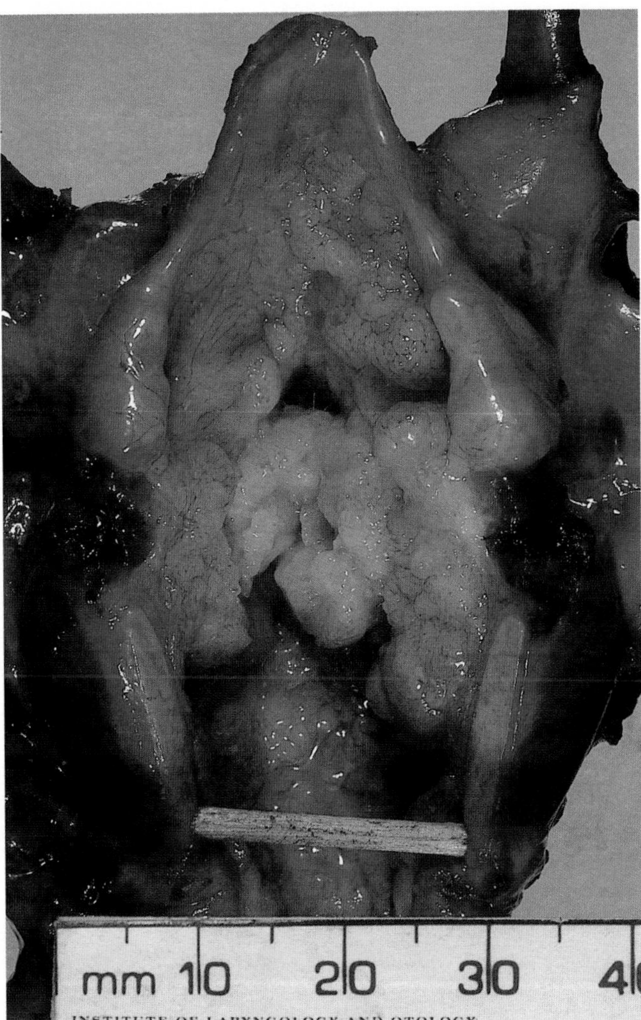

Fig. 43.48 Photograph showing a total laryngectomy specimen with transglottic tumour.

approximately 90 and 70 per cent, respectively, and the patient has an excellent voice following this type of treatment. If modern megavoltage radiotherapy is not available then early tumours may be excised by means of endoscopic laser surgery or open partial laryngeal surgery. This latter may be in the form of a laryngofissure when the thyroid cartilage is opened anteriorly in the midline and the squamous carcinoma excised under direct vision from the vocal fold or supraglottis or, in the case of more extensive unilateral glottic and supraglottic growths, a vertical hemilaryngectomy may be undertaken. This leaves a defect on one side of the larynx which is usually reconstructed with adjacent strap muscles. With early bilateral supraglottic tumours a horizontal laryngectomy may be undertaken excising the supraglottic growth and the remainder of the glottis. The subglottic part of the larynx is then stitched to the tongue base to provide continuity. In most patients undergoing partial laryngeal surgery of this type the voice result is not as satisfactory as that with radiotherapy, although the cure rates are often comparable.

Advanced laryngeal disease

Once the squamous carcinoma has caused fixation of the vocal fold or has infiltrated outside the larynx into adjacent structures such as the thyroid gland and strap muscles, some form of subtotal or total laryngectomy is required to attempt to cure the disease. Total laryngectomy is frequently required when radiotherapy fails (Figs 43.49–43.51). After the larynx has been removed, the remaining trachea is brought out on to the lower part of the neck as a permanent tracheal stoma and the hypopharynx, which is opened at the time of the operation, is closed to restore the continuity for swallowing. Thus, the upper aerodigestive and digestive tracts are permanently disconnected. Part or all of the thyroid gland and associated parathyroid glands may also need to be removed depending on

Table 43.13 TNM classification of laryngeal cancer

T – Primary tumour	
TX	Primary tumour cannot be assessed
T0	No evidence of primary tumour
Tis	Carcinoma *in situ*
Supraglottis	
T1	Tumour limited to one subsite of supraglottis, with normal vocal cord mobility
T2	Tumour invades more than one subsite of supraglottis or glottis, with normal vocal cord mobility
T3	Tumour limited to larynx with vocal cord fixation and/or invades postcricoid area, medial wall of piriform sinus or pre-epiglottic tissues
T4	Tumour invades through thyroid cartilage and/or extends to other tissues beyond the larynx, e.g. to oropharynx, soft tissues of neck
Glottis	
T1	Tumour limited to vocal cord(s) (may involve anterior or posterior commissures) with normal mobility T1a – Tumour limited to one vocal cord T1b – Tumour involves both vocal cords
T2	Tumour extends to supraglottis and/or subglottis, and/or with impaired vocal cord mobility
T3	Tumour limited to the larynx with vocal cord fixation
T4	Tumour invades through thyroid cartilage and/or extends to other tissues beyond the larynx, e.g. to oropharynx, soft tissues of the neck
Subglottis	
T1	Tumour limited to the subglottis
T2	Tumour extends to vocal cord(s) with normal or impaired mobility
T3	Tumour limited to the larynx with vocal cord fixation
T4	Tumour invades through cricoid or thyroid cartilage and/or extends to other tissues beyond the larynx, e.g. to oropharynx soft tissues of the neck
N – Regional lymph nodes	
M – Distant metastasis	

Stage grouping			
Stage 0	Tis	N0	M0
Stage I	T1	N0	M0
Stage II	T2	N0	M0
Stage III	T1	N1	M0
	T2	N1	M0
	T3	N0, N1	M0
Stage IV	T4	N0, N1	M0
	Any T	N2, N3	M0
	Any T	Any N	M1

the extent of the disease, so patients after this type of radical surgery may require oral thyroxine and calcium supplements for the remainder of their lives. Laryngectomy patients must obviously avoid immersion in water as this would flow straight into their tracheal stoma. However, a rather complex form of snorkle device has been developed to allow laryngectomy patients to go swimming and simple protection of the stoma with a towel may allow them to take a careful shower.

Vocal rehabilitation

The loss of the larynx as a generator of sound does not prevent patients speaking as long as an alternative source of vibrating can be created in the pharynx. There are basically three ways of achieving this.

- An artificial device which produces sound when applied to the soft tissues of the neck which is turned into speech by the vocal tract comprising the tongue, the pharynx, oral cavity, lips, teeth and nasal sinuses. These devices are usually battery powered.
- Voice production may be restored in some patients by learning to swallow air into the pharynx and upper oesophagus. On regurgitating the air, a segment of the pharyngo-oesophageal mucosa vibrates to produce sound which is once again modified by the vocal tract into speech (Fig. 43.52).
- The most modern method is to gain use of the expired air from the lungs to power speech which is achieved by placing a small valve through the back wall of the tracheal stoma into the pharynx. This is a one-way valve allowing air from the trachea to pass into the pharynx but it does not allow food and liquid to pass into the airway (Fig. 43.53).

There is a variety of these type of valves, the best known being the Blom–Singer valve which was developed in the USA. With the restoration of expired air passing into the pharynx, the segment of vibrating pharyngeal mucosa has a much greater quantity of air than when it is simply swallowed into the pharynx and oeosophagus, and this gives an improved flow and quality to the speech of total laryngectomy patients. These valves are common nowadays in laryngectomy patients in many countries and they must not be confused with tracheostomy tubes. Like all foreign bodies, the speaking valves are associated with minor complications such as the formation of granulations, bleeding or leakage of pharyngeal contents.

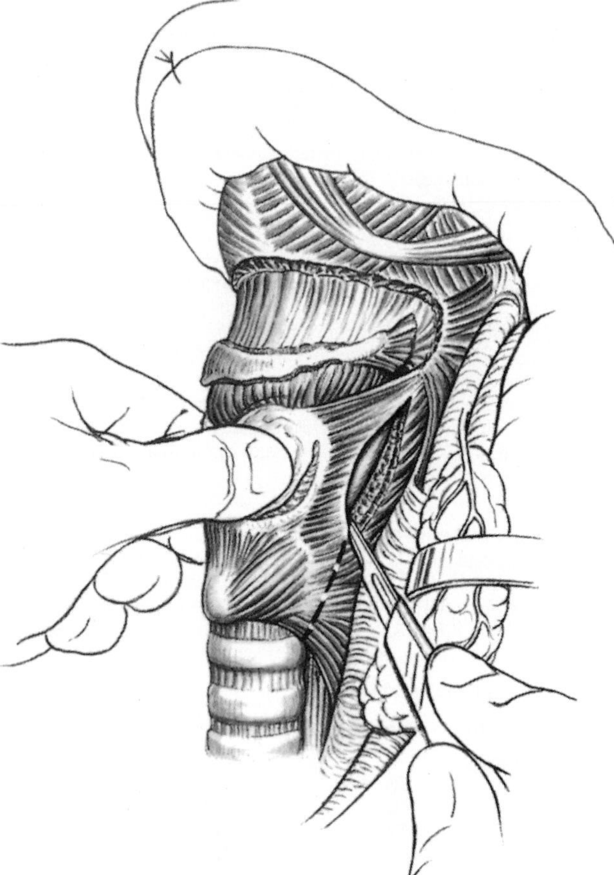

Fig. 43.49 Diagram showing the stages of a total laryngectomy. Freeing of the specimen by division of the inferior constrictor muscle, after division of the strap muscles. [Reproduced with permission from McGregor, I.A. and Howard, D.J. (eds), *Rob and Smith's Operative Surgery, Head and Neck Part 2*, Butterworth-Heinemann, Oxford, 1992, p. 486.]

The neck

Lump in the neck

The correct diagnosis of a lump in the neck can often be made with a careful history and examination. The clinical

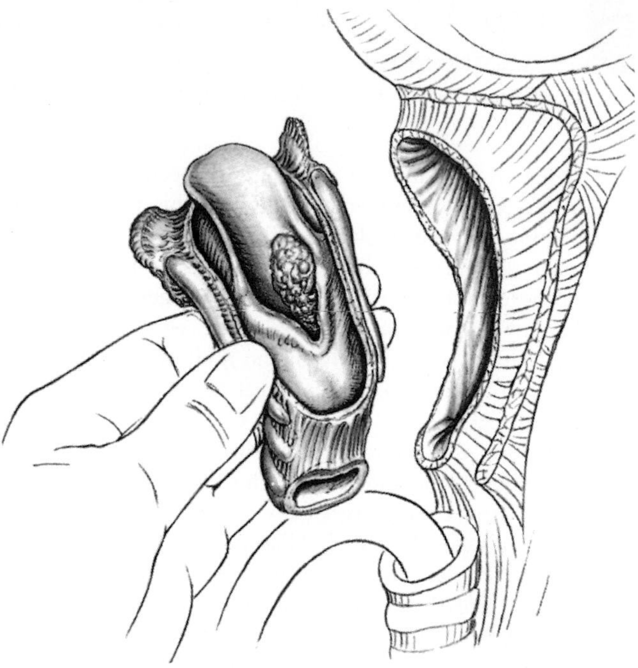

Fig. 43.50 Diagram showing removal of a laryngeal specimen. [Reproduced with permission from McGregor, I.A. and Howard, D.J. (eds), *Rob and Smith's Operative Surgery, Head and Neck Part 2*, Butterworth-Heinemann, Oxford, 1992, p. 487.]

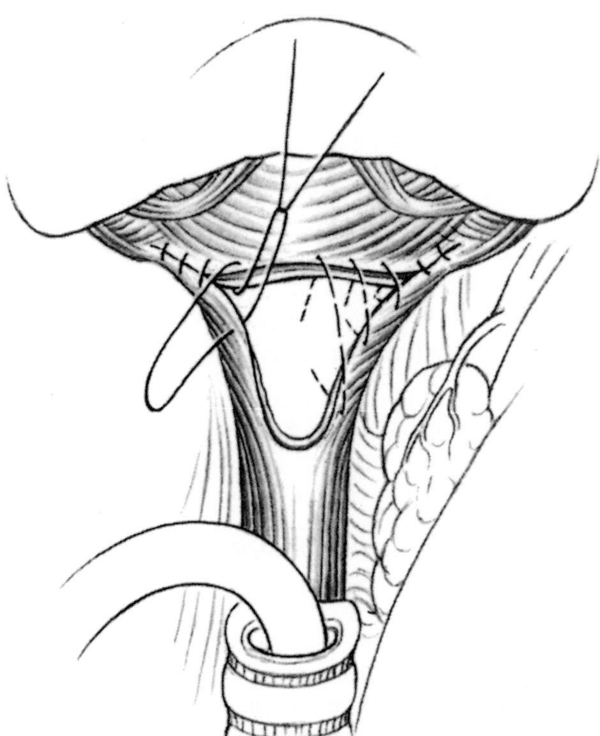

Fig. 43.51 Diagram showing transverse closure of the pharynx with an endotracheal tube in the end tracheostome. [Reproduced with permission from McGregor, I.A. and Howard, D.J. (eds), *Rob and Smith's Operative Surgery, Head and Neck Part 2*, Butterworth-Heinemann, Oxford, 1992, p. 488.]

signs of size, site, shape, consistency, fixation to skin or deep structures, pulsatility, compressability, transillumination or the presence of a bruit still remain as important as ever.

Branchial cyst

In the fifth week of foetal development four grooves can be seen on each side of the neck. These are the branchial clefts and the intervening bars are the branchial arches. Each arch contains a central cartilage and each cleft is composed of a groove on the outside and a pouch on the inside. The first cleft persists as the external auditory meatus, but the second, third and fourth normally disappear. A branchial cyst develops from the vestigial remnants of the second branchial cleft, is usually lined by squamous epithelium and contains thick turbid fluid full of cholesterol crystals (Fig. 43.54).

The branchial cyst usually presents in the upper neck in early or middle adulthood and is found at the junction of the upper third and middle third of the sternomastoid muscle at its anterior border. It is a fluctuant swelling which may transilluminate and is often soft in its early stages so that it may be difficult to palpate. If infection occurs it may become markedly erythematous and tender, and on occasions

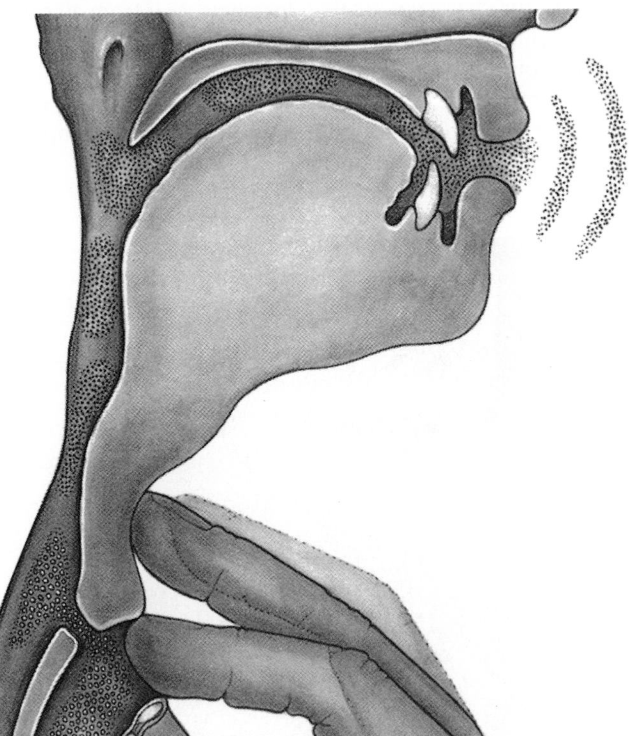

Fig. 43.52 Diagram showing production of oesophageal speech. [Reproduced with permission from McGregor, I.A. and Howard, D.J. (eds), *Rob and Smith's Operative Surgery, Head and Neck Part 2*, Butterworth-Heinemann, Oxford, 1992, p. 518.]

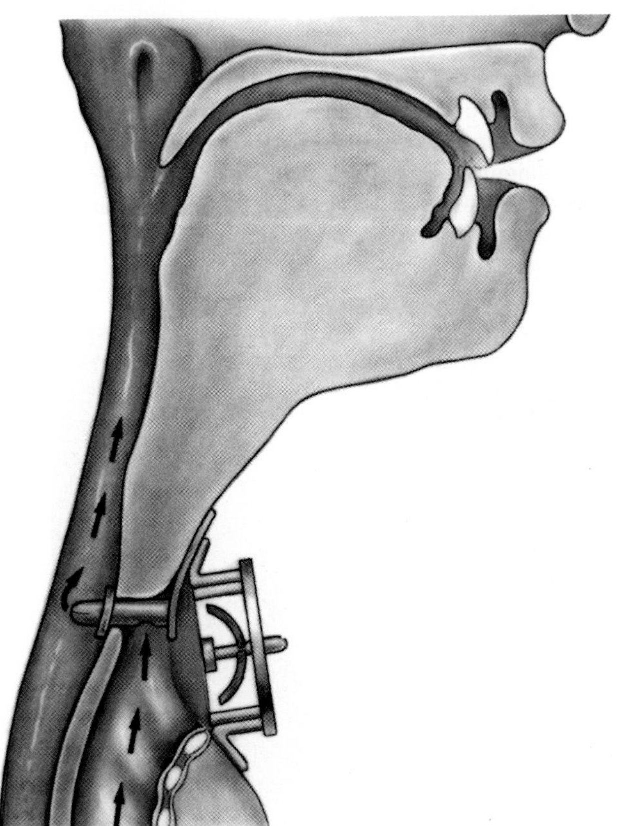

Fig. 43.53 Diagram showing a Blom–Singer valve with a tracheo-oesophageal fistula and an outer stoma valve. [Reproduced with permission from McGregor, I.A. and Howard, D.J. (eds), *Rob and Smith's Operative Surgery, Head and Neck Part 2*, Butterworth-Heinemann, Oxford, 1992, p. 521.]

it may be difficult to differentiate from a tuberculous abscess. Ultrasound and fine needle aspiration both aid with diagnosis, and treatment is by complete excision. This is best undertaken when the lesion is quiescent as attempted excision of an acutely inflammed cyst may convert it into a branchial sinus which may be more troublesome. Although the anterior aspect of the cyst is easy to dissect, it may pass backwards and upwards through the fork of the common carotid artery as far as the pharyngeal constrictors. It passes superficial to the hypoglossal and glossopharyngeal nerves but deep to the posterior belly of the diagastric. The hypoglossal and spinal accessory nerve are encountered in the operative field and must be positively identified to avoid damage. Microscopic examination of these cysts commonly shows a layer of lymphoid tissue suggesting that these cysts may arise as a result of branchial epithelium entrapped within a lymph node.

Branchial fistula

A branchial fistula (Fig. 43.55) may be unilateral or bilateral and are thought to represent a persistent second branchial cleft. Their external orifice is nearly always situated in the lower third of the neck near the anterior border of the sternocleiodomastoid, whilst the internal orifice is located on the anterior aspect of the posterior faucial pillar just behind the tonsil. However, the internal aspect of the tract may well end blindly at or close to the lateral pharyngeal wall, constituting a sinus rather than a fistula. The tract is lined by ciliated columnar epithelium and as such there may be a small amount of recurrent mucous or mucopurulent discharge on to the neck. The tract follows the same path as a branchial cyst and requires complete excision often by more than one transverse incision in the neck.

Branchogenic carcinoma

It is doubtful whether a primary carcinoma occurs in association with a branchial cyst and it is almost certainly due to cystic degeneration in a lymph node containing a deposit of squamous carcinoma. The primary focus giving rise to the squamous carcinoma may not be apparent, but is usually in the nasopharynx, tonsil, tongue base, piriform fossa or supraglottic larynx. Full examination, scanning and biopsy of these areas is necessary to exclude the occult primary.

Cystic hygroma (cavernous lymphangioma)

Around the sixth week of embryonic life, the primitive lymph sacs develop in the mesoblast, the principal pair being situated in the neck between the jugular and subclavian veins; these, which correspond to the lymph parts of lower animals, are known as the jugular lymph sacs. Sequestration of a portion of the jugular lymph sac from the lymphatic system accounts for the appearance of these swellings (Fig. 43.56).

Cystic hygroma usually manifests itself in the neonate or in early infancy, and occasionally may be present at birth and be so large as to obstruct labour. Swelling usually occurs in the lower third of the neck and as it enlarges it passes upwards towards the ear. Often the posterior triangle of the neck is mainly involved. As a result of the intercommunication of its many compartments, the swelling is soft and partially compressible, it visibly increases in size when the child coughs or cries, but the characteristic that distinguishes it from all other neck swellings is that it is brilliantly translucent. The cheek, axilla, groin and mediastinum are other, although less frequent, sites for a cystic hygroma. Cystic hygromas of the neck can on rare occasions be associated with lymphangiomatous lesions of the tongue.

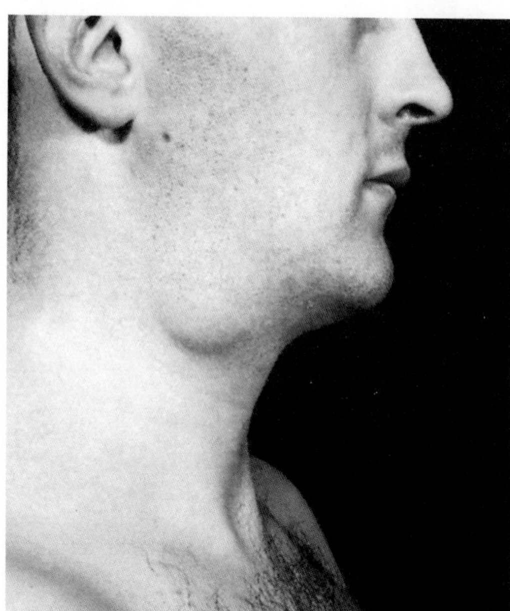

Fig. 43.54 Branchial cyst.

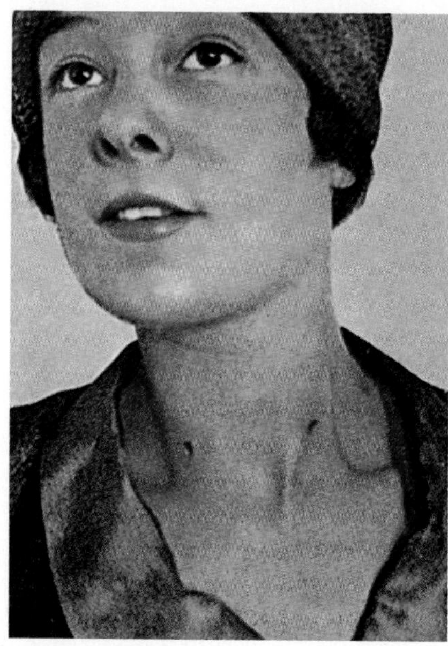

Fig. 43.55 Bilateral branchial fistula.

The behaviour of cystic hygromas during infancy is so uncertain that it is impossible at that age to predict what will happen. They sometimes expand rapidly and occasionally respiratory difficulty ensues demanding immediate aspiration of much of the cyst's contents and even, on occasion, a tracheostomy. The lesion may become infected when it becomes inflamed and painful. Spontaneous regression may occur. The cysts are filled with clear lymph and lined by a single layer of epithelium with a mosaic appearance.

Definitive treatment is excision of all of the cyst at an early stage. This requires a meticulous conservative neck dissection with excision of all lymphatic-bearing tissues whilst preserving the normal neurovascular structures if possible. A preliminary injection of sclerosing agents is not advisable as it destroys normal tissue planes making the curative surgery more difficult.

Thyroglossal duct cysts

Embryology. The thyroid gland descends early in foetal life from the base of the tongue towards its position in the lower neck with the isthmus lying over the second and third tracheal ring. At the time of its descent the hyoid bone has not been formed and the track of the descent of the thyroid gland is variable passing in front, through or behind the eventual position of the hyoid body. Thyroglossal duct cysts represent a persistence of this track and may therefore be found anywhere in or adjacent to the midline from the tongue base to the thyroid isthmus. Rarely, a thyroglossal cyst may be the only functioning thyroid tissue in the body.

Clinical features. The cysts almost always arise in the midline but when they are adjacent to the thyroid cartilage they may lie slightly to one side of the midline (Fig. 43.57). Classically, the cyst moves upwards on swallowing and notably with tongue protrusion but this may occur with other midline cysts, such as dermoid cysts, as it merely indicates attachment to the hyoid bone. Thyroglossal cysts may become infected and rupture on to the skin of the neck presenting as a discharging sinus. Whilst they often occur in children they may also present in adults even as late as the sixth or seventh decade of life.

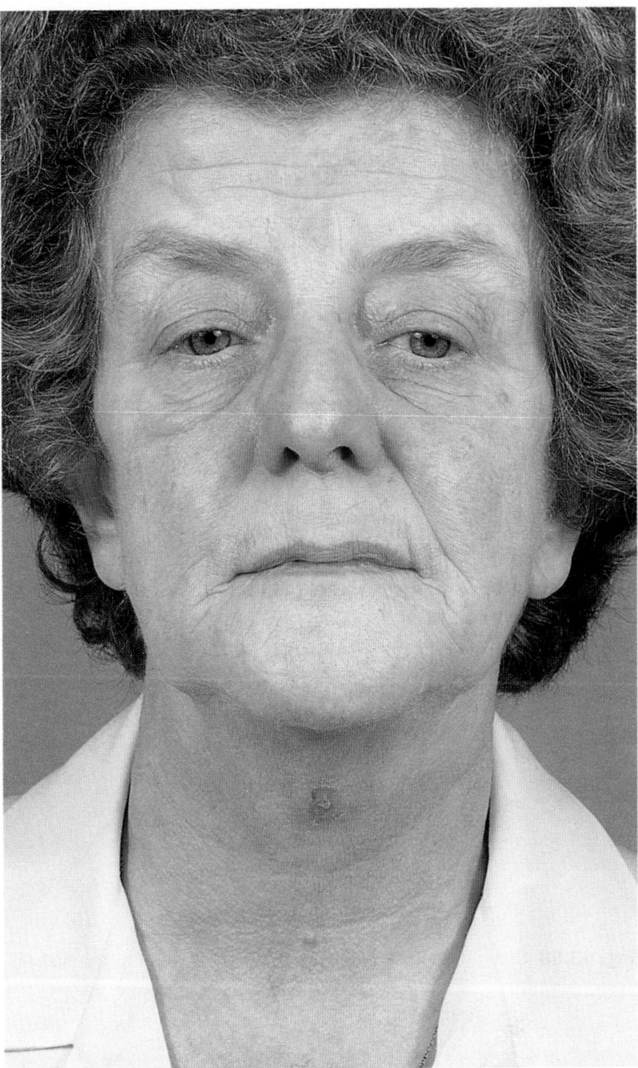

Fig. 43.57 Photograph of a patient with thyroglossal fistula from a cyst in the midline of the neck.

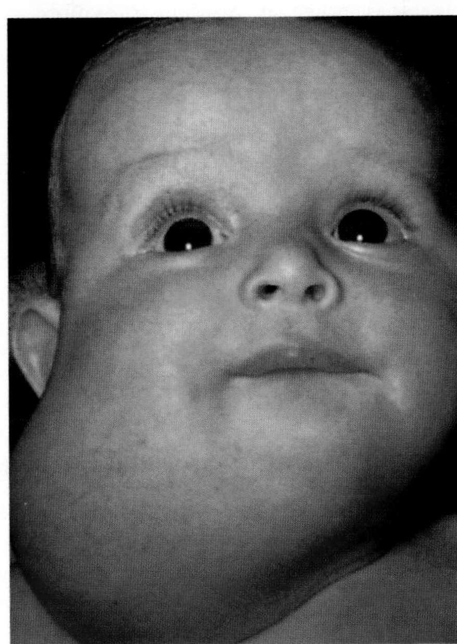

Fig. 43.56 Cystic hygroma.

Treatment. Treatment must include excision of the whole thryoglossal tract which involves removal of the body of the hyoid bone and the suprahyoid tract through the tongue base to the vallecula at the site of the primitive foramen caecum together with a core of tissue on either side. This operation is known as Sistrunk's operation and prevents recurrence, most notably from small side branches of the thyroglossal tract.

Walter Ellis Sistrunk, Jr, 1880–1933. Professor of Clinical Surgery, Baylor University College of Medicine, Dallas, Texas, USA.

Cervical rib and the scalene syndrome

Approximately 0.5 per cent of people have a seventh cervical rib, of which approximately half are unilateral and more commonly found on the right side. The cervical rib may give rise to nerve pressure symptoms and Fig. 43.58 shows the four main varieties of cervical rib. At their exit from the neck, the brachial plexus and subclavian artery pass through a narrow triangle and, if the base of the triangle is raised by the height of one vertebra due to the interposition of a cervical rib, the subclavian artery and the fourth first dorsal nerve are bound to be angulated or compressed. The artery may become constricted with a fusiform dilation of the first 2–4 cm distal to the constriction. Clotting may occur and portions of a mural thrombus may become detached and give rise to an embolus or emboli (Fig. 43.59). Three clinical situations are encountered with cervical ribs, the simplest being the patient presenting with a lump in the lower part of the neck which may be visible, bony hard and fixed. It may cause tenderness in the supraclavicular fossa. A cervical rib with vascular symptoms occurs only when the rib is complete, and pain in the forearm, but in some instances radiating to the upper arm, is the prevailing symptom. The pain is brought on by use of the arm and the pain is accelerated if the arm is in a raised position at the time of exercise. The pain is relieved by rest and is due to ischaemic changes in the muscles of the arm. The hand on the affected side may be colder than the opposite side, may become unduly pale when it is held aloft and may become blue when it is dependent for a time. The radial pulse may be less than on the normal side and sometimes absent. This will depend on the level of collateral circulation. The distal part of the subclavian artery should be auscultated and the systolic bruit will be significant. Numbness of the fingers may occur, followed by ulceration and very occasionally gangrene.

Treatment is by prompt extraperiostal excision of the cervical rib together with any bony prominence from the first rib. It may be advisable to perform sympathetic denervation of the upper limb. True cervical rib with nerve pressure symptoms is probably a rare occurrence as most cases have been found to be related to cervical spondylosis with pressure on the cervical roots in the region of the intervertebral foramina or by carpal tunnel syndrome which may cause wasting of the thenar eminence. Other conditions such as motor neuron disease and syringomyelia may cause similar symptoms. If a cervical rib needs excision it is essential to remove it with its periosteum or it will regenerate. Care must be exercised to avoid damage to the brachial plexus and phrenic nerves.

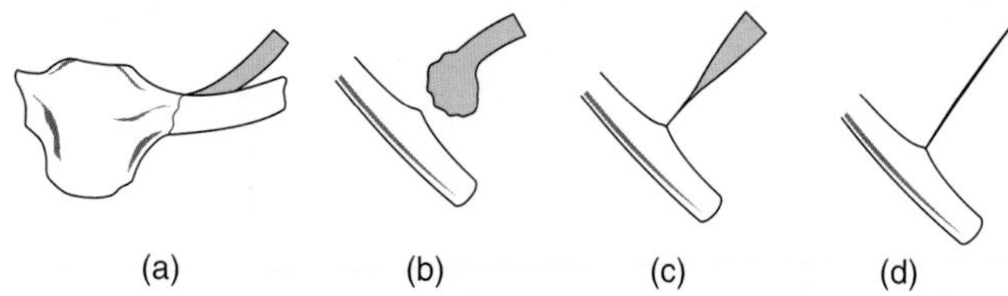

Fig. 43.58 Cervical rib showing variations in attachment to the first rib.

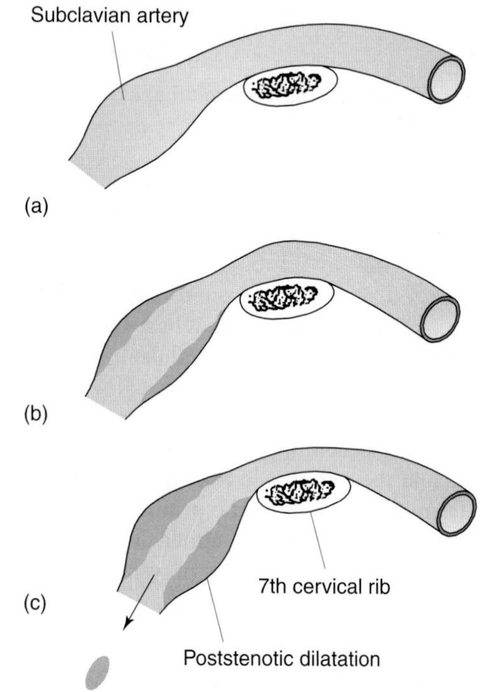

Fig. 43.59 Vascular narrowing due to a cervical rib.

Trauma to the neck

Cut throat

In the majority of cases admitted to accident and emergency centres the wound does not involve important neurovascular structures but only skin, platysma and sternocleidomastoid or strap muscles. It is, however, prudent to explore all of these wounds formally.

Wounds above the hyoid bone

The cavity of the mouth or pharynx may have been entered and the epiglottis may be divided via the pre-epiglottic space. These wounds require repair with absorbable sutures on a formal basis under a general anaesthetic. If there is any degree of associated oedema or bleeding, particularly in relation to the tongue base or laryngeal inlet, it is advisable to perform a tracheostomy to avoid any subsequent respiratory distress.

Wounds of the thyroid and cricoid cartilage

Blunt crushing injuries or severe laceration injuries to the laryngeal skeleton can cause marked haematoma formation and rapid loss of the airway. There may be significant disruption of the laryngeal skeleton. These patients should not have an endotracheal intubation for any length of time, even if this is the initial emergency way of protecting the airway. The larynx is a delicate three-tiered sphincter and the presence of a foreign body in its lumen after severe disruption gives rise to major fibrosis and loss of laryngeal function. These injuries are frequently an absolute indication for a low tracheostomy, following which the larynx can be carefully explored and damaged cartilages repositioned and sutured, and the paraglottic space drained. An indwelling stent of soft sponge shaped to fit the laryngeal lumen and held by a nylon retaining suture through the neck may be left in place for approximately 5 days. This stent can be removed endoscopically after cutting the retaining suture and as the laryngeal damage heals the patient may then be decannulated.

Division of the trachea

Wounds of the trachea are fortunately rare but they should all be formally explored, and in order to obtain adequate exposure it is usually necessary to divide and ligate the thyroid isthmus. A small tracheostomy below the wound and then repair of the trachea with a limited number of submucosal sutures is appropriate. In self-inflicted wounds the recurrent laryngeal nerves, which lie protected in the tracheo-oesophageal grooves, are rarely injured. However, in stab wounds to the neck any nerve may be involved including the vagus, recurrent laryngeal nerve or cervical sympathetic chain. Primary repair is rarely possible but may be undertaken at the time of formal exploration of a major neck wound.

Vascular complications of cut throat

In contrast to nerve damage, vascular damage can be severe. Major haemorrhagic shock may occur as a consequence of injury to the common carotid, external or internal carotid, or a venous air embolism as a result of damage to one of the major veins, most commonly the internal jugular. Infection of large neck wounds is not uncommon, and cellulitis may supervene and spread inferiorly to the mediastinum. Surgical emphysema may result if damage to the trachea is not recognised and air escapes into the neck. Oesophageal and pharyngeal fistula may occur but usually heal spontaneously. Aphonia or dysphonia may follow injury to the vocal folds or division of the recurrent laryngeal nerves. Stenosis of the trachea or larynx may be caused by scarring from major injuries due to road traffic accident or attempted hanging.

Wounds of the cervical portion of the thoracic duct

Wounds to the thoracic duct are fortunately rare and most often occur in association with dissection of lymph nodes in the left supraclavicular fossa. When damage to the duct is not recognised at the time of operation, chyle may subsequently leak from wound in amounts up to 2 litres/day and, as a result, the patient may waste rapidly.

Treatment

Should the damage be recognised during an operation, the proximal end of the duct must be ligated. Ligation of the duct is not harmful because there is a number of anastomotic channels between the lymphatic and venous system in the lower neck. If undetected, chyle usually starts to discharge from the neck wound within 24 hours of the operation. On occasions firm pressure by a pad and bandage to the lower neck may stop the leakage but frequently this is unsuccessful and it is best to re-explore the wound and locate and ligate the damaged duct. If the patient is given some cream to drink 2 hours before the operation the cut end of the duct is more easily found just lateral to the lower 4 cm of the left internal jugular vein. If it proves impossible to find the duct, particularly in an area of oedematous and fragile tissue, the wound can be packed firmly with a Whitehead's varnish pack and allowed to heal by granulation.

Inflammatory conditions of the neck

Parapharyngeal and retropharyngeal abscess formation has been covered earlier in this chapter.

Ludwig angina

Ludwig described a clinical entity characterised by a brawny swelling of the submandibular region combined with inflammatory oedema of the mouth. It is these combined cervical and intraoral signs that constitute the characteristic feature of the lesion, as well as the putrid halitosis that is always present. The infection is often caused by a virulent streptococcal infection associated with anaerobic organisms and sometimes with other lesions of the floor of the mouth such as carcinoma. The infection encompasses both sides of the mylohyoid muscle causing oedema and inflammation such that the tongue may be displaced upwards and backwards giving rise initially to dysphagia and subsequently to potential obstruction of the airway.

Clinical cause

Unless the infection is controlled cellulitis may extend down the neck beneath the deep fascial layers to involve the larynx causing glottic oedema.

Treatment

Antibiotic therapy should be instituted as soon as possible using intravenous broad-spectrum antibiotics such as amoxycillin or cefuroxime combined with metronidazole to combat the anaerobes. In advanced cases where the swelling does not subside rapidly with such treatment, a curved submental incision may be used to drain both submandibular triangles. The mylohyoid muscle may be incised to decompress the floor of the mouth. Simple but generous corrugated drains may be placed in the wound which is then lightly sutured. This operation may be conducted under local anaesthesia and on rare occasions an additional tracheostomy may be necessary.

Cervical lymphadenitis (Table 43.14)

There are approximately 800 lymph nodes in the body; no fewer than 300 of them lie in the neck. Inflammation of the lymph nodes of the neck is exceedingly common. Infection occurs from the oral and nasal cavities, the pharynx, larynx, ear, scalp and face. The source of the infection must be sought systematically.

Acute lymphadenitis

The affected lymph nodes are enlarged and tender, and there may be varying degrees of general constitutional disturbance of the patient with pyrexia, anorexia and general malaise. The treatment in the first instance is directed to the primary focus of infection, for example tonsillitis or a dental abscess. If, despite antibiotic therapy, the pain continues or abscess formation occurs in the lymph nodes, parapharyngeal or retropharyngeal space then surgical drainage may be required.

Chronic lymphadenitis

Chronic painless lymphadenopathy may be either tuberculous, in children or young adults, or due to secondary malignant metastases most commonly from a squamous carcinoma in older people. Lymphoma also commonly presents in cervical nodes in young adults.

Careful inspection of the upper airways and food passages is essential to exclude primary malignancy of the nasopharynx, tonsil, tongue base, piriform fossa or larynx. Fine needle aspiration of enlarged cervical lymph nodes is preferable to any form of open biopsy.

Tuberculous adenitis

Tuberculosis (TB) remains a problem throughout the world and is still a common cause of cervical lymphadenopathy. The condition most commonly affects children or young adults, but can occur at any age. The deep upper cervical nodes are most commonly affected, but there may be a widespread cervical lymphadenitis and the matching together of a substantial number of lymph nodes may be evident.

In most instances the tubercular bacilli gain entrance through the tonsil of the corresponding side of the lymphadenopathy. Both bovine and human TB may be responsible. In approximately 80 per cent of cases the tuberculous process is limited to the clinically affected group of lymph nodes but a primary focus in the lungs must always be suspected and investigated. As renal and pulmonary TB occasionally coexist, the urine should be examined carefully. Rarely, the patient may develop a natural resistance to the infection and the nodes may be detected at a later date as evidenced by calcification on an X-ray. This can also be seen after appropriate general treatment of tuberculous adenitis. If treatment is not instituted, the caseated node may liquefy and break down with the formation of a cold abscess in the neck (Fig. 43.60). The pus is first confined by the deep cervical fascia but after weeks or months this may become eroded at one point and the pus flows through the small opening into the space beneath the superficial fascia. The process has now reached the well-known stage of a 'collar stud' abscess. The superficial abscess enlarges steadily and, unless suitable treatment is adopted, the skin will soon become reddened over the centre of the fluctuating swelling and before long a discharging sinus occurs in the neck.

Treatment. The patient should be treated by appropriate chemotherapy, as confirmed by assessment of abscess contents for sensitivities to the antituberculous drugs. If an abscess fails to resolve despite appropriate chemotherapy and general measures, occasionally excision of the abscess and its surrounding fibrous capsule is necessary together with the relevant lymph nodes. If there is active TB of another system, for example pulmonary, then removal of tuberculosis lymph nodes in the neck is inappropriate. The nodes are commonly related to the internal jugular vein, common carotid and vagus nerve, and they may be associated with a great deal of surrounding fibrosis. Surgery can be difficult and a portion of the internal jugular vein may require excision with considerable care to avoid damage to the vagus or the cervical sympathetic trunk. A good view and access should be obtained at all times during this surgery and the sternocleidomastoid muscle divided to facilitate access, particularly if the disease is adjacent to the spinal accessory nerve or the hypoglossal nerve. The resected nodes should be sent for both pathological and microbiological analysis.

Table 43.14 Causes of cervical lymphadenopathy

1. Inflammatory
   - Reactive hyperplasia
2. Infective
   - Viral, e.g. infectious mononucleosis, HIV
   - Bacterial
     - streptococcus, staphylococcus
     - actinomycosis
     - TB
     - brucellosis
   - Protozoan – toxoplasmosis
3. Neoplastic
   - Malignant
   - primary, e.g. lymphoma
   - secondary, e.g. squamous cell carcinoma
     - known primary
     - occult primary

Wilhelm von Ludwig, 1790–1865. Professor of Surgery and Midwifery in Tubingen, Germany.

Primary tumours of the neck

Neurogenous tumours

Chemodectoma (carotid body tumour). This is a rare tumour but there is a higher incidence in areas where people live at high altitudes, for example in Peru and Mexico where increased numbers have been reported as a consequence of chronic hypoxia leading to carotid body hyperplasia. The tumours

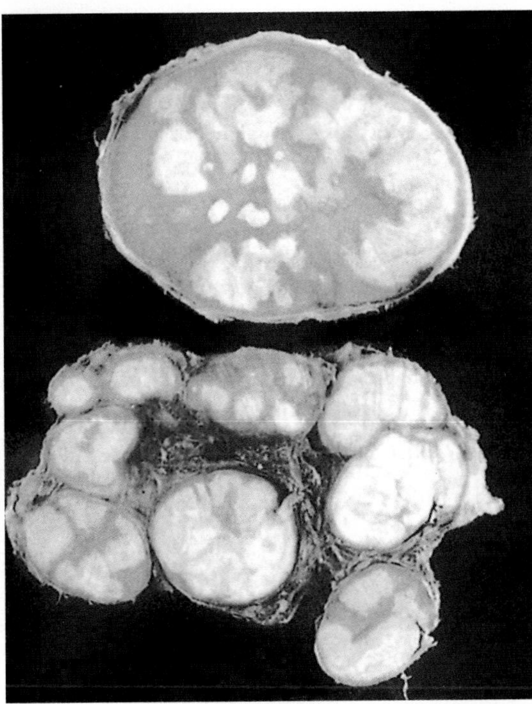

Fig. 43.60 Caseating tuberculous cervical lymph nodes.

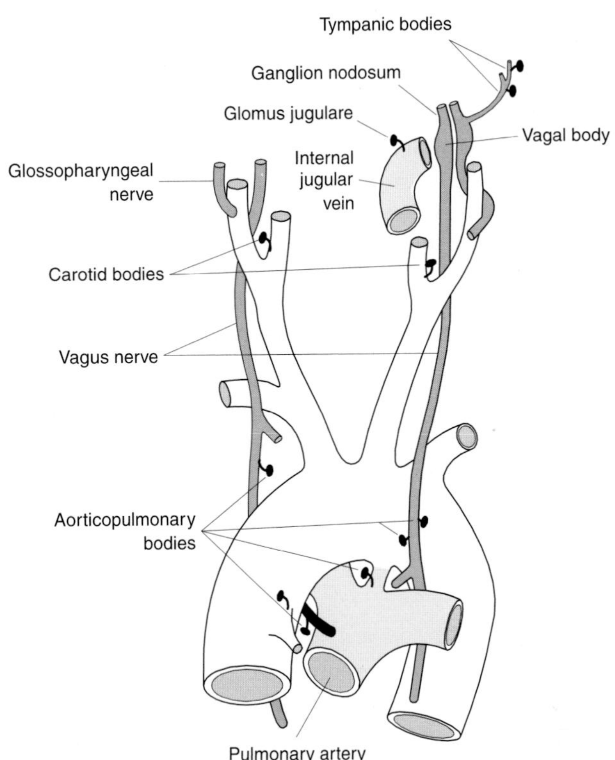

Fig. 43.61 Sites for chemodectomas.

most commonly present in the fifth decade and approximately 10 per cent of patients have a family history. There is an association with phaeochromocytoma. The tumours arise from the chemoreceptor cells on the medial side of the carotid bulb and at this point the tumour is adherent to the carotid wall (Fig. 43.61). The cells of the chemodectoma are not hormonally active and the tumours are usually benign with only a few proven metastases in a small number of cases.

Clinical features. The patients often present with a long history of several years of a slowly enlarging painless lump at the carotid bifurcation. About one-third of patients present with a pharyngeal mass pushing the tonsil medially and anteriorly. The mass is firm, rubbery, pulsatile and is mobile from side to side but not up and down, and can sometimes be emptied by firm pressure, after which it will slowly refill in a pulsatile manner. A bruit may also be present.

Swellings in the parapharyngeal space which often displace the tonsil medially should not be biopsied from within the mouth.

Investigations. When a chemodectoma is suspected a duplex study and, if indicated, a carotid angiogram should be carried out to demonstrate the carotid bifurcation which is usually splayed and a blush which outlines the normal tumour vessels. This tumour must not be biopsied and fine needle aspiration is also contraindicated.

Treatment. Because these tumours rarely metastasise and their overall rate of growth is slow, the need for surgical removal must be considered carefully as complications of surgery are potentially serious. The operation is best avoided in elderly patients. Radiotherapy has no effect. In some cases it may be possible to dissect the tumour away from the carotid bifurcation, but at times when the tumour is large it may not be separable from the vessels and resection will be necessary such that all appropriate facilities should be available to establish a bypass whilst a vein autograft is inserted to restore arterial continuity in the carotid system.

Vagal body tumours. Vagal paragangliomas arise from nests of paraganglionic tissue of the vagus nerve just below the base of the skull near the jugular foramen. They may also be found at various sites along the nerve down to the level of the carotid artery bifurcation.

Clinical features. They also present as slowly growing and painless masses in the anterolateral aspect of the neck, and may also have a long history commonly of 2–3 years before diagnosis. Diagnosis is confirmed by CT and MRI scanning and additional arteriography if necessary.

They may spread into the cranial cavity and surgery may be required.

Peripheral nerve tumours. Schwannomas are solitary and encapsulated tumours attached to or surrounded by a nerve. Paralysis of the associated nerve is unusual. The vagus nerve is the commonest site for these tumours within the neck. Neurofibromas also arise from the Schwann cell and may be part of von Recklinghausen syndrome of multiple neurofibromatosis. Multiple neurofibromatosis is an autosomal

Theodor Schwann, 1810–82. Professor of Anatomy, Louvain and Liège, Belgium.

Friedrich Daniel von Recklinghausen, 1833–1910. German histologist and pathologist. Professor at Würzeburg and Strasbourg, Germany.

dominant hereditary disease and the neurofibromata may be present at birth and often multiple. These lesions may occur in the neck and in about 10 per cent of these tumours malignant change occurs, although they usually enlarge slowly over a period of many years and the painless neck mass is the only sign. As with the lesions above, diagnosis requires angiography and scanning to differentiate them from other parapharyngeal tumours, but on occasions the diagnosis must wait until excision.

Secondary carcinoma of the neck

Secondary carcinomatous infiltration of the cervical lymph nodes is a common occurrence from important primary sites in the head and neck. These are nasopharynx, tonsil, tongue, piriform fossa and supraglottic larynx. All of these areas must be carefully assessed to search for the primary growth before considering biopsy or any surgery on the neck. Investigation is further assisted by fine needle aspirate of the neck node.

Management

The management of the involved cervical lymph nodes depends on the overall treatment regime to be given to the patient.

- If surgery is being used to treat the primary disease and the cervical nodes are palpable, and in excess of 3 cm, they may be excised *en bloc* with the primary lesion.
- If radiotherapy is used initially, as is always the case in carcinoma of the nasopharynx, then radiotherapy may also be given to the neck nodes whatever their stage. In the case of tongue, pharynx or larynx, however, if the node exceeds 3 cm in diameter then surgery may be necessary for the neck nodes even if the primary is treated by radiotherapy.
- If radiotherapy is used initially, as is always the case in carcinoma of the nasopharynx, then radiography may also be given to the neck nodes, whatever their stage. In the case of the tongues, pharynx or larynx however, if the node exceeds 3 cm in diameter then surgery may be necessary for the neck nodes, even if the primary is treated by radiotherapy. If radiotherapy is used initially with resolution of the primary but there is subsequent residual or recurrent nodal disease then this situation will require cervical lymph node dissection.

Types of neck dissection

- Classical radical neck dissection (Crile) – the clas/sic operation involves resection of the cervical lymphatics, the lymph nodes and those structures closely associated such as the internal jugular vein, the accessory nerve, the submandibular gland and the sternamastoid muscle. These structures are all removed *en bloc* and in continuity with the primary disease if possible. The main disability that follows the operation is the drooping of the shoulder due to paralysis of the trapezius muscle as a consequence of excision of the accessory nerve.
- Modified radical neck dissection – in selected cases one or more of the three following structures are preserved, the accessory nerve, the sternocleidomastoid muscle or the internal jugular vein, but otherwise all major lymph node groups and lymphatics are excised. Whichever structures are preserved at this dissection should be clearly noted.
- Selective neck dissection – in this type of dissection one or more of the major lymph node groups is preserved along with sternomastoid muscle, accessory nerve and internal jugular vein. Under these circumstances the exact groups of nodes excised must be documented.

Further reading

Hibbert, J. (ed.) (1997) *Scott Brown's Otolaryngology, Laryngology and Head and Neck Surgery*, 6th edn, Butterworth-Heinemann, Oxford.

Maran, A.G.D., Gaze, M. and Wilson, J.A. (1993) *Stell and Maran's Head and Neck Surgery*, Butterworth-Heinemann, Oxford.

McGregor, I.A. and Howard, D.J. (eds) (1992) *Rob and Smith's Operative Surgery, Head and Neck Part 1*, Butterworth-Heinemann, Oxford.

van Hasselt, C.A. and Gibb, A.G. (eds) (1991) *Nasopharyngeal Carcinoma*, Chinese University Press, Hong Kong.

George Washington Crile, 1864–1943. Professor of Surgery, Western Reserve University and one of the Founders of the Cleveland Clinic, Cleveland, Ohio, USA.

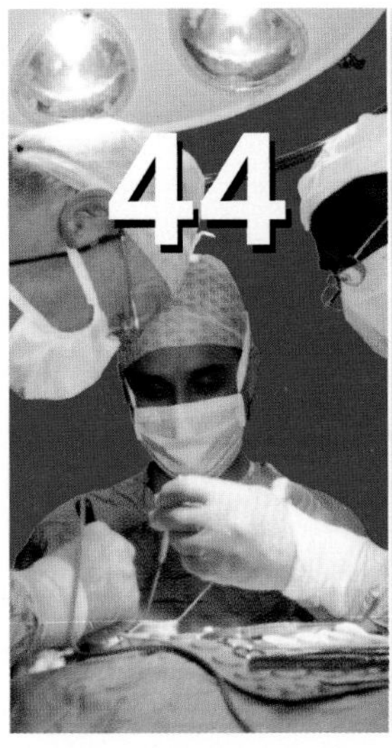

The thyroid gland and the thyroglossal tract

Embryology

The thyroid gland develops from the median bud of the pharynx (the thyroglossal duct) which passes from the foramen caecum at the base of the tongue to the isthmus of the thyroid. The ultimobranchial body which arises from a diverticulum of the fourth pharyngeal pouch of each side amalgamates with the corresponding lateral lobe. Parafollicular cells (C-cells) are derived from the neural crest and reach the thyroid via the ultimobranchial body. Recently, consideration has been given to the possibility that some C-cells are of endodermal rather than neural crest origin. It is doubtful whether the branchial apparatus itself contributes to the thyroid follicular cells.

Surgical anatomy (Figs 44.1 and 44.2)

The normal gland weighs 20–25 g. The functioning unit is the lobule supplied by a single arteriole and consisting of 24–40 follicles which are lined by cuboidal epithelium. The resting follicle contains colloid in which thyroglobulin is stored. The arterial supply is rich, and extensive anastomoses occur between the main thyroid arteries and branches of tracheal and oesophageal arteries. There is an extensive lymphatic network within the gland. Although some lymph channels pass directly to the deep cervical nodes, the subcapsular plexus drains principally to the juxtathyroid nodes, i.e. pretracheal (Delphic)[1] and paratracheal nodes, and nodes on the superior and inferior thyroid veins, and thence to the deep cervical and mediastinal group of nodes.

[1]*Pythia, the snake-woman oracle of Delphi, sat on her tripod, clutching the ribbons of the monolithic 'omphalos' of the world. She inhaled sulphurous fumes and laurel, and uttered a meaningless jargon which was interpreted equivocally by the attendant priests for those who came to consult her. Formerly, the purpose of these lymph nodes was uncertain and they were therefore called 'Delphic'.*

Bailey & Love's Short Practice of Surgery, 23rd edition. Edited by R.C.G. Russell, N.S. Williams and C.J.K. Bulstrode. Published in 2000 by Arnold Publishers.

Ectopic thyroid and anomalies of the thyroglossal tract

Some residual thyroid tissue along the course of the thyroglossal tract is not uncommon, and may be lingual, cervical or intrathoracic. Very rarely the whole gland is ectopic.

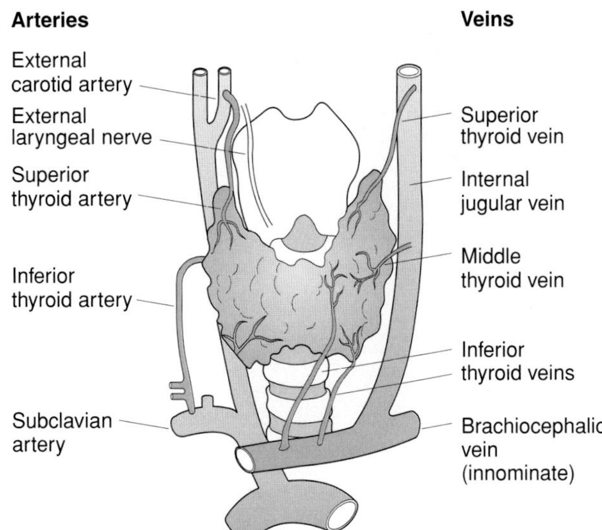

Fig. 44.1 The thyroid gland from the front.

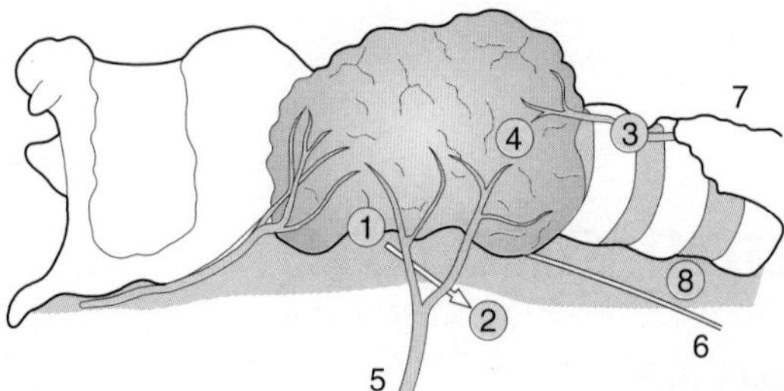

Fig. 44.2 Surgical anatomy of the thyroid. The situation after mobilisation of the right lobe, and the relationships of the recurrent laryngeal nerve, inferior thyroid artery and the parathyroid glands as they are usually found. 1 and 2: Common sites for superior parathyroid gland – the arrow shows the tendency for an enlarged gland to migrate from position 1 to position 2, i.e. in an inferior direction, to lie posterior to the inferior thyroid artery (5) and oesophagus (8); 3 and 4: common sites for inferior parathyroid gland[1]; 5: inferior thyroid artery; 6: recurrent laryngeal nerve; 7: thymus; 8: oesophagus.

[1]The upper horn of the thymus points like an index finger to the inferior parathyroid which may lie under the fingernail.' Per-Ola Grandberg, Formerly Chief of Endocrine Surgery, Karolinska Hospital, Stockholm, Sweden.

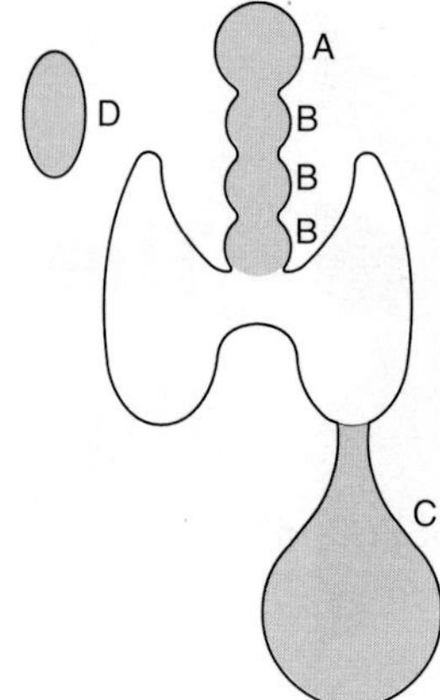

Fig. 44.4 Ectopic and aberrant thyroids. A and B are ectopic, C is an intrathoracic aberrant thyroid (nearly always acquired), D 'lateral aberrant thyroid' is well-differentiated thyroid cancer.

Lingual thyroid

This forms a rounded swelling at the back of the tongue at the foramen caecum (Figs 44.3 and 44.4) and it may represent the only thyroid tissue present. It may cause dysphagia, impairment of speech, respiratory obstruction or haemorrhage. It is best treated by full replacement with thyroxine when it should get smaller, but excision or ablation with radioiodine is sometimes necessary.

Median (thyroglossal) ectopic thyroid

This forms a swelling in the upper part of the neck (Fig. 44.4) and is usually mistaken for a thyroglossal cyst. Again, this may be the only normal thyroid tissue present.

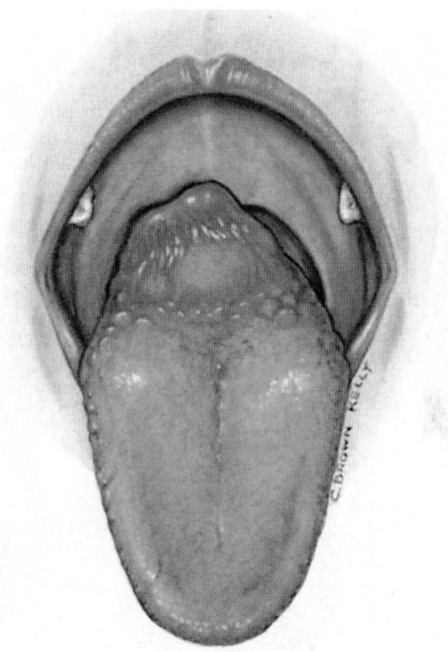

Fig. 44.3 Lingual thyroid (*courtesy of H. Wapshaw, FRCS, Glasgow*).

Rupert Allan Willis, 1898–1980. Professor of Pathology, Leeds, England.

Lateral aberrant thyroid

There is no evidence that aberrant thyroid tissue ever occurs in a lateral position (Willis). 'Normal thyroid tissue' found laterally, separate from the thyroid gland, must be considered and treated as a metastasis in a cervical lymph node from an occult thyroid carcinoma, almost invariably of papillary type. Struma ovarii is not ectopic thyroid tissue, but part of an ovarian teratoma. Very rarely, neoplastic change occurs or hyperthyroidism develops.

Thyroglossal cyst

This may be present in any part of the thyroglossal tract (Fig. 44.5). The common situations, in order of frequency, are beneath the hyoid, in the region of the thyroid cartilage, and above the hyoid bone. Such a cyst occupies the midline, except in the region of the thyroid cartilage, where the thyroglossal tract is pushed to one side, usually to the left. It is to be remembered that the swelling moves upwards on protrusion of the tongue as well as on swallowing because of the attachment of the tract to the foramen caecum.

A thyroglossal cyst should be excised because infection is inevitable, owing to the fact that the wall contains nodules of lymphatic tissue

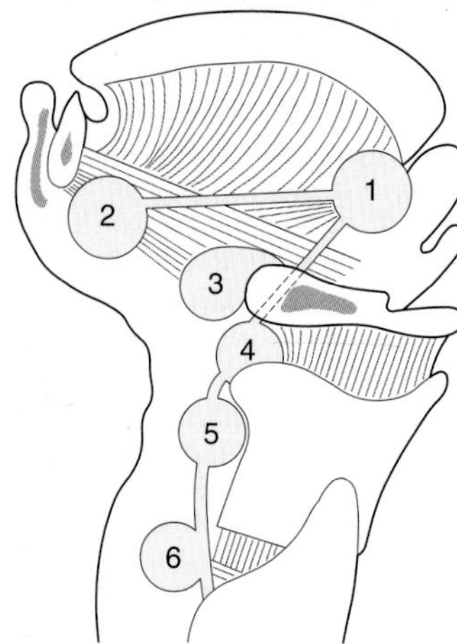

Fig. 44.5 Possible sites of a thyroglossal cyst. 1: Beneath the foramen caecum; 2: in the floor of the mouth; 3: suprahyoid; 4: subhyoid; 5: on the thyroid cartilage; 6: at the level of the cricoid cartilage.

which communicate by lymphatics with the lymph nodes of the neck. An infected cyst is often mistaken for an abscess and incised, which is one way in which a thyroglossal fistula arises.

Thyroglossal fistula

Thyroglossal fistula (Fig. 44.6a, b) is never congenital: it follows infection or inadequate removal of a thyroglossal cyst. Characteristically the cutaneous opening of such a fistula is drawn upwards on protrusion of the tongue. A thyroglossal fistula is lined by columnar epithelium, discharges mucus, and is the seat of recurrent attacks of inflammation.

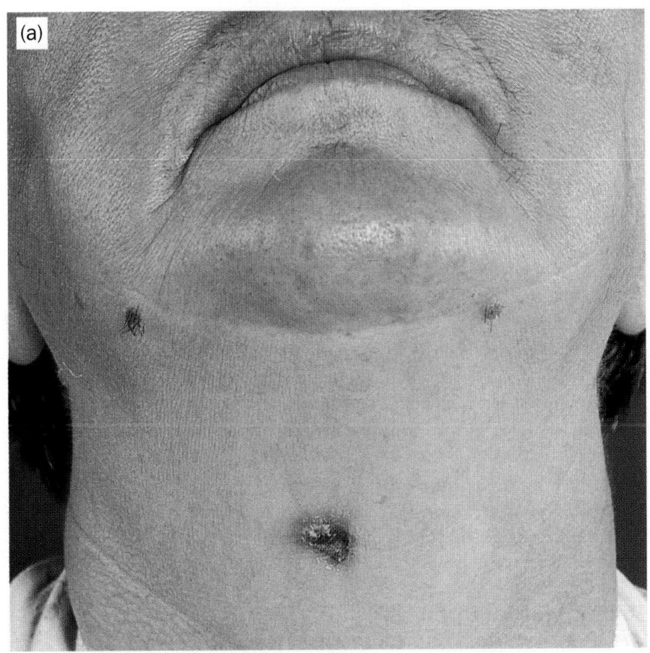

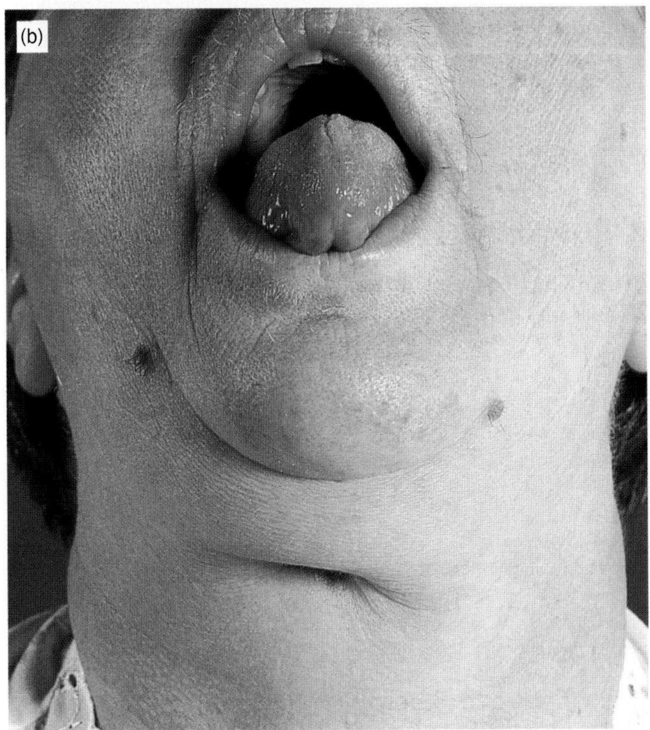

Fig. 44.6 (a) and (b) Thyroglossal fistula. Characteristic indrawing of the external opening of a thyroglossal fistula on protrusion of the tongue.

Treatment. Because the thyroglossal tract is so closely related to the body of the hyoid bone, this central part must be excised, together with the cyst or fistula, or recurrence is certain. When the thyroglossal tract can be traced upwards towards the foramen caecum, it must be excised with the central section of the body of the hyoid bone, and a central core of lingual muscle (Sistrunk's operation).

Physiology. The hormones tri-iodothyronine (T_3) and thyroxine (T_4) (extracted by E.C. Kendall in 1916) are bound to thyroglobulin within the colloid. Synthesis within the thyroglobulin complex is controlled by several enzymes, in distinct steps:

- trapping of inorganic iodide from the blood;
- oxidation of iodide to iodine;
- binding of iodine with tyrosine to form iodotyrosines;
- coupling of mono-iodotyrosines and di-iodotyrosines to form T_3 and T_4;
- when hormones are required the complex is resorbed into the cell and thyroglobulin broken down; T_3 and T_4 are liberated and enter the blood where they are bound to serum proteins: albumin and thyroxine binding globulin (TBG) and prealbumin (TBPA). A small amount of hormone remains free in the serum in equilibrium with the protein-bound hormone and is biologically active.

The metabolic effects of the thyroid hormones are due to unbound free T_4 and T_3 (0.03 per cent and 0.3 per cent of the total circulating hormones, respectively). T_3 is quick acting (within a few hours) whereas T_4 acts more slowly (4–14 days). T_3 is the more important physiological hormone and is also produced in the periphery by conversion from T_4.

Therapeutic notes: L-thyroxine (T_4) is the official name; trade name Eltroxin; tablet size 0.1 mg and 0.05 mg. Tri-iodothyronine (T_3), official name liothyronine; trade names Cynomel, Tertroxin; tablet size 20 μg.

Thyrocalcitonin

See calcitonin, Chapter 45.

The pituitary thyroid axis

Synthesis and liberation of thyroid hormones from the thyroid is controlled by thyroid-stimulating hormone (TSH) from the anterior pituitary. Secretion of TSH depends upon the level of circulating thyroid hormones and is modified in a classic negative feedback manner. In hyperthyroidism, where hormone levels in the blood are high, TSH production is suppressed whereas in hypothyroidism it is stimulated. Regulation of TSH secretion also results from the action of thyrotrophin-releasing hormone (TRH) produced in the hypothalamus.

Thyroid-stimulating antibodies

A family of IgG immunoglobulins binds with TSH receptor sites (TRAbs) and activate TSH receptors on the follicular cell membrane. They have a more protracted action than TSH (16–24 hours versus 1.5–3 hours) and are responsible for virtually all cases of thyrotoxicosis not due to autonomous toxic nodules. Serum concentrations are very low and not routinely measured.

Walter Ellis Sistrunk, Jr, 1880–1933. Professor of Clinical Surgery, Baylor University College of Medicine, Dallas, Texas, USA
Edward Calvin Kendall, 1886–1972. Professor of Physiological Chemistry, Mayo Clinic, Rochester, Minnesota, USA.

Table 44.1 Results of thyroid function tests in normal and pathological states

Thyroid functional state	*Free T_4 (nmol/litre)*	*Free T_3 (pmol/litre)*	*TSH (mU/litre)*
Euthyroid	10–30	3.5–7.5	0.3–3.3
Thyrotoxic	40*	12.0*	<0.1*
Myxoedema	3*	<1.0*	>45.0*
Developing thyroid failure	9*	3.0*	15*
Suppressive T_3 therapy	<1*	12.0*	<0.1*

*Representative value.

Tests of thyroid function

There is a variety of tests of thyroid function available, some of which are now only of historic interest and others in the province of the endocrinologist rather than the endocrine surgeon. The number of investigations requested should be the minimum necessary to reach a diagnosis and formulate a management plan. Only a small number of parameters needs to be measured as a routine although this may require supplementation or repeat when inconclusive.

Serum thyroid hormones

Serum TSH. TSH levels can be measured accurately down to very low serum concentrations and if the serum TSH level is in the normal range it is redundant to measure the T_3 and T_4 levels. Interpretation of deranged TSH levels however depends on knowledge of the T_3 and T_4 values (Table 44.1). In the euthyroid state, T_3, T_4 and TSH levels will all be within the normal range. Florid thyroid failure results in depressed T_3 and T_4 levels with gross elevation of the TSH. Incipient or developing thyroid failure is characterised by low normal values of T_3 and T_4 and elevation of the TSH. In toxic states the TSH level is suppressed and undetectable. *Thyroxine (T_4) and tri-iodothyronine (T_3)* are transported in plasma bound to specific proteins (thyroxine-binding globulin, TBG). Only a small fraction of the total (0.03 per cent of T_4 and 0.3 per cent of T_3) is free and physiologically active. Assays of both total and free hormone are available but the total values depend on the level of circulating proteins which are affected by the level of circulating oestrogen. Thus, pregnant women and those on the oral contraceptive pill have elevated total T_4 and T_3 levels without evidence of toxicity. The free hormone levels are unaffected. Similarly some patients have low levels of TBG either as a primary phenomenon or secondary to a reduction in serum protein levels as a result of systemic or liver disease and the total level of circulating hormone may be low. For these reasons the free levels are more meaningful. Highly accurate radioimmunoassays of free T_3 and free T_4 are now routine. T_3 toxicity (with a normal T_4) is a distinct entity and may only be diagnosed by measuring the serum T_3, although a suppressed TSH level with a normal T_4 is suggestive.

Various combinations of these tests are used in different laboratories. An appropriate combination is to establish the functional thyroid status at initial assessment, with TSH supplemented by free T_4, and T_3 evaluation when TSH is abnormal.

Isotope scanning (Fig. 44.7)

The uptake by the thyroid of a low dose of either radiolabelled iodine (^{123}I) or technetium-99m (^{99m}Tc, which is normally taken up like ^{123}I) will demonstrate the distribution of activity in the whole gland. This test is inappropriate for distinguishing benign from malignant lesions because the majority (80 per cent) of 'cold' swellings is benign and some (5 per cent) functioning or 'warm' swellings will be malignant. Its principal value is in the toxic patient with a nodule or nodularity of the thyroid. Localisation of overactivity in the gland will differentiate between a toxic nodule with suppression of the remainder of the gland and toxic multinodular goitre with several areas of increased uptake with important implications for therapy. Routine isotope scanning is unnecessary.

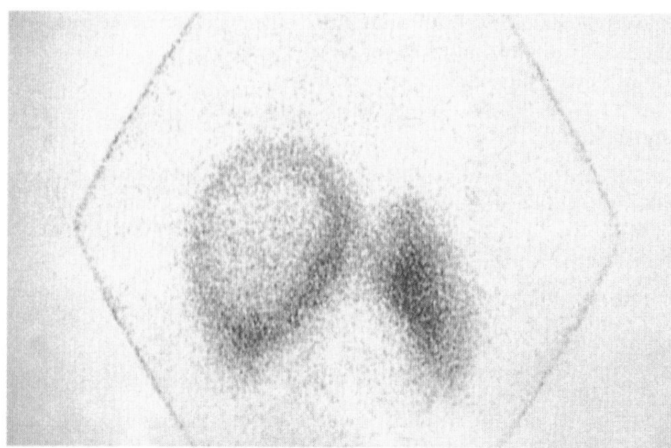

Fig. 44.7 Technetium thyroid scan showing a 'cold' nodule which does not take up isotope expanding the left thyroid lobe (*courtesy of Dr F.W. Smith, Aberdeen, Scotland*).

Whole body scanning is used to demonstrate metastases but the patient must have all normally functioning thyroid tissue ablated either by surgery or by ablation with high-dose radioiodine before the scan is performed because thyroid cancer cannot compete with normal thyroid tissue in the uptake of iodine.

Thyroid autoantibodies

Serum titres of antibodies against thyroid peroxidase and thyroglobulin are useful in determining the cause of thyroid dysfunction and swellings. Autoimmune thyroiditis may be associated with thyroid toxicity, failure or euthyroid goitre. Titres of greater than 1:100 are considered significant but a proportion of patients with histological evidence of lymphocytic (autoimmune) thyroiditis is seronegative.

Hypothyroidism

A scheme for classifying hypothyroidism is given in Table 44.2.

Cretinism (foetal or infantile hypothyroidism) (Figs 44.8 and 44.9)

Sporadic cretinism is due to complete or near complete failure of thyroid development (partial failure causes juvenile myxoedema): the parents and other children may be perfectly normal. In endemic areas, goitrous cretinism is common, and is due to maternal and foetal iodine deficiency. Immediate diagnosis and treatment with thyroxine within a few days of birth are essential if physical and mental development are to be normal, or if further deterioration is to be prevented when damage has already occurred *in utero*. Hypothyroidism occurs in 1 in 4000 live births and for this reason, in the UK, there is routine biochemical screening of neonates for hypothyroidism using TSH assay on a simple heel-prick blood sample. Women under treatment with antithyroid drugs may give birth to a hypothyroid infant.

Adult hypothyroidism

The term myxoedema should be reserved for severe thyroid failure and not applied to the much commoner mild

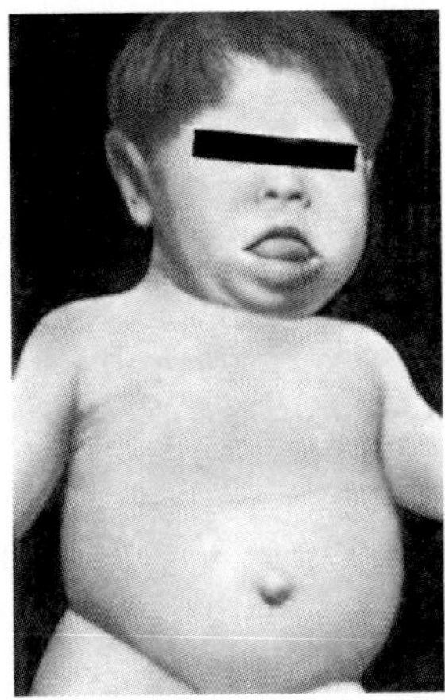

Fig. 44.8 An infant cretin with a pot belly, umbilical hernia, protruding tongue and pale, puffy face (*courtesy of the late Professor de Quervain, Berne, Switzerland*).

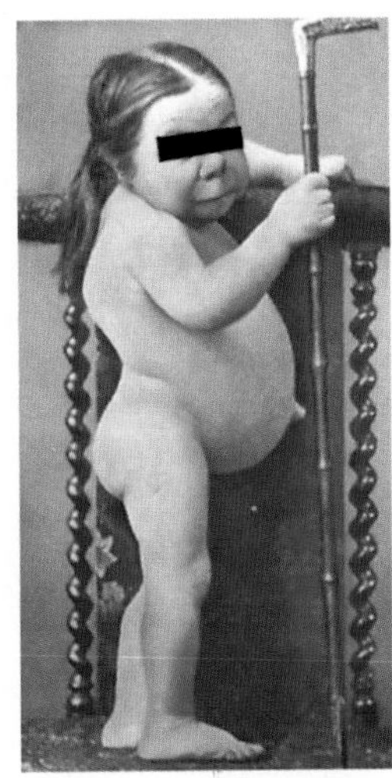

Fig. 44.9 A cretin woman, aged 22, mentally and physically retarded, with dry, wrinkled skin and supraclavicular pads of fat.

Table 44.2 Classification of hypothyroidism

- Autoimmune thyroiditis (chronic lymphocytic thyroiditis)
  - nongoitrous: primary myxoedema
  - goitrous: Hashimoto's disease
- Iatrogenic
  - after thyroidectomy
  - after radioiodine therapy
  - drug induced (antithyroid drugs, PAS and iodides in excess)
- Dyshormonogenesis
- Goitrogens
- Secondary to pituitary or hypothalamic disease
- Thyroid agenesis
- Endemic cretinism: often goitrous and due to iodine deficiency

thyroid deficiency. The signs of thyroid deficiency are:

- bradycardia;
- cold extremities;
- dry skin and hair;
- periorbital puffiness;
- hoarse voice;
- bradykinesis – slow movements;
- delayed relaxation phase of ankle jerks.

The symptoms are:

- tiredness;
- mental lethargy;
- cold intolerance;
- weight gain;
- constipation;
- menstrual disturbance;
- carpal tunnel syndrome.

Comparison of the facial appearance with a previous photograph may be helpful. *Delayed relaxation of the ankle jerk reflex is the most useful clinical sign in making the diagnosis.*

Thyroid function tests

Thyroid function tests (Table 44.1) show low T_4 and T_3 levels with a high TSH (except in the rare event of pituitary failure). High serum titres of antithyroid antibodies are characteristic of autoimmune disease.

Treatment

Oral thyroxine (0.10–0.20 mg) as a single daily dose (because of its prolonged action) is curative. Caution is required in the elderly or those with cardiac disease and the replacement dose is then commenced at 0.05 mg daily and cautiously increased. If a rapid response is required, tri-iodothyronine (20 mg three times a day) may be used.

Myxoedema[2] (Fig. 44.10)

The signs and symptoms of hypothyroidism are accentuated. The facial appearance (Fig. 44.11) is typical, and there is

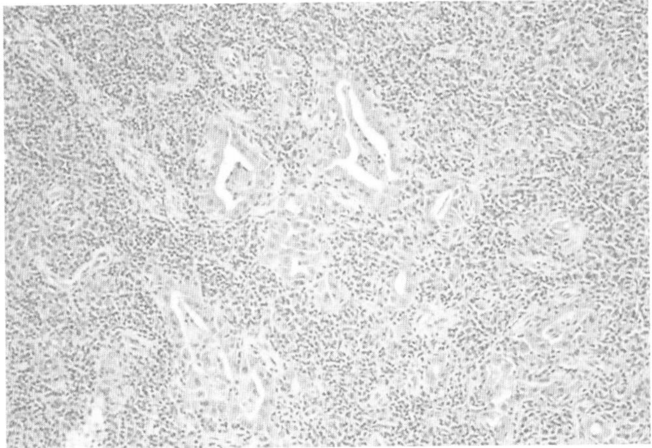

Fig. 44.10 Myxoedema (histology ×1000). Fibrosis, lymphocytic infiltration and atrophy of acini. Compare with normal histology in Fig. 44.24 (*courtesy of Dr S.W.B. Ewen, Aberdeen, Scotland*).

[2] *The first account of myxoedema was written in 1873 by Sir William Withey Gull (1816–90), physician to Guy's Hospital, London, England.*

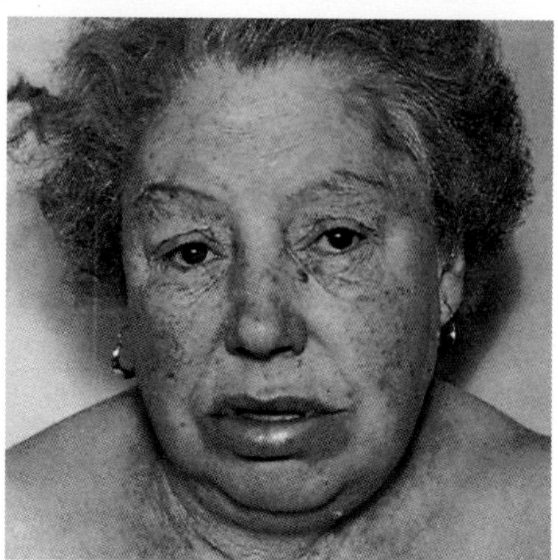

Fig. 44.11 Myxoedema. Note the bloated look, the pouting lips and the dull expression (*courtesy of Dr V.K. Summers, Liverpool, England*).

often supraclavicular puffiness, a malar flush and a yellow tinge to the skin. Myxoedema coma occurs in neglected cases and carries a high mortality; the body temperature is low and the patient must be warmed slowly: 1 g of intravenous hydrocortisone (in divided doses) should be given daily, and intravenous tri-iodothyronine in slowly increasing doses.

Autoimmune thyroiditis

The so-called primary or atrophic myxoedema is now considered to be an autoimmune disease similar to chronic lymphocytic (Hashimoto's) thyroiditis (see below) but without goitre formation from TSH stimulation. Because of the delay in diagnosis the hypothyroidism is usually much more severe than in goitrous autoimmune thyroiditis.

Dyshormonogenesis and goitrogens

Genetically determined deficiencies in the enzymes controlling the synthesis of thyroid hormones, if severe, are responsible for goitre formation with hypothyroidism. If of moderate degree, a simple (euthyroid) goitre results. Similarly goitrogens may produce a goitre with, or without, hypothyroidism.

A number of nonendemic goitrous cretins has been born to a group of itinerant tinkers living in Scotland who intermarry (Hutchison, Scotland). This was due to a deficiency of the enzyme dehalogenase. When thyroglobulin is broken down, uncoupled iodotyronines are liberated as well as T_3 and T_4. They are broken down by the enzyme dehalogenase and the iodine retained within the thyroid. If dehalogenase is deficient, iodotyrosines pass into the blood, and are excreted in the urine and this may result in iodine deficiency and goitre formation. Another classic example of dyshormonogenesis is Pendred's syndrome, where goitre is associated with congenital deafness. This is due to a deficiency of peroxidase, the enzyme responsible for organification of trapped iodine. Defects in thyroglobulin synthesis are also recognised in dyshormonogenesis.

James Holmes Hutchison. Emeritus Professor of Child Health, Glasgow, Scotland.

Vaughan Pendred, 1869–1946. General practitioner, East Sheen, Surrey, England. Described this syndrome in 1896 when practising in Durham city.

Thyroid enlargement

The normal thyroid gland is impalpable. The term goitre (Latin, *guttur* = the throat) is used to describe *generalised* enlargement of the thyroid gland. A discrete swelling (nodule) in one lobe with no palpable abnormality elsewhere is termed an *isolated (or solitary)* swelling. Discrete swellings with evidence of abnormality elsewhere in the gland are termed *dominant*.

A scheme for categorising thyroid enlargement is given in Table 44.3.

Simple goitre

Aetiology

Simple goitre may develop as a result of stimulation of the thyroid gland by TSH, either as a result of inappropriate secretion from a microadenoma in the anterior pituitary (which is rare), or in response to a chronically low level of circulating thyroid hormones. The most important factor in endemic goitre is dietary deficiency of iodine (see below) but defective hormone synthesis probably accounts for many sporadic goitres (see below).

Table 44.3 Classification of thyroid swellings

Simple goitre (euthyroid)
- Diffuse hyperplastic
  - physiological
  - pubertal
  - pregnancy
- Multinodular goitre

Toxic
- Diffuse
  - Graves' disease
- Multinodular
- Toxic adenoma

Neoplastic
- Benign
- Malignant

Inflammatory
- Autoimmune
  - chronic lymphocytic thyroiditis
  - Hashimoto's disease
- Granulomatous
  - de Quervain's thyroiditis
- Fibrosing
  - Riedel's thyroiditis
- Infective
  - acute (bacterial thyroiditis, viral thyroiditis, 'subacute thyroiditis')
  - chronic (tuberculous, syphilitic)
- Other
  - amyloid

TSH is not the only stimulus to thyroid follicular cell proliferation and other growth factors including immunoglobulins exert an influence. The heterogeneous structural and functional response in the thyroid resulting in characteristic nodularity may be due to the presence of clones of cells particularly sensitive to growth stimulation.

Iodine deficiency

The daily requirement of iodine is about 0.1–0.15 mg. In nearly all districts where simple goitre is endemic, there is a very low iodide content in the water and food. Endemic areas are in the mountainous ranges, such as the Rocky Mountains, the Alps, the Andes and the Himalayas. In Great Britain endemic goitre is found in the Mendips, Chilterns, Cotswolds and the Pennine chain of Derbyshire and Yorkshire. Endemic goitre is also found in lowland areas where the soil lacks iodide or the water supply comes from far away mountain ranges, e.g. the Great Lakes of North America, the Plains of Lombardy, the Struma valley[3], the Nile valley and the Congo.

Calcium is also goitrogenic and goitre is common in low-iodine areas on chalk or limestone, e.g. Derbyshire and Southern Ireland. Although iodides in food and water may be adequate, failure of intestinal absorption may produce iodine deficiency (McCarrison).

Defective hormone synthesis

Enzyme deficiency/dyshormonogenesis. It is probable that enzyme deficiencies of varying severity are responsible for many sporadic goitres, i.e. in nonendemic areas. There is often a family history suggesting a genetic defect. Environmental factors may compensate in areas of high iodine intake, for example goitre is almost unknown in Iceland where the fish diet is rich in iodine. Similarly a low intake of iodine encourages goitre formation in those with a metabolic predisposition.

Goitrogens. Well-known goitrogens are the vegetables of the brassica family (cabbage, kale and rape) which contain thiocyanate, drugs such as para-aminosalicylic acid (PAS) and, of course, the antithyroid drugs. Thiocyanates and perchlorates interfere with iodide trapping; carbimazole and thiouracil compounds interfere with the oxidation of iodide and the binding of iodine to tyrosine.

Surprisingly enough, iodides in large quantities are goitrogenic because they inhibit the organic binding of iodine and produce an iodide goitre.

The natural history of simple goitre

Stages in goitre formation are:

- persistent growth stimulation causes diffuse hyperplasia; all lobules are composed of active follicles and iodine uptake is uniform. This is a diffuse hyperplastic goitre, which may persist for a long time but is reversible if stimulation ceases;
- later, as a result of fluctuating stimulation, a mixed pattern develops with areas of active lobules and areas of inactive lobules;
- active lobules become more vascular and hyperplastic until haemorrhage occurs, causing central necrosis and leaving only a surrounding rind of active follicles;
- necrotic lobules coalesce to form nodules filled with either iodine-free colloid or a mass of new but inactive follicles;
- continual repetition of this process results in a nodular goitre. Most nodules are inactive and active follicles are present only in the internodular tissue.

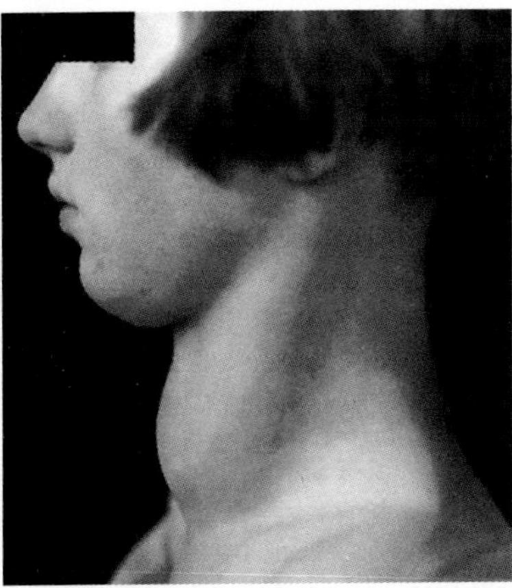

Fig. 44.12 Physiological hyperplasia of the thyroid gland (goitre of puberty).

Diffuse hyperplastic goitre

Diffuse hyperplasia corresponds to the first stages of the natural history. The goitre appears in childhood in endemic areas but, in sporadic cases, it usually occurs at puberty when metabolic demands are high – puberty goitre (Fig. 44.12). If TSH stimulation ceases, the goitre may regress, but tends to recur later at times of stress such as pregnancy. The goitre is soft, diffuse and may become large enough to cause discomfort. A colloid goitre is a late stage of diffuse hyperplasia when TSH stimulation has fallen off and when many follicles are inactive and full of colloid (Fig. 44.13).

Nodular goitre

Nodules are usually multiple, forming a multinodular goitre. Occasionally, only one macroscopic nodule is found, but microscopic changes will be present throughout the gland: this is one form of a clinically solitary nodule. Nodules may be colloid or cellular, and cystic degeneration and haemorrhage are common, as is subsequent calcification. Nodules appear early in endemic goitre and later (between 20 and 30 years) in sporadic goitre, although the patient may be unaware of the goitre until the late 40s or 50s. All types of simple goitre are far more common in the female than in the male and the presence of oestrogen receptors in normal thyroid tissue and in nodular goitre is relevant.

Diagnosis is usually straightforward. The patient is euthyroid: the nodules are palpable and often visible; they are smooth, usually firm and not hard, and the goitre is painless and moves freely on swallowing. Hardness and irregularity, due to calcification, may simulate carcinoma. A painful nodule, sudden appearance or rapid enlargement of a nodule raises suspicion of carcinoma but is usually due to

[3]*Struma. In the mountains of Bulgaria arises the river Struma, which flows into the Aegean Sea. Along its banks, and those of its tributaries, dwell persons of several nationalities among whom endemic goitre has long been prevalent. Struma is a European continental term for goitre.*

Sir Robert McCarrison, 1878–1960. Indian Medical Service. Director of the Nutrition Research Laboratories, Coonoor, Madras, India.

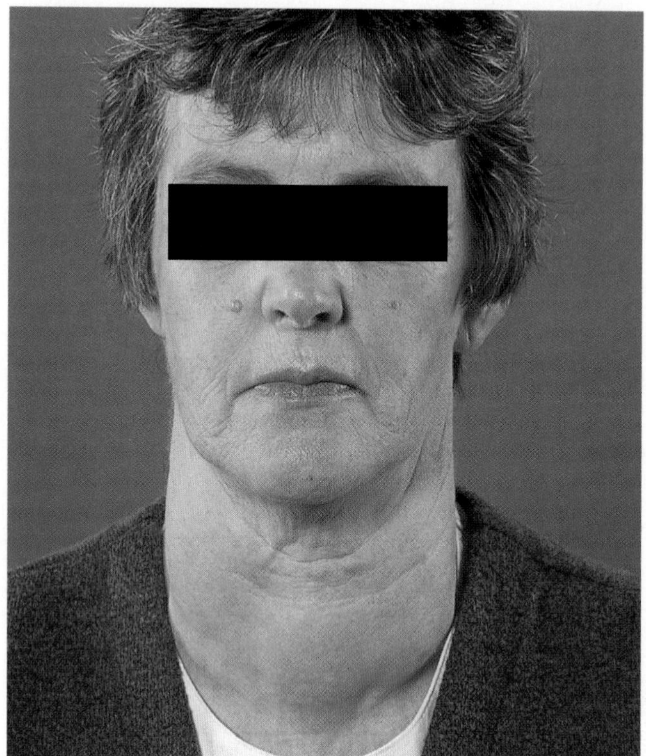

Fig. 44.13 Colloid goitre.

haemorrhage into a simple nodule. Differential diagnosis from autoimmune thyroiditis may be difficult.

Investigations. Tests of thyroid function are necessary to exclude mild hyperthyroidism, and the estimation of titres of thyroid antibodies to differentiate from autoimmune thyroiditis. Plain radiographs of the chest and thoracic inlet may show calcification and tracheal deviation or compression.

Complications. *Tracheal obstruction* is due to gross lateral displacement, or compression in a lateral or anteroposterior plane by retrosternal extension of the goitre (Fig. 44.14). Acute respiratory obstruction may follow haemorrhage into a nodule impacted in the thoracic inlet.

Secondary thyrotoxicosis. Many patients with nodular goitres experience transient episodes of mild hyperthyroidism. The incidence is difficult to estimate, but figures as high as 30 per cent have been suggested.

Carcinoma, which is usually of follicular pattern. It is uncommon but an increased incidence has been reported from endemic areas.

Prevention and treatment of simple goitre

In endemic areas, e.g. Switzerland, parts of the USA and Argentina, the incidence of goitre has been strikingly reduced by the introduction of iodised salt.

In the early stages a hyperplastic goitre may regress if thyroxine is given in a dose of 0.15–0.2 mg daily for a few months.

The nodular stage of simple goitre is irreversible. Most patients with multinodular goitre are asymptomatic and do not require operation. Operation may be indicated on cosmetic grounds if the goitre is unsightly. Retrosternal extension with actual or incipient tracheal compression is an indication for operation, as is the presence of a dominant area of enlargement which may be neoplastic.

There is a choice of surgical treatment: (a) total thyroidectomy with immediate and life-long replacement of thyroxine; or (b) some form of partial resection to conserve sufficient

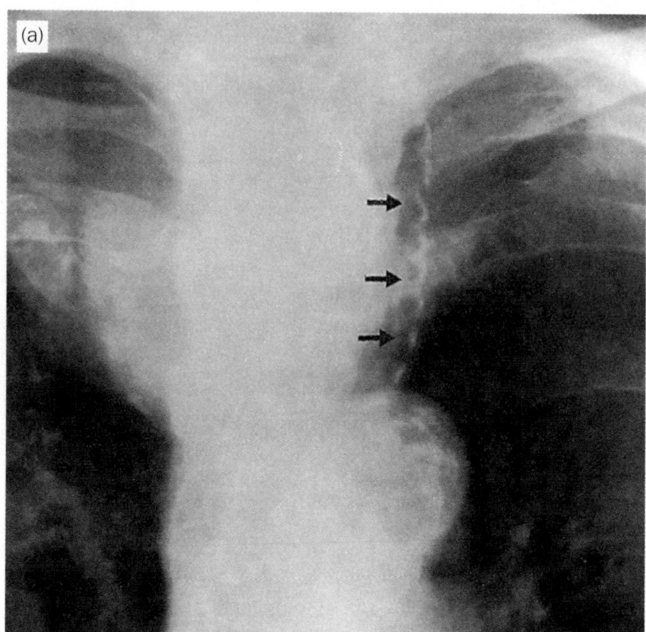

(b)

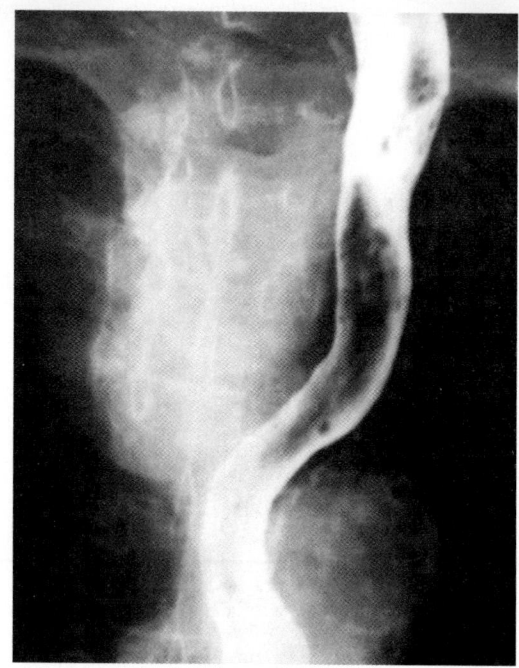

Fig. 44.14 Retrosternal goitre causing deviation of (a) the trachea and (b) oesophagus (barium swallow).

functioning thyroid tissue to subserve normal function whilst eliminating the risk of hypoparathyroidism which accompanies total thyroidectomy. Partial resection aims to remove the bulk of the gland, leaving up to 8 g of relatively normal tissue in each remnant. The technique is essentially the same as described for toxic goitre, as are the postoperative complications. More often, however, the multinodular change is asymmetrically distributed, with one lobe more significantly involved than the other. Under these circumstances total lobectomy on the more affected side is the appropriate management with either subtotal resection or no intervention on the less affected side. In many cases the causative factors persist and recurrence is likely. Reoperation for recurrent nodular goitre is more difficult and hazardous and for this reason many thyroid surgeons favour total thyroidectomy in younger patients. When a unilateral lobectomy alone has been performed for asymmetric goitre, reoperation is straightforward should it become necessary on the remaining lobe.

After subtotal resection it has been customary to give thyroxine to suppress TSH secretion with the aim of preventing recurrence. Whether this is either necessary or effective is uncertain, although the evidence of benefit in endemic areas is better than elsewhere. There is some evidence that recurrence after surgery may reduce in size after treatment with radioactive iodine.

Clinically discrete swellings

Discrete thyroid swellings (thyroid nodules) are common and are present in 3–4 per cent of the adult population in the UK and USA. They are three to four times more frequent in women than men.

Diagnosis

A discrete swelling in an otherwise impalpable gland is termed isolated or solitary, whereas the preferred term for a similar swelling in a gland with clinical evidence of generalised abnormality in the form of a palpable contralateral lobe or generalised mild nodularity is *dominant*. About 70 per cent of discrete thyroid swellings are clinically isolated and about 30 per cent dominant. The true incidence of isolated swellings is somewhat less than the clinical estimate. Clinical classification is inevitably subjective and overestimates the frequency of truly isolated swellings. When such a gland is exposed at operation or examined by ultrasonography, computed tomography (CT) or magnetic resonance imaging (MRI), clinically impalpable nodules are often detected. The true frequency of thyroid nodularity compared with the clinical detection rate by palpation is shown in Fig. 44.15. Establishing the presence of such minor abnormality is unnecessary because the management of discrete swellings, be they isolated or dominant, is similar.

The importance of discrete swellings lies in the risk of neoplasia compared with other thyroid swellings. Some 15 per cent of isolated swellings prove to be malignant, and an additional 30–40 per cent are follicular adenomas. The remainder are non-neoplastic largely consisting of areas of colloid degeneration, thyroiditis or cysts. Although the incidence of malignancy or follicular adenoma in clinically dominant swellings is approximately half that of truly isolated swellings, it is substantial and cannot be ignored.

Investigation

Thyroid function. The thyroid functional status should be established by estimation of serum thyroid hormones and TSH. If hyperthyroidism associated with a discrete swelling is confirmed biochemically, it indicates either a 'toxic adenoma' or a manifestation of toxic multinodular goitre. The combination of toxicity and nodularity is important and constitutes the only indication for isotope scanning to localise the area(s) of hyperfunction.

Autoantibody titres. The autoantibody status is important in determining which swellings may be a manifestation of chronic lymphocytic thyroiditis.

Isotope scan. Isotope scanning used to be the mainstay of investigation of discrete thyroid swellings to determine the functional activity relative to the surrounding gland according to isotope uptake.

On scanning, swellings are categorised as 'hot' (overactive), 'warm' (active) or 'cold' (underactive). A hot nodule is one that takes up isotope, while the surrounding thyroid tissue does not. Here the surrounding thyroid tissue is inactive because the nodule is producing such high levels of thyroid hormones that TSH secretion is suppressed. A warm nodule takes up isotope and so does normal thyroid tissue about it. A cold nodule takes up no isotope (Fig. 44.7).

About 80 per cent of discrete swellings are cold but only 15 per cent prove to be malignant and the use of this criterion as an indication for operation lacks discrimination. Routine isotope scanning has been abandoned except when toxicity is associated with nodularity.

Ultrasonography was formerly widely used as a noninvasive supplement to clinical examination in determining the physical characteristics of thyroid swellings. Although ultra-

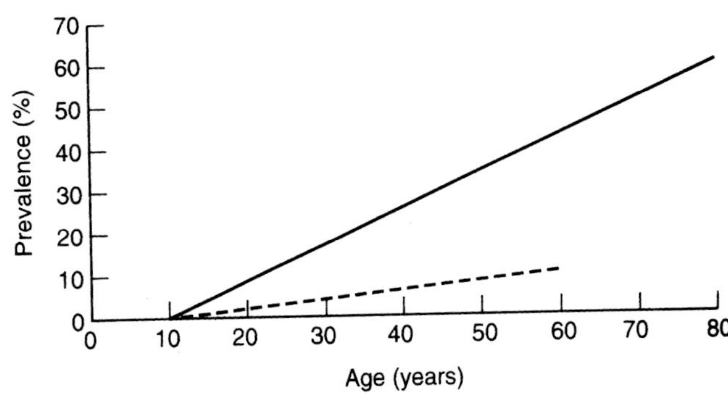

Fig. 44.15 The prevalence of thyroid nodules detected on palpation (broken line) or by ultrasonography or postmortem examination (solid line) (*after Mazzaferri*).

Ernest Mazzaferri. Ohio State University, Columbia, Ohio, USA.

sonography can demonstrate subclinical nodularity and cyst formation, the former is clinically irrelevant and the latter apparent at aspiration, which should be routine in all discrete swellings.

Fine-needle aspiration cytology (FNAC). FNAC has become established as the investigation of choice in discrete thyroid swellings. FNAC has excellent patient compliance, is simple and quick to perform in the out-patient department and is readily repeated. This technique, developed in Scandinavia some 30 years ago, has become popular in the rest of Europe and North America in the last 20 years.

Thyroid conditions that may be diagnosed by FNAC include colloid nodules (Fig. 44.16), thyroiditis, papillary carcinoma (Fig. 44.17), medullary carcinoma, anaplastic carcinoma and lymphoma. FNAC cannot distinguish between a benign follicular adenoma (Fig. 44.18) and follicular carcinoma as this distinction is dependent not on cytology but on histological criteria, which include capsular and vascular invasion.

Although FNAC has been reported as highly accurate by Lowhagen and his colleagues at the Karolinska Hospital, who were its pioneers, and by other authors, high accuracy has not always been reproducible, especially when results are analysed critically. There are very few false positives with respect to malignancy but there is a definite false-negative rate with respect to both benign and malignant neoplasia.

FNAC is less reliable in cystic than in solid swellings, often yielding only cyst fluid with macrophages and degenerate cells. After aspiration a further sample should be taken from the cyst wall, for cytology. Relatively few cysts are permanently abolished by one or more aspirations and, because of the risk of malignancy, recurrent cysts should be removed.

Radiology. Chest and thoracic inlet radiographs are only necessary when there is clinical evidence of tracheal deviation or compression or retrosternal extension.

Other scans. CT and MRI scans give excellent anatomical detail of thyroid swellings but have no role in the first line of investigation. They are occasionally useful in assessing recurrent and retrosternal swellings. The increased use of these imaging modalities in other head and neck swellings has created a new clinical conundrum which has been termed the '*Thyroid Incidentaloma*'. These are clinically unsuspected and impalpable thyroid swellings which with few exceptions require no further investigation or surgery.

Indirect laryngoscopy to determine the mobility of the vocal cords is widely used preoperatively, although usually for medicolegal rather than clinical reasons.

Large-bore needle (Trucut) biopsy. Trucut biopsy has a high diagnostic accuracy but has poor patient compliance and may be associated with complications such as pain, bleeding, tracheal and recurrent laryngeal nerve damage. It has little application in routine assessment except in locally advanced, surgically unresectable malignancy (either anaplastic carcinoma or lymphoma) when Trucut biopsy may avoid operation.

The main indication for operation is the risk of neoplasia which includes follicular adenoma as well as malignant swellings. The reason for advocating the removal of all follicular neoplasms is that it is seldom possible to distinguish between a follicular adenoma and carcinoma cytologically. The distinction usually depends on histological evidence of capsular or vascular invasion and FNAC cannot make this distinction, although on occasion cellular nuclear features may be so abnormal as to suggest malignant change. On this basis, some 50 per cent of isolated and

---

Torsten Lowhagen, Division of Cytology, Department of Tumour Pathology, Karolinska Hospital, Stockholm, Sweden.

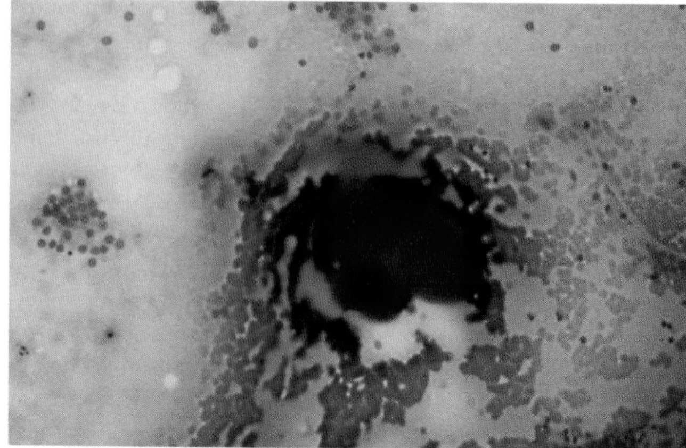

Fig. 44.16 Aspiration cytology – non-neoplastic appearances with scanty normal follicular cells together with colloid (= colloid nodule).

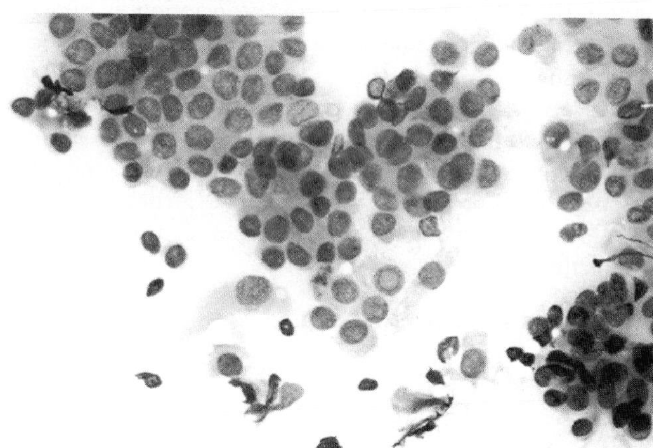

Fig. 44.17 Aspiration cytology. Papillary carcinoma with typical cellular variability and nuclear inclusions (*courtesy of Dr M. McKean, Aberdeen, Scotland*).

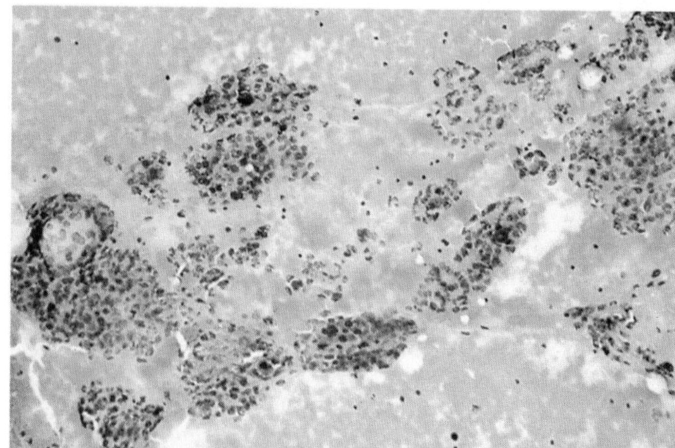

Fig. 44.18 Aspiration cytology. Follicular neoplasm showing increased cellularity with a follicular pattern (*courtesy of the late Dr V.M.M. Williams, Aberdeen, Scotland*).

25 per cent of dominant swellings should be removed on the grounds of neoplasia. Even when the cytology is negative, the age and sex of the patient and the size of the swelling may be relative indications for surgery, especially when a large swelling is responsible for symptoms. Some patients are happier to have a swelling removed even when cytology is negative.

There are useful clinical criteria to assist in selection for operation according to the risk of neoplasia and malignancy. Hard texture alone is not reliable since tense cystic swellings may be suspiciously hard but a hard, irregular swelling with any apparent fixity, which is unusual, is highly suspicious. Evidence of recurrent laryngeal nerve paralysis, suggested by hoarseness and a nonocclusive cough, and confirmed by indirect laryngoscopy, is almost pathognomonic. Deep cervical lymphadenopathy along the internal jugular vein in association with a clinically suspicious swelling is almost diagnostic of papillary carcinoma. In most patients, however, such features are absent but there are risk factors associated with sex and age. The incidence of thyroid carcinoma in women is about three times that in men, but a discrete swelling in a male is much more likely to be malignant than in a female and it is seldom justifiable to avoid removing such a swelling in a man. The risk of carcinoma is increased at either end of the age range and a discrete swelling in a teenager of either sex must be provisionally diagnosed as carcinoma. The risk increases as age advances beyond 50 years, and more so in males.

Thyroid cysts

Routine FNAC (or ultrasonography) shows that over 30 per cent of clinically isolated swellings contain fluid and are cystic or partly cystic. Tense cysts may be hard and mimic carcinoma. Bleeding into a cyst often presents with a history of sudden painful swelling which resolves to a variable extent over a period of weeks if untreated. Aspiration yields altered blood but reaccumulation is frequent. About 50 per cent of cystic swellings are the result of colloid degeneration, or of uncertain aetiology, because of an absence of epithelial cells in the lining. Although most of the remainder are the result of involution in follicular adenomas (Fig. 44.19) some 10–15 per cent of cystic follicular swellings are histologically malignant (30 per cent in males and 10 per cent in females). Papillary carcinoma is often associated with cyst formation (Fig. 44.20).

Most patients with discrete swellings, however, are females aged 20–40 years in whom the risk of malignancy, although significant, is low and the indications for operation are not clear cut. FNAC is the most appropriate investigation to aid selection.

The indications for operation in isolated or dominant thyroid swellings are listed in Table 44.4.

Retrosternal goitre

Very few retrosternal goitres arise from ectopic thyroid tissue; most arise from the lower pole of a nodular goitre. If the neck is short and the pretracheal muscles are strong, as in men, the negative intrathoracic pressure tends to draw these nodules into the superior mediastinum.

Clinical features

A retrosternal goitre is often symptomless and is discovered on a routine chest radiograph. There may, however, be severe symptoms:

- dyspnoea, particularly at night, cough and stridor (harsh sound on inspiration). Many of these patients may attend a chest clinic with a diagnosis of asthma before the true nature of the problem is discovered;
- dysphagia;
- engorgement of neck veins and superficial veins on the chest wall. In severe cases there may be obstruction of the superior vena cava (Fig. 44.21);
- recurrent nerve paralysis is rare. The goitre may also be malignant or toxic.

Radiographs show a soft-tissue shadow in the superior mediastinum – sometimes with calcification – and often causing deviation and compression of the trachea (Fig. 44.14). Radiographs of the thoracic inlet give better definition than a chest radiograph. Significant tracheal compression and obstruction may be demonstrated objectively by a flow–volume loop pulmonary function test in which the rate of flow is plotted against the volume of air inspired and then expired. Deterioration in flow due to increase in tracheal compression either acutely or in the long term may be used to monitor progression of the disease and indicate the need for surgery. The changes are reversed by operation (Fig. 44.22).

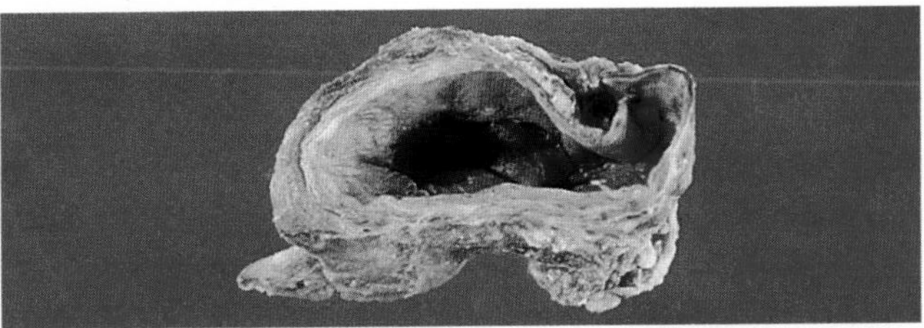

Fig. 44.19 Apparently simple cystic thyroid swelling, the wall of which comprised follicular neoplastic tissue.

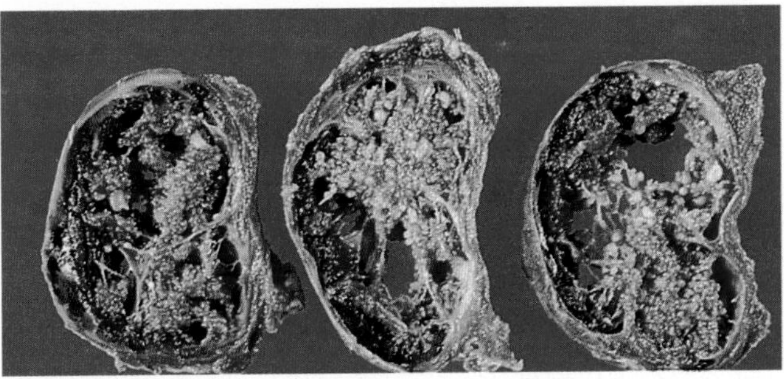

Fig. 44.20 Cyst formation in a papillary carcinoma.

Table 44.4 Indications for operation in thyroid swellings

- Neoplasia (FNAC positive, clinical suspicion)
  - age
  - male sex
  - hard texture
  - fixity
  - recurrent laryngeal nerve palsy
  - lymphadenopathy
  - recurrent cyst
- Toxic adenoma
- Pressure symptoms
- Cosmesis
- Patient's wishes

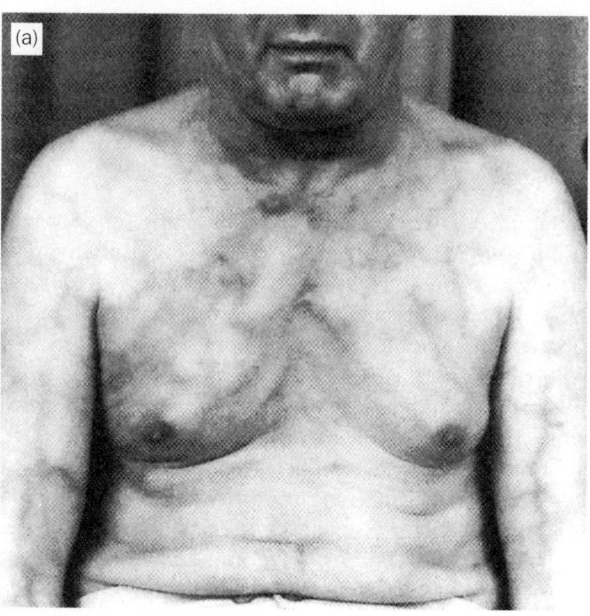

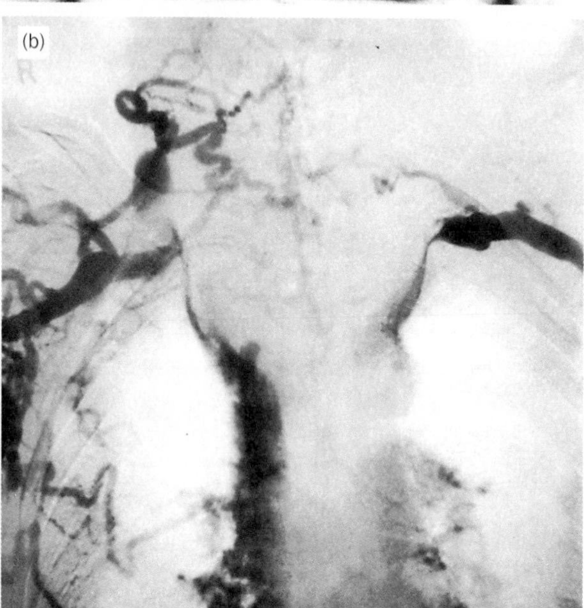

Fig. 44.21 (a) Infrared photograph of patient with enormous retrosternal goitre producing superior vena cava obstruction – dilated superior veins seen on trunk and arms; (b) venogram showing obstruction of superior vena cava.

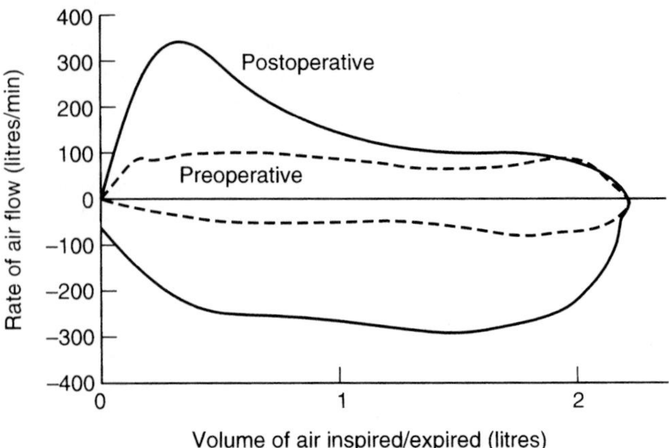

Fig. 44.22 Flow–volume loops before and after operation on a goitre causing tracheal obstruction.

Treatment

If obstructive symptoms are present in association with thyrotoxicosis it is unwise to treat a retrosternal goitre with antithyroid drugs or radioiodine as these may enlarge the goitre. Resection can almost always be carried out from the neck and a midline sternotomy is hardly ever necessary. The cervical part of the goitre should first be mobilised by ligation and division of the superior thyroid vessels, and by ligature and division of the middle thyroid veins and the inferior thyroid artery. The retrosternal goitre can then be delivered by traction and finger mobilisation. Haemorrhage is rarely a problem because the goitre takes its blood supply with it from the neck. The recurrent laryngeal nerve should be identified if possible before delivering the retrosternal goitre, as it may be abnormally displaced and is particularly vulnerable to injury from traction or tearing. If a large multinodular goitre cannot be delivered intact from the retrosternal position it may be broken with the fingers and delivered piecemeal, but this should never be done if the lesion is solitary and there is the possibility of carcinoma.

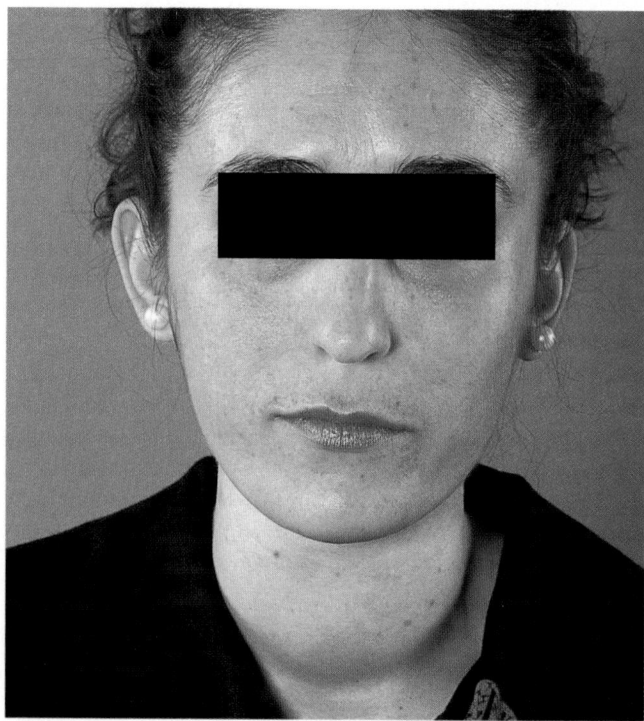

Fig. 44.23 Primary toxic goitre (Graves' disease) (*courtesy of Dr J.S. Bevan, Aberdeen, Scotland*).

Robert James Graves, 1796–1853. Physician, Meath Hospital, Dublin, Ireland. Published his account of exophthalmic goitre in 1835, 5 years before K.A. Von Basedow.

Hyperthyroidism

Thyrotoxicosis

The term thyrotoxicosis is retained because hyperthyroidism, i.e. symptoms due to a raised level of circulating thyroid hormones, is not responsible for all manifestations of the disease.

Clinical types are:

- diffuse toxic goitre (Graves' disease);
- toxic nodular goitre;
- toxic nodule;
- hyperthyroidism due to rarer causes.

Diffuse toxic goitre

Graves' disease – a diffuse vascular goitre appearing at the same time as the hyperthyroidism, usually in the younger woman and frequently associated with eye signs. The syndrome is that of primary thyrotoxicosis (Fig. 44.23). The whole of the functioning thyroid tissue is involved, and the hypertrophy and hyperplasia are due to abnormal thyroid-stimulating antibodies (TsAb).

Toxic nodular goitre

A simple nodular goitre is present for a long time before the hyperthyroidism, usually in the middle-aged or elderly and very infrequently associated with eye signs. The syndrome is that of secondary thyrotoxicosis.

In many cases of toxic nodular goitre, the nodules are inactive, and it is the internodular thyroid tissue that is overactive. However, in some toxic nodular goitres, one or more nodules are overactive and here the hyperthyroidism is due to autonomous thyroid tissue as in a toxic adenoma.

Toxic nodule

This is a solitary overactive nodule, which may be part of a generalised nodularity or a true toxic adenoma. It is autonomous and its hypertrophy and hyperplasia are not due to TsAb. *Because TSH secretion is suppressed by the high level of circulating thyroid hormones, the normal thyroid tissue surrounding the nodule is itself suppressed and inactive.*

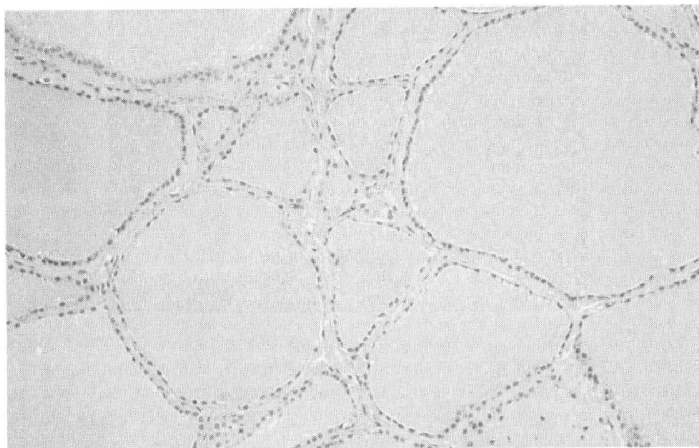

Fig. 44.24 Normal thyroid.

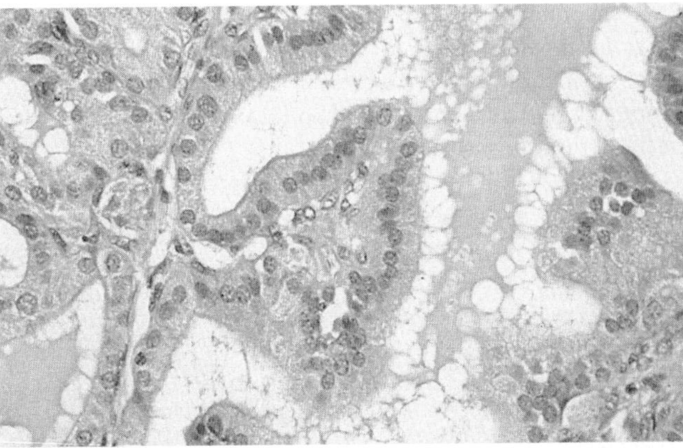

Fig. 44.25 Thyrotoxicosis.

Histology

The normal thyroid gland (Fig. 44.24) consists of acini lined by flattened cuboidal epithelium and filled with homogeneous colloid. In hyperthyroidism (Fig. 44.25) there is hyperplasia of acini, which are lined by high columnar epithelium. Many of them are empty and others contain vacuolated colloid.

Clinical features

The symptoms are:

- tiredness;
- emotional lability;
- heat intolerance;
- weight loss;
- excessive appetite;
- palpitations.

The signs of thyrotoxicosis are:

- tachycardia;
- hot, moist palms;
- exophthalmos;
- lid lag/retraction;
- agitation;
- thyroid goitre and bruit.

Symptomatology

Thyrotoxicosis is eight times commoner in females than in males. It may occur at any age. The most significant symptoms are loss of weight in spite of a good appetite, a recent preference for cold, and palpitations. The most significant signs are the excitability of the patient, the presence of a goitre, exophthalmos, and tachycardia or cardiac arrhythmia.

The goitre in primary thyrotoxicosis is diffuse and vascular, it may be large or small, firm or soft, and a thrill and a bruit may be present. The onset is abrupt, but remissions and exacerbations are not infrequent. Hyperthyroidism is usually more severe than in secondary thyrotoxicosis but cardiac failure is rare. Manifestations of thyrotoxicosis not due to hyperthyroidism per se, e.g. orbital proptosis, ophthalmoplegia and pretibial myxoedema, may occur in primary thyrotoxicosis.

In secondary thyrotoxicosis the goitre is nodular. The onset is insidious and may present with cardiac failure or atrial fibrillation. It is characteristic that the hyperthyroidism is not severe. Eye signs other than lid lag and lid spasm (due to hyperthyroidism) are very rare.

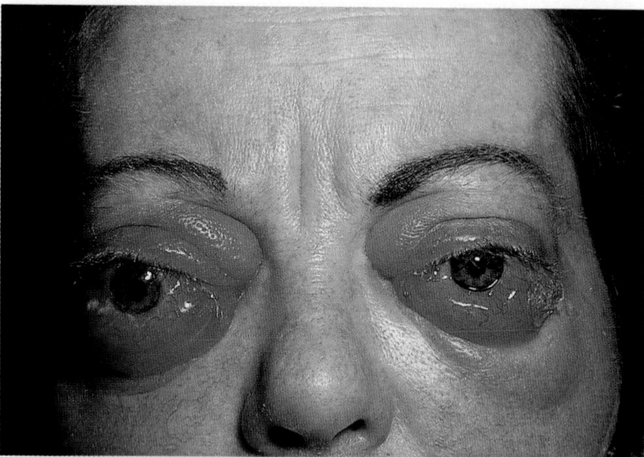

Fig. 44.26 Severe Graves' ophthalmopathy (*courtesy of Dr J.S. Bevan, Aberdeen, Scotland*).

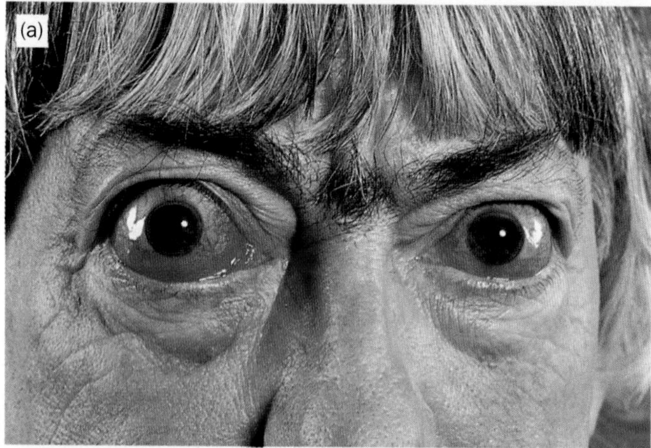

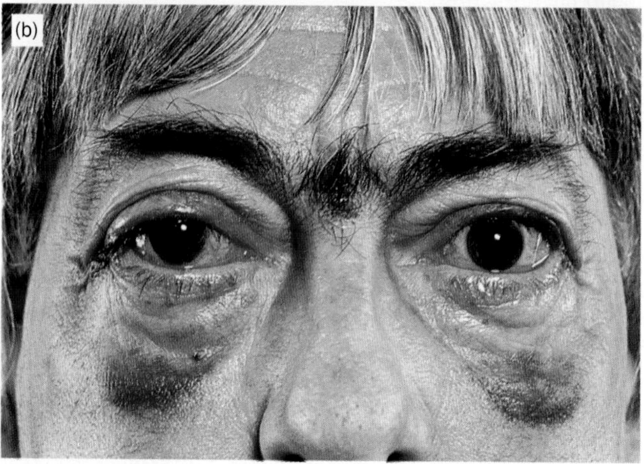

Fig. 44.27 (a) Progressive (malignant) exophthalmos. (b) Five weeks later following treatment with steroids, orbital radiotherapy and bilateral tarsorraphy (accounting for the bruising below the eyes) (*courtesy of Dr J.S. Bevan, Aberdeen, Scotland*).

Cardiac rhythm. A fast heart rate, which persists during sleep, is characteristic. Cardiac arrhythmias are superimposed on the sinus tachycardia as the disease progresses, and they are commoner in older patients with thyrotoxicosis because of the prevalence of coincidental heart disease. Stages of development of thyrotoxic arrhythmias are:

- multiple extrasystoles;
- paroxysmal atrial tachycardia;
- paroxysmal atrial fibrillation;
- persistent atrial fibrillation, not responsive to digoxin.

Myopathy. Weakness of the proximal limb muscles is commonly found if looked for. Severe muscular weakness (thyrotoxic myopathy) resembling myasthenia gravis occurs occasionally. Recovery proceeds as hyperthyroidism is controlled.

Eye signs. Some degree of exophthalmos is common (Fig. 44.23). It may be unilateral. True exophthalmos is a proptosis of the eye, caused by infiltration of the retrobulbar tissues with fluid and round cells, with a varying degree of retraction or spasm of the upper eyelid. (Lid spasm occurs because the levator palpebrae superioris muscle is partly innervated by sympathetic fibres.) This results in widening of the palpebral

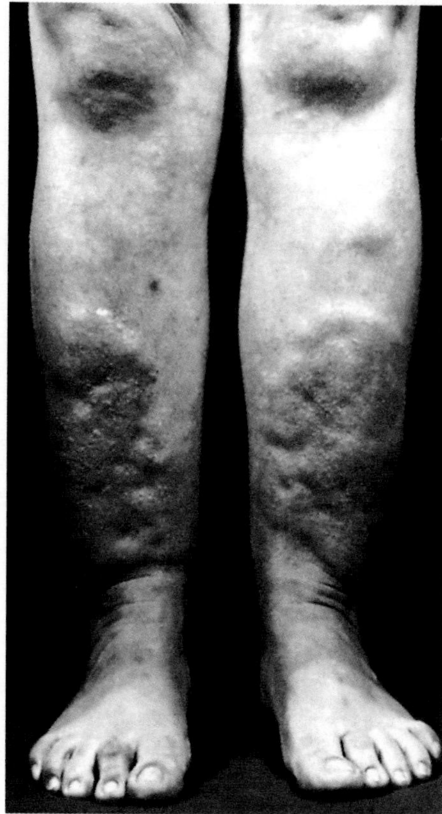

Fig. 44.28 Pretibial myxoedema. It is usually symmetrical, and minor degrees are not uncommon but are easily missed. The earliest stage is a shiny red plaque of thickened skin with coarse hair, which may be cyanotic when cold. In severe cases, the skin of the whole leg below the knee is involved, together with that of the foot and the ankle, and there may be clubbing of the fingers and toes (thyroid acropachy).

fissure so that the sclera may be seen clearly above the upper margin of the iris and cornea (above the 'limbus').

Spasm and retraction usually disappear when the hyperthyroidism is controlled. They may be improved by β-adrenergic blocking drugs, e.g. guanethidine eye drops. Oedema of the eyelids, conjunctival injection and chemosis are aggravated by compression of the ophthalmic veins (Fig. 44.26). Weakness of the extraocular muscles, particularly the elevators (inferior oblique), results in diplopia. In severe cases, papilloedema and corneal ulceration occur. When severe and progressive, it is known as malignant exophthalmos (Fig. 44.27) and the eye may be destroyed. Graves' ophthalmopathy is an autoimmune disease in which there are antibody-mediated effects on the ocular muscles.

Exophthalmos tends to improve with time. Sleeping propped up and lateral tarsorrhaphy will help to protect the eye but will not prevent progression. Hypothyroidism increases proptosis by a few millimetres and should be avoided.

Improvement has been reported with massive doses of prednisone. Intraorbital injection of steroids is dangerous because of the venous congestion, and total thyroid ablation has not proved effective. When the eye is in danger, orbital decompression may be required (see Dysthyroid exophthalmos).

Pretibial myxoedema (Fig. 44.28) is a thickening of the skin by a mucin-like deposit, nearly always associated with true exophthalmos, past or present hyperthyroidism, and high levels of TsAb.

Diagnosis of thyrotoxicosis

Most cases are readily diagnosed clinically. Difficulty is most likely to arise in the differentiation of mild hyperthyroidism from an anxiety state when a goitre is present. In these cases, the thyroid status is determined by the diagnostic tests described earlier. A TRH test is rarely indicated.

T_3 thyrotoxicosis is diagnosed by estimating the free T_3. It should be suspected if the clinical picture is suggestive but routine tests of thyroid function are within the normal range. A thyroid scan is essential in the diagnosis of an autonomous toxic nodule.

Thyrotoxicosis should always be considered in:

- children with a growth spurt, behaviour problems or myopathy;
- tachycardia or arrhythmia in the elderly;
- unexplained diarrhoea;
- loss of weight.

Principles of treatment of thyrotoxicosis

Nonspecific measures are rest and sedation and, in established thyrotoxicosis, should be used only in conjunction with specific measures – the use of antithyroid drugs, surgery and radioiodine.

Antithyroid drugs

Those in common use are carbimazole and propylthiouracil. Beta-adrenergic blockers, such as propranolol and nadolol, may also be used. Iodides, once thought to reduce the vascularity of the thyroid, should only be used as immediate preoperative preparation in the 10 days before surgery. Antithyroid drugs are used to restore the patient to a euthyroid state and to maintain this for a prolonged period in the hope that a permanent remission will occur, i.e. that production of TsAb will diminish or cease. *It should be noted that antithyroid drugs cannot cure a toxic nodule.* The overactive thyroid tissue is autonomous and recurrence of the hyperthyroidism is certain when the drug is discontinued.

Advantages

No surgery and no use of radioactive materials.

Disadvantages

- Treatment is prolonged and the failure rate after a course of 1.5–2 years is at least 50 per cent. Recently there has been a trend towards the use of shorter courses (6 months) of these drugs.
- It is impossible to predict which patient is likely to go into a remission. [Attempts have been made to predict which patients might relapse after a 6-month course of antithyroid drugs on the basis of human leucocyte antigen (HLA) status and the presence of TsAb production.]
- Some goitres enlarge and become very vascular during treatment – even if thyroxine is given at the same time. This is probably due to TsAb stimulation during the prolonged course of treatment and not a direct effect of the drug.
- Very rarely, there is a dangerous drug reaction, e.g. agranulocytosis or aplastic anaemia. In the event of agranulocytosis, the patient should be instructed to discontinue treatment, if a sore throat develops, until the white cell count has been checked.

Initially, 10 mg of carbimazole[4] is given three or four times a day, and there is a latent interval of 7–14 days before any clinical improvement is apparent. It is most important to maintain a high concentration of the drug throughout the 24 hours by spacing the doses at 8- or 6-hourly intervals. When the patient becomes euthyroid, a maintenance dose of 5 mg two or three times a day is given for another 12–18 months. If tri-iodothyronine (20 µg up to four times daily) or thyroxine (0.1 mg daily) is given in conjunction with antithyroid drugs, there is less danger of producing iatrogenic thyroid insufficiency or an increase in the size of the goitre ('*block and replacement treatment*').

Surgery

In diffuse toxic goitre and toxic nodular goitre with overactive internodular tissue, surgery cures by reducing the mass of overactive tissue. Cure is probable if the thyroid tissue can be reduced below a critical mass. This may result in a reduction of TsAb or it may be that circulating TsAb, however

[4]*Carbimazole also has an immunosuppressive action on TsAb production.*
Saul Hertz, Director of Radioactive Istope Research Institute, Boston, Massachusetts, USA.
A. Roberts, Isotope Department, Massachusetts Institute of Technology, Boston, Massachusetts, USA.

high its level, can only produce limited hypertrophy and hyperplasia when the mass of thyroid tissue is small. In the autonomous toxic nodule, and in toxic nodular goitre with overactive autonomous toxic nodules, surgery cures by removing all of the overactive thyroid tissue: this allows the suppressed normal tissue to function again.

Advantages

The goitre is removed, the cure is rapid and the cure rate is high if surgery has been adequate.

Disadvantages

- Recurrence of thyrotoxicosis occurs in approximately 5 per cent of cases.
- Every operation carries a morbidity but with suitable preparation and an experienced surgeon the mortality is negligible.
- Postoperative thyroid insufficiency occurs in 20–45 per cent of cases.
- Long-term follow-up is highly desirable as the few patients who develop recurrence may do so at any time in the future. In addition, although it is usually apparent within a year or two, thyroid failure may also be a late development.
- Parathyroid insufficiency: this should be permanent in less than 0.5 per cent.

Radioiodine

Radioiodine[5] destroys thyroid cells and, as in thyroidectomy, reduces the mass of functioning thyroid tissue to below a critical level.

Advantages

No surgery and no prolonged drug therapy.

Disadvantages

- Isotope facilities must be available.
- There is a high and progressive incidence of thyroid insufficiency which may reach 75–80 per cent after 10 years. This is due to sublethal damage to those cells not actually destroyed by the initial treatment and this eventually causes failure of cellular reproduction.
- Indefinite follow-up is essential.

There is no convincing evidence that radioiodine has been responsible for genetic damage, leukaemia, damage to the foetus if given inadvertently in early pregnancy, or carcinoma in the adult. In some clinics, radioiodine is given to almost all patients over the age of 25, i.e. when development is complete. Follow-up requirements are reduced if a total ablative dose of radioiodine is administered followed by routine replacement treatment with thyroxine. In the UK, reluctance to prescribe radioiodine under the age of 45 has faded. The dose of radioiodine varies between 300 and 600 MBq. Response is slow, but a substantial improvement is to be expected in 8–12 weeks. Accurate dosage is difficult and, should there be no clinical improvement after 12 weeks, a further dose is given. Two or more doses are necessary in 20–30 per cent of cases.

[5] *Radioactive iodine was first used in the treatment of thyrotoxicosis by Hertz and Roberts in 1942. Isotope – Greek,* isos = *equal,* topos = *place.*

Choice of therapeutic agent

Each case must be considered individually. Below are listed guiding principles on the most satisfactory treatment for a particular toxic goitre at a particular age; these must however be modified according to the facilities available and the personality, intelligence and wishes of the individual patient, business or family commitments and any other coexistent medical or surgical condition.

Diffuse toxic goitre

Over 45: radioiodine. Under 45: surgery for the large goitre, antithyroid drugs for the small goitre. As mentioned above, radioiodine is being increasingly used in younger patients, particularly when their families are complete.

Large goitres are uncomfortable and remission with antithyroid drugs is less likely than in the small goitre.

Toxic nodular goitre

Surgery. Toxic nodular goitre does not respond as well or as rapidly to radioiodine or antithyroid drugs as does a diffuse toxic goitre, and the goitre itself is often large and uncomfortable and enlarges still further with antithyroid drugs.

Toxic nodule

Surgery or radioiodine. Resection is easy, certain and without morbidity. Radioiodine is a good alternative over the age of 45 because the suppressed thyroid tissue does not take up iodine and there is thus no risk of delayed thyroid insufficiency.

Recurrent thyrotoxicosis after surgery

In general radioiodine, but antithyroid drugs may be used in young women intending to have children. Further surgery has no place.

Failure of previous treatment with antithyroid drugs or radioiodine. Surgery or thyroid ablation with ^{123}I.

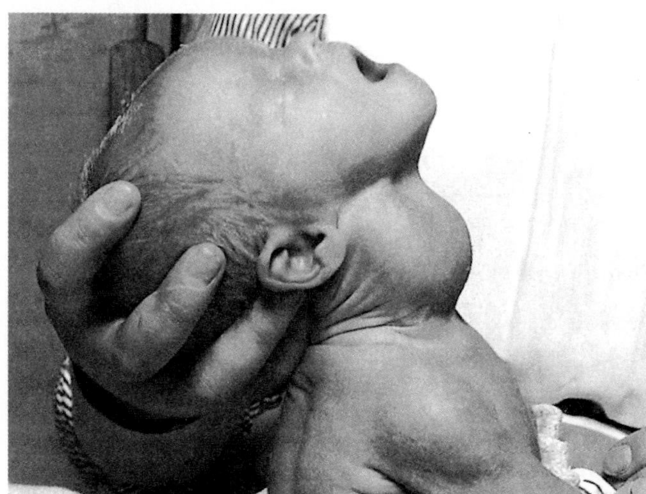

Fig. 44.29 Transmitted thiouracil goitre. This does not occur if T3 is given with antithyroid drugs as it, too, crosses the placenta.

In advising treatment, intelligence and compliance are important: unintelligent patients cannot be trusted to take drugs regularly if they feel well, and are unlikely to attend follow-up clinics indefinitely, which is essential after radioiodine or surgical therapy.

Special problems in treatment

Pregnancy. Radioiodine is absolutely contraindicated because of the risk to the foetus. The danger of surgery is miscarriage; and that of antithyroid drugs is of inducing thyroid insufficiency in the mother, and because both TSH and antithyroid drugs cross the placenta, of the baby being born goitrous (Fig. 44.29) and hypothyroid. The risk of either surgery in the second trimester, in competent hands, or careful administration of antithyroid drugs, is very small and the choice is exactly as in the uncomplicated case.

Postpartum hyperthyroidism. Pregnancy may lead to an exacerbation of a variety of autoimmune diseases in the postpartum period. Postpartum hyperthyroidism may be a problem in a patient previously diagnosed with hyperthyroidism or may occur in a patient without any previous history of thyroid disease.

Children. Radioiodine is contraindicated because of the theoretical risk of inducing thyroid carcinoma. There is an increased risk of recurrence after thyroidectomy because thyroid cells are highly active in the young. Children and adolescents should be treated with antithyroid drugs until the late teens, failing which total or near-total thyroidectomy by an expert surgeon should be undertaken.

The thyrocardiac. This is a patient with severe cardiac damage due wholly or partly to hyperthyroidism. The patient is usually middle aged or elderly with secondary thyrotoxicosis and the hyperthyroidism is not very severe. The cardiac condition is far more significant than the hyperthyroidism, but this must be rapidly controlled to prevent further cardiac damage. Beta-blockade (propranolol) can assist rapid control of cardiac effects.

Radioiodine is the treatment of choice together with antithyroid drugs started either before or after and continued until the radioiodine has had an effect (usually 6 weeks).

High titres of thyroid antibodies. Their presence indicates lymphatic infiltration of the goitre, i.e. a diffuse or focal thyroiditis, and a liability to spontaneous remission.

These patients are best treated conservatively but if medical treatment fails, definitive treatment by operation or radioiodine is not contraindicated. Steroids may help to reduce pain and swelling.

Proptosis of recent onset. There is a conventional view that to terminate thyrotoxicosis abruptly by thyroidectomy or radioiodine when proptosis is recent may induce malignant exophthalmos. Whilst there is no real proof of this it is reasonable to treat these patients with antithyroid drugs until the proptosis has been static for 6 months.

Hyperthyroidism due to other causes

Thyrotoxicosis factitia. (Usually seen in health 'cranks' or those given thyroid extract as 'a tonic'.) Hyperthyroidism may be induced by taking thyroxine, but only if the dosage exceeds the normal requirements of 0.15–0.25 mg a day. Doses below the normal requirements simply suppress normal hormone production by the thyroid.

Jod-Basedow thyrotoxicosis. (*Jod* = German for iodine + Basedow. In European countries diffuse toxic goitre is often called Basedow's disease.) Large doses of iodide given to a hyperplastic endemic goitre which is iodine avid may produce temporary hyperthyroidism, and very occasionally persistent hyperthyroidism.

In subacute or acute forms of autoimmune thyroiditis or of de Quervain's thyroiditis (see later), mild hyperthyroidism may occur in the early stages due to liberation of thyroid hormones from damaged tissue.

A large mass of secondary carcinoma will rarely produce sufficient hormone to induce mild hyperthyroidism.

Neonatal thyrotoxicosis occurs in babies born to hyperthyroid mothers or to euthyroid mothers who have had thyrotoxicosis. High TsAb titres are present in both mother and child because TsAb can cross the placental barrier. The hyperthyroidism gradually subsides after 3–4 weeks' time as the TsAb titres fall in the baby's serum.

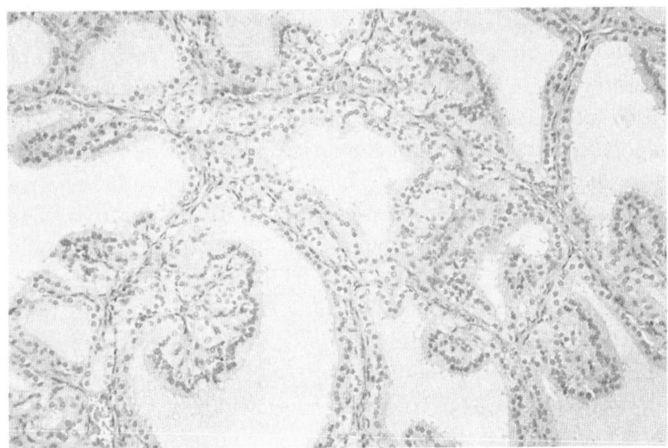

Fig. 44.30 'Prepared' thyrotoxicosis with acini lined by low cuboidal epithelium lacking the typical 'scalloping' of colloid seen in the untreated state. The pseudopapillary formation of the epithelium is retained. Compare with Fig. 44.25 (*courtesy of Dr S. Ewen, Aberdeen, Scotland*).

Surgery for thyrotoxicosis

Preoperative preparation (Fig. 44.30)

Traditional preparation aims to make the patient euthyroid or near euthyroid at operation. The thyroid state is determined by clinical assessment, i.e. by improvement in previous symptoms and by objective signs such as gain in weight and lowering of the pulse rate, and by serial estimations of the thyroid profile.

Preparation is as an out-patient and only rarely is admission to hospital necessary on account of severe symptoms at presentation or failure to control the hyperthyroidism. Failure to control with antithyroid drugs is unusual but may be due to uneven dosage, i.e. not taking the drug at 6- or 8-hourly intervals.

Carbimazole 30–40 mg a day is the drug of choice for preparation. When euthyroid – after 8–12 weeks – the dose may be reduced to 5 mg 8-hourly and the addition of thyroxine may facilitate maintenance of the euthyroid state. The last dose of carbimazole may be given on the evening before surgery. Iodides[6] are not used alone because, if the patient needs preoperative treatment, a more effective drug

Carl Adolph von Basedow, 1799–1854. General practitioner, Merseburg, Germany. Published his account of exophthalmic goitre in 1840.
Fritz de Quervain, 1868–1940. Professor of Surgery, Berne, Switzerland. Described this form of thyroiditis in 1902.
Jean Guillaume Auguste Lugol, 1786–1851. Physician, Hopital Saint-Louis, Paris, France.

[6]*Lugol's iodine. It is claimed that iodides reduce the vascularity of the goitre and make it firmer and easier to handle. It is traditional to prescribe these as Lugol's iodine 5 drops three times daily in milk. Potassium iodide tablets 60mg three times daily may be used as an alternative.*

should be given. Iodides may be given with carbimazole for 10–14 days immediately before operation but their use is of doubtful value and has been given up in many centres.

An alternative method of preparation that appears to be safe is to abolish the clinical manifestations of the toxic state, using beta-blocking drugs. This results in very rapid control and operation may be arranged within a week or two. The appropriate drugs are propranolol 40 mg three times daily or, preferably, the longer acting nadolol 160 mg once daily. Clinical response to beta-blockade is rapid and the patient may be reassessed within days: if clinically euthyroid, an operation date may be arranged; if not, the dose of beta-blocker is increased with early reassessment. Quite often larger doses are necessary.

Beta-blockers act on the target organs and not on the gland itself. Propranolol inhibits the peripheral conversion of T_4 to T_3. Long-acting beta-blockers, e.g. nadolol, are now also available and are administered once daily. They do not interfere with synthesis of thyroid hormones, so that hormone levels remain high during treatment and for some days after thyroidectomy. *It is, therefore, important to continue to give the drug for 7 days postoperatively.*

The addition of iodine for 10 days before operation gives an additional measure of safety in case the early morning dose of beta-blocker on the day of operation is mistakenly omitted (Plummer).

Propranolol or nadolol control symptoms very rapidly and have additional value in combination with carbimazole in the immediate treatment of patients with very severe hyperthyroidism.

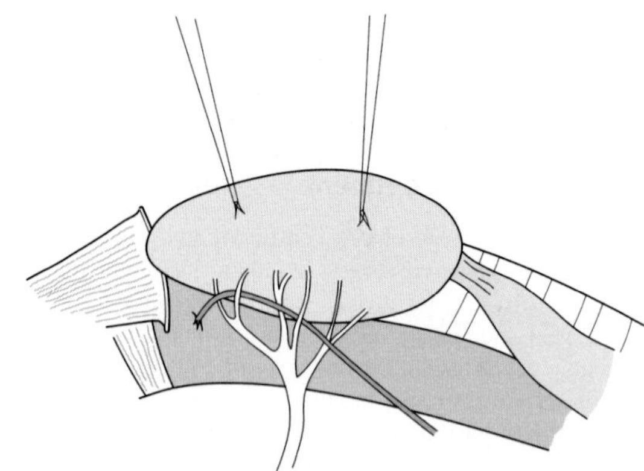

Fig. 44.31 Identification of the recurrent laryngeal nerve. Note how rotating the gland anteriorly kinks the nerve which is normally intimately related to the terminal branches of the inferior thyroid artery.

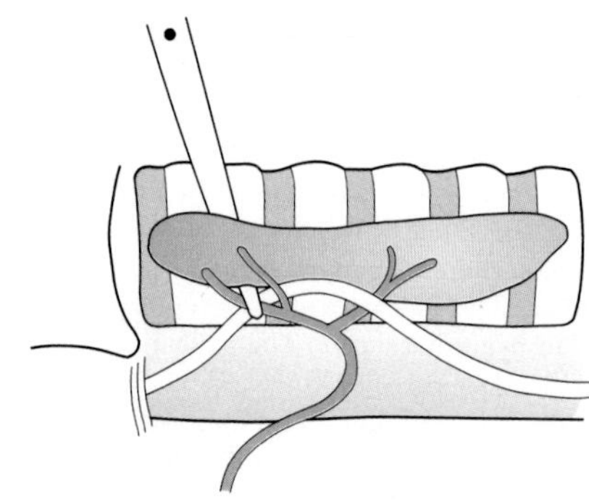

Fig. 44.32 On obtaining haemostasis, special care should be exercised on the medial side of the thyroid remnant, as the nerve can be easily damaged by haemostats or diathermy.

Subtotal thyroidectomy

Preoperative investigations to be carried out and recorded are:

- thyroid function tests;
- indirect laryngoscopy – it is a matter for local protocols whether this is routine. The outcome should have little impact on the operation because every recurrent laryngeal nerve must be routinely and obsessionally preserved;
- thyroid antibodies;
- serum calcium estimation;
- an isotope scan before preoperative preparation is necessary in patients with toxic nodular goitre if total thyroidectomy is not planned. The surgeon should know which nodules, if any, are autonomous and active in order to ensure their resection. A scan is of no value in diffuse toxic goitre when uptake, for practical purposes, is uniform. The diagnosis of a single toxic nodule can only be made by demonstrating that the nodule is active and the remaining thyroid tissue suppressed.

The extent of the resection depends on the size of the gland, the age of the patient, the experience of the surgeon, the need to minimise the risk of recurrent toxicity and the wish to avoid postoperative thyroid replacement. Thus young patients with small glands are at greatest risk of recurrence even with very small remnant sizes. There is an increasing trend towards total thyroidectomy which simplifies subsequent management and rapidly achieves a permanent euthyroid state on thyroxine replacement. In contrast, a patient with a large goitre who wishes to avoid postoperative medication is suitable for subtotal thyroidectomy.

Technique. General anaesthesia is administered through an endotracheal tube and good muscle relaxation obtained. The patient is supine on the operating table with the table tilted 15° at the head end to reduce venous engorgement. A sandbag is placed transversely under the shoulders and the neck extended (with care particularly in the elderly) to make the thyroid gland more prominent. A skin crease incision is made midway between the notch of the thyroid cartilage and the suprasternal notch. Flaps of skin, subcutaneous tissue and platysma are raised upwards to the superior thyroid notch and downwards to the suprasternal notch. The deep cervical fascia is divided in the midline between the sternothyroid muscles down to the plane of the thyroid capsule. The muscles are not divided as a routine but may be if greater exposure is required. The sternothyroid muscle is mobilised off the thyroid lobes. In 30 per cent of patients, middle thyroid veins passing directly into the internal jugular vein require ligation and division. The main blood supply is the superior thyroid artery which must be ligated securely. The lobe is then free to rotate out of its bed. The inferior thyroid arteries are not routinely ligated to preserve parathyroid blood supply. The recurrent

Henry Stanley Plummer, 1874–1937. Physician, Mayo Clinic, Rochester, Minnesota, USA, was the first to use iodine for preparing thyrotoxic patients for operation.

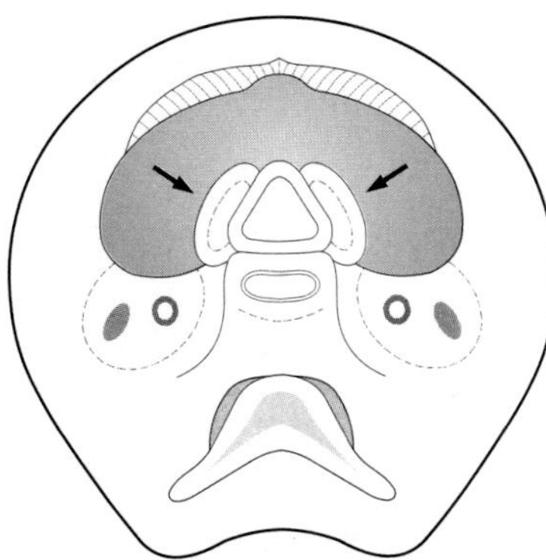

Fig. 44.33 Tension haematoma deep to pretracheal muscles (*after V.H. Riddell FRCS, London, England*).

laryngeal nerve should be identified in its course in the operative field. It should first be sought below the level of the inferior thyroid artery as it passes obliquely upwards and forwards. This course (Fig. 44.31), oblique to the trachea and oesophagus, is accentuated by mobilisation of the thyroid lobe. If not immediately seen, the nerve can usually be palpated as a taut strand. At a higher level the nerve lies between the branches of the inferior thyroid artery. The nerve passes into the larynx immediately behind the inferior cornu of the thyroid cartilage which is therefore a very important landmark. If the right nerve cannot be found in its usual course, an anomalous (nonrecurrent) nerve, present in 1 per cent of cases, should be suspected; this arises from the vagus trunk and usually passes from behind the carotid sheath, curving medially, forwards and upwards, and may be mistaken for the inferior thyroid artery. The parathyroid glands are protected by identification on careful inspection of the goitre before resection and by avoiding ligatures and sutures close to the hilum of identified glands. The use of diathermy in this area should be avoided as heat conduction may devascularise the parathyroids or damage the recurrent laryngeal nerves (Fig. 44.32). If a parathyroid gland is inadvertently excised or devascularised, it should be autotransplanted in several fragments within the sternomastoid muscle. Subtotal resection of each lobe is carried out, leaving a remnant of between 4 and 5 g on each side. Absolute haemostasis is secured by ligation of individual vessels and by suture of the thyroid remnants to the tracheal fascia. The pretracheal muscles and cervical fascia are sutured and the wound is closed with or without suction drainage to the deep cervical space.

Postoperative complications

Haemorrhage. A tension haematoma deep to the cervical fascia (Fig. 44.33) is usually due to slipping of a ligature on the superior thyroid artery: occasionally haemorrhage from a thyroid remnant or a thyroid vein may be responsible. It may, on rare occasions, be necessary to open the wound in the ward to relieve tension before taking the patient to theatre to evacuate the haematoma and to tie off a bleeding vessel.

A small subcutaneous haematoma or collection of serum may form under the skin flaps and should be evacuated or aspirated in the following 72 hours. This should not be confused with the potentially life-threatening deep tension haematoma.

Respiratory obstruction. This is very rarely due to collapse or kinking of the trachea. Most cases are due to laryngeal oedema. The most important cause of laryngeal oedema is a tension haematoma. However, trauma to the larynx by anaesthetic intubation and surgical manipulation is an important contributory factor – particularly if the goitre is very vascular – and may cause laryngeal oedema without a tension haematoma. Unilateral or bilateral recurrent nerve paralysis will not cause immediate postoperative respiratory obstruction unless laryngeal oedema is also present, but they will aggravate the obstruction.

If releasing the tension haematoma does not immediately relieve airway obstruction, the trachea should be intubated at once. An endotracheal tube can be left in place for several days; steroids are given to reduce oedema and a tracheostomy is rarely necessary. Intubation in the presence of laryngeal oedema may be very difficult and should be carried out by an experienced anaesthetist; repeated unsuccessful attempts may increase obstruction and cause serious cerebral anoxia (Wade). In an emergency, it is far safer for the inexperienced surgeon to perform a needle tracheostomy as a temporary measure; a Medicut 12G needle (diameter 2.3 mm) is highly satisfactory.

Recurrent laryngeal nerve paralysis may be unilateral or bilateral, transient or permanent (Chapter 43). Transient paralysis occurs in about 3 per cent of nerves at risk and recovers in 3 weeks to 3 months. Permanent paralysis is extremely rare if the nerve has been identified at operation.

Thyroid insufficiency. This usually occurs within 2 years, but it is sometimes delayed for 5 years or more. It is often insidious and difficult to recognise. The incidence is considerably higher than used to be thought and figures of 20–45 per cent have been reported after operations on diffuse toxic goitres and toxic nodular goitres with internodular hyperplasia. It represents a change in the autoimmune response from stimulation to destruction of thyroid cells. There is, however, a definite relationship between the estimated weight of the thyroid remnant and the development of thyroid failure after subtotal thyroidectomy for Graves' disease. Thyroid insufficiency is rare after surgery for a toxic adenoma because there is no autoimmune disease present.

Parathyroid insufficiency is due to removal of parathyroid glands, or infarction through damage to the parathyroid end-artery; often both factors occur together. Vascular injury is probably far more important than inadvertent removal. The incidence of this condition should be less than 0.5 per cent and most cases present dramatically 2–5 days after operation, but very rarely the onset is delayed for 2–3 weeks or a patient with marked hypocalcaemia is asymptomatic.

Thyrotoxic crisis (storm) is an acute exacerbation of hyperthyroidism. It occurs if a thyrotoxic patient has been inadequately prepared for thyroidectomy, and is now extremely rare. Very rarely, a thyrotoxic patient presents in a crisis and this may follow an unrelated operation. Symptomatic and supportive treatment is for dehydration, hyperpyrexia and restlessness. This requires the administration of intravenous fluids, cooling the patient with ice packs, administration of oxygen, diuretics for cardiac failure, digoxin for uncontrolled atrial fibrillation, sedation and intravenous hydrocortisone. Specific treatment is by carbimazole 10–20 mg 6-hourly, Lugol's iodine 10 drops 8-hourly by mouth or sodium iodide 1 g intravenously (i.v.). Propranolol 40 mg 6-hourly orally will block adverse beta-adrenergic effects. This agent may be given by careful intravenous administration (1–2 mg) under precise electrocardiographic control.

Wound infection. A subcutaneous or deep cervical abscess should be drained.

Hypertrophic or keloid scar is more likely to form if the incision overlies the sternum. Intradermal injections of corticosteroid should be given at once and repeated monthly if necessary.

Stitch granuloma. This may occur with or without sinus formation and is seen after the use of nonabsorbable suture material. Absorbable ligatures and sutures must be used throughout thyroid surgery. Some surgeons use a subcuticular absorbable skin suture rather than the traditional skin clips or staples. Skin staples should be removed in less than 48 hours.

Postoperative care

Indirect laryngoscopy has been advised as a routine before leaving hospital. Alternatively, it may be avoided when the voice is normal and the cough occlusive.

James Stanley Hilary Wade. Former Consultant Surgeon, University Hospital of Wales, Cardiff, Wales.

Table 44.5 Classification of thyroid neoplasms

Benign
- Follicular adenoma

Malignant
Primary
  Follicular epithelium: differentiated
  - follicular
  - papillary
  Follicular epithelium: undifferentiated
  - anaplastic
  Parafollicular cells
  - medullary
  Lymphoid cells
  - lymphoma
Secondary
  - metastatic
  - local infiltration

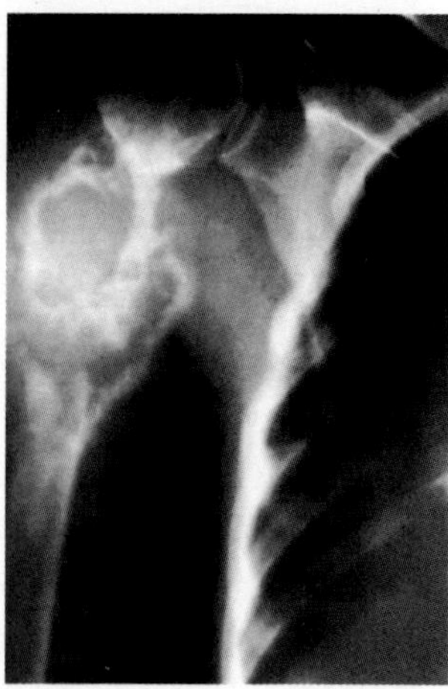

Fig. 44.34 Metastasis from a carcinoma of a thyroid in a humerus (*courtesy of D.S. Devadatta, Vellore, India*).

About 25 per cent of patients develop transient hypocalcaemia and, if associated symptoms are severe, intravenous calcium gluconate or oral calcium may be necessary, although this is unusual. To screen for parathyroid insufficiency, the serum calcium should be measured at the first review attendance 4–6 weeks after operation.

After operation, stability in terms of thyroid function takes time. It is important that biochemical (subclinical) thyroid failure should not be an indication for treatment during the first year as the majority of patients with early subclinical failure, which is common, ultimately regains normality. Even when there are clinical features of failure, thyroxine should be withheld if possible during the first 6 months. Most patients who develop thyroid failure do so within the first 2 years, but there is a continuing incidence thereafter. Recurrent thyrotoxicosis may occur at any time after operation. Follow-up should therefore be for life.

Once a stable situation has been achieved, follow-up after thyroid surgery may be carried out by an automated computer-activated system. Such systems in Scotland and Wales have been shown to be extremely cost-effective and dramatically reduce the number of patient attendances at the thyroid clinic.

The incidences quoted for thyroid failure (20–45 per cent) and recurrent thyrotoxicosis (5 per cent) after subtotal thyroidectomy for Graves' disease refer to UK experience and may be different elsewhere in the world. In Iceland, for example, an area of high dietary iodine intake, the incidence of thyroid failure is much lower and that of recurrent toxicity much higher than in the UK.

Neoplasms of the thyroid

Thyroid neoplasms are classified in Table 44.5.

Table 44.6 Relative incidence of primary malignant tumour of the thyroid gland

Relative incidence	%
Papillary carcinoma	60
Follicular carcinoma	17
Anaplastic carcinoma	13
Medullary carcinoma	6
Malignant lymphoma	4

Benign tumours

Follicular adenomas present as clinically solitary nodules and the distinction between a follicular carcinoma and an adenoma can only be made by histological examination: in the adenoma there is no invasion of the capsule or of pericapsular blood vessels. Treatment is, therefore, by wide excision – preferably a lobectomy. The remaining thyroid tissue is normal so that prolonged follow-up is unnecessary. It is doubtful whether there is such an entity as a papillary adenoma and all papillary tumours should be considered as malignant even if encapsulated.

Malignant tumours

The vast majority of primary growths is carcinomas (Table 44.6). Dunhill classified them histologically as differentiated and undifferentiated: and the differentiated carcinomas are

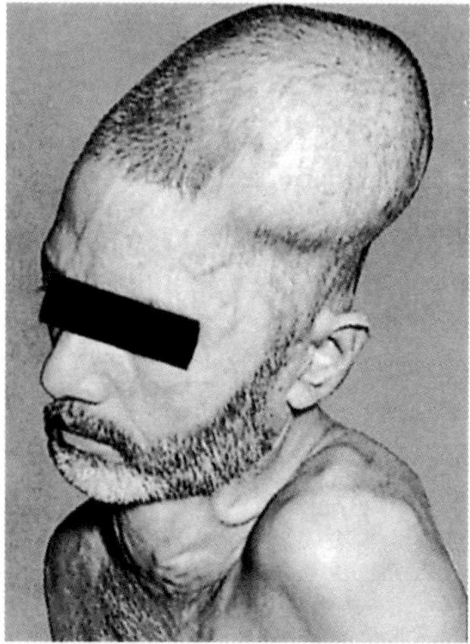

Fig. 44.35 Metastasis in the left parietal bone from a carcinoma of the thyroid (*courtesy of Professor A.K. Toufeeq, Lahore, Pakistan*).

Sir Thomas Peel Dunhill, 1876–1957. Surgeon, St Bartholomew's Hospital, London, England.

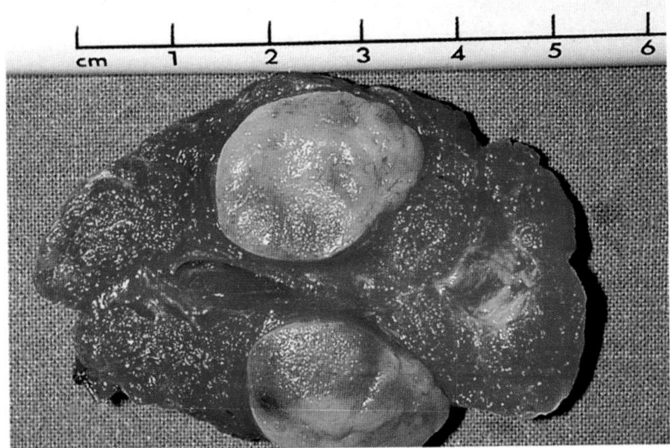

Fig. 44.36 Follicular neoplasm of thyroid presenting as an isolated swelling.

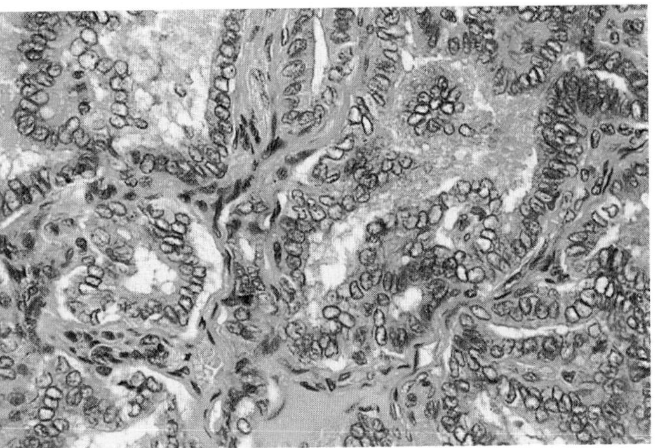

Fig. 44.37 Histology of papillary thyroid carcinoma showing typical papillary projections and empty (Orphan Annie-eyed) nuclei (*courtesy of Dr S.W.B. Ewen, Aberdeen, Scotland*).

now subdivided into follicular and papillary. Secondary growths are rare but blood-borne metastases occur (Figs 44.34 and 44.35). Blood-borne metastases more usually occur from primary carcinomas of breast, colon and kidney and from melanomas.

Aetiology of malignant thyroid tumours

Differentiated thyroid carcinoma, particularly papillary, frequently follows accidental irradiation of the thyroid in childhood[7]. The incidence of follicular carcinoma is high in endemic goitrous areas, possibly owing to TSH stimulation. Malignant lymphomas can present in a patient known to have autoimmune thyroiditis, so that the lymphocytic infiltration in the autoimmune process may be an aetiological factor. Indeed, it is likely that all lymphomas of the thyroid arise in glands affected by such thyroiditis.

Clinical features of thyroid neoplasms

The annual incidence is about 3.7 per 100 000 of the population and the sex ratio is three females to one male. The mortality should only be of the order of 2–3 per cent. The commonest presenting symptom is a thyroid swelling (Fig. 44.36) and a 5-year history is far from uncommon in differentiated growths. Enlarged cervical lymph nodes may be the presentation of papillary carcinoma. Recurrent laryngeal nerve paralysis may be a presenting feature of locally advanced disease.

Anaplastic growths are usually hard, irregular and infiltrating. A differentiated carcinoma may be suspiciously firm and irregular, but is often indistinguishable from a benign swelling. Small papillary tumours may be impalpable (occult carcinoma) – even when lymphatic metastases are present (so-called lateral aberrant thyroid). Pain, often referred to the ear, is frequent in infiltrating growths.

Diagnosis of thyroid neoplasms

Diagnosis is obvious on clinical examination in most cases of anaplastic carcinoma, although Riedel's thyroiditis (see later) is indistinguishable. The localised forms of granulomatous thyroiditis and lymphadenoid goitre may simulate carcinoma. It is not always easy to exclude a carcinoma in a multinodular goitre, and solitary nodules, particularly in the young male, are always suspect. Failure to take up radioiodine is characteristic of almost all thyroid carcinomas [only very rarely will differentiated carcinoma (primary or secondary) take up ^{123}I in the presence of normal thyroid tissue], but occurs also in degenerating nodules and all forms of thyroiditis. Thyroid antibody titres are often raised in carcinoma. The role of FNAC in preoperative diagnosis has already been discussed. No diagnostic test is absolutely certain, and exploration with excision in the form of lobectomy is essential when in doubt. Incisional biopsy may cause seeding of cells and local recurrence, and is most inadvisable in a resectable carcinoma. In an anaplastic and obviously irremovable carcinoma, however, incisional or needle biopsy is justified.

Papillary carcinoma

Most papillary tumours contain a mixture of papillary and colloid-filled follicles, and in some the follicular structure predominates. Nevertheless, if any papillary structure is present, the tumour will behave in a predictable fashion as a papillary carcinoma. Histologically the tumour shows papillary projections and characteristic pale, empty nuclei (Orphan Annie-eyed[8] nuclei) (Fig. 44.37). Papillary carcinomas are very seldom encapsulated.

[7] *The incidence of childhood thyroid cancer in the town of Gomel which was exposed to high levels of radioactive fallout following the Chernobyl nuclear incident in 1986 has risen from 0.5/million in 1984 to 96.4/million in 1994.*

Bernhard Moritz Carl Ludwig Riedel, 1846–1916. Professor of Surgery, Lena, Germany. Described this form of thyroiditis in 1896.

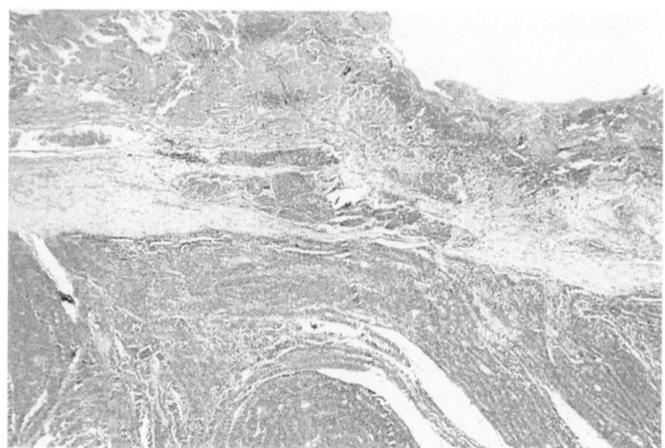

Fig. 44.38 Histology of follicular thyroid carcinoma showing vascular and capsular invasion (*courtesy of Dr S.W.B. Ewen, Aberdeen, Scotland*).

Multiple foci may occur in the same lobe as the primary tumour or, less commonly, in both lobes. They may be due to lymphatic spread in the rich intrathyroidal lymph plexus, or to multicentric growth. Spread to the lymph nodes is common but blood-borne metastases are unusual unless the tumour is extrathyroidal. The term extrathyroidal indicates that the primary tumour has infiltrated through the capsule of the thyroid gland.

Occult carcinoma

Papillary carcinoma may present as an enlarged lymph node in the jugular chain with no palpable abnormality of the thyroid. The primary tumour may be no more than a few millimetres in size and is termed occult. Such primary foci of papillary carcinoma may also be discovered in thyroid tissue resected for other reasons, e.g. Graves' disease. The term occult is now applied to all papillary carcinomas less than 1.5 cm in diameter. These have an excellent prognosis and are regarded as of little clinical significance.

Follicular carcinoma

These appear to be macroscopically encapsulated but microscopically there is invasion of the capsule and of the vascular spaces in the capsular region (Fig. 44.38). Multiple foci are seldom seen and lymph node involvement is much less common than in papillary carcinoma. Blood-borne metastases are almost twice as common and the eventual mortality rate is twice as high (Fig. 44.39). *Hurthle cell tumours are a variant of follicular neoplasm in which oxyphil (Hurthle, Askanazy) cells predominate histologically. It is doubtful whether Hurthle cell neoplasms are ever benign and they may be associated with a poorer prognosis.*

Differences between papillary and follicular carcinoma

The major differences between papillary (including mixed papillary and follicular) and follicular carcinoma have been set out by Cady on the basis of an analysis of 40 years' experience at the Lahey Clinic (Table 44.7).

Prognosis in differentiated thyroid carcinoma

The prognosis of differentiated thyroid carcinoma, although influenced by histological type, is much more dependent on

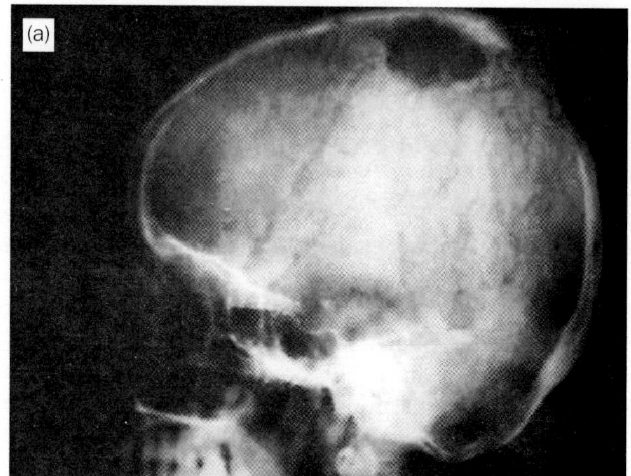

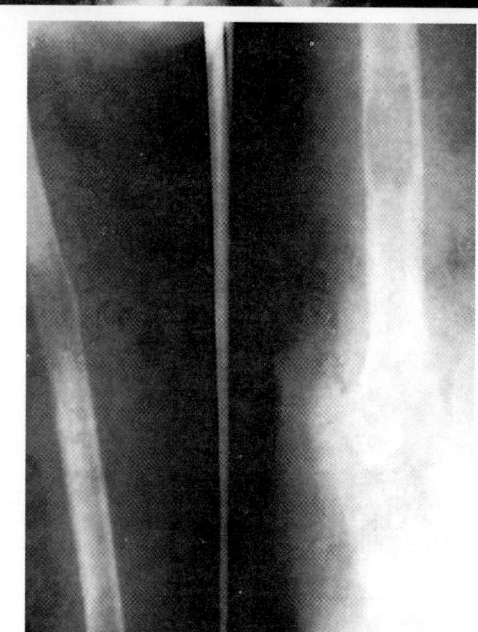

Fig. 44.39 Follicular carcinoma of thyroid with skeletal secondaries: (a) skull; (b) left femur (*courtesy of Dr M. Vasuderam, Tamil Nadu, India*).

[8]*Orphan Annie-eyed nuclei are named after the strip cartoon character who, along with other characters (such as Daddy Warbucks), was drawn with empty circles for eyes.*

Karl Hurthle, 1866–1945. German histopathologist who first drew attention to these tumours.

Max Askanazy, 1865–1940. Described these cells while working at the Pathological Anatomy Institute, Tubingen, Germany.

Blake Cady, Surgeon, New England Deaconess Hospital, Boston, Massachusetts, USA.

Table 44.7 Major differences between papillary and follicular carcinoma (*after Cady*)

	Papillary (%)	*Follicular* (%)
Male incidence	22	35
Lymph node metastases	35	13
Blood vessel invasion	40	60
Recurrence rate	19	29
Overall mortality rate	11	24
Location of recurrent carcinoma		
Distant metastases	45	75
Nodal metastases	34	12
Local recurrence	20	12

age, the presence of extrathyroidal spread or major capsular transgression (in follicular carcinoma), and the size of the tumour. Recently, several scoring systems based on multifactorial analysis of risk factors from retrospectively gathered data have been devised. On the basis of age, tumour spread, size and histology, these allow separation of patients into low- and high-risk groups with 25-year mortality rates of 2 per cent and 46 per cent, respectively. With regard to age, the prognosis is much worse in males over the age of 40 years and in females over 50 years. Distant metastatic disease is obviously an adverse prognostic factor but lymph node metastases are not associated with worse prognosis. Definitions of low- and high-risk groups based on data from the Lahey Clinic are given in Table 44.8.

Patients in the low-risk group account for 90 per cent of cases of differentiated thyroid carcinoma.

Surgical treatment

There is continuing disagreement on the most appropriate operation for differentiated thyroid carcinoma. The conservative approach advocates lobectomy with isthmusectomy in most patients with total thyroidectomy reserved for

Table 44.8 Differentiated thyroid carcinoma: risk group definitions

Low-risk group
- Men of 40 years and younger, women of 50 years and younger, without distant metastases
- All older patients with
  - intrathyroid papillary carcinoma or
  - follicular carcinoma with minor capsular involvement
  - tumours <5 cm in diameter
  - no distant metastases

High-risk group
- All patients with distant metastases
- All older patients with
  - extrathyroid papillary carcinoma or
  - follicular carcinoma with major capsular involvement
  - tumours 5 cm in diameter or larger regardless of extent of disease

Ian D. Hay, Physician, The Mayo Clinic, Rochester, Minnesota, USA.

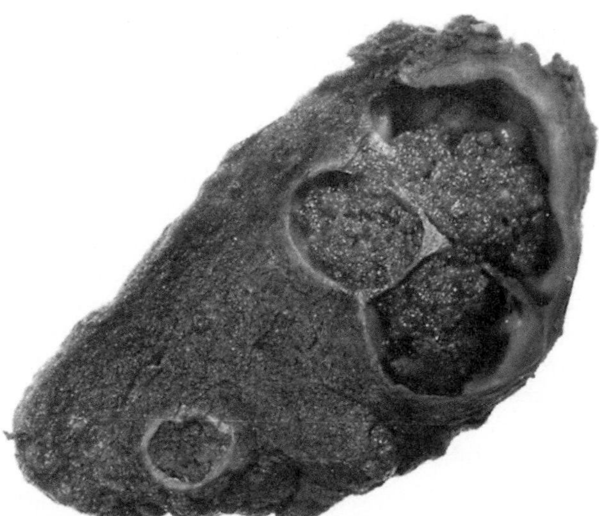

Fig. 44.40 Papillary carcinoma of the thyroid, showing multifocal tumour. This specimen demonstrates how necessary it is to remove the whole lobe (*courtesy of F.F. Rundle, FRCS, Sydney, Australia*).

specific indications (*viz.* those with bilateral disease or judged to be in a high-risk category). The more radical approach advocates routine total thyroidectomy often as a staged procedure depending on the pathological findings of the initial lobectomy.

The case for a policy of total thyroidectomy is theoretically based on the prevalence of multifocality in papillary carcinoma and on the feasibility thereafter of using radioiodine scanning to detect metastases, the thyroid having been ablated (Fig. 44.40). However, the clinical significance of multifocality is low as local recurrence is infrequent after unilateral resection. In addition, in those selected patients in whom scanning may be indicated, the remaining thyroid tissue may be ablated safely with a preliminary dose of radioiodine. Most importantly there is no evidence that the long-term results of routine total thyroidectomy as a policy are better than those of more conservative operations, and there is a substantial risk of permanent hypoparathyroidism. Clearly the risk of parathyroid damage varies according to expertise and the frequency with which the operation is done but, even at the Mayo Clinic, where thyroid surgery is frequently and expertly done, the rate of hypoparathyroidism is significant (Hay).

The large majority of patients with differentiated carcinoma, particularly since 90 per cent fall into a group with a 2 per cent mortality rate, is appropriately treated by lobectomy with isthmusectomy on the affected side. At the same time clinically obvious nodes, which may be pretracheal, paratracheal or in the jugular chain, are removed. If the jugular nodes are extensively involved, a modified neck dissection with preservation of the accessory nerve and sternomastoid muscle may be carried out through extension of the thyroidectomy incision. Very occasionally it may be necessary to sacrifice the recurrent laryngeal nerve if it is completely encircled and, on even more rare occasions, extrathyroidal spread may require resection of part of the trachea.

When there is clinically obvious bilateral disease at operation, bilateral resection is clearly indicated and bilateral resection may also be indicated in the few patients classified as high risk, although the evidence at present for improved prognosis is rather weak. Retrospective analysis of outcome in 860 patients with papillary carcinoma treated at the Mayo Clinic between 1946 and 1970 showed improved survival in high-risk patients undergoing bilateral resection, compared with lobectomy alone, although the difference was not statistically significant (Hay). There was no advantage for total compared with near-total thyroidectomy in which 1–2 g of thyroid tissue is preserved on the contralateral side to protect the blood supply to one or more parathyroid glands.

Surgical operations

Isthmusectomy. Swellings confined to the thyroid isthmus, including small differentiated carcinomas, may be appropriately removed by resection of the isthmus alone. Isthmusectomy is also an effective method of relieving tracheal obstruction and obtaining tissue for diagnosis in anaplastic carcinoma and lymphoma.

Thyroid lobectomy. Total lobectomy on the affected side together with isthmusectomy is the appropriate operation for removal of a discrete thyroid swelling and for most patients with differentiated carcinoma. The procedure, if performed meticulously by an experienced surgeon, is associated with very little risk of postoperative complications such as recurrent laryngeal nerve injury. The parathyroid glands should be seen and preserved *in situ* if possible; although the intact glands on the contralateral side will ensure normal function, removal of the contralateral lobe may occasionally be necessary in the future. It is unnecessary to ligate the main trunks of the inferior thyroid arteries. Instead, the individual arterial branches supplying the thyroid gland should be ligated close to the thyroid, preserving the parathyroid blood supply. The recurrent laryngeal nerve is carefully exposed throughout the dissection. It is particularly vulnerable close to where it angulates posteriorly to enter the larynx, at which site it is intimately related to the lateral thyroid ligament (ligament of Berry).

Near-total thyroidectomy. This consists of total thyroid lobectomy on the affected side, with conservation of 1–2 g of thyroid tissue on the contralateral side, which preserves the blood supply to one or both parathyroids.

Total thyroidectomy. The technique is essentially that of bilateral lobectomy and, if meticulous, the risk of complications is very low except for permanent hypoparathyroidism. The risk of hypoparathyroidism is variable but may be appreciable even in experienced hands.

Additional measures

Thyroxine. It is standard practice to prescribe thyroxine in a dose of 0.1–0.2 mg daily, to suppress endogenous TSH production, for all patients after operation for differentiated thyroid carcinoma on the basis that some tumours are TSH dependent. Suppression of the TSH level should be confirmed by measurement. Failure of suppression to a level of <0.1 µ/litre may indicate an inadequate dose of thyroxine or more usually that the patient is noncompliant. However, suppressive thyroxine is probably not of value in follicular carcinoma, and is unlikely to be of benefit in low-risk patients treated by lobectomy.

Sir James Berry, b. 1860. Surgeon, London, England.

Thyroid hormone replacement is obviously necessary after total thyroidectomy and in the majority of patients after near-total thyroidectomy, and is usually given in the form of thyroxine. Patients with potential or actual distant metastases who may require repeated radioiodine administration for scanning and therapy should be given tri-iodothyronine (60–80 mg/day) because it is much shorter acting, and on stopping it, increased TSH secretion and thyroid avidity for iodine recover quickly so that radioiodine may be given after several days. The patient is thereby spared weeks of developing thyroid insufficiency after stopping thyroxine before radioiodine may be given.

Radioiodine. If metastases take up radioiodine they may be detected by scanning and may be treated with large doses of radioiodine. For effective scanning, all thyroid tissue must have been ablated by either surgery or preliminary radioiodine and the patient must be hypothyroid to improve uptake. The indications for scanning after operations for differentiated carcinoma are disputed, but it is probably only indicated in patients with unresectable local recurrence or metastatic disease, high-risk patients, and in those with a rising serum thyroglobulin level. In addition, if metastases take up radioiodine they are likely to be suppressed as effectively by treatment with thyroxine as by radioiodine. Cases in which suppression has failed and radioiodine has given permanent control appear to be uncommon.

If metastases have been treated, the scan should be repeated at annual intervals and further therapeutic doses of radioiodine given as necessary. Solitary distant metastases may be treated by external radiotherapy.

Thyroglobulin. The measurement of serum thyroglobulin is of value in the follow-up and in the detection of metastatic disease in patients who have undergone surgery for differentiated thyroid cancer. This measurement may obviate the need for serial radioactive iodine scanning but when a rise occurs, a scan will be indicated to confirm and locate the metastatic disease. Thyroglobulin levels are, however, only an adjunct to careful clinical palpation of the neck because local recurrence detectable clinically may be present with a low thyroglobulin.

Undifferentiated (anaplastic) carcinoma

This occurs mainly in elderly women and is much less often diagnosed now than in the past when many thyroid lymphomas were mistakenly classified histologically as anaplastic carcinomas. Local infiltration is an early feature of these tumours with spread by lymphatics and by the bloodstream. They are extremely lethal tumours and survival for more than 1–2 years after presentation is most unusual. In most cases death occurs within months rather than within years. An attempt at curative resection is only justified if there is no infiltration through the thyroid capsule and no evidence of metastases. Many of these aggressive lesions present in an advanced stage with tracheal obstruction and require urgent

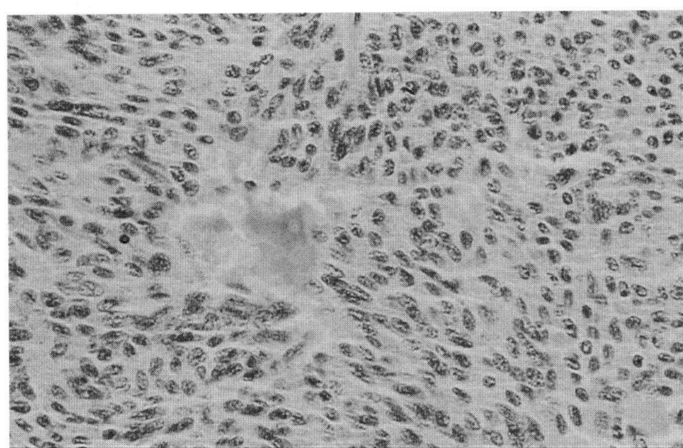

Fig. 44.41 Histology of medullary carcinoma showing characteristic 'cell balls' and amyloid (*courtesy of Dr S.W.B. Ewen, Aberdeen, Scotland*).

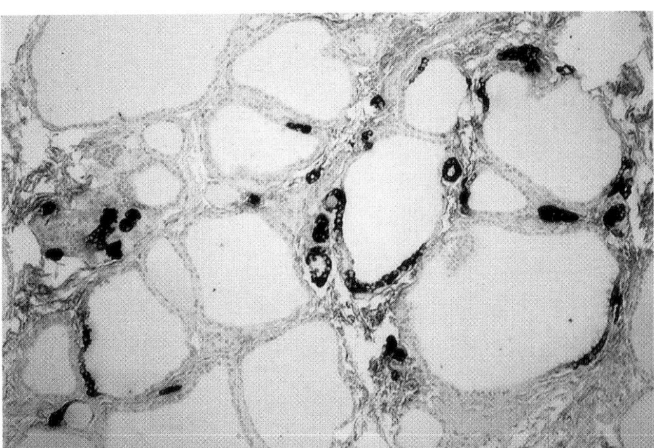

Fig. 44.43 Hyperplasia of parafollicular 'C' cells in a child from a family with medullary cancer (*courtesy of Dr S.W.B. Ewen, Aberdeen, Scotland*).

tracheal decompression. The trachea may be decompressed and tissue obtained for histology by isthmusectomy. Tracheostomy is best avoided. Radiotherapy should be given in all cases and may provide a worthwhile period of palliation as may combination chemotherapy [including doxorubicin (Adriamycin)].

Medullary carcinoma

These are tumours of the parafollicular (C)-cells derived from the neural crest and not from the cells of the thyroid follicle as are other primary thyroid carcinomas. The cells are not unlike those of a carcinoid tumour and there is a characteristic amyloid stroma (Fig. 44.41). High levels of serum calcitonin (>0.08 ng/ml) are produced by many medullary tumours. These levels fall after resection of a tumour and will rise again if the tumour recurs. This is a valuable tumour marker in the follow-up of patients with this disease. Diarrhoea is a feature in 30 per cent of cases and this may be due to 5-hydroxytryptamine or prostaglandins produced by the tumour cells.

Some tumours are familial and may account for 10–20 per cent of all cases. Medullary carcinoma may occur in combination with adrenal phaeochromocytoma and hyperparathyroidism (usually due to hyperplasia) in the syndrome known as multiple endocrine neoplasia type IIa (MEN IIa). The familial form of the disease frequently affects children and young adults whereas the sporadic cases occur at any age with no sex predominance. When the familial form is associated with prominent mucosal neuromas involving the lips, tongue (Fig. 44.42) and inner aspect of the eyelids, with occasionally a Marfanoid habitus, the syndrome is referred to as MEN type IIb.

Involvement of lymph nodes occurs in 50–60 per cent of cases of medullary carcinoma and blood-borne metastases are common. As would be expected, tumours are not hormone dependent and do not take up radioactive iodine. The course of the tumour is unpredictable; in general, life expectancy

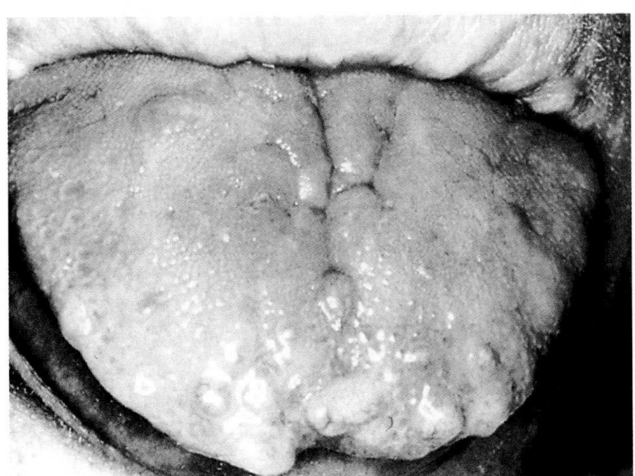

Fig. 44.42 Typical appearance of tongue and lips in patient with multiple endocrine neoplasia type IIb showing projecting ganglioneuromas (*courtesy of Professor E.D. William, Cardiff, Wales*).

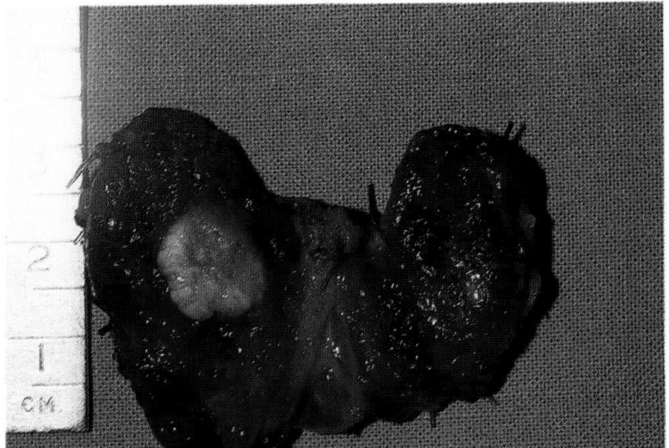

Fig. 44.44 Total thyroidectomy specimen from a young girl undergoing surgery following genetic screening and positive calcitonin stimulation tests showing a small medullary cancer in the right lobe.

Antoine Bernard-Jean Marfan, 1858–1942. French paediatrician.

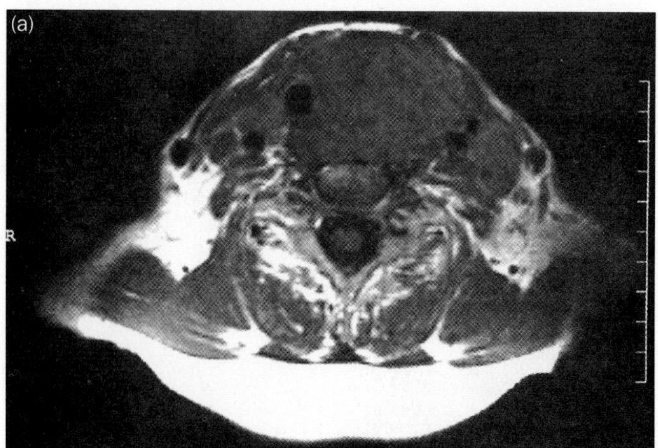

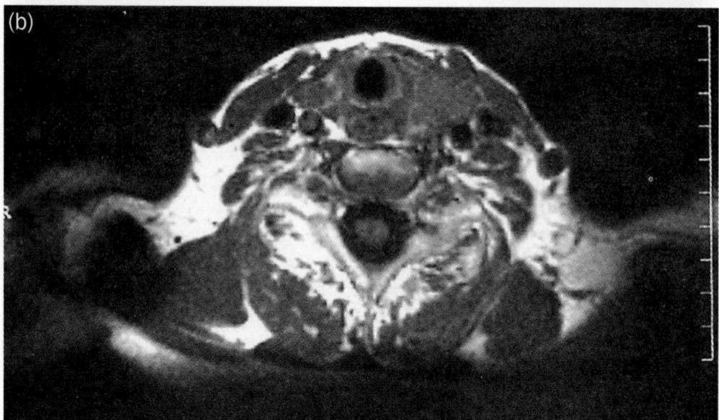

Fig. 44.45 Magnetic resonance imaging scans of extensive malignant lymphoma (a) before and (b) after 7 days of external beam radiotherapy (*courtesy of Dr F.W. Smith, Aberdeen, Scotland*).

is excellent if the tumour is confined to the thyroid gland, good as long as metastases are confined to the cervical lymph nodes and poor once blood-borne metastases are present.

Treatment is by total thyroidectomy and resection of involved lymph nodes with either a radical or modified radical neck dissection. Familial cases are now detected by genetic screening for the RET oncogene mutations which identifies individuals who will develop medullary cancer later in life (Fig. 44.43). The genetic tests are supplemented by estimating serum calcitonin levels in the basal state and after stimulation by either calcium or pentagastrin. A rise in calcitonin levels under these circumstances should lead to a prophylactic thyroidectomy but even then the disease may be beyond the preinvasive C-cell hyperplasia stage (Fig. 44.44).

Phaeochromocytoma must be excluded by measurement of urinary catecholamine levels (Chapter 45) in all cases before embarking upon thyroid surgery to avoid the potential hazards associated with this condition.

Malignant lymphoma

In the past, many malignant lymphomas were diagnosed as small round-cell anaplastic carcinomas. Response to irradiation is good (Fig. 44.45) and radical surgery is unnecessary once the diagnosis is established by biopsy. Although the diagnosis may be made or suspected on FNAC, sufficient material is seldom available for immunocytochemical classification, and large-needle (Trucut) or open biopsy is usually necessary. In patients with tracheal compression, isthmusectomy is the most appropriate form of biopsy. The prognosis is good if there is no involvement of cervical lymph nodes. Rarely the tumour is part of widespread malignant lymphoma disease, and the prognosis in these cases is worse.

Thyroiditis

Chronic lymphocytic (autoimmune) thyroiditis[9]

This common condition is usually associated with raised titres of thyroid antibodies. Not infrequently there is a family history of other autoimmune disease. It commonly presents as a multinodular goitre with established or subclinical thyroid failure, although it may present as a discrete swelling. Features of chronic lymphocytic (focal) thyroiditis are commonly present on histological examination in association with other thyroid disease – notably toxic goitre. Primary myxoedema without detectable thyroid enlargement represents the end stage of the pathological process.

Clinical features

As might be expected from the varied histological picture (above), the onset, the thyroid status and the type of goitre vary profoundly from case to case. The onset may be insidi-

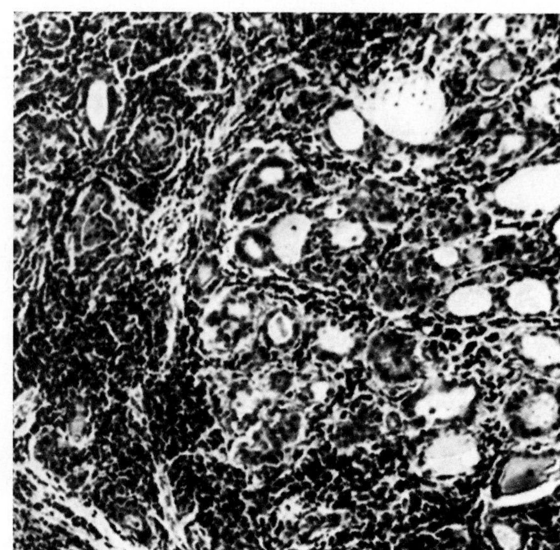

Fig. 44.46 Autoimmune thyroiditis (Hashimoto's disease; struma lymphomatosa). Intense lymphocytic-plasma cell infiltration, acinar destruction and fibrosis. Compare the normal histology (Fig. 44.24).

[9]*Chronic lymphocytic thyroiditis was described by Hakaru Hashimoto (1881–1934), Director of the Hashimoto Hospital, Mie, Japan, in 1912. The link to an autoimmune basis was first defined by Professor Roitt and co-workers at the Middlesex Hospital, London, England.*

ous and asymptomatic, or so sudden and painful that it resembles the acute form of granulomatous thyroiditis. Mild hyperthyroidism may be present initially, but hypothyroidism is inevitable and may develop rapidly or extremely slowly. The goitre is usually lobulated, and may be diffuse or localised to one lobe. It may be large or small, and soft, rubbery or firm in consistency – depending upon the cellularity and the degree of fibrosis. The disease is commonest in women at the menopause, but may occur at any age. Papillary carcinoma and malignant lymphoma are occasionally associated with autoimmune thyroiditis.

Diagnosis

Biochemical tests of thyroid function vary with the thyroid status and are of diagnostic value only if hypothyroidism is present. Significantly, raised titres of one or more thyroid antibodies are present in over 85 per cent of cases. Nevertheless, differential diagnosis from nodular goitre, carcinoma and malignant lymphoma of the thyroid is not always easy. FNAC is the most appropriate investigation although abundant lymphocytes may make the cytological distinction between autoimmune thyroiditis and lymphoma difficult (Fig. 44.46). When there is doubt about neoplastic disease, which may coexist with thyroiditis, operation is necessary.

Treatment

Full replacement dosage of thyroxine should be given for hypothyroidism and if the goitre is large or symptomatic, because some (under TSH stimulation) may subside with hormone therapy. More minor manifestations of the condition such as a small goitre with raised antibody titres, or histological evidence of thyroiditis in association with other thyroid disease, do not justify thyroxine replacement if thyroid function is biochemically normal; however, long-term surveillance is necessary because of the risk of late thyroid failure. Occasionally the goitre increases in spite of hormone treatment and in these circumstances there may be a favourable response to steroid therapy. Thyroidectomy may be necessary if the goitre is large and causes discomfort. The clinician must, however, be cautious when a lymphocytic goitre increases in size and becomes unresponsive to thyroxine as this may be due to the development of malignant lymphoma.

Granulomatous thyroiditis (subacute thyroiditis – de Quervain's thyroiditis)

This is due to a virus infection. (An epidemic reported from Israel was due to a mumps virus.) In a typical subacute presentation there is pain in the neck, fever, malaise and a firm, irregular enlargement of one or both thyroid lobes. There is a raised erythrocyte sedimentation rate and absent thyroid antibodies, the serum T_4 is high, normal or slightly raised, and the ^{123}I uptake of the gland is low. The condition is self-limiting and in a few months the goitre has subsided; subsequent hypothyroidism is rare. In 10 per cent of cases the onset is acute, the goitre very painful and tender, and there may be symptoms of hyperthyroidism. Thirty-five per cent of cases are asymptomatic but for the presence of the goitre. If diagnosis is in doubt, it may be confirmed by FNAC, radioactive iodine uptake and by a rapid symptomatic response to prednisone. The specific treatment for the acute case with severe pain is to give prednisone 10–20 mg daily for 7 days and the dose is then gradually reduced over the next month.

Riedel's thyroiditis

This is very rare, accounting for 0.5 per cent of goitres. Thyroid tissue is replaced by cellular fibrous tissue which infiltrates through the capsule into adjacent muscles, paratracheal connective tissue and the carotid sheaths. It may occur in association with retroperitoneal and mediastinal fibrosis and is most probably a collagen disease. The goitre may be unilateral or bilateral and is very hard and fixed. The differential diagnosis from anaplastic carcinoma can only be made with certainty by biopsy, when a wedge of the isthmus should also be removed to free the trachea. If unilateral, the other lobe is usually involved later and subsequent hypothyroidism is common.

Further reading

Cohn, K.H., Backdahl, M., Forsslund, C. *et al.* (1984) Biologic considerations and operative strategy in papillary thyroid cancer: arguments against the routine performance of total thyroidectomy. *Surgery*, **96**, 957–70.

Cusick, E.L., Krukowski, Z.H. and Matheson, N.A. (1987) Outcome of surgery for Graves' disease revisited. *British Journal of Surgery*, **74**, 780–3.

Harness, J.K., Fung, L., Thompson, N.W. *et al.* (1986) Total thyroidectomy: complications and technique. *World Journal of Surgery*, **10**, 781–8.

Hay, I.D., Grant, C.S., Taylor, W.F. and McConahey, W.M. (1987) Ipsilateral lobectomy versus bilateral lobe resection in papillary thyroid carcinoma: a retrospective analysis of surgical outcome using a novel prognostic scoring system. *Surgery*, **102**, 1088–95.

Matheson, N.A. (1985) *A Colour Atlas of Thyroid Lobectomy*, Wolfe Medical, London.

Mazzaferri, E.L. (1993) Management of a solitary thyroid nodule. *New England Journal of Medicine*, **328**, 55–9.

Wheeler, M.H. and Lazarus, J.H. (1994) *Diseases of the Thyroid. Pathophysiology and Management*, Chapman & Hall, London.

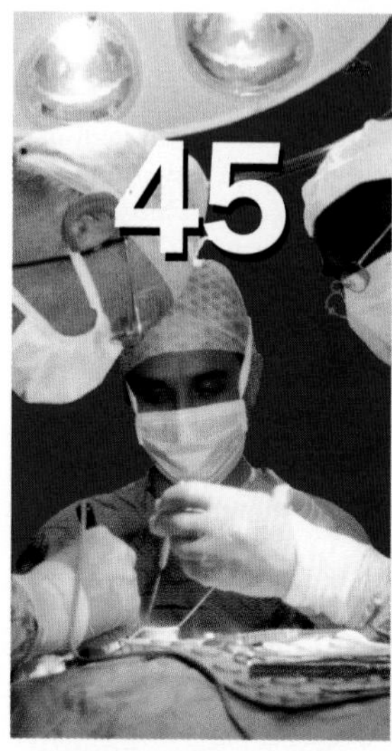

45 The parathyroid and adrenal glands

Parathyroid glands

Anatomy. The parathyroid glands, four in number, are small, oval in shape, commonly about 0.5 cm in size, soft, mobile, yellowish brown in colour and arranged in pairs – most often closely applied to the thyroid gland, either within or closely applied to its capsule. The upper pair is more constant in position than the lower: 80 per cent are found on the posterolateral aspect of the thyroid, immediately above the termination of the inferior thyroid artery, close to the cricothyroid articulation. Most of the remaining 20 per cent are posterolateral to the upper pole of the thyroid lobe. The lower pair is more variable in position: 40 per cent are found at the lower pole of the thyroid and 40 per cent are within the thymic tongue (Fig. 45.1). The remaining 20 per cent are variable in site, most often some distance lateral to the thyroid, and less often in the mediastinal thymus a few centimetres below the sternal notch or, very occasionally, ectopically situated near the carotid sheath, sometimes as high as the carotid bifurcation. On rare occasions, a parathyroid, usually the upper gland, may be retropharyngeal, retro-oesophageal or actually within the thyroid substance and, in 1–2 per cent of individuals, there is one or more supernumerary glands usually associated with a lobule of thymic tissue. Each gland has a delicate capsule and is supplied by a single leash of blood vessels clearly seen running in the subcapsular plane (Fig. 45.2). Very often, parathyroid glands are associated with or embedded within a pad of fat, which gives a useful clue to identification.

Histology. The stroma consists of a rich sinusoidal capillary network with islands of secretory cells interspersed with fat cells. The glandular cells are of two types. The 'chief' or 'principal' cells are small with vesicular nuclei and poorly staining cytoplasm. 'Water-clear' cells, derived from the chief cells, are found in hyperplastic and neoplastic glands. The 'oxyphil' cells are less numerous and larger, with granular cytoplasm and deeply staining nuclei.

Bailey & Love's Short Practice of Surgery, 23rd edition. Edited by R.C.G. Russell, N.S. Williams and C.J.K. Bulstrode. Published in 2000 by Arnold Publishers.

Physiology. The chief cells of the parathyroids produce parathormone, the hormone being released directly into the bloodstream. The circulating level of parathormone can be measured by radioimmunoassay, which is sufficiently reliable to distinguish between high and low levels. Facilities for obtaining the estimation are widely available.

Parathormone:

- stimulates osteoclastic activity, thereby increasing bone resorption by mobilising calcium and phosphate;
- increases the reabsorption of calcium by the renal tubules, thus reducing the urinary excretion of calcium;
- augments the absorption of calcium from the gut;
- reduces the renal tubular reabsorption of phosphate, thus promoting phosphaturia.

Parathyroid hormone is an 84 amino acid peptide which has a short half-life before degradation into amino-terminal and carboxy-terminal

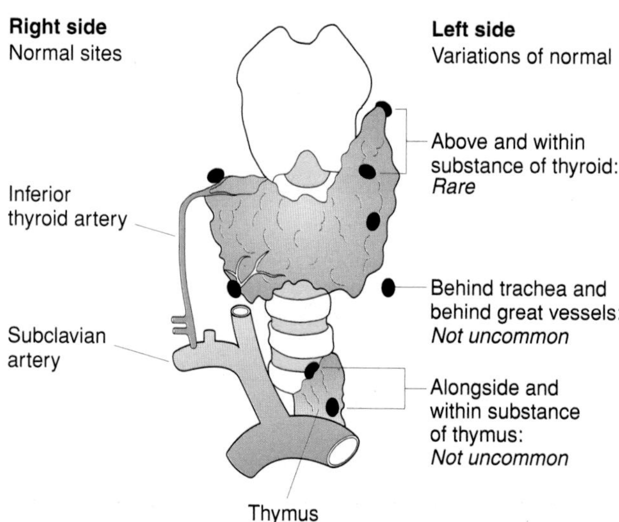

Fig. 45.1 Parathyroid gland. Normal and uncommon sites.

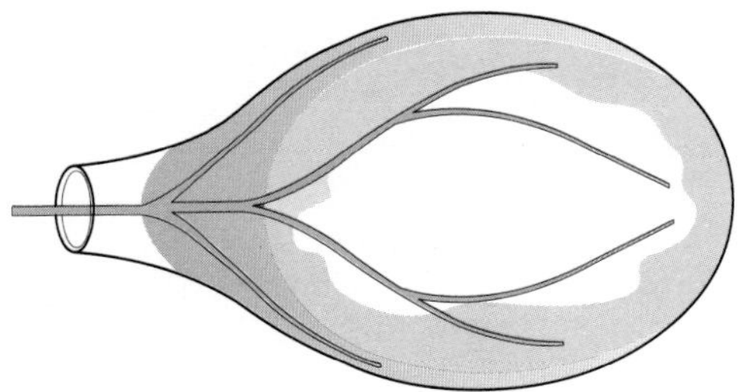

Fig. 45.2 The blood supply of a parathyroid gland.

fragments, with the amino-terminal fragment having biological activity. The amino-terminal fragment retains biological activity with a half-life of minutes and the carboxy-terminal fragment a half-life of hours. Available assays measure either the intact hormone, the amino- or carboxy-terminal or 'mid-portion' fragments.

Calcitonin (Copp) is secreted by the parafollicular cells of the thyroid (thyrocalcitonin). It lowers the serum calcium and affects calcium storage in bones; quite the opposite action of parathormone.

Parathyroid hormone-related protein (PTH-rP) is a hypercalcaemic factor with similar bioactivity to that of parathyroid hormone. Since its isolation from cancer cell lines and carcinoma of the breast, strong evidence has emerged that it is an important hormonal mediator of cancer-associated hypercalcaemia in patients with solid tumours. Plasma PTH-rP 1–86 concentrations may be measured by a two-site immunoradiometric assay.

Hypoparathyroidism

Parathyroid tetany, due to hypocalcaemia, is a rare complication of subtotal thyroidectomy (less than 1 per cent) but a more common complication of total thyroidectomy. At these operations, some of the parathyroid glands may be removed or have their blood supply temporarily embarrassed. It may also occur after surgery to the parathyroids themselves. Symptoms usually appear on the second or third postoperative day, and are temporary. Milder forms of hypoparathyroidism have been described in the follow-up of thyroidectomised patients. Permanent hypoparathyroidism, most commonly encountered following radical thyroidectomy for cancer, requires constant supervision and treatment. Tetany in the newborn may occur within the first few days of life in the child born of a mother with undiagnosed hypoparathyroidism.

Spontaneous hypoparathyroidism is an unusual form of autoimmune disease.

Clinical features

The first symptoms are tingling and numbness in the face, fingers and toes. In extreme cases, cramps in the hands and feet are very painful; the extended fingers are flexed at their metacarpophalangeal joints, with the thumb strongly adducted (Fig. 45.3); the toes are plantar-flexed and the ankle joints extended – the so-called carpopedal spasm. Spasm of the muscles of respiration results in not only pain and stridor, but also dread of suffocation. In infancy, the symptoms of tetany may be mistaken for epilepsy, although there is no loss of consciousness.

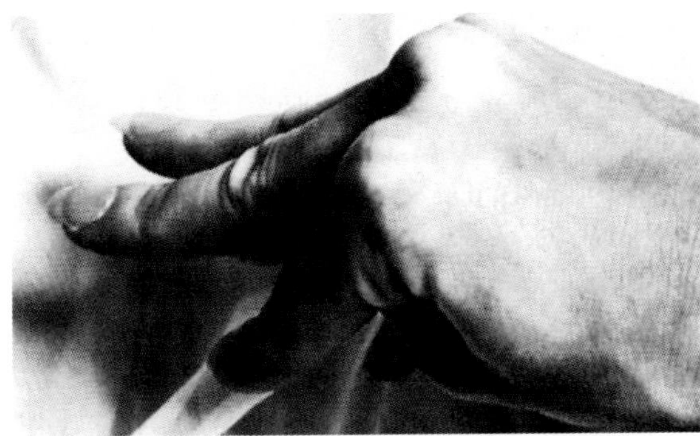

Fig. 45.3 The 'obstetrician's hand' seen in parathyroid tetany.

Latent tetany may be demonstrated by the following.

- **Chvostek's sign.** Tapping over the branches of the facial nerve at the angle of the jaw will produce twitching at the corner of the mouth, the ala of the nose and the eyelids.
- **Trousseau's sign.** A sphygmomanometer cuff applied to the arm and inflated above the systolic blood pressure for not more than 2 minutes will produce carpal spasm.

Treatment

In acute cases the symptoms may be relieved speedily by the slow intravenous injection of 10–20 ml of a 10 per cent solution of calcium gluconate. This may be repeated until the patient's circulating calcium level has been stabilised. For longer-term management, the absorption of calcium is enhanced by oral administration of the most active metabolite of vitamin D – 1,25-dihydroxycholecalciferol [$1,25(OH)_2D3$]. Its major action is on the gut, promoting active absorption of calcium and phosphorus, raising calcium levels to normal within a week. Magnesium supplements may occasionally be needed. Serum calcium levels must be estimated daily and the dosage adjusted as appropriate.

Hyperparathyroidism

Hyperparathyroidism is a more common condition than had been previously believed

- The symptomatic presentation may vary but the increased use of autoanalysers has resulted in 'asymptomatic' hypercalcaemic patients being the largest group.
- A corrected serum calcium concentration above the upper limit of normal and a simultaneous elevation of serum

Douglas Harold Copp. Professor of Physiology, University of British Columbia, Vancouver, British Columbia, Canada.

Frantisek Chvostek, 1835–84. Physician, Josefsakademie, Vienna, Austria.
Armand Trousseau, 1801–67. Physician, Hôtel Dieu, Paris, France.

parathyroid hormone level are mandatory for the diagnosis.
- Surgery should only be performed by an experienced parathyroid surgeon.

Long-term follow-up is essential as there is a significant increase in risk of death from cardiovascular disease.

Hyperparathyroidism is associated with an increased secretion of parathyroid hormone. This occurs in:

- **Primary** hyperparathyroidism, which is an unstimulated and inappropriately high parathyroid hormone secretion for the concentration of plasma-ionised calcium, and is due to adenoma or hyperplasia, and very rarely carcinoma.

  A single adenoma is the commonest finding (multiple in 6 per cent). The whole gland is usually considerably enlarged, darker in colour, firmer and more vascular than normal; in some a rim of normal parathyroid tissue may be seen surrounding the adenoma. The histological appearances are the same as in hyperplasia, with a predominance of chief and water-clear cells. Carcinoma of the parathyroids is extremely rare, less than 1 per cent. It tends to invade locally and recur after operation. Blood-borne metastases have been described.
- **Secondary** hyperparathyroidism is associated with chronic renal failure or malabsorption syndromes. The stimulus for the hyperplasia is chronic hypocalcaemia. All four glands are involved.
- **Tertiary** hyperparathyroidism is a further stage in the development of reactive hyperplasia where autonomy occurs as the parathyroids no longer respond to physiological stimuli.

Cinical features

Hyperparathyroidism, rarely found in the first decade of life, is commoner in women than men, and most commonly found between the ages of 20 and 60 years. The clinical features vary enormously, even when the biochemical changes are similar.

Asymptomatic cases

The most common presentation is the detection of unsuspected and asymptomatic hypercalcaemia by routine biochemical screening.

'Bones, stones, abdominal groans and psychic moans'

Only 50 per cent of patients suffer from any of these.

Nonspecific symptoms

Nonspecific symptoms include muscle weakness, thirst, polyuria, anorexia and weight loss – a challenge to the astute clinician!

Bone disease

There may be generalised decalcification of the skeleton, as in osteitis fibrosa cystica (von Recklinghausen's disease), single or multiple cysts, or pseudotumours of any bone. The latter are particularly common in the jaw bones. Early

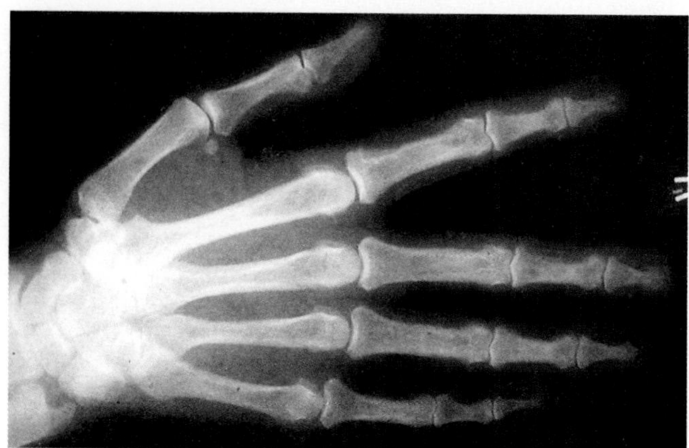

Fig. 45.4 Loss of density and subperiosteal resorption of the phalanges in a case of primary hyperparathyroidism (*courtesy of Professor Anthony W. Goode*).

radiological changes first appear in the skull and in the phalanges (Fig. 45.4), with loss of density and subperiosteal erosions. Many patients presenting with vague pains in the bones and joints are mistakenly diagnosed as rheumatic.

Renal stones

Hyperparathyroidism must be considered in every patient presenting with renal tract stone or nephrocalcinosis (Fig. 45.5), and even in those cases of renal colic where no stone can be demonstrated.

Dyspeptic cases

Patients with nausea, vomiting and anorexia are relatively common. Peptic ulcer and pancreatitis are not infrequently found in association with hyperparathyroidism, but the relationship is not as yet fully understood.

Psychiatric cases

Psychiatric cases are not uncommon; women, complaining of tiredness, listlessness and with obvious personality changes,

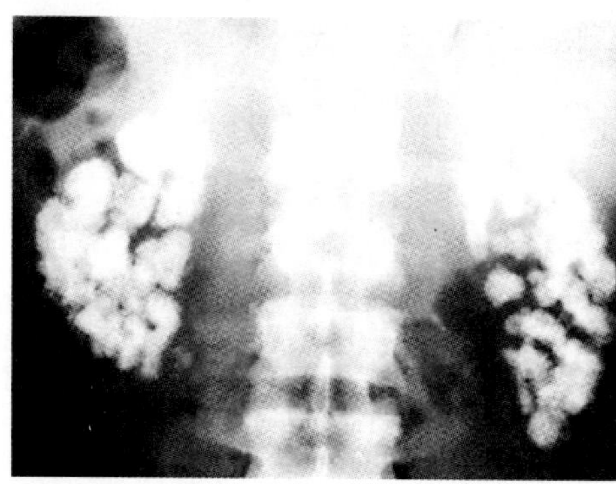

Fig. 45.5 Nephrocalcinosis.

Friedrich Daniel von Recklinghausen, 1833–1910. Professor of Pathology, Strasbourg, France.

are often wrongly labelled 'neurotic' or 'menopausal'. Patients have been admitted to mental institutions because of irrational behaviour.

Acute hyperparathyroidism

This diagnosis is difficult and only too often made after death. Nausea and abdominal pain is followed by severe vomiting, dehydration, oliguria and finally coma. The serum calcium is very high. Treatment is urgent after rehydration, which is vital. Biphosphonates (disodium etidronate and pamidronate) are specific inhibitors of bone resorption. They are highly effective given parenterally and may also be used in the preoperative, short-term medical management of severe hypercalcaemia in primary hyperparathyroidism.

Clinical examination and investigation

Clinical examination may be unrewarding but the cause of dehydration or confusion may be found in the eyes. *Corneal calcification* may be detected. It begins on the lateral and medial borders of the limbus (which distinguishes it from arcus senilis) and is best seen through a hand lens by the light of a bright torch reflected off the iris. Less common is *band keratopathy* in which a transverse band of calcification forms across the front of the cornea, and *conjunctival calcification* where redness of the eye also occurs. Hypertension may be present in up to 50 per cent of cases. There may be electrocardiographic changes with a shortened QT interval, primarily by an effect on the length of the S–T segment. A parathyroid adenoma is very seldom palpable in the neck. The diagnosis is confirmed with the following biochemical findings:

- elevation of serum calcium (upper limit of normal 2.6 mmol/litre). Serum calcium occurs as calcium ions complexed to citrate and bound to albumin. Therefore the serum albumin concentration should be known in order to apply a correction factor: corrected serum calcium (mmol/litre) = measured serum Ca (mmol/litre) + (40 – A) × 0.02, where A = serum albumin (g/litre);
- diminution of serum phosphorus (lower limit of normal 0.8 mmol/litre);
- increased excretion of calcium in the urine (upper limit of normal 62 mmol per 24 hours for females, 75 mmol for males);
- elevation of the serum alkaline phosphatase in cases with bone disease;
- elevation of serum parathormone concentration.

The diagnosis of hyperparathyroidism largely depends on confirmed hypercalcaemia, exclusion of other causes of hypercalcaemia (see below) and a raised parathormone level. Present-day immunoradiometric assays (upper limit of normal varies according to the laboratory) for biologically active intact parathormone are highly reliable and a raised level is even more reliable. Detectable levels of parathormone within the normal range, in the presence of hypercalcaemia, are suggestive of the diagnosis.

Preoperative localisation

Provided the surgeon is experienced in parathyroid surgery, preoperative localisation tests may do little to enhance the ability to detect 95 per cent of abnormal glands at surgery. However, a multimodal approach combining thallium–technetium isotope scanning, neck ultrasonography and magnetic resonance imaging (MRI) may yield precise information which will clearly facilitate surgery and reduce unnecessary dissection of tissue. Localisation tests are particularly indicated before re-exploration when the initial operation has failed, but may also be helpful to less experienced surgeons.

- The simplest localisation test is an ultrasonic scan but results vary according to the skill and experience of the investigator.
- Computerised tomography is of most value in localising a lesion in the mediastinum rather than the neck.
- Thallium–technetium isotope subtraction imaging may locate up to 90 per cent of parathyroid adenomas before surgery (Fig. 45.6). Like ultrasonography, subtraction scintigraphy is more accurate the larger the adenoma, and is inaccurate in parathyroid hyperplasia.
- MRI is improving rapidly with some centres reporting up to 64 per cent detection prospectively. A low signal is obtained from the parathyroid glands on a T_1-weighted image while a T_2-weighted image appears in early studies to produce good contrast resolution from the surrounding tissues.
- Invasive techniques such as selective angiography and selective venous sampling may be helpful in locating an abnormally situated gland after a failed initial exploration.

Differential diagnosis

Other causes of hypercalcaemia must be remembered and excluded. They are:

- secondary cancer in bone (breast, prostate, bronchus, kidney and thyroid);
- carcinoma with endocrine secretion (bronchus, kidney and ovary);

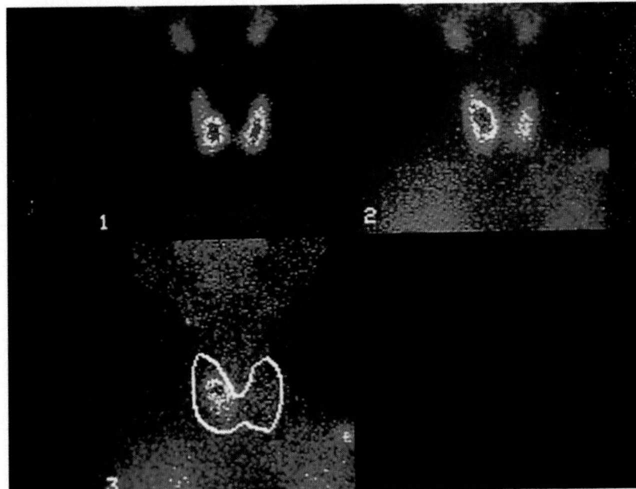

Fig. 45.6 The preoperative localisation of a parathyroid adenoma by Tl and Tc subtraction scintigraphy. The technique is first to outline the thyroid with Tc and then to administer an isotope such as Tl which is taken up by both thyroid and parathyroid tissue. The two images are captured by a gamma camera and by computer subtraction of the two images, the enlarged parathyroid remains as a 'hot spot' (Tl: thallium; Tc: technetium).

- multiple myeloma;
- vitamin D intoxication;
- sarcoidosis;
- thyrotoxicosis;
- immobilisation;
- medication: thiazide diuretics, lithium.

The differential diagnosis presents *no* problem if the parathormone level is estimated. In none of the above-mentioned conditions will parathormone be detectable in the blood.

Treatment

The only corrective treatment is surgical removal of the overactive gland or glands. In symptomatic patients, the indications for operation are clear-cut. Many patients, however, in whom hypercalcaemia has been discovered incidentally, are not overtly symptomatic and a decision in favour of operation is more difficult.

Preoperative treatment is not usually necessary except in acute cases, when rapid correction of dehydration and electrolyte imbalance is necessary, with a careful daily check on the serum calcium. Drugs used would have been discussed earlier.

A recent international survey of operative strategy shows that the approach is changing. Removal of the adenoma with biopsy of the other glands has been supplanted by removal of the adenoma, a peroperative histological diagnosis and then biopsy of one normal gland. If the peroperative biopsy is that of a hyperplastic gland, then removal of all four glands with autotransplantation is indicated. Approximately 90 per cent of cases of primary hyperparathyroidism are associated with single-gland disease (adenoma). Ten per cent of cases are associated with multiple-gland disease, either hyperplasia or more than one adenoma. Adenomas, single or multiple, are removed.

In approximately 10 per cent of cases even the most experienced surgeon in this field may find difficulty in locating a parathyroid adenoma.

Parathyroid tissue can be successfully autotransplanted into the arm, a useful technique to avoid repeated potentially difficult explorations of the neck. The indications are tertiary hyperparathyroidism in patients undergoing chronic renal dialysis, and recurrent hyperparathyroidism. The technique is to excise all of the parathyroid tissue from the neck and to implant eight 1-mm^3 fragments into a pocket in the forearm muscle mass, marking the site with nonabsorbable sutures. Postoperative vitamin D and calcium replacement therapy is required for varying periods. Recurrent hypercalcaemia is an indication for exploration of the implantation site and to excise further parathyroid tissue.

Prognosis

With successful surgery in severe cases, bones will recalcify and pseudotumours resolve. Renal stones will not disappear, but the incidence of recurrence after surgical removal is reduced and deterioration in renal function is prevented. Psychiatric patients show an early and often remarkable recovery. Many patients who are not overtly symptomatic beforehand are aware of an improvement in well-being after correction of hypercalcaemia. In a small minority of cases, hyperparathyroidism recurs after several years and may warrant further surgery. In some of these, autotransplantation (above) offers reasonable prospects of control; Wells has reported excellent results when autotransplantation has been used for recurrent and familial hyperparathyroidism.

Hypertension associated with hyperparathyroidism is common, but the mechanism is unclear.

Long-term survival has been studied in 900 patients in Sweden. Despite successful surgery for primary hyperparathyroidism, the risk of premature death from cardiovascular and malignant diseases remained significant. Thus long-term follow-up is important as this indicates that primary hyperparathyroidism causes damage that is not reversed by surgery.

Patients with persistent and recurrent primary hyperparathyroidism are a difficult management problem. For patients in whom initial exploration fails, reoperation is associated with a higher morbidity and a greater chance of failure. Accurate diagnosis and review of the initial pathology are essential, a family history of multiple endocrine neoplasia should be excluded, together with occult malignancy. Preoperative venous sampling of the neck and thorax is particularly valuable in localising a missed adenoma which is the most common cause of failure at the first operation.

Mild asymptomatic hypercalcaemia is a relative contraindication to further surgery but regular follow-up is mandatory. With an experienced surgeon, up to 90 per cent of missed lesions may be found but persistent postoperative hypocalcaemia may occur in up to 10 per cent of patients and recurrent laryngeal nerve injury is seen in about 6 per cent.

Parathyroid carcinoma

Parathyroid carcinoma is a rare condition to be considered when a high serum calcium is associated with a palpable lump in the neck. At operation it has a characteristic grey–white colour and is adherent because of local invasion of adjacent soft tissue. The best results are obtained by early recognition, avoiding rupture of the tumour capsule, and aggressive surgical management including ipsilateral thyroid lobectomy. Surgical clips should be used to outline the tumour bed for postoperative radiotherapy.

Multiple endocrine neoplasia syndrome – APUD cells

Always consider that a patient with hyperparathyroidism may also have multiple endocrine adenomas. The cells involved, irrespective of the site, have the common chemical characteristics of amine precursor uptake and decarboxylation and are thus known as APUD cells. The disorder is inherited as an autosomal dominant, the manifestations in any one family tend to be similar and all members of the family should be investigated.

Samuel A. Wells, Jr, Brixby Professor of Surgery and Chairman, Department of Surgery, Washington University School of Medicine, St Louis, Missouri, USA.

Type I

This most common variant involves the parathyroid glands (90 per cent), pancreatic islets (80 per cent), pituitary (65 per cent), thyroid and adrenal cortex. There is hyperplasia of the parathyroid glands and a chromophobe adenoma of the pituitary which may result in increased prolactin production or acromegaly. The pancreatic tumour may produce gastrin (the Zollinger–Ellison syndrome) or insulin, glucagon, somatostatin or vasoactive intestinal peptide (VIP) causing watery diarrhoea. Treatment is surgical excision.

Type IIa

A genetic abnormality located on chromosome 10 has been identified in MEN type IIa syndrome. Fifty per cent have parathyroid hyperplasia. The associated lesions may be a medullary carcinoma of thyroid, which produces calcitonin, and a phaeochromocytoma. The latter should be excluded or be the first priority for treatment before exploration of the neck (see also Chapter 44).

Type IIb

This is differentiated from type IIa because of additional neurological abnormalities. Mucosal neuromas produce 'lumpy and bumpy' lips (Fig. 44.42) or eyelids, and there is a characteristic Marfanoid facial appearance. Megacolon and ganglioneuromatosis are also found (see also Chapter 44).

Adrenal glands

Surgical anatomy

At birth, the adrenal glands have attained nearly adult proportions. Fully developed, each weighs about 4 g, but the left is a little larger than the right. A deeper yellow colour and a firmer consistency enable the gland to be distinguished from the adjacent fat. Each rests on the superior, anterior and medial aspects of the superior pole of the corresponding kidney, and presents the appearance of a French Liberty cap worn at a rakish angle.

Although intimately related anatomically, the adrenal cortex and the adrenal medulla are quite separate internal secretory glands.

The adrenal glands are supplied by several adrenal arteries, rendering them remarkably vascular, but only one vein drains each gland. On the right side the adrenal vein is short and enters the inferior vena cava, while on the left it empties into the left renal vein [which communicates through the azygos vein with the left intercostal, internal mammary and vertebral veins (Anson)]. This dissimilarity of the right and left venous flow determines, to some extent, the location of metastases from malignant tumours of these glands.

Robert Milton Zollinger, 1903–90. Formerly Professor of Surgery, Ohio State University, Columbus, Ohio, USA.
Edwin Holmer Ellison, 1918–70. Professor of Surgery, Marquette University, Milwaukee, Wisconsin, USA.
Antonin Bernard Jean Marfan, 1858–1942. Professor of Paediatrics, Paris, France.

Diagnostic investigations

Computerised tomography (CT) has been a significant advance in imaging the adrenal glands and in the detection of adrenal masses with an accuracy of 90 per cent (Fig. 45.7). Ultrasonography can detect most adrenal masses larger than 2 cm in diameter, but is operator and machine dependent and less accurate, especially in obese patients. CT has made invasive techniques, such as selective retrograde venography and selective arteriography, almost obsolete. In those cases where CT findings are inconclusive and functional information is required, isotope scanning (see below) and differential venous sampling for hormone levels may be indicated.

A radiograph or CT scan of the pituitary fossa showing an enlarged pituitary fossa is suggestive of a basophil adenoma of the pituitary gland with excess adrenocorticotrophic hormone (ACTH) pituitary secretion.

Adrenal gland scintigraphy using NP-59 [^{131}I-6(-iodomethyl-19 Norchest-5(10)EN-3β-ol] is of value in addition to CT. In a benign functioning adrenal tumour there is uptake with suppression of the contralateral gland. By contrast adrenocortical carcinoma does not usually concentrate the isotope and, as a result of contralateral gland suppression, there is little uptake. Bilateral adrenal hyperplasia produces the opposite result with a prominent bilateral image.

MRI is of value particularly for small lesions.

Adrenal cortex

The adrenal cortex is made up of the following layers from without inwards: the zona glomerulosa, the zona fasciculata and the zona reticularis.

Physiology. At least 50 steroid compounds have been isolated from the adrenal cortex. These hormones exhibit various types of activity which, for practical purposes, can be arranged in three groups.

Mineralocorticoids are concerned in the maintenance of water and electrolytic balance. A deficiency of these hormones produces sodium diuresis, potassium retention and dehydration; an excess results in hypertension, oedema, cardiac dilatation and hypokalaemia. *Aldosterone* is the most important of these 'salt-regulating' hormones (see Conn's syndrome later).

Glucocorticoids are concerned with the metabolism of proteins and carbohydrates, favouring the formation of the latter from the body's storehouse of the former. This conversion is known as gluconeogenesis.

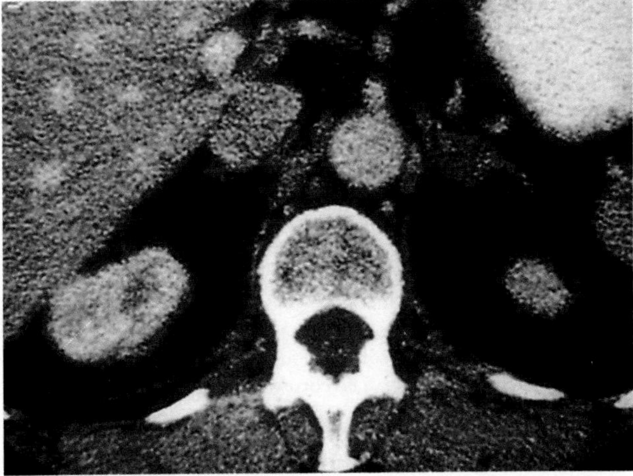

Fig. 45.7 Computerised tomography scan of adrenal glands showing a 1.5-cm left adrenal adenoma (courtesy of Professor Anthony W. Goode).

Barry J. Anson. Research professor, Department of Otolaryngology and Maxillofacial Surgery, College of Medicine, University of Iowa, Iowa City, Iowa, USA.

The best known of these are *hydrocortisone* (also known as *cortisol*) and *cortisone* (which is converted in the body to hydrocortisone). The therapeutic application of these hormones falls under two headings.

- *In endocrine deficiencies.* Hydrocortisone is the logical need in adrenocortical insufficiency and after bilateral adrenalectomy.
- *In nonendocrine disease.* Hydrocortisone or synthetic analogues, such as prednisone and betamethasone, are used in the treatment of a diversity of diseases, including allergic conditions, granulomatous disorders, blood diseases and the collagenoses. Hydrocortisone is used in the treatment of hypocorticism and shock (Chapter 4) and is an effective antiallergic agent in a number of skin diseases and eye conditions.

Sex hormones. Androgenic and oestrogenic hormones are produced by the adrenal cortex. Excessive secretion of androgens due to adrenal enzyme deficiencies or tumours causes virilism in females or, rarely, excessive secretion of oestrogens brings about effeminacy in males.

Interhormonic action. The anterior lobe of the pituitary gland secretes ACTH which stimulates the adrenal cortex, whereas the cortisol of the adrenal cortex inhibits the secretion of ACTH. ACTH secretion is also controlled by higher cerebral centres and the hypothalamic corticotrophin-releasing hormone (CRH).

Tests of adrenocortical activity

The tests are of two types, those that confirm the presence of a change in cortisol production and those that indicate a cause. No tests should be interpreted in isolation but all the results of the investigations should be considered together.

Plasma electrolytes. Sodium levels are raised and potassium is low in a hyperfunctioning adrenocortical lesion with the opposite in Addison's disease, but changes in Addison's disease may not occur until the patient is approaching crisis.

Plasma cortisol levels. Diurnal variation with a maximum value at 8.00 a.m. may be lost both in Cushing's syndrome, where all levels are high, and in insufficiency when levels are low.

Plasma ACTH levels. Low plasma levels are found with adrenal tumours and high levels with a pituitary lesion or ectopic ACTH production. The ratio of ACTH to related peptides such as β-lipotrophin may facilitate the distinction between pituitary Cushing's and ectopic ACTH production.

Plasma aldosterone levels. The concentration of aldosterone is only one-thousandth that of cortisol, and both dietary sodium and posture may change the value. Plasma renin levels should be measured along with aldosterone to differentiate between primary and secondary hyperaldosteronism.

Urinary steroid excretion. ***Cortisol secretion rate.*** The daily output of cortisol is a precise measure of adrenocortical activity, but is routinely performed in only a few centres. Adult levels are reached by 18 years of age and after 40 years fall gradually, to be halved by 70 years of age. The average excretion is higher in Caucasian males. The daily output may be determined by the administration of a small amount of radioactive-labelled cortisol, which is metabolised and excreted, and the urinary radioactivity measured. The normal range is 5–28 mg per 24 hours, with high levels in Cushing's syndrome and low levels in adrenal insufficiency.

Urinary cortisol excretion. The cortisol excretion in a 24-hour urine sample is probably the best screening test for adrenocortical oversecretion.

17-Oxosteroids or ketosteroids. These reflect androgen output, and excretion is increased in many women with virilising syndromes.

Dexamethasone suppression test. Dexamethasone is 25 times more potent than cortisol. Dexamethasone 0.5 mg is administered 6-hourly for 2 days and causes a marked decrease in urinary steroid excretion by inhibiting ACTH production, and thus cortisol, without contributing greatly to the total urinary steroid output. In Cushing's syndrome, no effect is produced by the dose. Larger doses of up to 2 mg 6-hourly will, over several days, reduce urinary steroid excretion if the overactivity is secondary to bilateral adrenal hyperplasia, but not with an adrenal tumour, which is autonomous. Measurement of the plasma cortisol at 9.00 a.m. after the administration of 2 mg dexamethasone the previous midnight serves as a convenient screening test for Cushing's syndrome.

Metyrapone test. This differentiates between excess ACTH production and a lesion in the adrenal cortex causing Cushing's syndrome. Metyrapone inhibits the biosynthesis of cortisol so plasma levels fall. If the pituitary–adrenal axis is intact, this results in an increase in ACTH production and stimulation of the adrenal cortex. The basal levels of 17-oxosteroids and ketosteroids in the urine are measured for 2 days, 750 mg of metyrapone is given per 4 hours and a 24-hour urine collection completed. A normal response is a two to fourfold increase in the urinary steroids over basal levels. A diminished response in Cushing's syndrome indicates a primary adrenal lesion.

Synacthen test. Tetracosactrin (Synacthen) 250 μg is given intramuscularly and blood cortisol measured at 30 and 60 minutes. In normal subjects the basal plasma cortisol should be greater than 60 μg/litre and be at least 70 μg/litre after stimulation. In Addison's disease the response is impaired.

Disorders of adrenocortical function

Acute hypocorticism. ***Adrenal apoplexy in the newborn.*** Extensive haemorrhage into one or both adrenals may be a cause of death in infants within the first few days of birth. The condition may occur after a long and difficult labour, and particularly when resuscitative procedures have to be employed to combat asphyxia neonatorum. The haemorrhage into the adrenals follows necrosis of the innermost layer of the cortex, which always occurs at birth, possibly as a result of sudden withdrawal of the female sex hormone (oestrogen). Adrenal crisis in the newborn produces signs of profound shock. A mass may be palpable in one or both renal regions. Intravenous fluid therapy with hydrocortisone, or failing the latter, cortisone intramuscularly, offers the only hope.

Waterhouse–Friderichsen syndrome. Massive bilateral adrenal cortical haemorrhage occurs in cases of fulminating meningococcal septicaemia and in some cases of streptococcal, staphylococcal or pneumococcal septicaemia. Most cases occur in infants and young children, but it can happen in adults with severe haemorrhage or burns. The onset is catastrophic, with rigors, hyperpyrexia, cyanosis and vomiting. Petechial haemorrhages into the skin which coalesce rapidly into purpuric blotches are a constant feature. Profound shock follows, and before long the patient passes into coma. The condition is one of overwhelming sepsis that pursues a galloping course, death occurring in most cases within 48 hours of the onset of symptoms unless correct treatment is given without delay.

Unilateral haemorrhage causing a lesser degree of systemic upset and not associated with infections has been described. This type of case resembles a perinephric abscess or other upper abdominal acute condition.

Thomas Addison, 1793–1860. Physician, Guy's Hospital, London, England. Described the effects of disease of the suprarenal capsules in 1849.

Harvey Cushing, 1869–1939. Professor of Surgery, Harvard University, Boston, Massachusetts, USA (1912–32). Described this syndrome in 1932.

Rupert Waterhouse, 1873–1958. Clinical Pathologist and Physician, Royal United Hospital, Bath, England. Described this syndrome in 1911.

Carl Friderichsen, b. 1886. Former Medical Superintendent, Children's Department, Sundby Hospital, Copenhagen. Wrote his account of this syndrome in 1918.

Confirming the diagnosis. It is futile to await the result of a blood culture. Bilateral tenderness 5 cm below the costal margin, clear urine (oliguria is often present) and an absence of signs in the lungs help to call attention to the adrenal glands. In meningococcal infection the diplococcus may be demonstrated by smears obtained from a punctured petechial spot in the skin.

Treatment. Antibiotic therapy must be given intensively by the intravenous route. Hydrocortisone 100 mg is given intravenously (i.v.), or intramuscularly (i.m.) if venous access is difficult. Up to 400 mg hydrocortisone may be required in the first 24 hours. No mineralocorticoid is needed as the weak intrinsic salt-retaining action of hydrocortisone suffices at this dosage. Oral medication may be commenced after the first day and then over about 4 days reduced to a maintenance level. Oxygen should also be administered. Following such treatment, improvement often sets in within 3 hours, and a number of patients has recovered.

Crises of infantile hypercortism. See later.

Following bilateral adrenalectomy. If precautions are taken, acute hypocorticism is unusual in the postoperative period. Treatment is to give 300 mg hydrocortisone on the first day. Most patients achieve a maintenance dose of 30 mg/day. After about 3 weeks fludrocortisone 0.1 mg may be given.

Postoperative adrenal haemorrhage. Adrenal haemorrhage is a rare unexpected cause of deterioration and sudden death in the postoperative period. In some cases the left adrenal gland is damaged during radical gastrectomy for carcinoma (Fox). In other cases, when adrenal haemorrhage is bilateral, there is no evidence of operative injury, they are usually associated with intra-abdominal sepsis, pneumonia, coagulation defects and cancer. Thrombosis of the adrenal veins is the cause of infarction of glands.

Chronic hypocorticism (Addison's disease)

This is due to adrenocortical insufficiency consequent upon progressive destruction with lymphocytic infiltration of the zona reticularis, the zona fasciculata, the zona glomerulosa and the medulla of the adrenal glands, in that order. In about 60 per cent of cases the condition is believed to be due to an autoimmune disease, sometimes in association with autoimmune thyroiditis (Chapter 44) and pernicious anaemia. Tuberculosis, metastatic carcinoma and amyloidosis account for the remaining 40 per cent.

Clinical features

Addison's disease usually commences in the third or fourth decade. Sometimes it is the terminal event in cases of adrenogenital hyperplasia. The sex distribution is about equal. The leading features are muscular weakness and a low blood pressure. Irregular dusky pigmentation of the skin, due to deposits of melanin, appears at points of pressure, e.g. garter or belt, and in the flexion creases. Pigmentation of mucous membranes, particularly of the mouth, is often striking. When fully established, the course of the disease is punctuated by crises of acute adrenocortical insufficiency (see above).

Bernard Fox. Pathologist, Charing Cross Hospital, London, England.

Treatment

Treatment is medical. In long-term management, most patients require 20–30 mg hydrocortisone in divided doses, with fludrocortisone 0.1 mg daily as mineralocorticoid replacement. Signs of overtreatment include hypertension, hypokalaemia and oedema; those of undertreatment, fatigue and hypotension. Where relevant, chemotherapy is mandatory for tuberculosis (Chapter 8).

Prognosis

By the use of replacement corticosteroids, the expectation of life of a patient suffering from Addison's disease has been extended from up to 3 years to many years.

Hypercorticism

The various forms of adrenal cortical hyperfunction are classified according to the age at onset:

- infantile;
- prepubertal;
- adult, otherwise known as Cushing's syndrome – the commonest type;
- postmenopausal;
- primary aldosteronism (Conn's syndrome) can occur at any age.

Infantile hypercorticism

Androgenic excess during intrauterine life is one form of pseudohermaphroditism in the *female child*. The condition is present at birth; sometimes the enlarged clitoris and a varying degree of hypospadias make it difficult to determine the infant's sex. The 17-ketosteroid content of the urine may be sufficiently elevated to substantiate a diagnosis of a female with adrenal hyperfunction. If this is not the case, it is justifiable to perform sex determination by a skin biopsy before the age of 1 year. Female pseudohermaphroditism with virilism is invariably associated with disease of the adrenal cortex, usually bilateral hyperplasia of the cortex. Hormonal studies have shown that there is a congenital failure of the adrenal glands to synthesise glucocorticoids. Owing to this lack, these infants are liable to acute phases of adrenal insufficiency during stress or infection, or to suffer from periodic hypoglycaemic attacks. They need corticosteroid replacement, not only in the emergency, but as long-term therapy, thereby inhibiting the secretion of excessive androgens. In the absence of such treatment, the epiphyses join early, the patients are dwarfed, menstruation does not occur and the breasts do not develop. These tendencies are corrected by hydrocortisone given orally, 25 mg or more daily, the dose being determined by 17-ketosteroid estimations (Simpson). Hirsutism is moderated, but not necessarily abolished. The treatment should be commenced early if good results are to be obtained.

Prepubertal hypercorticism

There is never any doubt as to the sex of the infant at birth and during the very early years of life the child is normal. The symptoms commence at about the age of 5 or 6 years.

Jerome W. Conn, b. 1907. American physician who was Professor of Internal Medicine at the University Hospital, Ann Arbor, Michigan, USA.
Samuel Leonard Simpson, 1900–83. Consulting Endocrinologist, St Mary's Hospital, London, England.

In the female. Pubic and axillary hair appear, but there is no gross enlargement of the clitoris. The child is short in stature, the legs being especially stunted, but she looks much older than she is. Puberty is often precocious, menstruation, if it occurs, being scanty. There is a deepening of the voice at this time.

In the male. The term 'infant Hercules' is descriptive. He is extremely short, muscular and hirsute. The genitalia assume adult proportions and spermatozoa are often present in the seminal fluid.

In both sexes, 17-ketosteroid content of the urine is increased. A very high reading supports the diagnosis of an adrenocortical tumour, which must always be excluded. In both males and females, with a later onset or the passage of time, the features of Cushing's syndrome become superadded.

Treatment. This is identical to that of Cushing's syndrome.

Postpubertal or adult hypercorticism (Cushing's syndrome)

Postpubertal or adult hypercorticism (Cushing's syndrome) is due to an excessive endogenous production of glucocorticoids, mainly hydrocortisone. It is an uncommon condition, often suspected but seldom confirmed. Pituitary-dependent Cushing's syndrome is the commonest form of endogenous hypercorticism accounting for up to two-thirds of all cases. An adrenal adenoma accounts for 20 per cent and carcinoma (which may be bilateral) 5 per cent. In the remainder there is no discernible structural alteration in the glands and the condition is due to an ectopic source of an ACTH-like substance being secreted, by either a benign tumour (e.g. bronchial carcinoid) or a malignant tumour of bronchus, mediastinum or pancreas. NonACTH-dependent primary adrenocortical hyperplasia is a rare cause of Cushing's syndrome. Alcoholism also must be considered.

In its most typical form, Cushing's syndrome is exogenous and is seen in patients treated with large doses of cortisone over long periods for nonendocrine diseases, particularly rheumatoid arthritis, and in patients receiving transplants.

Clinical features. The female to male ratio is at least 3:1. The great majority of cases (excluding those induced by cortisone therapy) occurs in females between 15 and 30 years of age, in whom it produces highly characteristic features. Although the patient's weight is not necessarily increased, there is a deposition of fat in certain situations. The face becomes rubicund, rounded like a full moon, and the lips are pursed. The abdomen becomes protuberant, the neck thick, the supraclavicular fossae obliterated and a roll of fat appears over the region of the vertebra prominens (buffalo hump). The arms, and especially the legs, are relatively thin, the muscular development is poor, and the patient complains of increasing weakness. As the disease progresses, so the general contour becomes more and more that of a 'lemon on matchsticks' (Fig. 45.8). Consequent upon the inhibitory effect of the hypercorticism on fibrous tissue, the skin becomes of tissue-paper consistency and inelastic. Exceedingly characteristic are purple-red striae distentiae, mostly on the abdomen (Fig. 45.9), of a texture that can be likened to an overstretched garter. Ecchymoses are frequent and bruising occurs on the slightest trauma. Acne is common and there is a low resistance to skin infections. Often there is increased growth of lanugo hair, but hirsutism is usually absent. Amenorrhoea is usual or, in the male, impotence. Owing to a negative calcium balance, the matrix of bone becomes thin and severe osteoporosis results. Pathological fractures, particularly compression fracture of a vertebra, are common, and this is sometimes the first reason for the patient seeking advice. Mild glycosuria is often present. Hypertension is

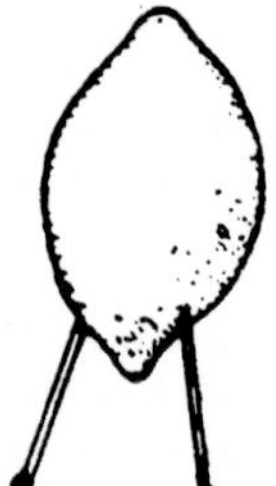

Fig. 45.8 Cushing's syndrome contour – lemon on matchsticks.

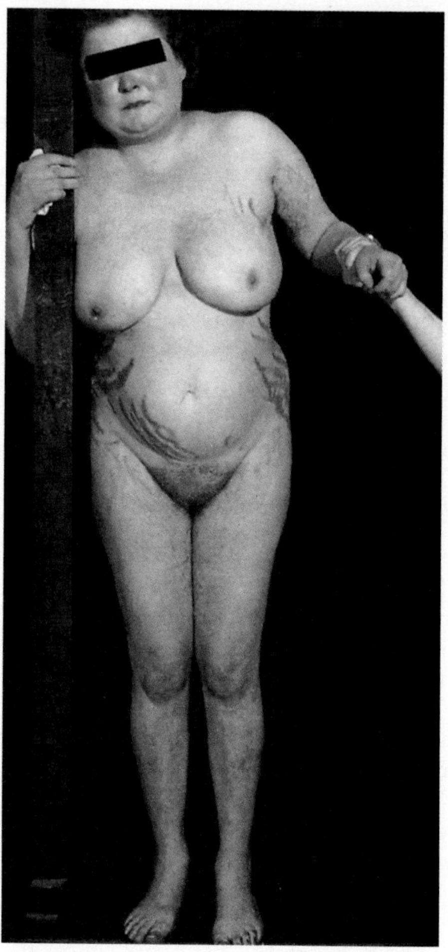

Fig. 45.9 Cushing's syndrome in a woman aged 23 years. Adrenal hyperplasia (*courtesy of Dr Leonard Simpson, London*).

Hercules, one of the most famous of the heroes of Greek mythology, was noted for his prodigious strength.

frequent and eventually congestive heart failure supervenes. In about 60 per cent of cases, various psychoses occur.

Cushing's syndrome is rare in children; when it occurs, the patient is nearly always a female and an adrenal tumour is usually the cause.

A subgroup, probably due to an excessive secretion of adrenal androgens (*adrenogenital syndrome*), commences between the ages of 15 and 25 and is confined to females. One of the first indications of its onset is amenorrhoea or oligomenorrhoea. There follows an excessive growth of hair on the face (Fig. 45.10), acne, atrophy of the breasts, alteration in bodily contour and muscular development, deepening of the voice and enlargement of the clitoris. Jewish and Spanish women are more prone to this affliction than those of other races.

Arrhenoblastoma of the ovary

This rare condition occurs between puberty and the menopause and also causes hirsutism. It may also arise in a suprarenal 'rest'.

Screening tests. There are three simple tests (see above) which may be used to screen patients suspected to have Cushing's syndrome:

- plasma cortisol levels and diurnal rhythm;
- 24-hour urinary free cortisol excretion;
- overnight dexamethasone suppression test.

Each of these tests is highly discriminating with false-positive and false-negative results in only about 5 per cent of cases. However, patients with severe or chronic illness or alcoholism may have elevated midnight plasma cortisol levels and may fail to show overnight suppression after dexamethasone.

Definitive diagnosis. Suspected Cushing's syndrome may be confirmed by the low-dose dexamethasone suppression test (see above), which is highly reliable.

Differential diagnosis. After the diagnosis of Cushing's syndrome has been established, it is necessary to determine the cause of adrenocortical hyperfunction. In general, adrenal hyperfunctioning tumours and ectopic ACTH-secreting tumours function autonomously and are unaffected by hormonal manipulation. In contrast, the feedback mechanism in pituitary Cushing's is functioning although it is abnormal. Thus appropriate investigations (see above) are the high-dose dexamethasone suppression test, measurement of plasma ACTH levels and the metyrapone test, which has largely been replaced by plasma ACTH assay. Nearly all patients with adrenal tumours and with the ectopic ACTH syndrome, in contrast to pituitary Cushing's, fail to suppress with a high dose of dexamethasone and suppression is indicative of Cushing's disease. In addition, patients with Cushing's disease or the ectopic ACTH syndrome have detectable or elevated plasma ACTH levels, whereas cortisol-producing adrenal tumours suppress pituitary ACTH secretion and plasma levels are extremely low. A high plasma ACTH level after high-dose dexamethasone indicates autonomous ACTH secretion by a nonpituitary tumour, whereas if the ACTH level is low it indicates the presence of an adrenocortical tumour that has suppressed ACTH secretion by the normal pituitary.

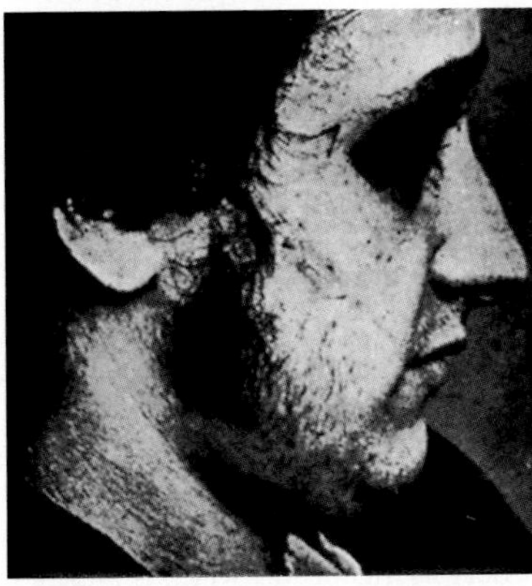

Fig. 45.10 Adrenogenital syndrome in a woman of 28 (courtesy of *Dr Leornard Simpson, London*).

Localisation studies. CT accurately identifies virtually all adrenal tumours in patients with Cushing's syndrome and has replaced other techniques. It is also the most reliable method of detecting nodules in the lungs, mediastinum and pancreas, which are potential sites of ectopic ACTH production. Pituitary CT has also replaced other techniques for the detection of pituitary microadenomas in Cushing's disease, although only 50 per cent of such adenomas are identified. Bilateral selective inferior petrosal venous sampling for ACTH levels is a valuable but technically difficult method of confirming and localising pituitary-dependent Cushing's disease if CT is unhelpful.

Treatment. Trans-sphenoidal pituitary adenectomy in skilled hands is now the treatment of choice for pituitary lesions. External pituitary irradiation is less reliable in terms of long-term remission but is more successful in children. Yttrium-90 implantation is an alternative form of pituitary irradiation. Bilateral total adrenalectomy is a reliable procedure for patients with Cushing's disease in whom pituitary treatment has failed.

The treatment of an adrenal tumour is surgical resection and resection of benign ectopic ACTH-secreting tumour is curative. Many, however, are malignant and widely disseminated when Cushing's syndrome becomes clinically apparent.

Nelson's syndrome

Hyperpigmentation and pituitary enlargement occur in about 20 per cent of cases after bilateral adrenalectomy and are avoided by selective pituitary microsurgery.

Prognosis. Most patients are alive 20 years after successful resection of an adrenal adenoma, but survival beyond 5 years is rare with a carcinoma (Welbourn). Pituitary microadenectomy in expert hands results in cure in about 80 per cent of patients.

Don H. Nelson, b. 1925. American internist.
Richard Burkewood Welbourn. Former Professor of Surgical Endocrinology, Royal Postgraduate Medical School, London, England.

Very rarely, the *adrenogenital syndrome* appears in youths and men. Owing to excessive production of oestrogenic hormones by the adrenal cortex, gynaecomastia, atrophy of the testicles and psychical signs of effeminacy appear (adrenal feminism).

Postmenopausal hypercorticism

Postmenopausal hypercorticism is usually characterised by the growth of a beard (the bearded woman of the circus) and is often accompanied by mental aberration. A lesser degree of hirsutism is almost a natural accompaniment of the ageing process, particularly in dark-haired females, and it is difficult to draw the line between the normal and the pathological. Thus it is that operative treatment is usually disappointing.

Primary aldosteronism

Primary aldosteronism (Conn's syndrome) is a surgically correctable type of hypertension found in 1–2 per cent of all hypertensive patients. It is characterised by autonomous excessive aldosterone secretion which leads to sodium retention and a fall in serum potassium. The latter causes the typical associated features of the syndrome, namely episodes of muscular weakness associated with polyuria and polydipsia. The plasma sodium is high and the potassium is low, but simple administration of potassium does not relieve the condition. Renin and angiotensin levels are depressed. The cause is either an aldosterone-secreting adrenal adenoma or bilateral adrenocortical hyperplasia (less common). CT and adrenal scanning with radioactive-labelled cholesterol are the appropriate localisation tests to distinguish between them. When these fail, adrenal venous sampling with measurement of aldosterone to cortisol ratios is the next step. Unilateral adrenalectomy is the treatment for an aldosterone-producing adenoma and has a high cure rate, whereas surgery has been disappointing in adrenocortical hyperplasia and these patients are generally managed medically.

Secondary aldosteronism

Secondary aldosteronism is associated with cirrhosis of the liver, and renal artery stenosis with high levels of renin and angiotensin.

The incidental adrenal mass – 'incidentaloma'

CT and MRI have resulted in increasing numbers (up to 1 per cent) of adrenal tumours being identified in the course of abdominal imaging for the investigation of other conditions. The finding may represent an adrenal tumour but more probably a benign lesion. Opinion is divided about management but essentially functioning lesions are excised whereas nonfunctioning lesions are managed according to size. Lesions less than 3 cm in size should be followed 3-monthly for a time by CT and excised if they enlarge, whereas those larger than 3 cm should be excised to exclude malignancy.

Adrenalectomy for hypercorticism

It is essential that all patients who are to be subjected to adrenalectomy are supported intraoperatively and postoperatively by adrenocortical hormone replacement therapy, irrespective of the extent of adrenal resection.

Corticosteroid therapy

Corticosteroids are started when anaesthesia is induced. There is no advantage of one steroid over another except for their different durations of action. Hydrocortisone is very short acting, prednisolone intermediate and dexamethasone long acting. Each may be given intravenously or intramuscularly.

During the first 24 hours after induction of anaesthesia, the patient should receive no more than 300 mg hydrocortisone, 60 mg prednisolone or 6 mg dexamethasone. The dosage should be halved each day until a maintenance dose orally (hydrocortisone 30 mg, prednisolone 5 mg or dexamethasone 0.5 mg) is reached. Fludrocortisone 0.1 mg daily (replacing aldosterone) is usually added to the maintenance dose of corticosteroid to regulate fluid and salt balance.

After total adrenalectomy the patient should always carry a card stating the dosage of corticosteroid being received. Any stress (e.g. further operation or infection) is an indication to increase the dosage.

Operation

When an adrenal tumour has been demonstrated preoperatively, excision of that adrenal gland alone is carried out.

Posterior approach

An ample posterolateral incision, such as is used for nephrectomy (Chapter 64), is used. After subperiosteal resection of the 12th rib, the lower border of the pleura is defined and protected. The incision is extended through the bed of the 12th rib to reveal the perinephric fat, within which the adrenal gland is identified, as described below. Sometimes an approach through the bed of the 11th rib, reflecting the pleura upwards, is preferred. (See also Anterior approach, below.)

On the right side the suprarenal vein is short and may be torn from the vena cava if it is not identified and ligated at an early stage of the dissection. By finger and gauze dissection, keeping close to the gland, the gland is freed from below and behind, upwards, ligating and dividing bleeding vessels as they are encountered, until it is suspended only by its main vascular pedicle near its apex.

Anterior approach

The adrenal glands are approached through either a curved transverse incision or a long midline incision. The *left adrenal gland* is approached first by cutting along the lateral leaf of the lienorenal ligament and then curving downwards and medially, so as to enable a wide peritoneal flap to be reflected. By retracting the spleen downwards and medially, the adrenal gland comes into view. The fascia over its lateral border is incised, and by gauze dissection the blood vessels of the gland are defined, ligated and divided, thus freeing the gland, which is removed. Alternative approaches can be made by an 'up and under' dissection of the mesocolon and pancreas, or through the lesser sac. The *right adrenal gland* is more deeply situated. The peritoneum is incised lateral to the duodenum and above the upper pole of the kidney. The flap of peritoneum is raised to expose the anterior surface of the adrenal gland as it lies against the bare surface of the liver. The fascia covering the lateral surface of the gland is incised. A finger can then be inserted above the upper pole of the gland into the space between the two layers of fascia enclosing the gland (Fig. 45.11). This prevents the gland from becoming displaced upwards, which otherwise it is prone to do. The anterior fascial layer is then incised transversely and the gland can be dissected under vision, as on the left side. After removal, each gland should be inspected to check its completeness, and each adrenal bed must be searched for the presence of accessory adrenal tissue, which is present in 32 per cent of cases. If this important step is omitted, failure of the operation is not unlikely.

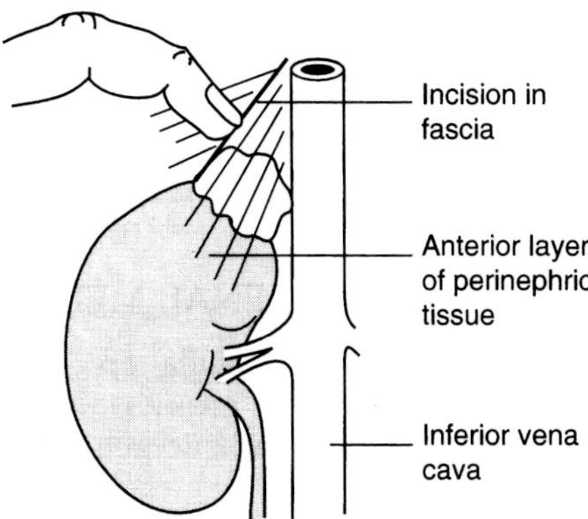

Fig. 45.11 Incision in the fascia lateral to the right adrenal gland. Insertion of the finger into the space above the gland prevents its upward displacement (*courtesy of J.C. McKeown and A. Ganguli*).

Thoracoabdominal approach

For removal of a large adrenal tumour (>10–15 cm in diameter) a thoracoabdominal incision gives the wide exposure necessary for radical resection *en bloc* which may involve removal of the ipsilateral kidney or spleen and tail of the pancreas.

Laparoscopic adrenalectomy

Laparoscopic adrenalectomy is a developing technique which may in selected patients, particularly patients with Conn's syndrome, provide an alternative operative approach using a full lateral decubitus transperitoneal flank approach. It is claimed that such a technique offers a less painful postoperative recovery, with the in-patient stay reduced from a mean of 8 days for open surgery to 3–4 days. This must be offset against a doubling of the operating time, a possible increased incidence of wound infection and port site hernia formation.

Left adrenalectomy. Start by dissecting the splenoparietal ligament close to the diaphragm to permit a complete mobilisation of the spleen to the right with the tail of the pancreas. Dissection of 5 cm of the splenic vein, when used as a landmark, permits exposure of the renal vein: which leads to the main and accessory adrenal veins. They can be safely divided between clips. The right side of the gland is dissected up to the diaphragm with clipping of the middle and upper arterial pedicles. The adrenalectomy is achieved by dissection of the fat and the gland is extracted in a bag.

Right adrenalectomy. The fundamental step of the procedure is the section of the hepatoparietal ligament far to the right allowing an upwards mobilisation of the liver. Then dissect towards the vena cava using this structure as a landmark to find the renal vein which is the inferior limit of the dissection. The main adrenal vein is doubly clipped and divided. The third step is to look for an accessory adrenal vein joining a subhepatic vein above the main adrenal vein. The adrenal arteries, superior, middle and the main inferior one coming from the renal artery, are dissected on the right side of the vena cava. The last step is straightforward coagulation, vessel clipping and dividing as on the left side.

Adrenal medulla

Physiology. The medulla of the adrenal glands (chromaffin tissue), which is developed, together with sympathetic nerves, from ectoderm, is grey in colour and connected intimately, both anatomically and functionally, with splanchnic nerves. Chromaffin tissue is so called because the large polyhedral cells of which it is composed contain granules that stain yellow with chromic acid. These granules are the internal secretion of the adrenal medulla itself, for they can be observed being extruded *in toto* into radicles of the adrenal vein. The secretion consists of the catecholamines[1], adrenaline and noradrenaline. In health, 80 per cent of the output is adrenaline and 20 per cent is noradrenaline. However, in hyperfunctioning medullary tumour (phaeochromocytoma) this ratio is completely reversed. Fear, anger, pain and effort give rise to an increased output in response to the stimuli received via the splanchnic nerves.

An amino acid peptide adrenomedullin has recently been isolated from human phaeochromocytoma. It has a structure similar to calcitonin gene-related peptide and amylin. Intravenous administration elicits a strong, long-lasting hypotensive effect. It has been detected in human plasma and vascular smooth muscle cells with specific receptors. It decreases blood pressure by lowering total peripheral resistance and increasing urine flow and urinary sodium excretion.

Actions of catecholamines. Catecholamines exert their effects through specific cell-surface receptors: alpha-receptors and beta-receptors (Table 45.1). These mediate the actions of the endogenously released catecholamines, noradrenaline and adrenaline, and some of the actions of dopamine. The receptors have quite different pharmacological properties and an organ may have more than one type. The complex actions of catecholamines include altering enzyme activity, metabolic pathways and the permeability of cell membranes to ions.

Pharmacological inhibitors of alpha stimulation (alpha-blockers) include the long-acting phenoxybenzamine (Dibenyline) and short-acting phentolamine (Rogitine). Beta-blockers include propranolol (Inderal) and practolol (Eraldin).

Tumours of the adrenal medulla

Tumours of the adrenal medulla are classified as follows:

- neoplasms of the sympathetic neurons:
  - ganglioneuroma,
  - neuroblastoma (sympatheticoblastoma);
- neoplasm of chromaffin cells: phaeochromocytoma.

Table 45.1 Effects of catecholamines mediated by alpha- and beta-adrenergic receptors

Effect on	*Alpha-receptor*	*Beta-receptor*
Cardiac output	Nil	Increase
Heart rate	Nil	Increase
Force of myocardial contraction	Nil	Increase
Myocardial excitability	Increase	Increase^{++}
Blood pressure – systolic	Increase	Nil
Blood pressure – diastolic	Increase	Decrease
Blood vessels – in skin	Constrict	Dilate
Blood vessels – in muscle	Constrict	Dilate
Smooth muscle – in bronchi	Nil	Relax
Smooth muscle – in intestine	Relax	Relax
Smooth muscle – in bladder	Relax	Relax
Smooth muscle – in sphincters	Constrict	Constrict

[1]*Synthesis of catecholamines: tyrosine → 3,4-dihydrophenylamine (DOPA) → 3,4-dihydroxyphenylethylamine (dopamine) → noradrenaline → adrenaline.*

Those occurring at any age

A **ganglioneuroma** is relatively benign. This neoplasm is symptomless, grows to a large size and constitutes one of the varieties of retroperitoneal 'sarcoma' (Chapter 56). Only 15 per cent involve the adrenal, the remainder occurring in any position along the sympathetic chain. If removed completely at a comparatively early stage, a cure may be expected.

Those occurring in infants and children

Neuroblastoma

Neuroblastoma is a malignant tumour of neural crest origin arising from sympathetic nervous tissue from the orbit to the pelvis. Three-quarters arise in the abdomen and half of these from the adrenal gland. It is the most common solid tumour of infancy and childhood, and by far the most common in the newborn. The incidence is approximately 1 per 10 000 live births. Ninety per cent of cases of neuroblastoma occur under the age of 8; over half occur in children under 2 years.

Clinical features. Three-quarters of patients present with an abdominal mass. Metastatic spread, via lymphatics and bloodstream, occurs at an early stage, and approximately 70 per cent of cases have metastases at the time of initial diagnosis (Fig. 45.12). Weight loss, failure to thrive, abdominal pain and distension, fever and anaemia may be present. Excessive catecholamine production may cause hypertension, flushing, sweating and general irritability. Some of these tumours produce VIP, which results in watery diarrhoea and hypokalaemia. Acute cerebellar ataxia characterised by opsomyoclonus and chaotic nystagmus or the 'dancing eye' syndrome is an unusual manifestation of neuroblastoma of unknown cause.

Diagnosis. Over 80 per cent of patients excrete catecholamine metabolites in the urine. The most common by-products assayed in the urine are vanillylmandelic acid (VMA) and homovanillic acid (HVA), and such measurements may be useful in monitoring the course of the disease.

Plain radiography shows fine, stippled calcification in 50 per cent of cases. Abdominal ultrasound examination shows the anatomical margins and extent of the disease, and is particularly helpful in evaluating the results of treatment.

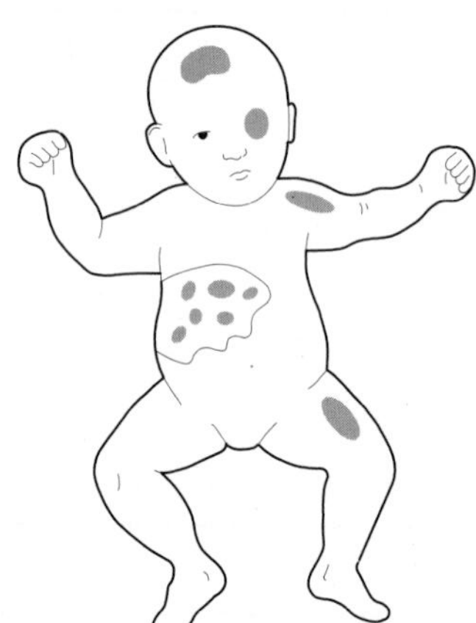

Fig. 45.12 The common sites for metastases from neuroblastoma of the adrenal. Bones are involved more frequently than the liver.

CT demonstrates calcium in 80 per cent of cases and accurately evaluates intraspinal extension as well as hepatic and renal metastatic disease. MRI is a promising technique which may supersede CT in many patients. It will also evaluate bone marrow metastases.

Meta-iodobenzyl-guanidine (MIBG, see below) is metabolised by neuroblastoma cells and may be used for imaging, especially in small residual tumours not evident on other conventional imaging studies.

Bone-seeking isotope (technetium-99m), as well as demonstrating bone involvement, is also concentrated by 60 per cent of adrenal lesions.

Treatment. Although surgical excision is the mainstay of cure in localised disease, widespread disease at presentation often makes surgery inappropriate as the primary form of treatment. Multidrug chemotherapy and radiotherapy are instituted in advanced disease. Surgical excision is appropriate in disease confined to one side of the midline, or as a delayed treatment following control by chemotherapy and radiotherapy. However, the cure rate remains low with an overall survival rate of 30–35 per cent. Age has an important favourable influence on prognosis – the younger the patient the better the prognosis, and children in the first year of life have a long-term survival rate of 70 per cent.

Phaeochromocytoma

Phaeochromocytoma has been called the '10 per cent tumour' because approximately 10 per cent are bilateral, malignant, extra-adrenal, multiple, familial and occur in children. Although 90 per cent of phaeochromocytomas arise in the adrenal medulla, they may be found anywhere along the paraganglionic system. The most common extra-adrenal site is the organ of Zuckerkandl at the aortic bifurcation and less common sites are the urinary bladder, renal hilum, chest and neck. Extra-adrenal tumours have a higher incidence of malignancy of 25–40 per cent. A phaeochromocytoma is a soft, vascular tumour usually less than 5 cm in diameter but occasionally very much larger. It is usually pink-tan in colour and is composed of large, differentiated, sympathetic ganglion cells and a few fibres, enclosed in a delicate capsule. It owes its name to the presence of chromaffin granules. This tumour occurs in both sexes, usually during early adult life or middle age. It produces, either intermittently or continuously, an excess of adrenaline, and especially of noradrenaline: the ratio of the latter to the former often being as high as 20:1 causing *hypertension* which is either *paroxysmal* or *persistent*. The latter predominates statistically and probably indicates a late stage of the disease. Consequently all patients under 60 years of age who suffer from sustained arterial hypertension deserve routine tests to confirm or exclude a phaeochromocytoma. Although not more than 0.5

Emil Zuckerkandl, 1849–1910. Anatomist, Vienna, Austria.

per cent of cases of hypertension are caused by a phaeochromocytoma, at the Mayo Clinic[2], where routine diagnostic procedures are undertaken to confirm or exclude the presence of this tumour in all cases of hypertension, the percentage has been stated to be nearly 3 per cent. Untreated, it progresses to a fatal termination from cardiac dysrhythmia or cerebral haemorrhage.

The importance of phaeochromocytoma as a component of the multiple endocrine neoplasia syndromes MEN IIa and MEN IIb should be remembered (see earlier and Chapter 44).

Clinical features. A typical complaint is that of fear – 'I thought I was going to die'. The most common symptoms, in order of frequency, are: headache (55 per cent), palpitation, vomiting, sweating, dyspnoea, weakness and pallor – i.e. the symptoms of adrenal overdosage. The paroxysmal attack may vary from a few minutes to some hours. The blood pressure may be very high and hyperglycaemia present. The symptoms may be mistaken for hyperthyroidism, hypocalcaemia, an acute anxiety state, paroxysmal atrial tachycardia and carcinoid syndrome. The main obstacle to the diagnosis of a phaeochromocytoma is the failure to think of it as a cause of the observed symptoms.

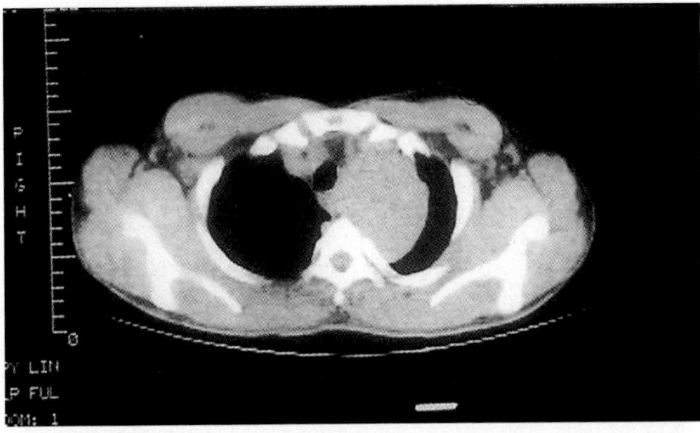

Fig. 45.13 Computerised tomography scan of upper thorax showing a solid medisatinal mass compressing the left lung and displacing the trachea to the right. A case of ectopic phaeochromocytoma (*courtesy of Professor Anthony W. Goode*).

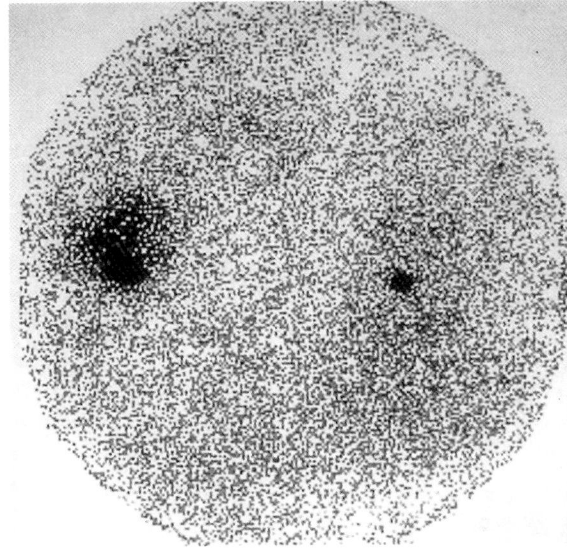

Fig. 45.14 Same case as Fig. 45.13 A metaliodobenzyl-guanidine (MIBG) scan confirming the presence of an ectopic phaeochromocytoma of the adrenal (*courtesy of Professor Anthony W. Goode*).

Diagnostic tests

The basis of the laboratory diagnosis is measurement of elevated catecholamines and their metabolites in urine and blood.

- **Urine studies.** Confirmation of the diagnosis is usually readily made by measurement of free catecholamines, VMA and metadrenalines (metanephrines) in 24-hour collections of urine. Patients with phaeochromocytoma usually excrete free catecholamines in excess of 100 μg/24 hours, VMA in excess of 7 mg/24 hours and metadrenalines in excess of 1.3 mg/24 hours. Laboratories vary in the reliance they place on these various estimations; at the Mayo Clinic, for example, most reliance is placed on urinary metadrenalines. False-positive elevations of metadrenaline excretion may occur in patients taking monoamine oxidase-inhibiting drugs, and in those who have recently had angiographic contrast studies.
- **Plasma catecholamines.** Sensitive assays are now available for plasma catecholamines and patients with phaeochromocytoma usually have total plasma catecholamines in excess of 1000 μg/ml. Such assays may be highly accurate in confirming the diagnosis, but plasma catecholamines may not be continuously elevated and many factors, including exercise, severe illness and the drug methyldopa, may influence the levels.

Localisation tests

- **Computerised tomography** (Fig. 45.13) is the method of choice for localisation with an accuracy of 90–95 per cent and has largely replaced more invasive and hazardous techniques such as arteriography and selective venous sampling. Because of their size, most adrenal phaeochromocytomas are also visible on ultrasound scanning.
- **Radionuclide imaging.** The development of a specific radionuclide for catecholamine precursors, iodine-labelled MIBG, has been a significant recent advance in the localisation of adrenal and ectopic phaeochromocytomas. Only abnormal areas of adrenergic tissue show uptake of MIBG and normal adrenals do not visualise. MIBG scanning may be particularly valuable in locating an ectopic phaeochromocytoma when CT shows normal adrenals (Fig. 45.14).

Preoperative preparation

Catecholamine-secreting tumours are a challenge to both the surgeon and anaesthetist. A patient with phaeochromocytoma is hypovolaemic because of the contraction of the vascular bed by excess circulating catecholamines. During surgery handling of the tumour may increase circulating catecholamine levels up to 600-fold causing large swings in blood pressure and cardiac arrhythmias. Severe hypotension may follow removal of the tumour. These dangers may be minimised by careful preoperative preparation. Effective blockade of the effects of high circulating catecholamines has significantly reduced the operative mortality and is mandatory. The alpha-adrenergic blocking drug

[2] *The Mayo Clinic, Rochester, Minnesota, USA, was founded in 1889 by William Worrall Mayo (1819–1911) and his two sons, William James Mayo (1861–1939) and Charles Horace Mayo (1865–1939).*

phenoxybenzamine in an initial dose of 20–40 mg/day is increased until hypertension is controlled and mild orthostatic hypotension induced. Such preparation takes 1–3 weeks. In most centres a beta-blocking drug such as propranolol is added for 3–7 days before operation to control tachycardia and arrythmias. Extra fluids should be given i.v. to occupy the sudden expansion of the vascular bed when the tumour is removed, and a preoperative fluid 'overload' is advisable.

Operation

During surgery, intravenous infusions of alpha- and beta-blocking drugs are given, if required, as determined by the blood pressure, pulse rate and central venous pressure. The hazardous phases in the operation are during the induction of anaesthesia, positioning of the patient on the operating table, when the tumour is manipulated, and immediately after removal of the tumour. Sodium nitroprusside, a direct peripheral vasodilator, is the drug of choice for the management of significant intraoperative hypertension.

Even though preoperative localisation is highly accurate, the possible multiplicity of tumours (intra- and extra-adrenal) and the need to avoid excessive tumour manipulation necessitate a generous transabdominal approach. The tumour should be manipulated as little as possible and the main adrenal vein ligated as a first step. Inadvertent rupture of the tumour should be avoided as this may result in local spread and recurrence of even apparently benign tumours.

Further reading

Brook, C.G.P. and Marshall, N.J. (eds) (1996) *Essential Endocrinology*, Blackwell Science, Oxford.

Clark, O.H. Siperstein, A.E. and Duh, Q.-Y. (eds) (1997) *Textbook of Endocrine Surgery*, W.B. Saunders, Philadelphia, PA.

Greenspan, F.S. and Strewler, G.J. (1997) *Basic and Clinical Endocrinology*, McGraw-Hill, New York.

Thanner, R.V. (ed.) (1997) *Molecular Genetics of Endocrine Disorders*, Chapman & Hall, London.

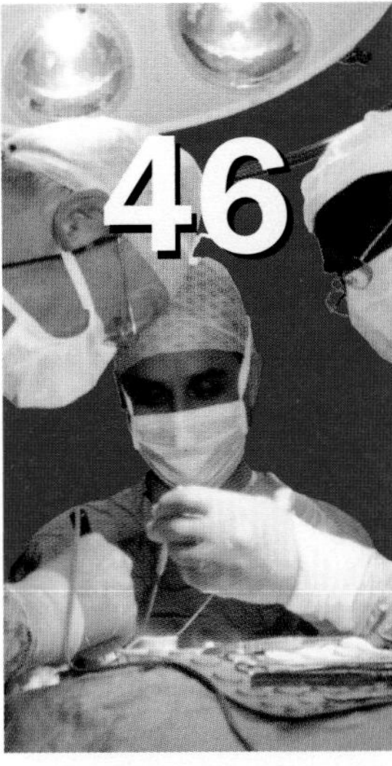

46 The breast

Subjects covered in this chapter include anatomy, investigations of the breast, the nipple, benign and malignant disorders of the breast, breast reconstruction, screening for breast cancer, breast cancer genetics and the male breast.

Comparative and surgical anatomy

The protuberant part of the human breast is generally described as overlying the 2nd to the 6th ribs, and extending from the lateral border of the sternum to the anterior axillary line. Actually, a thin layer of mammary tissue extends considerably farther from the clavicle above to the 7th or 8th ribs below, and from the midline to the edge of latissimus dorsi posteriorly. This fact is important when performing a mastectomy, the aim of which is to remove the whole breast. The anatomy of the breast is illustrated in Fig. 46.1

The axillary tail of the breast is of considerable surgical importance. In some normal cases it is palpable, and in a few it can be seen premenstrually or during lactation. A well-developed axillary tail is sometimes mistaken for a mass of enlarged lymph nodes or a lipoma.

The lobule is the basic structural unit of the mammary gland. The number and size of the lobules vary enormously: they are most numerous in young women. From 10 to over 100 lobules empty via ductules into a lactiferous duct of which there are from 15 to 20. Each lactiferous duct is lined by a spiral arrangement of contractile myoepithelial cells and is provided with a terminal ampulla – a reservoir for milk or abnormal discharges.

The ligaments of Cooper are hollow conical projections of fibrous tissue filled with breast tissue, the apices of the cones being attached firmly to the superficial fascia and thereby to the skin overlying the breast. These ligaments account for the dimpling of the skin overlying a carcinoma.

The areola contains involuntary muscle arranged in concentric rings as well as radially in the subcutaneous tissue. The areolar epithelium contains numerous sweat glands and sebaceous glands, the latter of which enlarge during pregnancy and serve to lubricate the nipple during lactation (Montgomery's tubercles).

The nipple is covered by thick skin with corrugations. Near its apex lie the orifices of the lactiferous ducts. The nipple contains smooth muscle fibres arranged concentrically and longitudinally; thus is an erectile structure which points outwards.

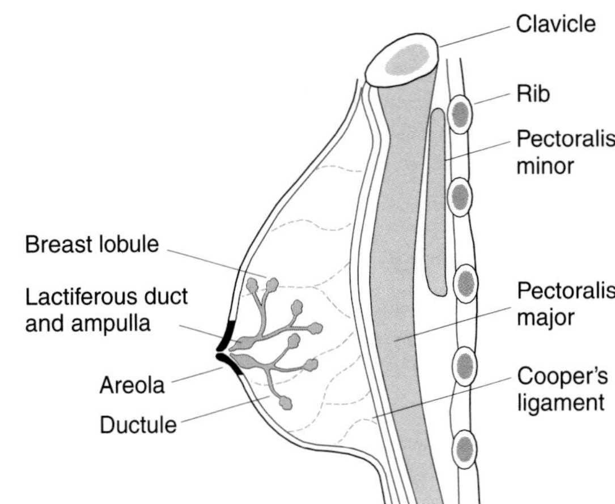

Fig. 46.1 Cross-sectional anatomy of the breast.

Bailey & Love's Short Practice of Surgery, 23rd edition. Edited by R.C.G. Russell, N.S. Williams and C.J.K. Bulstrode. Published in 2000 by Arnold Publishers.

Lymphatics of the breast drain predominantly into the axillary and internal mammary lymph nodes. The axillary nodes receive approximately 75 per cent of the drainage and are arranged in the following groups:

- **lateral**, along the axillary vein;
- **anterior**, along the lateral thoracic vessels;
- **posterior**, along the subscapular vessels;
- **central** embedded in fat in the centre of the axilla;
- **interpectoral**, a few nodes lying between the pectoralis major and minor muscles;
- **apical**, which lie above the level of the pectoralis minor tendon in continuity with the lateral nodes and receive the efferents of all the other groups.

The apical nodes are also in continuity with the supraclavicular nodes and drain into the subclavian lymph trunk which enters the great veins directly or via the thoracic duct or jugular trunk. The sentinal node is that lymph node designated as the first axillary node draining the breast.

The internal mammary nodes are fewer in number and lie along the internal mammary vessels deep to the plane of the costal cartilages.

Investigation of the breast

Although an accurate history and clinical examination are still the most important methods of detecting breast disease there are a number of investigations which can assist in the diagnosis as follows.

Mammography (Fig. 46.2)

Soft tissue X-rays are taken by placing the breast in direct contact with ultrasensitive film and exposing it to low-voltage, high-amperage X-rays. The dose of radiation is approximately 0.1 Gy and therefore mammography is a very safe investigation.

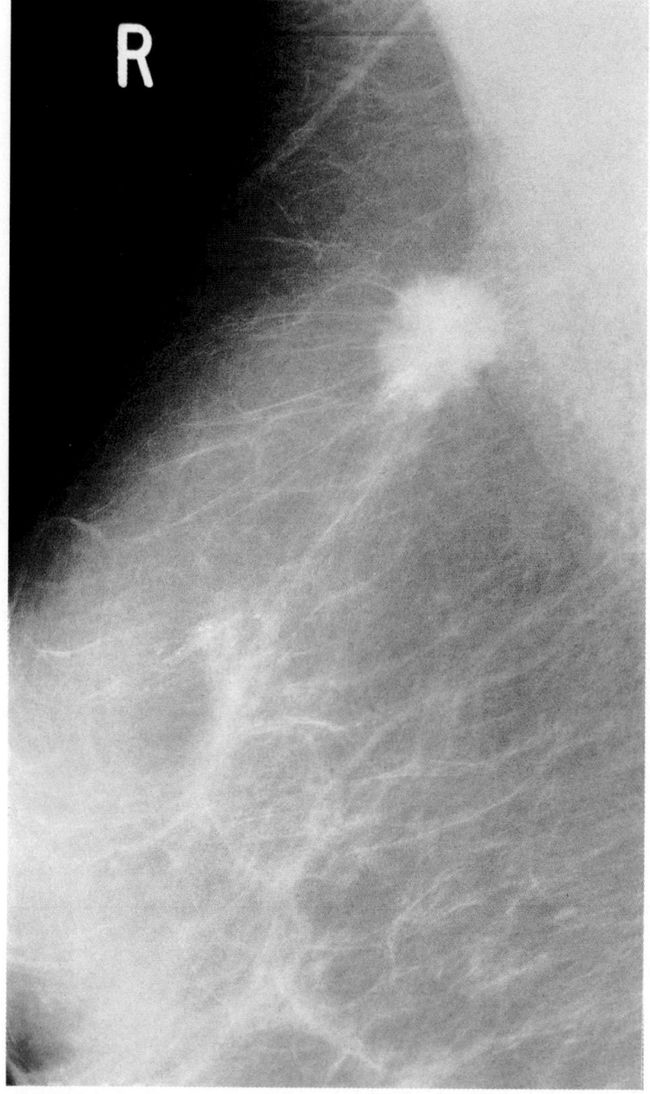

Fig. 46.2 Mammogram showing a carcinoma.

Ultrasound

Ultrasound is particularly useful in young women with dense breasts in whom mammograms are difficult to interpret, and in distinguishing cysts from solid lesions (Figs 46.3 and 46.4). It can also be used to localise impalpable breast lumps.

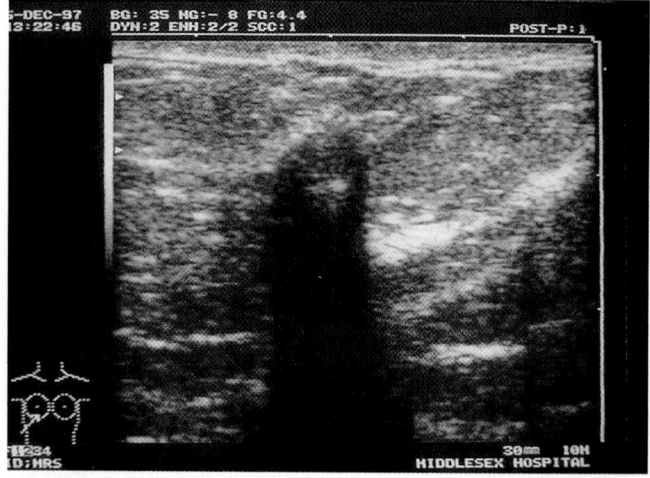

Fig. 46.3 Ultrasound of breast showing carcinoma.

Magnetic resonance imaging

Magnetic resonance imaging (MRI) is of increasing interest to breast surgeons in a number of settings: it can be useful to distinguish scar from recurrence in women who have had previous breast conservation therapy for cancer (although it is not accurate within 9 months of radiotherapy because of abnormal enhancement); it is the gold standard for imaging the breasts of women with implants; it may prove useful as a screening tool in high-risk women; and it is being evaluated in the management of the axilla in both primary breast cancer and recurrent disease (Fig. 46.5).

Needle biopsy/cytology

Histology can be obtained using a fine needle such as a Trucut or Corecut biopsy device under local anaesthesia (Fig. 46.6). Cytology is obtained using a 21 or 23 Gauge needle and 10-ml syringe with multiple passes

---

William Fetherston-Haugh Montgomery, 1797–1859. Dublin obstetrician. The glands to which he gave his name are also known as 'Montgomery's tubercles'.

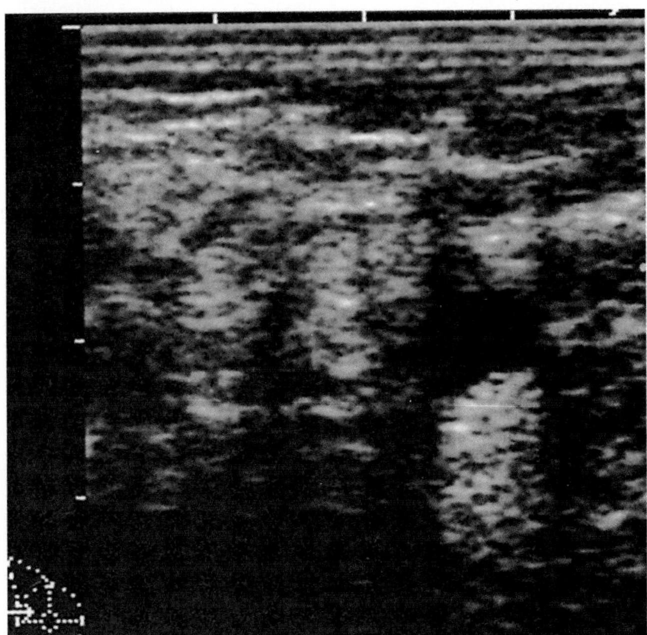

Fig. 46.4 Ultrasound of breast showing cyst.

throughout the lump without releasing the negative pressure in the syringe. The aspirate is then smeared on to a slide which is air dried (Fig. 46.7). Fine needle aspiration cytology (FNAC) is the least invasive technique of obtaining a cell diagnosis and is very accurate if both operator and cytologist are experienced. However, false negatives do occur, mainly through sampling error, and invasive cancer cannot be distinguished from *in situ* disease.

Triple assessment

In any patient who presents with a breast lump or other symptoms suspicious of carcinoma, the diagnosis should be made by a combination of clinical assessment, radiological imaging and a tissue sample taken for either cytological or histological analysis (Fig. 46.8): the so-called triple assessment.

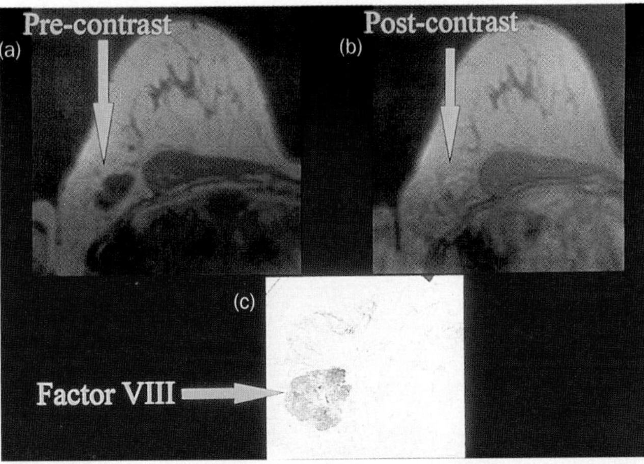

Fig. 46.5 (a) Precontrast and (b) postcontrast breast MRI showing a breast cancer in the right upper outer quadrant. (c) When tumour sections were stained with an endothelial marker (monoclonal antibody to factor VIII), high vascularity was evident within the tumour suggesting that tumour-induced angiogenesis is responsible for the enhancement seen with intravenous dimeglumine gadopentetate contrast (Magnavist, Schering).

The nipple

Absence of the nipple is rare, and usually associated with amazia (congenital absence of the breast).

Supernumerary nipples not uncommonly occur along a line extending from the anterior fold of the axilla to the fold of the groin (Fig. 46.9). This constitutes the milk line of lower mammals.

Nipple retraction

This may occur at puberty or later in life. Retraction occurring at puberty, also known as **simple nipple inversion**, is of

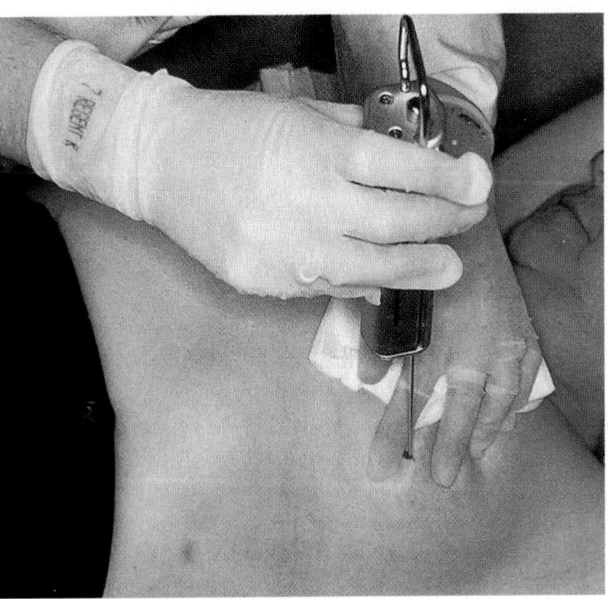

Fig. 46.6 Corecut biopsy of breast.

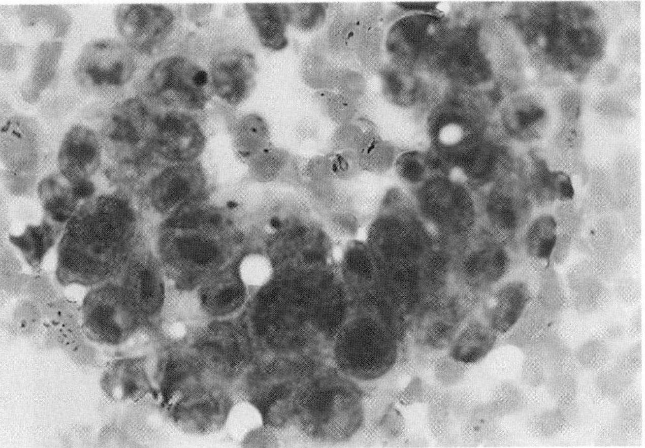

Fig. 46.7 Fine needle aspiration cytology showing grade III ductal carcinoma cells.

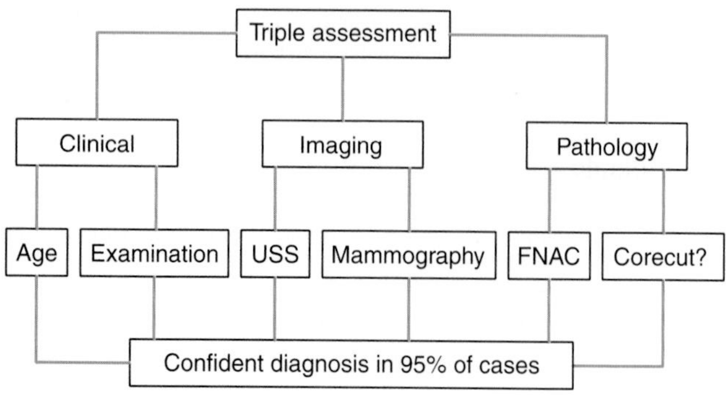

Fig. 46.8 Triple assessment of breast symptoms.

unknown aetiology. In about 25 per cent of cases it is bilateral. It may cause problems with breastfeeding and infection can occur, especially during lactation, owing to retention of secretions.

Treatment

Treatment is usually unnecessary, and it may spontaneously resolve during pregnancy or lactation.

Simple cosmetic surgery can produce an adequate correction but has the drawback of dividing the ducts. Mechanical suction devices have been used to attempt to evert the nipple with some effect.

Recent retraction of the nipple may be of considerable pathological significance. A slit-like retraction of the nipple may be due to duct ectasia and chronic periductal mastitis (Fig. 46.10a), but circumferential retraction, with or without an underlying lump, may well indicate an underlying carcinoma (Fig. 46.10b).

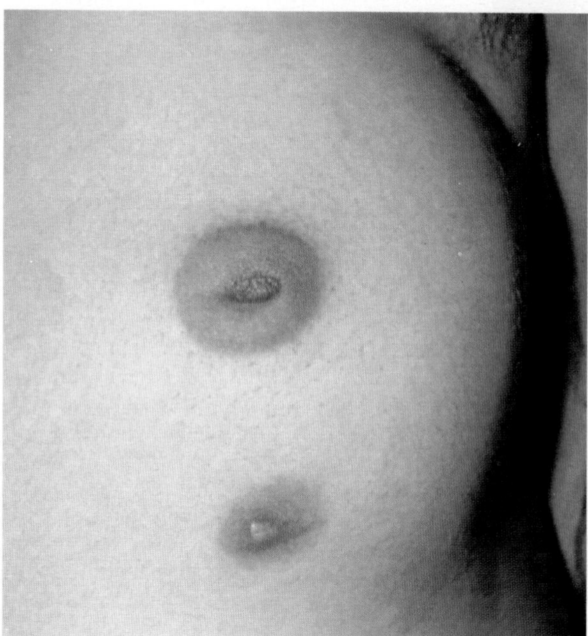

Fig. 46.9 Accessory nipple with congenital retraction of normal nipple (*courtesy of Dr Jitendra Goyal, Agra, India*).

Cracked nipple

This may occur during lactation and be the forerunner of acute infective mastitis. If the nipple becomes cracked during lactation, it should be rested for 24–48 hours and the breast emptied with a breast pump. Feeding should be resumed as soon as possible.

Papilloma of the nipple

Papilloma of the nipple has the same features of any cutaneous papilloma (Fig. 46.11) and should be excised with a tiny disc of skin.

Retention cyst of a gland of Montgomery

These glands, situated in the areola, secrete sebum, and if they become blocked a sebaceous cyst forms.

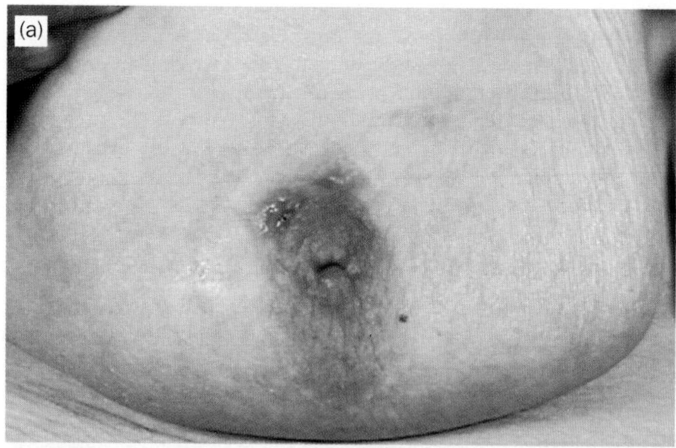

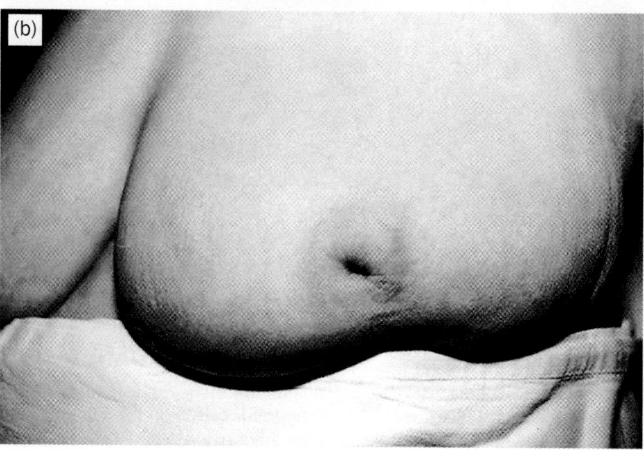

Fig. 46.10 Recent nipple retraction. (a) Slit-like retraction of duct ectasia with mammary duct fistula; (b) circumferential retraction with underlying carcinoma.

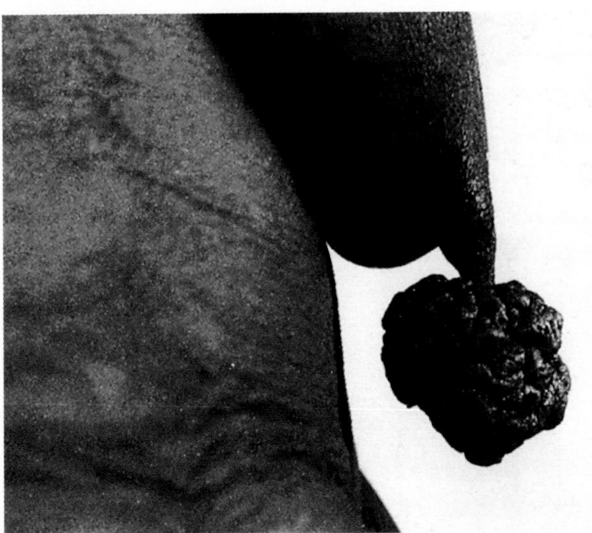

Fig. 46.11 Papilloma of the nipple (*courtesy of R.R. Deshmukh, M.S. Dhantoli, Nagpur, India*).

Chancre of the nipple

This very rare condition usually occurs by infection from a syphilitic buccal ulcer in the mouth of the partner, although can be seen in the wet-nurse of a syphilitic baby. The mother of such an infant is immune to reinfection from her own child.

Eczema

Eczema of the nipples is a rare condition and is bilateral, and usually associated with eczema elsewhere on the body.

Paget's disease

Paget's disease of the nipple must be distinguished from the eczema.

Abnormal discharges from the nipple

Discharge can occur from one or more lactiferous ducts. Management depends on the presence of a lump (which should always be given priority in diagnosis and treatment) and of the presence of blood in the discharge or discharge from a single duct. Mammography is rarely useful except to exclude an underlying impalpable mass. Cytology may reveal malignant cells but a negative result does not exclude a carcinoma.

A clear, serous discharge may be 'physiological' in a parous woman or may be associated with a duct papilloma or mammary dysplasia.

A blood-stained discharge may be caused by duct ectasia or less commonly a duct papilloma or carcinoma. A duct papilloma is usually single and situated in one of the larger lactiferous ducts and is sometimes associated with a cystic swelling beneath the areola.

A black or green discharge is usually due to duct ectasia and its complications.

Treatment

Treatment must firstly be to exclude a carcinoma by occult blood test and cytology. Simple reassurance may then be sufficient, but if the discharge is proving intolerable an operation to remove the affected duct or ducts can be performed. Figure 46.12 illustrates some causes of nipple discharge.

Microdochectomy. It is important not to express the blood before the operation as it may then be difficult to identify the duct in theatre. A lacrimal probe or length of stiff nylon suture is inserted into the duct from which the discharge is emerging. A tennis raquet incision can be made to encompass the entire duct, or a periareolar incision used and the nipple flap dissected to reach the duct. The duct is then excised. A papilloma is nearly always situated within 4–5 cm of the nipple orifice.

Cone excision of the major ducts (after Hadfield). When the duct of origin of nipple bleeding is uncertain or when there is bleeding or discharge from multiple ducts, the entire major duct system can be excised for histological examination without sacrifice of the breast form. A periareolar incision is made and a cone of tissue is removed with its apex just deep to the surface of the nipple and its base on the pectoral fascia. The resulting defect is obliterated by a series of purse-string sutures. It is important to warn the patient that she will be uanable to breast feed after this and may lose nipple sensation.

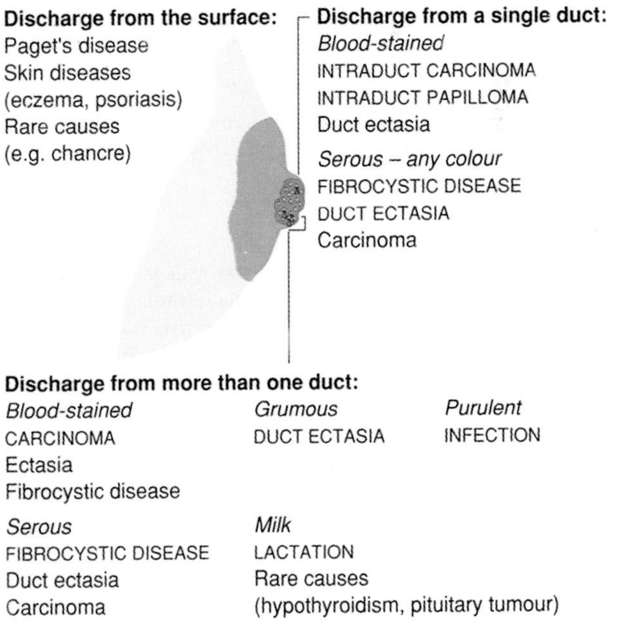

Discharge from the surface:
Paget's disease
Skin diseases
(eczema, psoriasis)
Rare causes
(e.g. chancre)

Discharge from a single duct:
Blood-stained
INTRADUCT CARCINOMA
INTRADUCT PAPILLOMA
Duct ectasia
Serous – any colour
FIBROCYSTIC DISEASE
DUCT ECTASIA
Carcinoma

Discharge from more than one duct:
Blood-stained
CARCINOMA
Ectasia
Fibrocystic disease
Grumous
DUCT ECTASIA
Purulent
INFECTION
Serous
FIBROCYSTIC DISEASE
Duct ectasia
Carcinoma
Milk
LACTATION
Rare causes
(hypothyroidism, pituitary tumour)

Fig. 46.12 Discharges from the nipple. The principal causes of the various discharges are in capitals.

Sir James Paget, 1814–99. Surgeon, St Bartholomew's Hospital, London, England.

Geoffrey John Hadfield. Former Surgeon, Stoke Mandeville Hospital, Aylesbury, England.

Benign breast disease

This is the most common cause of breast problems – up to 30 per cent of women will suffer from a benign breast disorder requiring treatment at some time in their lives. The most common symptoms are pain, lumpiness or a lump. The aim of treatment is to exclude cancer and, once this has been done, to treat any remaining symptoms.

Benign breast disorders can be classified in the following way:

- ANDI[1] (lumpy breasts, tenderness or a smooth lump):
  cyclical nodularity and mastalgia,
  cysts,
  fibroadenoma;
- duct ectasia/periductal mastitis;
- pregnancy related:
  galactocoele,
  peurperal abscess;
- congenital disorders:
  inverted nipple,
  supernumary breasts/nipples;
- nonbreast disorders:
  Tietze's disease;
  sebaceous cysts and other skin conditions.

Congenital abnormalities

Amazia

Congenital absence of the breast may occur on one (Fig. 46.13) or both sides. It is sometimes associated with absence of the sternal portion of the pectoralis major (Poland's syndrome). It is more common in males.

Polymazia

Accessory breasts (Fig. 46.14) have been recorded in the axilla (the most frequent site), groin, buttock and thigh. They have been known to function during lactation.

Mastitis of infants

Mastitis of infants is at least as common in the male as in the female. On the 3rd or 4th day of life, if the breast of an infant is pressed lightly, a drop of colourless fluid can be expressed; a few days later there is often a slight milky secretion, which disappears during the 3rd week. This is popularly known as 'witch's milk'. It is due to stimulation of the foetal breast by maternal prolactin, thus is essentially physiological.

Diffuse hypertrophy

Diffuse hypertrophy of the breasts occurs sporadically in otherwise healthy girls at puberty and, much less often, during the first pregnancy.

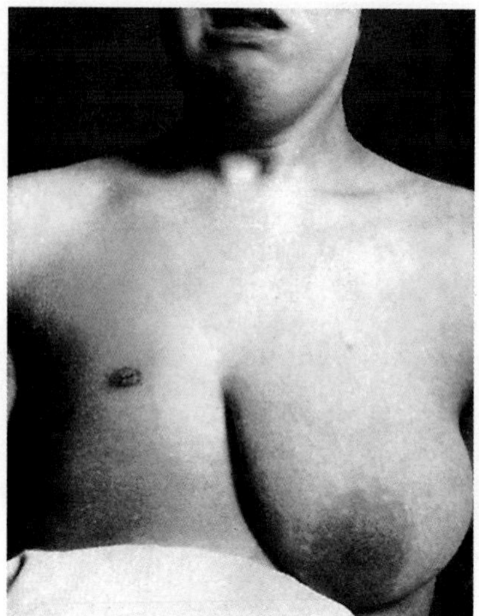

Fig. 46.13 Congenital absence of the right breast.

The breasts attain enormous dimensions (Fig. 46.15) and may reach the knees when the patient is sitting. The condition is rarely unilateral. This tremendous overgrowth is apparently due to an alteration in the normal sensitivity of the breast to oestrogenic hormones, and some success in treating it with antioestrogens has been reported. Treatment is otherwise by reduction mammoplasty.

Injuries of the breast

Haematoma

Haematoma, particularly a resolving haematoma, gives rise to a lump which, in the absence of overlying bruising, is difficult to diagnose correctly unless it is aspirated or incised.

Traumatic fat necrosis

Traumatic fat necrosis may be acute or chronic, and usually occurs in stout, middle-aged women. Following a blow, or

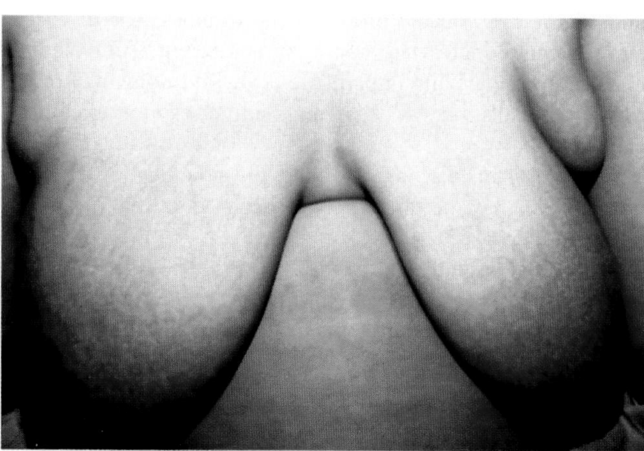

Fig. 46.14 Bilateral accessory breasts (courtesy of *Dr S.S. Rawat, Riyadh, Saudi Arabia*).

[1]*ANDI – aberrations of normal development and involution. A term approved by the senior author to encompass this difficult group of pathophysiological conditions.*

Alexander Tietze, 1864–1927. German surgeon.

Alfred Poland, b. 1920. London surgeon.

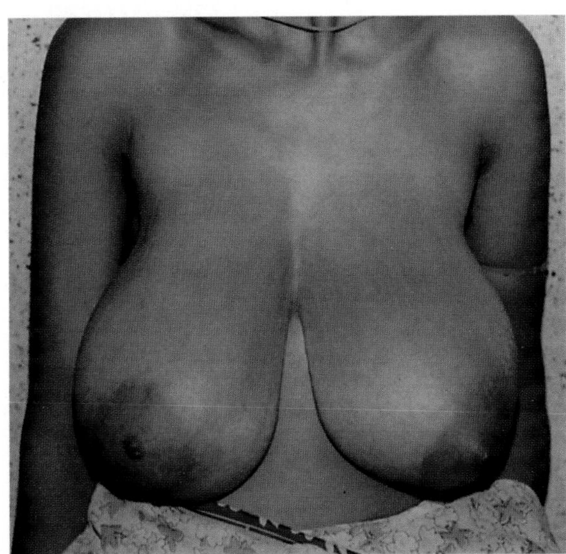

Fig. 46.15 Diffuse hypertrophy (*courtesy of Dr M. Vasuderan, Tamil Nadu, India*).

even indirect violence (e.g. contraction of the pectoralis major), a lump, often painless, appears. This may mimic a carcinoma, even displaying skin tethering and nipple retraction, and biopsy is required for diagnosis. A history of trauma is not diagnostic as this may merely have drawn the patient's attention to a pre-existing lump.

Acute and subacute inflammations of the breast

Bacterial mastitis

Bacterial mastitis is the commonest variety of mastitis and nearly always commences acutely. Although associated with lactation in the majority of cases, it is not necessarily so. Of 100 consecutive cases of breast abscess, 32 occurred in women who were not lactating (De Jode). Some of these will be associated with an infected haematoma or with periductal mastitis and this will be discussed later.

Aetiology. Lactational mastitis is seen far less frequently than in former years. Most cases are caused by *Staphylococcus aureus* and, if hospital-acquired, are likely to be penicillin resistant. The intermediary is usually the infant; after the second day of life 50 per cent of infants harbour staphylococci in the nasopharynx.

'Cleansing the baby's mouth' with a swab is also an aetiological factor. The delicate buccal mucosa is excoriated by the process; it becomes infected, and organisms in the infant's saliva are inoculated on to the mother's nipple.

Whilst ascending infection from a sore and cracked nipple may initiate the mastitis, in many cases the lactiferous ducts will first become blocked by epithelial debris leading to stasis – this theory is supported by the relatively high incidence of mastitis in women with a retracted nipple. Once within the ampulla of the duct, staphylococci cause clotting of milk and within this clot organisms multiply.

Clinical features. The affected breast, or more usually a segment of it, presents the classical signs of acute inflammation. Early on this is a generalised cellulitis, but later an abscess will form.

Treatment. During the cellulitic stage the patient should be treated with an appropriate antibiotic, e.g. flucloxacillin, and the breast rested, with feeding on the opposite side only. The infected breast should be emptied of milk using a breast pump. Support of the breast, local heat and analgesia will help to relieve pain.

If an antibiotic is used in the presence of undrained pus, an 'antibioma' may form. This is a large, sterile brawny oedematous swelling which takes many weeks to resolve.

The breast should be incised and drained if the infection does not resolve within 48 hours, or if, after being emptied of milk, there is an area of tense induration or other evidence of an underlying abscess.

The presence of pus can be confirmed with a needle aspiration, and the pus analysed for the infection and for cytology. This has the advantage of allowing diagnosis on the smear of a rare inflammatory carcinoma (Fig. 46.16). In contrast to the majority of localised infections, fluctuation is a late sign and incision must not be delayed until it appears. Usually the area of induration is sector-shaped, and in early cases about one-quarter of the breast is involved (Fig. 46.17); in many late cases the area is more extensive (Fig. 46.18). When in doubt an ultrasound scan may clearly define an area 'ripe' for drainage.

Drainage of an intramammary abscess. The usual incision is sited in a radial direction over the affected segment, although if a circumareolar incision will allow adequate access to the affected area this should be preferred because of a better cosmetic result. The incision passes through the skin and the superficial fascia. A long haemostat is then inserted into

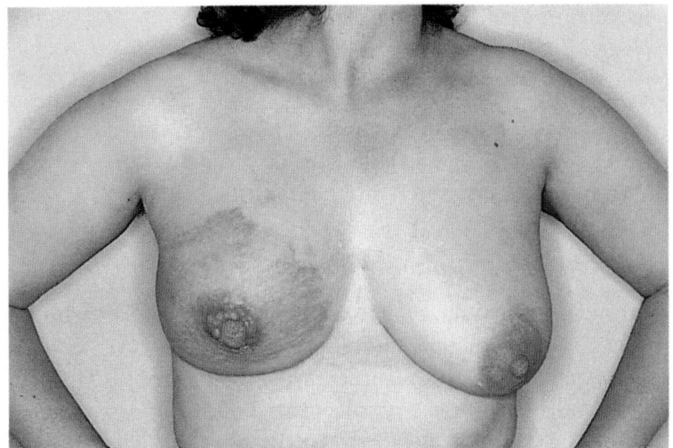

Fig. 46.16 Inflammatory carcinoma of the right breast.

Louis Rene Julien De Jode, 1926–82, Surgeon. Whipps Cross Hospital, Leytonstone, London, England. Established the best-known fellowship course.

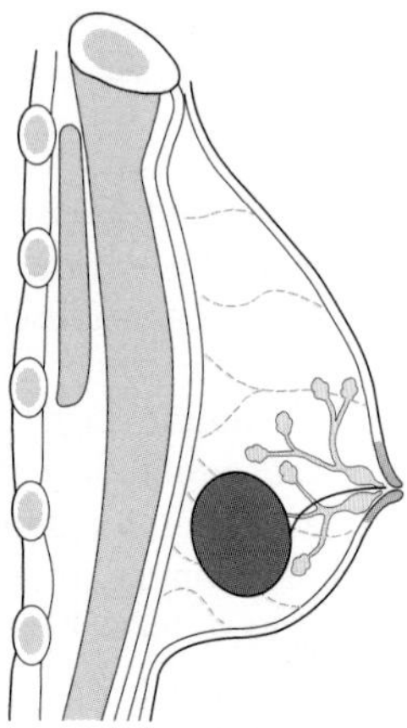

Fig. 46.17 Intramammary breast abscess.

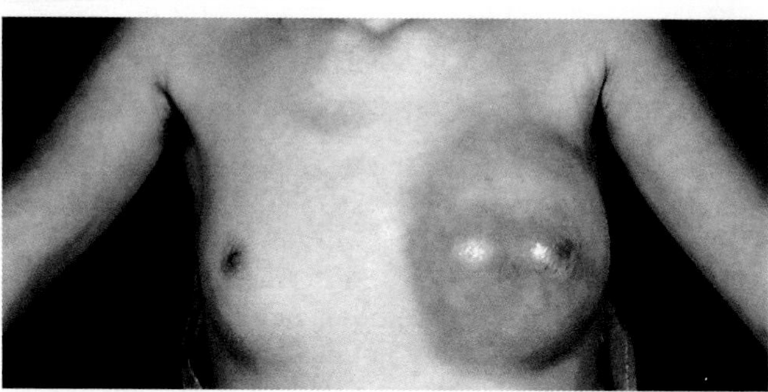

Fig. 46.18 Extensive intramammary breast abscess (*courtesy of T.A. Boucher-Hayes, Dublin*).

the abscess cavity. Every part of the abscess is palpated against the point of the haemostat and its jaws are opened. All loculi that can be felt are entered.

Finally, the haemostat having been withdrawn, a finger is introduced and any remaining septa are disrupted. The wound may then be lightly packed with ribbon gauze or a drain inserted to allow dependent drainage.

Mastitis from milk engorgement

Mastitis from milk engorgement is liable to occur around weaning time, and sometimes in the early days of lactation when one of the lactiferous ducts becomes blocked with epithelial debris. In the latter instance only a sector of the breast becomes indurated and tender.

Chronic intramammary abscess

Chronic intramammary abscess which follows inadequate drainage or injudicious antibiotic treatment is often a very difficult condition to diagnose: when encapsulated within a thick wall of fibrous tissue, the condition cannot be distinguished from a carcinoma without the histological evidence from a biopsy.

Tuberculosis of the breast

Tuberculosis of the breast, which is comparatively rare, is usually associated with active pulmonary tuberculosis or tuberculous cervical adenitis.

Tuberculosis of the breast (Fig. 46.19) occurs more often in parous women and usually presents with multiple chronic abscesses and sinuses and a typical bluish attenuated appearance of the surrounding skin. The diagnosis rests on bacteriological and histological examination. Treatment is with antituberculous chemotherapy. Healing is usual although often delayed, and mastectomy should be restricted to patients with persistent residual infection.

Actinomycosis

Actinomycosis of the breast is rarer still. The lesions present the essential characteristics of faciocervical actinomycosis.

Syphilis of the breast

A primary chancre of the nipple has been referred to (above). Secondary lesions of syphilis include diffuse syphilitic mastitis.

Mondor's disease

Mondor's disease is thrombophlebitis of the superficial veins of the breast and anterior chest wall (Fig. 46.20) although it has also been encountered in the arm.

In the absence of injury or infection, the cause of thrombophlebitis – like that of spontaneous thrombophlebitis in other sites – is obscure. The pathognomonic feature is a thrombosed subcutaneous cord, usually attached to skin. When the skin over the breast is stretched by raising the arm, a narrow, shallow subcutaneous groove alongside the cord becomes apparent. The differential diagnosis is lymphatic permeation from an occult carcinoma of the breast. The only treatment required is restricted arm movements, and in any case the condition subsides within a few months without recurrence, complications or deformity.

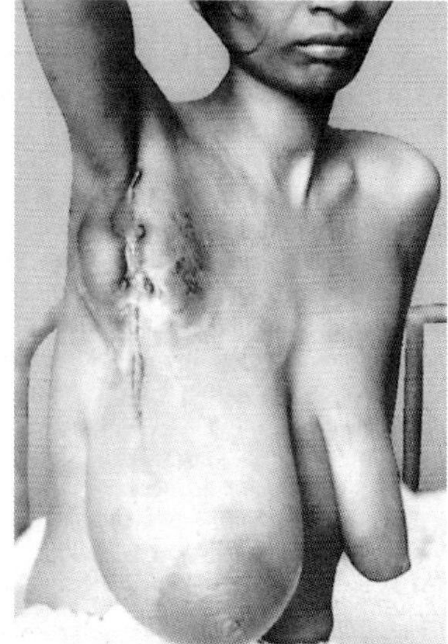

Fig. 46.19 Tuberculosis of the breast with secondary suppurating axillary lymph nodes (*courtesy of Professor A.K. Toufeeq, Lahore, Pakistan*).

Henri Mondor, 1885–1962. Surgeon, Paris, France.

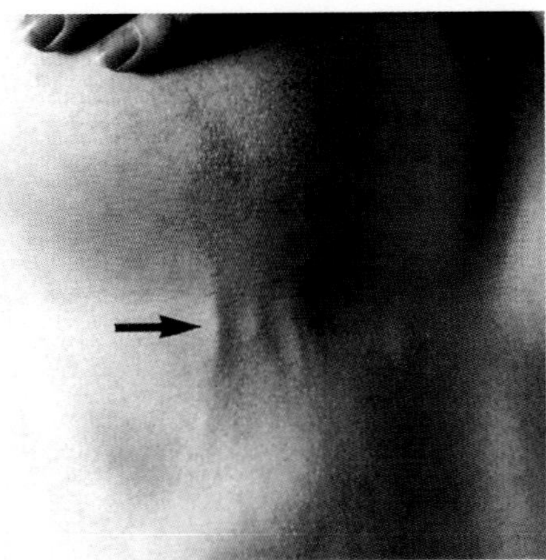

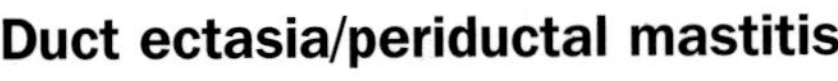

Fig. 46.20 Mondor's disease under the right breast.

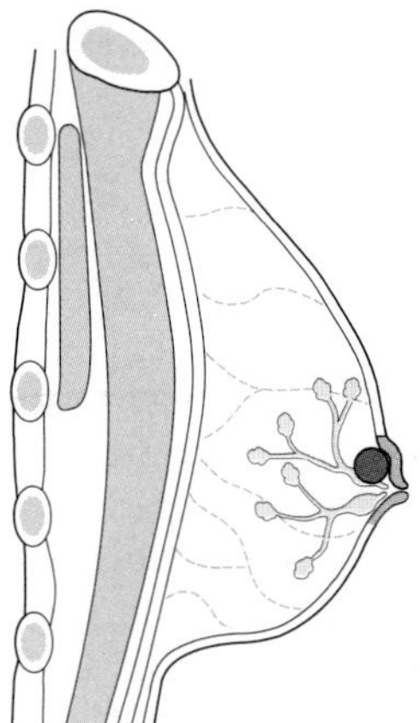

Fig. 46.21 Subareolar abscess in duct ectasia.

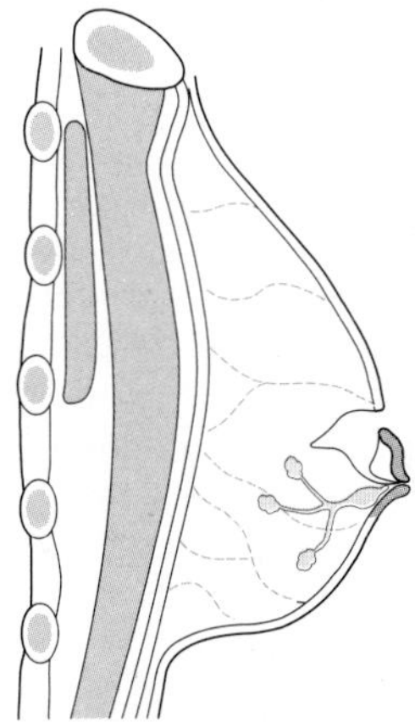

Fig. 46.22 Mammilliary fistula originating in a chronic subareolar abscess.

Duct ectasia/periductal mastitis

Pathology

This is a dilatation of the breast ducts associated with periductal inflammation, the pathogenesis of which is obscure and almost certainly not uniform in all cases, although the disease is much more common in smokers.

The classical description of the pathogenesis of duct ectasia asserts that the first stage in the disorder is a dilatation in one or more of the larger lactiferous ducts which fill with a stagnant brown or green secretion. This may discharge. These fluids then set up an irritant reaction in surrounding tissue leading to periductal mastitis or even abscess and fistula formation (Figs 46.21 and 46.22). In some cases a chronic indurated mass forms beneath the areola which mimics a carcinoma.

Fibrosis eventually develops which may cause slit-like nipple retraction.

An alternative theory suggests that periductal inflammation is the primary condition and anaerobic bacterial infection is found in some cases.

An association between recurrent periductal inflammation and smoking has been demonstrated which may suggest that arteriopathy is a contributing factor in its aetiology.

Clinical features

Nipple discharge (of any colour), a subareolar mass, abscess, mammary duct fistula and/or nipple retraction are the commonest symptoms (Fig. 46.23).

Treatment

In the case of a mass or nipple retraction, a carcinoma must be excluded by obtaining a mammogram and negative cytology or histology. If any suspicion remains the mass should be excised.

Antibiotic therapy may be tried, the most appropriate agents being flucloxacillin and metronidazole. However, surgery is often the only option likely to bring about cure of this notoriously difficult condition, and consists of excision of all of the major ducts (the Hadfield's operation).

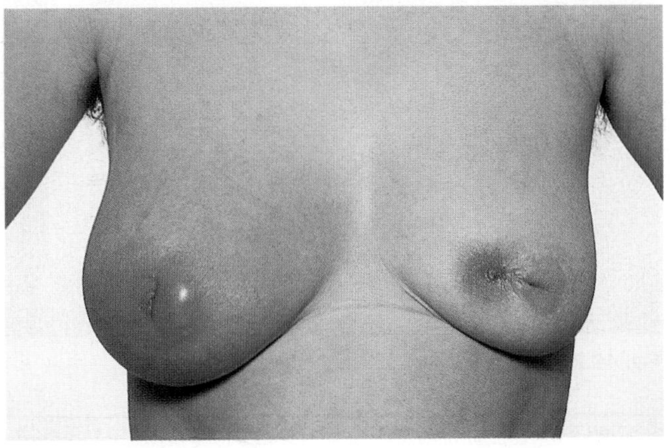

Fig. 46.23 Bilateral duct ectasia with fistula, abscess and nipple retraction.

Aberrations of normal development and involution (ANDI)

Nomenclature

The nomenclature of benign breast disease is very confusing. This is because over the last century a variety of clinicians and pathologists has chosen to describe a mixture of physiological changes and disease processes according to a variety of clinical, pathological and aetiological terminology. As well as leading to confusion, patients were often unduly alarmed or overtreated by ascribing a pathological name to a variant of physiological development. To sort out this confusion, a new system has been developed and described by the Cardiff Breast Clinic[2] – ANDI. (Many alternative terms have been applied to this condition including fibrocystic disease, fibroadenosis, chronic mastitis and mastopathy.)

Aetiology

The breast is a dynamic structure which undergoes changes throughout a woman's reproductive life, and superimposed upon this, cyclical changes throughout the menstrual cycle. This is illustrated in Fig. 46.24. The pathogenesis of ANDI involves disturbances in the breast physiology extending from an extreme of normality to well-defined disease processes. There is often little correlation between the histological appearance of the breast tissue and the symptoms.

Risk of malignancy developing in association with benign breast pathology

These relative risks according to different histological features found at biopsy are illustrated in Table 46.1.

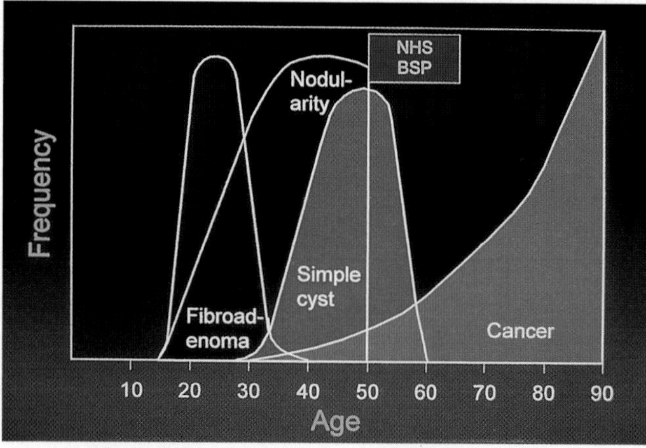

Fig. 46.24 Normal breast changes throughout life.

[2]*Cardiff – the capital of Wales. Surgical centre long been famous for the study of breast disease under the professorships of L.E. Hughes and R. Mansell.*

Table 46.1 Relative risk for invasive breast carcinoma based on pathological examination of benign breast tissue (American College of Pathologists Consensus Statement)

No increased risk	
Adenosis, sclerosing or florid	Hyperplasia
Apocrine metaplasia	Mastitis (inflammation)
Cysts macro and/or micro	Periductal mastitis
Duct ectasia	Squamous metaplasia
Fibroadenoma	
Fibrosis	
Slightly increased risk (1.5–2 times)	
Hyperplasia, moderate or florid, solid or papillary	
Papilloma with a fibrovascular core	
Moderately increased risk (5 times)	
Atypical hyperplasia (ductal or lobular)	
Insufficient data to assign a risk	
Solitary papilloma of lactiferous sinus	
Radial scar lesion	

After Page and DuPont (1978) by kind permission of *Journal of the National Cancer Institute, USA.*

Pathology

The disease consists essentially of four features which may vary in extent and degree in any one breast.

1. *Cyst formation*. Cysts are almost inevitable and very variable in size.
2. *Fibrosis*. Fat and elastic tissue disappears and is replaced by dense white fibrous trabeculae. The interstitial tissue is infiltrated with chronic inflammatory cells.
3. *Hyperplasia* of epithelium in the lining of the ducts and acini may occur with or without atypia.
4. *Papillomatosis*. The epithelial hyperplasia may be so extensive that it results in papillomatous overgrowth within the ducts.

Clinical features

The symptoms of ANDI include an area of lumpiness (seldom discrete) and/or breast pain (mastalgia).

A benign discrete lump in the breast is commonly a cyst or fibroadenoma. True lipomas occur rarely.

Lumpiness may be bilateral, commonly in the upper outer quadrant, or less commonly confined to one quadrant of one breast. The changes may be cyclical, with an increase in both lumpiness and often tenderness before a menstrual period.

Noncyclical mastalgia is commoner in perimenopausal and postmenopausal women. It may be associated with ANDI or with periductal mastitis, or referred from, for example, a musculoskeletal disorder. About 10 per cent of breast cancers exhibit pain at presentation. Common breast symptoms are illustrated in Table 46.2.

Table 46.2 Common breast symptoms

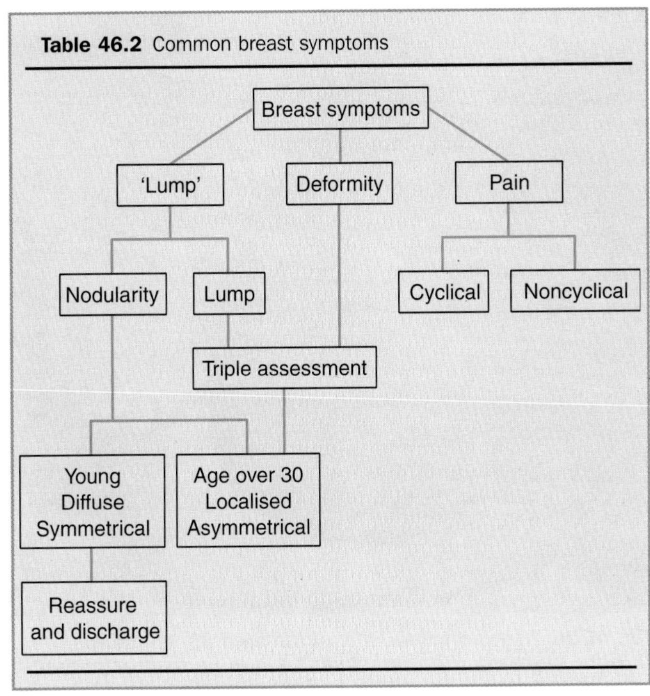

Table 46.3 Treatment of breast pain

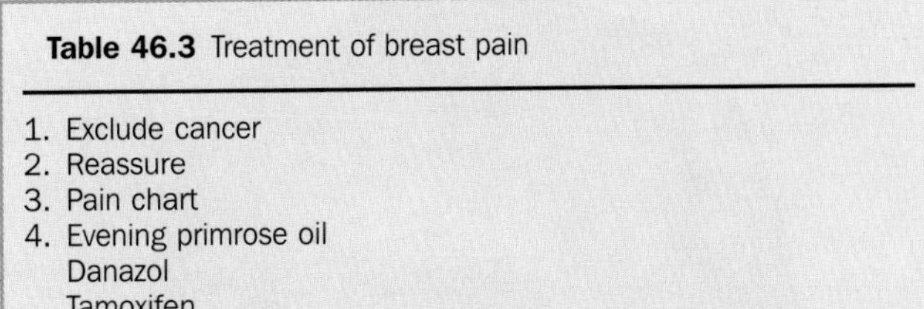

1. Exclude cancer
2. Reassure
3. Pain chart
4. Evening primrose oil
   Danazol
   Tamoxifen

Treatment of lumpy breasts

If the clinician is confident that he or she is not dealing with a discrete abnormality (and clinical confidence may be buttressed by mammography or ultrasound scanning if appropriate), then initially the woman can be offered firm reassurance. It is perhaps worthwhile reviewing the patient at a different point in the menstrual cycle, say 6 weeks after the initial visit, and often the clinical signs will have resolved by that time. There is a tendency for women with lumpy breasts to be rendered unnecessarily anxious and to be submitted to multiple random biopsies because the clinician lacks the courage of his or her convictions.

Treatment of mastalgia

Pronounced cyclical mastalgia may become a significant clinical problem where the pain and tenderness interfere with the woman's life, disturb her sleep and impair sexual activity. Initially, firm reassurance that the symptoms are not associated with cancer will help the majority of women. A patient symptom diary will help her to chart the pattern of pain throughout the month and thus determine whether this is cyclical mastalgia. If reassurance is inadequate, then a planned escalation of treatment (as shown in Table 46.3) could be advised. Oil of evening primrose, in adequate doses given over 3 months, will help more than half of these women. For those with intractable symptoms a prolactin inhibitor such as danazol may be given. Very rarely it is necessary to prescribe an antioestrogen, e.g. tamoxifen or a luteinizing hormone-releasing hormone (LHRH) agonist, to deprive the breast epithelium of oestrogenic drive.

For noncyclical mastalgia it is important to exclude extramammary causes such as chest wall pain, and it may be necessary to carry out a biopsy on a very localised tender area which might be harbouring a subclinical cancer. Treatment may be with nonsteroidal analgesics or by injection with local anaesthetic of a 'trigger spot'.

Breast cysts

These occur most commonly in the last decade of reproductive life due to a nonintegrated involution of stroma and epithelium. They are often multiple, may be bilateral and can mimic malignancy. Diagnosis can be confirmed by aspiration and/or ultrasound.

Treatment

A solitary cyst or small collection of cysts can be aspirated. If they resolve completely, and if the fluid is not bloodstained, no further treatment is required. However, 30 per cent will recur and require reaspiration. Cytological examination of cyst fluid is no longer practised routinely. If there is a residual lump or if the fluid is bloodstained, a local excision for histological diagnosis is advisable, as is also the case if the cyst repeatedly reforms.

Galactocele

Galactocele, which is rare, usually presents as a solitary, subareolar cyst, and always dates from lactation. It contains milk and in long-standing cases its walls tend to calcify. It can become enormous (Fig. 46.25).

Fibroadenoma

These usually arise in the fully developed breast during the 15–25-year period, although occasionally they occur in much older women. They arise from hyperplasia of a single lobule, and usually grow up to 2–3 cm in size. They are surrounded by a well-marked capsule and can thus be enucleated through a cosmetically appropriate incision. However, in a patient under 30 years these do not require excision unless associated with suspicious cytology, or if they become very large, or if the patient expressly desires the lump to be removed.

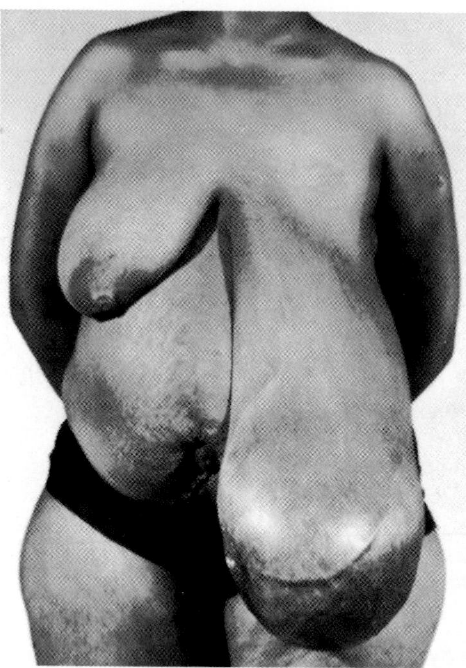

Fig. 46.25 Galactocoele. A 27-year-old multipara (3) with progressive breast enlargement following confinement (*courtesy of O.O. Ajayi and O. Adekunle, Ibadan, Nigeria*).

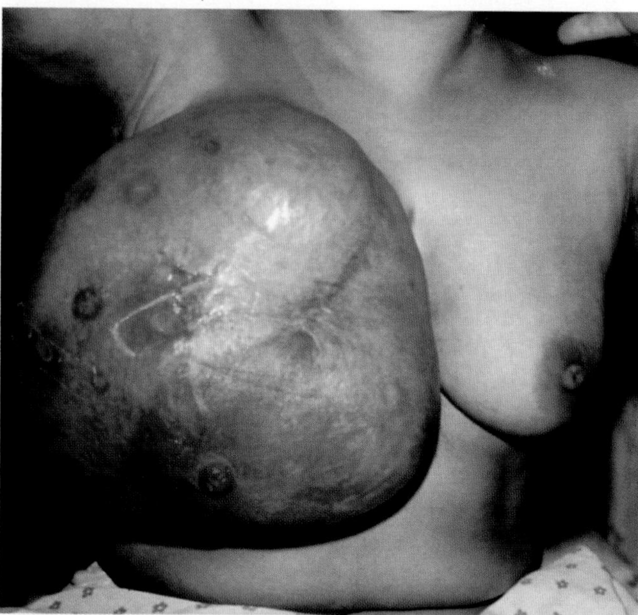

Fig. 46.26 Phyllodes tumour in a woman aged 28. It weighed 4.9 kg. Note the ulceration due to pressure. It should be possible to insert a probe freely between skin and tumour – not so in carcinoma of the breast (*courtesy of Dr S.R. Karmarkar, Bombay, India*).

Giant fibroadenomas occur occasionally during puberty. They are over 5 cm in diameter and are often rapidly growing, but in other respects are similar to smaller fibroadenomas and can be enucleated through a submammary incision.

Phyllodes tumour[3]

These benign tumours, previously sometimes known as serocystic disease of Brodie or cystosarcoma phyllodes, usually occur in women over the age of 40 but can appear in younger women (Fig. 46.26). They present as a large, sometimes massive tumour, with an unevenly bosselated surface. Occasionally ulceration of overlying skin occurs owing to pressure necrosis. In spite of their size they remain mobile on the chest wall. Histologically there is a resemblance to a fibroadenoma, but despite the name of cystosarcoma phyllodes they are rarely cystic and only very rarely develop features of a sarcomatous tumour. These may metastasise via the bloodstream.

Treatment

Treatment for the benign type is enucleation in very young women or wide local excision. Massive tumours, recurrent tumours and those of the malignant type will require mastectomy.

[3]*Phyllodes – from the Greek = leaf-like. There are branching projections of the tumour tissue into the cystic cavities of this neoplasm.*
Sir Benjamin Collins Brodie, 1783–1862. Surgeon, St George's Hospital, London, England. Described this disease in 1840.

When the diagnosis of carcinoma is in doubt

There will always be cases where the clinician cannot be sure whether a particular lump in the breast is an area of mammary dysplasia, a benign tumour or an early carcinoma.

If there is doubt on either clinical, cytological or radiological examination it is essential to obtain a tissue diagnosis. This is often possible by needle biopsy. In the advent of a negative result, open biopsy of the mass is necessary. Because of the possibility of reporting errors, the authors suggest that frozen section reporting should rarely be used and certainly should not form the basis for a decision to undertake a

Table 46.4 Investigation of a breast lump

Lump in the breast				
Cystic		*Solid*		
		Clinically benign		Clinically malignant
FNA		FNA		FNA
Cytology	Cytology	Cytology	Cytology	Cytology
Benign, lump disappears	Malignant lump persists or bloody	Benign	Malignant	Benign
Follow-up	Urgent biopsy	Follow-up or excise	Treat cancer	Urgent biopsy

Table 46.5 Three common breast lumps

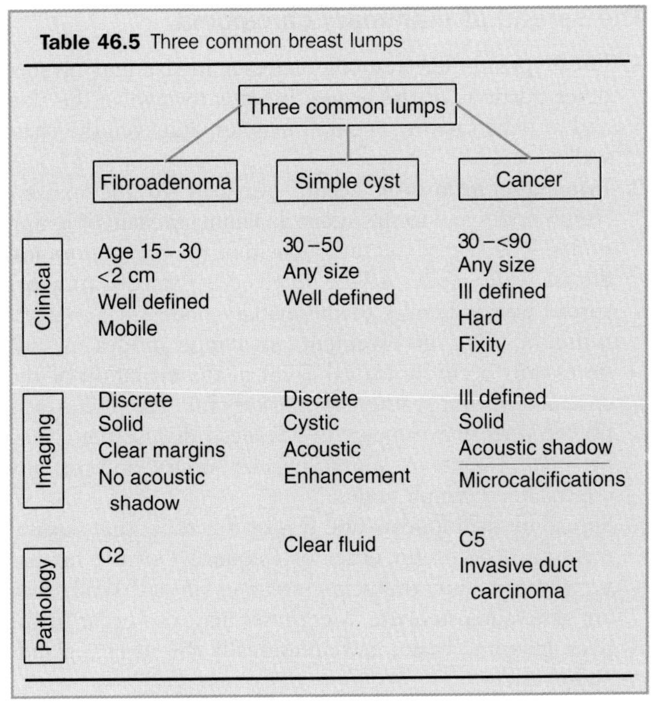

Three common lumps

	Fibroadenoma	Simple cyst	Cancer
Clinical	Age 15–30 <2 cm Well defined Mobile	30–50 Any size Well defined	30–<90 Any size Ill defined Hard Fixity
Imaging	Discrete Solid Clear margins No acoustic shadow	Discrete Cystic Acoustic Enhancement	Ill defined Solid Acoustic shadow Microcalcifications
Pathology	C2	Clear fluid	C5 Invasive duct carcinoma

mastectomy. Table 46.4 gives an algorithm for investigating any breast lump. Table 46.5 illustrates the features of three common lumps.

Carcinoma of the breast

Breast cancer is the commonest cause of death in middle-aged women in Western countries. In 1985, 719 000 new cases were diagnosed world-wide. In England and Wales one in 12 women will develop the disease during their lifetime.

Aetiological factors

1. **Geographical.** It occurs commonly in the Western world accounting for 3–5 per cent of deaths, yet is a rare tumour in Japan. In developing countries it accounts for 1–3 per cent of deaths.
2. **Age.** Carcinoma of the breast is extremely rare below the age of 20, but thereafter the incidence steadily rises so that by the age of 90 nearly 20 per cent of women are affected (Fig. 46.27).

By age 25	1 in 19 608	By age 60	1 in 24
By age 30	1 in 2525	By age 65	1 in 17
By age 35	1 in 622	By age 70	1 in 14
By age 40	1 in 217	By age 75	1 in 11
By age 45	1 in 93	By age 80	1 in 10
By age 50	1 in 50	By age 85	1 in 9
By age 55	1 in 33	Ever	1 in 8

1987–1988 Cancer incidence rates, NCI, USA.

Fig. 46.27 Chances of developing breast cancer related to age.

3. **Gender.** Less than 1 per cent of patients with breast cancer are male.
4. **Genetic.** It occurs more commonly in women with a family history of breast cancer than in the general population. Breast cancer related to a specific mutation accounts for about 5 per cent of breast cancers, yet has far-reaching repercussions in terms of counselling and attempted prevention in these women. This will be discussed more fully in a subsequent section.
5. **Diet.** Because breast cancer so commonly affects women in the 'developed' world, dietary factors may play a part in its causation. There is some evidence that there is a link between diets low in phyto-oestrogens. A high intake of alcohol is associated with an increased risk of developing breast cancer.
6. **Endocrine.** Breast cancer is commoner in nulliparous women and breastfeeding in particular appears to be protective. Also protective is having a first child at an early age, especially if associated with late menarche and early menopause. It is known that in postmenopausal women, breast cancer is more common in the obese. This is thought to be because of an increased conversion of steroid hormones to oestradiol in the body fat. The role of exogenous hormones, in particular the oral contraceptive pill and hormone replacement therapy, in the development of breast cancer is more controversial, but it can be said with some authority that for most women the benefits of these treatments will far outweigh the small putative risk.

The increase in the likelihood of developing breast cancer associated with the above risk factors is usually quantified in terms of the relative risk (RR). Thus a RR of 2.0 means that the individual has twice the chance of developing breast cancer as the average for the population, whilst a RR of 0.5 indicates a risk reduction of 50 per cent.

Pathology

Breast cancer may arise from the epithelium of the duct system anywhere from the nipple end of major lactiferous ducts to the terminal duct unit which is in the breast lobule. It may be entirely *in situ* – an increasingly common phenomenon with the advent of breast cancer screening – or may be invasive cancer. The degree of differentiation of the tumour is usually described by three grades – well differentiated, moderately or poorly differentiated. **Ductal carcinoma** is the most common variant, but **lobular carcinoma** occurs in up to 10 per cent of cases, although this may be mixed. Rarer histological variants, usually carrying a better prognosis, include **colloid carcinoma** whose cells produce abundant mucin, **medullary carcinoma** with solid sheets of large cells often associated with a marked lymphocytic reaction and **tubular carcinoma.** Invasive lobular carcinoma is commonly multifocal and/or bilateral.

Inflammatory carcinoma is a fortunately rare, highly aggressive cancer which presents as a painful, swollen breast, which is warm with cutaneous oedema. This is due to blockage of the subdermal lymphatics with carcinoma cells. Inflammatory cancer usually involves at least one-third of the breast and may mimic a breast abscess. A biopsy will confirm the diagnosis and show undifferentiated carcinoma cells.

***In situ* carcinoma** is preinvasive cancer which has not breached the epithelial basement membrane. This was previously a rare, usually asymptomatic finding in breast biopsy specimens but is becoming increasingly common owing to the advent of mammographic screening – it accounts for 20 per cent of cancers detected by screening. *In situ* carcinoma may be ductal (DCIS) or lobular (LCIS), the latter often multifocal and bilateral. Both are markers for the later development of invasive cancer which will go on to develop in at least 20 per cent of cases. Although mastectomy is curative, this is overtreatment in many cases and the best treatment for *in situ* carcinoma is the subject of a number of clinical trials.

Paget's disease of the nipple

Paget's disease of the nipple (Fig. 46.28a and b) is a superficial manifestation of an underlying breast carcinoma. It presents as an eczema-like condition of the nipple and areola which persists in spite of local treatment. The nipple is eroded slowly and eventually disappears. If left, the underlying carcinoma will sooner or later become clinically evident. Thus nipple eczema should be biopsied if there is any doubt about its cause. Microscopically Paget's disease is characterised by the presence of large, ovoid cells with abundant, clear, pale-staining cytoplasm in the Malpighian layer of the epidermis.

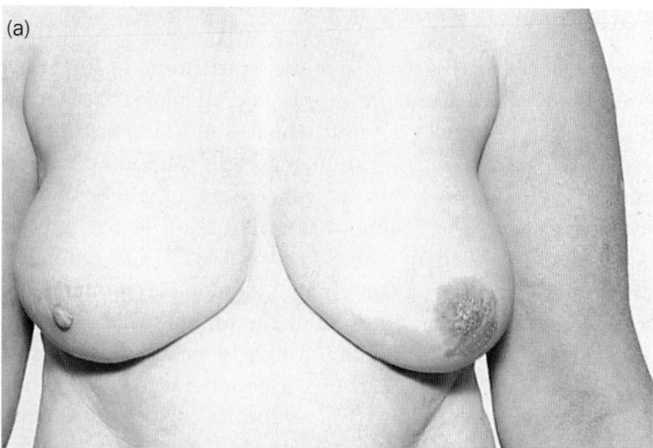

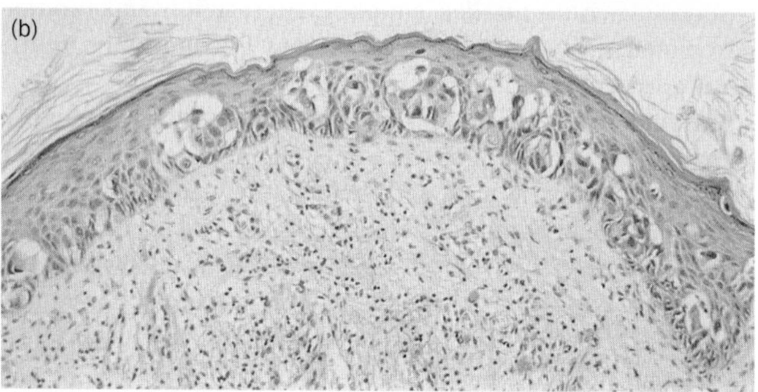

Fig. 46.28 (a) Paget's disease of the nipple. (b) Histological appearance of Paget's disease.

The spread of mammary carcinoma

1. **Local spread.** The tumour increases in size and invades other portions of the breast. It tends to involve the skin and to penetrate the pectoral muscles, and even the chest wall.
2. **Lymphatic metastasis** occurs primarily to the axillary lymph nodes and to the internal mammary chain of lymph nodes. The site of the tumour within the breast does not dictate which nodes will be involved, e.g. medial tumours spread just as readily to the axillary nodes as do lateral tumours. The involvement of lymph nodes is not necessarily a chronological event in the evolution of the carcinoma, but rather a marker for the metastatic potential of that tumour. In advanced disease there may be involvement of supraclavicular nodes and of any contralateral lymph nodes.
3. **Spread by the bloodstream.** It is by this route that skeletal metastases occur (in order of frequency) in the lumbar vertebrae, femur, thoracic vertebrae, rib and skull; they are generally osteolytic. Metastases may also occur in the liver, lung and brain, and occasionally the adrenal glands and ovaries.

Clinical presentation

While any portion of the breast, including the axillary tail, may be involved, breast cancer commences most frequently in the upper, outer quadrant (Figs 46.29 and 46.30). Most breast cancers will present as a hard lump, which may be

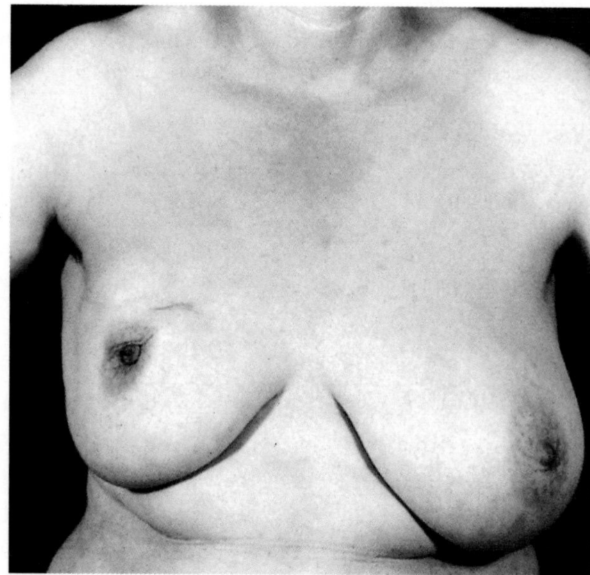

Fig. 46.29 Invasive duct (scirrhous) carcinoma of the right breast, upper outer quadrant and stage III. Note shrinking and elevation of the breast with nipple retraction.

Marcello Malpighi, 1628–94. Italian histologist.

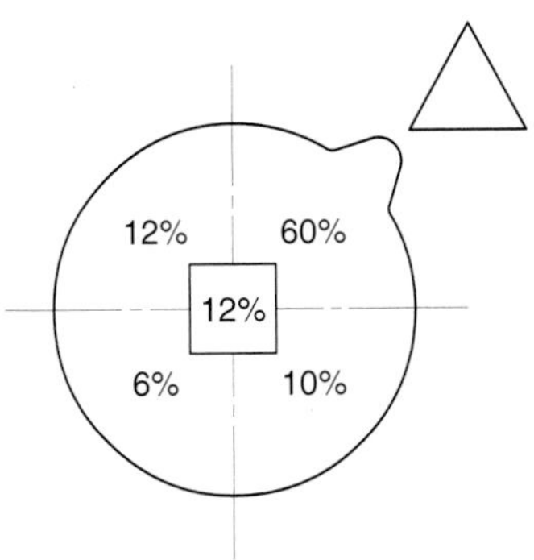

Fig. 46.30 The relationship of carcinoma of the breast to the quadrants of the breast (*courtesy of Marshall and Higginbotham's statistics*).

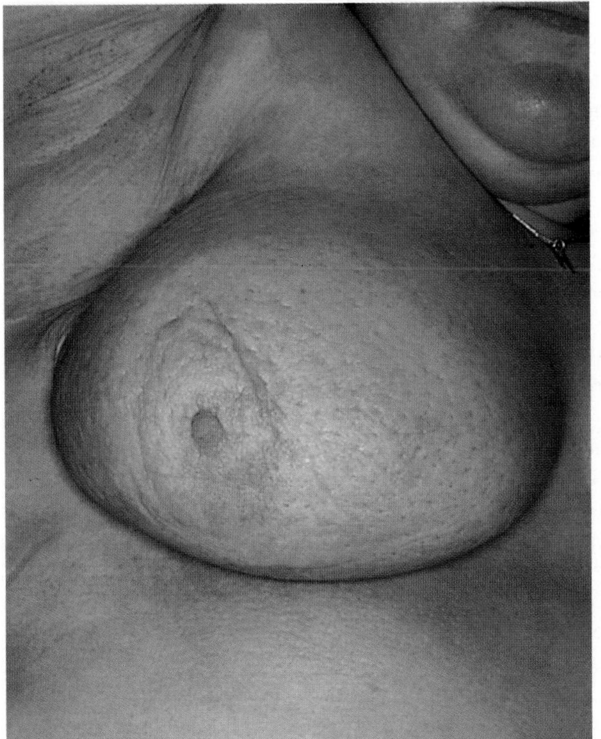

Fig. 46.31 Peau d'orange of the breast.

associated with indrawing of the nipple. As the disease advances locally there may be skin involvement with peau d'orange (Fig. 46.31) or frank ulceration and fixation to the chest wall (Fig. 46.32). This is described as cancer-en-cuirasse. About 5 per cent of breast cancers in the UK will present with either locally advanced disease or symptoms of metastatic disease. This figure is nearer 20 per cent in the developing world. These patients must then undergo a staging evaluation so that the full extent of their disease can be ascertained. This will include a careful clinical examination, chest X-ray, serum alkaline phosphatase and gamma glutamine transaminase (GGT), with liver ultrasound if these are abnormal, and an isotope bone scan (Fig. 46.33). This is important for both prognosis and treatment – a patient with widespread visceral metastases may obtain an

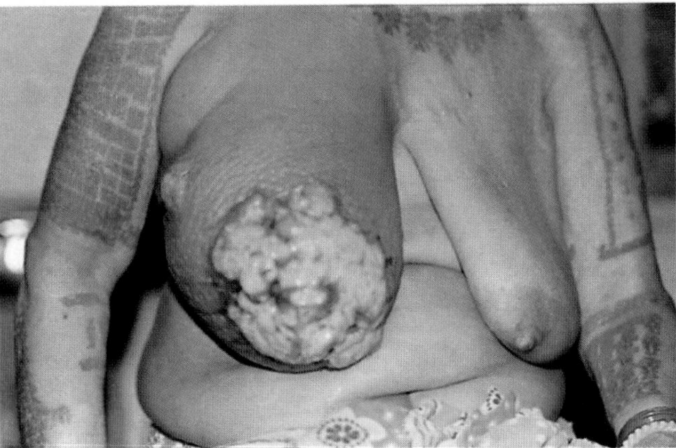

Fig. 46.32 Stage III. Enormous fungating carcinoma of right breast with enlarged axillary lymph nodes (*courtesy of Sanjay P. Thakur, Patna, India*).

increased length and quality of survival from systemic hormone or chemotherapy, but she is not likely to benefit from surgery as she will die from her metastases before local disease becomes a problem. In contrast, patients with relatively small (less than 5 cm in diameter) tumours confined to the breast and ipsilateral lymph nodes rarely need staging beyond a good clinical examination as the pick-up rate for distant metastases is so low.

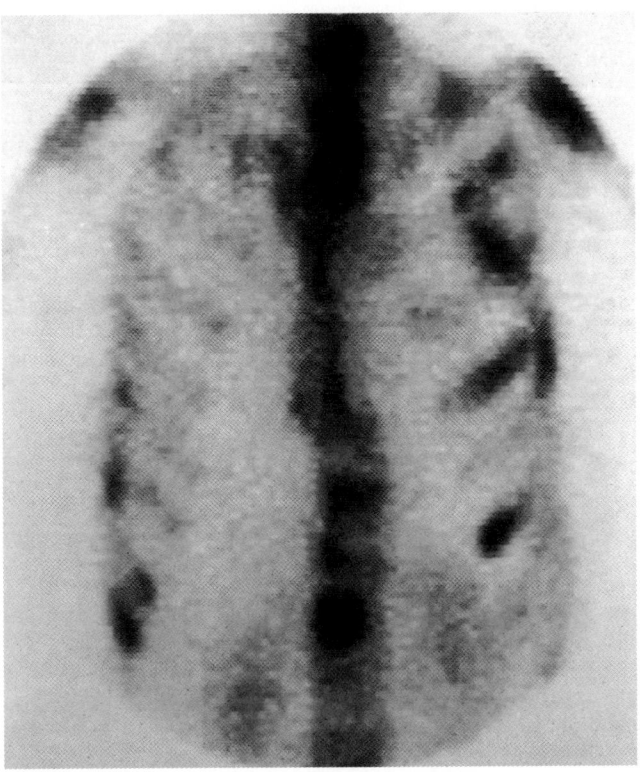

Fig. 46.33 Skeletal isotope bone scan showing multiple 'hot spots' due to metastases.

Table 46.6 Staging of breast cancer

		Manchester			
Stage	*Tumour grade*	*Clinical extent*	*Node grade*	*Clinical extent*	*Distant metastases*
TIS	T_{IS}	No palpable tumour	N_0	No nodal metastases	M_0 = no known distant metastases
I	T_1	<2 cm	N_0	No nodal metastases	
II	T_2	2–5 cm	N_1	Mobile axillary nodes	
III	T_3	>5 cm	N_2	Fixed axillary nodes	
IIIb	T_4	Any size invading skin or chest wall	N_3	Supraclavicular ipsilateral nodes	
IV					M_1 = distant metastases

Phenomena resulting from lymphatic obstruction in advanced breast cancer

Peau d'orange is due to cutaneous lymphatic oedema. Where the infiltrated skin is tethered by the sweat ducts it cannot swell, leading to an appearance like orange skin. Occasionally the same phenomenon is seen over a chronic abscess.

Late oedema of the arm is a troublesome complication of breast cancer treatment fortunately seen less often now that radical axillary dissection and radiotherapy are rarely combined. It does however occasionally still occur after either modality of treatment alone and appears anytime from months to years after treatment. There is usually no precipitating cause but recurrent tumour should be excluded as neoplastic infiltration of the axilla can cause arm swelling due to both lymphatic and venous blockage. This neoplastic infiltration is often painful due to nerve involvement.

An oedematous limb is susceptible to bacterial infections following quite minor trauma, and these require vigorous antibiotic treatment. Treatment of late oedema is difficult but limb elevation, elastic arm stockings and pneumatic compression devices can be useful.

Cancer-en-cuirasse[4]. The skin of the chest is infiltrated with carcinoma and has been likened to a coat.

It may be associated with a grossly swollen arm. This usually occurs in cases with local recurrence after mastectomy, and occasionally is seen to follow the distribution of irradiation to the chest wall. The condition may respond to palliative systemic treatment but prognosis in terms of survival is poor.

Lymphangiosarcoma (Fig. 46.34) is a rare complication of lymphoedema with an onset many years following the original treatment. It takes the form of multiple subcutaneous nodules in the upper limb and must be distinguished from recurrent carcinoma of the breast. The prognosis is poor but some cases respond to cytotoxic therapy or irradiation. Interscapulothoracic (forequarter) amputation is sometimes indicated.

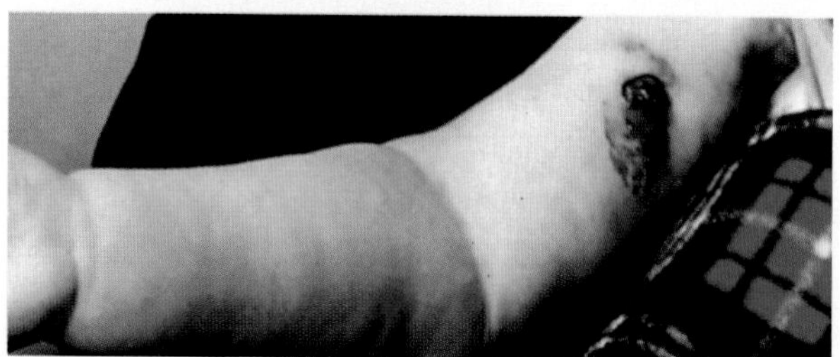

Fig. 46.34 Lymphangiosarcoma developed 3 years after radical mastectomy. Patient well many years after forequarter amputation (courtesy of *R.P. Singh, Karchana, India*).

[4]*Cuirasse = leather or metal breastplate worn by soldiers.*

Staging of breast cancer

There are two traditional systems of classification for breast carcinoma which predominantly rely on clinical staging of the disease. These are the Manchester system and the International Union Against Cancer TNM (tumour, nodes, metastases) staging system. These are illustrated in Table 46.6.

The TNM system was an attempt to allow a common language amongst oncologists world-wide, thus allowing accurate information exchange and evaluation of studies of treatment, as well as providing prognostic information to aid in the planning of treatment for the individual patient. However, this refinement of taxonomy in fact contributes little to any of these activities.

Further subdivisions in the TNM system now mean that there are seven T-stages, four N-stages and three M-stages, allowing for 180 possible combinations. Pathological lymph node staging depends on both the number of lymph nodes removed, thus the extent of surgery, and how assiduous the pathologist is in looking for deposits of tumour within the nodes. 'M' staging depends on what investigations have been performed – thus will vary between centres. Consequently staging is observer biased.

Although prognosis broadly correlates with stage, other factors also influence prognosis and should be assessed, for example the Nottingham Prognostic Index includes not only tumour size and lymph node status but tumour grade.

Conventional staging will indicate broadly which treatment is required but again other factors may be equally important. For example, surgical treatment of a small stage I, or II (T_1 or T_2) breast tumour usually requires only wide local excision rather than mastectomy – but the latter may have to be performed if the breast is very small, the tumour central or multifocal, or for patient preference. Equally the use of adjuvant systemic therapy is decided on not only tumour size and lymph node status but also biological measures such as oestrogen receptor status, patient age and menopausal status, and in the case of tamoxifen this can be recommended irrespective of clinicopathological variables.

Thus as we gain more knowledge of the biological variables which affect prognosis it becomes increasingly clear that it is these factors (discussed in more detail below) rather than anatomical mapping which influence outcome and

Table 46.7 A pragmatic classification for breast cancer

Group	Approx. 5-year survival	Examples	Treatment
'Very low risk' primary breast cancer	>90%	Screen detected DCIS, tubular or special types	Local
'Low risk' primary breast cancer	70–90%	Node negative with favourable histology	Locoregional ± systemic
'High risk' primary breast cancer	<70%	Node positive or unfavourable histology	Locoregional + systemic
Locally advanced	<30%	Large primary or inflammatory	Primary systemic
Metastatic	–		Primary systemic

treatment. Perhaps a more pragmatic approach would be to classify patients according to the treatment that they require. This is shown in Table 46.7.

Prognosis of breast cancer

The best indicators of likely prognosis in breast cancer are still tumour size and lymph node status (Fig. 46.35). However, it is realised that some large tumours will remain confined to the breast for decades whereas some very small tumours are incurable at diagnosis. Hence the prognosis of a cancer depends not on its chronological age but on its invasive and metastatic potential. In an attempt to define which tumours will behave aggressively, and thus require early systemic treatment, a host of prognostic factors has been described. These include histological grade of the tumour, hormone receptor status, measures of tumour proliferation such as S-phase fraction and thymidine-labelling index, growth factor analysis and oncogene or oncogene product measurements. Many others are under investigation but have proved of little practical value in patient management.

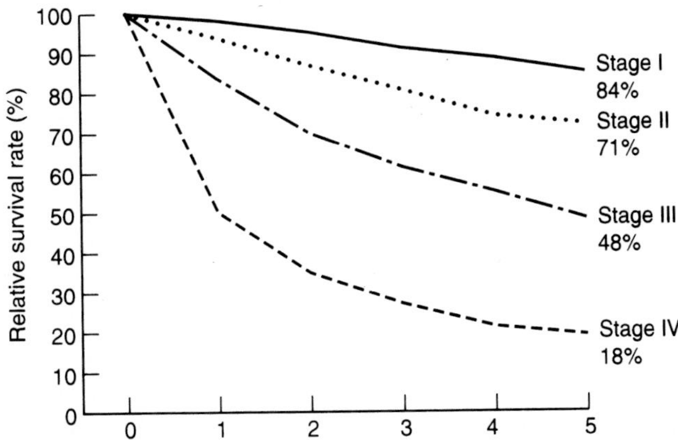

Fig. 46.35 Relative survival depending on stage of breast cancer at presentation.

Treatment of cancer of the breast

As has been indicated above, treatment will largely depend upon clinical stage of the disease at presentation including not only classical TMN staging but often other tumour characteristics such as tumour grade. Treatment of early breast cancer will usually involve surgery with or without radiotherapy. Systemic therapy such as chemotherapy or hormone therapy is added if there are adverse prognostic factors such as lymph node invasion indicating a high likelihood of metastatic relapse. At the other end of the spectrum locally advanced or metastatic disease is usually treated by systemic therapy to palliate symptoms, with surgery playing a much smaller role.

The multidisciplinary team approach

As in all branches of medicine good doctor–patient communication plays a vital role in helping to alleviate patient anxiety. Participation of the patient in treatment decisions is of particular importance in breast cancer where there may be uncertainty as to the best therapeutic option and the desire to treat the patient within the protocol of a controlled clinical trial. As part of the preoperative and postoperative management of the patient it is often useful to employ the skills of a trained breast counsellor and also to have available advice on breast prostheses, psychological support and physiotherapy, where appropriate. In many specialist centres the care of breast cancer patients is undertaken as a joint venture between the surgeon, medical oncologist, radiotherapist and allied health professionals such as the clinical nurse specialist.

Treatment of early breast cancer

The aims of treatment are:

1. 'cure': possible in some patients but recurrence up to 20 years after initial treatment is not uncommon;
2. control of local disease in the breast and axilla;
3. conservation of local form and function;
4. prevention or delay of the occurrence of distant metastases.

Local treatment of early breast cancer

Local control is achieved through surgery and/or radiotherapy.

Surgery

Surgery still has a central role to play in the management of breast cancer but there has been a gradual shift towards more conservative techniques, backed up by clinical trials which have shown equal efficacy between mastectomy and local excision followed by radiotherapy. This followed a change in the model of breast cancer spread, which is no longer thought of as a centrifugal anatomical spread but rather that it is the presence of micrometastases which predetermines the outcome of the disease.

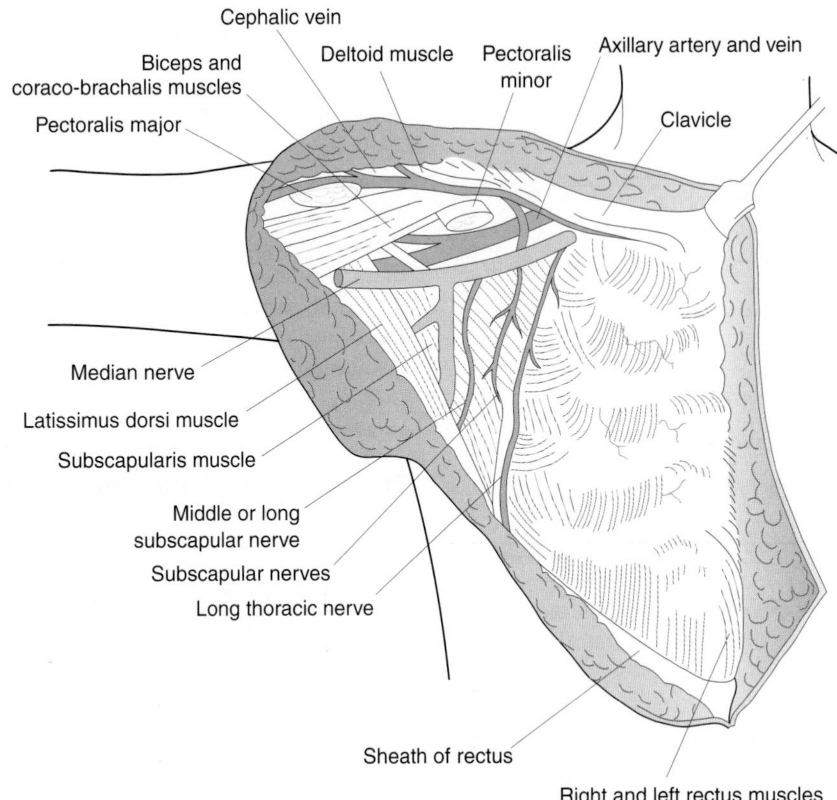

Fig. 46.36 Radical mastectomy completed – the modified radical leaves the pectoralis major muscle intact.

It was initially hoped that avoiding mastectomy would help to alleviate the considerable psychological morbidity associated with breast cancer, but recent studies have shown that over 30 per cent of women develop significant anxiety and depression following both radical and conservative surgery. After mastectomy they tend to worry about the effect of the operation on their appearance and relationships whilst after conservative surgery women may remain fearful of a recurrence.

Mastectomy is now only strictly indicated for large tumours (in relation to the size of the breast), central tumours beneath or involving the nipple, multifocal disease, local recurrence or for patient preference. The radical Halstead mastectomy which included excision of the breast, axillary lymph nodes, pectoralis major and minor muscles is no longer indicated as it causes excessive morbidity with no survival benefit. Modified radical ('Patey') mastectomy is more commonly performed and thus is described below. Simple mastectomy involves removal of the breast only with no dissection of the axilla, except for the region of the axillary tail of the breast which usually has attached to it a few nodes low in the anterior group. Because no pathological staging of the axilla is performed with a simple mastectomy, it is often followed by radiotherapy to the axilla.

'Patey' mastectomy. The breast and associated structures are dissected *en bloc* (see Fig. 46.36) and the excised mass is composed of:

- the whole breast;
- a large portion of skin, the centre of which overlies the tumour, but always includes the nipple;
- all of the fat, fascia and lymph nodes of the axilla. The pectoralis minor muscle is either divided or removed to gain access to the upper two-thirds of the axilla. The axillary vein and nerves to serratus anterior and latissimus dorsi should be preserved.

The wound is drained using a wide-bore suction tube.

Early mobilisation of the arm is encouraged and physiotherapy helps normal function to return very quickly – most patients are able to resume light work or housework within a few weeks.

William Stewart Halstead, 1852–1922. Professor of Surgery, Johns Hopkins University, Baltimore, Maryland, USA, was responsible for evolving the radical amputation of the breast. The operation is often known as 'a complete Halstead'.

David Howard Patey, 1899–1976. Surgeon, Middlesex Hospital, London, England.

Conservative breast cancer surgery is aimed at removing the tumour plus a rim of at least 1 cm of normal breast tissue. This is commonly referred to as a wide local excision or lumpectomy. A quadrantectomy involves removing the entire segment of the breast which contains the tumour. These are usually combined with axillary surgery, usually via a separate incision in the axilla, to either sample the axilla, remove nodes behind and lateral to pectoralis minor (level II) or perform a full axillary dissection (level III). A quadrantectomy, axillary dissection and radiotherapy is known as QUART and has been popularised by Professor Umberto Veronesi from Milan. Whilst it is recognised that there is a somewhat higher rate of local recurrence following conservative surgery, even if combined with radiotherapy, the long-term outlook in terms of survival is unchanged.

The role of axillary surgery is still debated, but it is accepted that the presence of metastatic disease within the axillary lymph nodes is still the best marker for prognosis. However, treatment of the axilla does not affect long-term survival, suggesting that the axillary nodes act not as a 'reservoir' for disease but as a marker for metastatic potential. An acceptable way to approach this problem in premenopausal women is to stage the axilla by operation as there is a good case for giving chemotherapy to lymph node-positive patients. In postmenopausal patients, tamoxifen is usually given regardless of axillary lymph node status. If mastectomy is performed it is reasonable to clear the axilla as part of the operation, but if a wide local excision is planned the surgeon may choose either operative dissection or postoperative radiotherapy. Axillary surgery should not be combined with radiotherapy to the axilla because of excess morbidity. Removal of the internal mammary lymph nodes is unnecessary.

Sentinal node biopsy is a technique currently under evaluation which may well prove the way forward in the future in the management of the axilla in patients with clinically node-negative disease. The sentinal node is localised perioperatively by the injection of patent blue dye and/or radioisotope-labelled albumin near the tumour. The marker will pass to the primary node draining the area, be detected visually or with a hand-held gamma camera, and sent for frozen section histological analysis. In patients in whom there is no tumour involvement of the sentinal node, it is hoped that further axillary dissection can be avoided as skip lesions are thought to occur in less than 3 per cent of patients.

Radiotherapy

Radiotherapy to the chest wall after mastectomy has been largely abandoned except in cases of extensive local disease with infiltration of the chest wall. It is conventional to combine conservative surgery with radiotherapy to the remaining breast tissue. However, there is currently doubt as to whether all patients undergoing conservative surgery should receive radiotherapy as most will not develop local recurrence and thus will be overtreated by adjuvant radiotherapy, which is not without morbidity and even long-term mortality from inadvertent irradiation to the myocardium. A UK national clinical trial is currently underway to try to ascertain whether there is a survival advantage with radiotherapy and to identify which patients are at highest risk of local relapse, and thus would benefit most from postoperative breast irradiation. Currently those thought to be at highest risk include those with extensive *in situ* carcinoma (or of course invasive cancer) at the margins of excision, patients under 35 years and those with multifocal disease.

Adjuvant systemic therapy

Over the last 25 years there has been a revolution in our understanding of the biological nature of carcinoma of the breast. It is now widely accepted that the outcomes of treatment are predetermined by the extent of micrometastatic disease at the time of diagnosis. Variations in the radical extent of local therapy might influence local relapse, but probably do not alter long-term mortality from the disease. However, systemic therapy targeted at these putative micrometastases might be expected to delay relapse and prolong survival. As a result of many international clinical trials and recent world overview analyses, it can be stated with extreme statistical confidence that the appropriate use of adjuvant chemotherapy or hormone therapy will improve relapse-free survival by approximately 30 per cent, which ultimately translates into an absolute improvement in survival of the order of 10 per cent at 15 years. Bearing in mind how common the disease is in Northern Europe and the USA, this translates into figures of major public health importance.

Who to treat and with what are still questions for which absolute answers have yet to found, but the data from an overview of recent trials suggest that lymph node-positive and poor prognosis node-negative premenopausal women should be recommended adjuvant combined chemotherapy and that postmenopausal women will obtain a worthwhile benefit from about 5 years of tamoxifen, 20 mg daily.

Hormone therapy

Tamoxifen is the most widely used 'hormonal' treatment in breast cancer. Its efficacy as an adjuvant therapy was first reported in 1983 and it has now been shown to reduce the annual rate of recurrence by 25 per cent, with a 17 per cent reduction in the annual rate of death. The effect of tamoxifen is favourable in most cases except for oestrogen receptor ER-negative premenopausal women; postmenopausal women with oestrogen receptor-rich (positive) tumours achieve a greater reduction in the relative risk of relapse than oestrogen receptor-negative cases. The beneficial effects of tamoxifen in reducing the risk of tumours in the contralateral breast have also been observed. Trials studying the optimal duration of treatment are close to maturity and suggest that 5 years of treatment may be preferable to 2 years.

Other hormonal agents are being developed which may prove beneficial as adjuvant therapy, such as the LHRH agonists which induce a reversible ovarian suppression and thus are hoped to have the same beneficial effects as surgical or radiation-induced ovarian ablation in premenopausal women, and the oral aromatase inhibitors for postmenopausal women.

Chemotherapy

Chemotherapy using a regimen such as a 6-monthly cycle of cyclophosphamide, methotrexate and 5-fluorouracil (CMF) will achieve a 30 per cent reduction in the risk of relapse over a 10–15-year period. This treatment has been confined to premenopausal poor prognosis women (where its effects are likely to be due in part to a chemical castration effect) but is being increasingly offered to postmenopausal women with poor prognosis disease as well. Chemotherapy may be considered in node-negative patients if other prognostic factors such as tumour grade infer a high risk of recurrence. The effect of combining hormone and chemotherapy is still under investigation and is beginning to look promising.

High-dose chemotherapy with stem cell rescue for patients with heavy lymph node involvement is still considered experimental and should not be offered outside controlled trials.

Primary chemotherapy is being used in many centres for large but operable tumours that would traditionally require a mastectomy (and almost certainly postoperative adjuvant chemotherapy). The aim of this treatment is to shrink the tumour to enable breast-conserving surgery to be performed. This approach is successful in up to 80 per cent of cases, but is not associated with improvements in survival compared with conventionally timed chemotherapy.

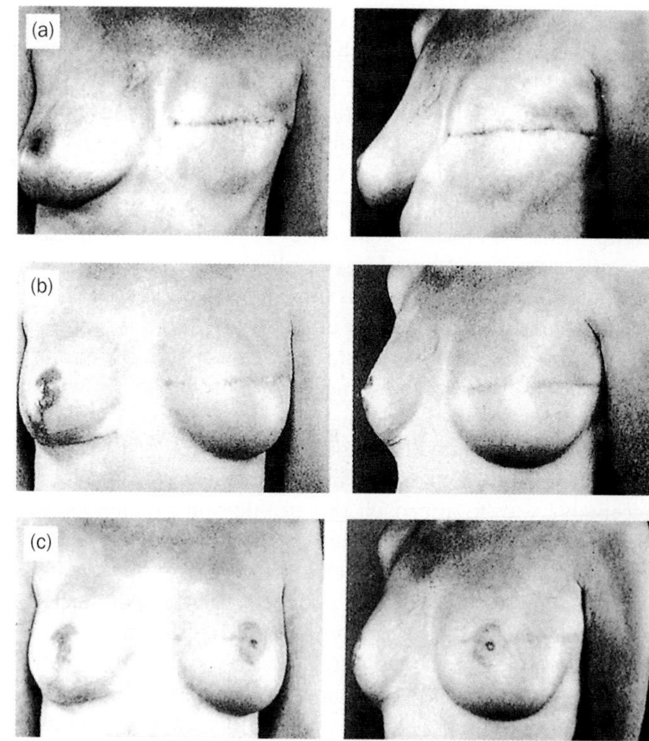

Fig. 46.37 Stages of reconstruction with silicone tissue expander including nipple reconstruction and right reduction mastopexy.

Breast reconstruction

Despite an increasing trend toward conservative surgery, up to 50 per cent of women still require, or want, a mastectomy. These women can now be offered immediate or delayed reconstruction of the breast. Few contraindications to breast reconstruction exist – even those with a limited life expectancy may benefit from the improved quality of life, however patients do require counselling before this procedure so that their expectations of cosmetic outcome are not unrealistic.

The most common type of reconstruction is using a silicone gel implant under the pectoralis major muscle.

This may be combined with prior tissue expansion using an expandable saline prosthesis first (or a combined device – Fig. 46.37) which creates some ptosis of the new breast. If the skin at the mastectomy site is poor (for example following radiotherapy) or if a larger volume of tissue is required, a musculocutanous flap can be constructed from either the latissimus dorsi muscle (an LD flap) or the contralateral transversus abdominis muscle (a TRAM flap – shown in Fig. 46.38). The latter gives an excellent cosmetic result in experienced hands but is a lengthy procedure and requires careful patient selection.

Nipple reconstruction is a relatively simple procedure which can be performed under a local anaesthetic. Alternatively the patient can be fitted with a prosthetic nipple. To achieve symmetry, the opposite breast may require a cosmetic procedure such as reduction or augmentation

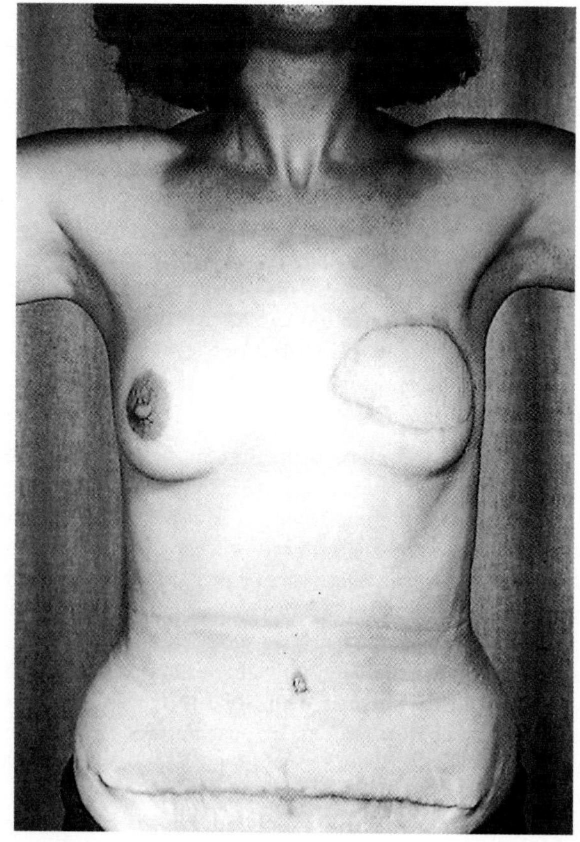
Fig. 46.38 TRAM flap.

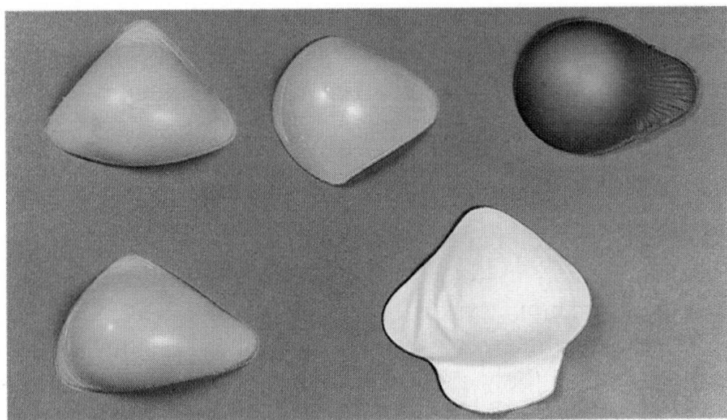

Fig. 46.39 A selection of external breast prostheses.

mammoplasty, or mastopexy. A breast reconstructive service can be offered by a suitably trained breast surgeon, a plastic surgeon or ideally a combined oncoplastic approach.

External breast prostheses which fit within the bra may also be recommended and some of these are illustrated in Fig. 46.39.

Screening for breast cancer

Because the prognosis of breast cancer is closely related to stage at diagnosis, it would seem reasonable to hope that a population screening programme which could detect tumours before they come to the patient's notice may reduce mortality from breast cancer. A number of studies has indeed shown that breast screening by mammography in women over the age of 50 will reduce cause-specific mortality by up to 30 per cent. Following the publication in 1987 of the Forrest report the National Health Service in the UK has launched a programme of 3-yearly mammographic screening for women between the ages of 50 and 64. The introduction of this programme has undoubtedly improved the quality of breast cancer services but a number of questions remains unanswered including the value of screening women under 50 and the ideal interval between screenings. The psychological consequences of false alarms or false reassurances still need to be addressed and self-examination programmes which have failed to show any benefit for the population in terms of earlier or decreased mortality from breast cancer still remain controversial. Figure 46.40 illustrates some benefits and disadvantages of screening. The senior author remains doubtful regarding the value of a screening programme in terms of the wider implications of healthcare planning.

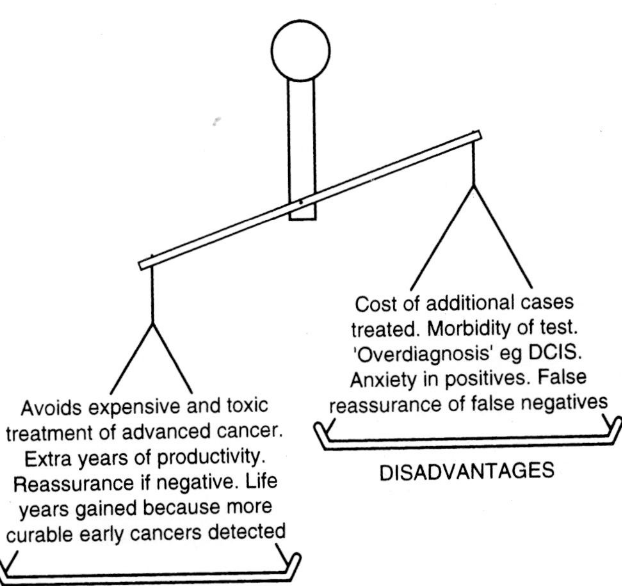

Fig. 46.40 Benefits and disadvantages of breast cancer screening.

Professor A.P.M. Forrest. Regius Professor of Surgery, Edinburgh, Scotland (1970–89).

Familial breast cancer

Recent developments in molecular genetics and the identification of a number of breast cancer predisposition genes (*BRCA1*, *BRCA2* and *TP53*) have done much to stimulate interest in this fascinating area. Yet women whose breast cancer is due to an inherited genetic change actually account for less than 5 per cent of all breast cancers – that is about 1250 cases per year in the UK and 9000 cases in the USA. A much larger number of women will have a risk elevated above normal due to an as yet unspecified familial inheritance. These women have a risk of developing breast cancer two to 10 times above baseline.

The risks associated with family history are summarised in Table 46.8.

The *BRCA1* gene has been cloned and is located on the long arm of chromosome 17 (17q). The gene frequency in the population is approximately 0.0006. *BRCA2* is located on chromosome 13q. Women who are thought to be gene carriers may be offered breast screening (and ovarian screening in the case of *BRCA1*, which is known to impart a 50 per cent lifetime risk of ovarian cancer), usually as part of a research programme, or may be offered genetic counselling and mutation analysis. Those who prove to be 'gene positive'

Table 46.8 Likelihood of genetic mutation with family history

No. family cases <50 years old	*BRCA1**	*BRCA2***
2	4%	3%
3	17%	13%
4	41%	33%
5	55%	44%

*BRCA1 also associated with colorectal and prostate cancer.
**BRCA2 associated with familial male breast cancer.

have an 80 per cent risk of developing breast cancer, predominantly whilst premenopausal. Many will opt for prophylactic mastectomy, although this does not completely eliminate the risk.

For those with a positive family history who are unlikely to be carriers of a breast cancer gene, which will comprise the great majority of women, there is no currently proven preventive or screening manoeuvre, although these are under investigation. Thus these women are best served by being assessed and followed up, if necessary, in a properly organised research family history clinic.

Pregnancy

The effects of pregnancy on breast cancer are not well studied but it is thought that breast cancer presenting during pregnancy or lactation tends to be at a later stage – presumably because the symptoms are masked by the pregnancy – but in other respects it behaves in a similar way to breast cancer in a nonpregnant young woman, and should be treated accordingly. Thus treatment is similar with some provisos: radiotherapy should be avoided during pregnancy, making mastectomy a more frequent option than breast conservation surgery; chemotherapy should be avoided during the first trimester but is probably safe subsequently; most tumours are hormone receptor negative and so hormone treatment, which is potentially teratogenic, is not required. Becoming pregnant subsequent to a diagnosis of breast cancer appears not to alter likely outcome, but women are usually advised to wait at least 2 years, as it is within this time that recurrence most often occurs.

The risk of developing breast cancer with **oral contraceptive** use is only slight, and disappears 10 years after stopping the Pill.

Hormone-replacement therapy

Hormone-replacement therapy (HRT) does not appear to increase significantly the risk of developing breast cancer unless taken for prolonged periods (over 10 years), and perhaps in certain high-risk groups. HRT may, however, prolong symptoms of benign breast disorder and make mammographic appearances more difficult to interpret.

Patients who develop breast cancer whilst on HRT appear to have a more favourable prognosis. The consequences in terms of recurrence in women using HRT following breast cancer are unknown.

Treatment of advanced breast cancer

Breast cancer may occasionally present as metastatic disease without evidence of a primary tumour (that is with an occult primary). The diagnosis is made partly by exclusion of another site for the primary and may be confirmed by histology of the metastatic lesions. Treatment should be aimed at palliation of the symptoms and treating the breast cancer, usually by endocrine manipulation.

Locally advanced inoperable breast cancer

Locally advanced inoperable breast cancer, including inflammatory breast cancer, is usually treated with systemic therapy – either chemotherapy or hormone therapy.

Occasionally 'toilet mastectomy' or radiotherapy is required to control a fungating tumour, but often incision through microscopically permeated tissues makes the outcome worse than the original.

Metastatic carcinoma of the breast

Metastatic carcinoma of the breast will also require some form of palliative systemic therapy to alleviate symptoms. Hormone manipulation is often the first line because of its minimal side effects. It is particularly useful for bony metastases. However, only about 30 per cent of these tumours will be hormone responsive, and unfortunately even these will in time become resistant to this treatment. First-line hormone therapy for postmenopausal women is tamoxifen, and for premenopausal women ovarian suppression, but where resistance to these has developed, other hormonal agents can prove useful, with about half of the response rate seen in the first-line therapy. Synthetic progestagens such as medroxyprogesterone acetate ('Provera') aromatase inhibitors or the newer agents such as antiprogestins and pure antioestrogens are all candidates for this role.

Cytotoxic therapy is used, particularly in younger women or those with visceral metastases and rapidly growing tumours. A variety of regimens is available and although none prolongs survival, contrary to expectations quality of life and symptom control is often better with more aggressive treatments, responses being seen in up to 70 per cent of patients.

Local treatment may also prove useful for some metastatic disease such as radiotherapy for painful bony deposits and internal fixation of pathological fractures.

The male breast

Gynaecomastia

Idiopathic

Hypertrophy of the male breast may be unilateral or bilateral. The breasts enlarge at puberty and sometimes present the characteristics of female breasts (Fig. 46.41).

Hormonal

Enlargement of the breasts often accompanied stilboestrol therapy for prostate cancer – now rarely used. It may also occur as a result of a teratoma of the testis, in anorchism and after castration. Rarely it may be a feature of ectopic hormonal production in bronchial carcinoma and in adrenal and pituitary disease.

Associated with leprosy

Gynaecomastia is very common in men suffering from leprosy. This is possibly because of bilateral testicular atrophy, which is a frequent accompaniment of leprosy.

Associated with liver failure

Gynaecomastia sometimes occurs in patients with cirrhosis due to failure of the liver to metabolise oestrogens. It is associated with drugs that interfere with the hepatic metabolism of oestrogens, such as cimetidine.

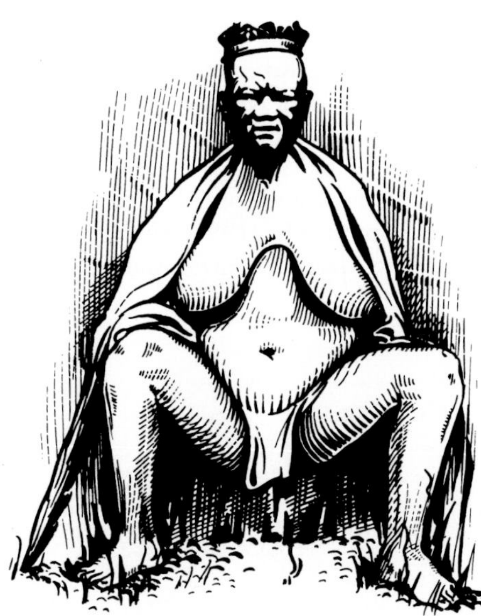

Fig. 46.41 Chief Chengwayo, from a photograph by Schujelot.

Associated with Klinefelter's syndrome

Gynaecomastia may occur in patients with Klinefelter's syndrome, a sex chromosome anomaly having XXY trisomy. It is also seen with certain drugs such as cimetidine, digitalis and spironolactone.

Treatment

Provided the patient is healthy and comparatively young, reassurance may be sufficient. If not mastectomy with preservation of the areola and nipple can be performed.

Carcinoma of the male breast

Carcinoma of the male breast (Figs 46.42 and 46.43) accounts for less than 2 per cent of all cases of breast cancer. The known predisposing causes include gynaecomastia and excess endogenous or exogenous oestrogen. As in the female it tends to present as a lump and is most commonly an infiltrating ductal carcinoma.

Treatment

Stage for stage the treatment is the same as for carcinoma in the female and prognosis depends upon stage at presentation. Adequate local excision, because of the small size of the breast, should always be with a 'mastectomy'.

Other tumours of the breast

Lipoma

A true lipoma is very rare.

Sarcoma of the breast

Sarcoma of the breast is usually of the spindle-cell variety, and accounts for 0.5 per cent of malignant tumours of the breast. Some of these growths arise in an intracanalicular fibroadenoma or may follow

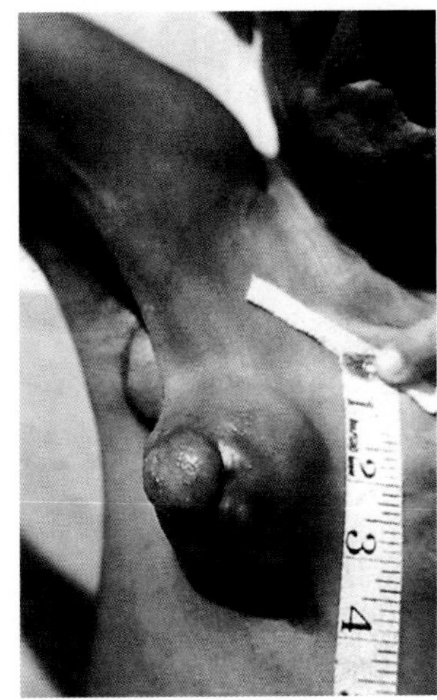

Fig. 46.42 Carcinoma of the male breast (*courtesy of Dr Y.V. Shah, Vamnagar, India*).

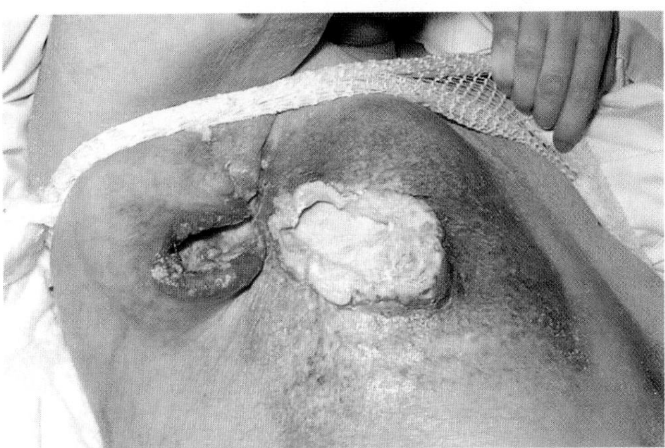

Fig. 46.43 Advanced carcinoma of the male breast (*courtesy of C.V. Mann, Royal London Hospital*).

previous radiotherapy, e.g. for Hodgkin's lymphoma many years previously. It may be impossible to distinguish clinically a sarcoma of the breast from a medullary carcinoma, but areas of cystic degeneration suggest a sarcoma and on incising the neoplasm it is pale and friable. Sarcoma tends to occur in younger women between the ages of 30 and 40. Treatment is by simple mastectomy followed by radiotherapy. The prognosis depends on the stage and histological type.

Metastases

On rare occasions, cancer elsewhere may present with a metastasis in the breast. The breast is also occasionally infiltrated by Hodgkin's disease and other lymphomas.

Harry Fitch Klinefelter, b. 1912. American physician practising in Baltimore, Maryland, USA. Described his syndrome in 1942.

Thomas Hodgkin, 1798–1866. Curator of the museum and demonstrator of morbid anatomy, Guy's Hospital, London, England.

Further reading

Dixon, M. and Sainsbury, R. (1993) *Diseases of the Breast*, Churchill Livingstone, Edinburgh.

Harris, J.R., Hellman, S., Henderson, I.C. and Kinne, D.W. (1987) *Breast Disease*, Lippincott, Philadelphia, PA.

Hayes, D.F. (1993) *Atlas of Breast Cancer*, Wolfe, London.

Hughes, L.E., Mansel, R.E. and Webster, D.J.T. (1989) *Benign Disorders and Diseases of the Breast*, Balliere Tindall, London.

Mansel, R.E. and Bundred, N.J. (1996) *Colour Atlas of Breast Diseases*, Mosby-Wolfe, London.

Powles, T.J. and Smith, I.E. (1991) *Medical Management of Breast Cancer*, Martin Dunitz, London.

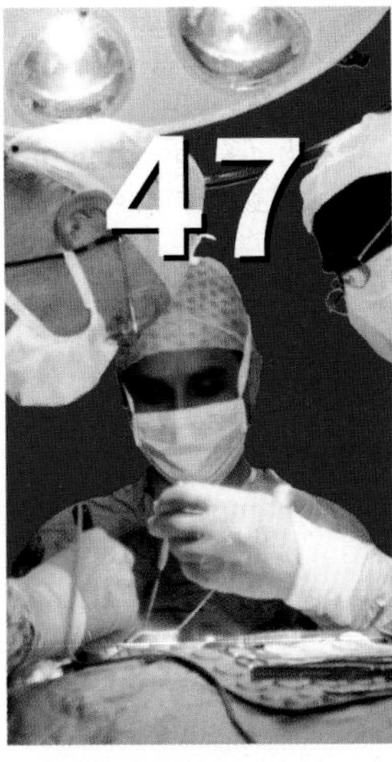

47 The thorax

Thoracic trauma

Many of the surgically treatable conditions of the lung are treated at specialist thoracic centres and the only exposure to thoracic surgery that most surgeons have is dealing with thoracic trauma. The approach to treatment must be methodical and exact because the signs, particularly in the presence of other injury, may easily be missed. The guidelines produced by the American College of Surgeons Advanced Trauma Life Support (ATLS®) Group provide a thorough and unambiguous approach to trauma. The general principles of resuscitation and need for priorities are extensively discussed and will not be repeated here. However, the specific aspects of trauma management related to the thorax will be covered. Thoracic trauma is responsible for over 70 per cent of all deaths following road traffic accidents. Blunt trauma to the chest in isolation is fatal in 10 per cent of cases, rising to 30 per cent if other injuries are present. An increasing number of penetrating thoracic wounds is also seen from domestic and civil violence, with a mortality rate of 3 per cent for simple stabbing to 15 per cent for gunshot wounds.

Initial management

Early deaths after thoracic trauma are caused by hypoxaemia, hypovolaemia and tamponade. The first steps in treating these patients should be to diagnose and treat these problems as early as possible because they may be readily corrected. Young patients have a large physiological reserve and serious injury may be overlooked until this reserve is used up; then the situation is critical and may be irretrievable. The best approach is to maintain a high index of suspicion and suspect the worst if life-threatening conditions are to be anticipated and treated. Early consultation with a regional thoracic centre is advised in cases of doubt. In an emergency it is essential that experienced help is summoned immediately.

The basic principles of resuscitation are securing the airway and restoring the circulating volume. Blood and secretions are removed from the oropharynx by suction. If the patient is unable to maintain his or her airway then an oropharyngeal airway followed by tracheal intubation (once a cervical spine injury is excluded) may be necessary.

A thorough inspection of the chest wall includes noting the frequency and pattern of breathing, external evidence of trauma and structural defects of the thorax. Palpation will detect surgical emphysema, paradoxical movement and a stove-in chest. Auscultation and percussion should reveal the existence of a pneumothorax (there is decreased movement on the affected side with a hyperresonant percussion note, reduced breath sounds in the axilla and shift of the trachea to the opposite side) which requires emergency drainage (see Pneumothorax for a more detailed appraisal and see Chest drainage for advice on technique of drain insertion).

Once the patient has been stabilised then radiographs of the chest should be taken and further treatment decided on the basis of the patient's condition and the radiographic result. It

Bailey & Love's Short Practice of Surgery, 23rd edition. Edited by R.C.G. Russell, N.S. Williams and C.J.K. Bulstrode. Published in 2000 by Arnold Publishers.

is rarely necessary to perform a thoracotomy in the resuscitation room but, in the case of tamponade from a penetrating injury, it might be life saving. However, the fact is that, even in experienced hands, the yield in terms of survival in this group of patients is very small. If there is profound hypotension as a result of cardiac tamponade, needle aspiration of the pericardium is life saving and may hold the situation long enough for more controlled surgery to be performed.

The components of chest injury in blunt trauma

Any combination of structures may be involved in varying degrees of severity. If the skeletal injuries are severe, underlying parenchymal injuries are likely to be in proportion; however, in young flexible chests, or those restrained by seat belts, there may be little external evidence of the severity of internal damage.

Chest wall

Localised rib fracture due to direct trauma. A simple rib fracture may be serious in elderly people or in those with chronic lung disease who have little pulmonary reserve. Uncomplicated fractures require sufficient analgesia to encourage a normal respiratory pattern and effective coughing. Oral analgesia may suffice but intercostal nerve blockade with local anaesthesia may be very helpful. Chest strapping or bed rest is no longer advised and early ambulation with vigorous physiotherapy (and oral antibiotics if necessary) is encouraged. A chest radiograph is always taken to exclude an underlying pneumothorax. It is useful to confirm the skeletal injuries but routine chest radiography may miss rib fractures. However, once a pneumothorax and major skeletal injuries are excluded, the management is the same – the local control of chest pain.

Major chest wall trauma. *Flail chest* (Fig. 47.1). This occurs when several adjacent ribs are fractured in two places either on one side of the chest or either side of the sternum. The flail segment moves paradoxically, that is, inwards during inspiration and outwards during expiration, thereby reducing effective gas exchange. The net result is poor oxygenation from injury to the underlying lung parenchyma and paradoxical movement of the flail segment. The underlying lung injury with loss of alveolar function may result in deoxygenated blood passing into the systemic circulation. This creates a right-to-left shunt and prevents full saturation of arterial blood. In the absence of any other injuries and, if the segment is small and not embarrassing respiration, the patient may be nursed on a high-dependency unit with regular blood gas analysis and good analgesia until the flail segment stabilises. In the more severe case, endotracheal intubation is required with positive pressure ventilation for up to 3 weeks, until the fractures become less mobile. Thoracotomy with fracture fixation is occasionally appropriate if there is an underlying lung injury to be treated at the same time. An anterior flail segment with the sternum moving paradoxically with respiration can be stabilised by internal fixation but operative management is not usual for either.

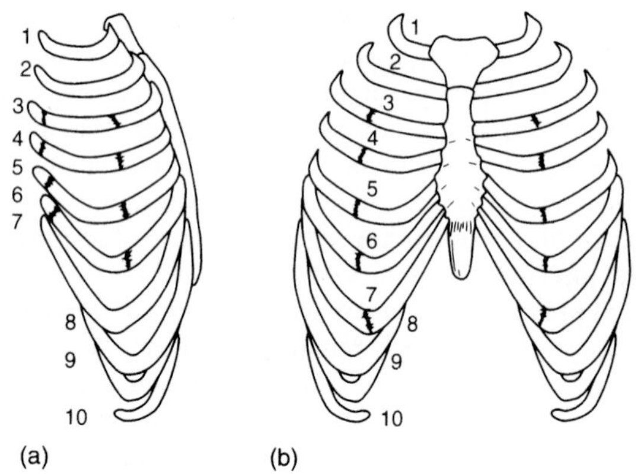

Fig. 47.1 Diagram of flail chest: (a) lateral flail; (b) anterior flail ('stove-in' chest).

First rib fracture. Fracture of the first rib should alert the clinician to a potentially serious chest injury. This rib is well protected and requires a considerable force to fracture and associated injuries to the great vessels, abdomen, head and neck are common. The mortality rate associated with a fracture of the first rib exceeds 30 per cent. Similar suspicions are raised when fractures of the sternum and scapula are seen. Fractures of the lower ribs may involve underlying abdominal viscera (spleen on the left and liver on the right). Intercostal artery bleeding may still be severe, resulting in haemothorax.

Fractures of the sternum (Fig. 47.2). This injury is now seen as a result of deceleration on to seat belts. Steering wheel injuries are now much less common. The injury is very painful even in the mild case where only the external plate of the sternum is fractured. However, there is a real risk of underlying myocardial damage and the patient should be observed in hospital with constant electrocardiogram (ECG) monitoring, analgesia and serial cardiac enzymes. Rupture of the aorta and associated cervical spine injuries also need to be excluded. Most cases need no specific treatment but paradoxical movement or instability of the chest may need more active management. It should be remembered that sternal fracture may occur during closed cardiac massage.

Vertebrae. The thoracic spine may be injured as one component of multiple injury or in isolation. It is more usual for the cervical spine to be injured and this must be excluded before any manipulations or movements take place. Damage to the thoracic spine is likely to be associated with injuries to other thoracic viscera. The assessment and treatment of spinal injury are discussed in Chapter 33. However, the thoracic spine injury is a reminder that, in patients where the chest injury predominates, a quick screening neurological examination confirming the integrity of the nerve supply to the lower limbs should be performed and documented.

Pleura. If the visceral pleura is breached (most commonly by a rib fracture) pneumothorax follows. Generation of positive pressure in the airways by coughing, straining, groaning

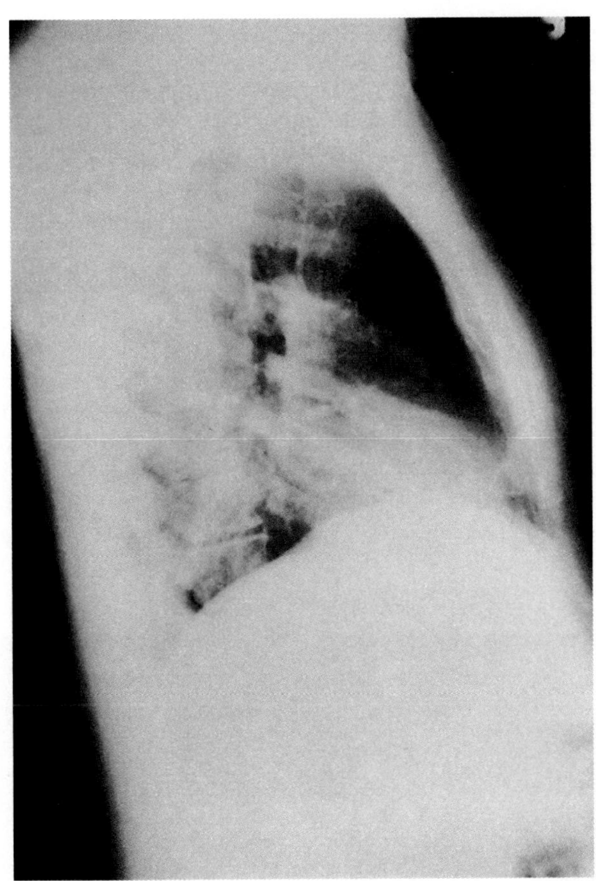

Fig. 47.2 Radiograph of sternal fracture.

or positive pressure ventilation will result in tension pneumothorax. The pleural space may also fill with blood as a result of injury anywhere in its vicinity. Remember that an erect chest radiograph is the only sure way to confirm or exclude the diagnosis of pneumothorax and should be obtained if at all possible. Early management of tension pneumothorax is life saving. Good management of the pleural space pre-empts many later complications from clotted haemothorax, constriction of the lung and empyema. The diagnosis and management of a simple pneumothorax are discussed in detail later, but in the trauma situation it is imperative to consider tension pneumothorax and haemothorax.

Traumatic pneumothorax. Blunt trauma to the chest wall may result in a lung laceration from a rib fracture. All traumatic pneumothoraces require drainage through an underwater seal drain because of the possibility that they may become a tension pneumothorax with mediastinal shift and circulatory collapse. There is decreased air entry on the affected side and the trachea may be pushed over to the opposite side. There is an increased percussion note and reduced breath sounds. If a tension pneumothorax is suspected on clinical grounds, treatment is necessary before radiographs can be taken. A wide-bore needle introduced into the affected hemithorax will release any air under tension and is life saving. A wide-bore intercostal tube is introduced laterally and directed to the apex of the pleural cavity. A second drain may be introduced basally to drain blood.

Chest drain insertion. Insertion of a chest drain is indicated when there is air or fluid in the pleural cavity (Fig. 47.3). The site of insertion is in the triangle of safety which is defined as the anterior border of the latissimus dorsi, the posterior border of the pectoralis major and the superior border of the fifth rib. The area chosen is infiltrated with local anaesthetic and an incision is made in the skin and subcutaneous tissues, sufficient to admit a finger easily. The intercostal muscles are separated with artery forceps and the pleura is punctured. The intercostal drainage tube is inserted with the stylette withdrawn, so as not to damage the underlying lung tissue. A large-bore tube is used for the drainage of blood and fluids, whereas a smaller-bore tube may be used for the removal of air.

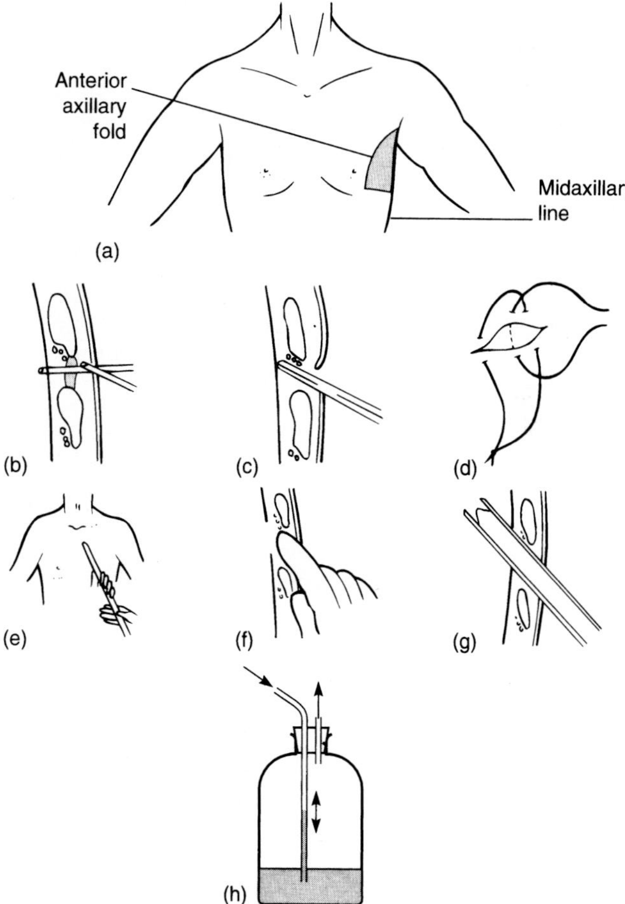

Fig. 47.3 Insertion of chest drain. (a) Triangle of safety; (b) penetration of the skin, muscle and pleura; (c) blunt dissection of the parietal pleura; (d) suture placement; (e) gauging the distance of insertion; (f) digital examination along the tract into the pleural space; (g) withdrawal of central trochar and positioning of drain; (h) underwater seal chest drain bottle.

Traumatic haemothorax. Drainage is essential because re-expansion of the lacerated lung compresses the torn vessels and reduces further blood loss. Drainage will also allow the mediastinal structures to return to the midline and relieve compression of the contralateral lung. If left, a dense fibrothorax will result, with the possibility of an added empyema. The procedure is similar to drainage for pneumothorax but a wide-bore tube (>28 Fr) is required and a basal drain is sometimes necessary. Continuing blood loss in excess of 200 ml/hour may require urgent thoracotomy within the first few hours.

Lung parenchyma

Lung contusion. The underlying lung is often injured in moderate-to-severe blunt thoracic trauma and the area of contusion may be extensive. This usually resolves but lacerations with persistent air leak may require exploration by thoracotomy. It is important to prevent infection of the underlying lung by early mobilisation (if the patient's condition permits), prophylactic antibiotics, suction drainage and physiotherapy. The importance of a good-quality posteroanterior erect chest radiograph following any trauma to the lung cannot be overemphasised (Fig. 47.4).

Major airways

Injuries to major bronchi are infrequently seen as the patient rarely survives the insult leading to major airway disruption. There is usually a combination of surgical emphysema, haemoptysis and pneumothorax. Chest drainage in spite of the addition of suction fails to reinflate the lung and a persistent air leak may be present. Injury to the trachea requires considerable force and consequently less than a quarter of patients survive to reach hospital. The injury may be from direct trauma or the result of high intratracheal

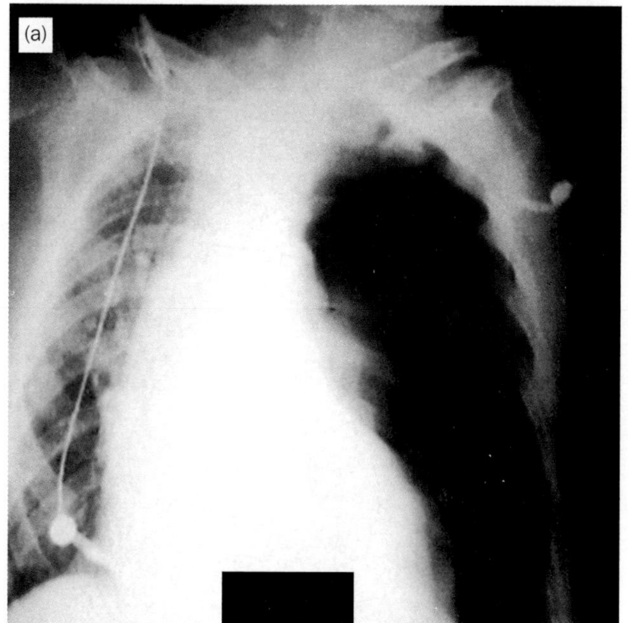

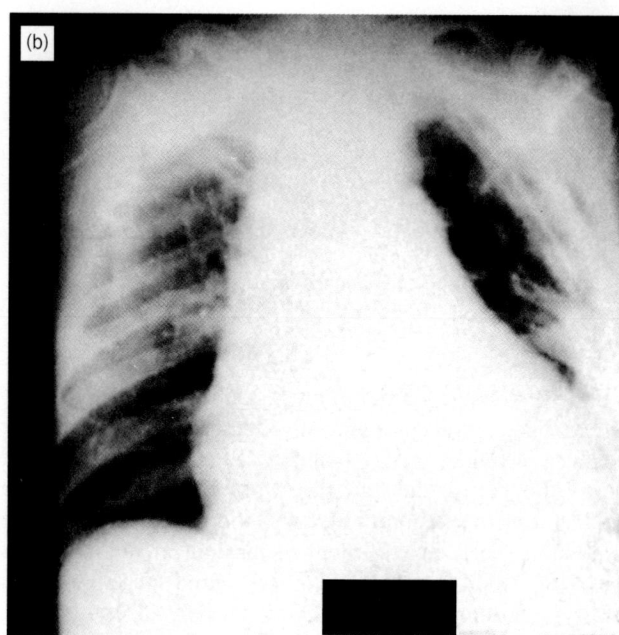

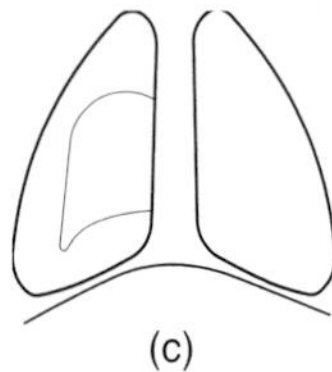

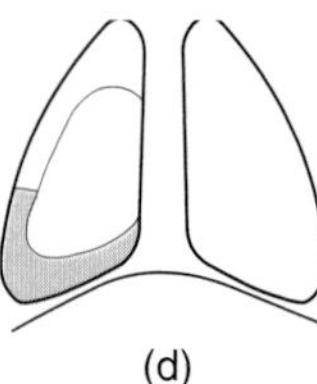

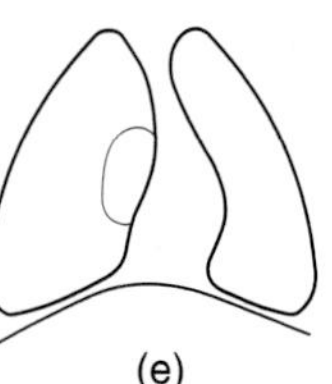

Fig. 47.4 (a) Traumatic tension pneumothorax showing mediastinal shift and compression of the contralateral lung; (b) resolution of the radiographic appearances following insertion of intercostal tube. Diagrammatic appearances of haemothorax: (c) minor pneumothorax; (d) haemopneumothorax; and (e) tension pneumothorax.

pressure against a closed glottis. There is hoarseness, dyspnoea and surgical emphysema. The exact pattern of signs will depend on the site of the injury and whether or not the pleura has been breached. The treatment is exploration and repair if possible. Resection of lung should be avoided as a surprising degree of recovery may occur.

Diaphragm

Diaphragmatic rupture. The mechanism for diaphragmatic rupture is high-speed blunt abdominal trauma with a closed glottis. The sudden rise in intra-abdominal pressure breaches the weakest part of the abdominal wall, namely the diaphragm. This occurs much more commonly on the left hemidiaphragm (the right is protected by the liver). Colon and stomach may herniate into the thorax, displacing the lung. Bowel sounds may be heard in the chest and the chest radiograph may reveal bowel gas in the lung fields. A contrast study will confirm the diagnosis. Occasionally, the injury is overlooked and the patient presents some time later with a diaphragmatic hernia. Cases presenting acutely should be explored by thoracotomy not only to repair the diaphragm and prevent respiratory embarrassment, but to exclude injury to an underlying abdominal viscus such as the spleen. Penetrating injuries below the level of the eighth rib may penetrate the diaphragm and injure an underlying abdominal viscus.

Oesophageal injury

The oesophagus is rarely injured in blunt trauma. The management of penetrating trauma to the oesophagus is discussed in Chapter 50.

Cardiac injury

Major injuries to the heart and great vessels from blunt trauma are frequently fatal and the patient rarely survives long enough to reach hospital. The injuries that are encountered in the accident and emergency department are the following.

Myocardial contusion. This must be suspected when the sternum is fractured, although the true incidence is not known. Myocardial damage from trauma will give an ECG pattern similar to myocardial infarction and enzyme changes may occur. In severe trauma there may be arrhythmias and signs of heart failure. Patients with ECG changes and enzyme rises even in the absence of any problems should be nursed in a high-dependence area with full monitoring and resuscitation equipment available. There is no specific treatment in the uncomplicated case but the risk of fatal arrhythmia diminishes after 48 hours or until the enzymes have returned to normal and any ECG changes have resolved. Occlusion of the coronary arteries progressing to discrete, localised myocardial infarction has been documented.

Chamber rupture and valve blow-out. This is well described and is thought to occur if the ventricle is compressed just before systole at the point of maximal diastolic filling. Chamber rupture is likely to be fatal and those that do survive are likely to have an atrial rupture. Rupture of the mitral or tricuspid valve may not be immediately apparent, but a loud pansystolic murmur should arouse suspicion. Surgical treatment usually results in dramatic improvement in these patients.

Aorta

Aortic transection (Fig. 47.5). This is usually the result of a major deceleration injury (road traffic accident or a fall from a height) and the patient often has other injuries. However, only about 15 per cent of patients with aortic transection survive long enough to reach hospital. Of these, two-thirds would die of late rupture within 14 days and the remainder

(a)

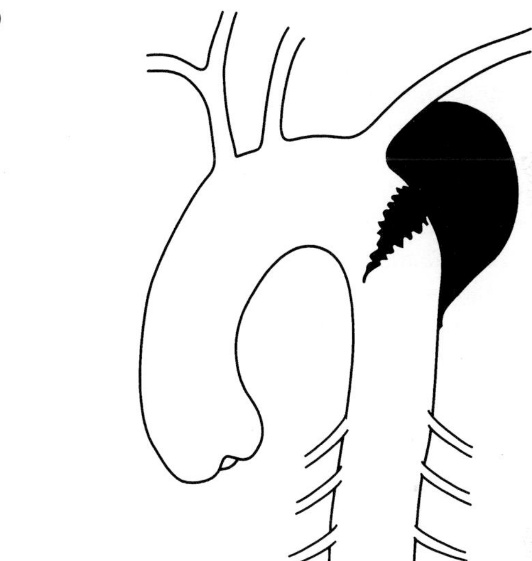

(b)

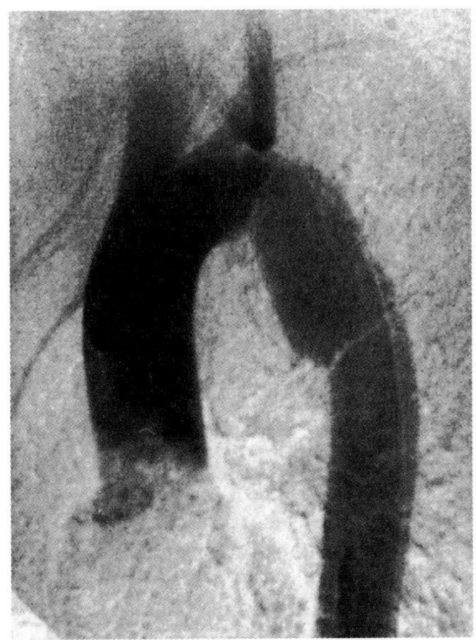

Fig. 47.5 (a) Diagram of aortic transection; (b) aortogram of transection.

would be at risk from rupture of a developing chronic false aneurysm. The site is remarkably consistent (Fig. 47.5a), presumably the anatomy of the aorta determining the site of rupture. The vessel is relatively fixed at the site of the ligamentum arteriosum, just distal to the left subclavian artery, and from there down is tethered to the vertebral column by intercostal arteries and mediastinal pleura. The shear forces from a sudden impact disrupt the intima and media, resulting in retraction. If the intima is not breached, the patient may be stable but the development of a left-sided pleural effusion is an ominous sign. Transection of the aorta must be suspected in all high-speed deceleration incidents. The clinical signs may be masked by concurrent injury but include intrascapular pain, a murmur, hoarseness and radiofemoral delay of the arterial pulse. The condition may be completely asymptomatic. A good-quality posteroanterior chest radiograph showing widening of the mediastinum is very suspicious. Portable chest radiographs taken from the front (anteroposterior) always magnify the mediastinal shadow and cause uncertainty. Aortography is the diagnostic investigation and should be available at most hospitals. Computerised tomography (CT) maybe unhelpful and misleading because transections have little length and intimal lesions are missed on 1-cm slices (in marked contrast to aortic dissection where CT is a valuable investigation). Once the diagnosis is made the treatment is urgent exploration via a left thoracotomy through the fourth intercostal space. Control above and below the transection is vital and the aorta is repaired by direct suture or interposition graft (Fig. 47.6). There is a risk of paraplegia (15 per cent) with this procedure and this should be specifically mentioned to the patient and the relatives before surgery. A heparin-bonded shunt (Gott) to maintain lower body perfusion may reduce the risk of paraplegia. Cardiopulmonary bypass is unsafe because systemic heparinisation is required in an already multiply injured patient.

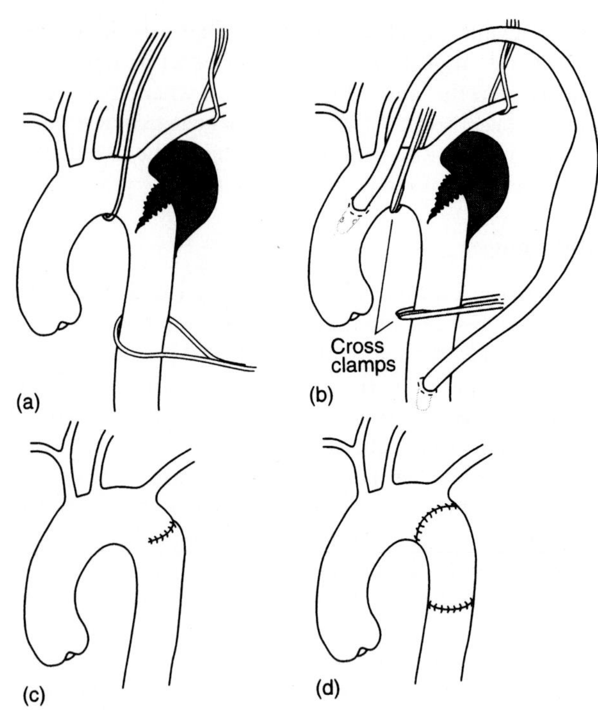

Fig. 47.6 (a)–(c) Diagram of repair transection; (d) insertion of interposition graft if primary repair not possible.

Management of blunt chest trauma

Most chest injuries where the heart is not injured are managed conservatively with underwater seal drainage if necessary, and oxygen and physiotherapy to help the patient to expectorate while the underlying lung parenchyma heals. In about 10 per cent of cases a thoracotomy is required. The indications for thoracotomy following blunt thoracic trauma are the following:

- 50–1000 ml of blood at the time of initial drainage is common and may need no further action, but greater volumes, especially if the blood is fresh, require intervention;
- continued brisk bleeding (>100 ml/15 minutes) from the intercostal drains indicates a serious breach of the lung parenchyma and urgent exploration is required;
- continued bleeding of >200 ml/hour for 3 or more hours may require thoracotomy under controlled conditions;
- rupture of the bronchus, aorta, oesophagus or diaphragm;
- cardiac tamponade (if needle aspiration is unsuccessful).

All explorations following trauma should have double-lumen tube endotracheal intubation to facilitate surgery on the injured side and to protect the undamaged lung.

If transfer is undertaken, the patient *must* be stabilised before the journey. All lines must be secured and ECG monitoring available. Chest drains must *not* be clamped during transfer and a medically qualified person should accompany the patient.

Penetrating injury

In some aspects, penetrating thoracic injury is simpler to deal with than blunt trauma because the wound is visible and the structures at risk can be quickly assessed. A defect in the chest wall through to the pleura is a 'sucking wound'. The underlying lung collapses and air moves in and out of the thorax with each breath. Emergency treatment involves sealing the wound and intercostal drainage. Definitive treatment may then follow. It is important to establish the path or track of bullet and stab wounds in the chest as there may be damage to the heart, great vessels, and the diaphragm and abdominal viscera in addition to the lung injury.

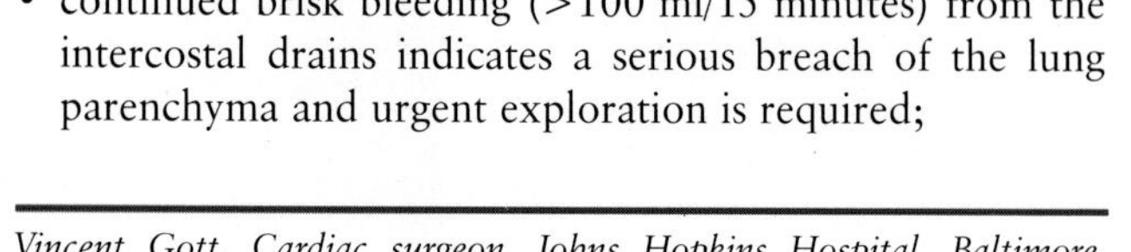

Vincent Gott. Cardiac surgeon, Johns Hopkins Hospital, Baltimore, Maryland, USA.

They are bringing him down,
He looks at me wanly.
The bandages are brown,
Brown with mud, red only –
But how deep a red in the breast of the shirt,
Deepening red too, as each whistling breath
Is drawn with the suck of a slow filling squirt
While waxen cheeks waste to the pallor of death.
From *Casualty*, 1917

by Robert Nichols, 1893–1944, one of the World War I poets.

Bullet wounds create a cavitating defect in the tissues that they pass through. The tissue damage may be very extensive with high-velocity missiles, and entry and exit wounds should be noted. Lung tissue is more compliant than the bone and muscles that comprise the limbs, and enthusiastic resection along the track can be avoided in most cases. Tetanus prophylaxis and high-dose antibiotics (to cover anaerobic organisms) should be given. Bullets lodged in the lung do not require removal if they are not causing any problems.

Penetrating wound of the heart

This is usually the result of a stabbing or shooting incident, but can also be iatrogenic from central line placement, cardiac catheterisation and endomyocardial biopsy. Cardiac tamponade may occur rapidly even with small amounts of blood in the pericardium and the condition is recognised by low blood pressure, tachycardia, a high central venous pressure, pulsus paradoxus and faint heart sound (Fig. 47.7). Emergency treatment includes aspiration of the pericardium by advancing a wide-bore needle to the left of the xiphisternum towards the heart. This may hold the situation until surgical repair is performed. The heart is exposed via a median sternotomy with incision of the pericardium in the midline. For the more generally trained surgeon or those without the necessary equipment to saw the sternum, a left anterior thoracotomy may be preferred. The pericardial cavity is evacuated and the cardiac defect repaired using buttressed sutures. Bullets in cardiac chambers should be removed under cardiopulmonary bypass.

How to do a thoracotomy

All surgeons dealing with trauma victims should be able to perform a thoracotomy if required. The standard route into the thoracic cavity is through a posterolateral thoracotomy. The incision is used for access to:

- the lung and major bronchi;
- the thoracic aorta (aneurysm resection, repair of transection, coarctation repair and ligation of patent ductus arteriosus);
- the oesophagus (resection and repair);
- the posterior mediastinum (for mediastinal mass resection).

Following induction of anaesthesia, a preoperative rigid bronchoscopy is performed, especially if a resection for cancer is contemplated. A double-lumen tube is used to control the lungs separately, if desired. Ventilation may be maintained by ventilating one lung while the other is collapsed to facilitate surgery. However, remember that they were devised to protect the underlying lung from pus and blood, and to stay under the anaesthetist's control. The

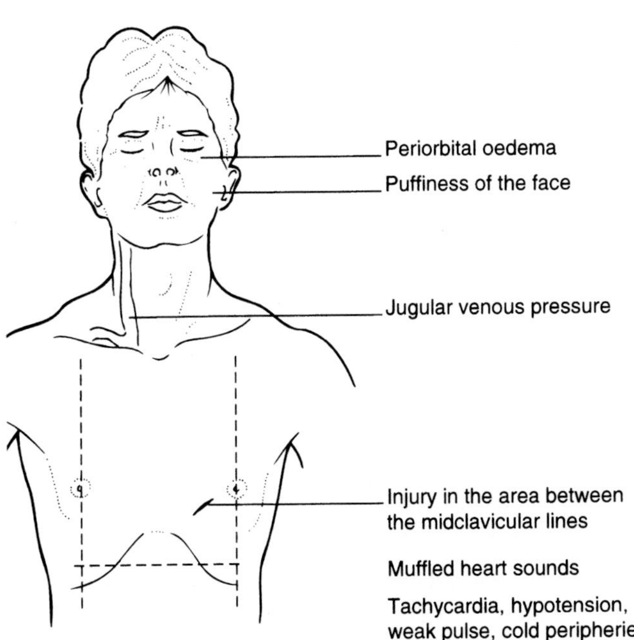

Fig. 47.7 Diagram for suspicion of cardiac injury.

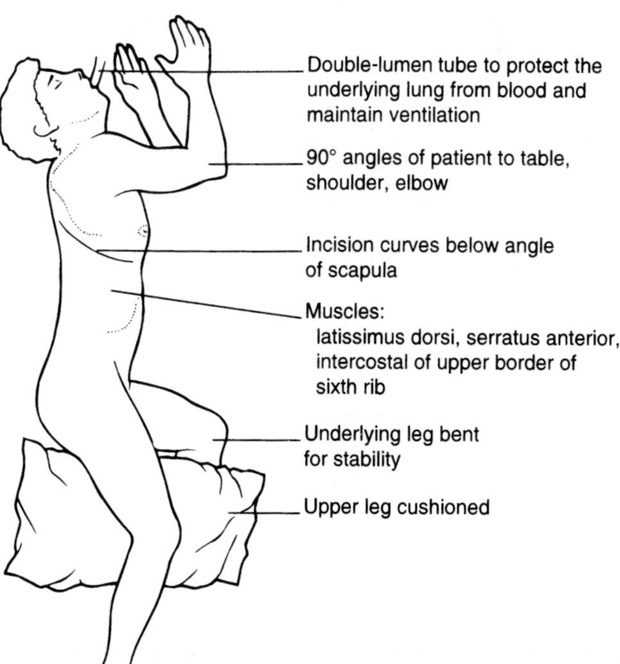

Fig. 47.8 Diagram of correct positioning for thoracotomy.

patient is turned on to the unaffected side in the lateral position (Fig. 47.8). The lower leg is flexed at the hip and the knee with a pillow between the legs. Table supports are used to maintain the position and additional strapping is used at the hips for stability. The upper arm is supported by a bracket in a position of 90° flexion. The lower arm is flexed and positioned by the head. It is important for the surgeon to be completely satisfied with the position of the patient at this stage.

The incision is made from 1 to 2 cm inferolateral to the nipple in men and the inframammary fold in women. The incision extends along 1–2 cm below the tip of the scapula and extends posteriorly and superiorly between the medial border of the scapula and the spine. The incision is deepened through the subcutaneous tissues until the latissimus dorsi is met. This muscle is divided with coagulating diathermy taking care over haemostasis. The line of division is the same as for the skin. A plane of dissection is developed by hand under the scapula and serratus anterior. The ribs can be counted down from the highest palpable rib (which is usually the second) and the sixth rib periosteum is scored with the diathermy near its upper border. A periosteal elevator is used to lift the periosteum off the superior border of the rib. This reveals the pleura which may be entered by blunt dissection. A rib spreader is inserted between the ribs and opened gently to prevent fracture. Exposure may be facilitated by dividing the rib at the costal angle or by dividing the costotransverse ligament. Routine resection of a rib is an uncommon practice. The anaesthetist is now able to deflate the affected lung to allow a better view of the intrathoracic structures. In an emergency thoracotomy for penetrating wounds of the heart, a more anterior approach is used and no specialised supporting equipment is required (Fig. 47.9).

Large-calibre (28–32 Fr) intercostal drains are usually inserted at the end of the procedure. It is common practice to site them through the seventh or eighth intercostal space anterior to the midaxillary line so that the patient does not lie on them. For chronic management, such as closed drainage of empyema, the drains are tunnelled to come out more anteriorly for easier management. Traditionally, the more anteriorly sited drain goes to the apex and the posteriorly placed drain goes to the lung base. A rib approximator is used to realign the ribs and the stripped periosteum and intercostal muscle is sutured to the intercostal muscle below the stripped rib using a continuous absorbable suture. A nonabsorbable suture may be used to maintain the closure if healing is likely to be compromised. The fascia and muscle layer are closed in layers using an absorbable suture (Fig. 47.10). Skin closure is a matter of personal preference.

Analgesia is an important aspect of postoperative care and the process may be started intraoperatively by infiltrating the intercostal nerves in the region of the incision with a long-acting local anaesthetic. Various strategies have been developed to deliver analgesics postoperatively to facilitate a normal breathing pattern.

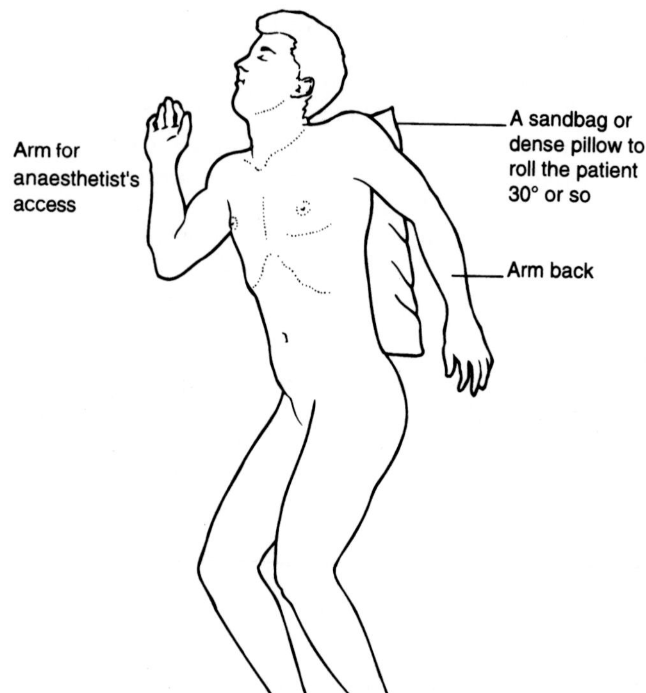

Fig. 47.9 Emergency left anterior thoracotomy for access to the heart. Requires no special supports or devices.

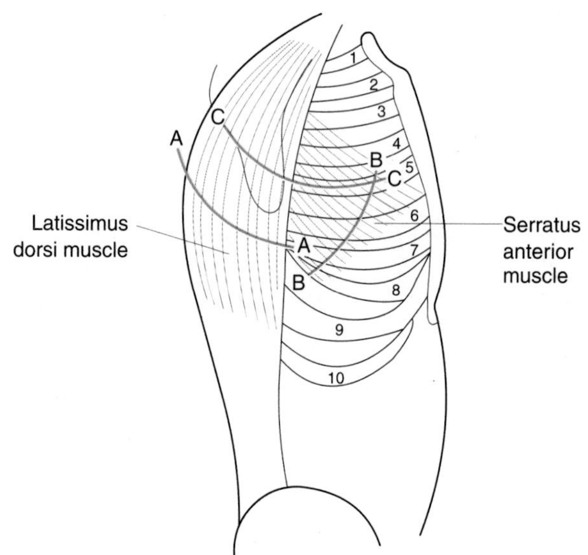

A– A The latissimus dorsi is divided in line with the skin incision
B– B The serratus anterior is divided close to its attachment to ribs 6, 7 and 8
C– C The intercostal muscles are stripped off the upper border of the rib

Fig. 47.10 Diagram of incision and layers encountered during antero-lateral thoracotomy.

Postoperative care

Lung function is rarely assessed before urgent thoracotomy for trauma but it is a vital part of the patient's preoperative work-up before elective thoracotomy. A description of lung function testing is given in Appendix 2 at the end of this chapter. These patients have limited respiratory reserve following lung resection, so infection and fluid overload are to be avoided. Chest drains placed at the time of surgery drain blood collections and cope with air leaks if present. Once the air leaks have settled and any remaining lung is re-expanded, the drains are removed. Mobilisation, breathing exercises and regular physiotherapy are begun as soon as the patient's condition permits.

Postoperative pain

It is important to deal with post-thoracotomy pain effectively so that a normal breathing pattern and gas exchange are achieved in the early postoperative period. Patient-controlled analgesia is an important development but still requires regular nursing and anaesthetic supervision. Internally placed catheters delivering local anaesthetic into the wound and beneath the pleura may also be effective. Long-term post-thoracotomy pain can be avoided by careful attention to detail during the operation. Sources of avoidable chronic pain include rib fracture and entrapment of intercostal nerves during wound closure.

Trauma accounts for most of the emergency workload of the thoracic surgeon but other situations are encountered that demand prompt investigation and treatment.

Airway obstruction

Tracheal obstruction may present acutely as a life-threatening emergency or insidiously with little in the way of symptoms until critical narrowing and stridor occur. The more common causes of airway narrowing are outlined in Table 47.1.

Treatment depends on the underlying cause. Tracheal resection is a very specialised problem but in expert hands up to 6 cm of trachea may be resected without undue tension on the anastomosis. Tracheostomy may be required to overcome the obstruction but there are few indications to do this as an emergency and, in this situation, a crico-thyroidotomy is probably preferable. Tracheal replacement with artificial sub-stitutes has so far been unsuccessful. Sleeve resections of the major bronchi are also possible. Reversible airway obstruction (e.g. asthma) is the domain of respiratory physicians.

Table 47.1 Causes of airway narrowing

Intraluminal
Inhaled foreign body
Neoplasm
Intramural
Congenital stenosis
Fibrous stricture (postintubation or tuberculosis)
Extramural
Neoplasm (thyroid cancer, secondary deposits)
Aortic arch aneurysm

Inhaled foreign bodies

This is a regrettably common occurrence in small children and is often marked by a choking incident which then apparently passes. Surprisingly large objects can be inhaled and become lodged in the wider calibre and more vertically placed right main bronchus. If not removed, an obstructive emphysema may result but, if there is total occlusion of the bronchus, the air distally will be absorbed and the secretions may become infected. There are three possible presentations:

1. asymptomatic;
2. wheezing (from airway narrowing) with a persistent cough and signs of obstructive emphysema;
3. pyrexia with a productive cough from pulmonary suppuration.

A chest radiograph is vital as the object may be radio-opaque. Often it is not radio-opaque or is obscured by the cardiac shadow or the inflammatory response. Bronchoscopy is required by an experienced operator with an experienced anaesthetist to administer the anaesthetic. The procedure may be very difficult if there is a severe inflammatory reaction. The rigid bronchoscope is best for retrieving inhaled foreign bodies. Failure to remove the object may necessitate a bronchotomy through a formal thoracotomy. If the object has caused chronic lung damage it may be necessary to remove the affected lobe.

Haemoptysis

There is a variety of conditions giving rise to repeated haemoptysis, including carcinoma, bronchiectasis, carcinoid tumours and certain infections. Severe rheumatic mitral stenosis is a rare cause. All patients with haemoptysis should be investigated at the very least by chest radiography and bronchoscopy and those with normal findings carefully followed up. Haemoptysis following trauma may be from a lung contusion or injury to a major airway. Severe haemoptysis is unusual and the treatment depends on the underlying cause.

Pulmonary neoplasms

Carcinoma of the bronchus is the most common malignancy in men and the second most common (after carcinoma of the breast) in women. A number of neoplasms affects the airways and suspicion of carcinoma of the bronchus should prompt thorough investigation to make the diagnosis at an early and therefore treatable stage.

Benign tumours

Benign tumours of the lung are uncommon and account for less than 15 per cent of solitary lesions seen on chest radiographs. They are usually an incidental finding on a chest radiograph done for some other reason, but symptoms, when present, depend on the site of the lesion. A peripheral tumour may produce little in the way of symptoms, whereas a centrally placed tumour may present with haemoptysis and signs of bronchial obstruction at a relatively early stage. A tumour is likely to be benign if it has not increased in size on chest radiograph for more than 2 years or has some degree of calcification. However, a tissue diagnosis is advisable as a noncalcified solitary lesion may be a primary carcinoma.

Most benign nodules are granulomas (tuberculosis or histoplasmosis), which give the appearance of a high-density lesion on CT. Low-density appearances are suspicious and the nodule should be removed by excision biopsy. Less than 50 per cent of solitary nodules are benign, underlining the importance of accurate diagnosis.

The most common benign tumour is the pulmonary hamartoma which is really a developmental abnormality containing mesothelial and endothelial elements. They may be lobulated and, although unlikely to undergo malignant transformation, they may be multicentric. Diagnosis (and definitive treatment) is achieved by excising the lesion.

Epithelial tumours

Epithelial tumours of the airways are a particularly troublesome problem. The airways become infected with a papilloma virus at birth and small stalk-like papillomas develop, initially in the larynx and then down into the major airways. Regular endoscopic follow-up is required following bronchoscopic resection, because recurrence is common and malignant change may occur.

Fibroma

Fibroma is the most common mesodermal tumour and tends to occur in the bronchi rather than the trachea. Fibromas are often pedunculated and therefore easily removed at bronchoscopy.

Hamartoma

Hamartoma is a disorganised mass of tissue within the lung substance containing respiratory structures. It is the result of a developmental abnormality and malignant change is rare.

Any of the mesodermal elements of the lung may form a mesodermal tumour (chondroma, lipoma, leiomyoma). Deposits of amyloid may give similar radiographic appearances of a nodule (pseudotumour).

Bronchial adenomas

Bronchial adenomas are mainly carcinoid tumours derived from the neuroendocrine cells of bronchial glands. Most (80 per cent) are found in the major bronchi and are characteristically slow growing and highly vascular. Occasionally these tumours secrete hormones [adenocorticotrophic hormone (ACTH), melanocyte-stimulating hormone or insulin]. This may be the first presentation but usually there are recurrent chest infections, persistent cough, haemoptysis and occasionally chest pain. Carcinoid tumours belong to a class of tumours that are benign at one end of the scale, to those that are locally aggressive and to the highly malignant oat cell tumour at the other end of the scale. Surgical excision is the most appropriate treatment and regular follow-up is advised.

Malignant tumours

Carcinoma of the bronchus, as stated earlier, is the most common malignancy in men and the second most common in women (following carcinoma of the breast), resulting in over 30 000 deaths per year in the UK (Fig. 47.11). There is only a 20 per cent 1-year survival for all cases after diagnosis and surgery represents the best chance of prolonged survival.

Accurate diagnosis and staging of the tumour are vital if surgery is to be considered. The real incidence of carcinoma of the bronchus earlier in the twentieth century was probably masked by the presence of tuberculosis. Once a cure for tuberculosis became available, the importance of carcinoma of the lung became apparent. Cigarette smoking is undoubtedly one of the major risk factors for developing bronchial carcinoma. To a lesser extent, atmospheric pollution and certain occupations (radioactive ore and chromium mining) also contribute to the problem. In the UK, the mortality from lung cancer for individuals smoking more than 40 cigarettes per day is over 210/100 000. This compares to a mortality of less than 4/100 000 in nonsmokers. Regular smoking causes characteristic changes in the bronchial epithelium from hyperplasia through squamous metaplasia to preinvasive carcinoma *in situ*. These changes are to some extent reversible if smoking is stopped.

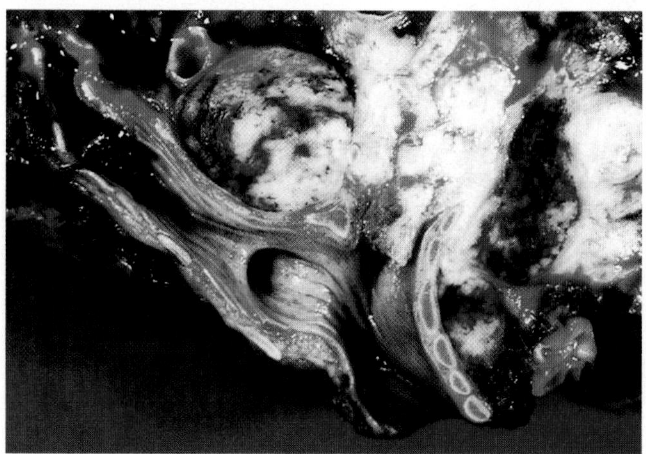

Fig. 47.11 Operative specimen of a carcinoma occluding a bronchus.

Histological types

Many bronchial and lung tumours have more than one cell type, and the behaviour and prognosis depend largely on the dominant cell type seen. There are several histological types which have an important bearing on prognosis and response to treatment.

Squamous cell carcinoma (SCC) accounts for the majority (over 60 per cent) of lung cancers. It is uncommon in nonsmokers and tends to be centrally placed. There is a tendency to cavitate and metastasise outside the thoracic cavity.

Adenocarcinoma is less common than SCC (15 per cent) in the UK but the incidence can vary in different countries. It is more common in females and nonsmokers, and tends to be sited in the periphery of the lung. Adenocarcinomas often metastasise widely to the liver, brain and adrenals. The typical histological appearance is that of gland formation and the only worthwhile treatment, if feasible, is surgical excision (Fig. 47.12). It is important to exclude secondary adenocarcinoma from other sites such as colon, breast and ovary.

Small cell carcinoma metastasises widely early in its course and is therefore rarely amenable to surgical resection. If discovered early then surgical removal has led to increased survival, but palliative chemotherapy and radiotherapy are the most appropriate treatment. These tumours are often associated with ectopic hormone production and paraneoplastic syndromes. The 5-year survival is less than 5 per cent, even with treatment.

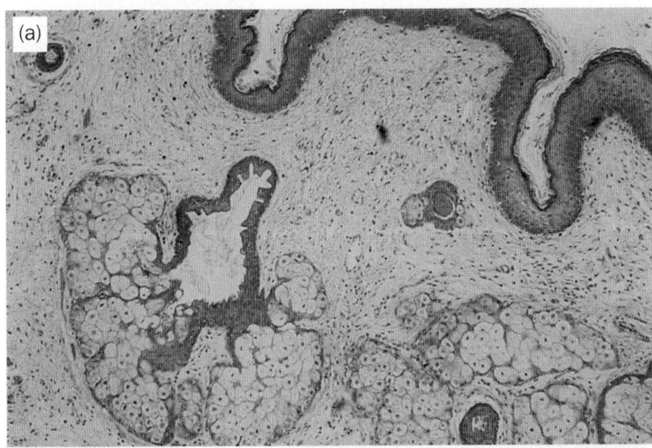

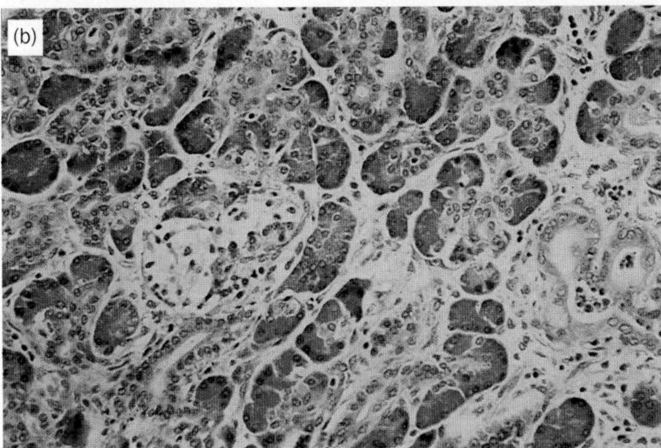

Fig. 47.12 Photomicrograph showing a moderately well-differentiated adenocarcinoma. (Hematoxylin and eosin.)

Alveolar cell carcinoma arises in the distal airways. Resection of a solitary nodule is associated with a good prognosis but the occurrence of a multicentric pneumonic type of alveolar cell carcinoma is associated with a poor prognosis.

Clinical features

Clinical features of lung carcinoma depend on:

- the site of the lesion;
- invasion of neighbouring structures;
- the extent of metastases.

Common symptoms include a persistent cough, weight loss, dyspnoea and nonspecific chest pain. Haemoptysis occurs in less than 50 per cent of patients presenting for the first time. Severe localised pain suggests chest wall invasion with the infiltration of an intercostal nerve. Invasion of the apical area may involve the brachial plexus leading to Pancoast's syndrome. Dyspnoea may come from loss of functioning lung tissue, lymphatic invasion or the development of a large pleural effusion. Clubbing and hypertrophic pulmonary osteoarthropathy are sometimes seen, particularly with squamous cell lesions. These features may resolve with excision of the primary lesion. The presence of blood in a pleural effusion suggests that the pleura is invaded. Invasion of the mediastinum may result in hoarseness (due to recurrent laryngeal nerve involvement), dysphagia (due to involvement of, or extrinsic pressure on, the oesophagus) and superior vena caval obstruction. Hormonal secretion by a tumour will have predictable pathological and physiological effects depending on the nature of the hormone. Small cell carcinoma is associated with the development of myopathies including the Eaton–Lambert syndrome, which is similar to myaesthenia gravis although the weakness tends to improve with repeated movement.

Diagnosis and staging

There are three keys to diagnosis:

- detection of the primary lesion;
- tissue diagnosis;
- assessment of spread (Table 47.2).

Detection of the primary lesion. ***Chest radiography.*** The principal investigation in detecting pulmonary pathology is a good-quality posteroanterior chest radiograph with an additional lateral view. The radiographic appearance will vary according to the site of the lesion and its effects (pleural effusion, lobar collapse, raised hemidiaphragm) (Fig. 47.13).

Henry Khunrath Pancoast, 1875–1939. Philadelphia radiologist.
Lee McKendree Eaton, 1905–58. American physician.
Edward Howard Lambert, b. 1915. American physiologist.

Table 47.2 The international TNM staging system

Primary tumour (T)
- TX – tumour proven by the presence of malignant cells and bronchial secretions but not visualised by radiography or by bronchoscopy
- T_0 – no evidence of primary tumour
- TIS – carcinoma *in situ*
- T_1 – a tumour that is 3 cm or less in greatest dimension, surrounded by lung or visceral pleura and without evidence of invasion proximal to a lobar bronchus at bronchoscopy
- T_2 – a tumour more than 3 cm in greatest dimension or a tumour of any size that either invades the visceral pleura or has associated atelectasis or obstructive pneumonitis that extends to the hilar region, but does not involve an entire lung; at bronchoscopy, the proximal extent of demonstrable tumour must be within a lobar bronchus or at least 2 cm distal to the carina
- T_3 – a tumour of any size, with direct extension into the chest wall (including superior sulcus tumours), diaphragm, mediastinal pleura or pericardium without involving the heart, great vessels, trachea, oesophagus or vertebral body, or a tumour in the main bronchus within 2 cm of the carina without involving the carina
- T_4 – a tumour of any size, with invasion of the mediastinum, or involving the heart, great vessels, trachea, oesophagus, vertebral body or carina, or the presence of malignant pleural effusion

Nodal involvement (N)
- N_0 – no demonstrable metastasis or regional lymph node
- N_1 – metastasis to lymph nodes in the peribronchial or the ipsilateral hilar region or both, including direct extension
- N_2 – metastasis to the ipsilateral mediastinal and subcarinal lymph nodes
- N_3 – metastasis to contralateral mediastinal lymph nodes, contralateral hilar lymph nodes, ipsilateral or contralateral scalene or supraclavicular lymph nodes

Distant metastasis (M)
- M_0 – no known distant metastasis
- M_1 – distant metastasis present

Computerised tomography (CT). This is more sensitive and reproducible than tomography, and has become almost routine in the assessment of these patients. The questions that the surgeon wants answered are (1) is the lesion resectable and (2) are the mediastinal lymph nodes involved? These two questions determine the prognosis (Fig. 47.14). Unfortunately, CT cannot always provide the answers. Lymph nodes more than 2 cm in diameter are likely to be involved in the disease (70 per cent) but those smaller than this (1–2 cm) may or may not be involved. Mediastinal lymph nodes of less than 1 cm in the longest axis are very unlikely to be involved. Visualisation of the liver by CT is a useful means of excluding metastases. Involvement of the mediastinal lymph nodes is usually regarded as a contraindication to surgery, but this view is continually debated. Enthusiasts of resection still seek to cure lung cancer by more extensive resection in N_2 disease. Resection is only justified in the presence of metastases if there is chronic debilitating sepsis from a cavitating tumour or uncontrolled haemoptysis.

Sputum cytology may reveal malignant cells but the false-negative rate is high, particularly in poorly differentiated lesions.

Bronchoscopy is used to visualise the bronchial tree and is useful in a number of ways (Table 47.3).

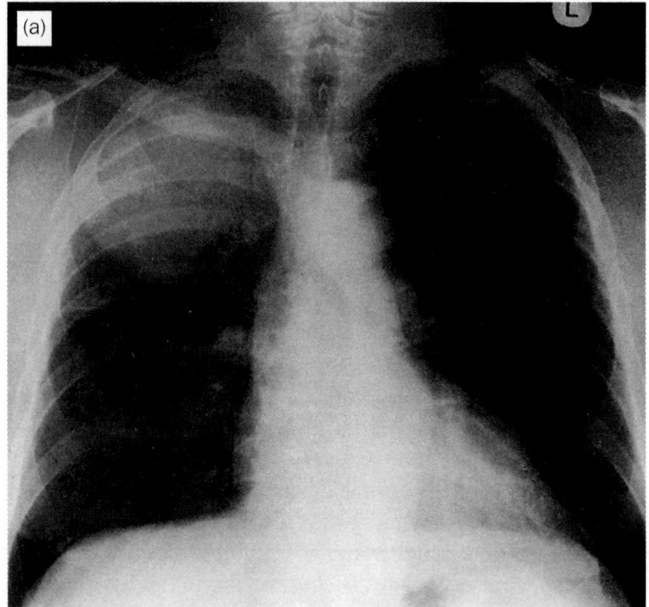

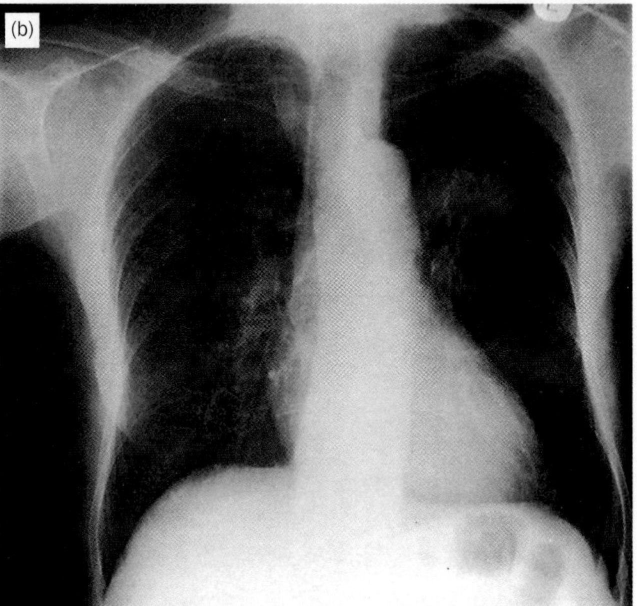

Fig. 47.13 Chest radiographs of carcinoma of the lung. (a) This patient has a large mass in the right upper lobe causing Horner's syndrome. (b) This patient has a left hilar mass and presented with haemoptysis.

Flexible bronchoscopy may be performed with the patient awake and the oropharynx anaesthetised with topical lignocaine (Fig. 47.15). The bronchoscope is passed into the nose and through the vocal folds under direct vision. As the scope is flexible its tip can be directed into the segmental bronchi with ease. Tissue and sputum samples may be obtained for diagnostic purposes. There is a greater range of movement with this instrument but the biopsies are relatively small and the suction facility may not be adequate. Nearly 40 per cent of biopsy diagnoses require modification following resection.

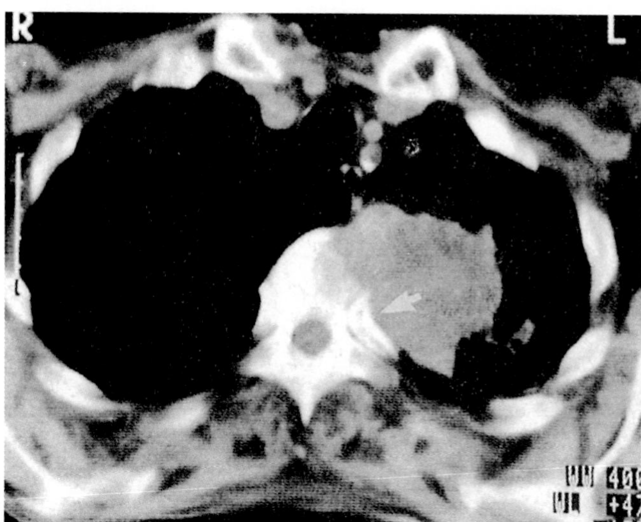

Fig. 47.14 Computerised tomogram of the upper thorax showing a Pancoast tumour invading the adjacent vertebra, making the tumour inoperable.

Table 47.3 Uses of bronchoscopy

Diagnostic
Confirmation of disease
Carcinoma of the bronchus
Vocal cord palsy
Inflammatory process
Infective process
Investigative
Tissue biopsy
Sputum
Preoperative assessment
Before lung resection
Before oesophageal resection
Persistent haemoptysis
Therapeutic
Removal of secretions
Removal of foreign bodies
Stent placement, endobronchial resection, etc.

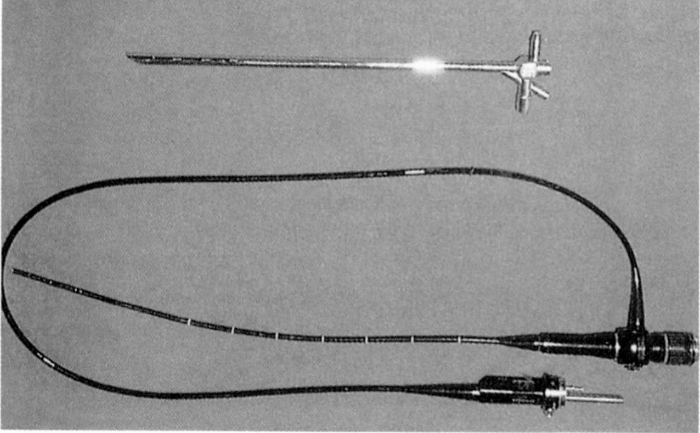

Fig. 47.15 Rigid and flexible rigid bronchoscope.

Rigid bronchoscopy. The rigid bronchoscope requires a general anaesthetic in most cases. However, it is ideal for therapeutic manoeuvres such as removal of foreign bodies, aspiration of blood and thick secretions, and intraluminal surgery (laser resection or stent placement). This instrument, introduced under general anaesthesia, allows visualisation and generous biopsy of the lesion (Fig. 47.15). The surgeon and the anaesthetist share control of the airway. The view is improved by using muscarinic premedication and paralysing agents. Continuous ECG and pulse oximetry monitoring are now mandatory. The operator stands behind the patient and lifts the maxilla by the upper teeth with the middle and forefinger of the left hand. The bronchoscope rests on the left thumb as it is introduced over the tongue in the midline. As the bronchoscope is passed under direct vision into the oropharynx, the neck is extended and the bronchoscope is lowered and advanced to visualise the larynx. Turning the instrument through 90° will help to negotiate the vocal cords. Care must be taken not to trap the lips or tongue between the teeth and the bronchoscope and the fulcrum should be the left thumb and not the teeth. The tracheal rings and the carina should be easily seen. Advancing the bronchoscope into the main bronchus reveals the orifices of the more peripheral bronchi. Operability is determined by the proximity of a lesion to the carina and whether or not the carina is widened (indicating inoperability from subcarinal lymph node involvement). If the bronchoscopy is for diagnosis rather than preoperative assessment, a biopsy may be taken. This should be done when the anaesthetist is satisfied that the anaesthetic can be quickly reversed. The biopsy is taken and a check made for bleeding. The anaesthetic is reversed and the patient turned on the side. This will allow drainage and easy expectoration of any blood or secretions.

Biopsy is hazardous under the following conditions:

- bleeding disorders;
- systemic anticoagulation;
- pulmonary hypertension.

Complications are rare in experienced hands but include bleeding, pneumothorax, laryngospasm and arrhythmia.

Bronchoscopy may not visualise the lesion unless it is in the main airways, and is inadequate for staging operable disease. More invasive techniques of biopsy of intrathoracic lesions are often necessary to confirm diagnosis, stage disease and plan treatment. The options range from percutaneous needle biopsy under radiological control to open lung biopsy (see below).

Needle biopsy. A thin needle passed into a lesion through the chest wall under local anaesthesia gives a good yield of malignant cells. It is best reserved for large or peripheral lesions and is performed under radiological CT control. Pneumothoraces are common (30 per cent) but rarely require intercostal tube drainage. Seeding in the biopsy track and haemorrhage are also reported complications. This procedure is also used in the diagnosis of life-threatening pneumonia where other attempts to establish a diagnosis have failed. The contraindications are similar to those of bronchoscopy but include those with poor respiratory reserve in whom even a small pneumothorax would be fatal.

The more invasive techniques of thoracoscopy, mediastinoscopy, mediastinotomy and open lung biopsy, are aimed at establishing a tissue diagnosis and assessing the degree of spread (staging) which determines resectability. Mediastinoscopy or mediastinotomy is advisable on all patients who have enlarged lymph nodes (>1 cm) on CT of the mediastinum to avoid futile thoracotomy without hope of cure. Smaller nodes are not likely to be involved and thoracotomy may be done based on the benefit of doubt. Whatever staging procedure is used, there will inevitably be a small rate (<5 per cent) of nonresective thoracotomies.

Mediastinoscopy. This procedure is performed under general anaesthesia with the patient supine and the neck extended (Fig. 47.16). A transverse incision is made 2 cm above the sternal notch and deepened until the strap muscles are reached. These are retracted laterally and the thyroid isthmus superiorly to reveal the pretracheal fascia. Careful blunt dissection in this plane allows direct palpation of the paratracheal and subcarinal nodes. A mediastinoscope may be introduced for direct visualisation and biopsy. Care must be taken to avoid damage to the brachiocephalic vessels anteriorly.

Mediastinotomy. An incision is made through the second intercostal space to gain access to some of the mediastinal lymph nodes on the affected side (Figs 47.17 and 47.18). Damage to the internal mammary artery and great vessels must be avoided. Biopsy of the mediastinal lymph nodes is possible and the medial extension of tumour can be assessed, so this technique has important application in the staging of lung cancer.

Great caution should be used in the presence of superior vena caval obstruction and previous exploration is a relative contraindication. Complications include pneumothorax and haemorrhage. These techniques may also be used in the diagnosis of other mediastinal conditions, including:

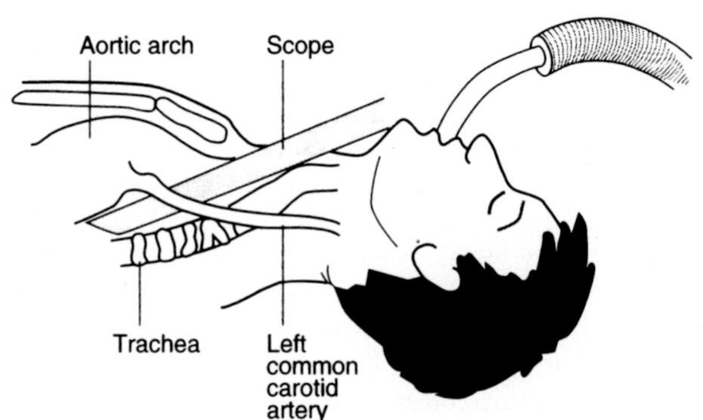

Fig. 47.16 Diagram of mediastinoscopy. The mediastinoscope slides down immediately in front of the trachea behind the aortic arch and behind and between the great vessels of the head and neck.

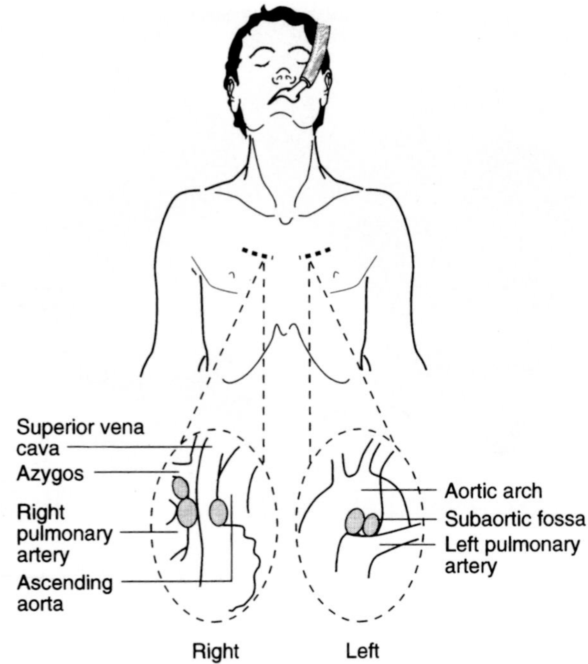

Fig. 47.17 Diagram of mediastinotomy. Structures accessible through anterior mediastinotomy.

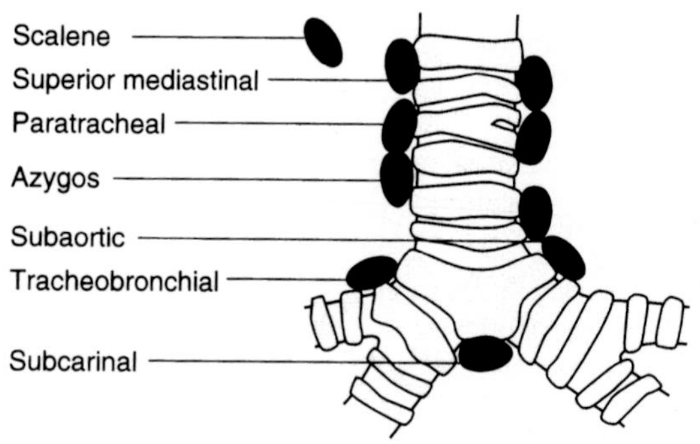

Fig. 47.18 Lymph node sites accessible by the techniques of mediastinotomy and mediastinoscopy.

- lymphoma;
- anterior mediastinal tumours;
- thymoma;
- sarcoid or any other cause of lymphadenopathy.

Thoracoscopy. A thoracoscope may be introduced through a small stab incision and a peripheral lesion biopsied. This requires general anaesthesia and double-lumen intubation. The technique has more application in the diagnosis of suspected metastatic disease and malignant pleural effusion (see Pleura).

Open lung biopsy. This requires a thoracotomy and is rarely performed to diagnose carcinoma. The site of the incision is dictated by the site of the lesion.

Table 47.4 Staging of carcinoma of the lung

Stage	*Tumour*	*Nodal involvement*	*Distant metastasis*	
Occult carcinoma	TX	N_0	M_0	Operable
Stage 0	TIS			
Stage I	T_1	N_0	M_0	
Stage II	T_1	N_1	M_0	
	T_2	N_1	M_0	
Stage IIIa	T_3	N_0	M_0	Inoperable
	T_3	N_1	M_0	
	T_{1-3}	N_2	M_0	
Stage IIIb	Any T	N_3	M_0	
	T_4	Any N	M_0	
Stage IV	Any T	Any N	M_1	

Treatment of lung cancer

Only 10 per cent of patients have potentially curable lesions on presentation, so careful investigation is required to determine which patients are operable and will benefit from a major thoracic resection. The internationally agreed staging system [tumour, node, metastasis (TNM)] gives some prognostic information on the natural history of the disease but it assumes that lung cancer behaves and spreads in a progressive manner by local invasion of the lymph nodes and then into the bloodstream. Tumours graded T_2, N_1, M_0 or less have a better prognosis when treated surgically. This means that the tumour must be staged as accurately as possible before resection (Table 47.4). Unfortunately, most lung cancers are beyond curative treatment at the time of presentation. However, palliation is a skilled process from which patients may benefit in terms of quality of life and disease-free survival. If preoperative investigations suggest that a lesion is localised and resectable then surgery should be undertaken. A number of factors including general fitness of the patient and the lung function tests determines the nature of treatment. Many patients are smokers and elective physiotherapy before the operation may be worthwhile.

Surgical management

The principle of surgery is to remove all cancer (the primary and the regional lymph nodes) but to conserve as much lung as possible. This is usually done by lobectomy but there is evidence that small peripheral lesions have as good an outcome if subjected to segmentectomy or simple wedge excision. A double-lumen tube for separate control of the lungs is used to facilitate dissection. It should be remembered, however, that techniques of one-lung anaesthesia were developed by anaesthetists to protect the nonoperated lung and to retain their control (Fig. 47.19).

Following exploration of the fissure, the lobar artery is isolated and ligated. The vein is then divided and oversewn leaving the affected bronchus, which is divided so as not to leave a stump. The divided bronchus is oversewn or stapled according to preference (Fig. 47.20).

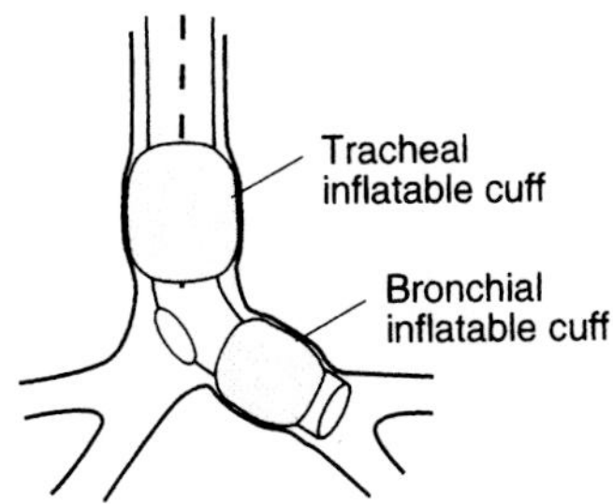

Fig. 47.19 The theory behind single lung anaesthesia.

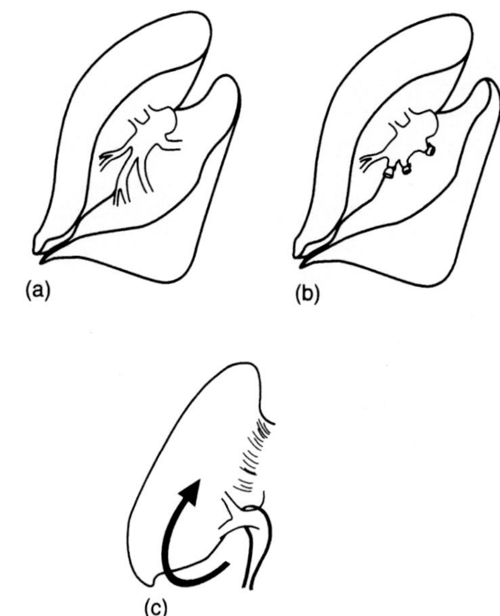

Fig. 47.20 Diagram of stages in lobectomy. (a) Pulmonary branches in fissure; (b) apical lower and basal divided, upper and lingula conserved; (c) inferior vein found inferiorly by turning lung up.

At the completion of the operation, the remaining lung is reinflated. Air leak is common and usually settles within a number of days. Intercostal drains are inserted to lie basally and apically. The patient is extubated in the recovery area once ventilation is deemed adequate.

Pneumonectomy is removal of the whole lung. This is a major undertaking and has a high mortality rate (5–10 per cent). The surgeon must be satisfied that the patient is fit enough to tolerate this procedure from the preoperative work-up. This procedure is reserved for either centrally placed tumours involving the main bronchus or those that straddle the fissure. At thoracotomy, an inspection of the lung and direct palpation of the mass will determine resectability and lymph node spread. Fixation of the tumour to the aorta, heart or oesophagus implies irresectability. Involvement of the mediastinal lymph chain is associated with a poor prog-

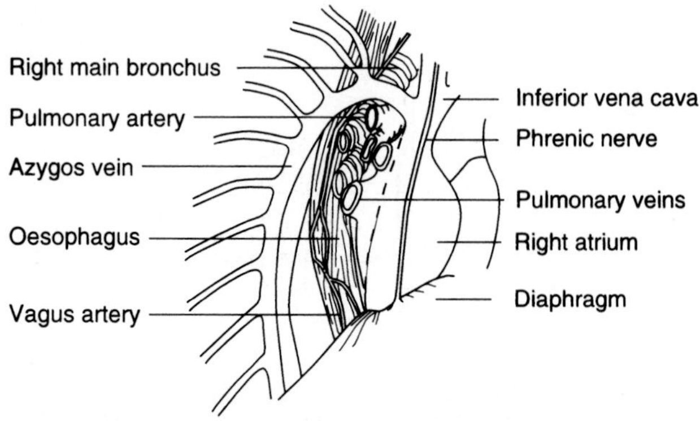

Fig. 47.21 Mediastinal structures after removal of right lung.

nosis. In all, 5–10 per cent of thoracotomies are exploratory only with no resection. The objective is to keep this to a minimum but extensive conservation would deny the patient a chance of cure.

Pneumonectomy, if performed, involves isolation of the main pulmonary artery after the initial exploration. An occlusive clamp is placed across the artery and, if this is tolerated, the resection proceeds. The artery is divided and oversewn. The pulmonary veins are then isolated and clamped. They too are divided and oversewn. This leaves the main bronchus which is divided so that no blind stump remains (Fig. 47.21). The technique of stump closure is important if a bronchopleural fistula is to be avoided. The tissues are carefully handled and the stump is closed with good apposition of the sides. Topical antibiotics may be used to prevent infection. The chest cavity is irrigated with warm saline to remove any blood clots or debris. Some saline is left in the hemithorax to cover the bronchial stump. The anaesthetist manually ventilates after the clamp is removed from the tube serving the affected side. The inflation pressures are gradually increased until the surgeon is satisfied that there is no leak present (by the absence of bubbles in the saline). Haemostasis is vital because there is a large space left after pneumonectomy. Drainage is a matter of preference. Some prefer to insert drains and unclamp them for 1 minute every hour until the drainage ceases; others prefer not to drain. The critical point is that no suction should be applied as there is now a sealed space with the mobile mediastinum on one side of it. The air in the pneumonectomy space is gradually absorbed and the fluid level within the space rises (Fig. 47.22).

Thoracoscopic lung resection. Minimally invasive surgery has become fashionable in recent years in all forms of sur-

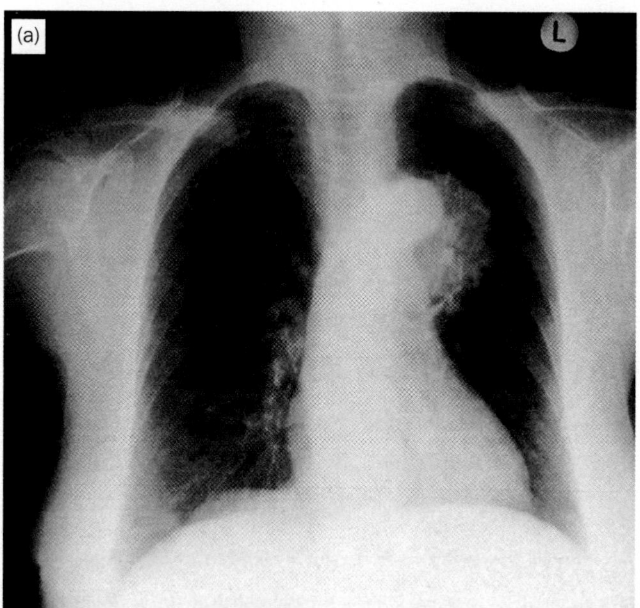

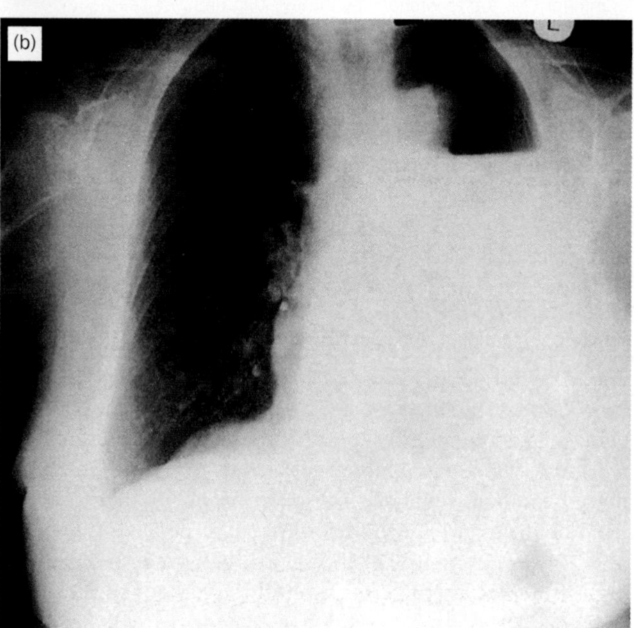

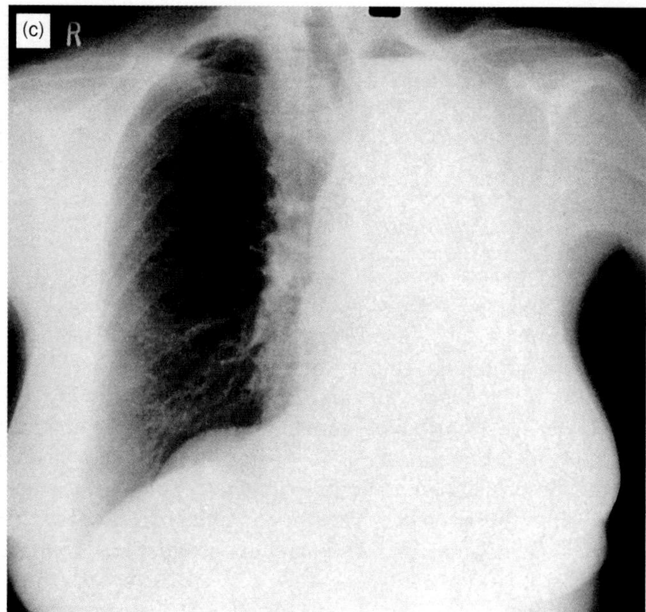

Fig. 47.22 Chest radiographs pre- and postpneumonectomy with rising fluid level in the left haemothorax.

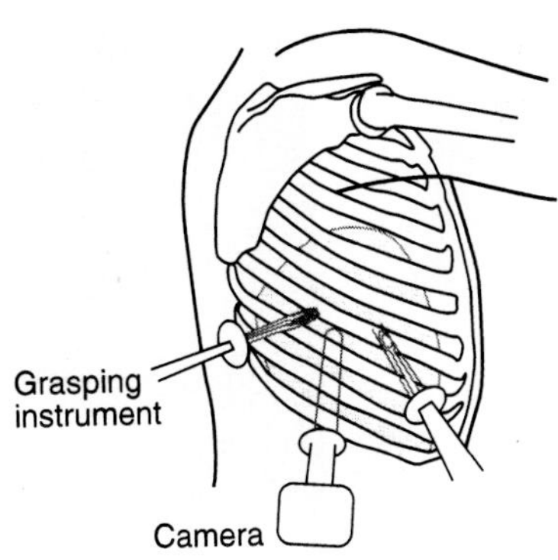

Fig. 47.23 Video-assisted thoraoscopic surgery (VATS). In general three ports are used. One is for the camera attached to a more remote video screen. This allows the surgeon to manipulate the lung with instruments introduced via two further ports.

gery. The thoracoscope has been used for many years but its use was limited mainly to performing biopsies. The instrument had a limited view and was uncomfortable to use for any length of time. All this has changed since the advent of video-assisted thoracoscopy (Fig. 47.23). The surgeon's hands are freed because the camera is attached to the thoracoscope which can be operated by an assistant; and the image is displayed on a television screen. The surgeon is able to manipulate instruments with both hands to perform an impressive variety of procedures. Pneumonectomy, lobectomy and empyema drainage are all possible, but thoracoscopic procedures for common, more minor problems is the area providing clear justification for this technique. Lung biopsy and the treatment of recurrent pneumothorax are the most frequent indications for this technique of operation. The principal advantage is that a large incision is not required and therefore less postoperative pain and a more rapid recovery should result. The scope of thoracoscopic surgery is increasing with the modern trend of less invasive surgery. Thoracoscopic lobectomy is now a feasible and reproducible procedure although the long-term results remain unproven. The thoracoscope is used in staging lung and oesophageal malignancy and in sympathectomy. Port access coronary artery surgery will be discussed in Chapter 48.

Complications of lung resection

Bleeding should be avoidable by use of careful surgical technique but may be very severe in the presence of dense adhesions.

Respiratory infection. Many of these patients are ex-smokers so basal collapse and hypoxaemia are common postoperatively.

Persistent air leak. Chest drains placed at the time of surgery should deal with this problem, but occasionally the air leak becomes chronic and the remaining lung does not expand. Rethoracotomy may then be necessary to seal the leak.

Bronchopleural fistula. Following pneumonectomy, the space left behind is initially filled with air. This is slowly reabsorbed and the space fills with tissue fluid. The fluid level rises until the air is finally reabsorbed. Dehiscence of the bronchial stump leads to the development of a bronchopleural fistula and the tissue fluid (which is almost inevitably infected) is expectorated in large quantities. This is a catastrophic complication with high morbidity and mortality. The patient is laid flat with the affected side down (to prevent infected fluid from entering the remaining lung) while arrangements are made to site a pleural drain. Bronchopleural fistulas are unlikely to resolve with conservative treatment and therefore some operative strategy must be tried. There is a number of ways of sealing the fistula, from tissue glue down the rigid bronchoscope to thoracotomy and a muscle flap to cover the bronchial stump. Bronchoscopic sealing with tissue glue may be successful but is difficult. Resuturing the bronchial stump may lead to healing and the thoracotomy will allow evacuation and thorough irrigation of the pneumonectomy space. Closure is more successful if viable tissue can be brought over the bronchial stump. This is achieved by dissecting a pedicle of intercostal muscle off the chest wall leaving its artery and vein intact and suturing it over the repair. Omentum is an alternative source of pedicled tissue. If closure is not possible or the patient will not tolerate closure, then a fenestration procedure may be performed to allow drainage of the fluid, usually including rib resection. Suturing the skin to the pleural surface to form a Clagett window provides chronic management in desperate circumstances.

Hypoxaemia. Poor oxygenation, as a result of pre-existing lung damage, pulmonary oedema from overenthusiastic crystalloid replacement, atelectasis and bronchopneumonia, may occur. Treatment is aimed at the underlying cause but great care must be taken in pneumonectomy patients who are very susceptible to hypoxaemia.

Survival

Carcinoma of the bronchus generally has a low survival rate after diagnosis (Table 47.5). Important factors in determining prognosis are the histological type of tumour, the spread

Table 47.5 Survival table for carcinoma of the bronchus

Five-year survival according to presurgical staging	%
Stage I	56–67
Stage II	39–55
Stage IIIa	23
Stage IIIb	<10
Five-year survival according to cell type	%
Squamous cell carcinoma	35–50
Adenocarcinoma	25–45
Adenosquamous carcinoma	20–35
Undifferentiated carcinoma	15–25
Small cell carcinoma	0–5

(stage) and the general condition of the patient. The 5-year survival rate is less than 2 per cent if no treatment is offered at the time of diagnosis and ipsilateral lymph nodes are involved. Those with mediastinal lymph nodes discovered and removed at thoracotomy have a better prognosis (15–30 per cent 5-year survival). Early detection and surgical resection offer the best hope for cure.

The mediastinum

Primary tumours of the mediastinum (Fig. 47.24)

Secondary involvement from direct infiltration of an intrathoracic primary or metastatic disease from elsewhere occurs more frequently than primary mediastinal tumours. Thymoma, neurogenic tumours and lymphoma account for most primary tumours of the mediastinum. Rarer conditions such as germ cell tumours, mesenchymal and endocrine tumours account for the remainder.

Thymoma

This is the most common mediastinal tumour accounting for 25 per cent of the total. These are tumours of the thymic epithelial cells of Hassall's corpuscles and are sited in the anterior and superior compartments. They generally occur after childhood and present as lobulated, occasionally calcified, masses in the anterior mediastinum (Fig. 47.25). They may appear encapsulated and are often associated with the autoimmune disease myasthenia gravis. The tumours vary in their behaviour from completely benign to aggressively invasive. The only reliable indicator of malignancy is capsular invasion. Diagnosis and treatment are best achieved by complete thymectomy, but radiotherapy may be the only treatment option if the lesion is advanced.

Eighty per cent of thymomas are benign and the prognosis is good. There is, however, a small risk of recurrence. A rarer type of thymoma has similar histological appearance to the benign thymoma, but it has capsular invasion and is occasionally aggressive with widespread metastases. Rarer still is the thymic carcinoma. This is not associated with myasthenia and resembles an SCC or an undifferentiated large cell tumour. The prognosis is generally poor in spite of combination treatment of excision, radiotherapy and cytotoxic therapy.

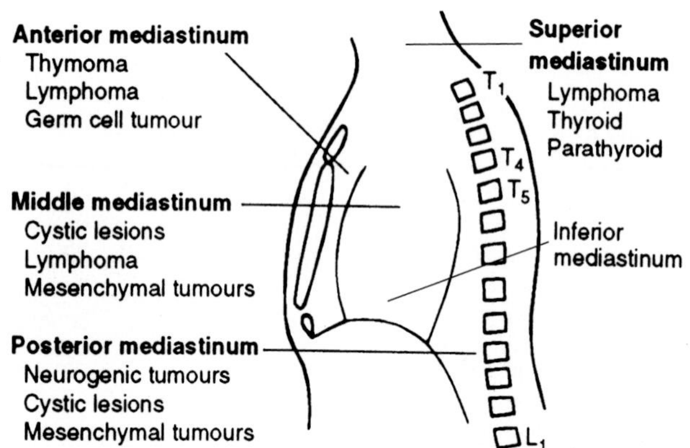

Fig. 47.24 Mediastinal pathology. Subdivisions of the mediastinum with the most common mediastinal masses.

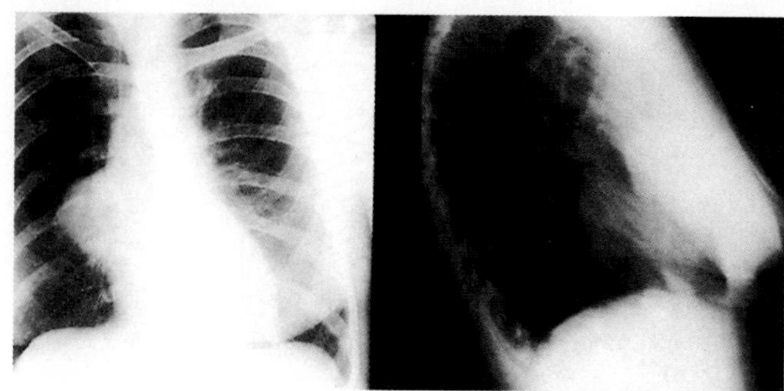

Fig. 47.25 Thymoma presenting as a mediastinal mass (chest radiograph).

Germ cell tumour

Germ cell tumours account for 13 per cent of all mediastinal masses and cysts, and are usually found in the anterior mediastinum (Fig. 47.26). They tend to occur in young adults and 75 per cent are benign and cystic, although they may cause compression of neighbouring structures. They contain elements from all three cell types (mesoderm, endoderm and ectoderm) and are best treated by surgical excision in case malignant transformation should occur. Malignancy is suspected if elevated levels of serum α-fetoprotein, human chorionic gonadotrophin and carcinoembryonic antigen are detected.

Lymphoma

Lymphoma is a common cause of a mediastinal mass lesion, particularly the anterior mediastinum, leading to obstruction of the superior vena cava. Lymphomas arise from the thymic lymph tissue or the lymph nodes of the mediastinum. They can be classified into Hodgkin's and non-Hodgkin's types but details of the pathological differences and their implications are outside the scope of this chapter. Hodgkin's lymphomas presenting in the thymus tend to be localised and usually have favourable histology and a favourable response to treatment. Non-Hodgkin's lymphomas are usually high grade and are more common in young to middle-aged females. A tissue diagnosis is essential so that the appropriate treatment can be planned. The overall prognosis in non-Hodgkin's lymphomas is poor.

Arthur Hill Hassall, 1817–94. English chemist and physician.
Thomas Hodgkin, 1798–1866. English physician.

(a)

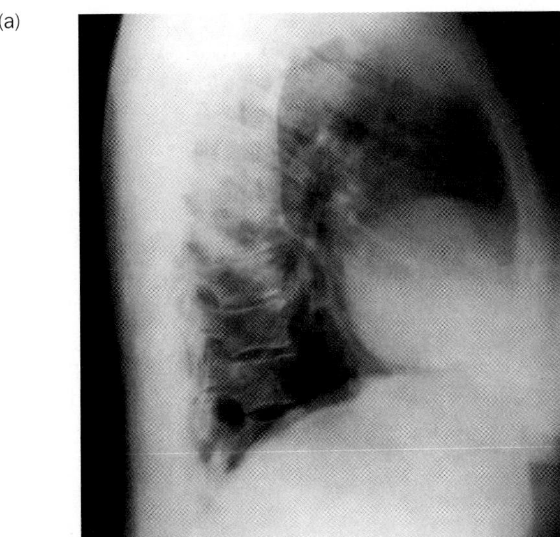

(b)

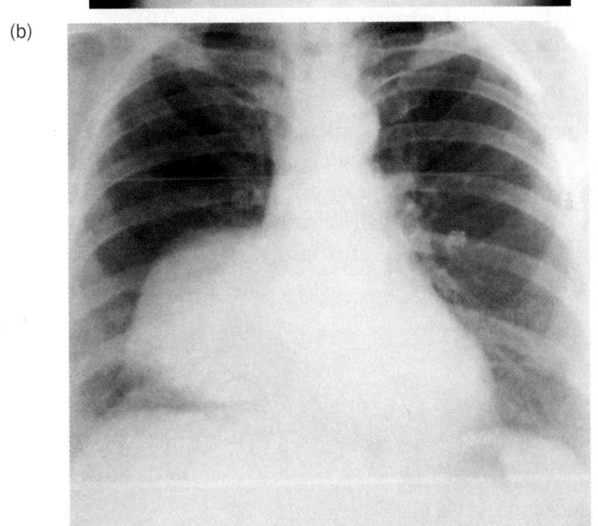

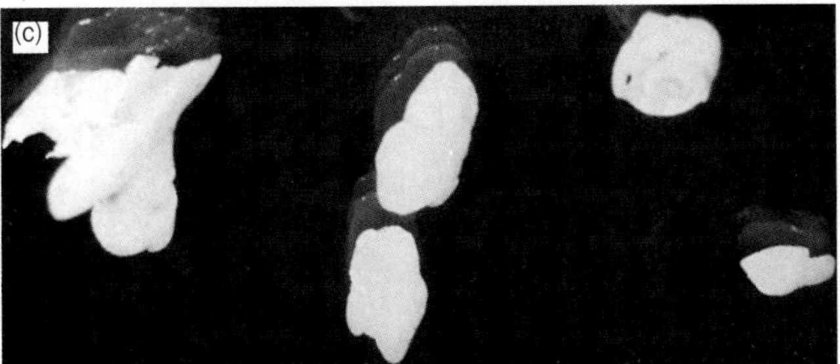

Fig. 47.26 (a) and (b) Lateral and posteroanterior radiographs of patient with a mediastinal teratoma. The tumour lies anteriorly and with a pedicle attached beneath the aortic arch. (c) Radiograph of excised tumour showing formation of teeth.

Mesenchymal tumours

A small number of mesenchymal tumours occurs within the mediastinum and approximately half are malignant. Lipomas are common in the anterior mediastinum, whereas the malignant form, liposarcoma, tends to occur posteriorly. Fibrosarcoma and mesothelioma may also occur.

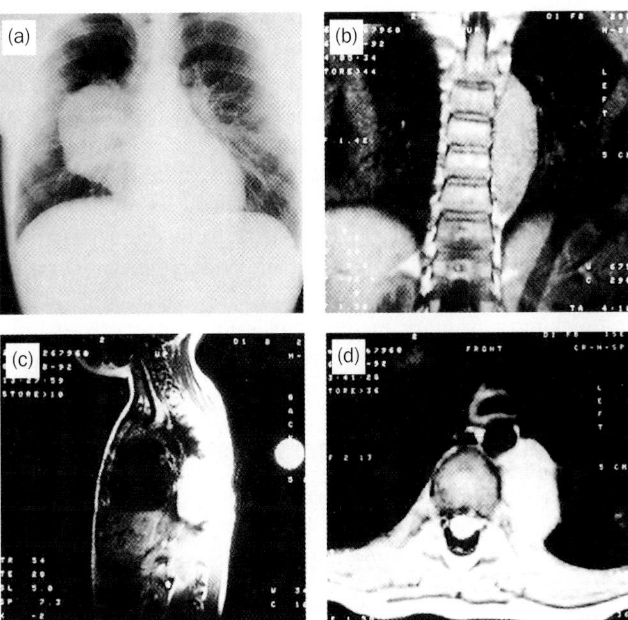

Fig. 47.27 (a) Radiograph; and (b)–(d) magnetic resonance images of a neural tumour.

Thyroid

Ectopic thyroid tissue (and parathyroid) may be found in the anterior mediastinum. Neoplasia and hyperplasia may occur but these are uncommon. More often the tumour is merely a mediastinal extension of a thyroid lesion.

Neural tumours

These may derive from the sympathetic nervous system or the peripheral nerves and are more prevalent in the posterior mediastinum. They may be painful but are more often discovered accidentally on routine chest radiography (Fig. 47.27).

Tumours of the sympathetic nervous system are more common in young patients less than 10 years of age.

Neuroblastoma. This rare childhood tumour consists of poorly differentiated primitive neural cells. It metastasises widely and has a poor prognosis.

Ganglioneuroma. This is a mixture of mature ganglion cells and spindle cells which does not progress after puberty and generally has a good prognosis.

Ganglioneuroblastoma. This tumour has a mixed pattern of mature and immature cell types and has an intermediate prognosis.

Adults are more prone to develop Schwannomas and neurofibromas. The histological appearances are similar to those found in conventional sites and they present as a mass lesion with pressure effects or as asymptomatic radiographic findings.

Theodor Schwann, 1810–82. German anatomist and physiologist; Professor of Anatomy at Louvain.

Tumours of the nerve sheath and fibres (neurofibromas and Schwannomas) have a wide range of presentations and behaviours. Multiple neurofibromas may be part of a familial syndrome (von Recklinghausen's disease, neurofibromatosis). Tumours in the paravertebral gutter may have a component within the intervertebral canal (a so-called 'dumb-bell' tumour).

Phaeochromocytomas. These arise from the sympathetic chain and produce the characteristic endocrine syndrome.

The mediastinum may be involved by metastatic tumour mimicking a primary mediastinal lesion. In elderly people, this is the most common cause of mediastinal lymphadenopathy.

Symptoms of mediastinal masses

Most asymptomatic mediastinal masses discovered by routine chest radiography will be benign. In contrast, masses presenting with symptoms, in particular pain, are much more likely to be malignant.

Symptoms are generally secondary to compression or invasion of a structure within the mediastinum.

Superior vena caval obstruction

Tumours located behind the sternum have little space in which to grow and consequently the low-pressure superior vena cava is the first to be compressed. Venous engorgement of the upper extremities and face occurs and persists even when the patient sits upright. The most common cause of this syndrome is carcinoma of the bronchus and radiotherapy usually provides good symptomatic relief.

Tracheal and oesophageal compression

This may be extrinsic or from mural invasion; symptoms include dysphagia, dyspnoea and occasionally stridor. Radiotherapy or intraluminal stenting may provide some relief.

Neural invasion

A left-sided hilar lesion may infiltrate the recurrent laryngeal nerve and paralyse the vocal cords leading to hoarseness and a bovine cough. Paralysis of the phrenic nerve causes a raised hemidiaphragm on the affected side and indicates irresectability if bronchial carcinoma is present. Horner's syndrome is a result of invasion of the sympathetic chain superiorly.

Pericardial invasion

Direct invasion may cause changes similar to pericarditis with arrhythmias and ECG changes. Chronic tamponade may occur from the slow accumulation of fluid in the pericardium.

Friedrich Daniel von Recklinghausen, 1833–1910. German pathologist.
Johann Friedrich Horner, 1831–86. Swiss ophthalmologist.

Neural tumours

Invasion of the spinal cord may lead to progressive paraplegia.

Investigation and treatment

Investigation of a mediastinal lesion follows the same pattern as investigation for pulmonary lesions with more emphasis on radiology, and mediastinotomy and mediastinoscopy. If a resection is planned, the best approach to the anterior and superior mediastinum is through a median sternotomy. The posterior mediastinum can be reached through a posterolateral thoracotomy at the appropriate level. Any operation must be carefully planned because the pitfalls are numerous and may be difficult or impossible to counter.

Pleural conditions

Normal pleural physiology (Fig. 47.28)

There is a potential space between the parietal and visceral pleura that contains only about 5 ml of pleural fluid at any one time. The amount of pleural fluid is governed by the factors producing and absorbing it (capillary hydrostatic pressure, capillary permeability, lymphatic drainage and colloid osmotic pressure). The turnover of fluid in the human pleural space is about 1 litre in 24 hours. Protein-depleted

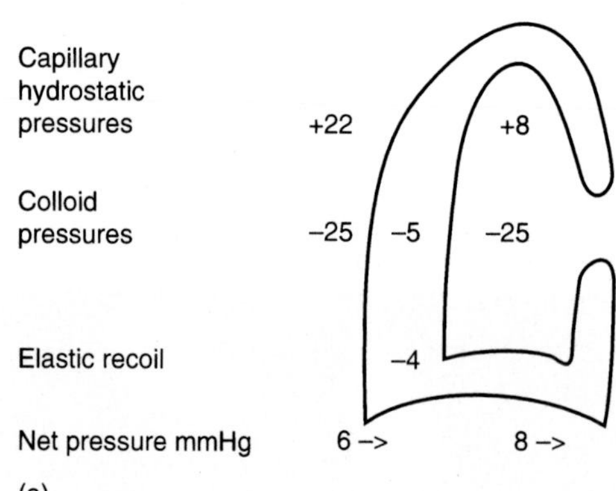

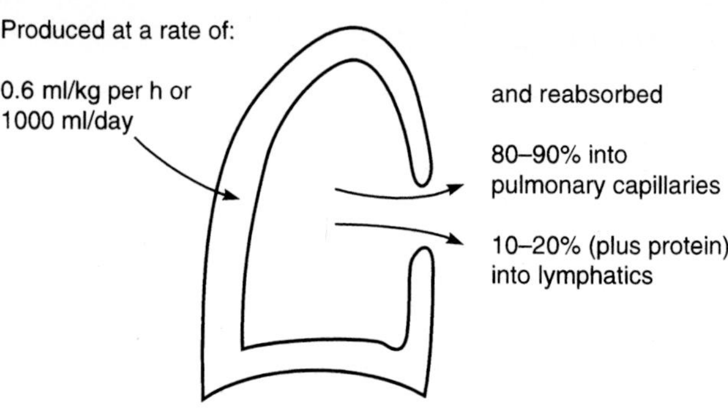

Fig. 47.28 Diagram of normal pleural physiology.

fluid is filtered into the pleural space from the capillaries in the parietal pleura. The fluid is then mostly absorbed into the pulmonary capillaries, with only about 10 per cent being absorbed by the pleural lymphatics.

Any disturbance of the equilibrium will lead to the development of a pleural effusion. There are two described types depending on the protein content of the fluid, although the distinction is not always clear.

Accumulation of protein in the pleural space results if the lymphatic drainage is deranged. This alters the osmotic pressure within the space and leads to the formation of an effusion. There is usually in excess of 30 g of protein per litre and this is termed an effusion. The underlying pathological mechanisms are:

- increased capillary permeability – capillary damage or inflammation;
- lymphatic obstruction;
- venous obstruction.

The most common pathologies associated with exudative effusions are:

- malignancy;
- infection;
- connective tissue disease;
- pulmonary infarction.

A transudate has less than 30 g/litre of protein and is the result of low colloid osmotic pressure from liver cirrhosis or high hydrostatic pressure from cardiac failure or a combination of both.

Presentation

The clinical signs depend on the rate of effusion growth. Rapidly developing effusions may cause severe dyspnoea, whereas slowly developing ones may be very large but asymptomatic. On clinical examination there are reduced breath sounds on the affected side with tracheal deviation to the opposite side. The chest is stony dull to percussion. A pleural effusion may be the initial presentation of a systemic malignancy in up to 30 per cent of cases.

Investigation

Radiology

A chest radiograph will determine the size of the effusion and may give a clue as to the aetiology (coexistent tuberculosis, hilar shadow, etc.). Further information about the lung may be obtained by CT it the lung is the primary pathology. Pleural thickening is best distinguished from fluid by ultrasonography.

Aspiration

Pleurocentesis (Fig. 47.29) is performed under local anaesthesia using aseptic precautions. The needle is introduced just above a rib (to avoid the neurovascular bundle) at the point of maximal dullness. Fluid is drawn for diagnosis (cytology and biochemistry) and symptomatic relief. It is important not to remove too much fluid because pulmonary oedema may ensue. Biochemistry will determine whether the fluid is an exudate. If it is then diagnostic efforts must be directed at finding the cause.

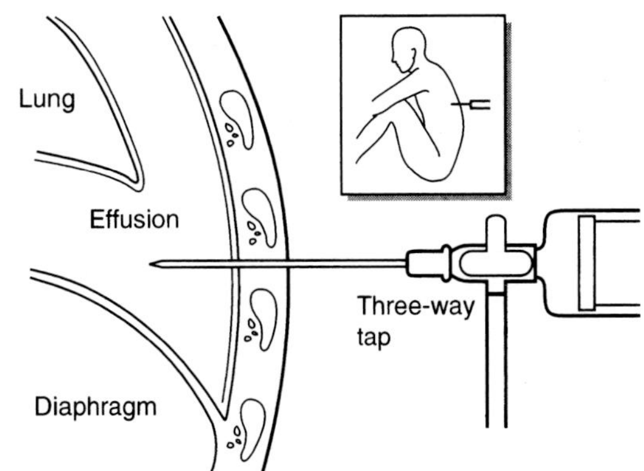

Fig. 47.29 Diagram of pleurocentesis.

Cytology

Histological examination of the aspirated fluid may be useful but the absence of malignant cells does not rule out malignancy. The yield may be increased by pleural biopsy (using an Abram's needle) taken at the same time.

Thoracoscopy

This is a more invasive technique performed under general anaesthesia. The patient is positioned and draped as for a thoracotomy. A small incision is made over an intercostal space down to the pleura. The pleura is opened and the effusion drained by suction. The thoracoscope is introduced and the parietal pleural and lung are inspected thoroughly. Any suspicious nodules or plaques may be biopsied and in the case of a recurrent malignant pleural effusion, definitive pleurodesis may be done.

Treatment

The prognosis for malignant pleural effusion is very poor and therefore the treatment should be simple and effective if the patient is to enjoy a reasonable quality of life. Simple aspiration is a temporary solution in the symptomatic patient, because the effusion usually reaccumulates and repeated aspiration merely results in loculation of the fluid. Treatment of the underlying malignancy may lead to resolution of the effusion but the distressing dyspnoea will be prolonged. A much better method of palliation is aspiration of the effusion and pleurodesis. Three requirements must be met for successful pleurodesis: the pleura must be aspirated to dryness, the pleural surfaces must be kept apposed and the fluid must not be allowed to reaccumulate. This can be achieved by tube drainage with underwater seal and 5 mmHg of suction pressure, and the introduction of a sclerosing agent. There is a variety of sclerosing agents, including tetracycline, bleomycin and iodised talc. Pleurodesis may be carried out on the ward but the success rate is higher if the procedure is performed under general anaesthesia with talc insufflation and thoracoscopic inspection to ensure that the pleural surface is completely covered. At the end of the procedure, basal and apical drains are inserted and left on suction to ensure that the pleural surfaces are apposed. There is an intense inflammatory reaction which is very uncomfortable for the patient. Adequate analgesia (avoiding nonsteroidal anti-inflammatory drugs) is therefore essential while the drains are in place. The success rate is over 75 per cent for this form of treatment and failures usually result from failure of the underlying lung to expand, lung metastases or lymphangitis. Pleurectomy is hard to justify because it is a major procedure in a patient with a very limited life expectancy.

Tumours of the pleura

The pleura is often secondarily involved as a result of direct or transcoelomic spread of lung or breast malignancy resulting in a malignant pleural effusion. However, there is one malignant tumour of the pleura that deserves mention.

Mesothelioma

Fibrous plaques overlying the pleura are often seen at thoracotomy and are benign in most cases. The most important malignant tumour affecting the pleura is a mesothelioma. This is an aggressive tumour that grows in diffuse layers, encapsulating and compressing the lung substance. It is associated with asbestos exposure and is a notifiable condition because sufferers may be eligible for compensation. There are several different cell types seen within the tumour (adenomatous, squamous or sarcomatous), although there is usually a predominance of one cell type.

Clinical features. The patients often present with large unilateral pleural effusions and dyspnoea and occasionally chest pain. Advanced disease is heralded by weight loss, pyrexia and night sweats.

Investigation. Chest radiography suggests the diagnosis but CT will show marked pleural thickening with compression of the lung. Pleural aspiration may reveal atypical cells but the diagnosis is more certain if thoracoscopic biopsy is performed. This also allows pleurodesis at the same time.

Treatment. The disease follows a progressive course over 12–24 months. Cure is rarely possible because the tumour is unresponsive to radiotherapy or chemotherapy, and palliation is difficult. Pain relief and appropriate supportive measures are best arranged at an early stage.

Pneumothorax

Pneumothorax is the presence of air in the thoracic space, outside the lung, that is, between the visceral and parietal layers of pleura which are normally only separated by a thin film of fluid. The lung is collapsed to the extent that it is displaced by the pneumothorax.

Classification of pneumothorax

Spontaneous – primary. The only abnormality is superficial blebs at the apex of one or more lobes, typically the upper lobes, which either leak spontaneously or are triggered by an otherwise unremarkable event such as exertion. It is more common in males, occurs predominantly in the 'teens or twenties, may be bilateral and may be familial.

Spontaneous – secondary. Any lung disease that breaches the pleura may cause a pneumothorax so probably every possible lung disease will, at one time or another, cause a pneumothorax. The most common causes are obstructive airways disease in any form and bullous emphysema.

Traumatic. See Thoracic trauma section.

Iatrogenic. This is commonly seen in general hospital practice as a result of insertion of central lines for central venous pressure monitoring, intravenous feeding or cardiac pacing.

Open. The air may come from a penetrating injury (stabbing or shooting) and passes in and out of the chest wall with each breath, but no effective ventilation occurs (see Thoracic trauma section).

Closed. Rib fracture – see Thoracic trauma section.

When air in the pleura is under pressure the situation is called 'tension pneumothorax' and is a medical emergency. This depends on the nonreturn valve-like mechanism, which is inherent in the structure of the lung. Positive pressure, generated within the airways with coughing or groaning in pain, forces air out which then cannot return through the collapsible peripheral alveoli (Fig. 47.30).

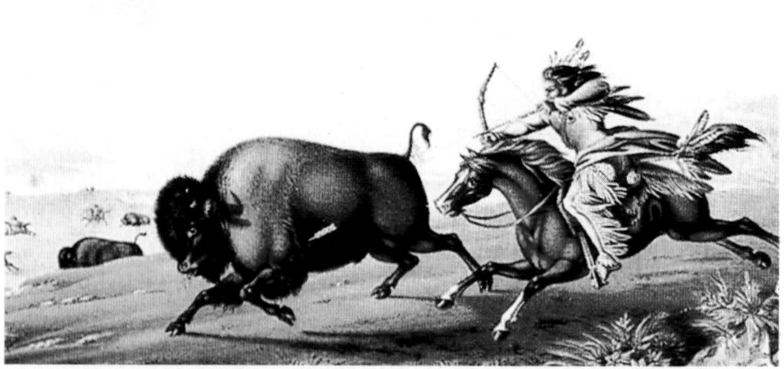

Fig. 47.30 The buffalo has a single pleural space – a fact that was advantageous to the Native American Indians who knew that a single arrow in a buffalo's chest would ultimately lead to the animal's death. Conversely, the elephant spontaneously develops a pleurodesis around the time of parturition as described at the start of the twentieth century. *'Les poumons adherient partout à la cage thoracique par du tissue conjunctif... mais la couer était libre dans son enveloppe'* (A. Giard, Comptes Redu de l'Academie des Sciences, 1907).

Diagnosis

The first thing is to suspect a pneumothorax and look for it deliberately in patients at risk:

- following needling of central veins;
- sudden deterioration in a ventilated patient;
- any trauma case;
- patients with obstructive airways disease.

On examination the affected side is more resonant and the breath sounds, listened for laterally in the axilla, are markedly different and reduced on the affected side. Shifts of the cardiac apex and trachea require severe distortion and are unreliable signs.

Chest radiography should be diagnostic but beware the supine film. Standard films are taken in inspiration. A small pneumothorax is exaggerated by expiration because the pneumothorax occupies proportionally more of the chest cavity.

Management

Tension pneumothorax is relieved by insertion of a large-bore intravenous cannula in a convenient intercostal space (with the usual precaution – see Chest drains) and then the situation can be managed as for a simple pneumothorax.

Spontaneous pneumothorax in a fit individual may cause little in the way of symptoms but in someone with poor respiratory reserve (chronic obstructive airway disease) it may be life threatening.

The natural elastic recoil of the lung is balanced by the negative pressure within the pleural space. Disruption of this equilibrium by air in the pleural space results in collapse of the lung to some extent. If the chest wall remains intact but the lung is punctured by a fractured rib the situation is termed a 'closed pneumothorax'. The danger is that, if this injury is part of a multiple injury, then positive pressure ventilation may lead to the development of a tension pneumothorax. If the chest wall is breached then this is termed an 'open pneumothorax', with the result that air moves in and out of the chest through the wound with each breath and there is no gas exchange across the alveolar surface.

Spontaneous pneumothorax may occur in any individual but is more common in young, slim men. The condition is often associated with apical blebs and there is a 30 per cent chance of recurrence.

Iatrogenic pneumothorax occurs when the lung parenchyma is breached by a medical procedure such as thoracocentesis, lung biopsy, liver biopsy or central venous cannulation.

Treatment

The initial treatment depends on the nature and severity of the pneumothorax; small pneumothoraces causing little disability may be observed with serial radiographs or may be aspirated. Large symptomatic or traumatic pneumothoraces require the insertion of a chest drain. Repeated spontaneous pneumothoraces are an indication for definitive treatment to prevent recurrence. This depends on the age of the patient, their general condition and the underlying aetiology of the pneumothorax. In older patients, talc pleurodesis has a good chance of success (>60 per cent) but many feel uncomfortable about this procedure in the young. Procedures such as thoracoscopic abrasion and partial pleurectomy or thoracotomy and pleurectomy (often with stapling of bullae) have a higher success rate. Old patients with severe obstructive airway disease (who may be receiving steroid therapy) present a major management problem.

Pleurectomy. Pleurectomy is the definitive treatment for recurrent pneumothorax. A small posterolateral thoracotomy is performed and as much of the parietal pleura as possible is stripped off the chest wall, particularly at the apex of the hemithorax. There are often apical bullas that may require stapling or oversewing. The parietal surface is abraded with a swab to induce an inflammatory reaction. Large-calibre suction drains are inserted to drain the apex and diaphragmatic surfaces of the lung. It is essential that suction is maintained long enough for the lung surface to become firmly adherent to the chest wall (usually 2–3 days). The thoracoscopic method of pleurodesis is becoming commonplace, with comparable results to open pleurodesis.

The chest wall

Tumours of the chest wall

These can be tumours of any component of the chest wall, i.e. bone, cartilage and soft tissue. They are treated similarly to those that occur in other sites and only require specialist input if major resection and chest wall reconstruction are contemplated.

The most common tumour is that of the rib (chondroma or osteoma) and presentation is as a hard swelling over the rib. Malignant tumours are painful and destructive and require wide resection. Even so, there is a tendency for tumours to recur and histological classification is difficult. Tumours of the sternum are usually malignant. Lung and pleural tumours may involve ribs and destroy them.

Most lesions may be seen on a chest radiograph but occasionally CT or isotope bone scanning is required. Excision biopsy is often the best way to deal with a rib neoplasm because the differentiation between benign and malignant growths may be difficult. This avoids the risk of 'spillage' and tumour seeding in the wound of an incision biopsy. If a major resection is to be planned, it may be preferable to know the nature of the lesion before surgery. The principle of surgery is to remove the rib along with the rib immediately above and below, and a length well past the margins of the tumour. Reconstruction is possible using a prosthetic material (Marlex or acrylic plates) to provide some stability to the chest wall. Myocutaneous flaps are occasionally employed to cover extensive tissue defects and therefore prior discussion with a plastic and reconstructive surgeon may be useful.

For lesions that are not amenable to resection, chemotherapy or radiotherapy, although unlikely to be curative, may provide symptomatic relief.

Other diseases of the chest wall

Congenital abnormalities are often incidental findings on chest radiography (bifid rib) but there are some important exceptions.

Cervical rib

This rib is usually represented by a fibrous band originating from the seventh cervical vertebra and inserting on to the first thoracic rib. It may be asymptomatic but because the axillary artery and brachial plexus course over it a variety of symptoms may occur. The lower trunk of the plexus (mainly T_1) is compressed, leading to wasting of the interossei and altered sensation in the T_1 distribution. Compression of the axillary artery may result in a poststenotic dilatation with thrombus and embolus formation. Treatment is by division or removal of the rib by a supraclavicular or an axillary approach.

Pectus excavatum

The sternum is depressed, with a dish-shaped deformity of the anterior portions of the ribs on one or both sides. It is probably never a cause of respiratory problems but may coexist with asthma, which is a common condition of children and young people. It may come to light during the growth spurt at adolescence when, of course, the teenager is particularly sensitive about appearance. Most patients are asymptomatic and the only justification for treatment is on cosmetic grounds. Some surgeons, and their referring doctors, make a very good case for this but the risk of morbidity and of a less than perfect result must be clearly spelt out to the patients and their parents.

The operation involves mobilising the sternum with the costal cartilages and holding this central panel anteriorly with a steel bar. Surgery is best left until the late 'teens when further growth of the chest wall is unlikely. It is worth recommending some body-building exercises because muscle development not only masks the skeletal deformity but boosts confidence.

Pectus carinatum (pigeon chest)

In this condition the sternum is elevated above the level of the ribs and treatment is offered for cosmetic reasons. The sternum is mobilised and allowed to fall back into place.

Pulmonary sepsis

Infections of the chest wall

These are unusual but may occur following osteomyelitis of the underlying rib. An empyema of the underlying thoracic cavity may discharge through the chest wall (empyema necessitans) leaving a chronic sinus. Sterile pus should alert the clinician that tuberculosis is present. Treatment of the chest wall infection depends on adequate treatment of the underlying condition.

Empyema

This is the end point of a number of conditions that result in the presence of pus in the pleural space, pleural thickening surrounding the walled-off infection and finally restricted lung movement on the affected side as a result of fibrosis. The presence of white cells and organisms is not sufficient to make the diagnosis of empyema.

The classic aetiology and still probably the most common is postpneumonic. A 'syn-pneumonic effusion' becomes colonised by bacteria and, at this stage, there is turbid but thin fluid, minimal pleural thickening and a mobile underlying lung. This is not properly called an empyema, an important point because the old-fashioned methods of rib resection would be fatal if applied to this condition and simpler treatments are effective. Untreated, this infected effusion develops into an empyema with thick pus in the pleural space surrounded by inflamed pleura thickened by deposition of fibrin. Finally, the cortex organises to form dense scar tissue or a 'fibrothorax'. Any cause of fluid collection, once contaminated, can evolve to reach this same end point (Table 47.6). Once established, any contaminated collection in the chest can result in empyema.

Symptoms. There are symptoms of pus at any site, namely swinging pyrexia with general malaise. Finger clubbing and weight loss are signs of chronicity. Progressive dyspnoea occurs as the hemithorax becomes more rigid. There may also be signs and symptoms of various predisposing conditions (see above). Pus may discharge into the overlying skin (empyema necessitans). Since the introduction of antibiotics, chronic empyema is not often seen but it is still a serious problem when it occurs.

Treatment. The management depends on the stage of the empyema.

Table 47.6 Conditions that predispose to empyema formation

Pulmonary infection
Unresolved pneumonia
Bronchiectasis
Tuberculosis
Fungal infections
Lung abscess
Aspiration of pleural effusion of any aetiology
Trauma
Penetrating injury
Surgery
Oesophageal perforation
Extrapulmonary spread
Subphrenic abscess
Bone infections
Osteomyelitis of ribs or vertebrae

Early empyema (thin pus, mobile lung and thin pleura). At this stage a brief period of pleural drainage, with underwater seal and adequate dosage of appropriate antibiotics, should result in resolution but inadequate treatment or no treatment will lead to a chronic empyema – a much more serious problem. Complete drainage and re-expansion of the lung should be achieved before the drains are removed. This need not take more than 2–3 days. Pus should be sent for microscopy and culture before antibiotic therapy.

Established empyema (adherent lung caused by inflamed and thickened pleura with thick pus in the empyema space). At this stage the old treatment of rib resection with open drainage is safe in that the lung is tethered. However, it is inelegant, protracted and incomplete in its results. It is better to insert drains, through a small thoracotomy (with resection of rib) if practical. This is best done under a general anaesthetic, except in desperate circumstances, and all the loculi are broken down, ensuring free drainage and the siting of one or two carefully situated tubes. The drains should span the cavity, have the last side hole just within the ribs, and be tracked to lie anterior to the midaxillary line so that they are comfortable and do not kink as the patient lies back.

Video-assisted thoracoscopic placement of drains is an increasingly appropriate alternative approach. Suction drainage is employed on chest closure and this is continued until the patient is ready for mobilisation. Provided there is no air leak (and there is usually none) portable vacuum drains, which the patient is able to manage at home, are inserted. Appropriate antibiotics are also given. A daily record of the amount drained is kept by the patient and, once the drainage is less than 25–50 ml/24 hours of serous fluid (it never becomes zero), the drain is removed.

Chronic empyema. If progression to a chronic fibrothorax has occurred, aspiration or drainage of pus will not lead to expansion of the lung because there is considerable fibrosis constricting the lung parenchyma.

Thoracotomy and decortication. A formal thoracotomy is performed and the thickened parietal pleura and the fibrin peel overlying the lung are painstakingly removed, piecemeal if necessary. This allows the lung to expand but there is often considerable blood loss from the raw surfaces. Wide-bore drains are inserted and connected to an underwater drainage system. Protracted air leak is common. When the leak has stopped (often up to 10 days later), the drains are removed. Antibiotics are given to cover organisms grown from the pus.

Postpneumonectomy empyema

This is discussed in the section concerning lung resections.

Lung abscess

Abscesses in the lung do not occur unless the underlying infection has caused thrombosis of the segmental artery and vein leading to infection with tissue necrosis. The most common causes are secondary to a chronic upper respiratory tract infection (sinusitis, dental abscess) or following bronchial obstruction from a neoplasm (Table 47.7).

Table 47.7 Causes of lung abscess

Specific pneumonia
Streptococcal
Staphylococcal
Pneumococcal
Klebsiella sp.
Anaerobic
Bronchial obstruction
Carcinoma
Carcinoid
Intramural foreign body
Postoperative atelectasis
Chronic respiratory sepsis
Sinusitis
Tonsillitis
Dental infection
Septicaemia
Penetrating lung injury

Diagnosis and treatment. The chest radiograph usually demonstrates a cavitating shadow which is similar in appearance to a necrotic bronchial carcinoma or less commonly a fungal infection. The diagnosis is confirmed with a combination of sputum culture, bronchoscopy and radiography. Most acute abscesses resolve with appropriate antibiotic therapy and postural drainage. The course of antibiotics is usually the highest permitted dose for a prolonged period. The virulent organism may change with such a prolonged antibiotic assault and the sputum must therefore be regularly monitored. Surgery is not usually part of the treatment. It is better for a lung abscess to drain via the bronchus and the contents are coughed up. Inserting a percutaneous drain creates a particularly difficult form of bronchopleural fistula.

Other thoracic disorders

The lungs

Lung cysts

Developmental. These may develop from the primitive lung buds near the trachea or main bronchi. There are no communications with the bronchi even though they are lined with respiratory epithelium and have a tendency to become infected. Removal is advised for this very reason.

Acquired. Lung cysts may contain air or fluid and may be single or multiple. The most common cause of multiple lung cysts is pulmonary hydatid disease, although this is unusual except in endemic areas. Air cysts (bullae) may be spontaneous but may be secondary to emphysematous degeneration (Fig. 47.31). In either case the cysts may become infected or compress functioning lung tissue and therefore some form of treatment is required.

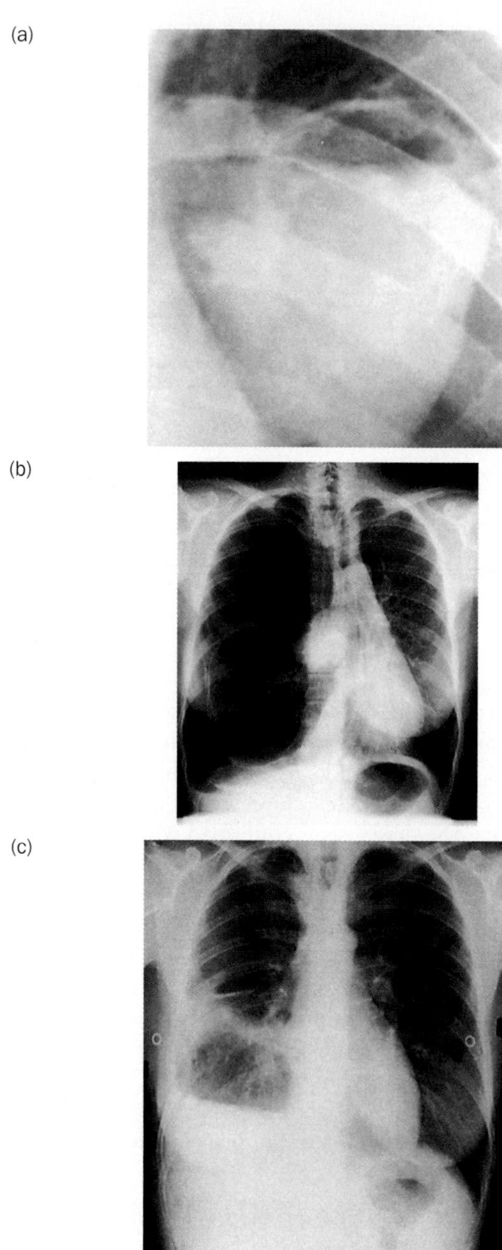

Fig. 47.31 Chest radiographs of hydatid cyst and large bulla. (a) Hydatid cyst; (b) giant bulla affecting the right lung; and (c) chest radiograph postbullectomy.

Pulmonary sequestration

This describes a section of lung supplied by the aorta and draining into the systemic circulation. There is no communication with the remainder of the lung and the segment becomes multicystic and infected, therefore compromising the surrounding healthy lung tissue. An interlobar sequestration occurs within the lung substance and commonly presents in younger patients.

Many cases are discovered on routine chest radiography but others may present with recurrent chest infections and occasionally bloodstained sputum. The chest radiograph normally shows a rounded opacity and the lesion cannot be seen at bronchoscopy (Fig. 47.32). Arteriography demonstrates the abnormal communication from the aorta and treatment involves removing the affected lobe, taking care to divide the abnormal artery (which usually runs in the inferior pulmonary ligament) as the first stage in the resection.

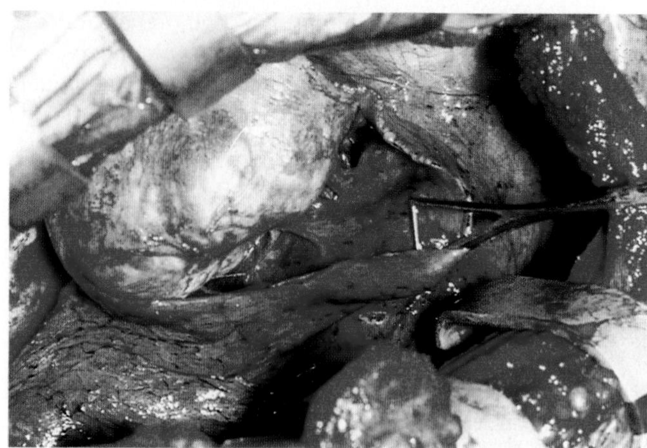

Fig. 47.32 Pulmonary sequestration.

Bronchiectasis

This is defined as chronic irreversible dilatation of the medium-sized bronchi. There are several causes but there are two basic mechanisms that account for this dilatation:

1. a weakening of the bronchial walls;
2. outward tension on the lung substance.

These may occur following a suppurative pneumonia or bronchial obstruction. The process often starts in childhood following a respiratory infection and slowly progresses during adult life. It is rarely confined to one lobe or even one lung, which precludes surgery in many cases. The incidence of severe bronchiectasis is falling thanks to the reduction in cases of whooping cough, measles and tuberculosis, and the improved management of infantile bronchiolitis. Inhalation of foreign bodies remains a potential cause of bronchiectasis and this possibility should be borne in mind.

Presentation. Some patients remain asymptomatic and the problem is discovered by chance on chest radiograph or *post mortem*. Usually there is a history of frequent chest infections from infancy with the production of copious volumes of sputum. In advanced cases foul-smelling sputum is produced with pain over the affected area, and there is weight loss and cachexia. Physical examination may be normal but often there is finger clubbing (in advanced disease), wheezing and consolidation over the affected lobe. Chronic nasal sinusitis may be a presentation and, in severe cases, amyloidosis may occur.

Investigation. A good posteroanterior chest radiograph will often show crowding of the lung markings on the affected side. A series of chest radiographs taken over two to three exacerbations may show persistent collapse or recurrent consolidation affecting the same area of lung. CT is now the investigation of choice.

Bronchography. This is rarely necessary to define which lobe(s) are affected; most surgeons would be satisfied with a CT scan. This investigation may need to be preceded by intensive physiotherapy and postural drainage to obtain adequate images.

Treatment. Removal of the bronchiectatic part of the lung is indicated when the disease is localised, and the respiratory function is adequate to cope with a reduced lung volume. Conservative surgery to preserve functioning lung tissue should be employed at all times.

Tuberculosis

This infection remains a major health problem in less developed countries but is increasing in frequency in Western countries as a result of immigration and immunosuppression [human immunodeficiency virus (HIV) and chemotherapy]. It commonly presents in the lungs and, if untreated or inadequately treated, can lead to serious complications. There is commonly a chronic cough with haemoptysis, weight loss and night sweats. The diagnosis should be firmly established by Ziehl–Neelsen staining of bacteria in the sputum or culture in Löwenstein–Jensen medium before starting antituberculous chemotherapy. Characteristic chest radiographic changes in symptomatic patients may be diagnostic if cultures are persistently negative; as a very last resort chemotherapy may be tried for 2 weeks. An improvement in symptoms indicates that tuberculosis is the problem.

The mainstay of treatment is antituberculous chemotherapy for the individual and bacille Calmette–Guérin (BCG) immunisation for contacts, attention to hygiene and housing in the community. Combination chemotherapy is usually successful in treating the infection. Inadequate treatment or noncompliance leads to the development of resistant organisms. The course of treatment is often over 6 months and in some less developed countries this can result in noncompliance. Surgery is rarely indicated for tuberculosis in developed countries but, when it is, it must be combined with adequate antitubercular chemotherapy or the benefit of surgery will be lost.

Indications for surgery. Indications are:

- suspicious lesion on chest radiograph in which neoplasia cannot be excluded;
- chronic tuberculous abscess, resistant to chemotherapy;
- aspergilloma within a tuberculous cavity;
- life-threatening haemoptysis.

Franz Ziehl, 1857–1926. German bacteriologist.
Friedrich Adolf Neelsen, 1854–94. German pathologist
Ernst Löwenstein, b. 1878. Pathologist, Vienna, Austria.
Johannes Hans Daniel Jensen, 1907–73. German physicist.
Albert Léon Charles Calmette, 1863–1933. French bacteriologist.
Camille Guérin, b. 1872. French bacteriologist.

Surgery is indicated for certain situations and is always used in conjunction with chemotherapy. With effective treatment and earlier diagnosis, the role of surgery is gradually decreasing in the management of this condition.

Diagnosis. Surgical procedures may be necessary to establish the diagnosis if the disease is suspected clinically, but sputum or pus cultures are persistently negative.

Bronchoscopy. This has a higher diagnostic yield than expectorated sputum.

Open lung biopsy. Tissues from intrathoracic lymph nodes, lung and pleura may be found to contain tuberculous material.

The formation of a tuberculous empyema can result in fibrosis of the affected lung and its functional destruction. A tube thoracostomy may suffice in the early stages of empyema, but once a fibrous rim has formed an exploratory thoracotomy with decortication, evacuation of pus and effective postoperative suction will be required. Complications such as aspergilloma in a chronic cavity, haemoptysis and localised carcinoma arising from a tuberculous scar may require lobectomy. Operations designed to collapse the lung, such as thoracoplasty, are occasionally used to collapse cavities.

Pulmonary vascular disease

A detailed discussion of all the diseases of pulmonary vasculature is beyond the scope of this book. However, pulmonary embolus is a major cause of morbidity and mortality and is discussed here, as is lung and heart–lung transplantation, which is indicated for end-stage pulmonary vascular disease.

Pulmonary embolus. This occurs following dislodgement of venous thrombi, generally from the femoral and iliac veins, and their subsequent impaction in the pulmonary vasculature. More unusual causes are fat embolus from multiple trauma, tumour embolus (renal carcinoma) and amniotic fluid. Pulmonary embolism accounts for over 20 000 deaths per year in the UK. Strategies aimed at preventing the development of thrombi in those at high risk (postsurgical patients, postmyocardial infarction and those who have previously had pulmonary embolus) include early mobilisation, low-dose subcutaneous heparin and compression stockings. The presentation can vary according to the size, number and timing of embolic episodes.

Small emboli may pass unnoticed, giving rise to minor pleuritic chest pain. Pulmonary vascular hypertension may develop with repeated episodes. Larger emboli may give rise to pleurisy and haemoptysis with signs of pleural rub and crackles on auscultation. Massive emboli lead to haemodynamic collapse if the outflow to the right ventricle is obstructed. There is severe chest pain and acute shortness of breath. The clinical signs are of right heart failure with raised central venous pressure and tachycardia, and there may be some changes on the ECG. A chest radiograph is often not helpful in the early stages but a ventilation–perfusion scan may show a mismatch, thereby confirming the diagnosis. A contrast-enhanced CT scan is the most accurate diagnostic technique.

Treatment: acute minor pulmonary embolus. Small emboli do not require specific treatment but preventive measures are needed to prevent further episodes. These take the form of systemic heparinisation in the first instance and then oral anticoagulation with warfarin or its derivatives. Recurrent emboli, even with adequate anticoagulation, may require treatment with an inferior vena caval filter.

Treatment: acute massive embolus. This occurs when a large embolus obstructs the pulmonary vasculature and results in haemodynamic disturbance. There is often a history of one or more minor emboli before the current episode. The haemodynamic problems dominate the clinical picture of acute right heart failure with corresponding low cardiac output and acute ventilation–perfusion mismatch. There is peripheral vasoconstriction, tachycardia with a small volume pulse and tachypnoea. Blood gas analysis usually reveals a low Po_2 from the ventilation–perfusion mismatch and a low Pco_2 from the associated hyperventilation. The patient will usually be more comfortable lying flat, in contrast to the patient with myocardial infarction who prefers to sit upright. Once the diagnosis has been made, treatment with thrombolytic agents (streptokinase and tissue plasminogen activator) is started. The emboli are seen as filling defects in the pulmonary artery (Fig. 47.33). The immediate priority is to resuscitate the patient by administering intravenous fluids to increase the right ventricular filling pressure and to avoid venodilators. Oxygen is administered via a face mask (100 per cent) and intravenous heparin is administered to prevent any further propagation of thrombi. Thrombolytic agents may be given directly into the pulmonary artery to ensure high concentrations at the appropriate site. Occasionally pulmonary embolectomy may be required. This may be done without cardiopulmonary bypass using caval inflow occlusion and extracting the embolus through a pulmonary arteriotomy. Better results are likely if the patient is fit enough for cardiopulmonary bypass to be established.

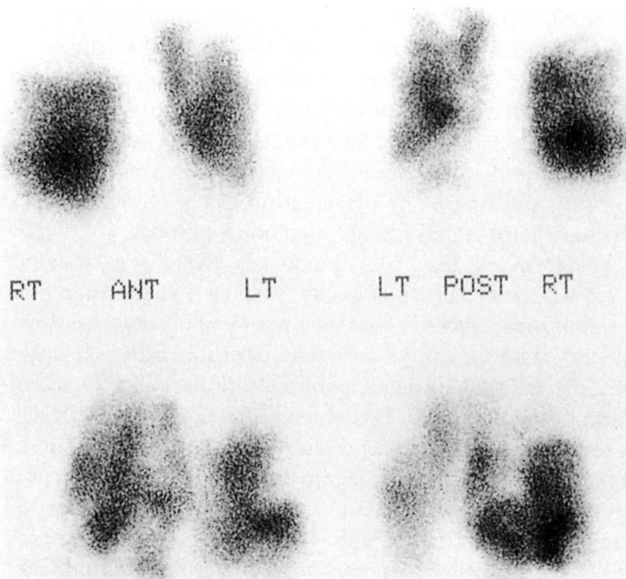

Fig. 47.33 Ventilation–perfusion scan showing multiple filling defects in both lungs suggesting multiple emboli.

Lung transplantation. Lung transplantation is becoming an established therapy for those with end-stage parenchymal or pulmonary vascular disease. The indications for lung transplantation are varied and may involve the use of one donor lung, two donor lungs or the heart–lung block. Cystic fibrosis and irreversible pulmonary hypertension with right ventricular failure are the main indications for heart–lung transplantation but there is now a trend towards single and sequential bilateral lung transplantation, leaving the native heart *in situ*. This reduces the risk of airway dehiscence which is common with a tracheal anastomosis. Pulmonary fibrosis and obstructive airway disease in young people are indications for single lung transplantation. Donor selection is much the same as for cardiac transplantation except that there must be good respiratory function and no evidence of pulmonary oedema, contusion or infection at the time of harvesting. Matching of donor and recipient and cytomegaloviral (CMV) status is more important than in heart transplantation in trying to avoid the development of CMV pneumonitis.

The recipient operation depends on the nature of the transplant. Heart–lung transplantation requires a median sternotomy and cardiopulmonary bypass. The recipient heart (in the absence of right heart failure) may be suitable for transplantation into another recipient. Single lung transplantation is performed through a thoracotomy with cardiopulmonary bypass if required. Vigorous physiotherapy and judicious antibiotic use are important in the early postoperative period. Opportunist infections may develop secondary to the immunosuppressive drugs and carry a high mortality unless treated aggressively. One-year survival following heart–lung, double lung and single lung transplantations stands at between 60 and 70 per cent.

There is a current shortage of suitable donors for organ transplantation, therefore alternative treatments for end-stage disease are being explored. One recent development in the field of thoracic surgery is lung volume reduction. This involves excising areas of lung in emphysematous patients with often surprising degrees of subjective and objective improvement. It is unsure whether this procedure restores the mechanics of breathing by altering the chest wall dimensions or improves respiratory function by minimising ventilation–perfusion mismatching.

The diaphragm

The diaphragm is the fibromuscular structure separating the thorax from the abdomen (Fig. 47.34). There are two well-recognised congenital sites where abdominal viscera can herniate into the chest. Traumatic rupture of the diaphragm may also lead to herniation. Congenital hernia tend to be apparent shortly after birth, with over 80 per cent presenting on the left side (Fig. 47.35). There is respiratory distress, apparent dextrocardia, a scaphoid abdomen and radiological appearances of bowel in the hemithorax. Treatment involves urgent nasogastric suction (to prevent distension of the bowel

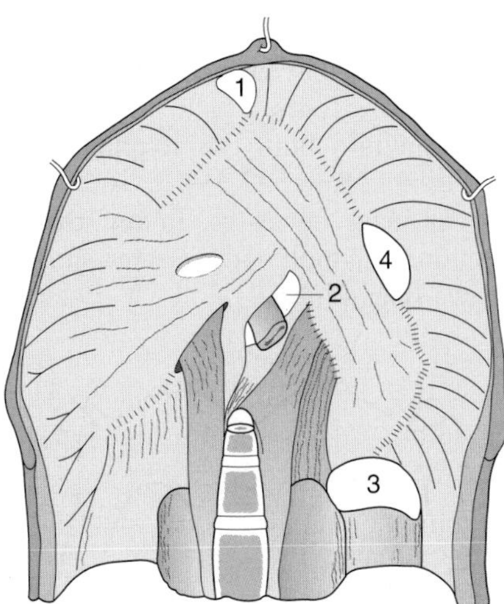

Fig. 47.34 Diagram of sites of hernias. The usual sites of congenital diaphragmatic hernia. (1) Foramen of Morgagni; (2) oesophageal hiatus; (3) foramen of Bochdalek (pleuroperitoneal hernia) (this is usually situated more anteriorly); (4) dome.

and further compression of the lung) and general resuscitation before surgical repair. Hernias manifesting later in life present with vague dyspeptic symptoms or a feeling of fullness in the chest.

Repair is advised and is undertaken through a left upper transverse abdominal approach or by thoracotomy through the seventh intercostal space with nonabsorbable sutures to repair the defect once the hernia has been reduced.

Oesophageal hiatus hernia is a common problem and is dealt with in Chapter 50.

Hernia through the foramen of Morgagni

This is an anteriorly placed hernia with the defect between the sternal and costal attachments of the diaphragm. The most commonly involved viscus is the transverse colon.

Hernia through the foramen of Bochdalek

This is really the persistence of the pleuroperitoneal canal and the opening is in the dome of the diaphragm posteriorly. It is the most common diaphragmatic hernia in children and presents with severe respiratory distress. There is a classic triad of respiratory distress, apparent dextrocardia and a scaphoid abdomen.

Eventration of the diaphragm

This is an abnormally elevated position of one or both hemidiaphragms from paralysis or atrophy of the muscle fibres. There may be some spontaneous improvement if the condition occurs in the perinatal period but long-standing cases with paradoxical respiration may benefit from operation.

Giovanni Morgagni, 1682–1771. Professor of Anatomy, Padua, Italy.
Vincent Alexander Bochdalek, 1801–83. Anatomist in Prague, now in the Czech Republic.

(a)

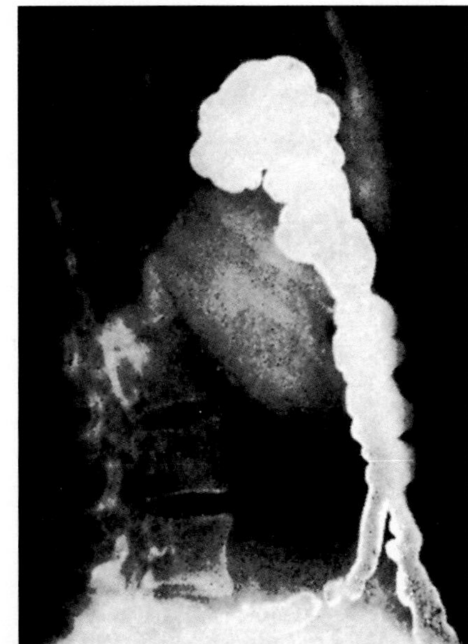

(b)

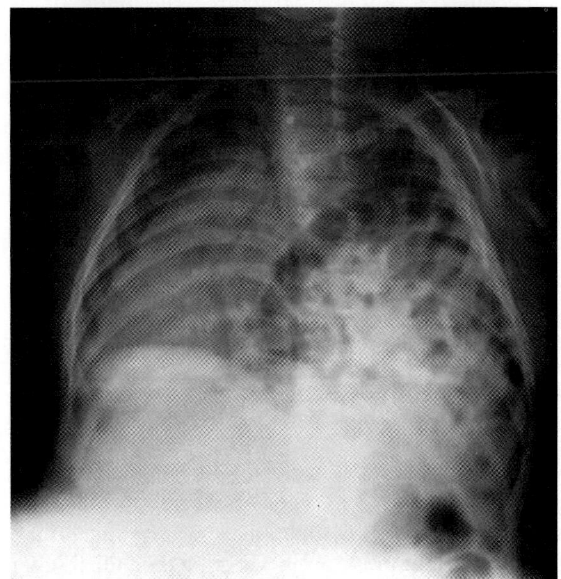

Fig. 47.35 Chest radiograph of congenital diaphragmatic hernia. (a) Colon occupying a Morgagni hernia (*courtesy of Dr Oliver Smith, Birmingham*). (b) Foramen of Bochdalek hernia on the left side in an infant. The left pleural cavity is occupied by intestine, the mediastinum is displaced to the right, and right lung is aerated very little.

The aim of surgery is to fix the diaphragm in inspiration so that paradoxical movement and mediastinal shift are minimised. This is achieved by plication of the redundant diaphragm, taking care not to damage the branches of the phrenic nerve.

Appendix 1: Anatomy and development of the lungs (Fig. 47.36)

During the fourth week of intrauterine growth the lung bud develops from the ventral surface of the primitive foregut.

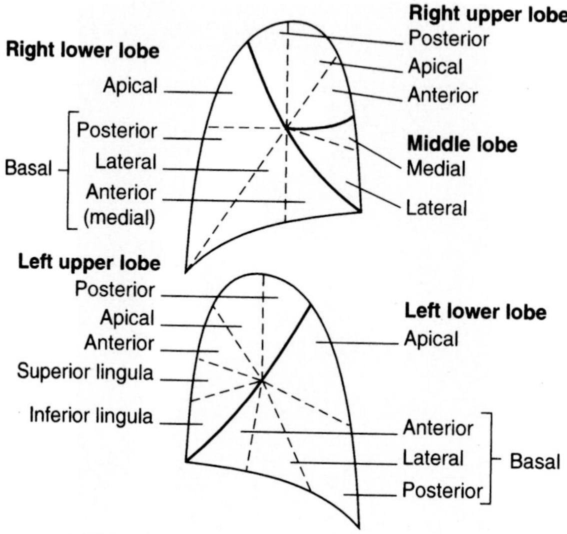

Fig. 47.36 The segmental arrangement of the lungs.

This becomes a bilobed structure, the ends of which ultimately become the lungs. The trachea and bronchi derive their blood supply from the bronchial arteries coming from the aorta. Although development is initially symmetrical in each lung bud, the typical lobar arrangement is defined early in foetal life. Congenital abnormalities may occur during development, the most important ones being agenesis (nonformation) or accessory lobes.

The primitive lungs drain into the cardinal veins which ultimately become the pulmonary veins draining into the left atrium. Abnormalities of venous drainage may occur at this stage of development (compare anomalous venous drainage).

Surgical anatomy of the lungs

There are three lobes to the right lung and two to the left, although the two sides are basically very similar (Fig. 47.37). Each lobe is composed of segments (see above) with its own discrete blood supply of pulmonary artery and pulmonary vein: an important point when resecting individual segments. No bronchi or arteries cross the intersegmental plains.

The right main bronchus is shorter, wider and nearly vertical compared with the left. As a consequence, inhaled foreign bodies are more likely to enter the right main bronchus than the left. The bronchi are supplied with blood from the bronchial arteries which arise directly from the aorta. They drain into both the systemic and pulmonary circulations (Figs 47.38 and 47.39).

Lymphatic drainage tends to follow the bronchi and certain collections of lymph nodes are recognised around the hila and trachea (Fig. 47.40).

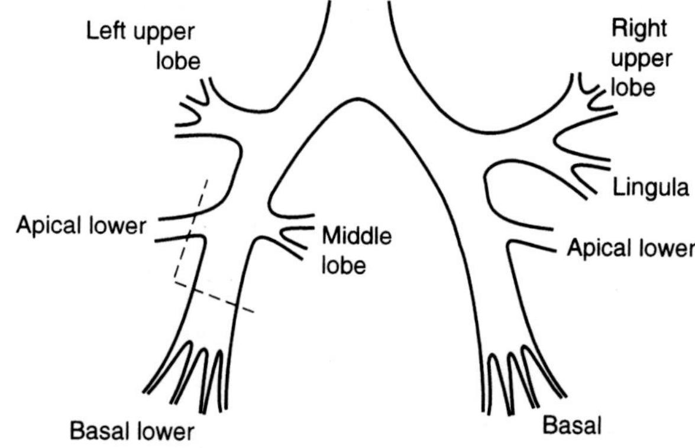

Fig. 47.37 Diagrammatic surgical anatomy of the bronchial tree.

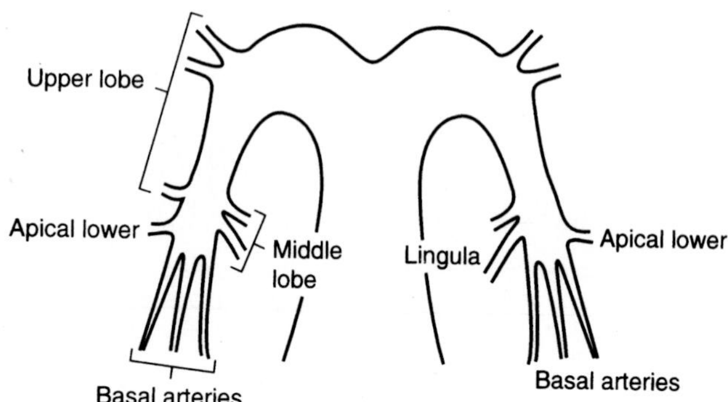

Fig. 47.38 The distribution of the pulmonary arteries.

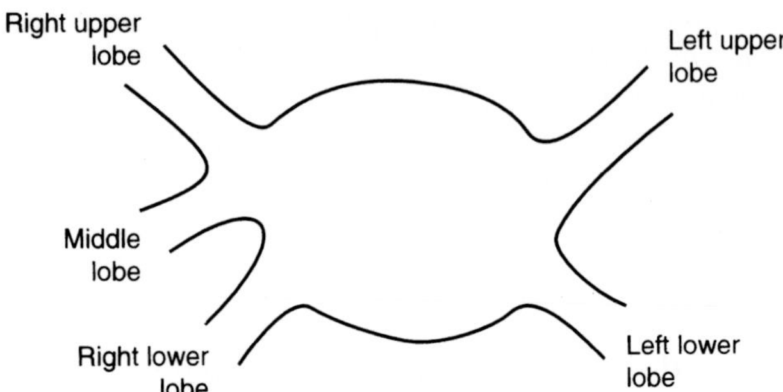

Fig. 47.39 The distribution of the pulmonary veins.

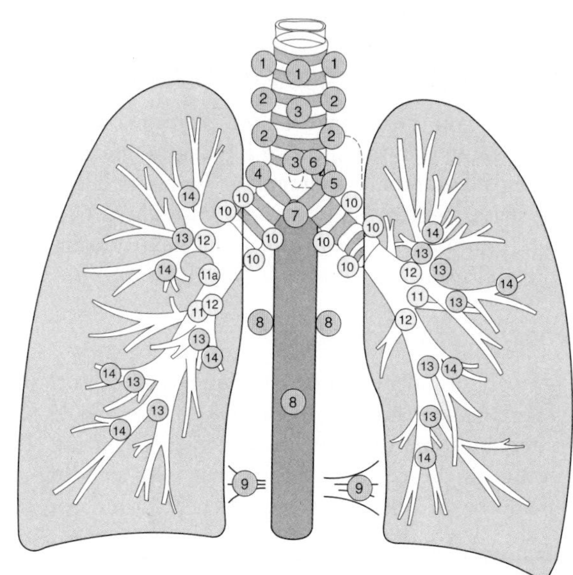

Fig. 47.40 The lymphatic drainage of the lung. Recognised lymph node situations for perioperative sampling during resection for malignant disease.

These are important as their presence or absence is useful in staging malignant disease (noninvasively by radiography or invasively by needle biopsy, mediastinotomy or mediastinoscopy). They are also important in determining prognosis following resection of a lung neoplasm.

Appendix 2: Investigation of the respiratory system

Any patient undergoing general anaesthesia requires some assessment of respiratory function. This is especially important in patients who are undergoing thoracotomy and lung resection, and in patients with limited pulmonary reserve undergoing any surgery.

There is a range of lung function tests available to provide objective evidence of pulmonary disease. These tests are useful in determining the functional capacity of the patient and the severity of the disease, and in predicting the response to various treatment options. The tests range from those that are simple and can be done at the bedside to those that are only available in specialist centres.

The simpler tests are the following (Table 47.8).

Table 47.8 Respiratory values in lung disease

	Obstructive pattern	*Restrictive pattern*
PEFR	↓↓	Normal or ↓
FEV_1	↓↓	Normal or ↓
FVC	Normal or ↓	↓↓
FEV_1/FVC (%)	<70	>80

Peak expiratory flow rate (PEFR)

This is measured by a Wright peak flowmeter or a peak flow gauge. This is a reliable and reproducible test,

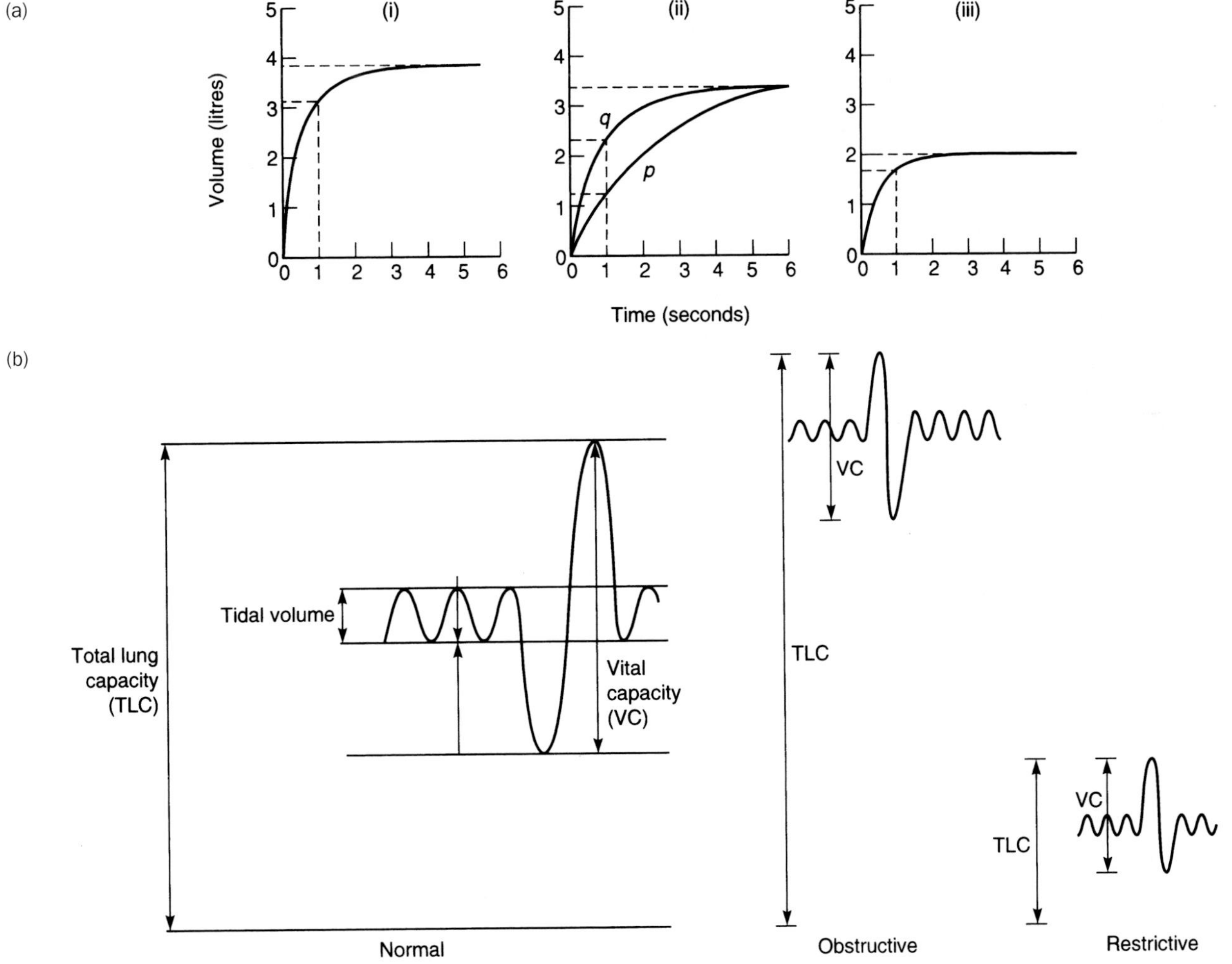

Fig. 47.41 Diagram of spirometry. (a) Spirogram drawings obtained from a Vitallograph. (i) Normal FEV_1 3.1 litres, FVC 3.8 litres, FEV_1/FVC 82%. (ii) Obstructive defect (reversible) asthma, *p* before a bronchodilator FEV_1 1.4 litres, FVC 3.5 litres, FEV_1/FVC 40% ; *q* after a bronchodilator FEV_1 2.5 litres, FVC 3.5 litres, FEV_1/FVC 71%. (iii) Restrictive defect, fibrosing alveolitis FEV_1 1.8 litres, FVC 2.0 litres, FEV_1/FVC 90%. No change with bronchodilators. (b) Changes in lung volume in obstructive and restrictive lung disease. (Reproducted from Gray H.H. Pulmonary emoblism, *Medicine International* 1993; 21:12:477 by kind permission of the Medicine Group (Journals) Ltd.)

Table 47.9 Blood gases

	Pao_2	$Paco_2$
Asthma		
Mild	↓	↓
Moderate	↓↓	Normal
Severe	↓↓↓	↑
Chronic bronchitis	↓↓	↑
Emphysema	Normal or ↓	↓
Fibrosing alveolitis	↓↓	↓ or Normal
Left ventricular failure or pulmonary embolus		
Type I respiratory failure	↓↓↓	Normal
Type II respiratory failure	↓↓↓	↓↓

Pao_2: arterial oxygen tension;
$Paco_2$: arterial carbon dioxide tension.

but has the disadvantage of being effort dependent and therefore it may be affected by abdominal or thoracic wound pain.

Forced expiratory volume in 1 second (FEV_1)

This is the amount of air forcibly expired in 1 second. It is low in obstructive lung disease and may be normal in restrictive lung disease.

Forced vital capacity (FVC)

This is the volume of air forcibly displaced following maximal inspiration to maximal expiration. The FEV_1 and the FVC can be measured using a Vitallograph and a ratio (FEV_1/FVC) can be calculated (Fig. 47.41). A low ratio indicates obstruction and the test should be repeated after bronchodilators. A normal ratio (FVC and FEV_1 reduced to the same extent) indicates a restrictive pathology.

Blood gases

A simple noninvasive probe will measure the oxygen saturation of haemoglobin but it should be borne in mind that the oxygen content of blood may fall precipitously at saturations of less than 90 per cent (as an effect of the oxygen dissociation curve). Arterial blood gases give a great deal of information; this is summarised in Table 47.9. Changing trends in the data provided by blood gas analysis are as important as the absolute values.

The risks and benefits of lung surgery should be discussed with the patients in the light of these tests. There are no absolute guidelines but, in general, a patient with the following values should tolerate a major lung resection:

- FEV_1 >1 litre;
- FVC >2 litres;
- normal carbon dioxide tension (Pco_2);
- age <70 years.

Further reading

Baum, P.A. (ed.) (1991) *Current Topics in Lung Cancer,* Springer, Berlin.

Beattie, E.J., Bloom, N. and Harvey, J. (1992) *Thoracic Surgical Oncology,* Churchill Livingstone, New York.

Hurt, R. and Bates, M. (1986) *Essentials of Thoracic Surgery,* Butterworths, London.

Paneth, M., Goldstraw, P. and Hyams, P. (1987) *Fundamental Techniques in Pulmonary and Oesophageal Surgery,* Springer, London.

Sheilds, T.W. (ed.) (1994) *General Thoracic Surgery*, 4th edn, Williams and Wilkins, Philadelphia, PA.

Wells, F. and Milstein, B.B. (1990) *Thoracic Surgical Techniques,* Baillière Tindall, London.

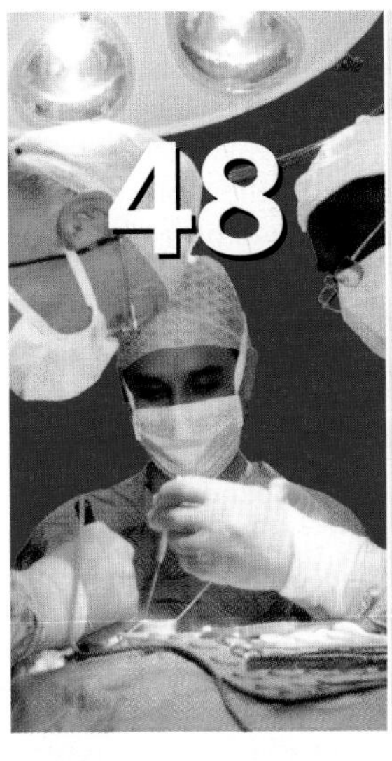

48 Heart and pericardium

Heart surgery

Congenital, valvular and coronary heart disease all have a largely mechanical component and lend themselves particularly well to surgical correction. This was predicted in 1925 by Henry Souttar of the London Hospital, Whitechapel, who wrote in the *British Medical Journal,* in the introduction to his report of the first mitral commissurotomy, that the heart should be as amenable to surgery as any other organ and that many of the problems in heart disease were to a large extent mechanical. He saw the main problem as being maintenance of blood flow, particularly to the brain, while surgery was being performed. The first real steps in surgery in and around the heart came in the late 1940s and early 1950s, driven by surgeons who had gained confidence and experience under the pressures and opportunities provided by war. Further progress had to wait until the development of cardiopulmonary bypass in the mid 1950s. Now the number, range and technical complexity of heart operations are remarkable; with the pump restored to good working order, the well-being and lifespan of patients with congenital, valvular and degenerative heart disease can be very much improved.

Henry Souttar, 1875–1964. Surgeon to the Royal London Hospital, Whitechapel, London, England.

Bailey & Love's Short Practice of Surgery, 23rd edition. Edited by R.C.G. Russell, N.S. Williams and C.J.K. Bulstrode. Published in 2000 by Arnold Publishers.

In this chapter those cardiac diseases that can be helped by surgery are included. The surgical management of heart disease is particularly appropriate to illustrate some principles in the logic of surgical decision making.

The purpose of an operation should be to relieve symptoms, to improve prognosis or both. As far as symptoms are concerned the surgeon should help the patient towards an informed appraisal of the risks and benefits applicable to the particular case, as with any other operation. For prognosis, the matter is one in which the surgeon should provide the patients with advice based on the best available knowledge. Ideally, three numerical pieces of information are required:

1. the outlook if the condition remains unoperated on;
2. the risk of the operation itself, including failure to deal with the disease;
3. the outlook following successful surgery.

The approach is illustrated diagrammatically (Fig. 48.1).

Cardiopulmonary bypass

Cardiopulmonary bypass allows the surgeon to manage the circulation while operating on a still heart in a bloodless field. Valve surgery under direct vision would not have been possible had it not been for the introduction of cardiopulmonary bypass in the 1950s by Gibbon. Before this, valve surgery was performed using closed techniques (mostly

John Gibbon Jr, 1904–73. Surgeon, Minnesota, USA.

commissurotomies or valvotomies performed with dilators). There is still a role for these procedures, but now most valve procedures are performed on a still heart with the aid of cardiopulmonary bypass, which has undergone many modifications since its first development (Figs 48.2–48.4).

Today it is a very safe way to manage the circulation during surgery, although there are still some associated problems that cause morbidity. For most operations, the heart is approached by a median sternotomy. An incision is made from the jugular notch to the lower end of the xiphisternum. The sternum is divided and retracted to expose the pericardium. The patient is fully heparinised and the pericardium is opened, taking care not to damage the brachiocephalic vein. The great vessels are exposed and a purse string is inserted into the adventitia of the ascending aorta proximal to the brachiocephalic artery. A second purse-string suture is inserted into the right atrium by the appendage. A 1-cm cannula is inserted into the ascending aorta and held in place by the purse-string suture. Air is excluded and the cannula is connected to the bypass circuit. Venous drainage is established from a cannula placed in the right atrium. Alternatively, the superior and inferior caval veins may be cannulated separately to gain better control over the venous return and to facilitate surgery within the right atrium. Once the circuit is connected, the cardiopulmonary bypass machine (the 'pump') takes over the circulation and ventilation can be discontinued. The core temperature may be lowered to reduce the metabolic demands of the tissues, and the surgeon can now isolate the heart from the rest of the circulation.

At the end of the procedure air must be meticulously excluded from the cardiac chambers. Once perfusion is restored to the coronary arteries, the heart may beat spontaneously or, if ventricular fibrillation is present, it may require a shock by a direct current (DC). Epicardial pacing wires may be placed to treat postoperative bradycardia or heart block. The patient is rewarmed, acidosis or hypokalaemia is corrected, ventilation is restarted and venous blood is allowed to fill the right atrium by clamping the venous line of the bypass machine. The heart gradually takes over the circulation while the arterial flow from the cardiopulmonary bypass machine is reduced. When the blood pressure is acceptable and the surgeon is confident that the heart function is adequate, cardiopulmonary bypass is discontinued and the venous

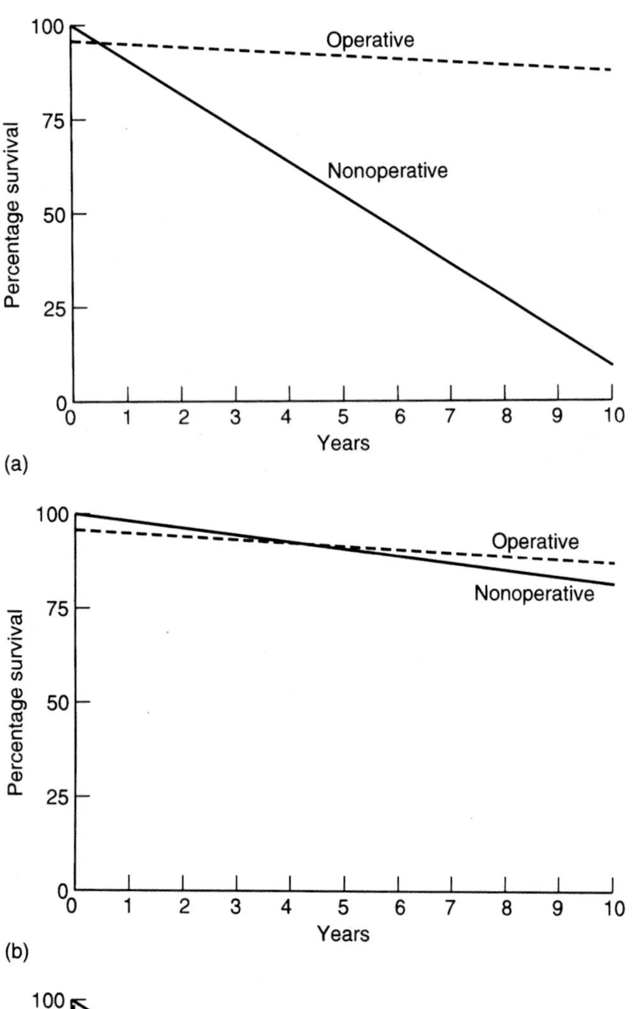

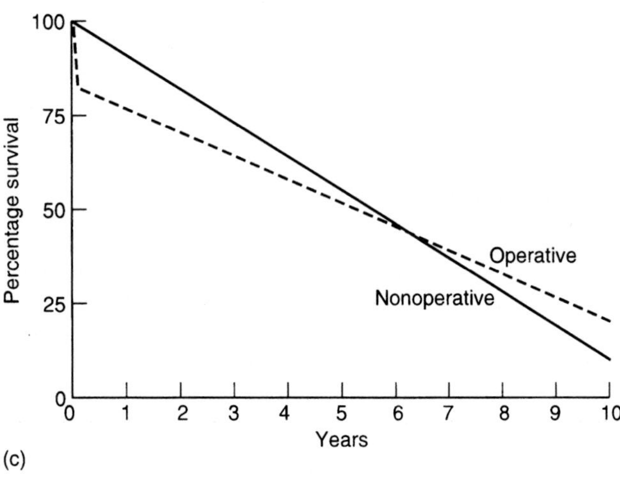

Fig. 48.1 Three graphs to illustrate the logic that should be employed when we operate to improve prognosis. (a) Hypothetical survival plots for medically and surgically managed patients where surgery offers improved prognosis over the poor natural history. Natural history: only about 10 per cent survival at 10 years; operative risk: 5 per cent; surgical outcome: about 90 per cent survival at 10 years. Ideal cases of aortic stenosis or left main-stem coronary artery disease behave like this. (b) A situation where surgery does not improve prognosis because the natural history is good. Natural history: over 85 per cent survive at 10 years; operative risk: low; surgical outcome: about 90 per cent survive at 10 years. The short-term risk and operative morbidity might not justify the marginal gain in survival. Single- and double-vessel coronary disease behave like this. (c) Here surgery may not be appropriate because it makes insufficient impact on the bad natural history. Natural history: only about 10 per cent survive at 10 years; operative risk: high; surgical outcome: only about 20 per cent survive at 10 years even with surgery. Advanced valve or coronary disease with a failing left ventricle and/or elevated pulmonary vascular resistance might behave like this.

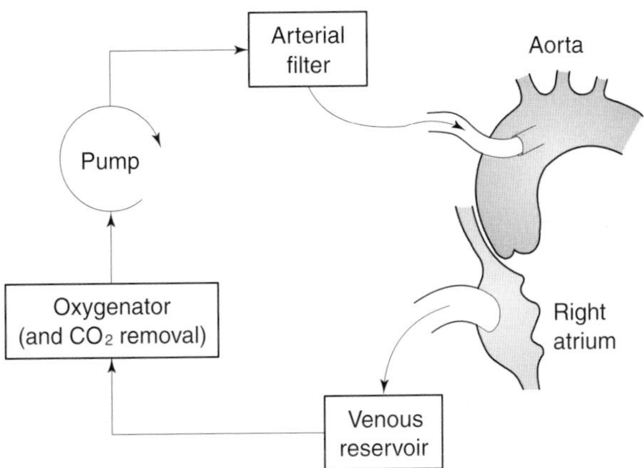

Fig. 48.2 Basic elements of the cardiopulmonary bypass circuit.

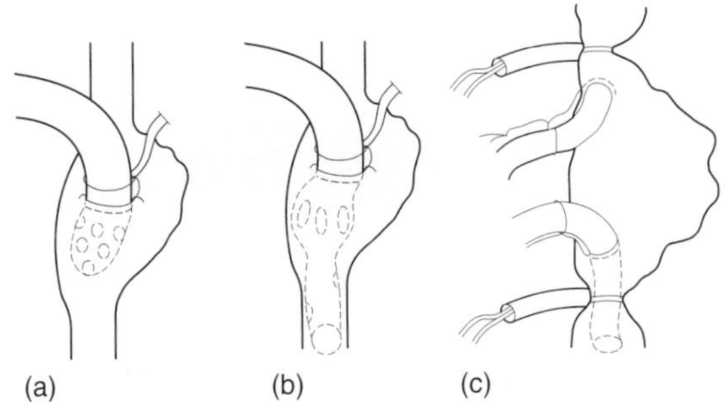

Fig. 48.3 Technical options for venous cannulation of the heart: (a) single venous cannula or 'Ross basket'; (b) two-stage (right atrial/inferior vena caval) cannula; (c) separate superior and inferior caval cannulae with snares to isolate the right atrium.

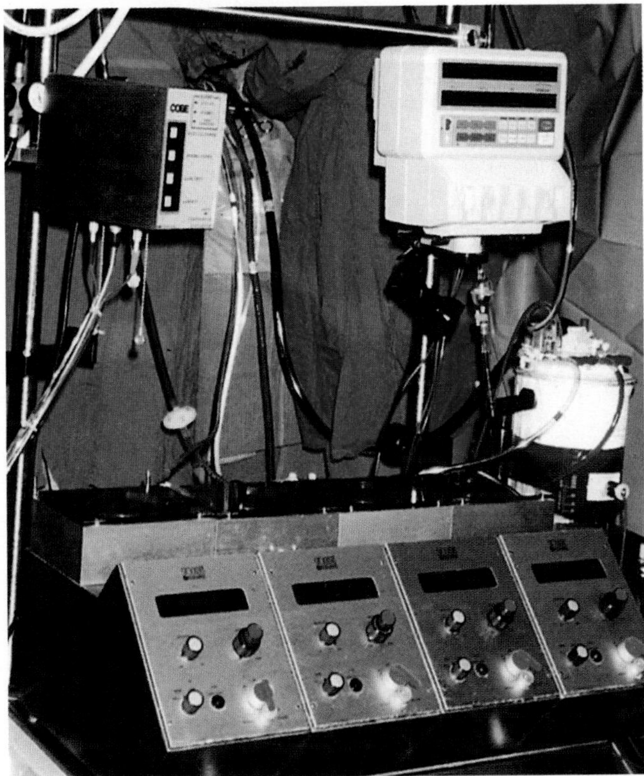

Fig. 48.4 The cardiopulmonary bypass machine.

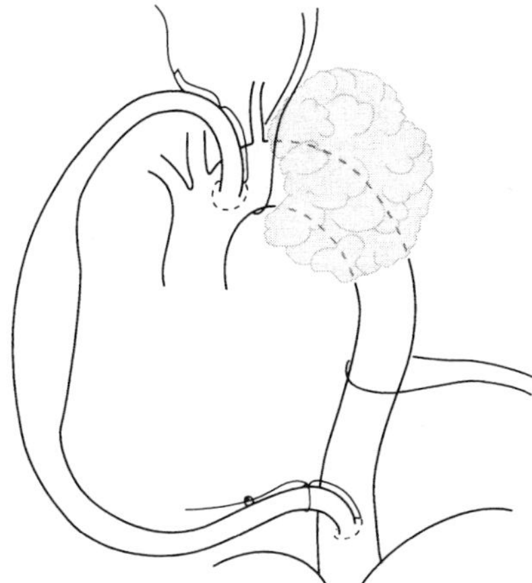

Fig. 48.5 Gott shunt: secured by purse-string sutures in the aortic arch and in the descending aorta. When the aorta is cross-clamped proximal and distal to the operative site, distal perfusion is maintained.

cannula removed. Blood from the bypass reservoir may be given through the arterial cannula while protamine is given to reverse the effects of heparinisation.

Femorofemoral bypass

This is a form of cardiopulmonary bypass that is used when it is difficult or impossible to enter the chest until bypass has been established. Venous drainage may be from the femoral vein or the right atrium. Arterial return is via the femoral artery which has to be surgically exposed.

Vascular shunts

Heparin-bonded shunts are used to bypass a section of aorta requiring resection or repair. They are particularly useful for aortic transection repair following a high-speed deceleration injury when cardiopulmonary bypass would be inadvisable. The shunt perfuses the aorta distal to the site of injury and therefore protects against paraplegia (Fig. 48.5).

Valvular heart disease

The proper functioning of the atrioventricular valves depends on the integrity of the valve annulus, the leaflets, the chordae tendineae and the papillary muscles. Malfunction of one or more components will adversely affect the performance of the valve. The semilunar valves allow blood to leave the ventricle during systole and prevent its regurgitation during diastole. The intrinsic shape of the valve allows this and disruption of the leaflets or the annulus can affect valve function. In the normal state a heart valve presents no resistance to forward flow but prevents regurgitation into the chamber proximal to it (Figs 48.6 and 48.7).

Vincent Gott. Surgeon, Johns Hopkins Hospital, Baltimore, Maryland, USA.

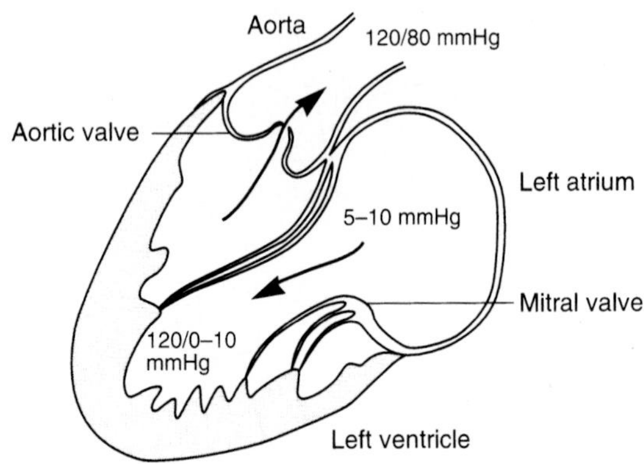

Fig. 48.6 Left-sided cardiac chambers as viewed from the left.

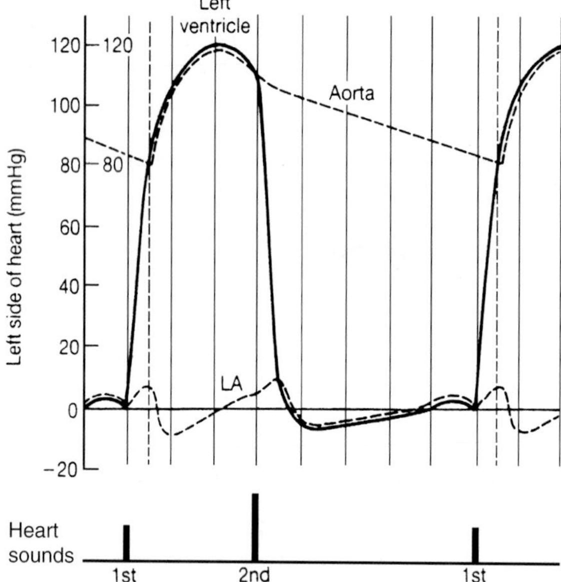

Fig. 48.7 Pressure changes on the left side of the heart. Vertical marks are at 0.2 s intervals. LA, left atrium.

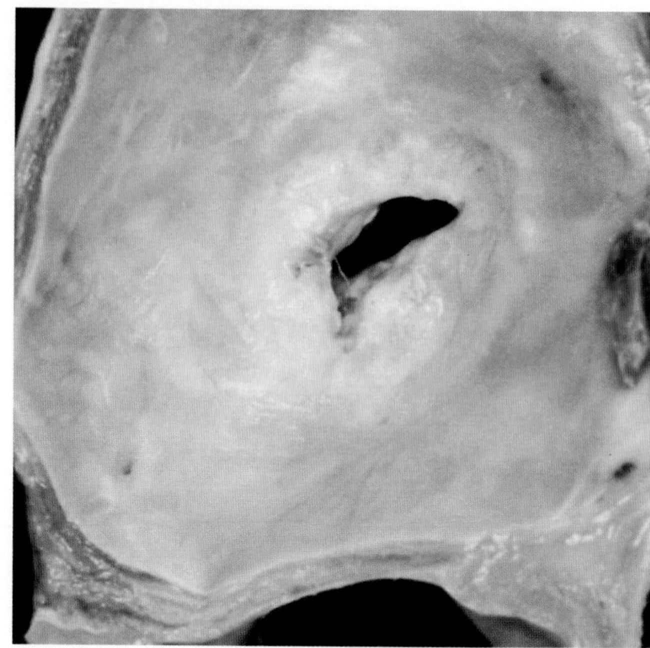

Fig. 48.8 Severe rheumatic mitral stenosis resulting in a 'fish-mouth' orifice. Note the dilated and thickened left atrium (*courtesy of Professor M.J. Davies*).

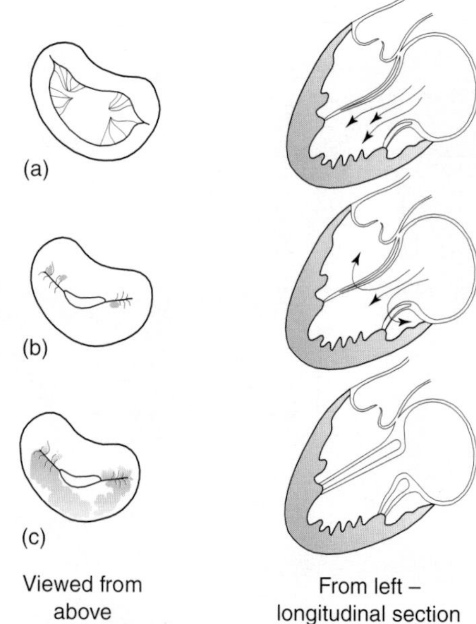

Fig. 48.9 The mitral valve viewed from the left atrial aspect (left) and in a longitudinal section (right). (a) The valve is normal, mobile and opens widely in diastole. (b) The commissures are fused but the cusps still pliable and the chordae free. At the onset of diastole the cusps tense abruptly (the so-called 'opening' snap), blood enters through the restricted orifice making a rumbling murmur, and the valve closes with a loud first sound. Commissurotomy, whether by surgical closed valvotomy, balloon dilatation or open operation, is effective. (c) The valve is rigid and calcified and the mechanism is funnel shaped. Valve replacement is the only practical solution.

Mitral valve disease

Mitral stenosis

Apart from rare congenital anomalies which present in infancy, mitral stenosis is a consequence of rheumatic fever (Figs 48.8 and 48.9). During the healing phase of acute rheumatic fever, the valve leaflets become adherent to each other at their free border so that the commissures become obliterated. This narrows the valve orifice and further obstruction ensues when the cusps become thickened and stiff. There may be a degree of regurgitation if the valve is unable to close during systole. This is the most common inflammatory disease affecting the heart valves world-wide, but the incidence has fallen over the last few decades probably as a result of a combination of improved housing, early treatment of streptococcal infections with antibiotics and possibly a change in the virulence of the organism. The acute condition affects all parts of the heart but the major residual haemodynamic effects are the result of involvement of the valves. The mitral valve is most frequently involved with the aortic, tricuspid and pulmonary valves affected less often. The characteristic pathological finding in chronic rheumatic valve disease is thickened valve cusps with fused leaflets and fused chordae.

Haemodynamics. The passage of blood is obstructed from the left atrium to the left ventricle and the pressure in the left atrium rises. The pressure in the pulmonary veins and capillaries rises and, if it exceeds the oncotic pressure, there is acute pulmonary oedema. With time, the lungs are protected against pulmonary oedema by contraction of proximal pulmonary arterioles, but this leads to an increased demand on the right ventricle which ultimately fails. Raised systemic venous pressure leads to peripheral oedema.

A serious complication of mitral stenosis is the development of atrial fibrillation. This may herald the onset of symptoms and the enlargement of the left atrium may predispose to the formation of thrombus. Infective endocarditis is a further hazard (Fig. 48.10).

Clinical features. There may be signs of right heart failure and the pulse may be irregular if atrial fibrillation has occurred. The heart sounds may reveal an opening snap if the valve is still pliable and in pure mitral stenosis, a low rumbling diastolic murmur will be heard. The pulmonary component of the second heart sound may be loud depending on the severity of the pulmonary hypertension.

Investigation. ***Chest radiography.*** There is a small aortic outline and a prominent pulmonary artery. The left atrium enlarges (sometimes to an enormous degree) and the right ventricle also appears enlarged. The left ventricle is spared if there is no aortic valve disease and is of normal size or small (Figs 48.11 and 48.12).

Electrocardiography (ECG). The right ventricular hypertrophy results in tall QRS complexes in the right ventricular leads (combined height of Q and R>30 mm in leads V1–V3). There may also be a characteristic notched P wave (P mitrale) if sinus rhythm is present. In long-standing mitral stenosis there is usually atrial fibrillation and no P waves are seen.

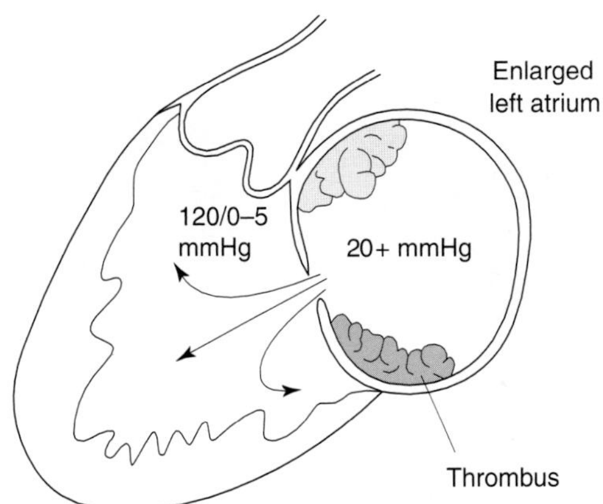

Fig. 48.10 Mitral stenosis. The aorta and left ventricle are relatively small owing to chronically reduced cardiac output. The atrium is enlarged and may fibrillate, become stagnant and contain thrombus. The ventricle fills with a turbulent jet which may be detected as a diastolic murmur or a thrill at the apex.

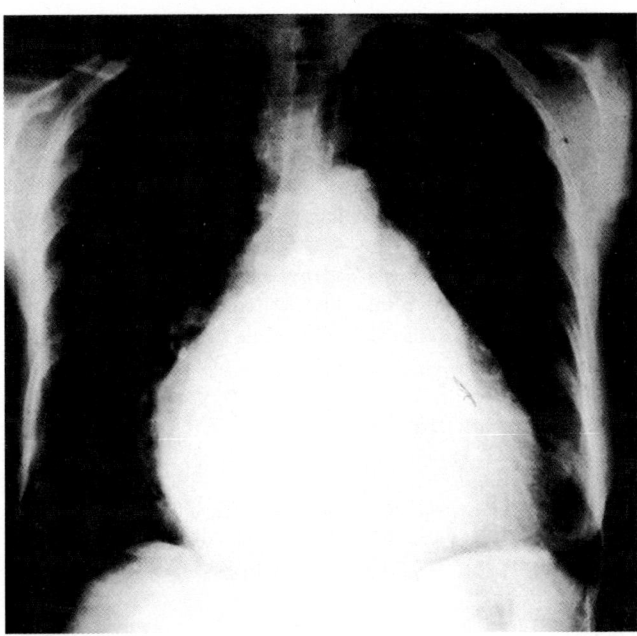

Fig. 48.11 Chest radiograph of long-standing mitral stenosis showing a massive left atrium.

Indications for surgery. Surgery is indicated for severe symptoms which are usually present if the pressure difference across the valve (during diastole) is 10 mmHg or more. Surgery is also indicated to protect the patient's future under certain circumstances, even if the patient is uncomplaining. Prognosis is determined by the severity of the stenosis, the size of the atrium, the onset of atrial fibrillation, rising pulmonary artery pressure and the unpredictable risk of

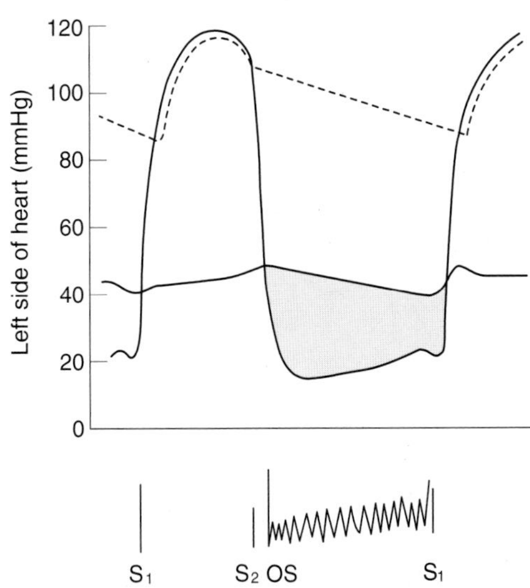

Fig. 48.12 Pressures in the left heart in mitral stenosis. S_1 and S_2 are the first and second heart sounds; OS is the 'opening snap'. The shaded area represents the pressure difference across the valve.

embolism from a large fibrillating atrium. The operation carries a low risk, particularly if the valve can be conserved rather than replaced; there is a high prospect of success and improved prognosis thereafter.

Surgery is best avoided during pregnancy but may be necessary if the heart cannot meet the extra demands placed on it. Other valves may be affected and their relative importance to the patient's condition must be assessed. Age is not a contraindication but the risks from surgery increase with age. A pliant, mobile valve may benefit from balloon valvotomy but restenosis is likely. Stiff, calcified valves require replacement.

Mitral regurgitation

Any pathology affecting the integrity of the valve apparatus (annulus, leaflets, chordae tendineae and papillary muscles) will lead to mitral regurgitation. There are many causes of regurgitation but they can be broadly classified into four headings:

1. degenerative (floppy valve – myxomatous degeneration of the leaflets);
2. ischaemic (papillary muscle rupture);
3. rheumatic (stiffened leaflets unable to coapt);
4. endocarditis (leaflet destruction by the infective process).

Mild degrees of regurgitation are well tolerated and even severe regurgitation which has slowly progressed may cause little disability (Fig. 48.13). The ventricle ejects into a large compliant left atrium and the pulmonary capillary pressure may be little affected. There is a pansystolic murmur over the apex, but there may be no other clinical signs if the process has progressed slowly and the left ventricle has adapted to the volume load placed on it. In contrast, acute mitral regurgitation is not well tolerated because the atrium is small and it may be associated with left ventricular ischaemia (for example, with papillary muscle rupture). There may then be clinical and radiological evidence of acute pulmonary oedema.

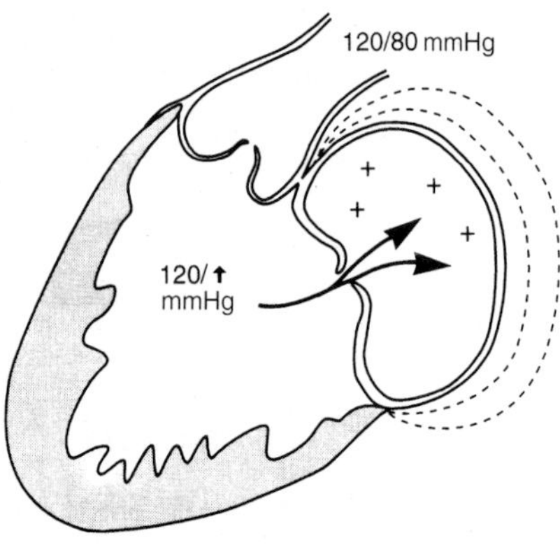

Fig. 48.13 Haemodynamics of mitral regurgitation. There is a loud pansystolic murmur and the left atrium enlarges. The left ventricle enlarges as a consequence of volume overload.

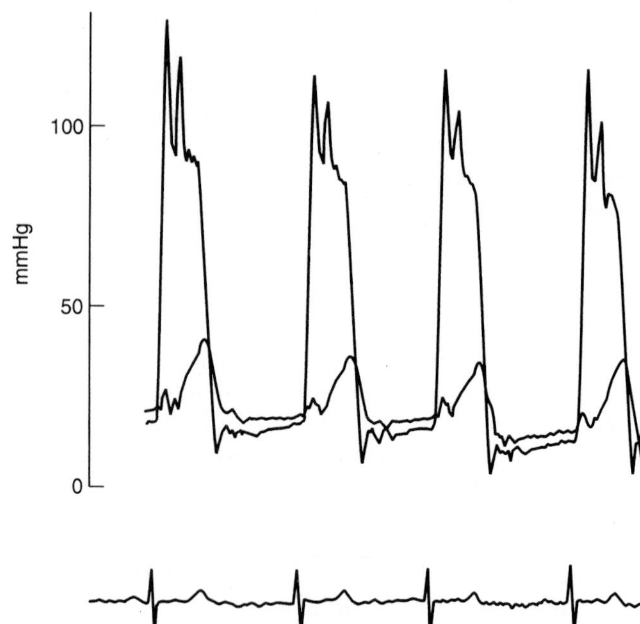

Fig. 48.14 An example of simultaneous left ventricular and left atrial pressure monitoring in a patient with mitral regurgitation.

Investigations. *Electrocardiography.* This does not really contribute to the diagnosis although there may be left ventricular hypertrophy (Fig. 48.14).

Chest radiography. There may be cardiomegaly and plethoric lung fields (Fig. 48.15).

Echocardiography. This will confirm the diagnosis and assess the degree of regurgitation.

Indications for operation. Patients with similar haemodynamics may have very different symptoms. Definite indications include severe symptoms, increasing pulmonary hypertension and uncontrolled endocarditis. Even in an

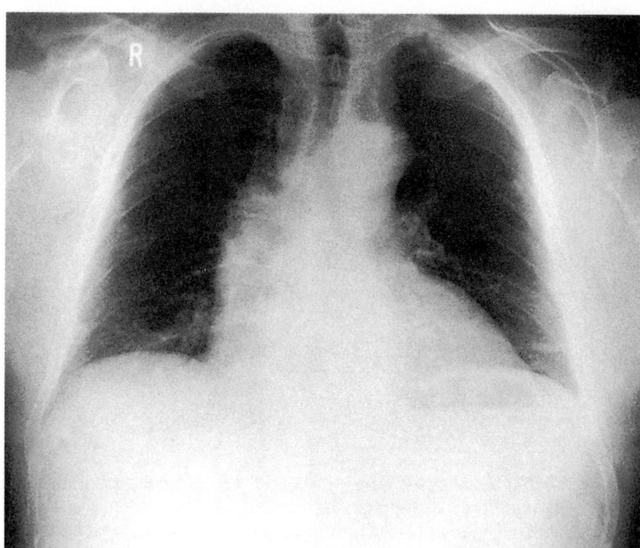

Fig. 48.15 Chest radiographic appearance of mitral regurgitation.

asymptomatic patient it may be important to operate to protect the future if the left ventricle is beginning to dilate. The aim is to conserve the valve but, if it cannot be made competent by surgical valvuloplasty, replacement is necessary.

Mitral valve operations

Closed mitral valvotomy

This procedure was the first commonly performed valve operation which effectively and reproducibly relieved the obstruction of mitral stenosis. The heart is approached through a left thoracotomy, and purse-string sutures are placed at the apex of the left ventricle and in the left atrial appendage. A finger is introduced into the left atrial appendage and the mitral valve is assessed by direct palpation. A special dilator (Tubbs) is inserted through the left ventricular apex and across the mitral valve (Fig. 48.16). The dilator is opened and the fused commissures are split. Some regurgitation may occur and the process may have to be repeated after 10–15 years. For the best results, the valve should be pliant, judged clinically by its loud first sound and opening snap; the characteristics of the valve are now ascertained by two-dimensional echocardiography. In experienced hands, the mortality rate is less than 1 per cent. It is uncommonly performed at present as similar results can be achieved with percutaneous balloon valvotomy (Fig. 48.17).

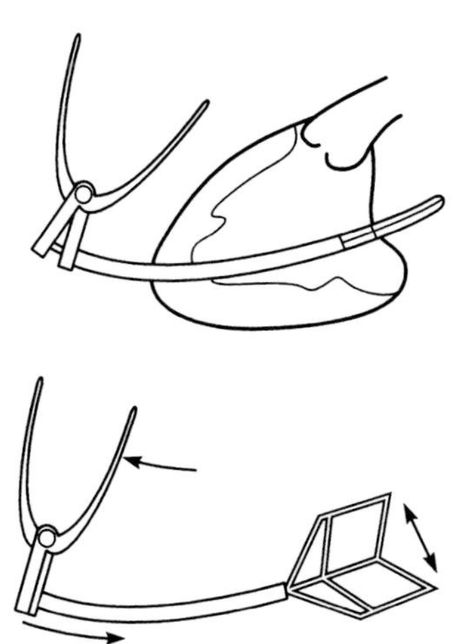

Fig. 48.16 The Tubbs' dilator for closed mitral valvotomy.

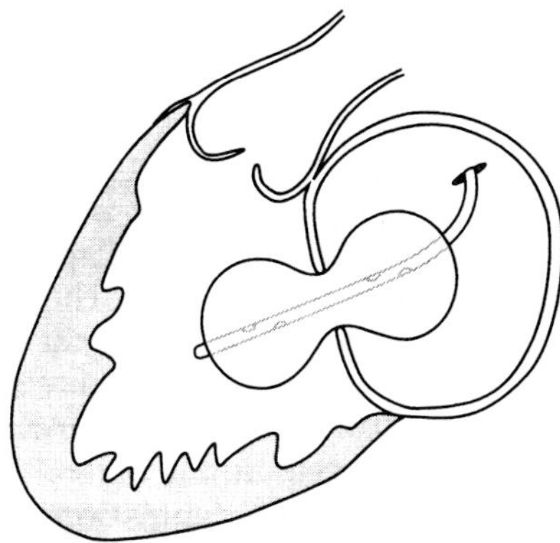

Fig. 48.17 Percutaneous balloon mitral valvotomy. The INOVE balloon is introduced transvenously and across the interatrial septum. Once across the mitral valve, the balloon is inflated.

Oswald Sidney Tubbs. Former Surgeon, St Bartholomew's Hospital, London, England.

Open repair

The current preference is to perform an open valvotomy with cardiopulmonary bypass under direct vision. This allows more accurate division of the commissures. In regurgitation, the valve can be repaired with a variety of techniques depending on the underlying pathology. Annular dilatation may be corrected by the use of an annuloplasty ring (Fig. 48.18). Leaflet destruction can be repaired with autologous pericardium and redundant tissue can be excised with direct repair to ensure leaflet apposition. Chordae can also be reconstructed. There is a trend to try and preserve the patient's native valve but if the valve is irreparable then it requires replacement.

Valve replacement

Valve replacement has undergone many modifications since it was introduced in the 1950s. There are two basic categories of replacement valve: biological and mechanical.

Biological valves. The most commonly used valve is the glutaraldehyde-preserved porcine valve, mounted on a

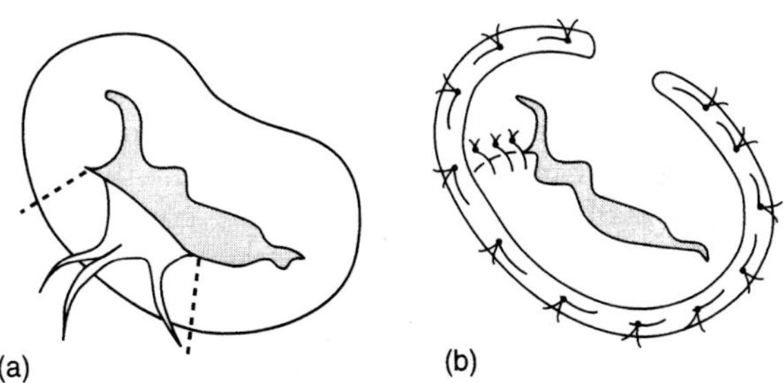

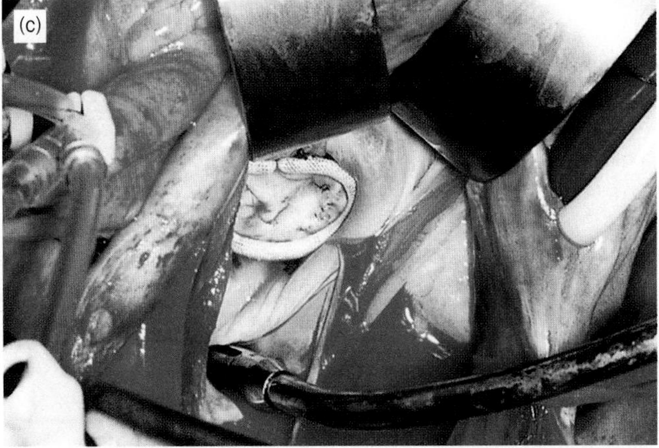

Fig. 48.18 Repair of the mitral valve using a Carpentier annuloplasty ring. Operative view of completed repair (*courtesy of A. Murday, FRCS*).

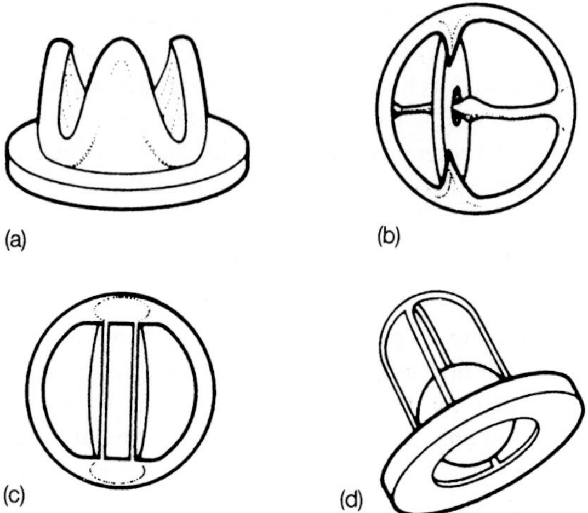

Fig. 48.19 A selection of valve types: (a) porcine; (b) disc valve; (c) bileaflet; (d) ball and cage (from *Disorders of the Cardiovascular System*, Edward Arnold).

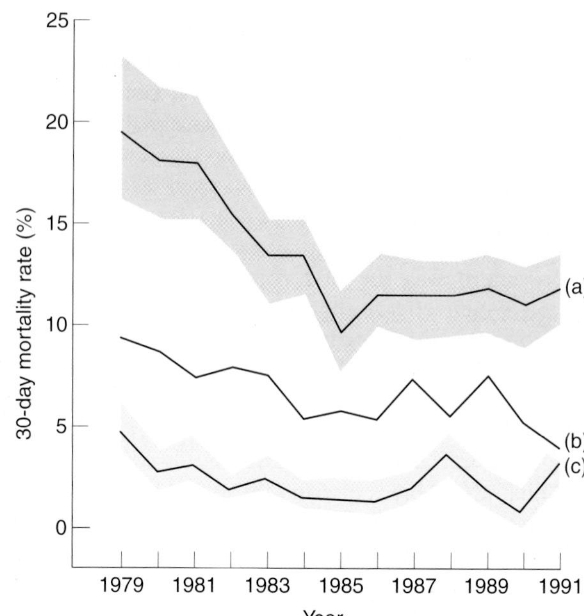

Fig. 48.20 Mortality associated with aortic and mitral valve surgery in the UK. (a) Valve replacement including coronary surgery; (b) mitral valve replacement alone; (c) mitral valve repair. The wide bands indicate confidence limits.

sewing ring and frame (Carpentier). It has very similar haemodynamics to a human valve but it degenerates with time. Its main advantage is that it is not thrombogenic and therefore anticoagulants are not required. Its limited lifespan and nonthrombogenicity make it suitable for elderly patients. Other indications include women of child-bearing age and those in whom warfarin is contraindicated; however, a further valve replacement will become necessary within 10–15 years.

Human valves (homograft) may be used particularly in the aortic position in young patients. There is an increasing trend to remove the native pulmonary valve and place it in the aortic position, using a homograft to replace the pulmonary valve (Ross). This operation is technically difficult and involves two valve operations (aortic and pulmonary) but the results are impressive with a low valve degeneration rate.

Mechanical valves. There are three commonly used designs: the cage and ball, the tilting disc and the bileaflet (Fig. 48.19). They are composed of a sewing ring and moving component(s) and have the advantage of durability. The main disadvantage is that the components of the valve are thrombogenic and therefore the patient requires systemic anticoagulation, usually with warfarin. This subjects the patients to a lifetime of blood tests, medication and the constant threat of haemorrhagic complications (intracerebral, epistaxis, gastrointestinal bleed). All patients with prosthetic valves are at risk of developing endocarditis.

Results of treatment

The operative mortality rate for elective mitral valve replacement is about 5 per cent (Fig. 48.20). This depends largely on the state of the myocardium and the general condition (including age) of the patient. Any associated pathology such as endocarditis or ischaemic heart disease increases the risk.

The aortic valve

Aortic valve disease

The normal aortic valve has three cusps corresponding to the sinuses of Valsalva, and named according to the relationships of the coronary orifices – right, left and noncoronary. Its surgical anatomy is challenging as it sits in the middle of the heart surrounded by the neighbouring three cardiac chambers: the right atrium (RA) and right ventricular (RV) outflow and the left atrium. The anterior leaflet of the mitral with the conducting tissue lies in continuity with the aortic valve annulus.

Stenosis

In young patients, stenosis is almost always congenital. In middle age, pathology is usually extensive calcification in a congenitally bicuspid valve. Senile stenosis is a result of thickening and calcification of the valve cusps but with no commissural fusion (unlike the appearances in rheumatic stenosis) (Figs 48.21–48.23). The left ventricle hypertrophies to overcome the stenosis but eventually the ventricular muscle fails. Patients are often asymptomatic until decompensation occurs. Dyspnoea, angina and exercise syncope are common complaints. There is an ejection systolic murmur over the aortic area radiating to the carotids. The pulse is slow rising in character and the apex beat may be displaced.

Alain Carpentier. Cardiac surgeon, Hospital Broussais, Paris, France.
Sir Donald Ross. Former Surgeon, National Heart Hospital, London, England.

Antonio Maria Valsalva, 1666–1723. Italian anatomist.

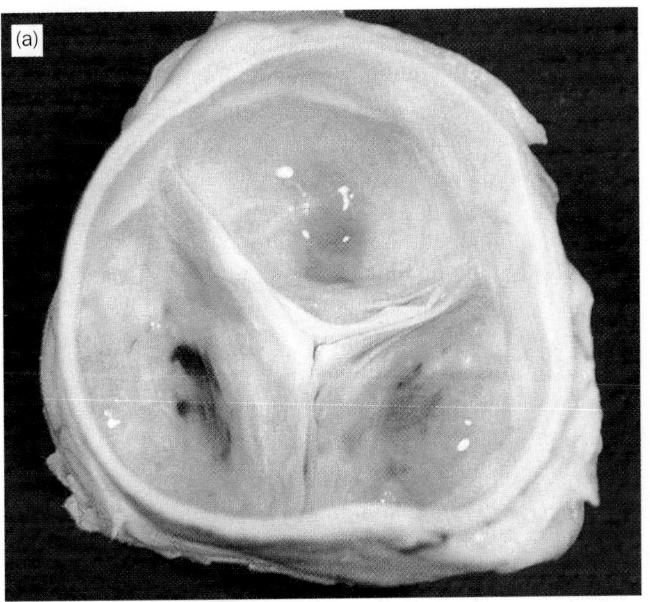

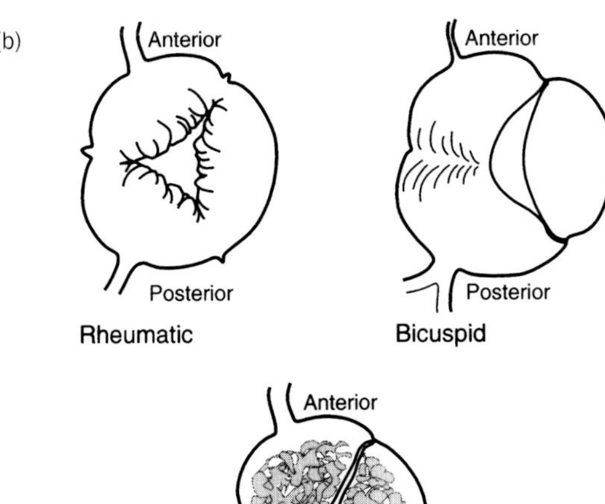

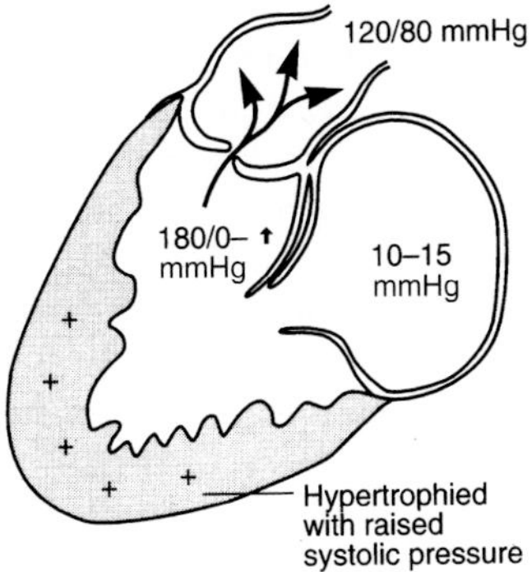

Fig. 48.21 (a) Formaldehyde-treated aortic valve (normal tricuspid configuration); (b) aortic stenosis – different pathologies.

Fig. 48.22 Aortic stenosis – haemodynamic changes. Aorta with poststenotic dilatation.

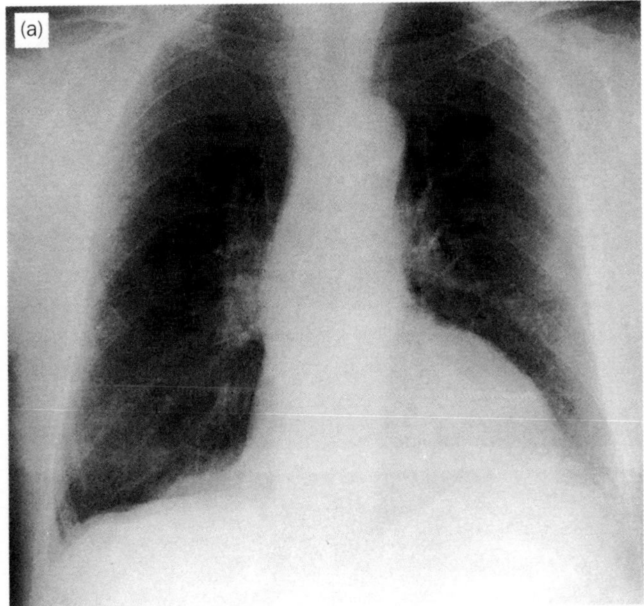

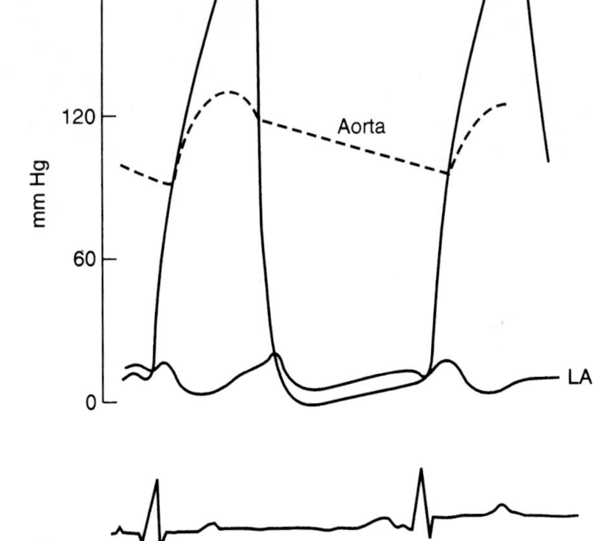

Fig. 48.23 (a) Chest radiograph in aortic stenosis; (b) a pressure diagram showing changes in aortic stenosis.

Investigations. ***Chest radiography.*** There is cardiomegaly in the advanced case and poststenotic dilatation of the aorta (Fig. 48.23).

Electrocardiography. There is left ventricular hypertrophy with tall R waves in the lateral leads and sometime a 'strain pattern' (ST depression in the lateral leads).

Echocardiography. This confirms the diagnosis and estimates the gradient.

Coronary angiography is often undertaken to exclude concurrent coronary artery disease and a direct measurement

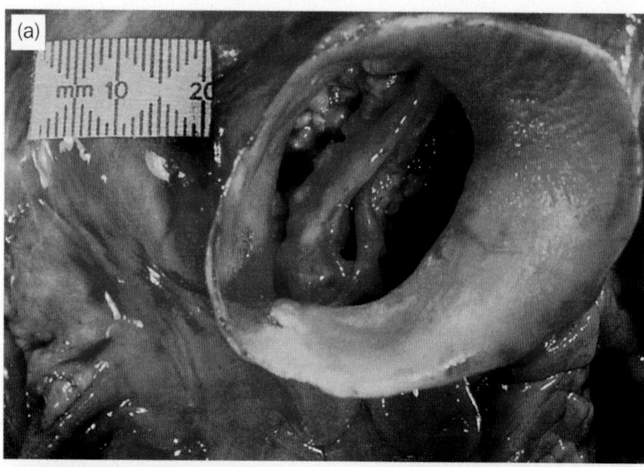

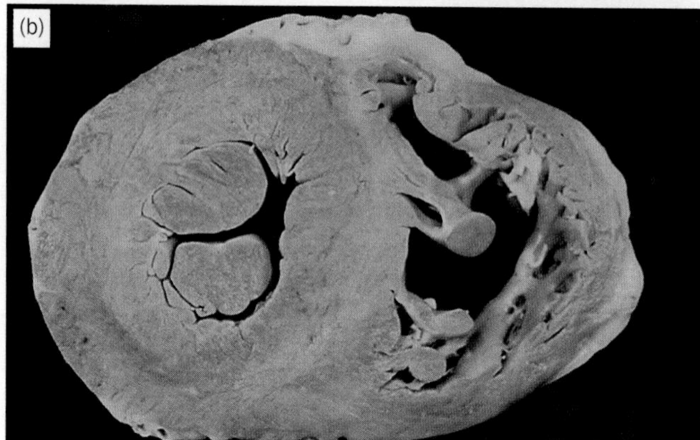

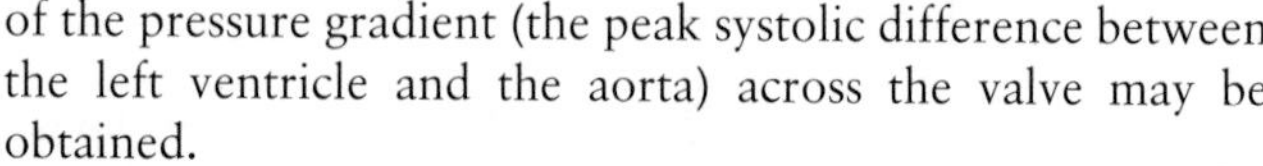
Fig. 48.24 (a) A bicuspid stenosed aortic valve; (b) a *post mortem* specimen demonstrating a grossly hypertrophic left ventricle in a patient with severe aortic stenosis.

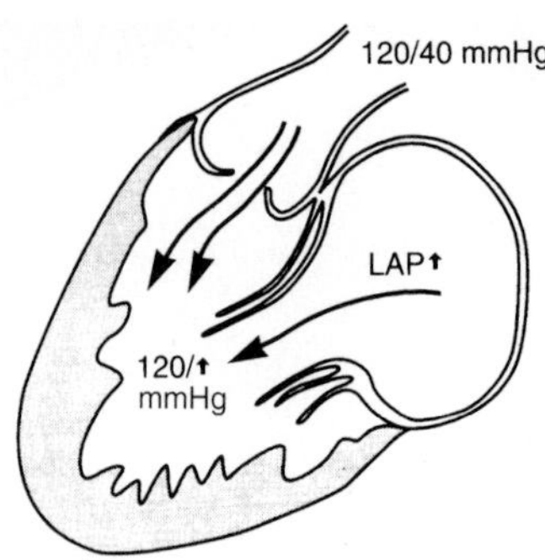

Fig. 48.25 Haemodynamic consequences of aortic regurgitation. The left ventricle dilates and hypertrophies and there is a diastolic mumur. LAP, left atrial pressure.

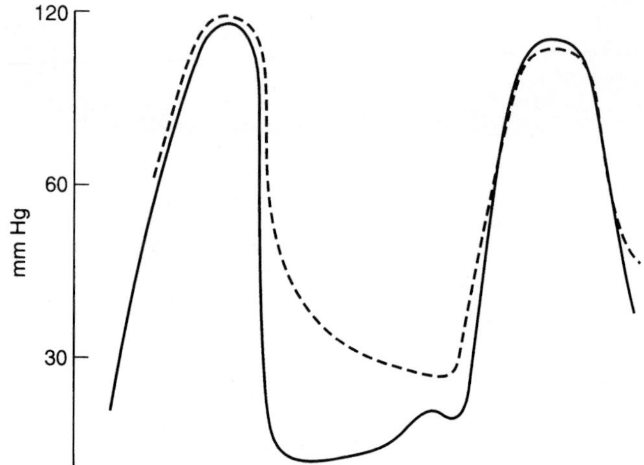

Fig. 48.26 The pressure changes in aortic regurgitation.

of the pressure gradient (the peak systolic difference between the left ventricle and the aorta) across the valve may be obtained.

Indications for operation. Operation is indicated for symptoms. In asymptomatic patients the stenosis should be relieved before irretrievable left ventricular failure occurs. The natural history is poor with a median survival of less than 2 years once symptoms occur. The patient is at risk of sudden death related to the severity of the stenosis. An estimated or actual gradient of over 60 mmHg is sufficient indication for replacement, but it should be remembered that, as the left ventricular function deteriorates, the stroke volume falls and the measurable gradient becomes less.

Aortic regurgitation

This may be caused by a number of conditions which disrupt the integrity of the aortic valve by affecting the cusps or their ability to coapt (Figs 48.25 and 48.26). Marfan's syndrome causes dilatation of the aortic root thus preventing closure of the valve. Other causes include rheumatic fever, connective tissue disorders, aortic dissection, tertiary syphilis and endocarditis. The increased stroke volume results in left ventricular dilatation. The pulse is large volume and collapsing in character.

Slowly progressive regurgitation may be well tolerated for years but the patient may complain of progressive dyspnoea on exertion and angina. Up to 70 per cent of the ejection fraction may return to the left ventricle in aortic regurgitation.

Investigations. *Chest radiography.* The disease may be severe without overall increase in the cardiac dimensions and increasing size is an indication that the left ventricle is dilating.

Electrocardiography. There are enlarged R waves in the lateral chest leads denoting left ventricular hypertrophy and a 'strain' pattern (ST depression) but the rhythm is normally regular.

Echocardiography with a Doppler probe will confirm the regurgitation.

Bernard-Jean Antonin Marfan, 1858–1942. French paediatrician.

Christian Johann Doppler, 1803–53. Austrian physicist and mathematician.

Coronary angiography may be required if coexistent ischaemic heart disease is suspected.

Indications for operation. Minor degrees of aortic regurgitation are well tolerated but if the ventricle deteriorates and dilates it may be too late to retrieve the situation. The end-systolic dimension, as measured by echocardiography, is often the best serial measure of worsening left ventricular dilatation and a figure of over 5.5 cmHg indicates severe pathology warranting valve replacement. Patients with severe symptoms or worsening left ventricular dilatation are candidates for surgery.

Aortic valve surgery

Unlike mitral valve surgery, there are few occasions where the aortic valve can be repaired and usually the valve requires replacement. This is performed through a median sternotomy on cardiopulmonary bypass. The aorta is cross-clamped and opened proximally to reveal the diseased valve. Cardioplegic solution is infused into the coronary arteries to arrest the heart in diastole. The valve is then excised leaving the annulus *in situ* but removing as much calcific debris as possible. The replacement valve is then sutured into position at the level of the native annulus and the aortotomy is closed. The heart is de-aired and the cross-clamp released, thus reperfusing the myocardium.

Results of treatment

The operative mortality rate for elective aortic valve surgery is less than 5 per cent, but emergency surgery, surgery for endocarditis or surgery in older patients results in a higher operative mortality rate (Fig. 48.27).

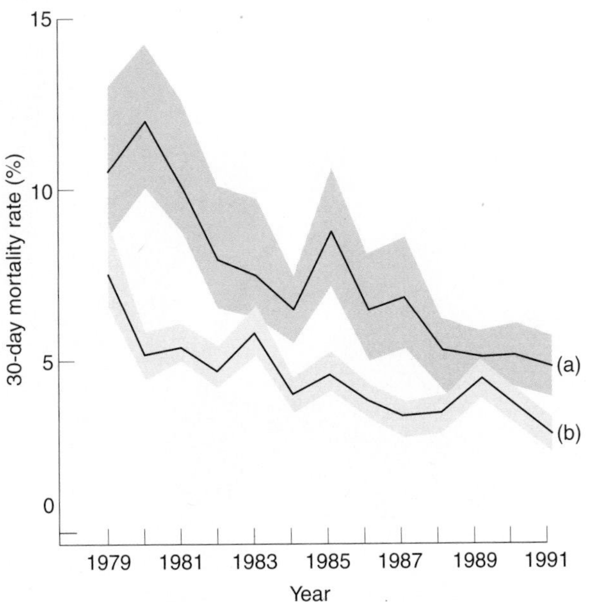

Fig. 48.27 Mortality rates from aortic valve surgery, based on data from the UK Cardiac Surgery Register. (a) Valve replacement and coronary surgery; (b) valve replacement alone.

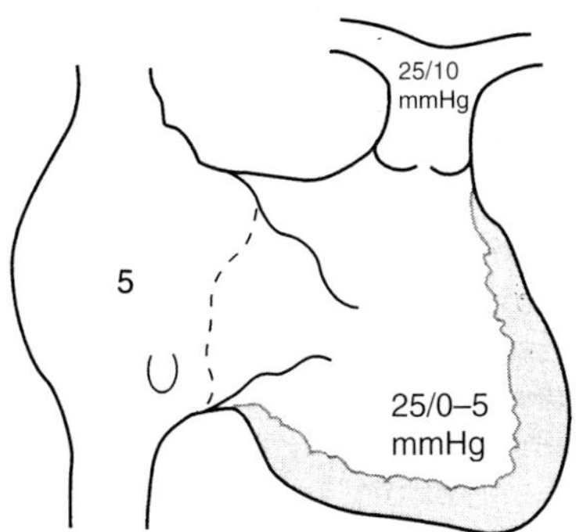

Fig. 48.28 Normal right-sided pressures.

Tricuspid valve

Tricuspid valve disease

This valve is rarely involved in isolation by a disease process (Fig. 48.28). In rheumatic fever, the aortic and mitral valves are usually affected as well, with stenosis more common than regurgitation. The carcinoid syndrome may produce isolated stenosis.

Isolated tricuspid regurgitation is almost exclusively caused by endocarditis in drug addicts who inject intravenously. There is characteristic venous pulsation in the neck and systolic pulsation of the liver, leading to abdominal pain and ascites.

It may be possible to perform a valvotomy for stenosis but this usually leads to severe incompetence. In these cases it is necessary to replace the valve. For regurgitation there are numerous ways to perform valvuloplasty, all of which seem to produce reasonable results. The mortality from tricuspid valve surgery is high, largely as a result of the associated pathology from other valve lesions.

Pulmonary valvular disease

Acquired pulmonary valve disease is rare and usually results from the carcinoid syndrome or rheumatic fever. In both diseases, other valve lesions usually dominate the clinical picture. Pulmonary valvotomy is usually feasible for stenosis. Replacement is almost never performed.

Prosthetic valve

Prosthetic valve disease

There is now a large cohort of patients who are long-term survivors after prosthetic valve surgery and a number of problems and complications can occur. Some of these problems may be technical and related to the valve itself and others are the result of valve replacement in general (Fig. 48.29).

Valve failure. From about 7 years after implantation, cases begin to come back for reoperation with increasing frequency. The deterioration results in stenosis, incompetence or both. This usually progresses slowly, allowing planned replacement in most cases (Fig. 48.30).

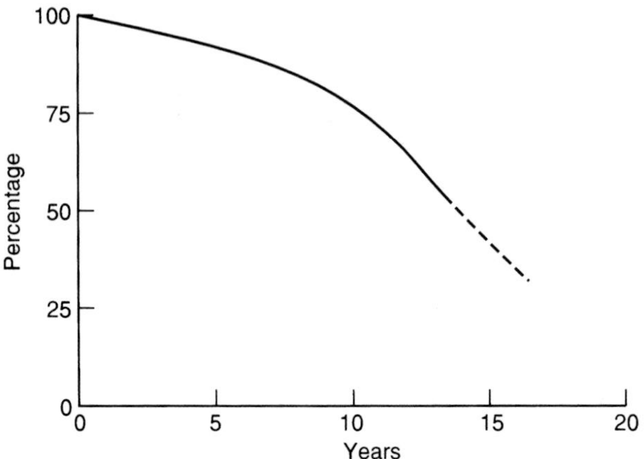

Fig. 48.29 Failure rate for biological valves. Tissue valve failure accelerates at 10 years; median is about 12–13 years.

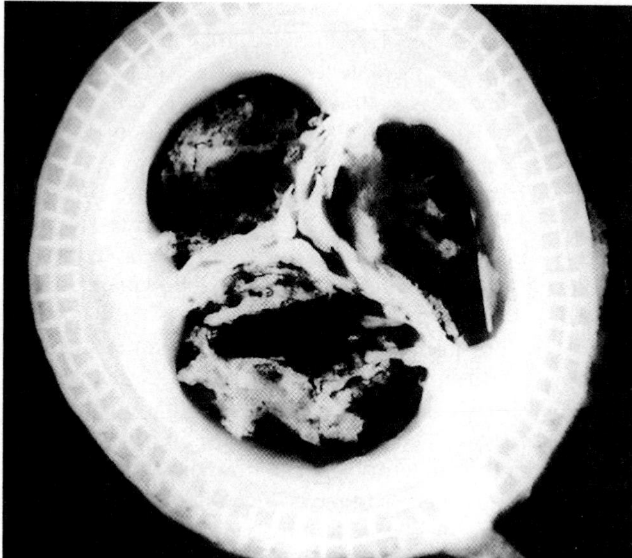

Fig. 48.30 Radiograph of a calcified, stenosed porcine valve showing large areas of calcification in the valve cusps and apposing edges.

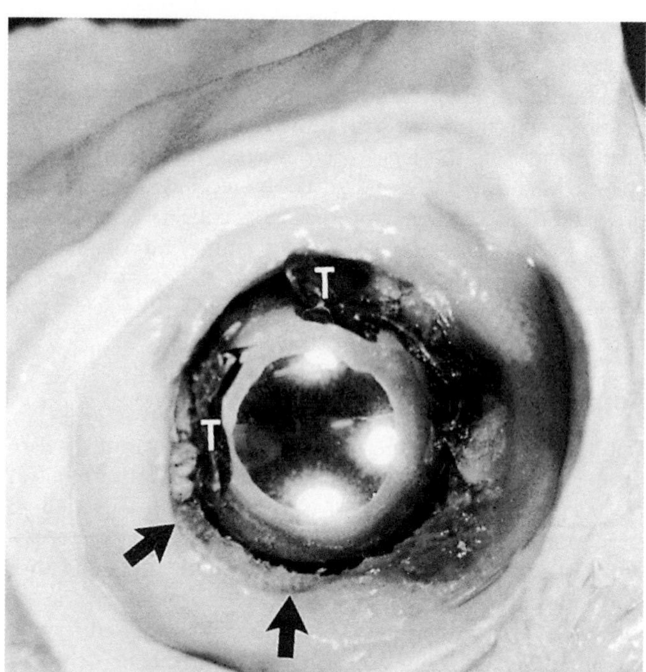

Fig. 48.31 Thrombus (T) on the moving component of a ball and cage valve.

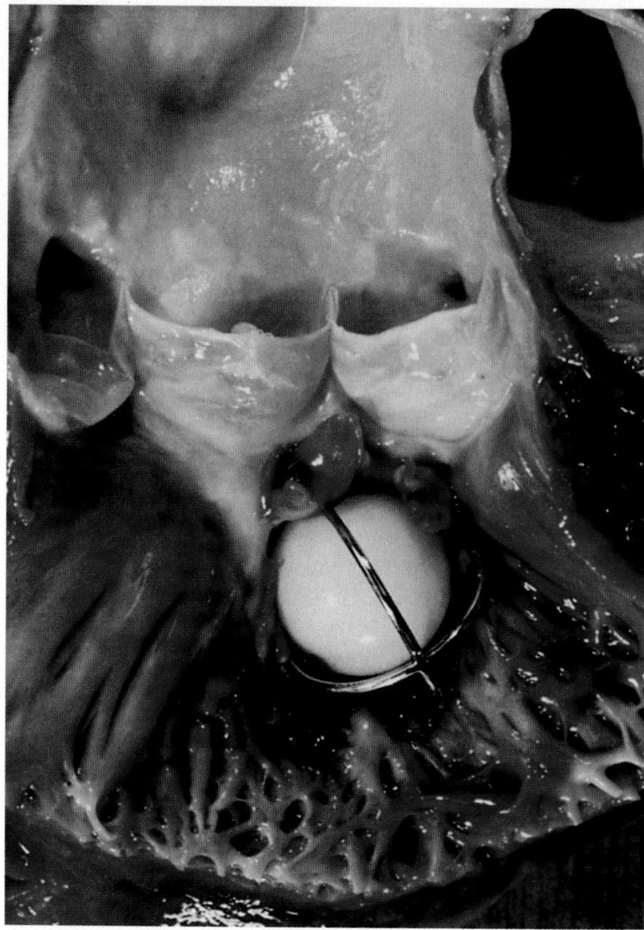

Fig. 48.32 A paraprosthetic leak by a cage and ball mitral valve prosthesis, just inferior to the aortic annulus.

Failure of a mechanical prosthesis can be sudden and catastrophic, resulting in a rapid demise.

Thromboembolism. This is always a risk with foreign material in the circulation (Fig. 48.31). The risk is low with the biological valves and anticoagulation is unnecessary. This makes this type of valve suitable for elderly patients. Anticoagulation is mandatory for mechanical valves and this results in frequent blood tests and the associated bleeding problems.

Paravalvular leak. This is usually a technical problem resulting in a leak between the valve ring and the native annulus (Fig. 48.32). It may also be the result of infection. The leak can cause haemolytic anaemia or haemodynamic compromise and the valve may need replacement.

Endocarditis is a serious complication. All patients must be made aware of this potential complication and must have prophylactic antibiotics for any type of surgical or dental procedure. There are marked systemic symptoms and the infective process may progress rapidly to destroy the native valve annulus, leading to abscess formation.

The mortality rate from this condition is very high (>50 per cent) even with antibiotics, and early surgery to remove the infected prosthesis is recommended. Aggressive surgical therapy using a homograft wherever possible has reduced the mortality rate to less than 20 per cent. Management should be a joint approach with involvement of the surgeon, physician and microbiologist.

Infective endocarditis

Endocarditis of a heart valve occurs when a suitable organism is exposed to a vulnerable intracardiac site. Most commonly, this is the patient's own abnormal valve or a valve replacement. Rarely it can occur in an intracardiac shunt (ventricular septal defect or patent ductus arteriosus). The bloodstream is often exposed to transient bacteraemias, particularly during dental treatment, but any microorganism, except viruses, can lead to endocarditis.

The most common organisms are:

- *Streptococcus viridans*;
- staphylococci;
- enterococci.

Endocarditis seems to become established in regions of turbulent flow in the heart. Fibrinous deposits containing platelets and the organisms develop to form characteristic vegetations. These may invade the surrounding tissue and destroy it, leading to valve incompetence and abscess formation (Fig. 48.33). Embolic debris may become lodged in the peripheries causing a variety of clinical features.

Presentation. There is often an influenza-type illness with generalised pain. The symptoms may fluctuate over several weeks, but once the endocarditis begins to destroy tissue then the patient's condition may markedly worsen.

An important part of the history is the presence of an underlying congenital or valvular anomaly. Anaemia may be present together with splinter haemorrhages and tender nodules (Osler's nodes) in the finger pulps. A detailed examination of the cardiovascular system should note any murmurs or change of murmur from those heard previously. Splenomegaly may occur and retinal emboli should be specifically excluded. Daily examination is mandatory to detect any deterioration in the patient's condition.

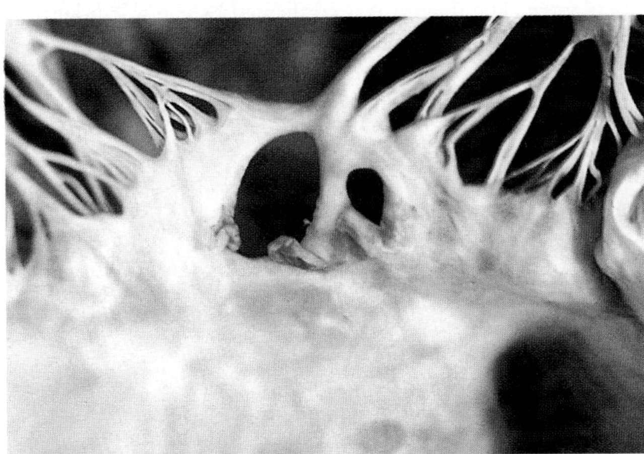

Fig. 48.33 Infective endocarditis leading to perforation of a mitral valve leaflet.

Blood cultures are taken from up to six different sites *before* antibiotics are given. Once an organism is grown, the antibiotics can be tailored to the organism isolated. About 80 per cent of blood cultures will grow an organism in this condition. The chest radiograph is often normal but the cardiac outline may enlarge if valve regurgitation is present and metastatic lung abscesses may occur. The ECG may show a lengthened P–R interval or degrees of heart block if an aortic root abscess has formed. Echocardiography is an important investigation because it will demonstrate the motion of the heart, the state of the valves and any vegetations present. Serial echocardiograms will monitor response to treatment.

In spite of the introduction of antibiotics, the 1-year mortality rate of this condition is 25–30 per cent. Cure is often possible if a sensitive organism is present and treatment started early. A delay in the diagnosis, inadequate treatment, prosthetic valve endocarditis and resistant organisms all reduce the likelihood of cure. Urgent surgery may be necessary if the haemodynamic state deteriorates while infection is still present. If the patient is haemodynamically stable, he or she needs 6 weeks of intravenous antibiotics. Indications for surgical intervention are:

- an important mechanical lesion that can be corrected (regurgitant valve or acquired shunt);
- development of an abscess resulting in heart block;
- uncontrolled infection in spite of seemingly adequate antibiotic regimens.

Congenital heart disease

Development of the heart

The primitive vascular tube is apparent by the third week of foetal life and over the next weeks it folds in on itself, becomes septated and begins to beat (Fig. 48.34). By 12 weeks it has fully developed. Abnormalities may arise from the persistence of normal foetal channels (patent ductus arteriosus, patent foramen ovale), failure of septation [atrial septal defect (ASD), ventricular septal defect, tetralogy of Fallot], stenosis (intracardiac – supravalulvar, valvular, infravalvular; or extracardiac – coarctation of the aorta), atresia or abnormal connections (transposition of the great arteries, total anomalous venous drainage). Echocardiography is now sufficiently sensitive to detect intracardiac lesions in the second trimester.

Sir William Osler, 1849–1919. Canadian-born physician; Professor of Medicine, McGill University, Canada, University of Pennsylvania, Johns Hopkins University, USA, and University of Oxford, England.

Etienne Louis Arthur Fallot, 1850–1911. Professor of Medicine, Marseille, France.

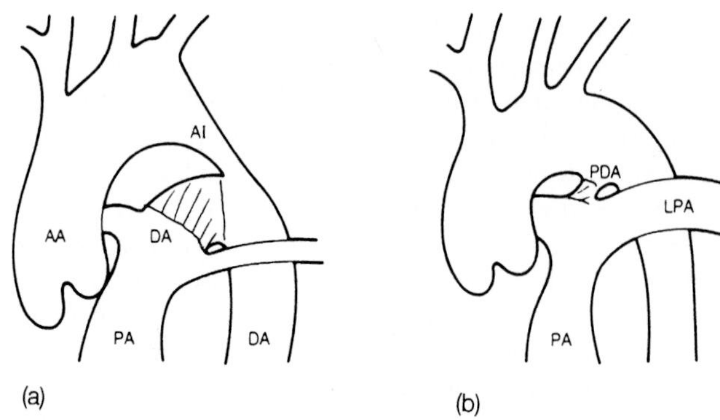

Fig. 48.34 (a) Relative sizes of the great vessels and the ductus arteriosus in the foetus. Oxygenated blood from the umbilical venous return passes from the hepatic vein, predominantly through the foramen ovale, and is ejected from the left heart to be distributed to the upper body. Desaturated blood passes through the right heart, out through the pulmonary artery (PA), bypasses the airless lungs, to pass via the ductus arteriosus into the descending aorta (DA). Note that the ductus arteriosus is large but the aortic isthmus (AI) and the right and left pulmonary arteries are relatively small. AA, ascending aorta. (b) Soon after birth the duct closes and the relative sizes of the great vessels gradually change to adult proportions. LPA, left pulmonary artery, PDA, persistent ductus arteriosus.

The incidence of congenital heart disease is about 1 per cent for live births. There is often no obvious aetiology but well-recognised associations include:

- maternal illness:
  - systemic lupus,
  - diabetes,
  - rubella,
  - alcohol abuse,
  - certain drugs (warfarin, phenytoin);
- chromosomal anomalies:
  - trisomy 21 (atrial septal defect – primum type, atrioventricular septal and atrioventricular canal defects),
  - trisomy 13 and 18,
  - Turner's syndrome (coarctation).

If the haemodynamic abnormality is tolerated, elective definitive operation is planned at an appropriate time in childhood but in some cases the infant is very ill and requires surgery in the neonatal period. Close co-operation between the paediatric cardiologist and the cardiothoracic surgeon is essential to define the anatomy of the defect, the degree of compromise and the necessary treatment.

Investigation of a child suspected of having a congenital defect begins with an accurate history from the parents and specific questions about maternal health and drug intake during pregnancy. A detailed family history is important because some defects are familial. Clinical examination may reveal a murmur, evidence of heart failure, failure to thrive and cyanosis. Investigation is much the same as for the adult patient and, with echocardiography available, catheterisation is now avoided whenever possible.

Henry Hubert Turner, b. 1892. American endocrinologist.

Classification

Congenital heart disease is broadly classified into cyanotic and acyanotic, although the distinction is not often clear cut. Only the more commonly encountered anomalies will be described.

There are three groups of cyanotic congenital heart disease and a representative example from each group will be described in detail.

1. A right-to-left shunt (compare Fallot's tetralogy): desaturated blood enters the systemic circulation before it passes through the lungs.
2. Parallel systemic and pulmonary blood flows (transposition of the great vessels): some mixing must occur or this situation would be incompatible with life.
3. Defects in the connections of the heart where there is mixing of the systemic and pulmonary blood flows [total anomalous pulmonary venous drainage (TAPVD)].

Tetralogy of Fallot

This is a range of conditions in which there is a ventriculoseptal defect with an overriding aorta, pulmonary artery stenosis and right ventricular hypertrophy making up the tetralogy (Fig. 48.35).

It is a relatively common condition accounting for about 10 per cent of all congenital heart defects. The large ventriculoseptal defect results in equal pressures within both ventricles. As a result of the pulmonary stenosis, more blood is discharged into the aorta but this blood is only partially saturated and cyanosis results. The lungs are only partially perfused and the total oxygenation is poor. The right ventricle is the dominant chamber in the circulation. One clinical feature of Fallot's tetralogy is squatting. This increases systemic vascular resistance and consequently blood is diverted into the pulmonary circulation with increased oxygenation. Lethargy and tiredness are common presenting symptoms but cyanosis is the most obvious clinical feature.

There is usually polycythaemia and the chest radiograph reveals a boot-shaped heart with poorly developed lung vasculature. The diagnosis is confirmed by echocardiography and cardiac catheterisation.

Indications for operation. These include severe cyanosis, dyspnoea on exertion and syncopal attacks. The choice of

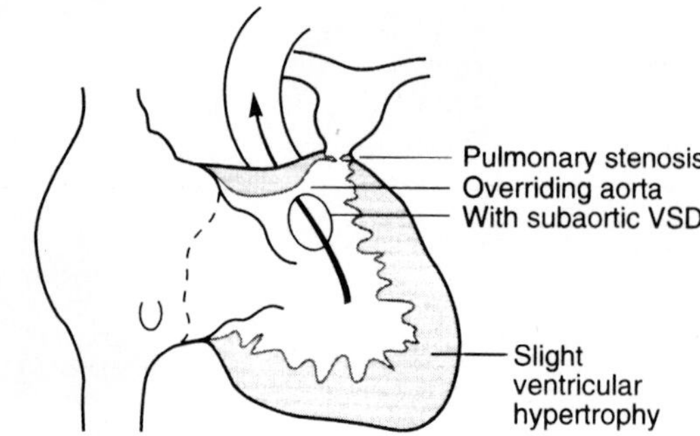

Fig. 48.35 Tetralogy of Fallot. VSD, ventricular septal defect.

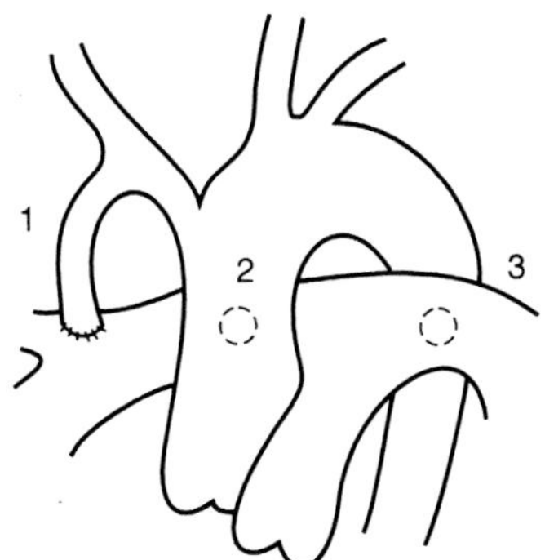

Fig. 48.36 Systemic to pulmonary shunts. 1, Blalock–Taussig subclavian artery to pulmonary artery; 2, Waterston ascending aorta to right pulmonary artery; 3, Potts descending aorta to left pulmonary artery.

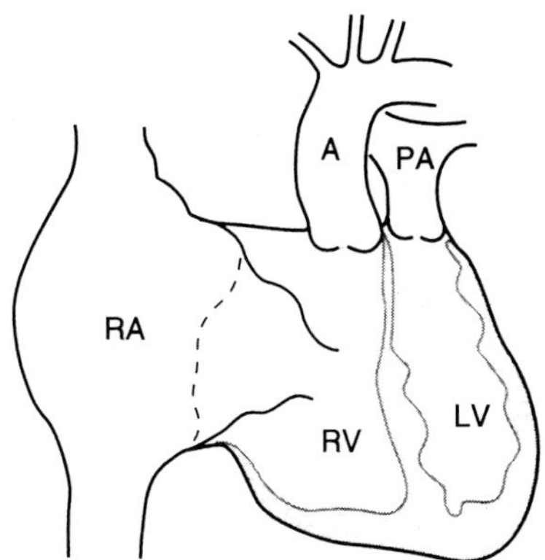

Fig. 48.37 Transposition of the great arteries. A, aorta; PA, pulmonary artery; RA, right atrium; RV, right ventricle; LV, left ventricle.

operation depends on anatomical considerations and the age and general condition of the patient.

There are two approaches to the operative treatment of Fallot's tetralogy (Fig. 48.36). Palliative procedures to divert systemic blood into the pulmonary circulation may be used to improve oxygenation. These include right subclavian to pulmonary artery anastomosis (Blalock–Taussig) or a modification in which an interposition graft is used or an aortic-pulmonary artery anastomosis (Potts). Definitive repair may be performed as the first procedure, or some years after a palliative shunt.

Total correction is via a median sternotomy and can include dealing with a previously constructed shunt. The correction is performed using cardiopulmonary bypass and the ventricular septal defect is closed (often with autologous pericardium), the stenotic infundibulum or pulmonary valve is dealt with and the right ventricular outflow tract is widened using a pericardial or a synthetic patch. Repair is often undertaken in the third year and ideally before the child reaches school age.

Transposition of the great vessels

In this condition the aorta arises from the right ventricle and the pulmonary artery from the left ventricle (Fig. 48.37). Oxygenated blood from the lungs is returned to the lungs and desaturated blood is pumped around the systemic circulation. Obviously, if the pulmonary and systemic circulations are separate, the situation is compatible with life. Mixing of blood must occur via an atrial or ventricular septal defect or patent ductus arteriosus. The condition was first described by Morgagni. Palliation was achieved by initially creating an ASD (Blalock) but both Senning and Mustard devised operations to redirect atrial blood into the appropriate ventricle so that oxygenated blood reaches the systemic circulation and deoxygenated blood goes into the pulmonary circulation.

The most obvious presentation is severe cyanosis in the neonatal period, but there is little in the way of respiratory symptoms. Cardiac catheterisation and echocardiography confirm the diagnosis and delineate the anatomy.

Treatment. The initial treatment for this condition is balloon septostomy (Rashkind). A balloon-tipped catheter is advanced from a large vein and manipulated across the atrial septum. The balloon is inflated and forcibly retracted thus producing a large tear in the intra-atrial septum. This allows adequate mixing of the two circulations and provides excellent palliation until a corrective procedure can be performed. Total anatomical correction has become popular and can be carried out even in the neonatal period. This involves disconnecting the pulmonary artery from the left ventricular outflow and the aorta from the right ventricular outflow. The coronary arteries are reimplanted into the aorta which now arises from the left ventricle (as it should). The mortality rate is 10 per cent but the long-term results for those who survive are good.

Total anomalous pulmonary venous drainage

This condition accounts for only 1–2 per cent of congenital heart disease. In this condition the pulmonary venous drainage has become disconnected from the left atrium and drains into the systemic venous circulation at some point (inferior vena cava, superior vena cava, coronary sinus or right atrium). There is mixing of the systemic and pulmonary circulations through a patent foramen ovale.

Alfred Blalock, 1899–1964. Professor of Surgery, Johns Hopkins University, Baltimore, Maryland, USA.

Helen Brooke Taussig, 1898–1986. American paediatrician and Professor, Johns Hopkins University, Baltimore, Maryland, USA.

Willis John Potts, 1895–1968. Surgeon, Children's Memorial Hospital, Chicago, Illinois, USA.

David James Waterston, former Surgeon, Hospital for Sick Children, Great Ormond Street, London, England.

Giovanni Morgagni, 1682–1771. Professor of Anatomy, Padua, Italy.

A. Senning, Professor of Surgery, Zurich, Switzerland.

William Mustard, 1914–87. Former Professor of Cardiovascular Surgery, Hospital for Sick Children, Toronto, Canada.

William Jacobson Rashkind, Surgeon, Children's Hospital, Philadelphia, Pennsylvania, USA.

Diagnosis. There is cyanosis on exertion, often with failure to thrive and feeding difficulties. The chest radiographic appearances depend on the anatomy but may be normal. There is right axis deviation and right ventricular hypertrophy on the ECG. Echocardiography and cardiac angiography are necessary to confirm the diagnosis and establish the location of the anomalous drainage.

Indications for surgery. Prognosis without operation is poor and the exact operative technique depends on the anatomy. The surgical principle is to re-establish the pulmonary venous drainage into the left atrium. Operative mortality is higher in younger patients and in those with complex lesions. The long-term results for survivors of the operation are generally good.

Eisenmenger's syndrome

This occurs following the reversal of a left-to-right shunt. There is a number of conditions resulting in a left-to-right shunt (atrial and ventricular septal defects, patent ductus arteriosus, etc.), but eventually the right ventricle hypertrophies and the pressure in the pulmonary artery increases as a result of the increased flow. Increasing pulmonary hypertension leads to equalisation of pressures either side of the shunt but, at some point, the right-sided pressures will exceed those on the left side and desaturated blood enters the left side of the circulation. Cyanosis and dyspnoea are the most common clinical features. This state of affairs is termed 'Eisenmenger's syndrome' and is irreversible. Closure of the shunt is contraindicated if pulmonary hypertension is irreversible because the right-to-left shunt now serves to decompress the pulmonary circulation.

Acyanotic congenital heart disease

Persistent ductus arteriosus

This anomaly accounts for 5–10 per cent of congenital heart disease. Following birth, the ductus arteriosus, which facilitates the transfer of oxygenated blood in the foetal circulation from the pulmonary artery to the aorta, begins to close. The trigger for this is poorly understood but the drop in the resistance of the pulmonary circulation as the lungs expand may contribute. The mechanism of ductus closure involves prostaglandins and prostaglandin analogues may be used therapeutically to keep the ductus open in the first few weeks of life. There may be occasions when a patent ductus is necessary for survival as in some forms of congenital heart defects (such as coarctation of the aorta), where the ductus provides the only means of oxygenated blood reaching the systemic circulation. The ductus may be closed during the first few weeks of life by administering indomethacin. In the isolated case of patent ductus, there is a left-to-right shunt of blood resulting in a high pulmonary blood flow. This may lead to respiratory difficulties in the preterm child in addition to heart failure. If medical treatment to close the ductus is unsuccessful, the lesion may be treated by interventional cardiology (i.e. an umbrella occlusion device inserted percutaneously) or by surgery via a left thoracotomy (Fig. 48.38). Treatment for asymptomatic ductus arteriosus should be considered because of the risk of endocarditis.

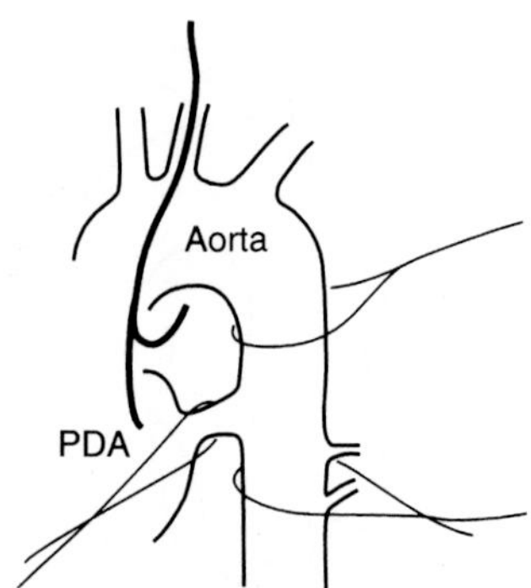

Fig. 48.38 Surgical exposure for closure of persistent ductus arteriosus (PDA). The tape is passed around the aorta above and below the duct, and the ductus is then either tied with a stout ligature or formally divided and either end sutured. In neonates a single liga clip can be used, usually with secure closure. The recurrent laryngeal nerve, and severe haemorrhage, are the surgical pitfalls.

Coarctation of the aorta

This accounts for 5 per cent of congenital heart disease. In this condition the arch of the aorta around the area of the ductus arteriosus is narrowed (Figs 48.39 and 48.40). The coarctation puts a pressure load on the left ventricle which can ultimately fail. The upper body is well perfused but the lower body, including the kidneys, is poorly perfused

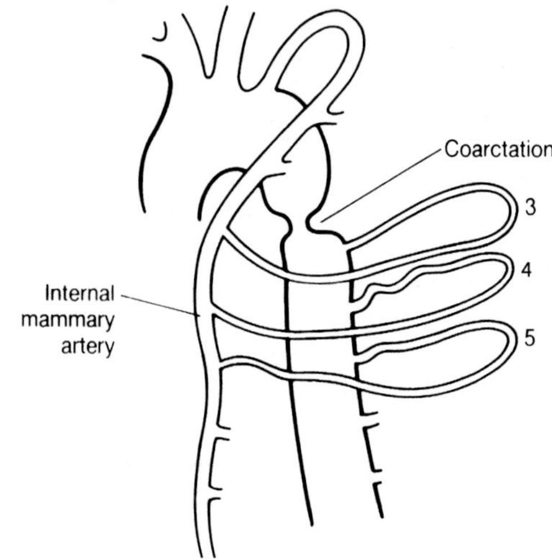

Fig. 48.39 The intercostal arteries (from the third down) become very much enlarged in coarctation. They connect the internal mammary artery, which arises well above the coarctation, to the aorta below it. The ribs are notched owing to the increased size and tortuosity of the intercostal arteries (from *Disorders of the Cardiovascular System,* Edward Arnold).

Victor Eisenmenger, 1822–1909. German physician.

(a)

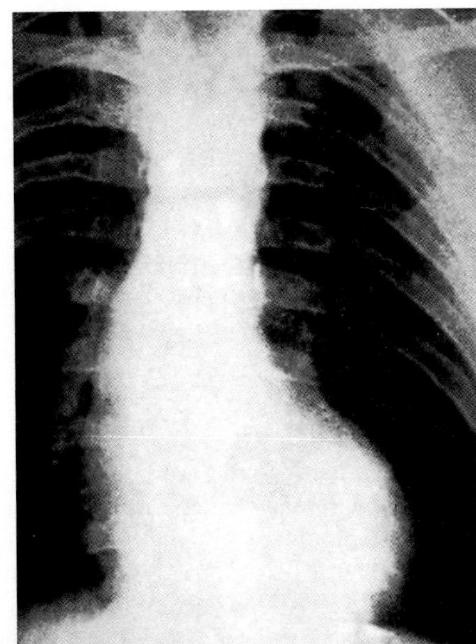

(b)

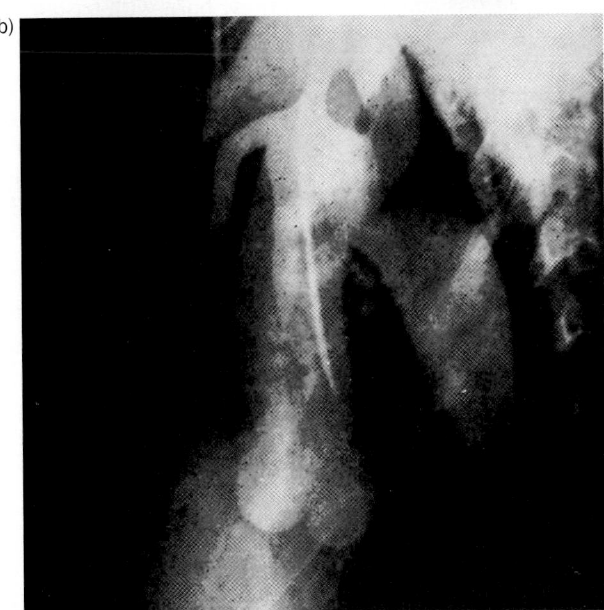

Fig. 48.40 (a) Coarctation of aorta showing a prominent ascending aorta, double aortic knuckle and rib notching; (b) aortogram showing the stenosis and the marked collateral vessels.

leading to fluid overload, excess renin secretion and acidosis. There is often radiofemoral delay when examining the pulses. The child often appears well in the first few days of life because the coarctation is bypassed by the ductus arteriosus and oxygenated blood reaches the entire systemic circulation.

As the ductus closes, the child becomes progressively more unwell. Emergency treatment includes the administration of prostaglandin analogues to keep the ductus open and general resuscitation before corrective treatment, which includes balloon dilatation or open operation via a left thoracotomy.

Operative options include resection of the coarctation and end-to-end anastomosis or the use of the left subclavian artery as an onlay flap. In older children, there is upper body hypertension with development of enormous collateral vessels which may cause rib notching and flow murmurs over the scapula. Treatment is advised because of the risk of endocarditis and heart failure, but the preoperative hypertension may not resolve. In the older patient, the subclavian flap operation is not feasible and resection with end-to-end anastomosis, interposition graft or a 'jump' graft are the surgical options.

Vascular rings

Abnormalities of the great vessels can constrict the structures in the mediastinum, namely the trachea and the oesophagus. Many vascular rings can be explained by the persistence or failure to regress of parts of the aortic arch system during embryonic development. Investigations include a barium swallow, bronchoscopy or angiography. Treatment is indicated for the relief of symptoms and is usually directed at dividing the nondominant vascular component of the ring.

Congenital valvular abnormalities

Among the obstructive lesions are aortic, mitral and pulmonary valve stenoses, as well as supravalvular and infravalvular obstructions.

Pulmonary stenosis. There is an incomplete obstruction in this condition to the flow from the right ventricle. This accounts for about 10 per cent of all congenital heart disease. The obstruction is often at valve level and there may be an associated ASD.

The right ventricle hypertrophies in an effort to overcome the obstruction and pulmonary artery pressures may exceed systemic pressure (Fig. 48.41). The defect is often asymptomatic and a murmur is detected at preschool screening. On chest radiographs the lung fields will be oligaemic and there is often poststenotic dilatation of the pulmonary artery. Treatment is directed at relieving the obstruction and this may be done under direct vision or by balloon dilatation.

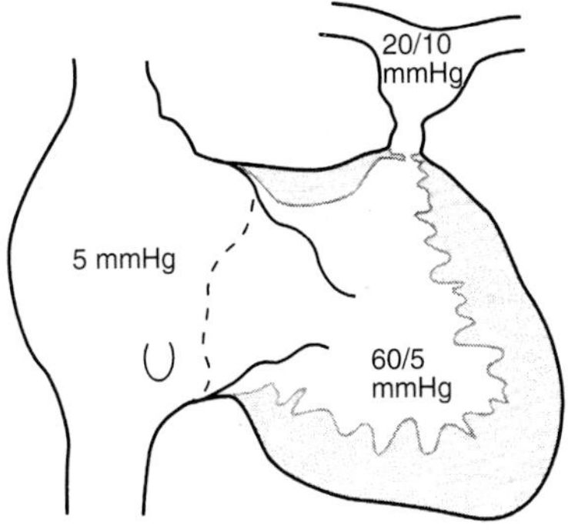

Fig. 48.41 Pressure consequences of pulmonary stenosis.

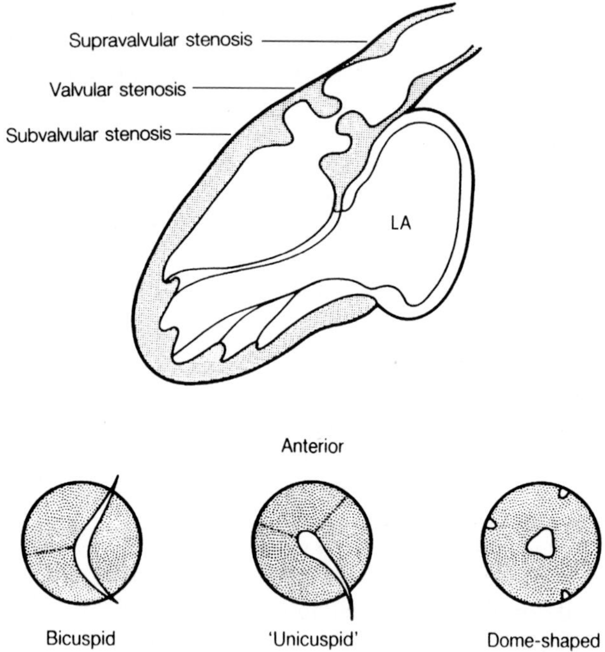

Fig. 48.42 Sagittal section of the left heart, showing subvalvular, valvular and supravalvular aortic stenosis. The abnormal valve may have two rudimentary cusps, an eccentric comma-shaped orifice, or a central orifice in a doming valve. The first two tend to be tolerated at least through infancy and childhood. LA, left atrium. (From *Disorders of the Cardiovascular System,* Edward Arnold.)

Congenital aortic stenosis. This may be valvular, subvalvular or supravalvular but in all cases there is a pressure load on the left ventricle leading to hypertrophy (Fig. 48.42). The most common defect is a bicuspid valve where one of the cusps has not developed; however, this is rarely a problem until adulthood. There may be a lot of calcification by the time initial symptoms present. There may be a regurgitant element to the problem. Echocardiography demonstrates the site of obstruction.

Indications for operation. Unfortunately the condition is well advanced once symptoms occur and therefore treatment may be indicated to safeguard the patient's future. The operation relieves the obstruction by repairing the cusps, excising obstructing hypertrophic myocardium or replacing the valve. Infravalvular obstruction is dealt with by excising the obstructing membrane and supravalvular obstruction is repaired using a patch graft. There is a high mortality for emergency procedures, but in the elective situation the mortality rate should be less than 5 per cent.

Atrial septal defect

The development of the atrial septum is complex and abnormalities of development lead to three commonly recognised ASDs.

Fossa ovalis defect (syn. ostium secundum ASD)

This is the most common type of ASD and is a defect in the floor of the fossa ovalis. Symptoms develop insidiously and may be no more than a tendency to chest infections. Rarely it presents early as a result of a paradoxical embolus from the venous circulation traversing the patent foramen ovale and reaching the systemic circulation. Symptoms appear when pulmonary hypertension develops, usually in the fourth decade, but may appear earlier under conditions of increased cardiac output (i.e. pregnancy).

Should the shunt reverse (i.e. become right to left) because of the pulmonary hypertension, then closure of the ASD is contraindicated. The development of a reversed shunt is termed 'Eisenmenger's syndrome'.

Atrioventricular septal defect (syn. primum defects)

When abnormalities of this type are confined to the atrial septum they are commonly called ostium primum ASD. Failure of the development of the septum primum is uncommon, but when it occurs it is associated with abnormalities of the mitral valve. A more extreme version may lead to an atrioventricular canal defect. There is a relatively high incidence of this abnormality in those born with trisomy 21 (Down's syndrome).

Sinus venosus

This is a rare defect and is the result of failure of partition of the pulmonary and systemic venous circulations. It is associated with anomalous pulmonary venous drainage (Fig. 48.43).

Treatment of atrial septal defect

Echocardiography will define the anatomy and any other abnormalities including the direction of the shunt. Pressure measurements may be required if pulmonary hypertension is suspected. Treatment is aimed at closing the defect. This may be from simple closure or patch graft in the primum type to an extensive closure and reconstruction of the mitral valve in the secundum type.

Ventricular septal defect (VSD)

This accounts for 15–20 per cent of congenital heart disease and affects 2 in 10 00 live births (Fig. 48.44). There is a high spontaneous closure rate and only 25 per cent persist. There is communication between the ventricles and this may occur in isolation or as part of a more complex set of cardiac abnormalities. Blood ejected from the heart tends to go into the pulmonary circulation where the resistance to flow is lower. If no compensation occurs, severe pulmonary oedema results. The pulmonary circulation may adapt by increasing the resistance to flow but this may lead to irreversible pulmonary oedema if the defect is not corrected. Small defects may close or cause little systemic disturbance (maladie de Roger).

John Langdon Haydon Down, 1828–96. English physician.
Henri Louis Roger, 1809–91. French physician.

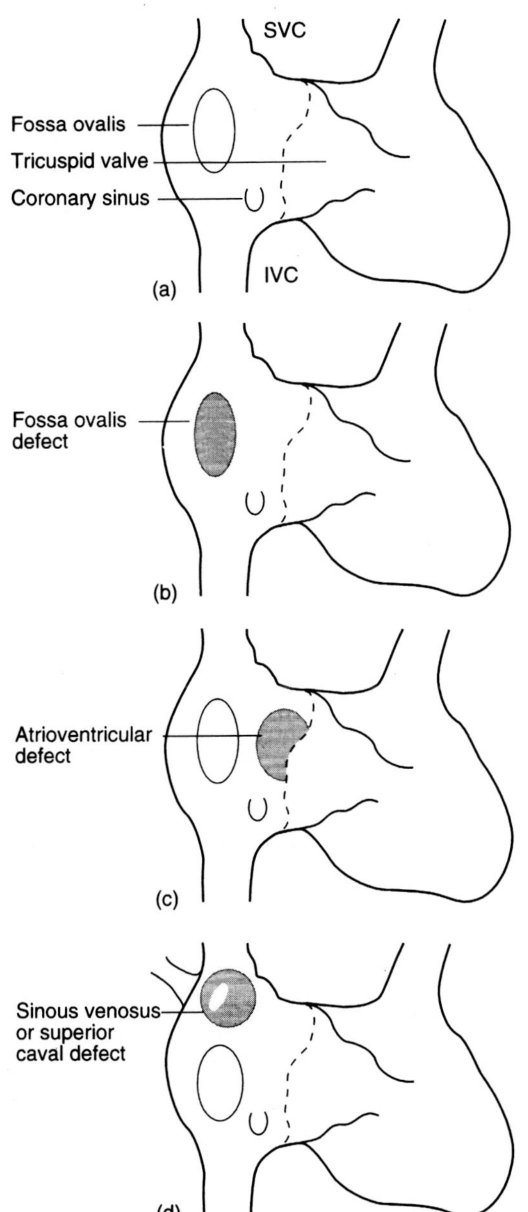

Fig. 48.43 The atrial septum viewed from the right. (a) The fossa ovalis is a useful reference point; (b) the commonest defect is in this area and is called a fossa ovalis (or ostium secundum) defect; (c) a defect near the atrioventricular junction may be part of the spectrum of atrioventricular septal defects; (d) if the defect is near the entry of the superior vena cava (SVC), it is commonly associated with anomalies of venous drainage into the atria. IVC, inferior vena cava.

In the case of larger defects the infant may have frank pulmonary oedema, failure to thrive and recurrent chest infections. In older children, pulmonary hypertension may be the predominant clinical feature with cyanosis present if the left-to-right shunt reverses (Eisenmenger's syndrome).

Echocardiography confirms the diagnosis and can estimate the degree of shunting across the defect. Catheterisation is recommended to quantify the various pressures within the cardiac chambers.

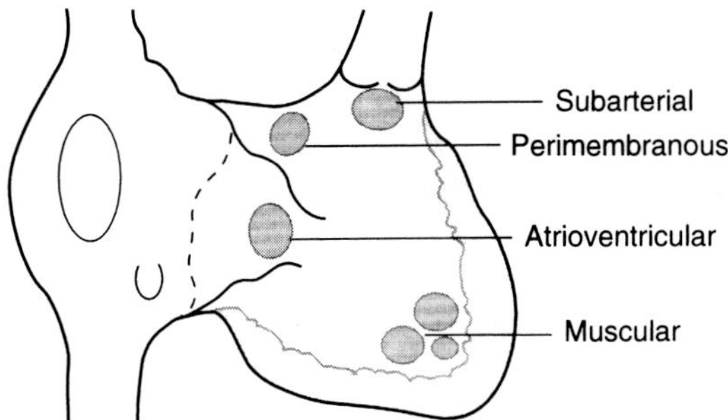

Fig. 48.44 The ventricular septum viewed from the right, showing the characteristic sites of ventricular septal defects.

Most VSDs will close spontaneously within the first year of life, but some will lead to death or irreversible pulmonary hypertension if not treated quickly. If the infant is severely symptomatic, the defect should be closed urgently otherwise elective repair is advised between 1 and 3 years of age. Very sick infants can be 'tided over' by banding the pulmonary artery. This protects the lungs from pulmonary hypertension and diverts the blood into the aorta. Elective surgery can then be carried out at a later stage when the child has grown.

Ischaemic heart disease

Ischaemic heart disease is a major cause of morbidity and mortality in developed countries. The underlying pathology is usually atherosclerosis of the coronary arteries. The coronary anatomy is such that each of the three major arteries (the right, the left anterior descending and the circumflex) supplies a similar proportion of the myocardium (Fig. 48.45). Triple-vessel disease refers to significant stenosis in these three vessels.

Presentation

Coronary artery disease may be (1) asymptomatic until it presents as sudden death or an acute myocardial infarction as the first manifestation, or (2) symptomatic with angina, typically on exertion and relieved by rest.

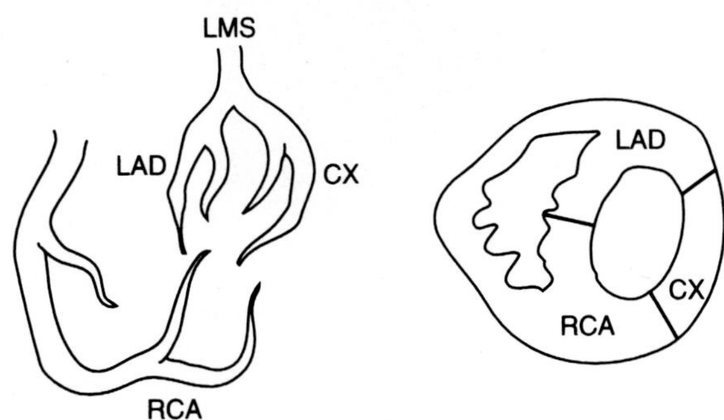

Fig. 48.45 The essential anatomy of the coronary arteries. LMS, left main stem. LAD, left anterior descending or anterior interventricular artery. CX, circumflex. RCA, right coronary artery. The three major distributing arteries supply the ventricle approximately in thirds, anteroseptal, lateral and inferoseptal, respectively.

Pathophysiology

The starting point in atherosclerosis is believed to be endothelial injury. This may be mechanical or biochemical and the result is platelet aggregation at the site of injury. There is consequent migration of smooth muscle cells into the intima. The risk factors are the following:

- hypercholesterolaemia;
- hypertension;
- cigarette smoking;
- diabetes mellitus;
- advancing age;
- family history of ischaemic heart disease.

An elevated plaque forms within the lumen and, with time, progressive thickening with ulceration, plaque rupture, thrombus formation or calcium deposition will further narrow the lumen. With a narrowing of over 70 per cent, the lumen is critically stenosed (Fig. 48.46).

Slow progression of this process encourages the formation of collateral vessels whereas sudden occlusion results in myocardial infarction. The rate of progression is highly variable and the distribution patchy, but to have only one vessel involved is unusual. Plaques tend to form in the proximal areas of the artery or branches.

Symptomatic patients with ischaemic heart disease can usually be helped by medical treatment in the first instance. Attention is paid to the elimination of risk factors wherever possible.

Pharmacological agents that relieve angina include nitrates, calcium antagonists and β-blockers. These agents reduce the vascular tone and therefore reduce preload and/or afterload of the left ventricular muscle, reduce the work of the heart and therefore reduce the metabolic demand.

Surgical involvement occurs when the symptoms are severe and not adequately controlled on a reasonable trial of medication or when the prognosis is adversely affected by continuing medical treatment.

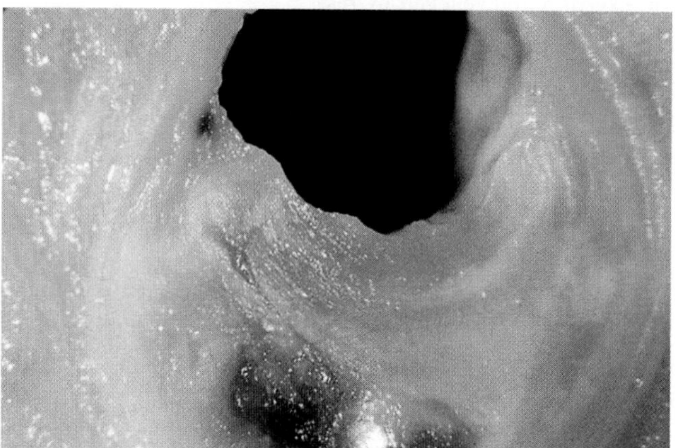

Fig. 48.46 Atheroma within a coronary artery. Concentric layers of atheroma are seen with haemorrhage at the base (*courtesy of Professor M.J. Davies*).

Investigations

Clinical examination is typically normal (although stigmata of diabetes or hypercholesterolaemia may be evident) and objective evidence of myocardial ischaemia must be sought.

Electrocardiography

The simplest test to demonstrate ischaemia is an exercise ECG. The patient is asked to undergo an increasing amount of exercise on a treadmill according to a carefully described protocol. Every 2 minutes the work rate increases. Full resuscitative equipment is available and the patient is continually monitored by ECG. The test is stopped if the patient experiences chest pain or arrhythmias or becomes dyspnoeic. If there is evidence of ischaemia on the ECG (>2 mm ST depression) then the test is positive.

Radionucleotide studies including thallium scanning also provide objective evidence of reversible ischaemia but the equipment is not always available.

Coronary angiography

This is an invasive test performed under radiographic screening. The arterial circulation is entered via the femoral or brachial artery and a catheter is advanced into the aorta to the coronary sinuses. The coronary ostia are located and iodine-containing dye is infused to outline the coronary anatomy. At least two views of the coronary anatomy are filmed in different planes to give a three-dimensional impression of the arterial system. A left ventriculogram is performed to estimate the ejection fraction, and a measurement of the left ventricular end-diastolic pressure is taken. This test only outlines the coronary anatomy and does not demonstrate ischaemia.

Indications for surgery

Many patients can be managed medically and there is an increasing trend for cardiologists and interventional radiologists to palliate the symptoms of angina by the technique of coronary angioplasty. This involves passing a small balloon-tipped catheter into the femoral or radial artery and feeding it retrogradely into the aortic root. Soluble dye is injected into the coronary ostia to delineate the coronary anatomy; the catheter is then passed across the stenosis and inflated so as to crush the atheromatous plaque with a 90 per cent initial success rate. If successful, this procedure provides symptomatic relief but restenosis occurs in 30 per cent within 3–6 months. The long-term benefits are unclear and the process may have to be repeated with up to 40 per cent of patients coming to definitive coronary artery bypass grafting within 2.5 years. Coronary artery stenting following angioplasty has improved the medium-term patency rate but the long-term benefits remain unclear. Several trials (RITA, BARI and CABRI) show that the early morbidity for angioplasty is less than that for coronary artery bypass graft (CABG) but the patients in the angioplasty groups are more likely to have more interventions and require more medication in the short term. A detailed discussion of these points is outside the scope of this chapter.

Angina can be relieved by surgical revascularisation in most patients and symptomatic improvement can be expected for over 10 years. Patients with lesions in one or two vessels may benefit from balloon angioplasty, but triple-vessel disease or left main stem stenosis is an indication for surgery.

Data from prospective, randomised trials demonstrate that patients with angina and left main stem stenosis or triple-vessel disease have a poor natural history which is significantly improved by surgery. Survival in patients with single-vessel disease is equally good when medical and surgical treatment are compared. Survival is further increased if an internal mammary artery is used to bypass a proximal stenosis of the left anterior descending (LAD) artery. Acute unstable angina usually settles with medical treatment but continuing pain in spite of adequate therapy is an indication for surgery. Surgery should be considered for chronic stable angina when a reasonable trial of medication has failed to control symptoms.

The history of surgical revascularisation

The earliest surgical proposal for the relief of angina was in 1899 by Franck when he suggested cervical sympathectomy to divide the cardiac afferents and cause coronary vasodilatation. It was not until the 1930s that augmentation of coronary blood flow was suggested as a treatment for angina.

Various attempts to provide additional blood to the myocardium were tried (omentopexy and induced pericardial adhesions) but were of little benefit. Vineberg pioneered an operation in which the internal mammary artery was dissected from its bed and the distal end implanted in the myocardium. This procedure was successful in some cases but gave inconsistent results and it is no longer performed. Cardiopulmonary bypass meant that it was possible to operate directly on the coronary arteries. The development of coronary angiography by Mason Somes led to the first CABG performed by Favorolo at the Cleveland Clinic in 1967. This was found to be an effective and reliable way to revascularise the myocardium. The long saphenous vein is the most commonly used conduit, but the internal mammary artery is now used for the left anterior descending graft in over 60 per cent of cases.

Vessels with 70 per cent stenosis or more require bypassing. Stenoses of less than 50 per cent may not progress and there is no evidence that grafting is beneficial. The usual procedure is three to four grafts.

Arthur Vineberg, 1903–88. Surgeon, Royal Victoria Hospital, Montréal, Canada.

Rene Favorolo. Cardiac surgeon, Buenos Aires, Argentina.

Choice of conduit

The patient's own saphenous vein and internal mammary artery are the conduits of choice but there is a small trend towards using other arterial conduits such as the gastroepiploic artery and the inferior epigastric artery. Other conduits such as human umbilical vein, bovine internal mammary artery and prosthetic grafts (Dacron and polytetrafluoroethylene) have disappointing patency rates of less than 50 per cent at 1 year.

The long saphenous vein graft (Fig. 48.47)

Although this graft has been used for over 25 years, there is a significant occlusion rate of 10–15 per cent at 1 year. Thereafter there is an occlusion rate of 2–3 per cent per annum. Low-dose aspirin from the time of operation reduces the graft occlusion rate.

The internal mammary graft (Fig. 48.48)

This graft has been accepted as the conduit of choice in terms of reliability, low occlusion rate and long-term patency. It can be adapted to the demands placed on it and provides excellent symptomatic relief.

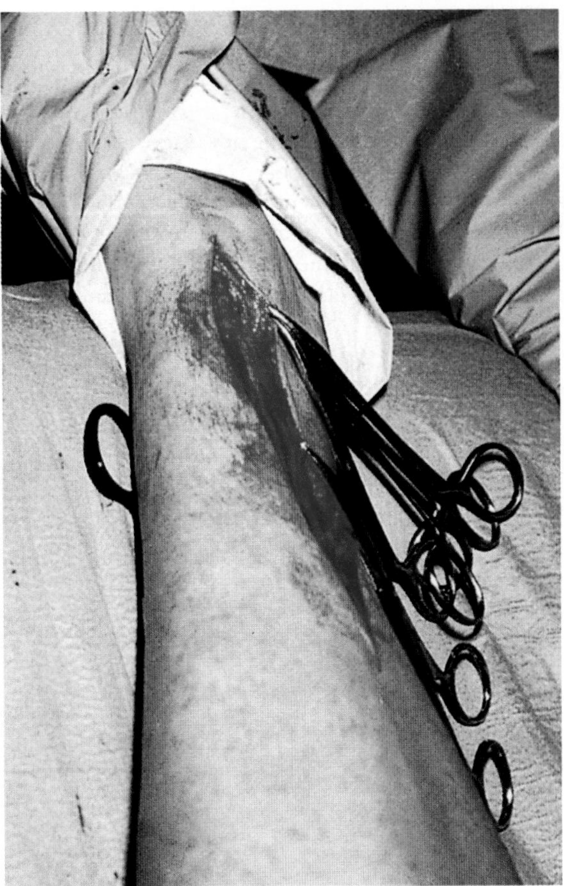

Fig. 48.47 The long saphenous vein is exposed at the ankle anterior to the medial malleolus.

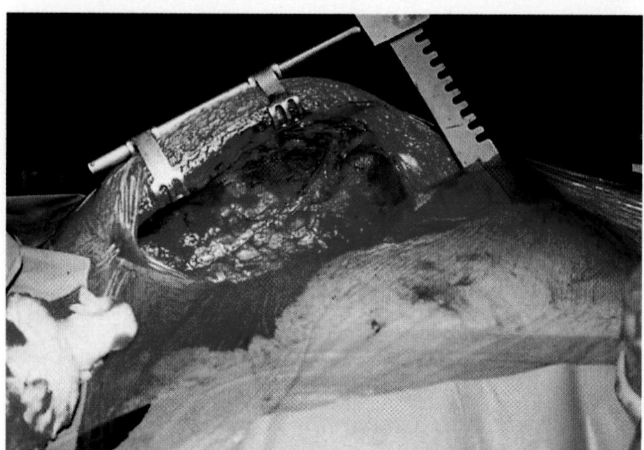

Fig. 48.48 The left internal mammary artery is dissected off the chest wall and divided inferiorly.

The operation is usually performed with cardiopulmonary bypass (Fig. 48.49). The distal anastomosis is performed beyond the narrowing in the coronary vessel. Application of the aortic cross-clamp facilitates this by preventing blood flow down the coronary arteries. This renders the myocardium ischaemic but there are ways of minimising this which are discussed in the Myocardial protection section. Once the final distal anastomosis is completed, the cross-clamp is removed and the heart is reperfused with oxygenated blood. Rewarming is commenced and the final proximal anastomosis is completed. The patient is returned to the intensive care unit at the completion of the operation. There is a trend to try and avoid cardiopulmonary bypass in coronary artery surgery altogether. Coronary anastomoses are possible on the beating heart with the aid of appropriate stabilising devices. The advantage is that the patient avoids the potential damaging effects of cardiopulmonary bypass and therefore has a shortened hospital stay. There is concern that the quality of the anastomosis may not be as good as those done on a completely still heart in a bloodless field. An extension of this principle is the development of port access surgery, where the operation is carried out through a small incision. The early results appear encouraging but the techniques have yet to gain widespread acceptance.

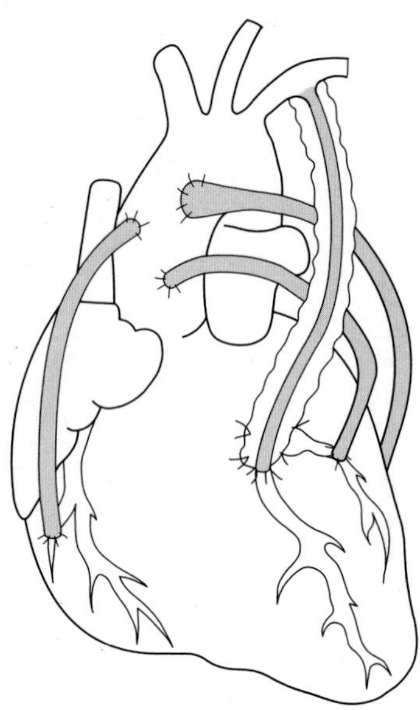

Fig. 48.49 Completed coronary artery bypass grafts.

Postoperative complications are not uncommon following cardiac surgery. Many patients are ex-smokers or diabetic so respiratory infections and basal collapse are common after surgery, and should be treated aggressively with antibiotics and physiotherapy. Minor wound infections may need little attention, but major wound infections leading to sternal dehiscence and mediastinitis may be very difficult to treat. The risk of serious sternal infection increases in elderly and diabetic patients and in those undergoing bilateral internal mammary artery grafting.

Results of treatment

Relief of symptoms and functional capacity are significantly improved following surgery when compared with medical therapy alone. Patients with impaired left ventricular function have a poor natural history, and it is this group that benefits most from surgical revascularisation. The hospital mortality rate has increased slightly to 3–4 per cent as a result of operating on older patients and those with impaired ventricular function. There is no doubt that the internal mammary artery improves patient survival and has a superior long-term patency over other conduits.

Up to 80 per cent of patients have complete relief of symptoms and require no further medication. Unfortunately, angina may return as a result of the following:

- graft thrombosis;
- anastomotic stenosis;
- conduit atherosclerosis;
- progression of native disease.

Attention is paid to secondary prevention of progressive disease and return of symptoms requires careful evaluation. There is clear evidence that cholesterol lowering (even in those who have a normal cholesterol) significantly reduces the progression of atherosclerosis in saphenous vein grafts. Developments in cardiology and therapeutics mean that patients have a wide range of options before reoperation is considered. Many patients respond to medical treatment but some require redo surgery. This is associated with an increased operative mortality and is only recommended for patients with severe symptoms. It is hoped that the use of arterial conduits will reduce the need for redo surgery, although this remains to be seen.

Surgery for the complications of myocardial infarction

Myocardial infarction leads to myocyte necrosis which may heal to form scar tissue or rupture if the ventricular wall gives way. Free rupture of the ventricle is usually fatal in spite of treatment, but intramyocardial rupture gives rise to a number of mechanical problems that have a very high mortality without surgery. The myocardial rupture rate is less than 2 per cent with the distribution in proportion to the relative risk. Free wall rupture is the most common, followed by ventricular septal rupture and then papillary muscle rupture.

Ventricular septal rupture (Fig. 48.50)

This occurs following an anterior or inferior infarct affecting the ventricular septum. The patient typically presents with an infarction and 3–7 days later develops pulmonary oedema with a pansystolic murmur and hypotension. The prognosis is dismal without surgery but operation carries a mortality rate of up to 40 per cent. The diagnosis is confirmed by trans-oesophageal echocardiography or Swan–Ganz catheterisation (the degree of left-to-right shunting can be calculated using this technique). The patient requires stabilisation and myocardial support (inotropes, renal dopamine and intra-aortic balloon pump counterpulsation) before surgical repair if this is indicated. The repair is undertaken with the aid of cardiopulmonary bypass and a pericardial patch or an artificial graft may be used to facilitate repair.

Papillary muscle necrosis (Fig. 48.51)

This occurs with full-thickness myocardial papillary muscle necrosis. The patient develops a pansystolic murmur and pulmonary oedema. Unlike chronic mitral regurgitation, where the left ventricle has time to adapt to the increased volume load, the left ventricle is acutely overloaded and failure results. Diagnosis is made by echocardiography and right heart catheterisation (showing large V waves). Mitral valve replacement is usually necessary, but the mortality is higher than in valve replacement for rheumatic heart disease as a result of the associated coronary artery disease.

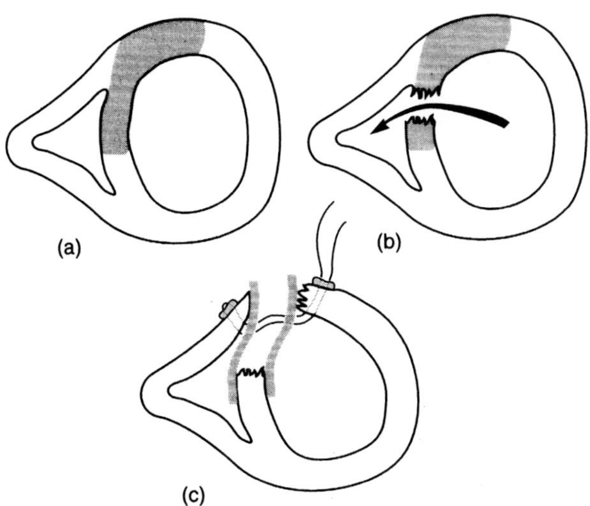

Fig. 48.50 Ischaemic ventriculoseptal rupture. (a) Transverse section of ventricles to show territory of arteroseptal infarction following LAD occlusion; (b) site of rupture with left-to-right shunt; (c) one approach to surgical repair with a double patch.

Harold Swan, b. 1922. American cardiologist.
William Ganz, b. 1919. American cardiologist.

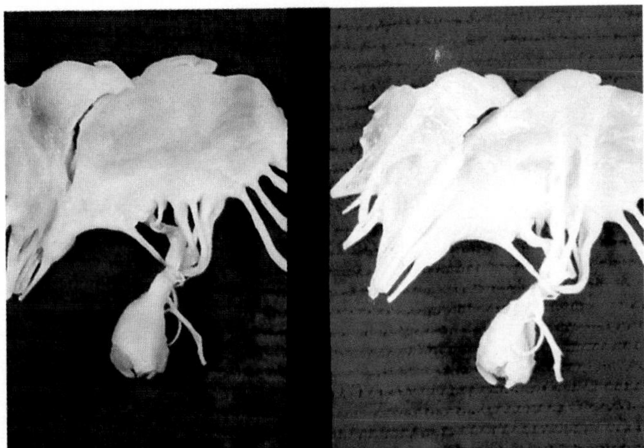

Fig. 48.51 Papillary muscle rupture following myocardial infarction.

Ventricular aneurysm (Fig. 48.52)

Partial-thickness necrosis of the ventricular wall may result in the development of a ventricular aneurysm if the free wall is replaced by noncontractile fibrous tissue. Left ventricular function is affected because the fibrous wall balloons out during systole and reduces the actual stroke volume. Repair is undertaken using cardiopulmonary bypass and CABG is undertaken at the same time if necessary.

Some patients develop refractory cardiac failure from a variety of causes that are not amenable to surgery because of poor left ventricular function. These patients should be considered for heart transplantation.

The thoracic aorta

The intrathoracic aorta, although, strictly speaking, not a cardiac structure for most of its course, is the domain of the cardiothoracic surgeon. The most common pathology affecting the aorta is aneurysm formation or dissection.

Aneurysm

A true aneurysm involves all layers of the vessel whereas a false aneurysm has compressed supporting tissue as its wall, and it is usually the result of a defect in the vessel intima (from trauma, dissection or previous surgery).

Aneurysms are described as fusiform when the whole circumference is affected or saccular when only part of the circumference is involved (Fig. 48.53).

The most common aetiology is atherosclerosis but connective tissue disorders (e.g. Marfan's syndrome) account

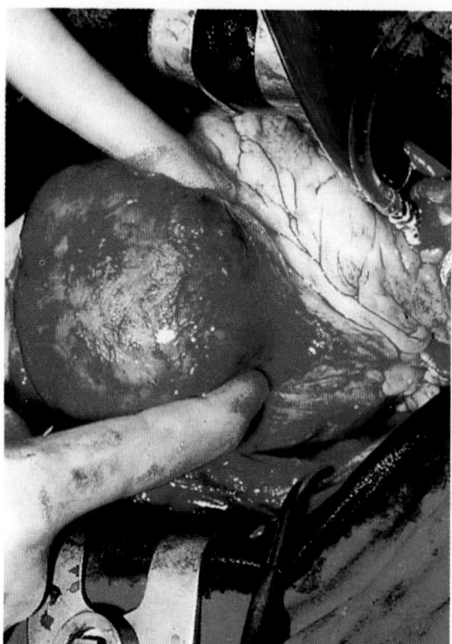
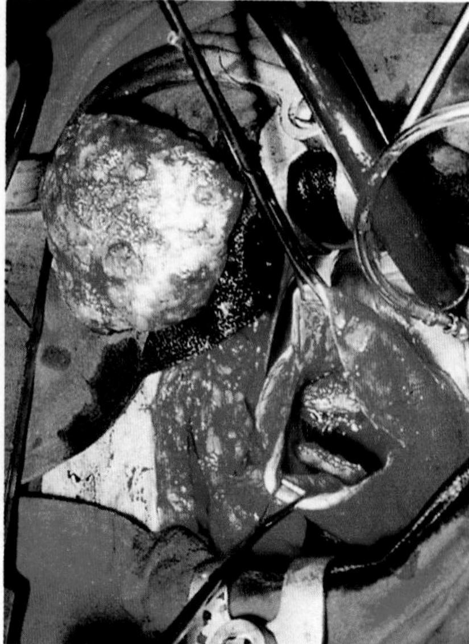
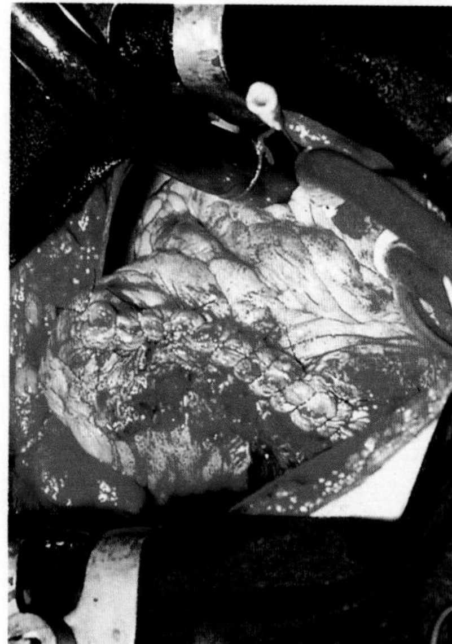

Fig. 48.52 The typical surgical left ventricular aneurysm in LAD territory bulges in the anteroapical region of the heart and is a thin-walled fibrous structure lined with thrombus. The most common surgical approach is resection and repair of the left ventricle by direct suture of the margins of the aneurysm.

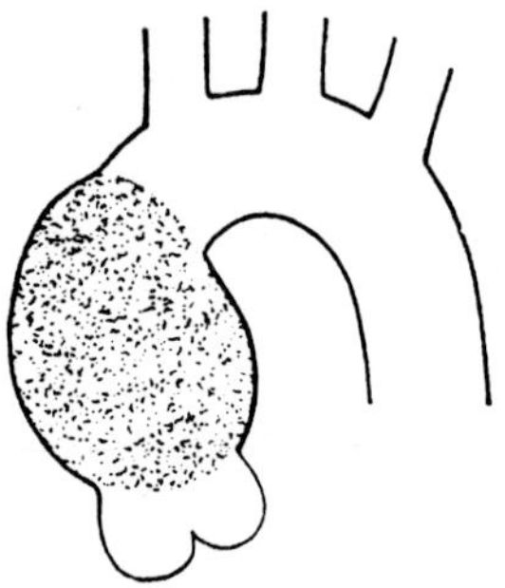

Fig. 48.53 Fusiform aneurysm of the ascending aorta.

for many aneurysms in the aortic root and ascending aorta now that syphilis is rare. Many aneurysms are asymptomatic and discovered incidentally on routine chest radiograph. Others are symptomatically related to a space-occupying lesion in the thorax. Pressure on adjacent structures may cause pain (vertebra), hoarseness (recurrent laryngeal nerve), dysphagia (oesophagus) and respiratory symptoms (left main bronchus). Aortic root aneurysm may lead to dilatation of the aortic root annulus and aortic regurgitation. Otherwise there are often no clinical features.

The diagnosis is confirmed by computerised tomography (CT) or magnetic resonance imaging (MRI), which will often show the extent of the aneurysm. Arteriography is not necessary for diagnosis but is often required to demonstrate the relation of the arch vessels to the aneurysm.

Without treatment the aneurysm is likely to expand and ultimately rupture so surgical treatment is advised. The important factors taken into consideration when planning treatment are the age and general condition of the patient and coexistence of coronary disease. The approach adopted for surgical treatment depends on the location of the aneurysm.

Aortic root

A median sternotomy is performed and cardiopulmonary bypass is established between the right atrium and the common femoral artery. The patient is cooled down to 18°C and the aorta cross-clamped above the aneurysm. The aorta is opened and the coronary ostia are perfused with a cardioplegic solution to protect the myocardium and to arrest the heart in diastole. The aorta, together with its annulus and valve, is resected and a composite graft is sutured to the aortic root. The circulation is arrested and after removal of the aortic cross-clamp, the distal anastomosis is completed. The coronary ostia require reimplantation into the graft (Bentall's operation) (Fig. 48.54). The patient is rewarmed, air is excluded from the heart and cardiac activity returns.

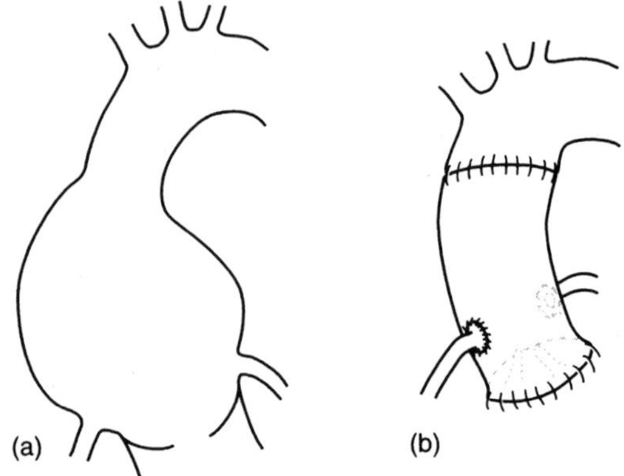

Fig. 48.54 Bentall's operation (modified). (a) Preoperative appearance of a dilated aortic root; (b) postoperative appearance showing complete root replacement with a bileaflet aortic valve, aortic conduit and coronary reimplantation.

Hugh Henry Bentall. Former Professor of Cardiac Surgery, Hammersmith Hospital, London, England.

Ascending aorta

The procedure involves resecting the affected aorta with graft replacement. The circulation and myocardium are managed in a similar way to the aortic root replacement.

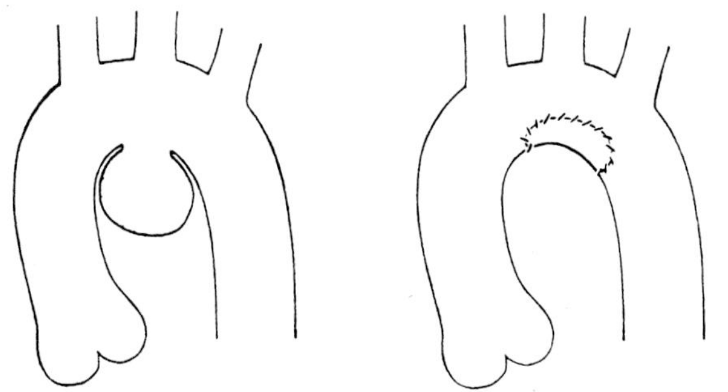

Fig. 48.55 Aneurysm of the aortic arch. Localised excision and plastic repair.

Aortic arch aneurysms (Fig. 48.55)

Surgery on this section of the aorta is a formidable undertaking because the cerebral and subclavian vessels have to be anastomosed to the graft, either separately or *en bloc*.

Descending aorta

Excision of the aneurysm is frequently necessary with graft replacement. This may be done under cardiopulmonary bypass with exposure via a left thoracotomy or by using a heparin-bonded shunt.

Aortic dissection (Fig. 48.56)

This occurs when there is a defect in the intima of the aorta resulting in blood tracking into the aortic tissues and creating a false lumen. It is often associated with systemic hyper-

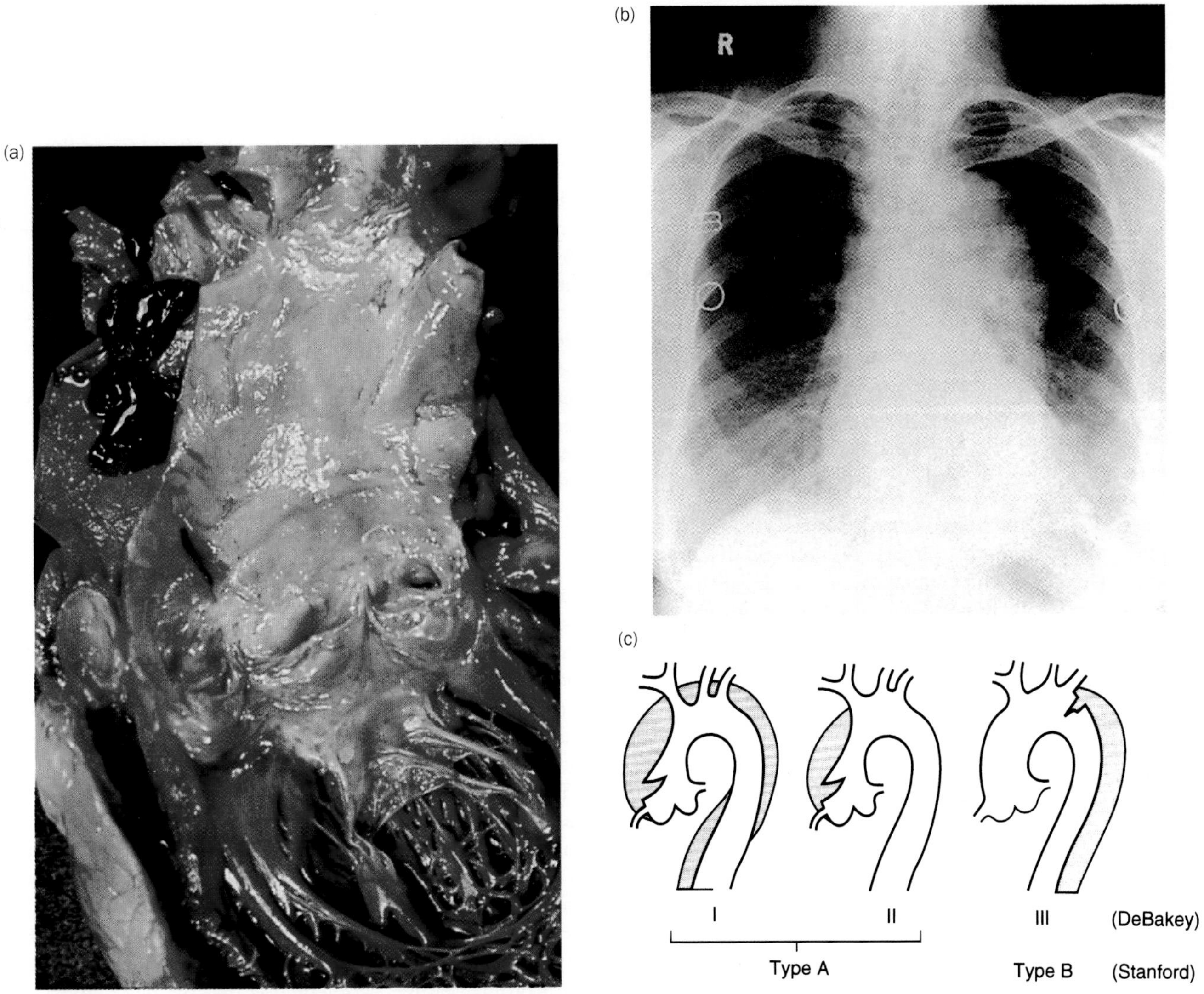

(a)

(b)

(c)

I II III (DeBakey)

Type A Type B (Stanford)

Fig. 48.56 (a) *Post mortem* appearance of an aortic dissection with an intimal tear just superior to the junction of the right and noncoronary aortic cusps. Note the *ante mortem* thrombus in the dissected media; (b) chest radiograph showing mediastinal widening from a dissection affecting the ascending aorta and the arch; (c) classification of aortic dissections according to whether the ascending aorta is involved (type A) or not (type B). This is simpler than the DeBakey classification (types I, II and III).

tension or Marfan's syndrome, and blood insinuates itself between the intima and the overlying adventitia. The diagnosis is suspected when chest radiography demonstrates a widened mediastinum. The dissection may extend distally down the aorta to involve the renal, spinal and iliac arteries, causing renal failure, paraplegia and leg ischaemia. The dissection may track proximally to involve the head and neck vessels and the coronary vessels, and the aortic root, leading to aortic regurgitation. The aneurysm may rupture back into the lumen or externally into the pericardium or mediastinum.

There are two classifications, the DeBakey classification based on the pattern of dissection and the Stanford classification based on whether the ascending aorta is involved.

Treatment (Fig. 48.57). In the emergency situation, the blood pressure (which is usually high at presentation) should be brought under control to prevent extension of the dissection. Once stabilised, arrangements are made to discover the origin of the dissection. The tests required depend on the facilities available; CT, MRI, transoesophageal echocardiography or an aortic angiogram are all appropriate.

Types 1 and 2 dissections, involving the ascending aorta, usually require surgical intervention. The chest is opened through a median sternotomy and an arterial cannula is inserted into the femoral artery. Venous drainage is from the right atrium or the femoral vein.

Cardiopulmonary bypass is started with core cooling down to 18°C. The aorta is cross-clamped as high as possible and opened. Cardioplegia solution is infused into the coronary ostia to arrest the heart in diastole. If the intimal tear is present and localised, the ascending aorta is excised with the tear and replaced with a synthetic graft. The distal anastomosis is performed with circulatory arrest. If the tear is more proximal than the innominate, the ascending aorta is still replaced to prevent the dissection extending to involve the coronary ostia.

Type 3 dissections are best managed medically with antihypertensive medication. Surgery is indicated if the pain increases (signalling impending rupture), the aneurysm is expanding on serial chest radiographs or neurological symptoms develop. The operation may be performed with a heparin-bonded shunt or under cardiopulmonary bypass. There is a real risk of paraplegia from this operation, which should be mentioned specifically to the patient before operation.

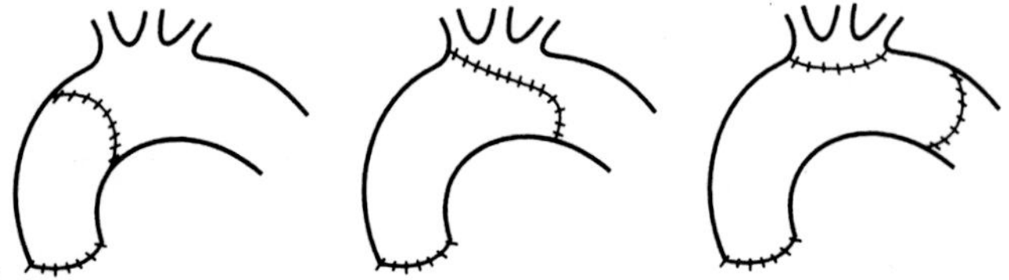

Fig. 48.57 Technical options in aortic replacement for disease involving the transverse arch.

Cardiac trauma

Trauma to the heart often involves the lungs or other mediastinal structures and is therefore best dealt with in a structured manner. Cardiothoracic injuries and their treatment are discussed in detail in Chapter 47.

The pericardium

This is a fibrous envelope covering the heart and separating the heart from the mediastinal structures. It is a fibrous structure with a parietal layer and it allows the heart to move with each beat. It is not essential for life because it can be left wide open after cardiac surgery without any ill effects. There is, however, a number of conditions affecting the pericardium which may present to the surgeon.

Pericardial effusion

There is a continuous production and resorption of pericardial fluid. This is a balanced system and only a few millilitres of fluid are present at any one time. A disease process that disturbs this balance by increasing production or interfering with resorption will lead to a build-up of fluid in the pericardium. If the pressure exceeds the pressure in the atria, compression will occur, venous return will fall and the circulation is compromised. This state of affairs is called tamponade. A gradual build-up of fluid (e.g. malignant infiltration) may be well tolerated for a long period before tamponade occurs, and the pericardial cavity may contain 2 litres of fluid. Acute tamponade (penetrating wounds or post-operatively) may occur in minutes with small volumes of blood. The clinical features are low blood pressure with a raised jugular venous pressure (JVP) and pulsus paradox. Kussmaul's sign is a characteristic pattern when the JVP rises with inspiration as a result of the impaired venous return to the heart.

Emergency treatment of pericardial tamponade is aspiration of the pericardial space and therefore relief of the compression on the cardiac chambers. A wide-bore needle is inserted under local anaesthesia to the left of the xiphisternum between the angle of the xiphisternum and the ribcage (Fig. 48.58). The needle is advanced towards the tip of the scapula into the pericardial space. An ECG electrode attached to the needle will indicate when the heart has been touched.

This will hold the situation temporarily until the cause of the tamponade is established. It is occasionally possible to drain the pericardium with a percutaneous drainage system. To prevent recurrence of a chronic tamponade, it is sometimes necessary to fashion a pericardial window between the pericardial space and the pleural or peritoneal space. This may be done through a subxiphoid incision, anterolateral thoracotomy, either thoracoscopically or percutaneously. Penetrating wounds of the heart usually require exploration

Adolf Kussmaul, 1822–1902. German physiologist.

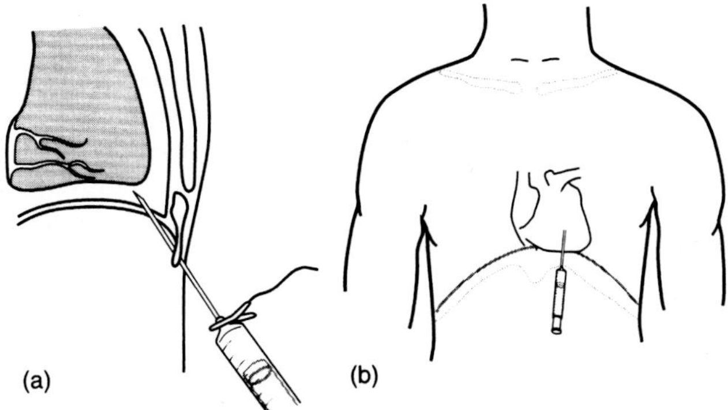

Fig. 48.58 (a) Pericardial aspiration through the subxiphoid region; (b) site of needle insertion for pericardial aspiration.

through a median sternotomy. Emergency room thoracotomy is rarely required.

Causes of acute tamponade

The causes include:

- trauma;
- aortic dissection;
- penetrating cardiac injury (usually of the atria as ventricular and aortic wounds tend to be fatal);
- iatrogenic: penetration of the right ventricle following central venous cannulation, endomyocardial biopsy, etc.;
- postoperative: blocked drains or inability of the drains to cope with excessive blood loss.

Chronic tamponade is usually a result of malignant infiltration of the pericardium (usually secondary carcinoma from breast or bronchus) or very occasionally uraemia or connective tissue diseases.

Pericarditis

Infection and inflammation may also affect the pericardium. Acute pericarditis usually occurs following a viral illness. There is a sensation of heaviness in the chest which may be positional. Treatment is with nonsteroidal anti-inflammatory drugs and bed rest (in case there is an underlying myocarditis). Acute purulent pericarditis is uncommon but requires urgent drainage and intravenous antibiotics with attention to the underlying cause.

Chronic pericarditis is an uncommon condition in which the pericardium becomes thickened and noncompliant. The heart cannot move freely and the stroke volume is reduced by the constrictive process. The central venous pressure is raised and the liver becomes congested. Peripheral oedema and ascites are also a feature. Establishing the diagnosis may not be easy because the chest radiograph and echoradiograph may be normal. Cardiac catheterisation demonstrates a 'reversed square root sign'. Treatment is aimed at relieving the constriction. The heart is approached through a median sternotomy and the pericardium is carefully stripped off the left ventricle, followed by the right ventricle. Cardiopulmonary bypass may be required if haemodynamic instability occurs.

Heart transplantation

Much of the pioneering work into human heart transplantation was done by Shumway and Lower in the early 1960s but the first successful human heart transplantation was performed by Barnard in 1967. The early results were very poor and, in spite of the initial optimism for the technique, the number of centres declined to only a few. Better patient and donor selection, together with the introduction of cyclosporin A, has led to a revival of the technique and it is now established as a treatment for end-stage cardiac failure in certain groups.

The main indication for heart transplantation is advanced terminal cardiac disease classified as New York Heart Association (NYHA) 4, with no alternative conventional medical or surgical treatment, and with a mortality rate higher than 90 per cent per year if transplantation is not carried out. Indeed, death commonly occurs while on the waiting list. Most cases referred for transplantation have either an ischaemic or a dilated cardiomyopathy. Rarer causes include postviral and hypertrophic obstructive cardiomyopathy. The patient needs careful preoperative assessment to determine the suitability for transplantation and counselling to prepare for the demands of life after transplantation. Younger patients tend to benefit most but the indications for transplantation have broadened since it was first introduced. Unfortunately, the limiting factor on the number of transplantations performed per year is the availability of donor hearts.

Absolute contraindications to transplantation include:

- active infection [or human immunodeficiency virus (HIV) positive];
- irreversible pulmonary hypertension;
- malignancy;
- another life-threatening illness.

Relative contraindications include:

- age >60 years;
- active duodenal ulceration;
- significant pulmonary vascular disease;
- creatinine clearance <30 mmol/litre;
- drug or alcohol abuse;
- psychiatric illness.

Donor selection is critically important if early postoperative problems are to be avoided. Potential donors will be certified as brain dead if two separate brain-stem function tests show no activity. Most donors have had head injuries or an intracerebral haemorrhage. Injuries to other organs may be present, but if the heart shows no evidence of injury then

---

Norman. E. Shumway. Cardiovascular surgeon, Stanford University Hospital, Stanford, California, USA.
Richard Lower. Cardiac surgeon, University of Virginia, Richmond, USA.
Christiaan Nelthling Barnard. Formerly Professor of Cardiac Surgery, Groote Schuur Hospital, Cape Town, South Africa.

it may be used. Haemodynamic instability can occur at any time in these patients, and skilled intervention with judicious use of inotropes, ventilation and diuretics may be required to keep the patient stable until the organs are harvested. Ideal criteria for the donor include the following:

- age (<45 years for males, <50 years for females) – the incidence of coronary artery disease rises after these ages;
- weight (within 25 per cent of the recipient);
- ABO compatibility;
- no evidence of cardiac injury (normal ECG, normal chest radiograph);
- no increased requirements for inotropes;
- no evidence of active infection (HIV, hepatitis B or bacterial);
- no palpable coronary artery disease.

The donor operation is usually performed in conjunction with other transplant teams. If the liver and kidneys are to be used, they require some preliminary dissection before removal of the heart. The heart is exposed by a median sternotomy and the cavae are dissected from the pericardial reflections to expose more of their length. Heparin is given and the aorta cannulated with a perfusion catheter. The aorta is clamped and the inferior vena cava divided to allow venous blood to escape into the chest. Cold cardioplegic solution is infused under pressure into the aortic root and the heart arrests in diastole. A pulmonary vein is then divided to allow blood in the left atrium to escape. Once the cardioplegic solution is infused, the pulmonary veins are divided followed by the pulmonary artery. The aorta is then divided just below the cross-clamp, leaving only the superior vena cava to be divided. This is divided as high as possible to avoid damage to the sinoatrial node. Care should be taken that all central venous cannulae are withdrawn to avoid possible embolism in the donor heart. The heart is then stored in cardioplegic solution and transported in ice to the recipient hospital.

The recipient operation

Once it is clear that the donor heart is satisfactory then the recipient operation is started. The heart is approached through a median sternotomy and heparin is given intravenously. The cavae are cannulated separately and the aorta is cannulated just proximal to the innominate artery. Cardiopulmonary bypass is not started until the donor heart is in the operating room. The recipient heart is excised leaving a generous cuff of atria and interatrial septum. The donor heart is trimmed appropriately and suturing begins with the left atria, the right atria, the pulmonary artery and finally the aorta. The heart is then de-aired and the cross-clamp released. Ventricular activity usually starts spontaneously but occasionally temporary pacing is required. The heart is allowed to beat on bypass until rewarming is complete and haemostasis is achieved. Ventilation is commenced and cardiopulmonary bypass is slowly weaned until the donor heart is supporting the circulation.

Postoperative care

In common with all forms of allogeneic transplantation, the normal host response is to mount an immune response to the donor organ. To combat this problem, regimens of immunosuppressive therapy have been developed. Intravenous methylprednisolone and azathioprine are given at the time of operation and these are converted to the oral forms once the patient is able to tolerate oral or nasogastric fluids. Cyclosporin A is added if the renal function is satisfactory. Cyclosporin A is nephrotoxic and regular trough levels are required to avoid excessive toxicity. Treatment with azathioprine can result in liver dyscrasias and neutropenia. The incidence of rejection is greatest in the first year post-transplantation. The only reliable way of monitoring the presence or absence of rejection is by endomyocardial biopsy. This is an invasive procedure requiring cannulation of a major vein and taking small biopsies of the ventricular septum from the right ventricle. The presence of a lymphocytic infiltrate suggests rejection and myocyte necrosis implies severe rejection. A pulse of intravenous steroids is usually given as first-line treatment but other therapies include antilymphocyte globulin and the monoclonal antibody preparation OKT3. Most rejection episodes resolve with treatment but occasionally the rejection is refractory to treatment and the allograft fails.

Another important cause of morbidity and mortality in these patients is infection. Immunosuppression lowers the host's resistance to infection and opportunist infections in addition to common infections may occur. The most common site for infection is the chest. Antibiotics should not be commenced until a full infection screen (throat swabs, midstream urine, sputum and venous blood cultures) has been taken. Viral, protozoal and fungal infections may also occur. Late complications include accelerated graft vascular disease and systemic malignancy.

Alternatives to transplantation are being explored. Novel operations such as skeletal myoplasty, left ventricular reduction surgery and implantable ventricular assist devices have had some notable success but these procedures have yet to gain widespread acceptance.

Results

The perioperative mortality rate is about 10 per cent but patients surviving to leave hospital may have a 90 per cent 1-year survival. This falls to 70 per cent at 5 years and 60 per cent at 10 years. Patients surviving more than 1 year usually have a good exercise capacity and are able to return to work (Fig. 48.59).

Future prospects

Heart transplantation is limited by donor availability. Increasing the donor pool by widening donor criteria and increasing public awareness have helped, but demand exceeds supply. The use of xenografts is one possibility but ethical, logistic and rejection problems mean that this prospect is a long way off. Artificial hearts have a role to play

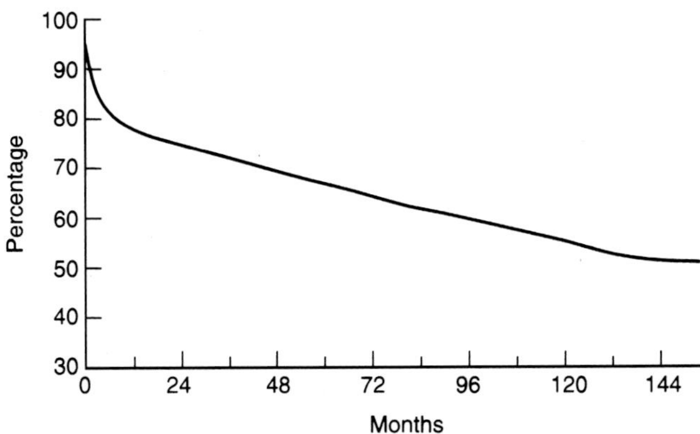

Fig. 48.59 Survival following orthotopic heart transplantation.

in supporting the circulation until a heart becomes available for transplantation but they do not seem practical for long-term use.

Appendix A: Myocardial management during aortic occlusion

The ideal situation for the surgeon operating on the heart is to have a still heart in a bloodless field. To render the heart bloodless, the aorta must be cross-clamped to prevent coronary perfusion. The heart is then rendered ischaemic and there are two ways of coping with this ischaemia without causing lasting myocardial damage.

Cardioplegic arrest

There are various cardioplegic solutions which arrest the heart in diastole and preserve adenosine triphosphate (ATP) levels. They all have high potassium levels and may be crystalloid or contain blood. Blood cardioplegia has become popular because it can act as a buffer with a high oncotic pressure and because it can also supply oxygen to the ischaemic myocardium at a rate sufficient to meet its metabolic demands. With the patient on full cardiopulmonary bypass, the core temperature is reduced to 26–28°C and the aorta is cross-clamped. Cardioplegic solution is infused into the aortic root and topical cooling with iced slush may also be employed to increase myocardial protection. The heart can be kept arrested for up to 2 hours with this technique.

There are many permutations with the type of cardioplegia, the temperature of cardioplegia, its route of delivery and whether it is given continuously or intermittently. There is no consensus agreement and the reader should refer to a specialist text for more information.

Ventricular fibrillation and intermittent aortic occlusion

This is a technique where ventricular fibrillation is induced by a small electrical charge. The heart does not eject and is relatively still but not bloodless. To perform an operative procedure (e.g. CABG) the aorta is cross-clamped to render the heart ischaemic. The heart can tolerate short periods of intermittent ischaemia providing the heart is reperfused and allowed to beat in-between. For CABG the choice between this technique and cardioplegia depends on the surgeon's preference.

Total circulatory arrest

Cardiopulmonary bypass is instituted and the core temperature reduced to 12–18°C. The metabolic rate of all the organs of the body is so low that periods of up to 30 minutes of total circulatory arrest with the pump switched off are tolerated. This technique has its main role in paediatric surgery and surgery of the ascending aorta.

Appendix B: Investigations in cardiac surgery

ECG

A resting ECG may provide valuable information but a cardiological textbook should be consulted for ECG changes associated with all of the conditions discussed in the text.

Chest radiography

Many patients with ischaemic heart disease are ex-smokers so pulmonary lesions may be noted in addition to the aortic and cardiac dimensions, although the chest radiograph is usually normal. Chamber hypertrophy, valve calcification and abnormalities of the great vessels may point to congenital or valvular heart disease but the chest radiograph may again be normal (Fig. 48.60).

Exercise ECG

To obtain objective evidence of myocardial ischaemia, an exercise ECG may be performed in patients with suspected ischaemic heart disease. Under carefully controlled conditions with full resuscitation equipment available, the patient is asked to perform a graded series of treadmill exercises. The work rate is increased every 2 minutes and continuous ECG recording is performed. The test is terminated when the patient complains of pain or dyspnoea, or there are significant ST segment changes or arrhythmia on the ECG. This test is potentially dangerous in patients with valvular lesions and other tests (e.g. isotope scanning) may be required to demonstrate ischaemic myocardium in these patients.

Isotope scanning

The radioisotope thallium is taken up by perfused myocardium and therefore ischaemic myocardium is shown up as a 'cold spot'. A myocardial uptake gated acquisition (MUGA) scan uses labelled erythrocytes to demonstrate left ventricular function and the ejection fraction (Fig. 48.61).

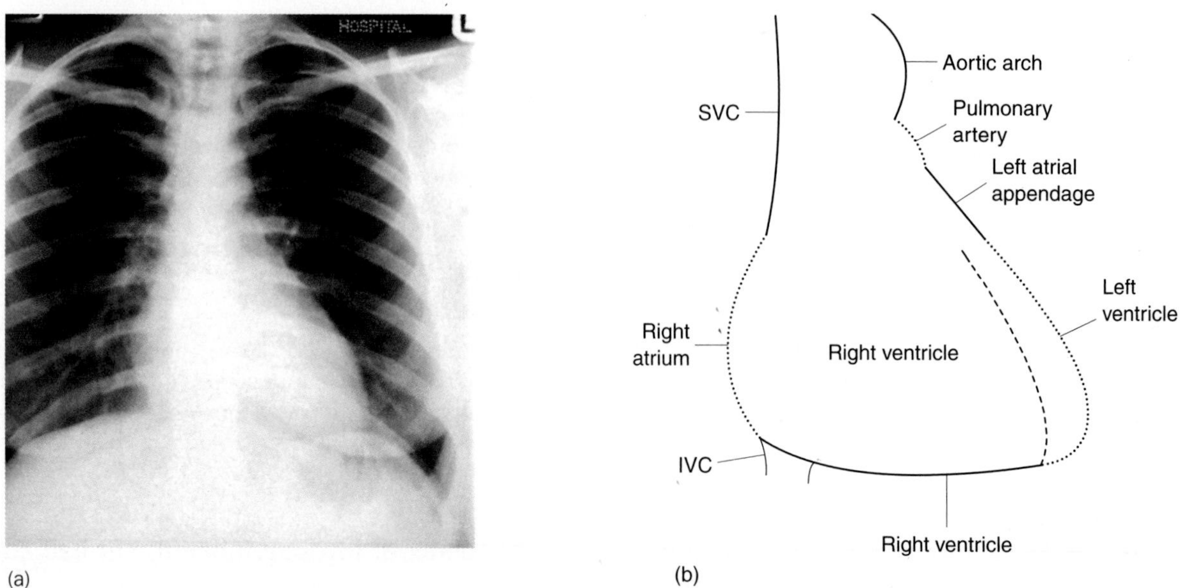

Fig. 48.60 (a) Normal plain posteroanterior chest radiograph; (b) drawing of outline of the heart with the structures that are represented.

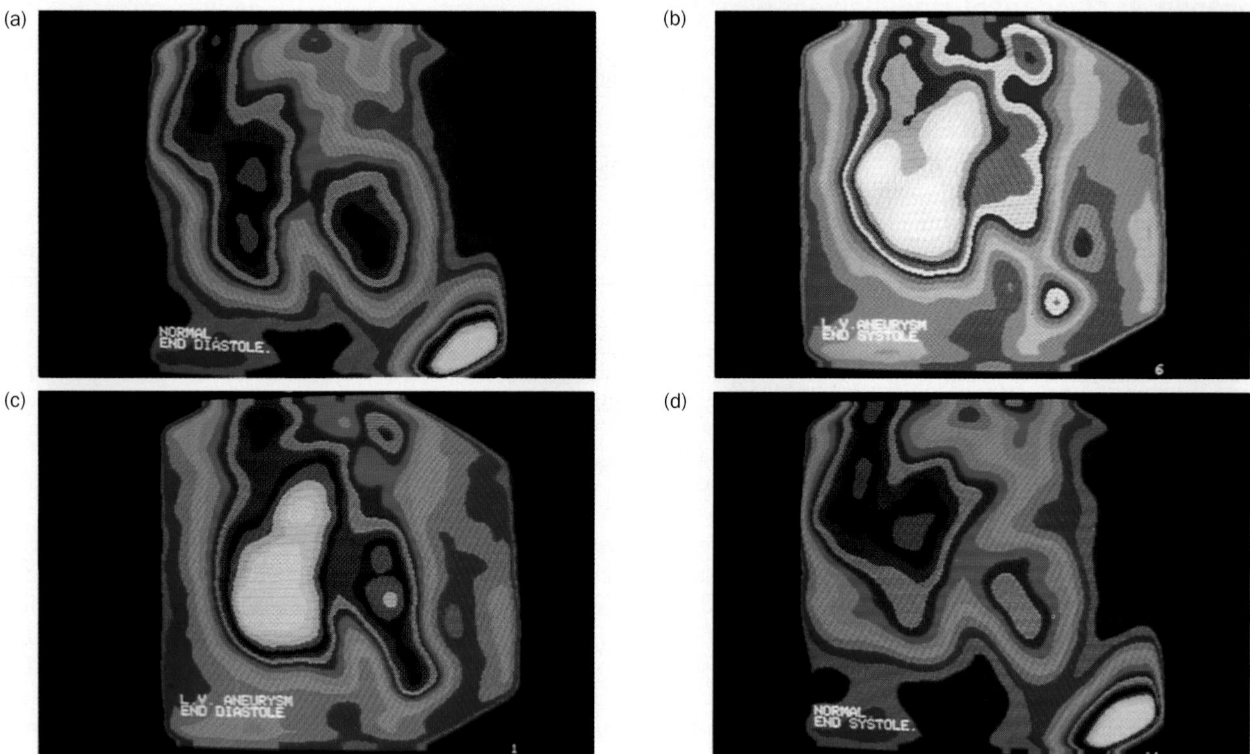

Fig. 48.61 Gated radionuclide blood pool images (MUGA scans). The intensity of radioactivity is represented by the colours. Red represents a very 'hot' region whereas the various shades of green represent less radioactivity. The greater the volume of blood the greater will be the intensity of the radioactivity. (a) A normal left ventricle at the end of diastole; (b) the same ventricle at the end of systole – the decrease in volume of the left ventricle can be seen, indicating that the ventricle is functioning well; (c) this scan is of a patient with a left ventricular aneurysm and the elongated appearance of the aneurysmal ventricle is well seen; (d) at the end of systole in the same ventricle a pool of blood can be seen remaining at the apex of the heart. This is within the aneurysmal sac.

Coronary angiography (Fig. 48.62)

This is an invasive test performed under radiographic screening. The arterial circulation is entered via the femoral or brachial artery, and a catheter is advanced into the aorta to the coronary sinuses. The coronary ostia are located and iodine-containing dye is infused to outline the coronary anatomy. At least two views of the coronary anatomy are

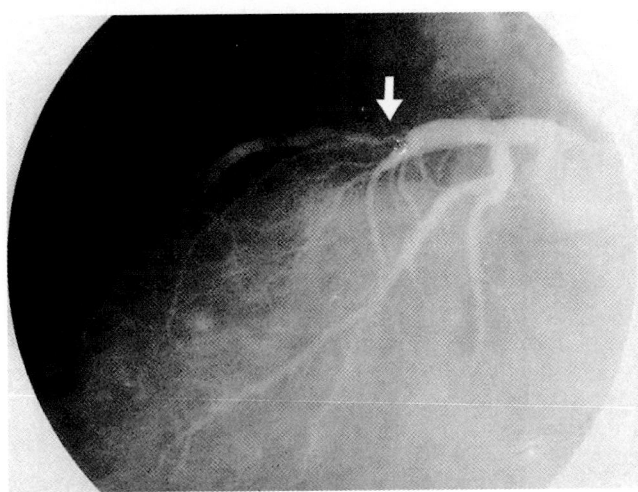

Fig. 48.62 Coronary angiogram demonstrating severe stenosis in the left anterior descending artery (arrow).

filmed in different planes to give a three-dimensional impression of the arterial system. A left ventriculogram is performed to estimate the ejection fraction and a measurement of the left ventricular end-diastolic pressure is taken. Direct pressure measurements of all of the cardiac chambers may be taken during this investigation.

Cardiac catheterisation

Cardiac catheterisation involves the introduction of a balloon flotation catheter (Swann-Ganz) into the right atrium, across the tricuspid valve and into the pulmonary artery. The pressure changes as the catheter passes through the cardiac chambers are characteristic. An estimate of the left atrial pressure can be obtained by wedging the balloon in a peripheral pulmonary artery. The cardiac output and other parameters can be calculated using a thermodilution technique.

Echocardiography

This is an extremely valuable examination because it can demonstrate valve thickness, calcification and motion, in addition to ventricular wall thickness, motion and chamber dilatation. Ultrasonic waves are transmitted through the heart until they reach an interface. They are reflected back to a probe and an image of the cardiac chambers, wall movement and valve motion can be made. The gradient across the stenotic valve can be estimated by a Doppler probe and regurgitation may also be demonstrated. Coronary angiography is used in patients suspected of having coexistent ischaemic heart disease and the actual gradient across the aortic valve may be shown during this procedure.

Other investigations

CT and MRI are not widely used for myocardial investigations but are useful in visualising the great vessels (aneurysms and dissection) and for demonstrating mediastinal and thoracic pathology.

Appendix C: Postoperative complications in cardiac surgery

Postoperative problems common to all patients occur following cardiac surgery (chest infection, wound infection, etc.) but some are characteristically seen in cardiac patients.

Neurological sequelae

For most patients, cardiopulmonary bypass leaves no obvious neurological deficit but, on detailed psychological testing, subtle abnormalities may be detected that often persist for up to 1 year. There is a risk of permanent stroke in the order of 1–2 per cent depending on age and carotid disease. This fact should be mentioned to all patients undergoing any cardiac surgery.

Poor cardiac output

There are several mechanisms for this complication in the early postoperative period, namely:

- poor myocardial function;
- infarction;
- tamponade or bleeding;
- intravascular volume depletion.

The diagnosis is usually simple as the patient is peripherally cold, with a low blood pressure and poor urine output.

Treatment

In the absence of tamponade, any underfilling should be corrected. Rhythm disturbances are treated and, if the low output state persists, the heart may require pharmacological or mechanical support.

Pharmacological support. Inotropic drugs act in a variety of ways to alter the systemic vascular resistance, increase the heart rate and increase the force of myocardial contraction. Commonly used inotropes indude isoprenaline, dopamine, dobutamine, adrenaline and noradrenaline; they are commonly used in conjunction with vasodilating agents which decrease the afterload.

Dobutamine is a β-agonist with chronotropic and inotropic properties and limited vasodilatation. The dose is titrated to the haemodynamic response and the usual range is 5–15 mg/kg per minute. Dopamine at low doses (<5 mg/kg per minute) has the beneficial effect of augmenting renal blood flow. At higher doses it constricts the renal arteries and has an inotropic effect (Table 48.1).

Judicious use of inotropes and vasodilators, with the use of physiological measures (heart rate, blood pressure, central venous pressure and Swan-Ganz measurements), help to optimise the cardiac output.

Rhythm disturbances. Atrial arrhythmias are common after cardiac surgery and must be treated if persistent or causing haemodynamic compromise. The most common

Table 48.1 Inotropic drugs

	Inotropic action	*Constriction*	*Chronotrope*	*Effect on renal blood flow*
Dobutamine	++	–	+	–
Isoprenaline	+	–	++	–
Adrenaline	++	+	+	–
Dopamine	+	–	+	+
Noradrenaline	+	++	+	–

arrhythmia is atrial fibrillation which occurs in 20–30 per cent of postoperative patients. Digoxin is a common treatment but calcium channel blockers or membrane stabilisers may be used. DC shock is only used if urgent control is necessary. Bradycardia is seldom seen, but temporary followed by permanent pacing may be required. Any arrhythmias may occur and the surgeon must be familiar with their cause, pattern, treatment and prevention.

Cardiac support. There is a number of ways to support the failing heart in the anticipation that it will (1) recover some or all of its function or (2) maintain the circulation long enough for cardiac transplantation.

There are circumstances when conventional cardiopulmonary bypass (from right atrium to aorta) is either not feasible, as in aortic dissection, or not advisable (multiple injury), and other means of supporting the circulation are employed.

Left and right heart bypass. This employs a similar technique to cardiopulmonary bypass except oxygenation is not employed and the returning blood is channelled into the same side of the circulation. In right ventricular dysfunction, blood is drained from the venous system, passed through the pump and returned to the pulmonary artery, thereby bypassing the right ventricle. It is useful when temporary dysfunction of a ventricle occurs and full recovery is expected. It has also been used on occasions to support the heart until transplantation.

Mechanical support (Fig. 48.63). If low cardiac output persists in spite of inotropic support, the heart may require mechanical support while it recovers its function. The intra-aortic balloon pump is a device that is inserted, either percutaneously or under direct vision, into the common femoral artery. It is threaded into the aorta until its tip lies just distal to the arch vessels. The balloon is triggered by the ECG to deflate in ventricular systole (thus reducing afterload) and inflate in diastole (displacing blood which perfuses the coronary arteries retrogradely). When the heart has recovered sufficiently, the balloon is removed. Complications include damage to the femoral artery, leg ischaemia and haemolysis.

Other means of augmenting ventricular performance

Intra-aortic balloon counterpulsation may not be sufficient to support the failing ventricle and is only suitable for the left-sided circulation. The ventricle (right or left or both) may be bypassed by draining blood from the proximal atrium, passing it through a centrifugal pump and returning it to the distal great vessel thereby bypassing the affected ventricle altogether. As the ventricle recovers, the flow in the pump is gradually reduced so that the ventricle slowly takes over the circulation. Once weaning is complete, the assist device is removed. Biventricular support is possible as a bridge to transplantation.

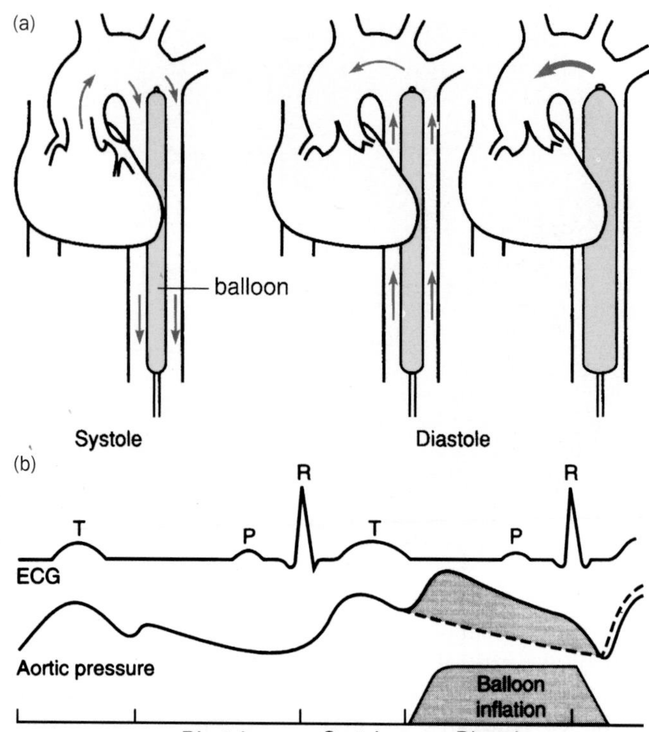

Fig. 48.63 Intra-aortic balloon pump counterpulsation. (a) The balloon deflates during systole and thereby lowers systemic resistance. It inflates during diastole and increases coronary perfusion in addition to augmenting the systemic blood pressure. (b) The pressure changes and phases of the ECG are shown.

Artificial hearts

It has proved impossible to find a perfect mechanical substitute for the native heart. The totally artificial heart is limited by thrombosis and infection, although survival of over 3 months has been documented. The energy supply to drive the implanted heart often weighs more than the patient and therefore mobility is restricted. The Jarvik total artificial heart has had limited success in temporarily supporting the circulation while heart transplantation is awaited. Further research is required before the expense of this technology can be justified for routine use.

Robert Jarvik, b. 1946. Implanted first permanent artificial heart in 1982.

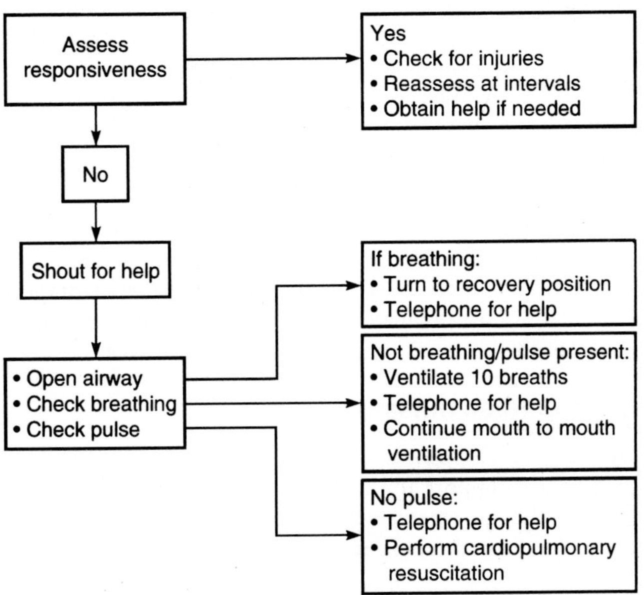

Fig. 48.64 Flow chart showing action plan for initial assessment and management of an apparently lifeless casualty (from *British Medical Journal,* with permission).

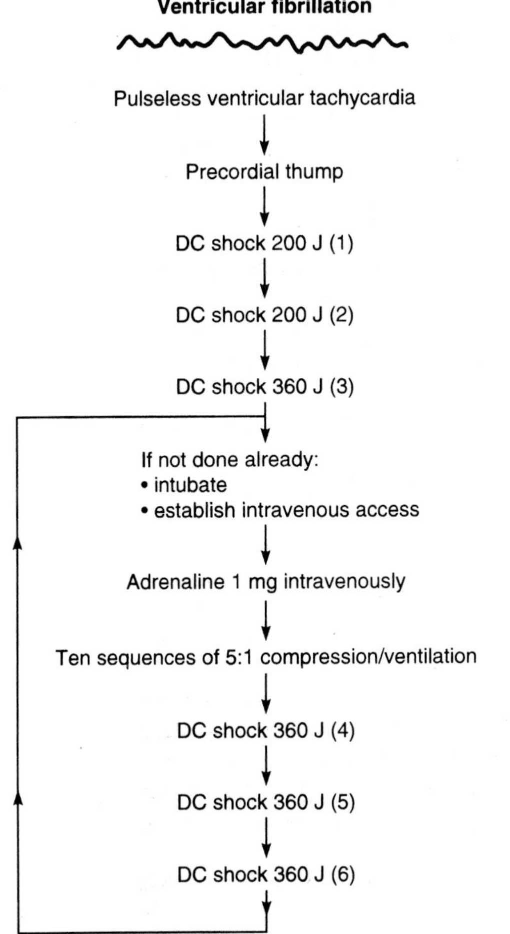

Fig. 48.65 Algorithm for managing ventricular fibrillation or pulseless ventricular tachycardia (from *British Medical Journal,* with permission).

Appendix D: Cardiopulmonary resuscitation

Cardiopulmonary resuscitation begins with basic life support before more advanced techniques can be employed. A logical approach to resuscitation has been produced in detail by the European Resuscitation Council in the *British Medical Journal* (Vol. 306, 1993, pp. 1587–1593). An outline of the steps involved using algorithms and flow charts in basic and advanced resuscitation (currently under review) are taken from this article (reproduced with permission) (Fig. 48.64).

Cardiac arrest is the cessation of cardiac mechanical activity, confirmed by the absence of a detectable pulse, unresponsiveness and apnoea (or agonal respirations). In adults the most common cause is primary ischaemic heart disease. Cardiac arrest may be associated with any of four heart rhythms: ventricular fibrillation, pulseless ventricular tachycardia, asystole or electromechanical dissociation.

Management of ventricular fibrillation or pulseless ventricular tachycardia – see Fig. 48.65.

Management of asystole – see Fig. 48.66.

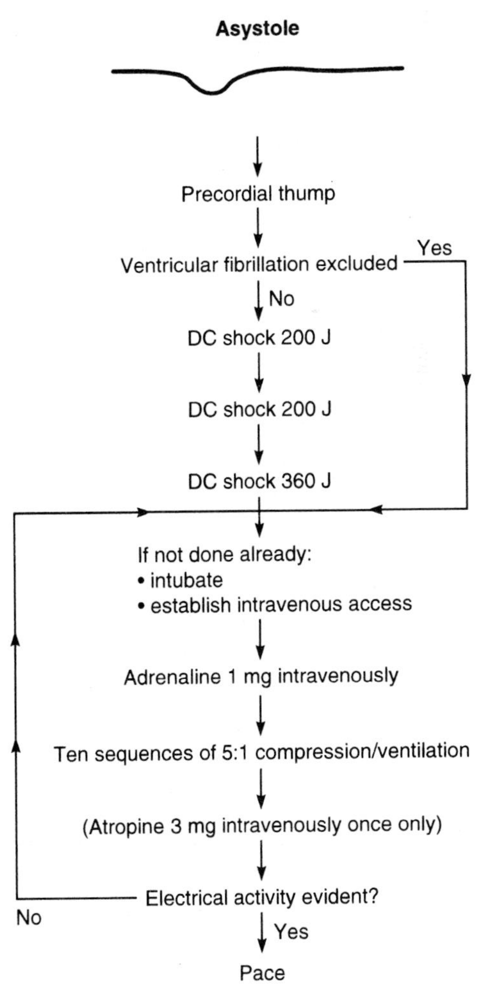

Fig. 48.66 Algorithm for managing asystole (from *British Medical Journal,* with permission).

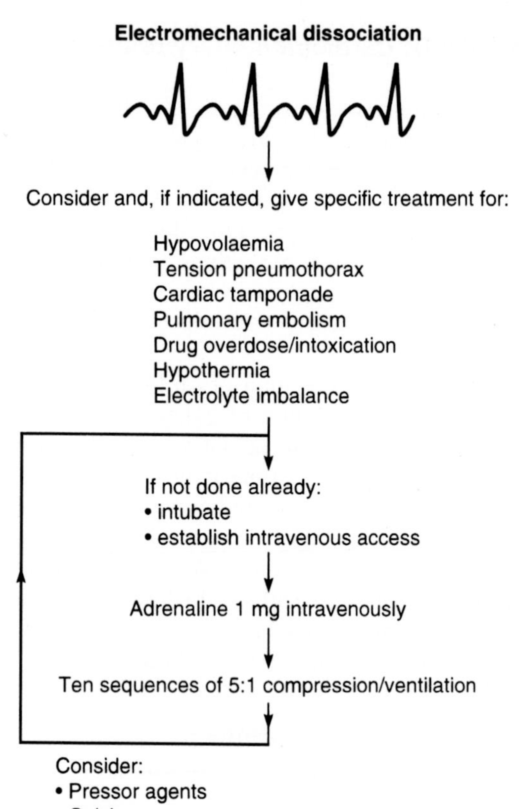

Fig. 48.67 Algorithm for managing electromechanical dissociation (from *British Medical Journal*, with permission).

Management of electromechanical dissociation – see Fig. 48.67.

Airway management

Tracheal intubation is the preferred technique for airway control during cardiopulmonary resuscitation. Advantages include isolation of the airway, prevention of aspiration and avoidance of gastric dilatation, facilitation of mechanical ventilation and the delivery of high oxygen concentrations. Suction of the trachea and major bronchi and delivery of drugs via the endobronchial route are also possible.

Drug delivery routes

The venous route is recommended for drug delivery during cardiac arrest. Peripheral venous cannulation is rapid, safe and does not interfere with cardiopulmonary resuscitation. Cannulation of an antecubital vein is the site of choice, although the external jugular vein is an alternative.

Open cardiac massage

Open chest massage is only rarely indicated in advanced cardiac life support for a patient with a 'medical' cardiac arrest, although emergency thoracotomy in cases of trauma is a well-validated procedure for which clear indications exist.

Further reading

Gravelee, G.P., Davis, R.F. and Utley, J.R. (eds) (1993) *Cardiopulmonary Bypass – Principles and Practice*, Williams & Wilkins, Baltimore, MD.

Hallman, G.L., Cooley, D.A. and Gutgesell, H.P. (1987) *Surgical Treatment of Congenital Heart Disease*, 3rd edn, Lea & Febiger, Philadelphia, PA.

Jamieson, S.W. and Shumway, N.E. (eds) (1986) *Rob and Smith's Operative Surgery: Cardiac Surgery*, Butterworths, London.

Kapoor, A.S., Laks, H., Schroeder, J.S. and Yacoub, M.H. (1991) *Cardiomyopathies and Heart-Lung Transplantation*, McGraw-Hill, New York.

Kirklin, J.W. and Barrat Boyes, B.G. (1993) *Cardiac Surgery*, 2nd edn, Churchill Livingstone, New York.

Milner, R. and Treasure, T. (1995) *Explaining Cardiac Surgery*, BMJ Publishing, London.

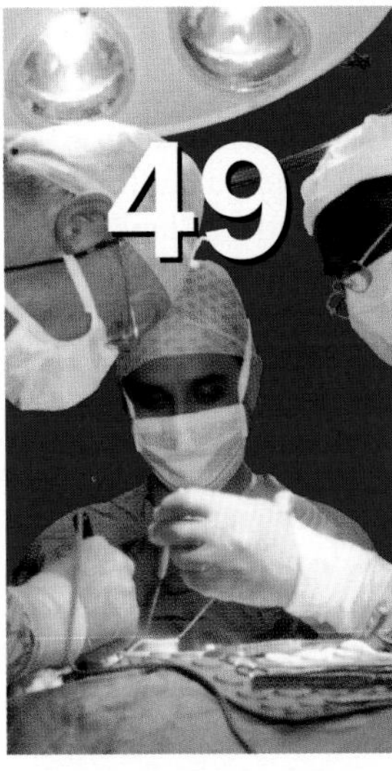

49 Anastomoses

Background

The experience of bowel surgery until the latter part of the nineteenth century was limited to dealing with protruding intestine following abdominal injury usually sustained during wars. If a laceration of the bowel was encountered attempts were made to repair it using the jaws of ants (described by Sushruta and Albucasis) or by suturing (Celsus). Probably the first surgeon to describe a suture made from animal gut was Albucasis. In Salerno, Italy, between the twelfth and thirteenth centuries, it was advised that if a piece of bowel had to be repaired it should be done over a stent of elder wood or animal trachea. Alternatives for dealing with injured intestine were to suture it to the abdominal wall to create a fistula or do nothing and let nature take its course. The latter management was frequently considered safer.

For centuries, no attempt was made to define the process of healing of the gastrointestinal tract. However, in 1812, Travers reported that intestinal wounds healed as a result of 'adhesive inflammation' binding down the peritoneal ('serosal') coat. Fourteen years later Lembert described a suturing technique in which serosa apposition was obtained.

As a consequence of the adoption of the Listerian principles of wound care and antiseptic surgery (Chapter 1) (together with general anaesthesia) surgeons in the second half of the nineteenth century began to perform laparotomies with the express purpose of resecting a piece of intestine and subsequently restoring continuity. Gastrointestinal surgery expanded rapidly and with it various methods of suturing the bowel together. All were modifications of Lembert's basic principles and were reviewed by Senn in 1893. A year earlier Murphy introduced his button but an adverse report appeared in the surgical literature citing colocolic anastomotic stricture which resulted in the patient's death.

Sushruta, fourth century AD. Indian surgeon.
Aulus Aurelius Cornelius Celsus, first century AD. Roman writer on medicine.

Bailey & Love's Short Practice of Surgery, 23rd edition. Edited by R.C.G. Russell, N.S. Williams and C.J.K. Bulstrode. Published in 2000 by Arnold Publishers.

In 1893, Senn advised two-layer interrupted anastomoses. His suture was of fine aseptic silk applied with ordinary sewing needles. Halsted favoured a one-layer anastomosis without penetration of the lumen. In contrast, Connell in 1903 strongly recommended a single layer of interrupted sutures which passed through all coats of the bowel and with the knots ligated intraluminally. Kocher also suggested an all-coats suture technique in two layers using catgut and silk. In 1907 Kerr and Parker used a temporary suture to close the bowel whilst the permanent sutures were inserted; once the anastomosis was completed these preliminary sutures were removed. Schoemaker and Remkin (1928) performed end-to-end anastomoses over narrow crushing clamps.

In 1922 Halsted described a closed colorectal technique in which the bowel was crushed, ligated and divided at the resection margins. Next submucosal buttress sutures joined the two ends of the bowel and finally an instrument with a knife blade was passed per rectum through the anastomotic diaphragm to divide the two sutures which had closed the lumen: the forerunner of our contemporary stapling devices. Stapling techniques have been 'reinvented' recently.

The closed method of anastomosis has been replaced by the open method for four major reasons (Table 49.1):

- the introduction of antibiotics;
- improved preoperative bowel cleaning;
- the use of atraumatic sutures;
- better on-table control of suture-line bleeding.

Benjamin Travers, b. 1783. English surgeon.
Antoine Lembert, 1802–51. French surgeon.
Joseph Lister, 1827–1912. British surgeon.
Nicholas Senn, b. 1844. Surgeon, Chicago, Illinois, USA.
John B. Murphy, 1857–1916. American surgeon.
William Stewart Halsted, 1852–1922. American surgeon.
F. Gregory Connell, 1875–1968. American surgeon.
E. Theodor Kocher, 1841–1917. Swiss surgeon and Nobel laureate.
Harry Hyland Kerr, b. 1881. American surgeon.
Edward Mason Parker, 1860–1941. American surgeon.
Jan Schoemaker, b. 1871. Surgeon, The Hague, The Netherlands.

Table 49.1 Reasons for change from closed method of anastomosis to open method

The introduction of antibiotics
Improved preoperative bowel cleansing
The use of atraumatic sutures
Better on-table control of suture-line bleeding

Alexis Carrel was a recognised revolutionist in vascular surgery. In 1902 he described a suture technique that he had developed that created a perfect end-to-end anastomosis of blood vessels. His method employed three retaining sutures which, when drawn taut, pulled the edges into an equilateral triangle which could then be easily sutured. This technique preserved the full patency of the lumen, and gave a smooth interior surface to reduce platelet and fibrin deposition.

Factors influencing anastomoses

Anastomotic healing is influenced by many factors and it is difficult to assess the influence of any single factor especially in the clinical situation. Healing depends on fibroblastic response and on the formation of plentiful collagen in the submucosa round the anastomosis. The general, specific and local factors influencing anastomotic healing are listed in Table 49.2.

The surgeon should be aware of good techniques relating to the main sites of anastomoses (Table 49.3).

Techniques for the commoner anastomoses

Gastrointestinal anastomoses

Certain important generalisations can be made as follows.

Table 49.2 Factors influencing anastomotic healing

General	*Specific*	*Local*
Age	Antibiotics	Mucosal inversion
Elective surgery		Suture material
		Good blood supply
		No tension
		?Drain

Table 49.3 Sites of anastomoses

Gastrointestinal	*Urological*	*Vascular*
Oeosphagus	Ureter	Aorta
Stomach	Bladder	Peripheral artery, e.g. femoral
Small intestine	Urethra	Vein, e.g. portal
Biliary and pancreatic	Vas deferens	Lymphatic
Large intestine		Coronary artery
		Microvascular, e.g. cerebral

Exposure

Any anastomosis becomes difficult if the surgical access and exposure are poor. This may be caused by inadequate anaesthesia and muscle relaxation, poor assistance, a badly placed and/or too short incision, and less than perfect illumination. Poor access may also result from inadequate mobilisation of the viscera and this is more likely to occur in oesophageal, colonic and rectal anastomoses as these parts of the gastrointestinal tract are anatomically fixed and deeply situated.

Blood supply

The only absolute criterion of an adequate blood supply prior to anastomosis is free bleeding from the cut edges of the bowel. The blood supply can be compromised by undue tension on the suture line, devascularisation of the bowel during mobilisation, strangulation of the tissues by tightly knotted sutures and the excessive use of diathermy.

Suture technique

Experimental work and clinical trials have shown that inverted suture lines are superior to everted ones, although this principle has been challenged by Ravitch. The vast majority of surgeons uses an open method of intestinal anastomosis. One aspect which remains a controversy is the use of one or two layers. The latter was devised by Czerny and is probably still the most popular technique today. It is alleged that a single layer results in less ischaemia and tissue necrosis, and less narrowing of the lumen. Studies in both experimental animals and humans have shown no great difference between the two techniques. Anastomoses involving the extraperitoneal portion of the rectum and also the oesophagus are better performed using a single-layer, full-thickness technique, as this preserves the blood supply and full lumen width better than a two-layer technique. Gastrointestinal anastomoses can be performed end-to-end, end-to-side or side-to-side and can be either 'open' or 'closed'. Generally the method used in any one operation is standard. In the UK the majority of surgeons employs the open method, removing the clamps following the placement of the outer, posterior, serosal layer of sutures. The techniques used for uniting parts of the gastrointestinal tract are as follows.

The open, end-to-end, two-layer technique (Fig. 49.1). The divided ends of the bowel are held in crushing clamps and light occlusion clamps are applied across the bowel, avoiding the mesentery. The outer posterior layer of sutures is usually placed in a continuous manner (Fig. 49.1a) but interrupted sutures can also be used. The crushing clamps are then cut away.

The inner layers of sutures are then inserted commencing at the antimesenteric border with the knot on the serosal surface. A continuous over-and-over technique is used, care

Alexis Carrel, 1873–1944. French–American surgeon and Nobel laureate.

Vincenz Czerny, 1842–1916. American surgeon.

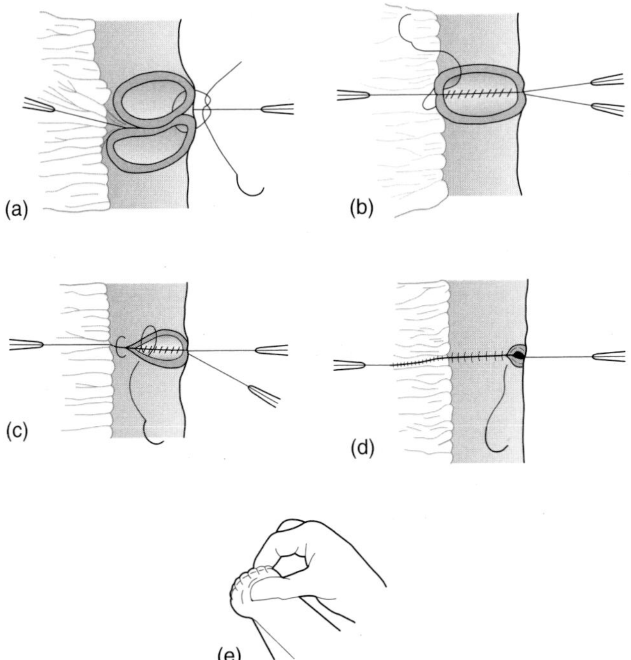

Fig. 49.1 The open, end-to-end, two-layer method. (a) Outer posterior serosa-to-serosa continuous layer; (b) inner continuous all-coats posterior layer; (c) anterior inner all-coats continuous layer inverting the mucosa (Connell technique); (d) final anterior serosa-to-serosa continuous layer; (e) test the lumen with finger and thumb.

being taken to include all coats of the bowel wall and avoiding grasping the mucosa with forceps.

The mesenteric corner of the anastomosis is securely invaginated using a Connell suture (Fig. 49.1b) and the anterior aspect closed using a continuous Connell technique (Fig. 49.1c) or a simple over-and-over technique. The suture is then tied to its other end. The anastomosis is completed by an anterior row of serosal sutures either continuous from the posterior layer or interrupted (Fig. 49.1d). The mesentery of the small intestine must be closed in every case and the anastomosis checked for patency (Fig. 49.1e).

An alternative to the above procedure is to place the inner all-coats first and then the outer layer, rotating the anastomosis to complete the posterior aspect. This is not recommended when the mesentery is very fat laden.

If there is disparity of the bowel ends, the smaller lumen orifice can be widened by cutting along its antimesenteric border (Cheatle's manoeuvre).

The open, end-to-end, one-layer technique (Fig. 49.2). This method is increasingly favoured for end-to-end anastomoses in areas of the gastrointestinal tract where the blood supply is poor, where there is no serosal coat or the lumen is small. In infants, a one-layer technique is the rule. Most surgeons favour the use of a one-layer open technique for the oesophagus and lower rectum.

Sir George Lenthal Cheatle, 1835–1910. Surgeon, London, England.

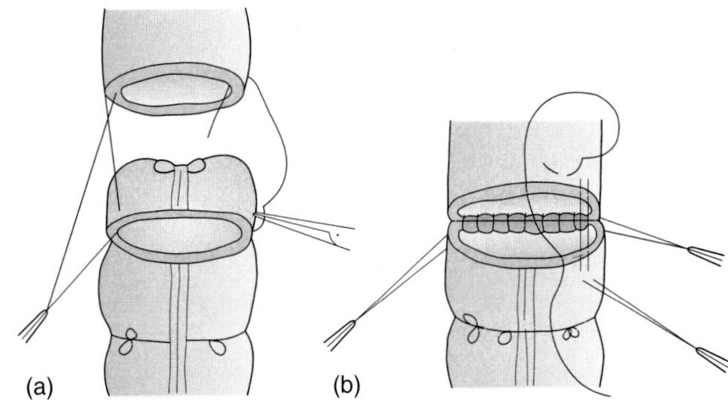

Fig. 49.2 The open, end-to-end, one-layer technique. (a) Stay sutures at corners to approximate and steady the posterior walls; (b) after completing the posterior layer, the anterior layer is continued by interrupted Lembert sutures.

After preliminary corner stitches are inserted to steady and approximate the posterior wall of the anastomosis (Fig. 49.2a), a series of interrupted deep 'all-coats' sutures of absorbable material (Dexon, Vicryl or PDS) is inserted 5 mm apart. After the corners have been reached, the suturing is continued along the anterior walls as interrupted Lembert stitches with a wide margin of muscle coat as shown (Fig. 49.2b): some surgeons use interrupted Connell sutures, but these are less haemostatic and turn in more tissue than the technique illustrated. The different single-row suture techniques are demonstrated in Fig. 49.3a–h.

The closed, end-to-end, single-layer technique (Fig. 49.4). The single-layer, inverting, closed anastomosis with interrupted nonabsorbable sutures was first advised by Halsted. The technique has been modified to incorporate the submucosa so that only the mucosa is excluded. It is commenced by inserting two angle stitches which are held untied. Posterior sutures are then placed longitudinally approximately 5 mm apart. Once finished, the anterior layer is inserted in a similar fashion. When this layer is in place the clamps are slipped out, the angle sutures tied and lastly the anterior ones. Patency must always be checked with finger and thumb (Fig. 49.1e).

End-to-end anastomosis (Fig. 49.5). This technique is used particularly in surgery of the oesophagus and stomach, and when there is significant disparity between two ends of intestine.

One end of the bowel must be closed and this is usually performed with a two-layer technique or alternatively by a row of staples. The anastomosis is performed as for an end-to-end one (Fig. 49.1).

Side-to-side anastomosis. This is usually performed to bypass an obstruction. Both ends are closed before the side-to-side anastomosis is carried out.

Stapling techniques (Figs 49.6 and 49.7).

1. Preliminary closure of the bowel ends can be performed using linear staples (Fig. 49.6) which can be cut away once the purse-string suture is in place.

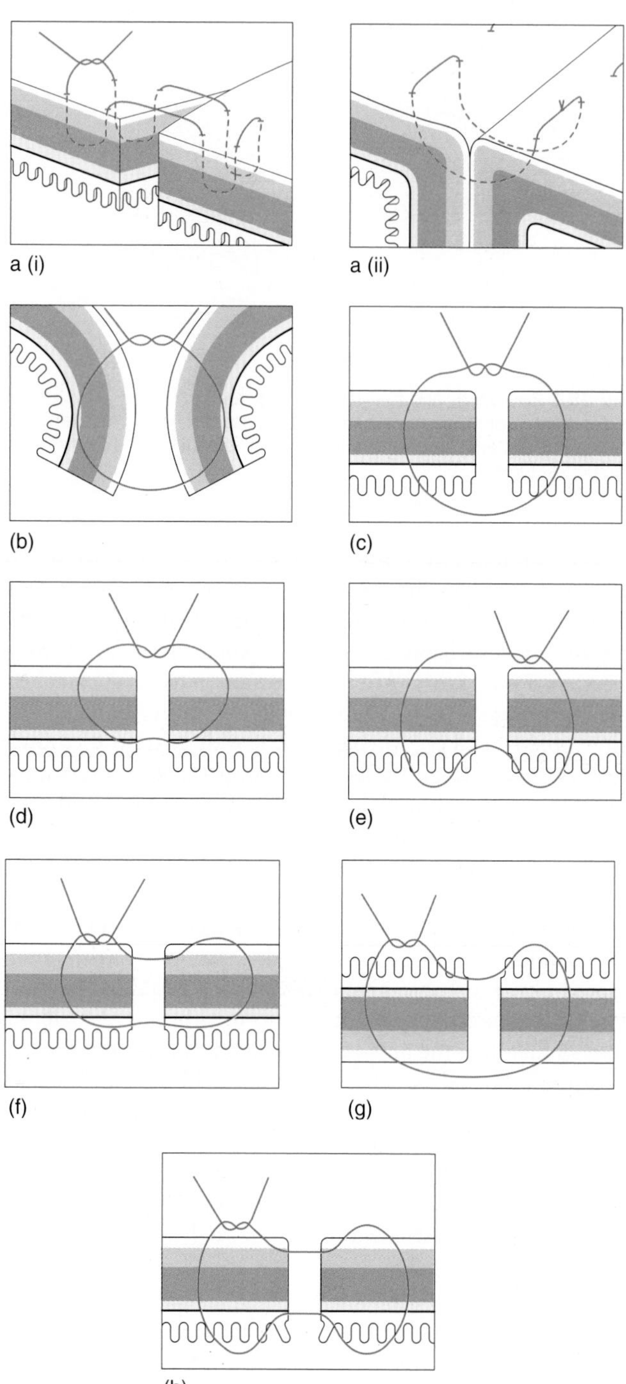

Fig. 49.3 The different single-row structures. (a) Halsted suture: (i) open and (ii) knotted; (b) Lembert suture; (c) all-layer suture (Albert); (d) extramucosal suture; (e) Gambee stitch – full thickness with mucosa backstitch; (f) extramucosal suture – backstitch through serosa; (g) backwall suture (Donati) – full thickness from inside with mucosa backstitch; (h) Herzog stitch – full thickness from outside, backstitch through mucosa and serosa.

Eduard Albert, 1841–1900. Austrian surgeon.
Donati, 1826–73. Italian surgeon.

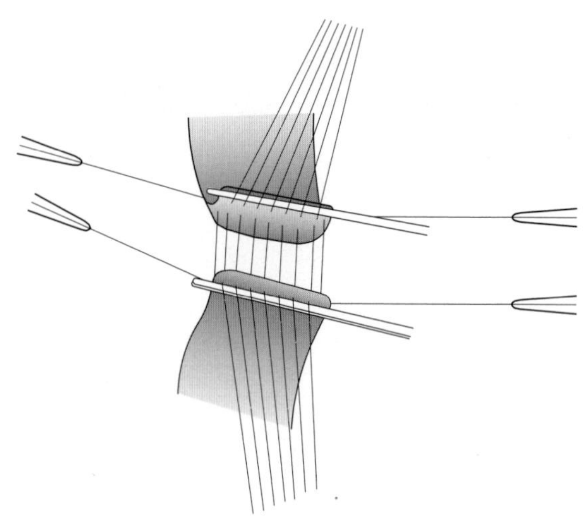

Fig. 49.4 Closed technique.

2. End-to-end anastomosis is performed using circular stapling devices [Premium CEEA (Autosuture) and ILS (Ethicon)]. Purse-string sutures must be carefully placed and for this the Furness clamp can be utilised (Fig. 49.6a). Circular staples are very useful for oesophageal and rectal anastomoses. A rectal anastomosis is illustrated in Fig. 49.6.
3. **The double-stapling technique.** The availability of an adjustable-angle linear stapler, the Roticulator (Autosuture), has added a new dimension to stapling techniques, further facilitating low rectal anastomoses. Together with the Premium CEEA (Autosuture) a low rectal anastomosis is technically easier and safer. The anastomosis of colon to rectum is effected using the Premium CEEA circular stapler through the rectal Roticulator linear staple line (see also Chapter 60).
4. Side-to-side anastomoses can be performed using the GIA stapler and this is useful for small-bowel and ileocolic anastomoses (Fig. 49.7).

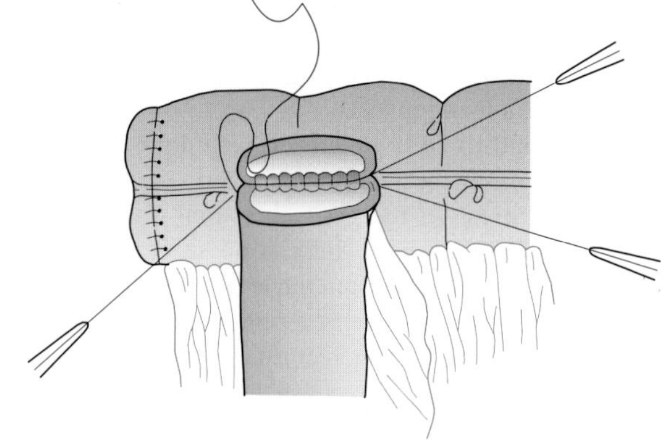

Fig. 49.5 End-to-end technique.

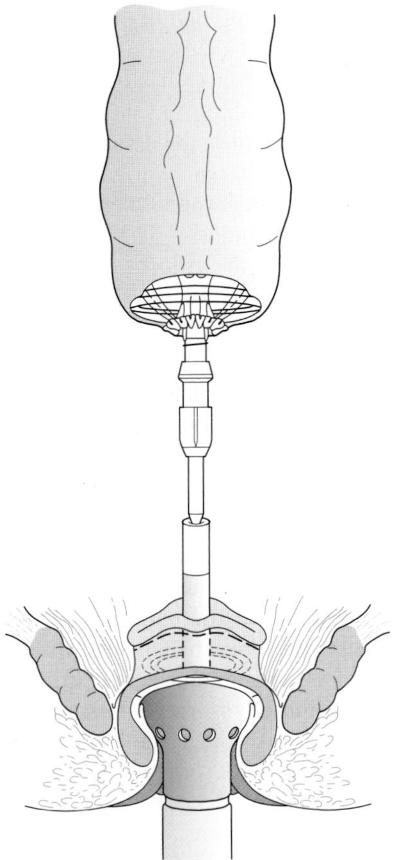

Fig. 49.6 Circular stapling device.

Special sites (Table 49.3)

Oesophageal anastomoses

When suturing the oesophagus, horizontal mattress sutures can be used as they have less tendency to cut through the oesophageal muscle than vertical mattress sutures. The cervical oesophagus can be anastomosed to stomach, colon or jejunum. Providing there is no tension and the blood supply to the intestine brought up to the neck is adequate, these anastomoses heal well.

The stomach is the simplest method of reconstruction but reflux can be a problem. The sutures are placed as horizontal or vertical mattress sutures in one layer. The author uses PDS for all intestinal anastomoses. The thoracic oesophagus is usually anastomosed to stomach (the Ivor Lewis operation) or jejunum. The technique is the same although the circular stapling device can also be used. The abdominal oesophagus is almost always anastomosed to jejunum either as a Roux-en-Y or to a loop and the circular stapling device is increasingly used in this situation.

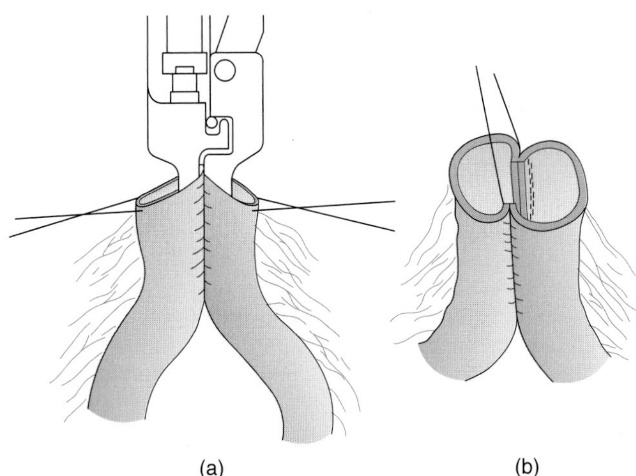

Fig. 49.7 GIA linear stapling device: (a) applying the staples; (b) the bowel ends must be closed over when the linear stapling device has been 'fired' and removed.

Gastric anastomoses

Following partial gastrectomy continuity is restored either to duodenum (Billroth I partial gastrectomy) or to jejunum [Polya partial gastrectomy (Fig. 49.8)]. The latter can be antecolic or retrocolic and should be performed by joining lesser curve to afferent loop, the latter being kept as short as possible. Because of the excellent blood supply absorbable sutures can be used and placed in a continuous manner. If the operation has been for carcinoma, e.g. a radical subtotal gastrectomy, it is advisable to make the anastomosis antecolic in case of recurrence and to use nonabsorbable sutures or PDS for the outer layer. Closure of the duodenum or stomach can be performed using a linear stapling device.

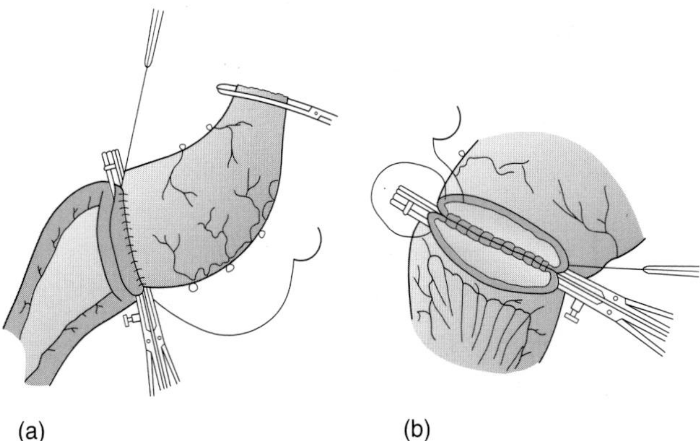

Fig. 49.8 Showing the gastrojejunal anastomosis during a Polya-type gastrectomy. (a) The posterior continuous layer being inserted – the gastric area to be removed is being used as a retractor before being cut away; (b) the stomach has been cut away and the anterior layer is started.

Ivor Lewis, 1895–1982. Former surgeon, North Middlesex Hospital, London, England.
Cesar Roux, 1857–1934. Swiss surgeon.
C.A. Theodor Billroth, 1829–94. Surgeon, Vienna, Austria.
Jeno Polya, 1876–1944. Hungarian surgeon.

Small-intestinal anastomoses

Jejunojejunal, jejunoileal, ileoileal, ileocolic and ileorectal anastomoses are all performed following resections for different disease processes. Like the stomach, the small intestine has an excellent blood supply and therefore continuous sutures can be used, although following right hemicolectomy and total colectomy the ileocolic and ileorectal anastomoses are best performed with an outer layer of interrupted sutures. It is always advisable to slant the clamps so that less antimesenteric border is left. The GIA stapling device can be used for any of these anastomoses.

Colocolic and colorectal anastomoses

Because (a) the vascular supply is less good, (b) distension from gas occurs and (c) the contents are faecal, large intestinal anastomoses may not heal well. Prior to resection, tapes are placed round the bowel and tied to ensure that no exfoliated malignant cells are reimplanted. Two layers of interrupted sutures may be used although most surgeons use only one layer. It is the author's practice to use one layer only for extraperitoneal anastomoses following anterior resection but for very low rectal anastomoses the circular stapling device is usually used (Fig. 49.6). No anastomosis should be performed if the colon has been poorly prepared as a low rectal anastomosis will be placed in jeopardy. The advent of 'on-table' lavage popularised at St Mary's Hospital, London (Dudley), is employed by the author, which ensures an empty colon above the subsequent anastomosis. A self-retaining catheter is inserted into the caecum usually via the base of the appendix following appendicectomy, or via the terminal ileum, and scavenger tubing tied in place over the cut colon (Fig. 49.9). Hartmann's solution is then passed via the catheter until all faecal matter has been expelled from the colon via the scavenger tubing and the effluent is clear.

In the emergency situation, the catheter can be retained as a tube caecostomy which acts as a gas vent. The terminal portion of the colon tied round the scavenger tubing is resected prior to anastomosis. The rectal stump is also lavaged from above and the effluent collected via a proctoscope in the anus. It is usual practice in cancer cases to employ a cytocidal fluid (mercuric perchloride, Noxythiolin and Povidone iodine are all used).

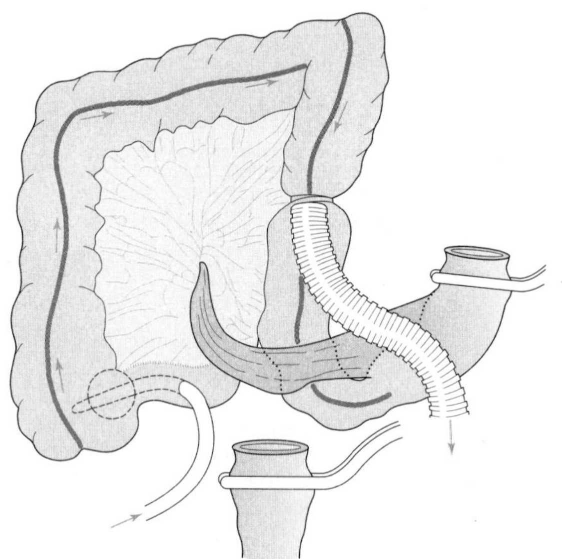

Fig. 49.9 Diagram of 'on-table' colonic lavage.

Hugh Dudley. Emeritus Professor of Surgery, St Mary's Hospital, London, England.
Alexis Hartmann, 1898–1964. American surgeon.

Biliary and pancreatic anastomoses

Either cholecystojejunostomy or choledochojejunostomy is used to bypass unresectable carcinoma of the head of the pancreas. Following cholecystojejunostomy a jejunojejunostomy distal to it is often performed. If there is danger of duodenal occlusion a gastrojejunostomy is also performed.

For benign strictures of the common bile duct, excision and primary anastomosis may be possible. Otherwise a Roux-en-Y loop is used as for some malignant strictures. Surgeons splint these anastomoses bringing the stent out well away from the anastomosis through the Roux loop on to the abdominal wall. This Roux loop should be sutured to the peritoneum and the place marked for subsequent radiological identification so as to provide access if necessary. Alternatively an access loop can be constructed and this sutured to the skin marking the site with a ring. Pancreatic duct anastomosis to jejunum is performed in a single layer and for all these anastomoses PDS is advocated. A nonabsorbable suture in the biliary tree can lead to stone formation.

Urological

Most anastomoses are ureterovesical but ureteroureteric and ureteroileal (Fig. 49.10) are also performed. Ureterocolic anastomoses are performed less commonly as an ileal bladder is preferable. The ureter should always be spatulated to increase

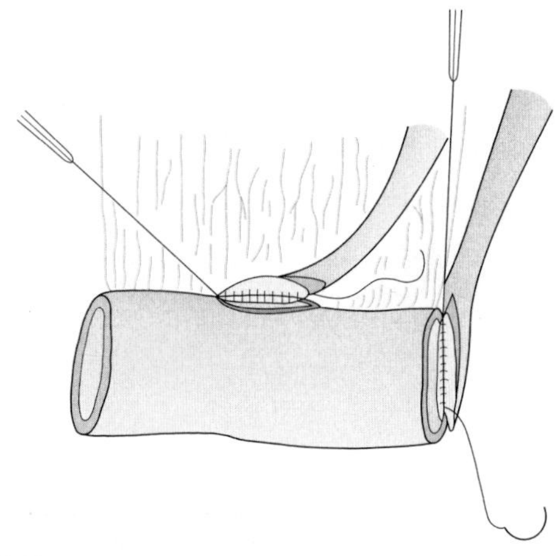

Fig. 49.10 Ureteroileal anastomosis.

the size of the anastomosis and splinting is usual. Sutures are usually absorbable and placed either continuously or interrupted. As in the biliary tree, nonabsorbable material, especially if braided, can lead to stone formation (see also Chapter 64).

Vascular

Except rarely (e.g. following trauma, when a severed vessel can be repaired primarily) most anastomoses are made to autografts or to veins (Fig. 49.11). The suture material used must be nonabsorbable and continuous, although occasionally with small vessels (e.g. fistula formation for haemodialysis) interrupted sutures are used. When placed end to end, the graft or vein should be stretched to increase the orifice size. Microvascular anastomoses are always done with interrupted sutures. If a vascular anastomosis is close to a joint, e.g. to the hip joint in the groin, excessive movements at that joint should be avoided until the anastomosis is healed (see also Chapter 15). Small clips/staples have been developed for vascular anastomoses which are proving very quick and useful especially for small vessels and for fistula formation.

New techniques

Biofragmental anastomosis rings have been proven to be safe anastomotic devices in elective surgery. These can be used throughout the intestine but it must be pointed out the cost is substantially higher than for a hand-sewn anastomosis.

Sutureless laser anastomoses have been performed experimentally using the neodymium: yttrium-aluminium-garnet (Nd:YAG) laser to create tissue welding. Tissue glue has also been used experimentally to anastomose small intestines.

Protecting an anastomosis

All anastomoses should be made without tension in an area of good blood supply. Colonic anastomoses can be protected from the faecal stream by a proximal colostomy or ileostomy. If drains are used they should lie alongside and not on the suture line. Gastrointestinal movement can be delayed or reduced by a policy of gastric suction, intravenous feeding and antispasmodic drugs (Buscopan). Oesophageal and rectal anastomoses should be checked by water-soluble contrast examination. Drains can be a source of sepsis and should be removed immediately they have ceased to drain significant quantities of fluid (or until a track has formed – usually after 7 or 8 days). If adverse healing factors are present (Table 49.3) precautions should be taken against breakdown, e.g. a diverting colostomy/ileostomy.

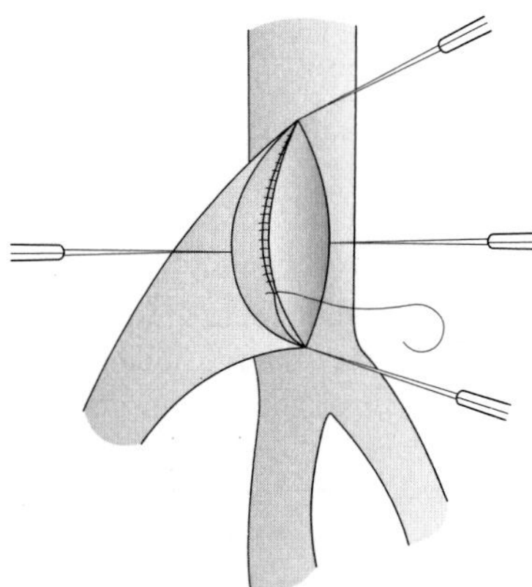

Fig. 49.11 A typical end-to-side vascular anastomosis. In this case a vein is being anastomosed to the common femoral artery (to bypass an obstruction to the superficial femoral artery in Hunter's canal).

John Hunter, 1728–93. Scottish surgeon, anatomist, physiologist and pathologist.

Table 49.4 Adverse factors influencing anastomotic healing

General	*Specific*	*Local*
Infancy and old age	Suture line disease	Oesophageal
Emergency surgery	Intradiated tissue	Rectum
Obstructed bowel	Infected anastomosis	Extraperiteal
Malignancy		Proximal faecal loading
Sepsis		Dilated proximal bowel
Corticosteroids		?Drain
Malnutrition		Enteral feeding
Anaemia		Drugs
Jaundice		
Uraemia		
Irradication		

Minimal access knotting and suturing

The performance of knotting and suturing during laparoscopic and thoracoscopic surgery is difficult because as well as working in a three-dimensional cavity looking at a two-dimensional screen, one is working with a needle and suture at some distance from one's fingers. Large needles cannot be introduced into the peritoneal cavity through a small port and long sutures become difficult to control whilst the instruments are less perfect than those used conventionally.

Endoloop ligation

Endoloop ligatures can be used to ligate tissue pedicles and vessels during laparoscopic and thoracoscopic procedures. They can also be used to close defects in structures, e.g. gall bladders and ovaries, thus preventing spillage of contents. The placement of an endoloop is a two-handed procedure. Pretied commercial ligatures are available in plain and chromic catgut, Vicryl and PDS; however they are expensive and they can be easily made out of the same ligatures utilising a Roeder or similar knot (Fig. 49.12).

Procedure

The endoloop ligature is 'back-loaded' into the introducer and the loop is completely retracted to protect the knot (Fig. 49.13). This introducer is then inserted via a 5-mm port and the endoloop advanced until the loop is exposed, resting it directly on the tissue with the pedicle centred in the loop. This pedicle is then held with a second grasper through the loop utilising it to pull the tissue upwards. The plastic shaft should be perpendicular to the knot, which helps to prevent suture breakage and ensures knot security. The endoloop is

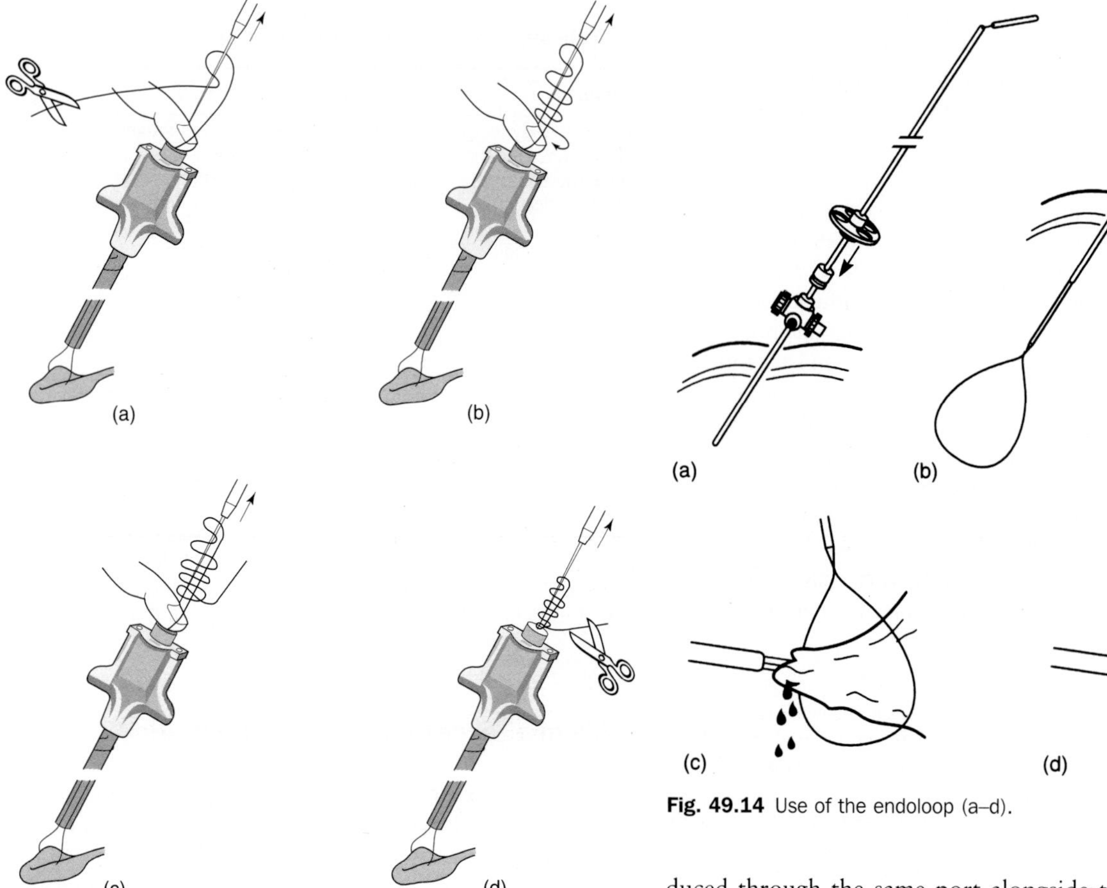

Fig. 49.12 The Roeder knot (a–d).

Fig. 49.14 Use of the endoloop (a–d).

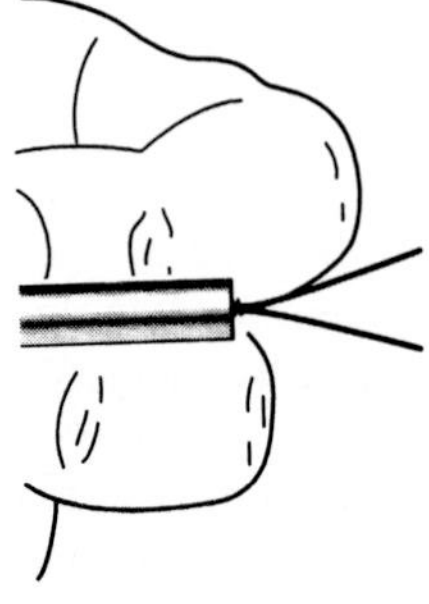

Fig. 49.13 Back-loading the endoloop correctly. The knot should be centred in the introducer cannula.

tightened by first snapping off the top end of the plastic shaft if a commercial endoloop is used and then pulling back on the small end piece whilst sliding the shaft forwards (Fig. 49.14a–c).

This movement allows the knot to slide forwards closing the loop. Once the knot has been moved down, the ligated tissue is released from the grasper. The knot is locked down securely, the plastic shaft withdrawn from the knot and the suture then cut at the required length. Alternatively, the small plastic end can be cut off by dividing the ligature at this point, the plastic pusher then removed and scissors introduced through the same port alongside the suture which is then cut and removed (Fig. 49.14d).

Extracorporeal knotting

This technique differs from intracorporeal knot-tying in one basic respect: once the needle/suture has been passed through the tissue, the suture is then brought outside the body and the knot is tied. The completed knot is then reintroduced into the abdominal cavity and then secured into position. Extracorporeal knot-tying can be used to ligate vessels, reconstruct organs, approximate opposing tissue surfaces and suture anastomoses.

Procedure

The needle/suture is loaded into the jaws of the needle holder by lightly grasping the needle below the swage point so that the needle will collapse into the introducer. The loaded introducer is then inserted through a 5-mm port (Fig. 49.15a, b). Once the needle appears in the peritoneal cavity it is passed to a grasper introduced from another port. The needle is steadied and then it is regrasped in the desired position by the needle holder. The needle and suture are then passed through the tissue and the tip of the needle is then regrasped with the needle holder. The suture will not be pulled out of the tissue if it is controlled with the second grasper; additional suture length is pulled into the peritoneal cavity. One must be careful not to bring the whole suture intraperitoneally as one

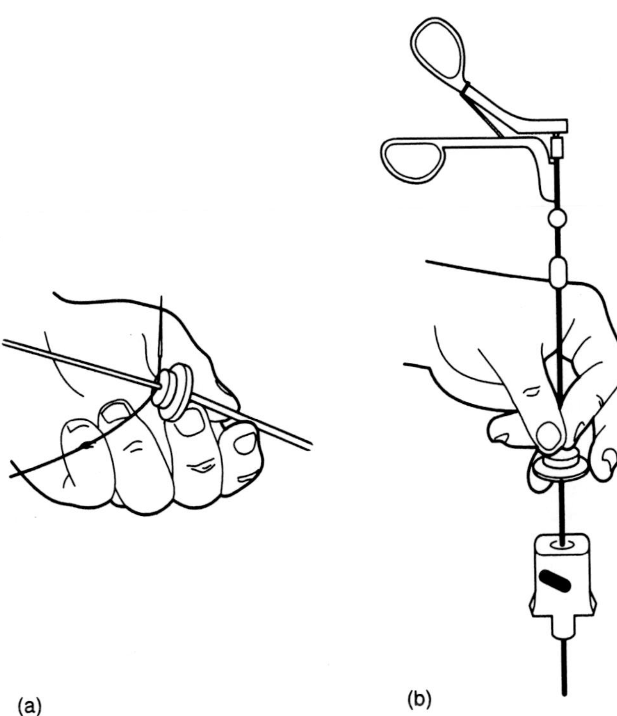

Fig. 49.15 Loading a suture into an introducer and inserting both via a 5-mm port. (a) Hold the needle holder and insert it into the introducer so that the needle is inside the cannula; (b) advance the loaded introducer through a 5-mm trocar.

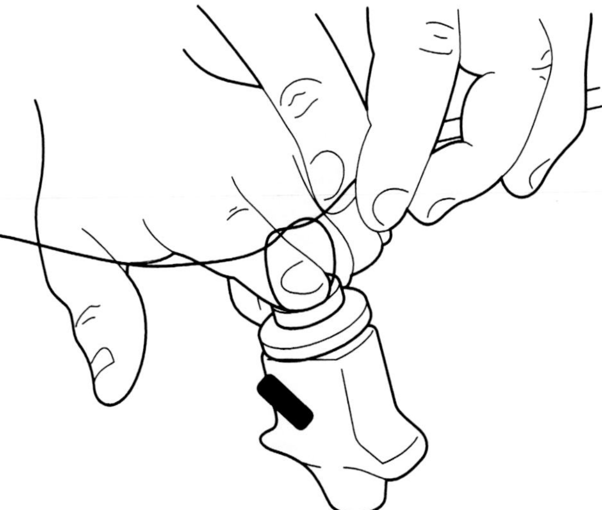

Fig. 49.16 Formation of a single-throw knot with the two suture ends.

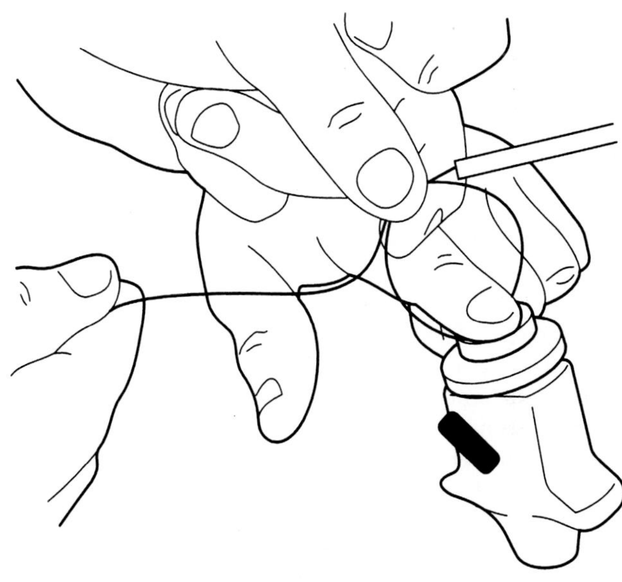

Fig. 49.17 Hold the knot with the thumb and third finger to hold it securely in place.

needs the end of the suture outside the port for knotting. The needle is then released and once again regrasped below the swage point with the needle holder so that it can then be withdrawn through the port removing the excess suture with it.

An assistant then covers the introducer channel with a finger to prevent loss of pneumoperitoneum. With both suture ends outside the body, the needle is cut off and a single throw knot made with the two suture ends (Fig. 49.16). The knot is held securely with the thumb and third finger of one hand (Fig. 49.17) whilst with the other a Roeder or Melzer knot (Fig. 49.18a–b) is completed. The suture tail is then cut off and a pusher used to slide the knot down as with the endoloop knot. An alternative is to make the first throw of the knot as described and then pass the suture ends through the jaws of a knot pusher which is introduced through the 5-mm port and the knot slid down on to the tissues. The knot pusher is then removed and a second conventional part of the knot fashioned, the ends of the sutures again being passed through the knot pusher. This second throw is then pushed down in a like manner to the first and the third knot can also be fashioned and slid down in a like manner. The suture is then cut using the scissors through the same port.

Intracorporeal suturing

Straight needle technique

A commercially available ski needle is available with different suture materials. The ski needle is a straight needle with a slight bend at its point. The suture should be cut to its desired length prior to introducing it into the peritoneal cavity. The suture/needle is held in the needle holder as previously described, holding it below the swage and then introducing the needle into an introducer. The needle and suture are manipulated in the same manner as for extracorporeal suturing, being careful to keep the swage point of the needle orientated towards the needle holder. Once the needle has been passed through the tissue to be sutured, two loops of suture are wrapped around the needle shaft utilising the

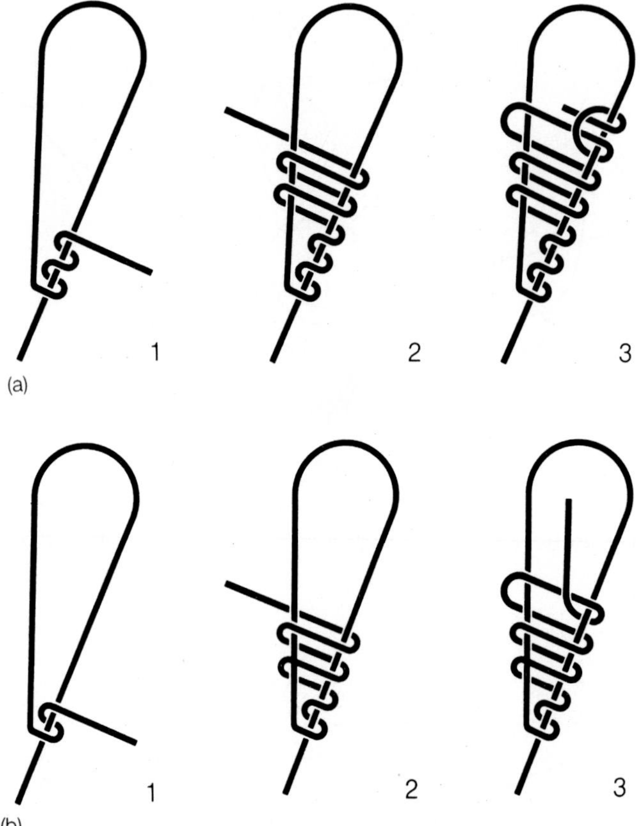

Fig. 49.18 (a) Melzer extracorporeal knot; (b) the Roeder extracorporeal knot.

second grasper. This is most easily performed by depressing the 5-mm grasper down around the tip of the needle holder and back up around its shaft. This motion is repeated to make the second loop (Fig. 49.19). After completing the two loops, one must be sure to keep the swage point of the needle orientated towards the needle holder.

The tail of the suture is then pulled through the two loops creating a knot which is slid down. Whilst holding the needle in a 5-mm grasper, two additional loops in the opposite direction are made by bringing the grasper around the needle holder shaft and then down around the needle holder tip.

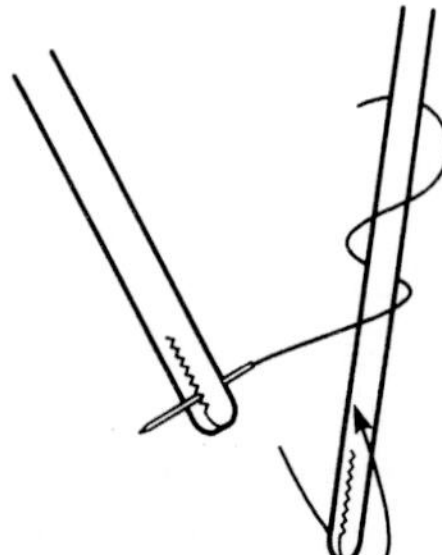

Fig. 49.19 Intracorporeal straight needle technique. To loop the suture around the needle holder, dip the 5-mm grasper down around the tip of the needle holder and back up around its shaft. Repeat this motion to make the second loop.

Once again the tail of the suture is grasped and pulled through the loops to tighten the knot. The suture is then cut at the desired length and the needle removed through the port.

Intracorporeal suturing using a curved needle

Endoscopic suturing with a curved needle offers the surgeon many of the same benefits experienced when suturing at laparotomy: precise needle placement and control in confined areas, rotational needle passage through tissue and a wide variety of needles and different suture materials from which to choose.

Technique. A needle holder is passed through an introducer and the end of the suture grasped. The entire length of the suture is then pulled back through the introducer leaving the needle free at its distal end. The tail of the suture is released and the needle holder then advanced again down the length of the introducer taking care not to crimp or damage the suture. The needle/suture is then grasped at the swage point keeping the needle curve parallel to the needle holder and introducer. The needle is then pulled into the distal end of the introducer (Fig. 49.20a–b). Excess suture is excised. A loaded needle holder and introducer is then introduced through a 10-mm port and it lies in the same fashion as for a straight needle. A different type of intracorporeal knot can be performed using the Topel or twist knot (Fig. 49.21). If the needle is too large for the port, then the cannula is removed and the needle passed through the incision and reintroduced through the port (Figs 49.20 and 49.21). Autosuture has developed a disposable straight needle 'endo-stitch' that uses a short straight needle which passes from jaw to jaw (Fig. 49.22). Knotting with this method is very easy.

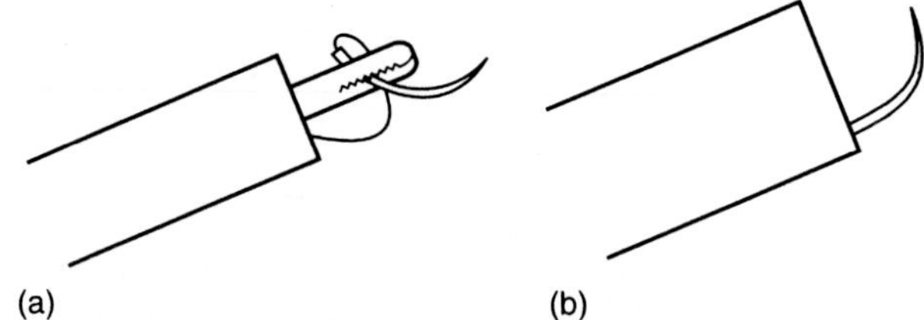

Fig. 49.20 Introduction of a curved needle into an introducer (a–b). (a) Grasp the needle/suture at the swage point, keeping the needle curve parallel to the needle holder and introducer; (b) pull the needle into the distal end of the introducer.

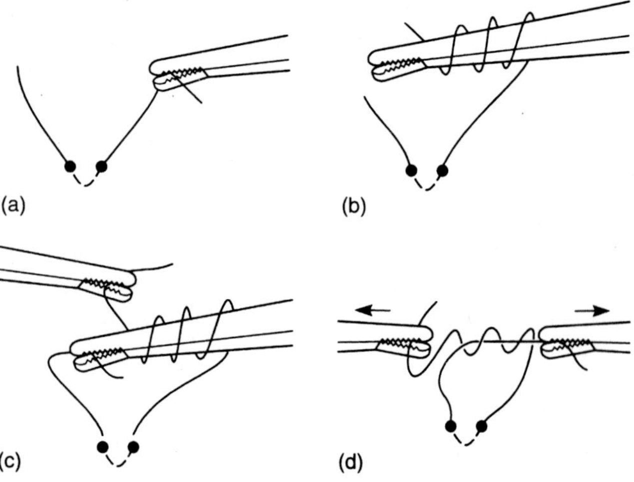

Fig. 49.21 The Topel 'twist' technique (H.C. Topel and J.V. Libretti).

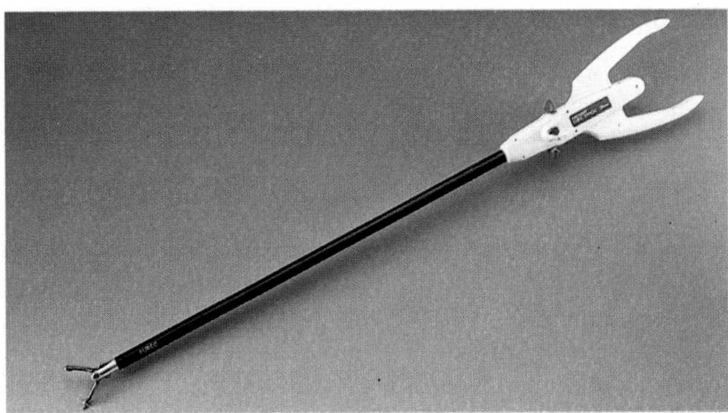

Fig. 49.22 The autosuture endo-stitch device.

Stapling

Linear stapling

An endo-GIA can be introduced through a 12-mm port and used thoracoscopically and laparoscopically. It is a haemostatic staple giving three rows of staples on either side of the tissue which is divided. Thoracoscopically it is used to divide the azygos vein and to staple off the lung. Intraperitoneally, it can be used on vascular pedicles and across the intestine. It is produced with different sizes of staples and in both 3-cm and 6-cm lengths. Further cartridges can be applied so that multiple uses of a disposable instrument can be effected during one operation. The resulting stapled ends are exactly the same as fashioned with the conventional GIA stapler.

It can also be used to anastomose two organs or loops of intestine together in the same manner as it is used conventionally at open operation. The defects left for the introduction of each jaw of the stapler then have to be closed either using a further stapler or closing it with a running suture.

The circular stapling devices are used at laparoscopic anterior resection and it is possible to place purse-string sutures across the divided colon and rectum. The anvil of the stapling device can be inserted through the rectum with its spike attached and then the purse string tightened. However, most surgeons performing laparoscopic colorectal surgery have moved towards laparoscopic-assisted colectomies and anterior resection so that the specimen would be brought out through a small iliac fossa or Pfannenstiel incision, which makes the placement of a purse-string suture in the proximal end of the colon and insertion of the anvil very much easier and quicker. The rectum can either be closed using a stapler or oversewn. At laparoscopic-assisted right hemicolectomy, the specimen is removed through a right hypochondrial or right iliac fossa incision and the anastomosis is most easily performed extracorporeally.

New innovations

Anastomosis can be performed using single staples and the peritoneum after a transabdominal preperitoneal hernia repair is usually closed with these staples, loaded in a multifire instrument. Absorbable staples are being manufactured.

Another innovation is to have a stopper applied to the end of a suture so that a knot is not required.

Suture materials

The different types and ideal properties of sutures are described in Tables 49.5 and 49.6.

A suture can be chosen with different properties in mind as follows.

Absorbable

Catgut is the oldest suture material known and is made from the submucosa of sheep intestines. It can be chromic or plain and is still the most frequently used suture material for intestinal anastomoses.

Table 49.5 Types of suture materials

Absorbable	*Nonabsorbable*
Catgut, collagen Homopolymer of glycolide Copolymers of glycolide and lactide Homopolymer of polydioxanone	Polyester, polyamide Polypropylene, polyethylene Steel, silk Cotton, linen
Biological	*Artificial*
Catgut, collagen Silk, linen, cotton	Polyester, polyamide, polypropylene Polyglycolide, polylactide Polydioxanone, steel
Monofilament	*Multifilament*
Polyamide, polypropylene Polyethylene, polydioxanone Catgut, steel	Polyester, polyamide Polyglycolide, polylactide Silk, cotton, linen, steel
Braided	*Twisted*
Polyester, polyamide Polyglycolide, polylactide, silk	Cotton, linen
Coated	*Uncoated*
Polyester, polyglycolide Polylactide, cotton, linen Polyethylene, catgut, collagen, steel	Polyamide, polypropylene

Table 49.6 Ideal properties of sutures

Strength
Minimal reaction
Easy handling properties
Good knotting security

Hermann Johann Pfannenstiel, 1862–1909. German gynaecologist.

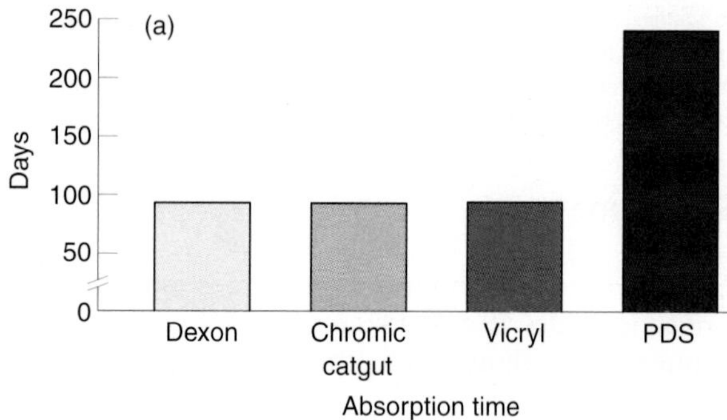

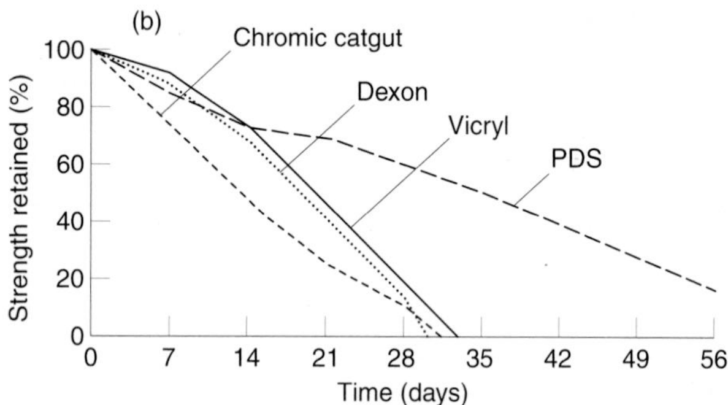

Fig. 49.23 (a) Absorption time and (b) *'in vivo'* breaking strength of sutures.

Suture material is absorbed in one of two ways. The first applies to catgut and collagen where the absorption mechanism is by enzymatic digestion. The other method is one of preliminary hydrolysis which is the effect of water on the suture material and does not require the same cellular involvement as does catgut with its proteolytic digestive enzymes. Hydrolysis is increased with rise in temperature or pH changes. Figure 49.23a demonstrates in general terms the comparative absorption times for catgut, Dexon (homopolymer of glycolide), Vicryl (copolymer of glycolide and lactide) and PDS (polydioxanone). Once a suture has been broken up by hydrolysis, polymorphonuclear cells and other macrophages (e.g. giant cells) can digest even so-called unabsorbable material. As the material absorbs it loses its tensile strength (Fig. 49.23b).

Delayed or nonabsorbable

Very few sutures are truly completely nonabsorbable. Silk is derived from the cocoon of the silkworm larva. The suture is braided round a core and coated with wax to reduce capillary action. Tissue reaction is greater than to the synthetic nonabsorbables because silk is a foreign protein. For this reason silk is not now used in anastomoses, and most surgeons prefer to use a monofilament synthetic suture if a nonabsorbable suture is deemed necessary. Wire sutures are ideal for qualities of inertness and permanence but working with them is difficult and they are virtually absolete.

Staples

Circular, linear and linear-cutting stapling devices are used to form anastomoses. The devices carrying these staples can be disposable or reusable. Until 1986 the staples were always nonabsorbable, being made of stainless steel. However, absorbable staples have now been developed. The circular stapling device is used for oesophageal and rectal anastomoses. Their use is not a short cut to the joining of two pieces of intestine. The preparation of the bowel ends and the placement of the purse-string sutures must be carefully executed. They do, however, help in situations where the placement of sutures can be difficult, e.g. a low colorectal or anal anastomosis in a patient with a narrow pelvis (Fig. 49.6).

Linear stapling for anastomoses may leave awkward edges and ends (Fig. 49.6). Linear-cutting staplers can save time if very long closures or multiple anastomoses are necessary but have little benefit over hand-sutured anastomoses.

It is necessary to choose suture material that has the best characteristics for carrying out an anastomosis in a particular site. Vascular anastomoses require fine suture materials with minimal tissue reaction – strength is a secondary consideration – and Prolene is commonly used. Gut anastomoses require sutures with good handling qualities with secure knotting; pliancy is also important, as is strength when the intestine begins to contract. Plain catgut is unsuitable for intestinal anastomoses, but chromic catgut can be used for gastric and small intestinal unions. Rectal and oesophageal anastomoses should employ unabsorbable, or long-delayed absorbable sutures (e.g. PDS), because these areas combine many adverse factors with the requirement to withstand powerful contractile activity.

Complications

There are four main complications, as follows (Table 49.7).

Haemorrhage

This can occur at the suture line or from the mesentery. The Connell suture is nonhaemostatic and therefore should not be used if the cut intestine has a profuse blood supply, e.g. the stomach.

Haemorrhage can be immediate (reactionary) or late (secondary), although this is rare. If the bleeding causes systemic effects, a laparotomy must be performed and the anastomosis resected and refashioned.

Table 49.7 Complications

Haemorrhage
Leakage
Stenosis
Diverticular formation
(Aneurysmal at vascular anastomoses)

Leakage

Oesophageal and colonic anastomoses are most prone to leak. The outcome depends on the size of the leak and its anatomical site. As already stated, the healing of anastomoses depends on good blood supply and no tension. With colonic anastomoses a clean bowel is also necessary.

Stenosis

Stenosis can be caused by excessive inversion especially with two-layer anastomoses. An inadequate stoma in the first place or ischaemia can also lead to subsequent stenoses. Circular staples, especially double rows, are prone to cause narrowing due to rigidity.

Diverticular formation

Caused by either a weakness of the wall or from a poor blood supply, a 'blow-out' occurs which is contained, i.e. perforation does not occur.

Although anastomoses depend on the many factors mentioned, a good technique is probably the most important one. Gentle handling of the tissues will ensure better healing. Anastomoses should never be rushed or performed if the above conditions cannot be fulfilled. A few extra minutes spent pays handsome dividends and may save the patient's life. An insecure anastomosis is an unacceptable iatrogenic hazard.

Further reading

Arregui, M.E. and Fitzgibbons, R.J. Jr (1994) *Principles of Laparoscopic Surgery: Basic and Advanced Techniques*, Springer, New York.

Rosin, R.D. (1993) *Minimal Access Medicine and Surgery: Principles and Techniques*, Radcliffe Medical Press, Oxford.

Rosin, R.D. (1994) *Minimal Access General Surgery*, Radcliffe Medical Press, Oxford.

Sabiston, D.C. Jr (1997) *Textbook of Surgery*, 15th edn, W.B. Saunders, Philadephia, PA.

Zucker, K.A. (1991) *Surgical Laparoscopy*, Quality Medical Publishing, St Louis, MO.

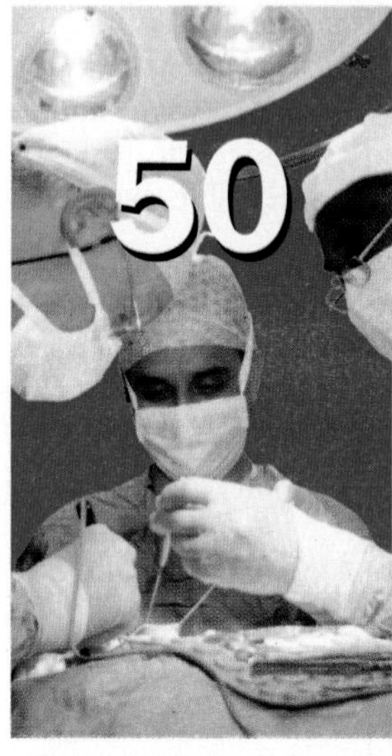

50 The oesophagus

Background

Surgical anatomy

The oesophagus is a muscular tube approximately 25 cm long occupying the posterior mediastinum and extending from the cricopharyngeal sphincter to the cardia of the stomach; 2 cm of this tube lies below the diaphragm. The musculature of the upper 5 per cent, including the upper oesophageal sphincter, is striated; the middle 40 per cent has mixed striated and smooth muscle with the proportion of smooth muscle increasing distally; the distal 55 per cent is entirely smooth muscle. It is lined by squamous epithelium. The parasympathetic nerve supply is mediated by the vagus which has synaptic connections to the myenteric (Auerbach's) plexus. Meissner's submucous plexus is very sparse in the oesophagus.

There is an upper and a lower oesophageal sphincter. The upper sphincter is powerful striated muscle, while the lower sphincter is much more subtle, but the elegant studies of Liebermann-Meffert have shown that there is an anatomical sphincter at the gastro-oesophageal junction. The arch of the

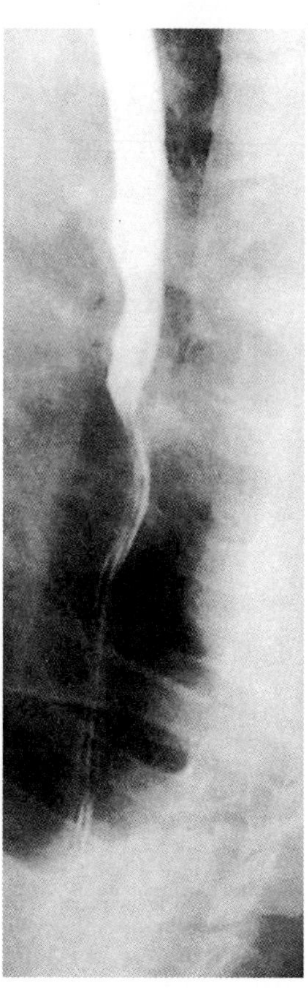

Fig. 50.1 The barium can show the indentation of the arch of the aorta and the left bronchus.

Leopold Auerbach, 1828–97. Professor of Neuropathology, Breslau, Germany (now Wroclaw, Poland).
George Meissner, 1829–1905. Professor of Physiology, Göttingen, Germany.
Dorothea Liebermann-Meffert. Surgical anatomist, Munich, Germany.

Bailey & Love's Short Practice of Surgery, 23rd edition. Edited by R.C.G. Russell, N.S. Williams and C.J.K. Bulstrode. Published in 2000 by Arnold Publishers.

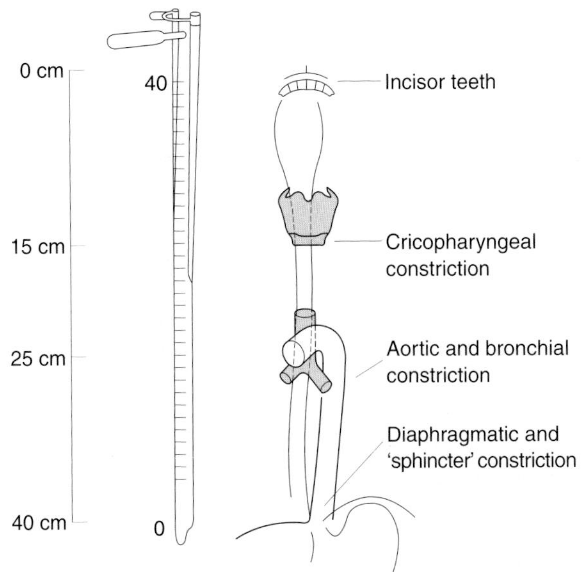

Fig. 50.2 Endoscopic landmarks. Distances are given from the incisor teeth. They vary slightly with the build of the individual.

aorta makes a definite impression on the oesophagus that can be seen on a radiograph (Fig. 50.1) or during endoscopy. It is helpful to remember the distances 15, 25 and 40 for anatomical location during endoscopy (Fig. 50.2).

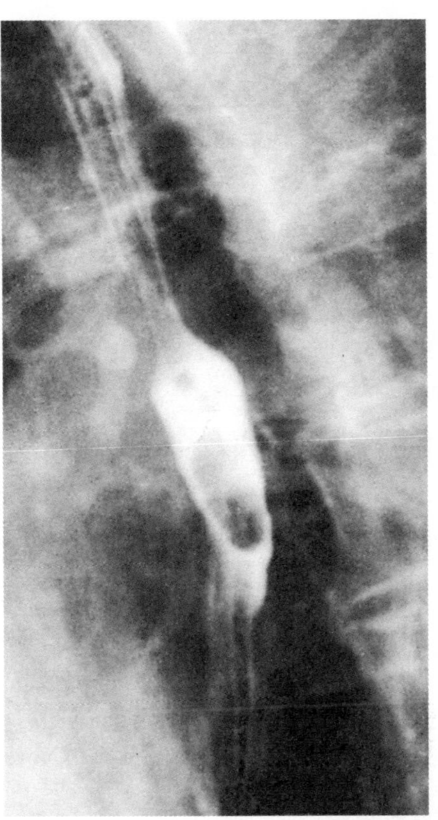

Fig. 50.3 A bolus of barium or food usually takes air with it into the stomach.

Physiology

The main function of the oesophagus is to transfer food from the mouth to the stomach in a co-ordinated fashion. The initial movement of food from the mouth is voluntary. The pharyngeal swallow response is triggered by stimulation of the pharynx and involves sequential contraction of the oropharyngeal musculature, together with simultaneous

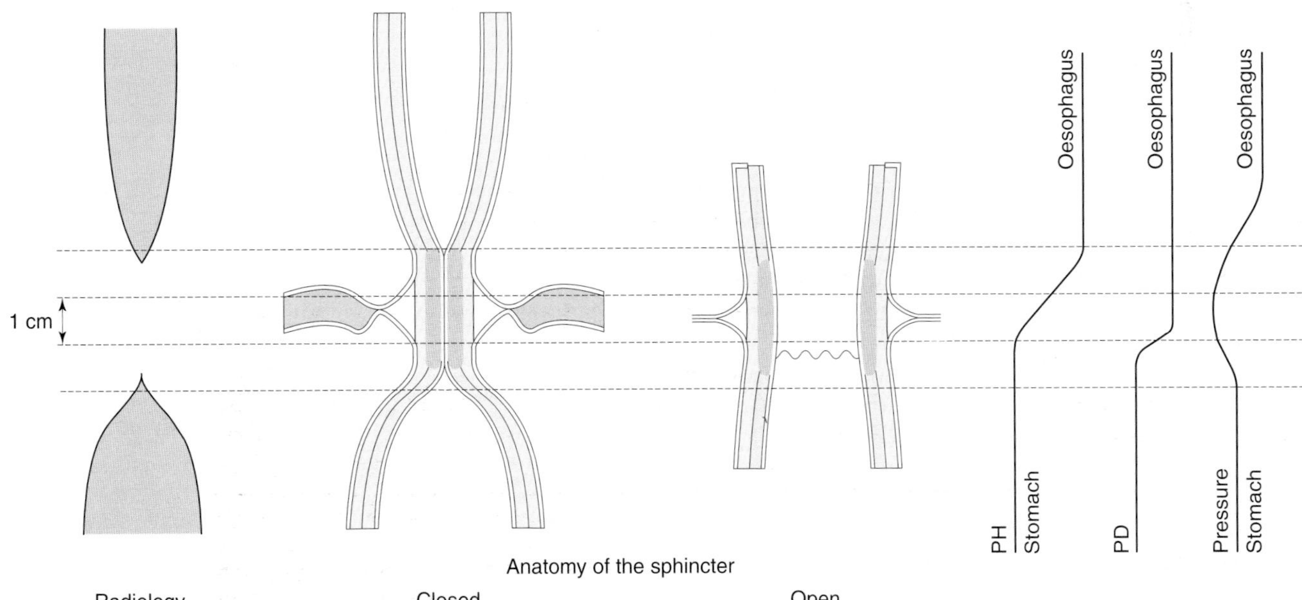

Fig. 50.4 Correlation between the radiological appearances of a barium column and the lower oesophageal sphincter open and closed. The three curves on the right, set up vertically, show the pH gradient, the mucosal potential difference (PD) marking the junction of squamous and columnar epithelium, and the high pressure zone of the sphincter.

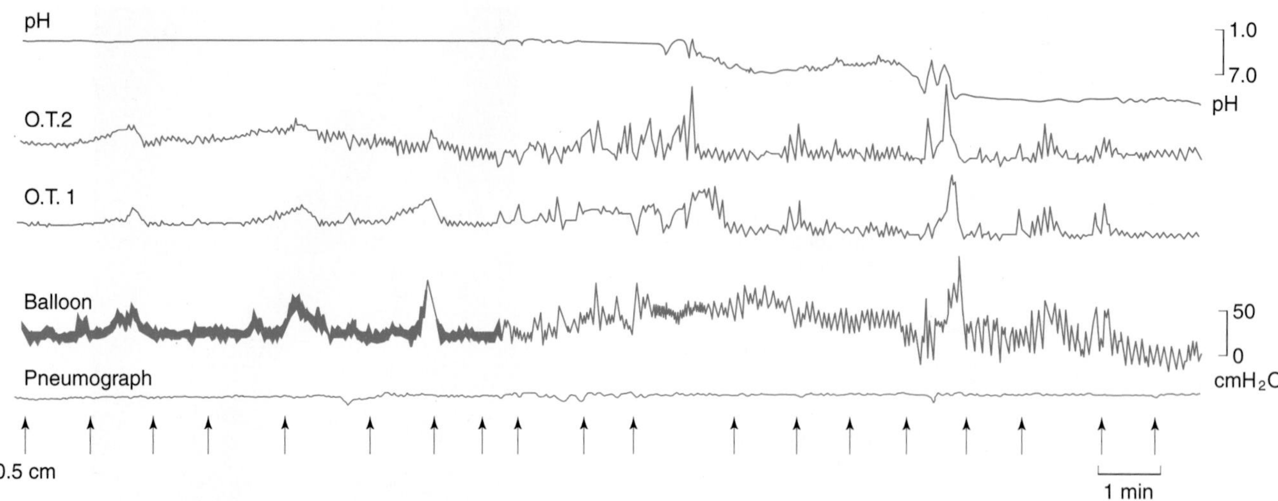

Fig. 50.5 Manometric recording from a pull-through examination of normal lower oesophagus. The balloon recording shows a zone of elevated pressure at the gastro-oesophageal sphincter.

closure of the nasal and respiratory passages, and opening of the upper oesophageal sphincter. The body of the oesophagus then propels the food bolus by *primary* peristalsis, through a relaxed lower oesophageal sphincter, into the stomach, taking air with it (Fig. 50.3). Primary peristalsis is under vagal control.

The upper oesophageal sphincter is normally closed at rest and serves as a protective mechanism against regurgitation of oesophageal contents into the respiratory passages, but it also serves to stop air entering the oesophagus other than the small amount that enters during swallowing. Failure to relax on swallowing may predispose to the development of a pharyngeal pouch (pulsion diverticulum).

The lower oesophageal sphincter (LOS) prevents gastric and duodenal contents from refluxing into the lower oesophagus (Fig. 50.4). The tone of the sphincter is influenced by many things including food, gastric distension, smoking and gastrointestinal hormones. The diaphragm also contributes to the action of the LOS. The function of the physiological sphincter was first demonstrated by Code by manometry using small balloons (Fig. 50.5). Nowadays LOS pressure is measured by perfused tubes or microtransducers. The normal LOS is 3–4 cm long and has a pressure of 10–25 mmHg (or cmH_2O).

Manometry may also be used to assess peristalsis (Fig. 50.6). The LOS relaxes in advance of the peristaltic wave. Primary peristalsis is induced by a swallow. *Secondary* peristalsis is the normal response to a stubborn food bolus or refluxed material and also clears the oesophagus (Fig. 50.7). Clearance and neutralisation of refluxed gastric acid is mainly achieved by primary peristalsis which carries saliva with its high bicarbonate content down to the lower oesophagus. *Tertiary* contractions occur occasionally and are non-peristaltic waves (Fig. 50.8).

Charles Code. Emeritus Professor of Physiology, Mayo Clinic, Rochester, Minnesota, USA.

Symptoms

Dysphagia

Dysphagia is the term used to describe difficulty, but not necessarily pain, on swallowing. The localisation of the hold-up may help to differentiate between an obstruction at the cricopharyngeal sphincter in the body of the oesophagus or at the lower end. The type of dysphagia is important. It may be dysphagia for solids or fluids, intermittent or progressive, precise or vague in its appreciation.

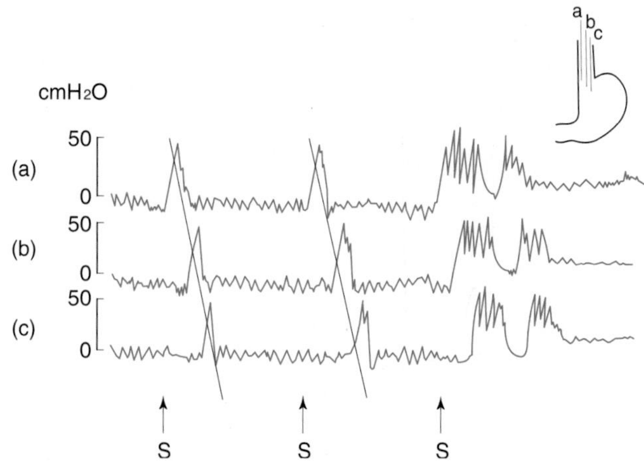

Fig. 50.6 Triple water perfused tube study of normal lower oesophagus and LOS. Note that the swallowing contractions in the body of the oesophagus are sequential, i.e. peristaltic. The tubes are recording at 1-cm intervals. The sphincter (at the right of the record) relaxes normally in sequence with each peristaltic contraction.

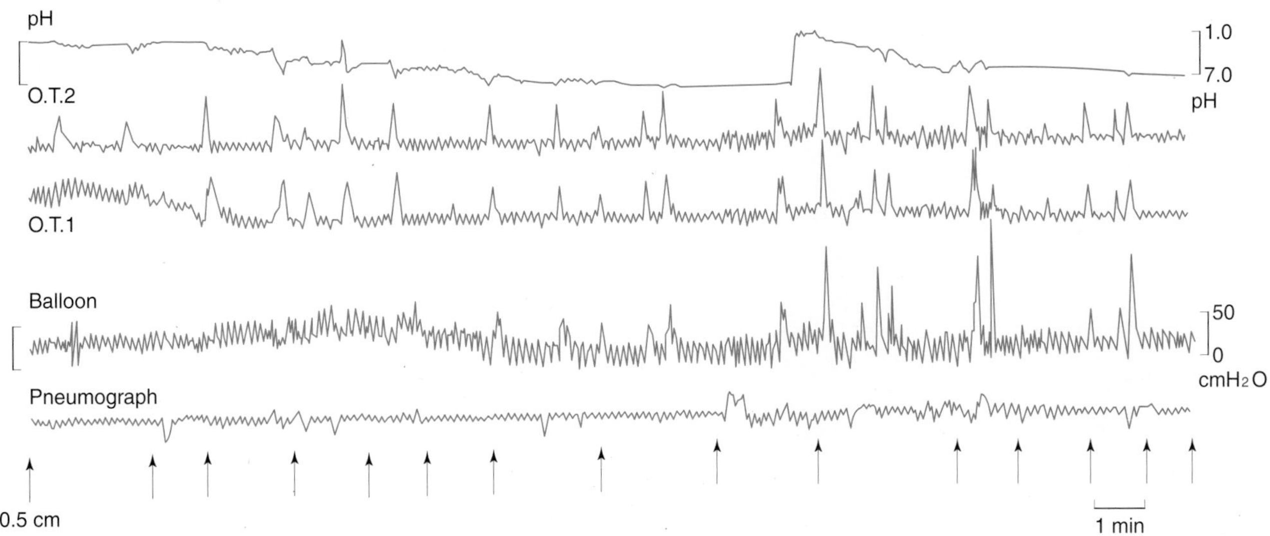

Fig. 50.7 pH trace from the lower oesophagus. Oesophageal acid clearance is demonstrated by the top recording line for pH. The pH moves to 1.0 due to acid reflux and then subsequent secondary peristaltic contractions induced by fluid in the lower oesophagus change the pH towards 7.0.

Odynophagia

Odynophagia refers to pain on swallowing. Patients with reflux oesophagitis often feel burning retrosternal discomfort within a few seconds of swallowing hot beverages, citrus drinks or alcohol. Odynophagia may be particularly severe in chemical injury of the oesophagus.

Regurgitation and reflux

Regurgitation and reflux are terms that are often used synonymously. It is helpful to differentiate between the two symptoms although it is not always possible. Regurgitation should strictly refer to the return of oesophageal contents from above an obstruction in the oesophagus that may be functional or mechanical. Reflux is the passive return of gastroduodenal contents to the mouth as part of the symptomatology of gastro-oesophageal reflux disease. Loss of weight, anaemia, cachexia, change of voice due to refluxed material irritating the vocal cords or recurrent laryngeal nerve palsy, and cough or dyspnoea due to tracheal aspiration are all important symptoms of oesophageal disorders.

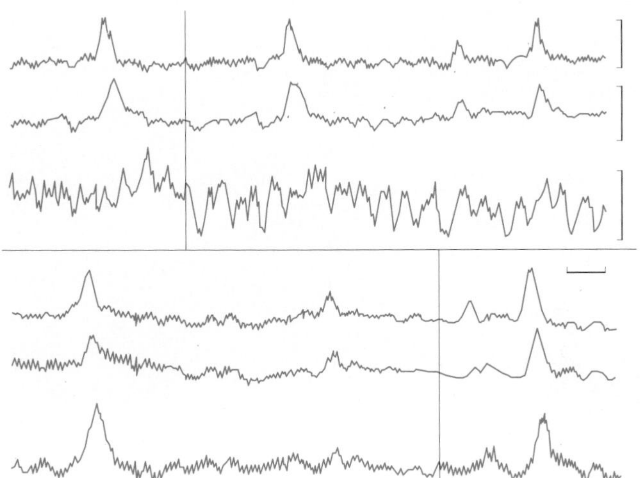

Fig. 50.8 Manometric recording from body of normal oesophagus. Peristalsis is seen in the first and last panels, but other waves are simultaneous. Nonperistaltic simultaneous contractions are called tertiary contractions.

Chest pain

Chest pain similar in character to angina pectoris may arise from an oesophageal cause, especially gastro-oesophageal reflux and motility disorders.

Investigations

Radiography

Contrast radiography has been somewhat overshadowed by endoscopy, but remains a very useful investigation for demonstrating narrowing, space-occupying lesions, anatomical distortion or abnormal motility. An adequate barium swallow takes time to do and should be tailored to the problem under investigation. It may be helpful to give a solid bolus (bread or marshmallow) if a motility disorder is suspected. Video recording is also useful to allow subsequent replay and detailed analysis. However, it should be stressed that barium radiology is very inaccurate in the diagnosis of gastro-oesophageal reflux, unless the reflux is gross, and should not be used for this purpose. Plain radiographs will show opaque foreign bodies.

Endoscopy

Endoscopy is necessary for the investigation of most oesophageal conditions. It is required to view the inside of

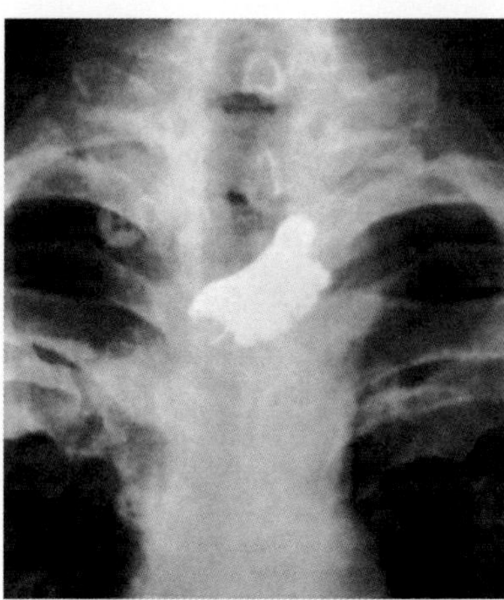

Fig. 50.9 False teeth impacted in the oesophagus. (NB. modern dentures are usually radiolucent.)

the oesophagus and the oesophagogastric junction, to obtain a biopsy or cytology specimen, for the removal of foreign bodies and to dilate strictures. Traditionally there are two types of instrument available – the rigid oesophagoscope and the flexible fibre-optic endoscope.

Rigid oesophagoscopy

Rigid oesophagoscopy is now virtually obsolete, but some surgeons still cling to this traditional method. The most commonly used instrument is the Negus oesophagoscope although there are newer varieties with better quality distal lighting, such as the Earlam oesophagoscope which is circular in cross-section. Passage of a rigid oesophagoscope is a skilful business and is relatively safe in the hands of an expert, but there is still a significant risk of perforation. There may be something to be said for the occasional use of a rigid instrument to examine the lower pharynx and the cricopharyngeal area, since the view can be rather poor with a flexible endoscope, in which case a shorter (and safer) laryngoscope is used. Most foreign bodies may be removed with a flexible gastroscope and an overtube to protect the oesophagus, but some may prefer to use the rigid instrument and large grasping forceps especially for a large foreign body such as a set of dentures (Fig. 50.9). It should be noted that most modern dentures are not radio-opaque. Dilatation of oesophageal strictures has been done for many years with the rigid instrument and the classic Chevalier Jackson bougie (Fig. 50.10), but dilators that are passed over a guidewire are much safer and they are now in general use.

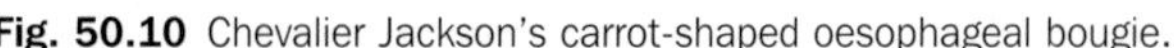

Fig. 50.10 Chevalier Jackson's carrot-shaped oesophageal bougie.

Sir Victor Negus, 1887–1974. Surgeon, Ear, Nose and Throat Department, King's College Hospital, London, England.
Richard Earlam. Retired surgeon, The Royal London Hospital, London, England.
Chevalier Jackson, 1865–1958. Professor of Bronchoscopy and Esophagoscopy, Jefferson Medical College, Philadelphia, Pennsylvania, USA.

Fibre-optic endoscopy (see Chapter 51)

The flexible fibre-optic gastroduodenoscope has virtually supplanted the rigid instrument for diagnostic and therapeutic endoscopy of the oesophagus because it has many advantages. General anaesthesia is not required, most examinations can be done on an out-patient basis, the quality of the magnified image is superb, especially with modern videoendoscopes, the instrument is much safer to pass and there is a greater range of therapeutic devices. The technology of fibre-optic endoscopy continues to improve at a steady pace.

As a matter of routine the stomach and duodenum are examined as well as the oesophagus. If a stricture is encountered if may be helpful to dilate it to allow a complete inspection of the upper gastrointestinal (GI) tract, but this advice should be tempered by clinical common sense. All endoscopic manipulations involve a degree of risk and it is prudent to keep risks to a minimum.

Therapeutic procedures

Dilatation of strictures

The advent of guidewire directed dilatation of the oesophagus in the 1970s has been a major advance. The Eder–Puestow dilator (Fig. 50.11) was the first to be used. This had

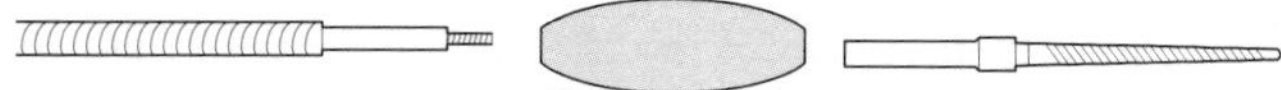

Fig. 50.11 Eder–Puestow dilator with interchangeable olive of increasing size.

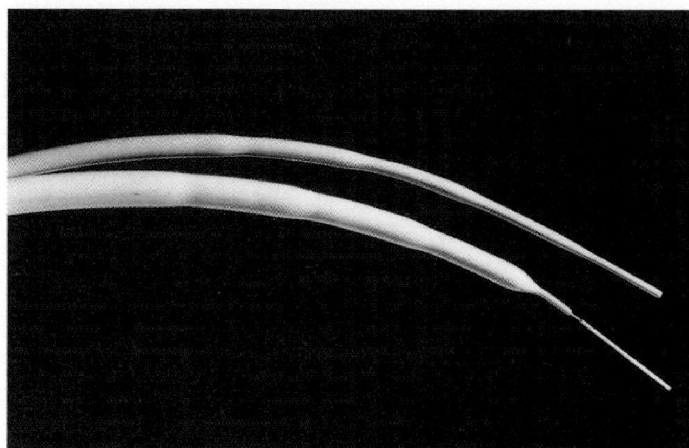

Fig. 50.12 Celestin dilators. The diameter increases in steps.

Charles B. Puestow, 1902–73. American surgeon.
Joseph Charrière, 1803–76. French instrument maker.
Roger Celestin. Surgeon, Frenchay Hospital, Bristol, England.

been produced by the Eder instrument company many years previously. The guidewire was intended to be passed blindly, but the method did not become popular until it was realised that the guidewire could be passed down the biopsy channel of an endoscope and through a stricture under vision. The endoscope is withdrawn leaving the guidewire in place and the dilators are passed over the guidewire. X-ray screening can be used to check that the wire is in satisfactory position and the dilators pass safely. With experience X-ray screening is rarely required, but may be reserved for difficult cases. To restore normal swallowing the stricture should be dilated to at least 16 mm diameter or 50 Fr. Charrière, a French instrument maker, originally measured dilators in millimetres circumference, hence the use of French gauge. Guidewire directed dilatation of oesophageal strictures is now normal practice in most units and there are many different types of dilator. The Celestin stepped dilators (Fig. 50.12) are widely used in the UK and have the merit of being easy to pass since only two are required for complete dilatation.

Balloons may also be used for dilatation of strictures. They come in many varieties. Some are designed for passage down the biopsy channel, others for passage in the X-ray department. In general balloons achieve rather less effective dilatation than solid dilators, but they may be useful to begin dilatation of difficult strictures.

Laser therapy

Lasers may be used to core a channel through a cancer for palliation of dysphagia. Similar effects may be produced by bipolar diathermy, injection of absolute alcohol or argon beam plasma coagulation.

Oesophageal manometry

Manometry is now widely used to diagnose oesophageal motility disorders. Recordings are usually made by passing a multilumen catheter with three to eight recording orifices at different levels down the oesophagus and into the stomach. The catheter channels are perfused with water by a low compliance pneumohydraulic pump for accurate measurement of rapid pressure changes. The catheter is withdrawn progressively up the oesophagus and recordings are taken at intervals of 0.5–1.0 cm to measure the length and pressure of the LOS and to assess motility in the body of the oesophagus during swallowing. Catheters with solid-state transducers are easier to use and are becoming more popular, but are still rather expensive.

24-hour pH recording

Prolonged measurement of oesophageal pH is now accepted as the most accurate method for the diagnosis of gastro-oesophageal reflux. A small pH probe is passed into the distal oesophagus and positioned 5 cm above the upper margin of the LOS as defined by manometry. The probe is then connected to a miniature digital recorder which is worn on a belt and allows most normal activities. A 20–24-hour recording period is usual and the pH record is analysed by an automated computer program using DeMeester's criteria. In some cases with atypical symptoms it is useful to compare the relationship between symptoms and reflux episodes.

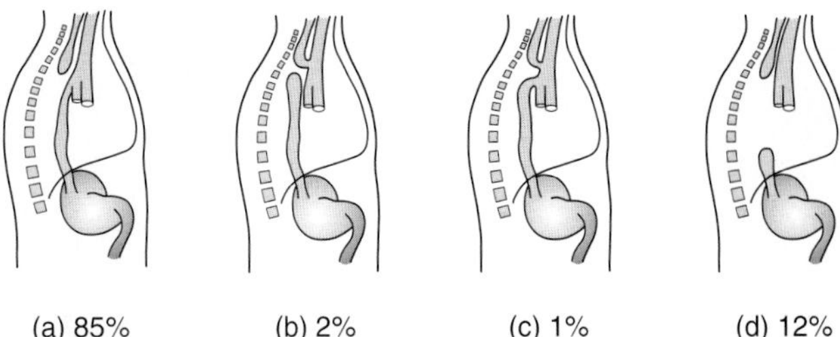

Fig. 50.13 Congenital oesophageal atresia: (a) lower segment opens into the trachea; (b) upper segment opens into the trachea; (c) both segments open into the trachea; (d) both segments end blindly and the mid-oesophagus is absent.

Congenital abnormalities

Atresia and tracheo-oesophageal fistula

Congenital atresia of the oesophagus is usually associated with a tracheo-oesophageal fistula. In 85 per cent of cases it is the *lower* segment that communicates with the trachea (Fig. 50.13).

It is important to be aware of this abnormality because its recognition within 48 hours of birth, and subsequent surgical correction, is the only hope of survival.

Suspect atresia in early feeding problems

Clinical features

The newborn baby regurgitates all of its first and subsequent feeds. Saliva pours almost continuously from its mouth. This is *the* sign of oesophageal atresia – it does not occur in any other condition. Attacks of coughing and cyanosis occur on feeding. It should be suspected in all cases of hydramnios, a condition that is present in 50 per cent of cases of atresia. Oesophageal atresia may occur as part of the VACTER group of anomalies (V – vertebral body segmentation defects; A – anal atresia; C – cardiovascular: patent ductus arteriosus, ventricular septal defect; TE – tracheo-oesophageal fistula; R – radial ray hypoplasia, unilateral renal agenesis).

Clinical confirmation of the diagnosis

A nasogastric tube typically comes against an obstruction within 10 cm. If this occurs the diagnosis is virtually certain.

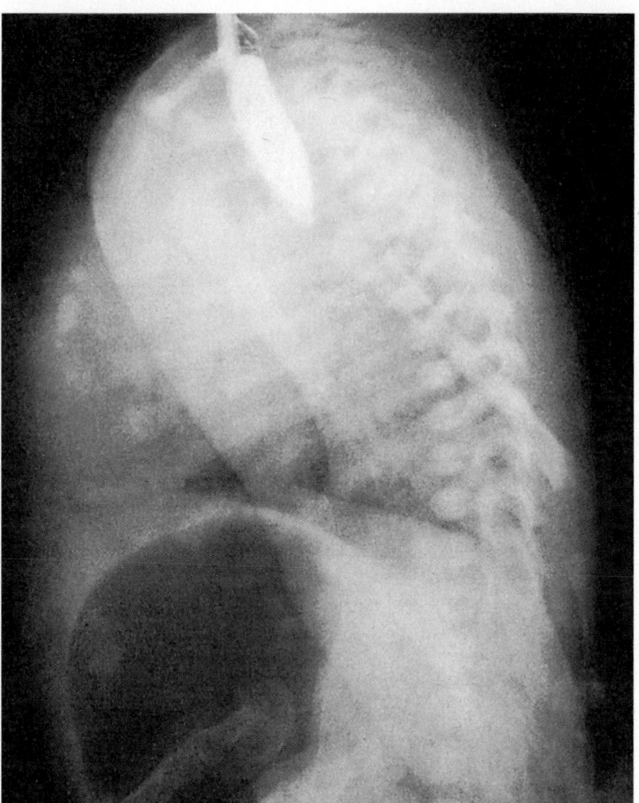

Fig. 50.14 Tracheo-oesophageal fistula with radio-opaque material in the proximal blind end. Gas in the stomach confirms that there is a fistula between the trachea and distal oesophagus.

Radiological confirmation

A lateral chest X-ray shows a lucent proximal pouch that may displace the trachea anteriorly. If bowel gas is present there must be a fistula to the distal oesophagus (Fig. 50.14). In cases of doubt air (preferred) or a small amount of contrast can be injected through the nasogastric tube. If contrast is injected it should be remembered that there may be a fistula between the upper segment and the trachea.

> Remember to locate the aortic arch

The side that the aortic arch is on needs to be determined because a thoracotomy will be done on the side opposite to the aortic arch. If the position of the aorta is not clear from the chest X-ray an echocardiogram should be done.

Treatment

Corrective surgery is normally performed shortly after the diagnosis is made. If there is a long distance between the two ends there is no need for hurry because there is no fistula to the trachea. It is usual to wait for several weeks so that the two ends of the oesophagus can grow towards each other to reduce the distance between them. In the meantime the child is fed through a gastrostomy tube.

Operation

The best approach is through a thoracotomy on the side opposite to the aortic arch, usually the right, at the level of the fifth intercostal space. The lower segment is divided at its entrance into the trachea and the fistula closed. It is usually possible to perform an anastomosis between the blind upper segment and the lower segment. If this is not possible part of the colon may be interposed.

Prognosis

The two most feared complications are pneumonia and leakage from the anastomosis. Following recovery from the immediate postoperative period the long-term prognosis is excellent. Most enter adult life with an essentially normal upper GI tract. Some have problems with gastro-oesophageal reflux and there can sometimes be a problem with aperistalsis of the distal segment giving rise to dysphagia.

Oesophageal stenosis

This is a rare congenital organic narrowing of the lumen of the oesophagus and is a cause of dysphagia. It occurs anywhere in the oesophagus.

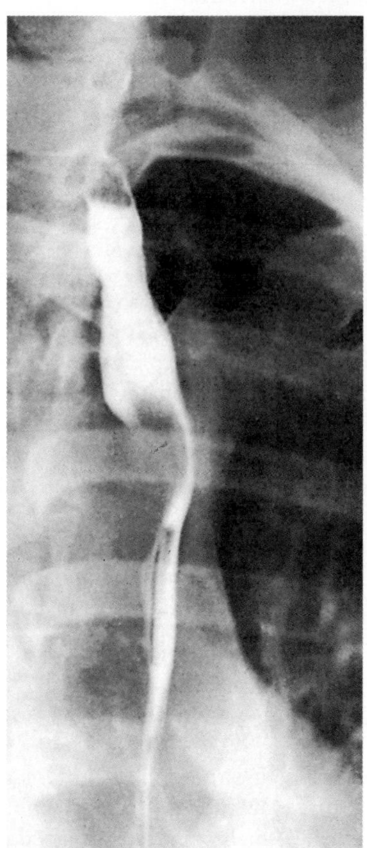

Fig. 50.15 Aberrant right subclavian artery causing oesophageal constriction. The words dysphagia lusoria are derived from the Latin *lusus naturae*, meaning sport of nature.

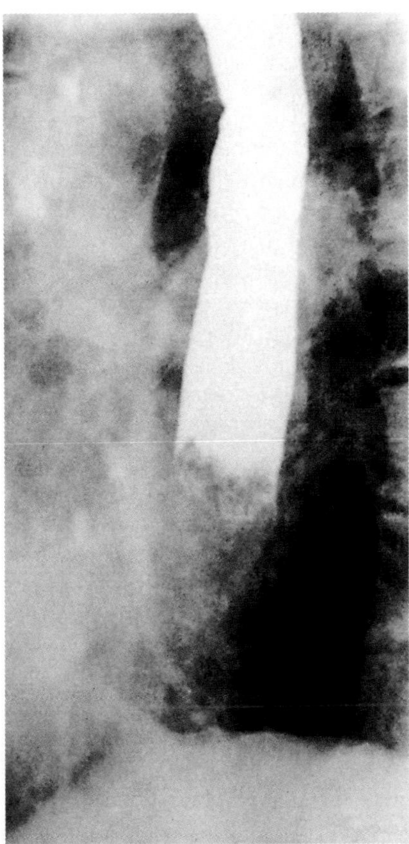

Fig. 50.16 An impacted meat bolus at the lower end of the oesophagus. This may be the first presentation of a benign stricture or a malignant tumour.

Dysphagia lusoria

Several vascular anomalies may produce dysphagia by compression of the oesophagus. Classically this is due to an aberrant right subclavian artery [arteria lusoria (Fig. 50.15)]. However, the oesophagus is more commonly compressed by vascular rings, such as a double aortic arch. Dysphagia occurs in only a minority of cases and usually presents early in childhood, although it can occur in the late teens. Treatment is usually by division of the nondominant component of the ring.

'Short' oesophagus with hiatus hernia is mentioned only to say that it is not a congenital abnormality. True shortening of the oesophagus is secondary to severe reflux oesophagitis (see below).

Foreign bodies in the oesophagus

All manner of foreign bodies have become arrested in the oesophagus such as coins, pins and dentures. Button batteries may be a troublesome problem in children. The commonest impacted material is food (Fig. 50.16). Plain radiographs are the most useful examination. A contrast examination is not usually required and may make endoscopy more difficult. Food impaction is almost always a sign of underlying pathology, most commonly a stricture or carcinoma.

> Beware of button batteries in the oesophagus

Foreign bodies that have become stuck in the oesophagus should be removed by endoscopy. Flexible endoscopy is now the method of choice and the majority of objects can be extracted with suitable grasping forceps, a snare or a basket. If the object may injure the oesophagus on withdrawal an overtube should be used, and the endoscope and object withdrawn into the overtube before removal. Button batteries can be a particular worry as they are difficult to grasp and it is tempting to push them on into the stomach. However, an exhausted battery may rapidly corrode in the GI tract and is best extracted. An impacted food bolus will often break up and pass on if the patient is given fizzy drinks and confined to fluids for a short time. The cause of the impaction can then be investigated. If symptoms are severe or the bolus does not pass on it can be extracted or broken up at endoscopy.

Perforation

Perforation of the oesophagus is a serious condition that requires prompt diagnosis and treatment.

Barotrauma – Boerhaave's syndrome

So-called 'spontaneous' perforation of the oesophagus is usually due to severe barotrauma when a person vomits against a closed glottis. The pressure in the oesophagus rapidly increases and the oesophagus bursts at its weakest point in the lower third, sending a stream of material into the mediastinum and often the pleural cavity as well. The condition was first reported by Boerhaave who reported the case of a grand admiral of the Dutch fleet who was a glutton and practised the habit of autoemesis. Boerhaave's syndrome is the most serious type of perforation because of the volume of infected material that is released under pressure.

> Suspect perforation if pain follows vomiting

The clinical history is of severe pain in the chest or upper abdomen following a meal or a bout of drinking. Many cases are misdiagnosed as myocardial infarction or as a perforated peptic ulcer or pancreatitis if the pain is confined to the upper abdomen. There may be a surprising amount of rigidity on examination of the upper abdomen even in the absence of any peritoneal contamination.

Herman Boerhaave, 1668–1738. Physician, Leiden, The Netherlands.

Pathological perforation

Perforation of ulcers, such as a Barrett's ulcer (see below) or tumours of the oesophagus are unusual, but do occur. They may also erode into the aorta or ventricle with rapidly fatal results.

Penetrating injury

Perforation by knives and bullets is uncommon, even in war, since the oesophagus is a relatively small target surrounded by other vital organs.

Foreign bodies

The oesophagus may be perforated during removal of a foreign body, but occasionally an object that has been left in the oesophagus for several days will erode through the wall.

Instrumental perforation

Instrumentation is by far the commonest cause of oesophageal perforation. Modern instrumentation is remarkably safe, but perforation remains a risk that should never be forgotten. The virtual demise of the rigid oesophagoscope has been a major factor in improving safety. It can readily be imagined that passing a rigid metal tube down the oesophagus of an elderly patient with a kyphotic spine is a hazardous undertaking. The pharynx may be perforated above the cricopharyngeal sphincter; the oesophagus may be crushed against osteophytes in the cervical spine (Fig. 50.17), particularly during the extension of the neck that is necessary to get the instrument down to the distal oesophagus. Perforations caused by rigid endoscopes are often large and generally require more energetic surgical treatment than those that occur during flexible endoscopy.

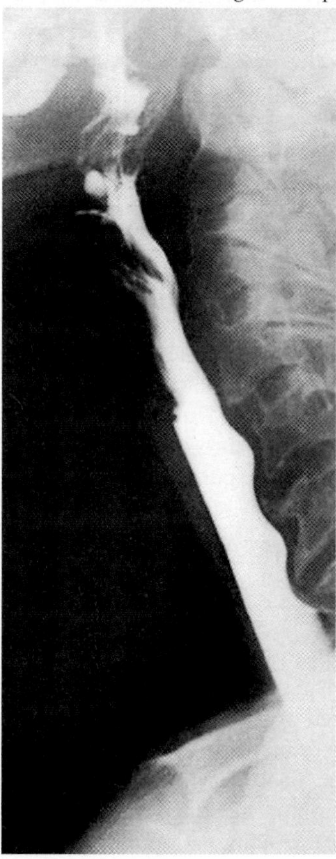

Fig. 50.17 Osteoarthritic cervical spine looks very impressive on the radiograph, but does not cause dysphagia. However, it emphasises the risks of rigid oesophagoscopy and the dangers of hyperextension of the neck.

Norman Barrett, 1903–79. Surgeon, St Thomas's Hospital, London, England.

Prevention of perforation is better than cure

Perforation during diagnostic flexible endoscopy of the upper GI tract is unusual, but occurs at a frequency of one in 4000 examinations. Therapeutic endoscopy increases the risk, but the overall risk should remain low. Dilatation of the oesophagus increases the risk significantly, but biopsy does not. The oesophagus may be perforated by a guidewire or dilator above or below a stricture. Splitting of a benign stricture during dilatation is exceedingly rare and is not a significant risk. Most perforations that occur during dilatation of benign strictures are probably due to movement of the guidewire that allows the dilator to move in an unpredictable direction. For this reason guidewires should always be held firmly against an unmoving object during the passage of dilators. This single act provides the greatest protection against injury. If dilatation of a stricture is done during rigid endoscopy the unconstrained dilator may be passed through the oesophagus above or, less commonly, below the stricture. Cancers may be dilated safely, but it should be remembered that they are unpredictably friable and may split as the dilator passes. It is therefore prudent to limit the dilatation of a cancer to the extent that is necessary for the matter in hand, such as passage of the endoscope for laser treatment of a cancer. A side-viewing duodenoscope [for an endoscopic retrograde cholangiopancreatography (ERCP)] that forms a loop in the oesophagus during insertion may cause a split. This is a particularly unpleasant situation because if a loop does form there is no safe method of undoing the loop. The oesophagus may be perforated by the large balloons that are used for the treatment of achalasia by forceful dilatation since these are inflated to a diameter (30–40 mm, 94–125 Fr) that is greater than that of the normal oesophagus. The incidence of perforation appears greater with the larger balloons and these should probably be reserved for repeat dilatations if a smaller balloon has failed to achieve the desired effect. Perforation may occur during the insertion of plastic tubes or expanding stents for the palliation of cancer. In such cases the leak may be sealed partially or completely once the stent is in place.

Diagnosis

Beware and be aware of perforation
Look for surgical emphysema

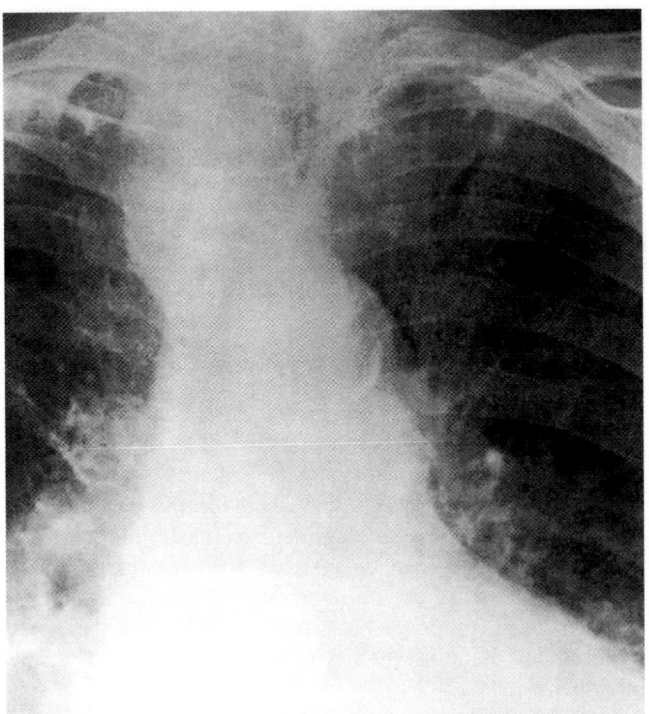

Fig. 50.18 Oesophageal perforation demonstrated by a gas shadow in the mediastinum or around the arch of the aorta. A pneumothorax or pleural 'effusion' may occur. The first clinical sign is pain. Prompt treatment is essential.

Perforation of the oesophagus usually produces severe chest pain and should be suspected if this occurs after instrumentation. Subcutaneous emphysema may be present in the neck and sometimes over the upper chest as well. Emphysema is more likely to appear if the oesophagus is perforated during flexible endoscopy because of the air insufflation that is an essential part of the procedure. Emphysema around the pericardium can sometimes be detected on auscultation as a mediastinal 'crunch' which sounds like footsteps in soft snow. A chest X-ray may show gas in the mediastinum, a pleural effusion or a pneumothorax (Fig. 50.18).

> Water-soluble contrast media may miss small perforations

It is essential to obtain a contrast swallow whenever a perforation is suspected. The only possible exception to this rule is when the diagnosis is obvious, for example when subcutaneous emphysema is present, and the management policy is nonoperative. In such cases it may be reasonable to avoid the additional small risk of worsening the contamination of the mediastinum by giving contrast. Contrary to popular opinion Gastrografin should *not* be used. This agent is hypertonic and can cause severe lung injury if aspirated. Modern nonionic contrast media are safer, but still give poorer images than barium suspension. In the author's opinion barium is the contrast material of choice. There is no evidence that the judicious use of barium suspension is clinically harmful in this setting and it is important to obtain good quality images. It should also be emphasised that water-soluble contrast media may miss small perforations of the oesophagus or small anastomotic disruptions.

Treatment

Perforation of the oesophagus usually leads to mediastinitis which is a very dangerous condition. The loose areolar tissues of the posterior mediastinum allow rapid spread of gastrointestinal contents. There may be marked systemic disturbance with cardiovascular collapse. Dysrhythmias are common, especially atrial fibrillation. The aim of treatment is to limit mediastinal contamination and deal with the existing infection. Operative repair deals with the injury directly, but imposes risks of its own. Nonoperative treatment aims to limit the effects of mediastinitis and provide an environment in which healing can take place.

> Prompt diagnosis and treatment is essential for the best results

The management of oesophageal perforation remains controversial with strong opinions in favour of operative and nonoperative treatment. Both schools of thought have their merits. The majority of perforations can nowadays be managed nonoperatively, but it is still important to keep an open mind, to tailor management to the individual patient and to be prepared to change the treatment plan in the light of clinical progress. The essential determinants of management are the septic load, the response of the patient to the septic challenge, the age and general condition of the patient and whether the perforation is confined to the mediastinum. Perforations of the abdominal oesophagus are probably best managed by operative repair as is Boerhaave's syndrome in which the septic load is high. Most endoscopic perforations involve minimal contamination and are ideal for nonoperative management, particularly if the patient is a poor risk for a thoracotomy. The relative indications for the two forms of management are listed in Table 50.1.

The key elements of nonoperative management are analgesia, nil by mouth, antibiotics and general supportive care. When the patient is stable enteral or parenteral nutrition is started. Enteral feeding is best given by feeding jejunostomy.

Table 50.1 Management options in perforation of the oesophagus

Factors that favour: *Nonoperative management*	*Operative repair*
Small septic load	Large septic load
Minimal cardiovascular upset	Septic shock
Perforation confined to mediastinum	Pleura breached
Perforation by flexible endoscope	Boerhaave syndrome
Perforation of cervical oesophagus	Perforation of abdominal oesophagus

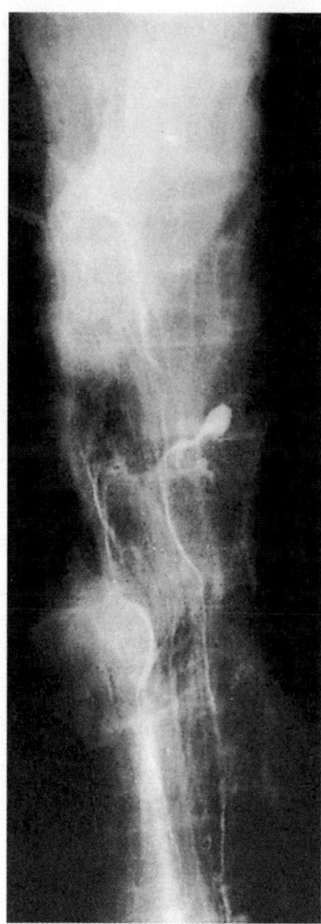

Fig. 50.19 Tracheo-oesophageal fistula following perforation by a rigid oesophagoscope. The ensuing abscess, which had burst into the trachea, eventually healed with nonoperative management.

Some authorities advocate a double-lumen suction catheter in the oesophagus, but this is not universally agreed. There is nothing to commend the use of a nasogastric tube which simply encourages gastro-oesophageal reflux and increases the risk of respiratory infection. Rather surprisingly even a perforated cancer will heal, given adequate time.

Nonoperative management of perforatred oesophagus
- Analgesia
- Nil by mouth
- Antibiotics
- Intravenous fluids/nutrition

The management of oesophageal perforation can be difficult and it is important to be prepared for complications, such as the tracheo-oesophageal fistula in Fig. 50.19.

Operative management usually involves thoracotomy and repair of the perforation. This is best done within a few hours of perforation. After 12 hours the tissues become swollen and friable, and less suitable for direct suture. The hole in the mucosa is always bigger than the hole in the muscle and the muscle should be incised to see the mucosal edges clearly. It is essential that there should be no obstruction distal to the repair. Ideally the repair should be strengthened with adjacent gastric fundus, diaphragm or intercostal muscle. If the site of the perforation is not healthy, oesophageal resection should be performed.

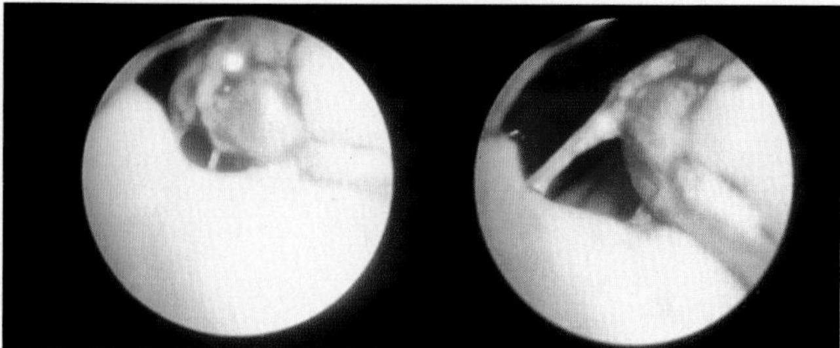

Fig. 50.20 The endoscopic appearance of a mucosal tear at the cardia (Mallory–Weiss).

An intermediate form of management is the insertion of a stent. This is now well established for the treatment of perforated cancers. Expanding metal stents are ideal for this purpose since they can be inserted with minimal trauma. Some clinicians use the more traditional plastic or silicone tubes for this purpose, but additional dilatation may be required for their insertion with the risk of worsening the injury.

There is a wide range of options for salvage following late diagnosis or failed nonoperative management including multiple tube drainage, oesophageal exclusion and resection, oesophagostomy, gastrostomy and delayed reconstruction. The management of such cases is challenging and highly specialised.

Mallory–Weiss syndrome

Forceful vomiting may produce a mucosal tear at the cardia rather than a full perforation of the oesophagus. The mechanism of injury is different. In Boerhaave's syndrome vomiting occurs against a closed glottis and pressure builds up in the oesophagus. In the Mallory–Weiss syndrome vigorous vomiting produces a vertical split which is in the gastric mucosa

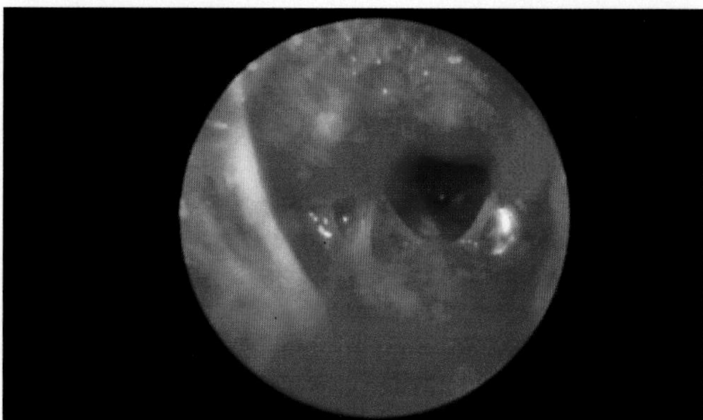

Fig. 50.21 Acute caustic burn in the haemorrhagic phase.

Kenneth Mallory. Pathologist, Boston, USA.
Sorna Weiss, 1898–1942. American physician.

immediately below the squamocolumnar junction at the cardia in 90 per cent of cases. In only 10 per cent is the tear in the oesophagus (Fig. 50.20). The condition presents with haematemesis. Usually the bleeding is not severe, but endoscopic injection therapy may be required for the occasional case with severe bleeding. Surgery is rarely required.

Corrosive injury

Skilled early endoscopy is useful in corrosive injury

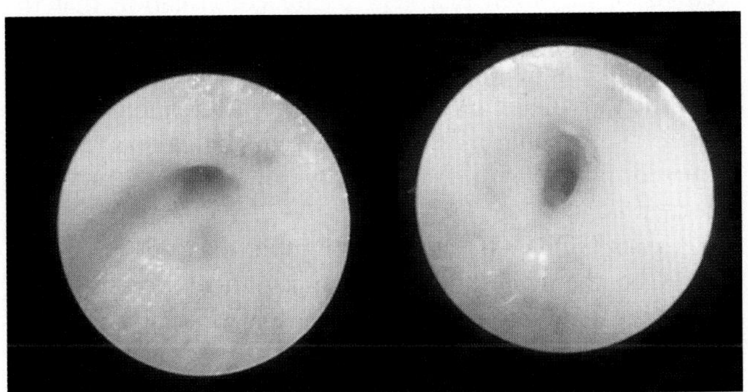

Fig. 50.22 The late result of a caustic alkali burn with a high oesophageal stricture.

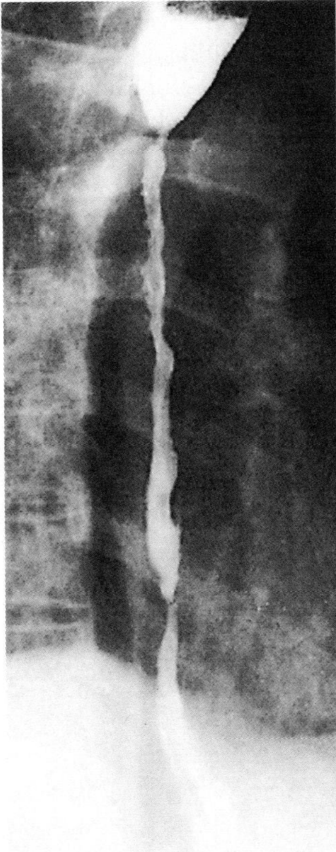

Fig. 50.23 Caustic or lye stricture with marked stenosis high in the body of the oesophagus. The strictures are frequently multiple and difficult to dilate unless treated energetically at an early stage.

Corrosives such as sodium hydroxide (lye) or sulphuric acid may be taken in attempted suicide. Bleach may be drunk by young children. All can cause severe damage to the pharynx, larynx, oesophagus and stomach. The oesophagus is usually worst affected by sodium hydroxide. The key to management is early endoscopy *by an experienced endoscopist* to inspect the whole of the oesophagus and stomach unless there is a severe necrotising lesion. Air insufflation should be kept to a minimum. Minor injuries resolve rapidly with no late *sequelae*. Severe mucosal injury (Fig. 50.21) should be treated with steroids for 3 weeks and a programme of regular dilatations started thereafter. If full-thickness necrosis is suspected resection should be done at an early stage.

Cases that present late may have extensive stricturing of the oesophagus that is difficult to dilate (Figs 50.22 and 50.23). Oesophageal resection may be required. Some advocate surgical bypass rather than resection as there may be a very marked fibrous perioesophagitis in late cases.

Drug-induced injury

Many medications, such as antibiotics and potassium preparations, are potentially damaging to the oesophagus as tablets may lie in the oesophagus for a long time, especially if taken without an adequate drink. Acute injury presents with dysphagia and odynophagia which may be very severe. The inflammation usually resolves within 2–3 weeks and no specific treatment is required apart from appropriate nutritional support. A stricture may follow the acute injury.

Gastro-oesophageal reflux disease

Aetiology

Normal competence of the gastro-oesophageal junction is maintained by the LOS. There has been considerable controversy about the relative importance of the *physiology* of the LOS and the *anatomy* of the cardia. This controversy is not completely resolved, but it is currently accepted that the most important factor in gastro-oesophageal competence is the function of the LOS, which is augmented by a normally functioning diaphragmatic hiatus.

Loss of competence of the LOS leads to gastro-oesophageal reflux disease (GORD). This rather clumsy name and inelegant acronym has come into common use because the alternatives do not describe the condition. *Sliding hiatus hernia* has a variable association with GORD. In general patients with the more severe stages of GORD tend to have a hernia, but most GORD sufferers do not have a hernia and many of those with a hernia do not have GORD. It should be noted that rolling or paraoesophageal hiatus hernia is a quite different and potentially dangerous condition (see below). *Reflux oesophagitis* is a complication of GORD that occurs in a minority of sufferers. It occurs in 40–50 per cent of those referred to hospital, but a much lower proportion of those who suffer from symptoms of GORD in the community as a whole.

A degree of gastro-oesophageal reflux is normal, particularly after meals when there is a need to regurgitate swallowed air to maintain comfort. *Physiological* reflux mostly occurs during transient lower oesophageal sphincter relaxations (TLOSRs) that are quite separate from swallow-induced relaxation. In the early stages of GORD most of the *pathological* reflux occurs as a result of an increased number of TLOSRs. In severe GORD a greater proportion of reflux occurs across a LOS that has lost its basal tone and has a shorter length exposed to intra-abdominal pressure. Understanding of the function of the LOS has been largely elucidated by Dent, who discovered the importance of TLOSRs, and by DeMeester, who clarified the importance of the basic competence of the LOS which is governed by basal LOS pressure, the overall length of the LOS and the length that is exposed to intra-abdominal pressure.

TLOSRs, the most important factor in gastro-oesophageal reflux

Length and pressure of the LOS is also important

In westernised countries GORD is by far the commonest condition affecting the upper GI tract. This is in part a relative change due to the declining incidence of peptic ulcers as the incidence of infection with *Helicobacter pylori* has reduced due to improved socioeconomic conditions. However, there has almost certainly been an absolute increase in the incidence of GORD in the last 20–30 years. The cause of the increase is unclear, but may be due in part to increasing obesity. In a curious way it may also be an effect of the reduced incidence of *Helicobacter* infection. Since chronic infection of the gastric *corpus* decreases acid secretion, and infection of the *antrum* increases acid secretion the overall effect of reduced infection on gastric acid secretion in the community is a matter of conjecture. Some suggest that the net effect is increased secretion that may increase the incidence of GORD. The epidemiology of upper GI disease is a fascinating topic of research that is evolving rapidly. It is a particularly important topic since medication for GORD is now the largest single item on the healthcare budget of many countries, and the incidence of cancer of the lower oesophagus and cardia is also increasing, possibly as a result of the changed incidence of GORD (see below).

Clinical features

Dyspepsia with fatty foods is more common in GORD than gallstone disease

Retrosternal burning pain (heartburn) and epigastric pain are the commonest symptoms. These are usually provoked by food, particularly fatty food. Indeed 'fatty dyspepsia' is a much more common feature of GORD than of gallstones with which the association is rather questionable. As the condition becomes more severe gastric acid may reflux to the mouth and produce an unpleasant taste. In gross cases food may reflux to the mouth and this can be a particularly trying symptom. It is in the more advanced cases there is a history of pain and reflux when lying flat or on stooping. A proportion of cases has odynophagia with hot beverages, citrus drinks or alcohol. This symptom which occurs within a few seconds of ingestion is a very useful confirmation that the patient is suffering from an oesophageal disorder and not a peptic ulcer. Some patients present with less typical symptoms such as angina-like chest pain, pulmonary or laryngeal symptoms. Dysphagia is usually a sign that a stricture has occurred, but may be caused by an associated motility disorder.

Because GORD is such a common disorder it should always be the first thought when a patient presents with oesophageal symptoms that are unusual or that defy diagnosis after a series of investigations.

Diagnosis

In the majority of cases the diagnosis is assumed rather than proven and treatment is empirical. Endoscopy is done mainly to exclude more serious pathology such as cancer. If the typical appearance of reflux oesophagitis, peptic stricture or Barrett's oesophagus is seen the diagnosis is clinched, but oesophagitis is not present in most cases. The endoscopic appearances of the normal oesophagus, hiatus hernia, oesophagitis and stricture are shown in Figs 50.24–30. In patients with severe or persistent symptoms in whom it is judged that an objective diagnosis is essential, oesophageal manometry and 24-hour oesophageal pH recording should

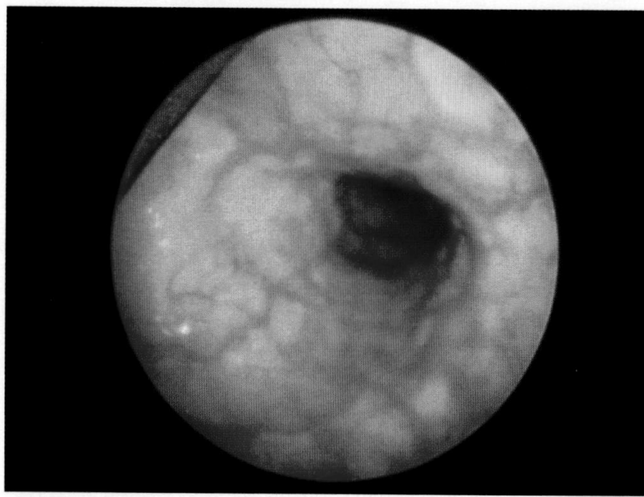

Fig. 50.24 The endoscopic appearance of the normal squamous mucosa in the body of the oesophagus.

John Dent. Gastroenterologist, Royal Adelaide Hospital, Adelaide, Australia.

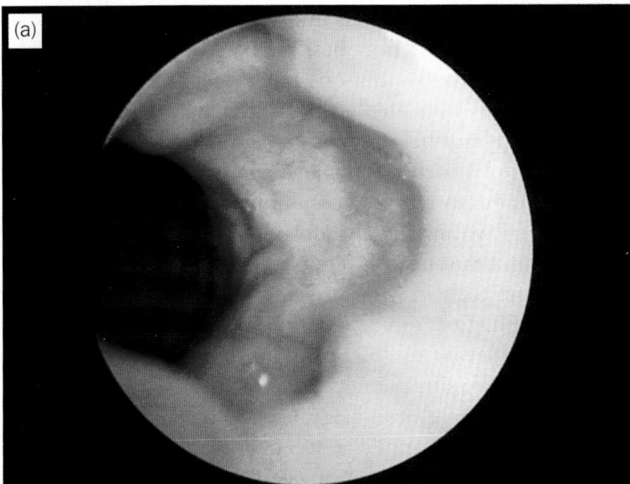

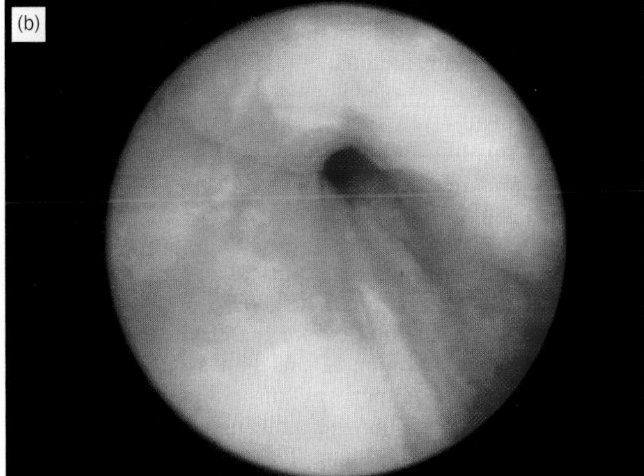

Fig. 50.25 The normal lower oesophageal sphincter: (a) open; and (b) closed.

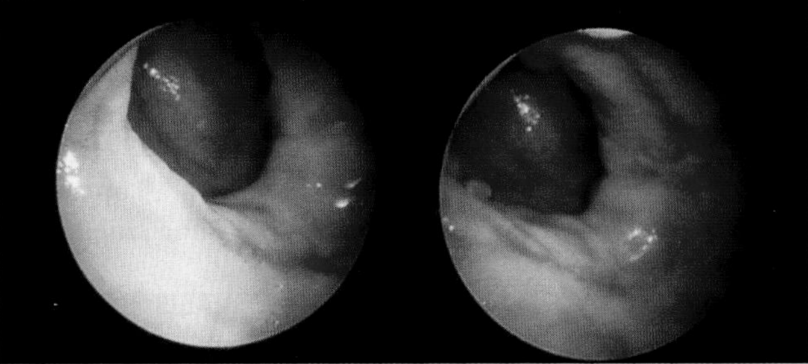

Fig. 50.27 Sliding hiatus hernia. The diaphragm can be seen constricting the upper stomach.

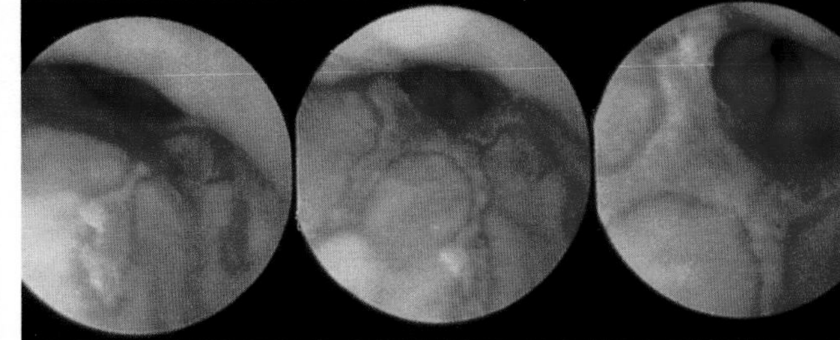

Fig. 50.28 Reflux oesophagitis.

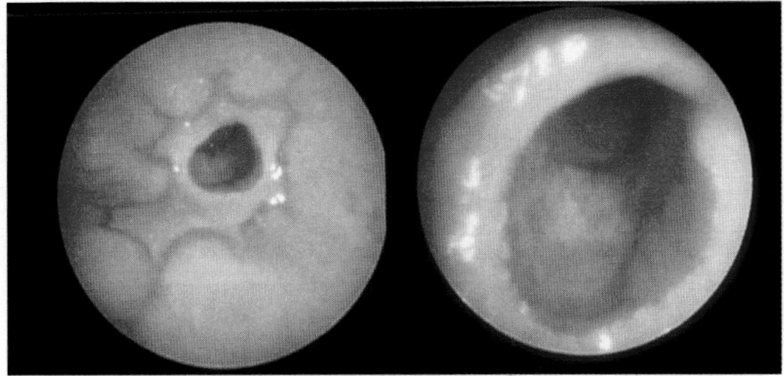

Fig. 50.29 Benign stricture: (a) with active oesophagitis; and (b) healed with columnar epithelium.

be done. It is essential to have an objective diagnosis before embarking on an antireflux operation. It is important that manometry is done at the same sitting as a pH study since fermentation of food residue in an achalasic oesophagus produces lactic acid surprisingly rapidly, and a significant proportion of patients with achalasia has abnormal acid exposure of the lower oesophagus. Usually the form of the pH trace in achalasia is different from that of GORD with slow undulations of pH rather than rapid bursts of reflux.

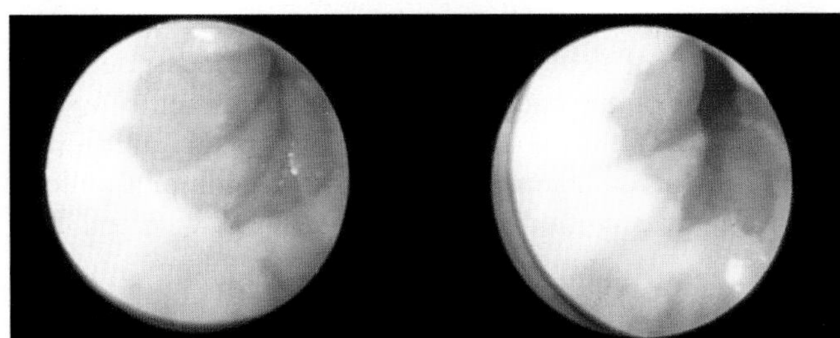

Fig. 50.26 The squamocolumnar junction is clearly seen in the lower oesophagus with a normal sharp demarcation.

However, the author has seen cases of achalasia with a pH recording identical to that of GORD and in whom the symptoms of achalasia have been completely relieved by Heller's myotomy without a concurrent antireflux procedure and without the onset of GORD on prolonged follow-up.

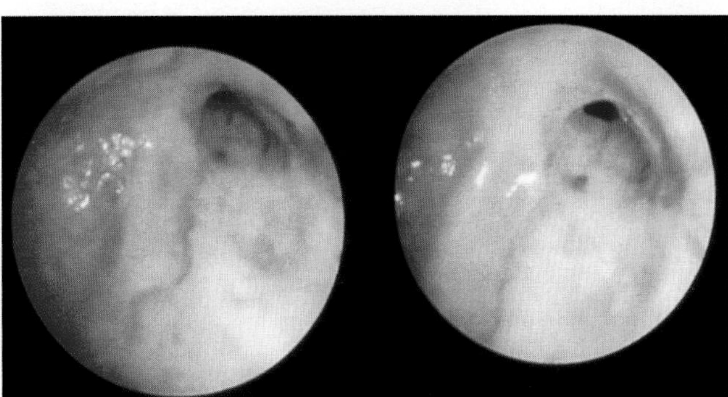

Fig. 50.30 Ulceration associated with a benign peptic stricture.

Ernst Heller, 1877–1964. Surgeon, Leipzig, Germany.

24-hour pH recording is the 'gold standard' for diagnosis of GORD

Barium swallow and meal examinations give the best appreciation of gastro-oesophageal anatomy (Fig. 50.31). This may be important to the surgeon planning an operation that may be complicated by oesophageal shortening or a rolling hiatus hernia, but it is not important for the diagnosis of GORD. Radiology is at best 50 per cent accurate in the diagnosis of GORD so that one might just as well toss coins. The use of the Trendelenburg position may give good pictures, but does not help the assessment of reflux.

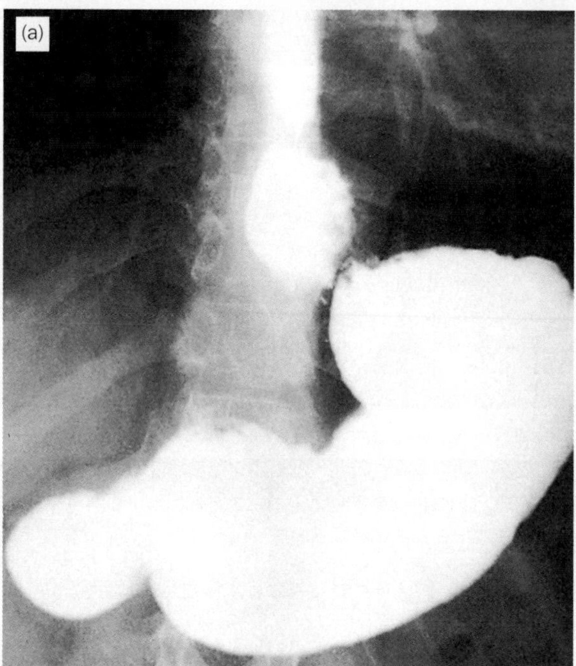

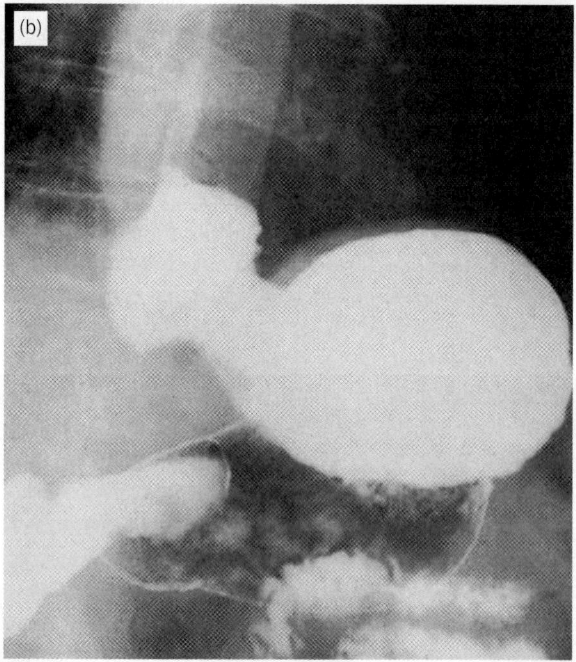

Fig. 50.31 (a) Sliding hiatus hernia with a sphincter and diaphragmatic crural narrowing clearly shown; (b) another sliding hernia in which the sphincter is lax and the diaphragm is wide open. The patient is in the Trendelenburg position to demonstrate barium in the fundus. This unphysiological position may stimulate 'reflux' in those who do not have GORD.

For the most part making a diagnosis of GORD is not difficult, but because it is so common there is a large number of people in whom the diagnosis is obscure. It should be borne in mind that proton pump inhibitors (PPIs), which are now quite properly in widespread use by family doctors, heal reflux oesophagitis rapidly so that there may be nothing abnormal to see at endoscopy. The effect of PPIs on acid secretion may be surprisingly prolonged, in some cases leading to false-negative oesophageal pH studies. As a matter of routine, PPIs are stopped a week before oesophageal pH recording, but acid secretion is sometimes reduced for 2 weeks or more. In cases of doubt 24-hour pH recording should be repeated and it is sometimes useful to stop PPIs 4 weeks before pH recording.

Achalasia and GORD are easily confused

A further perversity in the diagnosis of GORD is the ease with which its symptoms may be confused with those of achalasia. With the more widespread use of oesophageal manometry achalasia is often diagnosed at a much earlier stage than previously, long before the classic symptom pattern is established and long before the classic X-ray appearances are seen. It is perhaps surprising that the early symptoms of achalasia may be indistinguishable from those of GORD even with hindsight. This is especially important when patients are being considered for antireflux surgery.

Management of uncomplicated GORD

Medical management

Most sufferers from GORD do not consult a doctor and do not need to do so. They self-medicate with over-the-counter medicines such as simple antacids, antacid-alginate preparations and H_2 receptor antagonists. Consultation is more likely when symptoms are severe or prolonged. By the time a patient comes to consultation, and particularly hospital consultation, it is highly likely that simple treatment will have been tried and found wanting. Nevertheless it is always worth checking. Simple measures that may have been neglected include advice about weight loss, smoking, excessive consumption of alcohol, tea or coffee and a modest degree of head up tilt of the bed. Tilting the bed has been shown to have an effect that is similar to taking an H_2 antagonist. However, the common practice of using additional pillows has no significant effect apart from causing discomfort.

Friedrich Trendelenburg, 1844–1924. Professor of Surgery, Leipzig, Germany.

PPIs are the most effective medication for severe GORD

PPIs, such as omeprazole, lansoprazole and pantoprazole are by far the most effective drug treatment for GORD. Indeed they are so effective that, once started, patients are very reluctant to stop taking them. The PPIs have been a major advance in the treatment of GORD. Given an adequate dose oesophagitis heals in the majority of cases and even most strictures respond well to one or two dilatations and long-term PPI treatment. The only reservation is whether there will be serious side effects with long-term consumption. Thus far the PPIs have an excellent safety record, but doubts have been expressed as to whether the increased incidence of adenocarcinoma of the lower oesophagus and cardia in many countries may be due in part to the long-term treatment of GORD with powerful acid suppression.

Surgery

Strictly speaking the need for surgery should have been reduced since medication has improved so much. Paradoxically, the number of antireflux operations has remained relatively constant and may even be increasing. This is probably partly due to increased patient expectations and partly to the advent of minimal access surgery that has improved the acceptability of surgical procedures.

The results of antireflux surgery are generally good

The indication for surgery in uncomplicated GORD is essentially patient choice. The risks and possible benefits of surgery need to be discussed in detail. The risks include a small mortality rate (0.1–0.5 per cent, depending on patient selection), the risk of a failed operation (5–10 per cent) and the risk of side effects such as dysphagia, gas bloat or abdominal discomfort (10 per cent). With current operative techniques 85–90 per cent of patients should be satisfied with the result of an antireflux operation. Patients who are asymptomatic on a PPI need a careful discussion of the risk side of the equation. Those who are symptomatic on a PPI need a careful clinical review to make sure that they will benefit from an operation. Reasons for failure on a PPI include 'volume' reflux (good indication for surgery), 'hermit' lifestyle in which the least deviation from lifestyle rules leads to symptoms (good indication), psychological distress with intolerance of minor symptoms (bad indication – these patients are likely to be dissatisfied with surgery), poor compliance (good indication if the reason for poor compliance is the side effects of treatment, otherwise bad indication) and misdiagnosis of GORD. Clinical trials are now in progress to compare the relative efficacy of long-term medication and surgery, and it is hoped that the results will simplify clinical decision making.

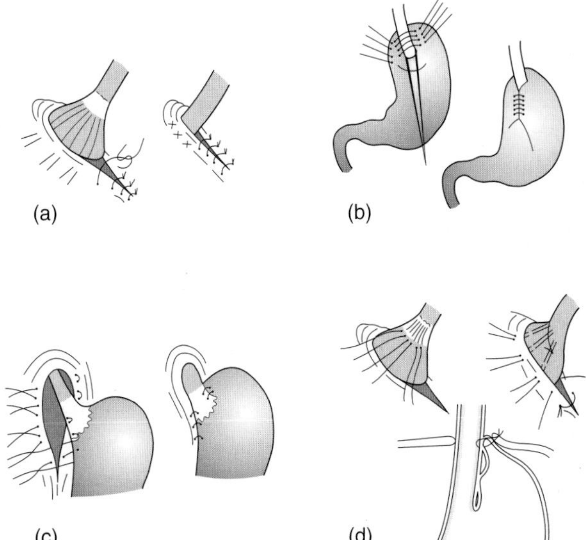

Fig. 50.32 Various operations for the surgical correction of GORD: (a) the original Allison repair of hiatus hernia (this is ineffective and is no longer done); (b) Nissen fundoplication; (c) Hill procedure; (d) Belsey Mark IV operation.

What operation?

There are many operations for GORD, but essentially the choice is between total and partial fundoplication. The major types of antireflux operation were all developed in the 1950s (Fig. 50.32). Anatomical repair of hiatus hernia has been abandoned as it is ineffective. Nissen described total fundoplication in which the fundus of the stomach is wrapped completely around the lower oesophagus. The Belsey operation is a thoracic procedure in which the oesophagus is sutured to the diaphragm and to the fundus of the stomach to reduce any hiatus hernia and produce a 240° anterior fundoplication. The Hill procedure is an operation in which the cardia is tightened and fixed to the preaortic fascia. The completed operation looks very like a fundoplication.

Total or partial fundoplication?

Done correctly these are all effective operations. The disadvantage of the Nissen fundoplication is that that it can produce an overcompetent cardia resulting in dysphagia or the gas bloat syndrome in which belching is prevented. As a result the stomach fills with air and the patient feels very full after meals and passes excessive flatus. The problem of the overcompetent cardia has been largely overcome by the *floppy* Nissen in which the fundoplication is made very loose

Rudolph Nissen. Emeritus Professor of Surgery, Istanbul, Turkey and Basle, Switzerland.

Ronald Belsey. Emeritus Consultant Thoracic Surgeon, Frenchay Hospital, Bristol, England.

Lucius Hill. Surgeon, Mason Clinic, Seattle, Washington, USA.

around the oesophagus and also by making a short fundoplication of 1 cm or so. Partial fundoplication is less prone to side effects, but has tended to have a higher recurrence rate. This tendency seems to have been partly overcome by improved suture materials. There are now many different partial fundoplication operations, but the principles of antireflux surgery remain the same.

The *Angelchik prosthesis* is a different type of antireflux procedure in which a silastic prosthetic collar is placed around the lower oesophagus. It probably acts by limiting distension of the cardia which is the trigger zone for TLOSRs and undoubtedly prevents reflux in the majority of cases in which it is implanted. However, it has a tendency to cause troublesome dysphagia and is much less popular than formerly.

> Roux-en-Y diversion reduces reflux

In some complicated cases, such as reoperative problems, the effects of reflux can be greatly reduced by performing a partial gastrectomy with a Roux-en-Y reconstruction. This reduces gastric acid secretion and diverts bile and pancreatic secretions away from the stomach. Thus the volume of potential refluxate in the stomach is reduced and because of its changed composition it is less damaging to the oesophagus.

What operative approach?

For many years the relative merits of the thoracic and abdominal approaches were hotly debated. The advent of minimal access surgery has overshadowed this debate and most antireflux operations are now done with a laparoscopic approach. A small number of surgeons has used a thoracoscopic or *video-assisted* thoracic approach. In general the abdominal approach is preferred unless there is a particular indication for opening the chest for safe surgery. Nowadays this is seldom required since there are excellent on-table retractors that allow access to the upper abdomen and lower mediastinum if necessary.

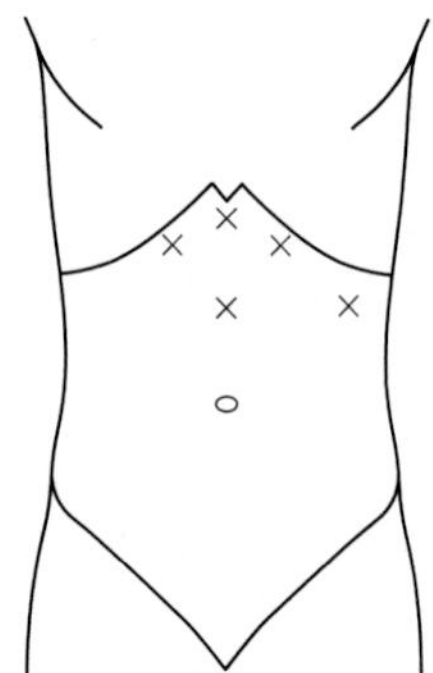

Fig. 50.33 Laparoscope cannula sites for laparoscopic fundoplication.

César Roux, 1857–1934. Professor of Surgery and Gynaecology, Lausanne, Switzerland.

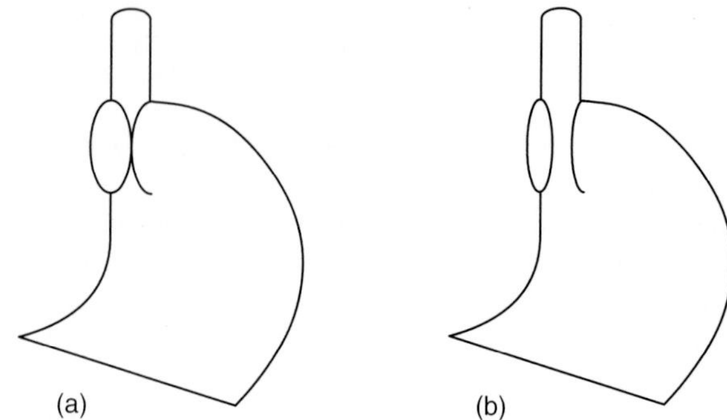

Fig. 50.34 (a) Total (Nissen) fundoplication; (b) partial fundoplication (Toupet).

Laparoscopic fundoplication

Five cannulae are inserted in the upper abdomen (Fig. 50.33). The cardia and lower oesophagus are separated from the diaphragmatic hiatus. The fundus may be mobilised by dividing the short gastric vessels that tether the fundus to the spleen. The hiatus is narrowed by sutures placed behind the oesophagus. The fundus is drawn behind the oesophagus and then sutured in front of the oesophagus. In the Nissen fundoplication fundus is sutured to fundus to encircle the oesophagus completely (Fig. 50.34a). In the Toupet partial fundoplication, which is a popular procedure, the fundus is sutured to the oesophagus on each side leaving a strip of exposed oesophagus anteriorly (Fig. 50.34b). If the operation cannot be completed safely or effectively by the laparoscopic method the abdomen is opened with an upper midline incision and the procedure is completed.

Complications of GORD

Stricture

Reflux-induced strictures (Fig. 50.30) are common, usually in late middle age and the elderly, but they may occur even in children. It is important to distinguish a benign reflux-induced stricture from a carcinoma. This is not usually difficult, but sometimes a cancer spreads under the oesophageal mucosa at its upper margin producing a surprisingly benign looking stricture on first sight.

> Day-case dilatation and PPI for peptic stricture

Peptic strictures generally respond well to dilatation and long-term treatment with a PPI. Since most of the patients are elderly antireflux surgery is not usually considered. However, it is an alternative to long-term PPI treatment just as in uncomplicated GORD in younger and fitter patients. It should be borne in mind that antireflux surgery may be difficult technically in stricture patients because of associated oesophageal shortening.

A.M. Toupet. Surgeon, France.

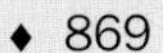

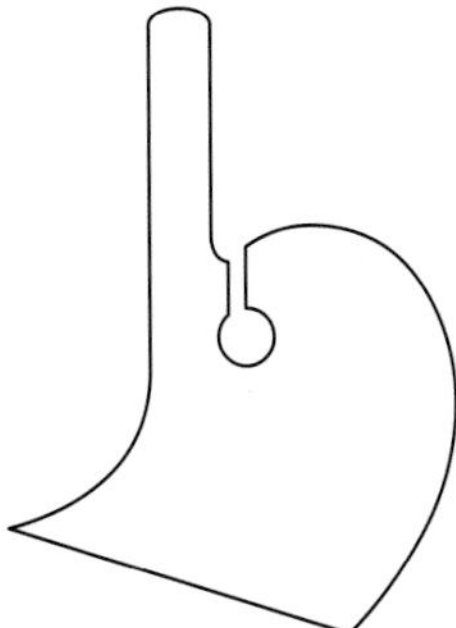

Fig. 50.35 Collis gastroplasty to produce a *neo-oesophagus* around which a Nissen fundoplication is done. The operation may be performed by an abdominal approach using circular and linear staplers.

Oesophageal shortening

With long-standing reflux oesophagitis the oesophagus has a tendency to contract longitudinally producing a secondary hiatus hernia. This does not matter in a patient being treated by medication, but it may cause difficulty during antireflux surgery. The shortening may be a minor problem that simply requires mobilisation of the oesophagus. If a good segment of intra-abdominal oesophagus cannot be restored without tension a Collis gastroplasty can be done (Fig. 50.35). This produces a *neo-oesophagus* around which a fundoplication can be done (Collis–Nissen operation).

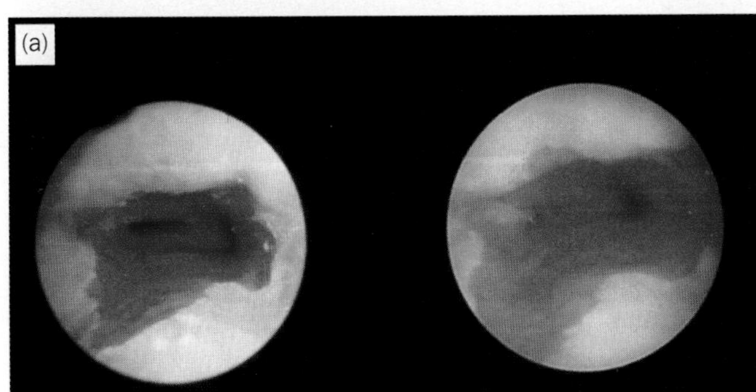

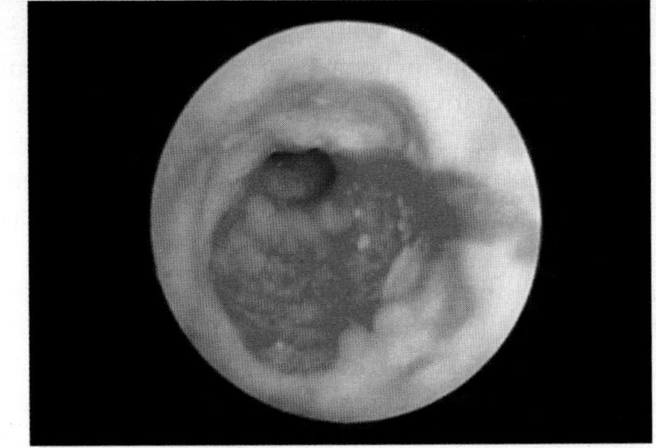

Fig. 50.36 Barrett's oesophagus with proximal migration of the squamocolumnar junction: (a) and (b) with a view of the distal oesophagus.

J. Leigh Collis. Surgeon, Birmingham, England.

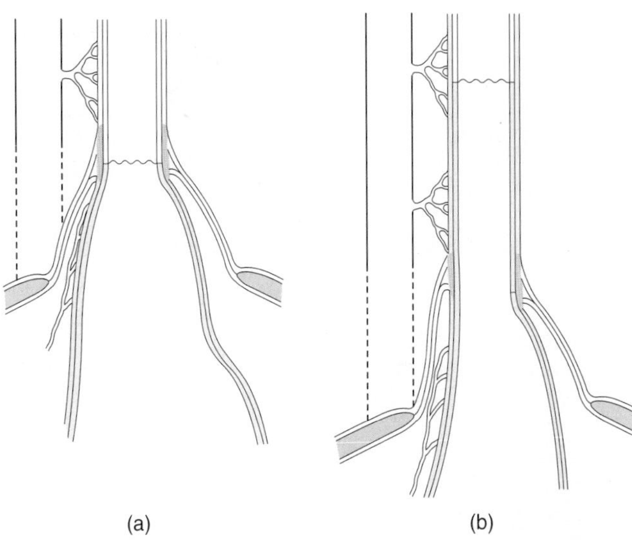

Fig. 50.37 (a) The relationship between the LOS, the squamocolumnar junction and the diaphragm in sliding hiatus hernia; (b) Barrett's oesophagus and sliding hernia.

Barrett's oesophagus (columnar-lined lower oesophagus)

Barrett's oesophagus is a metaplastic change in the lining mucosa of the oesophagus in response to chronic gastro-oesophageal reflux (Fig. 50.36). One of the great mysteries of GORD is why some people develop oesophagitis and others develop Barrett's oesophagus often without significant oesophagitis. In Barrett's oesophagus the junction between squamous oesophageal mucosa and gastric mucosa moves proximally. It may be difficult to distinguish a Barrett's oesophagus from a tubular sliding hiatus hernia during endoscopy since the two often coexist (Fig. 50.37). The key is where the gastric mucosal folds end. The mucosa in the body of the stomach has longitudinal folds. The columnar lining in Barrett's oesophagus is smooth. If a peptic stricture occurs in Barrett's oesophagus it always occurs at the new squamo-columnar junction (Fig. 50.38). A different type of stricture may occur in the columnar segment after healing of a Barrett's ulcer (see below).

Intestinal metaplasia, the important factor

Several types of gastric-type mucosa may be found in the lower oesophagus. When *intestinal metaplasia* occurs there is an increased risk of adenocarcinoma of the oesophagus of the order of 25 times that of the general population (Figs 50.39 and 50.40). Patients who are found to have Barrett's oesophagus may be submitted to regular screening endoscopy with multiple biopsies every year or two in the hope of finding dysplasia or *in situ* cancer rather than allowing invasive can-

(a)

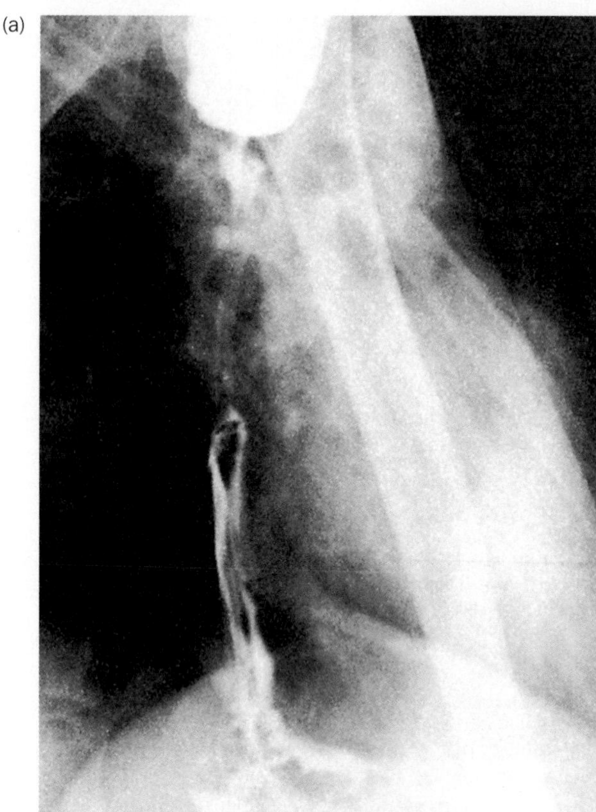

(b)

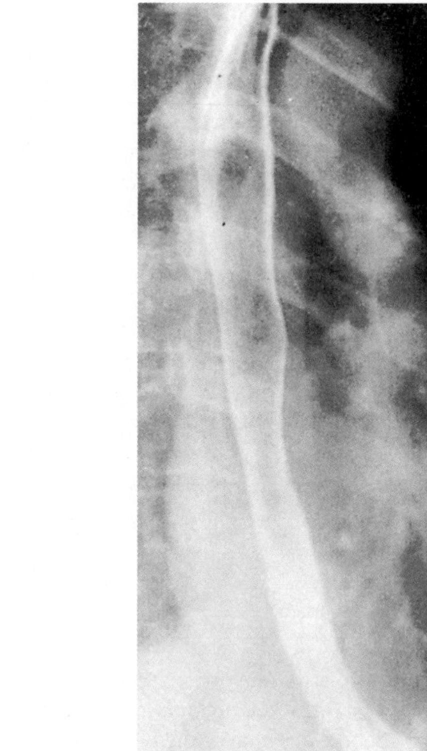

Fig. 50.38 (a) The radiological appearances of a mid-oesophageal stricture in a patient with Barrett's oesophagus; (b) normal lumen following dilatation.

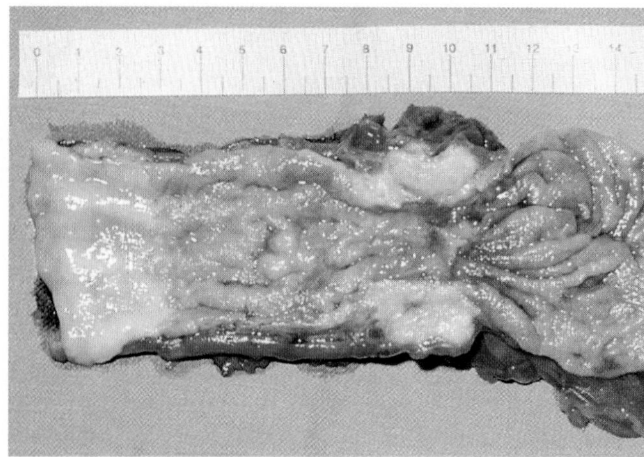

Fig. 50.39 The macroscopic appearances of an adenocarcinoma in Barrett's oesophagus.

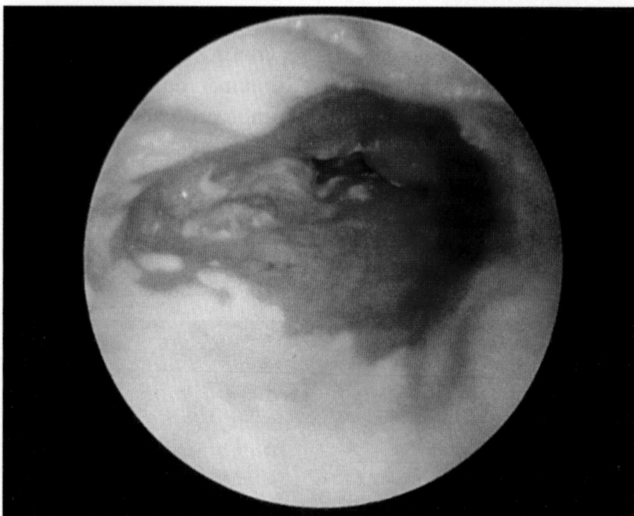

Fig. 50.40 Endoscopic view of carcinoma in Barrett's oesophagus.

cer to develop and cause symptoms. There is as yet no general agreement about the benefits of screening endoscopy, nor about the ideal frequency of endoscopy. A significant problem is that the incidence of Barrett's oesophagus in the community is estimated to be at least 10 times the incidence discovered by endoscopy in dyspeptic patients referred for endoscopy. Thus adenocarcinoma in Barrett's oesophagus often presents with invasive cancer without any preceding reflux symptoms.

Until recently Barrett's oesophagus was not diagnosed until there was at least 3 cm of columnar epithelium in the distal oesophagus. With the better appreciation of the importance of intestinal metaplasia Barrett's oesophagus may be diagnosed if there is *any* intestinal metaplasia in the oesophagus.

When Barrett's oesophagus is discovered the treatment is that of the underlying GORD. Several methods of ablation of Barrett's mucosa are under active study, including laser,

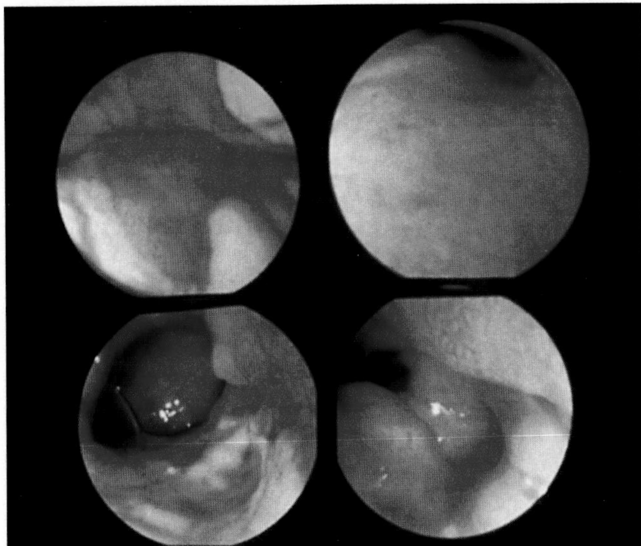

Fig. 50.41 Barrett's ulcer in the columnar cell-lined oesophagus.

photodynamic therapy and argon beam plasma coagulation. In conjunction with high-dose PPI treatment or an antireflux operation these endoscopic methods can restore the squamous lining of the oesophagus. It is not yet known whether this reduces the risk of malignant transformation since there are often remnants of glandular mucosa underneath the new squamous lining.

Don't confuse Barrett's ulcer with oesophagitis

Barrett's ulcer is an ulcer in the columnar-lined portion of a Barrett's oesophagus (Fig. 50.41). These are distinct from the more usual erosions of reflux oesophagitis that always occur at or just above the squamocolumnar junction. Barrett's ulcers may be deep and prone to bleeding or, rarely, perforation. Uncomplicated reflux oesophagitis almost never gives rise to severe haemorrhage.

Paraoesophageal ('rolling') hiatus hernia

Rolling hiatus hernias are dangerous

Unlike sliding hiatus hernia a rolling hiatus hernia is a true hernia that is prone to complications. True paraoesophageal hernias in which the cardia remains in its normal anatomical position are very rare and confined to museum exhibits and personal collections of interesting cases. The vast majority of rolling hernias is mixed hernias in which the cardia is displaced into the chest and the greater curve of the stomach rolls into the mediastinum (Fig. 50.42). Sometimes the whole of the stomach lies in the chest (Fig. 50.43) and may undergo volvulus with perforation or gangrene. Colon or small intestine may sometimes lie in the hernia sac, but rarely

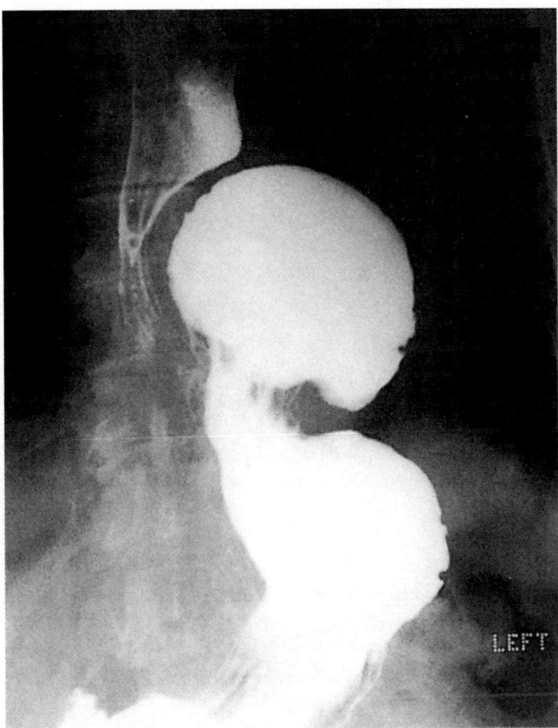

Fig. 50.42 A paraoesophageal hernia showing the gastro-oesophageal junction just above the diaphragm and the fundus alongside the oesophagus compressing the lumen.

causes additional complications. The hernia is commonest in the elderly, but may occur in young fit people.

The symptoms of rolling hernia are mostly due to twisting and distortion of the oesophagus and stomach. Dysphagia is common. Chest pain may occur due to distension of an obstructed stomach. Classically the pain is relieved by a loud

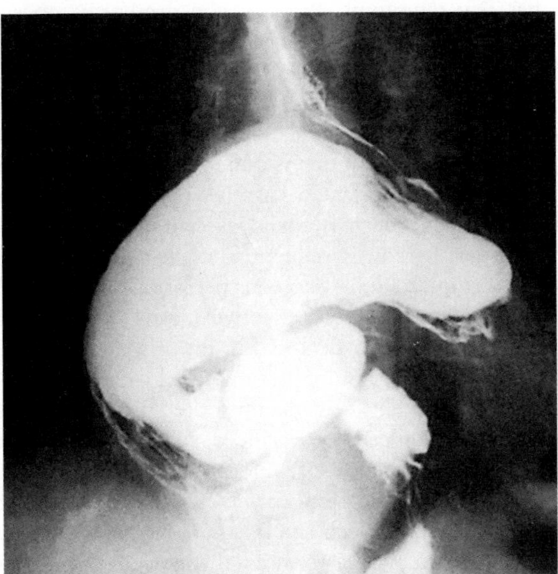

Fig. 50.43 A huge paraoesophageal hernia with an upside-down stomach and the pylorus just below the hiatus.

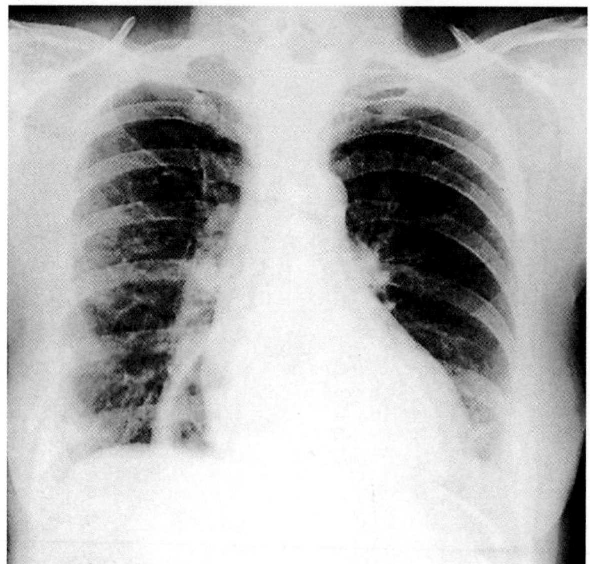

Fig. 50.44 A gas bubble seen on a plain chest X-ray showing the fundus of the stomach in the chest.

belch. Symptoms of GORD are variable. They may be present in the early stages of evolution of the hernia, but disappear as distortion of the cardia increases.

The hernia may be visible on a plain X-ray of the chest as a gas bubble, often with a fluid level behind the heart (Fig. 50.44). Fluid levels are not seen in sliding hernias. A barium meal is the best method of diagnosis. The endoscopic appearances may be confusing, especially in large hernias when the endoscopist feels as if they have lost their sense of direction.

Rolling hernias *always* require surgical repair as they are potentially dangerous. However, major surgery may not be an attractive prospect in frail elderly patients or in someone who has few symptoms. Patients who present as an emergency with acute chest pain may be treated initially by nasogastric tube to relieve the distension that causes the pain, followed by operative repair. If the pain is not relieved or perforation is suspected immediate operation is mandatory.

The type of operation that is done is somewhat controversial because of the variable occurrence of GORD. A thoracic or abdominal approach is equally acceptable. The essential part of the operation is reduction of the hernia and some form of *gastropexy*. Some surgeons perform a fundoplication arguing that this is a very effective means of maintaining reduction and that it deals with the associated GORD. Others argue that a fundoplication should only be done if reflux can be conclusively demonstrated beforehand. Surprisingly, both philosophies achieve good results. Laparoscopic repair has recently become popular. Full anatomical repair of a large rolling hernia can be tedious and difficult by the laparoscopic approach and it is more common simply to reduce the hernia and perform a gastropexy. Some surgeons lay a sheet of prosthetic mesh across the hiatal opening to stop the bowel entering it.

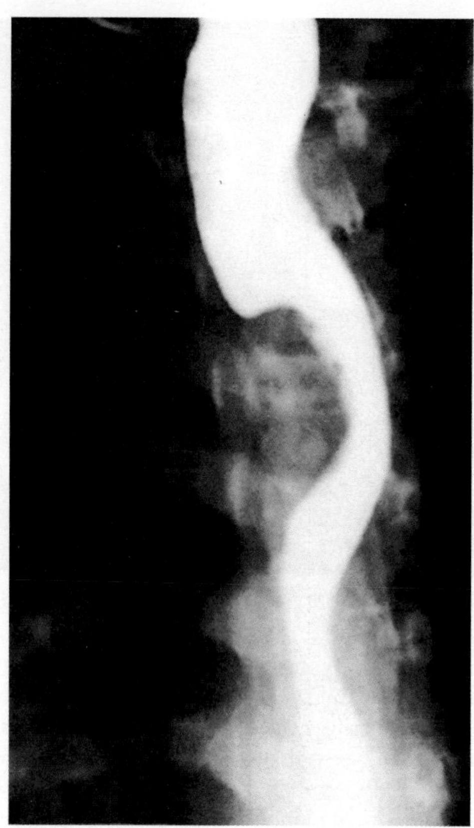

Fig. 50.45 Classic appearance of a benign leiomyoma on barium swallow.

Neoplasms of the oesophagus

Benign tumours

Benign tumours of the oesophagus are rare. The commonest is a leiomyoma (Fig. 50.45). Even a large leiomyoma may produce surprisingly mild symptoms. It is usually possible to enucleate the tumour at thoracotomy without breaching the mucosa. Small polyps of the oesophagus, such as granular cell tumours and fibrovascular polyps, may be found in the course of endoscopy for other conditions.

Malignant tumours

Sarcoma

Sarcoma of the oesophagus is exceedingly rare, but leiomyosarcoma (Fig. 50.46) and rhabdomyosarcoma have been reported. Other types of sarcoma have been reported, but are confined to individual case reports.

Malignant melanoma

Malignant melanoma of the oesophagus is rare. It may represent secondary spread, but primary melanoma of the oesophagus does occur. It has a very poor prognosis.

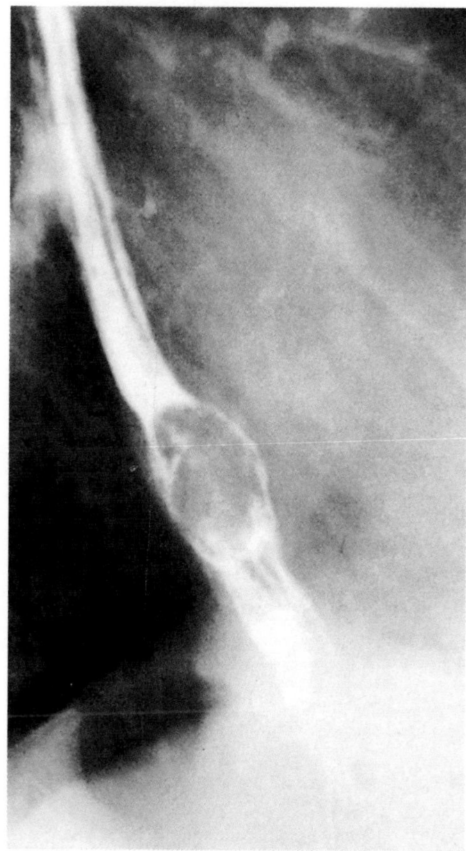

Fig. 50.46 Intraluminal polyp which proved to be a leiomyosarcoma.

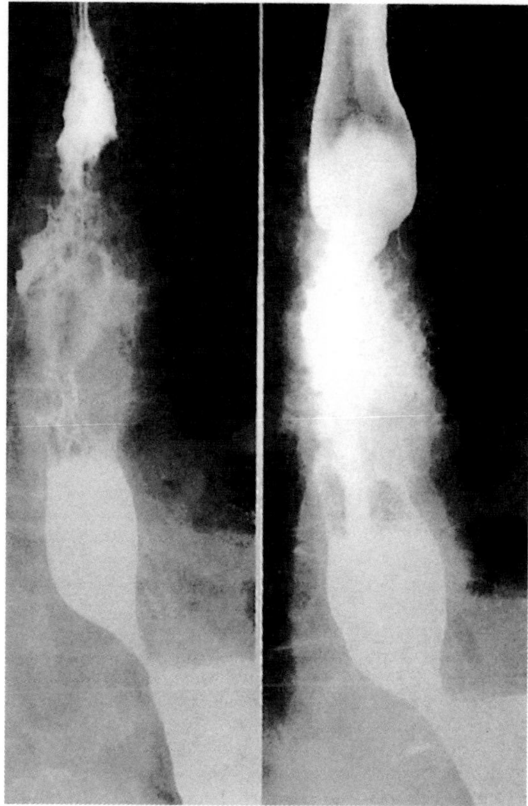

Fig. 50.47 The classic appearances of a mid-oesophageal proliferative squamous cell carcinoma.

Carcinoma of the oesophagus

Cancer of the oesophagus is the ninth most common cancer in the world. It is in general a disease of mid to late adulthood with a poor survival rate. Only 5–10 per cent of those diagnosed will survive for 5 years. Despite this gloomy prognosis there are some encouraging signs of change.

Pathology and aetiology. Squamous cell cancer (Figs 50.47 and 50.48) and adenocarcinoma (Figs 50.49 and 50.50) are the commonest types. Squamous cell carcinoma usually affects the upper two-thirds of the oesophagus and adenocarcinoma affects the lower one-third, but there are frequent exceptions to this rule. Oat cell cancer occurs occasionally. World-wide, it is squamous cell cancer that is commonest, but adenocarcinoma is the commonest type in most westernised countries and is increasing in incidence.

Geographical variation of oesophageal cancer

The incidence of oesophageal cancer varies more than any other cancer and its epidemiology provides a fascinating story. Squamous cell cancer is endemic in the Transkei region of South Africa and in the Asian 'cancer belt' that extends across the middle of Asia from the shores of the Caspian Sea in northern Iran to China. The highest incidence in the world is in Linxian in Henan province in China where it is the commonest single cause of death with more than 100 cases per 100 000 population per annum. The cause of the disease in the endemic areas is not definitely known, but is probably due to a combination of fungal contamination of food with the production of a carcinogenic mycotoxin, together with nutritional deficiencies in the population. In Linxian, supplementation of the diet with beta-carotene, vitamin E and selenium has been shown to reduce the incidence of cancer.

Away from the endemic areas tobacco and alcohol are the major factors in the occurrence of squamous cancer. Incidence rates vary from less that five per 100 000 in whites in the USA to 26.5 per 100 000 in some regions of France. Contrary to popular opinion Japan does *not* have a particularly high incidence of oesophageal cancer.

The incidence of adenocarcinoma of the oesophagus is increasing

In many westernised countries the incidence of squamous cell cancer has fallen or remained relatively static, but the incidence of adenocarcinoma of the oesophagus has increased since the mid-1970s by 5–10 per cent per annum. The change is greater than that of any other neoplasm in this time. Adenocarcinoma now accounts for 60–75 per cent of

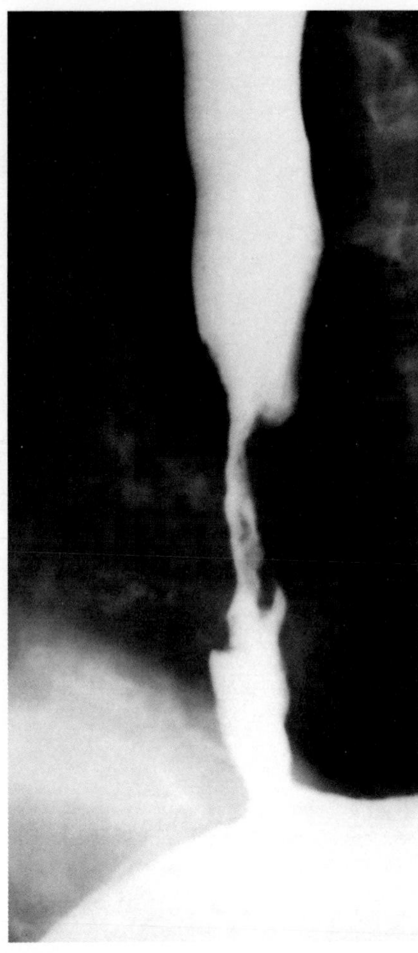

Fig. 50.48 Squamous cell carcinoma of the oesophagus producing an irregular stricture with shouldered margins.

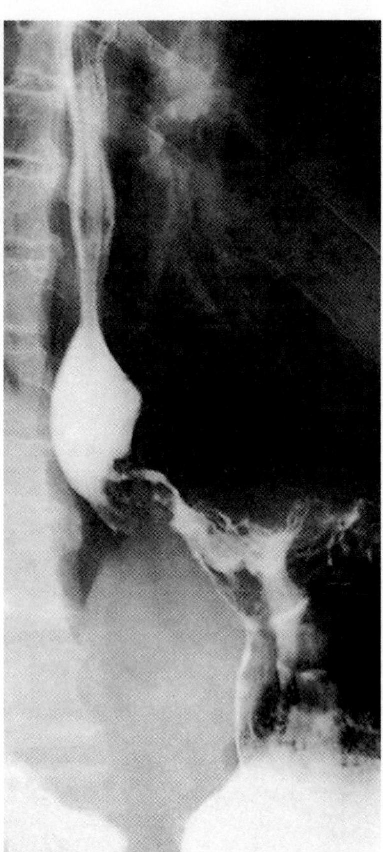

Fig. 50.49 Adenocarcinoma of the lower oesophagus spreading upwards from the cardia.

all oesophageal cancers in several countries. The reason for the change is not understood, but is thought to be due to a changed incidence of Barrett's oesophagus. There has been a similar increase in the incidence of carcinoma of the cardia of the stomach. This epidemiological change suggests that cancer of the cardia and adenocarcinoma of the oesophagus are, in fact, the same disease. The incidence of cancer of the gastric antrum has decreased markedly over the same period and now more than 60 per cent of all upper GI cancers involve the cardia or distal oesophagus. Survival rates remain poor although in several regions of the UK there has been a modest improvement in 5-year survival from 5 per cent to 10 per cent.

> Involvement of coeliac axis nodes is a bad prognostic sign

The poor prognosis of oesophageal cancer is proof of its ability to spread. This may be *locoregional* or *systemic*. Locoregional spread occurs through the wall of the oesophagus into adjacent structures, along the length of the oesophagus in the submucosal lymphatics, and to regional

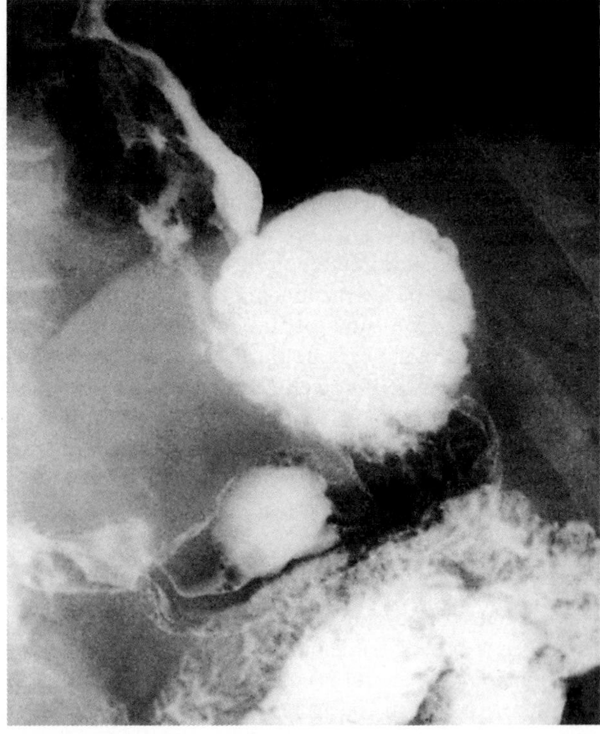

Fig. 50.50 An adenocarcinoma in a hiatus hernia. This lesion arises in the upper stomach and involves the cardia.

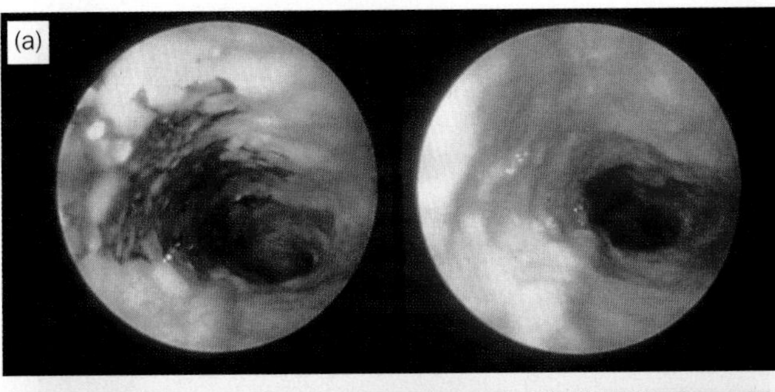

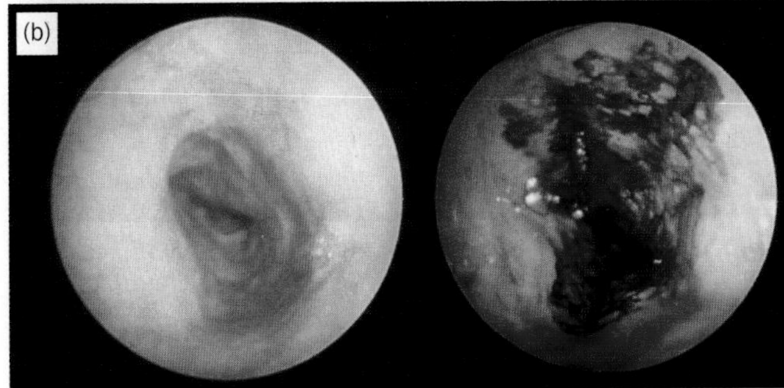

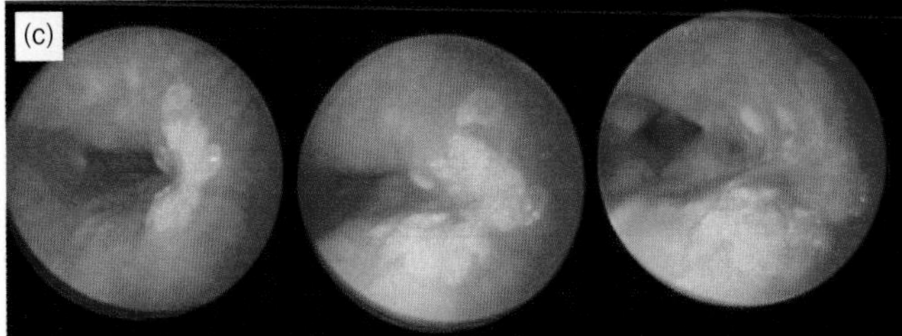

Fig. 50.51 Carcinoma *in situ* showing the varied presentations: (a) occult form; (b) erythroplakia; and (c) leucoplakia. The right-hand picture in (a) and (b) demonstrates the use of vital staining with methylene blue.

lymph nodes. Locoregional spread is often discontinuous, i.e. distant regional lymph nodes may be invaded even when local nodes are free of tumour, and there may be satellite nodules in the oesophagus proximal to the main tumour. Spread to the coeliac axis nodes from a lesion in the intrathoracic oesophagus is a bad prognostic sign and is regarded as metastatic (M) rather than nodal (N) disease in the TNM classification. Systemic spread is mainly to the liver and lungs, but practically any organ can be involved including brain, bone and skin.

Early endoscopic diagnosis is the key to good results

Clinical features. Dysphagia is the usual presenting feature and is generally a sign of advanced disease. Weight loss is likewise a sign of advanced disease. An increasing number of cancers is diagnosed at a relatively early stage when the chances of cure are greater. Patients with early disease may present with rather nonspecific dyspeptic symptoms or a vague feeling of 'something that is not quite right' during swallowing. Some are diagnosed during screening of Barrett's

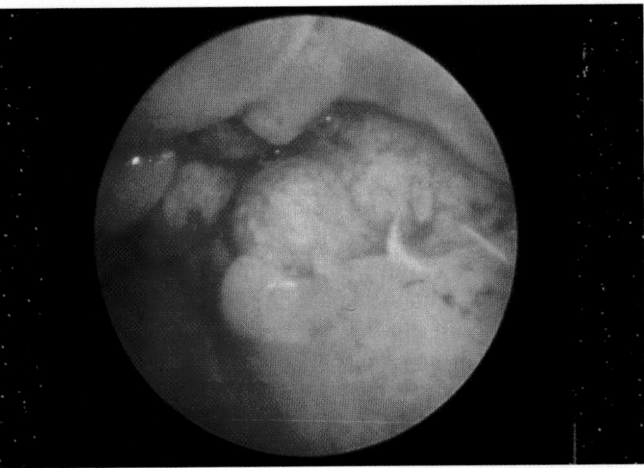

Fig. 50.52 Endoscopic appearances of a mid-oesophageal squamous cell carcinoma.

oesophagus, but it has to be confessed that the results of formal screening are still disappointing. The widespread use of endoscopy as a diagnostic tool is the major contributor to early diagnosis (Fig. 50.51). It should be emphasised that biopsies should be taken of all lesions (Fig. 50.52) no matter how trivial they appear. Small cancers are curable. Large ones

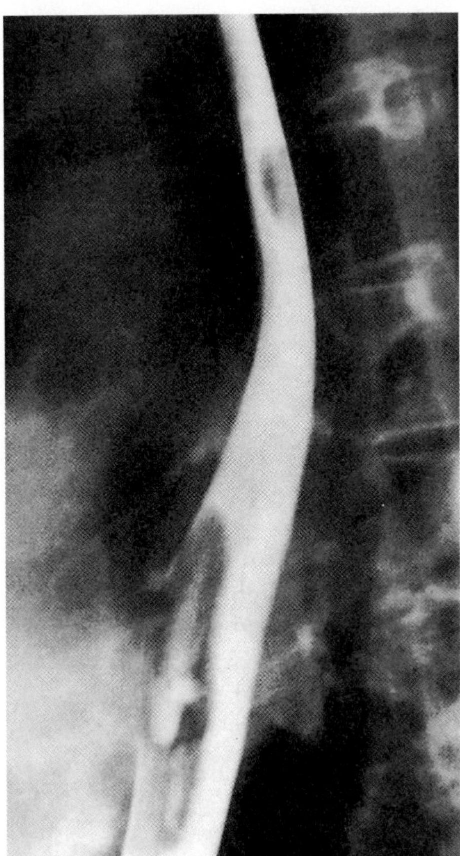

Fig. 50.53 Beware the differential diagnosis of infection, for what appears to be a tumour. This mid-oesophageal mass was actually tuberculosis.

usually are not. Some benign lesions can look surprisingly 'malignant' (Fig. 50.53).

Hoarseness due to recurrent laryngeal nerve palsy is a sign of advanced and incurable disease. Palpable lymphadenopathy in the neck is likewise a sign of advanced disease.

Staging and general assessment. Methodical assessment of the patient and the cancer is essential if the best results are to be achieved. Some patients are quite obviously not candidates for radical treatment even on the most superficial inspection and common humanity must always take precedence. Staging must not delay effective palliation.

The most important aspect of staging is a careful search for metastatic disease. Ultrasonography of the liver and computerised tomography (CT) scanning of the chest and abdomen is mandatory before resection. The purpose of CT scanning is to exclude metastatic disease from the lungs and liver. Despite considerable improvements in CT and magnetic resonance imaging these methods are still inaccurate for staging the primary lesion and for staging lymph nodes. Endoscopic ultrasonography, if available, is the best method for preoperative staging of oesophageal cancer. Bronchoscopy should be done in lesions of the upper or middle thirds where there is potential for tracheobronchial invasion (Fig. 50.54). Laparoscopy is useful for assessing adenocarcinoma of the distal oesophagus (Fig. 50.55), particularly if it is likely to extend below the *phreno-oesophageal* ligament. Laparoscopy is at its best for detecting transperitoneal spread and liver metastasis. It is an inexpensive technology that deserves to be widely used. At the cost of some time and effort it is also possible to sample lymph nodes.

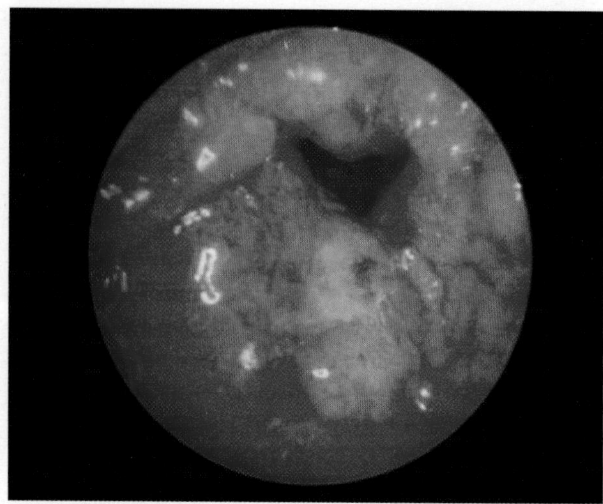

Fig. 50.55 Adenocarcinoma of the cardia. Transcoelomic spread may occur with this type of lesion.

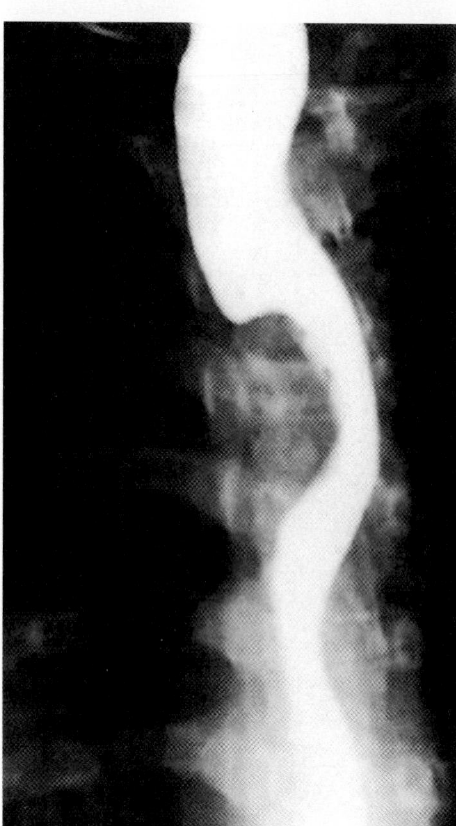

Fig. 50.54 Invasion into the posterior wall of the trachea from an oesophageal carcinoma.

> Short-term nutritional support has doubtful benefits

It is also important to assess the fitness of the patient to withstand major surgery. Respiratory and cardiovascular function are the most important aspects of the assessment. Nutritional assessment is also an important part of general care, but the value of preoperative nutritional support remains somewhat controversial. It is not possible to postpone treatment for several weeks to allow full nutritional 'resuscitation' and short periods of nutritional support are of questionable benefit for reducing postoperative morbidity and mortality. If food intake is impaired the simplest means of providing adequate nutrition is by withdrawing all solid food and starting the patient on a high-protein liquid diet. It is surprising how much severe dysphagia improves when obstructing food material in the oesophagus has been cleared.

Treatment of malignant tumours

Principles

A gastrostomy should *never* be carried out as the 'palliation' for oesophageal cancer. Palliation in this disease demands relief of dysphagia. It is important that staging and general assessment are carried out speedily and humanely. Those who have incurable disease should not be submitted to needlessly aggressive treatment that simply prolongs the process of dying. Palliation of dysphagia can be achieved in a number of ways that do not unduly stress the patient. Pain is also a surprisingly common feature of advanced oesophageal cancer and requires careful attention. Curative treatment involves radical surgery or radiotherapy. This should be carried out in a specialist centre with the necessary expertise. The role of palliative resection is debatable. It is wise not to embark on resection if it is clear beforehand that palliation is all that can be achieved. However, palliative resection may be appropriate if incurable disease is found when an operation is already well under way.

Surgical resection probably gives the best results for all forms of oesophageal cancer. Radical radiotherapy can cure both types of cancer, but poses technical problems at the lower end of the oesophagus. Tumours that involve the stomach are not generally accepted for radiotherapy. The results of radiotherapy have been improved by concurrent chemotherapy, so-called *chemoradiotherapy*. Some have suggested that this development may challenge the dominant place of surgery for cure.

Surgery

Beware of satellite nodules proximal to the primary lesion

Curative surgery involves resection of an appropriate length of the oesophagus together with any involved stomach and the locoregional lymphatics. There is controversy about the length of oesophagus that should be resected. Some surgeons feel that operative trauma should be reduced to the minimum by resecting only enough oesophagus to clear the tumour. Others advocate subtotal oesophagectomy pioneered in the UK by McKeown on the grounds that generous proximal clearance gives the best chance of clearing satellite nodules in the submucosal lymphatics and gives the best postoperative function with the least tendency to gastro-oesophageal reflux. Restoration of continuity is almost always achieved by transposition of the stomach and oesophagogastric anastomosis. Colon or, less commonly, small intestine may be interposed between the oesophageal remnant and the stomach, but is a more major undertaking with a higher postoperative mortality. There is also controversy about the extent of lymph node dissection that should be done. Akiyama has pioneered the concept of *three field lymph node dissection*, an ultraradical operation involving extensive removal of the regional lymph nodes in the abdomen, chest and neck.

Lesions of the cardia that do not involve the oesophagus to any significant extent may be dealt with by extended total gastrectomy to include the distal oesophagus or by proximal gastrectomy and distal oesophagectomy.

Subtotal oesophagectomy. A variety of approaches is possible. The most commonly used is the Ivor Lewis (or

Kenneth McKeown, 1912–95. Surgeon, Darlington, England.
Hiroshi Akiyama. Surgeon, Toranomon Hospital, Tokyo, Japan.
Ivor Lewis, 1895–1982. Surgeon, North Middlesex Hospital, London and Rhyl, North Wales.
Norman Cecil Tanner, 1906–82. Surgeon, Charing Cross Hospital, London, England.

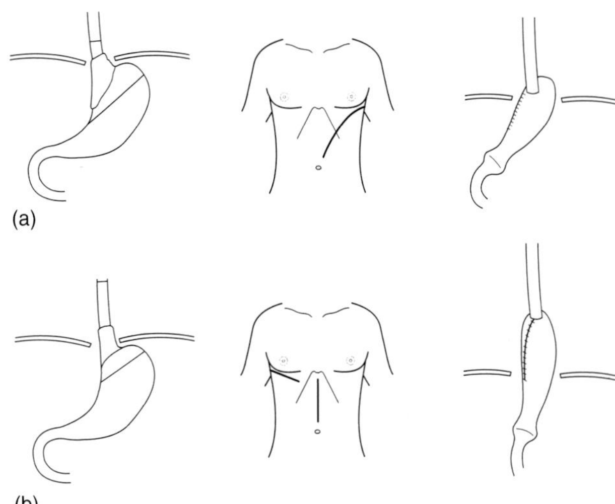

Fig. 50.56 The two usual approaches for surgery of the oesophagus are: (a) the thoracoabdominal which opens the abdominal and thoracic cavities together; and (b) the two-stage Ivor Lewis approach where the abdomen is opened first, closed and then the thoracotomy is performed. In the McKeown operation, a third incision in the neck is made to complete the cervical anastomosis.

Lewis–Tanner) approach. The stomach is first mobilised through a midline incision and then the oesophagus is approached from a right thoracotomy (Fig. 50.56). This approach is preferred by most surgeons because the access for resection and anastomosis is not hampered by the aortic arch as it is through a left thoracotomy. In the classic McKeown operation a third incision is made in the neck. However, in practice it is possible to remove just as much oesophagus by dividing the oesophagus in the chest at the thoracic inlet. A neck incision is required if a lymph node dissection is to be done or if there are technical difficulties with an anastomosis at the thoracic inlet. It is often stated that an oesophagogastric anastomosis is safest when done in the neck. In fact this only applies to an anastomosis that lies in the *anterior* part of the neck as for reconstruction with stomach or colon that has been brought up retrosternally or subcutaneously. The usual oesophagogastric anastomosis in the posterior neck drops back into its normal anatomical position and usually lies at the thoracic inlet. Any leak therefore has consequences that are just as serious as any other intrathoracic anastomosis.

Carefully preserve the blood supply of the stomach – venous and arterial

Mobilisation of the stomach must be done with care as it is essential to have a tension-free, well-vascularised stomach for transposition. The left gastric artery, the short gastric vessels and the left gastroepiploic are all divided. The viability of the transposed stomach mainly depends on the right gastroepiploic artery and vein with a small contribution from the right gastric. It should be noted that venous drainage is as important as arterial supply and it is essential to perform an accurate anatomical dissection that preserves the right gastroepiploic vein as well as the artery. The stomach is divided to remove the cardia and the upper part of the lesser curve including the whole of the left gastric artery and its associated lymph nodes.

> Right thoracic approach gives easy access to the oesophagus

The approach to the oesophagus through the right chest is relatively straightforward. The azygos vein is divided and this allows easy access to the whole of the intrathoracic oesophagus. A thoracotomy with entry above the fifth rib gives best access to the mid-mediastinum and the thoracic inlet. The oesophagus is divided just below the thoracic inlet. Since most lesions are in the lower third or middle third this usually gives adequate proximal clearance of at least 5 cm. If there is any doubt about clearance frozen sections should be taken from the resection margins and it may be helpful to open the oesophagus and assess whether the lesion is well circumscribed or whether it is diffusely infiltrating. Carcinomas of the upper thoracic oesophagus are almost always incurable at the time of diagnosis and invasion of the trachea is common. If one of these lesions is resectable it is essential to use an incision in the neck and to resect more of the oesophagus than is customary in the operation of subtotal oesophagectomy.

Oesophagogastric anastomosis may be performed equally well by hand or stapler. Both methods require attention to detail. In experienced hands serious anastomotic leakage should be uncommon (significantly less than 5 per cent). Minor leakage detectable by contrast radiology is more common, but should not disturb the patient. The significance of these minor leaks is debated. Most surgeons still prefer to keep the patient nil by mouth for 5–7 days and then perform a contrast swallow. If small leaks are to be detected it is essential to use barium for the examination. Water-soluble contrast media miss 50 per cent of anastomotic leaks. If leakage is detected the patient is kept nil by mouth until it has sealed.

Postoperative nutritional support remains controversial. There is general agreement that parenteral feeding is associated with more *nosocomial* infection, including pneumonia, than enteral feeding. It is also expensive. If nutritional support is given a feeding jejunostomy is probably the best method.

Transhiatal oesophagectomy (without thoracotomy). This approach has been popularised by Orringer in the USA and Pinotti in Brazil. The stomach is mobilised through a midline abdominal incision and the cervical oesophagus is mobilised through an incision in the neck. The diaphragm is then opened from the abdomen and the posterior mediastinum is entered. The lower oesophagus and the tumour are mobilised under direct vision and the upper oesophagus is mobilised by blunt dissection. This approach can provide an adequate removal of the tumour and lymph nodes in the lower mediastinum, but it is not possible to remove the nodes in the mid- or upper mediastinum. It may be a useful procedure for lesions of the lower oesophagus, but may be hazardous for a middle third lesion that may be adherent to the bronchus or to the azygos vein.

Left thoracoabdominal approach. A long skin and muscle incision is made on the left side with entry into the chest above the seventh rib and removal of a short segment of costal cartilage (Fig. 50.56). The diaphragm is incised and the oesophagus and stomach are removed. Some surgeons advocate a left thoracoabdominal approach together with an incision in the neck for subtotal oesophagectomy, the 'Birmingham' approach popularised by Matthews.

Thoracoscopic oesophagectomy. Oesophagectomy may be done by thoracoscopy or by the hybrid technique of video-assisted thoracic surgery (VATS) in which a combination of endoscopic and conventional instruments is used through small thoracic incisions. Thoracoscopic oesophagectomy in the prone position to minimise injury to the collapsed lung has been pioneered by Cuschieri. At present this is still an evolving technique and its place is not yet established. The procedure takes longer than open surgery and postoperative morbidity is still a problem.

Gastro-oesophageal reflux following oesophagogastric resection. Gastro-oesophageal reflux may be a major problem following any operation that involves resecting the cardia. Postoperative reflux may present with the typical symptoms of GORD or with a peptic stricture at the site of the anastomosis. However, the presentation may be different with a miserable patient who fails to thrive following the operation and who is then suspected of having recurrent cancer. This atypical presentation is particularly common following total gastrectomy with an inadequate reconstruction.

> Reflux may be a problem following resection
> Symptoms may be atypical

Reflux may be limited or avoided by:

1. subtotal oesophagectomy and gastric transposition high in the chest. The vertical stomach empties rapidly and functions as a barrier to reflux;
2. resection of a generous portion of proximal stomach if an anastomosis is made to the lower oesophagus. This reduces gastric secretion;
3. Roux-en-Y reconstruction with a long ascending jejunal limb (50–60 cm);
4. interposition of jejunum or colon (Fig. 50.57).

Mark Orringer. Surgeon, Ann Arbor, Michigan, USA.
Walter Pinotti. Surgeon, São Paulo, Brazil.

Hugoe Matthews. Thoracic surgeon, Birmingham, England.
Professor Sir Alfred Cuschieri. Professor of Surgery, Ninewells Hospital and Medical School, Dundee, Scotland.

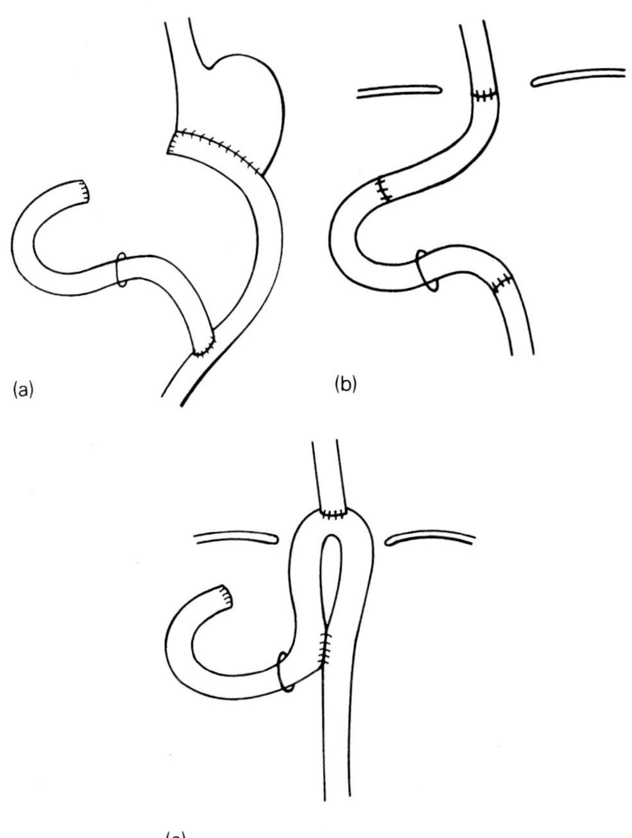

Fig. 50.57 Procedures using jejunum that may be used to re-establish continuity after resection of the stomach and cardia, and to prevent bile reflux into the lower oesophagus: (a) Roux-en-Y with partial or total gastrectomy; (b) Roux interposition loop and (c) Braun anastomosis. The last is ineffective in practice and should not be used.

The old Braun or *omega* reconstruction with an entero-enteroanastomosis below an oesophagojejunostomy is mentioned only to be condemned. The side-to-side anastomosis does not divert bile and pancreatic secretion satisfactorily from the oesophagus and several studies have shown that these patients fare badly.

Pyloroplasty. Pyroplasty or pyloromyotomy is an option following oesophageal resection. It may avoid early problems with gastric emptying, but the stomach always seems to recover its function even without pyloroplasty. If delayed gastric emptying is a problem in the early postoperative period erythromycin, which is a motilin agonist, seems to be the best therapy.

Radiotherapy for cure

Radiotherapy may be a useful alternative to surgery, especially in unfit patients

Radical radiotherapy can produce long-term survival in oesophageal cancer (Fig. 50.58). Although traditionally used for

Heinrich Braun, 1862–1934. Surgeon, Germany.

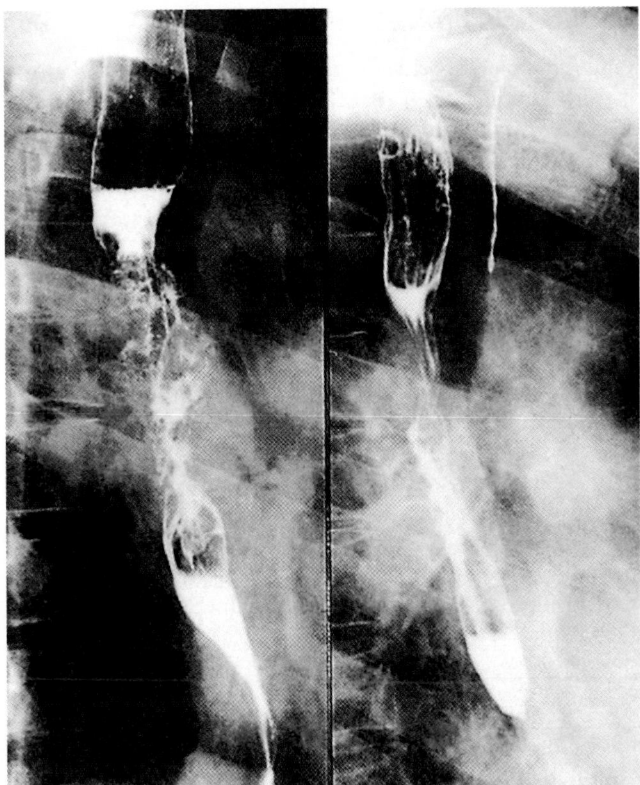

Fig. 50.58 Mid-oesophageal squamous cell carcinoma treated by radical radiotherapy (a) pretreatment and (b) post-treatment.

squamous cell cancer radiotherapy may also be effective for adenocarcinomas. There has been no formal comparison of the results of radiotherapy and surgical resection and it is therefore impossible to make dogmatic statements about the relative merits of each form of treatment. At present surgical resection is generally regarded as producing the best survival rates and quality of life. Many surgical series have reported 5-year survival rates between 20 per cent and 35 per cent, with an average figure of 25 per cent. Survival following radiotherapy with a typical UK case mix is between 9 per cent and, exceptionally, 19 per cent. The average appears to be about 10 per cent. However, the technology of radiotherapy continues to improve and the advent of chemoradiotherapy is a significant advance, if at the cost of significant morbidity. The survival figures make it abundantly clear that neither surgery nor radiotherapy is a particularly effective treatment. There is therefore a real need for improvements in early diagnosis, at present the best hope of improving survival, and improvements in treatment with the use of *multimodality* treatment.

Chemotherapy

With the advent of regimens containing cis-platinum, chemotherapy' for oesophageal cancer has improved considerably. Chemotherapy never cures the disease, but can produce worthwhile shrinkage of disease in up to 60 per cent of cases. The best responses are seen in squamous cell cancers. Survival is extended modestly.

Multimodality treatment

Randomised prospective studies of preoperative and postoperative radiotherapy have not shown any improvement in survival. Thus far there is no evidence that perioperative chemotherapy improves survival, but the results of studies using modern combination chemotherapy are awaited. Significant improvement in survival will only be achieved by a treatment that has a powerful effect on systemic disease.

Palliative treatment

Surgical resection and external beam radiotherapy may be used for palliation, but are not suitable when the expected survival is short, as most of the remainder of life will be spent recovering from the 'treatment'. Surgical bypass is likewise too major a procedure for use in a patient with a limited life expectancy. A wide variety of relatively simple methods of palliation is now available that will produce worthwhile relief of dysphagia with minimal disturbance to the patient.

> Palliation should be simple and effective

Intubation has been used for many years following the invention of the Souttar tube made of coiled silver wire (Fig. 50.59). This was superseded by the Celestin tube whose design gave a better quality of swallowing and was safer to insert. The Celestin tube was originally designed to be inserted by oesophagoscopy, to place a plastic rod in the stomach, followed by laparotomy and gastrostomy, to retrieve the rod and pull the tube down into place. The development of methods of intubation that could be used with a flexible endoscope was a major advance pioneered by Atkinson of Nottingham. The Atkinson tube is still in use. It is made of silastic with a nylon spiral reinforcement and has a distal retaining flange to prevent proximal displacement. It is inserted over a guidewire with a specially designed introducer. There are now many other designs of semirigid tubes for palliation including the Procter–Livingstone tube which is popular in South Africa where there is a very high incidence of oesophageal cancer.

The technology of intubation has now moved on with the invention of various types of expanding metal stent (Fig. 50.60). These are inserted under X-ray or endoscopic control. The stent is restrained in the collapsed state during insertion and then released when it is in the correct position. Expanding stents produce a better lumen for swallowing than rigid tubes, but are relatively expensive.

Endoscopic laser treatment may be used to core a channel through the tumour. It produces worthwhile improvement in swallowing, but has the disadvantage that it has to be repeated every few weeks. Lasers may also be used to unblock a stent that has been blocked by tumour overgrowth.

Brachytherapy is a method of delivering intraluminal radiation with a short penetration distance (hence the term *brachy*) to a tumour. An introduction system is inserted through the tumour and the treatment is then delivered in a single session lasting for 20 minutes or so. The equipment is expensive to purchase, but running costs are low.

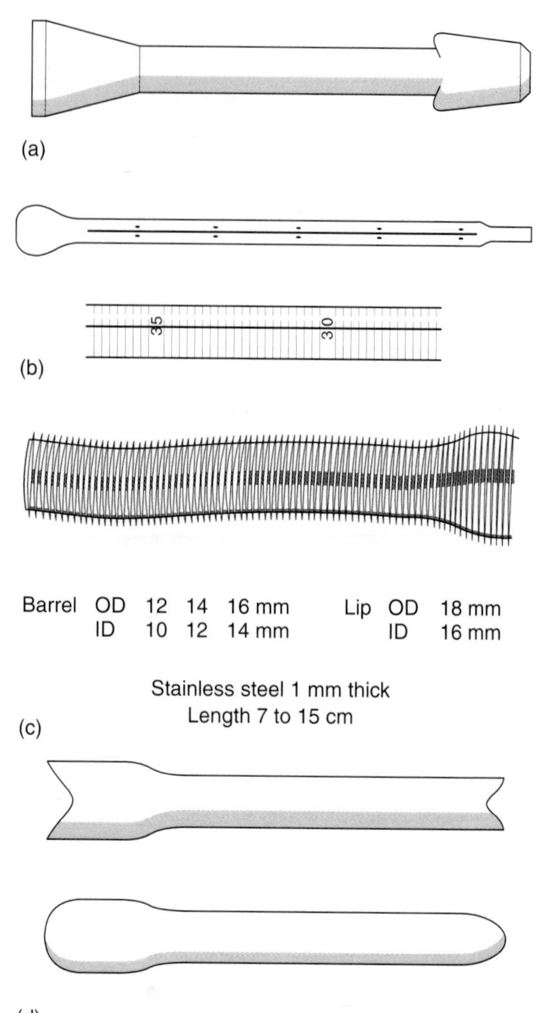

Fig. 50.59 Examples of palliative intubation tubes: (a) Atkinson; (b) Celestin; (c) Souttar; and (d) Procter–Livingstone.

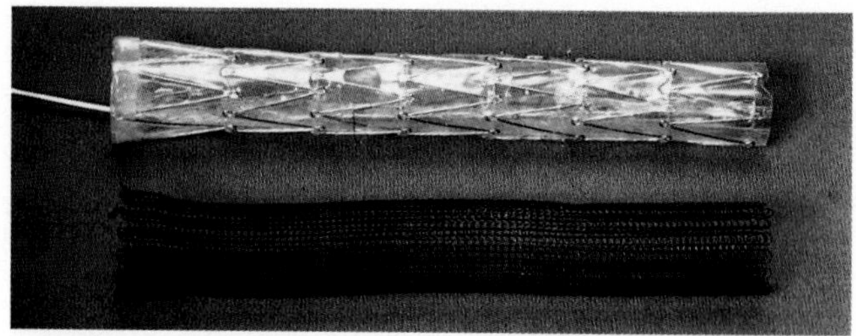

Fig. 50.60 Expanding metal stents – covered and uncovered.

Sir Henry Souttar, 1875–1964. Surgeon, The London Hospital, London, England.

Michael Atkinson. Emeritus Professor of Gastroenterology, University of Nottingham, Nottingham, England.

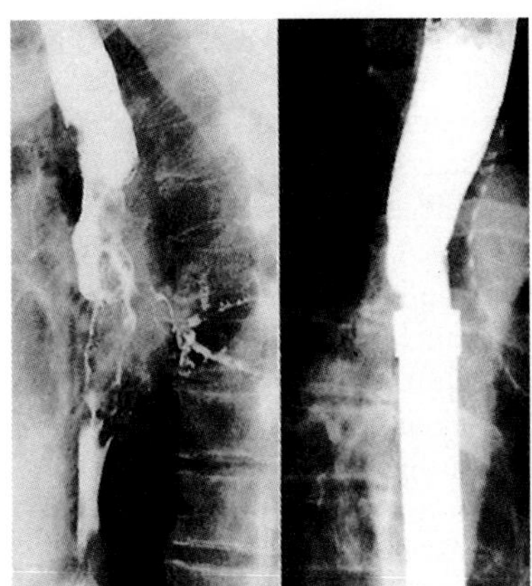

Fig. 50.61 Tracheo-oesophageal fistula treated by intubation with a Souttar tube: (a) before; and (b) after.

Other methods of palliation that can be given endoscopically include bipolar diathermy (the BICAP probe), argon beam plasma coagulation and alcohol injection.

Malignant tracheo-oesophageal fistula

Malignant tracheo-oesophageal fistula is a sign of incurable disease and life expectancy is short. Some have advocated surgical bypass and oesophageal exclusion, but this is a major procedure. An expanding metal stent is probably the best treatment, but semirigid prosthetic tubes may also be used (Fig. 50.61).

Postcricoid carcinoma

Postcricoid carcinoma is considered in the section on neoplasms of the pharynx (Chapter 43).

Motility disorders and diverticula

Oesophageal motility disorders

> Motility disorders may affect the whole gut

An oesophageal motility disorder can be readily understood when a patient has dysphagia in the absence of a stricture; a barium impregnated food bolus is seen to stick in the oesophagus and oesophageal manometry shows abnormal contractions in the oesophagus. The problem with oesophageal motility disorders is that the symptoms often seem disproportionately severe in comparison to the abnormality that can be demonstrated by objective investigation and the response to treatment may be so poor that the clinician is driven to questioning the very existence of motility disorders. The greatest difficulty arises when pain is the only symptom. Since surgery is advocated as a treatment for some motility disorders it is essential that the surgeon understands the nature of the condition. Much harm may be done by inappropriate enthusiastic surgery for ill-defined conditions.

Table 50.2 Classification of oesophageal motility disorders

Disorders of the pharyngo-oesophageal junction
Stroke
Myasthenia
Cricopharyngeal 'achalasia'
Disorders of the body of the oesophagus
Diffuse oesophageal spasm
Nutcracker oesophagus
Hypoperistalsis:
Systemic sclerosis (CREST)
Reflux-associated
Idiopathic
Allergic:
Eosinophilic oesophagitis
Nonspecific oesophageal dysmotility
Disorders of the lower oesophageal sphincter
Achalasia
Hypertensive lower sphincter
Incompetent lower sphincter (i.e. GORD)

CREST: calcinosis, Raynaud's syndrome, (o)esophageal motility disorders, sclerodactyly and telangiectasia.

It should also be remembered that there may be a general disturbance of GI function.

It is convenient to classify oesophageal motility disorders as in Table 50.2.

Pain in functional gastrointestinal disorders

Pain that is assumed to arise from dysfunction of the GI tract has three components, namely, abnormal motility and 'spasm', visceral hypersensitivity in which the gut is relatively intolerant of distension, and psychosocial factors. All three components are still poorly understood and it is therefore impossible to give dogmatic guidelines for treatment. Dealing with these conditions involves more art than science, but scientific understanding is slowly increasing.

Achalasia

Pathology and aetiology

> Selective loss of inhibitory neurons in achalasia

Achalasia is uncommon, but merits prominence because it is reasonably well understood and responds well to treatment. It is due to loss of the ganglion cells in Auerbach's plexus. The cause of the ganglion cell loss is unknown, but may be due to neurotropic viruses such as *Varicella zoster*. In South America chronic infection with the parasite *Trypanosoma Cruzi* causes Chagas' disease which has marked similarities to achalasia. Achalasia differs from Hirschsprung's disease of

Carlos Chagas, 1879–1934. Professor of Tropical Medicine, Rio de Janeiro, Brazil.
Harald Hirschsprung, 1830–1916. Danish physician.

(a)

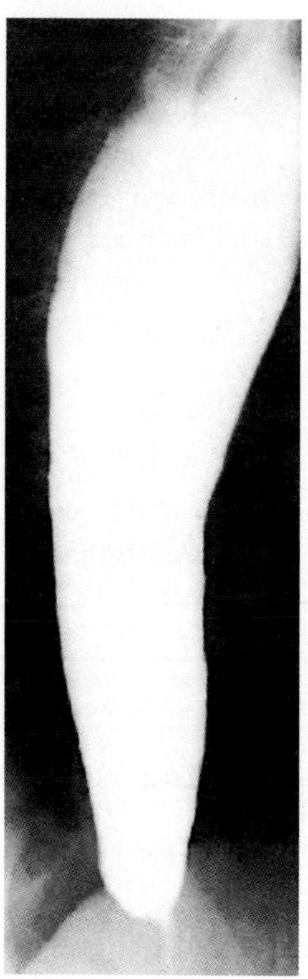

the colon because the dilated oesophagus usually contains few ganglion cells, whereas the dilated colon contains normal ganglion cells proximal to a constricted aganglionic segment. Histology of muscle specimens shows reduction of ganglion cells with a variable degree of chronic inflammation. In so-called vigorous achalasia, which may be an early stage of achalasia, there is inflammation and neural fibrosis, but normal numbers of ganglion cells. The neural damage in achalasia is somewhat selective since there is particularly severe loss of inhibitory neurons. The observation of selective loss of inhibitory innervation prompted the first attempts at treatment with botulinum toxin (see below). The term achalasia is derived form the Greek word αχαλασια which means failure to relax and was coined by Sir Arthur Hurst in 1910. The physiological abnormalities are incomplete or absent relaxation of the lower oesophageal sphincter and absent peristalsis in the body of the oesophagus. The oesophagus empties incompletely, almost always containing residual food and fluid. There is no gas bubble in the stomach because no bolus with its accompanying normal gas bubble ever passes through the sphincter. The oesophagus becomes dilated ('mega-oesophagus') and tortuous with a persistent retention oesophagitis due to fermentation of food residues (Fig. 50.62). There is an increased incidence of carcinoma of the oesophagus in patients with achalasia.

> Beware pseudoachalasia
> Look for tumour

(b)

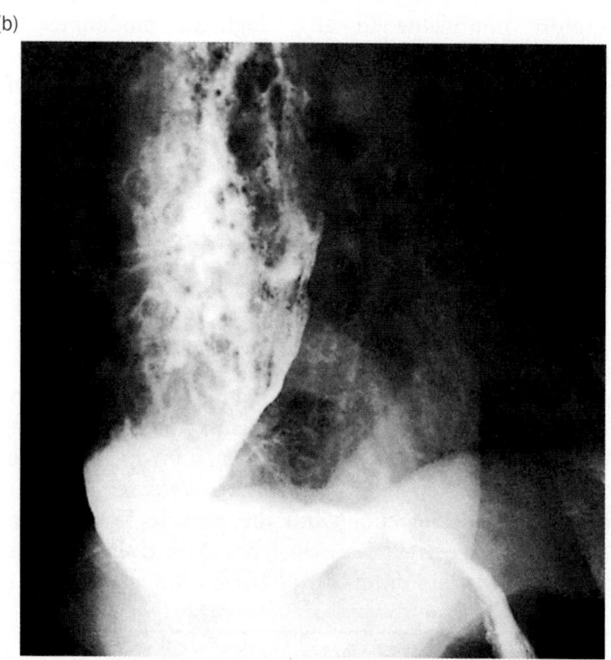

(c)

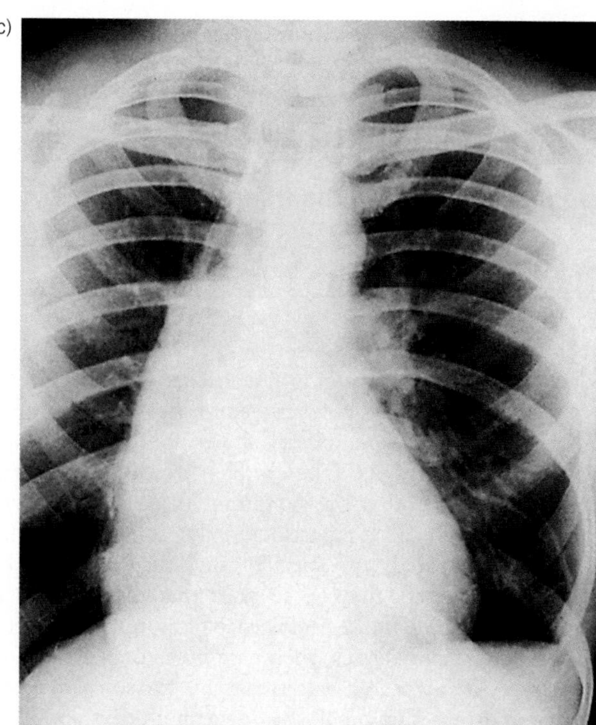

Fig. 50.62 Achalasia of the oesophagus. (a) Barium swallow showing smooth outline of the stricture, which narrows to a point at its lower end; (b) tortuosity and sigmoid appearance of lower oesophagus; (c) mediastinal shadow due to large fluid-filled oesophagus.

Pseudoachalasia is an achalasia-like disorder which is usually produced by adenocarcinoma of the cardia (Fig. 50.63) and sometimes also by cancers outside the oesophagus such as bronchogenic cancer, especially oat cell cancer, and pancreatic cancer.

Clinical features

The disease is commonest in middle life, but can occur at any age. It typically presents with dysphagia. In patients who have remained untreated for many years regurgitation is frequent and there may be overspill into the trachea, especially at night. In the early stages achalasia may present with retrosternal discomfort and this may lead to a mistaken diagnosis of GORD.

Diagnosis

Achalasia may be suspected at endoscopy by finding a tight cardia and food residue in the oesophagus. Barium radiology may show hold-up in the distal oesophagus, peristaltic dysfunction and a tapering stricture in the distal oesophagus often described as a bird's beak (Fig. 50.62). The gastric gas

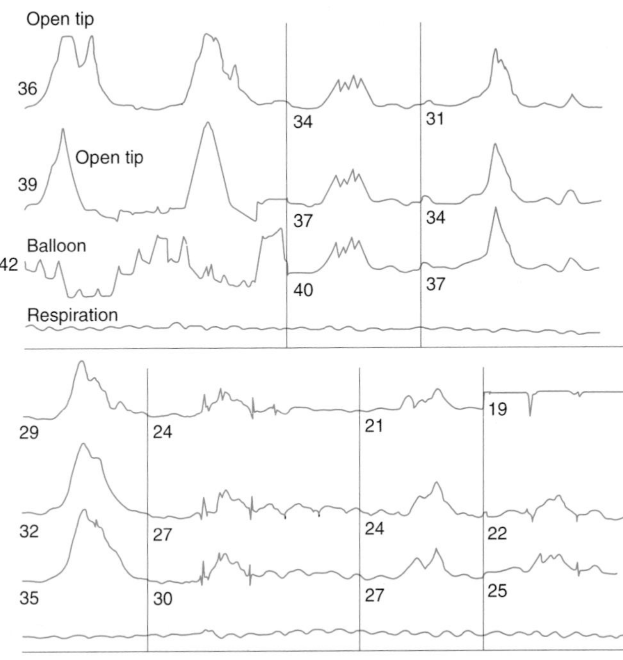

Fig. 50.64 Manometry in achalasia showing simultaneous contractions in the body of the oesophagus and incomplete relaxation of the LOS in response to swallowing.

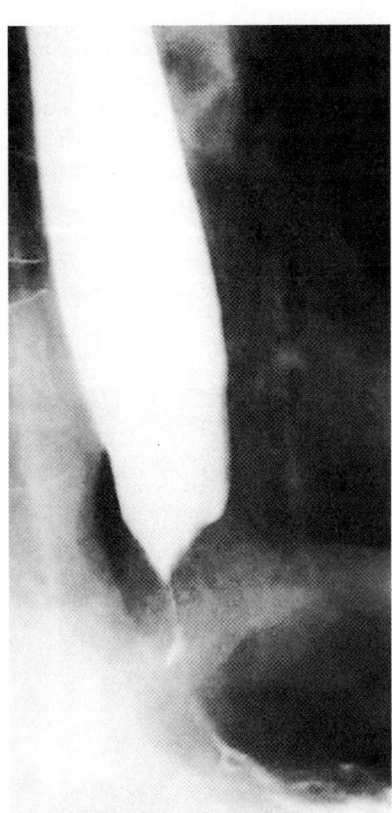

Fig. 50.63 Almost achalasia, but note the irregularity of the taper which indicates carcinoma of the cardia.

bubble is usually absent. However, these typical features of well-developed achalasia are often absent, and endoscopy and radiology are often normal. The barium meal may even be reported as showing gastro-oesophageal reflux. A firm diagnosis can only be made by oesophageal manometry. Classically there is a hypertensive lower oesophageal sphincter that does not relax completely on swallowing, aperistalsis of the oesophageal body and a raised resting pressure in the oesophagus (Fig. 50.64). In practice the LOS pressure is often normal.

Treatment

Alone among motility disorders achalasia responds well to treatment. The two main methods are forceful dilatation of the cardia and Heller's myotomy.

Beware perforation

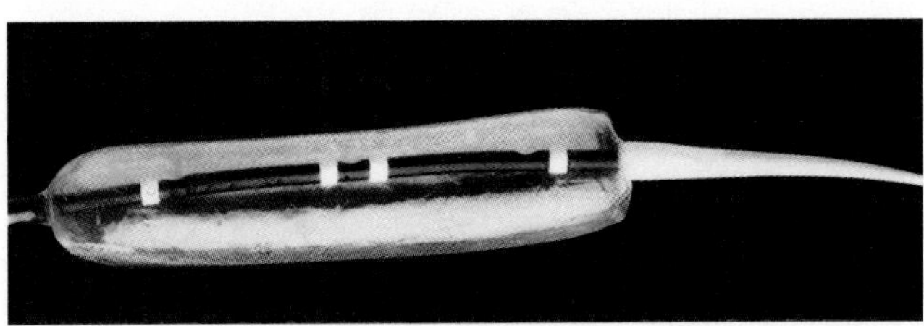

Fig. 50.65 Balloon dilator for treatment of achalasia by forceful dilatation.

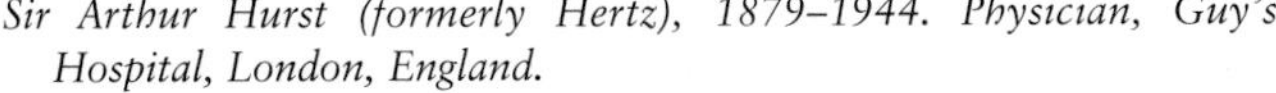

Sir Arthur Hurst (formerly Hertz), 1879–1944. Physician, Guy's Hospital, London, England.

Forceful dilatation. This involves stretching the cardia with a balloon to disrupt the muscle and render it less competent. The treatment was first described in the Mayo Clinic by Plummer. Many varieties of balloon have been available in the past, but nowadays plastic balloons with a precisely controlled external diameter are used. If the pressure in the balloon is too high the balloon is designed to split along its length rather than expanding further. Balloons of 30–40 mm diameter are available and are inserted over a guidewire (Fig. 50.65). Perforation is the major complication. With a 30-mm balloon the incidence of perforation should be less than 0.5 per cent. The risk of perforation increases with the bigger balloons and they should be used cautiously for progressive dilatation over a period of weeks. Forceful dilatation is curative in 75–85 per cent of cases. The results are best in patients aged more than 45 years.

Beware postoperative reflux

Heller's myotomy. This involves cutting the muscle of the lower oesophagus and cardia (Fig. 50.66). The major complication is gastro-oesophageal reflux. Reflux may be avoided by limiting the incision to the lower oesophagus and not more than 1 cm of the stomach. If the myotomy is carried further on to the stomach a prophylactic antireflux operation should be done. It is customary to perform a partial rather than a total fundoplication in this situation because of the risk of causing dysphagia in the presence of an aperistaltic oesophagus. However, a total fundoplication may be done provided that great care is taken to produce a very short and floppy fundoplication that does not cause obstruction. The proximal extent of the myotomy does not seem to matter provided that the obstructing segment is divided.

Heller's myotomy is ideally suited to a minimal access approach by either thoracoscopy or laparoscopy. It is successful in more than 90 per cent of cases and may be used after failed myotomy.

Botulinum toxin. This may be given by endoscopic injection into the LOS. This is a new form of treatment whose place is not yet established. It acts by interfering with cholinergic excitatory neural activity at the LOS.

Drugs. Drugs, such as calcium channel antagonists, have been used but are ineffective for long-term use. Sublingual nifedipine may, however, be useful for transient relief of symptoms if definitive treatment has to be postponed.

Other oesophageal motility disorders

Disorders of the pharyngo-oesophageal junction

These are for the most part neurological disorders and surgery has very little place in their management. Rarely, cricopharyngeal myotomy may be performed to reduce dysphagia in a myopathy affecting the pharyngeal muscles. For this to be successful there must be some preserved contraction of the pharynx and a stable neurological condition.

Cricopharyngeal 'achalasia' is a condition in which the upper oesophageal sphincter does not open adequately during swallowing. A cricopharyngeal 'bar' may be visible on a barium swallow. The disorder is probably caused by degeneration of the cricopharyngeal muscle with consequent loss of elasticity. The condition is rare, but responds well to cricopharyngeal myotomy. A similar abnormality of the

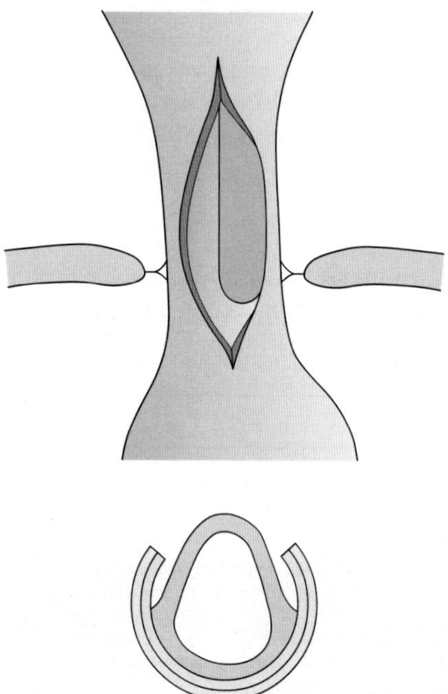

Fig. 50.66 Heller's myotomy weakens the sphincter, but should not completely destroy it. The incision should not go too far on to the stomach. The lateral extent must enable mucosa to pout out to prevent the edges healing together again.

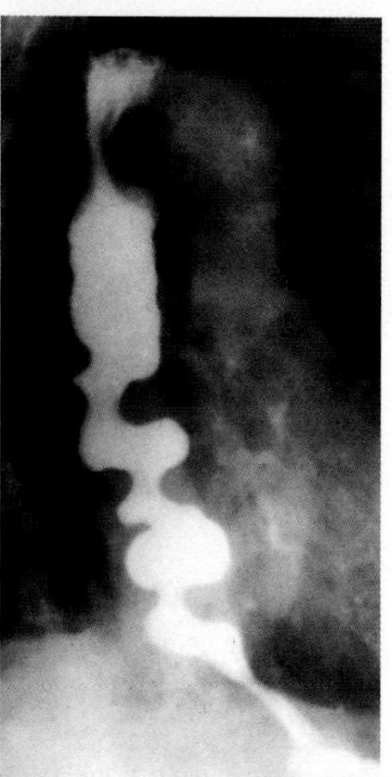

Fig. 50.67 Corkscrew oesophagus in diffuse oesophageal spasm.

cricopharyngeal muscle occurs in Zenker's diverticulum (see below).

Disorders of the body of the oesophagus

Diffuse oesophageal spasm is a condition in which there are incoordinate contractions of the oesophagus causing dysphagia and chest pain. The condition may be dramatic with spastic pressures on manometry of 400–500 mmHg, marked hypertrophy of the circular muscle and a corkscrew oesophagus on barium swallow (Fig. 50.67). If chest pain is the only symptom and the abnormality is not particularly dramatic it may be difficult to be sure that the disorder is the cause of the pain and not an epiphenomenon. Prolonged ambulatory oesophageal manometry with a detailed record of the timing of episodes of chest pain may help to make a diagnosis.

Dysphagia due to diffuse spasm may respond to forceful dilatation of the cardia, but the results are not as predictable as in achalasia. In very severe cases extended oesophageal myotomy up to the aortic arch may be required. Surgical treatment of diffuse spasm is more successful in improving dysphagia than chest pain and caution should be exercised in patients in whom chest pain is the only symptom.

Nutcracker oesophagus is a condition in which peristaltic pressures greater than 180 mmHg are developed. It is said to cause chest pain, but there is still some debate as to whether it is a real disorder.

Hypoperistalsis of the oesophagus occurs in the CREST variant of systemic sclerosis (Fig. 50.68), in severe GORD and sometimes for no obvious cause. Simultaneous oesophageal manometry and radiological studies have shown that a peristaltic pressure of about 30 mmHg is required to propel a bolus down the oesophagus. Peristaltic failure may cause dysphagia in its own right, but can also increase dysphagia if there is any organic obstruction. This is common in the CREST syndrome in which reflux is common as a result of the weak muscle in the lower oesophagus and even the must subtle peptic stricture causes severe dysphagia. Treatment aims at excluding organic obstruction and trying to improve the force of peristalsis with prokinetic agents such as cisapride. However, once peristaltic failure occurs it is usually irreversible.

When GORD and dysmotility occur together it is best to treat the reflux and ignore the dysmotility. It is commonly held that weak peristalsis is a contraindication to total fundoplication, but the author has not found this to be the case provided that care is taken with the construction of the fundoplication.

Eosinophilic oesophagitis is a distinct pathological entity described in patients who have intermittent dysphagia without GORD and without anatomical obstruction. Episodes of dysphagia may be severe and painful with bolus obstruction. Between episodes swallowing may be completely normal.

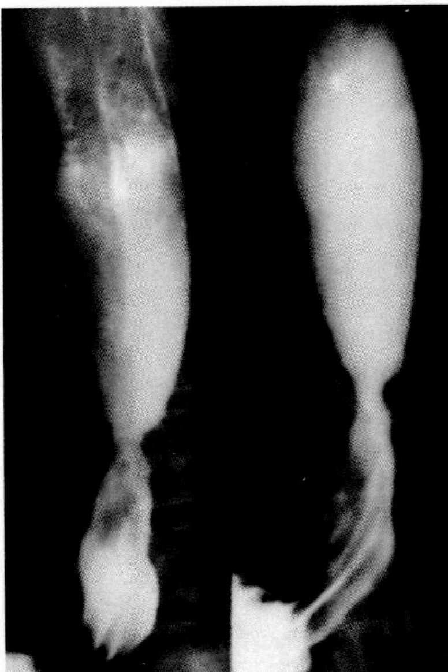

Fig. 50.68 Advanced scleroderma of the oesophagus. The oesophagus dilates and the LOS is widely incompetent.

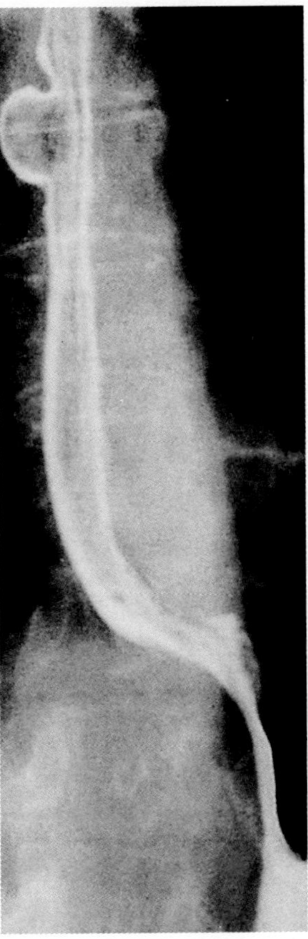

Fig. 50.69 Mid-oesophageal traction diverticulum with the mouth facing downwards.

Friedrich Albert von Zenker, 1825–98. German pathologist.

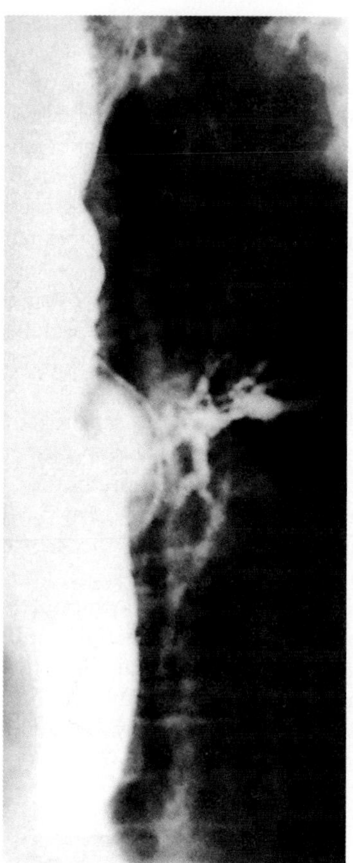

Fig. 50.70 Mid-oesophageal diverticulum with a tracheo-oesophageal fistula.

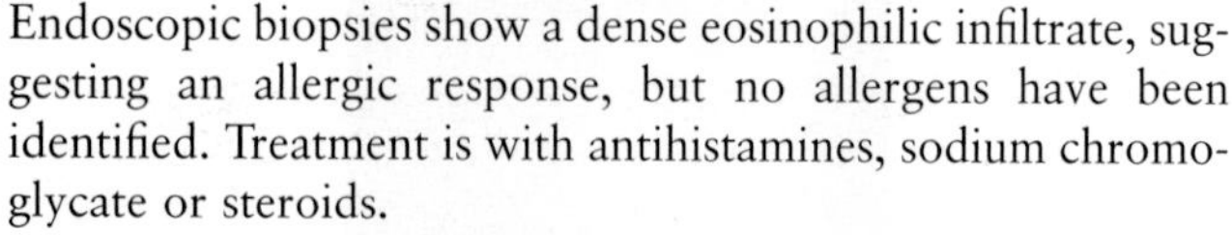

Endoscopic biopsies show a dense eosinophilic infiltrate, suggesting an allergic response, but no allergens have been identified. Treatment is with antihistamines, sodium chromoglycate or steroids.

Hypertensive lower oesophageal sphincter is defined as an LOS pressure greater than 45 mmHg with normal relaxation during swallowing. It is said to be associated with chest pain and dysphagia.

Oesophageal diverticula

Most oesophageal diverticula are *pulsion* diverticula that develop at a site of weakness as a result of chronic pressure against an obstruction. The symptoms are mostly caused by the underlying disorder unless the diverticulum is particularly large. *Traction* diverticula (Fig. 50.69) are much less common. They are mostly a consequence of chronic granulomatous disease affecting the tracheobronchial lymph nodes due to tuberculosis, atypical mycobacteria or histoplasmosis. Fibrotic healing of the lymph nodes exerts traction on the oesophageal wall and produces a focal outpouching that is usually small and has a conical shape. There may be associated broncholithiasis and additional complications may occur such as oesophagobronchial fistulation (Fig. 50.70) and bleeding.

(a)

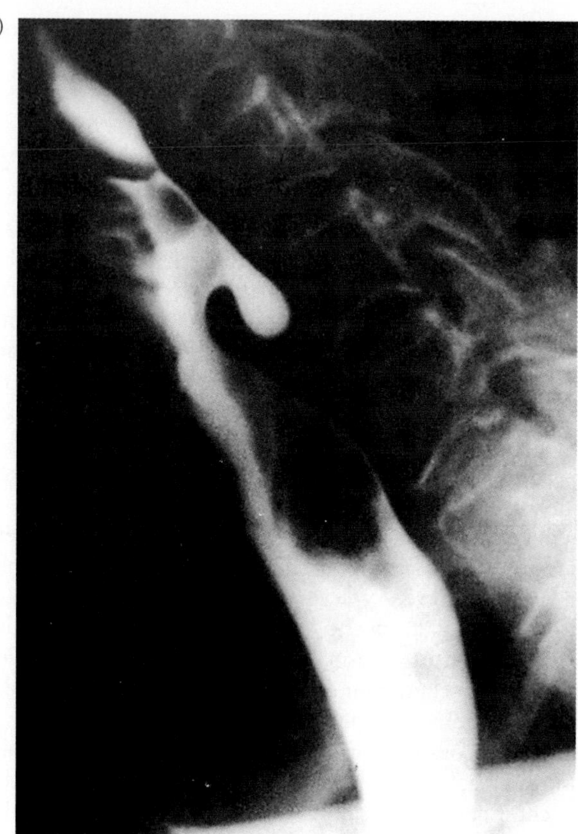

(b)

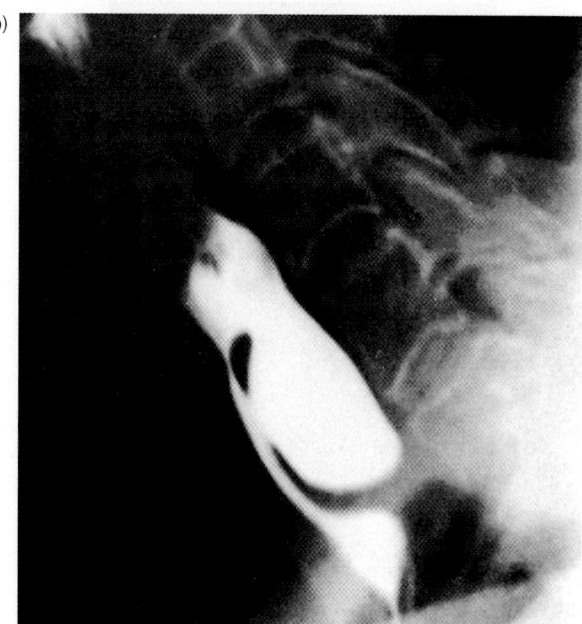

Fig. 50.71 The typical appearances of: (a) a small pharyngeal pouch with a prominent cricopharyngeal impression and 'streaming' of barium indicating partial obstruction; (b) a large pouch extending behind the oesophagus towards the thoracic inlet.

Zenker's diverticulum (pharyngeal pouch) is not really an oesophageal diverticulum as it protrudes posteriorly above the cricopharyngeal sphincter through the natural weak point between the oblique and horizontal fibres of the inferior pharyngeal constrictor (Figs 50.71 and 50.72). Nevertheless it is the commonest diverticulum affecting the region of the oesophagus. The underlying abnormality is the same as in cricopharyngeal achalasia. The diverticulum may be large and extend into the posterior mediastinum. Treatment is always necessary sooner or later. The optimum treatment is excision of the diverticulum combined with cricopharyngeal myotomy to deal with the underlying obstruction. In frail patients or those who decline formal operation an endoscopic linear cutting staple gun may be inserted through the mouth and fired to divide the septum between the diverticulum and the upper oesophagus producing a diverticulo-oesophagostomy.

Excision and myotomy for Zenker's diverticulum

Mid-oesophageal diverticula are usually small pulsion diverticula of no particular consequence. The underlying motility disorder does not usually require treatment. The exception to this rule is in areas of the world in which granulomatous diseases of the mediastinum are common, such as parts of the USA, where the possibility of a traction diverticulum should be considered. Some pulsion diverticula may fistulate into the trachea (Fig. 50.70), but this is much more common in granulomatous disease.

Epiphrenic diverticula are situated in the lower oesophagus above the diaphragm (Fig. 50.73). They may be quite large, but cause surprisingly few symptoms. If surgical

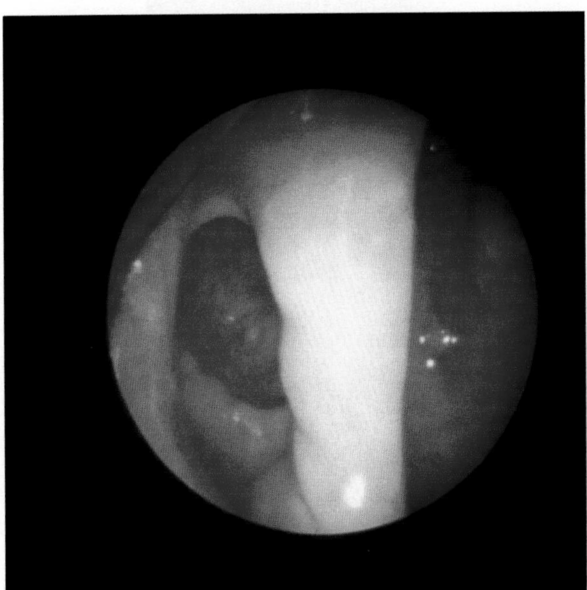

Fig. 50.72 The endoscopic appearance of the mouth of a pharyngeal pouch posterior to the normal opening (left of picture) of the oesophagus.

(a)

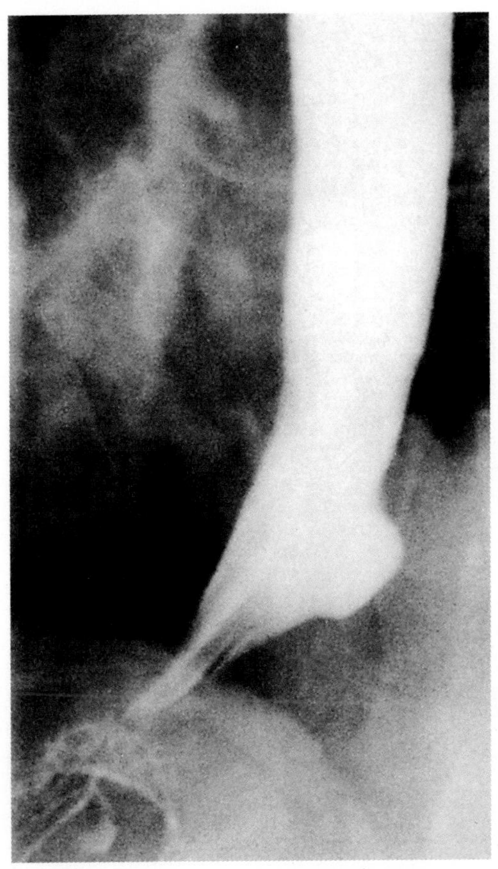

(b)

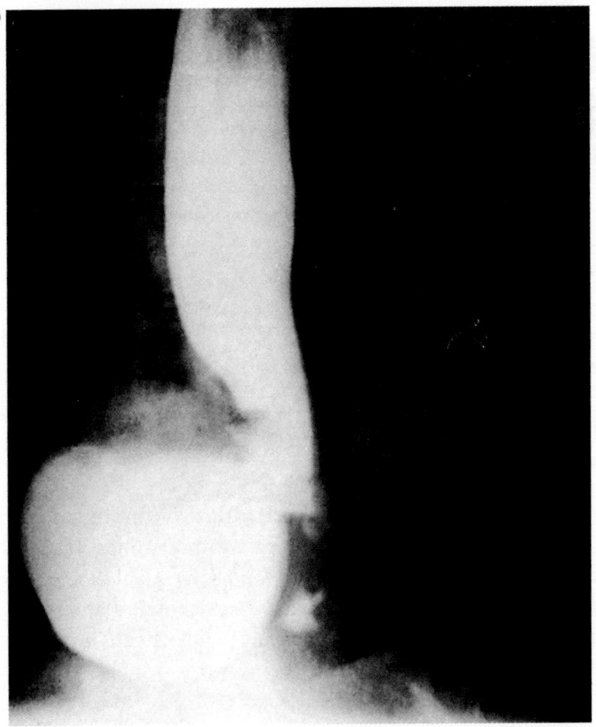

Fig. 50.73 Epiphrenic diverticulum proximal to the gastro-oesophageal sphincter: (a) small and asymptomatic; (b) large, symptomatic and appearing as a gas-filled bubble on chest X-ray.

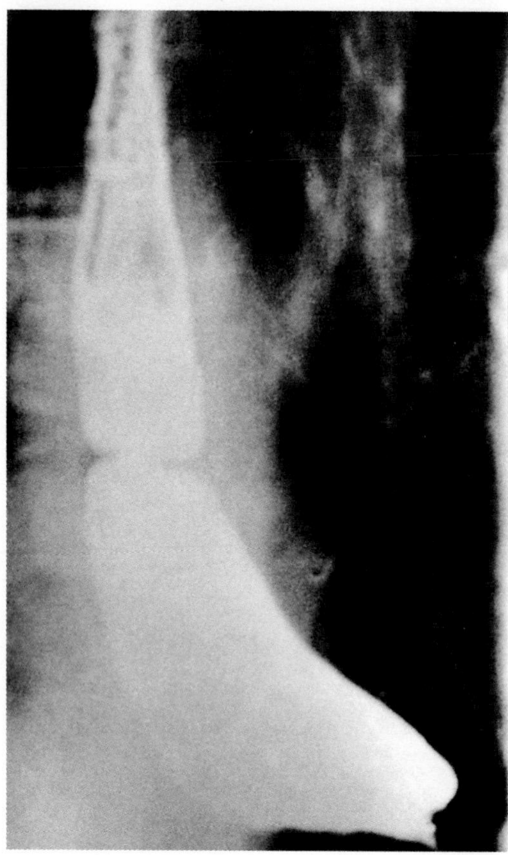

Fig. 50.74 Schatzki's ring, a thin submucosal web completely encircling the whole of the lumen usually situated at the squamocolumnar junction.

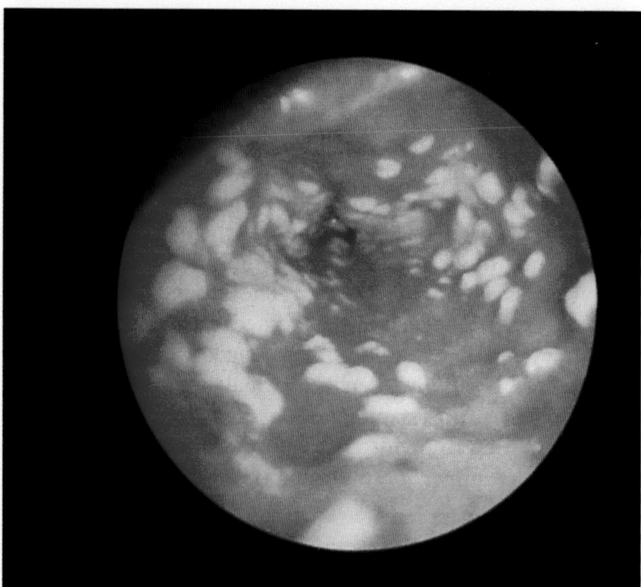

Fig. 50.75 Endoscopic appearance of oesophageal candidiasis.

treatment is required the precise cause of the symptoms, such as GORD, must be defined and corrected at the same time. The diverticulum cannot be assumed to account for the patient's illness just because it looks dramatic on an X-ray. Large diverticula may be excised and it is usual to perform a myotomy from the site of the diverticulum down to the cardia to relieve the functional obstruction and to reduce the risk of dehiscence of the suture line in the oesophagus.

The diverticulum may not be the cause of the symptoms

Diffuse intramural pseudodiverticulosis is a rare condition in which there are multiple tiny outpouchings from the lumen of the oesophagus. The pseudodiverticula are dilated excretory ducts of oesophageal sebaceous glands. It is questionable whether the condition produces any symptoms in its own right.

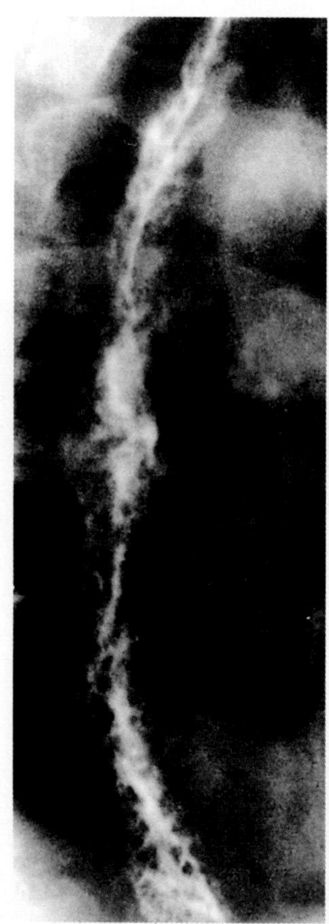

Fig. 50.76 Oesophageal candidiasis with shaggy appearance of mucosal defects.

Richard Schatzki, b. 1901. American radiologist.

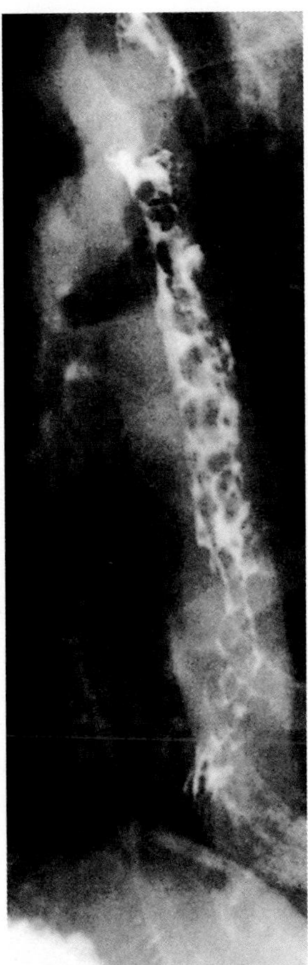

Fig. 50.77 Oesophageal varices with smooth outline of the filling defects.

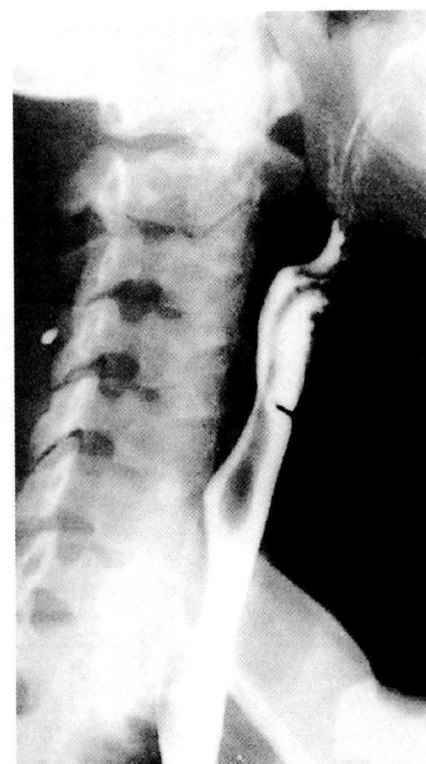

Fig. 50.78 Postcricoid web. This is a thin submucosal fibrotic narrowing that can be easily dilated.

Other non-neoplastic conditions

Schatzki's ring

Schatzki's ring is a circular ring in the distal oesophagus (Fig. 50.74), usually at the squamocolumnar junction. The cause is obscure. The core of the ring consists of variable amounts of fibrous tissue and cellular infiltrate. Most rings are incidental findings on barium examination. Some are associated with dysphagia and a single dilatation is curative.

Monilial oesophagitis

Oesophagitis due to *Candida albicans* is relatively common in patients taking steroids, including steroid inhalers for asthma. It may present with dysphagia or odynophagia. There may be visible thrush in the throat. Endoscopy shows numerous white plaques that cannot be moved, unlike food residues (Fig. 50.75). Biopsies are diagnostic. In severe cases a barium swallow may show dramatic mucosal ulceration and irregularity that is surprisingly similar to the appearance of oesophageal varices (Figs 50.76 and 50.77). Treatment is with nystatin lozenges or other antifungal agents.

Acquired immunodeficiency syndrome (AIDS) and the oesophagus

Dysphagia and odynophagia may occur in immune deficiency due to infection with a variety of agents including *Candida*, *herpes simplex* virus and *cytomegalovirus*. Similar infections may arise in immune suppression due to any other cause.

Crohn's disease

The oesophagus is not commonly affected by Crohn's disease. Rarely, it may be the *only* site of Crohn's disease. When it occurs symptoms are severe and may be mistaken for unusually severe reflux oesophagitis with retrosternal pain and dysphagia. Endoscopy shows extensive oesophagitis that extends much further proximally than is the case with reflux oesophagitis. Biopsies may be diagnostic, but may show only nonspecific inflammation. In severe cases a barium swallow may show deep sinuses in the oesophagus. Crohn's oesophagitis responds poorly to medical treatment and resection may be required. Reconstruction can be a challenging problem in a patient with widespread Crohn's disease at other sites.

Burrill Bernard Crohn, b. 1884. Gastroenterologist, Mount Sinai Hospital, New York, USA.

Plummer–Vinson syndrome

Also called the Brown Kelly–Paterson syndrome or *sideropenic dysphagia*, this may be a pathological relic. The original descriptions are vague and poorly supported by evidence of a coherent syndrome. They describe young women with iron deficiency anaemia and dysphagia referred high in the neck. The dysphagia was said to be caused by spasm or a web in the postcricoid area. The patients were said to have an increased tendency to postcricoid cancer.

Webs certainly occur in the upper oesophagus (Fig. 50.78), but their connection with any particular syndrome is questionable. The pathology is uncertain. More recently it has been noted that there is often a patch of heterotopic gastric mucosa in the upper oesophagus. It is probably congenital and may be seen in up to 4 per cent of endoscopic examinations. Most are small, less than 1 cm^2, and are easily missed. Occasional complications have been reported, such as ulceration, stricture and adenocarcinoma. Perhaps the Plummer–Vinson syndrome is a case of mistaken identity.

Henry Stanley Plummer, 1874–1957. Physician, Mayo Clinic, Rochester, Minnesota, USA.

Porter Paisley Vinson, 1890–1959. Physician, Mayo Clinic, Rochester, Minnesota, USA.

Adam Brown Kelly, 1865–1941. Surgeon, Ear, Nose and Throat Department, Victoria Infirmary, Glasgow, Scotland.

Donald Rose Paterson, 1862–1939. Surgeon, Ear, Nose and Throat Department, Royal Infirmary, Cardiff, Wales.

Further reading

Akiyama, H. (1990) *Surgery for Cancer of the Esophagus*, Williams and Wilkins, Baltimore, MD.

Castell, D.O. (1995) *The Esophagus*, 2nd edn, Little, Brown, Boston, MA.

Griffin, S.M. and Raimes, S.A. (1997) *Upper Gastrointestinal Surgery*, W.B. Saunders, London.

Hennessy, T.P.J. and Cuschieri, A. (1992) *Surgery of the Oesophagus*, 2nd edn, Butterworth-Heinemann, Oxford.

Jamieson, G.G. (1988) *Surgery of the Oesophagus*, Churchill Livingstone, Edinburgh.

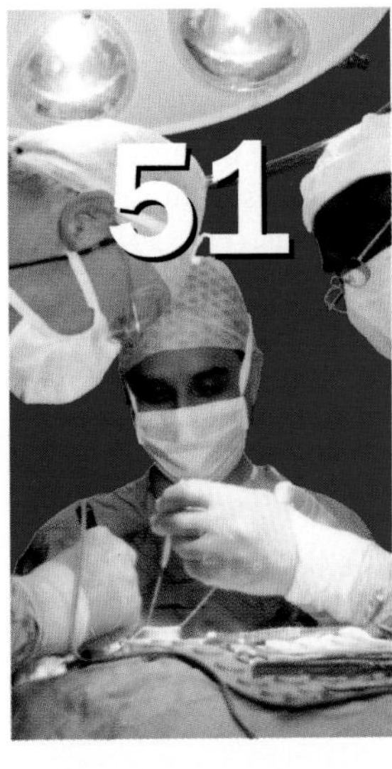

Stomach and duodenum

Surgical anatomy

Introduction

The function of the stomach is to act as a reservoir for ingested food. It also serves to break down foodstuffs mechanically and commence the processes of digestion before these products are passed on into the duodenum. The surgical anatomy must be viewed in this context.

Blood supply

Arterial supply

The stomach is richly endowed with an arterial supply on both lesser and great curves (Fig. 51.1). On the lesser curve the left gastric artery, a branch of the coeliac axis, forms an anastomotic arcade with the right gastric artery which arises from the common hepatic artery. Branches of the left gastric artery pass up towards the cardia. The gastroduodenal artery, which is also a branch of the hepatic artery, passes behind the first part of the duodenum, highly relevant with respect to the bleeding duodenal ulcer. Here it divides into the superior pancreaticoduodenal artery and the right gastroepiploic artery. The superior pancreaticoduodenal artery supplies the duodenum and pancreatic head, and forms an anastomosis

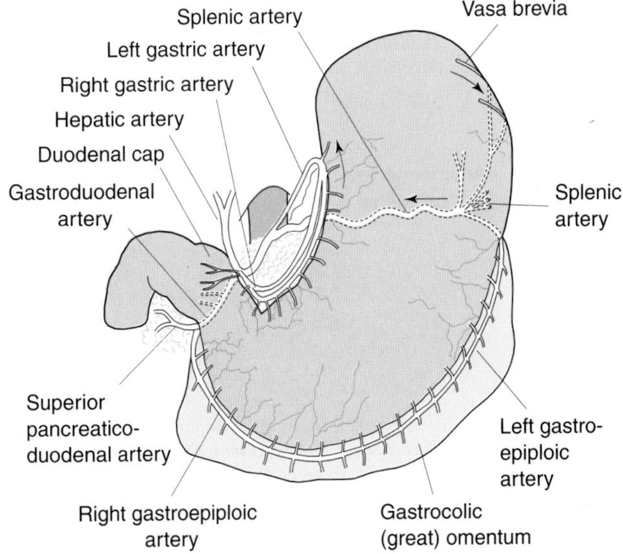

Fig. 51.1 The arterial blood supply of the stomach.

Bailey & Love's Short Practice of Surgery, 23rd edition. Edited by R.C.G. Russell, N.S. Williams and C.J.K. Bulstrode. Published in 2000 by Arnold Publishers.

with the inferior pancreaticoduodenal artery, a branch of the superior mesenteric artery. The right gastroepiploic artery runs along the greater curvature of the stomach eventually forming an anastomosis with the left gastroepiploic artery, a branch of the splenic artery. This vascular arcade, however, is often variably incomplete. The fundus of the stomach is supplied by the vasa brevia (or short gastric arteries) which arise from near the termination of the splenic artery.

Veins

In general the veins are equivalent to the arteries, those along the lesser curve ending in the portal vein and those on the greater curve joining via the splenic vein. On the lesser curve the coronary vein is particularly important. It runs up the lesser curve towards the oesophagus and then passes left to right to join the portal vein. This vein becomes markedly dilated in portal hypertension.

Lymphatics

The lymphatics of the stomach are of considerable importance in the surgery of gastric cancer and are therefore described in detail in that section (later).

Innervation

As with all of the gastrointestinal tract, the stomach and duodenum possess both intrinsic and extrinsic nerve supplies. The intrinsic nerves exist principally in two plexuses, the myenteric plexus of Auerbach and the submucosal plexus of Meissner. Compared with the rest of the gut the submucosal plexus of the stomach contains relatively few ganglionic cells as does the myenteric plexus in the fundus. However, in the antrum the ganglia of the myenteric plexus are well developed. The extrinsic supply is derived mainly from the vagus nerves, fibres of which originate in the brainstem. The vagal plexus around the oesophagus condenses into bundles which pass through the oesophageal hiatus (Fig. 51.2), the posterior bundle being usually identifiable as a large nerve trunk. Vagal fibres are both afferent (sensory) and efferent. The efferent fibres are involved in the receptive relaxation of the stomach and the stimulation of gastric motility, as well as the well-known secretory function. The sympathetic supply is derived mainly from the coeliac ganglia.

Histological anatomy of the stomach and duodenum

Stomach

The gastric epithelial cells are mucous producing and are turned over rapidly. In the pyloric part of the stomach and also the duodenum mucus-secreting glands are found. Most of the specialised cells of the stomach (parietal and chief cells) are found in the gastric crypts (Fig. 51.3). The stomach is also richly endowed with endocrine cells.

Parietal cells

These are in the body (acid-secreting portion) of the stomach and line the gastric crypts, more abundant distally. These are responsible for the production of hydrogen ions to form hydrochloric acid, which has a pH of around 1. The hydrogen ions are actively pumped by the proton pump, a hydrogen–potassium APTase (Sachs) which exchanges intraluminal

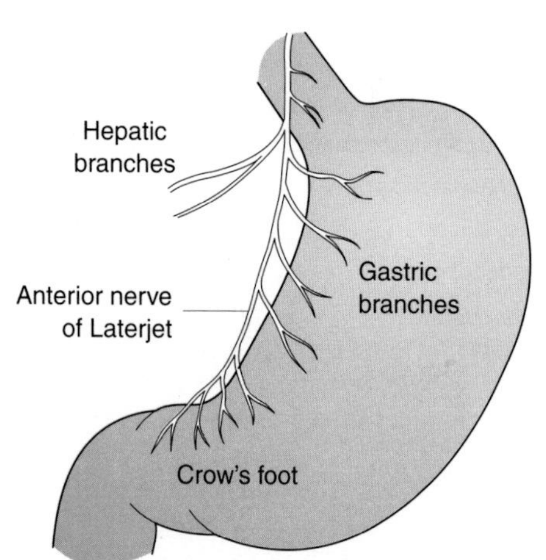

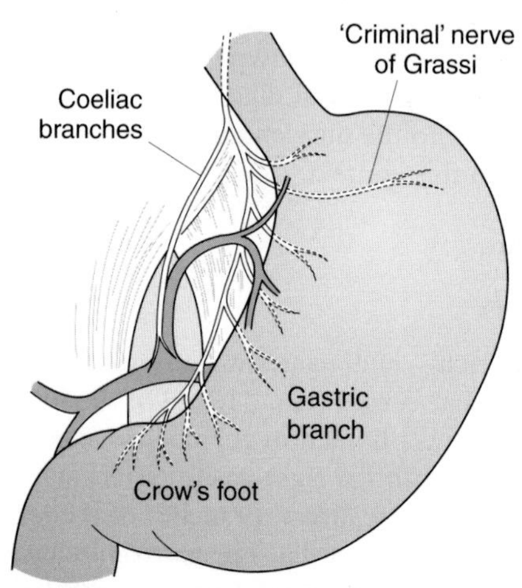

Fig. 51.2 The anatomy of the anterior and posterior vagus nerves in relation to the stomach. [Reproduced with permission from *Rob and Smith's Operative Surgery. Surgery of the Upper Gastrointestinal Tract*, 5th edn (eds G. Jamieson and H. Debas), Chapman & Hall, London, 1994, pp. 357–358.]

Leopold Auerbach, 1828–97. Professor of Neuropathology, Breslau, Germany.
Georg Meissner, 1829–1905. German physiologist.

George Sachs. Discoverer of the proton pump, Professor of Medicine, CURE, Los Angeles, California, USA.

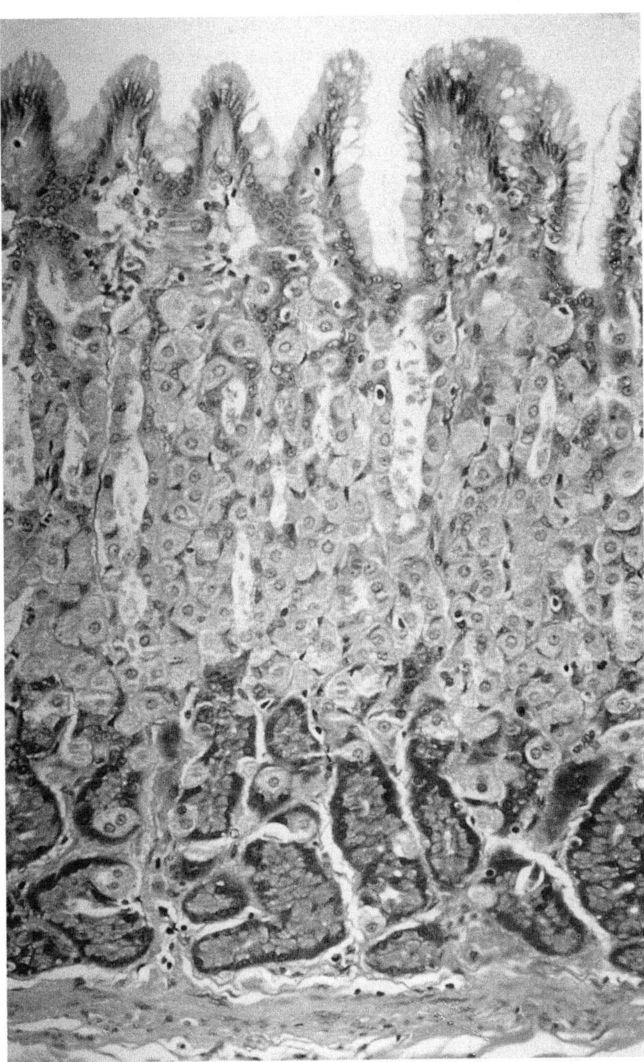

Fig. 51.3 The histological appearance of a gastric gland. The mucus-secreting cells are seen at the mucosal surface, the eosinophilic parietal cells superficially in the glands and the basophilic chief cells in the deepest layer.

potassium for hydrogen ions. The potassium ions enter the lumen of the crypts passively but the hydrogen ions are pumped against an immense concentration gradient (1 000 000:1), explaining the fact that this is an energy-consuming process.

Chief cells

These lie principally proximally in the gastric crypts and produce pepsinogen. Two forms of pepsinogen are described: pepsinogen I and pepsinogen II. Both are produced by the chief cell but pepsinogen I is produced only in the stomach. The ratio between pepsinogens I and II in the serum decreases with gastric atrophy, and this has been investigated as a means of selecting patients who are at higher risk of suffering from gastric cancer for screening. Pepsinogen is activated in the stomach to produce pepsin, the active enzyme.

Endocrine cells

The stomach is richly endowed with endocrine cells, which are critical to its function. In the gastric antrum the mucosa contains G cells which produce gastrin. Throughout the body of the stomach enterochromatin-like (ECL) cells are abundant and produce histamine, a key factor in gastric acid secretion. In addition, there are large numbers of somatostatin-producing D cells throughout the stomach, and somatostatin has a negative regulatory role. The peptides and neuropeptides produced in the stomach are discussed later.

Duodenum

The duodenum is lined by a mucus-secreting columnar epithelium. In addition, Brunner's glands lie beneath the mucosa and are similar to the pyloric glands in the pyloric part of the stomach. Endocrine cells in duodenum produce cholecystokinin and secretin.

Physiology of the stomach and duodenum

Introduction

The stomach mechanically breaks up ingested food and, together with the actions of acid and pepsin, forms chyme that passes into the duodenum. In contrast to the acidic environment of the stomach, that of the duodenum is alkaline, as a result of the secretion of bicarbonate ions from both the pancreas and the duodenum. This neutralises the acid chyme and adjusts the osmolarity to approximately that of plasma. Endocrine cells in the duodenum produce cholecystokinin that stimulates the pancreas to produce trypsin and the gall bladder to contract. Secretin is also produced by the endocrine cells of the duodenum. This hormone inhibits gastric acid secretion and promotes production of bicarbonate by the pancreas.

Gastric acid secretion

The secretion of gastric acid and pepsin tends to run in parallel, although the understanding of the mechanisms of gastric acid secretion is considerably greater than that of pepsin. Numerous factors are involved to some degree in the production of the gastric acid. These include neurotransmitters, neuropeptides and peptide hormones, and several other factors. This complexity need not detract from the fact that there are basic principles that are relatively easily understood (Fig. 51.4). As mentioned above, hydrogen ions are produced by the parietal cell by the proton pump. Although there is a multiplicity of factors that can act on the parietal cell, it is now widely accepted that the most important of these transmitters is histamine, which acts via the H_2 receptor. Histamine in turn is produced by the ECL cells of the stomach and acts in a paracrine (local) fashion on the

---

Johann Conrad Brunner, 1653–1729. Anatomist, Basel, Switzerland.

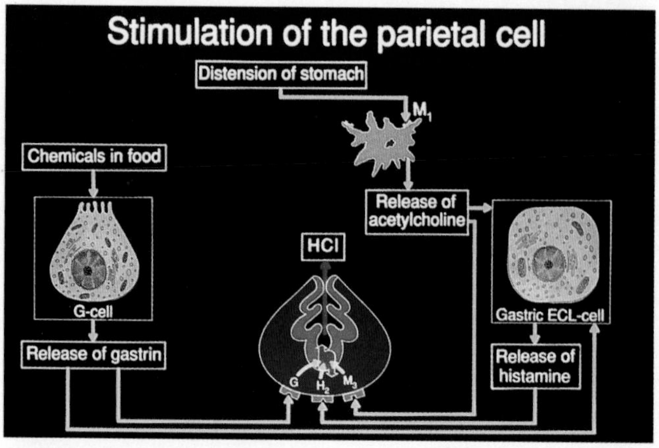

Fig. 51.4 The parietal cell in relation to the mechanism of gastric acid secretion.

parietal cells. These relationships explain why proton pump inhibitors can abolish gastric acid secretion, as they act on the final common pathway secretion, and why H_2-receptor antagonists have such profound effects on gastric acid secretion, even though this is not insurmountable (Fig. 51.4). The ECL cell produces histamine in response to a number of stimuli that include the vagus and gastrin. Gastrin is released by the G cells in response to the presence of the food in the stomach. The production of gastrin is inhibited by acid, hence creating a negative-feedback loop. Various other peptides, including secretin, inhibit gastric acid secretion.

Classically, three phases of gastric secretion are described. The cephalic phase is mediated by vagal activity secondary to sensory arousal as first demonstrated by Pavlov. The gastric phase is a response to food within the stomach that is mediated principally, but not exclusively, by gastrin. In the intestinal phase, the presence of chyme in the duodenum and small bowel inhibits gastric emptying and, as mentioned above, the acidification of the duodenum leads to the production of secretin that also inhibits gastric acid secretion, along with numerous other peptides originating from the gut. The stomach also possesses somatostatin-containing D cells. Somatostatin is released in response to a number of factors including acidification. This peptide acts probably on the G cell, the ECL cell and the parietal cell itself to inhibit the production of acid both directly and via intermediate pathways.

Gastric mucus and the gastric mucosal barrier

The gastric mucous layer is essential to the integrity of the gastric mucosa. It is a viscid layer of mucopolysaccharides produced by the mucus-producing cells of the stomach and the pyloric glands. Gastric mucus is an important physiological barrier to protect the gastric mucosa from mechanical damage, and also the effects of acid and pepsin. Its considerable buffering capacity is enhanced by the presence of bicarbonate ions within the mucous. Many factors can lead to the break down of this gastric mucous barrier. These include bile, nonsteroidal anti-inflammatory drugs (NSAIDs), alcohol, trauma and shock. Tonometry studies have shown that of all the gastrointestinal tract the stomach is the most sensitive to ischaemia following a hypovolaemic insult and also the slowest to recover. This may explain the high incidence of stress ulceration in the stomach.

Ivan Pavlov, b. 1849. Russian physiologist.

Peptides and neuropeptides in the stomach and duodenum

As with most of the gastrointestinal tract, the stomach is richly endowed with sources of peptide hormones and neurotransmitters. Previously nerves and endocrine cells were considered distinct in terms of their products. However, it is increasingly realised that there is enormous overlap within these systems. Many peptides recognised as hormones may also be produced by neurons, hence the term neuropeptides. The term 'messenger' can be used to describe all such products. There are three conventional modes of action which overlap.

- *Endocrine* – the messenger is secreted into the circulation where it affects tissues which may be remote from the site of origin (Bayliss and Starling).
- *Paracrine* – messengers are produced locally and have local effects on tissues. Neurons and endocrine cells both act in this way.
- *Neurocrine* (classical neurotransmitter) – messengers are produced by the neuron via the synaptic knob and pass across the synaptic cleft to the target.

The *autocrine* mode of action should be mentioned for completeness. Here messengers are released from cell to act on receptors on the same cell's surface membrane. Many growth factors such as epidermal growth factor and transforming growth factors α and β work in this way.

Many peptide hormones act on the intrinsic nerve plexus of the gut (see later) and influence motility. Similarly, neuropeptides may influence the structure and function of the mucosa. Some of these peptides, neuropeptides and neurotransmitters are shown in Table 51.1.

Gastroduodenal motor activity

The motility of the entire gastrointestinal tract is modulated to a large degree by its intrinsic nervous system. Critical in this discussion is the migrating motor complex (MMC). In the fasted state and after food has cleared the small bowel there is a period of quiescence lasting in the region of 40 minutes (phase I). There follows a series of waves, also lasting for about 40 minutes, of electrical and motor activity propagated from the fundus of the stomach in a caudal direction at a rate of about three per minute (phase II). These

William Maddock Bayliss, 1860–1924. Physiologist, University College, London, England. Discovered the first hormone, secretin, with Starling.

Ernest Henry Starling, 1866–1927. Physiologist, University College, London, England. Discovered the first hormone, secretin, with Bayliss.

Table 51.1 Function and source of peptides and neuropeptides in the stomach

Stimulate secretion	*Source*	*Inhibit secretion*	*Source*
Gastrin	G cells	Somatostatin	D cells and neurons
Histamine	ECL cells	Secretin	Duodenal endocrine cells
Acetylcholine	Neurons	Enteroglucagon	Small intestinal endocrine cells
Gastrin releasing peptide	Neurons and mucosa	Prostaglandins	Mucosa
Cholecystokinin (CCK)	Duodenal endocrine cells	Neurotensin	Neurons
		GIP	Duodenal and jejunal endocrine cells
		PYY	Small intestinal endocrine cells
Stimulate motility	*Source*	*Inhibit motility*	*Source*
Acetylcoline	Neuron	Somatostatin	D cells and neurones
5-HT	Neuron	VIP	Neurons
Histamine	ECL cell	Nitric oxide	Neurons and smooth muscle
Substance P	Neuron	Noradrenaline	Neurons
Substance K	Neuron	Encephalin	Neurons
Motilin	Neuron	Dopamine	Neurons
Gastrin	G cells		
Angiotensin			

ECL, enterochromatin-like cells; GIP, gastric inhibitory polypeptide; PYY, peptide YY; VIP, vasoactive intestinal peptide.

pass as far the pylorus but not beyond. Duodenal slow waves are generated in the duodenum at a rate of about 10 per minute that carry down the small bowel. The amplitude of these contractions increases to a maximum in phase III that lasts for about 10 minutes. This 90-minute cycle of activity is then repeated. From the duodenum the MMC moves distally at 5–10 cm/minute reaching the terminal ileum after 1.5 hours.

Following a meal the stomach exhibits receptive relaxation which lasts for a few seconds. Following this adaptive relaxation occurs which allows the proximal stomach to act as a reservoir. Most of the peristaltic activity is found in the distal stomach (the antral mill) and the proximal stomach demonstrates only tonic activity. The pylorus, which is most commonly open, contracts with the peristaltic wave and allows only a few millilitres through at a time. The antral contraction against the closed sphincter is important in the milling activity of the stomach. Although the duodenum is capable of generating 10 waves per minute, after a meal it only contacts after an antral wave reaches the pylorus. The co-ordination of the motility of the antrum, pylorus and duodenum means that only small quantities of food reach the small bowel at a time. Motility is influenced by numerous factors including mechanical stimulation and neuronal and endocrine influences.

Investigation of the stomach and duodenum

Flexible endoscopy

Amongst all of the methods used to investigate and image the stomach and duodenum, flexible endoscopy is now the 'gold standard'. The original gastroscopes were fibre-optic (Hirschowitz), but now most use a solid-state camera mounted at the instrument's tip (Figs 51.5). The main

Basil Hirschowitz. Professor of Medicine, Birmingham, Alabama, USA.

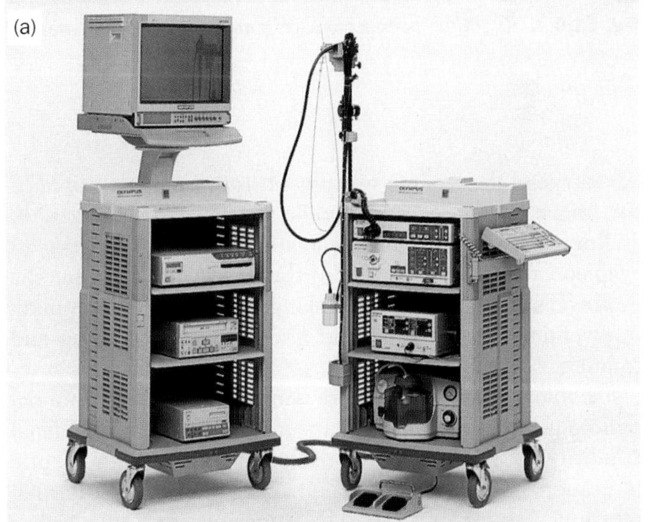

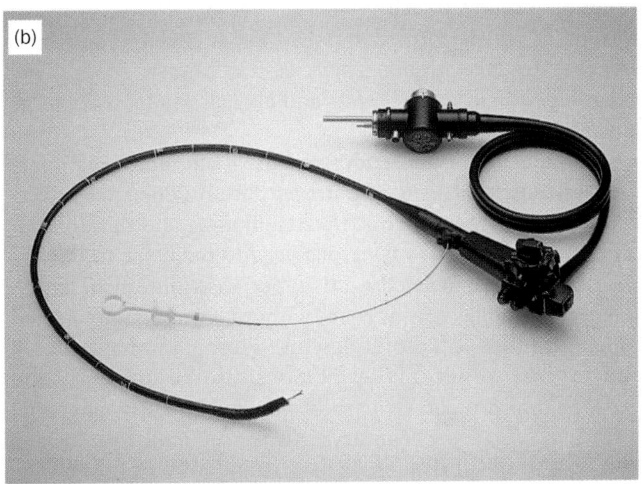

Fig. 51.5 A video gastroscope [*courtesy of KeyMed (Medical and Industrial Equipment) Ltd*].

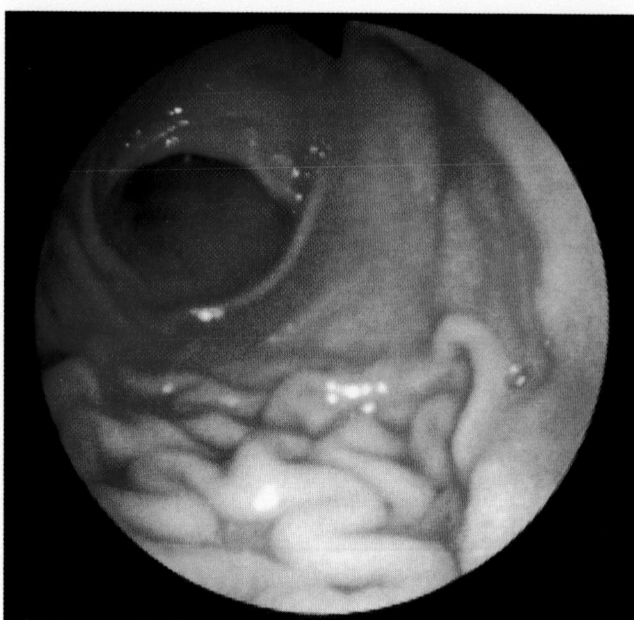

Fig. 51.6 A view of the normal stomach during endoscopy (*courtesy of Dr G.N.J. Tytgat, Amsterdam*).

advantage of the modern instruments is that they do not need the fragile fibre-optic fibre bundle to transmit the image. In addition, as the output is via a monitor rather than an eyepiece, the other members of the endoscopy team see the image. This is useful when taking biopsies or performing interventional techniques, and also facilitates teaching and training.

Flexible endoscopy is more sensitive than conventional radiology in the assessment of the majority of gastroduodenal conditions. This is particularly the case with peptic ulceration, gastritis and duodenitis. In upper gastrointestinal bleeding endoscopy is far superior to any other investigation and in most circumstances is the only imaging required. Although in Japan double-contrast barium meals performed by very experienced radiologists are able to detect quite small gastric cancers, endoscopy is far superior in most centres and also allows biopsies to be taken.

Although fibre-optic endoscopy is a safe and commonly used investigation, it is important that all personnel undertaking this procedure are adequately trained and that resuscitation facilities are always available. Although the morbidity and mortality associated with upper gastrointestinal endoscopy is extremely low, it is not without hazard. Careless and rough handling of the endoscope during intubation of a patient may result in perforations of the pharynx and oesophagus. Any other part of the upper gastrointestinal tract may also be perforated. An inadequately performed endoscopy is also dangerous as a serious condition may be overlooked. This is particularly the case in respect of early and curable gastric cancer, the appearances of which may often be extremely subtle and may be missed by inexperienced endoscopists with tragic consequences. In general, a more experienced endoscopist will have a higher index of suspicion for any mucosal abnormalities and will take more biopsies.

Upper gastrointestinal endoscopy is normally carried out under sedation usually with incremental doses of diazepam or midazolam until the patient is adequately sedated. Midazolam is often preferred for its amnesic effect. Sedation is of particular concern in the case of gastrointestinal bleeding as it may have a more profound effect on the patient's cardiovascular stability. It has now become the standard to use pulse oximetry to monitor patients during upper gastrointestinal endoscopy, and nasal oxygen is often also administered. Opiates are not usually necessary, although they are commonly used for endoscopic retrograde cholangiopancreatography (ERCP). Buscopan is useful to abolish duodenal motility for examinations of the second and third parts of the duodenum. Examinations of this type are best carried out using a side-viewing endoscope such as is used for ERCP.

Some patients are relatively resistant to sedation with benzodiazipenes, particularly those who are accustomed to alcoholic beverages. Increasing the dose of benzodiazepines in these patients may not afford any useful sedation but merely make the patient more restless and confused. Such patients are sometimes better endoscoped fully awake using a local anaesthetic throat spray and a narrow-gauge endoscope. Whatever the circumstances, it is important that resuscitation facilities are available including agents that reverse the effects of benzodiazepines, such as flumazenil.

The technology associated with upper gastrointestinal endoscopy is continuing to advance. Instrumentation is now available in many centres which allows both endoscopy and endoluminal ultrasound to be performed simultaneously (see later). Intervention via the endoscope is also developing rapidly. A variety of haemostatic measures is used in the treatment of bleeding ulcers such as injection with various substances, diathermy, heater probes and lasers. These approaches appear to have utility in the treatment of bleeding ulcers, although good controlled trials in this area are not abundant. There is no good evidence that such interventional procedures at the moment work in patients who are bleeding from very large vessels, such as the gastroduodenal artery or splenic artery.

Contrast radiology

Upper gastrointestinal radiology is not used as much as in previous years as endoscopy is a more sensitive investigation for most gastric problems. There is, however, a number of circumstances where the barium meal is of great value and augments the value of endoscopy. These include large hiatus hernias of the rolling type and chronic gastric volvulus where it may be difficult for the endoscopist to determine exactly the anatomy or, indeed, negotiate the deformity to see the

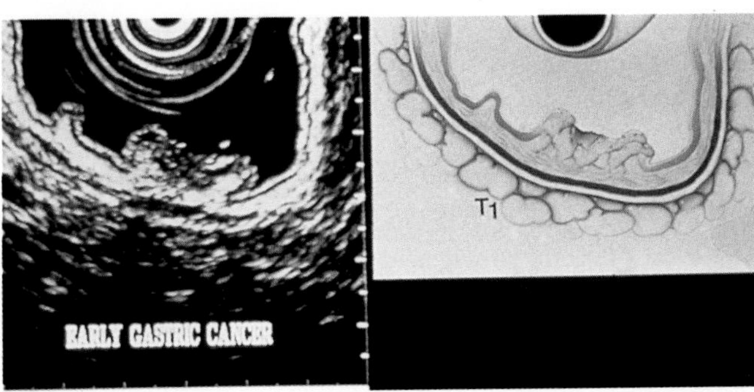

Fig. 51.7 Endoscopic ultrasound of the stomach. Five layers can be identified in the normal stomach. A gastic cancer is shown invading the muscle of the gastric wall (*courtesy of KeyMed (Medical and Industrial Equipment) Ltd*).

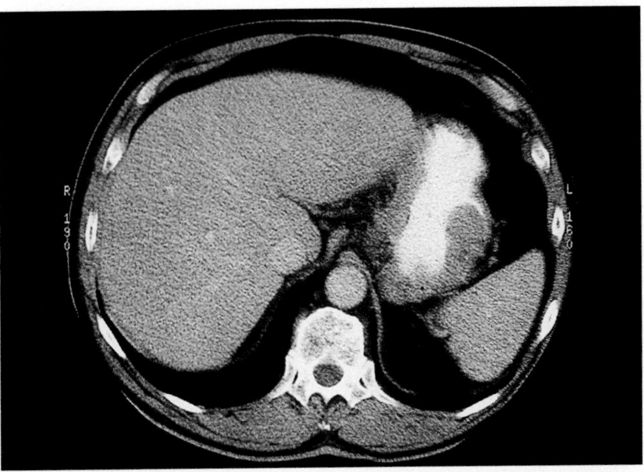

Fig. 51.8 A CT scan of the abdomen showing a gastric cancer arising in the body of the stomach.

distal stomach. Linitus plastica may be missed by even relatively experienced endoscopists as the mucosal aspect of the stomach may not look particularly abnormal. This condition may be diagnosed more easily by using contrast radiology, although this is of limited value to the patient as the outlook is so poor.

Ultrasonography

Standard ultrasound imaging can be used to investigate the stomach, particularly in patients with neoplasia. Thickening of the gastric wall can be seen in malignancy, some assessment made of local invasion, and liver and peritoneal disease is often detected. However, used conventionally, it is less sensitive than other modalities. By contrast, endoluminal ultrasound and laparoscopic ultrasound are probably the most sensitive techniques available in the preoperative staging of gastric cancer. In endoluminal ultrasound the transducer is usually attached to the distal tip of the instrument. However, devices have been developed which may be passed down the biopsy channel, albeit with poorer image quality. Five layers (Fig. 51.7) of the gastric wall may be identified on endoluminal ultrasound and the depth of invasion of a tumour can be assessed with exquisite accuracy (90 per cent accuracy for the 'T' component of the staging). Enlarged lymph nodes can also be identified and the technique's accuracy in this situation is about 80 per cent. Finally, it may be possible to identify liver metastases not seen on axial imaging. Laparoscopic ultrasound is also a very sensitive imaging modality, especially when combined with the laparoscopy (see later). It is one of the most sensitive methods of detecting liver metastases from gastric cancer.

An additional use of ultrasound is in the assessment of gastric emptying. Swallowed contrast is utilised which is designed to be easily seen using an ultrasound transducer. The emptying of this contrast is then followed directly. The accuracy of the technique is similar to that of radioisotope gastric emptying studies (below).

Computerised tomography (CT) scanning and manetic resonance imaging (MRI)

The resolution of the CT scanners is continuing to improve and this form of axial imaging is of increasing value in the investigation of the stomach, especially gastric malignancies (Fig. 51.8). The presence of gastric wall thickening associated with a carcinoma of any reasonable size can be easily detected by CT but the investigation lacks sensitivity in detecting smaller and curable lesions. It is much less accurate in 'T' staging than endoluminal ultrasound. Lymph node enlargement can be detected and, based on the size and shape of the nodes, it is possible to be reasonably accurate in detecting nodal involvement with tumour. However, as with all imaging techniques, it is limited. Microscopic tumour deposits in lymph nodes cannot be detected when the node is not enlarged and, by contrast, lymph nodes may undergo reactive enlargement but not contain tumour. These problems apply to all imaging techniques. The detection of small liver metastases is improving, although in general terms metastases from gastric cancer are less easy to detect using CT than those, for instance, from colorectal cancer. This is because metastases from gastric cancer may be of the same density as liver and may not handle the intravenous contrast any differently. MRI scanning does not at present offer any specific advantage in assessing the stomach, although it has a higher sensitivity for the detection of gastric cancer liver metastases than conventional CT imaging.

Laparoscopy

This technique is now well used in the assessment of patients with gastric cancer. Its particular value is in the detection of peritoneal disease that is difficult by any other technique, unless the patient has ascites or bulky intraperitoneal disease. Its main limitation is in the evaluation of posterior extension but other techniques are available to evaluate posterior

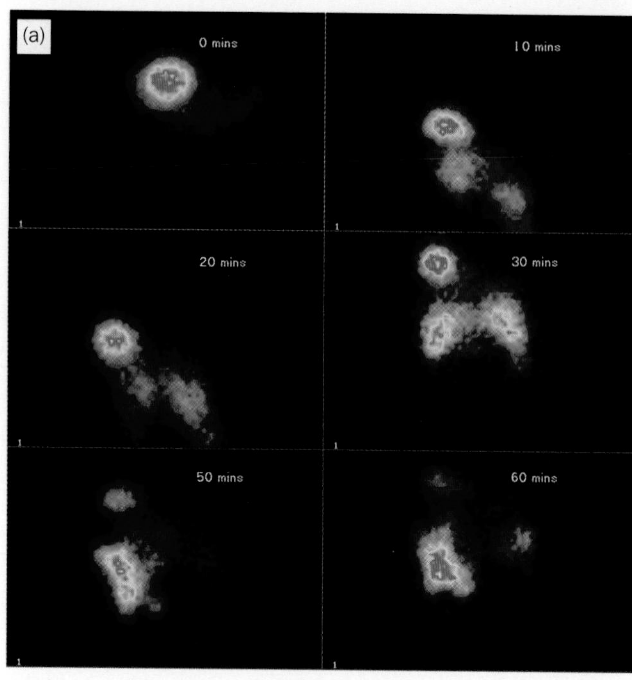

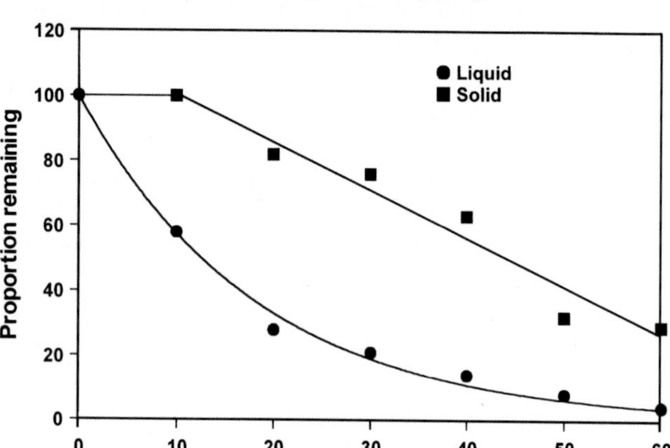

Fig. 51.9 Dual-phase solid and liquid gastric emptying. The use of two isotopic labels allows the liquid and solid phases of the emptying to be followed separately. (a) Anterior image acquisition. (b) Gastric emptying curves in a normal individual showing typical lag period in solid-phase emptying phase before linear emptying (Dr V. Lewington, Southampton).

invasion, especially CT and endoluminal ultrasound. Usually laparoscopy is combined with peritoneal cytology unless laparotomy follows immediately.

Gastric emptying studies

These are useful in the study of gastric dysmotility problems, particularly those that follow gastric surgery. The principle of the examination is that a radioisotope-labelled liquid and solid meal are ingested by the patient and the emptying of the stomach is followed on a gamma camera. This allows the proportion of activity in the remaining in the stomach to be assessed numerically, and it is possible to follow liquid and solid gastric emptying independently (Fig. 51.9).

Tests of gastric acid secretion and of pH monitoring

In the past tests of gastric acid secretion were frequently performed, particularly by surgeons. Recent advances, however, have made these tests virtually redundant except in the context of physiological and pharmacological studies. Part of the interest in these tests related to the higher levels of gastric acid secretion commonly found in patients with duodenal ulcer disease (see later).

Traditionally, basal and maximal acid output is measured. A nasogastric tube is passed into the stomach, the basal secretion collected over 1 hour and the acid output in millimoles calculated. To obtain the maximal acid output intramuscular injection of the gastrin analogue pentagastrin is given at a dose of 6 μg/kg body weight and the secretions are collected over the ensuing hour. The maximal acid output is calculated as the peak 15-minute collection multiplied by 4 or twice the peak 30-minute collection in two consecutive collections.

A wealth of data exists on the acid outputs in a whole range of populations. Ultimately, the peak acid output is related to the parietal cell mass; larger stomachs produce more acid. Although traditionally patients with duodenal ulcers do secrete more acid than normal, there is considerable overlap between normal and duodenal ulcer populations. Patients with gastric ulcers produce acid at approximately normal levels. In a patient with a gastrinoma the basal acid output is unusually high and there may be little response to pentagastrin, the parietal cell mass already being near maximally stimulated by the gastrin produced by the tumour. It is now known that other nongastrin peptide products also may result in the Zollinger–Ellison syndrome.

The insulin test was previously beloved of gastric surgeons, particularly those interested in the quality of vagotomy. The test was originally described by Hollander and involves the induction of hypoglycaemia in a postvagotomy patient using an intravenous soluble dose of insulin of 0.2 units/kg body weight. Gastric acid secretion is then measured in the 2 hours following insulin injection. The theoretical basis of the test is that the hypoglycaemia stimulates the hypothalamic nuclei inducing a parasympathetic response. If the vagus is intact to any degree this is reflected in a rise in gastric acid secretion. Various criteria are used to determine whether a test is positive or not. Distinction is often made between an 'early' positive test, thought to mean that a substantial vagal innervation remains, and a 'late' positive test, the significance of which is less clear.

Robert M. Zollinger, b. 1903. American surgeon.
Edwin H. Ellison, b. 1918. American surgeon.
Fredrick Hollander. Surgeon, San Diego, California, USA.

Although in these tests they did correlate to some degree with ulcer relapse following vagotomy, their use in patient management was always limited as they are performed postoperatively and therefore could not influence patient management. In this respect the intraoperative Grassi test may have been a more useful method of controlling the quality of vagotomy. However, all of these tests are virtually redundant as vagotomy is now uncommonly performed on the elective situation.

24-hour intragastric pH monitoring

Studies of this type became very popular during the 1980s, particularly in the investigation of new gastric antisecretory agents. The pH within the stomach is measured over a 24-hour period either by the passage of a nasogastric tube and regular aspiration or by placing a radiotelemetry capsule on a tether within the stomach and monitoring the pH with an externally worn aerial. The median daytime, night-time or 24-hour intragastric pH can thus easily be calculated and, by converting the pH to hydrogen ion concentration, the median intragastric acidity over various periods can be studied. This latter manoeuvre allows the percentage reduction in acidity produced by a pharmacological agent to be measured (the step of converting pH to hydrogen ion concentration is obviously vital as pH is a logarithmic scale). Although of great physiological and pharmacological interest, these tests have little clinical relevance.

Measurement of plasma gastrin

The measurement of plasma gastrin by radioimmunoassay is of use in the diagnosis of gastrinoma (Zollinger–Ellison syndrome). In most assays the normal fasting gastrin level is about 50 ng/litre, but in gastrinomas very high levels, sometimes many thousands of ng/litre, can be found. However, the other common cause of hypergastrinaemia is hypochlorhydria associated with gastric atrophy and very high gastrin levels are found in pernicious anaemia. Antral gastrin is released to excess as a result of the negative feedback loop. A condition is said to exist when there is autonomous production of gastrin by the antrum but this condition, if it exists, is of little clinical importance.

Paediatric disorders

Hypertrophic pyloric stenosis of infancy

Aetiology

The incidence of this condition is approximately three cases per 1000 births. It is four times as common in males as in females and the aetiology is unknown. It may be that the condition is analogous to achalasia of the oesophagus in which there is a failure of the pylorus to relax, leading to the muscular hypertrophy. In some cases there seems to be a familial association. In such families the mother has suffered from the condition in 50 per cent of cases, and 10 per cent of male siblings and 2 per cent of female siblings are affected.

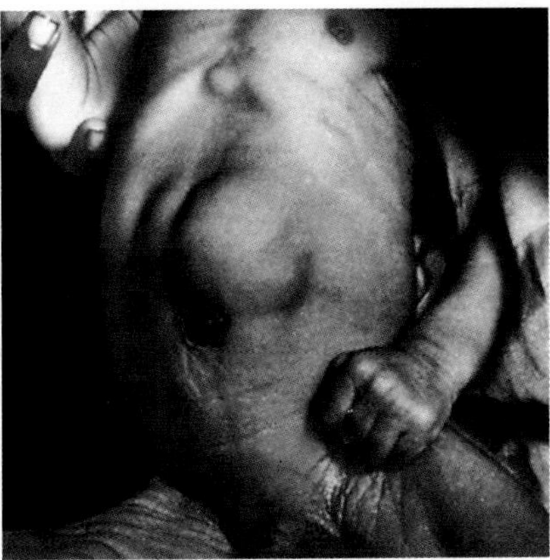

Fig. 51.10 Visible peristalsis in an infant with hypertrophic pyloric stenosis. This was induced by a test feed.

Pathology

The classical feature is that the musculature of the pylorus and adjacent antrum is grossly hypertrophied, the hypertrophy being maximum in the pylorus itself. The mucosa is compressed such that only a probe can be inserted.

Clinical features

Characteristically it is a first-born male child that is most commonly affected. The condition is most commonly seen at 4 weeks after birth ranging from the third week to, on rare occasions, the seventh. Inexplicably, it is the time following birth that seems important and not the child's gestational age. A premature infant will also develop the condition at about 4 weeks after birth. Vomiting is the presenting symptom that after 2–3 days becomes forcible and projectile. The child vomits milk and no bile is present. Immediately after vomiting the baby is usually hungry. Weight loss is a striking feature and rapidly the infant becomes emaciated and dehydrated. Diagnosis can usually be made with a test feed. This may produce characteristic peristaltic waves that can be seen to pass across the upper abdomen. At the same time, using a warm hand, the abdomen is palpated to detect the lump (Fig. 51.10).

Imaging

Ultrasonography is the investigation of choice as it can, without difficulty, detect the classical features in the pyloric canal. Contrast radiology is not now necessary.

Differential diagnosis

The common conditions from which pyloric stenosis must be differentiated are gastro-oesophageal reflux, feeding problems, urinary tract infection and raised intracranial pressure. The condition cannot normally be confused with duodenal atresia or intestinal obstruction because of the absence of bile in the milk vomit.

Treatment

Following diagnosis the first concern is to correct the metabolic abnormalities. Essentially this is the same situation that pertains in adults with the patient being dehydrated, with low sodium, chloride and potassium, and a metabolic alkalosis. The child should be rehydrated with dextrose–saline and potassium (2.5 per cent dextrose plus 0.45 per cent sodium chloride plus 1 g of potassium chloride per 500 ml of fluid). This will restore the infant's clinical condition and electrolytes to normal. Following this operation is required. Conservative treatment has little place in the management of this condition as with appropriate surgical treatment recovery is virtually 100 per cent.

Ramstedt's operation

In preparing the child for operation it is important that the stomach is emptied and washed out with saline, and that hypothemia is avoided. To achieve this the patient is encased in cotton wool allowing exposure of the upper abdomen. Operation is performed under general anaesthesia, although it is possible to perform the procedure under a local anaesthetic. The skin is opened through a transverse incision placed in the upper abdomen over the right rectus sheath, which is opened in the same line. The rectus muscle is then split along the line of its fibres and the posterior rectus sheath opened in the line of the skin incision. The hypertrophied pylorus is delivered and rotated so that its superior surface comes into view (Fig. 51.11). Thus, the least vascular portion can be selected for incision. To ascertain the distal limit of the hypertrophy the surgeon invaginates the duodenum with the index finger. The incision is made through the serosa only and from this point along the whole length of the pylorus and, importantly, the distal antrum. The hypertrophied pylorus has the consistency of an unripe pear, hence splitting the muscle coats can be accomplished by blunt dissection (Fig. 51.11). On separating the edges with artery forceps the pyloric mucosa bulges into the cleft which has been made in the muscle. Great care is taken not to penetrate the mucosa. When this injury occurs it is almost always in dividing the most distal part of the constricting fibres which are in the vicinity of the duodenal fornix. To be sure that there is no perforation some air is squeezed from the stomach into the duodenum. If a perforation has occurred it is closed and a piece of omentum placed over the closure. Haemostasis should be meticulous.

After operation the nasogastric tube can be removed and feeding commenced on the morning after operation. If the infant manages to feed without difficulty it can be discharged early from hospital. If the mucosa is inadvertently opened it is wise to delay feeding for 48 hours and to retain the child in hospital longer.

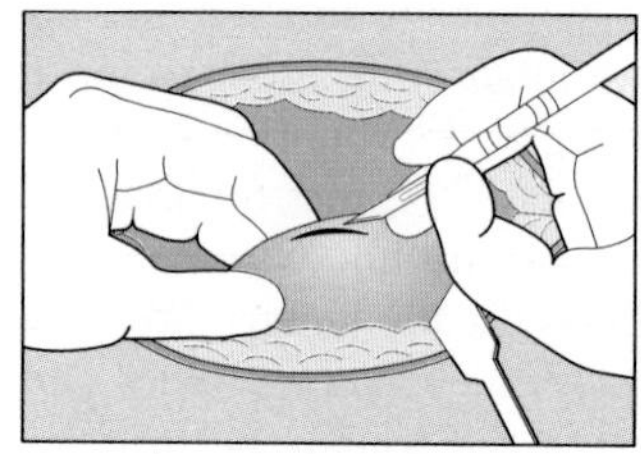

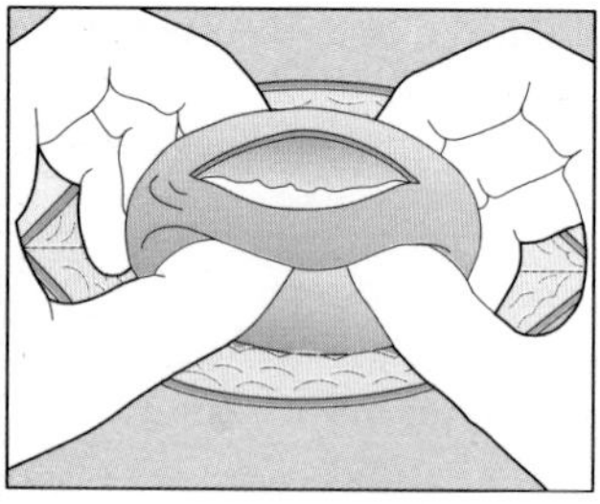

Fig. 51.11 Ramstedt's operation, showing the mucosa bulging into the incision in the hypertrophied muscle.

Complications of operation

Postoperative pyrexia is common and usually treated with paracetomol elixir. Wound disruption is rare and is more liable to occur in emaciated subjects. The incidence of wound infection is around 5 per cent, and 1 per cent will suffer wound disruption.

Duodenal atresia

This occurs at the point of fusion between the foregut and midgut, and therefore lies in the neighbourhood of the ampulla of Vater. There is a diaphragm, which is usually complete, across the duodenum at this point (Fig. 51.12) and the condition is frequently accompanied by other defects. The diagnosis is now made antenatally in most cases through the use of ultrasound. This shows the characteristic

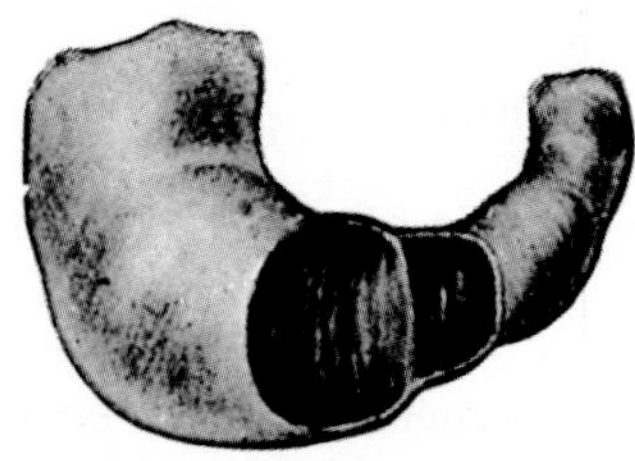

Fig. 51.12 Congenital septum of duodenal obstruction at the commencement of the third part of the duodenum. The proximal gut is enormously dilated (*after W.E. Ladd*).

Wilhelm Conrad Ramstedt, 1867–1963. Surgeon, Rafael Clinic, Munster, Germany. Performed his first pyloroyotomy in 1911. He discovered in church records that his grandfather had misspelt the family name with two 'm's, so in 1920 he reverted to the original spelling.

Abraham Vater, 1684–1751. Professor of Anatomy and Biology, Wittenburg, Germany.

William Edwards Ladd, 1880–1967. Professor of Child Surgery, Harvard, Boston, Massachusetts, USA.

appearance of a dilated stomach and first part of the duodenum (double bubble). The child vomits from birth and the vomitus is bile stained. The differential diagnosis includes high intestinal obstruction. Occasionally, however, the diaphragm may be proximal to the ampulla and in these circumstances the condition can be confused with pyloric stenosis, although in pyloric stenosis vomiting does not start from birth. Treatment is by the operation of the duodenoduodenostomy in which the dilated proximal duodenum is anastomosed to the atrophic distal duodenum (Ladd). This disparity in luminal size can produce delays in emptying and some surgeons have advocated the use of a transanastomotic tube. However, this has been demonstrated to delay emptying and is not now commonly used.

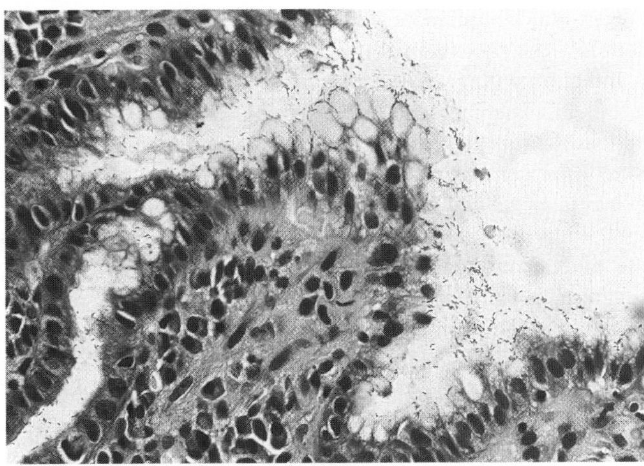

Fig. 51.13 Antral mucosa showing colonisation with *Helicobacter pylori* (modified Giemsa stain).

Helicobacter pylori

Over the last 20 years this organism has proved to be of overwhelming importance in the aetiology of a number of common gastroduodenal diseases such as chronic gastritis, peptic ulceration and gastric cancer. The organism had unquestionably been observed by a number of workers since Bircher's first description in 1874, but it was not until 1980 that Warren and Marshall, with enthusiasm but perhaps a lack of caution, ingested the organism to confirm that Koch's postulates could be fulfilled with respect to the gastritis that they succeeded in causing in themselves. Eradication therapy was then employed with mixed success. The organism is spiral shaped and is fastidious in its requirements, being difficult to culture outside the mucous layer of the stomach.

One of the characteristics of the organism is its ability to hydrolyse urea, resulting in the production of ammonia, a strong alkali. The effect of ammonia on the antral G cells is to cause the release of gastrin via the previously described negative-feedback loop. This is probably responsible for the modest but inappropriate hypergastrinaemia in patients with peptic ulcer disease which, in turn, may result in gastric acid hypersecretion. The organism's obligate urease activity is utilised by various tests used to detect the presence of the organism, including the C13 and C14 breath tests and the CLO test (which is a commercially available urease test kit), which is performed on gastric biopsies. The organism can also be detected histologically (Fig. 51.13), using the Giemsa or the Ethin–Stary silver stains, and cultured using appropriate media. Previous or current infection with the organism may also be detected serologically.

C.S. Warren. Perth, Australia, now Chicago, Illinois, USA. Credited with awakening the current interest in Helicobacter.
Barry Marshall. Perth, Australia, now Charlottesville, USA. Credited with awakening the current interest in Helicobacter.
Robert Koch, b. 1843. German bacteriologist.
Gustav Giemsa, b. 1867. German chemist.
Jean Crabtree. Biologist, Leeds, England.

Infection leads to the disruption of the gastric mucous barrier by the enzymes produced by the organism, and the inflammation induced in the gastric epithelium is the basis of many of the associated disease processes. The association of the organism with chronic (type B) gastritis is not in doubt as Koch's postulates have been fulfilled, most notably by Marshall and Warren. Some strains of *H. pylori* produce cytotoxins, and the production of cytotoxin seem to be associated with the ability of the organism to cause both gastritis and peptic ulceration (Crabtree). The effect of the organism on the gastric epithelium is to incite a classical inflammatory response that involves the migration and degranulation of acute inflammatory cells, such as neutrophils, and also the accumulation of chronic inflammatory cells, such as macrophages and lymphocytes.

It is evident how *H. pylori* infection results in chronic gastritis and also how this may progress to gastric ulceration, but it remained for a while an enigma how the organism could be involved in duodenal ulceration as the normal duodenum is not colonised. As mentioned above, the production of ammonia does increase the level of circulating gastrin and it has subsequently been shown that eradication of the organism in patients with duodenal ulcer disease will reduce the acid levels to normal. However, the overlap in gastric acid secretion between normal subjects and those with duodenal ulcers is considerable and the modestly increased acid levels in patients with *Helicobacter*-associated antral gastritis are insufficient to explain the aetiology of duodenal ulceration.

The explanation can probably be found in the phenomenon of duodenal gastric metaplasia. Gastric metaplasia is the normal response of the duodenal mucosa to excess acidity. It can be thought of as any other metaplasia in the gastrointestinal tract: an attempt by the mucosa to resist an injurious stimulus. Although normal duodenal mucosa cannot be infected with *H. pylori*, gastric metaplasia in the duodenum is commonly infected and this infection results in the same inflammatory process that is observed in the gastric mucosa

(Wyatt and Dixon). The result is duodenitis, which is almost certainly the precursor of duodenal ulceration.

Infection with *H. pylori* may be the most common human infection. The incidence of infection within a population increases with age, and in many populations infection rates of 80–90 per cent are not unusual. The possibility of infection is inversely related to socioeconomic group. The means of spread has not been identified, but the organism can occur in the faeces and faecal–oral spread seems most likely. The organism is not normally found in saliva or dental plaque. There is evidence in different environments and in different population groups that the manifestations of the infection may be different. Predominantly antral gastritis, which is commonly seen in the West, results initially in increased levels of acid production and peptic ulcer disease whereas gastritis affecting the body, common in the developing world, may lead to hypochlordria and gastric neoplasia.

It has been known since 1984 that *Helicobacter* infection is amenable to treatment with antibiotics and, in addition, that bismuth compounds are toxic for the organism. The profound hypochlorhydria produced by proton pump inhibitors combined with antibiotics is also effective in eradicating the organism. Commonly used eradication regimes include a bismuth compound and two antibiotics, such as metronidazole and amoxycillin, or a proton pump inhibitor, such as omeprazole, again in combination with antibiotics. High eradication rates in the region of 90 per cent can be achieved with combinations which include the antibiotic clarithromycin, although it may be that in the future antibiotic resistance becomes a problem.

At present eradication therapy is recommended for patients with duodenal ulcer disease but not for patients with nonulcer dyspepsia or in asymptomatic patients who are infected. However, recent data show that a proportion of patients with nonulcer dyspepsia does respond to treatment. *Helicobacter pylori* is now classed by the World Health Organisation as a class 1 carcinogen and it may be that the further epidemiological studies on the risk of gastric cancer change the current advice on treatment.

Gastritis

The understanding of gastritis has increased markedly following elucidation of the role of *H. pylori* in chronic gastritis.

Type A gastritis

This is an autoimmune condition in which there are circulating antibodies to the parietal cell. This results in the atrophy of the parietal cell mass, hence hypochlorhydria and ultimately achlorhydria. As intrinsic factor is also produced by the parietal cell there is malabsorption of vitamin B_{12} which, if untreated, may result in pernicious anaemia. In type A gastritis the antrum is not affected and the hypochlorhydria leads to the production of high levels of gastrin from the antral G cells. This results in chronic hypergastrinaemia. This in turn results in hypertrophy of the ECL cells in the body of the stomach which are not affected by the autoimmune damage. Over time it is apparent that microadenomas develop in the ECL cells of the stomach, sometimes becoming identifiable tumour nodules. Very rarely these tumours can become malignant. Patients with type A gastritis are predisposed to the development of gastric cancer and screening such patients endoscopically may be appropriate.

Michael Dixon. Professor of Pathology, Leeds, England.
Judy Wyatt. Consultant pathologist, Leeds, England.

Type B gastritis

There are abundant epidemiological data to support the association of this type of gastritis with *H. pylori*. Most commonly type B gastritis affects the antrum, and it is these patients who are prone to peptic ulcer disease. *Helicobacter*-associated pangastritis is also a very common manifestation of infection, but gastritis affecting the corpus alone does not seem to be associated. However, there are some data to suggest that *Helicobacter* may be involved in the initiation of the process. Patients with pangastritis seem to be most prone to the development of gastric cancer.

Intestinal metaplasia is associated with chronic pangastritis with atrophy. Although intestinal metaplasia per se is common, intestinal metaplasia associated with dysplasia has significant malignant potential and if this condition is identified the patient should be regularly screened endoscopically.

Reflux gastritis

This is caused by enterogastric reflux and is particularly common after gastric surgery. Its histological features are distinct from other types of gastritis. Although commonly seen after gastric surgery, it is occasionally found in patients with no previous surgical intervention or who have had a cholecystectomy. Bile chelating or prokinetic agents may be useful in treatment and as a temporising measure to avoid consideration of revisional surgery. Operation for the condition should be reserved for the most severe cases.

Erosive gastritis

This is caused by agents which disturb the gastric mucosal barrier; NSAIDs and alcohol are common causes. The nonsteroidal-induced gastric lesion is associated with inhibition of the cyclo-oxygenase type 1 (Cox 1) receptor enzyme, hence reducing the production of cytoprotective prostaglandins in the stomach. Fortunately, many of the beneficial anti-inflammatory activities of NSAIDs are mediated by Cox 2, and there is at present much activity to produce Cox 2 inhibitors which will spare some of the side effects of these agents.

Stress gastritis

This is a common sequel of serious illness or injury and is characterised by a reduction in the blood supply to superficial mucosa of the stomach. Although common, this is not usually recognised unless stress ulceration and bleeding supervene, in which case treatment can be extremely difficult. The condition also sometimes follows cardiopulmonary bypass. Prevention of the stress bleeding from the stomach is much easier than treating it, and hence the routine use of H_2 antagonists with or without barrier agents, such as sucralfate, in patients who are on intensive care. These measures have been shown to reduce the incidence of bleeding from stress ulceration.

Ménétrier's disease

This is an unusual condition characterised by gross hypertrophy of the gastric mucosal folds, mucus production and hypochlorhydria. The condition is premalignant and may present with hypoproteinaemia and anaemia. There is no treatment other than a gastrectomy. The disease seems to be caused by overexpression of transforming growth factor alpha (TGF-α). Like epidermal growth factor (EGF), this peptide also binds to the EGF receptor. The histological features of Ménétrier's disease may be reproduced in transgenic mice overexpressing TGF-α (Coffey).

Lymphocytic gastritis

This type of gastritis is seen rarely. It is characterised by the infiltration of the gastric mucosa by T cells and is probably associated with *H. pylori* infection.

Other forms of gastritis

Eosinophilic gastritis appears to have an allergic basis, and is treated with steroids and chromoglycate. Granulomatous gastritis is seen rarely in Crohn's disease and also may be associated with tuberculosis. Acquired immunodeficiency syndrome (AIDS) gastritis is secondary to infection with cryptospirodiosis. Phlegmonous gastritis is a rare bacterial infection of the stomach found in patients with severe intercurrent illness. It is usually an agonal event.

Peptic ulcer

Peptic ulcers are so named because, in addition to acid being a requirement for their occurrence, pepsin is probably also required. Certainly, it is clear that patients with duodenal ulcers tend to have a higher than average pepsin level within the gastric juice. However, this is of little practical importance as in the absence of acid, for instance in type A gastritis with atrophy, peptic ulcers do not occur. All peptic ulcers can be healed by using proton pump inhibitors, such as omeprazole, that can render a patient virtually achlorhydric.

Common sites for peptic ulcers are the first part of the duodenum and the lesser curve of the stomach, but they also occur on the stoma following gastric surgery, the oesophagus and even in a Meckel's diverticulum, which contains ectopic gastric epithelium. In general, the ulcer occurs at a junction between different types of epithelia, the ulcer occurring in the epithelium least resistant to acid attack.

In the past much distinction has been made between acute and chronic peptic ulcers, but this difference can sometimes be difficult to determine clinically. It is probably best to consider that there is a spectrum of disease from the superficial gastric and duodenal ulceration, frequently seen at endoscopy, to deep chronic penetrating ulcers. This does not minimise the importance of acute stress ulceration. These ulcers can both perforate and bleed (see 'Stress ulceration' later).

For many years and despite enormous research endeavour the cause of peptic ulceration remained an enigma. Acid, which is so easy to measure, was studied incessantly, such studies being particularly beloved by gastric surgeons. However, it is clear that although acid levels are higher comparing groups of patients with duodenal and prepyloric peptic ulcers with normal subjects the overlap is very considerable. Patients with gastric ulceration have normal levels of gastric acid secretion or, in the view of some, lower levels. As peptic ulceration will occur in the presence of very high acid levels, such as those found in patients with a gastrinoma (Zollinger–Ellison syndrome, see the section on 'Duodenal tumours' later), and as all ulcers can be healed in the absence of acid it is clear that acid is important. In some cases it may be the only aetiological factor. This is clearly not the case in the majority of patients. As with most diseases there clearly are genetic components as exemplified by the often quoted and clinically irrelevant finding that patients with blood group O are over-represented amongst the duodenal ulcer population. Similarly, social stress has also been implicatated, falsely (Asher).

It is now widely accepted that infection with *H. pylori* is the most important factor in the development of peptic ulceration. The other factor of major importance at present is ingestion of NSAIDs. Cigarette smoking predisposes to peptic ulceration and increases the relapse rate after

Pierre Ménétrier, 1859–1935. French physician.
Robert Coffey. Professor of Medicine, Nashville, Tennessee, USA.
Burrill B. Crohn, b. 1884. American physician.
Johann F. Meckel (The Younger), 1781–1833. Professor of Anatomy and Surgery, Halle, Germany.

Richard Asher, 1912–69. Physician, Central Middlesex Hospital, London, England. Described Munchausen's syndrome. Ridiculed the concept that the stress of modern living caused peptic ulceration by pointing out that the same claim was made for syphilis! It is an interesting coincidence that both diseases have strong aetiological associations with spiral organisms.
Baron von Munchausen. Legendary sixteenth century conflabulator.

treatment with either gastric antisecretory agents or, in the past, elective surgery. Although other factors exist, and multiple other factors may be involved in transition between the superficial and the deep penetrating chronic ulcer, they are of lesser importance.

Duodenal ulceration

Incidence

There have been marked changes in the last two decades in the demography of patients presenting with duodenal ulceration in the West. First, even before the introduction of H_2-receptor antagonists, the incidence of duodenal ulceration and the frequency of elective surgery for the condition were falling. This trend has continued and now, in the West, dyspeptic patients presenting with a duodenal ulcer at gastroscopy are uncommon. In part, this may relate to the liberal prescription of gastric antisecretory agents and eradication therapy for patients with dyspepsia. Secondly, the peak incidence is now in a much older age group than previously and, although it is still more common in men, the difference is less marked. These changes, at least in part, mirror the changes in the epidemiology of *H. pylori* infection. A cohort effect can be demonstrated (Susser), the age group in whom *Helicobacter* infection was prevalent in the early part of the twentieth century was ageing and suffering the complications of the infection late in life. This probable relationship with *H. pylori* can also be seen in relation gastric to ulceration and, indeed, gastric cancer. Similarly, the incidence of perforation and bleeding duodenal ulcers in young and middle-aged patients appears to be falling but, by contrast, there is currently a marked increase in the numbers of elderly and often infirm patients suffering these complications. This latter trend can be explained not only by the *H. pylori* cohort effect but also by the increased use of NSAIDs in the elderly. In Eastern Europe the disease remains common and, from having been uncommon in some developing nations, it is now observed more frequently. Again, the relationship with *H. pylori* appears compelling.

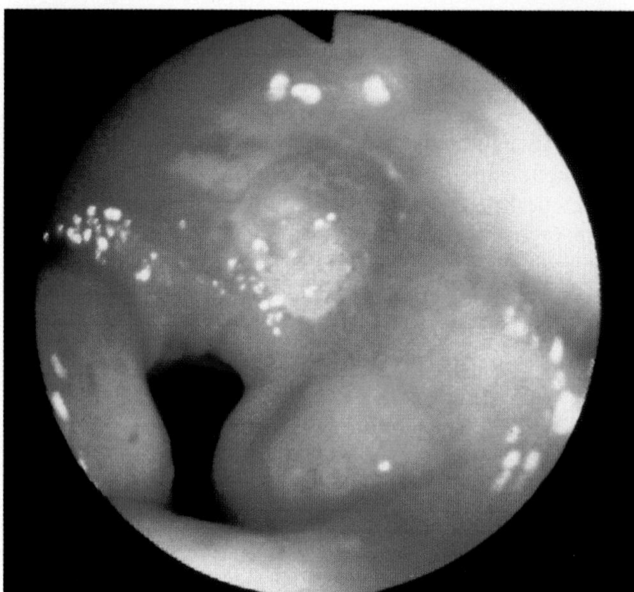

Fig. 51.14 Duodenal ulcer at gastroduodenoscopy (*courtesy of Dr G.N.J. Tytgat, Amsterdam*).

Mervyn Susser. Epidemiologist, Columbia, New York, USA.

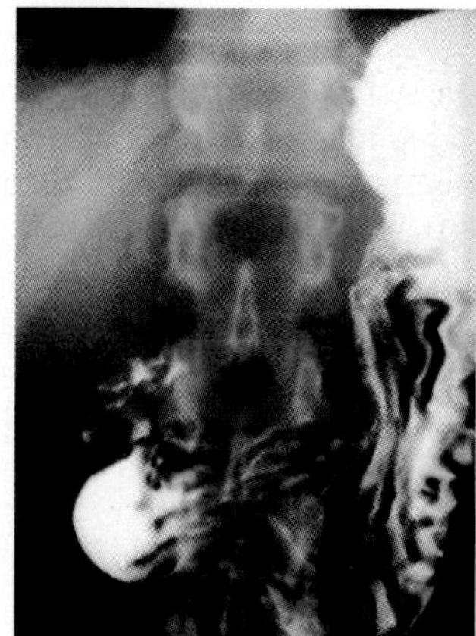

Fig. 51.15 Duodenal ulcer shown by barium meal.

Pathology

Most occur in the first part of the duodenum (Figs 51.14 and 51.15). A chronic ulcer penetrates the mucosa and into the muscle coat leading to fibrosis. The fibrosis causes deformities such as pyloric stenosis. When an ulcer heals a scar can be observed in the mucosa. Sometimes there may be more than one duodenal ulcer. The situation in which there is both a posterior and an anterior duodenal ulcer is referred to as 'kissing ulcers'. Anteriorly placed ulcers tend to perforate and, by contrast, posterior duodenal ulcers tend to bleed, sometimes by eroding a large vessel such as a gastroduodenal artery. Occasionally the ulceration may be so extensive that the entire duodenal cap is ulcerated and devoid of mucosa. With respect to the giant duodenal ulcer, malignancy in this region is so uncommon that under normal circumstances surgeons can be confident that they are dealing with benign disease even though from external palpation it may not appear so. In the stomach the situation is different.

Histopathology

Microscopically, destruction of the muscular coat is observed and the base of the ulcer is covered with granulation tissue, the arteries in this region showing the typical changes endarteritis obliterans. Sometimes the terminations of nerves can be seen amongst the fibrosis. The pathological appearances of the healing ulcer must be carefully interpreted as some of the epithelial down-growths can be misinterpreted as invasion. This is unlikely to be important in duodenal ulcers when malignancy rarely, if ever, occurs but it is much more important with gastric ulcers.

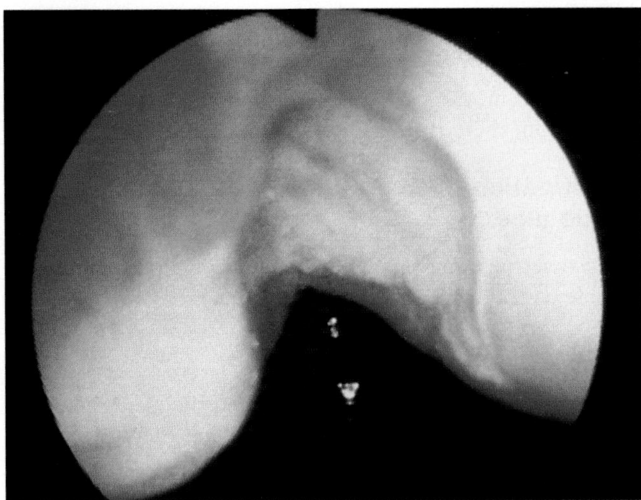

Fig. 51.16 Benign incisural gastric ulcer shown at gastroscopy (*courtesy of Dr G.N.J. Tytgat, Amsterdam*).

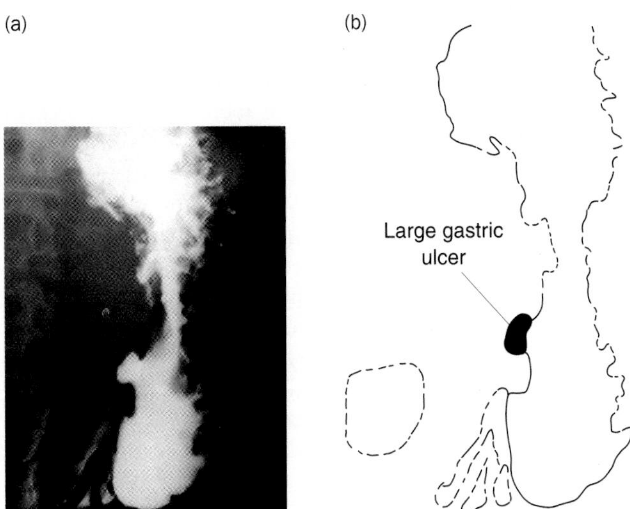

Fig. 51.17 Benign gastric ulcer shown on barium meal.

Gastric ulcers

Incidence

As with duodenal ulceration, *H. pylori* and NSAIDs are the important aetiological factors. Gastric ulceration is also associated with smoking, other factors are of lesser importance.

There are marked differences between the populations afflicted by chronic gastric ulceration compared with duodenal ulceration. First, gastric ulceration is substantially less common than duodenal ulceration. The sex incidence is equal and the population with gastric ulcers tends to be older. It is more prevalent in low socioeconomic groups and is considerably more common in the developing world than in the West.

Pathology

This is essentially similar to that of a duodenal ulcer, except that gastric ulcers tend to be larger. Fibrosis, when it occurs, may result in the now rarely seen hour-glass contraction of the stomach. Large chronic ulcers may erode posteriorly into the pancreas and on other occasions into major vessels such as the splenic artery. Less commonly, they may erode into other organs such as the transverse colon. Chronic gastric ulcers are much more common on the lesser curve, especially at the incisura angularis (Figs 51.16 and 51.17), than the greater curve, and even when high on the lesser curve they tend to be at the boundary between the acid-secreting and the non acid-secreting epithelia. With atrophy of parietal cell mass nonacid-secreting epithelium migrates up the lesser curvature.

Malignancy in gastric ulcers

Chronic duodenal ulcers are not associated with malignancy and, by contrast, gastric ulcers are. Widely varying estimates are made of the incidence of gastric malignancy in gastric ulcers. The reason for this is that the authors reporting such diverse incidences are describing different clinical situations. Two clinical extremes must be distinguished to understand this problem properly. First, there is the situation in which a benign chronic gastric ulcer undergoes malignant transformation. This is known to happen, albeit rarely, and can be observed histologically in specimens in which there are the classical histological features of benign gastric ulceration associated with an area of malignant transformation. It is impossible to estimate the incidence of such an occurrence but it is uncommon. The contrasting clinical extreme is the patient identified as having an ulcer in the stomach, either endoscopically or on contrast radiology, which is assessed as benign but biopsies reveal malignancy. In this situation the patient does not have, and probably never has had, chronic peptic ulceration in the stomach but has presented with an ulcerated cancer. This situation is common, although whether a lesion found in the stomach is described as being benign or malignant on clinical grounds depends very much on the skill and experience of the endoscopist or radiologist.

It is fundamental that any gastric ulcer should be regarded as being malignant no matter how classical the features of a benign gastric ulcer. Multiple biopsies should always be taken, perhaps as many as 10 well-targeted biopsies, before an ulcer can be tentatively accepted as being benign. Even then it is important that further biopsies are taken whilst the ulcer is healing and when healed. Modern antisecretory agents can frequently heal the ulceration associated with gastric cancer but clearly are ineffective in treating the malignancy itself. At operation even experienced surgeons may have difficulty distinguishing between the gastric cancer and a benign ulcer. Operative strategies differ so radically that it is essential, if at all possible, that a confident diagnosis be made before operation. The patechial haemorrhages found on the serosa of the patient with peptic ulceration are a useful sign but not entirely reliable. If, at operation, it are determined that the ulcer is probably benign it should, none the less, be excised, in totality if possible, and submitted for histological examination. It is not known whether a patient's survival is compromised by this approach if the ulcer turns out to be malignant on biopsy as convincing data are not available.

Other peptic ulcers

Prepyloric gastric ulcers require special mention. In terms of acid secretion they are similar to duodenal ulcers and in the past have proved to be more difficult to treat, a problem overcome with the advent of proton pump inhibitors. Pyloric channel ulcers are similar to duodenal ulcers. Both prepyloric and pyloric ulcers may be malignant, and biopsy is essential. Stomal ulcers occur after a gastroenterostomy or a gastrectomy of the Billroth II type. The ulcer is usually found on the jejunal side of the stoma.

Clinical features of peptic ulcers

Whilst many textbooks try and create differences in the clinical feature of gastric and duodenal ulceration, detailed analysis has shown that they cannot be differentiated on the basis of symptoms. Certainly, the demographic characteristics of groups of patients with gastric and duodenal ulceration do differ but this does not allow discrimination.

Pain

The pain is epigastric, often described as gnawing and may radiate to the back. Eating may sometimes relieve the discomfort. The pain is normally intermittent rather than intractable.

Periodicity

One of the classical features of untreated peptic ulceration is periodicity. Symptoms may disappear for weeks or months to return again. This periodicity may be related to the spontaneous healing of the ulcer.

Vomiting

Whilst this occurs, it is not a notable feature unless the stenosis has occurred.

Alteration in weight

Weight loss or, sometimes, weight gain may occur. Patients with gastric ulceration are often underweight but this may precede the occurrence of the ulcer.

Bleeding

All peptic ulcers may bleed. The bleeding may be chronic and presentation with anaemia is not uncommon. Acute presentation with haematemesis and melaena is discussed later.

Clinical examination

Examination of the patient may reveal epigastric tenderness but except in extreme cases (for instance gastric outlet obstruction) there is unlikely to be much else to find.

Investigation of the patient with suspected peptic ulcer

In the investigation of such patients, imaging, preferably with flexible gastroduodenoscopy, is required.

Gastroduodenoscopy

This is the most sensitive investigation in the management of suspected peptic ulceration and in the hands of a well-trained operator is highly sensitive and specific.

In the stomach any abnormal lesion should be multiply biopsied, and in the case of a suspected benign gastric ulcer numerous biopsies must be taken in order to exclude, as far as possible, the presence of a malignancy. Commonly biopsies of the antrum will be taken to see whether there is histological evidence of gastritis and a CLO test performed to determine the presence of *H. pylori*. A 'U' manoeuvre should be performed to exclude ulcers around the gastro-oesophageal junction. This is important as the increasing incidence of cancer at the gastro-oesophageal junction requires that all mucosal abnormalities in this region should undergo multiple biopsy. Similarly, if a stoma is present, for instance after gastroenterostomy or Billroth II gastrectomy, it is important to enter both afferent and efferent loops. Almost all stomal ulcers will be very close to the junction between the jejunal and gastric mucosa. Attention should be given to the pylorus to note whether there is any prepyloric or pyloric channel ulceration and also whether it is deformed, which is often the case with chronic duodenal ulceration. In the duodenum care must be taken to view all of the first part. It is not infrequent for an ulcer to be just beyond the pylorus and easily overlooked.

Treatment of peptic ulceration

The vast majority of uncomplicated peptic ulcers is treated medically. Surgical treatment of uncomplicated peptic ulceration has decreased markedly since the 1960s and in the West is now seldom performed. Surgical treatment was aimed principally at reducing gastric acid secretion and, in the case of gastric ulceration, removing the diseased mucosa. When originally devised medical treatment also aimed to reduce gastric acid secretion, initially using the highly successful H_2-receptor antagonist and subsequently proton pump inhibitors. This has now largely given way to eradication therapy.

Christian Albert Theodore Billroth, 1829–94. Professor of Surgery, Vienna, Austria.

Medical treatment

It is reasonable that a doctor managing a patient with an uncomplicated peptic ulcer should suggest modifications to the patient's lifestyle, particularly the cessation of cigarette smoking. This advice is rarely followed and pharmacological measures form the mainstay of treatment.

H_2-receptor antagonists

H_2 antagonists (Black) revolutionised the management of peptic ulceration. Most duodenal ulcers and gastric ulcers can be healed by a few weeks of treatment with these drugs provided that they are taken and absorbed. There remained, however, a group of patients who were refractory to conventional doses of H_2-receptor antagonists. This is largely now irrelevant as proton pump inhibitors can effectively render a patient achlorhydric and all benign ulcers will heal using these drugs. The problem with H_2-receptor antagonists alone, as with other gastric antisecretory agents, is that relapse is virtually inevitable once treatment is discontinued.

Proton pump inhibitors

All ulcers will heal on proton pump inhibitors, such as omeprazole, the majority within 2 weeks. Symptom relief is impressively rapid, most patients being asymptomatic within a few days. Like H_2 antagonists, omeprazole is safe and relatively devoid of serious side effects. As with H_2-receptor antagonists relapse following cessation of therapy is almost universal.

Eradication therapy

Eradication therapy is now routinely given to patients with peptic ulceration, and this is described earlier in this chapter. Evidence suggests that if a patient has a peptic ulcer and *H. pylori* is the principal aetiological factor (essentially the patient not taking NSAIDs) then complete eradication of the organism will cure the disease and reinfection as an adult is uncommon. Eradication therapy is therefore the mainstay of treatment with peptic ulceration. It is extremely economical by comparison with prolonged courses of antisecretory agents or surgery. It is also considerably safer than surgical treatment.

There are some patients with peptic ulcers in whom eradication therapy may not be appropriate and this includes patients with NSAID-associated ulcers. Such patients should avoid these drugs if possible and if not they should be co-prescribed with a potent antisecretory agent. Similarly, patients with stomal ulceration are not effectively treated with eradication therapy and require prolonged prescription of antisecretory agents. Patients with Zollinger–Ellison syndrome should be treated long term with omeprazole, unless the tumour can be adequately managed by surgery.

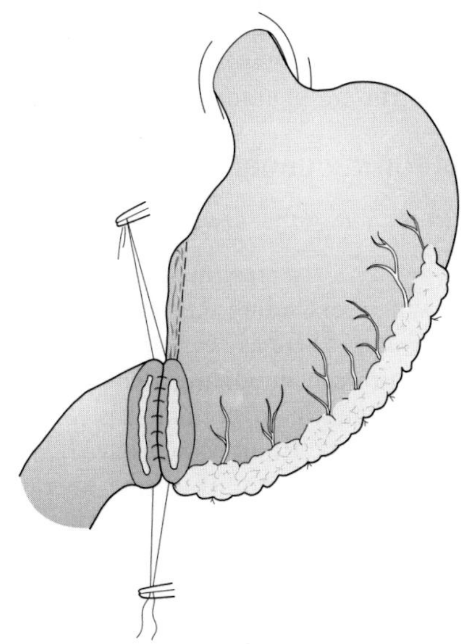

Fig. 51.18 Billroth I gastrectomy. [Reproduced with permission from *Rob and Smith's Operative Surgery. Surgery of the Upper Gastrointestinal Tract*, 5th edn (eds G. Jamieson and H. Debas), Chapman & Hall, London, 1994, p. 418.]

Surgical treatment of uncomplicated peptic ulceration

From its peak in the 1960s the incidence of surgery for uncomplicated peptic ulceration has fallen markedly, to the extent that peptic ulcer surgery is now of little more than historical interest. A description of operations used in the treatment of peptic ulcers is still necessary because surgery is

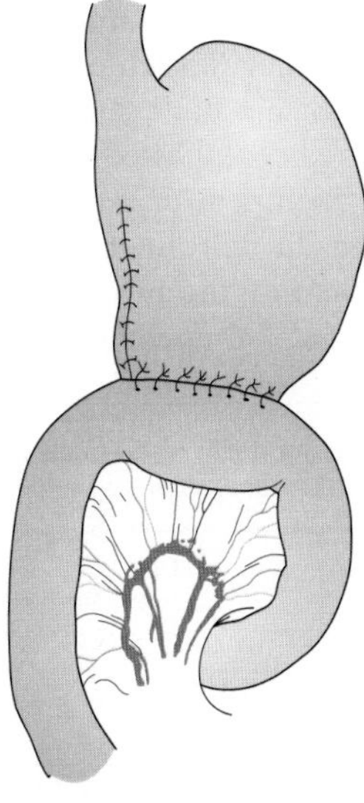

Fig. 51.19 Billroth II gastrectomy. [Reproduced with permission from *Rob and Smith's Operative Surgery. Surgery of the Upper Gastrointestinal Tract*, 5th edn (eds G. Jamieson and H. Debas), Chapman & Hall, London, 1994, p. 102.]

Sir James Black. London pharmacologist and discoverer of the H_2 receptor amongst other notable achievements.

commonly employed for the complicated ulcer and, in addition, many patients are left suffering from the consequences of the more destructive operations.

Operations for duodenal ulceration

Duodenal ulcer surgery – rationale

Procedures devised for the treatment of duodenal ulcers have the common aim of excluding the damaging effects of acid from the duodenum. This has been achieved by diversion of the acid away from the duodenum, reducing the secretory potential of the stomach, or both. It has long been known that patients with duodenal ulceration have higher than average levels of gastric secretion. All of the operations devised achieved their aim to some extent, but with varying degrees of morbidity, mortality and postoperative side-effects. The operations are described in historical sequence.

Billroth II gastrectomy

The first successful gastrectomy was performed by Billroth in January 1881 (Fig. 51.18) and Wolfer performed the first gastroenterostomy in the same year. The original Billroth operations consisted of a gastric resection with gastroduodenal anastomosis (Billroth I technique) (Fig. 51.18). The Billroth II operation was devised more by accident than design (Fig. 51.19). A gastroenterostomy (Fig. 51.20) was performed on a gravely ill patient with a pyloric cancer who was not expected to survive. Contrary to expectations the patient improved and the stomach distal to the anastomosis was resected. It soon became evident that the use of gastrojejunal anastomosis after gastric resection could be safer and easier than the Billroth I procedure, and it became popular and effective in the surgical treatment of duodenal ulcer. Because of its disadvantages, such as higher operative mortality and morbidity, it has not been used for many years in the patient with an uncomplicated ulcer but it is still used occasionally in the treatment of a complicated ulcer with a 'difficult' duodenum. In Billroth II gastrectomy, or its close relation Polya gastrectomy, the antrum and distal body of the stomach are mobilised by opening the greater and lesser omentum and dividing the gastroepiploic arteries, (right) gastric artery and the (left) gastric artery arcade at the limit of the resection. The duodenum is closed off either by suture or using staples, sometimes with difficulty in patients with a very deformed duodenum. Various techniques are available to close the difficult duodenum and *in extremis* a catheter may be placed in the duodenal stump, the duodenum closed around it and a catheter brought out through the abdominal wall. Following resection the distal end of the stomach is narrowed by the closure of the lesser curve aspect of the remnant. The greater curve aspect is then anastomosed, usually in a retrocolic fashion, to the jejunum leaving as short an afferent loop as feasible (Fig. 51.19). Even when well performed this procedure has an operative mortality rate of a few per cent and morbidity is not unusual. A common cause of morbidity is leakage from the duodenal stump, which is particularly associated with kinking of the afferent loop. Leakage from the gastrojejunal anastomosis is unusual unless either it is under tension or the stomach has been devascularised during the mobilisation. The incidence of side effects following gastrectomy is considerable, as shown in Table 51.2. Recurrence of the ulcer at the stoma is uncommon but can occur, especially as this procedure is traditionally not combined with the vagotomy.

Table 51.2 Operative mortality, side effects and incidence of recurrence following duodenal ulcer operations

Operation	*Operative mortality (per cent)*	*Significant side effects (per cent)*	*Recurrent ulceration (per cent)*
Gastrectomy	1–2	20–40	1–4
Gastroenterostomy alone	< 1	10–20	50
Truncal vagotomy and drainage	< 1	10–20	2–7
Selective vagotomy and drainage	< 1	10–20	5–10
Highly selective vagotomy	< 0.2	< 5	2–10
Truncal vagotomy and antrectomy	1	10–20	1

Anton Wolfer, 1850–1917. Professor of Surgery, Prague, Czechoslovakia.
Eugen Alexander Polya, 1876–1944. Surgeon, Budapest, Hungary.

Gastrojejunostomy

Because of the potential for mortality after gastrectomy the use of gastrojejunostomy alone in the treatment of duodenal ulceration was developed (Fig. 51.20). Reflux of alkali from the small bowel into the stomach reduced duodenal acid exposure and was often successful in healing the ulcer. However, because the jejunal loop was exposed directly to gastric acid stomal ulceration was extremely common, hence the procedure in isolation was ineffective.

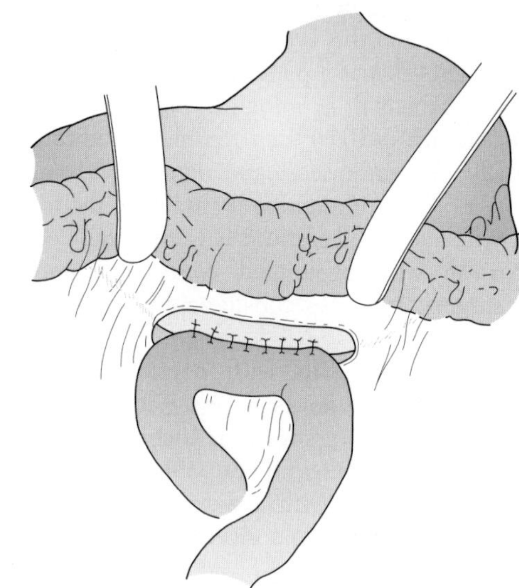

Fig. 51.20 Gastroenterostomy. [Reproduced with permission from *Rob and Smith's Operative Surgery. Surgery of the Upper Gastrointestinal Tract*, 5th edn (eds) G. Jamieson and H. Debas), Chapman & Hall, London, 1994, p. 406.]

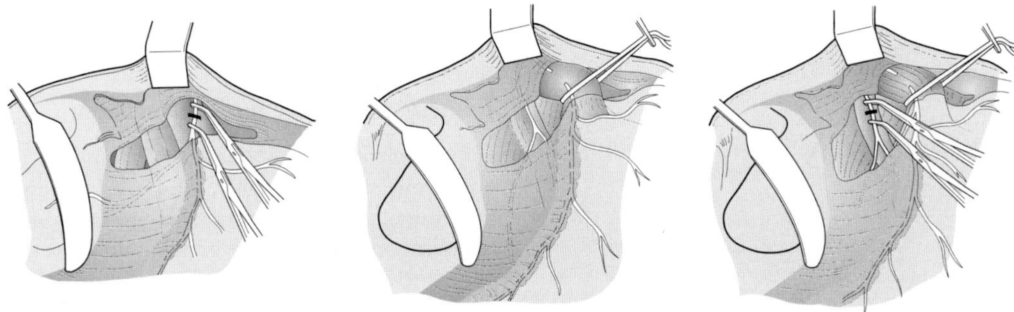

Fig. 51.21 Truncal vagotomy. [Reproduced with permission from *Rob and Smith's Operative Surgery. Surgery of the Upper Gastrointestinal Tract*, 5th edn (eds G. Jamieson and H. Debas), Chapman & Hall, London, 1994, p. 362.]

Truncal vagotomy and drainage

Truncal vagotomy was first introduced in 1943 by Dragstedt, and for many years this truncal vagotomy combined with drainage was the mainstay in the treatment of duodenal ulceration. The principle of the operation is that section of the vagus nerves, which are critically involved in the secretion of gastric acid, reduces the maximal acid output by approximately 50 per cent. This is similar to the effect of conventional doses of H_2-receptor antagonists. Because the vagal nerves are motor to the stomach, denervation of the antro-pyloro-duodenal segment results in gastric stasis in a substantial proportion of patients on whom truncal vagotomy alone is performed. This was first noted by Dragstedt who, when he first introduced the operation, did not perform a drainage procedure.

In performing truncal vagotomy the lower oesophagus is exposed by division of the overlying peritoneum. By gentle blunt dissection the oesophagus, which should contain a nasogastric tube, is encircled and slung with a tape. The posterior vagal trunk can be felt as a tight cord posteriorly and is divided between ligatures as it may be accompanied by blood vessels. On the front of the oesophagus the anterior vagus consists of a plexus which is divided. The lower 7 cm of oesophagus should be completely cleared of nerve fibres to achieve an adequate vagotomy (Fig. 51.21). The most popular drainage procedure is the Heineke–Mikulicz pyloroplasty (Fig. 51.22). It is simple to perform and involves the longitudinal section of the pyloric ring. This need not be an extensive excision when performed in the elective situation. The incision is closed transversely, usually with a single layer of interrupted sutures. Gastrojejunostomy (Fig. 51.20) is the alternative drainage procedure to pyloroplasty. This is performed through opening the lesser sac and an anastomosis performed between the most dependent part of the antrum and the first jejunal loop. An isoperistaltic anastomosis is most commonly performed. The operation of truncal vagotomy and drainage is substantially safer than gastrectomy (Table 51.2). However, the side effects of surgery are, in fact, little different from those that follow gastrectomy.

Lester Dragstedt, 1893–1975. Professor of Surgery, Chicago, Illinois, USA.
Walther Hermann Heineke, 1834–1901. Surgeon, Erlangen, Germany.
Johann von Mikulicz-Radecki, 1850–1905. Professor of Surgery, Breslau, formerly Germany, now Poland (Wroclaw).
David Johnston. Emeritus Professor of Surgery, Leeds, England.
Eric Amdrup, died 1998. Professor of Surgery, Aarhus, Denmark.

Selective vagotomy and drainage

In an attempt to reduce the side effects of truncal vagotomy, selective vagotomy was developed. In contrast to truncal vagotomy, where a complete vagal denervation is performed, in selective vagotomy the hepatic and coeliac nerves are preserved but the stomach is still completely vagally denervated. Drainage is required and, as this operation had all the disadvantages of truncal vagotomy but not the merit of simplicity, it was abandoned in favour of highly selective vagotomy.

Highly selective vagotomy

In 1968 Johnston and Amdrup independently devised the operation of highly selective vagotomy in which only the parietal cell mass of the stomach was denervated. This proved to be the most satisfactory operation for duodenal ulceration with a low incidence of side effects and acceptable recurrence rates when performed to a high technical standard. This operation became the gold standard for operations on duodenal ulceration in the 1970s. The operative

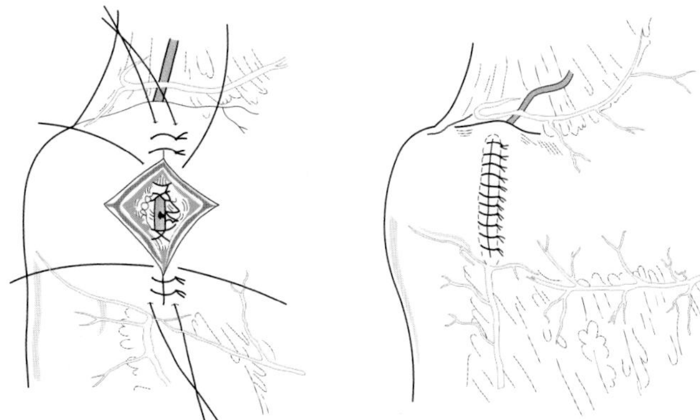

Fig. 51.22 Pyloroplasty. [Reproduced with permission from *Rob and Smith's Operative Surgery. Surgery of the Upper Gastrointestinal Tract*, 5th edn (eds G. Jamieson and H. Debas), Chapman & Hall, London, 1994, p. 396.]

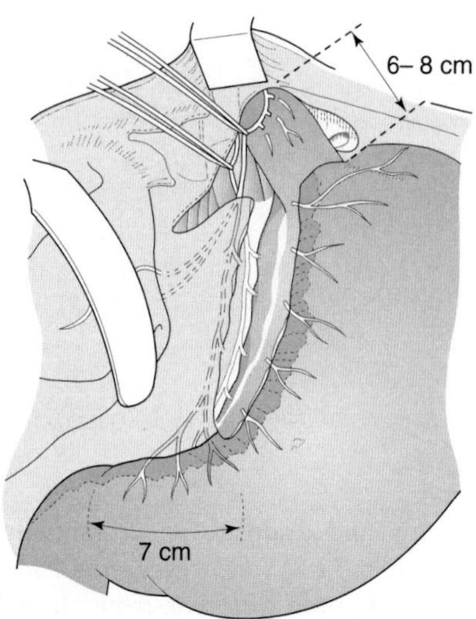

Fig. 51.23 Highly selective vagotomy. [Reproduced with permission from *Rob and Smith's Operative Surgery. Surgery of the Upper Gastrointestinal Tract*, 5th edn, (eds G. Jamieson and H. Debas), Chapman & Hall, London, 1994, p. 379.]

mortality was lower than any other definitive operation for duodenal ulceration, in all probability because the gastrointestinal tract is not opened during this procedure. The untoward effects of peptic ulcer surgery are largely avoided, although loss of receptive relaxation of the stomach does occur, leading to epigastric fullness and sometimes mild dumping. However, the severe symptoms that occur after other more destructive gastric operations do not occur. It is often said that recurrent ulceration is the Achilles' heel of this operation, although when performed well recurrence should be no more common than after truncal vagotomy.

In highly selective vagotomy the nerves of Latarjet supplying the antrum are preserved and a complete neurovascular clearance of the proximal lesser curve is carried out (Fig. 51.23). This is achieved by commencing the dissection from the anterior aspect and then opening the lesser sac through the greater omentum to perform the posterior dissection. Dissection is continued up to the oesophagogastric junction and the lower 7 cm of oesophagus cleared of nerve fibres. Particular attention must be paid to the nerve of Grassi which passes posteriorly to the greater curve, but the greater curvature itself need not be cleared. Attention must also be given to 'adhesions' within the lesser sac as these may carry nerve fibres. Using 24-hour pH-monitoring studies it has been demonstrated that this operation will achieve a reduction in the 24-hour intragastric acidity greater than can be obtained with conventional doses of H_2-receptor antagonists.

The advent of laparoscopic surgery renewed some interest in the surgery for duodenal ulceration but the technical difficulties in performing a full highly selective vagotomy laparoscopically are considerable. For this reason some centres adopted the procedure of anterior highly selective vagotomy and posterior truncal vagotomy as an alternative. However, as surgery for uncomplicated duodenal ulceration is to all intents and purposes unnecessary, there is now little interest in developing operations further.

Truncal vagotomy and antrectomy

For completeness this operation should be mentioned as it was at one stage popular in the USA. In addition to a truncal vagotomy, the antrum of the stomach is removed thus removing the source of gastrin, and the gastric remnant joined to the duodenum. The recurrence rates after this procedure are exceedingly low. However, the operative mortality is higher than after vagotomy and drainage (Table 51.2) and the incidence of unpleasant side effects is similar.

Operations for gastric ulcer

By contrast with duodenal ulcer surgery, where the principal objective is to reduce duodenal acid exposure, in gastric ulceration the diseased tissue is usually removed as well. This has the advantage that malignancy can then be confidently excluded. Although levels of gastric acid secretion are not abnormally high in the patients with gastric ulceration, acid is still a prerequisite and hence operations to lower acid secretion have been commonly employed.

Billroth I gastrectomy

This was the standard operation (Fig. 51.18) for gastric ulceration until medical treatments became prevalent. The distal stomach is mobilised and resected in the same way as in the Billroth II gastrectomy. This resection should include the ulcer that is usually situated on the lesser curve. The cut edge of the remnant is then partially closed from the lesser curve aspect leaving a stoma at the greater curve aspect which should be similar in size to the duodenum. Reconstruction may be facilitated by mobilising the duodenum using Kocher's manoeuvre. The incidence of recurrent ulceration after this operation is low, but it carries with it the morbidity and mortality associated with any gastric resection.

Billroth II gastrectomy

This may be used for the high and lesser curve gastric ulcer where a gastroduodenostomy is technically difficult.

Vagotomy, pyloroplasty and ulcer excision

Truncal vagotomy, drainage and ulcer excision was developed because of the concerns about morbidity and mortality following gastric resection for gastric ulcer. Highly selective vagotomy and gastric excision has a similar rationale, although is much more favourable in terms of side effects compared with truncal vagotomy and drainage. As with duo-

Theodore Kocher, 1841–1917. Professor of Surgery, Berne, Switzerland. One of the few surgeons to win the Nobel Prize for Medicine and Physiology 'for his work on the physiology, pathology and surgery of the thyroid gland'.

denal ulcers, most operations for uncomplicated gastric ulcers are of historical significance.

The complications of peptic ulceration

The common complications of peptic ulcer are perforation, bleeding and stenosis. Bleeding and stenosis are considered below in the relevant sections on 'Haematemesis and melaena' and 'Gastric outlet obstruction'.

Perforated peptic ulcer

Epidemiology

Overall and despite the widespread use of gastric antisecretory agents and eradication therapy, the incidence of perforated peptic ulcer has changed little. There has, however, been a considerable change in the epidemiology of perforated peptic ulcer over the last two decades. Previously, most patients were middle aged, with a ratio of 2:1 of male:female. With time there has been a steady increase in the age of the patients suffering this complication and an increase in the numbers of females, such that now perforations most commonly occur in elderly female patients. NSAIDs appear to be responsible for most of these perforations.

Clinical features

The classical presentation of perforated duodenal ulcer is instantly recognisable (Fig. 51.24). The patient, who may have a history of peptic ulceration, develops sudden onset severe generalised abdominal pain due to the irritant effect of gastric acid on the peritoneum. Although the contents of an acid-producing stomach are relatively low in bacterial load, bacterial peritonitis supervenes over a few hours usually accompanied by a deterioration in the patient's condition. Initially, the patient may be shocked with a tachycardia but a pyrexia is not usually observed until some hours after the event. The abdomen exhibits a board-like rigidity and the patient is disinclined to move because of the pain. The abdomen does not move with respiration. Patients with this form of presentation need an operation without which the patient will deteriorate with a septic peritonitis.

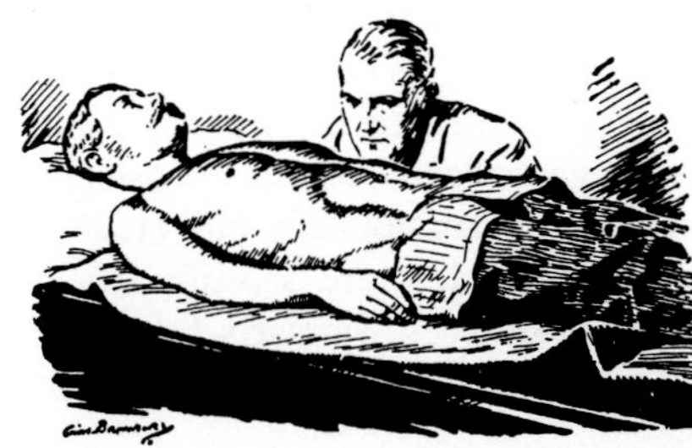

Fig. 51.24 A sketch of Mr Hamilton Bailey watching for abdominal movement on respiration. In the case of a classically presenting perforated ulcer the abdominal movement is restricted or absent.

Hamilton Bailey, 1894–1961. Surgeon, Royal Northern Hospital, London, England.

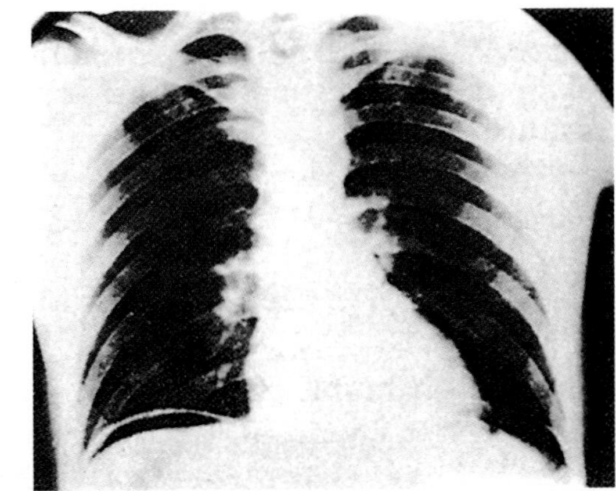

Fig. 51.25 Plain abdominal radiograph of a perforated ulcer showing air under the diaphragm.

This classical presentation of the perforated peptic ulcer is observed less commonly than in the past. Very frequently the elderly patient who is taking NSAIDs will have a less dramatic presentation, perhaps because of the use of potent anti-inflammatory drugs. The board-like rigidity seen in the abdomen of younger patients may also not be observed and a higher index of suspicion is necessary to make the correct diagnosis. In other patients the leak from the ulcer may not be massive. They may present only with pain in the epigastrium and right iliac fossa as the fluid may track down the right paracolic gutter. Sometimes perforations will seal owing to the inflammatory response and adhesion within the abdominal cavity and so the perforation may be self-limiting. All of these factors may combine to make the diagnosis of perforated peptic ulcer difficult.

By far the most common site of perforation is the anterior aspect of the duodenum. However, the anterior or incisural gastric ulcer may perforate and, in addition, gastric ulcers may perforate into the lesser sac, which can be particularly difficult to diagnose. These patients may not have obvious peritonitis.

Investigations

An erect plain chest radiograph will reveal free gas under the diaphragm in excess of 50 per cent of cases with perforated peptic ulcer (Fig. 51.25). All patients should have serum amylase performed, as distinguishing between peptic ulcer, perforation and pancreatitis can be difficult. Measuring the serum amylase, however, may not remove the diagnostic difficulty. It can be elevated following perforation of a peptic ulcer although, fortunately, the levels are not usually as high as the levels commonly seen in acute pancreatitis. Several other investigations are useful if doubt remains. A water-soluble contrast swallow will show a free peritoneal leak. Diagnostic peritoneal lavage will usually easily distinguish between perforation and pancreatitis, and a CT scan will normally be diagnostic in both conditions, although this is seldom necessary.

Treatment

The initial priorities are resuscitation and analgesia. Analgesia should not be withheld for fear of removing the signs of an intra-abdominal catastrophe. If anything, adequate analgesia makes the clinical signs more obvious. It is important, however, to titrate the analgesia so that the patient is not rendered unconscious. Following resuscitation and the diagnosis being established the treatment is principally surgical. Laparotomy is performed usually through an upper midline incision if the diagnosis of perforated peptic ulcer can be made with confidence. This is not always possible, and hence it may be better to place a small incision around the umbilicus to localise the perforation with more certainty. Alternatively, laparoscopy may be employed. The most important component of the operation is a thorough peritoneal toilet to remove all of the fluid and food debris. If the perforation is in the duodenum it can usually be closed by several well-placed sutures, closing the ulcer in a transverse direction as with a pyloroplasty. It is important that sufficient tissue is taken in the suture to allow the edges to be approximated, and the sutures should not be tied so tight that they tear out. It is common to place an omental patch over the perforation in the hope of enhancing the chances of the leak sealing. Gastric ulcers should, if possible, be excised and closed, so that malignancy can be excluded. Occasionally a patient is seen who has a massive duodenal or gastric perforation such that simple closure is impossible and in these patients a Billroth II gastrectomy is a useful operation.

All patients should be treated with systemic antibiotics and there may be some advantage in washing out the abdominal cavity with tetracycline, 1 g in 1 litre of isotonic saline. In the past many surgeons performed definitive procedures such as either truncal vagotomy and pyloroplasty or, more recently and probably more successfully, highly selective vagotomy during the course of an operation for a perforation. Studies show that in well-selected patients and in expert hands this is a very safe strategy. However, most commonly nowadays surgery is confined to first-aid measures and the peptic ulcer treated medically as described earlier in this chapter. Following operation gastric antisecretory agents should be started immediately.

Perforated peptic ulcers can often be managed by minimally invasive techniques if the expertise is available. The principles of operation are, however, the same; thorough peritoneal toilet is performed and the perforation closed by intracorporeal suturing. Whatever technique is used it is important that the stomach be kept empty postoperatively by nasogastric suction, and gastric antisecretory agents commenced to promote healing in the residual ulcer.

A great deal has been written about the conservative management of perforated ulcer. Some writers say that virtually all patients can be managed conservatively, whereas most surgeons have difficulty in understanding how a patient who is ill with widespread peritonitis and who has food debris widely distributed through the abdominal cavity will improve without an operation. However, there are undoubtedly patients who have small leaks from perforated peptic ulcer and relatively mild peritoneal contamination who may be managed with intravenous fluids, nasogastric suction and antibiotics. These patients are in the minority.

Patients who have suffered one perforation may suffer another one. They should therefore be managed aggressively to ensure that this does not happen. In patients with *Helicobacter*-associated ulcers, eradication therapy is appropriate. Patients on NSAIDs, who now form the majority of such patients, should have the drug withdrawn and another analgesic substituted. If it is necessary to continue the NSAIDs the patient should have concomitant treatment with a proton pump inhibitor such as omeprazole.

Sequelae of peptic ulcer surgery

There is a number of sequelae of peptic ulcer surgery which include recurrent ulceration, small stomach syndrome, bilious vomiting, early and late dumping, diarrhoea and malignant transformation. These sequelae principally follow from the more destructive operations that are now seldom performed. However, a substantial number of patients suffers from side effects from operations undertaken in the past. Approximately 30 per cent of patients can expect to suffer a degree of dysfunction following peptic ulcer surgery, and in about 5 per cent of such patients the symptoms will be intractable.

Recurrent ulceration

Although mentioned first, this is by far the easiest problem to treat. Just as all peptic ulcers will heal with potent antisecretory agents so will ulcers that are recurrent after ulcer surgery. The incidence of recurrent ulceration after the various operations is shown in Table 51.2.

The recurrent ulcer normally presents with pain, although some may develop a complication without any prior warning. Following an operation such as highly selective vagotomy the ulcer is in a similar position to the original ulcer, usually the first part of the duodenum. In patients with gastrojejunostomy, recurrent ulcer will commonly be at the anastomosis but on the jejunal side. Jejunal mucosa is much more sensitive to acid digestion compared with the stomach. Similarly, following gastrectomy the recurrent ulcer will be normally found on the jejunal side of the stoma.

A number of factors has been convincingly related to the development of recurrent ulceration. First and foremost, if the original operation was technically inadequate, such as the vagotomy being incomplete, then the incidence of recurrent ulceration is much higher. In this respect it is noteworthy that recurrent ulceration after, for instance, highly selective vagotomy is highly surgeon dependent. Cigarette smoking has been convincingly associated with an increased incidence of recurrent ulceration, and it has been shown that patients who had ulcers that are resistant to treatment with pharmacological agents before operation are more likely to develop recurrence afterwards.

If recurrent ulceration is diagnosed electively then long-term antisecretory agents are probably the treatment of choice if the patient has had an anatomically destructive operation. In patients with recurrent ulcer after highly selectively vagotomy, then eradication therapy may be effective. As with other peptic ulcers, recurrent ulcers may present with complications, particularly bleeding and perforation. In this respect the complication of gastrojejunal colic fistula requires a particular mention. In this rare condition the anastomotic ulcer penetrates into the transverse colon. The patient suffers from diarrhoea that is severe and follows every meal. They have foul breath and may vomit formed faeces. Severe weight loss and dehydration are rapid in onset, and for this reason the condition may be mistaken for malignancy. The major factor producing the nutritional disturbance is the severe contamination of the jejunum with colonic bacteria. A number of imaging techniques can be used to detect the fistula. A barium enema will normally demonstrate the problem, and CT scanning is also accurate. Endoscopy may not convincingly demonstrate the fistula and, in about half of such cases, the barium meal will not reveal the problem. The treatment of gastrocolic fistula consists of, first, correcting the dehydration and malnutrition and then performing revisional surgery.

Small stomach syndrome

Early satiety follows most ulcer operations to some degree, including highly selective vagotomy. In this latter circumstance, although there is no anatomical disturbance of the stomach there is loss of receptive relaxation. Fortunately, this problem does tend to get better with time and revisional surgery is not necessary.

Bile vomiting

Bile vomiting can occur after any form of vagotomy with drainage or gastrectomy. Commonly, the patient presents with vomiting a mixture of food and bile or sometimes some bile alone after a meal. Often eating will precipitate abdominal pain and reflux symptoms are common. Bile chelating agents can be tried but are usually ineffective. In intractable cases revisional surgery may be indicated. The nature of that revisional surgery depends very much on the original operation. Following gastrectomy Roux-en-Y diversion is probably the best treatment. In patients with a gastroenterostomy, this can be taken down and in most circumstances a small pyloroplasty performed. In patients with a pyloroplasty, reconstruction of the pylorus has been attempted but in general terms the results of this operation have been rather poor. Antrectomy and Roux-en-Y reconstruction may be the better option.

Early and late dumping

Although considered together because the symptoms are similar, early and late dumping have different aetiologies (Table 51.3). A common feature, however, is early rapid gastric emptying. Many patients have both early and late dumping.

Early dumping. Early dumping consists of abdominal and vasomotor symptoms that are found in about 10 per cent of patients following gastrectomy or vagotomy and drainage. It also affects a few per cent of patients following highly selective vagotomy due to the loss of receptive relaxation of the stomach. The small bowel is filled with foodstuffs from the stomach which have a high osmotic load and this leads to the sequestration of fluid from the circulation into the gastrointestinal tract. This can be observed by the rise in the packed cell volume while the symptoms are present. All of the symptoms shown in Table 51.3 can be related to this effect on the gut and the circulation.

Treatment. The principal treatment is dietary manipulation. Small dry meals are best, and avoiding fluids with a high carbohydrate content also helps. Fortunately, with time following operation the syndrome tends to improve. For some reason, however, there is a group of patients who suffer intractable dumping regardless of any of these measures. The somatostatin analogue octreotide given before meals has been shown to be useful in some individuals and the long-acting preparation may also be useful. However, this treatment can lead to the development of gallstones and it does not help the diarrhoea from which many patients with dumping also suffer.

Revisional surgery may be occasionally required. In patients with a gastroenterostomy, the drainage may be taken down or, in the case of a pyloroplasty, repaired. Alternatively, antrectomy with Roux-en-Y reconstruction is often effective, although the procedure is of greater magnitude. Following gastrectomy it is the revisional procedure of choice.

Table 51.3 Features of early and late dumping

	Early	*Late*
Incidence	5–10 per cent	5 per cent
Relation to meals	Almost immediate	Second hour after meal
Duration of attack	30–40 minutes	30–40 minutes
Relief	Lying down	Food
Aggravated by	More food	Exercise
Precipitating factor	Food, especially carbohydrate rich and wet	As early dumping
Major symptoms	Epigastric fullness, sweating, light headedness, tachycardia, colic, sometimes diarrhoea	Tremor, faintness, prostration

Cesar Roux, 1857–1934. Professor of Surgery, Lausanne, Switzerland. First described this method of forming a jejunal conduit, which has a multiplicity of uses in abdominal surgery.

Late dumping. This is reactive hypoglycaemia. The carbohydrate load in the small bowel causes a rise in the plasma glucose which in turn causes insulin levels to rise causing a secondary hypoglycaemia. This can be easily demonstrated by serial measurements of blood glucose in a patient following a test meal. The treatment is essentially the same as for early dumping. Octreotide is very effective in dealing with this problem.

Postvagotomy diarrhoea

This can be the most devastating symptom to afflict patients having peptic ulcer surgery. Most patients will suffer some looseness of bowel action to some degree (with the exception of highly selective vagotomy) but in about 5 per cent it may be intractable. In spite of much investigation the precise aetiology of the problem is uncertain. It is related, to some degree, to rapid gastric emptying. In all probability, the denervation of the upper gastrointestinal tract as a result of the vagotomy is also important. Exaggerated gastrointestinal peptide responses may also aggravate the condition.

The diarrhoea in postvagotomy patients may take several forms. It may be severe and explosive, the patient experiencing a considerable degree of urgency. The patients sometimes describe the diarrhoea as feeling like passing boiling water. At the other extreme some patients only have minor episodes of diarrhoea which are not as directly related to food.

Many authors regard diarrhoea and dumping as being essentially the same problem. However, many patients with severe diarrhoea do not have any of the other symptoms of dumping, and likewise some patients with dumping do not experience any significant diarrhoea.

The condition is difficult to treat. The patient should be managed as for early dumping and antidiarrhoeals may be of some value. Octreotide is not effective in this condition and the results of revisional surgery are too unpredictable to make this an attractive treatment option.

Malignant transformation

Many large studies now confirm that operations such as gastrectomy or vagotomy and drainage are independent risk factors for the development of gastric cancer. The increased risk appears to be approximately four times compared with the control population. It is interesting to note that this phenomenon is seen only in areas with already a significant incidence of gastric cancer; in areas such as Scandinavia with a low incidence it is difficult to observe such a phenomenon.

It is not difficult to understand the increased incidence of gastric cancer as bile reflux gastritis, intestinal metaplasia and gastric cancer are linked. The lag phase between operation and the development of malignancy is at least 10 years Highly selective vagotomy does not seem to be associated with an increased incidence of gastric cancer in the long term.

Nutritional consequences

Nutritional disorders are more common after gastrectomy than after vagotomy and drainage. Weight loss is common after gastrectomy and the patient may, in fact, never return to their original weight. Nutritional advice advising the taking of small meals is often more useful. Anaemia may be due to either iron or B_{12} deficiency.

Iron deficiency anaemia occurs after both gastrectomy and vagotomy and drainage and is probably multifactorial in origin. Reduced iron absorption is probably the most important factor, although the loss of blood from the gastric mucosa may also be important. B_{12} deficiency is prone to occur after total gastrectomy. However, because of the very large B_{12} stores that most patients have, this may be very late in occurring. B_{12} supplementation after total gastrectomy is, however, sensible. B_{12} deficiency may rarely occur after lesser forms of gastrectomy. In such patients the cause is probably a combination of reduced intrinsic factor production and also the fact that some patients have bacterial colonisation which results in the destruction of the B_{12} in the gut.

Bone disease is seen principally after Polya gastrectomy and mainly in women. The condition is essentially indistinguishable from the osteoporosis commonly seen in postmenopausal women. It is only the frequency and magnitude of the disorder that distinguish it. Treatment is by dietary supplementation, with calcium and vitamin D, and exercise.

Gallstones

The development of gallstones is strongly associated with truncal vagotomy. Following truncal vagotomy the biliary tree, as well as the stomach, is denervated leading to stasis and, hence, stone formation. Patients developing symptomatic gallstones will require cholecystectomy. This, however, may induce or worsen other postpeptic ulcer surgery syndromes such as bilious vomiting and postvagotomy diarrhoea.

Table 51.4 Causes of upper gastrointestinal bleeding

Condition	*Percentage*
Ulcers	60
– Oesophageal	6
– Gastric	21
– Duodenal	33
Erosions	26
– Oesophageal	13
– Gastric	9
– Duodenal	4
Mallory–Weiss tear	4
Oesophageal varices	4
Tumour	0.5
Vascular lesions, e.g. Dieulafoy's disease	0.5
Others	5

Haematemesis and melaena

Upper gastrointestinal haemorrhage remains a major medical problem and in spite of improvements in diagnosis and the proliferation in treatment modalities over the last few decades is still attended by significant mortality. A hospital mortality in the region of 5 per cent can be expected. In patients in whom the cause of bleeding can be found the most common causes are bleeding peptic ulcer, erosions, Mallory–Weiss tear and bleeding oesophageal varices (Table 51.4).

Whatever the cause the principles of management are identical. First, the patient should be adequately resuscitated and following this investigated urgently to determine the cause of the bleeding. Only then should treatment of a definitive nature be instituted. For any significant gastrointestinal bleed intravenous access should be established and, for those with severe bleeding, central venous pressure monitoring set up and bladder catheterisation performed. Blood should be cross-matched and the patient transfused as clinically indicated. As a general rule most gastrointestinal bleeding will stop, albeit temporarily, but there are sometimes instances when this is not the case. In these circumstances resuscitation, diagnosis and treatment should be carried out in quick succession. There are occasions when life-saving manoeuvres have to be undertaken without the benefit of an absolute diagnosis. For instance, in patients with known oesophageal varices and uncontrollable bleeding, a Sengstaken–Blakemore tube may be inserted before an endoscopy has been carried out. This practice is not to be encouraged, except *in extremis*. In some patients bleeding is secondary to a coagulopathy. The most important current causes of this are liver disease and inadequately controlled warfarin therapy. In these circumstances the coagulopathy should be corrected, if possible, with fresh frozen plasma.

Upper gastrointestinal endoscopy should be carried out by an experienced operator as soon as practicable after the patient has been stabilised. In patients in whom the bleeding is relatively mild, endoscopy may be carried on the morning after admission. In all cases of severe bleeding it should be carried out immediately.

Bleeding peptic ulcers

The epidemiology of bleeding peptic ulcers exactly mirrors that of perforated ulcers. The population affected has in recent years become much older and the bleeding is commonly associated with the ingestion of NSAIDs. Diagnosis can normally be made endoscopically, although occasionally the nature of the blood loss precludes accurately identifying the lesion. However, the more experienced the endoscopist the less likely this is to be a problem.

Medical and minimally interventional treatments

Medical treatment has limited efficacy. All patients are commonly started on either an H_2 antagonist or a proton pump antagonist, but well-performed studies have failed to show that such treatments influence rebleeding, operation rate or mortality. Meta-analysis of studies, however, does suggest that tranexamic acid, an inhibitor of fibrinolysis, reduces the rebleeding rate. Octreotide, a somatostatin analogue, has not proved effective.

Numerous endoscopic devices are now available which can be used to achieve haemostasis ranging from expensive lasers to inexpensive injection apparatus. There are few conclusive studies available but a review of the literature suggests that these modalities may have some utility, although they will probably never be effective in patients who are bleeding from large vessels and with which the majority of the mortality associated with the condition is associated.

Surgical treatment

Criteria for surgery are well worked out. A patient who continues to bleed requires surgical treatment. The same applies to a significant rebleed. Patients with a visible vessel in the ulcer base, a spurting vessel or an ulcer with a clot in the base are statistically likely to require surgical treatment to stop the bleeding. Elderly and unfit patients are more likely to die as a result of bleeding than younger patients. Ironically, they should have early surgery. A patient who has required more than 6 units of blood in general needs surgical treatment. Various scoring systems have been devised which predict the probability of rebleeding and mortality with some degree of accuracy.

The aim of the operation is to stop the bleeding. The advent of endoscopy has greatly helped in the management of upper gastrointestinal bleeding as a surgeon can usually be confident about the site of bleeding prior to operation. The most common site of bleeding from a peptic ulcer is the duodenum. In tackling this it is most important essential that the duodenum is fully Kocherised. This should be done before the duodenum is opened as it makes the ulcer much more accessible and also allows the surgeon's hand to be placed behind the gastroduodenal artery that is commonly the source of major bleeding. Following mobilisation, the duodenum and usually the pylorus are opened longitudinally as in a pyloroplasty. This allows good access to the ulcer, which is usually found posteriorly or superiorly. Accurate haemostasis is important. It is the vessel within the ulcer that is bleeding and this should be controlled using well-placed sutures which under run the vessel. The placing of more and more inaccurately positioned sutures is counter-productive. Following

George Kenneth Mallory, b. 1926. Professor of Pathology, Boston, Massachusetts, USA.

Soma Weiss, 1899–1942. Professor of Medicine, Boston, Massachusetts, USA.

Robert W. Sengstaken, b. 1923. American neurosurgeon.

under-running it is possible often to close the mucosa over the ulcer. The pyloroplasty is then closed with interrupted sutures in a transverse direction as in the usual fashion.

The principles of management of bleeding gastric ulcers are essentially the same. The stomach is opened at an appropriate position anteriorly and the vessel in the ulcer underrun. If the ulcer is not excised then a biopsy of the edge needs to be taken to exclude malignant transformation. Sometimes the bleeding is from the splenic artery and if there is a lot fibrosis present then the operation may be challenging. Most patients, however, can be managed by conservative surgery. Gastrectomy for bleeding has been widely practised in the past but is attended by higher levels of perioperative mortality even if the incidence of recurrent bleeding is less.

Much argument still remains about the use of definitive acid-lowering operations versus haemostatic surgery alone. Bearing in mind that most patients nowadays are elderly and unfit, the minimum surgery that stops the bleeding is probably optimal. Acid can be inhibited by pharmacological means and appropriate eradication therapy will prevent ulcer recurrence. Patients on long-term NSAIDs can be managed as outlined earlier.

Stress ulceration

This commonly occurs in patients with major injury or illness, who have undergone major surgery or who have major comorbidity. Previously, many such patients were to be found in intensive care units. There seems little doubt that the incidence of this problem has reduced in recent years owing to the widespread use of prophylaxis. Ranitidine has been shown to reduce the incidence of stress ulceration, as has the nasogastric administration of sulcrafate. There is no doubt that the prevention of this condition is far better than trying to treat it once it occurs. Endoscopic means of treating stress ulceration may be ineffective and operation required. The principles of management are the same as for the chronic ulcer.

Gastric erosions

Erosive gastritis has a variety of causes, especially NSAIDs. Fortunately, most such bleeding settles spontaneously but when it does not it can be a major problem to treat. In general terms, although there is a diffuse erosive gastritis, there is one (or more) specific lesion which has a significant sized vessel within it. This should be dealt with appropriately, preferably endoscopically, but sometimes surgery is necessary.

Mallory–Weiss tear

This is a longitudinal tear below the gastro-oesophageal junction, which is induced by repetitive and strenuous vomiting. Doubtless, many such lesions occur and do not cause bleeding. When it is a cause of haematemesis the lesion may often be missed as it can be difficult to see as it is just below the gastro-oesophageal junction, a position that can be difficult for the inexperienced endoscopist. Occasionally these lesions continue to bleed and require surgical treatment. Often the situation arises that the surgeon does not have guidance from the endoscopists as regards the site of bleeding, and a high index of suspicion in such circumstances is important. The stomach is opened by longitudinal gastrotomy and carefully inspected high up. It is normally possible to palpate the longitudinal mucosal tear with a little induration at the edges which gives a clue to the lesion's location. Under-running is all that is required.

Dieulafoy's disease

This is essentially a gastric arterial venous malformation that has a characteristic histological appearance. Bleeding due to this malformation is one of the most difficult causes of upper gastrointestinal bleeding to treat. The lesion itself is covered by normal mucosa and, when not bleeding, it may be invisible. If it can be seen whilst bleeding all that may be visible is profuse bleeding coming from an area of apparently normal mucosa. If this occurs cause is instantly recognisable. If the lesion can be identified endoscopically there are various means of dealing with it, including injection of sclerosant. If it is identified at operation then only a local excision is necessary. Occasionally a lesion is only recognised after gastrectomy and sometimes not even then. The pathologist, as well as the endoscopist, may have difficulty in finding it.

Tumours

All of the gastric tumours described below may present with chronic or acute upper gastrointestinal bleeding. Bleeding is not normally torrential but can be unremitting. Gastric smooth muscle tumours commonly present with bleeding and have a characteristic appearance, as the mucosa breaks down over the tumour in the gastric wall (Fig. 51.26). Whatever the nature, the tumours should be dealt with as appropriate.

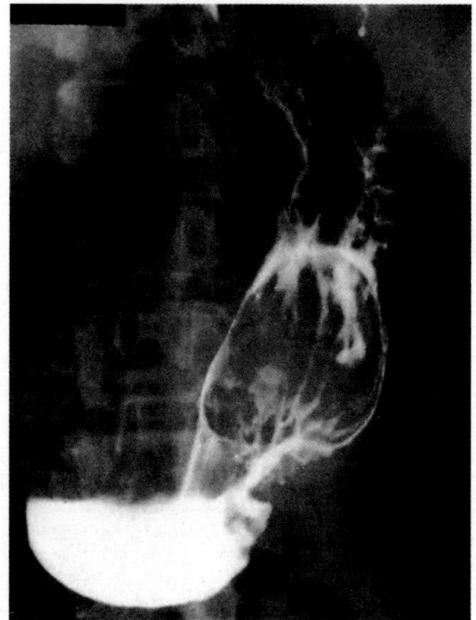

Fig. 51.26 Smooth muscle tumour of the stomach with ulceration.

Portal hypertension and portal gastropathy

The management of bleeding gastric varices is very challenging. Fortunately, most bleeding from varices is oesophageal and this is much more amenable to sclerotherapy, banding and balloon tamponade. Gastric varices may also be injected, although this is technically more difficult. Banding can also be used, again with difficulty. The gastric balloon of the Sengastaken–Blakemore tube can be used to arrest the haemorrhage if it is occurring from the fundus of the stomach. Octreotide is a somatostatin analogue which reduces portal pressure in patients with varices and trials suggest that it is of value in arresting haemorrhage in these patients, although its overall effect on mortality remains in doubt. Glypressin is also said to be of use.

Most surgeons prefer to avoid acute surgery on bleeding varices as, by contrast with elective operations for portal hypertension, acute shunts are attended by considerable operative mortality. For this reason the acute TIPSS procedure (transjugular intrahepatic portosystemic shunt) which is described in Chapter 52 can be an extremely useful, although technically demanding, procedure.

Portal gastropathy

Portal gastropathy is essentially the same disease process as described above. The mucosa is affected by the increased portal pressure and may exude blood even in the absence of well-developed visible varices. The treatment is as above.

Aortic enteric fistula

This diagnosis should be considered in any patient with haematemesis and melaena which cannot be otherwise explained. Contrary to expectation, the bleeding from such patients is not always massive, although it can be. Very often there is nothing much to distinguish the bleeding from the aortic enteric fistula from any other recurrent upper gastrointestinal bleeding. The vast majority of patients will have had an aortic graft and in the absence of this the diagnosis is unlikely. However, it is occasionally seen in patients with an untreated aortic aneurysm. A well-performed CT scan will commonly allow the diagnosis to be made with certainty. The condition should be managed by an expert vascular surgeon as, whether secondary or primary, the morbidity and mortality are high.

Gastric outlet obstruction

The two common causes of gastric outlet obstruction are gastric cancer (see below) and pyloric stenosis secondary to peptic ulceration. Previously the latter was more common. Now, with the decrease in the incidence of peptic ulceration and the advent of potent medical treatments, gastric outlet obstruction should be considered malignant until proven otherwise, at least in the West.

The term pyloric stenosis is normally a misnomer. The stenosis is seldom at the pylorus. Commonly, when the condition is due to underlying peptic ulcer disease, the stenosis is found in the first part of the duodenum, the most common site for a peptic ulcer. True pyloric stenosis can occur due to fibrosis around a pyloric channel ulcer. However, in recent years the most common cause of gastric outlet obstruction has been gastric cancer. In this circumstance the metabolic consequences may be somewhat different from those of benign pyloric stenosis because of the relative hypochlohydria found in patients with gastric cancer.

Clinical features

In benign gastric outlet obstruction there is usually a long history of peptic ulcer disease. Nowadays, as most patients with peptic ulcer symptoms are treated medically, it is easy to understand why the condition is becoming much less common. In some patients the pain may become unremitting and in other cases may largely disappear. The vomitus is characteristically unpleasant in nature and is totally lacking in bile. Very often it is possible to recognise foodstuff taken several days previously. The patient commonly complains of losing weight, and appears unwell and dehydrated. Examining the patient it may be possible to see the distended stomach and a succussion splash may be audible on shaking the patient's abdomen.

Metabolic effects

These are most interesting, as the metabolic consequences of benign pyloric stenosis are unique. The vomiting of hydrochloric acid results in hypochloraemic alkalosis. Initially the sodium and potassium may be relatively normal. However, as dehydration progresses more profound metabolic abnormalities arise, partly related to renal dysfunction. Initially the urine has a low chloride and high bicarbonate content reflecting the primary metabolic abnormality. This bicarbonate is excreted along with sodium, and so with time the patient becomes progressively hyponatraemic and more profoundly dehydrated. Because of the dehydration, a phase of sodium retention follows and potassium and hydrogen are excreted in preference. This results in the urine becoming paradoxically acidic and hypokalaemia ensues. Alkalosis leads to a lowering in the circulating ionised calcium, and tetany can occur.

Management

Treating the patient involves correcting the metabolic abnormality and dealing with the mechanical problem. The patient should be rehydrated with intravenous isotonic saline with potassium supplementation. Replacing the sodium chloride and water allows the kidney to correct the acid–base abnormality. Following rehydration it may become obvious that the patient is also anaemic, the haemoglobin being spuriously high on presentation.

It is noteworthy that the metabolic abnormalities may be

less if the obstruction is due to malignancy as the acid–base disturbance is less pronounced.

The stomach should be emptied using a wide-bore gastric tube. A large nasogastric tube may not be sufficiently large to deal with the contents of the stomach and it may be necessary to pass an orogastric tube and lavage the stomach until it is completely emptied. This then allows investigation of the patient with endoscopy and contrast radiology. Biopsy of the area around the pylorus is essential to exclude malignancy. The patient should also have a gastric antisecretory agent such as ranitidine, given initially intravenously to ensure absorption.

Early cases may settle with conservative treatment, presumably as the oedema around the ulcer diminishes as the ulcer is healed. Traditionally severe cases are treated surgically, usually with a gastroenterostomy rather than a pyloroplasty. The addition of a vagotomy in these circumstances may be appropriate. Endoscopic treatment with balloon dilatation has been practised and may be most useful in early cases. This treatment is, however, not devoid of problems. Dilating the duodenal stenosis may result in perforation. The dilatation may have to be performed several times and sometimes may not be successful in the long term.

Other causes of gastric outlet obstruction

Adult pyloric stenosis

This is a rare condition and its relationship to the childhood condition unclear, although some patients have a long history of problems with gastric emptying. It is commonly treated by pyloroplasty rather than pyloromyotomy.

Pyloric mucosal diaphragm

The origin of this rare condition is unknown. It usually does not become apparent until middle life. When found simple excision of the mucosal diaphragm is all that is required.

Gastric polyps

A number of conditions manifests as gastric polyps. Their main importance is that they may actually represent early gastric cancer. Biopsy is essential.

The most common type of gastric polyp is metaplastic. These are associated with *H. pylori* infection and regress following eradication therapy. Inflammatory polyps are also common. Fundic gland polyps deserve particular attention. They seem to be associated with the use of proton pump inhibitors and are also found in patients with familial polyposis. None of the above polypoid lesions has proven malignant potential. True adenomas have malignant potential and should be removed, but account for only 10 per cent of polypoid lesions. Gastric carcinoids, arising from the ECL cells, are seen particularly in patients with pernicious anaemia, and usually appear as small polyps.

Gastric cancer

Carcinoma of the stomach has been described as one of the 'Captains of the men of death'. Examining the survival statistics from the UK it is not hard to agree with this gloomy view. Some series demonstrate overall 5-year survival statistics in the region of 5 per cent. These data obscure the fact that gastric cancer is an eminently curable disease provided that it is detected at an appropriate stage and treated adequately. Gastric cancer rarely disseminates widely before it has involved the lymph nodes and therefore there is an opportunity to cure the disease prior to dissemination. Early diagnosis is therefore the key to success with this disease. The only treatment modality able to cure the disease is resectional surgery.

Incidence

There are marked variations in the incidence of gastric cancer worldwide. In the UK it is approximately 15 per 100 000 per year, in the USA 10 per 100 000 per year and in Eastern Europe 40 per 100 000 per year. In Japan the disease is much more common with an incidence of approximately 70 per 100 000 per year, and there are small geographical areas in China where the incidence is double that in Japan. These underlying epidemiological data make it clear that this is an environmental disease. In general men are more affected by the disease than women and, as with most solid organ malignancies, the incidence increases with age.

Currently marked changes are being observed in the West in terms of both the incidence and site of gastric cancer and the population affected, changes that to date have not been observed in Japan. First, the incidence of gastric cancer is continuing to fall at about 1 per cent per year. This reduction exclusively affects carcinoma arising in the body and distal stomach. By contrast, there appears to be an increase in the incidence of carcinoma in the proximal stomach, particularly the oesophagogastric junction. Carcinoma of the distal and body of the stomach is most common in low socioeconomic groups, whereas the increase in proximal gastric cancer seems to affect principally higher socioeconomic groups. Proximal gastric cancer does not seem to be associated with *H. pylori* infection, in contrast to carcinoma of the body and distal stomach.

Aetiology

Gastric cancer is a multifactorial disease (Correa). Epidemiological studies point to a role for *H. pylori*, although there is argument about how important this factor is. Certainly the EUROGAST study revealed a correlation between the incidence of gastric cancer in various populations and the prevalence of *H. pylori* infection, although there was a

P. Correa. Pathologist, New Orleans, Louisiana, USA. Produced a cogent hypothesis to explain the development of the intestinal type of gastric cancer.

considerable scatter about the regression line indicating that other factors were also important. There is insufficient evidence at the moment to support eradication programmes in asymptomatic patients who are infected with *Helicobacter* with a view to reducing the population incidence of gastric cancer. However, clinical trials may subsequently change this view. As mentioned above *Helicobacter* seems to be principally associated with carcinoma of the body, stomach and distal stomach rather than the proximal stomach. As *Helicobacter* is associated with gastritis, gastric atrophy and intestinal metaplasia the association with malignancy is perhaps not surprising.

Several other risk factors have been identified as being important in the aetiology of gastric cancer. Patients with pernicious anaemia and gastric atrophy are at increased risk, as are those with gastric polyps. Patients who have had peptic ulcer surgery, particularly those who have had drainage procedures such as Billroth II or Polya gastrectomy, gastro-enterostomy or pyloroplasty are at approximately four times the average risk. There is no direct evidence to date that highly selective vagotomy is associated with an increased risk of gastric cancer. Presumably duodenogastric reflux and reflux gastritis are related to the increased risk of malignancy in these patients. Intestinal metaplasia is a risk factor. Carcinoma is associated with cigarette smoking and dust ingestion from a variety of industrial processes. Diet appears to be important, as illustrated by the often quoted example of the change in the incidence of gastric cancer as Japanese families moved to the USA. The high incidence of gastric cancer in some pockets in China is probably environmental and probably diet related. The ingestion of substances such as spirits may induce gastritis and, in the long term, cancer. Excessive salt intake, deficiency of antioxidants and exposure to N-nitroso compounds are also related. The aetiology of proximal gastric cancer remains an enigma. Genetic factors are also important but imperfectly elucidated (see below).

The molecular pathology of gastric cancer

In contrast to colorectal cancer, the molecular pathology of gastric cancer is less well worked out. However, it is likely that with time the importance of the genetic events in gastric cancer will similarly be realised. The oncogenes H-ras and c-erb B2 have both been studied. Evidence suggests that *H-ras* mutations occur at an early stage of gastric carcinogenesis and it is not clear that *ras* mutations are of importance in tumour progression. *c-erb B2* encodes for a transmembrane tyrosine kinase receptor which has sequence homology with epidermal growth factor receptor. *c-erb B2* is amplified and overexpressed in well-differentiated gastric carcinomas of the intestinal type and, as it is commonly seen in metastases, it may therefore be important in tumour progression.

The role of tumour supressor genes has also been examined. The APC gene that is responsible for familial polyposis is mutated in 25 per cent of moderately/well-differentiated carcinomas, and loss of heterozygosity of this region is seen in about 60 per cent of tumours. However, loss of the APC gene has not been detected in poorly differentiated gastric cancers making its role unclear. p53 is the archetypal tumour supressor gene. p53 protein is overexpressed in many transformed cells and this overexpression is often related to a p53 mutation, the protein product of the mutant gene being more stable. Again, the role of p53 in gastric cancer is unclear. Abnormalities in p53 have been found in intestinal metaplasia in the stomach but not in the primary tumours except at a late stage.

Microsatellite instability is a form of genetic instability resulting from deficiencies in the mismatch repair genes. The result of this phenotype is the rapid accumulation of mutations within the genome (mutator phenotype), hence predisposing to malignant transformation. Inherited mismatch repair deficiency is responsible for hereditary nonpolyposis colorectal cancer (HNPCC). Gastric cancers are also found in families with this phenotype. Microsatellite instability is found in about 15 per cent of sporadic colorectal cancers and apparently in a similar per centage of sporadic gastric cancers.

Clinical features

The features of advanced gastric cancer are usually obvious. However, curable gastric cancer has no specific features to distinguish it symptomatically from benign dyspepsia. The key to improving the outcome of gastric cancer is early diagnosis and, although in Japan there is a screening programme, most curable cases are picked up by the liberal use of gastroscopy in patients with dyspepsia. Present guidelines suggest gastroscopy for any new dyspepsia, however mild, in a patient over 40 years of age. The same advice applies to a patient of any age with persistent dyspepsia or any unusual feature. It is important to note that gastric antisecretory agents will improve the symptoms of gastric cancer so the disease must be excluded, preferably before therapy is started.

In advanced cancer early satiety, bloating, distension and vomiting may occur. The tumour frequently bleeds resulting in iron deficiency anaemia. Obstruction leads to dysphagia, epigastric fullness or vomiting. With pyloric involvement the presentation may be of gastric outlet obstruction, although the alkalosis is usually less pronounced or absent compared to when duodenal ulceration leads to obstruction. In recent years gastric outlet obstruction is more commonly associated with malignancy than benign disease. Nonmetastatic effects of malignacy are seen, particularly thromboplebitis (Trousseau's sign) and deep venous thrombosis. These feature result from the effects of the tumour on thrombotic and haemostatic mechanisms.

Armand Trousseau, 1801–67. Physician, Hotel Dieu, Paris, France. This sign led him to suspect himself of having gastric cancer. He actually had pancreatic cancer, diagnosed post mortem.

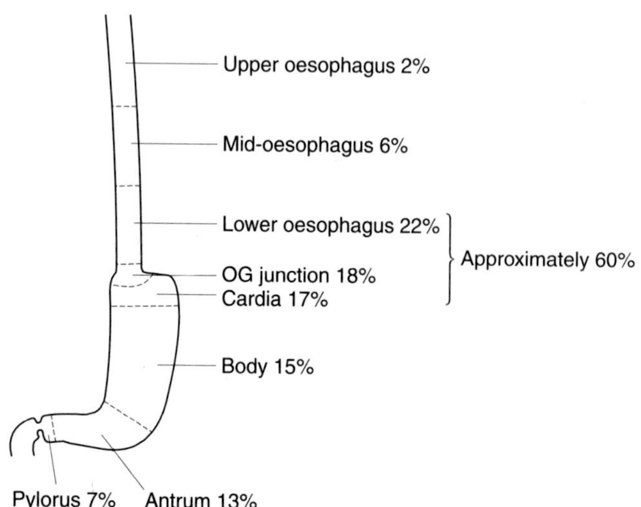

Fig. 51.27 The incidence of cancer in the various parts of the upper gastrointestinal tract in the UK. OG, oesophagogastric.

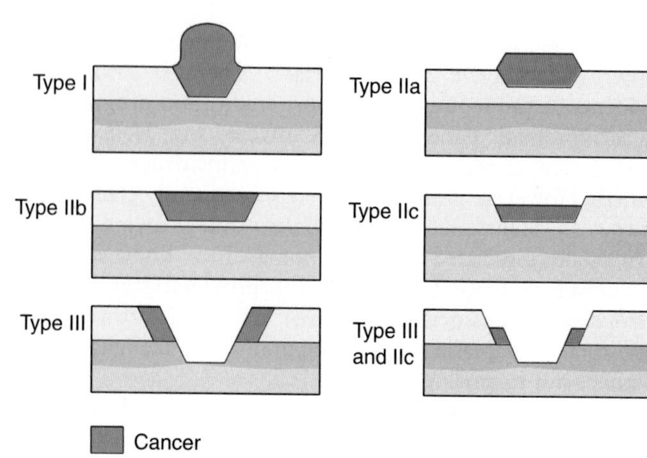

Fig. 51.28 Early gastric cancer, Japanese classification.

Site

The proximal stomach is now the most common site for gastric cancer in the UK. Because so many malignancies occur at the oesophageal–gastric junction and because the lower oesophagus is also a very common site of adenocarcinoma it is artificial to separate the stomach from the oesophagus. It is therefore best to consider the whole of the upper gastrointestinal tract from the cricopharyngeus to the pylorus. The incidence of cancer at these various sites is shown in Fig. 51.27. It can be seen that just under 60 per cent of all of the malignancies occurring in the oesophagus and stomach occur in proximity to the oesophagogastric junction. This high prevalence of proximal gastric cancer is not seen in Japan where distal cancer still predominates.

Pathology

The most useful classification of gastric cancer is the Lauren classification. In this system there are principally two forms of gastric cancer: intestinal gastric cancer and diffuse gastric cancer. In intestinal gastric cancer the tumour resembles a carcinoma elsewhere in the tubular gastrointestinal tract and forms polypoid tumours or ulcers. It probably arises in areas of intestinal metaplasia. By contract, diffuse gastric cancer inflitrates deeply into the stomach without forming obvious

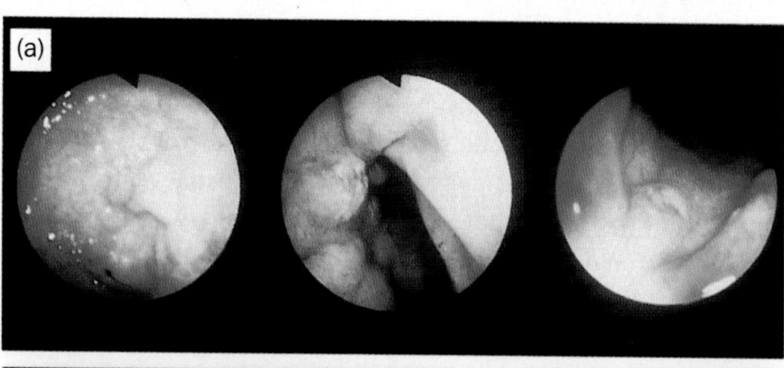

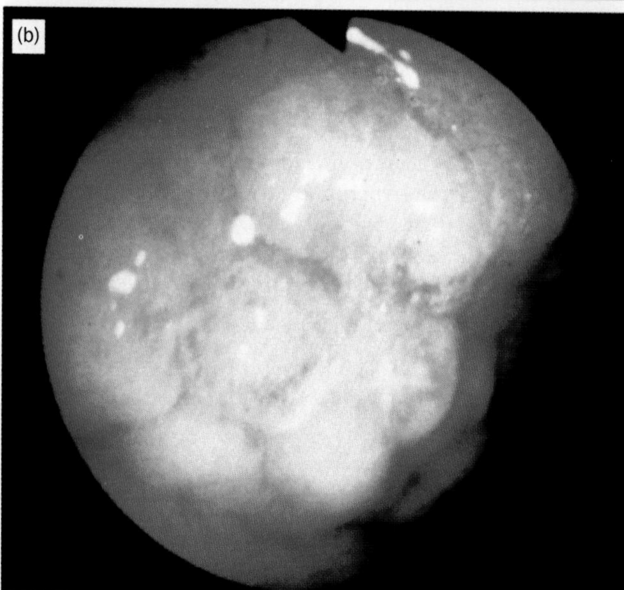

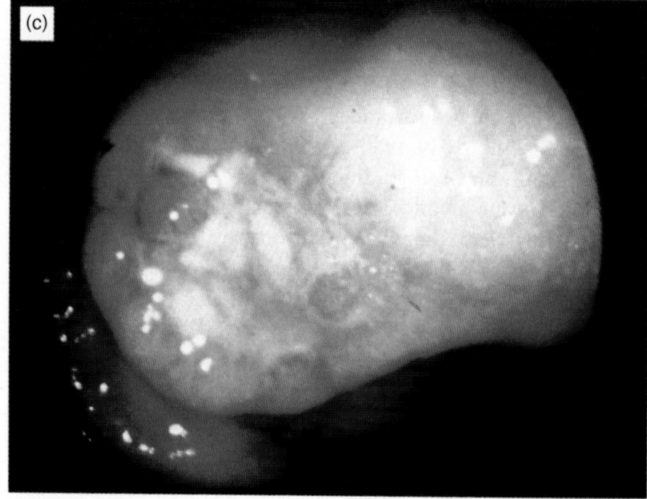

Fig. 51.29 Early gastric cancer. (a) Type I. (b) Type Iia. (c) Type III (*courtesy of Dr G.N.J. Tytgat, Amsterdam*).

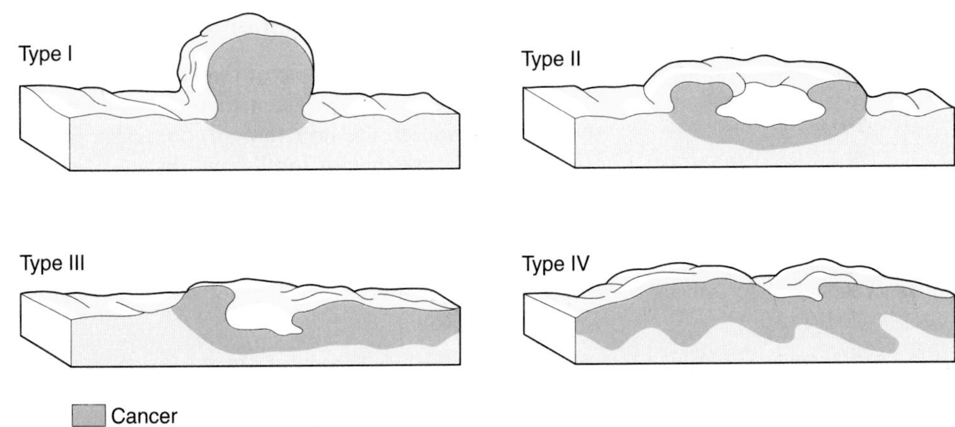

Fig. 51.30 Bormann classification of advanced gastric cancer.

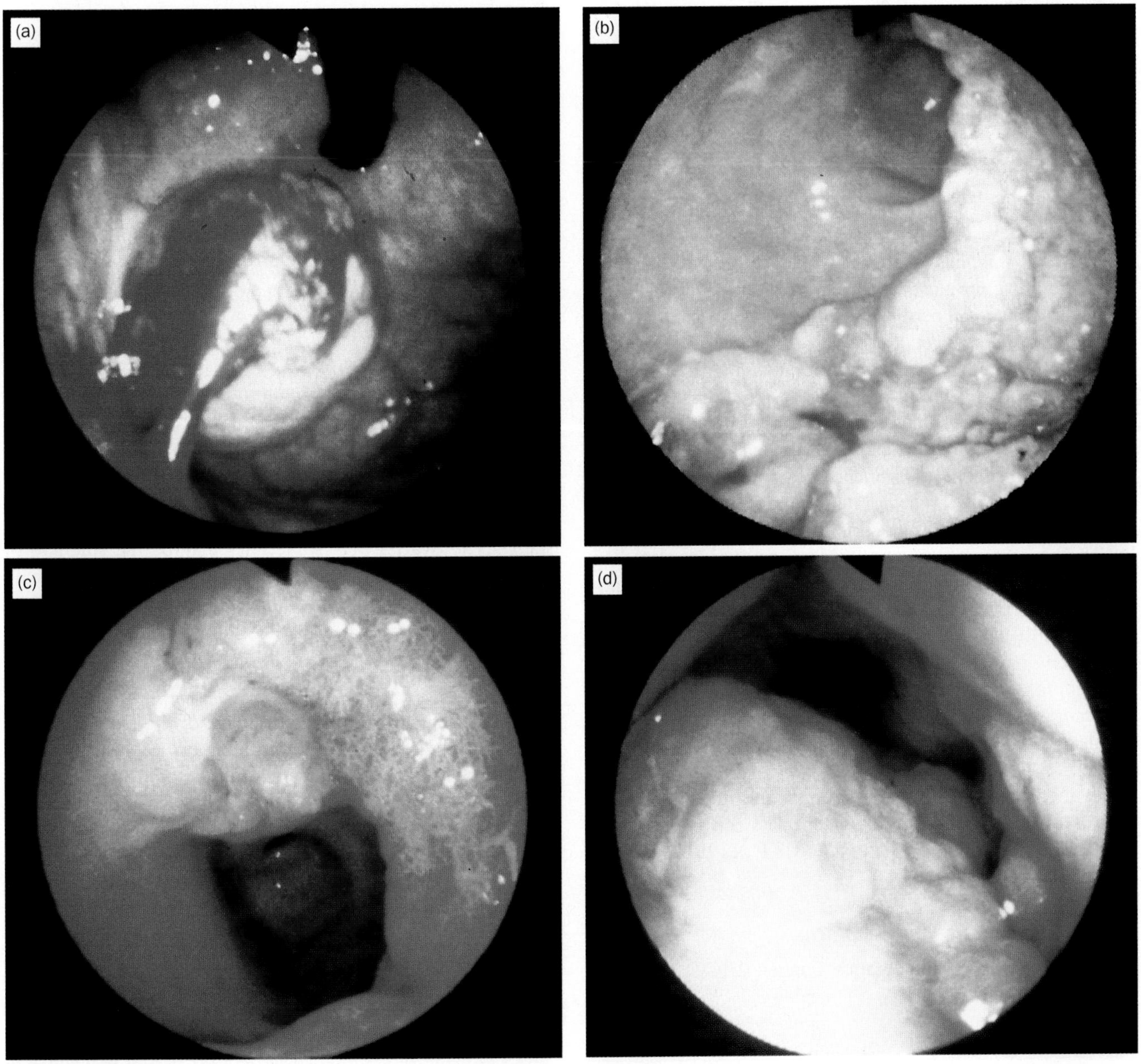

Fig. 51.31 Advanced gastric cancer. (a) Type I. (b) Type II. (c) Type III. (d) Type IV (linitus plastica) (*courtesy of Dr G.N.J. Tytgat, Amsterdam*).

Table 51.5 Staging of gastric cancer

T1	Tumour involves lamina propria or submucosa
T2	Tumour invades muscularis or subserosa
T3	Tumour involves mucosa
T4	Tumour invades adjacent organs
N0	No lymph node metastases
N1	Metastasis in perigastic nodes
N2	Metastasis in nodes along main arterial trunks
M0	No distant metastasis
M1	Distant metastasis (this includes peritoneum and N3/N4 nodes)

Staging			
IA	T1	N0	M0
IB	T1	N1	M0
	T2	N0	M0
II	T1	N2	M0
	T2	N1	M0
	T3	N0	M0
IIIA	T2	N2	M0
	T3	N1	M0
	T4	N0	M0
IIIB	T3	N2	M0
	T4	N1	M0
IV	T4	N2	M0
	Any T	Any N	M1

mass lesions but spreads widely in the gastric wall. Not surprisingly, this has a much worse prognosis. A small proportion of gastric cancers are of mixed morphology.

Gastric cancer can be divided into early gastric cancer and advanced gastric cancer. Early gastric cancer is defined as cancer limited to the mucosa and submucosa with or without lymph node involvement (T1, any N). The classification is shown in Fig. 51.28. This can be either protruding, superficial or excavated in the Japanese classification (Fig. 51.29). This type of cancer is eminently curable and even early gastric cancers associated with lymph node involvement have 5-year survival rates in the region of 90 per cent (Fig. 51.29). In Japan approximately one-third of gastric cancers diagnosed are in this stage. However, in the UK it is uncommon to detect gastric cancers at this stage. A number of reasons probably still accounts for this. First, because gastric cancer is less common in the UK dyspeptic patients are not always referred for endoscopy at an appropriate stage. Secondly, endoscopists are unfamiliar with the appearances of early gastric cancer and in all probability many such cases are missed.

Advanced gastric cancer involves the muscularis. Its macroscopic appearances have been classified by Bormann into four types (Figs 51.30 and 51.31). Types III and IV are commonly incurable.

Staging

The International Union Against Cancer (UICC) staging is shown in Table 51.5.

Charles Emile Trosier, 1844–1919. Professor of Pathology, Paris, France.

Spread of carcinoma of the stomach

No better example of the various modes by which carcinoma spreads can be given than the case of stomach cancer. It is important to note that this distant spread is unusual before the disease spreads locally and distant metastases are uncommon in the absence of lymph node metastases. The intestinal and diffuse types of gastric cancer spread differently. The diffuse type spreads via the submucosal and subserosal lymphatic plexus and it penetrates the gastric wall at an early stage.

Direct spread

The tumour penetrates the muscularis, serosa and ultimately adjacent organs such as the pancreas, colon and liver.

Lymphatic spread

This is both by permeation and emboli to the affected tiers (see below) of nodes. This may be extensive, the tumour even appearing in the supraclavicular nodes (Trosier's sign). Unlike malignancies such as breast cancer, nodal involvement does not imply systemic dissemination.

Blood-borne metastases

This occurs first to the liver and subsequently to other organs including lung and bone. This is uncommon in the absence of extensive nodal disease.

Transperitoneal spread

This is a common mode of spread once the tumour has reached the serosa of the stomach and indicates incurability. Tumours can manifest anywhere in the peritoneal cavity and commonly give rise to ascites. Advanced peritoneal disease may be palpated either abdominally or rectally as a tumour 'shelf'. The ovaries may sometimes may be the sole site of transcoelomic spread (Krukenberg's tumours). Tumour may spread via the abdominal cavity to the umbilicus (Sister Joseph's nodule).

Lymphatic drainage of the stomach

Understanding the lymphatic drainage of the stomach is the key to comprehending the radical surgery of gastric cancer. The lymphatics of the antrum drain into the right gastric lymph node superiorly, and right gastroepiploic and subpyloric lymph nodes inferiorly. The lymphatics of the pylorus drain into the right gastric suprapyloric nodes superiorly and the subpyloric lymph nodes situated around

Fredrich Ernst Krukenberg, 1870–1946. Ophthalmologist, Halle, Germany. Wrote a classic paper on malignant tumours of the ovary in 1896.
Sister Mary Joseph. Operating theatre sister who worked with the Mayo brothers at the eponymous clinic, Rochester, Minnesota, USA. Noted the presence of an umbilical nodule in many patients who proved to have advanced gastric cancer.

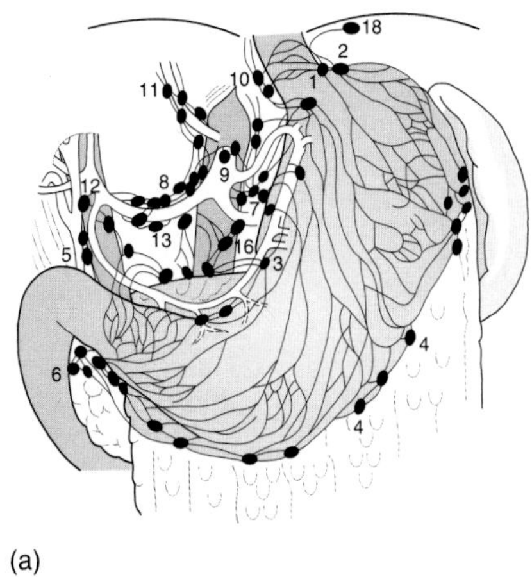

(a)

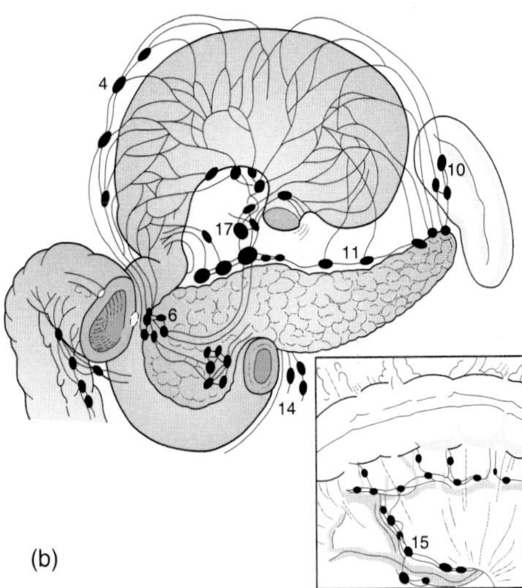

(b)

Fig. 51.32 Lymphatic drainage of the stomach and nodal stations by the Japanese classification. [Reproduced with permission from *Rob and Smith's Operative Surgery. Surgery of the Upper Gastrointestinal Tract*, 5th edn (eds G. Jamieson and H. Debas), Chapman & Hall, London, 1994, p. 451.]

the gastroduodenal artery inferiorly. The efferent lymphatics from suprapyloric lymph nodes converge on the para-aortic nodes around the coeliac axis, while the efferent lymphatics from the subpyloric lymph nodes pass up to the main superior mesenteric lymph nodes situated around the origin of the superior mesenteric artery. The lymphatic vessels related to the cardiac orifice of the stomach communicate freely with those of the oesophagus.

Whether or not there is histological evidence of regional lymph node involvement affects the prognosis of operable cases of carcinoma of the stomach. Retrograde (downward) spread may occur if the upper lymphatics are blocked. In Japan the lymph node dissection is highly advanced and the Japanese Research Society for Gastric Cancer has assigned a number to each lymph node station to aid the pathological staging (Fig. 51.32). Many centres in the West now perform surgery that involves a radical lymphadenectomy, but in others both the staging and surgery are inadequate.

Operability

It is important that patients with incurable disease are not subjected to radical surgery that cannot help them. Unequivocal evidence of incurability is haematogenous metastases, involvement of the distant peritoneum, N4 nodal disease and disease beyond the N4 nodes, and fixation to structures that cannot be removed. It is important to note that involvement of another organ per se does not imply incurability provided that it can be removed. Controversies with respect to operability include N3 nodal involvement and involvement of the adjacent peritoneum. Curative resection should be considered on the remaining patients.

Total gastrectomy

This is best performed through a long upper midline incision. The stomach is removed *en bloc* including the tissues of the entire greater omentum and lesser omentum (Fig. 51.33). In commencing the operation the transverse colon is completely separated from the greater omentum. The dissection may then be commenced either proximally or, more usually, distally. The subpyloric nodes are dissected and the first part of the duodenum is divided, usually with a surgical stapler. The hepatic nodes are dissected down to clear the hepatic artery; this dissection also includes the suprapyloric nodes. The right gastric artery is taken on the hepatic artery. The lymph node dissection is continued to the origin of the left gastric artery which is divided flush with its origin. The dissection is continued along the splenic artery taking all of the nodes at the superior aspect of the pancreas and in the splenic hilum. Separation of the stomach from the spleen, if this organ is not going to be removed, is carried out and this then allows access to the nodal tissues around the upper stomach and oesophagogastric junction. The oesophagus can then be divided at an appropriate point using a combination of stay sutures and a soft noncrushing clamp, usually of the right-angled variety. It is important that the resection margins are well clear of the tumour. Involvement of either proximal or distal resection margin carries an appalling prognosis and if in doubt frozen section should be performed. There is some controversy regarding the management of the spleen and distal pancreas in this procedure and this is discussed below.

Gastrointestinal continuity is reconstituted by means of a Roux loop. Other methods of reconstruction should be discouraged because of poor functional results. The Roux loop should be at least 50 cm long to avoid bile reflux oesophagitis. The simplest means of effecting the oesophagojejunostomy is to place a purse string in the cut end of the oesophagus and, using a circular stapler introduced through the blind end of the Roux loop, staple the end of the oesophagus on to the side of the Roux loop. The blind open end of the Roux loop may then be closed either with sutures or, alternatively, with a linear stapler. The anastomosis can also be fashioned end to end. The Roux loop may placed in either an anticolic or retrocolic position. The jejunojejunostomy is undertaken at a convenient point in the usual fashion (end to side, Fig. 51.34).

There remains some controversy about the extent of the lymphadenectomy required for the optimal treatment of curable gastric cancer. In Japan a D2 gastrectomy (removal of the second tier of nodes) at least is performed on all operable gastric cancer and some centres are practising more radical surgery (D3 and even D4 resections). Certainly, the results of surgical treatment stage for stage in Japan are much better than commonly reported in the West, and the Japanese contention is that the difference is principally related to the staging and the quality of the surgery. It is observed that the build of the average Japanese patient favours the performance of more radical procedures compared with the average patient in the West. However, radical lymphadenectomies above D2 have not been subjected to any randomised controlled trials. In the

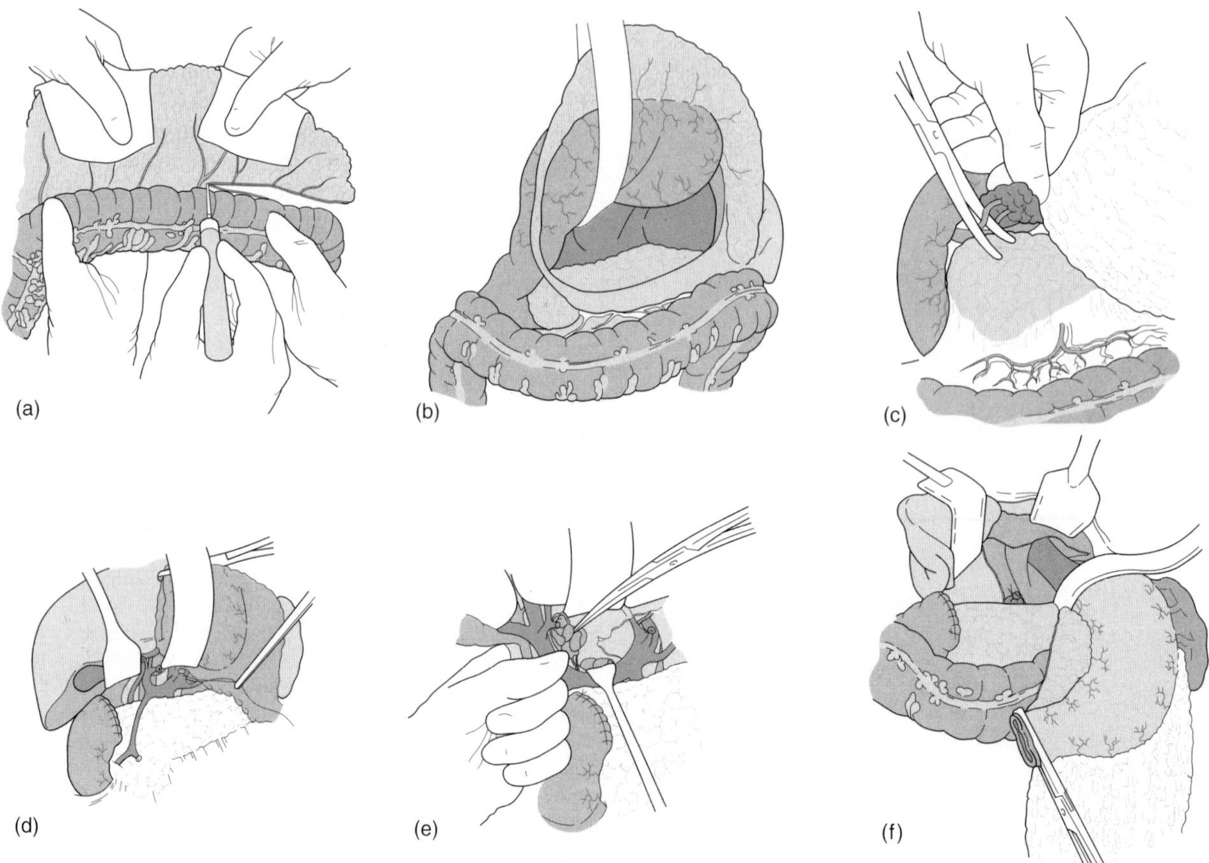

Fig. 51.33 Radical total gastrectomy. [Reproduced with permission from *Rob and Smith's Operative Surgery. Surgery of the Upper Gastrointestinal Tract*, 5th edn (eds G. Jamieson and H. Debas), Chapman & Hall, London, 1994, p. 452.]

UK and Europe randomised trials have been set up to compare D1 and D2 gastrectomy but the results are difficult to interpret. One of the problems relates to standardisation of the operation. Overall, it seems that the oncological outcome may be better following a D2 gastrectomy but this operation is associated with higher levels of morbidity and perioperative mortality. It is clear that most of this morbidity and mortality relates to the removal of the spleen with or without the distal pancreas. The traditional radical gastrectomy removes the spleen and distal pancreas *en bloc* with the stomach and, although this is indeed an adequate means of performing clearance of the lymph nodes around the splenic artery, there seems now little doubt that adding this substantially increases the complication rate. The Japanese D2 gastrectomy will commonly preserve spleen and pancreas.

The differentiation between a D1 and a D2 operation depends upon the tiers of nodes removed. Different tiers need to be removed depending on the positions of primary tumour and this is outlined in Table 51.6. In general, a D1 resection involves the removal of the perigastric nodes and a D2 resection involves the clearance of the major arterial trunks.

Subtotal gastrectomy

For tumours distally placed in the stomach it appears unnecessary to remove the whole stomach. The operation, however, is very similar to that of a total gastrectomy except that the proximal stomach is preserved, the blood supply being derived from the short gastric arteries. Following the resection the simplest form of reconstruction is to close the stomach from the lesser curve near the oesophagogastric junction

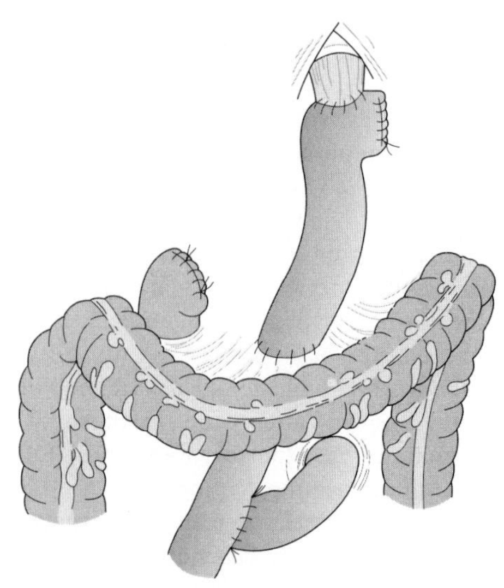

Fig. 51.34 Oesophagojejunostomy Roux-en-Y. [Reproduced with permission from *Rob and Smith's Operative Surgery. Surgery of the Upper Gastrointestinal Tract*, 5th edn (eds G. Jamieson and H. Debas), Chapman & Hall, London, 1994, p. 462.]

Table 51.6 The lymph node stations (see Fig. 51.32) which need to be removed in a D1 (N1 nodes removed) or a D2 (N2 nodes removed) resection. The nodes in stations 12–18 are not routinely removed in a D1 or D2 gastrectomy

LN number		Site of cancer: Antrum	Middle	Cardia	Cardia + oesophagus
1	Right cardial	N2	N1	N1	N1
2	Left cardial		N1	N1	N1
3	Lesser curve	N1	N1	N1	N1
4sa	Short gastric	N1	N1	N1	N1
4sb	Left gastroepiploic	N1	N1	N1	N1
4d	Right gastroepiploic	N1	N1	N2	N2
5	Suprapyloric	N1	N1	N2	N2
6	Infrapyloric	N1	N1	N2	N2
7	Left gastric artery	N2	N2	N2	N2
8a	Anterior hepatic artery	N2	N2	N2	N2
9	Coeliac artery	N2	N2	N2	N2
10	Splenic hilum		N2	N2	N2
11	Splenic artery		N2	N2	N2
19	Infradiaphragmatic				N2
20	Oesophageal hiatus			N2	N1
110	Lower oesophagus				N2
111	Supradiaphragmatic				N2

with either sutures or staples and then perform an anastomosis of the greater curve to the jejunum. Although this can be performed as in a Billroth II/Polya-type gastrectomy, this reconstruction results in quite marked enterogastric reflux and bile reflux oesophagitis, and the preferred reconstruction is to perform the reconstruction using a Roux loop.

Palliative surgery

In patients suffering from significant symptoms of either obstruction or bleeding, palliative resection is appropriate. A palliative gastrectomy need not be radical and it is sufficient to remove the tumour and reconstruct the gastrointestinal tract. Sometimes it is impossible to resect an obstructing tumour in the distal stomach and other palliative procedures need to be considered, although the prognosis in such patients, even in the short term, is poor. A high gastroenterostomy is a bad operation that very frequently does not allow the stomach to empty adequately but may produce the additional problem of bile reflux. A Roux loop with a wide anastomosis between the stomach and jejunum may be a better option, although even this may not allow the stomach to empty particularly well. Gastric exclusion and oesophagojejunostomy is practised by some surgeons. For inoperable tumours situated in the cardia either palliative intubation, stenting or another form recanalisation can be used (Chapter 50).

Postoperative complications of gastrectomy

Radical gastrectomy is complex major surgery and predictably there is a large number of potential complications of the operation. Leakage of the oesophagojejunostomy should be uncommon in experienced hands. When it occurs it can often be managed conservatively as the Roux-en-Y reconstruction means that it is mainly saliva and ingested food that leaks. Some patients may establish a fistula from the wound or drain site and others may need radiological or surgically placed drains. It is unclear whether a nasoenteric tube should be used routinely. Many surgeons use such tubes routinely but this is not supported by any evidence base. It is common practice to perform a water-soluble contrast swallow at 5–7 days after the operation to determine whether the anastomosis is intact, and finding a small radiological leak is not uncommon. It is unusual to detect a major leak in the absence of clinical signs.

As with any gastrectomy, leakage from the duodenal stump can occur. This is usually due to a degree of distal obstruction and care must be taken when performing the Roux-en-Y anastomosis that there is no kinking. Paraduodenal collections can be drained radiologically which will often convert the collection into an external fistula. Biliary peritonitis requires a laparotomy and peritoneal toilet, and in this circumstance it is best to leave a Foley catheter in the duodenum to establish a controlled duodenal fistula. If it is established that there is no distal obstruction, or any such obstruction is dealt with, then with time the fistula will close.

The presence of septic collections along with a very radical vascular dissection may lead to catastropic secondary haemorrhage from the exposed or divided blood vessels. This situation may be very difficult to manage whether reoperation or interventional radiology is employed.

Long-term complications of surgery

It is surprising that, considering the radical nature of the total gastrectomy, many patients, particularly the younger ones, have a good functional results. Most patients, however, will have a reduced capacity particularly in the short term. They need to be given detailed nutritional advice, the substance of which is to eat small meals and often while the jejunum or small gastric remnant adapts. There is, in fact, very little functional difference between patients who have a total and subtotal gastrectomy. Various attempts have been made to try and improve the short-term functional results by a forming a jejunal pouch and attaching this to the oesophagus. Most surgeons do not perform this as in the long term there seems little functional advantage. It is surprising that these patients only infrequently suffer from the complications of gastric surgery such as dumping and diarrhoea. Nutritional deficiencies may occur and the patient should be monitored with this in view. The loss of the parietal mass leads to vitamin B_{12} deficiency and replacement should be given routinely.

Outlook after surgical treatment

The outlook after surgical treatment varies considerably between the West and Japan. In Japan approximately 75 per cent of patients will have a curative resection and of these the overall 5-year survival rate will be in the region of 50–70 per cent. By contrast, in the West most series show that only 25–50 per cent of patients undergoing surgery will have a

Frederic E.B. Foley, 1891–1966. American urologist, Ankher Hospitals, St Paul, USA.

curative operation and the 5-year survival rate in such patients is only about 25–30 per cent, although in some series it approaches Japanese levels. These figures need some qualification to explain the differences in outcome between patients with gastric cancer in the West and in Japan. The allegation by some authors, not surprisingly all in the West, that gastric cancer is a somewhat different disease in Japan and that such differences explain the better outcome has no basis in evidence. Indeed, all of the studies in which the molecular pathology of gastric cancer has been studied suggest quite the reverse. A combination of differences in staging and a higher standard of surgery in Japan probably accounts for the differences. Staging is clearly crucial when survival figures are being compared. The more thorough the staging the higher the stage is likely to be and therefore stage for stage the outcome seems better in patients who are adequately staged pathologically. This phenomenon is termed 'stage migration'. Studies in the UK have shown that the lymph node yield after gastrectomy is minute in comparison to Japan. The pathologist will have considerable difficulty orientating a fixed specimen and finding lymph node groups, and therefore the optimal approach is for the surgeon to dissect the nodes from the specimen and send them separately to the pathologist, a practice commonly followed in Japan. Only in this way can an accurate staging be achieved.

Other treatment modalities

Because of the failure of radical surgery to cure advanced gastric cancer there has been an interest in the use of radiotherapy and chemotherapy.

Radiotherapy

The routine use of radiotherapy has not been supported by clinical trials. There is a number of radiosensitive tissues in the region of the gastric bed which limit the dose that can be given; this may partly explain the disappointing results. Radiotherapy has a role in the palliative treatment of painful bony metastases.

Chemotherapy

Gastric cancer may respond well to combination cytotoxic chemotherapy, and interest now focuses on the utility of such treatment in improving outcome. In treating advanced gastric cancer there is a number of well-investigated regimes but the best results are currently obtained using a combination of epirubacin, cisplatinum and 5-FU (5-fluorouracil) (ECF) by continuous infusion. A significant proportion of patients will respond to this regimen and, although studies comparing best supportive care with chemotherapy are not abundant, there is a consensus that improvement in survival of several months at least can be achieved by treatment. However, combination chemotherapy of this type is quite intensive and such benefits have to be set against the morbidity associated with chemotherapy. Systemic adjuvant chemotherapy has been investigated in a number of trials and has proved disappointing. However, many patients in these studies have not actually completed the course of chemotherapy and the total dose given was rather low compared with the regimens used for advanced disease. Good results have been obtained in Japan from the use of mitomycin C-impregnated charcoal given by the intraperitoneal route. The rationale for this is that this is taken up by the peritoneal lymphatics and may target the principal site of recurrence, which is the gastric bed. This treatment has not been widely used in the West. There is current interest in neoadjuvant chemotherapy given with a view to down-staging gastric cancer prior to surgical resection. Whether treatment of this type is effective awaits the results of randomised trials.

Pattern of relapse following surgical treatment

As might be expected, the most common site of relapse following radical gastrectomy is the gastric bed and represents inadequate extirpation of the primary tumour. Widespread nodal intraperitoneal metastases, distant nodal metastases and liver metastases are all common. Dissemination to the lung and bones usually only occurs after liver metastases are already established.

Gastric stromal tumours

Previously named leiomyoma and leiomyosarcoma, the rather bland name of stromal tumour is now used because the biological behaviour of these tumours is unpredictable. Although it is reasonably straightforward for a pathologist to say that one particular lesions has a benign appearance and, at the other extreme, a tumour is highly malignant, there is a large number of tumours in which the distinction between benign and malignant is unclear. In general terms the larger the tumour and the greater mitotic activity the more likely it is to metastasise. Within the gastrointestinal tract the stomach is the commonest site for such tumours.

The incidence of the condition is unclear as small stromal tumours of the stomach are probably quite common and remain unnoticed. Clinically obvious tumours are considerably less common than gastric cancer. The aetiology is unknown.

The only way that many stromal tumours are recognised is either that the mucosa overlying the tumour ulcerates (Fig. 51.26) leading to bleeding or that they are noticed incidentally at endoscopy. Because the mucosa overlying the tumour is normal, endoscopic biopsy can be uninformative unless the tumour has ulcerated. The appearance on barium meal is usually typical. Larger tumours present with nonspecific gastric symptoms and in many instances may initially be thought to be gastric cancer.

As the biological behaviour is difficult to predict the best guide is to consider the size of the tumour. Smaller tumours can be treated by wedge excision but larger ones require a gastrectomy. By their nature these tumours spread via the blood, and lymphatic metastases are relatively uncommon.

Common sites of spread include the liver, lungs and bone. Surgery is the only treatment modality that can cure the disease; adjuvant chemotherapy has not been shown to be beneficial. These tumours sometimes respond to systemic chemotherapy, but this is palliative.

Gastric lymphoma

Gastric lymphoma is an interesting disease and some aspects of the management are controversial. It is first important to distinguish primary gastric lymphoma from involvement in the stomach in a generalised lymphomatous process. This latter situation is more common than the former. Unlike gastric carcinoma, the incidence of lymphoma seems to be increasing. Primary gastric lymphoma accounts for approximately 5 per cent of all gastric neoplasms.

Gastric lymphoma is the most common in the sixth decade and the presentation is no different from gastric cancer, the common symptoms being pain, weight loss and bleeding. Acute presentations of gastric lymphoma such as haematemesis, perforation or obstruction are not common. Primary gastric lymphomas are B-cell-derived, the tumour arising from the mucosa-associated lymphoid tissue (MALT). Primary gastric lymphoma remains in the stomach for a prolonged period before involving the lymph nodes. At an early stage the disease takes the form of a diffuse mucosal thickening which may ulcerate. Diagnosis is made as a result of the endoscopic biopsy and seldom on the basis of the endoscopic features alone, which are not specific.

Following diagnosis adequate staging is necessary, primarily to establish whether the lesion is a primary gastric lymphoma or part of more generalised process. A CT scan of the chest and abdomen and bone marrow aspirate are required, as well as a full blood count.

Although the treatment of primary gastric lymphoma is somewhat controversial, it seems most appropriate to use surgery alone for the localised disease process. No benefit has been shown from adjuvant chemotherapy, although some oncologists contend that primary gastric lymphoma can be treated by chemotherapy alone. Chemotherapy alone is appropriate for patients with systemic disease.

Some of the more controversial aspects of gastric lymphoma concern the role of *H. pylori*. Lymphocytes are not found to any degree in normal gastric mucosa but are found in association with *Helicobacter* infection. It has also been shown that early gastric lymphomas may regress and disappear when the *Helicobacter* infection is treated (Issacson). This is an extremely surprising finding as it suggests that the neoplasm, which is demonstrably monoclonal, may be a response to the infective agent. It may be that the immunological response to the organism, probably a T-cell-related process, is important in maintaining the B-cell malignancy.

Peter Issacson. Professor of Pathology, University College, London, England.

Gastric involvement with the diffuse lymphoma

These patients are treated with chemotherapy, sometimes with dramatic and rapid responses. Surgeons are frequently asked to deal with the complications of gastric involvement. The two common complications are bleeding and perforation. Both may occur at presentation but more usually may follow the chemotherapy when there is rapid regression and necrosis of the tumour. These operations can be technically very challenging and normally require gastrectomy.

Duodenal tumours

Benign duodenal tumours

Duodenal villous adenomas occur principally in the periampullary region. Although generally uncommon, they are often found in patients with familial adenomatous polyposis. Indeed, malignant transformation in such adenomas is the commonest cause of death in patients with polyposis who have had the colon removed. The appearances are similar to those adenomas arising in the colon and, as they have malignant potential, should be locally excised with histologically clear margins.

Endocrine tumours

A number of endocrine neoplasms occurs in the duodenum. It is a common site for primary gastrinoma (Zollinger–Ellison syndrome). Other endocrine tumours include carcinoid tumours that, by comparison with ileal carcinoids, are uncommon.

Zollinger–Ellison syndrome

This syndrome is mentioned here because the gastrin-producing endocrine tumour is often found in the duodenal loop, although it also occurs in the pancreas, especially the head. It is a cause of persistent peptic ulceration. Before the development of potent gastric antisecretory agents the condition was recognised by the sometimes fulminant peptic ulceration which did not respond to gastric surgery short of total gastrectomy. It was also recognisable from gastric secretory studies in which the patient had a very high basal acid output but no marked response to pentagastrin, as the parietal cell mass was already near maximally stimulated by pathological levels of gastrin. The advent of proton pump inhibitors such as omeprazole has rendered this extreme endocrine condition fully controllable, but also less easily recognised.

Gastrinomas may be either sporadic or associated with the autosomal dominantly inherited multiple endocrine neoplasia (MEN) type I (in which a parathyroid adenoma is almost invariable). The tumours are most commonly found in the 'gastrinoma triangle' (Passaro) defined by the junction of the cystic duct and common bile duct superiorly, the junction of the second and third parts of the duodenum inferiorly, and the junction of the neck and body of the pancreas medially (essentially the superior mesenteric artery). Many are found in the duodenal loop, presumably arising in the G cells found in Brunner's glands. It is extremely important that the duodenal wall is very carefully inspected

Edward Passaro. Professor of Surgery, Los Angeles, California, USA.

endoscopically and also at operation. Very often all that can be detected is a small nodule which projects into the medial wall of the duodenum.

Even malignant sporadic gastrinomas may have a very indolent course. The palliative resection of liver metastases may be beneficial and liver transplantation is practised in some centres, as for other gut endocrine tumours, with reasonable long-term results. However, the minority of tumours found to the left of the superior mesenteric artery (outside the 'triangle') seems to have a worse prognosis, more having liver metastases at presentation. In MEN type I the tumours may be multiple and the condition is incurable. Even in this situation, as with sporadic gastrinoma, surgical treatment should be employed to remove any obvious tumours and associated lymphatic metastases as the palliation achieved may be extremely gratifying.

Duodenal adenocarcinoma

Although uncommon, this is the commonest site for adenocarcinoma arising in the small bowel. Most tumours originate in the periampullary region and commonly arise in pre-existing villous adenomas. Patients present with anaemia due to ulceration of the tumour or obstruction as the polypoid neoplasm begins to obstruct the duodenum. Direct involvement in the ampulla leads to obstructive jaundice. Histologically, the lesion is a typical adenocarcinoma and the metastases are commonly to regional lymph nodes and the liver. At presentation about 70 per cent of the patients have resectable disease and for those who survive operation the 5-year survival rate is in the region of 20 per cent, this approximately equating to cure. Poor prognostic features in the resected specimen include regional lymph node metastases, transmural involvement and perineural invasion. Curative surgical treatment will normally involve a pancreaticoduodenectomy (Whipple's procedure). Patients with familial polyposis, which is due to a mutation in the *APC* gene on chromosome 5, are predisposed to periampullary cancer which is one of the most common causes of death in patients who have had their colon removed.

Other duodenal malignancies are rare.

Duodenal obstruction

Duodenal obstruction in the adult is usually due to malignancy, and cancer of the pancreas is the most common cause. About one-third of patients with pancreatic cancer treated by endoscopic stenting will develop obstruction. Treatment is by gastroenterostomy. In patients having a surgical biliary bypass for pancreatic cancer gastric drainage may be necessary.

A variety of other malignancies can cause duodenal obstruction including metastases from colorectal and gastric cancer. Primary duodenal cancer is much less common as a cause of obstruction than these other malignancies.

Annular pancreas may rarely cause duodenal obstruction. Obstruction usually follows an attack of pancreatitis and on occasions the obstruction may be mistaken for malignancy.

Arteriomesenteric compression is an ill-defined condition in which it is proposed that the fourth part of the duodenum is compressed between the superior mesenteric artery and the vertebral column. Where it is convincingly demonstrated and causing weight loss duodenojejunostomy may be performed.

Gastroplasty for morbid obesity

A number of surgical treatments has been devised for morbid obesity, but of these the most commonly used is the vertical banded gastroplasty (Mason). Some surgeons prefer a gastric bypass operation which has some similarities. Indeed, gastric bypass can be used as a revisional procedure following stomal obstruction, one of the more common complications of gastroplasty.

Indications for operation

Selection of patients for operation should ideally be made by a team that includes a nutritionist/endocrinologist and a psychiatrist, as well as a surgeon, as it is important that major metabolic problems and severe psychiatric disorders are elucidated before operation. The patient should be 100 per cent over their ideal weight for height or have a body mass index [weight (kg)/height (m)^2] of greater than 45. This figure is selected because the increase in morbidity and mortality at this level of obesity is excessive. Very often the patient will have some of the morbidity associated with severe obesity such as hypertension, diabetes or osteoarthritis. Preoperative counselling should include discussion of the possibility of perioperative mortality (which is in the region of 1–4 per cent). This is very much an elective procedure and the patient is at risk of postoperative respiratory problems and pulmonary thromboembolism. Intensive or high-dependency care facilities must be available.

Operation

The operation is performed under general anaesthesia and the addition of an epidural greatly aids both the perioperative and postoperative management. The procedure should be undertaken by an anaesthetist very experienced in this area.

The abdomen is opened from the midline incision and adequate retraction provided to gain access to the upper part of the stomach. Approximately 50 per cent of patients will already have gallstones and, if this is the case, cholecystectomy should be carried out. Some surgeons advocate prophylactic cholecystectomy but this is difficult to substantiate. A large orogastric tube is placed in the stomach and the lesser sac is opened through the greater omentum by careful blunt dissection. A window is made between the lateral side of oesophagus and the lesser sac (Fig. 51.35). It is important to take great care during this part of the operation to avoid damaging the spleen or short gastric arteries. Once this has been carried out it is convenient to place a tape through this window to avoid losing access. A position is selected on the anterior wall of the stomach above the level of the incisura. A circular stapler with the head removed and the spike inserted is placed in the lesser sac with edge of the instrument up against the tube in the stomach. The handle of the stapler is then rotated to introduce the spike through the front and back wall of the stomach. Once this has been done the spike can be removed and the anvil of the stapler inserted in the usual fashion. Tightening up and firing the stapler produces a stapled circular defect in the midbody of the stomach with the space about 15 mm between the lesser curve and the window. Following this a stapler, such as the Autosuture TA90B, is inserted through the circular window and through the gap made at the lateral side of the oesophagus. This instrument is particularly recommended as it places four rows of staples

Allen Oldfather Whipple, 1881–1963. Professor of Surgery, Columbia University, New York, USA.

Edwin Mason. Professor of Surgery, Iowa City, USA.

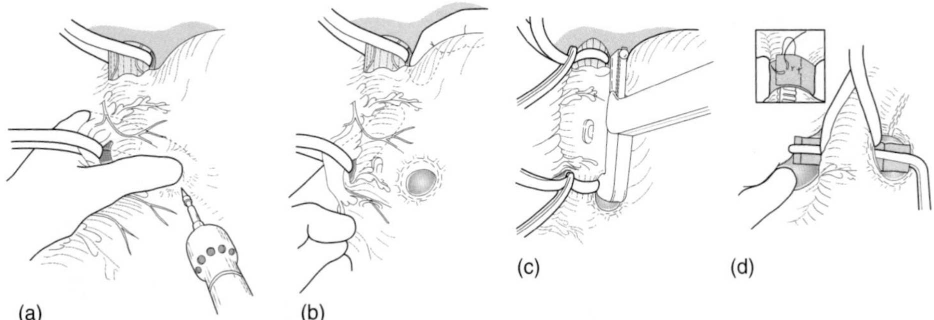

Fig. 51.35 Vertical banded gastroplasty for morbid obesity. [Reproduced with permission from *Rob and Smith's Operative Surgery. Surgery of the Upper Gastrointestinal Tract*, 5th edn (eds G. Jamieson and H. Debas), Chapman and Hall, London, 1994, p. 554.]

in the stomach (Fig. 51.35) which greatly reduces the possibility of staple line disruption. These manoeuvres lead to the creation of a pouch of about 30 ml, the volume being checked before the linear stapler is fired. It is then important to band the outlet of this pouch to avoid dilatation with time. A number of materials may be used including polypropylene mesh and expanded polytetrafluoroethylene (PTFE). Whatever material is used, the width should be approximately 1.5 cm and the circumference of the band about 5 cm. It has been shown in a variety of studies that if the band has a larger circumference than this there is a high incidence of inadequate weight loss, and if it made as small as 4.5 cm there is a high incidence of stomal stenosis. The exact dimensions of the band, however, are a critical part of the operation and the experience of the surgeon will often subtly alter the band circumference.

Postoperatively the patients should be managed on an intensive care or a high-dependency care unit until the possibility of apnoea and other complications is diminished. Epidural anaesthesia is useful as it avoids the amount of opiate given to the patient. The patient may be introduced to fluids on the first postoperative day and small quantities of food around the fourth or fifth day. Dietary advice is very important at this point. It is important that the patient understands that liquidised food or high-calorie supplements are to be avoided and that only small quantities of food are to be eaten to avoid blocking the narrow pouch outlet.

Patients can be expected to lose between a third and a half of their body weight in the 2 years following operation. Over this period it is advisable to take a vitamin supplement to avoid deficiencies which may otherwise occur. Following the first 2 years it is possible for the patient to begin weight gain, and it is important that they understand that moderation and self-control will be necessary in the long term. This is often possible because after 2 years the patient's eating habits have been quite radically changed and the apparently insurmountable task of losing almost a half of their body weight has been overcome.

Complications

Pulmonary embolism is a risk for all such patients and hence they should be managed with adequate doses of prophylaxis (5000 units of heparin tid). Although it might be expected that wound herniation would be a common sequel of this operation, in practice if the abdominal wound is repaired well with a continuous nonabsorbable suture such problems are uncommon. As with any procedure that involves opening the gastrointestinal tract, prophylactic antibiotics are important. Unlike small bowel bypass, vertical banded gastroplasty is not associated with major metabolic consequences or liver disease. The two commonest long-term complications are inadequate weight loss, which usually relates either to technical aspects of the procedure or to patient noncompliance, and stomal stenosis which may occur if the band is too tight or if fibrosis occurs in this region. The former complication can be dealt with only by revisional surgery. Stomal stenosis can be treated endoscopically by balloon dilatation, although very often this is unsuccessful in the long term.

Other gastric conditions

Acute gastric dilatation

This condition usually occurs in association with some form of ileus which is not treated by nasogastric suction. The stomach, which may also be atonic, dilates enormously. Often the patient is also dehydrated and has electrolyte disturbances. Failure to treat this condition can result in a sudden massive vomit with aspiration into the lungs. The treatment is nasogastric suction, fluid replacement and treatment of the underlying condition.

Trichobezoar and phytobezoar

Trichobezoar (hair balls) (Fig. 51.36) are unusual and are virtually exclusively found in female psychiatric patients, often young. It is caused by the pathological ingestion of hair which remains undigested in the stomach. The hair ball can lead to ulceration and gastrointestinal bleeding, perforation or obstruction. The diagnosis is made easily at endoscopy or, indeed, from a plain radiograph. Treatment consists of removal of the bezoar which may require open surgical treatment. Phytobezoars are made of the vegetable matter and found principally in patients who have gastric stasis.

Foreign bodies in the stomach

A variety of ingested foreign bodies reaches the stomach and very often these can be seen on a plain radiograph. If possible they should be removed endoscopically but if not most can be left to pass normally. Even objects such as needles, with which there is understandable anxiety, will seldom cause harm. In general, an object which leaves the stomach will pass spontaneously. By contrast, attempted removal at

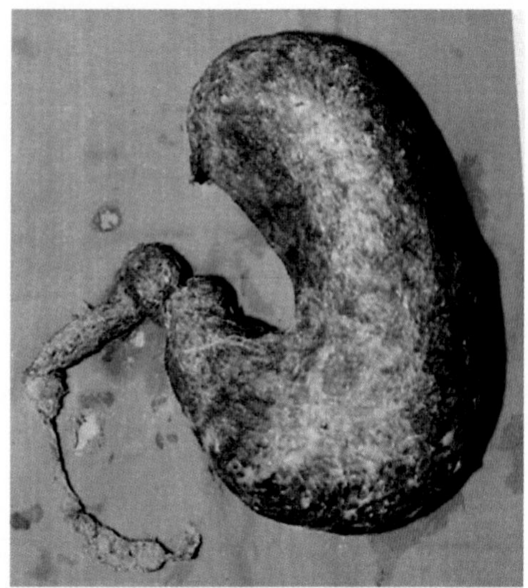

Fig. 51.36 Trichobezoar of the stomach in a girl aged 15 years.

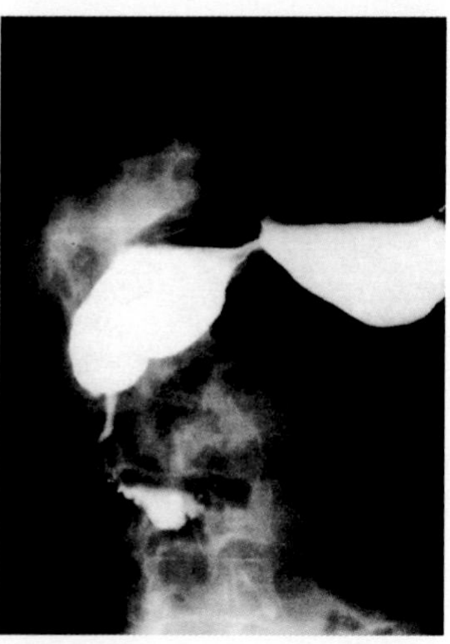

Fig. 51.37 Barium meal showing organoaxial volvulus of the stomach associated with eventration of the diaphragm.

laparotomy can be very difficult as the object may be much more difficult to find than might be expected. Most adults who swallow foreign bodies have ill-defined psychiatric problems and may appear to relish the attention associated with serial laparotomies. The treatment should therefore be expectant and intervention reserved for patients with symptoms in whom the foreign body is failing to progress.

Volvulus of the stomach

Rotation of the stomach usually occurs around the axis and between its two fixed points, i.e. the cardia and the pylorus. In theory, rotation can occur in the horizontal (organoaxial) or vertical (mesenterioaxial) direction but commonly it is the former which occurs. This condition is usually associated with a large diaphragmatic defect around the oesophagus (paraoesophageal herniation) (Fig. 51.37). What commonly happens is that the transverse colon moves upwards to lie under the left diaphragm, thus taking the stomach with it, and the stomach and colon may both enter the chest through the eventration of the diaphragm. The condition is commonly chronic, the patient presenting with difficulty in eating. An acute presentation with ischaemia may occur. Endoscopically, it can be extremely difficult to sort out the anatomy and this is one situation in which the contrast radiograph is superior.

Treatment

If the problem is causing symptoms then surgical treatment is the only satisfactory approach. Traditionally open surgery has been employed but this problem is suitable for laparoscopic treatment if appropriate skill is available. If there is a hernia, the sac and its contents (usually the stomach) should be reduced. The defect in the diaphragm should be closed, if necessary, with a mesh. It is advisable to separate the stomach from the transverse colon and then perform an anterior gastropexy to fix the stomach to the anterior abdominal wall. The results from this treatment are good.

Further reading

Jamieson, G. and Debas, H. (eds) (1994) *Rob and Smith's Operative Surgery. Surgery of the Upper Gastrointestinal Tract*, 5th edn, Chapman & Hall, London.

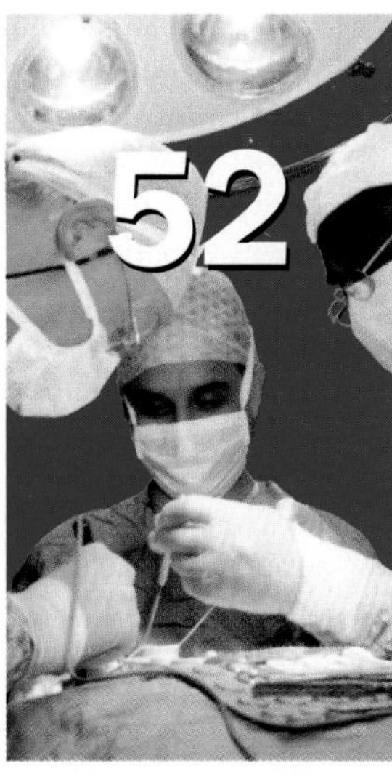

52 The liver

Anatomy of the liver

General

The liver is the largest organ in the body, weighing 1.5 kg in the average 70-kg male. Its position under the right hemidiaphragm allows it to be protected from trauma by the costal margin. The liver parenchyma is entirely covered by a thin capsule and by visceral peritoneum in all but the posterior surface of the liver, termed the 'bare area'. At first appearance the liver is divided into two main lobes: a large right lobe which comprises three-quarters of the liver parenchyma and a smaller left lobe the remaining quarter. Surgical resection of these lobes would be termed a right or left lobectomy.

Ligaments and peritoneal reflections

The liver is fixed in the right upper quadrant by peritoneal reflections which form ligaments. On the superior surface of the left lobe is the left triangular ligament. Dividing the anterior and posterior folds of this ligament allows the left lobe to mobilised from the diaphragm and the left lateral wall of the inferior vena cava (IVC) to be exposed. Large veins drain venous blood from the diaphragm to the hepatic veins and IVC at this level. The right triangular ligament fixes the entire right lobe of the liver to the undersurface of the right hemidiaphragm. Division of this ligament allows the liver to be mobilised from under the diaphragm and rotated to the left. Another major supporting structure is the falciform ligament, which runs from the umbilicus to the liver between the right and left lobes, passing into the interlobar fissure. Embryologically this ligament contained the umbilical vein which carried maternal nutrients to the liver of the foetus. From the fissure it passes anteriorly on the surface of the liver attaching it to the posterior aspect of the anterior abdominal wall. On the superior aspect of the liver the falciform ligament divides into two leaves, between which is loose areolar tissue and some small vessels. Division of this layer allows exposure of the suprahepatic IVC lying within a thin sheath of fibrous tissue. The final peritoneal reflection is between the stomach and the liver. This lesser omentum is often thin and fragile but contains the hilar structures in its free edge.

Liver blood supply

The blood supply to the liver is unique, being derived 80 per cent from the portal vein and 20 per cent from the hepatic artery. The arterial blood supply in most individuals is derived from the coeliac trunk of the aorta where the hepatic artery arises along with the splenic artery. After branching to form the gastroduodenal artery it branches at a very variable level to produce the right and left hepatic arteries. The right artery supplies the majority of liver parenchyma and is therefore the larger of the two arteries. There are many anatomical variations which are essential knowledge for safe surgery on the liver. The blood supply to the right lobe of the liver may be partly or completely supplied by a right hepatic artery arising from the superior mesenteric artery. This vessel passes posterior to the uncinate process and head of pancreas, and runs to the liver on the posterior wall of the

Bailey & Love's Short Practice of Surgery, 23rd edition. Edited by R.C.G. Russell, N.S. Williams and C.J.K. Bulstrode. Published in 2000 by Arnold Publishers.

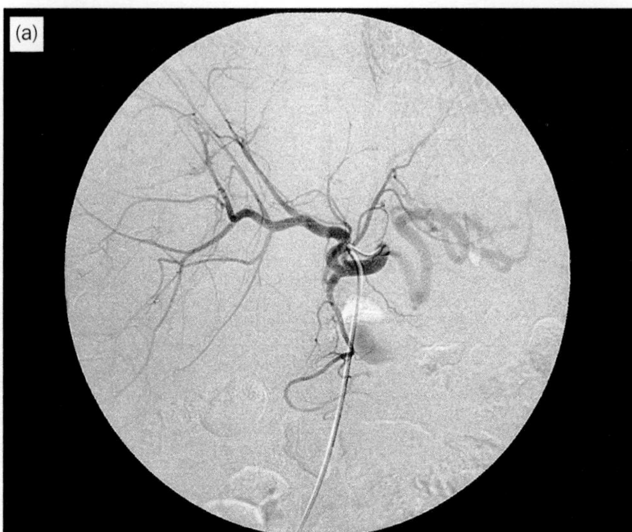

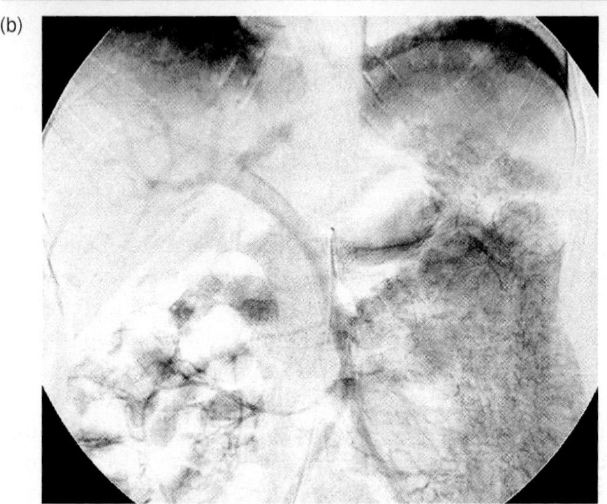

Figure 52.1 Hepatic angiography – conventional arterial anatomy. Arterial (a) and venous (b) phase of a selective hepatic angiogram. The hepatic artery usually arises from the coeliac trunk along with the splenic artery and gives rise to the gastroduodenal artery before dividing into a right and left hepatic artery. The portal vein forms from the superior mesenteric and splenic and divides into right and left branches in the hilum of the liver.

bile duct. Similarly, the arterial blood supply to the left lobe of liver may be derived from the coeliac trunk via its left gastric branch. This vessel runs between the lesser curve of the stomach and the left lobe of the liver in the lesser omentum (Fig. 52.1).

Structures in the hilum of the liver

The hepatic artery, portal vein and bile duct are present within the free edge of the lesser omentum or the 'hepatoduodenal ligament'. To expose these structures requires the peritoneum overlying the hilar triad to be divided followed by division of small vessels and an extensive lymphatic plexus. The standard relationship of these three structures is for the bile duct to be within the free edge, the hepatic artery to be above and medial, and for the portal vein to lie posteriorly. Within this ligament the common hepatic duct is joined by the cystic duct at varying levels to form the common bile duct. The common hepatic artery branches at a variable level within the ligament to form two or often three main arterial branches to the liver. The right hepatic artery often crosses the bile duct anteriorly or posteriorly before giving rise to the cystic artery. Multiple small hepatic arterial branches provide blood to the bile duct, principally from the right hepatic artery. The portal vein arises from the joining of the splenic vein with the superior mesenteric vein behind the neck of pancreas. It rarely branches until close to the liver parenchyma but has some important tributaries, including the left gastric vein joining just above the pancreas and a tributary anteriorly from the head of pancreas.

Division of structures at the hilum

At the hilum the major structures are divided into right and left branches. The right and left hepatic ducts arise from the hepatic parenchyma and join to form the common hepatic duct. The left duct has a longer extrahepatic course of approximately 2 cm. Once within the liver parenchyma the duct accompanies the branches of the hepatic artery and portal vein within a fibrous sheath. The portal vein often gives off two large branches to the right lobe which are accessible outside the liver for a short length before giving a left portal vein branch which runs behind the left hepatic duct.

Venous drainage of the liver

The venous drainage of the liver is via the hepatic veins into the IVC. The vena cava lies within a groove in the posterior wall of the liver. Above the liver it immediately penetrates the diaphragm to join the right atrium, whereas below the liver parenchyma there is a short length of vessel before the insertion of the renal veins. The inferior hepatic veins are short vessels which pass directly between the liver parenchyma and the anterior wall of the IVC. The major venous drainage is through three large veins which join the IVC immediately below the diaphragm. Outside the liver these vessels are surrounded by a thin fibrous layer. The right hepatic vein can be exposed fully outside the liver, but the middle and left veins usually join within the liver parenchyma. Immediately adjacent to the retrohepatic IVC lies the right kidney and adrenal gland. The right adrenal vein drains into the IVC at this level, usually via one main branch. The IVC can be mobilised fully from the retroperitoneal tissues and in the healthy state there are no significant vessels in this tissue plane. The right inferior phrenic vein often drains to the IVC via the right hepatic vein.

The internal anatomy of the liver

Safe liver surgery has been enormously facilitated by a better understanding of the internal anatomy of the liver which has been extensively investigated by the French anatomist Couinaud. He described the liver as being divided into eight

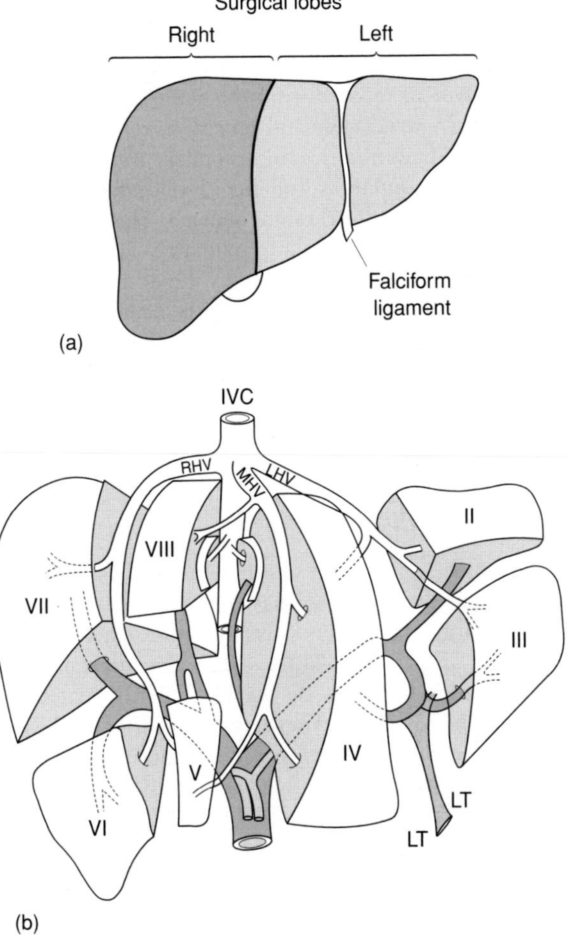

Figure 52.2 (a) Surgical labels of the liver. The 'surgical' labels of the liver compared with the usual anatomical division into tight and left lobes by the falciform ligament. (b) Segments of the liver (after Couinaud). IVC = interior vena cava; RHV = right hepatic vein; LHV = left hepatic vein; MHV = middle hepatic vein; LT = ligamentum teres.

segments (Fig. 52.2). Each of these segments can be considered as functional units, each with a branch of hepatic artery, portal vein and bile duct, and drained by a branch of the hepatic vein. The overall anatomy of the liver is divided into a functional right and left along the line between the gallbladder fossa and the middle hepatic vein. Liver segments (v–viii) to the right of this line are supplied by the right hepatic artery and the right branch of portal vein, and drain bile via the right hepatic duct. The liver parenchyma to the left of this line (segments i–iv) is functionally the left liver and is supplied by the left branch of the hepatic artery and the left portal vein branch, and drains bile via the left hepatic duct.

The hepatic lobules

The functional units within the liver segments are the liver lobules. These comprise plates of liver cells separated by the hepatic sinusoids, large thin-walled venous channels which carry blood to the central vein, a tributory of the hepatic vein from the portal tracts which contains branches of the hepatic artery and portal vein. During passage through the sinusoids the many functions of the liver take place, including bile formation which is channelled in an opposite direction to the blood flow to drain via the bile duct tributaries within the portal tracts.

Embryology

The liver is a foregut structure and forms as a small endodermal bud early in gestation. The cell population within the bud grows rapidly and forms two cell populations which differentiate into the liver and extrahepatic biliary tree and gallbladder. The liver cells are bipotential and may develop into hepatocytes or intrahepatic ductal cells. The liver endothelium is derived from the vitelline and umbilical veins which merge with the endodermal bud to form the liver sinusoids. The supporting connective tissue, haemopoetic cells, which are important during intrauterine life, and the Kupffer cells are derived from the mesoderm of the septum transversum.

Signs and tests of acute and chronic liver disease

Liver function and tests

Adequate liver function is essential to survival; humans will survive for only 24–48 hours in the anhepatic state despite full supportive therapy. The main functions of the liver are shown in Table 52.1. Routinely available tests of liver function are shown in Table 52.2. Bilirubin is synthesised in the liver and excreted in the bile. Increased levels may be associated with increased haemoglobin breakdown, hepatocellular dysfunction resulting in impaired bilirubin transport

Table 52.1 Main functions of the liver

- Maintaining core body temperature
- pH balance and correction of lactic acidosis
- Synthesis of clotting factors
- Glucose metabolism, glycolysis and gluconeogenesis
- Urea formation from protein catabolism
- Bilirubin formation from haemoglobin degradation
- Drug and hormone metabolism
- Removal of gut endotoxins and foreign antigens

Table 52.2 Routinely available tests of liver function

Test	*Normal range*
Bilirubin (Bil)	5–17 μmol/litre (conjugated < 5 μmol/litre)
Alkaline phosphatase (ALP)	35–130 IU/litre
Aspartate transaminase (AST)	5–40 IU/litre
Alanine transaminase (ALT)	5–40 IU/litre
Gamma-glutamyl transpeptidase (GGT)	10–48 IU/litre
Albumin (Alb)	35–50 g/litre
Prothrombin time (PT)	12–16 seconds

Karl Wilhelm von Kupffer, 1829–1902. Bavarian anatomist and embryologist.

Table 52.3 Common causes of acute liver failure

- Viral hepatitis – hepatitis A, B, (?)C, D, E
- Drug reactions – halothane, isoniazid-rafampicin, antidepressants, nonsteroidal anti-inflammatory drugs (NSAIDs), valproic acid
- Paracetamol overdose
- Mushroom poisoning
- Shock and multiorgan failure
- Acute Budd–Chiari syndrome
- Wilson's disease
- Fatty liver of pregnancy

Table 52.4 King's College criteria for orthotopic liver transplantation (OLT) in acute liver failure

Paracetamol induced:
- pH < 7.30 (irrespective of grade of encephalopathy)

or

- Prothrombin time (PT) > 100 seconds + serum creatinine > 300 μmol/l (with grade 3 or 4 encephalopathy)

Nonparacetamol induced (any three of the following):
- Age less than 10 years or more than 40 years
- Aetiology nonA, nonB, halothane or idiosyncratic drug reaction
- More than 7 days' jaundice before encephalopathy
- PT > 50 seconds
- Bilirubin > 300 μmol/litre

and excretion or from biliary obstruction. In patients with known parenchymal liver disease progressive elevation of bilirubin level in the absence of a secondary complication suggests deterioration in liver function. The serum alkaline phophatase is particularly elevated with cholestatic liver disease or biliary obstruction. The transaminase levels [aspartate transaminase (AST) and alanine transaminase (ALT)] reflect acute hepatocellular damage, as does the gamma-glutamyl transpeptidase (GGT) level which may be used to detect the liver injury associated with acute alcohol ingestion. The synthetic functions of the liver are reflected in the ability to synthesise proteins (albumin level) and clotting factors (prothrombin time). The standard method of monitoring liver function in patients with chronic liver disease is serial measurements of bilirubin, albumin and prothrombin time.

Signs of impaired liver function

The clinical signs associated with impaired liver function depend on the severity of dysfunction and whether it is acute or chronic.

Acute liver failure

The main causes of acute liver failure are shown in Table 52.3. In the early stages there may be no objective signs, but with severe dysfunction the onset of clinical jaundice may be associated with neurological signs of liver failure consisting of a liver flap, drowsiness, confusion and, eventually, coma. Treatment in the majority of cases is supportive therapy to allow the liver to recover from the acute damage. This may include intravenous fluids and nutrition, renal support with haemofiltration, antibiotics for secondary infective episodes, sedation and ventilation for the development of hepatic coma, and mannitol for cerebral oedema. The overall mortality for acute liver failure is approximately 50 per cent, even with the best the supportive therapy. Liver transplantation is appropriate for some patients with acute liver failure, although the overall results are poor in comparison to liver transplantation for chronic liver disease. Indications for orthotopic (OLT) liver transplantation, based on the King's College London transplant experience, are given in Table 52.4.

Chronic liver disease

Because of the many diverse functions of the liver, patients with chronic liver disease may present in many different ways. Lethargy and weakness are common features irrespective of the underlying cause. Often this precedes clinical jaundice which indicates the liver's inability to metabolise bilirubin. The serum level reflects the severity of the underlying liver disease. Progressive deterioration in liver function is associated with a hyperdynamic circulation involving a high cardiac output, large pulse volume, low blood pressure and flushed warm extremities. Fever is a common feature which may be related to underlying inflammation and cytokine release from the diseased liver or due to bacterial infection to which patients with chronic liver disease are predisposed. Skin changes may be evident, including spider naevi, cutaneous vascular abnormalities which blanch on pressure, palmar erythema and white nails (leuconychia). Endocrine abnormalities are responsible for hypogonadism and gynaecomastia. The mental derangement associated with chronic liver disease is termed 'hepatic encephalopathy'. This is associated with memory impairment, confusion, personality changes, altered sleep patterns and slow slurred speech. The most useful clinical sign is the flapping tremor demonstrated by asking the patient to extend his arms and hyperextend the wrist joint. Abdominal distension due to ascites is a common late feature. This may be suggested clinically by the demonstration of a fluid thrill or shifting dullness. Protein catabolism produces loss of muscle bulk and wasting, and a coagulation defect is suggested by the presence of skin bruising. A patient with the typical features of end-stage chronic liver disease is shown in Fig. 52.3. The Child's classification allows an easy method of describing the severity of liver disease and allows comparison of treatments for patients with chronic liver disease (Table 52.5).

Samuel A.K. Wilson, b. 1877. English neurologist.

C.G. Child. Professor and Chairman, Department of Surgery, Michigan, USA.

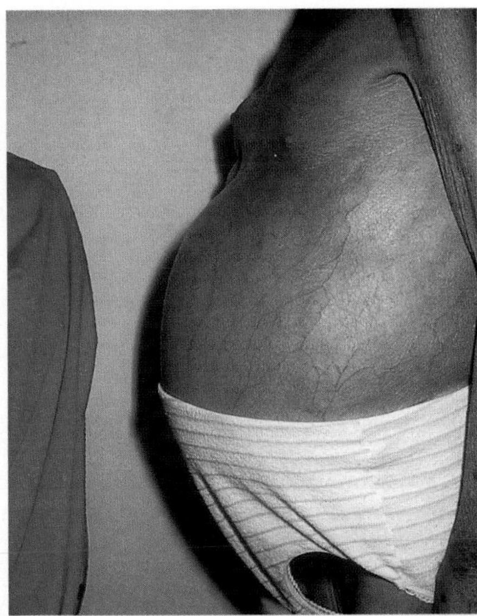

Figure 52.3 End stage liver cirrhosis. A patient with end stage liver disease demonstrating muscle wasting and gross abdominal distension due to ascites.

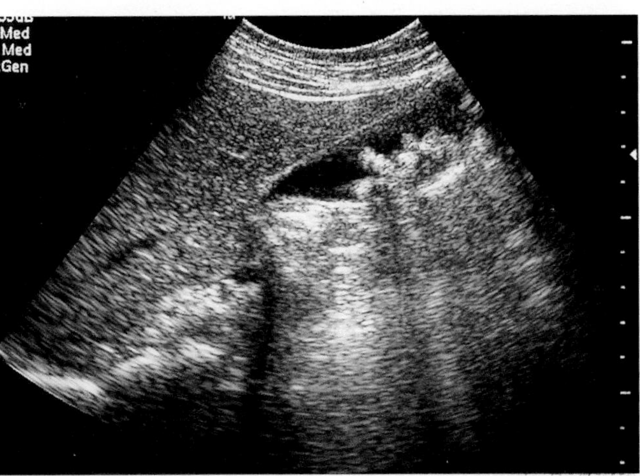

Figure 52.4 Ultrasound scan of the upper abdomen showing the liver on the left and a gallbladder containing multiple gallstones centrally. The stones can be seen to cast an acoustic 'shadow'.

Table 52.5 Child's classification of hepatocellular function in cirrhosis

Group designation	*A*	*B*	*C*
Bilirubin (mg/dl)	< 2.0	2.0–3.0	> 3.0
Albumin (g/dl)	> 3.5	3.0–3.5	< 3.0
Ascites	None	Easily controlled	Poorly controlled
Neurological disorder	None	Minimal	Advanced
Nutrition	Excellent	Good	Wasting

Imaging the liver

The major advances which have taken place over recent years in surgical approaches to the liver and the enormous improvement in the safety of liver surgery are due to the careful individualised planning of surgery which is possible owing to the information obtained by preoperative imaging. The ideal choice of imaging modality is determined by the likely liver pathology and the locally available equipment and radiological expertise.

Ultrasound

This is the first-line test owing to its safety and availability. It is entirely operator dependent. It is useful for determining bile duct dilatation, the presence of gallstones (Fig. 52.4) and the presence of liver tumours. Doppler ultrasound allows flow in the hepatic artery, portal vein and hepatic veins to be assessed. In some countries it is used as a screening test for the development of primary liver tumours in a high-risk population. Ultrasound is useful in guiding the percutaneous biopsy of a liver lesion.

Computerised tomography (CT)

The current 'gold standard' for liver imaging is triple-phase spiral CT. This provides fine detail of liver lesions down to less than 1 cm in diameter and gives information on their nature (Fig. 52.5). Oral contrast enhancement allows visualisation of the stomach and duodenum in relation to the liver hilum. The early arterial phase of the intravenous contrast vascular enhancement is particularly useful for detecting small liver tumours owing to their preferential arterial blood supply. The venous phase maps the branches of the portal vein within the liver and the drainage via the hepatic veins. Inflammatory liver lesions often exhibit rim enhancement with intravenous contrast, whereas the common haemangioma characteristically shows late venous enhancement. The density of any liver lesion can be measured, which can be useful in establishing the presence of a cystic lesion.

Magnetic resonance imaging (MRI)

MRI (Fig. 52.6) would appear to be as effective an imaging modality as CT in the majority of patients with liver disease. It does, however, offer several advantages. First, many patients are precluded from iodine-containing intravenous contrast agents because of a history of allergy. These patients should be offered MRI rather than contrast CT. Second, *magnetic resonance cholangiopancreatography* (MRCP) can produce excellent quality imaging of the biliary tract noninvasively. The image quality is currently below that available from endoscopic retrograde cholangiopancreaography (ERCP) or percutaneous transhepatic cholangiography (PTC) but this is rapidly improving. Currently, it should be considered for diagnostic questions where ERCP has failed or is impossible due to previous surgery. *Magnetic resonance angiography* (MRA) similarly provides high-quality images of the hepatic artery and portal vein without the need for arterial cannulation. It is used as an alternative to

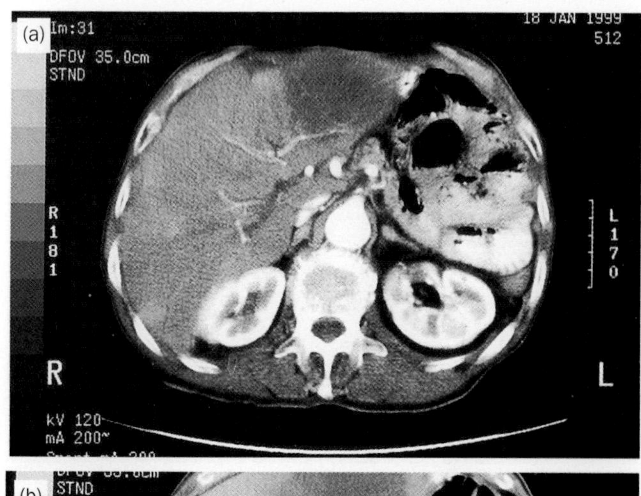

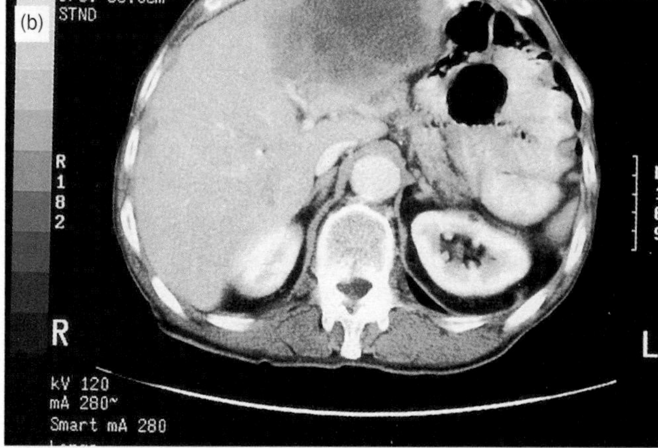

Figure 52.5 Computed tomography of liver tumour. Computed tomography scan of a patient with a liver tumour in the left lobe of the liver using intravenous contrast enhancement. The vascularity of the lesion and hence its possible nature can be determined from the (a) arterial and (b) venous phases of the scan.

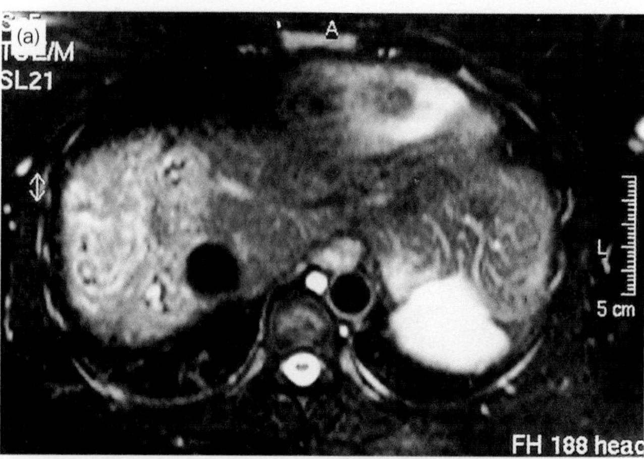

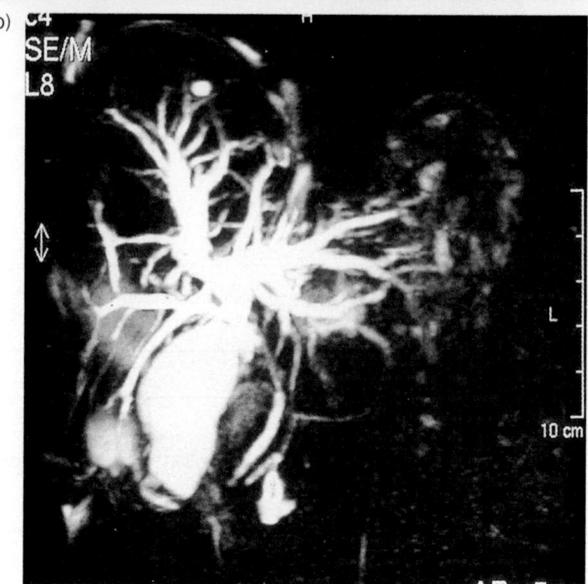

Figure 52.6 The role of magnetic resonance (MR) in liver disease. MR is increasingly used for imaging the liver. It may be used for cross-sectional imaging for staging liver cancers (magnetic resonance imaging, MRI), (a) for noninvasive cholangiography to demonstrate a hilar stricture (magnetic resonance cholangio-pancreatography MRCP), or (b) for the noninvasive assessment of blood vessels, magnetic resonance angiography, MRA.

selective hepatic angiography for diagnosis. It is particularly useful in patients with chronic liver disease and a coagulopathy in whom the patency of the portal vein and its branches is in question.

Endoscopic retrograde cholangiopancreatography

ERCP (Fig. 52.7) is required in patients with an obstructive pattern of liver function tests or in whom imaging has suggested an abnormality of the biliary tract. A preoperative check of coagulation is essential, along with prophylactic antibiotics and an explanation of the main complications which include pancreatitis, cholangitis and bleeding or perforation of the duodenum related to sphincterotomy. *Endoluminal ultrasound* of the biliary tract is possible using a 'baby' scope, and may provide additional information on the extent of hilar tumours. Therapeutic interventions are also possible at the time of ERCP and include stone retrieval, balloon dilatation of strictures, endoprosthesis insertion and brush cytology of tumours to provide a tissue diagnosis.

Percutaneous transhepatic cholangiography

PTC is indicated where endoscopic cholangiography has failed or is impossible, as in patients with previous polya gastrectomy. It is often required in patients with hilar bile duct tumours where endoscopic cholangiography fails to visualise the intrahepatic bile ducts (Fig. 52.7).

Angiography

Selective visceral angiography (Fig. 52.1) may be required both for diagnostic purposes and for therapeutic intervention. Prior to liver resection it may be used to visualise the anatomy of the hepatic artery to the right and left sides of the liver and to confirm patency of the portal vein. It can also

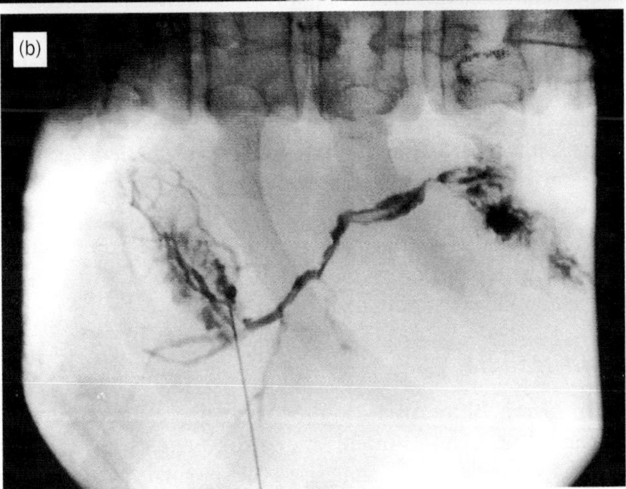

Figure 52.7 (a) Endoscopic retrograde cholangio-pancreatography (ERCP). ERCP demonstrating the biliary tract with multiple stones in the distal common bile duct. (b) Percutaneous cholangiography (PTC). Some contrast has extravasated at the site of hepatic puncture of the percutaneously placed needle but the biliary tract is clearly demonstrated and shows the multiple strictures typical of primary sclerosing cholangitis (PSC).

provide additional information on the nature of a liver nodule, primary liver tumours having a well-developed arterial blood supply. Therapeutic interventions include the occlusion of arteriovenous malformations, embolisation of bleeding sites in the liver and the treatment of liver tumours (chemoembolisation).

Nuclear medicine scanning

Radioisotope scanning can provide diagnostic information which cannot be obtained by other imaging modalities. Iodoida is a technetium-99m (^{99m}Tc)-labelled radionuclide which is administered intravenously, removed from the circulation by the liver, processed by hepatocytes and excreted in the bile. Imaging under a gamma camera allows its uptake and excretion to be monitored in real time. These data are particularly useful where a bile leak or biliary obstruction is suspected and a noninvasive screening test is required. A sulphur colloid liver scan allows the liver's Kupffer cell activity to be determined. This may be particularly useful to confirm the nature of a liver lesion, adenomas and haemangiomas having a lack of Kupffer cells and hence no uptake of sulphur colloid.

Laparoscopy and laparoscopic ultrasound

Laparoscopy is useful for the staging of hepatopancreatobiliary cancers. Lesions which have failed to be detected by conventional imaging are mainly peritoneal metastases and superficial liver tumours. Approximately 30 per cent of patients may have additional lesions detected by laparoscopy which have not been shown on good-quality planar imaging by CT or MRI. Laparoscopic ultrasound may increase this figure and provides additional information with liver tumours on their proximity to the major vessels and bile duct branches.

Fluorodeoxyglucose–position emission tomography (FDG–PET)

This new imaging modality depends on the avid uptake of glucose by cancerous tissue in comparison to benign or inflammatory tissue. At present it is mainly used to determine the nature of a mass lesion demonstrated on another form of imaging. Deoxyglucose is labelled with the positron emitter fluorine-18 (^{18}FDG) and this is administered to the patient prior to imaging by positron emission tomography (PET). A three-dimensional image of the whole body is obtained, highlighting areas of increased glucose metabolism (Fig. 52.8).

Liver trauma

General

Liver injuries are fortunately uncommon because of the liver's position under the diaphragm protected by the chest wall. However, when they do occur they are serious injuries

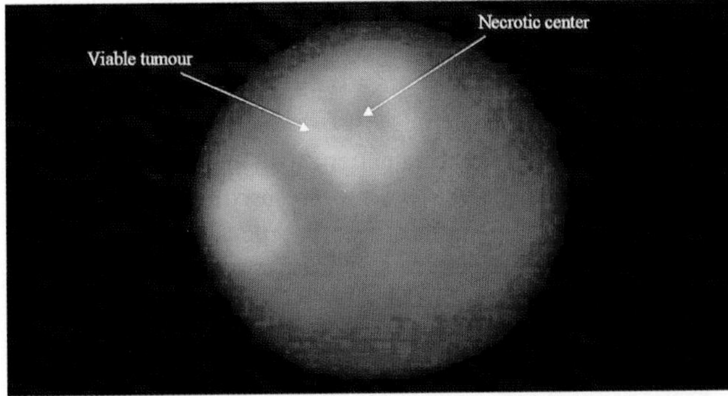

Figure 52.8 ^{18}Fluoro-deoxy-glucose-positron emission tomography (^{18}FDG–PET). The uptake of ^{18}fluorine-labelled glucose can be used as a tissue-specific imaging method, cancers showing an avid uptake in comparison to normal tissues. It can also be used as a method of assessing response to treatment, such as chemotherapy.

associated with a significant morbidity and mortality, even with prompt and appropriate management. Liver trauma can be divided into blunt traumatic injuries which produce contusions, lacerations and avulsion injuries to the liver, and penetrating injuries, such as stab and gunshot wounds. The liver is typically one of many organs to be damaged, the chest or pericardium often being involved with penetrating injuries and the spleen or kidney with blunt trauma.

Diagnosis of liver injury

The liver is an extremely well-vascularised organ and blood loss is therefore the major early complication of liver injuries. Clinical suspicion of a possible liver injury is essential as a laparotomy by an inexperienced surgeon with inadequate preparation preoperatively is doomed to failure. All lower chest and upper abdominal stab wounds should be suspect, especially if considerable blood volume replacement has been required. Similarly, severe crushing injuries to the lower chest or upper abdomen often combine rib fractures, haemothorax and damage to the spleen and/or liver. Patients with a penetrating wound will require a laparotomy and/or thoracotomy once active resuscitation is underway. Owing to the opportunity for massive ongoing blood loss and the rapid development of a coagulopathy, the patient should be directly transferred to the operating suite whilst blood products are obtained and volume replacement is ongoing. Patients with blunt trauma who are haemodynamically stable but have objective clinical signs, such as upper abdominal tenderness and guarding, should have an oral and intravenous contrast enhanced CT scan of the chest and abdomen. This will demonstrate evidence of parenchymal damage to the liver or spleen as well as associated traumatic injuries to their feeding vessels. Free fluid can also be clearly established and a diagnostic aspirate performed. The chest scan will help to exclude injuries to the great vessels and demonstrate damage to the lung parenchyma. Additional investigations which may be of value include peritoneal lavage, which can confirm the presence of haemoperitoneum, and laparoscopy, which can demonstrate an associated diaphragmatic rupture.

Initial management of liver injuries

Penetrating

The initial management of a patient with an upper abdominal penetrating injury is the basis of resuscitation. The initial survey assesses the patients airway patency, breathing pattern and circulation. Peripheral venous access is gained with two large-bore cannulae and blood sent for cross match of 10 units of blood, full blood count, urea and electrolytes, liver function tests, clotting screen, glucose and amylase. Initial volume replacement should be with colloid or O-negative blood if necessary. Arterial blood gases should be obtained and the patient intubated and ventilated if the gas exchange is inadequate. Intercostal chest drains should be inserted if associated pneumothorax or haemothorax is

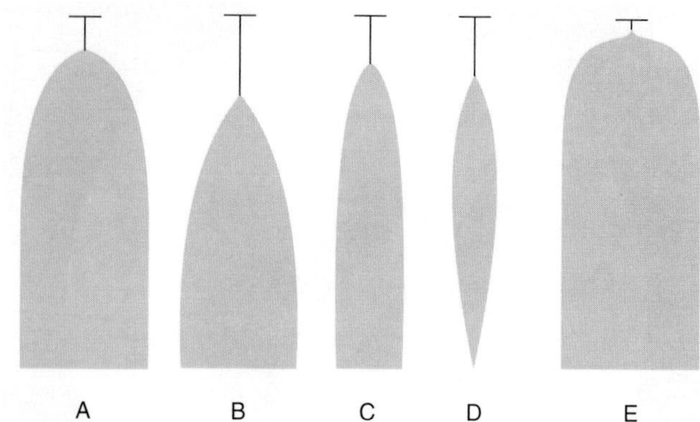

Figure 52.9 Thromboelastography (TEG). This dynamic form of assessing the coagulation status is being increasingly used for intra-operative monitoring. The shape of the TEG trace defines the nature of the underlying coagulation deficiency as shown.

suspected. Once initial resuscitation has been commenced the patient should be transferred to the operating theatre with further resuscitation being performed on the operating table. The necessity for fresh frozen plasma and cryoprecipitate should be discussed with the blood transfusion service immediately the patient arrives, as these patients rapidly develop irreversible coagulopathies due to a lack of fibrinogen and clotting factors. Standard coagulation profiles are inadequate to evaluate this acute loss of clotting factors, and factors should be given empirically, aided by the results of thromboelastography (TEG), if available (Fig. 52.9).

Blunt trauma

With severe blunt injuries the plan for resuscitation and management is as outlined above for penetrating injuries. For the patient whose vital signs are normal, imaging may be performed to evaluate further the nature of the injury. The basic surgical management differs between penetrating and blunt injuries thought to involve the liver. Penetrating injuries should be explored, whereas blunt injuries can be treated conservatively. The indication for discontinuing conservative treatment for blunt trauma would be evidence of ongoing blood loss despite correction of any underlying coagulopathy and the development of signs of generalised peritonitis.

The surgical approach to liver trauma

The surgical approach is partly dictated by the nature of the suspected injury. Good access is vital. A rooftop incision gives excellent visualisation of the liver and spleen and, if necessary, can be extended upwards for a median sternotomy. A stab incision in the liver can be sutured with a fine absorbable monofilament suture. If necessary, this may be facilitated by producing vascular inflow occlusion by placing an atraumatic clamp across the foramen of Winslow (the Pringle manoeuvre). Lacerations to the hepatic artery should be identified by

Sir John Pringle, b. 1772. British physician.

placing an atraumatic bulldog clamp on the proximal vessel prior to repair with 5/0 or 6/0 Prolene suture. If unavoidable the hepatic artery may be ligated, although parenchymal necrosis and abscess formation will result in some individuals. Portal vein injuries should be repaired with 5/0 Prolene, again with exposure of the vessel being facilitated by the placement of an atraumatic vascular clamp. The blunt trauma of deceleration injuries often produces lacerations of the liver parenchyma adjacent to the anchoring ligaments of the liver. These may be amenable to suture with an absorbable monofilament suture. Again, inflow occlusion may facilitate this suturing and, if necessary, the sutures can be buttressed to prevent them cutting through the liver parenchyma. With more severe deceleration injuries a portion of the liver may be avulsed from anterior to posterior. These injuries are more complex as they are associated with a devitalised portion of the liver and often major injuries to the hepatic veins and IVC. The initial management of liver injuries is to pack the liver to produce haemostasis. This is effective for the majority of liver injuries if the liver is packed against the natural contour of the diaphragm by packing from below. Large abdominal packs should be used to ease their removal, and the abdomen closed to facilitate compression of the parenchyma. Care should be taken to avoid over-zealous packing as this may produce pressure necrosis on the liver parenchyma. Crush injuries to the liver often result in large parenchymal haematomas and diffuse capsular lacerations. Suturing is usually ineffective, and packing is the most useful method of providing haemostasis. Necrotic tissue should be removed, but poorly perfused but viable liver left *in situ*. If packing is necessary the patient should have the packs removed after 48 hours, and commonly no further surgical intervention is required. Antibiotic cover is advisable and full reversal of any coagulopathy is essential. If a major liver vascular injury was suspected at the time of the initial laparotomy then referral to a specialist centre should be considered. A common surgical approach under these circumstances would be to place the patient on veno-venous bypass using cannulae in the femoral vein via a long saphenous cutdown and being returned, via a roller pump, to the superior vena cava (SVC) via an internal jugular line. Veno-venous bypass allows the IVC to be safely clamped to facilitate caval or hepatic vein repair. A rapid-infuser blood transfusion machine facilitates the delivery of a large volume of blood instantaneously. Once prepared, the patient is relaparotomised via the rooftop incision with a midline extension to the xiphisternum. The liver is mobilised by division of the supporting ligaments, and complete vascular isolation of the liver achieved by occluding the hilar inflow and the IVC above the renal veins and at the level of the diaphragm with atraumatic vascular clamps. Venous return is provided by the veno-venous bypass. Warm ischaemia of the liver is tolerated for up to 45 minutes, allowing sufficient time in a blood-free field for repair of injuries to the IVC or hepatic veins.

Jakob Benignus Winslow, 1669–1760. Danish anatomist.
Robert W. Sengstaken, b. 1923. American neurosurgeon.
Arthur H. Blakemore. American surgeon.

Other complications of liver trauma

By far the most important complication of blunt or penetrating trauma to the liver is sudden massive blood loss. There are, however, other presentations and complications which require specific investigation and treatment. A subcapsular or intrahepatic *haematoma* requires no specific intervention and should be allowed to resolve spontaneously. Attempts to aspirate these lesions may result in the development of a *liver abscess* due to contamination. Abscesses may also form as a result of secondary infection of an area of extensive parenchymal ischaemia, especially after penetrating trauma. Treatment under these circumstances is with appropriate systemic antibiotics and aspiration under ultrasound guidance once the necrotic tissue has liquefied. *Biliary fistulae* are a rare but important complication of liver trauma and may be difficult to control. The main aspects to management are to drain any intraperitoneal bile collections externally by percutaneous drainage under ultrasound guidance. This is followed by endoscopic or percutaneous cholangiography to determine the site of the biliary fistula and decompress the biliary tree by nasobiliary drainage or endoprosthesis insertion. If this fails to control the fistula the affected portion of the liver may require to be resected. Late vascular complications include *hepatic artery aneurysms* and *arteriovenous and arteriobiliary fistulae* (Figure 52.10). These are best treated nonsurgically by a specialist hepatobiliary interventional radiologist. The feeding vessel can be embolised transarterially. Evidence of *liver failure* may

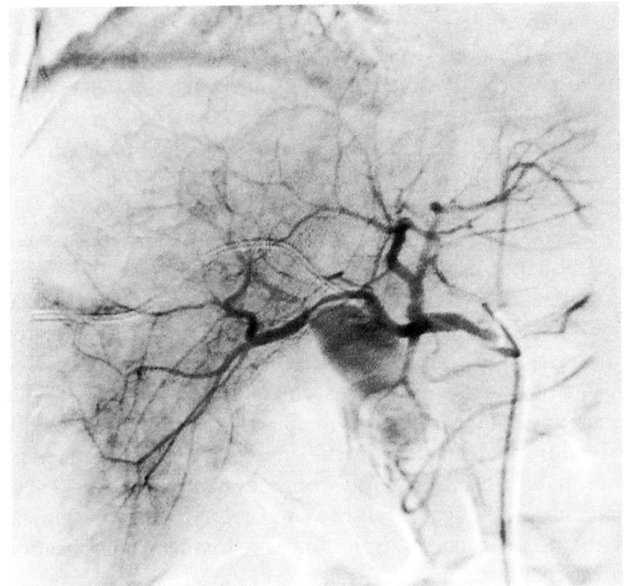

Figure 52.10 Hepatic aneurysm following liver trauma. An aneurysm arising from the right hepatic artery which can be optimally treated by the interventional radiologist using transarterial embolisation.

be seen with extensive liver trauma. If the blood supply and biliary drainage of the liver are intact this will usually reverse with conservative supportive treatment.

Long-term outcome of liver trauma

The capacity of the liver to recover from extensive trauma is remarkable, and parenchymal regeneration occurs rapidly. Late complications are rare but the development of biliary tract strictures many years after recovery from liver trauma has been reported. The treatment depends on the mode of presentation and the extent and site of stricturing. A segmental or lobar stricture associated with atrophy of the corresponding area of liver parenchyma and compensatory hypertrophy of the other liver lobe may be treated expectantly. A dominant extrahepatic bile duct stricture associated with obstructive jaundice may be treated initially with endobiliary balloon dilatation or stenting but will usually require surgical correction using a Roux-en-Y hepatodochojejunostomy.

Portal hypertension

An elevation in portal pressure is most commonly found accompanying liver cirrhosis, although it may be present in patients with extrahepatic portal vein occlusion, intrahepatic veno-occlusive disease or occlusion of the main hepatic veins [Budd–Chiari syndrome (BCS)]. As portal hypertension produces no symptoms it is usually diagnosed following presentation with decompensated chronic liver disease and encephalopathy, ascites or variceal bleeding.

Management of bleeding varices

General resuscitation

Varices usually present with the acute onset of a large volume haematemesis, the lower oesophagus being the most common site for variceal bleeding. The diagnosis may be suspected if the patient is known to have liver cirrhosis but needs to be confirmed following initial resuscitation of the patient. This involves obtaining peripheral and subsequently central venous access whilst adequate blood is obtained (initially 10 units). Liver function tests will reveal underlying liver disease and a coagulation profile will reveal any underlying coagulopathy. Vitamin K is administered (10 mg intravenously), but correction of a coagulopathy will require the administration of fresh frozen plasma. An associated thrombocytopenia is usually secondary to hypersplenism due to cirrhosis and is treated if the platelet count falls below 50 $\times 10^9$/litre. Variceal bleeding is often associated with hepatic encephalopathy, and endoscopic evaluation under these circumstances may require sedation and mechanical ventilation. Bronchial aspiration is a frequent complication of variceal bleeding.

George Budd, b. 1880. English physician.
Hans Chiari, b. 1851. Czech-French pathologist.

If the rate of blood loss prohibits endoscopic evaluation a Sengstaken–Blakemore tube may be inserted to provide temporary haemostasis. This is shown diagramatically in Fig. 52.11. Once inserted, the gastric balloon is inflated with 250 ml of air and retracted to the gastric fundus where the varices at the oesophagogastric junction are tamponaded by the subsequent inflation of the oesophageal balloon to a pressure of 40 mmHg. The two remaining channels allow gastric and oesophageal aspiration. An X-ray is used to confirm the position of the tube. The balloons should be temporarily deflated after 12 hours to prevent pressure necrosis of the oesophagus.

Drug treatment for variceal bleeding

Vasopressin has been the most extensively used drug for the initial control of variceal haemorrhage (20 units in 10 ml of 5 per cent dextrose intravenously over 10 minutes). Nitroglycerin (40 μg/min) may be as effective. Octreotide, the long-acting somatostatin analogue, has recently been evaluated and may have an important role.

Endoscopic treatment of varices

Initial treatment of oesophageal varices in most centres would be endoscopic sclerotherapy using 5 per cent ethanolamine oleate. Banding has recently produced encouraging results and is associated with a lower incidence of oesophageal ulceration. The majority of variceal bleeds will respond to a single course of sclerotherapy. An early re-bleed is less likely to be controlled by further sclerotherapy and a third bleed only rarely.

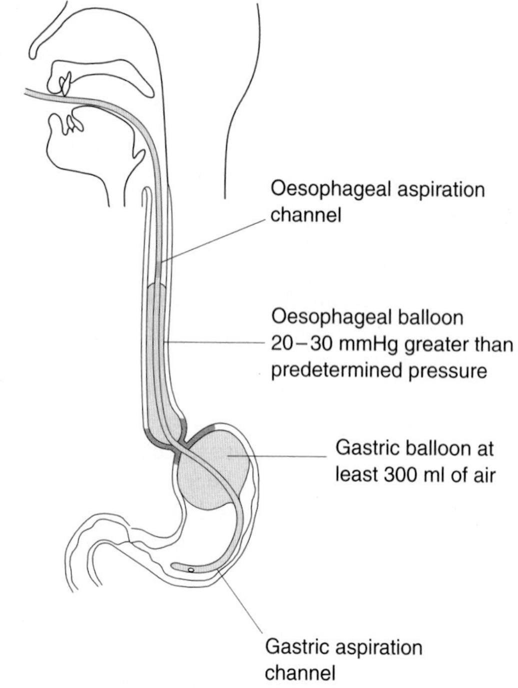

Figure 52.11 Oesophagal balloon tamponade.

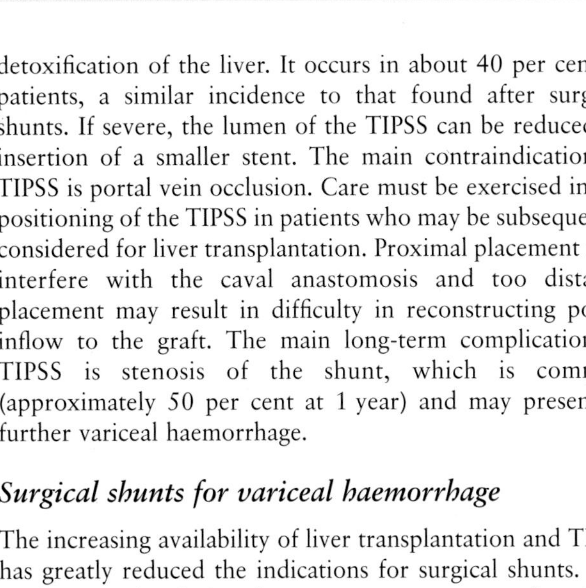

Figure 52.12 Insertion of a transhepatic portosystemic stent shunt (TIPSS). A check angiogram following insertion of a TIPSS shunt. Injection of contrast into the portal vein flows through the metallic stent and outlines the right hepatic vein. Pressure measurements are taken from within the portal vein before and after insertion.

Transjugular intrahepatic portosystemic stent shunts (TIPSS)

The emergency management of variceal haemorrhage has been revolutionised by the introduction of TIPSS in the early 1990s. Over a short period it has become the main treatment of variceal haemorrhage which has not responded to drug treatment and sclerotherapy. The shunts are inserted under local anaesthetic, analgesia and sedation using fluoroscopic guidance and ultrasonography. Via the internal jugular vein and SVC a guidewire is inserted into a hepatic vein and through the hepatic parenchyma into a branch of the portal vein. The track through the parenchyma is then dilated with a balloon catheter to allow insertion of a metallic stent which is expanded once a satisfactory position is achieved (Fig. 52.12). A satisfactory drop in portal venous pressure is usually associated with good control of the variceal haemorrhage. The main early complication of this technique is perforation of the liver capsule which can be associated with fatal intraperitoneal haemorrhage. TIPSS occlusion may result in further variceal haemorrhage and occurs more commonly in patients with well-compensated liver disease and good synthetic function. Postshunt encephalopathy is the confusional state caused by the portal blood bypassing the detoxification of the liver. It occurs in about 40 per cent of patients, a similar incidence to that found after surgical shunts. If severe, the lumen of the TIPSS can be reduced by insertion of a smaller stent. The main contraindication to TIPSS is portal vein occlusion. Care must be exercised in the positioning of the TIPSS in patients who may be subsequently considered for liver transplantation. Proximal placement may interfere with the caval anastomosis and too distal a placement may result in difficulty in reconstructing portal inflow to the graft. The main long-term complication to TIPSS is stenosis of the shunt, which is common (approximately 50 per cent at 1 year) and may present as further variceal haemorrhage.

Surgical shunts for variceal haemorrhage

The increasing availability of liver transplantation and TIPSS has greatly reduced the indications for surgical shunts. It is rarely considered for the acute management of variceal haemorrhage as the morbidity and mortality under these circumstances are high. The main current indication for a surgical shunt is a patient with Child's grade A cirrhosis in whom the initial bleed has been controlled by sclerotherapy. Long-term β-blocker therapy and chronic sclerotherapy or banding are the main alternatives.

Surgical shunts are an effective method of preventing rebleeding from oesophageal or gastric varices as they reduce the pressure in the portal circulation by diverting the blood into the low-pressure systemic circulation. Shunts may be divided into selective (e.g. splenorenal) and nonselective (e.g. portocaval), the former attempting to preserve blood flow to the liver whilst decompressing the left side of the portal circulation responsible for giving rise to the oesophageal and gastric varices. Selective shunts may be associated with a lower incidence of portal systemic encephalopathy (PSE), a confusional state commonly found in patients with chronic liver disease who have undergone radiological or surgical portosystemic shunts. The different types of surgical shunts are shown in Fig. 52.13. There is no evidence that prophylactic shunting is beneficial in patients with varices who have not bled.

Oesophageal stapled transection

This technique for the management of bleeding oesophageal varices utilised the circular stapling device initially employed for anastomosis of the rectum for stapling and resecting a ring of the lower oesophagus. As with surgical shunts in the acute situation, it was associated with a high perioperative mortality and has been largely abandoned in centres where TIPSS is available.

Management of varices secondary to splenic or portal vein thrombosis

Accurate angiography is an important aspect of the assessment of patients with suspected extrahepatic portal vein thrombosis. Therapeutic options are limited. Patients with

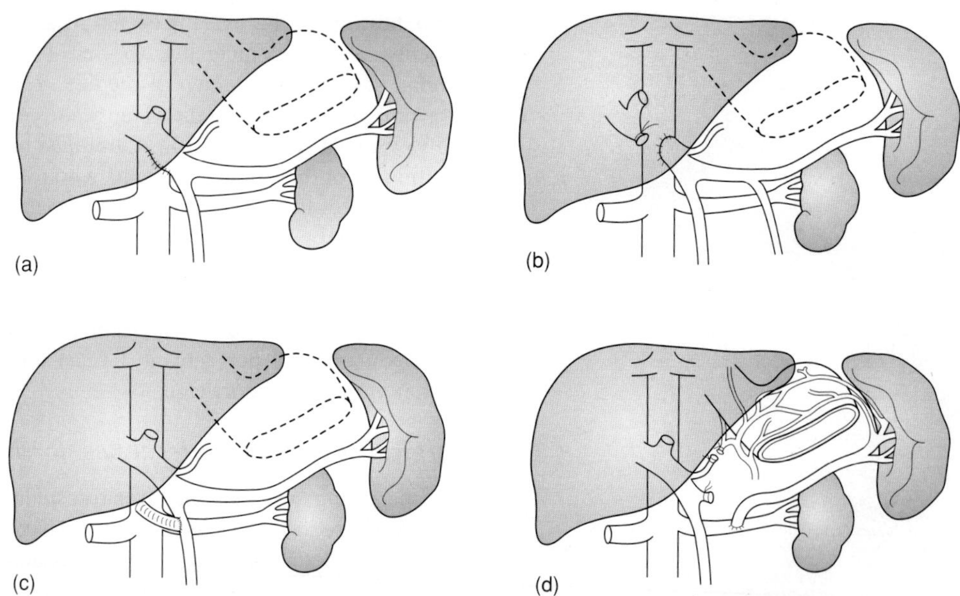

Figure 52.13 Surgical shunts (a–d). Surgical treatments for portal hypertension involve shunting portal blood into the systemic veins. This commonly involves (a) an end-to-side porto-caval anastomosis, (b) end-to-side porto-caval, (c) meso-caval or (d) spleno-renal.

oesophageal and/or gastric varices secondary to splenic or portal vein thrombosis can be effectively treated by splenectomy and gastro-oesophageal devascularisation, in which the blood supply to the greater and lesser curve of the stomach and lower oesophagus is divided. Splenic vein thrombosis may be seen secondary to chronic pancreatitis and portal vein thrombosis is a common late complication of liver cirrhosis.

Variceal bleeding and liver transplantation

The management of variceal bleeding should always take into account the possibility of liver transplantation where this is available. The patient's age or associated medical condition may be a contraindication. TIPSS would be the preferred management for bleeds resistant to sclerotherapy as long as placement is optimal. Previous surgical shunts greatly increase the morbidity associated with OLT and probably the mortality.

Ascites

The accumulation of free peritoneal fluid is a common feature of advanced liver disease independent of the aetiology. The fluid accumulation is usually associated with abdominal discomfort and a dragging sensation. Development is usually insidious. The aetiology of the ascites must be established. Imaging by CT will confirm the ascites and demonstrate the irregular and shrunken nature of a cirrhotic liver and associated splenomegaly. Intravenous contrast enhancement will allow abdominal varices to be demonstrated and patency of the portal vein, portal vein thrombosis being a common predisposing factor to ascites in chronic liver disease. In patients without evidence of liver disease malignancy is a common cause and a possible primary site may also be established on CT. Aspiration of the peritoneal fluid allows analysis for cytology, an amylase estimation to exclude pancreatic ascites, and both microscopy and culture to exclude primary bacterial peritonitis and tuberculous peritonitis. The urinary 24-hour sodium excretion is used as a guide to treatment.

Treatment of ascites in chronic liver disease

The initial treatment is to restrict additional salt intake and commence diuretics using either spironolactone or frusemide. This should be combined with advice on avoiding any precipitating factors for impaired liver function, such as alcohol intake in patients with alcoholic cirrhosis. Patients on diuretics should be monitored for the development of hyponatraemia and hypokalaemia.

Abdominal paracentesis

Patients failing to respond to diuretic treatment may require repeated percutaneous aspiration of the ascites (abdominal paracentesis) combined with volume replacement using salt-poor or standard human albumin solution dependent on the serum sodium level. This is an unsatisfactory treatment but may provide some short-term symptomatic relief.

Liver transplantation for ascites

Diuretic-resistant ascites is an indication for liver transplantation if associated with a deterioration in liver function (rising bilirubin, dropping albumin, prolonged PT). The patient's age, underlying aetiology of liver disease and associated medical problems will be the major factors determining suitability for liver transplantation. In those considered inappropriate for liver transplantation, management is aimed at symptomatic control of ascites.

Peritoneovenous shunting

The Le Veen shunt is designed for the relief of ascites due to chronic liver disease. One end of the silastic tube is inserted into the ascites within the peritoneal cavity and it is then tunnelled subcutaneously to the neck, where it is inserted under direct vision into the internal jugular vein and fed into the SVC. Owing to a one-way valve within the tubing, peritoneal fluid is drawn from the abdomen and drained to the circulation due to the lower pressure in the SVC in comparison to the abdomen during the respiratory cycle. Although often effective when combined with continued diuretic therapy they are prone to occlude and become displaced or infected. In an attempt to prevent the high occlusion rate a further development was the insertion of a chamber placed over the costal margin to allow digital pressure and evacuation of any debris within the peritoneovenous shunt (Denver shunt).

TIPSS for ascites

The procedure and its limitations are as outlined above for the emergency treatment of bleeding varices secondary to portal hypertension. The use of TIPSS for ascites is for symptomatic relief, and the procedure is associated with considerable risks including death from haemorrhage, renal failure or heart failure. Poststent encephalopathy is common (about 40 per cent) and the majority of stents will stenose on long-term follow-up (approximately 50 per cent by 1 year). Although a useful treatment modality, it has not become widely utilised because ascites is not life threatening. More encouraging results have been obtained in those with persistent chylothorax.

Chronic liver conditions

There are several chronic liver conditions which, although rare, are important to recognise because they require a specific plan for investigation and treatment, and may present mimicking a more common clinical condition.

Budd–Chiari syndrome

This is a condition principally affecting young females in which the venous drainage of the liver is occluded by hepatic venous thrombosis or obstruction from a venous web. As a result of venous outflow obstruction the liver becomes acutely congested with the development of impaired liver function and subsequently portal hypertension, ascites and oesophageal varices. In an acute thrombosis the patient may rapidly progress to fulminant liver failure, but in the majority of cases abdominal discomfort and ascites are the main presenting features. If chronic the liver progresses to established cirrhosis. The cause of the venous thrombosis needs to be established and an underlying myeloproliferative disorder or procoagulant state is commonly found, such as antithrombin 3, protein C or protein S deficiency. The diagnosis is commonly suspected in a patient presenting with ascites in whom CT scan shows a large congested liver (early stage, Fig. 52.14) or a small cirrhotic liver in which there is gross enlargement of segment I (the caudate lobe). This feature is due to preservation and hypertrophy of the segment with direct venous drainage to the IVC in the face of atrophy of the rest of the liver due to venous obstruction (Fig. 52.15). IVC compression or occlusion from the segment I hypertrophy is also commonly a feature, as is thrombosis of the portal vein. Confirmation of the suspected diagnosis is by hepatic venography via a transjugular approach which

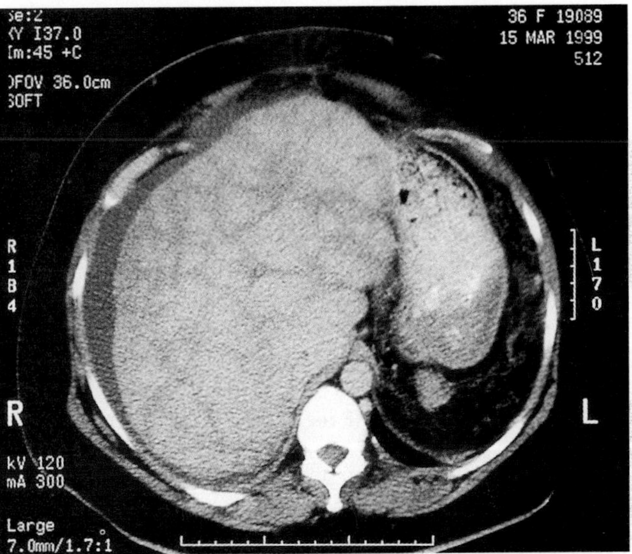

Figure 52.14 Early Budd–Chiari CT.

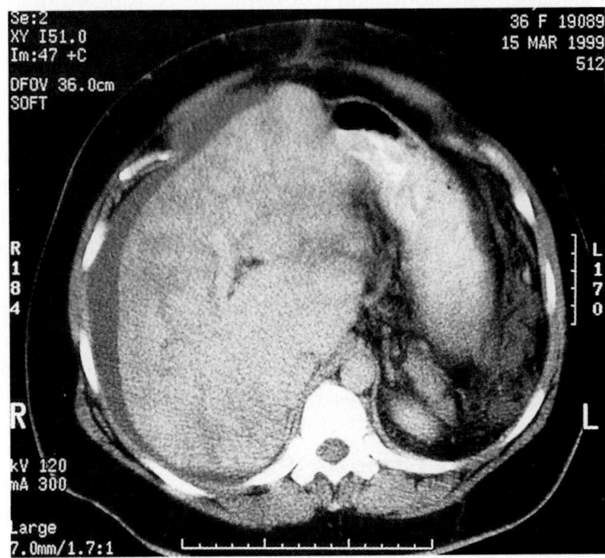

Figure 52.15 Segment I hypertrophy with BCS.

Harry le Veen. Professor of Surgery, University of South Carolina, USA.

demonstrates occlusion of the hepatic veins and may allow a transjugular biopsy. Treatment of BCS must be tailored to the individual patient and, in particular, the stage of disease at presentation. Patients presenting in fulminant liver failure should be considered for liver transplantation, as should those with established cirrhosis and the complications of portal hypertension. Those in whom cirrhosis is not established may be considered for portosystemic shunting by TIPPS, portocaval shunt or mesoatrial shunting. IVC compression may be relieved by the insertion of a retrohepatic expandable metallic stent. If the BCS is treated satisfactorily the prognosis of this patient group is largely dependent on the underlying aetiology and whether this is amenable to treatment. Patients are usually left on life-long anticoagulation with warfarin.

Primary sclerosing cholangitis (PSC)

This condition often presents in young adults with mild nonspecific symptoms, and biliary disease is suggested by the finding of abnormal liver function tests. Rarely the first presentation is with jaundice due to biliary obstruction. The disease process results in progressive fibrous stricturing and obliteration of both the intrahepatic and extrahepatic bile ducts. Although the aetiology is unknown, a genetic predisposition is likely owing to its association with chronic ulcerative colitis (UC). In patients with PSC and UC the condition usually progresses even if the diseased colon is removed. The diagnosis is principally based on the findings at cholangiography in which irregular, narrowed bile ducts are demonstrated in both the intrahepatic and extrahepatic biliary tree (Fig. 52.16). If the radiological appearances are equivocal a liver biopsy is required to demonstrate the fibrous obliteration of the biliary tracts. There is no specific treatment which can reverse the ductal changes, and the patients usually slowly progress to progressive cholestasis and death from liver failure. There is a strong prediposition to cholangiocarcinoma and this should be considered in any patient with PSC in whom a new or dominant stricture is demonstrated on cholangiography. Diagnosis of cancers in PSC is greatly facilitated by biliary brush cytology, as imaging rarely shows evidence of a mass lesion even in patients with advanced cancers. Patients with good liver function, no dominant strictures and negative biliary cytology may simply be monitored for disease progression. The only useful treatment modality is liver transplantation, which is associated with excellent results if carried out before bile duct cancer has developed. Temporary relief of obstructive jaundice due to a dominant bile duct stricture can be achieved by biliary stenting, although there is considerable risk of cholangitis from the introduction of bacteria to the biliary tract.

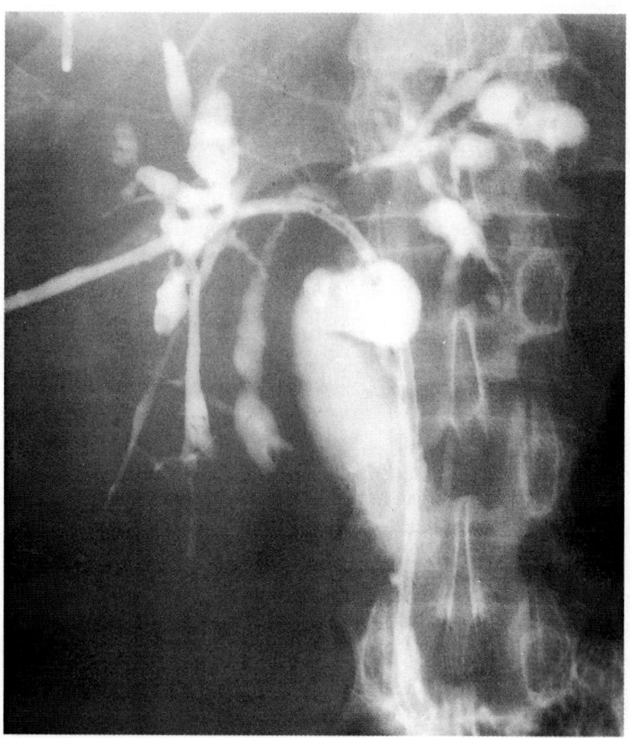

Figure 52.16 Primary sclerosing cholangitis (PSC). Percutaneous cholangiography showing the characteristic extensive bile duct strictures and dilatations associated with PSC.

Primary biliary cirrhosis (PBC)

As with PSC, the presentation of patients with PBC is often hidden with general malaise and lethargy prior to the development of clinical jaundice or the finding of abnormal liver function tests. The condition is largely confined to females. Diagnosis is suggested by the finding of circulating anti-smooth muscle antibodies and, if necessary, is confirmed by liver biopsy. The condition is slowly progressive with deterioration in liver function resulting in lethargy and malaise. It may be complicated by the development of portal hypertension and the secondary complications of ascites and variceal bleeding. The mainstay of treatment is liver transplantation, which should be considered when the patient's general condition starts to deteriorate with inability to lead a normal lifestyle.

Caroli's disease

This is congenital dilatation of the intrahepatic biliary tree which is often complicated by the presence of intrahepatic stone formation. Presentation may be with abdominal pain or sepsis. Imaging is usually diagnostic with the finding on ultrasound or CT of intrahepatic biliary lakes containing stones. Biliary stasis and stone formation combine to predipose to biliary sepsis which may be life threatening. Another well-recognised complication is the development of carcinoma. No specific treatment is available. Acute infective episodes are treated with antibiotics. Obstructed and septic bile ducts may be drained radiologically or surgically with some improvement. Malignant change within the ductal system results in cholangiocarcinoma which may be amenable to resection. Segmental involvement of the liver by Caroli's

Jaques Caroli. Professor of Medicine, Paris, France.

disease may be treated by resection of the affected part, although the ductal dilatation is usually diffuse. Transplantation is a radical but definitive treatment for a patient whose liver function is generally well preserved.

Simple cystic disease

Liver cysts are a common coincidental finding in patients undergoing abdominal ultrasound. Radiological findings to suggest that a cyst is simple are that it is regular, thin walled, unilocular, with no surrounding tissue response and no variation in density within the cyst cavity. If these criteria are confirmed and the cyst is asymptomatic no further tests or treatment are required. Large cysts may be associated with symptoms of abdominal discomfort, possibly related to stretching of the overlying liver capsule. Aspiration of the cyst contents under radiological guidance provides a sample for culture, microscopy and cytology, and allows the symptomatic response to cyst drainage to be assessed. Aspiration alone is usually associated with cyst and symptom recurrence, in which case more definitive treatment is required. Open or more recently laparoscopic deroofing is the treatment of choice for large symptomatic cysts and is associated with good long-term symptomatic relief.

Polycystic liver disease

This is a congenital abnormality associated with cyst formation within the liver and often other abdominal organs, principally the pancreas and kidney. Those associated with renal cysts may have autosomal dominant inheritance. The cysts are often asymptomatic and incidental findings on ultrasound. They usually have no effect on organ function and require no specific treatment. Occasionally, multiple liver cysts give rise to liver discomfort. This often responds to treatment with simple analgesics. Severe pain often indicates haemorrhage into a cyst which may be confirmed by ultrasound or CT scan. Cyst discomfort which is not adequately controlled by oral analgesics may be treated by open or laparoscopic fenestration of the liver cysts, although the results are less favourable than with simple cysts.

Liver infections

Viral hepatitis is a major world health problem. In addition to the well-recognised acute and chronic liver diseases produced by hepatitis A, B and C, other hepatitis viruses have been isolated including hepatitis D, which is usually detected only in patients with hepatitis B virus (HBV) infection, and hepatitis E, which produces a self-limiting hepatitis due to faecal–oral spread similar to hepatitis A.

Hepatitis A presents with anorexia, weakness and general malaise for several weeks prior to the development of clinical jaundice, often accompanied by tenderness on palpation of an enlarged liver. The condition is spread by the faecal–oral route and often spreads rapidly in closed communities. Liver function tests will be compatible with an acute hepatitis with elevation of bilirubin and transaminases. Diagnosis is confirmed by the antibody titre to hepatitis A. The condition is virtually always self-resolving, although rarely the viral hepatitis can lead to fulminant liver failure. Once the clinical condition resolves the liver tends to recover fully with no functional deficit and no long-term sequelae.

Hepatitis B is a more serious condition in most respects than hepatitis A. Although it can also produce an acute self-resolving hepatitis, the virus is often not cleared and produces long-term liver damage with the development of liver cirrhosis and primary liver cancers. Patients may therefore present acutely with malaise, anorexia, abdominal pain and clinical jaundice due to active hepatitis or may present at a late stage owing to the complications of cirrhosis, most commonly ascites or variceal bleeding. Treatment for acute hepatitis is supportive. In patients with cirrhosis, treatment is initially dictated by the specific complication at presentation (see subsections on the treatment of ascites and variceal bleeding earlier in this chapter). In established cirrhosis, liver transplantation may be considered if viral eradication or suppression can be achieved with antiviral agents (e.g. lamivudine). Without viral suppression death from reinfection of the transplanted liver is common. The hepatitis virus greatly increases the risk of primary liver cancers which usually appear at the stage when the liver parenchyma has become cirrhotic. The assessment and management of HBV cirrhosis with hepatocellular carcinoma (HCC) is discussed in the section on 'Liver tumours'.

Hepatitis C has become one of the commonest causes of chronic liver disease world-wide and in many countries a large percentage of the population has been exposed. One per cent of blood donors world-wide are hepatitis C virus (HCV) positive. Transmission is often related back to blood transfusion and routine screening of blood for HCV has only recently been introduced in many countries. As with hepatitis B, it may present as an acute hepatitis or remain hidden until the development of cirrhosis and the complications of portal hypertension. Acute hepatitis C proceeds to cirrhosis in about 20 per cent of cases. Deterioration in liver function, encephalopathy, ascites or bleeding in a patient with known HCV cirrhosis necessitates an urgent assessment for liver transplantation, if available. Although reinfection of the graft is common it generally results in a mild hepatitis from which the graft and patient fully recover and is associated with a good long-term outcome.

Ascending cholangitis

Ascending bacterial infection of the biliary tract is usually associated with obstruction, and presents with clinical jaundice, rigors and a tender hepatomegaly. The diagnosis is confirmed by the finding of dilated bile ducts on ultrasound, an obstructive picture of liver function tests and the isolation of an organism from the blood on culture. The condition is a medical emergency and delay in appropriate treatment results in organ failure secondary to septicaemia. Once the diagnosis has been confirmed the patient should be commenced on a first-line antibiotic (e.g. third-generation cephalosporin), rehydrated and arrangements made for endoscopic or percutaneous transhepatic drainage of the biliary tree. Biliary stone disease is a common predisposing factor and the causative ductal stones may be removed at the time of endoscopic cholangiography by endoscopic sphincterotomy.

Pyogenic liver abscess

The aetiology of a pyogenic liver abscess is unexplained in the majority of patients. It has an increased incidence in the elderly, diabetics and the immunosuppressed, who usually present with anorexia, fevers and malaise accompanied by right upper quadrant discomfort. The diagnosis is suggested by the finding of a multiloculated cystic mass on ultrasound or CT scan (Fig. 52.17) and is confirmed by aspiration for culture and sensitivity. The most common organisms are *Streptococcus milleri* and *Escherichia coli* but other enteric organisms such as *Streptococcus faecalis*, *Klebsiella* and *Proteus vulgaris* also occur and mixed growths are common. Opportunistic pathogens include *Staphylococci*. First-line antibiotics would be a penicillin, aminoglycoside and metronidazole or a cephalosporin and metronidazole. Treatment is with antibiotics and ultrasound-guided aspiration. Percutaneous drainage without ultrasound guidance should be avoided as an empyema may follow drainage through the pleural space. A source for the liver abscess should be sought, particularly from the colon. Atypical clinical or radiological findings should raise the possibility of a necrotic neoplasm.

Amoebic liver abscess

Entamoeba histolytica is endemic in many parts of the world. It exists in vegetative form outside the body and is spread by the faecal–oral route. The most common presentation is with dysentery but it may also present with an amoebic abscess, the common sites being paracaecal and in the liver. The amoebic cyst is ingested and develops into the trophozoite form in the colon which passes through the bowel wall and to the liver via the portal blood. Diagnosis is by isolation of the parasite from the liver lesion or the stool and confirming its nature by microscopy. Often patients with clinical signs of an amoebic abscess will be treated empirically with metronidazole (750 mg t.d.s. for 5–10 days) and investigated further only if they do not respond.

Hydatid liver disease

This is a very common condition in countries around the Mediterranean. The causitive tapeworm, *Echinococcus granulosus*, is present in the dog intestine and ova are ingested by humans and pass in the portal blood to the liver. Liver abscesses are often large by the time of presentation with upper abdominal discomfort or may present after minor abdominal trauma as an acute abdomen due to rupture of the cyst into the peritoneal cavity. Diagnosis is suggested by the finding of a multiloculated cyst on ultrasound and is further supported by the finding of a floating membrane within the cysts on CT scan (Fig. 52.18). Active cysts contain a large number of smaller daughter cysts (Fig. 52.19) and rupture can result in these implanting and growing within the peritoneal cavity. Liver cysts can also rupture through the diaphragm producing an empyema, into the biliary tract producing obstructive jaundice or into the stomach. Clinical and radiological diagnosis can be supported by serology for antibodies to hydatid antigen in the form of an enzyme-linked immunosorbent assay (ELISA). Treatment is indicated to prevent progressive enlargement and rupture of the cysts.

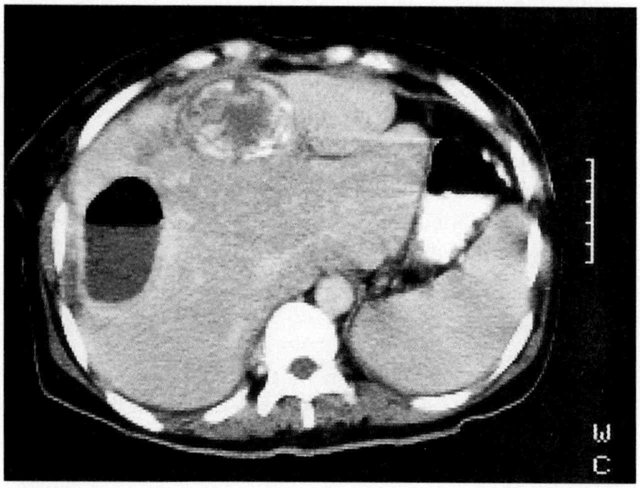

Figure 52.17 Liver abscess. CT scan showing an air/fluid level and rim enhancement with intravenous contrast typical of a liver abscess. In the adjacent liver is a calcified hydatid cyst.

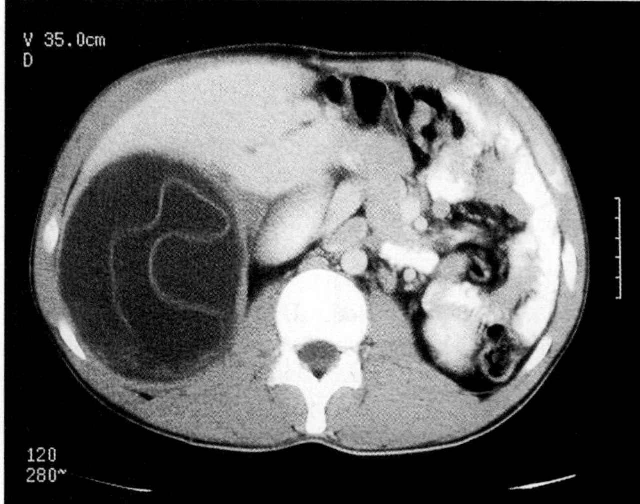

Figure 52.18 Hydatid liver cyst. Active hydatid disease usually produces a noncalcified liver cyst and within the cyst can be seen floating layers of the germinal membrane.

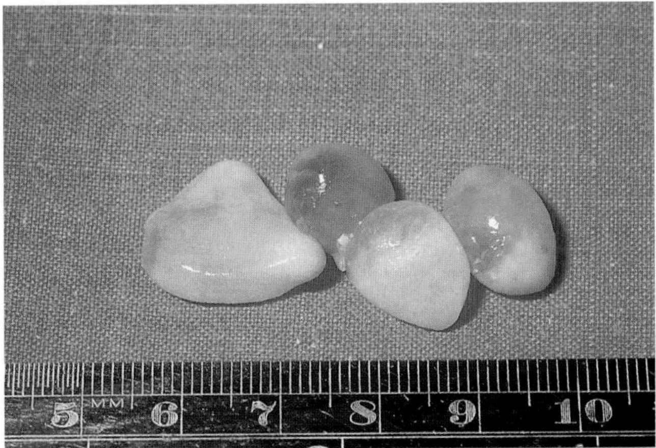

Figure 52.19 Hydatid 'daughter' cysts. These were removed from the bile duct of a patient presenting with obstructive jaundice due to a hydatid liver cyst communicating with the bile duct. Endoscopic removal should also be considered.

In the first instance a course of albendazole or mebendazole may be tried. Failure to respond to medical treatment usually requires surgical intervention, although percutaneous treatments with hypertonic saline and alcohol have been attempted. The surgical options range from liver resection or local excision of the cysts to deroofing with evacuation of the contents. Contamination of the peritoneal cavity at the time of surgery with active hydatid daughters should be avoided by continuing drug therapy with albendazole and adding perioperative praziquantel. This should be combined with packing of the peritoneal cavity with 2 N saline-soaked packs and instilling hypertonic (2 N) saline into the cyst before it is opened. A biliary communication should be actively sought and sutured. The residual cavity may become infected and this may be reduced, as may bile leakage, by packing the space with pedicled greater omentum (an omentoplasty). Calcified cysts may well be dead. If doubt exists as to whether a suspected cyst is active it can be followed on ultrasound, active cysts gradually becoming larger and more superficial in the liver. Rupture of daughter hydatids into the biliary tract may result in obstructive jaundice or acute cholangitis. This may be treated by endoscopic clearance of the daughter cysts prior to cyst removal from the liver.

Liver tumours

Surgical approaches to resection of liver tumours

Adequate exposure of the liver is an absolute prerequisite to safe liver surgery. A rooftop or transverse abdominal incision provides excellent access to the liver if adequate retraction of the costal margin is employed using a costal margin retractor. Thoracoabdominal incisions are no longer required. The procedure for complete mobilisation of the liver is described, although this will not be necessary in all cases. There are many variations in surgical technique.

Mobilisation of the liver

The falciform ligament is first divided and followed along the anterior surface of the liver towards the suprahepatic IVC. The left triangular ligament is divided, facilitated by placing an abdominal pack in front of the oesophagogastric junction. The right triangular ligament is then divided by retraction of the diaphragm away from the right lobe parenchyma. On exposure of the bare area of the liver the IVC can be seen as it passes behind the liver and this can be slung above the renal veins below the liver and at the level of the main hepatic veins. Mobilisation of the liver is completed by division of the lesser omentum. Removing the liver from the IVC is achieved by lifting the liver anteriorly to expose the multiple small veins passing between the liver parenchyma and the IVC. These should be suture ligated to ensure haemostasis. This proceeds from above the renal veins until the main hepatic veins are reached below the diaphragm.

Dissection of the hilum

The peritoneum overlying the hilar triad is divided. The common bile duct (CBD) is then exposed on the free edge of the lesser omentum, mobilisation being facilitated by ligation and division of the cystic duct and artery followed by removal of the gall bladder. Slinging the CBD with an elastic sling allows exposure of the common hepatic artery and dissection of the main right and left branches. These again may be slung to allow the remaining lymphatic tissue surrounding the portal vein to be ligated and divided. The possibility of an aberrant right hepatic artery should be sought lying posterior to the bile duct and an accessory left hepatic artery from the left gastric artery in the lesser omentum. Dissection of the hilar bile ducts requires careful retraction on segment IV of the liver, and division of the small vessels and bile duct branches passing between segment IV and the confluence of the right and left hepatic ducts.

Division of the parenchyma

Once the liver has been adequately mobilised and the hilar vessels have been exposed the main inflow vessels and bile duct can be divided to the liver lobe to be resected. The arterial branch may be ligated but the bile duct should be transfixed with 4/0 PDS and the portal vein branch with 4/0 Prolene suture. Division of the inflow vessels produces a line of demarcation between the right and left liver passing to the right and parallel with the falciform ligament. The parenchyma is divided along this plane of demarcation commencing by diathermy of the liver capsule. The ultrasound (Cusa) dissector is the most common method used for division of the parenchyma. This allows the parenchyma to be divided leaving the vessels and bile duct branches to be diathermied or ligated depending

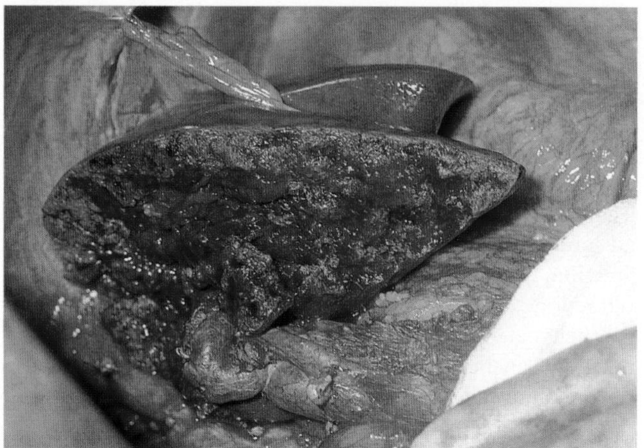

Figure 52.20 Hepatectomy post resection. Cut surface of the residual liver following a right hepatectomy in which segments viii–viii have been removed. On the lower edge the portal vein and bile duct can be visualised.

on their size. Dissection continues on an even plane until the hepatic vein branches are approached from within the liver parenchyma, where they are ligated and divided (Fig. 52.20).

Segmental and local resections

These are considered in patients whose liver tumours can be excised with an adequate margin (generally considered to be 1 cm) without a formal right or left lobe liver resection. The segments which can be removed individually are those shown in Fig. 52.2. Each carries its own blood supply, venous drainage and bile drainage. The extent of mobilisation of the liver required (described above) depends on the segment to be resected. Hilar dissection may not be necessary. Segmental resections are particularly used in patients with HCC and underlying liver disease (e.g. HBV or HCV) to minimise the risk of postoperative liver failure (Fig. 52.21). Local resections are principally used for patients with liver metastases where removal of the tumour mass with a minimum margin of 1 cm of normal liver parenchyma is required.

Blood loss and transfusion

The reduction of blood loss during liver surgery has been one of the major achievements in the last decade and resection without blood transfusion is often possible. The ultrasound dissector has been one of the main advances. Preoperative venesection, intraoperative haemodilution, reducing central venous pressure and the intraoperative cell saver have all helped to reduce the necessity for autologous blood transfusion. Better control of the coagulation cascade has been achieved using TEG (Fig. 52.9), and the antifibrinolytic drug aprotonin has significantly reduced bleeding in patients with liver disease and an underlying coagulopathy. Oozing from the resected surface can be reduced by the topical application of fibrin glue or fibrin-impregnated collagen fleece. The main alternative is the argon beam coagulator.

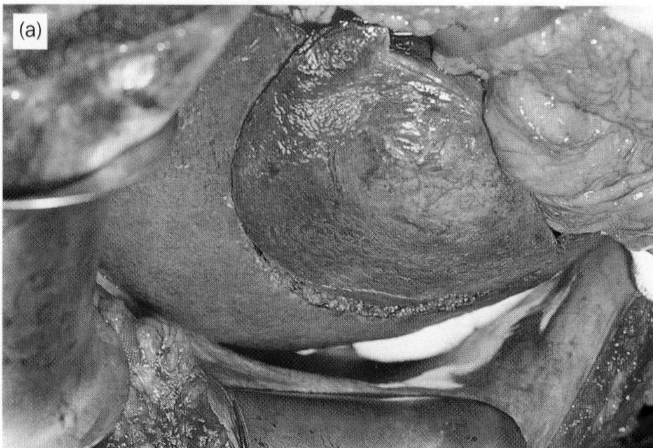

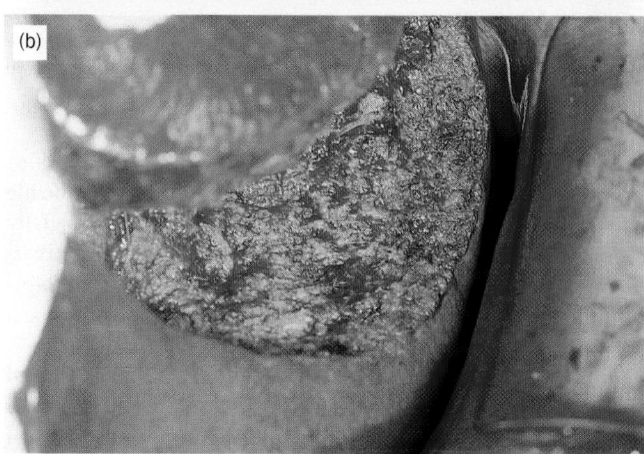

Figure 52.21 Segmental resection. Removal of a primary liver tumour (a) by resection of liver segment vi, (b) in a patient with well-compensated liver cirrhosis.

Benign liver tumours

Haemangiomas are most the common liver lesions and their reporting has increased with the widespread availability of diagnostic ultrasound. They consist of an abnormal plexus of vessels and their nature is usually apparent on ultrasound. If diagnostic uncertainty exists CT scanning with delayed contrast enhancement shows the characteristic appearance of slow contrast enhancement due to small vessel uptake in the haemangioma. Often haemangiomas are multiple. Lesions found incidentally require confirmation of their nature and no further treatment. The management of 'giant' haemangiomas is more controversial. Occasional reports of rupture of haemangiomas has led some to consider resection for the large lesions, especially if they appear to be symptomatic. They have little if any malignant potential and this is no indication for surgery. Percutaneous biopsy of these lesions should be avoided as they are vascular lesions and may bleed profusely into the peritoneal cavity.

Hepatic adenoma (Fig.52.22)

These are rare benign liver tumours. Imaging by CT demonstrates a well-circumscribed and vascular solid tumour. They usually develop in an otherwise normal liver. Unfortunately, there are no characteristic radiological features to differentiate these lesions from malignant tumours. Angiography will demonstrate a well-developed peripheral arterialisation of the tumour. Confirmation of the nature of these lesions is required by either percutaneous biopsy or resection with histological confirmation. These tumours are thought to have malignant potential and resection is therefore the treatment of choice. Owing to their vascularity, bleeding following percutaneous biopsy is well recognised. An association with sex hormones, including the oral contraceptive pill, is well recognised and regression of symptomatic adenomas on withdrawal of hormone stimulation is well documented.

Focal nodular hyperplasia (FNH)

This is an unusual benign condition of unknown aetiology in which there is a focal overgrowth of functioning liver tissue supported by fibrous stroma. Patients are usually middle-aged females, and there is no association with underlying liver disease. Ultrasound shows a solid tumour mass but does not help in discrimination. Contrast CT may show central scarring and evidence of a well-vascularised lesion. Again, these appearances are not specific for FNH. A sulphur colloid liver scan may be useful. FNH contain both hepatocytes and Kupffer cells. The latter takes up the colloid differentiating FNH from either a benign adenoma or a primary or metastatic cancer, none of which contains a significant number of Kupffer cells.

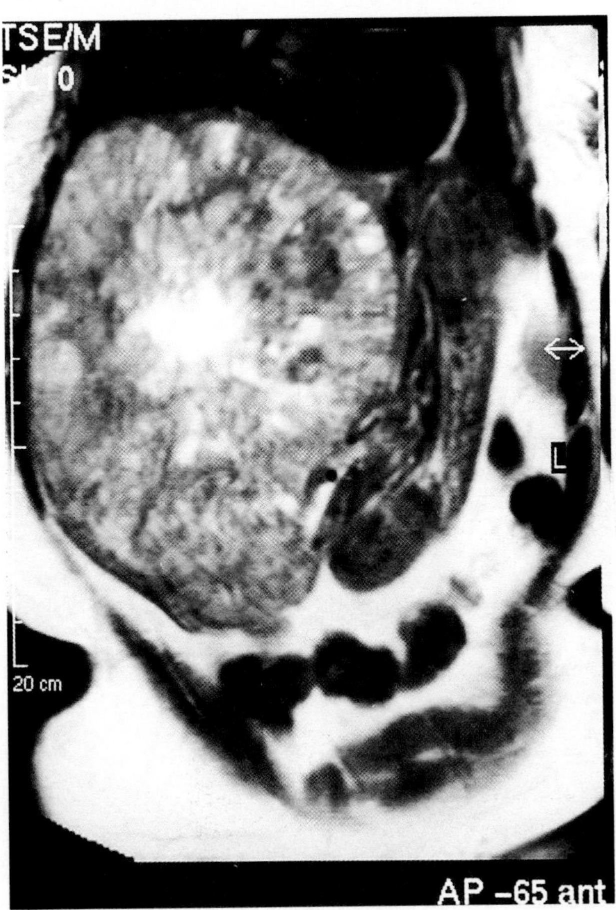

Figure 52.22 Hepatic adenoma. MRI scan of a giant hepatic adenoma. These lesions are thought to be premalignant, may haemorrhage and in some cases their growth is sex hormone sensitive. Withdrawal of hormone preparations may allow spontaneous regression.

Surgery for liver metastases

Outcome

The role of surgery in the treatment of colorectal liver metastases is now well established based on prospective data on resected patients compared with unresected patients with a similar stage of disease. The role of resection of liver metastases from other primary sites has not been defined. The expected patient survival rate for resection of solitary colorectal metastases is approximately 35 per cent at 5 years with few cancer-related deaths beyond this period. Multiple unilobar and bilobar liver metastases may also be considered for resection, although cure rates are significantly lower.

Staging

This involves defining the extent of the liver involvement with metastases and excluding extrahepatic disease. A standard work-up would involve oral and intravenous contrast CT scan of the liver and abdomen, chest CT scan, bone scan and colonoscopy, to look for locally recurrent or synchronous colonic cancers. This information should be taken in parallel with a general medical evaluation before deciding on the suitability for surgery of an individual patient. The typical appearance of colorectal liver metastases on contrast CT is shown in Fig. 52.23. These patients usually have normal liver parenchyma and therefore tolerate a 60–70 per cent resection of liver parenchyma without showing evidence of liver failure.

Surgical approach

The basic surgical approach for liver resection is outlined above. A search for local recurrent disease, peritoneal deposits and regional lymph node involvement should be made at the start of the laparotomy. Planar imaging often overlooks peritoneal or superficial liver metastatic deposits. Coeliac node involvement in patients with liver metastases considerably reduces the overall survival whether or not the liver and nodal disease is resected.

The treatment of unresectable disease

These patients may be offered systemic chemotherapy. First-line treatment is with 5-fluorouracil and folinic acid, which produces a response rate of 30 per cent and may improve the

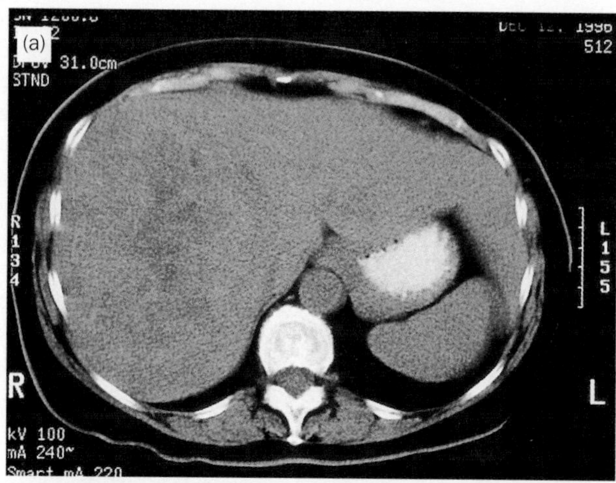

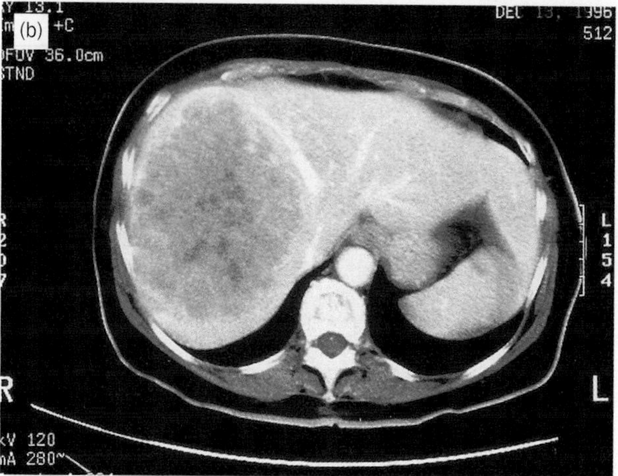

Figure 52.23 Colorectal liver metastases on computed tomography (CT). CT scanning in which a colorectal liver metastasis occupying the entire right lobe of the liver is difficult to visualise on oral contrast CT. The addition of intravenous contrast shows its lack of enhancement and its relationship to the hepatic veins.

quality of life. Other drug regimes are available and many studies are ongoing evaluating hepatic arterial administration of chemotherapy or radioactive microspheres. Many patients will have undergone previous adjuvant chemotherapy following resection of the large bowel primary. There is no proof as yet regarding further adjuvant treatment following resection of liver metastases.

Hepatocellular carcinoma

Primary liver cancer (HCC) is one of the world's commonest cancers and its incidence is expected to rise rapidly over the next decade. This rise is due to the association with chronic liver disease, particularly HBV and HCV. Owing to this association many patients who are known to have chronic liver disease are now being screened for the development of HCC by serial ultrasound scans of the liver or serum measurements of alpha fetoprotein (AFP). Patients often present in middle age either because of symptoms of the chronic liver disease (malaise, weakness, jaundice, ascites, variceal bleed, encephalopathy) or with the anorexia and weight loss of an advanced cancer. The surgical treatment options include resection of the tumour and liver transplantation. Which option is most appropriate for an individual patient depends on the stage of their underlying liver disease, the size and site of the tumour, the availability of organ transplantation and the management of the immunosuppressed patient.

Staging and clinical assessment of hepatocellular carcinoma

In addition to a general assessment of the patient's fitness for surgery, crucial information is the severity of the underlying liver disease based on Child's classification (Table 52.5) and the size and site of the tumour. As chronic liver disease predisposes to these tumours they are often multifocal by the time of diagnosis. Extensive liver resections in patients with advanced cirrhosis are associated with a high mortality due to liver failure and sepsis. In contrast, extensive resections for HCC in a noncirrhotic liver are associated with a low risk of liver failure, and resection rather than transplantation would be the treatment option of choice. Tumours often metastasise to the lung and bone, and a chest CT scan and bone scan are therefore useful staging investigations. Evidence of intraperitoneal disease is difficult to determine by CT scan, and laparoscopy may be useful for this purpose. The intrahepatic distribution of HCC is equally difficult to determine within the cirrhotic liver. Ultrasound, early arterial phase enhanced spiral CT scan and CT scan 2 weeks following intrahepatic administration of the contrast agent Lipiodol are the most useful that are currently available (Fig. 52.24).

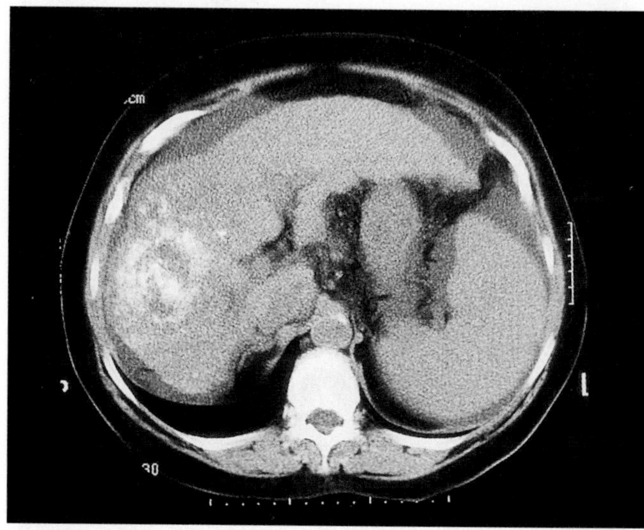

Figure 52.24 Lipiodol uptake in hepatocellular carcinoma (HCC). The poppy seed oil Lipiodol can be used a contrast material for imaging. It localises in primary liver cancers and, following its administration into the hepatic artery at selective mesenteric angiography, its uptake in HCC can be demonstrated at 2 weeks on CT.

Surgical approach to HCC

The surgical approach should remove the known cancer with a 1–2 cm margin of unaffected liver tissue. In patients with associated chronic liver disease the volume of liver resected should be minimised to reduce the incidence of postoperative liver failure. Local or segmental resections are preferred to major resections (Fig. 52.21).

Follow-up and adjuvant treatment

There is little evidence that adjuvant chemotherapy will improve the prognosis of patients following resection of HCC, and it may damage the function of the liver in those with underlying chronic liver disease. AFP is a clinically useful tumour marker for follow-up, although its low sensitivity would suggest that imaging should also be employed.

Cholangiocarcinoma

Presentation, pathology and natural history

Bile duct cancers typically present with painless obstructive jaundice. Elderly patients are frequently affected, but patients with primary sclerosing cholangitis (PSC) may develop these tumours at a much earlier age. These tumours are typically slow growing and often arise at the confluence of the right and left hepatic ducts, eventually invading the liver parenchyma. Cancers at this site are usually fibrous and produce tight duct strictures. Distal bile duct cholangiocarcinomas are more frequently polypoidal and obstruct the lumen of the duct. Both invade perineural planes and along lymphatics.

Investigation and staging

The diagnosis should be suspected when ultrasound examination of the jaundiced patient shows dilated intrahepatic but not extrahepatic bile ducts.

Cholangiography will usually show a hilar stricture (Fig. 52.25) and brush cytology will provide a tissue diagnosis in about two-thirds of patients. Polypoidal tumours may closely mimic CBD stones (Fig. 52.26). Spiral CT scan often shows little evidence of a mass lesion unless infiltration into the liver parenchyma has occurred. Regional lymphadenopathy may be apparent but cannot be assumed to be malignant. Evidence of local spread into the portal vein or evidence of hepatic arterial involvement may be obtained by angiography. Distal spread at presentation is unusual, as is peritoneal seeding. Hilar cholangiocarcinomas may be categorised using the system suggested by Bismuth (Fig. 52.27).

Treatment

Surgical resection offers the only possibility of cure and may also be the best form of palliation. Owing to local spread into lymphatics and the perineural space, local resection of a hilar cholangiocarcinoma is rarely curative, although some long-term survivors have been reported. Radical resection of the

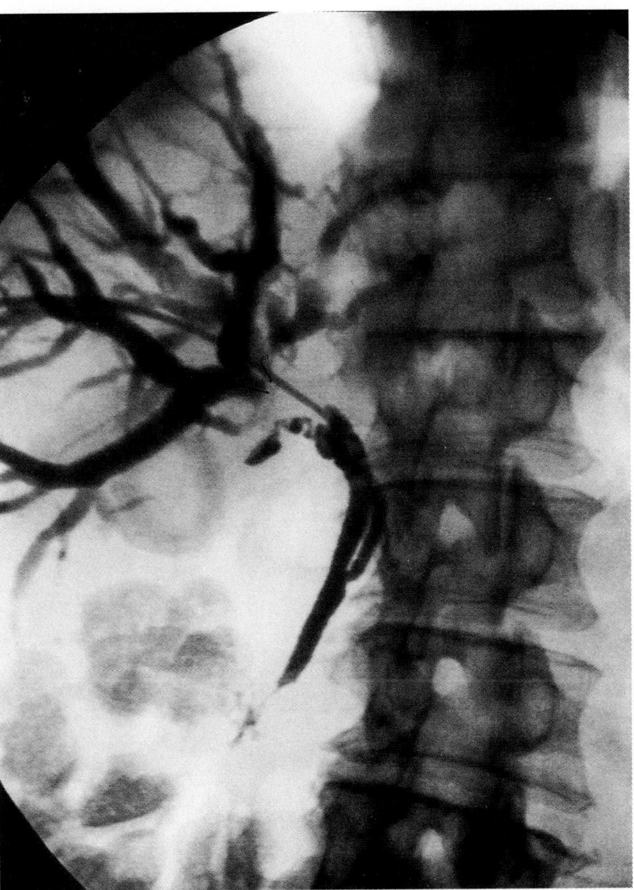

Figure 52.25 Hilar cholangiocarcinoma. Cholangiography demonstrating a short hilar stricture through which a drainage catheter has been inserted percutaneously.

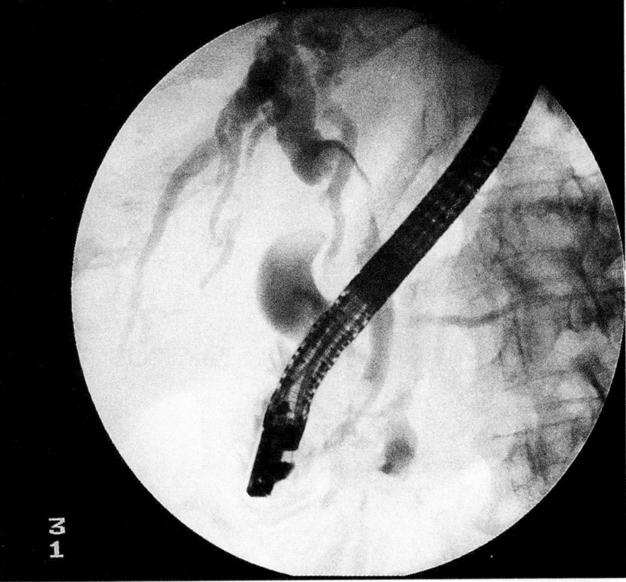

Figure 52.26 Polypoidal cholangiocarcinoma. ERCP demonstrating a filling defect of the mid bile duct due to a polypoidal carcinoma. These findings may be mistaken for ductal stone disease.

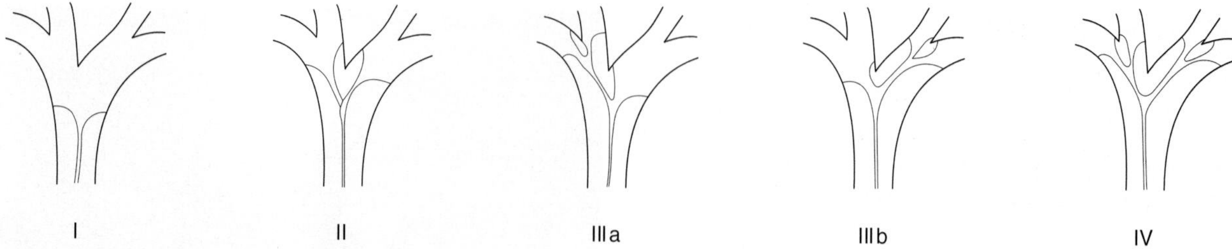

Figure 52.27 Bismuth staging of cholangiocarcinoma. This classification is a useful guide to the likelihood of resectability. Types I–III may be resectable based on angiography and staging investigations, whereas type IV is rarely resectable.

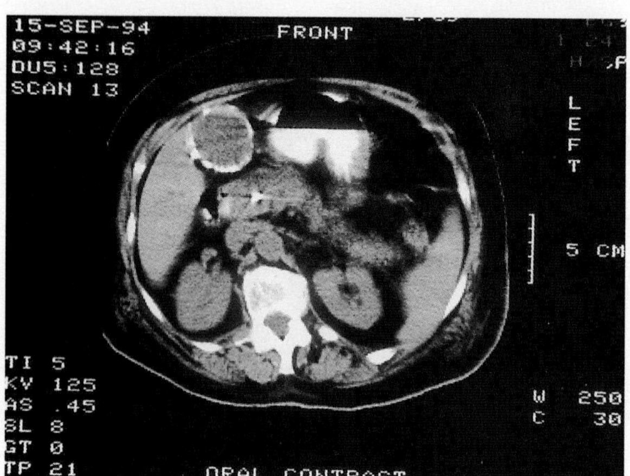

Figure 52.28 Porcelain gall bladder. Calcification of the gall-bladder wall strongly predisposes to gall-bladder cancer.

liver parenchyma associated with the affected bile duct has become the recognised treatment. Those patients in whom the volume of residual liver parenchyma following resection may be inadequate can be considered for transhepatic portal vein embolisation of the branch to the side of the liver to be removed, as described by Nimura and colleagues. This results in compensatory enlargement and functional improvement in the liver parenchyma.

Gall-bladder cancer

The aetiology of gall-bladder cancer is unknown but it almost invariably is associated with the presence of stones in the gall-bladder which may act as a chronic irritant to the gall bladder mucosa. Evidence of a field change in the gall bladder mucosa with areas of dysplasia would support this theory. It is also known to have a very high incidence in patients with gall-bladder wall calcification, the porcelain gall bladder (Fig. 52.28). Presentation is often with symptomatic gallstones where the gall-bladder cancer is an incidental finding. Alternatively, the patient may present with pain or obstructive jaundice and in these individuals the tumour is often advanced, having extended outside the liver or towards the hilum of the liver to produce ductal obstruction. Patients in whom the tumour is an incidental finding following cholecystectomy and is limited to the mucosa of the gall bladder have a good prognosis. Those in whom there is transmural spread or those presenting with obstructive jaundice have a poor prognosis. Staging of the tumour will decide the possibilities for management, and includes spiral CT scan of the chest and abdomen, cholangiography, selective hepatic angiography and staging laparoscopy. Radical surgery offers the only hope of cure for gall-bladder cancer and this may involve removing the right lobe liver parenchyma, the biliary tree, along with the hilar lymphatic drainage of the gall bladder by a hilar lymphadenectomy. There is little evidence for chemotherapy either as a sole treatment or in an adjuvant setting. Patients presenting with obstructive jaundice due to an unresectable gall-bladder cancer may have the symptoms relieved by insertion of a biliary endoprosthesis.

Further reading

Blumgart, L.H. (ed.) (1990) *Surgery of the Liver and Biliary Tract*, Churchill Livingstone Edinburgh.

Sherlock, S. and Dooley, J.S.D. (eds) (1993) *Diseases of the Liver and Biliary Tract*, 9th edn. Blackwell Scientific, Oxford.

McIntyre, N., Benhamou, J.-P., Bircher, J. *et al.* (eds) (1991) *Oxford Textbook of Clinical Hepatology*. Oxford University Press, Oxford.

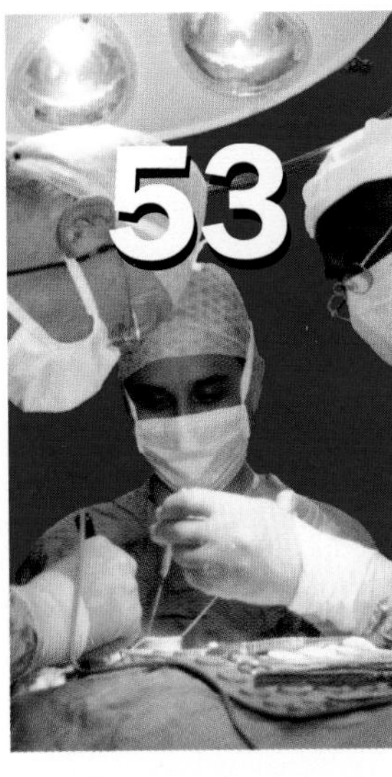

The spleen

Anatomy and physiology

The spleen arises by mesenchymal differentiation along the left side of the dorsal mesogastrium in the 8-mm embryo. The weight of the normal adult spleen is between 75 and 150 g. It is shaped like a segment of an orange, its convexity directed backwards and to the left. It lies between the tenth and eleventh ribs posteriorly. It abuts the diaphragm superiorly, anteriorly there is the gastric impression, posteriorly it is in contact with the kidney and the colon lies inferiorly. Within the hilum is the tail of the pancreas and the splenic vessels. It forms the apex of the lesser sac. Within the anterior leaf of the lesser sac the short gastrics pass to the greater curve of the fundus of the stomach. The splenic artery divides at the hilus into branches which run along the trabeculae of the spleen into the white pulp, where they give off branches which are almost perpendicular to the central trunk (Fig. 53.1). This produces a 'skimming effect' by which plasma tends to pass down the branches to the white pulp and most of the red cells pass in the trabecular artery to the red pulp. The white pulp has an immune function, whereas the red pulp filters abnormal red cells from the circulation. Phagocytosis of blood-borne particles occurs in both areas. On cutting the spleen areas of red pulp, within which can be seen pale ovoid nodules of white, are apparent.

Bailey & Love's Short Practice of Surgery, 23rd edition. Edited by R.C.G. Russell, N.S. Williams and C.J.K. Bulstrode. Published in 2000 by Arnold Publishers.

The white pulp consists of a central trabecular artery surrounded by nodules with germinal centres and periarterial lymphatic sheaths which provide a framework filled with lymphocytes and macrophages. At the edge of the white pulp is the marginal zone into which pass arteries from both the central artery and from the peripheral 'penicillar' arteries. Plasma-rich blood which has passed through the central lymphatic nodules is filtered as it passes through the sinuses within the marginal zone, and particles are phagocytosed. Immunoglobulins produced in the lymphatic nodules enter the circulation through the sinuses in the marginal zone. Beyond the marginal zone is the red pulp which consists of cords and sinuses. Cell-concentrated blood passes in the trabecular artery through the centre of the white pulp to the red pulp cords. To pass from the cords to the sinuses, the red cell must elongate and become thinner. This filters abnormally shaped or rigid cells out of the circulation.

Ninety per cent of blood passing through the spleen moves through an open circulation in which blood flows from arteries to cords and thence to sinuses. Thus, splenic pulp pressure reflects pressure throughout the portal venous system. The remaining 10 per cent bypasses the cords and sinuses by direct arteriovenous connections. The overall flow rate through the spleen is about 300 ml/minute.

Functions of the spleen

In the past the spleen was considered dispensable because it was found not to be essential to life. The surgeon therefore

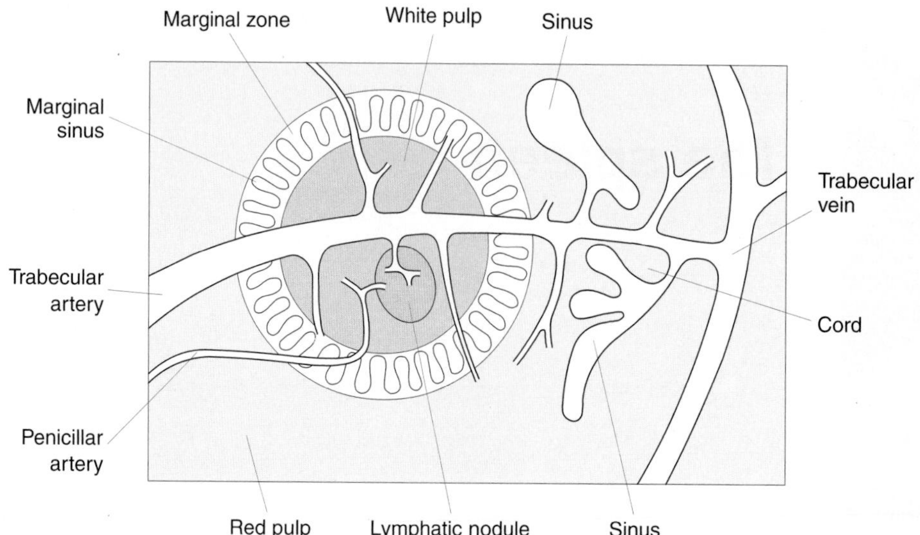

Fig. 53.1 A central trabecular artery passing through the white pulp into the surrounding red pulp. A blood flow skimming effect results in most of the plasma passing down branches of the artery while the cells pass in the central trabecular artery directly into the red pulp (*courtesy of Professor T.G. Allen-Mersh, Westminster and Charing Cross Hospitals, London, England*).

sacrificed the spleen with impunity. Increasing knowledge of the untoward effects of splenectomy has led to conservatism in the management of the spleen. Indeed, when splenectomy is performed as part of another operation, such as total gastrectomy, the incidence of complications increases and the mortality rises. For this reason the surgeon now tries to preserve the spleen and maintain the following functions.

- *Immune function* – the spleen processes foreign antigen and is a major site of specific immunoglobin M (IgM) production. The nonspecific opsonins tuftin and properdin are synthesised. These antibodies are of both B- and T-cell origin, and react with bacteria and fungi to make them more susceptible to phagocytosis.
- *Filter function* – macrophages in the reticulum capture cellular and noncellular material from the blood and plasma; this material includes bacteria, especially pneumococci.
- *Removal of effete, platelets and red cells* – this process is called '*culling*'.
- *Pitting* – this is the process of removing particulate inclusions from red cells and returning the repaired red cell to the circulation. Red blood cell nuclei or malarial parasites can be removed by this process without destroying the cell.
- *Iron reutilisation* – the phagocytic reticular cells remove iron from ingested degraded haemoglobin during red cell culling and return the iron to the plasma.
- *Pooling* – up to 30–40 per cent of blood platelets are sequestered within the spleen. In splenomegaly up to 80 per cent of the platelet pool can be sequestered in the spleen and this, together with accelerated platelet destruction, can result in thrombocytopenia.
- *Reservoir function* – in animals, especially the dog, up to one-third of the blood volume may be sequestered in the spleen during sleeping and returned to the circulation on waking. This does not occur in humans.
- *Haematopoiesis* – this only occurs up to the fifth intra-uterine month and thereafter in certain disease states.

Investigation of the spleen

Conditions that cause splenomegaly can be diagnosed by history, physical signs and laboratory examination. For instance in haemolytic anaemia a full blood count, reticulocyte count and tests for haemolysis will determine the type of anaemia. Similarly, splenomegaly associated with portal hypertension caused by hepatic cirrhosis is diagnosed by the physical signs of liver dysfunction, abnormal liver function tests and evidence of oesophageal varices. Many conditions that cause splenomegaly also cause lymphadenopathy. The cause of the splenomegaly should then be determined from investigations for diseases known to cause lymphadenopathy and splenomegaly. A lymph node biopsy can be helpful in this respect.

Plain radiography

This plays little part in investigation now, although calcification in the spleen may suggest an old infarct or hydatid disease. Multiple areas of calcification would suggest splenic tuberculosis.

Imaging

Ultrasonography of the spleen (Fig. 53.2) is of value in determining its size and consistency, and whether or not cysts are present. It can be used for diagnosis of a ruptured spleen. However, in this case a *computerised tomography* (CT) scan is more usually undertaken to exclude other intra-abdominal

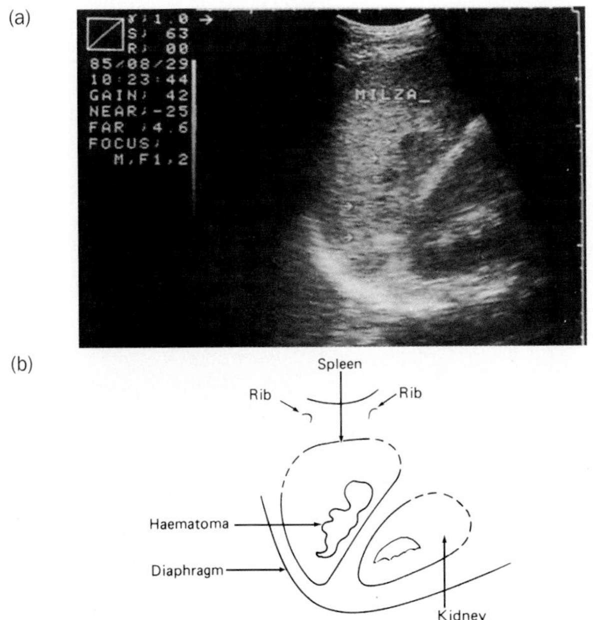

Fig. 53.2 Ultrasonogram obtained with a probe situated over the anterior aspect of the left lower ribs showing the spleen containing a haematoma. The left kidney is situated behind the spleen and the posterior diaphragm can be seen as it dips down posteriorly behind the left kidney. The subcapsular splenic haematoma is shown near the hilar surface of the spleen, as the drawing illustrates (*courtesy of Dr L. Solbiati, Ospidale Busto Arizio, Milan, Italy*).

problems. Similarly, a *spiral CT scan* with contrast enhancement will be preferable in the diagnosis of splenomegaly to determine both the extent of the disease and the associated problems such as the extent of lymphadenopathy.

Radioisotope scans

Technetium-99m (^{99m}Tc)-labelled colloid can provide information about the position and size of the spleen and, with appropriately labelled red cells, the life and place of their destruction can be determined.

Congenital abnormalities of the spleen

Absence of the spleen is rare, and when it occurs is often associated with congenital heart disease. Patients without a spleen are occasionally subject to fatal infection.

Splenunculi

These are single or multiple accessory spleens which are found near the hilum of the spleen in 50 per cent, related to the splenic vessels and behind the tail of the pancreas in 30 per cent, or in the splenic ligaments and mesocolon in the remainder. Up to 20 per cent of people have such splenunculi and most are no larger than 2 cm in diameter. Their importance lies in the fact that if not removed at the time of splenectomy they will undergo hyperplasia and may well be the site of persistent disease.

Hamartoma

Rarely, these are found in the spleen, usually being found incidentally at post-mortem examination. They vary in size from less than 1 cm in diameter to masses large enough to produce abdominal swelling. There are two varieties: one mainly lymphoid resembling the white pulp and the other resembling the red pulp. They are occasionally seen incidentally on CT scanning.

Splenic cysts

Nonparasitic cysts of the spleen are rare. They consist of true cysts formed from embryonal rests and include dermoids and mesenchymal inclusion cysts, or false cysts resulting from trauma which contain serous or haemorrhagic fluid. They can be clearly demarcated on scanning, punctured, drained and sclerosed. Operative removal is rarely, if ever, indicated.

Rupture of the spleen

Splenic rupture should be suspected after any trauma, but particularly if there has been direct injury to the left upper quadrant of the abdomen from any angle. Occasionally a fall without direct trauma to the trunk can rupture the spleen, especially if it is diseased or enlarged, for example in infectious mononucleosis or malaria. Advantage was once taken of the fragility of the enlarged spleen in Far Eastern countries where malaria is endemic. Murderers would achieve their purpose by digging a victim beneath the left ribs with a weapon known as the 'larang'; the enlarged malarial spleen would rupture. A splenic injury should be suspected if there are fractures of the overlying ribs. Iatrogenic rupture remains common and is a reminder of the need for care when dissecting in the left upper quadrant of the abdomen, especially if adhesions are present.

Cases of ruptured spleen may be divided into three groups.

- *The patient succumbs rapidly from massive haemorrhage* – this type rarely occurs in the normal spleen but is a reminder that a slipped pedicle suture can lead to rapid exsanguination.
- *Initial shock, recovery and signs of bleeding* – the initial shock is due to the blood loss, tamponade occurs and then further bleeding takes place. General signs of internal haemorrhage are variable but local signs show upper abdominal guarding and, later, local bruising and abdominal distension. Pain referred to the left shoulder is known as Kehr's sign. There may be hyperaesthesia in this area. The sign can often be demonstrated 15 minutes after elevation of the foot of the bed. It is due to blood in contact with the undersurface of the diaphragm, the pain being mediated through afferent fibres in the phrenic nerve. Shifting dullness may be present in the flanks and on rectal examination fullness in the pelvis is present. The

---

Hans Kehr, 1862–1916. Surgeon, Halberstädt, later Berlin. He died of septicaemia contracted during this work.

elicitation of these difficult signs should give way to appropriate ultrasonography or CT scanning to determine the site from which the bleeding is occurring.

- *The delayed case* – after initial signs have passed off and the concern about a serious intra-abdominal bleed has been postponed, late rupture can occur. Such cases should now be rare as scanning should delineate such patients and a haematoma around a spleen should be an indication for either laparotomy or, at the minimum, close observation. If ultrasonography cannot be performed and reliance has to be made on a plain X-ray of the abdomen it is important to ensure a high-quality soft-tissue X-ray so that the following signs can be elicited:
  - obliteration of the splenic outline;
  - obliteration of the psoas shadow;
  - indentation of the left side of the gastric air bubble;
  - fracture of one or more lower ribs of the left side;
  - elevation of the left hemidiaphragm;
  - free fluid between gas-filled intestinal coils.

Treatment of rupture of the spleen

Previously, immediate laparotomy has been the only reliable course. With better understanding of the problems associated with splenectomy, particularly in countries where malaria is common, splenic preservation should be undertaken where possible. Blood is evacuated and the spleen inspected. If by careful compression of the spleen the bleeding can be controlled a vicryl mesh bag can be constructed and the spleen placed in the bag which is then tightened to compress the spleen and to stop the bleeding. This manoeuvre is invaluable in children who are most at risk from splenectomy.

Rupture of a malarial spleen

As has been mentioned, in tropical countries this is not an infrequent catastrophe. The delayed type of rupture (following 'trivial' injury) is also very common and the patient is admitted with a perisplenic haematoma. If splenectomy can be performed before the haematoma bursts into the general peritoneal cavity, the prognosis is less grave. Enlarged spleens from any cause can rupture spontaneously or with mild trauma.

The operation is considerably more difficult than in the case of a ruptured normal spleen. Surgeons with tropical experience have surmounted these difficulties by ligating the splenic vessels as they run along the superior border of the body of the pancreas before disturbing the haematoma.

Aneurysm and infarction

Aneurysm of the splenic artery

This is an uncommon condition; estimates of its incidence at post-mortem examination vary between 0.04 and 1 per cent. Whereas aneurysms of other arteries are more common in men, in the splenic artery they are about twice as common in women. They are usually single and situated in the main trunk of the splenic artery (Fig. 53.3), but more than one are found in a quarter of cases.

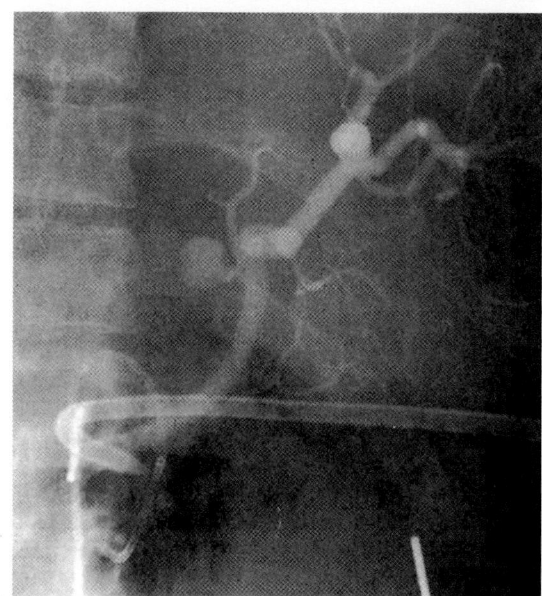

Fig. 53.3 Usual position of a splenic aneurysm.

The aneurysm is symptomless unless it ruptures. Occasionally it is palpable in the epigastrium or associated with a bruit over the left hypochondrium. It may be discovered accidentally, on plain radiograph of the upper abdomen, as a calcified ring situated to the left of the first lumbar vertebra. Rupture of the aneurysm is unsuspected in about half of all cases; it bursts into the peritoneal cavity and the symptoms resemble those of splenic rupture. Nearly half of all cases of rupture occur in patients less than 45 years of age, and a quarter of all cases are in pregnant women (usually in the third trimester of pregnancy or actually in labour).

The treatment of choice is splenectomy and removal of the length of artery bearing the aneurysm. If the aneurysm has eroded into the pancreas or is close to the origin of the splenic artery, then proximal and distal ligation of the sac is usually followed by thrombosis in the aneurysm. In younger

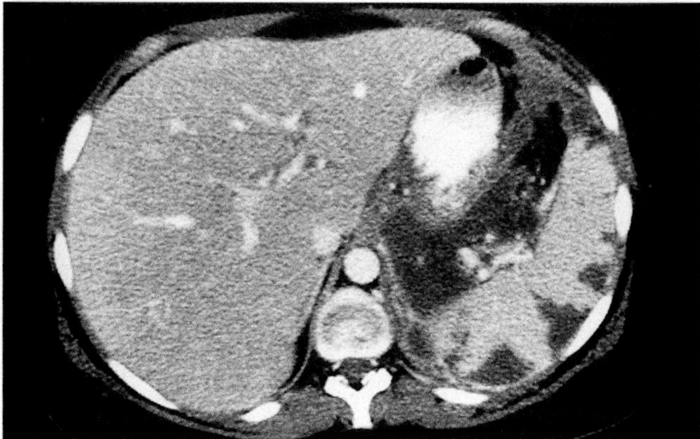

Fig. 53.4 CT scan showing splenic infarcts secondary to severe acute pancreatitis.

Table 53.1 Causes of enlargement of the spleen

Infective	Bacterial	Typhoid and paratyphoid
		Typhus
		Anthrax
		Tuberculosis*
		Septicaemia
		Abscess of the spleen†
	Spirochaetal	Weil's disease
		Syphilis
	Viral	Infectious mononucleosis
		Psittacosis
	Protozoal and parasites	Malaria
		Schistosomiasis (Egyptian splenomegaly)*
		Trypanosomiasis
		Kala-azar
		Hydatid cyst‡
		Tropical splenomegaly*
Blood disease	Myelofibrosis†	
	Acute leukaemia	
	Chronic leukaemia (lymphocytic or granulocytic)†	
	Pernicious anaemia	
	Polycythaemia vera	
	Erythroblastosis fetalis	
	Hereditary spherocytosis	
	Autoimmune haemolytic anaemia*	
	Idiopathic thrombocytopenic purpura‡	
	Mediterranean anaemia (thalassaemia)†	
	Sickle cell disease	
Metabolic	Rickets	
	Amyloid	
	Porphyria	
	Gaucher's disease† (Chapter 52)	
Circulatory	Infarct	Infective endocarditis†
		Mitral stenosis
	Occlusion of the portal vein	Portal hypertension† (Chapter 52)
		Thrombophlebitis*
		Neoplastic, e.g. carcinoma of the tail of pancreas†
Collagen diseases	Still's disease (Chapter 26)	
	Felty's syndrome* (this chapter)	
Nonparasitic cysts	Congenital‡	
	Acquired‡	
Neoplastic	Angioma‡	
	Primary fibrosarcoma‡	
	Hodgkin's lymphoma† (Chapter 17)	
	Other lymphomas†	

*Often benefited by splenectomy.
†Splenectomy sometimes indicated.
‡Benefited by splenectomy.

patients, particularly women, with an asymptomatic splenic artery aneurysm, surgery is indicated after the diagnosis has been confirmed by selective coeliac arteriography. The maternal mortality rate for surgery at the time of rupture, in late pregnancy, is over 70 per cent. In elderly patients, particularly men, where an asymptomatic calcified aneurysm is detected on plain radiograph, there is less risk of rupture and surgery is not indicated.

Infarction of the spleen (Fig. 53.4)

This occurs in patients with massive spleens resulting from myeloproliferative syndrome, or with vascular occlusion produced by sickle cell disease or an embolus from an infected heart valve in bacterial endocarditis. The infarct may be asymptomatic or may cause left upper quadrant abdominal pain radiating to the left shoulder with splinting of the hemidiaphragm and guarding and, at times, a friction rub may be heard over the splenic area. Sedation and bed rest are sufficient except rarely when a septic infarct causes an abscess necessitating splenectomy.

Adolph Weil, 1848–1916. Physician, Dorpat (Tartu), Estonia.
Sir George Frederick Still, 1868–1941. Professor of Diseases of Children, King's College Hospital, London, England.

Enlargement of the spleen

The spleen is a meeting place of medicine and surgery. Table 53.1 summarises the many causes of enlargement of the organ.

In connection with Table 53.1, the following points should be noted. In idiopathic thrombocytopenic purpura (ITP) the spleen, although somewhat enlarged, is seldom palpable. In psittacosis the enlarged spleen can be palpated regularly after the first few days of the illness; this enlargement is helpful to differentiate the condition from other varieties of pneumonia. In portal hypertension the spleen is enlarged secondary to hepatic cirrhosis or portal vein thrombosis (Chapter 52). As emphasised in Table 53.1, not all causes of splenomegaly will require splenectomy as part of their treatment. Elective splenectomy is required to treat haematological disease with medically uncontrolled hypersplenism, occasionally to stage and diagnose lymphoma, to treat splenic cysts, tumours and abscesses, and for the relief of the discomfort associated with splenomegaly.

Idiopathic thrombocytopenic purpura

Purpura

Not all cases of purpura (purpura = *porphyra* (Greek) = purple) benefit from splenectomy. Purpura is defined as local haemorrhage into the skin. A history of purpura and evidence of it on examination should be sought before any surgical procedure is undertaken. Purpura may result from the following.

1. Increased capillary fragility, as in steroid-induced or Henoch–Schönlein purpura.
2. Defective platelets (thrombocytopathies), for example, after taking aspirin which inhibits thromboxane and prostaglandin, and reduces their property of making the platelet adhesive.
3. A reduced number of normal platelets (thrombocytopenia). This can be a consequence of:
   (a) decreased platelet production by marrow megakaryocytes; for example, because of marrow suppression by cytotoxic chemotherapy or in aplastic anaemia;
   (b) increased platelet consumption, as seen in disseminated intravascular coagulation where the clotting cascade is triggered by septicaemia and platelets adhere to vascular endothelium, or in a large haemangioma in which platelets adhere to the abnormal endothelium;
   (c) increased platelet destruction by the spleen. This may be associated with autoimmune disease (e.g. systemic lupus erythematosus); with drug reactions, for example, to quinine; and with certain infections (e.g. mononucleosis). Alternatively, as in ITP, the platelet destruction may not be associated with any other condition;
   (d) increased splenic sequestration of platelets. This can be associated with any condition that produces gross splenic enlargement, e.g. portal hypertension.

Splenectomy may sometimes be helpful in purpura associated with splenic destruction or sequestration (points 3c and 3d, above). It is most reliably of use in the management of ITP.

Aetiology of idiopathic thrombocytopenic purpura

In most cases the low platelet count in ITP is due to the development of antibodies which damage the patient's own platelets (the normal blood platelet count is 250×10^9–400×10^9/litre). Transfused platelets have a short survival time after transfusion into patients with ITP, and the children born to mothers with ITP may have temporary maternal antibody-induced thrombocytopenia after birth.

Clinical features

Purpuric patches (ecchymoses) occur in the skin and mucous membranes which tend to be more prominent in dependent areas because of a higher, gravity aided, intravascular pressure. A tendency to spontaneous bleeding from mucous membranes (e.g. epistaxis), and in women to menorrhagia, and prolonged bleeding of minor wounds is common. Urinary and gastrointestinal haemorrhage and haemarthrosis are rare. Intracranial haemorrhage is also rare, but is the most frequent cause of death. Cutaneous ecchymoses may be found on examination and the tourniquet test is positive. The spleen is palpable in only 25 per cent of cases, and gross splenic enlargement suggests that the diagnosis is not ITP.

Investigations

The bleeding time is increased, but the clotting and prothrombin times are normal. The platelet count in the peripheral blood film is reduced (usually less than 60×10^9/litre). Bone marrow biopsy reveals a plentiful supply of platelet-producing megakaryocytes (the giant cells of bone marrow give origin to blood platelets).

Treatment

The behaviour of the disease is different in children and adults. In children, the disease regresses spontaneously in 75 per cent of cases after one attack. Short courses of corticosteroids or occasionally azothiaprine are usually followed by recovery. Splenectomy is reserved for severe cases which have relapsed or girls approaching menarche. In adults, the initial attack is less severe than in children, but the disease relapses and becomes more severe. Splenectomy is indicated where the ITP has persisted for more than 6–9 months.

Sixty per cent of patients can be regarded as cured, 20 per cent will be improved and 15 per cent or more will derive no benefit from the splenectomy. It is often, although not invari-

---

Eduard Heinrich Henoch, 1820–1910. Physician, Berlin, Germany.
Johannes Lucas Schönlein, 1793–1864. Physician, Berlin, Germany.

able, that a response to steroids predicts a good response to splenectomy. If severe bleeding has not been controlled by steroids, fresh blood transfusion or transfusion with platelet concentrates before operation is often necessary. Splenectomy is contraindicated during the acute phase of ITP; the disease should first be controlled by medical treatment. Occasionally, in resistant cases, the antiplatelet immune response can temporarily be blocked by IgG transfusion to saturate the splenic Fc binding sites and reduce platelet destruction to allow the platelet count to rise at the time of surgery.

Splenectomy for other causes of thrombocytopenic purpura

Occasionally, splenectomy is of benefit in thrombocytopenia due to systemic lupus erythematosus and in hypersplenism; also in purpura associated with points 3c and 3d above.

The haemolytic anaemias

There are five causes of haemolytic anaemia which are amenable to splenectomy:

- hereditary spherocytosis;
- acquired autoimmune haemolytic anaemia;
- thalassaemia;
- hereditary elliptocytosis;
- pyruvate kinase deficiency.

Hereditary spherocytosis

The essential lesion is an increase in permeability of the red cell membrane to sodium. As the sodium leaks into the red cell its osmotic pressure rises, it swells and becomes more spherical, and in consequence more fragile. The mechanism by which the cells rids itself of sodium – the sodium pump – has to work harder. This has two consequences: (1) there is greater loss of membrane phospholipid and so a weakening of the membrane which thus becomes more fragile; and (2) the energy and the oxygen requirements increase. These requirements are particularly difficult to satisfy in the spleen where there is deficiency of both glucose and oxygen. Thus, a large number of red cells is destroyed in the spleen, and splenectomy reduces this cell destruction. Splenectomy does not, of course, cure the congenital red cell membrane defect, but it lessens the anaemia and makes the red cell survival time normal. The defect is transmitted by either parent as a Mendelian autosomal dominant (in 1866 Mendel described 'dominant' and 'recessive' traits in hybrids; his work passed unnoticed for 35 years). Males and females are equally affected.

Gregor Johann Mendel, 1822–84. Augustinian monk and naturalist, who later became Abbot of Brunn, Austria (now Brn, Czech Republic). His work on inheritance was published in 1866 but passed almost unnoticed during his lifetime.

The circulating bilirubin is not conjugated with glycuronic acid. It is attached to albumin and is not excreted in the urine (acholuric jaundice). Although there is excessive breakdown of red cells with transformation of liberated haemoglobin to bilirubin, the bilirubin compound so produced is excreted by the liver and not the kidneys, thus favouring the formation of pigment gallstones.

Clinical features

Once the disease manifests itself, spontaneous remissions are almost unknown. As a rule the patient is pale and has jaundice. In established cases lassitude and undue fatigue are present, but they vary with the degree of haemolysis.

Sometimes the patient is born jaundiced or becomes so early in life. In certain families the disease is characterised by severe crises of red blood cell destruction; thus, with the onset of a crisis, an erythrocyte count may fall from 4.5×10^6 to 1.5×10^6 in less than a week. Such crises are characterised by the onset of pyrexia, abdominal pain, nausea, vomiting and extreme pallor, followed by increased jaundice. These crises may be precipitated by acute infection, and can be so severe as to cause death in infancy or childhood. More usually the jaundice, although variable, is very mild and may not appear until adolescence or even adult life. In adult cases there is often a history of attacks of biliary colic; indeed, 68 per cent of untreated patients over the age of 10 years have pigment stones in their gall bladder. Every child with gallstones should be investigated for hereditary spherocytosis, and enquiry should be made among relatives of patients with spherocytosis for evidence of similar disease.

On examination the spleen is large and, in thin patients, can be palpated easily. Sometimes the liver is also palpable. Chronic leg ulcers can occur in adults with the disease.

Haematological investigations

The fragility test. Increased fragility of erythrocytes characterises this disease. Normally, erythrocytes begin to haemolyse in 0.47 per cent saline solution. In this condition haemolysis occurs in 0.6 per cent or in even stronger solutions.

The reticulocyte count. To compensate for the loss of erythrocytes by haemolysis, the bone marrow discharges into the circulation immature red cells which differ from adult cells by possessing a reticulum.

Faecal urobilinogen. Faecal urobilinogen is increased, as most of the urobilinogen is excreted by this route.

Use of radioactive chromium. Labelling the patient's own red cells with ^{51}Cr will demonstrate the severity of red cell destruction, and if this is accompanied by daily scanning over the spleen it will show the degree of red cell sequestration by the spleen. If splenic radioactivity is high, splenectomy will be of value.

Treatment

All patients who have hereditary spherocytosis should be treated by splenectomy. In juvenile cases the age at which operation is recommended has been decreasing. If it is not imperative before, the optimum time seems to be about 7 years of age, before gallstones have had time to form but subsequent vulnerability to infection is reduced. Ultrasonography should be performed preoperatively to determine the presence or absence of gallstones.

Acquired autoimmune haemolytic anaemia

This may be due to a drug reaction (e.g. to α-methyldopa), to another disease (e.g. systemic lupus erythematosus) or its cause may be unknown. Red cell survival is reduced because of an immune reaction triggered by immunoglobulins or complement on the red cell surface. The red cell surface is damaged as a result of the binding of the Fc portion of the red cell antibody to a macrophage Fc receptor in the spleen. The red cell is thus rendered vulnerable to 'culling' within the red cell pulp.

Clinical features

Autoimmune haemolytic anaemias are more common after the age of 50 years and in women. The spleen is enlarged in 50 per cent and pigment gallstones are present in 20 per cent of cases.

Investigations

Anaemia is invariably present and may be associated with spherocytosis because of red cell membrane damage. The Coombs' test is usually, but not invariably, positive.

Treatment

Usually the disease has an acute, self-limiting course, and no treatment is necessary. Splenectomy should, however, be considered if:

- corticosteroids are ineffective;
- the patient is developing complications from long-term steroid treatment;
- corticosteroids are contraindicated, for example because of a history of peptic ulcer.

Eighty per cent of patients respond to splenectomy.

Thalassaemia (syn. Cooley's anaemia; Mediterranean anaemia)

Thalassaemia is the result of a defect in haemoglobin peptide chain synthesis which is transmitted as a dominant trait. The disease is really a group of related diseases α, β and γ, depending on the haemoglobin peptide chain whose rate of synthesis is reduced. Most patients suffer from β-thalassaemia in which a reduction in the rate of β-chain synthesis results in a decrease in haemoglobin A. In addition to a decrease in haemoglobin, intracellular precipitates (Heinz bodies) contribute to premature red cell destruction. The disease is no longer thought to be confined to those living around the Mediterranean.

Robin Royston Amos Coombs, b. 1921. Quick Professor of Biology, Cambridge, England.

Thomas Benton Cooley, 1871–1945. Professor of Paediatrics, Wayne University, Detroit, USA.

Robert Heinz, 1865–1924. German pathologist.

Clinical features

Graduations of the disease range from heterozygous thalassaemia minor to homozygous thalassaemia major which is associated with chronic anaemia, jaundice and splenomegaly. Patients with homozygous thalassaemia major frequently develop clinical signs within the first year of life: retarded growth, enlarged head with slanting eyes and depressed nose, leg ulcers, jaundice and abdominal distension (due to splenomegaly).

Investigations

Red cells are small, thin and misshapen, and have a characteristic resistance to osmotic lysis. In the more severe forms nucleated red cells and other immature blood cells are seen. The final diagnosis is by haemoglobin electrophoresis.

Treatment

Blood transfusion may be necessary to correct profound anaemia. Splenectomy is occasionally of benefit in patients who require frequent blood transfusion – particularly if they have developed haemolytic antibodies from repeated transfusion – and where the bulky spleen is uncomfortable or painful.

Sickle cell disease

Sickle cell disease is a hereditary haemolytic anaemia, occurring mainly among those of African origin, in which the normal haemoglobin A is replaced by haemoglobin S (HbS). The HbS molecule crystallises when the blood oxygen tension is reduced and this distorts and elongates the red cell. This increases blood viscosity and obstructs flow of blood through both the 'open' and 'closed' circulations in the spleen, and through other blood vessels. Splenic micro-infarcts, splenomegaly and, later, autosplenectomy develop. This is associated with reduced antibody production and a reduced ability to filter bacteria – especially *Streptococcus pneumoniae* – in the spleen.

Clinical features

The sickle cell trait can be detected in 9 per cent of those of African origin but most are asymptomatic; sickle cell disease occurs in about 1 per cent of Africans. Depending on the vessels affected by the vascular occlusion, patients may have bone or joint pain, priapism, neurological abnormalities, skin ulcers or abdominal pain due to visceral blood stasis.

Investigations

Characteristic sickle-shaped cells can be seen in a blood film, but this has been replaced by haemoglobin electrophoresis.

Treatment

Hypoxia, which provokes a sickling crisis, should be avoided, and particular care taken in patients with sickle cell anaemia undergoing general anaesthesia. Adequate hydration and partial exchange transfusion may help in a crisis. Splenectomy is of benefit in a few patients where excessive splenic sequestration of red cells aggravates the anaemia. This hypersplenism may be chronic, which usually occurs in late childhood or adolescence, or acute, which occurs in the first 5 years of life and may be precipitated by *Streptococcus pneumoniae* infection. Acute attacks of hypersplenism can usually be treated with packed red cell transfusion, but occasionally splenectomy is of benefit.

Hypersplenism

This is an indefinite term which includes splenic enlargement, any combination of anaemia, leucopenia or thrombocytopenia, compensatory bone marrow hyperplasia and improvement after splenectomy. The vagueness of the definition implies careful clinical judgement between surgeon and haematologist to determine when long- and short-term risks of splenectomy are less than those of continued conservative management.

Splenomegaly

Schistosomiasis

This is prevalent in Africa (particularly around the Nile delta), Asia and South America. It is caused by infection with *Schistosoma mansoni* in nearly 75 per cent of cases and by *Schistosoma haematobium* in the remainder. Splenic enlargement is produced by hyperplasia which is induced by phagocytosis of disintegrated worms, ova and toxins, and by portal hypertension which is the result of hepatic fibrosis.

Clinical features

Splenomegaly arising from schistosomiasis can occur at any age and is more prevalent in males. The degree of splenic enlargement reflects the extent of hepatic fibrosis and may be massive.

Investigations

The urine and faeces are examined for ova. Liver function tests reveal a varying degree of hepatic impairment. A hypochromic anaemia is always present.

Sir Patrick Manson, 1844–1922. Practised in Formosa and Hong Kong. Later physician, Dreadnought Hospital, Greenwich, London, England. He is regarded as the 'Father of Tropical Medicine'.

Treatment

Successful medical treatment of established cases does not result in regression of the splenomegaly. Removal of the painful and bulky spleen is indicated where there is no evidence of hepatic or renal insufficiency. If ascites is present, a portosystemic shunt should be combined with splenectomy.

Tropical splenomegaly

Massive enlargement of the spleen occurs frequently in the tropics, for example in malaria (especially in children), kala-azar and schistosomiasis (see above). In parts of Africa and New Guinea splenomegaly cannot be fully attributed to these diseases because tropical splenomegaly is restricted to only a few adults in areas where malaria is endemic. The most likely explanation is an abnormal immune response to malaria or unusual species of plasmodia. Malnutrition may also be a factor and there is a high incidence in lactating women.

The spleen is grossly enlarged (2000–4000 g). This is associated with anaemia due to shortened red cell life and thrombocytopenia due to splenic sequestration of platelets, which respond to splenectomy. Splenectomy is indicated for those disabled by anaemia or by the weight of an enormous spleen. Splenectomy reduces immunity to malaria and therefore antimalarial chemotherapy (e.g. proguanil) should follow splenectomy in malaria endemic areas and be maintained for life.

Hypersplenism due to portal hypertension

Splenomegaly invariably accompanies portal hypertension. This splenic enlargement results in thrombocytopenia (due to splenic sequestration of platelets) and granulocytopenia. These are permanently relieved when splenectomy accompanies operation for the relief of portal hypertension. Shunt surgery alone does not have the same effect.

Felty's syndrome

A moderate number of patients with chronic rheumatoid arthritis develops mild leucopenia; in a few of these, neutropenia becomes extreme and is usually associated with enlargement of the spleen; this combination is referred to as 'Felty's syndrome'. A remarkable characteristic of this syndrome is that the leucopenia and splenic enlargement are apparently unrelated to the severity of the arthritic changes; indeed, in some instances the arthritis has begun to improve or has become quiescent by the time the low white cell count and the splenomegaly become unmistakable. In those cases in which the arthritis is slight but the splenic enlargement and blood changes are much in evidence, a diagnosis of primary splenic neutropenia is sometimes made. The results of splenectomy are variable. Usually there is an improvement in the blood picture with increased neutrophils, but this

Augustus Roi Felty, 1895–1964. Physician, Hartford Hospital, Hartford, Connecticut, USA.

improvement is not maintained. However, the liability to infections seems to be decreased in many cases and rheumatoid arthritis that has become resistant to steroid therapy may, once again, react favourably to the administration of steroids.

Tuberculosis

Tuberculosis of the spleen is not so uncommon as is sometimes believed. It occurs chiefly in adults between 20 and 40 years of age. When a patient has splenomegaly with asthenia, loss of weight and an evening fever, it is well to bear in mind the possibility that the enlargement of the spleen may be due to tuberculosis. Too often the signs lead to erroneous diagnosis of leukaemia or some other disorder for which splenectomy is not indicated. Occasionally tuberculosis of the spleen produces portal hypertension. Another form is cold abscess, which is very rare. Splenic puncture followed by culture or guinea-pig inoculation will yield positive results. A therapeutic test with antituberculous drugs (Chapter 8) brings about some improvement, and there is less danger of dissemination of the tubercle bacilli if splenectomy is undertaken. The operation, which is usually rendered difficult because of adhesions, is contraindicated only if other active tuberculous lesions are found to be present. Otherwise, the results of splenectomy in the treatment of tuberculosis of the spleen are excellent.

Neoplasms

The most common benign tumour of the spleen is the haemangioma which may, on occasion, develop into a haemangiosarcoma. Splenectomy may be necessary. The commonest cause of neoplastic enlargement of the spleen is lymphoma. Splenectomy may play a part in the management of these conditions (Chapter 17), but the role is now limited.

Porphyria

Porphyria is a hereditary error of catabolism of haemoglobin in which porphyrinuria occurs. The abdominal crises, which are characterised by violent intestinal colic with constipation, are liable to be precipitated by the administration of barbiturates, for which these patients have an idiosyncrasy. The patient is anaemic, frequently suffers from photosensitivity and, in advanced stages of the disease, neurological or mental symptoms (from damage to the brain) are commonly present. On examination, the spleen will be found to be enlarged. On a number of occasions the splenic enlargement, which is usually well marked, has been overlooked and the abdomen has been opened on the presumptive diagnosis of intestinal or appendicular colic, with negative findings. Another manifestation of acute porphyria is spasmodic abdominal pain followed by jaundice.

Two methods of establishing the diagnosis are available.

- The urine is sometimes normal in colour – usually it is orange (often dismissed as 'concentrated'). If a urine specimen is left exposed to daylight for a few hours it develops a port wine colour, particularly near the surface where it is exposed to the air. There are several conclusive laboratory tests for porphyrinuria.
- Radiography of the abdomen – serial radiographs show areas of intestinal spasm causing short segments of gaseous dilatation of the small and large intestine, and especially of the caecum.

Treatment

Often there is a striking decrease in the serum sodium level and the patient is improved considerably by the infusion of isotonic saline solution with careful control of electrolyte balance. Methadone is the best drug to relieve the abdominal pain. If a sedative is required, one of the phenothiazines (e.g. chlorpromazine) should be given. Splenectomy is not of value except in the uncommon erythropoeitic type with splenomegaly.

Gaucher's disease

As mentioned, the spleen may take an active part in the storage of abnormal lipoids, as does the remainder of the reticuloendothelial system. In the case of Gaucher's disease the lipoid in question is glucocerebroside. Gaucher's disease, which is rare, is characterised by enormous enlargement of the spleen, which may weigh 8 or 9 lbs (3.6–4.1 kg). In most cases the splenic enlargement begins in early childhood, often before the age of 12 years, although the patient rarely seeks advice before adult life. Until the splenic enlargement becomes massive the symptoms are few. There is anaemia, a yellowish-brown discoloration of the skin of the hands and face, and a curious conjunctival thickening (pinguecula) that helps to clinch the clinical diagnosis. Slavonic and Jewish races appear to be more prone to the disease than other races. The diagnosis is confirmed by finding Gaucher's cells in the bone marrow.

Treatment

Splenectomy rids the patient of a large abdominal swelling, but the operation is difficult because of perisplenitis and friability of the splenic pulp. It does not greatly influence the course of the disease, but because it reduces the hypersplenism (anaemia, leucopenia and thrombocytopenia) and makes the patient more comfortable, the procedure may be indicated.

Leukaemia

Leukaemia is one of the conditions to be considered in the differential diagnosis of splenomegaly. The diagnosis can be made by examination of a blood or marrow film. The main treatment is chemotherapy or radiotherapy; occasionally

Philippe Charles Ernest Gaucher, 1854–1918. Physician, Hospital St Louis, Paris, France.

marrow transplantation may be necessary. Splenectomy during the chronic phase of chronic granulocytic leukaemia will not reduce the incidence of blastic transformation or improve survival. The procedure should be reserved for hypersplenism occurring during the chronic phase, or for when bone marrow transplantation might be necessary. In rare instances the removal of a symptomatic enlarged spleen during the blastic phase produces relief, but the period of relief is brief and the operation hazardous.

Splenectomy is occasionally indicated for palliation of a painful bulky spleen in chronic lymphocytic leukaemia, but only after consultation with an experienced haematologist.

Abscess of the spleen

If a splenic embolus is infected, and the primary condition does not prove fatal, a splenic abscess may be expected to follow. Other sources of metastatic abscess of the spleen are typhoid and paratyphoid fever, osteomyelitis, otitis media and puerperal sepsis. An abscess in the right upper pole of the spleen may rupture and form a left subdiaphragmatic abscess. If the abscess is in the lower pole, rupture results in diffuse peritonitis.

Treatment

As a rule, owing to dense adhesions, drainage of the abscess is the only course. Very rarely, splenectomy may be possible with the abscess *in situ*. The drainage may be performed percutaneously, under ultrasonic or CT guidance, so avoiding the need for operative intervention.

Splenectomy

The usual indications for splenectomy are:

- trauma – either following an accident or during a surgical operation, for example when mobilising the splenic flexure of the colon;
- removal *en bloc* with the stomach as part of a radical gastrectomy;
- removal as part of a staging laparotomy undertaken before treatment of a Hodgkin's lymphoma, a very rare indication with the advent of improved staging by imaging;
- to reduce anaemia or thrombocytopenia in spherocytosis, ITP or hypersplenism;
- in association with shunt or variceal surgery for portal hypertension.

Other indications for splenectomy are given in Table 53.1.

Technique of splenectomy

Most surgeons use a left paramedian or transverse left subcostal incision. For a large spleen adherent to the diaphragm a thoracoabdominal incision may be necessary. Before operation, the passage of a nasogastric tube enables the stomach to be emptied. This eases the identification of the abdominal oesophagus and decompresses the stomach during the procedure; however, it should be removed at the end of the operation.

If the operation is for traumatic rupture, a quick mobilisation is necessary. The hand is passed round the outer surface of the spleen, the posterior layer of the lienorenal ligament divided largely by blunt dissection and the spleen rotated medially into the incision. A large pack is inserted behind the spleen and the short gastric vessels, and those in the pedicle are ligated and divided. It is important to separate the tail of the pancreas from the vessels in the hilum before ligation (see below, and the subsection on 'Rupture of a malarial spleen' above).

For other conditions requiring splenectomy, the first step is to open the gastrosplenic ligament and divide the short gastric vessels (Fig. 53.5). The splenic vessels at the superior border of the pancreas are underrun with Vicryl and ligated. The posterior surface of the spleen is exposed, the posterior leaf of the lienorenal ligament divided by long curved scissors and the spleen rotated medially, together with the tail and body of the pancreas. The pancreas is separated from the hilum and the vessels are dissected out, ligated and divided. A careful search must be made for accessory spleens. The wound should not be drained, as haemostasis must be perfect before closure of the abdomen.

Postoperative complications

- Haemorrhage, if a ligature slips off the splenic artery.
- Gastric dilatation following partial mobilisation of the stomach when ligating the short gastric vessels.
- Haemetemesis may rarely occur – possibly due to mucosal damage to the stomach when ligating the short gastric vessels.
- Left basal atelectasis, sometimes with pleural effusion, is common. This may be due to damage or to irritation of the left hemidiaphragm or a subphrenic abscess, and may be accompanied by persistent hiccough.
- Damage to the tail of the pancreas during mobilisation of the splenic pedicle. This may produce a localised abscess or, if the area has been well drained, a pancreatic fistula. This may be associated with a left pleural effusion, a peritoneal effusion or abdominal wall dehiscence.
- Splenectomy is frequently followed by a rise in the white cell and platelet count a few days after operation. There may be a risk of thrombosis if the platelet count rises above 1000×10^9/litre and it is essential to anticoagulate prophylactically the patient should this level be attained.
- Gastric fistula due to damage of the greater curvature of the stomach when ligating the short gastric vessels.
- Postsplenectomy septicaemia. The spleen phagocytoses bacteria, particularly encapsulated bacteria. Splenectomised patients show reduced antibody production when challenged with particulate antigens, are deficient in tuftsin, and may have reduced IgM and properdin levels (see the subsection on 'Functions of the spleen' at the start of this chapter). Splenectomised patients are at increased risk of septicaemia due to *Streptococcus pneumoniae*, *Neisseria meningitidis*, *Haemophilus influenzae* and *Babesia microti*. The risk becomes ever greater in splenectomised patients treated with cytotoxic chemotherapy or radiation, and in patients who have undergone splenectomy for thalassaemia, sickle cell disease, and autoimmune anaemia or thrombocytopenia.

Opportunist postsplenectomy infection (OPSI) is now of major concern. Pneumococcal antitoxin (Pneumovax) should be given 2 weeks preoperatively. It is important to advise the patient of the dangers of OPSI and to prescribe antibiotics with all infections. As previously mentioned, splenectomised patients living in malaria endemic areas should receive antimalaria prophylaxis.

Thomas Hodgkin, b. 1798. English physician.

Table 53.2 Dosing regimens for antibiotic prophylaxis and treatment

Antibiotic	*Oral prophylaxis*	*Treatment for suspected infection**
Penicillin		
Adult	250–500 mg 12-hourly[†,‡]	1.2 g 4–6 hourly[§]
Child aged 5–14 years	250 mg 12-hourly[‡]	200–300 mg/kg per day in six divided doses (maximum 6 g)[§]
Child under 5 years[¶]	125 mg 12-hourly[‡]	200–300 mg/kg per day in six divided doses (maximum 6 g)[§]
Erythromycin (base)		
Adult and child over 8 years	250–500 mg daily	0.5–1.0 g 6-hourly by mouth or intravenously
Child aged 2–8 years	250 mg daily	250 mg 6-hourly by mouth *or* 12.5 mg/kg/day intravenously by infusion in four divided doses
Child under 2 years	125 mg daily	12.5 mg/kg/day orally or intravenously by infusion in four divided doses
Amoxycillin–coamoxiclav (doses according to amoxycillin content)		
Adult	250–500 mg daily	0.5–1.0 g 8-hourly by mouth or intravenously
Child aged 5–14 years	125 mg daily	250 mg 8-hourly by mouth *or* 90 mg/kg/day intravenously in three divided doses
Child aged 1–5 years	10 mg/kg/day	125 mg 8-hourly by mouth *or* 90 mg/kg/day intravenously in three divided doses
Child aged under 1 year	10 mg/kg/day	62.5 mg 8-hourly by mouth *or* 90 mg/kg/day intravenously in three divided doses
Cefotaxime		
Adult	Not suitable	2 g 8-hourly intravenously
Child under 14 years	Not suitable	100 mg/kg/day intravenously in three divided doses (maximum 12 g)
Ceftriaxone		
Adult	Not suitable	1–2 g once daily intravenously
Child under 14 years	Not suitable	80 mg/kg/day intraveously in a single dose (maximum 4 g)
Chloramphenicol (only patients allergic to penicillins and cephalosporins)		
All patients	Not suitable	Expert advice required

*Established infection may require much higher doses given in hosptial.
[†]If compliance is a problem 500 mg once daily is acceptable.
[‡]Phenoxymethyl penicillin.
[§]Benzylpenicillin (intravenous).
[¶]Seek expert advice for neonatal doses.

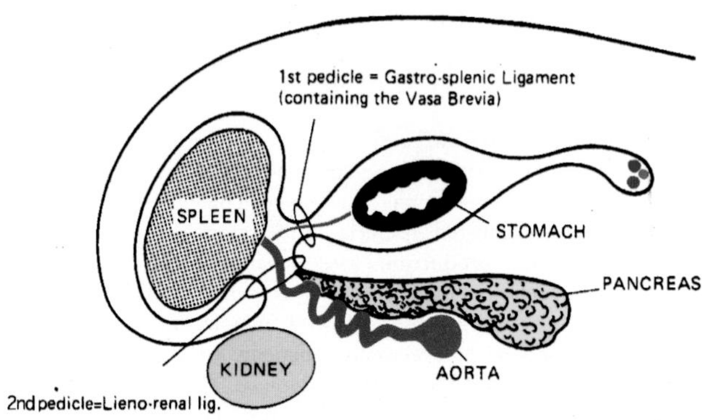

Fig. 53.5 From the surgical standpoint, the spleen may be said to have two pedicles; the gastrosplenic ligament and the lienorenal ligament. The splenic artery and vein lie in the latter (*courtesy of Professor T.G. Allen-Mersh, Westminster and Charing Cross Hospitals, London, England*).

Because of concern over correct management of patients following splenectomy, guidelines have been produced by a working party of the British Committee for Standards in Haematology. They are set out in Table 53.2. It should be noted where the recommendation is based on published evidence and that of expert opinion. The authors note that there are no randomised controlled trials or case-controlled studies on this issue, which is why the level of evidence is poor and emphasises the difficulty in making recommendations in a subject where the incidence of opportunist infection is not known.

Further reading

Weatherall, D.J., Ledingham, J.G.C. and Warrell, D.A. (eds) (1996) *Oxford Textbook of Medicine*, 3rd edn, Oxford University Press, Oxford, pp. 3587–96.

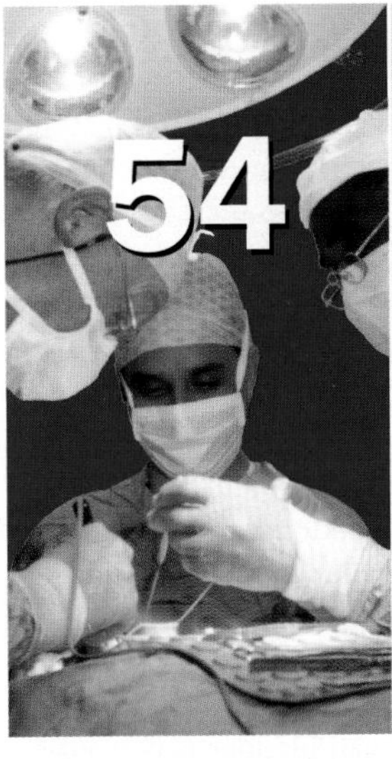

54 The gall bladder and bile ducts

Surgical anatomy and physiology

The gall bladder is pear-shaped, 7.5–12 cm long, with a normal capacity of about 50 ml, but capable of considerable distension in certain pathological conditions. The anatomical divisions are a fundus, a body and a neck that terminates in a narrow infundibulum. The muscle fibres in the wall of the gall bladder are arranged in a criss-cross manner, being particularly well developed in its neck. The mucous membrane contains indentations of the mucosa that sink into the muscle coat; these are the crypts of Luschka.

The *cystic duct* is about 3 cm in length but variable. Its lumen is usually 1–3 mm in diameter. The mucosa of the cystic duct is arranged in spiral folds known as the valves of Heister. Its wall is surrounded by a sphincteric structure called the sphincter of Lutkins. While the cystic duct joins the common hepatic duct in its supraduodenal segment in 80 per cent of cases, it may extend down into the retroduodenal or even retropancreatic part of the bile duct before joining. Occasionally the cystic duct may join the right hepatic duct or even a right hepatic sectorial duct.

The *common hepatic duct* is usually less than 2.5 cm long and is formed by the union of the right and left hepatic ducts.

Hubert Luschka, 1820–75. Professor of Anatomy, Tübingen, Germany.
Lorenz Heister, 1683–1758. Professor of Surgery and Botany, Helmstädt, Germany.

Bailey & Love's Short Practice of Surgery, 23rd edition. Edited by R.C.G. Russell, N.S. Williams and C.J.K. Bulstrode. Published in 2000 by Arnold Publishers.

The *common bile duct* is about 7.5 cm long and formed by the junction of the cystic and common hepatic ducts. It is divided into four parts:

- the *supraduodenal portion*, about 2.5 cm long, running in the free edge of the lesser omentum;
- the *retroduodenal portion*;
- the *infraduodenal portion* lies in a groove, but at times in a tunnel, on the posterior surface of the pancreas;

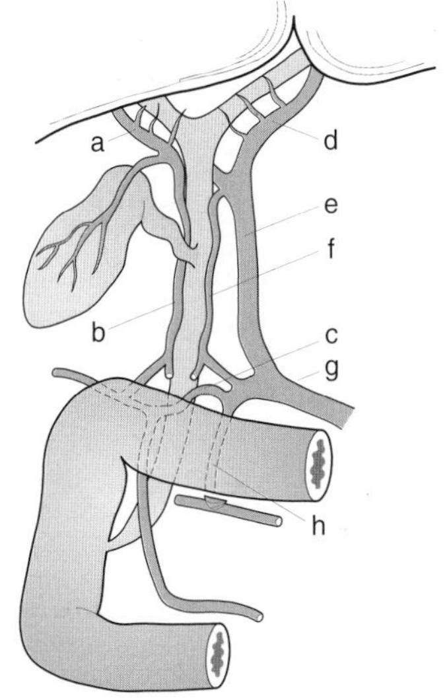

Fig. 54.1 The anatomy of the gall bladder and bile ducts. Note the arrangement of the arterial tree: (a) right hepatic artery; (b) right choledochal artery; (c) retroduodenal artery; (d) left branch of hepatic artery; (e) hepatic artery; (f) left choledochal artery; (g) common hepatic artery; (h) gastroduodenal artery.

- the *intraduodenal portion* passes obliquely through the wall of the second part of the duodenum where it is surrounded by the sphincter of Oddi. It terminates by opening on the summit of the papilla of Vater.

The *arterial supply* of the gall bladder is critical. It is proposed that arterial damage during cholecystectomy may cause ischaemia and result in postoperative bile-duct stricture. The cystic artery, a branch of the right hepatic artery, is usually given off behind the common hepatic duct (Fig. 54.1). Occasionally, an accessory cystic artery arises from the gastroduodenal artery. In 15 per cent of cases the right hepatic artery and/or the cystic artery cross in front of the common hepatic duct and the cystic duct. The most dangerous anomalies are where the hepatic artery takes a torturous course on the front of the origin of the cystic duct, or the right hepatic artery is torturous and the cystic artery short. The tortuosity is known as the 'caterpillar turn' or 'Moynihan's hump' (Fig. 54.2). This variation is the cause of many problems during a difficult cholecystectomy with inflammation in the region of the cystic duct. Inadvertent damage to the right hepatic artery is most difficult to control laparoscopically.

Lymphatics

The lymphatic vessels of the gall bladder (subserosal and submucosal) drain into the cystic lymph node of Lund (the sentinel lymph node), which lies in the fork created by the junction of the cystic and common hepatic ducts. Efferent vessels from this lymph node go to the hilum of the liver, and to the coeliac lymph nodes. The subserosal lymphatic vessels of the gall bladder also connect with the subcapsular lymph channels of the liver, and this accounts for the frequent spread of carcinoma of the gall bladder to the liver.

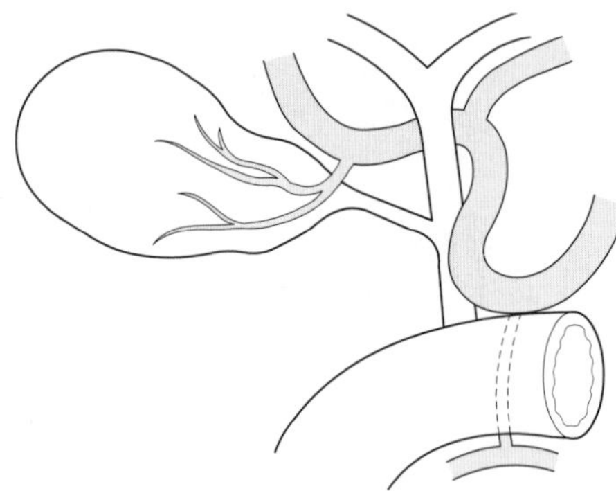

Fig. 54.2 Tortuous hepatic artery (so-called 'caterpillar turn' or 'Moynihan's hump').

Ruggero Oddi, 1845–1906. Physiologist, Perugia, Italy.

Abraham Vater, 1684–1751. Professor of Anatomy and Botany, Wittenberg, Germany.

Berkeley George Andrew Moynihan (Lord Moynihan), 1865–1936. Professor of Clinical Surgery, Leeds, England.

Fred Bates Lund, 1865–1950. Surgeon, Boston City Hospital, Boston, Massachusetts, USA.

Surgical physiology

Bile, as it leaves the liver, is composed of 97 per cent water, 1–2 per cent bile salts, and 1 per cent pigments, cholesterol and fatty acids. The liver excretes bile at a rate estimated to be approximately 40 ml/hour. The rate of bile secretion is controlled by cholecystokinin which is released from the duodenal mucosa. With feeding there is increased production of bile.

Functions of the gall bladder

The gall bladder is a reservoir for bile. During fasting resistance to flow through the sphincter is high, and bile excreted by the liver is diverted to the gall bladder. After feeding the resistance to flow through the sphincter of Oddi is reduced, the gall bladder contracts and the bile enters the duodenum. These motor responses of the biliary tract are in part effected by the hormone cholecystokinin.

The second main function of the gall bladder is concentration of bile by active absorption of water, sodium chloride and bicarbonate by the mucous membrane of the gall bladder. The hepatic bile which enters the gall bladder becomes concentrated 5–10 times, with a corresponding increase in the proportion of bile salts, bile pigments, cholesterol and calcium.

The third function of the gall bladder is the secretion of mucus – approximately 20 ml is produced per day. With total obstruction of the cystic duct in a healthy gall bladder, a mucocele develops on account of this function of the mucosa of the gall bladder.

Investigation of the biliary tract

Plain radiograph

The skilfully taken plain X-ray of the gall bladder will show radio-opaque gallstones in 10 per cent of patients (Fig. 54.3). It will also show the rare cases of calcification of the gall

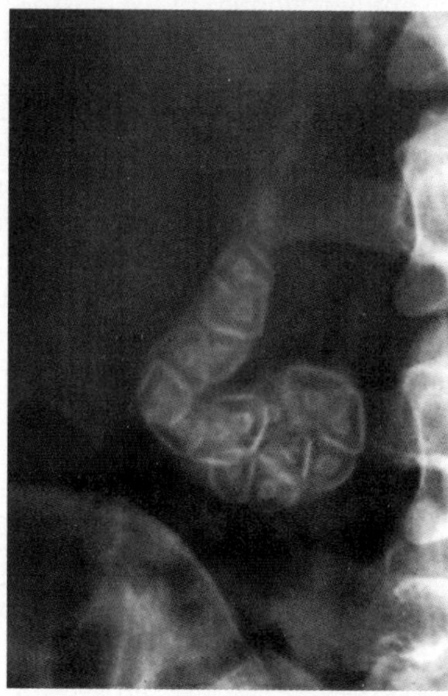

Fig. 54.3 Plain radiograph showing radio-opaque stones in the gall bladder. Radio-opaque stones are rare (10 per cent).

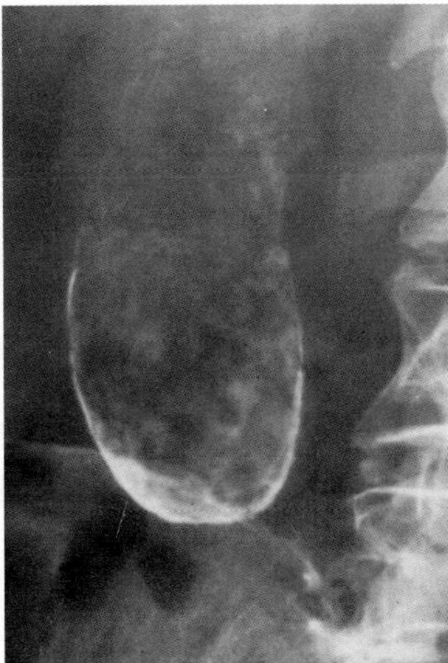

Fig. 54.4 Porcelain gall bladder.

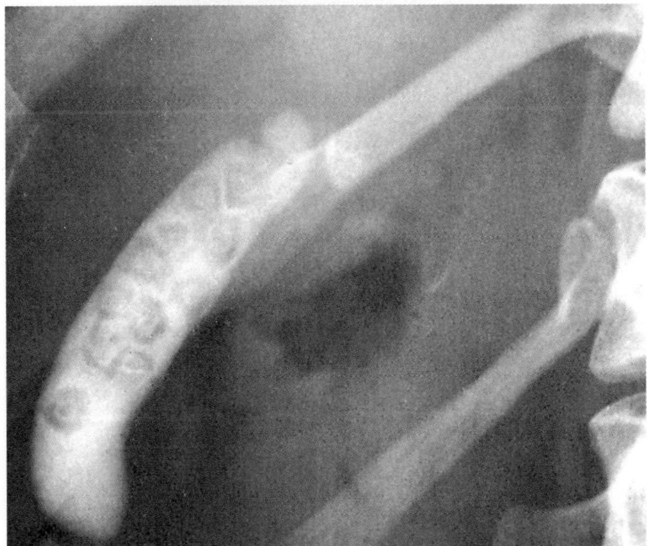

Fig. 54.5 Plain radiograph showing a gall bladder filled with limey bile. Gallstones are also present.

bladder, a so-called 'porcelain' gall bladder (Fig. 54.4). The importance of this appearance is that it is premalignant and an indication for cholecystectomy. Limey bile is a curiosity and is frequently related to multiple small stones (Fig. 54.5). This lesion is not a premalignant lesion.

Oral cholecystography (Graham–Cole test) (Figs 54.6 and 54.7)

Iopanoic acid BP is taken as tablets on the night before the examination. A control radiograph is taken before the tablets are given and a series of X-rays is taken on the following day, with further films after a fatty meal. The fatty meal stimulates gall-bladder contraction and reveals the adequacy of gall-bladder function.

This investigation has been discarded by most hospitals because of its inaccuracy except to show diverticulae and polyps, and to assess function; adequate films depend on the patient taking the tablets, and the tablets being absorbed,

Evarts Ambrose Graham, 1883–1957. Bixby Professor of Surgery, Washington University, St Louis, Missouri, USA.

Warren Henry Cole. Emeritus Professor of Surgery, University of Illinois, Chicago, Illinois, USA.

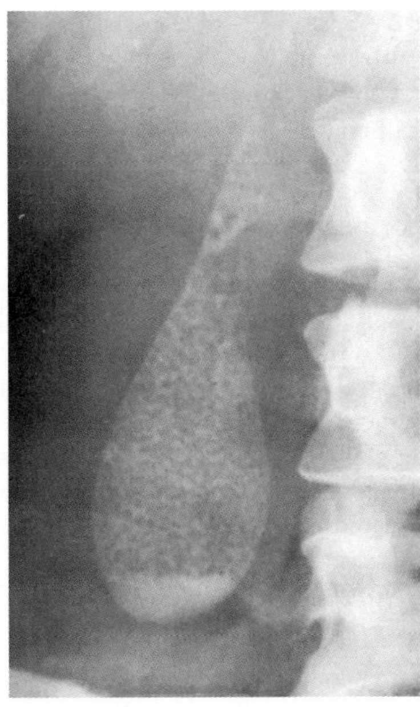

Fig. 54.6 Nonopaque stones rendered visible by oral cholecystography.

(a)

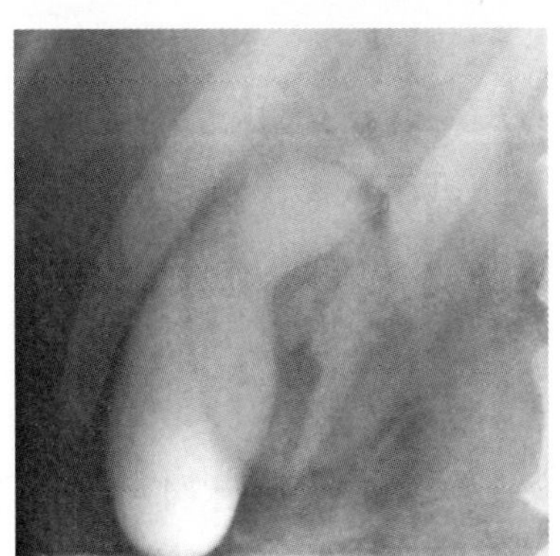

(b)

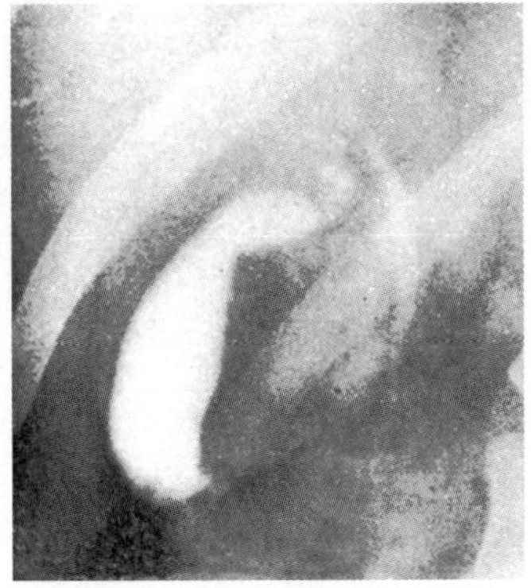

Fig. 54.7 (a) A normal cholecystogram; (b) same gall bladder after a fatty meal.

secreted by the liver and concentrated in the gall bladder after passing into the gall bladder through an unobstructed cystic duct. Thus, a cholecystogram which shows no concentration of contrast can result from many causes and is not diagnostic of gallstone disease.

Intravenous cholangiography

Intravenous cholangiography (biligram–meglumine ioglycamate) permits radiological visualisation of the bile ducts. The drug is given intravenously and is rapidly secreted by the liver into the biliary tree. Careful radiography with or without tomography can clearly define the ducts and the gall bladder delineating the presence of stone disease. The contrast agent can cause allergic reactions such that this test has been discarded in most units.

Ultrasonography

Ultrasonography (Figs 54.8–54.13) is noninvasive and is now the standard initial imaging technique for the investigation of the patient suspected of having a gallstone, and is also the prime investigation for the patient presenting with jaundice. It will demonstrate biliary calculi, the size of the gall bladder, the thickness of the gall-bladder wall, the presence of inflammation around the gall bladder, the size of the common bile duct and, occasionally, the presence of stones within the biliary tree. It may even show a carcinoma of the pancreas occluding the common bile duct.

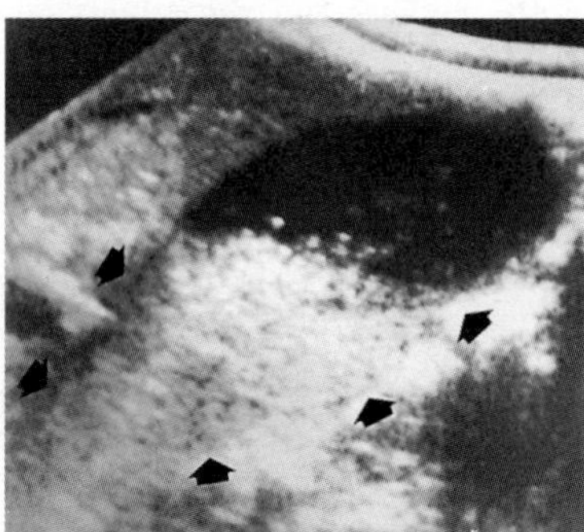

Fig. 54.8 Ultrasound examination. Multiple small gallstones filling part of the body and infundibulum of a large gall bladder (*courtesy of James McIvor, FDS, FRCR, London, England*).

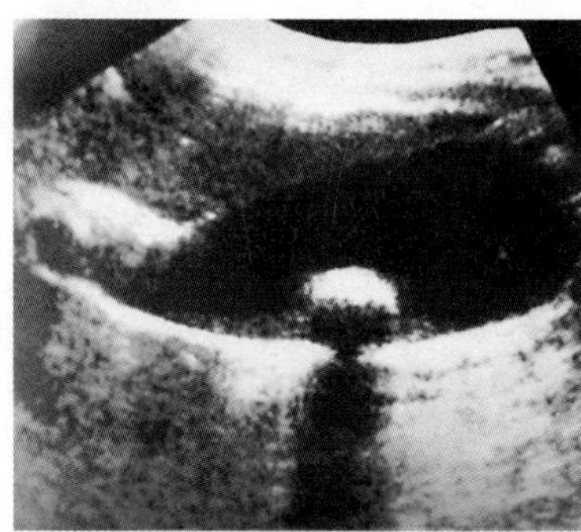

Fig. 54.9 Ultrasound examination. Single large gallstone casting an 'acoustic shadow' (*courtesy of James McIvor, FDS, FRCR, London, England*).

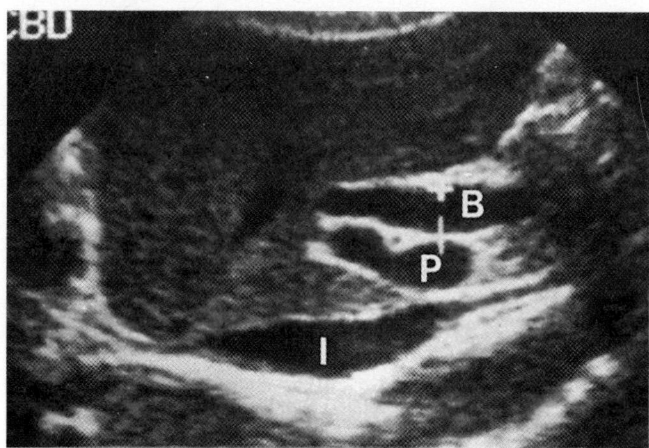

Fig. 54.10 Ultrasound examination. Longitudinal scan through the hilium of the liver showing the dilated common bile duct (B). P = portal vein; I = IVC (*courtesy of Dr J.E. Boultbee, Charing Cross Hospital, London, England*).

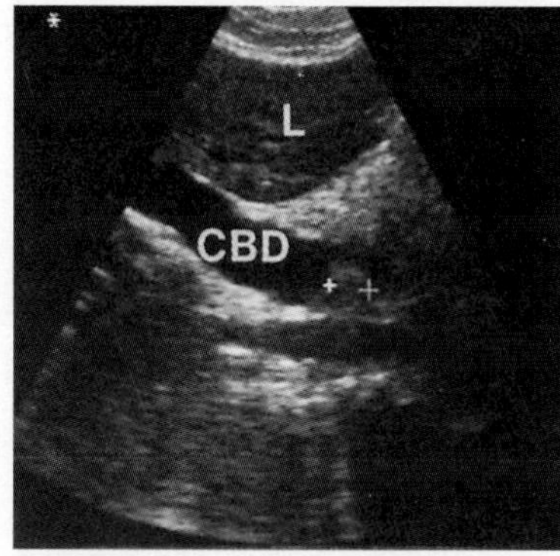

Fig. 54.11 Ultrasound examination. Longitudinal scan with obstruction of the common bile duct, which is dilated (*courtesy of Dr J.E. Boultbee, Charing Cross Hospital, London, England*).

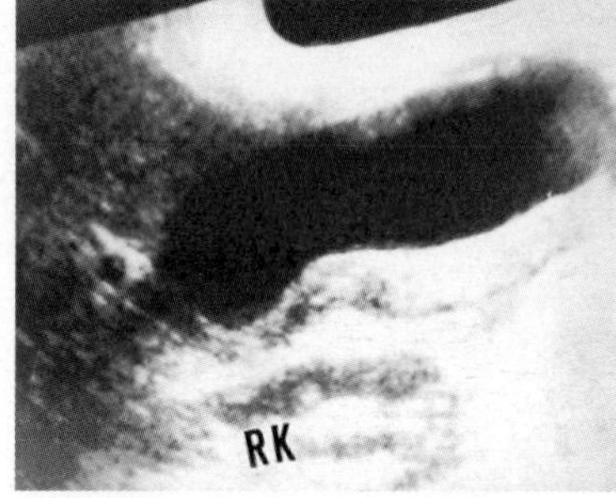

Fig. 54.12 Ultrasound examination. Mucocele of the gall bladder which is now larger than the right kidney (RK) (*courtesy of James McIvor, FDS, FRCR, London, England*).

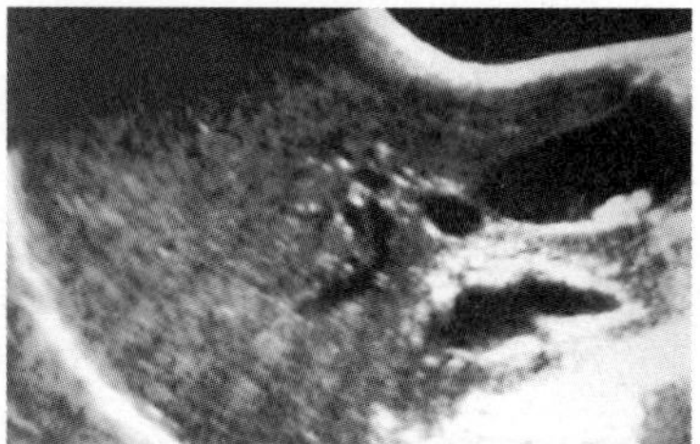

Fig. 54.13 Ultrasound examination. Dilation of the intrahepatic and common bile ducts due to a calculus impacted at the sphincter of Oddi. There are calculi visible in the gall bladder (*courtesy of James McIvor, FDS, FRCR, London, England*).

Radioisotope scanning

Technetium-99m (^{99m}Tc)-labelled derivatives of iminodiacetic acid (HIDA, PIPIDA) are excreted in the bile and are used to visualise the biliary tree. In acute cholecystitis the gall bladder is not seen. The technique is used when biliary-enteric anastomoses are functioning inadequately as it will show the extent of obstruction at the anastomosis and indicate the delay in excretion.

Computerised tomography (CT)

CT is not a useful technique in investigating the biliary tree. Its only value is in the investigation of patients who may have a cancer of the gall bladder or bile ducts, and in these patients will define its extent, the presence of lymphadenopathy and the presence of metastases.

Magnetic resonance cholangiopancreatography (MRCP)

MRCP is now becoming the standard technique for investigation of the biliary tree. Contrast is not necessary and, with appropriate computing, a clear outline of the biliary tree can be achieved with a sensitive and specific diagnosis of bile-duct stones. This technique will replace alternative diagnostic aids as the appropriate magnets with the specific software become more widely available (Fig. 54.14).

Endoscopic retrograde cholangiopancreatography (ERCP)

The ampulla of Vater can be cannulated with the aid of a fibre-optic duodenoscope. The bile ducts are visualised after injecting water-soluble contrast. Bile can be sent for cytological and microbiological examination, and brushings can be taken from strictures for cytological studies. Acute cholangitis may follow ERCP when contrast fills a dilated and obstructed duct; antibiotics are given as prophylaxis, and if obstruction is encountered relief of that obstruction by the placement of a stent must be undertaken. If drainage cannot be achieved then percutaneous transhepatic drainage should be performed. Diagnostic ERCP is now less commonly performed, but its value is its ability to remove stones and stent strictures, thus becoming a therapeutic rather than a diagnostic technique (Figs 54.15–20).

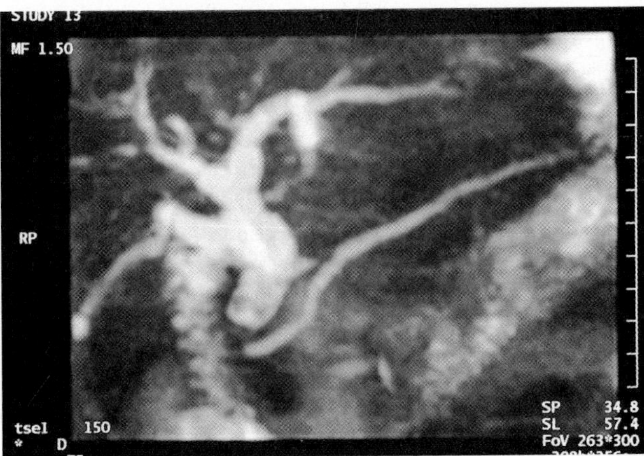

Fig. 54.14 A magnetic resonance cholangiopancreatogram (MRCP) showing stones within a dilated bile duct. The normal pancreatic duct is well visualised.

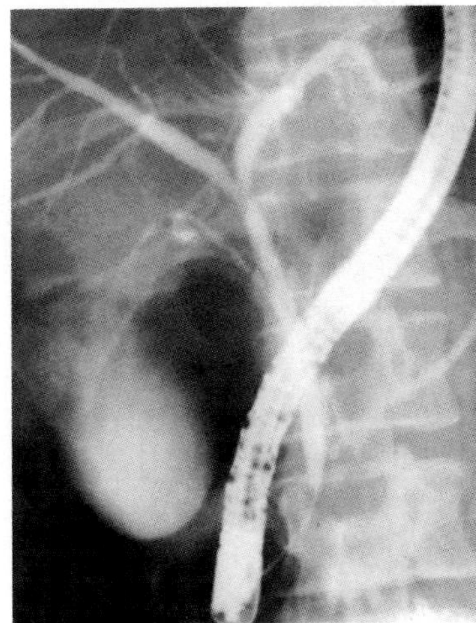

Fig. 54.15 ERC: normal cholangiogram.

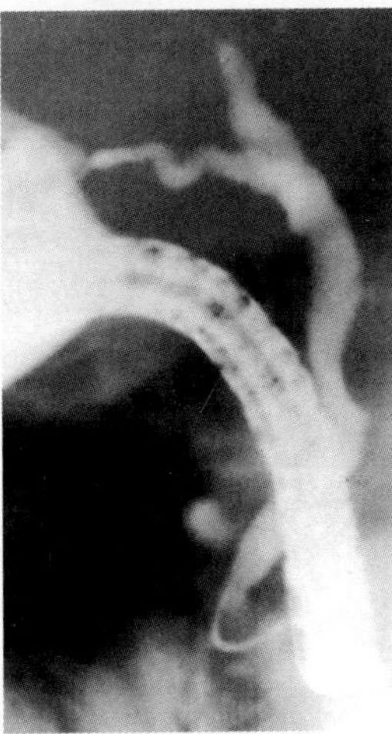

Fig. 54.16 ERC: complete occlusion of common hepatic duct due to cholangiocarcinoma.

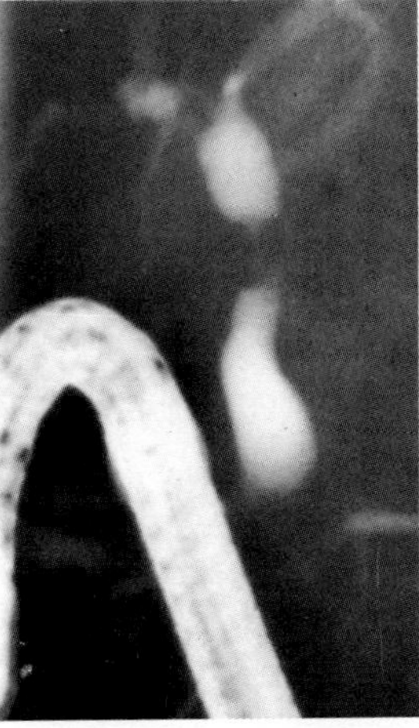

Fig. 54.17 ERC: partial occlusion of the bile duct by a malignant stricture.

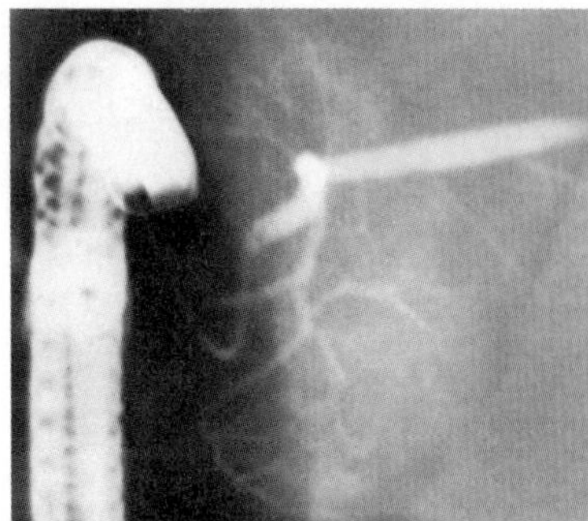

Fig. 54.18 ERC: same patient as Fig. 54.18. A complete block to the main pancreatic duct indicates a pancreatic carcinoma.

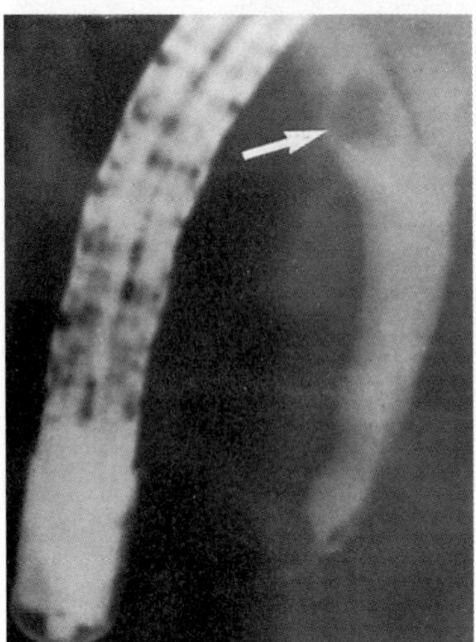

Fig. 54.19 ERC: a small solitary gallstone in the bile duct following cholecystectomy.

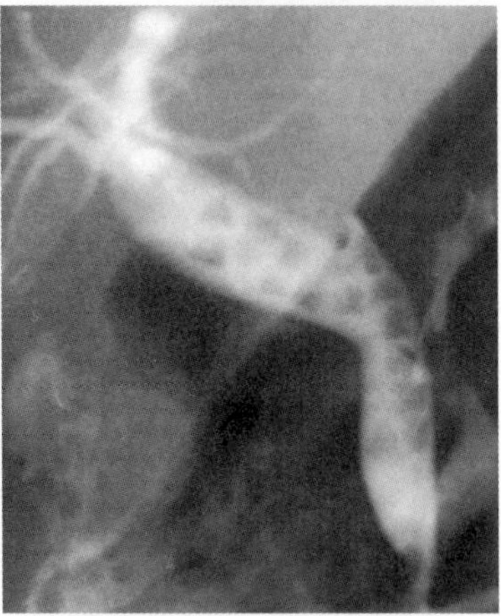

Fig. 54.20 ERC: small, multiple stones in a dilated common bile duct following cholecystectomy.

Percutaneous transhepatic cholangiography (PTC) (Figs 54.21 and 54.22)

This investigation is only undertaken once a bleeding tendency has been excluded and the patient's prothrombin time is normal. Antibiotics should be given prior to the procedure. Under fluoroscopic control, a needle (the Chiba or Okuda needle) 15 cm long and 0.7 mm in diameter is advanced into the liver through the eighth intercostal space in the mid-axillary line to a point about 2 cm short of the right margin of the vertebral column. The stilette is then removed and while injecting contrast (e.g. meglumine iothalamate 60 per cent, w/v) the needle is slowly withdrawn until contrast is seen entering a bile radical. Addition to this technique enables placement of a catheter into the bile ducts to provide external biliary drainage or the insertion of indwelling stents. The scope of this procedure can be further extended by leaving the drainage catheter *in situ* for a number of days and then dilating the track sufficiently for a fine flexible choledochoscope to be passed into the intrahepatic biliary tree in order to diagnose strictures, take biopsies and remove stones.

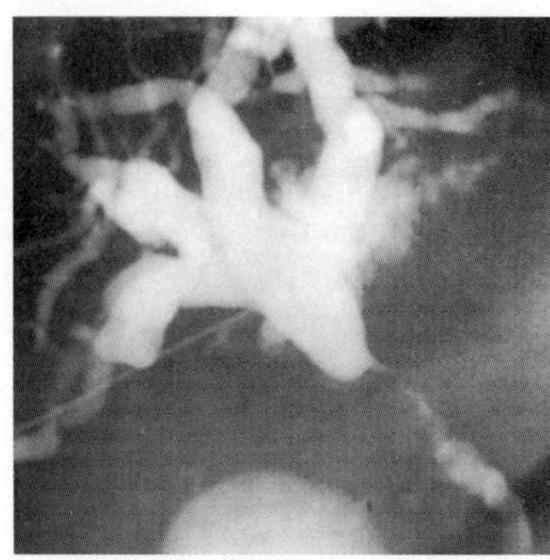

Fig. 54.21 Percutaneous transhepatic cholangiogram in the same patient as Fig. 54.16. It demonstrates the upper extent of the malignant stricture.

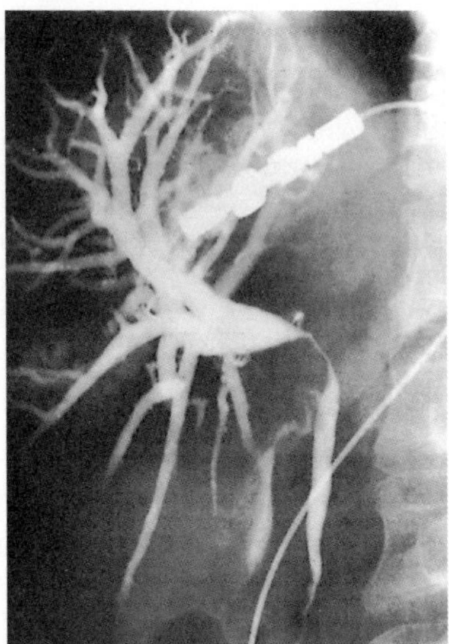

Fig. 54.22 Transhepatic cholangiogram showing a stricture of the common hepatic duct (*courtesy of Miss Phyllis George, FRCS, London, England*).

Kunio Okuda. Professor of Medicine, Chiba University, Japan.

Peroperative cholangiography

During cholecystectomy a catheter can be placed in the cystic duct and contrast injected into the biliary tree. The technique defines the anatomy and excludes the presence of stones. With improved preoperative imaging and a more careful operative approach the value of this technique is debatable. The limitation of the technique using single plates can be overcome by an X-ray image intensifier with a television monitor which enables a much more accurate diagnosis of biliary pathology (Figs 54.23–54.25).

Operative biliary endoscopy (choledochoscopy)

At operation a flexible fibre-optic endoscope can be passed down the cystic duct into the common bile duct enabling stone identification and removal under direct vision. The technique can be combined with an X-ray image intensifier to ensure complete clearance of the biliary tree. After exploration of the bile duct, a tube can be left in the cystic duct remnant or in the common bile duct (a T-tube) and drainage of the biliary tree established. After 7–10 days, a track will be established. This track can be used for the passage of a choledochoscope to remove residual stones in the awake patient in an endoscopy suite. This technique is invaluable in the management of difficult stone disease and prevents the excessive prolongation of an operative exploration of the common bile duct.

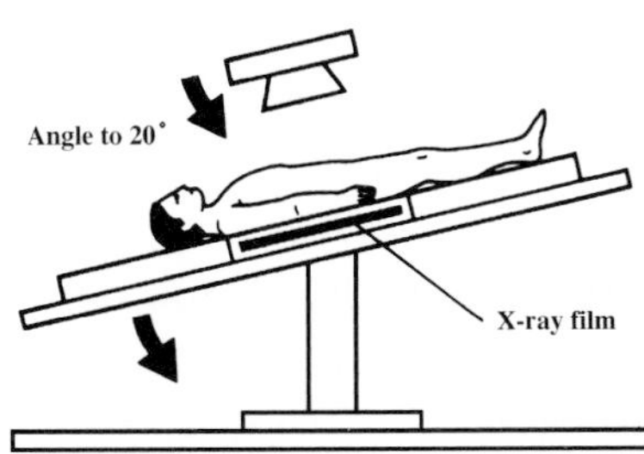

Fig. 54.23 Peroperative cholangiography using a radiolucent table-top.

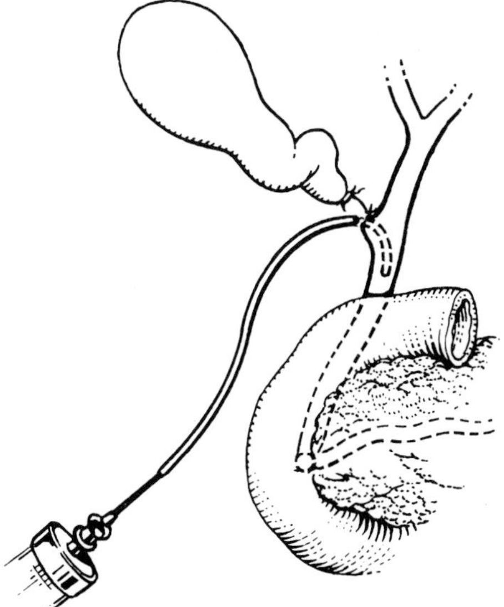

Fig. 54.24 Peroperative cholangiography. The method of introducing the medium.

(a)

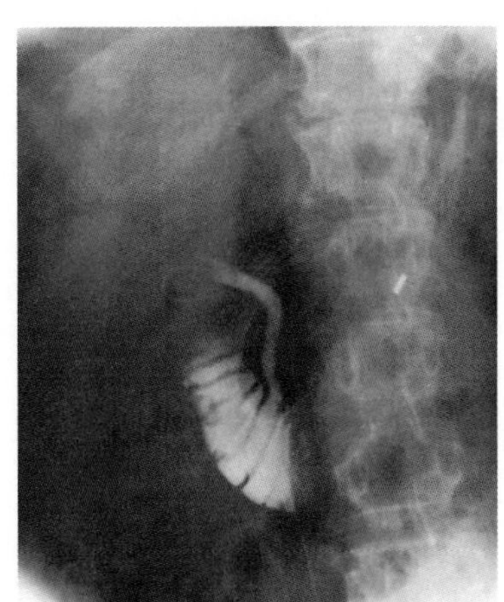

(b)

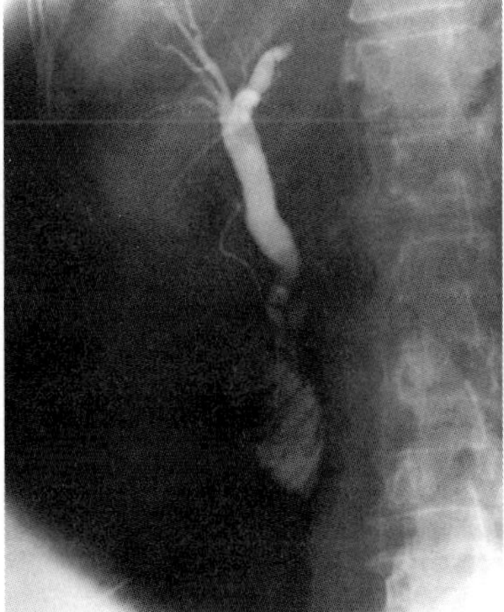

(c)

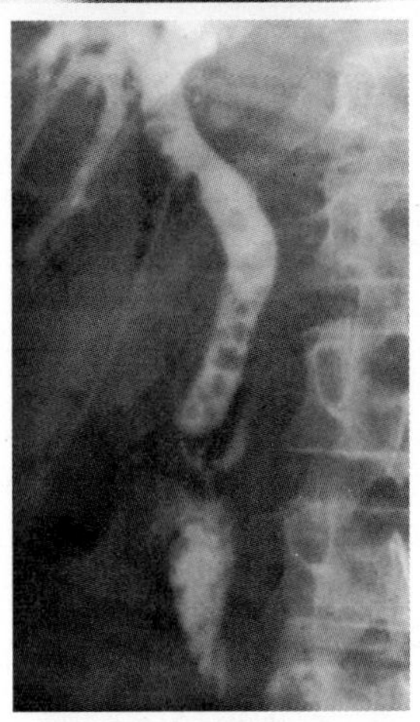

Fig. 54.25 Peroperative cholangiography. (a) Gentle infusion of contrast, passing without hindrance into the duodenum. A normal duct with no problems. (b) The duct is dilated and there is a slight hold-up of contrast. No stones and no real indication to operate on the sphincter of Oddi (see subsection on 'Transduodenal sphincterotomy'). (c) All of the ducts are dilated and contain many stones. There is narrowing of the lower end of the duct with reflux of contrast into the pancreatic duct. Sphincterotomy was performed.

Congenital abnormalities of the gall bladder and bile ducts

Embryology

The hepatic diverticulum arises from the ventral wall of the foregut and elongates into a stalk to form the choledochus. A lateral bud is given off which is destined to become the gall bladder and cystic duct. The embryonic hepatic duct sends out many branches which join up the canaliculi between the liver cells. As is usual with embryonic tubular structures, hyperplasia obliterates the lumina of this ductal system; normally recanalisation subsequently occurs and bile begins to flow. During early foetal life the gall bladder is entirely intrahepatic.

Absence of the gall bladder

Occasionally the gall bladder is absent. Failure to visualise the gall bladder is not necessarily a pathological problem.

The Phrygian cap

The Phrygian cap (Fig. 54.26) is present in 2–6 per cent of cholecystograms and may be mistaken for a pathological deformity of the organ. 'Phrygian cap' refers to hats worn by people of Phrygia, an ancient country of Asia Minor; it was rather like a liberté cap of the French Revolution.

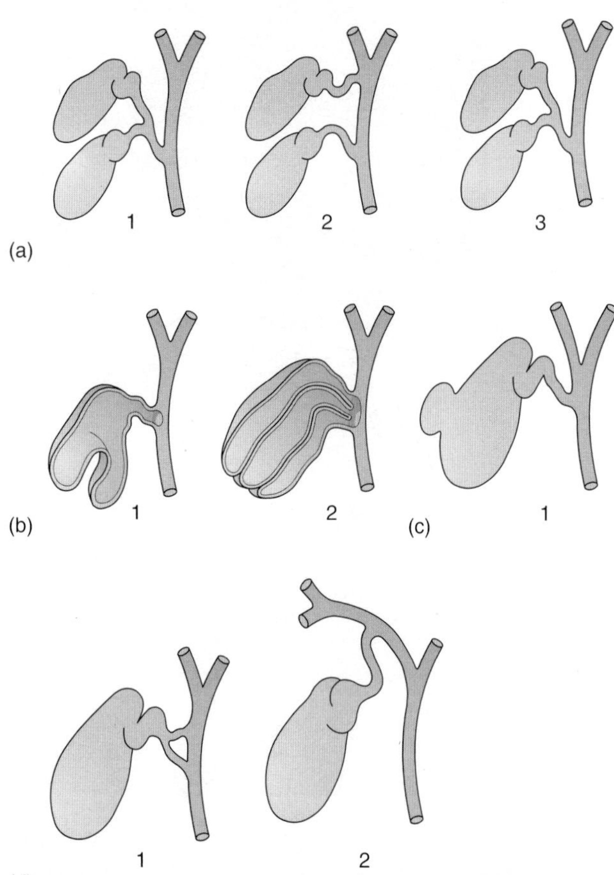

Fig. 54.26 The main variations in gall bladder and cystic duct anatomy. (a) Double gall bladder. (b) Septum of the gall bladder; 1 is the most common, the so-called 'Phrygian cap'. (c) Diverticulum of the gall bladder. (d) Variations in cystic duct insertion.

Floating gall bladder

The organ may hang on a mesentery which makes it liable to undergo torsion.

Double gall bladder

Rarely, the gall bladder is twinned. One of the twins may be intrahepatic.

Absence of the cystic duct

This is usually a pathological, as opposed to an anatomical anomaly and indicates the recent passage of a stone or the presence of a stone at the lower end of the cystic duct which is ulcerating into the common bile duct. The main danger at surgery is damage to the bile duct, and particular care to identify the correct anatomy is essential before division of any duct.

Low insertion of the cystic duct

The cystic duct opens into the common bile duct near the ampulla. All variations of this anomaly can occur. At operation they are not important. Dissection of a cystic duct which is inserted low in the bile duct should be avoided as removal will damage the blood supply to the common bile duct and can lead to stricture formation.

An accessory cholecystohepatic duct

Ducts passing directly into the gall bladder from the liver do occur and are probably not uncommon. Nevertheless, larger ducts should be closed but before doing so the precise anatomy should be carefully ascertained (Fig. 54.27).

Extrahepatic biliary atresia

Aetiology and pathology

Atresia is present in one per 14 000 live births, and affects male and females equally. The extrahepatic bile ducts are progressively destroyed by an inflammatory process which starts around the time of birth. Intrahepatic changes also occur and eventually result in biliary cirrhosis and portal hypertension. The untreated child dies before the age of 3 years of liver failure or haemorrhage.

The inflammatory destruction of the bile ducts has been classified into three main types (Fig. 54.28):

- type I – atresia restricted to the common bile duct;
- type II – atresia of the common hepatic duct;
- type III – atresia of the right and left hepatic ducts.

Associated anomalies include, in about 20 per cent of cases, cardiac lesions, polysplenia, situs inversus, absent vena cava and a preduodenal portal vein.

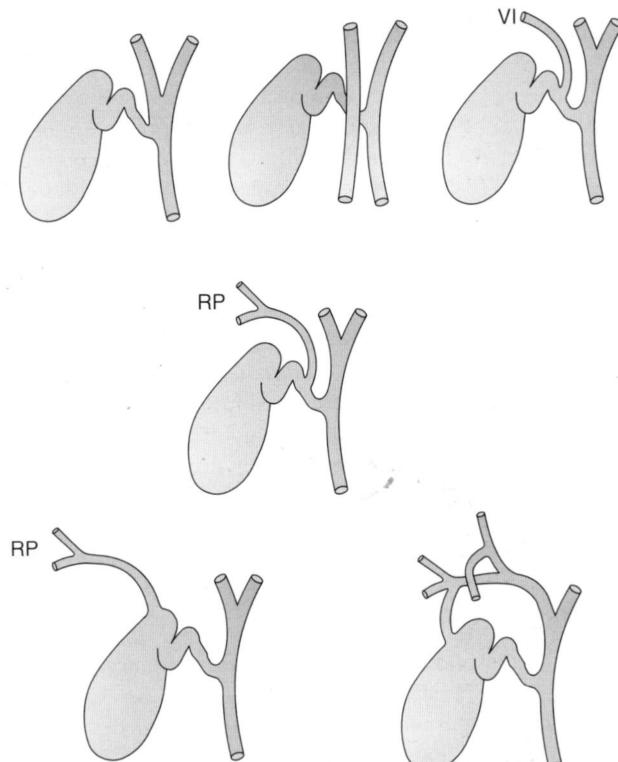

Fig. 54.27 Patterns of cystic duct anatomy – note segment VI drainage into the cystic duct and the drainage of the right posterior sectorial duct (RP) into the neck of the gall bladder.

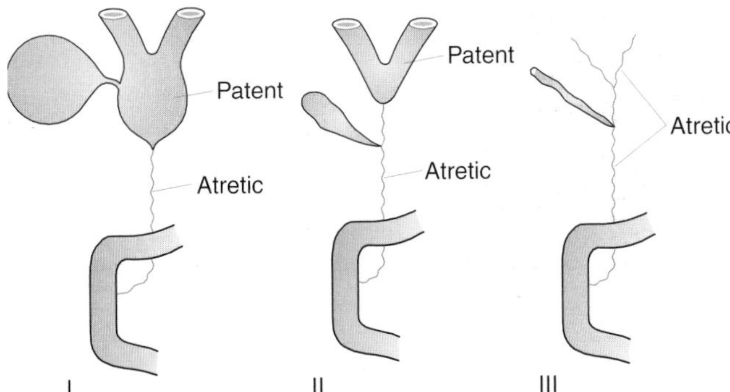

Fig. 54.28 Classification of biliary atresia. The gall bladder filling provides a clue to the type of atresia.

Clinical features

About one-third of cases are jaundiced at birth. In all, however, jaundice is present by the end of the first week and deepens progressively. The meconium may be a little bile stained but later the stools are pale and the urine is dark. Prolonged steatorrhoea gives rise to osteomalacia (biliary rickets). Pruritis is severe. Clubbing and skin xanthomas, probably related to a raised serum cholesterol, may be present.

Differential diagnosis

This includes any form of jaundice in a neonate giving a cholestatic picture. Examples are α_1-antitrypsin deficiency, cholestasis associated with intravenous feeding, choledochal cyst and inspissated bile syndrome. Neonatal hepatitis is the most difficult to differentiate. Both extrahepatic biliary atresia and neonatal hepatitis are associated with giant cell transformation of the hepatocytes. Liver biopsy and radionuclide excretion scans are essential.

Treatment

Patent segments of proximal bile duct are found in 10 per cent of type I lesions. A direct Roux-en-Y anastomosis will achieve bile flow in 75 per cent, but progressive fibrosis results in disappointing long-term results. Type II and III are treated by the Kasai procedure, in which radical excision of all bile-duct tissue up to the liver capsule is performed. A Roux-en-Y loop of jejunum is anastomosed to the exposed area of liver capsule above the bifurcation of the portal vein. The chances of achieving effective bile drainage after porto-enterostomy are maximal when the operation is performed before the age of 8 weeks, and approximately 90 per cent of children whose bilirubin falls to within the normal range can be expected to survive for 10 years or more. Early referral for surgery is critical.

Postoperative complications include bacterial cholangitis, which occurs in 40 per cent. Repeated attacks lead to hepatic fibrosis and 50 per cent of long-term survivors develop portal hypertension, with one-third having variceal bleeding. Liver transplantation may be considered in the failures.

Congenital dilatation of the intrahepatic ducts (Caroli's disease)

This rare, congenital, nonfamilial condition is characterised by multiple irregular sacular dilatations of the intrahepatic ducts separated by segments of normal or stenotic ducts. Biliary stasis leads to stone formation and cholangitis. The patients present in childhood or in early adult life. Associated conditions include congenital hepatic fibrosis, medullary sponge kidney and, rarely, cholangiocarcinoma. The mainstays of treatment are antibiotics for the cholangitis and the removal of calculi. As the condition can be limited to one lobe of the liver, lobectomy may be indicated.

Choledochal cyst

Choledochal cyst is due to a specific weakness in a part of or the whole of the wall of the common bile duct. Anomalous junctions of the biliary pancreatic junction are frequently observed and long common channels result in high levels of biliary amylase in 80 per cent of cases. Common pancreato-biliary channels may be associated with repeated attacks of pancreatitis (Fig. 54.29).

César Roux, 1857–1934. Professor of Surgery and Gynaecology, Lausanne, Switzerland.
Morio Kasai. Professor of Surgery, Tokyo University, Japan.
Jacques Caroli. Professor of Medicine, Paris, France.

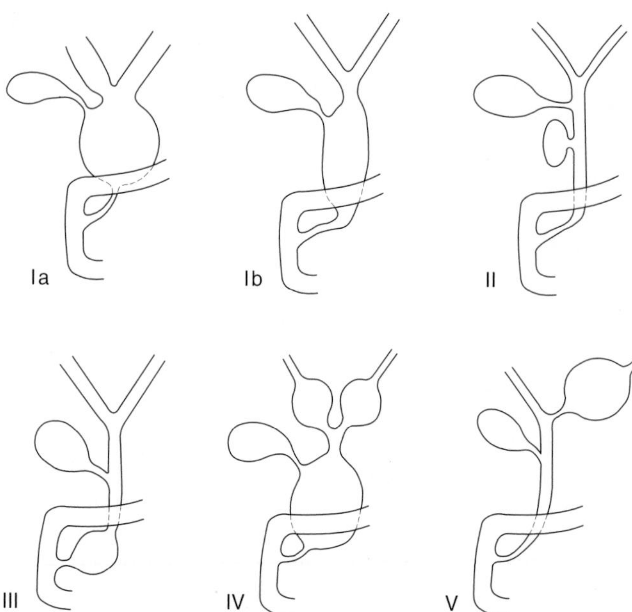

Fig. 54.29 Classification of types of choledochal cyst.

The patient may present at any age with attacks of jaundice of obstructive type, cholangitis and abdominal signs. In some patients a swelling may be detected in the upper abdomen. Ultrasonography will confirm the presence of an abnormal cyst and a magnetic resonance imaging (MRI) scan will reveal the anatomy; in particular, the relationship between the lower end of the bile duct and the pancreatic duct. It appears that the anomaly is premalignant; carcinoma of the biliary tract is a well-recognised complication and carries a poor prognosis, and therefore excision is the appropriate management.

Radical excision of the cyst is the treatment of choice with reconstruction of the biliary tract using a Roux-en-Y loop of jejunum. Other procedures have been shown to be ineffective and associated with recurrent attacks of cholangitis.

Trauma

Injuries to the gall bladder and extrahepatic biliary tree are rare. They occur as a result of a penetrating wound or a crush injury. Operative trauma is perhaps more frequent than external trauma. The physical signs are those of an acute abdomen. The treatment is cholecystectomy for gall bladder injuries and if the bile duct is damaged then drainage using a T-tube to the bile duct and a drain to the site of damage is appropriate. Many will stricture and these can be secondarily be repaired by a Roux-en-Y anastomosis.

Torsion of the gall bladder

This is very rare and relies on a long mesentery which often occurs in an older patient with a large mucocele of the gall bladder. The patient presents with extreme pain and an acute abdomen. Immediate exploration is indicated with cholecystectomy as the only treatment.

Gallstones (cholelithiasis)

Gallstones are the most common biliary pathology. Indeed, cholecystectomy is the commonest surgical procedure in the abdomen in the Western world. Gallstones are classified according to their chemical composition into cholesterol stones, mixed stones and pigment stones. Cholesterol stones consist almost entirely of cholesterol and are often solitary (cholesterol solitaire). Mixed stones account for 90 per cent of gallstones. Cholesterol is the major component. Other components include calcium bilirubinate, calcium phosphate, calcium carbonate, calcium palmitate and proteins. Usually they are multiple, and they are often faceted. Pigment stones are most common in the Far East and are composed almost entirely of calcium bilirubinate. They are mostly small and multiple. Some are hard and coral-like, whereas others are soft and really concretions of sludge rather than stones (Fig. 54.30).

Gas in gallstones

Rarely the centre of a stone may contain radiolucent gas in a triradiate or biradiate fissure and this gives rise to characteristic dark shapes on a radiograph – the 'Mercedes Benz' or 'seagull' signs.

Limey bile

'Lime-water' bile is revealed on a plain radiograph (Fig. 54.5) more clearly than if the gall bladder has been visualised by cholecystography. The opacity is the result of the gall bladder becoming filled with a mixture of calcium carbonate and calcium phosphate, usually the consistency of toothpaste. The condition tends to occur when there is a gradual obstruction of the cystic or common bile duct, for example due to chronic pancreatitis or carcinoma of the pancreas. Organisms are rarely grown from the emulsion.

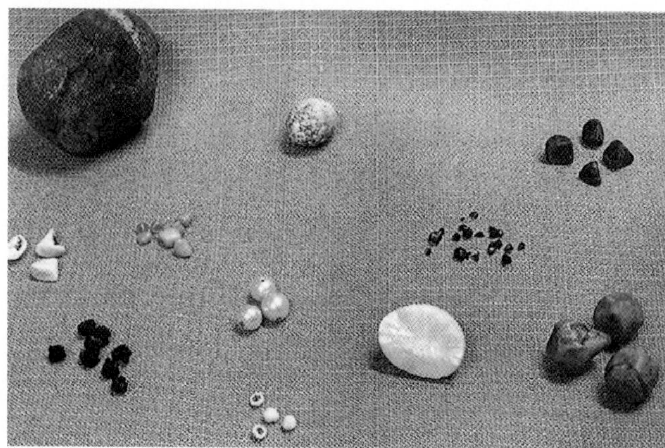

Fig. 54.30 Gallstones. Note, however, the three pearls, which are usually formed of calcium carbonate in the oyster around a parasite or a grain of sand.

Incidence of gallstones

A 'fat, fertile, flatulent, female of fifty' is the classical sufferer from symptomatic gallstones. Useful as this clinical memorandum is, it should be tempered with the knowledge that cholelithiasis occurs in both sexes from childhood to the centenarian. In men the disease tends to occur in the older age groups at which point the incidence is equal to that of women. Stones are rarer in Africa and in southern India, but not in north India.

Causal factors in gallstone formation

The aetiology of gallstones is probably multifactorial. Factors implicated are: (1) metabolic; (2) infective; and (3) bile stasis.

Cholesterol and mixed stones

Metabolic

Cholesterol, insoluble in water, is held in solution by a detergent action of bile salts and phospholipids with which it forms micelles (Fig. 54.31). Bile containing cholesterol stones has an excess of cholesterol relative to bile salts and phospholipids, thus allowing cholesterol crystals to form. Such bile is termed 'supersaturated' or 'lithogenic'. Bile cholesterol increases with age and is raised in women, particularly those taking the contraceptive pill, in obesity and by clofibrate – a drug used in the treatment of certain hyperlipoproteinaemias. The concentration of bile salts in bile is reduced by oestrogens, and also by factors which interrupt the intrahepatic circulation of bile salts (e.g. ileal disease, resection or bypass and cholestyramine therapy). These conditions are all associated with an increased incidence of stones, but there are still some people with cholesterol supersaturation who remain free of stones, suggesting that there are other factors of importance.

Infection

The role of infection in causing stones is unclear. Often bile from patients with gallstones is sterile, but organisms have been cultured from the centres of gallstones: the radiolucent centre of many gallstones may represent mucus plugs originally formed around bacteria (Moynihan's aphorism: 'A gallstone is a tombstone erected to the memory of the organism within it'). *Helicobacter pylori* antigens have been isolated within gall bladders containing stones.

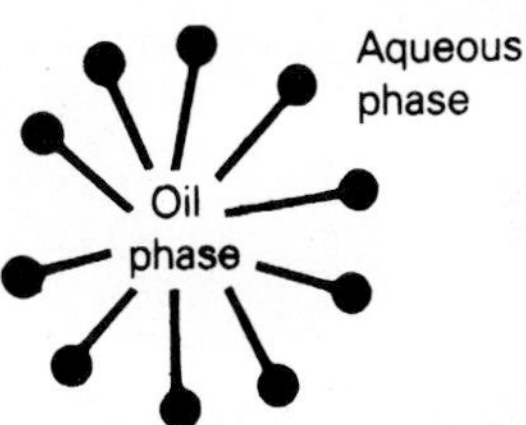

Fig. 54.31 Diagram representing a spherical micelle formed by aggregation of bile acid molecules. The rounded end of each molecule is water-loving (hydrophilic), whilst the stick end is the hydrophobic part to which the water-insoluble cholesterol is absorbed.

Bile stasis

Gall bladder contractility is reduced by oestrogens, in pregnancy and after truncal vagotomy, situations in which the incidence of gallstones is increased. Patients on long-term parenteral nutrition have a high incidence of stones. Lack of good oral intake precludes the release of cholecystokinin, the hormonal stimulant of gall-bladder contraction released from the duodenal mucosa.

Pigment stones are seen in patients with haemolysis in which bilirubin production is increased. Examples are hereditary spherocytosis, sickle cell anaemia, thalassaemia, malaria and mechanical destruction of red cells by prosthetic heart valves. Pigment stones are found in the ducts of patients with benign and malignant bile duct strictures. Pigment stones in Oriental countries are associated with infestations of the biliary tree by *Clonorchis sinensis* and *Ascaris lumbricoides*. *Escherichia coli* is often found in the bile of these patients. This bacterium produces the enzyme β-glucuronidase which converts the bilirubin into its unconjugated insoluble form. These stones are often present throughout the biliary tree including the intrahepatic ducts.

The effects and complications of gallstones

Stones are found throughout the biliary tract and their complications relate to obstruction of the cystic duct, of the intrahepatic radicals or of the ampulla of Vater. Obstructive complications may be aggravated by the presence of infection leading to cholangitis and abscess formation. Nevertheless, gallstones can be asymptomatic; it is estimated that between 85 and 90 per cent of patients who have gallstones remain asymptomatic. In the UK the prevalence of gallstones at the time of death is estimated to be 17 per cent and possibly increasing. Thus, the mere presence of gallstones is not an indication for a surgical approach. For this reason symptoms must be analysed with care. A typical patient may fulfil Saint's triad having gallstones, diverticulosis of the colon and a hiatus hernia, yet with symptoms that cannot be directly contributed to any of these. When considering management of a patient with gastrointestinal symptoms it is important to take a specific history and consider whether or not the pain from which the patient suffers is typical or not of biliary tract disease.

Effects and complications of gallstones
- *In the gall bladder*:
  - Silent stones
  - Chronic cholecystitis
  - Acute cholecystitis
  - Gangrene
  - Perforation
  - Empyema
  - Mucocele
  - Carcinoma
- *In the bile ducts*:
  - Obstructive jaundice
  - Cholangitis
  - Acute pancreatitis
- *In the intestine*:
  - Acute intestinal obstruction ('gallstone ileus')

Charles Frederick Morris Saint, 1886–1973. Emeritus Professor of Surgery, Cape Town, South Africa.

Cholecystitis

It is probably inappropriate, although classical, to subdivide chronic and acute calculous cholecystitis. They are part of the same spectrum of disease and are related to inflammation within the gall bladder secondary to obstruction of the cystic duct by stones. With stones in a gall bladder it appears that there is always some degree of inflammatory change, but there is insufficient evidence to suggest that this is a cause of symptoms. The concept of 'flatulent dyspepsia' being caused by gallstones in the absence of the classic symptoms of biliary colic is probably inappropriate. Nevertheless, some patients do complain of right hypochondrial pain of varying severity in association with nausea and occasional vomiting, and some tenderness in the right subcostal region. Flatulent dyspepsia is common in such patients yet many will not be relieved by cholecystectomy. Numerous investigations have been performed to determine whether those with symptoms of dyspepsia will benefit from cholecystectomy; all have proved ineffective and thus the surgeon must rely on clinical judgement.

Clinical features

The patient has specific episodes of right subcostal pain radiating to the back and to the shoulder. Occasionally the pain starts on the left subcostal side or even in the epigastrium, but at its most severe it is invariably on the right side. Pain may radiate to the chest. The pain is usually severe and may last for minutes or even several hours. Frequently, the pain starts during the night and wakes the patient. Minor episodes of the same discomfort may occur intermittently during the day. Dyspeptic symptoms may coexist and be worse after such an attack. As the pain resolves the patient improves and is able to eat and drink again, often only to suffer further episodes. It is of interest that the patient may have several episodes of this nature over a period of a few weeks and then no more trouble for some months.

If the pain does not resolve the patient will become more systemically unwell as infection supervenes. This is associated with a continuous pain, nausea, vomiting and pyrexia. On examination the patient will be tender in the right subcostal area and may develop guarding, even rigidity, and later a mass may be palpable as the omentum walls off an inflamed gall bladder.

Fortunately, this process is limited by the stone slipping back into the body of the gall bladder and the contents of the gall bladder escaping by way of the cystic duct. This achieves adequate drainage of the gall bladder and enables the inflammation to resolve.

If resolution does not occur the gall bladder may perforate with the development of localised peritonitis or an abscess may form; the abscess may then perforate into the peritoneal cavity with a septic peritonitis – this is uncommon, however, because the gall bladder is usually localised by omentum around the perforation.

When examining a patient with acute cholecystitis it should be noted whether the patient is pyrexial, is jaundiced or dehydrated. His or her respiration should be noted to determine whether there is pain on deep inspiration. On examining the abdomen it is important to determine whether the movement is normal or shallow breathing is present with intestinal distension. The abdomen should be palpated gently, working towards the subcostal area where tenderness with guarding may be noted. In some patients a mass may be palpable. Bowel sounds are usually present but reduced.

Differential diagnosis

Conditions commonly presenting similarly to acute cholecystitis are appendicitis, perforated peptic ulcer and acute pancreatitis. Occasionally acute pyelonephritis of the right kidney, myocardial infarction and right lower lobe pneumonia may lead to confusion. The diagnosis is confirmed by ultrasonography which should show the presence of stones in an inflamed gall bladder with oedema around the gall bladder wall (Fig. 54.32). The stone can often be observed impacted in the infundibulum. A serum amylase estimation should be performed to exclude pancreatitis, and liver functions tests performed to determine whether or not jaundice is present. A mild elevation of the bilirubin can merely be due to oedema around the porta hepatis or obstruction of the biliary tree by a stone escaping into the common bile duct. The distended bile duct should be noted on ultrasonography. A chest X-ray will exclude pneumonia, and if there is doubt concerning a cardiac origin then an electrocardiogram should be performed. Renal disease can be excluded by sending the urine for microscopy and culture.

Treatment

Conservative treatment followed by cholecystectomy

Experience shows that in more than 90 per cent of cases the symptoms of acute cholecystitis subside with conservative

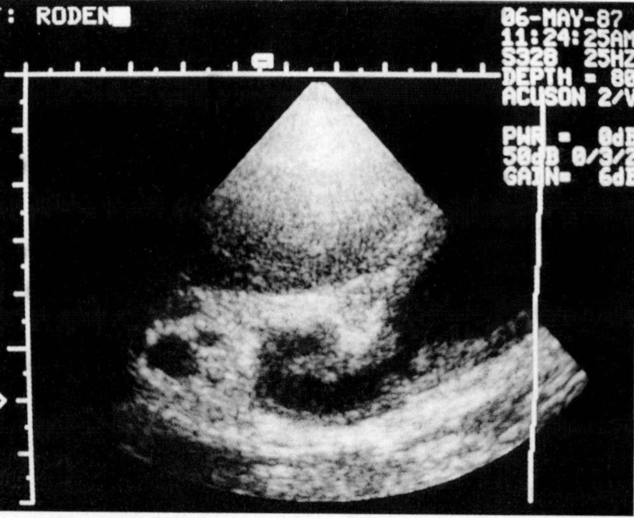

Fig. 54.32 An ultrasound scan of acute cholecystitis showing an obstructed infundibulum and marked oedema of the mucosa.

measures. Nonoperative treatment is based on four principles:

- nasogastric aspiration and intravenous fluid administration;
- administration of analgesics;
- administration of antibiotics – as the cystic duct is blocked in most instances, the concentration of antibiotic in the serum is more important than its concentration in bile. A broad-spectrum antibiotic effective against Gram-negative aerobes is most appropriate (e.g. cephazolin, cefuroxime or gentamycin);
- subsequent management – when the temperature, pulse and other physical signs show that the inflammation is subsiding, the nasogastric tube is removed and oral fluids followed by a fat-free diet are given. Ultrasonography is performed to ensure that no local complications have developed, that the bile duct is of a normal size and that no stones are contained in the bile duct. Cholecystectomy may either be performed on the next available list, or the patient is allowed home to return later when the inflammation has completely resolved.

Conservative treatment is not advised when there is uncertainty about the diagnosis and the possibility of a high retrocaecal appendix or a perforated duodenal ulcer cannot be excluded.

Conservative treatment must be abandoned if the pain and tenderness increase; in this case a percutaneous cholecystostomy performed by the radiologist under ultrasound control will rapidly relieve symptoms. Subsequent cholecystectomy will be required.

Routine early operations

Some surgeons advocate urgent operation as a routine measure in cases of acute cholecystitis. Provided that the operation is undertaken within 48 hours of the onset of the attack, the surgeon is experienced and excellent operating facilities are available, good results are claimed. Nevertheless, the conversion rate in laparoscopic cholecystectomy is five times higher in acute than in elective surgery.

Mucocele of the gall bladder

This occurs when the neck of the gall bladder becomes obstructed by a stone but the contents remain sterile. The bile is absorbed and replaced by mucous secreted by the gall bladder epithelium. The gall bladder may be palpable. Enormous sizes and shapes have been encountered. A mucocele also occurs in those cases of malignancy which occlude the cystic duct, for instance a cholangiocarcinoma.

Empyema of the gall bladder

The gall bladder appears to be filled with pus but, surprisingly in over half of cases, bacteria cannot be cultured from this pus. It may be a sequel of acute cholecystitis or the

Hans C.J. Gram, b. 1853. Danish physician.

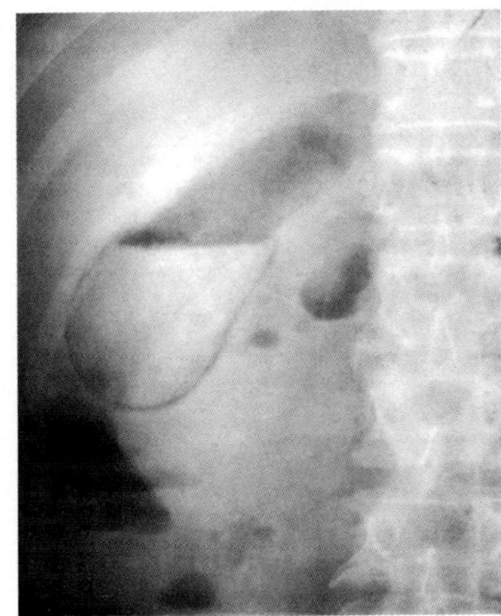

Fig. 54.33 Gas in a gall bladder and gall-bladder wall (*C. perfringens*). Emergency surgery is indicated.

result of a mucocele becoming infected. The treatment is drainage and, later, cholecystectomy (Fig. 54.33).

Acalculous cholecystitis

Acute and chronic inflammation of the gall bladder can occur in the absence of stones and give rise to a clinical picture similar to calculous cholecystitis. Some patients have nonspecific inflammation of the gall bladder, whereas others have one of the cholecystoses. Oral cholecystography is more useful than ultrasonography in the diagnosis of those patients presenting with chronic symptoms, and radioisotope scanning in those presenting acutely. The identification of cholesterol crystals in a duodenal aspirate may also help. Acute acalculous cholecystitis is particularly seen in patients recovering from major surgery, trauma and burns. In these patients the diagnosis is often missed and the mortality rate is 20 per cent.

The cholecystoses (cholesterosis, polyposis, adenomyomatosis and cholecystitis glandularis proliferans)

This is a not uncommon group of conditions affecting the gall bladder in which there are chronic inflammatory changes with hyperplasia of all tissue elements.

Cholesterosis ('strawberry gall bladder')

In the fresh state the interior of the gall bladder looks something like a strawberry; the yellow specks (submucous aggregations of cholesterol crystals and cholesterol esters) correspond to the seeds (Fig. 54.34). It may be associated with cholesterol stones.

Cholesterol polyposis of the gall bladder

Cholecystography shows negative shadows in a functioning gall bladder, or on ultrasound there is a well-defined polyp present. These are either cholesterol polyposis or adenoma-

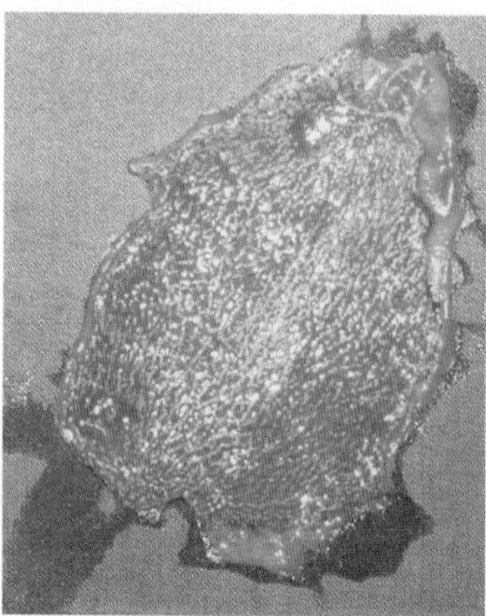

Fig. 54.34 The interior of a strawberry gall bladder (cholesterosis) (*courtesy of Dr Sanjay P. Thakur, Patna, India*).

tous change. With improving ultrasonography they are seen more frequently and surgery advised only if they change in size.

Cholecystitis glandularis proliferans (polyp, adenomyomatosis and intramural diverticulosis)

Figure 54.35 summarises the varieties of this condition. A polyp of the mucous membrane is fleshy and granulomatous. All layers of the gall bladder wall may be thickened but sometimes an incomplete septum forms which separates the hyperplastic from the normal. Intraparietal 'mixed' calculi may be present. These can be complicated by an intramural, and later extramural, abscess. If symptomatic, the patient is treated by cholecystectomy.

Diverticulosis of the gall bladder

Diverticulosis of the gall bladder is usually manifest as black pigment stones impacted in the out-pouchings of the lacunae of Luschka. Diverticulosis of the gall bladder may be demonstrated by cholecystography, especially when the gall bladder contracts after a fatty meal. There are small dots of contrast medium just outside the gall bladder (Fig. 54.36). A septum may also be present (to be distinguished from the Phrygian cap – Fig. 54.26) and the treatment is cholecystectomy.

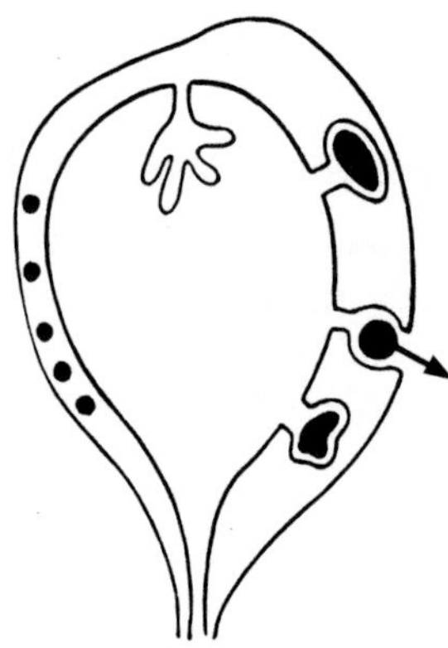

Fig. 54.35 Types of cholecystitis glandularis proliferans (polypus, intramural or diverticular stones and fistula).

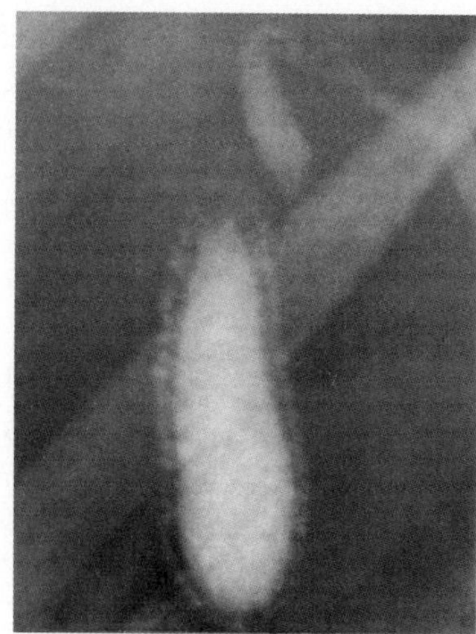

Fig. 54.36 Cholecystogram showing cholecystitis glandularis proliferans.

Typhoid gall bladder

Salmonella typhi ('Typhoid Mary', a cook-general who passed *Salmonella typhi* in her faeces and urine, was responsible for nearly a score of epidemics of typhoid in and around New York City) or, occasionally, *Salmonella typhimurium* can infect the gall bladder. Acute cholecystitis can occur. More frequently, chronic cholecystitis occurs, the patient being a typhoid carrier excreting the bacteria in the bile. Gallstones may be present (surgeons should not give patients their stones after their operation if there is any suspicion of typhoid!). It is debatable whether the stones are secondary to the salmonella cholecystitis or whether pre-existing stones predispose the gall bladder to chronic infection. Salmonellae can, however, frequently be cultured from these stones. Ampicillin and cholecystectomy are indicated.

Cholecystectomy

Preparation for operation

After appropriate history taking and assessment of the patient's fitness for the procedure, which will include investigation of the cardiovascular and respiratory systems if history suggests these to be a risk factor, a full blood count and biochemical profile are done to exclude abnormal liver function tests or anaemia. Blood coagulation is checked if there is a history of jaundice. The patient is given prophylactic antibiotics either with the premedication intramuscularly, or intravenously at the time of induction. A second-generation

Daniel Elmer Salmon, 1850–1914. Veterinary pathologist, Chief of the Bureau of Animal Industry, Washington, DC, USA.

cephalosporin is appropriate. Subcutaneous heparin or antiembolus stockings are prescribed. A consent form is signed ensuring that the patient is fully aware of the procedure being undertaken, the risks involved and complications that may occur.

Laparotomy

A short right upper transverse incision is made centred over the lateral border of the rectus muscle. A full laparotomy, inspecting all abdominal organs, is undertaken and the diagnosis of gallstones confirmed. The gall bladder is appropriately exposed and packs are placed on the hepatic flexure of the colon, the duodenum and the lesser omentum to ensure a clear view of the anatomy of the porta hepatis. These packs may be retracted using the hand of the assistant ('It is the left hand of the assistant that does all the work' – Moynihan) or a stabilised ring retractor used to keep the packs in position (Fig. 54.37). An artery forceps is placed on the infundibulum of the gall bladder and the peritoneum overlying Calot's triangle is placed on a stretch. The peritoneum is then divided close to the wall of the gall bladder and the fat in the triangle of Calot carefully dissected away to expose the cystic artery and the cystic duct. The cystic duct is cleaned down to the common bile duct whose position is clearly ascertained. The cystic artery is tied and divided. The whole of the triangle of Calot is displayed to ensure that the anatomy of the ducts is clear and the cystic duct is then divided between ligatures. The gall bladder is then dissected away from the gall-bladder bed.

Some golden rules in case of difficulty.

- When the anatomy of the triangle of Calot is unclear, blind dissection should stop.
- Bleeding adjacent to the triangle of Calot should be controlled by pressure and not by blind clipping or clamping.

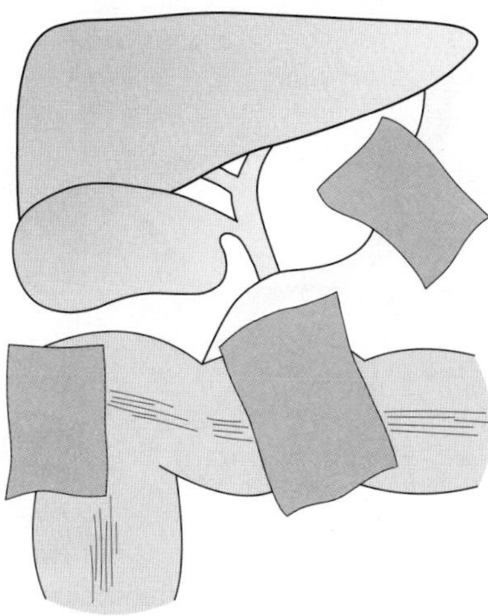

Fig. 54.37 Cholecystectomy. Positions of the packs after identifying the colon, the duodenum and the stomach.

Jean François Calot, 1861–1944. Surgeon, Paris, France.

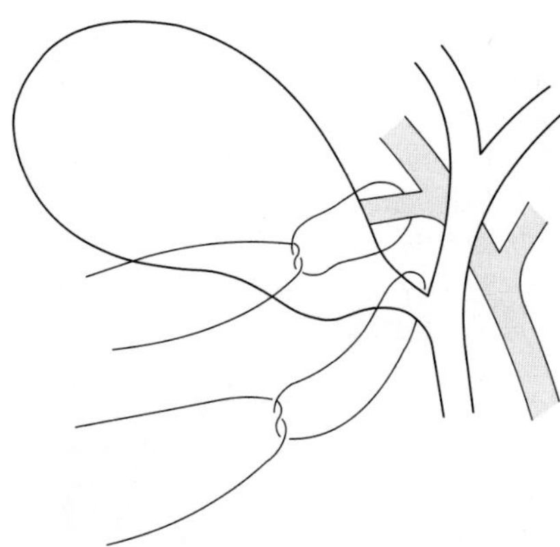

Fig. 54.38 Ligatures are passed and tied around the cystic artery and cystic duct.

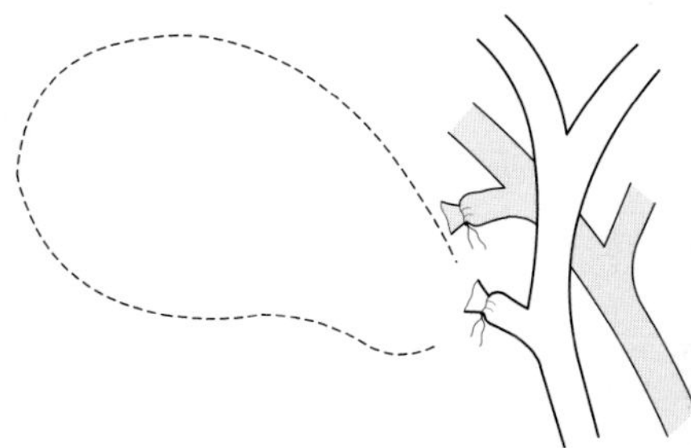

Fig. 54.39 The gall bladder has been removed.

- When there is doubt about the anatomy a 'fundus-first' cholecystectomy dissecting on the gall-bladder wall down to the cystic duct can be helpful.
- If the cystic duct is densely adherent to the common bile duct and there is the possibility of a Mirizzi syndrome (the stone ulcerating through into the common duct), the infundibulum of the gall bladder should be opened, the stone removed and the infundibulum oversewn.
- A cholecystostomy is almost never indicated, but if it has to be done as many stones as possible should be extracted and a large Foley catheter (14 French) placed in the fundus of the gall bladder with a direct track externally. By so doing, should stones be left behind in the gall bladder, these can be extracted with a choledochoscope.

The technique of open cholecystectomy has largely been superseded by laparoscopic cholecystectomy. Nevertheless, no surgeon undertaking laparoscopic cholecystectomy should lose the different technique of undertaking an open cholecystectomy as this may be required when difficulties are encountered laparoscopically.

Laparoscopic cholecystectomy

The preparation and indications for cholecystectomy are the same whether it is performed by laparoscopy or by open techniques. However, a laparoscopic cholecystectomy should

Frederic E. B. Foley, 1891–1966. American urologist, Ankher Hospitals, St Paul, USA.

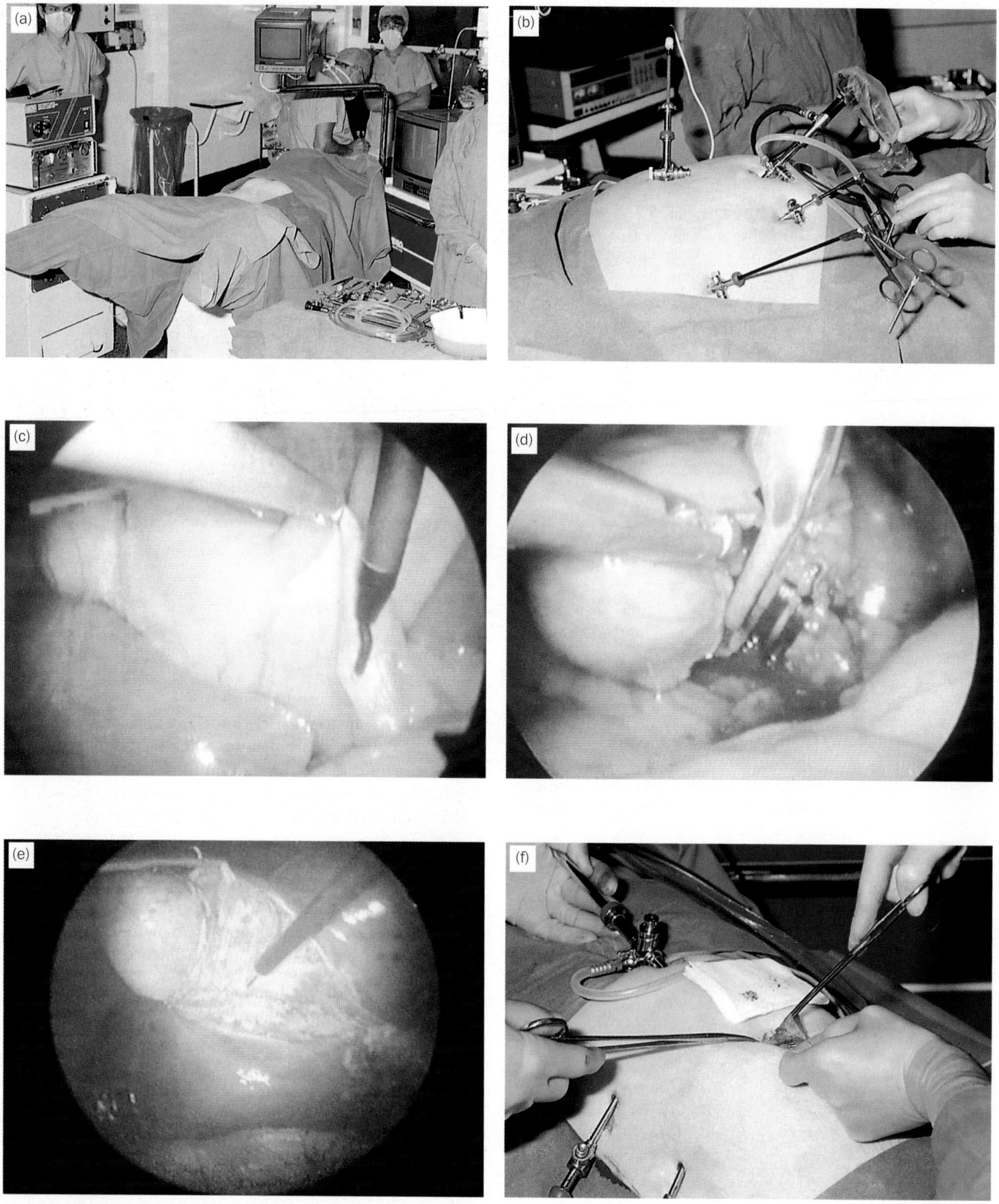

(a) (b)

(c) (d)

(e) (f)

Fig. 54.40 Laparoscopic cholecystectomy. (a) The patient is placed on the operating table in the modified Lloyd-Davies position with the legs apart. (b) The surgeon stands between the legs. After creating the pneumoperitoneum, an 11-mm trocar is placed in the umbilicus and epigastrium while two 5-mm trocars are placed in the right side of the abdomen. (c) Dissection of the gall bladder with a diathermy hook starts on the gall bladder near the triangle of Calot. (d) Absolok clips are placed on the cystic duct before division of the duct. (e) Dissection of the gall bladder from the gall-bladder bed with a diathermy hook. (f) The gall bladder is extracted from the umbilicus; large stones are removed from the gall bladder with foreceps before delivery of the whole gall bladder.

only be performed by a surgeon who is frequently undertaking laparoscopic procedures as the skills are different from those required in undertaking an open cholecystectomy.

The patient is positioned either in a Lloyd-Davies position or flat on the table depending on whether the French or American approach is used by the surgeon. A pneumoperitoneum is created and four ports are placed in the abdomen, usually at the umbilicus and the epigastrium, with two 5-mm ports laterally. The triangle of Calot is laid widely open by dividing the peritoneum on the posterior and on the anterior aspect. The cystic duct is carefully defined as is the cystic artery which is divided. Once the triangle of Calot has been laid widely open the cystic duct is clipped and divided. The gall bladder is then removed from the gall bladder bed and once free removed via the umbilicus (Fig. 54.40).

Indications for choledochotomy

In an environment where the modern diagnostic armamentarium described at the beginning of this chapter is not available and neither is peroperative cholangiography, it is well to rehearse the traditional indications for choledochotomy, which are: (1) palpable duct stones; (2) there is jaundice or a history of jaundice or cholangitis; (3) the common bile duct is dilated; and (4) the liver function tests are abnormal, in particular, the alkaline phosphatase is raised.

In centres where adequate facilities are available it is probably inadvisable to do a choledochotomy laparoscopically, but rather to rely on endoscopic techniques unless particular expertise has been achieved in laparoscopic exploration of the bile duct. The incidence of symptomatic stones in the bile duct varies from 5 to 8 per cent. These can, in the main, be dealt with endoscopically without resort to opening the duct. However, current trials suggest that in experienced hands the morbidity of the two techniques is identical.

Symptoms persisting after cholecystectomy

In 15 per cent of patients cholecystectomy fails to relieve the symptoms for which the operation was performed. Such patients may be considered to have a 'postcholecystectomy' syndrome. However, such problems are usually related to the preoperative symptoms and are merely a continuation of those symptoms. Full investigation should be undertaken to exclude the presence of a stone in the bile duct, a stone in the cystic duct stump or operative damage to the biliary tree. This is best performed by an MRCP or an ERCP which has the added advantage that if a stone remains it can be removed.

Management of bile-duct obstruction

Patients with symptoms after a cholecystectomy, particularly if jaundice is present, demand urgent investigation. Any patient who does not make an uneventful recovery following gall-bladder surgery should be investigated by ultrasound scanning as a matter of immediacy. If jaundice (either biochemical or clinical) is present emergency measures are required.

The first step in management is to undertake an immediate ultrasound scan. If there is evidence of fluid in the subhepatic space or obstruction of the biliary tree as shown by bile-duct dilatation then an immediate ERCP should be performed to ascertain whether a stone is present or there is obstruction of the common bile duct due to damage at the time of surgery (Fig. 54.41).

If a stone is present immediate removal endoscopically is indicated. If the common bile duct is obstructed by clips or there is leakage from the biliary tree due to a cystic duct leak then a drain should be placed in the subhepatic space percutaneously and a stent placed in the bile duct where possible. Small leaks will usually resolve spontaneously. Should the common bile duct be damaged the patient should be referred to an appropriate expert for reconstruction of the duct.

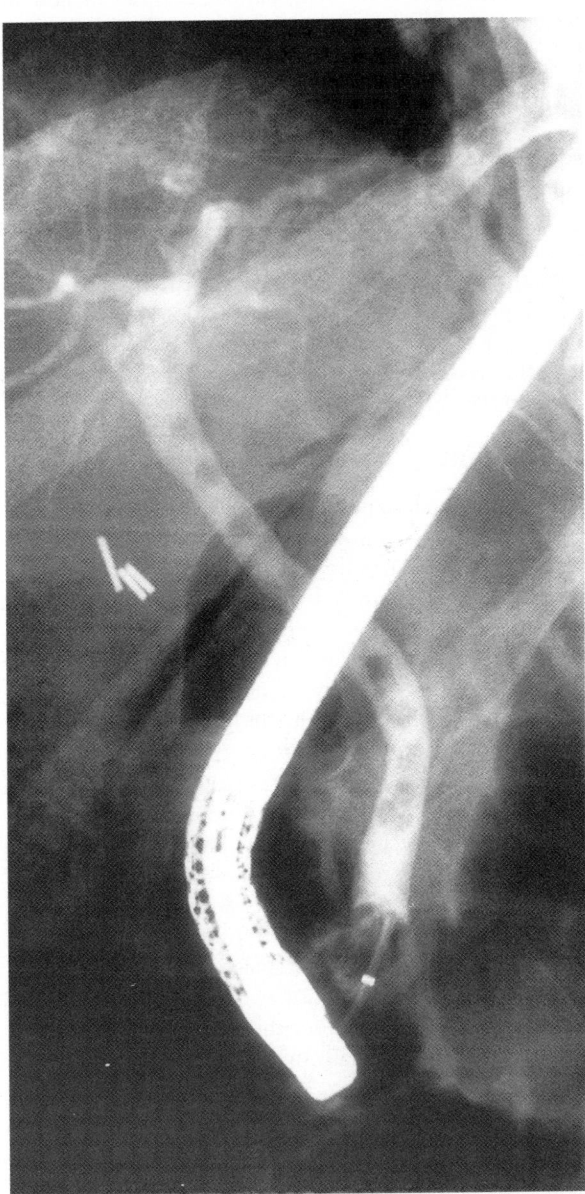

Fig. 54.41 This patient presented with jaundice 4 days after a cholecystectomy. The duct contained multiple stones.

Stones in the bile duct

Duct stones may occur many years after a cholecystectomy or be related to the development of new pathology, such as infection of the biliary tree or infestation by *Ascaris lumbricoides* or *Clinorchis sinensis*. Any obstruction to the flow of bile can give rise to stasis with the formation of stones within the duct. The consequences of duct stones are either obstruction to bile flow or infection-cholangitis. Stones in the bile ducts are more often associated with infected bile (80 per cent) than are stones in the gall bladder.

Symptoms

The patient may be asymptomatic but usually has bouts of pain, jaundice and fever. The patient is often ill and feels unwell. The term 'cholangitis' is given to the triad of pain, jaundice and fevers sometimes known as 'Charcot's triad'.

Signs

Tenderness may be elicited in the epigastrium and the right hypochondrium. In the jaundiced patient it is useful to remember Courvoisier's law – 'in obstruction of the common bile duct due to a stone, distension of the gall bladder seldom occurs; the organ usually is already shrivelled'. In obstruction from other causes distension is common by comparison. However, if there is no disease in the gall bladder and the obstruction is due to a cancer of the ampulla, pancreas or bile duct, then the gall bladder may well be distended.

Management

It is essential to determine whether the jaundice is due to liver disease, disease within the duct such as sclerosing cholangitis or obstruction. Ultrasound scanning, liver function tests, liver biopsy if the ducts are not dilated, and MRI or ERCP will demarcate the nature of the obstruction.

The patient may be ill. Pus may be present within the biliary tree and liver abscesses may be developing. Full supportive measures are required with rehydration, attention to clotting, exclusion of diabetes and starting the appropriate broad-spectrum antibiotics. As soon as resuscitation has taken place, relief of the obstruction is essential. Endoscopic papillotomy is the preferred first technique with a sphincterotomy, removal of the stones using a Dormia basket (Fig. 54.42) or the placement of a stent if stone removal is not possible. If this technique fails, a percutaneous transhepatic cholangiogram can be performed to provide drainage and subsequent percutaneous choledochoscopy. Surgery, in the form of choledochotomy, is now rarely used for this situation as most patients can be managed by minimally invasive techniques (Fig. 54.43).

Choledochotomy

If a stone (or stones) is present in the common bile duct,

Jean Marie Charcot, 1825–93. Physician, Hôpital Salpêtriere, Paris, France.
Ludwig Courvoisier, 1843–1918. Professor of Surgery, Basel, Switzerland.

(a) 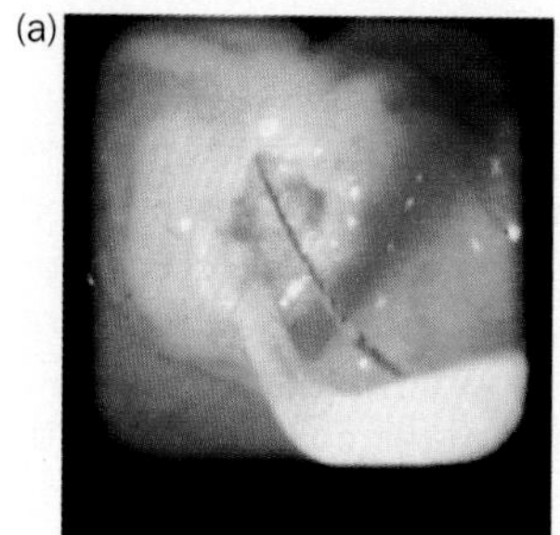 (b) 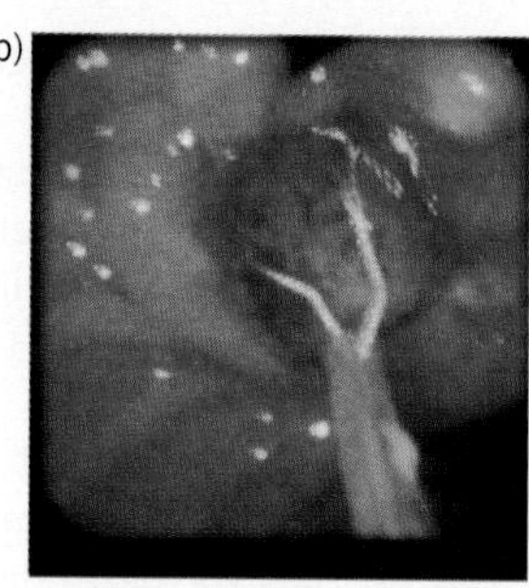

Fig. 54.42 (a) Endoscopic sphincterotomy; (b) extraction of a stone from the bile duct through the ampulla.

removal should have priority over cholecystectomy. Should the patient be unfit for cholecystectomy, or even cholecystostomy, the gall bladder should be removed on a future occasion ('a living problem is better than a dead "cert"' – Grey Turner). In particular, this may be the case in suppurative cholangitis. Recent evidence suggests that subsequent cholecystectomy may not be necessary. After endoscopic removal of stones, only 10 per cent of patients will have subsequent problems with their gall bladder.

Supraduodenal choledochotomy

Most stones in the common bile duct can be removed by this route. If, as is often the case, a stone can be felt, an attempt is made to manoeuvre it into a position midway between the entrance of the cystic duct and the superior border of the duodenum. The stone is steadied between the finger and thumb. The duct is opened longitudinally directly on to the stone, enabling it to be removed by a malleable scoop or Desjardin's gallstone forceps. The interior of the duct is then explored upwards and downwards with the scoop for further stones.

When the stone cannot be felt, or cannot be manipulated into the optimum position just described, 2 cm of the common bile duct is exposed, two stay sutures are placed in the duct and a longitudinal incision into the duct is made between them. Escaping bile is mopped up or removed by suction. Through this opening it may be possible to identify the stones and remove them with a scoop or forceps (Fig. 54.44). A balloon catheter, similar to that used for embolectomy, and irrigation of the ducts with saline are useful additional methods. Choledochoscopy may be employed to confirm that all calculi have been removed. Usually drainage of the common bile duct is carried out by means of a T-tube (Fig. 54.45); T-tubes should be made of latex or rubber and used only once – plastic tubes are hardened by the bile and are difficult to remove. Latex and rubber stimulate fibrinous adhesion of the omentum to liver and colon to form a safe track. There is very little reaction to a plastic tube and therefore the risk of biliary peritonitis is greater. The transverse

Dormia. Assistant Professor of Urology, University of Milan, Italy.
George Grey Turner, 1877–1951. Professor of Surgery, Postgraduate Medical School, London, England.
Abel Desjardins. Surgeon, Dispensaire Henri de Rothschild, Paris, France.

(a)

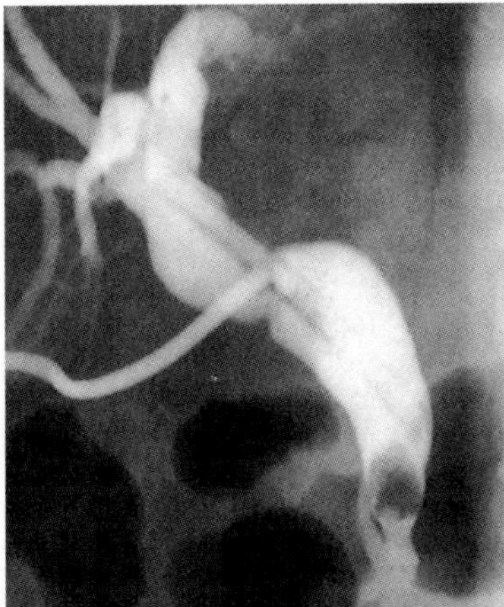

(b)

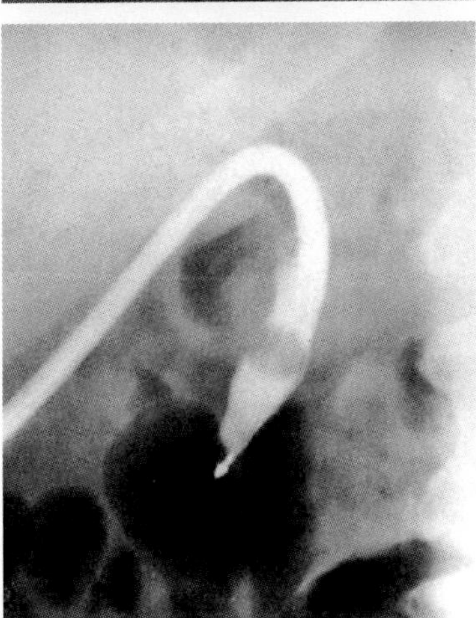

(c)

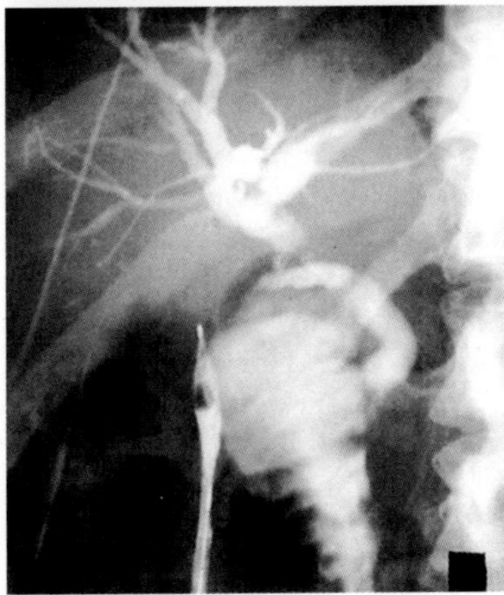

Fig. 54.43 Extraction of a stone from the common bile duct by the Burhenne technique. (a) A T-tube *in situ* with a stone in the duct. (b) A steerable catheter has been manipulated into the duct and a basket placed around the stone. (c) The stone being extracted from the bile duct along the T-tube track.

limb, shortened if necessary to about 5 cm long, is inserted in the duct which is closed snugly about the vertical limb, using fine catgut on an atraumatic needle. The long limb is brought out through a separate stab wound laterally, as this facilitates the Burhenne procedure should it subsequently be required for a retained stone. The bile draining from the tube is collected in a plastic bag by the side of the bed, its amount and character being noted. After 10 days the tube may be clamped for increasing periods, and the absence of pain and jaundice and the presence of bile in the stools indicate satisfactory flow into the duodenum. Sodium diatrizoate is injected down the tube to obtain a cholangiogram, and if there are no filling defects in a well-outlined duct, and the contrast enters the duodenum freely, the T-tube can be removed. Subsequent bile drainage is minimal and does not usually persist for more than 1 day.

Closure of the common duct without a T-tube

If this procedure is attempted, it is essential to provide drainage placed in apposition to the common duct.

Transduodenal sphincterotomy

Transduodenal sphincterotomy is indicated when a stone is found to be impacted near the ampulla of Vater (Fig. 54.46) and it cannot be retrieved from above. Other indications are when the common bile duct is dilated and contains multiple stones and biliary sludge, and when the papilla is fibrosed and stenosed secondary to the passage of stones through it. Some surgeons prefer the method to supraduodenal choledo-

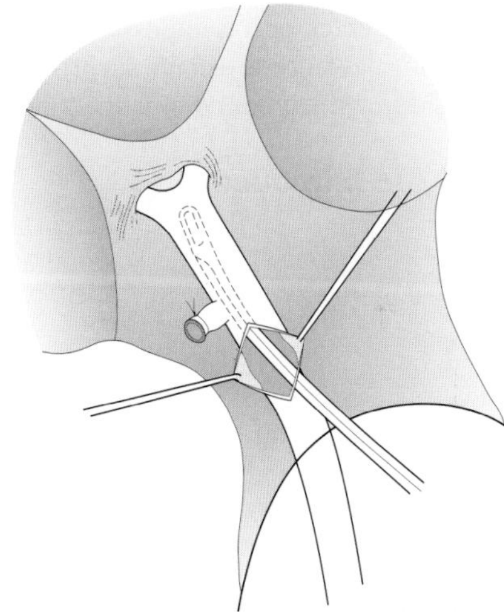

Fig. 54.44 Choledochotomy. The stone is seized with Desjardins' forceps.

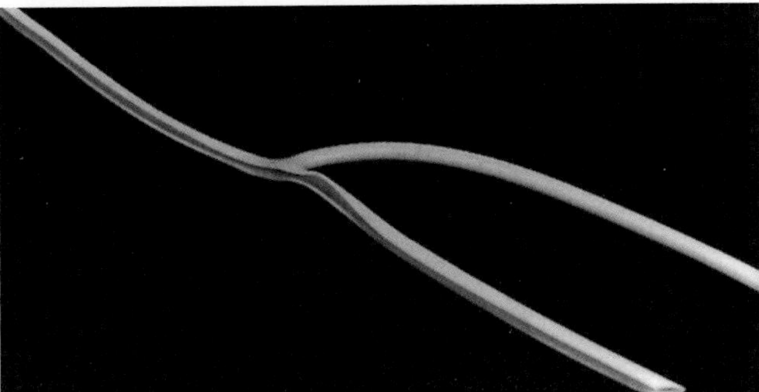

Fig. 54.45 A T-tube for draining the common bile duct.

Joachim Burhenne. Radiologist, Vancouver, Canada.

chotomy to remove all duct stones. If the supraduodenal approach fails to clear the duct, it is preferable to place a large T-tube in the duct (14 or 16 Fr) and close the abdomen. Subsequently, the stone can be removed by the Burhenne procedure or endoscopically. The combination of a supraduodenal approach with a transduodenal approach frequently leads to complications.

The duodenum is opened in its second part between stay sutures and the region of the ampulla brought into the opening by traction using tissue forceps. Removal of the stone or stones requires division of the duodenal papilla and the sphincter. A grooved director is passed through the papillary opening and up into the bile duct where *it must be palpated*. The papilla and part of all the sphincter are now divided at 10 o'clock. If the bile-duct mucosa is sutured to that of the duodenum, the procedure is called a sphincteroplasty. Before sutures are placed in the papilla, it is essential to identify the pancreatic duct.

Choledochoduodenostomy

Choledochoduodenostomy is an alternative to transduodenal sphincterotomy when the common bile duct is dilated and contains multiple stones and sludge, particularly in elderly people (Fig. 54.47).

The operation is contraindicated if the common duct is not 15 mm or more in diameter, or it is impossible to make a stoma of 2–3 cm. The convalescence is usually surprisingly placid. It is, indeed, a procedure which has commanded much support.

Stricture of the bile duct

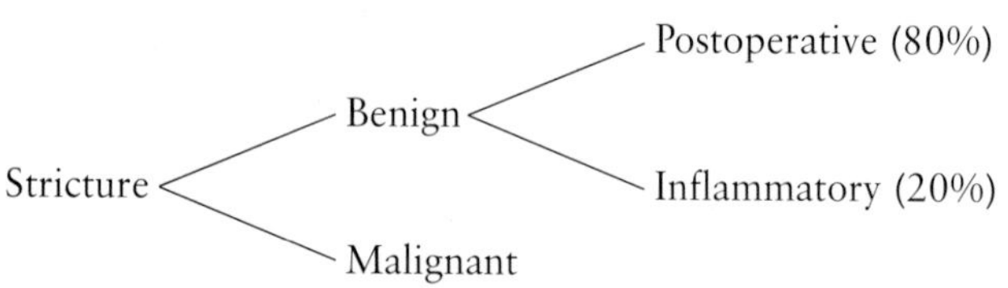

Postoperative stricture

Postoperative strictures concern either the common bile duct or the common hepatic duct. In a few cases only the right

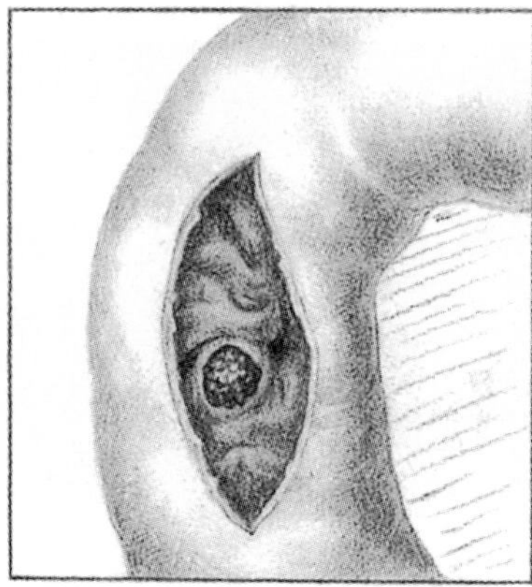

Fig. 54.46 The transduodenal approach to a stone in the ampulla of Vater.

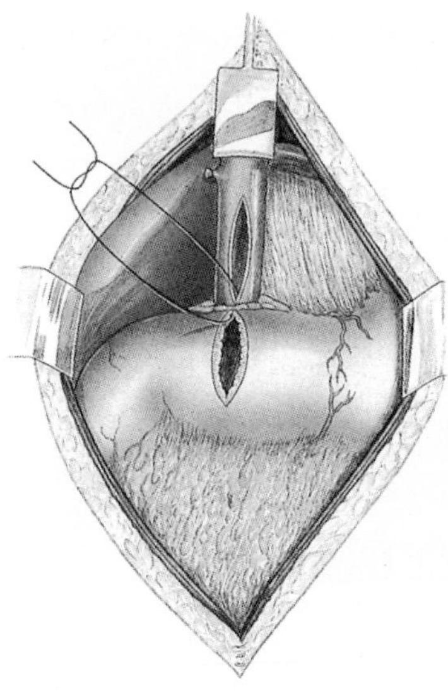

Fig. 54.47 Choledochoduodenostomy. The stoma must be 2–3 cm long. The stoma is fashioned to extend as low as possible in order to reduce the collection of sludge in the 'sump' necessarily left in the retroduodenal portion of the duct. It must permit free entry and egress of fluid, for if it is large enough regurgitant cholangitis does not occur and liver function is not impaired. The two openings are approximated with polydioxanone as a single layer.

hepatic duct is implicated. The stricture is the result of a preventable error in technique during the performance of cholecystectomy.

- Blind plunge application of a haemostat to a bleeding cystic or accessory cystic artery, or to the right hepatic artery, is likely to damage the common hepatic duct (Fig. 54.48). The prevention of this tragic happening is standardised. All unexpected haemorrhage in this region should be controlled initially by inserting an index finger into the foramen of Winslow, and pinching the free edge of the gastrohepatic omentum between the finger and thumb. Temporary compression of the hepatic artery in this way allows the bleeding point to be visualised and ligated securely (Hogarth Pringle's manoeuvre).
- Should cholecystectomy be performed by dissecting from the fundus (fundus-first procedure) too much traction applied to the freed gall bladder may so tent the common bile duct that any forceps intended for the cystic duct grasp the angulated main channel (Fig. 54.49) (forceps should not, in fact, ever be used for grasping the cystic duct prior to ligature – Fig. 54.38).
- Failure to identify the anatomy in Calot's triangle when there is much inflammation. The common hepatic duct is tied instead of the cystic duct.
- Ignorance of the anatomical anomalies of the bile ducts.
- Laceration of the common bile duct while exploring it for stones.

Jacob Benignus Winslow, 1669–1760. Professor of Anatomy, Physics and Surgery, Paris, France.

James Hogarth Pringle, 1863–1941. Surgeon, Royal Infirmary, Glasgow, Scotland.

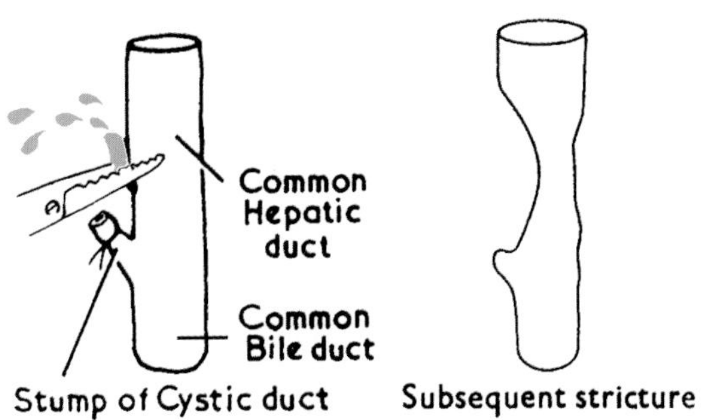

Fig. 54.48 One way of damaging the common hepatic duct and causing stricture.

- In 3 per cent of cases of stricture of the common bile duct, injury occurs during related surgical procedures.

About 15 per cent of injuries to the bile ducts are not recognised at the time of operation. In 85 per cent of cases the injury declares itself postoperatively by: (1) a profuse and persistent leakage of bile if drainage has been provided, or bile peritonitis if such drainage has not been provided; and (2) deepening obstructive jaundice. When the obstruction is incomplete, jaundice is delayed until subsequent fibrosis renders the lumen of the duct inadequate.

Radiological investigation of biliary strictures

- Ultrasonography
- Cholangiography via T-tube, if present
- ERCP
- Transhepatic cholangiography

Treatment

In the debilitated patient, temporary external biliary drainage may be achieved by passing a catheter percutaneously into an intrahepatic duct. Also, stents may be passed through strictures at the time of ERCP and left to drain into the duodenum. When the general condition of the patient has improved, definitive surgery can be undertaken. However, both of these methods may be complicated by cholangitis and are not recommended for all cases. For benign stricture or duct transection, the preferred treatment is immediate Roux-en-Y choledochojejunostomy by a surgeon well versed in managing benign postoperative strictures. For a stricture of recent onset through which a guidewire can be passed, balloon dilatation with insertion of a stent is an acceptable alternative provided that the services of an experienced endoscopist are available.

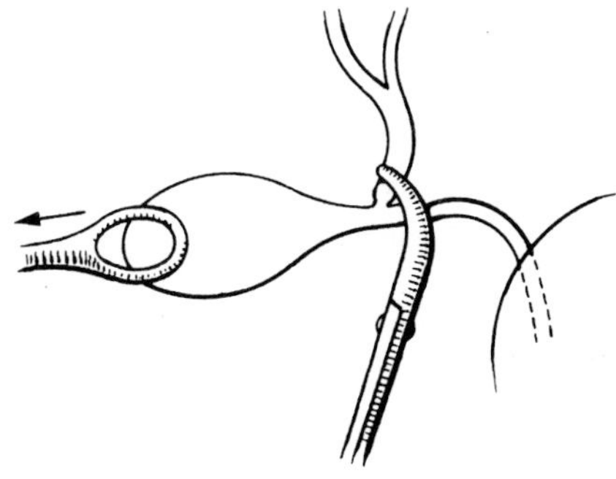

Fig. 54.49 Another way of damaging the duct!

Primary sclerosing cholangitis

This is a chronic fibrosing inflammatory condition of the biliary tree which affects both intrahepatic and extrahepatic ducts, and may involve the gall bladder and pancreas. It is of unknown origin and must be distinguished from secondary sclerosing cholangitis associated with choledocholithiasis. It is associated with inflammatory bowel disease, usually ulcerative colitis, in 50–70 per cent of cases, and these patients may be at greater risk of developing a bile-duct carcinoma. The patients are commonly young, being less than 50 years old. They present with a progressive cholestatic disorder and right upper quadrant discomfort, jaundice, pruritis and fever. Investigation reveals a considerable elevation of the alkaline phosphatase, and on cholangiography stricturing and beading of the bile ducts (Fig. 54.50). As the majority of patients has both intrahepatic and extrahepatic biliary tree involvement, surgical treatment is not appropriate. Primarily, these patients are managed with antibiotics, vitamin K, cholestyramine, steroids and azothiaprine, but with little benefit. Repeated dilatation of the strictures is helpful. Many go on to develop cirrhosis due to obstruction. If liver failure supervenes these patients are suitable candidates for liver transplantation.

Parasitic infestation of the biliary tract

Biliary ascariasis

The round worm, *A. lumbricoides,* commonly infests the intestine of inhabitants of Asia, Africa and Central America. It may enter the biliary tree through the ampulla of Vater and cause biliary pain. Complications include strictures, suppurative cholangitis, liver abscesses and empyema of the gall bladder. In the uncomplicated case, antispasmodics can be given to relax the sphincter of Oddi and the worm will return to the small intestine to be dealt with by antihelminthic drugs. Operation may be necessary to remove the worm or deal with complications. Worms can be extracted via the ampulla of Vater by ERCP.

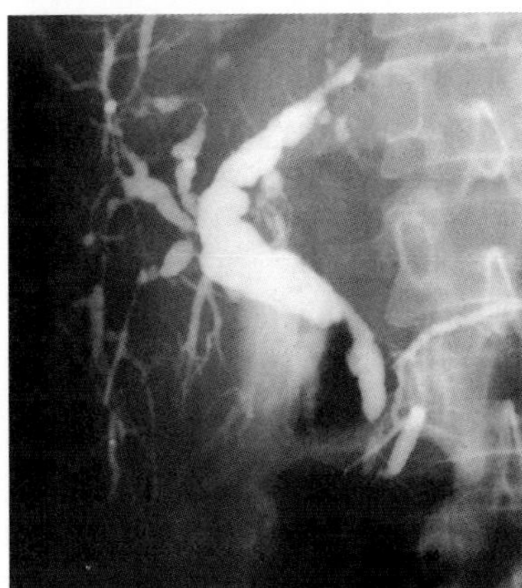

Fig. 54.50 Sclerosing cholangitis in a patient with ulcerative colitis visualised by ERCP.

Clonorchiasis (asiatic cholangiohepatis)

The disease is endemic in the Far East. The fluke, up to 25 mm long and 5 mm wide, inhabits the bile ducts, including the intrahepatic ducts. Fibrous thickening of the duct walls occur. Many cases are asymptomatic. Complications include biliary pain, stones, cholangitis, cirrhosis and bile-duct carcinoma. Choledochotomy and T-tube drainage and, in some cases, choledochoduodenostomy are required. Because a process of recurrent stone formation is set up, a choledochojejunostomy with Roux loop affixed to the abdominal parietes is performed in some centres to allow easy subsequent access to the duct system.

Hydatid disease

A large hydatid cyst may obstruct the hepatic ducts. Sometimes a cyst will rupture into the biliary tree and its contents cause obstructive jaundice or cholangitis, requiring appropriate surgery (see Chapter 52).

Tumours of the bile duct

Papillomatosis

This rare condition is characterised by the presence of multiple mucous-secreting tumours of the biliary epithelium. These tumours are low-grade papillary carcinomas and should be treated by choledochoscopy with obliteration of the papillary lesions. The malignancy tends to develop over a period of years and may require liver resection. If both lobes are affected then liver transplantation may be required.

Carcinoma of the bile duct

Incidence and aetiology

The incidence of bile-duct carcinoma varies markedly in different parts of the world. It is very rare in the UK, but high rates are found in parts of the world where biliary infection is common. It is associated with the presence of bile-duct stones in a quarter of patients, and is more frequent in patients with sclerosing cholangitis and ulcerative colitis. Anatomical abnormalities, particularly intrahepatic cystic change and choledochal cyst, are also associated with an increased incidence. Clinorchis sinensis is a recognised aetiological factor.

Pathology

Macroscopically, the tumour arises as a small nodule which rapidly encases the bile duct causing jaundice. The tumour invades locally spreading via the nerves, the lymphatics and the portal venous trunk. It may directly invade the portal vein or the surrounding liver. Microscopically, the majority of bile duct tumours are well- to poorly differentiated adenocarcinomas.

Clinical features

The patient presents with jaundice. The diagnosis is suspected when obstruction in the biliary tree with a characteristic stricture is demonstrated.

Local spread is frequent and metastases are common at the time of presentation. The diagnosis is confirmed by biopsy, either by the percutaneous transhepatic route or endoscopically, or by cytological brushings taken at endoscopy.

If the patient is under 70 years of age and the tumour is localised either to one lobe of the liver or to the extrahepatic bile duct then resection is possible in 10–20 per cent of patients. Such resections may involve excision of a lobe of the liver and reconstruction of the biliary tree. With the improved techniques associated with modern liver surgery the mortality is now 5 per cent. The median survival is 18 months, with 20 per cent of the patients surviving for 5 years.

Carcinoma of the gall bladder

This is rare in the Western world but there are areas where the incidence is high (in Patna, India, the incidence reaches as high as 9 per cent of biliary tract disease). The tumour is found in less than 1 per cent of gall-bladder operations. In over 90 per cent of instances gallstones are present. The patients are usually in their late 70s, with a female to male ratio of 5:1. The tumour is usually scirrhous, but squamous cell and mixed squamous adenocarcinomas are found. Spread is by direct invasion through the mucosa to the serosa and into the liver, the lymphatics and the veins.

Clinical features

Most present either with an extensive mass in the liver during investigations for jaundice, or at cholecystectomy at the time the histology is received, the tumour being unrecognised by the surgeon.

Treatment and prognosis

Those that are diagnosed at cholecystectomy and confined to the mucosa have a good prognosis. It is debated whether such patients should have a wide excision with resection of adjacent liver and lymph nodes. For those tumours that involve the serosa, the prognosis is poor and chemoradiotherapy is all that can be offered. The survival rate is less than 5 per cent at 5 years and the median survival is 12 months.

Further reading

Blumgart, L.H. (ed.) (1988) *Surgery of the Liver and Biliary Tract*, Churchill Livingstone, Edinburgh.

Carter, D.C., Russell, R.C.G., Pitt, H.A. and Bismuth, H. (eds) (1996) *Rob & Smith's Operative Surgery: Hepatobiliary and Pancreatic Surgery*, Chapman and Hall, London.

Sherlock, S. and Dooley, J. (eds) (1997) *Diseases of the Liver and Biliary System*, 10th edn, Blackwell Science, Oxford.

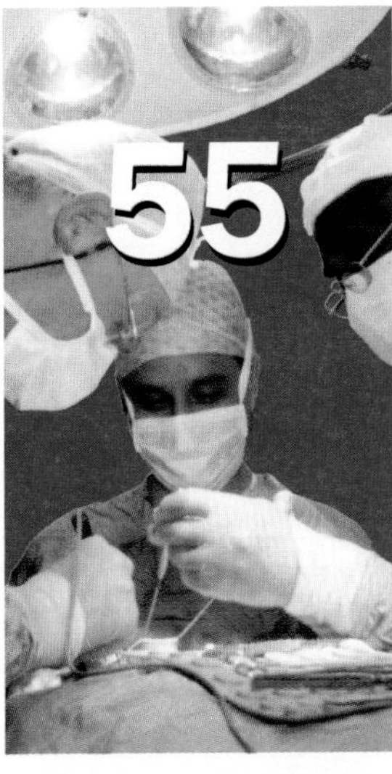

55 The pancreas

Anatomy and physiology

Surgical anatomy

The name 'pancreas' is derived from the Greek '*pan*' (all) and '*kreas*' (flesh). It was originally thought to act as a cushion for the stomach. The gland weighs approximately 80 g and is situated retroperitoneally. It is divided into a head, which occupies 30 per cent of the gland by mass, and a body and tail which comprises 70 per cent of the whole organ. The head lies within the curve of the duodenum overlying the body of the second lumbar vertebra and the vena cava, with more medially the aorta beneath the neck of the gland. The neck of the pancreas is that part which has the superior mesenteric vessels as a posterior relation. Coming off the side of the pancreatic head and passing to the left and behind the superior mesenteric vein is the uncinate process of the pancreas. Behind the neck of the pancreas, near its upper border, the superior mesenteric vein joins the splenic vein to form the portal vein (Figs 55.1 and 55.2).

Fig. 55.1 The posterior relationships of the pancreas.

There are nine key processes that occur during pancreatic embryogenesis (Table 55.1). Malrotation of the ventral bud in the fifth week results in an annular pancreas, while the mode of ductular fusion in the seventh week produces the

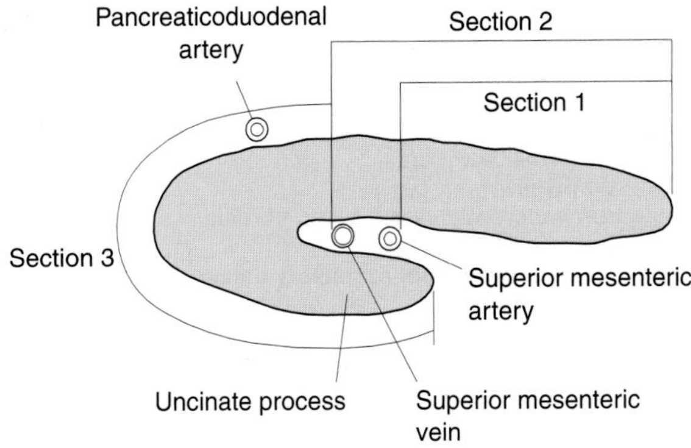

Fig. 55.2 Transverse section of the pancreas: section I – body and tail of pancreas; section II – neck of pancreas; section III – head of pancreas. Note the position of the uncinate process behind the vessels.

Bailey & Love's Short Practice of Surgery, 23rd edition. Edited by R.C.G. Russell, N.S. Williams and C.J.K. Bulstrode. Published in 2000 by Arnold Publishers.

Table 55.1 Steps in the development of the pancreas

1	Day 26	Dorsal pancreatic duct arises from the dorsal side of the duodenum
2	Day 32	Ventral bud arises from the base of the hepatic diverticulum
3	Day 37	Contact occurs between the two buds. Fusion by the end of week 6
4	Week 6	Ventral bud produces head and uncinate process
5	Week 6	Ducts fuse
6	Week 6	Ventral duct (duct of Wirsung) and distal portion of dorsal duct form main duct
7	Week 6	Proximal dorsal duct forms duct of Santorini
8	Month 3	Acini appear
9	Months 3–4	Islets of Langerhans appear and become biologically active

various possible ductular patterns. Between the 12th and 40th weeks of foetal life, the pancreas differentiates into exocrine and endocrine elements. Of the pancreatic mass, 80–90 per cent is composed of exocrine tissue. The primitive ducts and their ductules are responsible for the lobular arrangement of the pancreas. The main pancreatic duct is lined by columnar epithelium which becomes cuboidal in the ductules. Congenital anomalies of the pancreas are varied and arise during the early phase of development (Table 55.2).

Pancreatic acinar tissue is organised into lobules. The main duct ramifies into intralobular and interlobular ducts, ductules and, finally, acini. Acinar cells are clumped around a central lumen to form an acinus which communicates with the duct system. The pancreas thus consists of a network of fine ducts lined by secretory cells. The islets of Langerhans are distributed throughout the pancreas. Islet cells consist of differing cell types: 75 per cent are B cells (producing insulin), 20 per cent A cells (producing glucagon), and the remainder are D cells (producing somatostatin) and a small number of pancreatic polypeptide cells. Within an islet, the B cells form an inner core surrounded by the other cells. Capillaries draining the islet cells drain into the portal vein forming a pancreatic portal system.

'Normal' pancreatic ducts

60%

(a)

Suppression of the accessory duct

Supression of the main duct

(b) (c) (d) (e) (f) (g)

30% 10%

Pancreas divisum

Wirsung branch

Wirsung branch

Fig. 55.3 Variations in the pancreatic ducts: (a) the usual configuration; (b)–(d) progressive depression of the accessory duct (30 per cent); (e)–(g) progressive depression of the main duct (10 per cent); (f) pancreas divisum – the ventral duct drains only the uncinate process.

Table 55.2 Anomalies of the pancreas – those in bold type are the more frequent anomalies encountered in surgical practice

- Aplasia
- Hypoplasia
- Hyperplasia
- Hypertrophy
- Dysplasia
- **Variations and anomalies of the ducts**
  - pancreas divisum
  - rotational anomalies
- **Annular pancreas**
- Pancreatic gall bladder
- **Polycystic disease**
- **Congenital pancreatic cysts, cystic fibrosis**
  - von Hippel–Lindau syndrome
- **Ectopic pancreatic tissue, accessory pancreas**
- Vascular anomalies
- **Choledochal cysts**
- Horseshoe pancreas

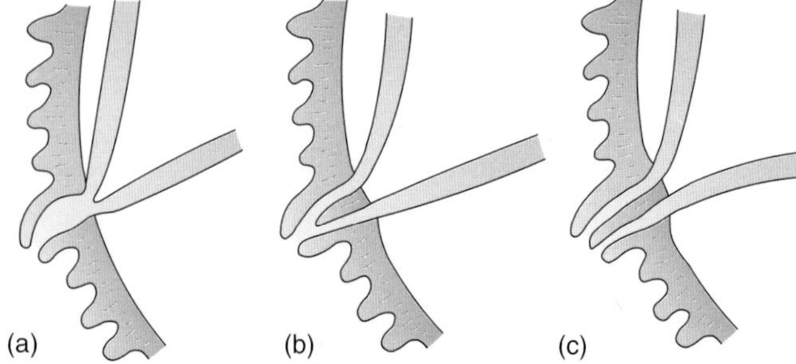

Fig. 55.4 Variations in the relationship of the common bile duct and main pancreatic duct at the duodenal papilla. In (a) there is a common channel with no sphincter mechanism protecting flow between the ducts. In (b) there is a partial common channel, while in (c) there is separation of the two channels. Gallstone pancreatitis is more likely with (a) and (b).

Paul Langerhans, 1847–88. Professor of Pathological Anatomy, Freiberg, Germany.
Johann Georg Wirsung, 1600–43. German physician.

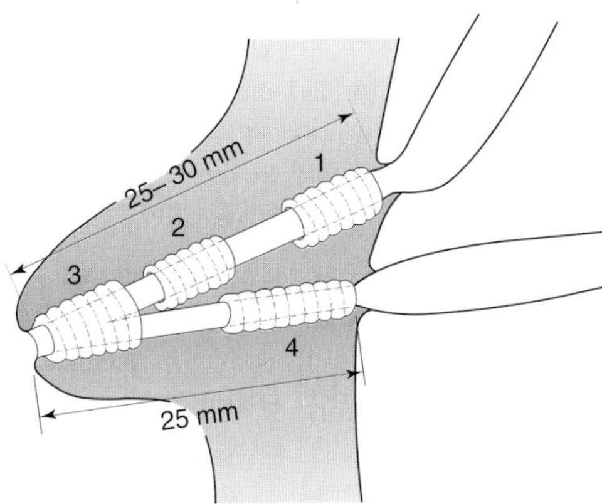

Fig. 55.5 The complexity of the sphincter: (1) superior choledochal sphincter; (2) inferior choledochal sphincter; (3) ampullary sphincter; (4) pancreatic sphincter.

The pancreatic duct anatomy is variable as a result of the primordial bud development. The dorsal duct is expressed in a variable manner in the adult, as outlined in Fig. 55.3. Approximately 10 per cent of patients will have a significant flow from the main duct through the accessory papilla. The anatomy of the main papilla is also variable (Fig. 55.4) with the outlet of each duct protected by a complex sphincter mechanism (Fig. 55.5). Pancreatic anatomy has an implication on disease, and thus a grasp of the development and variations is important in the assessment of the patient.

Surgical physiology

In response to a meal, the pancreas secretes digestive enzymes in an alkaline (pH 8.4) bicarbonate-rich fluid. Spontaneous secretion is minimal, the hormone secretin which is released from the duodenal mucosa evokes a bicarbonate-rich fluid. Cholecystokinin-pancreozymin (CCK) is released from the duodenal mucosa in response to food: CCK produces no increase in the volume of secretion, but is responsible for enzyme secretion. Vagal stimulation increases volume. Protein is synthesised at a greater rate (per gram of tissue) in the pancreas than in any other tissue, with the possible exception of the lactating mammary gland. About 90 per cent of this protein is exported from the acinar cells as a variety of digestive enzymes. Approximately 6–20 g of digestive enzymes enter the duodenum each day. Nascent proteins are synthesised as preproforms and during their transit through the rough endoplasmic reticulum and Golgi cisterni, the newly synthesised proteins undergo modification in a sequence of steps. The proteins move from the rough endothelial endoplasmic reticulum to the Golgi complex, where lysosomes and mature zymogen storage granules containing proteases are stored, and move to the ductal surface of the cell from which they are extruded by exostosis. During this phase the proteolytic enzymes are in an inactive form, the maintenance of which is important in preventing pancreatitis.

Camillo Golgi, 1843–1926. Italian pathologist.

Table 55.3 Investigation of the pancreas

- Serum enzyme levels
- Pancreatic function tests
- Morphology
  - Ultrasound scan
  - Computed tomography
  - Magnetic resonance imaging
  - Positron-emission tomography
  - Endoscopic retrograde cholangiopancreatography
- Plain X-ray
  - Chest
  - Upper abdomen

Investigations

It is possible to obtain information about: (1) pancreatic damage by measuring levels of pancreatic enzymes in body fluids; (2) pancreatic function by measuring bicarbonate and enzymes produced in the pancreatic juice; and (3) morphological abnormality of the parenchyma and duct system by ultrasonography, computerised tomography (CT), magnetic resonance imaging (MRI) and endoscopic retrograde cholangiopancreatography (ERCP) (Table 55.3).

Estimation of pancreatic enzymes in body fluids

When the pancreas is damaged, enzymes such as amylase, lipase, trypsin, elastase and chymotrypsin are released into the serum. Measurement of amylase is the most widely used test of pancreatic damage, and none of the other tests shows better specificity or sensitivity. The serum amylase rises within a few hours of pancreatic damage and declines over the next 4–8 days. A markedly elevated serum level is highly suspicious of acute pancreatitis. Urinary amylase and amylase–creatinine clearance ratios add little to diagnostic accuracy. If confirmation of the diagnosis is required, CT of the pancreas is of greater value.

Pancreatic function tests

Pancreatic secretion in response to a standardised stimulus can provide an assessment of the functional capacity of the gland. The tests can be divided into those where the stimulus to secretion is indirect – produced by the ingestion of a test meal – and those where secretion is directly stimulated by injection of a hormone. Previously, duodenal intubation with the introduction of a triple lumen tube was performed so that the gastric and duodenal juices could be aspirated, and a nonabsorbable marker such as polyethylene glycol used to assess the completeness of the aspiration. A meal stimulus can be used such as in the Lundh test, or secretin and CCK can be administered intravenously to produce both bicarbonate and enzyme stimulation. These tests have been largely abandoned because chronic pancreatitis cannot be diagnosed until

Göran Lundh, Department of Surgery, University of Lund, Lund, Sweden.

over 70 per cent of the gland has been destroyed or there is obstruction to the duct. The more practical test is the nitroblue tetrazolium–para-aminobenzoic acid (NBT PABA) test in which the recovery in the urine of PABA is measured after oral administration. The *p*-aminobenzoic acid is liberated by pancreatic chymotrypsin and excreted in the urine after absorption and liver conjugation. In the pancreolauryl test (PLT), the substrate is represented by fluorescein esterified with two molecules of lauric acid. This complex is hydrolysed by a specific pancreatic aryl-esterase and the fluorescein, liberated into the intestinal lumen, absorbed by the intestinal mucosa and then excreted by the kidneys. This test is cheap, is easy to perform and has a high reliability in recognising severe pancreatic exocrine insufficiency. Careful interpretation of the test results is required in postgastrectomy patients, in patients with extensive intestinal inflammatory disease, or in patients with gastrointestinal or hepatobiliary disease that markedly alters gastrointestinal transit and intestinal absorptive capacity.

A simpler test now available is one which measures faecal elastase levels. Absence indicates chronic pancreatitis and is specific.

Imaging investigations

Ultrasonography

In the hands of a skilled radiologist, ultrasonography can outline the pancreas with accuracy. However, in patients who are fat and those with much gas or fluid in the bowel, the images of the pancreas are poor and an accurate diagnosis cannot be achieved. In the investigation of jaundice ultrasonography remains the initial preferred investigation. Not only will ultrasound determine whether or not the bile duct is dilated, but it will also define the presence or absence of a mass in the pancreas and the coexistence of gallstones or gross disease within the liver such as metastases (Fig. 55.6).

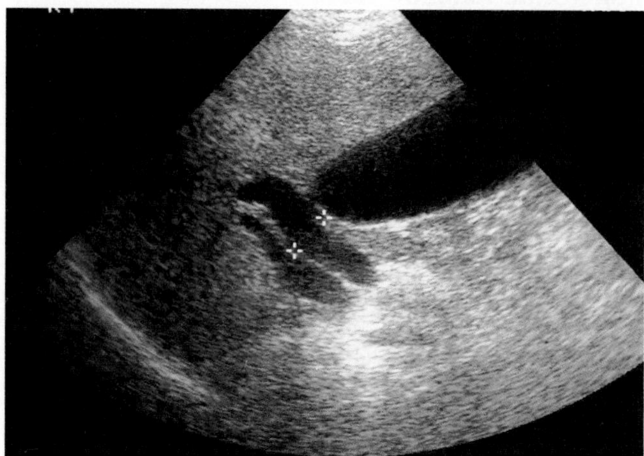

Fig. 55.6 Ultrasound of gall bladder containing biliary 'sand'. The common bile duct has a diameter at the upper end of the normal range. The sand is a possible cause of pancreatitis.

Computerised tomography (Figs 55.7–55.12)

Pancreatic carcinomas of 1–2 cm in size can usually be demonstrated whether in the head, body or tail of the pancreas. A specific pancreatic protocol should be followed using a spiral CT scanner. Following rapid injection of intravenous contrast, scanning is performed at 5-mm intervals in the arterial phase and 10-mm intervals during the venous phase. Prior to injection of contrast an unenhanced CT scan is essential to determine the presence of calcification within the pancreas and gall bladder. The stomach and duodenum

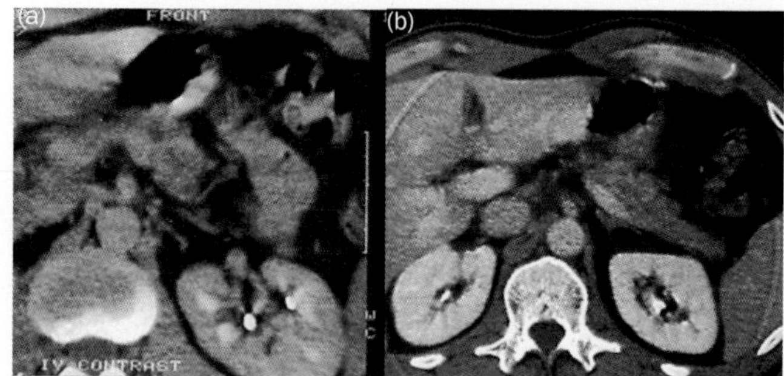

Fig. 55.7 (a) CT of a normal head of pancreas showing a bile duct of normal calibre. (b) CT of the tail of the pancreas with a normal size duct just discernible (*courtesy of Professor W.R. Lees*).

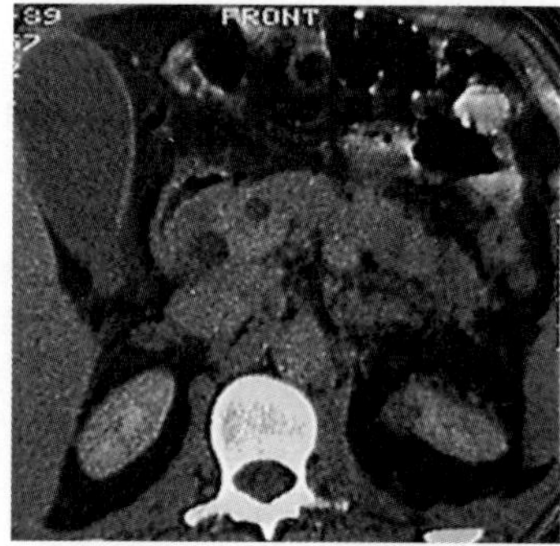

Fig. 55.8 CT of a carcinoma of the pancreas with a dilated bile duct infiltrated by tumour. The gall bladder is distended.

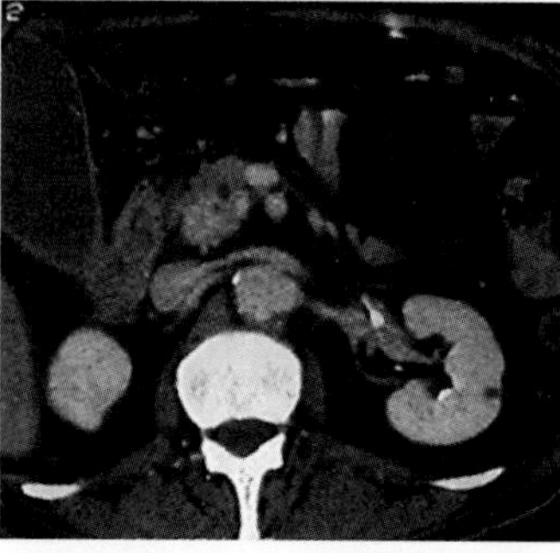

Fig. 55.9 CT of a carcinoma of the pancreas with a markedly enlarged gall bladder to obstruction of the common bile duct by the carcinoma.

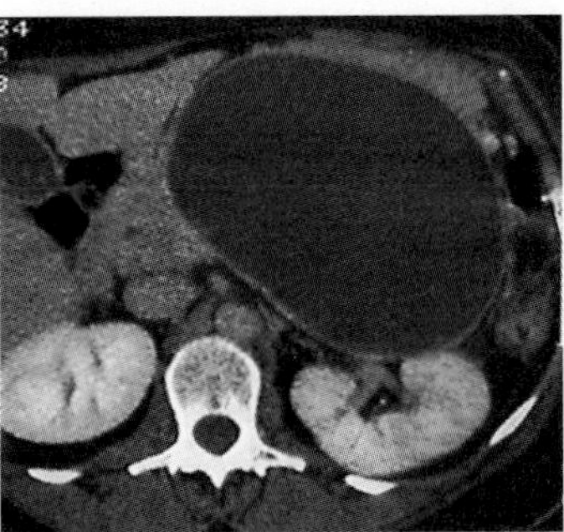

Fig. 55.10 CT of a pseudocyst of the tail of the pancreas.

should be outlined with water and distended to define the duodenal loop. All significant pathologies within the pancreas can be diagnosed on high-quality spiral CT scans. Endocrine tumours which previously could not be imaged can now be seen with clarity (Fig. 55.12) and this is now probably the preferred technique for defining such tumours. CT scanning is also of value in the therapeutic setting to drain cysts or abscesses, or to guide percutaneous biopsies.

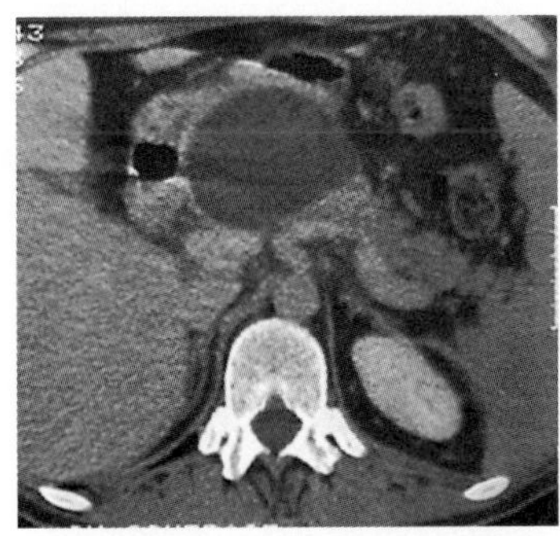

Fig. 55.11 CT of a pseudocyst of the head of the pancreas.

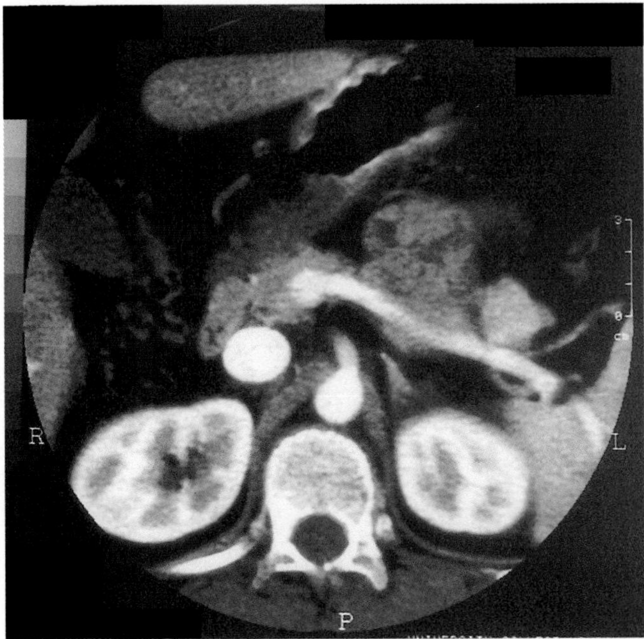

Fig. 55.12 Spiral CT showing a hypervascular insulinoma sitting adjacent to the splenic vein. Local excision of the tumour resulted in normoglycaemia.

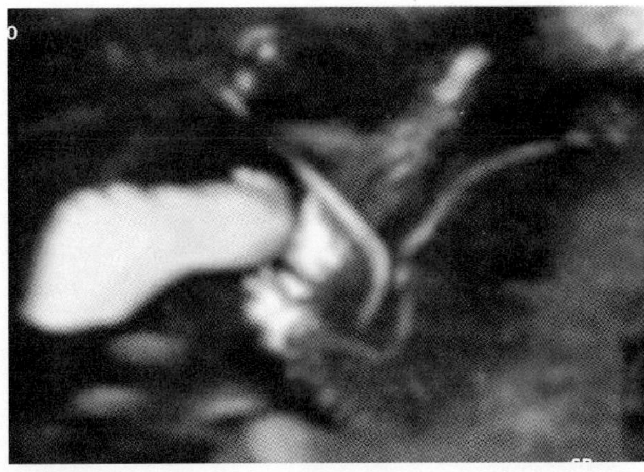

Fig. 55.13 MRI scan showing the bile duct, the gall bladder, the duodenum and the main pancreatic duct. The main duct enters the duodenum by the accessory papilla – pancreas divisum.

Magnetic resonance imaging

With the recent developments in MRI the pancreas can now be clearly displayed in a manner similar to the best CT image. In addition, clear images of the bile duct and the pancreatic duct, together with fluid collections, can be defined. Magnetic resonance pancreatography and cholangiography may well replace diagnostic endoscopic pancreatography and cholangiography. MRI is noninvasive and cheaper (Fig. 55.13). Using special contrast agents flow within a duct can be delineated; using the technique in conjunction with secretin emptying of the pancreatic duct can be demonstrated to show the absence or presence of obstruction.

Endoscopic retrograde cholangiopancreatography

By using this technique with a side-viewing fibre-optic duodenoscope the ampulla of Vater can be clearly seen. Images of contrast injected into the biliary and pancreatic ducts can display the anatomy and pathology of these ducts. Changes seen in chronic pancreatitis include pancreatic duct strictures, dilatation of the main pancreatic duct with stones (Figs 55.14–55.19), abnormalities of pancreatic duct side branches, communication of the pancreatic duct with cysts and bile-duct strictures. In pancreatic carcinoma, the main pancreatic duct may be narrowed or completely obstructed at the site of the tumour with dilatation upstream but with a normal duct system downstream. This, in conjunction with bile-duct obstruction or a stricture, results in the so-called

Abraham Vater, 1684–1751. Professor of Anatomy and Botany, Wittenberg, Germany.

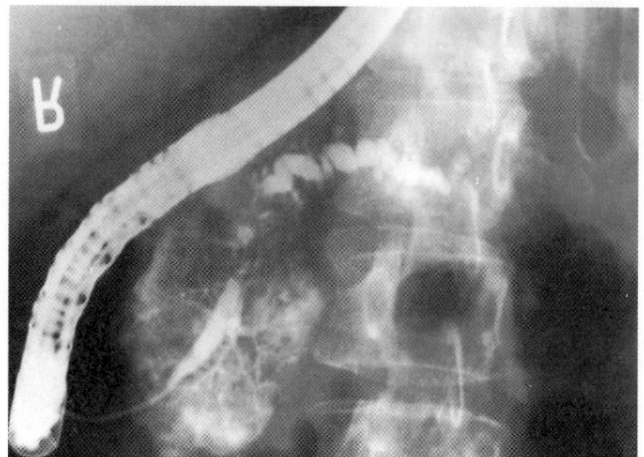

Fig. 55.14 ERCP: pancreatic carcinoma. Irregular stricture of the main pancreatic duct with dilation upstream of obstruction.

'double duct sign'. Collection of bile or pancreatic juice at endoscopy and brushing of these ducts can yield cells which confirm the suspected diagnosis of carcinoma (Fig. 55.20).

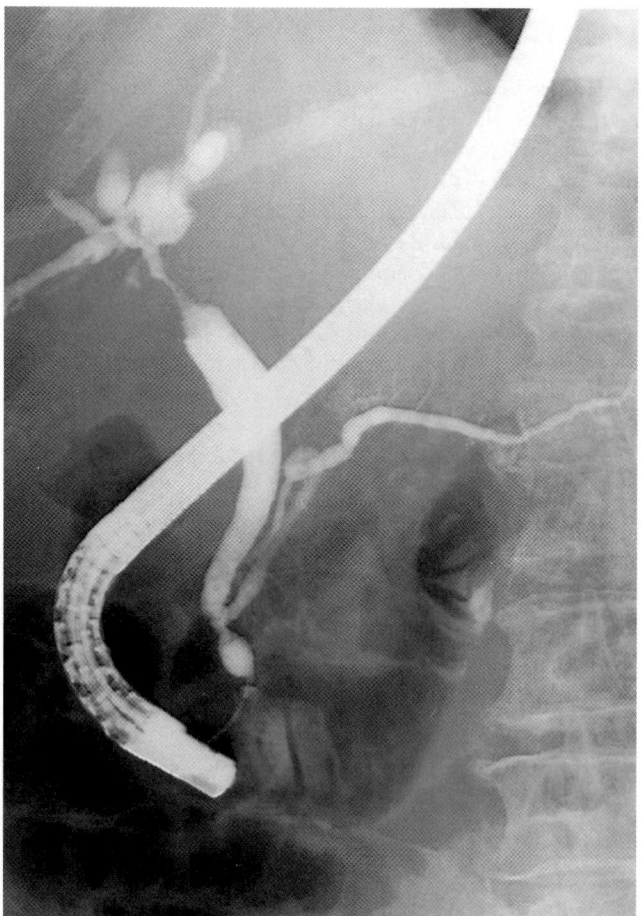

Fig. 55.15 Endoscopic retrograde cannulation of the pancreatic duct and biliary tree depicting a stricture (carcinoma) in the common hepatic duct just distal to the junction of the right and left hepatic ducts.

(a)

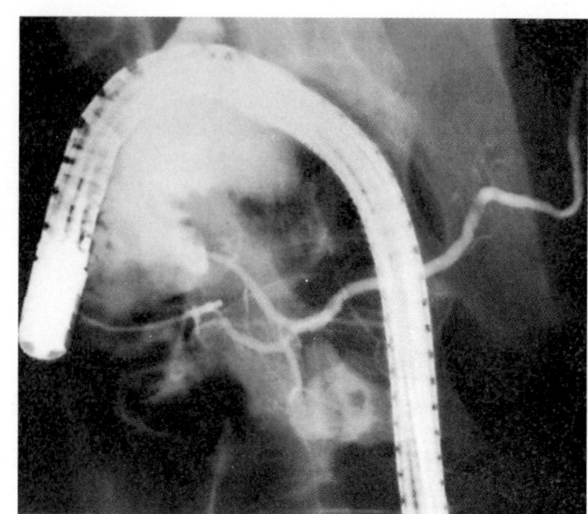

(b)

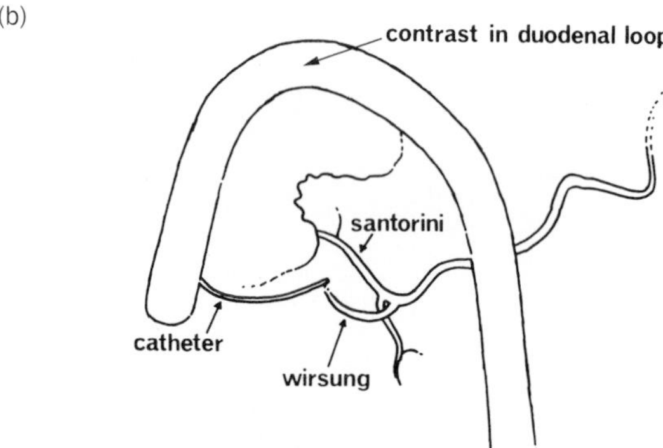

Fig. 55.16 ERCP: normal pancreatic duct with filling of duct of Santorini from the duct of Wirsung.

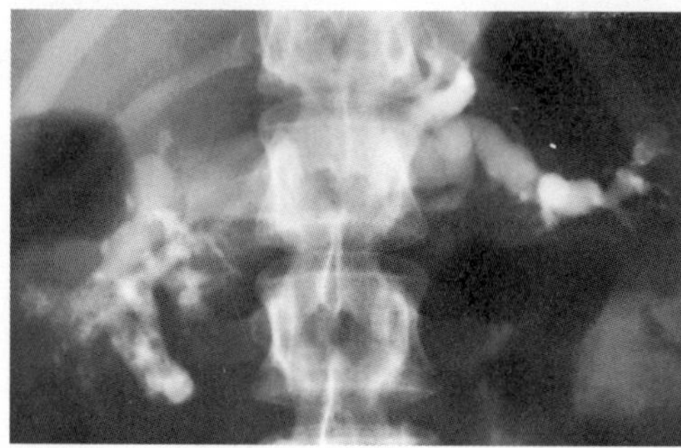

Fig. 55.17 ERCP: chronic pancreatitis. Most of the opacities lie within the duct system and are stones. Gross dilation of ducts in body and tail due to obstruction by stones in head of pancreas.

Plain X-ray

A chest X-ray should never be forgotten as it may show a complication of pancreatic disease (Fig. 55.21). A plain X-ray before contrast studies is essential to delineate calcification (Fig. 55.22)

(a)

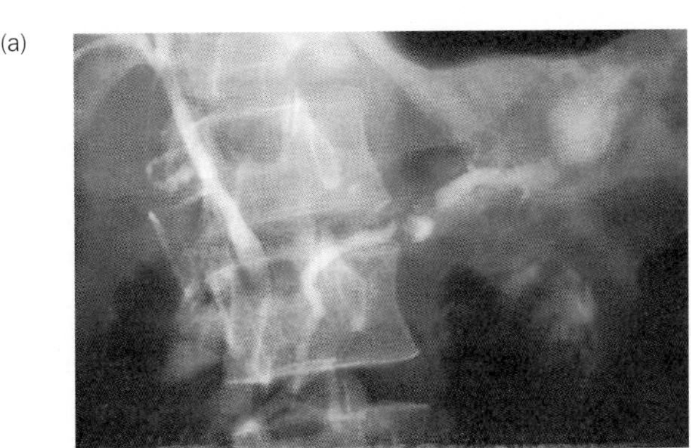

(b)

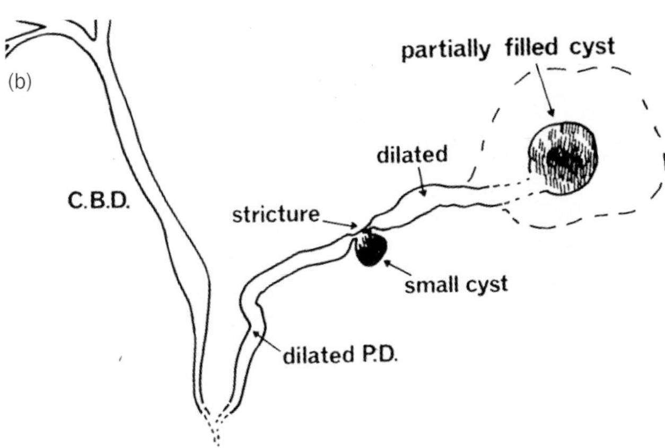

Fig. 55.18 ERCP: relapsing acute pancreatitis. Normal biliary tree. Pancreatogram shows stricture of main duct in the body with distal dilation and cyst formation.

(a)

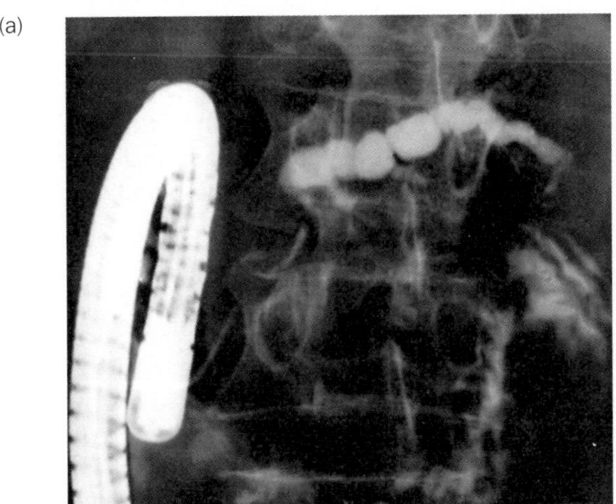

(b)

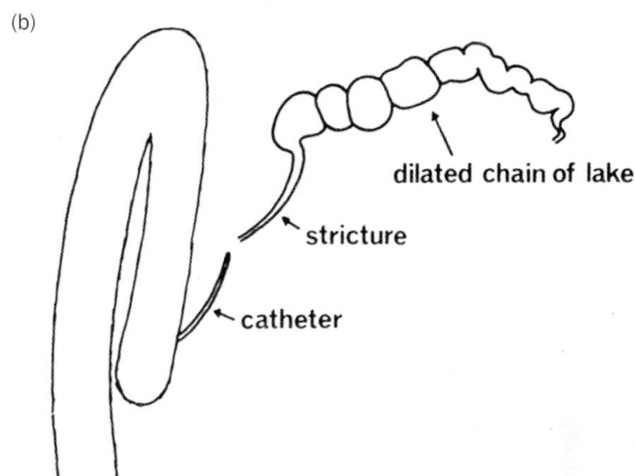

Fig. 55.19 ERCP: chronic pancreatitis. Long stricture of pancreatic duct in the head; distal pancreatic duct shows sacculation with intervening short strictures, 'chain of lakes'.

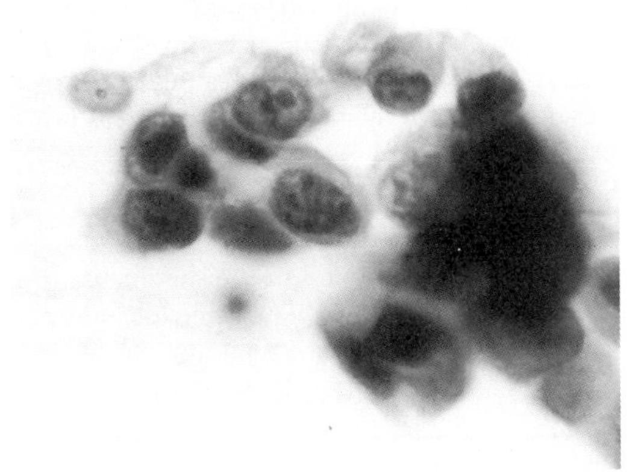

Fig. 55.20 A group of adenocarcinoma cells from the pancreatic juice, collected at the time of ERCP of the patient illustrated in Fig. 55.14.

Congenital abnormalities

See Table 55.2.

Cystic fibrosis

This is inherited as an autosomal recessive condition. The abnormal genes have been defined and diagnosis of the disorder can now be confirmed by DNA testing. It most frequently occurs amongst Caucasians, in whom it is the most commonly occurring inherited disorder (incidence one in 1800 live births). Heterozygous carriers of the gene are asymptomatic but can be identified by DNA analysis. Recent reports suggest that such patients may develop pancreatitis later in life. Such findings may give insight into mechanisms of pancreatic disease.

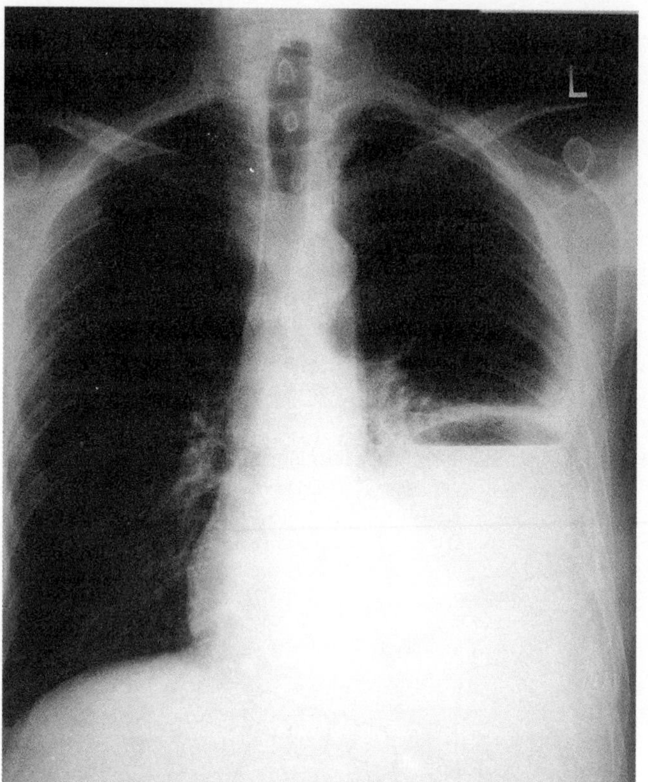

Fig. 55.21 Chest X-ray showing an abscess with a fluid level below the left diaphragm secondary to a pancreatic abscess.

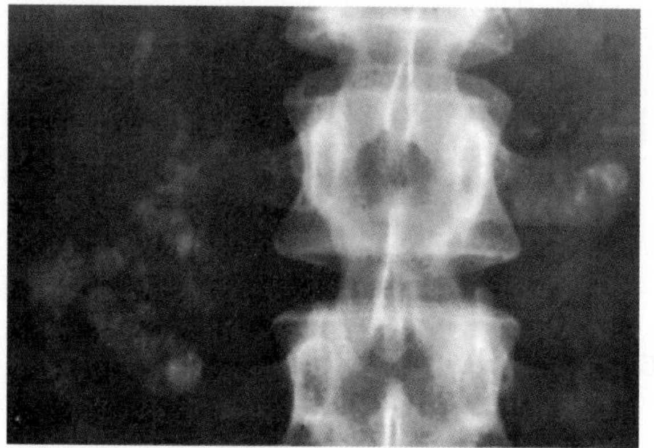

Fig. 55.22 Plain abdominal radiograph: chronic pancreatitis. Multiple opacities in the region of the head and tail of pancreas.

The disorder is the result of a generalised dysfunction of exocrine glands. Glandular secretions have abnormal physiochemical properties resulting in malabsorption caused by pancreatic insufficiency, chronic pulmonary disease arising from plugging of bronchi and bronchioles, and elevated sodium and chloride ion concentrations in sweat. It is the most common cause of chronic lung disease among children in developed countries.

Secretions precipitate in the lumen of the pancreatic duct causing blockage which results in duct ectasia and fatty replacement of exocrine acinar tissue. The islets of Langerhans usually appear normal, but diabetes mellitus can occur in older patients. Steatorrhoea is usually present from birth resulting in stools which are bulky, oily and offensive. At birth the meconium may set in a sticky mass and produce intestinal obstruction (meconium ileus). Although about 15 per cent of patients do not develop clinical steatorrhoea, most show complete exocrine insufficiency.

The earliest clinical signs of cystic fibrosis are poor growth, poor appetite, rancid greasy stools, abdominal distension, persistent cough, emphysematous chest and finger clubbing. Later the liver may become cirrhotic as a result of bile-duct plugging and signs of portal hypertension may appear; cor pulmonale may develop and the appearance of secondary sexual characteristics may be delayed. The mother may have noticed that the child is salty when kissed – levels of sodium and chloride ions in the sweat above 90 mmol/litre confirm the diagnosis.

Treatment is aimed at control of the secondary consequences of the disease. Malabsorption is treated by administration of pancreatic enzyme preparations, and pulmonary function preserved with aggressive physiotherapy and antibiotics. A suitable diet is low in fat but contains added salt to replace the high losses in the sweat. With optimal treatment 80 per cent of the patients diagnosed early should survive to beyond their 19th year.

Annular pancreas

This is the result of failure of complete rotation of the ventral pancreatic bud during development, so that a ring of pancreatic tissue surrounds the second or third part of the duodenum. It is more prevalent in the Down's syndrome child, and in infants with other congenital gut abnormalities. It is one of the causes of obstructive vomiting in the neonate. The vomiting can be bile stained if the duodenal obstruction is below the ampulla of Vater. Peristaltic waves and upper abdominal distension may be seen, and plain abdominal radiographs show the 'double bubble' sign of the interrupted gastroduodenal shadow produced by the rigid ring of pancreatic tissue. The usual treatment is bypass (duodeno-jejunostomy or duodenoduodenostomy). Attempts at resection of the band may result in a pancreatic fistula. The disease may occur in older life as one of the causes of pancreatitis, in which case resection of the head of the pancreas is preferable to lesser procedures.

Ectopic pancreas

Ectopic pancreas can be found in the submucosa in parts of the stomach, duodenum or small intestine (including Meckel's diverticulae), the gall bladder, adjoining the pancreas, for

---

John Langdon Down, 1826–96. English physician.

Johann Friedrich Meckel (The Younger), 1781–1833. Professor of Anatomy and Surgery, Halle, Germany.

example in the hilum of the spleen, or in 2 per cent of carefully conducted necropsies, within the liver. Ectopic pancreas in the wall of the intestine may give rise to symptoms and can be a cause of cysts, but this is extremely rare.

Congenital cystic disease of the pancreas

This sometimes accompanies congenital disease of the kidneys and liver, and occurs as part of the von Hippel–Lindau syndrome.

Injuries to the pancreas

External injury (Fig. 55.23)

Presentation and management

The most frequent presentation of blunt pancreatic trauma is epigastric pain which may be minor at first, with the progressive development of more severe pain due to the sequelae of leakage of pancreatic fluid into the surrounding tissues. A rise in pancreatic amylase occurs in 90 per cent of cases. A CT scan of the pancreas or ultrasound scan will delineate the damage that has occurred to the pancreas. Persisting abdominal pain with signs of peritonitis require careful assessment of the patient, and support by intravenous fluids and a nil oral regime should be instituted. Immediate operation is contraindicated because the bruising associated with the retroperitoneal damage will prevent clear visualisation of the pancreas. It is preferable to manage conservatively, investigate with ultrasound and, once the damage is ascertained, undertake appropriate action. Operation is only indicated if there is disruption of the main pancreatic duct; almost all other patients will resolve with conservative management unless duct stricturing develops leading to recurrent episodes of pancreatitis, in which case the appropriate treatment is resection of the tail of the pancreas up to the site of duct disruption. If the damage is purely confined to the head of the pancreas simple drainage is normally effective; should this fail, however, then a pancreatoduodenectomy may be necessary.

A pancreatic pseudocyst may develop (Fig. 55.24). If the main duct is intact, the cyst should be drained percutaneously. It is now rarely necessary to undertake a cystgastrostomy (Fig. 55.25). If the cyst develops in the presence of complete disruption of the pancreas, there is no alternative but to undertake a distal resection.

Prognosis

The most common cause of death in the immediate period is bleeding, but once the acute phase has passed the mortality and morbidity should be minimal with a complete return to normal activity. The mortality rate of penetrating injury to the pancreas with associated injuries to the surrounding viscera approaches 50 per cent.

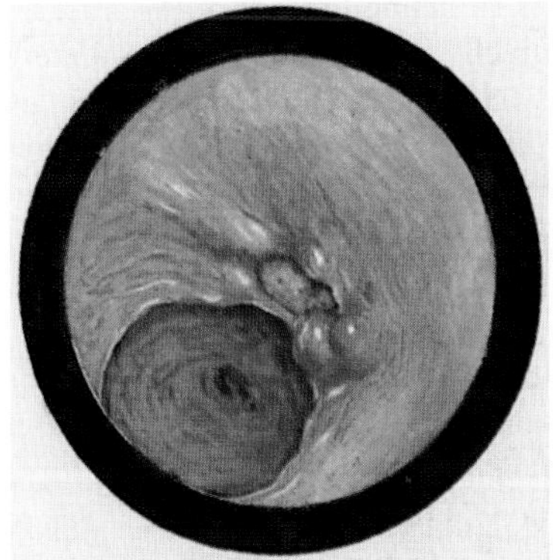

Fig. 55.24 Spiral CT scan showing a large pseudocyst arising as a result of blunt abdominal trauma. The pancreatic duct was found to be intact and the cyst resolved following endoscopic cystgastrostomy.

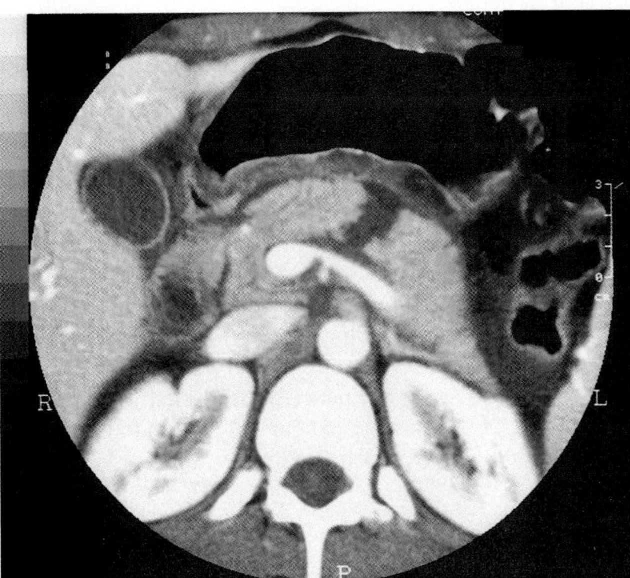

Fig. 55.23 Spiral CT scan showing a pancreatic transection due to a bicycle handlebar injury. A distal pancreatectomy was performed. The patient remains well 4 years later.

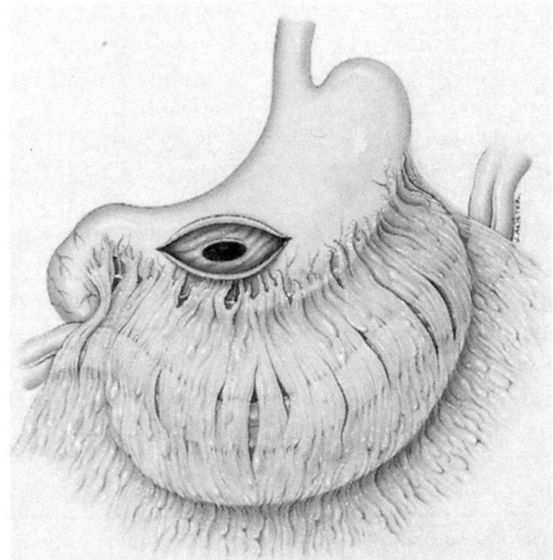

Fig. 55.25 Cystgastrostomy for a pseudopancreatic cyst.

Iatrogenic injury

This can occur in four ways.

- Injury to the tail of the pancreas during splenectomy resulting in a pancreatic fistula.
- Injury to the accessory pancreatic duct (Santorini) which is the main duct in 7 per cent of patients during Billroth II gastrectomy. A pancreatogram performed by cannulating the duct at the time of discovery of such an injury will demonstrate whether it is safe to ligate and divide the duct. If no alternative drainage duct can be demonstrated then the duct should be reanastomosed to the duodenum.
- Attempts at enucleation of islet cell tumours of the pancreas can result in fistulae.
- Duodenal or ampullary bleeding following sphincterotomy. This injury may require duodenotomy to control the bleeding.

Pancreatic fistula

This usually follows operative trauma to the gland, or may occur as a complication of acute or chronic pancreatitis. Management is to define the site of the fistula, the epithelial structure to which it communicates (e.g. external to skin or internal to bowel), and to correct metabolic and electrolyte disturbances. The danger of a pancreatic fistula is that there is digestion of surrounding structures by activated pancreatic enzymes causing local damage, perforation, bleeding and digestion of the skin. Immediate control of the fistula can be obtained by a nil by mouth regime, the use of octreotide and adequate drainage of the fistula with protection of the skin. Investigation of the cause of the fistula is required and, usually, once the cause is determined appropriate remedies can be introduced. Frequently the cause is related to obstruction within the pancreatic duct which can be overcome by the insertion of a stent or catheter endoscopically into the pancreatic duct, and waiting for closure of the fistula while supporting the patient by a conservative regime with parenteral nutritional support and good nursing. As a principle, in the management of any fistula, the underlying cause for the fistula must be treated before closure will be effective.

Pancreatitis

Pancreatitis is primarily due to the intracellular activation of trypsinogen to trypsin by numerous stimuli which, as yet, have not been fully elucidated. The recent discovery that hereditary pancreatitis is related to an abnormal cationic trypsinogen due to an abnormality in the long arm of chromosome 7, in which histidine replaces arginine allowing in certain instances intracellular activation of trypsinogen to trypsin, elucidates in a small way intracellular mechanisms which can occur to cause this disease. In hereditary pancreatitis the same defect can give rise both to acute and to chronic pancreatitis. It is probable that acute pancreatitis is but a phase of chronic pancreatitis; the two are inter-related. For clinical purposes it is useful to divide pancreatitis into acute, which presents as an emergency, and chronic which is a prolonged and frequently life-long disorder resulting from the development of fibrosis within the pancreas.

Acute pancreatitis is defined as an acute condition presenting with abdominal pain and usually associated with raised pancreatic enzyme levels in the blood or urine as a result of inflammatory disease of the pancreas. Acute pancreatitis may recur.

Chronic pancreatitis is defined as a continuing inflammatory disease of the pancreas characterised by irreversible morphological change typically causing pain and/or permanent loss of function. Many patients with chronic pancreatitis have exacerbations, but the condition may be completely painless.

Acute pancreatitis

Incidence

Acute pancreatitis accounts for 3 per cent of all cases of abdominal pain admitted to hospital in the UK. The incidence varies from 21 to 283 cases per million population. In Japan the best estimate is that of 121 cases per million population. The disease may occur at any age, with a peak in the young male and the older female. The mortality has remained unaltered at 10–15 per cent over the past 20 years. About one-third of patients die in the early phase of an attack from multiple organ failure, while deaths occurring after the first week of onset are due to infective complications. Eighty per cent of patients will have a mild attack of pancreatitis in which the mortality is around 1 per cent, while in those who have a severe attack of pancreatitis the mortality varies from 20 to 50 per cent.

Aetiology

The two major causes of acute pancreatitis are biliary calculi, which occurs in 50–70 per cent of patients, and alcohol, which occurs in 25 per cent. The remaining cases may be due to rare causes or be idiopathic (Table 55.4).

The importance of aetiology is that removal of the causative factor can avoid further episodes of pancreatitis. Thus, in a patient who has gallstone pancreatitis, the gallstones should be removed as soon as the patient is fit to undergo surgery and, preferably, before discharge from hospital.

Clinical presentation

There are no pathognomonic symptoms and signs, but pain is usually the cardinal symptom. It characteristically develops quickly, reaching maximum intensity within minutes rather than hours, and persists for hours or even days. The pain is

Giovanni Domenico Santorini, 1681–1737. Professor of Anatomy and Medicine, Venice, Italy.
Christian A. Billroth, b. 1829. Austrian surgeon.

Table 55.4 Clinical associations and acute pancreatitis

Clinical setting	*Proposed aetiologies*
Alcoholism	Diet, malnutrition Direct toxicity Hypersecretion Duct obstruction or reflux Hyperlipidaemia
Gallstone	Bile reflux (common channel) Pancreatic duct hypertension or obstruction Reflux of infected fluid Reflux of activated enzymes
Ischaemia	Hypoxaemia Free radical production Vascular endothelial injury
Drug induced	Direct toxicity Altered secretions
Hyperparathyroidism	Accelerated conversion of trypsinogen to trypsin
Hypercalcaemia	Calculus formation Direct toxicity Disordered secretion
Trauma	Disruption of parenchyma or ducts
ERCP	Ductal disruption and enzyme extravasation
Mechanical obstruction	Ductal hypertension and disruption
Pancreas divisum	Ductal obstruction
Autoimmune	(?) Vasculitis Drug effects
Hereditary	Unknown
Infectious	(?) Direct toxicity
Malnutrition	(?) Vitamin or mineral deficiency
Scorpion bite	(?) Anticholinergic effects
Idiopathic	None

frequently severe or even agonising, it is refractory to the usual doses of analgesics, and constant in nature and intensity. Pain is usually experienced first in the epigastrium but may be localised to either upper quadrant or felt diffusely throughout the abdomen. There is radiation to the back in about 50 per cent of patients and some patients may gain relief by sitting or leaning forwards. The suddenness of onset may simulate a perforated peptic ulcer, while biliary colic or acute cholecystitis can be mimicked if the pain is maximal in the right upper quadrant. Radiation to the chest can simulate myocardial infarction, pneumonia or pleuritic pain. In fact, acute pancreatitis can mimic most causes of the acute abdomen and should seldom be discounted in differential diagnosis. The diagnosis must always be considered in a patient who suddenly develops shock or anuria regardless of whether they have abdominal pain.

Acute pancreatitis should be suspected in the patient who:

- develops marked abdominal pain, fever or unexplained shock following abdominal surgery;
- presents with diabetic coma and shock;
- has clinical features suggesting myocardial infarction with abdominal distension.

Nausea, vomiting and retching are usually marked accompaniments. Vomiting is often frequent and persistent, and retching may persist despite the stomach being kept empty by nasogastric aspiration. Hiccoughs can be troublesome and may be due to gastric distension or irritation of the diaphragm.

On examination the appearance may be that of a patient who is well or, at the other extreme, one who is gravely ill with profound shock, toxicity and confusion. Tachypnoea is common, tachycardia is usual and hypotension may be present. The body temperature is often normal or even subnormal, but frequently rises as inflammation develops. Mild icterus can be caused by biliary obstruction in gallstone pancreatitis, and an acute swinging pyrexia suggests cholangitis. Bleeding into the fascial planes can produce blueish discoloration of the flanks (Grey Turner sign) or umbilicus (Cullen's sign). Neither sign is pathognomonic of acute pancreatitis; in fact Cullen's sign was first described with rupture of an ectopic pregnancy. Subcutaneous fat necrosis may produce small red tender nodules on the skin of the legs. Abdominal examination may reveal distension due to ileus or, more rarely, ascites with shifting dullness. A mass can develop in the epigastrium due to inflammation. There is usually muscle guarding in the upper abdomen, although marked rigidity is unusual. A pleural effusion is present in 10–20 per cent of patients. Pulmonary oedema and pneumonitis are also described and may give rise to the differential diagnosis of pneumonia or myocardial infarction. The patient may be confused and exhibit the signs of metabolic derangement together with hypoxaemia.

Investigations

A serum amylase four times above normal is indicative of the disease. Plain abdominal X-ray findings include a generalised or local ileus (sentinel loop), a colon 'cut-off' sign and a renal 'halo' sign. Occasional helpful, but nondiagnostic, signs include calcified gallstones and pancreatic calcification. A chest X-ray may show a spectrum of changes depending on the disease severity. A pleural effusion is present in 20 per cent, and in severe cases a diffuse alveolar interstitial shadowing may suggest an acute respiratory distress syndrome.

Ultrasound scanning. The swollen pancreas may be detected but the gland is poorly visualised in 25–50 per cent of cases. Ultrasound is valuable in detecting free peritoneal fluid, gallstones, dilatation of the common bile duct and, occasionally, other pathologies such as abdominal aortic aneurysm.

If doubt remains a CT scan should be performed in order to determine the diagnosis.

George Grey Turner, 1877–1951. Professor of Surgery, Postgraduate Medical School, London, England. Formerly Professor of Surgery, University of Durham, England.

Thomas Stephen Cullen, 1868–1953. Professor of Gynaecology, Johns Hopkins University, Baltimore, Maryland, USA.

Table 55.5 Basis of factor scoring systems to predict the severity of acute pancreatitis: in both systems disease is classified as severe when three or more factors are present

Ranson score	*Glasgow scale*
On admission	
Age > 55 years	Age > 55 years
White blood cell count = 16 × 10^9/litre	White blood cell count > 15 × 10^9/litre
Blood glucose > 10 mmol/litre	Blood glucose > 10 mmol/litre (no diabetic history)
LDH > 700 units/litre	Serum urea > 16 mmol/litre (no response to intravenous fluids)
AST > 250 Sigma Frankel units per cent	Arterial oxygen saturation (PaO_2) < 60 mmHg
Within 48 hours	
Blood urea nitrogen rise > 5 mg per cent	Serum calcium < 2.0 mmol/litre
Arterial oxygen saturation (PaO_2) < 60 mmHg	Serum albumin < 32 g/litre
Serum calcium < 2.0 mmol/litre	LDH > 600 units/litre
Haematocrit fall > 10 per cent	AST / ALT > 600 units/litre
Base deficit > 4 mmol/litre	
Fluid sequestration > 6 litres	

AST, aspartate aminotranferase; ALT, alanine aminotransferase; LDH, lactic dehydrogenase; PaO_2, arterial oxygen tension.

Laparotomy. To misdiagnose acute pancreatitis is not uncommon because the presentation is so variable that even the shrewdest clinician can be mistaken. The appearances at laparotomy are characteristic (Fig. 55.26).

Management

On account of the difference in outcome between patients with mild and severe disease it is important to define that group of patients who will develop severe pancreatitis. Various scoring systems have been introduced such as the Ranson and Glasgow scoring systems (Table 55.5). A C-reactive protein level greater than 210 mg/litre in the first 4 days of the attack or 120 mg/litre at the end of the first week has a predictive performance similar to that of the other criteria and has the added benefit of simplicity. Similarly, the Apache II scoring system, well used in intensive care units, can be applied; a score of 9 or more indicates a severe attack but excludes many with a lower score who will develop complications. An Apache score of 6 or more will include 95 per cent of all those who develop a complication.

If after initial assessment a patient is considered to have a mild attack of pancreatitis, a conservative approach is indicated with nil by mouth, intravenous fluid administration and frequent, but noninvasive, observation. However, if the patient develops a severe attack of pancreatitis then a more aggressive approach is required with the patient being admitted to a high-dependency or an intensive care unit. The patient is monitored invasively to ensure homeostasis of the cardiovascular, respiratory and renal systems. In the mild attack antibiotics are not indicated unless there is evidence of infection. There is no indication for pharmacological or therapeutic treatments, and CT scanning is unnecessary unless there is evidence of deterioration. The management of the severe attack involves full resuscitation, and strict asepsis should be observed in the placement of all monitoring lines. If there is evidence of cardiocirculatory compromise then a Swan–Ganz catheter should be inserted in order to measure

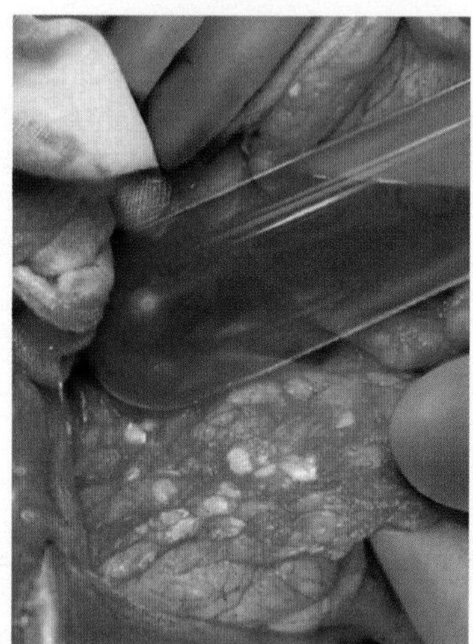

Fig. 55.26 Widespread fat necrosis of omentum. A test-tube has been filled with blood-stained peritoneal fluid. This specimen was rich in amylase. Fat necroses are dull, opaque, yellow-white areas suggestive of drops of wax. They are most abundant in the vicinity of the pancreas, but are widespread in the greater omentum and the mesentry. At necroscopy, they can sometimes be demonstrated beneath the pleura and pericardium, and even in the subsynovial fat of the knee joint. Fat necroses consist of small islands of saponification caused by the liberation of lipase, which splits into glycerol and fatty acids. Free fatty acids combine with calcium to form soaps = fat necrosis (*courtesy of G.D. Adhia, FRCS, Bombay*).

John Ranson. Professor of Surgery, New York University School of Medicine, New York, USA.

H.J.C. Swan, b. 1922. Professor of Medicine, UCLA School of Medicine, Director of Cardiology, Cedar Sinai Medical Center, Los Angeles, California, USA.

William Ganz, b. 1919. Professor of Medicine, UCLA School of Medicine, Senior Research Scientist, Cedars Sinai Medical Center, Los Angeles, California, USA.

pulmonary artery wedge pressure, cardiac output and systemic resistance (see Chapter 4). Regular arterial blood gas analysis is essential as the onset of hypoxia and acidosis may be detected late by clinical means alone. The techniques evolved in the critical care environment should be applied to the patient with pancreatitis. The patient should be made comfortable, appropriately sedated and adequate analgesics given. Specific therapy such as the administration of aprotinin, somatostatin and platelet-activating factor inhibitors has failed to improve prognosis in numerous clinical trials and should not be given. There is some evidence to support the use of prophylactic antibiotics in the prevention of local and other septic complications. Intravenous cefuroxime or imipenem is advised. If gallstones are the aetiology of severe pancreatitis, an urgent ERCP is indicated to exclude the presence of a stone stuck in the ampulla of Vater if there is no improvement in the general condition of the patient within 48 hours. The presence of cholangitis with abnormal liver function tests is an indication for urgent endoscopic intervention.

Table 55.6 Complications of acute pancreatitis

Systemic	*Local*
Cardiovascular	Phlegmon
Pulmonary	Oedema
Renal	Effusion
Haematological	Ascites
Metabolic	Infected effusion
Neurological	Pseudocyst
Gastrointestinal	Pancreatic abscess
	Necrosis

Table 55.7 Criteria for defining systems failure in acute pancreatitis

Systemic	*Local*
Cardiac	Hypotension, tachycardia > 130 beats/minute, arrhythmias; electrocardiogram changes
Pulmonary	PO_2 < 60 mmHg Adult respiratory distress syndrome
Renal	Urine output < 40 ml/hour Rising blood urea and creatinine
Metabolic	Low calcium, magnesium, albumin
Haematological	Falling haematocrit, disseminated intravascular coagulation
Neurological	Irritability, confusion, localising signs
Gastrointestinal	Severe ileus with fluid sequestration

Complications

General. Pancreatitis may involve all organs of the body (Tables 55.6 and 55.7) and present demands on the surgeon beyond his or her skills. Those patients who develop systemic complications should be managed by a multidisciplinary team. There is no role for surgery during the initial period of resuscitation and stabilisation. The full care associated with critical care medicine is applied to these patients, and surgical intervention is only contemplated in the patient who deteriorates following successful stabilisation. Once the presence of infected necrosis is suspected and confirmed, an appropriate débridement may be performed. The only other indication for intervention is the presence of cholangitis, in which case an endoscopic sphincterotomy should be performed.

Local. Once the acute phase has been survived, usually by the end of the first week, and major organ failure is under control, then local complications become pre-eminent in the management of these patients. An awareness of these complications is aided by carefully following the course of the patient, and if clinical resolution does not take place a CT scan should be performed to enable definition of any abnormality present. Such abnormalities should be re-imaged at intervals until there is clear evidence of regression. If a fluid collection or abscess persists then drainage, preferably under radiological control, is indicated.

Definitions

Acute fluid collection. This occurs early in the course of acute pancreatitis and is located in or near the pancreas. The wall encompassing the collection is ill defined.

Acute pseudocyst. A collection of pancreatic juice enclosed in a wall of fibrous or granulation tissue that arises following an attack of acute pancreatitis. Formation of a pseudocyst requires 4 weeks or more from the onset of acute pancreatitis (Figs 55.27 and 55.28).

Pancreatic necrosis. A diffuse or focal area of nonviable parenchyma which is typically associated with peripancreatic fat necrosis. The onset of infection results in infected necrosis which is associated with a trebling of the mortality rate.

Pancreatic abscess. A circumscribed intra-abdominal collection of pus, usually in proximity to the pancreas containing little or no pancreatic necrosis.

Pancreatic effusion. An encapsulated collection of fluid arising as a consequence of acute pancreatitis, typically in the pleural cavity.

Pancreatic ascites. Chronic generalised peritoneal enzyme-rich effusion usually associated with pancreatic duct disruption.

Pseudoaneurysm. Pseudoaneurysm is a false aneurysm of a major peripancreatic vessel confined as a clot by the surrounding tissues and often associated with infection. Recurrent bleeding is common, often culminating in fatal haemorrhage.

Management of local complications

Complications in pancreatic disease are serious and carry a significant mortality. The prime role in the management of acute pancreatitis is that of the conservative approach. If fluid collections cause symptoms or impair function then percutaneous or transgastric drainage is appropriate. Sterile necrotic material should not be drained. The only indication for

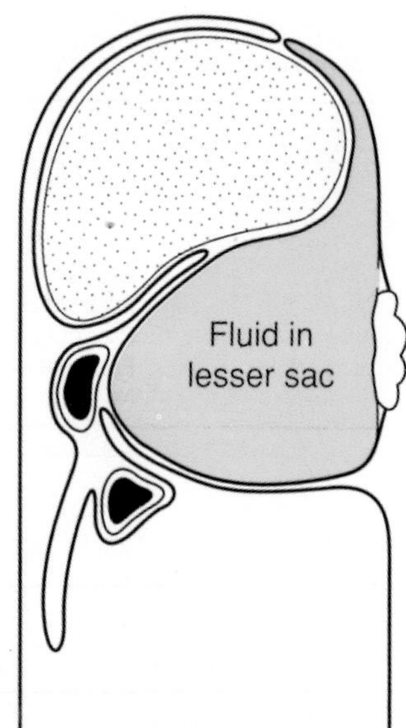

Fig. 55.27 Pseudopancreatic cyst.

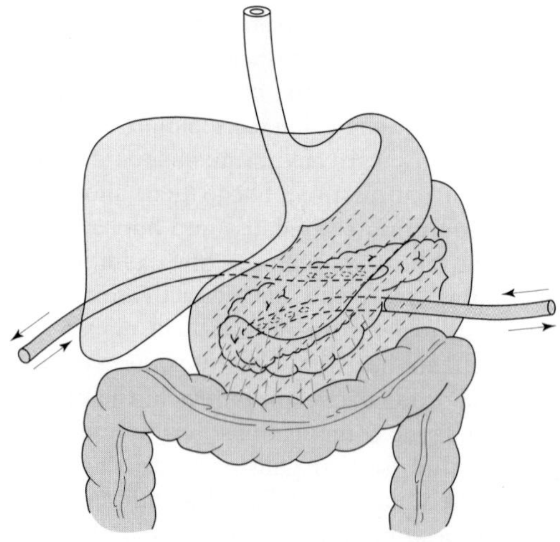

Fig. 55.29 Continuous postoperative closed lavage of the lesser sac as advised by Beger. Lavage is carried out through several double-lumen and single-lumen catheters. Each time 1 litre of saline is infused through and then drained over a period of hours, and the process repeated.

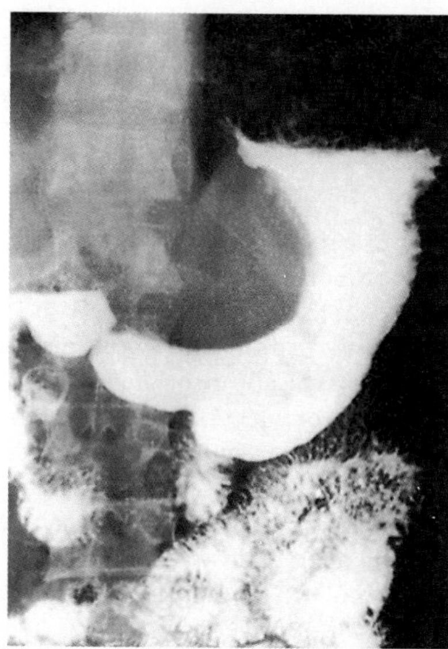

Fig. 55.28 Barium meal. Pseudocyst displacing stomach (*courtesy of Dr V.K. Kapoor, Delhi*).

operative intervention in acute pancreatitis is the presence of an abscess related to necrosis in or around the pancreas. All other complications can be managed conservatively and, indeed, some authorities suggest that even an infected necrotic pancreas can be managed conservatively with radiological drainage. To determine whether a collection of peripancreatic oedema and fluid is necrotic and infected, a CT scan should be performed and a needle passed into the necrotic area under CT guidance, choosing a path that does not traverse hollow viscera. If the aspirate is infected and the patient's condition deteriorating, then a laparotomy with débridement of the dead tissue around the pancreas is appropriate. Because the process is progressive further necrotic tissue may form, and the abscess cavity can either be drained and flushed (Beger) (Fig. 55.29) or repeated laparotomies performed until there is a clean granulating cavity (Bradley).

Some of these patients are ill for long periods of time. Nutritional support is essential. During the early phase of disease parenteral nutrition is important and no advantage has yet been shown for early enteral nutrition. However, once the phase of paralytic ileus has been passed it is appropriate to commence nasojejunal feeding or feeding via a jejunostomy placed in those who have undergone laparotomy. This has the effect of reducing the risk of sepsis from parenteral feeding, and enteral feeding restores the gut mucosal barrier preventing bacterial translocation through the damaged mucosa.

Prognosis of acute pancreatitis

For the patient with an acute mild episode the mortality should be less than 1 per cent, while for the patient with a severe attack 20–25 per cent mortality is anticipated. For those who have infected necrosis a mortality of up to 50 per cent can be anticipated. There is a clear responsibility before the patient is discharged to determine the aetiology of the attack of pancreatitis. Gallstones must be treated, and the other causes, listed in Table 55.4, must be excluded. The failure to remove a predisposing factor could lead to a second attack of pancreatitis, which could be fatal.

Chronic pancreatitis

Chronic pancreatitis is a chronic inflammatory disease in which there is irreversible progressive destruction of pancreatic tissue. Its clinical course is characterised by a dynamic progressive fibrosis of the pancreas. In the early stages of its evolution it is frequently complicated by attacks of acute pancreatitis that are responsible for recurrent pain which may be the only clinical symptom. The incidence of chronic pancreatitis in a prospective study in Copenhagen was 8.2 new cases per 100 000 population per year, with a prevalence of 27.4 cases per 100 000. The incidence rates in retrospective European, North American and Japanese studies range from two to 10 cases per 100 000 population per year. The disease occurs more frequently in men (male to female ratio of 4:1) and the mean age of onset is about 40 years.

Pathology and aetiology

At the onset of the disease when symptoms have developed the pancreas may appear normal. Later the pancreas enlarges and becomes hard as a result of fibrosis. The ducts become distorted and dilated with areas both of stricture formation and of ectasia. Calcified stones weighing from a few milligrams to 200 mg may form within the ducts. The ducts may become occluded with a gelatinous proteinaceous fluid and debris-deformed cysts. Histologically, the lesions affect the lobules producing ductular metaplasia and atrophy of acini, hyperplasia of duct epithelium and interlobular fibrosis. The most frequent cause of chronic pancreatitis is a high alcohol consumption. Other causes are pancreatic duct obstruction resulting from stricture formation after trauma, acute pancreatitis or even occlusion of the duct by pancreatic cancer. Hereditary pancreatitis, infantile malnutrition and a large unexplained idiopathic group make up the remainder. Amongst the idiopathic group there are those who live in warm climates such as Kerala in southern India, and appear to have a high incidence of pancreatitis. Here the pancreatitis begins at a young age, is associated with a high incidence of diabetes mellitus and stone formation is frequent. The importance of hereditary pancreatitis and pancreatitis occurring at a young age is that there is an undoubtedly increased risk of the development of pancreatic cancer, particularly if the patient smokes tobacco heavily.

Clinical features

Pain is the outstanding symptom in the majority of patients. The site of pain depends to some extent on the main focus of the disease. If the disease is mainly in the head of the pancreas then epigastric and right subcostal pain is common, while if it is limited to the left side of the pancreas then left subcostal and back pain are the presenting manifestations. In some patients the back pain predominates, while in others the pain is more diffuse. Radiation to the shoulder, usually the left shoulder, occurs. Nausea is common during attacks, and vomiting may occur. The pain is dull and gnawing. The pain is both continuous and episodic, in that severe bouts of pain may occur superimposed on background discomfort. All of the complications of acute pancreatitis can occur with chronic pancreatitis. Because of the pain weight loss is common, in that the patient does not feel like eating. The pain prevents sleep and time off work is frequent. The number of hospital admissions for acute exacerbations is a pointer towards the severity of the disease. Analgesic use–abuse is frequent. This, too, gives an indication of the severity of the disability. The patient's lifestyle will gradually be destroyed by pain, analgesic dependence, weight loss and inability to work. Complications frequently bring the patient to the attention of the surgeon. Infection is not infrequent, possibly related to the increasing incidence of diabetes mellitus with time. Loss of exocrine function will occur leading to steatorrhoea which can be debilitating without supplementation, whilst loss of endocrine function and the development of diabetes are not uncommon, and the incidence increases as the disease progresses.

Investigation

Only in the early stages of the disease will there be a rise in serum amylase. Pancreatic function tests merely confirm the presence of pancreatic insufficiency or that more than 70 per cent of the gland has been destroyed. Steatorrhoea affects more than 30 per cent of patients with chronic pancreatitis.

The prime investigation is either an MRI scan or a CT scan which will show the outline of the gland, the main area of damage and the possibilities for surgical correction. An MR cholangiogram will show the presence of biliary obstruction, and an MR pancreatogram the state of the pancreatic duct. An ERCP or a percutaneous pancreatogram (Fig. 55.30) can elucidate the anatomy of the duct and, in conjunction with the whole organ morphology, determine the type of operation required, if operative intervention is indicated.

Treatment

A diet low in fat and with no alcohol is advised. Pancreatic enzyme supplementation may reduce the frequency of painful crises. Attention must be paid to nutrition to ensure that the patient gains weight and takes an adequately varied and nutritionally appropriate diet. The use of morphine

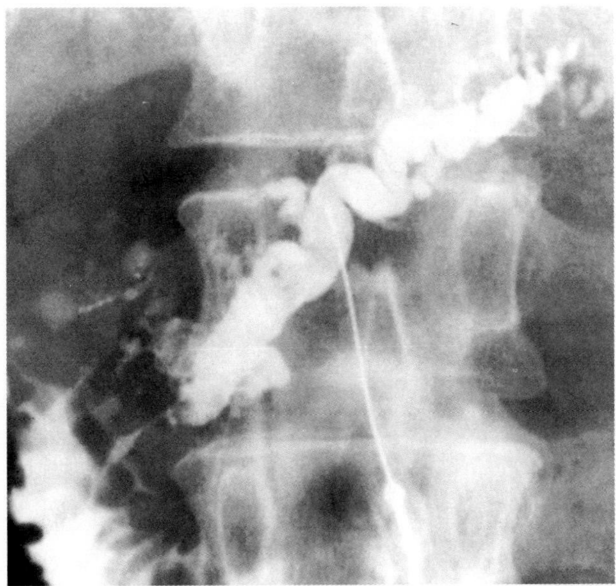

Fig. 55.30 A percutaneous pancreatogram showing a markedly dilated pancreatic duct with a stricture near the ampulla and stones in the duct.

should be avoided and tobacco smoking curtailed. There is no single therapeutic agent which has been shown to relieve symptoms, although the use of antioxidants to mop up free oxygen radicals has been tried.

The role of surgery is in overcoming obstruction and removing mass lesions. Most patients have a mass in the head of the pancreas, for which a resection of the head of the pancreas either by a pancreatoduodenectomy or a Beger procedure is appropriate. If the duct is markedly dilated, then a longitudinal pancreatojejunostomy or Frey procedure can be of value (Fig. 55.31). The rare patient with disease limited to the tail will be cured by a distal pancreatectomy.

Prognosis

Correctly chosen surgery will relieve symptoms in 75 per cent of patients provided that the aetiological factor is removed. Development of pancreatic cancer is a risk in those who have had the disease more than 20 years. New symptoms or a change in the pattern of symptoms should be investigated and development of cancer excluded.

Carcinoma of the pancreas

Pancreatic cancer is the eighth most common cancer causing death in the UK. The incidence is 10 cases per 100 000 population per year. The incidence has risen steadily over the last 25 years, until 5 years ago when it levelled off. The disease is a disease of ageing, with the average age of death in men being 74 years and that in women 79 years. It affects men and women to the same degree. Predisposing factors are tobacco smoking and chronic pancreatitis. No other relationships have been elucidated.

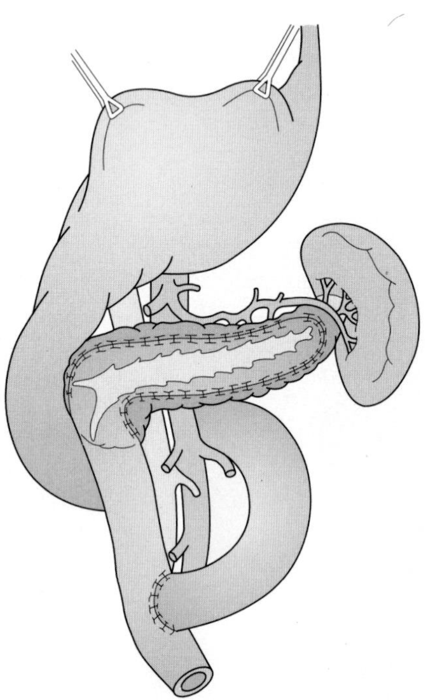

Fig. 55.31 Pancreatojejunostomy. The pancreatic duct is opened longitudinally and a loop of jejunum sutured to the duct. In the Frey procedure, the superficial part of the head of the pancreas is removed to achieve improved drainage.

Pathology

More than 85 per cent of cases are duct cell adenocarcinomas. The remaining tumours are a fascinating variety of pathologies, each with their own characteristics. The more common tumours are listed in Table 55.8. The importance of the pathology is that some tumours have a prolonged natural history, for instance, the cystadenocarcinomas, while those with an ampullary tumour (Fig. 55.32) or a neuroendocrine have an increased survival after resection.

Clinical features

The most frequent symptoms are nonspecific, namely epigastric discomfort, anorexia and weight loss. Often the patient is aware of their digestion for the first time in their life, and such is the mildness of the initial symptoms that they are frequently dismissed both by patient and by doctor. Jaundice is the commonest sign and symptom which brings the patient to the attention of his or her physician. Some 85 per cent of patients present with this symptom. It is characteristically painless jaundice but may be associated with nausea and epigastric discomfort. Change of bowel habit is rare.

On examination there is frequently evidence of weight loss, a palpable liver, a palpable gall bladder and even metastatic lymph nodes in the neck. Courvoisier first drew attention to the association of an enlarged gall bladder and a pancreatic tumour in 1890, when he stated that when the common duct is obstructed by a stone dilatation is rare; when the duct is obstructed in some other way, dilatation is common. In those days dilatation of the duct could not be determined and the dilatation, thus, refers to the gall bladder. Other signs of intra-abdominal malignancy should be looked for with care, such as a mass, ascites and tumour deposits in the pelvis.

Investigation

If the patient is jaundiced, the usual blood tests and ultrasound scan should be performed. This will determine whether or not the bile duct is dilated. If it is and there is a genuine suspicion of a tumour in the head of the pancreas, the preferred test is now a contrast-enhanced spiral CT scan specific for the pancreas. The next investigation is that of an endoscopic examination to determine whether the jaundice can be relieved endoscopically. If it can, a stent should be inserted through the stricture to relieve the jaundice. Attention should be paid to the coagulation to ensure that no bleeding occurs during this process. If the ERCP shows the characteristic features of a tumour and the CT scan shows that the tumour is small (less than 4 cm), and confined to the head of the pancreas without evidence of distant spread or

Ludwig Courvoisier, 1843–1918. Professor of Surgery, Basle, Switzerland.

Table 55.8 Classification of exocrine primary pancreatic neoplasia (Armed Forces Institute of Pathology)

Benign	*Malignant*
Epithelial origin	
Duct/ductile/centroductal (acinar) cell	Duct/ductule cell origin
Polyp?	Duct cell carcinoma
Papilloma, papillomatosis, villous papilloma	Giant cell carcinoma (incl. osteoclastoid)
Adenoma	Adenosquamous carcinoma (incl. spindle cell type)
Solid	Microadenocarcinoma (solid microglandular)
Duct (ductule)	Mucinous ('colloid') carcinoma
Centroductular (centroacinar)	Mucinous–carcinoid carcinoma
Cystadenoma	'Oat-cell' carcinoma
Serous – Simple	
Serous – Papillary	Papillary cystic tumour
Mucinous – Simple	Mucinous ('colloid') carcinoma
Mucinous – Papillary	
Carcinoid	Carcinoid
Oncocytoma	Oncocytic carcinoma/carcinoid
Ciliated cell?	Ciliated cell carcinoma?
Acinar cell	Acinar cell
Adenoma	Acinar cell carcinoma
Cystadenoma	Acinar cell cystadenocarcinoma
Mixed epithelial cells	Mixed cell
Duct/islet; duct/acinar	Duct/islet; duct/islet/acinar
Duct/acinar/islet;	Acinar/islet; carcinoid/islet
Acinar/islet; carcinoid/islet?	
Connective tissue origin	
Fibroma	Fibrosarcoma
Leiomyoma	Leiomyosarcoma
Neurilemmoma	Malignant neurilemmoma
Fibrous histiocytoma	Malignant fibrous histiocytoma
Vascular	
Lymphangioma	
Haemangioma	
Miscellaneous	Osteogenic/lipo-/rhabdomyosarcoma
Mixed epithelial–connective tissue origin	
Fibroadenoma?	
Uncertain histiogenesis/other	
	Pancreatoblastoma (simple and mixed types)
	Unclassified (large, small or clear cell type)

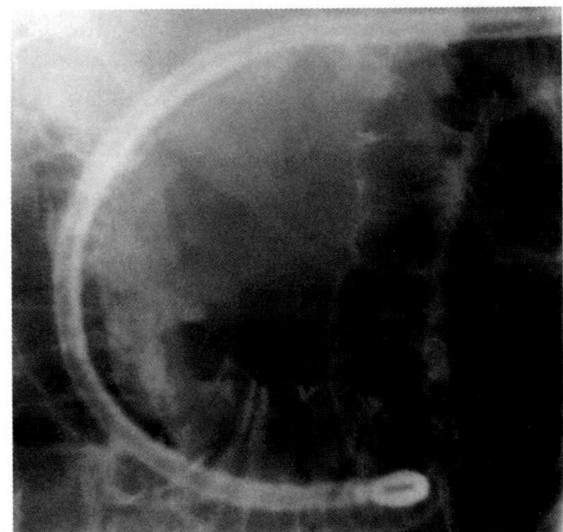

Fig. 55.32 Carcinoma of ampulla. Filling defect in region of ampulla.

vascular invasion, then the patient should be considered for operative intervention and their state of general fitness assessed. More accurate information can be obtained by endoscopic ultrasound in which the ultrasound probe on the end of an endoscope is used to obtain images of the tumour via the duodenum, giving good definition of the tumour and its extent. Unfortunately, lymphadenopathy is not well shown by this technique, but it is possible to determine with accuracy whether or not the portal vein is involved.

Management

At the time of presentation, 90–95 per cent of patients are unsuitable for resection because of either local spread into the superior mesenteric vein, paraaortic or mesenteric lymphadenopathy, or hepatic metastases. In some patients age precludes major operative intervention. For those patients who are inoperable palliative treatment should be offered.

Jaundice is relieved by stenting. Obstruction of the duodenum occurs in approximately 15 per cent; if this occurs early in the course of the disease surgical bypass by gastrojejunostomy is appropriate, but if it is late in the course of the disease then the use of expanding metal stents inserted endoscopically is preferred as many of these patients have prolonged delayed gastric emptying following surgery. If the patient is not a suitable candidate for endoscopic biliary stenting a percutaneous transhepatic stent can be placed. In younger patients who may have a better prognosis a laparotomy to assess the tumour can be appropriate; if the tumour is proved inoperable a choledochoduodenostomy and gastrojejunostomy is the preferred approach, but the simpler cholecystjejunostomy (Fig. 55.33) is more frequently performed. The disadvantage of the latter technique is that bile must drain through the cystic duct which is narrow, and if the cystic duct is inserted low into the bile duct it is vulnerable to occlusion by tumour growth. Any patient who has palliative treatment should have a biopsy performed to obtain histological verification. If operation is undertaken this can be done at the time of the operation, but if no operative procedure is undertaken a percutaneous trucut biopsy of the tumour should be performed.

The role of chemotherapy in the management of pancreatic cancer remains ill defined. If the tumour is a lymphoma then benefit is without doubt. Lymphomas of the pancreas are rare, however, comprising less than 3 per cent of the total number of pancreatic cancers. For the duct cell adenocarcinoma, 5-fluorouracil (5FU) or gemcitabine will produce a remission in 15–25 per cent of patients, whilst the remainder will have no benefit from the therapy. In those that have a remission prognosis is extended by approximately 6 months. No long-term cures have been described with oncological agents.

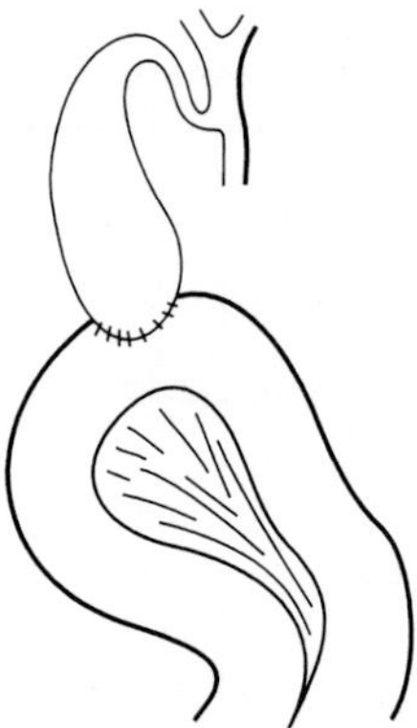

Fig. 55.33 Cholecystjejunostomy. Some surgeons also perform an enteroenterostomy lower down so that intestinal contents are diverted from the biliary tree.

Surgical resection

If a cystic tumour is encountered, no matter how large, most of these can be removed surgically with a reasonable chance of cure and with low operative mortality. Tumours of the ampulla have a good prognosis and should, if at all possible, be resected. Some of the rare tumours and the neuroendocrine lesions should also be resected if at all possible. Patients with duct cell cancers which are less than 4 cm in diameter, not involving the superior mesenteric or portal veins and with no evidence of multiple enlarged nodes or distant spread, should be considered for a resection. The appropriate resection is that of a pylorus-preserving pancreatoduodenectomy with a local lymphadenectomy. Extended resections have not been shown to be beneficial in improving survival and are associated with an increased morbidity.

The operation can now be performed safely with a mortality of 3–5 per cent. The morbidity remains high with some 40 per cent of patients developing a complication in the postoperative period. These complications are usually infective, but a leak from the pancreatic duct is known to occur in at least 10 per cent of patients and this may give rise to major complications. The role of adjuvant radiotherapy and chemotherapy with resection has not been elucidated.

Pancreatoduodenectomy – preoperative management. A full assessment of the patient's general condition should be carried out and a decision made whether or not to relieve the jaundice preoperatively. Occasionally, if the period of jaundice is short (2 weeks), it is safe to proceed to operation, but if the period of jaundice is prolonged and a more detailed preoperative assessment of operability is required then a stent allows more time and relieves the symptoms associated with jaundice. The clotting should be carefully checked preoperatively and adequate hydration ensured. A full explanation is made to ensure that the patient is aware of the diagnosis, the gravity of the operation and the risks involved, and consent taken.

Under general anaesthesia with adequate monitoring, the abdomen is explored and operability assessed. If the tumour is localised and without distant spread then resection is appropriate. A cholecystectomy is performed. The bile duct is dissected together with the structures in the porta hepatis, removing the lymphatic tissue in this area. This will expose the hepatic artery and enable division of the gastroduodenal artery which will expose the portal vein. The duodenum and right colon are mobilised from the retroperitoneal tissues and the fourth part of the duodenum is dissected and freed from the ligament of Treitz so that the upper jejunum can be brought into the supracolic compartment. The jejunum is divided and the mesentery of the proximal jejunum detached. The proximal duodenum is divided. The neck of the pancreas is divided and then the uncinate process separated from the superior mesenteric artery and vein working up towards the upper bile duct which is divided releasing the specimen (Fig. 55.34). Retroperitoneal lymph nodes are completely removed with the specimen as are those attached to the superior mesenteric vessels. Reconstruction is carried out as in Fig. 55.35. The operation should take between 3 and 6 hours. Blood loss should be low and transfusion unnecessary. Neither duct is stented and a single drain to the subhepatic space should be kept *in situ* for 4 days.

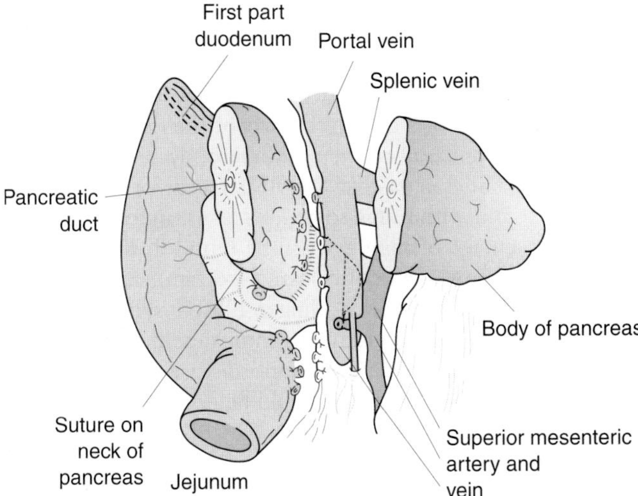

Fig. 55.34 Resection of the head of the pancreas.

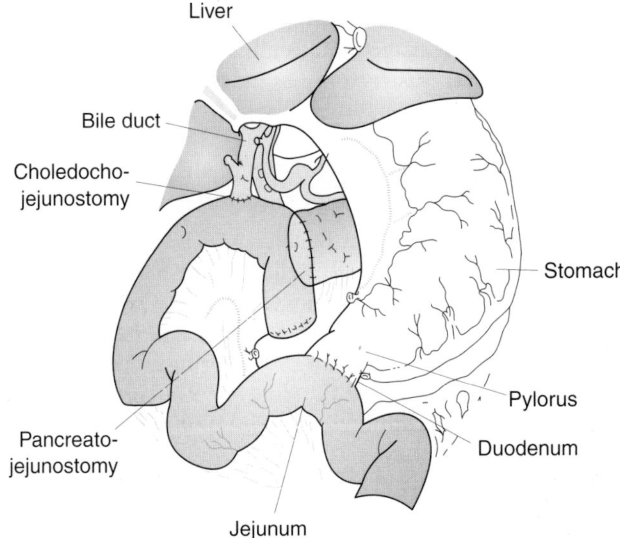

Fig. 55.35 Reconstruction after a pancreatoduodenectomy.

Prognosis

The overall median survival for patients with pancreatic cancer is 20 weeks. Less than 3 per cent of patients will survive for 5 years. Patients with a carcinoma of the ampulla of Vater who have had a resection will have a 5-year survival rate of 40 per cent, while those with a duct cell carcinoma will have a 5-year survival rate of 20 per cent. More 'benign' tumours will, of course, have a better prognosis. Following surgery all patients who have had palliative treatment require regular follow-up in order to care for steatorrhoea with enzyme supplementation, diabetes mellitus, if it develops, with oral hypoglycaemics or insulin as appropriate, and pain with either analgesics or an appropriate nerve block. The procedure of transthoracic splanchnicectomy is now the preferred procedure for relieving the pain and should be considered in preference to a coeliac plexus block.

Endocrine tumours of the pancreas

The islet of Langerhans contain three types of cells: α, β and δ, and of these the β-cell is most prevalent. Tumours of these endocrine cells comprise 1 per cent of all pancreatic tumours.

Pathology

The actual islet cell lesion may be one of the following: (1) generalised hyperplasia; (2) discrete adenoma; (3) generalised adenomatosis; and (4) carcinoma. In about one-third of cases they are multiple and in one-third they are malignant. As part of the multiple endocrine neoplasia syndrome they may be associated with tumours in other endocrine glands, especially the anterior pituitary, the parathyroids and the adrenal cortex. The neuroendocrine tumours may secrete hormones which give rise to the following conditions: insulinoma (insulin), gastrinoma (gastrin), watery diarrhoea hypokalaemia achlorhydria syndrome (WDHA) (vasoactive intestinal peptide), glucagonoma (glucagon), somatostatinoma (somatostatin), CCKoma (CCK), ectopic adrenocorticotrophic hormone syndrome (ACTH), hyperpigmentation syndrome (melanocyte-stimulating hormone), ectopic hyperparathyroidism (parathyroid hormone-related protein), carcinoid syndrome (5-hydroxytryptamine), pancreatic polypeptidoma (PPoma) (pancreatic polypeptide) and growth hormone secreting factor tumour. The commonest of these is the insulinoma.

Hyperinsulinism

Clinical features

The symptoms are many and varied, but the attacks are always associated with hypoglycaemia and occur at irregular intervals, often with progressively increasing frequency and severity. The symptoms include epigastric discomfort, nervousness, 'feeling unwell', trembling, sweating, dizziness, episodes of inarticulate speech and uncoordinated movements and, in extreme cases, fits indistinguishable from epilepsy. The age of the patient is variable.

Diagnosis

Diagnosis is made by the three criteria described by Whipple which consists of the signs and symptoms of hypoglycaemia, serum levels of less than 2.8 mmol/litre and the prompt relief of symptoms by the administration of glucose. The hypoglycaemia should be documented and associated with inappropriate levels of serum insulin (greater than 6 μunits/dl) and elevated C-peptide levels. Once the diagnosis has been made, the next step is to localise the tumour. The prime investigation is that of a high-quality CT scan of the pancreas with rapid injection (5–7 ml/second) of intravenous contrast (Fig. 55.12). The diagnosis of the

Alan 'Old Father' Whipple, 1881–1963. Valentine Mott Professor of Surgery, Columbia University College of Physicians and Surgeons, New York, USA.

characteristic 'blush' noted at the site of the tumour can be confirmed by endoscopic ultrasound. Angiography and selective sampling is no longer indicated. Further information is not required.

Treatment

The only curative treatment is extirpation of the tumour. Appropriate intravenous therapy with glucose and insulin is started preoperatively to maintain the blood sugar between 5 and 8 mmol/litre. The tumour is located usually with ease. Occasionally, the tumour cannot be palpated and then intraoperative ultrasound will invariably localise the tumour if present. Enucleation is the procedure of choice. Resection is rarely necessary unless the tumour is adjacent to the main duct in the head of the pancreas or there are multiple tumours in close proximity. The operative mortality rate is 1 per cent and the symptoms should be relieved in more than 95 per cent of patients.

Zollinger–Ellison syndrome

Diagnosis

The diagnosis should be suspected when peptic ulcer disease occurs at a very young age, there is virulent peptic ulcer disease, peptic ulcer disease occurs in unusual sites such as the jejunum, there is a marginal ulcer, unexplained diarrhoea, coexistent parathyroid disease or a family history of endocrinopathy.

The diagnosis of Zollinger–Ellison syndrome is confirmed by the demonstration of hypergastrinaemia and concurrent gastric hyperacidity. If there is doubt about the diagnosis a confirmatory secretin or calcium infusion test should be performed.

Location and localisation

In 1984 Stabile *et al.* described the 'gastrinoma triangle' (confluence of the cystic duct and common bile duct superiorly, junction of the second and third parts of the duodenum inferiorly, and the junction of the neck and body of the pancreas medially) and suggested that 80–90 per cent of gastrinomas would be found within this triangle. This is, indeed, the case. A high percentage of tumours will be found in the duodenal wall and these are often quite small (4–6 mm). As 50–60 per cent of patients with the Zollinger–Ellison syndrome have malignant tumours careful investigation should be performed preoperatively to exclude metastatic disease. If there is no metastatic disease exploration should be undertaken.

Treatment

If the tumour is localised then resection of the tumour should be undertaken. Unfortunately, the surgical cure rate is only 30 per cent. Nevertheless, if a single tumour is found and excised the patient is cured. If other problems coexist, the patient can be managed medically with omeprazole and octreotide. Total gastrectomy is advised only if medical therapy fails.

Further reading

Beger, H.G., Warshaw, A.L., Büchler, M.W., Carr-Locke, D.L., Neoptolemos, J.P.N., Russell, C. and Sarr, M.G. (eds) (1998) *The Pancreas*, Blackwell Science, Oxford.

Johnson, C.D. and Imrie, C.W. (eds) (1999) *Pancreatic Disease. Towards the Year 2000*, Springer, London.

Trede, M. and Carter, D.C. (eds) (1997) *Surgery of the Pancreas*, Churchill Livingstone, Edinburgh.

Robert Milton Zollinger, b. 1903. Former Professor of Surgery, Ohio State University, Columbus, Ohio, USA.

Edwin H. Ellison, b. 1918. Former Professor of Surgery, Marquette University, Milwaukee, Wisconsin, USA.

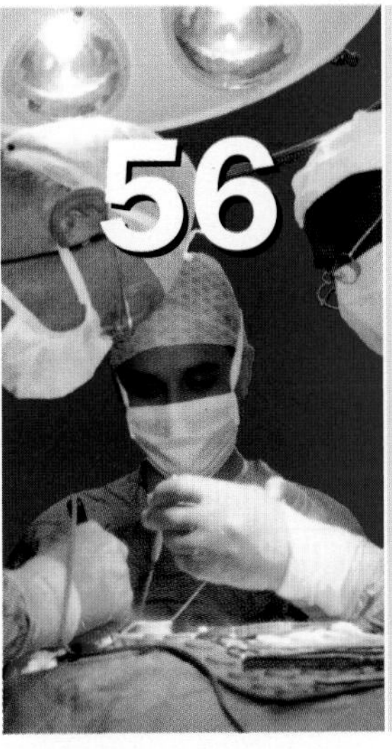

The peritoneum, omentum, mesentery and retroperitoneal space

The peritoneum

The peritoneal membrane is conveniently divided into two parts – the *visceral* surrounding the viscera and the *parietal* lining the other surfaces of the cavity. The peritoneum has a number of functions (Table 56.1). The parietal portion is richly supplied with nerves and, when irritated, causes severe pain accurately localised to the affected area. The visceral peritoneum, in contrast, is poorly supplied with nerves, and its irritation causes vague pain which is usually located to the midline.

Table 56.1 Functions of the peritoneum

Pain perception (parietal peritoneum)
Visceral lubrication
Fluid and particulate absorption
Inflammatory and immune responses
Fibrinolytic activity

Table 56.2 Causes of a peritoneal inflammatory exudate

Bacterial infection, e.g. appendicitis, tuberculosis
Chemical injury, e.g. bile peritonitis
Ischaemic injury, e.g. strangulated bowel, vascular occlusion
Direct trauma, e.g. operation
Allergic reaction, e.g. starch peritonitis

Bailey & Love's Short Practice of Surgery, 23rd edition. Edited by R.C.G. Russell, N.S. Williams and C.J.K. Bulstrode. Published in 2000 by Arnold Publishers.

The peritoneal cavity is the largest cavity in the body, the surface area of its lining membrane (2 m^2 in an adult) being nearly equal to that of the skin. The peritoneal membrane is composed of flattened polyhedral cells (mesothelium), one layer thick, resting upon a thin layer of fibroelastic tissue. Beneath the peritoneum, supported by a small amount of areolar tissue, lies a network of lymphatic vessels and rich plexuses of capillary blood vessels from which all absorption and exudation must occur. In health, only a few millilitres of peritoneal fluid is found in the peritoneal cavity. The fluid is pale yellow, somewhat viscid and contains lymphocytes and other leucocytes; it lubricates the viscera allowing easy movement and peristalsis.

In the peritoneal space mobile gas-filled structures float upwards under the influence of posture, as does free air ('gas'). In the erect position, when free fluid is present in the peritoneal cavity, pressure is reduced in the upper abdomen compared with the lower abdomen. When air is introduced it rises, allowing all of the abdominal contents to sink.

During expiration intra-abdominal pressure is reduced and peritoneal fluid, aided by capillary attraction, travels in an upward direction towards the diaphragm. Experimental evidence shows that particulate matter and bacteria are absorbed within a few minutes into the lymphatic network through a number of 'pores' within the diaphragmatic peritoneum. This upward movement of peritoneal fluids is responsible for the occurrence of many subphrenic abscesses.

The peritoneum has the capacity to absorb large volumes of fluid: this ability is used during peritoneal dialysis in the treatment of renal failure. But the peritoneum can also produce an inflammatory exudate when injured (Table 56.2). When a visceral perforation occurs the free fluid which spills into the peritoneal cavity runs downwards, largely directed by the normal peritoneal attachments. For example, spillage from a perforated duodenal ulcer may run down the right paracolic gutter.

When parietal peritoneal defects are created healing occurs, not from the edges, but by the development of new mesothelial cells throughout the surface of the defect. In this way large defects heal as rapidly as small defects.

Acute peritonitis

Most cases of peritonitis are due to an invasion of the peritoneal cavity by bacteria, so that when the term 'peritonitis' is used without qualification, bacterial peritonitis is implied. Bacterial peritonitis is usually polymicrobial, both aerobic and anaerobic organisms being present. The exception is primary peritonitis ('spontaneous' peritonitis) in which a pure infection with streptococcal, pneumococcal or haemophilus bacteria occurs.

Bacteriology

Bacteria from the gastrointestinal tract. The number of bacteria within the lumen of the gastrointestinal tract is normally low until the distal small bowel is reached, while high concentrations are found in the colon. However, disease (e.g. obstruction, achlorhydria, diverticula) may increase proximal colonisation. The biliary and pancreatic tracts are normally free from bacteria, although they may be infected in disease, e.g. gallstones. Peritoneal infection is usually caused by two or more bacterial strains. The commonest are *Escherichia coli*, aerobic and anaerobic streptococci, and the bacteroides. Less frequently *Clostridium welchii* is found; still less frequently staphylococci or *Klebsiella pneumoniae* (Friedländer's bacillus). Gram-negative bacteria contain endotoxins (lipopolysaccharides) in their cell walls which have multiple toxic effects on the host, primarily by causing the release of tumour necrosis factor (TNF) from host leucocytes. Systemic absorption of endotoxin may produce endotoxic shock with hypotension and impaired tissue perfusion. Other bacteria such as *C. welchii* produce harmful exotoxins.

Bacteroides are commonly found in peritonitis. These Gram-negative, nonsporing organisms, although predominant in the lower intestine, often escape detection because they are strictly anaerobic, and slow to grow on culture media unless there is an adequate carbon-dioxide tension in the anaerobic apparatus (Gillespie). In many laboratories, the culture is discarded if there is no growth in 48 hours. These organisms are resistant to penicillin and streptomycin but sensitive to metronidazole, clindamycin, lincomycin and cephalosporin compounds. Since the widespread use of metronidazole ('Flagyl') bacteroides infections have diminished greatly.

Nongastrointestinal causes of peritonitis

Nongastrointestinal causes of peritonitis include chlamydia, gonococcus, beta-haemolytic streptococcus, pneumococcus and *Mycobacterium tuberculosis*. Since the advent of antibiotics haemolytic streptococcal peritonitis has lost many of its dreaded lethal properties. In young girls and women, pelvic infection via the Fallopian tubes is responsible for a high proportion of 'nongastrointestinal' infections but bacteroides is also found in the female genital tract.

Immunodeficient patients, for example those with human immunodeficiency virus (HIV) infection (the acquired immunodeficiency syndrome – AIDS) or on immunosuppressive treatment, may present with opportunistic peritoneal infection, e.g. mycobacterium avis intracellulare (MAI).

Theodor Albrecht Edwin Klebs, 1834–1913. Professor of Bacteriology successively at Prague, Zurich and Rush Medical College, Chicago, Illinois, USA.

Hans Christian Joachim Gram, 1853–1938. Danish bacteriologist and Professor of Medicine, Copenhagen, Denmark.

Carl Friedländer, 1847–87. Prosector, Berlin-Friedrichshain Hospital, Germany.

William Alexander Gillespie. Former Professor of Clinical Bacteriology, University of Bristol, England.

Gabriele Fallopio (Fallopius), 1523–63. Professor of Anatomy, Surgery and Botany, Padua, Italy.

Table 56.3 Paths to peritoneal infection

Gastrointestinal perforation
e.g. perforated ulcer, diverticular perforation
Exogenous contamination
e.g. drains, open surgery, trauma
Transmural bacterial translocation (no perforation)
e.g. inflammatory bowel disease, appendicitis, ischaemic bowel
Female genital tract infection
e.g. pelvic inflammatory disease
Haematogenous spread (rare)
e.g. septicaemia

Route of infection

Infecting organisms may reach the peritoneal cavity via a number of routes (Table 56.3).

Even in patients with nonbacterial peritonitis (e.g. acute pancreatitis, intraperitoneal rupture of the bladder or haemoperitoneum) the peritoneum often becomes infected by transmural spread of organisms from the bowel, and it is not long (often a matter of hours) before a bacterial peritonitis develops. Most duodenal perforations are initially sterile for up to several hours, and many gastric perforations are also sterile at first; intestinal perforations are usually infected from the beginning. The proportion of anaerobic to aerobic organisms increases with the passage of time. Mortality reflects:

- the degree and duration of peritoneal contamination;
- the age of the patient;
- the general health of the patient;
- the nature of the underlying cause.

Localised peritonitis

Anatomical, pathological and surgical factors may favour the localisation of peritonitis.

Anatomical

The greater sac of the peritoneum is divided into (a) the subphrenic spaces, (b) the pelvis, and (c) the peritoneal cavity proper. The latter is redivided into a supracolic and an infracolic compartment by the transverse colon and transverse mesocolon, which deter the spread of infection from one to the other. When the supracolic compartment overflows, as is often the case when a peptic ulcer perforates, it does so over the colon into the infracolic compartment, or by way of the right paracolic gutter to the right iliac fossa, and thence to the pelvis. Posture can assist in directing collections into the pelvis, as in the 'Sherren' regime for perforated appendicitis.

Pathological

The clinical course is determined in part by the manner in which adhesions form around the affected organ. Inflamed

James Sherren, 1872–1945. Surgeon, The London Hospital, London, England.

peritoneum loses its glistening appearance and becomes reddened and velvety. Flakes of fibrin appear and cause loops of intestine to become adherent to one another and to the parieties. There is an outpouring of serous inflammatory exudate rich in leucocytes and plasma proteins that soon becomes turbid; if localisation occurs, the turbid fluid becomes frank pus. Peristalsis is retarded in affected bowel, and this helps in preventing distribution of the infection. The greater omentum, by enveloping and becoming adherent to inflamed structures, often forms a substantial barrier to the spread of infection.

Surgical

Drains are frequently placed during operation to assist localisation (and exit) of intra-abdominal collections: their value is disputed. They may act as conduits for exogenous infection. Collections detected postoperatively on ultrasound or computerised tomography (CT) scanning may be drained percutaneously.

Diffuse peritonitis

A number of factors may favour the development of diffuse peritonitis.

Speed of peritoneal contamination is a prime factor in the spread of peritonitis. If an inflamed appendix (Fig. 56.1) or other hollow viscus perforates before localisation has taken place, there is a gush of contents into the peritoneal cavity which may spread over a large area almost instantaneously. Perforation proximal to an obstruction, or from sudden anastomotic separation, is associated with severe generalised peritonitis and a high mortality.

Stimulation of peristalsis by the ingestion of food, or even water, hinders localisation. Violent peristalsis occasioned by the administration of a purgative or an enema may cause the widespread distribution of an infection that would otherwise have remained localised.

The virulence of the infecting organism may be so great as to render the localisation of infection difficult or impossible.

Young children have a small omentum.

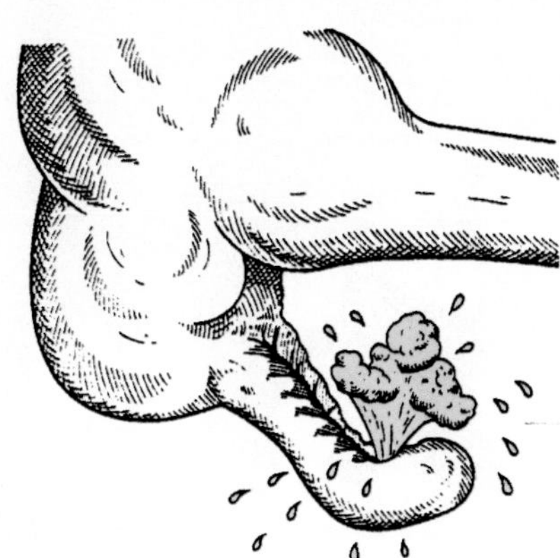

Fig. 56.1 Sudden perforation, especially if engendered by purgation, often results in an immediate, widespread bacterial peritonitis.

Disruption of localised collections may occur with injudicious and rough handling, e.g. appendix mass or pericolic abscess.

Deficient natural resistance ('immune deficiency') may result from drugs (e.g. steroids), disease (e.g. AIDS) or old age.

Clinical features

Localised peritonitis

Localised peritonitis is bound up intimately with the causative condition and the initial symptoms and signs are those of that condition. When the peritoneum becomes inflamed the temperature, and especially the pulse rate, rise. Abdominal pain increases and usually there is associated vomiting. The most important sign is guarding and rigidity of the abdominal wall over the area of the abdomen which is involved, with a positive 'release' sign (rebound tenderness). If inflammation arises under the diaphragm shoulder tip ('phrenic') pain may be felt. In cases of pelvic peritonitis arising from an inflamed appendix in the pelvic position or from salpingitis the abdominal signs are often slight, deep tenderness of one or both lower quadrants alone being present, but a rectal or vaginal examination reveals marked tenderness of the pelvic peritoneum. With appropriate treatment localised peritonitis usually resolves. In about 20 per cent of cases an abscess follows. Infrequently, localised peritonitis becomes diffuse. Conversely, in favourable circumstances diffuse peritonitis can become localised, most frequently in the pelvis or at multiple sites within the abdominal cavity. A large collection of bile localised to the subhepatic space can remain dangerously 'silent' until a late stage.

Diffuse (generalised) peritonitis

Diffuse (generalised) peritonitis may present in differing ways dependent on the duration of infection.

Early. Abdominal pain is severe and made worse by moving or breathing. It is first experienced at the site of the original lesion, and spreads outwards from this point. Vomiting may occur. The patient usually lies still. Tenderness and rigidity on palpation are typically found when the peritonitis affects the anterior abdominal wall. Abdominal tenderness and rigidity are diminished or absent if the anterior wall is unaffected, as in pelvic peritonitis or, rarely, peritonitis in the lesser sac. Patients with pelvic peritonitis may complain of urinary symptoms; they are tender on rectal or vaginal examination. Infrequent bowel sounds may still be heard for a few hours but they cease with the onset of paralytic ileus. The pulse rises progressively, but if the peritoneum is deluged with irritant fluid, there is a sudden rise. The temperature changes are variable and *can be subnormal*.

Late. If resolution or localisation of generalised peritonitis does not occur, the abdomen remains silent and increasingly distends. Circulatory failure ensues, with cold, clammy extremities, sunken eyes, dry tongue, thready (irregular) pulse, and drawn and anxious face (Hippocratic facies, Fig.

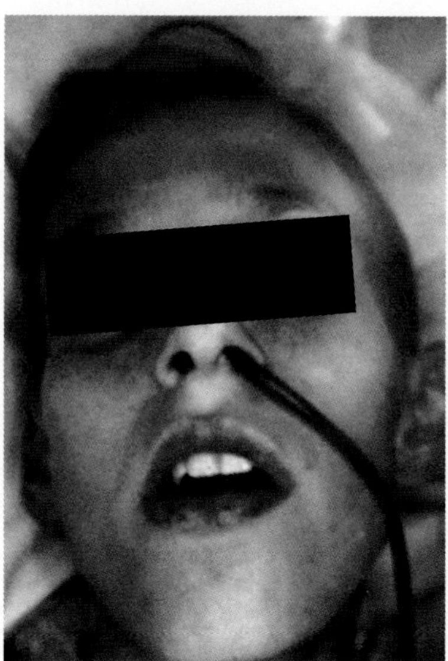

Fig. 56.2 The facies in terminal diffuse peritonitis.

56.2). The patient finally lapses into unconsciousness. With early diagnosis and adequate treatment, this condition is rarely seen in modern surgical practice.

Diagnostic aids

A number of investigations may elucidate a doubtful diagnosis, but the importance of a careful history and repeated examination must not be forgotten

A **leucocytosis** is usually seen in peritonitis but is often delayed for many hours.

Peritoneal diagnostic aspiration may be helpful but is usually unnecessary. After infiltrating the skin of the abdomen with local anaesthetic, the peritoneum is entered in one or more quadrants with a sterile needle an or intravenous cannula attached to a syringe into which is sucked any free fluid. Bile-stained fluid indicates perforated peptic ulcer or gall bladder, the presence of pus indicates bacterial peritonitis; blood is aspirated in a high proportion of patients with intraperitoneal bleeding. When aspiration fails, the introduction of a small quantity of sterile physiological saline, followed after a few minutes by peritoneal aspiration may produce fluid of diagnostic value. Microscopy of the fluid may show neutrophils (indicative of acute inflammation) and bacteria (confirming infection).

An **X-ray film of the abdomen** may confirm the presence of dilated gas-filled loops of bowel (consistent with a paralytic ileus) or show free gas, although the latter is best shown on *an erect chest X-ray* (Fig. 56.3). If the patient is too ill for an 'erect' film to demonstrate free air collecting under the diaphragm, a lateral decubitus film is just as useful showing gas beneath the abdominal wall.

Hippocrates, by common consent the Father of Medicine, was born on the Greek Island of Cos, off Turkey, about 460 BC and died in 375 BC.

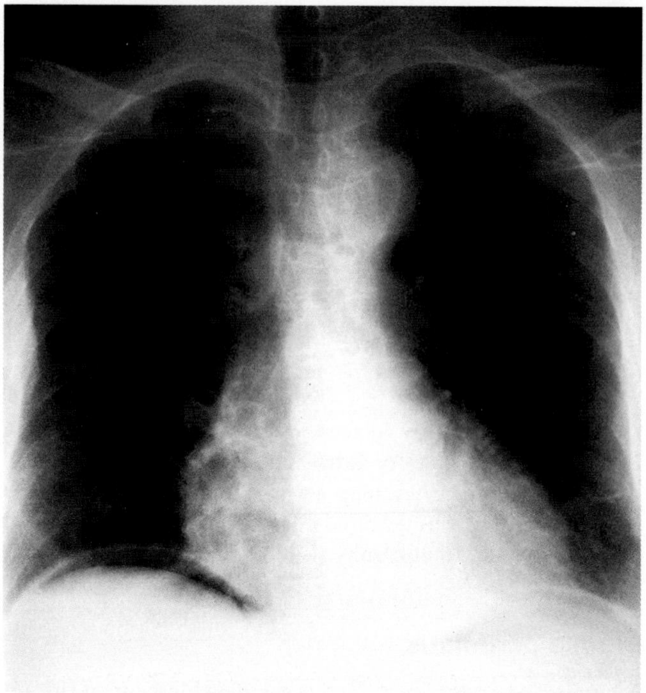

Fig. 56.3 Gas under the diaphragm in a patient with free perforation and peritonitis (*courtesy of Dr S. Padley, Chelsea and Westminster Hospital, London*).

Serum amylase estimation may uphold the diagnosis of acute pancreatitis provided it is remembered that moderately raised values are frequently found following other abdominal catastrophes and operations, e.g. perforated duodenal ulcer.

Ultrasound and CT scanning, when available, may also be helpful in some patients by identifying a cause of peritonitis e.g. perforated appendicitis, acute pancreatitis (Fig. 56.4). Such knowledge may influence operative approach or contraindicate operation.

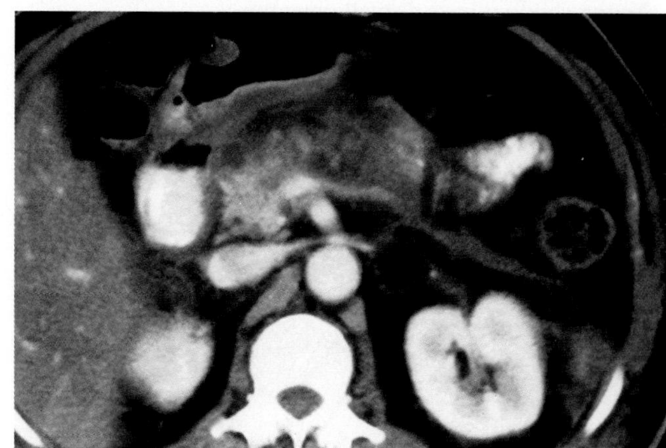

Fig. 56.4 Acute pancreatitis seen on CT scanning with swelling of the gland and surrounding inflammatory changes (*courtesy of Dr J. Healy, Chelsea and Westminster Hospital, London*).

Treatment

It cannot be stressed too strongly that in any case of doubt, early surgical intervention is to be preferred to a 'wait and see' policy; for greater numbers of patients die from delay than from an 'unnecessary' laparotomy. This rule is particularly true for postoperative peritonitis.

Treatment consists of:

- general care of the patient;
- specific treatment for the cause;
- peritoneal lavage when appropriate.

General care of the patient

Correction of circulating volume and electrolyte imbalance. Patients are frequently hypovolaemic with electrolyte disturbances. The plasma volume must be restored and the plasma electrolyte concentrations corrected. Central venous catheterisation and pressure monitoring may be helpful in correcting fluid and electrolyte balance particularly in patients with concurrent disease. Plasma protein depletion may also need correction as the inflamed peritoneum leaks large amounts of protein. If the patient's recovery is delayed for more than 7–10 days, intravenous feeding ('hyperalimentation' or 'total parenteral nutrition') is required.

Gastrointestinal decompression. A nasogastric tube is passed into the stomach and aspirated. Intermittent aspiration is maintained until the paralytic ileus resulting from peritonitis has recovered. Measured volumes of water are allowed by mouth when only small amounts are being aspirated. If the abdomen is soft and not tender, and bowel sounds return, oral feeding may be progressively introduced. It is important not to prolong the ileus by missing this stage.

Antibiotic therapy. Administration of antibiotics prevents the multiplication of bacteria and the release of endotoxins. As the infection is usually a mixed one, initially parenteral broad-spectrum antibiotics active against aerobic and anaerobic bacteria should be given.

A fluid balance chart must be started so that daily output by gastric aspiration and urine is known. Additional losses from the lungs, skin, and in faeces are estimated, so that the intake requirements can be calculated and seen to have been administered. Throughout recovery, the haematocrit and serum electrolytes and urea must be checked regularly.

Analgesia. The patient should be nursed in the sitting-up position and must be relieved of pain before and after operation. Once the diagnosis has been made morphine may be given, and continued as necessary. If appropriate expertise is available epidural infusion may provide excellent analgesia. Freedom from pain allows early mobilisation and adequate physiotherapy in the postoperative period which help to prevent basal pulmonary collapse, deep-vein thrombosis and pulmonary embolism.

Vital system support. Especially if septic shock is present, special measures may be needed for cardiac, pulmonary and renal support. Administration of oxygen postoperatively can help to prevent and mitigate the effects of septic shock, especially adult respiratory distress syndrome (ARDS) which may require a period of mechanical ventilation. If oliguria persists despite adequate fluid replacement, both diuretics and inotropic agents such as dopamine may be needed.

Specific treatment of the cause

If the cause of peritonitis is amenable to surgery, such as in perforated appendicitis, diverticulitis, peptic ulcer, gangrenous cholecystitis or in rare cases of perforation of the small bowel, operation must be carried out as soon as the patient is fit for anaesthesia. This is usually within a few hours. In peritonitis due to pancreatitis or salpingitis, or in cases of primary peritonitis of streptococcal or pneumococcal origin, nonoperative treatment is preferred (if the diagnosis can be made with certainty).

Peritoneal lavage

In operations for general peritonitis it is essential that after the cause has been dealt with the whole peritoneal cavity should be explored with the sucker and mopped dry, if necessary until all seropurulent exudate is removed. The use of a large volume of saline (1–2 litres) containing dissolved antibiotic (e.g. tetracycline) has been shown to be very effective (Matheson).

Prognosis

With modern treatment diffuse peritonitis carries a mortality of about 10 per cent. The systemic complications and lethal factors are listed in Table 56.4.

Complications of peritonitis

All of the complications of a severe bacterial infection are possible, but the specific abdominal complications of peritonitis are listed in Table 56.5.

Table 56.4 Systemic complications of peritonitis

Bacteraemic/endotoxic shock
Bronchopneumonia/respiratory failure
Renal failure
Bone marrow suppression
Multisystem failure

Table 56.5 Abdominal complications of peritonitis

Adhesional small bowel obstruction
Paralytic ileus
Residual or recurrent abscess
Portal pyaemia/liver abscess

N.A. Matheson. Surgeon, Aberdeen Royal Infirmary, Scotland.

Acute intestinal obstruction due to peritoneal adhesions

This usually gives central colicky abdominal pain with evidence of small bowel gas and fluid levels sometimes confined to the proximal intestine on X-ray. Bowel sounds are increased. It is more common with localised peritonitis. It is essential to distinguish this from paralytic ileus.

Paralytic ileus

There is usually little pain and gas-filled loops with fluid levels are seen distributed throughout the small and large intestines on abdominal X-ray. In paralytic ileus, bowel sounds are reduced or absent.

Abscesses

Abscess formation following local or diffuse peritonitis usually occupies one of the situations shown in Fig. 56.5. The symptoms and signs of a purulent collection may be very vague and consist of nothing more than lassitude, anorexia and failure to thrive; pyrexia (often low-grade), tachycardia, leucocytosis and localised tenderness are also common. Later on a palpable mass may develop. When palpable an intraperitoneal abscess should be monitored by marking out its limitations on the abdominal wall, and meticulous daily examination. More commonly its course is monitored by repeat ultrasound or CT scanning. In the majority of cases with the aid of antibiotic treatment, the abscess or mass becomes smaller and smaller, and finally is undetectable. In others, the abscess fails to resolve, or becomes larger, in which event it must be drained. In many situations, by waiting for a few days the abscess becomes adherent to the abdominal wall, so that it can be drained without opening the general peritoneal cavity. If facilities are available ultrasound or CT-guided drainage may avoid further operation. Open drainage of an intraperitoneal collection should be carried out by cautious blunt finger exploration to minimise the risk of an intestinal fistula.

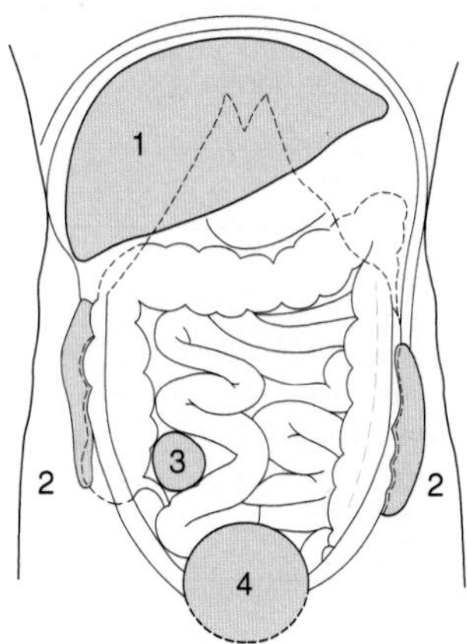

Fig. 56.5 Common situations for residual abscesses: (1) subphrenic; (2) paracolic; (3) right iliac fossa; (4) pelvic.

Pelvic abscess

The pelvis is the commonest site of an intraperitoneal abscess because the vermiform appendix is often pelvic in position and also the Fallopian tubes are frequent sites of infection. A pelvic abscess can also occur as a sequel to any case of diffuse peritonitis and is a common sequel of anastomotic leakage following large bowel and rectal surgery. Pus can accumulate in this area without serious constitutional disturbance and unless the patient is examined carefully from day to day, such abscesses may attain considerable proportions before being recognised. The most characteristic symptoms of a pelvic abscess are diarrhoea and the passage of mucus in the stools. It is no exaggeration to say that the *passage of mucus, occurring for the first time in a patient who has, or is recovering from, peritonitis, is pathognomonic of pelvic abscess*. Rectal examination reveals a bulging of the anterior rectal wall which, when the abscess is ripe, becomes softly cystic. Left to nature, a proportion of these abscesses bursts into the rectum, after which the patient nearly always recovers rapidly. If this possible happy termination does not readily occur the abscess should be drained deliberately. In women vaginal drainage through the posterior fornex is often chosen. In other cases, where the abscess is definitely pointing into the rectum, rectal drainage (Fig. 56.6) is employed. If any uncertainty exists, the presence of pus can be

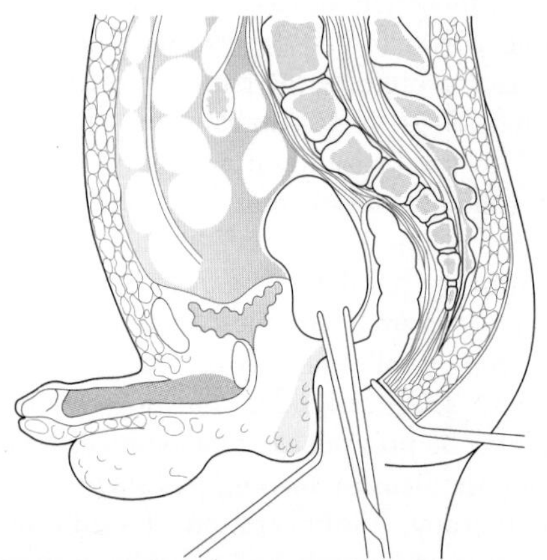

Fig. 56.6 Opening a pelvic abscess into the rectum.

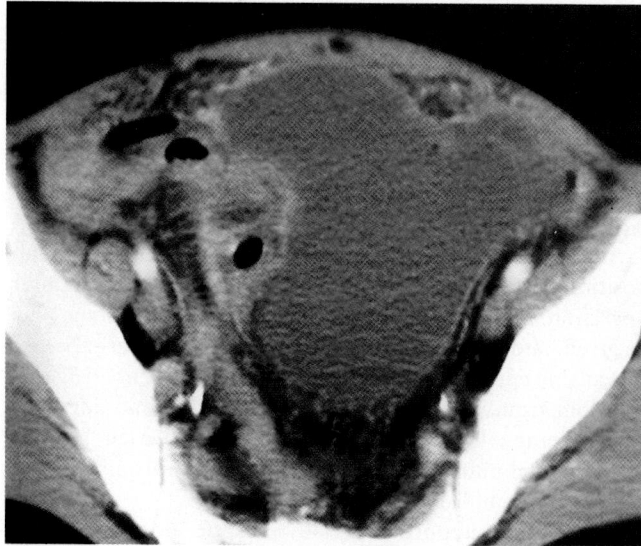

Fig. 56.7 A pelvic abscess seen on CT scanning (*courtesy of Dr J. Healy, Chelsea and Westminster Hospital, London*).

confirmed by ultrasound or CT scanning or by an aspirating needle introduced through the rectum or abdominal wall into the swelling. Laparotomy is almost never necessary. Rectal drainage of a pelvic abscess is far preferable to suprapubic drainage, which risks exposing the general peritoneal cavity to infection. Drainage tubes can also be inserted percutaneously or via the vagina or rectum under radiological (ultrasonic or CT) guidance (Fig. 56.7).

Subphrenic abscess

Anatomy

The complicated arrangement of the peritoneum results in the formation of four peritoneal and three extraperitoneal spaces in which pus may collect. Three of these spaces are on either side of the body, and one is approximately in the midline (Figs 56.8 and 56.9).

Left superior (anterior) intraperitoneal ('left subphrenic') is bounded above by the diaphragm, and behind by the left triangular ligament and the left lobe of the liver, the gastrohepatic omentum and anterior surface of the stomach. To the right is the falciform ligament and to the left the spleen, gastrosplenic omentum and diaphragm. The common cause of an abscess here is an operation on the stomach, the tail of the pancreas, the spleen or the splenic flexure of the colon.

Left inferior (posterior) intraperitoneal ('left subhepatic') is another name for the 'lesser' sac. The commonest cause of infection here is complicated acute pancreatitis. In practice a perforated gastric ulcer rarely causes a collection here because the potential space is obliterated by adhesions.

Right superior (anterior) intraperitoneal ('right subphrenic') lies between the right lobe of the liver and the diaphragm. It is limited posteriorly by the anterior layer of the coronary and the right triangular ligaments, and to the left by the falciform ligament. Common causes here are perforating cholecystitis, a perforated duodenal ulcer, a duodenal cap 'blow out' following gastrectomy and appendicitis.

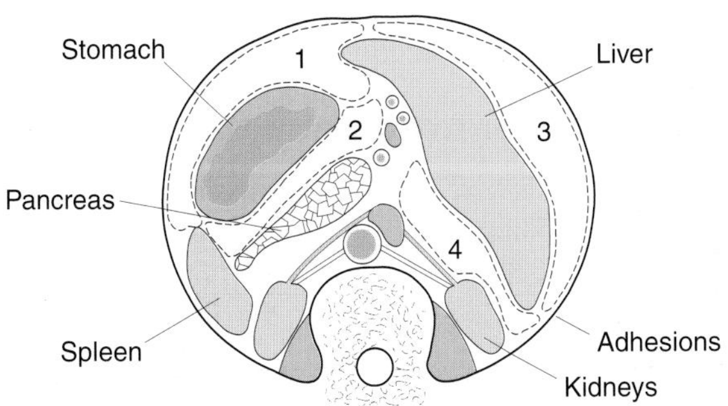

Fig. 56.8 Intraperitoneal subphrenic abscesses on transverse section. (1) The left superior space; (2) left inferior space (lesser sac); (3) right superior space which becomes shut off by adhesions from (4) right inferior space.

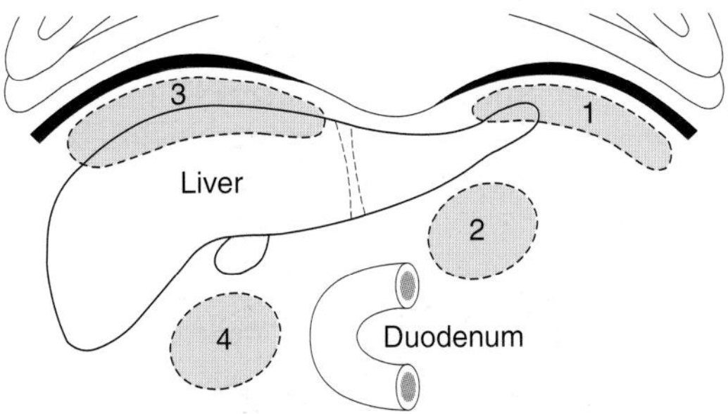

Fig. 56.9 Intraperitoneal subphrenic abscesses on sagittal section. (1) Left superior (anterior) abscess ('left subphrenic'); (2) left inferior (posterior) abscess ('left subhepatic); (3) right superior (anterior) abscess ('right subphrenic'); (4) right inferior (posterior) abscess ('right subhepatic').

Right inferior (posterior) intraperitoneal ('right subhepatic') lies transversely beneath the right lobe of the liver in Rutherford Morison's pouch. It is bounded on the right by the right lobe of the liver and the diaphragm. To the left is situated the foramen of Winslow and below this lies the duodenum. In front are the liver and the gall bladder, and behind, the upper part of the right kidney and diaphragm. The space is bounded above by the liver, and below by the transverse colon and hepatic flexure. It is the deepest space of the four and the commonest site of a subphrenic abscess which usually arises from appendicitis, cholecystitis, a perforated duodenal ulcer or following upper abdominal surgery.

Extraperitoneal. There are three of these:

- *right and left extraperitoneal* which are terms given to perinephric abscesses (Chapter 64);
- *midline extraperitoneal* which is another name for the 'bare' area of the liver which may develop an abscess in amoebic hepatitis (the commonest cause) or a pyogenic liver abscess (Chapter 52).

Clinical features

The symptoms and signs of subphrenic infection are frequently nonspecific, and it is well to remember the aphorism, 'pus somewhere, pus nowhere else, pus under diaphragm'.

Symptoms

A common history is that when some infective focus in the abdominal cavity has been dealt with, the condition of the patient improves temporarily, but after an interval of a few days or weeks, symptoms of toxaemia reappear. The condition of the patient steadily, and often rapidly, deteriorates. Sweating, wasting and anorexia are present. There is sometimes epigastric fullness and pain, or pain in the shoulder on the affected side, owing to irritation of sensory fibres in the phrenic nerve, referred along the descending branches of the cervical plexus. Persistent hiccup may be a presenting symptom.

Signs

A swinging pyrexia is usually present, unless antibiotics or drugs (steroids) have interfered. If the abscess is anterior, abdominal examination will reveal some tenderness, rigidity or even a palpable swelling. Sometimes the liver is displaced downwards, but more often it is fixed by adhesions. Examination of the chest is important, and in the majority of cases collapse of the lung or evidence of basal effusion or empyema is to be found.

Investigations

A number of these may be helpful as follows.

Blood count usually shows a leucocytosis.

James Rutherford Morison, 1853–1939. Professor of Surgery, Durham, England.

Jacob Benignus Winslow, 1669–1760. Professor of Anatomy, Physic and Surgery, Paris, France.

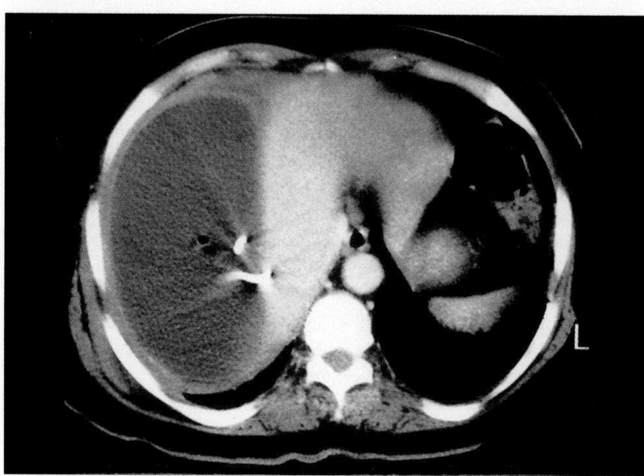

Fig. 56.10 A subphrenic abscess drained under CT guidance (*courtesy of Dr J. Healy, Chelsea and Westminster Hospital, London*).

A plain radiograph sometimes demonstrates the presence of gas or a pleural effusion. On screening, the diaphragm is often seen to be elevated (so-called 'tented' diaphragm) and its movements impaired.

Ultrasound or CT scanning is the investigation of choice and permits early detection of subphrenic collections (Fig. 56.10).

Radiolabelled white cell scanning may occasionally prove helpful when other imaging techniques have failed.

Differential diagnosis. Pyelonephritis, amoebic abscess, pulmonary collapse and pleural empyema give rise to most of the diagnostic difficulties.

Treatment

The clinical course of suspected cases is watched, and blood and imaging investigations are made at suitable intervals. If suppuration seems probable, intervention is indicated. If skilled help is available it is possible to insert a percutaneous drainage tube under ultrasound or CT control. The same tube can be used to instil antibiotic solutions or irrigate the abscess cavity. To pass an aspirating needle at the bedside through the pleura and diaphragm invites potentially catastrophic spread of the infection into the pleural cavity.

If an operative approach is necessary and a swelling can be detected in the subcostal region or in the loin, an incision is made over the site of maximum tenderness, or over any area where oedema or redness is discovered. The parietes usually form part of the abscess wall so that contamination of the general peritoneal cavity is unlikely.

If no swelling is apparent, the subphrenic spaces should be explored either by an anterior subcostal approach or from behind after removal of the *outer part* of the 12th rib according to the position of abscess on imaging. With the posterior approach the pleura must not be opened and after the fibres of the diaphragm have been separated a finger is inserted beneath the diaphragm so as to explore the adjacent area. The aim with all techniques of drainage is to avoid dissemination of pus into the peritoneal or pleural cavities.

When the cavity is reached, all of the fibrinous loculi must be broken down with the finger and one or two drains or drainage tubes must be fully inserted. These drains are withdrawn gradually during the next 10 days and the closure of the cavity is checked by sinograms or scanning. The appropriate antibiotics are also given.

Special forms of peritonitis

Postoperative

The patient is ill, with raised pulse and peripheral circulatory failure. Following an anastomotic dehiscence the general condition of a patient is usually more serious than if the patient had suffered leakage from a perforated peptic ulcer with no preceding operation. Local symptoms and signs are less definite. Abdominal pain may not be prominent and is often difficult to assess because of normal wound pain and postoperative analgesia. The patient's deterioration may be wrongly attributed to cardiopulmonary collapse which is usually concomitant.

Peritonitis follows abdominal operations more frequently than is realised. The principles of treatment do not differ from those of peritonitis of other origin. Antibiotic therapy alone is inadequate; no antibiotic can stay the onslaught of bacterial peritonitis due to leakage from a suture line, which must be dealt with by operation.

In patients under treatment with steroids

Pain is frequently slight or absent. Physical signs are similarly vague and misleading.

In children

The diagnosis is in some ways more difficult, in other ways easier, than in adults. If a history can be taken it is plain and unembroidered. Any physical signs elicited by a gentle, patient and sympathetic examiner are meaningful.

In senile patients

These can be as fractious as children and unable to give a reliable history. Abdominal tenderness is usually well localised, but guarding and rigidity are less marked because the abdominal muscles are thin and weak.

Bile peritonitis

Unless there is reason to suspect that a bile duct was damaged at an operation, it is improbable that bile as a cause of peritonitis will be thought of until the abdomen has been opened and bile is seen therein. The common causes of bile peritonitis are shown in Table 56.6. Unless the bile has extravasated slowly and the collection becomes shut off from the general peritoneal cavity there are signs of diffuse peritonitis. After a

Table 56.6 Causes of bile peritonitis

Perforated cholecystitis

Post cholecystectomy
- cystic duct stump leakage
- division of accessory duct in gall-bladder bed
- bile duct injury
- T-tube drain dislodgement (or tract rupture on removal)

Following other operations/procedures
- leaking duodenal stump post gastrectomy
- leaking biliary enteric anastomosis
- leakage around percutaneous placed biliary drains

few hours a tinge of jaundice is not unusual. Laparotomy (or laparoscopy) should be undertaken with evacuation of the bile and peritoneal lavage. The source of bile leakage should be identified. A leaking gall bladder is excised or a cystic duct ligated. An injury to the bile duct may simply be drained or alternatively intubated; later reconstructive operation is often required. Infected bile is more lethal than sterile bile. A 'blown' duodenal stump must be drained as it is too oedematous to repair, but sometimes it can be covered by a jejunal patch. The patient is often jaundiced from absorption of peritoneal bile, but the surgeon must ensure that the abdomen is not closed until any obstruction to a major bile duct has been either excluded or relieved. Post cholecystectomy bile leaks may be dealt with by percutaneous (ultrasound guides) drainage and endoscopic biliary stenting to reduce bile duct pressure. The drain is reduced when dry and the stent at 4–6 weeks.

Meconium peritonitis

Meconium is a sterile mixture of epithelial cells, mucin, salts, fats and bile and is formed when the foetus commences to swallow amniotic fluid. By the third month of intrauterine life the upper third of the small intestine has become filled with meconium; by the fourth month the accumulation has reached the ileocaecal valve; during the remainder of intrauterine life the colon becomes increasingly filled.

Meconium peritonitis is an aseptic peritonitis which develops late in intrauterine life or during, or just after, delivery. Meconium enters the peritoneal cavity through an intestinal perforation and in over 50 per cent of cases the perforation is the result of some form of neonatal intestinal obstruction; in the remainder no cause for the perforation is discernible. When meconium, which is sterile, enters the peritoneal cavity an exudate is secreted that organises rapidly; matting of intestinal loops occurs, and in many cases in a matter of weeks the extruded meconium becomes calcified.

Meconium remains sterile until about 3 hours after birth; thereafter, unless the perforation has become sealed, sterile meconium peritonitis gives place to acute bacterial peritonitis which, unless treated promptly, is rapidly fatal.

Clinical features. Meconium peritonitis should always be considered when a baby is born with a tense abdomen. There is vomiting and failure to discharge meconium. The differential diagnosis between neonatal intestinal obstruction and peritonitis is, in many cases, virtually impossible; indeed in half the cases both are present. Free fluid in the peritoneal cavity is often sufficient to give a fluid thrill. Meconium ileus occurs in 5–10 per cent of newborn babies with cystic fibrosis (mucoviscidosis) who have an inherited autosomal recessive abnormality of mucus secretion. This leads to secondary damage to the pancreas, lungs, liver and small bowel. Bronchial obstruction by mucus plugs can cause fatal pneumonia.

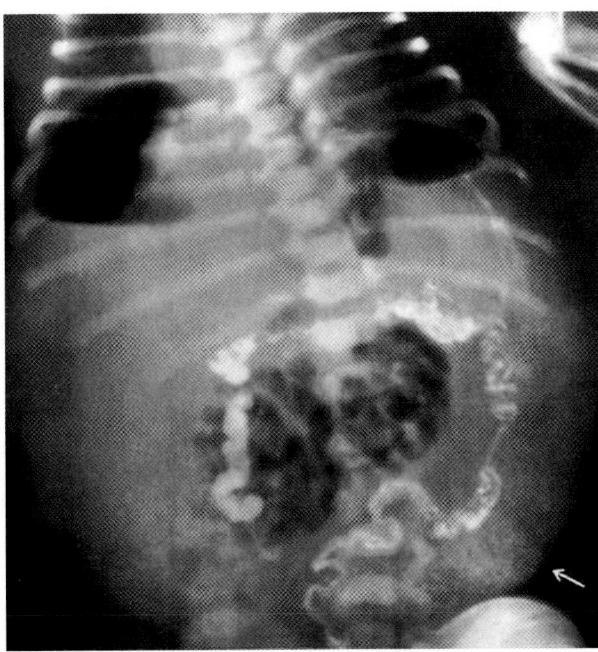

Fig. 56.11 Meconium peritonitis. Note the free air and fluid in the peritoneal cavity; intra-abdominal calcification (arrowed) and on the spleen; air in the small intestine; and microcolon shown by a barium enema (*courtesy of Dr Jack Lester, Copenhagen, Denmark*).

Radiography (Fig. 56.11). Free air in the peritoneal cavity, an abundant quantity of abdominal fluid, fluid levels, calcification (often most distinct on the surface of the liver or the spleen and most readily seen in a lateral view) are characteristic findings, all of which are unlikely to be present in every case. Meconium peritonitis has been diagnosed by radiography of the foetus *in utero* 2 days before birth.

Treatment. The prognosis is bad, but recovery may follow prompt operation. The greatest chance of survival is in those patients who have an intestinal perforation but no intestinal obstruction, in which case closure of the perforation and drainage of the peritoneal cavity are performed expeditiously. Intestinal lavage can prevent reformation of meconium bolus obstruction and supplements of pancreatic exocrine enzymes are often necessary throughout life. If there is an associated pulmonary problem, the condition requires special treatment (e.g. oxygen, bronchial lavage, nebulisers and long-term use of antibiotics).

Pneumococcal peritonitis

There are two forms of this disease: (1) primary, and (2) secondary to pneumonia.

Primary pneumococcal peritonitis is much more common. The patient is often an undernourished girl between 3 and 6 years of age, and it is probable that the infection sometimes occurs via the vagina and Fallopian tubes, for pneumococci have been cultured from patients' vaginas. At other times, and always in males, the infection is blood-borne from the upper respiratory tract or the middle ear. After the age of 10 years pneumococcal peritonitis is most unusual. Children with nephritis are more liable to this condition than others. During the past 30 years the instance of pneumococcal peritonitis has declined greatly and the condition is now rare.

Clinical features. The onset is sudden and the earliest symptom is pain localised to the lower half of the abdomen. The temperature is raised to 39.8°C or more and there is usually frequent vomiting. After 24–48 hours profuse diarrhoea, occasionally blood-stained, is characteristic. There is usually increased frequency of micturition. The last two symptoms are due to severe pelvic peritonitis. Herpes on the lip or nostril is often present. In acute forms of the disease, even in cases where there is no involvement of a lung, there is a tinge of cyanosis of the lips and cheeks and movement of the alae nasi is often discernible. On examination rigidity is usually bilateral but is less than in most cases of acute appendicitis with peritonitis.

Differential diagnosis. A leucocytosis of 30 000/mm^3 (30 × 10^9/1itre) or more with approximately 90 per cent polymorphs suggests pneumococcal peritonitis rather than appendicitis. Even so, it is often impossible, especially in males to exclude perforated appendicitis. The other condition which is extremely difficult to differentiate from primary peritonitis in its early stage is pneumonia. An unduly high respiratory rate and the absence of abdominal rigidity are the most important signs supporting the diagnosis of pneumonia, which is usually clarified by a chest X-ray.

Treatment. Early operation is always required. After starting antibiotic therapy and correcting dehydration and electrolyte imbalance, a short midline incision is made. The peritoneum is incised. Should the exudate be odourless and sticky, the diagnosis of pneumococcal peritonitis is practically certain, but it is essential to perform a routine laparotomy to exclude other lesions. Assuming that no other cause for the peritonitis is discovered some of the excudate is removed with a syringe and sent to the laboratory for culture and sensitivity tests. Thorough peritoneal lavage is carried out and the incision closed. The patient is returned to bed, and antibiotic and fluid replacement therapy continued. Nasogastric suction drainage is essential. Recovery is usual.

Primary streptococcal peritonitis of infants and children

Primary streptococcal peritonitis of infants and children is rather more frequent than pneumococcal peritonitis but still uncommon. When a streptococcus is the infecting organism the peritoneal exudate is thin and slightly clouded and contains flecks of fibrin. The clinical presentation and treatment of streptococcal peritonitis in infants and children are similar to those of pneumococcal peritonitis (see above), but the mortality is higher. An intravaginal foreign body should always be looked for in female patients.

Idiopathic streptococcal and staphylococcal peritonitis in adults

Idiopathic streptococcal and staphylococcal peritonitis in adults is fortunately rare, for prior to the antibiotic era it was nearly always fatal and the mortality is still very high. Rightly, in early cases the abdomen is opened, usually on a diagnosis of acute appendicitis. In streptococcal peritonitis the peritoneal exudate is odourless, thin, contains some flecks of fibrin and may be blood stained. In these circumstances pus is removed by suction, the abdomen closed with drainage and nonoperative treatment of peritonitis performed. Recently the use of intravaginal tampons has led to an increased incidence of *Staphylococcus aureus* infections: these can be associated with 'toxic shock syndrome' and disseminated intravascular coagulopathy.

Peritonitis following abortion/parturition

The abortionist has usually pushed an instrument through the uterine vault and streptococcal peritonitis follows. Peritonitis following puerperal infection is more common after first deliveries. Rigidity is seldom much in evidence; this, at any rate in part, is due to the stretched condition of the abdominal musculature. The lochia may be offensive but not necessarily so. Diarrhoea is common.

Treatment. Provided the infection is limited strictly to the pelvis, the correct treatment is to rest the gastrointestinal tract and provide intravenous fluids, the required antibiotics and attention to electrolyte balance. Posterior colpotomy may be necessary if a pelvic abscess forms. If the peritonitis is generalised, the patient is usually extremely ill and drainage is advisable. This may be carried out by making a small suprapubic incision under local anaesthesia and inserting a drain, which can be done with the patient in bed, if necessary.

In the preantibiotic era the mortality of general peritonitis following parturition or abortion was at least 50 per cent; with antibiotic therapy and timely operation, the mortality has fallen to less than 10 per cent (Brews).

Familial Mediterranean fever (periodic peritonitis)

Familial Mediterranean fever (periodic peritonitis) is characterised by abdominal pain and tenderness, mild pyrexia, polymorphonuclear leucocytosis and occasionally pain in the thorax and joints. The duration of an attack is 24–72 hours, when it is followed by complete remission but exacerbations recur at regular intervals. Most of the patients have undergone appendicectomy in childhood. This disease, often familial, is limited principally to Arabs, Armenians and Jews; other races are occasionally affected. The aetiology is unknown. Usually children are affected but it is not rare for the disease to make its first appearance in early adult life when females outnumber males by two to one. Exceptionally the disease becomes manifest in patients over 40 years of age. At laparotomy, which may be necessary to exclude other causes, the peritoneum – particularly in the vicinity of the spleen and the gall bladder – is inflamed. There is no evidence that the interior of these organs is abnormal. Colchicine may prevent recurrent attacks.

Differential diagnosis. Patients with abdominal epilepsy do not have positive physical signs of pyrexia and their attacks are usually controlled by anticonvulsive medication.

Tuberculous peritonitis

Acute tuberculous peritonitis

Tuberculous peritonitis sometimes has an onset that resembles so closely acute peritonitis that the abdomen is opened. Straw-coloured fluid escapes and tubercules are seen scattered over the peritoneum and greater omentum. Early tubercles are greyish and translucent. They soon undergo caseation, and appear white or yellow and are then less difficult to distinguish from carcinoma. Occasionally they appear like patchy fat necrosis. On opening the abdomen and finding tuberculous peritonitis the fluid is evacuated, some being retained for bacteriological studies. A portion of the diseased omentum is removed for histological confirmation of the diagnosis and the wound closed without drainage.

At other times, although acute abdominal symptoms arise, the presence of ascites makes diagnosis of acute tuberculous peritonitis reasonably evident.

Chronic tuberculous peritonitis

Although the incidence of tuberculous peritonitis has declined in Britain, in many parts of the world where

Richard Alan Brews, 1902–65. Obstetric and Gynaecological Surgeon, The London Hospital, London, England.

measures for eradicating tuberculosis (especially the disease in cows) are enforced less strictly, the condition still occurs. The condition presents with abdominal pain (90 per cent of cases), fever (60 per cent), loss of weight (60 per cent), ascites (60 per cent), night sweats (37 per cent) and abdominal mass (26 per cent).

Origin of the infection

Infection originates from:

- tuberculous mesenteric lymph nodes;
- tuberculosis of the ileocaecal region;
- a tuberculous pyosalpinx;
- blood-borne infection from pulmonary tuberculosis, usually the 'miliary' but occasionally the 'cavitating' form.

Varieties of tuberculous peritonitis

There are four varieties of tuberculous peritonitis: ascitic, encysted, fibrous and purulent.

Ascitic form

The peritoneum is studded with tubercules and the peritoneal cavity becomes filled with pale, straw-coloured fluid. The onset is insidious. There is loss of energy, facial pallor and some loss of weight. The patient is usually brought for advice because of enlargement of the abdomen. Pain is often completely absent; in other cases there is considerable abdominal discomfort which may be associated with constipation or diarrhoea. On inspection, dilated veins can be seen coursing beneath the skin of the abdominal wall. Shifting dullness can be elicited readily. In the male child congenital hydroceles sometimes appear, due to the patent processi vaginales becoming filled with ascitic fluid from the peritoneal cavity. Because of the increased intra-abdominal pressure an umbilical hernia commonly occurs. On abdominal palpation a transverse solid mass can often be detected. This is rolled-up greater omentum infiltrated with tubercules.

Diagnosis is seldom difficult except when it occurs in an acute form or when it first appears in an adult, in which case it has to be differentiated from other forms of ascites, especially from malignant secondary deposits. A positive Mantoux test in a child with ascites strongly suggests, and a negative test is good evidence against, tuberculosis. In adults this test is of negligible value. Laparoscopy is useful by allowing inspection of the peritoneal cavity, where the appearance is often diagnostic. Areas of caseation can be biopsied for histology and microbiological studies. The 'open' (Hassan) technique of trocar insertion should be used because of the risk of adhesions to the abdominal wall. The diagnosis of tuberculous peritonitis having been made, it is always important to look for tuberculous disease elsewhere. The possibility of tuberculous salpingitis in females should be remembered. A chest X-ray should always be taken before laparoscopy or laparotomy is performed.

The ascitic fluid is pale yellow, usually clear and rich in lymphocytes. The specific gravity is comparatively high, often 1.020 or over. Even after centrifugation, rarely can *M. tuberculosis* be found, but its presence can be demonstrated by culture or by guinea-pig inoculation.

Treatment. See guidelines, Chapter 8. If the general condition is good, the patient can return home and, if an adult, to light work, before the course of chemotherapy has been completed.

Encysted form

Encysted (syn. loculated) form is similar to the above, but one part of the abdominal cavity alone is involved. Thus, a localised intra-abdominal swelling is produced which gives rise to difficulty in diagnosis. In a female above the age of puberty when the swelling is in the pelvis, an ovarian cyst will probably be diagnosed. In the case of a child it is sometimes difficult to distinguish the swelling from a mesenteric cyst. For these reasons laparotomy is often performed, and if an encapsulated collection of fluid is found, it is evacuated and the abdomen is closed. The general treatment already detailed is required, but the response to this treatment is more rapid. Late intestinal obstruction is a possible complication.

Fibrous form

Fibrous (syn. plastic) form is characterised by the production of widespread adhesions, which cause coils of intestine, especially the ileum, to become matted together and distended. These distended coils act as a 'blind loop' and give rise to steatorrhoea, wasting and attacks of abdominal pain. On examination, the adherent intestine with omentum attached, together with the thickened mesentery, may give rise to a palpable swelling or swellings. The first intimation of the disease may be subacute or acute intestinal obstruction. Sometimes the cause of the obstruction can be remedied easily by the division of bands. Lateral anastomosis between an obviously dilated loop and a collapsed loop of small intestine should not be done, as the 'blind loop' syndrome is a certain outcome. If the adhesions are accompanied by fibrous strictures of the ileum as well it is best to excise the affected bowel, provided not too much of the small intestine needs to be sacrificed. If adhesions only are present a plication may be performed (see Chapter 58). Chemotherapy after adequate surgery will rapidly cure the condition.

Purulent form

The purulent form is rare. When it occurs, usually it is secondary to tuberculous salpingitis. Amidst a mass of adherent intestine and omentum, tuberculous pus is present. Sizeable cold abscesses often form, and point on the surface, commonly near the umbilicus, or burst into the bowel. In addition to prolonged general treatment, operative treatment

---

Charles Mantoux, 1877–1947. Physician, Le Cannet, Alpes Maritimes, France.

may be necessary for the evacuation of cold abscesses and possibly for intestinal obstruction. If a faecal fistula forms it usually persists because of distal intestinal obstruction. Closure of the fistula must therefore be combined with some form of anastomosis between the segment of intestine above the fistula and an unobstructed area below. The prognosis of this variety of tuberculous peritonitis is relatively poor.

Peritoneal bands and adhesions

Congenital bands and membranes. Congenital bands and membranes occur in the peritoneum at various sites as described in textbooks of anatomy. Intestinal obstruction is rarely seen except by an obliterated vitellointestinal duct.

Peritoneal adhesions. Peritoneal adhesions are abnormal deposits of fibrous tissue that form after peritoneal injury. They follow operation or peritonitis and are the commonest cause of small bowel obstruction and secondary female infertility in developed countries. They are discussed in detail in Chapter 58.

Talc granuloma. Talc (silicate of magnesium) should never be used as a lubricant for rubber gloves for it is a cause of peritoneal adhesions and granulomas in the Fallopian tubes. Potassium bitartrate which is completely soluble is free from these serious complications.

Starch peritonitis. Like talc, starch powder has found disfavour as a surgical glove lubricant. In a few starch-sensitive patients it causes a painful ascites, fortunately of limited duration. Should laparotomy be performed any small granulomas in, say, the omentum will be found to contain birefringent starch particles. Starch-free surgical gloves are now widely available.

Ascites

Ascites, an excess of serous fluid within the peritoneal cavity, can be recognised clinically only when the amount of fluid present exceeds 1500 ml; in the obese a greater quantity than this is necessary before there is clear evidence of the presence of intraperitoneal fluid. Ultrasound and CT scanning can detect much smaller volumes of ascitic fluid.

Mechanism of ascites

The balanced effects of plasma and peritoneal colloid osmotic and hydrostatic pressures determine the exchange of fluid between the capillaries and the peritoneal fluid. Normal intraperitoneal pressure and normal peritoneal fluid colloid osmotic pressure cannot be measured. Protein-rich fluid enters the peritoneal cavity when capillary permeability to protein is increased, as in peritonitis and carcinomatosis peritonei. Capillary pressure may be increased because of generalised water retention, cardiac failure, constrictive pericarditis or vena cava obstruction. Capillary pressure is raised selectively in the portal venous system in the Budd–Chiari syndrome, cirrhosis of the liver or extra-hepatic portal venous obstruction (see Chapter 52). Plasma colloid osmotic pressure may be lowered in patients with reduced nutritional intake, diminished intestinal absorption, abnormal protein losses, or defective protein synthesis as occurs in cirrhosis. Peritoneal lymphatic drainage may be impaired resulting in the accumulation of protein-rich fluid.

Table 56.7 Causes of ascites

Transudates (protein <25 g/litre)
Low plasma protein concentrations
Malnutrition
Nephrotic syndrome
Protein-losing enteropathy
High central venous pressure
Congestive cardiac failure
Constrictive pericarditis
Cirrhosis
Portal vein thrombosis
Exudates (protein >25 g/litre)
Tuberculous peritonitis
Peritoneal malignancy
Budd–Chiari syndrome (hepatic vein occlusion or thrombosis)
Pancreatic ascites
Chylous ascites
Meigs' syndrome

Clinical features

The abdomen is distended evenly, with fullness of the flanks, which are dull to percussion. Usually shifting dullness is present, but when there is a very large accumulation of fluid this sign is absent. In such cases, on flicking the abdominal wall, a characteristic fluid thrill is transmitted from one side to the other. In women, ascites must be differentiated from an enormous ovarian cyst. The causes of ascites are listed in Table 56.7.

Congestive heart failure, the commonest cause of ascites, causes increased venous pressure in the vena cava and consequent obstruction to the venous outflow from the liver. This increased pressure can be seen as engorgement of the veins of the neck – a striking sign in this condition. The ascitic fluid is light yellow and of low specific gravity, about 1.010, with a low protein concentration (<25 g/litre). Patients with constrictive pericarditis (syn. Pick's disease) have both peritoneal and pleural effusions due to engorgement of the venae cavae consequent upon the diminished capacity of the right side of the heart.

In cirrhosis there is obstruction to the portal venous system which is caused by obliterative fibrosis of the intrahepatic venous bed. Lymph flow may be increased. In the Budd–Chiari syndrome (Chapter 52), thrombosis or obstruction of the hepatic veins is responsible for obstruction to venous outflow from the liver.

The ascites seen in patients with peritoneal metastases is due to excessive exudation of fluid and lymphatic blockage. The fluid is dark yellow and frequently blood stained. The specific gravity, 1.020 or over, and the protein content

George Budd, 1808–82. Professor of Medicine, King's College Hospital, London, England.

Hans Chiari, 1851–1916. Professor of Pathological Anatomy, Prague and Strasbourg Universities.

Friedel Pick, 1876–1926. Professor of Laryngology, Prague, Czechoslovakia. Described this disease in 1896.

Joe Vincent Meigs, 1892–1964. Gynaecological Surgeon, Massachusetts General Hospital, Boston, Massachusetts, USA.

(>25 g/litre) are high. Microscopical examination often reveals cancer cells especially if large quantities of fluid are 'spun-down' to produce a concentrated deposit for sampling.

Ascites occurs with low plasma albumin concentrations; for example in patients with albuminuria or starvation. The ascites in this instance is due to alterations in the osmotic pressure of the capillary blood, and has a low specific gravity.

Rarely ascites and pleural effusion are associated with solid fibroma of the ovary (Meigs' syndrome). The effusions disappear when the tumour is excised.

Treatment

Ascites may be tapped (paracentesis abdominis) but unless other measures are taken, the fluid soon reaccumulates and repeated tappings remove valuable protein. Treatment of the specific cause is undertaken whenever possible, for example if portal venous pressure is raised, it may be possible to lower it by treatment of the primary condition (Chapter 52). Dietary sodium restriction to 200 mg per day may be helpful but diuretics are usually required.

Paracentesis abdominis

The bladder having been emptied by a catheter, under local anaesthesia puncture of the peritoneum is carried out with a moderate sized trocar and cannula at one of the points shown in Fig. 56.12. Alternatively a peritoneal drain may be inserted under ultrasound guidance to minimise the risk of visceral injury. In cases where the effusion is due to cardiac failure the fluid must be evacuated slowly. In other circumstances this precaution is unnecessary. If the cannula becomes blocked with fibrin it is cleared with a stylet or the drain is flushed. After the fluid has been evacuated the puncture is sealed and a tight binder is applied to the abdomen. Some surgeons prefer to perform the 'tap' over the liver beneath the costal margin or in the midline beneath the xiphisternum.

Permanent drainage of ascitic fluid

In rare cases where ascites accumulates rapidly after paracentesis and the patient is otherwise fit, permanent drainage of the ascitic fluid via a peritoneovenous shunt (e.g. LeVeen) may render the patient more comfortable. Similar in concept to shunts for hydrocephalus (Chapter 35), a catheter (e.g. of silicone) is constructed with a valve so as to allow one-way flow from the peritoneum to a central vein (e.g. internal jugular). A chamber placed subcutaneously over the chest wall may be included for manual compression. Insertion is relatively simple. The complications include overloading the venous system, cardiac failure and disseminated intravascular coagulopathy. The frequency of these complications may be reduced by evacuating ascitic fluid and partially replacing it with normal saline at the time of shunt insertion. The procedure may also be used for patients with terminal malignant ascites giving improved quality of life, despite the risk of further dissemination of malignant cells.

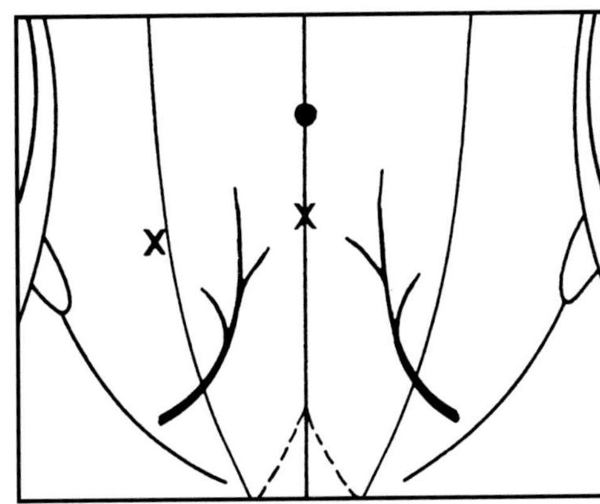

Fig. 56.12 Usual points of puncture for tapping ascites. The bladder must be emptied by a catheter before the puncture is made. Note the relationship of the sites of the puncture to the inferior epigastric artery (*courtesy of Drs V.C. and V.V. Shah, Jamnagar, India*).

Harry LeVeen. Professor of Surgery, University of South Carolina, USA.

Chylous ascites

In some patients the ascitic fluid appears milky due to an excess of chylomicrons (triglycerides). Most cases are associated with malignancy, usually lymphomas; other causes are cirrhosis, tuberculosis, filariasis, nephrotic syndrome, abdominal trauma (including surgery), constrictive pericarditis, sarcoidosis and congenital lymphatic abnormality. The condition is rare. The prognosis is poor unless the underlying condition can be cured. In addition to other measures used to treat ascites, patients should be placed on a fat-free diet with medium-chain triglyceride supplements.

Peritoneal loose bodies (peritoneal mice)

Peritoneal loose bodies almost never cause symptoms. One or more may be found in a hernial sac or in the pouch of Douglas. The loose body may come from an appendix epiploica that has undergone axial rotation followed by necrosis of its pedicle and detachment, but they are also found in those who suffer from subacute attacks of pancreatitis. These hyaline bodies attain the size of a pea or bean, and contain saponified fat surrounded by fibrin.

Neoplasms of the peritoneum

Carcinoma peritonei is a common terminal event in many cases of carcinoma of the stomach, colon, ovary or other abdominal organs and also of the breast and bronchus. The peritoneum, both parietal and visceral, is studded with secondary growths, and the peritoneal cavity becomes filled with clear, straw-coloured or blood-stained ascitic fluid.

The main forms of peritoneal metastases are:

- discrete nodules – by far the most common variety;
- plaques varying in size and colour;
- diffuse adhesions – this form occurs at a late stage of the disease, and gives rise, sometimes, to a 'frozen pelvis'.

Gravity probably determines the distribution of free malignant cells within the peritoneal cavity. Cells not caught in peritoneal folds along the attachments of mesenteries gravitate into the pelvic pouches or into a hernial sac, enlargement of which is occasionally the first indication of the condition. Implantation occurs also on the greater omentum, the appendices epiploicae and the inferior surface of the diaphragm. It is remarkable how often patients riddled with intraperitoneal carcinoma preserve their nutrition and look and feel comparatively well until the terminal stage.

James Douglas, 1675–1742. Anatomist and Obstetrician, London, England.

Differential diagnosis

Early discrete tubercles common in tuberculous peritonitis are greyish and translucent and closely resemble the discrete nodules of peritoneal carcinomatosis, but the latter feel hard when rolled between the finger and thumb, making the differential diagnosis tolerably simple. Fat necrosis usually can be distinguished from a carcinomatous nodule by its opacity. Peritoneal hydatids can also simulate malignant disease after rupture of a hydatid cyst, with seeding of daughter cysts.

Treatment

Ascites due to carcinomatosis of the peritoneum may respond to systemic chemotherapy. In other cases intraperitoneal chemotherapy with cisplatin, mitomycin C or methotrexate after drainage of ascites may be effective.

Tamoxifen (an oestrogen receptor site competitor) can dramatically reduce ascites due to breast cancers which are oestrogen dependent.

Pseudomyxoma peritonei

This rare condition occurs more frequently in females. The abdomen is filled with a yellow jelly, large quantities of which are often more or less encysted. The condition is associated with both mucinous cystic tumours of the ovary and appendix. Recent studies suggest that most cases arise from a primary appendiceal tumour with secondary implantation on to one or both ovaries. It is often painless and there is frequently no impairment of general health for a long time. Although an abdomen distended with what seems to be fluid that cannot be made to shift should raise the possibility, the diagnosis is more often suggested by ultrasound and CT scanning or made at operation. At laparotomy masses of jelly are scooped out. The appendix, if present, should be excised together with any ovarian tumour. Unfortunately recurrence is usual. Pseudomyxoma peritonei is locally malignant but does not give rise to extraperitoneal metastases. Occasionally the condition responds to radioactive isotopes or intraperitoneal chemotherapy which may be used in recurrent cases.

Mesothelioma

As in the pleural cavity, this is a highly malignant tumour. Asbestos is a recognised cause. It has a predilection for the pelvic peritoneum, but it is not radiosensitive. Alkylating agents have given remissions. Benign forms are reported. Recent regimens of multiple chemocytotoxic agents have been reported as curative for *early* forms of malignant mesothelioma.

Desmoid

This is considered under familial adenomatous polyposis (Chapter 57).

Laparoscopy (peritoneoscopy)

Laparoscopic surgery has developed rapidly over recent years (Chapter 70). Previously used largely as a diagnostic procedure, laparoscopy with the aid of modern video technology is now used to perform many 'minimally invasive' operations (Table 56.8).

The primary trocar for laparoscopy is inserted using either the 'open' or 'closed' technique. In the latter method a 'pneumoperitoneum' is created by the insertion of a special needle (e.g. Verres') through which carbon dioxide is delivered. Once the peritoneal cavity is adequately distended a sharp-ended trocar is inserted 'blindly' and the laparoscope then introduced. In the 'open' method, which is to be preferred, a small incision (usually subumbilical) is made through the abdominal wall down to the peritoneum which is opened under direct vision. This reduces the risk of visceral injury and eliminates the rare major vascular injuries (iliac, vena caval and aortic) that occur with the 'closed' method.

Table 56.8 Examples of laparoscopic surgery

Diagnostic
Ascites
Liver metastases/tumour
Staging investigations, e.g. stomach, pancreatic cancer
Acute abdominal pain, e.g. appendicitis, pelvic inflammatory disease
Therapeutic
Cholecystectomy
Appendicectomy
Operations for gastro-oesophageal reflux (e.g. fundoplication)
Closure of perforated peptic ulcer
Colostomy/ileostomy
Colorectal resection
Bile-duct exploration
Gastroenterostomy
Rectopexy

The greater omentum

Rutherford Morison called the greater omentum 'the abdominal policeman' [but it has not any feet, i.e. it does not move across the abdomen of its own volition, but passively due to peristalsis, and it may be pushed by the movements of the abdominal wall into an area of immobility (rigidity) where there is local peritoneal irritation]. Relatively larger and structurally more substantial in the adult than in the child, the discharge of its life-saving constabulary duties becomes more effective after puberty, and remains unabated throughout life. The greater omentum attempts, often successfully, to limit intraperitoneal infective and other noxious processes (Fig. 56.13). For instance, an acutely inflamed appendix is often found wrapped in omentum and this saves many patients from developing diffuse peritonitis. Some sufferers of herniae are also greatly indebted to this structure, for it often plugs the neck of a hernial sac and prevents a coil of intestine from entering and becoming strangulated.

Apart from a small portion of it becoming gangrenous while performing the last-mentioned duty (strangulated omentocele) this Good Samaritan[1] of the peritoneal cavity seldom itself becomes diseased; when it does become overwhelmed, as in tuberculous peritonitis and carcinomatosis peritonei, it becomes rolled like a scroll.

Torsion of the omentum. Torsion of the omentum is a rare emergency and consequently is seldom diagnosed correctly. It is usually mistaken for appendicitis with somewhat abnormal signs. It may be primary or secondary to an adhesion of the omentum, to an old focus of infection, or to a hernia. Successive herniations of a portion of the omentum into a hernial sac of irregular bore are credited with giving the necessary stimulus to omental torsion.

[1]*Samaritan, an inhabitant of Samaria, Jordan. The parable of the Good Samaritan is told in the Bible, Luke x, 30–7.*

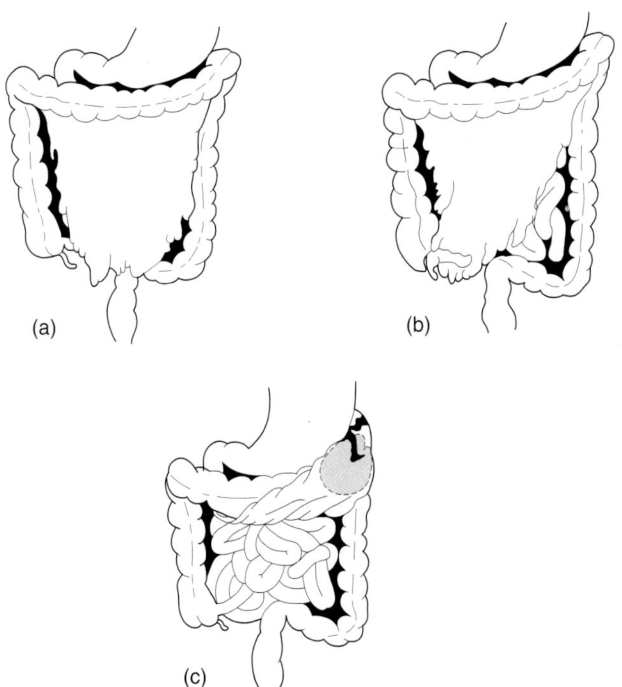

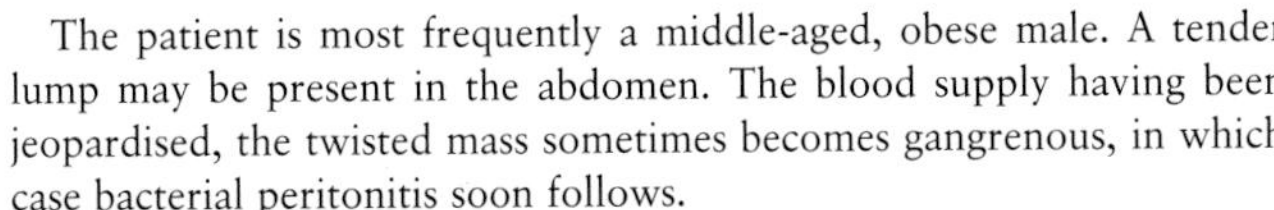

Fig. 56.13 The greater omentum. (a) Normal; (b) in appendicitis; (c) in a (comparatively small) laceration of the spleen.

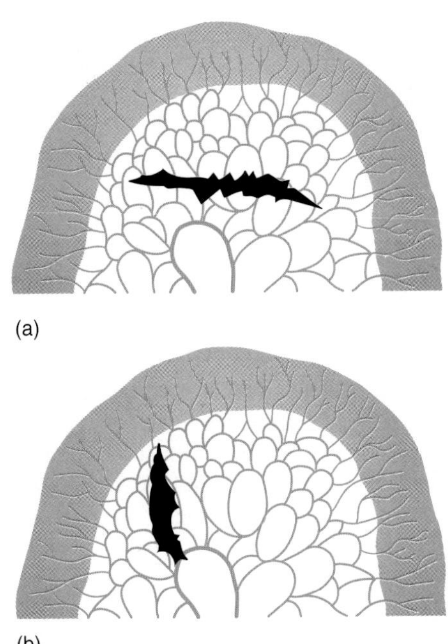

Fig. 56.14 Laceration of the mesentery, a common injury in driving accidents; (a) a transverse tear often imperils the blood supply of a segment of intestine, making resection necessary; (b) a longitudinal tear can also be closed by suture.

The patient is most frequently a middle-aged, obese male. A tender lump may be present in the abdomen. The blood supply having been jeopardised, the twisted mass sometimes becomes gangrenous, in which case bacterial peritonitis soon follows.

Treatment. The abdomen having been opened, the pedicle above the twist is ligated securely and the mass removed.

Omental cyst (see below).

The mesentery

A wound of the mesentery can follow a severe abdominal contusion and is a cause of haemoperitoneum.

Seat-belt syndrome

If a car accident occurs when a seat belt is worn, sudden de-acceleration can result in a torn mesentery. This possibility should be borne in mind particularly as multiple injuries may distract attention from this injury. If there is any bruising of the abdominal wall, or even marks of clothing impressed into the skin, laparotomy may be indicated.

Diagnostic peritoneal lavage

Diagnostic peritoneal lavage may be helpful in this situation (Chapter 4). Under local anaesthetic a subumbilical incision is made down to the peritoneum in a similar way to that used for 'open' laparoscopy (see above). A purse-string suture is placed in the peritoneum which is then incised. Free fluid, e.g. blood or intestinal contents, may be found, but if not a peritoneal dialysis catheter is inserted and the purse-string suture tied. A litre of normal saline is run into the peritoneum and then drained off by placing the bag and tubing below the patient's abdomen. The presence of blood ($>$100 000 red blood cells/mm^3), bile or intestinal contents is an indication for laparotomy. In about 60 per cent of cases, the mesenteric laceration is associated with a rupture of the intestine. If the tear is a large one and especially if it is transverse (Fig. 56.14a), the blood supply to the neighbouring intestine is cut off and a limited resection of gut is imperative. Small wounds and wounds in the long axis (Fig. 56.14b) should be sutured. If extensive damage to the mesenteric arcade of vessels is associated with damage to contiguous intestine, exteriorisation of the damaged segment is preferable to excision and suture.

Torsion of the mesentery

See volvulus neonatorum, and volvulus of the small intestine, Chapter 58.

Embolism and thrombosis of mesenteric vessels

See Chapters 57 and 58.

Acute nonspecific ileocaecal mesenteric adenitis

Aetiology

Nonspecific mesenteric adenitis was so named to distinguish it from specific (tuberculous) mesenteric adenitis. It is now very much more common than the tuberculous variety. Despite much investigation the aetiology often remains unknown although some cases are associated with Yersinia infection of the ileum. In other cases an unidentified virus is blamed. In about 25 per cent of cases a respiratory infection precedes an attack of nonspecific mesenteric adenitis. This self-limiting disease is never fatal but may be recurrent.

Pathology

There is a small increase in the amount of peritoneal fluid. The ileocaecal mesenteric lymph nodes are enlarged and can be seen and felt between the leaves of the mesentery. In very acute cases they are distinctly red and many of them are the size of a walnut. The nodes nearest the attachment of the mesentery are the largest. They are not adherent to their peritoneal coats and if a small incision is made through the overlying peritoneum, a node is extruded easily.

Clinical features

During childhood, acute nonspecific mesenteric adenitis is a common condition. It is unusual after puberty but is sometimes seen in teenage girls. The typical history is one of short attacks of central abdominal pain lasting from 10 to 30 minutes, and associated with circumoral pallor. They tend to come on when the patient is tired. Vomiting is common but there is no alteration of bowel habit. If vomiting is absent, it is more likely to be a case of mesenteric adenitis than appendicitis.

On examination

There are spasms of general abdominal colic, usually referred to the umbilicus, with intervals of complete freedom, which never appertains in obstructive appendicitis. The patient seldom looks ill. In more than half of the cases the temperature is elevated; in severe examples it exceeds 38.3°C. Abdominal tenderness is greatest along the line of the mesentery. When present, shifting tenderness is a valuable sign for differentiating the condition from appendicitis. After laying the patient on the left side for a few minutes, the maximum tenderness moves to the left of the original site.

The pelvic peritoneum is tender to rectal palpation in 30 per cent of cases. The neck, axillae and groins should be palpated for enlarged lymph nodes – if these nodes are enlarged, brucellosis should come to mind.

Leucocyte count

There is often a leucocytosis of 10 000–12 000/mm^3 (10–12 × 10^9/litre) or more on the first day of the attack, but this falls on the second day.

Treatment

When the diagnosis can be made with assurance, bed rest for a few days is the only treatment necessary. If at a second examination, an hour or two after confinement to bed, acute appendicitis cannot be excluded, it is safer to perform either appendicectomy or diagnostic laparoscopy.

Tuberculosis of the mesenteric lymph nodes

Tuberculous mesenteric lymphadenitis is considerably less common than acute nonspecific lymphadenitis. Tubercle bacilli, usually, but not necessarily, bovine, are ingested and enter the mesenteric lymph nodes by way of Peyer's patches. It is possible for one draught of raw milk to start the infection; it is equally possible that a toddler can become infected with human tubercule bacilli by placing one dust-covered small object in its mouth. Sometimes only one lymph node is infected; usually there are several; occasionally massive involvement occurs.

Presentation. ***Demonstrated radiologically.*** The shadows cast by one or more calcified tuberculous lymph nodes are seen in a plain radiograph of the abdomen. They must be distinguished from other calcified lesions, e.g. renal or ureteric stones. Their mobility on repeated plain abdominal radiographs can clinch the diagnosis but urography can be employed in doubtful cases. Often the shadow cast by such a lymph node or nodes is situated in the ileocaecal region, but nearly as many are displayed along the line of attachment of the mesentery. Usually, the radiological characteristics are unmistakable. Each node is round or oval, not homogeneous, but mottled, and its outline is not regular, but bosselated like a blackberry. Calcification of these lymph nodes occurs at the earliest in 18 months. It is often assumed, wrongly, that because a tuberculous lymph node is calcified, the infection is necessarily defunct. Especially in children, this assumption may not be valid.

As a cause of general symptoms. The patient, usually a child under 10 years of age, loses appetite, looks pale and there is some loss of weight; sometimes evening pyrexia occurs. In children with these symptoms, especially those who live in the country, if the Mantoux test is negative, brucellosis, the 'disease of mistakes' should be thought of and serological studies undertaken.

As a cause of abdominal pain. Sometimes abdominal pain is the cause of the patient being brought for advice; usually this pain is central, not severe but rather a discomfort and is often constant. On examination the abdomen is somewhat protuberant and there is tenderness on deep pressure to the right of the umbilicus. In these circumstances, the condition resembles acute nonspecific mesenteric lymphadenitis. On deep palpation inflamed mesenteric lymph nodes are sometimes palpable as firm, discrete, tender, bean-like objects most frequently to the right of and near the umbilicus. A normal leuococyte count favours tuberculosis and, in a child, a positive Mantoux test is confirmatory evidence of tuberculosis.

Symptoms indistinguishable from those of appendicitis. On occasions the abdominal pain is acute and may be accompanied by vomiting. This, combined with tenderness and some rigidity in the right iliac fossa, makes the diagnosis from appendicitis almost impossible. When, as is sometimes the case, the tuberculous infection of the mesenteric lymph nodes becomes reactivated in adolescent or adult life, the diagnostic difficulties are even greater. A radiograph may show calcified lymph nodes, but as such a condition can coexist with appendicitis, in some cases laparoscopy or laparotomy is necessary. If the mesentery is found to be in an inflamed state with caseation of some of the lymph nodes, the diagnosis of active tuberculosis is confirmed.

Sir David Bruce, 1855–1931. Major-General, Royal Army Medical Service. He described Malta fever ('brucellosis') in 1887.

Johann Conrad Peyer, 1653–1712. Professor of Logic, Rhetoric and Medicine, Schaffhausen, Switzerland.

As a cause of intestinal obstruction. Remote, rather than recent, tuberculous mesenteric adenitis can be the cause of intestinal obstruction. For instance, a coil of small intestine becomes adherent to a caseating node, and is thereby angulated, or a free coil may become imprisoned in the tunnel beneath the site of adherence and the mesentery.

As a cause of pseudomesenteric cyst. When tuberculous mesenteric lymph nodes break down, the tuberculous pus may remain confined between the leaves of the mesentery, and a cystic swelling having the characteristics of a mesenteric cyst is found. When such a condition is confirmed at operation, the tuberculous pus should be aspirated without soiling the peritoneal cavity, the wound closed, the sensitivity of the organism should be sought and medical treatment continued until the infection has been overcome.

As ileocaecal lymph nodes. At laparotomy hard, enlarged lymph nodes may be found limited to the ileocaecal mesentery as a result of previous tuberculous infection. If the nodes have a yellow colour, they may well arise from a carcinoid tumour of the appendix or ileum (Chapter 57).

Treatment. Therapy is similar to that of other tuberculous infections (Chapter 8). Most cases subside but from time to time a local abscess forms, usually in the right iliac fossa when the tuberculous pus should be evacuated and the abdomen closed without drainage.

Mesenteric cysts

Mesenteric cysts are classified as:

- chylolymphatic;
- enterogenous;
- urogenital remnant;
- dermoid (teratomatous cyst).

Chylolymphatic cyst, the commonest variety of mesenteric cyst, probably arises in congenitally misplaced lymphatic tissue that has no efferent communication with the lymphatic system; it arises most frequently in the mesentery of the ileum. The thin wall of the cyst, which is composed of connective tissue lined by flat endothelium, is filled with clear lymph or, less frequently, with chyle varying in consistency from watered milk to cream. Occasionally the cyst attains a great size. More often unilocular than multilocular, a chylolymphatic cyst is almost invariably solitary, although there is an extremely rare variety in which myriads of cysts are found in the various mesenteries of the abdomen. A chylolymphatic cyst has a blood supply independent of that of the adjacent intestine, thereby enucleation is possible without the necessity of resection of gut.

Enterogenous cyst is believed to be derived either from a diverticulum of the mesenteric border of the intestine, which has become sequestrated from the intestinal canal during embryonic life, or from a duplication of the intestine. An enterogenous cyst has a thicker wall than a chylolymphatic cyst, and it is lined by mucous membrane, sometimes ciliated. The content is mucinous, and is either colourless or yellowish-brown from bygone haemorrhage into the cyst. As can be seen at operation, the muscle in the wall of an enterogenous cyst and the bowel with which it is in contact have a common blood supply; consequently removal of the cyst always entails resection of the related portion of intestine.

Clinical features of a mesenteric cyst. A mesenteric cyst is encountered most frequently in the second decade of life, less often between the ages of 1 and 10 years and, exceptionally, in infants under 1 year.

The patient presents on account of:

- *a painless abdominal swelling.* A cyst of the mesentery presents characteristic physical signs:
  - there is a fluctuant swelling near the umbilicus (Fig. 56.15a),
  - the swelling moves freely in a plane at right angles to the attachment of the mesentery (Fig. 56.15b),
  - there is a zone of resonance around and, classically, a belt of resonance across the cyst;

(a)

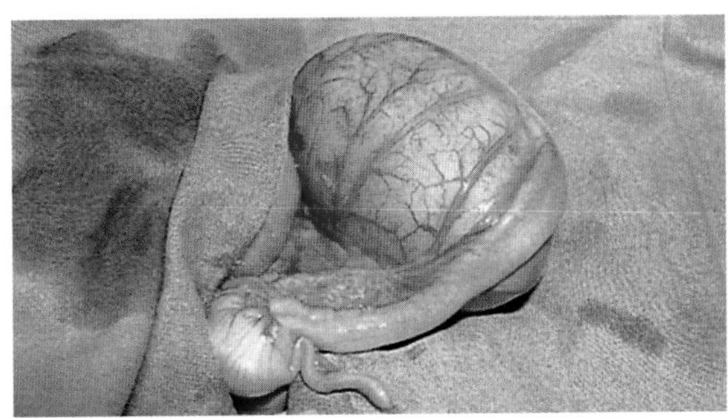

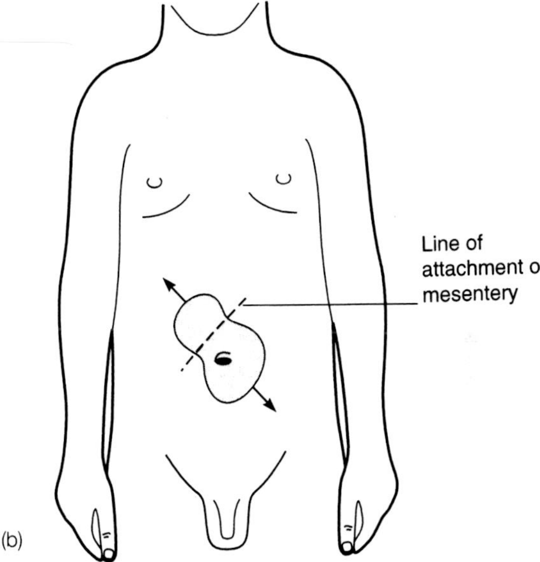

(b)

Fig. 56.15 A mesenteric cyst (a) moves freely in the direction of the arrows, i.e. at right angles to the attachment of the mesentery (b).

- *recurrent attacks of abdominal pain* with or without vomiting. The pain results from recurring temporary impaction of a food bolus in a segment of bowel narrowed by the cyst, or possibly from torsion of the mesentery;
- *an acute abdominal catastrophe* arises as a result of:
  - torsion of that portion of the mesentery containing the cyst,
  - rupture of the cyst, often due to a comparatively trivial accident,
  - haemorrhage into the cyst,
  - infection.

Radiography. In most instances, the patient should be submitted to a barium meal and follow through. The hollow viscera will be found to be displaced around the cyst and not infrequently some portion of the lumen of the small intestine will be narrowed. In order to exclude or confirm the diagnosis of a hydronephrosis, an ultrasound examination or a urogram should be performed. In cases of painless enlargement of the abdomen, an ultrasound scan should be undertaken first. Needle aspiration combined with instillation of radio-opaque water-soluble contrast media can transform doubt into certainty.

Treatment. As has been indicated already, many chylolymphatic cysts can be enucleated *in toto*.

When, after aspiration of about half the contents of the cyst, the major portion of the cyst has been dissected free, but one portion abutting on the intestine or a major blood vessel seems too dangerous to remove, this portion can be left attached and its lining destroyed by careful diathermy.

In the case of an enterogenous cyst, enucleation must not be attempted. If a comparatively short segment of the intestine is involved, resection of the cyst with the adherent portion of the intestine, followed by intestinal anastomosis, is the correct course. Should a very large segment of small intestine be implicated, an anastomosis should be made between the apex of the coil of small intestine and the cyst wall which, in this instance, holds sutures well.

The older treatment of marsupialisation of a mesenteric cyst has little to recommend it; a fistula or recurrence results. Occasionally, however, on account of its simplicity it is advisable in a poor-risk subject in whom surgery is necessary.

Omental cysts

Omental cysts occur nearly as frequently as mesenteric cysts. Preoperative differentiation is possible because a lateral radiograph, ultrasound or CT scan shows the cyst in front of the intestines. Treatment is omentectomy.

Cyst of the mesocolon

Cyst of the mesocolon is uncommon and it is differentiated from a mesenteric cyst only at operation. The treatment is similar.

Cysts arising from a urogenital remnant

Cysts arising from a urogenital (Wolffian or Müllerian) remnant are essentially retroperitoneal, but they are included in the classification because it is not impossible for such a cyst to project forward into the mesentery.

The following, while not being mesenteric cysts in the true meaning of the term, give rise to the same physical signs and, in practice, they *are* mesenteric cysts:

- *serosanguineous* cyst is probably traumatic in origin, but a history of an accident is seldom obtained;
- *tuberculous abscess of the mesentery*;
- *hydatid cyst of the mesentery*.

Neoplasms of the mesentery

Mesenteric tumours are classified as:

- benign:
  - lipoma,
  - fibroma,
  - fibromyxoma;
- malignant:
  - lymphoma,
  - secondary carcinoma.

Tumours situated in the mesentery give rise to physical signs similar to those of a mesenteric cyst, the sole exception being that they sometimes feel solid.

A benign tumour of the mesentery is excised in the same way as an enterogenous mesenteric cyst, i.e. with resection of the adjacent intestine. When possible, a malignant tumour of the mesentery is subjected to the same treatment. In inoperable cases, radiotherapy can be employed if the biopsy specimen reveals that the growth is radiosensitive.

Kasper Friedrick Wolff, 1733–94. Professor of Anatomy and Physiology, St Petersburg, Russia.

Johannes Peter Müller, 1801–58. Professor of Anatomy and Physiology, Berlin, Germany.

The retroperitoneal space

Pus or blood in the retroperitoneal space tends to track to the corresponding iliac fossa. If a retroperitoneal abscess develops, it should be evacuated by the nearest route through the abdominal wall, avoiding opening the peritoneum. Should the retroperitoneal collection be found at laparotomy, it must be drained by a counter-incision in the flank. Pus frequently develops from a renal or spinal source and is sometimes tuberculous ('cold abscess'): tracking can develop alongside the psoas muscle and appear in the groin, where it must be distinguished from other swellings (e.g. hernia, Chapter 62). Retroperitoneal haematoma may be caused by fractured spine, a leaking abdominal aneurysm, acute pancreatitis or a ruptured kidney.

Retroperitoneal cyst

A cyst developing in the retroperitoneal space often attains very large dimensions, and has at first to be distinguished from a hydronephrosis. Even after the latter condition has been eliminated by scanning or urography, a retroperitoneal cyst can seldom be diagnosed with certainty from a retroperitoneal tumour until displayed at operation. The cyst may be unilocular or multilocular. Many of these cysts are believed to be derived from a remnant of the Wolffian duct, in which case they are filled with clear fluid. Others are teratomatous and are filled with sebaceous material.

Excision of these and other retroperitoneal swellings is best performed through a transperitoneal incision.

Idiopathic retroperitoneal fibrosis

This is one of a group of fibromatoses (others being Dupuytren's contracture and Peyronies disease). Most cases are idiopathic, but many causes are known (Table 56.9). Familial cases are known, involving mediastinal fibrosis, sclerosing cholangitis, Riedel's thyroiditis and orbital pseudotumour. An autoimmune link has not been demonstrated. Extensive collagen deposition surrounds the ureters, mostly at the level

Table 56.9 Causes of retroperitoneal fibrosis

Causes
Benign
Idiopathic (Ormond's disease)
Chronic inflammation
Extravasation of urine
Retroperitoneal irritation by leakage of blood or intestinal content
Aortic aneurysm ('inflammatory type')
Trauma
Drugs
– chemotherapeutic agents
– methysergide
– beta-adrenoceptor antagonists
Malignant
Lymphoma
Carcinoid tumours
Secondary deposits (especially from carcinoma of stomach, colon, breast and prostate)

J.K. Ormond, an American urologist, described the typical findings in a case of retroperitoneal fibrosis in 1947.

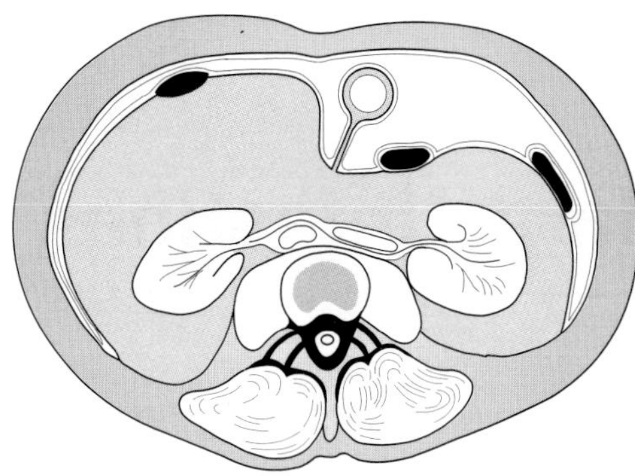

Fig. 56.16 Rapidly growing retroperitoneal liposarcoma.

of the pelvic brim or below. Most patients present with ureteric obstruction, often with renal failure (Chapter 64); cases due to malignancy are treated appropriately according to the cause, but the prognosis is often poor.

Primary retroperitoneal neoplasms arising from connective tissues

Retroperitoneal lipoma, in the first instance, is usually mistaken for a hydronephrosis, a diagnosis which is ruled out by ultrasonography, CT scan or urography. Women are more often affected. These swellings sometimes reach an immense size. A retroperitoneal lipoma sometimes undergoes myxomatous degeneration, a complication which does not occur in a lipoma in any other part of the body. Moreover, a retroperitoneal lipoma is often malignant (liposarcoma) (Fig. 56.16) and may increase rapidly in size.

Retroperitoneal sarcoma presents signs similar to a retroperitoneal lipoma. The patient may seek advice on account of a swelling or because of indefinite abdominal pain. On other occasions the tumour, by pressure on the colon, causes symptoms of subacute intestinal obstruction. On examination a smooth fixed mass, which is not tender, is palpated. The most probable original diagnosis is that of a neoplasm of the kidney. This is ruled out by scanning or urography. The ureter, however, is liable to become displaced by the tumour. Exploratory laparotomy should be performed and when possible the tumour is removed. Often it is found widely disseminated in the retroperitoneal space, rendering complete removal impossible, in which case a portion is excised for microscopy. Even when excised at a comparatively early stage, recurrence always takes place, and these tumours must be looked upon as being necessarily fatal. Radiotherapy sometimes keeps recurrences in abeyance for a time.

Removal of a retroperitoneal cyst or neoplasm. After the anterior abdominal wall has been opened and the diagnosis of a retroperitoneal tumour has been confirmed, the incision is extended as necessary. The small intestine is packed away in the upper abdomen or exteriorised and the caecum and the sigmoid colon are relegated to their respective fossae. The posterior peritoneum is then incised throughout its length over the area to be exposed, the incision being parallel to the left border of the aorta. The peritoneum is dissected from the tumour which is removed as completely as possible.

Baron Guillaume Dupuytren, 1777–1835. Surgeon, Hôtel Dieu, Paris, France.

François de la Peyronie, 1678–1747. Surgeon to Louis XIV and founder of the Royal Academy of Surgery, Paris, France.

Bernhard Moritz Carl Ludwig Riedel, 1846–1916. Professor of Surgery, Jena, Germany. Described form of thyroiditis in 1896.

J.K. Ormond, an American urologist, described the typical findings in a case of retroperitoneal fibrosis in 1947.

Retroperitoneal tumours arising from specific organs

These may arise from:

- lymph nodes (Chapter 17);
- adrenal gland (Chapter 45);
- kidney and ureter (Chapter 64);
- nervous tissue (Chapter 34).

Further reading

Jenkins, M.P., Alvaranga, J.C. and Thomas, J.M. (1996) The management of retroperitoneal soft tissue sarcomas. *European Journal of Cancer,* **32A**, 622–6.

Krukowski, Z.H. and Matheson, N.A. (1983) The management of peritoneal and parietal contamination in abdominal surgery. *British Journal of Surgery*, **10**, 440.

Paterson-Brown, S. (ed.) (1997) *Emergency Surgery and Critical Care*, W.B. Saunders, London.

Press, O.W., Press, N.O. and Kaufman, S.D. (1982) Evaluation and management of chylous ascites. *Annals of Internal Medicine*, **96**, 358.

Trentner, K.-H. and Schumpelick, V. (eds) (1997) *Peritoneal Adhesions*, Springer, Berlin.

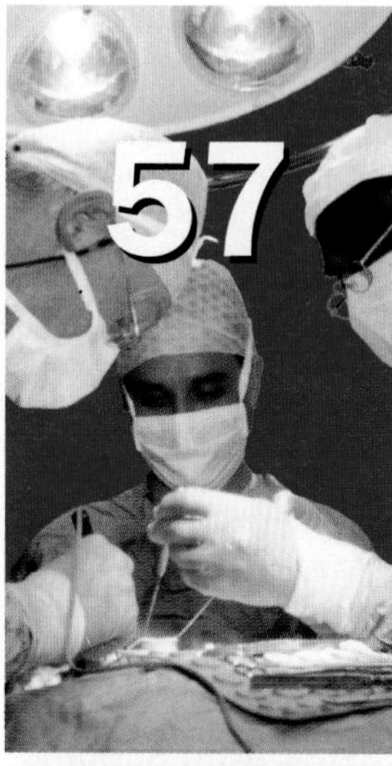

57 The small and large intestines

Abdominal pain

Abdominal pain arising from the alimentary canal is of two types.

1. **Visceral pain.** The alimentary tract is primarily a midline structure with a bilateral nerve supply. Although rotation about the midline occurs during development, nevertheless true visceral pain is referred to the midline as shown in Fig. 57.1. It is dull and poorly localised. For example, an obstructing stenosis of the terminal ileum, which is part of the midgut, would give rise to colicky periumbilical pain.
2. **Peritoneal pain** is of the somatic type and is much more precise, more severe and localised to the site of origin. These components account for the changes in character and site of pain which occur in appendicitis. Once the full thickness of the appendicular wall becomes inflamed the overlying peritoneum becomes involved and the patient has localised right iliac fossa pain (see Chapter 59).

Surgical anatomy

It is of great practical importance to be able to do the following:

1. distinguish various portions of the intestinal tract at sight;
2. know in which part of the abdomen the upper coils, as opposed to the lower coils, of small intestine lie in relationship to the anterior abdominal wall;
3. be able to decide which is the proximal and which is the distal end of any coil under consideration;
4. distinguish irrefutably large from small intestine.

The following are useful tips.

Bailey & Love's Short Practice of Surgery, 23rd edition. Edited by R.C.G. Russell, N.S. Williams and C.J.K. Bulstrode. Published in 2000 by Arnold Publishers.

- The mesentery of the jejunum has only two series of arcades of blood vessels, whereas the lower ileum has several series of arcades.
- The mesenteric attachment runs from left to right. Provided that the gut is not twisted, the proximal small bowel lies in the upper part of the abdomen and the lower small bowel lies in the lower part of the abdomen.
- The large intestine can be characterised by its taenia coli and appendices epiploicae.

Malformations and functional abnormalities

Congenital malformations

These malformations are described in the following:

- congenital atresia of the duodenum (see Chapter 58);
- congenital atresia of the small intestine (see Chapter 58);
- volvulus neonatorum (see Chapter 58);
- vascular anomalies (angiodysplasia) (see below);
- malrotation of the colon with failure of descent of the caecum which remains under the right lobe of the liver. This is clearly very important should the patient develop appendicitis (see Chapter 59).

Megacolon and nonmegacolon constipation

There is no single definition of constipation that can be described according to the character of the stools, the frequency of evacuation and the ease of evacuation. Generally speaking a bowel frequency of less than one every 3 days would be

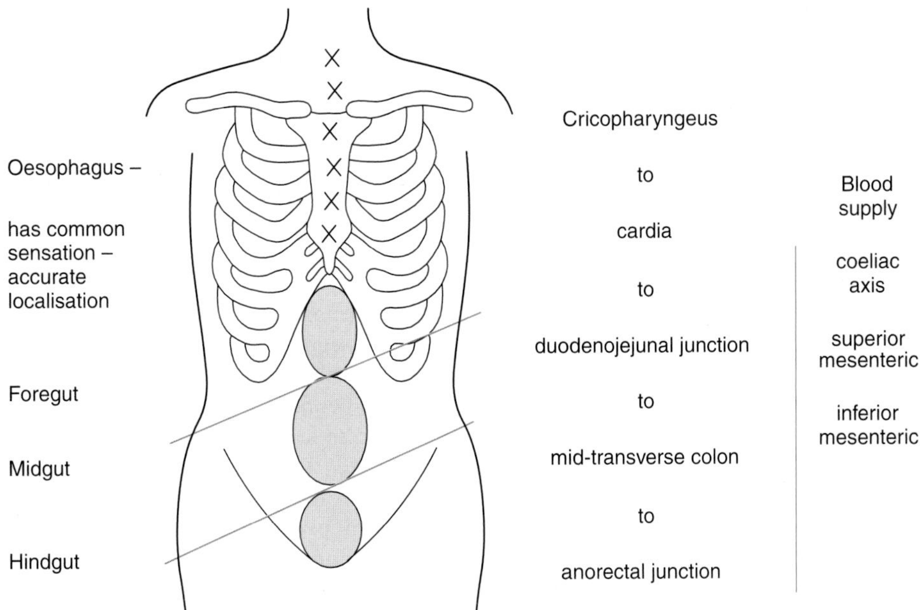

Fig. 57.1 Sites of origin of visceral pain.

considered abnormal. This group of conditions can be divided into:

1. megacolon:
   (a) Hirschsprung's disease,
   (b) non-Hirschsprung's megarectum and megacolon;
2. nonmegacolon:
   (a) slow transit,
   (b) normal transit.

Hirschsprung's disease

Pathology

The major feature of Hirschsprung's disease is an absence of ganglion cells in the neural plexus of the intestinal wall, together with hypertrophy of the nerve trunks. This is believed to result from a failure of migration of neuroblasts into the gut from vagal nerve trunks at the end of the first trimester of foetal life.

The loss of ganglion cells extends for a variable distance above the anorectal junction. In about two-thirds of patients the rectum and lower sigmoid colon are involved, but involvement of extremely short segments of the lower rectum or the whole intestinal tract have been described.

The severity of symptoms is not always consistent with the length of the intestinal segment involved and may be related to the number of acetylcholinesterase-positive nerve fibres.

The absence of ganglion cells gives rise to a contracted nonperistaltic segment with a dilated hypertrophied segment of normal colon above it (Fig. 57.2).

Clinical features

Hirschsprung's disease occurs in approximately one in 4500 live births. It shows a familial tendency and is more common in males than in females.

Harold Hirschsprung, 1830–1916. Physician, Queen Louise Hospital for Children, Copenhagen, Denmark.

The clinical picture varies from acute intestinal obstruction in neonates to chronic constipation in later life.

1. In neonates the delayed passage of meconium together with mild abdominal distension should alert the paediatrician to the diagnosis of Hirschsprung's disease. It is often complicated by enterocolitis which may result in perforation and septicaemia, and there is still a high mortality from Hirschsprung's disease at this age.

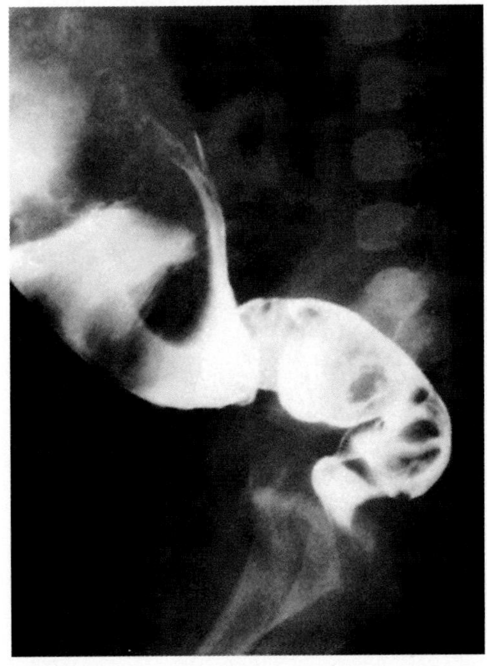

Fig. 57.2 Radiological appearances in Hirschsprung's disease; coning (the transitional zone) as well as dilation, above the contracted segment, is apparent.

2. Chronic constipation starting in the first few weeks of life. The classic picture of gross abdominal distension, chronic constipation and failure to thrive should be rare with a greater awareness of the diagnosis.
3. Severe constipation without soiling in otherwise healthy children and adults can be caused by a short segment of Hirschsprung's disease. Faecal soiling is not usually a feature of the condition.

Diagnosis

Rectal biopsy. Confirmation of the diagnosis depends on histological demonstration of aganglionosis and hypertrophic nerve fibres in the nerve plexus. The pathologist has to be able to see a representative area of at least one nerve plexus in the biopsy. In children this can be obtained by a suction rectal biopsy or, in adults, by a formal strip, full-thickness, rectal biopsy. Specimens are usually taken from just above the anorectal junction. One is sent for biochemistry and one for histochemistry and histopathology (Fig. 57.3).

Anorectal manometry. This is a useful screening test in the constipated young child or adult who is otherwise fit. The rectosphincteric inhibitory reflex is absent. It should not be carried out in ill neonates because of poor anal tone.

Radiology. Erect and supine abdominal radiographs are useful. If the large intestine is obstructed, they will show distended loops of small and large intestine with fluid levels consistent with a low intestinal obstruction. Intramural gas will indicate enterocolitis, and free peritoneal gas, a perforation.

An enema using a water-soluble contrast medium will often confirm the diagnosis and indicate the length and site of involved intestine. A rectal examination should not be performed before radiology because it may dilate the abnormal segment and modify the radiological features. The contrast is instilled through a fine 5 Fr catheter under screening control with the patient in the lateral position. The coning down of the transition zone, irregularity in the mucosa and abnormal contractions of the intestine are important positive findings.

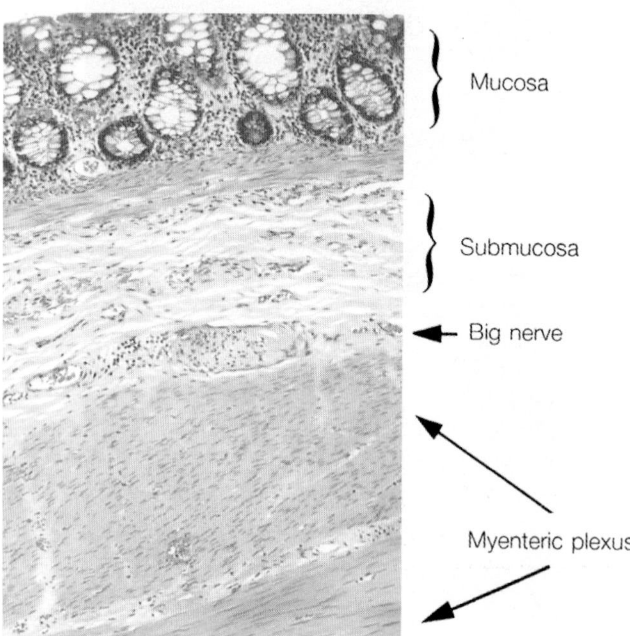

Fig. 57.3 Section of involved segment in Hirschsprung's disease. Note the large nerves but absence of ganglia. Haematoxylin and eosin.

Treatment

This depends on the age of the patient, the length of the involved segment, the severity of symptoms and the presence of enterocolitis.

In the neonate presenting with obstruction or any child or adult presenting with enterocolitis, an initial colostomy is performed. The site of the colostomy should be as low as possible in the ganglionated segment. A peroperative frozen section biopsy is taken to establish the presence of ganglia. This is important as the transition zone may be difficult to locate precisely.

In the child or adult with constipation alone, the dilated intestine can be evacuated with repeat rectal saline washouts and enemas as a first step. The choice of surgical procedure to follow will depend on the length of the involved segment.

Short segment disease with minimal symptoms may respond to an extended myectomy removing a strip of rectal wall up to the area where normal ganglion cells start.

Long segment disease may be helped by one of the four operations shown below. The definitive operation is preceded by a temporary colostomy for a few months which allows the proximal distended colon to return to its normal calibre. If a neonate requires a colostomy the definitive operation is delayed until the child weighs approximately 10 kg when the pelvis is still shallow but wide enough to give good access. The child will be between 10 months and 1 year of age and toilet training can usually start soon after the operation.

In some older children it may be possible to clear the retained faeces with enemas and laxatives; if so it may be possible to perform a one-stage operation.

Duhamel operation

The aganglionic segment is removed down to the level of the peritoneal reflection over the rectum. The rectum is divided and dosed. The sacral hollow is opened and the normal colon brought down to the posterior aspect of the rectal stump. With an anal retractor in place a transverse incision is made from the level in the posterial wall just above the anal sphincter. The normal colon is then grasped and sewn to the transverse incision in the rectum. The spur between the rectum and normal colon is then divided with a stapler.

Swenson's procedure

The rectum is mobilised from above taking care to dissect immediately outside the fascia propia, preserving autonomic nerves to the bladder

---

Orvar Swenson, Professor of Surgery, Northern University, Chicago, Illinois, USA.
Bernard Duhamel, Chief-Surgeon Hospital Saint-Denis, France.

and seminal vesicles. The intestine is transected proximally through normal colon, the presence of ganglion cells having first been checked for by frozen section biopsy. The mobilised aganglionic segment is then everted out through the anus, the everted rectal mucosa is cleaned, and the anterior half of the junction between the top of the anal canal and the rectum is opened transversely. The proximal normal colon is then pulled through this opening and an end-to-end anastomosis made between the colon and anal canal as the aganglionic segment is excised. Once the anastomosis is complete it is reduced back into the anal canal.

Coloanal anastomosis

This is usually reserved for older children, teenagers and adults. The rectum is mobilised as before and transected just above the level of the pelvic floor. The normal colon is then joined to the top of the anal canal either directly with a stapling tecnhique or by a sleeve technique following a mucosectomy of the upper anal canal and rectum, a procedure described by both Soave and Parks.

Restorative proctocolectomy

In cases of Hirschsprung's disease involving the entire colon, it is possible to reconstruct with an ileoanal pouch procedure (see Chapter 60).

Idiopathic megarectum and megacolon

This is a rare condition and the cause is not known although in some it may result from poor toilet training during infancy and in others by a congenital abnormality of the intestinal myenteric plexus.

Investigation

On clinical examination there may be a hard faecal mass arising out of the pelvis, and on rectal examination there is a large faecaloma in the lumen. The anus is usually patulous, perianal soiling is common, and sigmoidoscopy is usually impossible but may show melanosis coli if the patient has been taking laxatives over many years.

Radiology. As there is an enlarged rectum often with distention of the colon over a variable length, a radiograph should be taken without prior bowel preparation using a small quantity of water-soluble contrast to prevent barium impaction. There is usually gross faecal loading of the enlarged rectum and colon and, when a contrast examination is carried out, the width of the colon measured at the pelvic brim is usually more than 6.5 cm (Fig. 57.4).

Anorectal physiology tests show abnormally large volumes inflated in the rectum to induce a feeling of rectal fullness, and inhibition of the internal and external anal sphincters is present but at much larger volumes than normal. Full-thickness rectal biopsy shows normal ganglion cells which distinguishes this condition from Hirschsprung's disease.

Sarpi Paolo Soave, 1552–1663. Prelate, historian, scientist, theologian. Discovered function of venous valves, blood circulation and dilation of iris.

Sir Alan Parks, FRCS, 1920–82. Surgeon, St Mark's and The Hospitals, England.

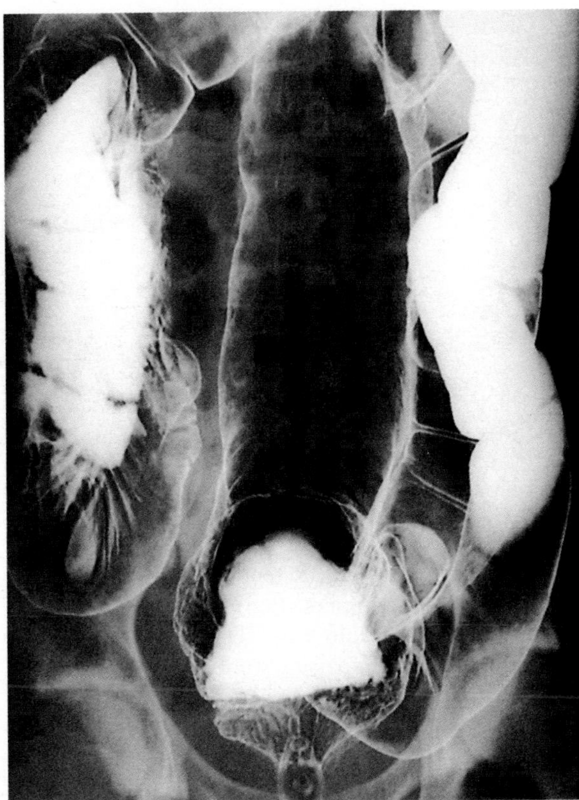

Fig. 57.4 Double-contrast barium enema showing megarectum and a huge megasigmoid with normal left colon alongside for comparison (*courtesy of Dr D. Nolan, John Radcliffe Hospital, Oxford*).

Medical treatment

This is directed at emptying the rectum and keeping it empty with enemas, washouts and sometimes manual evacuation under anaesthesia. Thereafter the patient is encouraged to develop a regular daily bowel habit with the use of laxatives and repeated enemas as necessary.

Surgical treatment

Surgical treatment is necessary sometimes if medical therapy fails. Resection of the dilated rectum and colon (Fig. 57.5) back to normal diameter colon with normal ganglion cells confirmed by frozen section at the time of surgery is followed by reconstruction with a coloanal anastomosis.

Nonmegacolon constipation

Although constipation is often regarded as a trivial symptom some patients are greatly disabled by abdominal pain, distension, reliance on laxatives and difficulty with defecation. These are usually otherwise healthy individuals who seek help for constipation but eat a normal diet and have a normal colon on endoscopy and barium enema.

Investigation

Whole gut transit time can be measured by asking the patient to stop all laxatives and take a capsule containing radio-

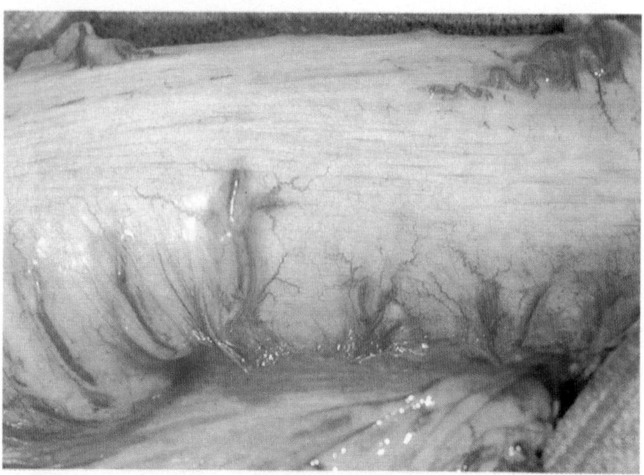

Fig. 57.5 Megacolon.

opaque markers (Fig. 57.6). Retention of more than 80 per cent of the shapes, 120 hours after ingestion, is abnormal.

Defecating proctography may be helpful if the main complaint is difficulty in passing stools.

Idiopathic slow transit constipation

This disorder is usually seen in women and results from infrequent bowel actions which may have been present since childhood or may suddenly follow abdominal or pelvic surgery. They have delayed transit using marker studies and may or may not be able to empty the rectum normally (Fig. 57.6).

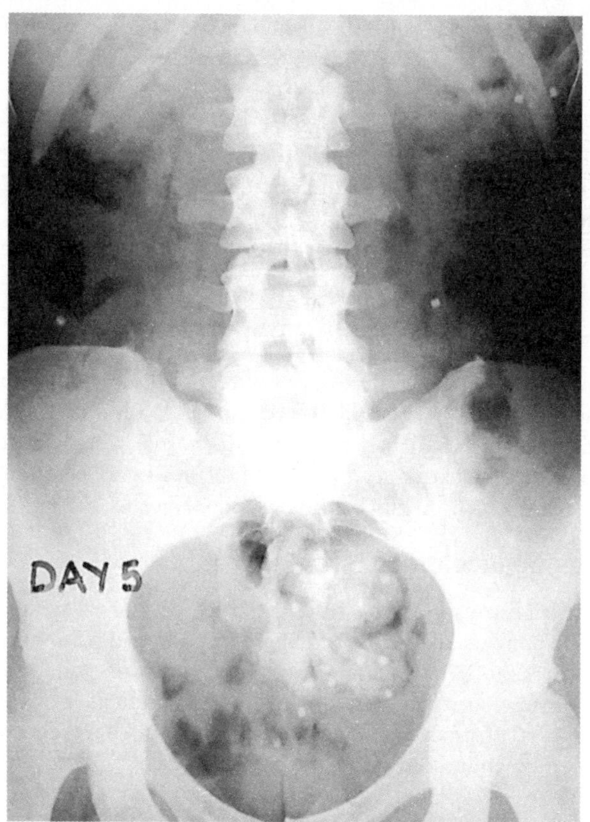

Fig. 57.6 Whole gut transit studied using radio-opaque markers. More than 80 per cent should have passed by day 5, demonstrating here delayed transit (*courtesy of Dr D. Nolan, John Radcliffe Hospital, Oxford*).

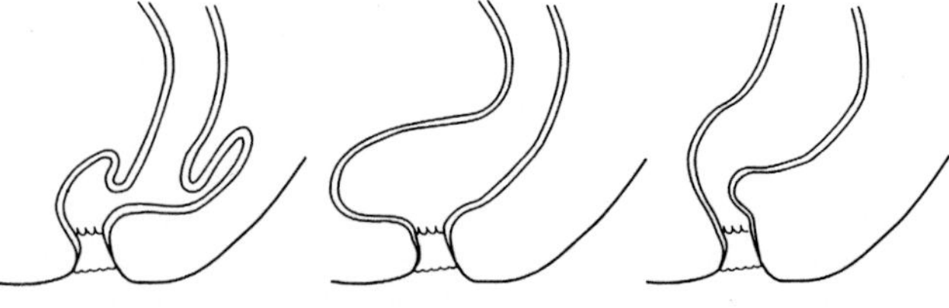

Fig. 57.7 Line diagram showing the common abnormalities seen during defecation proctography, lateral views.

This is a difficult condition to treat medically; dietary measures are usually unsuccessful and surgical treatment is only justified after careful studies and when medical treatment has been exhausted. Total colectomy and ileorectal anastomosis is the preferred procedure but the results are unpredictable. One-third of patients continues to have diarrhoea or constipation and two-thirds persisting abdominal pain. It is essential to exclude underlying psychiatric or psychological problems.

Obstructed defecation

Some patients complain of extreme difficulty in expelling stool. They may have repeated attempts at rectal evacuation and their transit is often normal. The common feature in these patients is weakness of the pelvic floor which descends on straining. Patients may resort to digital evacuation or pressure on the perineum or within the vagina to assist defecation. The cause is not known. It may arise from damage to pelvic nerves caused by prolonged straining at stool or childbirth.

Defecation proctography will show abnormal evacuation. There may be an intussusception with the upper rectum folding in to the lower rectum or an anterior rectocele where the rectum bulges forward into the posterior wall of the vagina (Fig. 57.7).

Biofeedback training may be helpful in some patients; dietary therapy and laxatives are usually unsuccessful. Surgery is a last resort, and either a defunctioning ileostomy or a colostomy with colostomy irrigation is used in intractable cases.

Vascular anomalies (angiodysplasia)

Capillary or cavernous haemangiomas are a cause of haemorrhage from the colon at any age presenting with colonic bleeding. In the middle-aged or elderly patient it needs to be distinguished from other causes of sudden massive haemorrhage, such as diverticulitis, ulcerative colitis or ischaemic colitis.

Angiodysplasia is a vascular malformation associated with ageing. It has been recognised since the introduction of intestinal angiography and colonoscopy. Angiodysplasias occur particularly in the ascending colon and caecum of elderly patients over the age of 60 years and are not associated with cutaneous lesions. The malformations consist of dilated tortuous submucosal veins and in severe cases the mucosa is replaced by massive dilated deformed vessels. On histological investigation, they are made up of dilated, distorted, thin-walled vessels with only a scanty amount of muscle in their walls.

Inspection of the mucosa is often unremarkable. The lesions are only a few millimetres in size and appear as reddish raised areas at endoscopy. Bleeding is usually chronic and intermittent and can be severe. Many patients previously thought to have bled from diverticular disease have probably been bleeding from angiodysplasia in the caecum. There is an association with aortic stenosis.

Barium enema is usually unhelpful and should be avoided. Provided the bleeding is not too brisk colonoscopy may show the characteristic lesion in the caecum or ascending colon. Selective superior and inferior mesenteric angiography shows the site and extent of the lesion by a blush. If this fails a radioactive test using technetium-99m (^{99m}Tc)-labelled red cells may confirm and localise the source of haemorrhage.

Some angiodysplastic lesions can be treated by colonoscopic diathermy, but if bleeding is brisk and the patient seriously ill emergency surgery will be necessary. Here a catheter is placed in the appendix stump and the colon irrigated progradely with saline or water. On-table colonscopy is carried out and the site of the bleeding can then be confirmed. Angiodysplastic lesions are sometimes demonstrated by transillumination through the caecum (Fig. 57.8). If it is still not clear exactly which segment of colon is involved then a total abdominal colectomy with ileorectal anastomosis may be necessary.

Blind loop syndrome

It has been shown in dogs that, if a blind loop of the small intestine is made (Fig. 57.9), defects of absorption will appear. If this occurs in the upper intestine the defect is chiefly of fat absorption; if in the lower intestine there is vitamin B_{12} deficiency. This has been found to occur in humans and is referred to as the blind loop syndrome.

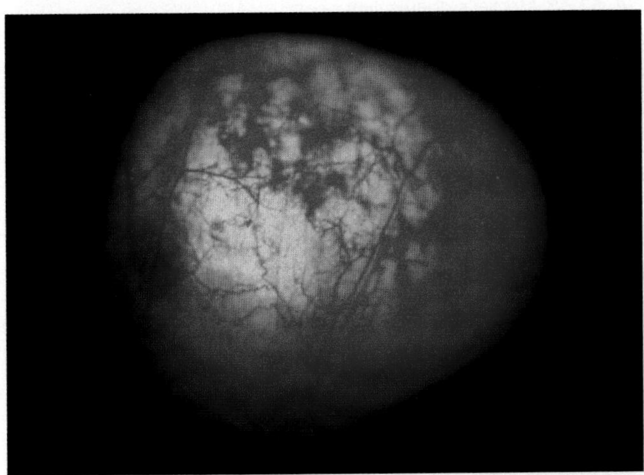

Fig. 57.8 Angiodysplasia of the caecum demonstrated by transillumination with a colonoscope intraoperatively.

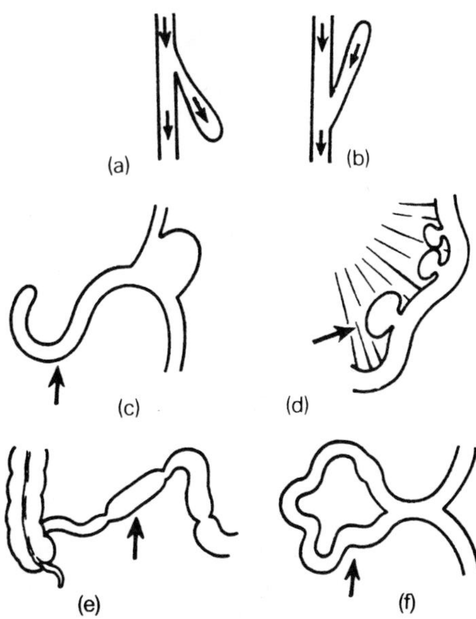

Fig. 57.9 Common types of blind loops. (a) Self-filling: deficiency occurs; (b) self-emptying: no deficiency occurs; (c) long afferent loop stasis in Polya gastrectomy; (d) jejunal diverticula; (e) intestinal stricture causing stasis; (f) 'stenosis–anastomosis loop' syndrome.

Essentially, the stasis produces an abnormal bacterial flora, which prevents proper breakdown of the food (especially fat) and mops up the vitamins that are present. Sometimes the only manifestation is anaemia, resulting from vitamin B_{12} deficiency, but if steatorrhoea appears, other serious malabsorption features follow. In general, high loops produce steatorrhoea, whereas low loops tend to produce anaemia.

Temporary improvement will follow the use of antibiotics to destroy the bacteria causing the trouble, but the main treatment is surgical extirpation of the cause of the stasis where applicable.

Diverticular disease

One meaning of diverticulum is a wayside house of ill-fame; certainly these 'wayside houses' live up to their evil reputation. Diverticula can occur from the stomach to the rectosigmoid. There are two varieties:

1. **Congenital.** All three coats of the bowel are present *in* the wall of the diverticulum, e.g. Meckel's.
2. **Acquired.** The wall of the diverticulum lacks a proper muscular coat. Most alimentary diverticula are thought to be acquired.

Small intestine

Most of these diverticula arise from the mesenteric side of the bowel probably as the result of mucosal herniation through the point of entry of blood vessels.

Johann Friedrich Meckel (The Younger), 1781–1833. Professor of Anatomy and Surgery, Halle, Germany.

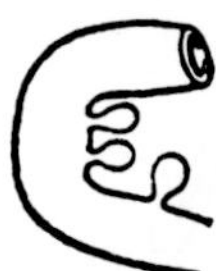

Fig. 57.10 Primary diverticula of second and third parts of duodenum.

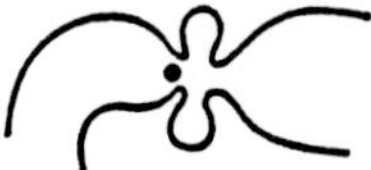

Fig. 57.11 Secondary diverticula of duodenal cap.

Duodenal diverticulum

There are two types:

1. **Primary**. Mostly in older patients on the inner wall of the second and third parts, these diverticula are found incidentally on barium meal and usually do not cause symptoms. They can cause problems locating the ampulla during endoscopic retrograde cholangiopancreatography (ERCP) (Fig. 57.10).
2. **Secondary**. Diverticula of the duodenal cap resulting from long-standing duodenal ulceration (Fig. 57.11).

Jejunal diverticula

These are usually of variable size and multiple (Fig. 57.12). Clinically they may (1) be symptomless, (2) give rise to abdominal pain, flatulence and borborygmi, (3) produce a malabsorption syndrome, or (4) present as an acute abdomen with acute inflammation and occasionally rupture. They are more common in patients with connective tissue disorders. In patients with major malabsorption problems giving rise to anaemia, steatorrhoea, hypoproteinaemia or vitamin B_{12} deficiency; resection of the affected segment with end-to-end anastomosis can be effective.

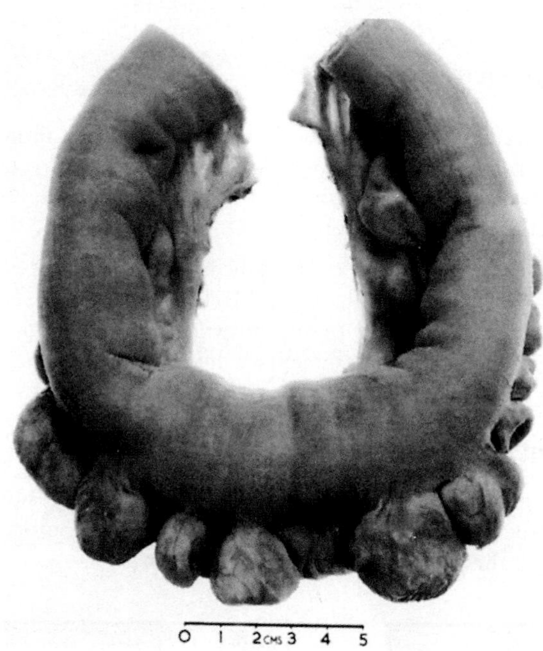

Fig. 57.12 Jejunal diverticula.

Meckel's diverticulum

Meckel's diverticulum is present in 2 per cent of the population; it is situated on the antimesenteric border of the small intestine, commonly 60 cm from the ileocaecal valve, and is usually 3–5 cm long. Many variations occur (2 per cent – 2 feet – 2 inches is a useful *aide mémoire*) (Figs 57.13 and 57.14).

A Meckel's diverticulum possesses all three coats of the intestinal wall and has its own blood supply. It is therefore vulnerable to infection and obstruction in the same way as the appendix. In 20 per cent of cases the mucosa contains heterotopic epithelium, namely, gastric, colonic or sometimes pancreatic tissue. When present, the abnormal mucosa lines the greater part of the proximal end of the pouch and extends sometimes for a short distance into the nearby ileum.

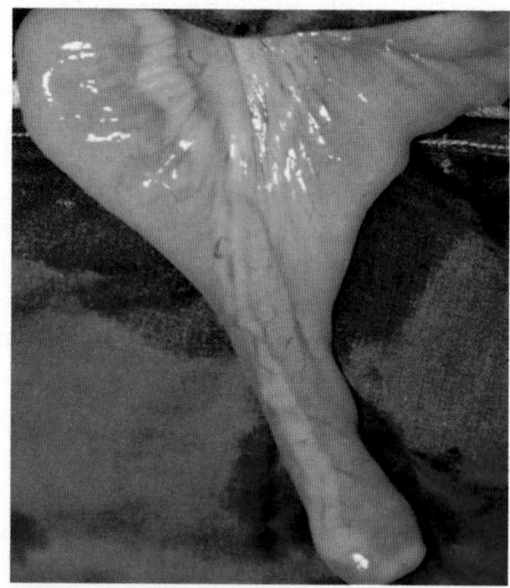

Fig. 57.13 Meckel's diverticulum.

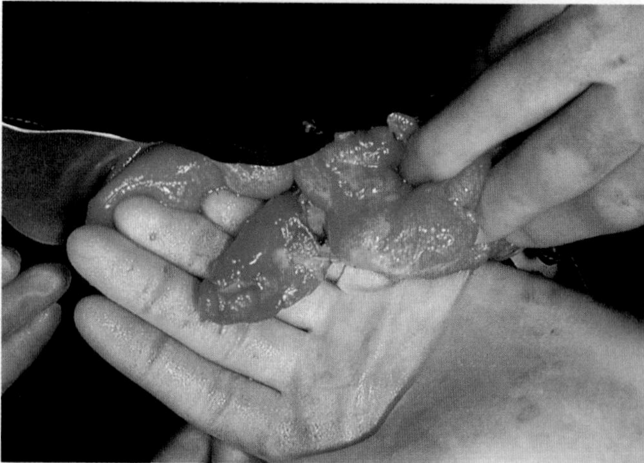

Fig. 57.14 Gangrenous Meckel's diverticulitis.

Although Meckel's diverticulum occurs with equal frequency in both sexes, symptoms usually resulting from the epithelium contained in the diverticulum predominantly occur in males. In order of frequency, these symptoms are as follows.

1. **Severe haemorrhage,** caused by peptic ulceration. The blood is passed per rectum, and is maroon in colour. Although the patient may vomit, the vomit does not contain blood. There is rarely any pain and sometimes the bleeding precedes perforation. An operation is required for serious progressive gastrointestinal bleeding. When no lesion in the stomach or duodenum can be found the terminal 150 cm of ileum should be carefully inspected.
2. **Intussusception.** In most cases, the apex of the intussusception is the swollen, inflamed, heterotopic epithelium at the mouth of the diverticulum.
3. **Meckel's diverticulitis,** with or without perforation, may result from obstruction by food residue. The symptoms are those of acute appendicitis and, unless the appendix has already been removed, the diagnosis is impossible before operation. When a diverticulum perforates the symptoms may simulate those of a perforated duodenal ulcer. Whether or not the diverticulum is perforated urgent surgery is required. In nonperforated cases an inflamed diverticulum should be sought as soon as it has been demonstrated that the appendix and Fallopian tubes are not at fault.
4. **Chronic peptic ulceration.** As the diverticulum is part of the midgut, the pain, although related to meals, is felt around the umbilicus.
5. **Intestinal obstruction.** The presence of a band between the apex of the diverticulum and the umbilicus may cause obstruction either by the band itself or by a volvulus around it.

Radiology

Meckel's diverticulum can be very difficult to demonstrate by contrast radiology; small bowel enema would be the most accurate investigation.

Technetium-99m scanning

In cases of repeated gastrointestinal haemorrhage of unknown cause where a Meckel's diverticulum is suspected the abdomen is imaged with gamma camera after the injection of 30–100 μCi (111–370 × 10^{10} Bq) of ^{99m}Tc-labelled pertechnetate intravenously. This may localise heterotopic gastric mucosa revealing the site of a Meckel's diverticulum in 90 per cent of cases.

'Silent' Meckel's diverticulum

An aphorism attributed to Dr Charles Mayo is: 'a Meckel's diverticulum is frequently suspected, often sought for and seldom found'. A Meckel's diverticulum usually remains symptomless throughout life and is found only at necropsy. When a silent Meckel's diverticulum is encountered in the course of an abdominal operation, provided it is wide-mouthed and the wall of the diverticulum does not feel thickened, it can be left. Where there is doubt and it can be removed without appreciable additional risk it should be resected.

Exceptionally a Meckel's diverticulum is found in an inguinal or a femoral hernia sac – Littre's hernia.

Gabriele Fallopio, 1523–62. Italian anatomist, Professor of Anatomy at Pisa and Padua, Italy.
Charles Mayo, 1865–1939. Surgeon and co-founder of the Mayo Clinic with his brother William.
Alexis Littre, 1658–1726. Surgeon and anatomist, Paris, France.

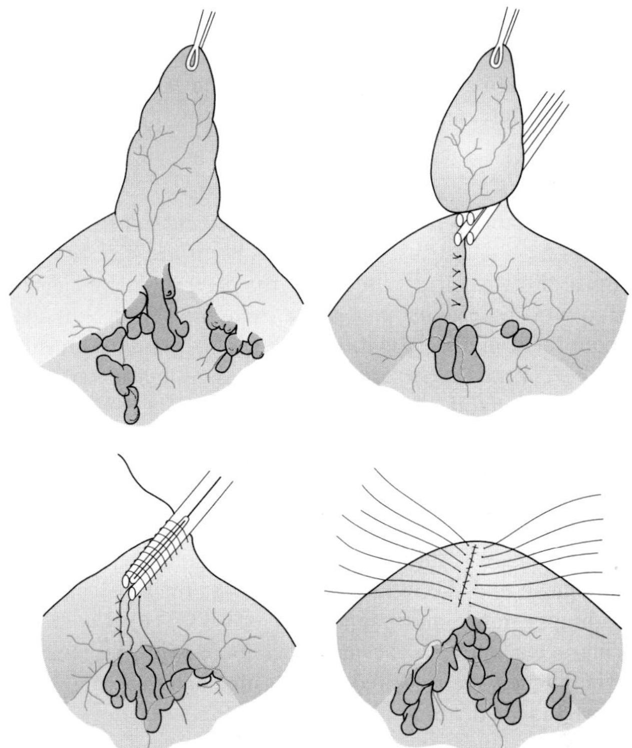

Fig. 57.15 Steps in the performance of Meckelian diverticulectomy.

Meckel's diverticulectomy

A Meckel's diverticulum which is broad based should not be amputated at its base and invaginated in the same way as a vermiform appendix, because of the risk of stricture. Furthermore this does not remove heterotopic epithelium where it is present. The steps of diverticulectomy are shown in Fig. 57.15. Alternatively, a linear stapler device may be used. Where there is induration of the base of the diverticulum extending into the adjacent ileum, it is advisable to resect a short segment of ileum containing the diverticulum, restoring continuity with an end-to-end anastomosis.

Colon

Diverticula of the colon are acquired herniations of colonic mucosa, protruding through the circular muscle at the points where the blood vessels penetrate the colonic wall. They tend to occur in rows between the strips of longitudinal muscle, sometimes partly covered by appendices epiploicae. The condition is most commonly found in the sigmoid colon but the caecum can also be involved and on occasion the entire large bowel can be affected. The rectum with its complete muscle layers is not affected. In 90 per cent of cases the sigmoid colon is involved and is almost always the site of inflammation, i.e. diverticulitis. Some 5 per cent of patients have associated gallstones and hiatus hernia (Saint's triad).

Diverticular disease is rare in Africans and Asians who eat a diet that contains natural fibre. In Western countries, where

Charles Fredrick Morris Saint, 1886–1973. Emeritus Professor of Surgery, Cape Town, South Africa.

the roughage has been removed from flour and refined sugar forms a large part of the diet, diverticula are found in 25 per cent of barium enemas of patients over the age of 40 and the incidence increases with age.

Diverticulosis

It is important to distinguish between diverticulosis and the presence of diverticula which may be asymptomatic, and clinical diverticular disease where the diverticula are causing symptoms. Diverticula probably arise as a result of muscular incoordination and spasm, resulting in increased segmentation and intraluminal pressures. Excessive segmentation in response to food, prostigmine and morphine is found in colonic motility studies, and this exaggerated response is more apparent in symptomatic than in asymptomatic individuals. On histological investigation the diverticulum consists of a protrusion of mucous membranes covered with peritoneum. There is thickening of the circular muscle fibres of the taeniae and the intestine develops a concertina or saw-tooth appearance on barium enema (Fig. 57.16). The diverticula occur between the muscle clefts making the mucosal surface appear trabeculated. The elastin content of the taenia coli is increased compared with controls.

Diverticulitis

Diverticulitis is the result of inflammation of one or more diverticula, usually with some pericolitis. Episodes of diverticulitis may be followed by years free of symptoms, but the condition is essentially progressive – the longer the duration the worse the symptoms and the greater the risk of complications. Diverticulitis is not a precancerous condition, but cancer may coexist.

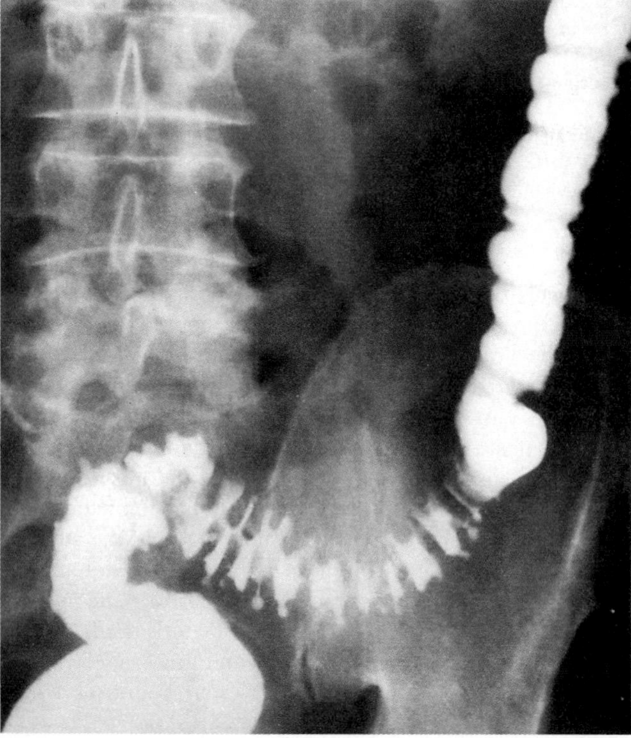

Fig. 57.16 Barium enema showing sigmoid diverticular disease 'saw teeth' and diverticula (*courtesy of Dr D. Nolan, John Radcliffe Hospital, Oxford*).

The **complications** are the following:

1. recurrent periodic inflammation and pain – in some patients these episodes may be clinically silent;
2. perforation leading to general peritonitis or local (pericolic) abscess formation;
3. intestinal obstruction:
   (a) in the sigmoid as a result of progressive fibrosis causing stenosis,
   (b) in the small intestine caused by adherent loops of small intestine on the pericolitis;
4. haemorrhage: diverticulitis may present with profuse colonic haemorrhage in 17 per cent of cases, often requiring blood transfusions;
5. fistula formation (vesicocolic, vaginocolic, enterocolic, colocutaneous) occurs in 5 per cent of cases, vesicolic being the most common.

Clinical features

Diverticulosis may be asymptomatic, but the disordered colonic function may cause symptoms of distension, flatulence and a sensation of heaviness in the lower abdomen, all of which may be indistinguishable from the symptoms of irritable bowel syndrome. Excessive colonic segmentation can cause severe pain in the left iliac fossa, but this must be distinguished from episodes of often subclinical inflammation in the sigmoid colon as a result of diverticulitis.

Diverticulitis. Persistent lower abdominal pain, usually in the left iliac fossa with or without peritonitis in patients of either sex over the age of 40, could be caused by diverticulitis. Fever, malaise and leucocytosis can differentiate diverticulitis from painful diverticulosis. The patient may pass loose stools or may be constipated; the lower abdomen is tender especially on the left but occasionally also in the right iliac fossa if the sigmoid loop lies across the midline. The sigmoid colon is often palpable, tender and thickened. Rectal examination may but does not usually reveal a tender mass. The condition has been likened to left-sided appendicitis. Any urinary symptoms may herald the formation of a vesicocolic fistula which leads to pneumaturia (flatus in the urine) and even faeces in the urine.

Diagnosis

Radiology. Diverticulosis, as for the 'irritable bowel' syndrome, is a diagnosis of exclusion and symptoms should not be attributed to diverticulosis unless other diseases have been excluded by barium enema, sigmoidoscopy or colonoscopy. Although the diagnosis of acute diverticulitis is made on clinical grounds it can be confirmed during the acute phase by computerised tomography (CT). This will demonstrate not only the diverticula but also any associated pericolic

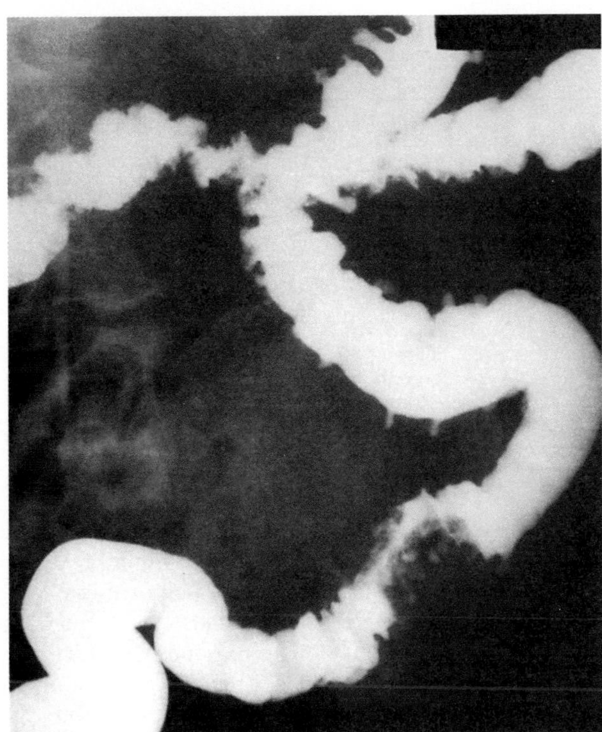

Fig. 57.17 Barium enema showing large tilling defect in sigmoid colon caused by pericolic abscess (*courtesy of Dr D. Nolan, John Radcliffe Hospital, Oxford*).

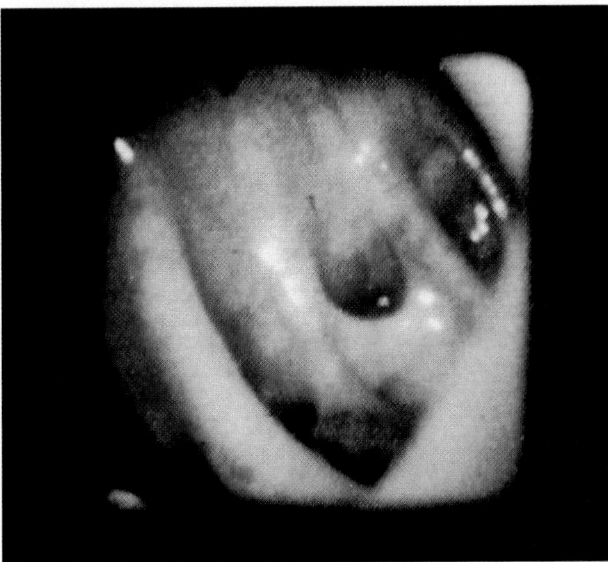

Fig. 57.18 Colonoscopic view of sigmoid diverticula. Note the mouths of diverticula between hypertrophied colonic wall.

abscess (Fig. 57.17). Barium enemas and sigmoidoscopy are usually reserved for patients who have recovered from an attack of acute diverticulitis for fear of causing perforation or peritonitis. Water-soluble contrast enemas may, however, be helpful in sorting out patients with large bowel obstruction. Barium radiology is carried out to exclude a carcinoma and to assess the extent of the disease. Where the sigmoid colon is thickened and narrowed, a 'saw-tooth' appearance may be seen. Some strictures can be very difficult to distinguish by radiology alone and in those circumstances colonoscopy will be necessary to rule out a carcinoma.

Sigmoidoscopy. The mucosa may be normal and in acute attacks the sigmoidoscopy will be painful and the mucosa inflamed. Colonoscopy or flexible sigmoidoscopy is more helpful (Fig. 57.18). The necks of diverticula can be seen and the narrowed area of diverticulitis can be entered, but on occasion not passed because of the severity of disease. The differential diagnosis from a carcinoma can be impossible if a tight stenosis prevents endoscopy.

Management

Diverticulosis should be treated with a high-residue diet containing roughage in the form of wholemeal bread, flour, fruit and vegetables. Bulk formers such as bran, Celevac, Isogel and Fybogel may be given until the stools are soft. Painful diverticular disease may require bed rest and antispasmodics.

Acute diverticulitis is treated by bed rest and intravenous antibiotics (usually cefuroxime and metronidazole). After the acute attack has subsided and if the diagnosis has not already been confirmed by CT, a barium enema should be carried out.

Operative procedures for diverticular disease. Some 10 per cent of patients require an operation either for recurrent attacks which make life a misery or for the complications of diverticulitis.

1. The ideal operation carried out as an interval procedure after careful preparation of the gut is a one-stage resection. This involves removal of the affected segment and restoration of continuity by end-to-end anastomosis. At this operation the sigmoid loop is often found adherent in the pouch of Douglas. Careful dissection will allow eventual mobilisation of the rectosigmoid out of the pelvis exposing the normal rectum, and greater mobility will allow an easier anastomosis.
2. If there is obstruction, inflammatory oedema and adhesions or the bowel is loaded with faeces, a Hartmann's operation is the procedure of choice. The involved area is resected. The rectum is closed at the peritoneal reflection, and the left colon brought out as a left iliac fossa colostomy. The once popular staged procedures using a preliminary transverse colostomy are now rarely used except by inexperienced surgeons because of the high mortality associated with them. In selected obstructed cases the bowel can be cleaned by on-table lavage, placing a urinary

James Douglas, 1675–1742. Scottish anatomist, London, England.
Henri Hartmann, 1860–1952. Professor of Surgery, Hôtel Dieu, Paris, France.

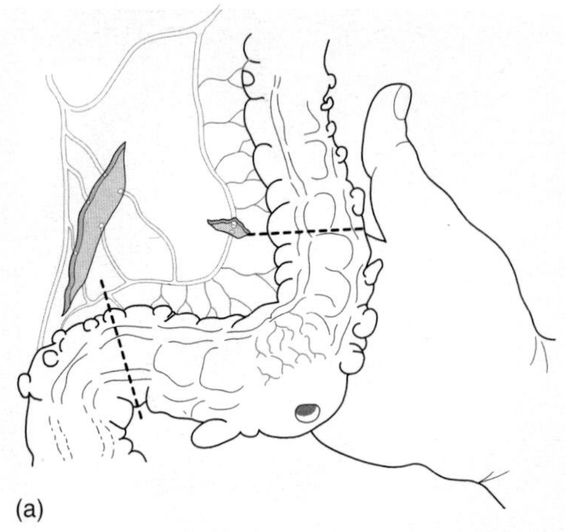
(a)

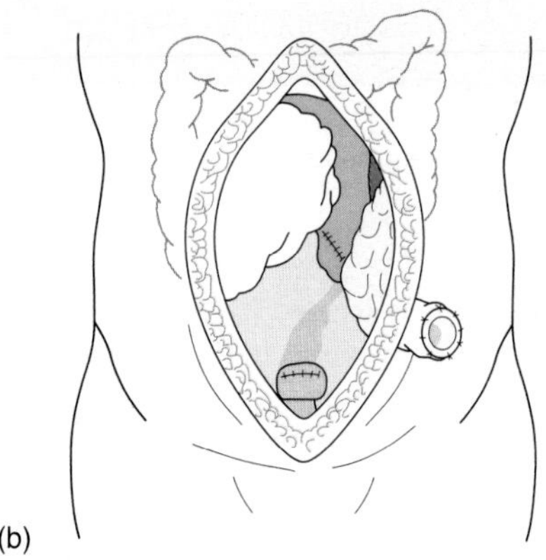
(b)

Fig. 57.19 (a) Drawing to show perforated sigmoid diverticular disease. (b) The Hartmann procedure – oversewn rectal stump and left iliac fossa colostomy.

catheter through the appendix stump and washing the colon with physiological saline or water for irrigation. This makes subsequent restoration and bowel continuity with an anastomosis much safer (Fig. 57.19a, b).

3. In acute perforation, peritonitis soon becomes general and may be purulent, which has a mortality rate of about 15 per cent. Gross faecal peritonitis carries more than a 50 per cent mortality rate and pneumoperitoneum is usually present; the diagnosis may not be confirmed until emergency laparotomy. There is a choice of procedures:
   (a) primary resection and Hartmann's procedure (see above);
   (b) primary resection and anastomosis after on-table lavage in selected cases;
   (c) exteriorisation of the affected bowel which is then opened as a colostomy, now rarely used;
   (d) suture of the perforation with drainage with or without proximal defunction. In selected cases with a small leak and minimal soiling.
4. Fistulae can only be cured by resection of the diseased bowel and closure of the fistula. In the case of a colovesical fistula it is usually possible to 'pinch off' the affected bowel from the bladder, close it and then resect the sigmoid. In very difficult cases a staged procedure with a preliminary defunctioning stoma may be necessary on occasion.
5. Haemorrhage from diverticulitis must be distinguished from angiodysplasia. It usually responds to conservative management and occasionally requires resection. On-table lavage and colonoscopy may be necessary to localise the bleeding site.

Table 57.1 Differentiation of diverticulitis from carcinoma of the colon

	Diverticulitis	*Carcinoma*
History	Long	Short
Pain	More common	25% painless
Mass	25% have tenderness	
Bleeding	17% often profuse, periodic	65% – usually small amounts persistently
Radiograph	Diffuse change	Localised: no relaxation with propantheline bromide
Sigmoidoscopy	Inflammatory change over an area	No inflammation until ulcer reached
Colonoscopy	No carcinoma seen	Carcinoma seen and biopsied

Diverticular disease and carcinoma coexist in 12 per cent of cases. Exploration may be necessary but, even then, differentiation may be difficult until histological investigations are available (Table 57.1). Weight loss, falling haemoglobin and persistently positive occult blood are sinister features.

Solitary diverticulum of the caecum and ascending colon is rare and is congenital, and may present with symptoms and signs identical to those of acute appendicitis.

Extensive diverticular disease can sometimes affect the right colon. This, however, is rare in the West but more common in Eastern countries. In Japan, China, Malaysia and Korea, right-sided disease is twice as common as left-sided disease.

Ulcerative colitis

Aetiology

The cause of ulcerative colitis is unknown; its prevalence among first-degree relatives of patients is 15 times that of the general population but there is no clear Mendelian pattern of inheritance. In spite of intensive bacteriological studies, no organisms or group of organisms can be incriminated. Relapse of colitis has, however, been reported in association with bacterial dysenteries. Some cases are allergic to milk protein. Smoking seems to have a protective effect and there have been anecdotal reports of remission of the disease with smoking or the use of nicotine chewing gum. Patients often

Gregor Johann Mendel, 1822–84. Austrian biologist and botanist.

comment that relapses are associated with periods of stress at home or at work, but personality and psychiatric profiles are the same as the normal population.

There remain three main hypotheses, none of which has been proved:

1. a mucosal immunological reaction;
2. a weakened mucous barrier;
3. defective mucosal metabolism of butyrates.

Epidemiology

There are 10–15 new cases per 100 000 population a year in the UK. The disease has been rare in Eastern populations but is now being reported more commonly, suggesting an environmental cause that has developed as a result of an increasing 'westernisation' of diet and/or social habits and better diagnostic facilities. The sex ratio is equal; it is uncommon before the age of 10 and most patients are between the ages of 20 and 40 at diagnosis.

Pathology

In 95 per cent of cases the disease starts in the rectum and spreads proximally. When the ileocaecal valve is incompetent, retrograde (backwash) ileitis involving the last 30 cm of the ileum is likely to occur. It is a nonspecific inflammatory disease, primarily affecting the mucosa and superficial submucosa, and only in severe disease are the deeper layers of the intestinal wall affected. There are multiple minute ulcers, and microscopic evidence proves that the ulceration is almost always more severe and extensive than the gross appearance indicates. When the disease is chronic, inflammatory polyps (pseudopolyps) occur in up to 20 per cent of cases and may be numerous. They result from previous episodes of ulceration leaving islands of spared mucosa which will remain prominent when the adjacent mucosa heals. In severe fulminant colitis a section of the colon, usually the transverse colon, may become acutely dilated and the intestinal wall then becomes extremely thin and may perforate ('toxic megacolon'). On microscopic investigation there is an increase of inflammatory cells in the lamina propia, the walls of crypts are infiltrated by inflammatory cells and there are crypt abscesses. There is depletion of goblet cell mucin. The crypts are reduced in number and appear to be atrophic and irregularly spaced. With time these changes become severe and precancerous changes can develop (= severe dysplasia or carcinoma *in situ*).

Symptoms

The first symptom is watery or bloody diarrhoea; there may be a rectal discharge of mucus which is either blood stained or purulent. Pain as an early symptom is unusual. In most cases the disease is chronic and characterised by relapses and remissions. In general, a bad prognosis is indicated by (1) a severe initial attack, (2) disease involving the whole colon and (3) increasing age, especially after 60 years. If the disease remains confined to the left colon the outlook is better.

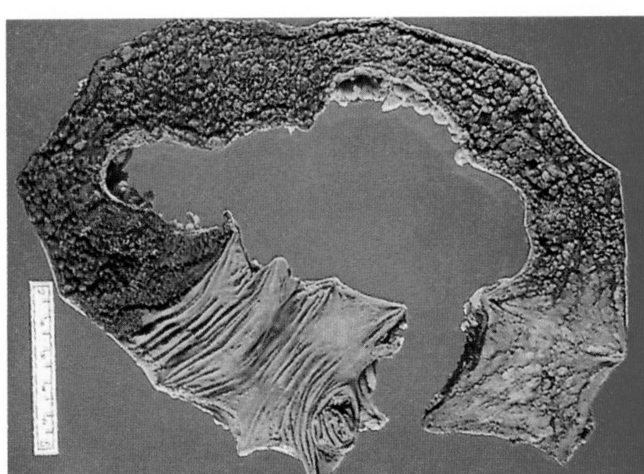

Fig. 57.20 Extensive, active ulcerative colitis (the rectum is spared, which is unusual in the absence of treatment) (*courtesy of Dr Ian Talbot, St Mark's Hospital, London*).

Proctitis

Inflammation confined to the rectum accounts for about 25 per cent of all cases. As most of the colon is healthy the stool is formed or semi-formed and the patient is often severely troubled by tenesmus and urgency. The risk of cancer in these cases is low. In 5–10 per cent there is spread to involve the rest of the colon.

Left-sided and total colitis (Fig. 57.20)

Diarrhoea usually implies that there is active disease proximal to the rectum. Approximately 15 per cent of patients have left-sided colitis, and 25 per cent have total colitis extending beyond the midtransverse colon. The clinical pattern is one of recurrent severe attacks of bloody diarrhoea up to 20 times a day, dehydration and fluid electrolyte losses. Anaemia and hypoproteinaemia are common.

Disease severity

Disease severity can be graded as:

1. mild – rectal bleeding or diarrhoea with four or fewer motions per day and the absence of systemic signs of disease;
2. moderate – more than four motions per day but no systemic signs of illness;
3. severe – more than four motions a day together with one or more signs of systemic illness: fever over 37.5°C, tachycardia more than 90/minute, hypoalbuminaemia less than 30 g/litre, weight loss more than 3 kg.

Complications of severe disease

Fulminating colitis and toxic dilatation (megacolon) (Fig. 57.21). Patients with severe disease should be admitted to hospital. Dilatation should be suspected in patients with active colitis who develop severe abdominal pain. It is an indication that inflammation has gone through all the muscle layers of the colon. The diagnosis is confirmed by the presence on a plain abdominal radiograph of the colon with a diameter more than 6 cm. The condition must be differentiated from dysentery, typhoid and amoebic colitis. Plain abdominal radiographs should be obtained daily in patients

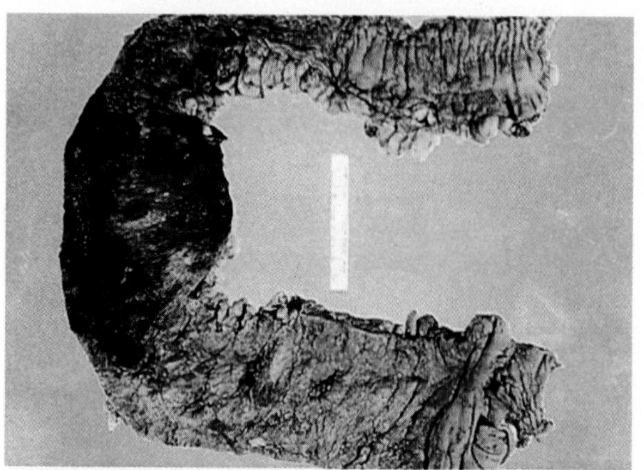

Fig. 57.21 Fulminating ulcerative colitis with toxic dilation of transvense colon (*courtesy of Dr Ian Talbot, St Mark's Hospital, London*).

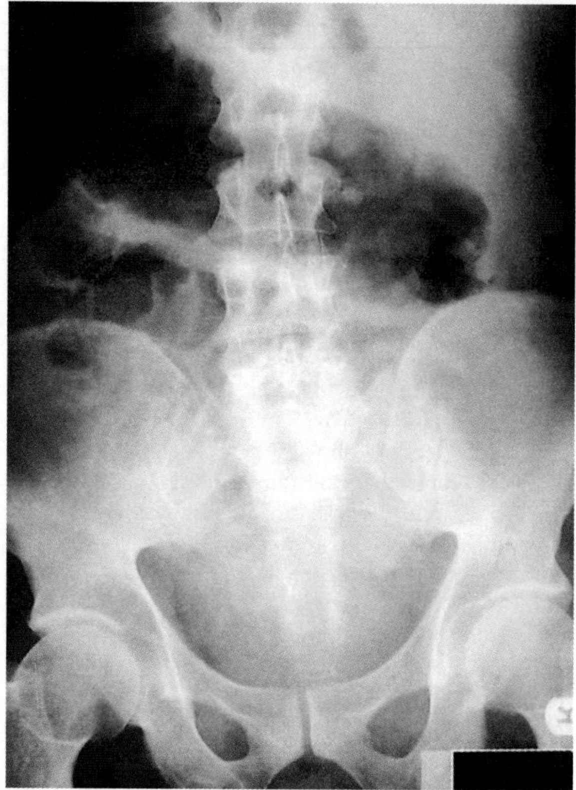

Fig. 57.22 Supine abdominal radiograph in toxic megacolon. The transverse colon is dilated (7 cm), there is no formed residue in the colon and large mucosal islands are present in the ascending colon and hepatic flexure. No haustration is present in the transverse colon, which distinguishes this from ileus of obstruction. Mucosal islands are due to oedematous remnants of mucosa where there has been extensive ulceration (*courtesy of Dr Clive Bartram, St Mark's Hospital, London*).

with severe colitis and a progressive increase in diameter in spite of medical therapy is an indication for surgery (Fig. 57.22).

Perforation. Colonic perforation in ulcerative colitis is a grave complication with a mortality rate of 50 per cent or more. Steroids may mask the physical signs. Perforation can sometimes occur without toxic dilatation. Generally patients with severe attacks should be managed so that they do not develop these complications.

Severe haemorrhage. Severe rectal bleeding is uncommon and may occasionally require transfusion and rarely surgery.

Investigations

A plain abdominal film can often show the severity of disease. Faeces are only present in parts of the colon that are normal or only mildly inflamed. Mucosal islands can sometimes be seen and have been mentioned. Small bowel loops in the right lower quadrant may be a sign of severe disease.

Barium enema

The principal signs are (Fig. 57.23):

- loss of haustration, especially in the distal colon;
- mucosal changes caused by granularity;
- pseudopolyps;
- in chronic cases, a narrow contracted colon.

In some centres an instant enema is used with a water-soluble medium for contrast instead of barium and no bowel preparation to avoid aggravating any underlying colitis (Fig. 57.24).

Sigmoidoscopy

Sigmoidoscopy is essential for diagnosis of early cases and mild disease not showing up on a barium enema. The initial findings are those of proctitis, the mucosa is hyperaemic, bleeds on touch and there may be a pus-like exudate. Later tiny ulcers may be seen and appear to coalesce. This is different from the picture of amoebic dysentery where there are large deep ulcers with intervening normal mucosa.

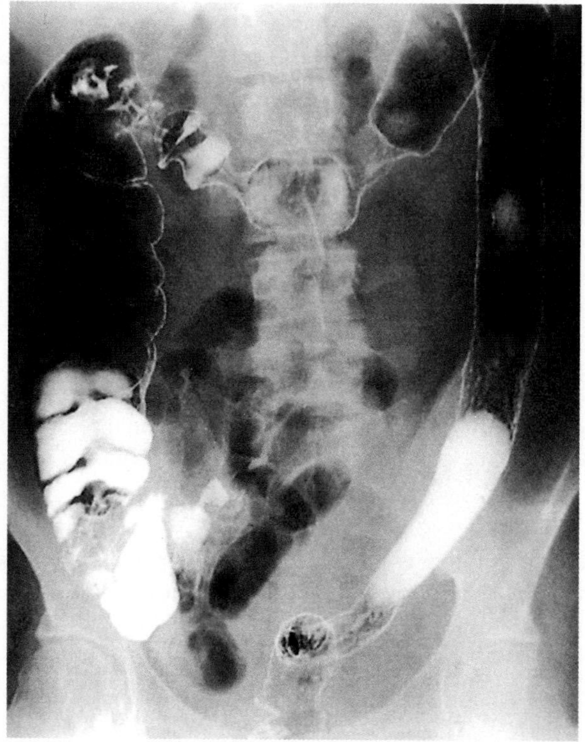

Fig. 57.23 Double-contrast barium enema showing left-sided ulcerative colitis with a tubular left colon compared with a normal right colon (*courtesy of Dr D. Nolan, John Radcliffe Hospital, Oxford*).

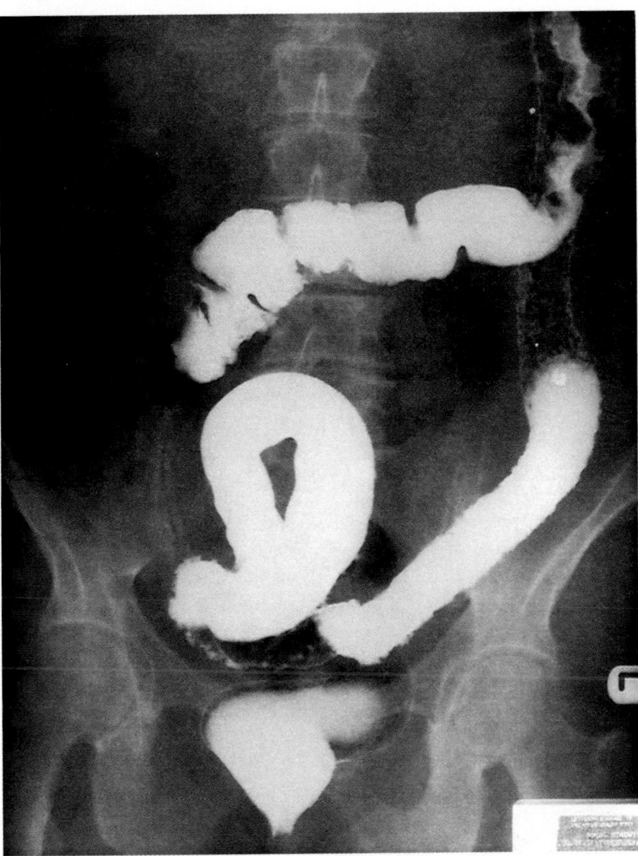

Fig. 57.24 Instant enema in acute ulcerative colitis. The rectum shows a granular mucosa with ulceration extending from the proximal sigmoid into the splenic flexure region. The ulcers are seen tangentially as collar-stud projections from the mucosal line. Formed residue is present in the ascending colon and hepatic flexure. The colitis extends into the midtransverse colon but is most active in the descending colon (*courtesy of Dr Clive Bartram, St Mark's Hospital, London*).

Colonoscopy and biopsy

This has an important place in management:

1. to establish the extent of inflammation;
2. to distinguish between ulcerative colitis and Crohn's colitis;
3. to monitor response to treatment;
4. to assess long-standing cases for malignant change.

Although it may occasionally be helpful, colonoscopy is not usually used in acute cases for fear of aggravating the disease or perforation.

The cancer risk in colitis

Although this is an important complication the overall risk is only about 3.5 per cent. It is much less in early cases but increases with duration of disease. Thus, after 20 years of colitis the risk may be as much as 12 per cent. Carcinoma is more likely to occur where the whole colon is involved and

Burrill Bernard Crohn, b. 1884. New York physician.

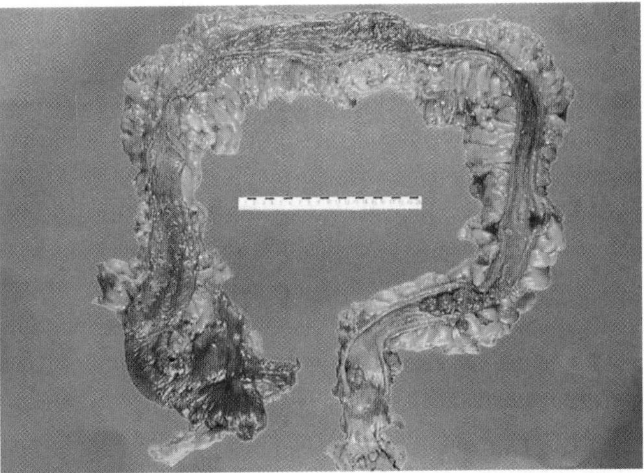

Fig. 57.25 Resection specimen from patient with long-standing ulcerative colitis showing a narrow tubular colon with areas of cancer change in the rectum and sigmoid (*courtesy of Dr B. Warren, John Radcliffe Hospital, Oxford*).

where the disease started in early life (Fig. 57.25). Carcinomatous change, often atypical and high grade, may occur at many sites at once. The colon is involved rather than the rectum and the maximal incidence is during the fourth decade.

The golden rule is that, when the disease has been present for 10 years or more, regular colonoscopic checks must be carried out, even if the disease is clinically quiescent. If on biopsy there is severe epithelial dysplasia, surgery is indicated. Annual colonoscopy and biopsy is then part of cancer surveillance. In the rare cases with a fibrous stricture these should be examined especially carefully for the presence of an underlying carcinoma.

Extraintestinal manifestations

Arthritis occurs in around 15 per cent of patients and is of the large joint polyarthropathy type, affecting knees, ankles, elbows and wrists. Sacroileitis and ankylosing spondylitis are 20 times more common in patients with ulcerative colitis.

Skin lesions: erythema nodosum, pyoderma gangrenosum or aphthous ulceration.

Eye problems: iritis.

Liver disease: sclerosing cholangitis has been reported in up to 70 per cent of cases. Diagnosis is by ERCP which demonstrates the characteristic alternating stricturing and bleeding of the intrahepatic and extrahepatic ducts.

Bile duct cancer is a rare complication and colectomy does not appear to reduce the risk of subsequent bile duct cancer or sclerosing cholangitis.

Treatment

Medical treatment of an acute attack

Corticosteroids are the most useful drugs and can be given either locally for inflammation of the rectum or systemically when the disease is more extensive. Sulphasalazine and other 5-aminosalicylic acid (5-ASA) derivates, for example, mesalazine and olsalazine, can be given both topically and systemically.

Their main function is in maintaining remission rather than treating an acute attack. Nonspecific antidiarrhoeal agents have no place in the routine management of ulcerative colitis.

Mild attacks

Patients with a mild attack and limited disease will usually respond to rectally administered steroids. In those with more extensive disease, oral prednisolone 20–40 mg/day is given over a 3–4-week period. Suiphasalazine 1 g three times a day or one of the newer 5-ASA compounds should be given concurrently.

Moderate attacks

These patients should be treated with oral prednisolone 40 mg/day, twice daily steroid enemas and 5-ASA. Failure to achieve remission as an out-patient is an indication for admission.

Severe attacks

These patients must be regarded as medical emergencies and require immediate admission to hospital. Their appearance is often misleading, and they must be examined at least twice a day with particular reference to the presence of signs of peritonism. Their abdominal girth is measured and liver dullness should be percussed regularly. A plain abdominal radiograph is taken daily and inspected for dilatation of the transverse colon of more than 5.5 cm. The presence of mucosal islands on plain radiographs (see Fig. 57.22), increasing colonic diameter or a sudden increase in pulse and temperature may indicate a colonic perforation. A stool chart helps in the assessment of response to therapy, and careful medical/surgical joint management is essential. Fluid and electrolyte balance is maintained, anaemia is corrected and adequate nutrition provided, sometimes in severe cases with intravenous nutrition. The patient is maintained nil by mouth and treated with intravenous hydrocortisone 100–200 mg four times daily. This can be supplemented with a rectal infusion of prednisolone. There is no evidence that antibiotics modify the course of a severe attack. Some patients are treated with azathioprine or cyclosporin A to induce remission. If there is failure to gain an improvement within 5–7 days then surgery must be seriously considered. Prolonged high-dose intravenous steroid therapy is fraught with danger. Patients who have had weeks of treatment, during which the colonic wall has become friable and disintegrates at laparotomy, are now fortunately rare.

Indications for surgery

The risk of colectomy is 20 per cent overall, ranging from 5 per cent in those patients with proctitis to 50 per cent in those patients with a very severe attack:

- severe or fulminating disease failing to respond to medical therapy;
- chronic disease with anaemia, frequent stools, urgency and tenesmus;
- steroid-dependent disease: here the disease is not severe but remission cannot be maintained without substantial doses of steroids;
- the risk of neoplastic change: patients who on review colonoscopy have severe dysplasia;
- extraintestinal manifestations;
- rarely, severe haemorrhage or stenosis causing obstruction.

Operations

1. In the emergency situation the 'first-aid procedure' is a total abdominal colectomy and ileostomy. The rectum can either be brought out at the lower end of the wound as a mucous fistula or closed just beneath the skin. This has the advantage that the patient recovers quickly, the histology of the resected colon can be checked, and restorative surgery can be contemplated at a later date when the patient is no longer on steroids and in optimal nutritional condition. The alternative, division of the rectum below the sacral promontory, can result in breakdown and pelvic abscess, and makes subsequent identification of the stump more difficult.
2. Proctocolectomy and ileostomy: this is the procedure associated with the least compilcation rate. The patient is left with a permanent ileostomy. There is, however, a 20 per cent long-term risk of adhesion obstruction, and 5–10 per cent of the perineal wounds are very slow to heal. The late result will be a chronic perineal sinus which may require repeated currettage or excision. The obvious disadvantage is an ileostomy and although many patients cope remarkably well there is a psychological and social 'cost'.

   Rectal and anal dissection. Refinements of the procedure have included a close rectal dissection to minimise damage to the nervi erigenti and hence erectile dysfunction which may occur in 0.5–2 per cent, and intersphincteric excision of the anus which results in a smaller perineal wound and fewer healing problems.
3. Restorative proctocolectomy with an ileoanal pouch (Parks). In this operation a pouch or reservoir is made out of ileum (Fig. 57.26) as a substitute for the rectum and sewn or stapled to the anal canal. Various pouch designs have been described, but the J is the most popular and the most easily made using staplers (Fig. 57.27). There is some controversy over the correct technique for ileoanal anastomosis. In the earliest operations, the mucosa from the dentate line up to midrectum was stripped off the underlying muscle, but it is now known that a long muscle cuff is not needed. A mucosectomy of the upper anal canal with an anastomosis at the dentate line is claimed to remove all of the at-risk mucosa and any problem of subsequent cancer. It may also result in imperfect continence with nocturnal seepage. The alternative is a double stapled anastomosis to the top of the anal canal preserving the upper anal canal mucosa. Continence appears to be better, but the theoretical risk of leaving inflamed mucosa remains.

   The procedure can be carried out in one, two or three stages. In selected cases a covering loop ileostomy is omitted but is usually used. Complications include pelvic sepsis – usually resulting from a leak of the ileoanal anastomosis, small bowel obstruction and pouch vaginal fistula. Frequency of evacuation is determined by pouch volume, completeness of emptying, reservoir inflammation and intrinsic small bowel motility, but can be between three and six evacuations daily. Although associated with a higher complication rate, it is rapidly becoming the operation of choice in younger patients, avoiding a permanent ileostomy. About 20 per cent of patients have an episode of pouchitis, that is, inflammation of the reservoir, at some time. It usually responds to treatment with metronidazole.
4. Colectomy and ileorectal anastomosis: if there is minimal rectal inflammation this can occasionally be used; it has largely been superseded by restorative proctocolectomy.

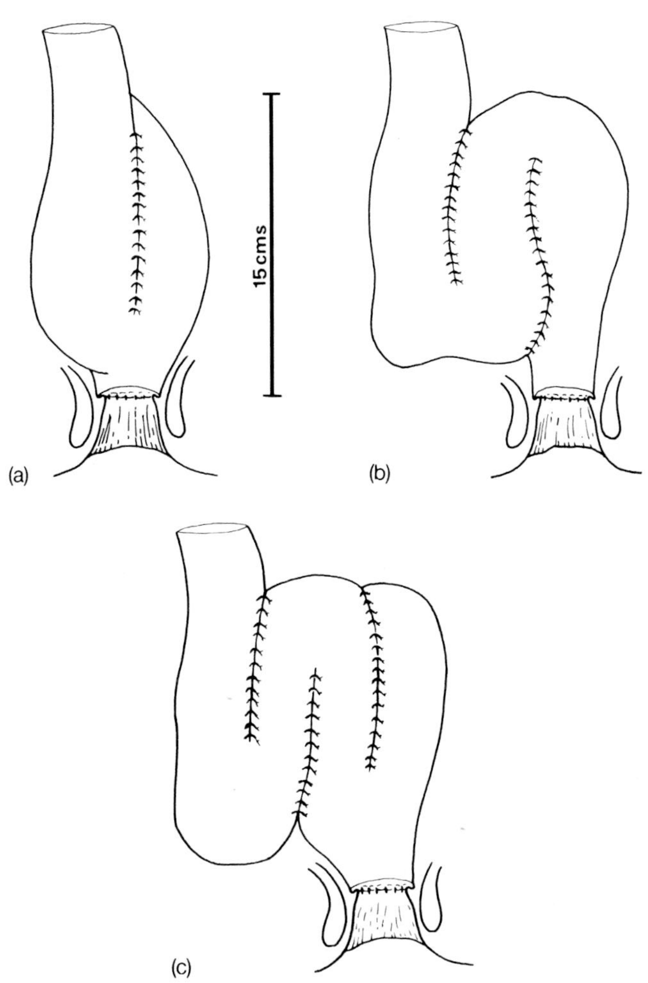

Fig. 57.26 Ileoanal anastomosis with pouch. A substitute rectum is made from joined folds of ileum to form an expanded pouch of small intestine. The pouch is then joined directly to the anus at the level of the dentate line, all other anal mucosa having been removed. Three ways of forming a pouch are illustrated: (a) a simple reversed 'J'; (b) an 'S' pouch; (c) a 'W' pouch.

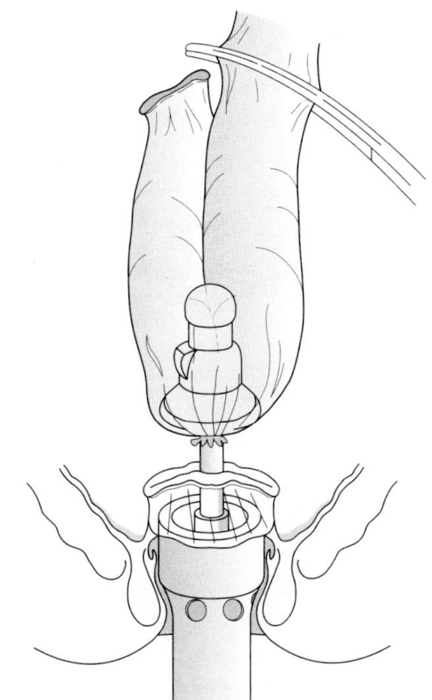

Fig. 57.27 Stapled J pouch with stapler creating a pouch anal anastomosis.

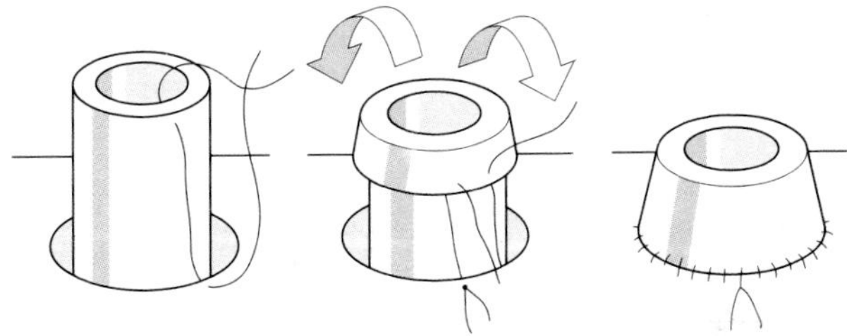

Fig. 57.28 Suturing the free extremity of the proximal ileum to the skin edges after eversion to form a spout (after Brooke).

5. Ileostomy with a continent intra-abdominal pouch (Kock's procedure). A reservoir is made of ileum and just beyond this a spout is made by inverting the efferent ileum into itself to give a continent valve just below skin level. The pouch is emptied by the patient inserting a catheter through the valve; now rarely used.

Ileostomy

End ileostomy (Brooke). In those patients with a permanent ileostomy there must be scrupulous attention to detail during the operation to ensure that the patient has a good functional result. The position of the ileostomy should be carefully chosen by the patient with the help of a stoma care nursing specialist. The ileum is normally brought through the lateral edge of the rectus abdominis muscle. The use of a spout (Fig. 57.28) was originally described by Bryan Brooke and it should project some 4 cm from the skin surface. A disposable appliance is placed over the ileostomy so that it is a snug fit at skin level.

Nils Kock. Surgeon, Güteborg, Sweden.

Bryan Brooke. Emeritus Professor of Surgery, St George's Hospital, London, England.

Ileostomy care

During the first few postoperative days, fluid and electrolyte balance must be adjusted with great care. There may be an 'ileostomy flux' while the ileum adapts to the loss of the colon, and the fluid losses can amount to 4 or 5 litres/day. The stools thicken in a few weeks and are semisolid in a few months. The help, skill and advice of the stoma care nursing specialist are essential. Modern appliances have transfonmed stoma care and skin problems are unusual (Fig. 57.29).

Complications of an ileostomy include prolapse, retraction, stenosis, bleeding and paraileostomy hernia.

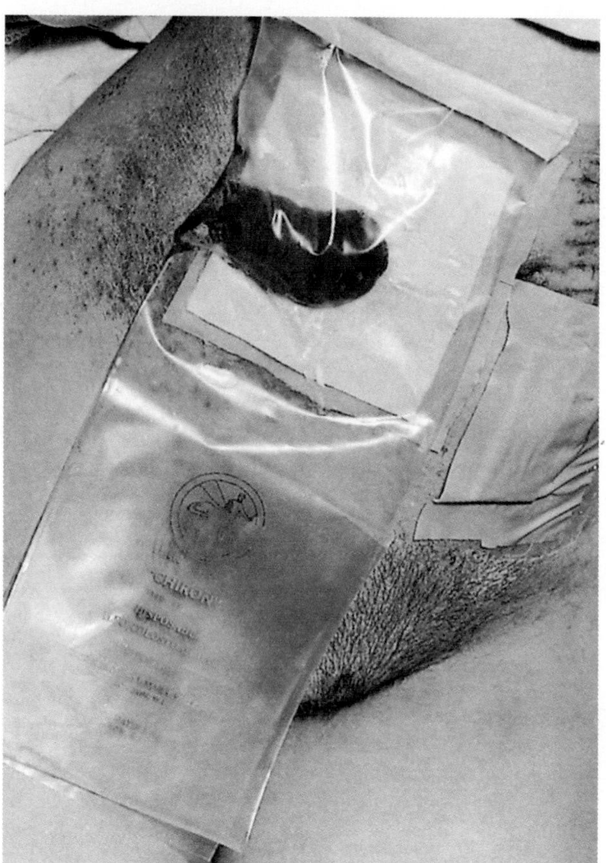

Fig. 57.29 Disposable ileostomy bag (*courtesy of Bryan N. Brooke, FRCS, London*).

Loop ileostomy. This is often used to defunction a pouch ileoanal procedure or even a low anterior resection. A knuckle of ileum is pulled out through a skin trephine in the right iliac fossa. An incision is made in the distal part of the knuckle and this is then pulled over the top of the more proximal part to create a spout on the proximal side of the loop with a flush distal side still in continuity. This allows near-perfect defunction, but also the possibility of restoration of continuity by taking down the spout and reanastomosing the partially divided ileum.

Crohn's disease (regional enteritis)

Crohn's disease became widely recognised following the report in 1932 by Crohn, Ginzburg and Oppenheimer describing young adults with a chronic inflammatory disease of the ileum. It can affect any part of the gastrointestinal tract from the lips to the anal margin, but ileocolonic disease is the most common presentation.

Leon Ginzburg, 1899–1988. Clinical Professor of Surgery, Beth Israel Hospital, New York, USA.

Julius Robert Oppenheimer, 1904–67. US nuclear physicist. Won Fermi Prize in 1963.

Epidemiology

It is most common in North America and northern Europe. Prevalence rates as high as 56 per 100 000 have been reported in the UK. Over the last four decades there seems to have been a rise in the incidence which cannot be accounted for by increased diagnosis. It is slightly more common in females than in males but is most commonly diagnosed in young patients between the ages of 25 and 40. There does, however, seem to be a second peak of incidence around the age of 17.

Aetiology

Although Crohn's disease has some features suggesting chronic infection, no causative organism has ever been found; similarities between Crohn's disease and tuberculosis have focused attention on mycobacteria. Focal ischaemia has also been postulated as a causative factor, possibly originating from a vasculitis arising through an immunological process. A wide variety of foods has now been implicated but none conclusively. Smoking increases the risk threefold.

About 10 per cent of patients have a first-degree relative with the disease and there is an association with ankylosing spondylitis. Cell-mediated immune function may be defective in patients with Crohn's disease but it is not known whether this is a consequence of the disease itself or the effects of malnutrition and medical therapy. As with ulcerative colitis it is now believed that Crohn's disease can predispose to cancer, although the incidence of malignant change is not nearly as high as in ulcerative colitis and is most manifest in the ileum.

Pathology

Ileal disease is the most common accounting for 60 per cent of cases; 30 per cent of cases are limited to the large intestine and the remainder consists of patients with ileal disease alone or more proximal small bowel involvement. Anal lesions are common. Crohn's disease of the mouth, oesophagus, and stomach and duodenum are uncommon. Resection specimens show a fibrotic thickening of the intestinal wall with a narrow lumen (Fig. 57.30). There is usually dilated gut just proximal to the stricture and, in the strictured area, there are deep mucosal ulcerations with linear or snake-like patterns. Oedema in the mucosa between the ulcers gives rise to a cobblestone appearance. The transmural inflammation leads to adhesions, inflammatory masses with mesenteric abscesses and fistulae into adjacent organs. The serosa is usually opaque, there is thickening in the mesentery and mesenteric lymph nodes are enlarged. The condition is discontinuous with inflamed areas separated from normal intestine; these are sometimes called skip lesions. Under the

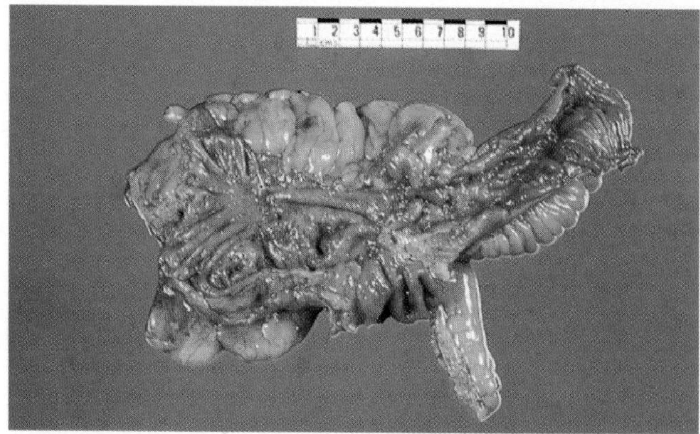

Fig. 57.30 Crohn's disease of the ileocaecal region showing typical thickening of the wall of the terminal ileum with narrowing of the lumen (*courtesy of Dr B. Warren, John Radcliffe Hospital, Oxford*).

microscope there are focal areas of chronic inflammation involving all layers of the intestinal wall. There are noncaseating giant cell granulomas but these are only found in 60 per cent of patients. They are most common in anorectal disease. The earliest mucosal lesions are discrete aphthous ulcers. Recent studies have also shown multifocal arterial occlusions in the muscularis propia.

Clinical features

Presentation depends upon the area of involvement.

Acute Crohn's disease

Acute Crohn's disease occurs in only 5 per cent of cases. Symptoms and signs resemble those of acute appendicitis but there is usually diarrhoea preceding the attack. Rarely there could be a free perforation of the small intestine, resulting in a local or diffuse peritonitis. Acute colitis with or without toxic megacolon can occur in Crohn's disease but is less common than in ulcerative colitis.

Chronic Crohn's disease

There is often a history of mild diarrhoea extending over many months occurring in bouts accompanied by intestinal colic. Patients may complain of pain, particularly in the right iliac fossa, and there may be a tender mass palpable. Intermittent fevers, secondary anaemia and weight loss are common. A perianal abscess or fissure may be the first presenting feature of Crohn's disease; the cause is often an infected anal crypt associated with concomitant diarrhoea, but as the disease becomes chronic specific fistulae resulting from the Crohn's disease itself can develop.

After months of repeated attacks with acute inflammation the affected area of intestine begins to narrow with fibrosis causing abdominal pain on eating, giving rise to what has been described as 'food fear'. Children developing the illness before puberty may have retarded growth and sexual development.

With progression of the disease adhesions and transmural fissuring, intra-abdominal abscesses and fistula tracts can develop.

1. Enteroenteric fistulae can occur into adjacent small bowel loops or the pelvic colon and enterovesical fistulae may cause repeated urinary tract infections and pneumaturia.
2. Enterocutaneous fistulae rarely occur spontaneously and usually follow previous surgery.

Anal disease (see Chapter 58)

In the presence of active disease, the perianal skin appears bluish. Three or more oedematous pinky-blue fleshy tags protrude from the anal margin; they may have superficial ulceration on the inner surface extending into the anal canal. Superficial ulcers with undermined edges are relatively painless and can heal with bridging of epithelium. Deep cavitating ulcers are usually found in the upper anal canal; they can be painful and cause perianal abscesses and fistulae, discharging around the anus and sometimes forwards into the genitalia.

The most distressing feature of anal disease is sepsis from secondary abscesses and perianal fistulae. Remarkably the rectal mucosa is often spared and may feel normal on rectal examination. If it is involved, however, it will feel thickened, nodular and irregular.

Investigation

Sigmoidoscopic examination

Sigmoidoscopic examination may be normal or show minimal involvement. Ulceration in the anal canal will, however, be readily seen.

Colonoscopy

As a result of the discontinuous nature of Crohn's disease there will be areas of normal colon or rectum. In between these there are areas of inflamed mucosa which are irregular, ulcerated with a mucopurulent exudate. The earliest appearances are aphthoid-like ulcers surrounded by a rim of erythematous mucosa. These become larger and deeper with increasing severity of disease. In colonic Crohn's disease there may be stricturing and it is important to exclude malignancy in these sites (Fig. 57.31). At the ileocolic anastomosis of a patient having had previous ileocaecal resection, recurrent disease is usually seen on the ileal side of the anastomosis.

Radiology

Barium enema will show similar features to those of colonoscopy in the colon. The best investigation of the small intestine is small bowel enema (Fig. 57.32). This will show up areas of delay and dilatation characterising partial obstruction. The involved areas tend to be narrowed, irregular and sometimes, when a length of terminal ileum is involved, there may be the string sign of Kantor. Sinograms are useful in patients with enterocutaneous fistulae. CT scans are used in patients with fistulae and those with intra-abdominal abscesses and complex involvement.

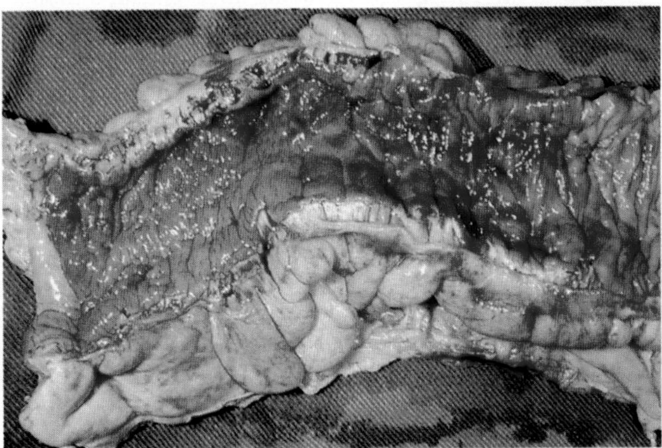

Fig. 57.31 Colonic Crohn's disease. Note the normal mucosa on either side of the inflammatory stricture (*courtesy of Dr B. Warren, John Radcliffe Hospital, Oxford*).

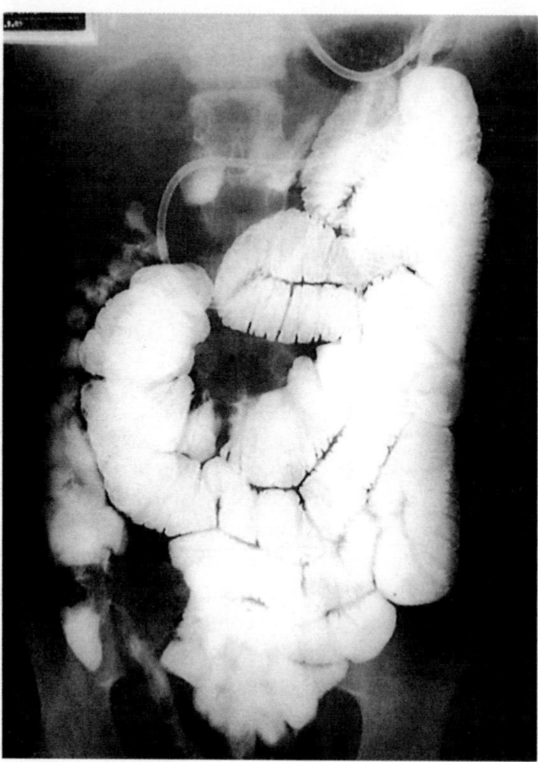

Fig. 57.32 Small bowel enema examination showing a narrow terminal involved with Crohn's disease – the 'string' sign of Kantor (*courtesy of Dr D. Nolan, John Radcliffe Hospital, Oxford*).

Magnetic resonance imaging (MRI) has been shown to be useful in assessing perianal disease.

Treatment

Medical therapy

Steroids are the mainstay of treatment. Patients with a relapse of their Crohn's disease are treated with up to 40 mg prednisolone orally, daily supplemented by 5-ASA compounds in those patients with colonic involvement, although there is some evidence that this may help small bowel disease as well. Those who have symptoms and signs of a mass or an abscess are also treated with antibiotics. Azathioprine is used for its additive and steroid-sparing effect. Nutritional support is essential. Severely malnourished people may require intravenous feeding or nasoenteric feeding regimens. Anaemia, hypoproteinaemia, electrolyte, vitamin and metabolic bone problems must all be addressed.

Indications for surgery

Surgical resection will not cure Crohn's disease. Surgery is therefore focused on complications of the disease. As many of these indications for surgery may be relative, joint management by an aggressive physician and a conservative surgeon is thought to be ideal. These complications include:

- recurrent intestinal obstruction;
- bleeding;
- perforation;
- failure of medical therapy;
- intestinal fistula;
- fulminant colitis;
- malignant change;
- perianal disease.

Surgery

To preserve functional gut length, resection is kept to a minimum so as to deal with the local problem. The whole of the gastrointestinal tract has to be examined carefully at the time of laparotomy. If on occasion Crohn's disease is diagnosed during the course of an operation for suspected appendicitis, the appendix should be removed. If the ileum is thick, rigid and pipe-like, senior help should be sought so that an ileocaecal resection can be carried out.

The course of the disease after surgery is unpredictable but recurrence is common. It does not seem to be related to the presence of disease at the resection line. Recurrence rates vary from site to site but the cumulative probability of recurrence requiring surgery for ileal disease is of the order of 20, 40, 60 and 80 per cent at 5, 10, 15 and 20 years, respectively, after previous resection. Restorative operations have a higher incidence of recurrence than, for example, proctocolectomy and ileostomy.

1. **Ileocaecal resection** is the usual procedure for ileocaecal disease with a primary anastomosis between the ileum and the transverse colon.
2. **Segmental resection**: short segments of small or large bowel involvement can be treated by segmental resection.
3. **Colectomy and ileorectal anastomosis.** In patients with widespread colonic disease with rectal sparing and a normal anus this can be a useful option.
4. **Temporary loop ileostomy.** This can be used either in patients with acute distal Crohn's disease allowing remission and later restoration of continuity or in patients with severe perianal or rectal disease.
5. **Proctocolectomy.** Patients with colonic and anal disease failing to respond to medical treatment or defunction will eventually require a permanent ileostomy.
6. **Strictureplasty.** Multiple strictured areas of Crohn's disease (Fig. 57.33) can be treated by a local widening procedure, strictureplasty, to avoid excessive small bowel resection (Fig. 57.34) (Lee).
7. **Anal disease** is usually treated conservatively by simple drainage of abscesses, placing setons around any fistulae, and occasionally in patients with inactive disease primary repair of a rectovaginal or high fistula *in ano* could be attempted.

Emanuel Lee, 1933–86. Surgeon, Oxford, England.

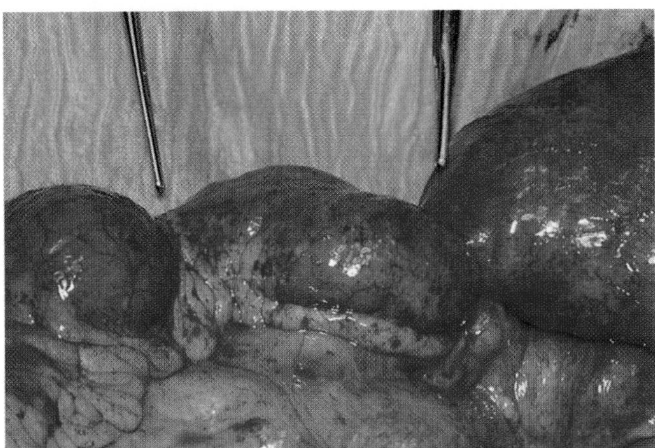

Fig. 57.33 Small bowel strictures in Crohn's disease with dilatation between strictures.

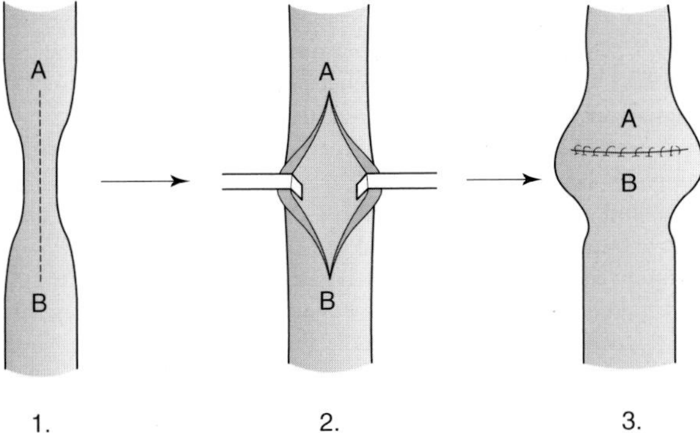

Fig. 57.34 Strictureplasty. (1) A strictured length of intestine is incised along its length. (2) The bowel is opened and the walls are retracted as shown. (3) The bowel is resutured transversely to widen the narrowed segment.

Infections

Intestinal amoebiasis. Amoebiasis is an infestation with *Entamoeba histolytica*. This parasite has a world-wide distribution.

Life history of the parasite. The active form of the parasite or trophozoite lives in the intestinal mucous membrane where it ingests red blood corpuscles and other cells and multiples by mitosis. Should the parasite become pathogenic, it makes its way into the follicles of Lieberkühn and, by dissolving into glandular tissue via the cytolysins, submucous loculi are produced. Some of these burst through the mucous membrane to become amoebic ulcers. While the trophozoites continue their activities in the base of the ulcer, others cease to feed, migrate towards the surface and become transformed into cysts which pass into the outer world with the faeces. Amoebiasis is transmitted mainly in contaminated drinking water.

Pathology. The ulcers, which have been described as 'bottlenecked' because of their considerably undermined edges, have a yellow necrotic floor, from which blood and pus exude. Although on rare occasions the ulcers are scattered throughout the large intestine, in 75 per cent they are confined to the lower sigmoid and upper rectum.

Biopsy. Endoscopic biopsies or fresh hot stools are examined carefully to look for the presence of amoebae. It is important to emphasise, however, that the presence of the parasite does not indicate that it is pathogenic (Fig. 57.35).

Johann Nathaniel Lieberkühn, 1711–57. German anatomist.

Clinical features. Dysentery is the principal manifestation of the disease but it may come in various other guises.

Appendicitis or amoebic caecal mass. In tropical countries where amoebiasis is endemic, this is a constantly recurring problem. To operate on a patient with amoebic dysentery without the precautions subsequently described is to invite an exacerbation of amoebiasis which may prove fatal. The bowel is friable and satisfactory closure of the appendix stump becomes difficult or impossible, especially in cases where a palpable mass is present. When there is an amoebic mass there tends to be tenderness on deep palpation over the caecum and the sigmoid.

Perforation. The most common sites are the caecum and rectosigmoid; usually perforation occurs into a confined space where adhesions have previously formed and a pericolic abscess results which eventually needs draining. When there is sudden faecal flooding in the general peritoneal cavity, drainage of the region of the perforation, gastrointestinal aspiration, intravenous fluid, antibiotics and a full course of emetine are sometimes successful.

Severe rectal haemorrhage as a result of separation of the slough is liable to occur.

Granuloma. Progressive amoebic invasion of the wall of the rectum or colon, with secondary inflammation, can produce a granulomatous mass indistinguishable from a carcinoma.

Fibrous stricture may follow the healing of extensive amoebic ulcers.

Intestinal obstruction is a common complication of amoebiasis, and the obstruction is the result of adhesions associated with pericolitis and large granuloma.

Paracolic abscess, ischiorectal abscess and fistula occur from perforation by amoebae of the intestinal wall followed by secondary infection.

Ulcerative colitis. A search for amoebae should always be made in the stools of patients believed to have ulcerative colitis.

Treatment. High-dose intravenous steroids in this situation can be catastrophic. Metronidazole (Flagyl) is the first-line drug, 800 mg three times daily for 7–10 days. Diloxanide furoate is best for chronic infections associated with the passage of cysts in stools. Intestinal antibiotics improve the results of the chronic stages, probably by coping with superadded infection.

Typhoid and paratyphoid. ***Surgical complications.*** *Paralytic ileus* is the most common complication of typhoid.

Intestinal haemorrhage may be the leading symptom.

Perforation. Perforation of a typhoid ulcer usually occurs during the third week and is occasionally the first sign of the disease. The ulcer is parallel to the long axis of the gut and is usually situated in the lower ileum.

Paratyphoid B. Perforation of the large intestine sometimes occurs. Vigorous intravenous antibiotic therapy is given; occasionally surgery is required to defunction the colon or in late cases remove the colon as for ulcerative colitis.

Cholecystitis. Acute typhoid cholecystitis is not uncommon and perforation can occur; gallstones occasionally contain typhoid bacilli and some patients may become typhoid carriers.

Phlebitis. Venous thrombosis, particularly of the left common iliac vein, is an occasional complication of typhoid fever.

Genitourinary complications. Typhoid cystitis, pyelitis and epididymo-orchitis may all occur.

Joints. All degrees of arthritis, from a mild effusion to suppuration, occur as a complication of this disease.

Bone. Typhoid osteomyelitis and typhoid of the spine occur.

Tuberculosis of the intestine. Tuberculosis can affect any part of the gastrointestinal tract from the mouth to the anus. The sites affected most often are the ileum, proximal colon and peritoneum. There are two principal types.

Ulcerative tuberculosis is secondary to pulmonary tuberculosis and arises as a result of swallowing tubercle bacilli. There are multiple ulcers in the terminal ileum, lying transversely, and the overlying serosa is thickened, reddened and covered in tubercles.

Clinical features. Diarrhoea and weight loss are the predominant symptoms and usually the patient will be receiving treatment for pulmonary tuberculosis.

Radiology. A barium meal and follow-through or small bowel enema will show the absence of filling of the lower ileum, caecum and most of the ascending colon as a result of narrowing and hypermotility of the ulcerated segment (Fig. 57.36).

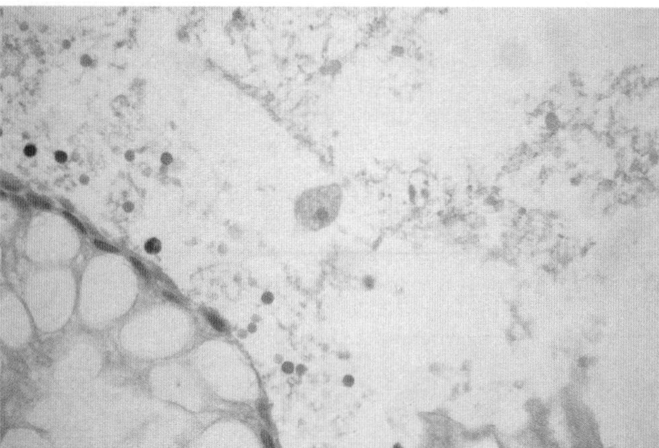

Fig. 57.35 An amoeba in a rectal biopsy.

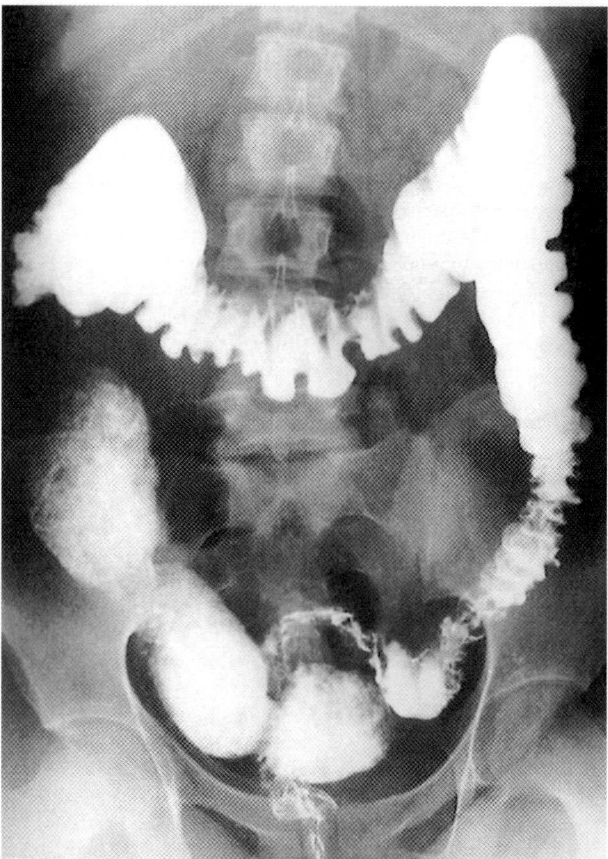

Fig. 57.36 Ileocaecal tuberculosis; absent ascending colon and caecum with dilatation of terminal ileum (*courtesy of Dr Vinay Kumar Kapoor, Delhi, India*).

Treatment. A course of chemotherapy is given. Healing often occurs provided the pulmonary tuberculosis is adequately treated. An operation is only required in the rare event of a perforation or intestinal obstruction.

Hyperplastic tuberculosis. This usually occurs in the ileocaecal region although solitary and multiple lesions in the lower ileum are sometimes seen. This is caused by the ingestion of *Mycobacterium tuberculosis* by patients with a high resistance to the organism. The infection establishes itself in lymphoid follicles, and the resulting chronic inflammation causes thickening of the intestinal wall and narrowing of the lumen. There is early involvement of the regional lymph nodes which may caseate. Unlike Crohn's disease, with which it shares many similarities, abscess and fistula formation is rare.

Untreated, sooner or later subacute intestinal obstruction will supervene often together with the impaction of an enterolith in the narrowed lumen.

Clinical features. Attacks of abdominal pain with intermittent diarrhoea are the usual symptoms. The ileum above the partial obstruction is distended, and the stasis and consequent infection lead to steatorrhoea, anaemia and loss of weight. Sometimes the presenting picture is of a mass in the right iliac fossa in a patent with vague ill health. The differential diagnosis is that of an appendix mass, carcinoma of the caecum, Crohn's disease, tuberculosis or actinomycosis of the caecum.

Radiology. A barium follow-through or small bowel enema will show a long narrow filling defect in the terminal ileum.

Treatment. When the diagnosis is certain and the patient has not yet developed obstructive symptoms, treatment with chemotherapy is advised and may cure the condition. Where obstruction is present, operative treatment is required and ileocaecal resection is best.

Actinomycosis of the ileocaecal region. Abdominal actinomycosis is rare. Unlike intestinal tuberculosis, narrowing of the lumen of the intestine does not occur and mesenteric nodes do not become involved. A local abscess, however, spreads to the retroperitoneal tissues and the adjacent abdominal wall, becoming the seat of multiple indurated discharging sinuses. The liver may become involved via the portal vein.

Clinical features. The usual history is that appendicectomy has been carried out for an appendicitis. Some 3 weeks after surgery a mass is palpable in the right iliac fossa and soon afterwards the wound begins to discharge. At first this is thin and watery, and then later it becomes thicker and malodorous. Other sinuses may form and a secondary faecal fistula develop. Pus should be sent for bacteriological examination where the characteristic sulphur granules can be seen.

Treatment. Penicillin or cotrimoxazole has to be prolonged and high dosage.

Tumours of the small intestine

Compared with the large intestine, the small intestine is rarely the seat of a neoplasm and these become progressively less common from the duodenum to the terminal ileum.

Benign. Adenoma, submucous lipoma and leiomyoma occur from time to time, and sometimes reveal themselves by causing an intussusception. The second most common complication is intestinal bleeding from an adenoma in which event the diagnosis is frequently long delayed because the tumour is overlooked at barium radiology, endoscopy and even surgery.

Peutz–Jeghers syndrome consists of:

- familial intestinal hamartomatous polyposis affecting the jejunum, where it is a cause of haemorrhage, and often intussusception;
- melanosis of the oral mucous membrane and the lips.

John Law Augustine Peutz, 1886–1957. Chief Specialist for Internal Medicine, St John's Hospital, The Hague, The Netherlands.

Harold Jos Jeghers. Professor of Internal Medicine, New Jersey College of Medicine and Dentistry, Jersey City, USA.

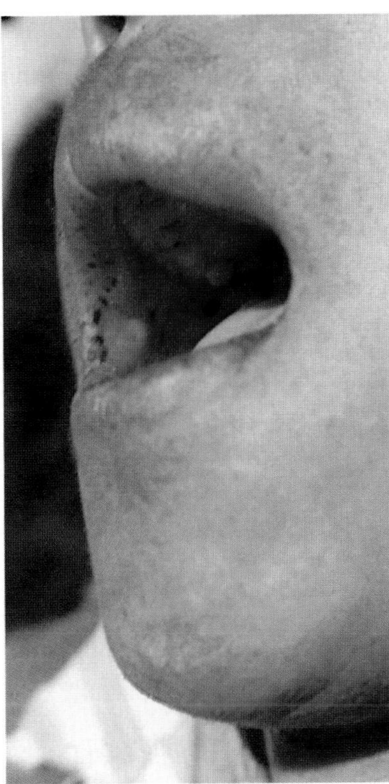

Fig. 57.37 Melanin spots on the lips of a patient afflicted with Peutz–Jeghers syndrome (*courtesy of Major P.C.M. Manta, Indian Medical Service*).

The melanosis takes the form of melanin spots sometimes present on the digits and the perianal skin, but the pigmentation of the lips is the *sine qua non* (Fig. 57.37).

Histology. The polyps can be likened to trees. The trunk and branches are smooth muscle fibres and the foliage is virtually normal mucosa.

Treatment. As malignant change rarely occurs, resection is necessary only for serious bleeding or intussusception. Large single polyps can be removed by enterotomy or short lengths of heavily involved intestine can be resected. Those lesions within reach can be snared by colonoscopy.

Malignant. ***Lymphoma***. There are three main types as follows.

1. *Western type lymphoma*. These are annular ulcerating lesions, which are sometimes multiple. They are now thought to be non-Hodgkin's B-cell lymphoma in origin. They may present with obstruction and bleeding, perforation, anorexia and weight loss.
2. *Primary lymphoma associated with coeliac disease*. There is an increased incidence of lymphoma in patients with coeliac disease; this is now regarded as a T-cell lymphoma. Worsening of the patient's diarrhoea, with pyrexia of unknown origin together with local obstructive symptoms, is the usual feature.
3. *Mediterranean lymphoma*. This is found mostly in North Africa and the Middle East and is associated with α-chain disease.

Unless there are particular surgical complications these conditions are usually treated with chemotherapy.

Carcinoma. As with other small bowel tumours these can present with obstruction, bleeding or diarrhoea. Complete resection offers the only hope of cure (Fig. 57.38).

Thomas Hodgkin, 1798–1866. Curator of the Museum and demonstrator of morbid anatomy, Guy's Hospital, London, England.

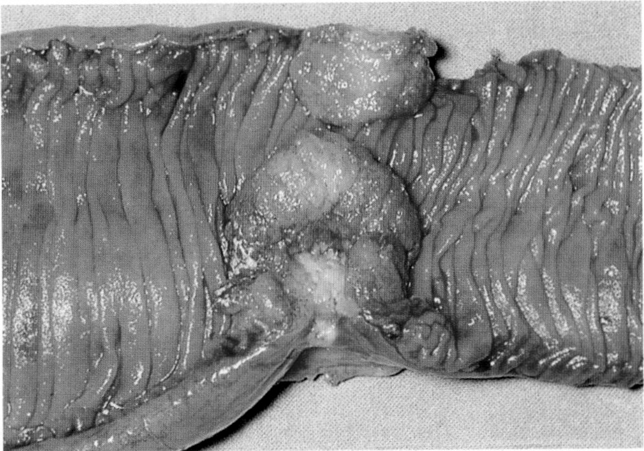

Fig. 57.38 Small bowel adenocarcinoma.

Carcinoid tumour. These tumours occur throughout the gastrointestinal tract, most commonly in the appendix, ileum and rectum in decreasing order of frequency. They arise from neuroendocrine cells at the base of intestinal crypts. The primary is usually small but when they metastasise, the liver is usually involved with numerous secondaries, which are larger and more yellow than the primary, and when this has occurred the carcinoid syndrome will become evident. The tumours can produce a number of vasoactive peptides, most commonly 5-hydroxytryptamine (serotonin), which may be present as 5-hydroxyindoleacetic acid in the urine during attacks.

The clinical syndrome itself consists of reddish-blue cyanosis, flushing attacks, diarrhoea, borborygmi, asthmatic attacks and, eventually, sometimes pulmonary and tricuspid stenosis. Classically the flushing attacks are induced by alcohol.

Treatment. Most patients with gastrointestinal carcinoids do not have carcinoid syndrome. Surgical resection is usually sufficient. In the cases found incidentally at appendicectomy nothing further is required. In patients with metastatic disease, multiple enucleations of hepatic metastases or even partial hepatectomy can be carried out. The treatment has been transformed by the use of octreotide (a somatostatin analogue) which reduces both flushing and diarrhoea, and octreotide cover is usually used in patients with a carcinoid syndrome who have surgery to prevent a carcinoid crisis. Carcinoid tumours generally grow more slowly than most metastatic malignancies; the patients may live with the syndrome of metatastic disease for many years.

Tumours of the large intestine

Benign

The term 'polyp' is a clinical description of any elevated tumour. It covers a variety of histologically different tumours shown in Table 57.2.

Polyps can occur either singly, synchronously in small numbers or as part of a polyposis syndrome. In familial adenomatous polyposis, more than 100 adenomas are present. It is important to be sure of the histological diagnosis because adenomas have significant malignant potential.

Adenomatous polyps

Adenomatous polyps vary from a tubular adenoma (Fig. 57.39), rather like a raspberry on a stalk, to the villous adenoma, a

Table 57.2 Classification of polyps of the large intestine

Class	*Varieties*
Inflammatory	Inflammatory polyps
Metaplastic	Metaplastic or hyperplastic polyps
Harmartomatous	Peutz–Jeghers polyp
	Juvenile polyp
Neoplastic	Adenoma – tubular
	Tubulovillous
	Villous
	Adenocarcinoma
	Carcinoid tumour

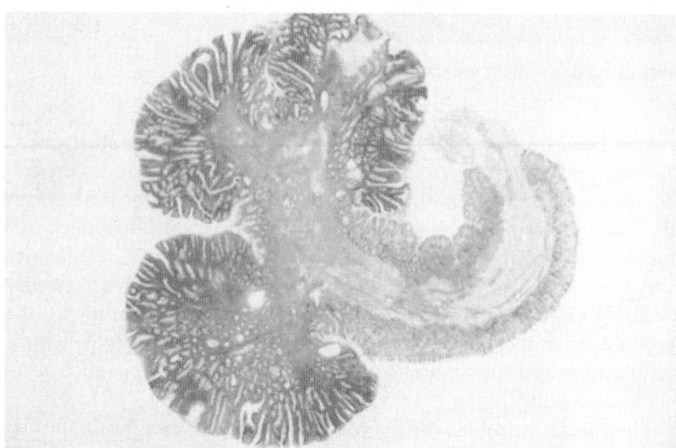

Fig. 57.39 Pedunculated adenomatous polyp of the large intestine, longitudinal section (*courtesy of Dr P. Millard, John Radcliffe Hospital, Oxford*).

flat spreading lesion. Solitary adenomas are usually found during the investigation of colonic bleeding or sometimes fortuitously. Villous tumours more usually give symptoms of diarrhoea, mucus discharge and occasionally hypokalaemia. The risk of malignancy developing in an adenoma increases with increasing size of tumour, for example, in 1-cm diameter tubular adenomas there is a 10 per cent risk of cancer, whereas in villous adenomas over 2 cm in diameter there may be a 15 per cent chance of carcinoma. Adenomas larger than 5 mm in diameter are usually treated because of their malignant potential. Colonoscopic snare polypectomy or diathermy obliteration with hot biopsy forceps can be used. Huge villous adenomas of the rectum can be difficult to remove even with techniques per anus and occasionally proctectomy is required; the anal sphincter can usually be preserved.

Harmartomatous polyps

Peutz–Jeghers polyps may occur in the colon as either solitary or multiple lesions. Juvenile polyps may occur as multiple lesions in the colon often associated with a congenital defect such as a malrotation or Meckels' diverticulum. They have minimal malignant potential and are only removed if they are causing troublesome pain, bleeding or hypoproteinaemia.

Haemangioma

A localised submucous telangiectasis is often the cause of bleeding which may be profuse. If bleeding is continuing, both angiography and colonoscopy can help to localise the source. If found by colonoscopy the lesion can be removed endoscopically, whereas arteriographic detection can be followed by the use of vasopressin or microspheres to stop the haemorrhage. Often the only method of detecting it is to operate while the bleeding is in progress. The distribution of blood within the intestine is noted; scrutiny of the blood-containing portion of the colon may reveal the lesion but on-table colonoscopy could be necessary. The tumour is resected once located.

Lipoma

Lipoma is less frequently encountered in the large than in the small intestine. In the large intestine it is almost always confined to the caecum. The tumour is submucous and in more than half the cases it is the cause of an intussusception. On occasion a lipoma at the ileocaecal valve can be confused with a caecal cancer.

Familial adenomatous polyposis

Familial adenomatous polyposis (FAP) is a general neoplastic disorder of the intestine. Although the large bowel is mainly affected polyps can occur in the stomach, duodenum and small intestine. The main risk is large bowel cancer, but duodenal and ampullary tumours have been reported. It is inherited as a Mendelian dominant and the gene responsible (APC gene) has now been identified on the short arm of chromosome 5 (Bodmer). Males and females are equally affected. It can also occur sporadically without any previous sign or history, presumably by new mutations. There is often, in these cases, a history of large bowel cancer occurring in young adulthood or middle age suggesting pre-existing adenomatosis.

FAP can be associated with benign mesodermal tumours such as desmoid tumours and osteomas. Epidermoid cysts can also occur (Gardner's syndrome); desmoid tumours in the abdomen invade locally to involve the intestinal mesentery and although nonmetastasising they can become unresectable.

Clinical features. Polyps are usually visible on sigmoidoscopy by the age of 15 years and will almost always be visible by the age of 30. Carcinoma of the large bowel occurs 10–20 years after the onset of the polyposis. One or more cancers will already be present in two-thirds of those patients presenting with symptoms.

Symptomatic patients. These are either new propositi or those from an affected family who have not been screened. They may have loose stools, lower abdominal pain, weight loss, diarrhoea and the passage of blood and mucus. Polyps are seen on sigmoidoscopy, and the number and distribution of polyps, and usually cancers if they are symptomatic, are shown on a double-contrast barium enema. If in doubt colonoscopy is performed with biopsies to establish the number and histological type of polyps. If over 100 adenomas (Fig. 57.40) are present the diagnosis can be made confidently but it is important not to confuse this with non-neoplastic forms of polyposis.

Sir Walter Bodmer. Director, Imperial Cancer Research Fund, London, England.

Eldon J. Gardner, b. 1909. American geneticist.

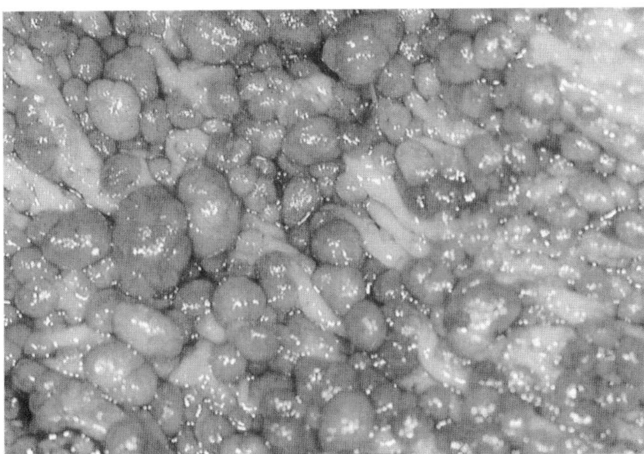

Fig. 57.40 Familial adenomatous polyposis.

Asymptomatic patients. Usually members of affected families attend for screening. As yet there is no reliable means of knowing whether an individual is affected unless adenomas develop. If there are no adenomas by the age of 30, FAP is unlikely. Pigmented spots in the retina (CHIRPES) and deoxyribonucleic acid (DNA) tests for the FAP gene should make screening more reliable in the future.

If the diagnosis is made during adolescence, operation is deferred usually to the age of 17 or 18.

Screening policy.

1. All members of the family should be examined at the age of 10–12 years, repeated every 1–2 years.
2. Most of those who are going to get polyps will have them at 20 and these require operation.
3. If there are no polyps at 20, continue with 5-yearly examination until age 50; if there are still no polyps there is probably no inherited gene. Carcinomatous change may exceptionally occur before the age of 20. Examination of blood relatives, including cousins, nephews and nieces, is essential and a family tree should be constructed and a register of affected families maintained.

Treatment. Colectomy with ileorectal anastomosis has in the past been the usual operation because it avoids an ileostomy in a young patient. The rectum is subsequently cleared of polyps by snaring or fulguration. The patients are examined by flexible sigmoidoscopy at 6-monthly intervals thereafter. In spite of this, a proportion of patients develops carcinoma in the rectal stump. The risk of carcinoma in the St Mark's series was 10 per cent over a period of 30 years.

The alternative and now more common operation is a restorative proctocolectomy with an ileoanal anastomosis. This has a higher complication rate than ileorectal anastomosis. It is indicated in patients with serious rectal involvement with polyps, those who are likely to be poor at attending for follow-up and those with an established cancer of the rectum or sigmoid. However, it is now used more frequently for less severe cases.

Malignant

Adenocarcinoma of the colon

Pathology. Microscopically, the neoplasm is a columnar cell carcinoma originating in the colonic epithelium. Macroscopically the tumour may take one of four forms (Fig. 57.41). Type 4 is the least malignant form. It is likely that all carcinomas start as a benign adenoma, the so-called 'adenoma–carcinoma sequence'. The annular variety tends to give rise to obstructive symptoms whereas the others more commonly will present with bleeding. Site and distribution of cases of cancer are shown in Fig. 57.42. Tumours are more common in the left colon and rectum.

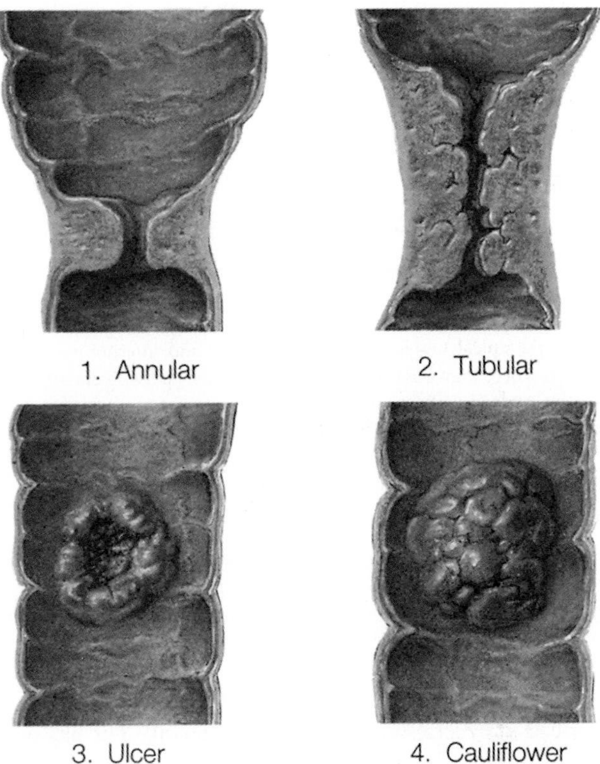

Fig. 57.41 The four common macroscopic varieties of carcinoma of the colon.

The spread of carcinoma of the colon. Generally this is a comparatively slow growing neoplasm.

Local spread

The tumour is limited to the bowel for a considerable time; it spreads round the intestinal wall and usually causes intestinal obstruction before it invades adjacent structures. The ulcerative type more commonly

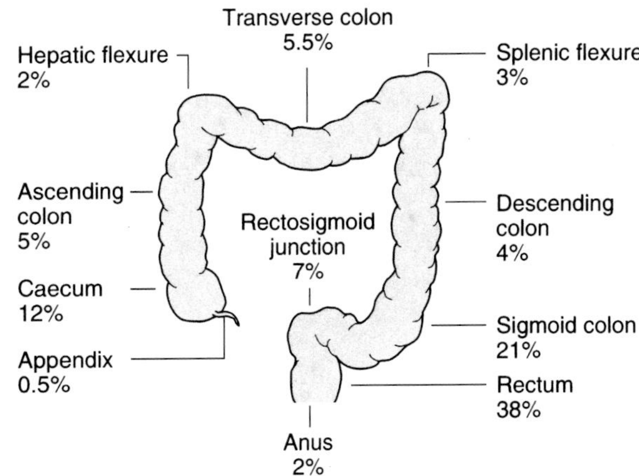

Fig. 57.42 Drawing showing distribution of colorectal cancer by site.

invades locally and an internal fistula may result, for example, into the bladder. There may also be a local perforation with an abscess or even an external faecal fistula. The progression of invasion occurs across the submucosa into the muscularis propia and thence out into the serosa and fat, lymphatics and veins in the mesentery alongside the bowel wall.

Lymphatic spread

Lymph nodes draining the colon are grouped as follows:

- N1 – nodes in the immediate vicinity of the bowel wall;
- N2 – nodes arranged along the ileocolic, right colic, midcolic, left colic and sigmoid arteries;
- N3 – the apical nodes around the superior and inferior mesenteric vessels where they arise from the abdominal aorta. Involvement of the lymph nodes by the tumour progresses in a gradual manner from those closest to the growth along the course of the lymphatic vessels to those placed centrally.

Bloodstream spread

This accounts for a large proportion (30–40 per cent) of late deaths. Metastases are carried to the liver via the portal system sometimes at an early stage before clinical or operative evidence is detected (occult hepatic metastases).

Staging colon cancer. Dukes' classification was originally described for rectal tumours (see Chapter 60) but has been adopted for histopathological reporting of colon cancer as well. There have been numerous modifications of the original system leading to some confusion but in its most basic form Dukes' classification for colon cancer is as follows.

Dukes'

A – confined to bowel wall;
B – through the bowel wall but not involving the free peritoneal serosal surface;
C – lymph nodes involved.

Dukes himself never described a D stage, but this is often used to describe either advanced local disease or metastases to the liver.

TNM classification. The TNM classification is more detailed and accurate but more demanding.

T – tumour stage:
T_1 – into submucosa;
T_2 – into muscularis propria;
T_3 – into pericolic fat but not breaching serosa;
T_4 – breaches serosa or directly involving another organ.
N – nodal stage:
N_0 – no nodes involved;
N_1 – 1–2 nodes involved;
N_2 – 3 or more nodes.
M – metastases:
M_0 – no metastases;
M_1 – metastases.
Ly – lymphatic invasion:
L_0 – no lymphatic vessels involved;
L_1 – lymphatics involved.
V – venous invasion:
V_0 – no vessel invasion;
V_1 – vessels invaded.
R – residual tumour:
R_0 – no residual tumour;
R_1 – margins involved, residual tumour present.

Cuthbert Esquire Dukes, 1890–1977. Pathologist, St Mark's Hospital, London, England.

Clinical features. Carcinoma of the colon usually occurs in patients over 50 years of age but it is not rare earlier in adult life. Twenty per cent of cases present as an emergency with intestinal obstruction or peritonitis. In any case of colonic bleeding in patients over the age of 40 a complete investigation of the colon is required. A careful family history should be taken. Those with first-degree relatives who have developed colorectal cancer at the age of 45 or below are at high risk and may be part of one of the colorectal cancer family syndromes.

Carcinoma of the left side of the colon

Most tumours occur in this location. They are usually of the stenosing variety. The main symptoms are those of increasing intestinal obstruction.

Pain is referred to the suprapubic area. Patients will have episodes of colic; a constant ache may suggest an advanced tumour.

Alteration of bowel habit. An adult previously having a predictably regular bowel habit suddenly develops irregularity. There may be increasing difficulty in getting the bowels to move, requiring laxatives. The episodes of constipation may be followed by attacks of diarrhoea.

Palpable lump. The lump that is felt on abdominal, rectal or bimanual palpation is sometimes not the tumour itself, but impacted faeces above it. When the tumour is situated in a pendulous pelvic colon, a hard movable swelling may be felt in the rectovesical pouch on rectal examination.

Distension. Lower abdominal distension is not uncommon and, as with the pain, is relieved by passing flatus.

Carcinoma of the sigmoid

This follows the general pattern of the above, with these differences.

Pain is usually colicky from the outset.

Tenesmus. Low tumours may give rise to a feeling of the need for evacuation which may result in tenesmus accompanied by the passage of mucus and blood, especially in the early morning.

Bladder symptoms are not unusual and in some instances may herald a colovesical fistula.

Carcinoma of the transverse colon

This may be mistaken for a carcinoma of the stomach because of the position of the tumour together with anaemia and lassitude.

Carcinoma of the caecum and ascending colon

This may present with the following.

- Anaemia, severe and unyielding to treatment; there may be a palpable tumour present.
- The presence of a mass in the right iliac fossa. Colonoscopy may be needed to confirm the diagnosis.
- Caecal carcinoma is sometimes discovered unexpectedly at operation for acute appendicitis or for an appendix abscess failing to resolve. On rare occasions the appendix is inflamed, or even gangrenous, from the obstruction to its lumen by the tumour.
- A carcinoma of the caecum can be the apex of an intussusception presenting with the symptoms of intermittent obstruction.

Metastatic disease

Patients may present for the first time with liver metastases and an enlarged liver, ascitis from carcinomatosis peritonei and, more rarely, metastases to the lung, skin, bone and brain.

Methods of investigation

Sigmoidoscopy. This is part of the routine investigation of patients passing blood and mucus that is really limited to the rectum.

Flexible sigmoidoscopy. The 60-cm, fibre-optic, flexible sigmoidoscope is being used increasingly in the out-patient clinic or in special rectal bleeding clinics. The patient is prepared with a disposable enema and sedation is not usually necessary.

Colonoscopy. This has the advantage of not only picking up a primary cancer but also having the ability to detect synchronous polyps or even multiple carcinomas which occur in 5 per cent of cases. It tends to be used in patients with bleeding as their main presenting symptom, those with known polyps and those in whom there is doubtful radiology. Ideally every case should be proven histologically before surgery. Full bowel preparation and sedation are necessary.

Radiology. Double-contrast barium enema is used routinely now. It shows a cancer of the colon as a constant irregular filling defect (Fig. 57.43). It is the investigation of choice in patients with predominant change in bowel habit as their presenting symptom. Ultrasonography is often used as a screening investigation for liver metastases, and CT is used in patients with large palpable abdominal masses to determine local invasion and is particularly used in the pelvis in the assessment of rectal cancer.

Treatment

Preoperative preparation. Full mechanical bowel preparation before colonic surgery is essential. The most commonly used method is dietary restriction to fluids only for 48 hours before surgery; on the day before operation two sachets of Picolax (sodium picosulphate) are taken to purge the colon.

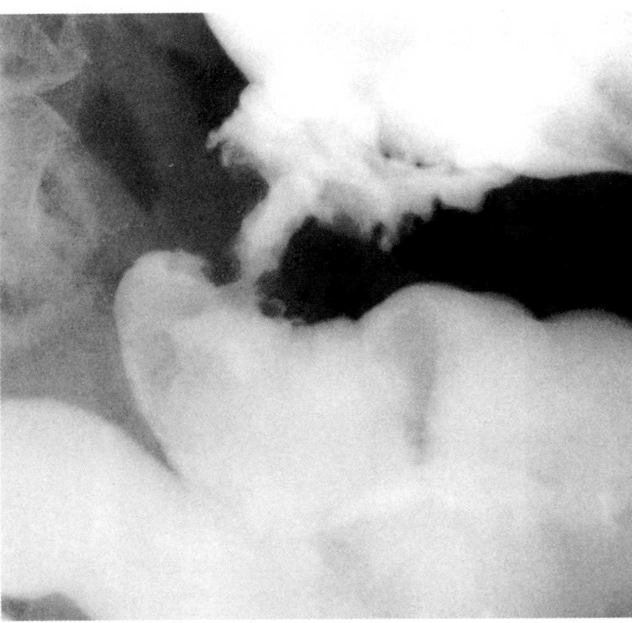

Fig. 57.43 Barium enema showing a carcinoma of the sigmoid colon. It may have an 'apple core' appearance, i.e. a short, irregular stenosis with sharp shoulders at each end.

In addition a rectal washout may be necessary. Alternatives include prograde lavage via a nasogastric tube using water or balanced electrolyte solutions. A stoma site is carefully discussed with the stoma care nursing specialist and antiembolus stockings are fitted; the patient is started on prophylactic subcutaneous heparin and intravenous prophylactic antibiotics are given at the start of surgery.

When intestinal obstruction is present, preparation in this way may precipitate abdominal pain and it may be safer to save preparation to the time of the operation using an on-table lavage technique.

Operations

The test of operability. The abdomen is opened and the tumour assessed for resectability.

1. The liver is palpated for secondary deposits, the presence of which is not necessarily a contraindication to resection because the best palliative treatment for carcinoma of the colon is removal of the tumour.
2. The peritoneum, particularly the pelvic peritoneum, is inspected for signs of small, white, seed-like, neoplastic implantations. Similar changes can occur in the omentum.
3. The various groups of lymph nodes that drain the involved segment are palpated. Their enlargement does not necessarily mean that they are invaded by metastases because the enlargement may be inflammatory.
4. The neoplasm is examined with a view to mobility and operability. Local fixation, however, does not always imply local invasion because some tumours excite a brisk inflammatory response.

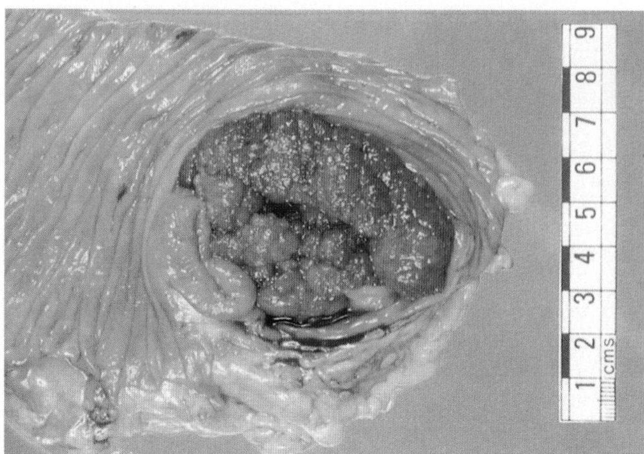

Fig. 57.44 Large villous tumour of the caecum with cancer change.

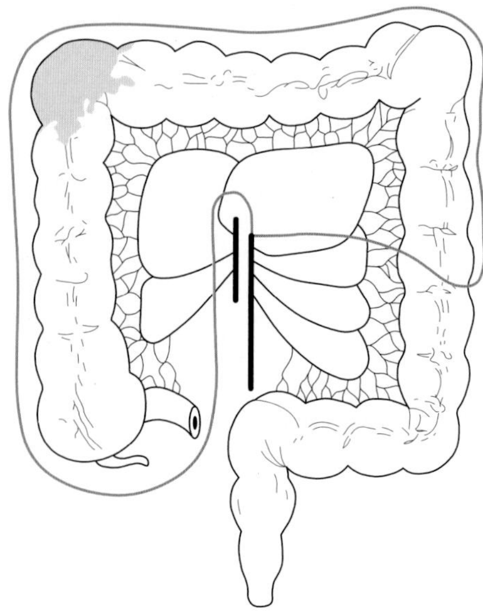

Fig. 57.46 Area to be resected when the growth is situated at the hapatic flexure.

The operations to be described are designed to remove the primary tumour and its draining locoregional lymph nodes which may be involved by metastases. Lesser resections are indicated, however, should hepatic metastases render the condition curable nonsurgically. There is some evidence that early division of major blood vessels supplying the involved colon (no-touch technique – Turnbull) can slightly improve the number of curative operations.

Carcinoma of the caecum or ascending colon (Fig. 57.44) is treated when resectable by right hemicolectomy (Fig. 57.45).

The abdomen is opened, the peritoneum lateral to the ascending colon is incised and the incision carried around the hepatic flexure. The right colon is elevated, with the leaf of peritoneum containing its vessels and lymph nodes, from the posterior abdominal wall, taking care not to injure the ureter, spermatic vessels in the male or the duodenum. The peritoneum is separated medially near the origin of the ileocolic artery, which is divided together with the right colic artery when this has a separate origin from the superior mesenteric. The mesentery of the last 30 cm of ileum, and the leaf of raised peritoneum attached to the caecum, ascending colon and hepatic flexure, after ligation of the mesenteric blood vessels, is divided as far as the proximal third of the transverse colon. When it is clear that there is an adequate blood supply at the resection margins, the right colon is resected and an end-to-end anastomosis fashioned between the ileum and transverse colon.

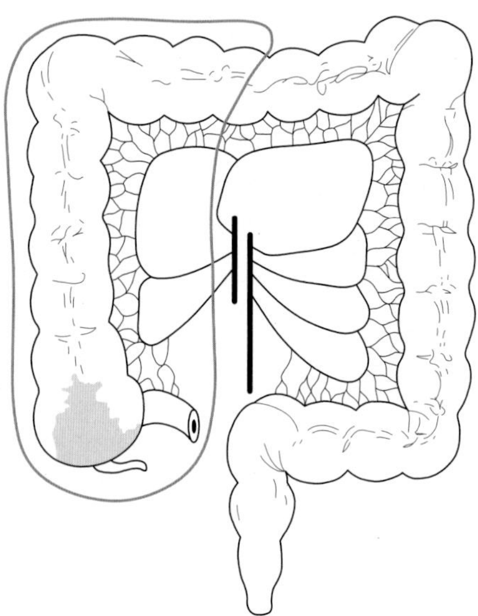

Fig. 57.45 Area to be resected when the growth is situated in the caecum.

R. Turnbull. Surgeon, Cleveland Clinic, Cleveland, Ohio, USA.

Carcinoma of the hepatic flexure. When the hepatic flexure is involved the resection must be extended correspondingly (Fig. 57.46).

Carcinoma of the transverse colon. When there is no obstruction, excision of the transverse colon and the two flexures together with the transverse mesocolon and the greater omentum, followed by end-to-end anastomosis, can be used. An alternative is an extended right hemicolectomy (Fig. 57.46).

Carcinoma of the splenic flexure or descending colon. The extent of the resection is from right colon to descending colon. Sometimes removal of the colon up to the ileum, with an ileorectal anastomosis, is preferable.

Carcinoma of the pelvic colon. The left half of the colon is mobilised completely (Fig. 57.47). So that the operation is radical, the inferior mesenteric artery below its left colic branch, together with the related paracolic lymph nodes, must be included in the resection. This entails carrying the dissection as far as the upper third of the rectum. Many surgeons advocate flush ligation of the inferior mesenteric artery on the aorta (high litigation). Provided that there is no obstruction primary anastomosis is the rule. Occasionally a

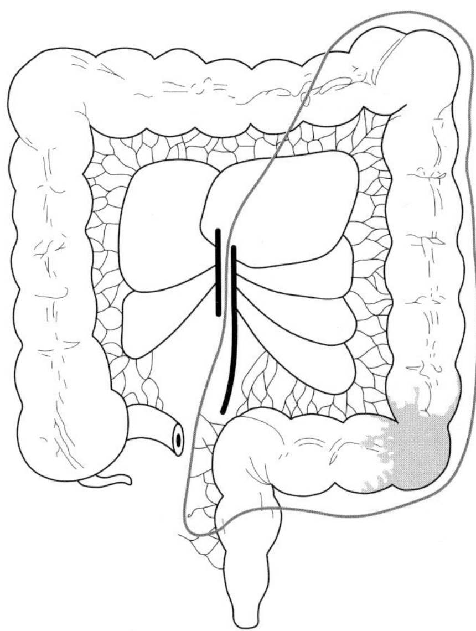

Fig. 57.47 Area to be resected in the case of a carcinoma of the pelvic colon.

protecting upstream stoma may be necessary. The methods of dealing with large bowel obstruction as a result of colon cancer are described in Chapter 58.

When a growth is found to be inoperable. In the upper part of the left colon, a transverse colostomy is performed. In the pelvic colon, a left iliac fossa colostomy is preferable. With an inoperable growth in the ascending colon a bypass using an ileocolic anastomosis is the best procedure. Over 95 per cent of colonic carcinomas can, however, be resected.

Adjuvant therapy

See Chapter 60.

Hepatic metastases

It is important to biopsy hepatic metastases for histological diagnosis. Unless they are on the very surface and edge of the liver, they are not usually resected at the time of colonic surgery. Patients with up to two or three liver metastases confined to one lobe of the liver may be offered hepatic resection. Multiple painful hepatic metastases can be palliated by cytotoxic drugs, cryosurgery or laser therapy (Fig. 57.48).

Other disorders

Traumatic rupture

The intestine can be ruptured with or without an external wound – so-called blunt trauma (Fig. 57.49). The most common cause of this is a blow on the abdomen which crushes the bowel against the vertebral column or sacrum; also a rupture is more likely to occur where part of the gut has been fixed, for example, in a hernia, or where a fixed part of the gut joins a mobile one such as the duodenojejunal flexure. Here the damage may be retroperitoneal and easily overlooked.

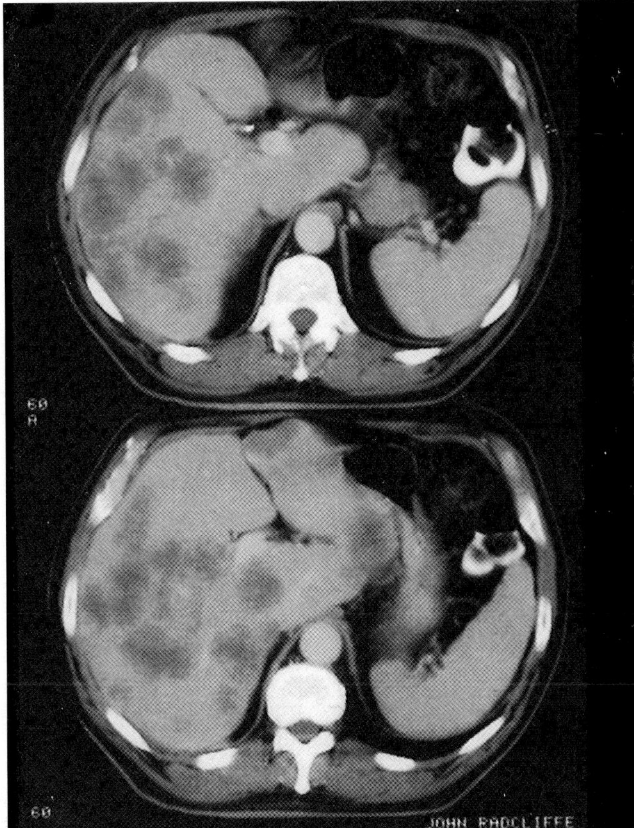

Fig. 57.48 CT scan of the liver showing multiple metastases from carcinoma of the colon.

In small perforations the mucosa may prolapse through the hole and partly seal it, making the early signs misleading. In addition there may be a laceration in the mesentery. The patient will then have a combination of intra-abdominal bleeding and release of intestinal contents into the abdominal cavity, giving rise to peritonitis.

Traumatic rupture of the large intestine is much less common. In blast injuries of the abdomen following the detonation of a bomb, the pelvic

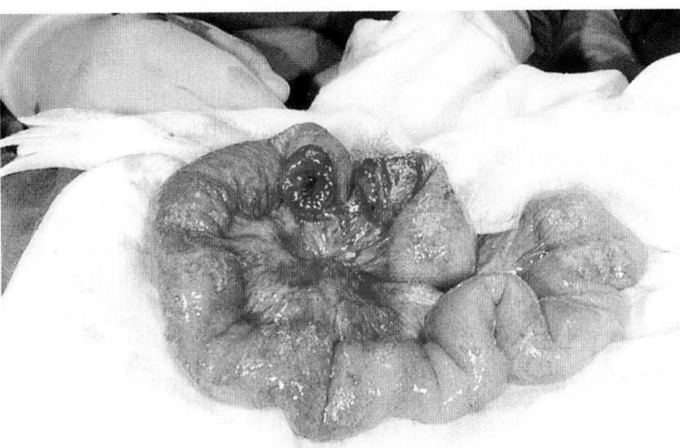

Fig. 57.49 Traumatic rupture of the small intestine as a result of blunt abdominal trauma.

colon is particularly at risk of rupture. Compressed air rupture can follow the dangerous practical joke where an air-line carrying compressed air is turned on near the victim's anus.

Rupture of the upper rectum can occur during sigmoidoscopy and occasionally during the placement of rectal catheters for barium radiology. Traumatic rupture of the colon can occur during colonoscopy. The most common site is the sigmoid colon where the formation of a sigmoid loop pushes against the antimesenteric border of the sigmoid colon, stretching it out and eventually perforating it.

Gun shot wounds and impalement injuries to the bowel have more serious consequences because of the introduction of debris from the patient's clothing or the missile itself mixing with the bacteria in the patient's gut. High-velocity missiles may cause extensive damage of the bowel over a much wider area than just the entry and exit wounds.

Treatment

Where rupture is suspected a plain radiograph in the erect or lateral decubitus position will demonstrate the presence of free air in the peritoneal cavity or indeed in the retroperitoneal tissues. In almost all cases an abdominal exploration must be performed and, in many instances, simple closure of the perforation is all that is required. In others, for example, where the mesentery is lacerated and the bowel is not viable, resection may be necessary. In the case of the large intestine small clean tears can be closed primarily, if there is a large tear with damage to the surrounding structures to the adjacent mesentery resection, exteriorisation may be used. Much depends on the amount of intra-abdominal soiling.

In the case of retroperitoneal portions of the intestine, for example, the duodenum, perforations can involve the front and back walls and the duodenum in particular has to be carefully mobilised to check that a concealed tear is not overlooked. In all cases the abdomen is washed out with saline and broad-spectrum intravenous antibiotics are given.

Pneumatosis cystoides intestinalis

This is a rare condition in which gas-filled cysts are found in the subserosa or submucosa of the small intestine or colon. They are usually translucent, thin-walled, range in size between 1 and 2 cm and contain gas, mainly nitrogen, but also an increased content of hydrogen, and have a lining of flattened cells. The cause is not known; there is an association with chronic obstructive pulmonary disease but an increased local production of intestinal gas is a more probable cause. It has been seen in patients with necrotising enteritis, enterocolitis and diverticulitis. The cysts are usually symptomless but occasionally can give rise to intestinal obstruction and rectal bleeding, diarrhoea or mucus in the stool. The cysts may be recognised at sigmoidoscopy or seen on plain abdominal films, barium studies (Fig. 57.50) and even CT scans. Management of the uncomplicated primary disease is conservative. When symptoms demand treatment the first line is intermittent high-flow oxygen therapy providing a concentration of 70 per cent continuously for 5 days by nasal specula. The cysts may also resolve with antibiotic treatment, particularly metronidazole. In resistant cases maintenance treatment with sulphasalazine may be helpful.

Enterocutaneous or faecal fistula

An external fistula communicating with the caecum sometimes follows an operation for gangrenous appendicitis or the draining of an appendix abscess. A faecal fistula can occur

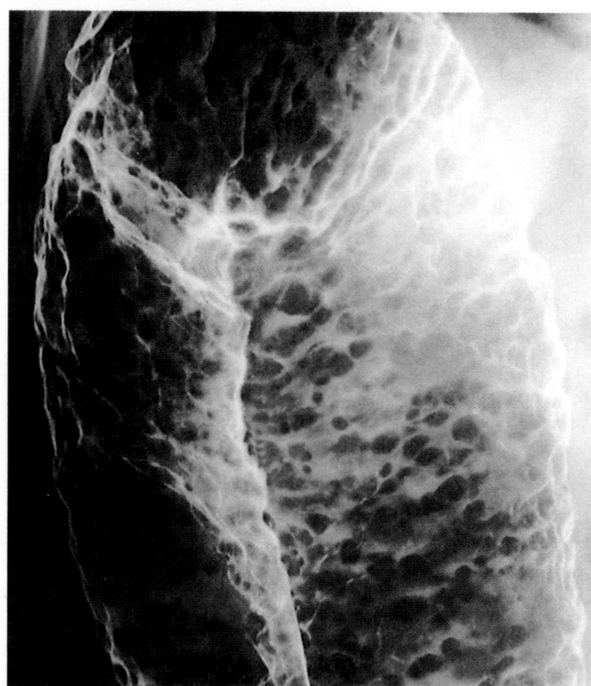

Fig. 57.50 Double-contrast barium enema showing multiple gas-filled submucosal cysts due to pneumatosis cystoides intestinalis.

from necrosis of a gangrenous patch of intestine after the relief of a strangulated hernia, or from a leak from an intestinal anastomosis. The opening of an abscess connected with chronic diverticulitis or carcinoma of the colon frequently results in faecal fistula. Radiation damage is also another cause of fistula formation. The most common cause of enterocutaneous fistula is, however, previous surgery. This happens most often in patients with adhesions following previous operations. Damage to the small intestine occurs inadvertently during dissection of the adhesions and, because of an associated subacute obstruction or abscess, the fistula 'blows' postoperatively. Enterocutaneous fistulae can be divided into:

- those with a high output, more than 1 litre/day;
- those with a low output, less than 1 litre/day.

They can also be described anatomically as simple, with a direct communication between the gut and the skin, or complex, that is, those with one or more tracts that are tortuous and sometimes associated with an intervening abscess cavity half-way along the tract.

The discharge from a fistula connected with the duodenum or jejunum is bile stained and causes severe excoriation of the skin. When the ileum or caecum is involved the discharge is fluid faecal matter; when the distal colon is the affected site it is solid or semisolid faecal matter. The site of leakage and the length of the fistula can be determined by small bowel enema and barium enema, by fistulography and most importantly CT of the abdomen will show up any associated abscesses (Fig. 57.51).

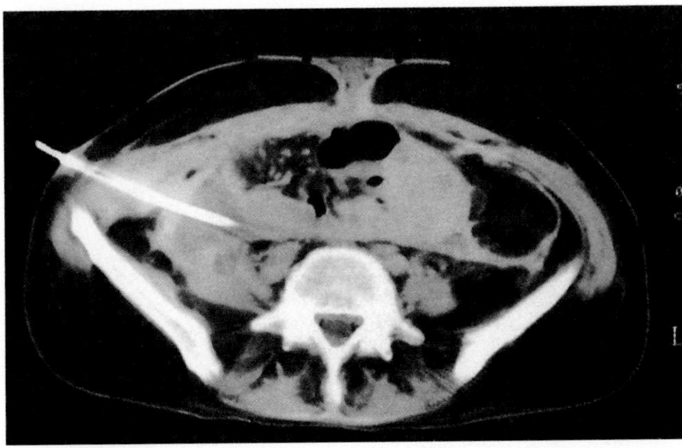

Fig. 57.51 CT scan in a patient with a complex enterocutaneous fistula and an intra-abdominal abscess being drained with a CT-guided catheter.

Treatment

This can be very challenging in patients with a high-output fistula. Low-output fistulae can be expected to heal spontaneously, provided there is no obstruction beyond the fistula opening. Reasons for failure of spontaneous healing also include:

- epithelial continuity between the gut and the skin;
- the presence of active disease where, for example, there is Crohn's disease or carcinoma at the site of the anastomosis or in the tract;
- an associated complex abscess.

The abdominal wall must be protected from erosion by the use of appliances. The patient must remain nil by mouth, intravenous nutrition is started and signs of a decrease in the fistula output are sought. The higher the fistula in the intestinal tract the more skin excoriation must be expected, and this is worst in the case of a duodenal fistula. High-output fistulae cause rapid dehydration and hypoproteinaemia. Vigorous fluid replacement and nutritional support are essential. The drainage of an intra-abdominal abscess can be life saving. This can be achieved by either CT-guided drainage or occasionally laparotomy. In patients with a complex fistula it may be necessary to bring out a defunctioning stoma upstream of the fistula site, even if this results in a high-output stoma.

Treatment with a somatostatin analogue (octreotide) may be useful in these cases to reduce fistula output and stoma output.

Operative treatment

Operative repair should only be attempted after a trial of conservative management. The surgery can on occasion be technically extremely demanding and anastomosis should not be fashioned in the presence of continuing intra-abdominal sepsis or when the patient is hypoproteinaemic.

Stomas

Colostomy

A colostomy is an artificial opening made in the large bowel to divert faeces and flatus to the exterior, where it can be collected in an external appliance. Depending on the purpose for which the diversion has been necessary a colostomy may be temporary or permanent.

Temporary colostomy

This is most commonly established to defunction an anastomosis after an anterior resection, to prevent faecal peritonitis developing following traumatic injury to the rectum or colon, and to facilitate the operative treatment of a high fistula *in ano*. It is now less commonly used for patients with distal obstruction of the sigmoid colon as a result of carcinoma or diverticular disease.

A temporary colostomy is made bringing a loop of colon to the surface (loop colostomy) where it is held in place by a plastic bridge passed through the mesentery. Once the abdomen has been closed the colostomy is opened and the edges of the colonic incision are sutured to the adjacent skin margin (Fig. 57.52). When firm adhesion of the colostomy to the abdominal wall has taken place, after 7 days the bridge can be removed.

A loop of colon can most easily be brought to the surface using large bowel that has a mesentery. Most loop colostomies are made in the transverse colon but the sigmoid colon can also be suitable. Following the surgical cure or healing of the distal lesion for which the temporary stoma was constructed, the colostomy can be closed. It is usual to perform a contrast examination (distal loopogram) to check that there is no distal obstruction or continuing problem at the site of previous

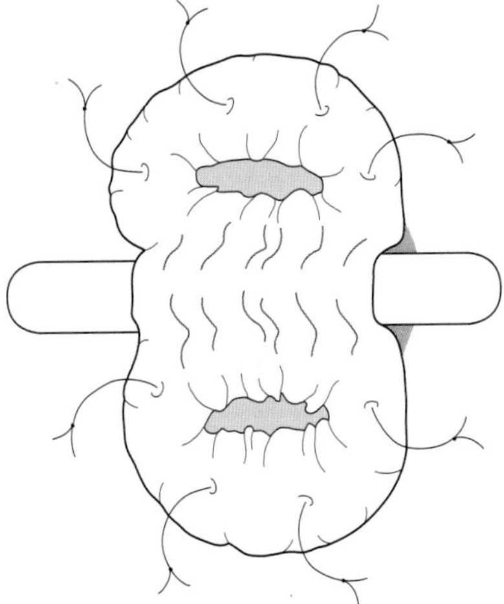

Fig. 57.52 Usual temporary (loop) colostomy opened over a rod, and immediate suture of colon wall to surrounding skin (many new rods are designed to lie beneath the skin's surface; alternatively a skin bridge is used).

surgery. Colostomy closure is most easily and safely accomplished if the stoma is mature, that is, after the colostomy has been established for 2 months. Closure is usually performed by an intraperitoneal technique which is accompanied by fewer closure breakdowns with faecal fistulae.

Double-barrelled colostomy

This colostomy was designed so that it could be closed by crushing the intervening 'spur' using an enterotome or a stapling device. It is rarely used now but occasionally the colon is divided so that both ends can be brought separately to the surface ensuring that the distal segment is completely defuntioned.

Permanent colostomy

This is usually formed after excision of the rectum for a carcinoma by the abdominoperineal technique.

It is formed by bringing the distal end (end colostomy) of the divided colon to the surface in the left iliac fossa, where it is sutured in place joining the colonic margin to the surrounding skin.

The point at which the colon is brought to the surface must be carefully selected to allow a colostomy bag to be applied without impinging on the bony prominence of the antero-superior iliac spine. The best site is usually through the lateral edge of the rectus sheath, 6 cm above and medial to the bony prominence (Fig. 57.53).

An important point after the colostomy has been made is to close the lateral space between the intraperitoneal segment of the sigmoid colon and the peritoneum of the pelvic wall, to prevent internal herniation of strangulation of loops of small bowel through the deficiency. Alternatively a retroperitoneal tunnel for the colostomy avoids creating lateral space.

Colostomy bags and appliances (Fig. 57.54)

Faeces from a permanent colostomy are collected in disposable adhesive bags. A wide range of such bags is currently available. Many now incorporate a stomahesive backing, which can be left in place for several days. In most hospitals a stoma care service is available to offer advice to patients and to acquaint them with the latest appliances, and the appropriate psychological and practical help.

(a)

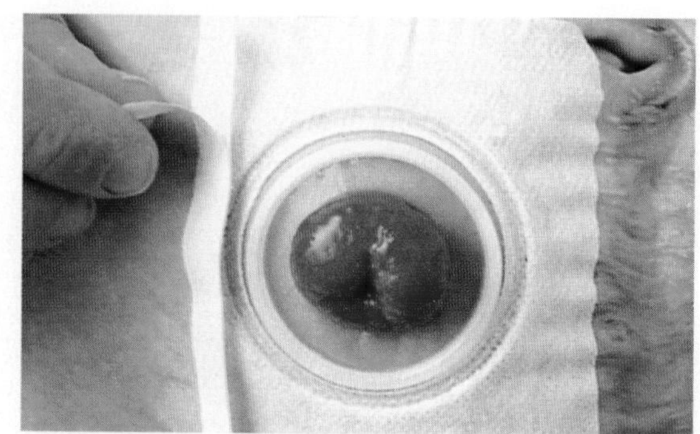

(b)

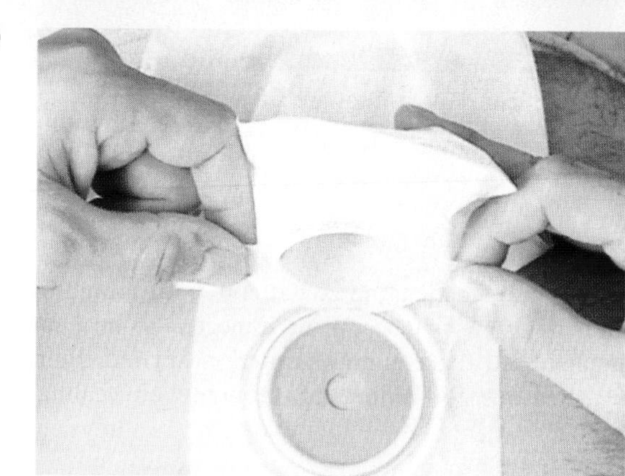

(c)

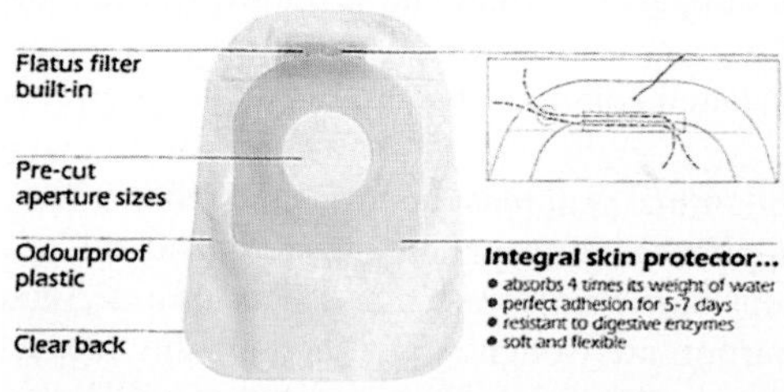

Fig. 57.54 (a) Shows the usual long-term backing ('stomahesive') and flange, on to which the bag is placed (b). (c) Draws attention to the desirable features incorporated in modern systems.

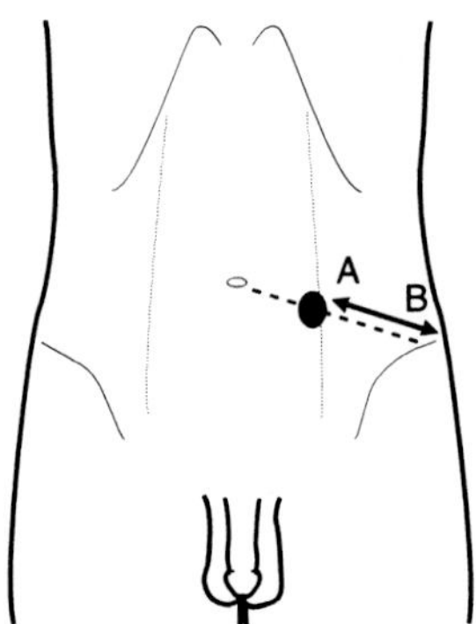

Fig. 57.53 Usual site of a permanent (end) colostomy in the left iliac fossa. Note distance A–B, 2.5 cm at least.

Complications of colostomies

The following complications can occur to any colostomy but are more common after poor technique:

- prolapse;
- retraction;
- necrosis of the distal end;
- stenosis of the orifice;
- colostomy hernia;
- bleeding (usually from granulomas around the margin of the colostomy);
- colostomy 'diarrhoea': this is usually an infective enteritis and will respond to oral metronidazole 200 mg three times daily.

Many of these complications require revision of the colostomy. Sometimes this can be achieved with an incision immediately around the stoma but on occasion reopening the abdomen and freeing up the colostomy may be necessary. Occasionally transfer to the opposite side of the abdomen may be necessary.

Loop ileostomy

An ileostomy is used by some surgeons as an alternative to colostomy, particularly for defunctioning a low rectal anastomosis. The creation of a loop ileostomy from a knuckle of terminal ileum has already been described. The advantages of a loop ileostomy over a loop colostomy are the ease with which the bowel can be brought to the surface and the absence of odour. Care is needed, when the ileostomy is closed, that suture line obstruction does not occur.

Caecostomy

This is rarely used now. In desperately ill patients with advanced obstruction, a caecostomy may be useful. In late cases of obstruction the caecum may become so distended and ischaemic that rupture of the caecal wall may be anticipated. This can occur spontaneously giving rise to faecal peritonitis or at operation when an incision in the abdominal wall reduces its supportive role and allows the caecum to expand. In such a situation it should be decompressed by suction as soon as the abdomen is opened. In thin patients it may then be possible to carry out direct suture of the incised or perforated caecal wall to the abdominal skin of the right iliac fossa, although a resection of this area is really the best treatment. Following on-table lavage, via the appendix stump the irrigating catheter can be left in place as a tube caecostomy. Caecostomy is only a short-term measure to allow a few days for the condition of the patient to improve. Reoperation should normally follow fairly soon thereafter and a proper surgical procedure carried out.

Further reading

Allan, R.N., Keigliley, M.R.B., Alexander, J. and Hawkins, E. (1990) *Inflammatory Bowel Diseases,* Churchill Livingstone, Edinburgh.

Keighley, M.R.B. and Williams, N.S. (1999) *Surgery of the Anus, Rectum and Colon*, 2nd edn, W.B. Saunders, London.

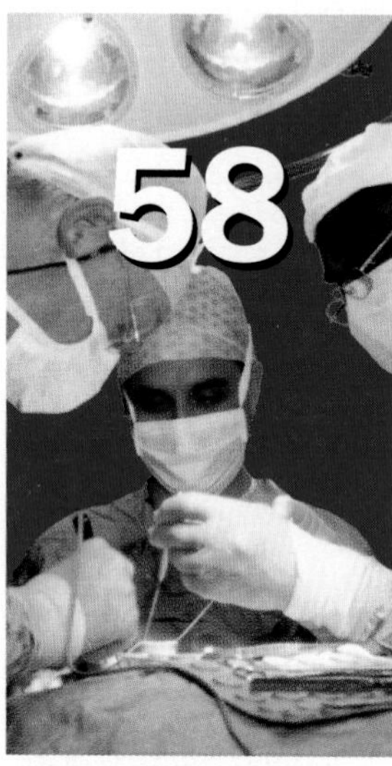

58 Intestinal obstruction

Introduction

Intestinal obstruction may be classified into two types.

- *Dynamic* – where peristalsis is working against a mechanical obstruction. The obstructing lesion may be:
  - intraluminal, for example impacted faeces, foreign bodies, bezoar, gallstones;
  - intramural, for example malignant or inflammatory strictures;
  - extramural, for example intraperitoneal bands and adhesions, hernias, volvulus or intrassusception.
- *Adynamic* – this may occur in two forms. Peristalsis may be absent (e.g. paralytic ileus) or it may be present in a non-propulsive form (e.g. mesenteric vascular occlusion or pseudo-obstruction). In both types a mechanical element is absent.

Dynamic obstruction

The diagnosis of intestinal obstruction is based on the classic quartet of pain, distension, vomiting and absolute constipation.

Obstruction may be classified clinically into two types:

- small bowel obstruction – high or low;
- large bowel obstruction.

Bailey & Love's Short Practice of Surgery, 23rd edition. Edited by R.C.G. Russell, N.S. Williams and C.J.K. Bulstrode. Published in 2000 by Arnold Publishers.

In *high small bowel obstruction* vomiting occurs early and is profuse with rapid dehydration. Distension is minimal with little evidence of fluid levels on abdominal radiography.

In *low small bowel obstruction* pain is predominant with central distension. Vomiting is delayed. Multiple central fluid levels are seen on radiography.

In *large-bowel obstruction* distension is early and pronounced. Pain is mild and vomiting and dehydration are late. The proximal colon and caecum are distended on an abdominal radiograph.

The nature of presentation will also be influenced by whether the presentation is:

- acute;
- chronic;
- acute on chronic;
- subacute.

Acute obstruction usually occurs in small bowel obstruction with sudden onsets of severe colicky central abdominal pain, distension, with early vomiting and constipation.

Chronic obstruction is usually seen in large bowel obstruction with lower abdominal colic and absolute constipation, followed by distension.

In *acute on chronic obstruction* there is a short history of distention and vomiting against a background of pain and constipation.

Subacute obstruction implies an incomplete obstruction.

Presentation will be further influenced by whether the obstruction is:

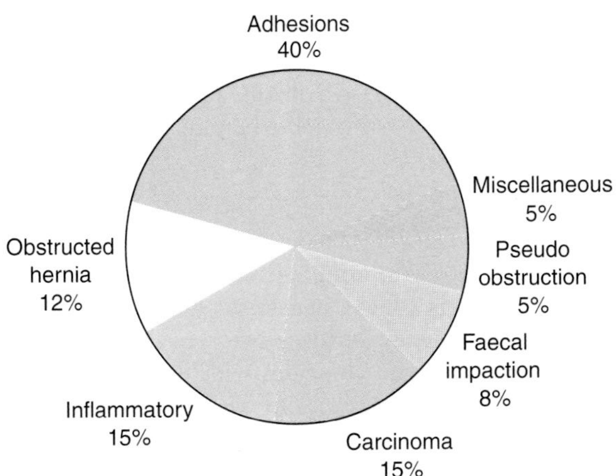

Fig. 58.1 Pie chart showing the relative frequency of the underlying diagnosis of intestinal obstruction.

Table 58.1 Mechanism of obstruction

- Volvulus
- Incarceration
- Obstruction
- Intussusception

- simple – where the blood supply is intact;
- strangulating/strangulated – where there is direct interference to blood flow, usually by hernial rings or intraperitoneal adhesions/bands.

The common causes of intestinal obstruction in Western countries and their relative frequency are shown in Fig. 58.1. The underlying mechanisms are shown in Table 58.1.

Pathophysiology

Irrespective of aetiology or acuteness of onset, the proximal bowel dilates and develops an altered motility. Below the obstruction, the bowel exhibits normal peristalsis and absorption until it becomes empty, when it contracts and becomes immobile. Initially, proximal peristalsis is increased to overcome the obstruction, with the length of time it remains vigorous being proportional to the distance of the obstruction. If the obstruction is not relieved the bowel begins to dilate causing a reduction in peristaltic strength, ultimately resulting in flaccidity and paralysis. This is a protective phenomenon to prevent vascular damage secondary to increased intraluminal pressure.

The distension proximal to an obstruction is produced by two factors:

- Gas – regardless of the level of obstruction, there is a significant overgrowth of both aerobic and anaerobic organisms resulting in considerable gas production. Following the reabsorption of oxygen and carbon dioxide, the majority is made up of nitrogen (90 per cent) and hydrogen sulphide.
- Fluid – this is made up of the various digestive juices (Table 58.2). Following obstruction, fluid accumulates within the bowel wall and any excess is secreted into the lumen, whilst absorption from the gut is retarded. Dehydration and electrolyte loss are therefore due to:
  - reduced oral intake;
  - defective intestinal absorption;
  - losses due to vomiting;
  - sequestration in the bowel lumen.

Table 58.2 Approximate volumes of digestive juices produced by the gut in 24 hours

Saliva	1000–1500 ml
Gastric juice	1500–2500 ml
Bile	1000 ml
Pancreatic juice	1500 ml
Succus enterricus	3000 ml

Strangulation

When strangulation occurs the viability of the bowel is threatened secondary to a compromised blood supply. This may be due to:

- external compression (hernial orifices/adhesions/bands);
- interruption of mesenteric flow (volvulus, a twist of bowel loop on its mesenteric pedicle or intussusception where a segment of bowel invaginates into an adjacent segment);
- rising intraluminal pressure (closed-loop obstruction);
- primary obstruction of intestinal circulation (mesenteric infarction).

The venous return is compromised before the arterial supply unless primary obstruction is present. The resultant increase in capillary pressure leads to local mural distension with loss of intravascular fluid and red blood cells intramurally and intra- and extraluminally. Once the arterial supply is impaired, haemorrhagic infarction occurs. As the viability of the bowel wall is compromised there is marked translocation and systemic exposure to aerobic and anaerobic organisms with their associated toxins. The associated danger is far greater for intraperitoneal strangulation than that of an external hernia where there is a smaller absorptive surface.

The morbidity and mortality associated with strangulation are dependent on age and extent. In strangulated external hernias the segment involved is short and the resultant blood and fluid loss is small. When bowel involvement is extensive the loss of blood and circulatory volume will cause peripheral circulatory failure.

Closed-loop obstruction

This occurs when the bowel is obstructed at both the proximal and distal point (Fig. 58.2). It is present in many cases of intestinal strangulation. Unlike cases of nonstrangulating obstruction, there is no early distension of the proximal intestine. When gangrene of the strangulated segment is imminent, retrograde thrombosis of the mesenteric veins results in distension on both sides of the strangulated segment.

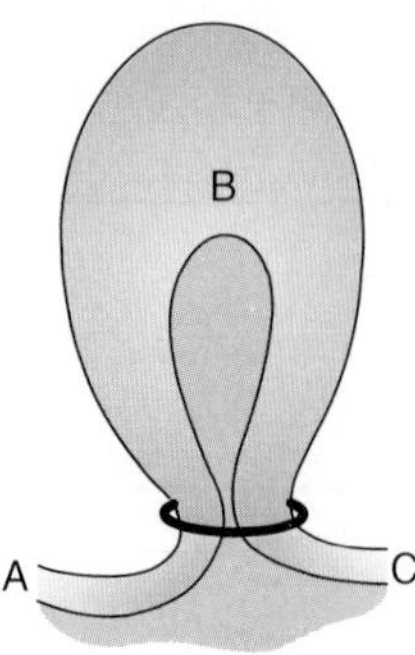

Fig. 58.2 Distension. Closed loop obstruction with no proimal (A) or distal (C) distension and impending strangulation (B).

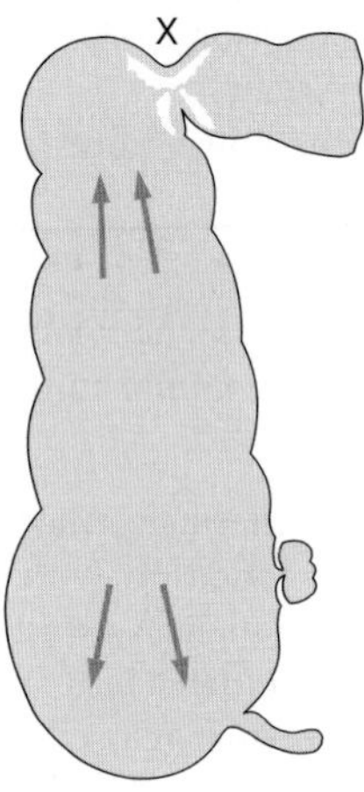

Fig. 58.3 Carcinomatous stricture (X) of the hepatic flexure: closed-loop obstruction.

A classic form of closed-loop obstruction is seen in the presence of a tight carcinomatous stricture of the colon with a competent ileocaecal valve (present in up to a third of individuals). The inability of the distended colon to decompress itself into the small bowel results in an increase in luminal pressure, greatest at the caecum, with subsequent impairment of blood supply. Unrelieved, this results in necrosis and perforation (Fig. 58.3).

Acute intestinal obstruction

Clinical features

There are four cardinal features:

- pain;
- vomiting;
- distension;
- constipation.

These features vary according to:

- the location of the obstruction;
- the age of the obstruction;
- the underlying pathology;
- the presence or absence of intestinal ischaemia.

Late manifestations which may be encountered include dehydration, oliguria, hypovolaemic shock, pyrexia, septicaemia, respiratory embarrassment and peritonism. In all cases of suspected intestinal obstruction, all hernial orifices must be examined.

Pain

Pain is the first symptom, it occurs suddenly and is usually severe. It is colicky in nature and is usually centred around the umbilicus (small bowel) or lower abdomen (large bowel). The pain coincides with increased peristaltic activity. With increasing distension, the colicky pain is replace by a mild constant diffuse pain. The development of severe pain is indicative of the presence of strangulation. Pain may not be a significant feature in postoperative simple mechanical obstruction and does not occur in paralytic ileus.

Vomiting

The more distal the obstruction, the longer the interval between the onset of symptoms and the appearance of nausea and vomiting. As obstruction progresses the character of the vomitus alters from digested food to faeculent material due to the presence of enteric bacterial overgrowth.

Distension

In the small bowel the degree of distension is dependent on the site of the obstruction and is greater the more distal the lesion. Visible peristalsis may be present (Fig. 58.4). It is delayed in colonic obstruction and may be minimal or absent in the presence of mesenteric vascular occlusion.

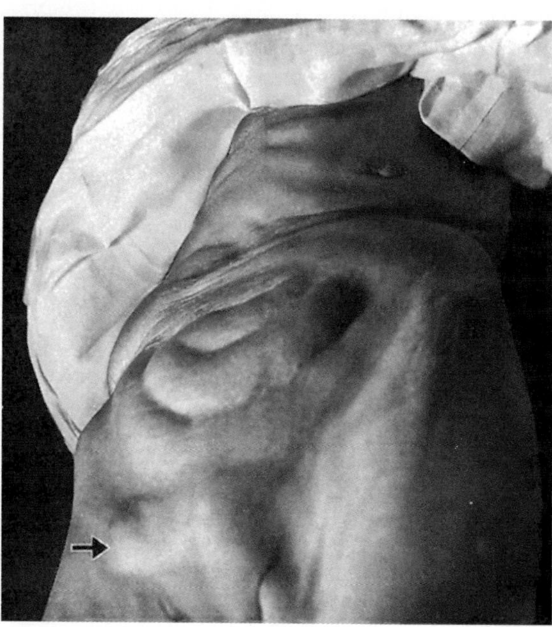

Fig. 58.4 Visible peristalsis. Intestinal obstruction due to the strangulated right femoral hernia, to which the arrow points.

Constipation

This may be classified as absolute (i.e. neither faeces nor flatus is passed) or relative (where flatus only is passed). Absolute constipation is a cardinal feature of complete intestinal obstruction. Some patients may pass flatus or faeces after the onset of obstruction owing to the evacuation of distal bowel contents.

The rule that constipation is present in intestinal obstruction does not apply in:

- Richter's hernia;
- gallstone obturation;
- mesenteric vascular occlusion;
- obstruction associated with a pelvic abscess;
- partial obstruction (faecal impaction/colonic neoplasm) where diarrhoea may often occur.

Other manifestations

Dehydration

This is seen most commonly in small bowel obstruction due to repeated vomiting and fluid sequestration. This results in dry skin and tongue, poor venous filling and sunken eyes with oliguria. The blood urea level and haematocrit rise giving a secondary polycythaemia.

Hypokalaemia

This is not a common feature in simple mechanical obstruction. An increase in serum potassium, amylase or lactate dehydrogenase may be associated with the presence of strangulation, as may leucocytosis or leucopenia.

Pyrexia

Pyrexia in the presence of obstruction may indicate:

- the onset of ischaemia;
- intestinal perforation;
- inflammation associated with the obstructing disease.

Hypothermia indicates septicaemic shock.

Abdominal tenderness

Localized tenderness indicates pending or established ischaemia. The development of peritonism or peritonitis indicates overt infarction and/or perforation.

Clinical features of strangulation

It is vital to distinguish strangulating from nonstrangulating intestinal obstruction, as the former is a surgical emergency. The diagnosis is entirely clinical. In addition to the features outlined above, the following should be noted:

- the presence of shock indicates underlying ischaemia;
- in impending strangulation, pain is never completely absent;
- symptoms usually commence suddenly and recur regularly;
- the presence and character of any local tenderness are of great significance and, however mild, tenderness requires frequent reassessment.

In nonstrangulated obstruction there may be an area of localized tenderness at the site of the obstruction; in strangulation there is always localized tenderness associated with rigidity/rebound tenderness.

- Generalized tenderness and the presence of rigidity are indicative of the need for early laparotomy.
- In cases of intestinal obstruction where pain persists despite conservative management, even in the absence of the above signs, strangulation should be diagnosed.
- When strangulation occurs in an external hernia the lump is tense, tender, irreducible, there is no expansile cough impulse and it has recently increased in size.

Radiological diagnosis

Erect abdominal films are no longer routinely provided and the radiological diagnosis is based on a supine abdominal film (Fig. 58.5).

When distended with gas the jejunum, ileum, caecum and remaining colon have a characteristic appearance that allows them to be distinguished radiologically. The diameter of the distended viscus is not diagnostic.

- The obstructed small bowel is characterized by straight segments that are generally central and lie transversely. No gas is seen in the colon.
- The jejunum is characterized by its valvulae conniventes that completely pass across the width of the bowel and are regularly spaced giving a 'concertina' or ladder effect.

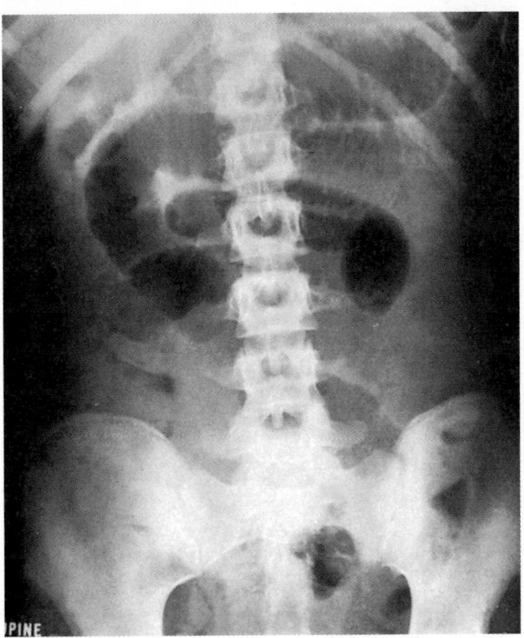

Fig. 58.5 Gas-filled small bowel loop; patient supine.

August Richter, 1742–1812. German surgeon.

- Ileum – the distal ileum has been piquantly described by Wangensteen as featureless.
- Caecum – a distended caecum is shown by a rounded gas shadow in the right iliac fossa.
- Large bowel – except for the caecum shows haustral folds which, unlike valvulae conniventes, are spaced irregularly and the indentations are not placed opposite one another.

Volvulus of the sigmoid colon has a characteristic radiological appearance with a grossly dilated loop of colon, with or without visible haustrae which arises from the pelvis and extends obliquely across the spine to the upper abdomen.

In intestinal obstruction fluid levels appear later than gas shadows as it takes time for gas and fluid to separate (Fig. 58.6). In infants less than 2 years of age, a few fluid levels in the small bowel may be physiological. In adults, two inconstant fluid levels may be regarded as normal – one at the duodenal cap and the other in the terminal ileum.

During the obstructive process, fluid levels become more conspicuous and more numerous when paralysis has occurred. When fluid levels are pronounced the obstruction is advanced. In the small bowel, the number of fluid levels is directly proportional to the degree of obstruction and to its site; the number increasing the more distal the lesion.

In contrast, low colonic obstruction does not commonly give rise to small bowel fluid levels unless advanced, whilst high colonic obstruction may do in the presence of an incompetent ileocaecal valve. Colonic obstruction is usually associated with a large amount of gas in the caecum. A limited water-soluble enema may be undertaken to differentiate large bowel obstruction from pseudo-obstruction. A barium follow-through is contraindicated in the presence of acute obstruction and may be life threatening.

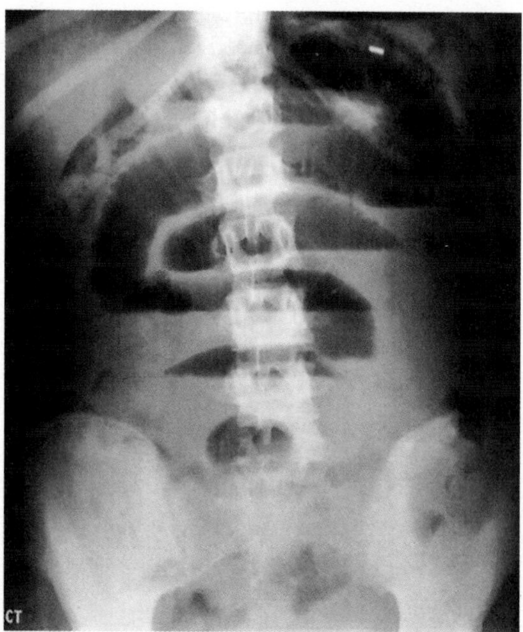

Fig. 58.6 Fluid levels with gas above; 'stepladder pattern'. Ileal obstruction by adhesions; patient erect.

Impacted foreign bodies may be seen on abdominal radiographs. In gallstone ileus, gas may be seen in the biliary tree with the stone visible, usually in the right iliac fossa, in 25 per cent of cases.

It is noteworthy that gas-filled loops and fluid levels in the small and large bowel can also be seen in established paralytic ileus and pseudo-obstruction. The former can, however, normally be distinguished on clinical grounds whilst the latter can be confirmed radiologically. Fluid levels may also be seen in nonobstructing conditions such as inflammatory bowel disease, acute pancreatitis and intra-abdominal sepsis.

Treatment of acute intestinal obstruction

There are three main measures:

- gastrointestinal drainage;
- fluid and electrolytic replacement;
- relief of obstruction, usually surgical.

The first two steps are always necessary prior to the surgical relief of obstruction and are the mainstay of postoperative management. In a proportion of cases, particularly adhesive obstruction, they may be used exclusively.

Surgical treatment is necessary for most cases of intestinal obstruction, but should be delayed until resuscitation is complete, provided there is no:

- sign of strangulation;
- evidence of closed-loop obstruction.

There are three principles of surgical intervention (Table 58.3).

Table 58.3 Principles of surgical intervention for obstruction

- Management of segment at site of obstruction
- The distended proximal bowel
- Underlying cause of obstruction

Supportive management

- Nasogastric decompression is achieved by the passage of a nonvented (Ryle) or vented (Salem) tube. The tubes are normally placed on free drainage, with 4-hourly aspiration, but may be placed on continuous or intermittent suction. As well as facilitating decompression proximal to the obstruction, they also reduce the risk of subsequent aspiration during induction of anaesthesia and postextubation.
- The basic biochemical abnormality is sodium and water loss, and therefore the appropriate replacement is Hartmann's solution or normal saline. The volume required

Owen Harding Wangensteen, b. 1898. Formerly Emeritus Professor of Surgery, University of Minnesota, Minnesota, USA.

Abdus Salam, b. 1926. Pakistani physicist and Nobel Laureate.
Henri Hartmann, 1860–1952. French surgeon.

varies and should be determined by clinical haematological and biochemical criteria.
- Antibiotics – whilst not mandatory, many clinicians initiate broad-spectrum antibiotic early in therapy because of bacterial overgrowth. Antibiotic therapy is mandatory for all patients undergoing small or large bowel resection.

Surgical treatment

The timing of surgical intervention is dependent on the clinical picture with the indications of early operation being:

- obstructed or strangulated external herniae;
- internal intestinal strangulation;
- acute obstruction.

The classic clinical advice that 'the sun should not both rise and set' on a case of unrelieved intestinal obstruction is sound and should be followed unless there are positive reasons for delay. Such cases may include obstruction secondary to adhesions where there is no pain or tenderness, despite continued radiological evidence of obstruction. Under these circumstances, conservative management may be continued for up to 72 hours in the hope of spontaneous resolution.

If the site of obstruction is unknown, adequate exposure is best achieved by a midline incision. Operative assessment is directed to:

- the site of obstruction;
- the nature of the obstruction;
- the viability of the gut.

Identification and assessment of the caecum is the best initial manoeuvre. If it is collapsed, the lesion is in the small bowel and may be identified by careful retrograde assessment. A dilated caecum indicates large bowel obstruction. To display the cause of obstruction, distended loops of small bowel should be displaced with care and covered with warm moist abdominal packs.

Operative decompression may be required if dilatation of bowel loops prevents exposure, the viability of the bowel wall is compromised or subsequent closure will be compromised. Its benefits should be balanced against potential risk of septic complications from spillage. Decompression may be performed using Savage's decompressor within a seromuscular purse-string suture (Fig. 58.7). Alternatively, with a large-bore nasogastric tube in place the small bowel contents may be gently milked in a retrograde manner to the stomach for aspiration. All volumes of fluid removed should be accurately measured and appropriately replaced.

The type of surgical procedure required will depend upon the nature of the cause – division of adhesions (enterolysis), excision, bypass or proximal decompression.

Following relief of obstruction, the viability of the involved bowel should be carefully assessed (see Table 58.4). Whilst frankly infarcted bowel is obvious, the viability status in many cases may be difficult to discern. If in doubt, the bowel should be wrapped in hot packs for 10 minutes with increased oxygenation and reassessed. The state of the mesenteric vessels and pulsation in adjacent arcades should be sought. Nevertheless, nonocclusive vascular insufficiency may occur despite adequate pulsation. In doubtful cases, following resection, both ends of the bowel should be raised as stomas. This is not only safe but also allows regular assessment of the bowel. Where no resection has been undertaken or there are multiple ischaemic areas (mesenteric vascular occlusion) a second look laparotomy at 24–48 hours may be required.

Special attention should always be paid to the sites of constriction at each end of an obstructed segment. If of doubtful viability they should be infolded by the use of a seromuscular suture and covered with omentum.

The surgical management of massive infarction in the form of superior mesenteric artery occlusion is dependent on the patient's overall prognostic criteria. In the elderly, infarction of the small bowel from the duodenojejunal flexure and the right colon may be considered incurable, whilst in the young, with potential for long-term intravenous alimentation and small bowel transplantation, a less conservative policy may be justified.

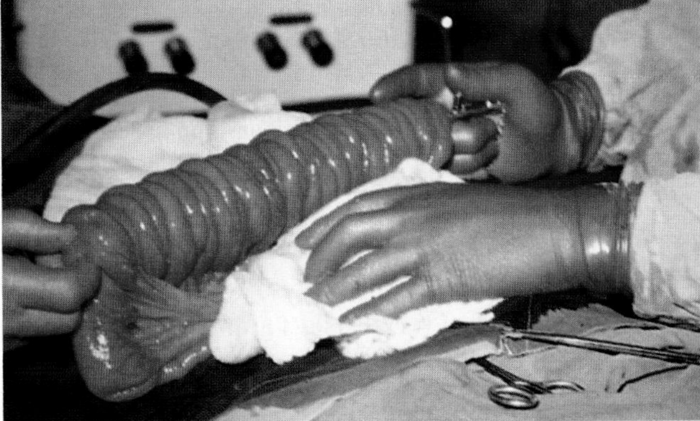

Fig. 58.7 Small intestine obstruction. Savage's decompressor is introduced into the small intestine which is plicated over it.

Table 58.4 Differentiation between viable and nonviable intestine

Intestine	*Viable*	*Nonviable*
Circulation	Dark colour becomes lighter; mesentery bleeds if pricked	Dark colour remains; no bleeding if mesentery is pricked
Peritoneum	Shiny	Dull and lustreless
Intestinal musculature	Firm. Pressure rings may or may not disappear. Peristalsis may be observed.	Flabby, thin and friable. Pressure rings persist. No peristalsis

Whenever small bowel is resected, the exact site of resection, the length of the resected segment and that of the residual bowel should be recorded.

Large bowel obstruction

This is usually due to underlying carcinoma or occasionally diverticular disease, and presents in an acute or chronic form. The condition of pseudo-obstruction should always be considered and excluded by a limited contrast study or air computerised tomography (CT) scan to confirm organic obstruction.

After full resuscitation the abdomen should be opened through a midline incision. Distension of the caecum will confirm large bowel involvement. Identification of a collapsed distal segment of the large bowel and its sequential proximal assessment will readily lead to identification of the cause. When a removable lesion is found in the caecum, ascending colon, hepatic flexure or proximal transverse colon an emergency right hemicolectomy should be performed. If the lesion is irremovable, a proximal stoma (colostomy or ileosotomy if the ileocaecal valve is incompetent) or ileotransverse bypass should be considered. Obstructing lesions at the splenic flexure should be treated by an extended right hemicolectomy with ileodescending colonic anastomosis.

For obstructing lesions of the left colon or rectosigmoid junction, immediate resection should be considered unless there are clear contraindications such as:

- inexperienced surgeon;
- moribund patient;
- advanced disease.

In rare instances, or where caecal perforation is imminent, time to improve the patient's clinical condition can be bought by performing an emergency caecostomy (or ileosotomy in the presence of an incompetent ileocaecal valve).

In the absence of senior clinical staff, it is safest to bring the proximal colon to the surface as a colostomy. Where possible the distal bowel should be brought out at the same time (Paul–Mikulicz procedure) to facilitate subsequent extraperitoneal closure. In the majority of cases the distal bowel will not reach and is closed and returned to the abdomen (Hartmann's procedure). A second-stage colorectal anastomosis can be planned when the patient is fit.

If an anastomosis is to be considered using proximal colon, in the presence of obstruction, it must be decompressed and cleaned by an on-table colonic lavage. Nevertheless, the subsequent anastomosis should still be protected with a covering stoma.

Frank Thomas Paul, 1851–1941. English surgeon, Liverpool, England.
Johannes Mikulicz, 1850–1905. Surgeon, Breslau, Poland.

Table 58.5 The common causes of intra-abdominal adhesions

Ischaemic areas	Sites of anastomoses Reperitonealisation of raw areas Trauma Vascular occlusion
Foreign material	Talc, starch, gauze, silk
Infection	Peritonitis, tuberculosis
Inflammatory conditions	Crohn's disease
Radiation enteritis	
Drugs	Practolol

Obstruction by adhesions and bands

In Western countries where abdominal operations are common, adhesions and bands are the commonest cause of intestinal obstruction. Furthermore, in the early postoperative period, the onset of such a mechanical obstruction may be difficult to differentiate from paralytic ileus.

The causes of intraperitoneal adhesions are shown in Table 58.5.

Any source of peritoneal irritation results in local fibrin production which produces adhesions between opposed surfaces. Early fibrinous adhesions may disappear when the cause is removed or they may become vascularised and replaced by mature fibrous tissue.

Prevention. The following factors may limit adhesion formation:

- good surgical technique;
- washing of the peritoneal cavity with saline to remove clots, etc.;
- minimize contact with gauze;
- cover anastomosis and raw peritoneal surfaces.

Numerous substances have been instilled in the peritoneal cavity to prevent adhesion formation, including hyaluronidase, hydrocortisone, silicone, dextran, polyvinylpropylene (PVP), chondroitin and streptomycin, anticoagulants, antihistamines, nonsteroidal anti-inflammatory drugs and streptokinase. Currently no single agent has been shown to be safe and effective, and their use is not recommended.

Adhesions may be classified into various types by virtue of whether they are early (fibrinous) or late (fibrous) or by the underlying aetiology. From a practical perspective, there are only two types – 'easy' flimsy ones and 'difficult' dense ones.

Postoperative adhesions giving rise to intestinal obstruction usually involve the lower small bowel. Operations for appendicitis and gynaecological procedures are the most common precursors and are an indication for early intervention.

Bands

Usually only one band is culpable. This may be:

- congenital, for example obliterated vitellointestinal duct;
- a string band following previous bacterial peritonitis;
- a portion of greater omentum usually adherent to the parietes.

Treatment. Initial management is based on intravenous rehydration and nasogastric decompression. Occasionally it is curative. Whilst an initial conservative regime is considered appropriate, regular assessment is mandatory to ensure that strangulation does not occur. Conservative treatment should not be prolonged beyond 72 hours.

When, as is usual, laparotomy is required, although multiple adhesions may be found, only one may be causative. This should be divided and the remaining adhesions left *in situ* unless severe angulation is present. Division of these adhesions will only cause further adhesion formation.

When obstruction is caused by an area of multiple adhesions, they should be freed by sharp dissection. To prevent recurrence the bare area should be covered with omental grafts.

Following release of band obstruction, the constriction sites that have suffered direct compression should be carefully assessed and if they show residual colour changes, invaginated.

Treatment of recurrent intestinal obstruction due to adhesions

Several procedures may be considered in the presence of recurrent obstruction, including:

- repeat adhesiolysis (enterolysis) alone;
- Noble's plication operation;
- Charles–Phillips transmesenteric plication;
- intestinal intubation.

Their relative efficacy remains unclear.

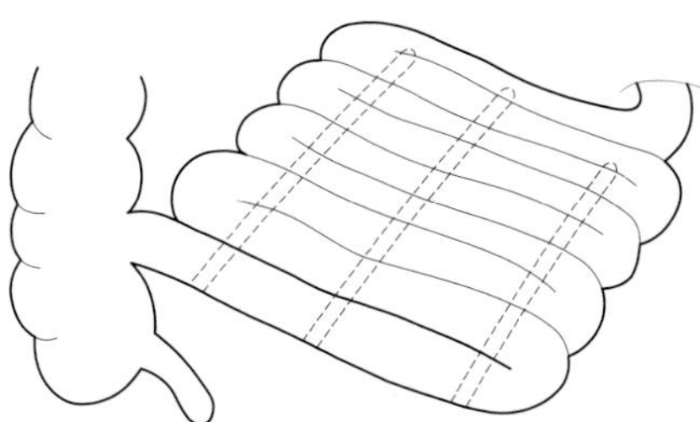

Fig. 58.9 The Charles–Phillips procedure.

In Noble's intestinal plication (Fig. 58.8) all involved intestine is freed. Adjacent coils (average length 15–20 cm) are sutured with serosal sutures to form gentle curves. If only a proportion of the small bowel is plicated, the mesentery must be united to prevent internal hernias. This procedure is time-consuming, and associated with a high morbidity and recurrent symptoms.

In the Charles–Phillips operation (Fig. 58.9), following adhesiolysis, the bowel is placed in an orderly fashion and three long synthetic sutures are passed through the mesentery of the plicated bowel, each doubled back upon itself and tied loosely. The stitch should pass a few centimetres from the bowel wall and not be adjacent to it. The resultant bowel should look like a packet of sausages. Results from this procedure are relatively good.

Intraluminal tube insertion (Baker), via a Witzel jejunostomy or gastrostomy, may facilitate the formation of gentle curves. Most tubes have an inflatable balloon near the tip to facilitate placement within the caecum. This procedure is associated with a long postoperative ileus, and reports of outcome are conflicting (Figs 58.10 and 58.11).

Postoperative intestinal obstruction

Differentiation between persistent paralytic ileus and early mechanical obstruction may be difficult in the early postoperative period. In practice, the latter is probably more common. Early evidence of obstruction (days 1–5) is usually

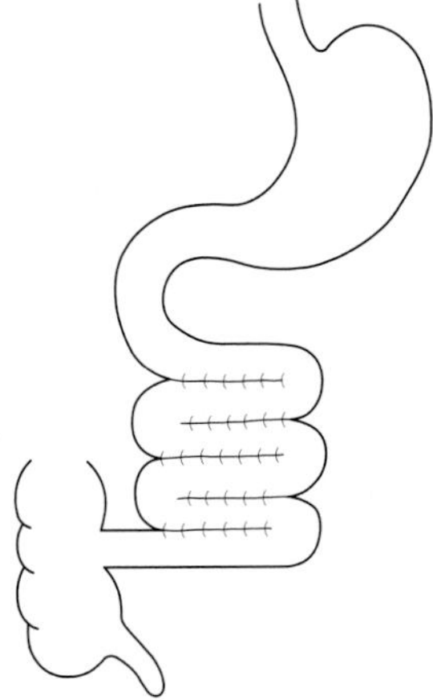

Fig. 58.8 Noble's plication.

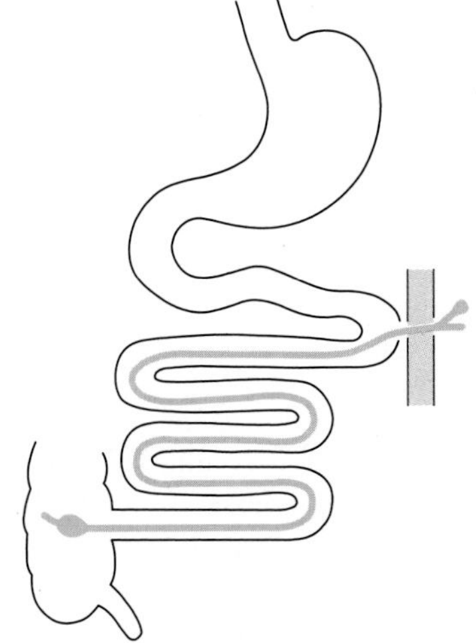

Fig. 58.10 Baker's tube inserted via a Witzel jejunostomy.

Thomas Benjamin Noble, 1895–1958. Surgeon, Community Hospital, Indianapolis, Indiana, USA.

Richard V. Phillips. Surgeon, Albuquerque, New Mexico, USA.

Friedrich Oskar Witzel, 1856–1925. Surgeon, Bonn, Germany.

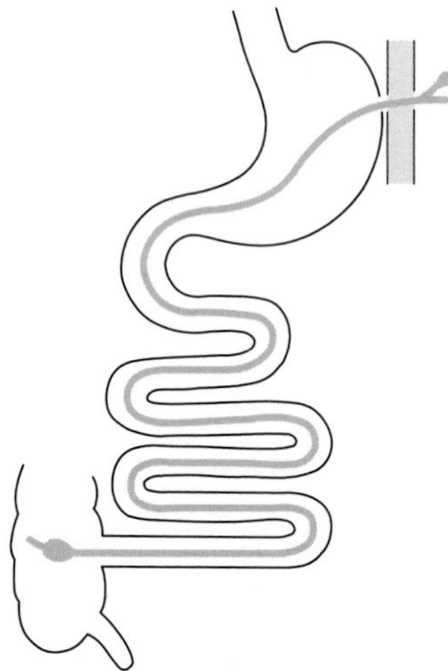

Fig. 58.11 Insertion via a gastrostomy.

due to nonstrangulating causes such as fibrinous adhesions and oedema. Obstruction is usually incomplete and the majority settles with continued conservative management. Late postoperative obstruction (greater than 7 days) is usually more significant in nature and timely surgical intervention is usually required.

Special types of mechanical intestinal obstruction

Internal hernia

Internal herniation occurs where a portion of the small intestine becomes entrapped in one of the retroperitoneal fossae or into a congenital mesenteric defect.

The following are potential sites of internal herniation:

- the foramen of Winslow;
- a hole in the mesentery;
- a hole in the transverse mesocolon;
- defects in the broad ligament;
- congenital or acquired diaphragmatic hernia;
- duodenal retroperitoneal fossae – left paraduodenal and right duodenojejunal;
- caecal/appendiceal retroperitoneal fossae – superior, inferior and retrocaecal;
- intersigmoid fossa.

Internal herniation in the absence of adhesions is uncommon and a preoperative diagnosis is unusual. The standard treatment for a hernia is to release the constricting agent by division. This should not be undertaken in cases of herniation involving the foramen of Winslow, mesenteric defects and the paraduodenal/duodenojejunal fossae as major blood vessels run in the edge of the constriction ring. The distended loop in such circumstances must first be decompressed with minimal contamination and then reduced.

Obstruction from enteric strictures

Small bowel strictures usually occur secondary to tuberculosis or Crohn's disease. Malignant strictures associated with lymphoma are common, whilst carcinoma and sarcoma are rare. Presentation is usually subacute or chronic. Standard surgical management consists of resection and anastomosis. In Crohn's disease strictureplasty may be considered in the presence of short multiple strictures without active sepsis.

Bolus obstruction

Bolus obstruction in the small bowel may be caused by food, gallstones, trichobezoar, phytobezoar, stercoliths and worms.

Gallstones. These tend to occur in the elderly secondary to erosion of a large gallstone through the gall bladder into the duodenum. Classically, there is impaction about 60 cm proximal to the ileocaecal valve. The patient may have recurrent attacks as the obstruction is frequently incomplete or relapsing due to a ball-valve effect. A radiograph will show evidence of small bowel obstruction with a diagnostic air–fluid level in the biliary tree. The stone may or may not be visible. At laparotomy it may be possible to crush the stone within the bowel lumen if it is soft, after milking it proximally. If not, the intestine is opened and the gallstone disimpacted, milked back and removed. If the gallstone is faceted a careful check for other enteric stones should be made. The region of the gall bladder should not be explored.

Food. Bolus obstruction may occur after partial or total gastrectomy when unchewed articles can pass directly into small bowel. Apple, coconut, brussels sprouts, dried fruit and orange pips are particularly liable to cause obstruction. The management is similar to a gallstone with intraluminal crushing usually being successful.

Trichobezoars and phytobezoars. These are firm masses of undigested hair balls and fruit/vegetable fibre, respectively. The former is due to persistent hair chewing and sucking, and may be associated with an underlying psychiatric abnormality. Phytobezoars are predisposed to by high fibre intake, inadequate chewing, previous gastric surgery, hypochlorhydria and loss of gastric pump mechanism. Where possible, the lesion may be kneaded into the caecum, otherwise open removal is required.

Stercoliths. Usually found in the small bowel in association with a jejunal diverticulum or ileal stricture. Presentation and management are identical to gallstones.

Worms. *Ascaris lumbricoides* may cause low small bowel obstruction particularly in children, the institutionalized and those near the tropics (Fig. 58.12). An attack frequently follows initiation of antihelminthic therapy. Debility is frequently out of proportion to that produced by the obstruction. If worms are not seen in stool or vomitus, the diagnosis may be indicated by eosinophilia or the sight of worms within gas-filled small bowel loops on a plain radiograph (Naik). At laparotomy it may be possible to knead the tangled mass into the caecum; if not it should be removed. Occasionally worms may cause a perforation and peritonitis, especially if the enteric wall is already weakened by such conditions as ameobiasis.

Jacob Benignus Winslow, 1669–1760. Danish anatomist.

Burrill Bernard Crohn, b. 1884. Gastroenterologist, Mount Sinai Hospital, New York, USA.

Vinod C. Naik. Doctor, Nansari, India.

Acute intussusception

This occurs when one portion of the gut becomes invaginated within an immediately adjacent segment; invariably it is the proximal into distal bowel.

Aetiology. The condition is encountered most commonly in children, where it occurs in an idiopathic form with a peak incidence at 3–9 months. Seventy to 95 per cent of cases are classed as idiopathic, and an associated illness such as gastroenteritis or urinary tract infection is found in 30 per cent. It is believed that hyperplasia of Peyer's patches in the terminal ileum may be the initiating event. This may occur secondary to weaning. In light of the seasonal variation with peak incidence in spring and summer, it may be related to upper respiratory tract infection pathogens such as adenovirus or rotavirus.

(a)

(b)

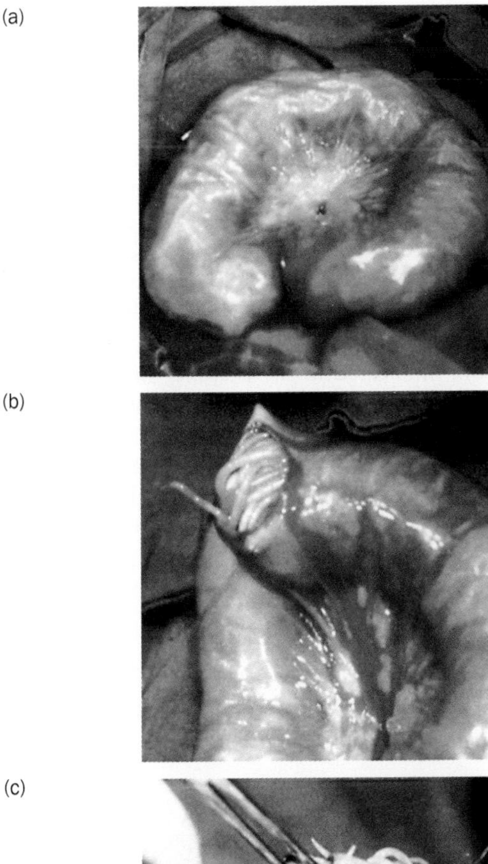

(c)

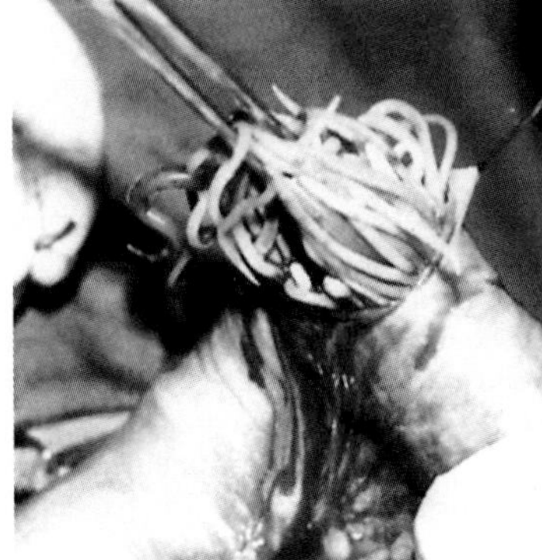

Fig. 58.12 Obstruction of the small intestine due to *Ascaris lumbricoides* (*courtesy of Asal. Y, Izzidien, Nenavah, Iraq*).

Children with intussusception associated with a lead point – such as Meckel's diverticulum, polyp, duplication, Henoch–Schönlein purpura or appendix – are usually older than the idiopathic cases. Adult cases are invariably associated with a lead point which is usually a polyp (e.g. Peutz–Jegher syndrome), a submucosal lipoma or tumour, the exception being after periods of long fasting (Moro). The colocolic variety is common in adults.

Pathology. An intussusception is composed of three parts (Fig. 58.13):

- the entering or inner tube;
- the returning or middle tube;
- the sheath or outer tube (intussuscipiens).

The part which advances is the apex; the mass is the intussusception and the neck is the junction of the entering layer with the mass.

An intussusception is an example of strangulating obstruction as the blood supply of the inner layer is usually impaired. The degree of ischaemia is dependent on the tightness of the invagination, which is usually greatest as it passes through the ileocaecal valve.

Intussusception may be anatomically defined as ileoileal, ileocaecal and ileocolic depending on the site and extent of invagination (Table 58.6).

Clinical features. The presentation of intussusception in a child is classical. An otherwise fit and well male child of 6 months develops sudden onset of screaming associated with drawing up of the legs. The attacks last for a few

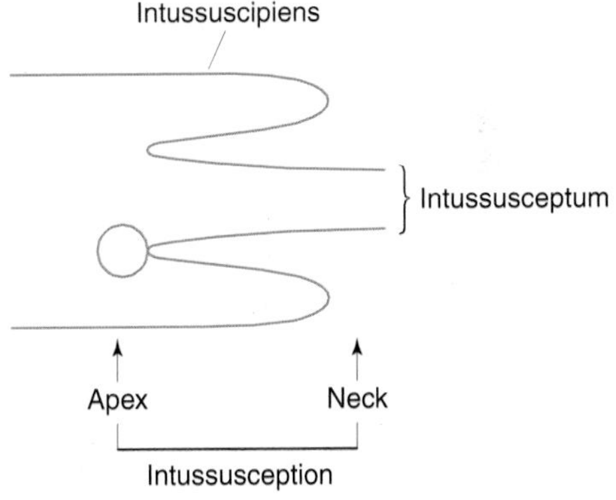

Fig. 58.13 Mechanism and nomenclature of intussusception.

Johan Conrad Peyer, 1653–1712. Professor of Logic, Rhetoric and Medicine, Schaffhausen, Switzerland.

Johann F. Meckel (The Younger), 1781–1833. Professor of Anatomy and Surgery, Halle, Germany.

Edward Heinrich Henoch, 1820–1910. Professor of Diseases of Children, Berlin, Germany.

Johann Lucas Schönlein, 1793–1864. German physician.

John Law Augustine Peutz, 1886–1957. Chief Specialist for Internal Medicine, St John's Hospital, The Hague, The Netherlands.

Harold Jos Jegher. Professor of Internal medicine, New Jersey College of Medicine and Dentistry, Jersey City, USA.

Table 58.6 Types of intussusception (after Gross) (in 702 cases)

	Percentage of series
Ileoileal	5
Ileocolic	77
Ileo-ileo-colic	12
Colocolic	2
Multiple	1
Retrograde	0.2
Others	2.8

minutes, recur every 15 minutes and become progressively severe. During attacks the child has facial pallor whilst between episodes he is listless and drawn.

Vomiting may or may not occur at the outset but becomes conspicuous with time. Initially the passage of stool may be normal, whilst later blood and mucus are evacuated – the 'redcurrent' jelly stool.

Examination should be undertaken, wherever possible, between episodes without disturbing the child. Classically, the abdomen is not distended, a lump may be felt which hardens on palpation but this is present in only 50–60 per cent of cases (Fig. 58.14). There may be an associated feeling of emptiness in the right iliac fossa (the sign of Dance). On rectal examination blood-stained mucus may be found on the finger. Occasionally, in extensive ileocolic or colocolic intussusception, the apex may be palpable or even protrude from the anus.

Unrelieved, the pain will become continuous with abdominal distension and profound vomiting. Ultimately death occurs from small bowel obstruction or peritonitis secondary to gangrene. Rarely, natural cure may occur due to sloughing of the intussusceptium.

Radiography. A plain abdominal film usually reveals evidence of small or large bowel obstruction with an absent caecal gas shadow in ileoileal or ileocolic cases. A barium enema may be used to diagnose the presence of an ileo-colic

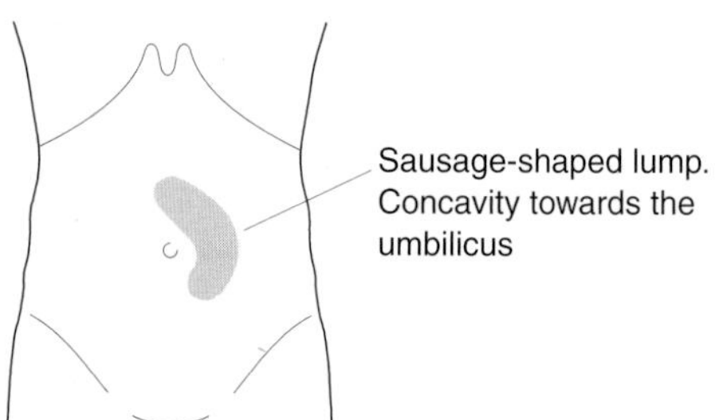

Fig. 58.14 The physical signs as recorded by Hamilton Bailey in a typical case of intussusception in an infant.

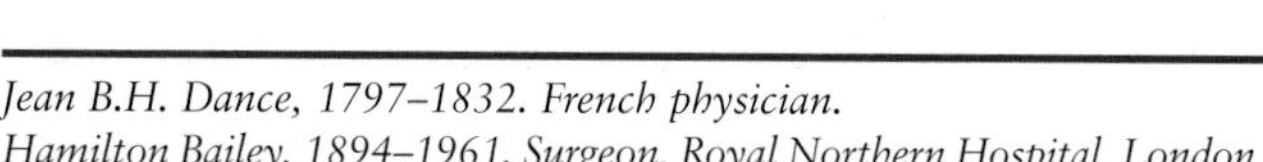

Jean B.H. Dance, 1797–1832. French physician.
Hamilton Bailey, 1894–1961. Surgeon, Royal Northern Hospital, London.

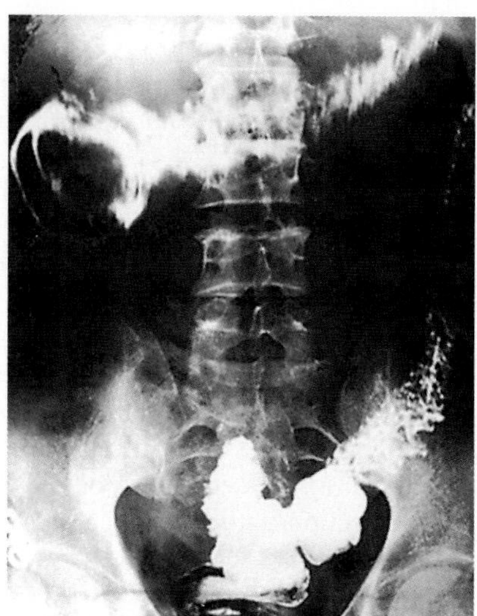

Fig. 58.15 'Claw' sign of ileocolic intussusception. The barium in the intussuscipiens is seen as a claw around the negative shadow of the intussusception (*courtesy of R.S. Naik, Durg, India*).

or colocolic form (the claw sign) (Fig. 58.15) but would be negative for the ileoileal variant in the presence of a competent ileocaecal valve. Equivocal cases of ileoileal intussusception may be further evaluated by CT scan which should reveal the presence of a small bowel mass.

Barium enema may also be used therapeutically in selected cases to reduce an infant intussusception. Hydrostatic reduction is contraindicated in the presence of obstruction, peritonism or a prolonged history (greater than 48 hours) and is unlikely to succeed where a lead point is likely. It is successful in 50 per cent of cases with a recurrence rate in the order of 5 per cent. Complete reduction must be confirmed by the visualization of contrast entering the terminal ileum. In cases where complete reduction is not possible, the intussusception may be so reduced in size and near its origin that only a grid-iron incision is required for surgical management.

Unfortunately, in many cases the clinical scenario is not clear-cut enough for an early diagnosis to be made and the bowel is already ischaemic by the time treatment in hospital is instituted.

Differential diagnosis.

- Acute enterocolitis – whilst abdominal pain and vomiting are common with occasional blood and mucus in the stool, diarrhoea is a leading symptom and faecal matter or bile is always present in the stool.
- Henoch–Schöenlein purpura (HSP) – HSP is associated with a characteristic rash and abdominal pain but intussusception may also occur. Laparotomy should be considered in equivocal cases.
- Rectal prolapse – this may be easily differentiated by the fact that the projecting mucosa can be felt in continuity with the perianal skin whereas in intussusception the finger may pass indefinitely into the depths of a sulcas.

Operative management. This is required where hydrostatic reduction has failed or is contraindicated.

A midline incision is used after complete preoperative resuscitation with nasogastric decompression and intravenous rehydration. Reduction is achieved by squeezing the most distal part of the mass in a cephalad direction (Fig. 58.16). *Do not* pull. The last part of the reduction is the most difficult and the majority of cases is achieved by squeezing the apex. After reduction, the terminal part of the small bowel and the appendix will be seen to be reddened and stiffened with oedema. The viability of all bowel should be checked carefully.

In difficult cases the little finger may be gently inserted into the neck of the intussusception to try and separate adhesions (Cope's method). Subsequently, the thumb and forefinger are placed in such a way as to deinvaginate the apex. Gentle pressure is applied and gradually increased to reduce the oedema around the ileocaecal valve (Fig. 58.17). After reduction the underlying cause requires appropriate treatment.

In the presence of an irreducible or gangrenous intussusception the mass should be excised *in situ* and an anastomosis or temporary end stoma created.

Postoperative care. In the uncomplicated cases, gastric aspiration and intravenous rehydration should be continued for 24 hours. Oral fluids or breast feeding may be restarted on day 2 or when postoperative ileus shows signs of resolving.

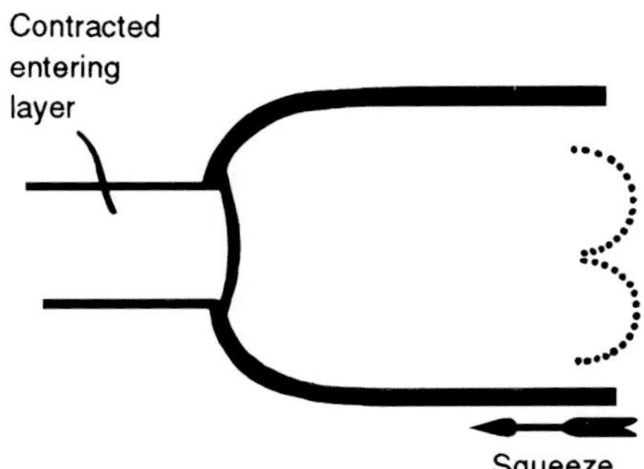

Fig. 58.16 Diagram showing the method of reducing an intussusception.

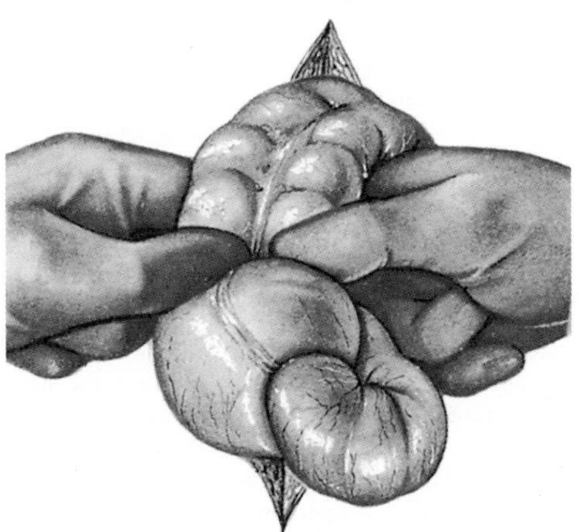

Fig. 58.17 Reducing the terminal part of the intussusception (*after R.E. Gross*).

Recurrent intussusception. This rare complication may occur in 5 per cent of idiopathic cases. Anchorage of the last part of the terminal ileum to the ascending colon has been advocated where repeat surgery is required.

Volvulus

A volulus is a twisting or axial rotation of a portion of bowel about its mesentery. When complete it forms a closed loop of obstruction with resultant ischaemia secondary to vascular occlusion.

Volvuli may be primary or secondary. The primary form occurs secondary to congenital malrotation of the gut, abnormal mesenteric attachments or congenital bands. Examples include volvulus neonatorum, caecal and sigmoid volvulus. A secondary volvulus, which is the more common variety, is due to actual rotation of a piece of bowel around an acquired adhesion or stoma.

Volvulus neonatorum is predisposed to by arrested gut rotation with a resultant narrow mesentery of the small bowel and caecum. The symptoms are similar to arrested rotation (*vide infra*) with repeated vomiting, but the onset is more catastrophic with abdominal distention and rapid dehydration. Abdominal radiography reveals evidence of duodenal obstruction. Laparotomy reveals a distended stomach and coils of small bowel (Fig. 58.19). The whole midgut should be delivered to the wound and wrapped in warm, moist towels, in order to demonstrate the volvulus which usually occurs in a clockwise direction. The operation consists of reduction by untwisting and division of any secondary obstructive lesions – such as the transduodenal band of Ladd.

Volvulus of the small intestine

This may be primary or secondary and usually occurs in the lower ileum. It may occur spontaneously in Africans, particularly following consumption of a large volume of vegetable matter, whilst in the West it is usually secondary to adhesions passing to the parietes or female pelvic organs. Treatment consists of reduction of the twist and is then directed to any underlying cause.

Caecal volvulus

This may occur as part of volvulus neonatorum or *de novo* and is usually a clockwise twist. It is more common in females and usually presents acutely with the classic features of obstruction. At first the obstruction may be partial with the passage of flatus and faeces. In 25 per cent of cases, examination may reveal a palpable tympanic swelling in the midline or left side of the abdomen. Plain radiograph may reveal a gas-filled ileum and occasionally a distended caecum. A barium enema may be used to confirm the diagnosis with an absence of barium in the caecum and a bird beak deformity.

At operation the volvulus should be reduced. Sometimes this can only be achieved after decompression of the caecum by a needle. Further management consists of either fixation of the caecum to the right iliac fossa (caecopexy) and/or a caecostomy. If the caecum is ischaemic or gangrenous a right hemicolectomy should be performed.

Sigmoid volvulus

This is rare in Europe and the USA but more common in Eastern Europe and Africa; indeed it is the commonest cause of large bowel obstruction in indigenous black Africans (Loefler). The predisposing cause is

Sir Zachary Cope, 1881–1975. Surgeon, St Mary's Hospital, London, England.

William Edwards Ladd, 1880–1967. Professor of Child Surgery, Harvard University, Boston, Massachusetts, USA.

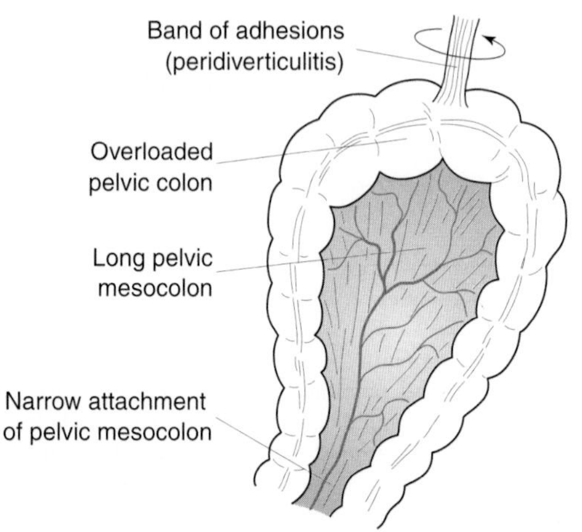

Fig. 58.18 Predisposing causes of volvulus of the sigmoid colon. Idiopathic megacolon usually precedes the volvulus in Africans.

summarised in Fig. 58.18. Rotation nearly always occurs in an anticlockwise direction. Predisposing factors include high residue diet and chronic constipation.

(a)
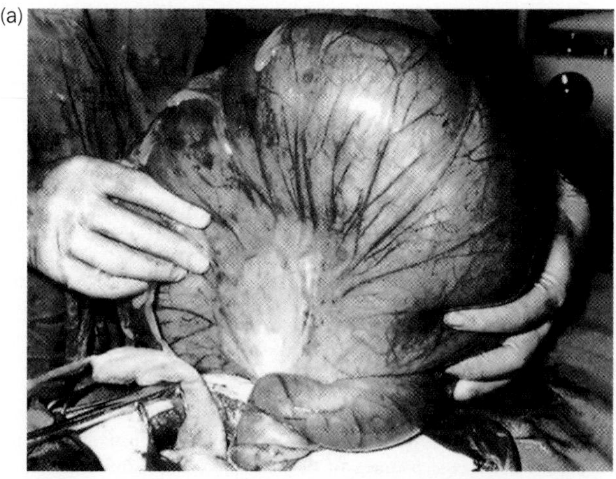

(b)
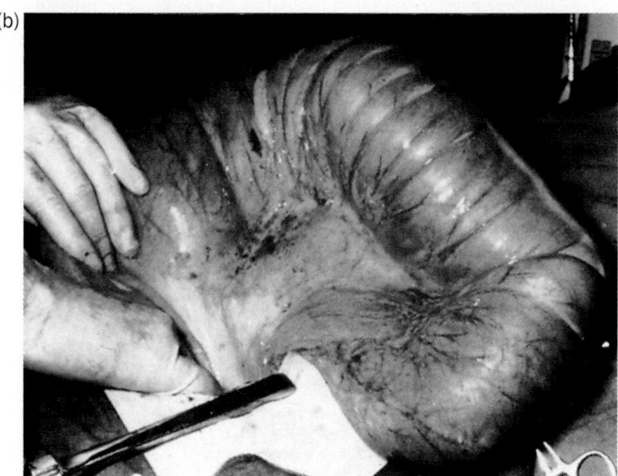

Fig. 58.19 Volvulus of the sigmoid colon (a) before and (b) after untwisting (*courtesy of S.U. Rahman, Manchester, UK*).

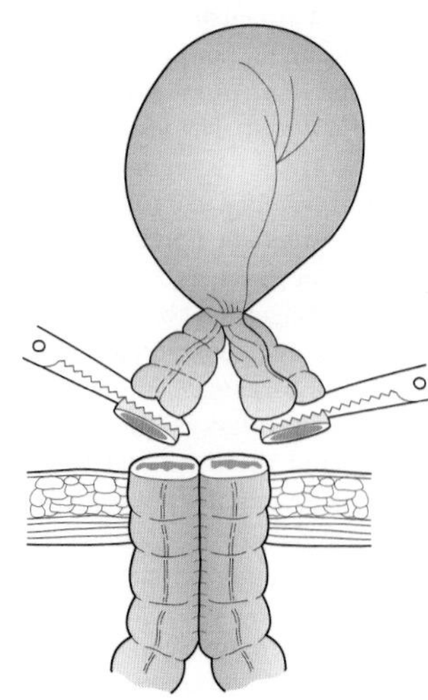

Fig. 58.20 The Paul–Mikulicz operation applied to volvulus of the pelvic colon.

The symptoms are of large bowel obstruction which may initially be intermittent, followed by the passage of large quantities of flatus and faeces. Presentation varies in severity and acuteness, with younger patients appearing to develop the more acute form. Abdominal distension is an early and progressive sign which may be associated with hiccough and wretching; vomiting occurs late. Constipation is absolute. In the elderly a more chronic form may be seen. A plain radiograph shows massive colonic distension. The classic appearance is of a dilated loop of bowel running diagonally across the abdomen from right to left with two fluid levels seen, one within each loop of bowel.

Treatment

Flexible sigmoidoscopy or rigid sigmoidoscopy and insertion of a flatus tube should be carried out to allow deflation of the gut. Success, as long as ischaemic bowel is excluded, will provide temporary respite allowing resuscitation and an elective procedure. Failure results in an early laparotomy, with untwisting of the loop and per-anal decompression (Fig. 58.19). When the bowel is viable, fixation of the sigmoid colon to the posterior abdominal wall may be a safer manoeuvre in inexperienced hands. Resection is preferable if it can be achieved safely. A Paul–Mikulicz procedure is a useful procedure particularly if there is suspicion of impending gangrene (Fig. 58.20). An alternative is a sigmoid colectomy and, where anastomosis is considered unwise, a Hartmann's procedure with subsequent reanastomosis.

Compound volvulus

This is a rare condition also known as ileosigmoid knotting. The long pelvic mesocolon allows the ileum to twist around the sigmoid colon resulting in gangrene of either or both segments of bowel. The patient presents with acute intestinal obstruction, but distension is comparatively mild. Plain radiography reveals distended ileal loops in a distended sigmoid colon. At operation decompression, resection and anastomosis are required.

Acute intestinal obstruction of the newborn

Neonatal intestinal obstruction has an approximate incidence of 1:2000 live births. Congenital atresia and stenosis are the commonest causes. Volvulus neonatorium, meconium ileus and Hirschpring's disease may also be responsible.

Congenital atresia

The incidence of atresia varies with anatomical site:

- duodenum – 35 per cent;
- jejunum – 15 per cent;
- ileum – 25 per cent;
- ascending colon – 10 per cent;
- multiple sites – 15 per cent.

The high incidence of multiple sites makes peroperative assessment of the whole small and large bowel mandatory. Except in the case of duodenal atresia there are frequently associated abnormalities of the heart and great vessels.

Atresia/stenosis of the duodenum

Atresia and stenosis occur with equal frequency. In most cases, except for the oesophagus, duodenum and rectum, the atresia is a result of an intrauterine vascular accident occurring late in pregnancy such as volvulus, intussusception or strangulation at the umbilical ring. As the foetus is germ-free the ischaemic portion is absorbed and disappears. In the presence of complete obstruction, persistent vomiting occurs from birth. The presence or absence of bile is dependent on the relationship of the septum to the duodenal papilla. Bile-stained vomiting is nearly always organic in origin. Distension is often absent but visible peristalsis may be seen in the left upper quadrant. Atresia of the duodenum occurs at the level of the ampulla of Vater. Thirty per cent of babies have associated Down's syndrome. Radiography reveals a classic so-called double stomach due to gross distention of the stomach and upper part of the duodenum with two air–fluid levels (Fig. 58.21).

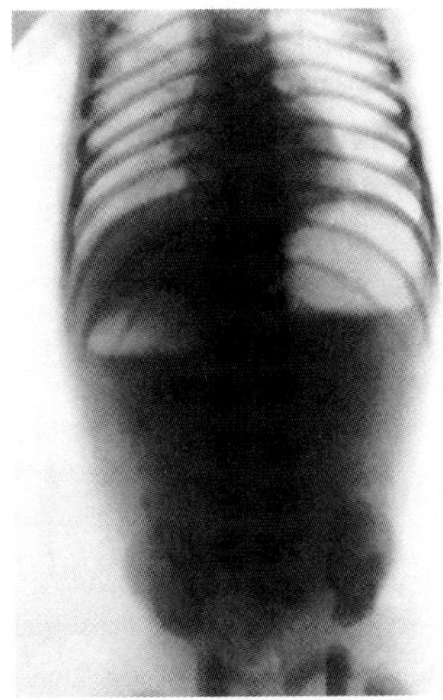

Fig. 58.21 Duodenal atresia. 'Double stomach' appearance on erect film. Gas and fluid levels in both stomach and duodenum.

Harold Hirschsprung, 1830–1916. Physician, Queen Louise Hospital for Children, Copenhagen, Denmark.

In cases of partial obstruction the location of the lesion may be confirmed by installation, via a nasogastric tube, of a small volume of gastrografin. Once the lesion is confirmed the medium must be aspirated. Suprapapillary duodenal atresia may be distinguished from oesophageal atresia by the absence of dribbling saliva, and from infantile pyloric stenosis by the absence of a lump.

Duodenal obstruction in infancy may also be due to midgut volvulus, a band obstruction or an annular pancreas.

Treatment

Surgery is required as soon as resuscitation is complete. Duodeno-jejunostomy is the operation of choice. A silastic catheter is introduced through a stab incision in the antrum and guided through the anastomosis. A Witzel gastrostomy is constructed around the proximal tube which is brought out through a stab incision. Early enteral feeding through this tube is recommended.

Atresia/stenosis of the jejunum/ileum

There are four main types:

- type 1 – diaphragm with continuity of the bowel wall;
- type 2 – gap between the two ends (may be connected by fibrous cord) plus a mesenteric defect;
- type 3 – multiple atresias;
- type 4 – apple peel atresia with loss of dorsal mesentery.

The vital importance of a diagnosis lies in the fact that proximal distention of the bowel may be so great that the vascular integrity of the bowel wall is compromised leading to gangrene and perforation (Fig. 58.22).

In ileal atresia the child is born with abdominal distension or it presents within 24 hours of birth. In jejunal atresia early distention is lacking but vomiting occurs early. In both conditions the vomit contains bile and some meconium is likely to be evacuated.

Radiography

Plain radiographs are only diagnostic when air–fluid levels are seen. When they are present the obstruction is usually well advanced.

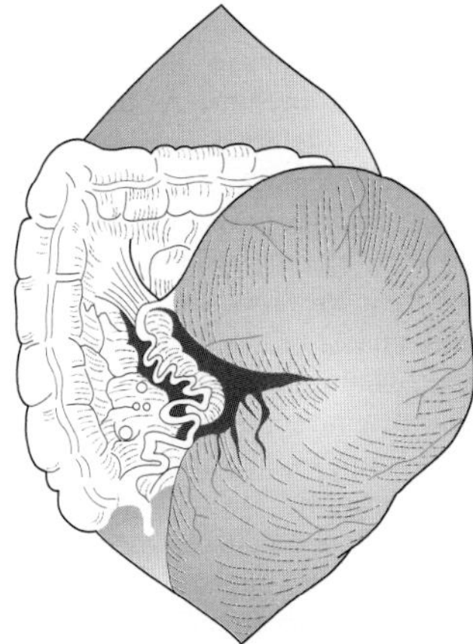

Fig. 58.22 Congenital atresia of the ileum (*courtesy of V. Swain, London, UK*).

Abraham Vater, 1684–1751. Professor of Anatomy and Botany, Wittenburg, Germany.
John Langdon Haydon Down, 1828–96. British physician.

Surgery

If the stenosis is ileal and the discrepancy in bowel diameter above and below the obstruction is marked the two limbs may be brought out in a manner similar to the Paul–Mikulicz procedure. The proximal limb will need to be proud of the abdominal wall (usually by eversion) in order to prevent skin excoriation. Secondary closure by circumstomal mobilization and anastomosis, rather than use of crushing clamps, is recommended. When the stenosis is jejunal, the impact of the high jejunostomy output can make subsequent management difficult and wherever possible an end-to-end anastomosis is recommended.

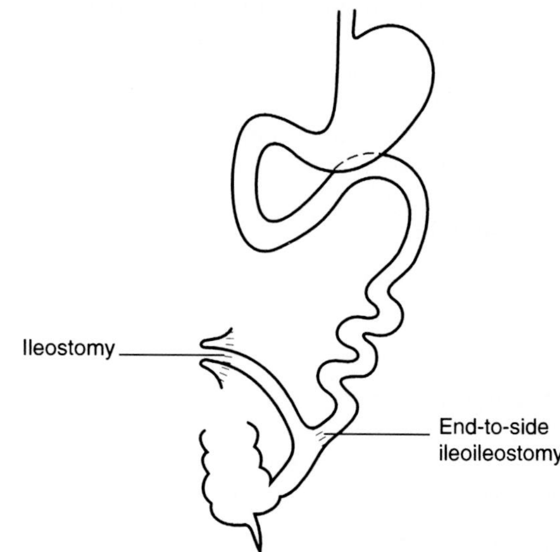

Fig. 58.23 Bishop–Koop operation. This shows the completed procedure after grossly distended ileum has been resected. Because intestinal continuity is preserved, early closure of the ileostomy is not essential.

Arrested rotation

Up to 10 weeks of gestation the gut lies outside the abdominal cavity. The orderly return may be arrested at any stage resulting in four major types of arrest.

The whole bowel may remain free as a narrow-based mesentery. The caecum may be displaced with transduodenal bands. The intestine may return in a clockwise direction producing a reversed intestinal rotation or a failure of rotation altogether, with the small bowel on the right and the large bowel on the left.

The most common anomaly is where the caecum remains in the left hypochondrium and a peritoneal band is found running from the caecum to the right side of the abdomen and then across the second part of the duodenum – the transduodenal band of Ladd. The symptoms of repeated vomiting, due to pressure on the duodenum, and the radiographic appearances are identical to those of duodenal stenosis. Treatment consists of early laparotomy after appropriate resuscitation. The band is divided near its attachment to the parietal peritoneum. Often there is a second band which must also be divided, extending from the midline to the commencement of the caecum. The caecum and the colon are centred on the left of the abdominal cavity with the small bowel on the right (Nixon).

Meconium ileus

This is the neonatal manifestation of cystic fibrosis. Meconium is normally kept fluid by the action of pancreatic enzymes. The terminal ileum becomes filled with meconium and viscid mucus resulting in progressive inspissation *in utero* and neonatal obstruction. Inspissated meconium may be palpated as a rubbery swelling. Abdominal radiography may reveal a distended small intestine, with mottling. Fluid levels are generally not seen. Unlike ileal atresia there is no abrupt termination of the gas-filled intestine. As the condition is due to an autosomal recessive genetic defect a family history may be present. Further assessment includes absence of trypsin from stool or bile and a concentration of sodium chloride in sweat greater than 80 mmol/litre, or a negative immunoreactive blood trypsin estimation.

Forty per cent of cases are associated with complications such as volvulus neonatorium, atresia or meconium peritonitis (Dickson). Any evidence to suggest an acute intra-abdominal process due to twisting of the grossly distended proximal bowel indicates the need for urgent laparotomy. When this is not so, a gastrografin or mypaque enema may be given to confirm the diagnosis. The radio-opaque fluid will pass easily to the ileum where it may disperse the obstructing meconium and relieve the condition owing to its high osmolarity and detergent action. As the instilled solution is markedly hypertonic, the rapid loss of fluid into the bowel lumen must be corrected by replacement. If conservative management fails, laporotomy is indicated. The only condition with which meconium ileus may be confused is Hirschsprung's disease affecting the whole colon. The standard treatment is resection of the most dilated segment with an end-to-side anastomosis of the colon to the ileum. The distal ileal opening is formed into an ileostomy, through which the meconium may be irrigated postoperatively (the Bishop–Koop operation). The ilesotomy becomes a mucus fistula which usually requires subsequent closure (Fig. 58.23).

Necrotising enterocolitis

This is a common phenomenon amongst sick premature neonates. The risk is inversely proportional to birth weight and may be associated with hypoxia, hypothemia, hypotension and umbilical artery cannulation. The ileum, caecum, distal colon and total colon are affected with a complete spectrum from mucosal to transmural necrosis.

The usual presentation is bilious vomiting, abdominal distension, colour change and lethargy in a high-risk neonate. The abdomen is usually soft. Abdominal radiographs may show pneumatosis intestinalis or free intraperitoneal air. Management consists of aggressive resuscitation with intravenous feeding. The optimal time for surgery is not in the acute phase as the baby can withstand the pressure of necrosis better than an adult but not the stress of laparotomy. At laparotomy excision of all necrotic bowel with primary anastomosis is usual. The overall mortality is 25 per cent with 10–30 per cent of neonates developing a colonic stricture.

Chronic intestinal obstruction

The symptoms of chronic intestinal obstruction may arise from two sources – the cause and the subsequent obstruction.

The causes of obstruction may be organic:

- intramural – faecal impaction;
- mural – colorectal cancer, diverticulitis, strictures (Crohn's disease, ischaemia), anastomotic stenosis;
- extramural – adhesion (small bowel only), metastatic deposits, endometriosis;

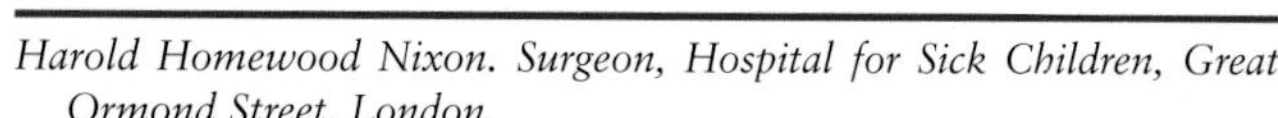

Harold Homewood Nixon. Surgeon, Hospital for Sick Children, Great Ormond Street, London.

James Alexander Scott Dickson. Emeritus Consultant Surgeon, Sheffield.

or

- functional – Hirschsprung's disease, idiopathic megacolon, pseudo-obstruction.

The symptoms of chronic obstruction differ in their predominance, timing and degree from acute obstruction. Constipation appears first. It is initially relative and then absolute, associated with distension. In the presence of large bowel disease, the point of greatest distension is in the caeum and this is heralded by the onset of pain. Vomiting is a late feature and therefore dehydration is exceptional. Examination is unremarkable, save for confirmation of distension and the onset of peritonism in late cases. Rectal examination may confirm the presence of faecal impaction or a tumour.

Investigation

Plain abdominal radiography may confirm the presence of large bowel obstruction. All such cases should be confirmed by a subsequent single contrast water-soluble enema study to rule out functional disease. Organic disease requires a laparotomy, whilst functional disease requires colonoscopic decompression and conservative management.

In the presence of organic obstruction, after resuscitation surgical management depends on the underlying cause and the relevant chapters in this book should be consulted.

Hirschsprung's disease

This is due to failure of complete migration of the ganglion cells of the large bowel to the anus. This results in an aganglionic segment producing physiological obstruction. Eighty per cent present in the neonatal period with acute large bowel obstruction, whilst 20 per cent present with failure to thrive or severe constipation.

Barium enema reveals a characteristic narrow segment, whilst a full-thickness rectal strip biopsy will show absence of ganglion cells. The rectoanal inhibitory reflex is absent on physiological testing.

Treatment consists of an initial loop colostomy followed by a definitive pull-through procedure.

Adynamic obstruction

Paralytic ileus

This may be defined as a state in which there is failure of transmission of peristaltic waves secondary to neuromuscular failure [i.e. in the myenteric (Auerbach) and the submucous (Meissner) plexuses]. The resultant stasis leads to accumulation of fluid and gas within the bowel with associated distension, vomiting, absence of bowel sounds and absolute constipation.

Varieties

The following varieties are recognised.

- Postoperative – a degree of ileus usually occurs after any abdominal procedure and is self-limiting with a variable duration of 24–72 hours. Postoperative ileus may be prolonged in the presence of hypoproteinaemia or metabolic abnormality (*vide infra*).
- Infection – intra-abdominal sepsis may give rise to localized or generalised ileus. Resultant adhesions may contribute a mechanical element to the initial neurogenic aetiology.
- Reflex ileus – may occur following fractures of the spine or ribs, retroperitoneal haemorrhage or even the application of a plaster jacket.
- Metabolic – uraemia and hypokalaemia are the commonest contributory factors.

Clinical features

Paralytic ileus takes a clinical significance if 72 hours after laparotomy:

- there has been no return of bowel sound on auscultation;
- there has been no passage of flatus.

Abdominal distension becomes more marked and tympanitic. Pain is not a feature. In the absence of gastric aspiration, effortless vomiting may occur. Radiologically, the abdomen shows gas-filled loops of intestine with multiple fluid levels.

Management

The essence of treatment is prevention, with the use of nasogastric suction and restriction of oral intake until bowel sounds and the passage of flatus return. Electrolyte balance must be maintained.

Specific treatment is directed towards the cause, but the following general principles apply:

- the primary cause must be removed;
- gastrointestinal distension must be relieved by decompression;
- close attention to fluid and electrolyte balance is essential;
- there is no place for routine use of peristaltic stimulants. Rarely, medical therapy with the adrenergic blocking agent in association with cholenergic stimulation, e.g. neostigmine (the Catchpole regime), may be used in resistant cases provided that an intraperitoneal cause has been excluded;
- if paralytic ileus is prolonged and threatens life, a laparotomy should be considered to exclude a hidden cause and facilitate bowel decompression.

Pseudo-obstruction

This condition describes an obstruction, usually of the colon, in the absence of a mechanical cause or acute intra-abdominal disease. It is associated with a variety of syndromes where there is an underlying neuropathy and/or myopathy. A variety of causes has been described (Table 58.7).

Small intestinal pseudo-obstruction

This condition may be primary (i.e. idiopathic or associated

Table 58.7 Factors associated with pseudo-obstruction

Idiopathic
- Metabolic:
  - Diabetes – acute intermittent porphyria
  - Hypokalaemia
  - Uraemia
  - Myxoedema
- Severe trauma (especially to lumbar spine and pelvis)
- Shock
  - Burns
  - Myocardial infarct
  - Stroke

Septicaemia
- Retroperitoneal irritation:
  - Blood
  - Urine
  - Enzymes (pancreatitis)
  - Tumour
- Drugs:
  - Tricyclic antidepressants
  - Phenothiazines
  - Levadopa
  - Laxatives
- Secondary gastrointestinal involvement:
  - Scleroderma
  - Chagas' disease

with familial visceral myopathy) or secondary. The clinical picture consists of recurrent subacute obstruction. The diagnosis is made by the exclusion of a mechanical cause. Treatment consists of initial correction of any underlying disorder. Metoclopramide and erythromycin may be of use but cisapride, which increases the local concentration of acetylchlorine with the smooth muscle, is the drug of choice.

Colonic pseudo-obstruction

This may occur in an acute or a chronic form. The former, also known as Ogilvie syndrome, presents as acute large bowel obstruction. Abdominal radiographs show evidence of colonic obstruction with marked caecal distension being a common feature. Indeed, caecal perforation is a well-recognised complication. The absence of a mechanical cause requires urgent confirmation by colonoscopy or a single contrast water-soluble barium enema. Once confirmed, pseudo-obstruction should be treated by colonoscopic decompression. This may recur in 25 per cent of cases requiring further colonoscopy with simultaneous placement of a flatus tube. When colonoscopy fails or is unavailable, a tube caecostomy may be required. The chronic form may respond to cisapride but continued symptoms may benefit from surgical intervention with subtotal colectomy and ileorectal anastomosis.

Carlos Chagas, 1879–1934. Brazilian physician.
Sir William Ogilvie, 1887–1971. British physician.

Acute mesenteric ischaemia

Mesenteric vascular disease may be classified as acute intestinal ischaemia – with or without occlusion – venous, chronic arterial, central or peripheral. The superior mesenteric vessels are likeliest of the visceral vessels to be affected by embolisation or thrombosis, with the former being most common. Occlusion at the origin of the superior mesenteric artery (SMA) is almost invariably the result of thrombosis, whilst emboli lodge at the origin of the middle colic artery. Inferior mesenteric involvement is usually clinically silent owing to a better collateral circulation.

Possible sources for the embolisation of the SMA include the left atrium associated with fibrillation, a mural myocardial infarct, an atheromatous plaque from an aortic aneurysm and a mitral valve vegetation associated with endocarditis.

Primary thrombosis is associated with atherosclerosis or thromboangitis obliterans.

Primary thrombosis of the superior mesenteric veins may occur in association with factor V leiden, portal hypertension, portal pyaemia, sickle cell disease and in women taking the contraceptive pill.

Irrespective of whether the occlusion is arterial or venous, haemorrhagic infarction occurs. The mucosa is the only layer of the intestinal wall to have little resistance to ischaemic injury. The intestine and its mesentery become swollen and oedematous. Blood-stained fluid exudes into the peritoneal cavity and bowel lumen. If the main trunk of the SMA is involved the infarction covers an area from just distal to the duodenojejunal flexure to the splenic flexure. Usually a branch of the main trunk is implicated and the area of infarction is less.

Clinical features

The most important clue to an early diagnosis is the sudden onset of severe abdominal pain in a patient with atrial fibrillation or atherosclerosis. The pain is typically central and out of all proportion to physical findings. Persistent vomiting and defecation occur early with the subsequent passage of altered blood. Hypovolaemic shock rapidly ensues. Abdominal tenderness may be mild initially with rigidity being a late feature.

Investigation will usually reveal a profound neutrophil leucocytosis with an absence of gas in the thickened small intestine on abdominal radiograph. The presence of gas bubbles in the mesenteric veins is rare but pathognomnonic.

Treatment needs to be tailored to the individual. In conjunction with full resuscitation, in early embolic cases emabolectomy via the ileocolic artery or revascularisation of the SMA may be considered. The majority of cases, however, is diagnosed late. In the young all affected bowel should be resected, whilst in the elderly or infirm the situation may be deemed incurable. Anticoagulations should be implemented early in the postoperative period.

After extensive enterectomy it is usual for patients to require intravenous alimentation. The young, however, may sometimes develop sufficient intestinal digestive and absorptive function to lead relatively normal lives. In selected cases, consideration may be given to small bowel transplantation, but at present this must be considered experimental.

Infarction of the large intestine alone is relatively rare. Involvement of the middle colic artery territory should be treated by transverse colectomy and exteriorisation of both ends, with an extended right hemicolectomy in selected cases.

Ischaemic colitis describes the structural changes which occur in the colon as a result of the deprivation of blood. They are commonest in the splenic flexure whose blood supply is particularly tenuous. They have been classified by Marston into gangrenous, stricturing and transient forms. Acute presentation is with lower abdominal pain and the passage of blood per rectum. The differential diagnosis is usually from a carcinoma, Crohn's disease or ulcerative colitis. In those patients without evidence of peritonism, most cases resolves spontaneously. In a few, a permanent stricture develops requiring elective resection.

Jeffrey Adrian Priestly Marston. Retired surgeon, Middlesex Hospital, London.

Further reading

Bizer, L.S., Liebling, R.W., Delaney, H.M. and Gliedman, M.L. (1981) Small bowel obstruction: the role of non-operative treatment in simple intestinal obstruction and predictive criteria for strangulation obstruction. *Surgery*, **89**, 407–13.

Dudley, H.A.F., Radcliffe, A.G. and McGeehan, D. (1980) Intra-operative irrigation of the colon to permit primary anastomosis. *British Journal of Surgery*, **67**, 80–81.

Ellis, H, (1971) The causes and prevention of postoperative intraperitoneal adhesions. *Surgery, Gynaecology and Obstetrics*, **133**, 497–511.

Fielding, L.P. (1993) Colonic surgery for acute conditions: obstruction. In *Rob & Smith's Operative Surgery*, 5th edn (eds L.P. Fielding and S.M. Goldberg), Butterworth-Heinemann, Oxford, pp. 397–415.

Omas, S. and Shirazi, S.S. (1984) Colonic pseudo-obstruction. *American Journal of Gastroenterology*, **79**, 525–32.

Jones, P.F. (1993) Stomas. In *Rob & Smith's Operative Surgery*, 5th edn (eds L.P. Fielding and S.M. Goldberg), Butterworth-Heinemann, Oxford, pp. 240–301.

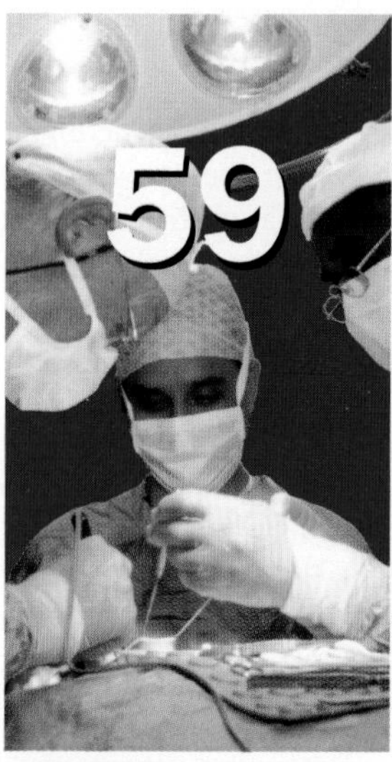

59 The vermiform appendix

Introduction

The vermiform appendix is considered by most to be a vestigial organ, its importance in surgery due only to its propensity for inflammation which results in the clinical syndrome known as acute appendicitis. Acute appendicitis is the most common cause of an 'acute abdomen' in young adults, and as such the associated symptoms and signs have become a paradigm for clinical teaching. Appendicitis is sufficiently common that appendicectomy (termed appendectomy in North America) is the most frequently performed urgent abdominal operation, and is often the first major procedure performed by a surgeon in training. Yet, despite extraordinary advances in modern radiographic imaging and diagnostic laboratory investigations, the diagnosis of appendicitis remains essentially clinical requiring a mixture of observation, clinical acumen and surgical science. In an age accustomed to early and accurate preoperative diagnosis, acute appendicitis remains an enigmatic challenge and a reminder of the art of surgical diagnosis.

Anatomy

The vermiform appendix is present only in humans, certain anthropoid apes and the wombat (a nocturnal, burrowing Australian marsupial). It is a blind muscular tube with mucosal, submucosal, muscular and serosal layers. Morphologically, it is the undeveloped distal end of the large caecum found in many lower animals. At birth, the appendix is short and broad at its junction with the caecum, but differential growth of the caecum produces the typical tubular structure by about the age of 2 years (Condon). During childhood, continued growth of the caecum commonly rotates the appendix into a retrocaecal but intraperitoneal position (Fig. 59.1). In approximately a quarter of cases, rotation of the appendix does not occur resulting in a pelvic, subcaecal or paracaecal position. Occasionally, the tip of the appendix becomes extraperitoneal lying behind the caecum or ascending colon. Rarely, the caecum does not migrate during development to its normal position in the right lower

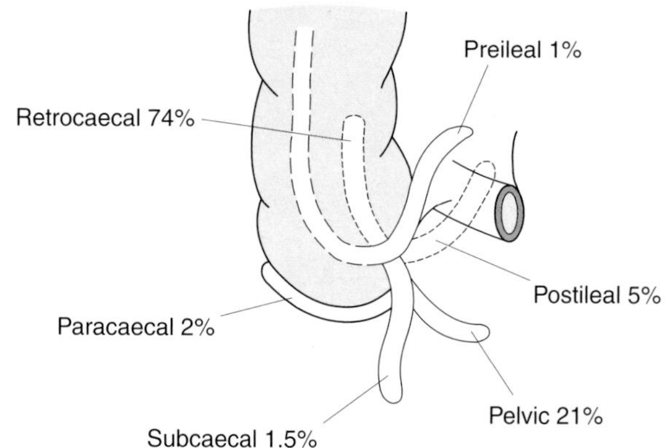

Fig. 59.1 The various positions of the appendix (*after Sir Cecil Wakeley, London, formerly PRCS*).

Robert E. Condon. Professor of Surgery, Medical College of Wisconsin, USA.

Bailey & Love's Short Practice of Surgery, 23rd edition. Edited by R.C.G. Russell, N.S. Williams and C.J.K. Bulstrode. Published in 2000 by Arnold Publishers.

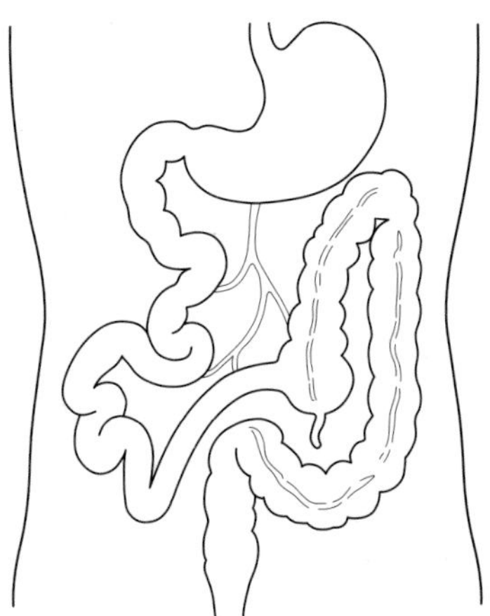

Fig. 59.2 Left-sided caecum and appendix due to an intestinal malrotation (*after Findlay and Humphreys*).

quadrant of the abdomen. In these circumstances the appendix can be found near the gall bladder or, in the case of *situs inversus viscerum*, in the left iliac fossa causing diagnostic difficulty if appendicitis develops (Fig. 59.2).

The position of the base of the appendix is constant, being found at the confluence of the three taeniae coli of the caecum which fuse to form the outer longitudinal muscle coat of the appendix. At operation, use can be made of this to find an elusive appendix, as gentle traction on the taeniae coli, particularly the anterior taenia, will lead the operator to the base of the appendix.

The mesentery of the appendix or *mesoappendix* arises from the lower surface of the mesentery of the terminal ileum, and itself is subject to great variation. Sometimes as much as the distal third of the appendix is bereft of mesoappendix. Especially in childhood, the mesoappendix is so transparent that the contained blood vessels can be seen (Fig. 59.3). In many adults it becomes laden with fat, which obscures these vessels. The *appendicular artery*, a branch of the lower division of the ileocolic artery, passes behind the terminal ileum to enter the mesoappendix a short distance from the base of the appendix. It then comes to lie in the free border of the mesoappendix. An *accessory appendicular artery* may be present but, in most people, the appendicular artery is an 'end-artery', thrombosis of which results in necrosis of the appendix (syn. gangrenous appendicitis). Four, six or more lymphatic channels traverse the mesoappendix to empty into the ileocaecal lymph nodes.

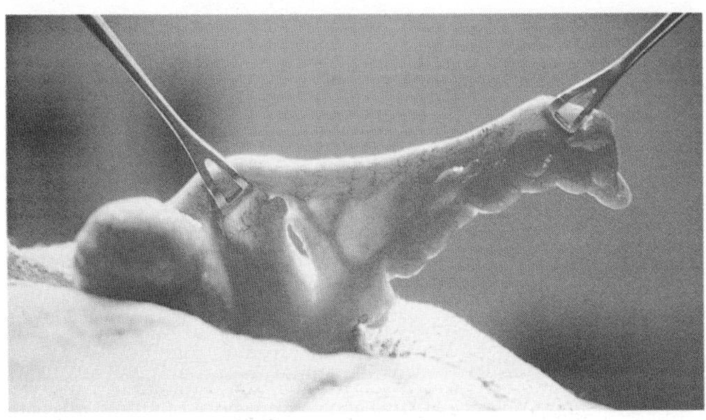

Fig. 59.3 Mesoappendix displayed demonstrating appendicular artery.

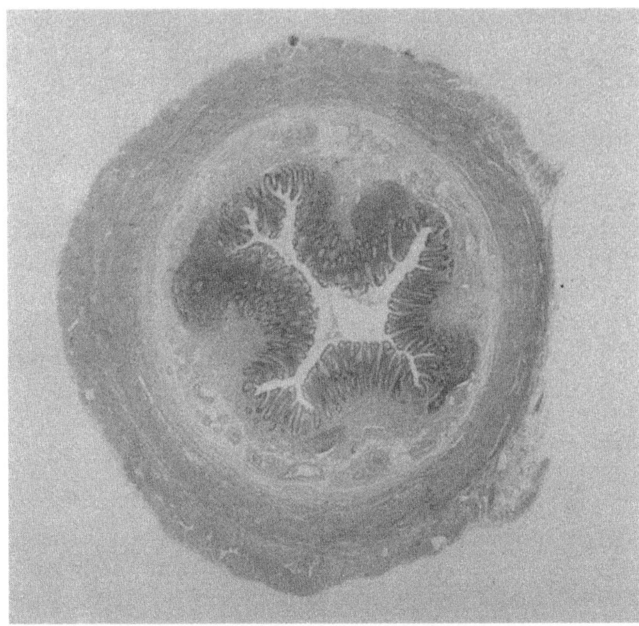

Fig. 59.4 Normal vermiform appendix. The narrow lumen is bounded by mucosa which may be arranged in folds, There is usually abundant lymphoid tissue in the mucosa, especially in younger individuals. This may encroach on and further narrow the lumen. The mucosa is bounded by a relatively thin muscularis propria (*courtesy of Dr Peter Kelly, Dublin, Ireland*).

Microscopic anatomy

The appendix varies considerably in length and circumference. The average length is between 7.5 and 10 cm. The lumen is irregular, being encroached upon by multiple longitudinal folds of mucous membrane lined by columnar cell intestinal mucosa of colonic type (Fig. 59.4). Crypts are present but are not numerous. In the base of the crypts lie argentaffin cells (Kultschitzsky cells) which may give rise to carcinoid tumours (*vide infra*). The appendix is the most frequent site for carcinoid tumours which may present with appendicitis due to occlusion of the appendiceal lumen.

The submucosa contains numerous lymphatic aggregations or follicles. This profusion of lymph tissue has promoted the concept that the appendix is the human equivalent of the avian bursa of Fabricius as a site of maturation of thymus-independent lymphocytes. While no discernible change in immune function results from appendicectomy, the prominence of lymphatic tissue in the appendix of young adults seems important in the aetiology of appendicitis (*vide infra*).

Acute appendicitis

While there are isolated reports of perityphlitis (fatal inflammation of the caecal region) from the late 1500s, recognition of acute appendicitis as a clinical entity is attributed to

Nikolai Kulschitzsky, 1856–1925. Professor of Histology, Krakov, Ukraine.

Fabricius of Acquapendente, 1537–1619. Professor of Anatomy, Padua.

Reginald Fitz who presented a paper to the first meeting of the Association of American Physicians in 1886 entitled 'Perforating inflammation of the vermiform appendix'. Soon afterwards Charles McBurney described the clinical manifestations of acute appendicitis including the point of maximum tenderness in the right iliac fossa that since bears his name. The incidence of appendicitis seems to have risen greatly in the first half of the twentieth century, particularly in Europe, America and Australasia, with up to 16 per cent of the population undergoing appendicectomy. In the past 30 years the incidence has fallen dramatically in these countries, with the number of operations in England and Wales declining from 113 000 in 1966 to 48 000 in 1990. In developing countries, which are adopting a more refined Western-type diet, the incidence continues to rise. No reason has been established for these changes in the incidence of acute appendicitis.

Acute appendicitis is relatively rare in infants, and becomes increasingly common in childhood and early adult life, reaching a peak incidence in the teens and early 20s. After middle age the risk of developing appendicitis in the future is quite small. The incidence of appendicitis is equal amongst males and females before puberty. In teenagers and young adults the male:female ratio increases to 3:2 at the age of 25 years, thereafter the greater incidence in males declines.

Aetiology

There is no unifying hypothesis regarding the aetiology of acute appendicitis. While appendicitis is clearly associated with bacterial proliferation within the appendix, no single organism is responsible, indeed a mixed growth of aerobic and anaerobic organisms is usual. The initiating event causing bacterial proliferation is controversial. Obstruction of the appendix lumen has been widely held to be important, and indeed some form of luminal obstruction by either a faecolith or stricture is found in the majority of cases.

A faecolith is composed of inspissated faecal material, calcium phosphates, bacteria and epithelial debris. Rarely a foreign body is incorporated into the mass. The incidental finding of a faecolith is a relative indication for prophylactic appendicectomy (Fig. 59.5). A fibrotic stricture of the appendix usually indicates previous appendicitis which resolved without surgical intervention (Fig. 59.6). Obstruction of the appendiceal orifice by tumour, particularly carcinoma of the caecum, is an occasional cause of acute appendicitis in middle age and the elderly. Intestinal parasites, particularly *Oxyuris vermicularis* (syn. pinworm), can proliferate in the appendix and occlude the lumen.

Pathology

Obstruction of the appendiceal lumen seems to be essential for development of appendiceal gangrene and perforation. Yet, in many cases of early appendicitis the appendix lumen is patent despite the presence of mucosal inflammation and lymphoid hyperplasia. Occasional clustering of cases amongst children and young adults suggests an infective agent, possibly viral, which initiates an inflammatory response, which within the narrow lumen of the appendix leads to luminal obstruction. Once obstruction occurs, continued mucus secretion and inflammatory exudation increase intraluminal pressure, obstructing lymphatic drainage. Oedema and mucosal ulceration develop with bacterial translocation to the submucosa. Resolution may occur at this point either spontaneously or in response to antibiotic therapy. Where the condition progresses, further distension of the appendix may cause venous obstruction and ischaemia of the appendix wall. With ischaemia, bacterial invasion occurs through the muscularis propria and submucosa producing acute appendicitis (Fig. 59.7). Finally, ischaemic necrosis of the appendix wall produces gangrenous appendicitis, with free bacterial contamination of the peritoneal cavity. Alternatively, the greater omentum and

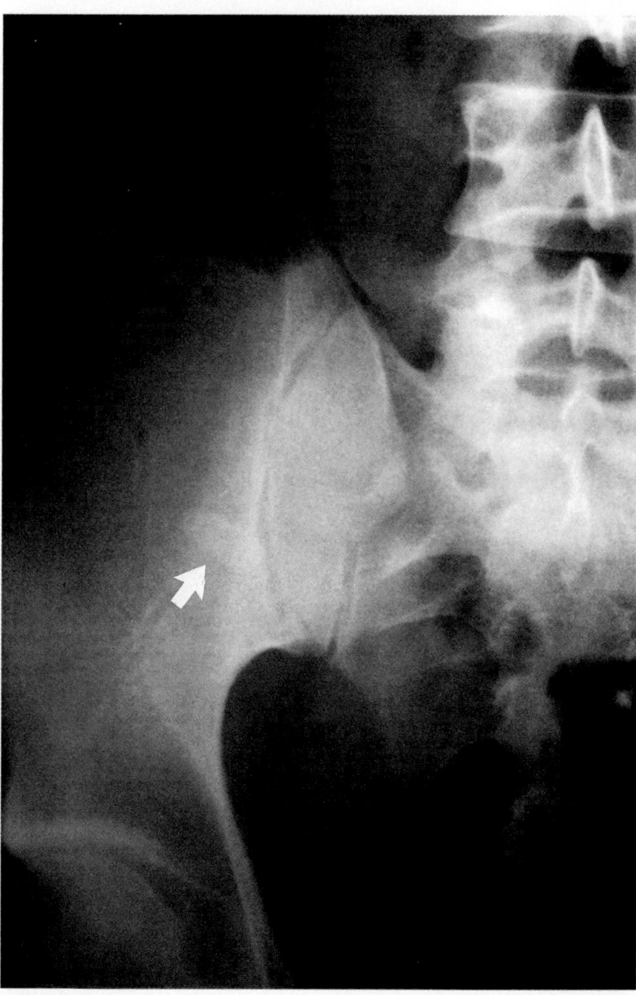

Fig. 59.5 Supine abdominal X-ray showing presence of a large faecolith in right iliac fossa (arrow).

Reginald Heber Fitz, 1843–1913. Professor of Medicine, Harvard University, Boston, Massachusetts, USA.

Charles McBurney, 1845–1913. Professor of Surgery, Columbia University, New York, USA.

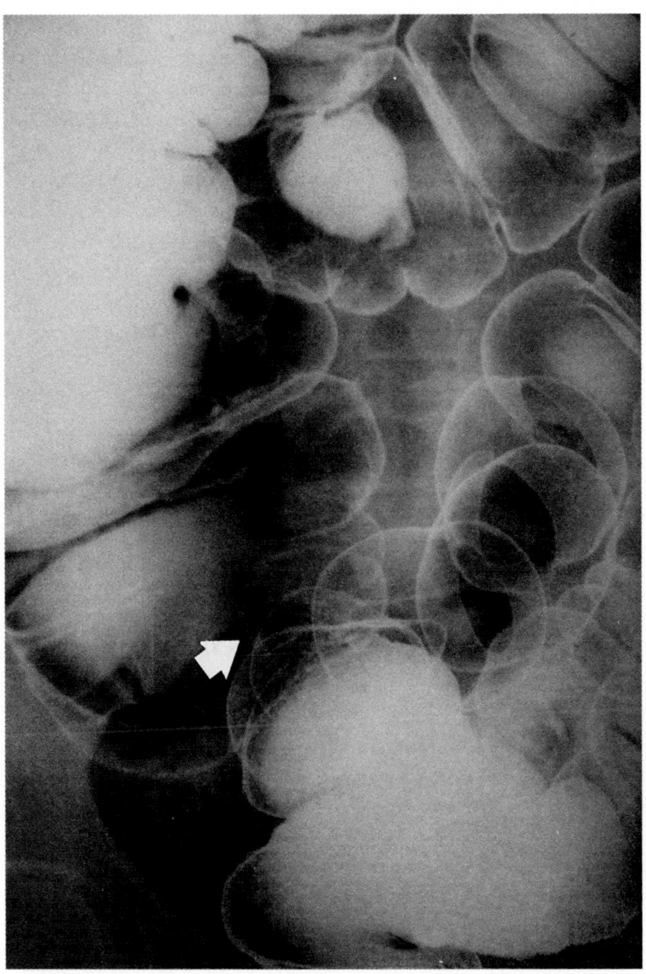

Fig. 59.6 Barium enema radiograph demonstrating faecoliths of the appendix (arrow) with distal stricture of the appendix.

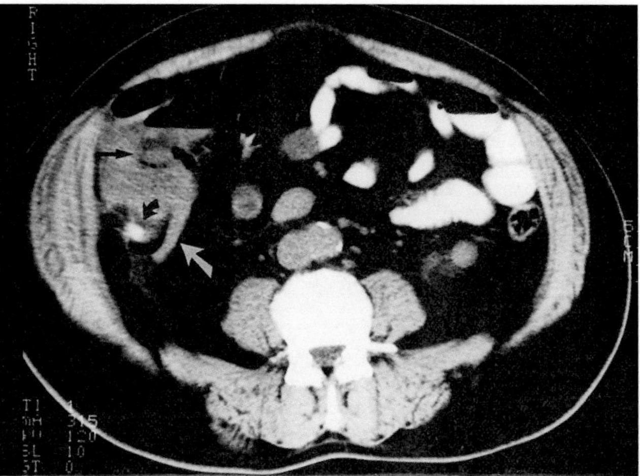

Fig. 59.8 Abdominal CT showing faecolith of the appendix (black curved arrow), distended appendix (white arrow) and phlegmonous mass surrounding tip of the appendix (straight arrow) (*courtesy of Dr Denis O'Connell, Dublin, Ireland*).

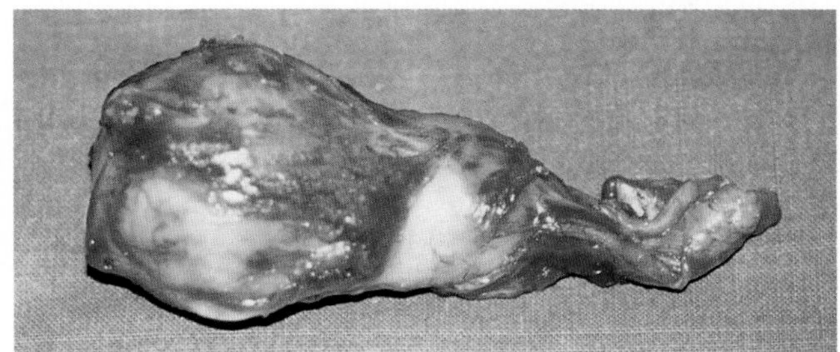

Fig. 59.9 Mucocele of the appendix, following excision.

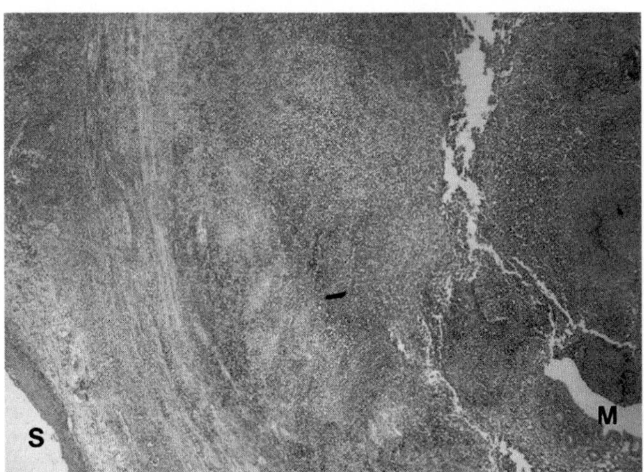

Fig. 59.7 Acute appendicitis. A heavy acute inflammatory infiltrate extends through the full thickness of the wall of the appendix, destroying the mucosa, of which only a small island (M) remains, and the smooth muscle. The Inflammation extends to involve the serosa (S) (*courtesy of Dr Peter Kelly, Dublin, Ireland*).

loops of small bowel become adherent to the inflamed appendix, walling off the spread of peritoneal contamination resulting in a phlegmonous mass or paracaecal abscess (Fig. 59.8). Rarely, appendiceal inflammation resolves leaving a distended mucus-filled organ termed a mucocele of the appendix (Fig. 59.9).

It is the potential for peritonitis that is the great threat of acute appendicitis. Peritonitis occurs as a result of free migration of bacteria through an ischaemic appendicular wall, through frank perforation of a gangrenous appendix or delayed perforation of an appendix abscess. Factors which promote this process include extremes of age, immunosupression, diabetes mellitus, faecolith obstruction of the appendix lumen, a free-lying pelvic appendix and previous abdominal surgery which limits the ability of the greater omentum to wall off the spread of peritoneal contamination (Table 59.1). In these situations a rapidly deteriorating clinical course is accompanied by signs of diffuse peritonitis and systemic sepsis syndrome.

Table 59.1 Risk factors for perforation of the appendix

- Extremes of age
- Immunosuppression
- Diabetes mellitus
- Faecolith obstruction
- Pelvic appendix
- Previous abdominal surgery

Clinical diagnosis – history

The classical features of acute appendicitis begin with poorly localised colicky abdominal pain (Table 59.2). This is due to midgut visceral discomfort in response to appendiceal inflammation and obstruction. The pain is frequently first noticed in the periumbilical region and is similar to, but less intense than, the colic of small bowel obstruction. Central abdominal pain is associated with anorexia, nausea and usually one or two episodes of vomiting which follow the onset of pain (Murphy). Anorexia is a useful and constant clinical feature, particularly in children. The patient often gives a history of similar discomfort which settled spontaneously.

With progressive inflammation of the appendix, the parietal peritoneum in the right iliac fossa becomes irritated producing more intense, constant and localised somatic pain which begins to predominate. This is often reported by the patient as an abdominal pain which has shifted and changed in character. Typically, coughing or sudden movement exacerbates the right iliac fossa pain.

The classical visceral–somatic sequence of pain is present in only about half those patients subsequently proven to have acute appendicitis. Atypical presentations include pain which is predominantly somatic or visceral and poorly localised. Atypical pain is more common in the elderly in whom localisation to the right iliac fossa is unusual. An inflamed appendix in the pelvis may never produce somatic pain involving the anterior abdominal wall, but may instead cause suprapubic discomfort and tenesmus. In this circumstance, tenderness may only be elicited on rectal examination and is the basis for the recommendation that a rectal examination should be performed on every case of lower abdominal pain.

During the first 6 hours there is rarely any alteration in temperature or pulse rate. After that time, slight pyrexia (37.2–37.7°C) with corresponding increase in the pulse rate to 80 or 90 is usual. However, in 20 per cent of cases there is no pyrexia or tachycardia in the early stages. In children a temperature greater than 38.5°C suggests other causes, for example mesenteric adenitis (*vide infra*).

Table 59.2 Clinical features of appendicitis

- Periumbilical colic
- Pain shifts to right iliac fossa
- Anorexia
- Nausea

Typically, two clinical syndromes of acute appendicitis can be discerned, acute *catarrhal* (*nonobstructive*) appendicitis and *acute obstructive* appendicitis. The latter is characterised by a much more acute course. The onset of symptoms is abrupt and there may be generalised abdominal pain from the start. The temperature may be normal and vomiting is common, so that the clinical picture may mimic acute intestinal obstruction. Once recognised, urgent surgical intervention is required because of the more rapid progression to perforation.

Clinical diagnosis – signs (Tables 59.3 and 59.4)

The diagnosis of appendicitis rests more on thorough clinical examination of the abdomen than on any aspect of the history or laboratory investigation. The cardinal features are those of an unwell patient with low-grade pyrexia, localised abdominal tenderness, muscle guarding and rebound tenderness. Inspection of the abdomen may show limitation of respiratory movement in the lower abdomen. The patient is then asked to point to where the pain began and to where it moved (*the pointing sign*). Gentle superficial palpation of the abdomen, beginning in the left iliac fossa moving anticlockwise to the right iliac fossa, will detect muscle guarding over the point of maximum tenderness, classically McBurney's point. Asking the patient to cough or gentle percussion over the site of maximum tenderness will elicit rebound tenderness.

Deep palpation of the left iliac fossa may cause pain in the right iliac fossa (Rovsing's sign), which is helpful in supporting a clinical diagnosis of appendicitis. Occasionally

Table 59.3 Clinical signs in appendicitis

- Pyrexia
- Localised tenderness in the right iliac fossa
- Muscle guarding
- Rebound tenderness

Table 59.4 Signs to elicit in appendicitis

- Pointing sign
- Rovsing's sign
- Psoas sign
- Obturator sign

John B. Murphy, 1857–1916. Surgeon, Mercy Hospital, Chicago, Illinois, USA.

Thorkild Rovsing, 1862–1937. Professor of Surgery, Copenhagen, Denmark.

an inflamed appendix lies on the psoas muscle and the patient, often a young adult, will lie with the right hip flexed for pain relief (*the psoas sign*). Spasm of the obturator internus is sometimes demonstrable when the hip is flexed and internally rotated. If an inflamed appendix is in contact with the obturator internus, this manoeuvre will cause pain in the hypogastrium (*the obturator test*) (Zachary Cope). Cutaneous hyperaesthesia may be demonstrable in the right iliac fossa, but is rarely of diagnostic value.

Special features, according to position of the appendix

Retrocaecal

Rigidity is often absent and even on deep pressure tenderness may be lacking (silent appendix), the reason being that the caecum, distended with gas, prevents the pressure exerted by the hand from reaching the inflamed structure. However, deep tenderness is often present in the loin, and rigidity of the quadratus lumborum may be in evidence. Psoas spasm, due to the inflamed appendix being in contact with that muscle, may be sufficient to cause flexion of the hip joint. Hyperextension of the hip joint may induce abdominal pain when the degree of psoas spasm is insufficient to cause flexion of the hip.

Pelvic

Occasionally early diarrhoea results from an inflamed appendix being in contact with the rectum. When the appendix lies entirely within the pelvis there is usually complete absence of abdominal rigidity, and often tenderness over McBurney's point is lacking as well. In some instances deep tenderness can be made out just above and to the right of the symphysis pubis. In either event, a rectal examination reveals tenderness in the rectovesical pouch or the pouch of Douglas, especially on the right side. Spasm of the psoas and obturator internus muscles may be present when the appendix is in this position. An inflamed appendix in contact with the bladder may cause frequ``zency of micturition.

Postileal

Although this is rare, it accounts for some of the cases of 'missed appendix'. Here the inflamed appendix lies behind the terminal ileum. It presents the greatest difficulty in diagnosis because the pain may not shift, diarrhoea is a feature and marked retching may occur. Tenderness, if any, is ill-defined, although it may be present immediately to the right of the umbilicus.

Special features, according to age

Infants

Appendicitis is relatively rare in infants under 36 months of age and for obvious reasons the patient is unable to give a history. Because of this, diagnosis is often delayed and thus the incidence of perforation and postoperative morbidity is considerably higher than in older children. Diffuse peritonitis can develop rapidly due to the underdeveloped greater omentum, which is unable to give much assistance in localising the infection.

Sir Vincent Zachary Cope, 1881–1975. Surgeon, St Mary's Hospital, London, England.

James Douglas, 1675–1742. Anatomist and Obstetrician, London, England.

Children

It is rare to find a child with appendicitis who has not vomited. Children with appendicitis usually have complete aversion to food. In addition, they do not sleep during the attack and very often bowel sounds are completely absent in the early stages.

The elderly

Gangrene and perforation occur much more frequently in elderly patients. Elderly patients with lax abdominal walls or obesity may harbour a gangrenous appendix with little evidence of it, and the clinical picture may simulate subacute intestinal obstruction. These features coupled with coincident medical conditions produce a much higher mortality for acute appendicitis in the elderly.

The obese

Obesity can obscure and diminish all the local signs of acute appendicitis. Delay in diagnosis coupled with the technical difficulty of operating in the obese make it wiser to consider operating through a midline abdominal incision.

Pregnancy

Appendicitis is the most common extrauterine acute abdominal condition in pregnancy with a frequency of from one in 1500 to one in 2000 pregnancies. Diagnosis is complicated by delay in presentation; early nonspecific symptoms are often attributed to the pregnancy, and the changing location of the appendix during pregnancy. As pregnancy develops during the second and third trimesters, the caecum and appendix are progressively pushed to the right upper quadrant of the abdomen. This displacement can result in flank or back pain, and may be confused with pyelonephritis, while lower abdominal pain may be confused with torsion of an ovarian cyst. Foetal loss occurs in 3–5 per cent of cases, increasing to 20 per cent if perforation is found at operation.

Differential diagnosis

Although acute appendicitis is the most common abdominal surgical emergency, the diagnosis at times can be extremely difficult. It is important to remember that many conditions which mimic appendicitis also require surgical intervention, or if they do not are rarely made worse by appendicectomy. However, there is a number of common conditions that it is wise to consider carefully and, where possible, exclude. The differential diagnosis differs in patients of different ages and in adult life, females have the added differential of diseases of the female genital tract (Table 59.5).

Children

The diseases most commonly mistaken for acute appendicitis are *acute gastroenteritis* and *mesenteric lymphadenitis*. In acute gastroenteritis there is intestinal colic together with diarrhoea and vomiting, but localised tenderness does not usually occur. There is often a history of other family members being affected. Postileal appendicitis may mimic this condition, thus hospital admission and careful observation are warranted. Where serious doubt persists laparoscopy or surgical exploration may be indicated. In mesenteric

Table 59.5 Differential diagnosis of acute appendicitis

Children	*Adult*	*Adult female*	*Elderly*
Gastroenteritis	Regional enteritis	Mittelschmerz	Diverticulitis
Mesenteric adenitis	Ureteric colic	Salpingitis	Intestinal obstruction
Meckel's diverticulitis	Perforated ulcer	Pylonephritis	Colonic carcinoma
Intussusception	Torsion testis	Ectopic pregnancy	Torsion appendix epiploicae
Henoch–Schönlein purpura	Pancreatitis	Torsion/rupture of an ovarian cyst	Mesenteric infarction
Lobar pneumonia	Rectus sheath haematoma	Endometriosis	Aortic aneurysm

lymphadenitis, the pain is colicky in nature and the patient may be completely free from pain between attacks, which last for a few minutes. Cervical lymph nodes may be enlarged. If present, shifting tenderness when the child turns on to his or her left side is convincing evidence. The condition presents a common diagnostic difficulty in children and if doubt exists exploration is advisable.

It may be impossible clinically to distinguish *Meckel's diverticulitis* from acute appendicitis. The pain is similar, however signs may be central or left-sided. Occasionally, there is a history of antecedent abdominal pain or anaemia.

It is important to distinguish between acute appendicitis and *intussusception*. Appendicitis is uncommon before the age of 2 years, whereas the median age for intussusception is 18 months. A mass may be palpable in the right lower quadrant and the preferred treatment of intussusception is reduction by careful barium enema.

Henoch–Schönlein purpura

This is often preceded by a sore throat or respiratory infection. Abdominal pain can be severe and be confused with intussusception or appendicitis. There is nearly always an ecchymotic rash, typically affecting the extensor surfaces of the limbs and on the buttocks. The face is usually spared. The platelet count and bleeding time are within normal limits.

Lobar pneumonia and pleurisy

Lobar pneumonia and pleurisy, especially at the right base, may give rise to right-sided abdominal pain and mimic appendicitis. Abdominal tenderness is minimal, pyrexia is marked and chest examination may reveal a pleural friction rub or altered breath sounds on auscultation. A chest radiograph is diagnostic.

Adults

Terminal ileitis

In its acute form terminal ileitis may be indistinguishable from acute appendicitis unless a doughy mass of inflamed ileum can be felt. An antecedent history of abdominal cramping, weight loss and diarrhoea suggests regional ileitis rather than appendicitis. The ileitis may be nonspecific, due to Crohn's disease or *Yersinia* infection. *Yersinia enterocolitia* causes inflammation of the terminal ileum, appendix and caecum with mesenteric adenopathy. If suspected, serum antibody titres are diagnostic and treatment with intravenous tetracycline antibiotic is appropriate. If *Yersinia* infection is suspected at operation, a mesenteric lymph node should be excised, divided, and half submitted for microbiological culture (including tuberculosis) and half for histological examination.

Ureteric colic

Ureteric colic does not commonly cause diagnostic difficulty as the character and radiation of pain differ from those of appendicitis. Urinalysis should always be performed and the presence of red cells should prompt a supine abdominal X-ray. Renal ultrasound or an intravenous urogram is diagnostic.

Right-sided acute pyelonephritis

This is accompanied and often preceded by increased frequency of micturition. It may cause difficulty in diagnosis, especially in women. The leading features are tenderness confined to the loin, fever (temperature 39°C), and possibly rigors and pyuria.

Perforated peptic ulcer

(Duodenal contents pass along the paracolic gutter to the right iliac fossa.) There is usually a history of dyspepsia and a very *sudden* onset of pain, which starts in the epigastrium and passes down the right paracolic gutter. In appendicitis the pain starts classically in the umbilical region. Rigidity and tenderness in the right iliac fossa are present in both conditions, but in perforated duodenal ulcer the rigidity is usually greater in the right hypochondrium. Radiography may show gas under the diaphragm.

Johann Friedrich Meckel (the Younger), 1781–1833. Professor of Anatomy and Surgery, Halle, Germany.
Eduard Heinrich Henoch, 1820–1910. German paediatrician.
Johann Lucas Schönlein, 1793–1864. German physician.
Burrill Bernard Crohn, b. 1884. Gastroenterologist, Mount Sinai Hospital, New York, USA.

Testicular torsion

Testicular torsion in a teenager or young adult male is easily missed. Pain can be referred to the right iliac fossa, and shyness on the part of patient may lead the unwary to suspect appendicitis unless the scrotum is examined in all cases.

Acute pancreatitis

Acute pancreatitis should be considered in the differential diagnosis of all adults suspected of acute appendicitis and when appropriate excluded by serum or urinary amylase measurement.

Rectus sheath haematoma

This is a relatively rare but easily missed differential diagnosis. It usually presents with acute pain and localised tenderness in the right iliac fossa, often after an episode of strenuous physical exercise. Localised pain without gastrointestinal upset is the rule. Occasionally, in an elderly patient, particularly those on anticoagulant therapy, a rectus sheath haematoma may present with a mass and tenderness in the right iliac fossa following minor trauma (Fig. 59.10).

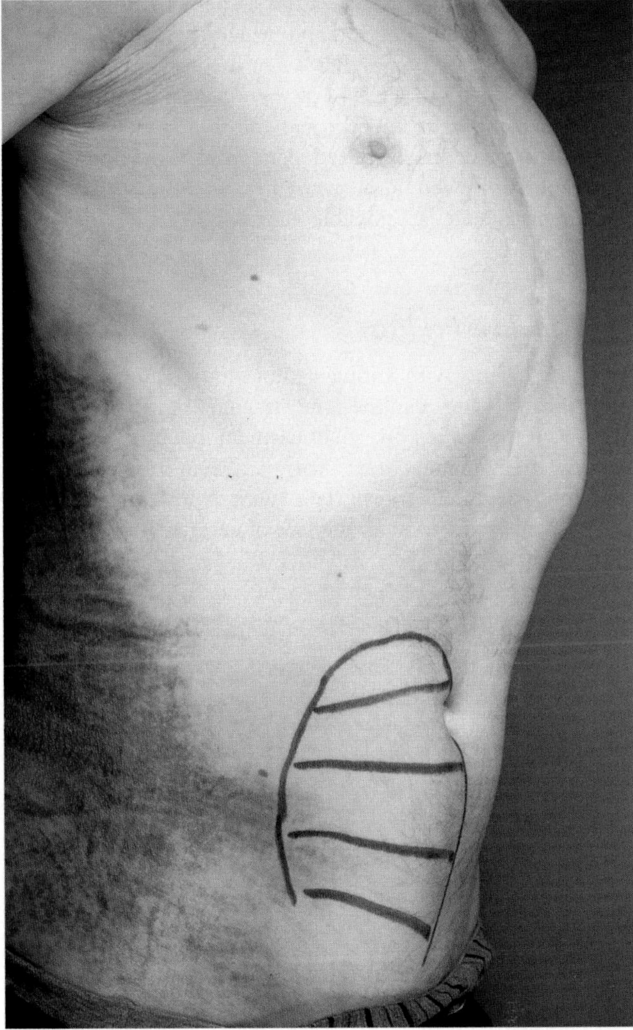

Fig. 59.10 Rectus sheath haematoma in an elderly patient taking anticoagulants, which presented as a tender mass in the right iliac fossa thought to be an appendix mass. Bruising in the flanks appeared several days later.

Adult females

It is in women of child-bearing age that pelvic disease most often mimics acute appendicitis. A careful gynaecological history should be taken in all women with suspected appendicitis concentrating on menstrual cycle, vaginal discharge and possible pregnancy. The most common diagnostic mimics are salpingitis, mittelschmerz, torsion or haemorrhage of an ovarian cyst and ectopic pregnancy.

Salpingitis

This is the condition which poses greatest diagnostic difficulty in young women. Typically, the pain is lower than in appendicitis and is bilateral. A history of vaginal discharge, dysmenorrhoea and burning pain on micturition are all helpful differential diagnostic points. There may be a history of contact with sexually transmitted disease. When suspected, the opinion of a gynaecologist should be obtained, and high vaginal swab taken for *Chlamydia* culture. When serious diagnostic uncertainty persists, diagnostic laparoscopy should be undertaken.

Mittelschmerz

Midcycle rupture of a follicular cyst with bleeding produces lower abdominal and pelvic pain, typically midcycle. Systemic upset is rare, pregnancy test is negative and symptoms usually subside within hours. Occasionally, diagnostic laparoscopy is required.

Torsion/haemorrhage of an ovarian cyst

This can prove a difficult differential diagnosis. When suspected, pelvic ultrasound and a gynaecological opinion should be sought. If encountered at operation, ovarian cystectomy should be performed, if necessary, in women of child-bearing years. Documented visualisation of the contralateral ovary is an essential medicolegal precaution.

Ectopic pregnancy

It is unlikely that a *ruptured* ectopic pregnancy, with its well-defined signs of haemoperitoneum, will be mistaken for acute appendicitis, but the same cannot be said for a right-sided tubal abortion, or still more for a right-sided unruptured tubal pregnancy. In the latter, the signs are very similar to those of acute appendicitis, except that the pain *commences* on the right side and stays there. The pain is severe and continues unabated until operation. Usually there is a history of a missed menstrual period and urinary pregnancy test may be positive. Severe pain is felt when the cervix is moved on vaginal examination. Signs of intraperitoneal bleeding usually become apparent and the patient should be questioned specifically regarding referred pain in the shoulder. Pelvic ultrasonography should be carried out in all cases where an ectopic pregnancy is a possible diagnosis.

Elderly

Sigmoid diverticulitis

In some patients with a long sigmoid loop, the colon lies to the right of the midline and it may be impossible to differentiate between diverticulitis and appendicitis. A trial of conservative management with intravenous fluids and antibiotics is often appropriate, with a low threshold for exploratory laparotomy in the face of deterioration or lack of clinical response.

Intestinal obstruction

The diagnosis of intestinal obstruction is usually clear, the subtlety lies in recognising acute appendicitis as the occasional cause in the elderly. As with diverticulitis, intravenous fluids, antibiotics and nasogastric decompression should be instigated with early resort to laparotomy.

Carcinoma of the caecum

When obstructed or locally perforated, carcinoma of the caecum may mimic or cause obstructive appendicitis in adults. A history of antecedent discomfort, altered bowel habit or unexplained anaemia should raise suspicion. A mass may be palpable (*vide infra*) and barium enema or colonoscopy is diagnostic.

Rare differential diagnoses

Preherpetic pain of the right 10th and 11th dorsal nerves is localised over the same area as that of appendicitis. It does not shift and is associated with marked hyperaesthesia. There is no intestinal upset or rigidity. The herpetic eruption may be delayed for 3–8 hours. *Tabetic crises* are now rare. Severe abdominal pain and vomiting usher in the crisis. Other signs of tabes confirm the diagnosis. *Spinal conditions* are sometimes associated with acute abdominal pain, especially in children and the elderly. These may include tuberculosis of the spine, metastatic carcinoma, osteoporotic vertebral collapse and multiple myeloma. The pain is due to compression of nerve roots and may be aggravated by movement. There is rigidity of the lumbar spine and intestinal symptoms are absent. The abdominal crises of *porphyria and diabetes mellitus* need to be remembered. A urinalysis should be tested in every abdominal emergency. In *cyclical vomiting* of infants or young children there is a history of previous similar attacks, and abdominal rigidity is absent. Acetone is found in the urine but is not diagnostic as it may accompany starvation. *Typhlitis* or *leukaemic ileocaecal syndrome* is a rare but potentially fatal enterocolitis occurring in immunosuppressed patients. Gram-negative or *clostridial* (especially *C. septicum*) septicaemia can be rapidly progressive. Treatment is with appropriate antibiotics and haematopoetic factors. Surgical intervention is rarely indicated.

Investigation

The diagnosis of acute appendicitis is essentially clinical. A full blood count and urinalysis should be performed in all cases. In women of reproductive years, it is wise to obtain a urinary pregnancy test before proceeding to exploration. Pelvic ultrasound is of value in excluding tubal or ovarian disease if suspected. Abdominal ultrasound examination is a useful diagnostic tool, particularly in children, with a diagnostic accuracy of appendicitis in excess of 90 per cent (Fig. 59.11).

In dehydrated or elderly patients or where comorbid conditions dictate, serum urea and electrolytes should be checked. If a diagnosis of intestinal obstruction, intussusception or ureteric colic is being entertained, a supine abdominal X-ray should be performed (Table 59.6).

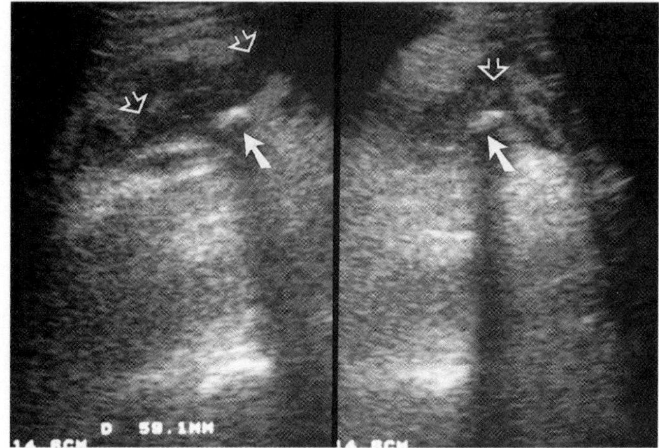

Fig. 59.11 Abdominal ultrasound examination showing features of acute appendicitis, distended oedmatous appendix (open arrows), longitudinal scan (left) and transverse scan (right). A faecolith is seen (closed arrow) (*courtesy of Dr Michael Behan, Dublin, Ireland*).

Table 59.6 Preoperative investigations in appendicitis routine

- Routine:
  - Full blood count
  - Urinalysis
- Selected cases:
  - Pregnancy test
  - Urea and electrolytes
  - Supine abdominal X-ray
  - Ultrasound abdomen/pelvis

Hans Christian Joachim Gram, 1853–1938. Professor of Medicine, Copenhagen, Denmark.

Treatment

The treatment of acute appendicitis is appendicectomy. There is a perception that urgent operation is essential to prevent the increased morbidity and mortality of peritonitis. While there should be no unnecessary delay, all patients, particularly those most at risk of serious morbidity, benefit from a short period of intensive preoperative preparation. Intravenous fluids sufficient to establish adequate urine output (catheterisation is needed only in the very ill) and appropriate antibiotics should be given. There is ample evidence that a single perioperative dose of antibiotics reduces the incidence of postoperative wound infection. When peritonitis is suspected, therapeutic intravenous antibiotics to cover Gram-negative bacilli, as well as anaerobic cocci, should be given. Hyperpyrexia in children should be treated with salicylates in addition to antibiotics and intravenous fluids. With appropriate use of intravenous fluids and parentral antibiotics, a policy of deferring appendicectomy after midnight to first case on the following morning does not increase morbidity. However, when acute obstructive appendicitis is recognised, operation should not be deferred longer than it takes to optimise the patient's condition.

Appendicectomy

Appendicectomy may be performed by conventional open operation or by using laparoscopic techniques. The first surgeon to perform deliberate appendicectomy for acute appendicitis was Lawson Tait, in May 1880. The patient recovered. It is recorded in 1736 that Claudius Amyand successfully removed an acutely inflamed appendix from the hernial sac of a boy.

Appendicectomy should be performed under general anaesthetic with the patient supine on the operating table. When a laparoscopic technique is to be used, a nasogastric tube should be inserted and the bladder must be empty (ensure the patient has voided before leaving the ward). Prior to preparing the entire abdomen with an appropriate antiseptic solution, the right iliac fossa should be palpated for a mass. If a mass is felt, it may, on occasion, be preferable to adopt a conservative approach (*vide infra*). Draping of the abdomen is in accordance with the planned operative technique, taking account of any requirement to extend the incision or convert a laparoscopic technique to open operation.

Conventional appendicectomy

When the preoperative diagnosis is considered reasonably certain, the incision that is widely used for appendicectomy is the so-called *grid-iron incision* (a grid-iron was a frame of cross-beams to support a ship during repairs). The grid-iron incision (described first by McArthur) is made at right angles to a line joining the anterior superior iliac spine to the umbilicus, its centre being along the line at McBurney's point (Fig. 59.12). In the subcutaneous tissues an arterial twig from the superficial circumflex iliac artery usually requires ligation. The external oblique is incised in the line of its fibres along the length of the incision. The fibres of the internal oblique and transversus abdominis are split, and with suitable retraction the peritoneum is opened. If better access is required, it is possible to convert the grid-iron to a Rutherford Morrison incision (*vide infra*) by cutting the internal oblique and transversus muscles in the line of the incision.

In recent years, a transverse *skin crease* (Lanz) incision has become more popular, as the exposure is better and extension, when needed, is easier. The incision, appropriate in length to the size and obesity of the patient, is made approximately 2 cm below the umbilicus centred on the midclavicular–midinguinal line (Fig. 59.13). The external oblique aponeurosis, internal oblique and transversus muscles are split in the direction of the fibres and the peritoneum is opened. When necessary the incision may be extended medially, with retraction or suitable division of the rectus abdominis muscle.

When the diagnosis is in doubt, particularly in the presence of intestinal obstruction, a lower midline abdominal incision is to be preferred over a right lower paramedian incision. The latter, although widely practised in the past, is difficult to extend, more difficult to close and provides less good access to the pelvis and peritoneal cavity.

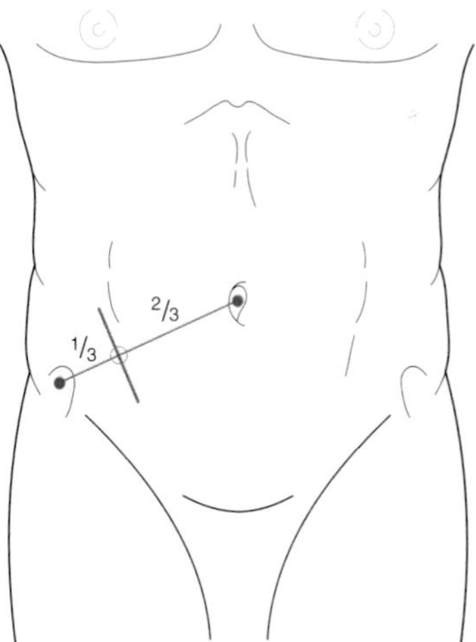

Fig. 59.12 Grid-iron incision for appendicitis, at right angles to the line joining anterior superior iliac spine and umbilicus, centred on McBurney's point (*courtesy of Mr Michael Earley, Dublin, Ireland*).

Lawson Tait, 1845–99. Surgeon, Hospital for Diseases of Women, Birmingham, England.

Claudius Amyand, 1685–1740. Surgeon, St George's Hospital, London, England.

Lewis Linn McArthur, 1858–1934. Surgeon, St Luke's Hospital, Chicago, Illinois, USA.

James Rutherford Morrison, 1853–1939. Professor of Surgery, University of Durham, England.

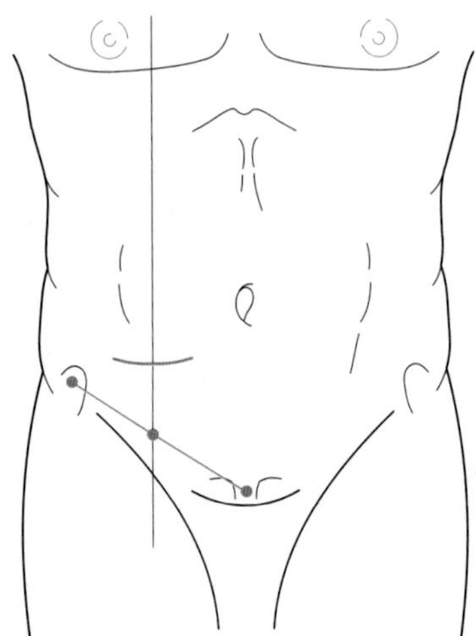

Fig. 59.13 Transverse or skin crease incision for appendicitis, 2 cm below the umbilicus, centred on the midclavicular–midinguinal line (*courtesy of Mr Michael Earley, Dublin, Ireland*).

Rutherford Morrison's incision is useful if the appendix is paracaecal or retrocaecal and fixed. It is essentially an oblique muscle-cutting incision with its lower end over McBurney's point and extending obliquely upwards and laterally as necessary. All layers are divided in the line of the incision.

Removal of the appendix

It will be assumed that the abdomen has been opened by a skin crease incision. A retractor is placed under the medial side of the wound and the peritoneum, and the abdominal wall is elevated. Serous exudate is removed with a sucker. Pus, if present, is likewise removed having first retained a specimen for microbiological culture. The caecum is identified by the presence of teniae coli, and using a finger or a swab the caecum is withdrawn. A turgid appendix may be felt at the base of the caecum. Inflammatory adhesions must be gently broken with a finger which is then hooked around the appendix to deliver it into the wound. The appendix is conveniently controlled using a Babcock or Lane's forceps applied in such a way as to encircle the appendix and yet not damage it. The base of the mesoappendix is clamped in a haemostat, divided and ligated (Fig. 59.14a). When the mesoappendix is broad the procedure must be repeated with a second, or rarely, a third haemostat. The appendix, now completely freed, is crushed near its junction with the caecum in a haemostat, which is removed and reapplied just distal to the crushed portion. An absorbable 2/0 ligature is tied around the crushed portion close to the caecum. The appendix is amputated between the haemostat and the ligature (Fig. 59.14b). An absorbable 2/0 or 3/0 purse-string or 'Z' suture may then be inserted into the caecum about 1 cm from the base (Fig. 59.14c). The stitch should pass through the muscle coat, picking up the taeniae coli. The stump of the appendix is invaginated (Fig. 59.14d) while the purse-string or 'Z' suture is tied, thus burying the appendix stump. Many surgeons believe that invagination of the appendiceal stump is unnecessary.

William Wayne Babcock, 1872–1963. American surgeon.
Sir William Arbuthnot Lane, 1856–1943. British surgeon.

Methods to be adopted in special circumstances

When the caecal wall is oedematous, the purse-string suture is in danger of cutting out. If the oedema is of limited extent this can be overcome by inserting the purse-string suture into more healthy caecal wall at a greater distance from the base of the appendix. Occasions may arise when, because of the extensive oedema of the caecal wall, it is better not to attempt invagination.

When the base of the appendix is inflamed, it should not be crushed but ligated close to the caecal wall just tightly enough to occlude the lumen, after which the appendix is amputated and the stump invaginated. Should the base of the appendix be gangrenous, neither crushing nor ligation must be attempted. Two stitches are placed through the caecal wall close to the base of the gangrenous appendix, which is amputated flush with the caecal wall, after which these stitches are tied. Further closure is effected by means of a second layer of interrupted seromuscular sutures.

Retrograde appendicectomy

When the appendix is retrocaecal and adherent, it is an advantage to divide the base between haemostats. The appendiceal vessels are then ligated, the stump is ligated and invaginated, and gentle traction on the caecum will enable the surgeon to deliver the body of the appendix which is then removed from base to tip. Occasionally, this manoeuvre requires division of the lateral peritoneal attachments of the caecum.

Drainage of the peritoneal cavity

This is usually unnecessary provided adequate peritoneal toilet has been done. If, however, there is considerable purulent fluid in the retrocaecal space or the pelvis, a soft silastic drain may be inserted through a separate stab incision. The wound should be closed using absorbable sutures to oppose muscles and aponeurosis. In the presence of soiling or if a gangrenous appendix has been delivered through the wound, it is often wise to leave open or to delay primary closure by inserting a gauze wick between interrupted skin sutures (Brady) (Fig. 59.15).

Laparoscopic appendicectomy

The most valuable aspect of laparoscopy in the management of suspected appendicitis is as a diagnostic tool, particularly in women of child-bearing age. In general, an open technique should be used to establish a pneumoperitoneum, and for insertion of the laparoscopic ports as it is safer than the closed techniques using a Verres needle. The placement of the operating port may vary according to operator preference and previous abdominal scars. The operator stands to the patient's left and faces a video monitor placed at the patient's

Michael P. Brady. Professor of Surgery, University College Cork, Ireland.

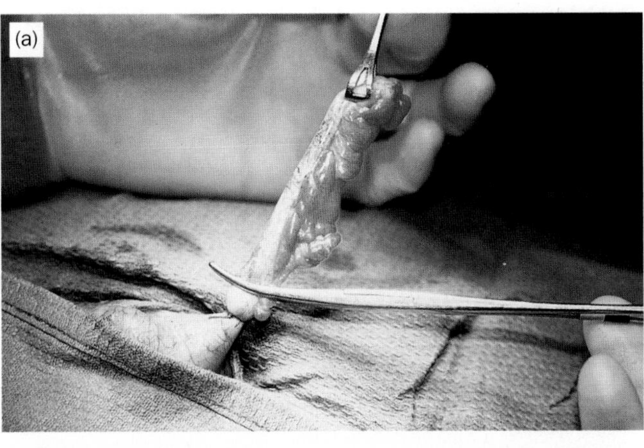

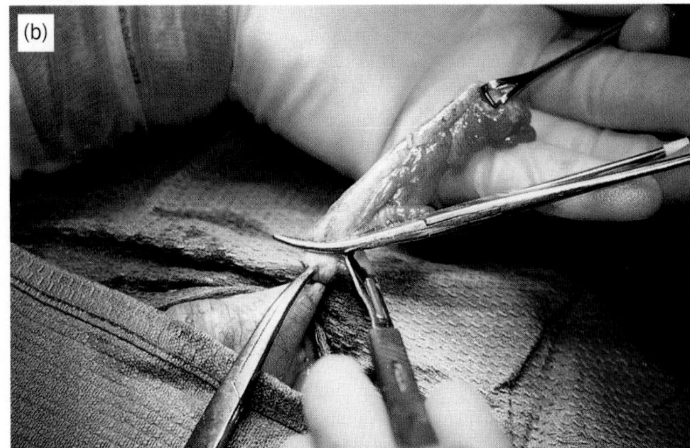

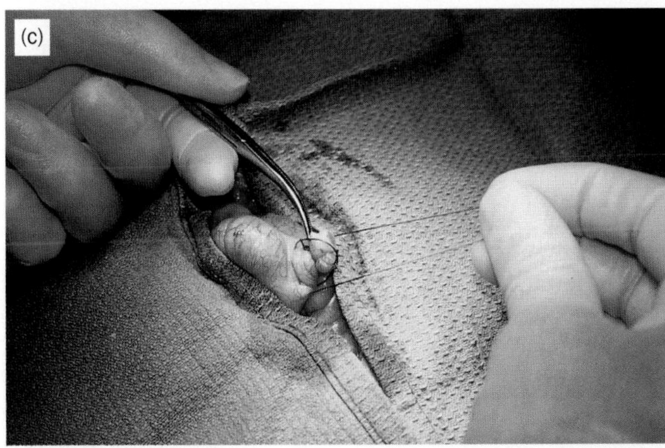

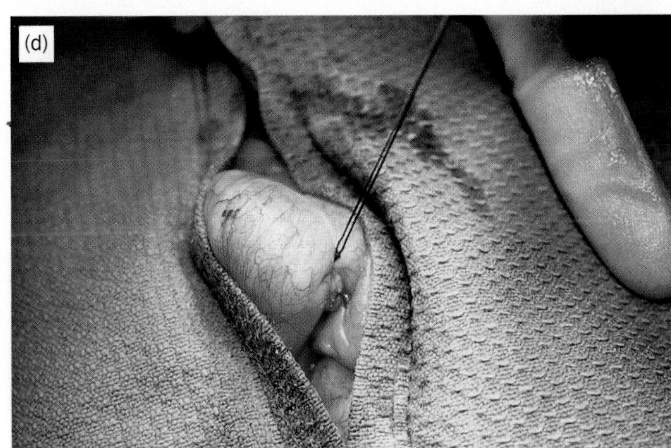

Fig. 59.14 (a) Mesoappendix divided between haemostats and ligated. (b) Appendix crushed and ligated at its base and about to be divided. (c) 'Z' suture inserted prior to inversion of the appendiceal stump. (d) Appendiceal stump inverted, the 'Z' suture having been tied.

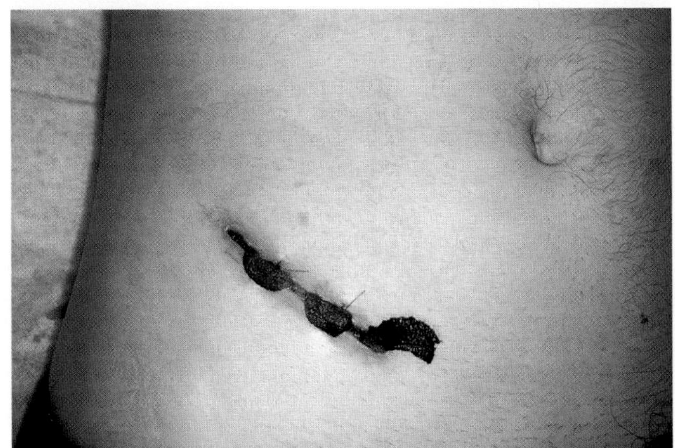

Fig. 59.15 Appendicectomy wound following excision of gangrenous appendix. Wound drainage and delayed primary closure achieved by use of a gauze wick, soaked in dilute povodone iodine solution.

right foot (Fig. 59.16). A moderate Trendelenberg tilt of the operating table assists delivery of loops of small bowel from the pelvis. The appendix is found in the conventional manner by identification of the caecal taeniae and is controlled using laparoscopic tissue-holding forceps. By elevating the appendix the mesoappendix is displayed (Fig. 59.17a). A dissecting forceps is used to create a window in the mesoappendix to allow the appendicular vessels to be coagulated or ligated using a clip applicator. The appendix, free of its mesentery, can be ligated at its base with an absorbable loop ligature (Fig. 59.17b), divided (Fig. 59.17c) and removed through one of the operating ports. It is not usual to invert the stump of the appendix (Fig. 59.17d). A single absorbable suture is used to close the linea alba at the umbilicus and the small skin incisions may be closed with a subcuticular suture (Fig. 59.18).

Patients who undergo laparoscopic appendicectomy are likely to be discharged from hospital and return to work slightly sooner than those who have undergone open appendicectomy, but it remains to be seen whether this justifies the slightly longer operating time and higher costs involved.

Fredrich Trendelenburg, 1844–1924. German surgeon.

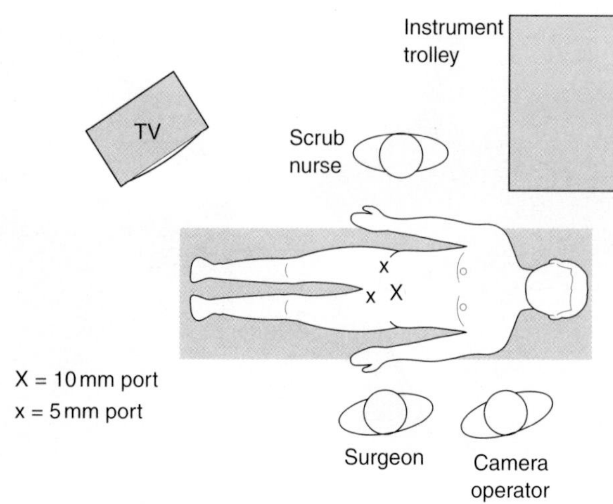

Fig. 59.16 Position of surgeon, assistants and equipment for laparoscopic appendicectomy.

Problems encountered during appendicectomy

- *A normal appendix is found* – this demands careful exclusion of other possible diagnoses, particularly terminal ileitis, Meckel's diverticulitis and tubal or ovarian causes in women. It is usual to remove the appendix to avoid future diagnostic difficulties, even though the appendix is macroscopically normal, particularly if a skin crease or grid-iron incision has been made. A case can be made for preserving the macroscopically normal appendix seen at diagnostic laparoscopy, although approximately a quarter of seemingly normal appendices show microscopic evidence of inflammation.
- *The appendix cannot be found* – the caecum should be mobilised and the taenia coli should be traced to their confluence on the caecum before the diagnosis of 'absent appendix' is made.
- *An appendicular tumour is found* – small tumours (under 2.0 cm in diameter) can be removed by appendicectomy; larger tumours should be treated by a right hemicolectomy.
- *An appendix abscess is found* and the appendix cannot be removed easily – this should be treated by local peritoneal toilet, drainage of any abscess and intravenous antibiotics. Very rarely a caecectomy or partial right hemicolectomy is required. (The first recorded operation for an appendix abscess was by Henry Hancock of Charing Cross Hospital, London, in 1848.)

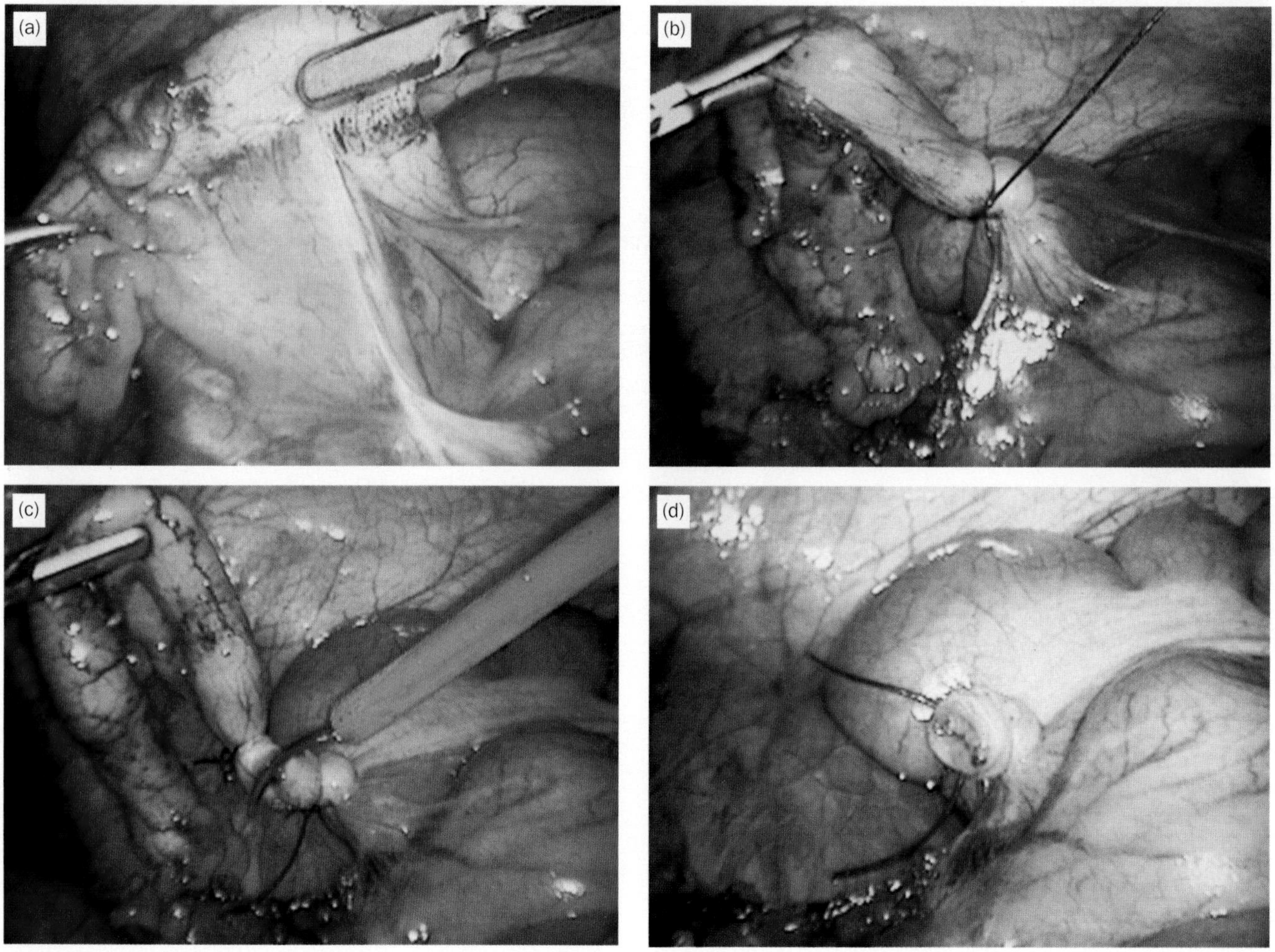

Fig. 59.17 Laparoscopic appendicectomy: (a) mesoappendix displayed; (b) ligation at the base of the appendix; (c) division of base; and (d) appendicectomy complete (*courtesy of Mr Oliver McAnena, Galway, Ireland*).

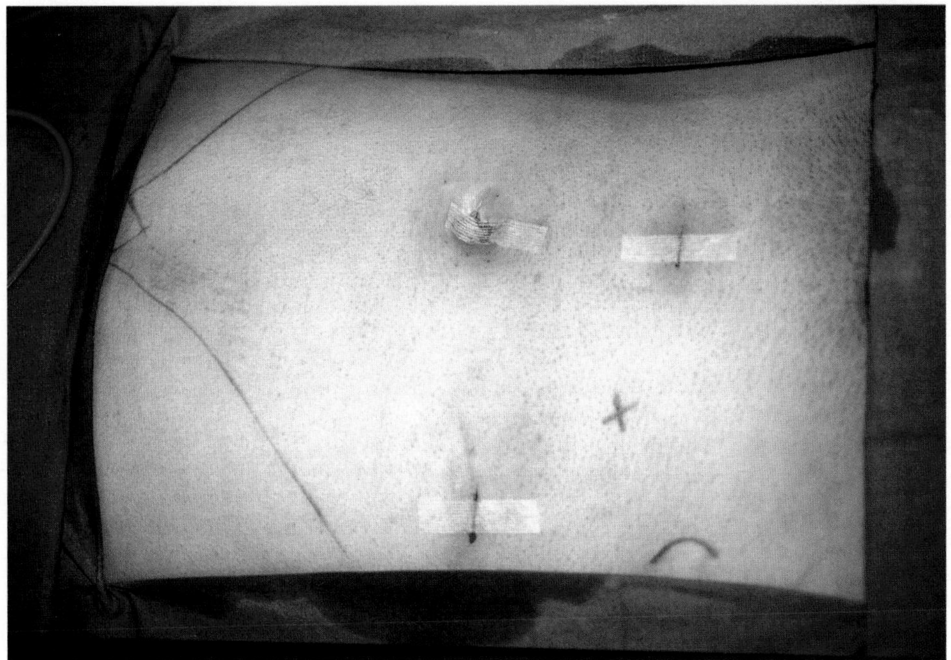

Fig. 59.18 Abdominal wall following completion of laparoscopic appendicectomy (*courtesy of Mr Conor Delaney, Dublin, Ireland*).

Appendicitis complicating Crohn's disease

Occasionally, a patient is operated on for acute appendicitis who is found to have concomitant Crohn's disease of the ileo-caecal region. Providing the caecal wall is healthy at the base of the appendix, appendicectomy can be performed without increasing the risk of an enterocutaneous fistula. Rarely, the appendix is involved with the Crohn's disease. In this situation a conservative approach may be warranted, and a trial of intravenous corticosteroids and systemic antibiotics used to resolve the acute inflammatory process.

Appendix abscess

Failure of resolution of an appendix mass or continued spiking pyrexia usually indicates that there is pus within the phlegmonous appendix mass. Ultrasound or abdominal CT scan may identify an area suitable for insertion of a percutaneous drain. Should this prove unsuccessful, laparotomy through a midline incision is indicated.

Pelvic abscess

Pelvic abscess formation is an occasional complication of appendicitis and can occur irrespective of the position of the appendix within the peritoneal cavity. The most common presentation is a spiking pyrexia several days following appendicitis; indeed the patient may have already been discharged from hospital. Pelvic pressure or discomfort associated with loose stool or tenesmus is common. Rectal examination reveals a boggy mass in the pelvis, anterior to the rectum, at the level of the peritoneal reflection (Fig. 59.19). Pelvic ultrasound or CT scan will confirm. Treatment is transrectal drainage under general anaesthetic.

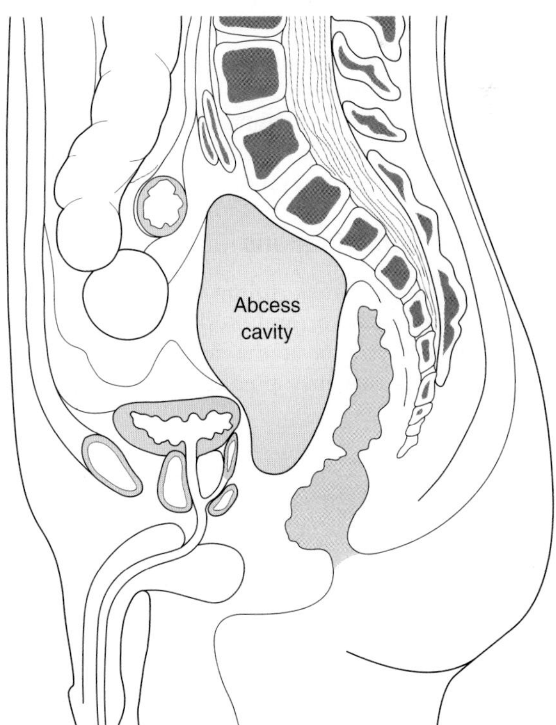

Fig. 59.19 Appendix abscess involving the pelvis. Note the relationship to the rectum.

Table 59.7 Criteria for stopping conservative treatment of appendix mass

- A rising pulse rate
- Increasing or spreading abdominal pain
- Increasing size of the mass
- Vomiting or copious gastric aspirate

Management of an appendix mass

If an appendix mass is present and the condition of the patient is satisfactory, the standard treatment is the conservative Ochsner–Sherren regimen. This strategy is based on the premise that the inflammatory process is already localised and that inadvertent surgery is difficult and may be dangerous. It may be impossible to find the appendix and, occasionally, a faecal fistula may form. For these reasons it is wise to observe a nonoperative programme, but to be prepared to operate should clinical deterioration occur (Table 59.7).

Careful record of the patient's condition and the extent of the mass should be made, and the abdomen regularly re-examined. It is helpful to mark the limits of mass on the abdominal wall using a skin pencil. A nasogastric tube should be passed and intravenous fluid and antibiotic therapy instigated. Temperature and pulse rate should be recorded 4-hourly and a fluid balance record maintained. Clinical deterioration or evidence of peritonitis is indication for early laparotomy. Clinical improvement is usually evident within 24–48 hours at which time the nasogastric tube can be removed and oral fluids introduced. Failure of the mass to resolve should raise suspicion of a carcinoma or Crohn's disease. Using this regime approximately 90 per cent of cases resolve without incident. It is advisable to remove the appendix usually after an interval of 6–8 weeks.

Postoperative complications

Postoperative complications following appendicectomy are relatively uncommon and reflect the degree of peritonitis that was present at the time of operation and intercurrent diseases that may predispose to complications (Table 59.8).

Wound infection

This is the most common postoperative complication which occurs in 5–10 per cent of all cases. This usually presents with pain and erythema of the wound on the fourth or fifth postoperative day, often soon after hospital discharge.

Albert John Ochsner, 1858–1925. Professor of Clinical Surgery, University of Illnois, Chicago, Illinois, USA.

James Sherren, 1872–1945. Surgeon, The London Hospital, London, England.

Table 59.8 Checklist for an unwell patient following appendicectomy

- Examine the wound and abdomen for an abscess
- Consider a pelvic abscess, and perform a rectal examination
- Examine the lungs – pneumonitis or collapse
- Examine the legs, consider venous thrombosis
- Examine the conjunctivae for an icteric tinge and the liver for enlargement, and enquire if the patient has had rigors (pylephlebitis)
- Examine the urine for organisms (pyelonephritis)
- Suspect subphrenic abscess

Treatment is by wound drainage and antibiotics when required. The organisms responsible are usually a mixture of Gram-negative bacilli and anaerobic bacteria, predominantly *Bacteroides* species and anaerobic streptococci.

Intra-abdominal abscess

Intra-abdominal abscess has become a relatively rare complication after appendicectomy with the use of perioperative antibiotics. Postoperative spiking fever, malaise and anorexia, developing 5–7 days after operation, suggest an intraperitoneal collection. Interloop, paracolic, pelvic and subphrenic sites should be considered. Abdominal ultrasonography and CT scanning greatly facilitate diagnosis and allow percutaneous drainage. Laparotomy should be considered in patients suspected to have intrabdominal sepsis in whom imaging fails to show a collection, particularly those with continuing ileus.

Ileus

A period of adynamic ileus is to be expected after appendicectomy, and may last for a number of days following removal of a gangrenous appendix. Ileus persisting for more than 4–5 days, particularly in the presence of a fever, is indicative of continuing intra-abdominal sepsis and should prompt further investigation (see above).

Respiratory

In the absence of concurrent pulmonary disease, respiratory complications are rare following appendicectomy. Adequate postoperative analgesia and physiotherapy, when appropriate, reduce the incidence.

Venous thrombosis and embolism

These are rare after appendicectomy except in the elderly and women taking the oral contraceptive pill. Appropriate prophylactic measures should be taken in such cases.

Portal pyaemia (pylephlebitis)

Pylephlebitis is a rare but very serious complication of gangrenous appendicitis associated with high fever, rigors and jaundice. It is due to septicaemia in the portal venous system and may leads to the development of intrahepatic abscesses (often multiple). Treatment is with systemic antibiotics and percutaneous drainage of hepatic abscesses as appropriate.

Faecal fistula

Leakage from the appendicular stump rarely occurs, but may follow if the encircling stitch has been put in too deeply or if the caecal wall was involved by oedema or inflammation. Occasionally, a fistula may result following appendicectomy in Crohn's disease.

Adhesive intestinal obstruction

Adhesive intestinal obstruction is the most common late complication of appendicectomy. At operation often a single band adhesion is responsible. Occasionally, chronic pain in the right iliac fossa is attributed to adhesion formation after appendicectomy. In such cases laparoscopy is of value in confirming the presence of adhesions and allowing division.

Right inguinal hernia

This is said to be more common following a grid-iron incision for appendicitis due to injury to the iliohypogastric nerve.

Recurrent acute appendicitis

Appendicitis is notoriously recurrent. It is not uncommon for patients to attribute such attacks to 'biliousness' or dyspepsia. The attacks vary in intensity, may occur every few months and the majority of cases ultimately culminate in severe acute appendicitis. If a careful history is taken from patients with acute appendicitis many remember having had milder but similar attacks of pain. The appendix in these cases shows fibrosis indicative of previous inflammation (Fig. 59.20). Chronic appendicitis, per se, does not exist. Patients labelled thus are usually examples of the recurrent form of the disease.

Less common pathological conditions

Mucocele of the appendix

Mucocele of the appendix may occur when the proximal end of the lumen slowly becomes completely occluded, usually by a fibrous stricture, and the pent-up secretion remains sterile. The appendix is greatly enlarged and sometimes it contains several millilitres of mucus (Fig. 59.9). The symptoms produced are those of mild subacute appendicitis unless infection supervenes, when the mucocele is converted into an *empyema*. Rupture of a mucocele of the appendix is a cause of *pseudomyxoma peritonei*. Occasionally, the mucocele is caused by a mucus-secreting adenocarcinoma, in which case a right hemicolectomy is the correct treatment.

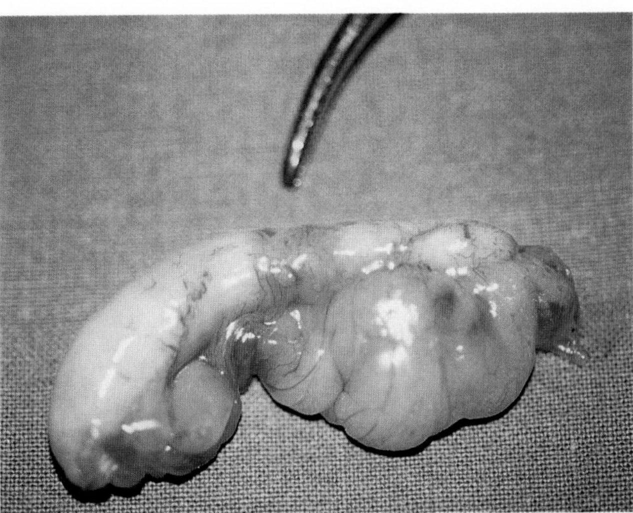

Fig. 59.20 Excised appendix showing point of luminal obstruction with distal fibrosis.

Diverticulae of the appendix

Diverticulosis of the appendix is relatively rare and the diverticulae may be true congenital (all coats) or acquired (no muscularis layer). The condition may occur in conjunction with mucocele, in which case the intramural pressure rises sufficiently to cause herniation of the mucous membrane through the muscle coat at several points. More often, there is no demonstrable obstruction to the lumen. The patient usually gives a history of previous recurrent attacks of appendicitis. If encountered during the course of an operation for another condition, a diverticulae-bearing appendix should be removed because of a propensity to perforate if inflamed.

Intussusception of the appendix

This is rare and occurs mostly in childhood. It can be diagnosed only at operation. The symptoms usually are not acute. Untreated, the condition may pass on to an appendiculocolic intussusception. The appendix may slough, and this accounts for most of the very rare cases in which the appendix is absent. The treatment is appendicectomy.

Neoplasms of the appendix

Carcinoid tumour (syn. argentaffinoma)

Carcinoid tumours arise in argentaffin tissue (Kulschitzsky cells of the crypts of Lieberkuhn) and are most commonly found in the vermiform appendix. Carcinoid tumour is found once in every 300–400 appendices subjected to histological examination and is 10 times more common than any other neoplasm of the appendix. In many instances the appendix had been removed because of symptoms of subacute or recurrent appendicitis. The tumour can occur in any part of the appendix, but it frequently does so in the distal third. The neoplasm feels moderately hard, and on sectioning the appendix it can be seen as a yellow tumour

Johann Nathaniel Lieberkühn, 1711–56. German anatomist.

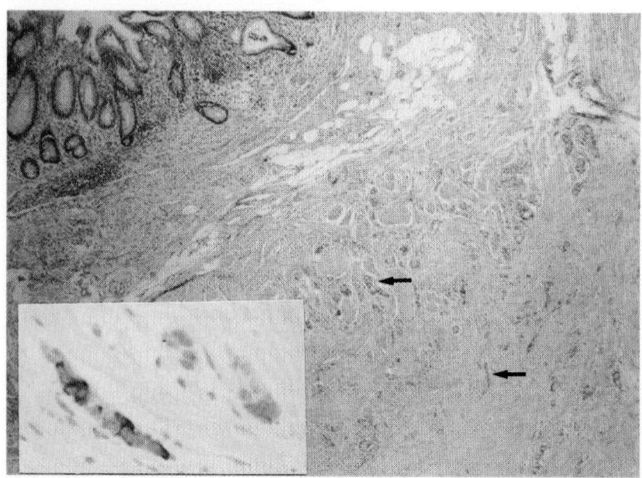

Fig. 59.21 Carcinoid tumour. A small incidental carcinoid tumour of the appendix. The tumour cells infiltrate through the muscle arranged in small nests and trabeculae (arrows). Tumour cells are small and have inconspicuous nuclei. Inset: higher magnification of an immunohistochemical stain for Chromogranin B shows a strong positive reaction (brown) of tumour cells (*courtesy of Dr Peter Kelly, Dublin, Ireland*).

between the intact mucosa and the peritoneum. Microscopically, the tumour cells are small, arranged in small nests within the muscle and have a characteristic pattern using immunohistochemical stain for Chromogranin B (Fig. 59.21). Unlike carcinoid tumours arising in other parts of the intestinal tract, carcinoid tumour of the appendix rarely gives rise to metastases. Appendicectomy has been shown to be sufficient treatment, unless the caecal wall is involved, the tumour is 2 cm or more in size, or involved lymph nodes are found, otherwise right hemicolectomy is indicated.

Primary adenocarcinoma

Primary adenocarcinoma of the appendix is extremely rare. It is usually of the colonic type and should be treated by right hemicolectomy (as a second-stage procedure if the condition is not recognised at the first operation).

Further reading

Berry, J. and Malt, R.A. (1984) Appendicitis near its centenary. *American Journal of Surgery*, **200**, 567–75.

Krukowski, Z.H., Irwin, S.T., Denholm, S.D. and Matheson, N.A. (1988) Preventing infection after appendicectomy: a review. *British Journal of Surgery*, 75, 102–33.

McAnenna, O.J., Austin, O., O'Connell, P.R., Hederman, W.P., Gorey, T.F. and Fitzpatrick, J.M. (1992) Laparoscopic versus open appendicectomy: a prospective evaluation. *British Journal of Surgery*, 79, 818–20.

Ramachandran, P., Sivit, C.J., Newman, K.D. and Schwartz, M.Z. (1996) Ultrasonography as an adjunct in the diagnosis of acute appendicitis: a 4-year experience. *Journal of Pediatric Surgery*, **31**, 164–7.

Savage, P.E.A. (1991) Appendicectomy. In *Rob and Smith's Operative Surgery. Alimentary Tract and Abdominal Wall*, 4th edn, Vol. 1 (eds H. Dudley, W. Pories and D. Carter), Butterworth-Heinemann, Oxford, pp. 373–9.

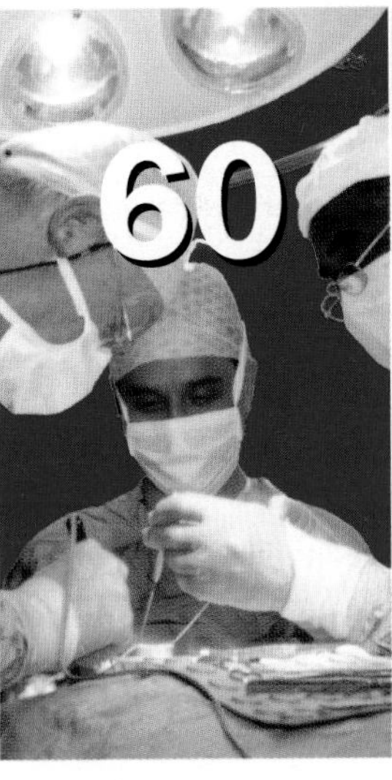

60 The rectum

Anatomy

Surgical anatomy

The rectum has an ill-defined anatomical beginning, but *surgically* the rectosigmoid junction lies opposite the sacral promontory. From here the rectum follows the curve of the sacrum to end at the anorectal junction. At this point, the puborectalis muscle encircles the posterior and lateral aspects of the junction, creating the anorectal angle (normally 120°). The rectum has three lateral curvatures: the upper and lower are convex to the right, and the middle convex to the left: on the mucosal (lumen) aspect these three curves are marked by semicircular folds (Houston's valves) (Fig. 60.1). That part of the rectum that lies below the middle valve has a much wider diameter than the upper third, and is known as the ampulla of the rectum.

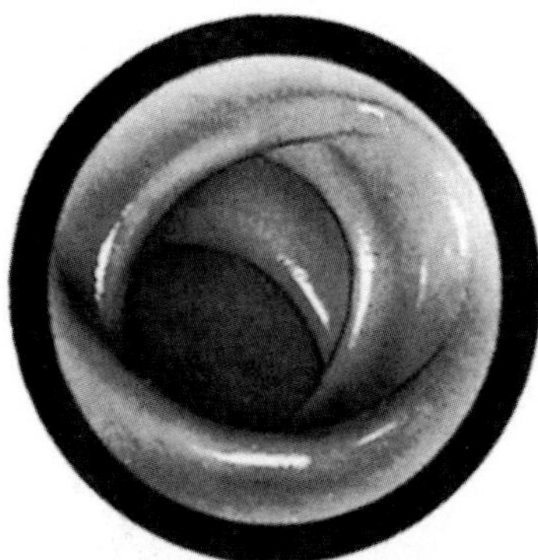

Fig. 60.1 Houston's valves as seen through a sigmoidoscope.

The adult rectum is approximately 18–20 cm in length and is conveniently divided into three equal parts: the upper third, which is mobile and has a peritoneal coat except near to the middle third where the peritoneum only covers the anterior and part of the lateral surfaces; the middle third, which is the widest part of the rectum and is confined within the diameter of the bony pelvis; and the lowest third, which lies within the muscular floor of the pelvis and has important relations to fascial layers.

The lowest part of the rectum is separated by a fascial condensation – Denonvilliers' fascia – from the prostate in front, and behind by another fascial layer – Waldeyer's fascia – from the coccycx and last two sacral vertebrae (Table 60.1). *These fascial layers are surgically important as they are a barrier to malignant penetration, and are valuable guides at operation.*

Blood supply

The superior rectal artery is the direct continuation of the inferior mesenteric artery and is the main arterial supply of the rectum. Opposite the third sacral vertebra, the artery divides again behind the lower third of the rectum into two – an anterior and a posterior branch. The arteries and their

John Houston, 1802–45. Physician, City of Dublin Hospital and Lecturer in Surgery, Dublin, Ireland.
Charles Pierre Denonvilliers, 1808–72. French surgeon.
Heinrich Wilhelm Gottfried Waldeyer-Hartz, 1836–1921. Professor of Pathological Anatomy, Berlin, Germany.

Bailey & Love's Short Practice of Surgery, 23rd edition. Edited by R.C.G. Russell, N.S. Williams and C.J.K. Bulstrode. Published in 2000 by Arnold Publishers.

Table 60.1 Relations of the rectum

	Male	Female
Anterior	Bladder Seminal vesicles Ureters Prostate Urethra	Pouch of Douglas Uterus Cervix Posterior vaginal wall
Lateral	Lateral ligaments Middle rectal artery Obturator internus muscle Side wall of pelvis Levator ani muscle	Lateral ligaments Middle rectal artery Obturator internus muscle Side wall of pelvis Levator ani muscle
Posterior	Sacrum and coccyx Loose areolar tissue Fascial condensation Superior rectal artery Lymphatics	Sacrum and coccyx Loose areolar tissue Fascial condensation Superior rectal artery Lymphatics

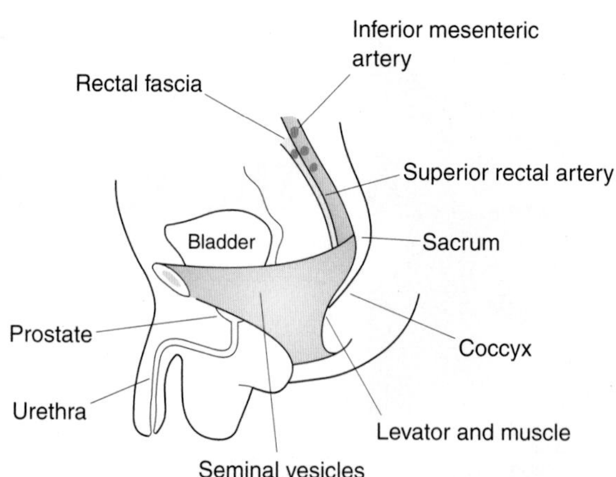

Fig. 60.3 Diagram showing the rectum lying in the male pelvis (sagittal view). Note the lymph nodes along the path of the superior rectal artery (Gerota's nodes).

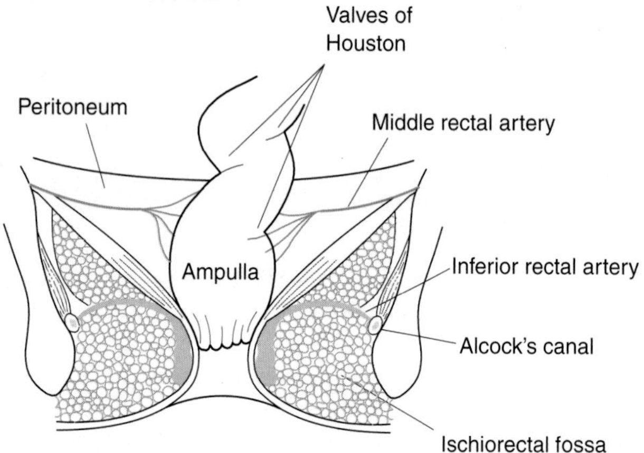

Fig. 60.2 Diagram showing the rectum lying in the pelvis (coronal view). Note the curvatures corresponding to Houston's valves.

accompanying lymphatics are kept applied to the back of the rectum by dense connective tissue (the mesorectum or 'rectal fascia').

The middle rectal artery arises on each side from the internal iliac artery (Fig. 60.2) and passes to the rectum in the lateral ligaments. It is usually small and breaks up into several terminal branches.

The inferior rectal artery arises on each side from the internal pudendal artery as it enters Alcock's canal. It hugs the inferior surface of the levator ani muscle as it crosses the roof of the ischiorectal fossa to enter the anal muscles (Fig. 60.2).

Venous drainage

The superior haemorrhoidal veins draining the upper half of the anal canal above the dentate line pass upwards to become the rectal veins: these unite to form the *superior rectal vein* which later becomes the *inferior mesenteric vein*. This forms part of the portal venous system, and ultimately drains into the splenic vein. Middle rectal veins exist, but are small, unimportant channels unless the normal paths are blocked.

Lymphatic drainage

The lymphatics of the mucosal lining of the rectum interchange freely with those of the muscular layers. The usual drainage flow is *upwards*, and only to a limited extent laterally and downwards. For this reason, surgical ablation of malignant disease concentrates mainly on achieving wide clearance of proximal lymph nodes. However, if the usual upwards routes are blocked (e.g. by carcinoma) flow can reverse, and it is then possible to find metastatic lymph nodes on the side walls of the pelvis (along the middle rectal vessels) or even in the inguinal region (along the inferior rectal artery).

Superior rectal nodes

These are an important group of nodes on the back of the rectal ampulla above the levator ani muscle (Fig. 60.3), also known as the pararectal lymph glands of Gerota.

Middle rectal nodes

These lie close to the middle rectal arteries and pass to lymph nodes around the internal arteries. The Japanese have stressed the importance of removing these lymph glands when operating on rectal cancer.

Clinical features of rectal disease

Symptoms

Rectal diseases are common and serious, and can occur at any age. The symptoms of many of them overlap. In general, the inflammations affect younger age groups, while the tumours

Benjamin Alcock, 1849–55. Professor of Anatomy, Cork, Ireland. He was dismissed from his post for a breach of the Anatomy Acts, and disappeared in America.

James Douglas, 1675–1742. Anatomist and obstetrician, London, England.

Dumitru Gerota, 1867–1939. Professor of Surgery, Bucharest, Rumania.

occur in the middle-aged and elderly. But no age is exempt from any of the diseases, however young: ulcerative colitis has been reported in the newborn, and rectal cancer is not rare in young people. The common symptoms of rectal disease are the following.

Bleeding

This demands at least digital examination at any age.

Altered bowel habit

Early morning stool frequency ('spurious diarrhoea') is a symptom of rectal carcinoma, while blood-stained frequent loose stools characterise the inflammatory diseases.

Discharge

Mucus and pus are associated with rectal pathology.

Tenesmus

Often described by the patient as 'I feel I want to go but nothing happens'; this is normally an ominous symptom of rectal cancer.

Prolapse

This usually indicates either mucosal (partial) or full-thickness (complete) rectal wall descent.

Pruritis

This may be secondary to a rectal discharge.

Loss of weight

This usually indicates serious or advanced disease, e.g. hepatic metastases.

> Main symptoms of rectal disease
> - Bleeding per rectum
> - Altered bowel habit
> - Mucus discharge
> - Tenesmus
> - Prolapse

Signs

Because the rectum is accessible via the anal orifice these can be elicited by systematic examination. The patient is either positioned in the left-lateral (Sims) position or examined in the knee–elbow position (Fig. 60.4).

Inspection

Visual examination of the anus precedes rectal examination to exclude the presence of anal disease, e.g. fissure, haemorrhoids or fistula.

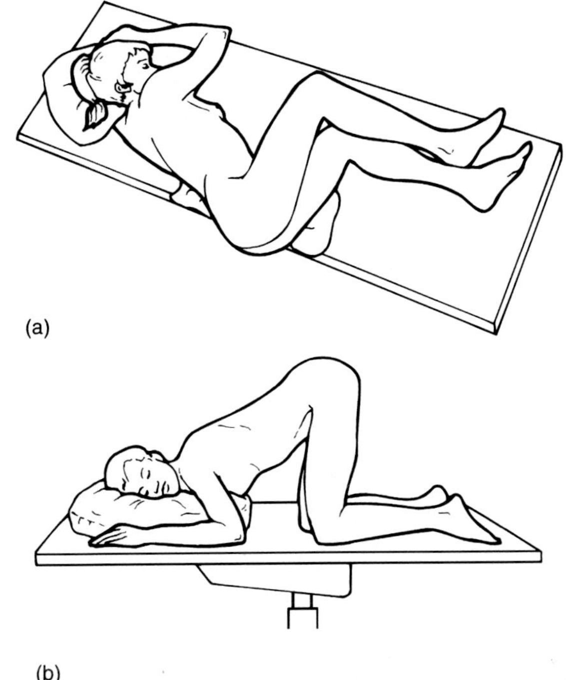

Fig. 60.4 Positions for digital rectal examination. (a) Left lateral (Sims); (b) Knee–elbow. (Redrawn with permission from *Colon and Rectal Surgery*, 3rd edn, J.B. Lippincott Co., London.)

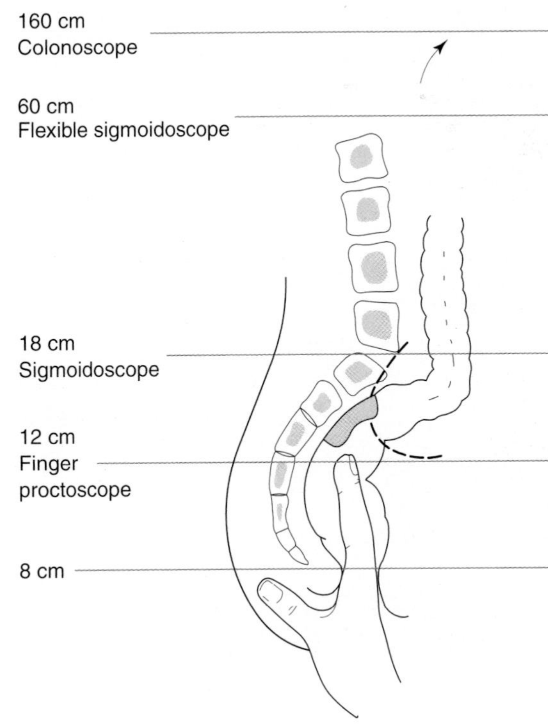

Fig. 60.5 Illustration showing how the various methods of examining the rectum reach different levels. Note that even cancers in the upper part of the rectum can be felt with the index finger, especially if the patient is asked to 'strain down' (*courtesy of C.V. Mann*).

J. Marion Sims, 1813–83. American gynaecologist.

Digital examination

The index finger used with gentleness and precision remains the most valuable test for rectal disease (Fig. 60.5). Tumours in the lower and middle thirds of the rectum can be felt and assessed; by asking the patient to strain, even some tumours in the upper third can be 'tipped' with the finger. After it is removed the finger should be examined for tell-tale traces of mucus, pus or blood. It is always useful to note the normal as well as the abnormal findings on digital examination, e.g. the prostate in the male. Digital findings can be recorded as intraluminal (e.g. blood, pus), intramural (e.g. tumours, granular areas, strictures) or extramural (e.g. enlarged prostate, uterine fibroids).

Proctoscopy

This can be used to inspect the anus, anorectal junction and the lower rectum (up to 10 cm) (Fig. 60.6). Biopsy can be performed of any suspicious areas.

(a)

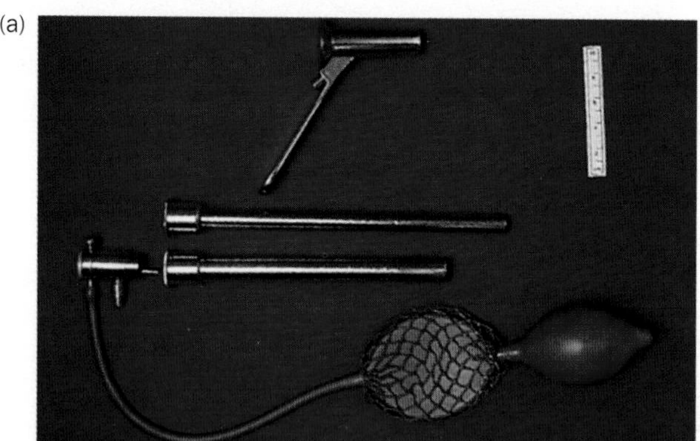

(b)

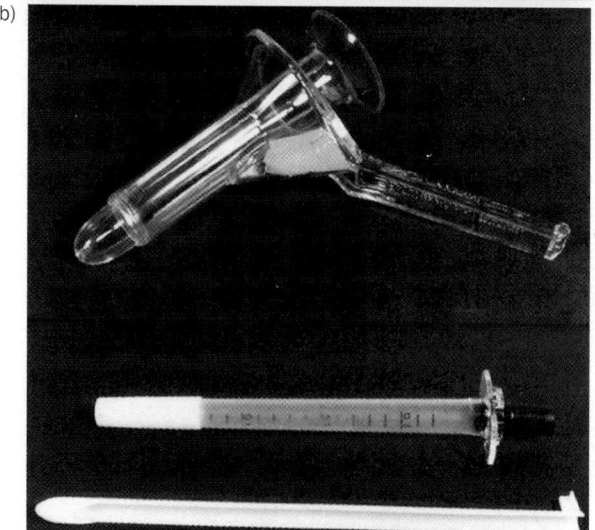

Fig. 60.6 (a) A metal protoscope and two different-sized metal Lloyd-Davies rigid sigmoidoscopes – small (diameter 15 mm) and large (diameter 20 mm). Since the prevalence of human immunodeficiency virus (HIV) infection, disposable protoscopes and sigmoidoscopes (b) have replaced the reusable metal types.

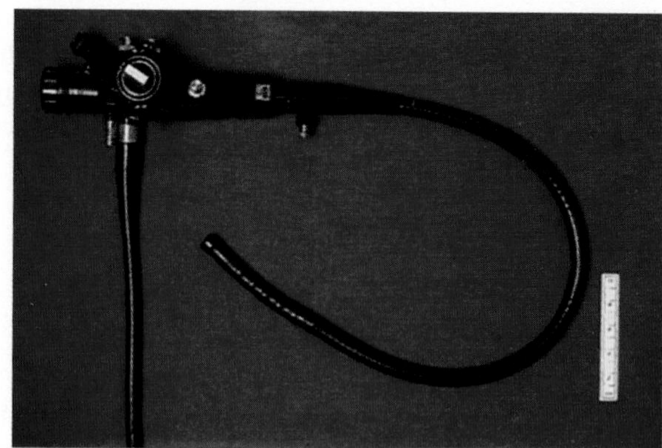

Fig. 60.7 The flexible (60-cm) endoscope ('flexiscope').

Sigmoidoscopy

The sigmoidoscope was in the past a rigid stainless-steel instrument of variable diameter and was normally 25 cm in length (Fig. 60.6). This has in the main been replaced by a disposable Perspex instrument which has major advantages when considering transmittable disease. The rectum must be empty for proper inspection with a sigmoidoscope. Gentleness and skill are required for its use, and perforations can occur if care is not exercised.

Flexible sigmoidoscope

The 'flexiscope' can be used to supplement or replace rigid sigmoidoscopy (Fig. 60.7). It requires special skill and experience, and the lower bowel should be cleaned out with preliminary enemas. In addition to the rectum, the whole sigmoid colon is within visual reach of this instrument. The instrument is expensive and requires careful maintenance.

Injuries

The rectum or anal canal may be injured in a number of ways, all uncommon.

- By falling in a sitting posture on to a spiked or blunt-pointed object. The upturned leg of a chair, handle of a broom, floor-mop, pitchfork or a broken shooting stick have all resulted in rectal impalement.
- By the fetal head during childbirth, especially forceps-assisted.

Diagnosis. When there is a history of rectal impalement, the first interrogation should be, 'Has the patient passed urine since the accident?' The anus having been inspected, the abdomen should be palpated. If rigidity or tenderness is present, early laparotomy is imperative. Prior to the operation, a urethral catheter is passed. If the urine is bloodstained and/or the quantity recovered is unexpectedly small, it is wise to suspect ruptured bladder or urethra (see Chapters 65 and 67).

Treatment. After the patient has been anaesthetised, the rectum is examined with a finger and a speculum, especial attention being directed to the anterior wall. A lower laparotomy is then performed. If an intraperitoneal rupture of the rectum is found, the perforation is closed with sutures. Should blood be present beneath the pelvic peritoneum, it is necessary to mobilise the rectosigmoid, which allows the rectum to be drawn upwards, thus permitting the perforation below the pelvic diaphragm to be closed securely. A perforation in the bladder can also be sutured via this avenue. After closing the laparotomy wound, a defunctioning colostomy is constructed in the left iliac fossa. In cases where the bladder has been injured, a self-retaining urethral catheter is placed in position. If the rectal injury is below the pelvic floor, wide drainage from below is indicated. A 'protective' colostomy is advisable. If the defect in the rectum is very large, resection may have to be contemplated. In such circumstances, a Hartmann's procedure is indicated. Care must be taken to preserve sphincter function during the débridement of the perineal wounds. Antibiotic cover should be provided against both aerobic and anaerobic organisms.

Foreign bodies in the rectum

The variety of foreign bodies which have found their way into the rectum is hardly less remarkable than the ingenuity displayed in their removal (Fig. 60.8). A turnip has been delivered *per anum* by the use of obstetric forceps. A stick firmly impacted has been withdrawn by inserting a gimlet into its lower end. A tumbler, mouth looking downwards, has been extracted by filling the interior with a wet plaster of Paris bandage, leaving the end of the bandage protruding, and allowing the plaster to set.

If insurmountable difficulty is experienced in grasping any foreign body in the rectum, a laparotomy is necessary, which allows that object to be pushed from above into the assistant's finger in the rectum. If there is considerable laceration of the mucosa, a temporary colostomy is advisable.

Prolapse

Partial prolapse

The mucous membrane and submucosa of the rectum protrude

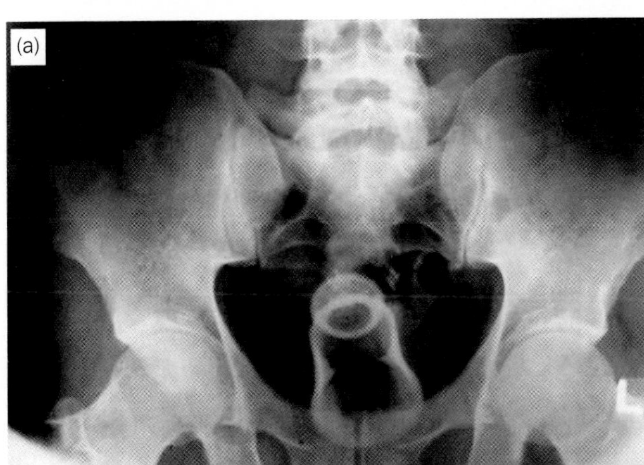

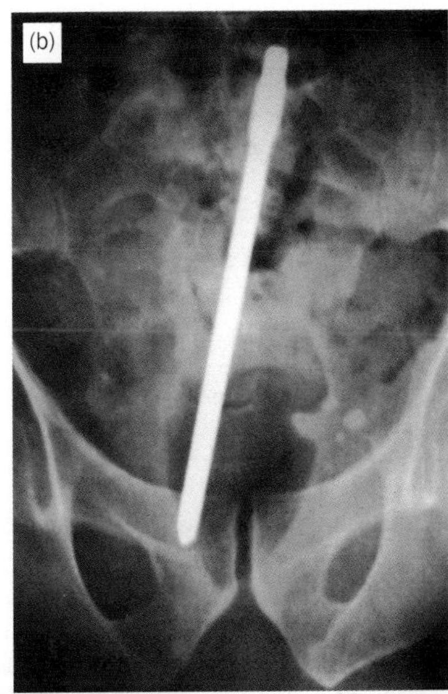

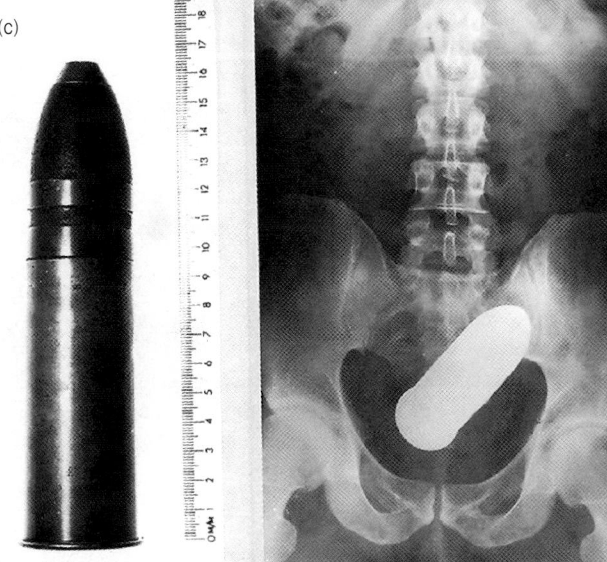

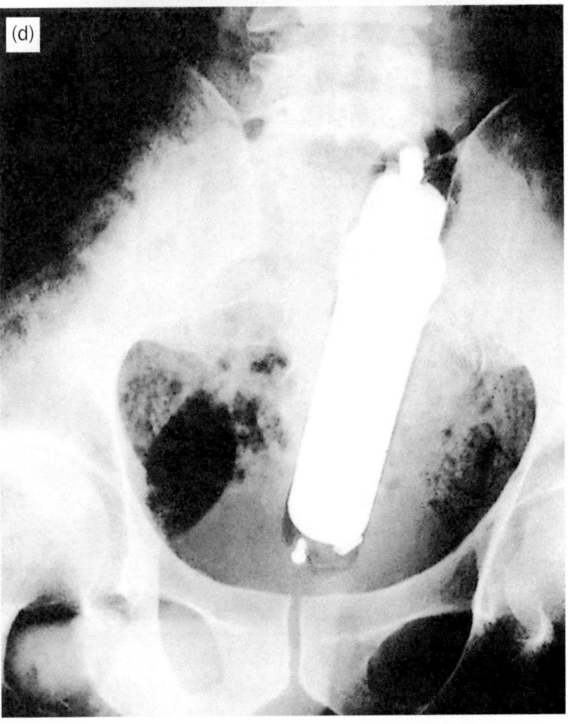

Fig. 60.8 (a) Pepper pot in the rectum. On removal it was found to be inscribed 'A present from Margate'! (*Dr L.S. Carstairs, Royal Northern Hospital, London, UK*); (b) a screwdriver with a plastic handle (*Dr A.K. Sharma, Agra, India*); (c) a live shell, which needed careful handling; and (d) a large vibrator which had pierced the lateral intraperitoneal rectal wall and caused peritonitis.

Henri Albert Charles Antoine Hartmann, 1860–1952. Professor of Surgery, Paris, France.

outside the anus for approximately 1–4 cm. When the prolapsed mucosa is palpated between the finger and thumb, it is evident that it is composed of no more than a double layer of mucous membrane (cf. complete prolapse). There is some confusion as to its exact nature. Some believe that partial rectal prolapse represents the head of a rectal intussusception, and is the early manifestation of a complete rectal prolapse. Others consider that it is a separate entity. The probable truth is that both types exist. The condition occurs most often at the extremes of life – in children between 1 and 3 years of age, and in elderly people.

In infants

The direct downward course of the rectum, due to the as yet undeveloped sacral curve (Fig. 60.9), predisposes to this condition, as does the reduced resting anal tone which offers diminished support to the mucosal lining of the anal canal (Mann).

In children

Partial prolapse often commences after an attack of diarrhoea, as a result of severe whooping cough, or from loss of weight and consequent diminution in the amount of fat in the ischiorectal fossae.

In adults

The condition in adults is usually associated with third-degree haemorrhoids. In the female, a torn perineum predisposes to prolapse, and in the male straining from urethral obstruction. In old age, both partial and complete prolapse are associated with atony of the sphincter mechanism but whether this is the cause of the problem or secondary to it is unknown.

Partial prolapse may follow an operation for fistula-in-ano where a large portion of muscle has been divided. Here the prolapse is usually localised to the damaged quadrant and is seldom progressive.

Prolapsed mucous membrane is pink; prolapsed internal haemorrhoids are plum coloured and more pedunculated.

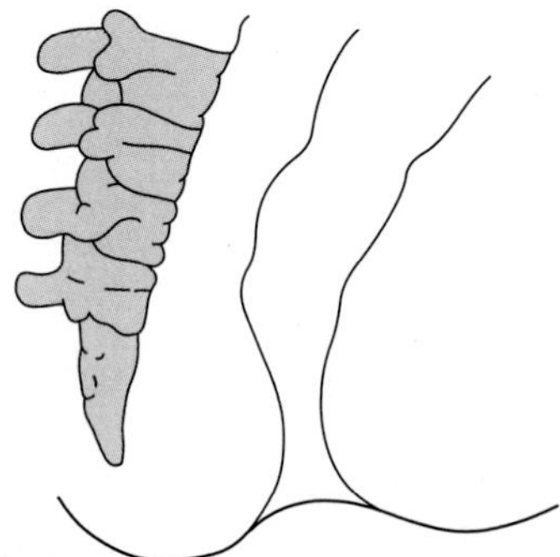

Fig. 60.9 The absence of the normal sacral curve predisposes to rectal prolapse in an infant.

Treatment

In infants and young children

Digital reposition. The parent must be taught to replace the protrusion. The distal two-thirds of the index finger is wrapped in tissue paper. The finger is inserted into the protrusion and the mass is eased into place. Gently, the finger is withdrawn, leaving the tissue paper to disintegrate. In cases of malnutrition, dietetic adjustments are necessary.

Submucous injections. If digital reposition fails after 6 weeks' trial, injections of 5 per cent phenol in almond oil are carried out under general anaesthesia. As a result of the aseptic inflammation following these injections, the mucous membrane becomes tethered to the muscle coat.

Technique. The submucosa at the apex of the prolapse is injected circularly, so as to form a raised ring, up to 10 ml of the solution being injected. A similar injection is made at the base of the prolapse. Alternatively, if the prolapse cannot be brought down, the injections are given through a proctoscope.

Thiersch's operation. When the prolapse persists in spite of these measures, Thiersch's operation (below) may succeed. In infants, insertion of the little finger into the anus before the stitch is tied is recommended. In infants and young children, strong chromic catgut should be used for the stitch instead of silver wire: if wire were employed (or any other retained unabsorbable material) as growth proceeded, the stitch would have to be removed or anal stenosis would result. As the procedure is designed only as a *temporary* measure in the young, chromic catgut is adequate for the purpose.

In adults

Submucous injections. Submucous injections of phenol in almond oil occasionally are successful in cases of early partial prolapse.

Excision of the prolapsed mucosa. When the prolapse is unilateral the redundant mucosa can be excised after inserting and tying Goodsall's ligature (Fig. 60.10) which, after the needles have been cut off, permits the base of the prolapsed mucous membrane to be ligated in three portions lying in juxtaposition. When necessary, the operation is combined with haemorrhoidectomy, and if the pedicle of one or more of the haemorrhoids is broad, Goodsall's ligature is applied. Alternatively, an endoluminal stapling technique can now be used.

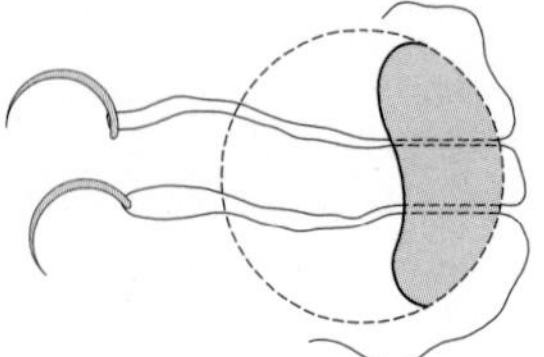

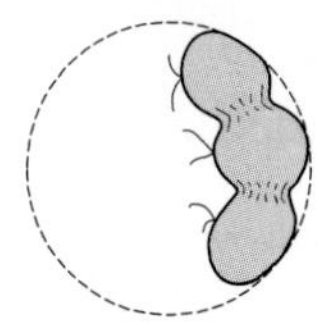

Fig. 60.10 Goodsall's ligature.

Charles Victor Mann. Consulting surgeon, St Mark's Hospital for Diseases of the Rectum and Colon, London, and The Royal London Hospital, London, England.

Karl Thiersch, 1822–95. Professor of Surgery, Leipzig, Germany.

Goodsall, 1843–1906. Surgeon, St Mark's Hospital for Diseases of the Rectum and Colon, London, England.

Complete prolapse

Complete prolapse (syn. procidentia) is less common than the partial variety. The protrusion consists of all layers of the rectal wall and is a descending hernia-en-glissade of the rectum downwards through the levator ani. As the rectum descends, it intussuscepts upon itself. The process starts with the anterior wall of the rectum where the supporting tissues are weakest, especially in women. It is more than 4 cm and commonly as much as 10–15 cm in length. On palpation between the finger and the thumb, the prolapse feels much thicker than a partial prolapse, and obviously consists of a double thickness of the entire wall of the rectum. Any prolapse over 5 cm in length contains anteriorly between its layers a pouch of peritoneum (Fig. 60.11). When large, the peritoneal pouch contains small intestine, which returns to the general peritoneal cavity with a characteristic gurgle when the prolapse is reduced. The prolapsed mucous membrane (Fig. 60.12) is often arranged in a series of circular folds. The anal sphincter is characteristically patulous and gapes widely on straining to allow the rectum to prolapse. Complete prolapse is uncommon in children. In adults, it can occur at any age, but is more common in the elderly. Women are six times more often affected than men. In women, prolapse of the rectum is commonly associated with prolapse of the uterus, or a past history of a gynaecological operation, e.g. hysterectomy. In the Middle East and Asia, complete rectal prolapse is not uncommon in young males. In approximately 50 per cent of adults, faecal incontinence is also a feature.

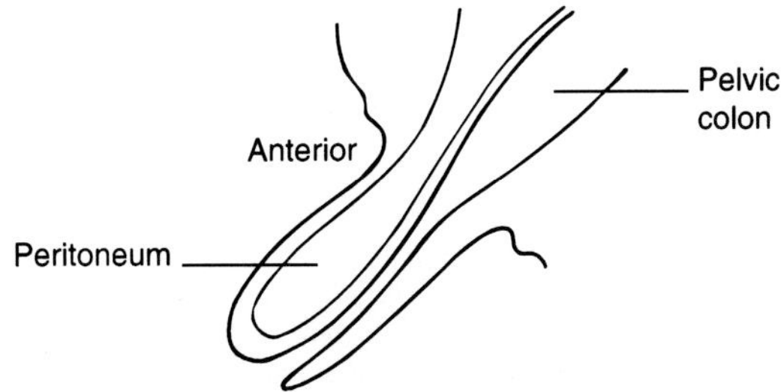

Fig. 60.11 Rectal prolapse containing a pouch of peritoneum.

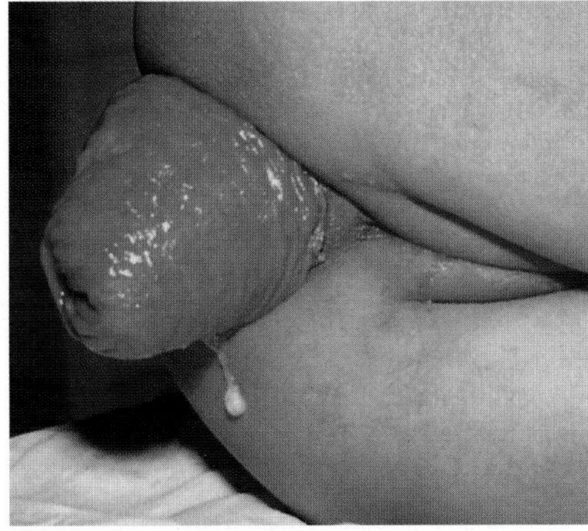

Fig. 60.12 Complete rectal prolapse (*courtesy of G.D. Adhia, Bombay*).

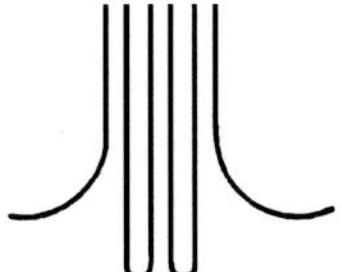

Fig. 60.13 Partial prolapse of the rectum.

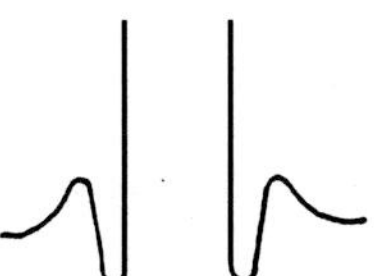

Fig. 60.14 Intussusception protruding from the anus.

Differential diagnosis. In the case of a child with abdominal pain, prolapse of the rectum must be distinguished from *ileocaecal intussusception* protruding from the anus. Figures 60.13 and 60.14 make the differential diagnosis clear. In *rectosigmoid intussusception* in the adult, there is a deep groove (5 cm or more) between the emerging protruding mass and margin of the anus, into which the finger can be entered.

Treatment

Surgery is required and the operation can be performed via the perineal or the abdominal approaches. Whenever possible, an abdominal rectopexy is recommended, but when the patient is elderly and very frail, or is suffering from injury or disease of the spinal cord, or in very early life, a perineal operation is indicated.

Perineal approach. Two procedures have been used most commonly.

Delorme's operation (Fig. 60.15). In this procedure, the rectal mucosa is removed circumferentially from the prolapsed rectum over its length, apart from 0.5-cm strips at its proximal end and at its tip. The underlying muscle is then imbricated with a series of chromic catgut sutures, such that, when these are tied, the rectal muscle is concertinaed towards the anal canal. The anal canal mucosa is then sutured

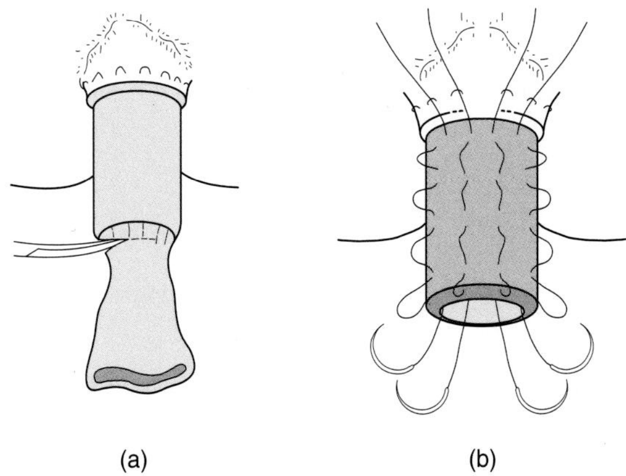

Fig. 60.15 Delorme's operation for rectal prolapse. (a) The mucosa has been removed from the prolapse; (b) interrupted sutures have been placed in the underlying muscle so that, when tied, the muscle is plicated. (Redrawn with permission from Keighley, M.R.B.K. and Williams, N.S., *Surgery of the Anus, Rectum and Colon*, W.B. Saunders, London, 1999.)

circumferentially to the rectal mucosa remaining at the tip of the prolapse. This manoeuvre has the effect of reducing the prolapse and creating a ring of muscle within the anal canal, which narrows the orifice and prevents recurrence.

Thiersch operation. This procedure, which aims to place a steel wire or, more commonly now, a silastic or nylon suture, around the anal canal has in the past been the most frequently performed perineal procedure. However, it has become obsolete for the treatment of rectal prolapse in adults, although it still does have a place in the treatment of partial prolapse in children. The reasons for its lack of popularity are that the suture would often break or cause chronic perineal sepsis, or both, or the anal stenosis so created would produce severe functional problems. Delorme's operation is now the preferred perineal operation.

If an abdominal repair must be avoided (e.g. in a young man in whom sexual potency must be preserved by avoiding damage to the pelvic nerves) more extensive perineal procedures are available. These include strengthening the puborectalis and external anal sphincters by an approach through the intersphincteric plane (see above), the so-called *postanal repair* (Parks) and perineal rectosigmoidectomy (Altemeier) in which the prolapsed rectum is exised from below.

Abdominal approach. The principle of all abdominal operations for rectal prolapse is to replace and hold the rectum in its proper position. Of the many operations described, the following are relatively simple. They are recommended in patients with complete prolapse, who are otherwise in good health.

Wells' operation. In this operation the rectum is fixed firmly to the sacrum by inserting a sheet of polyvinyl alcohol sponge or, more commonly now, polypropylene mesh between them (Fig. 60.16). The rectum is separated from the sacrum in the usual way. The mesh is fixed by a series of sutures to the periosteum over the midline of the sacrum and is then wrapped loosely about the rectum covering all except the anterior wall. The free margins of the mesh are sutured to the lateral margins of the anterior wall of the rectum. The peritoneal floor is resutured so that the mesh is excluded from the peritoneal cavity. The mesh does not give rise to a foreign body reaction, but it does produce very marked fibrous tissue formation. Many proctologists regard this as the method of choice. Recently, the technique has been performed laparoscopically, thus reducing the operative trauma and limiting the time in hospital (Fig. 60.17).

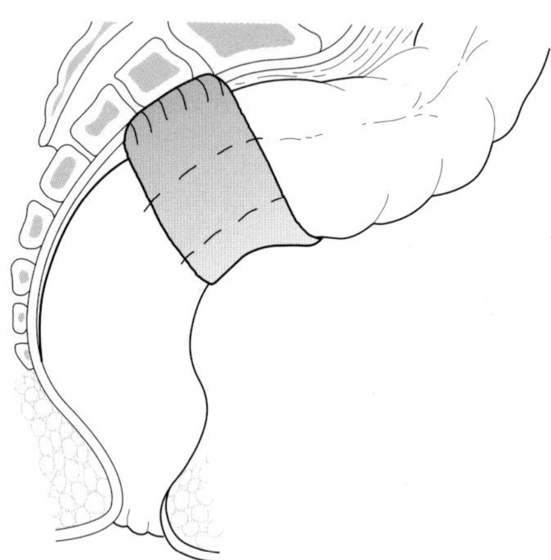

Fig. 60.16 Wells' operation for rectal prolapse. The rectum is mobilised and fixed to the sacrum with a sheet of polyvinyl sponge or polypropylene mesh. (Redrawn with permission from *Colon and Rectal Surgery*, 3rd edn, J.B. Lippincott, London, 1992.)

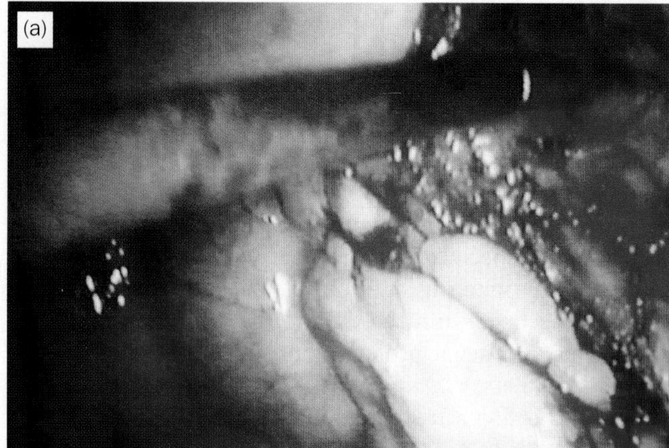

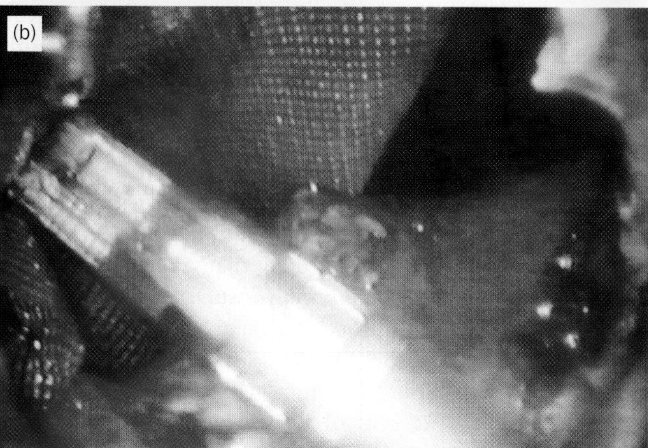

Fig. 60.17 (a) The rectum is mobilised laparoscopically by division of the lateral ligaments and dissection in the presacral plane; (b) a polypropylene mesh is stapled posteriorly to the sacrum and to the serosa of the lateral wall of the rectum using the endostapler.

Ripstein's operation. In this operation, the rectosigmoid junction is hitched up by a Teflon sling to the front of the sacrum just below the sacral promontory. The operation is very safe and simple, and the results are good. Some surgeons recommend combining this procedure with resection of the sigmoid colon (Goldberg).

Lahaut's operation. This operation depends entirely upon mobilising the rectum and lower sigmoid colon, and holding it up by taking it through the rectus sheath. The results are moderate and few surgeons use this method.

Edmond Delorme, 1847–1929. Chief of Surgery in the French Army.
The late Sir Alan Parks, PRCS, was the first to popularise this operation.

Charles Alexander Wells. Professor Emeritus of Surgery, Liverpool, England.
Charles Benjamin Ripstein. Surgeon, Brookdale Hospital Center, New York, USA.
Stanley Goldberg. Professor of Colo-Rectal Surgery, University of Minneapolis, Minnesota, USA.
Jules Lahaut. Surgeon-in-Chief, Hôpital du Pont Canal, Jemappes (Hainault), Belgium.

It should be noted that approximately 50 per cent of adult patients with a complete rectal prolapse are incontinent, and rectopexy cures only about one-third. Consequently, it may be necessary to perform a subsequent procedure to correct the incontinence.

Proctitis

Inflammation is sometimes limited to the rectal mucosa; in others it is associated with a similar condition in the colon (proctocolitis). The inflammation can be acute or chronic. The symptoms are tenesmus, the passage of blood and mucus and, in severe cases, of pus also. Although the patient has a frequent intense desire to defecate, the amount of faeces passed at a time is small. Acute proctitis is usually accompanied by malaise and pyrexia. On rectal examination the mucosa feels swollen and is often exceedingly tender. Proctoscopy is seldom sufficient and sigmoidoscopy is the more valuable method of examination. If the diagnosis is confirmed, colonoscopy with multiple biopsies is mandatory, so as to determine the extent of the inflammatory process. Skilled pathological assistance is required to establish or exclude the diagnosis of specific infection by bacteriological examination and culture of the stools, examination or scrapings or swabs from ulcers, and serological tests. When early carcinoma cannot be excluded, biopsy is necessary.

Nonspecific proctitis is an inflammatory condition affecting the mucosa and, to a lesser extent, the submucosa, confined to the terminal rectum and anal canal. It is the most common variety. In 10 per cent of cases the condition extends to involve the whole colon (total ulcerative colitis).

Aetiology. This is unknown. The concept that the condition is a mild and limited form of ulcerative colitis (although actual ulceration is often not present) is the most acceptable hypothesis.

Clinical features. The patient is usually middle-aged, and complains of slight loss of blood in the motions. Often the complaint is one of diarrhoea, but on closer questioning it transpires that usually one relatively normal action of the bowels occurs each day, although it is accompanied by some blood. During the day the patient attempts to defecate, with the passage of flatus and a little blood-stained faecal matter, which is mistakenly interpreted as diarrhoea. On rectal examination, the mucosa feels warm and smooth. Often there is some blood on the examining finger. Protoscopic and sigmoidoscopic examination shows inflamed mucous membrane of the rectum, but usually no ulceration. The inflammation usually extends for only 12.5–15 cm from the anus, the mucosa above this level being quite normal.

Treatment. Although, fortunately, the condition is usually self-limiting, much relief may be obtained from the use of sulphasalazine (Salazopyrin) and its more active component 5-ASA (Asacol), acetarsol suppositories or prednisolone retention enemas. Milk should be rigidly excluded from the diet. In very severe resistant cases, oral steroids may have to be used to obtain remission. Rarely, surgical treatment is used as a last resort when the patient is desperate for relief of symptoms.

Ulcerative proctocolitis. Proctitis is present in a high percentage of cases of ulcerative colitis, and the degree of severity of the rectal involvement may influence the type of operative procedure (see Chapter 57).

Proctitis due to Crohn's disease. Crohn's disease can occasionally affect the rectum, although classically it is spared. Sigmoidoscopic characteristics differ from those in nonspecific proctitis. The inflammatory process tends to be patchy rather than confluent and there may be fissuring, ulceration and even a cobblestone appearance. Rectal Crohn's disease is often associated with severe perineal disease characterised by fistulation. Skip lesions are also often present in the rest of the colon or small bowel, or both.

Proctitis due to specific infections

Clostridium difficile. An acute form of proctocolitis by infection with *C. difficile* can follow broad-spectrum antibiotic administration (especially lincomycin). A 'membrane' can sometimes be seen on proctoscopy ('pseudomembranous' enterocolitis).

Bacillary dysentery. The appearance is that of an acute purulent proctitis with multiple small, shallow ulcers. The examination of a swab taken from the ulcerated mucous membrane is more certainly diagnostic than is a microscopical examination of the stools. Proctological examination is painful; agglutination tests may render it unnecessary.

Amoebic dysentery. The infection is more liable to be chronic, and exacerbations after a long period of freedom from symptoms often occur. Proctoscopy and sigmoidoscopy are not painful. The appearance of an amoebic ulcer is described in Chapter 57. Scrapings from the ulcer should be immersed in warm isotonic saline solution and sent to the laboratory for immediate microscopical examination.

Amoebic granuloma. This presents as a soft mass, usually in the rectosigmoid region. This lesion is frequently mistaken for a carcinoma. Sigmoidoscopy shows an ulcerated surface, but the mass is less friable than a carcinoma. A scraping should be taken, preferably with a small, sharp spoon on a long handle, and the material sent for immediate microscopical examination, as detailed above. If doubt exists, a provocative dose of emetine may cause cysts of the amoebae to appear in the stools. A biopsy can also help. Treatment is as described in Chapter 57.

Amoebic granuloma of the rectum is from time to time encountered in a patient who has never visited a country in which the disease is endemic. Persons living in old people's institutions are liable to harbour this deceptive lesion.

Tuberculous proctitis. This is nearly always associated with active pulmonary tuberculous ulceration of the anus. Submucous rectal abscesses burst and leave ulcers with an undermined edge. A hypertrophic type of tuberculous proctitis occurs in association with tuberculous peritonitis, or tuberculous proctitis occurs in association with tuberculous peritonitis or tuberculous salpingitis. This type of tuberculous proctitis requires biopsy for confirmation of the diagnosis.

Gonococcal proctitis. Gonococcal proctitis occurs in both sexes as the result of rectal coitus, and in the female from direct spread from the vulva. In the acute stage, the mucous membrane is hyperaemic and thick pus can be expressed as the proctoscope is withdrawn. In the early stages, the diagnosis can be readily established by bacteriological examination, but later, when the infection is mixed, it is more difficult to recognise. Specific treatment is so effective that local treatment is unnecessary.

Lymphogranuloma inguinale. The modes of infection are similar to those of gonococcal proctitis, but in the female infection spreading from the cervix uteri via lymphatics to the pararectal lymph nodes is common. The proctological findings are similar to those of gonococcal proctitis. The diagnosis of lymphogranuloma in inguinale should be suspected when the inguinal lymph nodes are greatly enlarged, although the enlargement may be subsiding by the time proctitis commences (Chapter 67).

Primary syphilis. A primary chancre may occur inside the anus (Chapter 64) – a paradox – 'a painless anal fissure'.

Burrill Bernard Crohn, b. 1884. Gastroenterologist, Mount Sinai Hospital, New York, USA.

Acquired immunodeficiency syndrome (AIDS). AIDS may present with a particularly florid type of proctitis. In such patients unusual organisms such as cytomegalovirus (CMV) are often found on culture.

'Strawberry' lesion of the rectosigmoid. This is due to an infection by *Spirochaeta vincenti* and *Bacillus fusiformis*. The leading symptom is diarrhoea, often scantily blood stained. Occasionally the diagnosis can be made by the demonstration of the specific organisms in the stools. More often sigmoidoscopy is required. The characteristic lesion is thickened, somewhat raised mucosa with superficial ulceration in the region of the rectosigmoid. The inflamed mucous membrane oozes blood at numerous pin-points, giving the appearance of an over-ripe strawberry. A swab should be taken from the lesion and examined for Vincent's and fusiform organisms. Swabs from the gums and the throat are also advisable.

Treatment. Acetarsol suppositories together with vitamin C are almost specific.

Rectal bilharziasis. Rectal bilharziasis is caused by *Schistosoma mansomi*, which is endemic in many tropical and subtropical countries, and particularly in the delta of the Nile.

Stage 1. A cutaneous lesion develops at the site of entrance of the cercariae (parasites of freshwater snails).

Stage 2 is characterised by pryrexia, urticaria and a high eosinophilia. Both of these stages are frequently overlooked.

Stage 3 is due to deposition of the ova in the rectum (much more rarely in the bladder, Chapter 65) and is manifested by biharzial dysentery. On examination in the later stages, papillomas are frequently present. The papillomas, which are sessile or pedunculated, contain the ova of the trematode, the life-cycle of which resembles that of *Schistosoma haematobium*.

Untreated, the rectum becomes festooned, and prolapse of the diseased mucous membrane is usual. Multiple fistulae-in-ano are prone to develop.

General treatment of bilharziasis mansomi. *Compounds not containing antimony* include niridazole (Ambilhar) in cases of infestation with *S. haematobium* or *S. mansomi* (not *S. japonicum* or in those with heart, mental or liver disease). Dose is 25 mg/kg body weight daily in two divided doses for 5–7 days. Hycanthone, lucanthone and oxamniquine are other compounds with weight-related single doses given by deep intramuscular (i.m.). injection, and all have toxic side effects. Metriphonate is an organophosphorous compound, effective against *S. haematobium* only and must be handled with care. Praziquantel (Biltricide) has proved a major advance in drug therapy, and is highly effective against all schistosome species. It is generally given as a single oral dose of 40 mg/kg for *S. haematobium* and *S. mansomi*, and for *S. japonicum* a higher dose of 60 mg/kg is given as two or three divided doses throughout 1 day.

Compounds containing antimony, either as the salts, *tartar emetic* (antimony potassium tartrate) and sodium salt given intravenously (i.v.)., or antimony lithium thiomalate, sodium antimonygluconate, stibogluconate and stibocaptate (Astiban) may still be required.

Local treatment. When the papillomas persist in spite of general treatment, they must be treated in the same manner as other papillomas by local destruction.

Proctitis due to herbal enemas. This is a well-known clinical entity to those practising in tropical Africa. Following an enema consisting of a concoction of ginger, pepper and bark, administered by a witch doctor, a most virulent proctitis sets in. Pelvic peritonitis frequently supervenes. Not infrequently, a complete gelatinous cast of the mucous membrane of the rectum is extruded. Very large doses of morphine, together with streptomycin, often prevent a fatal issue if commenced early (Bowesman). Temporary colostomy is often advisable.

Treatment

General treatments should include bed rest in extreme cases. The stools should be kept soft with Isogel. Suppositories of 5-ASA are often beneficial. The specific treatments for the dysenteries, tuberculosis, gonorrhoea, lymphogranuloma inguinale and syphilis are described in the appropriate sections of this book.

Solitary rectal ulcer

This is becoming a more commonly diagnosed problem. Classically, it takes the form of an ulcer on the anterior wall of the rectum. In this form it must be differentiated from a rectal carcinoma or inflammatory bowel disease, particularly Crohn's disease. In recent years, it has been appreciated that the ulceration may heal, leaving a polypoid appearance. A variety of explanations as to its cause has been suggested, including persistent trauma by sexual malpractices. However, recent proctographic studies indicate that the cause may be due to a combination of internal intussusception or anterior rectal wall prolapse, and an increase in intrarectal pressure. This combination of factors is usually due to chronic straining as a result of constipation. The histological appearances confirm the diagnosis (Morson) and they are similar to the appearances of biopsies from a full-thickness overt rectal prolapse. The condition, although benign, is difficult to treat. Symptomatic relief from bleeding and discharge may sometimes be achieved by preventing the internal prolapse by an abdominal rectopexy. In rare cases rectal excision may be required.

Benign tumours

The rectum, along with the sigmoid colon, is the most frequent site of polyps (and cancers) in the gastrointestinal tract. All neoplastic polyps of the colon and rectum (with rare exceptions) have a tendency to become malignant. This tendency is greatly enhanced if the polyp is more than 1 cm in diameter, shows obvious signs of increasing size and has a sessile rather than a penduculated shape. For these reasons, removal of all polyps is recommended, and *total* removal is mandatory. Only total removal will give complete histological examination and exclude (or confirm) localised carcinoma *in situ*, and also prevent local recurrence. For these reasons, destruction of anorectal tumours by fulguration is

---

Jean Hyacinthe Vincent, 1862–1950. Professor of Epidemiology, Val-de-Grace Military Hospital, Paris, France.

Theodor Maximilian Bilharz, 1825–62. Professor of Zoology, Cairo, Egypt.

Sir Patrick Manson, 1844–1922. Practised in Formosa and Hong Kong. Later Physician, Dreadnought Hospital, Greenwich, London, England. He is regarded as the 'Father of Tropical Medicine'.

Charles Bowesman. Former Surgical Specialist, Colonial Medical Service, Kumasi, Ghana.

Basil Clifford Morson CBE. Consulting Pathologist, St Mark's Hospital, London, England.

not the best treatment, and should be used for only the tiniest polyps. If one or more rectal polyps are discovered on sigmoidoscopic examination, a colonoscopy must be performed as further polyps are frequently found in the colon and treatment may be influenced. *No rectal tumour should be removed until the possibility of a proximal carcinoma has been ruled out, otherwise local implantation of cancer cells may occur in the distally situated rectal wound.*

The rectum shares substantially the same spectrum of polyps as the colon. Polyps are described chiefly in terms of their tissue organisation. For further clinical details the reader is referred to Chapter 67. Certain polyps which have features relevant to the rectum are now described.

Polyps relevant to the rectum

Juvenile polyp

This is a bright red glistening pedunculated sphere ('cherry tumour') which is found in infants and children. Occasionally it persists into adult life. It can cause bleeding, or pain if it prolapses during defecation. It often separates itself, but can be removed easily with forceps or a snare. It has virtually no tendency to malignant change but should be treated if it is causing symptoms. It has a unique histological structure of large mucus-filled spaces covered by a smooth surface of thin rectal cuboidal epithelium (Fig. 60.18).

Metaplastic polyps

These are small, pinkish, sessile polyps 2–4 mm in diameter and frequently multiple. They are harmless.

Pseudopolyps

These are oedematous bosses of mucous membrane. They are usually associated with colitis in the UK, but most inflammatory diseases (including tropical diseases) can cause them. They are more likely to cause radiological difficulty as the sigmoidoscopic appearances are usually associated with obvious signs of the inflammatory cause.

Villous adenomas

These have a characteristic frond-like appearance. They are often of very large size, and occasionally fill the entire rectum. The large tumours have an enhanced tendency to become malignant – a change that can be detected most easily by palpation with the finger; any hard area should be assumed to be malignant and should be biopsied.

Rarely, the profuse mucous discharge from these tumours, which is high in potassium content, causes dangerous electrolyte and fluid losses (Fig. 60.19).

Provided cancerous change has been excluded, these tumours can be removed either by submucous dissection per anum, or by sleeve resection from above. Only very unusually is rectal excision required, and then only when malignant change has occurred. A recent technique known as transanal endoscopic microsurgery (TEM) has been developed (Buess) which has improved the endoanal approach for the local removal of villous adenomas. The method requires the insertion of a very large operating sigmoidoscope. The rectum is distended by carbon dioxide insufflation, the operative field is magnified by a camera inserted via the sigmoidoscope, and

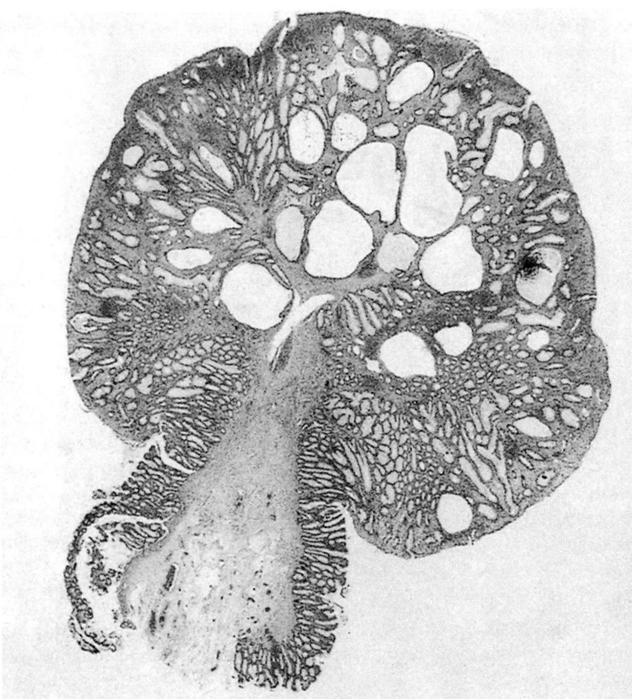

Fig. 60.18 Microscopic appearance of juvenile polyp.

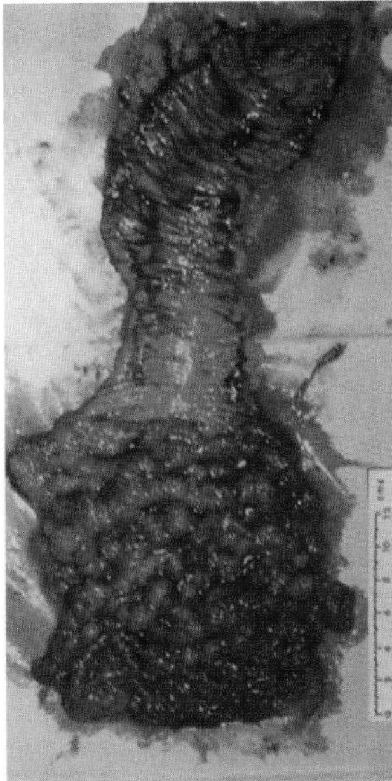

Fig. 60.19 Huge villous adenoma which occupied the lower half of the rectum and caused hypokalaemia.

Gerhardt Buess. Professor of Surgery, Tubingen, Germany.

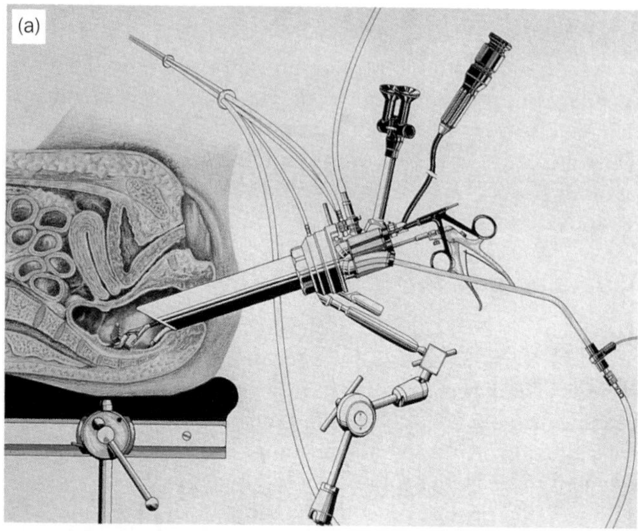

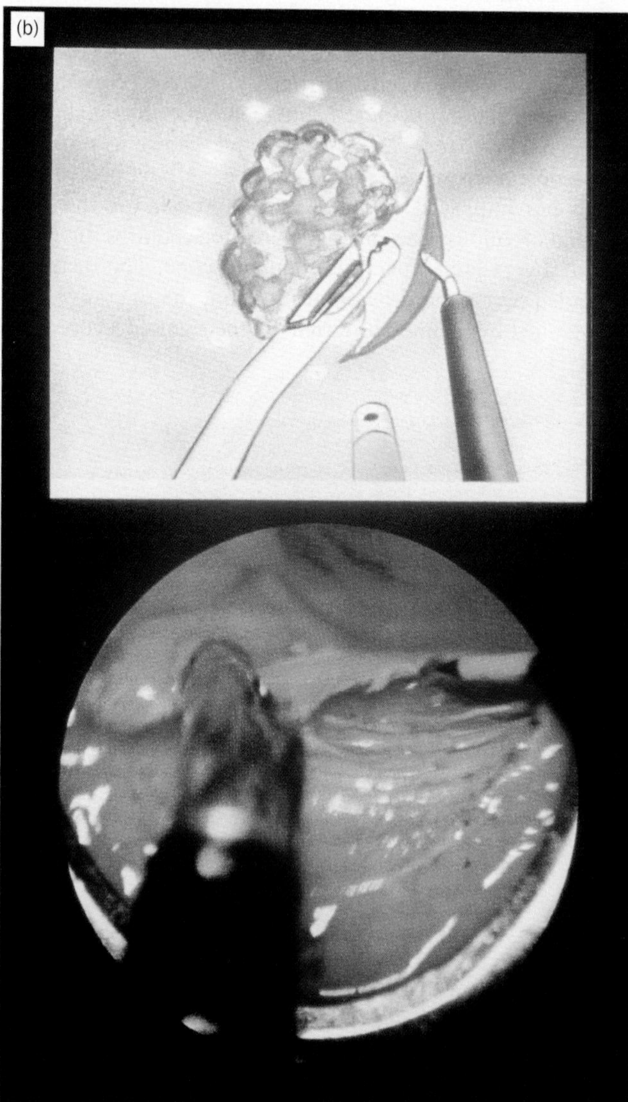

Fig. 60.20 Transanal endoscopic microsurgery technique.

the image is displayed on a monitor (Fig. 60.20). The lesion is excised using specially designed instruments with the surgeon observing the monitor screen. The technique is highly specialised and takes a considerable amount of time to master.

All neoplastic polyps can be solitary or multiple. Small colonic polyps (under 5 cm in size) can now be snared through the colonoscope. This instrument has revolutionised the treatment of multiple polyps.

Familial adenomatous polyposis (formerly known as familial polyposis coli)

This disease usually manifests itself by the development of multiple rectal and colonic polyps around puberty. A colonoscopy and biopsy will confirm the presence of multiple colonic adenomatous polyps. Recently the adenomatous polyposis cell (APC) gene responsible for the disease has been isolated on chromosome 5 (Bodmer). This discovery should make screening of affected families far more cost-effective than at present. As this condition is premalignant, a total colectomy must be performed, but often the rectum can be preserved by regular fulguration of polyps before they develop carcinoma. The operation of restorative proctocolectomy with pouchanal anastomosis is now being used in most centres of coloproctology: the rectum is replaced by a 'pouch' of folded ileum (Chapter 57). A pan-proctocolectomy with permanent ileostomy is necessary in some instances, especially when patient follow-up may be impractical.

Differential diagnosis

Bilharzia

In patients who have lived in Egypt, or any country where bilharzial infestation is rife, bilharzial papilloma must be excluded.

Treatment. Diathermy coagulation is satisfactory in the case of a small papilloma, but the patient must be examined at regular intervals as recurrence is common, as in the case of the bladder. For large papillomas, especially the sessile variety, excision of the rectum may be the only curative treatment. Some cases (not, as a rule, those invading the anal canal) are suitable for conservative resection of the rectum. In a few cases intestinal continuity can be restored by a low coloanal 'sleeve' anastomosis or one achieved by the circular stapling gun.

Benign lymphoma. This occurs as a circumscribed movable nodule, firm but not hard, greyish-white to pink in colour, and is essentially submucosal. This neoplasm, which occurs at all ages and in both sexes, has no definite capsule. Notwithstanding, complete local excision is curative.

Endometrioma. Endometrioma is rare, and as a rule is diagnosed as a carcinoma. This neoplasm produces either a constricting lesion of the rectosigmoid or a tumour invading the rectum from the rectovaginal septum. The latter variety gives rise to a very tender submucous elevation of the rectal wall. Endometrioma occurs usually between 20 and 40 years of age; less often at the menopause. Dysmenorrhoea with rectal bleeding are the main symptoms. On sigmoidoscopy endometriosis

Walter Bodmer. Former Director, Imperial Cancer Research Fund, UK.

involving the rectosigmoid junction usually presents as a stricture with the mucous membrane intact. Bilateral öophorectomy may be followed by regression of the tumour, rendering resection unnecessary. The contraceptive pill is also effective as it inhibits ovulation.

Haemangioma. Haemangioma of the rectum, which is an uncommon tumour, is a cause of serious and, if the neoplasm is large, sometimes fatal haemorrhage. When localised in the lower part of the rectum or anal canal, a haemangioma can be excised after applying. Goodsall's ligature. When the neoplasm is diffuse, or lying in the upper part of the rectum, the symptoms simulate ulcerative colitis, and often the diagnosis is missed for a long period. At other times, the neoplasm is mistaken for a vascular carcinoma, an error which, fortunately, is not often a cause for serious regret because the correct treatment of an extensive haemangioma is excision of that portion of the anorectum bearing the neoplasm. Lesser procedures are followed nearly always by recurrence and renewed loss of blood.

Leiomyoma. Benign smooth muscle tumours of the rectum are rare. They consist of spindle cells. It is often difficult to predict how they will behave. If the mitotic rate is high, and if there is variation in number, size and shape, hyperchromasia and frequent bizarre cells, these tumours are likely to metatasise. In these circumstances, they should be classified as leiomyosarcomas. This uncertainty in their behaviour means that treatment should, whenever possible, be by radical excision.

Carcinomas

Colorectal carcinoma is the fourth most common variety of malignant tumour found in women, and its frequency in men is surpassed only by carcinoma of the bronchus and stomach. Overall, it is the second most common carcinoma in the Western countries, with approximately 18 000 patients in the UK dying per annum. The rectum is the most frequent site involved.

Origin

In many cases, operation specimens show that in some part of the bowel that has been removed, in addition to the carcinoma, there are one or more synchronous adenomas or papillomas, proof indeed that adenoma and papilloma of the rectum are precarcinomatous conditions. In approximately 5 per cent of cases, there is more than one carcinoma present. It is now believed that most rectal cancers start as an adenoma and this is due to a series of genetic changes which progressively change the adenoma from one that is not dysplastic to one that shows severe dysplasia and finally becomes a carcinoma (the adenoma–carcinoma sequence) (Vogelstein) (Chapter 67).

Pathological histology

Three types are recognised:

- well-differentiated adenocarcinoma;
- averagely differentiated adenocarcinoma;
- anaplastic, highly undifferentiated adenocarcinoma.

The more malignant varieties frequently contain large numbers of mucin-producing cells. The prognosis after treatment is greatly influenced by the histological grading of the tumour (see below).

Usually these carcinomas present as an ulcer, but papilliferous and infiltrating types are common.

B. Vogelstein. Scientist, USA.

Types of carcinoma spread

Local spread

Local spread occurs circumferentially rather than in a longitudinal direction. Usually a period of 6 months is required for involvement of a quarter of the circumference, and 18 months to 2 years for complete encirclement, the annular variety being common at the rectosigmoid junction. After the muscular coat has been penetrated, the growth spreads into surrounding mesorectum, but is still limited by the fascia propria (perirectal fascia). Eventually, the fascia propria is penetrated but this occurrence is rare before 18 months from the commencement of the disease. If penetration occurs anteriorly, the prostate, seminal vesicles or the bladder become involved in the male; in the female the vagina or the uterus is invaded. In either sex, if the penetration is lateral, a ureter may become implicated, while posterior penetration invoves the sacrum and the sacral plexus. Downward spread for more than a few centimetres is rare except in anaplastic tumours.

Lymphatic spread

Enlargement of lymph nodes from bacterial infection is more frequent than enlargement from metastasis, and microscopical examination is required to detect carcinomatous involvement of the nodes.

Lymphatic spread from a carcinoma of the rectum above the peritoneal reflection occurs almost exclusively in an *upward* direction; below that level to within 1–2 cm of the anal orifice the lymphatic spread is still *upwards*, but the first halting place is in the pararectal lymph nodes of Gerota. The exception to this rule is when the neoplasm lies within the field of the middle rectal artery, i.e. between 4 and 8 cm from the anus, in which case primary *lateral* spread along the lymphatics that accompany the middle rectal vein is not infrequent.

Downward spread is exceptional, drainage along the subcutaneous lymphatics to the groins being confined, for practical purposes, to the lymph nodes draining the perianal rosette and the epithelium lining the distal 1–2 cm of the anal canal.

Metastasis at a higher level than the main trunk of the superior rectal artery occurs only late in the disease. A radical operation should ensure that the high-lying lymph nodes are removed by ligating the inferior mesenteric artery and vein at the highest possible level.

Atypical and widespread lymphatic permeation can occur in highly undifferentiated neoplasms.

Venous spread

As a rule, spread via the venous system occurs late, except in that portion of the anal canal where the anoderm is firmly adherent to deeper structures. Anaplastic and rapidly growing tumours in younger patients are much more liable to spread in this way than tumours of relatively low malignancy. The principal sites for blood-borne metastases are: liver (34 per cent), lungs (22 per cent) and adrenals (11 per cent).

The remaining 33 per cent is divided among the many other locations where secondary carcinomatous deposits are wont to lodge, including the brain.

Peritoneal dissemination

This may follow penetration of the peritoneal coat by a high-lying rectal carcinoma.

Stages of progression

As a rule, carcinoma of the rectum does not metastasise early. Dukes classified carcinoma of the rectum into three stages (Fig. 60.21).

A The growth is limited to the rectal wall (15 per cent). Prognosis excellent.

B The growth is extended to the extrarectal tissues, but no metastasis to the regional lymph nodes (35 per cent). Prognosis reasonable.

C There are secondary deposits in the regional lymph nodes (50 per cent). These are subdivided into C^1 where the local pararectal lymph nodes alone are involved, and C^2 where the nodes accompanying the supplying blood vessels are implicated up to the point of division. This does not take into account cases that have metastasised beyond the regional lymph nodes or by way of the venous system. Prognosis bad.

A stage D is often included which was not described by Dukes. This stage signifies the presence of widespread metastases, usually hepatic. Other staging systems have been developed (e.g. Astler–Coller TNM) to improve prognostic accuracy. The TNM classification has become popular internationally. T represents the extent of local spread and there are four grades, T_1, T_2, T_3 and T_4, depending on whether the tumour (T) is confined to the mucosa or has penetrated the rectal wall. N describes nodal involvement and M indicates the pressure of distant metastases.

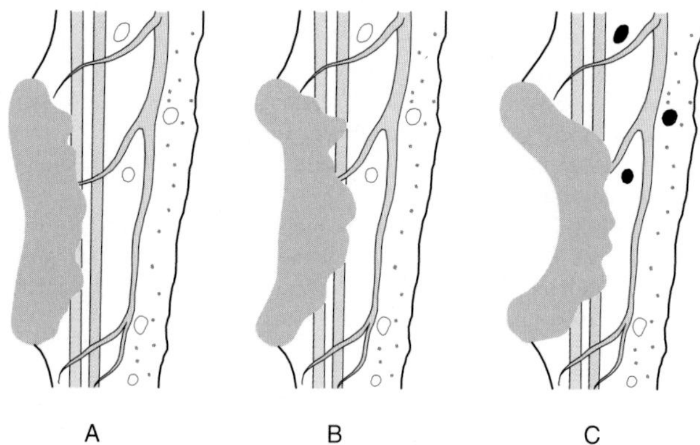

Fig. 60.21 The three cardinal stages of progression of the neoplasm (*after Cuthbert Dukes, FRCS*).

Histological grading. In the great majority of cases, carcinoma of the rectum is a columnar-celled adenocarcinoma. The more nearly the tumour cells approach normal shape and arrangement, the less malignant is the tumour. Conversely, the greater the percentage of cells of an embryonic or undifferentiated type, the more malignant is the tumour:

Low grade = well-differentiated tumours	11 per cent	Prognosis good
Average grade	64 per cent	Prognosis fair
High grade = anaplastic tumours	25 per cent	Prognosis poor

Colloid carcinoma. This type of carcinoma is present in 12 per cent of cases. There are two forms: primary and secondary; much the more frequent is secondary mucoid degeneration of an adenocarcinoma. Histologically the glandular arrangement is preserved and mucus fills the acini. This type is of average malignancy. In a small number of cases the tumour is a primary mucoid carcinoma. The mucus lies within the cells, displacing the nucleus to the periphery, like the seal of a signet ring. Primary mucoid carcinoma gives rise to a rapidly growing bulky growth which metastasises very early and the prognosis of which is very bad.

Clinical features

Carcinoma of the rectum is not uncommon early in life, and when the disease commences in youth, in spite of radical treatment, death usually results within a year. However, the adult age of presentation is above 55 years. Often the early symptoms are so slight that the patient does not seek advice for 6 months or more.

Bleeding

Bleeding is the earliest and most common symptom. There is nothing characteristic about the time at which it occurs, neither is the colour or the amount of blood distinctive; often the bleeding is slight in amount, and occurs at the end of defecation, or is noticed because it has stained underclothing. Indeed, more often than not, the bleeding in every respect simulates that of internal haemorrhoids (haemorrhoids and carcinoma sometimes coexist) and it is lamentable that, in spite of oft-repeated exhortations, the patient's doctor sometimes fails to examine the rectum but prescribes a salve while the growth advances to inoperability (see footnote, Chapter 59).

Sense of incomplete defecation

The patient's bowels open but there is the sensation that there are more faeces to be passed (*tenesmus*, a painful straining to empty the bowels without resultant evacuation). This is a very important early symptom and is almost invariably present in tumours of the lower half of the rectum. The patient may endeavour to empty the rectum several times a day (spurious diarrhoea), often with the passage of flatus and a little blood-stained mucus ('bloody slime').

Cuthbert Esquire Dukes, 1890–1977. Pathologist, St Mark's Hospital, London, England.

V.B. Astler. Highland Park, New Jersey, USA.

F.A. Coller. University of Michigan, Chicago, Michigan, USA.

Alteration in bowel habit

This is the next most frequent symptom. The patient may find it necessary to start taking an aperient, or to supplement the usual dose, and as a result a tendency towards diarrhoea ensues. A patient who has to get up before the accustomed hour in order to defecate, and one who passes blood and mucus in addition to faeces ('early morning bloody diarrhoea'), is usually found to be suffering from carcinoma of the rectum. Usually, it is the patient with an annular carcinoma at the pelvirectal junction who suffers with increasing constipation, and the one with a growth in the ampulla of the rectum with early morning diarrhoea (Bruce).

Pain

Pain is a late symptom, but pain of a colicky character accompanies advanced growths of the rectosigmoid, and is due to some degree of intestinal obstruction. When a deep carcinomatous ulcer of the rectum erodes the prostate or bladder, there is severe pain. Pain in the back, or sciatica, occurs when the growth invades the sacral plexus. *Weight loss* is suggestive of hepatic metastases.

> Early symptoms of rectal cancer
>
> - Bleeding per rectum
> - Tenesmus
> - Early morning diarrhoea

Abdominal examination

Abdominal examination is negative in early cases. Occasionally, when an advanced annular growth is situated at the rectosigmoid junction, signs of obstruction to the large intestine are likely to be present. By the time the patient seeks advice, metastases in the liver may be palpable. When the peritoneum has become studded with secondary deposits, ascites results.

Rectal examination

In approximately 90 per cent of cases, the neoplasm can be felt digitally: in early cases as a plateau or as a nodule with an indurated base. When the centre ulcerates, a shallow depression will be found, the edges of which are raised and everted; this, combined with induration of the base of the ulcer, is a frequent and unmistakable finding. On bimanual examination, it may be possible to feel the lower extremity of a carcinoma situated in the rectosigmoid junction. After the finger has been withdrawn, if it has been in direct contact with a carcinoma, it is smeared with blood or mucopurulent material tinged with blood. When a carcinomatous ulcer is situated in the lower third of the rectum, involved lymph nodes can sometimes be felt as one or more hard, oval swellings in the extrarectal tissues posteriorly or posterolaterally above the tumour. In females, a vaginal examination should be performed, and when the neoplasm is situated on the anterior wall of the rectum, with one finger in the vagina and another in the rectum, very accurate palpation can be carried out.

Sir John Bruce, 1905–75. Professor of Surgery, Edinburgh, Scotland.

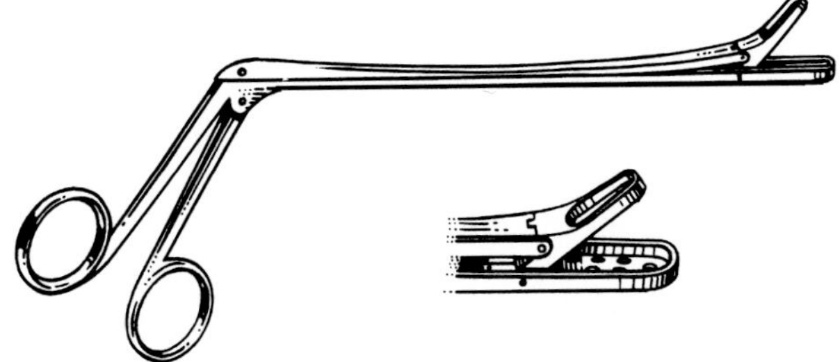

Fig. 60.22 Yeoman's biopsy forceps.

Proctosidmoidoscopy

Proctosidmoidoscopy will always show a carcinoma, if present – provided that the rectum is emptied of faeces beforehand.

Biopsy

Employing biopsy forceps (Fig. 60.22) by way of a sigmoidoscope, a portion of the edge of the tumour is removed. If possible, another specimen from the more central part of the growth is also obtained. Expert histological examination will not only enable the diagnosis of carcinoma to be confirmed, but the tumour can be graded as to its relative malignancy, although not always with complete accuracy.

Barium enema. Barium enema or, preferably, *a colonoscopy* is required if possible in all patients to exclude a synchronous tumour, be it an adenoma or a carcinoma. If an adenoma is found, it can be conveniently snared and removed via the colonoscope. If a synchronous carcinoma is present, the operative strategy will need changing.

When a stenosing carcinoma is present, it may not be possible using these investigations, especially colonoscopy, to visualise the proximal colon. However, in view of the high incidence of synchronous tumours, it is imperative that a colonoscopy is always performed either before or after surgical resection.

Differential diagnosis. When a seemingly benign *adenoma* shows evidence of induration or unusual friability, it is almost certain that malignancy has occurred, even in spite of biopsy findings to the contrary. On the other hand, biopsy is invaluable in distinguishing carcinoma from an *inflammatory stricture* or an *amoebic granuloma*, which simulates a carcinoma very closely. The possibility of a neoplasm being an *endometrioma* should always be entertained in patients with dysmenorrhoea. The possibility of a *carcinoid tumour* in atypical cases must be remembered. In the last four instances biopsy should establish the correct diagnosis. The *solitary ulcer* syndrome has already been alluded to above.

Treatment

Some form of excision of the rectum is essential, if at all possible, because of the extreme suffering entailed if the neoplasm remains. However, before surgery is embarked upon, it is necessary to assess:

- the fitness of the patient for operation;
- the extent of spread of the tumour.

The findings will affect the surgical approach.

Assessment of spread should include ultrasonography or computed tomography (CT) of the liver, and a chest radiograph to exclude distant metastases (Fig. 60.23).

Endoluminal ultrasound whereby a probe is placed in the rectal lumen can be used to assess the local spread of the tumour (Fig. 60.24), as can CT and, more recently, magnetic resonance imaging (MRI).

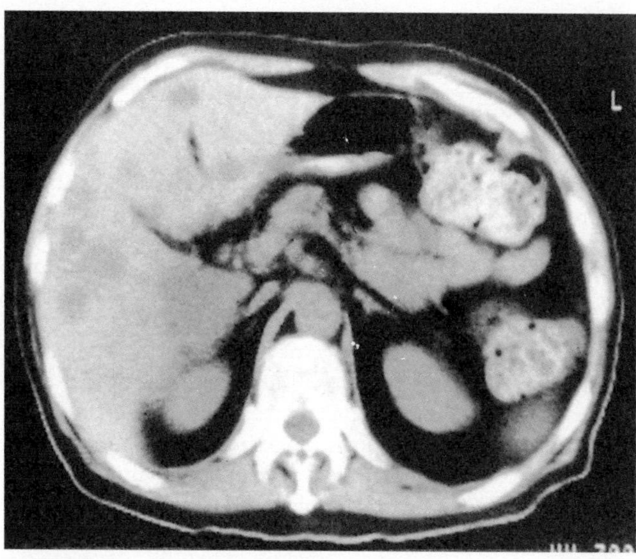

Fig. 60.23 Computerised tomography scan of the liver in a patient with a rectal cancer showing multiple liver metastases.

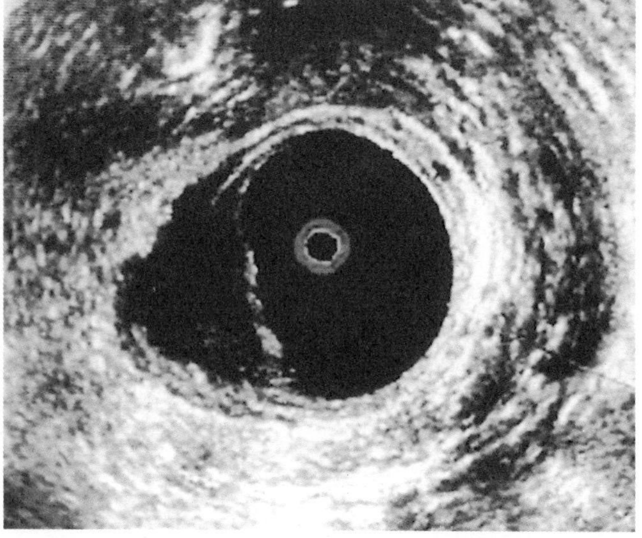

Fig. 60.24 Endoluminal ultrasound. The probe is in the rectal lumen and shows a rectal tumour invading through the rectal wall.

Principles of surgical treatment

Radical excision of the rectum, together with the mesorectum and associated lymph nodes, should be the aim. Even in the presence of widespread metastases a rectal excision should be considered, as this is often the best means of palliation. The presence of a solitary liver metastasis does not necessarily rule out the feasibility of a radical excision. Many instances have been reported where a presumed solitary liver metastasis has been resected either at the time of excision of the rectum or subsequently with long-term survival being achieved.

When a tumour appears to be locally advanced, the administration of a course of preoperative radiotherapy may reduce its size and make it more amenable to radical excision. Indeed, recent evidence suggests that the administration of preoperative adjacent radiotherapy in all rectal cancer cases reduces the incidence of local recurrence significantly (Pahlman).

For patients who are unfit for radical surgery or who have widespread metastases, a local procedure such as transanal excision, laser destruction or interstitial radiation should be considered.

When a rectal excision is possible, whenever feasible, the aim should be to restore gastrointestinal continuity and continence by preserving the anal sphincter. A sphincter-saving operation (*anterior resection*) is usually possible for tumours of the upper two-thirds of the rectum. Although removal of the rectum with a permanent colostomy (*abdominoperineal excision*) is often required for tumours of the lower third of the rectum, the introduction of the stapling gun has enabled many more of these patients to be treated by a sphincter-saving procedure. Provided a minimum distal margin of clearance of 2 cm can be secured, it is safe to restore gastrointestinal continuity (Williams). Because of the much wider degree of local spread by anaplastic tumours and the high risk of local recurrence, it has been customary not to perform restorative operations when these carcinomas are in the lower third of the rectum. However, with the realisation that a preoperative biopsy is often inaccurate with respect to the degree of histological differentiation, coupled with the more widespread use of preoperative and postoperative radiotherapy, many more anaplastic lesions are being treated by sphincter-saving procedures. Anterior resection is now applied to at least two-thirds of cases presenting with carcinoma of the rectum. The principles of the operation involve radical excision of the neoplasm, with at least a 2 cm margin of normal bowel below the lower edge of the tumour, removal of all the mesorectum, i.e. total mesorectal excision (TME) (Heald) and high proximal ligation of the inferior mesenteric lymphovascular pedicle. Once the

---

Lars Pahlman. Surgeon, Sweden.
Norman S. Williams. Professor of Surgery, The Royal London Hospital, London, England.
R.J. Heald. Surgeon, Basingstoke, England.

rectum has been mobilised adequately, and the bowel washed out proximally and distally, it is removed. Restoration of continuity by direct end-to-end anastomosis (manually or by stapling) must be carried out by a meticulous technique to reduce risks of suture line breakdown. If a perfect union is achieved, a protecting colostomy is not necessary (see later).

Preoperative preparation of the alimentary tract

This is usually achieved by a combination of mechanical cleansing (purgatives, enemas or 'whole-gut irrigation') and antibiotics. The antibiotic regime must be active against both aerobic and anaerobic organisms. At present a suitable prescription would be cefuroxime 750 mg plus metronidazole 500 mg 1 hour before surgery, plus another two doses of each drug at 6 and 12 hours after the operation. If a patient comes to surgery with a loaded colon, perioperative washouts can be performed provided the rest of the wound is scrupulously protected. Detergent preparations are available for this.

Blood and electrolyte deficiencies are corrected. Before commencing the operation, an indwelling catheter is inserted into the bladder.

Combined (abdominal and perineal) excision of the rectum. This operation is still required for large extensive tumours of the lower third of the rectum, which are unsuitable for a sphincter-saving procedure. It has the advantage for difficult tumours of the lower rectum of two surgeons operating from the abdominal and perineal approaches simultaneously. This considerably reduces the time expended in performing the operation, and obviates turning the patient. A large catheter is passed and with the patient in Trendelenburg lithotomy position, the legs being supported in special crutches designed by Lloyd-Davies, access is afforded to the abdomen and the perineum at the same time.

The *abdominal surgeon* makes a midline incision, extending it well above the umbilicus. The liver and the peritoneum are examined for metastases and the degree of fixity of the growth is established. The small intestine is packed away from the pelvis. A self-retaining retractor is placed in the wound and the pelvic colon freed by dividing any congenital adhesions on the left side. The peritoneum and the pelvic floor are divided with a knife by an icision which runs from the colon at the proposed site of division over the mesocolon and across the base of the bladder or near the cervix on the pelvic floor and then upwards on the right side of the mesocolon. The peritoneum is now raised, using the points of the scissors to expose the ureters and testicular or ovarian artery. The mesocolon is now divided at the site of the proposed division of the colon and the trunk of the inferior mesenteric artery (Fig. 60.25), is ligated and divided distal to the first branch. (Some surgeons emphasise 'flush ligation' of the artery at its origin from the aorta.) The rectosigmoid mesentery is further divided and separated from the sacrum by blunt dissection with the fingers. In this way, the sacrum is cleared almost down to the coccyx. The peritoneal incision anterior to the rectum is now deepened and the seminal vesicles or the vaginal wall

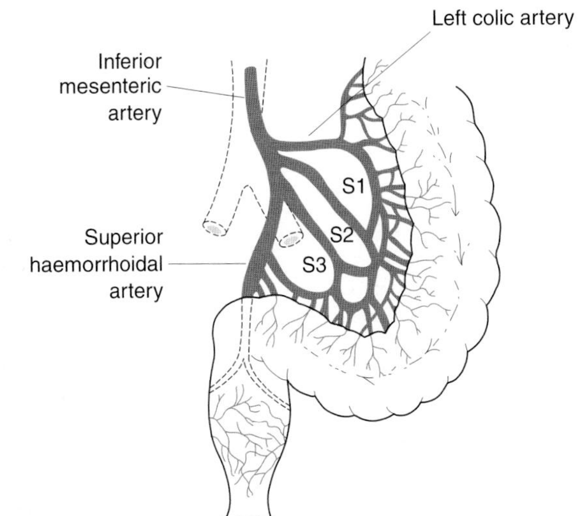

Fig. 60.25 The inferior mesenteric artery. S_1, S_2 and S_3 are sigmoid branches.

are identified so that Denonvilliers' fascia behind them is cleared by a dissection leading down to the prostate or perineal body. The middle rectal vessels usually lying anterior to the lateral ligaments on each side are now seized with clamps, divided and ligated. The site of division of the pelvic colon is cleared of fat and the colon divided between clamps with diathermy.

By this time, the *perineal surgeon* working from below has mobilised the anus and the lower rectum so that the whole of the bowel together with a clamp can be passed through the perineal wound by the abdominal surgeon. Haemostasis over the sacrum may be difficult, but it is achieved by diathermy and a hot saline pack left in position for a few

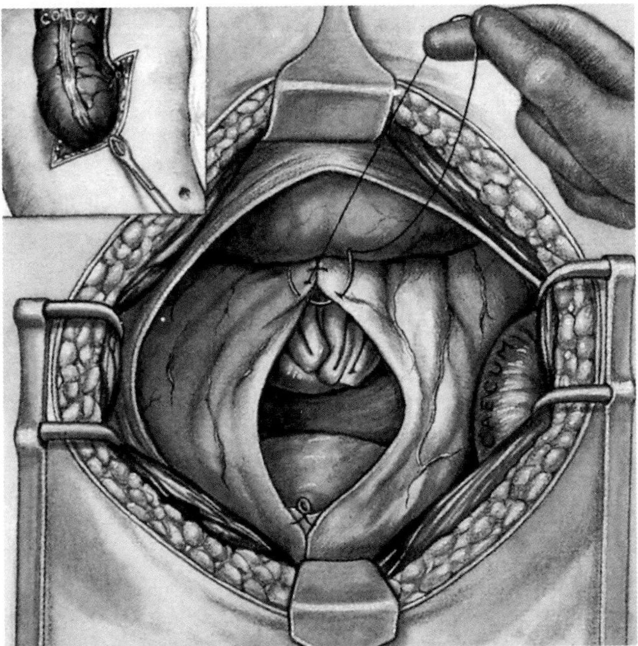

Fig. 60.26 The cut edges of the pelvic peritoneum are being united over the space (filled by packing) where the 'perineal' surgeon is working. *Inset.* The pelvic colon drawn through the left iliac incision to form a terminal colostomy.

Friedrich Trendelenburg, 1844–1924. Professor of Surgery, Leipzig, Germany.

O. *Lloyd-Davies, 1905–87. Consultant Surgeon, St Mark's Hospital, London, England.*

minutes. The pelvic peritoneum is now united by continuous catgut stitches from the bladder right back over the promontory of the sacrum (Fig. 60.26).

The site in the left iliac fossa for the colostomy should have been marked preoperatively by the stoma care nurse in consultation with the patient. If this has not been possible it should be sited equidistant from the umbilicus and the left anterior superior iliac spine at the linea semi-lunaris about 2.5 cm above the spinoumbilical line. A circular piece of skin and fascia, about 3 cm in diameter, is excised and this hole deepened to excise similar layers of fascia and peritoneum. The protected end of the colon with the clamp is now passed through this incision and the colostomy performed by suturing the colon to the peritoneum and the mucosa directly to the skin. The paracolic gutter is closed with sutures – this will close the 'lateral space'. The abdomen is closed and the layers of the incision are protected from the colostomy. An adherent plastic colostomy bag is then fitted in position and the dressings are placed on the abdominal wound.

When the abdominal surgeon has made certain that the condition is operable, the *perineal surgeon* closes the anus with pursestring sutures of stout silk. An elliptical incision between the tip of the coccyx and the central perineal point is made around the anus and deepened. The left forefinger is insinuated into the levator ani which is divided lateral to the finger first on one side and then on the other. The dissection is deepend posteriorly by incising Waldeyer's fascia which is a thick condensation of pelvic fascia lying between the rectum and the sacrum. Contact is made with the abdominal surgeon. The apex of skin anterior to the anus is grasped in a haemostat, which serves as a retractor, and by scissors and gauze dissection the wound is deepened, when the catheter within the membranous urethra will be felt. In both the male and the female, a plane of cleavage will be found between the rectum and the prostate of the rectum and the vagina, respectively. This plane having been carefully determined, Denonvilliers' fascia is divided, after which the rectum can be stripped from the prostate or the vagina. The posterior wall of the vagina is frequently excised with the rectum. When the abdominal surgeon has cleared the rectum laterally, the whole of the anus and rectum can be drawn downwards and removed. Haemostasis must be secured and the perineal wound closed anteriorly and posteriorly in layers around a large drainage tube or closed entirely around suction drains. Large dressings of gauze and wool are applied over the area and a triangular bandage is used to keep the dressing in place. It is usual to employ *primary closure* of the perineal wound, and to use laterally situated suction drains brought out through each ischiorectal fossa to keep the large perineal cavity from filling up with blood and serous exudate. These drains can be removed after 5 days.

After treatment. The patient is returned to bed, blood transfusion being continued as necessary. The catheter is connected to a closed drainage system and left in for 5 days. It may have to be reinserted if voluntary micturation is not re-established.

Reactionary haemorrhage from the perineal wound may demand return to the theatre to open and pack the wound with gauze. The colour of the colostomy must be watched to make sure that the blood supply is adequate. Small-bowel obstruction may occur by herniation through the lateral space of the colostomy or through the pelvic peritoneal closure line. Discharge of urine from the perineal wound demands immediate investigation for bladder, ureteric or urethral damage.

Care of the colostomy. This is much the same as the care of an ileostomy (Chapter 57). Within a very short time, the colostomy acts once or twice a day. The patient soon learns which foods cause diarrhoea and therefore avoids them. Many patients are now taught to empty their lower colon by irrigations through the colostomy: this has many advantages for the patient who requires an inactive colostomy while at work. Occlusive caps are also available which fit in the end of the stoma and allow some degree of continence.

Stenosis of colostomy is usually avoided by the removal of the circle of skin and subcutaneous tissues at the colostomy site. Dilators may be necessary if there is any tendency for stenosis to occur.

Laparoscopic abdominoperineal excision. Recently, it has been demonstrated that the operation can be carried out laparoscopically. The rectum is mobilised completely from above using the laparoscope. A small circular perineal incision is made around the anal canal, and via a limited perineal dissection the rectum and anal canal are completely mobilised. After transecting the midsigmoid colon with an Endo GIA instrument, the specimen containing the carcinoma is delivered through the perineal wound. A trephine incision is made in the left iliac fossa and the sigmoid colon is brought out as an end colostomy. Although the operative technique has been shown to be quite feasible and reduces postoperative pain and time in hospital, there is concern that it may not be as curative as the standard 'open' technique. The concern surrounds the degree of clearance that can be achieved via the laparoscope, and the risk of free cancer cells being disseminated around the peritoneal cavity and implanting, particularly at the 'port' sites. Controlled trials will be needed to determine whether the laparoscopic approach is safe.

Anterior resection

In cases of carcinoma of the rectum situated above the peritoneal reflection, lymphatic spread is virtually confined to the upward path. Here a wide resection of the bowel with its lymphatic field, followed by end-to-end anastomosis and preservation of the sphincter mechanism is both justifiable and highly desirable.

As discussed previously, in the last two decades there has been a move to extend sphincter-saving operations to treat most tumours of the middle third of the rectum, and indeed many of the lower third. The introduction of the stapling

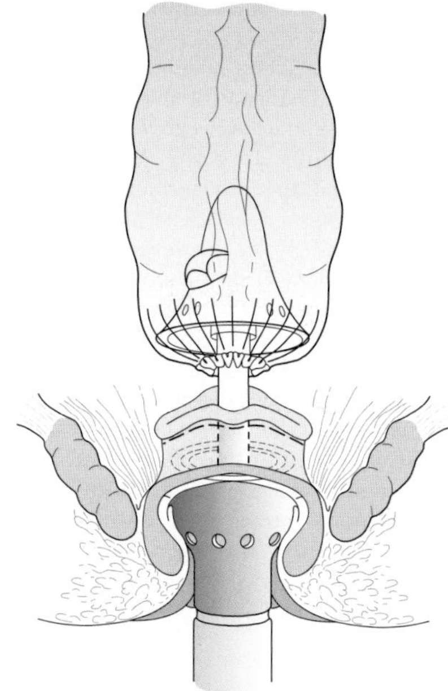

Fig. 60.27 Low anterior resection by the double stapling method. The rectum has been excised and the distal anorectal stump has been transected with the transverse stapling device. Colorectal anastomosis is achieved by the use of the Premium CEEA mechanical stapling gun.

instruments, particularly the new Premium CEEA instrument with its detachable head, has made such procedures far more feasible.

The operation of low anterior resection proceeds in the same manner as the abdominal part of abdominoperineal excision. The rectum is mobilised to such an extent that a right-angled clamp can be placed at least 2 cm below the tumour. The rectal stump can then be stapled transversely, using a TA instrument. After the rectum and sigmoid colon have been excised, continuity is re-established by the method depicted in Fig. 60.27. Some surgeons are concerned that the anastomotic leakage rate will be increased if the technique of cross-stapling of the rectal stump is used. They prefer to place a pursestring suture in the rectal stump lumen, as well as in the proximal colon. After the stapling gun is fired and removed, it is essential that the head of the instrument is detached and the 'doughnuts' are examined. A break in the circumference of one or both 'doughnuts' signifies a defect in the anastomosis, and the latter should be sought and repaired with interrupted sutures. In these circumstances, a covering stoma will also be required to allow safe healing of the anastomosis. Some surgeons believe that such a stoma is required for all colorectal and coloanal anastomoses which are constructed below the peritoneal reflection.

Occasionally, although the rectum, together with its tumour, can be removed adequately, continuity cannot be restored by a stapling technique. In such cases, it may still be possible to restore continuity by bringing the colon down to the anal canal and constructing a coloanal anastomosis via the transanal route (Fig. 60.28) (the so-called *abdominotransanal–coloanal operation* first described by Parks).

In each of the procedures, it is essential to ensure that any free tumour cells released by mobilisation of the rectum are destroyed by irrigation of the colonic and rectal lumens with a cancercidal solution such as 1 per cent centrimide. By so doing, the implanatation of such cells and subsequent local recurrence is prevented. However, it should be realised that, although a small percentage of local recurrences is due to implantation of shed cells, the majority is due to inadequate removal of the tumour at the time of the initial operation. Although it is usual for the surgeon to remove all macroscopic tumour, he or she is often unable to remove all microscopic tumour. Particular interest has recently focused on local microscopic spread. It is now known that micrometastases are present in the mesorectum, and these are the most likely cause of local recurrence after rectal excision (Quirke). Heald has emphasised how important it is to remove all of

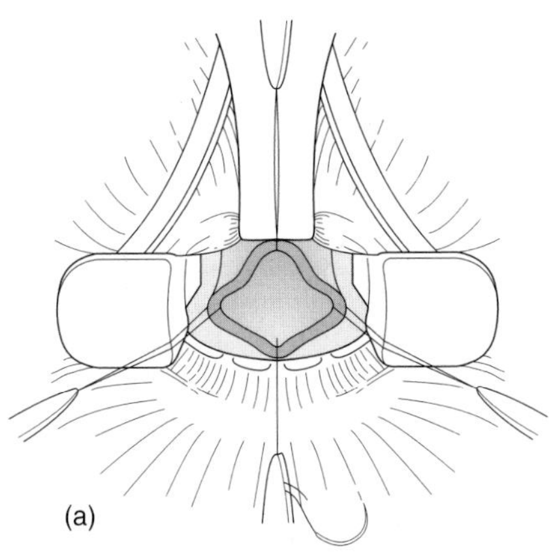

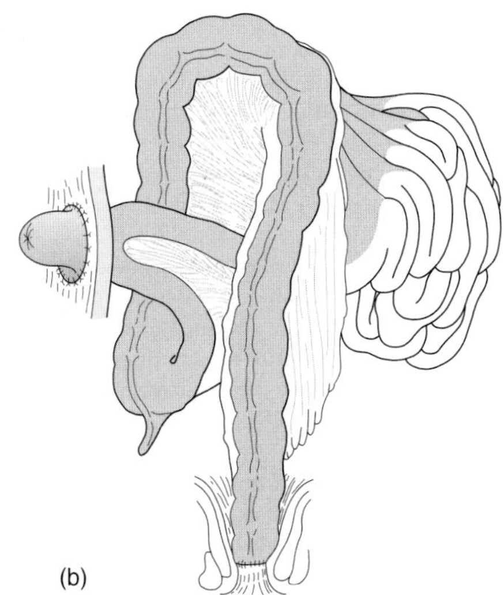

Fig. 60.28 Abdomino-transanal–coloanal anastomosis. (a) The rectum has been excised and the mucosa from the distal anorectal stump has been removed, leaving the rectal muscle intact. The proximal colon has been brought down through the rectal muscular cuff, to be anastomosed to the anal mucosa via the transanal route. (b) The completed coloanal anastomosis. A covering ileostomy has been performed, so as to allow the anastomosis to heal.

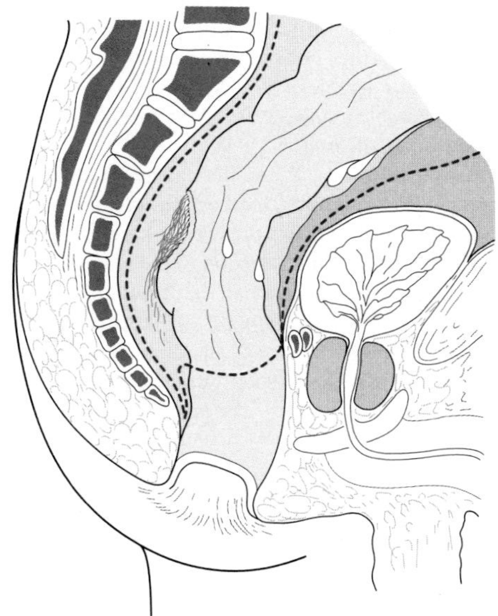

Fig. 60.29 Plane of dissection for total mesorectal excision.

Phillip Quirke. Professor of Pathology, Leeds, England.

the mesorectum during anterior resection or abdominoperineal excision. TME is now being practised world-wide and appears to reduce the risks of local recurrence substantially (Fig. 60.29). However, it is unlikely that surgery alone will deal adequately with the micrometastases in the pelvis. Consequently, adjuvant radiotherapy may have added benefit (see below).

Laparoscopic anterior resection

It is now possible to perform a high anterior resection using the laparoscope, the anastomosis being performed intraperitoneally using a slightly modified circular stapling gun. Laparoscopic anastomoses below the peritoneal reflection are feasible, but are much more difficult. However, with improvements in technology such procedures may become more commonplace. Nevertheless, like laparoscopic abdominoperineal excision, there is concern that these operations may be less curative than the standard operations.

Hartmann's operation. This is an excellent procedure in an old and feeble patient who would not stand a lengthy anterior resection or an abdominoperineal procedure. Through an abdominal incision the rectum is excised, if possible, to within 2.5 cm of the anus, the anorectal stump is transected usually with a stapler, a colostomy is performed and the peritoneum oversewn to cover the pelvic defect in the usual way. In an old patient, where the neoplasm is usually slow growing and spread is late, this is a most useful operation.

Palliative colostomy. This is indicated *only* in cases giving rise to intestinal obstruction, or where there is gross infection of the neoplasm. It is often possible to resect the growth later, and in some cases cure, rather than palliation, is achieved.

Local operations. For small, low-grade mobile lesions, which are often Dukes' A tumours, local removal should be curative. For these tumours, especially in the unfit or patients who will not accept a colostomy, local removal has been used. Such operations are only suitable for lesions within 10 cm of the anal verge. Turnbull advocated local diathermy removal while York-Mason developed a trans-sphincteric approach, but a peranal approach is usually possible, with full-thickness excision of the lesion. More recently, the TEM technique has been used for these tumours. There is considerable doubt whether such techniques should be used for potential curable lesions as they do not deal with the mesorectal or lymphatic spread of the tumour.

More extensive operations. When the carcinoma of the rectum has spread to contiguous organs, the radical operation can often be extended to remove these structures. Thus in the male, where the spread is usually to the bladder, a cystectomy and resection of the rectum can be effected. In the female, the uterus acts as a barrier preventing spread from the rectum to the bladder. Accordingly, a hysterectomy should be undertaken in addition to excision of the rectum. Should the bladder base be involved, then pelvic exenteration must include that structure. Pelvic evisceration for carcinoma of the rectum is justifiable only when the surgeon is reasonably confident that the growth can be removed *in toto*.

R. Turnbull. Surgeon, Cleveland Clinic, Cleveland, Ohio, USA.

Aubrey York-Mason. Surgeon, St Helier Hospital, Carshalton, Surrey, England.

Alexander Brunschwig, 1901–69. Surgeon, Memorial Hospital for the Treatment of Cancer, New York, USA.

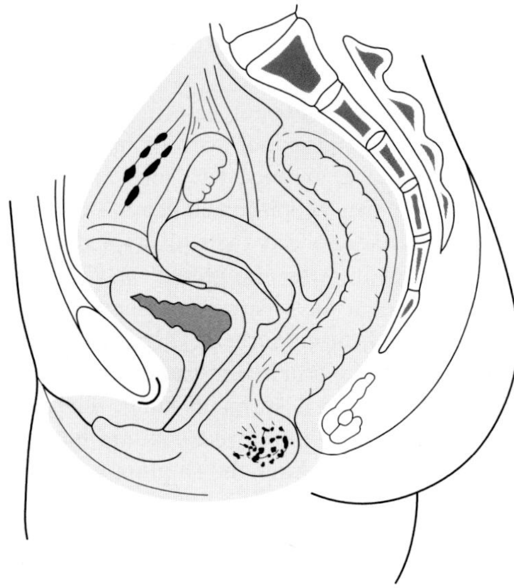

Fig. 60.30 Radical pelvic exenteration, indicating the extent of the dissection and the viscera removed. (Redrawn with permission from Keighley, M.R.B.K. and Williams, N.S., *Surgery of the Anus, Colon and Rectum*, 2nd edn, W.B. Saunders, London, 1999.)

Pelvic exenteration (Brunschwig's operation). The aim is to remove all of the pelvic organs, together with the internal iliac and the obturator groups of lymph nodes (Fig. 60.30). The Trendelenburg lithotomy position facilitates the procedure, and ligation of both internal iliac arteries diminishes the blood loss. The small intestine fills the empty pelvis. Special care must therefore be taken to suture accurately the perineal skin, and to avoid pressure necrosis of the perineal incision by nursing the patient on alternate sides. Some form of urinary diversion is necessary (Chapter 65), usually an ileal conduit.

Radiotherapy. With modern techniques (MV cobalt therapy or neutron beam irradiation) some adenocarcinomas now respond to radiotherapy. Various controlled trials have recently been performed to investigate the effect of adjuvant radiotherapy given either preoperation or postoperatively. The overall results of these trials suggest that provided an adequate dose is given (4000–5000 Gy) adjuvant radiotherapy can reduce the incidence of local recurrence; however, long-term survival is not affected. Surprisingly, with modern techniques morbidity from the radiation is not a major problem. Another advantage of preoperative radiotherapy is often its ability to reduce the size of a large tumour and make its subsequent removal easier. Palliative irradiation can be given for inoperable primary tumours or local recurrence, especially when painful. Papillon perfected a technique of intracavity radiation which applies the treatment direct to the tumour from the rectal lumen. In a selected series of early cases, the results were good (more than 70 per cent 5-year survival rates). Intraoperative irradiation is also being evaluated.

Chemotherapy and immunotherapy. A variety of drugs has been tried both as an adjuvant therapy and for the treatment of disseminated disease. The most frequently used drug is 5-fluorouracil (5FU). Up until recently, the results of various trials using 5FU either alone or in combination were disappointing. However, some optimism has recently

J. Papillon. Professor of Radiotherapy, Lyons, France.

been aroused by studies which have infused 5FU into the portal vein during and immediately after the primary operation (Taylor). Such adjuvant therapy is thought to kill malignant cells which are released into the circulation during operative manipulation of tumour, and thus prevent the formation of metastases. Initial results suggest that such therapy does reduce the incidence of metastases and can prolong survival.

There is also evidence that systemic folinic acid (leucovorin) has an effect as an adjuvant therapy when used in combination with 5FU. Similarly, studies from both the UK and the USA suggested that the combination of 5FU and levamisole (a nonspecific stimulator of the immune process) was effective as an adjuvant therapy for Dukes' C carcinomas. A variety of studies is now being conducted world-wide to examine which are the best forms of adjuvant therapy that should be used for both rectal and colon cancer. At the present it is generally accepted that the combination of 5FU and folinic acid given for a 6-month period in patients who are at high risk of recurrence can reduce cancer specific mortality.

There is considerable interest at present in immunotherapy for the treatment of disseminated colorectal cancer. Various monoclonal antibodies to carcinoembryonic antigen have been developed, which theoretically can be targeted to malignant deposits. When these antibodies are conjugated to cancericidal agents, they have the ability to destroy the cancerous cells. Unfortunately, the antibodies are not sufficiently specific and, therefore, normal tissue is likely to be damaged. Nevertheless, the search continues for more selective antibodies.

Results of surgery for rectal cancer. In specialised centres, the resectability rate may be as high as 95 per cent, with an operative mortality of less than 5 per cent. Overall, 5-year survival rates in these centres is about 50 per cent, but the rate falls to approximately 25 per cent when the results of nonspecialised centres are included. The most likely reason for this difference is the higher proportion of advanced and emergency cases treated in nonspecialised hospitals. However, another contributing reason is that in specialised centres there is a concentration of expertise which is not readily available in district hospitals. Survival rates are influenced by Dukes' stage, with C cases doing worse than A and B lesions (Fig. 60.31). The degree of mobility also influences survival, with fixed lesions having a worse prognosis than mobile lesions. The lower the tumour is in the rectum, the worse the outlook. Histological grade also influences outcome, anaplastic lesions having the worse prognosis. Interestingly, despite the more frequent use of sphincter-saving resection compared with abdominoperineal excision, survival has not been affected.

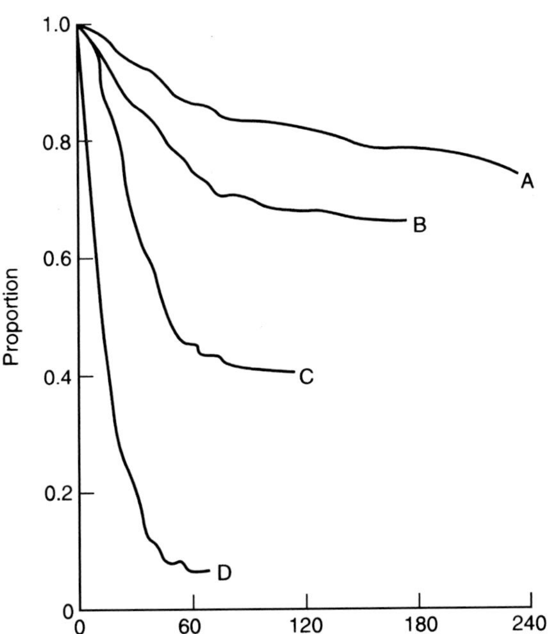

Fig. 60.31 Cancer specific survival rates following surgery for rectal cancer according to Dukes' stage. (Redrawn with permission from *Surgery of the Anus, Rectum and Colon*, 2nd edn, W.B. Saunders, London, 1999.)

Local recurrence. Local recurrence after rectal excision is a major problem. The patient often presents with persistent pelvic pain, which radiates down the legs if sacral roots have been involved. Bladder problems may occur. If recurrence develops after abdominoperineal excision, a swelling or induration may be present in the perineum, or an abscess or discharging sinus may develop. Occasionally, the presence of a large recurrence in the pelvis may lead to bilateral leg oedema, from either from pressure or invasion of lymphatics or veins. After sphincter-saving resection, local recurrence may produce a change in bowel habit, or the passage of blood per rectum. Sigmoidoscopic examination after sphincter-saving resection may reveal friable tissue at the anastomosis which, when biopsied, confirms the diagnosis. However, usually the recurrence is situated extrarectally, and is detected either as induration on digital examination or by endoluminal ultrasonography or CT. These investigations can also detect recurrence before it causes symptoms. Local recurrence rates vary between 2 and 25 per cent and seem to occur with equal frequency after sphincter-saving resection an abdominoperineal excision. The most common cause is inadequate removal of all the tumour at the initial operation. This is due to the presence of microscopic tumour deposits in the tissues surrounding the rectum. Heald has shown that if the mesorectum is removed in its entirety, the local recurrence rate can be reduced to less than 5 per cent.

Other possible causes for local recurrence include implantation of viable cells on the suture line and the development of a new primary tumour. Although both mechanisms may occur, inadequate removal of the tumour is by far and away the most important reason for recurrence. Eighty per cent of all local recurrences develop within 2 years following surgery and are very difficult to treat. The best prospect of salvage is by surgical resection. However, it is only possible to achieve apparent complete removal in a minority of cases. It was hoped that serial measurements of carcinoembryonic antigen might identify those patients who might benefit by early radical surgery, but this has been found not to be the case (Northover).

The mainstay of therapy for local recurrence is radiotherapy, which is invariably palliative. Occasionally, a neodymium:yttrium-aluminium-garnet (Nd:Yag) laser can be used to deal with an obstructing or bleeding lesion.

Carcinoid tumour. Carcinoid tumour of the rectum, as far as its lethal properties are concerned, can be looked upon as a gradation between a benign tumour and a carcinoma. A latter-day aphorism is 'keep carcinoid in mind when an atypical neoplasm (ulcer) of the rectum is encountered'. Like benign lymphoma, carcinoid tumour originates in the submucosa, the mucous membrane over it being intact. Consequently, it seldom produces evidence of its presence in the early stages, when it presents as a small plaque-like elevation. The incidence of clinical malignancy, i.e. the occurrence of metastases, is 10 per cent. This is much less than that for carcinoid tumour of the small intestine, but it is greater than that of

I. Taylor. Professor of Surgery, University College Hospital, London, England.

J.M.A. Northover. Surgeon, St Mark's Hospital, England.

carcinoid tumour of the vermiform appendix. Multiple primary carcinoid tumours of the rectum are not infrequent. The neoplasm is of slow progression, and usually metastasises late. Large carcinoids (over 2 cm) are almost always malignant.

Treatment. Local excision is sufficient treatment. Resection of the rectum is advisable if the growth is more than 2.5 cm in diameter, if recurrence follows local excision or if the growth is fixed to the perirectal tissues. Even when metastases are present, resection may prolong life.

Further reading

Keighley, M.R.B.K. and Williams, N.S. (1999) *Surgery of the Anus, Rectum and Colon*, 2nd edn, W.B. Saunders, London.

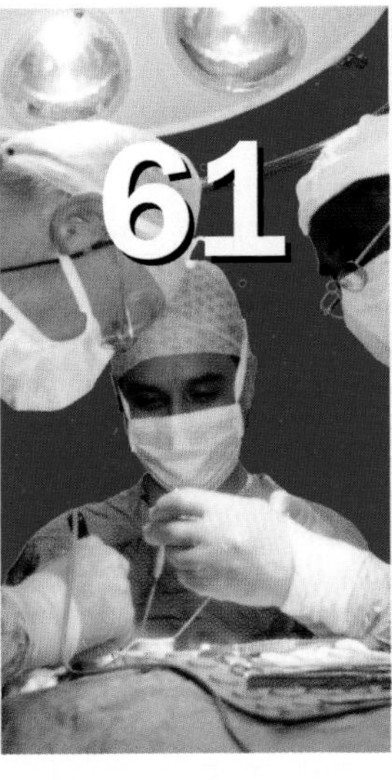

61 The anus and anal canal

Anatomy and physiology

Surgical anatomy

The anal canal commences at the level where the rectum passes through the pelvic diaphragm and ends at the anal verge (the external or distal boundary of the anal canal). The muscular junction between the rectum and anal canal can be felt with the finger as a thickened ridge – the anorectal 'bundle' or 'ring'.

Anal canal musculature (Fig. 61.1)

The internal sphincter is a thickened continuation of the circular muscle coat of the rectum. This involuntary muscle commences where the rectum passes through the pelvic diaphragm and ends at the anal orifice, where its lower border can be felt. The internal anal sphincter is 2.5 cm long and 2–5 mm thick. When exposed during life, it is pearly white in colour, and its individual, transversely placed fibres can be seen clearly. Spasm and contracture of this muscle play a major part in fissure and other anal affections.

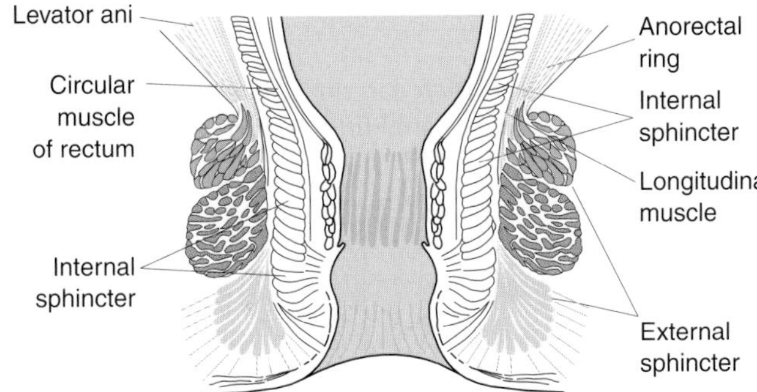

Fig. 61.1 The musculature of the anal canal (*after Sir Clifford Naunton Morgan, London, England*).

The longitudinal muscle is a continuation of the longitudinal muscle coat of the rectum intermingled with fibres from the puborectalis. Its fibres fan out through the lowest part of the external sphincter, to be inserted into the true anal and perianal skin. The longitudinal muscle fibres that are attached to the epithelium provide pathways for the spread of perianal infections, and mark out tight 'compartments' that are responsible for the intense pressure and pain that accompany many localised perianal lesions.

Beneath the anal skin lie the scanty fibres of the corrugator cutis ani muscle.

The external sphincter, formerly subdivided into a deep, superficial and subcutaneous portion is now considered to be one muscle (Goligher). Some of its fibres are attached posteriorly to the coccyx, while anteriorly they are inserted into the midperineal point in the male, whereas in the female they fuse with the sphincter vaginae. In life the external sphincter is pink in colour and homogeneous. Unlike the pale internal sphincter muscle, which is involuntary, the red external sphincter is composed of voluntary (somatic) muscle.

Between the internal (involuntary) sphincter and the external (voluntary) sphincter muscle mass is found a potential space, the *intersphincteric plane*. This plane is important as it contains the basal parts of eight to 12 apocrine glands, which can cause infections, and it is also a route for the spread of pus. It can also be opened up by a surgeon to provide access for operations on the sphincter muscles.

The puborectalis plays a key role in maintaining the angle between the anal canal and rectum and, hence, is essential for the preservation of continence (Fig. 61.2). There is a close association between the puborectalis portion of the levator ani and the external sphincter muscle.

The mucous membrane. The *pink* columnar epithelium lining the rectum extends through the anorectal ring into the surgical anal canal.

John Cedric Goligher. Professor of Surgery, Leeds, England.

Bailey & Love's Short Practice of Surgery, 23rd edition. Edited by R.C.G. Russell, N.S. Williams and C.J.K. Bulstrode. Published in 2000 by Arnold Publishers.

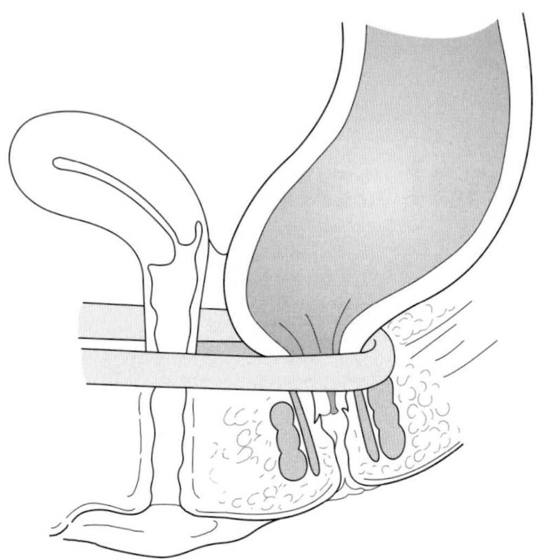

Fig. 61.2 The disposition of the puborectalis muscle. Note how it maintains the rectoanal angle.

The mucosa of the upper anal canal is attached loosely to the underlying structures, and covers the internal rectal plexus. Passing downwards where it clothes the series of eight to 12 longitudinal folds known as the columns of Morgagni, the mucous membrane becomes cubical, and *red* in colour (Fig. 61.3); above the anal valves the mucous membrane becomes *plum coloured*. Just below the level of the anal valves there is an abrupt, albeit wavy, transition to squamous epithelium, which is *parchment colour*. This wavy junction constitutes the dentate line. The squamous epithelium lining the lower anal canal is thin and shiny, and is known as the anoderm. This squamous epithelium differs from the true skin in that it has no epidermal appendages, i.e. hair and sweat glands. The anoderm passes imperceptibly into the pigmented skin of the anus. At the dentate line the anoderm is attached very firmly indeed to deeper structures.

The dentate line is a most important landmark both morphologically and surgically. It represents the site of fusion of the proctodaeum and postallantoic gut, and the position of the anal membrane, remnants of which may frequently be seen as anal papillae situated on the free margin of the anal valves. The dentate line separates:

above

- cubical epithelium;
- autonomic nerves (insensitive);
- portal venous system;

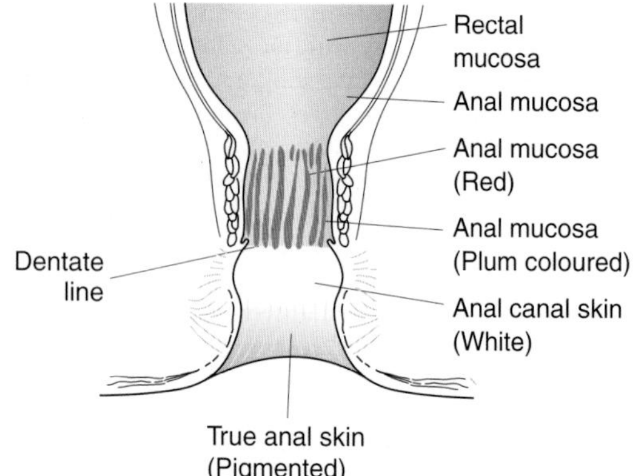

Fig. 61.3 The lining membrane of the anal canal (*after Sir Clifford Naunton Morgan, London, England*).

Giovani Battista Morgagni, 1682–1771. Professor of Anatomy, Padua, Italy.

below

- from squamous epithelium;
- from spinal nerves (very sensitive);
- from systemic venous system.

The anal valves of Ball are a series of transversely placed semilunar folds linking the columns of Morgagni. They lie along and actually constitute the waviness of the dentate line. They are functionless remnants of the fusion of the postallantoic gut with the proctodaeum.

The crypts of Morgagni (syn. anal crypts) are small pockets between the inferior extremities of the columns of Morgagni. Into several of these crypts, mostly those situated posteriorly, opens one *anal gland* by a narrow duct. This duct bifurcates, and the branches pass outward to enter the internal sphincter muscle, in 60 per cent of people (Fig. 61.4). Issuing from this ampula there are three to six tubular sub-branches that extend into the intermuscular connective tissue, where they end blindly. In some lower animals, these glands secrete an odoriferous substance during the rutting season; in humans, their function, if any, is obscure. Some of their cells have been shown to give a positive staining reaction for mucin, but as the lining epithelium is mainly cubical, the mucus-secreting propensity of the anal glands must be extremely small. Infection of an anal gland can give rise to an abscess, and in the opinion of a number of surgeons, infection of an anal gland is the most common cause of anorectal abscesses and fistulae.

The anorectal ring marks the junction between the rectum and the anal canal. It is formed by the joining of the puborectalis muscle (Fig. 61.2), the deep external sphincter, conjoined longitudinal muscle and the highest part of the internal sphincter. The anorectal ring can be clearly felt digitally, especially on its posterior and lateral aspects. Division of the anorectal ring results in permanent incontinence of faeces. The position and length of the anal canal, as well as the angle of the anorectal junction, depend to a major extent on the integrity and strength of the puborectalis muscle sling.

Arterial supply

The anal canal is supplied by branches from the superior, middle and inferior haemorrhoidal arteries. The most important is the superior haemorrhoidal, whose left branch supplies the left half of the canal by a single terminal branch, while its right has two terminal branches. All of the arteries contribute to a rich submucous and intramural plexus, so that interruption of the arterial supply from above by division of the superior and middle rectal arteries does not deprive the anus of its blood supply.

Venous drainage

The anal veins are distributed in similar fashion to the arterial supply. The superior and middle haemorrhoidal veins drain

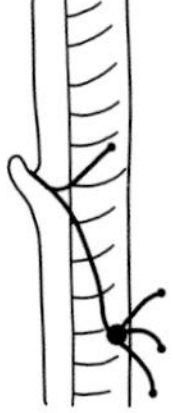

Fig. 61.4 Anal gland with duct opening into a crypt of Morgagni.

Sir Charles Bent Ball, 1851–1916. Regius Professor of Surgery, Dublin, Ireland.

via the inferior mesenteric vein into the portal system, having become the superior rectal vein *en route*. The superior haemorrhoidal vein drains the upper half of the anal canal. The inferior haemorrhoidal veins drain the lower half of the anal canal and the subcutaneous perianal plexus of veins: they eventually join the external iliac vein on each side.

Lymphatic drainage

Lymph from the upper half of the anal canal flows upwards to drain into the postrectal lymph nodes and from there goes to the para-aortic nodes via the inferior mesenteric chain. Lymph from the lower half of the anal canal drains on each side first into the superficial and then into the deep inguinal group of lymph glands. However, if the normal flow is blocked, e.g. by tumour, the lymph can be diverted into the alternative route.

Surgical physiology of the anal muscles and pelvic floor

The function of the anal canal and pelvic floor muscles is not only to contain the contents of the rectum, but also to allow effortless, unimpeded voiding at defecation. Interference with the integrity of the anatomy or physiology of the muscles of the anus and pelvic floor can lead to the extremes of intractable constipation or incontinence. If the muscles of the pelvic floor become too floppy, the entire anorectal mechanism can drop down ('perineal descent'), or alternatively can gape open, so allowing intussusception and prolapse of the rectum.

If the puborectalis and anorectal ring of muscles fail to relax appropriately (so-called 'inappropriate function' or anismus) to allow the rectum to empty at defecation, obstructed defecation ensues: this can usually be overcome by excessive voluntary straining efforts, but frequently ends in intractable constipation. Excessive straining can cause both partial and complete rectal prolapse. When a patient presents with incontinence caused by weak or damaged anorectal musculature, or if bizarre or extreme complaints of constipation are elicited, it is now possible to investigate these symptoms to obtain objective data on which to base a management protocol (Swash and Henry). The length, resting tone and the

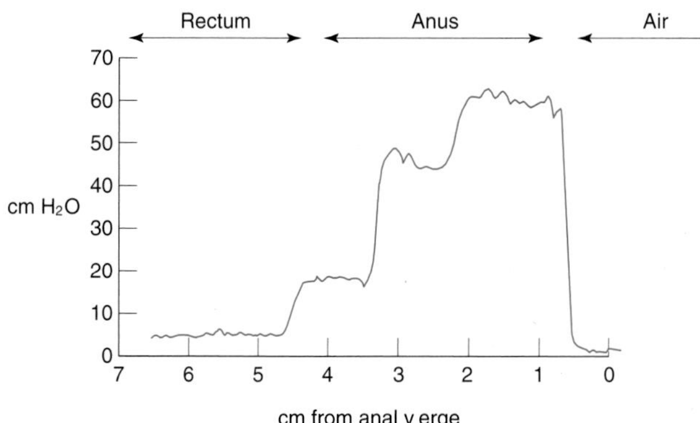

Fig. 61.5 A typical, normal 'pull-through' manometric study of the anal canal (3.5 cm long; maximal pressure 60 cmH_2O approx.).

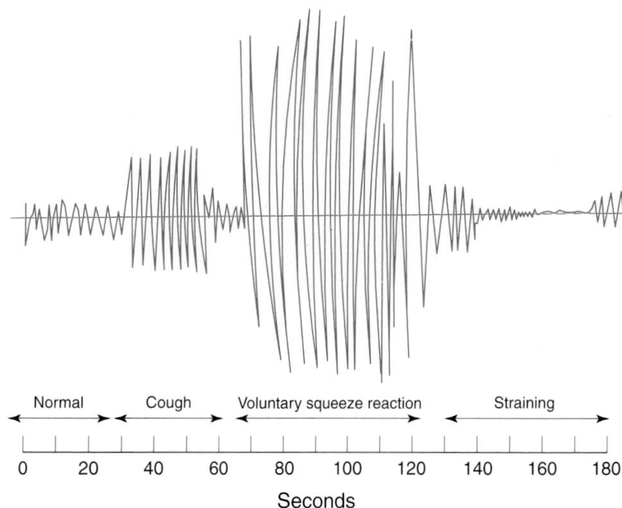

Fig. 61.6 A typical, normal electromyographic study of the external sphincter during various activities.

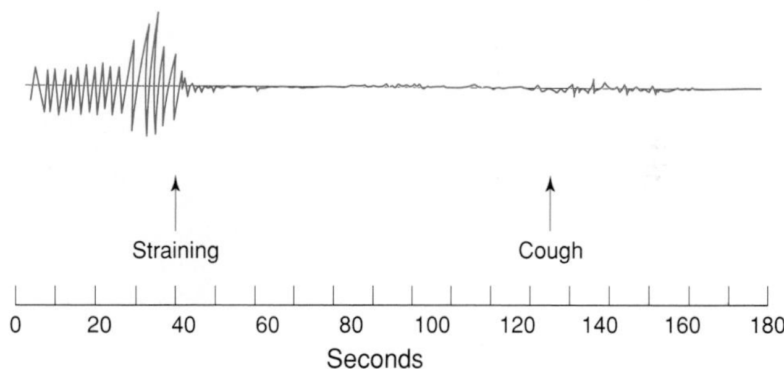

Fig. 61.7 An electromyographic study of the external sphincter showing prolonged inhibition on straining and absent cough reflex. This is typical of a denervated patulous sphincter.

power to relax and contract the anal sphincter muscles can be assessed by manometry and electromyography (Figs 61.5, 61.6 and 61.7): these studies can be combined with delineation of rectal sensibility and function by balloon distension and radiology ('defecatory proctography') and the abnormalities identified. In addition to the intrinsic defects, mechanical deviations can be mapped: the level and angle of the anorectal junction can be established by clinical observation and by an appliance ('perineometer'). Furthermore, it is possible to take radiographs of the acts of straining and evacuation while simultaneously recording electromyographs of the sphincter muscles and intrarectal pressure (Williams) (Fig. 61.8). This technique is known as dynamic integrated protography. Endoluminal ultrasound can also be used to visualise the integrity of both the internal and external anal sphincters (Fig. 61.9). The above techniques provide information which enables many patients with incontinence and constipation to be treated effectively.

Professor M. Swash. Physician to the Royal London Hospital and St Mark's Hospital, London, England.

M. Henry. Surgeon, Central Middlesex Hospital and St Mark's Hospital, London, England.

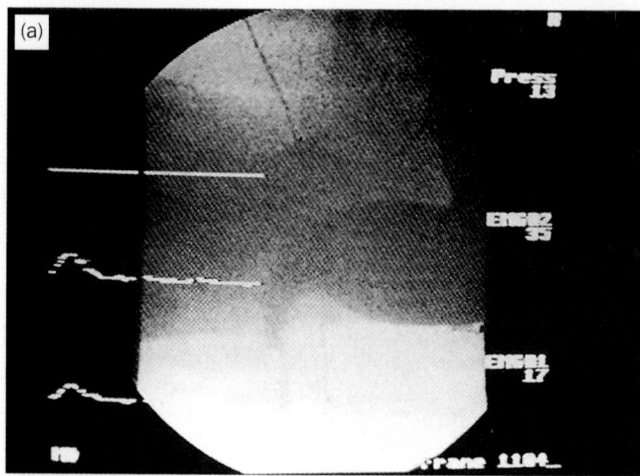

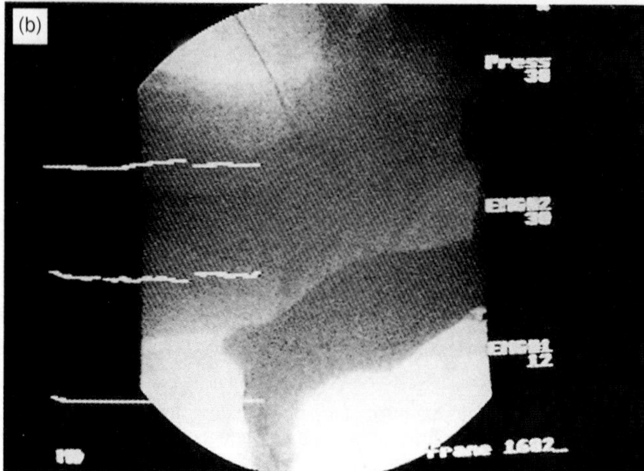

Fig. 61.8 Integrated dynamic proctography. (a) At rest; (b) during evacuation. Visualisation of the rectum is achieved by using barium impregnated 'synthetic stool'. The effects of straining and evacuation on the EMG activity of the sphincter muscles and intrarectal pressure can be simultaneously recorded (Williams).

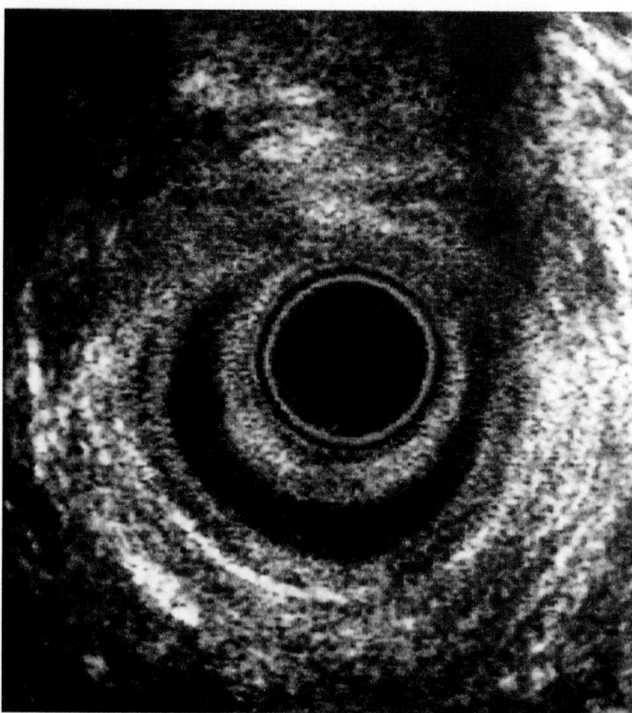

Fig. 61.9 Endoluminal ultrasound showing defect in anterior aspect of external anal sphincter (white outer band) and internal anal sphincter (dark inner band).

Examination of the anus

This requires careful attention to circumstances. The examining couch should be of sufficient height to allow easy inspection and access for any necessary manoeuvres. A good light is mandatory. The Sims (left lateral) or the lithotomy position is satisfactory: the latter is less convenient for an elderly patient and can cause social embarrassment to young women. A protective glove should be worn. The patient should be relaxed and able to co-operate. A few quiet words from the doctor can prevent many loud ones from the patient.

Inspection

With the buttocks opened, the anus is inspected. Note is made of any lesions, e.g. inflammatory skin changes, haemorrhoids, fissure ('sentinel pile') or fistula. The patient is asked to strain down before inspection is concluded.

Digital examination with the index finger

A good lubricant is necessary – neither too little nor too much. Any secretions should be sampled before applying lubricant to the anal verge.

Extreme gentleness should be the rule so that pain is not caused. Painful spasm of the anal sphincters is confirmation of a hidden fissure if the history is suggestive.

The examination should check normal, as well as abnormal, structures according to the following plan:

- intraluminal:
  - normal: faeces,
  - abnormal: polyp or carcinoma;
- intramural:
  - normal: sphincter muscles and anorectal angle,
  - abnormal: carcinoma or leiomyoma;
- extramural:
  - normal: perianal structures,
  - abnormal: abscess.

At the same examination, the rectum is examined according to the same system. Before withdrawing the finger, the patient is asked again to strain down, and a note is made regarding the prostate in a male patient and the cervix, uterus and pouch of Douglas in a female.

Norman S. Williams. Professor of Surgery, The Royal London Hospital, London, England.

J. Marion Sims, 1813–83. American gynaecologist.

James Douglas, 1675–1742. Anatomist and obstetrician, London, England.

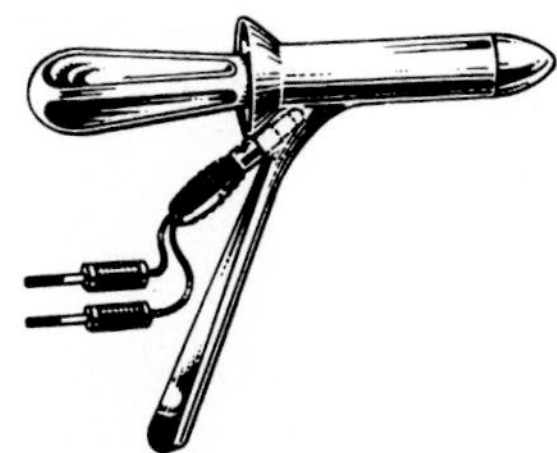

Fig. 61.10 An illuminated proctoscope.

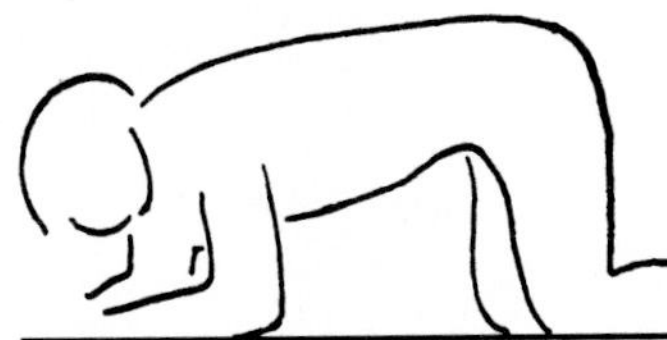

Fig. 61.11 Knee–elbow position for proctoscopy.

Discharge

After withdrawal, the finger is examined for mucus, pus, blood and abnormal faecal material.

Proctoscopy (Fig. 61.10)

This examination is of great importance. Either the Sims position with the buttocks elevated on a small cushion, or the knee–elbow position (Fig. 61.11) may be used. The lower third of the rectum, the anorectal junction and the anal canal can be inspected as the instrument is withdrawn slowly. The patient should also be asked to strain during withdrawal as by so doing an internal intusussception may be made visible. Minor procedures can be carried out through this instrument, e.g. treatment of haemorrhoids by injection or banding (see below) and biopsy.

Sigmoidoscopy (Chapter 60)

Although this is a strictly an examination of the rectum and lower sigmoid colon, it should be carried out even when an anal lesion has been confirmed. Rectal pathology, e.g. colitis or carcinoma, is frequently the cause of an anal lesion, e.g. fissure or haemorrhoids. Not infrequently, rectal pathology is found that is independent of the anal lesion and which requires treatment.

Special investigations

These are discussed above.

Physiological studies
Manometry Electrophysiology Proctography Endoluminal ultrasound

Congenital abnormalities

Early in embryonic life there is a common chamber – the cloaca – into which open the hind gut and the allantois. The cloaca becomes separated into the bladder and postallantoic gut (rectum) by the downgrowth of a septum. About this time an epiblastic bud, the proctodaeum, grows in towards the rectum. Normally fusion between these two structures occurs during the third month of intrauterine life.

Imperforate anus

(The term is used as a well-recognised description. Strictly it should be 'agenesis' and 'atresia' of the rectum and anus.) One infant in 4500 is born with an imperforate anus, or with imperfect fusion of the postallantoic gut with the proctodaeum. The condition is divided into two main groups: the high and the low, depending on whether the termination of the bowel is above or below the pelvic floor. The low varieties are easy to diagnose and relatively simple to treat, and the outlook is good. The high varieties often have a fistula into the urinary tract together with a deficient pelvic floor, and are difficult to treat.

Low abnormalities (Fig. 61.12)

Covered anus. The underlying anal canal is covered by a bar of skin with a track running forwards to the perineal raphe. The track should be opened with scissors, followed by routine dilatation of the anus.

Ectopic anus. The anus is situated anteriorly and may open in the perineum in boys, or more commonly in the vulva in girls, or rarely into the vagina. A plastic 'cut-back' operation is required (Pena).

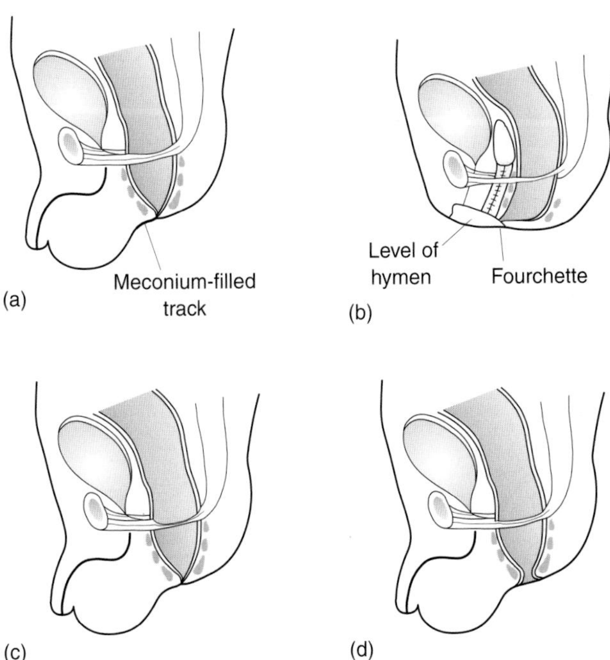

Fig. 61.12 Low abnormalities of the anus: (a) covered anus; (b) vulval ectopic anus; (c) anal stenosis; and (d) anal membrane (*courtesy of J.P. Partridge, Barnstaple, and M.H. Gough, London, England*).

A. Pena. Paediatric surgeon, New York, USA.

Stenosed anus. The anus is microscopic, but careful examination usually reveals a minute opening which responds to regular dilatation.

Membranous stenosis. Here the anus is normally sited, but is covered with a thin membrane which bulges with retained meconium. It is rare, and an incision will cure the condition.

High abnormalities (Fig. 61.13)

These are often associated with a fistulous connection between the blind rectal stump and the bladder, or other abnormalities of the pelvic structures.

Anorectal agnesis. A blind rectal pouch lies just above the pelvic floor – its anterior aspect in the male is attached to the bladder and often there is a rectovesical fistula manifested by the passage of gas or meconium in the urine. In the female, the fistula is usually into the posterior fornix.

Rectal atresia. The anal canal is normal but ends blindly at the level of the pelvic floor. The bowel also ends blindly above the pelvic floor without a fistulous opening. This anomaly is rare but must be treated by mobilisation of the rectum and excision of the stricture. After that, end-to-end anastomosis of the anus and rectum must be attempted. More conservative measures are followed by an intractable stricture.

Cloaca. This occurs only in females and here the bowel, urinary and genital tracts all open into a common wide cavity. Commonly severe malformations of the area are associated with other developmental abnormalities, e.g. tracheobronchial fistula.

Clinical management

As congenital abnormalities are frequently multiple, very careful general examination of the baby must be made to exclude any other anomalies. It is urgent and important to determine whether the abnormality is high or low, and a radiograph will help.

Radiological examination

Six hours after birth sufficient air may have collected in the large intestine to cast an X-ray shadow. With a metal button or a coin strapped to the site of the anus, or a metal bougie inserted into the blind anal canal, the infant is held upside down for 3–4 minutes and radiographed in the inverted position (Fig. 61.14). The gas in the rectum will rise to the top and indicates the distance between the site of the metal indicator and the blind end of the rectum. If the distance is over 2.5 cm, the abnormality is 'high'. This method, although useful, is sometimes vitiated by a plug of meconium in the rectum causing an apparent gap far in excess of that actually present. It may be necessary to wait until the baby is 24 hours old before rectal gas appears.

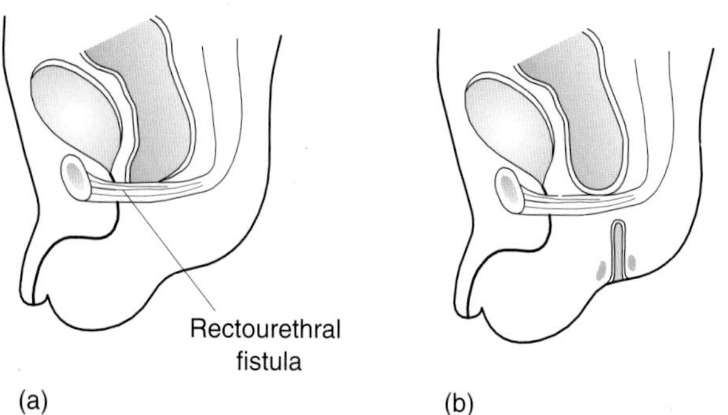

Fig. 61.13 High abnormalities: (a) anorectal agensis with recto-urethral fistula; and (b) rectal atresia (*courtesy of J.P. Partridge, Barnstaple, and M.H. Gough, London, England*).

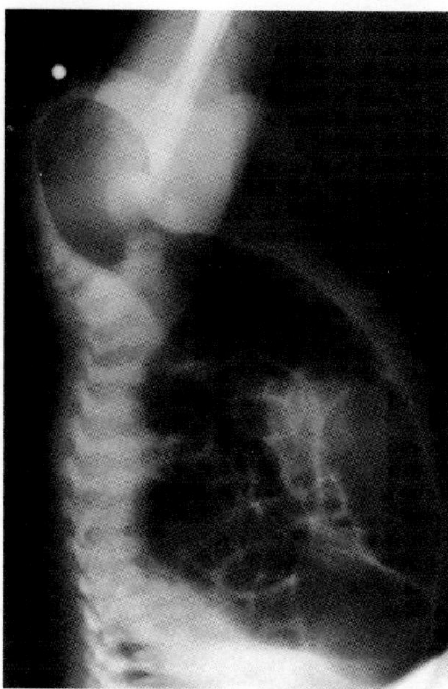

Fig. 61.14 Radiograph of neonate whilst held upside down to show gas in the rectum. Anal dimple is marked by a piece of lead shot (*courtesy of Graham Airth, Bristol, England*).

Where a 'high' lesion is suspected, an effort must be made to obtain a specimen of urine – the presence of *proteus* or *pyocynaneus* usually signifies that a fistula is present. An intravenous (i.v.) urogram is recommended by some, even though there is a definite radiation risk. There may be gas in the bladder. A diagnostic perineal exploration is usually unwise – it may prejudice the chances of further surgery.

Treatment

In the *low* abnormalities, this is usually simple and has been outlined when each condition was described above. The *high* abnormalities present a very difficult problem and each case must be considered on its merits. On the whole, newborn babies stand surgery very well, provided compatible blood is available, a clear airway is maintained postoperatively and inhalation of vomit prevented by nasogastric suction. The presence of other congenital abnormalities is also a most important factor to consider. The possibilities are:

- laparotomy, division of rectourethral fistula and transverse colostomy. A rectal 'pull-through' operation can be done later;
- laparotomy, division of fistula and 'pull-through' operation in one stage;

- division of the fistula and rectal 'pull-down' operation through the perineum (this method is now rarely used);
- post-sagittal rectoplasty (PSARP) (Pena). Similar to above but via posterior approach;
- colostomy only (for the cloacal variety).

For the 'pull-through' operation the lower bowel is mobilised, and a new passage is created through the pelvic floor by passing a pair of curved forceps through it, keeping close to the urethra, to the site of the future anus. This is dilated by Hegar's dilators so that the bowel can be pulled down and its mucosa stitched to the skin of the newly formed anus. (For details the reader is referred to the standard textbooks of operative surgery and the publications of Swenson, Duhamel and Nixon.)

In general, daily dilatation will be required for at least 3 months and it may be necessary for years.

In a high percentage of cases, imperforate anus is associated with other congenital abnormalities, especially of the urinary organs, and nearly half the deaths in cases of imperforate anus are due to other malformations.

Sacrococcygeal teratoma

Sacrococcygeal teratoma, although rare, is among the most common of the large tumours seen during the first 3 months of life. The frequency of the precoccygeal region for the development of a teratoma is explained by the fact that this area is the site of the 'primitive knot', a group of totipotent cells that retain their totipotentiality longer than any others save the sex anlage. Females are more often affected than males.

The tumour, which arises between the sacrum and the rectum, is firmly attached to the coccyx and, occasionally, to the last piece of the sacrum. At the time of birth some of these tumours are huge, and in 20 per cent of cases the infant is stillborn. The tumour tends to be large (Fig. 61.15), but it can be small enough to pass unnoticed until it enlarges or a complication ensues. It is this variety that is prone to become malignant, usually at about 10 months of age.

Treatment. Removal should be soon after birth; delay is liable to result in fatal ulceration, infection, rectal or urinary obstruction, or malignant change.

Operation: excision is undertaken through a longitudinal elliptical incision, the coccygeal attachment being left until the last. The coccyx must always be excised; occasionally the last piece of the sacrum must be removed also. There may be a fistula between the tumour and the rectum, but as a rule this is small, and can be closed safely without performing a colostomy. The dead space in the pelvis is drained, the skin united and a pressure dressing applied.

When the operation is undertaken soon after birth, the prognosis is good.

Postanal dermoid

The space in front of the lower part of the sacrum and coccyx is occupied by a soft, cystic swelling – a postanal dermoid cyst – which is

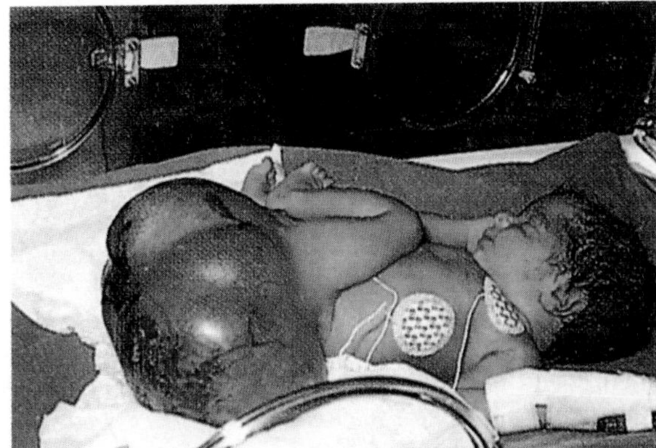

Fig. 61.15 Sacrococcygeal teratoma (*courtesy of Professor Asal Al-Samarrai, Riyadh, Saudi Arabia*).

regarded as a simple form of teratoma. Hidden in the hollow of the sacrum, it is unlikely to be discovered unless a sinus communicating with the exterior is present, or develops as a result of inflammation. Such a cyst usually remains symptomless until adult life, when it is prone to become infected. Exceptionally, by its very size, it gives rise to difficulty in defecation. The cyst is easily palpable on rectal examination.

Differential diagnosis. Especially in a child, an anterior sacral meningocele must be excluded. The latter enlarges when the child cries, and is frequently associated with paralysis of the lower limbs and incontinence. When a discharging sinus is present, a postanal dermoid will probably be mistaken for a pilonidal sinus, unless pressure over the sacrococcygeal region with a finger in the rectum causes a flow of sebaceous material, and injection of contrast and radiography reveals a bottle-necked cyst in front of the coccyx.

Treatment is complete excision of the cyst, and sinus if present. In the case of large cysts it is necessary to remove the coccyx in order to gain access.

Postanal dimple (syn. fovea coccygea)

A dimple, sometimes amounting to a short blind pit, in the skin beneath the tip of coccyx, is noticed from time to time in the course of a clinical examination.

Pilonidal sinus

Pilonidal means 'appertaining to a nest of hair' (Latin: *pilus* = hair, *nidus* = nest).

Aetiology

The army of supporters of the congenital theory of the origin of pilonidal sinus has become reduced to a corporal's guard.

That, in rare instances, a sinus in the anococcygeal area *is* congenital must be allowed, but in these cases of proven congenital origin the sinus is not necessarily pilonidal. It could be a sinus connected with a postanal dermoid, referred to above, or a sinus resulting from a persistent caudal remnant of the original neural canal. The latter occurs in the sacral rather than the coccygeal region, and is definitely connected with the spinal theca. On this account, meningitis from an extradural abscess may occur in a child.

Alfred Hegar, 1830–1914. Professor of Obstetrics and Gynaecology, Freiburg, Germany.

O. Swenson. Surgeon, USA.

B. Duhamel. Surgeon, France.

H.H. Nixon. Surgeon, Royal Hospital for Sick Children, Great Ormond Street, London, England.

The reasons which support the acquired theory of origin of pilonidal sinus can be summarised as follows.

- Interdigital pilonidal sinus is an occupational disease of hairdressers, the hair within the interdigital cleft or clefts being the customers'. Pilonidal sinuses of the axilla and umbilicus have also been reported.
- The age incidence of the appearance of pilonidal sinus (82 per cent occur between the ages of 20 and 29 years) is at variance with the age of onset of congenital lesions.
- Hair follicles have almost never been demonstrated in the walls of the sinus.
- The hairs projecting from the sinus are dead hairs, with their pointed ends directed towards the blind end of the sinus.
- The disease mostly affects men, and hairy men most frequently.
- Recurrence is common, even though adequate excision of the track is carried out.

The mode of origin of a pilonidal sinus is now believed to be as follows: on sitting, the buttocks take the weight of the body, and move independently, or together. Hairs broken off by friction against clothing, and shed short hairs, whether originating from the nape of the neck, back, or buttocks, tend to collect in the cleft of the nates and/or a postanal dimple. Furthermore, it is suggested that the use of toilet paper may contribute to hair entangled in faecal matter being swept into the cleft; pilonidal sinus is extremely rare in those races that employ ablution after defecation. By reason of the shearing action of the buttocks, which is increased by sitting on a hard seat, and especially by vibration of a vehicle, loose hair travels down the intergluteal furrow, to penetrate the skin or the open mouth of a sudoriferous gland, such glands being more active in early manhood. It is not yet clear whether the initial entry of hairs through the skin is a primary event, or follows the softening of the skin due to pustular or other forms of dermatitis. Once a sinus has formed, intermittent negative pressure of the area may suck other loose hairs into the pit. So common was pilonidal sinus among jeep riders in the 1935–45 war, that it became known as 'jeep bottom'.

Pathology

The sinus extends into the subcutaneous planes as an infected track. Branching side channels are not infrequent. A stratified squamous epithelial lining, of varying degrees of integrity, is found in about half the cases. Hair shafts are found either lying loose in the sinus, embedded in granulation tissue, or deep in mature scar tissue in three-quarters of the cases. Foreign-body giant cells are common.

Clinical features

There is a chronic or recurring sinus in the midline about the level of the first piece of the coccyx. Typically, a tuft of hair projects from its mouth. The discharge from the sinus or sinuses is often bloodstained, and contains foul sebum and sometimes hairs. Secondary openings may be present on either side of the midline, often far out on to the buttocks or in the perineum.

As has been indicated already, symptoms usually commence during the third decade; patients presenting later in life nearly always give a history dating back to this period.

Males with this condition outnumber females by four to one, the females being on an average 3 years younger than the males; this corresponds to the earlier maturation of the female. The condition rarely occurs in blonds; many of the patients are exceptionally hairy and are usually obese. In spite of the preponderance in dark-haired persons, whose hair is stiffer than the silky blond (Oldham), the condition is practically confined to white races. The complaint is of a discharge, pain or a tender swelling at the bottom of the spine. Even at the height of an attack of inflammation the constitutional symptoms are slight. Often there is a history of repeated abscesses in the region that have discharged spontaneously or have been incised. The primary sinus may have one, or as many as six openings, all of which are strictly in the midline between the level of the sacrococcygeal joint and the tip of the coccyx. Unlike a fistula in ano, the sinus passes upwards and forwards towards the sacrum. It does not reach bone, but ends blindly near the bone. When an abscess forms it may discharge through a primary sinus; more frequently it points and bursts, or is incised to one side of the midline (usually the left), thus forming a secondary sinus.

Conservative treatment

Patients reporting for the first time with mild symptoms can sometimes be cured by conservative measures, which consist of cleaning out the track, removing all hairs from the area, followed by frequent washing of the parts with a detergent and water, and applying equal parts of witch hazel (liq. ext. hamamelis) and alcohol. Long sitting, e.g, driving a car, is avoided if possible. These measures, tried on a large scale in the US Army, proved tolerably successful – more successful than similar attempts in civil life, because the sufferer could be relegated to duties that were unlikely to aggravate the condition.

Treatment of an acute exacerbation (abscess)

If rest, baths, local antiseptic dressings and the administration of a broad-spectrum antibiotic fail to bring about resolution, the abscess should be opened through a comparatively small incision. Provided all hairs and granulation tissue are removed from the abscess cavity, there is some prospect of curing the lesion (Millar). After it has been cleaned out, the track can be destroyed by careful instillation of pure phenol solution (Maurice). In all other circumstances, an elective operation must be planned.

Operation should be performed only when the inflammation has been controlled by the measures indicated already.

The patient is placed on the operating table, for preference in the 'jack-knife' position. Methylene blue is injected into the sinus to colour

---

James Bagot Oldham, 1899–1977. Surgeon, United Liverpool Hospitals, Liverpool, England.

Douglas Malcolm Millar. Retired surgeon, Essex County Hospital, Colchester, England.

Brian Armstead Maurice. Surgeon, Tunbridge Wells, Kent, England.

all the tracks, the nozzle of the syringe being pressed against the opening to obtain some pressure. Variations in operative technique include the following.

- Lay open the tracks, remove all debris and hair, and suture the edges to the skin, thus marsupialising the sinus. This procedure yields a good, hairless scar.
- Excise all of the tracks, as stained by blue dye, meticulously secure haemostasis by diathermy and catgut ligature and, using sutures, coapt the subcutaneous fat and skin very accurately and institute a drain and suction (i.e. Redivac) for 48 hours to remove blood and serum. In cases of extensive sinus formation, primary cover may be achieved by rotating a flap of skin and fat.
- Excise all of the tracks as stained by the blue dye and, after securing haemostasis as above, pack the wound. The following day the whole dressing is removed, and daily baths and moist dressing are instituted until the wound heals by granulation. A silastic elastomer pack is particularly useful for dressing the wound as it can be removed, washed and reinserted by the patient, and ensures that the wound heals from below. Epithelialisation can sometimes be speeded up by skin grafting.

Immediately after operation, the patient should avoid sitting on the wound. Subsequently, the scar may require protection from further incursions of hair by selective hair-trimming. The recurrence rate after primary closure may be as high as 50 per cent without meticulous technique.

Recurrent pilonidal sinus. Three possibilities account for this disappointment:

- a diverticulum of the main channel has been overlooked at the primary operation;
- new hairs enter the skin or the scar;
- when the natal fold is deformed by scarring, the least trauma causes tearing of the scar, and the resulting crevice becomes contaminated with coliform and cutaneous bacteria.

An alternative approach to circumvent the incident of recurrence has been to ensure that the sound closure is to one side of the midline (Karydakis); this method has been reported as having a high rate of success. Yet another recently described technique said to have a high incidence of success is that described by Bascom. The procedure involves an incision lateral to the midline which allows the chronic abscess cavity

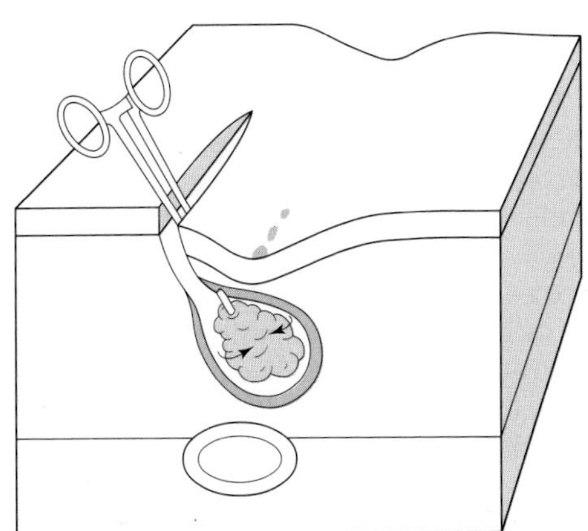

Fig. 61.16 Bascom technique for pilonidal sinus.

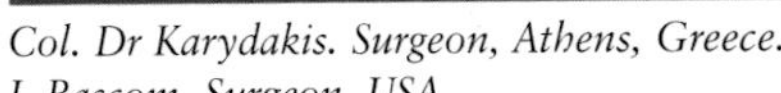

Col. Dr Karydakis. Surgeon, Athens, Greece.
J. Bascom. Surgeon, USA.

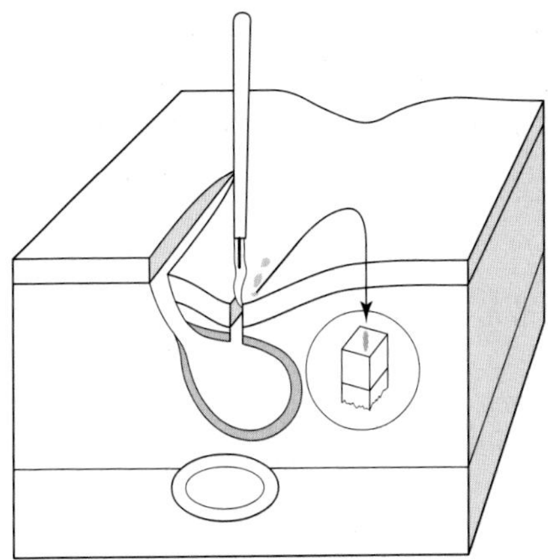

Fig. 61.17 Bascom technique for pilonidal sinus.

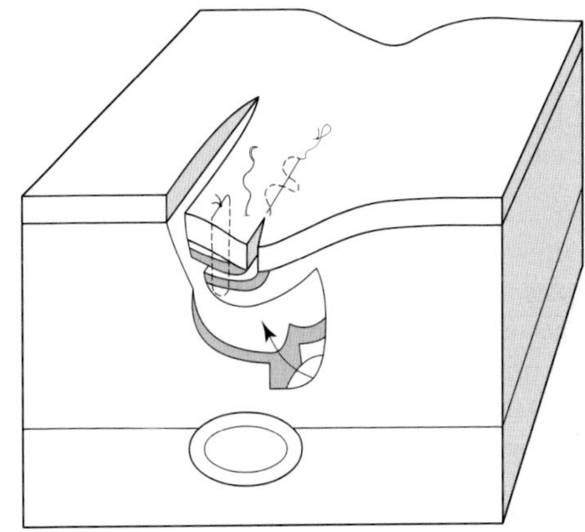

Fig. 61.18 Bascom technique for pilonidal sinus.

to be scrubbed free of hair and granulation tissue (Fig. 61.16). Removal of the small midline pits is carried out with small (7 mm) incisions (Fig. 61.17). The lateral wound is then left open, but the midline incisions are closed (Fig. 61.18).

Anal incontinence

Aetiology

Aetiology of incontinence
Descent
Destruction
Debility
Deficiency
Damage
Denervation
Dementia

The origins of anal incontinence may derive from causes relating to:

- descent:
  - perineal descent,
  - rectal prolapse;

- destruction:
  - malignant tumours,
  - irradiation;
- debility:
  - illness,
  - old age;
- deficiency:
  - congenital abnormalities;
- damage:
  - wounds,
  - surgical procedures,
  - childbirth;
- denervation:
  - spinal injuries,
  - neurosurgical procedures,
  - spina bifida,
  - neurological disorders, e.g. multiple sclerosis;
- dementia:
  - senility,
  - psychological abnormality.

Of these causes, geriatric, traumatic and obstetric cases predominate – with anal surgical procedures an important contributor to the traumatic group. Another major cause in women is pudendal nerve neuropathy which results from chronic straining, perineal descent and a traction injury to the nerve. This type of incontinence used to be termed idiopathic but neurophysiological studies have determined its true nature. In particular, the latency of pudendal nerve transmission can now be measured by stimulating the pudendal nerve per rectum and measuring the time taken for an electromyographic (EMG) response to be detected in the external and sphincter. A latency above 2 ms is usually diagnostic of pudendal nerve neuropathy.

Once the cause of the incontinence has been precisely defined by a careful history and meticulous examination, supported by special investigations as indicated (see above), treatment may be possible. Surgical procedures have been developed to repair and support damaged or weak sphincter muscles. These may be classified as follows.

Operations to reunite divided sphincter muscles

The sphincter muscles may have been divided as a result of direct trauma, operations for fissure and fistula or by obstetrical injury. The ends of the divided muscle are found and reunited by a *double overlap repair* (Fig. 61.19).

Operations to reef the external sphincter and puborectalis muscle

If the sphincter muscles are stretched and patulous (as they often are in old age and cases of rectal prolapse) they may be tightened by a *postanal repair*. These operations use darns of absorbable material to narrow down and plicate the external sphincter and the puborectalis sling (Fig. 61.20). They restore length to the anal canal, strength to the anal sphincter and angulation to the anorectal junction. The approach is usually through the intersphincteric plane.

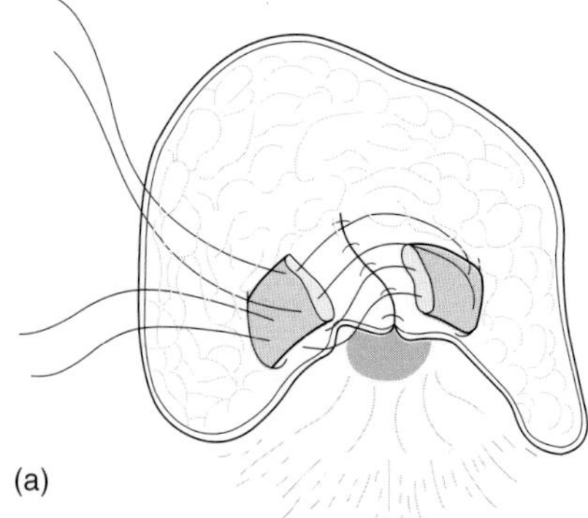

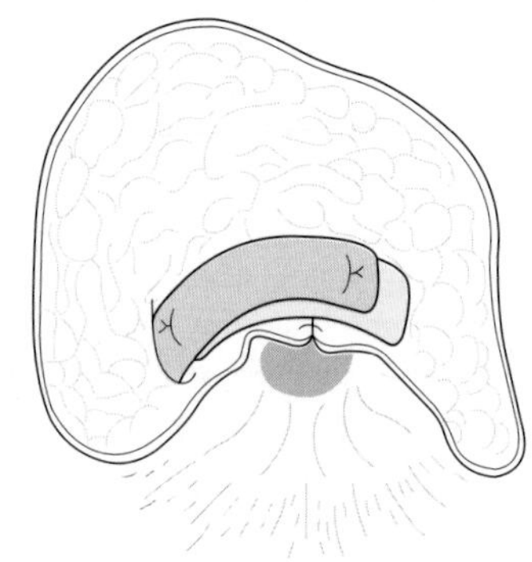

Fig. 61.19 Direct sphincter repair in which (a) the sphincter defect is excised; and (b) the remaining muscle is overlapped. (Redrawn from Mann, C.V. and Glass, R.E., *Surgical Treatment of Anal Incontinence*, Springer, New York, 1991.)

Operations to support the anal canal

If the anal canal is gaping and has feeble muscles that cannot be strengthened by direct means, support can be given by encircling stitches or Mersilene strands after the *Thiersch operation pattern* (Chapter 53). However, these techniques are not popular since the sutures may erode into the anal canal or cause an impediment to satisfactory evacuation and have now been abandoned. Recently, attempts have been made to create a new anal sphincter by transposing the gracilis muscle around the anal canal and stimulating it electrically by a pacemaker (Williams) (Fig. 61.21). This appears a promising technique and is effective in approximately 60 per cent of patients who have previously had more conventional operations.

More recently an artificial sphincter has been developed from that used in urology. It consists of a silastic cuff which is inflated around the anal canal and occludes it. When evacuation is required, the cuff is deflated by squeezing a small balloon attached to a reservoir (Fig. 61.22). Since this device is a foreign body which exerts pressure on the bowel wall, there is concern that erosion and infection will be a common problem.

Karl Thiersch, 1822–95. Professor of Surgery, Leipzig, Germany.

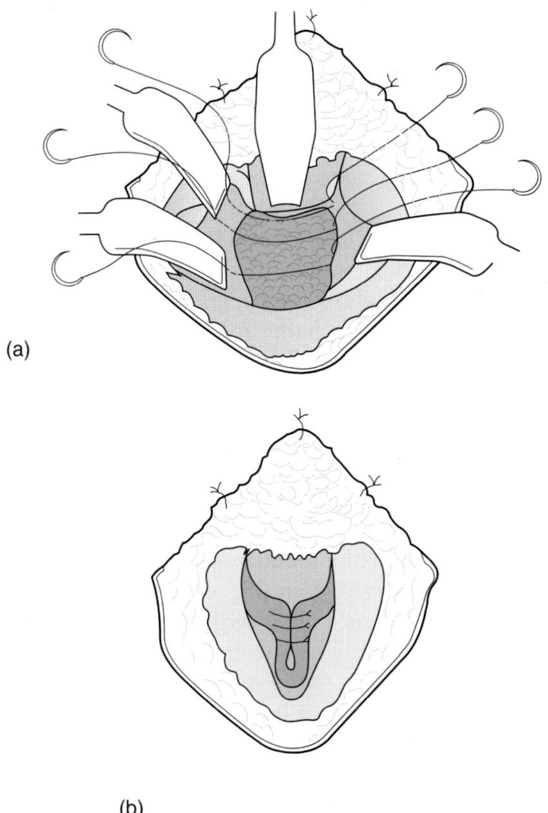

Fig. 61.20 Postanal repair in which (a) the sphincter muscle is plicated posterior to the anal canal, thus restoring the anorectal angle; (b) the completed repair. (Redrawn from Mann, C.V. and Glass, R.E., *Surgical Treatment of Anal Incontinence*, Springer, New York, 1991.)

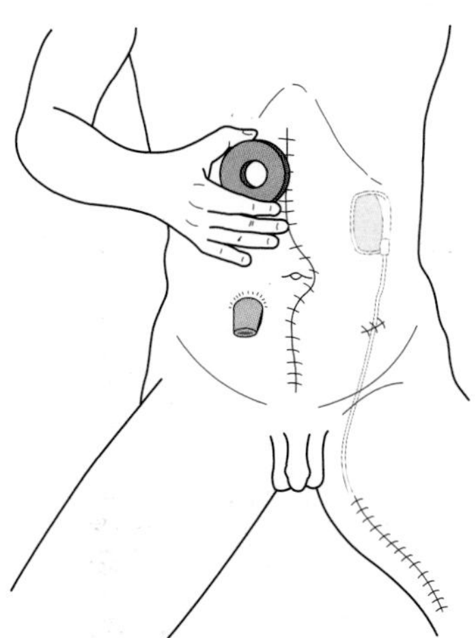

Fig. 61.21 Electrically stimulated gracilis neosphincter in which the gracilis muscle is transposed around the anal canal and the muscle is stimulated via a totally implanted 'pacemaker'. In this way, the muscle is converted from a fast-twitch fatiguable muscle to a slow-twitch nonfatiguable muscle. The stimulator can be turned off by use of a magnet. (Redrawn with permission from Williams *et al.*, Development of an electronically stimulated neoanal sphincter, *Lancet*, **338**, 1167, 1991.)

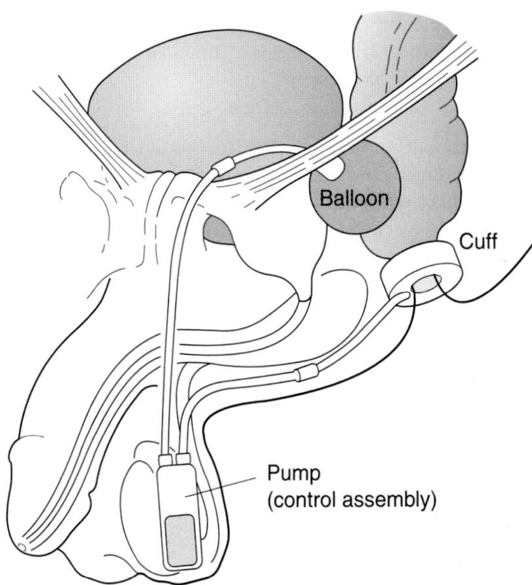

Fig. 61.22 Artificial bowel sphincter. A cuff is placed around the anal canal. An inflatable pump control assembly is placed in the scrotum and the balloon reservoir under the symphysis pubis.

All of these procedures achieve best results if the bowel habit is regulated and a normal defecatory pattern established over the preoperative and postoperative periods. The operations should be covered by antibiotics active against both aerobic and anaerobic organisms to reduce the risk of septic complications. If any of these procedures fail or are contraindicated, the patient may require a permanent colostomy.

Anal fissure

Definition

An anal fissure (syn. fissure in ano) is an elongated ulcer in the long axis of the lower anal canal.

Location

The site of election for an anal fissure is the midline posteriorly (90 per cent overall). The next most frequent situation is the midline anteriorly.

Aetiology

The cause of anal fissure, and particularly the reason why the midline posteriorly is so frequently affected, is not completely understood. A probable explanation is as follows: the posterior wall of the rectum curves forwards from the hollow of the sacrum to join the anal canal, which then turns sharply backwards. During defecation the pressure of a hard faecal mass is mainly on the posterior anal tissues, in which event the overlying epithelium is greatly stretched and, being relatively unsupported by muscle, is placed in a vulnerable position when a scybalous mass is being expelled. Possibly some cases are due to tearing down of an anal valve of Ball. An anterior anal fissure is much more common in women, particularly in those who have borne children. This can be explained by the lack of support of the anal mucous membrane by a damaged pelvic floor and an attenuated perineal body. A more recent suggestion supported by Doppler flow studies is that a fissure is due to ischaemia. It may be that the cause is a combination of trauma initially perpetuated by a poor blood supply.

Some causes of anal fissure are certain:

- an incorrectly performed operation for haemorrhoids in which too much skin is removed. This results in anal stenosis and tearing of the scar when a hard motion is passed;
- inflammatory bowel disease – particularly Crohn's disease;
- sexually transmitted diseases.

Pathology

An anal fissure is either acute or chronic. The upper internal end of the fissure stops at the dentate line. Because the fissure occurs in the stratified sensitive epithelium of the lower half of the anal canal, pain is the most prominent symptom (see below).

Acute anal fissure is a deep tear through the skin of the anal margin extending into the anal canal. There is little inflammatory induration or oedema of its edges. There is accompanying spasm of the anal sphincter muscle.

Chronic anal fissure is characterised by inflamed indurated margins, and a base consisting of either scar tissue or the lower border of the internal sphincter muscle. The ulcer is canoe-shaped, and at the inferior extremity there is a tag of skin, usually oedematous. This tag is known picturesquely as a sentinel pile – 'sentinel' because it guards the fissure. There may be spasm of the involuntary musculature of the internal sphincter. In long-standing cases, this muscle becomes organically contracted by infiltration of fibrous tissue. Infection is common and may be severe, ending in abscess formation. A cutaneous fistula may follow.

Chronic fissure in ano may have a specific cause – often a granulomatous infection, e.g. Crohn's disease. Biopsy examination is advisable of any tissue removed at operation for a chronic fissure. Specific fissures of this type are often less painful than the appearances of the lesion would suggest.

Clinical features

Symptoms of anal fissure
Pain on defecation
Bright red bleeding
Mucus discharge
Constipation

The condition is more common in women and generally occurs during the meridian of life. It is uncommon in the aged, because of muscular atony, whereas anal fissure is not rare in children, is sometimes encountered during infancy and may cause acquired megacolon (Chapter 57).

- *Pain* is *the* symptom – sharp, agonising pain starting during defecation, often overwhelming in intensity and lasting for an hour or more. As a rule, it ceases suddenly, and the sufferer is comfortable until the next action of the bowel. Periods of remission occur for days or weeks. The patient tends to become *constipated* rather than go through the agony of defecation. (One patient accustomed himself to take a generous dose of senna on Saturday night, and retire to the toilet on Sunday morning with a bottle of whisky and the newspaper.)
- *Bleeding* – this is usually slight and consists of bright streaks on the stools or the paper.
- *Discharge*. A slight discharge accompanies fully established cases.

On examination

In cases of some standing, a sentinel skin tag can usually be displayed. This, together with a typical history and a tightly closed, puckered anus, is almost pathognomonic of the condition. By gently parting the margins of the anus, the lower end of the fissure can be seen (Fig. 61.23).

Because of the intense pain it causes, digital examination of the anal canal should not be attempted *at this stage* unless the fissure cannot be seen, or it seems imperative to exclude major intrarectal pathology. In these circumstances, the local application of a surface anaesthetic such as 5 per cent xylocaine on a pledget of cotton wool, left in place for about 5 minutes, will enable the necessary examination to be made. In early cases, the edges of the fissure are impalpable; in fully established cases, a characteristic crater which feels like a vertical buttonhole can be palpated. *The diagnosis must be established beyond doubt, for which a general anaesthetic may be required.*

Differential diagnosis

Carcinoma of the anus in its very early stages easily simulates a fissure. If real doubt exists, the lesion must be excised under general anaesthesia and submitted to histological examination.

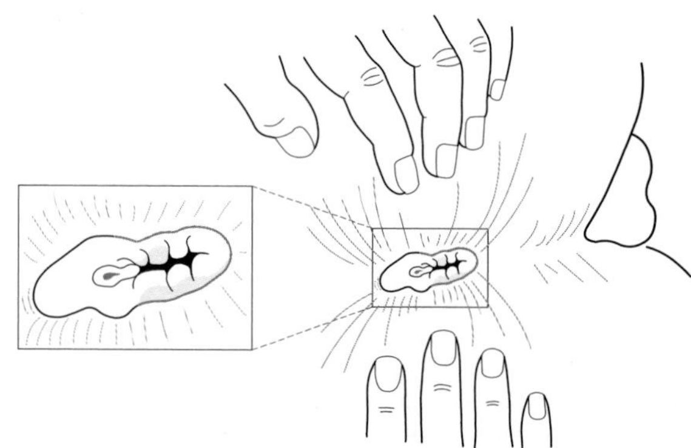

Fig. 61.23 The appearances of an anal fissure. If the buttocks are gently parted, the presence of an anal fissure can usually be detected as an ulcer of variable depth with a skin tag and an anal papilla. (Redrawn with permission from Keighley, M.R.B. and Williams, N.S., *Surgery of the Anus, Colon and Rectum*, 2nd edn, W.B. Saunders, 1999.)

Christian Johann Doppler, 1803–53. Austrian physicist.
Burill Bernard Crohn, b. 1884. Gastroenterologist, Mount Sinai Hospital, New York, USA.

Multiple fissures in the perianal skin are commonly seen as a complication of skin diseases, scratching and inflammatory bowel disease, as well as homosexual practices (sodomy, fisting and the use of anorectal sex toys; Fig. 60.8) and anorectal sexually transmitted disease such as herpes. Admitted homosexuals, should, after appropriate counselling, be offered a human immunodeficiency virus (HIV) test as they may have acquired immunodeficiency syndrome (AIDS) (Chapter 9).

Tuberculous ulcer has an undermined edge.

Proctalgia fugax (see below) causes severe episodic pain.

Treatment

The pain of an anal fissure is so great that usually the patient demands relief, and consequently many patients with an acute fissure present early. The object of all treatment for this condition is to obtain *complete relaxation* of the internal sphincter. Provided the complications are dealt with, the fissure will slowly heal as soon as all spasm has disappeared.

Conservative treatment

Because of the risks of incontinence associated with sphincterotomy, it is now usual practice to treat anal fissures conservatively in the first instance using a chemical sphincterotomy. Nitric oxide has been shown to be the neurotransmitter which induces relaxation of the internal sphincter. Glyceryl trinitrate, being a nitric acid donor, when applied as an ointment (0.2 per cent by weight) to the anal canal produces sufficient relaxation of the sphincter to allow the fissure to heal in up to two-thirds of patients (Scholefield). In addition, glyceryl trinitrate ointment improves blood flow to the area, and this aids healing. Unfortunately, glyceryl trinitrate ointment may produce severe headaches and other agents with fewer side effects should be available soon. Other measures include laxatives to ensure the motions are soft, but the stools should not be made watery. Celevac tablets give a soft stool of good bulk which is ideal. Anal dilators used in conjunction with xylocaine ointment are difficult to insert because of pain and are rarely effective.

Operative measures. The simplest procedure in the past has been gentle dilatation of the sphincter. Under general anaesthesia, the index and middle finger of each hand were inserted simultaneously into the anus and carefully pulled apart dilating the anus so that its diameter was no greater than four finger breadths. Great care and judgement had to be exercised, so that the anal sphincter was not overstretched. The risks of incontinence following this procedure have now made it unpopular. Although it might still be used for young men with high pressure sphincters who understand the slight risk, it is definitely contraindicated in those patients with weak sphincters.

Should these measures prove ineffective, or if the fissure is chronic with fibrosis, a skin tag or a mucous polyp, then surgical measures are advisable. General anaesthesia is best, although some surgeons use a local anaesthetic in the form of xylocaine or lignocaine introduced into the ischiorectal fossa on each side, in order to anaesthetise the nerves passing towards the rectum. In other situations, a caudal anaesthetic is suitable.

Lateral anal sphincterotomy (Notaras). In this operation, the internal sphincter is divided away from the fissure itself – usually either in the right or the left lateral positions. The procedure can be done by an open or a closed method. Healing is usually complete within 3 weeks. The operation is more successful for acute than chronic fissures. Seventy-five per cent of cases are suitable for treatment by this method, which can be done as an out-patient procedure under local anaesthesia by an experienced surgeon. However, there is a definite yet small risk of incontinence and it is imperative that patients are appraised of this risk preoperatively.

Dorsal fissurectomy and sphincterotomy. The essential part of the operation is to divide the transverse fibres of the internal sphincter in the floor of the fissure. If a sentinel pile is present, this is excised. The ends of the dividend muscle retract and a smooth wound is left. The after-treatment consists of attention to bowels, a daily bath and the passage of an anal dilator until the wounds have healed, which usually takes about 3 weeks. Despite the presence of the wound, there is little or no pain and the results are good. The disadvantage of this operation is the prolonged healing time – usually not less than 3 weeks and often longer – and, occasionally, a mild, persistent and permanent mucus discharge. It is now reserved only for the most chronic or recurrent anal fissures, the majority being treated by lateral sphincterotomy. Once again incontinence might be a postoperative complication.

Hypertrophied anal papilla

Anal papillae occur at the dentate line, and are remnants of the ectodermal membrane that separated the hindgut from the proctodaeum. As these papillae are present in 60 per cent of patients examined proctologically, they should be regarded as normal structures. Anal papillae can become elongated, as they frequently do in the presence of an anal fissure. Occasionally, an elongated anal papilla may be the cause of pruritus. An elongated anal papilla associated with pain and/or bleeding at defecation is sometimes encountered in infancy. Haemorrhage into a hypertrophied anal papilla can cause sudden rectal pain. A prolapsed papilla may become nipped by contraction of the sphincter mechanism after defecation. Occasionally, a red oedematous papilla is encountered with local pain and a purulent discharge from the associated crypt. This condition of 'cryptitis' may be cured by laying open the mouth of the infected anal gland and removing the papilla.

Treatment. Using a slotted proctoscope, elongated papillae without haemorrhoids should be crushed and excised after injecting the base with local anaesthetic. When large papillae complicate internal haemorrhoids, this is an indication for operative treatment of the haemorrhoids, as well as excision of the elongated papillae.

Proctalgia fugax

This disease is characterised by attacks of severe pain arising in the rectum, recurring at irregular intervals and apparently unrelated to organic disease. The pain is described as cramp-like, often occurs when the patient is in bed at night, usually lasts only for a few minutes and disappears spontaneously. It may follow straining at stool, sudden explosive bowel action or ejaculation. It seems to occur more commonly in patients suffering from anxiety or undue stress, and also it is said to afflict young doctors. The pain may be unbearable – it is possibly due to segmental cramp in the pubococcygeus muscle. It is unpleasant, incurable, but fortunately harmless and gradually subsides. A more chronic form of the disease has been termed the 'levator syndrome' and can be associated with severe constipation. Biofeedback techniques have been used to help such patients: some surgeons have been willing to sever the puborectalis muscle, but this can cause incontinence.

John Scholefield. Surgeon, Nottingham, England.

Mitchell James Notaras. Surgeon, Barnet General Hospital, London, England.

Haemorrhoids

Haemorrhoids (Greek: *haima* = blood, *rhoos* = flowing) syn. piles[1] (Latin: *pila* = a ball) are dilated veins occurring in relation to the anus. Such haemorrhoids may be **external** or **internal**, i.e. external or internal to the anal orifice. The external variety is covered by skin, while the internal variety lies beneath the anal mucous membrane. When the two varieties are associated, they are known as **interoexternal** haemorrhoids.

The veins which form internal haemorrhoids become engorged as the anal lining descends and is gripped by the anal sphincters. The mucosal lining is gathered prominently in three places (the 'anal cushions'), which can be in the areas of the three terminal branches of the superior haemorrhoidal artery, but this is exceptional (Thomson). The anal cushions are present in embryonic life and are necessary for full continence. Straining causes these cushions to slide downwards and internal haemorrhoids develop in the prolapsing tissues.

Haemorrhoids may be **symptomatic** of some other condition, and this important fact must be remembered. Symptomatic haemorrhoids may appear:

- in *carcinoma of rectum*. This, by compressing or causing thrombosis of the superior rectal vein, gives rise to haemorrhoids (Fig. 61.24) sufficiently often to warrant examination of the rectum and the rectosigmoid junction for a neoplasm in every case of haemorrhoids;
- during *pregnancy*. Pregnancy piles are due to compression of the superior rectal veins by the pregnant uterus and the relaxing effect of progesterone on the smooth muscle in the walls of the veins, plus an increased pelvic circulating volume;
- from *straining at micturition* consequent upon a stricture of the urethra – or an enlarged prostate;
- from chronic constipation.

NB. Contrary to the usual belief, in 128 consecutive cases of portal hypertension, Macpherson did not encounter a single example of haemorrhoids that could be attributed to portal cirrhosis, although bleeding oesophageal varices often complicate portal hypertension.

The great majority of haemorrhoids is not symptomatic. The description that follows concerns symptomatic haemorrhoids that are *not* secondary to an underlying cause.

Internal haemorrhoids

Internal haemorrhoids, which include interoexternal haemorrhoids, are exceedingly common. Essentially, the condition is a dilatation of the internal venous plexus with an enlarged displaced anal cushion. Because of the communication between the internal and external plexuses, if the former becomes engorged, the latter is liable to become involved also.

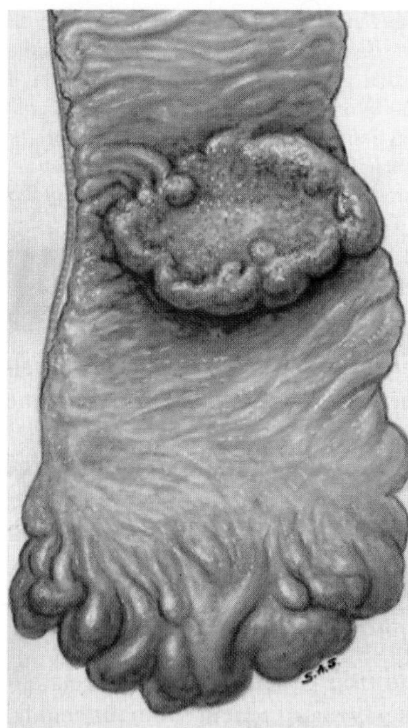

Fig. 61.24 Carcinoma of the rectum associated with haemorrhoids. A not infrequent diagnostic pitfall.

Aetiology

Hereditary. The condition is so frequently seen in members of the same family that there must be a predisposing factor, such as a congenital weakness of the vein walls or an abnormally large arterial supply to the rectal plexus.

Varicose veins of the legs and haemorrhoids often occur concurrently.

Morphological. In quadrupeds, gravity aids, or at any rate does not retard, return of venous blood from the rectum. Consequently venous valves are not required. In humans, the weight of the column of blood unassisted by valves produces a high venous pressure in the lower rectum, unparallelled in the body. Except in a few fat old dogs, haemorrhoids are exceedingly rare in animals.

Anatomical. The collecting radicles of the superior haemorrhoidal vein lie unsupported in the very loose submucous connective tissue of the anorectum. These veins pass through muscular tissue and are liable to be constricted by its contraction during defecation. The superior rectal veins, being tributaries of the portal vein, have no valves.

Exacerbating factors. Straining accompanying constipation or that induced by overpurgation is considered to be a potent cause of haemorrhoids. Less often, the diarrhoea of enteritis, colitis or the dysenteries aggravates latent haemorrhoids. In both instances, descent and swelling of the anal cushions are prominent features.

Pathology

Internal haemorrhoids are frequently arranged in three groups at 3, 7, and 11 o'clock with the patient in the lithotomy position [in which patients used to be put for the

[1] *'The common people call them piles, the aristocracy call them haemorrhoids, the French call them figs – what does it matter so long as you can cure them?' John of Arderne, 1370.*

John of Arderne, 1306–90. The first English surgeon. He practised in Newark and later in London, England.

William Hamish Fearon Thomson. Surgeon, Gloucestershire Royal Hospital, Gloucester, England.

Archibald Ian Stewart Macpherson. Surgeon, Royal Infirmary, Edinburgh, Scotland.

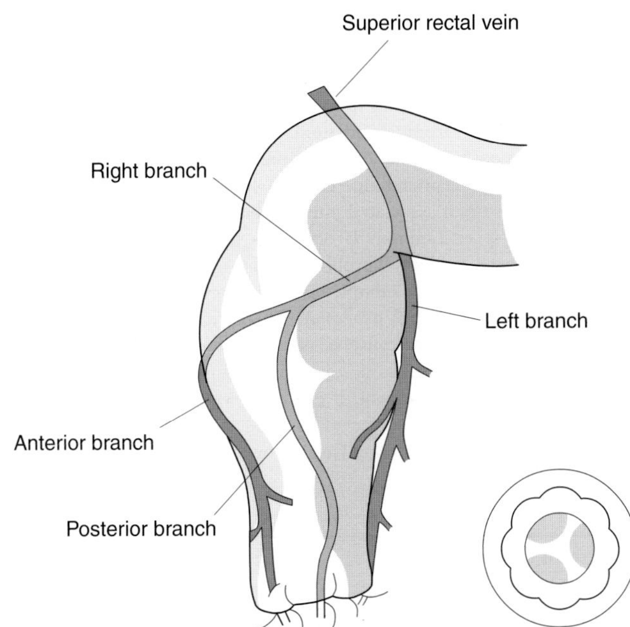

Fig. 61.25 Disposition of anal vasculature illustrating why haemorrhoids are classically sited at 3, 7 and 11 o'clock.

classical operation of 'cutting' for bladder stone via the urethral or the perineal route (Chapter 62)]. This distribution has been ascribed to the arterial supply of the anus whereby there are two subdivisions of the right branch of the superior rectal artery, but the left branch remains single (Fig. 61.25), but this is now known to be atypical. In between these three primary haemorrhoids there may be smaller secondary haemorrhoids. Each principal haemorrhoid can be divided into three parts.

- The *pedicle* is situated at the anorectal ring. As seen through a proctoscope, it is covered with pale pink mucosa. Occasionally, a pulsating artery can be felt in this situation.
- The *internal haemorrhoid*, which commences just below the anorectal ring. It is bright red or purple, and covered by mucous membrane. It is of variable size.
- An *external associated haemorrhoid* lies between the dentate line and the anal margin. It is covered by skin, through which blue veins can be seen, unless fibrosis has occurred. This associated haemorrhoid is present only in well-established cases.

Entering the pedicle of an internal haemorrhoid may be a branch of the superior rectal artery. Very occasionally there is a haemangiomatous condition of this artery – an 'arterial pile'—which leads to ferocious bleeding at operation.

Clinical features

Symptoms of haemorrhoids
Bright red painless bleeding Mucus discharge Prolapse Pain only on prolapse

Bleeding, as the name haemorrhoid implies, is the principal and earliest symptom. At first the bleeding is slight; it is bright red and occurs during defecation (a 'splash in the pan'), and it may continue intermittently thus for months or years. Haemorrhoids that bleed but do not prolapse outside the anal canal are called *first-degree haemorrhoids*.

Prolapse is a much later symptom. In the beginning the protrusion is slight and occurs only at stool, and reduction is spontaneous. As time goes on the haemorrhoids do not reduce themselves, but have to be replaced digitally by the patient. Haemorrhoids that prolapse on defecation but return or need to be replaced manually and then stay reduced are called *second-degree haemorrhoids*. Still later, prolapse occurs during the day, apart from defecation, often when patients are tired or exert themselves. Haemorrhoids that are permanently prolapsed are called *third-degree haemorrhoids* (Fig. 61.26). By now, the haemorrhoids have become a source of great discomfort and cause a feeling of heaviness in the rectum but are not usually acutely painful.

Discharge. A mucoid discharge is a frequent accompaniment of prolapsed haemorrhoids. It is composed of mucus from the engorged mucous membrane, sometimes augmented by leakage of ingested liquid paraffin. *Pruritus* will almost certainly follow this discharge.

Pain is absent unless complications supervene. For this reason, any patient complaining of 'painful piles' must be suspected of having another condition (possibly serious) and examined accordingly.

Anaemia can be caused very rarely by persistent profuse bleeding from haemorrhoids.

Investigation

On inspection there may be no evidence of internal haemorrhoids. In more advanced cases, redundant folds or tags of

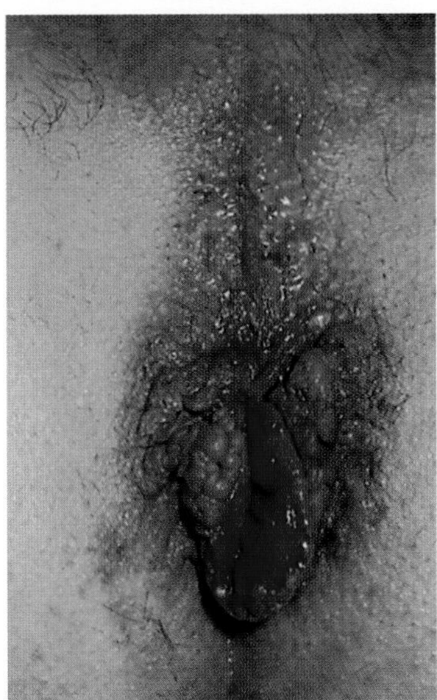

Fig. 61.26 Third-degree haemorrhoids (*courtesy of C.V. Mann, The Royal London Hospital*).

skin can be seen in the position of one or more of the three primary haemorrhoids. When the patient strains, internal haemorrhoids may come into view transiently or, if they are of the third degree, they are, and remain, prolapsed.

Digital examination. Internal haemorrhoids cannot be felt unless they are thrombosed.

Proctoscopy. A proctoscope is passed to its fullest extent and the obturator is removed. The instrument is then slowly withdrawn. Just below the anorectal ring internal haemorrhoids, if present, will bulge into the lumen of the proctoscope.

Sigmoidoscopy should be done as a precaution in every case (Chapter 60 and Fig. 60.5).

Complications

Profuse haemorrhage is not rare. Most often it occurs in the early stages of the second degree. The bleeding occurs mainly externally, but it may continue internally after the bleeding haemorrhoid has retracted or has been returned. In these circumstances, the rectum is found to contain blood.

Strangulation. One or more of the internal haemorrhoids prolapse and become gripped by the external sphincter. Further congestion follows because the venous return is impeded. Second-degree haemorrhoids are most often complicated in this way. Strangulation is accompanied by considerable pain, and is often spoken of by the patient as an 'acute attack of piles' [a phrase that also embraces a thrombotic pile (see below) or an inflamed anal skin tag]. Unless the internal haemorrhoids can be reduced within an hour or two, strangulation is followed by thrombosis.

Thrombosis. The affected haemorrhoid or haemorrhoids become dark purple or black (Fig. 61.27) and feel solid. Considerable oedema of the anal margin accompanies thrombosis. Once the thrombosis has occurred, the pain of strangulation largely passes off, but tenderness persists.

Ulceration. Superficial ulceration of the exposed mucous membrane often accompanies strangulation with thrombosis.

Gangrene occurs when strangulation is sufficiently tight to constrict the arterial supply of the haemorrhoid. The resulting sloughing is usually superficial and localised. Occasionally, a whole haemorrhoid sloughs off, leaving an ulcer which heals gradually. Very occasionally, massive gangrene extends to the mucous membrane within the anal canal and rectum, and can be the cause of spreading anaerobic infection and portal pyaemia.

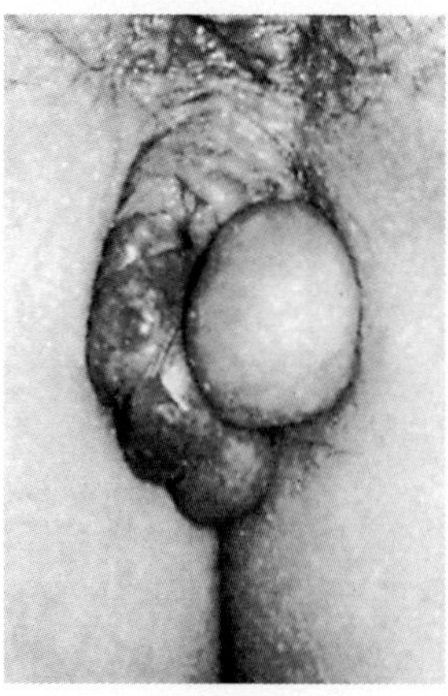

Fig. 61.27 An attack of piles. Prolapsed strangulated piles, as commonly seen, on the left. A less common mass on the right with a fibrofatty covering.

Fibrosis. After thrombosis, internal haemorrhoids sometimes become converted into fibrous tissue. The fibrosed haemorrhoid is at first sessile, but by repeated traction during prolapse at defecation, it becomes pedunculated and constitutes a fibrous polyp that is readily distinguished by its white colour from an adenoma, which is bright red. Fibrosis following transient strangulation commonly occurs in the subcutaneous part of a primary haemorrhoid. Fibrosis in an external haemorrhoid favours prolapse of an associated internal haemorrhoid.

Suppuration is uncommon. It occurs as a result of infection of a thrombosed haemorrhoid. Throbbing pain is followed by perianal swelling, and a perianal or submucous abscess results.

Pylephlebitis (syn. portal pyaemia). Theoretically, infected haemorrhoids should be a potent cause of portal pyaemia and liver abscesses (Chapter 52). Although cases do occur from time to time, this complication is surprisingly infrequent. It can occur when patients with strangulated haemorrhoids are subjected to ill-advised surgery and has even been reported to follow banding (see below).

Treatment

Treatment of haemorrhoids

- Symptomatic
- Injection of sclerosant
- Banding
- Photocoagulation
- Haemorrhoidectomy

Nonoperative treatment is recommended when the haemorrhoids are a symptom of some other condition or disease except, of course, when a carcinoma is present. The bowels are regulated by hydrophyllic colloids (Isogel, etc.) and if necessary a small dose of Senokot at night. Various proprietary creams can be inserted into the rectum from a collapsible tube fitted with a nozzle, at night and before defecation. Suppositories are also useful.

Active treatment. This consists of injection or treatment by elastic band applications to the base of each haemorrhoid or formal operation, each with specific indications. Treatment should not be withheld because the patient is elderly or infirm.

Injection treatment (Mitchell). ***Indications.*** This is ideal for first-degree internal haemorrhoids which bleed. Early second-degree haemorrhoids are often cured by this method but a proportion relapses.

Technique. The patient should have an empty rectum, but no special preparation is necessary. A proctoscope is introduced and the haemorrhoids are displayed. The proctoscope is introduced further in until the haemorrhoid has almost disappeared from the lumen and only its upper end is visible. The injection is made at this point above the main mass of each haemorrhoid (Fig. 61.28) into the submucosa at, or just above, the anorectal ring. Using Gabriel's syringe or more commonly a disposable instrument (Fig. 61.29) with the bevel of the needle directed towards the rectal wall, from 3 to 5 ml of 5 per cent phenol in almond oil is injected. The injection should produce elevation and pallor of the mucosa. The solution spreads in the submucosa upwards to the pedicle, and

---

Clinton Mitchell. Illinois, USA. He first used carbolic acid for injecting haemorrhoids in 1871. Itinerant irregular practitioners exploited the method.

Williams Bashall Gabriel, 1893–1975. Surgeon, Royal Northern and St Mark's Hospitals, London, England.

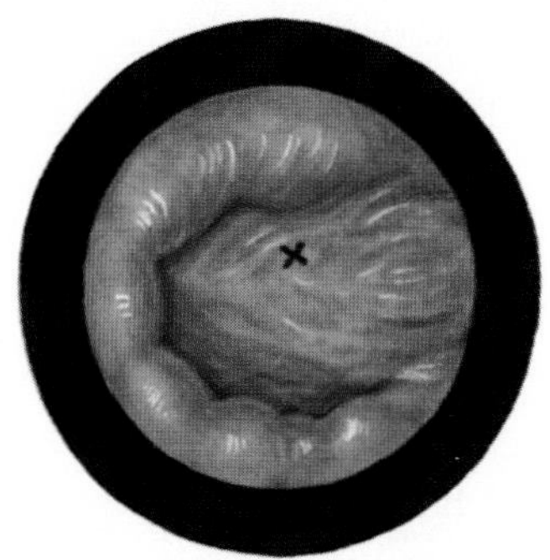

Fig. 61.28 Correct site for injecting a haemorrhoid (*after W.B. Gabriel, London*).

(a)

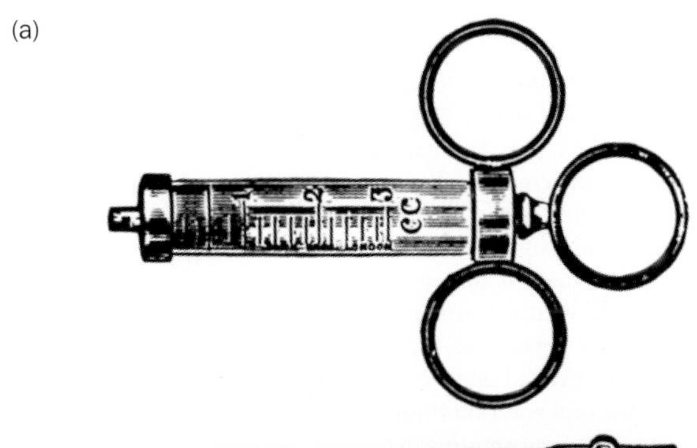

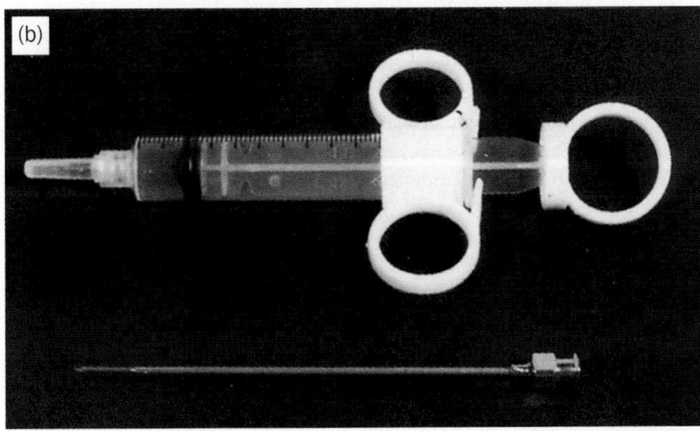

Fig. 61.29 Gabriel's syringe (a) has now been replaced by disposal syringes. (b) The instrument shown is produced by Rocket of London.

downwards to the internal haemorrhoid and to secondary haemorrhoids if present, but it is prevented by the intermuscular septum from reaching the external haemorrhoid. There is slight, transient bleeding from the point of puncture. The injection is painless, but a dull ache is common for a few hours. There is no special after-treatment. If there is only one haemorrhoid present, it may be cured by one injection; if all three haemorrhoids are equally enlarged, each is injected at the same session. Often three sessions at 6-weekly intervals are required. Care should be taken not to inject into the prostate anteriorly, for the resulting prostatitis can be crippling.

Banding treatment (Barron)

For second-degree haemorrhoids which are too large for successful handling by injections, treatment is available by slipping tight elastic

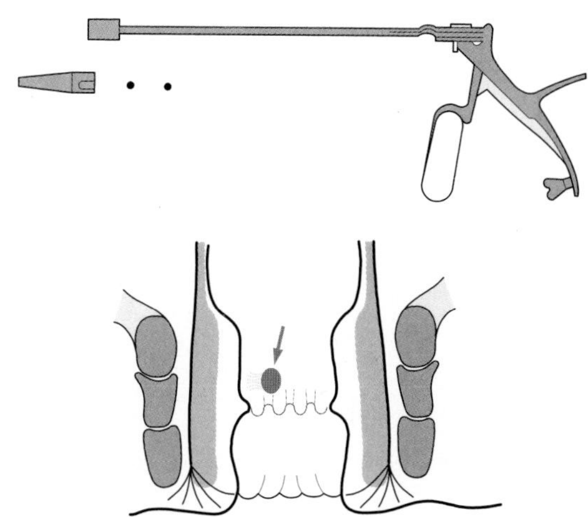

Fig. 61.30 Barron's banding apparatus with the appearance of a typical 'banded' haemorrhoid.

bands on to the base of the pedicle of each haemorrhoid with a special instrument (Fig. 61.30). The bands cause ischaemic necrosis of the piles, which slough off within a few days. The procedure should be painless if done properly, and can be performed in the out-patient department. Not more than two haemorrhoids should be banded at each session and 3 weeks at least should elapse between each treatment.

Cryosurgery

The application of *liquid nitrogen* has been evaluated in some centres. The extreme cold (–196°C) of the application causes coagulation necrosis of the piles, which subsequently separate and drop off. Although some encouraging early results were reported (Lloyd-Williams), the technique often caused troublesome mucus discharge and pain, and has now been abandoned.

Photocoagulation

The application of infrared coagulation by a specially designed instrument has recently been advocated for the treatment of haemorrhoids that do not prolapse (Leicester). This is said to be an effective and painless method of treatment.

Operation. ***Indications.*** Cases unsuitable for injection or banding treatment are:

- third-degree haemorrhoids;
- failure of nonoperative treatments of second-degree haemorrhoids;
- fibrosed haemorrhoids;
- interoexternal haemorrhoids when the external haemorrhoid is well defined.

These are indications for haemorrhoidectomy.

Haemorrhoidectomy

Some preoperative treatment is necessary. An aperient is given on the evening before the operation and an enema is administered. The anal

John Barron. Surgeon, Chicago, Illinois, USA.
Kenneth Lloyd-Williams. Surgeon, Royal United Hospitals, Bath, England.
Roger Leicester. Surgeon Commander, St George's Hospital, London, England.

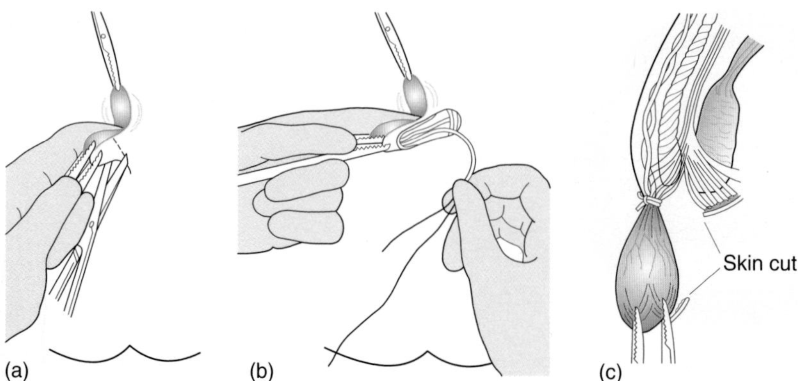

Fig. 61.31 Ligation and excision of haemorrhoids. Open technique: (a) the skin is cut to the left lateral haemorrhoid; (b) transfixion of the pedicle; (c) ligation.

region is shaved. On the morning of the operation the rectum is evacuated with the aid of a disposable enema.

Haemorrhoidectomy can be performed using an open or a closed technique. The open technique is most commonly used in the UK, and is known as the Milligan–Morgan operation – named after the surgeons who described it. The closed technique is the popular technique in the USA. Both involve ligation and excision of the haemorrhoid, but in the open technique the anal mucosa and skin are left open to heal by secondary intention, and in the closed technique, the wound is sutured.

Open technique. With the patient in the lithotomy position, the sphincter is gently stretched, and the internal haemorrhoids are then prolapsed by traction on the skin tags, or on the skin of the anal margin. Each haemorrhoid is dealt with as follows: it is picked up with dissecting forceps and traction is exerted. Traction displays a longitudinal fold (the pedicle) above the haemorrhoid. Each pedicle is grasped in a fine-pointed haemostat, as also is each external haemorrhoid or skin tag connected with each internal haemorrhoid. These pairs of haemostats, when held out by the assistants, form a triangle. The operator takes the left lateral pair of haemostats in the palm of his hand and places the extended forefinger in the anal canal to support the internal haemorrhoid. In this way traction is applied to the skin of the anal margin. With scissors, a V-shaped cut is made (Fig. 61.31a), each limb of which is placed on either side of the skin-holding haemostat. This cut transverses the skin and the corrugator cutis ani. Exerting further traction a little blunt dissection exposes the lower border of the internal sphincter. A transfixion ligature of no. 3 chromic catgut is applied to the pedicle at this level (Fig. 61.31b). Each haemorrhoid, having been dealt with in this manner (Fig. 61.31c), is excised 1.25 cm distal to the ligature, the ends of which are cut about 1 cm from the knot. The stumps of the ligated haemorrhoids are returned to the rectum by tucking a piece of gauze into the anal canal.

The margins of the skin wounds are trimmed so as not to leave overhanging edges (Fig. 61.32). Bleeding subcutaneous arteries having been secured, the corners of three pieces of petroleum-jelly gauze are tucked into the anus so as to cover the areas denuded of skin. A pad of gauze and wool and a firmly applied T-bandage complete the operation.

Closed technique (Fig. 61.33). The patient is placed in the prone jack-knife position with the buttocks strapped apart. A suitable retractor, such as the Hill–Ferguson type, is placed within the anal canal, and the anus is infiltrated with 20 ml of a 1 in 300 000 adrenaline–saline solution. The haemorrhoid is excised, together with the overlying mucosa, as illustrated in Fig. 61.33a. The haemorrhoid is dissected carefully from the underlying sphincter and haemostatis is achieved. The pedicle is transfixed and ligated with 3.0 chromic catgut or Dexon. Any residual small haemorrhoids should be removed by filleting them out after undermining the edges of the cut mucosa. The mucosal defect is then closed completely with a continuous suture using the same stitch that was employed to ligate the haemorrhoid pedicle. The remaining haemorrhoids are excised and ligated in similar fashion, ensuring there are adequate mucosal and skin bridges between each area of excision, so as to avoid a subsequent stenosis.

Edward T. Campbell Milligan, 1925–51. Surgeon, St Martin's Hospital, London, England.
Sir Clifford Naunton-Morgan, 1932–67. Surgeon, St Martin's Hospital, London, England.

Postoperative care. In these days of economic stringencies, the patient is discharged from hospital within a day or two of the operation. In the USA, the procedure is often performed on a day-care basis. The patient is instructed to take two warm baths a day, and is given a bulk laxative to take twice daily, together with appropriate analgesia. Dry dressings are applied as necessary, a sterile sanitary towel usually being ideal. The patient is seen again 3–4 weeks after discharge and a rectal examination is performed. If there is evidence of stenosis, the patient is encouraged to use a dilator.

Postoperative complications may be early or late.

Complications of haemorrhoidectomy

Early	*Late*
Pain	Secondary haemorrhage
Acute retention of urine	Anal stricture
Reactionary haemorrhage	Anal fissure

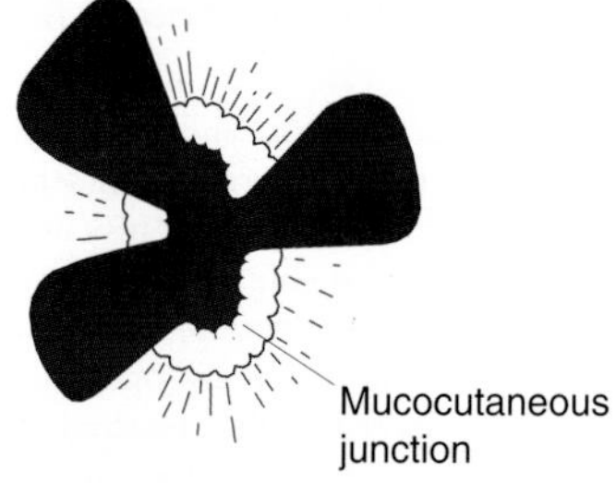

Fig. 61.32 The appearance of the anus at the conclusion of the operation. (NB. To avoid stricture formation it is necessary to ensure that a bridge of skin and mucous membrane remains between each wound.) If it looks like a clover the trouble is over, if it looks like a dahlia, it's surely a failure.

James A. Ferguson. Ferguson Clinic, Grand Rapids, Michigan, USA.

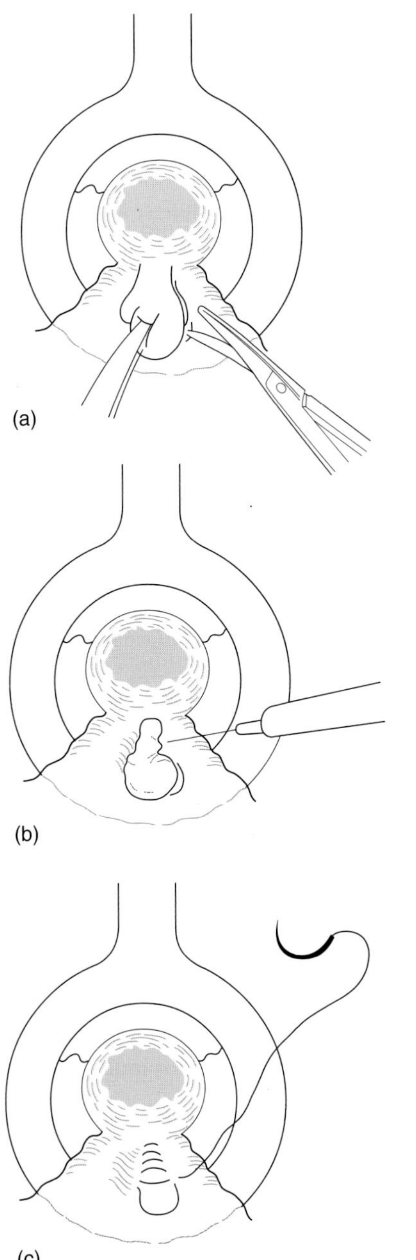

Fig. 61.33 Closed technique of haemorrhoidectomy. (a) The haemorrhoidal tissue is excised; (b) bleeding is controlled by diathermy; (c) the defect is closed with a continuous suture after first undermining the anoderm on each side. (Redrawn with permission from Keighley, M.R.B. and Williams, N.S., *Surgery of the Anus, Colon and Rectum*, 2nd edn, W.B. Saunders, 1999.)

Early. *Pain* may demand repeated pethidine. Xylocaine jelly introduced through a fine nozzle into the rectum, as necessary, is of considerable value.

Retention of urine is not unusual after haemorrhoidectomy in male patients, and frequently it is precipitated by the presence of a rectal tube or pack, or both. Before resorting to catheterisation, the patient should be reassured, given an analgesic, allowed to stand at the side of the bed in privacy or be assisted to a hot bath into which he may be able to void urine.

Reactionary haemorrhage is much more common than secondary haemorrhage. The haemorrhage may be mainly or entirely concealed, but will become evident on examining the rectum.

Treatment. A suitable dose of morphine is given intravenously. If the bleeding persists, the patient must be taken to the operating theatre and the bleeding point secured by diathermy or under-running with a ligature on a needle. Should a definite bleeding point not be found, suspected areas are under-run in this way and the anal canal and rectum are packed.

Late. *Secondary haemorrhage* is uncommon; when it occurs, it does so about the 7th or 8th day after operation. It is usually controlled by morphia but, if the haemorrhage is severe, an anaesthetic should be given and a catgut stitch inserted to occlude the bleeding vessel.

Anal stricture. This must be prevented at all costs (Fig. 61.32 and legend). A rectal examination at the 10th day will indicate whether stricturing is to be expected. It may then be necessary to give a general anaesthetic and dilate the anus. After that, daily use of the dilator should give a satisfactory result.

Anal fissure and submucous abscesses may also occur.

Treatment of complications

Strangulation, thrombosis and gangrene. In these cases, it was formerly believed that surgery would promote pylephlebitis. If adequate antibiotic cover is given from the start, this is not found to be so and immediate surgery can be justified in many patients. Besides adequate pain relief, bed rest with frequent, hot sitz baths and warm saline compresses with firm pressure usually cause the pile mass to shrink considerably in 3–4 days when standard ligation and excision of the piles can be carried out. Some surgeons consider that the operation at this stage increases the risk of postoperative stenosis and delay surgery for a month or so. They then review the situation and only carry out haemorrhoidectomy if necessary. In spite of the low risk of pylephlebitis, caution should dictate a 'noninterventionist' policy whenever this is practical. An anal dilation technique has in the past been used as an alternative treatment to surgery for painful 'strangulated' haemorrhoids. However, the stretching should be far more circumspect than that recommended by Lord in his original description and the patient must be warned about other risks of incontinence. Once again an anal stretch must be avoided in patients with a weak or potentially weak anal sphincter. Many colorectal surgeons have abandoned the use of anal stretch in any circumstances.

Severe haemorrhage. The cause usually lies in a bleeding diathesis or the use of anticoagulants. If such are excluded, a local compress containing adrenaline solution, with an injection of morphine and blood transfusion if necessary, will usually control the haemorrhage. After blood replacement is adequate, ligation and excision of the piles may be required.

External haemorrhoids

Unlike internal haemorrhoids, external haemorrhoids consists of a conglomerate group of distinct clinical entities.

Peter Lord. Emeritus Consultant, High Wycombe, England.

A thrombosed external haemorrhoid is commonly termed a *perianal haematoma*. It is a small clot occurring in the perianal subcutaneous connective tissue, usually superficial to the corrugator cutis ani muscle. The condition is due to back pressure on an anal venule consequent upon straining at stool, coughing or lifting a heavy weight.

The condition appears suddenly and is very painful, and on examination a tense, tender swelling which resembles a semiripe blackcurrant is seen. The haematoma is usually situated in a lateral region of the anal margin. Untreated it may resolve, suppurate, fibrose and give rise to a cutaneous tag, or burst and extrude the clot, or continue bleeding.

In the majority of cases resolution or fibrosis occurs. Indeed, this condition has been called 'a 5-day, painful, self-curing lesion' (Milligan).

Provided it is seen within 36 hours of the onset, a perianal haematoma is best treated as an emergency. Under local anaesthesia the haemorrhoid is bisected and the two halves are excised together with 1.25 cm of adjacent skin. This leaves a pear-shaped wound which is allowed to granulate. The relief of pain is immediate and a permanent cure is certain. On the rare occasions in which a perianal haematoma is situated anteriorly or posteriorly, it should be treated conservatively because of the liability of a skin wound in these regions to become an anal fissure.

Associated with internal haemorrhoids = interoexternal haemorrhoids. These have been discussed.

Dilatation of the veins of the anal verge becomes evident only if the patient strains, when a bluish, cushion-like ring appears. This variety of external haemorrhoid is almost a perquisite of those who lead a sedentary life. The only treatment required is an adjustment in habits of the patient.

A 'sentinel' pile is associated with an anal fissure (see above).

Genital warts – see Chapter 67.

Pruritis ani

This is intractible itching around the anus. Usually the skin is reddened hyperkeratotic and may become cracked and moist. The causes are numerous. A useful mnemonic is: 'pus, polypus, parasites, piles, psyche'.

- **Lack of cleanliness**, excessive sweating, and wearing rough or woollen underclothing are common causes.
- **An anal or perianal discharge** which renders the anus moist. The causative lesions include an anal fissure, fistula in ano, prolapsed internal or external haemorrhoids, genital warts and excessive ingestion of liquid paraffin. A mucous discharge is an intense pruritic agent and a polyp can be the cause.
- **A vaginal discharge**, especially due to the *Trichomonas vaginalis*.
- **Parasitic causes.** Threadworms should be excluded, especially in young subjects. Children suffering from threadworms should wear gloves at night, less they scratch the perianal region and are reinfested with ova by nail biting – 'parasites lost, parasites regained'. Scabies and pediculosis pubis may infest the anal region.
- **Epidermophytosis** is a common cause especially if the skin between the toes is also infected. Microscopic and cultural examinations are essential. Half-strength Whitfield's ointment quickly gives relief and is the sheet anchor of treatment.
- **Allergy** is sometimes the cause, in which case there is likely to be a history of other allergic manifestations, such as urticaria, asthma or hay fever. Antibiotic therapy may be the precipitating factor.
- **Skin diseases** localised to the perianal skin – psoriasis, lichen planus and contact dermatitis.
- **Bacterial infection.** Intertrigo due to a mixed bacterial infection. Erythrasma due to *Corynebacterium minutissimum* is responsible for some cases and its presence is detected by ultraviolet light which induces a pink fluorescence.
- **A psychoneurosis.** It is alleged that in a few instances neurotic individuals become so immersed in their complaint that a pain–pleasure complex develops, the pleasure being the scratching. Possibly this is true, but such a syndrome should not be assumed without firm grounds for coming to this conclusion.
- **Diabetes.** Diabetes can sometimes present with pruritus ani and the urine should be tested in all patients.

Treatment. The cause is treated. Other methods include the following.

- *Hygienic measures.* Cotton wool should be substituted for toilet paper. Soap is avoided and replaced by a detergent. These measures alone, combined with wearing cotton cellular underwear and applications of calamine lotion, are all that is necessary to cure some cases. If there is much anal hair trapping the moisture and discharge, shaving can be very helpful.
- *Hydrocortisone.* In cases with dermatitis, and only in cases with dermatitis, prednisolone, applied topically in a cream of 1 per cent is often beneficial; sometimes after discontinuation of the therapy, the pruritus is liable to return, in which event 5 per cent xylocaine ointment can be substituted for a time.
- Strapping the buttocks apart is a most useful procedure, especially when the pruritus is acute, and in chronic cases when the opposing surfaces are moist. The strapping is worn so long as the patient finds it beneficial.

Operative treatment

This may be necessary for a concomitant lesion of the anorectum which is thought to initiate or contribute to the pruritis. Otherwise, surgery is not indicated.

Anorectal abscesses

In 60 per cent of cases the pus from the abscess yields a pure culture of *Escherichia coli*; in 23 per cent a pure culture of *Staphylococcus aureus* is obtained. In diminishing frequency, pure cultures of *Bacteroides*, a *Streptococcus* or *Proteus* strain are found. In many cases the infection is mixed. In a high percentage of cases – some estimate it as high as 90 per cent – the abscess commences as an infection of an anal gland (Figs 61.34 and 61.35). Other causes are penetration of the rectal wall, e.g. by a fish bone, a blood-borne infection or an extension of a cutaneous boil. Underlying rectal disease, such as neoplasm and particularly Crohn's disease, may be the cause. Similarly patients with generalised disorders, such as diabetes and more recently AIDS, may present with an anorectal abscess. The latter patients usually have abscesses which run an aggressive course.

Arthur Whitfield, 1868–1947. Professor of Dermatology, King's College Hospital, London, England.

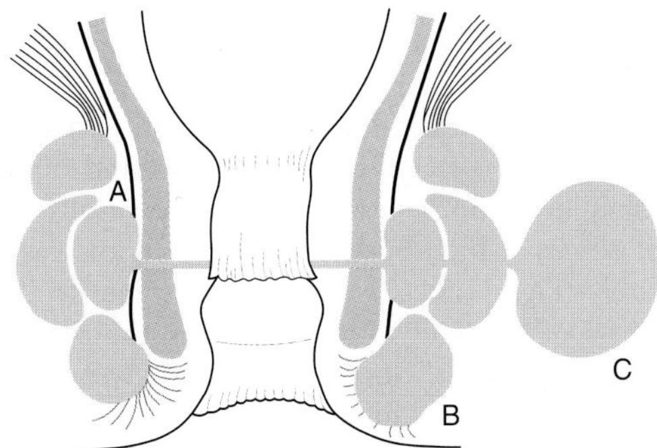

Fig. 61.34 Spread of infection from the primary anal gland abscess (A) to the perianal region (B) and the ischiorectal fossa (C) (*after Sir Alan Parks, London, England*).

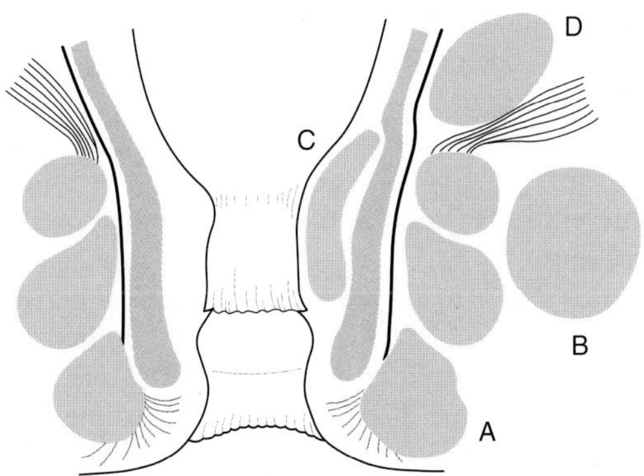

Fig. 61.35 The four types of anorectal abscess: (A) perianal; (B) ischiorectal; (C) submucous; and (D) pelvirectal (*after W.F.W. Southwood, Bath, England*).

A large percentage of anorectal abscesses coincides with a fistula in ano. For this reason, anorectal abscess becomes a highly important subject. Moreover, as antibiotics cannot reach the contents of an abscess in adequate concentration, no reliance can be placed on antibiotic therapy alone. A fistula is much more likely if bacterial culture of the pus discloses bowel (as opposed to skin) organisms (Grace).

Differential diagnosis

The only conditions with which an anorectal abscess is likely to be confused are an abscess connected with a pilonidal sinus, Bartholin's gland or Cowper's gland.

Classification

A clear understanding of suppuration in this area is dependent on a concise knowledge of the anatomy (Figs 61.34 and 61.35). There are four main varieties: perianal, ischiorectal, submucous and pelvirectal.

Roger Grace. Professor of Colorectal Surgery, Wolverhampton, England.
Caspar Bartholin, 1655–1738. Professor of Medicine, Anatomy and Physics, Copenhagen, Denmark.
William Cowper, 1666–1709. Surgeon, London, England.

Perianal (60 per cent)

This usually occurs as the result of suppuration in an anal gland, which spreads superficially to lie in the region of the subcutaneous portion of the external sphincter (Fig. 61.35a). It may also occur as a result of a thrombosed external pile. If the haematoma is not evacuated, it may become infected and a perianal abscess results. This is the most common abscess of the region. Persons of all ages are affected and the condition is not uncommon, even in infancy and childhood. The constitutional symptoms and the pain are less pronounced than in the ischiorectal abscess because the pus can expand the walls of this part of the intermuscular space comparatively easily. Early diagnosis is made by inspecting the anal margin, when an acutely tender, rounded, cystic lump about the size of a cherry is seen and felt at the anal verge below the dentate line.

Treatment. No time should be lost in evacuating the pus.

Operation. Thorough drainage is achieved by making a cruciate incision over the abscess and excising the skin edges – this completely removes the 'roof' of the abscess.

Ischiorectal abscess (30 per cent)

Commonly, this is due to an extension laterally through the external sphincter of a low intermuscular anal abscess (Fig. 61.35b). Rarely, the infection is either lymphatic or blood borne. The fat, which fills the ischiorectal fossa (Fig. 61.36), is particularly vulnerable because it is poorly vascularised; consequently it is not long before the whole space becomes involved. The ischiorectal fossa communicates with that of the opposite side via the postsphincteric space, and if an ischiorectal abscess is not evacuated early, involvement of the contralateral fossa is not uncommon. Should an internal opening into the anal canal ensue, a 'horseshoe' abscess develops enveloping the whole of the posterior part of the circumference of the anal canal (cf. horseshoe fistula).

An ischiorectal abscess gives rise to a tender, brawny induration palpable on the corresponding side of the anal canal and the floor of the fossa. Constitutional symptoms are severe, the temperature often rising to 38–39°C. Men are affected more often than women.

Treatment. Operation should be undertaken early – as soon

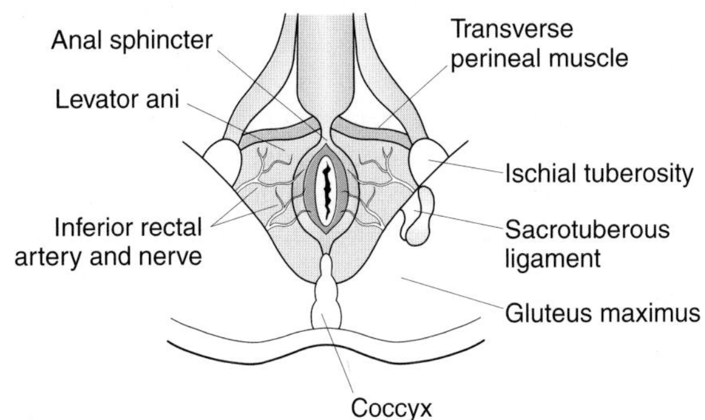

Fig. 61.36 The ischiorectal fossa (*after V.C. Shah and Y.V. Shah*).

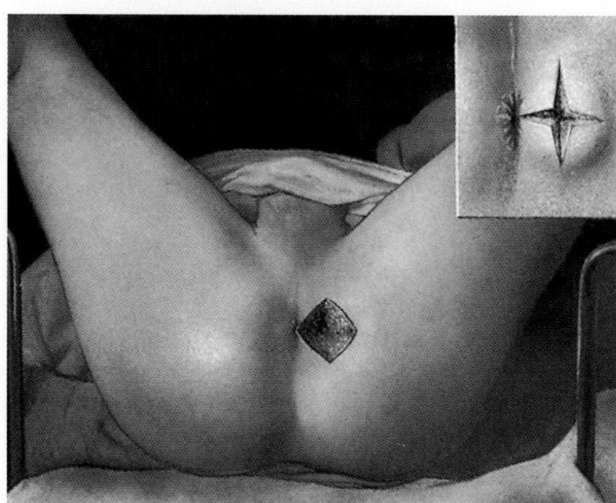

Fig. 61.37 Incision of an ischiorectal abscess. The cavity is explored and, if septa exist, they should be broken down gently with a finger, and the necrotic tissue lining the walls of the abscess should be removed by the finger wrapped in gauze. It is wise to biopsy the wall and send the pus for culture. Nothing further is done at this stage.

as it is certain that an abscess is present in this area – remembering that antibiotic therapy often masks the general signs.

Operation. *Stage 1.* A cruciate incision (Fig. 61.37 inset) is made into the abscess. A portion of skin is sometimes excised (Fig. 61.37) but deroofing is not necessary in every case.

Stage 2. As soon as the acute infection has subsided, the wound should be re-examined, preferably under general anaesthesia. A careful search is made for a fistulous opening communicating with the anal canal. If such is found, the treatment should be as for fistula. If no fistula is found, the cavity should be lightly packed with gauze wrung out in any weak antiseptic favoured by the operator. A T-bandage is applied. When the cavity has become covered with granulation tissue, skin grafting may help to expedite final epithelialisation.

Submucous abscess

Submucous abscess (5 per cent) occurs above the dentate line (Fig. 61.35c). When it occurs after the injection of haemorrhoids, it always resolves. Otherwise, it can be opened with sinus forceps when adequately displayed by a protoscope.

Pelvirectal abscess

Pelvirectal abscess is situated between the upper surface of the levator ani and the pelvic peritoneum (Fig. 61.35d). It is nothing more or less than a pelvic abscess and, as such, is usually secondary to appendicitis, salpingitis, diverticulitis or parametritis. *Abdominal Crohn's disease is an important cause of pelvic disease that can present as perianal sepsis* (cf. fistula in ano). A relevant point to remember is that, rarely, a supralevator abscess/fistula may be due to overenthusiastic attempts to drain an ischiorectal abscess or to display a fistula, when a probe is forced through the levator ani/rectal wall from below.

Fissure abscess

This is the name given to a subcutaneous abscess lying in immediate association with an anal fissure. Drainage is achieved at the same time as the fissure is treated by sphincterotomy.

Fistula in ano

A fistula in ano[2] is a track, lined by granulation tissue, which connects deeply in the anal canal or rectum and superficially on the skin around the anus. It usually results from an anorectal abscess which burst spontaneously or was opened inadequately (Fig. 61.34). The fistula continues to discharge and, because of constant reinfection from the anal canal or rectum, seldom, if ever, closes permanently without surgical aid. An anorectal abscess may produce a track, the orifice of which has the appearance of a fistula, but it does not communicate with the anal canal or the rectum. By definition this is *not* a fistula, but a sinus.

Types of anal fistulae

These are divided into two groups, according to whether their internal opening is below or above the anorectal ring.

Low-level fistulae open into the anal canal below the anorectal ring.

High-level fistulae open into the anal canal at or above the anorectal ring.

As an alternative to the common anatomical classification illustrated in Fig. 61.38, Parks produced another based on the origin of the fistula from an abscess in an anal gland situated in the plane between the internal and external sphincters (the 'anal intersphincteric plane') (Fig. 61.39).

The importance of deciding whether a fistula is a low- or a high-level type is that a low-level fistula can be laid open usually without fear of permanent incontinence (from damage to the anorectal bundle), while a high-level fistula can be treated only by 'staged' operations, often with the use of a protective colostomy to prevent septic complications and to shorten healing time between the stages.

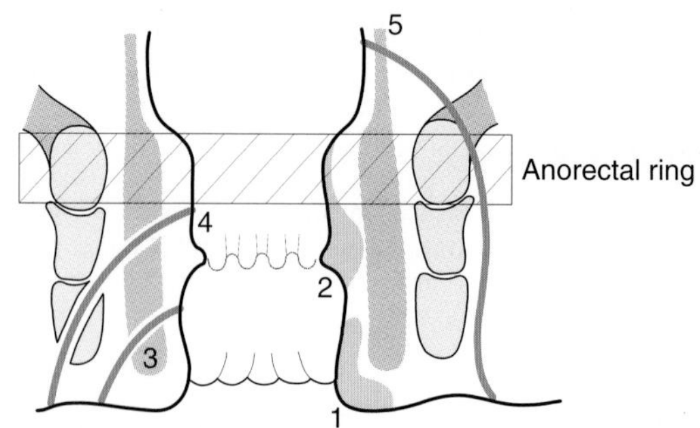

Fig. 61.38 Types of anal fistula (standard classification): (1) subcutaneous; (2) submucous; (3) low anal; (4) high anal; and (5) pelvirectal.

[2]*For treating successfully Louis XIV's fistula in ano, Charles Félix, barber – surgeon to the Court, received a gift of a farm, 300 000 livres and a title. Today, 300 000 livres would be worth about £25 000.*

Sir Alan Guyatt Parks, 1920–82. Surgeon, The London Hospital and St Mark's Hospital, London, England.

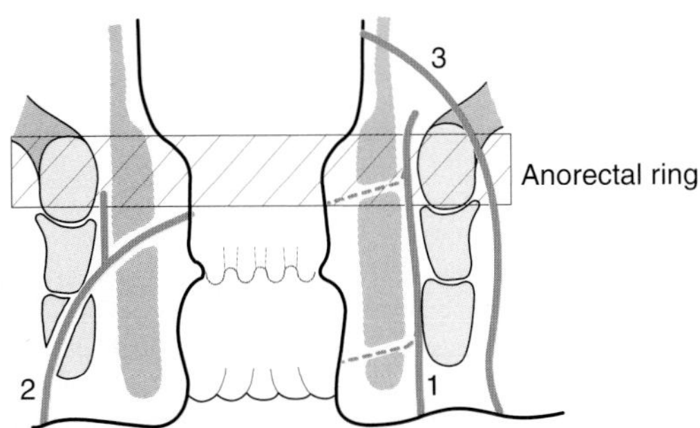

Fig. 61.39 Types of anal fistula: (1) intersphincteric; (2) trans-sphincteric (which may be high or low); and (3) supralevator (after Sir Alan Parks).

In probing a high fistulous track, great care must be taken not to create an internal opening into the rectum where none existed previously. Such a disaster could convert a relatively straightforward 'intersphincteric' track into a high 'pelvirectal' fistula that might prove very difficult to cure.

By the standard classification, a *high* fistula refers to both a high anal [Fig. 61.38(4)] and a pelvirectal fistula [Fig. 61.38(5)]. By the Parks' classification, both a high trans-sphincteric and a supralevator fistula would qualify as high, with the intersphincteric falling into either category depending on whether an internal opening was present at all, and at what level it entered the anal canal [see Fig. 61.38(1)].

Low-level fistulae

Clinical features. Commonly, the principal symptom is a persistent seropurulent discharge that irritates the skin in the neighbourhood and causes discomfort. Often the history dates back for years. So long as the opening is large enough for the pus to escape, pain is not a symptom, but if the orifice is occluded pain increases until the discharge erupts. Frequently, there is a solitary external opening, usually situated within 3.5–4 cm of the anus, presenting as a small elevation with granulation tissue pouting from the mouth of the opening. Sometimes superficial healing occurs, pus accumulates and an abscess reforms and discharges through the same opening or a new opening. Thus there may be two or more external openings, usually grouped together on the right or left of the midline but, occasionally, when both ischiorectal fossas are involved, an opening is seen on each side, in which case there is often intercommunication between them (Fig. 61.40). As a rule there is much induration of the skin and subcutaneous tissues around the fistula.

Goodsall's rule. Fistulae with an external opening in relation to the anterior half of the anus tend to be of the direct type (Fig. 61.41). Those with an external opening or openings in relation to the posterior half of the anus, which are much more common, usually have curving tracks, and may be of the horseshoe variety. Note that posteriorly situated fistulae may have multiple external openings which always connect to a solitary internal orifice, usually midline (Fig. 61.41).

David Henry Goodsall, 1843–1906. Surgeon, St Mark's Hospital for Diseases of the Rectum and Colon, London, England.

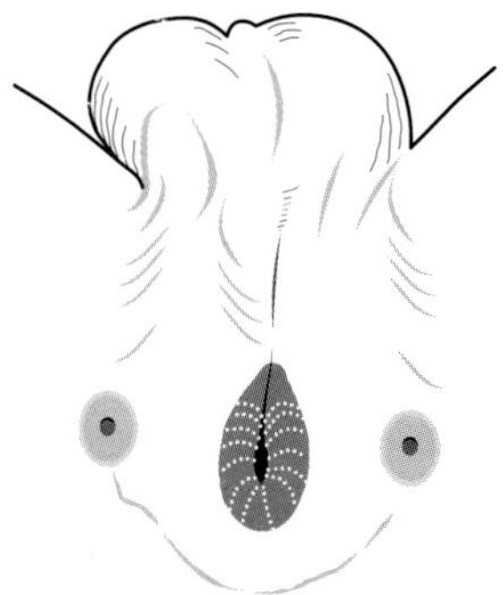

Fig. 61.40 Horseshoe fistula in ano. Both ischiorectal fossae involved. Usually there is only one internal orifice.

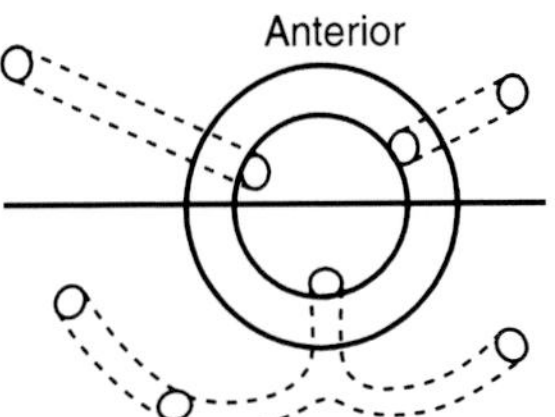

Fig. 61.41 Goodsall's rule.

Digital examination. Not infrequently an internal opening can be felt as a nodule on the wall of the anal canal. Irrespective of the number of external openings, there is almost invariably only one internal opening.

Proctoscopy sometimes will reveal the internal opening of the fistula. A hypertrophied papilla is suggestive that the internal orifice lies within the crypt related to the papilla (Fig. 61.42).

Probing. In the past, it was the universal practice to probe a fistula in the ward or the out-patient department. *Such manoeuvres accomplish nothing*, are painful and are liable to reawaken dormant infection. Furthermore, if probing is performed without the utmost gentleness, or if the patient, experiencing pain, makes a sudden jerk, a false passage may result which complicates the condition still further. Probing should be postponed until the patient is under an anaesthetic in the operating theatre.

The injection of lipiodol, or other opaque medium, along the sinus, before radiography *has little to recommend it*. The radiographs thus obtained are seldom illuminating, and the procedure is likely to cause a recrudescence of inflammation. Endoluminal ultrasonography and magnetic resonance imaging are being developed as techniques for 'mapping' complex fistulae.

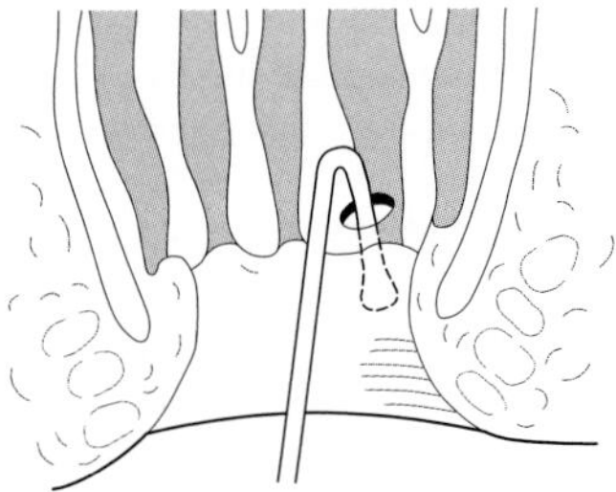

Fig. 61.42 Retrograde probing of an anal canal sometimes reveals the internal orifice of the fistula.

Radiography of the thorax should be undertaken and the possibility of pulmonary tuberculosis considered, despite the fact that today it will be found in only a small proportion of patients with fistula in ano – usually of Asian origin (see below).

Special clinical types of fistulae in ano

Fistula connected with an anal fissure. Unlike the usual fistula in ano, pain (due to the fissure) is a leading symptom. The fistula is very near the anal orifice, usually posterior, and the external opening is often hidden by the sentinel pile.

Fistula with an internal opening above the anorectal ring is due, almost invariably, to penetration by a foreign body or probing and interference with a high abscess. A supralevator fistula arising spontaneously will be seen only once or at most twice in a surgical career.

Granulomatous infections and Crohn's disease. If induration around a fistula is lacking, if the opening is ragged and flush with the surface, if the surrounding skin is discoloured and the discharge is watery, or if the external openings are multiple, tuberculous or Crohn's disease should be considered. In more than 30 per cent of patients suffering from pulmonary tuberculosis, virulent tubercle bacilli are present in the rectum. About 2–3 per cent of fistulae in the UK are due to Crohn's disease or tuberculosis. In Asian communities, the incidence of tuberculosis is higher. Crohn's disease should also be suspected if there are other stigmata, and a small bowel meal may be necessary. If tuberculosis is suspected, a chest radiograph and sputum cultures are mandatory. However, the diagnosis can usually only be made on histological examination of biopsy material from the track. If due to tuberculosis, the fistula will usually respond to antituberculous drugs alone.

Fistulae with many external openings may arise from tuberculous proctitis, Crohn's disease of colon or ileum, bilharziasis and lymphogranuloma inguinale with a fibrous rectal stricture. Crohn's disease is the most frequent cause seen in this country from this group.

Carcinoma arising within perianal fistulae. Colloid carcinoma may complicate fistulae in ano and a colloid carcinoma of the rectum is notoriously liable to be complicated by perianal fistulae. In some instances, the fistulous condition, with its discharge of colloid material, overshadows the primary carcinoma, and not a few unfortunate patients have had their condition diagnosed for a time as an inflammatory fistula in ano. If a primary tumour is present in the rectum, usually it can be detected and its nature established by biopsy. Dukes established conclusively that colloid carcinomatous fistulae can develop without a primary neoplasm in the rectum. He regarded such cases as examples of colloid carcinoma developing in a reduplicated portion of the intestinal tract. Both adenocarcinoma and squamous-cell carcinoma are known to arise within chronic fistulous tracks. The former can develop from the anal granular tissue; the latter is an example of true malignant change of squamous epithelium lining the wall of the track.

Hidradenitis suppurativa. This is a chronic infection of apocrine glands around the anal margin giving rise to numerous sinuses. The mons pubis and groin can also be affected. After excision of the area, granulation and healing are accelerated by using Silastic foam dressing (Hughes).

Treatment. That the fistulous track must be laid open from its termination to its source was a rule promulgated by John of Arderne more than 600 years ago.

The operation can best be described in stages:

Step 1. Preoperative cleaning enemas are necessary. When the patient has been anaesthetised, he or she is placed in the lithotomy position or in the prone jack-knife position, according to the preference of the operator. Using bidigital palpation under anaesthesia, it is often possible to obtain more information concerning a fistula than can be learned from probing; it is surprisingly easy to push a probe through the wall of the track. Unfortunately, many inexperienced operators find it more reassuring to create a false passage than to risk criticism for not being able to demonstrate the internal opening. Careful bidigital palpation of the perianal tissue will often reveal a cord-like induration, representing the track, which will lead the intra-anal finger towards the proximal opening. Rather than insert a probe through the distal orifice at this stage, it is better to endeavour to find the internal opening via a proctoscope. If the internal opening still cannot be seen, the insertion of a probe retrogradely into an anal crypt, especially one with a nearby hypertrophied papilla, often reveals the internal portion of the track (Fig. 61.42). The injection of dilute methylene blue or other dye into the external mouth of the fistula to establish the site of the internal opening is occasionally necessary, but is not recommended as a routine.

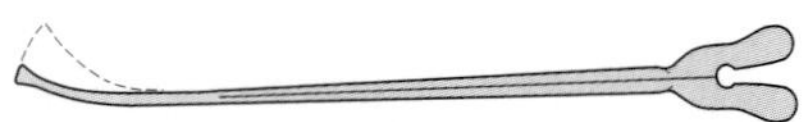

Fig. 61.43 A director with a probe-pointed malleable extremity is a useful instrument.

Step 2. A probe-pointed director (Fig. 61.43) is inserted into the distal orifice, and it is advanced delicately until it reaches a point where it does not pass readily. The track is opened along the director and bleeding is controlled.

Step 3. If it is not at once evident in which direction the track passes, granulations are wiped away with gauze (it is seldom necessary to use a curette). Often this will leave a granulation-filled spot at one site only. Gentle probing at this spot frequently will give the clue to the continuation of the fistula. The director is reinserted, and again followed with the knife for a short distance. This procedure is repeated until the entire track, and any side channels, are laid open. As far as possible, all muscle is divided at right angles to its fibres. In the rare event of the track passing above the anorectal ring, cutting should cease at the level of the dentate line, and from thenceforth the operation is conducted as suggested below. In most instances, probing and laying open the track can be repeated until the entire track is laid open. Pursuing this course, if there is no internal opening, the track will become bereft of granulations on wiping it. As a rule, the internal opening can be demonstrated either by direct inspection through a proctoscope, or by a bent probe inserted into an anal crypt. In the latter circumstance, the internal portion of the track is excised in continuity.

Step 4. The edges of the track are trimmed, 1–3 mm of tissue being removed – a step that makes postoperative packing unnecessary after the first 24–36 hours. Hughes advocated primary split skin grafting of the wound resulting from fistulotomy. The grafts are taken from the inner aspect of the thigh and applied to the anal wound, being stitched to the skin edges and to each other in the depths of the wound. Tulle gras is then superimposed and a firm pack of cotton wool applied. The first dressing is done on the 5th postoperative day.

When skin grafting is not employed, digital dilatation of the anus, or the passage of a St Mark's Hospital[3] dilator every other day, prevents pocketing or bridging of the granulating wound.

Biopsy. Always send a piece of track for biopsy.

High-level fistulae

The treatment of these cases is difficult. If the track is laid open as for low-level fistulae, incontinence will follow. There are four types (Parks).

Cuthbert Esquire Dukes, 1890–1977. Pathologist, St Mark's Hospital, London, England.

Leslie Ernest Hughes. Emeritus Professor of Surgery, Welsh National School of Medicine, Cardiff, Wales.

[3]*St Mark's Hospital for Diseases of the Rectum and Colon, London, founded in 1835 as St Mark's Hospital for Fistula.*

Supralevator fistula – secondary to local disease [Fig. 61.39(3)]. It occurs as a result of Crohn's disease, ulcerative colitis, carcinoma, a foreign body perforating the rectal ampulla from above or trauma. This fistula is quite unrelated to the ordinary type and the treatment is that of the cause. A traumatic fistula usually needs a colostomy. None of these fistulae requires to be laid open, which would in any case cause incontinence.

Trans-sphincteric fistula [Fig. 61.39(2)] with *perforating secondary track*. The condition starts as an *intersphincteric* track [Fig. 61.39(1)], often with a high secondary track in the ischiorectal fossa up to the levator ani. Here lies the danger. Although the anal opening may be low, during exploration of the high secondary track, unless great care is taken, the probe can be pushed through the levator ani into the rectal ampulla, thus converting a low fistula into a high-level type. Treatment should first of all be directed to the low trans-sphincteric fistula and healing of the upper track may follow. If it fails to do so, or if the opening into the rectum is of any size or near the anorectal bundle, a colostomy must sometimes be done before sound healing will take place. High tracks often require staged operations.

A *seton* – a time-honoured device – (i.e. a ligature of silk, nylon, silastic or linen) is helpful when the internal opening is near the anorectal ring. Insertion of a seton and subsequent re-examination of the patient without anaesthesia will establish whether the internal opening is situated so near to the anorectal ring that incontinence would result if the track were laid open. Under these conditions, a staged operation and a covering colostomy would be the proper treatment. While the seton remains *in situ* it acts as a wick/drain and allows the acute inflammatory reaction around the track to subside: this can greatly simplify subsequent surgery. In expert hands, primary repair of divided sphincter muscle can preserve continence when a high-level track is laid open.

Intersphincteric fistula. The track starts as a primary anal gland abscess (Fig. 61.34a), and it runs between the internal and external sphincter along the plane of the longitudinal muscle fibres (see Fig. 61.39, Type 1). It may have an opening into the rectum above the anorectal ring and below at the site of a perianal abscess (Fig. 61.34b). Providing it is recognised it is easy to treat. The internal sphincter is divided and the whole track is laid open without fear of incontinence.

Suprasphincteric fistula. Occasionally, the intersphincteric track passes over the top of the sphincter before passing down again in the ischiorectal fossa. Treatment of this type is very difficult and is sometimes best done by an indwelling seton.

Nonmalignant strictures

Congenital

- A stricture at the level of the anal valves, due to incomplete obliteration of the proctodeal membrane, sometimes does not give rise to symptoms until early childhood.
- Patients who have had an operation for imperforate anus in infancy may require periodic anorectal dilatation.

Spasmodic

- An anal fissure causes spasm of the internal sphincter.
- Rarely, a spasmodic stricture accompanies secondary megacolon (Chapter 57), possibly due to chronic use of laxatives.

Organic

- **Postoperative stricture** sometimes follows haemorrhoidectomy performed incorrectly. Low coloanal anastomoses, especially if a stapling gun is used, can narrow down postoperatively.
- **Irradiation stricture** is an aftermath of irradiation.
- **Senile anal stenosis** – a condition of chronic internal sphincter contraction is sometimes seen in the aged. Increasing constipation is present with pronounced straining at stool. Faecal impaction is liable to occur. The muscle is rigid and feels like a tight umbrella-ring. There is no evidence of a fissure in ano. The treatment is internal sphincterotomy or dilatation at frequent intervals.
- **Lymphogranuloma inguinale** (Chapter 67). This is by far the most frequent cause of a *tubular* inflammatory stricture of the rectum and 80 per cent of the sufferers are women. Frei's reaction is usually positive. This variety of rectal stricture is particularly common in black races, and may be accompanied by elephantiasis of the labia majora. In the early stages, antibiotic treatment may lead to cure. In advanced cases excision of the rectum is required.
- **Inflammatory bowel disease.** Stricture of the anorectum also complicates ulcerative proctocolitis and most commonly large-bowel Crohn's disease; in this instance the stricture is annular and often more than one is present. A carcinoma should be suspected if a stricture is found, until a biopsy is obtained.
- **Endometriosis** of the rectovaginal septum may present as a stricture. There is usually a history of frequent menstrual periods with the appearance of severe pain during the first 2 days of the menstrual flow.
- **Neoplastic.** When free bleeding occurs after dilatation of a supposed inflammatory stricture, carcinoma should be suspected (Grey Turner) and a portion of the stricture should be removed for biopsy. Sometimes in these cases repeated biopsies show inflammatory tissue only. If, however, the symptoms show a marked progression, malignancy should be strongly suspected.

Clinical features

Increasing difficulty in defecation is the leading symptom. The patient finds that increasingly large doses of aperients are required, and if the stools are formed, they are 'pipe-stem' in shape. In cases of inflammatory stricture, tenesmus, bleeding

---

Wilhelm Siegmund Frei, 1885–1943. Professor of Dermatology, Berlin, who later settled in New York, USA.

George Grey Turner, 1877–1951. Professor of Surgery, Postgraduate Medical School, London. Formerly Professor of Surgery, University of Durham, England.

and the passage of mucopus are superadded. Sometimes the patient comes under observation only when subacute or acute intestinal obstruction has supervened.

Rectal examination. The finger encounters a sharply defined shelf-like interruption of the lumen. If the calibre is large enough to admit the finger, it should be noted whether the stricture is annular or tubular. Sometimes this point can be determined only after dilatation. A biopsy of the stricture must be taken.

Treatment

Prophylactic

The passage of an anal dilator during convalescence after haemorrhoidectomy greatly reduces the incidence of postoperative stricture. Efficient treatment of lymphogranuloma inguinale in its early stages should lessen the frequency of stricture from that cause.

Dilatation by bougies

For anal and many rectal strictures dilatation by bougies at regular intervals is all that is required.

Anoplasty

The stricture is incised and a rotation or advancement flap of skin and subcutaneous tissue replaces the defect and enlarges the anal orifice (Fig. 61.44). This technique is particularly useful for postoperative strictures.

Colostomy

Colostomy must be undertaken when a stricture is causing intestinal obstruction, and in advanced cases of stricture complicated by fistulae in ano. In selected cases, this can be followed by restorative resection of the stricture-bearing area. If this step is anticipated, the colostomy is placed in the transverse colon.

Rectal excision and coloanal anastomosis

When the strictures are at or just above the anorectal junction, and are associated with a normal anal canal, but irreversible changes necessitate removal of the area, excision can be followed by a coloanal anastomosis with good functional results. A similar procedure can be done for an otherwise incurable supralevator fistula, especially postirradiation.

Malignant tumours

Malignant lesions of the anus and anal canal
Squamous cell carcinoma
Basaloid carcinoma
Mucoepidermal carcinoma
Basal cell carcinoma
Malignant melanoma
Anal intraepithelial neoplasia (AIN)

Carcinoma of the anus differs from carcinoma of the rectum in histological structure, behaviour and types of treatment. This is mainly because of its accessibility, its sensitivity and its abundant lymph drainage, both superficial and deep. Seventy per cent of anal tumours arise in the anal canal: 30 per cent are squamous cell carcinomas of the anal verge.

Squamous cell carcinoma

Because of its superficial situation, the presence of this lesion is frequently recognised by the patient, who often presents early. However, there are exceptions.

- Radiation carcinoma sometimes develops in the anal and perianal skin of a patient unwisely treated with lightly filtered radiographs for pruritus ani. The chronic radiation dermatitis becomes so familiar to the patient that too often he or she does not perceive the superimposition of carcinoma.
- Anal warts sometimes take on a carcinomatous change (Fig. 61.45). This is particularly likely in HIV-positive individuals.
- Occasionally, a squamous cell carcinoma develops in the track of a long-standing fistula in ano.

The following malignant tumours of the anal canal are also found, but they are rare.

Basaloid carcinoma

This is also known as cloacogenic carcinoma and is a form of nonkeratinising squamous carcinoma. It can metastasise to lymph nodes and can be highly malignant. It is not very sensitive to irradiation.

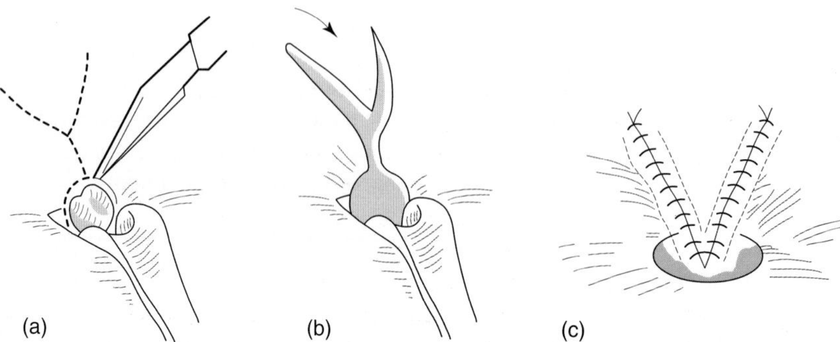

Fig. 61.44 Y-V advancement flap for anal stenosis.

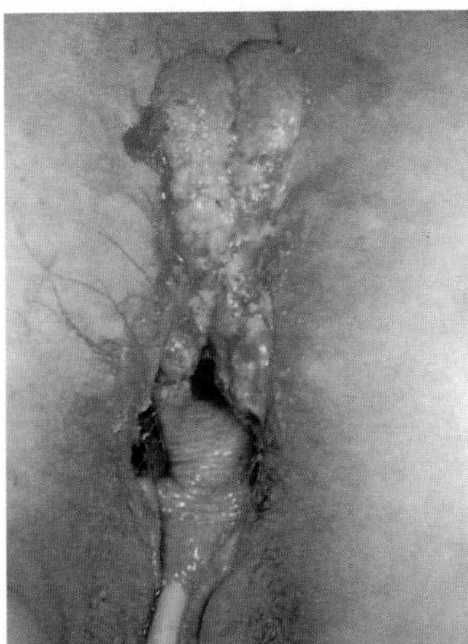

Fig. 61.45 Neglected papillomas of the anus which have become malignant.

Mucoepidermoid carcinoma

This tumour arises near the squamocolumnar cell junction and is of average malignancy. It is not well keratinised and is radiosensitive.

Basal cell carcinoma

Like the true squamous cell carcinomas of the anal verge and lower anal canal these are 'skin tumours' and behave accordingly.

Melanoma

Melanoma of the anus presents as a bluish-black soft mass that is apt to be confused with a thrombotic pile, and therefore unfortunately incised. Such trauma, followed by the trauma of defecation, incites the tumour to rapid metastasis. Left undisturbed, it ulcerates and the colour of the tumour changes from blue to black. The inguinal lymph nodes are soon involved. Unless a melanoma is excised at an early stage, it disseminates by the bloodstream. The tumour is radioresistant and has a very poor prognosis (Fig. 61.46).

Lymphoma

This may rarely affect the anal region and may be part of a more widespread lymphomatous condition.

Clinical features

Anal cancer can occur at almost any age, but is usually found in the 6th and 7th decades. It is a rare condition, accounting for approximately 2 per cent of all colorectal cancers. Symptoms include rectal bleeding, mucus discharge, tenesmus, the sensation of a lump in the anus and a change in bowel habit. Occasionally, a patient may present with a mass in the inguinal region due to metastatic lymph nodes.

Rectal examination may reveal an ulcerating, hard, tender, bleeding mass in the anal canal or at the anal verge. The lesion may fungate through the anal canal and appear on the perianal skin, or present through a chronic draining anal fistula.

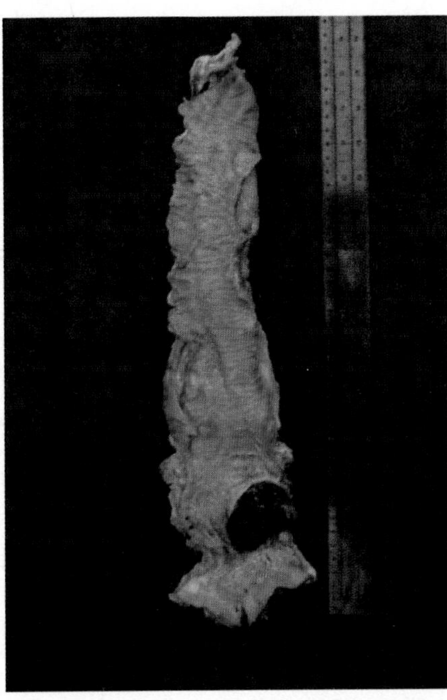

Fig. 61.46 Malignant melanoma of the anal canal (*courtesy of Mr B. Thomas, Kalushi, Zambia*).

Predisposing conditions

There appears to be a relationship between anal condylomata caused by the human papilloma virus, particularly type 16, and anal cancer. Similarly, the disease is more prevalent in patients infected with the human immunodeficiency virus and those with anal intraepithelial neoplasia (AIN) (see later). Several reports suggest a significantly higher incidence of anal cancer in patients with Crohn's disease.

Treatment of squamous carcinoma of the anus and anal canal

Tumours of the anal verge

For small squamous cell lesions of the anal verge, wide local excision leaving a margin of at least 2.5 cm of tissue all round is often sufficient to effect a cure. Lymphatic dissemination will be to the inguinal nodes, which should be watched carefully. If they become involved, block dissection removal of the glands of one or both groins will be necessary and carries a fair prognosis for cure.

Tumours of the anal canal

The traditional treatment for carcinoma of the anal canal has been abdominoperineal excision, removing the growth and perianal area widely. If and when the inguinal lymph nodes became involved, a radical dissection of the groins was carried out. Although this operation is based on sound pathological principles, the need for a permanent colostomy and the morbidity associated with it have encouraged surgeons to try a more conservative approach first.

Radiotherapy alone was used for selected small tumours for a long time. This was applied by external beam, interstitial and intracavitary techniques (Pack). Approximately 50 per cent of tumours treated in this way were said to be eradicated, making subsequent abdominoperineal excision unnecessary (Quan). In patients who presented with inguinal lymph node metastases, block dissection of the groin was indicated in addition to the radiotherapy.

A combination of chemotherapy and radiotherapy, so-called chemoradiation (Nigro) has now become the preferred initial therapy for all anal canal tumours. The patient is given a combination of 5-fluorouracil (5-FU) and mitomycin for approximately 1 week. Some authors have used a combination of bleomycin, cisplatinum and adriamycin. The chemotherapy is followed by radiotherapy given over 3–7 weeks. The patient is then examined 4–6 weeks after cessation of treatment. If there is obvious tumour remaining, an abdominoperineal excision is performed. If there has been a good response to therapy, the scar is excised; and if no microscopic carcinoma is present, the patient is followed up carefully. The therapy does have unpleasant side effects: most patients suffer proctitis and perineal dermatitis from the radiotherapy, and leucopenia and thrombocytopenia are frequent with the chemotherapy; all patients must be warned about the possibility of alopecia. Nevertheless, approximately two-thirds of patients respond to chemoradiation and avoid a major surgical procedure, and 90 per cent of patients are alive and well 2 years after treatment. This therapy is applicable for all tumours, but those with a diameter of 5 cm or more have a higher failure rate. Although many of these are likely to result in eventual abdominoperineal excision, it is probably best to treat them initially by chemoradiation, as this may make subsequent surgery easier.

In the frail patient with an advanced lesion, a defunctioning colostomy may be the only therapy available to relieve the patient of distressing symptoms such as incontinence.

Anal intraepithelial neoplasm

AIN appears to be a premalignant lesion of the anal region. The term describes a dysplastic change which is histologically characterised by a loss of epithelial cellular maturation with associated nuclear hyperchromasia, pleomorphism, cellular crowding and abnormal mitoses within the anal epithelium. These features are identical to those of similar cervical and vulval lesions, and AIN is classified according to nomenclature used for genital intraepithelial neoplasia. Thus:

- AIN I – cellular and nuclear abnormalities are restricted to the lower third of the epithelium;
- AIN II – the lower two-thirds of the epithelium are affected;
- AIN III – the full thickness of the epithelium is affected. This is synonymous with carcinoma *in situ* of the anus (sometimes termed Bowen's disease).

AIN seems to be aetiologically linked with human papilloma virus (HPV), type 16, and is more prevalent in women with genital intraepithelial neoplasia and those individuals who are systemically immunosuppressed (Scholefield). The natural history is unknown, but there is circumstantial evidence that in certain cases AIN may lead to invasive squamous cell carcinoma.

AIN I and II are considered low grade and probably have minimal malignant potential and therefore do not require treatment. In contrast, AIN III is considered high grade, but treatment is difficult because the surgeon is often dealing with a wide field change. Options include simple excision, excision with grafting, laser ablation, cryoablation or the application of cytotoxic creams (such as 5FU).

Further reading

Fielding, L.P. and Goldberg, S. (eds) (1999) *Robb and Smith's Operative Surgery, Surgery of the Colon, Rectum and Anus*, 2nd edn, Chapman and Hall, London.

Keighley, M.R.B. and Williams, N.S. (1999) *Surgery of the Anus, Rectum and Colon*, 2nd edn, W.B. Saunders, London.

George Thomas Pack. Former Clinical Professor of Surgery, New York Medical College, New York, USA.

S.H.Q. Quan. Surgeon, Memorial and Sloan-Kettering Cancer Centre, New York, USA.

N. Nigro. Surgeon, Wayne State University, Detroit, Michigan, USA.

John T. Bowen, 1857–1940. American dermatologist.

John Scholefield. Surgeon, Nottingham, UK.

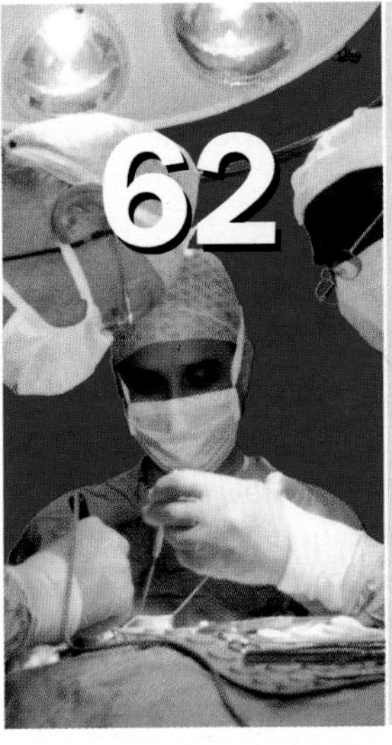

62 Hernias. Umbilicus. Abdominal wall

Hernias

> No disease of the human body, belonging to the province of the surgeon, requires in its treatment a better combination of accurate anatomical knowledge with surgical skill than Hernia in all its varieties. (Sir Astley Paston Cooper, 1804)

A hernia is a protrusion of a viscus or part of a viscus through an abnormal opening in the walls of its containing cavity. The external abdominal hernia is the commonest form, the most frequent varieties being the inguinal, femoral and umbilical, respectively, 75, 8.5 and 15 per cent (Fig. 62.1). The rarer forms comprise 1.5 per cent, excluding incisional hernias.

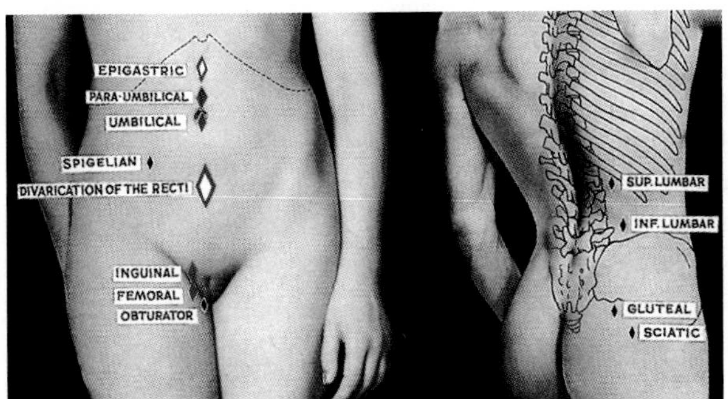

Fig. 62.1 External hernias. Red = common; white = not unusual; black = rare.

Sir Astley Paston Cooper, 1768–1841. Anatomist and surgeon, Guy's Hospital, London, England.

Bailey & Love's Short Practice of Surgery, 23rd edition. Edited by R.C.G. Russell, N.S. Williams and C.J.K. Bulstrode. Published in 2000 by Arnold Publishers.

General features common to all hernias

Aetiology

Any condition which raises intra-abdominal pressure, such as a powerful muscular effort, may produce a hernia. Whooping cough is a predisposing cause in childhood, whilst a chronic cough, straining on micturition or straining on defecation may precipitate a hernia in an adult. Hernias are more common amongst smokers, which may be the result of an acquired collagen deficiency increasing an individual's susceptibility to the development of hernias. It should be remembered that the appearance of a hernia in an adult can be a sign of intra-abdominal malignancy. Stretching of the abdominal musculature because of an increase in contents, as in obesity, can be another factor. Fat acts to separate muscle bundles and layers, weakens aponeuroses and favours the appearance of paraumbilical, direct inguinal and hiatus hernias. A femoral hernia is rare in nulliparous women and men, but more common in multiparous women owing to stretching of the pelvic ligaments. An indirect hernia may occur in a congenital preformed sac – the remains of the processus vaginalis.

Peritoneal dialysis can cause the development of a hernia from a previously occult weakness or enlargement of a patent processus vaginalis.

Composition of a hernia

As a rule, a hernia consists of three parts – the sac, the coverings of the sac and the contents of the sac.

The sac

The sac is a diverticulum of peritoneum consisting of mouth, neck, body and fundus. The neck is usually well defined, but in some direct inguinal hernias and in many incisional hernias there is no actual neck. The diameter of the neck is important because strangulation of bowel is a likely complication where the neck is narrow, as in femoral and paraumbilical hernias.

The body of the sac

The body of the sac varies greatly in size and is not necessarily occupied. In cases occurring in infancy and childhood the sac is gossamer thin. In long-standing cases the wall of the sac may be comparatively thick.

The covering

Coverings are derived from the layers of the abdominal wall through which the sac passes. In long-standing cases they become atrophied from stretching and so amalgamated that they are indistinguishable from each other.

Contents

These can be:

- omentum = omentocele (syn. epiplocele);
- intestine = enterocele. More commonly small bowel, but may be large intestine or appendix;
- a portion of the circumference of the intestine = Richter's hernia;
- a portion of the bladder (or a diverticulum) may constitute part of or be the sole contents of a direct inguinal, a sliding inguinal or a femoral hernia;
- ovary with or without the corresponding fallopian tube;
- a Meckel's diverticulum = a Littré's hernia;
- fluid – as part of ascites or as a residuum thereof.

Classification

Irrespective of site, a hernia can be classified into five types.

Classification of hernias

1. Reducible
2. Irreducible
3. Obstructed
4. Strangulated (complication of irreducible hernias)
5. Inflamed

August Gottlieb Richter, 1742–1812. Lecturer on Surgery, Göttingen, Germany.

Gabriele Fallopio (Fallopius), 1523–63. Professor of Anatomy, Surgery and Botany, Padua, Italy.

Johann Friedrich Meckel (The Younger), 1781–1833. Professor of Anatomy and Surgery, Halle, Germany.

Alexis Littré, 1658–1726. Surgeon and anatomist, Paris, France. Littré described 'Meckel's' diverticulum in a hernia sac in 1700, 81 years before Meckel was born.

Reducible hernia

The hernia either reduces itself when the patient lies down, or can be reduced by the patient or the surgeon. The intestine usually gurgles on reduction and the first portion is more difficult to reduce than the last. Omentum, in contrast, is described as doughy and the last portion is more difficult to reduce than the first. A reducible hernia imparts an expansile impulse on coughing.

Irreducible hernia

Here the contents cannot be returned to the abdomen, but there is no evidence of other complications. It is usually due to adhesions between the sac and its contents or from overcrowding within the sac. Irreducibility without other symptoms is almost diagnostic of an omentocele, especially in femoral and umbilical hernias. Note: any degree of irreducibility predisposes to strangulation.

Obstructed hernia

This is an irreducible hernia containing intestine which is obstructed from without or within, but there is no interference to the blood supply to the bowel. The symptoms (colicky abdominal pain and tenderness over the hernia site) are less severe and the onset more gradual than is the case in strangulation, but more often than not the obstruction culminates in strangulation. Usually there is no clear distinction clinically between obstruction and strangulation, and the safe course is to assume that strangulation is imminent and treat accordingly.

Incarcerated hernia. The term 'incarceration' is often used loosely as an alternative to obstruction or strangulation, but is correctly employed only when it is considered that the lumen of that portion of the colon occupying a hernial sac is blocked with faeces. In that event the scybalous contents of the bowel should be capable of being indented with the finger, like putty.

Strangulated hernia

A hernia becomes strangulated when the blood supply of its contents is seriously impaired, rendering the contents ischaemic. Gangrene may occur as early as 5–6 hours after the onset of the first symptoms. Although inguinal hernia may be 10 times more common than femoral hernia, a femoral hernia is more likely to strangulate because of the narrowness of the neck and its rigid surrounds.

Pathology. The intestine is obstructed and its blood supply impaired. Initially, only the venous return is impeded, the wall of the intestine becoming congested and bright red with the transudation of serous fluid into the sac. As congestion increases, the wall of the intestine becomes purple in colour. The intestinal pressure increases distending the intestinal loop and impairing venous return further. As venous stasis increases, the arterial supply becomes more and more impaired. Blood is extravasated under the serosa and is effused into the lumen. The fluid in the sac becomes blood stained and the shining serosa dull due to a fibrinous, sticky exudate. At this stage the walls of the intestine have lost their tone and become friable. Bacterial transudation occurs secondary to the lowered intestine viability and the sac fluid becomes infected.

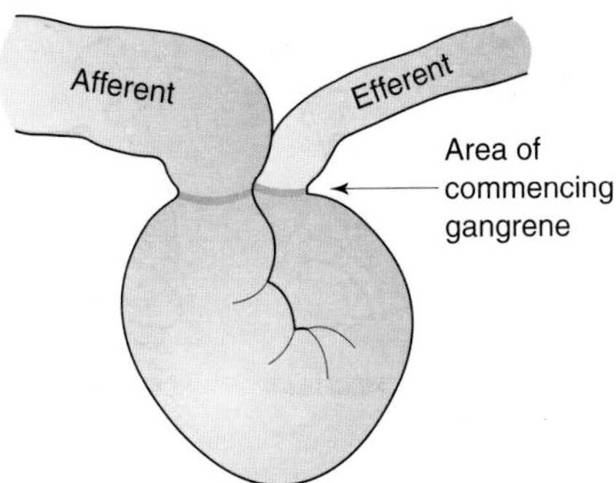

Fig. 62.2 Gangrene commences at the areas of constriction and then at the antimesenteric border.

Gangrene appears at the ring of constriction (Fig. 62.2), which become deeply indented and grey in colour. The gangrene then develops in the antimesenteric border, the colour varying from black to green depending on the decomposition of blood in the subserosa. The mesentery involved by the strangulation also becomes gangrenous. If the strangulation is unrelieved, perforation of the wall of the intestine occurs, either at the convexity of the loop or at the seat of constriction. Peritonitis spreads from the sac to the peritoneal cavity.

Clinical features. Sudden pain at first situated over the hernia is followed by generalised abdominal pain, colicky in character and often located mainly at the umbilicus. Nausea and subsequently vomiting ensue. The patient may complain of an increase in hernia size. On examination, the hernia is tense, extremely tender and irreducible, and there is no expansile cough impulse.

Unless the strangulation is relieved by operation, the spasms of pain continue until peristaltic contractions cease with the onset of ischaemia when paralytic ileus (often the result of peritonitis) and septicaemia develop. Spontaneous cessation of pain must be viewed with caution as this may be a sign of perforation.

Richter's hernia

Richter's hernia is a hernia in which the sac contains only a portion of the circumference of the intestine (usually small intestine). It usually complicates femoral and, rarely, obturator hernias.

Strangulated Richter's hernia

Strangulated Richter's hernia (Fig. 62.3) is particularly noteworthy as operation is frequently delayed because the clinical features mimic gastroenteritis. The local signs of strangulation are often not obvious, the patient may not vomit and, while colicky pain is present, the bowels are often opened normally or there may be diarrhoea; absolute constipation is delayed until paralytic ileus supervenes. For these reasons, gangrene of the knuckle of bowel and perforation have often occurred before operation is undertaken.

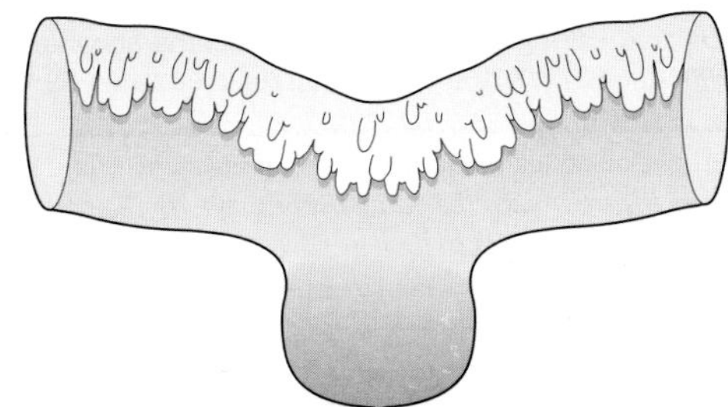

Fig. 62.3 Gangrenous Richter's hernia from a case of strangulated femoral hernia.

Strangulated omentocele. The initial symptoms are in general similar to those of strangulated bowel. Vomiting and constipation may be absent as omentum, unlike intestine, can exist on a very meagre blood supply. The onset of gangrene is therefore delayed, occurring first in the centre of the fatty mass. Unrelieved, a bacterial invasion of the ischaemic contents of the sac will occur and an abscess eventually develops. In an inguinal hernia, infection usually terminates as a scrotal abscess, but extension from the sac to the general peritoneal cavity is always a possibility.

Inflamed hernia. Inflammation can occur from inflammation of the contents of the sac (e.g. acute appendicitis or salpingitis) or from external causes (e.g. the trophic ulcers which develop in the dependent areas of large umbilical or incisional hernias). The hernia is usually tender but not tense, and the overlying skin red and oedematous. Treatment is based on treatment of the underlying cause.

Individual features of hernias

Inguinal hernia

Surgical anatomy

The *superficial inguinal ring* is a triangular aperture in the aponeurosis of the external oblique and lies 1.25 cm above the pubic tubercle. The ring is bounded by a superomedial and an inferolateral crus joined by the criss-cross intercrural fibres. Normally, the ring will not admit the tip of the little finger.

The *deep inguinal ring* is a U-shaped condensation of the transversalis fascia and it lies 1.25 cm above the inguinal (Poupart's) ligament, midway between the symphysis pubis and the anterior superior iliac spine. The transversalis fascia is the fascial envelope of the abdomen and the competency of the deep inguinal ring depends on the integrity of this fascia.

The inguinal canal. In infants the superficial and deep inguinal rings are almost superimposed and the obliquity of the canal is slight. In adults the inguinal canal, which is 3.75 cm long, is directed downwards and medially from the deep to the superficial inguinal ring. In the male the inguinal canal transmits the spermatic cord, the ilio-inguinal nerve and the genital branch of the genitofemoral nerve. In the female the round ligament replaces the spermatic cord.

Boundaries of the canal. Figure 62.4 illustrates the canal, viewing the structures from superficial to deep as is seen at operation. The *anterior* boundary comprises mainly the external oblique aponeurosis with the conjoined muscle laterally. The *posterior* boundary is formed by the fascia transversalis and the conjoined tendon (internal oblique and transversus abdominus medially). The inferior epigastric vessels lie posteriorly and medially to the deep inguinal ring.

François Poupart, 1661–1708. Surgeon, Hôtel Dieu, Paris, France.

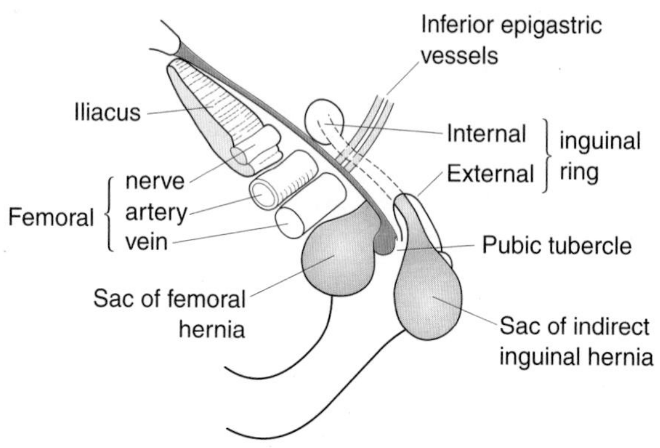

Fig. 62.4 The relationship of an indirect inguinal and a femoral hernia to the pubic tubercle; the inguinal hernia emerges above and medial to the tubercle, the femoral hernia lies below and lateral to it.

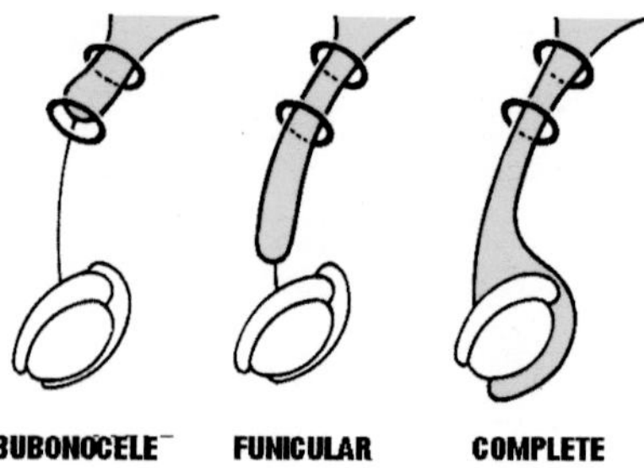

Fig. 62.5 Types of oblique inguinal hernia. *Bubon* (Greek) = groin; *funiculus* (Latin) = a small cord.

The *superior* boundary is formed by the conjoined muscles (internal oblique and transversus) and the *inferior* boundary is the inguinal ligament.

An indirect hernia travels down the canal on the outer (lateral and anterior) side of the spermatic cord. A direct hernia comes out directly forwards through the posterior wall of the inguinal canal. While the neck of the indirect hernia is lateral to the inferior epigastric vessels, the direct hernia usually emerges medial to this except in the saddle-bag or pantaloon type, which has both a lateral and a medial component. An inguinal hernia can be differentiated from a femoral hernia by ascertaining the relation of the neck of the sac to the medial end of the inguinal ligament and the pubic tubercle, i.e. in the case of an inguinal hernia the neck is above and medial, while that of a femoral hernia is below and lateral (Fig. 62.4). Digital control of the internal ring may help in distinguishing between an indirect and a direct inguinal hernia, although some reports have found the preoperative diagnosis to be incorrect as often as correct.

Indirect (syn. oblique) inguinal hernia

This is the most common of all forms of hernia (see 'Aetiology'). It is most common in the young, whereas a direct hernia is most common in the old. In the first decade of life inguinal hernia is more common on the right side in the male. This is no doubt associated with the later descent of the right testis and a higher incidence of failure of closure of the processus vaginalis. In adult males, 65 per cent of inguinal hernias are indirect and 55 per cent are right-sided. The hernia is bilateral in 12 per cent of cases[1].

Three types of indirect inguinal hernia occur (Fig. 62.5).

- **Bubonocele** – when the hernia is limited to the inguinal canal.
- **Funicular** – the processus vaginalis is closed just above the epididymis. The contents of the sac can be felt separately from the testis, which lies below the hernia.
- **Complete** (syn. scrotal) – a complete inguinal hernia is rarely present at birth but is commonly encountered in infancy. It also occurs in adolescence or adult life. The testis appears to lie within the lower part of the hernia.

[1]*If both sides are explored in an infant presenting with one hernia, the incidence of a patent processus vaginalis on the other side is 60 per cent.*

Clinical features[2]

Occurring at any age, males are 20 times more commonly affected than females. The patient complains of pain in the groin or pain referred to the testicle when performing heavy work or taking strenuous exercise. When asked to cough a small transient bulging may be seen and felt together with an expansile impulse. When the sac is still limited to the inguinal canal, the bulge may be better seen by observing the inguinal region from the side or even looking down the abdominal wall while standing behind the respective shoulder of the patient.

As an indirect inguinal hernia increases in size it becomes apparent when the patient coughs and persists until reduced (Fig. 62.6). As time goes on the hernia comes down as soon

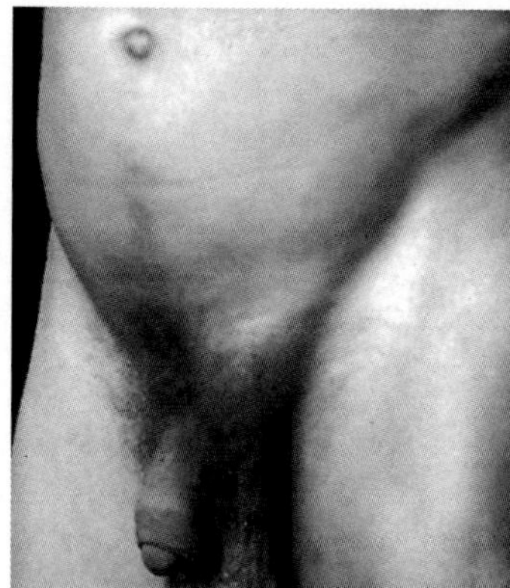

Fig. 62.6 Oblique left inguinal hernia which became apparent when the patient coughed, and persisted until it was reduced when he lay down.

[2]Notes on the clinical examination. *The clinician should examine the patient from the front with the patient standing with their legs apart. The patient should be instructed to look at the ceiling and cough. If the hernia is to come down, it usually does. The examiner should look and feel for the impulse, and then satisfies him/herself on the following points. (1) Is the hernia right, left or bilateral? (2) Is it an inguinal or femoral hernia? (3) Is it a direct or an indirect hernia? (4) Is it reducible or irreducible? (The patient may have to lie down for this to be ascertained.) (5) Is the inguinal hernia incomplete or complete? (6) What are the contents?*

as the patient stands up. In large hernias there is a sensation of weight, and dragging on the mesentery may produce epigastric pain. If the contents of the sac are reducible, the inguinal canal will be found to be commodious.

In infants the swelling appears when the child cries. It can be translucent in infancy and early childhood, but never in an adult. In girls an ovary may prolapse into the sac.

Differential diagnosis in the male.

- A *vaginal hydrocele* (Fig. 62.7);
- an *encysted hydrocele of the cord*;
- *spermatocele*;
- a *femoral hernia*;
- an *incompletely descended testis in the inguinal canal* – an inguinal hernia is often associated with this condition;
- a *lipoma of the cord* – this is often a difficult, but unimportant, diagnosis. It is usually not settled until the parts are displayed by operation.

NB. Examination using finger and thumb across the neck of the scrotum will help to distinguish between a swelling of inguinal origin and one which is entirely intrascrotal.

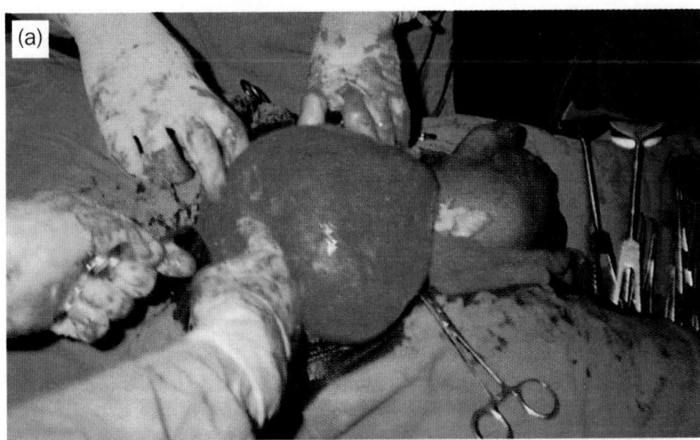

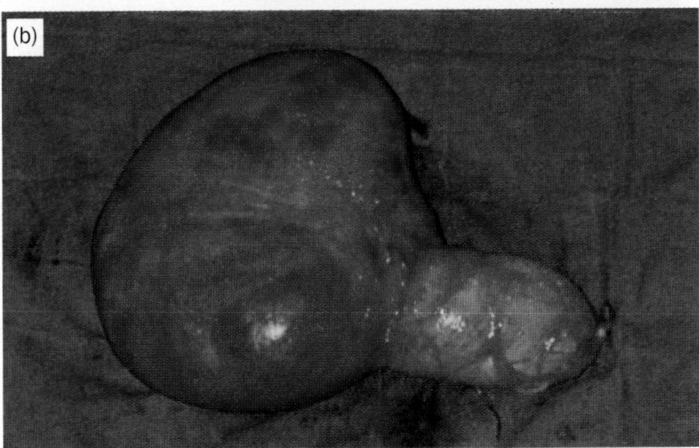

Fig. 62.7 Large transilluminant cystic swelling present in the lower abdomen, extending down the inguinal canal into the scrotum. (a) Lesion being removed; (b) excised specimen. It is not possible to distinguish between a complex scrotal hernia, a hydrocele of the cord and a vaginal hydrocele in such a case before exposing the anatomy; in this case the lesion was an abdominoscrotal hydrocele (hydrocele-en-bisac) (*courtesy of Drs D. Pratep and R. Sahai, Jhansi, India*).

Anton Nuck, 1650–92. Professor of Anatomy and Medicine, Leiden, The Netherlands.

Differential diagnosis in the female.

- A *hydrocele of the canal of Nuck* is the commonest differential diagnostic problem;
- a *femoral hernia*.

Treatment of indirect inguinal hernia

Operative treatment. *Operation is the treatment of choice.* It must be remembered that patients who have a bad cough from chronic bronchitis should not be denied an operation, for these are the very people who are in danger of getting a strangulated hernia. In adults, local, epidural or spinal, as well as general, anaesthesia can be used.

Inguinal herniotomy. This is the basic operation which entails dissecting out and opening the hernial sac, reducing any contents, and then transfixing the neck of the sac and removing the remainder. It is employed either by itself or as the first step in a repair procedure (herniorrhaphy). By itself it is sufficient for the treatment of hernia in infants, adolescents and young adults. Any attempts at repair in such cases may, in fact, do more harm than good.

In infants it is not necessary to open the canal, as the internal and external rings are superimposed. Excellent results are obtained. The operation is usually now performed as a day case unless there are additional medical or social problems.

Herniotomy and repair (herniorrhaphy). This operation consists of: (l) excision of the hernial sac; plus (2) repair of the stretched internal inguinal ring and the transversalis fascia; and (3) further reinforcement of the posterior wall of the inguinal canal. (2) and (3) must be achieved without tension resulting in the wound and various techniques exist to achieve this, e.g. Shouldice operation, fascial flaps or polypropylene mesh implants.

Operative procedures

1. **Excision of the hernal sac (adult herniotomy).** An incision[3] is made in the skin and subcutaneous tissue 1.25 cm above and parallel to the medial two-thirds of the inguinal ligament. In large irreducible hernias the incision may be extended laterally or into the upper part of the scrotum. After dividing the superficial fascia and securing haemostasis, the external oblique aponeurosis and the superficial inguinal ring are identified. The external oblique aponeurosis is incised in the line of its fibres and the structures beneath are carefully separated from its deep surface before completing the incision through the superficial inguinal ring. In this way, the ilio-inguinal nerve is safeguarded. With the inguinal canal thus opened, the upper leaf of the external oblique is separated from the internal oblique by blunt dissection. In the same way, the lower leaf is separated from the contents of the inguinal canal until the inner aspect of the inguinal ligament is seen. The cremasteric muscle fibres may be divided longitudinally to display the spermatic cord, but this is by no means essential.

Edward Earle Shouldice, 1890–1965. Founder of the Shouldice Clinic specialising in hernia repair, Toronto, Canada.

[3]*Prior to the skin incision in large inguinoscrotal hernias, the usual antiseptic preparation of the skin should not be extended to the perineal aspect of the scrotum for, by so doing, severe bacterial contamination of the operation site is likely.*

Excision of the sac. The indirect sac may be distinguished as a pearly white structure lying on the outer side of the cord and, when the internal spermatic fascia has been incised longitudinally, it can usually be dissected out and then opened between haemostats.

Variations in dissection. If the sac is small, it can be freed *in toto*. If it is of the long funicular or scrotal type, or is extremely thickened and adherent, the fundus must not be sought, for in so doing the blood supply to the testis may be compromised. The sac is freed within the inguinal canal and divided circumferentially such that the fundus remains in the scrotum. Care must be taken to avoid damage to the vas and spermatic artery when freeing the sac posteriorly.

An adherent sac can be separated from the cord by first injecting saline under the posterior wall from within (hydrodissection). A similar tactic is employed when dissecting the gossamer sac of infants and children.

Reduction of contents. Intestine or omentum is returned to the peritoneal cavity. Omentum is often adherent to the neck or fundus of the sac: if to the neck, it is freed, and if to the fundus of a large sac, it may be transfixed, ligated and cut across at a suitable point. The distal part of the omentum, like the distal part of a large scrotal sac, can be left *in situ* (the fundus should, however, not be ligated).

Isolation and ligation of the neck of the sac. Whatever type of sac is encountered, it is necessary to free its neck by blunt dissection until the parietal peritoneum can be seen on all sides. The dissection is only considered complete when the extraperitoneal fat has been encountered and the inferior epigastric vessels are seen on the medial side. It used to be considered essential to open the sac to ensure that no bowel or omentum was adherent to the neck. If the sac is obviously empty, it is sufficient simply to reduce it, close the internal ring and perform a herniorrhaphy if required. If the sac is opened, all contents should be reduced and the neck transfixed as high as possible before excising the sac.

2. **Repair of the transversalis fascia and the internal ring.** When the internal ring is weak and stretched, and the transversalis is bulging, the repair should include a technique of narrowing the deep ring, for example the Lytle method of narrowing the ring with lateral displacement of the cord (Fig. 62.8) or the Shouldice method, whereby the ring and fascia are incised and carefully separated from the deep inferior epigastric vessels and extraperitoneal fat before an overlapping repair ('double breasting') of the lower flap behind the upper flap is performed. In the classic Shouldice operation, a third and fourth layer of tension-free suturing, using monofilament materials, polypropylene, polyamide or wire, is placed between the internal oblique aponeurosis arch and the inguinal ligament (Fig. 62.9).

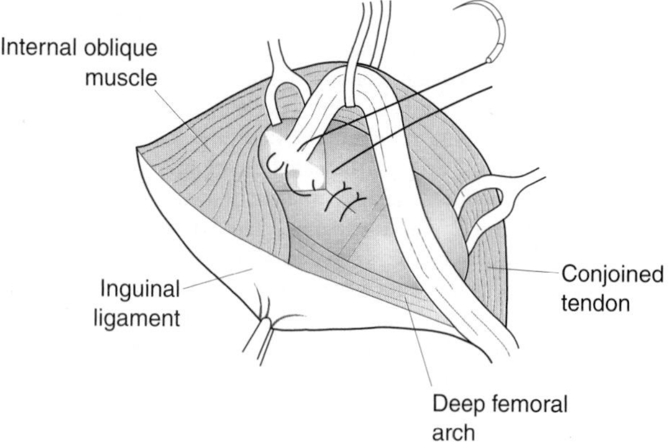

Fig. 62.8 The Lytle method of repair of the stretched internal inguinal ring which should be narrowed to admit the tip of the little finger. Lateral displacement of the cord is often advantageous (*after F.S.A. Doran, FRCS, Bromsgrove, England*).

William James Lytle, 1896–1986. Surgeon, Royal Infirmary, Sheffield, England.

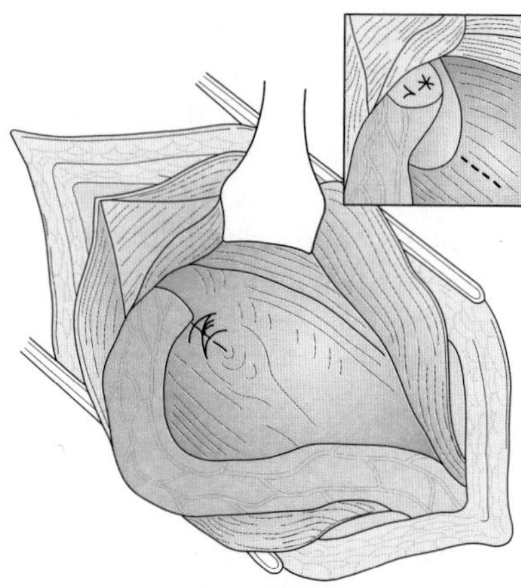

Fig. 62.9 After the neck of the sac has been divided at the deep inguinal ring the fascia transversalis of the deep opening is identified and assessed. If the ring is normal sized the stump of the sac is reduced and no more need be done. If the ring is marginally dilated (stretched) it should be carefully dissected and possibly divided slightly (inset), and then sutured tightly around the medial side of the cord with polypropylene to reconstitute a competent deep inguinal ring.

3. **Reinforcement of the posterior inguinal wall.** This is achieved by suturing without tension between the tendinous aponeurotic arch of internal oblique to the under surface of the inguinal ligament and to the pubic tubercle (as described above in the Shouldice operation) or by reinforcing the posterior wall of the canal with a prosthetic mesh. Care is taken when suturing not to pick up the same tendinous bundle for each suture. Suturing of muscle bundles is of no value. The suturing method can include a rectus-relaxing incision (Halsted–Tanner). The Lichtenstein tension-free hernioplasty involves placement of an approximately 16 × 8 cm (tailored to the individual patient's requirements) mesh as an extra lamina, anterior to the posterior wall and overlapping it generously in all directions, including medially over the pubic tubercle. Other historical techniques, which should now be abandoned because of poor results, include overlapping the external oblique behind the cord (making it lie subcutaneously). Special care was needed to avoid excessive narrowing of the new external ring which could jeopardise the vascular supply to and the venous return from the testis.
4. **Completion of operation.** If desired, the cremasteric muscle can be reconstituted: the external oblique is directly sutured or overlapped leaving a new external ring which should accommodate the tip of a finger (Fig. 62.10).

A truss. A truss may be used when operation is contraindicated or when operation is refused. Its use should be mainly historical as there are very few contraindications to surgery with today's variety of anaesthetic techniques. If a truss is to be worn, the hernia must be reducible. A rat-tailed spring truss with a perineal band to prevent the truss slipping will, with due care and attention, control a small or moderate size inguinal hernia. A truss must be worn continuously during waking hours, kept

William Stuart Halsted, 1852–1922. Surgeon, Johns Hopkins Hospital, Baltimore, Maryland, USA.

Norman Cecil Tanner, 1906–82. Surgeon, Charing Cross Hospital, London, England.

Irving Lichtenstein. Pioneered the use of mesh for inguinal hernioplasty.

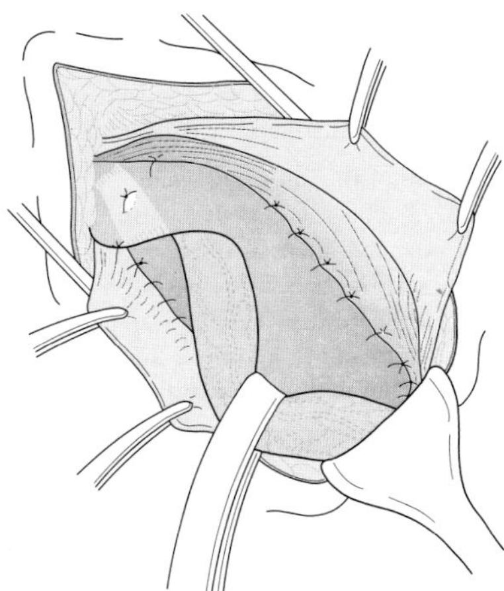

Fig. 62.10 'Tails' are overlapped and crossed, and a single suture is placed to create a new 'internal' ring.

clean and in proper repair, and renewed when it shows signs of wear. It must be applied before the patient gets up and while the hernia is reduced. A properly fitting truss must control the hernia when the patient stands, with his legs apart, stoops and coughs violently. If it does not it is a menace, for it increases the risk of strangulation.

There is no place for trusses in the management of infant hernias. If an infant hernia becomes suddenly irreducible, urgent operative repair is indicated. Otherwise, the infant hernia can be left alone until the child is over 3 months old when routine day-case repair can be performed.

Direct inguinal hernia

In adult males, 35 per cent of inguinal hernias are direct. At presentation, 12 per cent of patients will have a contralateral hernia in addition and there is a four-fold increased risk of future development of contralateral hernia if one is not present at the original presentation.

A direct inguinal hernia is always acquired. The sac passes through a weakness or defect of the transversalis fascia in the posterior wall of the inguinal canal. In some cases the defect is small and is represented by a discrete defect in the transversalis fascia, while in others there is a generalised bulge. Often the patient has poor lower abdominal musculature, as shown by the presence of elongated bulgings (Malgaigne's bulges). Women practically never develop a direct inguinal hernia (Brown). Predisposing factors are smoking, and occupations that involve straining and heavy lifting. Damage to the ilio-inguinal nerve (previous appendicectomy) is another cause, due to resulting weakness of the conjoined tendon.

Direct hernias do not often attain a large size or descend into the scrotum (Fig. 62.11). In contrast to an indirect inguinal hernia, a direct inguinal hernia lies behind the spermatic cord. The sac is often smaller than the hernial mass would indicate, the protruding mass mainly consisting of extraperitoneal fat. As the neck of the sac is wide, direct inguinal hernias do not often strangulate.

Joseph François Malgaigne, 1806–65. Professor of Surgery, Paris, France.
Francis Brown, 1889–1967. Surgeon, Royal Infirmary, Dundee, Scotland.

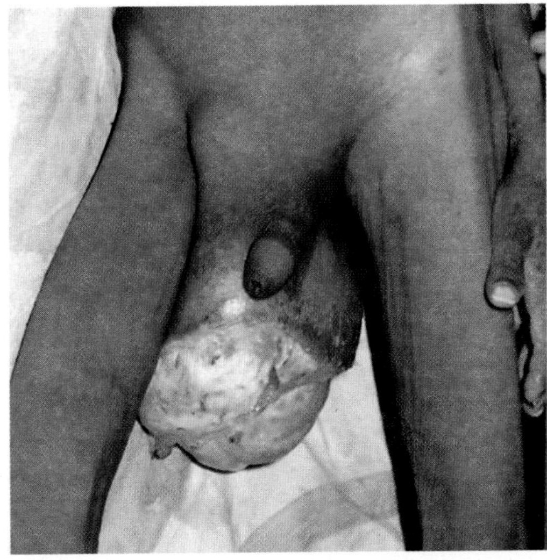

Fig. 62.11 A huge inguinal hernia (direct) which has descended into the scrotum, and the overlying skin has become gangrenous and sloughed away (*courtesy of Dr Anupam Rai, Jabalpur, India*).

Funicular direct inguinal hernia (syn. prevesical hernia). This is a narrow-necked hernia with prevesical fat and a portion of the bladder that protrudes through a small oval defect in the medial part of the conjoined *muscle* just above the pubic tubercle. It occurs principally in elderly males and occasionally becomes strangulated. Unless there are definite contraindications, operation should always be advised.

Dual (syn. saddle-bag; pantaloon) hernia. This type of hernia consists of two sacs which straddle the inferior epigastric artery, one sac being medial and the other lateral to this vessel. The condition is not rare and is a cause of recurrence, one of the sacs having been overlooked at the time of operation.

Operation for direct hernia. The principles of repair of direct hernias are the same as those of an indirect hernia with the exception that the hernia sac can usually be simply inverted after the sac has been dissected free and the transversalis fascia reconstructed in front of it. This reconstruction of the posterior wall of the inguinal canal should be undertaken by the Shouldice repair or mesh implant using the Lichtenstein technique (Figs 62.9 and 62.10). The darn operation is no longer acceptable because of its high recurrence rate and slow rehabilitation.

Strangulated inguinal hernia

Pathological and clinical features are described earlier in this chapter. Strangulation of an inguinal hernia occurs at any time during life and in both sexes. Indirect inguinal hernias strangulate more commonly, the direct variety not so often owing to the wide neck of the sac. Sometimes a hernia strangulates on the first occasion that it descends; more often strangulation occurs in patients who have worn a truss for a long time, and in those with a partially reducible or irreducible hernia.

In order of frequency, the constricting agent is: (a) the neck of the sac; (b) the external inguinal ring in children; and (c), rarely, adhesions within the sac.

Contents

Usually, the small intestine is involved in the strangulation; the next most frequent is the omentum; sometimes both are involved. It is rare for the large intestine to become strangulated in an inguinal hernia, even when the hernia is of the sliding variety.

Strangulation during infancy

The incidence of strangulation is 4 per cent (Gross) and the ratio of females to males is 5:1. More frequently the hernia is irreducible but not strangulated. In most cases of strangulated inguinal hernia occurring in female infants the content of the sac is an ovary or an ovary plus its fallopian tube.

Treatment of strangulated inguinal hernia

The treatment of strangulated hernia is by emergency operation ('The danger is in the delay not in the operation', Sir Astley Paston Cooper). Vigorous resuscitation with intravenous fluids, nasogastric aspiration and antibiotics is essential, although operation should not be unduly delayed in moribund patients. It is also advisable to empty the bladder, if necessary by catheterisation.

Inguinal herniotomy for strangulation. An incision is made over the most prominent part of the swelling. The external oblique aponeurosis is exposed and the sac, with its coverings, is seen issuing from the superficial ring. In all but very large hernias, it is possible to deliver the body and fundus of the sac together with its coverings and (in the male) the testis on to the surface. Each layer covering the anterior surface of the body of the sac near the fundus is incised and, if possible, stripped off the sac. The sac is then incised and any fluid, which may be highly infective, drained effectively. The external oblique aponeurosis and the superficial inguinal ring are divided. A finger is then passed into the opening in the sac and, employing the finger as a guide, the sac is slit along its length. If the constriction lies at the superficial inguinal ring, or within the canal, it is readily divided by this procedure. When the constriction is at the deep ring, by applying haemostats to the cut edge of the neck of the sac and drawing them downwards, and at the same time retracting the internal oblique upwards, it may be possible to continue slitting the sac over the finger towards the point of constriction. When the constriction is too tight to admit a finger, a grooved dissector is inserted and the neck of the sac is divided with a knife in an upward and inward direction, i.e. parallel to the inferior epigastric vessels, under vision. Once the constriction has been divided, the strangulated contents can be drawn down. Devitalised omentum is excised after being securely ligated. Viable intestine is returned to the peritoneal cavity. Doubtfully viable and gangrenous intestine is excised by localised resection. If the hernial sac is of moderate size and can be separated easily from its coverings, it is excised and closed by a purse-string suture. When the sac is large and adherent, much time is saved by cutting across the sac as described earlier. Having tied or sutured the neck of the sac, a repair can be made if the condition of the patient permits. In those circumstances where the incision has been soiled or gangrenous bowel resected, prosthetic mesh is best avoided, although some authorities have successfully utilised polypropylene mesh with antibiotic cover.

Conservative measures. These are only indicated in infants. The child is given analgesias and placed in gallow's traction (the judgement of Solomon position). In 75 per cent of cases reduction is effected and there appears to be no danger of gangrenous intestine being reduced (Irvine Smith).

NB. *Vigorous manipulation* (taxis) has no place in modern surgery and is mentioned only to be condemned. Its dangers include:

- contusion or rupture of the intestinal wall;
- *reduction-en-masse*: 'The sac together with its contents is pushed forcibly back into the abdomen; as the bowel will still be strangulated by the neck of the sac, the symptoms are in no way relieved' (Treves);
- reduction into a loculus of the sac;
- the sac may rupture at its neck and the contents are reduced, not into the peritoneal cavity but extraperitoneally.

Maydl's hernia (syn. hernia-in-W). Maydl's hernia is rare. The strangulated loop of the W lies within the abdomen, thus local tenderness over the hernia is not marked. At operation two comparatively normal-looking loops of intestine are present in the sac. After the obstruction has been relieved, the strangulated loop will become apparent if traction is exerted on the middle of the loops occupying the sac.

Results of operations for inguinal hernia – recurrence. Reported recurrence rates vary between 0.2 and 15 per cent depending on the technique employed. Only by using a meticulous technique, principally concentrating on reinforcement of the posterior wall of the inguinal canal, with the Shouldice technique or mesh hernioplasty, can a recurrence rate of less than 2 per cent be achieved. Only 50 per cent of recurrences will become apparent within 2 years. In a few cases 'false' recurrences occur, i.e. another type of hernia occurs – direct after indirect, femoral after inguinal. To the patient it is a recurrence!

The spermatic cord as a barrier to effective closure of the inguinal canal. Even in the elderly patient, removal of the testis and cord is very rarely required for effective repair even in cases of recurrent inguinal hernia. In operations for multiple recurrences or when previous surgery has been associated with infections or excessive scarring, the operation should be approached through virgin territory, i.e. the preperitoneal route, by an experienced surgeon.

Sliding hernia (syn. *hernia-en-glissade*) (Fig. 62.12)

As a result of slipping of the posterior parietal peritoneum on the underlying retroperitoneal structures, the posterior wall of the sac is not formed of peritoneum alone, but by the sigmoid colon and its mesentery on the left, the caecum on the right and, sometimes, on either side by a portion of the bladder. It should be clearly understood that the caecum, appendix or a portion of the colon *wholly* within a hernial sac does not constitute a sliding hernia. A small bowel sliding hernia occurs approximately once in 2000 cases; a sacless hernia once in 8000 cases.

Clinical features

A sliding hernia occurs almost exclusively in males. Five out of six sliding hernias are situated on the left side; bilateral sliding hernias are rare. The patient is nearly always over 40 years of age, the incidence rising with age. There are no

Robert Edward Gross. Ladd Professor of Children's Surgery, Harvard University Medical School, Boston, Massachusetts, USA.

Solomon, King of Israel. The story of the judgement of Solomon is told in the Bible, I Kings III, 16–28.

Irvine Battinson Smith. Surgeon, Burton-on-Trent General Hospital, Staffordshire, England.

Sir Frederick Treves, 1853–1923. Surgeon, The London Hospital, London, England.

Karel Maydl, 1853–1903. Professor of Surgery, Prague, now the Czech Republic.

(a)

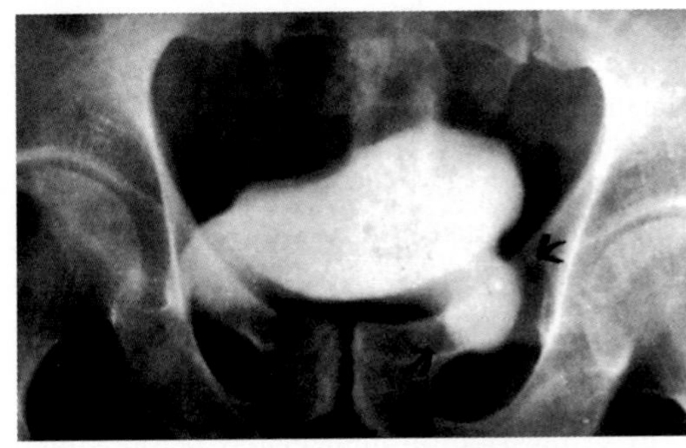

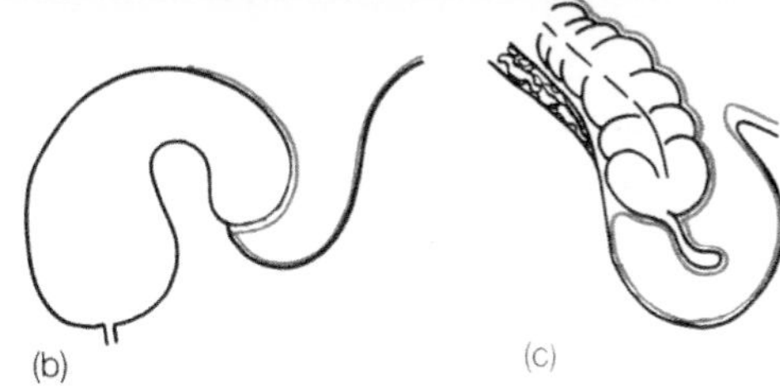
(b) (c)

Fig. 62.12 Sliding hernia. (a) Cystogram showing a bladder involving a left inguinal hernia. (b) Diagram of the same. (c) Caecum and appendix in a right sliding hernia.

clinical findings that are pathognomonic of a sliding hernia, but it should be suspected in a very large globular inguinal hernia descending well into the scrotum. Occasionally large intestine is strangulated in a sliding hernia; more often nonstrangulated large intestine is present behind the sac containing strangulated small intestine.

Treatment

A sliding hernia is impossible to control with a truss, and as a rule the hernia is a cause of considerable discomfort. Consequently, operation is indicated and the results are very good.

Operation. It is unnecessary to remove any of the sliding hernial sac provided that it is freed completely from the cord and the abdominal wall, and that it is replaced deep to the repaired fascia transversalis. In many circumstances it is desirable to perform orchidectomy in order to effect a secure repair. No attempt should be made to dissect the caecum or colon free from the peritoneum under the impression that these are adhesions, in which case peritonitis or a faecal fistula resulting from necrosis of a devascularised portion of the bowel may occur. This is especially liable to occur on the left side, as vessels in the mesocolon may be injured.

Femoral hernia

Femoral hernia is the third most common type of primary hernia. It accounts for about 20 per cent of hernias in women and 5 per cent in men. The overriding importance of femoral hernia lies in the facts that it cannot be controlled by a truss and that of all hernias it is the most liable to become strangulated, mainly because of the narrowness of the neck of the sac and the rigidity of the femoral ring. Strangulation is the initial presentation of 40 per cent of femoral hernias.

Surgical anatomy. The femoral canal occupies the most medial compartment of the femoral sheath and it extends from the femoral ring above to the saphenous opening below. It is 1.25 cm long and 1.25 cm wide at its base, which is directed upwards. The femoral canal contains fat, lymphatic vessels and the lymph node of Cloquet. It is closed above by the septum crurale, a condensation of extraperitoneal tissue pierced by lymphatic vessels, and below by the cribriform fascia.

The femoral ring is bounded:

- *anteriorly* by the inguinal ligament;
- *posteriorly* by Astley Cooper's (ileopectineal) ligament, the pubic bone and the fascia over the pectineus muscle;
- *medially* by the concave knife-like edge of Gimbernat's (lacunar) ligament, which is also prolonged along the iliopectineal line as for Astley Cooper's ligament;
- *laterally* by a thin septum separating it from the femoral vein.

Sex incidence. The female to male ratio is about 2:1, but it is interesting that whereas the female patients are frequently elderly, the male patients are usually between 30 and 40 years of age. The condition is more prevalent in women who have borne children than in nulliparae.

Pathology. A hernia passing down the femoral canal descends vertically as far as the saphenous opening. While it is confined to the inelastic walls of the femoral canal the hernia is necessarily narrow but, once it escapes through the saphenous opening into the loose areolar tissue of the groin, it expands, sometimes considerably. A fully distended femoral hernia assumes the shape of a retort and its bulbous extremity may be above the inguinal ligament. By the time the contents have pursued so tortuous a path they are usually irreducible and apt to strangulate.

Clinical features. Femoral hernia is rare before puberty. Between 20 and 40 years of age the prevalence rises and continues to old age. The right side (Fig. 62.13) is affected twice as often as the left, and in 20 per cent of cases the condition is bilateral. The symptoms to which a femoral hernia gives rise are less pronounced than those of an inguinal hernia; indeed, a small femoral hernia may be unnoticed by the patient or disregarded for years, perhaps until the day it strangulates. Adherence of the greater omentum sometimes causes a dragging pain. Rarely, a large sac is present.

Differential diagnosis. A femoral hernia has to be distinguished from the following.

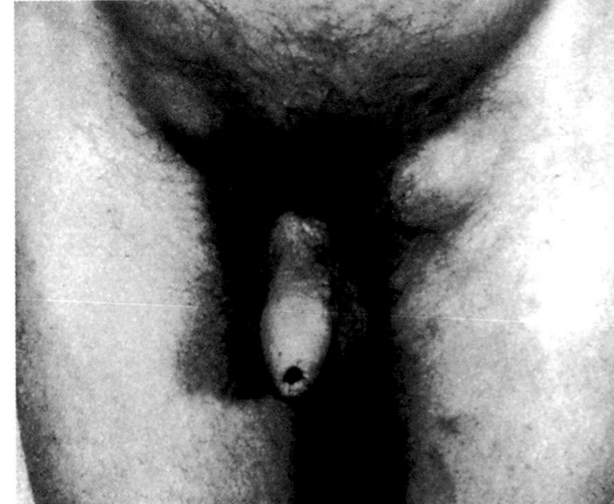

Fig. 62.13 The patient has a left inguinal and a right femoral hernia (as in Fig. 62.14).

Jules Germain Cloquet, 1790–1883. Professor of Anatomy and Surgery, Paris, France.

Don Antonio de Gimbernat, 1734–1816. Professor of Anatomy, Barcelona, Spain, and later Director of the Royal College of Surgeons in Spain.

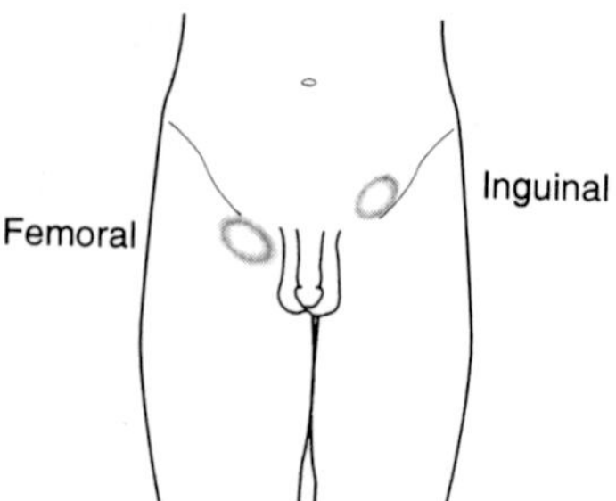

Fig. 62.14 The essentials of differential diagnosis between a femoral and an inguinal hernia (as in Fig. 62.13).

An inguinal hernia. The neck of the sac lies above and medial to the medial end of the inguinal ligament at its attachment to the pubic tubercle. The neck of the sac of a femoral hernia lies below this (Fig. 62.14). The fundus of an inguinal or a femoral hernia may follow the line of least resistance and occupy a variety of places, for instance, occasionally the fundus of a femoral hernia sac overlies the inguinal ligament.

A saphena varix. A saccular enlargement of the termination of the long saphenous vein, usually accompanied by other signs of varicose veins. The swelling disappears completely when the patient lies flat, while a femoral hernia sac is usually still palpable. In both, there is an impulse on coughing. A saphena varix will, however, impart a fluid thrill to the examining fingers when the patient coughs or when the saphenous vein below the varix is tapped with the fingers of the other hand. Sometimes a venous hum can be heard when a stethoscope is applied over a saphena varix.

An enlarged femoral lymph node. There may be other enlarged lymph nodes to aid the diagnosis. If Cloquet's lymph node alone is affected, it may be impossible to distinguish from a femoral hernia sac unless there are other clues, such as an infected wound or abrasion on the corresponding limb or on the perineum.

Lipoma.

A femoral aneurysm. See Chapter 15.

A psoas abscess. There is often a fluctuating swelling – an iliac abscess – which communicates with the swelling in question. If suspected, an examination of the spine and an X-ray will confirm the diagnosis.

A distended psoas bursa. The swelling diminishes when the hip is flexed and osteoarthritis of the hip is present.

Rupture of the adductor longus. Rupture of the adductor longus with haematoma formation – suspected on clinical history.

Hydrocele of a femoral hernial sac. The neck of the sac becomes plugged with omentum or by adhesions, and a hydrocele of the sac results.

Laugier's femoral hernia. This is a hernia through a gap in the lacunar (Gimbernat's) ligament. The diagnosis is based on unusual medial position of a small femoral hernia sac. The hernia has nearly always strangulated.

Narath's femoral hernia. This occurs only in patients with congenital dislocation of the hip and is due to lateral displacement of the psoas muscle. The hernia lies hidden behind the femoral vessels.

Cloquet's hernia. Cloquet's hernia is one in which the sac lies under the fascia covering the pectineus muscle. Strangulation is likely. The sac may coexist with the usual type of femoral hernia sac.

Strangulated femoral hernia

A femoral hernia strangulates frequently and gangrene rapidly develops. This is explained by the narrow, unyielding femoral ring. In 40 per cent of cases the obstructing agent is not the lacunar ligament but the neck of the femoral sac itself. A Richter's hernia is a frequent occurrence (see above).

Treatment of a femoral hernia. The constant risk of strangulation is sufficient reason to recommend operation, which should be carried out soon after the diagnosis has been made. A truss is contraindicated because of this risk.

Operative treatment. Several approaches to the femoral hernia have been advocated including the low operation (Lockwood), the high operation (McEvedy) and the inguinal operation (Lotheissen). In all cases the bladder must be emptied by catheterisation immediately before commencing surgery.

The low operation (Lockwood). The sac is dissected out below the inguinal ligament via a groin-crease incision. It is essential to peel off the anatomical layers which cover the sac. These are often thick and fatty. After dealing with the contents (e.g. freeing adherent omentum) the neck of the sac is pulled down, ligated as high as possible and allowed to retract through the femoral canal. The canal may be closed by suturing the inguinal ligament to the iliopectineal line using three nonabsorbable sutures. An alternative method of closure is to roll a sheet of polypropylene mesh into a cylinder and anchor the cylinder in the canal with nonabsorbable sutures placed medially, superiorly and inferiorly.

The high (McEvedy) operation. Classically, a vertical incision is made over the femoral canal and continued upwards above the inguinal ligament. An acceptable alternative that heals well and with less pain is to use a 'unilateral' Pfannenstiel incision, which can be extended to form a complete Pfannenstiel incision if formal laparotomy is required. This incision provides good access to the preperitoneal space. Through the lower part of the incision the sac is dissected out. The upper part of the incision exposes the inguinal ligament and the rectus sheath. The superficial inguinal ring is identified and an incision 2.5 cm above the ring and parallel to the outer border of the rectus muscle is deepened until the extraperitoneal space is identified. By gauze dissection in this space the hernial sac entering the femoral canal can be easily identified. Should the sac be empty and small, it may be drawn upwards; if it is large, the fundus is opened below and its contents, if any, dealt with appropriately before delivering the sac upwards from its canal. The sac is then freed from the extraperitoneal tissue and its neck ligated. An excellent view of the iliopectineal ligament is obtained and the conjoined tendon is sutured to it with nonabsorbable sutures. An alternative repair, particularly suitable for recurrent femoral hernias, is to suture a sheet of polypropylene mesh over the femoral canal orifice, anchoring the mesh inferiorly to the iliopectineal ligament and medially to the rectus sheath.

An advantage of this approach is that if resection of intestine is required, ample room can be obtained by opening the peritoneum. The disadvantage of this approach is that if infection occurs, an incisional hernia may develop.

Lotheissen's operation. The inguinal canal is opened as for inguinal herniorrhaphy. The transversalis fascia is incised to the medial side of the epigastric vessels and the opening is enlarged. The peritoneum is now in view; one must be certain that it is the peritoneum and not the bladder or a diverticulum thereof. The peritoneum is picked up with dissecting

Stanislas Laugier, 1799–1872. Surgeon, Hôtel Dieu, Paris, France.
Albert Narath, 1864–1924. Professor of Surgery, Heidelberg, Germany.

Charles Barret Lockwood, 1856–1914. Surgeon, St Bartholomew's Hospital, London, England.
Peter George McEvedy, 1890–1941. Surgeon, Ancoats Hospital, Manchester, England.
Hermann John Pfannenstiel, 1862–1909. Gynaecologist, Breslau, Germany.
Georg Lotheissen, 1868–1941. Surgeon, Kaiser Franz Joseph Hospital, Vienna, Austria.

forceps and incised. It is now possible to ascertain whether any intraperitoneal structure is entering the femoral sac. Should the sac be empty, haemostats are placed upon the edges of the opening into the peritoneum and, by gauze dissection, the sac is withdrawn from the femoral canal. An empty sac can be delivered easily. If strangulation is suspected, as soon as the external oblique has been exposed, the inferior margin of the wound is retracted, thereby displaying the swelling. The coverings of the sac are incised and peeled off, until the sac, dark from contained blood-stained fluid, is apparent. The sac is incised and the fluid that escapes is mopped up with care. The retractor is removed and the operation is continued above the inguinal ligament as described above. Once the peritoneum has been opened above the inguinal ligament, one can see exactly what is entering the sac. Should the obstruction lie in a narrow neck of the sac, the neck of the sac may be gently stretched by insertion of a haemostat. (An abnormal obturator artery is present either on the medial or the lateral side of the neck of the sac in 28 per cent of cases.) The contents of the sac are delivered and dealt with appropriately. Sometimes, in order to facilitate reduction of the hernial contents, it becomes necessary to divide or digitally dilate part of the lacunar (Gimbernat's) ligament.

The Lotheissen repair is effected by suturing the conjoined tendon to the iliopectineal line to form a shutter. While protecting the external iliac/femoral vein with the forefinger, nonabsorbable sutures are passed through the periosteum and Cooper's ligament overlying the iliopectineal line. The retractor is removed and the long ends of the sutures are passed from within, outwards, through the conjoined tendon and tied, thus approximating the conjoined tendon to the iliopectineal line. If there is any tension, a Tanner's slide will facilitate this step. The incised external oblique is sutured.

An alternative repair is to buttress the femoral canal with a sheet of polypropylene mesh. Once the sac has been dealt with, a sheet of mesh is inserted into the preperitoneal space and anchored inferiorly to the iliopectineal line, inferomedially to Cooper's ligament and superomedially to the rectus sheath. The transversalis fascia may then be approximated in front of the mesh and the incised external oblique repaired. It should be noted that the peritoneum must be closed before placement of the mesh.

NB. Throughout operations for the repair of a femoral hernia, on the lateral side, the external iliac/femoral vein must be protected, and on the medial side, great care must be taken not to injure the bladder, particularly as a portion of the bladder may form part of the wall of the sac (a sliding femoral hernia).

Umbilical hernia

Exomphalos (syn. omphalocele) occurs once in every 6000 births; it is due to failure of all or part of the midgut to return to the coelom during early foetal life. There is some debate as to whether gastroschisis represents a separate entity or is simply an exomphalos with ruptured membranes, but the debate has little practical importance because the principles of treatment are similar. When the sac remains unruptured, it is semitranslucent (Fig. 62.15) and, although very thin, it consists of two layers – an outer layer of amniotic membrane and an inner layer of peritoneum. Omphaloceles may be divided into those with a fascial defect of less than or greater than 4 cm. The former are termed herniation of the umbilical cord. In smaller defects, a single loop of intestine may not be obvious and ligation of what was thought to be a normal umbilical cord will result in transection of the intestine, leaving the embarrassing problem of an umbilicoenteric fistula.

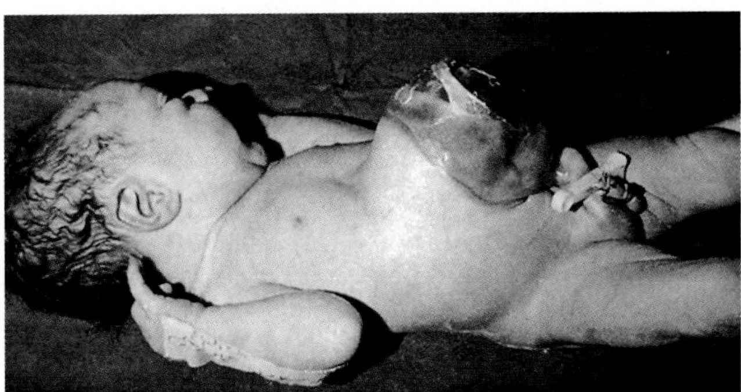

Fig. 62.15 Exomphalos. The delicate sac ruptured soon afterwards.

In large defects the liver, spleen, stomach, pancreas, colon or bladder may be seen through the membrane. The intestine lies freely mobile within the intact sac without evidence of adhesions or inflammation. In contrast, the liver has dense adhesions to the sac, a fact which must be remembered during surgical repair.

Treatment

Small defects may be closed primarily soon after birth as there is usually no difficulty with disproportion between the size of the abdominal cavity and the volume of the sac contents.

Large defects present a more substantial problem and four techniques have been described: nonoperative therapy, skin flap closure, staged closure, and primary closure.

Nonoperative therapy. This is appropriate for premature infants with a gigantic intact sac or those in whom associated anomalies make survival of a major operation unlikely. The intact sac is painted daily with a desiccating antiseptic solution and, if successful, an eschar forms over the sac. Eventually granulisation grows in from the periphery and the subsequent ventral hernia can be repaired later.

Skin flap closure. The sac is gently trimmed away enabling inspection of the abdominal contents. The skin is freed from the fascial edges and undermined laterally. The umbilical vessels are ligated or one artery is cannulated for monitoring. The skin flaps are approximated in the midline with simple sutures and the ventral hernia is then closed at a later date (months to years later).

Staged closure. The sac is gently trimmed away from the skin edge and the skin further freed from the fascial attachments. The prosthetic material [polypropylene mesh or expanded polytetrafluoroethylene (PTFE)] is sutured with interrupted nonabsorbable sutures circumferentially to the full thickness of the musculofascial abdominal wall to form a silo. The top of the silo is gathered and tied with umbilical tape. At daily intervals, the silo is opened under strict aseptic conditions and the contents are examined for infection or dehiscence. The viscera are pushed gently back in to the abdominal cavity and the infant is observed for signs of raised intra-abdominal pressure. The silo is then tied at a reduced level and the cycle repeated until the sac is flush with the abdominal wall. At this stage, the fascia may be closed with interrupted sutures and skin closed over the top.

Primary closure. The sac is gently dissected away from the skin edge and the underlying fascia. The intestine is then evacuated completely of meconium and fluid distally and proximally through a nasogastric tube. The abdominal wall is stretched gradually and repeatedly in quadrants, usually achieving a doubling of volume. The viscera are then replaced and the fascial layer is closed primarily, usually under moderate tension. Intragastric pressure monitoring is helpful to prevent undue vena caval compression.

Congenital umbilical hernia. Rarely, a fully developed umbilical hernia is present at birth, presumably due to intra-uterine epithelialisation of a small exomphalos.

Umbilical hernia of infants and children

This is a hernia through a weak umbilicus which may partially result from failure of the round ligament (obliterated umbilical vein) to cross the umbilical ring and partially from absence of the Richet fascia. Both sexes seem to be equally affected, although there are significant racial differences, with the incidence in black infants reported as up to eight times higher than in white infants. The hernia is often symptomless but increases in size on crying and assumes a classical conical shape (Fig. 62.16). Obstruction or strangulation below the age of 3 years is extremely uncommon.

Treatment. Conservative treatment is indicated under the age of 2 years. When the hernia is symptomless, reassurance of the parents is all that is necessary and 95 per cent of hernias will disappear spontaneously. If the hernia persists at 2 years of age or older, it is unlikely to resolve and herniorrhaphy is indicated.

Operation. A small curved incision is made immediately below the umbilicus. The skin cicatrix is dissected upwards and the neck of the sac isolated. After ensuring that the sac is empty of contents, it is either inverted into the abdomen or ligated by transfixion and excised. The defect in the linea alba is closed with interrupted *absorbable* sutures.

Paraumbilical hernia (syn. supraumbilical or infraumbilical hernia)

In adults the hernia does not occur through the umbilical scar. It is a protrusion through the linea alba just above or sometimes just below the umbilicus (Fig. 62.17). As it enlarges it

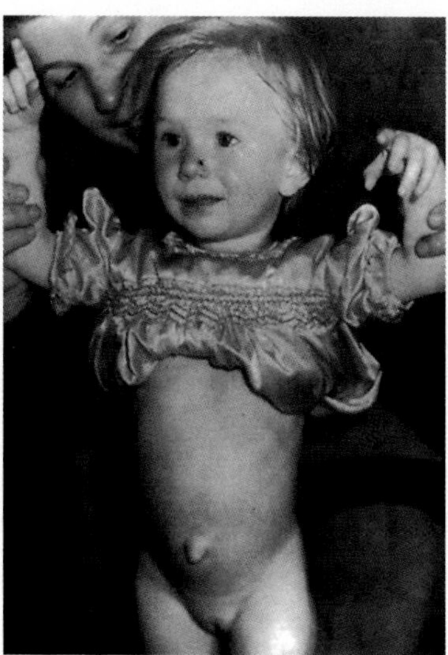

Fig. 62.16 Infantile umbilical hernia.

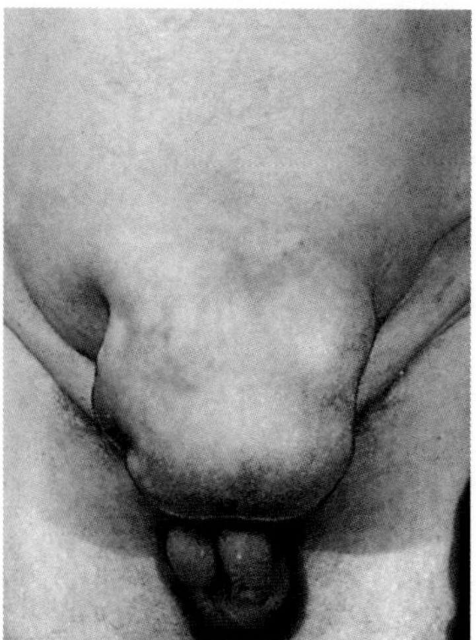

Fig. 62.17 A large paraumbilical hernia.

becomes rounded or oval in shape, with a tendency to sag downwards. Paraumbilical hernias can become very large. The neck of the sac is often remarkably narrow compared with the size of the sac and the volume of its contents, which usually consist of greater omentum often accompanied by small intestine and, alternatively or in addition, a portion of transverse colon. In long-standing cases the sac sometimes becomes loculated owing to adherence of omentum to its fundus.

Clinical features. Women are affected five times more frequently than men. The patient is usually overweight, and between the ages of 35 and 50 years. Increasing obesity, with flabbiness of the abdominal muscles, and repeated pregnancy are important aetiological factors. These hernias may become irreducible owing to the formation of omental adhesions within the sac. Symptomatically, a large umbilical hernia causes a dragging pain by its weight. Gastrointestinal symptoms are common and are probably due to traction on the stomach or transverse colon. Often there are transient attacks of intestinal colic due to partial intestinal obstruction. In long-standing cases intertrigo of the adjacent surfaces of skin and trophic ulcers of the fundus are troublesome complications.

Treatment. Untreated, the hernia increases in size and more and more of its contents become irreducible. Eventually, strangulation may occur. Therefore operation should be advised in nearly all cases. If the patient is obese and the hernia is symptomless, operation can be postponed until the patient has lost weight.

Epigastric herniorrhaphy. If the defect is small, a primary herniorrhaphy can be performed. If the defect is large, the repair is best performed with prosthetic buttressing of the abdominal wall. The classic primary repair is that described by Mayo. A transverse elliptical incision is made around the umbilicus and the subcutaneous tissues are dissected off the rectus sheath to expose the neck of the sac. The neck is incised to expose the contents. Intestine is returned to the abdomen and any adherent omentum freed. Excess adherent omentum can be removed

Charles-Robert Richet, 1850–1935. French physiologist, Professor, University of Paris.

William James Mayo, 1861–1939. Surgeon, The Mayo Clinic, Minnesota, USA, described this operation in 1901.

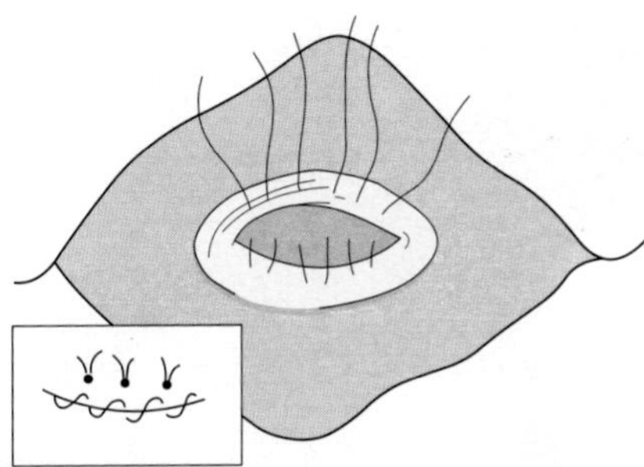

Fig. 62.18 Mayo's operation for umbilical hernia. Interrupted sutures to provide an overlap are first inserted. *Inset*: The overlap has been made and completed with a continuous suture. It is important to denude the area of fat before stitching the flap in position.

with the sac if necessary. The sac is then removed and the peritoneum closed with an absorbable suture. The aponeurosis on both sides of the umbilical ring is mobilised from underlying tissue sufficiently to allow an overlap of 5 or 7.5 cm. Interrupted mattress sutures are then inserted into the aponeurosis, as shown in Fig. 62.18. When this row of mattress sutures has been tied, the overlapping upper margin is stitched to the sheath of the rectus abdominis and the midline aponeurosis. A suction drain should be placed in the wound in fat patients, who ooze blood and liquid fat. The subcutaneous fat and skin are then approximated with deep sutures.

Paraumbilical hernioplasty. In the case of very large primary paraumbilical hernias (fascial defect > 4 cm) or for recurrent paraumbilical hernias, the use of prosthetic material (polypropylene mesh) is recommended.

Additional lipectomy. In patients with a paraumbilical hernia associated with a large, pendulous, fat-laden abdominal wall the operation can, with great advantage, be combined with panniculectomy by fashioning the incisions to embrace a larger area of the fat-laden superficial layers of the abdominal wall.

Strangulation is a frequent complication of a large paraumbilical hernia in adults. Owing to the narrow neck and the fibrous edge of the linea alba, gangrene is liable to supervene unless early operation is carried out. It should also be remembered that in large hernias the presence of loculi may result in a strangulated knuckle of the bowel in one part of an otherwise soft and nontender hernia.

Operation. In early cases, the operation does not differ from that for nonstrangulated cases. Gangrenous contents are dealt with as in other situations. If a portion of the transverse colon is gangrenous, it should be exteriorised by the Paul–Mikulicz method and the gangrenous portion excised. If the ring is large enough to transmit the colon unhampered, it is left alone; otherwise it is enlarged. It is important that the small intestine be thoroughly scrutinised as a small loop may have been trapped and slipped back when the constriction was relieved. If nonviable gut is overlooked, peritonitis quickly supervenes and the symptoms are ascribed to postoperative discomfort. The condition of the patient steadily deteriorates until they succumb after a few days.

Epigastric hernia (syn. fatty hernia of the linea alba)

An epigastric hernia occurs through the linea alba anywhere between the xiphoid process and the umbilicus, usually midway between these structures. Such a hernia commences as a protrusion of extraperitoneal fat through the linea alba, and it was hypothesised that this protrusion occurs at the site where small blood vessels pierced the linea alba. However, only a minority of epigastric hernias is accompanied by blood vessels, and it is more likely that the defect occurs as a result of a weakened linea alba due to abnormal decussation of the fibres of the aponeurosis. More than one hernia may be present and the commonest cause of 'recurrence' is failure to identify a second defect at the time of original repair.

A swelling the size of a pea consists of a protrusion of extraperitoneal fat only (fatty hernia of the linea alba). If the protrusion enlarges, it drags a pouch of peritoneum after it and so becomes a true epigastric hernia. The mouth of the hernia is rarely large enough to permit a portion of hollow viscus to enter it; consequently, either the sac is empty or it contains a small portion of greater omentum.

It is probable that an epigastric hernia is the direct result of a sudden strain tearing the interlacing fibres of the linea alba. The patients are often manual workers between 30 and 45 years of age.

Clinical features

- *Symptomless* – a small fatty hernia of the linea alba can be felt better than it can be seen and may be symptomless, being discovered only in the course of routine abdominal palpation.
- *Painful* – sometimes such a hernia gives rise to attacks of local pain, worse on physical exertion, and tenderness to touch and light clothing. This may be because the fatty contents become nipped sufficiently to produce partial strangulation.
- *Referred pain* – it is not uncommon to find that the patient, who may not have noticed the hernia, complains of pain suggestive of a peptic ulcer. However, as the majority of these hernias is asymptomatic, symptoms should not be ascribed to the hernia until any gastrointestinal pathology has been excluded.

Treatment

If the hernia is giving rise to symptoms, operation should be undertaken.

Operation. An adequate vertical or transverse incision is made over the swelling, exposing the linea alba. The protruding extraperitoneal fat is cleared from the hernial orifice by gauze dissection. If the pedicle passing through the linea alba is slender, it is separated on all sides of the opening by blunt dissection. After ligating the pedicle, the small opening in the linea alba is closed by nonabsorbable sutures in adults and with absorbable sutures in children. When a hernial sac is present, it is opened and any contents are reduced, after which the sac neck is transfixed and the sac excised before repairing the linea alba. If smaller protrusions of fat are found above or below the hernia, these should also be dealt with. If the hernia is large (defect greater than 4 cm in diameter), the repair should be reinforced with polypropylene mesh positioned in the retromuscular plane.

Frank Thomas Paul, 1851–1941. English surgeon, Liverpool, England.

Rare external hernias

Interparietal hernia (syn. interstitial hernia). An interparietal hernia has a hernial sac which passes between the layers of the anterior abdominal wall. The sac may be associated with, or communicate with, the sac of a concomitant inguinal or femoral hernia. Lack of knowledge of this condition is the cause of misdiagnosis and mismanagement.

Other varieties.

- *Preperitoneal* (20 per cent) – usually the sac takes the form of a diverticulum from a femoral or inguinal hernia.
- *Intermuscular* (60 per cent) – the sac passes between the muscular layers of the anterior abdominal wall, usually between the external oblique and internal oblique muscles. The sac is nearly always bilocular and is associated with an inguinal hernia.
- *Inguinosuperficial* (20 per cent) – the sac expands beneath the superficial fascia of the abdominal wall or the thigh. This type is commonly associated with an incompletely descended testis.

Clinical features. The patients (mostly male) present with intestinal obstruction, due to obstruction or strangulation of the hernia. In the preperitoneal variety, as no swelling is likely to be apparent, delays in diagnosis occur and consequently the mortality in this variety is high.

Treatment. Operation is imperative because of intestinal obstruction.

Spigelian hernia. This is a variety of interparietal hernia occurring at the level of the arcuate line. It is very rare with only 1000 cases reported in the literature. The fundus of the sac, clothed by extraperitoneal fat, may lie beneath the internal oblique muscle where it is virtually impalpable. More often it advances through that muscle and spreads out like a mushroom between the internal and external oblique muscles, and gives rise to a more evident swelling. The patient is often corpulent and usually over 50 years of age, men and women being equally affected. Typically, a soft, reducible mass will be encountered lateral to the rectus muscle and below the umbilicus. Diagnosis is confirmed by computerised tomography (CT) or ultrasound scanning, the latter having the advantage of being able to stand the patient upright if no defect is visible in the reclining position. Owing to the rigid fascia surrounding the neck, strangulation may occur.

Treatment. Operation. If a defect is palpable, a muscle-splitting approach is used. After isolating the sac, dealing with any contents, and ligating and excising it, the transversus, internal oblique and external oblique muscles are repaired by direct apposition. If no sac is palpable, a paramedian approach is used and the sac sought in the extraperitoneal space. The repair then proceeds as described above.

Lumbar hernia. Most primary lumbar hernias occur through the inferior lumbar triangle of Petit (Fig. 62.19), bounded below by the crest of the ilium, laterally by the external oblique and medially by the latissimus dorsi. Less commonly, the sac comes through the superior lumbar triangle which is bounded by the twelfth rib above, medially by the sacrospinalis and laterally by the posterior border of the internal oblique. Primary lumbar hernias are very rare with only 300 cases reported. More commonly lumbar hernias are secondary to renal operations, when extensive incisional sacs may be present.

Differential diagnosis. A lumbar hernia must be distinguished from:

- lipoma;
- a cold abscess pointing to this position;
- phantom hernia due to local muscular paralysis. Lumbar phantom hernia can result from any interference with the nerve supply of the affected muscles (e.g. poliomyelitis).

Treatment. A primary lumbar hernia, being small, is easily repaired. As the natural history is for these hernias to increase in size with time, any primary lumbar hernia should be repaired at presentation. Incisional lumbar hernias may be large and the defect is impossible to repair unless fascial flaps are used. The repair can be reinforced with a sheet of polypropylene mesh.

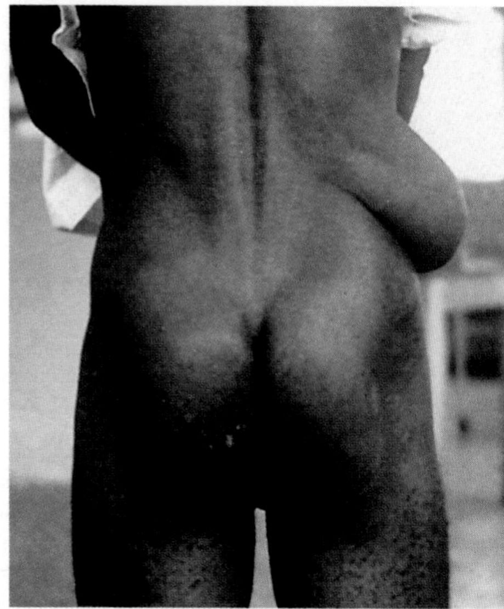

Fig. 62.19 Inferior lumbar hernia. It contained caecum, appendix and small bowel. Note filarial skin rash on the buttocks (*courtesy of V.J. Hartfield, formerly of S.E. Nigeria*).

Perineal hernia. This type of hernia is very rare. Varieties include:

- *postoperative hernia through a perineal scar* may occur after excision of the rectum;
- *median sliding perineal hernia* is a complete prolapse of the rectum (Chapter 60);
- *anterolateral perineal hernia* occurs in women and presents as a swelling of the labum majus;
- *posterolateral perineal hernia,* which passes through the levator ani to enter the ischiorectal fossa.

Treatment. A combined operation is generally the most satisfactory for the last two types of hernia. The hernia is exposed by an incision directly over it. The sac is opened and its contents are reduced. The sac is cleared from surrounding structures and the wound closed. With the patients in semi-Trendelenburg position, the abdomen is opened and the mouth of the sac is exposed. The sac is inverted, ligated and excised and the pelvic floor repaired by muscle apposition and, if indicated, buttressing of the repair with prosthetic mesh.

Obturator hernia. The hernia, which passes through the obturator canal, occurs six times more frequently in women than in men. Most of the patients are over 60 years of age. The swelling is liable to be overlooked because it is covered by the pectineus. It seldom causes a definite swelling in Scarpa's triangle, but if the limb is flexed, abducted and rotated outwards, sometimes the hernia becomes more apparent. The leg is usually kept in a semiflexed position and movement increases the pain. In more than 50 per cent of cases of strangulated obturator hernia, pain is referred along the obturator nerve by its geniculate branch to the knee. On vaginal or rectal examination the hernia sometimes can be felt as a tender swelling in the region of the obturator foramen.

Cases of obturator hernia which present themselves have usually undergone strangulation, which is frequently of the Richter type.

Treatment. Treatment consists of the following:

- perform lower laparotomy (on the side of the lesion, if known). Confirm the diagnosis and then adopt full Trendelenburg's position;

Jean Louis Petit, 1644–1750. Director of the Academy of Surgery, Paris, France.

Freidrich Tredelenberg, 1844–1924. Professor of Surgery, Leipzig. Germany.
Antonio Scarpa, 1747–1832. Professor of Anatomy, Parvia, Italy. Elected FRS in 1791.

- the constricting agent is the obturator fascia. Taking every precaution to avoid spilling infected fluid from the hernial sac into the peritoneal cavity, this fascia can be stretched to allow reduction by inserting suitable forceps through the gap in the fascia and opening the blades with care. If incision of the fascia is required, it should be made parallel to the obturator vessels and nerve;
- the contents of the sac are dealt with;
- the broad ligament is stitched over the opening to prevent recurrence.

Gluteal and sciatic hernias. A *gluteal hernia* passes through the greater sciatic foramen, either above or below the piriformis. A *sciatic hernia* passes through the lesser sciatic foramen. Differential diagnosis must be made between these conditions and:

- a lipoma or fibrosarcoma beneath the gluteus maximus;
- a tuberculous abscess;
- a gluteal aneurysm.

All doubtful swellings in this situation should be explored by operation.

Umbilicus

Diseases of the umbilicus

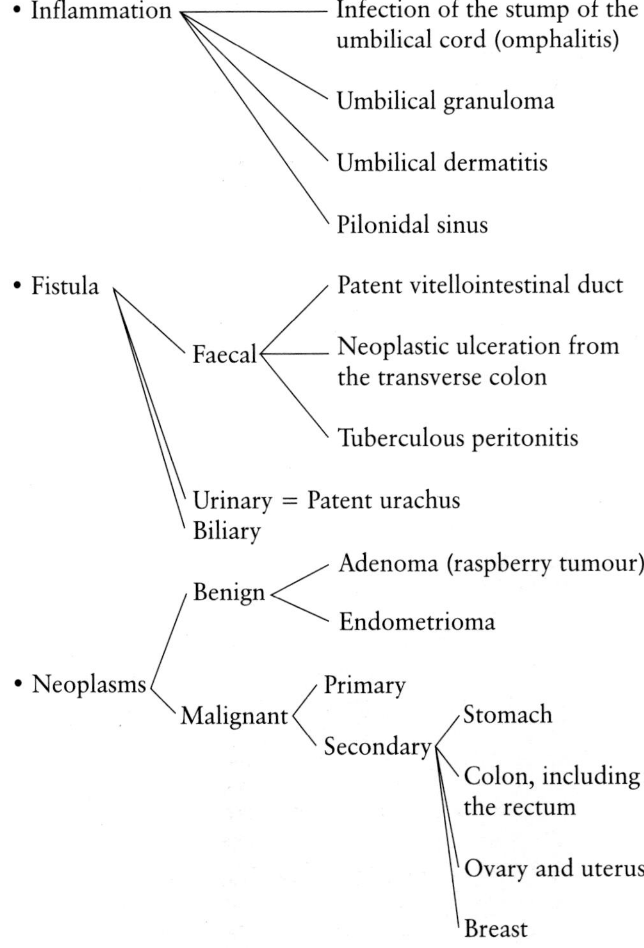

- Hernia
- Umbilical calculus
- Eversion (in ascites)

Inflammation of the umbilicus

Infection of the umbilical cord

By the third or fourth day postdelivery the stump of the umbilical cord is found to be carrying staphylococci in over 50 per cent of babies born in maternity hospitals. Less commonly, the stump of the cord harbours streptococci, and epidemics of puerperal sepsis in maternity hospitals have been traced to the umbilical cord of one infant in the nursery thus infected. *Escherichia coli* and *Clostridium tetani* (causing neonatal tetanus) are other possible invaders. The chief prophylaxis is strict asepsis during severance of the cord and the use of 0.1 per cent chlorhexidine, locally, for a few days.

Omphalitis. The incidence of an infected umbilicus is much higher in communities that do not practise aseptic severance of the umbilical cord. When the stump of the umbilical cord becomes inflamed, antibiotic therapy usually localises the inflammation. By employing warm moist dressings, the crusts separate, giving exit to pus. Exuberant granulation tissue requires a touch of silver nitrate. In more serious cases infection is liable to spread along the defunct hypogastric arteries or umbilical vein when, in all probability, one or other of the following complications will supervene.

Abscess of the abdominal wall. If gentle pressure is exerted above or below the navel, and a bead of pus exudes at the navel, a deep abscess associated with one of the defunct umbilical vessels is present. This must be opened. A probe is passed into the sinus to determine its direction and this is followed by a grooved director on to which the skin and overlying tissues are incised in the midline.

Extensive ulceration of the abdominal wall. Extensive ulceration of the abdominal wall due to synergistic infection is treated in the same way as postoperative subcutaneous gangrene (*vide infra*).

Septicaemia. Septicaemia can occur from organisms entering the bloodstream via the umbilical vein. Jaundice is often the first sign. An abscess in the abdominal wall above the umbilicus should be sought. In other respects the treatment of this grave complication follows the usual lines (Chapter 4).

Jaundice in the newborn. Infection reaching the liver via the umbilical vein may cause a stenosing intrahepatic cholangiolitis, appearing some 3–6 weeks after birth.

Portal vein thrombosis. Portal vein thrombosis and subsequent portal hypertension.

Peritonitis. Peritonitis carries a bad prognosis.

Umbilical hernia.

Umbilical granuloma. Chronic infection of the umbilical cicatrix which continues for weeks causes granulation tissue to pout at the umbilicus. There is no certain means of distinguishing this condition from an adenoma. Usually an umbilical granuloma can be treated by one application of silver nitrate followed by dry dressings, but an adenoma soon recurs in spite of these measures.

Dermatitis of and around the umbilicus. This is common at all times of life. Fungal and parasitic infections are more difficult to eradicate from the umbilicus than from the skin of the abdomen. Sometimes the dermatitis is consequent upon a discharge from the umbilicus, as is the case when an umbilical fistula or a sinus is present. In overweight women intertrigo occurs.

A deep, tender swelling in the midline below the umbilicus signifies an abscess present in the extraperitoneal fat and is usually due to an infected urachal remnant. Exploration and proper drainage are necessary.

Pilonidal sinus. Pilonidal sinus (a sinus containing a sheath of hairs) is sometimes encountered. It should be excised.

Umbilical calculus (umbolith). This is often black in colour, and is composed of desquamated epithelium which becomes inspissated and collects in the deep recess of the umbilicus. The treatment is to dilate the orifice and extract the calculus but, to prevent recurrence, it may be necessary to excise the umbilicus.

Umbilical fistulae

The umbilicus being a central abdominal scar, it is understandable that a slow leak from any viscus is liable to track to the surface at this point. Added to this, very occasionally, the vitellointestinal duct or the urachus remains patent; consequently it has been aptly remarked that the umbilicus is a creek into which many fistulous streams may open.

For instance, an enlarged inflamed gallbladder perforating at its fundus may discharge gallstones through the umbilicus. Again, an unremitting flow of pus from a fistula at the umbilicus of a middle-aged women led to the discovery of a length of gauze overlooked during a hysterectomy 5 years previously.

The vitellointestinal duct. The vitellointestinal duct occasionally persists and gives rise to one of the following conditions.

- It remains patent (Fig. 62.20a). The resulting umbilical fistula discharges mucus and, rarely, faeces. Often a small portion only of the duct near the umbilicus remains unobliterated. This gives rise to a sinus that discharges mucus. The epithelial lining of the sinus often becomes everted to form an adenoma.
- Sometimes both the umbilical and the intestinal ends of the duct close, but the mucous membrane of the intervening portion remains and an intra-abdominal cyst develops (Fig. 62.20b).
- With its lumen obliterated or unobliterated, the vitellointestinal duct provides an intraperitoneal band (Fig. 62.20c) which is a potential danger, for intestinal obstruction is liable to occur. The obstruction results from a coil of small intestine passing under or over or becoming twisted around the band.
- Such a band may contract and pull a Meckel's diverticulum into a congenital umbilical hernia (Fig. 62.20d).
- A vitellointestinal cord connected to a Meckel's diverticulum, but not attached to the umbilicus, becomes adherent to, or knotted around, another loop of small intestine and so causes intestinal obstruction.

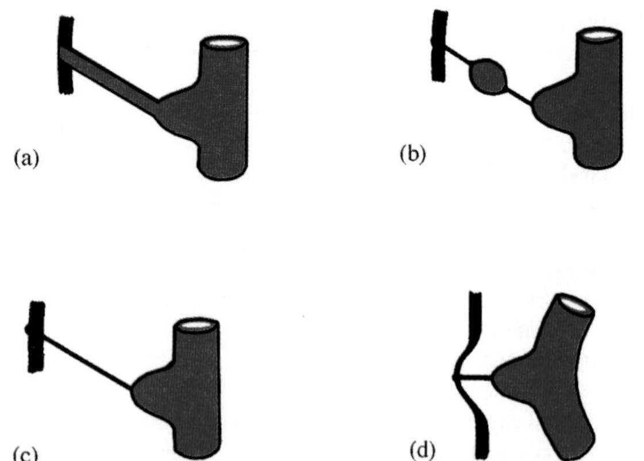

Fig. 62.20 Anomalies connected with the vitellointestinal duct. (a) Umbilical fistula; (b) intra-abdominal cyst; (c) intraperitoneal band; (d) Meckel's diverticulum with a band adherent to the sac of a congenital umbilical herna.

Johann Friedrich Meckel (The Younger), 1781–1833. Professor of Anatomy and Surgery, Halle, Germany.

- Sometimes a band extending from the umbilicus is attached to the mesentery near its junction with a distal part of the ileum. In this case the band is probably an obliterated vitelline artery and is not necessarily associated with a Meckel's diverticulum.

Treatment. A patent vitellointestinal duct should be excised together with a Meckel's diverticulum, if one is present, preferably when the child is about 6 months old. When a vitellointestinal band gives rise to acute intestinal obstruction, after removing the obstruction by dividing the band, it is expedient, where possible, to excise the band and bury the cut ends.

Patent urachus. A patent urachus seldom reveals itself until maturity or even old age. This is because the contractions of the bladder commence at the apex of the organ and pass towards the base. A patent urachus, because it opens into the apex of the bladder, is closed temporarily during micturition and so the potential urinary stream to the bladder is cut off. Therefore the fistula remains unobtrusive until a time when the organ is overfull, usually due to some form of obstruction.

Treatment. Treatment is directed to removing the obstruction to the lower urinary tract. If, after this has been remedied, the leak continues or a cyst develops in connection with the urachus, umbilectomy and excision of the urachus down to its insertion into the apex of the bladder, with closure of the latter, is indicated.

Neoplasms of the umbilicus

Umbilical adenoma or *raspberry tumour* is commonly seen in infants (Fig. 62.21), but only occasionally later in life. It is due to a partially (occasionally a completely) unobliterated vitellointestinal duct. Mucosa prolapsing through the umbilicus gives rise to a raspberry-like tumour, which is moist and tends to bleed.

Treatment

If the tumour is pedunculated, a ligature is tied around it and, in a few days, the polypus drops off. Should the tumour reappear after this procedure, umbilectomy is indicated. Sometimes a patent vitellointestinal duct, or more often a vitellointestinal band, will be found associated with a Meckel's diverticulum. The Meckel's diverticulum and the

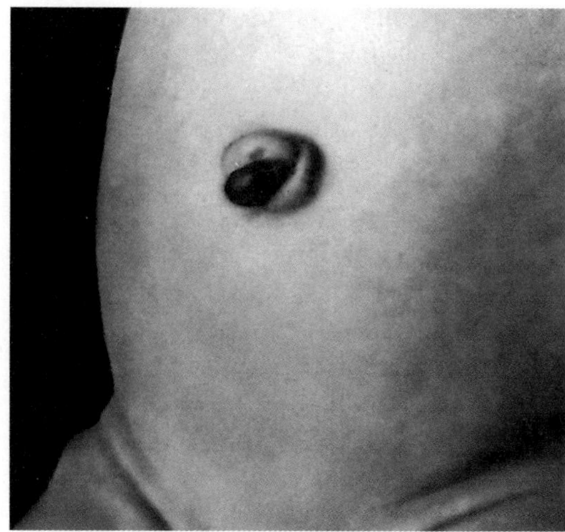

Fig. 62.21 Adenoma (raspberry tumour) of the umbilicus.

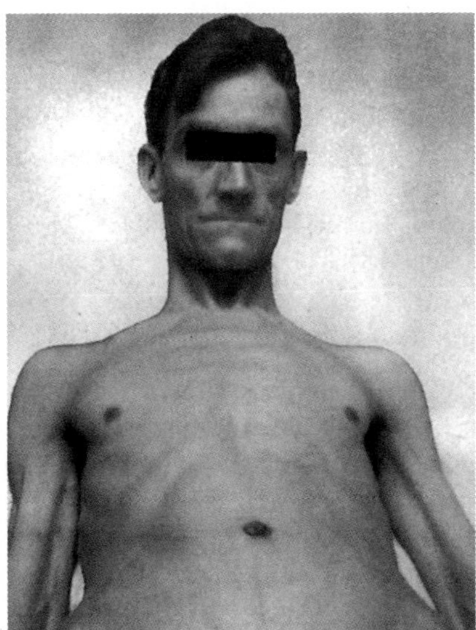

Fig. 62.22 Secondary nodule at the umbilicus in a case of carcinoma of the stomach.

attached cord or duct should be excised at the same time as the umbilicus. Histologically, the tumour at the umbilicus consists of columnar epithelium rich in goblet cells.

Endometrioma. Endometrioma occurs in women between the ages of 20 and 45 years. On histological examination it is found to consist of endometrial glands occupying the same plane in the dermis as the sudoriferous glands and opening on to the surface in the same way. The umbilicus becomes painful and bleeds at each menstruation, when the small fleshy tumour between the folds of the umbilicus becomes more apparent. Occasionally an umbilical endometrioma is accompanied by endometriomas in the uterus or ovary. When, as is usually the case, the tumour is solitary, umbilectomy will cure the condition.

Secondary carcinoma. Secondary carcinoma at the umbilicus (or Sister Joseph's nodule)[4] (Fig. 62.22) is not very uncommon, but it is always a late manifestation of the disease. The primary neoplasm is often situated in the stomach, colon or ovary, but a metastasis from the breast, probably transmitted along the lymphatics of the round ligament of the liver, is sometimes located here.

The abdominal wall

Burst abdomen (syn. abdominal dehiscence) and incisional hernia (syn. ventral hernia)

In 1–2 per cent of cases, mostly between the 6th and 8th day after operation, an abdominal wound bursts open and viscera are extruded. The disruption of the wound tends to occur a few days beforehand when the sutures apposing the deep layers (peritoneum, posterior rectus sheath) tear through or even become untied. An incisional hernia usually starts as a symptomless partial disruption of the deeper layers during the immediate or early postoperative period, the event passing unnoticed if the skin wound remains intact after the skin sutures have been removed.

Factors relating to the incidence of burst abdomen and incisional hernia.

Technique of wound closure.

- *Choice of suture material* – catgut leads to a higher incidence of bursts than the use of nonabsorbable monofilament polypropylene, polyamide or wire, and should never be used;
- *method of closure* – interrupted suturing has a low incidence. Through and through suturing is good for the obstructed case. A one-layer closure has a low incidence, but it is higher than that following a two-layered closure. Interrupted 'far and near' sutures are a recommended technique for single-layer mass closures. When continuous suturing of layers (one or two) is performed a particular fault is the use of a short length of material, pulled tightly, for in an anaesthetised relaxed patient the incision is shortened thereby, and made taut so that the material will act as if it were a cheese wire-cutter when the patient is conscious and coughing. The golden rule is to insert a length of suture at least four times the length of the incision but less than five times the length of the incision. This ensures that the layers are gently apposed;
- *drainage* directly through a wound leads to a higher incidence of 'bursts' than employing drainage through a separate (stab) incision.

Factors relating to incisions. Midline and vertical incisions have a tendency to burst which is higher than those which are transverse. Since the widespread use of nonabsorbable suture materials even midline vertical incisions have a very low incidence of disruption.

Reasons for operation. Infected case; deep wound infection has a notorious reputation for causing burst abdomen and/or late incisional hernias. Operations on the pancreas, with leakage of enzymes, and on obstructed cases are other reasons for disruption.

Coughing; vomiting; distension. At the completion of an operation any violent coughing set off by the removal of an endotracheal tube and suction of the laryngopharynx strains the sutures; likewise cough, vomiting and distension (e.g. due to ileus) in the early postoperative period. Over-vigorous postoperative ventilation in sedated patients can lead to wound disruption.

General condition of the patient. Obesity, jaundice, malignant disease, hypoproteinaemia and anaemia are all factors conducive to disruption of a laparotomy wound (Chapter 1); abdominal wounds in pregnancy are notorious for a high risk of disruption; steroids delay wound healing.

Burst abdomen (syn. abdominal dehiscence)

Clinical features

A serosanguinous (pink) discharge from the wound is a forerunner of disruption in fully 50 per cent of cases. It is the most pathognomonic sign of impending wound disruption and it signifies that intraperitoneal contents are lying extraperitoneally. Patients often volunteer the information that they 'felt something give way'. If skin sutures have been removed, omentum or coils of intestine may be forced through the wound and will be found lying on the skin. Pain and shock are often absent. It is important to note that there may be symptoms and signs of intestinal obstruction.

Treatment

An emergency operation is required to replace the bowel, relieve any obstruction and to resuture the wound. While

[4]*Sister Joseph of the Mayo Clinic imparted this clinical observation to the late Dr William Mayo. The first reports of this clinical sign were from the Walshe in 1846 (Dr M.R. Shetty, Northwestern Community Hospital, Arlington, Illinois, USA).*

awaiting operation, reassure the patient and cover the wound with a sterile towel. The stomach should be emptied using a nasogastric tube and intravenous fluid therapy commenced.

Operation. Each protruding coil of intestine is washed gently with saline solution and returned to the abdominal cavity. Then protruding greater omentum is treated similarly and spread over the intestine. The abdominal wall having been cleaned, all layers are approximated by through and through sutures of monofilament nylon, each passed through a soft rubber or plastic tuber collar. The abdominal wall may be supported by strips of adhesive plaster encircling the anterior two-thirds of the circumference of the trunk. Antibiotic therapy should be started.

Contrary to what might be thought, peritonitis rarely supervenes and, although the skin wound may become infected, healing is satisfactory. A second dehiscence rarely occurs. There is biochemical evidence that healing after disruption produces a stronger wound. This is due to the improvement in collagen metabolism under these circumstances. An incisional hernia is often a later sequel (see below).

Incisional hernia (syn. ventral hernia; postoperative hernia)

Aetiology

Incisional hernia occurs most often in obese individuals, and a persistent postoperative cough and postoperative abdominal distension are its precursors. There is a high incidence of incisional hernia following operations for peritonitis because, as a rule, the wound becomes infected. The placing of a drainage tube through a separate stab incision, as opposed to bringing such a tube through the laparotomy wound, reduces the frequency (see also the section 'General features common to all hernias').

An incisional hernia usually starts as a symptomless partial disruption of the deeper layers of a laparotomy wound during the immediate or very early postoperative period. Often the event passes unnoticed if the skin wound remains intact after the stitches have been removed (or because subcuticular stitches have been used which remain in place). A serosanguinous discharge is often the signal of dehiscence, and resuture of the deeper layers of the incision obviates the more difficult repair of an established and much larger hernia later on.

Clinical features

There are great variations in the degree of herniation. The hernia may occur through a small portion of the scar, often the lower end. More frequently, there is a diffuse bulging of the whole length of the incision. A postoperative hernia, especially one through a lower abdominal scar, usually increases steadily in size and more and more of its contents become irreducible. Sometimes the skin overlying it is so thin and atrophic that normal peristalsis can be seen in the underlying intestine. Attacks of partial intestinal obstruction are common and strangulation is liable to occur at the neck of a small sac or in a loculus of a large one. Nevertheless, most cases of incisional hernia are asymptomatic and broad-necked, and do not need treatment.

Treatment

Palliative. An abdominal belt is sometimes satisfactory, especially in cases of a hernia through an upper abdominal incision.

Operation. Many procedures have been advocated, which is testimony to the fact that the repairs may be difficult to accomplish, but it is now clear that one technique is superior to all of the others.

Preoperative measures

In order to obtain a lasting repair, very special preparation is required. If the patient is obese, weight reduction by dieting should precede the operation. To attempt to return the contents of a very large hernia to the main abdominal cavity if they have not been there for several years is to court danger, particularly if weight reduction has not been effected. In these circumstances, not only is there a risk of failure of the hernioplasty, but there is a greatly increased risk of paralytic ileus from visceral compression and of pulmonary complications from elevation of the diaphragm. The repair of these large hernias is highly specialised surgery and should only be performed in centres with considerable experience in dealing with them. For example, one technique employed to enlarge the abdominal cavity is that of prolonged pneumoperitoneum in which the intra-abdominal pressure is raised to 15–18 cmH_2O for up to several weeks preoperatively. The technique requires careful monitoring and patient counselling to be effective but, if employed correctly, can enable a primary repair to be successful.

Operation. Three techniques have been described: simple and complex apposition and plastic fibre mesh or net closures.

Simple apposition. The hernial sac is dissected. It is then formally, if not already inadvertently, opened and the contents are reduced. Adherent omentum and bowel have to be freed by dissection before the mouth of the sac can be defined. The layers are repaired usually with nonabsorbable sutures: first the peritoneum, then the fascial (aponeurotic) layers. The lateral edges of the fascia are freed from the overlying muscles for some distance and this fascial layer is approximated with interrupted sutures at the upper and lower ends of the wound. The muscles and the remaining fascial layer are approximated. Tension-relaxing incisions may be required and should be placed well laterally.

Complex apposition. These consist of various types of layered closures (Mayo, 'Keel', da Silva) and should be considered obsolete and of historical interest only.

Plastic fibre mesh or net closures. These techniques are now the method of choice for all but the smallest defects (< 4 cm). The sac is dealt with as above. The layers of the fascia are dissected out and, if above the umbilicus, the posterior rectus sheath edges apposed. A sheet of polypropylene mesh is then inserted between the posterior rectus sheath and the muscle fibres, and anchored in place. If below the umbilicus, the mesh is placed in the preperitoneal space. The anterior rectus sheath is then apposed as above. If the defect is too large to close by apposition of the rectus sheath, the deficiency in the abdominal wall can be bridged by sewing the mesh to the fascia on either side of the defect, ensuring at least a 4-cm overlap of the fascial edges.

Careful haemostasis and meticulous asepsis are essential during these operations. Postoperative collections of serum can be removed by drainage, using plastic tubing led, via skin punctures lateral to the wound, into closed suction drainage bottles (e.g. Redi-vac).

Postoperative treatment. Gastric decompression and intravenous fluids are employed, and nothing by mouth allowed until the bowels have functioned. Early ambulation and gentle physical exercise are to be encouraged. The patient should not resume strenuous exercise for several weeks.

Results of treatment. Most series report recurrence of the hernia in between 30 and 50 per cent of cases except where mesh inlay techniques have been employed in specialist centres, where recurrence rates may be as low as 10 per cent.

Divarication of the recti abdominis

Divarication of the recti abdominis is seen principally in elderly multiparous patients. When the patient strains, a gap can be seen between the recti abdominis through which the abdominal contents bulge. When the abdomen is relaxed, the fingers can be introduced between the recti.

Treatment. An abdominal belt is all that is required. There is no risk of strangulated intestinal contents. A similar condition is seen in babies, only the divarication exists above the umbilicus. No treatment is necessary; as the child grows a spontaneous cure results.

Tearing of the inferior epigastric artery

Tearing of the inferior epigastric artery occurs in three dissimilar types of individual, namely elderly women, often thin and feeble; athletic, muscular men, usually below middle age; and pregnant women, mainly multiparas late in pregnancy. The site of the haematoma is usually at the level of the arcuate line, where the posterior sheath of the rectus abdominis is lacking.

Clinical features. The possibility of tearing of the epigastric vessels should always be considered when, following a bout of coughing or a sudden blow to the abdominal wall, an exquisitely tender lump appears in relation to the rectus abdominis. Occasionally, a haematoma occurs within the muscles lateral to the rectus sheath. Unless there is bruising of the overlying skin, the diagnosis may be difficult.

Differential diagnosis. The conditions for which the haematoma is frequently mistaken are, in the female, a twisted ovarian cyst, and in both sexes, when the lump is on the right side, an appendix abscess. The sign most likely to be of value in differentiating a haematoma of the abdominal wall from these conditions, namely tensing the abdominal musculature, is often unsatisfactory because of the pain it causes. Again, the differential diagnosis between the haematoma and a strangulated Spigelian hernia may be difficult. The absence of vomiting suggests a haematoma and the presence of resonance over the swelling favours a Spigelian hernia, while a plain radiograph of the abdomen sometimes gives positive evidence of the latter.

As a complication of pregnancy. Rupture of the inferior epigastric artery occurs occasionally during pregnancy. Surprisingly to relate, the haemorrhage into this closed space from this comparatively small artery has proved fatal.

Treatment. With rest, a comparatively small haematoma may resolve, but sometimes renewed haemorrhage causes the haematoma to rupture into the peritoneal cavity. Therefore it is safer to operate early, evacuate the clot and ligate the artery.

Infections

Cellulitis can occur in any of the planes of the abdominal wall.

Superficial cellulitis is usually discovered when an abdominal wound is inspected following pyrexia. The earliest sign is when the stitches become embedded in the oedematous skin. Later there is a blush extending for a variable distance from the incision or the stitch holes. On palpation with the gloved hand usually one area is found to be more indurated and tender than the remainder. A stitch should be removed from the immediate vicinity, and if pus or seropus escapes it should be sent for bacteriological examination; treatment should then be commenced with a broad-spectrum antibiotic.

Deep cellulitis is characterised by brawny oedema towards one or both flanks, and not infrequently of the scrotum or vulva as well. Antibiotic therapy is the mainstay of treatment. When tenderness persists, an anatomical incision dividing the muscles carefully, layer by layer, until pus or purulent fluid is encountered is often advisable.

Progressive postoperative bacterial synergistic gangrene. This is, fortunately, a rare complication after laparotomy, usually for a perforated viscus (notably perforated appendicitis). It has also occurred after gallbladder operations, colectomy for ulcerative colitis and even after drainage of an empyema thoracis. The condition is due to the synergistic action of microaerophilic nonhaemolytic streptococci and, usually, a staphylococcus. The skin in the immediate vicinity of the wound exhibits signs of cellulitis. Within a few hours, a central purplish zone with an outer brilliant red zone can be distinguished and the whole region is extremely tender. The condition advances with various degrees of rapidity (Fig. 62.23). The gangrenous skin liquefies exposing underlying granulation tissue. If the condition persists, overwhelming septicaemia and associated multiorgan failure supervene.

Treatment. Identification of the organisms and a report on their sensitivity to antibiotics is essential. Metronidazole should be given together with a powerful broad-spectrum antibiotic. Without vigorous and effective treatment the gangrene spreads to the flanks and the patient may die of toxaemia. If the infection has become established, surgical débridement of all the necrotic and infected tissue should be performed. Hyperbaric oxygen, if available, can be life-saving. Cellulitis due to bacteroides may give no bacterial growth by conventional techniques and may be missed.

Amoebic cutis. The possibility of this potentially lethal complication of amoebic colitis, liver abscess or empyema being present should always be considered (see Chapter 52). Confirmation may be difficult and an immunofluorescence test necessary.

Subcutaneous gas-forming infection. This is described in Chapter 7 (under 'Gas gangrene').

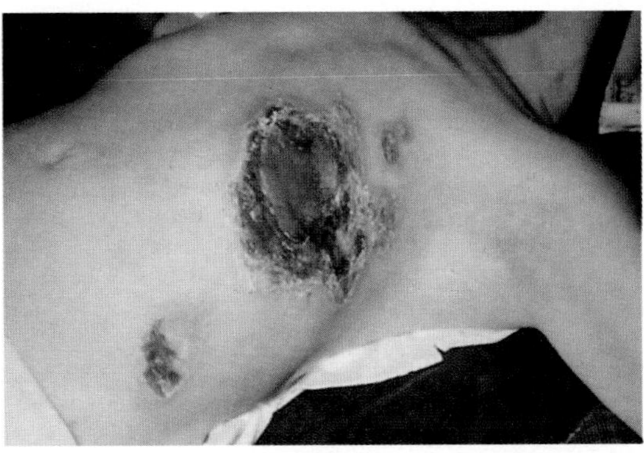

Fig. 62.23 Bacterial synergistic gangrene of the chest and abdominal wall. The area has become gangrenous and looks like suede leather. Beware of amoebiasis cutis.

Neoplasms of the abdominal wall

A *desmoid tumour* is a tumour arising in the musculoaponeurotic structures of the abdominal wall, especially below the level of the umbilicus. It is a completely unencapsulated fibroma and is so hard that it creaks when it is cut. Some cases recur repeatedly in spite of apparently adequate excision.

Aetiology. Eighty per cent of cases occur in women, many of whom have borne children, and the neoplasm occurs occasionally in scars of old hernial or other abdominal operation wounds. Consequently, trauma, for example the stretching of the muscle fibres during pregnancy or possibly a small haematoma of the abdominal wall, appears to be an aetiological factor. They can occur in cases of familial polyposis coli (Gardner's syndrome).

Pathology. The tumour is composed of fibrous tissue containing multinucleaterd plasmodial masses resembling foreign-body giant cells. Usually of very slow growth, it tends to infiltrate muscle in the immediate neighbourhood. Eventually it undergoes a myxomatous change; it then increases in size more rapidly. Metastasis does not occur. Unlike fibroma elsewhere, no sarcomatous change occurs.

Treatment. Unless the tumour is excised widely, with a surrounding margin of at least 2.5 cm of healthy tissue, recurrence commonly takes place. After removal of a large tumour, repair of the defect in the abdominal wall by nylon mesh is required. These tumours are moderately radiosensitive. (Intraperitoneal desmoids are best left alone when possible.)

Eldon J. Gardner, b. 1909. American geneticist.

Fibrosarcoma of the abdominal wall is rare. It is resistant to radiotherapy and only in some cases can a wide excision, with nylon mesh repair, offer hope of a cure.

Adenocarcinoma of the colon or of other viscera may invade the abdominal wall. In such cases, the resection of this extension, along with the primary growth, may require special repair of the resulting defect.

Secondary implantation in the wound may follow any abdominal operation for carcinoma, and bladder cancer is notorious for this propensity.

Further reading

Devlin, B. and Kingsnorth, A.N. (1998) *The Management of Abdominal Hernias*, 2nd edn, Arnold, London.

Leaper, D.J. (1985) Laparotomy closure. *British Journal of Hospital Medicine*, 33, 37.

Mudge, M. and Hughes, L.E. (1985) Incisional hernia: a 10 year prospective study of incidence and attitudes. *British Journal of Surgery*, 72, 70.

Nyhus, L.M. and Condon, R.E. (eds) (1995) *Hernia*, 4th edn, J.B. Lippincott, Philadelphia.

Poole, G.V. (1985) Mechanical factors in abdominal wall closure. The prevention of fascial dehiscence. *Surgery*, 97, 631.

Raffensperger, J.G. (1980) In *Swenson's Paediatric Surgery*, 4th edn, Appleton Century Crofts, New York.

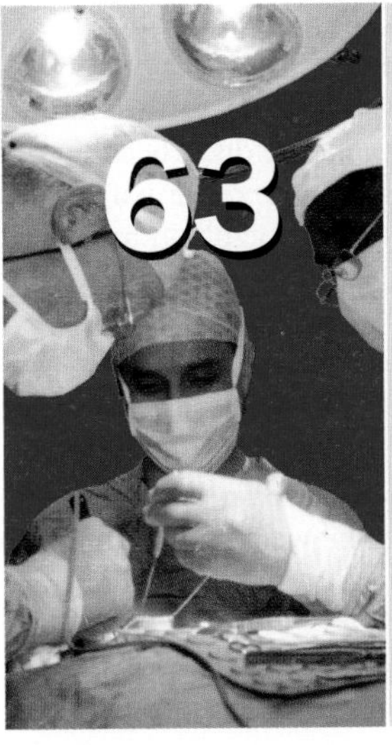

63 Urinary symptoms. Investigation of the urinary tract. Anuria

Urinary symptoms

Haematuria

The presence of blood in the urine (haematuria) is always abnormal and may be the only indication of pathology in the urinary tract (Fig. 63.1). Tiny amounts of blood that are insufficient to stain the urine (microscopic haematuria) may be detected by dipstick testing as part of a routine health check. A substantial haemorrhage into the urinary tract will give the urine a red or brownish tinge (macroscopic haematuria) and the patient may pass blood clots. False-positive stick tests and the discoloured urine caused by beetroot and certain drugs (e.g. dindevan, pyridium and furadantin) can be distinguished from haematuria by the absence of red blood cells on urinary microscopy.

Haematuria may be intermittent or persistent. Blood appearing at the beginning of the urinary stream indicates a lower urinary tract cause, while uniform staining throughout the stream points to a cause higher up. Terminal haematuria is typical of severe bladder irritation by stone or by infection. If the patient experiences pain with haematuria, the characteristics of the pain may help to identify the source of the bleeding. Commonly, there is no pain.

None of these variations in the presentation of haematuria is sufficient in itself to diagnose the cause of bleeding, and all patients with haematuria need investigation *even if they are taking anticoagulant drugs*. In a significant proportion, all tests will be negative: the chance of finding a urological cause in patients under 40 years of age who are found to have micro-

Fig. 63.1 The more common causes of haematuria.

Bailey & Love's Short Practice of Surgery, 23rd edition. Edited by R.C.G. Russell, N.S. Williams and C.J.K. Bulstrode. Published in 2000 by Arnold Publishers.

scopic haematuria is particularly small. However, bleeding into the urinary tract may be caused by an occult nephropathy so it is important to check for hypertension in these patients.

Pain

Renal pain

Inflammation and acute obstruction to the flow of urine from the renal pelvis are liable to cause pain that is typically felt as a deep-seated, sickening ache in the loin. It is probably the result of stretching the capsule of the kidney. However, calculi in the kidney can also be painful in the absence of infection, although they may be too small or peripherally placed to cause obstruction. Slow-growing masses such as tumours or cysts are not usually painful unless they are very large. When the cause is inflammatory, there may be local deep tenderness and occasionally spasm of the psoas muscle.

Ureteric colic

This is an acute pain felt in the loin and radiating to the ipsilateral iliac fossa and genitalia. The patient often rolls around in agony as waves of excruciating sharp pain are imposed upon a continuing background of discomfort. Contrast this with the patient suffering from peritoneal pain who lies still to avoid exacerbating the pain by movement.

Ureteric colic is caused by the passage of a foreign body, usually a stone. The site of the pain can be a guide to the progress of the stone: the more the pain radiates into the groin, the more distal the stone. Local tenderness is much less than would be expected from the severity of the pain.

Bladder pain

Bladder pain is felt as a suprapubic discomfort made worse by bladder filling. In men, a sharp pain misleadingly referred to the tip of the penis may be the result of irritation of the trigone of the bladder. Severe inflammation of the bladder can cause an extreme wrenching discomfort at the end of micturition. This symptom of bladder stone was recognised by the old lithotomists who called it *strangury*.

Prostatic and seminal vesicle pain

This is felt as a penetrating ache in the perineum and rectum. There may be associated discomfort in the groin. The patient is characteristically exasperated and depressed by pain that has a peculiarly relentless nature. Pelvic pain is often blamed on 'chronic prostatitis' but it occurs in both men and women and is notoriously difficult to treat successfully.

Urethral pain

Urethral pain is a scalding or burning felt in the vulva or penis especially during voiding.

Altered bladder function

The normal bladder has two distinct phases of function. During the *filling phase* the bladder acts as a reservoir to collect urine until it is emptied in the *voiding phase*. Inappropriate contraction of the bladder detrusor muscle during filling (instability) is perceived as a sensation of *urgency* to pass urine. The patient may have *frequency* of micturition and a tendency to *urge incontinence*. Sleep may be disturbed by *nocturia*. Instability may be idiopathic in both sexes or part of the bladder response to outflow obstruction, notably in men with enlargement of the prostate. When detrusor instability has a demonstrable neurological cause, it is known as hyperreflexia.

Symptoms of impaired emptying are most commonly the result of bladder outflow obstruction, but detrusor failure or atony presents a similar picture. The patient has difficulty initiating voiding (*hesitancy*) and the stream is variable or slow. Abdominal straining improves the weak flow. When the act of micturition is completed there may be a feeling that urine remains in the bladder so the patient tries again (*pis-en-deux*). With time, the bladder becomes chronically overfilled and is unable to act as an effective reservoir. Urine spills out, typically at night when sleep halts constant trips to the lavatory (*chronic retention with overflow*).

Investigation of the urinary tract

With the exception of renal and scrotal masses or tenderness, a palpable bladder or an abnormal prostate on digital rectal examination, urological conditions are most likely to be diagnosed from the history or by investigations.

Urine

Dipsticks impregnated with chemicals which change colour in the presence of blood, protein or nitrites (Multistix; Labstix) are a convenient way to screen urine for the presence of abnormalities. When the urine is macroscopically clear and negative on dipstick testing the chances of finding an abnormality on microscopy and culture of a midstream clean-catch specimen are small. Indeed, some bacteriological laboratories decline further examination of the urine in these circumstances on the grounds that it is not cost-effective. The presence of protein and nitrites (which are a product of the activity of organisms in the urine) indicates the likelihood of infection. The significance of microscopic haematuria is discussed above. Some dipsticks also give an indication of the pH and specific gravity of the urine.

Microscopy is essential to confirm the presence of white and red blood cells in the urine, and bacteria may also be

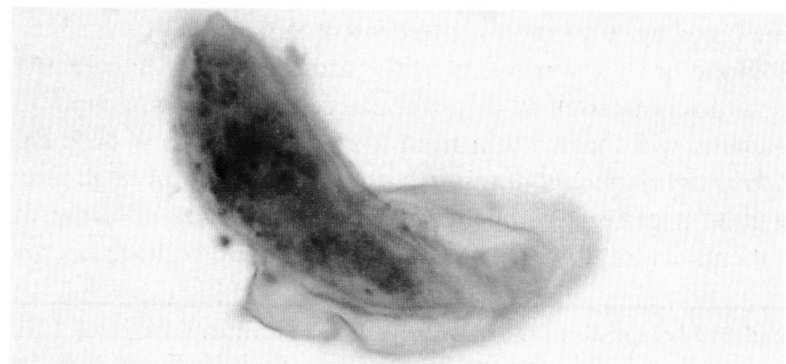

Fig. 63.2 Schistosoma ovum (*courtesy of Dr Nawal Derius*).

visible under light microscopy. The presence of protein casts suggests disease affecting the renal parenchyma, as does red cell dysmorphia seen on phase contrast microscopy. Schistosoma ova have a typical appearance (Fig. 63.2), and vegetable or meat fibres may be present if there is a fistula connecting the bowel with the urinary tract.

Cytological examination of the urinary sediment is sensitive and specific for poorly differentiated transitional cell tumours anywhere in the urinary tract. However, false negatives are common in the 50 per cent of these cancers that are well differentiated. A new chemical test (BTA-Bard©) detects a bladder tumour antigen in the urine, and its findings can complement cytological examination of the urine.

Bacteriological culture of a clean-catch midstream specimen of the urine is the standard means of identifying urinary pathogens. The presence of organisms at a level of 10^5/ml is deemed to indicate the presence of infection rather than contamination of the urine by bacteria. If there are pus cells in the urine but there is no growth on the routine culture media (sterile pyuria) it is worth testing for more fastidious organisms. The centrifuged sediment of multiple early-morning urine specimens must be cultured on Löwenstein–Jensen medium to detect urinary tract tuberculosis. Chlamydia is another common urinary pathogen that will not be detected on routine culture.

Biochemical examination for electrolytes, glucose, bilirubin, haemoglobin and myoglobin is essential to detect abnormal amounts of these substances in urine. Analysis of a 24-hour specimen of urine will quantify the rate of loss, and is especially useful in the investigation of calculus disease due to abnormal excretion of calcium, oxalate, uric acid and other products of metabolism.

Tests of renal function

More than 70 per cent of the kidney function must be lost before renal failure becomes evident: there is a large functional reserve. It follows that renal damage must be extensive before changes occur in blood constituents whose level is controlled by renal excretion. Such damage is of three main types: reduction of renal plasma flow, destruction of glomeruli or impairment of tubular function. In severe hypertension or renal artery stenosis, the plasma flow is impaired. In glomerulonephritis or acute cortical necrosis, there is a loss of glomeruli, while in pyelonephritis tubular function is most severely affected. In obstructive nephropathy, back-pressure on the renal parenchyma causes all three types of damage.

Levels of blood urea and serum creatinine can be affected by various factors but in practice, when taken together, they serve as a useful clinical guide to overall renal function. A creatinine clearance will give an approximate value for glomerular filtration rate but is prone to error. A more accurate assessment of glomerular function can be obtained from an estimate of the clearance of chromium-51-labelled ethylenediaminetetra-acetic acid. Surgeons will usually call on their nephrological colleagues for more detailed investigation of tubular function and renal blood flow.

The specific gravity of the urine is fixed at a low level when the kidney loses the power to concentrate because of renal tubular dysfunction. Estimation of urinary loss of sodium, β_2-microglobulin or the tubular enzyme *N*-acetyl-β-D-glucosamine (NAG) will further define the nature of functional impairment.

Radiology–contrast studies

A plain abdominal X-ray showing the kidneys, ureters and bladder (the KUB) can disclose a wealth of useful information. With the film properly orientated (with the liver on the right and gastric air-bubble on the left unless there is situs invertus!) a glance at the spine and bony structures may reveal the presence of scoliosis, spina bifida, degenerative disease of the spine, metastases, fractures and arthritis. All of these may have a relevance to the urological diagnosis. The soft-tissue shadows of the kidneys, outlined to a greater or lesser extent by their more radiolucent fatty coverings, overlie the upper attachments of the psoas muscles. A full bladder often presents a hazy outline arising from the pelvis.

Most urinary calculi absorb X-rays and should be sought in the region of the renal shadows and along the course of each ureter. This normally follows the tips of the transverse processes of the vertebrae, crosses the sacroiliac joints and heads for the ischial spine before hooking medially towards the bladder base. Stones with a low calcium content and those overlying bony structure may be difficult to see on the plain film. Pelvic phleboliths are very common and can look like lower ureteric calculi. Uric acid stones are the most common radiolucent calculi.

Intravenous urogram (urography; IVU) (Fig. 63.3)

Excretion renography has been a mainstay of urological investigation since the introduction of intravenous contrast

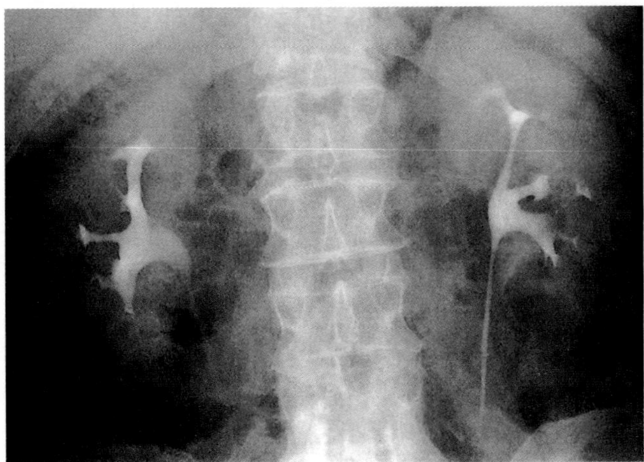

Fig. 63.3 Normal intravenous urogram showing the outline of both kidneys with the collecting system and upper ureters highlighted by the contrast medium.

Ernst Löwenstein, b. 1878. Pathologist, Vienna, Austria.
Carl Oluf Jensen, (1864–1934). Pathologist, Copenhagen, Denmark.

media in the 1930s. These are organic chemicals to which iodine atoms are attached to absorb X-rays. When injected, usually into a vein in the antecubital fossa, the substance is filtered from the blood by the glomeruli and does not undergo tubular absorption. As a result, it rapidly passes through the renal parenchyma into the urine which it renders radio-opaque.

Although the IVU gives excellent images of the urinary tract, its use should be restricted because in a few patients the iodine in the contrast medium may provoke a potentially life-threatening anaphylactic reaction. Patients with a history of allergy, atopy and eczema are particularly vulnerable, but severe reactions may occur without warning. Less invasive and dangerous imaging techniques are clearly to be preferred where they give comparable diagnostic information.

Preparation

It is usual to give a laxative to clear faeces that might otherwise obscure details of urinary tract anatomy. Modest fluid restriction is permissible but dehydration is dangerous because it may precipitate acute renal failure.

Technique

The patient is observed carefully while the first few drops of contrast medium (Urografin or Niopam 370) are injected. The earliest films, taken within minutes of the injection, show the renal parenchyma opacified by contrast medium – the nephrogram phase. A delayed nephrogram on one side indicates unilateral functional impairment. Distortion of the renal outline or failure of part of the kidney to function suggests a space-occupying lesion.

After a few minutes, the contrast is excreted into the collecting system opacifying the calyces and the renal pelvis. Later films show the ureters and, at the end of the study, the patient is asked to pass urine and a final film is taken to show detail of the bladder area. It is important to bear in mind that the static images of the IVU provide only snapshots of dynamic events in the urinary tract. The appearance of a normal ureter changes as peristaltic waves of contraction pass along it.

An IVU is particularly valuable to demonstrate tumours and calculi within the urinary tract which are sometimes difficult to see on ultrasonography. It may also be useful to show details of abnormal anatomy which are difficult to interpret on an ultrasonogram.

As ultrasonography and other forms of scanning have become more sophisticated, the indications for the urogram are fewer. Obstruction to the upper urinary tract interferes with transport of contrast medium into the urine which will show up as a nonfunctioning kidney on the standard urogram films. In these circumstances, a further radiograph taken many hours after injection of the contrast medium may show hazy opacification of a dilated system. Distortion of the calyces or the renal outline can equally be caused by a tumour or by harmless simple cysts. In each of these cases, more information can be obtained from ultrasonography or computerised tomography (CT).

Retrograde ureteropyelography (syn. retrograde ureterogram)

A fine ureteric catheter can be passed into the ureteric orifice through a cystoscope (Fig. 63.4). Contrast medium injected through the catheter will demonstrate the anatomy of the upper urinary tract. The procedure is particularly useful if there is doubt about an intraluminal lesion (Fig. 63.5) or if renal function is deficient (before surgery for pelviureteric junction obstruction, for instance). When a transitional tumour is found it can be sampled by aspiration of urine from

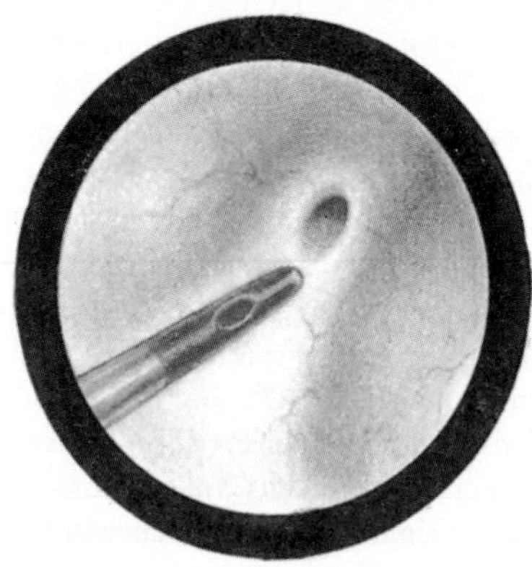

Fig. 63.4 A ureteric catheter about to enter the left ureteric orifice. Cystoscopic view.

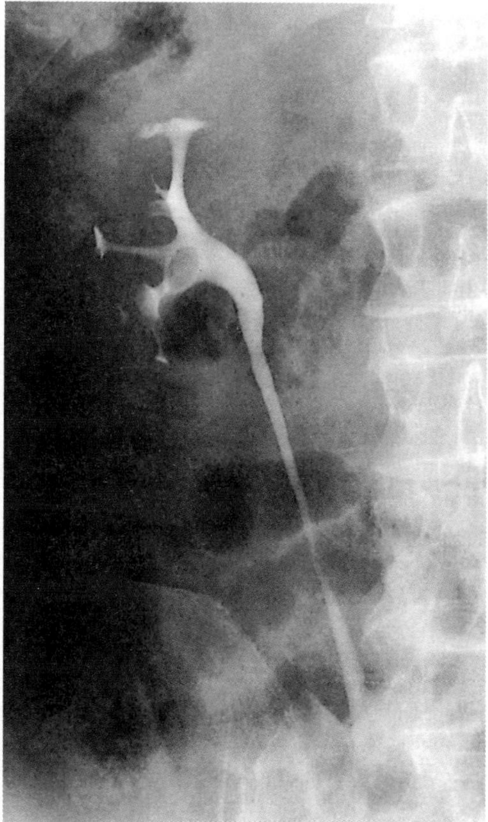

Fig. 63.5 Retrograde ureterogram demonstrating the collecting system. The radiolucent filling defect in the renal pelvis is caused by a uric acid calculus.

the upper tract or by brush biopsy. Retrograde ureteropyelography is possible under topical urethral anaesthesia using the flexible cystoscope.

Antegrade pyelography

Percutaneous puncture of a dilated renal collecting system is a reasonably simple procedure for the experienced interventional radiologist. The most common indication is the placement of a nephrostomy tube to drain an obstructed infected kidney or to provide access for percutaneous nephrolithotomy. Antegrade pyelography – where contrast medium is introduced through the nephrostomy – can be helpful when retrograde studies are prevented by obstruction at the extreme lower end of the ureter.

Digital subtraction arteriography (DSA)

Refinements in radiological imaging have now almost eliminated the need for translumbar aortography. Satisfactory imaging of the renal vessels can even be achieved by digital subtraction angiography after intravenous injection of contrast medium. More precise information can be obtained by intra-arterial injection through a fine catheter inserted into the femoral artery using the Seldinger technique. Arterography is now rarely used to demonstrate tumour vasculature in a hypernephroma (Fig. 63.6), but a flush venogram is useful when CT suggests tumour invasion of the renal vein and vena cava.

Cystography

Cystography is now most commonly a component of video-urodynamic assessment (see Chapter 65). Its role in assessing ureteric reflux in children has been largely superseded by radioisotope scanning and dynamic ultrasonography.

Urethrography

Ascending urethrography is valuable to demonstrate the extent of a urethral stricture (Fig. 63.7) and the presence of false passages and diverticula associated with it. A urethrogram can be used to assess the extent of urethral trauma, but there is a serious danger that contrast medium may pass into the circulation. Lipiodol carries the danger of fat embolus and should never be used, and death has followed the use of barium emulsion. Umbradil viscous V is a radio-opaque water-soluble gel that contains the local anaesthetic lignocaine. It can be injected gently and safely using Knutsson's apparatus even if the urotheium is breached.

Venography

Because extension of a renal carcinoma from the renal vein into the vena cava can usually be demonstrated by ultrasound or, venography is now infrequently used for this purpose.

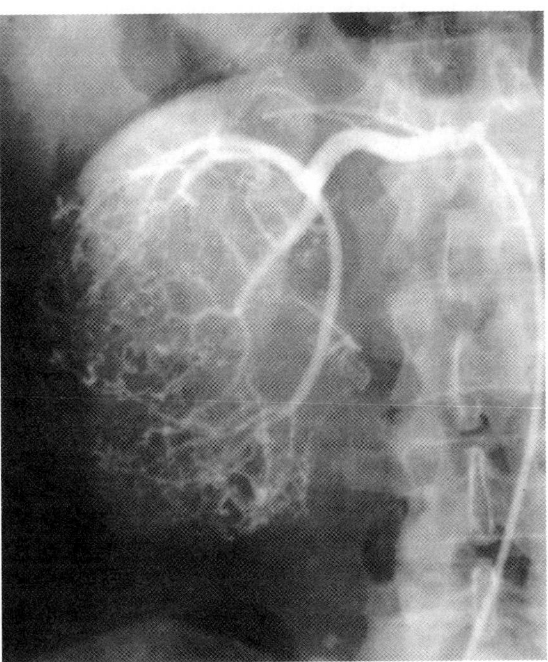

Fig. 63.6 A selective renal arteriogram showing abnormal vessels in a renal cell carcinoma.

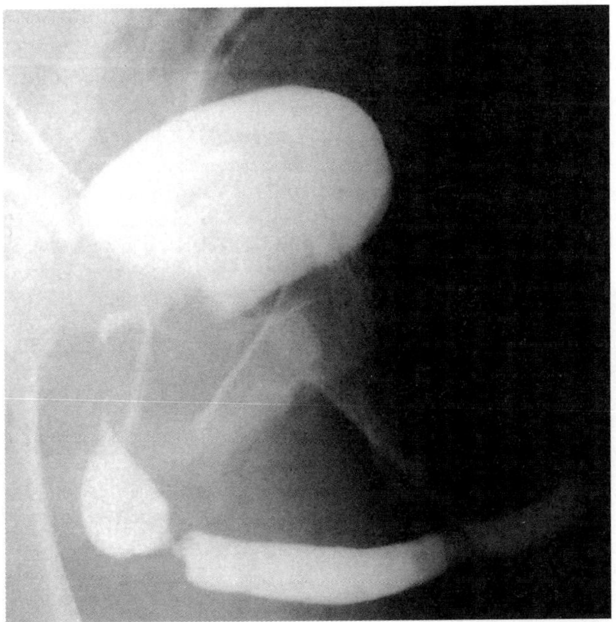

Fig. 63.7 Ascending urethrogram demonstrating a tight stricture in the bulbar urethra. Above the stricture the contrast outlines the prostatic urethra and bladder.

S.I. Seldinger, b. 1921. Swedish radiologist.

Folke Knutsson. Director, Roentgen Department, University Hospital, Uppsala, Sweden.

Ultrasonography

High-resolution ultrasonography is perhaps the imaging technique most widely used in urology. The size of the kidney, the thickness of its cortex, and the presence and degree of hydronephrosis can be measured with great accuracy. Intrarenal masses can be diagnosed as smooth walled and fluid filled (simple cysts) or solid and complex (possible tumours). The volume of urine in the bladder before and after micturition can be calculated, and even tiny filling defects within it detected. Scrotal contents can be displayed in great detail. Only the lower ureter resists effective investigation by transabdominal ultrasonography because of its small calibre and its proximity to the large bones of the pelvis and spine.

Transrectal ultrasonography

This has become a routine component of the investigation of suspected carcinoma of the prostate. Most commonly, suspicion has arisen because the patient has a raised prostate specific antigen or there is an abnormality of the texture or outline of the prostate on digital rectal examination. The features of carcinoma or benign enlargement of the prostate, while not absolutely specific, are sufficiently well recognised to allow an experienced ultrasonographer to identify promising sites for transrectal fine-needle biopsy.

Computerised tomography

CT is particularly useful to assess structures in the retroperitoneum (Fig. 63.8). In renal carcinoma it will show:

- the size and site of the tumour and the degree of invasion of adjacent tissue;
- the presence of enlarged lymph nodes at the renal hilum;
- invasion of the renal vein and vena cava.

CT is of crucial importance in the initial staging and follow-up of men with testicular cancer in whom the presence of retroperitoneal lymph node masses is a feature of advanced disease. It has also been used to stage bladder and prostate cancer, but its value is less clear cut in these diseases.

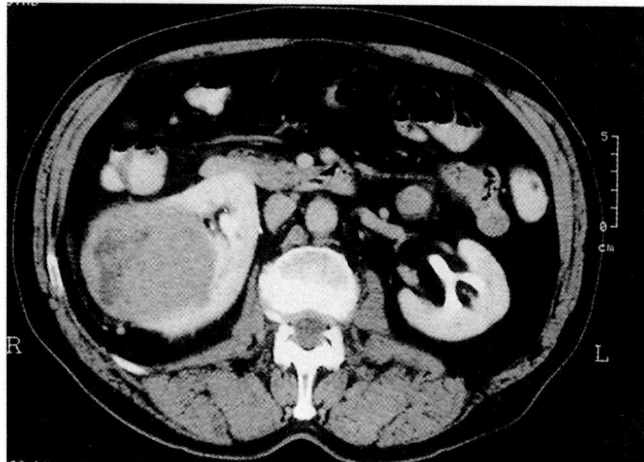

Fig. 63.8 Computerised tomography showing a renal cell carcinoma of the right kidney. (Note: scans are read as viewed from the feet of the patient.)

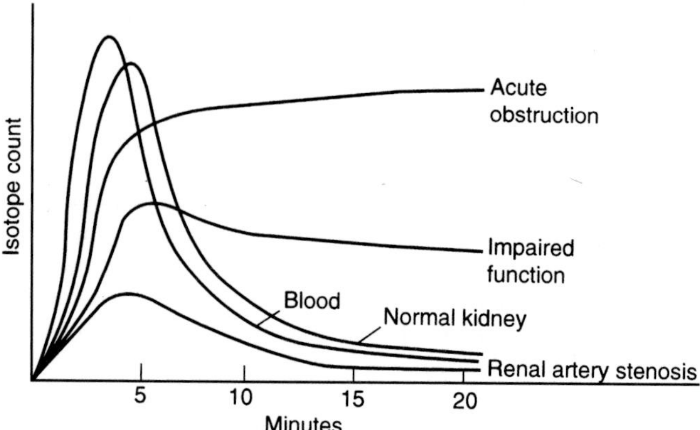

Fig. 63.9 Radioisotope renogram.

Magnetic resonance imaging

In the investigation of renal, bladder and prostatic disease, magnetic resonance imaging is not clearly superior to good-quality CT. Positron emission tomography may prove to be more valuable in staging urological maligancies.

Radioisotope scanning

Radioisotope scanning is used in particular to obtain information about function in individual renal units. Diethyltriaminepentacetic acid (DTPA) behaves in the kidney like inulin: it is filtered by the glomeruli and not absorbed by the tubules. Using a gamma camera, DTPA labelled with technetium-99m can be followed during its transit through individual kidneys to give dynamic representation of renal function. A ^{99m}Tc-DTPA scan is particularly useful to prove that collecting system dilatation is due to obstruction. In obstruction, radioactivity will remain in the kidney even if urine flow is stimulated by administration of a diuretic. Other substances (DMSA, MAG-3 and Hippuran) labelled with suitable radioactive isotopes have similarly been used to investigate renal function (Fig. 63.9).

Isotope bone scanning is fundamental to staging kidney and prostate cancers which typically metastasise to the skeleton.

Endoscopy

Effective visual inspection of the lower urinary tract has been possible since 1877 when Nitze invented his cystoscope. A second leap forward in urological endoscopy came with the introduction by Hopkins of the rod-lens telescope and fibre-optic illumination. This permitted the development of a family of endoscopes which allow the urologist to visualise the upper and lower urinary tract for diagnosis and therapy. Finally, in the early 1980s, the small-calibre flexible fibrescopic cystoscope was introduced. This allows simple diagnostic cystourethroscopy, bladder biopsy and retrograde ureterography to be performed under topical urethral anaesthesia with minimal discomfort to the patient.

Anuria

Anuria is defined as the complete absence of urine production. Oliguria is present when less than 300 ml of urine is excreted in a day.

Max Nitze, Professor of Urology, Berlin, Germany. In 1877, Nitze, in conjunction with Beneche, an optician of Vienna, produced the first cystoscope.

Sir Frederick Gowland Hopkins, 1861–1947. British biochemist.

The maintenance of renal function and urine production depends upon perfusion of the kidneys with oxygenated blood. Reduced renal blood flow or hypoxia impairs renal function. When both are present, the danger of acute renal failure is even greater.

Renal failure is traditionally divided into:

- prerenal;
- renal;
- postrenal (obstructive).

Prerenal

Prerenal cause of acute renal failure include:

- hypovolaemia;
- blood loss;
- sepsis;
- cardiogenic shock;
- anaesthesia;
- hypoxia.

Hypovolaemia

This may result from inadequate fluid intake or from excessive loss of body water. Dehydration, prolonged vomiting, diarrhoea and other abnormal gastrointestinal fluid losses, burns and excessive sweating are all common causes of hypovolaemia.

Blood loss

This is usually caused by trauma or surgery, but acute blood loss from the gastrointestinal tract or associated with childbirth may be sufficient to cause hypovolaemic renal impairment.

Sepsis

Gram-negative septicaemia from a urinary tract source is a particularly potent cause of bacteraemic shock. Sepsis from the biliary tract and overwhelming infection from other sites, especially in the immunocompromised individual, are also associated with acute renal failure.

Cardiogenic shock

Acute dysrhythmia secondary to myocardial infarction, cardiac tamponade and pulmonary embolus may all result in the reduced cardiac output of often poorly oxygenated blood.

Anaesthesia

Hypotension is a hazard of epidural and spinal anaesthesia.

Hypoxia

Prolonged hypoxia from any cause may occasionally be responsible.

Hans Christian Joachim Gram, 1853–1938. Professor of Medicine, Copenhagen, Denmark.

Renal

Renal causes of acute renal failure include:

- drugs;
- poisons;
- contrast media;
- eclampsia;
- myoglobinuria;
- incompatible blood transfusion;
- disseminated intravascular coagulation.

It is uncommon for patients with established glomerulo-nephritis to develop acute oliguria; however, such patients are more prone to rapid deterioration of remaining renal function should any renal insult occur.

Drugs

Aminoglycosides, cephalosporins and diuretics can be nephrotoxic particularly if used in combination. They are quite commonly used in patients whose renal function is already compromised by sepsis or circulatory abnormalities. Prolonged use of nonsteroidal anti-inflammatory drugs (NSAIDs) can cause a chronic interstitial nephritis and papillary necrosis; they also reduce renal plasma flow and therefore have nephrotoxic properties. Angiotensin-converting enzyme inhibitors used for the control of hypertension can cause a rapid reduction in the glomerular filtration rate; this is particularly liable to occur in patients who have a reduced renal blood flow.

Poisons

Some of these are nephrotoxic.

Contrast media

Even modern contrast media may cause renal failure when injected into a dehydrated patient with compromised renal function.

Eclampsia

The early recognition of pre-eclampsia is vital to avoid the nephrotoxic consequences of toxaemia and uncontrolled hypertension.

Myoglobinuria

The presence of myoglobin in the urine is associated with the 'crush' syndrome after major trauma. Less severe injuries can also cause the syndrome, especially if a compartment syndrome is unrecognised or pressure areas break down.

Incompatible blood transfusion

This may lead to renal failure with myoglobinuria.

Disseminated intravascular coagulation

Disseminated intravascular coagulation usually follows major sepsis or massive blood transfusion and may occur postpartum.

Obstructive

Obstructive causes of acute renal failure include:

- calculi;
- pelvic malignancy;
- surgery;
- retroperitoneal fibrosis;
- bilharzia;
- crystaluria.

Calculi

Renal calculus disease is probably the most common cause of acute obstruction leading to anuria. The patient is likely to have unilateral renal colic against a background of nonfunction of the contralateral kidney, often due to previous surgery or pre-existing obstruction by calculus.

Pelvic malignancy

Carcinomas arising from the bladder, prostate, cervix, ovary or rectum can all lead to obstruction of one or both ureters. A history of haematuria and vaginal or rectal bleeding signpost the diagnosis. A large pelvic mass is commonly palpable on bimanual examination.

Surgery

The ureters are vulnerable to damage during pelvic and retroperitoneal surgery but injury should be avoided if proper care is taken. It is unusual, but not impossible, to damage both ureters.

Retroperitoneal fibrosis

For details of retroperitoneal fibrosis see Chapter 64 on 'The kidneys and the ureters'.

Bilharzia

Schistosomiasis may lead to ureteric fibrosis and stenosis, and may be responsible for the development of squamous cell carcinoma of the bladder.

Crystaluria

Crystaluria causing urinary tract obstruction used to be associated with sulphonomide medications. This is now rare. However, uric acid crystaluria can develop in patients receiving chemotherapy for leukaemia or lymphoma unless they are given prophylactic treatment with allopurinol.

Clinical aspects

Answers to the following questions should indicate the probable cause of reduced urine output.

Is urine being produced? Catheterisation of the bladder is mandatory if a voided sample cannot be obtained. If urine is available check the specific gravity, look for the presence of casts (implying a renal cause), test for myoglobinuria and send some for culture and microscopy.

Is there an obvious prerenal cause? This can usually be answered by clinical examination, assessment of the patient's vital signs, examination of the fluid balance chart and measurement of the arterial oxygen concentration.

Is there ureteric obstruction? Hydronephrosis may not be marked in acute obstruction, but ultrasonography will usually show some degree of ureteric dilatation. A plain abdominal radiograph should be checked for calculi.

What drugs have been given recently? If a drug is thought to be responsible for renal impairment it should obviously be withdrawn unless its use is vital.

Is this a progression to chronic renal failure? The presence of shrunken kidneys on ultrasound, normochromic anaemia and hypertension suggest progression to a chronic state even if a previous history of renal failure is not available.

Management and treatment

Renal failure caused by acute tubular necrosis may progress through three recognisable phases:

- oliguria;
- the diuretic phase;
- recovery.

The initial management is aimed at prompt restoration of circulating volume deficit and correction of tissue hypoxia. Most patients will require a level of care available only in a specialised unit. As a minimum, monitoring with a pulse oximeter and central venous pressure measurement will supplement basic observations. For patients with hypovolaemia or sepsis, inotropic support with dopamine may improve cardiac efficiency and increase renal blood flow. If urine production is not promptly restored, frusemide can be given but this is not always successful and the drug is itself associated with nephrotoxicity. Mannitol may be used as a plasma expander and osmotic diuretic, but care must be taken not to overload the circulation. The aim is to achieve the best possible blood pressure with a central venous pressure of 7–9 cmH_2O. One-hundred per cent oxygen may be needed to maintain the oxygen tension (PO_2).

If these measures fail, acute tubular necrosis has supervened. Excess fluid loads must be avoided and fluid input restricted to match the reduced output plus insensible losses (500–800 ml per 24 hours depending on ambient conditions). Abnormal losses due to vomiting, nasogastric aspiration, diarrhoea or fistulae will be monitored and replaced.

A hyperkalaemic acidosis is the characteristic metabolic abnormality of the oliguric phase of renal failure. Correction of the metabolic acidosis with intravenous bicarbonate is tempting but not always advisable. Rising serum potassium is life threatening and requires effective intervention. A calcium resonium enema is the simplest remedy. The ion-exchange resin can also be administered orally but is unpalatable. Cautious use of intravenous dextrose and insulin should be considered if ion exchange fails. The help of a renal physician is highly desirable.

The diuretic phase traditionally occurs between the 8th and 10th day but may be delayed as long as 6 weeks. Glomerular filtration recommences but tubular function takes longer to recover. A heavy loss of sodium and potassium can be expected, and fluid and electrolyte requirements must be carefully judged. In most patients, the diuretic phase is followed by the recovery phase but some never recover and will need renal replacement therapy if they are to survive.

Factors that influence the outcome of acute renal failure include the need for artificial ventilation, the need for inotropic support and the presence of jaundice. There is a significant mortality.

Nutritional support

Many of these patients are unable to eat. If enteral feeding is impossible, parenteral nutrition must be administered with extreme care to avoid circulatory overload.

Infection

These patients are at increased risk of generalised infection. Swabs taken from the nose and throat, sputum specimens and urine, if available, should be sent for culture. If antibiotics are required, they should be nonnephrotoxic.

General nursing care

Meticulous recording of fluid balance is obviously central to successful management of these patients. Patients who are seriously ill or comatose need regular turning and care to pressure areas if they are to avoid pressure sores. Physiotherapy to the chest and extremities will aid recovery.

Renal support

Renal replacement is needed for those patients in whom the oliguric or anuric phase is associated with significant uraemic symptoms (vomiting, muscular twitching, itching and altered states of consciousness) or uncontrollable hyperkalaemia.

Peritoneal dialysis. Provided that the patient has not had recent abdominal surgery, peritoneal dialysis can be performed by insertion of a fenestrated catheter under local anaesthesic. This is placed just inferior to the umbilicus in the mid-line. Sterile dialysis fluid is then run into the peritoneal cavity where it equilibrates with the extracellular fluid using the peritoneum as a dialysis membrane. After a variable time, the fluid is drained into a closed drainage system. The process is repeated in cycles. Occasionally, when anuria is prolonged, a Tenckhoff cuffed catheter needs to be inserted, as used in chronic ambulatory peritoneal dialysis. The disadvantages of acute peritoneal dialysis are the potential for introducing infection into the peritoneum and the rather slow rate of correcting metabolic imbalance, particularly hyperkalaemia.

Haemodialysis. A few sessions of haemodialysis may be life saving. A double-lumen catheter is placed over a guidewire into the one of the great veins (jugular, subclavian or femoral). Between sessions of dialysis, the lines are kept patent by filling them with heparin solution. Haemodialysis can result in a rapid correction of metabolic abnormalities but also tends to result in considerable fluctuations of the overall fluid balance. The other disadvantage is that heparinisation is necessary, and this may be undesirable after a recent surgical procedure.

Haemofiltration. This, like haemodialysis, requires the use of an extracorporeal machine but causes much less haemodynamic upset. This may be of critical importance for the acutely ill patient.

Obstructive renal failure

When the patient is too ill for surgery to remove the cause of obstruction to the upper urinary tract, the treatment of obstructive renal impairment is drainage either externally using a nephrostomy or internally using an indwelling stent.

Percutaneous nephrostomy. Under ultrasonographic guidance and local anaesthetic, a fine-bore hollow needle is introduced via the flank through the parenchyma and into the expanded collecting system of the obstructed kidney. Once it penetrates the system, contrast medium can be

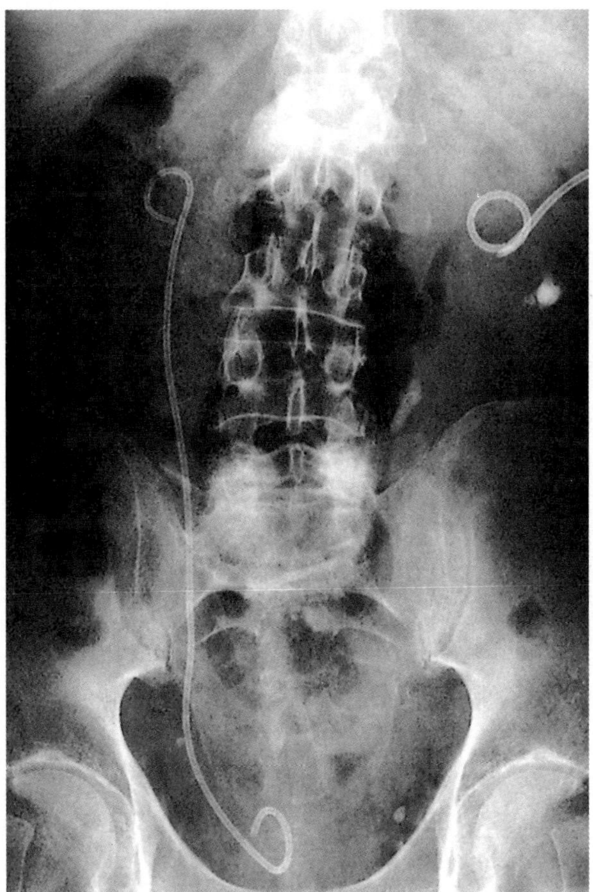

Fig. 63.10 Radiograph showing left-sided, pigtail nephrostomy tube draining a kidney obstructed by a ureteric calculus seen at the level of L3–4. A J-stent is in the right ureter, which has been cleared of stones.

injected through the needle to define its exact position. A wire passed through the lumen of the needle is used to guide the insertion of a series of dilators which enlarge the track until it will accept a suitably sized nephrostomy tube (Fig. 63.10). This will drain urine and pus, provided that the latter is not too viscous. The tube is anchored firmly in place to allow continued drainage as renal function recovers.

Insertion of a J-stent. The ureter can be drained into the bladder by the insertion of a pigtail- or J-stent (see Fig. 63.10). The procedure begins with a retrograde ureterogram under fluoroscopic control to provide an image of ureter. This will often give an indication of the cause of the obstruction. A guidewire is introduced through the ureteric orifice and guided up the ureter into the renal pelvis. The stent is rail-roaded over the guidewire until its distal end also lies within the renal pelvis above the obstruction. When the guidewire is removed, the ends of the stent curl to form a J-shape or a pigtail to secure the device against migration. Stents can be placed under topical urethral anaesthesia using the flexible cystoscope and may be safely left in position for several months. They are a foreign body in the urinary tract and are prone to infection and encrustation if neglected. It is vital to keep careful records to account for all stents inserted.

If the J-stent cannot be inserted cystoscopically, it may be placed from above through a nephrostomy.

Open surgery. This is a rarity when the minimally invasive methods described above are available. Retrograde insertion of a nephrostomy through an incision in the renal pelvis is the preferred method because it can be surprisingly difficult to locate even dilated calyces by blind puncture of the renal parenchyma.

Further reading

Blandy, J.P. (1995) *Lecture Notes in Urology,* 5th edn, Blackwell Science, Oxford.

Walsh, P.C., Retik, A.B., Darracott Vaughan, E. and Wein, A.J. (1998) *Campbell's Urology*, 7th edn, W.B. Saunders, Philadelphia, PA.

Whitfield, H.W., Hendry, W.F., Kirby, R.S. and Duckett J. (1998) *Textbook of Genito-urinary Surgery*, 2nd edn, Blackwell Science, Oxford.

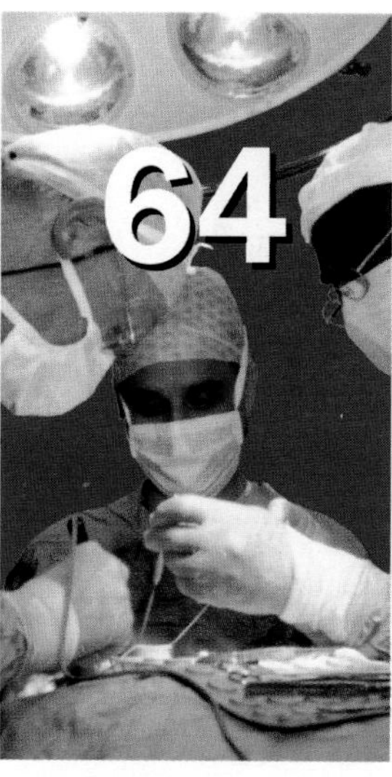

64 The kidneys and ureters

Embryology

A bud from the lower end of the mesonephric (Wolffian) duct grows backwards behind the peritoneum to the sacral region. The stalk of the bud forms the ureter and its dilated upper extremity the renal pelvis. From 6 weeks to 8 months, the primitive pelvis bifurcates repeatedly to form first the calyces and, after several subsequent divisions, the collecting ducts.

The renal parenchyma is derived from the metanephros which is the last in a series of embryonic renal masses: the primitive pronephros is supplanted by the mesonephros which is in turn succeeded by the metanephros. The continuity of glomerular apparatus and nephric tubules formed within the metanephros is established through connection with the collecting ducts. Between weeks 5 and 8 of embryonic development, each kidney ascends the posterior abdominal wall to reach its normal position in the loin. At the same time, it rotates so that its hilum faces medially instead of forwards as it did previously.

In humans the lobulation of the foetal kidney is usually lost as the lobules become bonded together by the growth of new cortex and the renal capsule. In some mammals, e.g. oxen and bears, foetal lobulation is retained.

Surgical anatomy

The parenchyma of each kidney usually drains into seven calyces, three in the upper and two each in the middle and lower calyces (Fig. 64.1). Each of the three segments represents an anatomical and physiologically distinct unit with its own blood supply.

Kaspar Friedrich Wolff, 1733–94. Professor of Anatomy and Physiology, St Petersburg, Russia.

Bailey & Love's Short Practice of Surgery, 23rd edition. Edited by R.C.G. Russell, N.S. Williams and C.J.K. Bulstrode. Published in 2000 by Arnold Publishers.

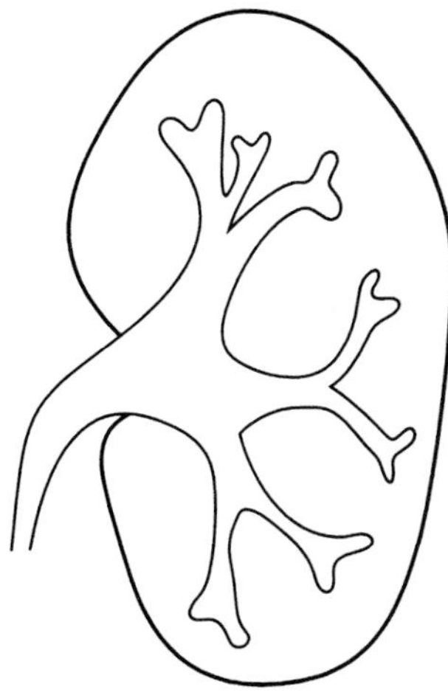

Fig. 64.1 The arrangement of renal calyces.

Congenital abnormalities of the kidney (Table 64.1)

Absence of one kidney

Congenital aplasia of one kidney is usually discovered incidentally on intravenous urography, computerised tomography (CT) scan or renal ultrasonography. If the mesonephric duct has failed to bud, the ureter will be absent and on cystoscopy no ureteric orifice is visible on that side. Alternatively, the ureter and renal pelvis are present but the kidney is

Table 64.1 Congenital abnormalities of the kidney and ureter

Renal aplasia	
Renal ectopia	Pelvic kidney
	Horseshoe kidney
	Crossed dystopia
Cystic disease	Polycystic kidneys
	Infantile polycystic disease
	Unilateral multicystic disease
	Solitary cyst
Aberrant renal vessels	Multiple renal arteries and veins
Duplication	Duplex kidney
	Duplex renal pelvis
	Duplex kidney and ureter
Others	Retrocaval ureter
	Congenital megaureter

absent or almost so. In either case the solitary contralateral kidney is likely to be hypertrophied. An absent or grossly atrophic kidney is found in about 1:1400 individuals.

Renal ectopia

In approximately 1:1000 people the kidney does not ascend. Ectopic kidneys are usually found near the pelvic brim and, for reasons which are not understood, they are usually left sided. The contralateral kidney is generally present and in its normal position. Renal ectopia may present diagnostic problems when acute disease develops in the kidney and there is always a danger that an unwary surgeon may be tempted to remove it as an unexplained pelvic mass.

Horseshoe kidney

If the most medial subdivisions of the mesonephric bud meet and fuse in the midline, the normal ascent of the kidneys is impeded by structures arising in the midline. The result is a pair of ectopic kidneys that are usually fused at their lower poles with the junction in front of the fourth lumbar vertebra. Horseshoe kidney is found in 1:1000 necropsies and is more common in men. Fusion of the upper poles is uncommon.

Clinical features

Horseshoe kidneys are liable to become diseased, possibly because the ureters are angulated as they pass over the fused isthmus (Fig. 64.2). This may lead to urinary stasis with consequent infection and nephrolithiasis. More commonly, there is a true pelviureteric junction obstruction as an associated abnormality, with the same consequences. Presentation as a fixed mass below the umbilicus is uncommon and horseshoe kidney is usually a radiological diagnosis. The most frequent appearance on the urogram shows the lower pole calyces on both sides being directed towards the midline. More rarely, all or most of the calyces are reversed (Fig. 64.3). The ureters characteristically have vase-like curves. Although horseshoe kidney is not a contraindication to pregnancy, urinary complications are more frequent.

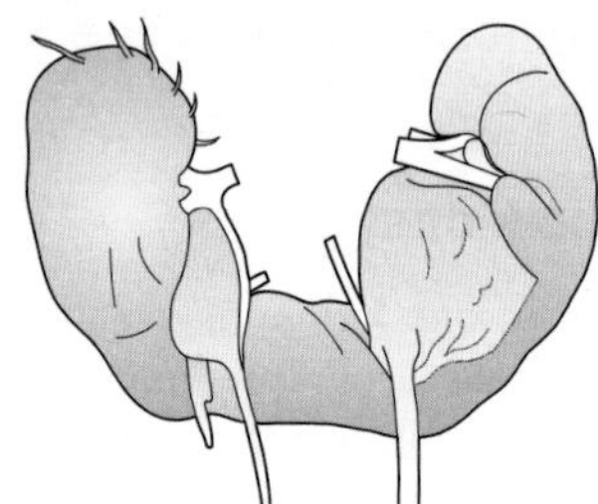

Fig. 64.2 Horseshoe kidney. Note the ureters passing in front of the fused lower poles.

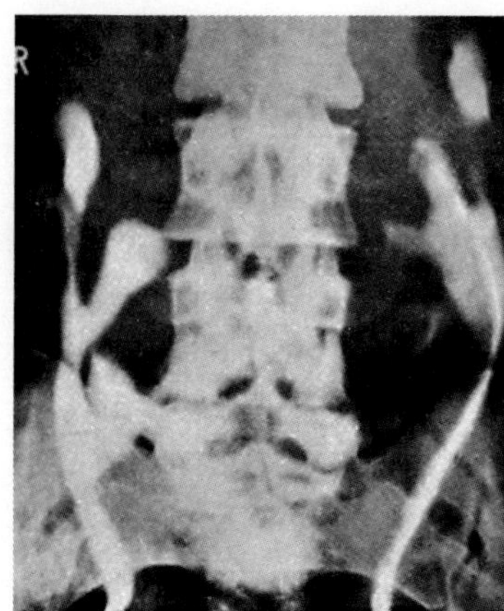

Fig. 64.3 Urogram of a horseshoe kidney. Only rarely are all the calyces directed towards the spinal column.

Division of the isthmus between the kidneys is usually only indicated in the course of surgery for abdominal aortic aneurysm. Although the tissue is likely to be less vascular than normal renal parenchyma, care must be taken to avoid the vascular supply of the horseshoe which is typically eccentric, springing unpredictably from adjacent major vessels.

Unilateral fusion

Unilateral fusion (syn. crossed dystopia) is rare but the urogram appearance is striking. Both kidneys are in one loin and are usually fused. The ureter of the lower kidney crosses the midline to enter the bladder on the contralateral side. Both renal pelves can lie one above each other medial to the renal parenchyma (unilateral long kidney) or the pelvis of the crossed kidney faces laterally [unilateral S-shaped kidney (Fig. 64.4)].

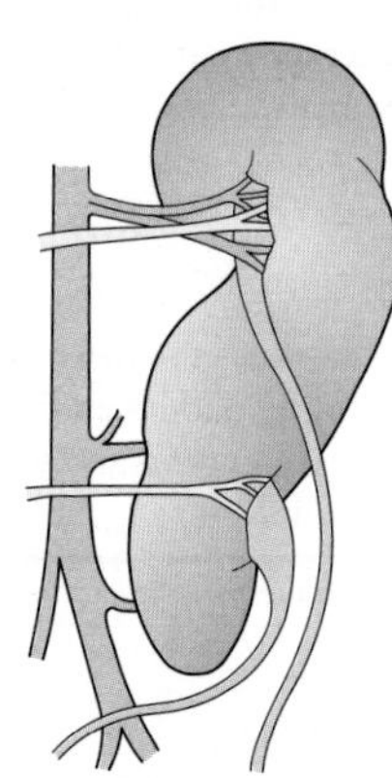

Fig. 64.4 Unilateral S-fusion of the kidneys.

Congenital cystic kidneys (syn. polycystic kidneys)

Polycystic kidneys are hereditary and can be transmitted by either parent as an autosomal dominant trait. This is important in genetic counselling because the risk of an offspring inheriting the condition can be as high as one in two depending upon the penetrance of the gene. The disease is not usually detectable on standard imaging until the second and third decades of life and does not usually manifest itself clinically before the age of 30 years.

Pathology

The kidneys become enormously enlarged, the cysts giving the appearance of a collection of bubbles below the renal capsule. On histological section the renal parenchyma is riddled with cysts of varying size, containing clear fluid, thick brown material or coagulated blood. In 18 per cent of cases there is a congenital cystic liver disease. The pancreas and lungs are occasionally affected as well. The aetiology of all renal cysts is uncertain although theories abound.

Clinical features in the adult

The condition is slightly more common in women than men. There are six clinical features:

- irregular upper quadrant abdominal mass;
- loin pain;
- haematuria;
- infection;
- hypertension;
- uraemia.

Renal enlargement. The bilateral knobbly enlargement can hardly be mistaken when discovered in the course of a routine examination. Less florid examples may be revealed at laparotomy or abdominal imaging for some other condition. *Unilateral renal swelling,* in which one kidney contains larger cysts than the other, may be confused clinically with a cystic renal tumour.

Pain, felt as dull loin ache, is thought to be caused by the weight of the organ dragging upon its pedicle or by stretching of the renal capsule by the cysts. Haemorrhage into a cyst may cause more severe pain, as may the passage of a calculus from the diseased kidney.

Haematuria. Rupture of a cyst into the renal pelvis may cause haematuria which is typically moderate, lasts for a few days and recurs at intervals. Profuse haematuria is uncommon.

Infection. Pyelonephritis is common in patients with congenital cystic kidney, presumably because of urinary stasis.

Hypertension is present in up to 75 per cent of patients over the age of 20 years with polycystic kidneys. Why some escape this complication is not clear; the high blood pressure could possibly result from a separate genetic factor linked to the gene for congenital cystic kidneys.

Uraemia. Patients with congenital cystic kidneys pass large volumes of urine of low specific gravity (1.010 or less) which contains a trace of albumin but no casts or cells. Chronic renal failure develops as functioning renal tissue is replaced progressively by cysts. The patient complains of anorexia, headache and vague abdominal discomfort. As the symptoms are nonspecific the diagnosis may be missed until drowsiness and vomiting result from the biochemical derangement. Severe anaemia is common. Signs of end-stage renal failure often begin suddenly during middle life and the patient is unlikely to survive without renal replacement by dialysis or renal transplantation.

Imaging

Ultrasound and CT will show multiple cysts in both kidneys, and sometimes cysts in the liver and other organs. The presence of blood and debris in the cysts may mimic the heterogeneity of a cystic adenocarcinoma. By contrast, simple (acquired) cysts are usually solitary and have smooth thin walls and homogeneous contents (Fig. 64.5). Doubt about the diagnosis can be resolved by cytological examination of cyst fluid obtained by fine needle aspiration.

Polycystic kidneys have a typical appearance on excretory urography: the renal shadows are enlarged in all directions; the renal pelvis is compressed and elongated; and the calyces are stretched over the cysts and are often narrow (like spiders' legs) or bell-like (Fig. 64.6).

Treatment

Renal failure. As kidney failure develops, a low protein diet will help to postpone the need for renal replacement. Infection, anaemia and disturbances of calcium metabolism need appropriate treatment, usually by a nephrologist.

Surgical treatment to uncap the cysts (Rovsing's operation) is rarely indicated because few surgeons now accept that this can preserve renal function by relieving pressure on the parenchyma. If cysts are to be decapped in the hope of reducing pain, the operation can be done laparoscopically.

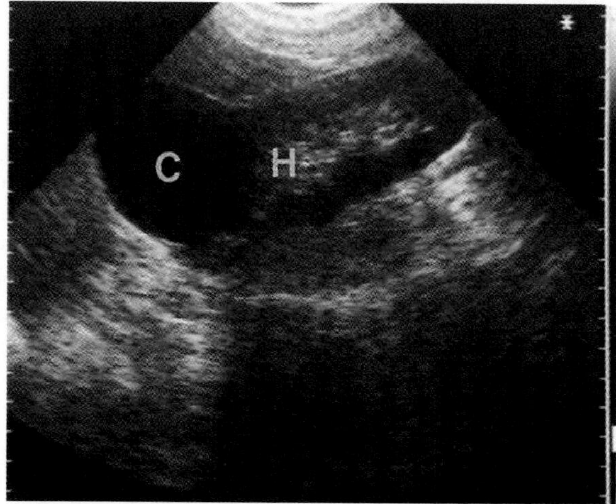

Fig. 64.5 Simple cyst of lower pole shown on longitudinal ultrasound scan of the kidney.

Nils Thorkild Rovsing, 1862–1927. Professor of Surgery, Copenhagen, Denmark.

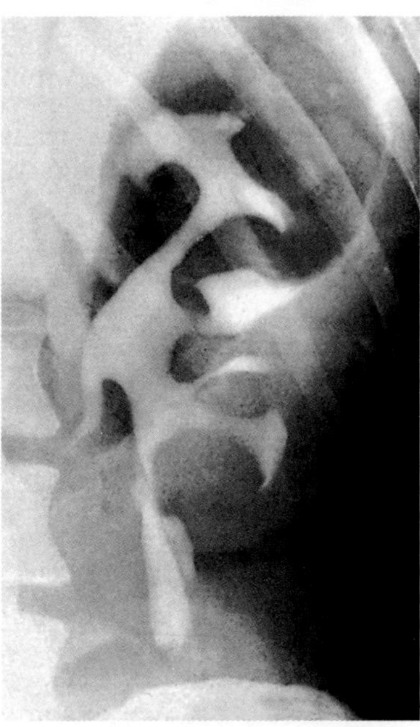

Fig. 64.6 Polycystic kidney: urographic appearance. Note length of the kidney and bell-like calyces stretched over the cysts.

Infantile polycystic disease

Infantile polycystic disease is an unrelated and much rarer condition. The kidneys are large and may obstruct birth. Many cases are stillborn and most of the others die from renal failure early in life. The condition is inherited as an autosomal recessive.

Unilateral multicystic disease

Unilateral multicystic disease is much more common. It presents as a nonfunctioning mass in the flank. Exploration and removal is the treatment of choice. In the differential diagnosis, Wilms' tumour (see below), neuroblastoma and congenital hydronephrosis are all rarer conditions.

Solitary renal cyst (syn. simple cyst of the kidney) (Fig. 64.5)

The term 'solitary' cyst serves to distinguish the condition from congenital cystic disease of the kidneys, but more than one cyst is often present in one or both kidneys. Simple cysts are most frequently discovered incidentally on imaging of the upper abdomen: they rarely give symptoms. A palpable mass, pain from haemorrhage into the cyst and infection are relatively uncommon presentations. Occasionally a cyst in the hilum of the kidney (a parapelvic cyst) presses on the pelviureteric junction and causes obstructive symptoms.

When discovered as a filling defect on excretion urography the true nature of a solitary cyst will be apparent by its characteristic appearance on ultrasound or CT. Percutaneous cyst puncture will yield fluid for cytological examination but this is rarely necessary with sophisticated modern imaging.

Max Wilms, 1867–1918. Professor of Surgery, Heidelberg, Germany.

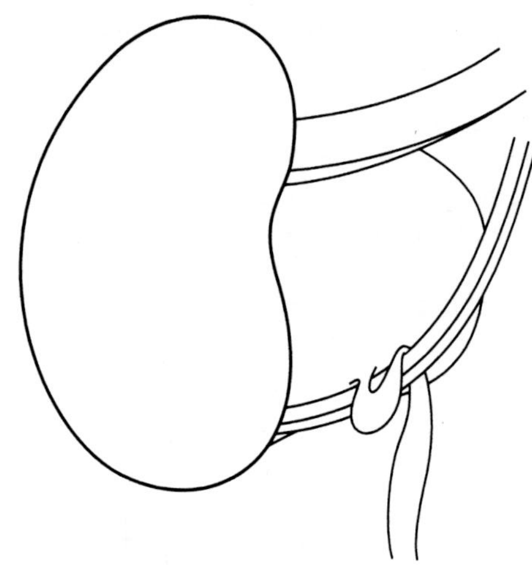

Fig. 64.7 Aberrant accessory renal artery with hydronephrosis. The dilated renal pelvis bulges over the vessel.

Differential diagnosis

In sheep-rearing districts, *hydatid cyst of the kidney* is common. On the right side if hydatid disease is suspected the swelling is liable to be mistaken for hydatid cyst of the liver. Occasionally, the patient complains of passing 'grape skins' (ruptured daughter cysts) in the urine. Removal of the cyst must follow the principles used in excision of hydatid cyst of the liver, i.e. the scolices must be killed by injection of a scolicide-like formalin solution before the cyst is handled. If the cyst is large nephrectomy may be the safest course.

Aberrent renal vessels

Two or more renal arteries are most common on the left. The main importance of the abnormality is as a source of potential error during operations in the retroperitoneum, especially those on the kidney. The renal arteries are functional end arteries so division of an aberrant lower pole artery will lead to infarction of the section of parenchyma that it supplies. Renal veins, by contrast, have extensive collaterals and an aberrant *vein* can be divided with impunity. Aberrant vessels probably do not cause hydronephrosis, although a hydronephrotic renal pelvis may bulge between renal vessels, making them particularly noticeable (Fig. 64.7).

Congenital abnormalities of the renal pelvis and ureter

Duplication of a renal pelvis

Duplication of a renal pelvis (Fig. 64.8) is the most common congenital abnormality of the upper renal tract and is found in about 4 per cent of patients. It is usually unilateral and is slightly more common on the left. The upper renal pelvis is relatively small and drains the upper group of calyces; the larger lower renal pelvis drains the middle and lower groups of calyces.

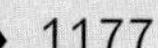

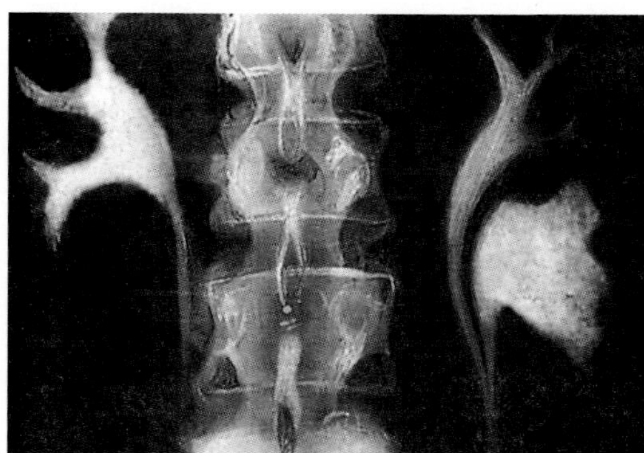

Fig. 64.8 Urograms showing left kidney with double pelvis.

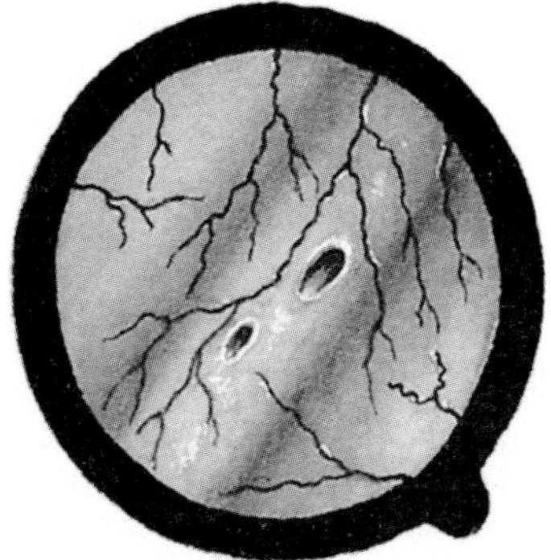

Fig. 64.10 Complete ureteric duplication. Two ureteric orifices seen on cystoscopy: the lower and more medial drains the upper renal pelvis.

Duplication of a ureter

Duplication of a ureter is found in about 3 per cent of excretion urograms. The ureters often join before they reach the bladder, usually in the lower third of their course (Fig. 64.9) and have a common ureteric orifice. Less commonly the ureters open independently into the bladder, in which case the ureter from the upper pelvis opens distal and medial to its fellow (Fig. 64.10).

Clinical features

Duplication of the renal pelvis or ureter is often a chance finding on renal imaging but infection, calculus formation and pelviureteric junction obstruction are more common than in normal kidneys. One of the moieties may be dysplastic and nonfunctioning. Where the two ureters open separately, the lower orifice is liable to be abnormal in function or position. Failure of the normal valvular mechanism at the ureterovesical junction may lead to urinary reflux and, if there is associated infection, damage to the parenchyma of the upper moiety. An ectopic second ureteric opening is a rarity but it may cause puzzling symptoms.

In the female an ectopic ureter opens either into the urethra below the sphincter (Fig. 64.11) or into the vagina. The diagnosis can often be made from the history alone and is confirmed by excretion urography. A girl or woman who has dribbled urine for as long as she can remember, despite the fact that she has a desire to void and indeed voids normally, probably has an ectopic ureteric orifice. The orifice is often difficult to see because it is guarded by a valve: it may help to give an intravenous injection of a dye such as indigocarmine to colour the urine leaking from it.

In the male patient the aberrant opening is above the external urethral sphincter so the patient is continent. The ureteric orifice at the apex of the trigone, the posterior urethra, in a seminal vesicle or in an ejaculatory duct is likely to be functionally abnormal and infection is the most common complication.

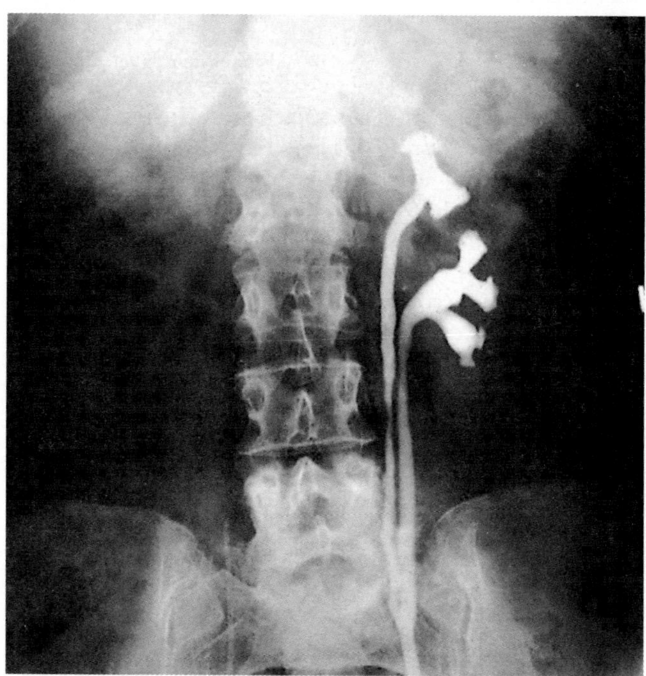

Fig. 64.9 Retrograde ureterogram showing double ureter on the left.

Treatment

Asymptomatic duplication of the kidney is a harmless variant and does not require treatment. If one moiety is severely

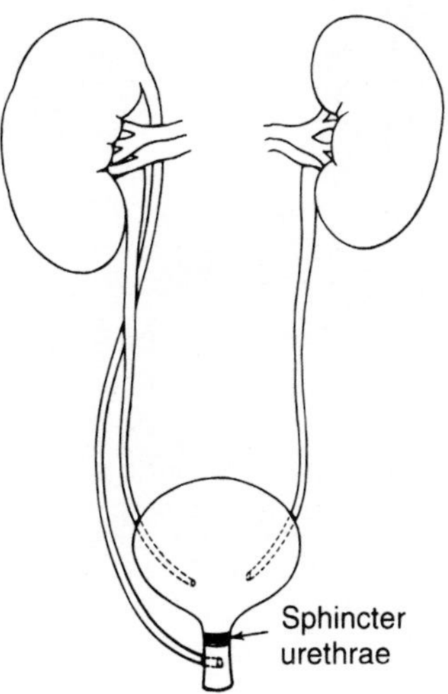

Fig. 64.11 In women one ureteric orifice may open below the sphincter causing intractable incontinence of urine.

diseased or atrophic, partial nephrectomy is usually simple and effective. An ectopic ureter in the female frequently drains hydronephrotic and chronically infected renal tissue, which is best excised. Rarely, the incontinence can be cured and renal function preserved by implanting the ectopic ureter into the bladder or by joining it to its fellow.

Congenital megaureter

Congenital megaureter is a curious and uncommon condition which may be bilateral and is often associated with other congenital anomalies. A functional obstruction at the lower end of the ureter leads to progressive dilatation and a tendency to infection. The ureteric orifice appears normal and a ureteric catheter passes easily. Reflux is not a feature of the untreated condition but is almost inevitable if the ureteric orifice is opened endoscopically to make it drain. Definitive surgical treatment involves refashioning the lower end of the affected ureter so that a tunnelled reimplantation into the bladder can be done to prevent reflux.

Postcaval ureter

The right ureter passes behind the inferior vena cava instead of lying to the right of it. If this causes obstructive symptoms, the ureter can be divided and rejoined in front of the cava using a long oblique anastomosis without tension. Unusually, the retrocaval portion of the ureter is fibrotic and must be excised.

Ureterocele

Ureterocele is a cystic enlargement of the intramural portion of the ureter thought to result from congenital atresia of the ureteric orifice. Although present from childhood, the condition is often unrecognised until adult life. The 'adder head' on excretory urography (Fig. 64.12) is typical. Usually the cyst wall is composed of urothelium only and the diagnosis is confirmed by the cystoscopic appearance of a translucent cyst enlarging and collapsing as urine flows in from the upper ureter (Fig. 64.13). Treatment should be avoided unless there are symptoms arising from infection and/or stone formation. Ureterocele is most common in women; occasionally the cyst may cause obstruction to the bladder outflow by prolapsing into the internal urethral opening.

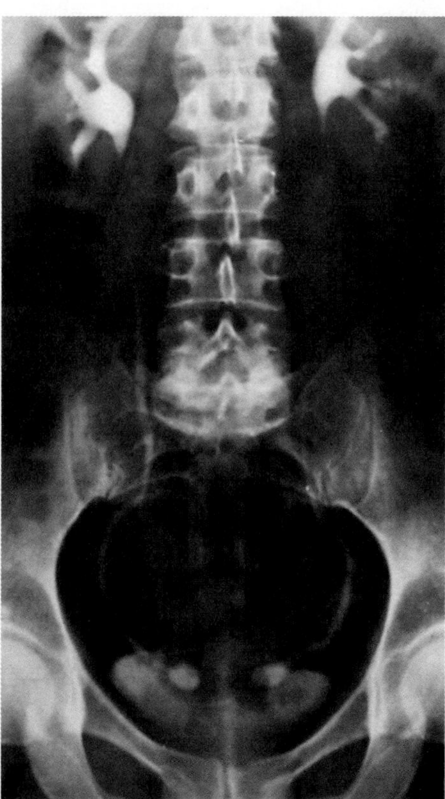

Fig. 64.12 Adder head appearance of ureterocele.

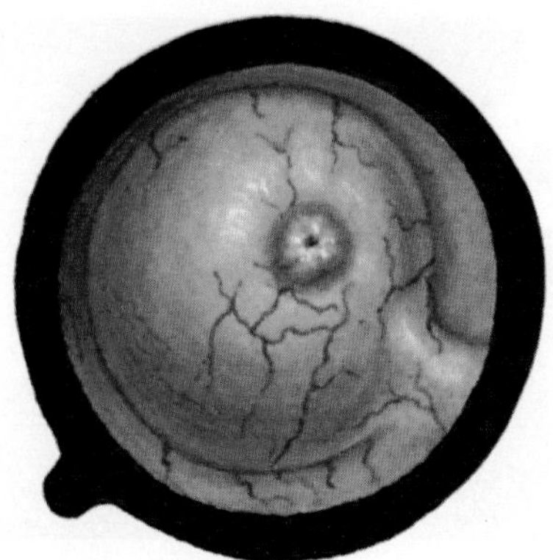

Fig. 64.13 Ureterocele on cystoscopy.

Endoscopic diathermy incision is usually all that is required for treatment of a symptomatic ureterocele, although a micturating cystogram is advisable to detect postoperative urinary reflux. In advanced unilateral cases with hydronephrosis or pyonephrosis, nephrectomy may be appropriate.

Injuries to the kidney

In civilian life injuries to the kidney result most often from either blows or falls on the loin or crushing injury to the abdomen, typically in a road traffic accident. Haematuria after trivial injury to the kidney should suggest the possibility of a pre-existing abnormality, e.g. calculus, hydronephrosis or tuberculosis.

The degree of injury varies considerably from a small subcapsular haematoma to a complete tear involving the whole thickness of the kidney (Fig. 64.14). The kidney may be partially or wholly avulsed from its vascular pedicle; one pole may be completely detached.

Closed renal injury is almost always extraperitoneal. The exception is seen occasionally in young children who have very little extraperitoneal fat. The peritoneum, which is closely applied to the kidney, can tear with the renal capsule allowing blood and urine to leak into the peritoneum.

Clinical features

Superficial soft tissue bruising may testify to the severity of the blow but is often absent. There is likely to be local pain and tenderness.

Haematuria

Haematuria is the cardinal sign of a damaged kidney, but it may not appear until some hours after the injury. Profuse bleeding may be accompanied by clot colic.

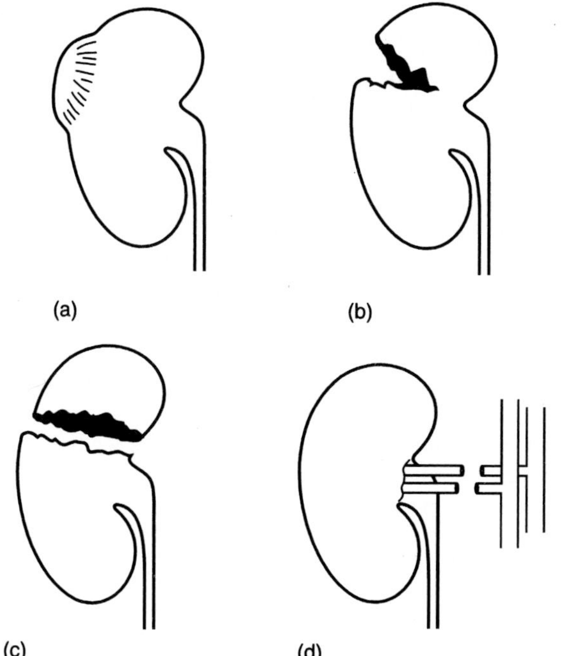

Fig. 64.14 Types of closed renal trauma: (a) subcapsular haematoma; (b) laceration; (c) avulsion of one pole; (d) avulsion of renal pedicle.

Severe delayed haematuria

Sudden profuse haematuria can occur between the third day and the third week after the accident in a patient who appears to be progressing favourably. It is due to a clot becoming dislodged.

Meteorism

Abdominal distension 24–48 hours after renal injury is probably due to retroperitoneal haematoma implicating splanchnic nerves.

Management and treatment

Conservative treatment of closed renal trauma is usually successful but appropriate measures must be instituted without delay. The possibility of injury to other organs must be considered at an early stage.

1. Blood should be cross-matched and available for transfusion if there is evidence of hypovolaemic shock or continuing haemorrhage. Intravenous access should be established.
2. The patient must be confined to bed while there is macroscopic haematuria and physical activity must be curtailed for at least 1 week after the urine clears.
3. Morphine should be given as an analgesic and sedative.
4. Hourly pulse and blood pressure charts must be kept.
5. Antibiotics should be given to prevent infection of the haematoma.
6. Each sample of urine passed should be checked for haematuria and the result charted.
7. An intravenous urogram (IVU) should be obtained urgently (a) to assess the damage to the kidney and (b) to show that the other kidney is normal.

Surgical exploration

Surgical exploration is necessary in less that 10 per cent of closed injuries and is indicated if either there are signs of progressive blood loss or there is an expanding mass in the loin. The aim is to stop bleeding while conserving as much renal tissue as possible; and a renal arteriogram performed preoperatively can be helpful in framing a strategy for doing this. There is also a chance that a skilled radiologist will be able to stop the haemorrhage by embolisation if a bleeding vessel can be identified.

The approach to the kidney should be transperitoneal to exclude the possibility of damage to other abdominal organs. The danger is that release of the tamponading effect of the perirenal haematoma will result in massive uncontrollable haemorrhage and this eventuality must be prepared for. When the kidney is irretrievably ruptured or avulsed from its pedicle, nephrectomy is the only course. Small tears can be sutured over a haemostatic sponge or a piece of detached muscle. Large single rents in the kidney are best dealt with by passing a tube nephrostomy through the defect and suturing the renal tissue around it. If the laceration is confined to one pole of the kidney, partial nephrectomy may be practicable.

When a solitary existing kidney is sufficiently damaged to need exploration, it must be repaired. Failing this, the wound is packed firmly with gauze to stop the bleeding in the hope that some renal function may be retained when the ruptured kidney heals.

Multiple injuries

The mortality of cases of ruptured kidney with damage to the liver spleen or hollow intra-abdominal organs is high.

Complications

1. Heavy haematuria may lead to clot obstruction of the bladder outflow and bladder washout through a catheter or a cystoscope may be necessary.
2. Pararenal pseudohydronephrosis may occur in the course of a few weeks as a result of a combination of complete cortical tear and ureteric obstruction caused by scarring.
3. Hypertension resulting from renal fibrosis may occur 3 months or more after injury. It is often refractory to medical treatment and nephrectomy may be necessary.
4. Aneurysm of the renal artery (Fig. 64.15) is a rare but striking complication of severe renal trauma. There is pain in the loin and a nontender swelling may be felt if the aneurysm is large. Congestion of the parenchyma leads to intermittent haematuria. Aortography is diagnostic. Rupture of a renal artery aneurysm is liable to be fatal and excision or nephrectomy is urgently indicated.

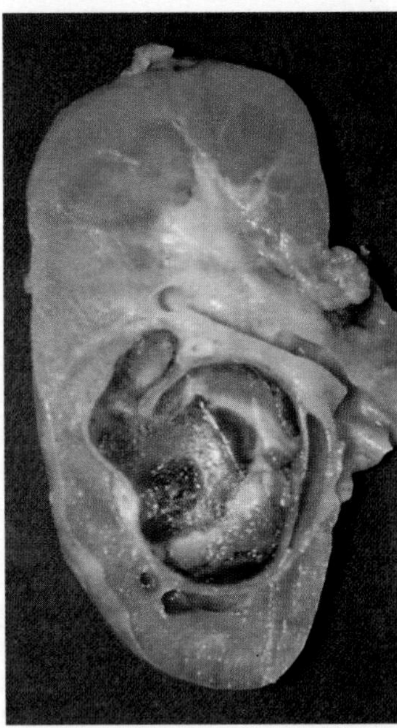

Fig. 64.15 Aneurysm of the renal artery containing lamellated thrombus.

Injuries to the ureter

Rupture of the ureter

This is an uncommon result of a hyperextension injury of the spine. The diagnosis is rarely made until there is swelling in the loin or iliac fossa associated with a reduction of urine output. An excretion urogram shows extravasation of contrast from the ureter on the injured side.

Injury to one or both ureters during pelvic surgery

This is far more common and occurs most often during vaginal or abdominal hysterectomy. Typically there is a failure to recognise the ureter, which is divided, ligated, crushed or excised. Preliminary catheterisation of the ureters prevents such accidents as the catheters make it easy to see and feel the ureters.

Injury recognised at the time of operation

Ureterovesical continuity should be restored by one of the methods described below unless the patient's condition is poor when deliberate ligation of the proximal end of the ureter is the best course. If the patient rallies within 2 days, temporary nephrostomy is carried out with a view to repair of the injury later.

Injury not recognised at the time of operation

Unilateral injuries. There are three possibilities.

No symptoms. Secure ligation of a ureter may simply lead to silent atrophy of the kidney that it drains. If the other kidney is functioning, the injury may be unsuspected until the patient undergoes urological imaging some time later.

Loin pain and fever, possibly with pyonephrosis occurs with infection of the obstructed system. Excretory urography shows no function, a state that will be permanent unless urgent steps are taken to relieve the obstruction, usually by inserting a percutaneous nephrostomy.

A urinary fistula develops through the abdominal or vaginal wound. The urogram shows extravasation of contrast with or without obstruction to one or both ureters. Temporary nephrostomies may be inserted and repair postponed until oedema and inflammation have subsided. The traditional delayed repair, however, leaves the patient incontinent and demoralised. Early repair is now regarded as safe provided that the patient is fit and the surgeon has the necessary experience.

Bilateral injury. Ligation of both ureters leads to anuria. Ureteric catheters will not pass and urgent relief of obstruction is mandatory.

Repair of the injured ureter (Table 64.2)

1. If there is no loss of length and the cut ends of the ureter can be brought together *without tension*, they should be joined by a spatulated anastomosis over a double pigtail catheter. (A pigtail catheter is a plastic tube with preformed coils at each end. The catheter is inserted over a guidewire which straightens its ends. When the wire is removed, the coils reform to anchor the ends of the catheter.)
2. If the division is very low down, the bladder wall may be hitched up so that the ureter can be reimplanted into it. Extra length may be obtained by mobilising the kidney.
3. *Boari's operation* (Fig. 64.16). A flap of bladder wall is fashioned into a tube to replace the lower ureter.
4. The ureter may be implanted end to side into the contralateral ureter. The disadvantage of a transureteroureterostomy is that it risks converting a unilateral injury into a bilateral one.
5. Occasionally, when conservation of all renal tissue is vital, replacement of the damaged ureter by a segment of ileum is necessary.
6. Nephrectomy may be the best course when the patient's outlook is poor and the other kidney is normal.

Table 64.2 Methods for repairing a damaged ureter

If there is no loss of length	Spatulation and end-to-end anastomosis without tension
If there is little loss of length	Mobilise kidney Psoas hitch of bladder Boari operation
If there is marked loss of length	Transureteroureterostomy Interposition of isolated bowel loop or mobilised appendix Nephrectomy

Achille Boari. Nineteenth-century Italian surgeon.

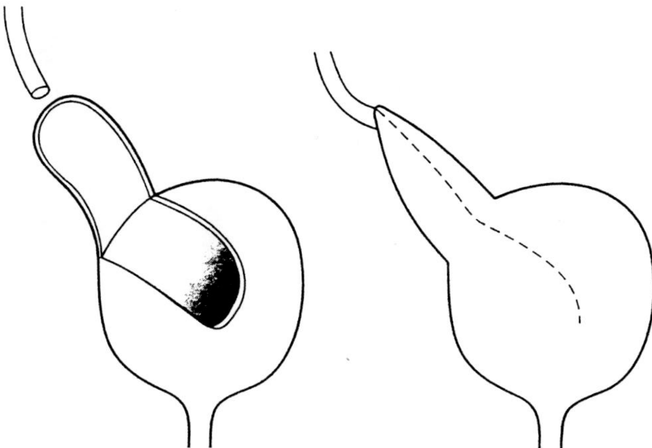

Fig. 64.16 Boari's operation: a strip of bladder wall is fashioned into tube to bridge the gap between the cut ureter and the bladder.

Hydronephrosis

Hydronephrosis is an aseptic dilatation of the kidney due to a partial or complete obstruction to the outflow of urine.

Unilateral hydronephrosis

Unilateral hydronephrosis (Table 64.3) is caused by some form of ureteric obstruction, with the ureter above the obstruction being dilated.

Bilateral hydronephrosis

Bilateral hydronephrosis is usually the result of urethral obstruction, but it may be caused by one of the lesions described above occurring on both sides.

When due to lower urinary obstruction, the cause may be:

1. **Congenital:**
   (a) congenital stricture of the external urethral meatus or, rarely, phimosis;
   (b) congenital valves of the posterior male urethra or congenital contracture of the bladder neck.

Table 64.3 Causes of unilateral ureteric obstruction

Extramural obstruction
Tumour from adjacent structures, e.g. carcinoma of the cervix, prostate, rectum, colon or caecum
Idiopathic retroperitoneal fibrosis
Retrocaval ureter
Intramural obstruction
Congenital stenosis, physiological narrowing of the pelviureteric junction leading to pelviureteric junction obstruction
Ureterocele and congenital small ureteric orifice
Inflammatory stricture following removal of a calculus, repair of a damaged ureteric segment or tuberculous infection
Neoplasm of the ureter or bladder cancer involving the ureteric orifice
Intraluminal obstruction
Calculus in the renal pelvis or ureter
Sloughed papilla in papillary necrosis (especially in diabetics, analgesic abusers and those with sickle cell disease, may obstruct the ureter)

2. **Acquired:**
   (a) benign prostatic enlargement or carcinoma of the prostate; postoperative bladder neck scarring;
   (b) inflammatory or traumatic urethral stricture, phimosis.

Urethral obstruction tends to lead to hypertrophy of the bladder detrusor muscle which can lead to obstruction to the ureters in the intramural part of their course.

Pathology

In a kidney with an extrarenal pelvis, the dilatation first affects the pelvis alone (pelvic hydronephrosis). If the obstruction is not relieved, the calyces become increasingly dilated and the renal parenchyma is progressively destroyed by pressure atrophy. In a kidney with a predominantly intrarenal pelvis, destruction of the parenchyma occurs more rapidly. A kidney destroyed by long-standing hydronephrosis is a thin-walled lobulated sac containing pale uriniferous fluid of low specific gravity.

Clinical features

Unilateral hydronephrosis

The female:male ratio of unilateral hydronephrosis (most commonly caused by idiopathic pelviureteric junction obstruction or calculus) is 2:1; the right side is more commonly affected.

Presenting features include the following.

1. **Insidious onset** of mild pain or dull aching in the loin. There is often a sensation of dragging heaviness which is made worse by excessive fluid intake. An enlarged kidney may be palpable if the cause is pelviureteric junction obstruction.
2. **Attacks of acute renal colic** may occur with no palpable swelling.
3. **Intermittent hydronephrosis.** After an attack of acute renal pain a swelling in the loin is found. Some hours later, following the passage of a large volume of urine, the pain is relieved and the swelling disappears (Dietl's crisis).

Bilateral hydronephrosis

From lower urinary obstruction. There is little to call attention to the hydronephrosis except, perhaps, a dull loin ache. Symptoms of bladder outflow obstruction predominate. The kidneys are unlikely to be palpable because renal failure intervenes before the kidneys become sufficiently large.

From bilateral upper urinary tract obstruction. This is rare compared with unilateral lesions although idiopathic retroperitoneal fibrosis commonly affects both ureters. Although both systems are obstructed, symptoms may be referred to one side only.

From pregnancy. Dilatation of the ureters and renal pelves occurs early in pregnancy and becomes more marked until the 20th week. The condition results from the effects of high

Joseph Dietl, 1804–78. Professor of Pathology and Therapeutics, Krakau, Poland. In his later years he achieved fame as a politician.

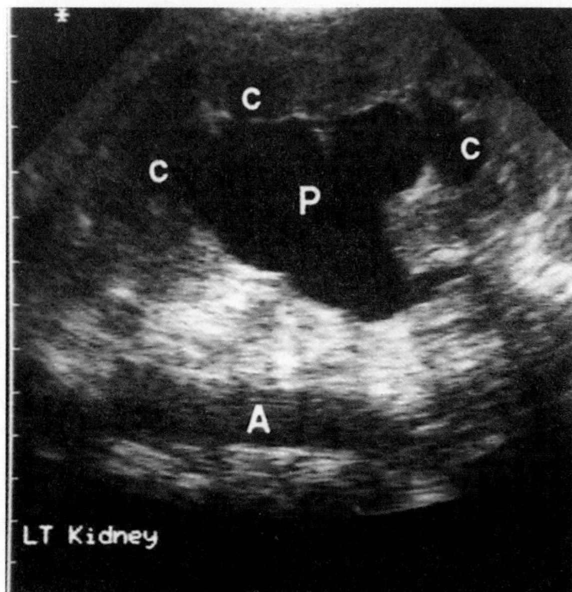

Fig. 64.17 Ultrasound of hydronephrotic kidney.

levels of circulating progesterone on the ureteric smooth muscle and it may be considered as part of normal pregnancy. The ureters return to their normal size within 12 weeks of delivery. The main importance of the condition is an increased liability to infection and the possibility that abdominal pain during pregnancy may be erroneously ascribed to ureteric obstruction.

Imaging

Ultrasound scanning (Fig. 64.17) is the least invasive means of detecting hydronephrosis and has been used to diagnose pelviureteric junction obstruction *in utero*.

Excretion urography is helpful if there is still significant function in the obstructed kidney. The extrarenal pelvis is dilated and the minor calyces lose their normal cupping and become '*clubbed*'. In very advanced cases, the thin rim of poorly functioning renal parenchyma may give a faint nephrogram around the dilated calyces – a '*soap-bubble*' appearance. If the level of obstruction is in doubt it can help to take follow-up films up to 24 hours after the contrast has been injected. The radio-opaque medium slowly diffuses to fill the obstructed system down to the block.

Isotope renography is the most helpful test to establish that dilatation of the renal collecting system is due to obstruction. A substance [usually diethylenetriaminepenta-acetic acid (DTPA) or MAG-3] which is filtered by the glomeruli and not absorbed is injected intravenously. The DTPA is labelled with technetium 99m, a γ-ray emitter, so that the passage (of ^{99m}Tc-labelled DTPA) through the kidneys can be tracked using a gamma camera. ^{99m}Tc-DTPA is quickly cleared from a normal kidney but if the ureter is obstructed the marker is trapped in the renal pelvis and will not be washed out even if the flow of urine is increased by administering frusemide (Fig. 64.18).

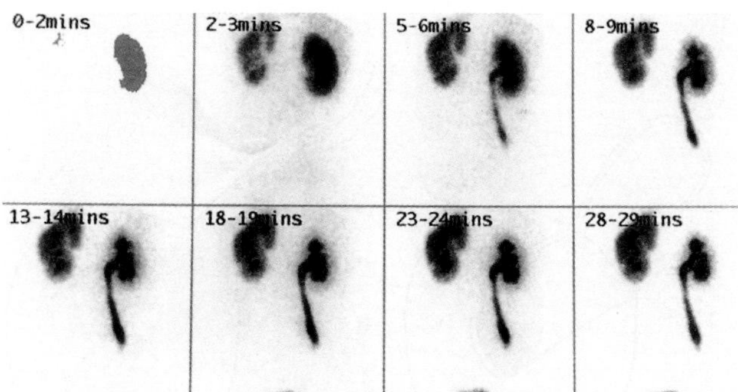

Fig. 64.18 MAG-3 renogram: marker persists in the left kidney and will not be washed out when frusemide is administered.

Very occasionally, doubt still persists and a Whitaker *test* is indicated. A percutaneous puncture of the kidney is made through the loin and fluid is infused at a constant rate with monitoring of intrapelvic pressure. An abnormal rise in pressure confirms obstruction. *Retrograde pyelography* (Fig. 64.19) is rarely indicated but will confirm the site of obstruction immediately before corrective surgery.

Treatment

The indications for operation are bouts of renal pain, increasing hydronephrosis, evidence of parenchymal damage and infection. *Conservation* of renal tissue is the aim; nephrectomy should be considered only when the renal parenchyma has been largely destroyed. Mild cases should be followed by serial ultrasound scans and operated upon if dilatation is increasing.

Pyeloplasty

The Anderson–Hynes operation (Fig. 64.20) is appropriate in cases of pelviureteric junction obstruction where a reasonable thickness of functioning parenchyma remains. The affected kidney is displayed and the upper third of the ureter and the renal pelvis carefully mobilised. A renal vein overlying the distended pelvis can be divided but an artery in this situation should be preserved to avoid infarction of the territory that it supplies. The anastomosis is made in front of such an artery using absorbable stitches to avoid calculus formation on the suture line. It is usual to protect the anastomosis with a nephrostomy tube or a ureteric stent.

Endoscopic pyelolysis

Disruption of the pelviureteric junction by a specially designed balloon passed up the ureter and distended under radiographic control has been used to treat idiopathic pelviureteric junction obstruction. The long-term benefit of this and other minimal access techniques still has to be proved.

Robert Whitaker. Consultant Urologist, Addenbrook's Hospital, Cambridge, England.

James Christie Anderson. Consulting Surgeon, Royal Hospital, Sheffield, England.

Wilfred Hynes. Surgeon, Plastic and Jaw Department, United Sheffield Hospitals, Sheffield, England.

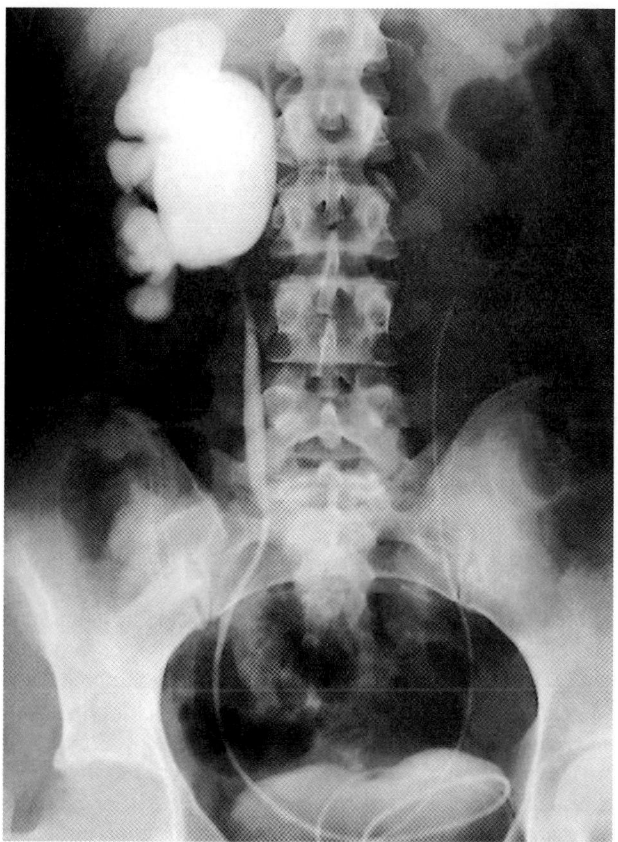

Fig. 64.19 Retrograde ureteropyelogram showing hydronephrosis with greatly enlarged renal pelvis and dilated 'clubbed' calyces.

Renal calculi

Aetiology

The subject is complex and the following represents a brief summary of current opinion.

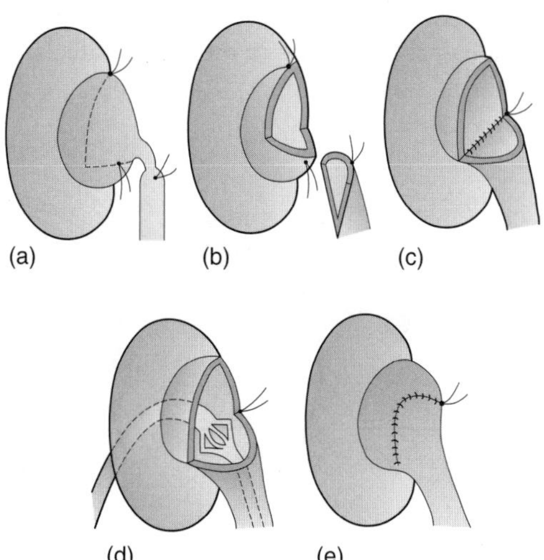

Fig. 64.20 Anderson–Hynes disjunction pyeloplasty.

Dietetic. Deficiency of vitamin A causes desquamation of epithelium. The cells form a nidus around which stone is deposited. From a study of economic conditions in places where stones are common, it is evident that the inhabitants do suffer dietary imbalance. It is uncertain whether this mechanism is of importance other than in the formation of bladder calculi.

Altered urinary solutes and colloids. Dehydration leads to an increased concentration of urinary solutes and tends to cause them to precipitate. It has been postulated that reduction of urinary colloids which adsorb solutes or mucoproteins which chelate calcium will also result in a tendency for stone components to come out of solution.

Decreased urinary citrate. The presence of citrate in urine, 300–900 mg/24 hours (1.6–4.7 mmol/24 hours) as citric acid, tends to keep otherwise relatively insoluble calcium phosphate and citrate in solution. The urinary excretion of citrate is under hormonal control and decreases during menstruation.

Renal infection. Infection favours the formation of urinary calculi. Both clinical and experimental stone formation are common when urine is infected with urea-splitting streptococci, staphylococci and especially *Proteus* sp. The predominant bacteria found in the nuclei of urinary stones are staphylococci and *Escherichia coli.*

Inadequate urinary drainage and urinary stasis. Stones are liable when urine does not pass freely.

Prolonged immobilisation from any cause, e.g. paraplegia, is liable to result in skeletal decalcification and an increase in urinary calcium favouring the formation of calcium phosphate calculi.

Hyperparathyroidism leading to hypercalcaemia and hypercalciuria is found in 5 per cent or less of those who present with radio-opaque calculi. In cases of recurrent or multiple stones this cause should be eliminated by appropriate investigations (see Chapter 45). Hyperparathyroidism results in a great increase in the elimination of calcium in the urine. These patients 'pass their skeletons in their urine'. A parathyroid adenoma should be removed before definitive treatment for the urinary calculi.

Randall's plaque and microliths. Randall suggested that the initial lesion in some cases of kidney stone was an erosion at the tip of a renal papilla. Deposition of calcium on this erosion produced a lesion which has been called Randall's plaque. It has further been shown that minute concretions (microliths) regularly occur in the renal parenchyma and Carr postulated that these particles are carried by lymphatics to the subendothelial region where they may accumulate. Ulceration of the epithelium exposes the potential calculus to the urine with the result that a stone forms. The importance of Randall's plaques and Carr's microliths in most patients with stones is a matter for debate.

Types of renal calculus

Oxalate calculus (calcium oxalate) (Fig. 64.21). Oxalate stones are irregular in shape and covered with sharp projections which tend to cause bleeding. The surface of the calculus is discoloured by the pigments of altered blood. A calcium oxalate monohydrate stone is very hard and absorbs X-rays well; it is easy to see radiologically.

Phosphate calculus [usually calcium phosphate, although sometimes combined with ammonium magnesium phosphate (struvite)] is smooth and dirty white (Fig. 64.22). The stone tends to grow in alkaline urine especially when proteus organisms are present which split urea to ammonium. As a result, the calculus may enlarge to fill all or most of the renal collecting system forming a *stag-horn calculus* (Fig. 64.22). Even a

Alexander Randall, 1883–1951. Professor of Urology, University of Pennsylvania, Pennsylvania, USA.

Reginald Joseph Carr. Radiologist, Bradford Royal Infirmary, Bradford, England.

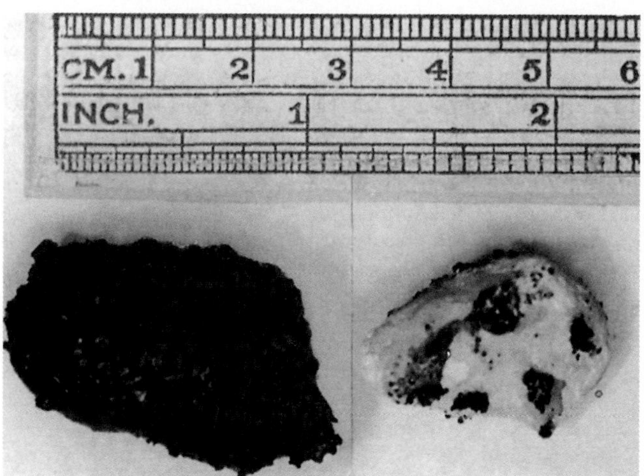

Fig. 64.21 Oxalate calculi. The larger one removed from the right kidney is blackened by the deposition of altered blood. The sharp edges of the smaller calculus removed from the left side are also discoloured.

very large stag horn may be clinically silent for years until it signals its presence by causing intractable urinary infection or haematuria. Because they are large, phosphate calculi are usually easy to see on X-ray films.

Uric acid and urate calculi are hard, smooth and often multiple. Their colour varies from yellow to reddish brown and they sometimes have an attractive multifaceted appearance. Pure uric acid stones are radiolucent and appear on an excretion urogram as a filling defect, which can be mistaken for a transitional tumour of the upper urinary tract. In practice most uric acid stones contain some calcium so they cast a faint radiological shadow. In children mixed stones of ammonium and sodium urate are sometimes found. They are yellow, soft and friable. They are radiolucent unless they are contaminated with calcium salts.

Cystine calculi are uncommon. They appear in the urinary tract of patients with a congenital error of metabolism which leads to cystinuria. Cystine crystals are hexagonal, translucent white and appear only in acid urine. Cystine stones are often multiple and may grow to form a cast of the renal pelvis and calyces. They are pink or yellow when first removed but they change colour to a greenish hue when exposed to air. Cystine stones are radio-opaque because of the sulphur that they contain, and they are very hard.

Xanthine calculi are extremely rare. They are smooth and round, brick red in colour and show lamellation on cross-section.

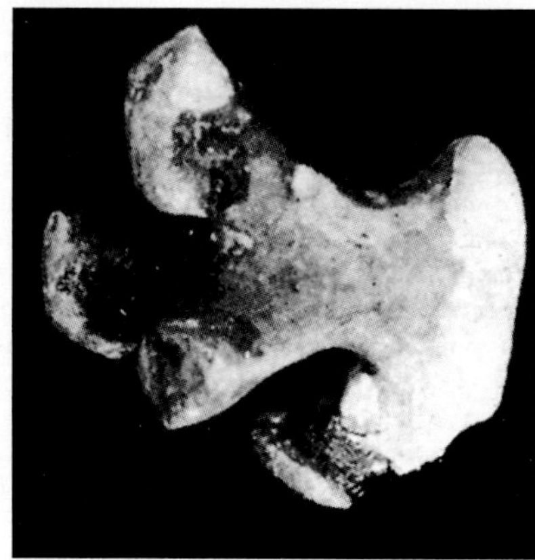

Fig. 64.22 Stag-horn calculus.

Clinical features

Renal calculi are very common. Fifty per cent of patients present between the ages of 30 and 50 years. The male:female ratio is 4:3.

The symptoms are variable and the diagnosis sometimes remains obscure until the stone is discovered on a radiograph.

Silent calculus

Some stones, even large stag-horn calculi, cause no symptoms for long periods during which there is progressive destruction of the renal parenchyma. If the calculi are bilateral, uraemia may be the first indication of their presence, although secondary infection usually gives symptoms first.

Pain

Pain is the leading symptom in 75 per cent of people with urinary stone disease.

Fixed renal pain is located posteriorly in the renal angle (Fig. 64.23), anteriorly in the hypochondrium, or in both. It may be worse on movement, particularly on climbing stairs.

Ureteric colic is an agonising pain passing from the loin to the groin. Typically it starts suddenly causing the patient to move around trying in vain to find comfort. Strangury, the painful passage of a few drops of urine, may occur if the stone is in the intramural ureter. An attack of colic rarely lasts more than 8 hours. It is not associated with pyrexia, although the pulse rate usually rises as a reflex response to the severe pain.

Ureteric colic is often caused by a stone entering the ureter but it may also occur when a stone becomes lodged in the pelviureteric junction. The severity of the colic is not related to the size of the stone.

Abdominal examination. During an attack of ureteric colic there is rigidity of the lateral abdominal muscles but not, as a rule, of the rectus abdominis. Percussion over the kidney produces a stab of pain and there may be tenderness on gentle deep palpation. Hydronephrosis or pyonephrosis leading to a palpable swelling in the loin is rare.

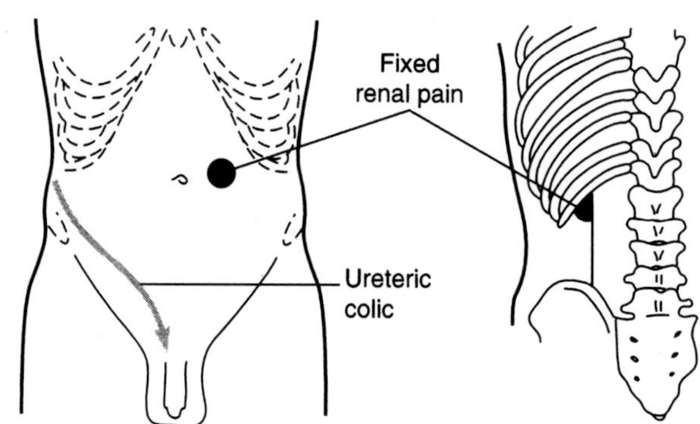

Fig. 64.23 The usual distribution of renal pain.

Haematuria

Haematuria is sometimes a leading symptom of stone disease and occasionally the only one. As a rule the amount of bleeding is small.

Pyuria

Infection is likely in the presence of stones and is particularly dangerous when the kidney is obstructed. As pressure builds in the dilated collecting system, organisms are injected into the circulation and a life-threatening septicaemia can quickly develop.

The mechanical effect of stones irritating the urothelium may cause pyuria even in the absence of infection.

Investigation of suspected urinary stone disease

Radiography

Calculi are easier to see if the bowel is empty and it is helpful to administer a vegetable laxative. The 'scout' film must show the kidney, ureters and bladder (a 'KUB' film). When a renal calculus is branched, there is no doubt about the diagnosis (Fig. 64.24). An opacity that keeps a constant position relative to the urinary tract during respiration is likely to be a calculus within it.

A doubtful opacity can sometimes be shown to be anterior to the vertebral bodies on a *lateral radiograph* and hence outside the urinary tract (Table 64.4); such is the finding with calcified mesenteric nodes and opacities within the alimentary tract.

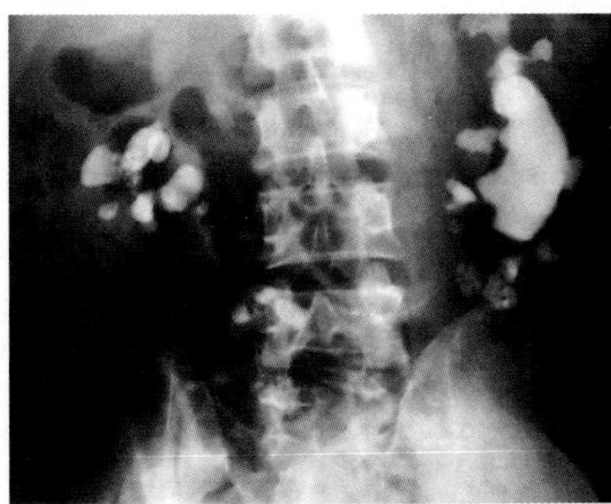

Fig. 64.24 Plain abdominal X-ray showing complete stag-horn calculi.

Table 64.4 Opacities on a plain abdominal radiograph which may be confused with renal calculus

Calcified mesenteric lymph node
Gallstone or concretion in the appendix
Tablets or foreign bodies in the alimentary canal (e.g. Navidrex-K)
Phleboliths – calcification in the walls of veins especially in the pelvis
Ossified tip of the 12th rib
Calcified tuberculous lesion in the kidney
Calcified adrenal gland

Excretion urography

Excretion urography is the most useful investigation to establish the presence of a calculus. It also shows where the stone is and gives important information about the function of the other kidney.

Ultrasound scanning

Ultrasound scanning is of most value in locating stones for treatment by extracorporeal shock wave treatment (see below).

Surgical treatment of urinary calculi

Conservative management

Calculi which are smaller than 0.5 cm are likely to pass spontaneously unless they are impacted. Any surgical intervention carries the risk of complication and needless intervention should be avoided. Small renal calculi may cause symptoms by obstructing a calyx or acting as a focus for secondary infection. However, most can be safely observed until they pass.

Preoperative treatment

If urinary infection is present, appropriate antibiotic treatment is started and continued during and after surgery as necessary.

Operation for stone

In developed countries, open surgery for renal calculus disease is uncommon. Most stones are treated by specialist urologists using minimal access and minimally invasive techniques. Open operations are still needed when the appropriate expertise is not available or newer techniques have failed to clear the calculus. The following account should be read with this in mind.

Modern methods of stone removal

Kidney stones

Percutaneous nephrolithotomy (Fig. 64.25). This involves the placement of a hollow needle into the renal collecting system through the soft tissue of the loin and the renal parenchyma. A wire inserted through the needle is used to guide the passage of a series of dilators which expand the track into the kidney until it is large enough to take the nephroscope used to look for the stone. Small stones may be grasped under vision and extracted whole. Larger stones must be fragmented by an ultrasound or electrohydraulic probe and removed piecemeal.

The aim of the procedure is to remove all fragments if possible and this may take quite a long time if the calculus is large. When the operation is finished a nephrostomy tube is left to drain the system. This decompresses the kidney and

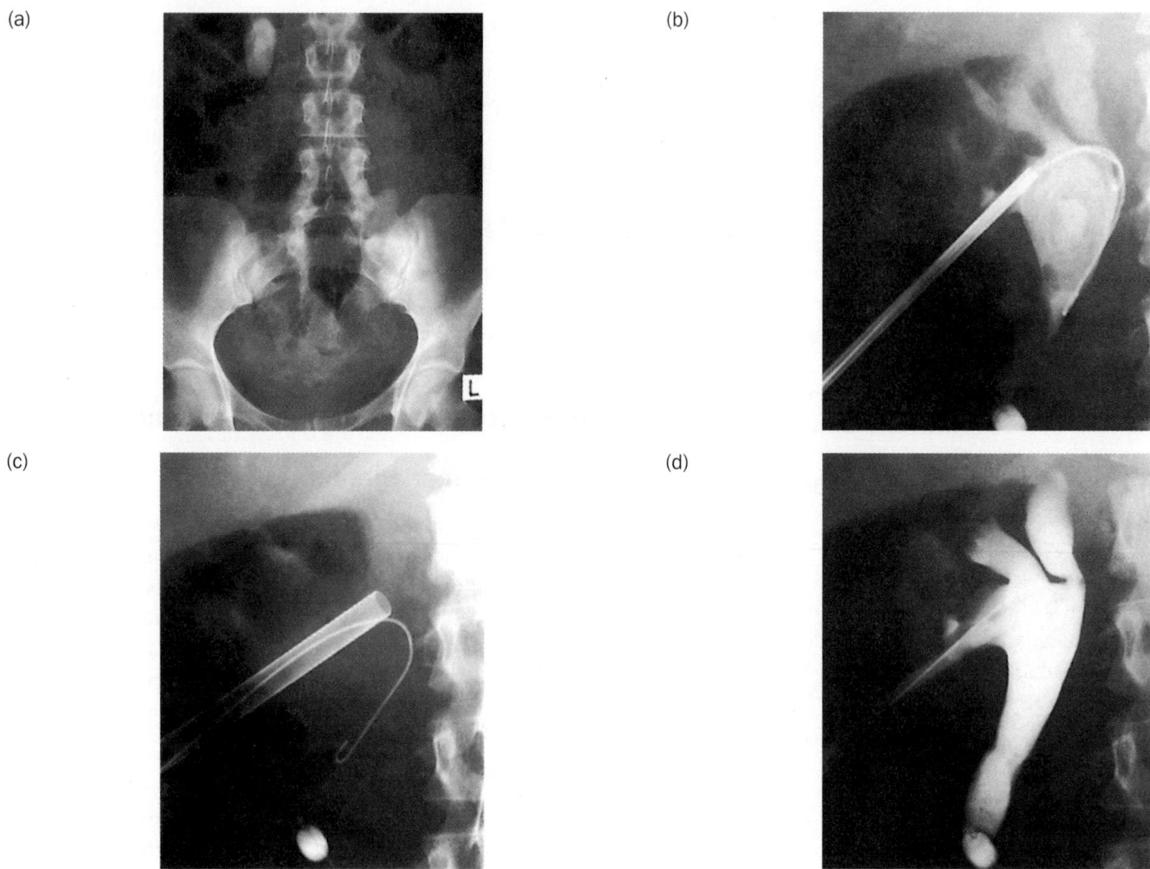

Fig. 64.25 Percutaneous renal stone removal: (a) the stone is in the right renal pelvis; (b) shows placement of a balloon catheter to stop fragment migrating into the upper ureter; (c) shows that the stone fragments have been successfully removed by irrigation; (d) a nephrostogram confirm that the renal pelvis is intact.

allows repeated access to the system if stone particles remain. Percutaneous nephrolithotripsy is sometimes combined with extracorporeal shock-wave lithotripsy (ESWL) in the treatment of complex (stag-horn) calculi. The surgeon removes the central part of the stone percutaneously and the more peripheral fragments are treated by ESWL.

Complications of percutaneous nephrolithotripsy include (1) haemorrhage from the punctured renal parenchyma – this may be profuse and difficult to control; (2) perforation of the collecting system with extravasation of irrigant (which should be saline); (3) perforation of the colon or pleural cavity during placement of the percutaneous track.

Extracorporeal shock-wave lithotripsy. The management of kidney stones has been revolutionised by the development of lithotriptors. The first of these was made in Germany by the Dornier Company. Many machines of different design are now available.

A urinary calculus is a crystalline structure. If it is bombarded with shock waves of sufficient energy it will disintegrate into fragments. The principle is seen at its simplest in the original Dornier machine where shock waves were generated by an electrical discharge placed at one focus of an ellipsoid mirror. The patient was positioned, under radiographic control, so that the calculus was subjected to the full force of the shock waves where they were concentrated at the second focus of the mirror. As shock waves are poorly transmitted through air, both the patient and the shock-wave generators were immersed in a bath of water.

Modern ESWL machines do not have a water bath; the fluid is confined to the path that the shock waves must follow to reach the kidney. The shocks may be generated by the discharge of an array of piezoelectric cells and they may be aimed by ultrasound rather than X-ray imaging (Fig. 64.26). The devices also differ in the strength of the disruptive force which they can develop. Less powerful machines are less effective in breaking stones and several treatments may be necessary to achieve clearance of a calculus. Weaker shocks hurt less, however, and treatment can be given without general anaesthesia.

When ESWL is successful, the stone fragments have to be passed down the ureter. Ureteric colic is common after ESWL and the patient must be given appropriate analgesia, usually in the form of a nonsteroidal anti-inflammatory drug such as diclofenac. If the stone is large the bulky fragments may become impacted in the ureter, causing obstruction. To avoid this, a self-retaining stent should be placed in the ureter so

(a)

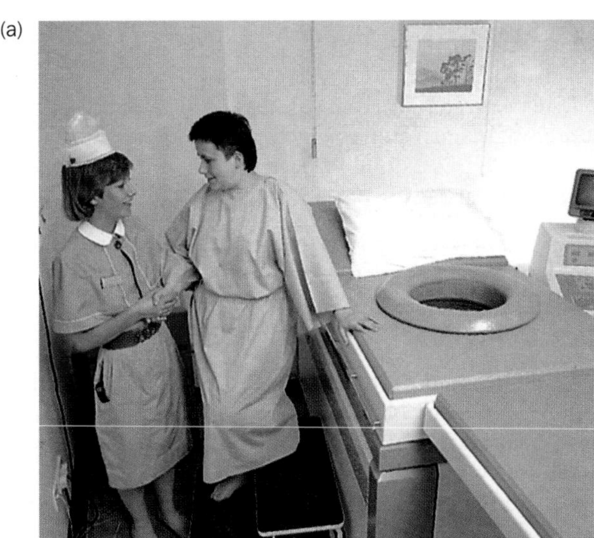

(b)

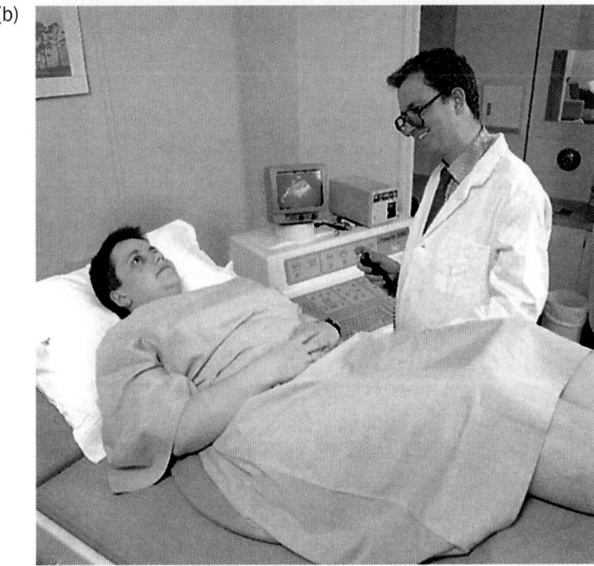

Fig. 64.26 Extracorporeal shock wave lithotripsy.

that the kidney can drain while the pieces of stone pass. Occasionally impacted fragments have to be removed ureteroscopically (see below).

In addition to pain and fragment impaction, the principal complication of ESWL is infection. Many calculi contain bacteria which are released when the stone is broken. It is wise to give prophylactic antibiotics before ESWL and an obstructed system should be decompressed by the insertion of a ureteric stent or percutaneous nephrostomy before treatment.

The clearance of stone from the kidney will depend upon the consistency of the stone and its site. Most oxalate and phosphate stones fragment well and, if lying in the renal pelvis, will clear within days. The results with harder stones, especially cystine stones, are less satisfactory. When treating calyceal stones, the patients should be warned that the clearance of fragments may take months.

There is currently great interest in the long-term outcome of patients treated by ESWL. Certainly some stones recur, especially if small fragments remain after treatment. Long-term renal damage now seems unlikely.

Open surgery for renal calculi (Fig. 64.27)

Operations for kidney stone are usually performed via a loin or lumbar approach. All of the procedures are difficult unless the kidney is fully mobilised and its vascular pedicle controlled. A sling should be placed around the upper ureter to stop stones migrating downwards.

Pyelolithotomy is indicated for stones in the renal pelvis. When the wall of renal pelvis has been dissected free from its surrounding fat, an incision is made in its long axis directly on to the stone. The stone is removed with gallstone forceps, care being taken not to break it because fragments may be difficult to retrieve. Stone fragments in peripheral calyces may be detected by direct palpation or by intraoperative radiography or nephroscopy. If there is no infection, the pelvic incision is closed with interrupted absorbable sutures. If there is gross sepsis, it is wise to place a nephrostomy to drain the system.

Extended pyelolithotomy. The plane between the renal sinus and the wall of the collecting system is developed on the posterior surface of the kidney. This avoids major vessels and allows incisions to be made into the calyces so that even large stag-horn stones can be removed intact.

Nephrolithotomy. If there is a complex calculus branching into the most peripheral calyces, it may be necessary to make incisions into the renal parenchyma to clear the kidney. Nephrolithotomy may also be necessary when the adhesions resulting from previous surgery make access to the renal pelvis difficult. The renal pedicle must be temporarily cross-clamped to reduce bleeding from the highly vascular renal tissue. Incisions are made just posterior and parallel to the most prominent part of the convex renal border where the territories of the anterior and posterior branches of the renal artery meet (Brödel's line). Cooling the kidney with ice packs or cooling coils extends the time that the kidney can remain ischaemic without permanent damage. All the incisions must be carefully closed with haemostatic sutures and the patient observed after the operation for signs of reactionary haemorrhage.

Partial nephrectomy is sometimes preferable when the stone is present in the lowermost calyx and there is associated infective damage to the adjacent parenchyma.

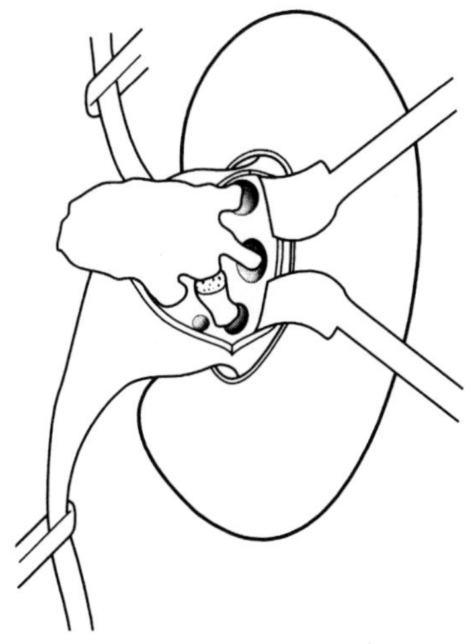

Fig. 64.27 Open operations for renal calculus.

Max Brödel, 1870–1941. Baltimore physician.

Nephrectomy is indicated when the kidney has been destroyed by obstruction and infection associated with stone disease. This is particularly the case when there is xanthogranulomatous pyelonephritis. This stone-related inflammatory mass must be removed with particular care because it is liable to be attached to adjacent structures such as the colon.

Treatment of bilateral renal stones. Usually the kidney with better function is treated first, the operation on the contralateral side being deferred for 2–3 months. Exceptions are if either one kidney is more painful, suggesting an obstruction, or there is pyonephrosis in one kidney – this must be drained by percutaneous nephrostomy.

In cases of silent bilateral stag-horn calculi in the elderly and infirm, it may be best not to operate. The patient should be encouraged to maintain a high fluid intake.

Prevention of recurrence

Frère Jacques, that famous lithotomist of the Middle Ages, used to say, 'I have removed the stone, but God will cure the patient'. When a renal stone has been removed, steps must be taken to prevent recurrence.

Ideally all stone formers should be investigated to exclude metabolic factors. In practice the pick-up rate in patients with a single small stone is very small. The urine of all patients with stones should be screened for infection. The following investigations are appropriate in bilateral and recurrent stone formers:

- serum calcium, measured fasting on three occasions to exclude hyperparathyroidism;
- serum uric acid;
- urinary urate, calcium and phosphate in a 24-hour collection. The urine should also be screened for cystine;
- analysis of any stone passed.

Dietary advice is not usually helpful in avoiding stone recurrence in people who have a normal balanced diet. Those who consume excessive amounts of milk products (calcium stones), rhubarb, strawberries, plums, spinach and asparagus (calcium oxalate stones) should be advised to be more moderate.

Patients with hyperuricaemia should avoid red meats, offal and fish, which are rich in purines and should have treatment with allopurinol. Eggs, meat and fish are high in sulphur-containing proteins and should be restricted in those with cystinuria.

The most effective dietary advice is that originally offered to stone sufferers by Hippocrates. They should *drink plenty* to keep their urine dilute. Fluid intake should be increased appropriately to take account of increased losses.

Drug treatment has not been shown to be effective other than in those few patients who are shown to have idiopathic hypercalciuria. Bendrofluazide 5 mg and a calcium-restricted diet reduces urinary calcium.

Frère Jacques, 1651–1719. Itinerant Italian lithotomist, after serving as a trooper in the French army, adopted semireligious habit and cut for stone in the bladder.

Hippocrates, by common consent the father of medicine, was born on the Greek Island of Cos, off Turkey, about 460 BC *and died in 375* BC.

Ureteric calculus

A stone in the ureter nearly always has its birth in the kidney. Most are single small stones which pass spontaneously.

Clinical features

The presence of a stone passing down the ureter often causes intermittent attacks of ureteric colic.

Ureteric colic

A stone in the upper ureter produces symptoms identical with those of a stone blocking the pelviureteric junction. As the stone progresses to the lower ureter, the waves of agonising pain are typically referred more to the groin, external genitalia and the anterior surface of the thigh. In a man, the testis may be retracted by spasm of the cremaster and tenderness may persist for some days after the colic has ceased. When the stone is in the intramural ureter, the pain is referred to the tip of the penis. In both sexes there may be strangury.

Impaction

Most stones pass spontaneously from the ureter but there are five sites of anatomical narrowing where the stone may be arrested (Fig. 64.28). When the stone becomes impacted the attacks of colic give way to a more consistent dull pain, often felt in the iliac fossa. The pain is increased by exercise and lessened by rest. Distension of the renal pelvis due to obstruc-

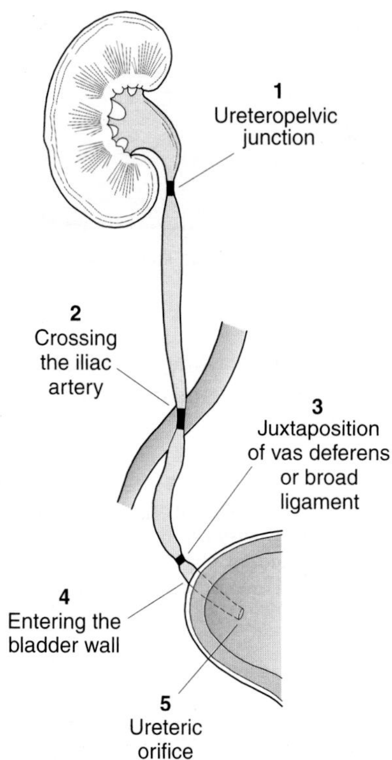

Fig. 64.28 Normal anatomical narrowings of the ureter.

tion may cause pain and discomfort in the loin. As time goes by the stone may become imbedded as the adjacent ureteric wall becomes eroded and oedematous due to pressure ischaemia. Perforation of the ureter and extravasation of urine is a rare complication.

Severe renal pain persisting for 1 or 2 days and then subsiding suggests that the ureter is completely obstructed by the stone. If urography (IVU) or ultrasonography suggests that obstruction persists after 1–2 weeks, the calculus should be removed because prolonged distension of the kidney will lead eventually to atrophy of the renal parenchyma.

Haematuria

Almost every attack of ureteric colic is associated with microscopic haematuria which lasts for a day or so. More profuse bleeding is uncommon and should raise the suspicion that the colic is due to passage of a clot.

Abdominal examination

There is tenderness and some rigidity over some part of the course of the ureter. The principal difficulty on the right side is to distinguish symptoms and signs of ureteric colic from those of acute appendicitis or acute cholecystitis. The presence of haematuria does not rule out appendicitis, because an inflamed appendix lying near the ureter can give rise to a local ureteritis which will result in some red cells in the urine. In practice, the patient with acute renal colic is usually in greater pain and less systemically ill.

Imaging

Most urinary calculi are radiodense and visible on a plain abdominal radiograph. The stone may not be seen along the line of the ureter if it is very small or if it is obscured by contents of the gut or the shadows of nearby bones. An intravenous urogram performed while the patient has pain can confirm the diagnosis. During and for some time after an attack of renal colic there will probably be little or no excretion on the affected side. Occasionally, there is an extravasation of contrast from the dilated system. Late radiogaphs, taken up to 36 hours after the injection of contrast, may show dilatation of the ureter down to an obstructing calculus. A radiolucent uric acid stone may be demonstrated as a filling defect in the contrast.

Analgesic abusers occasionally simulate symptoms to obtain drugs and the urogram is useful in excluding renal colic. *If the urogram is normal during an attack, the patient does not have renal colic.*

Cystoscopy is not indicated routinely but may reveal oedema and petechiae of the urothelium around the ureteric orifice when the stone is in the lower ureter. The stone may be visible in the orifice as it makes its passage into the bladder.

Retrograde ureterography is usually performed as an immediate preliminary to an endoscopic operation to remove a calculus but it may be of use if doubt remains after the intravenous urogram.

Treatment

Pain

Nonsteroidal anti-inflammatory drugs such as diclofenac and indomethacin have replaced opiates as the first line of treatment for renal colic. The value of smooth muscle relaxants such as propantheline (Pro-Banthine) is debateable.

Removal of the stone (Table 64.5)

Expectant treatment is appropriate for small stones that are likely to pass naturally. This may take many months and, as long as the patient is not disabled by recurrent attacks of colic, the progress of the stone can be followed by radiographs repeated every 6–8 weeks.

Endoscopic stone removal. *Dormia basket.* The use of wire baskets under image intensifier control has been replaced by ureteroscopic techniques, but may be useful when the necessary instruments and expertise are not available. There is a significant danger of ureteric injury, and basketry under radiographic control should only be used for small stones that are within 5 or 6 cm of the ureteric orifice (Fig. 64.29).

Ureteric meatotomy. Stones often lodge in the intramural part of the ureter. Careful endoscopic incision using a diathermy knife can enlarge the opening and free the stone. The procedure may lead to urinary reflux but it is rare for this to cause problems.

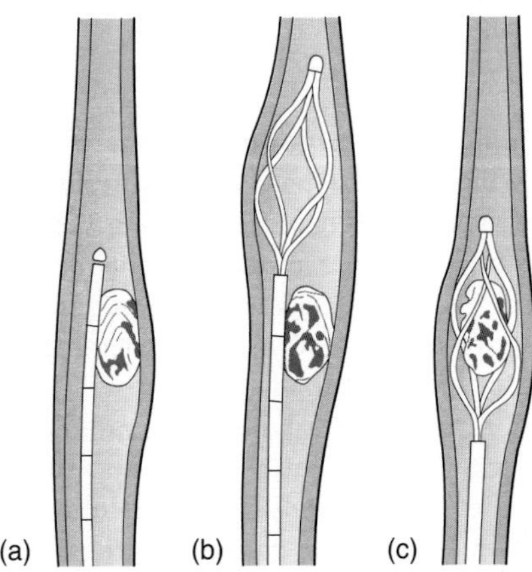

Fig. 64.29 Dormia stone-catching basket in use: (a) basket introduced past stone; (b) opened; and (c) enclosing stone ready for withdrawal.

Table 64.5 Indications for surgical removal of a ureteric calculus

Repeated attacks of pain and the stone is not moving
Stone is enlarging
Complete obstruction of the kidney
Urine is infected
Stone is too large to pass
Stone is obstructing a solitary kidney or there is bilateral obstruction

Dormia. Assistant Professor of Urology, University of Milan, Italy.

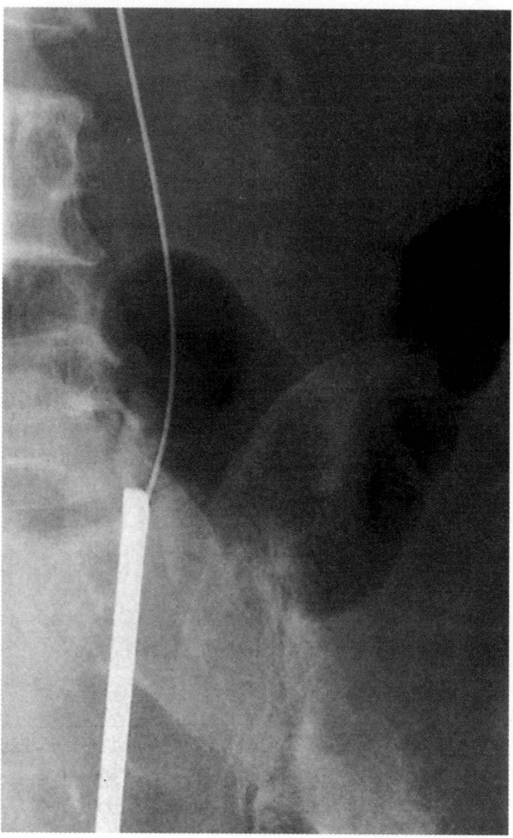

Fig. 64.30 Ureteroscopy. A radiograph showing a ureteroscope and guidewire in the lower ureter.

Ureteroscopic stone removal. A ureteroscope is a long endoscope which can be passed transurethrally across the bladder into the ureter (Fig. 64.30). The ureteroscope is used to remove stones which are impacted in the ureter. Stones that cannot be caught in baskets or endoscopic forceps under direct vision are fragmented using an electrohydraulic, percussive or laser lithotriptor.

Push bang. A stone that is lying in the middle or upper part of the ureter can often be flushed back into the kidney using a ureteric catheter. The repositioned calculus is 'secured' in the kidney by a J-stent. The patient can then be referred for ESWL.

Lithotripsy *in situ*. Provided the stone is in a part of the ureter that can be identified by the imaging system of the lithotriptor, it can be fragmented *in situ*. This form of treatment is not appropriate if there is complete obstruction or if the stone has been impacted for a long time.

Open surgery

Ureterolithotomy. A radiograph should be taken to confirm the position of the stone immediately before surgery.

The incision must be appropriate for the position of the stone. Calculi in the upper third of the ureter are approached through a loin or upper quadrant transverse incision as used for a stone in the renal pelvis. Access to midureteric stones is through a muscle-cutting iliac fossa incision; lower ureteric stones are best reached through a Pfannenstiel incision. For stones close to the bladder exposure is improved by ligating and dividing the superior vesicle vascular pedicle. The ureter is exposed in the retroperitoneum and slings are applied above and below the calculus to stop it from migrating from the operative field. The ureter is incised longitudinally, directly on to the stone, which is freed from adhesions by blunt dissection, and removed with stone forceps. Soft catheters are passed upwards and downwards to ensure that the ureter is clear. The ureterotomy is closed with interrupted absorbable sutures and a drain left in place for a day or so to drain urine leakage.

Idiopathic retroperitoneal fibrosis

This is a rare condition in which one or both ureters become bound up in a progressive fibrosis of the retroperitoneal tissues. The cause is unknown although some cases may be drug related. A similar clinical picture occurs in patients with leaking aortic aneurysm and infiltrating retroperitoneal malignancy.

The patient complains of backache which is unremitting for several months. The onset of anuria and renal failure prompts investigation of the renal tract which reveals hydronephrosis. The excretion urogram typically shows displacement of the obstructed ureters towards the midline and the appearances on CT are diagnostic. The sedimentation rate is markedly raised.

Treatment. It may be possible to insert ureteric stents as a temporary measure while renal function recovers. If not, percutaneous nephrostomies will allow the obstructed kidneys to drain. Some patients need renal replacement by dialysis. Some advocate that these patients should be treated conservatively with high-dose steroids. Surgical treatment involves careful dissection of the ureters from their entrapment (ureterolysis). Wrapping omentum around the freed ureters make recurrent obstruction less likely.

Kidney infections (Table 64.6)

Aetiology

Renal infections arise in the following ways.

- *Haematogenous infection* from a primary site in the tonsils or carious teeth, or from cutaneous infections, particularly boils or a carbuncle. Renal tuberculosis occurs by blood-borne spread from lymph nodes in the neck, chest or abdomen.

Table 64.6 Kidney infection

Acute pyelonephritis – in childhood – in pregnancy – with urinary obstruction
Chronic pyelonephritis – reflux nephropathy
Pyonephrosis
Renal abscess
Perinephric abscess

Hermann Johann Pfannenstiel, 1862–1909. Gynaecologist, Breslau, Germany.

- *Ascending infection* in the urinary tract is the most common route, and it is most likely to occur when there is vesicoureteric reflux. Urinary stasis and the presence of calculi are common contributory factors.

Bacteriology. *Escherichia coli* and other Gram-negative organisms are commonly responsible. When *Streptococcus faecalis* is present it is usually accompanied by other organisms. In *E. coli* and streptococcal infections the urine is acid. *Proteus* sp. and staphylococci split urea, forming ammonia which makes the urine alkaline and promotes the formation of calculi.

Acute pyelonephritis

Acute pyelonephritis is more common in females, especially during childhood, at puberty, soon after marriage (as a complication of 'honeymoon cystitis'), during pregnancy and during menopause. It occurs more on the right and is frequently bilateral.

Clinical features

There may be prodromal symptoms of headache, lassitude and nausea but the onset of pain is usually sudden, often with a rigor and vomiting. There is acute pain in the flank and hypochondrium. In a few cases the pain resembles renal colic. The temperature rises to 38.8 or 39.5°C and is remitting. The symptoms of cystitis set in soon after the onset with urgency, frequency and scalding dysuria. On examination, there is tenderness in the hypochondrium and in the loin. Rarely in cases of severe bilateral pyelonephritis, especially when there is an associated obstruction, the damage to renal function may be sufficient to cause uraemia.

Bacteriological examination of the urine

A midstream urine should be collected into a sterile container; the urine is centrifuged and the sediment examined microscopically. In early acute pyelonephritis there are usually a few pus cells and many bacteria. The macroscopic appearance of the urine may be misleadingly clear, until the infection becomes established when the urine is cloudy and full of pus. Culture and sensitivity testing of the causative organisms allows a rational choice of antibiotic, but parenteral treatment with a broad-spectrum antibiotic should be started before the results are available.

Severe cases

There are repeated rigors and the temperature rises to 40°C or more, often without a corresponding rise in pulse rate. There is vomiting, sweating and thirst; the patient feels awful. The blood culture is usually positive, especially if the specimen has been taken during a rigor.

Differential diagnosis

When the symptoms and signs are typical the diagnosis is straightforward. In other circumstances it may be difficult to be sure that the patient does not have pneumonia, acute appendicitis or acute cholecystitis. The urgent need is to distinguish acute pyelonephritis from appendicitis, and the site of pain and the presence of marked peritonism are usually helpful in identifying the latter. A plain abdominal radiograph may show the outline of a swollen kidney and, if the infection is severe, a skilled ultrasonographer may be able to detect the typical appearances of pyelonephritis.

Hans Christian Joachim Gram, 1853–1938. Danish bacteriologist and Professor of Medicine, Copenhagen, Denmark.

Pyelonephritis of pregnancy

Pyelonephritis of pregnancy usually occurs between the fourth and sixth month of gestation in women who have a past history of recurrent urinary infection. In about 10 per cent of cases the disease runs a severe and protracted course and occasionally leads to abortion or premature birth.

Urine infection in childhood

Urine infection in childhood is important to recognise because it may endanger the function of the growing kidney. In young children, there may be few symptoms but the child passes cloudy or offensive urine. The possibility of urinary sepsis should always be considered if a child fails to thrive, fails to eat or suffers unexplained pyrexia. Pain or screaming on micturition may occur. The older child may complain of loin pain and may develop urinary frequency and nocturnal incontinence.

Up to 50 per cent of children with urinary infection have an underlying anatomical abnormality. Once the diagnosis has been confirmed by examination of a clean-catch specimen or by a specimen obtained by suprapubic needle puncture, a full urological investigation is essential.

Vesicoureteric reflux of urine is detectable in about 35 per cent of children with recurrent urinary infection. In some patients the reflux is caused by high pressure in a neuropathic bladder. It may be intermittent and is often more marked when there is active infection. Renal damage results from the combination of reflux and urinary infection early in life and reflux nephropathy is the most common cause of end-stage renal failure in the UK. Once the diagnosis has been confirmed by micturating cystography, the urine should be cleared by means of an appropriate antibiotic. Long-term prophylactic antibiotic treatment has become the favoured treatment for recurrent urinary infections resulting from reflux. Surgical reimplantation of the ureters is reserved for those in whom conservative measures fail. Reimplantation in these patients often fails to cure reflux.

Acute pyelonephritis associated with urinary retention

Acute pyelonephritis is a relatively uncommon complication of chronic urinary retention. Often the organisms are introduced during instrumentation and, in the days of unsterile catheterisation, the condition was known as 'surgical kidneys'. Patients who have significant postmicturition urinary residue should be given prophylactic antibiotics to cover transurethral procedures.

Treatment of acute pyelonephritis

The treatment of acute pyelonephritis should be *prompt, appropriate and prolonged.* A full investigation to exclude underlying abnormalities in the urinary tract should be undertaken as soon as the attack is controlled.

The patient will usually feel like lying in bed. While awaiting the bacteriological report and the results of sensitivity tests, an antimicrobial with a wide range of activity, such as amoxycillin or gentamicin, should be administered, parenterally if necessary. If the urine is acid, as it is in the common coliform infections, alkalinisation of the urine by potassium citrate may help by inhibiting the growth of these organisms and relieving dysuria. When pain is severe a morphine-like analgesic drug may be necessary if nonsteroidal anti-inflammatory agents are not effective. The patient should be encouraged to drink copiously; if this is not possible because of nausea and vomiting, an intravenous infusion should be set up.

Most urinary infections acquired outside hospital are sensitive to relatively cheap agents such as *trimethoprim and amoxycillin.* Hospital-acquired infections are much more likely to be resistant and more expensive second-line antibiotics may be needed. *Gentamicin* and *carbenicillin* are suitable for combating infections with more resistant strains of *Pseudomonas pyocyanea, Proteus* sp. and *Klebsiella* sp. *Ciprofloxacin* is particularly useful against *Pseudomonas* sp. in patients who do not have septicaemia. Despite the efficacy of modern antibacterial drugs, recurrent infection is likely if there is an untreated underlying abnormality of the urinary tract such as a stone, vesicoureteric reflux or retention of urine.

Chronic pyelonephritis

Chronic pyelonephritis is so often associated with vesicoureteric reflux that some feel that it is better named *'reflux nephropathy'*. It is an important cause of renal damage and death from end-stage renal failure.

Pathology

There is interstitial inflammation and scarring of the renal parenchyma with a patchy distribution. The renal tubules bear the brunt of the destruction – they are atrophic and dilated. The glomeruli retain their normal structure until the final stages of the disease.

Clinical features

The condition is almost three times as common in women as it is in men. Two-thirds of affected females are under 40 years of age, whereas 60 per cent of the males are over 40.

It is possible, but unusual, for chronic pyelonephritis to remain clinically silent until the symptoms of advanced renal insufficiency appear.

Lumbar pain, dull and nonspecific in character, is present in 60 per cent of cases.

Increased urinary frequency and **dysuria** are common.

Hypertension is present in 40 per cent of cases and may be of the accelerated ('malignant') type. It develops slowly and is most in evidence in long-standing disease.

Constitutional symptoms of lassitude, malaise, anorexia, nausea and headache constitute the main complaint in 30 per cent of cases. The true cause of these nonspecific symptoms may elude diagnosis for years.

Pyrexia. Attacks of low-grade fever often prompt the urinary tract investigations which bring the condition to light.

Anaemia. Normochromic anaemia due to unsuspected renal impairment is an occasional presenting feature.

Investigations

As the glomeruli are relatively preserved, proteinuria is less marked than in glomerulonephritis (<3 g daily). Casts are not usually present but white cells are plentiful.

Bacteriological examination of the urine commonly reveals the presence of *E. coli, S. faecalis, Proteus* sp. or *Pseudomonas* sp.

Treatment

Treatment may be difficult and is aimed at eradicating predisposing contributory factors such as obstruction or stones and treating the infection with appropriate antibiotics, often as repeated courses of treatment. Unfortunately, once the parenchyma has been scarred it becomes vulnerable to blood-borne organisms and reinfection is likely, sometimes with a different and resistant organism. Consequently, antibiotics confer only temporary benefit and progressive renal damage is common.

Surgical treatment is only indicated when the disease is confined to one kidney. This is unusual but in such cases nephrectomy or partial nephrectomy may stop the symptoms of infection and make hypertension easier to control. Some patients with end-stage renal failure require renal transplantation.

Hypertension and a unilateral renal lesion

Ischaemia of the renal parenchyma leads to the release of pressor agents which cause arterial hypertension. Where a renal lesion is discovered during the investigation of hypertension, nephrectomy may not bring the pressure to normal but it may make the hypertension more amenable to drug treatment.

Pyonephrosis

The kidney is converted into a multilocular sac containing pus or purulent urine. Pyonephrosis can result from infection of a hydronephrosis, follow acute pyelonephritis or, most commonly, arise as a complication of renal calculus disease. Pyonephrosis is usually unilateral.

Clinical features

The classical triad of symptoms is anaemia, fever and a swelling in the loin. When the condition arises as an infected hydronephrosis, the swelling may be very large and the pyrexia very high and associated with rigors. Symptoms of cystitis may be prominent.

Investigations

The plain radiograph may show a calculus and an ultrasonogram will demonstrate dilatation of the renal pelvis and calyces. The intravenous urogram will show poor function and the features of hydronephrosis on the affected side.

Treatment

Pyonephrosis is a surgical emergency because the patient is threatened with permanent renal damage and a potentially lethal septicaemia. Parenteral antibiotics should be given immediately and the kidney drained. If the pus is too thick to be aspirated through a large percutaneous nephrostomy, it may be necessary to consider open nephrostomy. In cases where there is a stone, the stone should be removed. Nephrectomy may be considered when long-standing obstruction is known to have destroyed the kidney, and function on the other side is good.

Renal carbuncle

An abscess may form in the renal parenchyma as the result of blood-borne spread of organisms, especially coliforms or *Staphylococcus aureus*, from a focus elsewhere in the body. Occasionally the condition results from infection of a haematoma following a blow to the kidney. Renal carbuncle is most commonly seen in diabetic patients, intravenous drug abusers, those debilitated by chronic disease and patients with acquired immunodeficiency.

Pathology. The renal parenchyma contains an encapsulated necrotic mass.

Clinical features. There is an ill-defined tender swelling in the loin, persistent pyrexia and leucocytosis, signs that closely simulate those of perinephric abscess. In early cases there is no pus or bacteria in the urine but they appear after a day or so. Urography shows a space-occupying lesion in the kidney which may be confused with a renal adenocarcinoma on ultrasonography and CT (Fig. 64.31).

Treatment. Resolution by antibiotic treatment alone is unusual. Formal open incision of the abscess may be necessary if the pus is too thick to be drained by percutaneous aspiration.

Perinephric abscess

The common causes of perinephric abscess are shown in Fig. 64.32. Other causes are infection of a perirenal haematoma and perinephric discharge of an untreated pyonephrosis or renal carbuncle. A mycobacterial perinephric abscess may arise by extension from a nearby tuberculosis vertebra.

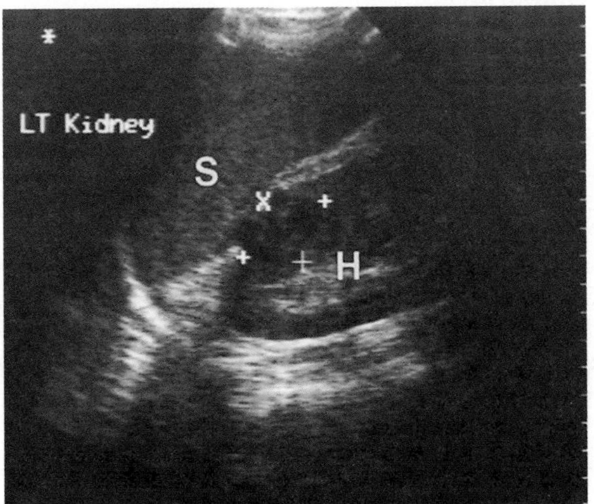

Fig. 64.31 Longitudinal ultrasound scan through the upper pole of the left kidney demonstrates a renal carbuncle, outlined by crosses. S = spleen.

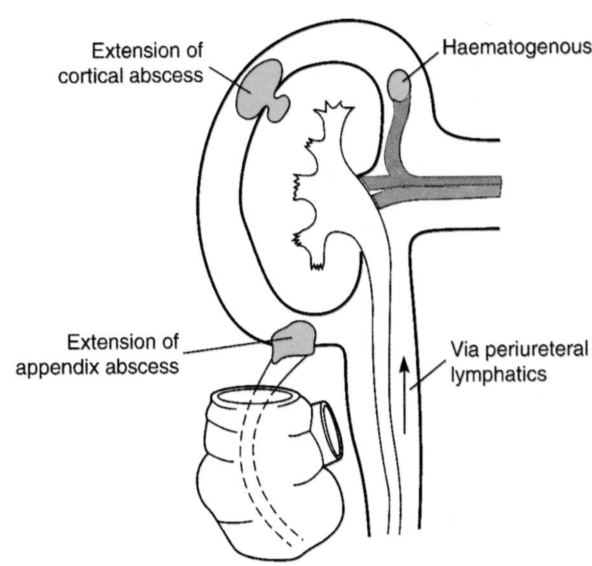

Fig. 64.32 Sources of perinephric abscess.

Clinical features

The classical symptoms and signs of perinephric abscess are a high swinging pyrexia, abdominal tenderness and fullness in the loin (Fig. 64.33). Local signs present early if the infection starts in the lower part of the perinephric fat. Infection at the upper pole is masked by the lower ribs and the signs in the loin are much less marked. The white cell count is always markedly raised but there are characteristically no pus cells or organisms in the urine.

Imaging

The psoas shadow is obscured on the plain abdominal radiograph. There may be a reactionary scoliosis – with the concavity toward the abscess – and elevation and immobility of the diaphragm on the affected side. A calculus may be present. Ultrasonography and CT are diagnostic.

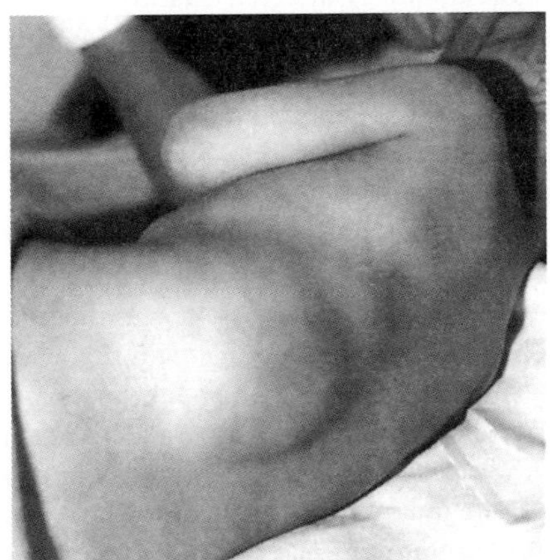

Fig. 64.33 A large perinephric abscess.

Treatment

Open drainage may be necessary if the abscess cannot be aspirated through a large percutaneous needle. A lumbar incision is made under antibiotic cover. This should be large enough to allow the surgeon to open pockets of pus and to explore for an unruptured cortical abscess which may also be present. A specimen of pus is sent for culture and the wound is closed over a tube drain.

Renal tuberculosis

Aetiology and pathology

Tuberculosis of the urinary tract arises from haematogenous infection from a distant focus which is often impossible to identify. The lesions are usually confined to one kidney. A group of tuberculous granulomas in a renal pyramid coalesces and forms an ulcer. Mycobacteria and pus cells are discharged into the urine. Untreated, the lesions enlarge and a *tuberculous abscess* may form in the parenchyma. The necks of the calyces and the renal pelvis stenosed by fibrosis confine the infection so that there is *tuberculous pyonephrosis* which is sometimes localised to one pole of the kidney. Extension of pyonephrosis or tuberculous renal abscess leads to *perinephric abscess* and the kidney is progressively replaced by caseous material (*putty kidney*) which may be calcified (*cement kidney*). At any stage the plain radiograph may show areas of calcification (*pseudocalculi*). Less commonly the kidneys may be bilaterally affected as part of the generalised process of miliary tuberculosis (Fig. 64.34).

Renal tuberculosis is often associated with tuberculosis of the bladder and typical tuberculous granulomas may be visible in the bladder wall. In the male, tuberculous epididymo-orchitis may occur without apparent infection of the bladder.

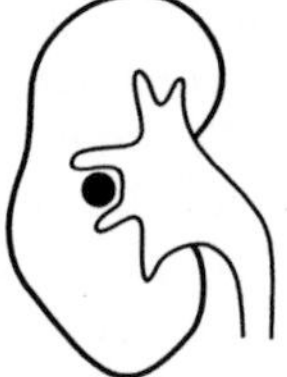
(a) Tuberculous papillary ulcer

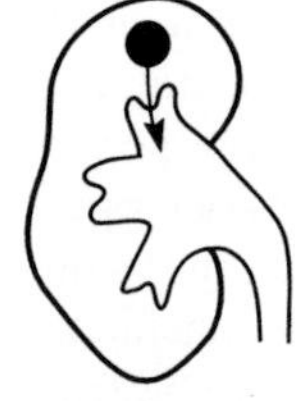
(b) Cavernous form
'It tends to burst like a bombshell'

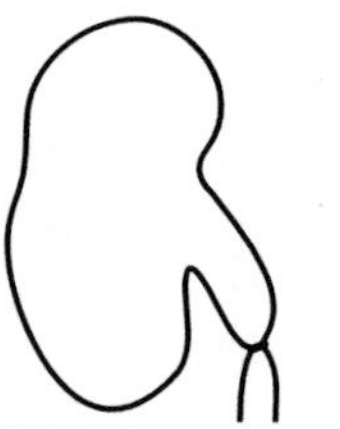
(c) Hydronephrosis (rare)

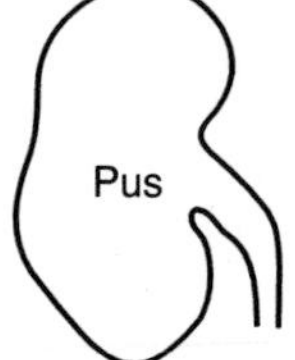

(d) Pyonephrosis
Secondary infection. E. coli. etc. very prone to supervene

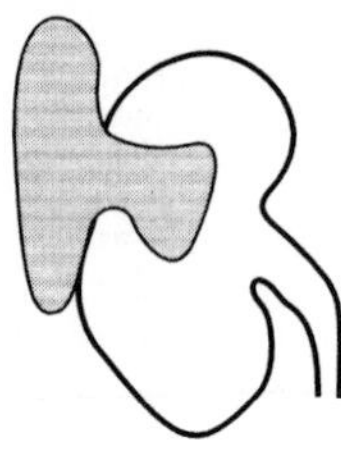
(e) Tuberculous perinephric abscess

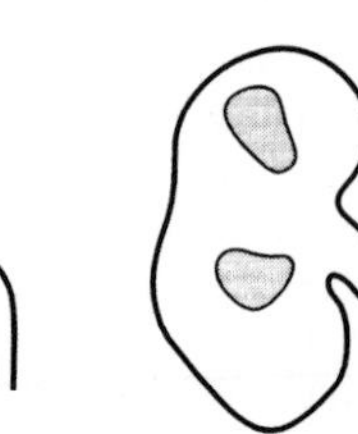
(f) Pseudocalculi
On X-ray examination, calcified tuberculous areas in the kidney simulate calculi

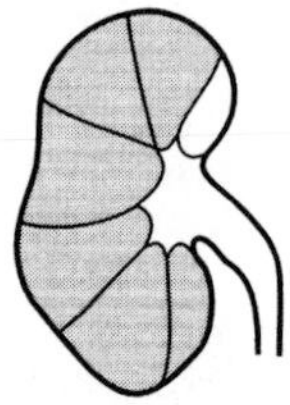
(g) Caseous kidney
Divided by fibrous septa

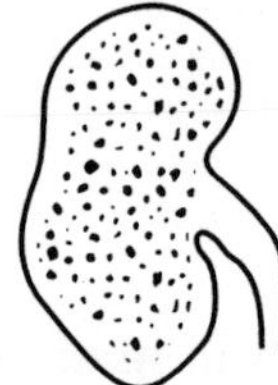
(h) Miliary
A part of a general tuberculous process

Fig. 64.34 Types of lesion in renal tuberculosis.

Clinical features

Renal tuberculosis usually occurs between 20 and 40 years of age, and is twice as common in men as in women; also, the right kidney is affected slightly more often than the left.

Urinary frequency is often the earliest symptom and may be the only one. The patient complains that, over a period of months, there has been a progressive increase in both daytime and night-time frequency.

'Sterile' pyuria. In early cases the urine is pale and slightly opalescent. Routine urine culture is negative.

Painful micturition is a feature as soon as tuberculous cystitis sets in. First there is a suprapubic pain if voiding is delayed; later a burning pain accompanies micturition. When there is secondary infection a superadded agonising pain referred to the tip of the penis or to the vulva is often associated with haematuria and strangury.

Renal pain is often minimal but there may be a dull ache in the loin.

Haematuria

In 5 per cent of cases the first symptom is haematuria occurring from an ulcer on a renal papilla. The tuberculous lesion may be difficult to detect radiologically and mycobacteria may not be cultured from the urine until the onset of more suggestive symptoms some months later.

A tuberculous kidney is oedematous and friable and is more liable to damage than a normal kidney.

Constitutional symptoms are common. Weight loss is usual and a slight evening pyrexia is typical. A high temperature suggests secondary infection or dissemination, i.e. miliary tuberculosis.

On examination

It is unusual for a tuberculous kidney to be palpable. The prostate, seminal vesicles, vasa and scrotal contents should be examined for nodules or thickening.

Investigation

Bacteriological

Bacteriological examination of at least three full specimens of early-morning urine should be sent for microscopy and culture before specific chemotherapy is started. Staining of the urine sediment with the Ziehl–Neilsen stain occasionally shows the presence of acid-fast bacilli but proof that these are pathological mycobacteria must await prolonged culture on Löwenstein–Jensen medium. Where the clinical picture is convincing it is permissible to start antituberculous therapy in anticipation of the culture results which will come some 6 weeks later.

Radiography

A plain abdominal radiograph may show the calcified lesions described above.

Intravenous urography

In the very earliest stages of the disease the normally clear-cut outline of a renal papilla may be rendered indistinct by the presence of ulceration. Later there may be evidence of calyceal stenosis (Fig. 64.35) and/or hydronephrosis caused by stricture of the renal pelvis or the ureter draining the affected kidney; this may be more easily demonstrable by retrograde ureterography (Fig. 64.36). A tuberculous abscess appears as a space-occupying lesion which causes adjacent calyces to splay out. The bladder may appear shrunken with its wall irregular or thickened. In late stages there may be dilatation of the contralateral ureter from obstruction where the ureter passes through a thickened and oedematous bladder wall.

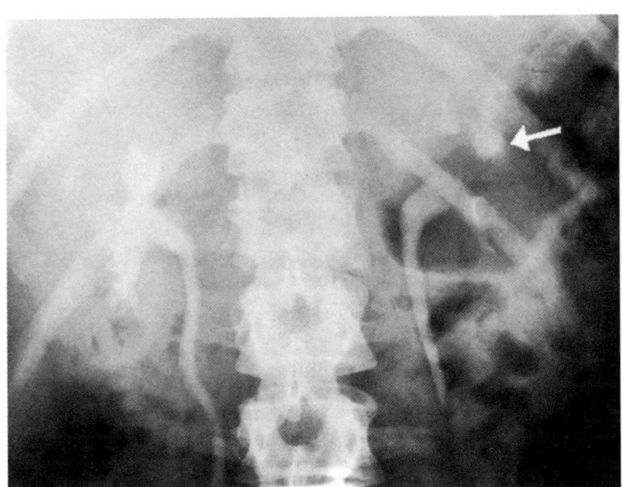

Fig. 64.35 Intravenous urogram showing a small localised tuberculous lesion with hydrocalyx. Healing took place with conservative treatment.

Franz Ziehl, 1857–1926. Neurologist, Lubeck, Germany.
Friedrich Karl Adolf Neilson, 1854–94. Prosector, Stadt-Krankenhaus, Dresden, Germany.
Ernst Löwenstein, b. 1878. Pathologist, Vienna, Austria.
Carl Oluf Jensen, (1864–1934). Pathologist, Copenhagen, Denmark.

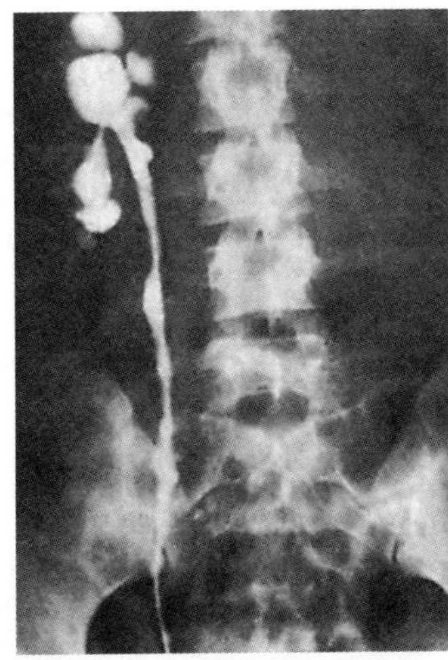

Fig. 64.36 Retrograde ureterogram showing advanced tuberculosis of the right kidney and ureter.

Cystoscopy

Cystoscopy is not indicated as a routine part of the investigation of urinary tuberculosis but is often performed because there has been haematuria or unexplained bladder symptoms. There may be little to see in the first stages of the disease but later the bladder urothelium is found to be studded with granulomas which cluster particularly around the ureteric orifices. The tubercules may coalesce to produce a tuberculous ulcer. As the bladder wall fibroses the bladder capacity decreases. Contraction of the fibrosed ureter tugs at the ureteric orifice which is displaced upwards, its mouth wide open (the so-called 'golf-hole' ureteric orifice).

Chest radiograph

A chest radiograph is indicated to exclude an active lung lesion.

Treatment

Antituberculous chemotherapy is best managed by a physician with experience of the most modern drug regimens and their potential adverse effects. The surgeon must ensure that the state of the urinary tract is reviewed during the first few weeks of therapy because *stricturing of the renal pelvis and ureter may continue after treatment has started.*

Prognosis in renal tuberculosis is good and there should be no recrudescence of the disease if the patient completes the course of chemotherapy.

Operative treatment

Operative treatment should be as conservative as possible. The aim is to remove large foci of infection, which are difficult to treat with drugs, and to correct the obstruction caused by fibrosis. The optimum time for surgery is between 6 and 12 weeks of the start of antituberculous chemotherapy.

The surgeon needs a repertoire of procedures to deal with various potential effects of urinary tuberculosis. An obstructed lower pole calyx may be drained into the upper ureter. A strictured renal pelvis needs a pyeloplasty. Ureteric stenosis and shortening may require a Boari operation or a bowel interposition, depending on the level and extent of the fibrosis. If the kidney has no function it is best to perform a nephroureterectomy (Fig. 64.37). A bladder which is so contracted that it can no longer function as a reservoir for urine may need to be replaced with a neobladder fashioned from a loop of bowel in a *substitution cystoplasty*.

(a)

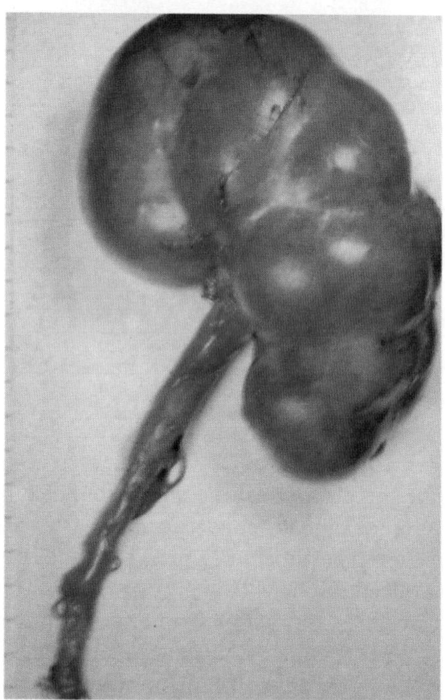

(b)

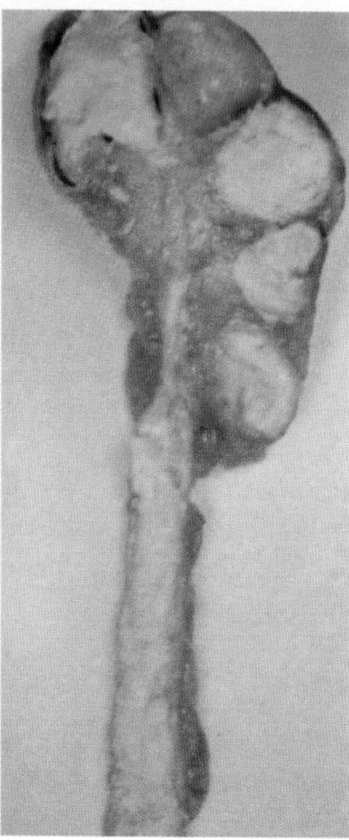

Fig. 64.37 Nephroureterectomy specimen from a patient with kidney destroyed by tuberculous pyonephrosis.

Table 64.7 Renal neoplasms

Benign neoplasms
Adenoma
Angioma
Angiomyolipoma
Malignant neoplasms
Wilms' tumour (nephroblastoma in children)
Grawitz tumour (adenocarcinoma, hypernephroma)
Transitional cell carcinoma of the renal pelvis and collecting system
Squamous carcinoma of the renal pelvis

Neoplasms of the kidney (Table 64.7)

Benign neoplasms

Adenoma. Pea-like cortical adenomas are occasionally discovered at *post mortem* examination or incidentally during radiological imaging. They are asymptomatic and by definition benign.

Angioma may cause profuse haematuria, often in young adults. The source of the bleeding may be difficult to diagnose without renal angiography.

Angiomyolipoma is an unusual tumour of the kidney which is often but not always associated with tuberous sclerosis. Its high fat content gives it a typical appearance on CT. Malignant elements are present in about a quarter of them and may lead to metastasis.

Malignant neoplasms

Benign tumours of the kidney are rare and it is a good rule that all neoplasms of the kidney which are recognised clinically should be treated as malignant. They are uncommon between the ages of 7 and 40.

Renal neoplasms in children

Wilms' tumour (syn. nephroblastoma)

This is a mixed tumour containing epithelial and connective tissue elements arising from embryonic nephrogenic tissue. The tumours are usually discovered during the first 4 years of life. They are normally in one or other pole of one kidney, but bilateral tumours occasionally pose a difficult clinical problem.

Pathology. The cut surface of the tumour is greyish or pinkish white. A rapidly growing tumour is likely to be soft and friable in consistency (Fig. 64.38).

Microscopically the tumour is composed of epithelial and connective tissue cells, occasionally with islands of bone, cartilage and muscle fibre. Some of the elements in this cellular mixture may be less sensitive to radiotherapy than others.

Clinical features. ***Abdominal tumour.*** An abdominal tumour appears which grows rapidly while the general well being of the child deteriorates. The mass may be enormous compared with the tiny patient.

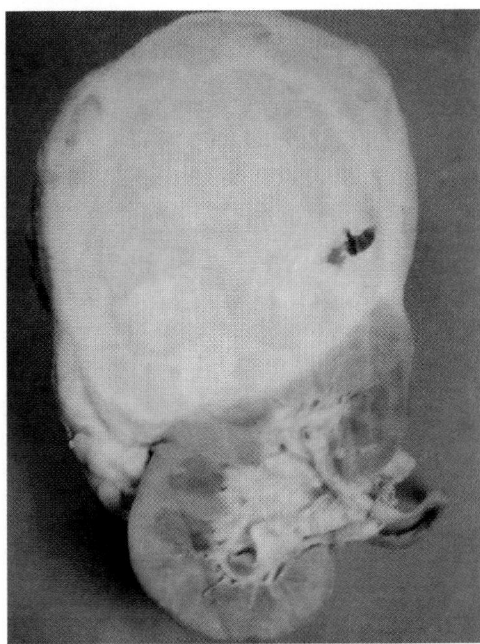

Fig. 64.38 Wilms' tumour.

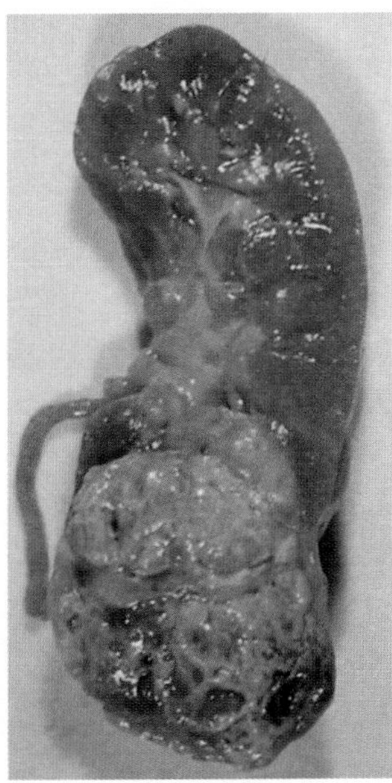

Fig. 64.39 Adenocarcinoma of the kidney (Grawitz's tumour).

Pyrexia, which is a feature in half of these patients, disappears when the tumour is removed.

Haematuria denotes extension of the tumour into the renal pelvis and the prognosis is not so good.

Imaging by ultrasonography, urography or CT confirms a solid space-occupying lesion in the kidney.

Metastasis occurs early, mainly by the bloodstream to the lungs. Liver and bone metastases are rare, and brain metastases even more so. Lymphatic spread is uncommon.

The presence of bone secondaries favours a diagnosis of nephroblastoma, another renal tumour of childhood which is treated in the same way as Wilms' tumour.

Treatment. These children do best when treated in specialist units. *Nephrectomy* should be performed as soon as possible and followed by radiotherapy with or without chemotherapy. *Partial nephrectomy* may be possible in patients with bilateral disease.

Prognosis. Under 1 year of age 80 per cent survive for 5 years, but the prognosis is less good in older children. Recurrences usually occur within a year, so a child surviving for 18 months or more is probably cured.

Renal neoplasm in adults

Hypernephroma (syn. Grawitz's tumour)

This is an adenocarcinoma and is the most common neoplasm (75 per cent) of the kidney. It arises from renal tubular cells. Whether carcinoma arises in pre-existing adenomas is a matter for dispute.

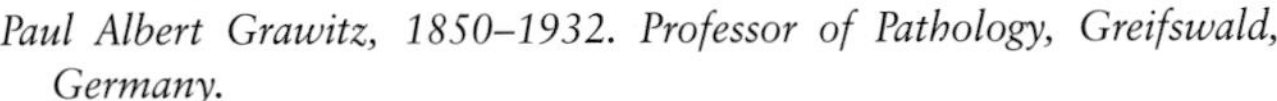

Paul Albert Grawitz, 1850–1932. Professor of Pathology, Greifswald, Germany.

Pathology. Moderate sized tumours are spherical and often occupy the poles of a single kidney, most commonly the upper pole. Tumours in the hilum are less common. The cut surface of the tumour is usually yellowish or dull white, semitransparent, with areas of haemorrhage (Fig. 64.39). The tumour is often divided into lobules by fibrous septa, some of which are cystic. Larger tumours are irregular in shape with central haemorrhage and necrosis.

Microscopical structure. The most common pattern is of solid areas of polyhedral or cubical clear cells with deeply stained small rounded nuclei and abundant cytoplasm containing lipids, cholesterol and glycogen. The cells are occasionally arranged as papillary cysts or tubules. Less commonly the cells are granular (dark), and both clear and dark cells may be represented in the same tumour. In all cases the stroma is scanty but rich in large blood vessels.

Spread. The tumour is prone to grow into the renal vein. Pieces of growth are swept into the circulation and end up in the lungs where they grow to form **cannonball** secondary deposits (Fig. 64.40). Metastasis to bone also occurs and a secondary deposit in a long bone may remain the only sign of distant spread for a year or more. Highly vascular metastases may pulsate. If the tumour extends beyond the renal capsule it is liable to metastasise via the lymph nodes in the hilum of the kidney to the para-aortic nodes and beyond.

Clinical features. Hypernephroma is twice as common in men as in women. Haematuria is usually the presenting symptom, sometimes with clot colic. There may be a dragging discomfort in the loin or the patient may detect a mass. In men, a rapidly developing varicocele is a rare but impressive sign, occurring most often on the left side because the left gonadal vein is obstructed where it joins the left renal vein.

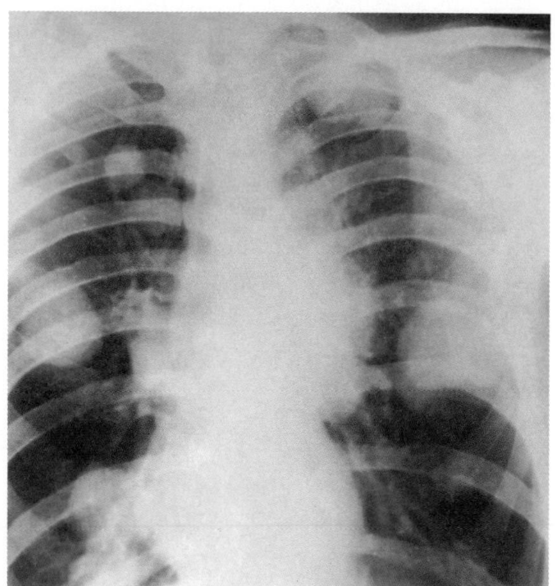

Fig. 64.40 Cannonball secondaries from a hypernephroma.

Atypical presentations.

1. In 25 per cent of cases there are no local symptoms. The patient presents with symptoms due to secondary deposits such as a painful enlargement of a long bone (Fig. 64.41), a pathological fracture, persistent cough or haemoptysis.
2. Occasionally persistent pyrexia (37.8–38.9°C) is the only symptom. There is no evidence of infection. Persistence of the pyrexia after nephrectomy suggests the presence of metastases.
3. A small number of patients presents with constitutional symptoms and is found to be extremely anaemic.
4. Polycythaemia occurs in 4 per cent of cases as a result of the production of erythropoietin by tumour cells. The erythrocyte sedimentation rate is always raised above the 1–2 mm found in idiopathic polycythaemia vera. The blood count returns to normal after nephrectomy unless there are metastases. Other hormones, such as renin and calcitonin, may be produced by the tumour. Hypercalcaemia is common.
5. Nephrotic syndrome has been reported as a rare presentation of hypernephroma.

Investigation. ***Intravenous urography*** is still an important component of the investigation of haematuria. The plain radiograph may show abnormal calcification in the tumour and distortion of the renal outline which will be confirmed on the nephrogram film. The calyces may be stretched and distorted. It is important to know whether the contralateral kidney is working (Fig. 64.42).

Ultrasound and CT. Once a mass has been demonstrated in the kidney a scan is needed to decide whether it is solid or cystic. Modern high-definition ultrasound will give this information. CT with enhancement will demonstrate the extent of the lesion more clearly and will show whether there is hilar lymphadenopathy or renal vein involvement (Fig. 64.43).

Renal angiography is used less since CT became available. Enthusiasm for preoperative embolisation of hypernephroma has waned. Occasionally a flush inferior cavagram is helpful to show the extent of caval involvement by tumour growing in from the renal vein.

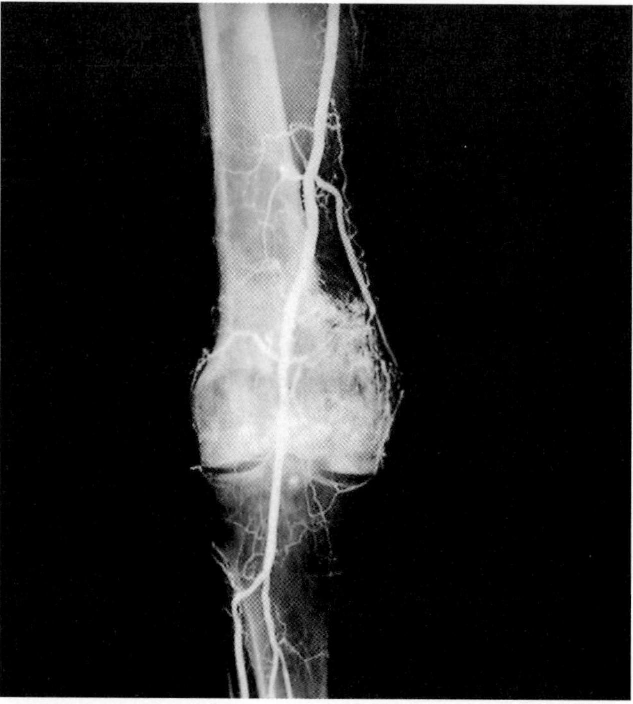

Fig. 64.41 Arteriogram showing vascular 'blush' due to metastasis from a Grawitz's tumour.

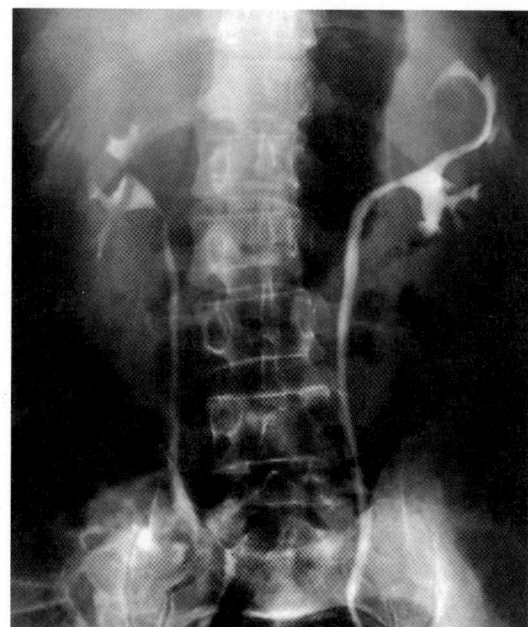

Fig. 64.42 Intravenous urogram in a case of hypernephroma of the left kidney. The only symptom was one attack of painless haematuria. Note displacement of upper pole calyces by the mass.

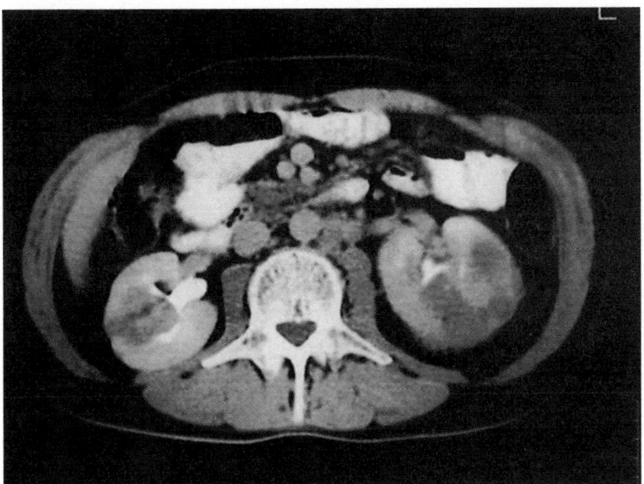

Fig. 64.43 CT scan showing large bilateral renal adenocarcinomas.

A chest radiograph is essential to detect lung secondaries. An **isotope bone scan** will reveal deposits in the skeleton.

Treatment. If the tumour is confined to the kidney treatment is nephrectomy with removal of the perinephric fat.

Nephrectomy can be performed through a loin or a transverse or oblique upper abdominal incision. The transabdominal approach has the advantage that the renal pedicle and the inferior vena cava can be widely exposed.

The vascular pedicle should be ligated before the kidney is mobilised because handling the tumour may cause malignant cells to be released into the circulation. The first step in the procedure is to clean the renal artery and ligate it in continuity. This may be more difficult from an anterior approach because the vessel lies *behind* the vein. However, once the artery is occluded the tumour loses most of its profuse blood supply and massive bleeding during mobilisation becomes less likely. The renal vein should be gently palpated to be sure that it does not have tumour in its lumen. If it is empty, it can be divided between ligatures. The renal artery is then divided and the kidney mobilised within its fascial and fatty coverings. Troublesome bleeding can still occur when aberrant vessels feeding the tumour are divided, and these must be carefully ligated or coagulated. The ureter is then traced downwards as far as is safe and divided between ligatures.

If the renal vein or the inferior vena cava is invaded the surgeon must obtain control of the cava above and below as a first priority. If there is extension into the thorax, the cardiac team may be needed to put the patient on cardiac bypass so that tumour can be removed from the right side of the heart if necessary.

Adenocarcinoma of the kidney does not respond well to radiotherapy or conventional chemotherapy. There have been early promising results from clinical trials of the cytokine interleukin-2 in this condition.

Prognosis. Removal of even the largest neoplasm may cure the patient. In operable cases 70 per cent of patients are well after 3 years and 60 per cent after 5 years. Macroscopic involvement of the renal vein or its tributaries, tumour invasion beyond the capsule and lymph node involvement all worsen the prognosis.

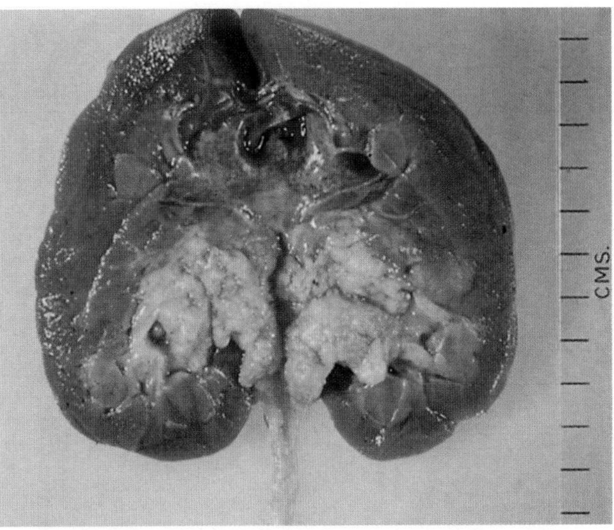

Fig. 64.44 Papillary transitional cell tumour of the renal pelvis.

Papillary transitional cell tumours of the renal pelvis (Fig. 64.44)

These resemble those of the bladder but are much less common. They tend to invade the renal parenchyma and have a tendency to distant spread. There is a strong tendency for the tumours to be multifocal. Seeding down the lumen of the urinary tract may give rise to multiple ureteric tumours, but the condition is thought to arise from a field change which renders the whole urothelium liable to metaplasia. Whether the carcinogen is chemical or viral is uncertain in most cases.

Clinical features. Haematuria is the most common symptom and usually causes the patient to seek help before the tumour mass becomes palpable.

Urine cytology. Examination of the urine for the presence of malignant cells may indicate whether the tumour is well or poorly differentiated. There is some evidence that those with poorly differentiated tumours do better if they have a short course of radiotherapy before surgery. It is therefore useful to obtain cells from the tumour by sampling using a brush or catheter passed up the ureter under radiological control.

Intravenous urography usually demonstrates the tumour (Fig. 64.45). Retrograde pyelography may be helpful if the urogram is indistinct.

Treatment. Conventional surgical treatment is by nephroureterectomy. The ureter must be disconnected with a cuff of bladder wall. If this is done by open surgery a second incision is needed to remove the kidney. Alternatively, the ureteric orifice can be widely resected with a resectoscope and the ureter delivered by a somewhat perilous blunt dissection from the upper abdominal wound used to remove the kidney. This pluck operation is not for the inexperienced. Some urologists argue that well-differentiated upper urinary tract transitional tumours should be treated conservatively like superficial bladder tumours. However, percutaneous resection of these cancers is controversial and steps must be taken to avoid the growth of tumour seeded in the percutaneous track.

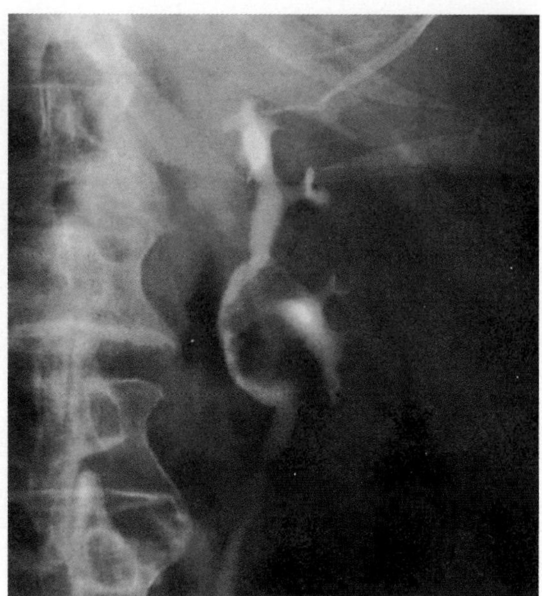

Fig. 64.45 Intravenous urogram shows a filling defect in the left renal pelvis due to transitional cell carcinoma.

Squamous cell carcinoma of the renal pelvis

This is rare and often associated with chronic inflammation and leucoplakia resulting from stone. The tumours are radiosensitive but metastasise at an early stage and the prognosis is poor.

Transitional cell tumours of the ureter

These are rare. They behave like tumours of the renal pelvis. Treatment is by nephroureterectomy.

About one half of patients with tumours of the upper urinary tract will have tumours in the bladder at some stage. Follow-up by cystoscopy with regular urography is therefore necessary to detect recurrent tumours.

Balkan nephropathy. Transitional cell tumours of the upper urinary tract have a very high incidence in certain areas of the former Yugoslavia. They also have a high incidence of a form of primary nephropathy. The causative agent has not been identified with certainty but there seems to be an association with the consumption of grain products stored in a damp environment. Tumours which develop against a background of Balkan nephropathy should be treated by conservative surgery in view of the impaired overall renal function.

Nephrectomy for benign disease

Nephrectomy is now rarely performed for benign disease but may be necessary if the kidney is atrophic or dysplastic or the cause of accelerated hypertension. Nonfunctioning kidneys resulting from long-standing obstruction or stone disease are a potential site for infection and even malignancy. Because they do not excrete they cannot be properly seen on an excretion urogram and it is often wisest to perform a simple nephrectomy. In a **simple nephrectomy** the kidney is dissected free though the convenient plane between the capsule and its fatty coverings. If this plane is obscured by the scarring of previous surgery a **subcapsular nephrectomy** may be safer. **Laparoscopic nephrectomy** is sometimes possible for small kidneys destroyed by benign disease but the technique requires special skills and the costs and benefits are under evaluation.

Further reading

Blandy, J.P. and Fowler, C.G. (1995) *Urology,* 2nd edn, Blackwell Scientific, Oxford.

Walsh, P.C., Retik, A.B., Darracott Vaughan, E. and Wein, A.J. (1998) *Campbell's Urology,* 7th edn, W.B. Saunders, Philadelphia, PA.

Whitfield, H.W., Hendry, W.F., Kirby, R.S. and Duckett J. (1998) *Textbook of Genito-urinary Surgery,* 2nd edn, Blackwell Science, Oxford.

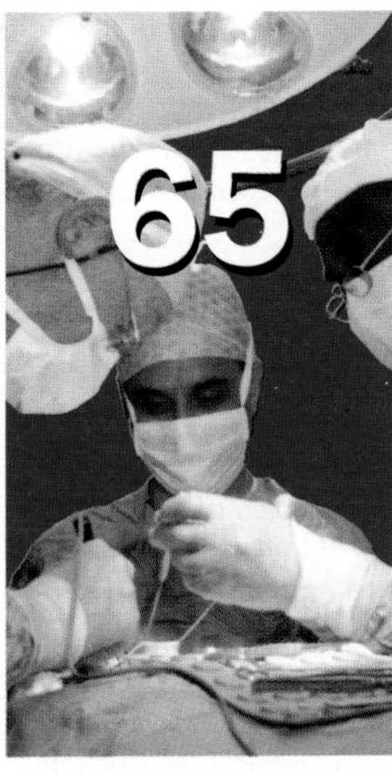

65 The urinary bladder

Surgical anatomy and physiology

Surgical anatomy

- Lined by transitional epithelium which covers a connective tissue known as the lamina propria
- The fibres of the detrusor smooth muscle are intermingled and not arranged in distinct layers
- When the detrusor hypertrophies from bladder outlet obstruction, neurological bladder dysfunction or detrusor instability, the fasciculi of the inner layer, covered by urothelium, stand out to give rise to the endoscopic and radiological appearance of trabeculation
- Lining the trigone is a separate, thin layer of smooth muscle to which the epithelium is closely adherent and which extends as a sheath around the lower ureters and also passes into the proximal urethra
- Around the male bladder neck is the smooth muscle internal sphincter which fulfils a sexual function, it is innervated by α-adrenergic fibres and prevents retrograde ejaculation
- The distal urethral sphincter is a horseshoe-shaped mass of striated muscle which lies anterior and distal to the prostate or proximal two-thirds of the female urethra
- The distal sphincter is a somatic, striated muscle, quite distinct from the pelvic floor and is supplied by S2–S4 fibres via the pudendal nerve and also by somatic fibres passing directly through the inferior hypogastric plexus

Bailey & Love's Short Practice of Surgery, 23rd edition. Edited by R.C.G. Russell, N.S. Williams and C.J.K. Bulstrode. Published in 2000 by Arnold Publishers.

Fascial and ligamentous supports of the bladder

Several parts of the surrounding pelvic fascia are of surgical importance. Posteriorly, there are condensations of the endopelvic fascia which are continuous with the lateral ligaments of the rectum; these pass forward medial to the ureter to join with the fascia surrounding the prostate: these sheets of fascia need to be divided during radical cystectomy. The anterior *puboprostatic ligaments* are well defined, are condensations of the anterior part of the endopelvic fascia and are of great surgical importance. Each stretches from the front of the prostate to the lower part of the periosteum of the pubis. They lie lateral to the dorsal vein complex of the penis and in their deep parts are closely adherent to large veins. When they are divided it is important to stay laterally and very close to the periosteum of the pubis.

The urachus and obliterated hypogastric arteries, together with the folds of peritoneum overlying these structures, are called the *false (median and lateral umbilical) ligaments of the bladder*. Condensations of fascia around the blood vessels passing to the bladder are known as the *superior and inferior vascular pedicles*.

Arteries

The superior and inferior vesical arteries are derived from the anterior trunk of the internal iliac artery. Branches from the obturator and inferior gluteal arteries (and in the female from the uterine and vaginal arteries) also help to supply the bladder.

Veins

The veins form a plexus on the lateral and inferior surfaces of the bladder; in the male the prostatic plexus is large and continuous with the vesical plexus, which drains into the internal iliac vein.

Lymphatics

These accompany the veins, and drain into the lymph nodes along the internal iliac vessels and thence to the obturator and external iliac chains. Some lymphatics pass to nodes which are situated posterior to the internal iliac artery lying directly on the sacral fascia.

Physiology (Fig. 65.1)

The nerves concerned in micturition are as follows.

The parasympathetic input

This innervation is the most important component and is derived from the anterior primary divisions of the second, third and fourth sacral segments (mainly S2 and S3). These fibres pass through the pelvic splanchnic nerves to the inferior hypogastric plexus, from which they are distributed to the bladder. The pelvic plexus is easily damaged during excisions of the rectum, following which disturbances of micturition and sexual function may occur.

The sympathetic input

These nerves arise in the 11th thoracic to the second lumbar segments. These fibres pass via the presacral hypogastric nerve and the sympathetic chains to the inferior hypogastric plexus, which is situated lateral to the rectum, and thence to the bladder.

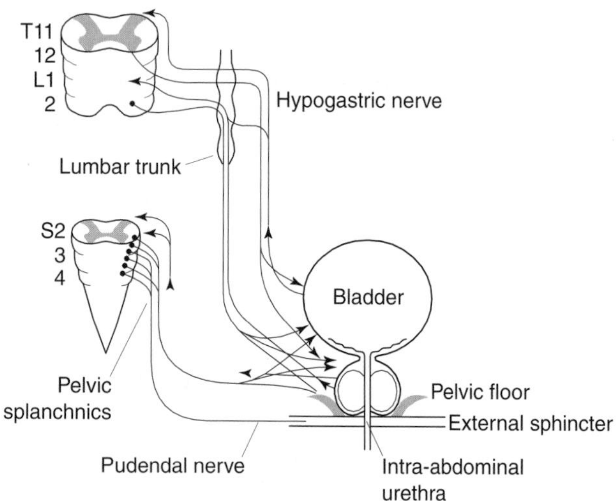

Fig. 65.1 The nervous control of the bladder. Micturition is partly a reflex and partly a voluntary act.

Somatic innervation

A somatic innervation also passes to the distal sphincter mechanism via the pudendal nerves and also via fibres which pass through the inferior hypogastric plexus without synapsing to the distal sphincter.

The sympathetic nerves convey afferent painful stimuli following overdistension of the fundus. Other afferents arise from the mucosa where they respond to touch, temperature and pain, and also from the muscle of the detrusor and lamina propria where they convey stretch information. These afferents pass via the inferior hypogastric plexus to the posterior roots of S2–S4. Efferent fibres pass via the pelvic parasympathetics. Normal micturition is co-ordinated in the pons in the midbrain where detrusor contraction is timed with inhibition of the distal sphincter mechanism. Interruption of this pathway with preservation of the function of the sacral cord is therefore likely to result in a contractile detrusor but with a tonically active distal sphincter mechanism which does not relax during voiding (detrusor-sphincter dyssynergia).

Ectopia vesicae (syn. exstrophy of the bladder)

This is thought to be caused by the incomplete development of the infra-umbilical part of the anterior abdominal wall, associated with incomplete development of the anterior wall of the bladder owing to delayed rupture of the cloacal membrane.

Clinical features of ectopia vesicae

- One in 50 000 births (four male:one female)
- Characteristic appearance (Fig. 65.2) because of the pressure of the viscera behind it
- Edges of abdominal wall can be felt
- Umbilicus is absent

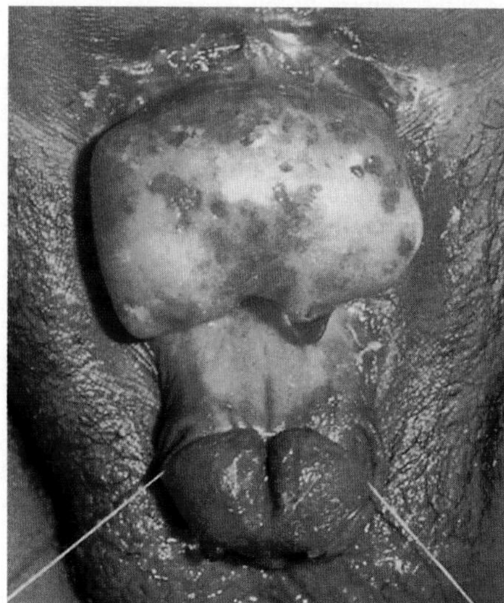

Fig. 65.2 Ectopia vesicae in a male. A drop of urine is seen at the left ureteric orifice, the corona glandis being retracted by threads (*courtesy of G.D. Adhia, Bombay*).

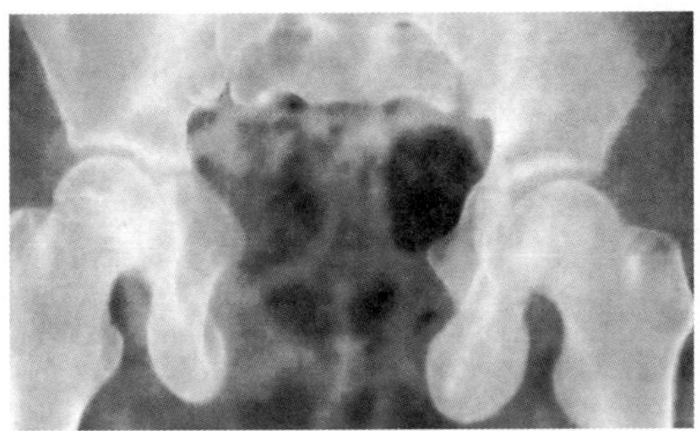

Fig. 65.3 Separation of the pubes in a case of ectopia vesicae (*courtesy of the late Professor Grey Turner, London*).

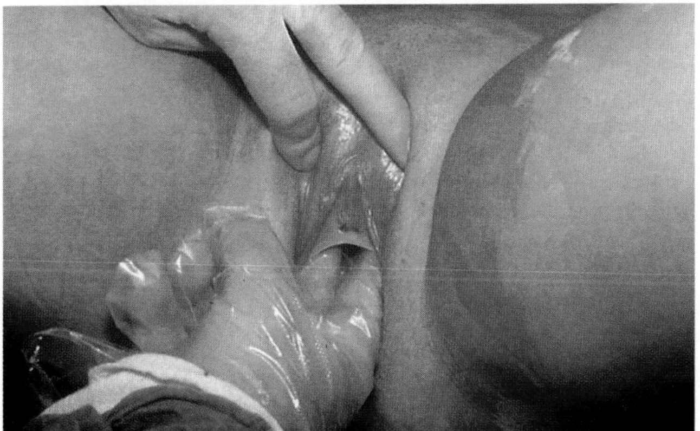

Fig. 65.4 Photograph of female epispadias showing deficient sphincter and bifid clitoris.

In the male the completely epispadiac penis is broader and shorter than normal, and bilateral inguinal herniae may be present; the prostate and seminal vesicles are rudimentary, whereas the testes are normal and have usually descended.

In the female the clitoris is bifid and the labia minora are separated anteriorly, exposing the vaginal orifice. In both sexes, there is separation of the pubic bones (Fig. 65.3), which are connected by a strong ligament. This bony defect causes no disability and subsequent delivery is normal. The linea alba is also broad. In the rare, incomplete form of penile epispadias or female epispadias, the pubes are united and the external genitalia are almost normal, although in the female the clitoris is bifid (Fig. 65.4).

Treatment

Iliac osteotomy, closure of the bladder and closure of abdominal wall

In the first year of life, the bladder is closed following osteotomy of both iliac bones just lateral to the sacroiliac joints. Later reconstruction of the bladder neck and sphincters is required. In some patients, the reconstructed bladder remains small and requires augmentation.

Another option is urinary diversion which may be necessary if continence is poor following bladder reconstruction. This can be done by means of a ureterosigmoid anastomosis or the formation of an ileal conduit, colonic conduit or continent urinary diversion. Long-term complications are frequent after ureterosigmoidostomy. These include: (1) stricture at the site of anastomosis with bilateral hydronephrosis and infection; (2) hyperchloraemic acidosis; and (3) there is an increased risk (20-fold) of tumour formation (adenomas aid adenocarcinoma) at the site of the ureterocolic anastomosis.

Rupture of the bladder

This may be intraperitoneal (20 per cent) or extraperitoneal (80 per cent) (Figs 65.5 and 65.6). Intraperitoneal rupture may be secondary to a blow, kick or fall on a fully distended bladder and it is more common in the male than in the female, and usually follows a bout of beer drinking. More rarely, it is due to surgical damage. Extraperitoneal rupture is usually caused by a fractured pelvis or is secondary to major trauma or surgical damage.

Intraperitoneal rupture

Intraperitoneal rupture

- Sudden, agonising pain in the hypogastrium, often accompanied by syncope
- The shock later subsides and the abdomen commences to distend
- No desire to micturate
- Varying degrees of abdominal rigidity and abdominal distension are present on examination
- No suprapubic dullness, but there is tenderness
- There may be shifting dullness
- If the urine is sterile, symptoms and signs of peritonitis are delayed

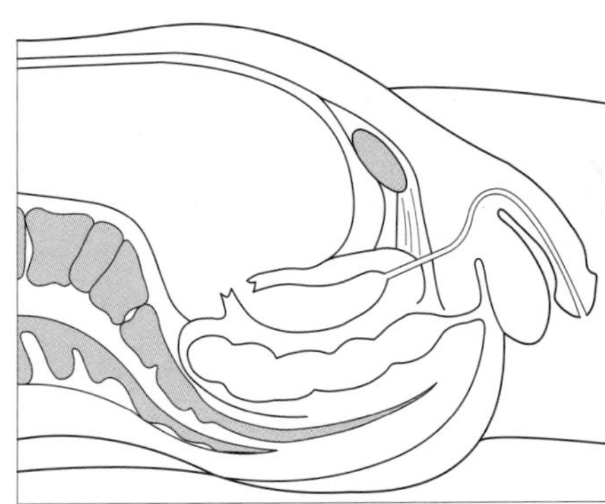

Fig. 65.5 Intraperitoneal extravasation of urine.

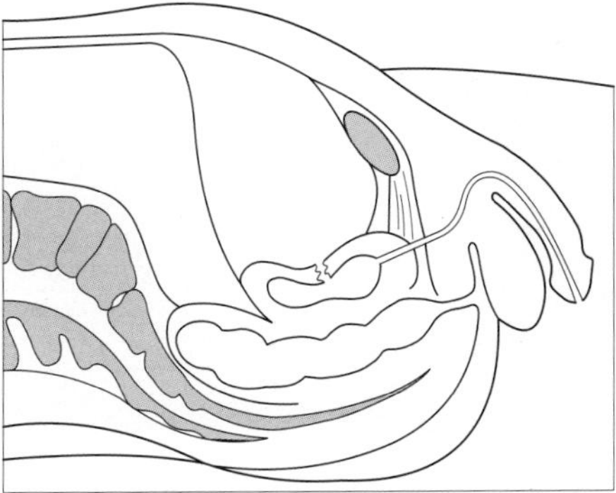

Fig. 65.6 Extraperitoneal extravasation of urine.

Extraperitoneal rupture

In many cases of pelvic trauma, this is difficult to distinguish from rupture of the membranous urethra. This injury is dealt with in Chapter 66 on 'The prostate and seminal vesicles'.

> Confirming a suspected diagnosis of intraperitoneal rupture
>
> - Plain X-ray in the erect position may show the ground-glass appearance of fluid in the lower abdomen
> - Intravenous urography (IVU) may confirm a leak from the bladder
> - A peritoneal 'tap' may be of value if facilities for radiological examination are not available
> - If doubt still exists and if there is no sign of fracture then retrograde cystography can be performed safely. With careful asepsis a small [14 French gauge (FG)] catheter is passed. Usually some blood-stained urine will drain. A solution made from 60 ml of 35 per cent Hypaque® or Conray® with 120 ml of sterile isotonic saline is injected into the bladder and radiographs are taken (Fig. 65.7)

Treatment of intraperitoneal rupture

The mainstay is to provide adequate drainage of the bladder. The standard treatment is to perform a lower midline laparotomy, urine is removed by suction, after which the patient is placed in Trendelenberg's position. The edges of the rent, which are usually situated in the posterior part of the dome of the bladder, are trimmed and sutured with two layers of interrupted catgut stitches, and the operation completed by placement of a suprapubic and urethral catheter. The peritoneum should be irrigated with copious amounts of warm saline. Very rarely, the bladder will rupture through an unsuspected tumour and it is perhaps wise in atypical cases to take a biopsy before suturing the defect.

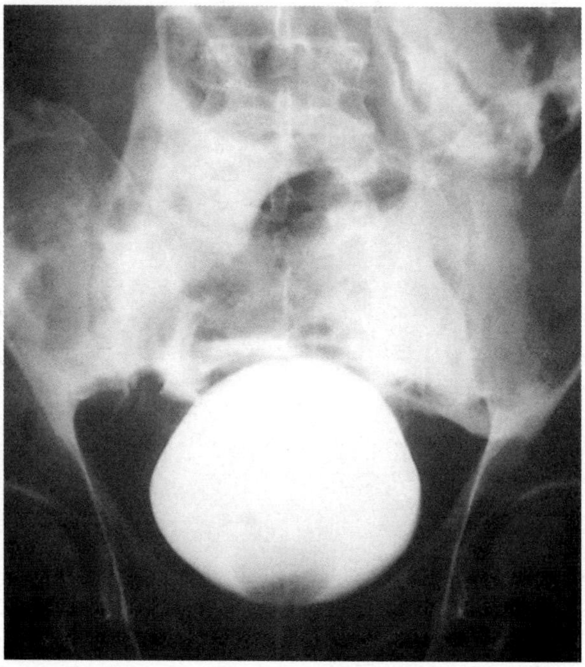

Fig. 65.7 Cystogram of a patient who has fallen over and developed severe abdominal pain. Leakage of contrast into the peritoneal cavity is seen.

Wounding of the bladder during operation

Operations in which the bladder is liable to be injured are: (1) inguinal or femoral herniotomy; (2) hysterectomy by either the abdominal or vaginal route; and (3) excision of the rectum. In the latter two operations, the bladder should be catheterised prior to operation to minimise the risks of this accident. If the injury is recognised at the time, the bladder must be repaired in two layers and urethral catheter drainage maintained for 7 days. If it is not recognised, the treatment is similar to that of rupture of the bladder.

When accidental perforation of the bladder occurs during endoscopic resection of a bladder tumour, or the prostatic capsule is perforated during transurethral prostatectomy, the perforation is usually extraperitoneal. When the accident is recognised at the time, drainage of the bladder with a large urethral catheter and the administration of antibiotics usually suffice. If, however, a mass of extravasated fluid is palpable *per abdomen* it is best to place a small drain into the extraperitoneal perivesical space through a small stab incision. A laparotomy will usually be required if an intraperitoneal perforation is caused by transurethral resection of a large bladder tumour on the dome of the bladder.

Retention of urine

Retention of urine is either acute or chronic, the latter leading ultimately to retention-with-overflow (see Chapter 66 on 'The prostate and seminal vesicles').

Acute retention

> The most frequent causes of acute retention
>
> - In the male:
>   - Bladder outlet obstruction
>   - Urethral stricture
>   - Postoperative
> - In the female:
>   - Retroverted gravid uterus
>   - Multiple sclerosis
> - In the male child:
>   - Meatal ulcer with scabbing
> - Other causes:
>   - Spinal anaesthesia
>   - Acute urethritis or prostatitis
>   - Blood clot in the bladder
>   - Urethral calculus
>   - Rupture of the urethra
>   - Phimosis
>   - Neurogenic (injury or disease of the spinal cord)
>   - Smooth muscle cell dysfunction associated with ageing
>   - Faecal impaction
>   - Anal pain (haemorrhoidectomy)
>   - Intensive postoperative analgesic treatment
>   - Certain drugs

Fredrich Trendelenberg, 1844–1924. Professor of Surgery, Leipzig, Germany.

Clinical features

Clinical features of acute retention urine

- No urine passed for several hours
- The bladder may be visible and is tender to palpation (Fig. 65.8) and dull to percussion
- Rarely, a prolapsed lumbar disc causing a cauda equina lesion will be the cause – exclude this by checking the reflexes in the lower limb and perianal sensation

Treatment

In most patients, the correct treatment is to pass a fine urethral catheter (14 FG – French guage is defined as the circumference in millimetres) and to arrange further urological management. Occasionally, a patient with postoperative retention may pass urine if he or she is sedated and placed in a warm bath. If the patient gives a good history of bladder outflow obstruction there seems little point in attempting conservative measures and a catheter should be passed; this should be carried out using full aseptic technique. Following a thorough wash of the hands and arms, sterile gloves should be donned. The external genitalia are gently cleaned using soapy antiseptic solution (Savlon®). A tube of local anaesthetic (Lidothesin®) is then carefully inserted down the urethra (Figs. 65.9–65.12) warning the patient that this will create a stinging sensation, but if the jelly is injected slowly through the plastic nozzle it should cause no pain. The jelly should be massaged well posteriorly in the urethra in an attempt to anaesthetise the sphincter and prostatic urethra, and it is of advantage to place a penile clamp for 10 minutes. A small (12–14 FG) Foley self-retaining catheter should then gently be passed down the urethra while the penis is held taut. In a female patient, the labia should be parted using the middle and index finger of the left hand, which should not be moved once the cleaning process has been performed to prevent contamination. Providing a stricture is not the cause of the retention, the catheter should normally pass freely into the bladder. Once urine begins to drain down the catheter it is wise to pass a few more centimetres of catheter into the bladder before the self-retaining balloon is inflated to avoid inflation of the balloon in the prostatic urethra. *Force should not be necessary*. Occasionally, a large obstructing middle lobe of the prostate may prevent a simple catheter entering the bladder; in this instance a coudé catheter should pass without difficulty. The bladder is then allowed to drain and the catheter attached to a closed drainage system. In the male, if the catheter will not pass into the bladder, it is usually due to poor technique, lack of anaesthesia, traumatisation of the urethra or because there is a urethral stricture. The usual reason is that the local anaesthetic has not been left long enough.

If, after a reasonable attempt with catheters, the bladder has not been entered, the following plan should be pursued according to circumstances.

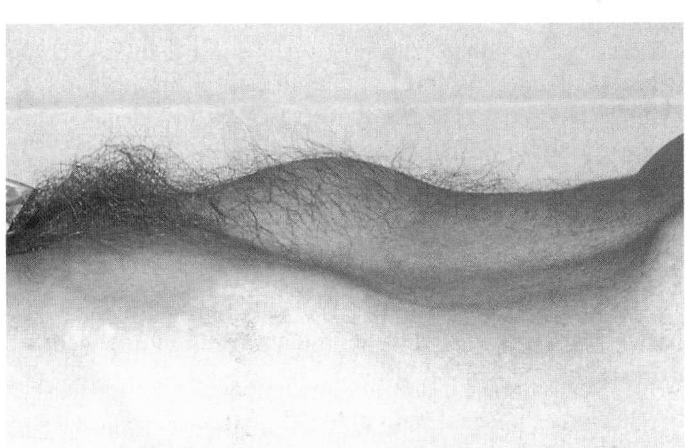

Fig. 65.8 Drawing of a man who presented with retention of urine showing a distended bladder.

Frederic Eugene Basil Foley, 1891–1966. Urologist, Ancker Hospitals, St Paul, USA.

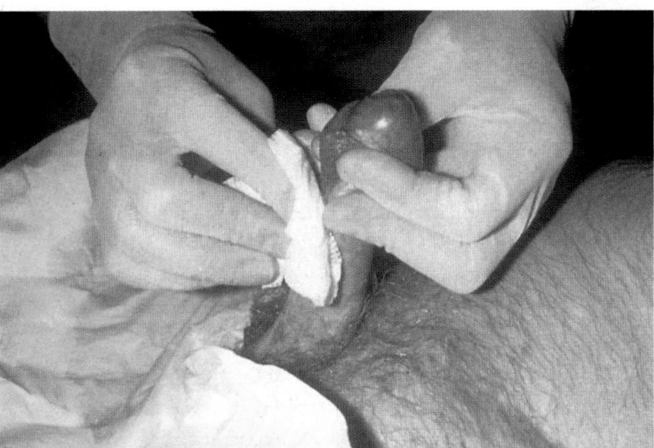

Fig. 65.9 Photograph showing cleaning of the penis before catheterisation.

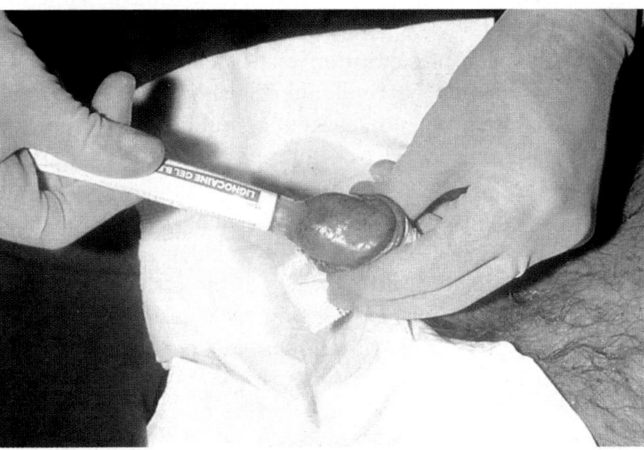

Fig. 65.10 Insertion of local anaesthetic before insertion of a catheter.

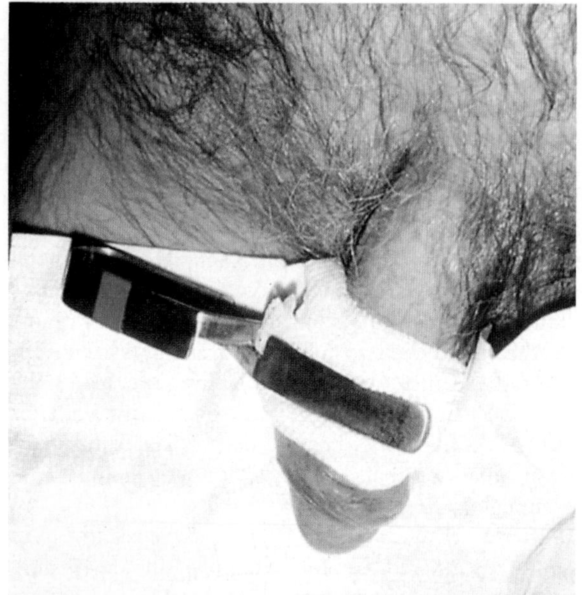

Fig. 65.11 The use of a penile clamp to ensure that sufficient time is given to allow the anaesthetic to work before the catheter is inserted.

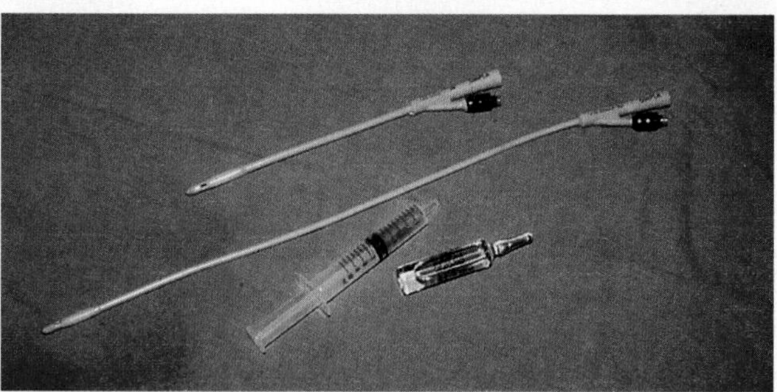

Fig. 65.12 A selection of silicone catheters.

Suprapubic puncture. Suprapubic puncture with commercially available catheters such as Cystofix® or a 'Bonnano' catheter is straightforward provided that the bladder is palpable. If such devices are not available a lumbar puncture needle or an Abbocath® is a useful method of relieving acute retention when catheterisation has failed. However, if the bladder is allowed to refill after it has been punctured, leakage into the prevesical space may follow.

The best plan is to place a suprapubic catheter after anaesthetising the skin, the fascia and the retropubic space with 0.5 per cent lignocaine. Correct placement of the needle can be confirmed by aspiration of the bladder. A large-bore needle is then placed, down which a fine catheter is passed (Cystofix) and secured in position by suturing. The other option is to place a plastic suprapubic trochar and cannula which has a removable plastic strip on the side so that a standard 12 FG Foley catheter can be passed down it, the balloon inflated, the strip pulled off and the plastic cannula pulled away from the catheter (Addacath).

If these devices are not available, a catheter can be placed in the bladder under direct vision through a small incision under local anaesthetic, although this has nothing to recommend it if percutaneous devices are available.

Urethral instrumentation. In a patient with a known urethral stricture, an experienced urologist may elect to dilate the stricture or the patient may be taken to theatre, a urethroscopy carried out, the stricture divided using a urethrotome under direct vision and a urethral catheter placed (see Chapter 66).

Whenever the bladder is catheterised for urinary retention it is important to record the volume drained and to examine the patient's abdomen a few minutes after the procedure to exclude some other intra-abdominal pathology. Conditions such as rupture of an aortic aneurism, ureteric colic or inflamed colonic diverticula can cause confusion as they present with a low urine output (mistaken as retention) and abdominal pain.

Chronic retention

Chronic retention

- Chronic retention differs from acute retention in that the distension of the bladder is almost painless
- These patients are at risk of upper tract dilatation because of the high intravesical tension due to the large residual urine and the high resting bladder pressure
- Men with chronic retention owing to bladder outlet obstruction require urgent referral for prostatectomy
- Those with a serum creatinine level greater than 200 μmol/litre are at risk of developing a postobstructive diuresis following catheterisation and may need careful monitoring with replacement of inappropriate urine losses by intravenous saline; they are also at risk of haematuria as the previously distended urinary tract suddenly shrinks. Slow decompression by means of intermittent spigotting of the catheter does not prevent haematoma

Retention with overflow

In this condition the patient has no control of his or her urine, small amounts passing involuntarily from time to time from a distended bladder. It may follow a neglected acute retention or chronic retention.

Retention with overflow is referred to also under 'incontinence' and 'prostatic enlargement'. The general principles which govern the treatment of this condition are similar to those of acute retention.

Indwelling catheters and closed systems of catheter drainage

The incidence of ascending infection following catheterisation is decreased by connecting the catheter (urethral, suprapubic or perineal) to sterile tubing connected to a sterile collecting bag and employing irrigations only if clot retention occurs (Fig. 65.13). When a catheter has been *in situ* for 5 days or more some degree of urethritis and bacteriuria is likely. Changing a catheter in the presence of active urethritis entails a risk of severe infection spreading from the anterior to the posterior urethra and thence to other parts of the urogenital system – not to mention the risk of bacteraemia,

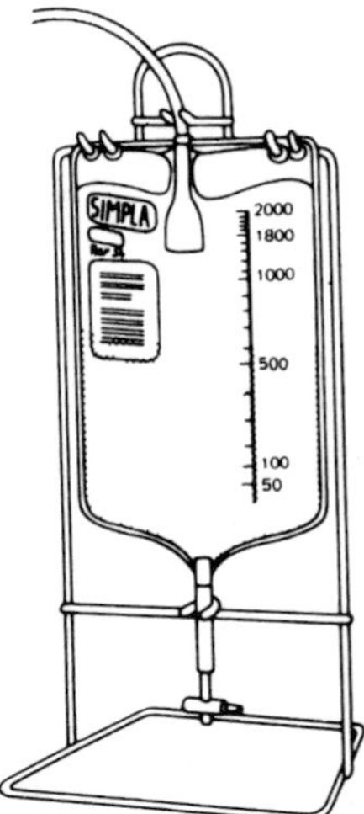

Fig. 65.13 Modern Simpla bag used for continuous bladder drainage. (The nurse who is emptying the bag should be wearing disposable gloves to avoid contaminating the hands with organisms.) A disadvantage is that the plastic tube may be too stiff to 'milk'.

septicaemia and abscess formation elsewhere. In such patients, the change of catheter should be covered by appropriate prophylactic antibiotics.

Special forms of retention of urine

Postoperative retention of urine

Retention of urine can occur after any operation, but is common after operations on the anal canal and perineal region. After operations on the pelvic viscera, retention of urine is so common (sometimes owing to damage to the pelvic autonomic plexus or to nonspecific causes) that it is usual to forestall it by inserting a catheter before or at the conclusion of the operation.

When the patient is an elderly male, prostatic obstruction, hitherto latent, should be suspected. Many patients cannot urinate while lying or sitting in bed. In a heavily sedated patient, urinary retention may be missed and patients may suffer from severe over-distension of the bladder which can result in long-term impairment of voiding function. This is particularly common after hip replacement in elderly patients as there may be reluctance to catheterise them.

Treatment. First of all, reassure the patient and provide privacy. If the male patient, while supported, is permitted to sit on the edge of his bed he is often able to empty his bladder. The sound of running water is often helpful. When circumstances permit, a warm bath is often helpful. If after a reasonable trial patients cannot pass urine they must be catheterised temporarily.

Acute retention due to drugs

A number of drugs is prone to induce or precipitate retention of urine. Antihistamine drugs, antihypertensive drugs, anticholinergics and tricyclic antidepressants may be responsible for producing acute retention of urine.

Management of the neuropathic bladder

Immediately after a spinal cord injury, *spinal shock* occurs (see Chapter 33 on 'The spine'), which may last for days, weeks or even months, and in this state the detrusor is paralysed, the bladder distends and overflow incontinence will occur. This will lead to damage to the detrusor muscle, infection and ultimately renal failure. Management is as follows.

1. The bladder must be kept empty either by intermittent catheterisation with an aseptic technique performed two or three times daily, or by the use of an indwelling urethral catheter on continuous drainage and making sure that the patient has a high urinary output (3 litres/day) to combat infection. Currently, the use of intermittent catheterisation is preferred as soon as the patient can be moved when the spinal injury is stable.
2. The upper level of the neurological lesion must be assessed by the level of sensory and motor loss. Ischaemic necrosis of the cord may extend a variable distance below the upper level of cord injury. Where sensory loss below the upper level of cord injury is total, recovery is unlikely. Incomplete lesions, in contrast, may recovery somatic and bladder function.
3. Demonstration of intact bulbocavernosus and anal reflexes indicates that the sacral cord and nerves are intact. In such circumstances reflex bladder contractions are likely to develop, although they may be insufficient to empty the bladder completely. If these reflexes are absent and there is persistent total loss of perineal sensation it means that either the sacral cord or cauda equina is damaged. In such circumstances an acontractile bladder is likely to develop. In cauda equina lesions there may be sensory, motor or mixed loss.
4. Full urodynamic assessment of bladder function should be undertaken when the injury is stable (see below). A *urodynamic study* allows accurate assessment of detrusor and sphincter activity, and the sensation. Various aspects of bladder function can be checked including *adequacy of bladder emptying*, *bladder capacity*, *pressure during filling* and *continence* related to the extent and level of neurological damage. Many types of bladder dysfunction can occur.

The results of these studies should enable decisions to be made as to the further management of the bladder, the prime aim being to prevent upper tract damage by promoting good bladder emptying and to avoid infection. The following situations represent only the *typical* pattern of bladder function.

Lesions above cord segment T10

The common situation is an upper motor neuron bladder with all reflexes intact but isolated from higher control and inhibition. Such patients are at risk of autonomic dysreflexia.

Emptying. The bladder is usually contractile, but because co-ordinated inhibition of the distal sphincter mechanism does not occur (detrusor-sphincter dyssynergia), the contractions are often high pressure and ineffective in producing complete bladder emptying. The bladder neck is normally open in these patients. If left untreated, the upper tracts suffer at the hands of the chronically full bladder and raised intravesical pressure. Hydronephrosis and renal failure may result.

Capacity. This is usually decreased after some years with the development of trabeculation and a typical 'fir-tree' appearance of the bladder. The bladder pressure is often increased and demonstrates marked phasic increases as the bladder tries to contract and empty against the spastic sphincter mechanism.

Control. The patients are incontinent during the high-pressure phasic contractions because the sphincter resistance suddenly diminishes, allowing urinary leakage.

The treatment of these patients depends on urodynamic assessment. Constant vigilance is required, a watch being kept for hydronephrosis. This may be done by serial intravenous urography (IVU) or ultrasound scanning. Regular follow-up urodynamic investigations are necessary. The patient with complete bladder emptying and reasonable capacity with normal upper tracts may be managed by means of condom drainage. The patient with incomplete bladder emptying and good capacity may be managed by means of clean intermittent catheterisation (CISC). Patients with poor emptying, low capacity and upper tract dilatation require additional treatment. This may range from endoscopic sphincterotomy and condom drainage in the male, which will allow complete bladder emptying at low pressure, to complete bladder reconstruction with bladder substitution using intestinal segments and the fitment of artificial urinary sphincters, depending on the mobility and motivation of the patient and available services.

Lesions involving the sympathetic outflow, T11, T12, L1, L2

These patients are usually similar to the above group, but may have increased outflow resistance. α-Adrenergic blockers may help.

Damage to the sacral centre S2, 3, 4 and cauda equina lesions

This is essentially a lower motor neuron bladder.

Emptying. The detrusor is acontractile because there is injury to the parasympathetic innervation. Abdominal straining and pressure on the bladder through the abdominal wall can produce reasonable emptying in some patients. Nowadays, the mainstay of management is the use of clean intermittent self-catheterisation popularised by Lapides (CISC), which involves the patient passing themselves a clean, but not sterile, catheter 2- or 3-hourly to ensure adequate bladder emptying. Some patients may have a sensation of filling through the hypogastric nerves if *T11 and T12* are intact.

Capacity. The bladder capacity may be good, but these patients may have high resting bladder pressures and high tonic increases during bladder filling, which means that if bladder emptying is incomplete there is a risk to the upper urinary tract. The bladder neck is usually open and the distal sphincter mechanisms may be paralysed, but the fixed urethral resistance prevents good bladder emptying by means of straining. Vesico-ureteric reflux is common and upper tract damage is frequent in neglected cases.

Control. Patients who can achieve satisfactory bladder emptying by means of CISC usually have reasonable continence.

Persistent retention of urine following excision of the rectum or radical hysterectomy

Ten to 15 per cent of patients undergoing radical rectal excision for cancer sustain damage to the inferior hypogastric plexus leading to impotence in the male and neurogenic bladder dysfunction. This type of bladder dysfunction is similar to the cauda equina lesion, but the pressures during filling tend to be greater, leading to more incontinence and a greater risk to the upper tracts. Postoperative retention in other patients is simply caused by bladder outlet obstruction. The best plan is to catheterise the patient with a 14 Fr silicone catheter, to allow a period for postoperative recovery, and then carry out a urodynamic investigation which will distinguish these two conditions. One requires treatment by means of prolonged CISC, while the other will respond well to transurethral prostatectomy.

Jack Lapides. American urologist.

Incontinence of urine

Normal urinary continence is dependent on several factors. These include normal mobility and normal brain function allowing a perception of when it is socially acceptable to void, normal bladder sensation, normal voluntary detrusor contraction producing good bladder emptying, a normally competent sphincter mechanism which relaxes appropriately during a voluntary detrusor contraction allowing good bladder emptying and good bladder capacity with normally low pressures during filling. This is clearly a fine balance and several factors can cause incontinence.

In the diagnosis of urinary incontinence, a careful history and physical examination may help, but it will be necessary to carry out urodynamic testing in most patients if surgical intervention is proposed. The urine should be cultured to exclude infection and the serum creatinine should be measured. It may be appropriate to have anatomical visualisation of the urinary tract by means of IVU if one suspects a ureteric fistula, although ultrasound examination will often provide adequate details.

Urodynamic testing

The key to the practical management of lower urinary tract dysfunction lies with urodynamic investigation. The principle is artificially to simulate bladder filling and emptying whilst obtaining pressure measurements (Fig. 65.14).

The patient attends with a full bladder and is allowed to void in private to measure maximum urinary flow rate. After voiding, the residual urine is measured by means of ultrasound to assess the completeness of bladder emptying. Urodynamic testing involves the aseptic passage of a small pair of catheters or a twin-lumen catheter into the bladder; this allows the bladder to be filled with saline or contrast medium at a rate of 50 ml/minute whilst a continuous recording of the intravesical

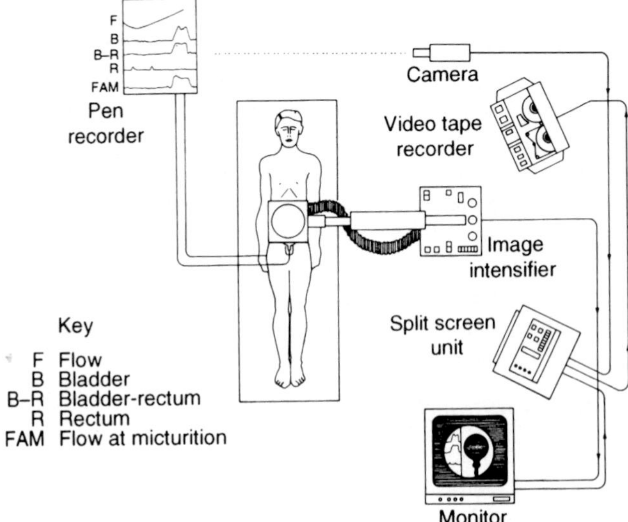

Fig. 65.14 Urodynamic study.

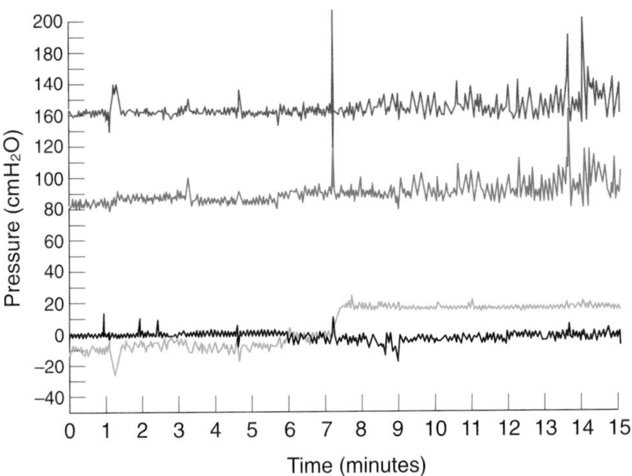

Fig. 65.15 A section of an ambulatory, natural fill urodynamic trace. The rectal pressure is in red, the bladder pressure in blue, the subtracted detrusor trace in black. The orange trace is the output of an electronic nappy which records urinary leakage. A cough is shown which results in urinary leakage with no rise in subtracted detrusor pressure: this is genuine stress incontinence.

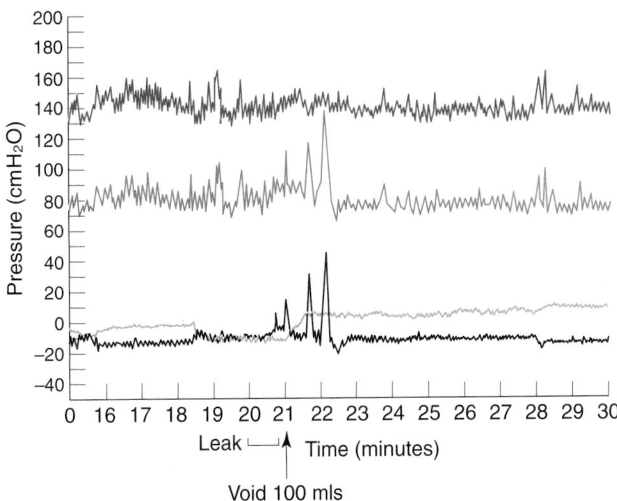

Fig. 65.16 A section of an ambulatory, natural fill urodynamic trace. The rectal pressure is in red, the bladder pressure in blue, the subtracted detrusor trace in black. The orange trace is the output of an electronic nappy which records urinary leakage. Phasic activity is shown which is detrusor instability resulting in urge incontinence.

pressure is made via a transducer. To obtain true detrusor pressure, a second pressure channel is required to assess intra-abdominal pressure which is usually measured by means of a small intrarectal or intravaginal balloon. The bladder is filled until the patient states that their bladder is full. Screening by means of radiographic imaging may be carried out to assess bladder neck closure, and urinary leakage during voiding or during bouts of phasic detrusor pressure (detrusor instability). The patient is then asked to void at the end of bladder filling after the filling catheter has been removed.

Usefulness of urodynamic testing

- Distinguishing genuine stress incontinence (due to sphincter weakness) from detrusor instability in women (Fig. 65.15)
- Classification of neurogenic bladder dysfunction
- Distinguishing bladder outflow obstruction from idiopathic detrusor instability in men
- Investigation of incontinence

The normal bladder will accept approximately 400–550 ml when filled with saline at room temperature at filling rates of 50 ml/minute. The pressure increase in the bladder should be less than 15 cmH_2O. In addition, phasic pressure increases should not be seen. The normal voiding pressure should not exceed 60 cmH_2O in men and about 40 cmH_2O in women, with a flow rate of between 20 and 25 ml/second.

Common abnormalities identified during urodynamic testing in incontinence

- Phasic increases giving rise to sensations of urgency of micturition and urge incontinence (detrusor instability; Fig. 65.16). This abnormality is found in patients with several types of neurogenic bladder dysfunction such as multiple sclerosis (MS), Parkinson's disease, or following a stroke or certain types of spinal injury when it is known as detrusor hyperreflexia. In addition, about 50 per cent of men with bladder outflow obstruction have detrusor instability, and in about half of these men the instability resolves after prostatectomy. Idiopathic detrusor instability is common and must be distinguished from genuine stress incontinence in women before performing bladder neck suspension procedures.
- Genuine stress incontinence is defined as urinary leakage occurring during increased bladder pressure when this is solely due to increased abdominal pressure and not due to increased true detrusor pressure (Fig. 65.15). It is caused by sphincter weakness.
- Chronic urinary retention with overflow incontinence. This is recognised by a large residual volume of urine (Fig. 65.17) and is usually associated with high pressures during bladder filling.

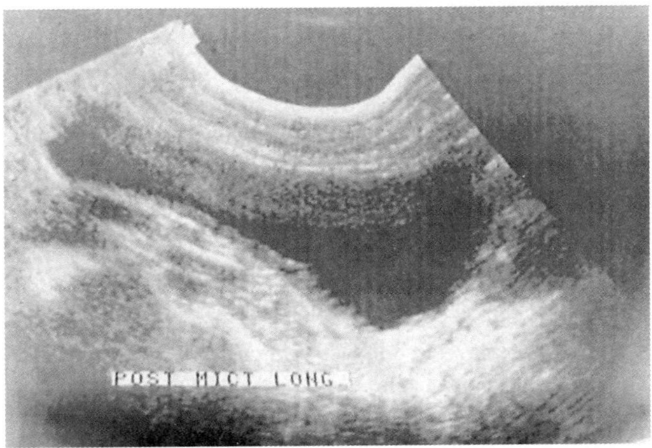

Fig. 65.17 An ultrasound scan showing a large postvoid residual urine.

James Parkinson, 1755–1824. English physician.

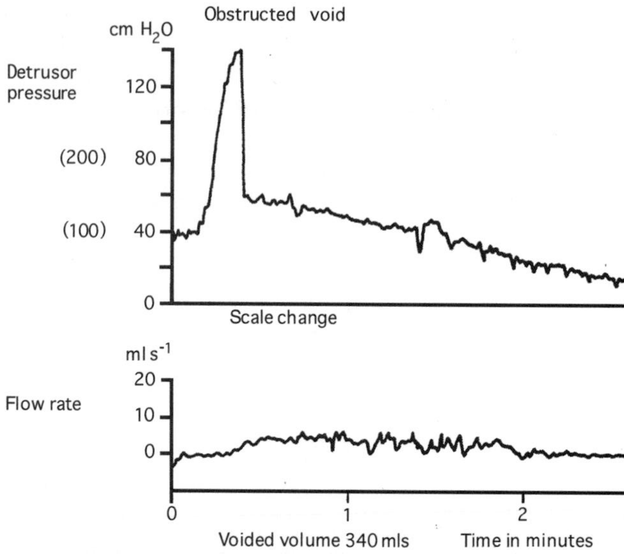

Fig. 65.18 A conventional urodynamic trace showing detrusor pressure during voiding. There has been a change of scale because the pressure was so high; voiding pressures are increased with a low flow rate, which is diagnostic of bladder outflow obstruction.

- Bladder outflow obstruction, which is associated with increased voiding pressures often being in excess of 90 cmH_2O (Fig. 65.18), coupled with low urinary flow rates.
- Neurogenic bladder dysfunction.

Causes of incontinence

There are various ways of classifying causes of incontinence. A good functional method is as follows.

- *Problems of social control* – patients with Alzheimer's disease, Parkinson's disease or multi-infarct dementia often have urinary incontinence owing to a combination of uninhibited detrusor hyperreflexia and impaired social perception.
- *Storage problems* – patients with a small capacity owing to fibrosis from tuberculosis or interstitial cystitis can develop incontinence. Patients with a small functional capacity owing to severe idiopathic detrusor instability, neurogenic bladder dysfunction or urinary infection also can develop incontinence.
- *Severe impairment of emptying* – patients with chronic retention or some types of neurogenic bladder dysfunction often have small *functional* bladder capacities with detrusor overactivity causing incontinence, despite having large residual volumes of urine.
- *Weak sphincter* – patients with genuine stress incontinence owing to previous prolonged labour or with damage to the distal sphincter mechanism secondary to prostatectomy or with neurogenic bladder dysfunction often have impaired sphincter function which leads to stress incontinence. Congenital causes such as epispadias also result in sphincter weakness.
- *Fistulae* – leakage from fistulae or upper tract duplication with an ectopic ureter.

The common causes may be classified into male, female or mixed sex groups.

Male

Chronic urinary retention with overflow. This is a common cause of incontinence and may be due to benign prostatic hypertrophy, carcinoma of the prostate, urethral stricture and, in younger men, hypertrophy of the bladder neck. The key to the diagnosis lies with the history of prolonged hesitancy and a poor urinary stream with both daytime and nocturnal 'dribbling incontinence' coupled with the finding of a distended bladder. Examination may reveal that the bladder is visibly distended, the transverse suprapubic crease is lost and the painless distension of the bladder may be palpated or percussed. It may easily be diagnosed by means of ultrasound measurement of residual urine volume. The treatment is discussed in Chapter 66.

Postprostatectomy. Postprostatectomy incontinence may result from injury to the external sphincter mechanism which may be caused by clumsy surgery – urodynamic evaluation will demonstrate genuine sphincter weakness. The other cause of incontinence is idiopathic detrusor instability, although such patients often have significant irritative symptoms prior to prostatectomy and should be identified and investigated by means of urodynamic studies prior to prostatectomy.

Female

Stress incontinence. The commonest cause of leakage of urine in women is genuine stress incontinence (GSI), although in some parts of the world vesicourethral fistulae owing to neglected labour are very common. GSI occurs secondary to weakness of the distal sphincter mechanism associated with laxity of the pelvic floor. It is usually found in multiparous women with a history of difficult labour often accompanied by the use of forceps. It can be found in normal young women who indulge in competitive trampolining and also in patients with epispadias. The classical symptoms are complaints of urine loss during coughing, laughing, sneezing or sudden change of posture. The symptoms may change with the menstrual cycle. The volume of urine loss can be measured during an exercise test which is performed by putting the patient through a standard set of tests with 300 ml of fluid in the bladder; in GSI the fluid losses usually range from 10 to 50 ml. Urinary frequency and urgency are, however, often found in such patients as they try to avoid incontinence by frequent voiding.

Idiopathic detrusor instability can closely mimic GSI and indeed can coexist with it. It is important to make a correct

Aloïs Alzheimer, 1864–1915. German neurologist.

preoperative diagnosis by urodynamic measurements, as the outcome of surgery is significantly worse in women with idiopathic detrusor instability.

Minor degrees of stress urinary incontinence often can be controlled by means of teaching the patient a series of pelvic floor exercises. However, if this fails then surgery is indicated. The best standard operation is the Burch colposuspension.

This operation is carried out with the patient in the Lloyd-Davies position through a Pfannenstiel incision. The vaginal fascia is identified by sweeping the bladder off the vagina and three sutures are placed on each side between the vaginal fascia and the iliopubic ligament. A suprapubic catheter is placed. The operation corrects minor degrees of cystocoele. Voiding difficulties are frequent, but usually temporary. It is best to warn women with large bladder capacities and low voiding pressures that this complication may occur and that they may require to carry out CISC for a period. The operation is very successful in the treatment of GSI with 90 per cent 1-year good results, which are maintained in about 80 per cent at 5 years. Endoscopic needle bladder neck suspension can now be carried out, but is less successful than open operation.

Common to both sexes

Idiopathic detrusor instability (DI). This condition is very common. Phasic increases in bladder pressure may occur during filling in otherwise normal patients (idiopathic) or it may be found in several conditions including neurogenic bladder dysfunction (then known as detrusor hyperreflexia) and bladder outflow obstruction. Idiopathic detrusor instability may be symptomless, but usually results in symptoms of frequency, urgency, urge incontinence, nocturia or nocturnal incontinence (enuresis) depending on the severity of the instability. It must be distinguished from GSI and from bladder outflow obstruction as colposuspension or prostatectomy have poor results in patients with severe idiopathic DI. Most urologists will want to exclude infection, tuberculosis or carcinoma *in situ* by urine culture, cytological examination, cystoscopy and confirmation of the diagnosis by means of urodynamic investigation. The mainstay of treatment is the use of various anticholinergic medication (propantheline, oxybutinine, tolteroclise, and amytryptiline). Severe symptoms resistant to conventional conservative treatment resulting in major impairment of quality of life may need more aggressive treatment such as enterocystoplasty.

Ageing. In both sexes ageing can result in smooth muscle cell dysfunction that can cause combinations of small functional capacities, detrusor instability, impaired bladder emptying and symptoms of lower urinary tract dysfunction.

Reynold E. Burch. American gynaecologist.
R.W. Lloyd-Davies. British surgeon.
Hermann Johann Pfannensteil, 1862–1909. Gynaecologist in Breslau, Germany.

Congenital. Ectopic vesicae and severe epispadias. The abnormal entry of an ectopic ureter distal to the sphincter complex or into the vagina in a female should theoretically result in total urinary incontinence. This is discussed in Chapter 62.

Trauma. Trauma, whether from pelvic surgery or associated with pelvic fracture, may result in disruption of the nerve supply to the bladder or urethra or in fistula formation.

Infection. Simple lower urinary tract infection may be sufficient, particularly in a woman, to induce urinary incontinence. A history of frequency, burning and a fever should prompt the diagnosis. The bladder may be tender whether palpated suprapubically or *per vaginam*. Symptoms will usually settle with a course of antibiotics, but in the case of recurrent infection further investigation of the urinary tract will clearly be indicated.

Neoplasia. Locally advanced cancers in the pelvis, particularly carcinoma of the cervix in a woman and prostate in a man, may result in direct invasion of the sphincter mechanism causing incontinence; occasionally, fistula formation may occur in women.

Other causes

Neurogenic incontinence

Neurogenic incontinence
This has been dealt with in the previous section. The common causes include:

- myelodysplasia;
- multiple sclerosis;
- spinal cord injuries;
- cerebral dysfunction [cerebrovascular accident (CVA), dementia];
- Parkinson's disease (paralysis agitans).

These conditions lead to a combination of neurogenic vesical dysfunction often associated with loss of mobility. Careful investigation of the whole urinary tract is always required, and the treatment needs to strike a fine balance between preventing hydronephrosis from abnormally high bladder pressures yet at the same time maintaining continence.

The mainstay of management is accurate urodynamic assessment to assess bladder emptying, incontinence and the risks to the upper tract. The upper tracts should be assessed with regular ultrasound scanning, and assessment of the patient's mobility, intelligence and motivation is vital. The important factors to assess urodynamically are:

- bladder emptying;
- bladder capacity and bladder pressure during filling;
- continence.

The standard way of dealing with impaired bladder emptying is the use of CISC. Occasionally, in an elderly immobile patient an indwelling urethral or suprapubic catheter or an ileal conduit external urinary diversion may be justified, or the performance of an endoscopic sphincterotomy followed by the use of a condom appliance should be considered.

Patients with a small functional bladder capacity (< 150 ml), a high-pressure increase during filling (> 25 cmH_2O) and a large residual volume of urine are at high risk of developing upper tract dilatation, and in the past would have undergone endoscopic sphincterotomy. However, there have been major changes in the management of mobile, well-motivated patients with impaired bladder emptying or with high-risk bladders. Such treatment will often involve major bladder reconstruction with replacement of the high-pressure bladder with a low-pressure substitute made of a detubularised bowel segment, often accompanied by surgery to the bladder outflow using artificial urinary sphincters or a colposuspension. Such treatment will usually need to be accompanied by the patient carrying out CISC afterwards.

Small bladder capacity

The capacity of the bladder may be considerably diminished in several conditions. This can cause crippling urinary frequency and incontinence. It may follow tuberculosis, radiotherapy or interstitial cystitis. Radiotherapy for pelvic cancer can also cause this problem.

Drug-induced incontinence

The detrusor muscle is basically under postganglionic parasympathetic control and the main neurotransmitter system is cholinergic. Recent studies have established the presence of a number of neuro-transmitters including α-adrenergic fibres in the region of the bladder neck and other neuropeptides, whose function is uncertain as yet, are present throughout the bladder. A number of drugs can induce urinary retention (anticholinergic agents, tricyclic antidepressants, lithium and some antihypertensives). Overflow incontinence may ensue. Drugs giving extrapyramidal side-effects may induce urinary frequency and incontinence, for example phenothiazine.

Constant dribbling of urine coupled with normal micturition

This occurs when there is a ureteric fistula or an ectopic ureter associated with a duplex system opening into the urethra beyond the urethral sphincter in females, or into the vagina. The history is diagnostic, and intravenous pyelography or ultrasound scanning may reveal the upper pole segment which is often poorly functioning. These segments are very liable to infection. Treatment is by excision of the aberrant ureter and portion of kidney which needs it. A ureteric fistula can be difficult to diagnose and may require retrograde ureterography and a high degree of suspicion to demonstrate.

Nocturnal enuresis

This is a condition of young children and young adults. The time at which children become dry at night varies, of course, and in some of them it is merely a delayed onset of continence. In others it persists until late adolescence and is classified into primary and secondary nocturnal enuresis.

Primary nocturnal enuresis occurs in patients with nocturnal enuresis alone and with no daytime symptoms. Often, they have been dry for a period and the vast majority of patients will eventually become dry. In the meantime a sympathetic approach to these children is essential. They often respond to a system of rewards using a 'star' chart. In addition, the use of DDAVP (vasopressin analogues) can produce increased urinary concentration at night with a decrease in nocturnal incontinence. Other treatments include the use of amytriptiline and alarms which wake the child (or at least the child's parents) when incontinence occurs.

Patients with secondary nocturnal enuresis have daytime symptoms of urinary frequency, urgency and urge incontinence. Essentially, these patients have idiopathic detrusor instability and should be treated in a similar way (see subsection on 'Treatments for incontinence').

Treatments for incontinence

Treatments are listed below. Management is dependent on making a correct working diagnosis. The treatment depends on the cause. The aim is to keep the patient dry, free of odour, to lessen the incidence of skin excoriation, and to protect the kidneys from the effects of infection and back pressure.

Management and treatment

Problems of social functioning. Patients with Alzheimer's disease, Parkinson's disease and multi-infarct dementia are difficult to treat. Often these patients will respond to regular toileting. Anticholinergic agents can cause confusion in these patients and often, in severe cases, an indwelling catheter is needed.

Storage problems. Patients with a small capacity owing to fibrosis may require augmentation cystoplasty. Patients with a small functional bladder capacity owing to detrusor overactivity from neurogenic bladder dysfunction or idiopathic detrusor instability should be tried on anticholinergic medication, but in severe cases, particularly in neuropathic patients at high risk of upper tract dilatation, bladder substitution (near-total supratrigonal cystectomy followed by the need for detubularised ileocaecal segment bladder substitution) or augmentation (enterocystoplasty) may be needed. These procedures should only be carried out after careful assessment in units used to dealing with these problems. Patients with very impaired mobility and MS may require ileal conduit diversion.

Impaired bladder emptying. Patients with overflow incontinence owing to bladder outflow obstruction will respond well to prostatectomy, after an initial period of catheterisation to allow bladder and renal function to recover to some extent. Patients with impaired bladder emptying owing to neurogenic bladder dysfunction should be treated in the first place by means of CISC.

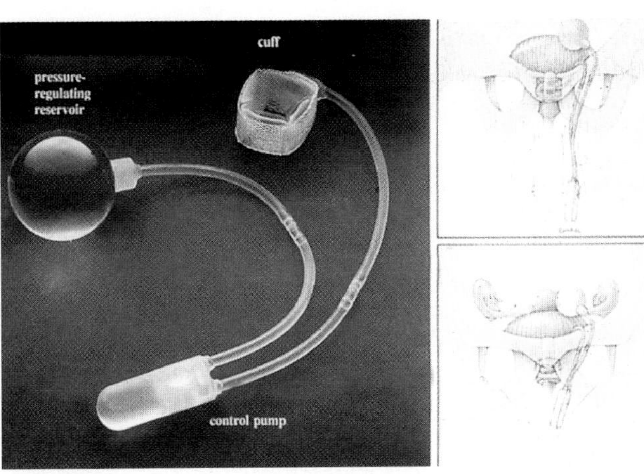

Fig. 65.19 The artificial urinary sphincter made by American Medical Systems.

Weak sphincter. Patients with genuine stress incontinence owing to previous prolonged labour should be treated by means of pelvic floor exercises or colposuspension. Those with postprostatectomy incontinence or with neurogenic bladder dysfunction may require fitment of an artificial urinary sphincter (Fig. 65.19) if they are well motivated and mobile.

Leakage from fistulae or upper tract duplication with an ectopic ureter. This will require the appropriate surgical treatment.

Appliances in women are usually unsatisfactory. In elderly, immobile or mentally impaired patients, an indwelling catheter drained constantly into a leg urinal is usually a satisfactory solution, although in some instances diversion via an ileal conduit is necessary. In men, a condom urinary appliance may be satisfactory, and can avoid an indwelling catheter.

More major surgical treatments

Various types of urinary diversion. This may be required for the treatment of end-stage incontinence that is not otherwise treatable (see later in this chapter).

Bladder substitution procedures. The principle behind these operations is the creation of a low-pressure, large-capacity reservoir. These can be made using any segment of bowel isolated on its vascular pedicle (Figs 65.20–65.22). This is then detubularised by dividing its antimesenteric border and suturing this into a plate. This can then be reconfigured into a spherical structure. This reservoir can then be anastomosed to the bladder remnant after excision of the fundus above the trigone. If necessary, the ureters can be reimplanted into the bowel segment. This new bladder (Fig. 65.23) will almost certainly need to be emptied by means of intermittent self-catheterisation (CISC).

'Clam' enterocystoplasty. This procedure was originally described by Bramble for the treatment of nocturnal enuresis. It is now being used more frequently in the treatment of idiopathic detrusor instability. It involves the isolation of a 16-cm segment of ileum on its vascular pedicle. This is

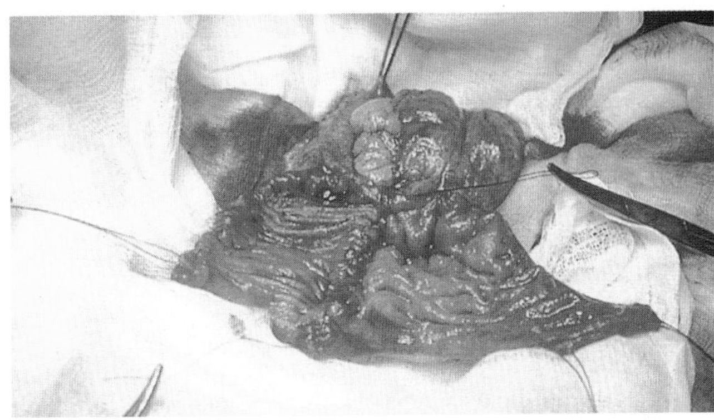

Fig. 65.20 A vascularised ileocaecal segment being detubularised.

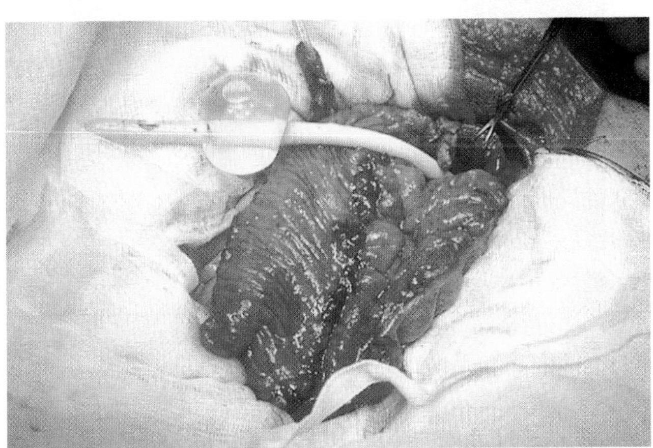

Fig. 65.21 An ileocaecal segment being anastomosed to the trigone after near-total cystectomy; the left ureter is about to be implanted by means of a Camay–Le Duc anastomosis.

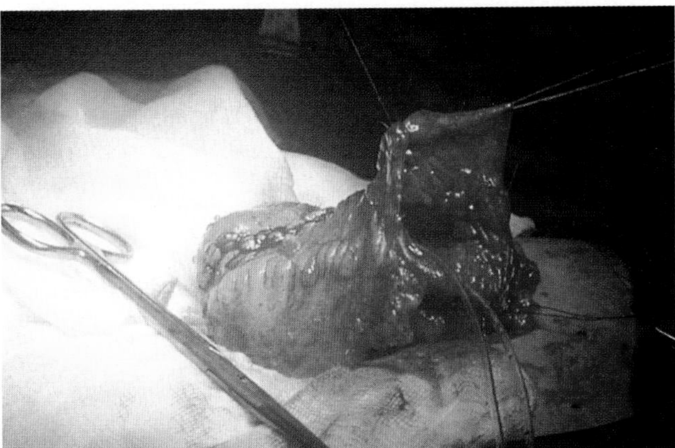

Fig. 65.22 A capacious ileocaecal reservoir to be used in a patient requiring bladder substitution. These segments may be used for: total bladder replacement, bladder substitution and the construction of continent diversion with a Mitrofanoff-type anti-incontinence mechanism (see later in this chapter).

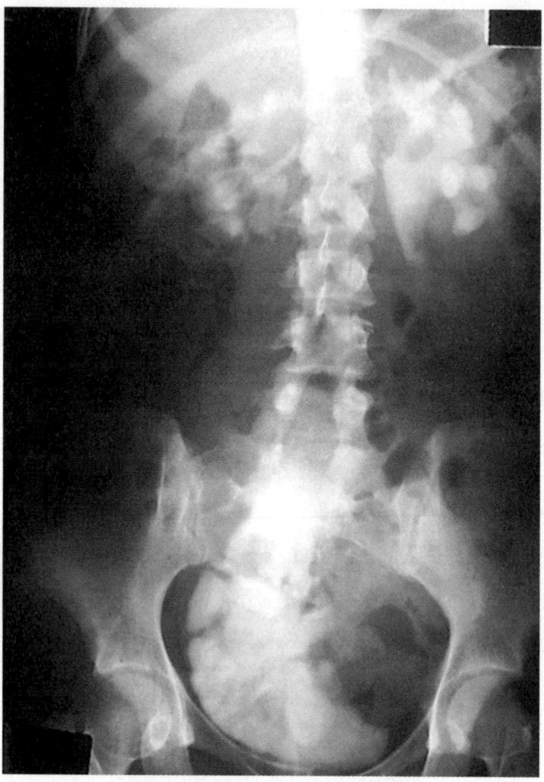

Fig. 65.23 A patient with spinal bifida who had undergone urinary undiversion with bladder substitution using an ileocaecal pouch. Although CISC is necessary, the patient is continent.

Treatments for incontinence	
1. Devices for collection or control	External penile condom, indwelling catheter, penile clamps
2. Drugs	To increase the strength of the bladder neck (e.g. α-adrenergic agonists), to decrease the strength of the bladder neck (e.g. α-adrenergic blockers), mixed action on the bladder neck and central nervous system (e.g. tricyclic drugs), inhibit bladder activity (e.g. anticholinergic drugs)
3. Intermittent self-catheterisation to improve emptying	
4. Surgery to decrease outlet resistance	Prostatectomy, urethrotomy in females with obstruction
5. Increasing outlet resistance	Pelvic floor physiotherapy, colposuspension or slings, periurethral collagen or silicone particles, artificial urinary sphincter
6. Denervation of bladder (to inhibit bladder activity and improve functional capacity)	Neurectomy procedures, transection of bladder
7. Augmentation of bladder capacity	'Clam' enterocystoplasty, bladder substitution with detubularised bowel segment
8. Urinary diversion	Ileal conduit, continent urinary diversion

divided on its antimesenteric border and sutured into the opened out bladder. The bladder is divided along a circumference from bladder neck at 3 o'clock to 9 o'clock in the coronal plane (Fig. 65.24). This procedure can also be used as an augmentation procedure in patients with neurogenic bladder dysfunction and a reasonable preoperative bladder capacity (approximately 300 ml).

Fitment of artificial urinary sphincter. See Fig. 65.19.

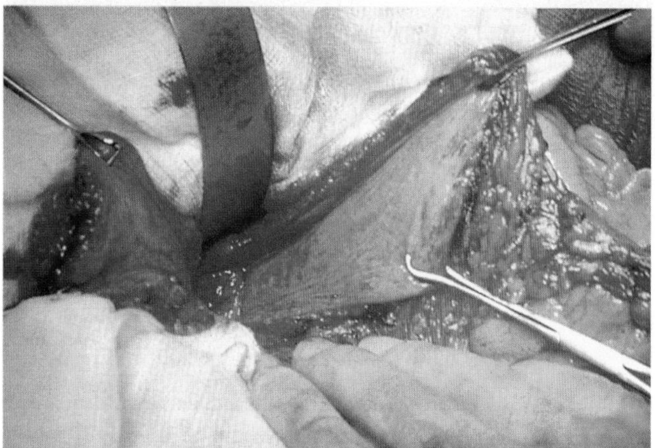

Fig. 65.24 A 'clam' cystoplasty being performed. The ureteric orifices can be seen with the interureteric bar; the defect will be filled by a segment of detubularised ileum, performing a bladder augmentation.

Bladder stones

Definition

A *primary bladder stone* is one that develops in sterile urine; it often originates in a kidney and passes down the ureter to the bladder, where it enlarges.

A *secondary bladder stone* occurs in the presence of infection, bladder outflow obstruction, impaired bladder emptying or a foreign body such as nonabsorbable sutures, metal staples or catheter fragments.

Incidence

Until the twentieth century, bladder stone was one of the most prevalent disorders among the poor, and the incidence was especially high in childhood and adolescence. Owing to improved diet, especially an increased protein–carbohydrate ratio, primary vesical calculus is rare in Western society – particularly among children.

Composition and cystoscopic appearance

Most vesical calculi are mixed but have one component in excess, and assume the appearance of that variety.

Oxalate calculus is a primary calculus that grows slowly. Usually, it is of moderate size and is solitary. Its surface is uneven (mulberry type); sometimes it bristles with spines (Fig. 65.25). Although calcium oxalate is white, the stone is usually dark brown or black because of the incorporation of blood pigment on to it.

Uric acid and urate calculi are round or oval, fairly smooth, and vary in colour from pale yellow to light brown: they may be single or multiple (Fig. 65.26). They may occur in patients with gout, but are also found in patients with ileostomies or with bladder outflow obstruction.

Cystine calculus occurs only in the presence of cystinuria and is radio-opaque owing to its high sulphur content.

Triple phosphate calculus is composed of ammonium, magnesium and calcium phosphates, and occurs in urine infected with urea-splitting organisms. It tends to grow rapidly. In some instances, it occurs on a nucleus of one of the foregoing types of calculus; much more rarely on a foreign body (Figs 65.27 and 65.28). In others, the nucleus is composed of desquamated epithelium and bacteria. It is dirty white in colour and of chalky consistency.

A bladder stone is usually free to move in the bladder. It gravitates to the lowest part of the bladder which is the outflow when the patient is erect or sitting. In the recumbent position (and at cystoscopy) the stone occupies a position behind the interureteric ridge. Less commonly, the stone is wholly or partially in a diverticulum where it may be hidden from view.

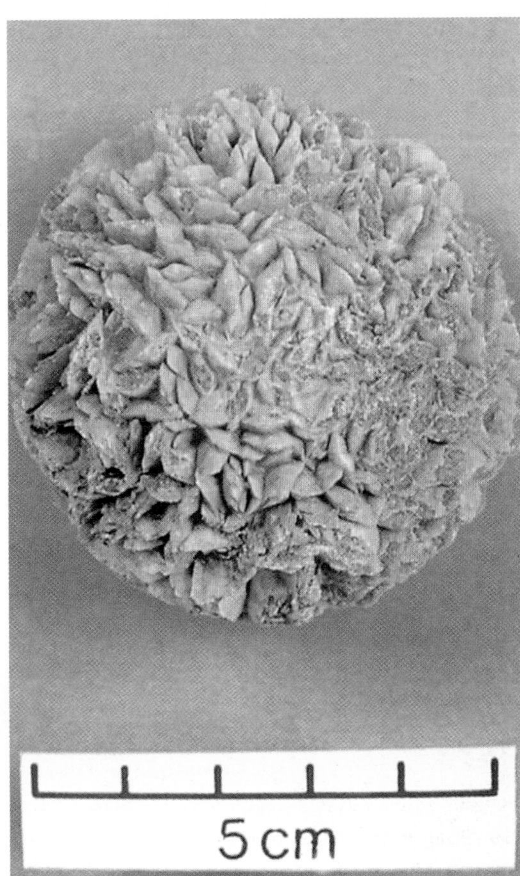

Fig. 65.25 A rough bladder stone.

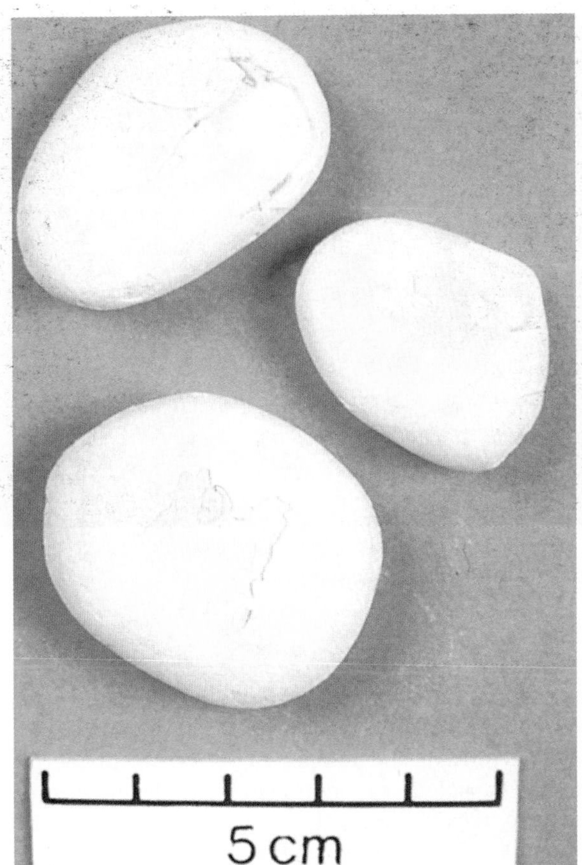

Fig. 65.26 Smooth uric acid type stones.

Clinical features

Males are eight times more often affected than females. It may be asymptomatic and found incidentally during cystoscopy before a prostatectomy is carried out.

Symptoms

Frequency is the earliest symptom, although it is often more common during the daytime. There may be a sensation of incomplete bladder emptying.

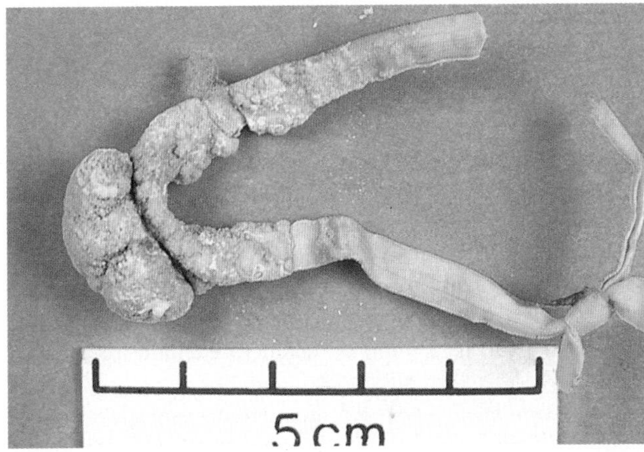

Fig. 65.27 Stone on a vaginal sling which had eroded into the bladder.

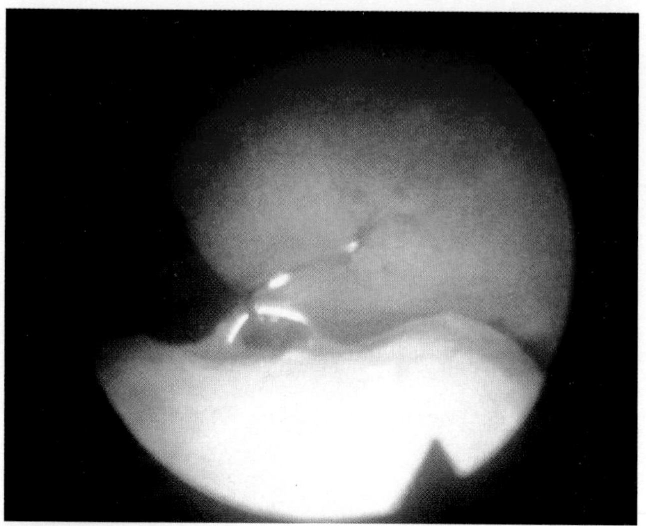

Fig. 65.28 Uric acid stones which had formed on metal staples used to construct a colonic bladder augmentation.

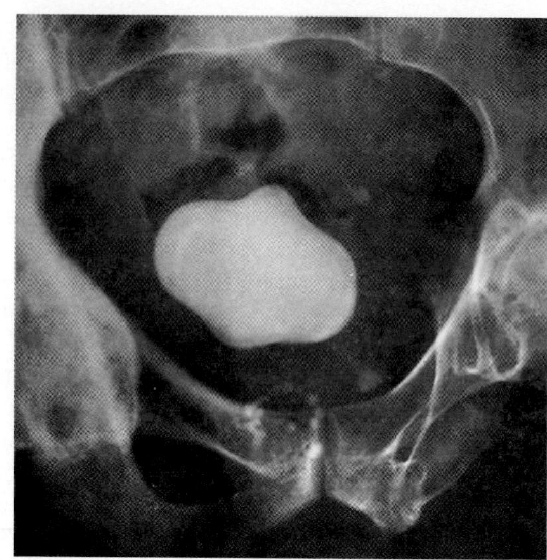

Fig. 65.29 Radiograph showing a vesical calculus (no contrast has been used).

Pain (*strangury*) is most often found in patients with a spiculated oxalate calculus. It usually occurs at the end of micturition and is referred to the tip of the penis or to the labia majora, more rarely to the perineum or suprapubic region. The pain is worsened by movement. In young boys, screaming and pulling at the penis with the hand at the end of micturition are indicative of bladder stone.

Haematuria is characterised by the passage of a few drops of bright red blood at the end of micturition, and is due to the stone abrading the vascular trigone – a fact that also accounts for the pain.

Interruption of the urinary stream is due to the stone blocking the internal meatus and may develop into *acute retention of urine* which occurs infrequently in adults.

Symptoms of urinary infection. Urinary infection is a common presenting symptom.

Examination

Rectal or vaginal examination is usually normal, occasionally a large calculus is palpable in the female.

Examination of the urine usually reveals microscopic haematuria, pus or crystals typical of the calculus, for example envelope-like in the case of an oxalate stone, or hexagonal plates with cystine calculi.

Radiography – in most patients, the stone is visible on a plain X-ray (Fig. 65.29). If the stone is radiolucent, a filling defect may be visualised on IVU. Radiographs of the whole of the urinary tract should be taken to exclude upper tract stone.

Cystoscopy is essential and most stones nowadays can be dealt with endoscopically. Frequently, on introducing the sheath of the cystoscope, a significant 'click' will be felt when a free-lying stone comes in contact with the instrument.

The whole of the bladder should be inspected: basal or generalised inflammation may be seen. In men with bladder outflow obstruction endoscopic resection of the prostate should be performed at the same time as the stone is dealt with.

Treatment

In most patients, the cause of the underlying stone should be sought and treated. This may include bladder outflow obstruction plus infection and incomplete bladder emptying in patients with neurogenic bladder dysfunction. In most patients, treatment can be delivered endoscopically.

Litholapaxy

Historically, the blind lithotrite (Fig. 65.30) was an early type of minimally invasive technique. Other methods include the optical lithotrite and the electrohydraulic probe or ultrasound probe (Fig. 65.31). Nevertheless, the blind lithotrite is still a satisfactory instrument in the right hands for the treatment of a large, hard stone. Other devices include the stone punch which is useful to crush small fragments further so that they can be evacuated with an Ellik evacuator.

Contraindications to perurethral litholopaxy are given below.

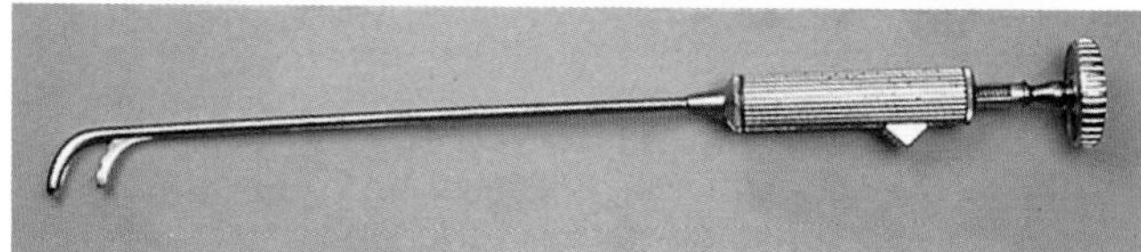

Fig. 65.30 'Blind' lithotrite used to crush bladder stones.

Milo Ellik, b. 1905. American urologist.

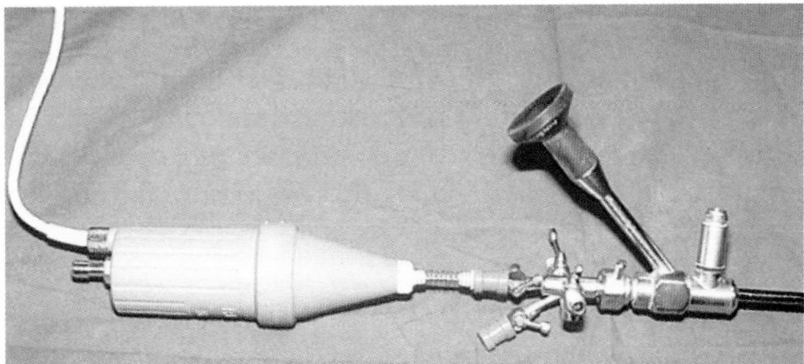

Fig. 65.31 An endoscopic ultrasound probe which is used to fragment bladder or kidney stones.

Contraindications to per-urethral litholopaxy

- Urethral:
  - A urethral stricture that cannot be dilated sufficiently
  - When the patient is below 10 years of age
- Bladder:
  - A contracted bladder
- Stone characteristics:
  - A very large stone

Technique. The patient should receive appropriate antibiotics treatment before operation. The major advantage of the blind lithotrite is that, because of its solidity and strength, harder stones can be crushed than is the case with the optical instrument. A cystoscopic lithotrite, stone punch or stone loop enables the stone or stone fragments to be seized under vision. To carry out litholapaxy, the bladder is filled with about 200–300 ml of saline and the instrument is introduced with its obturator in place so that its closed jaws point downwards. After irrigation of the bladder and insertion of the telescope, the stone is seen. The distal blade is hooked over the centre of the stone and grasped. After withdrawing the telescope slightly to prevent damage to the optics, the screw is turned slowly, breaking the stone. Large fragments are crushed into small ones by repeating the manoeuvre. With the jaws closed the lithotrite is rotated so that the jaws point upwards, and after removing the telescope and allowing the saline and stone fragments to escape, the instrument is withdrawn. The use of an Ellik evacuator is necessary to ensure complete removal of all stone fragments.

Mechanohydraulic lithotripsy

The lithoclast generates energy by purely mechanical means using a steel ball which is fired in a closed chamber at the proximal end of the endoscopic probe. Also, an energy source is generated between paired or concentric electrodes. With repeated discharges, the stone is broken into small pieces. The probes come in two or three sizes and it is sensible to use the largest (9 F) for bladder calculi. The patient is cystoscoped and the probe placed close to the stone, but away from the end of the telescope, and fired. It is important not to damage the bladder wall by discharging the electrode on the mucosa. A newly developed device

Evacuation of the fragments. Fluid (200 ml) is introduced into the bladder. The evacuator, filled with solution, is fitted on to the sheath. The bulb is compressed slowly and then permitted to expand. The returning solution carries with it fragments of stone which sink into the glass receptacle. Alternate compression of the bulb and aspiration is continued until no further fragments fall. The beak of the cannula is turned to the left and to the right, and suction is applied in these situations. After checking that no fragments are left in the bladder, a Foley catheter is introduced and left *in situ* for 24 hours.

Suprapubic lithotomy

The alternative to litholapaxy is removal of the stone through a suprapubic incision, after which the bladder is closed and drained by a urethral catheter.

Percutaneous suprapubic litholapaxy

It is possible to insert a needle into the bladder and then pass a guidewire. As in percutaneous nephrolithotomy, Alken metal dilators can be passed over the guidewire to dilate the track, an Amplatz sheath is inserted and a large-bore nephroscope can be inserted. This is the best method to use if it is not possible to carry out litholapaxy *per urethram* because of a narrow urethra.

Extracorporeal shock wave lithotripsy (ESWL)

These devices can be used in the treatment of bladder calculi, but if the stone is large endoscopic litholopaxy is preferable.

Removal of a retained Foley catheter

This is not an uncommon problem and is usually caused by the channel which connects the balloon to the side arm becoming blocked, usually at the very distant end. The best way of dealing with this problem is to further inflate the balloon with 20 ml of water and then burst the balloon percutaneously using a spinal needle under ultrasound screening. The instillation of fluid such as ether to dissolve the balloon is not recommended because fragments of balloon may be left behind. However the balloon is burst, it is important to subsequently cystoscope the patient to ensure that any fragments are removed before they can form a foreign body calculus.

Foreign bodies in the bladder

The commonest foreign body is a fragment of catheter balloon (see above). The variety of foreign bodies which have been removed from the bladder is astonishing, for example manicure stocks, hair clasps, hairpins and candle wax. Occasionally, a foreign body enters through the wall of the bladder, for example nonabsorbable sutures used in an extravesical pelvic operation. The diagnosis rests on cystoscopy, and in the case of radio-opaque foreign bodies on radiography.

Complications of a foreign body in the bladder

- Lower urinary tract infection
- Perforation of the bladder wall
- Bladder stone

Treatment

A small foreign body can usually be removed per urethram by means of an operating cystoscope. Occasionally, a suprapubic approach using the percutaneous insertion of a cystoscope is needed.

P. Alken. Urologist, University of Heidelburg, Germany.

Diverticula of the bladder

Definition

The normal intravesical pressure during voiding is about 35–50 cmH_2O. Pressures as great as 150 cmH_2O may be reached by a hypertrophied bladder endeavouring to force urine past an obstruction. This pressure causes the mucous lining between the inner layer of hypertrophied muscle bundles to protrude, so forming multiple saccules. If one or more, but usually one, saccule is forced through the whole thickness of the bladder wall, it becomes a diverticulum (Fig. 65.32). Congenital diverticula are due to developmental defect.

> Aetiology of diverticulum
>
> - *Congenital diverticulum* – This is rare. It may be situated in the midline anterosuperiorly and represent the unobliterated vesical end of the urachus. It empties with the bladder and is symptomless. Others in the usual situation on the base of the bladder can occur without obstruction, and may require excision because of the risk of chronic infection or stone formation in a young adult
> - *Pulsion diverticulum* – the usual causative obstructive lesion is bladder outflow obstruction

Pathology

Usually the mouth of the diverticulum is situated above and to the outer side of one ureteric orifice. Exceptionally, it is near the midline behind the interureteric ridge. The size varies from 2 to 5 cm, but may be larger. It is lined by bladder mucosa and the wall is composed of fibrous tissue only (compare traction diverticulum). A large diverticulum enlarges in a downward direction and sometimes may obstruct a ureter – probably because of peridiverticular inflammation.

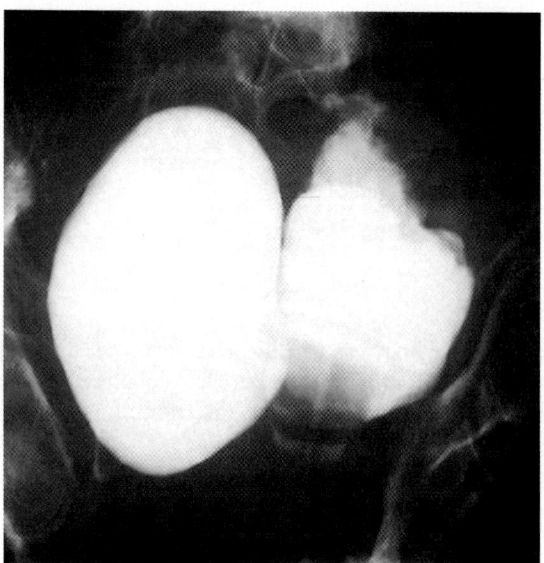

Fig. 65.32 Cystogram showing a large diverticulum of the bladder.

Complications

Most patients who develop a small bladder diverticulum secondary to bladder outflow obstruction develop no symptoms after the prostate is resected. The presence of a diverticulum per se is not an indication for open resection and surgical treatment.

Recurrent urinary infection

As the pouch cannot empty itself there remains a stagnant pool of urine within it. Once infected, the infection persists. In long-standing cases, peridiverticulitis causes dense adhesions between the diverticulum and surrounding structures. Squamous cell metaplasia and leucoplakia are infrequent complications.

Bladder stone

This develops as a result of stagnation and infection. The stone often protrudes into the bladder.

Hydronephrosis and hydroureter

This is extremely rare and is a consequence of peridiverticular inflammation and fibrosis.

Neoplasm

Neoplasm arising in a diverticulum is an uncommon complication (< 5 per cent). The prognosis is dependent on the stage of the tumour (see a later section).

Clinical features

An uninfected diverticulum of the bladder usually causes no symptoms. The patient is nearly always male (95 per cent) and over 50 years of age.

There are no pathognomonic symptoms; they are those of lower urinary tract obstruction, recurrent urinary infection and pyelonephritis. Haematuria (due to infection, stone or tumour) is a symptom in about 30 per cent. In a few patients, micturition occurs twice in rapid succession (the second act may follow a change of posture).

Cystoscopy

This is the usual means of discovering the diverticulum. Most often its orifice is seen as a clear-cut hole about 5 mm in diameter, the depths of which are black and unilluminated (Fig. 65.33). With inadequate distension of the bladder, the mouth of the diverticulum is closed with epithelium thrown into radiating pleats (Fig. 65.34). Full distension of the bladder is needed if searching for a diverticulum.

Intravenous urography

IVU may give information regarding the size of the diverticulum.

Retrograde cystography

In practice, this is only used during a video urodynamic investigation which may have been carried out in the investigation of voiding dysfunction. This test will also give information about the emptying characteristics of the bladder and diverticulum.

Ultrasonography

A diverticulum may be detected during an ultrasound scan carried out to measure the residual urine after voiding (Fig. 65.35).

Indications for operation

Operation is only necessary for the treatment of complications. Provided the diverticulum is small and the associated outflow obstruction has been dealt with, there is no reason to resect the diverticulum. Even a large diverticulum may not require treatment in the absence of infection or other complications.

Preoperative treatment

When the urine is infected, suitable preoperative antibiotic treatment is given. In the presence of gross sepsis and retention of urine, it is necessary to resort to an indwelling urethral catheter for a period.

Combined intravesical and extravesical diverticulectomy

This is the standard operation. Cystoscopy is performed, a ureteric stent is passed up the ureter on the affected side, as damage or devascularisation of the ureter is the most common serious complication. The anterior bladder wall is exposed through a suprapubic incision, the peritoneum is displaced upwards and the side of the bladder bearing the diverticulum is cleared from surrounding structures until the pouch is identified. The bladder is then incised in the mid-line and the diverticulum is packed with a strip of gauze. Usually the neck of the diverticulum can be separated from the ureter and when the pouch is free it is severed from its attachment to the bladder with a diathermy knife. The resulting defect is closed in two layers. A suprapubic catheter is left in place and an extravesical drain is inserted.

An alternative method, if the sac is densely adherent, is to carry the incision in the bladder down to the rim of the diverticular orifice, then to detach the diverticulum, together with its fibrous rim. The incision in the bladder is closed and the diverticulum left in position with a corrugated drain into it for 2–3 days. The track fibroses rapidly after removal of the drain.

If bladder outlet obstruction is part of the picture, prostatectomy should be carried out at the same time as the diverticulectomy.

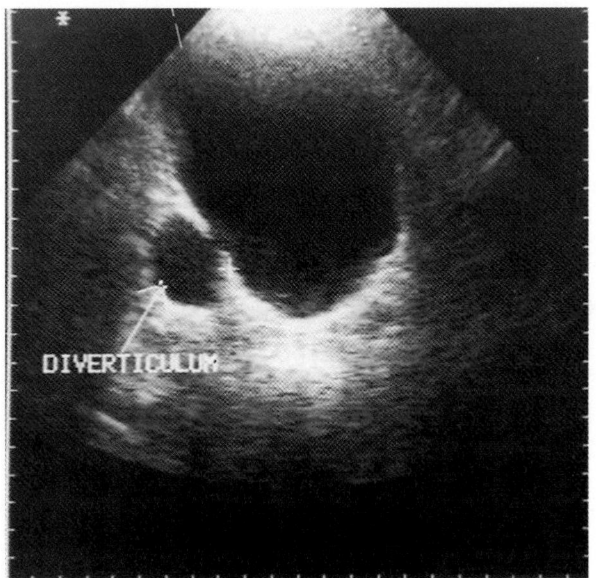

Fig. 65.35 Bladder diverticulum demonstrated by ultrasound.

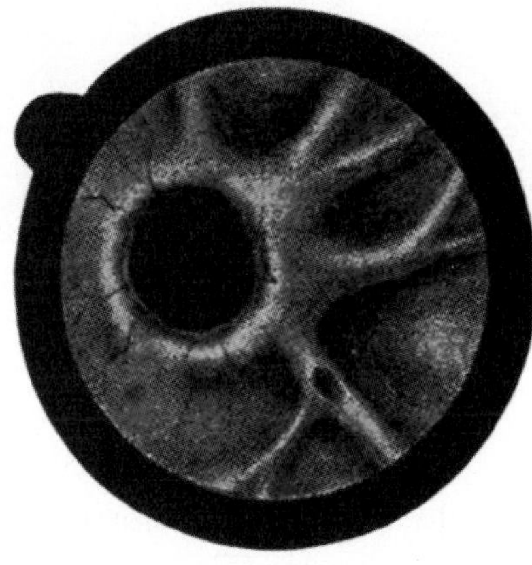

Fig. 65.33 Cystoscopic appearance of the orifice of a diverticulum and trabeculation of the bladder.

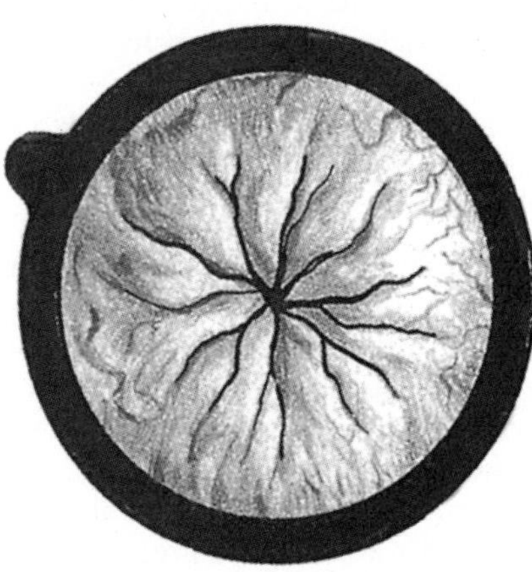

Fig. 65.34 Occasional appearance with inadequate distension of the bladder.

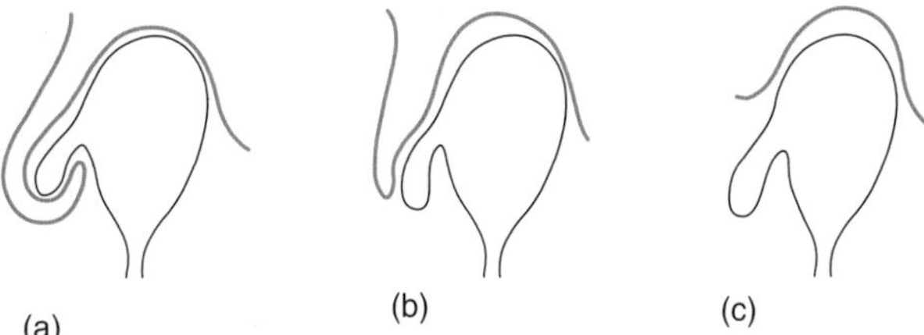

Fig. 65.36 (a) Intraperitoneal, (b) paraperitoneal and (c) extraperitoneal hernia of the bladder, in relation to a hernial sac.

Traction diverticulum (syn. hernia of the bladder)

A portion of the bladder protruding through the inguinal or femoral hernial orifice occurs in 1.5 per cent of such herniae treated by operation (Fig. 65.36).

Urinary fistulae

A urinary fistula is an abnormal communication between any part of the urinary system and the skin or some internal hollow viscus. The persistence of a fistula on the skin implies the presence of distal obstruction or the presence of chronic infection, such as tuberculosis, or a foreign body, such as a stone or nonabsorbable ligature.

Congenital urinary fistula

- Ectopia vesicae;
- from a patent urachus – the presence of a urinary leak from the umbilicus present at birth or commencing soon after suggests this diagnosis. In adult life infection in a urachal cyst may produce a fistula and adenocarcinoma may occur (Figs 65.37 and 65.38). Treatment is by means of excision of the urachal tract and closure of the bladder once distal obstruction has been excluded;
- in association with imperforate anus (see Chapter 61).

Traumatic urinary fistula

Perforating or penetrating wounds, damage not recognised during surgery, or poor healing and avascular necrosis following a combination of radiotherapy and surgery may lead to fistula formation. Also, clot retention occurring after a transvesical prostatectomy or diverticulectomy may lead to dehiscence of the bladder wound and a temporary fistula, which will heal quickly, provided the bladder is kept empty with an indwelling catheter.

Vesicovaginal fistula

This is a common condition which rapidly leads to loss of morale and serious social disruption in countries where surgical treatment is not readily available.

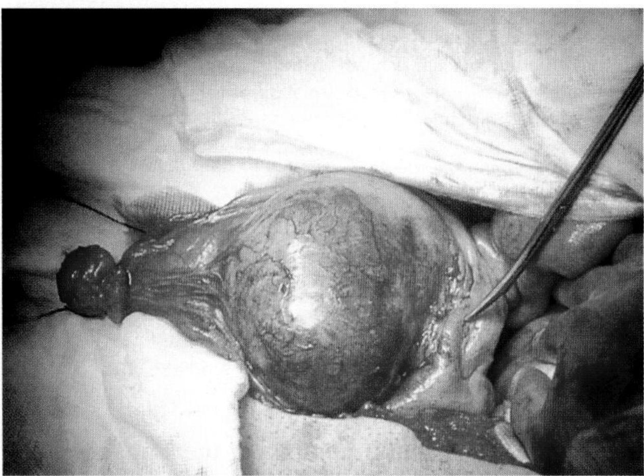

Fig. 65.37 An operative photograph showing a large urachal cyst in which adenocarcinoma formation had occurred. A partial cystectomy with total removal of the urachal remnant is about to be carried out.

(a)

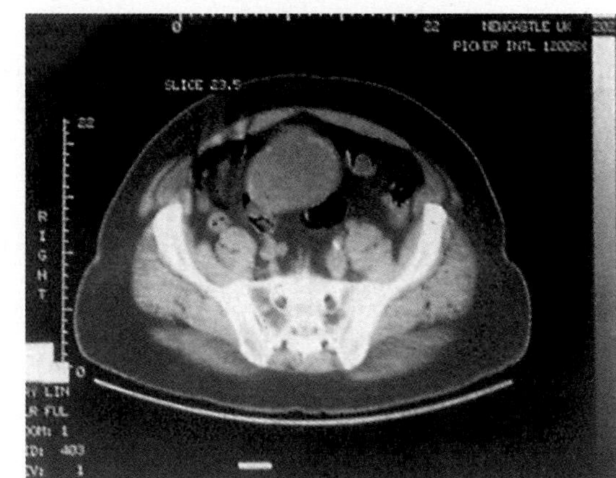

(b)

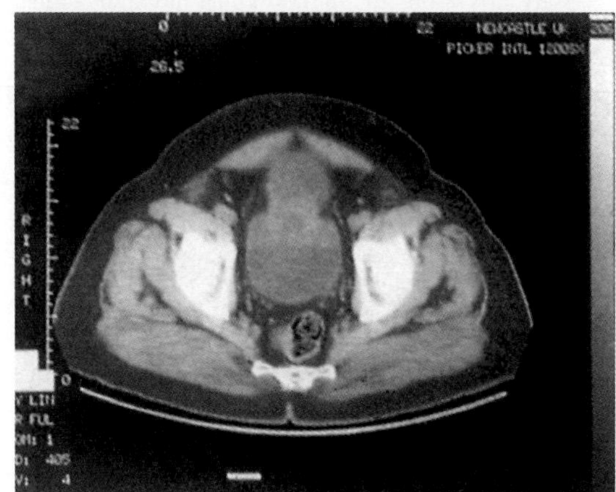

Fig. 65.38 A CT scan for the same patient as in Fig. 65.37, showing a large urachal cyst closely approximated to the dome of the bladder.

Aetiology

- Obstetrics – the usual cause is protracted or neglected labour;
- gynaecological – the operations chiefly causing this complication are total hysterectomy and anterior colporrhaphy;
- radiotherapy – the main cause is radiotherapy used in the treatment of carcinoma of the cervix; to a lesser extent external beam irradiation of the pelvic viscera for other reasons is responsible;
- direct neoplastic infiltration – exceptionally, carcinoma of the cervix ulcerates through the anterior fornix to implicate the bladder.

When a wound of the bladder is recognised and repaired at once, leakage is uncommon, but escape of urine will quickly follow if such damage passes unnoticed. However, most vesicovaginal fistulas are the result of ischaemic necrosis of the bladder wall due to prolonged pressure of the foetal head in obstetric cases. In gynaecological cases, the ischaemia is brought about by grasping the bladder wall in a haemostat, including the bladder wall in a suture, or perhaps even by local oedema or haematoma. Leakage due to necrosis of tissue seldom manifests itself before 7 days after the operation.

An intractable fistula following radium treatment of carcinoma of the cervix uteri may arise from avascular necrosis years after the apparent cure of the original lesion.

Clinical features

There is leakage of urine from the vagina and as a consequence excoriation of the vulva occurs. Digital examination of the vagina may reveal a localised thickening on its anterior wall, or in the vault in the case of posthysterectomy fistula. On inserting a vaginal speculum, urine will be seen escaping from an opening in the anterior vaginal wall. It is usually possible to pass a bent probe from the vagina into the bladder. Cystoscopy may be difficult, owing to the contraction of the bladder from cystitis and the escape of urine from the fistula. However, usually the tip of the probe that has been passed can be seen emerging through an area of granulation tissue.

Differential diagnosis between a ureterovaginal and vesicovaginal fistula can be made if a swab is placed in the vagina and a solution of methylene blue is injected through the urethra; the vaginal swab becomes coloured blue if a vesico-vaginal fistula is present. With the advent of good, portable X-ray image intensifiers, a cystoscopy and bilateral retrograde ureterograms provide a more reliable demonstration of the anatomy. Ureterovaginal fistula is discussed in Chapter 62. An IVU should be performed to exclude a coincidental ureterovaginal fistula. Usually it demonstrates some upper tract dilatation owing to partial obstruction.

Treatment

Just occasionally, conservative management of a vesicovaginal fistula following hysterectomy by urethral bladder drainage is successful. Usually, operative treatment is required and the traditional teaching has been to delay surgery for some months. This has recently been questioned. The low fistula (subtrigonal) is best repaired *per vaginam.* The fistula is exposed with dissection of the edges which are freshened. The bladder is then closed using absorbable sutures and the vagina subsequently closed with a separate layer. A urethral catheter should be left *in situ* for at least 10 days. For the higher (supratrigonal) fistula, a transvaginal approach can be extremely difficult. These patients should always be cystoscoped prior to a repair procedure and bilateral ureterograms performed as occasionally one of the ureters is also involved. For the high fistula, a suprapubic approach is the best method in most hands. The Pfannenstiel incision should be re-opened, the bladder should be dissected free from the peritoneum and bisected posteriorly in the midline down to the level of the fistula. The bladder is then separated from the vagina and, occasionally, careful dissection from the rectum is also required. The vagina is then closed with a heavy catgut suture and omentum brought down to lie between the closed vagina and the bladder anteriorly. This is lightly sutured in place and the bladder then closed. A urethral and suprapubic catheter should be left *in situ* for 10–14 days.

For the patient with a ureterovaginal fistula, an extraperitoneal approach to the ureter via the previous Pfannenstiel incision is made. Considerable adhesions will be encountered but the ureter can usually be found above the level of the injury and followed down. Fibrosed or strictured ureter should be discarded and then reimplantation into the bladder is required. Depending on the amount of ureter lost, it may be possible to achieve a simple reimplantation with a psoas hitch procedure. If the gap is too large to be bridged by this manoeuvre, a Boari flap of anterior bladder wall should be cut and brought over to meet the ureter and a reimplant performed. The most important principle of ureteric reimplantation is that there should be no tension on the anastomosis. Results from these repairs need to be good as a failure will cause despair and further enrage the already litigious patient.

Fistula from renal pelvis to skin or gut

Tuberculosis of a kidney may result in caseation and a chronic sinus leading to duodenum, colon or skin in the iliac fossa or lumbar triangle. Similarly, a pyonephrosis may spontaneously discharge into the gut or on to the skin. Cases of duodenal ulcer involving the pelvis of the right kidney and Crohn's disease involving either renal pelvis or ureter, or cases of xanthogranulomatous pyelonephritis may cause fistulae.

Fistulae arising as a result of infection

The commonest cause is diverticulitis of the colon. They may also follow Crohn's disease, appendix abscess or pelvis sepsis in association with acute salpingitis, or may be the result of surgery and radiotherapy within the pelvis.

The onset may not be dramatic and may well be treated as a simple urinary infection. The diagnosis can be difficult to make, but on cystoscopy a patch of oedema on the left side of the vault is suggestive and bubbles of gas may be seen (Fig. 65.39). A cystogram may reveal the fistula. However, as the track is not always patent the test may be negative. A contrast enema may be helpful not only to demonstrate the fistula, but also to define the cause. The passage of gas *per urethram* in a patient is most suggestive (provided that diabetes resulting in urinary infection with a gas-forming organism is excluded).

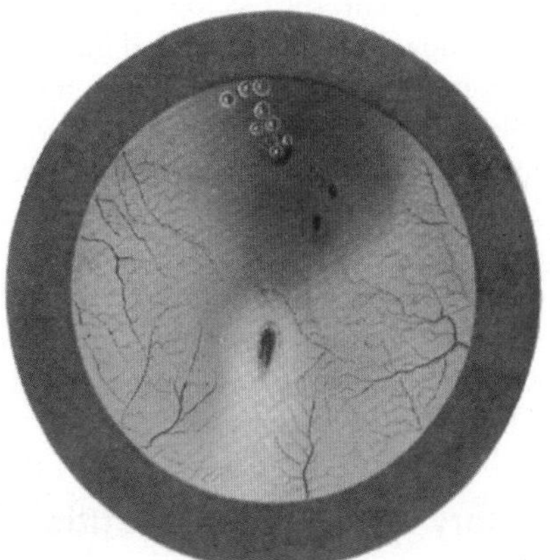

Fig. 65.39 Cystoscopic view of a vesicointestinal fistula. Bubbles of gas can be seen issuing from the orifice of the fistula.

Achille Boari. Nintenth-century Italian surgeon.
Burrill Bernard Crohn, b. 1884. New York physician.

Treatment

In most patients, a single-stage operation is indicated provided that the surgeon is experienced in colonic surgery. In some cases, a defunctioning colostomy is made above the fistula as the first step and inflammation is allowed to subside over 2–3 months. At laparotomy, the communication is separated, the hole in the bladder being closed and patched with omentum, and the segment of diseased bowel resected; the main feature is to ensure that the left colon, and if necessary the splenic flexure, is fully mobilised to facilitate a tension-free, well-vascularised anastomosis. The bladder is drained by a urethral catheter. The colostomy is closed several weeks later provided that a barium enema revels no leaks.

Cases due to carcinoma

By the time a fistula between the bowel and the bladder has developed the tumour is usually locally advanced, but may be operable.

Urethral fistulae

These occur as the result of infection above a stricture producing a paraurethral abscess which ruptures into the urethra, allowing extravasation to occur suddenly into the scrotum and perineum. Urine and infection extend into the upper 2.5 cm of thigh and lower abdominal wall. Widespread cellulitis and tissue necrosis (which may lead to Fournier's gangrene) may occur unless drainage of urine is achieved by suprapubic cystotomy, and the tissue planes are freely drained by inguinal and scrotal incisions.

Neoplastic fistulae

Primary bladder tumours very rarely fungate through the abdominal wall unless an open cystotomy has been performed without further treatment, such as low-dose irradiation being performed to cut down the risk of wound implantation. Only palliative treatment is possible in most of such cases. Involvement of the bladder by tumours of cervix, uterus, colon and rectum can produce fistulae, as may lymphosarcoma of the small gut. Carcinoma of the prostate rarely produces a rectal fistula. Treatment in most such cases is difficult and prolonged, and in most only palliative relief can be given. It is rarely in the patient's interest to carry out urinary diversion, although minimally invasive techniques such as placement of ureteric stents can be helpful in palliating symptoms.

Lower urinary infection and cystitis

Infection of the bladder gives rise to symptoms of frequency, urgency, suprapubic discomfort, dysuria and cloudy offensive urine. These symptoms are often known as 'cystitis'. Lower urinary tract infections (UTI) are much more common in women than in men, particularly in the under 50s. Recurrent lower urinary infection occurs in some healthy women after intercourse, without any demonstrable abnormality of the urinary tract. Repeated attacks of UTI in women, or a single attack in a man or a child of either sex, should always be followed by investigation to discover and treat the predisposing cause; sometimes, however, no cause can be found. Asymptomatic bacteriuria is found commonly (in approximately 5–10 per cent of cases), particularly in women, and investigation may fail to demonstrate any underlying cause.

Predisposing causes

- Incomplete emptying of the bladder which may be secondary to bladder outflow obstruction caused by prostatic obstruction, urethral stricture or meatal stenosis, bladder diverticulum, neurogenic bladder dysfunction or decompensation of the detrusor muscle.
- The presence of a calculus, foreign body or neoplasm.
- Incomplete emptying of the upper tract caused by dilatation of the ureters associated with pregnancy or vesicoureteric reflux. In childhood, the mainstay of treatment of vesicoureteric reflux is antibiotic therapy; operation is reserved for those with recurrent infection despite antibiotics or severe upper tract dilatation.
- Oestrogen deficiency which may give rise to lowered local resistance.
- Colonisation of the perineal skin by strains of *Escherichia coli* expressing molecules that facilitate adherence to mucosa.

Avenues of infection

Ascending infection from the urethra is the commonest route (see Chapter 66). The organisms originate in the bowel, contaminate the vulva and reach the bladder because of the shortness of the female urethra. The passage of urethral instruments may cause urinary infection in either sex, especially when the bladder contains residual urine. This happens because it carries organisms from the urethra into the bladder (Fig. 65.40).

Other routes are less common. These include: *descending* from the kidney (tuberculosis), *haematogenous spread*, *lymphogenous* and from *adjoining structures* (fallopian tube, vagina or gut).

Bacteriology

Escherichia coli is the commonest organism, followed by *Proteus mirabilis*, *Staphylococcus epidermidis* and *Streptococcus faecalis*. Infection with other organisms or mixed organisms is found in patient with neurogenic bladder dysfunction or those with a long-standing indwelling urethral catheter. These organisms include *Pseudomonas*, *Klebsiellae*, *Staphylococcus aureus* and various streptococci. Tuberculous infection is considered below.

Jean Alfred Fournier, 1832–1914. Dermatologist in Paris, France.

The presence of pus cells without organism calls for repeated examination for *Mycobacterium tuberculosis* and *Neisseria gonorrhoeae*. Having eliminated these possibilities, the underlying condition may be abacterial cystitis, carcinoma *in situ*, renal papillary necrosis, stones or incomplete treatment of a urinary infection.

Clinical features

Symptoms

The severity of the symptoms varies greatly.

Frequency. This occurs during the day and night, it may occur every few minutes and may cause incontinence.

Pain. Pain varies from mild to severe. It may be referred to the suprapubic region, the tip of the penis, the labia majora or the perineum.

Haematuria. The passage of a few drops of blood-stained urine or blood-stained debris at the end of micturition is a frequent accompaniment. Less often the whole specimen is blood stained.

Pyuria. This is usually present.

Examination

On examination there is tenderness over the bladder. Initial and midstream urine specimens should be collected in a male as acute prostatitis may be present (see below) which will lead to threads in the initial specimen. The midstream specimen must be subjected to microscopy and culture, and the sensitivity of any organisms assessed.

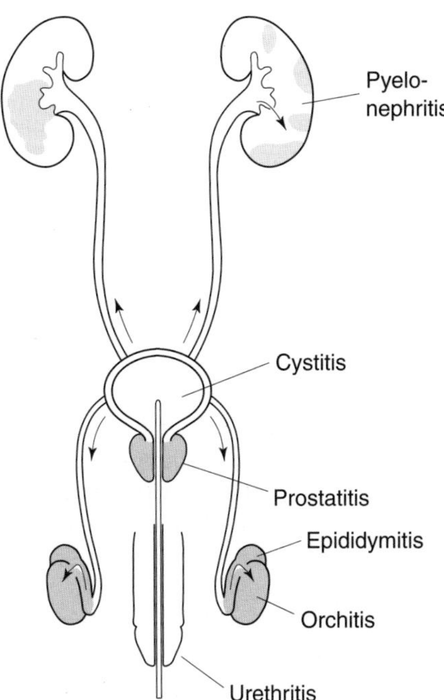

Fig. 65.40 Complications liable to follow the changing of a urethral catheter in the presence of urethritis (*courtesy of C.G. Scorer, FRCS, London*).

Treatment

Treatment should be commenced forthwith, and modified if necessary when the bacteriological report is to hand. The patient is urged to drink. Appropriate first-line antibiotics include trimethoprim, amoxycillin or one of the quinolones. Failure to respond indicates the necessity for further investigation to exclude predisposing factors.

Investigation

Cystoscopy. This is not necessary in the acute phase.

Other investigations. These include measurement of urinary flow rates and postvoid residual urine. An IVU will usually be carried out together with cystoscopy. Difficult cases may require urodynamic investigation.

Special forms of lower urinary tract infection

Acute abacterial cystitis (acute haemorrhagic cystitis)

The patient presents with symptoms of severe UTI. Pus is present in the urine, but no organism can be cultured. It is sometimes associated with abacterial urethritis and is commonly sexually acquired. Tuberculous infection and carcinoma *in situ* must be ruled out. The underlying causative organism may be mycoplasma or herpes.

Frequency–dysuria syndrome (urethral syndrome)

This is common in women. It consists of symptoms suggestive of urinary infection, but with negative urine cultures and absent pus cells. Carcinoma *in situ*, tuberculosis and interstitial cystitis should be excluded. No significant abnormalities in these patients have been found and most urologists advise patients to adopt general measures such as wearing cotton underwear, using simple soaps, general perineal hygiene and voiding after intercourse. Other treatments include cystoscopy and urethral dilatation, although the benefits remain doubtful.

Tuberculous urinary infection

Tuberculous urinary infection is secondary to renal tuberculosis. Cystoscopy shows that early tuberculosis of the bladder commences around the ureteric orifice or trigone, the earliest evidence being pallor of the mucosa due to submucous oedema. Subsequently tubercles may be seen, and in long-standing cases there is much fibrosis and the capacity of the bladder is greatly reduced (Fig. 65.41).

Treatment

Tuberculous infection usually responds rapidly to antituberculous drugs (see Chapter 7), but occasionally, in cases with advanced renal changes, may not subside until the involved kidney and ureter have been removed.

If the bladder remains of low capacity, patients will have severe symptoms and the upper tracts are at risk of dilatation because of high filling pressures plus vesicoureteric reflux. Such patients after appropriate chemotherapy respond very well to bladder augmentation. The ureters may need reimplantation into the neo-bladder.

Bladder augmentation by ileocystoplasty or caecocystoplasty. The fibrosed supratrigonal bladder is removed and the bladder augmented with a segment of bowel. This may consist of an intact segment of caecum, a detubularised segment of ileum or a detubularised ileocaecal segment. After preoperative preparation bowel preparation (see Chapter 56) a segment of bowel with an ample blood supply as demonstrated by transillumination is disconnected, leaving its mesentery intact, and the continuity of the intestine is restored by anastomosis. The segment of bowel is opened longitudinally and sutured together as a 'U' shape. This can then be anastomosed to the trigone of the bladder. Alternatively, an intact segment of caecum may be used (Figs 65.20–65.23).

Interstitial cystitis (Hunner's ulcer)

For practical purposes, this is confined to women. The symptoms commence when the patient is in her 40s and cause significant distress.

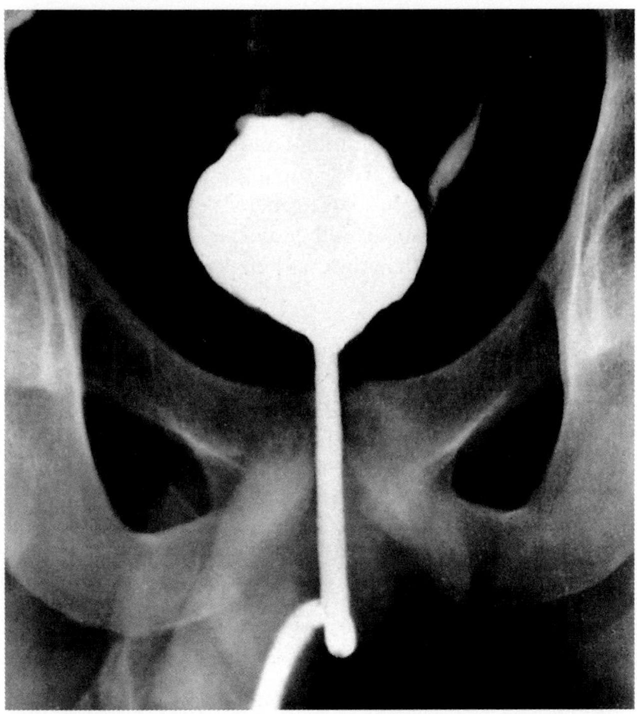

Fig. 65.41 Retrograde cystograph showing exceedingly contracted ('thimble') bladder in a case of tuberculous cystitis.

Aetiology

This is as obscure as it was when Guy Hunner first described the condition in 1914. It does not appear to start as an ordinary UTI, but consists of a chronic pan-cystitis, often with marked infiltration with lymphocytes and macrophages.

Pathology

As a result of the pan-cystitis, fibrosis of the vesical musculature ensues, leading to contracture of the bladder and areas of avascular atrophy of the epithelium. Ulceration of the mucosa occurs in the fundus of the bladder. In severe cases, the bladder capacity is reduced to 30–60 ml. The characteristic linear bleeding ulcer is due to splitting of the mucosa when the bladder is distended under anaesthesia for cystoscopy.

Microscopically, inflammation of all coats of the bladder is present with granulation tissue in the submucosa underlying the ulcer. The muscularis is hypertrophied and the peritoneum in proximity to the area of maximum disease is thickened. The inflammation may involve the trigone, the urethra and, in severe cases, the peritoneum. Pronounced mast cell infiltration is seen, but is not specific to the condition.

Clinical features

The first symptom is increased frequency. Pain, relieved by micturition and aggravated by jarring and over-distension of the bladder, is a characteristic symptom. In most patients pyuria and urinary infection are absent. Haematuria also occurs.

Cystoscopy

The characteristic ulcer is found in the fundus, but it may be absent. This area bleeds readily as the bladder is decompressed.

Treatment

Treatment is difficult and unsatisfactory. Hydrostatic dilatation under anaesthesia may give relief for some months. Light diathermy fulguration of the ulcer may help. Instillation of dimethylsulphoxide (Rimso 50®) improves some patients. Other drugs that have been tried include ranitidine. Patients with severe symptoms may well come to bladder substitution. In patients with severe inflammation involving the trigone and urethra, this operation may not result in complete relief and some type of urinary diversion may be needed.

Guy LeRoy Hunner, 1868–1951. Gynaecological surgeon, Johns Hopkins University, Baltimore, Maryland, USA.

Alkaline encrusting cystitis

Alkaline encrusting cystitis is rare and is due to urea-splitting organisms causing phosphatic encrustations on the bladder mucosa of elderly women. There are symptoms of chronic UTI and a plain X-ray shows the bladder outline. The encrustations may be removed by bladder irrigation and the infection treated with appropriate antibiotics.

Cystitis cystica

Glands are not found in the normal bladder mucosa. Under the influence of chronic inflammation, the surface epithelium sends down buds, resulting in minute cysts filled with clear fluid, most abundant on the trigone. This is frequently found in patients with recurrent frequency and dysuria. Whilst very rarely cases of adenocarcinoma of the bladder may arise in these areas of glandular metaplasia, there is no doubt that cystitis cystica is usually completely innocuous.

Schistosomiasis of the bladder

Geographical distribution

The disease is endemic in many parts of Africa, in Israel, Syria, Saudi Arabia, Iran, Iraq and along the shores of China's great lakes. Dwellers of the Nile valley have suffered for centuries. Marshes or slow-running fresh water provide a favourable habitat for the particular freshwater snail (*Bulinus truncatus*) which is the intermediate host.

Mode of infestation

The disease is acquired while bathing in infected water. The free-swimming, bifid-tailed embryos (cercariae) of the trematode *Schistosoma haematobium* penetrate the skin. Shedding their tails, they enter blood vessels and are swept to all parts of the body, but flourish in the liver where they live on erythrocytes. They develop into male and female worms. The female is long, smooth and slender, and is furnished with two weak suckers anteriorly. The male is broader, shorter (11 mm in length), bosselated and provided with a strong sucker at either end. Sexual maturity having been attained, the nematodes leave the liver and enter the portal vein. The male bends into the shape of a gutter (the gynaecophoric canal), into which a female nestles and the pair makes its way towards the inferior mesenteric vein. *Schistosoma haematobium* has an affinity for the vesical venous plexus which they reach through the portosystemic anastomotic channels.

Having reached the bladder, the female moves forward until she enters a submucous venule so small that she completely blocks it. She now proceeds to lay about 20 ova in a chain. Each ovum is provided with a terminal spine which penetrates the vessel wall. A heavily infected subject passes many hundreds of ova a day. If the ova reach fresh water, the low osmotic pressure causes their envelope to burst and the ciliated miracidium emerges. To survive, it must reach and penetrate the intermediate host within 36 hours. Within the snail's liver the miracidium enlarges and gives rise to myriads of daughter cysts which are set free on the death of the snail. A single miracidium begets thousands of cercariae to complete the life cycle.

Clinical features

After penetration of the skin, urticaria lasting for about 5 days can occur (swimmer's itch). After an incubation period ranging from 4 to 12 weeks, high evening temperature, sweating and asthma, together with leucocytosis and eosinophilia, occur. Usually, an asymptomatic period of several months supervenes before the ova are released, causing the typical early sign and symptom of intermittent, painless, terminal haematuria. Men are three times more often affected than women. Patients often present at a very late stage.

Examination of the urine

The last few millilitres of an early-morning urine specimen are collected and centrifuged in a dry container. Examination on several consecutive days may be required, but a negative result does not exclude bilharziasis, especially in patients no longer resident in bilharzial districts.

Cystoscopy

Dependent on the length of time for which the disease has remained untreated, cystoscopy will reveal one or more of the following.

1. *Bilharzial pseudotubercles* are the earliest specific appearance. The pseudotubercles are larger, more prominent, more numerous, more yellow and more distinctly grouped (Fig. 65.42) than those of tuberculosis.
2. *Bilharzial nodules* (Fig. 65.43) are due to the fusion of tubercles in the presence of secondary infection. They are larger and greyer than those in 1.
3. *'Sandy patches'* are the result of calcified dead ova with degeneration of the overlying epithelium. They occur in the first instance around one or both ureteric orifices (Fig. 65.44). Considerable calcification of this nature is visible on the radiograph.
4. *Ulceration* is the result of sloughing of mucous membrane containing dead ova or, what is even more common, sloughing of a bilharzial papilloma. The ulcer is shallow (Fig. 65.45) and bleeds readily, and its common position is the posterior wall of the bladder.
5. *Fibrosis* is mainly the result of secondary infection. The capacity of the bladder becomes much reduced and contracture of the bladder neck may be found.
6. *Granulomas*. Bilharzial masses are due to an aggregation of nodules. They are sessile and soft, and bleed readily when touched.
7. *Papillomas* are distinguished from those in 6, above, by being more pedunculated (Fig. 65.46). They vary in size and may be single or multiple.
8. *Carcinoma* is a common end result in grossly infected bilharziasis of the bladder which has been neglected for years. It usually commences, not in a papilloma, but in an ulcer, and is therefore a squamous-celled carcinoma (due to metaplasia). It is usually advanced and will require radical cystectomy (see the section on 'Carcinoma of the bladder').

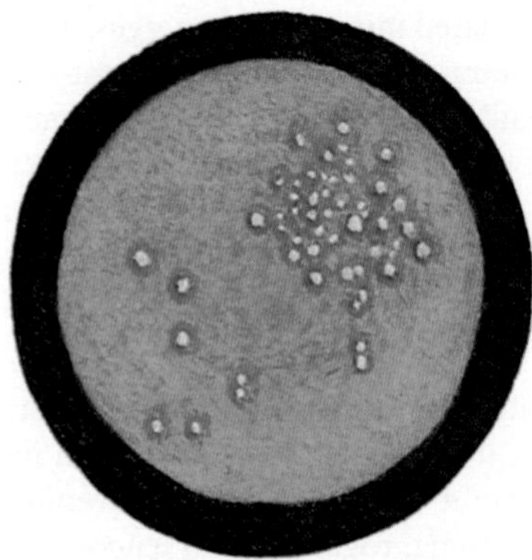

Fig. 65.42 Bilharzial tubercles (*courtesy of N. Makar*).

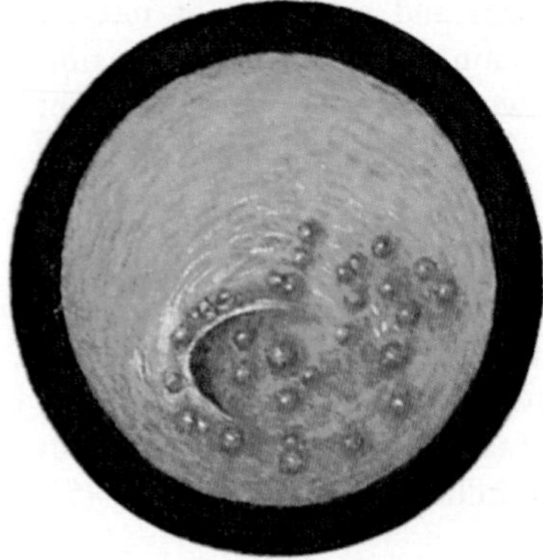

Fig. 65.43 Bilharzial nodules (*courtesy of N. Makar*).

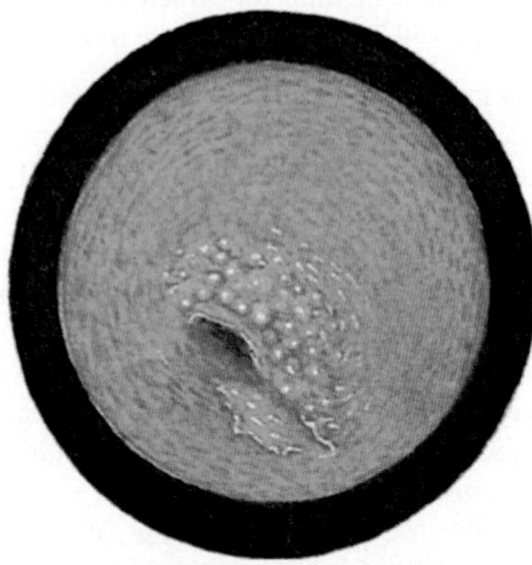

Fig. 65.44 'Sandy patches' (*courtesy of N. Makar*).

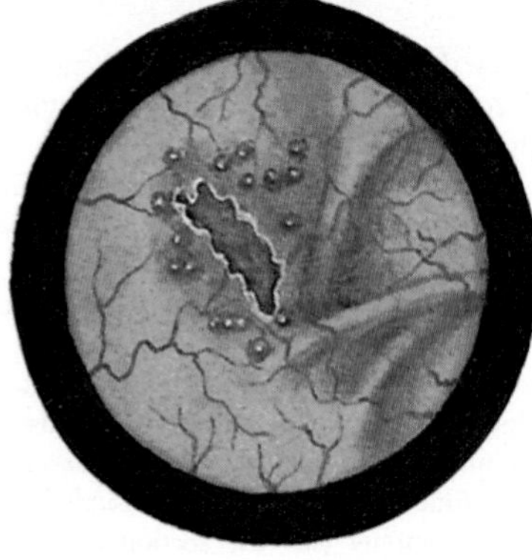

Fig. 65.45 Bilharzial ulcer (*courtesy of N. Makar*).

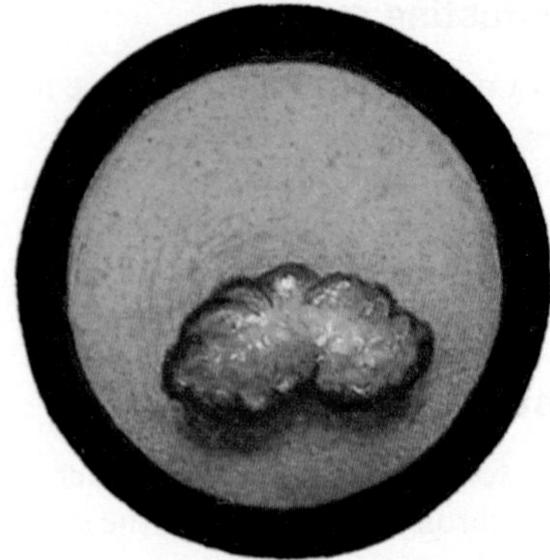

Fig. 65.46 Bilharzial papilloma (*courtesy of N. Makar*).

Treatment

Lesions 1–6, inclusive, can be expected to heal in response to systemic treatment by antimony or other preparations (e.g. praziquantel and metriphonate). It takes many months for dead ova to be expelled, and even after repeated courses and healing of the bladder lesion living bilharzial worms have been found at necropsy in the portal system. In addition to general treatment, healing of bilharzial ulcers and granulomas is expedited by light diathermy coagulation. Bilharzial papillomas and carcinomas do not respond and require the same surgical measures as nonbilharzial papillomas and carcinomas.

Other complications and their treatment

- Secondary bacterial cystitis is commonly present and requires treatment.
- Urinary calculi, especially vesical and ureteric, occur more frequently when bilharzial lesions of the bladder are present.
- Stricture of the ureters affects the last inch of the ureters. These often respond to dilatation, but sometimes reimplantation of the affected ureter is necessary.
- Prostatoseminal vesiculitis.
- Fibrosis of the bladder and bladder neck (Fig. 65.47) should be treated in the same way as that of nonbilharzial origin.
- Bilharzial urethral strictures are often accompanied by fistulae, and can be cured only by excision of the fistulous tracks and urethroplasty.

Neoplasms of the bladder

Ninety-five per cent of primary bladder tumours originate in the epithelium; the remainder arise from connective tissue (angioma, myoma, fibroma and sarcoma) or are extra-adrenal phaeochromocytomas.

Secondary tumours of the bladder are not rare and most commonly arise from a neighbouring organ, particularly the sigmoid and rectum, the prostate, the uterus or ovary, although bronchial neoplasms also may spread to bladder.

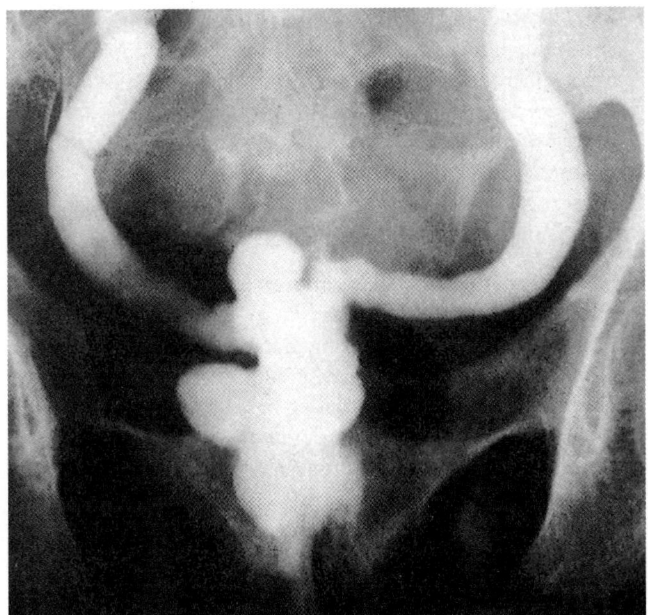

Fig. 65.47 Bilharzial contracture of the bladder, with ureteric reflux (*courtesy of H. Talib, Baghdad, Iran*).

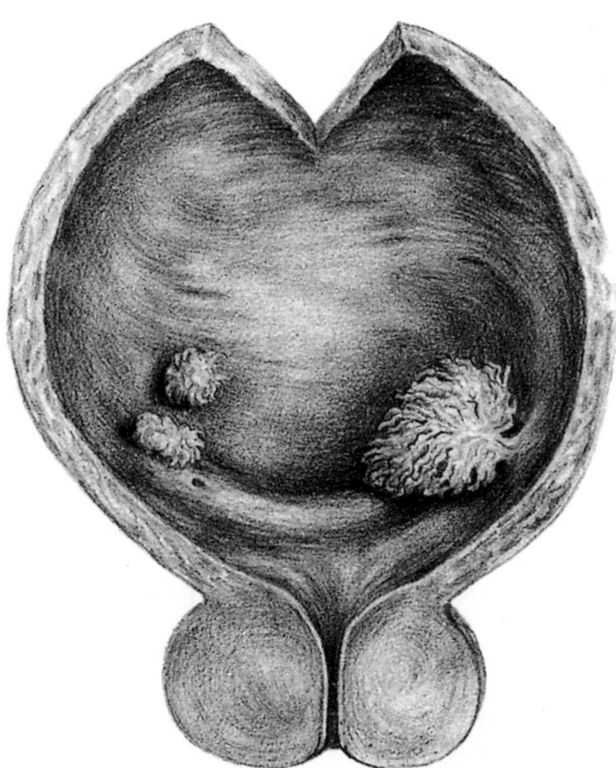

Fig. 65.48 Papillary tumour with daughter implantation ('kiss' cancer).

Pathology

Benign papillary tumours. Many histopathologists will not diagnose benign papillomas of the bladder, stating that most of them are merely better differentiated types of superficial bladder cancer. The papilloma consists of a single frond with a central vascular core with villi; it looks like a red sea-anemone (Figs 65.48 and 65.49). Inverted papilloma is a condition where the proliferative cells penetrate under normal mucosa so that the lesion is covered with smooth urothelium – it is benign.

Carcinoma of the bladder

Carcinoma arising within the bladder may be of three cell types: transitional, squamous and adenocarcinoma [or mixed owing to metaplasia in a transitional cell carcinoma (TCC)]. Over 90 per cent are transitional cells in origin. Pure squamous carcinoma is uncommon (approximately 5 per cent), apart from areas where bilharzia is endemic. Primary adenocarcinoma, which arises either from the urachal remnant or from areas of glandular metaplasia, accounts for 1–2 per cent of cases.

Transitional cell carcinoma

Aetiology. The first suspicion of a chemical cause for bladder cancer was raised by Rehn in 1894 when he recorded a series of tumours in workers in aniline dye factories. Hueper was able to show that 2-naphthylamine was carcinogenic in dogs. Subsequent investigation demonstrated that the following compounds may be carcinogenic:

- 2-naphthylamine;
- 4-aminobiphenyl;
- benzidine;
- chlornaphazine;
- 4-chloro-o-toluidine;
- o-toluidine;
- 4,4′-methylene bis(2-choloraniline);
- methylene dianiline;
- benzidine-derived azo dyes.

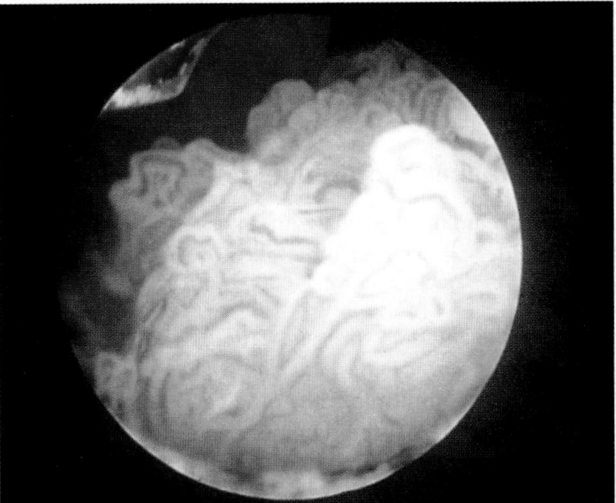

Fig. 65.49 Endoscopic photograph of a pTa bladder tumour about to be resected.

Ludwig Rehn, 1849–1930. Surgeon, Frankfurt on Main, Germany.

Occupations which have been reported to have a significantly excess risk of bladder cancer are shown below.

Occupations with an excess risk of bladder cancer

- Textile workers
- Dye workers
- Tyre rubber and cable workers
- Petrol workers
- Leather workers
- Shoe manufacturers and cleaners
- Painters
- Hairdressers
- Lorry drivers
- Drill press operators
- Chemical workers
- Rodent exterminators and sewage workers

Bladder cancer became a prescribed industrial disease (No. 39) in 1953 and ex-workers may be entitled to compensation. Cigarette smoking is associated with a two- to three-fold excess risk, and certain genetic polymorphisms for *N*-acetyl tranferase, glutathione transferase and one of the cytochrome P450s (CYP2D6) may increase the risk of occupationally acquired bladder cancer. In areas where *S. haematobium* is endemic bladder cancer is more common, and this tends to be squamous in type. Balkan nephropathy has been associated with an increased incidence of upper tract urothelial tumours (see Chapter 63).

A series of genetic events has been clearly implicated in cancer formation that is outside the remit of this chapter. Activation of dominantly acting oncogenes such as *ras* and c-*erbB-2* has been reported in bladder cancer, as has the inactivation of tumour suppressor genes such as *p53*, *p16* and retinoblastoma. Activation of other genes is responsible for the phenotypic changes seen in the cancer cell. These include the activation of enzymes which may dissolve the basement membrane such as the metalloproteinases (stromelysin, collagenases and elastase), lysosomal enzymes such as the cathepsins and others including urinary plasminogen activators; angiogenic factors [vascular endothelial growth factor (VEGF)] and other peptide growth factors such as the epidermal growth factor and its receptor also have a role to play. These changes are common to several tumour types including prostate cancer.

Tumour staging and grading (Fig. 65.50)

Study of the biological behaviour of transitional cell cancer of the bladder shows that they fall into the three following groups.

- *Nonmuscle invasive tumours (pTa) and pT1 account for 70 per cent of all new cases.* These tumours may be single or multiple. Histological examination may reveal invasion of the lamina propria (pT1) but not of the muscle or no invasion of lamina propria (pTa) – single papillary pTa tumours account for a significant proportion of bladder cancers and carry an excellent prognosis.
- *Muscle invasive disease (accounts for 25 per cent of new cases).* Such tumours carry a much worse prognosis as they are subject to local invasion and distant metastasis.
- *Flat, noninvasive carcinoma* in situ *(primary cis – accounts for 5 per cent of new cases).* Unless diagnosed and treated promptly, this carries a poor prognosis.

Superficial bladder cancer (pTa and pT1)

These are usually papillary tumours which grow in an exophytic fashion into the bladder lumen. They may be single or multiple and may appear pedunculated arising on a stalk with a narrow base, but if the tumours are less well differentiated they are more solid with a wider base. The mucosa around the tumour is often rather oedematous with angry-looking, dilated blood vessels. These areas may contain *in situ* changes (concomitant cis).

Some patients with bladder cancer have urinary infection, although this is more common with muscle invasive disease. Occasionally, calcium salts are deposited on these tumours, giving them a crusted exterior. The urothelium elsewhere in the bladder may also appear rather oedematous and velvety; this suggests a generalised 'field change' with the presence of widespread carcinoma *in situ*. The most common sites for superficial tumours are the trigone and lateral walls of the bladder.

After initial complete treatment by endoscopic transurethral resection (TURT) patients with pTa or pT1 disease may develop two problems:

- 50–70 per cent develop recurrent tumours which may be single or multiple, and the recurrences may occur on one or on many occasions. Usually the recurrent tumours are of the same stage or grade as the primary tumour. High-

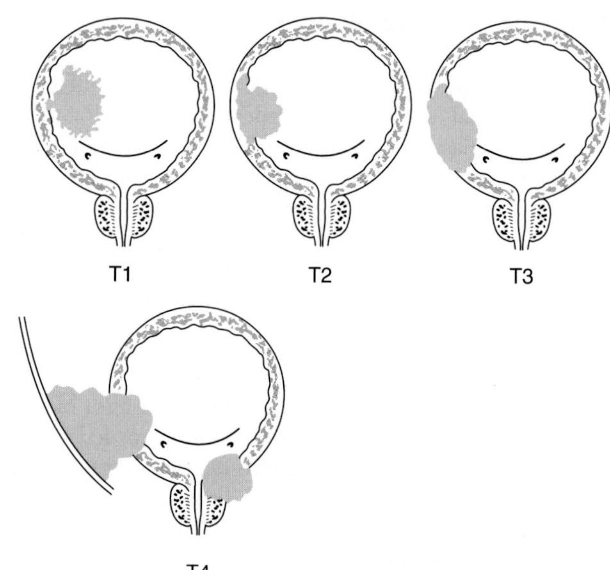

Fig. 65.50 Clinical assessment of the stage of progression of a bladder tumour by bimanual palpation (*courtesy of D.M. Wallace*).

grade, multiple tumours with concomitant cis are most likely to develop recurrent disease;
- about 15 per cent will develop a recurrent tumour which is invading the bladder muscle. The risk of such *progression* increases with high grade, with pT1 disease, with multiple primary disease and with concomitant cis. Many urologists now regard the presence of pT1 G3 tumours as an indication for more radical treatment.

This behaviour provides the rationale for performing check cystoscopies. The factors which result in an increased recurrence and progression rates are:

- high grade;
- pT1 disease;
- concomitant cis;
- multiple primary tumours;
- recurrent disease at the first check cystoscopy.

Patients presenting with a solitary grade 1 or grade 2 pTa tumour, without concomitant cis and which do not recur within the first 6 months have an excellent outcome.

Muscle invasive transitional cell carcinoma

The tumour with muscle invasion is nearly always solid (Fig. 65.51), although there may be a low tufted surface. These tumours are often large and broad based, having an irregular, ugly, sometimes ulcerated, appearance within the bladder. The incidence of metastases, whether from lymphatic invasion in the pelvis or blood-borne to the lung, liver or bones, is much more common and will cause the death of 30–50 per cent of patients.

In situ carcinoma

The histological appearance of irregularly arranged cells with large nuclei and a high mitotic index replacing the normally well-ordered urothelium is known as carcinoma *in situ*. This may occur alone (primary cis) or in association with a new tumour (concomitant cis) or occur later in a patient who has previously had a tumour (secondary cis). This change may be appreciated macroscopically at the time of cystoscopy, although often is only diagnosed when a biopsy is examined under the microscope. The association of *in situ* carcinoma with papillary tumours increases the chance of recurrent disease and progression. It may cause severe symptoms of dysuria, suprapubic pain and frequency (hence its old name of malignant cystitis).

World-wide experience of this condition seems to indicate that symptomatic cis carries a high malignant potential. Fifty per cent of patients will die of bladder cancer.

Pure squamous cell carcinoma of the bladder

Squamous cell tumours tend to be solid and are nearly always associated with muscle invasion. This is the most prevalent form of bladder cancer in areas where bilharzia is endemic. Squamous cell tumours may be associated with chronic irritation caused by stone disease in the bladder as a result of metaplasia.

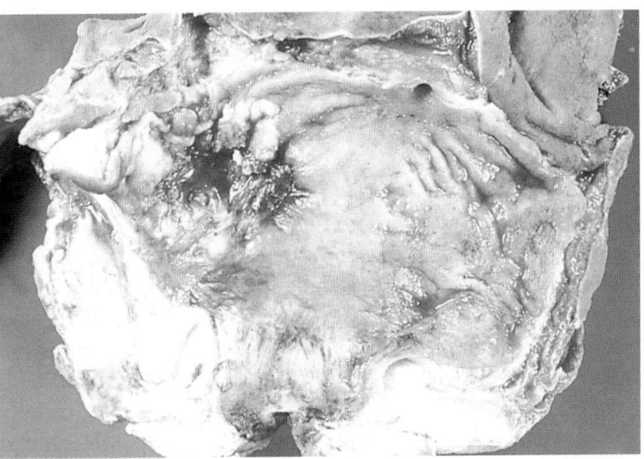

Fig. 65.51 Radical cystectomy specimen showing a large solid bladder cancer with total removal of the bladder and prostate.

Pure adenocarcinoma

This accounts for approximately 1–2 per cent of bladder cancer. It usually arises in the fundus of the bladder at the site of the urachal remnant. Occasionally, primary adenocarcinomas arise at other sites and probably originate from areas of glandular metaplasia. Such tumours need to be distinguished from secondary cancer.

Clinical features

Painless haematuria is by far the most common symptom and should be regarded as indicative of a bladder carcinoma until proven otherwise. The haematuria may occur on only one or two occasions, and because the urine once again becomes clear patients only too often fail to declare the symptom to their general practitioner. Many months may elapse before it recurs and causes concern. The bleeding if more severe may give rise to clot formation and subsequent clot retention. It is fairly uncommon for the bleeding to be so profuse that emergency admission to hospital and blood transfusion is necessary. Occasionally, a pedunculated tumour or clot may occlude the bladder neck, causing retention of urine. The development of recurrent urinary tract infections, particularly in women in the later decades of life, should also arouse one's suspicions.

Constant pain in the pelvis usually heralds extravesical spread. There is often frequency and discomfort associated with urination. Pain in the loin or pyelonephritis may indicate ureteric obstruction and hydronephrosis. A late manifestation is nerve involvement causing pain referred to the suprapubic region, groins, perineum, anus and into the thighs.

It is also important to assess the patient as a whole. Many are elderly men who have been life-long smokers and suffer from chronic obstructive airways disease or cardiovascular disease. Their suitability for anaesthesia must be borne in mind.

Investigation

Urine. Urine should be cultured and examined cytologically for malignant cells. This is not a good screening test for patients with haematuria as, particularly with low-grade tumours, malignant cells may not be identified unless a specimen obtained from a bladder washout is examined. False-positive results occur infrequently and are usually associated with stone disease. New tests are being developed based on the presence of antigens, such as nuclear matrix proteins, which may be good at detecting new or recurrent tumours.

Blood. Estimation of the haemoglobin and the serum electrolytes and urea should be carried out.

IVU. This should be performed on patients with haematuria. Occasionally, the preliminary film shows a faint shadow of an encrusted neoplasm of the bladder. The most common radiological sign is a filling defect. Occasionally, irregularity of the bladder wall may herald the presence of an invasive tumour (Fig. 65.52). Hydronephrosis may occur if a superficial tumour grows up the intramural ureter or if direct invasion of the ureteric wall occurs. Ultrasound scanning should be carried out if the kidney is nonfunctioning.

Cystourethroscopy. Cystourethroscopy is the mainstay of diagnosis and *should always* be performed on patients with haematuria. It can be done with a rigid instrument under general anaesthesia or with a flexible instrument under local anaesthesia. The urethra is inspected at the initial insertion of the instrument (urethroscopy) and the bladder is then examined in a systematic fashion (cystoscopy).

Bimanual examination. A bimanual examination with the patient fully relaxed under general anaesthesia should be performed both before and after endoscopic surgical treatment of these tumours. The bladder should be empty and the bimanual examination is executed with the right index finger in the rectum of a male and placed *per vaginam* in a female. The four fingers of the left hand push down on the anterior abdominal wall in the suprapubic region. Occasionally, a very large superficial fronded tumour may be felt as a soft but mobile thickening prior to resection. Superficial tumours are not usually palpable bimanually at the beginning and by definition are not palpable after resection. Once there is muscle invasion the differentiation between T2 and T3 disease depends on whether a mass is palpable bimanually at the end of the procedure (T3). Where invasion has spread into the prostate in a male or the vagina in a woman it is classified as T4a. If the tumour is fixed to the lateral pelvic side wall it is staged as T4b.

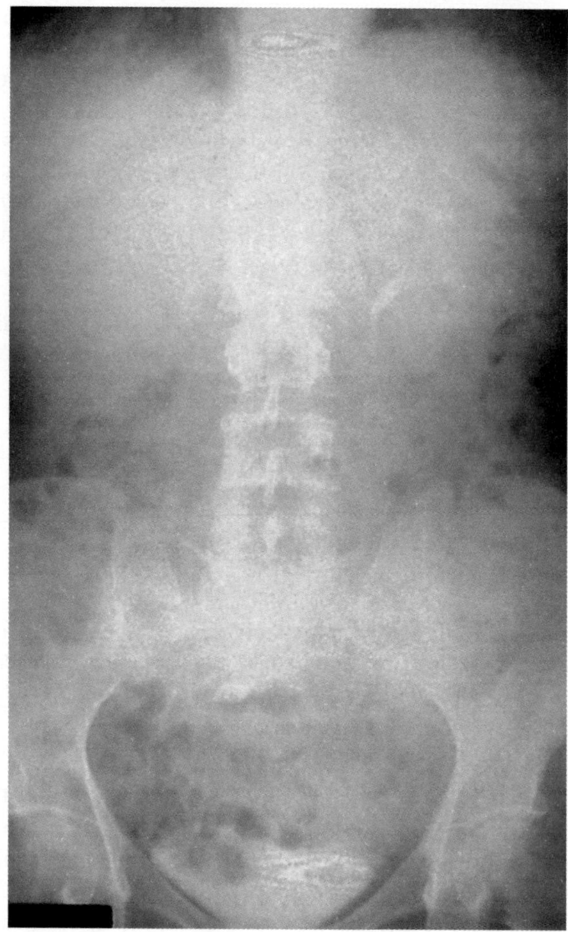

Fig. 65.52 IVU showing a filling defect in the region of the right ureteric orifice.

Treatment for carcinoma of the bladder

Noninvasive tumours

Endoscopic surgery

It is not acceptable to take a tiny biopsy from the top of a papillary tumour and apply a fulgurating coagulation current to the rest unless a small recurrence is being dealt with. The tumour should be carefully resected in layers using a resectoscope. The base of the tumour is sent separately for histological examination. Small biopsies are taken near to and distant from the primary lesion to diagnose unsuspected cis. After removal of the tumour, two or three further loops of tissue from the base should be sent separately so that the pathologist can accurately determine whether there is lamina propria or muscle invasion. The base of the tumour is then coagulated, so achieving haemostasis. The appearance of pale yellow glistening fat will indicate a perforation of the bladder. Should this occur before the resection is complete, it may be prudent to stop the resection and place a catheter in the bladder for a few days. In this instance the procedure could be completed some 2 weeks later. The bimanual examination is repeated at the end of each endoscopic procedure.

Patients with solid tumours should have adequate material resected for histological staging and grading. These patients will usually need some other form of treatment. It is likely that a debulking resection of these tumours is helpful prior to radiotherapy. Following these procedures an irrigating catheter is left *in situ* for 48 hours to prevent clot retention of urine. There is good evidence that *a single dose* of mitomycin C (40 mg in 60 ml of fluid) instilled into the bladder prior to catheter removal decreases the risks of recurrence in patients with pTa, PT1 grade 1 and 2 disease.

Follow-up. Most urologists agree that patients with a single, low- or medium-grade pTa tumour can safely be treated by resection alone and followed up by means of regular cystoscopies.

The treatment of patients with multiple low- or medium-grade pTa tumour can be by either means of resection alone or resection followed by a *6-week course* of intravesical chemotherapy with mitomycin C, adriamycin or epirubicin.

The treatment of pT1 disease is difficult. Many urologists, including many North American and European urologists, would offer immediate cystectomy to a patient with a high-grade pT1 tumour – particularly if it was multiple or accompanied by cis, because of the 30–50 per cent risk of progression to muscle invasion. Others will treat such patients by means of endoscopic treatment followed by intravesical immunotherapy with intravesical bacille Calmette–Guérin (BCG) – although there is no firm evidence that this decreases the risk of progression. The treatment of solitary medium-grade pT1 disease remains uncertain, but a reasonable approach would be endoscopic resection followed re-resection of the area in 6 weeks followed by intravesical chemotherapy with BCG.

Follow-up cystoscopies are essential; they may be carried out by means of local anaesthesia with a flexible cystoscope or by means of general anaesthesia if the urologist feels that the patient has a high risk of recurrence. They should initially be performed at 3-monthly intervals over the year; following this the time interval between cystoscopies can be determined according to the presence or absence of further disease. Thirty per cent of patients will never develop another tumour, so that after 2 years if the bladder has remained clear annual inspection may be adequate. For patients who go on to develop multiple recurrences within the bladder at each examination, the cystoscopies need to be maintained at frequent intervals so that the growths can be resected. These patients are at a greater risk from developing progression of their disease; whilst intravesical chemotherapy can decrease the recurrence rate, no reduction in progression rates has been found.

Albert Léon Charles Calmette, 1863–1933. French bacteriologist.
Camille Guérin, b. 1887. French bacteriologist.

Intravesical chemotherapy and immunotherapy

Various agents have been used. These include thiotepa (which may be absorbed because of its low molecular weight and cause blood dyscrasias), mitomycin C, epirubicin and adriamycin. They are of equal efficacy and the cheapest should be chosen. They are administered by means of a urethral catheter and held in the bladder for 1 hour, the patients are turned from side to side and try to hold their urine for as long as possible. Usually the patients are treated weekly for 8–10 weeks and then re-cystoscoped. BCG is now frequently used as intravesical immunotherapy. It carries a greater risk of local side effects such as 'cystitis-like' symptoms and also risks of systemic side effects – including systemic BCGosis. Nevertheless, it is probably more effective than intravesical chemotherapy and is the treatment of choice for cis. Currently, 'booster' doses of maintenance BCG treatment are being given in addition to the initial 6-week course.

Open surgical excision

This should be totally avoided. If by some error a bladder containing a tumour is entered, then the tumour may be removed with a diathermy needle and the base coagulated and the bladder closed. Postoperative radiotherapy to the wound will diminish the chance of tumour implantation.

Invasive tumours

The treatment of cancer with proven muscle invasion remains a subject for debate. Whatever the modality of treatment employed, few centres have 5-year survival figures of more than 40 per cent. The controversy is centred around whether primary surgery (radical cystectomy), radical radiotherapy, or a combination of the two, provides the best result. There is a move towards primary surgical treatment in most centres. The use of systemic chemotherapy by means of a combination of agents using cis-platinum, methotrexate, adriamycin and vinblastine (M-VAC) in addition to conventional treatment is presently being studied.

Radiotherapy

Deep external beam X-ray therapy. External beam radiotherapy is usually given by means of high-powered linear accelerators. Radical radiotherapy giving 60 Gy over a 4–6-week period will produce a 40–50 per cent complete response. The difficulty with radiotherapy is in patients who do not respond at all or those who have a partial response, having a bladder with pTa or pT1 tumour in it, and who are subject to recurrence. Patients with residual disease after radiotherapy should be offered 'salvage cystectomy' if they are fit. The protagonists of radiotherapy would claim that for most patients it saves the need to remove the bladder and allows men to retain potency. Radiotherapy is not always without complications, and during the course of treatment will cause urinary frequency and also diarrhoea. Late com-plications can leave the bladder contracted and fibrosed, in which case the bladder may need to be removed for palliative reasons. Late complications affecting the rectum should be uncommon, especially if lateral fields of irradiation are employed.

Local radiotherapy. For small invasive lesions, local radiotherapy can be delivered by open placement of a radioactive tantalum wire (^{182}Ta) or iridium wire or the implantation of gold grains (^{198}Au). It is used infrequently today.

Surgery

Partial cystectomy. This should be limited to the treatment of small adenocarcinomas of the bladder.

Radical cystectomy and pelvic lymphadenectomy. This is now standard treatment for localised pT2–pT3 disease without evidence of secondary spread or of cis which has not responded to BCG. Before contemplating radical surgery to remove the bladder, it is important to have evidence that surgical cure is attainable. A CT scan of the pelvis may overstage the bladder if a recent resection has been carried out, although the finding of grossly enlarged pelvic, iliac or para-aortic nodes or liver metastases will alter the decision for cystectomy. A bone scan [technetium-99m (^{99m}Tc)] will help to show whether there is spread to bone.

Operation

Alternative drainage for the urine is necessary following removal of the bladder. The standard procedure is to perform an ileal conduit. Patients should be counselled about the onset of erectile impotence and absent ejaculation following the operation; they should also be told about alternative forms of urinary diversion which include continent urinary diversions and orthotopic bladder replacement.

Patients should be seen by a stoma care therapist who will help to advise the patient and will try different ileostomy bags to ensure that the correct site is chosen avoiding skin creases so that one does not end up with the disaster of a leaking urinary ileostomy. A decision is made about whether the male urethra is to be removed (depending on the estimated risk of recurrence within the urethra); a urethrectomy is usually indicated in patients with primary cis or those with tumour invading the prostate stroma. Many surgeons are now offering total replacement of the bladder after cystectomy (Fig. 65.53).

Preoperatively, the bowel is prepared with a balanced solution of polyethylene glycol (Golytely or Kleanprep). The patient should receive prophylactic antibiotics including metronidazole, cefuroxime and amoxycillin, and low-dose heparin.

The abdomen is opened through a long lower midline incision extending down to the symphysis pubis. The liver and the retroperitoneum are checked for evidence of metastases and the operability of the bladder is assessed. A bilateral pelvic lymphadenectomy is performed removing external iliac nodes, internal iliac nodes and the nodes in the obturator fossae. The vessels passing to the bladder from the side wall are ligated in continuity; these include the obliterated hypogastric vessels, the superior vesical artery, the middle vesical veins, and the inferior vesical arteries and veins. The ureters are then divided. The posterior ligaments extending from the pararectal area to the back of the bladder are ligated and divided, and the layer posterior to Denonvillier's fascia is opened up. The endopelvic fascia is then divided on each side and the puboprostatic ligaments are divided. A ligature is passed between the dorsal vein complex and the urethra, and the former is ligated and divided. The urethra is then mobilised and divided. The ligaments lateral to the prostate are divided and the bladder is removed. In women, the uterus and anterior vaginal wall need to be included. *Women must be counselled about the loss of ovarian and uterine function.*

An isolated loop of ileum is then prepared on its own mesentery, and continuity of the small bowel restored. The ureters are then implanted into the bowel and the ileostomy is created. Meticulous care must be taken to close all mesenteric windows, thus avoiding internal hernias. If the bladder is to be replaced orthotopically, a reservoir made from detubularised bowel (usually an ileocaecal segment or ileum) is created and anastomosed to the urethra after implantation of the ureters.

The operative mortality associated with cystectomy used to be considerable, but should be in the order of 2 per cent. Late complications include urethral recurrence (about 5–8 per cent) which is increased in the presence of multifocal tumours, cis and, particularly, invasion of prostatic stroma (Fig. 65.54).

Leukoplakia

This condition is simply squamous metaplasia of the bladder. Profuse production of keratin may result in the passing of white particles in the urine. It cannot be treated easily. Localised areas may be resected endoscopically. Diffuse leucoplakia of the bladder is premalignant and results in squamous bladder cancer. Careful cystoscopic assessment is required. The condition may require cystectomy.

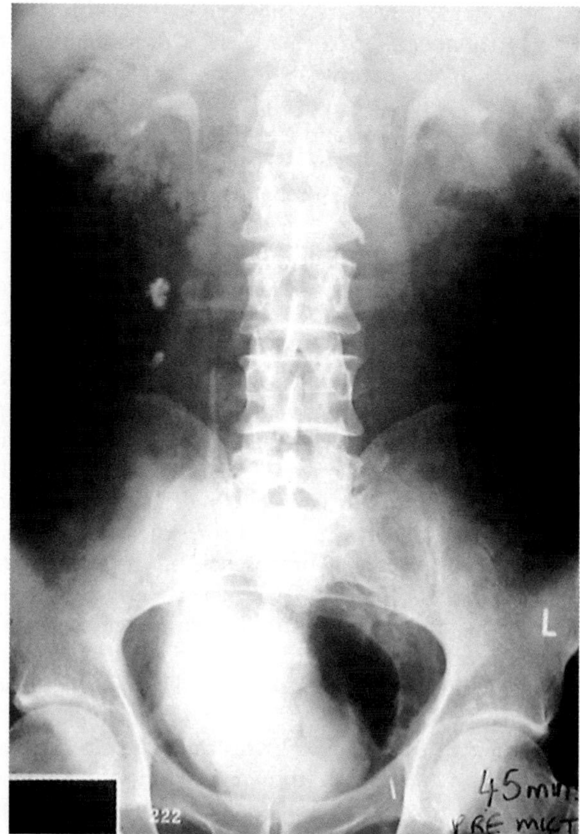

Fig. 65.53 IVU 6 months after radical cystoprostatectomy for a pT2 bladder cancer. The bladder has been replaced by a detubularised bowel segment. The patient is completely continent and voids by abdominal straining.

Charles Pierre Denonvillier, 1808–72. Surgeon in Paris, France.

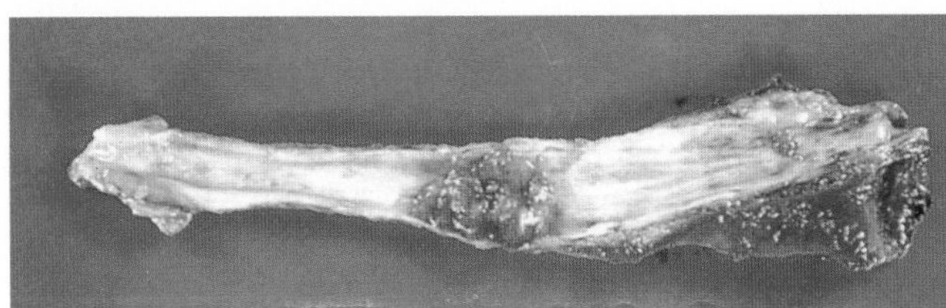

Fig. 65.54 Urethrectomy specimen from a patient who had previously undergone a radical cystectomy showing new transitional cell tumour formation in the urethra.

Endometriosis

Endometriosis within the bladder wall is rare, but can have the appearance of a vascular bladder tumour or a tumour which contains chocolate-coloured or bluish cysts. The swelling enlarges and bleeds during menstruation. If medical management fails, by means of danazol or luteinising hormone-releasing agonists (LHRH), further treatment is usually by means of partial cystectomy or full-thickness endoscopic resection, depending on its site. The condition may be part of more widespread disease. Endometriosis is also a cause of ureteric stricture.

Internal and external urinary diversion

This chapter closes with an account of the principles of this important subject, and includes indications, the methods employed and their attendant problems, and some operative details.

Indications

Diversion of the urine may be either a temporary expedient to relieve distal obstruction, or a permanent procedure when: (1) the bladder has been removed; (2) the sphincters of the bladder have been damaged or have lost their normal neurological control; (3) there is an incurable fistula; (4) there is an irremovable obstruction; and (5) in late cases of ectopia vesicae.

Methods of urinary diversion

The urinary tract may be diverted at most sites extending from the kidney, the ureter, the bladder and the urethra or it may involve the creation of new structures such as an ileal or colonic conduit, continent diversions or bladder substitutions (Fig. 65.55). The diversion may be achieved by any of the following methods, but the choice in each case will be decided largely by the primary disease, patient comorbidity and motivation:

- pyelostomy or nephrostomy (now carried out percutaneously by means of interventional percutaneous nephrostomy – Chapter 62) or catheter drainage (or urethrostomy);
- cutaneous ureterostomy or the use of indwelling 'double J' pigtail ureteric stents;
- suprapubic cystostomy (with indwelling catheter);
- cutaneous vesicostomy (cystostomy);
- ureterosigmoidostomy: (1) in continuity; (2) making a rectal bladder and colostomy; or (3) creating a rectal reservoir;
- external diversion of urine by a number of surgical techniques. The following problems may occur: (1) collection of the urine; (2) stricture formation at any anastomosis; and (3) reflux and reabsorption of urinary solutes. The problems of infection are intimately related to all three;
- internal urinary diversion by means of bladder replacement.

Collection of urine

Catheters

In the past, indwelling catheters have been used for permanent diversion. They invariably result in bacteriuria and carry a risk of infection, and they often become blocked by phosphate encrustation. Temporary nephrostomy drainage is very useful in the management of patients with acute upper tract obstruction. For temporary cutaneous ureterostomy drainage, the tubes should be of soft silicone.

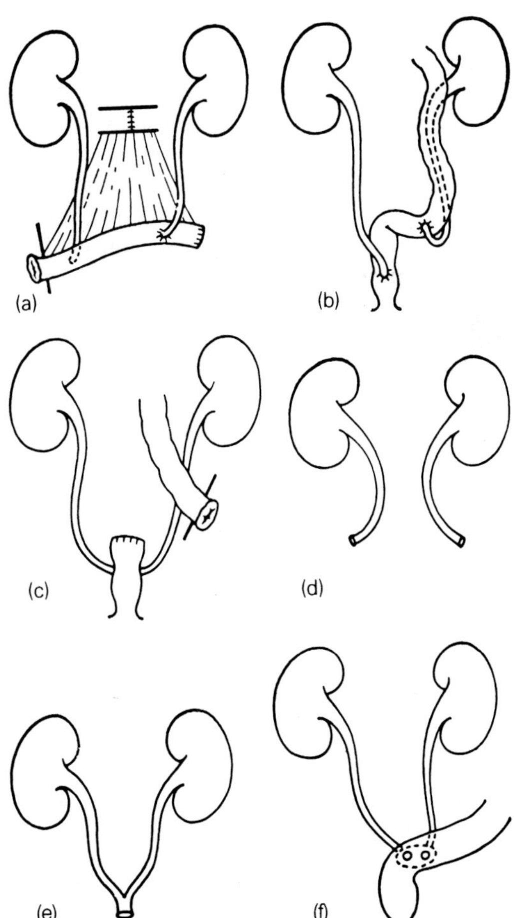

Fig. 65.55 Diversion of urine. Flavoured methods: (a) ileal conduit; (b) ureterosigmoidostomy; (c) rectal bladder with terminal colostomy; (d) bilateral cutaneous ureterostomies; (e) joined ureters – cutaneous openings; (f) trigonocolostomy.

Bladder drainage. In elderly patients unfit for prostatectomy and in some terminal cases of carcinoma of the prostate, an indwelling silicone urethral Foley catheter changed every 3 months is a satisfactory method of drainage. Other methods include the use of prostatic urethral stents passed under ultrasound or direct vision to hold open the prostatic urethra and bladder neck.

Cutaneous stomas

Suprapubic vesicostomy or urethrostomy. Collection from a formal suprapubic vesicostomy (cystostomy) is unsatisfactory because the local incisions result in skin creases which make it difficult to apply a water-tight collecting appliance.

Cutaneous ureterostomies. These are very liable to stricture formation. In addition, two openings (Fig. 65.55d) and appliances add to the patient's burden. Mobilisation of the ureters and the making of a central abdominal stoma may be useful in children with grossly dilated ureters as a temporary measure (Fig. 65.55e).

Ileal or colonic conduit. At present, the most generally useful form of external diversion is to implant each ureter with as little mobilisation as possible into an isolated segment of gut (ileum or colon), which conducts the urine onwards to a cutaneous stoma (Fig. 65.55a). Urine is then collected in an ileostomy bag. This form of diversion limits infection and avoids the problems of reabsorption of urine as contact time with the mucosa is minimal. In some cases in which the pelvic area has been subjected to radiation, the lower ureters may be unhealthy. A high division with insertion of the ureters into an ileal loop above the root of the mesentery may be wiser (Fig. 65.56).

Siting of stoma. The site for the stoma must be chosen before operation in consultation with a stoma care therapist. The site of the future stoma is marked indelibly on the skin.

Colon and rectum

The advantage of diverting urine into the colon is that no collecting apparatus is necessary (Fig. 65.55b and f). Clearly, however, the anal sphincter must be competent. Before ureterosigmoidostomy is undertaken, the patient must prove that he or she can control at least 200 ml of fluid in the rectum. The disadvantage of the operation is that the renal tract is exposed continuously to infection from the faeces. This can be minimised by performing some type of antireflux procedure or by establishing a terminal left iliac colostomy, and closing the upper rectum to make a rectal bladder (Fig. 65.55c). This prevents the urine refluxing retrogradely round the colon to the caecum, diminishes reabsorption (see below) and protects renal function. Cancer can develop at long-standing ureterocolic junctions (Fig. 65.57). More recent developments include the formation of a detubularised sigmoid segment that provides a low-pressure reservoir in continuity.

Stricture formation

Ureterosigmoidostomy was first used by Chaput (1894). Subsequent modifications included those made by Coffey and Grey Turner. In these methods, the ureters were cut obliquely and pulled into the gut by a stitch – the ends were not stitched to the gut wall. Stenosis was common. Nesbit, Cordonnier and Leadbetter all recognised that these strictures could be prevented by anastomosing mucosa to mucosa.

Reflux of urine and reabsorption of urinary solutes

Reflux of urine

High-pressure activity within a segment of gut can cause reflux of infected urine at high pressure to the kidneys. In the long term this can cause renal impairment.

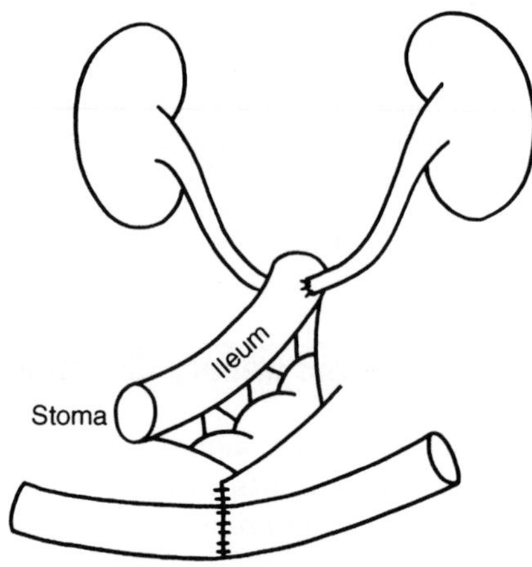

Fig. 65.56 Ureteroileostomy. (*After D. Wallace, FRCS.*)

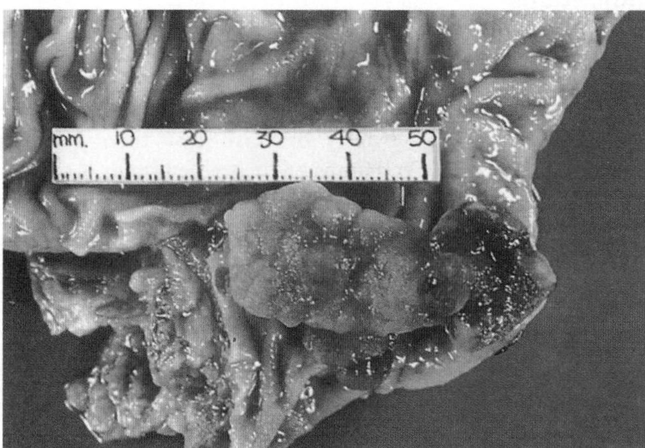

Fig. 65.57 An anterior resection of the rectum specimen in a patient aged 18 years who had previously undergone ureterosigmoidostomy in the treatment of bladder exstrophy.

Henri Chaput, 1857–1919. French surgeon.
Robert Calvin Coffey, 1869–1933. American surgeon.
George Grey Turner, 1877–1951. Professor of Surgery, Postgraduate Medical School, London. Formerly Professor of Surgery, University of Durham, England.
Robert R. Nesbit. American urologist.
James Cordonnier. American urologist.
Guy W. Leadbetter. American urologist.

Reabsorption of urinary solutes

This depends upon the following factors: (1) the area of bowel which is exposed to urine; and (2) the length of time for which the urine is in contact with the bowel epithelium.

The biochemical changes associated with urinary diversion are due to a combination of reabsorption of chloride and urea, and progressively diminishing tubular function as a result of chronically impaired tubular function due to pyelonephritis. Diarrhoea with loss of potassium-containing mucus may exacerbate the loss of potassium. The typical changes of a hyperchloraemic acidosis with potassium depletion occur frequently in patients with ureterosigmoid diversion. When severe, the patient develops loss of appetite, weakness, thirst and diarrhoea. Coma may ensue. Mild acidosis, unrecognised over a long period, produces osteomalacia. Bone pain and even pathological fracture can occur. Renal impairment from pyelonephritis and reabsorption from the mucosa are seen less frequently after ileal or colonic conduit formation, continent urinary diversion or orthotopic bladder substitution. In particular, they are seen very infrequently except in patients with pre-existing renal impairment and unsatisfactory emptying of the urinary reservoir.

Treatment

Prevention. Patients should be instructed to empty the rectum or continent reservoir or neo-bladder 3-hourly by day. In cases of ureterosigmoidostomy where acidosis is present a rectal tube should be inserted at night to drain the urine continuously. The patient should take a mixture of potassium citrate and sodium bicarbonate t.d.s. (2 g of each, either as crystals or as tablets). Regular serum biochemical analyses, including calcium, are required.

Established hyperchloraemic acidosis is usually associated with marked dehydration and the mainstay of treatment is intravenous saline. The patient may be given small doses of sodium bicarbonate to half-correct the pH deficit if it is severe and additional intravenous potassium. This should be coupled with appropriate systemic antibiotic treatment.

Operative details

Bowel preparation is by means of 3 litres of balanced polyethylene glycol solution (Golytely or Kleanprep). The abdomen is opened by a lower midline incision. The patient is then placed in the Trendelenberg position.

Ureterocolic anastomosis

The right ureter is sought at the pelvic brim and dissected towards its entry into the bladder. The ureter is divided and its distal stump ligated; the proximal end is trimmed obliquely and split for 1 cm. An incision 3 cm long is made in the anterior wall of the colon and the peritoneal and muscular coats are divided, but not the mucous membrane. An incision is made into the extreme lower end of the exposed mucous membrane and the full thickness of the ureteric wall is joined by interrupted 4/0 chromic catgut sutures to the mucosal opening. The incision in the outer coats of the bowel is approximated over the ureter. A drain is left down to the area. The left ureter is implanted into the colon above in a similar manner. A full-sized Foley's catheter is inserted through the anus no further than the rectal ampulla and the balloon is inflated, which permits urine output to be measured.

Ureteroileostomy (ileal loop conduit)

A coil of ileum, approximately 15–20 cm long and 30 cm from the ileocaecal valve, with its blood supply intact, is isolated. The left ureter is brought behind the mesorectum. The ureters may be joined to the ileum either end-to-side or end-to-end after anastomosing of the distal spatulated ureters to form a plate (Wallace). The ileal loop is tacked lightly to the peritoneum of the posterior abdominal wall at the level of the pelvic brim. The distal end of the coil is brought out through an incision at the site which had been identified before operation; a disc of skin and fat is removed, a cruciate incision is made in the fascia and the muscle is split. The stoma is made about 2–3 cm long. It is evaginated initially by means of four sutures passing through the skin, the ileal loop as it passes through the opening, and the cut edge of the ileum (Fig. 65.57).

Bladder replacement

Over the past decade, various techniques have become available to form a near-spherical urinary reservoir out of various lengths of bowel which are detubularised. These may consist of ileum, ileum and caecum or sigmoid colon. The ureters can then be reimplanted in these reservoirs in an antireflux manner and the reservoir can then be anastomosed to the membranous urethra in the male (Figs 65.20–65.23 and 65.53). These reservoirs usually need to be emptied by means of CISC. The results are good in selected younger men after radical cystectomy.

Continent urinary diversion

A similar concept is used in the construction of continent diversions. A urinary reservoir is made as described above and the ureters are attached to the reservoir. A continence mechanism is then made to connect the reservoir to the skin. This is the complication-prone part of the operation. The continence mechanism may be made of an invaginated loop of ileum supported by three rows of staples (Kock pouch) or made from the appendix buried in an antireflux manner in a submucosal tube (Mitrofanoff; Fig. 65.58) or a length of ileum can be made into a tube (of similar size to the appendix) after excision of the antimesenteric ileum and buried in a submucosal tunnel in an antireflux way. Clearly, these operations are complex, with the potential for increased postoperative complication.

David M. Wallace. Former surgeon to St Peter's Hospital and Professor of urology, University of Riyadh, Saudi Arabia.

Nils Kock. Twentieth century surgeon.

P. Mitrofanoff. French urologist, Hospitalier Universitaire Rouen, France.

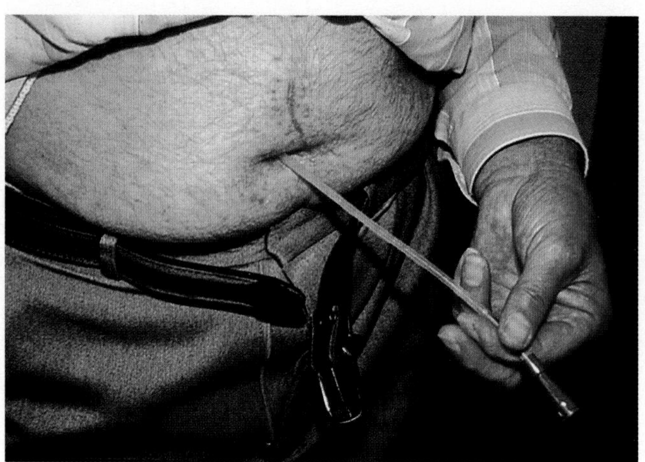

Fig. 65.58 A patient with pT3a bladder cancer who had previously undergone cystoprostatectomy and urethrectomy. A detubularised ileocaecal segment had been used to create a urinary reservoir and the appendix had been placed in a submucosal tunnel in the reservoir to provide a continence mechanism. The appendix had been brought to the umbilicus and is catheterised 4–6-hourly to empty the reservoir.

Bladder substitution and augmentation

In patients with contraction of the bladder due to tuberculosis or with neuropathic dysfunction and a small bladder capacity, the bladder may need to be augmented. Similar techniques to those used to perform a bladder replacement can be utilised to make a near-spherical pouch from detubularised bowel which can then be attached to the trigone or bladder neck after a near-total cystectomy (Figs 65.20–65.23). The ureters are then reimplanted. The facility to provide a continence mechanism must be available if needed in the neuropathic patient. This may comprise an artificial urinary sphincter or a colposuspension in the female.

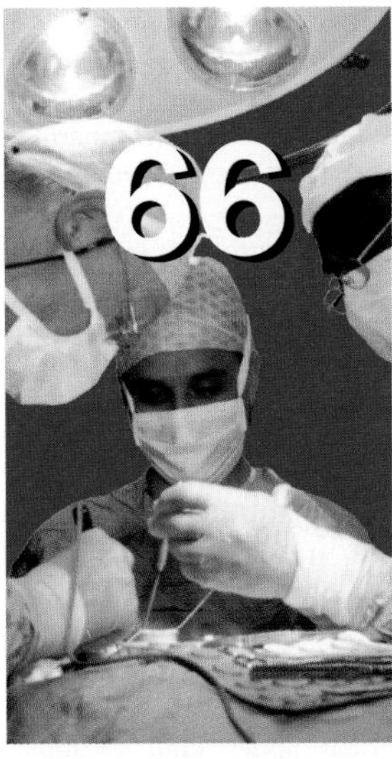

66 The prostate and seminal vesicles

Embryology

- From the primitive urethra as a series of solid epithelial buds which in a matter of weeks become canalised
- Surrounding mesenchyme forms the muscular and connective tissue of the gland and has a major role in differentiation (stromal epithelium interactions)
- Skene's tubules opening on either side of the female urethra are the homologue of the prostate

Surgical anatomy

The contemporary classification of the prostate into different zones was based on the work of McNeal (Fig. 66.1). He showed that it is divided into: the peripheral zone (PZ) which lies mainly posteriorly and from which most carcinomas arise, and a central zone (CZ) which lies posterior to the urethral lumen and above the ejaculatory ducts as they pass through the prostate; the two zones are rather like an egg in its egg-cup. There is a also periurethral transitional zone (TZ) from which most benign prostatic hyperplasia (BPH) arises. Smooth muscle cells are found throughout the prostate, but in the upper part of the prostate and bladder neck, there is a separate sphincter muscle that subserves a sexual function, closing during ejaculation. Resection of this tissue during prostatectomy is responsible for retrograde ejaculation. The distal striated urethral sphincter muscle is found at the junction of the prostate and the membranous urethra, it is horse-shoe shaped with the bulk lying anteriorly; it is quite distinct from the muscle of the pelvic floor (Fig. 65.1).

The glands of the peripheral zone (Fig. 66.2), lined by columnar epithelium, lie in the fibromuscular stroma and their ducts which are long and branched open into posterolateral grooves on either side of the verumontanum. The glands of the CZ and TZ are shorter and un-

Fig. 66.1 Sagittal diagram of prostate just lateral to the urethra showing the division into the different zones described by McNeal. The transitional zone is the area from which most BPH arises.

Alexander Johnson Chalmers Skene, 1828–1900. Professor of Gynaecology, Long Island Hospital, New York, USA.

Bailey & Love's Short Practice of Surgery, 23rd edition. Edited by R.C.G. Russell, N.S. Williams and C.J.K. Bulstrode. Published in 2000 by Arnold Publishers.

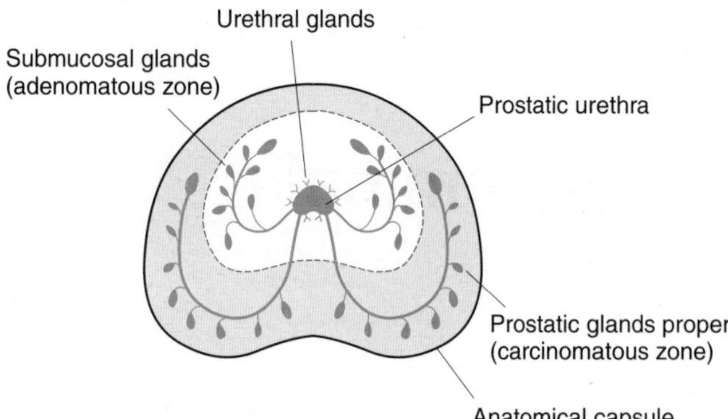

Fig. 66.2 A transverse section of the prostate. The peripheral zone is the area from which most prostate cancers arise. The 'adenomatous' zone comprises the central and transitional zones.

branched. All of these ducts, the common ejaculatory ducts and the prostatic utricle open into the prostatic urethra. No wonder that infection of the prostatic urethra is difficult to eradicate!

Benign prostatic hyperplasia (BPH) starts in the periurethral transitional zone and as it increases in size it compresses the outer PZ of the prostate which becomes the *false capsule*. There is also the outer true fibrous *anatomical capsule*; and external to this lie condensations of endopelvic fascia known as the *periprostatic sheath of endopelvic fascia*. Between the anatomical capsule and the prostatic sheath lies the abundant prostatic venous plexus. The prostatic sheath is contiguous with the strong fascia of Denonvillier that separate the prostate and its coverings from the rectum. The neurovascular bundles supplying autonomic innervation to the corpora of the penis are in very close relationship to the posterolateral aspect of the prostatic capsule and are at risk of damage during radical cystoprostatectomy or radical prostatectomy; inadvertent diathermy in the region of these nerves may be the cause of erectile impotence after transurethral prostatectomy.

Physiology

The prostate has a sexual function, but it is a little unclear how important its secretions are to human fertility. That the normal adult prostate undergoes atrophy after castration was known to John Hunter.

Systemic hormonal influences (endocrine) and local growth factors (paracrine and autocrine)

The growth of the prostate is governed by many local and systemic hormones whose exact functions are not yet known. The main hormone acting on the prostate is testosterone which is secreted by the Leydig cells of the testes under the control of luteinizing hormone (LH), which is secreted from the anterior pituitary under the control of hypothalamic luteinizing hormone-releasing hormone (LHRH). Testosterone is converted to 5-di-hydrotestosterone (DHT) by the enzyme 5α-reductase, which is found in high concentration in the prostate and the perigenital skin. Other androgens are secreted by the adrenal cortex, but their effects are minimal. Oestrogenic steroids are also secreted by the adrenal cortex and in the ageing male may play a part in disrupting the delicate balance between DHT and local peptide growth factors, and hence increase the risk of BPH. Increased levels of serum oestrogens, by acting on the hypothalamus, decrease the secretion of LHRH (and hence LH) and thereby decrease serum testosterone levels. Therefore, pharmacological levels of oestrogens cause atrophy of the testes and prostate by means of reductions in testosterone.

Other locally acting peptides are secreted by the prostatic epithelium and mesenchymal stromal cells in response to steroid hormones. These include epidermal growth factor, insulin-like growth factors, basic fibroblast growth factor and transforming growth factors α and β. These undoubtedly play a part in normal and abnormal prostatic growth, but as yet their functions are unclear.

Elaboration and secretion of prostate-specific antigen (PSA) and acid phosphatases

PSA is a glycoprotein which is a serine protease. Its function may be to facilitate liquefaction of semen, but it is a marker for prostatic disease. It is measured by an immunoassay and the normal range can differ a little from laboratory to laboratory. The normal upper limit is about 4 nmol/ml. Its level in men with metastatic prostate cancer is usually increased to >30 nmol/ml and falls to low levels after successful androgen ablation. Men with locally confined prostate cancer usually have serum PSA levels <~15 nmol/ml. Although PSA is a reliable marker for the progress of advanced disease it is neither specific nor sensitive in the differential diagnosis of early prostate cancer and BPH, as both diseases are compatible with PSA in the range of 4–12 nmol/ml. PSA measurement has superseded measurement of serum acid phosphatase.

Benign prostatic hyperplasia

BPH occurs in men over 50 years of age; by the age of 60 years 50 per cent of men have histological evidence of BPH and 15 per cent have significant lower urinary tract symptoms

Aetiology of benign prostatic hyperplasia

Hormones

Serum testosterone levels slowly but significantly decrease with advancing age; however, levels of oestrogenic steroids are not decreased equally. According to this theory the prostate enlarges because of increased oestrogenic effects. It is likely that the secretion of intermediate peptide growth factors plays a part in the development of BPH.

Pathology

BPH affects both glandular epithelium and connective tissue stromal to variable degrees. These changes are similar to those occurring in breast dysplasia (see Chapter 45), where adenosis, epitheliosis and stromal proliferation are seen in differing proportions. BPH typically affects the submucous group of glands in the transitional zone, forming a nodular enlargement. Eventually, this overgrowth compresses the PZ glands into a false capsule and causes the appearance of the typical 'lateral' lobes.

When BPH affects the subcervical central zone glands, a

Charles Pierre Denonvillier, 1808–72. Surgeon in Paris, France.
John Hunter, 1728–93. Scottish surgeon and anatomist.
Franz von Leydig, 1821–1908. German anatomist.

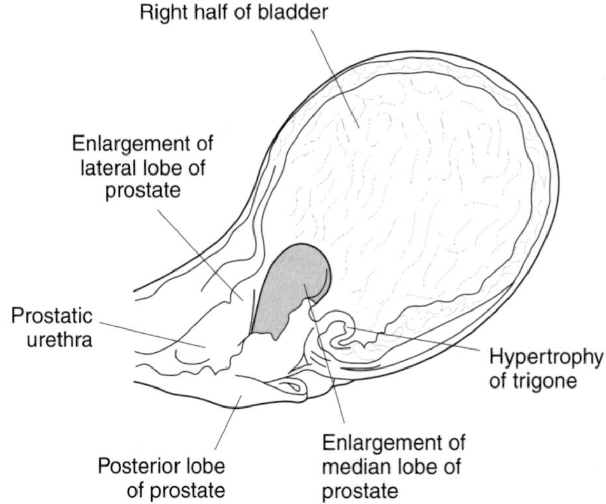

Fig. 66.3 Diagram of late-stage bladder outflow obstruction showing enlargement of the prostate from BPh, trabeculation of the bladder with smooth muscle hypertrophy and fibrosis.

'middle' lobe develops which projects up into the bladder within the internal sphincter (Fig. 66.3). Sometimes both lateral lobes also project into the bladder, so that when viewed from within, the sides and back of the internal urinary meatus are surrounded by an intravesical prostatic collar.

Effects of benign prostatic hyperplasia

It is important to realise that the relationship between anatomical prostatic enlargement (BPH), symptoms of prostatism and urodynamic evidence of bladder outflow obstruction (BOO) is complex (Fig. 66.4). Pathophysiologically, bladder outflow obstruction may be caused in part by increased smooth muscle tone which is under the control of α-adrenergic agonists.

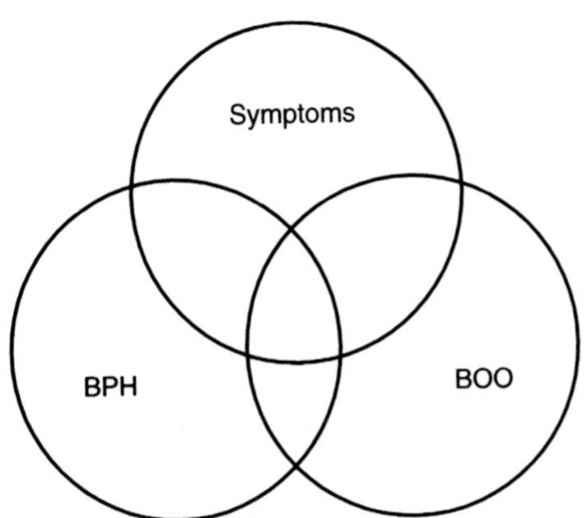

Fig. 66.4 Diagrammatic representation of the relation between symptoms of prostatism, benign prostatic hyperplasia (BPH) and urodynamically proven bladder outflow obstruction (BOO).

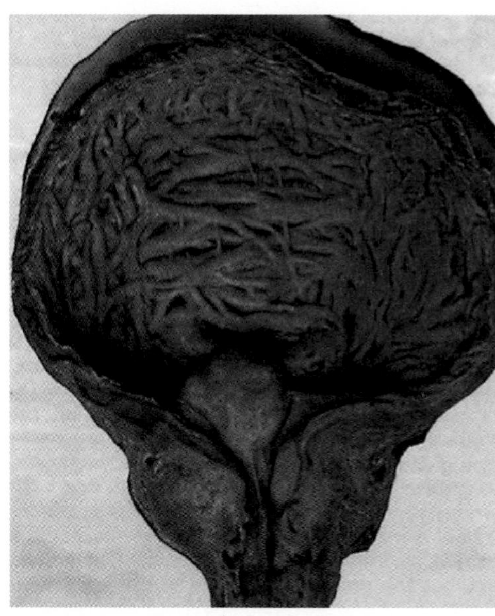

Fig. 66.5 Trabeculation of the bladder from prostatic obstruction. When viewed from within, bands of mucsle fibres can be seen – trabeculation. Between these hypertrophied bundles there are shallow depressions, i.e. sacculations. Sometimes one of the saccules (rarely two or more) continues to enlarge, and forms a diverticulum (*courtesy of the late Professor K.A.L. Aschoff, Freiburg*).

Box 66.3 Consequences of BPH

- No symptoms, no bladder outflow obstruction (BOO)
- No symptoms, but urodynamic evidence of BOO
- Symptoms of prostatism, no evidence of BOO
- Symptoms of prostatism and BOO
- Others (acute/chronic retention, haematuria, urinary infection and stone formation)

Anatomically, the effects are as follows.

Urethra

The prostatic urethra is lengthened, sometimes to twice its normal length, but it is not narrowed anatomically. The normal posterior curve may be so exaggerated that it requires a curved catheter to negotiate it. When only one lateral lobe is enlarged, distortion of the prostatic urethra occurs.

Bladder

If BPH causes bladder outflow obstruction, the musculature of the bladder hypertrophies to overcome the obstruction and appears trabeculated (Fig. 66.5). Significant BPH is associated with increased blood flow and the resultant veins at the base of the bladder are apt to cause haematuria.

Lower urinary tract symptoms or 'prostatism'

In both sexes nonspecific symptoms of bladder dysfunction become more common with ageing, probably owing to impairment of smooth muscle function and neurovesical co-ordination. Not all symptoms of disturbed voiding in ageing men should therefore be attributed to BPH causing BOO. Many urologists prefer the term 'lower urinary tract symptoms' (LUTS).

The following conditions can coexist with BOO, leading to difficulty in diagnosis and in predicting the outcome of treatment:

(a) idiopathic detrusor instability (see Chapter 65);
(b) neuropathic bladder dysfunction as a result of strokes, Alzheimer's disease or Parkinson's disease (see Chapter 65);
(c) degeneration of bladder smooth muscle giving rise to impaired voiding and detrusor instability;
(d) BOO due to BPH.

Symptoms of 'prostatism' or lower urinary tract symptoms (LUTS)	
Obstructive	*Irritative*
Hesitancy (worsened if the bladder is very full)	Frequency
Poor flow (unimproved by straining)	Nocturia
Intermittent stream – stops and starts	Urgency
Dribbling (including after micturition)	Urge incontinence
Sensation of poor bladder emptying	Nocturnal incontinence (enuresis)
Episodes of near retention	

The symptoms of prostatism are now usually assessed by means of scoring systems which give a semiobjective measure of severity. However, some symptoms do not give an accurate picture of the underlying pathophysiological problem. For instance, a man with severe detrusor instability may only void small volumes and hence he will have a sensation of poor flow because low voided volumes (<100 ml) are associated with low flow rates.

Severe irritative symptoms are usually associated with detrusor instability. **Postmicturition dribbling** is now realized **not** to be a consequence of bladder outflow obstruction and is usually not improved by prostatectomy.

Bladder outflow obstruction

This is a urodynamic concept based on the combination of low flow rates in the presence of high voiding pressures. It can be diagnosed definitively only by pressure–flow studies. This is because symptoms are relatively nonspecific and can result from detrusor instability, neurological dysfunction and weak bladder contraction. Even low measured peak flow rates (<10–12 ml/second) are not absolutely diagnostic because in addition to BOO, weak detrusor contractions or low voided volumes (owing to instability) can be the cause.

Alios Alzheimer, 1864–1915. German neurologist.
James Parkinson, 1755–1824. English physician.

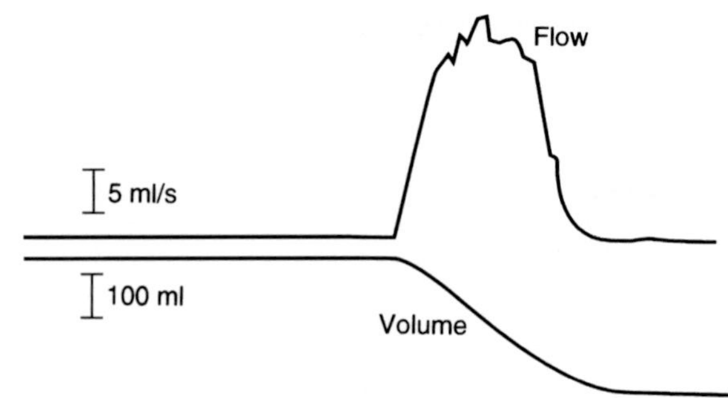

Fig. 66.6 Diagram of a normal flow rate. The voided volume is well in excess of 350 ml and the maximum flow rate is in excess of 25 ml/second.

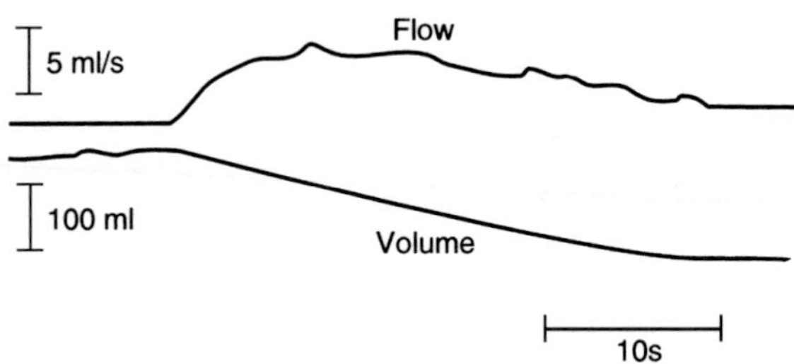

Fig. 66.7 Diagram of a low flow rate showing a rather low voided volume of about 200 ml, but with markedly decreased flow rate. Such a flow rate could be caused by a urethral stricture, bladder outflow obstruction or a weak detrusor.

Urodynamically proven bladder outlet obstruction may result from:
- BPH
- bladder neck stenosis
- bladder neck hypertrophy
- prostate cancer
- urethral strictures
- functional obstruction due to neuropathic conditions

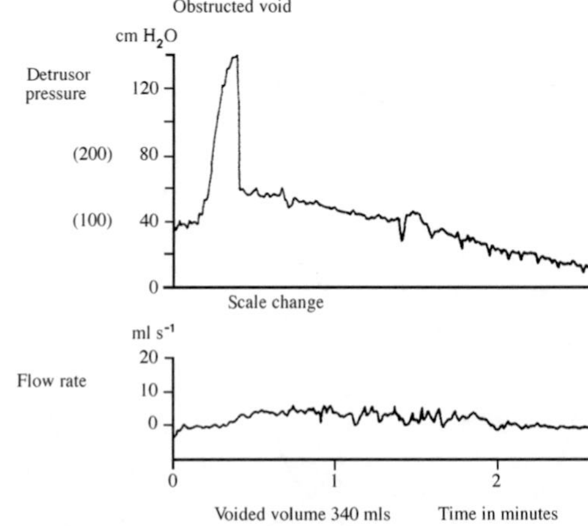

Fig. 66.8 Conventional urodynamic trace showing detrusor pressure during voiding. There has been a change of scale because the pressure was so high; voiding pressures are increased with a low flow rate. This is diagnostic of bladder outflow obstruction.

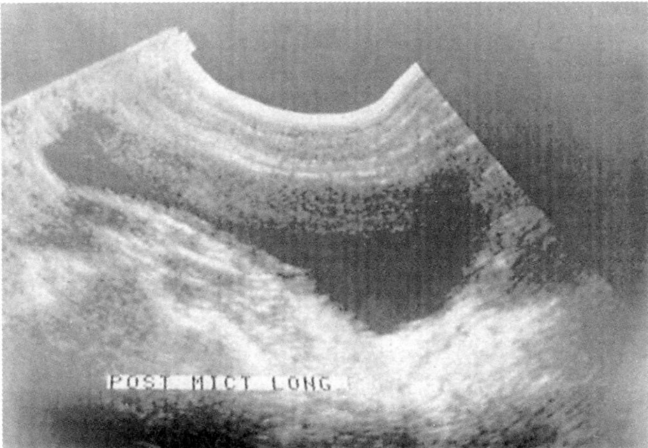

Fig. 66.9 An ultrasonogram showing a large postvoid residual urine.

Primary effects of BOO on the bladder

- Urinary flow rates decrease [for a voided volume >200 ml; a peak flow rate of >15 ml/second is normal (Fig. 66.6), one of 10–15 ml/second equivocal and one <10 ml/second low (Fig. 66.7)]
- Voiding pressures increase [pressures >80 cmH_2O are high (Fig. 66.8), pressures between 60 and 80 cmH_2O are equivocal, pressures <60 cmH_2O are normal]

The long-term effects of bladder outflow obstruction are as follows.

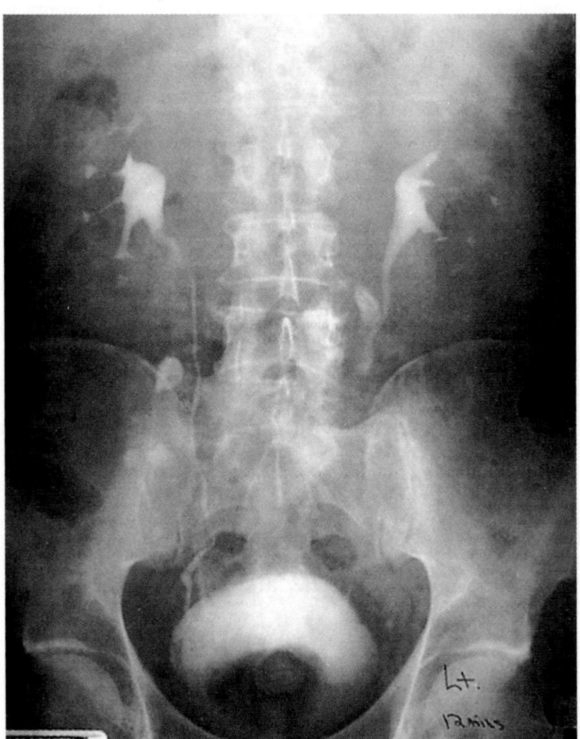

Fig. 66.10 IVU from a patient with symptoms of outflow obstruction and a moderate postmicturition residual urine. The patient did not undergo treatment.

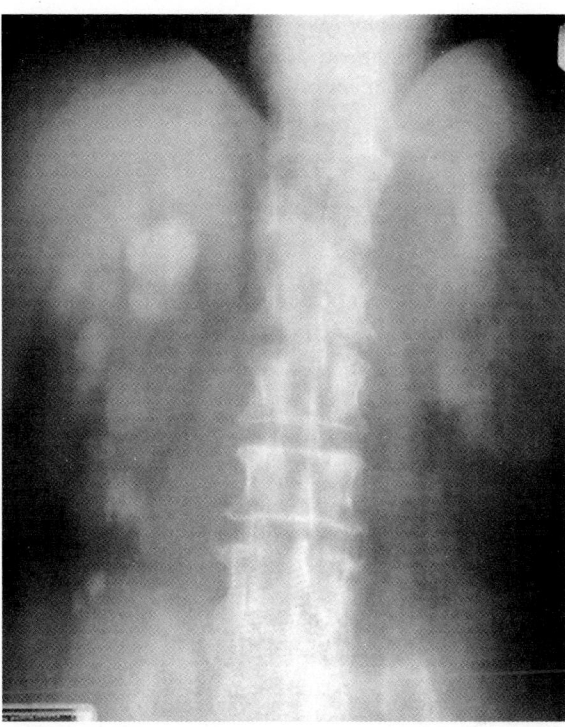

Fig. 66.11 IVU from the same patient as in Fig. 66.10 but carried out some years later. The patient had developed chronic urinary retention and renal impairment owing to upper urinary tract dilatation.

1. The bladder may decompensate so that detrusor contraction becomes progressively less efficient and a **residual urine** develops.
2. The bladder may become more irritable during filling with a decrease in functional capacity partly caused by **detrusor instability** (see Chapter 65) which may also be caused by neurological dysfunction or ageing, or be idiopathic.

Aside from symptoms, the complications of BOO are as follows.

1. *Acute retention of urine* is sometimes the first symptom of BOO. Postponement of micturition is a common precipitating cause; overindulgence in beer, confinement to bed on account of intercurrent illness or operation are other causes.
2. *Chronic retention.* In patients in whom the residual volume is >250 ml or so (Fig. 66.9), the tension in the bladder wall increases owing to the combination of a large volume of residual urine and increased resting and filling bladder pressures (a condition known as **high-pressure chronic retention.** The increased intramural tension results in functional obstruction of the upper urinary tract with the development of bilateral hydronephrosis (Figs 66.10 and 66.11). As a result, upper tract infection and renal impairment may develop. Such men may present with **overflow incontinence, enuresis** and **renal insufficiency.** These symptoms should alert the doctor to the presence of this condition.

3. *Impaired bladder emptying*. If the bladder decompensates with the development of a large volume of **residual urine**, **urinary infection** and **calculi** are prone to develop.
4. *Haematuria*. This may be a complication of BPH. Other causes **must** be excluded by carrying out an IVU, cystoscopy, urine culture and urine cytological examination.
5. *Pain* is not a symptom of BOO and its presence should prompt the exclusion of acute retention, urinary infection, stones, carcinoma of the prostate and carcinoma *in situ* of the bladder.

Assessment of the patient with prostatism

Abdominal examination is usually normal. In patients with chronic retention, a distended bladder will be found on palpation, percussion and sometimes on inspection with loss of the transverse suprapubic skin crease. General physical examination may demonstrate signs of chronic renal impairment with anaemia and dehydration. The external urinary meatus should be examined to exclude stenosis, and the epididymes are palpated for signs of inflammation.

Rectal examination

In benign enlargement, the posterior surface of the prostate is smooth, convex and typically elastic, but the fibrous element may give the prostate a firm consistency. The rectal mucosa can be made to move over the prostate. Residual urine may be felt as a fluctuating swelling above the prostate. It should be noted that if there is a considerable amount of residual urine present, it pushes the prostate downwards, making it appear larger than it is.

The nervous system

The nervous system is examined to eliminate a neurological lesion. Diabetes mellitus, tabes, disseminated sclerosis, cervical spondylosis, Parkinson's disease and other neurological states may mimic prostatic obstruction. If these are suspected then a pressure–flow urodynamic study should be carried out to diagnose BOO. Examination of perianal sensation and anal tone is useful in detection of an S2 to S4 cauda equina lesion.

Serum prostate-specific antigen

The difficulty here is the uncertain benefit of early detection and radical treatment of prostate cancer – this is dealt with in the section on prostate cancer. Certainly men should be informed about the test, the risks of the prostate biopsy that might be required and the risks of the detection of a cancer that we are not certain how best to treat. After suitable counselling, measurement of serum PSA may be helpful. Men in whom a diagnosis of early prostate cancer might influence treatment option – such as those under 60 or those with a positive family history who might be offered radical treatment – should be offered a PSA measurement. If this is in excess of 4 nmol/litre, then transrectal ultrasound scanning (TRUS) plus multiple transrectal biopsies should be considered.

If rectal examination is quite normal with no suspicion of cancer and if no change in treatment policy would result anyway from the diagnosis of early prostate cancer then there seems little point in the routine measurement of PSA in men with uncomplicated BOO.

Flow rate measurement

For this to be meaningful two or three voids should be recorded and the voided volume should be in excess of 150–200 ml. This usually means the patient attending a special flow rate clinic. A typical history and a flow rate <10 ml/second [for a voided volume of >200 ml (Fig. 66.7)] will be sufficient for most urologists to recommend treatment. Usually a flow rate measurement will be coupled with ultrasound measurement of postvoid residual urine.

There are pitfalls in the measurement of flow rates. The machine must be accurately calibrated. The patient must void volumes in excess of 150 ml and two or three recordings are needed to obtain a representative measurement. Decreased flow rates and symptoms of prostatism may be seen in:

- BOO;
- low voided volumes (characteristically in men with detrusor instability);
- men with weak bladder contractions (low pressure–flow voiding).

Pressure–flow urodynamic studies (Fig. 66.8)

Details of these studies are outlined in Chapter 65. They should be performed on the following patients:

- men with suspected neuropathy (Parkinson's disease, dementia, long-standing diabetes, previous strokes, multiple sclerosis)
- men with a dominant history of irritative symptoms and men with life-long urgency and frequency
- men with a doubtful history and those with flow rates in the near-normal range (~ or >15 ml/second)
- men with invalid flow rate measurements (because of low voided volumes)

Blood tests

Serum creatinine, electrolytes and haemoglobin should be measured.

Examination of urine

The urine is examined for glucose and blood, a midstream specimen should be sent for bacteriological examination and cytological examination may be carried out if carcinoma *in situ* is thought possible.

Upper tract imaging

Most urologists no longer carry out imaging of the upper tract in men with straightforward symptoms. Obviously if infection or haematuria is present then the upper tract should be imaged by means of an IVU or USS.

Cystourethroscopy

Inspection of the urethra, the prostate and the urothelium of the bladder should always be done immediately prior to prostatectomy, whether it is being done transurethrally or by the open route to exclude a urethral stricture, a bladder carcinoma and the occasional nonopaque vesical calculus. The decision whether to perform prostatectomy must be made before cystoscopy. This should be based on the patient's symptoms, signs and investigations. Direct inspection of the prostate is a poor indicator of BOO and need for surgery.

Transrectal ultrasound scanning

This increases the rate of detection of associated early prostate cancer but, as pointed out above, unless this would substantially affect treatment there is no need to carry it out routinely. Accurate estimation of prostatic size is possible by means of transrectal or transabdominal ultrasound scanning.

Management of men with benign prostatic hyperplasia or bladder outflow obstruction

Strong indications for treatment (usually prostatectomy) include:

1. *acute retention* (see Chapter 65) in fit men with no other cause for retention (drugs, constipation, recent operation, etc.) (accounts for 25 per cent of prostatectomies);
2. *chronic retention and renal impairment*: a residual urine of 200 ml or more, a raised blood urea, hydroureter or hydronephrosis demonstrated on urography, and uraemic manifestations (accounts for 15 per cent of prostatectomies);
3. *complications of bladder outflow obstruction*: stone, infection and diverticulum formation;
4. *haemorrhage*: occasionally, venous bleeding from a ruptured vein overlying the prostate will require prostatectomy to be performed;
5. *elective prostatectomy for severe symptoms of 'prostatism'*: this accounts for about 60 per cent of prostatectomies. Increasing difficulty in micturition, with considerable frequency day and night, delay in starting, and a poor stream are the usual symptoms for which prostatectomy is advised. *Frequency alone* is **never** an indication for prostatectomy. The natural progression of outflow obstruction is variable and rarely gets worse after 10 years. Severe symptoms, a low maximum flow rate (<10 ml/second) and an increased residual volume of urine (100–250 ml) are relatively strong indications for operative treatment. The exact cut-off for operative or nonoperative treatment will depend on careful discussion between patient and urologist.

Acute retention

The management of retention is discussed in detail in Chapter 65. Once the bladder has been drained by means of a catheter, the patient's fitness for treatment is determined. If retention was not caused by drugs or constipation then prostatectomy would usually be the correct management. Unfit men or those with dementia may be treated by means of indwelling prostatic stents or a catheter. Similar comments apply to men with chronic retention once renal function has been stabilized by catheterization.

Special problems in the management of chronic retention (see Chapter 65 for general management of retention)

Men who do not have symptoms suggestive of coexistent infection and with good renal function do not necessarily require catheterization before proceeding to prostatectomy on the next available list. For those who are uraemic, urgent catheterization is mandatory to allow renal function to recover and stabilize. Haematuria often occurs following catheterization owing to collapse of the distended bladder and upper tract, but settles within a couple of days.

Uraemic patients with chronic retention are often dehydrated at the time of admission. Owing to the chronic back pressure on the distal tubules within the kidney, there is loss of the ability to reabsorb salts and water. The result, following release of this pressure, may be an enormous outflow of salts and water which is known as postobstructive diuresis. It is for this reason that a careful fluid chart, daily measurements of the patient's weight and serial estimations of creatinine and electrolytes are mandatory. Intravenous fluid replacement is required if the patient is unable to keep up with this fluid loss. These patients are often anaemic and may require a blood transfusion once fluid balance is stabilised (if haemoglobin is <9 g/litre).

Indications for elective treatment in men with symptoms of prostatism

Following careful assessment (see section of assessment of men with prostatism), the following questions should be answered.

1. *Is bladder outflow obstruction present?*

   In many cases, the findings of significant symptoms (assessed by symptoms scoring), a benign prostate supplemented by the finding of a low maximum flow rate [<10–12 ml/second for a good voided volume (>200 ml)] will suffice to make a reasonable working diagnosis of BOO. Some men – particularly those with irritative symptoms, suspected neurological disease or those with technically imperfect flow rate measurements – will require pressure–flow studies to be performed.

2. *How severe are the symptoms and what are the risks of doing nothing?*

   Severe symptoms and a large residual volume of urine will usually require treatment. Men with mild symptoms, good flow rates (>10 ml/second) and good bladder emptying (residual urine <100 ml) may be safely managed by reassurance and review: such patients rarely develop severe complications such as retention in the long term.
3. *Is the man fit for operative treatment?*
4. *What treatments are available, what are the outcomes and do the side effects justify treatment?*

In men who do not have a strong indication for operative treatment the options for treatment are shown below.

> Nonoperative treatment for BPH
>
> - Conservative 'watchful waiting' – general advice about fluid intake, use of anticholinergic medication in men with mild symptoms
> - Use of prostatic stents in men with retention who are unfit or have dementia
> - Balloon dilatation of the prostate (experimental)
> - Drug treatment to supplement conservative treatment in men with mild symptoms (α-adrenergic blocking agents and 5α-reductase inhibitors)
> - Use of permanent indwelling catheters in unfit men with retention or associated dementia

Minimally invasive methods

These are new and their roles are not yet determined:

- contact laser of the prostate;
- microwave treatment of the prostate (thermotherapy);
- other new minimally invasive methods of prostate destruction including microwave hyperthermia and thermal ablation and high-energy ultrasound.

Conventional operative treatment

This includes:

- transurethral resection of the prostate (TURP);
- bladder neck incision for the small prostate (<20 g);
- open prostatectomy for the big gland (>~80–100 g).

Men with symptoms attending for elective treatment (excluding acute and chronic retention)

Conservative treatment

It is in men with relatively mild symptoms, reasonable flow rates (>10 ml/second) and good bladder emptying (residual urine <100 ml) that careful discussion over the merits and side effects of operative treatment is warranted. Waiting for a period of 6 months after careful discussion of the diagnosis is indicated. After this a repeat assessment of symptoms, flow rates and ultrasound scan is helpful; many men with stable symptoms will elect to leave matters be. Advice over limiting fluid intake in the evening and careful use of propantheline to help with irritative symptoms is also useful.

Drugs

In men who are very concerned about the development of sexual dysfunction after TURP, the use of drugs may be helpful. Two classes of drugs have been used in the treatment of men with BOO. These include α-adrenergic blocking agents which inhibit the contraction of smooth muscle which is found in the prostate. The other class of drug is the 5α-reductase inhibitors, which inhibit the conversion of testosterone to DHT, the androgen which is effective. These drugs, when taken for a year, result in a 25 per cent shrinkage of the prostate gland. On average, both drugs seem to be of similar efficacy, and although the 5α-reductase inhibitors have fewer side effects, α-blockers work more quickly. They result in improvements in maximum flow rates by about 2 ml/second greater than placebo and result in mild (20 per cent) improvement in symptom scores. TURP, however, results in improvements in maximum flow rates from 9 to 18 ml/second and 75 per cent improvements in symptom scores. These drugs are expensive in comparison to their effectiveness and a significant proportion of men who try these drugs will subsequently undergo TURP. Their role may be best targeted on men who have failed an initial trial of watchful waiting and who wish to avoid surgery for a period.

Operative treatment

Apart from the strong indications for operative treatment mentioned above, the commonest reason for TURP is a combination of severe symptoms and a low flow rate <12 ml/second. The key is to assess symptoms carefully and to counsel men about side effects and likely outcome before advising operative treatment.

Counselling men undergoing prostatectomy

Men undergoing prostatectomy need to be advised about the following.

1. *Retrograde ejaculation* occurs in about 65 per cent of men after prostatectomy.
2. *Erectile impotence* occurs in about 5 per cent of men, usually in those whose virility is waning.
3. *The success rate* – on the whole men with acute and chronic retention do well from the symptomatic point of view. Ninety per cent of men undergoing elective operation for severe symptoms and urodynamically proven BOO do well in terms of symptoms and flow rates. Only about 65 per cent of those with mild symptoms or those with weak bladder contraction as the cause of their symptoms do well. Men with unobstructed detrusor instability do not respond well to TURP. This is the reason for

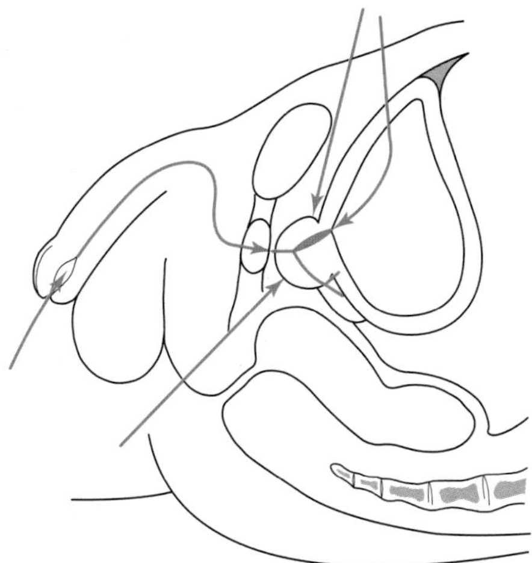

Fig. 66.12 The surgical approaches to the prostate.

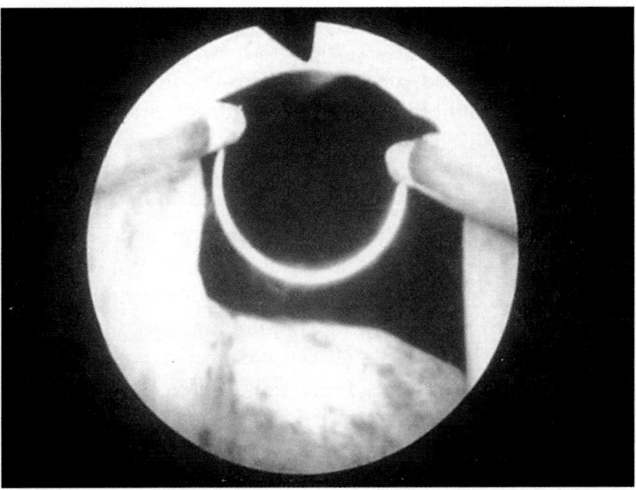

Fig. 66.13 Endoscopic photograph of transurethral prostatectomy.

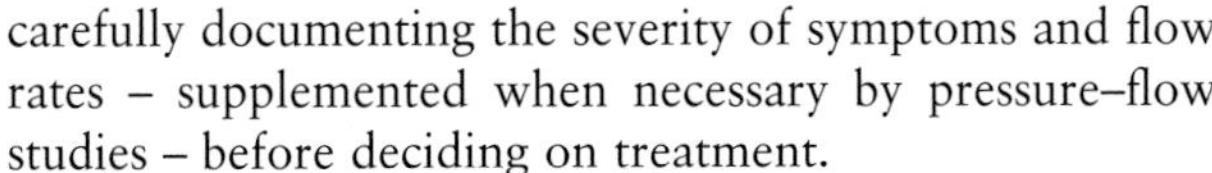

carefully documenting the severity of symptoms and flow rates – supplemented when necessary by pressure–flow studies – before deciding on treatment.

4. *The risk of reoperation* after TURP is about 15 per cent after 8–10 years.
5. **The morbidity rate**: death after TURP is infrequent (<0.5 per cent), severe sepsis is found in about 6 per cent and severe haematuria requiring transfusion >2 units is found in about 3 per cent. After discharge about 15–20 per cent of men subsequently require antibiotic treatment for symptoms of urinary infection. Risk factors for complications include admission with retention, prostate cancer, renal impairment and advanced age.

Methods of performing prostatectomy

The prostate can be approached (1) transurethrally – TURP, (2) retropubically – RPP, (3) through the bladder (transvesical – TVP) or (4) from the perineum (Fig. 66.12). *Preliminary vasectomy* is now no longer performed.

Transurethral resection of the prostate

TURP has largely replaced other methods unless diverticulectomy or the removal of large stones necessitates open operation; over 95 per cent of men being treated by trained urologists can be dealt with by TURP. The earlier instruments designed by McCarthy have been replaced by single-hand-operated instruments often being used under video control. Perhaps the greatest advance in the history of transurethral surgery was marked by the development of the rigid lens system of Professor Harold Hopkins. His lenses illuminated by a fibre-optic light source permit unparalleled visualisation of the working field. Men with indwelling catheters, those with recent urinary infection, those with chronic retention or those with prosthetic material or heart valves should receive broad-spectrum prophylactic antibiotics with amoxycillin plus cefuroxime intravenously at induction of anaesthesia.

Strips of tissue are cut from the bladder neck down to the level of the verumontanum (Fig. 66.13). Cutting is performed by a high-frequency diathermy current which is applied across a loop mounted on the hand-held trigger of the resectoscope. Coagulation of bleeding points can be accurately achieved and damage to the external sphincter is avoided provided one uses the verumontanum as a guide to the most distal point of the resection. The 'chips' of prostate are then removed from the bladder using an Ellik evacuator. Hyponatraemia is avoided by using 1.5 per cent isotonic glycine for irrigation and the recent introduction of continuous flow resectoscopes makes the procedure swift and safe in experienced hands. At the end of the procedure, careful haemostasis is performed and a three-way, self-retaining catheter irrigated with isotonic saline is introduced into the bladder to prevent any further bleeding from forming blood clots. Irrigation is continued until the outflow is pale pink and the catheter usually removed on the second or third post-operative day. In men with small prostates or bladder neck dyssynergia or stenosis, it is better to divide the bladder neck and prostatic urethra with a diathermy 'bee-sting' electrode.

Retropubic prostatectomy (Millin, 1945)

Using a low, curved transverse suprapubic Pfannenstiel incision, which includes the rectus sheath, the recti are split in the midline and retracted to expose the bladder with its typical appearance of pale brown muscle bundles with a loose covering of fatty tissue and veins. With the patient in the

McCarthy. American urologist who developed the endoscopic rectoscope.
Harold Hopkins. British physicist, University of Reading, who developed fibre-optic systems.

Terence Millin. Irish urologist who worked in London, England. Proposed retropubic prostatectomy in 1945.
Hermann Johann Pfannenstiel, 1862–1909. Gynaecologist, Breslau, Germany.

Trendelenberg position, the surgeon separates the bladder and the prostate from the posterior aspect of the pubis. In the space thus obtained the anterior capsule of the prostate is incised with diathermy below the bladder neck, care being taken to obtain complete control of bleeding from divided prostatic veins by suture ligation. The prostatic adenoma is exposed and enucleated with a finger. A wedge is taken out of the posterior lip of the bladder neck to prevent secondary stricture in this region. The exposure of the inside of the prostatic cavity is good, and control of haemorrhage is achieved with diathermy and suture ligation of bleeding points before closure of the capsule over a Foley catheter (inserted per urethram) draining the bladder.

Transvesical prostatectomy

The bladder is opened, and the prostate enucleated by putting a finger into the urethra, pushing forwards towards the pubes to separate the lateral lobes, and then working the finger between the adenoma and the false capsule. In Freyer's operation (1901) the bladder was left open widely and drained by a suprapubic tube with a 16-mm lumen, in order to allow free drainage of blood and urine. Harris (1934) advocated control of the prostatic arteries by lateral stitches inserted with his boomerang needle, the bladder wall was closed and the wound drained.

Perineal prostatectomy (Young)

This has now been abandoned for the treatment of BPH.

After-treatment

Most urologists irrigate the bladder with sterile saline by means of a three-way Foley catheter for 24 hours or so.

Complications

Local

Haemorrhage is a major risk following prostatectomy whatever the surgical approach. Care should be taken in diathermising arterial bleeding points after TURP; they are often better seen when the rate of inflow of fluid is decreased. In the recovery room one should check that the bladder is adequately draining, if it is not this may indicate that a clot is blocking the eye of the catheter. The bladder should be promptly washed out using strict aseptic technique. The catheter should be changed by the surgeon. Only rarely is it necessary to return the patient to the operating room.

Secondary haemorrhage tends to occur after the patient has been discharged. All men should be warned about this possibility and given appropriate advice to rest and to have a high fluid intake. It is usually minor in degree, but if clot retention occurs, the patient will need to be readmitted, a catheter will have to be passed and the bladder washed out.

Perforation of the bladder or the prostatic capsule can occur at the time of transurethral surgery. This usually occurs from a combination of inexperience in association with a large prostate or heavy blood loss. If the field of vision becomes obscured by heavy blood loss, it is often prudent to achieve adequate haemostasis and abandon the operation, swallowing one's pride on the understanding that a second attempt may be necessary. A large perforation with marked extravasation may require the insertion of a small suprapubic drain. Rectal perforation should be extremely rare.

Sepsis. Bacteraemia is common even in men with sterile urine and occurs in over 50 per cent of men with infected urine, prolonged catheterisation or chronic retention. Septicaemia can occur in these patients shortly after operation or when the catheter is removed. In men at high risk the use of prophylactic antibiotics is recommended. Wound infection following open prostatectomy is common if a urethral catheter has been *in situ* for a number of days before the operation. Perhaps the most worrying aspect of infection is the early rigor following surgery. If left undetected and untreated this may progress to frank septicaemia with profound hypotension. A blood culture should be taken and antibiotics given parenterally, e.g. amoxycillin plus cefuroxime.

Incontinence. Incontinence is inevitable if the external sphincter mechanism is damaged. The bladder neck is rendered incompetent by these operations and therefore an intact distal sphincter mechanism is essential for continence. Damage to the sphincter may occur at open prostatectomy and following transurethral surgery if the resection extends beyond the verumontanum. If pelvic floor physiotherapy is ineffective, then the only satisfactory treatment is the fitting of an artificial urinary sphincter. In some patients, detrusor instability contributes to the incontinence. The use of anticholinergic agents or imipramine may help.

Retrograde ejaculation and impotence – see previous section.

Urethral stricture. This may be secondary to prolonged catheterisation, the use of an unnecessarily large catheter, clumsy instrumentation or to the presence of the resectoscope in the urethra for too long a period. These strictures arise either just inside the meatus or in the bulbar urethra. An early stricture can usually be managed by simple bouginage but later on it may be necessary to cut the densely fibrotic stricture with the optical urethrotome. The routine use of an Otis urethrotomy prior to TURP reduces the incidence of postoperative stricture.

Friedrich Trendelenberg, 1844–1945. Professor of Surgery, Leipzig, Germany.

Frederic E.B. Foley, 1891–1966. American urologist, Ankher Hospitals, St Paul, USA.

Sir Peter Johnston Freyer, b. 1851. London surgeon of Irish extraction. He claimed priority in having originated the transvesical prostatectomy method in 1900.

Samuel Henry Harris, b. 1880. Australian surgeon.

Bladder neck contracture. Occasionally a dense fibrotic stenosis of the bladder neck occurs following overaggressive resection of a small prostate. It may be due to the overuse of the coagulating diathermy. Transurethral **incision** of the scar tissue is necessary.

Reoperation

It is now known that after 8 years, 15–18 per cent of men with BPH will undergo repeat TURP (the rate after open prostatectomy is about 5 per cent). The reasons include a technically imperfect primary procedure and a speculative repeat operation in men with symptoms who are cystoscoped after operation.

General complications

Death occurs in about 0.2–0.3 per cent of men undergoing elective prostatectomy. In very elderly men, in men with prostate cancer admitted as an emergency with acute or chronic retention, or those with very large prostates the 30-day death rate may be in the order of 1–1.5 per cent.

Cardiovascular. Pulmonary atelectasis, pneumonia, myocardial infarction, congestive cardiac failure and deep venous thrombosis are all potentially life-threatening conditions that can affect this elderly and often frail group of men.

Water intoxication. The absorption of water into the circulation at the time of transurethral resection can give rise to congestive cardiac failure, hyponatraemia and haemolysis. Accompanying this there is frequently confusion and other cerebral events often mimicking a stroke. The incidence of this condition has been reduced since the introduction of isotonic glycine for performing the resections and the use of isotonic saline for postoperative irrigation. The treatment consists of fluid restriction.

Osteitis pubis is rare.

Newer treatments

In general, newer, minimally invasive treatments occupy a position intermediate between TURP and drug treatment. As yet, there are no long-term data on duration of effectiveness.

Microwave and laser treatments and other methods of tissue destruction

Microwave treatment aims at providing an external source of microwaves which are then focused within the prostate gland. The source may be within the rectum or the urethra, although recent machines use the intraurethral route. With the first-generation machines, the prostate heats to between 40°C and 45°C (hyperthermia). There is very minimal tissue destruction and there is no rise in serum PSA, confirming that little of the prostate is damaged. Although there may be symptom improvement, there are no improvements in voiding pressures. The next generation of microwave machines is able to provide an increased source of energy which destroys some of the prostate (thermtherapy – temperature >50°C). The outcome appears to be better than hyperthermia.

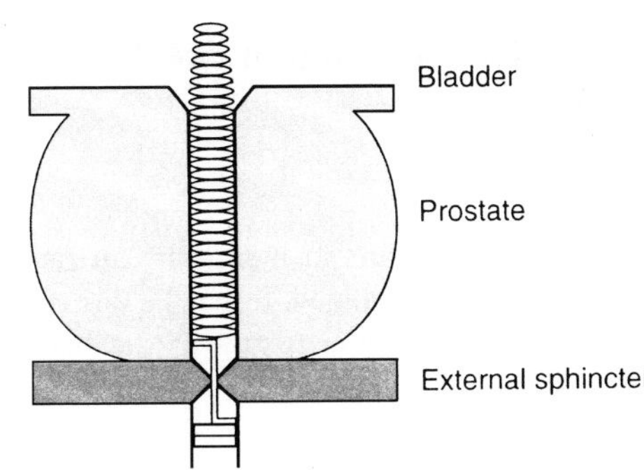

Fig. 66.14 Diagram showing one type of prostatic stent *in situ*.

Laser treatments can be of several types. In one a noncontact probe is used to vaporize prostatic tissue under direct vision. There is no bleeding and this treatment can be used to carry out bladder neck incisions in men with small prostate glands as day-case treatment and a catheter may not be necessary. Hence this treatment would be potentially cost-effective in this setting. The cost of the probes at present, however, is £500, which would balance out any cost saving in terms of hospital stay. These probes are not useful in the treatment of men with large glands as the treatment would take too long.

Another type of laser is a contact side-firing laser of lower energy but greater penetration. This energy results in necrosis of the prostate gland to a varying thickness. The energy can by applied transurethrally under direct vision or transurethrally under the control of ultrasound. The potential advantage of the latter technique is that it means that greater energy can be applied to thicker areas of BPH, ensuring a more complete treatment. A suprapubic catheter is inserted for several weeks whilst the necrotic prostate sloughs – significant symptoms can occur during this period. There is little or no bleeding and the treatment can be given as a short-stay procedure or day-case procedure. Laser treatment, however, requires a general anaesthetic. The cost of the probes is about £400. A laser can be purchased for about £45 000.

The outcome of contact laser treatment appears to be better than microwave hyperthermia, with improvement in flow rates from 9 to about 14 ml/second and improvement in symptom score by about 50 per cent. It is as yet unclear how effective it is in comparison to TURP in terms of cost-effectiveness, symptomatic and urodynamic outcome. Other types of laser treatment include interstitial laser therapy, which involves the insertion of laser probes into the substance of the prostate, and Holmium laser treatment. The latter approach involves excision of parts of the prostate using a cutting laser and then morcellating the excised prostate fragments which fall back into the bladder so that they can be removed.

There are newer methods of treatment becoming available including focused high-frequency ultrasound and direct treatment of the prostate with needles providing high-energy electromagnetic treatment. The outcome of these treatments is unknown.

Intraurethral stents (Fig. 66.14)

These devices are helpful in the management of men with retention and who are grossly unfit (classified by the American Society of Anesthesiologists as ASA grade IV or V). These men are rare cases.

Bladder outflow obstruction due to the bladder neck

Aetiology

This condition usually occurs in men, but can rarely affect children of both sexes and women. It may be due to muscular hypertrophy, or fibrosis of the tissues at the bladder neck following TURP.

Clinical syndromes

1. *Due to muscle hypertrophy or dyssynergia.* Marion described a series of cases in which muscular hypertrophy of the internal sphincter in a young person had resulted in the development of a vesical diverticulum or hydronephrosis (Marion's disease or *prostatism sans prostate*). It is thought that dyssynergic contraction of the smooth muscle of the bladder neck (bladder neck dyssynergia) may account for some cases of bladder outflow obstruction.
2. *Due to fibrosis.* The symptoms are similar to those of prostatic enlargement, but are a consequence of scarring after TURP.

Treatment

The management of these patients depends on achieving an accurate diagnosis. For this, urodynamic investigation is often necessary, which should demonstrate raised voiding pressures and diminished flow rate.

Drugs

The presence of α-adrenergic receptors in the region of the bladder neck and prostatic urethra allows pharmacological manipulation of the outflow to the bladder. Alpha-blocking drugs: alfuzosin – 2.5 mg b.d. to t.d.s. (to a total maximum of 10 mg/day); doxazosin – 1 mg nocte (up to maximum of 8 mg/day); indoramin – 20 mg b.d. (increased to total maximum of 100 mg/day in divided doses); prazosin 500 mg b.d. (maintenance up to 2 mg/day); and terazosin 1 mg nocte (to a total maximum of 10 mg/day) can be very useful, causing relaxation of the bladder neck. These drugs are not target specific and the patients must be warned of the possibility of possible postural hypotension.

Transurethral incision

Transurethral incision of the bladder neck is the operation of choice. Sometimes symptoms recur, but this is usually due to inadequate division of the fibres of the bladder neck.

Congenital valves of the prostatic urethra

See Chapter 60.

Georges Marion, 1869–1932. French urologist.

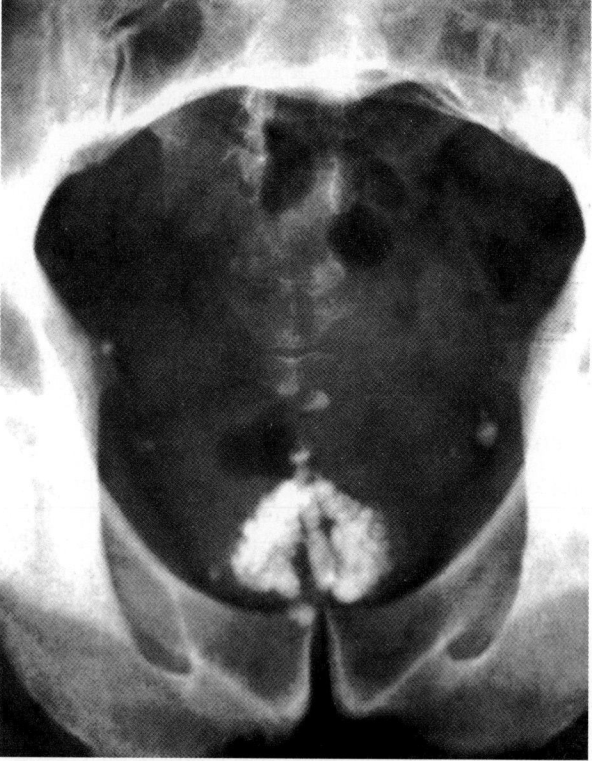

Fig. 66.15 Endogenous prostatic calculi.

Prostatic calculi

Prostatic calculi are of two varieties: endogenous, which are common, and exogenous, which are comparatively rare.

An exogenous prostatic calculus is a urinary (commonly ureteric) calculus that becomes arrested in the prostatic urethra. This is considered in Chapter 60.

Endogenous prostatic calculi are usually composed of calcium phosphate combined with about 20 per cent of organic material.

Clinical features

Prostatic calculi are usually symptomless, being discovered on TRUS, radiography of the pelvis, during prostatectomy, or associated with carcinoma of the prostate or chronic prostatitis. In cases associated with severe chronic prostatic infection, the associated fibrosis and nodularity are difficult to differentiate from carcinoma. On X-ray or ultrasound scanning, these stones often form a horseshoe (Fig. 66.15) or a circle.

Treatment of prostatic calculi

They usually require no treatment.

Conservative measures

Associated chronic prostatic infection may be treated by means of ciprofloxacin or trimethoprim.

Transurethral resection

Transurethral resection will often release small calculi as the strips of prostatic tissue are excised. Others are passed *per urethram* at a later date.

Corpora amylaceae

Corpora amylaceae are tiny calcified lamellated bodies found in the glandular alveoli of the prostates of elderly men and apes, but not in the prostates of animals lower in the phylogenetic scale than anthropoids. Corpora amylaceae are probably the forerunners of endogenous prostatic calculi.

Carcinoma of the prostate

Carcinoma of the prostate is the commonest malignant tumour in men over the age of 65 years. In England and Wales in 1998 11 000 men were registered and 8000 died from it; the corresponding figures in the USA were 130 000 and 25 000, respectively. If histological section of prostates at autopsy is performed increasingly frequent foci of microscopic prostate cancers are found with increasing age. These foci of prostate cancer have variable potential for progressing clinically to metastatic disease. About 10–15 per cent of younger men who develop prostate cancer have a positive family history of the disease, but the aetiology is unclear. Throughout the world, rates of microscopic foci of prostate cancer are constant, but rates of clinically evident disease are low in men in Japan and China. Carcinoma of the prostate usually originates in the peripheral zone of the prostate (Fig. 66.2), so 'prostatectomy' for benign enlargement of the gland confers no protection from subsequent carcinoma.

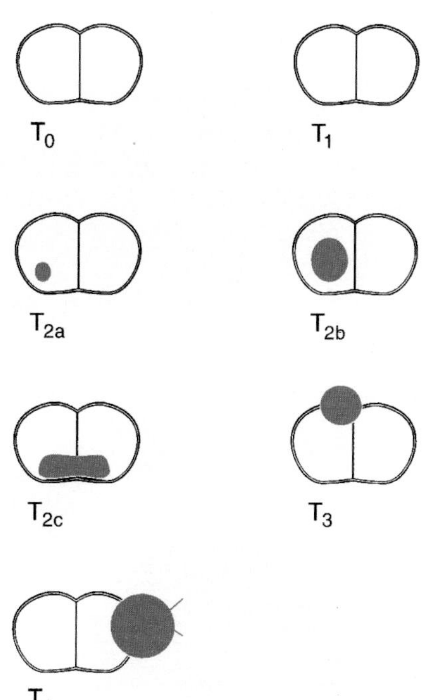

Fig. 66.16 Schematic representation of the present TNM system.

Types of prostate cancer

Latent carcinoma of the prostate

Serial sections of prostates obtained at routine necropsy demonstrate prostate carcinoma in 15–20 per cent of men between 50 and 65 years of age. The incidence in men over 80 is in the region of 50 per cent (Franks). Most of these neoplasms are tiny and (if life had continued) might have remained latent for years.

Types of prostate cancer

- Microscopic latent cancer found on autopsy or at cystoprostatectomy
- Tumours found incidentally during TURP (T1a and T1b); or following screening by PSA measurement – T1c
- Early, localised prostate cancer (T2)
- Advanced local prostate cancer (T3 and T4)
- Metastatic disease which may arise from a clinically evident tumour (T2, T3 or T4) or which may arise from an apparently benign gland (T0, T1), i.e. occult prostate cancer

It should be noted that only the last two groups cause symptoms and such tumours are not curable. Only screening or the treatment of incidentally found tumours can result in cure of the disease. The problem is that many such tumours would never progress during the patient's lifetime – herein lies the problem with prostate cancer.

Histological appearances

The prostate is a glandular structure consisting of ducts and acini; therefore the histological pattern is one of an adenocarcinoma. The prostatic glands are surrounded by a layer of myoepithelial cells. The first change associated with carcinoma is the loss of the basement membrane with glands appearing to be in confluence. As the cell type becomes less differentiated more solid sheets of carcinoma cells are seen. A classification of the histological pattern based on the degree of glandular de-differentiation and its relation to stroma has been devised by Gleason; this (and the volume of the cancer) appears to correlate well with the likelihood of spread and of prognosis.

Local spread

Locally advanced tumours tend to grow upwards to involve the seminal vesicles, the bladder neck, trigone and, later, the tumours tend to spread distally to involve the distal sphincter mechanism. Further upward extension obstructs the lower end of one or both ureters, the latter terminating in anuria. The rectum may become stenosed by tumour infiltrating around it, but direct involvement is rare.

Spread by the bloodstream

Spread by the bloodstream occurs particularly to bone; indeed the prostate is the most common site of origin

Gleason. American urologist.

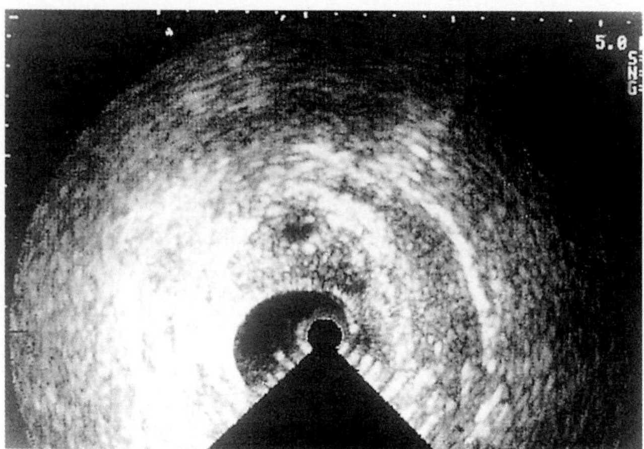

Fig. 66.17 Transrectal ultrasound scan of a T2 nodule in the prostate.

for skeletal metastases, being followed in turn by the breast, the kidney, the bronchus and the thyroid gland. The bones involved most frequently by carcinoma of the prostate are the pelvic bones and the lower lumbar vertebrae. The femoral head, rib cage and skull are other common sites.

Lymphatic spread

Lymphatic spread may occur (1) via lymphatic vessels passing to the obturator fossa or along the sides of the rectum to the lymph nodes beside the internal iliac vein and in the hollow of the sacrum and (2) via lymphatics which pass over the seminal vesicles and follow the vas deferens for a short distance to drain into the external iliac lymph nodes. From retroperitoneal lymph nodes, the mediastinal nodes and occasionally the supraclavicular nodes may become implicated.

Staging using the tumour, node, metastasis (TNM) system (Fig. 66.16)

1. *T1a, T1b and T1c*: these are incidentally found tumours in a clinically benign gland after histological examination of a prostatectomy specimen. T1a is a well or moderately well-differentiated tumour involving less than 5 per cent of the resected specimen. T1b is a poorly differentiated tumour or a tumour involving >5 per cent of the resected specimen. T1c tumours are impalpable tumours found following PSA screening
2. *T2a* disease presents as a suspicious nodule (Fig. 66.17) on rectal examination of <2 cm
   T2b disease is a nodule involving greater than 2 cm
   T2c is tumour in both lobes but still clinically confined
3. *T3* is a tumour involving the seminal vesicles or bladder neck
4. *T4* is a tumour involving the rectum or pelvic side wall

Clinical features

Only advanced cases give rise to symptoms, but even advanced cases may be asymptomatic. Symptoms of advanced disease include:

- BOO;
- pelvic pain and haematuria;

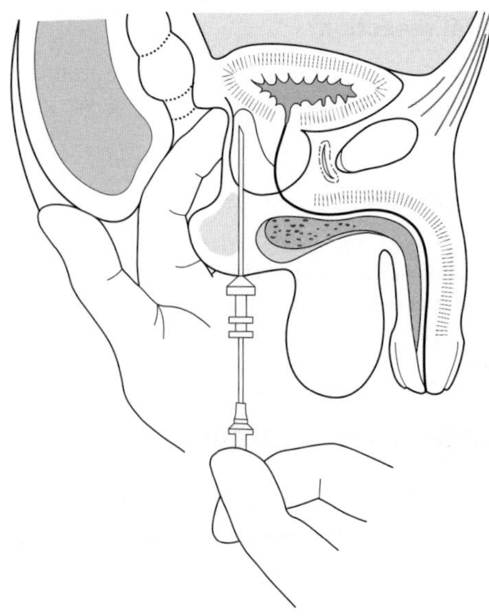

Fig. 66.18 Obtaining a specimen of prostatic tissue by means of Turkel's needle.

- bone pain, malaise, 'arthritis', anaemia or pancytopaenia;
- renal failure;
- locally advanced disease or even asymptomatic metastases may be found incidentally on investigation of other symptoms.

Early prostate cancer is asymptomatic and it may be found:

- incidentally following TURP for clinically benign disease (T1);
- as a nodule (T2) on rectal examination.

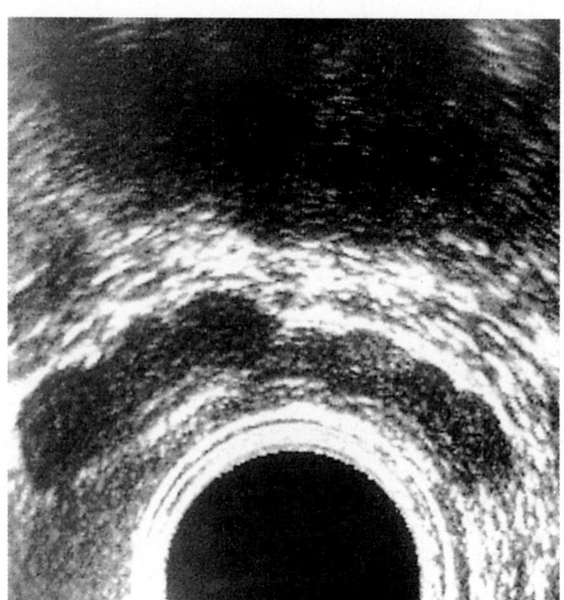

Fig. 66.19 Transrectal ultrasound scan showing normal seminal vesicles.

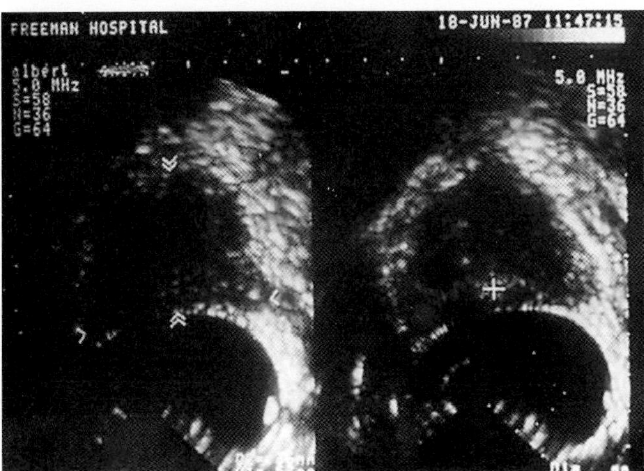

Fig. 66.20 Transrectal ultrasound scan showing local extension of a T3 prostate cancer.

Rectal examination

Examination under anaesthesia together with cystoscopy and needle biopsy (Fig. 66.18) or TRUS may be used to assess the local stage. Irregular induration, characteristically stony hard in part or in the whole of the gland – with obliteration of the median sulcus – suggests carcinoma. Extension beyond the capsule up into the bladder base and vesicles (Fig. 66.19) is diagnostic, as is deformity and projection outwards of the capsule (Fig. 66.20).

General blood tests

These are normal in early disease, but in metastatic disease there may be leucoerythroblastic anaemia secondary to extensive marrow invasion or anaemia may be secondary to renal failure. There may be thrombocytopenia and evidence of disseminated intravascular coagulopathy with increased fibrinogen degradation products (FDPs).

Liver function tests

These will be abnormal if there is extensive metastatic invasion of the liver. The alkaline phosphatase may be raised from either hepatic involvement or secondaries in the bone. These can be distinguished by measurement of isoenzymes or gamma-glutamyl transferase.

Prostate-specific antigen

This is discussed earlier in this chapter. It is good at following the course of advanced disease. It is lacking in sensitivity and specificity in the diagnosis of early localised prostate cancer. Nevertheless, the finding of a PSA >10 nmol/ml is suggestive of cancer and >35 ng/ml is diagnostic of advanced prostate cancer. A decrease of PSA to the normal range following hormonal ablation is a good prognostic sign.

Acid phosphatase

Acid phosphatase has been superseded by measurement of PSA.

Radiological examination

X-ray of the chest may reveal metastases either in the lung fields or the ribs. An abdominal X-ray may show the char-

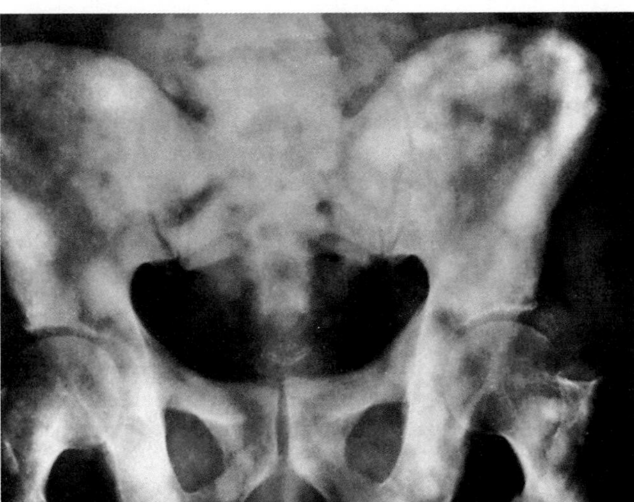

Fig. 66.21 Osseous metatases of the pelvic bones in carcinoma of the prostate (*courtesy of L.N. Pyrah, Leeds*).

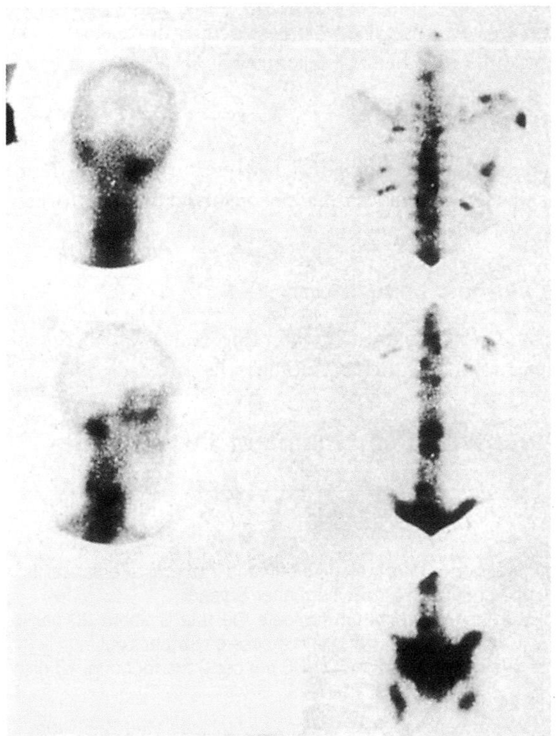

Fig. 66.22 Bone scan showing multiple hot spots suggestive of metastatic disease in a man with prostate cancer.

acteristic sclerotic metastases in lumbar vertebrae and pelvic bones (Fig. 66.21). The bone appears dense and coarse and sometimes difficulty is found distinguishing the change from that in Paget's disease of bone. Osteolytic metastases nevertheless are very common in prostate cancer and may coexist with sclerotic ones. Information about the upper urinary tracts can be obtained by excretion urography or ultrasound.

Ultrasonography

TRUS remains the most accurate method of staging the local disease. It can be used in the early detection of tumours in screening programmes. Local (T2) disease can be diagnosed with increased sensitivity by TRUS (Fig. 66.17) compared with rectal examination, but nevertheless many tumours will be missed. This problem remains a real one in screening for early prostate cancer; in comparison with breast cancer where mammography will detect 70–80 per cent of tumours, TRUS plus rectal examination and measurement of PSA will detect only 30–50 per cent of cancers that are known to be present on autopsy studies (although it may detect the larger, more significant cancers).

Bone scan

Once the diagnosis has been established, it would be normal to perform a bone scan as part of the staging procedure if the PSA is >20 nmol/ml. If the PSA is <20 nmol/ml then a bone scan would only be performed on clinical indications. The bone scan is performed by the injection of technetium-99m, which is then monitored using a gamma camera. It is more sensitive in the diagnosis of metastases (Fig. 66.22) than a skeletal survey, but false positives occur in areas of arthritis, osteomyelitis or a healing fracture.

Lymphangiography

This is no longer carried out. If accurate information is required then pelvic lymphadenectomy can be performed by means of laparoscopic surgery.

Bone marrow aspiration

Sometimes examination of the bone marrow will reveal the presence of metastatic carcinoma cells.

Treatment of carcinoma of the prostate

Natural history of prostate cancer

T1 and T2
The progression rate of well-differentiated T1a prostate cancer is very low, being about 10–14 per cent after 8 years
For moderately differentiated tumours the rate is about 20 per cent, but for T1b tumours the rate is in excess of 35 per cent
Similar rates of progression (20–30 per cent) are found for T2 disease

T3 and T4 (MO)
About 50 per cent progress to bony metastases after 3–5 years

M1
The median survival of men with metastatic disease is about 3 years

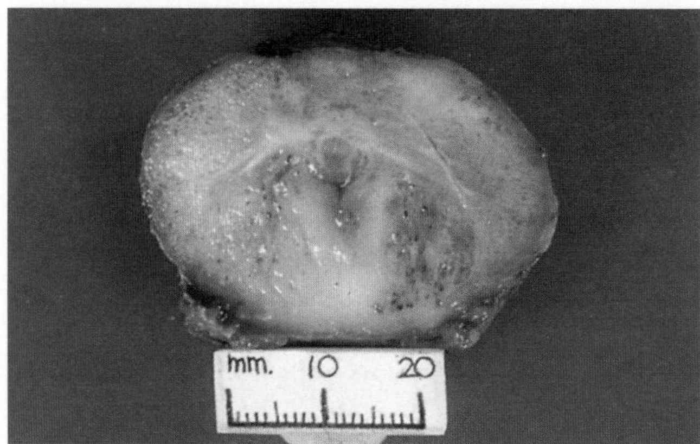

Fig. 66.23 Radical prostatectomy specimen for a T2a prostate cancer. Preoperative PSA was 6 nmol/litre; postoperative levels remained undetectable at 8 years. The patient is fully continent.

Prostatic biopsy

If there is suspicion of prostate cancer, because of either local findings, a raised PSA or metastatic disease, then a transrectal biopsy using an automated gun with appropriate antibiotic cover is indicated. Several cores may be needed to make a diagnosis. The incidence of sepsis from transrectal biopsy increases if more than three biopsies are taken. If there are associated symptoms of BOO then either:

- a TURP can be performed which will provide diagnostic material and symptomatic relief;
- transrectal biopsy can be carried out. If the diagnosis is positive and there is locally advanced disease, then hormone ablation can provide good symptomatic relief without the need for operation.

Early disease

Curative treatment can only be offered to patients with early disease (T1a, T1b, T1c and T2). The treatment of patients with advanced disease (T3, T4 or any M0) is only palliative.

Radical prostatectomy

Radical prostatectomy is only suitable for localised disease (T1 and T2) and should only be carried out in men with a life expectancy of >10 years. Exclusion of metastases would require a negative bone scan, chest X-ray and a serum PSA <20 nmol/ml. It is a major surgical procedure and should only be performed by experienced surgeons when there is a high chance of cure. It results in a high incidence of impotence, but a low incidence of severe stress incontinence (<5 per cent) which may require the fitting of an artificial urinary sphincter. It involves removal of the prostate down to the distal sphincter mechanism in addition to the seminal vesicles (Fig. 66.23). The bladder neck is reconstituted and anasto-

Sir James Paget, 1814–99. Surgeon, St Bartholomew's Hospital, London, England.

mosed to the urethra. Recent modifications to this operation by Professor Patrick Walsh of the Johns Hopkins Hospital in Baltimore have led to the realisation that careful dissection in early stage disease can lead to preservation of the neurovascular bundles which lie behind the prostate. This modification has led to the preservation of erectile function in about 60–70 per cent of cases.

Pelvic lymph node dissection

Pelvic lymph node dissection is carried out immediately prior to radical prostatectomy when radical treatment is being considered. In some centres this was combined with the open open implantation of ^{125}I seeds, although with recent surgical modification of radical prostatectomy this is now only rarely performed.

Radical radiotherapy for early prostate cancer

Radical radiotherapy to the prostatic bed and pelvic lymph nodes rather than radical surgery has tended to be the treatment of choice in the UK for locally confined prostate cancer. The survival rates in the treatment of T1 to T2 disease are not greatly different from radical prostatectomy, although histological evidence of persistent tumour is found within the prostate in about 30 per cent of treated patients. Patients with locally advanced disease (T3) may be treated by radiotherapy, but most urologists treat such patients by means of androgen ablation. The treatment requires the patient to attend hospital on a daily basis for between 4 and 6 weeks. Some local complications are inevitable, namely irritation of the bladder with urinary frequency, urgency and sometimes urge incontinence and similar problems affecting the rectum with diarrhoea and, occasionally, late radiation proctitis.

Advanced disease

There is still debate about the timing of androgen ablation treatment in patients with locally advanced or metastatic disease without symptoms. The options are androgen deprivation at diagnosis or careful review, reserving active treatment for the later development of symptoms. Patients with local or general symptoms should be offered androgen deprivation.

Orchidectomy

Orchidectomy is performed to carry out androgen ablation in the treatment of locally advanced (T3 or T4) disease or of metastatic disease. In 1941 prostate cancer was shown to be responsive to such treatment by Charles Huggins – the only urologist to win the Nobel Prize. Bilateral orchidectomy, whether total or subcapsular, will eliminate the major source of testosterone production.

Patrick C. Walsh. Professor of Urology, Johns Hopkins Hospital, Baltimore, Maryland, USA.

Charles Huggins, b. 1901. American surgeon and the only urologist to win the Nobel Prize.

Hypophysectomy and adrenalectomy

These treatments are no longer carried out. In the past, patients who had initially responded to hormone treatment but subsequently relapsed were thought to have a small chance of obtaining further relief if a hypophysectomy was performed.

General radiotherapy

General radiotherapy for symptomatic metastases is an excellent form of palliative treatment often producing dramatic pain relief in men with hormone-relapsed prostate cancer. More recently, hemi-body irradiation has been shown to decrease symptoms in men with widespread bony metastases.

Strontium

Strontium is now being employed as a bone-seeking isotope which delivers effective radiotherapy to metastatic areas. It appears to be as effective as hemibody irradiation in the treatment of men with metastatic hormone-relapsed disease.

Medical forms of androgen ablation

Medical forms of androgen ablation have been available since the discovery of stilboestrol. Initially there was great enthusiasm for this treatment and Honvan® (phosphorylated diethylstilboestrol) could be given intravenously. Both treatments are effective in producing regression of prostate cancer, but are associated with significantly increased thrombotic complications and cardiovascular mortality. Even if stilboestrol is used at a dose of 1 mg three times a day complications can occur. Other hormones that have been tried include progestogens and Provera®.

The other commonly available treatment to reduce testosterone levels to the castrate range is LHRH agonists. These agents initially stimulate hypothalamic LHRH receptors, but because of their constant presence (rather than the normal diurnal rhythm) they then down-regulate them, resulting in cessation of pituitary LH production and hence a decrease in testosterone production. In the first 10 days or so serum testosterone levels may increase and it is wise to give flutamide, bicalutamide (Casodex) or Cyproterone acetate for this period. LHRH agonists may be given by monthly or 3 monthly depot injection.

Other treatments have become available recently which block the androgen receptor. Cyproterone acetate also has some progestogenic effect, whilst flutamide and bicalutamide are pure antiandrogen. In general, oral monotherapy has not been shown to be as good as LHRH agonists or orchidectomy.

Complete androgen blockade

Complete androgen blockade has been advocated as being likely to result in increased life expectancy and an increased time to progression in a fitter subgroup of men with advanced prostate cancer. The concept is that of abolishing the testicular secretion of testosterone by means of orchidectomy or the use of LHRH therapy and then inhibiting the effects of adrenal androgenic steroids by means of androgen receptor blockade with flutamide, bicalutamide (Casodex) or the use of cyproterone acetate. Recent overviews of randomised trials do not confirm earlier reports of effectiveness.

Cytotoxic agents in the treatment of these elderly men have proved disappointing, but whether this is because the tumour is inherently insensitive or because these elderly men will not tolerate effective doses is uncertain.

Summary of treatment

1. *Incidentally diagnosed T1a and T1b disease.* For men in their 70s conservative treatment would usually be the correct approach. Radical surgical treatment might be considered in the younger (<65 years) man with this form of the disease, although even in this group some men will elect to pursue a conservative course when counselled about risks versus benefits.
2. *Localised T2 disease.* In younger fitter men (<65 years), this may be treated by radical prostatectomy or radical radiotherapy. Watchful waiting remains an option – particularly for more elderly patients. In the elderly patient with outflow obstruction transurethral resection with or without hormone therapy is indicated. The benefit of radical treatment over a conservative approach is likely to be at most 25 per cent, given that progression to metastatic disease is in this order of magnitude after 10 years.
3. *Locally advanced T3 and T4 disease.* These patients are at significant risk of disease progression. Early androgen ablation is favoured if close follow-up is not possible. For the sexually active a careful conservative approach with the adoption of androgen ablation when symptoms arise is reasonable.
4. *Metastatic disease.* Once metastases have developed the outlook is poor. For patients with symptoms there is no dilemma; androgen ablation will provide symptomatic relief in over two-thirds of the patients. For patients with asymptomatic metastases the timing of treatment is less clear.

There are few hard and fast rules in the treatment of this cancer, but the surgeon should avoid making the patients worse through creating more complications as a result of treatment than the disease would have caused in its own right.

Prostatitis

In both acute and chronic prostatitis the seminal vesicles and posterior urethra are usually also involved.

Acute prostatitis

Aetiology

Acute prostatitis is common, but underdiagnosed. The usual organism responsible is *Escherichia coli*, but *Staphylococcus aureus* and *albus*, *Streptococcal faecalis* and *Neisseria gonorrhoea* may be responsible. The infection may be haematogenous from a distant focus or it may be secondary to acute urinary infection.

Clinical features

General manifestations overshadow the local: the patient feels ill, shivers, may have a rigor, has 'aches' all over, especially in the back, and may easily be diagnosed as having influenza. The temperature may be up to 39°C. Pain on micturition is usual, but not invariable. The urine contains threads in the initial voided sample which should be cultured. Perineal heaviness, rectal irritation and pain on defecation can occur; a urethral discharge is rare. Frequency occurs when the infection involves the bladder. Rectal examination reveals a tender prostate, one lobe may be swollen more than the other and the seminal vesicles may be involved. A frankly fluctuant abscess is uncommon.

Treatment

Treatment must be rigorous and prolonged or the infection will not be eradicated and recurrent attacks may ensue. Spread of infection to the epididymes and testes may occur. Prolonged treatment with an antibiotic which penetrates the prostate well is indicated (trimethoprim or ciprofloxacin).

Prostatic abscess

In addition to the foregoing symptoms and signs, the advent of a prostatic abscess is heralded by the temperature rising steeply with rigors. Antibiotics disguise these features. Severe, unremitting perineal and rectal pain with occasional tenesmus often cause the condition to be confused with an anorectal abscess. Nevertheless, if a rectal examination is performed, the prostate will be felt to be enlarged, hot, extremely tender and perhaps fluctuant. Retention of urine is likely to occur and in such men suprapubic catheterization is best.

Treatment. The abscess should be drained without delay.

1. The abscess can be drained by perurethral resection – unroofing the whole cavity.
2. The perineal route is rarely indicated unless there is marked periprostatic spread.

Chronic prostatitis

Many urologists find the syndromes of chronic prostatitis and 'prostatodynia' very difficult, for many men present with perigenital pain, testicular pain, prostatic pain exacerbated by sexual intercourse or pain which apparently renders sexual intercourse out of the question. Psychosexual dysfunction in such patients may be the underlying problem. The diagnosis of chronic prostatitis has to be based on:

- persistent threads in voided urine;
- prostatic massage showing pus cells with or without bacteria in the absence of urinary infection.

Aetiology

This is thought to be sequel of inadequately treated acute prostatitis. While pus is present in the prostatic secretion, often the responsible organism is difficult to find. Other organisms such as *Chlamydia* species may be responsible for chronic abacterial prostatitis.

Clinical features

The clinical features are extremely varied. Only men with symptoms of posterior urethritis, prostatic pain and perigenital pain accompanied by intermittent fever and pus cells or bacteria in the postprostatic massage specimen should be diagnosed as having chronic prostatitis.

Diagnosis

1. *The three-glass urine test* is valuable. If the first glass with the initial voided sample shows urine containing prostatic threads, prostatitis is present.
2. *Rectal examination* of the prostate may be normal or may show a soft, boggy and tender prostate.
3. *Examination of the prostatic fluid* obtained by prostatic massage should show pus cells and bacteria.
4. *Urethroscopy* may reveal inflammation of the prostatic urethra, and pus may be seen exuding from the prostatic ducts. The verumontanum is likely to be enlarged and oedematous. In many men with the symptoms described above all investigations are normal.

Treatment

Antibiotic therapy should only be administered in accordance with bacteriological sensitivity tests. Trimethoprim penetrates well into the prostate. Where trichomonas or anaerobes are the responsible agent, a rapid response is obtained from administration of flagyl (metronidazole, 200 mg t.d.s. for 7 days to both partners). If *Chlamydia* is suspected, doxycycline is the antibiotic treatment of choice. It is uncertain whether prostatic massage helps in eradicating the infection.

Prostatodynia

This diagnosis is made by the presence of perigenital pain in the absence of any objective evidence of prostatic inflammation. Whether the syndrome has any relationship with the prostate is unclear.

Tuberculosis of the prostate and seminal vesicles

Tuberculosis of the prostate and seminal vesicles is rare and associated with renal tuberculosis. In 30 per cent of cases, there is a history of pulmonary tuberculosis within 5 years of the onset of genital tuberculosis.

Tuberculosis of one or both seminal vesicles may be found when examining a patient with chronic tuberculosis epididymitis, no symptoms being referable to the internal genitalia. On rectal examination, the affected vesicle is found to be nodular.

When the prostate is involved, rectal examination reveals nodules in one or both lateral lobes. Patients with tuberculous prostatitis usually present with the following:

- urethral discharge;
- painful, sometimes bloodstained, ejaculation;
- mild ache in the perineum;
- infertility;
- dysuria;
- abscess formation.

Special forms of investigation

Radiography sometimes displays areas of calcification in the prostate and/or the seminal vesicles.

Bacteriological examination of the seminal fluid yields positive cultures for tubercle bacilli.

Treatment

The general treatment is that for tuberculosis. If a prostatic abscess forms it should be drained transurethrally.

Seminal vesicles

Acute seminal vesiculitis

Acute seminal vesiculitis occurs in association with prostatitis. Prior to the antibiotic treatment of gonorrhoea, gonococcal vesiculitis was common.

Chronic seminal vesiculitis

Chronic seminal vesiculitis usually presents with haematospermia and pain on intercourse. TRUS demonstrates the features of distension, thickening and the presence of turbid fluid. The treatment is the same as for chronic prostatitis.

Tuberculous seminal vesiculitis

The clinical features and treatment have been discussed above.

Diverticulum of the seminal vesicle

Diverticulum of the seminal vesicle occurs occasionally. In such cases, the kidney of that side is absent and the diverticulum represents an abortive ureteric bud. It is a cause of persistent infection.

Cyst of the seminal vesicle

A cyst of the seminal vesicle is uncommon and rarely requires treatment. It may be removed by dissection through an incision similar to that for perineal prostatectomy, if it is large or giving rise to symptoms.

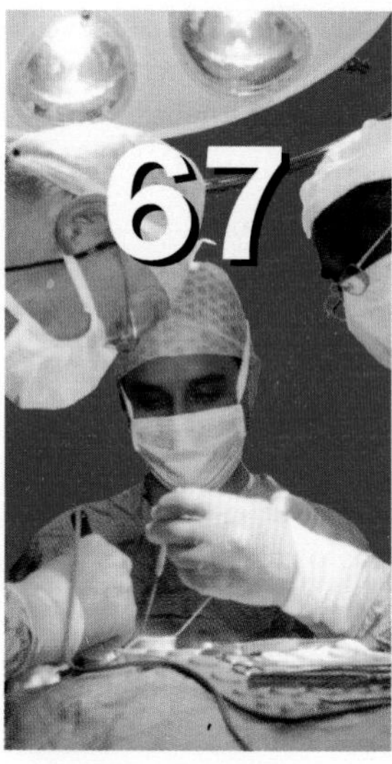

67 The urethra and penis

The male urethra

The most common congenital abnormalities of the male urethra are:

- meatal stenosis;
- congenital urethral stricture;
- congenital valves;
- hypospadias;
- epispadias.

Meatal stenosis

A congenital stenosis of the external urinary meatus, normally the narrowest part of the male urethra, is associated with phimosis. After circumcision, meatal ulceration may lead to stricturing of the meatus. When the meatal opening is reduced to a pinhole there may be chronic retention of urine with back-pressure effects and eventually chronic renal failure. Lesser degrees of stenosis lead to loss of the normal urinary stream with spraying or dribbling.

Treatment by meatotomy or meatal dilatation is indicated for symptomatic stenosis, if the stricture is sufficient to prevent free drainage of discharge in a patient with urethritis or there is a need to pass endoscopic instruments transurethrally.

Bailey & Love's Short Practice of Surgery, 23rd edition. Edited by R.C.G. Russell, N.S. Williams and C.J.K. Bulstrode. Published in 2000 by Arnold Publishers.

Meatotomy

The tightened meatus is opened by cutting down on to a fine probe placed in the anterior urethra. The cut edges of urothelium and skin are sewn together with absorbable suture. If the stenosis recurs a skin flap can be laid in as a *meatoplasty* to widen the meatus (Fig. 67.1).

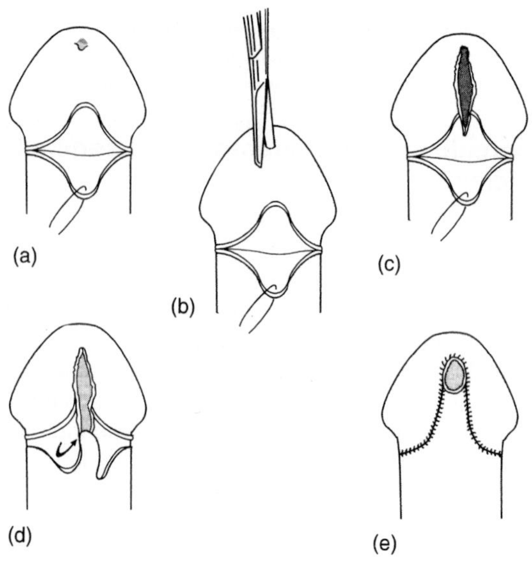

Fig. 67.1 Meatoplasty. The strictured meatus is incised and a flap of penile skin is laid to form a funnel-shaped meatal opening.

Congenital urethral stricture

This condition is rare. Some cases are associated with duplication of the urethra. Usually symptoms are delayed until adolescence, when it may be difficult to be sure that a supposedly congenital stricture of the bulbar urethra is not due to unrecognised urethral injury in childhood. A single treatment by optical urethrotomy or dilatation is usually effective.

Congenital valves of the posterior urethra

These are symmetrical folds of urothelium which can cause obstruction to the urethra of boys. They are usually found just distal to the verumontanum but they may be within the prostatic urethra. They behave as flap valves so, although urine does not flow normally, a urethral catheter can be passed without difficulty. In some instances, the valves are incomplete and the patient remains without symptoms until adolescence or adulthood. In such cases the prostatic urethra is grossly dilated and saccules and diverticula are present within it.

The valves are difficult to see on urethroscopy because the flow of irrigant sweeps them into the open position. If the bladder is filled with contrast medium, the dilatation of the urethra above the valves can be demonstrated on a voiding cystogram.

Treatment

A suprapubic catheter is inserted to relieve the back pressure and allow the effects of renal failure to subside before definitive treatment by transurethral resection of the valves using a paediatric resectoscope.

Hypospadias

Hypospadias occurs in one in 350 male births and is the most common congenital malformation of the urethra. The external meatus opens on the *underside* of the penis or the perineum, and the inferior aspect of the prepuce is poorly developed ('hooded prepuce').

Hypospadias is classified according to position of the meatus.

- *Glandular hypospadias* – this is the most common type and does not usually require treatment. The normal site of the external meatus is marked by a blind pit, although it occasionally connects by a channel to the ectopic opening on the underside of the glans.
- *Coronal hypospadias* – the meatus is placed at the junction of the underside of the glans and the body of the penis.
- *Penile and penoscrotal hypospadias* – the opening is on the underside of the penile shaft (Fig. 67.2).
- *Perineal hypospadias* — this is the most severe abnormality. The scrotum is split and the urethra opens between its two halves. There may be testicular maldescent which may make it difficult to determine the sex of the child.

The more severe varieties of hypospadias represent an absence of the urethra and corpus spongiosum distal to the ectopic opening. The absent structures are represented by a fibrous cord which deforms the penis in a downward direction (chordee). The more distant the opening from its normal position, the more pronounced the bowing.

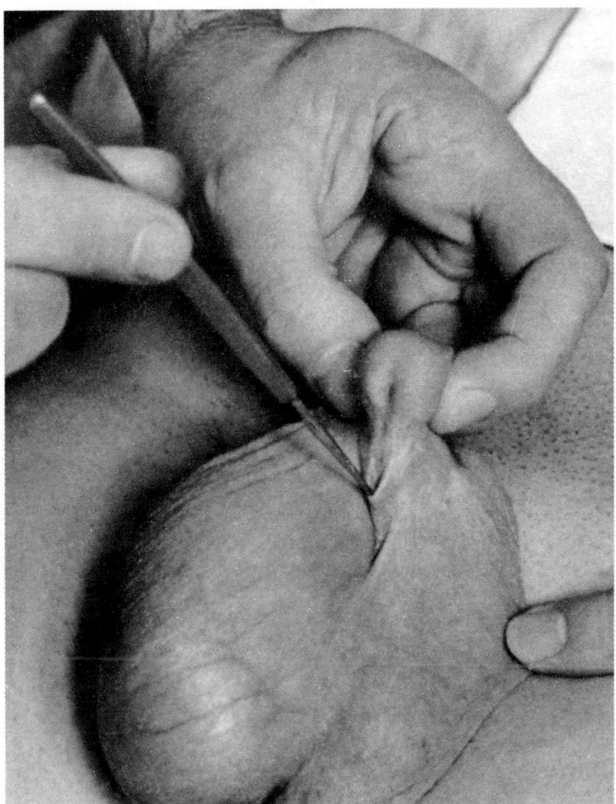

Fig. 67.2 Penile hypospadias. The patient passes urine through the orifice demonstrated by the probe.

Treatment

Glandular hypospadias does not need treatment unless the meatus is stenosed, in which case a meatotomy is performed. Surgery is indicated for other forms of hypospadias to improve sexual function and for cosmetic reasons. A bewildering variety of plastic surgical procedures is described to correct the chordee and to bring the urethra to an opening at the tip of the penis. Most of these procedures make use of prepuceal skin and so circumcision should be avoided until the hypospadias has been repaired. Operations for hypospadias are best performed by a specialist paediatric urologist and will not be detailed here.

Epispadias

Epispadias is very rare, occurring in one in 30 000 males and one in 400 000 females. In penile epispadias the opening on the dorsum is associated with upward curvature of the penis (Fig. 67.3). Total epispadias usually goes with ectopia vesicae and other severe developmental defects.

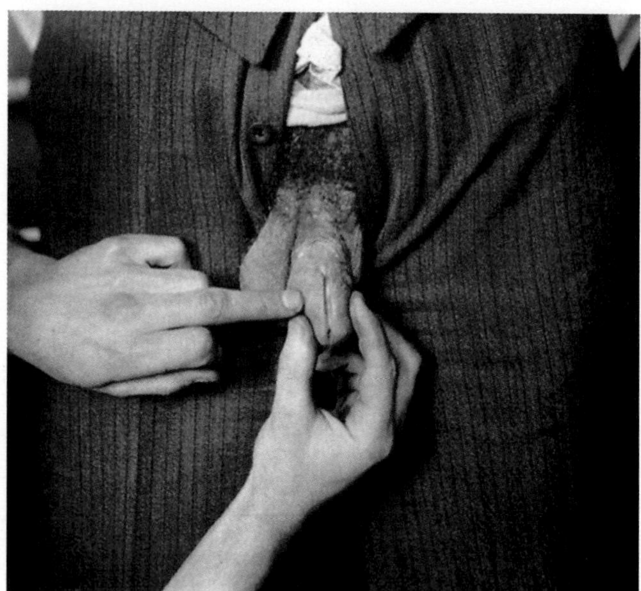

Fig. 67.3 Glandular epispadias.

Injuries to the male urethra

Rupture of the bulbar urethra

Rupture of the bulbar urethra is the most common urethral injury. There is a history of a blow to the perineum usually due to a fall astride a projecting object. In the days of sailing ships, the common cause was falling astride a spar; the modern equivalent is seen among workers losing their footing on scaffolding. Cycling accidents, loose manhole covers (Fig. 67.4) and gymnasium accidents astride the beam account for a number of cases.

Clinical features

The triad of signs of a ruptured bulbar urethra is retention of urine, perineal haematoma and bleeding from the external urinary meatus.

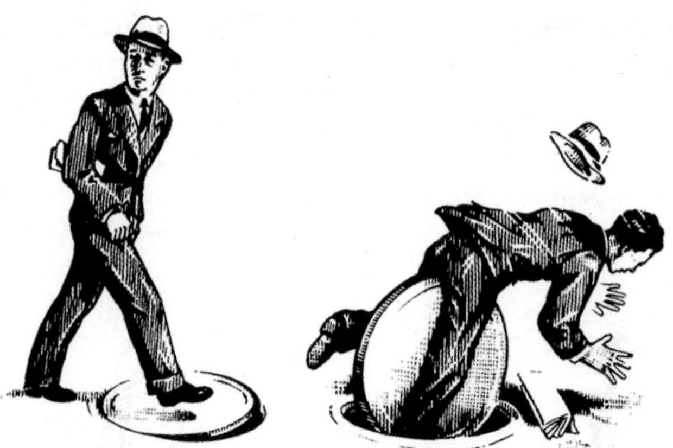

Fig. 67.4 The type of accident which results in ruptured bulbar urethra (*after V.J. O'Connor*).

Preliminary assessment and treatment

The patient will be in pain and should be treated with appropriate analgesic drugs. He should be discouraged from passing urine if rupture of the urethra is suspected. Instead, if the bladder is full, a simple percutaneous suprapubic puncture should be performed and a fine catheter inserted to drain it (Fig. 67.5). This will reduce the likelihood of urinary extravasation and allow appropriate investigations to establish the full extent of the urethral injury. If the patient has already passed urine when first seen and there is no extravasation, the rupture, if any, is partial and a catheter is not needed. In either case, it is probably wise to administer a course of prophylactic antibiotics.

Treatment. The initial management of bulbar urethral injuries has been controversial but a consensus is emerging. The main worry is that injudicious urethral catheterisation will convert a partial tear into a complete transection of the urethra. The initial treatment described above is to be recommended for most of those who go into urinary retention after the accident, especially if there is bleeding from the urethra. More information may be obtained by an ascending urethrogram or even a flexible cystoscopy to assess the injury. Very occasionally, if the facilities for passing a percutaneous suprapubic catheter are not available, it may be permissible to try to pass a soft, small-calibre urethral catheter *without force*. This may allow a few patients to avoid the open placement of a suprapubic tube into the bladder.

If investigations show a complete tear of the urethra, the suprapubic catheter should be left in place until arrangements can be made to repair it. Some surgeons advocate early open repair of the urethra with excision of the traumatised section and spatulated end-to-end reanastomosis of the urethra (Fig. 67.6). Others wait longer before embarking upon a repair operation but may attempt to find a way across the gap in the urethra using a urethroscope. This allows a urethral catheter to be placed so that the alignment of the urethra is as near as possible to normal while healing occurs.

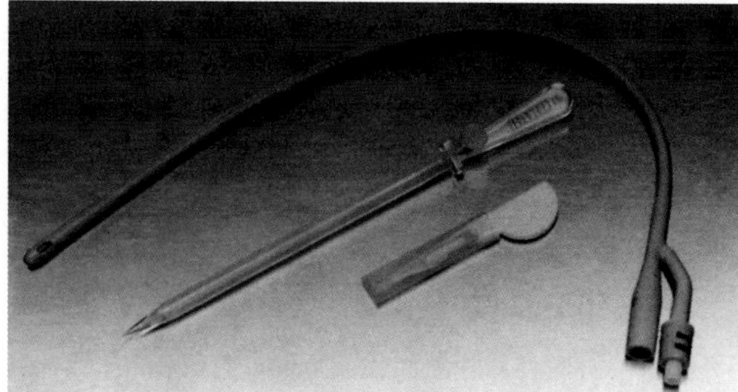

Fig. 67.5 Kit for percutaneous suprapubic drainage of the bladder.

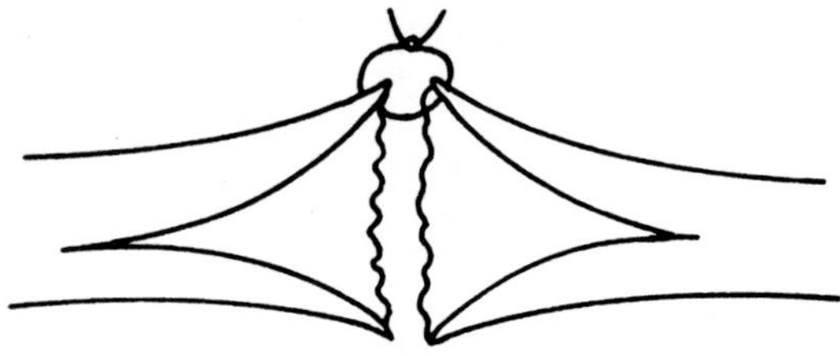

Fig. 67.6 Open repair of a ruptured bulbar urethra.

Complications

Subcutaneous extravasation of urine occurs in complete rupture if the patient attempts to pass urine.

Stricture is a common sequel to urethral trauma, whether there is a partial or complete tear or simply periurethral bruising. Infection may also play a part.

Rupture of the membranous urethra

Extraperitoneal rupture of the urethra

Intrapelvic rupture of the membranous urethra occurs near the apex of the prostate (Fig. 67.7). Like extraperitoneal rupture of the bladder, it may be due to penetrating wounds but in civilian life it is most usually a result of pelvic fracture.

Fracture of the pubic and ischial rami is most likely to result when sudden force is applied to one lower limb in a car accident or in landing on one leg after falling from a height. There is an associated disruption of the sacroiliac joint so that one half of the pelvis and ischiopubic ramus is pushed up above the other. This applies a traction force on the prostate which is firmly bound by ligaments to the back of the symphysis pubis. The torn ends of the urethra may be widely displaced by this type of injury.

In another type of pelvic fracture the patient suffers a front-to-back compression of the pelvis in a blow directly from the front. A 'butterfly fracture' of the pubic rami on each side occurs. When the compressive force is relieved, the pubic fragment springs back so that the ends of the torn urethra are close to each other. About 10–15 per cent of cases of fractured pelvis have associated urethral injury.

Clinical features

The most common causes of pelvic fracture are road traffic accidents, severe crush injuries and falls. There is often multiple trauma with injury to the head, thorax and abdomen, and fracture of long bones. Often the management of these injuries must take precedence and the over-riding priority is to keep the patient alive by appropriate resuscitation.

The urethral injury can be managed in the short term by inserting a suprapubic catheter, and this should be done as soon as it is practicable. The type of urethral injury can often be deduced from the plain radiograph – a major urethral disruption is almost certain if there is significant displacement of the pubic bones. If the prostate is displaced, it may be impossible to reach or appear to be very 'high' on rectal examination. An ascending urethrogram may be justified if there is doubt.

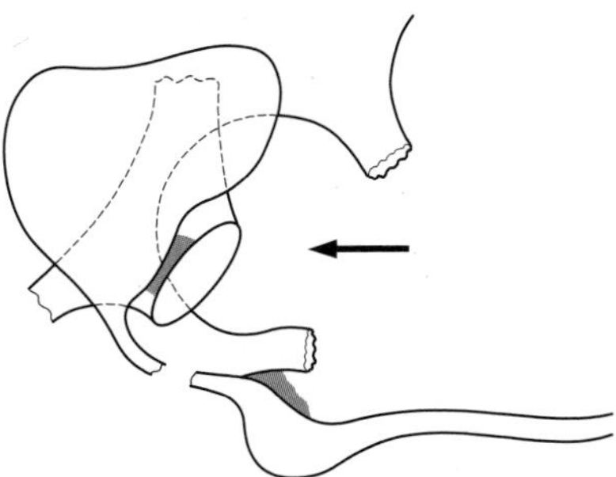

Fig. 67.7 Intrapelvic rupture of the urethra. Note the displacement of the bladder.

There may be associated injury to the bladder with either an intraperitoneal or extraperitoneal rupture. The former is associated with the onset of peritonitis and if suspected demands exploration and repair of the bladder even if laparotomy is not indicated by other injuries. Extraperitoneal rupture of the bladder causes symptoms which are difficult to distinguish from those of rupture of the membranous urethra. There is pain, bruising and dullness to percussion above the umbilicus. If there is a significant bladder rupture it must be repaired, a suprapubic catheter inserted and the retroperitoneal space drained.

Complications

Stricture. The main complication of urethral trauma is urethral stricture. When the injury is severe and the disrupted ends of the urethra are far apart the stricture is likely to be very difficult to treat. Because of this worry, some surgeons urge that an attempt should be made to realign the urethra as soon as the emergency is over and the patient is well enough to be taken to theatre. Often the orthopaedic surgeons will want to improve the position of the pelvic fragments at this stage with the possibility of external fixation. In some cases a urethral catheter can be inserted if a way through the stricture can be found with a flexible or rigid urethroscope. In others an open repair of the urethra can be attempted. Other surgeons feel that it is better to allow a longer period of recovery before attempting to correct the urethral injury.

If the urethra is relatively well aligned, an established urethral stricture may be treatable by optical urethrotomy (Sachse) but many of these patients need a full-scale urethroplasty. Sometimes the ends of the urethra are widely displaced and there is extensive fibrosis and even ectopic calcification where the urethra should be. Occasionally there is such a gap that the ends can only be brought together by cutting away the pubic bone. The management of a severe urethral stricture should be in the hands of a specialist urologist.

Urinary incontinence. If the external urethral sphincter is destroyed, continence of urine will depend upon the competence of the bladder neck mechanism. Subsequent surgical manoeuvres such as prostatectomy which destroy the bladder neck may cause incontinence.

Impotence. Erectile impotence is common after pelvic fracture with urethral injury. It is assumed that this is the result of damage to the nerve supply of the penis. The patients are usually able to achieve erection with prostaglandin injections or a vacuum device.

Orthopaedic

For management of the fractured pelvis, see Chapter 21 on 'Fractures and dislocations'.

Extravasation of urine

Superficial extravasation is likely with complete rupture of the bulbar urethra and in ruptured urethral abscess.

The extravasated urine is confined in front of the midperineal point by the attachment of Colles fascia to the triangular ligament, and by the attachment of Scarpa's fascia

---

Hans Sachse. Munich, Germany.
Abraham Colles, 1773–1843. Irish surgeon.
Antonio Scarpa, b. 1747. Italian anatomist and surgeon.

just below the inguinal ligament. The external spermatic fascia stops it getting into the inguinal canals. Extravasated urine collects in the scrotum and penis and beneath the deep layer of superficial fascia in the abdominal wall.

Treatment is by urgent operation to drain the bladder by suprapubic cystostomy. This prevents further extravasation.

Deep extravasation (Fig. 67.7) occurs with extraperitoneal rupture of the bladder or intrapelvic rupture of the urethra. It can also occur if the ureter is damaged or if there is perforation of the prostatic capsule or bladder during transurethral resection. Urine extravasates in the layers of the pelvic fascia and the retroperitoneal tissues.

Treatment is by suprapubic cytostomy and drainage of the retropubic space.

Inflammations of the urethra

Inflammatory conditions of the urethra include:

- meatal ulcer;
- urethritis:
  - gonoccoccal urethritis;
  - nonspecific urethritis;
  - Reiter's syndrome.

Ulceration of the urethral meatus

Meatal ulcer is quite common in circumcised boys. It may occur soon after the operation or may be delayed for up to 2 years from circumcision. Lack of protection by the prepuce seems to be the excitatory cause with friction from clothing and ammoniacal dermatitis as contributory factors. The ulcer forms a scab which blocks the meatus and the child can only pass urine by bursting the scab. This hurts so the boy screams and a tiny amount of blood may be passed as well. The process causes fibrosis which can result in an acquired pinhole meatus.

Treatment

Local measures to soften the scab and alkalinise the urine are often curative. A few need meatotomy.

Gonorrhoeal urethritis

Gonorrhoea is a sexually transmitted disease caused by *Neisseria gonorrhoeae* (gonococcus), a Gram-negative kidney-shaped diplococcus that infects the anterior urethra in the male, the urethra and cervix in females, and the oropharynx, rectum and anal canal in both sexes, but especially men.

Gonorrhoea in men usually declares itself by urethral discomfort and urethral discharge up to 10 days after exposure. There is often scalding dysuria. In some there may be no symptoms other than slight discharge.

Investigations. Pus and gonococci are present in the Gram-stained urethral smear. The passage of pus in the first part of the urinary stream can be demonstrated as haziness in the first glass of a *two-glass test*. Treatment should not wait upon the results of urethral culture when the clinical picture and urethral smear are typical.

Complications are uncommon in the UK and are all prevented by effective treatment. Local complications include posterior urethritis, prostatitis – acute or chronic, acute epididymo-orchitis, periurethral abscess and urethral stricture. Gonococcal arthritis, iridocyclitis, septicaemia and endocarditis are even more unusual.

Treatment is by antibiotics, usually penicillin. The effective concentration may be increased by probenicid and high doses may be needed for resistant strains. Completely resistant β-lactamase-producing strains, rare in the UK, will not respond to penicillin whatever the dose. Patients with these organisms and those allergic to penicillin must be treated with second-line drugs such as kanomycin.

Contact tracing is important in controlling the spread of the disease.

Gonorrhoea in women affects primarily the urethra and cervix, and is often symptomless. It can never be diagnosed on clinical grounds alone. Almost three-quarters of all female cases attend initially as a result of contact tracing. Symptoms which are present in 50 per cent or less often consist of a mild dysuria or slight urethral discharge which can go unnoticed by the patient. If Skene's tubules are emptied by milking the urethra against the posterior pubic ramus, a bead of pus may appear at the urethral meatus. There may be some reddening or erosion of the cervix with a mucopurulent cervical plug but copious vaginal discharge is more likely to be due to concomitant trichomonal vaginitis.

Complications. Gonococcal proctitis occurs in at least 60–70 per cent of cases and is usually symptomless. Ten per cent suffer from salpingitis which, if bilateral, may lead to infertility.

Gonorrhoea in the newborn is now rare. It used to be an important cause of blindness.

Nonspecific urethritis (syn. nongonococcal urethritis)

This is a form of urethritis which is diagnosed by exclusion when gonorrhoea and other known infections have been excluded. At present some 40 per cent of cases are due to *Chlamydia trachomatis* and some are shown to be caused by *Ureaplasma urealytica*. The causative agent in up to 50 per cent is unknown.

Clinical features. Dysuria and a mucopurulent urethral discharge appear up to 6 weeks after sexual intercourse. The urine is usually grossly clear but may contain 'threads' or pus cells. Epididymitis is not uncommon and urethral stricture rarely results. In women the condition presents as a form of urethrotrigonitis and may be very resistant to diagnosis.

Treatment with oxytetracycline or doxycycline is usually effective, although relapse is common especially in men in whom the prostate may act as a reservoir of infection. It is important to treat both partners as re-infection is probable if this is not done.

Reiter's disease

Reiter's disease (syn. sexually acquired reactive arthritis) is usually Sexually transmitted in the UK but abroad it is more commonly dysenteric in origin. Subacute urethritis 4–6 weeks after contact is associated with a clear, viscid discharge which is free from organisms.

Heins C. Reiter, 1861–1969. Physician, President of the Health Service and Honorary Professor of Hygiene, Berlin, Germany. Described Reiter's disease in 1916.

Hans C. J. Gram, 1853–1938. Danish physician and bacteriologist.

Alexander Johnson Chalmers Skene, 1828–1900. Professor of Gynaecology, Long Island Hospital, New York, USA.

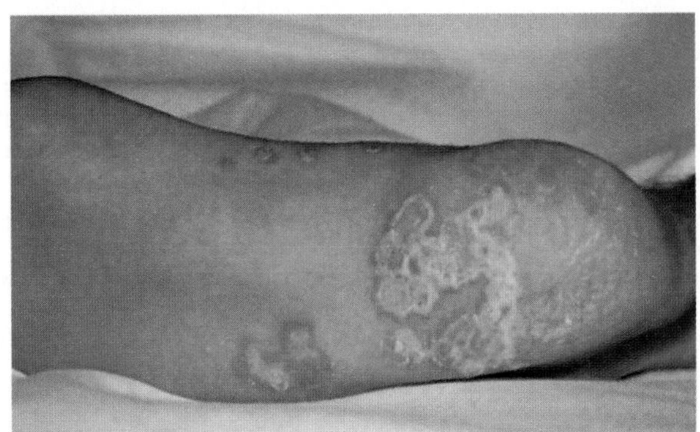

Fig. 67.8 Reiter's disease – keratoderma blennorrhagicum of the heel.

A few days later, conjunctivitis, unilateral then bilateral, occurs in 50 per cent. In more severe cases there is anterior uveitis. Usually in 10 days to 2 weeks arthritis supervenes but it is not an invariable feature of the condition. Another concurrent manifestation is keratoderma blennorrhagicum, consisting of nodules, vesicles and pustules frequently found on the sole of the foot (Fig. 67.8).

Differential diagnosis. This is principally from gonorrhoea, which must be excluded by blood culture. In Reiter's disease, the urethritis and arthritis are milder and the incubation period is longer than gonorrhoea.

Prognosis. The urethritis and conjunctivitis frequently subside in a few weeks but the arthritis may persist for months. Severe anterior uveitis and frequently recurrent attacks suggest a bad outlook.

Treatment. The ophthalmic complications are treated with eye baths and shades. Mydriatics and topical steroids are indicated for iritis. Other symptoms may prove difficult to control and severe cases should be under the care of a specialist in genitourinary medicine.

Urethral stricture

The causes of urethral stricture are:

- congenital;
- traumatic;
- inflammatory:
  - postgonorrhoeal;
  - posturethral chancre;
  - tuberculous;
- instrumental:
  - indwelling catheter;
  - urethral endoscopy;
- postoperative:
  - open prostatectomy;
  - amputation of penis.

Postgonorrhoeal stricture

This is less common since the introduction of effective antibiotic treatment for gonorrhoea. The stricture is most commonly in the bulbar urethra but postmeatal strictures are also seen.

Pathology. Infection in the periurethral glands persists after inadequately treated gonorrhoea. The infection spreads to cause a perurethritis which heals by fibrosis to result in a stricture. Most strictures appear within 1 year of infection but they may not cause difficulty in micturition for 10–15 years.

Clinical features

The first symptoms are usually those of bladder outflow obstruction with straining to void and poor urinary stream. The relative youthfulness of the patient often distinguishes these from the symptoms of prostatic enlargement which characteristically occur after the age of 50. As the stream becomes narrower, micturition is prolonged with dribbling after it seems to have ended. This is due to urine trickling from the dilated urethra proximal to the stricture. Increased urinary frequency by day and night is also common, and is due to incomplete bladder emptying or infection, or both.

When the stricture is well established, it may be possible to palpate the scarring along the line of the urethra. If the stricture is tight enough, the patient will go into acute retention. If this happens, there is a danger that ham-fisted attempts to pass a urethral catheter will result in a false passage. *If a patient has gone into retention because of a urethral stricture, the urethra will be too narrow to allow even a tiny catheter to pass safely.*

Urethroscopy allows the stricture to be viewed as a circumferential scar (Fig. 67.9). The openings of false passages may be seen if there have been misguided attempts to pass a urethral catheter.

Urethrography using a water-miscible gel containing contrast medium will show the extent and severity of the stricture or failure of the medium to pass beyond the tightness indicating complete stenosis (Figs 67.10 and 67.11).

Treatment of urethral stricture is by:

- dilatation:
  - gum-elastic bougie;
  - filiform and follower;
  - metal sounds;
  - self-dilatation with Nélaton catheter;

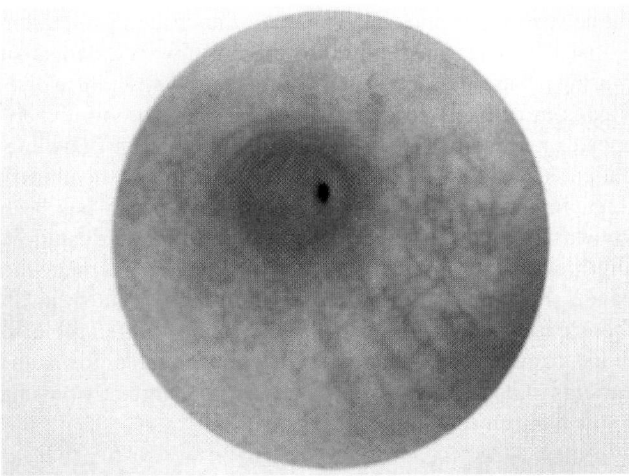

Fig. 67.9 Urethroscopic appearance of urethral stricture.

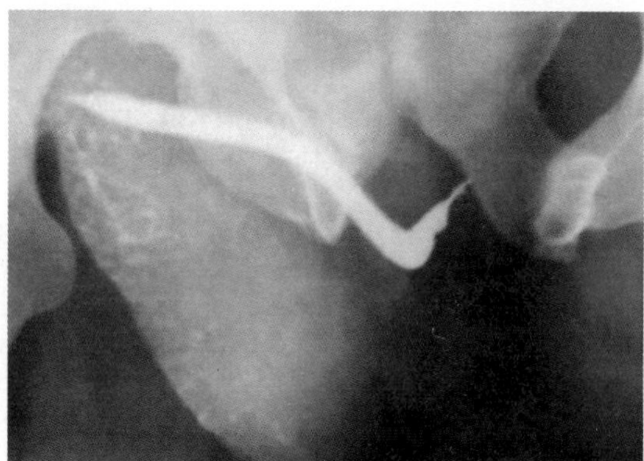

Fig. 67.10 Ascending urethrogram showing urethral stricture of the membranous urethra following fracture of the pelvis.

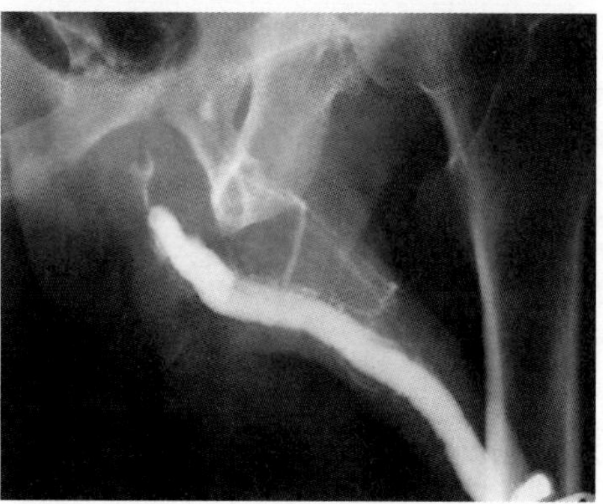

Fig. 67.11 Gonnorrhoeal stricture of the bulbar urethra. Note that some contrast has entered the penile veins.

- urethrotomy:
  - internal visual urethrotomy;
- urethroplasty:
  - excision and end-to-end anastomosis;
  - patch urethroplasty.

Intermittent dilatation is the traditional treatment for stricture. Under aseptic conditions, the urethra is stretched using a graduated series of dilators. With care and gentleness, the procedure can be performed under local urethral anaesthesia with lignocaine gel. The main drawback of dilatation is that it is performed 'blind' so there is always a danger of causing a false passage which will make the stricture worse. This is most likely to occur when the operator is inexperienced or unfamiliar with the complexities of an individual patient's urethra. As with any instrumentation of the urinary tract, infection is a danger and fatal septicaemia has been known to follow a supposedly straightforward dilatation. Urethral dilatation still has a place in elderly gentlemen who have a short stricture which recurs at infrequent intervals. In these patients, occasional bouginage may be preferable to more complex procedures. It may be possible for some patients to dilate their own urethras by intermittently passing a soft Nélaton catheter.

Auguste Nélaton, 1807–73. Surgeon, Paris, France.

Instruments. Strictures have been treated by surgeons for centuries and there are many different dilating instruments on the shelves of surgical museums, each with the name of the surgeon who invented it. A simple stricture may be dilated using metal *sounds* (Fig. 67.12), so called because they were originally used to 'sound' for stones in the bladder or gum-elastic *bougies* (French 'candle') (Fig. 67.13). These must be wielded with great care as it is easy to make a false passage with them. *Filiforms* are gum-elastic filaments which can be passed through the lumen of a urethral stricture (Fig. 67.15). This is usually best done under direct vision using a urethroscope, although the 'faggot method' may be helpful if endoscopes are not available (Fig. 67.14). Once the lumen has been located with its tip, the other end of the filiform is screwed on to a '*follower*': a gum-elastic bougie with a screw thread at its tip for the

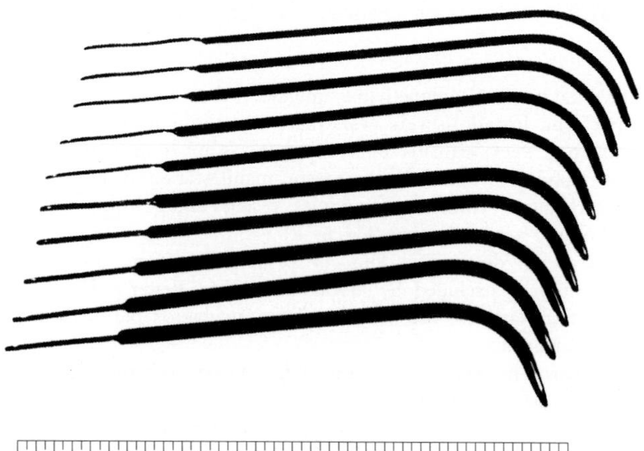

Fig. 67.12 Metal dilators ('sounds').

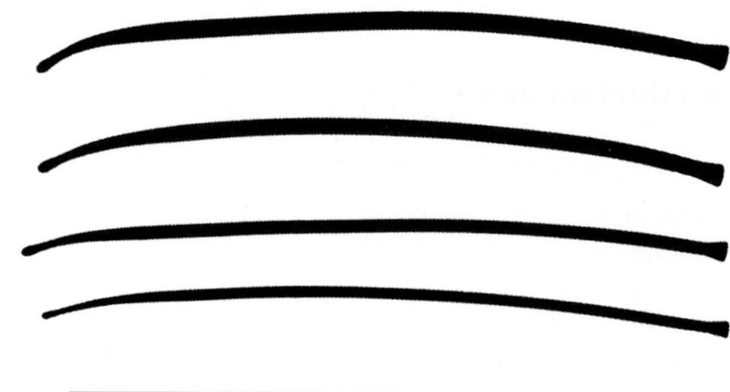

Fig. 67.13 Gum-elastic bougies.

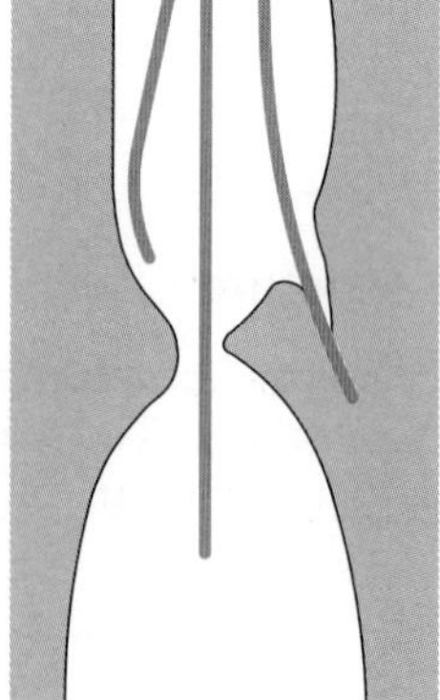

Fig. 67.14 'Faggot' method of introducing a bougie throught a stricture.

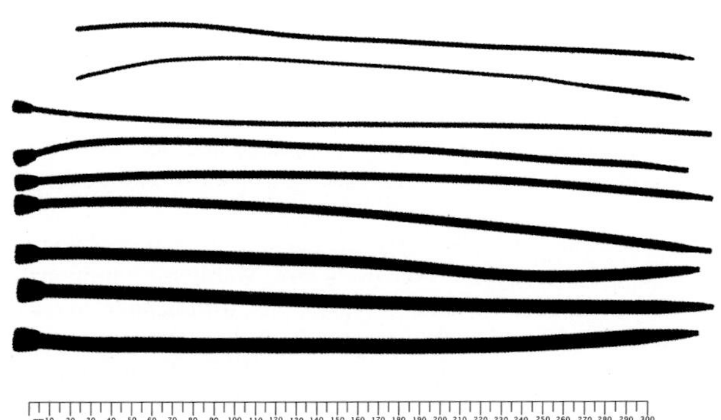

Fig. 67.15 Filiform bougies with followers.

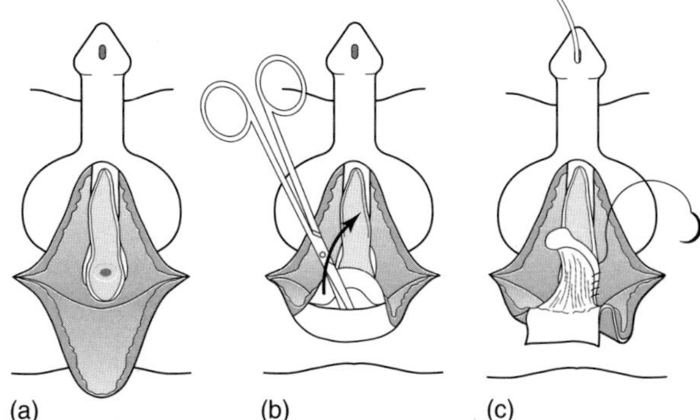

Fig. 67.16 The pedicled patch urethroplasty of Orandi and Blandy. (a) A 'U'-shaped incision in the perineum is developed to form a flap. The strictured urethra is incised. (b) A patch of skin attached to the underlying dartos muscle is separated from the tip of the 'U'-shaped flap. (c) The patch is sutured in place to widen the strictured urethra. The blood supply to the patch comes from the underlying dartos muscle.

purpose (Fig. 67.15). As the follower is advanced the filiform guides it safely through the stricture. Once the stricture has been partially dilated by followers of increasing size, it is often safe to change to metal dilators. Patients who have had an optical urethrotomy are sometimes taught to keep the stricture open by regular self-dilatation with a urethral catheter of a suitable size.

Operative treatment. *Internal urethrotomy* is performed using the Sachse optical urethrotome. The stricture is cut under visual control using a tiny knife passed through the sheath of a rigid urethroscope. The stricture is usually cut at the 12 o'clock position taking care not to cut too deeply into the vascular spaces of the corpus spongiosum which surrounds the urethra. If one cut is insufficient, others can be made until there is a wide passage through the strictured segment of urethra. After the procedure, many surgeons leave a catheter for 1–2 days, but there is no evidence that this makes a significant difference to the effectiveness of the procedure. A single urethrotomy seems to give a permanent cure of uncomplicated stricture in about 50 per cent of patients. The rest require further treatment by urethrotomy, dilatation or urethroplasty. The main complications are infection and bleeding. It is possible to get lost when trying to cut a way through a very tight stricture. This is especially true when there are false passages due to previous dilatation attempts. In these circumstances, it helps to pass a guidewire to establish the true lumen of the urethra.

Urethroplasty. The simplest urethroplasty involves excision of the stenosed length of urethra and reanastomosis of the spatulated cut end (Fig. 67.6). This operation is only possible if the stricture is relatively short because there must be no tension at the suture line. If end-to-end anastomosis is not feasible, there is a large number of different plastic surgical procedures to replace part or all of the wall of the strictured urethra using free full-thickness or pedicled skin grafts. The Orandi–Blandy operation makes use of a myocutaneous patch of perineal skin and dartos muscle (Fig. 67.16): Turner-Warwick favours penile skin.

Urethroplasty should be considered when more simple means fail to give lasting relief of symptoms. The procedure can be very demanding, especially when the stricture is the result of pelvic trauma and the urethra is encased in woody, hard fibrosis. A prolonged hospital stay is usual while the graft heals.

Other causes of urethral stricture

Congenital stricture has been considered previously.

Traumatic stricture. The stricture which follows neglected or untreated rupture of the membranous urethra is sometimes a complete loss of continuity. These patients often need a transpubic urethroplasty to bridge the gap.

Postinstrumental stricture. This follows endoscopy or catheterisation and may affect any part of the urethra. Some surgeons recommend prophylactic dilatation or urethrotomy before transurethral surgery to try to avoid this complication. Some cases of stricture seem to be due to a sensitivity to chemicals from the catheter but most are the result of a combination of trauma, infection and pressure necrosis.

Postoperative stricture. Postoperative stricture develops after about 4 per cent of prostatectomies, irrespective of the method employed. The stricture is usually in the proximal part of the prostatic urethra and is also known as bladder neck stenosis. If it cannot be managed by dilatation, bladder neck stenosis should be treated by transurethral incision and resection of the stricture.

Postoperative stricture is also a complication of amputation of the penis (see below).

Complications of urethral stricture

Complications include:

- retention of urine;
- urethral diverticulum;
- periurethral abscess;
- urethral fistula;
- hernia, haemorrhoids and rectal prolapse due to abdominal straining to void urine.

Diverticulum of the male urethra (syn. urethral pouch). This is usually congenital and represents a partial duplication of the urethra. Acquired cases are uncommon. They are sometimes seen as a result of increased intraurethral pressure behind a stricture. Others are due to the long-standing presence of a foreign body such as a stone or calculus in the urethra.

Treatment is by excision of the diverticulum and removal of the cause if possible.

Periurethral abscess. Periurethral abscesses can be either penile, bulbar or chronic.

A *penile periurethral abscess* usually arises as an acute gonococcal infection of one of the glands of Littré. The tender induration felt on the underside of the penis points and discharges externally, often leaving a fistula.

Ahmad Orandi. Urological surgeon, Fergus Falls, Minnesota, USA.

John Peter Bland. Emeritus Professor of Urology, The London Hospital Medical College, London, England.

Richard Trevor Turner-Warwick. Urologist, The Middlesex Hospital, London, England.

Alexis Littré, 1654–1725. French physician and anatomist. Described hernia and urethral mucous glands.

Treatment. An anterior urethrotomy will encourage the abscess to burst into the urethra. When the abscess lies behind a stricture, it should be opened externally.

A *bulbar periurethral abscess* is a spreading cellulitis due to infection with streptococci and anaerobic organisms. It may or may not be associated with a urethral stricture, and extravasation of urine is not unusual.

Clinical features. There is perineal pain with pyrexia, rigors and a rapid pulse rate. Tenderness and swelling rapidly spread from the perineum to the penis and the anterior abdominal wall.

Treatment. Appropriate antibiotics are essential. Collections of pus should be drained and the urethra should be defunctioned by inserting a suprapubic urinary catheter.

A *chronic periurethral abscess* sometimes results from a long-standing urethral stricture (Fig. 67.17). The multiple loculi of pus should be drained and the stricture treated appropriately. Urethral fistula may occur either spontaneously or as a result of incision of the abscess.

Urethral fistula. The most frequent cause of urethral fistula is bursting or incision of a periurethral abscess. If the fistulae arise behind a tight stricture, there may be multiple openings (watering-can perineum). A fistula can also follow urethroplasty if there is necrosis of part of the graft.

Treatment. If the stricture is cured, some fistulae heal themselves. Occasionally urethroplasty is indicated.

Urethral calculi. Urethral calculi can arise primarily behind a stricture or in an infected urethral diverticulum. More commonly, the stone is a renal calculus which has migrated to the urethra via the bladder.

Clinical features. Migratory calculi cause sudden pain in the urethra soon after an attack of ureteric colic. There is blockage to the flow of urine and, if the stone is small, the force of the jet will expel it from the external urethral meatus. Larger stones become stuck and have to be removed endoscopically. It is sometimes possible to feel the calculus as a hard lump in the urethra, but if there is doubt the diagnosis is confirmed by urethroscopy.

A stone formed within the urethra is less likely to cause recognisable symptoms and is usually detected during urethroscopy or bouginage.

Treatment. A stone in the *prostatic urethra* is displaced back into the bladder and treated by lithopaxy or suprapubic cystotomy as if it were a bladder stone. Calculi in more distal parts of the urethra are removed by basketing under vision or fragmented *in situ* using the electrohydraulic or ultrasonic lithotriptor. It may be necessary to perform a meatotomy to deliver the stone. Open removal by external urethrotomy is rarely necessary.

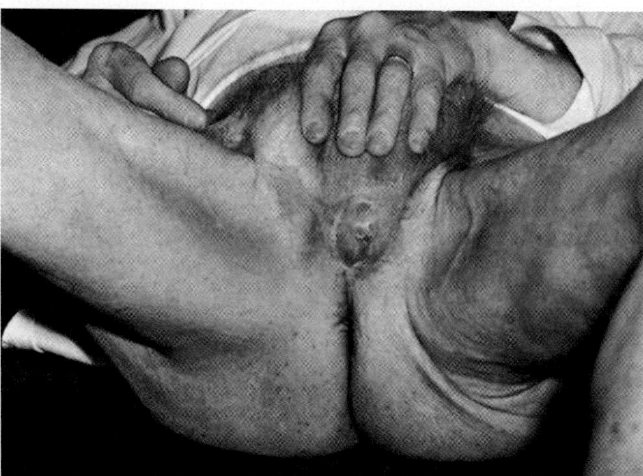

Fig. 67.17 Chronic periurethral abscess.

Neoplasms

Polyps are a relatively common finding in the prostatic urethra where they may result from chronic infection.

Genital warts acquired by sexually transmitted infection are sometimes found in the anterior urethra as an extension of warts on the skin of the glans penis.

Angioma of the urethra is a very rare cause of urethral bleeding.

Carcinoma of the urethra is relatively rare. Multifocal transitional cell cancers of the bladder are sometimes associated with tumours in the prostatic urethra and occasionally more distally. Although these tumours are usually superficial and can be destroyed locally by diathermy or laser, they seem to be associated with a tendency to distant spread. Squamous carcinoma can develop in an area of squamous metaplasia sometimes seen downstream of a urethral stricture. It carries a poor prognosis even if the patient is treated by radical surgery. A bloody discharge from the urethra in the absence of infection should raise the suspicion that the patient has a urethral tumour.

The female urethra

Abnormalities of the female urethra include:

- prolapse;
- stricture;
- diverticulum;
- caruncle;
- carcinoma.

Prolapse. Prolapse occurs in later life and is usually symptomless. Prolapse of the urethral lining also occurs as a congenital abnormality when it causes discomfort proportional to the degree of prolapse.

Stricture. This is uncommon in women but it may follow urethritis or, more commonly, the trauma of a difficult labour. Urinary retention, usually chronic, is an occasional result. True urethral strictures in women respond well to dilatation and should not be confused with a spasm of the urethral muscle of obscure cause which sometimes causes retention in women, particularly after they have had unrelated surgery. The condition, which was described by Fowler and Kirby, is associated with an abnormal myotonic discharge in the urethral sphincter which can be detected on an electromyogram. The patients remain in retention after urethral dilatation and many of them require intermittent self-catheterisation for life.

Diverticulum (syn. urethrocele). Diverticulum is more common in women than men. Some seem to be congenital. Others are acquired by rupture of a distended urethral gland or injury of the urethra during childbirth. Urine within the diverticulum becomes infected causing local pain and repeated bouts of cystitis. Purulent urine is discharged if the urethra is compressed with a finger placed in the vagina. Excision of the diverticulum through the anterior vaginal wall is effective but care must be taken not to damage the urethral sphincter.

Carbuncle. This is common in elderly women. It presents as a soft, raspberry-like, pedunculated granulomatous mass about the size of a pea attached to the posterior urethral wall near the external meatus. It is composed of highly vascular connective tissue stroma infiltrated with pus cells.

Clinical feature. There may be frequency of micturition and pain afterwards. Occasionally there is bleeding. A urethral prolapse is less tender and is not pedunculated.

Treatment. Treatment is by excision and diathermy coagulation of the base of the stalk. The patient should be given antibiotics to treat the underlying chronic urethritis.

Clare Juliet Fowler. Uro-neurologist, The National Hospital for Neurology and Neurosurgery, London, England.

Roger S. Kirby. Urologist, St George's Hospital, London, England.

Papilloma acuminata. Papilloma acuminata are the same as the sexually transmitted warts which occur on the penis. They are treated in the same way. In female Africans, papilloma accuminata are common and may grow to such a large size during pregnancy that they obstruct labour and necessitate a Caesarian section (Bowesman).

Carcinoma of the urethra. This occurs twice as often in women as in men. Whether a caruncle can become malignant is disputed but they often occur in a similar site. Malignant swellings of the urethra feel harder than benign ones.

Treatment by radiotherapy or radical surgery is often ineffective. The overall prognosis is poor.

The penis

Phimosis

Phimosis is sometimes congenital but is much over-diagnosed. The physiological adhesions between the foreskin and the glans penis may persist until the boy is 6 years of age or more, giving the false impression that the prepuce will not retract. Rolling back the prepuce causes its inner lining to pout and the meatus comes into view. This condition should not be confused with true phimosis in small boys where there is scarring of the prepuce which will not retract without fissuring. In these cases, the aperture in the prepuce may be so tight as to cause urinary obstruction. Urinary difficulty with residual urine and back-pressure effects on the ureters and kidney is more commonly due to meatal atresia which may be masked by the prepuce. Phimosis also occurs later in life as a result of *balanitis xerotica obliterans,* a curious condition in which the normally pliant foreskin becomes thickened and will not retract. It is difficult to keep the penis clean, and there is both a problem with hygiene and an increased susceptibility to carcinoma.

Treatment is by circumcision.

Circumcision

Apparently, circumcision did not originate among the Jews: they took the practice from either the Babylonians or the Negroes, probably the latter. It had been practised in West Africa for over 5000 years.

Indications. *In infants and young boys*, circumcision is most usually performed at the request of the parents for social or religious reasons. Occasionally, there is true phimosis with recurrent attacks of balanitis. As stated above, it is normal for the prepuce to be long and adherent to the glands during the first few years of life. Recurrent balanoprosthitis and phimosis may result from misguided attempts by parents to expose the glans forcibly.

In adults, circumcision is indicated because of inability to retract for intercourse, for splitting of an abnormally tight frenulum, balanitis and sometimes prior to radiotherapy for carcinoma of the penis.

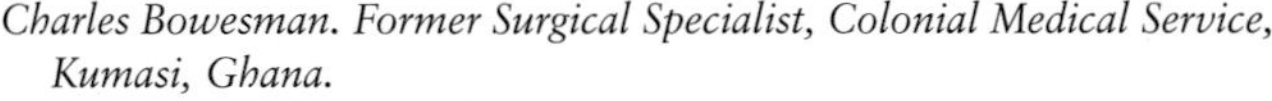

Charles Bowesman. Former Surgical Specialist, Colonial Medical Service, Kumasi, Ghana.

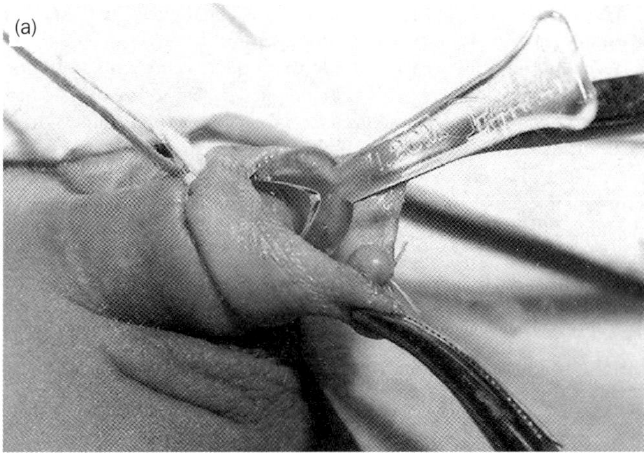

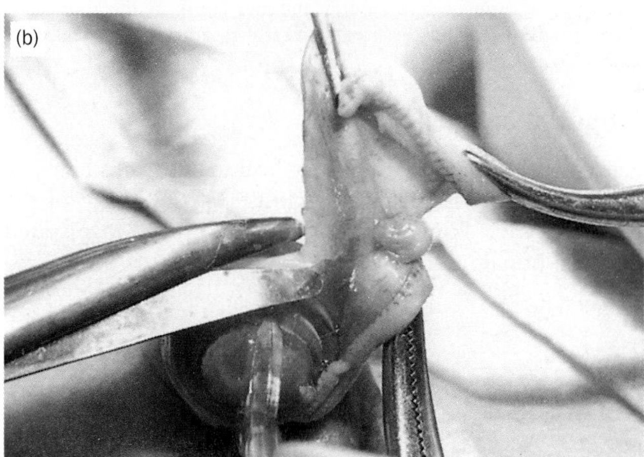

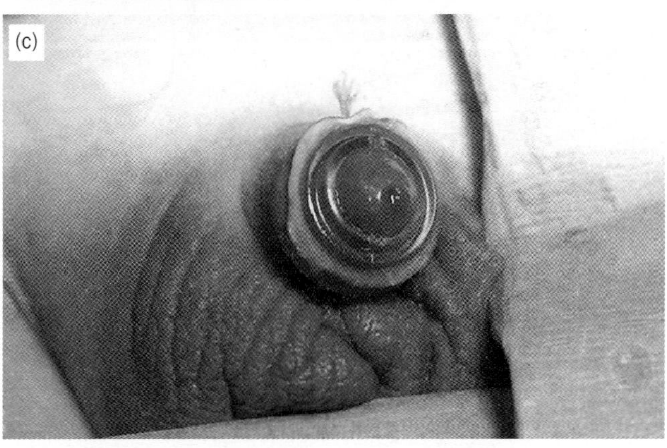

Fig. 67.18 The Plastibel (Hollister) device for circumcision in infants. (a) The foreskin is freed and retracted; (b) after the Plastibel device has been slipped into place over the glans penis, the foreskin is ligated over the groove of the bell and redundant foreskin is cut away; (c) shows the completed operation (*courtesy of Professor Asal Y. Izzidien Al-Samarrai, King Saud University, Riyadh, Saudi Arabia*).

Technique in an infant. The much advocated method of applying a clamp or bone forceps across the prepuce distal to the glans with blind division of the foreskin can no longer be condoned. To see one little boy with partial or total amputation of the glans is enough to realise the folly of this technique. It is far better to perform a proper circumcision under direct vision as in an adult.

The Plastibel (Hollister) is used as shown in Fig. 67.18: the ring separates between 5 and 8 days postoperatively.

Technique in adolescents and adults. In adolescents and adults the following method is preferable. The prepuce is held in haemostats and put on a gentle stretch. A circumferential incision in the penile skin is made at the level of the corona using a knife. The prepuce is then slit up the midline dorsally to within 1 cm of the corona. This converts the foreskin into two flaps connected at the midline anteriorly. When the undersurface of the prepuce has been separated from the glans, the inner layer of each flap is incised with a second circumferential incision leaving about 5 mm of the inner layer of the prepuce distal to the corona. Cutting the remaining connective tissue completes the excision (Fig. 67.19). Monopolar diathermy should be avoided in operations on the penis in small boys because there is a danger that the small current path will cause coagulation at the base of the penis. Haemostasis is important in circumcision, however, and should be secured by bipolar diathermy or ligated with catgut. The cut edges are approximated using catgut sutures and the layers in the immediate region of the frenulum are brought neatly together using a mattress suture (Fig. 67.20).

Preputial calculi

Late in life, chronic posthitis may lead to adhesions between the prepuce and the glans and closure of the orifice of the preputial sac. Preputial calculi result from inspissated smegma, urinary salts or both.

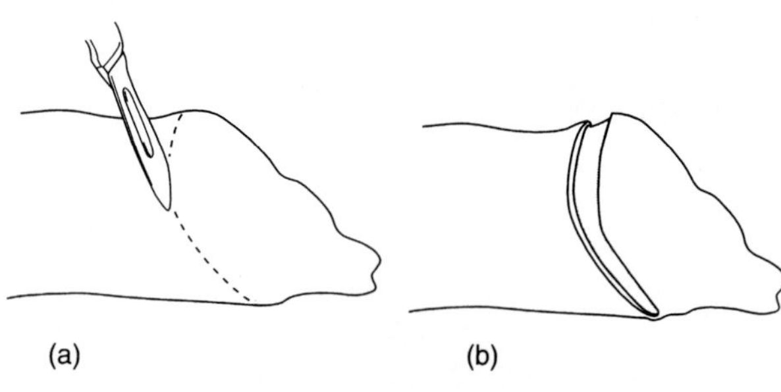

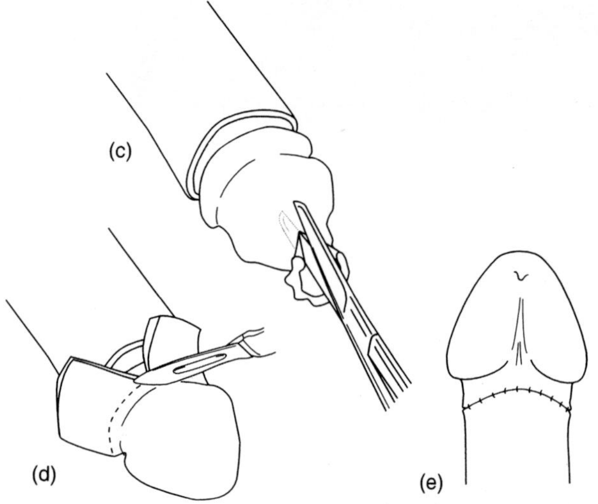

Fig. 67.19 Stages in a circumcision.

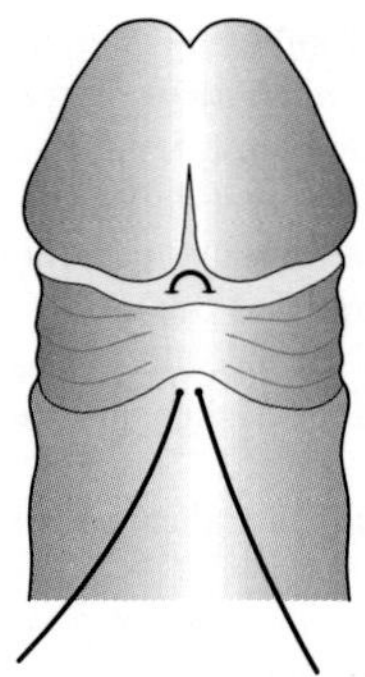

Fig. 67.20 The 'four in one' frenal stitch.

Injuries

Avulsion of the skin of the penis

Entanglement of clothing in rotating machinery is the usual cause. Repair is effected by burying the shaft of the penis in the scrotum (Fig. 67.21) with subsequent release at the time of a definitive plastic surgical repair. The prepuce is also at risk in the zip fastening of the trouser fly.

Fracture of the penis

Fracture of the penis is an uncommon accident usually occurring when the erect penis is bent violently downwards during over-enthusiastic intercourse. The extravasation of blood causes great pain and swelling. In early cases, incision and drainage of the clot with suture of the defect in the tunica of the ruptured corpus cavernosum give acceptable results.

Strangulation of the penis

Strangulation of the penis by rings placed on the penis, usually for sexual reasons, can cause venous engorgement which prevents their removal. It may help to aspirate the corpora cavernosa but often the ring must be cut off with a ring cutter or hacksaw.

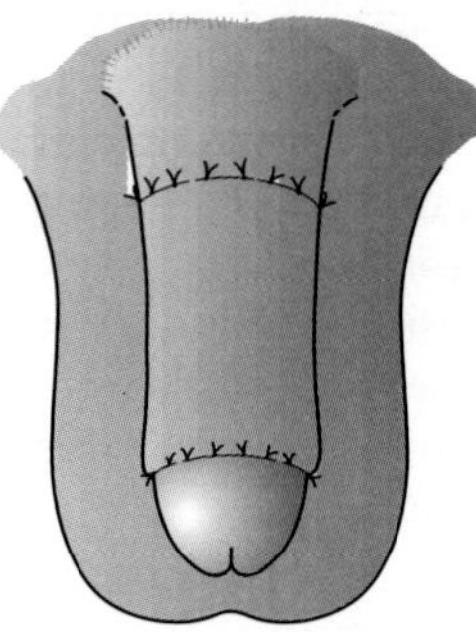

Fig. 67.21 Covering the denuded shaft of the penis by burying it in a scrotal tunnel.

Paraphimosis

When the tight foreskin is retracted, it may sometimes be difficult to return and a paraphimosis results. In this condition, the venous and lymphatic return from the glans and distal foreskin is obstructed and these structure swell alarmingly causing even more pressure within the obstructing ring of prepuce. Icebags, gentle manual compression and injection of a solution of hyaluronidase in normal saline may help to reduce the swelling. Such patients can be treated by circumcision if careful manipulation fails. A dorsal slit of the prepuce under local anaesthetic may be enough in an emergency.

Inflammations

Balanoposthitis

Inflammation of the prepuce is known as posthitis; inflammation of the glans is balanitis. The opposing surfaces of the two structures are often involved – hence the term balanoposthitis. Skin conditions such as lichen planus and psoriasis affect the penis and may indeed be localised there. Drug hypersensitivity reactions can affect the skin of the penis.

In mild cases, the only symptom is itching and some discharge. In more severe inflammation, the glans and foreskin are red-raw and pus exudes. Balanoposthitis is associated with penile cancer, diabetes and phimosis. Monilial infections are quite common under the prepuce.

Treatment is by broad-spectrum antibiotics and local hygienic measures.

Genital herpes

Genital herpes is caused by sexual transmission of the herpes virus hominis HPV (human papilloma virus type 2 – occasionally type 1). Recurrent attacks occur in 50 per cent or more. Pain along the distribution of the sensory nerve, usually genitofemoral, precedes the eruption by 2 days and may be particularly severe around the anus. A group of tiny vesicles rapidly erodes to form shallow yellow- or red-based ulcers. In females the ulcers often spread on to the thighs during the attack. Involvement of the urethra may cause retention of urine which may persist for up to 14 days if there is radiculitis of the S2 and S3 nerve roots. Acyclovir has been shown to be effective in treating genital herpes but it does not prevent recurrences.

A child born to a mother with active infection is liable to a fatal generalised herpes in the neonatal period. Caesarean section should be considered in these circumstances. There is an increased risk of carcinoma of the cervix and annual cytology for life is recommended.

Lymphogranuloma venereum

Lymphogranuloma venereum is a sexually transmitted tropical disease caused by *Clamydia trachomatis* (*Chlamydia A*) types L1–L3. The primary lesion is a fleeting, painless, genital papule or ulcer often unnoticed by the patient.

The inguinal glands become enlarged and painful in both sexes between 2 weeks and 4 months from infection. The masses of nodes mat together above and below the inguinal ligament to give the 'sign of the groove'. The overlying skin reddens and there may be fluctuation. In women, there may be a proctitis which can go on to produce a rectal stricture if untreated. Lymphatic obstruction leads to lymphoedema in the perineum and occasionally the lower limbs. Urethritis and urethral stricture occur in the male.

Confirmation is by isolating *Chlamydia A* from the lesion and by immunological tests to detect antibodies against the organism.

Treatment is by a combination of antibiotics which may include sulphonamide, oxytetracycline and erythromycin. The multilocular bubo should not be incised – aspiration is permissible to reduce discomfort.

Granuloma inguinale

This is a chronic and slowly progressive ulcerative tropical disease affecting the genitals and surrounding tissue but occasionally occurring elsewhere in the body. It is usually sexually transmitted and is most common among socially deprived people. The incubation period varies greatly but is frequently 7–30 days.

Clinical course

A painless vesicle or indurated papule usually on the external genitals but occasionally elsewhere on the skin gradually erodes into a slowly extending ulcer with a beefy red, granulomatous base. More chronic lesions may become greyish especially at the edges where, after months or years, malignant change may develop. The ulcerated area may bleed, if touched, but is surprisingly painless. Without treatment healing is only partial and keloid is common.

Diagnosis is by microscopy of material from the edges of the ulcer which shows the presence of short Gram-negative rods within the cytoplasm of the large mononuclear cells – Donovan bodies.

Treatment is by oxytetracycline, streptomycin or co-trimoxazole.

Condylomata acuminata (syn. genital warts)

Genital warts are caused by infection with human papilloma virus and are sexually transmitted. Ordinary skin warts can occur on the genitals by direct contact with a finger lesion but they are less moist, soft and less often pedunculated than the genital variety. The lesions most commonly occur under the prepuce in the coronal sulcus but may be found elsewhere, including inside the urinary meatus (Fig. 67.22). In women, genital warts are most commonly found on the vulva but they may line the vagina and occur on the cervix. Perianal warts are common.

Other associated sexually transmitted disease should be excluded – candidiasis and trichomonas mainly in women, and in men, syphilis or gonorrhoea. Genital warts may complicate human immunodeficiency virus (HIV) infection.

Treatment is by chemical or physical means. Podopyllin 25 per cent in spirit is often effective as a topical application. It is applied to the wart with great care to avoid the surrounding skin and washed off after 6 hours or so.

Charles Donovan, 1863–1951. Irish surgeon.

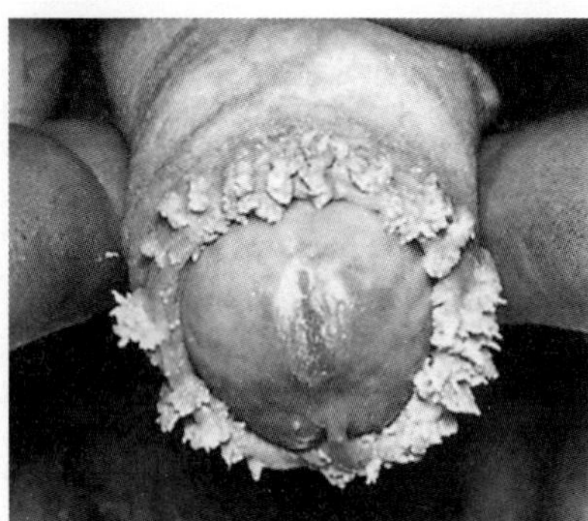

Fig. 67.22 Penile warts.

If chemical methods fail, the warts can be excised or they can be ablated with cryosurgery, electrosurgery or laser. Circumcision is sometimes advised if there are florid lesions under the foreskin.

Other abnormalities

Chordee. Chordee (French = corded) is a fixed bowing of the penis due to hypospadias or, more rarely, chronic urethritis. Erection is deformed and sexual intercourse may be impossible. Treatment is usually surgical.

Peyronie's disease. Peyronie's disease is a relatively common cause of deformity of the erect penis. On examination, hard plaques of fibrosis can be palpated in the tunica of one or both corpora cavenosa. The plaques may be calcified (Fig. 67.23). The presence of the unyielding plaque tissue within the normally elastic wall of the corpus cavernosum causes the erect penis to bend, often dramatically, towards the side of the plaque. The aetiology is uncertain, but it may be a result of past trauma – there is an association with Dupuytren's contracture (see Chapter 30).

Treatment is difficult. Some cases continue to progress. Others seem to remit after 3–5 years. Various drug treatments have been suggested but their beneficial effect is hard to prove in such a chronic condition. When the deformity of the penis is causing distress, it may be possible to straighten it by placing nonabsorbable sutures in the corpus cavernosum opposite the plaque. This reduces the elasticity in this region to balance that caused by the plaque (Nesbitt's operation).

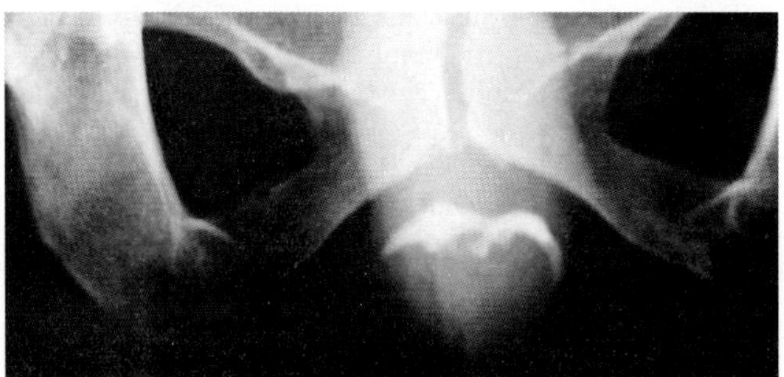

Fig. 67.23 Penile calcification in Peyronie's disease (*courtesy of Dr S.S. Rawat, Riyadh, Saudi Arabia*).

Persistent priapism. The penis remains erect and becomes painful. This is a pathological erection and the glans penis and the corpus spongiosum are not involved. The condition is usually seen as a complication of a blood disorder such as sickle cell disease or leukaemia. However, it can sometimes follow therapeutic injection of papaverine or even an abnormally prolonged bout of otherwise normal sexual activity. A tiny proportion is due to malignant disease in the corpora cavernosa or the pelvis. Priapism is rarely seen as a consequence of spinal cord disease.

Treatment. An underlying cause should be excluded. The patient should be referred for specialist urological care. If aspiration of the sludged blood in the corpora cavernosa fails to cause detumescence, and injection of metaraminol or 1:100 000 adrenaline solution is ineffective, it may be necessary to decompress the penis by an anastomosis between the corpus spongiosum and one of the corpora cavernosa. The outlook for normal erectile function is poor.

Carcinoma

Aetiology

Circumcision soon after birth confers almost complete immunity against carcinoma of the penis. Later circumcision does not seem to have the same effect and Moslems circumcised between the ages of 4 and 9 years are still liable to the disease. Chronic balanoposthitis in known to be a contributory factor and there are definite precarcinomatous states:

- *leucoplakia of the glans* is similar to the condition seen on the tongue;
- long-standing *genital warts* may rarely be the site of malignant change;
- *Paget's disease of the penis.*

Paget's disease of the penis (syn. *erythroplasia of Querat*) is 'a persistent rawness of the glans like a long-standing balanitis followed by cancer of the substance of the penis' (Sir James Paget). Treatment is by circumcision, observation and excision if the lesion does not resolve.

Pathology

Carcinoma of the penis may be flat and infiltrating or papillary (Fig. 67.24). The former often starts as leucoplakia and the latter results from an existing papilloma. Local growth continues for months or years. The earliest lymphatic spread is to the inguinal and then to the iliac nodes. Once the growth breaches the partial barrier formed by the fascial sheath of the corpora cavernosa it spreads rapidly and iliac lymph node involvement is common (Fig. 67.25). Distant metastatic deposits are infrequent.

François de la Peyronie, 1678–1747. Surgeon to Louis XIV and Founder of the Royal Academy of Surgery, Paris, France.
Baron Guillaume Dupuytren, 1777–1835. Surgeon, Hôtel Dieu, Paris, France.
Thomas Nesbitt. Urological surgeon, Nashville, Tennessee, USA.
Auguste Querat, b. 1872. Parisian dermatologist.
Sir James Paget, 1814–99. Surgeon, St Bartholomew's Hospital, London, England.

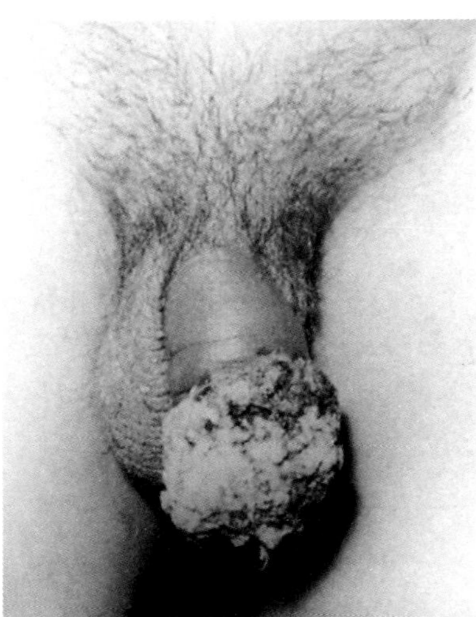

Fig. 67.24 Carcinoma of the penis (*courtesy of Dr V.K. Kapoor, All India Institute of Medical Sciences, Delhi, India*).

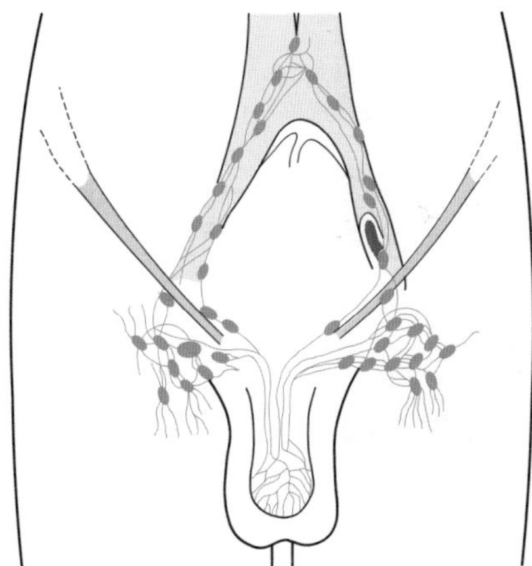

Fig. 67.25 The lymphatic drainage of the penis. Superficial lymphatics drain to the inguinal and deep lymphatics to the iliac lymph nodes (*after Archie L. Dean*).

Clinical features

Forty per cent of patients are under 40 years of age. The early symptoms of mild discomfort and light discharge are often neglected and the disease progresses slowly. By the time the patient presents, the growth is often large and secondary infection causes a foul bloody discharge. There is little or no pain.

Sixty per cent have inguinal lymph node enlargement when they present but in half this is reactive enlargement due to sepsis. In most the prepuce is nonretractile and must be split to view the lesion. A biopsy should be performed to make the diagnosis.

Untreated, the whole glans may be replaced by a fungating offensive mass. Later the inguinal nodes erode the skin of the groin and the death of the patient may be due to involvement of the femoral or external iliac artery with torrential haemorrhage.

Treatment

Radiotherapy is effective (60–70 per cent survival at 5 years) if the growth is small. Circumcision precedes treatment which may be delivered by implanted radioactive tantalum wires, external beam radiation or by means of a radioactive mould applicator applied externally to the penis.

Surgery is needed for large anaplastic growths, if there is infiltration of the shaft and when radiotherapy fails. *Partial amputation* is used for distal growths when adequate clearance of the tumour is possible. When an advanced, infiltrating or anaplasic lesion is present, *total amputation* is necessary.

Treatment of associated enlarged inguinal lymph nodes should usually be delayed until at least 3 weeks after local treatment to the primary lesion. Enlargement due to infection will usually show signs of subsiding with antibiotic treatment if necessary. Block dissection is indicated if there is persistent enlargement which needle aspiration biopsy shows to be due to tumour. The 5-year survival rate falls to 35 per cent in these cases. If surgery to the nodes is impossible, radiotherapy may cause a worthwhile temporary regression.

Buschke–Löwenstein tumour is uncommon. It has the histological pattern of a verrucous carcinoma. It is locally destructive and invasive, but appears not to spread to lymph nodes or to metastasise. Treatment is by surgical excision.

Secondary cancer of the penis is uncommon as a result of spread from a primary tumour of the bladder, rectum or prostate.

Further reading

Blandy, J.P. and Fowler, C.G. (1995) *Urology,* 2nd edn, Blackwell Scientific, Oxford.

Walsh, P.C., Retik, A.B., Darracott Vaughan, E. and Wein, A.J. (1998) *Campbell's Urology,* 7th edn, W.B. Saunders, Philadelphia, PA.

Whitfield, H.W., Hendry, W.F., Kirby, R.S. and Duckett J. (1998) *Textbook of Genito-urinary Surgery,* 2nd edn, Blackwell Science, Oxford.

Abraham Buschke, 1868–1943. Dermatologist, Berlin, Germany.
Ernst Löwenstein, b. 1878. Pathologist, Vienna, Austria.

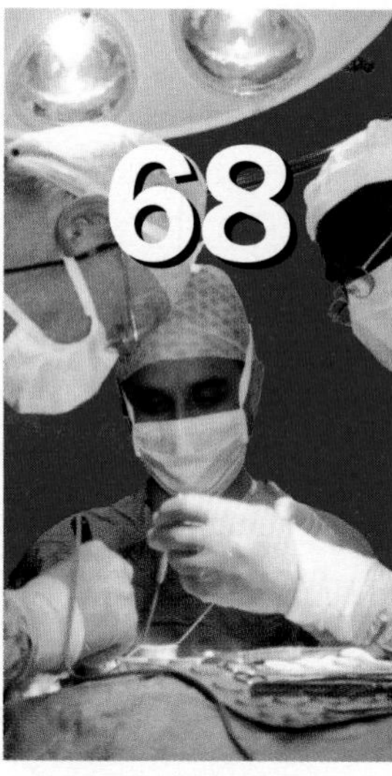

68 The testis and scrotum

Imperfect descent of the testis

Incomplete descent

The testis is arrested in some part of its path to the scrotum.

Ectopic testis

The testis is abnormally placed outside this path.

Development of the testis

The testes develop from the genital fold medial to the mesonephros (Wolffian body); in early foetal life, they lie in the retroperitoneum below the developing kidneys. The primitive testis is attached to the posterior abdominal wall by the mesorchium, a neurovascular pedicle derived from the lowermost thoracic segments. The mesonephros begins to disappear about the 10th week of intrauterine life but some of its tubules unite with the rete testis to become the vasa efferentia. The Wolffian duct becomes the epididymis and vas deferens. About the same time the precursor of the gubernaculum develops as a fold of peritoneum which can be traced from its attachment between the vas and the epididymis to the region of the developing phallus. The processus vaginalis starts as a dimple of peritoneum about the 10th week and precedes the testis in its journey through the abdominal wall down to the scrotum. The fully developed gubernaculum contains muscle fibres but there is still no certainty as to the part that it plays in testicular descent.

Maternal chorionic gonadotrophin stimulates growth of the testis and may stimulate its migration. Imperfectly developed testes tend to descend incompletely.

Kaspar Friedrich Wolff, 1733–94. Professor of Anatomy and Physiology, St Petersburg, Russia.

Bailey & Love's Short Practice of Surgery, 23rd edition. Edited by R.C.G. Russell, N.S. Williams and C.J.K. Bulstrode. Published in 2000 by Arnold Publishers.

Comparative anatomy

Most misplacements of the testis in man are seen as the normal arrangement elsewhere in the animal kingdom. The testes of the whale and the elephant are intra-abdominal throughout life. Rodents and creatures which hibernate, such as the hedgehog, the mole and the bat, have open inguinal canals. The testes descend into the scrotum ready for the breeding season.

Incompletely descended testis

Incidence

Scorer examined 2000 newborn boys. There was incomplete descent of one or both testes in 4 per cent of full-term infants and in 30 per cent of those born preterm. About 50 per cent of incompletely descended testes reached into the scrotum during the first month of life but full descent after that was uncommon. The incidence in later childhood and puberty is thus around 2 per cent. The genitals of all male infants are examined at birth but the condition is sometimes missed until the boy is examined by a school medical officer. In a few cases, the presence of a hernia, testicular pain or acute torsion directs attention to the abnormality. In an examination of 10 000 recruits during World War II, the incidence of incompletely descended testis was 0.28 per cent. In 10 per cent of unilateral cases there is a family history.

Pathology

Incompletely descended testes are often normal until the age of 6 years but by puberty the testis is flabby and poorly

Charles Gordon Scorer, 1918–85. Surgeon, Hillingdon Hospital, Uxbridge, Middlesex, England.

developed compared with its intrascrotal counterpart. Histologically the epithelial elements are grossly immature and by the age of 16 irreversible destructive changes have occurred which halt spermatogenesis and limit the production of androgens to around half of the normal output.

An incompletely descended testis brought down before puberty often develops and functions satisfactorily.

Clinical features

The condition is unilateral on the right in 50 per cent and on the left in 30 per cent. Arrested descent of both testes occurs in 20 per cent. Secondary sexual characteristics are normal but other abnormalities of the genitourinary tract may be present. The testis may be:

- *intra-abdominal*, lying extraperitoneally usually just above the internal inguinal ring;
- *in the inguinal canal,* where it may or may not be palpable. When both testes are impalpable, the condition is known as cryptorchidism (hidden testes) (Fig. 68.1);
- *in the superficial inguinal pouch*, where it must be distinguished from the much more common *retractile testis* which may be found in the same condition.

During childhood the testes are mobile and the cremasteric reflex is very active. In some boys, the least stimulation of the skin of the scrotum or thigh will result in the testis disappearing to the superficial ring or into the inguinal canal. Simply exposing the parts can have this effect so that the testis appears never to be in its proper intrascrotal position. Retractile testes should be suspected when the scrotum is normal as the scrotum is usually underdeveloped if there is true incomplete descent. After a while the cremaster relaxes and the telltale bulge of the testis reappears only to vanish when the scrotal skin is touched. A retractile testis can always be brought to the bottom of the scrotum by gently milking it from its position in the inguinal region. A diagnosis of true incomplete descent should be made only if this is not possible. In infancy, 80 per cent of inapparent testes are retractile. They are normal and require no treatment.

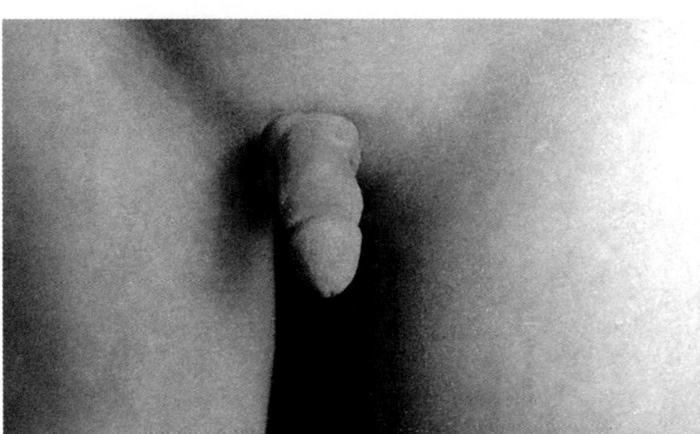

Fig. 68.1 A cryptorchid aged 12. Note the retracted underdeveloped scrotum. In cases of retractile testes, the scrotum is relatively well developed.

Hazards of incomplete descent are:

- *sterility* in bilateral cases;
- *pain* due to trauma;
- *an associated indirect inguinal hernia* that is often present and, in older patients, it is frequently the hernia which causes symptoms;
- *torsion;*
- *epididymo-orchitis* that, in an incompletely descended testis, is extremely rare but of interest because, on the right side, it mimics appendicitis;
- *atrophy* of an inguinal testis that can occur even before puberty, possibly due to recurrent minor trauma;
- *increased liability to malignant disease.* All types of malignant testicular tumour are more common in incompletely descended testes even if they have been brought down surgically. It has been estimated that the chance of a tumour is about 35 times that in a normally positioned testis. Testicular tumours are relatively rare and there are no reliable statistics as to whether orchidopexy diminishes the liability. *However, it does improve the prospect of early diagnosis.*

Surgical treatment

Operating on very small children needs the highly specialised skills of a paediatric surgeon so orchidopexy is not usually performed before the age of 2 years. Provided that safe anaesthetic services are available, however, testes should be brought down into the scrotum before the boy starts school. It is best to wait until he is dry because it is less easy to manage the inguinal wound if the child is wearing nappies. In cryptorchidism it is usual to operate on one side at a time.

Orchidopexy

Orchidopexy (syn. orchiopexy) consists firstly, of mobilisation of the testis and spermatic cord and secondly, retaining the testis in the scrotum. The operation is performed through a short groin incision over the deep inguinal ring. The inguinal canal is exposed by division of the external oblique aponeurosis in the direction of its fibres.

Mobilisation begins with isolation of the indirect inguinal hernial sac which is almost invariably present lying anterior to the cord. The sac is diaphanous and fragile but, with care, it can be swept laterally to reveal filmy fibrous strands which join the neck of the sac to the cord. The fibrous bands are divided and the spermatic vessels are dissected free of the peritoneum to which they are adherent until there is sufficient length of liberated cord to place the testis in the scrotum *without tension.* Division of the cremaster and the coverings of the cord may give a little more length but there is a risk of damage to the tiny vas and testicular artery. The empty half of the scrotum is stretched with a finger passed into it through the inguinal incision to give enough room for the testis.

Retaining the testis in the scrotum can be achieved by a number of means. In some cases it is enough simply to anchor it to the fundus of the scrotum with an absorbable suture. More commonly the testis is placed in a pouch constructed between the dartos muscle and the skin (Fig. 68.2). An alternative to the *dartos pouch* is to take the testis through the scrotal septum (*Ombrédan's operation*).

Louis Ombrédan, 1871–1956. Surgeon, Hôpital des Enfants Malades, Paris, France.

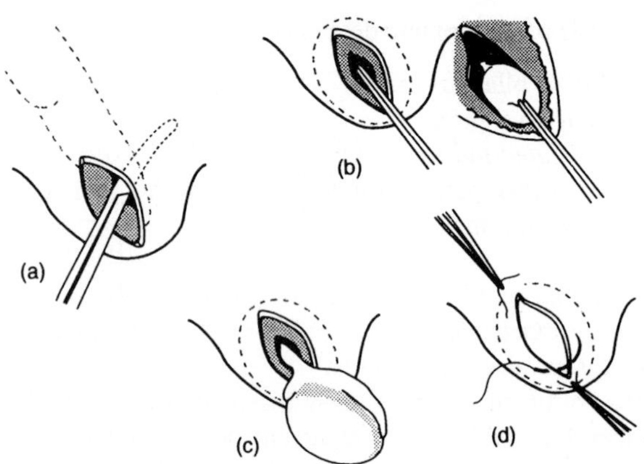

Fig. 68.2 The testis is mobilised and retained in a pouch constructed between the dartos muscle and the skin.

Failure to bring the testis down

Sometimes a two-stage procedure is successful: the testis is mobilised as far as possible and anchored with a suture. The mobilisation is completed 6 months later. *Orchidectomy* should be considered if the other testis is normal, especially if the incompletely descended testis is hopelessly atrophic or the patient is past puberty.

Hormone treatment with human chorionic gonadotrophin is only appropriate when there is established hypogonadism.

Ectopic testis

The sites of ectopic testis are:

- at the superficial inguinal ring;
- in the perineum;
- at the root of the penis;
- in the femoral triangle.

An ectopic testis is usually fully developed. Its main hazard is a liability to injury.

Injuries to the testis

Rupture by a blow is uncommon because of its mobility within the scrotum. Both severe contusion and rupture are associated with a collection of blood around the testis and cannot usually be demonstrated without exploration. The haematocele should be drained and the tunica albuginea repaired after evacuation of haematoma. A very severely damaged testis may have to be removed.

Haematocele. See Fig. 68.3.

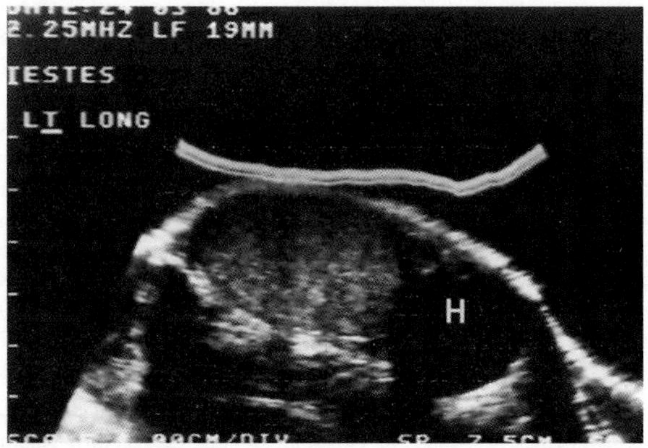

Fig. 68.3 Longitudinal scan of testicle with haematocele (H) at lower pole.

Traumatic displacement occasionally follows a blow. The displaced testis usually lies in one of the sites of ectopic testis and can be returned to its normal position by manipulation before it becomes anchored by fibrosis.

Torsion of the testis

Predisposing causes

Torsion of the testis (syn. torsion of the spermatic cord) is uncommon because the normal fully descended testis is well anchored and cannot rotate. For torsion to occur one of several abnormalities must be present.

- **Inversion of the testis** is the most common predisposing cause. The testis is rotated so that it lies transversely or upside down.
- **High investment of the tunica vaginalis** causes the testis to hang within the tunica like a clapper in a bell (Fig. 68.4). Very occasionally, torsion occurs outside the tunica vaginalis.
- **Separation of the epididymis** from the body of the testis permits torsion of the testis without involving the cord. The twisting is confined to the pedicle which connects the testis with the epididymis (Fig. 68.5).

Normally, when there is a violent contraction of the abdominal muscles, the cremaster contracts as well. The spiral attachment of the cremaster favours rotation around the vertical axis when this is made possible by one of the abnormalities described above. Straining at stool, lifting a heavy weight and coitus are all possible precipitating factors. Alternatively, torsion may develop spontaneously during sleep.

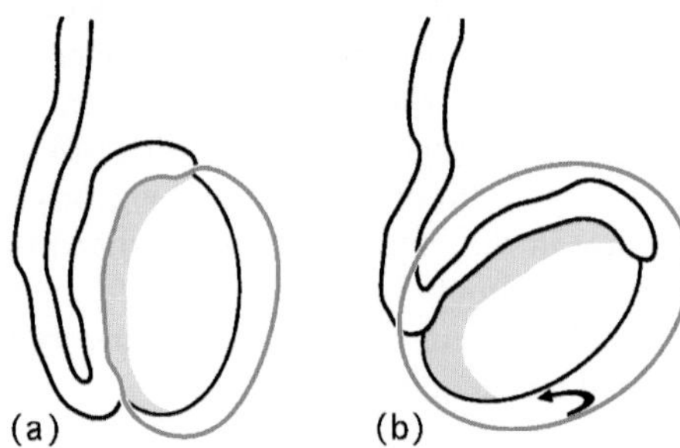

Fig. 68.4 Testicular torsion. (a) Normal attachment; (b) an abnormally high attachment of the tunica vaginalis predisposes to torsion – the 'bell-clapper'.

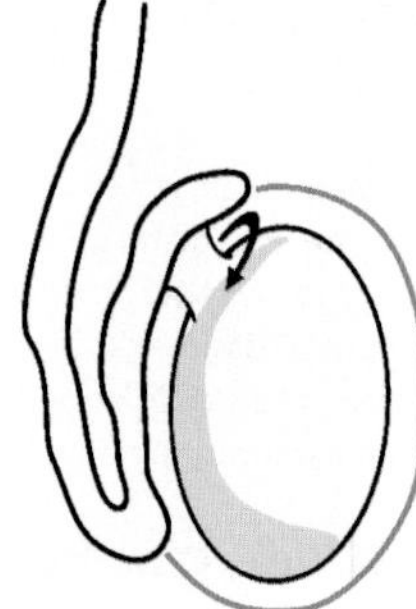

Fig. 68.5 Testicular torsion. Separation of the testis from the epididymis – torsion about the pedicle between them.

Clinical features

Testicular torsion is most common between 10 and 25 years of age and a few cases occur in infancy. Symptoms vary with the degree of torsion. Most commonly there is sudden agonising pain in the groin and the lower abdomen. The patient vomits.

Torsion of a fully descended testis is usually easy to recognise by the high lie of the testis and thickening of the tender twisted cord which can be palpated above it. In mumps orchitis the cord is not particularly thickened. The onset of redness of the skin after 6 hours or so and the onset of a mild pyrexia may cause confusion with epididymo-orchitis in the older patient but there will usually be an associated urethritis. Elevation of the testis reduces the pain of epididymo-orchitis and makes it worse in torsion. Very occasionally, the condition can be convincingly mimicked by a small tense strangulated inguinal hernia compressing the cord and causing compression of the pampiniform plexus. *If there is any doubt about the diagnosis*, the scrotum should be explored without delay.

It is almost impossible to distinguish *torsion of an imperfectly descended testis* until the parts are exposed at operation. An empty oedematous hemiscrotum on the side suggests that a tender lump at the external inguinal ring is a torted testis.

Treatment

In the first hour or so it may be possible to untwist the testis by gentle manipulation. If manipulation is successful pain subsides and the testis is out of danger. However, arrangements should be made for early operative fixation to avoid recurrent torsion.

Exploration for testicular torsion can be performed through a scrotal incision. If the testis is clearly viable when the cord is untwisted, it should be prevented from twisting again by fixation by nonabsorbable sutures between the tunica vaginalis and the tunica albuginea. The opposite testis should also be fixed because the anatomical variation responsible for the torsion is likely to be bilateral. A totally infarcted testis should be removed – the patient can be counselled later about a prosthetic replacement if this is appropriate. If it is clear that there has been an established torsion for several days it will not be possible to recover the testis and little is gained by exploration. The affected testis will become woody-hard and atrophy to a fibrous nodule. The other testis should be fixed at an early date.

Torsion of a testicular appendage is sometimes mistaken for acute epididymo-orchitis and cannot be distinguished with certainty from testicular torsion. The most common structure to twist is the appendix of the testis (the pedunculated hydatid of Morgagni) but other vestigial structures related to the testis and epididymis may also rotate. Immediate operation with ligation and amputation of the twisted appendage cures the condition.

Giovanni Battista Morgagni, 1682–1771. Professor of Anatomy, Padua, Italy. Held chair for 56 years and is regarded as the founder of pathological anatomy.

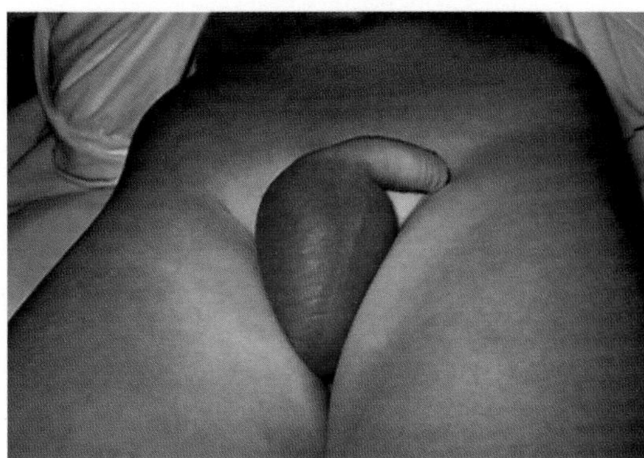

Fig. 68.6 Oedema of the scrotum.

Idiopathic scrotal oedema is a curious condition which occurs between the age of 4 and 12 years and has to be differentiated from torsion. The scrotum is very swollen but there is very little pain or tenderness. The swelling may extend into the perineum, groin and penis. It is thought to be an allergic phenomenon – occasionally there is eosinophilia. The swelling subsides after a day or so but may recur (Fig. 68.6).

Varicocele

A varicocele is a varicose dilatation of the veins draining the testis.

Surgical anatomy. The veins draining the testis and the epididymis form a bulky plexus called the pampiniform plexus. The veins become fewer as they traverse the inguinal canal and at or near the inguinal ring they join to form one or two testicular veins which pass upwards behind the peritoneum. The left testicular vein empties into the left renal vein, the right into the inferior vena cava below the right renal vein. The testicular veins may have valves near their terminations but these are often absent. There is an alternative (collateral) venous return from the testes through the cremasteric veins which drain mainly into the inferior epigastrics.

Aetiology

Most varicoceles are noticed in adolescence or early adulthood. The left side is affected in 95 per cent. In many cases the dilated vessels are cremasteric veins and not part of the pampiniform plexus.

Obstruction of the left testicular vein by a renal tumour or after nephrectomy is an occasional cause of varicocele in middle life and after. *Characteristically the varicocele does not decompress in the supine position.*

Clinical features

Varicocele is more frequent and more troublesome in hot climates: in all parts of the world, tall, thin men with pendulous scrota are frequently affected, whereas short, fat individuals are seldom so. Varicocele does not usually cause symptoms but there may be a vague and annoying dragging discomfort which is worse if the testis is unsupported by underwear. The scrotum on the affected side hangs lower than normal (Fig. 68.7) and on palpation, with the patient standing, the varicose plexus feels like a bag of worms. There may be a cough

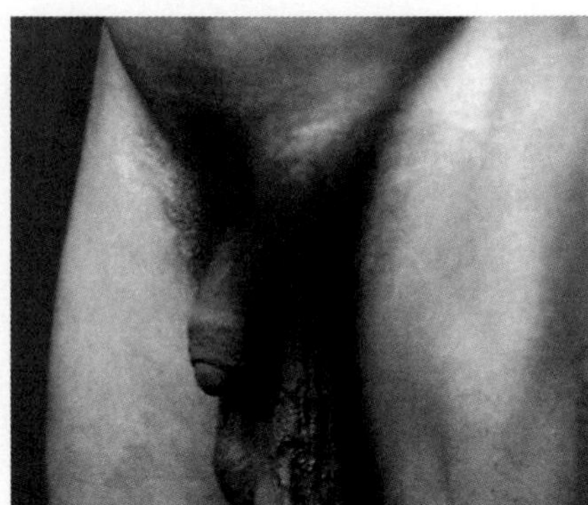

Fig. 68.7 Large varicocele in a pendulous scrotum. Note the left inguinal hernia.

impulse. If the patient lies down the veins empty by gravity and this provides an opportunity to ensure that the underlying testis is normal to palpation. In long-standing cases the affected testis is smaller and softer than its fellow owing to a minor degree of atrophy. It has been said that varicocele causes infertility but statistical evidence supporting the claim is lacking.

Varicocele and spermatogenesis

Of all the possible causes of primary infertility, oligospermia is one of the most difficult to treat. Because varicocele is relatively common, some of those with oligospermia have a varicocele and it is tempting to blame this for the infertility. It is suggested that the presence of the unilateral varicocele somehow interferes with the normal temperature control of the scrotum which keeps the testes at some 2.5°C below rectal temperature. Unfortunately, there is little evidence that varicocelectomy improves semen quality or the rate of conception.

Treatment

Operation is not indicated for varicocele unless it is causing symptoms. The simplest procedure is ligation of the testicular vein above the inguinal ligament where the pampiniform plexus has coalesced into one or two vessels. Recently this operation has been done laparoscopically. Because of the presence of plentiful potential collateral veins, recurrence is common after all types of surgery for varicocele.

Hydrocele

A hydrocele is an abnormal collection of serous fluid in some part of the processus vaginalis, usually the tunica. Four types of congenital hydrocele are encountered (Fig. 68.8). Acquired hydroceles are primary or idiopathic, or secondary to testicular disease.

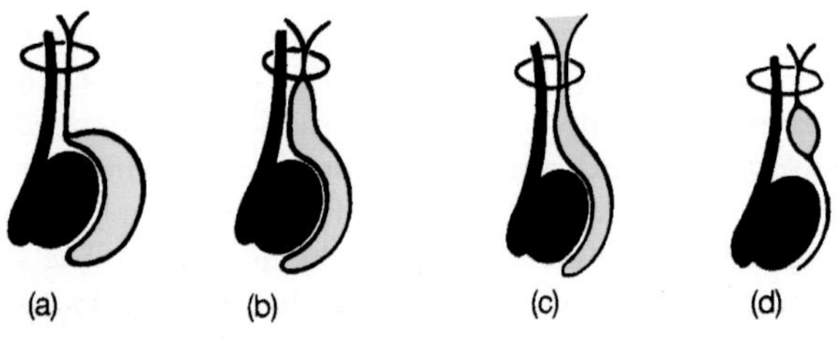

Fig. 68.8 (a) Vaginal hydrocele (very common); (b) 'infantile' hydrocele (unusual); (c) congenital hydrocele; (d) hydrocele of the cord.

Aetiology

A hydrocele can be produced in four ways:

- by excessive production of fluid within the sac, e.g. secondary hydrocele;
- by defective absorption of fluid. This appears to be the explanation for most primary hydroceles although the reason why the fluid is not absorbed is obscure;
- by interference with lymphatic drainage of scrotal structures;
- by connection with a hernia of the peritoneal cavity in the congenital variety.

Hydrocele fluid is amber coloured and sterile, and contains albumin and fibrinogen. If the contents of a hydrocele are allowed to drain into a collecting vessel, the liquid does not clot, but the fluid coagulates if it is mixed with even a small quantity of blood that has been in contact with damaged tissue. In long-standing cases, hydrocele fluid is sometimes opalescent with cholesterol and may occasionally contain crystals of tyrosine.

Clinical features

Hydroceles are almost invariably translucent and it is possible to 'get above the swelling' on examination of the scrotum.

Primary vaginal hydrocele

Primary vaginal hydrocele is most common in middle and later life but can also occur in early childhood. The condition is particularly common in hot countries. Because the swelling is usually painless it may reach a prodigious size before the man presents for treatment. The testis may be palpable within a lax hydrocele but an ultrasound may be necessary to visualise the testis if the hydrocele sac is tense. *Be wary of an acute hydrocele in a young man; there may be a testicular tumour* (Fig. 68.9).

About 5 per cent of inguinal hernias are associated with a vaginal hydrocele on the same side[1].

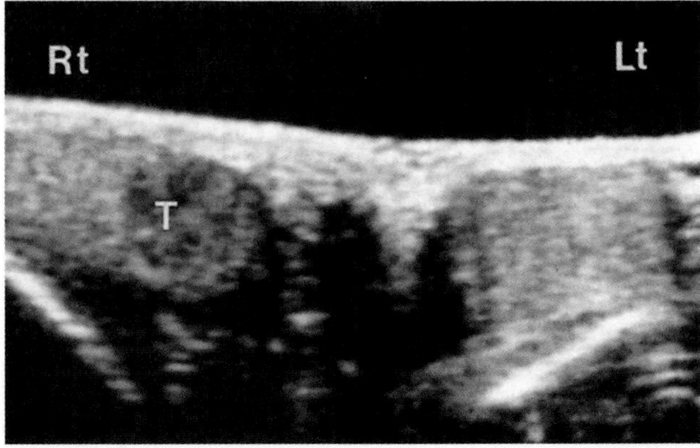

Fig. 68.9 Transverse ultrasound scan shows both testes. There is a small well-defined mass in the right testis which is a testicular teratoma.

[1]*Edward Gibbon, 1737–94, the English historian, who is best known for his 'History of the Decline and Fall of the Roman Empire' was greatly embarrassed by a large hydrocele. The second time it was tapped the hydrocele became infected and Gibbon died a few days later. There was a large associated scrotal hernia which was probably punctured.*

Infantile hydrocele

Infantile hydrocele does not necessarily appear in infants. The tunica and processus vaginalis are distended to the inguinal ring but there is no connection with the peritoneal cavity.

Congenital hydrocele

The processus vaginalis is patent and connects with the general peritoneal cavity. The communication is usually too small to allow herniation of intra-abdominal contents. Digital pressure on the hydrocele does not usually empty it but the hydrocele fluid may drain into the peritoneal cavity when the child is lying down. Ascites or even ascitic tuberculous peritonitis should be considered if the swellings are bilateral.

Encysted hydrocele of the cord

There is a smooth oval swelling near the spermatic cord which is liable to be mistaken for an inguinal hernia. The swelling moves downwards and becomes less mobile if the testis is pulled gently downwards.

Hydrocele of the canal of Nuck is a similar condition. It occurs in females and the cyst lies in relation to the round ligament. Unlike a hydrocele of the cord, a hydrocele of the canal of Nuck is always at least partially within the inguinal canal.

Complications of hydrocele

- **Rupture** usually occurs as a result of trauma but may be spontaneous. On rare occasions cure results after the fluid has been absorbed.
- **Herniation of the hydrocele sac** through the dartos muscle sometimes occurs in long-standing cases.
- **Transformation into a haematocele** occurs if there is spontaneous bleeding into the sac or as a result of trauma.
- The sac may calcify.

Treatment

A variety of surgical procedures is available. Congenital hydroceles are a special form of indirect inguinal hernia and are treated by herniotomy. The thin sac of an infantile hydrocele should be excised.

Established acquired hydroceles often have thickened walls. Unless great care is taken to stop bleeding after subtotal excision of the wall, haemorrhage from the cut edge is liable to cause a large scrotal haematoma, even if the wound is drained. *Lord's operation* is suitable when the sac is reasonably thin-walled (Fig. 68.10). There is minimal dissection and the risk of haematoma is reduced. Evertion of the sac with placement of the testis in a pouch prepared by blunt dissection in the fascial planes of the scrotum is an alternative (*Jaboulay's procedure*) (Fig. 68.11).

Drainage of the hydrocele fluid through a cannula is simple but the condition always recurs within a week or so. It may be suitable for very elderly infirm men who are unfit even for scrotal surgery under regional anaesthesia. Injection of sclerosants such as tetracycline is sometimes effective but tends to be very painful.

Secondary hydrocele is most frequently associated with acute or chronic epididymo-ochitis. It is also seen with torsion of the testis and with some testicular tumours. A secondary hydrocele is usually lax and of moderate size: the underlying testis is palpable. If a tumour is suspected, the hydrocele should not be punctured for fear of implantation of malignant cells in the needle track. A secondary hydrocele subsides when the primary lesion resolves.

Anton Nuck, 1650–92. Professor of Anatomy and Medicine, Leiden, The Netherlands.
Jaboulay, 1860–1913. Surgeon of Lyons.
Peter Lord. High Wycombe, England.

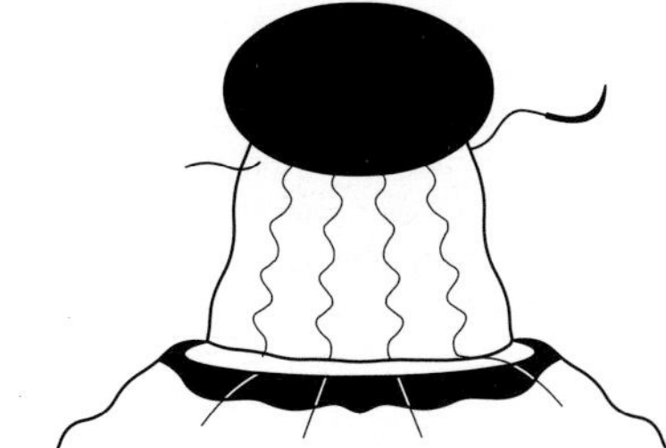

Fig. 68.10 Lord's operation. A series of interrupted absorbable sutures is used to plicate the redundant tunica vaginalis. When these are tied the tunica is bunched into a 'ruff' at its attachment to the testis.

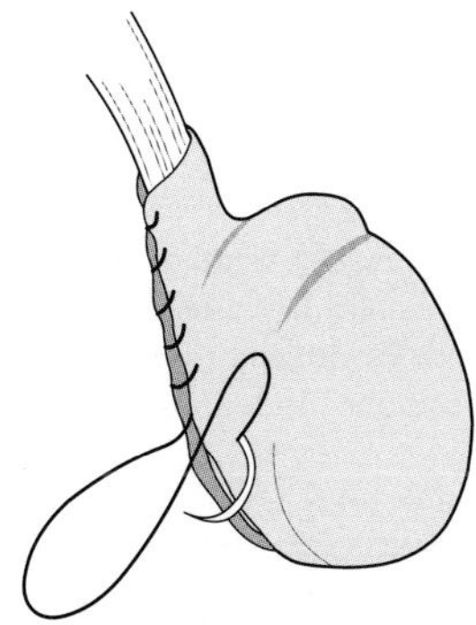

Fig. 68.11 Jaboulay's procedure. The hydrocele sac is everted and the opening snugged around the cord with sutures.

Postherniorrhaphy hydrocele

Postherniorrhaphy hydrocele is a relatively rare complication of inguinal hernia repair. It is possibly due to interruption to the lymphatics draining the scrotal contents.

Hydrocele of a hernial sac

Hydrocele of a hernial sac occurs when the neck is plugged with omentum or occluded by adhesions.

Filarial hydroceles and chyloceles

Filarial hydroceles and chyloceles account for up to 80 per cent of hydroceles in some tropical countries where the parasite is endemic. Filarial hydroceles follow repeated attacks of filarial epididymo-orchitis. They vary in size and may develop slowly or very rapidly. Occasionally the fluid contains liquid fat which is rich in cholesterol. This is due to rupture of a lymphatic varix with discharge of chyle into the hydrocele. Adult worms of the *Wuchereria bancrofti* have been found in the epididymis removed at operation or at necropsy. In long-standing chyloceles, there are dense adhesions between the scrotum and its contents. Filarial elephantiasis supervenes in a small number of cases.

Treatment is by rest and aspiration. The more usual chronic cases are treated by excision of the sac.

Haematocele

Haematocele usually results from damage to a small vessel during tapping of a hydrocele. Prompt refilling of the sac with pain, tenderness and poor or absent transillumination leave no doubt about the diagnosis. Acute haemorrhage into the tunica vaginalis sometimes results from testicular trauma and it may be difficult without exploration to decide whether the testis has been ruptured. If the haematocele is not drained, a clotted haematocele usually results.

Clotted hydrocele

Clotted hydrocele may result from a slow spontaneous ooze of blood into the tunica vaginalis. It is usually painless and by the time the patient seeks help, it may be difficult to be sure that the swelling is not due to a testicular tumour. Indeed a tumour may present as a haematocele.

Treatment is by orchidectomy unless the testis is indubitably benign. As a rule it is impossible to be certain of this until the mass has been bisected. The testis is often compressed and relatively useless (Fig. 68.12).

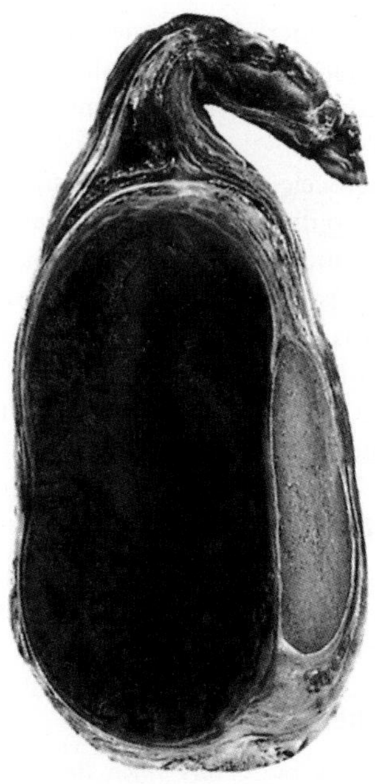

Fig. 68.12 A long-standing haematocele. The testis has been flattened by prolonged pressure.

Otto Edward Heinrich Wucherer, 1820–73. German physician who practised in Brazil.

Joseph Bancroft, 1836–94. Surgeon, General Hospital, Brisbane, Australia.

Cysts connected with the epididymis

Epididymal cysts

These are filled with a crystal-clear fluid (as opposed to the barley-water fluid of a spermatocele or the amber fluid of a hydrocele). They are very common, usually multiple and vary greatly in size at presentation. They represent cystic degeneration of the epididymis.

Clinical features

Cysts of the epididymis are usually found in middle age and the condition is often bilateral. The clusters of tense thin-walled cysts feel like a tiny bunch of grapes on palpation. They should be brilliantly transilluminable. The presence of a scrotal mass should always raise the possibility of a testicular neoplasm. Epididymal cysts are almost always quite separate from the testis proper and this is a reassuring sign.

Treatment

Aspiration is useless because the cysts are multilocular. If they are causing discomfort they should be excised. The man should be warned that excision may interfere with the export of sperms from the testis on that side.

Cyst of a testicular appendage

Cyst of a testicular appendage is usually unilateral and is felt as a small globular swelling at the superior pole. Such cysts are liable to torsion and should be removed if they cause symptoms.

Spermatocele

This is a unilocular retention cyst derived from some portion of the sperm-conducting mechanism of the epididymis.

Clinical features

A spermatocele nearly always lies in the head of the epididymis above and behind the upper pole of the testis. It is usually softer and laxer than other cystic lesions in the scrotum but like them it transilluminates. The fluid contains spermatozoa and resembles barley water in appearance. Spermatoceles are usually small and unobtrusive. Less frequently they are large enough to make the patient think that he has three testicles.

Treatment

Small spermatoceles can be ignored. Larger ones should be aspirated or excised through a scrotal incision.

Epididymo-orchitis

Acute disease

Inflammation confined to the epididymis is epididymitis; when infection spreads to the body of the testis, the condition is known as epididymo-orchitis.

Mode of infection

Infection reaches the globus minus of the epididymis via the lumen of the vas from a primary infection of the urethra, prostate or seminal vesicles. In men with outflow obstruction, epididymitis may result from a secondary urinary infection – a high pressure in the prostatic urethra causes reflux of infected urine up the vasa. A noninfective epididymitis sometimes arises from a similar cause when unusual exertion or violent strain when the bladder is full causes injection of urine into the vasa under pressure. In young men, the most common sexually transmitted infection causing epididymitis is now chlamydia but gonococcal epididymitis is still prevalent. Both are associated with urethritis. Blood-borne infections of the epididymis are less common but may be suspected when there is *Escherichia coli*, streptococcal, staphylococcal or proteus infection without evidence of urinary infection.

Clinical features

The initial symptoms are those of acute prostatitis. Some days later an ache in the groin and a fever herald the onset of epididymitis. The epididymis and testis swell rapidly and become exquisitely painful. The scrotal wall which is at first red, oedematous and shiny may become adherent to the epididymis. Resolution is signalled by scaling of the scrotal skin and may take 6–8 weeks to complete. Occasionally the infection may go on to abscess formation and discharge of pus may occur through the scrotal skin.

Acute epididymo-orchitis can follow any form of urethral instrumentation. It is particularly common when there is an indwelling catheter and an associated infection of the prostate. The incidence of acute postoperative epididymitis which was a serious and frequent complication of prostatectomy has been greatly reduced by closed drainage, catheter care and the early use of antibiotics.

Acute tuberculous epididymitis should come to mind when the vas is thickened and there is little response to the usual antibiotics.

Acute epididymo-orchitis of mumps develops in about 18 per cent of males suffering from mumps, usually as the parotid swelling is waning. The main complication is testicular atrophy which may cause infertility if the condition is bilateral (which is not usual). Partial atrophy is associated with persistent testicular pain. The epididymitis of mumps sometimes occurs in the absence of parotitis, especially in infants. The epididymis and testis may be involved by infection with other enteroviruses and in brucellosis and lymphogranuloma venereum.

Treatment

The patient should rest in bed while the acute symptoms persist. Doxycycline (100 mg daily) is the treatment of choice for young men with chlamydial infection. If an organism is isolated from the urine, this simplifies the choice of antibiotic. Otherwise treatment should be with an agent that is active across a broad spectrum of urinary tract pathogens. The patient should drink plenty of fluid. Local measures can help to reduce pain. The scrotum is supported on a sling made of broad adhesive tape attached between the thighs. The inflamed organ rests on a pad of cotton wool placed on the sling.

Antibiotic treatment should continue for 2 weeks or until the inflammation has subsided. If suppuration occurs, drainage is necessary. The patient should be warned that the testis may atrophy.

Chronic disease

Chronic tuberculous epididymo-orchitis usually begins insidiously.

Aetiology. The frequency with which the globus is first attacked indicates that the infection is retrograde from a tuberculous focus in the seminal vesicles.

Clinical features. Typically there is a firm discrete swelling of the lower pole of the epididymis which aches a little. The disease progresses until the whole epididymis is firm and craggy behind a normal-feeling testis. There is a lax secondary hydrocele in 30 per cent and in some a characteristic beading of the vas is apparent due to subepithelial tubercles. The seminal vesicle feels indurated and swollen. In neglected cases a tuberculous 'cold' abscess forms which may discharge. The body of the testis may be uninvolved for years but the contralateral epididymis often becomes diseased.

In two-thirds of cases there is evidence of renal tuberculosis or previous disease. The other patients appear healthy.

The urine and semen should be examined repeatedly for tubercle bacilli in all patients with chronic epididymo-orchitis. An intravenous urogram and a chest X-ray should be performed.

Treatment. When the epididymitis is secondary, it may resolve when the primary tuberculous focus is treated.

Treatment with antituberculous drugs is less effective in genital tuberculosis than in urinary tuberculosis. If resolution does not occur within 2 months, epididymectomy or orchidectomy is advisable. A full course of antituberculous chemotherapy should be completed even if there is no evidence of disease elsewhere.

Chronic nontuberculous epididymitis usually follows the failure of an acute attack to resolve fully. The condition is difficult to distinguish from tuberculosis but the swelling may be larger and smoother. It is essential to exclude urethral stricture causing reflux of urine down the vas. If alternative granulomatous conditions such as sarcoidosis have been eliminated, chronic epididymitis should be treated with antibiotics. Epididymectomy or orchidectomy should be considered if there is no resolution after 4–6 weeks of conservative treatment.

Orchitis. *Syphilitic orchitis* affects the body of the testis and is now uncommon. There are three varieties:

- *bilateral orchitis* is a feature of congenital syphilis;
- *interstitial fibrosis* causes painless destruction of the testis;
- *gumma* of the testis presents as a unilateral painless swelling of the testis which grows slowly. It feels hard and heavy and is very difficult to distinguish from a neoplasm without surgical exploration.

Leprous orchitis causes testicular atrophy in over 25 per cent of male lepers.

Tumours of the testes

The lymphatic drainage of the testes follows the spermatic cord to end in the para-aortic lymph nodes near the origin of the gonadal vessel. Lymphatics from the medial side of the testis may run with the artery to the vas and drain into a node at the bifurcation of the common iliac artery. The contralateral para-aortic lymph nodes are sometimes involved by tumour spread but the inguinal lymph nodes are only affected if the scrotal skin is involved.

Malignant

About 99 per cent of testicular neoplasms are malignant, and although they make up only about 1–2 per cent of malignant tumours in men, they are one of the commonest forms of cancer in the young male adult. Maldescent undoubtedly predisposes to malignancy. It is curious that despite the fact that the testis is usually easily palpable, a testicular tumour often escapes detection until after it has metastasised. There is a campaign to encourage men to perform regular testicular self-examination in the hope that tumours will be detected earlier but as yet this has not been as successful as a similar drive to get women to screen their own breasts for lumps.

Tumours of the testis are classified according to the predominant cellular type:

- seminoma (40 per cent);
- teratoma (32 per cent);
- combined seminoma and teratoma (14 per cent);
- interstitial tumours (1.5 per cent);
- lymphoma (7 per cent);
- other tumours (5.5 per cent).

Teratomas tend to occur in a younger age group, the peak incidence being between 20 and 35 while that of seminoma is between 35 and 45. Seminoma is extremely rare before puberty.

Seminoma

Seminoma compresses neighbouring testicular tissue as it grows (Fig. 68.13). The enlarged testis is smooth and firm. The cut surface is homogeneous and pinkish cream in colour. Occasionally fibrous septa give a lobulated appearance. In rapidly growing tumours there may be areas of necrosis of variable consistency.

Histologically, a seminoma is made of slightly oval cells with clear cytoplasm and large rounded nuclei with prominent acidophilic nucleoli. The cells are arranged in sheets separated by a fine fibrous stroma. Derived from seminiferous tubules, the cells resemble spermatocytes. Active infiltration of the tumour with lymphocytes suggests a good host response and a better prognosis.

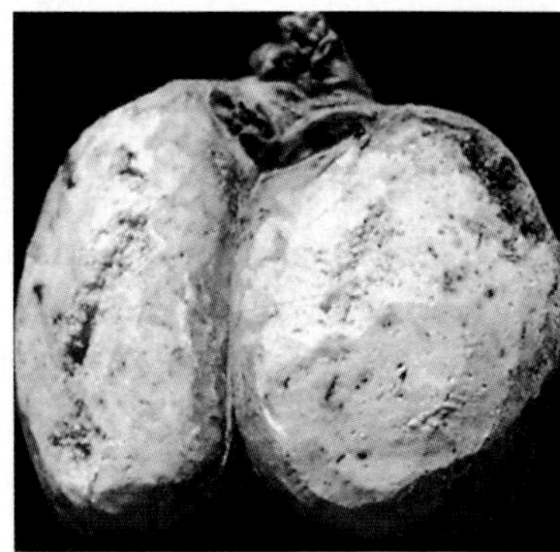

Fig. 68.13 Seminoma of the testis.

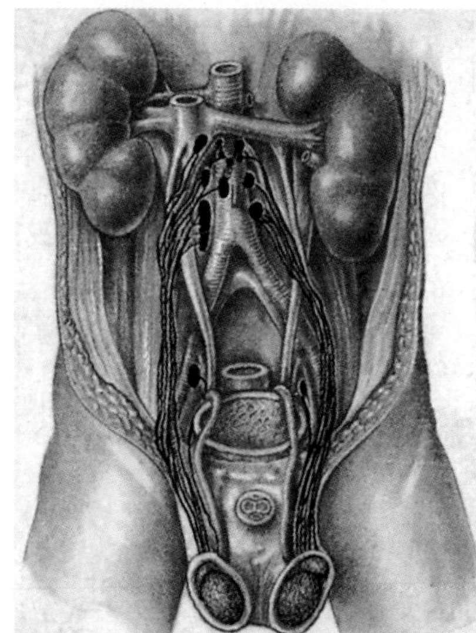

Fig. 68.14 Lymphatic drainage of the testes to para-aortic lymph nodes.

Seminomas spread via the lymphatics (Fig. 68.14) and metastasis via the bloodstream is uncommon.

Teratoma

Teratoma arises from totipotent cells in the rete testis and often contains a variety of cell types of which one or more predominate. The tumour may be as small as a peanut or as large as a coconut. Even when large, the tumour is moulded by the tunica albuginea so the overall outline of the testis is maintained although the surface may be slightly irregular.

The usual variety is yellowish in colour with cystic spaces containing gelatinous fluid (Fig. 68.15). Nodules of cartilage are often present.

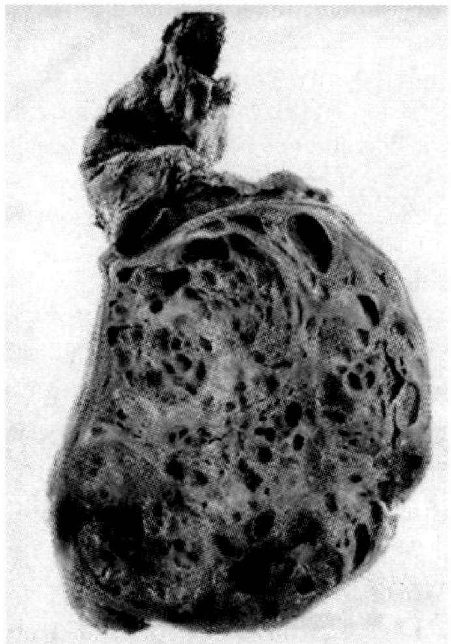

Fig. 68.15 Teratoma of the testis – note solid and cystic areas (*courtesy of Dr Keith Simpson, London*).

Histology. The Testicular Tumour Panel has classified teratomas as follows:

- *Teratoma differentiated (TD)* (uncommon) has no histologically recognisable malignant components but cannot be considered benign because such growth has metastasised. The best known variety is a dermoid cyst which may contain cartilage and muscle as well as glandular elements.
- *Malignant teratoma intermediate, teratocarcinoma (MTI – A and B)* (most common) contains definitely malignant and incompletely differentiated components. There is some mature tissue in type A but not in type B.
- *Malignant teratoma anaplastic (MTA), embryonal carcinoma* is composed of anaplastic cells of embryonal origin in parts. Cells presumed to be derived from yolk sac are often responsible for elevated α-fetoprotein levels. MTA is not always radiosensitive.
- *Malignant teratoma trophoblastic (MTT)* (uncommon) contains within other cell types a syncytial cell mass with malignant villous or papillary cytotrophoblast (chroriocarcinoma). It often produces human chorionic gonadotrophin (HCG). Spread by bloodstream and lymphatics is early. It is one of the most malignant tumours known.

Interstitial cell tumours

Interstitial cell tumours arise from Leydig or Sertoli cells. A Leydig cell tumour masculinises; a Sertoli cell tumour feminises.

Prepubertal interstitial cell tumours excrete androgens which cause sexual precocity and extreme muscular development. Regression of the symptoms after orchidectomy may be incomplete because of hypertrophy of the contralateral testis.

Postpubertal interstitial cell tumours usually arise from Sertoli cells with output of feminising hormones leading to gynaecomastia, loss of libido and aspermia. As a rule the tumour is benign and orchidectomy cures.

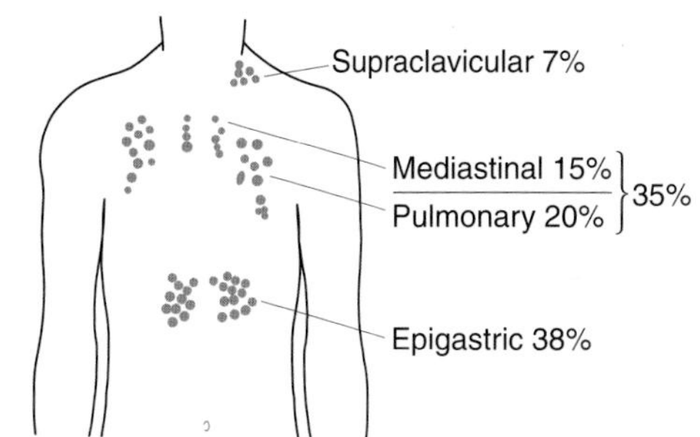

Fig. 68.16 Distribution of metastases in teratoma of the testis.

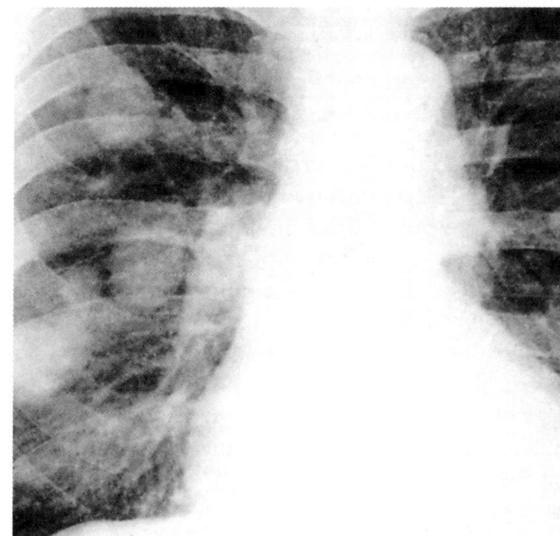

Fig. 68.17 Cannon ball metastases from carcinoma of the testis.

Clinical features

The patient may not seek advice for several months after first noticing that he has a testicular lump. A sensation of heaviness occurs when the testis is two or three times its normal size but there is pain in only 30 per cent or so. There is a history of trauma to the affected side in over 10 per cent. It is generally conceded that this merely calls attention to the testicular enlargement and in no way initiates the neoplasm.

On examination, the testis is enlarged, smooth, firm and heavy. Later one or more softer protruberances may be palpable. In no other disease is testicular sensation lost so early or so completely but the sign should be elicited with care for fear of disseminating the disease. Ten per cent have a lax secondary hydrocele which does not usually obscure the underlying tumour. The epididymis is normal at first but becomes more difficult to feel as it is flattened or incorporated in the growth. Thickening of the spermatic cord occurs later due to cremasteric hypertrophy and enlargement of the testicular vessels. The vas is never thickened and rectal examination shows the prostate and seminal vesicles to be normal.

Secondary retroperitoneal deposits may be palpable especially just above the umbilicus on the side of the tumour. There may be hepatic enlargement. Occasionally, an enlarged supraclavicular node is the presenting sign of a testicular tumour (Fig. 68.16). A chest radiograph is most likely to show pulmonary metastases when the primary tumour is a teratoma (Fig. 68.17).

Occasionally, the predominant symptoms are those of metastatic disease. Intra-abdominal disease may cause abdominal or lumbar pain and the mass may be discovered in the epigastrium. Lung metastases are usually silent but they can cause chest pain, dyspnoea and haemoptysis in the later stages of the disease. The primary tumour may not have been noticed by the patient and may indeed be so tiny that it can only be detected by sophisticated ultrasound imaging or operative exploration.

Atypical cases may simulate epididymo-orchitis; there may even be a urinary infection. *All testicular swellings should be treated with suspicion* and failure to respond to antibiotics should raise the possibility of a testicular tumour. Rarely, patients present with severe pain and acute enlargement of the testis due to haemorrhage into a neoplasm. Between 1 and 5 per cent have gynaecomastia (mainly the teratomas).

The hurricane tumour is a ferocious malignancy which kills in a matter of weeks. A few teratomas grow slowly with increasing enlargement of the testis over 2 or 3 years.

Franz von Leydig, 1821–1908. German anatomist.

Enrico Sertoli, 1842–1910. Professor of Experimental Physiology, Milan, Italy.

Treatment of testicular tumours

Staging is an essential first step in planning treatment.

- Blood is collected for radioimmunoassay of tumour markers (human chorionic gonadotrophin, α-foetoprotein and lactate dehydrogenase. Their level in the blood can be used to monitor the response to treatment.
- A chest radiograph will show whether there are pulmonary deposits.
- Orchidectomy is essential to remove the primary tumour and to obtain information about the histological type of the tumour.
- Computerised tomography and magnetic resonance imaging are the most useful means of detecting intra-abdominal and intrathoracic secondaries and for detecting their response to therapy.

Scrotal exploration and orchidectomy for suspected testicular tumour. The spermatic cord is displayed by dividing the external oblique aponeurosis through a groin incision. A soft clamp is placed across the cord to stop dissemination of malignant cells as the testis is mobilised into the wound. If there is doubt about the diagnosis at this stage, the testis should be bisected along its anterior convexity so that its internal structure can be examined. If there is a tumour or doubts still remain even after frozen section, the cord should be double ligated at the level of the inguinal ring and divided so that the testis can be removed.

Staging of testicular tumours

The stages are:

- stage 1: testis lesion only – no spread;
- stage 2: nodes below the diaphragm only;
- stage 3: nodes above the diaphragm;
- stage 4: pulmonary or hepatic metastases.

Management by staging and histological diagnosis (after orchidectomy)

Seminomas are radiosensitive and excellent results have been obtained by irradiating stage 1 and stage 2 tumours. More recently, the tumour has been shown to be highly sensitive to cisplatin, which is already being used for patients with metastatic disease. The experts are divided as to whether patients with stage 1 disease should have adjuvant chemotherapy.

Teratomas are less sensitive to radiation. Stage 1 tumours can be managed by watching the level of serum markers and by repeated computerised tomography. Teratomas at stages 2–4 are managed by chemotherapy. Cisplatin, methotrexate, bleomycin and vincristine have been used in combination with great success. There are those who advocate adjuvant chemotherapy for stage 1 teratoma arguing that effective prophylaxis is less troublesome to the patient than prolonged surveillance.

Retroperitoneal lymph node dissection is sometimes needed when retroperitoneal masses remain after chemotherapy (Fig. 68.18). The tissue removed may contain only necrotic tissue but a proportion of patients has foci of mature teratoma or active malignancy. The operations can be formidable if the tumour is large and retrograde ejaculation is likely unless steps are taken to preserve the sympathetic outflow to the bladder neck.

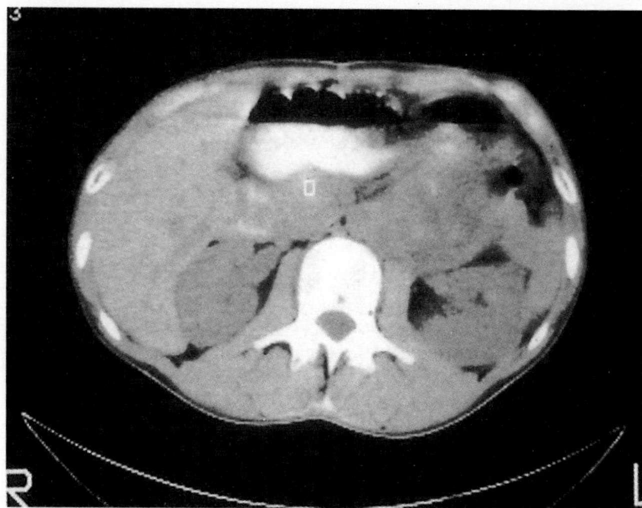

Fig. 68.18 Computerised tomography scan showing large residual retroperitoneal mass after chemotherapy.

Prognosis of testicular tumours depends on the histological type and the stage of the growth.

Seminoma. If there are no metastases 95 per cent will be alive 5 years after orchidectomy and radiotherapy or chemotherapy. If there are metastases survival drops to 75 per cent.

Teratoma. More than 85 per cent 5-year survival is achievable in stages 1 and 2 teratoma. In stages 3 and 4, the survival is about 60 per cent and getting better with improvements in chemotherapy.

Testicular tumours in children are usually anaplastic teratomas. They occur before the age of 3 years and are often rapidly fatal.

Tumours of the epididymis may be benign mesothelioma or malignant sarcoma or secondary carcinoma. They are extremely rare but should not be forgotten when the patient presents with a noncystic lump in the epididymis.

The scrotum

Prepenile scrotum

Prepenile scrotum is an exceedingly rare congenital condition in which the scrotum is suspended from the mons pubis in front of the penis.

Idiopathic scrotal oedema is described above.

Idiopathic scrotal gangrene

Idiopathic scrotal gangrene (syn. Fournier's gangrene) is an

Jean Alfred Fournier, 1832–1914. Dermatologist in Paris, France.

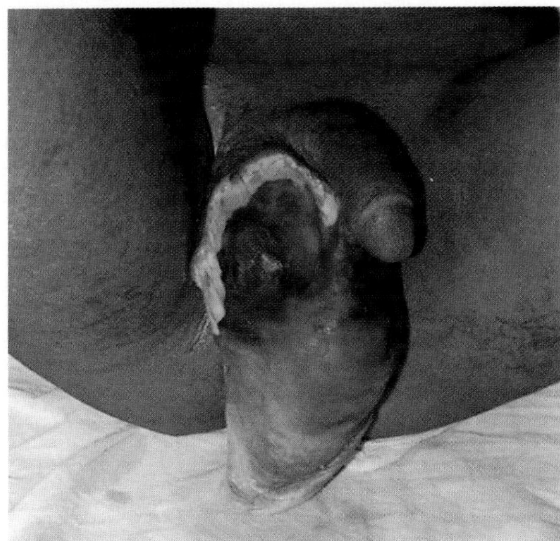

Fig. 68.19 Fournier's gangrene.

uncommon and nasty condition (Fig. 68.19). It is a vascular disaster of infective origin which is characterised by:

- sudden appearance of scrotal inflammation;
- rapid onset of gangrene leading to exposure of the scrotal contents;
- absence of any obvious cause in over half the cases.

It has been known to follow minor injuries or procedures in the perineal area, such as a bruise, scratch, urethral dilatation, injection of haemorrhoids or opening of a periurethral abscess.

The haemolytic streptococcus (sometimes microaerophilic) is associated with other organisms (staphylococcus, *E. coli*, *Clostridium welchii*) in a fulminating inflammation of the subcutaneous tissues which results in an obliterative arteritis of the arterioles to the scrotal skin (cf. gangrene of the abdominal wall, Chapter 62).

Clinical features

There is sudden pain in the scrotum, prostration, pallor and pyrexia. At first only the scrotum is involved but if unchecked, the cellulitis spreads until the entire scrotal coverings slough leaving the testes exposed but healthy.

Treatment. Expert microbiological advice should be obtained. The organisms are usually sensitive to gentamicin and a cephalosporin which should be given until the bacteriological report is available. Wide excision of the necrotic scrotal skin provides the best possible drainage and stops the spread of the gangrene. Many patients die despite active treatment.

Filarial elephantiasis of the scrotum

Filarial elephantiasis of the scrotum is due to obstruction of the pelvic lymphatics by *Wuchereria bancrofti* with superadded infection and lymphangitis. In long-standing cases, the enormously swollen scrotum may bury the penis (Fig. 68.20). There is no medical treatment for the condition. The principle of surgical treatment is the construction of new lymphatic pathways using plastic surgery. In very advanced cases excision of the affected skin with implantation of the testes into the thighs and a skin graft to the penis may be the only curative treatment.

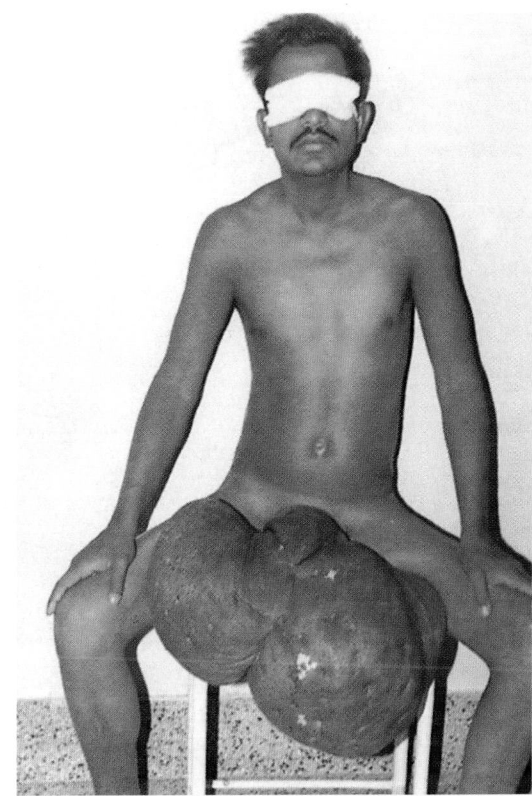

Fig. 68.20 Elephantiasis of the scrotum burying the penis (*courtesy of Mr S. Bhattacharjee, Lucknow, India*).

Nonfilarial elephantiasis

Nonfilarial elephantiasis can result from fibrosis of the lymphatics due to lymphogranuloma venereum.

Sebaceous cysts

Sebaceous cysts are common in the scrotal skin. They are usually small and multiple (Fig. 68.21).

Carcinoma of the scrotum

In the nineteenth century squamous epithelioma of the scrotum was the chimney sweep's cancer described by Percival Pott. With mechanisation of the cotton industry, impure lubricating oil from the spinning machine soaking the crutch of the mule spinners' trousers proved even more carcinogenic than soot. Today a few cases of scrotal cancer occur in tar and shale oil workers but the majority of cases arises with no

Percivall Pott, 1714–88. Surgeon, St Bartholomew's Hospital, London, England, first described this disease in 1775. In those days, the chimney sweep's apprentice climbed up inside the chimney.

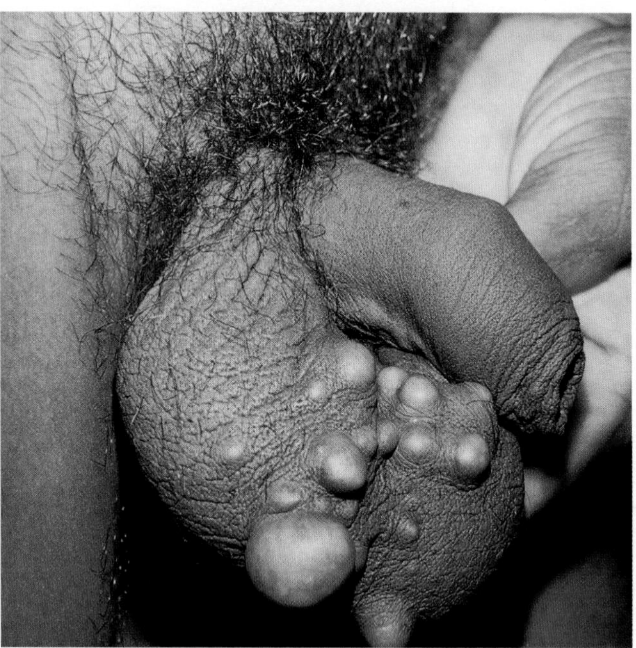

Fig. 68.21 Sebaceous cysts of the scrotum (*courtesy of Dr R. Kaje MS, Jimper, India*).

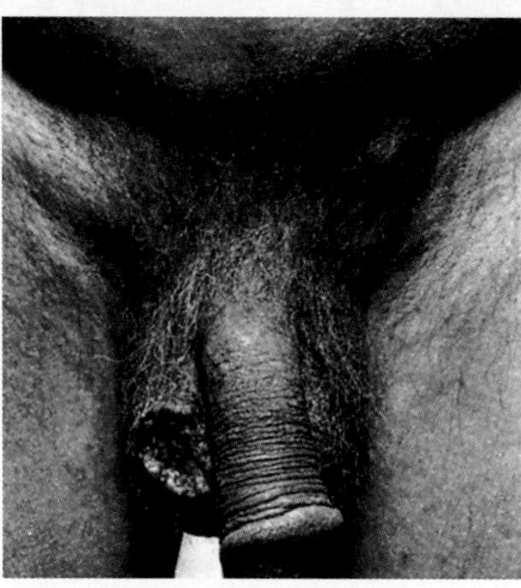

Fig. 68.22 Carcinoma of the scrotum with bilateral enlargement of the inguinal lymph nodes (*courtesy of Department of Medical Photography, Cardiff Royal Infirmary, Cardiff, Wales*).

obvious aetiological factor. It is remarkable that, unlike carcinoma of the penis, carcinoma of the scrotum is almost unknown in India and Asiatic countries.

Clinical features

The growth starts as a wart or ulcer (Fig. 68.22). As it grows it may involve the testis.

Treatment

The growth is excised with a margin of healthy skin. If associated enlargement of the inguinal nodes does not subside with antibiotics, a bilateral block dissection should be carried out up to the external nodes.

Male infertility

Testicular failure

The semen may contain no sperms (azoospermia), few sperms (oligospermia) or predominantly abnormal sperms. The cause is presumably some form of testicular dysfunction which may follow mumps infection, exposure to radiation or testicular trauma but is more often unknown. The normal feedback mechanism to control the production of gonadotrophic hormones is disturbed if there is testicular atrophy and the serum levels of luteinising hormone and follicle-stimulating hormone will be high. In some cases of azoospermia the testicular biopsy shows a failure of sperm development. Many treatments have been attempted but the results have been disappointing.

Obstruction

Azoospermia may also be due to obstruction to the pathway of spermatozoa from the testis via the epididymis to the ejaculatory ducts. The testicular biopsies will show active spermatogenisis. If the site of the obstruction can be identified by vasography it may be possible to perform a bypass operation. Unfortunately, even in the best hands, the results of epididymovasostomy are poor.

In some couples there appears to be an immunological cause for the infertility with clumping of sperms exposed to serum or cervical mucous.

Intracytoplasmic sperm injection

Intracytoplasmic sperm injection has revolutionised the management of male factor infertility. Spermatozoa harvested from the ejaculate, by aspiration of the epididymis or even from testicular biopsy, can be injected *in vitro* into ova obtained from the mother. Embryos are then transferred into the mother's uterus at the 4–6 cell stage.

Vasectomy for sterilisation

Vasectomy for sterilisation is one of the most commonly performed operations throughout the world. It should only be undertaken after the couple has been carefully counselled. They need to know that the operation is performed to make the man *permanently sterile*. They should be warned that they should continue with their normal contraceptive precautions until the success of the operation has been confirmed by semen analysis performed 12–16 weeks after surgery. They should also be warned of the remote but important possibility of spontaneous recanalisation which may restore fertility unexpectedly.

Vasectomy is easily and painlessly performed under local anaesthetic. The vasa are delivered through tiny bilateral or a single midline scrotal incision. For medicolegal reasons it is wise to remove a segment of each vas to prove that it has been successfully divided. Burying the cut ends or turning them back on themselves probably helps to prevent them rejoining.

Reversal of vasectomy may not restore fertility even if technically successful because of the presence of autoantibodies developed against the sequestered sperms. A success rate of 60–80 per cent may be possible if the operation is performed within 3–4 years of vasectomy.

Further reading

Blandy, J.P. and Fowler, C.G. (1995) *Urology,* 2nd edn, Blackwell Scientific, Oxford.

Walsh, P.C., Retik, A.B., Darracott Vaughan, E. and Wein, A.J. (1998) *Campbell's Urology,* 7th edn, W.B. Saunders, Philadelphia, PA.

Whitfield, H.W., Hendry, W.F., Kirby, R.S. and Duckett J. (1998) *Textbook of Genito-urinary Surgery,* 2nd edn, Blackwell Science, Oxford.

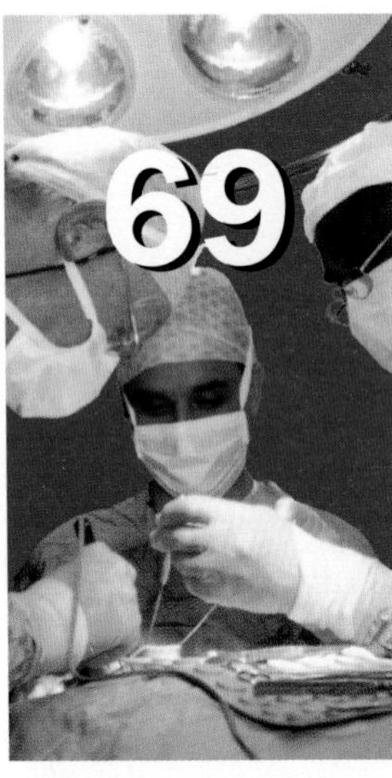

69 Day surgery

Introduction

Day surgery is an increasingly important part of elective surgery. It currently accounts for 50 per cent of elective surgery in the UK, and 60 per cent or more in the USA and Canada, with predictions of further increases. The impetus for this has been the high cost of keeping patients in in-patient beds, the reduction in availability of these beds and long surgical waiting lists in publicly funded healthcare systems. Improvements in anaesthesia and pain control, minimally invasive surgery and changing attitudes to recovery after surgery have all promoted the expansion of day surgery. Patients, particularly children, benefit from reduced stays in hospital and a rapid return to their home environment, provided that their surgery is uncomplicated and without significant pain or nausea. The quality of care in day surgery should be of the same high standard as that expected for in-patient surgery. Day Surgery Units (DSU) are the best way to achieve this.

Definition

Day surgery is defined as planned investigations or procedures on patients who are admitted and discharged home on the day of their surgery but require some facilities and time for recovery. Minor procedures in out-patient or accident and emergency departments are not included. In most countries, this means that the patient spends a few hours in hospital and does not stay overnight. However, in the USA, day surgery is termed 'ambulatory surgery' and includes patients who may spend up to 23 hours in hospital, allowing a greater range of procedures to be included.

Historical

Day surgery is not a new concept. In 1909 James Nicoll, a Scottish surgeon, reported operating on nearly 9000 children as day cases, for operations such as talipes, correction of hare lip, hernia repair and mastoid surgery. His motivation was to save money and use resources better – reasons which are equally valid today. In the USA Ralph Waters, an anaesthetist, founded his 'downtown anaesthesia clinic' for dental and minor surgery in 1912, the prototype for the free-standing DSU. Despite acclaim for these innovations at the time, the concept was slow to gain acceptance, and it was only when the disadvantages of prolonged bed rest after surgery were appreciated in the 1940s that day surgery could really progress.

In 1951 Eric Farquharson, an Edinburgh surgeon, carried out day-case adult hernia repairs under local anaesthesia in order to reduce long waiting lists in the newly introduced

Bailey & Love's Short Practice of Surgery, 23rd edition. Edited by R.C.G. Russell, N.S. Williams and C.J.K. Bulstrode. Published in 2000 by Arnold Publishers.

James H. Nicoll. Surgeon, Western Infirmary and Royal Hospital for Sick Children, Glasgow, Scotland.
Ralph Waters. Anaesthetist, Sioux City, Iowa, USA.
Eric Farquharson. Surgeon, Edinburgh, Scotland.

National Health Service (NHS). He initiated policies of careful patient assessment and cooperation with general practitioners (GPs) to ensure care after discharge. Hospital-based DSUs began to appear in the United States in the 1960s, and in 1969 Walter Reed, an American surgeon, set up the Phoenix Surgicenter, the first free-standing DSU. UK hospitals followed suit from the 1970s and DSUs became established in most hospitals, although the free-standing DSU is almost unknown in the UK.

Day surgery now began to take on a momentum of its own, and influential reports such as those from the Royal College of Surgeons of England in 1985 and 1992, and the Audit Commission in 1990, focused attention on the benefits of day surgery and set standards and guidelines.

The benefits and caveats of day-case surgery

Financial

Every healthcare system in the world is under financial pressure. Day surgery operations cost less, saving expensive out-of-hours nursing and in-patient beds, which may be closed or used for more major surgery. Extra capital and resources may be needed to set up DSUs.

Better use of resources

Efficient throughput of patients makes more effective use of operating theatre time. Good organisation, patient selection and assessment can virtually eliminate last-minute cancellations and expedite admission on the day of surgery. DSUs should be 'ring fenced' against use for emergency cases so that admission as arranged is guaranteed.

Table 69.1 Benefits of day surgery

- Reduced costs
- More efficient high-volume throughput of patients
- Reduced waiting lists for elective surgery
- In-patient beds freed for major and emergency surgery
- Fewer cancellations on the day of surgery
- Low incidence of serious postoperative morbidity
- Reduced thromboembolism and hospital-acquired infections
- Minimal disruption to patient's life
- Early return to work and normal activities
- Patients, particularly children, prefer it

Table 69.2 Potential problems of day surgery

- Initial costs of setting up Day Surgery Units
- Good organisation and management needed
- Resistance from senior medical staff
- Poor patient and procedure selection
- Morbidity from anaesthesia and surgery
- Provision of adequate information to patients
- Increased community workload

Walter Reed. Surgeon, Phoenix, Arizona, USA.

Care must be taken that complications do not increase owing to pressure to expand the range of day-case operations and that beds for the few inevitable patients who are unfit to go home are identified.

Reduction in waiting lists

Operations suitable for day surgery are usually those which can wait and so form a large part of waiting lists, which have usually been reduced where day surgery has been instituted. However, these more minor operations may be the first to be postponed or rationed when money runs out.

Patients

Day surgery would not have gained such widespread acceptance if patients did not prefer to go home after surgery, and numerous surveys have confirmed its acceptability to patients. Hospital-acquired infections, thromboembolism and pulmonary complications are reduced. For children in particular, day surgery is the ideal option because they spend as little time as possible away from their families and familiar surroundings, and most of the common operations of childhood lend themselves to day surgery.

This assumes that patients are not sent home in discomfort or to inadequate care. Day surgery may simply pass the expense and burden of care to relatives and GPs, although this has not been found to be true in practice. A small percentage of patients have commented that insufficient attention was paid to home circumstances, that more information should be given before admission and that they were sent home before they felt well enough.

The Day Surgery Unit

The DSU is a self-contained dedicated day surgery facility with its own reception, operating and recovery areas, designed to ensure that all of the essentials for good day surgery practice are carried out. While it is possible to use an in-patient ward, and mixed in-patient and day-case operating sessions, in practice this achieves neither efficient throughput nor good-quality care. A compromise is to have a day-case ward close to the operating suite with dedicated day-case operating sessions, with the same good organisation found in self-contained DSUs. Hospitals without a DSU never achieve high percentages of day cases.

The DSU is usually part of a general hospital, and ideally should be purpose built. Nearby parking for escorts collecting patients should be provided. The design should maximise efficient patient flow. The number of beds and theatres will be dictated by the workload of the specialities using the unit. In general, a throughput of 1.5 patients/bed day is possible, but may be less if more major procedures requiring longer recovery are undertaken. The balance of beds to operating theatres, and the scheduling of the operating sessions, should be planned with this in mind, but there should be flexibility for changing needs. The DSU may also be used for a variety of other procedures that require different facilities and

Table 69.3 Desirable features of a Day Surgery Unit

- Self-contained with its own reception, ward, theatre(s) and recovery area
- Adjacent parking
- Well laid out with good patient flow
- Equipped to the same high standards as in-patient wards and theatres
- Beds:theatre ratios related to surgical speciality
- Flexibility for changing needs
- Protocols for selection, analgesia and discharge criteria
- Good record keeping
- Support services readily available
- Trained experienced staff
- Consultant-led anaesthesia and surgery
- Organised training with close supervision of trainees
- Clinical Director in overall charge
- Teamwork between staff groups
- Liaison with community services

equipment such as gastrointestinal endoscopy, flexible cystoscopy, interventional radiology, and chronic pain or minor medical procedures.

Children-only days or sessions may be planned. Procedures needing longer recovery should be scheduled early in the day, and local anaesthetic cases later. Many units now stay open into the evening to allow later operating sessions.

The unit layout

The reception area

The reception area should be welcoming and large enough to accommodate patients and their escorts on arrival and discharge, with adequate space for secretarial and reception staff. Admission procedures are completed here before the patients go to the ward.

The day surgery ward

This may be equipped with beds or trolleys. Preoperative assessment and investigations will already have been carried out, but the patient must be assessed before surgery by the surgeon and the anaesthetist. Basic preoperative checks are carried out, site of surgery marked and consent for the procedure signed, if not already done. Time must be allowed for this assessment so that the patient does not meet the anaesthetist in the anaesthetic room when it is too late to address any problems. Sedative premedication is usually avoided as it may prolong recovery time, and unsedated patients can walk to the anaesthetic room. After leaving the recovery room, the patient will return to this ward area to recover sufficiently to have light refreshment and be taken home.

The anaesthetic room and operating theatres

These should have *precisely* the same high-quality specification, monitoring, safety and surgical equipment as in-patient operating suites. Trained assistance must be provided throughout the perioperative period. The use of operating trolleys, on which the patients can also recover, can save considerable time and manpower as patients do not have to be moved between trolley and operating table.

The recovery area

The recovery area should be fully equipped to in-patient standards and be adjacent to the theatre. In the UK, patients usually spend only a short time here before returning to the ward to recover, but in the USA this area, called the Post Anesthesia Recovery Unit (PACU), may be used until the patient is ambulant and can to be sent to a 'step-down area' where they remain in a chair until fit to go home. Patients who have had local anaesthesia with no or mild sedation may be able to bypass this area and go straight to the ward.

Personnel

Staffing of the Day Surgery Unit

Experienced day surgery nurses excel at dealing with problems and giving reassurance and information. In many units, multiskilling allows nurses and operating department personnel (ODP) to undertake ward, theatre and anaesthetic assistant duties. Specialised nurses may be needed for children or for certain types of surgery such as ophthalmic. Ancillary staff for portering and domestic duties are also needed.

Record keeping

This must be accurate and complete, often difficult with high-volume fast turnover. Unnecessary paperwork should be minimised while ensuring that vital information is logged. A folder containing all of the relevant records is ideal. Computerised systems can help greatly and are now commercially available.

Support services

Although the need for laboratory and radiology services is minimal, these should be available if required. In-patient and resuscitation back-up must be identified for the rare occasions when it will be needed.

Medical staff and training

Good-quality treatment with minimal complications means that day surgery must be consultant led and carried out by fully trained medical staff, surgical and anaesthetic, to achieve the best results and reduce complications and risk. However, senior staff may find the work unchallenging and be tempted to delegate it to trainees. Training in day surgery is essential, but trainees should be closely supervised and extra time allowed for this.

Clinical Director

The Clinical Director, usually a consultant surgeon or an anaesthetist, should manage the DSU and implement and audit good standards of care. Regular multidisciplinary meetings with all those using the unit are needed, as is liaison with GPs and community care.

Table 69.4 Morbidity after day surgery

Major	*Minor*
Myocardial infarction	Pain
Pulmonary embolus	Nausea and vomiting (PONV)
Respiratory failure	Dizziness, drowsiness
Cerebrovascular accident	Minor bleeding
Major postoperative haemorrhage	Infection
Unrecognised damage to viscus	Sore throat, headache

Postoperative morbidity after day surgery

Day surgery has an excellent safety record. Major morbidity with the potential for serious harm is rare. In a large study from the Mayo Clinic in 1993, Warner reported that the mortality and major morbidity in the 30 days after day surgery was 0.0007 per cent – lower than in the general population who had not had surgery.

Minor morbidity, however, is common and apparently minor problems can have significant consequences. For the hospital, it results in longer stays in the DSU and increased rates of overnight admission, which may cause problems if no bed is available or the bed is earmarked for another patient. For the patient, it is not only unpleasant but delays their recovery and return to normal life and is a cause of dissatisfaction. For GP, it may increase workload.

Postoperative morbidity is related to the type of anaesthesia used and the surgery itself. The procedure is generally the most important predictor of complications. The requirement to discharge patients within a relatively short time of their surgery demands meticulous and safe anaesthetic and surgical techniques to ensure good recovery with minimal postoperative morbidity.

The essentials of good day surgery

In order to achieve good results in day surgery and avoid the pitfalls described above the following are essential:

- selection of appropriate procedures and patients;
- preadmission assessment and information;
- anaesthesia and surgery with minimal morbidity and complications;
- postoperative and postdischarge analgesia;
- discharge criteria and postoperative instructions;
- follow-up and audit.

Day surgery selection

The aim of day surgery selection is to avoid predictable complications and morbidity. In selecting suitable procedures and patients, consider:

- the procedure to be undertaken;
- the social circumstances;
- the fitness of the patient.

Criteria for suitable day-case procedures

- Minimal physiological trespass;
- not associated with excessive blood loss or fluid shifts;
- very low risk of serious postoperative complications (e.g. bleeding or airway obstruction);
- duration of up to 1 hour, 2 hours maximum;
- pain must be controllable with oral analgesics after discharge;
- the patient should be reasonably ambulant afterwards.

The use of surgical drains is controversial; if needed, these are removed before the patient goes home. Urinary catheters are surprisingly well tolerated and may allow urology patients to go home. Absorbable sutures and improved wound closure methods may reduce the need for patients to return for stitch removal.

Relatively uncontroversial day-case procedures (Table 69.5) make up the bulk of day surgery. However, other more major operations may now be included as minimally invasive surgical techniques using laparoscopy and lasers reduce postoperative problems and pain. *Open* abdominal, intrathoracic, intracranial and major vascular procedures are still universally considered to be unsuitable.

In general, longer and more invasive operations are associated with more pain, bleeding or other complications, although this is not absolutely true – some may simply be time-consuming without increasing morbidity. Laparoscopic surgery in particular is associated with increased morbidity and overnight admission, particularly for procedures such as cholecystectomy. Tonsillectomy is also controversial: while routinely performed on a day-case basis in many centres, anxiety about the risk of bleeding deters others. The pathology is important – small haemorrhoids or incisional hernias are suitable, very large ones may not be.

The push to ambulatory surgery in the USA has led to the inclusion of major surgery, such as mastectomy and vaginal hysterectomy, often with little regard for patient comfort and preference. This has resulted in a backlash, with legislation to prohibit the 'drive-through' mastectomy.

The social circumstances

- Day surgery needs ready access to a hospital or GP after discharge, although the demand on these should be minimal.
- A responsible adult to escort the patient home and care for them at least until the following morning is mandatory. For more major day-case operations, longer care may be needed. Elderly or disabled partners may be unsuitable.
- Patients must have reasonable home circumstances with good toilet facilities, few stairs to climb and access to a telephone.

M.A. Warner. Anaesthetist, Mayo Clinic, Rochester, Minnesota, USA.

Table 69.5 Suitable day surgery procedures

- General surgery
  - 'Lumps and bumps': sebaceous cysts, lipomata, etc.
  - Breast lumps: excision or biopsy, subcutaneous mastectomy for gynaecomastia
  - Varicose veins: ligations, avulsions, stripping
  - Hernia repairs: inguinal, femoral, umbilical, epigastric, incisional (small)
  - Toenail avulsions
  - Anal procedures: anal stretch, lateral sphincterotomy, banding or injection of haemorrhoids
- Urology
  - Urethroscopy: dilation and resection of stenosis
  - Cystoscopy: diagnostic, resection/diathermy of bladder tumour, short bladder distension
  - Ureteroscopy: insertion of stent, stone breaking/removal procedures
  - Circumcision
  - Varicocele surgery
  - Orchidectomy
  - Orchidopexy
  - Scrotal lesions: hydrocele, spermatocele
  - Vasectomy and reversal of vasectomy
  - Extracorporeal shock wave lithotripsy
- Plastic surgery
  - Skin lesions: excision with small flaps and skin grafts
  - Minor hand surgery: synovectomy, tendon transfer, Dupuytren's contracture carpal tunnel decompression
  - Tendon repairs and transfers
  - Augmentation mammoplasty
  - Rhinoplasty, blepharoplasty and other cosmetic surgery
  - Limited liposuction
  - Otoplasty
- Orthopaedic surgery
  - Manipulation under general anaesthesia
  - Arthroscopy – knee, elbow, shoulder
  - Nerve and tendon repair and decompression
  - Ganglionectomy
  - Carpal tunnel decompression
  - Bunionectomy, hammer toe correction
  - Removal of orthopaedic hardware and foreign bodies
- Ophthalmic surgery
  - Cataract surgery ± intraocular lens implant
  - Trabeculectomy
  - Strabismus correction
  - Eyelid and lacrimal surgery
  - Vitreo-retinal surgery
  - Corneal surgery
- Ear, nose and throat surgery
  - Myringotomy + grommets
  - Myringoplasty
  - Tympanoplasty
  - Adenoidectomy
  - Laryngoscopy
  - Nasal polyps
  - Nasal fractures
  - Sinus procedures, especially endoscopic
  - Limited submucous resection (SMR)
  - Submandibular stones
- Oral surgery
  - Conservative dental treatment
  - Extraction of deciduous and wisdom teeth
  - Orthodontic treatment

Table 69.5 *(Continued)*

- Gynaecological surgery
  - Dilatation and curettage: diagnostic, evacuation of retained products of conception
  - Hysteroscopy
  - Termination of pregnancy
  - Endometrial ablation
  - Labial procedures: Bartholin's cysts
  - Laparoscopy: for investigation, sterilization, endometriosis, ovarian cysts

Baron Guillaume Dupuytren, 1777–1835. Surgeon, Hôtel Dieu, Paris, France.

- Patients should live within 60 minutes' travelling distance, both to reduce discomfort on the way home and to have ready access to hospital care if needed. Patients should not travel home by public transport.
- Other options have been used where home circumstances are not ideal, such as hospital hotels supplying overnight supervision at low cost or, more rarely, transfer to a community hospital. An overnight stay in hospital (the '23-hour admit') may permit more procedures and patients to be considered suitable 'day cases', but may not achieve the benefits of day surgery.
- Developing countries with long distances and difficult travelling conditions to reach medical care may find that these are obstacles to introducing day surgery.

The fitness of the patient for general anaesthesia

The patient should be medically stable and have been screened before admission to exclude major health problems. The American Society of Anesthesiologists (ASA) classification of patient fitness is often used, with the stipulation that ASA 1, 2 and stable 3 patients are suitable, although this may be difficult to define with accuracy. The aspects of patient fitness which have been shown to relate to complications during surgery and to unplanned overnight admission are severe symptomatic respiratory disease, symptomatic cardiac disease and hypertension.

Age. 70 is often taken as an upper age limit, but the physiological age of the patient is more important than actual age. Elderly patients may be suitable for day-case procedures under local or regional anaesthesia.

The lower age limit depends on the facilities available, the experience of the staff and the procedures undertaken. The

Table 69.6 ASA (American Society of Anesthesiologists) classification

ASA 1	A healthy patient
ASA 2	Mild systemic disease, no functional limitation
ASA 3	Severe systemic disease some functional limitation
ASA 4	Severe systemic disease, incapacitating and a constant threat to life
ASA 5	Moribund patient not expected to survive for 24 hours with or without operation

healthy full-term neonate is suitable for minor day-case procedures, provided that there is immediate access to in-patient neonatal care if needed. More caution is needed with preterm or ex-preterm babies, who should not be considered before 60 weeks' conceptual age because of the risk of perioperative apnoea.

Obesity. Weight limits expressed as body mass index (BMI) (weight in kg/height in m^2) are often imposed, although there is little hard evidence as to what is unacceptable. Surgery and anaesthesia are undoubtedly more difficult and have more complications in overweight patients, who may also have more health problems. Although a BMI of 30 is often taken as an upper limit, in otherwise fit patients problems do not really become apparent until the BMI exceeds 35.

Respiratory disease. Asthmatics with no history of hospital admission for their asthma, and patients with chronic obstructive airways disease, are suitable for day surgery if they have reasonable exercise tolerance, usually expressed as the ability to climb a flight of stairs.

Hypertension. Untreated or previously unrecognised hypertension in apparently fit patients is the commonest predictable reason for cancellation on the day of surgery, and 'white coat hypertension' on the patient's arrival in hospital is a recurring source of strife between surgeons, anaesthetists and GPs. However, this type of hypertension has been shown to be related to abnormal left ventricular function and to perioperative myocardial ischaemia. A preadmission blood pressure (BP) is mandatory, and BP ≥ 175/105 mmHg should be treated before surgery, together with electrocardiography (ECG) and full cardiac history to exclude more severe underlying cardiac disease.

Cardiac disease. Unsuitable conditions include cardiac failure, symptomatic valvular disease, severe or rest angina, fast ventricular arrythmias, unpaced second- or third-degree heart block, or myocardial infarction within the previous 6 months. In patients with lesser degrees of heart disease, further cardiac assessment may be required.

Diabetes. Well-controlled noninsulin-dependent diabetes (NIDDM) usually poses no problems. Although otherwise fit insulin-dependent diabetics have been considered suitable, in practice, even with a well-controlled and well-motivated patient, the stress of surgery and fasting can upset the patient's diabetic control, making their day surgery episode difficult and time-consuming for medical staff.

Drug therapy. Patients taking anticoagulants, systemic steroids, digoxin, drugs for dysrrhythmias and angina, and monamine oxidase inhibitors need individual anaesthetic evaluation before booking for day surgery. Oestrogen-containing oral contraceptives need not be discontinued except for lower limb operations, particularly where a tourniquet will be used.

This is only a guide. There are no absolute exclusions – the severity must be evaluated – and local or regional anaesthesia may be suitable for patients who cannot safely be given a general anaesthetic. Simple guidelines (Table 69.7) should be circulated to surgical staff and displayed in out-patient departments.

Table 69.7 Selection criteria for adult day surgery patients for general anaesthesia

Social criteria	
Responsible adult to escort home + supervise at home overnight	
Lives within 1 hour's drive *maximum*	
Reasonable social circumstances – consider stairs, telephone, toilet, heating, etc.	
Physical fitness	
Generally fit and ambulant	
Not grossly obese (BMI should be under 35)	
The patient should be able to climb one flight of stairs	
Do NOT book patients who have:	
Cardiovascular disease:	*Poorly controlled hypertension* (BP > 170/100 mmHg)
	Angina, CCF or peripheral vascular disease
	MI, TIA or CVA within last 6–12 months
	Symptomatic valvular disease
Respiratory disease:	Severe asthma or chronic obstructive airways disease
Diabetes:	Insulin-dependent or poorly controlled NIDDM
Renal or hepatic disease, alcoholism, narcotic addiction	
Multiple sclerosis (advanced), myasthenia, severe cervical spondylosis	
Severe psychiatric disease	
Drugs – do NOT book patients taking:	
Anticoagulants	Monoamine oxidase inhibitors
Digoxin	Systemic steroids
Antidysrhythmics	Oral contraceptive (lower limb surgery)
GTN	

Patients who do not meet these criteria may be suitable for day surgery but need to be arranged with the anaesthetist.
BMI, body mass index; CCF, congestive cardiac failure; MI, myocardial infarct; TIA, transient ischaemic attack; CVA: cerebrovascular accident; NIDDM, noninsulin-dependent diabetes mellitus, GTN, glycerol trinitrate.
(Reproduced with permission from Millar, J.M., Rudkin, G.E. and Hitchcock, M., *Practical Anaesthesia and Analgesia for Day Surgery*, BIOS Scientific, Oxford, 1997.)

Assessment before admission for surgery

This is an essential component of well-organised day surgery. The timing should allow any problems to be sorted out, but not be so far in advance that the patient develops new problems.

Methods of assessing patients

Surgeons are not good at assessing patients for anaesthetic fitness, particularly in the middle of a busy clinic. The ideal would be to have the patient seen by an anaesthetist, preferably the one who will anaesthetise the patient. This is usually impracticable in terms of time, cost and available anaesthetic time. The best alternative is a filtering process (Fig. 69.1) with specially trained nurses using patient questionnaires (Table 69.8) and locally agreed protocols of suitable criteria. Borderline cases are referred for anaesthetic opinions, and consultant anaesthetists involved in day surgery should be identified to advise.

Assessment clinics

A good assessment clinic prevents cancellation on the day of surgery for predictable reasons, particularly hypertension. It also speeds up the process of admitting the patient, and may reduce unplanned overnight admission for those who have not arranged for an escort home. It can reduce unnecessary investigations, perioperative complications and risk. Patient compliance may be improved – given information and the opportunity to discuss anxieties, they are more likely to turn up for their operations and to have obeyed their preoperative instructions (Fig. 69.2). It should also increase the number of suitable patients by addressing problems, and by arranging for borderline cases to be considered for local or regional anaesthesia. Assessment clinics are cost-effective (Table 69.9).

Preadmission information

This has been identified as a cause for patient dissatisfaction. Providing clear concise information means that patients arrive well prepared, having obeyed the fasting instructions, and knowing what to expect from the surgery and in the recovery period. The prolonged fluid fast of former times may be detrimental to recovery, and although a 4–6-hour fast from solid food is essential, clear fluids my be allowed up to 2–3 hours preoperatively. Information about expected levels of pain and restrictions on activity after specific procedures helps the patient to plan their care at home – for instance mothers of small children may need to arrange for help for longer than just overnight. All of the important information (Table 69.10) should be on one page, or patients may not read it. Separate leaflets on individual procedures are useful. Resist the temptation to overload the patient with information.

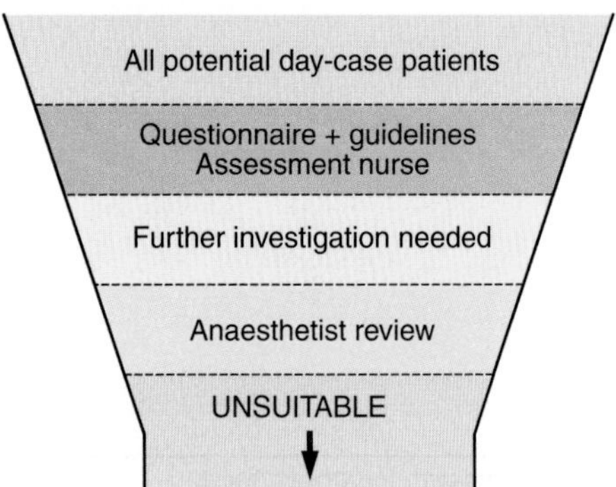

Fig. 69.1 Filtering patients using the assessment process. (Reproduced with permission from Millar, J.M., Rudkin, G.E. and Hitchcock, M., *Practical Anaesthesia and Analgesia for Day Surgery*, BIOS Scientific, Oxford, 1997.)

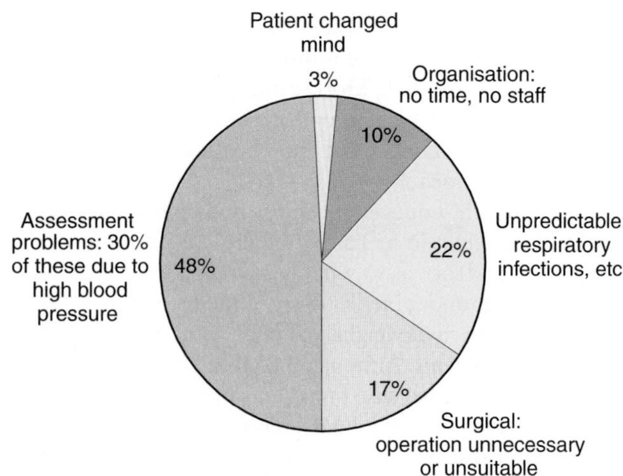

Fig. 69.2 Why are patients cancelled on the day of surgery?

Anaesthesia for day surgery

Anaesthetic morbidity is a major reason for unplanned admission, in particular sleepiness, dizziness and nausea (Fig. 69.3). The choice is between local or regional anaesthesia with or without mild sedation, or general anaesthesia with local anaesthetic where appropriate to provide postoperative analgesia.

Local or regional anaesthesia is perhaps the ideal, although it is not suitable for all procedures or patients. It is excellent for elderly patients and is usually economical, although it may be more time-consuming than general anaesthesia, and necessitates gentle surgery. Patients and surgeons may express a preference for general anaesthesia.

The type of local anaesthesia must be carefully chosen. Central anaesthetic blocks, epidural, spinal or caudal, may be less suitable because of the time taken to carry out the block and allow it to work, the time taken for the patient to mobilise and the high incidence of urinary retention.

Suitable blocks are listed in Table 69.11. The ideal choice of agent is a long-acting one, such as bupivacaine, and if speed of onset is important lignocaine may be mixed with this. Prilocaine will be needed for Bier's blocks

August Karl Gustav Bier, 1861–92. Berlin surgeon.

Table 69.8 Assessment questionnaire

Adult Day Surgery Assessment Questionnaire for General Anaesthesia

You may be able to have your operation as a day case.
To help us plan your treatment, please answer the following questions.

Can an adult take you home by car or taxi after your operation?	☐ Yes	☐ No
Is there a responsible and physically fit adult to look after you for the first night after your operation?	☐ Yes	☐ No
Would it take you less than 1 hour to get home from the Hospital/Day Surgery Unit?	☐ Yes	☐ No
Do you suffer from or have you ever suffered from:		
Heart disease or a heart murmur	☐ Yes	☐ No
High blood pressure	☐ Yes	☐ No
Chest pains or angina	☐ Yes	☐ No
Stroke	☐ Yes	☐ No
Asthma	☐ Yes	☐ No
Chronic cough or bronchitis	☐ Yes	☐ No
Too breathless to climb one flight of stairs	☐ Yes	☐ No
Diabetes	☐ Yes	☐ No
Epilepsy	☐ Yes	☐ No
Kidney problems	☐ Yes	☐ No
Jaundice	☐ Yes	☐ No
Bleeding problems	☐ Yes	☐ No
Heartburn or hiatus hernia	☐ Yes	☐ No
Any other diseases	☐ Yes	☐ No
If you answered YES to any of these questions, please tell us about it		
Are you taking any tablets, pills, inhalers or medicine?	☐ Yes	☐ No
If yes, please list them		
....		
Have you any allergies (including drug allergies)?	☐ Yes	☐ No
If yes, please list them		
....		
Do you smoke? If YES, how many per day?	☐ Yes	☐ No
....		
Do you have false, capped, crowned or loose teeth?	☐ Yes	☐ No
....		
Have you had any operations or anaesthetics before?	☐ Yes	☐ No
If yes, please list		
....		
Were there any problems? If so please give details		
....		
Have any of your family had problems with anaesthetics?	☐ Yes	☐ No
If so what were the problems?		

(Reproduced with permission from Millar, J.M., Rudkin, G.E. and Hitchcock, M., *Practical Anaesthesia and Analgesia for Day Surgery*, BIOS Scientific, Oxford, 1997.)

Table 69.9 Benefits of a preadmission assessment clinic

- Problems are sorted out before admission
- Unnecessary investigations are reduced
- Cancellation for predictable reasons is virtually eliminated
- Patients are better prepared and informed
- Nonattendance is reduced
- Admission on the day is expedited
- Perioperative complications may be reduced
- Unplanned overnight admission is reduced

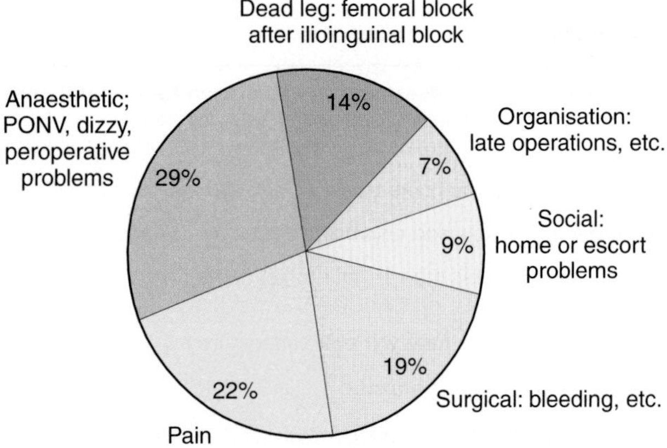

Fig. 69.3 Unplanned overnight admission after general surgery.

(intravenous regional anaesthesia). Care should be taken not to exceed safe doses, and if the surgeon administers the local anaesthetic, an anaesthetist should be available for anything more than very minor procedures, in case of complications.

General anaesthesia

Propofol, a newer anaesthetic agent, has established itself as the agent of choice for the induction, and often also the maintenance, of day-case patients because of its good anaesthetic conditions, rapid problem-free recovery and lack of postoperative nausea and vomiting (PONV). Indeed, it is antiemetic, a major advantage in day surgery. Children are increasingly induced intravenously. For inhalation induction sevoflurane has now replaced halothane in many countries because of its ease of use and speed of recovery.

Maintenance of anaesthesia is commonly with a volatile agent, such as isoflurane or enflurane, and nitrous oxide in oxygen. The newer volatile agents, desflurane and sevoflurane, with ultra-fast immediate recovery times, have proved disappointing, as like all volatile anaesthetic agents they have a high incidence of PONV which delays recovery, and little advantage has been shown to justify their increased cost. Many day surgery anaesthetists therefore use propofol by infusion to maintain anaesthesia, as well as for induction – total intravenous anaesthesia (TIVA). The increased cost may be justified in view of the excellent recovery, particularly after longer procedures and where the risk of PONV is high.

Short-acting opioids, such as alfentanil or fentanyl, are usually included in the general anaesthetic to reduce the dosage of other drugs and to provide some analgesia in the early postoperative period.

The laryngeal mask airway (LMA) has become popular in day surgery as it allows fast easy control of the airway, and endotracheal intubation and its hazards often can be avoided. It is now commonly used for straightforward laparoscopies, and for dental and head and neck procedures.

Table 69.10 Preadmission information

- On the front page – important information
  Time and date of the operation
  Contact telephone number if unable or unfit to keep the appointment
  The need for an escort and taxi or car to go home (not public transport)
  Instructions not to drive or operate machinery for 48 hours
  Fasting instructions
  Do not omit medication unless specifically requested to do so
  For women, ring the day surgery unit if you think that you might be pregnant
  Instructions for clothing, valuables and something to pass the time
- Other information on day surgery
  Map, parking and how to find the DSU
  A brief description of what will happen on the day
  Duration of stay and time for escort to come
  Postanaesthetic restrictions on driving, alcohol, taking decisions, etc.
  Who to contact about problems after discharge
- Procedure-specific information
  What the operation is, in simple nonfrightening terms ± diagrams/pictures
  Preoperative preparation, e.g. shaving
  Expected postoperative morbidity
  Time required off work and before resuming normal activities
  When to seek advice on postoperative problems
  Wound management, stitch removal and follow-up, if relevant

(Reproduced with permission from Millar, J.M., Rudkin, G.E. and Hitchcock, M., *Practical Anaesthesia and Analgesia for Day Surgery*, BIOS Scientific, Oxford 1997.)

Table 69.11 Suitable local and regional analgesia in day surgery

• Topical analgesia:	Skin surface, eyes, urethra
• Wound infiltration or dripping	
• Instillation into joints at arthroscopy	
• Instillation into peritoneum during laparoscopy	
• Peripheral nerve blocks:	Ilio-inguinal/genitofemoral Field block for hernia Penile Digit Wrist or ankle Axillary brachial plexus Peribulbar Dental, etc. and many more
• Intravenous regional analgesia (IVRA)	

Sedation

This is given ideally by an anaesthetist, but sometimes by other medically qualified personnel. The sedationist must not be involved in the procedure: the single-handed operator–sedationist is neither safe nor medicolegally defensible. Monitoring is required and supplemental oxygen is usually given. Sedation means that the patient is relaxed and calm while maintaining rational verbal contact. It is all too easy to oversedate the patient beyond this level, so that the patient is anaesthetised and airway control may be lost. Sedation is best left to experienced anaesthetists.

The use of midazolam, a short-acting benzodiazepine, is popular but its long-lasting postoperative amnesia may mean that postoperative instructions are forgotten. Propofol in low dose is very suitable for sedation, with faster wake-up and less amnesia, although some patients may prefer not to recall events in theatre. Small doses of opioids may also be used with caution, but may result in respiratory depression or apnoea.

Analgesia

Good pain control is essential. It is a major reason for delay in discharge (Fig. 69.3), unplanned overnight admission, GP consultations after discharge, and, not least, patient distress and dissatisfaction. It limits early patient mobilisation and prolongs return to normal function. The use of morphine, while successful in controlling pain, is less successful in day surgery because of its sedation and high incidence of nausea, which may only become apparent after the patient leaves the DSU. In order to avoid its use, a mixture of analgesic methods is needed – so-called balanced or multimodal analgesia. Nonsteroidal anti-inflammatory drugs (NSAIDs) plus local anaesthesia, where possible, form the basis, with additional short-acting opioids and other mild analgesics if needed. Although none of these methods is sufficient alone, in combination they are very effective.

The best local anaesthesia will not last longer than the evening of surgery, so it is important to provide sufficient oral analgesia for 3–5 days postdischarge. These should be prepared in packs supplied to the DSU and prescribed according to the expected pain for that operation (Table 69.12). Combinations of regular NSAIDs with simpler analgesics for break-through pain are successful. Unless clear instruction on their use is given, patients' compliance may be poor (Table 69.13).

Discharge

The patient must be seen before discharge by the surgeon and the anaesthetist, or their deputies. Formal discharge criteria are required, with documentation signed by the individual delegated to discharge the patient, usually a nurse. The patient and their escort must be given clear instructions on what to do after their general anaesthetic and surgery, including stitch removal and follow-up where needed (Tables 69.14 and 69.15).

Follow-up, audit and quality control

Good day surgery practice means that the incidence of non-attendance, cancellations, complications before and after discharge, overnight admission and readmission is audited, and improvements are made where needed. Where possible, a telephone call to the patient the next day reassures the patient and gives immediate feedback on the adequacy of analgesia and other problems. Specific audits should be conducted on patient satisfaction with their overall management, morbidity related to specific types of surgery and anaesthesia, and the adequacy of postoperative analgesia. The involvement of community services and GPs should be monitored.

Table 69.12 Expected pain and suitable analgesia to take home

Expected level of pain	*Analgesia*
Operations with mild pain e.g. minor gynaecological surgery, breast lump excision, minor lumps and bumps	Regular NSAID, e.g. ibuprofen or diclofenac **or** paracetamol with dextropropoxyphene (Coproxamol), or dihydrocodeine (Codydramol) or codeine 8 mg (Cocodamol)
Operations with moderate pain e.g. varicose vein surgery, knee arthroscopy	Regular NSAID, e.g. ibuprofen or diclofenac **plus**, as required if still in pain, paracetamol with dextropropoxyphene (Coproxamol) or dihydrocodeine (Codydramol) or codeine 8 mg (Cocodamol)
Operations with severe pain e.g. hernia repair, laparoscopic sterilisation, haemorrhoidectomy	Regular NSAID, e.g. ibuprofen or diclofenac **plus**, as required if still in pain, paracetamol 500 mg/codeine 30 mg 1–2 capsules 4-hourly (Cocodamol 30/500, Tylex®, Solpadol®) **or** Tramadol (Zydol®) 50–100 mg 4-hourly, if constipation must be avoided

Sufficient analgesia to last up to 5 days should be supplied before discharge.

Table 69.13 Example of patient instruction sheet for combination analgesia

Pain Killers to Take Home After Surgery
You have been given two types of pain killer to take home.

Diclofenac: 1 tablet every 8 hours.
Start as soon as you feel any pain or before you go to bed and continue to take them regularly. This means that you stay more comfortable.
If you still have pain, you make also take, in addition to the diclofenac:

Paracetamol 500 mg/codeine phosphate 30 mg*: 1–2 capsules every 4 hours. Do not take more than 8 capsules in 24 hours. (*Cocodamol 30/500, Tylex®, Solpadol®)

We recommend that you take both pain killers before going to bed on the first night after your operation to make sure that you have a pain-free night

Do Not Exceed The Recommended Doses
If you are still in pain despite taking the tablets you have been given, please contact your own doctor or telephone the Day Surgery Unit

NB: *Cocodamol 30/500/Tylex®/Solpadol® contains paracetamol, so do not take additional paracetamol
(Reproduced with permission from Millar, J.M., Rudkin, G.E. and Hitchcock, M., *Practical Anaesthesia and Analgesia for Day Surgery*, BIOS Scientific, Oxford, 1997.)

Table 69.14 Guidelines for safe discharge

- Vital signs stable for at least 1 hour
- The patient must be:
  orientated to person, time and place
  able to tolerate oral fluids*
  able to void†
  able to dress
  able to walk without assistance
- The patient must not have:
  more than minimal nausea or vomiting
  excessive pain
  bleeding
- The patient must be discharged by both the person who gave the anaesthesia and the person who performed the surgery or their designees‡
- Written instructions for the postoperative period at home, including a contact place and person who may be telephoned, need to be reinforced
- Patients must have a responsible 'vested' adult to escort them home and to stay with them at home

*Drinking is recommended before discharge but is not mandatory.
†Voiding is recommended as a criterion for discharge but is not mandatory. It should be required after spinal or epidural blocks, and after pelvic-related surgery.
‡It is not mandatory that these persons are physically present upon discharge if a discharge note has been signed and discharge is carried out following strict policy.
(Reproduced with permission from Korrtila, K., Recovery from outpatient anaesthesia. *Anaesthesia*, **50** (Suppl.), 22–8, 1995.)

Table 69.15 Instructions for patients who have had a general anaesthetic

Anaesthetic drugs remain in the body for some time and can have hangover effects even after you appear to be recovered. After your anaesthetic it is important to obey the following instructions:

- Do not drive a car, or any other vehicle including bicycles, or operate machinery for 48 hours
- Take great care with appliances such as kettles or cookers
- Avoid alcohol
- Do not lock the bathroom or toilet door, or make yourself inaccessible to the person looking after you
- Drink plenty of fluids and eat a light diet, avoiding heavy or greasy foods
- Take things easy the day after your operation and do not go to work or take strenuous exercise
- Do not make important decisions or sign important documents for 48 hours after your anaesthetic
- If there are problems after your return home,

  please telephone ....

  on (telephone number) and ask for ....

From the Day Surgery Unit, John Radcliffe Hospital, Oxford, UK.

Children in day surgery

Day surgery is the ideal for many paediatric surgical procedures, with well-documented psychological benefits for children. The principles for adults apply just as much to children, with a few crucial differences. Specially trained anaesthetic, surgical and nursing staff are required, and children should be kept separate from adults with designated children-only days or areas. A visit to the DSU beforehand to prepare the child and the provision of child-friendly areas and toys set the scene for stress-free surgery. Liaison with community services and the GP is essential, particularly for more major procedures. Children with single parents or in poor housing may need special assessment as to suitability.

The future of day surgery

Day surgery is no longer the fastest surgery on the fittest patients. The criteria for what is suitable are being stretched by the inclusion of older, less fit patients and more major procedures, enabled by developments in surgery and anaesthesia. Different modes of postdischarge care will be developed, although the cost-effectiveness of these must be established. Increasing attention will need to be paid to quality issues and to patients' attitudes as to what is actually acceptable. This underlines the importance of good day surgery practice.

Further reading

Audit Commission for Local Authorities and the National Health Service in England and Wales (1990) *A Short Cut to Better Services – Day Surgery in England and Wales*, HMSO, London.

Audit Commission for Local Authorities and the National Health Service in England and Wales (1991) *Measuring Quality: The Patients' View of Day Surgery*, HMSO, London.

National Association for the Welfare of Children in Hospital (1991) *Just for the Day: Children Admitted to Hospital for Day Treatment*, National Association for the Welfare of Children in Hospital, London.

NHS Management Executive (1993) *Day Surgery. Report by the Day Surgery Task Force*, BAPS Health Publications Unit, Heywood, Lancashire.

Royal College of Anaesthetists (1994) *Guidance for Purchasers on Perioperative Care*, Royal College of Anaesthetists, London.

Royal College of Surgeons of England (1992) *Guidelines for Day Case Surgery*, RCS, London.

White, P.F. (1997) *Ambulatory Anesthesia and Surgery*, W.B. Saunders, London.

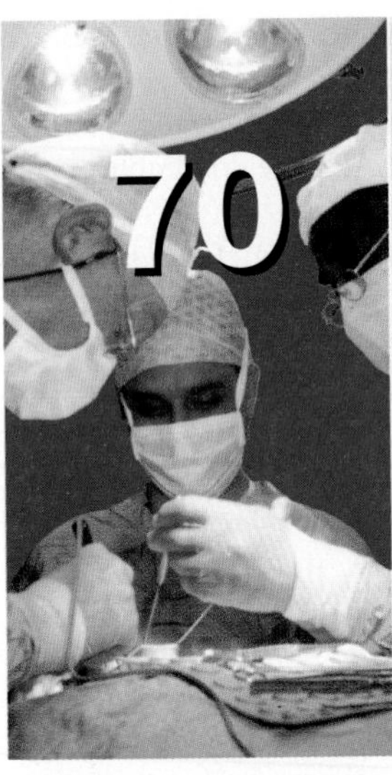

70 Principles of laparoscopic surgery

Definition

Minimal access surgery is a marriage of modern technology and surgical innovation which aims to accomplish surgical therapeutic goals with minimal somatic and psychological trauma. Minimal access techniques are less invasive and less disabling and disfiguring than conventional techniques. With increasing experience they offer cost-effectiveness both to health services and to employers by shortening operating times, shortening hospital stays and allowing faster recuperation.

Extent of minimal access surgery

Minimal access surgery has crossed all traditional boundaries of specialities and disciplines. Shared, borrowed and overlapping technologies and information are encouraging a multidisciplinary approach which serves the whole patient rather than a specific organ system. Broadly speaking, minimal access techniques can be categorised as follows.

Laparoscopy

A rigid endoscope is introduced through a metal sleeve into the peritoneal cavity which has been previously inflated with carbon dioxide to produce a pneumoperitoneum. There is little doubt that laparoscopic cholecystectomy has revolutionised the surgical management of cholelithiasis and has become the mainstay of management of uncomplicated gallstone disease. With improved instruments and more experience, it is likely that other advanced procedures, currently regarded as controversial, will also become fully accepted.

Thoracoscopy

A rigid endoscope is introduced through an incision in the chest to gain access to the thoracic contents. Many feel that the benefits of thoracoscopy will prove to be even greater than those of laparoscopy.

Endoluminal endoscopy

Flexible or rigid endoscopes are introduced into hollow organs or systems, such as the urinary tract, upper or lower gastrointestinal tract, and respiratory and vascular systems.

Perivisceral endoscopy

Body planes can be accessed even in the absence of a natural cavity. Examples are mediastinoscopy, retroperitoneoscopy and retroperitoneal approaches to the kidney, aorta and lumbar sympathetic chain. Other more recent examples include subfascial ligation of incompetent perforating veins in varicose vein surgery.

Arthroscopy and intra-articular joint surgery

Orthopaedic surgeons have long used arthroscopic access to the knee, and have now moved their attention to other joints including the shoulder, wrist, elbow and hip.

Bailey & Love's Short Practice of Surgery, 23rd edition. Edited by R.C.G. Russell, N.S. Williams and C.J.K. Bulstrode. Published in 2000 by Arnold Publishers.

Combined approach

The diseased organ is visualised and treated by an assortment of endoluminal and extraluminal endoscopes and other imaging devices.

Surgical trauma in open and laparoscopic surgery

Most of the trauma of an open procedure is inflicted because the surgeon must have a wound large enough to give adequate exposure for safe dissection at the target site. The wound is often the cause of morbidity including infection, dehiscence, bleeding, herniation and nerve entrapment. The pain of the wound prolongs recovery time, and by reducing mobility contributes to an increased incidence of pulmonary collapse, chest infection and deep venous thrombosis.

Mechanical and human retractors cause additional trauma. Body wall retractors tend to inflict localised damage which may be as painful as the wound itself. By contrast, during laparoscopy, the retraction is provided by the low-pressure pneumoperitoneum giving a diffuse force applied gently and evenly over the whole body wall, causing minimal trauma.

Exposure of any body cavity to the atmosphere also causes morbidity through cooling and fluid loss by evaporation. There is also evidence from the literature to suggest that the incidence of postsurgical adhesions has been reduced by the use of the laparoscope because there is less damage to delicate serosal coverings. In handling intestinal loops the surgeon and assistant disturb the peristaltic activity of the gut and provoke adynamic ileus.

In minimal access surgery the trauma of access and exposure is reduced while visualisation is magnified and improved.

Limitations of minimal access surgery

To perform minimal access surgery with safety, the surgeon must operate remote from the surgical field using an imaging system which provides a two-dimensional representation of the operative site. The endoscope offers a whole new anatomical landscape which the surgeon must learn to navigate without the usual cues which make it easy to judge depth. The instruments are longer and sometimes more complex to use than those common in open surgery. The result of all this is that the beginner in minimal access surgery is faced with significant problems of hand–eye co-ordination. Stereoscopic imaging for laparoscopy is still in its infancy. Future improvements in these systems will greatly enhance manipulative ability in critical procedures such as knot tying and dissection of closely underlying tissues. There are, however, some drawbacks, such as reduced display brightness and interference with normal vision due to the need to wear specially designed glasses. It is probable that brighter projection displays will be developed, at increased cost. However, the need to wear glasses will not be easily overcome. Looking further to the future, it is evident that the continuing reduction in costs of elaborate image processing techniques will make a wide range of transformed presentations available. It will ultimately be possible for a surgeon to call up any view of the operative region that is accessible to a camera and present it stereoscopically in any size or orientation, superimposed on past images taken in other modalities. It is for the medical community to decide which of these many imaginative possibilities will contribute most to effective surgical procedures.

Another problem occurs when there is intraoperative arterial bleeding. Haemostasis may be very difficult to achieve endoscopically because blood obscures the field of vision and there is a significant reduction of the image quality owing to light absorption.

Some of the procedures performed by this new approach are more technically demanding and are slower to perform. Indeed, on occasion a minimally invasive operation is so technically demanding that both patient and surgeon are better served by conversion to an open procedure. Unfortunately, there seems to be a sense of embarrassment or humiliation associated with conversion which is quite unjustified. It is vital for surgeons and patients to appreciate that the decision to close or convert to an open operation is not a complication but instead usually implies sound surgical judgement.

Another disadvantage of laparoscopic surgery is the loss of tactile feedback. Laparoscopic ultrasonography might be a substitute for the need 'to feel' in intraoperative decision making. Although ultrasonography has progressed significantly in the past several years, laparoscopic ultrasound remains in its infancy. The rapid progress in advanced laparoscopic techniques, including biliary tract exploration and surgery for malignancies, has provided a strong impetus for the development of laparoscopic ultrasound. Although incompletely developed, this technique already has advantages that far outweigh its disadvantages.

In more advanced techniques the large piece of resected tissue, such as the lung or colon, has to be extracted from the body cavity. Occasionally, the extirpated tissue may be removed through a nearby natural orifice, such as the rectum or the mouth. At other times a novel route may be employed. For instance, a benign colonic specimen may be extracted through an incision in the vault of the vagina. Although tissue 'morcellators, mincers and liquidisers' could be used in some circumstances, this has the disadvantage of reducing the amount of information available to the pathologist. Recent reports of tumour implantation in the sites of port holes have raised important questions about the future of the laparoscopic treatment of malignancy.

Hand-assisted laparoscopic surgery is a newly developed technique. It involves the intra-abdominal placement of a hand or forearm through a minilaparotomy incision whilst pneumoperitoneum is maintained. In this way the surgeon's hand can be used as in an open procedure. It can be used to palpate organs or tumours, to reflect organs atraumatically, to retract structures, to identify vessels, to dissect bluntly along a tissue plane and to provide finger pressure to bleeding points while proximal control is achieved. In addition, several reports have suggested that this approach is more economical than a totally laparoscopic approach, reducing both the number of laparoscopic ports and the number of instruments required. Some advocates of the technique claim that it is also easier to learn and perform than totally laparoscopic approaches, and that there may be increased patient safety.

There is a growing need for improvement in dissection techniques in laparoscopic surgery and, specifically, for improving the safe use of electrosurgery and lasers. Ultrasonic dissection and tissue removal has been utilised by a growing number of specialities for several years. The adaptation of the technology to laparoscopic surgery grew out of the search for alternative, possibly safer, methods of dissection. The current units combine the functions of three or four separate instruments, reducing the need for instrument exchanges during a procedure. This flexibility, combined with the ability to provide a clean, smoke-free field, improves safety while shortening operating times.

Although dramatic cost savings are possible with laparoscopic cholecystectomy, the position is less clear-cut with other procedures. There is another factor which may complicate the computation of cost–benefit. A significant rise in the rate of cholecystectomy followed the introduction of the laparoscopic approach as the threshold for referring patients for surgery lowered. The increase in the number of procedures performed has led to an overall increase in the cost of treating symptomatic gallstones.

Preoperative evaluation

Preparation of the patient undergoing laparoscopic surgery

Although the patient may only be in hospital for a few hours, careful preoperative management is essential to minimise morbidity.

Preparation is very similar to that for open surgery, and aims to ensure that:

- the patient is fit for the procedure;
- the patient is fully informed and consented;
- operative difficulty is predicted where possible;
- appropriate theatre time and facilities are available.

History

Patients must be fit for general anaesthesia and open operation if necessary. Potential coagulation disorders (for example, associated with cirrhosis) are particularly dangerous in laparoscopic surgery. As adhesions may cause problems, previous abdominal operations or peritonitis should be documented.

Examination

Routine preoperative physical examination is required as for any major operation. Although laparoscopic surgery in general allows quicker recovery, it may involve longer operating time and the establishment of the pneumoperitoneum may provoke cardiac arrythmias. Severe chronic obstructive airways disease and ischaemic heart disease may be contraindications to the laparoscopic approach.

Particular attention should be paid to the presence or absence of jaundice, abdominal scars, palpable masses or tenderness.

Moderate obesity does not increase operative difficulty significantly, but massive obesity may make pneumoperitoneum difficult, and standard instrumentation may be too short. Access may prove difficult in very thin patients, especially those with severe kyphosis.

Premedication

Premedication is the responsibility of the anaesthetist, with whom coexisting medical problems should be discussed, for example significant ischaemic heart disease.

Prophylaxis against thromboembolism

Venous stasis induced by the reversed Trendelenburg position during laparoscopic surgery may be a risk factor for deep vein thrombosis, as is a lengthy operation and the obesity of many patients. Subcutaneous heparin and TEDs should be used routinely in addition to pneumatic leggings during the operation. Patients already taking warfarin for other reasons should have this stopped temporarily or converted to intravenous heparin, depending on the underlying condition, as it is not safe to perform laparoscopic surgery in the presence of a significant coagulation deficit.

Urinary catheters and nasogastric tubes

In the early days of laparoscopic surgery routine bladder catheterisation and nasogastric intubation were advised. Most surgeons now omit these but it remains essential to check that the patient is fasted, and has recently emptied the bladder, before the blind insertion of a Verres needle.

Informed consent

The basis of many complaints and much litigation in surgery, especially laparoscopic surgery, relates to the issue of informed consent. It is mandatory that the patient understands the nature of the procedure, the risks involved and, where appropriate, what alternatives are available. A locally prepared explanatory booklet concerning the laparoscopic procedure to be undertaken is extremely useful.

Friedrich Trendelenberg, 1844–1924. Professor of Surgery, Leipzig, Germany.

In an elective case a full discussion of the proposed operation should take place in the out-patient department with a surgeon of appropriate seniority, preferably the operating surgeon, before the decision is made to operate. On admission it is the responsibility of the operating surgeon and anaesthetist to ensure that the patient has been fully counselled, although the actual witnessing of the consent form may have been delegated. The patient should understand what laparoscopic surgery involves and that there is a risk of conversion to open operation. If known, this risk should be quantified, for example the increased risk with acute cholecystitis or in the presence of extensive upper abdominal adhesions. The conversion rate will also vary with the experience and practice of the surgeon. Common complications should be mentioned, such as shoulder tip pain and minor surgical emphysema, as well as rare but serious complications including injury to the bile ducts and visceral injury from trochar insertion or diathermy.

A few patients may insist on having an open procedure (probably influenced by accounts of mishaps) and the surgeon should be prepared to offer this, although most will opt for laparoscopy if the surgeon offers an extensive experience and impressive safety record.

General intraoperative principles

Laparoscopic cholecystectomy is the treatment of choice for gallstone disease. The most accepted technique was outlined by Reddick and Olsen. The main drawback of the technique is the increased incidence of bile-duct injury compared with open cholecystectomy. However, with better understanding of the mechanisms of injury and with proper training, virtually almost all of these injuries can be avoided. This chapter highlights important technical steps that should be taken during any form of laparoscopic surgery to avoid complications.

Creating a pneumoperitoneum

The most common method of obtaining a pneumoperitoneum is by blind puncture using a Verres needle. Although this method is fast and relatively safe, there is a small but significant potential for intestinal or vascular injury on introduction of the needle or first trocar. The routine use of the open technique for creating a pneumoperitoneum avoids the morbidity related to a blind puncture. To do this, a 1-cm vertical or transverse incision is made at the level of the umbilicus. Two small retractors are used to dissect bluntly the subcutaneous fat and expose the midline fascia. Two sutures are inserted each side of the midline incision, followed by the creation of a 1 cm opening in the fascia. Free penetration into the abdominal cavity is confirmed by the gentle introduction of a finger. Finally, a Hasson (or other blunt-tip) trocar is inserted and anchored with the fascial sutures (Fig. 70.1). The open technique may initially appear time-consuming and even cumbersome. With practice, however, it is overall more efficient.

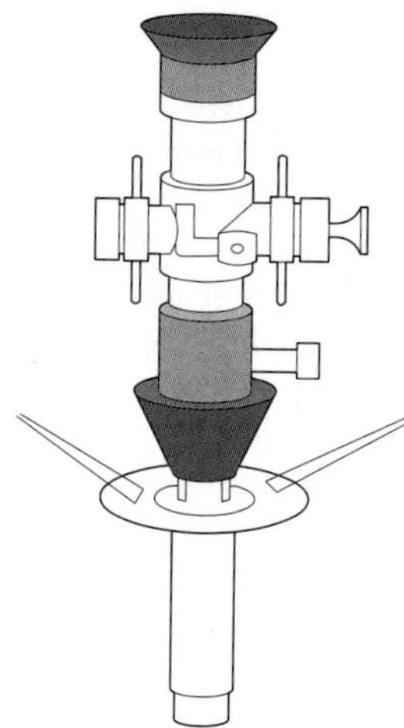

Fig. 70.1 Open technique with Hasson port. Apply safe principles of closed technique.

Preoperative problems

Previous abdominal surgery

Previous abdominal surgery is no longer a contraindication to laparoscopic surgery, but preoperative evaluation is necessary to assess the type and location of surgical scars. As mentioned earlier, the open technique for insertion of the first trocar is safer. Prior to trocar insertion, the introduction of a fingertip helps to ascertain penetration into the peritoneal cavity and also allows adhesions to be gently removed from the entry site. After the tip of the cannula has been introduced, a 0°-laparoscope is used as a blunt dissector to tease adhesions gently away and to form a tunnel towards the quadrant where the operation is to take place. This step is accomplished by a careful pushing and twisting motion under direct vision. With experience, the surgeon learns to differentiate visually between thick adhesions that may contain bowel and should be avoided, and thin adhesions that would lead to a window into a free area of the peritoneal cavity (Fig. 70.2).

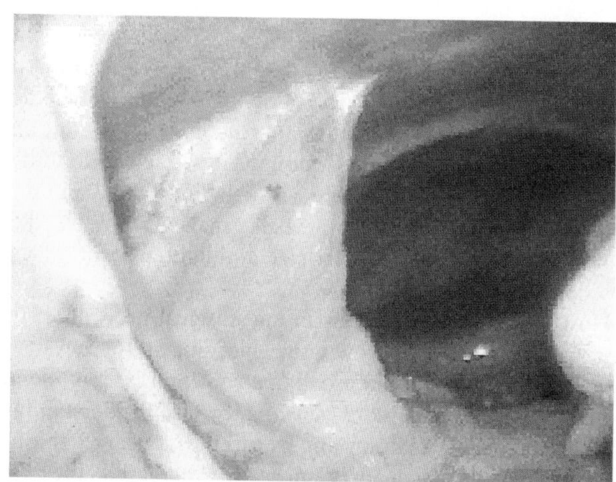

Fig. 70.2 Intra-abdominal adhesion.

Obesity

Laparoscopic surgery has proved to be a safe and effective procedure in the obese population. In fact, some procedures are less difficult than their open counterpart for the morbidly obese patient. Technical difficulties occur, however, in obtaining pneumoperitoneum, in reaching the operative region adequately and in achieving adequate exposure in the presence of an obese colon. Increased thickness of the subcutaneous fat makes insufflation of the abdominal cavity more difficult. With the closed technique, a larger Verres needle is often required for morbidly obese patients. Pulling the skin up for fixation of the soft tissues is better accomplished with towel clamps. Only moderate force should be used to avoid separating the skin farther away from the fascia. The needle should be passed at nearly a right angle to the skin and preferably above the umbilicus where the peritoneum is more firmly fixed to the midline. The open technique of inserting a Hasson trocar is easier and safer for obese patients. The main difficulty is reaching the fascia. A larger skin incision (1–3 cm) starting at the umbilicus and extending superiorly may facilitate this. To reach the operative area adequately, the location of some of the ports has to be modified, and in some instances, larger instruments are necessary. When the length of the laparoscope appears to be insufficient to reach the operative area adequately, the initial midline port should be placed nearer to the operative field.

Operative problems

Perforation of the gall bladder

Perforation of the gall bladder is more common with the laparoscopic technique than with the open technique. Some authors have reported an incidence of up to 30 per cent, but this did not appear to be a factor in increasing the early postoperative morbidity. However, it is well known that bile is not a sterile fluid and bacteria can be present in the absence of cholecystitis. Unless the perforation is small, closure with endoloops should be attempted to avoid contamination.

Bleeding

In some of the larger series, bleeding has been the most common cause for conversion to an open procedure. Bleeding plays a more important role in laparoscopic surgery because of factors inherent to the technique. These include a limited field that can easily be obscured by relatively small amounts of blood, magnification that makes small arterial bleeding look like a significant haemorrhage and light absorption that obscures the visual field.

How to avoid bleeding. As in any surgical procedure, the best way to handle intraoperative bleeding is to prevent it from happening. This can usually be accomplished by identifying patients at high risk of bleeding, by clear understanding of the laparoscopic anatomy and by careful surgical technique.

Risk factors which predispose to increased bleeding include:

- cirrhosis;
- inflammatory condition (acute cholecystitis, diverticulitis);
- coagulation defects: these are contraindications to a laparoscopic procedure.

Bleeding from a major vessel. Damage to a large vessel requires immediate assessment of the magnitude and type of bleeding. When the bleeding vessel is identified, a fine-tip grasper can be used to grasp it and apply either electrocautery or a clip, depending on the size of the vessel. When the vessel is not identified early and a pool of blood forms, compression should be applied immediately with a blunt instrument, a cotton swab or with the adjacent organ. Good suction and irrigation are of utmost importance. After the area has been cleaned, pressure should be released gradually to identify the site of bleeding. Insertion of an extra cannula may be required to achieve adequate exposure and at the same time to enable the concomitant use of a suction device and an insulated grasper. Although most of the bleeding vessels can be controlled laparoscopically, judgement should be used not to prolong bleeding but to convert to an open procedure at an early stage whenever control of bleeding is not achieved promptly.

Bleeding from the gall-bladder bed. Bleeding from the gall-bladder bed can usually be prevented by performing the dissection in the correct plane. When a bleeding site appears during detachment of the gall bladder, the dissection should be carried a little farther better to expose the bleeding point. After this step has been performed, direct application of the electrocautery usually controls the bleeding. If bleeding persists, indirect application of the electrocautery is useful because it avoids detachment of the formed crust. This procedure is accomplished by applying pressure to the bleeding point with a blunt insulated grasper and then applying electrocoagulation by touching this grasper with a second insulated grasper that is connected to the electrocautery. One must be careful to keep all conducting surfaces of the graspers within the visual field while applying the electrocautery current.

Bleeding from a trocar site. Bleeding from the trocar sites is usually controlled by applying upward and lateral pressure with the trocar itself. Considerable bleeding may occur if the falciform ligament is impaled with the substernal trocar or if one of the epigastric vessels is injured. If significant continuous bleeding from the falciform ligament occurs, haemostasis is achieved by percutaneously inserting a large straight needle at one side of the ligament. A monofilament suture attached to the needle is passed into the abdominal cavity, and the needle is exited at the other side of the ligament using a grasper (Fig. 70.3). The loop is suspended and compression is achieved. Maintaining compression throughout the procedure usually suffices. After the procedure has been completed, the loop is removed under direct laparoscopic visualisation to ensure complete haemostasis. When significant continuous bleeding from the abdominal wall occurs, haemostasis can be accomplished either by pressure or by suturing the bleeding site. Pressure can be applied using a Foley balloon catheter. The catheter is introduced into the abdominal cavity through the bleeding trocar site wound, the balloon is inflated, traction is placed on the catheter and it is bolstered in place to keep it under tension. The catheter is left *in situ* for 24 hours and then removed. Although this method is successful in achieving haemostasis, the author favours direct suturing of the bleeding vessel. This manoeuvre is accomplished by extending the skin incision by 3 mm at both ends of the bleeding trocar site wound. Two figure-of-eight sutures are placed in the path of the vessel at both ends of the wound.

Evacuation of blood clots. The best way of dealing with blood clots is to avoid them. As mentioned, careful dissection and identification of the cystic artery and its branches, as well as identifying and carrying out dissection of the gall bladder in the correct plane, avoid bleeding from the cystic vessels and the hepatic bed. Nevertheless, clot formation takes place when unsuspected bleeding occurs or when inflammation is severe and a clear plane is not present between the gall bladder and the hepatic bed. The routine use of 5000–7000 units of heparin per litre of irrigation fluid helps to avoid the formation of clots. When extra bleeding is foreseen, a small pool of irrigation fluid can be kept in the operative field to prevent clot formation. After clots have formed, a large-bore suction device should be used for their retrieval. Care should be taken to avoid suctioning in proximity to placed clips.

Principles of electrosurgery during laparoscopic surgery

Electrosurgical injuries during laparoscopy are potentially serious. The vast majority occurs following the use of monopolar diathermy. The overall incidence is between one and two patients per 1000 operations. Electrical injuries are usually unrecognised at the time they occur, with patients commonly presenting 3–7 days after injury with complaints of fever and abdominal pain. As these injuries usually present late, the reasons for their occurrence are largely speculative.

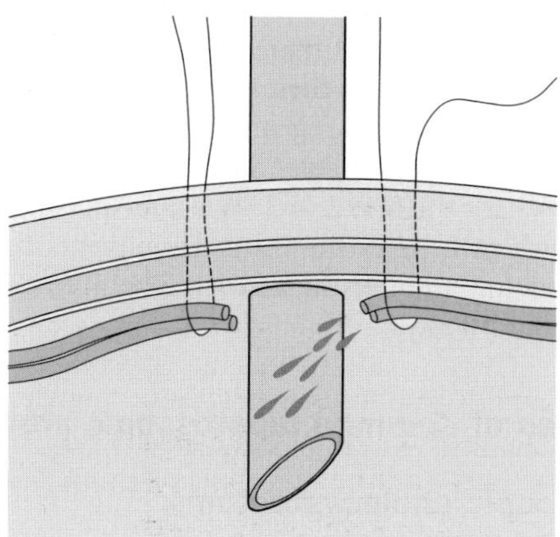

Fig. 70.3 Port side bleeding controlled with sutures.

Frederic E.B. Foley, 1891–1966. American urologist, Ankher Hospitals, St Paul, USA.

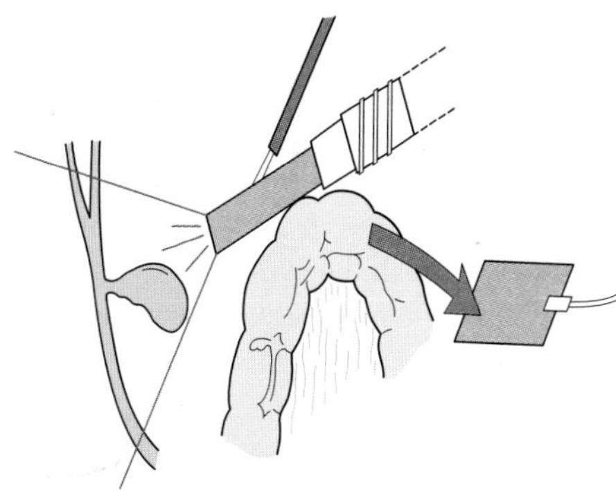

Fig. 70.4 Direct coupling between bowel and laparoscope, which is touching the activated probe.

The main theories are: (1) inadvertent touching or grasping of tissue during current application; (2) direct coupling between a portion of bowel and a metal instrument which is touching the activated probe (Fig. 70.4); (3) insulation breaks in the electrodes; (4) direct sparking to bowel from the diathermy probe; and (5) current passage to the bowel from recently coagulated, electrically isolated tissue. Bipolar diathermy is safer and should be used in preference to monopolar diathermy, especially in anatomically crowded areas. If monopolar diathermy is to be used important safety measures include attainment of a perfect visual image, avoiding excessive current application and meticulous attention to insulation. Alternative methods of performing dissection such as ultrasonic devices may improve safety.

Postoperative care

The postoperative care of patients after laparoscopic surgery is generally very straightforward with a very low incidence of pain or other problems. The most common routine postoperative symptoms are a dull upper abdominal pain, nausea and pain around the shoulders (referred from the diaphragm). It is a good general rule that if the patient develops a fever or tachycardia or complains of severe pain at the operation site, something is wrong and they should be kept under close observation. In that case routine investigation should include full blood count, liver function tests, amylase and, probably, an ultrasound of the upper abdomen to detect fluid collections. If bile duct leakage is suspected an endoscopic retrograde cholangiopancreatography (ERCP) may be needed. In cases of doubt, relaparoscopy or laparotomy should be performed earlier rather than later. Death following technical errors in laparoscopic cholecystectomy has often been associated with a long delay in deciding to re-explore the abdomen.

In the absence of problems the patient should be fit for discharge within 24 hours. They should be given instructions to telephone the unit or their general practitioner and to return to the hospital if they are not making satisfactory progress.

Nausea

About half of the patients after laparoscopic surgery experience some degree of nausea and rarely this is severe. It usually responds to an antiemetic such as ondansetron and settles within 12–24 hours. It is made worse by opiate analgesics and these should be avoided.

Shoulder pain

The patient should be warned about this preoperatively and told that the pain is referred from the diaphragm and not due to a local problem in the shoulders. It can be at its worse 24 hours after the operation. It usually settles within 2–3 days and is relieved by simple analgesics such as paracetamol.

Abdominal pain

Pain in one or other of the port site wounds is not uncommon and is worse if there is haematoma formation. It usually settles very rapidly. Increasing pain after 2 or 3 days may be a sign of infection and occasionally antibiotics are indicated.

Analgesia

A 100-mg diclofenae suppository should be given at the time of the operation. This may be repeated two or three times postoperatively for more severe pain. Otherwise paracetamol 500–1000 mg 4-hourly usually suffices. Opiate analgesics cause nausea and should be avoided unless the pain is very severe. In that case suspect a postoperative complication (as above). The majority of patients requires between one and four doses of 1 g of paracetamol postoperatively.

Orogastric tube

An orogastric tube may be placed during the operation if the stomach is distended and obscuring the view. It is not necessary in all cases. It should be removed as soon as the operation is over and before the patient regains consciousness.

Oral fluids

There is no significant ileus after laparoscopic surgery, except in resectional procedures such as colectomy or small bowel resection. Patients can start taking oral fluids as soon as they are conscious. They usually do so 4–6 hours after the end of the operation.

Oral feeding

Providing the patient has an appetite a light meal can be taken 4–6 hours after the operation. Some patients remain slightly nauseated at this stage but almost all eat a normal breakfast on the morning after the operation.

Patients will require advice about what they can eat at home. They should be told they can eat a normal diet but should avoid excess. It seems sensible to keep off high-fat meals for the first week, although there is no clear evidence that this is necessary.

Urinary catheter

If a urinary catheter has been placed in the bladder during the operation it should be removed before the patient regains consciousness. The patient should be warned of the possibility and symptoms of postoperative cystitis and told to seek advice in the unlikely event of these occurring.

Drains

Some surgeons drain the abdomen at the end of laparoscopic cholecystectomy, although there is controversy about this. If a drain is placed to vent the remaining gas and peritoneal fluid it should be removed within 1 hour of the operation. If it has been placed because of excessive hepatic bleeding or bile leakage it should be removed when that problem has resolved, usually after 12–24 hours. Continued blood loss from a drain is an indication for re-exploring the abdomen.

Discharge from hospital

Some surgeons discharge a proportion of their patients on the day of surgery but most are kept in overnight and discharged next morning. The patient should not be discharged until they are seen to be comfortable and eating and drinking satisfactorily. They should be told that if they develop abdominal pain or other severe symptoms they should return to the hospital or to their general practitioner.

Skin sutures

If nonabsorbable sutures or skin staples have been used these can be removed from the port sites after 48 hours.

Mobility and convalescence

Patients can get out of bed to go to the toilet as soon as they have recovered from the anaesthetic and they should be encouraged to do so. Such movements are remarkably pain free when compared with the mobility achieved after an open operation. Similarly, patients can cough actively and clear bronchial secretions and this helps to diminish the incidence of chest infections. Many patients are able to walk out of hospital on the evening of their operation, and almost all are fully mobile by the following morning. Thereafter the postoperative recovery is variable. Some patients prefer to take things quietly for the first 2 or 3 days interspersing increasing exercise with rest. After the third day patients have undertaken increasing amounts of activity. The average return to work is about 10 days.

Principles of common laparoscopic procedures

Laparoscopic cholecystectomy

Laparoscopic cholecystectomy is the treatment of choice for gallstone disease. The most accepted technique was outlined by Reddick and Olsen, and has been described extensively in the literature. The main drawback of the technique is the increased incidence of bile duct injury compared with open cholecystectomy. However, with better understanding of the mechanisms of injury and with proper training, virtually all of these injuries can be avoided. This chapter highlights important technical steps during routine laparoscopic cholecystectomy with particular emphasis on the safe performance of a difficult cholecystectomy.

Following introduction of the three working trocars, the operation is carried out using the surgical principles of open cholecystectomy. Most common bile-duct injuries can be avoided by adhering to the following steps.

1. Ensure maximum cephalic traction on the gall bladder. This step minimises redundancies in the gall bladder infundibulum for better visualisation of Calot's triangle (Fig. 70.5).
2. The gall bladder should be pulled away from the liver by maintaining lateral and inferior traction on Hartmann's pouch. This manoeuvre avoids alignment of the cystic and common bile duct, allowing more precise identification of both structures.
3. Dissection should begin high in the neck of the gall bladder and proceed in a lateral-to-medial direction. All dissection should be kept close to the gall bladder until the anatomy is well defined. The cystic duct node is a good landmark at which to start the dissection. The cystic duct should be the first spherical structure found in Calot's triangle when dissecting in a lateral-to-medial direction.
4. Hartmann's pouch should be turned medially for posterolateral dissection of the gall-bladder serosa. This manoeuvre aids identification of the junction between the neck of the gall bladder and the cystic duct. Dissection should proceed along the posterolateral aspect, dividing the serosal attachments of the neck of the gall bladder to the liver. The narrowing of the gall-bladder infundibulum into the cystic duct should be clearly defined in all of its circumference, particularly in the presence of acute inflammation or chronic scarring (Fig. 70.6).
5. Dissect the neck of the gall bladder from its hepatic bed. This approach, similar to that of the anterograde technique of open cholecystectomy, permits clear visualisation of the neck of the gall bladder as it narrows into the cystic duct. Identification of the cystic duct–common duct junction is no longer considered imperative if there is adequate visualisation of the gall-bladder–cystic duct junction. Extensive dissection in the region of the common duct may be a source of avoidable morbidity.
6. A clear view of the cystic duct should be obtained before the application of clips, which should be placed as close to the gall bladder as possible under direct vision. When a short cystic duct is present, an endoloop or ligature around the gall-bladder neck can be used instead of a clip. Diathermy should never be used to divide the cystic duct or artery.
7. Operative cholangiography – intraoperative cholangiography is helpful for definition of the anatomy, detecting the presence of calculi and preventing, recognising or decreasing the severity of a bile-duct injury. However, a significant percentage of surgeons does not perform cholangiography unless indicated. It is left to the surgeon's discretion to decide upon the use of cholangiography.
8. Following division of the cystic duct and artery, dissection should continue close to the gall-bladder wall and away from the liver hilum. Excessive use of electrocautery should be avoided in close proximity to the hilar structures. Bipolar diathermy is safer but less efficient than monopolar diathermy. Most surgeons use monopolar diathermy with lower voltage during dissection. Progressive detachment of the gall bladder is much easier

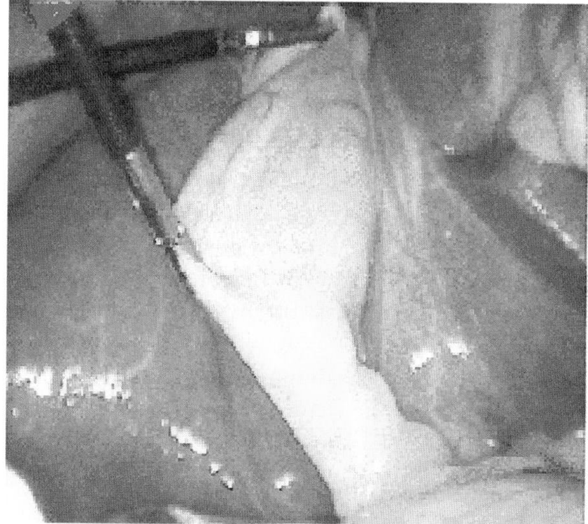

Fig. 70.5 Calot's triangle exposed by traction of the gall-bladder fundus upwards and Hartmann's pouch laterally.

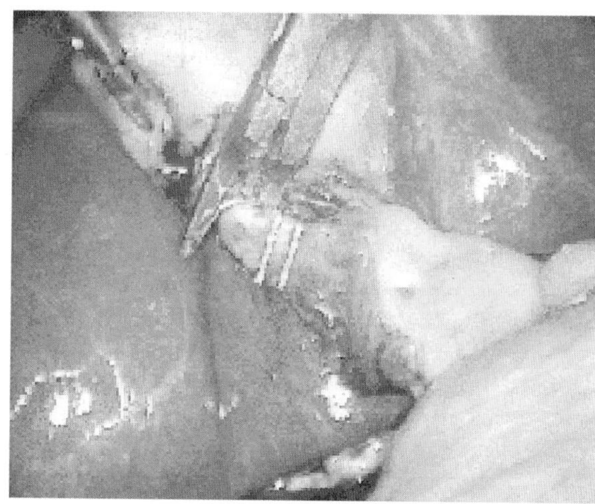

Fig. 70.6 Cystic cyst clipped.

Jean François Calot, 1861–1944. Surgeon, Paris, France.
Henri Albert Charles Antoine Hartmann, 1860–1952. Professor of Surgery, Paris, France.

and occurs with less bleeding if dissection is carried in the correct plane close to the gall-bladder wall.

9. Convert to open cholecystectomy – the surgeon should consider his or her limitations and be able to determine when the degree of difficulty or uncertainty necessitates conversion to open cholecystectomy. Conversion should not be considered as 'loss of face' and should be undertaken when 'progress no longer seems feasible'.
10. Removal of the dissected gall bladder from the abdominal cavity should be performed under direct vision from either the umbilical or the epigastric port. It is not uncommon for extraction to be complicated by a thickened gall-bladder wall or the presence of multiple large calculi. Enlarging the fascial incision by a few millimetres at each edge should not be left too late as this manoeuvre can prevent the spillage of calculi or bile into the abdominal cavity. Endoscopic retrieval bags can be used to prevent stone spillage if gall-bladder perforation has occurred (Fig. 70.7). Extending the incision by a small amount does not appear to increase postoperative pain and, overall, may save time. Reduction in postoperative shoulder-tip pain may be achieved if care is taken to remove any residual fluid or blood and to obtain complete deflation before closure.

Laparoscopic inguinal hernia repair

Inguinal hernia is one of the most common surgical problems seen in general practice, and accounts for 15 per cent of operating time in a typical district general hospital. Despite the existence of many well-established traditional hernia repairs, results have been variable with recurrence rates ranging from 0.2 to 18 per cent. These unsatisfactory results have led to surgeons developing and seeking new methods of hernia repair. The main factor contributing to hernia recurrence is the tension produced after the repair by the suturing together of structures not normally in apposition. This theory led to the use of mesh to repair the hernia, making it a 'tension-free' procedure. Today the tension-free hernioplasty is one of the most succesful variations of hernia repair.

Recently, with the introduction of minimal access techniques and the subsequent success of laparoscopic cholecystectomy, surgeons have investigated the possibility of repairing inguinal hernias using such an approach. The advantages to using a minimal access approach to hernia repair are mainly to do with patient comfort rather than hospital stay. Although laparoscopic hernia repair can be done as a day-case procedure, so can open hernia repair. Multiple hernias and recurrent hernias are more effectively dealt with using a laparoscopic approach.

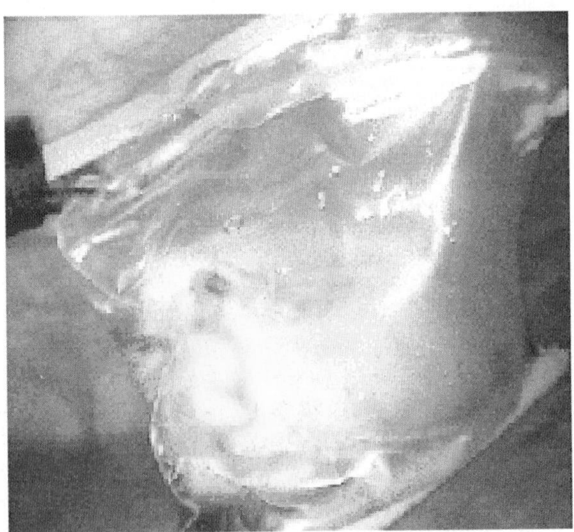

Fig. 70.7 Gall-bladder extraction bag.

Types of laparoscopic hernia repair

As with the open approach many variations on the laparoscopic approach have been developed, some of which have already fallen from favour.

Transabdominal preperitoneal repair (TAPP). The procedure is carried out under general anaesthesia, the patient's abdomen is inflated with carbon dioxide gas, the peritoneum is incised above the hernia and a prosthetic mesh is stapled over the defect. The peritoneum is once again apposed over the mesh by the use of a stapling device.

Extraperitoneal repair. In this repair the abdominal cavity is not entered but instead surgical balloons are inflated in the extraperitoneal space, and endoscopic trocars and instruments are placed in this operating tunnel (Fig. 70.8). Again a stapled prosthetic mesh is used for repair. By not incising the peritoneum this decreases the risk of mesh eroding into bowel and the occurrence of bowel obstruction due to herniation of the small bowel through the staple line in the peritoneum.

Results thus far have been encouraging: the repair has been shown to be effective and safe if it is carried out in a major laparoscopic centre with well-equipped and trained laparoscopic surgeons. Solid conclusions about recurrence rates cannot be made as the follow-up period is too short.

Laparoscopic antireflux surgery

Gastro-oesophageal reflux disease (GORD) is one of the most common disorders affecting the gastrointestinal system. Whilst the use of antacids, H_2-receptor antagonists and proton pump inhibitors may allow healing of oesophagitis to take place, GORD is often a chronic or recurrent problem requiring long-

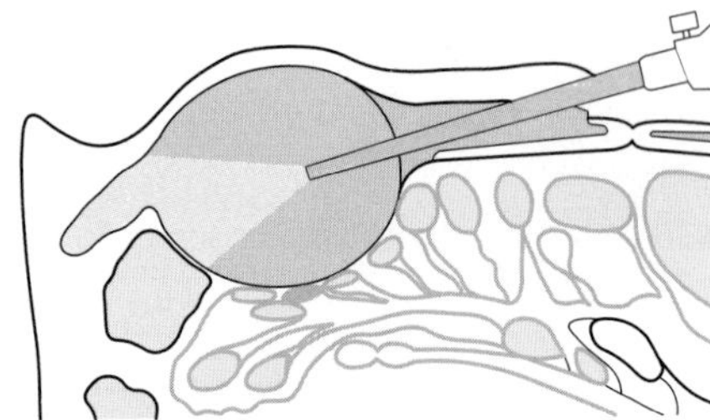

Fig. 70.8 Endoscopic extraperitoneal inguinal hernia repair using an endoscopic balloon dissector inflated under direct endoscopic view.

term medical management. Open surgery for selected patients has been shown to be effective, but is a major undertaking associated with considerable morbidity. Hence the possibility of treating this condition effectively whilst exploiting the benefits of a minimal access approach is very attractive.

Techniques of laparoscopic antireflux surgery

The advantages of laparoscopic cholecystectomy over open surgery in terms of postoperative pain, hospital stay, return to normal activity and cosmesis have led to the application of this approach to several gastrointestinal procedures. Whereas open antireflux surgery provides poor exposure using either abdominal or thoracic approaches, a laparoscopic approach provides an unparalleled view of the diaphragmatic hiatus. Indeed, the anatomical detail provided by this technique combined with the potential benefits of minimal access surgery have led to the reincarnation of several antireflux operations that were rarely performed in the past.

The laparoscopic Nissen fundoplication was introduced in 1991 and is the most widely performed laparoscopic antireflux procedure. The operation is essentially the same as the open version with a few exceptions. Access is achieved via a five-port arrangement with the surgeon standing to the left, right or between the legs of the patient, depending on preference. Whilst mobilisation of the oesophagus is underway it is important that the liver be adequately retracted, a process facilitated by the use of fan retractors. An enlaged left lobe of the liver is a relative contraindication to fundoplication as it may make retraction difficult and dissection hazardous.

The Rossetti modification of the Nissen repair involves using just the anterior fundus to perform the wrap (Rossetti). This reduces the amount of gastro-oesophageal dissection needed and also makes division of the short gastric vessels unnecessary. Division of all short gastric vessels may be required for a Nissen fundoplication to ensure a short, loose wrap to reduce the incidence of mechanical complications. The wrap is secured with four or five silk sutures which may be tied by an intracorporeal or extracorporeal technique. Nissen did not consider closure of the hiatus by bringing the crura together behind the oesophagus, an important step in the procedure. However, several authors advocate crural closure to promote physiological function of the lower oesophageal sphincter and prevent upward displacement of the wrap.

Given the recent introduction of the procedure and short follow-up times, results for the laparoscopic Nissen repair are promising. Operative times are, on average, less than 2.5 hours and conversion rates are low. The incidence of operative and postoperative complications is low and comparable to that reported from open series. Intraoperative complications include unrecognised pleural lacerations requiring chest drainage, hepatic laceration, gastric perforation and wrap necrosis with perforation. Most patients experience gastrointestinal side effects in the postoperative period, the commoner ones being early satiety, hyperflatuence, diarrhoea, nausea and odynophagia, but these become less common with time. A low incidence of postoperative dysphagia has been attributed by one author to the enforcement of a liquid diet for 3 weeks after surgery.

As with all laparoscopic surgery it can never be assumed that just because a procedure can be performed laparoscopically, it should be adopted. As none of the laparoscopic versions of antireflux operations represents a major departure from their open counterparts, there is no reason to expect better symptomatic results. There should, however, be a reduction in hospital stay and wound complications, and earlier return to normal activities. In the past, gastroenterologists have perhaps been reluctant to refer patients for antireflux surgery, perceiving it to be a major undertaking in a field where the procedure of choice is by no means agreed upon. However, if laparoscopic antireflux surgery shows itself to be safe and effective, one might see a lowering of the threshold for referral. The important point is that the selection criteria should not change. As to the question of which procedure, the answer lies in long-term randomised prospective trials. Assessment of symptomatic success should be done objectively, for example using Visick grading. pH studies should be performed preoperatively and postoperatively to document healing, and where possible, assessment should be performed by independent parties.

Laparoscopic splenectomy

Laparoscopic splenectomy has been reported as a feasible and attractive procedure on selective patients with haematological disorders. The criteria for the effectiveness of laparoscopic splenectomy include: technical feasibility, safety and, most importantly, long-term recurrence rates of thrombocytopenia. The ultimate aim is cure, through the removal of all splenic tissue including accessory spleen. Open splenectomy has already achieved these goals with a technical feasibility of 100 per cent and an operative mortality of 0–4 per cent. The postoperative complication rate is 10–20 per cent and long-term cure rate is 65–90 per cent in patients with idiopathic thrombocytopenia purpura (ITP).

The majority of reported series on laparoscopic splenectomy has essentially focused on the technical problem of laparoscopic feasibility. The purpose of this review is to describe a technical modification of laparoscopic splenectomy using the hand port system to facilitate hand-assisted laparoscopic splenectomy.

Selection of patients

Not all patients or all haematological disorders can be treated by a laparoscopic-assisted approach. In the author's experience, obesity, a previous history of upper abdominal surgery and the presence of an acute coagulation abnormality are relative contraindications to hand-assisted laparoscopic splenectomy. ITP represents the base indication, but patients with congenital spherocytosis, haemolytic anaemia, Hodgkin's disease, lymphoma, splenic tumour and thrombo-

Thomas Hodgkin, b. 1798. English physician.

cytopenia related to acquired immunodeficiency syndrome are all considered to be suitable. Although normal sized spleens are best suited for a laparoscopic approach, the hand-assisted method significantly facilitates the excision of large spleens where difficulties in laparoscopic access alone significantly complicate laparoscopic mobilisation, access to the splenic hilum and extraction. Abdominal computed tomography (CT) is the best preoperative investigation to measure the splenic volume in order to detect the pancreatic tail impacted within the splenic hilum, exclude lymph nodes at the splenic hilum and detect accessory spleens.

Preoperative management

All patients receive preoperative pneumoccocal vaccination, especially children. Patients with ITP receive high doses of immunoglobulin G to increase their platelet count to an almost normal value; however, in the remaining patients, platelet transfusions might need to be used at the time of surgery.

Operative steps

Exposure of the spleen and access to the splenic hilum are the most critical factors in achieving a safe dissection. The vertical approach to the splenic hilum is mandatory with:

- high insertion of the trocar along the left costal margin;
- rotation of the table to the right side;
- use of reverse Trendelenburg position for the operative table;
- use of a 30° laparoscope.

Dissection is then performed laterally and posteriorly by dividing the lateral peritoneal reflection of the spleen anteriorly upward in the inferior part of the gastrosplenic ligament. The splenic hilum is approached anteriorly and inferiorly. This approach is greatly facilitated if posterior, lateral mobilisation of the spleen up to the splenophrenic ligament is achieved, with the liberation of the upper part of the spleen. The hilar vessels are isolated with the fingers from the pancreatic tail and stapled using an endoscopic stapling device. Finally, the short gastric vessels are secured within the upper part of the gastrocolic ligament with complete mobilisation of the superior port of the spleen.

The second operative step is the extraction of the surgical specimen which is usually facilitated and greatly simplified in the presence of a hand inside, so the spleen can be placed in a heavy plastic bag and extracted through the hand port device. During all intraoperative manipulations, one must be careful to avoid parenchymal tear and spillage to prevent splenosis. Some authors have advocated the use of preoperative splenic embolisation before laparoscopic splenectomy.

Potential advantages are reported to be easier dissection, shrinkage of the enlarged spleen, and reduction of operative blood loss and a certain amount of autotransfusion before splenectomy.

Disadvantages include the invasiveness of the procedure, high cost, higher complication rates and lack of diagnosis of accessory spleen in its most unusual location.

Another disadvantage of the laparoscopic approach for splenectomy appears to be a significant increase in the operative time; however, with the use of the hand port device, in the author's experience, the operative time is no longer than that of an open splenectomy.

Laparoscopic splenectomy is technically feasible in both normal sized and enlarged spleens. In the hands of the experienced laparoscopic surgeon the procedure is safe and has a low complication rate. The most common intraoperative complication is haemorrhage, which is responsible for most cases of conversion. Careful intraoperative search for and removal of accessory spleen is essential during the procedure, which is once again enhanced with the use of the hand-assisted device.

The future

Although there is no doubt that minimal access surgery has changed the practice of surgeons, it has not changed the nature of disease. The basic principles of good surgery still apply, including appropriate case selection, excellent exposure, adequate retraction and a high level of technical expertise. If a procedure makes no sense with conventional access, it will make no sense with a minimal access approach.

Improvements in instrumentation and the development of structured training programmes are the key to the future of minimal access surgery. It is certain that there is much that is new in minimal access surgery. Time will tell how much of what is new is truly better.

> The cleaner and gentler the act of operation, the less the patient suffers, the smoother and quicker his convalescence, the more exquisite his healed wound. (Lord Moynihan of Leeds)

Further reading

Cadiere, G.B., Houben, J.J., Bruyns, J., Himpens, J., Panzer, J.M and Gelin, M. (1994) Laparoscopic Nissen fundoplication: technique and preliminary results. *British Journal of Surgery*, **81**, 400–3.

Cuschieri, A. (1992) A rose by any other name: minimal access or minimally invasive surgery. *Surgical Endoscopy*, **6**, 214.

Cuschieri, A. (1993) Laparoscopic anti-reflux surgery and repair of hiatal hernia. *World Journal of Surgery*, **17**, 40–5.

McKernan, J.B. and Laws, H.L. (1994) Laparoscopic Nissen fundoplication for the treatment of gastroesophageal reflux disease. *American Surgeon*, **60**, 87–93.

Mouiel, J. and Katkhouda, N. (1994) Laparoscopic Rossetti fundoplication. In *Principles and Practice of Laparoscopic Surgery* (eds S. Patterson-Brown and J. Garden), W.B. Saunders, London, pp. 262–76.

Nduka, C., Super, P., Monson, J.R.T. and Darzi, A. (1994) Cause and prevention of electrosurgical injury in laparoscopic surgery. *Journal of the American College of Surgeons*, **179**, 161–79.

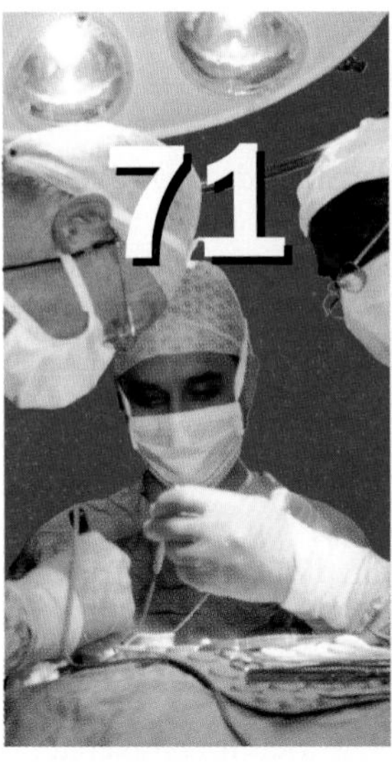

71 Audit in surgery

Learning objectives

- Audit is an obligatory activity in which all healthcare professionals must play a role.
- Audit can and will provide useful data about the outcome of clinical activity and will fulfil the requirements of ensuring that quality care is provided.
- Medical audit and resource management activities are inseparable.
- For audit to be undertaken properly and efficiently the acquisition of data must be part of normal everyday medical record keeping and must make full use of information technology as it becomes available.

The recent emphasis on quality of medical care (not just quantity) has made the importance of collecting good quality audit data more important than ever before.

Audit and the methods used to undertake audit allow us to gather simply information about our surgical activity. It allows us to look at what happens to our patients (outcomes) and it allows us to improve practice (completing the audit loop). A simple audit of the outcome of an operation can pick up variations from the expected at an early stage. This should reduce future damage to patients and any legal problems that might accompany disasters.

Bailey & Love's Short Practice of Surgery, 23rd edition. Edited by R.C.G. Russell, N.S. Williams and C.J.K. Bulstrode. Published in 2000 by Arnold Publishers.

The features of a 'simple' audit

- Define the type of audit (e.g. case record review)
- Identify a representative sample (random selection or consecutive cases)
- Define the questions to be answered
- Define the criteria for assessment
- Establish the standards for comparison
- Perform the audit
- Record the results
- Re-audit at a defined time in the future

What is audit?

Audit can be defined as a systematic review of aspects of practice that results in a change in that practice. Johnson defined medical audit as 'a means of quality control for medical practice by which the profession shall regulate its activities with the intention of improving overall patient care'. *'A First Class Service'* (Department of Health, 1998) states 'Clinical audit involves systematically looking at the procedures used for diagnosis, care and treatment, examining how associated resources are used and investigating the effect care has on the outcome and quality of life for the patient. Audit is a valuable tool to improve the quality of professional care and, ultimately, patient choice'.

Much of what is called audit is actually only fact gathering. The facts are essential to undertaking the audit, but unless

David Johnson. Professor of Surgery, Leeds, England.

the effects of the activity on patients are also included (i.e. outcome data) the facts alone cannot influence surgical practice.

Traditionally audit has been divided into medical and clinical audit. The term medical audit refers to an audit undertaken by doctors and consists of a review of clinical events; e.g. does one surgical procedure result in a better outcome compared with another? Clinical audit is usually taken as a review of all potential medical events surrounding the treatment of a patient. This will include nursing, physiotherapy, social aspects, etc. The boundaries between the two forms of audit are blurred and indeed 'medical' audit is merely a subset of clinical audit focusing only on the medical aspects. The majority of audits will consider aspects which are both medical and clinical.

The separation of the provision (and rationing) of resource from clinical audit is artificial. All medical activity costs money so an understanding of the management of the resources has to be included in the audit process. When healthcare resources are rationed, the limitation on funding is likely to have a direct effect on structure and process, and hence on outcome. 'Total' audit should include any activity which occurs in the delivery of healthcare to an individual patient or a group of patients.

It is, at least, a useful intellectual exercise to consider the financial implications of introducing a new technique. For example, arthroscopic stabilisation of the shoulder is a relatively new technique to appear in orthopaedic practice in the UK. If it is to be adopted by a hospital trust the following questions might need to be answered.

- Is there a surgeon who can perform the techniques?
- What training is required?
- What equipment is required? Is new equipment needed?
- What will the consumables cost and are they readily available?
- What are the operating theatre and 'hotel' requirements for the patients?
- What is the failure rate of the techniques, i.e. will there be a large number of patients who will need revision surgery or will be unsatisfied with the outcome?
- What is the rehabilitation time and when will the patients be able to return to work?
- And of course, how does this new technique compare with the usual accepted techniques when the same questions are asked?

Each and every surgical procedure could and probably should be examined in this way. In the example given above, data from prospective clinical trials comparing the new technique with the old are required to demonstrate a statistically significant improvement if the method is to be justified purely on the grounds of clinical benefit. For an individual surgeon, audit data showing that the results obtained by that surgeon are comparable to the results of the clinical trials are needed. The cost to the hospital, and the cost to the patient (in time off work, etc.) will also need to be calculated. Using data like these there are several ways of justifying the introduction of a new technique as follows.

- The new technique is clinically better than the old – better outcomes (including patient satisfaction), decreased failure and decreased morbidity.
- The technique is cheaper to patient, hospital or both.
- Patients can be treated more quickly using the new method, which produces the same results as the old method.

The components of audit

Audit is traditionally viewed as a loop, the components of which are structure–process–output. The term structure refers to the physical environment in which healthcare is provided; process refers to the activity of providing care; and output to the outcome of that care both for the individual and for the community as a whole. The loop is completed by the output feeding back on potentially both structure and process. Table 71.1 summarises what is needed to provide a quality service – structure, process, outcome data and feedback.

Both a quality service and an audit cycle need the feedback loop to be effective. The loop must be viewed as an unending sequence. Moreover, it is implicit in the definitions that a single clinician cannot perform audit alone; teamwork with finance managers and other clinical staff, etc., is obligatory.

All aspects of clinical audit must be compared with some form of standard and then retested against the standard on the next loop of the cycle. It is generally accepted that as far as specific surgical techniques are concerned the comparison must be against properly constructed prospective randomised clinical trials. Other independent and objective standards must be established for other comparisons.

Traditional methods of performing audit

Shaw in Frostick *et al.*'s *Medical Audit: Rationale and Practicalities* (1993) describes the traditional views of medical audit in terms of the 'characteristics of effective audit' and the 'methods'.

Table 71.1 Quality care and clinical audit

Provision of resources	*Structure*
Delivery of the resources (Treatment, support care, etc.)	Process
Assessment of the effect of utilisation of the resources	Outcome
Comparison with accepted standards of care (outcome measures, health economics)	
Adjusting the provision/delivery of the resources to improve the effect	Completing the loop
= Quality care	= Audit

The characteristics can be summarised as:

- explicit criteria for good clinical practice – guidelines for practice;
- objective measurement of patterns of current practice – looking at identified groups or activities;
- comparison of results amongst peers – acceptable published data;
- explicit identification of corrective action – agreed action and its implementation;
- documentation of procedure and results – a formal report of the proceedings and action required.

The methods that Shaw outlines are basically very simple and can be undertaken by a small group (i.e. a directorate) or on a larger scale. Examples of the usual types of audit that can and are performed include:

- workload and case mix;
- appropriateness of care;
- access to care;
- outcomes of care;
- quality of records;
- efficiency.

The advantages of a traditional approach to audit are as follows.

- It is simple and cheap.
- Data should be easy to acquire and their accuracy can be checked.
- The cycles and so the effectiveness of the audit can be repeated at short time intervals.
- There are simple educational outcomes which are derived from regular, small and well-run audit meetings.

The disadvantages of traditional audit are as follows.

- Meetings may occur but are not repeated so the audit cycle is not completed.
- Standards may not be easy to define in an objective way.
- The onus often falls on the most junior person on the firm to acquire and present the data.
- Morbidity and mortality meetings can be embarrassing and destructive.
- The education may be by guided 'shaming' not by guided learning.

Audit versus clinical research

Clinical research requires that a prospective controlled trial is performed. Such a trial requires a hypothesis, a control and an experimental group and will be the subject of rigorous statistical analysis.

Audit data should be acquired prospectively but there will be no comparison between defined groups. Care will be needed in interpreting the data because there will be many factors that are not controlled. In order to make use of these data they will need to be compared with a standard, i.e. what is acceptable practice prior to the audit? The standard should be established by examining the published data and using prospective clinical trials as the primary source. It is important to examine the clinical trials on which the standard is based. This is to ensure that the patient groups are similar to those which will be the subject of the audit, and that the surgical procedure and other treatment roughly match what is being audited, etc.

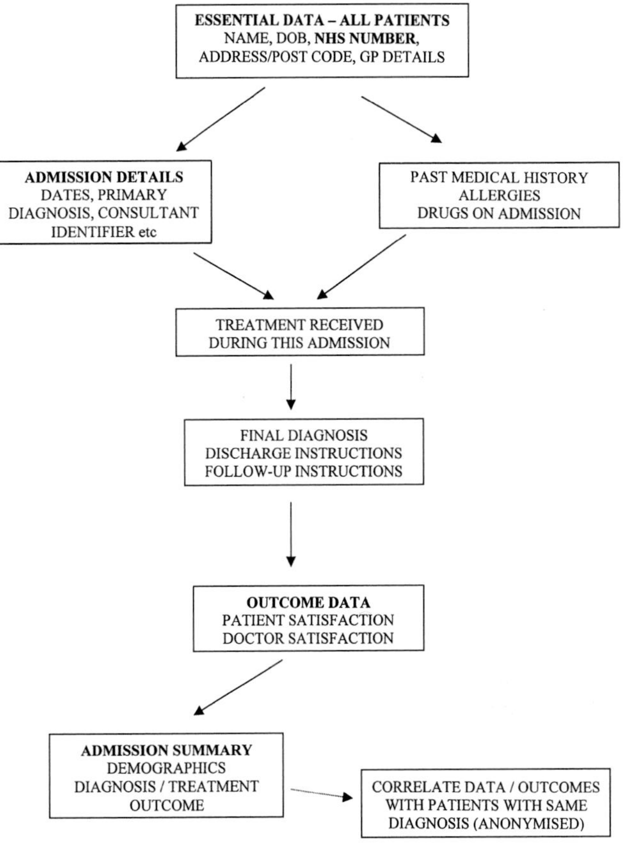

Fig. 71.1 The building blocks of data collection. DOB: date of birth; GP: general practitioner.

Minimum dataset

Probably the most essential data item is the (new) National Health Service (NHS) number. This number is unique to each individual andshould allow patients to be followed from birth to death. A number of audits in Scandinavia has been very successful at tracking patients over long periods and long distances because of the Swedish equivalent of the new NHS number. Outcome data on hip fractures and lower limb joint arthroplasty are examples of the type of long-term data collection that has occurred in Sweden (Thorngren, 1993).

Computers versus paper

How should audit be undertaken?

Traditionally we have been told that a simple paper-based exercise is the best and most effective way of performing an audit. This is only true if the goals of the audit are limited or a pro forma is created prior to commencing the audit and completed for each patient.

A 'common' type of audit has been a review of clinical records. This is a simple method of ensuring that the standard record keeping is adequate from a medical and medicolegal standpoint. A random selection of case records from an identified group is gathered and criteria are defined to determine the adequacy of the notes; the next stage should be to recommend changes and to re-audit. This type of audit does not require any detailed methodology; it requires that a record of the defects and recommendations is kept. This type of audit method has value in educating new housemen about the need to keep adequate records and so should probably be used early on in their employment in the firm.

Another simple audit is to choose a particular disease or treatment (surgical operation, for example). Data about the patients in this group are then used either to review aspects of process (stay length, time to operation, etc.) or to review the actual patient outcome – alive or dead, cured or recurrence, etc. This methodology may offer reasonable insight into the pathological process under consideration. However, a number of possible sources of error of interpretation and difficulty must be highlighted. These include the following.

- Patients are identified from an unreliable source resulting in either patients who did not have the condition or, more often, missing varying numbers of patients who did have the condition. Patients may also be lost at follow-up.
- Inappropriate statistical tests may be used or the correct test used wrongly.
- Historical controls may be used for comparison which are not comparable.

If paper-based audits are to be undertaken a few simple rules should be followed.

1. Develop a simple and comprehensible pro forma which will record the information upon which the audit is based. Avoid pro formas that require a lot of text entry. Wherever possible use a series of 'tick' boxes with either single or multiple choices. This type of pro forma can be completed speedily and accurately as the person placing the ticks is presented with all of the answers. The disadvantage of this type of form is that it can look complex and large, especially if there is a lot of choices for each field.
2. Undertake the audit **prospectively**. Retrospective data are helpful as a basis of a pilot study in the sense that the potential numbers under study might be predicted from a review of the admissions, etc., over the last months or years. There is usually very little sense in auditing a rare event as it will require many years of data acquisition in order to get a study of sufficient size to make any worthwhile comment. The retrospective data may also give a clue to the types of outcome measures that should be employed.
3. Choose outcome measures that can be readily assessed.
4. Choose a method of assessment that will be independent of bias that might be introduced by the initiator of the audit. Patients will often tell doctors what they wish to hear and therefore either an independent person needs to assess the outcome or a method that is neutral in its presentation needs to be used (e.g. a patient questionnaire).

Computer-based audits

Using modern information technology is very attractive and can be efficient and effective. Alternatively, there may be a tendency to develop such complexity that data will not be entered.

The main advantages of using a computer-based system for audits are as follows.

- Large numbers of entries can be analysed easily.
- In the future electronic patient records will automatically record information concerning a clinical event that will allow us to perform effective audits.

The main disadvantages are as follows.

- Knowledge of the construction and operation of a database is required.
- Commercial databases are often very expensive but increasingly on-line national databases are being created that make use of a central server.
- Appropriate fields for the database need to be created before data entry. If fields are added after data are captured it can be extremely difficult to complete the new fields.
- The level of complexity of the database needs to be determined at the outset and will be dependent upon the uses to which the database will be put.
- Entry of data will need to be checked (validated) against an independent source to ensure accuracy. It is usual to select randomly 10 per cent of cases and compare the computer records with the original case records held by the hospital.
- Methods of highlighting inappropriate entries into particular fields and the completion of obligatory fields will need to be considered.

Coding

Traditionally all patient diagnoses and treatments have been coded, i.e. given an alphanumeric code for the purposes of storing the diagnosis on computer. The International Classification of Diseases (ICD) coding system has been accepted as the international method of coding diagnoses and treatments. The codes (ICD version 10) are available on CD-ROM and are a fairly comprehensive system. Using this coding system allows easy international comparison of some aspects of data collection, especially disease incidence, geographic distribution of disease, etc. The Department of Health in the UK has invested in an alternative coding system, originated by Dr James Read. In the latest form of this coding system there is automatic mapping to ICD-10. The development of the Read Codes is attempting to unify an alphanumeric coding system with the use of familiar clinical terms in real language. With modern computers there is a real question as to whether coding is needed at all. Its main role seems to be in defining terms so that what one surgeon defines as an infection is the same as another surgeon. Without this audit data cannot be compared or combined and much of their power is lost.

Outcome measures

Defining and using appropriate outcome measures are the hardest parts of undertaking an audit that is going to achieve a worthwhile end. In general, there has to be a decision as to whether the outcome is doctor or patient orientated. Doctor-based outcomes look at such outcomes as mortality, complications and the cost of consumables. A patient-orientated outcome may measure patient satisfaction. In some situations the operation may be a technical failure but the patient is happy with the result, producing a poor result for doctor-orientated audit, but a good result for patient-based audit.

Whatever method of assessing outcome is to be used the surgeon must be certain that the instrument is measuring something relevant to the audit being undertaken. Moreover, the outcome measure must be recordable within a time frame that will be relevant but also achievable. For example, following laparascopic herniorraphy it would be reasonable to assess patient satisfaction with the process of the operation within a short, perhaps 3-month, time frame. The success of the operation in terms of recurrence of the hernia cannot be fully assessed for many months or perhaps several years after the procedure.

In order for outcome scores to be useful, they must be rigorously validated. The specific 'tests' that need to be used are as follows.

- Internal consistency (Cronbach's alpha) determines whether the questionnaire or score is measuring a single essential concept.
- Reproducibility (test–retest reliability) determines that the score will give a roughly similar result if repeated.
- Validity: does the score actually measure what the developers are interested in? This is divided into *content validity* (the questions deal with all aspects that they are intended to cover) and *construct validity* (whether the questionnaire supports the hypothesis).
- Sensitivity to change: will the score reveal small changes which are of clinical importance during the period of study?

To develop a score/questionnaire there are several ways of establishing the types of question and the specific questions to be asked. It is possible to ask a panel of experts what they think are the important issues to be assessed in a disease or operation or anatomical region (face validity). The list that is created is then collated to come up with groups of questions and specific questions within each group. Once the draft questionnaire has been created the validation tests will be applied. An alternative method in order to create a patient-orientated questionnaire is to ask the patients what they think is important, especially functional aspects. Again the responses are collated and can be refined by posing the questions to another group of patients. The questions should also be exposed to a panel of experts at an appropriate stage. Once again the validation tests will have to be applied before the questionaire can be used in a study.

Audit and statistics

Details of statistical tests will not be covered here but general comments are required so that statistics are not abused when performing an audit. Descriptive statistics are useful and acceptable – distribution of ages, operation type, etc. Many surgeons will quote a 'mean' and 'standard deviation' for items such as age; this assumes that the data are normally distributed which is not necessarily the case. It is often better to use median and range for ages, time after surgery, etc. It is unlikely that incidence or prevalence can be calculated from an audit as the size of the overall population (the denominator) will not be known. The use of tests of significance is not acceptable in audit data. Performing tests of significance requires a comparison between two groups, one of which represents a control group. A control group is one which is identical to the test group except in the one aspect that is being examined. Therefore, tests of probability can only be used where patients are entered into a prospective randomised clinical trial.

The presentation of data in a publication is a source of concern in many audit papers. Often the scenario arises that a surgeon will find that a certain number of patients underwent a specific procedure some years before. The surgeon will then try and find the details from records of those patients but for various reasons it is only possible to find, for example, 75 per cent of the original records. The surgeon will next try and contact this 75 per cent of patients to find out the 'outcome' of the operation (usually using an unvalidated questionnaire or score). Only, for example, 50 per cent of those contacted will reply to an enquiry (i.e. 50 per cent of 75 per cent of the original number). Some of the remainder may have died but many simply will not be traceable. In this process if the original number was 100, the assessment will be undertaken for only about 37 patients. Many authors will then make comments about the data that can only be applied to the 37 who were assessed but the report is written as if it refers to the total number.

National audits

Over the years a number of national enquiries has been undertaken. The *National Confidential Enquiry into Maternal Mortality* and the *National Confidential Enquiry into Perinatal Death* are the 'oldest' of these audits. The *National Confidential Enquiry into Perioperative Deaths* (NCEPOD), which first reported in 1988, has examined surgical and anaesthetic deaths and made various recommendations. The return of information to NCEPOD has, to some extent, been voluntary. Under the most recent NHS reforms NCEPOD and the other National Confidential Enquiries will be controlled by the National Institute for Clinical Excellence (NICE). Moreover, participation will be obligatory.

The Royal College of Surgeons of England established a comparative audit service in the early 1990s. Surgeons contributed data confidentially and voluntarily to the service based at the College. Surgeons were ranked in order of number of a particular operation or number of complications, etc. Only the surgeons themselves were able to identify their own position in the ranking. During the period for which the service was offered the audits were changed from retrospective to prospective. The main disadvantage of the audits was that few (about 20 per cent) surgeons responded to the audits – the enthusiasts took part but the others saw no benefit.

Clinical governance

In simple terms clinical governance tries to answer the following questions.

- Are we doing the right thing?
- Are we doing it right?
- Are we measuring what is going wrong?
- Are we responding to this to make things better?

The National Institute for Clinical Excellence

> A new National Institute for Clinical Excellence will be established to give new coherence and prominence to information about clinical and cost effectiveness.

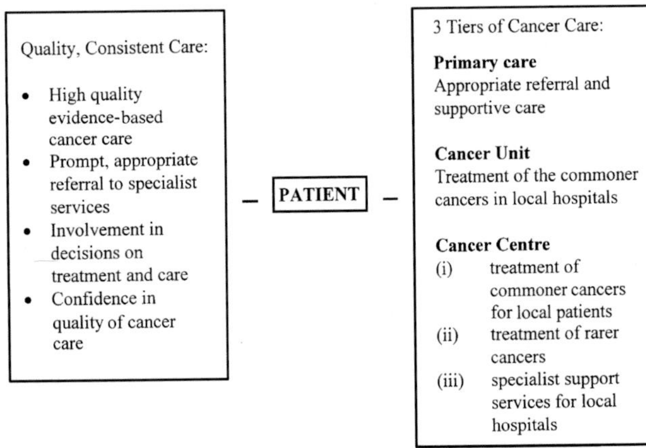

Fig. 71.2 The Calman–Hines Cancer Service Framework (from Department of Health, *A First Class Service*, 1998).

The main roles of NICE will be to produce guidelines for clinical practice based on clinical evidence and associated with cost effectiveness. A number of stages of the work of NICE has been identified:

- stage 1 – *identification* – which is subdivided into the introduction of new technologies into the NHS and their impact on healthcare, and examining current practice and to look for variations in quality;
- stage 2 – *evidence collection* – 'undertaking research to assess the clinical and cost-effectiveness of health interventions';
- stage 3 – *appraisal and guidance* – examining the evidence and producing guidelines;
- stage 4 – *dissemination* – distribution of guidelines and the methods required to audit their effect;
- stage 5 – *implementation* – at a local level, through **clinical governance** and other approaches;
- stage 6 – *monitoring* – the impact and keeping under review, taking into account the views of patients and their representatives and any new research findings.

It can be seen from these stages that the work of NICE is massive and far reaching and will have one of the greatest effects on healthcare delivery since the inception of the NHS.

Commission for Health Improvement (CHIP)

The Government identifies CHIP as an *independent* statutory body that will monitor quality issues. The commission will have extensive powers to act 'where there is evidence of systematic failure'. For clinicians to be able to justify their actions good-quality audit data will have to be available.

The future of audit in surgery

Over the years a number of attempts has been made to develop an audit system which will acquire data as a part of everyday activity. The advantage of this type of data acquisition is that we can derive outcome data, etc., as a part of normal working practice rather than having specifically to undertake audit projects. In order to achieve this it will be necessary to ensure that a few basic rules are followed.

- Standard pro formas will need to be developed to allow consistent data entry.
- There will be obligatory fields that have to be completed on all patients.
- Specific data fields will need to be created that are disease or speciality specific.
- Data validation will need to be undertaken to check correct data entry.
- Education of both healthcare workers to understand the electronic records and the general public to demonstrate confidentiality and accuracy of records will be necessary.
- The systems must be able to produce reports automatically for clinical purposes and for audit.

Using an electronic record does not eliminate the need to 'think' what audits to undertake but facilitates the acquisition and storage of useful data. An individual will still need to develop specific audit projects and apply the accepted rules to undertake the study. If the systems are successful the completeness of data should be high; patients will be traceable and surgeons will have direct and rapid access to understanding their own practice and how it affects their patients.

Further reading

Department of Health (1998) *A First Class Service in the New NHS*, Department of Health Service Executive, London.

Department of Health (1999) *Clinical Governance Quality in the New NHS*, Department of Health Service Executive, London.

Department of Health (1999) *The NHS Performance Assessment Framework*, Department of Health Service Executive, London.

Frostick S., Radford P. and Wallace, W. (eds) (1993) *Medical Audit: Rationale and Practicalities*, Cambridge University Press, Cambridge.

Johnson, R. (1991) *The Purpose and Conduct of Medical Audit – An Educational Perspective,* From the office of the Director of Postgraduate Educationand Training, Oxford University and Region.

Smith, R. (1992) *Audit in Action*, BMJ Publishing, London.

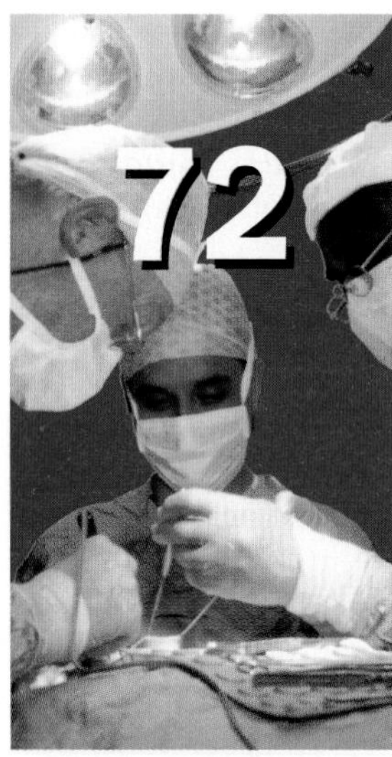

72 Clinical trials/statistics

Introduction

Vast numbers of clinical publications are printed in the surgical literature every year. Many are flawed and it is important that a surgeon trainee has the skills to examine critically research done by others. In addition, a surgeon should be able both to design and to complete an original study. Performing research can be arduous and time-consuming. However, surgical research is good for society as it advances medicine, it is good for patients as the clinical outcome is often improved for patients in clinical trials, and it is good for surgeons as it is a way of keeping track of personal clinical results. In addition, much clinical work is tedious and repetitive. Rigorous evaluation of even the simplest techniques and conditions can help to keep the surgical brain active throughout a long career and ensure a good outcome for the patient.

The earlier a surgeon develops skills in surgical research the better. The hardest trial to do, or article to write, is the first. The best way to develop a critical understanding of the research of others is to perform studies of your own. It is unlikely that the first piece written by any surgeon will be an earth-shattering randomised trial. Starting small is often the best way.

This chapter contains all the information required to complete a randomised trial. Using it, a surgeon will be armed to write a surgical paper and to evaluate research carried out by others.

Bailey & Love's Short Practice of Surgery, 23rd edition. Edited by R.C.G. Russell, N.S. Williams and C.J.K. Bulstrode. Published in 2000 by Arnold Publishers.

Identifying a topic

The hardest part of research is to come up with a good idea. It appears that all the best trials have already been completed, but a careful consideration of scientific support for surgical action reveals deficiencies in surgical knowledge. Facts commonly taken for granted often have no basis. The best research often answers the simplest question. Once an idea has been formed, or a question asked, it needs transforming into a hypothesis. It is helpful to approach surgeons who regularly publish research articles and who have a special interest in the surgical area being considered. As ideas are suggested, keep thinking whether the question posed by the proposed research really matters. Spend some time refining the question because this is probably the most important part of research. Choosing the wrong topic at this stage can lead to many wasted hours.

Once a topic has been identified do not rush into the study. It is worth spending a considerable time investigating the subject in question. The worst possible thing is to find at the end of a long arduous study that the research has already been done.

First port of call for information is the medical library. Avoid textbooks, as most are out of date as soon as they are published. Look for current articles about the proposed research; review articles and meta-analyses can be particularly helpful. At this stage most clinicians go to an electronic library and perform a database search. It is very important to learn how to do an accurate and efficient search as early as possible. Details are beyond the scope of this chapter, but most librarians will help out if a little interest and enthusiasm is shown. Current techniques involve searching on Medline

Table 72.1 Electronic information sites

Database	*Producer*	*Coverage*	*Availability**
MEDLINE http://www.docnet.org.uk/dr felix	US National Library of Medicine (NLM)	World-wide journals, 9 000 000 records, since 1966	Free of charge: Internet subscription: CD-ROM, Internet
EMBASE not free on-line	Electronic version of *Excerpta Medica*	Good European, drug/pharmacology, 6 000 000 records, since 1980	Subscription: CD-ROM, Internet
CINAHL not free on-line	Cumulated index to nursing and allied health literature	World-wide journals and books, 95 per cent English language, multidisciplinary: health psychology, community care, clinical guidelines and protocols, since 1982	Subscription: CD-ROM, Internet
ERIC http://www.askeric.org	Educational Resources Information Center, US Department of Education	Theory and practice of education, multidisciplinary, 1 000 000 records, since 1966	Free of charge: Internet subscription: CD-ROM and Internet
Cochrane Collaboration http://www.cochrane.co.uk	BMJ Publishing Group	Evidence-based healthcare, systematic reviews, methodology, trials register, since 1995	Free of charge: Internet subscription: CD-ROM, floppy disk, Internet
OMNI http://omni.ac.uk	UK healthcare libraries	Review web sites on the Internet	Free of charge: Internet

*Licensed to many organisations who provide their own interface. Main providers offering a 'pay as you go' service can be found: http://www.ovid.com or http://www.silverplatter.com.

or other collected databases but as electronic information advances and the world-wide web becomes more user-friendly new search strategies may emerge. Collections of reviews are becoming available – the Cochrane Collaboration brings together evidence-based medical information and is available in most libraries (Table 72.1).

Once a stack of articles on the subject has been obtained it is important that these are carefully perused. If the proposed research project is still looking good after some thorough reading it is worth further discussion with experts. Do not be afraid to contact authors who have written a paper on a similar subject. All scientists are flattered by interest in their work and most will not pilfer your ideas.

Now it should be possible to start to plan the research project. During the first phase it is very important to keep in the mind the following questions.

- Why do the study?
- Will it answer a useful question?
- Is it practical?
- Can it be accomplished in the available time and with available resources?
- What findings are expected?
- What impact will it have?

Robert Greenhill Cochrane. Former Medical Superintendent, Kola Ndoto Leprosarium, Shinyange, Tanzania.

Project design

Next to choosing the subject for study, time spent carefully designing a project is never wasted. There are many different types of scientific study. The design used depends totally on the study. Beloved of present scientists, the randomised controlled trial is regarded as the best method of scientific research. It must not be forgotten that much surgical practice has been advanced by other different types of study such as those listed in Table 72.2. For example, testing a new type of operation often requires a pilot study to assess feasibility followed by a formal randomised controlled trial.

Research can be qualitative or quantitative. Quantitative research uses hard data to speak for themselves. A medical condition is analysed systematically using hard objective end-points such as death or amputation. In qualitative research data often come from patient narratives, and the psycho-social impact of the disease and its treatment are analysed, for example narratives of breast cancer. This sort of data is often collected using quality of life measurements. A variety of different quality of life questionnaires exists to suit several different clinical situations. Much of the best research is both quantitative and qualitative.

As finances for healthcare are always stretched, it is also important to include a cost–benefit analysis in any major area of research so that the value of the proposed intervention or change in treatment can be assessed.

Table 72.2 Types of study

Type of study	*Definition*
Observational	Evaluating results of condition or treatment in a defined population
retrospective –	analysing past events
prospective –	collecting data contemporaneously
Case–control	Series of patients with a particular disease or condition contrasted with matched control patients
Cross-sectional	Measurements made on a single occasion, not looking at the whole population but selecting a small similar group and expanding results
Longitudinal	Measurements are taken over a period of time, not looking at the whole population but selecting a small similar group and expanding results
Experimental	Two or more treatments are compared. Allocation to treatment groups is under the control of the researcher
Randomised	Two randomly allocated treatments
Randomised controlled	Includes control group with no treatment

Sample size

Calculating the number of patients required to perform a satisfactory investigation is a very important prerequisite to the study. An incorrect sample size is probably the most frequent reason for research to be invalid. So often surgical trials are marred by the possibility of error caused by the inadequate number of patients investigated.

- Type I error – benefit is perceived when really there is none (false positive).
- Type II error – benefit is missed because study has small numbers (false negative).

Calculating the number of patients required in the study can overcome this bias. Unfortunately, it very often reveals that a larger number of patients is needed for the study than can possibly be obtained from available resources. This often means expanding enrolment by using a multicentre study. There is no point in embarking on a trial when it will never be possible to recruit an adequate sample size. Never forget that more patients will need to be randomised than the final sample size to take into account patients who die, drop out or are lost to follow-up.

The following is an example calculation for a study to recruit patients into two groups. In order to calculate a sample size it is common practice to set the level of power for the study at 80 per cent with a 5 per cent significance level. This means that if there is a difference between study groups, there is an 80 per cent chance of detecting it. Based on previous studies, realistic expectations of differences between groups should be used to calculate sample size. The formula below uses the figures of a reduction in event rate from 30 to 10 per cent (e.g. new treatment expected to reduce complication rate such as wound infection from 30 to 10 per cent):

$$8 \times \frac{r(100-r)+s(100-s)}{(r-s)^2}$$

$$8 \times \frac{30(100-30)+10(100-10)}{(30-10)^2} = 60 \text{ needed in each group}$$

Eliminating bias

It is important to imagine how a study could be invalidated by thinking of things that could go wrong. One way to eliminate any bias inherent in the data collection is to have observers or recorders who do not know which treatment has been used (single blind). In the best randomised studies neither patient nor researcher is aware of which therapy has been used until after the study has finished (double blind). Randomised trials are essential for testing new drugs. In practice, however, in some surgical trials randomisation may not be possible or ethical.

Study protocol

Now that the question to pose has been decided and it has been checked that sufficient patients will be available to enrol into the study, it is time to prepare the detail of the trial. At this stage a study protocol should be constructed to define the research strategy. It should contain a paragraph on the background of the proposed study, the aim and objectives, a clear methodology, definitions of population and sample sizes, and methods of proposed analysis. It should include the patient numbers, inclusion and exclusion criteria, and the time scale for the work. At this stage it is helpful to construct a flow diagram giving a clear summary of the research protocol and its requirements (Fig. 72.1). It is helpful to imagine the paper that will be written about the study, before it is performed. This may prevent errors of data collection.

When a study is planned, sufficient time should be reserved at the beginning for fund-raising and obtaining ethical approval if required, and afterwards for collecting the data and writing it up. A data collection form should be designed or a computer collection package developed. Do not forget that if data are collected on computer, appropriate safeguards for privacy and confidentiality will be necessary. It is important to ensure the co-operation of any other specialities or clinicians who will be involved in the study and to agree on the sharing of responsibility for the trial. This will also help to prevent disagreement about who takes the credit once a study is ready for presentation and publication.

Ethics

Common sense is the best guide to whether a study is ethical or not. If there is any doubt consult a local ethics committee, available in all hospitals. Whenever a patient has treatment chosen by chance, ethical approval is required. All multicentre trials need approval. Even for nonrandomised trials it is important to try and obtain written consent for any

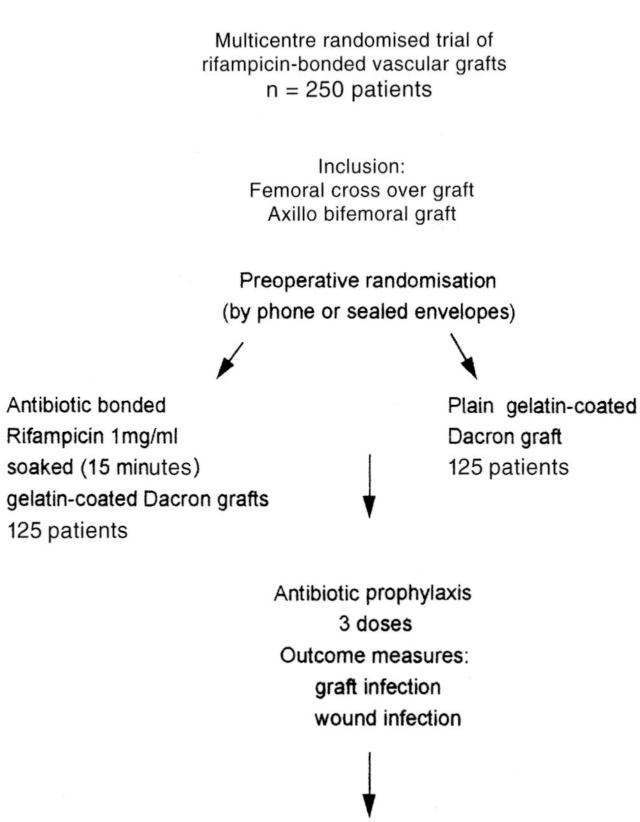

Fig. 72.1 The protocol for a recent study.

new or extraordinary procedure or therapy. All studies involving animals require approval from statutory licensing authorities.

Leave plenty of time for this to be obtained and do not embark on the study until approval has been granted. Ethics committees prefer to see fully developed trial protocols but it is often possible to get some preliminary advice from the committee chairman. Ethics committee forms are often long and detailed, and it is important that these are filled in correctly. All dealings with ethics committees should be intelligent and courteous.

Most ethics committees are briefed to ensure that a project does not incur hidden expenses to a hospital. The cost of nonroutine investigations and extra treatments should be covered by a grant application, or at least underwritten by a hospital finance department.

Statistical analysis

Many find the statistical analysis the most difficult part of research. It is also the most commonly criticised part of papers written by other clinicians.

There are many useful books about statistics which can be consulted; if in any doubt a statistician will be pleased to give assistance in analysing research. Statisticians like to be consulted before research has been conducted rather than being presented with the results at the end of the trial; they often give helpful advice over study design.

The following terms are frequently used when summarising statistical data:

Mean: the result of dividing the total by the number of observations (the average).
Median: the middle value with equal number of observations above and below – used for numerical or ranked data.
Mode: the value with the highest frequency observed – used for nominal data collection.
Range: the largest to the smallest value.

The most important decision for analysis is whether the distribution of results is normal (parametric). Normally distributed results have a symmetrical, bell-shaped curve, and the mean, median and mode all lie at the same value. Some types of data, such as blood group, are not normally distributed and require other methods of analysis (nonparametric).

Parametric tests

When the results are normally distributed a *t*-test can be used to compare the outcome between intervention and control groups. Confidence intervals are the best guide to the possible range in which the true differences are likely to lie. A confidence interval that includes zero usually implies a lack of statistical significance.

Nonparametric tests

Statistical tests such as the chi-squared test, Wilcoxon Signed Rank test (single sample) and the Mann–Whitney *U*-test (compares two samples) can be used because they make no assumptions about the underlying population distribution.

Scientists usually employ *P* values to describe statistical chance. A *P* value <0.05 is taken to imply a true difference. It is important not to forget that $P = 0.05$ simply means there is only a one in 20 chance that the differences between the variables happened by chance. If enough variables are examined in any study significant differences will occur simply due to chance.

Statistics simply deal with the chance that observations between populations are different. Clinical results should show clear differences. If statistics are required to demonstrate differences between results, they are unlikely to have major clinical significance.

Computer software packages available

Statistical computer packages offer a quick way to analyse descriptive statistics such as mean, median and the range, as well as the most commonly used statistical tests such as the chi-squared test. Various packages are available commercially and are useful tools in data analysis.

Table 72.3 Checklist for authors

Heading	*Subheading*	*Descriptor*
Title		Identify as randomised trial
Abstract		Structured format
Introduction		Prospectively defined hypotheses, clinical objective
Methods	Protocol	Study population
		Intervention, timing
		Primary and secondary outcome
		Statistical rationale
		Stopping rules
	Assignment	Unit of randomisation
		Method: allocation schedule
	Masking (blinding)	
Results	Participant flow and follow-up	Trial profile, flow diagram
	Analysis	Estimated effect of intervention
		Result in absolute numbers
		Summary data with appropriate inferential statistics
		Protocol deviation
Comment		Specific interpretation of study
		Sources of bias
		External validity
		General interpretation

Taken from the CONSORT statement. (Reproduced with permission from Begg *et al.*, Improving the quality of reporting of randomized controlled trials. The CONSORT statement. *Journal of the American Medical Association*, **276**, 637–9, 1996.)

Analysing a scientific article

The simplest way to analyse an article from a scientific journal is to look at the checklist of requirements for good scientific research. The CONSORT document has been produced as a guideline of how to conduct clinical trials. A good paper will look at a specific clinical problem for which improving the outcome would realise significant clinical benefits. Looking in detail at the study design will often be the best way of deciding whether or not a trial is a good one. The CONSORT document includes a checklist for the conduct of good randomised trials (Table 72.3). Often clinicians overlook biases which others find obvious to detect that can have a profound influence on the outcome of any study.

Presenting and publishing an article

There is no point in conducting a research project and then leaving the results unpresented. Even when results of a trial are negative they are worth distributing; few research projects are worthless. However, most studies do not provide dramatic results and few surgeons publish seminal articles.

The key to both presentation and publication is to decide on the message and then aim for an appropriate forum. Big important randomised studies merit presentation at national meetings and publication in international journals. Small observational studies are more often accepted for presentation at regional or hospital meetings and publication in smaller specialist journals. Help and advice from clinicians familiar with presentation and publication is invaluable at this stage. The most important piece of advice is to follow accurately instructions for journal submission. Most international meetings will accept presentations eagerly (especially by poster) as this increases the attendance at a conference.

Most surgeons publish research in peer-reviewed journals. The work that is submitted is checked anonymously by other surgeons before publication. If in doubt about whether to submit to a journal, many editors will give advice about the suitability of an article by letter or telephone.

Convention dictates that articles are submitted in IMRAD form – Introduction, Methods, Results and Discussion. Increasingly, electronic publication and the world-wide web may change the face of scientific publication and in the next decade these restrictions on style may disappear. For now the IMRAD format remains inviolable. The length of an article is important: a paper should be as long as the size of the message. Readers of big randomised multicentre trials wish to know as much detail about the study as possible; reports on small negative trials should be brief.

Introduction

This should always be short. A brief background of the study should be presented and then the aims of the trial outlined.

Methods

The methodology and trial design should be given in detail. It is important to own up to any biases. Any new techniques or investigations should be detailed in full; if they are common practice or have been described elsewhere this should be referenced instead of described.

Results

Results are always best shown diagrammatically using tables and figures if possible. Results shown in the form of a diagram need not then be duplicated in the text.

Discussion

It is important not to repeat the Introduction or reiterate the Results in this section. The study should be interpreted intelligently and any suggestions for future studies or changes in management should be made. It is important not to indulge in flights of fantasy or wild imagination about future possibilities; most journal editors will delete these.

References

This section should include all relevant papers recording previous studies on the subject in question. The number should reflect the size of the message and the importance of the work. The Reference section does not usually have to be exhaustive but should include up-to-date articles.

Evidence-based surgery

Surgical practice has been considered an art: ask 50 surgeons how to manage a patient and you will probably get 50 different answers. There is so much clinical information available that no surgeon can know it all. Evidence-based surgery is a move to find the best ways of managing patients using clinical evidence from collected studies. It was estimated that sufficient evidence to justify routine myocardial thrombolysis for heart attacks was available years before the ISIS studies which finally made it clinically acceptable. No one had gathered all the available information together. Centres such as the Cochrane Collaboration have been collecting randomised trials and reviews to provide up-to-date information for clinicians. The Cochrane Library presently includes a database of systematic reviews, reviews of surgical effectiveness and a register of controlled trials. It is expected that this will gradually smooth out the differences between clinicians as the best way of managing patients becomes more evident. Collecting published evidence together and analysing it often requires reviews of multiple randomised trials. These meta-analyses involve complex statistical analyses designed to interpret multiple findings and synthesise the results of multiple studies.

Further reading

Altman, D.G. (1991) *Practical Statistics for Medical Research*, Chapman and Hall, London.

Brown, R.A. and Swanson Beck, J. (1994) *Medical Statistics on Personal Computers*, BMJ Publishing Group, Plymouth.

Gardner, M.J. and Altman, D.G. (1989) *Statistics with Confidence*, BMJ Publishing Group, London.

Polgar, S. and Thomas, S.A. (1995) *Introduction to Research in the Health Sciences*, Churchill Livingstone, Edinburgh.

Swinscow, T.D.V. (1996) *Statistics at Square One*, 9th edn, BMJ Publishing Group, London.

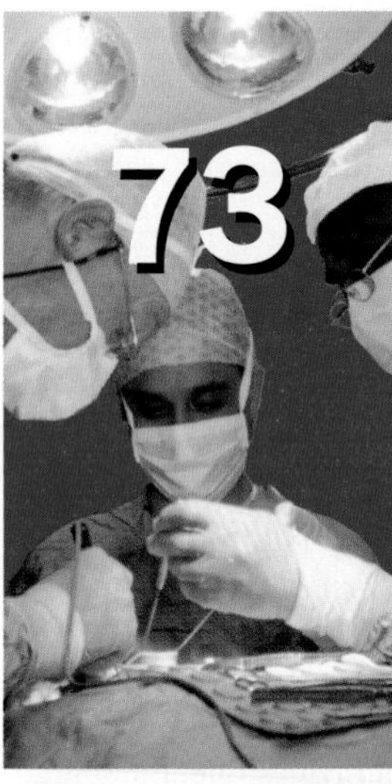

Theatre safety

Introduction

In addition to the overall design of the theatre, including good-quality, well-maintained equipment, the single most important aspect of theatre safety is the high performance of all theatre staff in their various roles. This requires careful protocols and guidelines which need to be adhered to, good initial training and on-going education, with good managerial aspects that include motivating staff.

The risks for the patient starts when he or she leaves the ward and continues until the safe return from theatre. All too often discussion of theatre safety is confined to procedures in the operating theatre, whereas in reality this is only part of the overall delivery of high-quality care.

Theatre design

Operating theatres should be sited near surgical wards and the main lifts, and they should be within easy access of the accident and emergency department and X-ray department; ideally the intensive therapy unit (ITU) and anaesthetic office should be close by.

Principles in design

The operating suite should include the following areas.

1. An outer reception area including:
   - the reception office;
   - the reception bay for patients to wait after checking in, for which there should be soft lighting and gentle music;
   - an area for storage of trolleys;
   - an area for hanging of clean gowns and overshoes for parents to wear when accompanying children to the anaesthetic room.
2. A 'clean zone' including a wide, clean corridor which allows access to and from the following:
   - the anaesthetic rooms;
   - the recovery bay;
   - the clean storage area;
   - the emergency autoclave;
   - staff relaxation rooms/changing rooms;
   - a storage area for large equipment including X-ray image intensifiers, etc.
3. The operating theatres.
   - There should be a dirty or 'back' corridor where there are adequate disposal areas for soiled linen, soiled disposable drapes, disposable instruments and cleaning of used instruments prior to their delivery by direct lift shaft to the Central Sterile Supplies Department (CSSD)
   - Laminar airflow is important in maintaining theatre asepsis; most theatres have between 20 and 40 air changes per hour, with the air being pumped in through filters in the ceiling and exiting through ventilation

Bailey & Love's Short Practice of Surgery, 23rd edition. Edited by R.C.G. Russell, N.S. Williams and C.J.K. Bulstrode. Published in 2000 by Arnold Publishers.

flaps adjacent to the floor. Humidity and air control are important both for patient safety and for staff comfort (a hot humid atmosphere leads to a reduction in concentration and performance by the operating surgeons).

- The operating theatres, recovery rooms and anaesthetic rooms must always be designed to have adequate power points, emergency electricity, piped gases, anaesthetic scavenging systems, ancillary lighting and wall suction. Cardiac resuscitation equipment must be readily available.
- Of considerable importance are the proper location of telephones and the use of internal vacuum tubes for the transportation of samples and specimens.

Preoperative preparations

Staff

Health and safety policies

The following health and safety policies should be implemented for all theatre staff:

- all staff should have a chest X-ray before commencing work;
- appropriate vaccination schedules, e.g. hepatitis B, and tetanus immunisation policies should be in place;
- policies for staff protection when handling patients with a high-risk transmittable disease, e.g. hepatitis B or C, human immunodeficiency virus (HIV);
- protocols for accident procedure;
- protocols for incident procedure;
- ionising irradiation guidelines with instructions for use for the X-ray image intensifier. All staff who use such instruments must be in possession of the Irradiation Protection Certificate;
- policy with regard to the adequacy of exhaustible anaesthetic gases;
- guidelines for the use of a laser;
- infection control policy with regular monitoring.

Staff facilities

- Changing area – this should be adequate inside with secure lockers, and with clean and adequate supplies of clean clothing, which should be of a close-woven coloured material with trousers for both sexes which should have elasticated ankles. Appropriate disposal bags for dirty linen, adequate toilets and washing facilities including hand basins and showers. Caps, masks and aprons should be available. Staff should have their own comfortable, regularly cleaned, antistatic footwear.
- Masks – these are important for staff protection and for operations involving splashing, such as drilling, there should be visor protection of the eyes. They are of questionable value in reducing infection rate. They should be:
  - fabric not cotton;
  - not touched by hands;
  - not put in pockets;
  - destroyed after single use.

Equipment

- Trolleys should be clean, have safety rails and have oxygen cylinders with well-fitting tubes and masks, all of which are regularly checked so that empty cylinders are replaced. Trollies must be able to be tipped into the Trendelenburg position in case of regurgitation of gastric contents.
- The operating table should be cleaned with regular checks to see that it can be raised and lowered smoothly with the appropriate gears for Trendelenburg tilt, lateral tilt and an adequate braking system. Accessories should be clean and available and fit well, and it is particularly important to ensure that stirrups fit well.
  - Settlement of negligence claims in this area is *very* costly.
- The lights should be modern and easily movable by members of the scrubbed team and by other theatre personnel.
- The suction apparatus should be clean and thoroughly checked, with spare suction tubes and catheters available.
- Anaesthetic machines should be in good working order – many of them are now supplied on a loan basis with a strict policy as to the correct connections and nontransferable piping. They must be regularly serviced and a record of this must be maintained.

  - All electrical equipment should be regularly checked and marked accordingly.
  - A fire policy, regular fire drills and weekly testing of fire doors are essential safety precautions.

Patient movement

Safety procedures

A fully filled-in request slip should be given to the theatre porters giving a clear indication of the name of the patient and the ward. The patient should be transferred from the bed to the trolley and safety rails raised; the patient is to be made comfortable and warm, during this procedure (it is important to ensure that the patient's dignity is preserved and that the patient's body is not unduly exposed) curtains should be drawn and doors closed where appropriate.

Before leaving the ward it is important to ensure that:

- the correct patient has been sent for, in accordance with the written operating list;
- the consent form is completed by the appropriate doctor (it is desirable that the surgeon performing the operation or senior member of the team has obtained the consent and this is preferably done in the out-patients' department before elective surgery);
- the site and side, e.g. right or left breast or right or left foot, has been marked where appropriate, preferably by the operating surgeon;
- the patient has been seen by the operating surgeon;

Friedrich Trendelenberg, 1844–1924. Professor of Surgery, Leipzig, Germany.

- any intraoperative investigations, such as X-rays or frozen section histology, have been booked;
- the full notes and X-rays are available and are transported with the patient;
- the wrist identification tag has been checked;
- the patient leaves the ward accompanied by an escort and the porter.

Transfer of the patient from reception to the anaesthetic room

Safe transfer from the bed to the trolley will have involved the patient either moving themselves or being transferred using a slide; the following points should be checked:

- worn canvasses, which may split, should be discarded;
- the patient should not be lifted but slid on a special sliding board which is correctly placed using handles on the canvas. Correct posture should be adopted by staff to avoid back strain;
- the position of the patient's head in relation to the canvas should be checked;
- the use of transferable trolley tops overcomes many of these problems.

With regard to the trolley the patient should be placed correctly so that the head end can be rapidly tipped into the Trendenlenburg position in an emergency. The patient should be positioned so that there is no pressure against the rails; intravenous lines and infusions should be correctly attached to the trolley and the patient's covers should be in place. The notes and X-ray should be stacked under the trolley.

An appropriate lifting and handling policy can virtually eliminate back strain amongst staff if properly designed protocols are followed. Back injury is expensive and debilitating. It is avoidable.

The reception area

This is an important area which must be designed to receive the incoming and existing patients on trolleys together with an office where there are telephones and where the receptionist can check in and record the patient's details, often with computer-recording facilities which permit reliable data collection for audit purposes.

Important safety aspects include:

- an appropriately trained reception clerk;
- the insistence of written lists at all times which cannot be changed by crossing out but must be rewritten;
- correct operative description;
- identification of the side to be operated on, i.e. right or left;
- the appropriate forms for sending for patients must contain specific details (never send for the 'next patient').

At reception. The patient should be greeted, the trolleys locked together and, wherever possible, lifting by canvas is avoided by the use of the sliding modules which are both smooth and comfortable. Preliminary identification of the patient and the checklist should include:

- name, including the name on the wrist band;
- the operation to be undertaken;
- the consultant in charge;
- the time at which the last meal and/or drink was taken;
- the presence of a valid consent form, the notes and X-rays.

A more extensive checklist is then carried out by the anaesthetic nurse in the anaesthetic room.

The anaesthetic room

On arrival at the anaesthetic room the patient is greeted, and once again a further full checklist and protocol must be undertaken, including:

- the presence of false teeth;
- the presence of a prothesis, especially with metal components;
- the wearing of any jewellery;
- allergies to drugs, plasters, dressings or disinfectants. These should all be checked. Allergies must be marked on the front of the notes, on the drug chart and on the anaesthetic form;
- the care plan is checked, the patient is watched, observed and engaged in appropriate conversation. Prior to the induction of the anaesthetic, the gowns are loosened in privacy, the patient is otherwise kept well covered;
- electrocardiogram (ECG) electrodes are applied;
- the diathermy indifferent electrode is applied correctly;
- the induction of the anaesthetic is carried out by the anaesthetist, assisted by the designated anaesthetic nurse or assistant. The operation site is appropriately exposed. The covers and drapes are removed and installed in a warmer;
- all drugs given are recorded;
- all drugs are kept locked;
- the patient is transferred into the operating room with all lines well secured and with the appropriate documents. *Ensure protection of the patient against trauma.*

Special points. Special points to note are:

- the full check must have been carried out;
- the patient is observed at all times, particularly during induction and transfer of the patient from the anaesthetic room to the operating theatre. Cross-matched blood, if required, is available and the correct units are in the storage fridge;
- the limbs are safeguarded, especially if paralysed;
- nerves are protected from pressure;
- eyes are protected, the lids must be closed on induction to avoid inversion of the eyelashes and to protect the cornea against abrasions, drying and foreign bodies.

Tourniquets. Pneumatic cuffs and tourniquets are usually applied in the anaesthetic room; they should be regularly checked by an engineer:

- the pressure and time should be recorded by the nurse or operating theatre assistant;

- the tourniquet width and position *must* be checked by the operating surgeon;
- Esmarch rubber bandages used must be applied with care to avoid burns;
- 'disinfectant' must not be allowed to run under the Esmarch bandage or tourniquet;
- the use of more sophisticated equipment must be carefully supervised, and its design understood by the surgeon.

Operating theatre

Regular maintenance will ensure correct air ventilation with 20–40 changes per hour in a general surgical theatre. Ultraclean air will be used in orthopaedic theatres. The temperature should range between 19 and 22°C with a humidity of 45–55 per cent. The lights should be of appropriate design and will therefore differ in orthopaedic and general surgical theatres.

Anaesthetic gases and suction should be piped with different colour coding. Cables on the floor should be kept to a minimum. Trolleys should be steel with no sharp corners.

The operating table should have a smooth action for raising and lowering the table, the appropriate handle and gears to alter the tilt giving Trendelenberg or reverse Trendelenberg positions, lateral roll and a bridging system for use in procedures such as nephrectomy. The function of electrically operated tables must be understood before starting the operation.

The mattresses must be well maintained, cleaned and sealed. The table should be checked to see that it is correctly orientated, particularly when an intraoperative X-ray is anticipated.

Diathermy

In surgical diathermy a high-frequency alternating current is passed through body tissue and the concentration of current producing an area of high current density liberates heat – temperatures may rise to 1000°C or above. Current frequencies in the range of 400 kHz–10 mHz are used, and in this range there is minimal muscular response.

Monopolar diathermy

A high-frequency current is generated from the diathermy machine and is delivered to the active electrode held by the surgeon. There is high current density where the electrode touches body tissue, producing local heating, and the current then spreads through the body and returns to the diathermy machine or generator via the patient electrode.

Bipolar diathermy

The surgeon holds a pair of forceps connected to the diathermy generator, the current passes down one limb of the forceps, through a small piece of tissue and then back through the other limb of the forceps to the generator. There is no requirement for a plate and the system uses considerably less power, but it cannot be used for cutting and tissue must not be squeezed between the diathermy forceps. As the bipolar current will only pass directly from one diathermy arm to the other it is very safe.

Safety measures. Certain safety measures are essential.

- The diathermy generator and accessories require a regular service with a full record being kept.
- Plugs, leads and sockets need to be checked to ensure that all are sound.
- The foot pedals should be checked to ensure that they are completely sealed and sensitive to light pressure.
- The alarm systems should all be in order.
- The appropriate mode of diathermy, whether it be monopolar or bipolar, should be selected prior to use and the correct setting to be used is checked. When monopolar diathermy is used care must be taken to ensure that the coagulation and cutting levels are correctly set (cutting and fulguration involve higher power current than coagulation; these are not applicable to bipolar).
- *Make sure that the indifferent electrode in the monopolar system uses a flat surface which is dry and there is no thick hair present, as this may interfere with conduction.*
- *Ensure that the patient is protected from metal, and that the skin is checked after removal of the plate.*
- *Ensure that the live electrode is always placed in the quiver and never on the drapes or on the tray. Insulation of the instruments should be checked regularly.*

If diathermy is ineffective, before increasing the current, look for:

- faulty connection;
- faulty active electrode;
- poor contact of plate;
- a disconnected or faulty cable.

Precautions. The following precautions should be taken:

- staff should understand the clear rules of operation of diathermy;
- the alarm system, generator and equipment should be checked regularly;
- the power should not be turned up if the diathermy appears to be ineffective without first carrying out a number of checks;
- diathermy should *never* be used in the presence of ether and should be kept at least 50 cm from the anaesthetic machine;
- alcoholic disinfectants must be dried before diathermy is used.

The commonest causes of diathermy injury are:

- incorrect application of the patient plate;
- the patient touching earth, metal objects such as parts of the table;
- careless technique, e.g. the electrode not being put back into the cover.

Johann Friedrich August von Esmarch, 1823–1908. Professor of Surgery, Kiel, Germany. Introduced his bandage in 1869 for use on the battlefield.

Positioning the patient

When the patient is transferred from the anaesthetic room to the operating theatre, the trolley should be positioned close to the operating table and the height of the latter should be adjusted. The optimal way of transfer is using the 'patient slide' as this avoids lifting at awkward angles which may cause back problems to the staff. It also avoids the use of a canvas which may be worn or defective or where the lifting poles have been inserted incorrectly. The patient should be positioned correctly in respect of the cushions, particularly if either the lithotomy or Lloyd-Davies position is used. The patient's legs should be supported so that undue pressure on the calf does not occur. Both surgeon and anaesthetist should be fully aware of the optimal position required during movement; the airway and intravenous drip lines should be protected and particular care taken to ensure that the patient's head is on the canvas, so that in the paralysed patient the head does not become unsupported with hyperextension of the neck. Lithotomy poles and Lloyd-Davies stirrups must be securely anchored to the table.

Protection of nerves

This is particularly important in thin patients.

- In the Lloyd-Davies stirrups, care must be taken to protect the lateral peroneal nerve. It is important to ensure that the stirrups are well padded so that there is no direct contact with metal.
- If the arms are by the patient's side or placed on an arm board, care must be taken to protect the ulnar nerve at the elbow.
- If the arm is placed above the head, as it may be in some breast biopsy procedures, then care should be taken to ensure that the shoulder is supported posteriorly, as failure to do this will result in a brachial plexus traction injury.
- In patients with rheumatoid arthritis the team should always be aware of the possibility of a fracture dislocation of the odontoid peg with subluxation. Endotracheal intubation in such patients is a risky procedure and patients should wear a protective cervical collar.
- Patients who have lumbar disc problems should be positioned particularly carefully if lithotomy is to be considered.
- In patients in whom hyperextension of the cervical spine is required, such as thyroidectomy, the surgeon should ensure that the weight of the head is not being taken on the unsupported hyperextended cervical spine.

Deep venous thrombosis prophylaxis must be considered. The calves should be protected against pressure by whatever means is chosen: graduated support stockings or intermittent flow compression. Subcutaneous low-dose heparin is widely used additionally (see Chapter 15 on 'Arterial disorders').

R.W. Lloyd-Davies. British Surgeon.

The patient

On entry to theatre the patient should be clean, the gown should be appropriately applied and, before anaesthesia is started, the ties at the back should have been loosened (the patient's modesty should be protected), fingernails should be clean and free from coloured varnish.

In theatre the appropriate area of skin should be disinfected with care taken to avoid splash (particularly adjacent to the diathermy plate) or pooling of alcoholic disinfectant, which must not be allowed to run under a tourniquet. The appropriate drapes should be used with attention to the possibility of allergy.

Tourniquets must be applied correctly with the appropriate time of starting noted.

Theatre staff

Although the number of persons in the theatre should be kept to a minimum from the point of view of infection, it is obviously important to have a clear policy whereby nurses of adequate seniority act as the scrub nurses. The circulating nurses must be aware of the importance of meticulous counting of swabs, needles and instruments, and also the handling of samples and specimens. Appropriate training with the possibility of advancement and promotion is considered important in the maintenance of morale and standards.

- Of particular importance are the counts at the beginning and the end of the procedure. It is essential to have an instrument, swab and needle count prior to closure after laparotomy, and a final count prior to removal of any equipment from the theatre. In this respect, swabs, packs, disposable equipment, instruments, needles and such items as tapes are to be recorded. The creation of swabs in bundles of five with a radio marker and red string bundles is helpful. Dirty swabs should be placed singly in the swab holders. It is important to stress that all swabs should be removed from the previous surgery before any current count is taken.
- It is important to have a count before body cavities, incised organs or joint spaces are closed.
- Rubber tubes and tapes should never be cut.
- *Nothing* should be removed from the operating theatre until the incision is closed and the scrub nurse indicates that all is correct.
- Particular care should be taken when there is a changeover of staff, which may occur during prolonged surgery, such as a oesophagectomy, pancreatectomy, spinal or neurosurgical procedures. At such a time:
  - the surgeons should stop;
  - the first scrub nurse only descrubs when the second scrub nurse and the surgeon have indicated. The time and the names of those who change should be noted in the theatre record.
- Nonradio-opaque swabs should not be used during surgery and radiopaque swabs should not be cut.

- Needles should be checked, both for number and the fact that they are complete.
- With regard to power tools, the nurse should check that all detachable parts are neither faulty nor loose.

The surgeon

The surgeon should be thoroughly familiar with the procedure and should have received appropriate training. If he or she is a doctor in training then appropriate senior cover must be present.

- He or she should be in good health with no upper respiratory chest infection and no septic lesions, and should not have a positive carrier state for *Staphylococcus aureus*.
- The scrub-up procedure should be carried out thoroughly, with brushes restricted to cleaning nails. Gowning, masking and gloving should proceed with aseptic precautions, and the amount of talking and movement should be cut to the minimum.
- Assistants should not lean on patients, as this may cause damage, bruising or neuropraxia.

Specimens

Great care should be taken with the handling of specimens.

- The specimens must be identified and, if multiple, should be placed into separate labelled specimen pots which should be appropriate for the study required, namely histology, cytology, microbiology or biochemistry.
- For histology and cytology the appropriate method of fixation should be selected and checked (all too often samples for microbiology are placed in formalin and vice versa).
- All specimens and all request forms should be labelled fully and clearly, and clinical details must be given.
- The circulating nurse should check with either the scrub nurse or the surgeon that the correct fixative or microbiological storage agent has been selected.

The samples should be checked for a good seal prior to transport.

- Specimens at high risk of infectivity should be identified and treated securely according to the policy.
- Formalin splashing when placing a large specimen in a container must be avoided.
- The record book must be signed with the full description of the specimen and the time that it left theatre.

Disposables

Those disposables such as drains should be secured to the patient and checked for patency. Those disposables to be discarded such as soiled linen, drapes and other waste should be disposed of appropriately, and material of high infectivity needs to be sealed and marked accordingly.

The record book

This should be kept in each theatre; if a surgical procedure is different from the one that was planned it is the responsibility of the surgeon to inform both the patient subsequently and the relatives.

Radiation and image intensification

All surgeons using X-ray equipment should be in possession of a certificate, to the effect that they have attended a course on Protection Against Ionising Radiation. Staff should reduce exposure to the minimum and good-quality aprons must be available.

- Random dose recording should be a part of quality control.
- Pregnant staff must not be in the vicinity of radiation.
- Sterility must not be compromised.

Lasers

Lasers should be used in a *designated* operating theatre by fully trained medical staff. In addition to this, further precautions are appropriate:

- warning signs must be present on the operation doors;
- no reflective or inflammable fixtures or furnishings must be present in that operating theatre;
- care with the direction of the laser beam is critical in safe usage;
- protective eye wear must be worn at all times;
- the surgeon should warn the staff before firing the laser.

The recovery room

All too often the recovery room has received too little attention and is often inadequate in terms of size and equipment. With increasing medicolegal considerations it is now imperative that each theatre suite has a fully equipped adequate recovery room in which patients recuperate to a stable level with regard to their cardiorespiratory system before transfer back to the ward. The recovery room should meet the following criteria:

- the temperature should be between 19 and 22°C, and the bed linen should be warmed;
- lighting should be adequate;
- fire doors should be free;
- piped oxygen should be available with a range of masks in appropriate sizes;
- suction apparatus should be attached to the wall, regularly checked and appropriate tubing and sucker attachments available;
- there should be *no* trailing tubes or wires;
- adequate monitoring equipment is essential.

Monitoring equipment should be available for every patient in the recovery room, screens and curtains are appropriate for those spending a longer time in the recovery room, and defibrillation equipment should be immediately accessible.

Management of the patient in recovery includes attention to the following:

- the airway, with monitoring of the oxygen saturation;
- pulse rate, blood pressure and respiratory rate which should be regularly recorded on charts. The patient should be easily accessible on a trolley which has brakes, safety rails and head-lowering facilities;
- pain relief is mandatory and if the patient is having a patient-controlled analgesic set up then adequate intravenous analgesics to overcome initial pain is important;
- pressure areas should not be overlooked;
- hand hygiene of the staff between patients is important;
- an emergency bell available to each bay should be clearly marked and in good working order;
- stands attachable to trolleys for intravenous infusions should be at hand and fit well;
- with regard to drug administration, this should be recorded on the patient's chart with both time and dosage and, of course, the controlled drugs register should be kept up to date and double signed;
- where a central venous pressure line is present, and particularly if there are multiple channels, these should be handled in a strict aseptic way and clearly labelled.

Before the patient leaves the recovery room a clear record of the readings should have been made and the line should be well secured. Additional observations should include:

- drains;
- the presence of a stoma;
- urine output;
- nasogastric aspiration in terms of both quality and quantity. The position of a drainage bag is checked (a leakage is all too common, stains the pillow and leads to the patient developing a sore rash on his or her cheek);
- chest (under water seal) drains should be monitored and be placed below the level of the chest.

Transfer of the patient to the ward

Prior to transfer, the ward nurse will come down and there should be a clear verbal handover between the nurse incharge of that patient in the recovery room and the ward nurse. The following documents should accompany the patient:

- nursing record;
- postoperative recovery chart;
- anaesthetic record;
- operation record;
- prescription chart;
- fluid balance and temperature charts.
- The patient should be clearly identified by both the recovery room nurse and the ward nurse to ensure the correct transfer of the patient to the correct ward. The linen should be clean, and the patient comfortable and well positioned on the trolley away from pressure points.

Management of the operating suite

There is good evidence that theatre safety is based on good management. This implies a good staff relationship with the appropriate training facilities and schedules to maintain morale. A good career structure will enhance standards and provide a good reputation, enhancing future recruitment. High standards and patient safety are at a premium. Additional points that must be considered in the safer running of theatres include:

- a ready supply of clean linen;
- safe disposal of dirty linen and waste products;
- rapid transfer of instruments to and from CSSD to avoid delay;
- adequate pharmaceutical supplies with close liaison with the pharmacy;
- monitoring of the medical and surgical supplies and requisitions so that excess stocks of items do not accumulate; conversely the amount of expensive emergency ordering must be cut to a minimum. It should be remembered that larger stores utilise much revenue; equipment may also go out of date and this is wasteful. Stock level checking is an important part of the theatre sister's role but does require time;
- transfer of specimens to the laboratory – this should take place on a regular basis. The use of sealed containers in a vacuum tube system for small specimens is highly efficient;
- instrument maintenance is essential and saves money;
- there should be close liaison with the electronics, central sterile supply and theatre infection control officer;
- health and safety rules and procedures should be understood by all staff;
- an accident record should be kept, and regular audit should take place.

Summary

In the delivery of a health service the proper provision of an operating suite with appropriate training of personnel is an essential but costly investment. Breakdown in safety and aseptic techniques will lead to increased patient mortality and morbidity, and increase costs. Septic complications and accidents in theatre are very expensive and potentially avoidable.

Further reading

Crumplin, M.K.H. (1999) Operating theatres and special equipment. In *Clinical Surgery in General*, 3rd edn (eds R.M. Kirk, A.O. Mansfield and J. Cochrane), Churchill Livingstone, London, pp. 189–203.

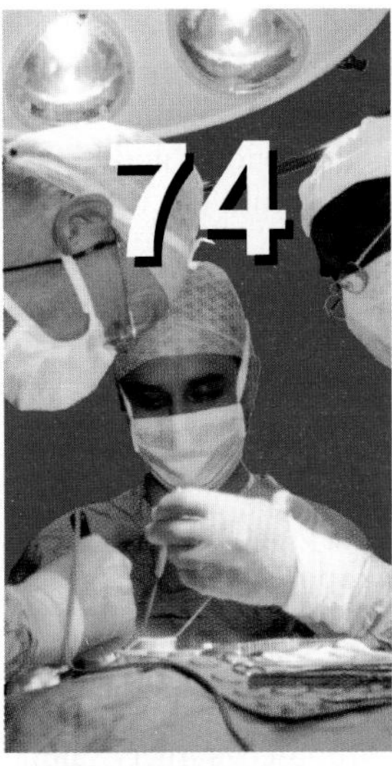

Surgical ethics

Introduction

Ethics and surgical intervention must go hand in hand. In any other arena of public or private life, if someone deliberately cuts another person, draws blood, causes pain, leaves scars and disrupts everyday activity then the likely result will be a criminal charge. If the person dies as a result, the charge could be manslaughter or even murder. Of course, it will be correctly argued that the difference between the criminal and the surgeon is that the latter causes harm only incidentally. The surgeon's intent is to cure or manage illness and any bodily invasion that occurs only does so with the permission of the patient.

Patients consent to surgery because they trust their surgeons. Yet what should such consent entail in practice and what should surgeons do when patients need help but are unable or unwilling to agree to it? When patients do consent to treatment, surgeons wield enormous power over them – the power not just to cure but to maim, disable and kill. How should such power be regulated to reinforce the trust of patients and to ensure that surgeons practise to an acceptable professional standard? Are there circumstances where it is acceptable to sacrifice the trust of individual patients in the public interest through revealing information that was communicated in what patients believed to be conditions of strict privacy?

Bailey & Love's Short Practice of Surgery, 23rd edition. Edited by R.C.G. Russell, N.S. Williams and C.J.K. Bulstrode. Published in 2000 by Arnold Publishers.

These questions about what constitutes good professional practice concern ethics rather than surgical technique. Surgeons may be expert in the management of specific diseases and yet have little understanding of how much and what sort of information is required for patients to give valid consent to treatment. Surgeons can understand the delicate techniques associated with specific types of procedures without knowing when these should be administered to patients who are unable to consent at all. Surgeons can recognise their own mistakes and those of colleagues without knowing how much should be said about them to others. And so it goes on.

Traditional surgical training offers little help in the resolution of such ethical dilemmas. This chapter provides guidance which is morally coherent, widely endorsed and legally justifiable. Our focus will be the practice of surgery within the United Kingdom, although much of the analysis will also apply to surgical work elsewhere.

Respect for autonomy

What is the difference between veterinary surgeons and surgeons who treat humans? Both are trained in anatomy, physiology, biochemistry, and the other clinical and surgical skills required to care for the bodies of their patients. As a by-product of employing these skills, both invade these bodies in ways which can cause harm in order to meet need. Finally, both work within the same duty of care – to protect their patient's life and health to an acceptable standard. To distinguish between the two types of surgeon, we must ask another question. What is the major difference between animals and humans, and how does this difference create special duties for human surgeons which are of no concern for those who work only with animals?

We can only wonder at the attributes and abilities of many animals, characteristics which humans can only aspire to. For example, we can respect the big cats of the sub-Saharan plains because of their strength and speed – for behaving in the unique ways that characterise their species. The same can be said of humans. What makes us unique as animals is our autonomy – our ability to formulate both goals and beliefs about how they should be achieved. Humans can attempt to plan their lives on the basis of reason and choice in ways which other animals cannot. Therefore, when we talk of the particular type of respect which it is appropriate to show to humans, the focus should primarily be on our autonomy rather than our particular physical characteristics. Respect for human dignity is respect for human autonomy.

It is for this reason that surgeons have a duty of care towards their human patients which goes beyond just protecting their life and health. Their additional duty of care is to respect the autonomy of their patients – their ability to make choices about their treatments and to evaluate potential outcomes in light of other life plans. Such respect is particularly important for surgeons because without it the trust between them and their patients may be compromised, along with the success of the surgical care provided. We are careful enough at the best of times about who we allow to touch us and to see us unclothed. It is hardly surprising that many people feel strongly about exercising the same discretion in circumstances where someone is not only going to do these things but to inflict what may be very serious wounds on them as well.

For all of these reasons, there is a wide moral and legal consensus that patients have the right to exercise choice over their surgical care. In this context a right should be interpreted as a claim which can be made on others and which they believe that they have a strict duty to respect, regardless of their own preferences. Thus, to the degree that patients have a right to make choices about proposed surgical treatment, it then follows that they should be allowed to refuse treatments that they do not want, even when surgeons think that they are wrong. For example, patients can even refuse surgical treatment which will save their lives – either at present or in the future through the formulation of advance directives specifing the types of life-saving treatments which they do not wish to have if they become incompetent to refuse them.

Informed consent

In surgical practice, respect for autonomy translates into the clinical duty to obtain informed consent before the commencement of treatment. The word 'informed' is important here. Because of the extremity of their clinical need, patients might agree to surgery on the basis of no information at all. Agreement of this kind, however, does not constitute a form of consent which is morally or legally acceptable. Unless such patients have some understanding of what they are agreeing to, their choices may have nothing to do with planning their lives and thus do not count as expressions of their autonomy. Worse still, if patients are given no information, their subsequent choices may be based on misunderstanding and lead to plans and further decisions which they would not otherwise have made.

For agreement to count as consent to treatment, patients need to be given appropriate and accurate information about:

- their condition and the reasons why it warrants surgery;
- what type of surgery is proposed and how it might correct their condition;
- what the proposed surgery entails in practice;
- the anticipated prognosis of the proposed surgery;
- the expected side effects of the proposed surgery;
- the unexpected hazards of the proposed surgery;
- any alternative and potentially successful treatments for their condition other than the proposed surgery, along with similar information about these;
- the consequences of no treatment at all.

With such information, patients can link their clinical prospects with the management of other aspects of their life and lives of others for whom they may be morally and/or professionally responsible.

Good professional practice dictates that obtaining informed consent should occur in circumstances which are designed to maximise the chances of patients understanding what is said about their condition and proposed treatment, as well as giving them an opportunity to ask questions and express anxieties. Where possible:

- a quiet venue for discussion should be found;
- written material in the patient's preferred language should be provided to supplement verbal communication;
- patients should be given time and help to evaluate their own understanding and to come to their own decision;
- the person obtaining the consent should ideally be the surgeon who will carry out the treatment. It should not be – as is sometimes the case – a junior member of staff who has never conducted such a procedure and thus may not have enough understanding to counsel the patient properly.

Surgeons should always attempt to approximate these conditions, even when they might not be completely achievable.

Good communication skills go hand in hand with properly obtaining informed consent for surgery. It is not good enough just to go through the motions of providing patients with information required for considered choice. Attention must be paid to:

- whether or not the patient has understood what has been stated;
- not using overly technical language in descriptions and explanations;
- the provision of translators for patients for whom English is not their first language;
- asking patients if they have further questions.

When there is any doubt about their understanding, surgeons should ask patients questions about what has supposedly been communicated to see if they can explain the information in question for themselves.

Surgeons have a legal, as well as moral, obligation to obtain consent for treatment based on appropriate levels of information. Failure to do so could result in one of two civil proceedings, assuming the absence of criminal intent. First, in law, intentionally to touch another person without their consent is a battery, remembering that we are usually touched by strangers as a consequence of accidental contact. Surgeons have a legal obligation to give the conscious and competent patient sufficient information 'in broad terms' about the surgical treatment being proposed and why. If the patient agrees to proceed, no other treatment should ordinarily be administered without further explicit consent.

Negligence is the second legal action which might be brought against a surgeon for not obtaining appropriate consent to treatment. Patients may have been given enough information about what is surgically proposed to agree to be touched in the ways suggested. However, surgeons may still be in breach of their professional duty if they do not provide sufficient information about the risks which patients will encounter through such treatment. While standards of how much information should be provided about risks vary between nations, as a matter of good practice, surgeons should inform patients of the hazards that in their view any reasonable person in the position of the patient would wish to know. In practice, this is probably best decided through surgeons asking themselves what they or a close relative or friend should be entitled to know in similar circumstances. Only through supporting this standard of disclosure of information linked to the requirements of a reasonable person can surgeons help to ensure that they, their relatives and friends will be treated with respect and dignity.

Finally, surgeons now understand that when they obtain consent to proceed with treatment then patients are expected to sign a consent form of some kind. The detail of such forms can differ but they often contain very little of the information supposedly communicated to patients, who signed it. Partly for this reason, the process of formally obtaining consent can become overly focused on obtaining the signature of patients rather than ensuring that appropriate types and amounts of information have been provided, and that they have been understood.

Both professionally and legally, it is important for surgeons to understand that a signed consent form is not proof that valid consent has been properly obtained. It is simply a piece of evidence that consent may have been attempted. Even when they have provided their signature, patients can and do deny that appropriate information has been communicated or that the communication was effective. Surgeons are therefore well advised to make brief notes of what they have said to patients about their proposed treatments, especially information about significant risks. These notes should be placed in the patient's clinical record.

Practical difficulties

Thus far, we have examined the moral and legal reasons why the duty of surgeons to respect the autonomy of patients translates into the specific responsibility to obtained informed consent to treatment. For consent to be valid, patients must:

- be competent to give it – to be able to understand, remember, deliberate about and believe whatever information is provided to them about treatment choices;
- not be coerced into decisions which reflect the preferences of others rather than themselves;
- be given sufficient information for these choices to be based on an accurate understanding of reasons for and against proceeding with specific treatments.

Surgeons will face four key practical difficulties in aspiring to these goals.

First, surgical care will grind to a halt if it is always necessary to obtain explicit informed consent every time a patient is touched in the context of their care. Fortunately, such consent is unnecessary because patients will have already given their implied consent to whatever bodily contact is required in order to fulfil the therapeutic goals when they gave their explicit consent to treatment. Yet, the fact that this is so underlines the importance of obtaining proper and explicit consent in the first place, along with taking care to note any sign of the patient withdrawing that consent or placing restrictions on it – say, through verbally refusing or physically resisting specific aspects of care.

Second, some patients will not be able to give consent because of temporary unconsciousness. This might be a by-product of their illness or injury, or it could simply be the result of the administration of general anaesthetic. The moral and legal rules which govern such situations are clear. If patients are at risk of death or of serious and permanent disability if surgery is not immediately performed then the situation is one of medical necessity and intervention can occur without consent. However, surgery not entailing such risks should be postponed until patients regain consciousness and are able to give informed consent for themselves. Surgeons must take care to respect this distinction between procedures which are therapeutically necessary and those which are done merely out of convenience, even when in the course of one operation they discover problems unknown to the patient which they believe to require further surgical work. For example, a surgeon was successfully sued for battery by a female patient for performing a hysterectomy thought to be in her best interests when all that she had explicitly consented to was a dilatation and curettage.

Third, informed consent may be made impossible by incompetence of other kinds. In the case of children, parents or someone with parental responsibility are ordinarily required to give explicit written consent on their behalf. This said, surgeons should:

- take care to explain to children what is being surgically proposed and why;
- always consult with children about their response;
- where possible, take their views into account and note that even young children can be competent to consent to treatment provided that they too can understand, remember, deliberate about and believe information relevant to their clinical condition.

When such competence is present, children under English law can provide their own consent to surgical care, although they cannot unconditionally refuse it until they are 18 years old. With the exception of the latter, these provisions illustrate the importance of respecting as much autonomy as is present among child patients and remembering that, for the purposes of consent to medical treatment, they may be just as autonomous as adults.

Where competence is severely compromised by psychiatric illness or mental handicap, other moral and legal provisions hold. If patients lack the autonomy to choose how to protect themselves then others charged with protecting them must assume the responsibility. Yet, care must be taken not to abuse this duty. For example, adult voluntary psychiatric patients have the same rights to consent to and refuse treatment as any other competent adult. Even when they have been legally detained for compulsory psychiatric care, it does not follow that such patients are unable to provide consent for surgical care. Their competence should be assumed and consent should be sought. If it is established with the help of their carers that such patients are also incompetent to provide consent for surgery and that they are at risk of death or serious and permanent disability then therapy can proceed. However, if treatment can be postponed then this should be done until, as result of their psychiatric care, patients become able either to consent to or refuse it. As with children, respect should always be shown for as much autonomy as is present.

If, for whatever clinical reason, adult patients are permanently incompetent to consent to surgery, therapy can again proceed if it is necessary to save life or to prevent serious and permanent injury. In the UK, the final decision to proceed with surgery which is elective and can be postponed rests ultimately with the surgeon and other doctors responsible for the patient's care. It does not depend on the views of the relatives of the patient. The moral justification for this is that the patient's professional carers are more likely to act consistently in their best interests than their relatives.

Thus, it is always a futile exercise in the UK to ask the relatives of incompetent patients to sign consent forms for surgery on adults who cannot do so for themselves. Indeed, to do so can be a great disservice to relatives who may feel an unjustified sense of responsibility if the surgery fails. This said, relatives should be treated with politeness and consulted about issues which pertain to determining the best interest of patients. In other legal jurisdictions, relatives can be given powers of guardianship to provide consent for surgical treatment, although even here surgeons should ensure that such powers are vested in the specific person asked to provide it.

Matters of life and death

It has been noted that the right of a competent adult to consent to and refuse treatment is unlimited, including the refusal of life-sustaining treatment. Probably the example most familiar to surgeons of this is Jehovah's Witnesses who refuse blood transfusions at the risk of their own lives. There can be no more dramatic example of the potential tension between the duties of care to protect life and health and to respect autonomy, with autonomy always constituting the trump card.

The tension does not stop here, however. For there will be some circumstances where the protection of the life and health of patients is judged to be inappropriate, where they are no longer able to be consulted and where they have not expressed a view about what their wishes would be under such circumstances. Here a decision may be made to withhold or to withdraw life-sustaining treatment on behalf of the incompetent patient. The fact that such decisions can be seen as omissions to act does not excuse surgeons from morally and legally having to reconcile them with their ordinary duty of care. Ultimately, this can only be done through arguing that such omissions to sustain life are in the patient's best interests.

The determination of best interests in these circumstances will rely on one of three objective criteria, over and above the subjective perception by the surgeon that the quality of life of the patient is poor. There is no obligation to provide or to continue life-sustaining treatment:

- if doing so is futile – when clinical consensus dictates that it will not achieve the goal of extending life. Thought of in this way, judgements about futility should not be linked to evaluations of a patient's quality of life;
- if patients are imminently and irreversibly close to death – in such circumstances it would not be in their best interest slightly to prolong life (e.g. through the application of intensive care) when, again, there is no hope of any sustained success. Not needlessly interfering with the process of a dignified death can be just as caring as the provision of curative therapy;
- if patients are so permanently and seriously brain damaged that, lacking awareness of themselves or others, they will never be able to engage in any form of self-directed activity. The argument here is backed up by morally and legally reasoning that further treatment other than effective palliation cannot be in the best interests of patients as it will provide them with no benefit.

When any of these principles are employed to justify an omission to provide or to continue life-sustaining treatment, the circumstances should be carefully recorded in the patient's medical record, along with a note of another senior clinician's agreement.

Finally, surgeons will sometimes find themselves in charge of the palliative care of patients whose pain is increasingly difficult to control. There will come a point in the management of such pain when effective palliation might only be possible at the risk of life because of the respiratory effects of the palliative drugs. In such circumstances, surgeons can with legal justification administer a dose which might be lethal. The argument employed to justify such action refers to its 'double effect' – that both the relief of pain and death might follow from such an action. As intentional killing – active euthanasia – is rejected as professional and legal medical practice throughout most of the world, a potentially lethal dose is only regarded as appropriate when it is motivated by palliative intent.

Debates rage about whether or not it is realistic in such circumstances to believe that surgeons can or should keep all ideas out of their minds about helping such unfortunate patients to die, especially as we have seen that clinical decisions are already made that foreshorten the lives of incompetent patients in specific circumstances. Deciding whether or not potentially lethal palliation is justified will require an evaluation – by either the patient, the clinician or both – of whether or not the life in question is too valuable on other grounds to risk. Once a negative conclusion is reached and the risks are incurred, it seems impossible in the face of continued and dramatic palliative failure then to purport to banish thoughts of the desirability of death from the scene. What is clear is that surgeons should document that their intent is purely palliative through only gradually and incrementally increasing doses of the drugs that they administer for this purpose.

Confidentiality

Respect for autonomy does not only entail the right of competent patients to consent to treatment. Their entitlement to exercise control over their life and future corresponds to the duty of surgeons to respect their privacy – not to communicate information revealed in the course of treatment to anyone else without consent. Generally speaking, such respect means that surgeons must not discuss clinical matters with relatives, friends, employers and others unless the patient explicitly agrees. To do otherwise is regarded by all of the regulatory bodies of medicine and surgery as a grave offence incurring harsh penalties. For breaches of confidentiality are not only abuses of human dignity; they again undermine the trust between surgeon and patient on which successful surgery and the professional reputations of surgeons depend.

Important as respect for confidentiality is, however, it is not absolute. Surgeons are allowed to communicate private information to other professionals who are part of the healthcare team – provided that the information has a direct bearing on treatment. Here the argument is that patients have given their implied consent to such communication when they explicitly consent to a treatment plan. Certainly, patients cannot expect strict adherence to the principle of confidentiality if it poses a serious threat to the health and safety of others. There will be some circumstances when confidentiality either must or might be breached in the public interest. For example, it must be breached as a result of court orders or in relation to the requirements of public health legislation. It may be ignored in attempts to prevent serious crime or to protect the safety of other known individuals who are risk of serious harm.

Research

As part of their duty to protect life and health to an acceptable professional standard, surgeons have a subsidiary responsibility to strive to improve operative techniques through research – to assure themselves and their patients that the care proposed is the best that is currently possible. Yet, there is moral tension between the duty to act in the best interests of individual patients and the duty to improve surgical standards through exposing patients to the unknown risks which any form of research inevitably entails.

The willingness to expose patients to such risks may be further increased by the professional and academic pressures on many surgeons to maintain a high research profile in their work. For this reason, surgeons, and physicians who face the same dilemmas, now accept that their research must be externally regulated to ensure that patients give their informed consent, that any known risks to patients are far outweighed by the potential benefits and that other forms of protection for the patient are in place (e.g. proper indemnity) in case they are unexpectedly harmed. The administration of such regulation is through research ethics committees, and surgeons should not participate in research which has not been approved by such bodies.

In practice, it is not always clear what is to count as surgical research which should be subjected to regulation and what constitutes a minor innovation dictated by the contingencies of a particular clinical situation. Surgeons must always ask themselves in such circumstances whether or not the innovation in question falls within the boundaries of standard procedures in which they are trained. If so, what may be a new technique for them will count not as research but as an incremental improvement on personal practice.

Yet, if the improvement is to be thought of in this way, no conclusions can be drawn from it to alterations in standard practice or to an evaluation of their efficacy. Equally, there will be no consequences for surgical training, as the innovation in question should only have been attempted against the background of the already existing training and experience of the surgeon in question. Where a proposed innovation exceeds these conditions then it does count as research and should be approved by a research ethics committee. Such surgical research should also be subject to a clinical trial designed to ensure that findings about outcomes are systematically compared with the best available treatment and that favourable results are not because of arbitrary factors (e.g. unusual surgical skill among researchers) which cannot be replicated.

Maintaining standards of excellence

To optimise success in protecting life and health to an acceptable standard, surgeons must only offer specialised treatment in which they have been properly trained. To do so will entail sustained further education throughout a surgeon's career in the wake of new surgical procedures. While training, surgery should only be practised under appropriate supervision by someone who has appropriate levels of skill. Such skill can only be demonstrated through appropriate clinical audit to which all surgeons should regularly submit their results. When these reveal unacceptable levels of success, no further surgical work of that kind should continue unless further training is undergone under the supervision of someone whose success rates are satisfactory. To do otherwise would be to place the interest of the surgeon above that of their patient, an imbalance which is never morally or professionally appropriate.

Surgeons also have a duty to monitor the performance of their colleagues. To know that a fellow surgeon is exposing patients to unacceptable levels of potential harm and to do nothing about it is to incur partial responsibility for such harm when it occurs. Surgical teams and the institutions in which they function should have clear protocols for exposing unacceptable professional performance and helping colleagues to understand the danger to which they may exposing patients. If necessary, offending surgeons must be stopped from practising until, again, they can undergo further appropriate training and counselling. Too often such danger has had to be reported by individuals whose anxieties have not been properly heeded and who have been professionally pilloried rather than congratulated for their pains. Surgeons and anyone else discovered to participate in such cover-up and ostracism should share the blame and punishment for any resulting harm to patients.

Conclusion

The two general duties of surgical care are to protect life and health and to respect autonomy, both to an acceptable professional standard. The specific duties of surgeons were shown to follow from these: acceptable practice concerning informed consent, confidentiality, decisions not to provide or to omit life-sustaining care, surgical research and the maintenance of good professional standards. The final duty of surgical care is to exercise all of these general and specific responsibilities with fairness and justice, and without arbitrary prejudice. The conduct of ethical surgery illustrates good citizenship: protecting the vulnerable and respecting human dignity and equality. To the extent that the practice of individual surgeons is a reflection of such sustained conduct, they deserve the civil respect which they often receive. To the extent that it is not, they should not practise the honourable profession of surgery.

Further reading

Beauchamp, T. and Childress, J. (1994) *Principles of Biomedical Ethics*, Oxford University Press, Oxford.

British Medical Association (1993) *Medical Ethics Today: Its Practice and Philosophy*, BMA, London.

Gilion, R. (ed.) (1994) *Principles of Healthcare Ethics*, John Wiley, Chicester.

McHale, J. and Fox, J. (1997) *Healthcare Law – Text and Materials*, Sweet and Maxwell, London.

Rosenthal, M. (1994) *The Incompetent Doctor*, Open University Press, Buckingham.

Royal College of Surgeons of England (1996) *Code of Practice for the Surgical Management of Jehovah's Witnesses*, Royal College of Surgeons, London.

Senate of Surgery of Great Britain and Ireland (1997) *The Surgeon's Duty of Care: Guidance For Surgeons on Ethical and Legal Issues*, Royal College of Surgeons, London.

Wear, S. (1993) *Informed Consent*, Kluwer, Dordrecht.

White, B. (1994) *Competence to Consent*, Georgetown University Press, Washington, DC.

Index